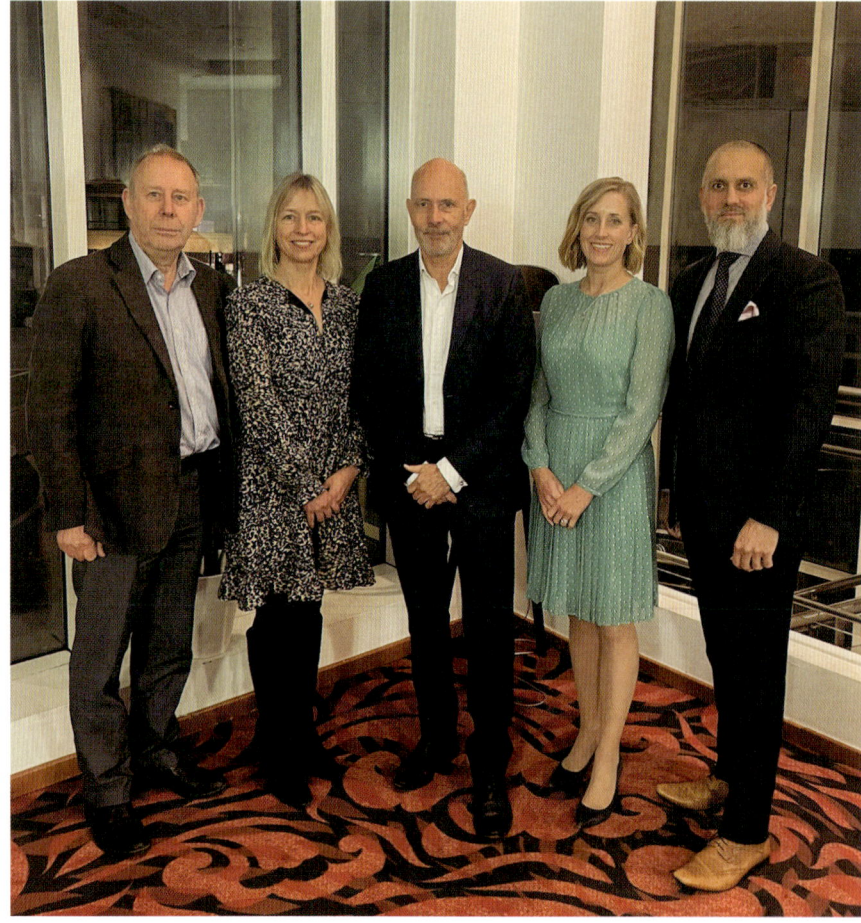

The Editors
From left to right: Jonathan Barker, Tanya Bleiker, Christopher Griffiths, Rosalind Simpson, Walayat Hussain

Rook's Textbook of Dermatology

TENTH EDITION

EDITED BY

Christopher Griffiths OBE, MD, FMedSci
Emeritus Professor of Dermatology
The University of Manchester
Manchester, UK

Adjunct Professor & Consultant Dermatologist
King's College London
London, UK

Jonathan Barker MD, FRCP
Professor of Medical Dermatology
St John's Institute of Dermatology
Faculty of Life Sciences and Medicine
King's College London
London, UK

Tanya Bleiker FRCP
Consultant Dermatologist
University Hospitals of Derby and Burton NHS Foundation Trust
Derby, UK

Walayat Hussain FRACP
Consultant Dermatological & Mohs Micrographic Surgeon
Dermatology Surgical & Laser Unit
Chapel Allerton Hospital
Leeds, UK

Rosalind Simpson MRCP, PhD
Associate Professor and Consultant Dermatologist
Centre of Evidence Based Dermatology
University of Nottingham
Nottingham, UK

IN FOUR VOLUMES

VOLUME 1

WILEY Blackwell

This edition first published 2024
© 2024 John Wiley & Sons Ltd

Edition History
John Wiley & Sons Ltd (9e, 2016); Blackwell Publishing, Ltd (1e, 1968, 2e, 1972, 3e, 1979, 4e, 1986, 5e, 1992, 6e, 1998, 7e, 2004, 8e, 2010)

All rights reserved. No part of this publication may be reproduced, stored in a retrieval system, or transmitted, in any form or by any means, electronic, mechanical, photocopying, recording or otherwise, except as permitted by law. Advice on how to obtain permission to reuse material from this title is available at http://www.wiley.com/go/permissions.

The right of Christopher E. M. Griffiths, Jonathan N. W. N. Barker, Tanya O. Bleiker, S. Walayat Hussain, Rosalind C. Simpson to be identified as the authors of the editorial material in this work has been asserted in accordance with law.

Registered Office(s)
John Wiley & Sons, Inc., 111 River Street, Hoboken, NJ 07030, USA
John Wiley & Sons Ltd, The Atrium, Southern Gate, Chichester, West Sussex, PO19 8SQ, UK

Editorial Office(s)
9600 Garsington Road, Oxford, OX4 2DQ, UK
The Atrium, Southern Gate, Chichester, West Sussex, PO19 8SQ, UK

For details of our global editorial offices, customer services, and more information about Wiley products visit us at www.wiley.com.

Wiley also publishes its books in a variety of electronic formats and by print-on-demand. Some content that appears in standard print versions of this book may not be available in other formats.

Limit of Liability/Disclaimer of Warranty
The contents of this work are intended to further general scientific research, understanding, and discussion only and are not intended and should not be relied upon as recommending or promoting scientific method, diagnosis, or treatment by physicians for any particular patient. In view of ongoing research, equipment modifications, changes in governmental regulations, and the constant flow of information relating to the use of medicines, equipment, and devices, the reader is urged to review and evaluate the information provided in the package insert or instructions for each medicine, equipment, or device for, among other things, any changes in the instructions or indication of usage and for added warnings and precautions. While the publisher and authors have used their best efforts in preparing this work, they make no representations or warranties with respect to the accuracy or completeness of the contents of this work and specifically disclaim all warranties, including without limitation any implied warranties of merchantability or fitness for a particular purpose. No warranty may be created or extended by sales representatives, written sales materials or promotional statements for this work. The fact that an organization, website, or product is referred to in this work as a citation and/or potential source of further information does not mean that the publisher and authors endorse the information or services the organization, website, or product may provide or recommendations it may make. This work is sold with the understanding that the publisher is not engaged in rendering professional services. The advice and strategies contained herein may not be suitable for your situation. You should consult with a specialist where appropriate. Further, readers should be aware that websites listed in this work may have changed or disappeared between when this work was written and when it is read. Neither the publisher nor authors shall be liable for any loss of profit or any other commercial damages, including but not limited to special, incidental, consequential, or other damages.

Library of Congress Cataloging-in-Publication Data has been applied for.

Set ISBN (4 Volumes): 9781119709213

Cover Design: Wiley
Cover Image: © khamkula/Adobe Stock

Set in 9.5/12pt, Palatino LT Std by Straive, Chennai, India

Printed in Great Britain by Bell & Bain Ltd, Glasgow

10 9 8 7 6 5 4 3 2 1

Contents

List of Associate Editors, x

List of Contributors, xi

Preface to the Tenth Edition, xxi

Preface to the First Edition, xxii

About the Companion Website, xxiii

VOLUME 1

Part 1 Foundations of Dermatology

1 History of Dermatology, 1.1
Nick J. Levell

2 Structure and Function of the Skin, 2.1
John A. McGrath and Jouni Uitto

3 Histopathology of the Skin: General Principles, 3.1
Eduardo Calonje and John Mee

4 Diagnosis of Skin Disease, 4.1
Ian H. Coulson, Emma C. Benton and Stephanie Ogden

5 Epidemiology of Skin Disease, 5.1
Hywel C. Williams and Sinéad M. Langan

6 Health Economics and Skin Disease, 6.1
Matthias Augustin

7 Global Health Dermatology, 7.1
L. Claire Fuller

8 Genetics and the Skin, 8.1
John A. McGrath

9 Inflammation, Immunology and Allergy, 9.1
Muzlifah Haniffa

10 Photobiology, 10.1
Antony R. Young

11 Cutaneous Response to Injury and Wound Healing, 11.1
Edel A. O'Toole

12 Topical Drug Delivery, 12.1
Richard H. Guy and Adrian F. Davis

13 Clinical Pharmacology, 13.1
Richard T. Woolf and Catherine H. Smith

14 Adverse Immunological Reactions to Drugs, 14.1
Michael R. Ardern-Jones

Part 2 Management

15 Psychological and Social Impact of Long-Term Conditions and Principles of Holistic Management, 15.1
Sandy R. McBride and Alexandra Mizara

16 Principles of Measurement and Assessment in Dermatology, 16.1
Andrew Y. Finlay and Faraz M. Ali

17 Principles of Evidence-based Dermatology, 17.1
Michael Bigby and Hywel C. Williams

18 Principles of Topical Therapy, 18.1
Deirdre A. Buckley

19 Principles of Systemic Therapy, 19.1
Andrew E. Pink, Richard T. Woolf and Catherine H. Smith

20 Principles of Skin Surgery, 20.1
S. Walayat Hussain, Christopher J. Miller and Timothy S. Wang

21 Principles of Phototherapy, 21.1
Kevin McKenna and Sally Ibbotson

22 Principles of Photodynamic Therapy, 22.1
Sally Ibbotson and Kevin McKenna

23 Principles of Cutaneous Laser Therapy, 23.1
Vishal Madan and Jill S. Waibel

24 Principles of Radiotherapy, 24.1
Charles G. Kelly, John Frew and Najibah Mahtab

Part 3 Infections and Infestations

25 Viral Infections, 25.1
Catherine A. Harwood and Jane C. Sterling

26 Bacterial Infections, 26.1
Catriona Wootton and Ivo Elliott

27 Mycobacterial Infections, 27.1
Stephen L. Walker and Richard O. Phillips

28 Leprosy, 28.1
Diana N. J. Lockwood and Stephen L. Walker

29 Syphilis and Congenital Syphilis, 29.1
George R. Kinghorn and Rasha Omer

30 Non-syphilitic Bacterial Sexually Transmitted Diseases, 30.1
George R. Kinghorn and Nadi K. Gupta

31 HIV and the Skin, 31.1
Christopher B. Bunker and Vincent Piguet

32 Fungal Infections, 32.1
Roderick J. Hay

33 Parasitic Diseases, 33.1
Austinn C. Miller, Alfredo Siller Jr. and Stephen K. Tyring

34 Arthropods, 34.1
Charlotte Bernigaud, Gentiane Monsel, Pascal Delaunay and Olivier Chosidow

Index

VOLUME 2

Part 4   Inflammatory Dermatoses

35 Psoriasis and Related Disorders, 35.1
Brian Kirby and A. David Burden

36 Pityriasis Rubra Pilaris, 36.1
Curdin Conrad

37 Lichen Planus and Lichenoid Disorders, 37.1
Felix Lauffer and Kilian Eyerich

38 Graft-versus-host Disease, 38.1
Tanya N. Basu

39 Eczematous Disorders, 39.1
Ayad A. Mughal and John R. Ingram

40 Seborrhoeic Dermatitis, 40.1
Sarah Wakelin and Anastasia Therianou

41 Atopic Eczema, 41.1
Michael R. Ardern-Jones, Carsten Flohr and Nick J. Reynolds

42 Urticaria, 42.1
Clive E. H. Grattan and Alison V. Sears

43 Recurrent Angio-oedema without Weals, 43.1
Clive E. H. Grattan and Marcus Maurer

44 Urticarial Vasculitis, 44.1
Karoline Krause and Clive E. H. Grattan

45 Autoinflammatory Diseases Presenting in the Skin, 45.1
Dan Lipsker, Clive E. H. Grattan and Christopher R. Lovell

46 Mastocytosis, 46.1
Clive E. H. Grattan and Deepti H. Radia

47 Reactive Inflammatory Erythemas, 47.1
Ruth Murphy

48 Adamantiades–Behçet Disease, 48.1
Christos C. Zouboulis

49 Neutrophilic Dermatoses, 49.1
Philip J. Hampton and Stephanie Ball

50 Immunobullous Diseases, 50.1
Enno Schmidt and Richard Groves

51 Lupus Erythematosus and Antiphospholipid Syndrome, 51.1
Jan Dutz and Touraj Khosravi-Hafshejani

52 Dermatomyositis, 52.1
Patrick Gordon and Daniel Creamer

53 Undifferentiated and Mixed Connective Tissue Disease and Dermatological Manifestations of Rheumatoid Disease, 53.1
Philip M. Laws

54 Systemic Sclerosis, 54.1
Catherine H. Orteu and Christopher P. Denton

55 Morphoea and Allied Scarring and Sclerosing Inflammatory Dermatoses, 55.1
Catherine H. Orteu

Part 5   Metabolic and Nutritional Disorders Affecting the Skin

56 Cutaneous Amyloidoses, 56.1
Stephan Schreml

57 Cutaneous Mucinoses, 57.1
Franco Rongioletti

58 Cutaneous Porphyrias, 58.1
Robert P. E. Sarkany

59 Calcification of the Skin and Subcutaneous Tissue, 59.1
Johnny Bourke and Matthew Murphy

60 Xanthomas and Abnormalities of Lipid Metabolism and Storage, 60.1
Paul D. Flynn

61 Nutritional Disorders Affecting the Skin, 61.1
Albert C. Yan and Netravali Michelle Oboite

62 Skin Disorders in Diabetes Mellitus, 62.1
Johnny Bourke and Matthew Murphy

Part 6   Genetic Disorders Involving the Skin

63 Inherited Disorders of Cornification, 63.1
Vinzenz Oji, Kira Süßmuth, Dieter Metze, Angela Hernandez Martin and Heiko Traupe

64 Inherited Acantholytic Disorders, 64.1
Mozheh Zamiri

65 Ectodermal Dysplasias, 65.1
Peter Itin

66 Inherited Hair Disorders, 66.1
Eli Sprecher

67 Genetic Defects of Nails and Nail Growth, 67.1
Samantha Gordon and Amy S. Paller

68 Genetic Disorders of Pigmentation, 68.1
Fanny Morice-Picard and Alain Taïeb

69 Genetic Blistering Diseases, 69.1
John A. McGrath

70 Genetic Disorders of Collagen, Elastin and Dermal Matrix, 70.1
Nigel Burrows

71 Disorders Affecting Cutaneous Vasculature, 71.1
Anne Dompmartin, Nicole Revencu, Laurence M. Boon and Miikka Vikkula

72 Genetic Disorders of Adipose Tissue, 72.1
George W. M. Millington

73 Congenital Naevi and Selected Naevoid Conditions, 73.1
Veronica A. Kinsler and Neil J. Sebire

74 Chromosomal Disorders, 74.1
Neil Rajan, Alan D. Irvine and Jemima E. Mellerio

75 Poikiloderma Syndromes, 75.1
Alan D. Irvine and Jemima E. Mellerio

76 DNA Repair Disorders with Cutaneous Features, 76.1
Hiva Fassihi

77 Syndromes with Premature Ageing, 77.1
Alan D. Irvine and Jemima E. Mellerio

78 Inherited Skin Tumour Syndromes, 78.1
Neil Rajan, Jemima E. Mellerio and Alan D. Irvine

79 Inherited Metabolic Diseases, 79.1
Andrew A.M. Morris

80 Inherited Immunodeficiency, 80.1
Tim Niehues and Andrew R. Gennery

Part 7   Psychological, Sensory and Neurological Disorders and the Skin

81 Pruritus, Prurigo and Lichen Simplex, 81.1
Sonja Ständer and Gil Yosipovitch

82 Mucocutaneous Pain Syndromes, 82.1
Jon Goulding and Anthony Bewley

83 Neurological Conditions Affecting the Skin, 83.1
Andrew G. Affleck

84 Psychodermatology, 84.1
Anthony Bewley and Ruth E. Taylor

85 Acquired Disorders of Epidermal Keratinisation, 85.1
Matthew J. Scorer and Graham A. Johnston

Index

VOLUME 3

Part 8   Skin Disorders Associated with Specific Cutaneous Structures

86 Acquired Pigmentary Disorders, 86.1
Nanja van Geel and Reinhart Speeckaert

87 Acquired Disorders of Hair, 87.1
Matthew J. Harries, Susan Holmes, Amy McMichael and Andrew G. Messenger

88 Acne, 88.1
Alison M. Layton, Christos C. Zouboulis and Heather Whitehouse

89 Rosacea, 89.1
Esther J. van Zuuren, Jerry Tan, Mireille M. D. van der Linden and Martin Schaller

90 Hidradenitis Suppurativa, 90.1
John R. Ingram, Hessel H. van der Zee and Gregor B. E. Jemec

91 Acquired Non-infective Disorders of the Pilosebaceous Unit, 91.1
Kapil Bhargava, Evangelos Christou and Christos Tziotzios

92 Disorders of the Sweat Glands, 92.1
Ian H. Coulson and Niall J. E. Wilson

93 Acquired Disorders of the Nails and Nail Unit, 93.1
Marcel C. Pasch, Bertrand Richert and Matilde Iorizzo

94 Acquired Disorders of Dermal Connective Tissue, 94.1
Caoimhe M. R. Fahy and Christopher R. Lovell

95 Granulomatous Disorders of the Skin, 95.1
John W. Frew and Saleem M. Taibjee

96 Sarcoidosis, 96.1
Joaquim Marcoval and Juan Mañá

97 Panniculitis, 97.1
Luis Requena and Lorenzo Cerroni

98 Non-inflammatory Disorders of Subcutaneous Fat, 98.1
Grace L. Lee, Amit Garg and Amy Y.-Y. Chen

Part 9   Vascular Disorders Involving the Skin

99 Purpura, 99.1
Nick J. Levell

100 Cutaneous Vasculitis, 100.1
Nick J. Levell and Chetan Mukhtyar

101 Dermatoses Resulting from Disorders of the Veins and Arteries, 101.1
Portia C. Goldsmith and Christina George

102 Ulceration Resulting from Disorders of the Veins and Arteries, 102.1
Jürg Hafner and Eberhard Rabe

103 Disorders of the Lymphatic System, 103.1
Peter S. Mortimer and Kristiana Gordon

104 Flushing and Blushing, 104.1
Elizabeth Keeling and Síona Ní Raghallaigh

Part 10 Skin Disorders Associated with Specific Sites, Sex and Age

105 Dermatoses of the Scalp, 105.1
Paul Farrant, Megan Mowbray and Anita Takwale

106 Dermatoses of the External Ear, 106.1
Cameron Kennedy and Ashish Sharma

107 Dermatoses of the Eye, Eyelids and Eyebrows, 107.1
Valerie P. J. Saw and Stuart N. Cohen

108 Dermatoses of the Oral Cavity and Lips, 108.1
Barbara Carey and Jane Setterfield

109 Dermatoses of the Male Genitalia, 109.1
Christopher B. Bunker and Richard E. Watchorn

110 Dermatoses of the Female Genitalia, 110.1
Fiona Lewis

111 Dermatoses of Perineal and Perianal Skin, 111.1
Eleanor Mallon

112 Cutaneous Complications of Stomas and Fistulae, 112.1
Calum Lyon

113 Dermatoses of Pregnancy, 113.1
Amy Stanway

114 Dermatoses of the Neonate, 114.1
Timothy H. Clayton and Jennifer C. Harrison Sharif

115 Dermatoses of Infancy, 115.1
Lea Solman and Mary T. Glover

116 Haemangiomas and Other Non-malignant Tumours of Infancy, 116.1
Lea Solman and Mary T. Glover

Index

VOLUME 4

Part 11 Skin Disorders Caused by External Agents

117 Benign Cutaneous Adverse Reactions to Drugs, 117.1
Michael R. Ardern-Jones

118 Severe Cutaneous Adverse Reactions to Drugs, 118.1
Daniel Creamer, Sarah Walsh and Haur Yueh Lee

119 Cutaneous Side Effects of Chemotherapy and Radiotherapy, 119.1
Louise Fearfield and Charlotte Edwards

120 Dermatoses Induced by Illicit Drugs, 120.1
Anthony Bewley and Iyas Assalman

121 Dermatological Manifestations of Metal Poisoning, 121.1
Rabindranath Nambi

122 Mechanical Injury to the Skin, 122.1
Saqib J. Bashir and Ai-Lean Chew

123 Pressure Injury and Pressure Ulcers, 123.1
Emily Haesler and Jan Kottner

124 Cutaneous Reactions to Cold and Heat, 124.1
Saqib J. Bashir and Ai-Lean Chew

125 Burns and Heat Injury, 125.1
Marc G. Jeschke

126 Cutaneous Photosensitivity Diseases, 126.1
Sally Ibbotson

127 Allergic Contact Dermatitis, 127.1
David Orton and Natalie Stone

128 Irritant Contact Dermatitis, 128.1
Jonathan M. L. White

129 Occupational Dermatology, 129.1
Jonathan M. L. White

130 Stings and Bites, 130.1
Alfredo Siller Jr., Austinn C. Miller and Stephen K. Tyring

Part 12 Neoplastic, Proliferative and Infiltrative Disorders Affecting the Skin

131 Benign Melanocytic Proliferations and Melanocytic Naevi, 131.1
Irene Stefanaki, Dimitris Sgouros and Alexander Stratigos

132 Benign Keratinocytic Acanthomas and Proliferations, 132.1
Edward Seaton and Vishal Madan

133 Cutaneous Cysts, 133.1
Vishal Madan and Edward Seaton

134 Lymphocytic Infiltrates, 134.1
Fiona Child and Sean J. Whittaker

135 Cutaneous Histiocytoses, 135.1
Thai Hoa Tran, Elena Pope and Sheila Weitzman

136 Soft-tissue Tumours and Tumour-like Conditions, 136.1
Eduardo Calonje and Zlatko Marušić

137 Tumours of Skin Appendages, 137.1
Eduardo Calonje and Zlatko Marušić

138 Kaposi Sarcoma, 138.1
Kenneth Y. Tsai

139 Cutaneous Lymphomas, 139.1
Sean J. Whittaker

140 Basal Cell Carcinoma, 140.1
Carl Vinciullo and Vishal Madan

141 Squamous Cell Carcinoma and its Precursors, 141.1
Girish Gupta and Thomas Dirschka

142 Melanoma Clinicopathology, 142.1
Jean Jacques Grob and Caroline Gaudy-Marqueste

143 Melanoma Surgery, 143.1
Noah R. Smith, Kelly B. Cha, Timothy M. Johnson and Alison B. Durham

144 Systemic Treatment of Melanoma, 144.1
Reinhard Dummer and Simone M. Goldinger

145 Dermoscopy of Melanoma and Naevi, 145.1
Natalia Jaimes and Ashfaq A. Marghoob

146 Merkel Cell Carcinoma, 146.1
Jürgen C. Becker, Isaac Brownell and Thibault Kervarrec

147 Skin Cancer in the Immunocompromised Patient, 147.1
Catherine A. Harwood, Rubeta N. Matin and Charlotte M. Proby

Part 13   Systemic Disease and the Skin

148 Cutaneous Markers of Internal Malignancy, 148.1
Lennart Emtestam and Karin Sartorius

149 The Skin and Disorders of the Haematopoietic and Immune Systems, 149.1
Tanya N. Basu and Austin Kulasekararaj

150 The Skin and Endocrine Disorders, 150.1
Ralf Paus and Yuval Ramot

151 The Skin and Disorders of the Heart, 151.1
Sonja Molin and Thomas Ruzicka

152 The Skin and Disorders of the Respiratory System, 152.1
Sonja Molin and Thomas Ruzicka

153 The Skin and Disorders of the Digestive System, 153.1
Sonja Molin and Thomas Ruzicka

154 The Skin and Disorders of the Kidney and Urinary Tract, 154.1
Sonja Molin and Thomas Ruzicka

155 The Skin and Disorders of the Musculoskeletal System, 155.1
Christopher R. Lovell

Part 14   Aesthetic Dermatology

156 Skin Ageing, 156.1
Elisabeth A. Pedersen, Gary J. Fisher, John J. Voorhees and Dana L. Sachs

157 Cosmeceuticals, 157.1
Neera R. Nathan, Eubee Koo, Alexandra B. Kimball and Molly Wanner

158 Soft-Tissue Augmentation (Fillers), 158.1
Berthold Rzany

159 Aesthetic Uses of Botulinum Toxins, 159.1
Nicholas J. Lowe and Philippa L. Lowe

160 Chemical Peels, 160.1
Chee-Leok Goh and Joyce Teng Ee Lim

161 Lasers and Energy-based Devices, 161.1
Nazanin Saedi and Christopher B. Zachary

Index

List of Associate Editors

Andrew Affleck
BSc (Hons), MBChB, MRCP (UK)
Consultant Dermatologist and Dermatological Surgeon, Ninewells Hospital and Medical School, Dundee, Scotland

Sarah T. Arron
MD, PhD
Dermatologist and Mohs Micrographic Surgeon
Peninsula Dermatology, Burlingame, CA, USA

Eduardo Calonje
MD, DipRCPath
Consultant Dermatopathologist, St John's Institute of Dermatology, Guy's and St Thomas' NHS Foundation Trust, London, UK

Mahbub M. U. Chowdhury
MBChB, FRCP, FAcadMed
Consultant Dermatologist, Honorary Senior Lecturer, Cardiff University, Welsh Institute of Dermatology, University Hospital of Wales, Cardiff, UK

Tamara W. Griffiths
BA, MD, FRCP
Consultant Dermatologist and Honorary Senior Lecturer, The Dermatology Centre, Salford Royal NHS Foundation Trust, The University of Manchester, Manchester, UK

John A. McGrath
MD, FRCP, FMedSci
Professor of Molecular Dermatology, St John's Institute of Dermatology, Division of Genetics and Molecular Medicine, Faculty of Life Sciences and Medicine, King's College London, London, UK

Dedee Murrell
MA (Cantab), BMBCh (Oxon), FAAD (USA), MD (UNSW), FACD
Professor, St George Hospital, The University of New South Wales, Sydney, NSW, Australia

Nick J. Reynolds
BSc, MBBS, MD, FRCP
Professor of Dermatology and Honorary Consultant, Department of Dermatology, Royal Victoria Infirmary and Institute of Translational and Clinical Medicine, Newcastle University, Newcastle upon Tyne, UK

Eli Sprecher
MD, PhD
Professor and Chair, Department of Dermatology, Tel Aviv Sourasky Medical Center; and Department of Human Molecular Genetics and Biochemistry, Sackler Medical School, Tel Aviv University, Tel Aviv, Israel

Jane C. Sterling
MBBChir, MA, FRCP, PhD
Senior Lecturer and Honorary Consultant, Dermatologist, Department of Dermatology, University of Cambridge, Addenbrooke's Hospital, Cambridge, UK

Sarah Walsh
MD
Consultant Dermatologist, Lead Clinician for Dermatology KCH, Department of Dermatology, King's College Hospital NHS Foundation Trust, London, UK

List of Contributors

Andrew G. Affleck
BSc, MBChB, MRCP
Department of Dermatology, Ninewells Hospital & Medical School, NHS Tayside, Dundee, UK
Chapter 83

Faraz M. Ali
MBBCh, PhD, MRCP (Derm), PGCert (Med Ed)
Dermatologist, Division of Infection and Immunity, Cardiff University School of Medicine, Cardiff, UK
Chapter 16

Michael R. Ardern-Jones
BSc, MBBS, DPhil, FRCP
Associate Professor in Dermatology / Consultant Dermatologist, Sir Henry Wellcome Laboratories, Clinical and Experimental Sciences, Faculty of Medicine, University of Southampton, Southampton General Hospital, Southampton, UK
Chapters 14, 41, 117

Iyas Assalman
MD, MRCPsych, CILT, CCT
Consultant Psychiatrist, East London NHS Foundation Trust, London, UK
Chapter 120

Matthias Augustin
MD
Director and Professor of Dermatology and Health Economics, Institute for Health Services Research in Dermatology and Nursing, University Medical Center Hamburg-Eppendorf, Hamburg, Germany
Chapter 6

Stephanie Ball
BMBS, MRCP, MSc
Consultant Dermatologist, Newcastle Hospitals NHS Trust, Newcastle upon Tyne, UK
Chapter 49

Saqib J. Bashir
BSc, MBChB, MD, FRCP
Consultant Dermatologist and Dermatological Surgeon, King's College Hospital, King's College Hospital NHS Foundation Trust, London, UK
Chapters 122, 124

Tanya N. Basu
MA, PhD, FRCP
Consultant Dermatologist, Department of Dermatology, King's College Hospital, London, UK
Chapters 38, 149

Jürgen C. Becker
MD, PhD
Translational Skin Cancer Research (TSCR), German Cancer Consortium (DKTK) Site Essen/Düsseldorf, Essen; Deutsches Krebsforschungsinstitut (DKFZ), Heidelberg, Germany
Chapter 146

Emma C. Benton
MBChB, FRCP
Consultant Dermatologist, St John's Institute of Dermatology, Guy's and St Thomas' NHS Foundation Trust, London, UK
Chapter 4

Charlotte Bernigaud
MD, PhD
Dermatologist, GrIDIST, Groupe Infectiologie Dermatologique – Infections Sexuellement Transmissibles, Société Française de Dermatologie; Research group Dynamyc, EA7380, Faculté de Médecine de Créteil, Ecole nationale vétérinaire d'Alfort, USC ANSES, Université Paris-Est Créteil, Créteil, France; UPEC-Université Paris-Est Créteil Val de Marne, Department of Dermatology, AP-HP, Hôpital Henri-Mondor, Créteil, France
Chapter 34

Anthony Bewley
BA, MBChB, FRCP
Consultant Dermatologist, Department of Dermatology, Barts Health NHS Trust, London; Queen Mary College of Medicine, University London, London, UK
Chapters 82, 84, 120

Kapil Bhargava
BSc, MBBS, FRCP (UK), FRCP (Derm)
Consultant Dermatologist and Dermatologic/Mohs Surgeon Department of Dermatology, St Bartholomew's and the Royal London Hospital, Barts Health NHS Trust and St. John's Institute of Dermatology, Guy's & St. Thomas' Hospitals NHS Foundation Trust, London, UK
Chapter 91

Michael Bigby
MD
Vice President for Research and Academics, Beth Israel Deaconess Medical Center, Associate Professor of Dermatology, Harvard Medical School and Beth Israel Deaconess Medical Center, Boston, MA, USA
Chapter 17

Laurence M. Boon
MD, PhD
Coordinator, Center for Vascular Anomalies, Cliniques Universitaires Saint-Luc, Université catholique de Louvain (a VASCERN VASCA European Reference Centre), Brussels, Belgium
Chapter 71

Johnny Bourke
MD, FRCPI
Consultant Dermatologist, South Infirmary-Victoria University Hospital, Cork; Clinical Senior Lecturer, University College, Cork, Ireland
Chapters 59, 62

Isaac Brownell
MD, PhD
Dermatology Branch, National Institute of Arthritis and Musculoskeletal and Skin Diseases, National Institutes of Health, Bethesda, MD, USA
Chapter 146

Deirdre A. Buckley
FRCP
Consultant Dermatologist, Department of Dermatology, Sulis Hospital, Bath, UK
Chapter 18

List of Contributors

Christopher B. Bunker
MA, MD, FRCP
Consultant Dermatologist and Honorary Professor, University College London Hospitals and Chelsea & Westminster Hospitals, London, UK
Chapters 31, 109

A. David Burden
MD, FRCP
Professor of Dermatology, Institute of Infection and Immunity, University of Glasgow, Glasgow, UK
Chapter 35

Nigel Burrows
MD, FRCP
Consultant Dermatologist, Department of Dermatology, Addenbrooke's Hospital, Cambridge University Hospitals NHS Foundation Trust, Cambridge, UK
Chapter 70

Eduardo Calonje
MD, DipRCPath
Consultant Dermatopathologist, St John's Institute of Dermatology, Guy's and St Thomas' NHS Foundation Trust, London, UK
Chapters 3, 136, 137

Barbara Carey
BDS NUI, MBBCh, BAO, FDS(OM) RCSI, FFDRCSI (Oral Medicine), FHEA
Consultant in Oral Medicine, Department of Oral Medicine, Guy's and St Thomas' NHS Foundation Trust, London, UK
Chapter 108

Lorenzo Cerroni
MD
Department of Dermatology, Medical University of Graz, Graz, Austria
Chapter 97

Kelly B. Cha
MD, PhD
Associate Professor, Michigan Medicine Department of Dermatology, Ann Arbor, MI, USA
Chapter 143

Amy Y.-Y. Chen
MD, FAAD
Founding partner, Central Connecticut Dermatology, Avon, Farmington, Southington, Bloomfield and Cromwell, CT USA
Chapter 98

Ai-Lean Chew
MBChB, MRCP
Consultant Dermatologist, Beckenham Beacon Hospital, King's College Hospital NHS Foundation Trust, London, UK
Chapters 122, 124

Fiona Child
BSc, MBBS, MD, FRCP
Consultant Dermatologist, St John's Institute of Dermatology, Guy's and St Thomas' NHS Foundation Trust, London, UK
Chapter 134

Olivier Chosidow
MD, PhD
Dermatologist, AP-HP, University Hospital La Pitié-Salpêtrière, Paris, France; GrIDIST, Groupe Infectiologie Dermatologique – Infections Sexuellement Transmissibles, Société Française de Dermatologie; Research group Dynamyc, EA7380, Faculté de Médecine de Créteil, Ecole nationale vétérinaire d'Alfort, USC ANSES, Université Paris-Est Créteil, Créteil, France
Chapter 34

Evangelos Christou
MD, PgCertMedEd, MRCP
St John's Institute of Dermatology, Guy's and St Thomas' NHS Foundation Trust, London, UK
Chapter 91

Timothy H. Clayton
MBChB, FRCP, MRCPCH
Consultant Adult and Paediatric Dermatologist, Royal Manchester Children's Hospital, Manchester; Salford Royal NHS Foundation Trust, Manchester; Honorary Senior Lecturer, University of Manchester, Manchester, UK
Chapter 114

Stuart N. Cohen
BMedSci, MMedSci, FRCP
Department of Dermatology, Liverpool University Hospitals NHS Foundation Trust; University of Liverpool School of Medicine, Liverpool, UK
Chapter 107

Curdin Conrad
MD
Professor, Department of Dermatology, Lausanne University Hospital CHUV, Lausanne, Switzerland
Chapter 36

Ian H. Coulson
BSc, FRCP
Consultant Dermatologist, Burnley General Teaching Hospital, East Lancashire NHS Trust IHC, Burnley, UK
Chapters 4, 92

Daniel Creamer
MD, FRCP
Consultant Dermatologist, Department of Dermatology, King's College Hospital, London, UK
Chapters 52, 118

Adrian F. Davis
PhD
Director Limeway Pharma Design, Ltd., Limeway Pharma Design Ltd, Dorking, UK
Chapter 12

Pascal Delaunay
MD
Parasitologist, Entomologist, Department of Parasitology-Mycology, Centre Hospitalier Universitaire de Nice, Hôpital de l'Ardet, Nice, France
Chapter 34

Christopher P. Denton
PhD, FRCP
Division of Medicine, University College London, London; Royal Free London NHS Foundation Trust, London, UK
Chapter 54

Thomas Dirschka
MD, PhD
Consultant Dermatologist and Medical Director and Associate Professor, CentroDerm Clinic, Wuppertal, Germany; Faculty of Health, University Witten-Herdecke, Witten, Germany
Chapter 141

Anne Dompmartin
MD, PhD
Coordinator, Consultation of Vascular Anomalies, Université de Caen Basse Normandie, Caen; Department of Dermatology, CHU Caen, Caen, France
Chapter 71

Reinhard Dummer
MD
Professor, Department of Dermatology, University Hospital Zurich, Zurich, Switzerland
Chapter 144

Alison B. Durham
MD
Associate Professor, Michigan Medicine Department of Dermatology, Ann Arbor, MI, USA
Chapter 143

Jan Dutz
MD, FRCPC
Professor, Skin Care Centre, Vancouver General Hospital, Vancouver; BC Children's Hospital Research Institute, Vancouver, BC, Canada
Chapter 51

Charlotte Edwards
MBChB, MRCP
Consultant Dermatologist, Chelsea & Westminster, London, UK
Chapter 119

Ivo Elliott
DPhil, MBChB, MRCP, FRCPath, DTM&H
Consultant in Infectious Diseases and Microbiology, Dermatology Department, Churchill Hospital, Oxford, UK; Department of Infection, John Radcliffe Hospital, Oxford, UK
Chapter 26

Lennart Emtestam
MD, PhD
Professor, Department of Medicine Huddinge, Karolinska Institutet, Stockholm, Sweden
Chapter 148

Kilian Eyerich
MD, PhD
Department of Dermatology and Allergy, Technical University of Munich, Munich; Department of Dermatology and Venerology, Medical Center, University of Freiburg, Freiburg, Germany; Division of Dermatology and Venereology, Department of Medicine Solna, Karolinska Institutet, Stockholm, Sweden
Chapter 37

Caoimhe M. R. Fahy
MBBCh, BAO, BMedSci, FRCPI, FRCP
Consultant Dermatologist, Department of Dermatology, Royal United Hospital, Bath, UK
Chapter 94

Paul Farrant
BSc, MBBS, MRCP
Consultant Dermatologist, Department of Dermatology, Brighton General Hospital, University Hospitals Sussex, Brighton, UK
Chapter 105

Hiva Fassihi
MA, MD, FRCP
Consultant Dermatologist, St John's Institute of Dermatology, Guy's and St Thomas' NHS Foundation Trust, London, UK
Chapter 76

Louise Fearfield
MA (Oxon), DM, FRCP
Consultant Dermatologist, Chelsea & Westminster, London, UK
Chapter 119

Andrew Y. Finlay
CBE, MBBS, FRCP
Professor of Dermatology, Division of Infection and Immunity, Cardiff University School of Medicine, Cardiff, UK
Chapter 16

Gary J. Fisher
PhD
Professor of Dermatology, University of Michigan Medical Center, Ann Arbor, MI, USA
Chapter 156

Carsten Flohr
MA, MPhil, DHSR, MSc, PhD, FRCP, FRCPCH
Chair in Dermatology and Population Health Sciences, St John's Institute of Dermatology, King's College London, London, UK; Honorary Consultant Dermatologist, Guy's & St Thomas' NHS Foundation Trust, London, UK
Chapter 41

Paul D. Flynn
PhD, FRCP
Consultant Physician, Acute and Metabolic Medicine, Addenbrooke's Hospital, Cambridge; Affliated Assitant Professor, School of Clinical Medicine, University of Cambridge, Cambridge, UK
Chapter 60

John Frew
MBChB, MRCP, FRCR
Consultant Clinical Oncologist, Northern Centre for Cancer Care, Freeman Hospital, Newcastle upon Tyne, UK
Chapter 24

John W. Frew
MBBS, MMed, MS, PhD, FACD
Department of Dermatology, Liverpool Hospital, University of New South Wales, Sydney, Australia
Chapter 95

L. Claire Fuller
MA, FRCP
Consultant Dermatologist, Chelsea and Westminster NHS Foundation Trust, London, UK
Chapter 7

Amit Garg
MD, FAAD
Professor & Founding Chair, Department of Dermatology, Zucker School of Medicine at Hofstra/Northwell; Professor, Center for Health Innovations & Outcomes Research, Feinstein Institutes for Medical Research; Director, Research Program for Outcomes in Dermatology; SVP, Dermatology Service Line, Northwell Health Hempstead, NT, USA; Department of Dermatology, Donald and Barbara Zucker School of Medicine at Hofstra Northwell, Hempstead, NY, USA
Chapter 98

Caroline Gaudy-Marqueste
MD, PhD
Professor of Dermatology, Service de Dermatologie et Cancérologie Cutanée, Hôpital de la Timone, Aix-Marseille Université, Marseille, France
Chapter 142

Nanja van Geel
PhD
Department of Dermatology, Ghent University Hospital, Ghent, Belgium
Chapter 86

Andrew R. Gennery
MD, PhD
Paediatric Immunologist and Haematopoietic Stem Cell Transplanter, Translational and Clinical Research Institute, Newcastle University, and Paediatric Haematopoietic Stem Cell Transplant Unit, Great North Children's Hospital, Newcastle upon Tyne, UK
Chapter 80

Christina George
MBBS, BSc, MRCP (Derm)
Consultant Dermatologist, Imperial College Healthcare NHS Trust, London, UK
Chapter 101

Mary T. Glover
MA, FRCP, FRCPCH
Consultant Paediatric Dermatologist, Great Ormond Street Hospital for Children NHS Foundation Trust, London, UK
Chapters 115, 116

Chee-Leok Goh
MD, MBBS, MRCP (UK), MMed (Int Med), FACD (Hon)
Senior Consultant Dermatologist, National Skin Centre, Singapore; Clinical Professor, National University of Singapore, Singapore
Chapter 160

Simone M. Goldinger
MD
Senior Physician, Department of Dermatology, University Hospital Zurich, Zurich, Switzerland
Chapter 144

Portia C. Goldsmith
MD, FRCP
Consultant Dermatologist, Barts Health and Homerton University Hospital, London, UK
Chapter 101

Kristiana Gordon
MBBS, MRCP, MD (Res)
Consultant in Dermatology and Lymphovascular Medicine, St George's Hospital, London, UK
Chapter 103

Patrick Gordon
FRCP, PhD, MBBS
Consultant Rheumatologist and Honorary Senior Lecturer, Department of Rheumatology, King's College Hospital, London, UK
Chapter 52

Samantha Gordon
MD
Pediatric Dermatology Fellow, Departments of Dermatology and Pediatrics, Northwestern University, Chicago, IL, USA
Chapter 67

Jon Goulding
BSc, BMBCh, MMedEd, FHEA, FRCP
Consultant Dermatologist, Department of Dermatology, Solihull Hospital, University Hospitals Birmingham NHS Foundation Trust, Birmingham, UK
Chapter 82

Clive E. H. Grattan
MA, MD, FRCP
Consultant Dermatologist, St John's Institute of Dermatology, Guy's and St Thomas' NHS Foundation Trust, London, UK
Chapters 42, 43, 44, 45, 46

Jean Jacques Grob
MD
Professor of Dermatology, Service de Dermatologie et Cancérologie Cutanée, Hôpital de la Timone, Aix-Marseille Université, Marseille, France
Chapter 142

Richard Groves
FRCP
Consultant Dermatologist, Clinical Immunodermatology, St John's Institute of Dermatology, Guy's and St Thomas' NHS Foundation Trust, London, UK
Chapter 50

Girish Gupta
MBChB, FRCP
Consultant Dermatologist and Honorary Clinical Senior Lecturer, University of Edinburgh, Edinburgh, UK; Department of Dermatology, Royal Infirmary of Edinburgh, Edinburgh, UK
Chapter 141

Nadi K. Gupta
MBChB, FRCP, DipGUM, DFFP, DipHIV, MFSRH
Honorary Senior Clinical Lecturer, University of Sheffield, Sheffield; Consultant Physician in Genitourinary Medicine, Rotherham Hospital NHS Foundation Trust, Rotherham, UK
Chapter 30

Richard H. Guy
PhD, DSc
Professor of Pharmaceutical Science, University of Bath, Department of Pharmacy and Pharmacology, University of Bath, Bath, UK
Chapter 12

Emily Haesler
PhD, BN, P Grad Dip Adv Nurs (Gerontics)
Adjunct Professor, Curtin Health Innovation Research Institute; Adjunct Associate Professor, Australian Centre for Evidence Based Aged Care; Curtin Health Innovation Research Institute, Curtin University Perth, Australia; Australian Centre for Evidence Based Aged Care, School of Nursing, La Trobe University, Melbourne, Victoria, Australia; Academic Unit of General Practice, ANU Medical School, The Australian National University, Canberra, Australia
Chapter 123

Jürg Hafner
MD
Professor, Dermatologist, Dermatologic Surgeon, Angiologist and Phlebologist and Senior Staff, Department of Dermatology, University Hospital of Zurich, Zurich, Switzerland
Chapter 102

Philip J. Hampton
MBBS, BMedSci, FRCP, PhD
Consultant Dermatologist, Newcastle Hospitals NHS Trust, Newcastle upon Tyne, UK
Chapter 49

Muzlifah Haniffa
MBBCh, PhD, FRCP, FMedSci
Wellcome Senior Research Fellow in Clinical Science, Senior Group Leader, Wellcome Sanger Institute, Cambridge; Department of Dermatology and NIHR Newcastle Biomedical Research Centre, Newcastle Hospitals NHS Foundation Trust, Newcastle upon Tyne; Professor of Dermatology and Immunology, Biosciences Institute, Newcastle University, Newcastle upon Tyne, UK
Chapter 9

Matthew J. Harries
PhD, FRCP
Consultant Dermatologist, University of Manchester, MAHSC and NIHR Manchester Biomedical Research Centre, Salford Royal Hospital, Northern Care Alliance NHS Foundation Trust, Salford, Greater Manchester, UK
Chapter 87

Catherine A. Harwood
MBBS, MA, PhD, FRCP
Centre for Cell Biology and Cutaneous Research, Blizard Institute, Barts and the London School of Medicine and Dentistry, Queen Mary University of London, London, UK; Department of Dermatology, The Royal London Hospital, Barts Health NHS Trust, London, UK
Chapters 25, 147

Roderick J. Hay
DM, FRCP, FRCPath, FMedSci
Professor (Emeritus) of Cutaneous Infection, St John's Institute of Dermatology, King's College London, UK
Chapter 32

Susan Holmes
BSc (Hons), MD, FRCP
Consultant Dermatologist, Alan Lyell Centre for Dermatology, Glasgow Royal Infirmary, Glasgow, UK
Chapter 87

S. Walayat Hussain
BSc, MBChB, MRCP, FRACP, FACMS
Consultant Dermatological Surgeon, Leeds Centre for Dermatology, Chapel Allerton Hospital, Leeds Teaching Hospitals NHS Trust, Leeds, UK
Chapter 20

Sally Ibbotson
BSc, MBChB, MD, FRCP
Professor of Photodermatology and Honorary Consultant Dermatologist, Photobiology Unit, University of Dundee, Ninewells Hospital and Medical School, Dundee, UK; Photobiology Unit, Dermatology Department, Ninewells Hospital and Medical School, University of Dundee, Dundee, UK
Chapters 21, 22, 126

John R. Ingram
MA, MSc, DM, MRCP (Derm), FAcadMEd
Clinical Reader and Consultant Dermatologist, Division of Infection and Immunity, Cardiff University, Cardiff, UK
Chapters 39, 90

Matilde Iorizzo
MD, PhD, FMH
Dermatologist, Private Dermatology Practice, Bellinzona/Lugano, Switzerland
Chapter 93

Alan D. Irvine
MD, FRCP, FRCPI
Consultant Dermatologist, Children's Health Ireland at Crumlin, Dublin; St James's Hospital, Dublin; Trinity College, Dublin, Ireland
Chapters 74, 75, 77, 78

Peter Itin
MD
Professor of Dermatology and Venerology and Head of Department of Dermatology, University Hospital of Basel, Basel, Switzerland
Chapter 65

Natalia Jaimes
MD
Assistant Professor, Dr Phillip Frost Department of Dermatology & Cutaneous Surgery and Sylvester Comprehensive Cancer Center, University of Miami Miller School of Medicine, Miami, FL, USA
Chapter 145

Gregor B. E. Jemec
MD, DMSc
Professor and Clinical Lead, Department of Dermatology, Zealand University Hospital, Roskilde; Faculty of Health and Medical Sciences, University of Copenhagen, Copenhagen, Denmark
Chapter 90

Marc G. Jeschke
MD, PhD, FACS, FCAHS, FCCM, FRCS (C)
Vice President Research, Hamilton Health Sciences, Hamilton Health Sciences, Hamilton; McMaster University, Hamilton; Department of Surgery, Plastic Surgery, Department of Immunology, University of Toronto, Toronto, Ontario, Canada
Chapter 125

Timothy M. Johnson
MD
Professor, Michigan Medicine Department of Dermatology, Ann Arbor, MI, USA
Chapter 143

Graham A. Johnston
MBChB, FRCP, FRSPH
Consultant Dermatologist, Leicester Royal Infirmary, University Hospitals of Leicester NHS Trust, Leicester, UK
Chapter 85

Elizabeth Keeling
MBBCh, BAO, LRCP&SI, MRCPI
Dermatology Specialist Registrar, Beaumont Hospital, Dublin, Ireland
Chapter 104

Charles G. Kelly
MBChB, MSc, FRCP, FRCR, FBIR, DMRT
Consultant Clinical Oncologist and Lead for Radiotherapy, Northern Centre for Cancer Care, Freeman Hospital, Newcastle upon Tyne; Deputy Degree Programme Director and Honorary Clinical Senior Lecturer, Northern Institute for Cancer Research, Newcastle University, Newcastle upon Tyne, UK
Chapter 24

Cameron Kennedy
MA, MBBChir, FRCP
Consultant Dermatologist, Bristol Royal Infirmary and Bristol Royal Hospital for Children, Bristol, UK; Honorary Clinical Senior Lecturer, University of Bristol, Bristol, UK
Chapter 106

Thibault Kervarrec
MD, PhD
Department of Pathology, University Hospital Center of Tours, Tours, France
Chapter 146

Touraj Khosravi-Hafshejani
MD
Senior Resident, Department of Dermatology and Skin Science, University of British Columbia, Vancouver, BC, Canada
Chapter 51

Alexandra B. Kimball
MD, MPH, FAAD
Harvard Medical Faculty Physicians, Beth Israel Deaconess Medical Center, Boston, MA, USA
Chapter 157

George R. Kinghorn
OBE, MD, FRCP
Formerly, Honorary Professor and Consultant Physician in Genitourinary Medicine, Sheffield Teaching Hospitals NHS Foundation Trust, Sheffield, UK
Chapters 29, 30

Veronica A. Kinsler
MA, MBBChir, MRCPCH, PhD
Professor of Paediatric Dermatology and Dermatogenetics, Great Ormond St Hospital for Children NHS Foundation Trust and UCL GOS Institute of Child Health; Senior Group Leader, Mosaicism and Precision Medicine Laboratory, The Francis Crick Institute, London, UK
Chapter 73

Brian Kirby
MD, FRCPI
Consultant Dermatologist, St Vincent's University Hospital and Charles Institute, University College Dublin, Dublin, Ireland
Chapter 35

Eubee Koo
BS
Permanente Medical Group, Oakland, CA, USA
Chapter 157

Jan Kottner
PhD
Professor, Charité-Universitätsmedizin Berlin, Institute of Clinical Nursing Science, Berlin, Germany; Professor, Ghent University, Faculty of Medicine and Health Sciences, Ghent, Belgium
Chapter 123

Karoline Krause
Institute of Allergology, Charité-Universitätsmedizin Berlin, corporate member of Freie Universität Berlin, Humboldt-Universität zu Berlin, and Berlin Institute of Health, Germany
Chapter 44

Austin Kulasekararaj
MRCP, MD, FRCPath
Consultant Dermatologist, Department of Haematology, King's College Hospital, London, UK
Chapter 149

Sinéad M. Langan
MSc, PhD, FRCP
Professor of Clinical Epidemiology, Department of Non-Communicable Disease Epidemiology, London School of Hygiene and Tropical Medicine, London, UK; Honorary Consultant Dermatologist, St John's Institute of Dermatology, Guy's and St Thomas' NHS Foundation Trust, London, UK
Chapter 5

Felix Lauffer
MD, PhD
Department of Dermatology and Allergy, Technical University of Munich, Munich, Germany
Chapter 37

Philip M. Laws
MBChB, BSc (Hons)
Consultant Dermatologist and Honorary Senior Lecturer, Department of Dermatology, Chapel Allerton Hospital, Leeds, UK
Chapter 53

Alison M. Layton
MBChB, FRCP
Professor, Dermatology Skin Research Centre, Hull York Medical School, University of York, York; Department of Dermatology, Harrogate and District NHS Foundation Trust, Harrogate, UK
Chapter 88

Grace L. Lee
MD, FAAD
Assistant Professor, Baylor College of Medicine, Department of Dermatology, Consultant Pediatric Dermatologist, Texas Children's Hospital, Department of Pediatrics, Houston, TX, USA; Department of Dermatology, Baylor College of Medicine, Houston, TX, USA
Chapter 98

Haur Yueh Lee
MBBS, MRCP (UK), MMed (IntMed), FAMS (Derm)
Head of Department and Consultant Dermatologist, Department of Dermatology, Singapore General Hospital; Adjunct Assistant Professor, DUKE-NUS Graduate Medical School, Singapore
Chapter 118

Nick J. Levell
MD, FRCP, MBA
Professor of Dermatology and Consultant Dermatologist, Norwich Medical School, Norfolk and Norwich University Hospital, Norwich, UK
Chapters 1, 99, 100

Fiona Lewis
MD, FRCP
Consultant Dermatologist, St John's Institute of Dermatology, Guy's and St Thomas' NHS Foundation Trust, London, UK
Chapter 110

Joyce T. E. Lim
MBBS, FRCPI, FAMS (Derm)
Senior Consultant Dermatologist, Joyce Lim Skin and Laser Clinic, Singapore
Chapter 160

Mireille M. D. van der Linden
MD
Department of Dermatology, Amsterdam University Centre, Amsterdam, the Netherlands
Chapter 89

Dan Lipsker
MD, PhD
Faculté de Medicine, Université de Strasbourg, Strasbourg, France
Chapter 45

Diana N. J. Lockwood
BSc, MD, FRCP
Emeritus Professor of Tropical Medicine, London School of Hygiene and Tropical Medicine, London; Retired Consultant Leprologist, Hospital for Tropical Diseases, University College Hospital NHS Trust, London, UK
Chapter 28

Christopher R. Lovell
MBChB, MD, FRCP
Consultant Dermatologist, Department of Dermatology, Royal United Hospital and Royal National Hospital for Rheumatic Diseases, Bath, UK
Chapters 45, 94, 155

Nicholas J. Lowe
MBChB, MD, FRCP, FACP
Fellow American Academy of Dermatology, Consultant Dermatologist and Honorary Lecturer, Department of Dermatology, University of Manchester, Manchester, UK; Clinical Professor of Dermatology, UCLA School of Medicine, Los Angeles, CA, USA
Chapter 159

Philippa L. Lowe
MBChB, Dip, Derm
Dermatology Specialist, Manchester, UK
Chapter 159

Calum Lyon
FRCP
Dermatologist and Honorary Clinical Lecturer, York Hospital NHS Trust, York; Salford Royal Hospital NHS Trust, Salford, UK
Chapter 112

Vishal Madan
MBBS, MD, FRCP
Consultant Dermatologist, Laser Division, Dermatology Centre, Salford Royal NHS Foundation Trust, Salford, UK
Chapters 23, 132, 133, 140

Najibah Mahtab
MBBS, BSc, MRCP, FRCR
Northern Centre for Cancer Care, Freeman Hospital, Newcastle upon Tyne, UK
Chapter 24

Eleanor Mallon
MBBS, MD, FRCP
Consultant Dermatologist, Department of Dermatology, St Mary's Hospital, Imperial College Healthcare NHS Trust, London, UK
Chapter 111

Juan Mañá
MD, PhD
Professor of Dermatology, Department of Dermatology, Bellvitge University Hospital; Professor of Dermatology, Barcelona University, Barcelona, Spain
Chapter 96

Joaquim Marcoval
MD, PhD
Professor of Dermatology, Department of Dermatology, Bellvitge University Hospital; Professor of Dermatology, Barcelona University, Barcelona, Spain
Chapter 96

Ashfaq A. Marghoob
MD
Attending Physician, Dermatology Service, Memorial Sloan-Kettering Cancer Center, New York, NY, USA
Chapter 145

Angela Hernandez Martin
MD
Dermatología, Hospital Infantil Universitario Niño Jesús, Madrid, Spain
Chapter 63

Zlatko Marušić
MD, PhD
Consultant Pathologist, Clinical Department of Pathology and Cytology, University Hospital Center Zagreb, Zagreb, Croatia
Chapters 136, 137

Rubeta N. Matin
PhD, BSc, MBBS, FRCP
Department of Dermatology, Churchill Hospital, Oxford University Hospitals NHS Foundation Trust, Oxford, UK
Chapter 147

Marcus Maurer
MD
Institute of Allergology, Charité – Universitätsmedizin Berlin, corporate member of Freie Universität Berlin and Humboldt-Universität zu Berlin and Fraunhofer Institute for Translational Medicine and Pharmacology ITMP, Allergology and Immunology, Berlin, Germany
Chapter 43

Sandy R. McBride
MBBS, FRCP, MD
Consultant Dermatologist, Royal Free Hospital, London, UK
Chapter 15

John A. McGrath
MD, FRCP, FMedSci
Mary Dunhill Chair in Cutaneous Medicine, St John's Institute of Dermatology, School of Basic and Medical Biosciences, Faculty of Life Sciences and Medicine, King's College London, London, UK
Chapters 2, 8, 69

Kevin McKenna
MD, FRCP
Consultant Dermatologist, Dermatology Department, Belfast Trust, Belfast, UK
Chapters 21, 22

Amy McMichael
MBBS, MD, FRCP
Professor of Dermatology, Wake Forest Baptist Medical Center, Winston-Salem, NC, USA
Chapter 87

John Mee
BSc, PhD
Clinical Scientist, Immunodermatology Laboratory, Synnovis Analytics, St Thomas' Hospital, London; St John's Institute of Dermatology, Guy's and St Thomas' NHS Foundation Trust, London, UK
Chapter 3

Jemima E. Mellerio
BSc, MD, FRCP
Consultant Dermatologist and Honorary Senior Lecturer, St John's Institute of Dermatology, Guy's and St Thomas' NHS Foundation Trust, London, UK
Chapters 74, 75, 77, 78

Andrew G. Messenger
MBBS, MD, FRCP
Professor of Dermatology, University of Sheffield, Sheffield, UK
Chapter 87

Dieter Metze
MD
Professor, Department of Dermatology, University Hospital Münster, Münster, Germany
Chapter 63

Austinn C. Miller
MD
University of Texas Health Science Center, Houston, TX, USA
Chapters 33, 130

Christopher J. Miller
MD
Director, Penn Dermatology Oncology Center, Hospital of the University of Pennsylvania, Philadelphia, PA, USA
Chapter 20

George W. M. Millington
PhD, FRCP
Consultant Dermatologist, Dermatology Department, Norfolk and Norwich University Hospital, Norwich, UK
Chapter 72

Alexandra Mizara
BA, MSc, DPsych
Counselling Psychologist/Highly Specialist Psychologist in Psychodermatology, Royal Free Hospital, London, UK
Chapter 15

Sonja Molin
MD
Division of Dermatology, Queen's University, Kingston, Canada
Chapters 151–154

Gentiane Monsel
MD
Dermatologist, Sorbonne Université, Department of Infectious and Tropical Diseases, AP-HP, Hôpital Pitié-Salpêtrière, Paris, France; GrIDIST, Groupe Infectiologie Dermatologique – Infections Sexuellement Transmissibles, Société Française de Dermatologie
Chapter 34

Fanny Morice-Picard
MD, PhD
Service de Dermatologie et Dermatologie Pédiatrique, Hôpital St André, Bordeaux, France
Chapter 68

Andrew A.M. Morris
BM, BCh, PhD, FRCPCH
Consultant in Paediatric Metabolic Diseases, Manchester Centre for Genomic Medicine, Manchester University Hospitals NHS Foundation Trust, Manchester, UK
Chapter 79

Peter S. Mortimer
MD, FRCP
Professor of Dermatological Medicine, St George's Hospital, London, UK
Chapter 103

Megan Mowbray
MBChB, DCH, FRCP, MD, BTEC
Consultant Dermatologist, Department of Dermatology, Queen Margaret Hospital, NHS Fife, Dunfermline, UK
Chapter 105

Avad A. Mughal
BSc, FRCP, MRCP (Derm), MAcadMEd, PGDip, MBBCh
Consultant in Dermatology, Cutaneous Allergy and Biologics, Dermatology Department, Neath and Port Talbot Hospital, Swansea Bay University Health Board, Port Talbot, Wales, UK
Chapter 39

Chetan Mukhtyar
MB, MSc, MD, FRCP, FRCP (Edin)
Norwich Medical School, Norfolk and Norwich University Hospital, Norwich, UK
Chapter 100

Matthew Murphy
MBBCh, BAO, BSc, FRCPI
Consultant Endocrinologist, South Infirmary-Victoria University Hospital, Cork, Ireland
Chapters 59, 62

Ruth Murphy
DTM&H, MMEdSci, PhD, FRCP
Honorary Professor in Dermatology, Sheffield University, Sheffield; Sheffield University Teaching Hospitals NHS Foundation Trust, Sheffield, UK
Chapter 47

Rabindranath Nambi
MD, FRCP
Consultant Dermatologist, University Hospitals of Derby and Burton NHS Foundation Trust, Derby, UK
Chapter 121

Neera R. Nathan
MD, MSHS, FAAD
Department of Dermatology, Harvard Medical School, Massachusetts General Hospital, Boston, MA, USA
Chapter 157

Tim Niehues
MD
Paediatric Immunologist, Immunologist, Rheumatologist and Haematologist/Oncologist, Centre for Child Health and Adolescence, HELIOS Klinikum, Krefeld; Academic Hospital, RWTH, Aachen; Immunodeficiency and Rheumatology Centre, Krefeld, Germany
Chapter 80

Edel A. O'Toole
MBBCh, PhD, FRCP
Professor of Molecular Dermatology and Centre Lead, Centre for Cell Biology and Cutaneous Research, Blizard Institute, Queen Mary University of London, UK
Chapter 11

Netravali Michelle Oboite
MDc
Attending Physician, Children's Hospital of Philadelphia, Pennsylvania, USA
Chapter 61

Stephanie Ogden
MRCP, PhD
Salford Royal Hospital, Greater Manchester, UK
Chapter 4

Vinzenz Oji
MD
Private Lecturer, Department of Dermatology, University Hospital Münster, Münster; Hautarztpraxis am Buddenturm, Münster, Germany
Chapter 63

Rasha Omer
MBBS, MRCP, DTM&H, DipGUM, DipHIV, DRFSH
Consultant Physician in Genitourinary Medicine, Rotherham NHS Foundation Trust, Rotherham, UK
Chapter 29

Catherine H. Orteu
MBBS, BSc, MD, FRCP
Department of Dermatology, Royal Free London NHS Foundation Trust, London, UK
Chapters 54, 55

David Orton
BSc, MSc (Allergy), MBBS, FRCP
Consultant Dermatologist, OneWelbeck Skin Health and Allergy, London, UK
Chapter 127

Amy S. Paller
MD
Walter J Hamlin Professor and Chair of Dermatology, Professor of Pediatrics, Departments of Dermatology and Pediatrics, Northwestern University, Chicago, IL, USA
Chapter 67

Marcel C. Pasch
MD, PhD
Dermatologist, Radboud University Medical Center, Department of Dermatology, Nijmegen, The Netherlands
Chapter 93

Ralf Paus
MD, DSc, FRSB
Research Professor, Dr Phillip Frost Department of Dermatology & Cutaneous Surgery, University of Miami Miller School of Medicine, Miami, FL, USA; Centre for Dermatology Research, Institute of Inflammation and Repair, University of Manchester, Manchester, UK; and Department of Dermatology, University of Münster, Münster, Germany
Chapter 150

Elisabeth A. Pedersen
MD, PhD
Clinical Instructor in Dermatology, University of Michigan Medical Center, Ann Arbor, MI, USA
Chapter 156

Richard O. Phillips
PhD, FWACP, FGCP
Kumasi Centre for Collaborative Research in Tropical Medicine, Kwame Nkrumah University of Science and Technology, Kumasi, Ghana
Chapter 27

Vincent Piguet
MD, PhD, FRCP
Professor and Department Division Director, Division of Dermatology, Department of Medicine, University of Toronto; Division of Dermatology, Women's College Hospital, Toronto, Ontario, Canada
Chapter 31

Andrew E. Pink
MD, FRCP
Consultant Dermatologist and Senior Lecturer, St John's Institute of Dermatology, Guy's and St Thomas' NHS Foundation Trust, London, UK
Chapter 19

Elena Pope
MSc, FRCPC
Pediatric Dermatologist, Hospital for Sick Children, Toronto, Ontario, Canada
Chapter 135

Charlotte M. Proby
MA, FRCP
Division of Molecular and Cellular Medicine, School of Medicine, University of Dundee, Ninewells Hospital, Dundee, UK
Chapter 147

Eberhard Rabe
MD
Professor, Dermatologist and Phlebologist, Emeritus President of the International Union of Phlebology (UIP) and retired Senior Staff, Department of Dermatology, University Hospital of Bonn, Bonn, Germany
Chapter 102

Deepti H. Radia
BSc (Hons), MRCPI, FRCPath, MSc (MedEd)
Haematology Consultant, St John's Institute of Dermatology, Guy's and St Thomas' NHS Foundation Trust, London; Department of Haematology, Guy's and St Thomas' NHS Foundation Trust, London, UK
Chapter 46

Síona Ní Raghallaigh
MBBCh, BAO, MRCPI, MD
Consultant Dermatologist, Beaumont Hospital, Dublin, Ireland
Chapter 104

Neil Rajan
MBBS, PhD
Senior Lecturer and Honorary Consultant Dermatologist, Translational and Clinical Research Institute, Newcastle University and Newcastle Hospitals NHS Foundation Trust, Newcastle upon Tyne, UK
Chapters 74, 78

Yuval Ramot
MD, MSc
Dermatologist, Department of Dermatology, Hadassah Medical Center and the Faculty of Medicine, Hebrew University of Jerusalem, Jerusalem, Israel
Chapter 150

Luis Requena
MD, PhD
Chairman of Dermatology and Professor of Dermatology, Department of Dermatology, Fundación Jiménez Díaz, Universidad Autónoma, Madrid, Spain
Chapter 97

Nicole Revencu
MD, PhD
Consultant Clinical Geneticist, Center for Vascular Anomalies, Cliniques Universitaires Saint-Luc, Université catholique de Louvain (a VASCERN VASCA European Reference Centre), Brussels, Belgium
Chapter 71

Nick J. Reynolds
MBBS, BSc, FRCP, MD
Professor of Dermatology, Institute of Translational and Clinical Medicine, Newcastle University, UK; Honorary Consultant Dermatologist, Department of Dermatology, Newcastle Hospitals NHS Foundation Trust, Newcastle upon Tyne, UK
Chapter 41

Bertrand Richert
MD, PhD
Dermatologist, Brugmann – St Pierre and Children's University Hospitals, Université Libre de Bruxelles, Brussels, Belgium
Chapter 93

Franco Rongioletti
MD
Professor of Dermatology, Dermatology Clinic, University Vita-Salute San Raffaele Hospital, Milan, Italy
Chapter 57

Thomas Ruzicka
MD
Department of Dermatology and Allergology, Ludwig Maximilian University, Munich, Germany
Chapters 151–154

Berthold Rzany
MD, ScM
Medizin am Hauptbahnhof, Wien, Austria
Chapter 158

Dana L. Sachs
MD
Professor of Dermatology, University of Michigan Medical Center, Ann Arbor, MI, USA
Chapter 156

Nazanin Saedi
MD
Clinical Associate Professor, Department of Dermatology and Cutaneous Biology, Thomas Jefferson University, Philadelphia, PA, USA
Chapter 161

Robert P. E. Sarkany
FRCP, MD
Consultant Dermatologist and Head of Photodermatology, St John's Institute of Dermatology, Guy's and St Thomas' NHS Foundation Trust, London, UK
Chapter 58

Karin Sartorius
MD, PhD
Consultant Dermatologist, Department of Clinical Sciences and Education, Karolinska Institutet, Stockholm; and Department of Dermatology, Södersjukhuset, Stockholm, Sweden
Chapter 148

Valerie P. J. Saw
MBBS (Hons), FRANZCO, PhD
Consultant Ophthalmologist, Imperial College Healthcare NHS Trust, University College London Institute of Ophthalmology, London, UK
Chapter 107

Martin Schaller
MD, PhD
Professor, Deputy Medical Director, Department of Dermatology, Universitätsklinikum Tübingen, Tübingen, Germany
Chapter 89

Enno Schmidt
MD, PhD
Professor of Dermatology, Department of Dermatology and Lübeck Institute of Experimental Dermatology, University of Lübeck, Lübeck, Germany
Chapter 50

Stephan Schreml
MD, PhD
Department of Dermatology, University Medical Centre Regensburg, Regensburg, Germany
Chapter 56

Matthew J. Scorer
BMBS, MRCP
Consultant Dermatologist, Leicester Royal Infirmary, University Hospitals of Leicester NHS Trust, Leicester, UK
Chapter 85

Alison V. Sears
St John's Institute of Dermatology, Guy's and St Thomas' NHS Foundation Trust, London, UK
Chapter 42

Edward Seaton
DM, FRCP
Consultant Dermatologist, OneWelbeck Skin Health and Allergy, London, UK
Chapters 132, 133

Neil J. Sebire
BSc, FRCPath, MD
Professor of Paediatric Pathology, Paediatric Pathology, Great Ormond Street Hospital for Children NHS Foundation Trust and UCL GOS Institute of Child Health, London, UK
Chapter 73

Jane Setterfield
BDS, DCH, DRCOG, MD, FRCP
Professor of Oral & Dermatological Medicine/Honorary Consultant, Centre for Host-Microbiome Interactions, King's College London Faculty of Dentistry, Oral & Craniofacial Sciences, London, UK; Department of Oral Medicine & St John's Institute of Dermatology, Guy's and St Thomas' NHS Foundation Trust, London, UK
Chapter 108

Dimitris Sgouros
MD
Consultant Dermatologist, 1st Department of Dermatology and Venereology, School of Medicine, National and Kapodistrian University of Athens, Andreas Sygros Hospital, Athens, Greece
Chapter 131

Jennifer C. Harrison Sharif
MbCHB, BmedSCI, MRCP (Derm)
Consultant Dermatologist, Salford Royal NHS Foundation Trust, Manchester, UK
Chapter 114

Ashish Sharma
MA, MBBS, MRCS, MRCP
Consultant Dermatologist and Mohs Surgeon, Nottingham University Hospital, Nottingham, UK
Chapter 106

Alfredo Siller Jr
MD
University of Texas Health Science Center, Houston, TX, USA
Chapters 33, 130

Catherine H. Smith
MD, FRCP
Professor of Dermatology and Therapeutics and Consultant Dermatologist, Skin Therapy Research Unit, St John's Institute of Dermatology, Guy's and St Thomas' Hospitals NHS Foundation Trust and King's College London, London, UK
Chapters 13, 19

Noah R. Smith
MD
Assistant Professor, Michigan Medicine Department of Dermatology, Ann Arbor, MI, USA
Chapter 143

Lea Solman
MD, MRCP, FRCPCH
Consultant Paediatric Dermatologist, Great Ormond Street Hospital for Children NHS Foundation Trust, London, UK
Chapters 115, 116

Reinhart Speeckaert
MD, PhD
Department of Dermatology, Ghent University Hospital, Ghent, Belgium
Chapter 86

Eli Sprecher
MD, PhD, MBA
Professor and Chair, Division of Dermatology, Deputy Director General for R&D and Innovation, Division of Dermatology, Tel Aviv Sourasky Medical Center, Tel Aviv, Israel
Chapter 66

Sonja Ständer
MD
Dermatologist and Dermatopathologist, Department of Dermatology, University Hospital Münster, Münster, Germany
Chapter 81

Amy Stanway
MBChB, FRACP
Consultant Dermatologist, Bethlehem Skin Clinic, Tauranga, New Zealand
Chapter 113

Irene Stefanaki
MD, PhD
Academic Consultant Dermatologist, 1st Department of Dermatology and Venereology, School of Medicine, National and Kapodistrian University of Athens, Andreas Sygros Hospital, Athens, Greece
Chapter 131

Jane C. Sterling
MBBChir, MA, FRCP, PhD
Consultant Dermatologist, Department of Dermatology, Cambridge University Hospitals NHS Foundation Trust, Addenbrooke's Hospital, Cambridge, UK
Chapter 25

Natalie Stone
BA, FRCP
Consultant Dermatologist, Aneurin Bevan University Health Board, Newport, Wales, UK
Chapter 127

Alexander Stratigos
MD
Professor of Dermatology-Venereology, 1st Department of Dermatology and Venereology, School of Medicine, National and Kapodistrian University of Athens, Andreas Sygros Hospital, Athens, Greece
Chapter 131

Kira Süßmuth
MD
Department of Dermatology, University Hospital Münster, Münster, Germany
Chapter 63

Saleem M. Taibjee
MBBCh, BMedSci, MRCPCH, DipRCPath
Consultant Dermatologist, Departments of Dermatology and Pathology, Dorset County Hospital, Dorchester, Dorset, UK
Chapter 95

Alain Taïeb
MD, PhD
Service de Dermatologie et Dermatologie Pédiatrique, Hôpital St André, Bordeaux, France
Chapter 68

Anita Takwale
MBBS, MD, MRCP
Consultant Dermatologist, Department of Dermatology, Gloucestershire Royal Hospital, Gloucestershire Hospitals NHS Foundation Trust, Gloucester, UK
Chapter 105

Jerry Tan
MD, FRCP
Adjunct Professor, Department of Medicine, Western University, Ontario, Canada
Chapter 89

Ruth E. Taylor
BSc, MBChB, MRC Psych, MSc (Psych), MSc (Epid), PhD
Consultant Liaison Psychiatrist, Department of Liaison Psychiatry, Barts Health NHS Trust, London; Senior Lecturer, Queen Mary College of Medicine, University of London, London, UK
Chapter 84

Anastasia Therianou
MBBS, PhD
Consultant Dermatologist, Imperial College Healthcare Trust, London, UK
Chapter 40

Thai Hoa Tran
MD, FRCPC
Pediatric Hematologist-Oncologist, CHU Sainte-Justine, Montreal, Quebec, Canada
Chapter 135

Heiko Traupe
MD
Assistant Professor, Department of Dermatology, University Hospital Münster, Münster, Germany
Chapter 63

Kenneth Y. Tsai
MD, PhD, FAAD
Senior Member, Departments of Anatomic Pathology and Tumor Biology, H. Lee Moffitt Cancer Center and Research Institute, Tampa, FL, USA
Chapter 138

Stephen K. Tyring
MD, PhD
University of Texas Health Science Center, Houston, TX, USA;
Chapters 33, 130

Christos Tziotzios
MA, MBBChir (Cantab), PhD, FHEA, FRCP
Senior Lecturer, Genetic Skin Disease Group, St. John's Institute of Dermatology, King's College London; Consultant Dermatologist, St. John's Institute of Dermatology, Guy's & St. Thomas' Hospitals NHS Foundation Trust, London, UK
Chapter 91

Jouni Uitto
MD, PhD
Professor and Chair, Department of Dermatology and Cutaneous Biology, Thomas Jefferson University, Philadelphia, PA, USA
Chapter 2

Miikka Vikkula
MD, PhD
Professor of Human Genetics, Human Molecular Genetics, de Duve Institute, Université catholique de Louvain, Brussels, Belgium; Center for Vascular Anomalies, Cliniques Universitaires Saint-Luc, Université catholique de Louvain (a VASCERN VASCA European Reference Centre), Brussels, Belgium
Chapter 71

Carl Vinciullo
MBBS, FACD
Emeritus Consultant, Department of Dermatology, Royal Perth Hospital, Perth, Western Australia, Australia
Chapter 140

John J. Voorhees
MD, FRCP
Duncan and Ella Poth Distinguished Professor of Dermatology and Chair of Department of Dermatology, University of Michigan Medical Center, Ann Arbor, MI, USA
Chapter 156

Jill S. Waibel
MD
Consultant Dermatologist, Miami Dermatology and Laser Institute, Miami, FL, USA
Chapter 23

Sarah Wakelin
BSc, MBBS, FRCP
Consultant Dermatologist, Imperial College Healthcare Trust, London, UK
Chapter 40

Stephen L. Walker
PhD, MRCP (UK), DTM&H
Clinical Lecturer, Faculty of Infectious and Tropical Diseases, London School of Hygiene and Tropical Medicine, London, UK
Chapters 27, 28

Sarah Walsh
MBBCh, BAO, BMedSci, MRCP
Consultant Dermatologist, Department of Dermatology, King's College Hospital, London, UK
Chapter 118

Timothy S. Wang
MD
Associate Professor, Department of Dermatology, Johns Hopkins Health System, Baltimore; Director, Cutaneous Surgery Unit and Micrographic Surgery and Dermatologic Oncology (Mohs) Fellowship Program, Johns Hopkins Health System, Baltimore, MD, USA
Chapter 20

Molly Wanner
MD, MBA
Assistant Professor, Department of Dermatology, Harvard Medical School, Massachusetts General Hospital, Boston, MA, USA
Chapter 157

Richard E. Watchorn
MBBCh, BAO, MD, FRCP
Consultant Dermatologist and Honorary Clinical Senior Lecturer, Beaumont Hospital, Dublin, Ireland; University College London Hospitals and Chelsea & Westminster Hospitals, London, UK
Chapter 109

Sheila Weitzman
MBBCh, FRCPC
Pediatric Hematologist-Oncologist, Hospital for Sick Children, Toronto, Ontario, Canada
Chapter 135

Jonathan M. L. White
PhD, MRCP (UK)
Consultant Dermatologist, Department of Dermatology, Hôpital Erasme, Brussels; Ecole de Santé Publique, Université libre de Bruxelles, Brussels, Belgium
Chapters 128, 129

Heather Whitehouse
MBBS, PGCert Health Research, MRCP (Derm)
Consultant Dermatologist, The Leeds Centre for Dermatology, Leeds Teaching Hospitals NHS Trust, Leeds, UK
Chapter 88

Sean J. Whittaker
MBChB, MD, FRCP
Consultant Dermatologist and Professor of Cutaneous Oncology (Skin Cancer), Division of Genetics and Molecular Medicine, King's College London, London, UK; St John's Institute of Dermatology, Guy's and St Thomas' NHS Foundation Trust, London, UK; School of Basic and Medical Biosciences, Kings College London, London, UK
Chapters 134, 139

Hywel C. Williams
DSc, FRCP, FMedSci
Professor of Dermato-Epidemiology and Co-Director, Nottingham University Hospitals NHS Trust, Nottingham, UK; Centre of Evidence-Based Dermatology, Population and Lifespan Sciences, School of Medicine, University of Nottingham, Nottingham; Centre of Evidence-Based Dermatology
Chapters 5, 17

Niall J.E. Wilson
FRCP
Consultant Dermatologist, Liverpool University Hospitals NHS Foundation Trust, UK
Chapter 92

Richard T. Woolf
PhD, MRCP
Consultant Dermatologist, St John's Institute of Dermatology, Guy's and St Thomas' Hospitals NHS Foundation Trust, London, UK
Chapters 13, 19

Catriona Wootton
MBChB, MRCP (Derm), DTM&H, MA (Hons)
Consultant Dermatologist, Dermatology Department, Churchill Hospital, Oxford, UK; Department of Infection, John Radcliffe Hospital, Oxford, UK
Chapter 26

Albert C. Yan
MD, FFAP, FFAD
Paediatric Dermatologist, Children's Hospital of Philadelphia, Pennsylvania, USA
Chapter 61

Gil Yosipovitch
MD
Dermatologist, Stiefel Chair in Medical Dermatology; Director, Miami Itch Center; Dr Phillip Frost Department of Dermatology and Cutaneous Surgery, Miller School of Medicine, University of Miami, Miamia, FL, USA
Chapter 81

Antony R. Young
BSc, MSc, PhD
Professor of Experimental Photobiology, St John's Institute of Dermatology, School of Basic and Medical Biosciences, Faculty of Life Sciences and Medicine, King's College London, London, UK
Chapter 10

Christopher B. Zachary
MBBS, FRCP
Professor and Chair Emeritus, Department of Dermatology, University of California, Irvine, CA, USA
Chapter 161

Mozheh Zamiri
MD, FRCP
Consultant Dermatologist, Department of Dermatology, Queen Elizabeth University Hospital, Glasgow, UK
Chapter 64

Hessel H. van der Zee
MD, PhD
Department of Dermatology, Erasmus Medical Center, Rotterdam, the Netherlands
Chapter 90

Christos C. Zouboulis
Prof.Dr.med., Prof.h.c., Dr.h.c.
Director and Professor of Dermatology and Venereology, Departments of Dermatology, Venereology, Allergology and Immunology, Staedtisches Klinikum Dessau, Brandenburg Medical School Theodor Fontane and Faculty of Health Sciences Brandenburg, Dessau, Germany
Chapters 48, 88

Esther J. van Zuuren
MD
Department of Dermatology, Leiden University Medical Centre, Leiden, the Netherlands
Chapter 89

Preface to the Tenth Edition

Eight years have elapsed since the publication of the last edition of Rook's Textbook of Dermatology – "Rook". The SARS-CoV-2 (COVID) pandemic delayed and disrupted our plans and enforced some workplace changes for our publishers, Wiley, but we are delighted that the tenth edition of Rook is finally on the shelves and available online. Despite being a disrupter, COVID inevitably makes an appearance in several of our chapters with particular mention in the one on viral diseases. The book retains the format introduced at the time of the complete overhaul and rewrite for the ninth edition but with an increase in the number of chapters to 161. We said goodbye to two of our senior editorial team Robert Chalmers and Daniel Creamer and thank them for their service to Rook. In their place we welcome Rosalind Simpson and Walayat Hussain who bring new perspectives and youthful dynamism to the team. The Associate Editor team has been refreshed and is now a team of 11 Section Editors with an expanded brief. The authorship is more international than ever before to reflect the worldwide reach of Rook, but at the same time retaining the book's quintessential Britishness. The global nature of dermatology is reflected by a new chapter devoted to the topic.

There is a long overdue recognition of the characteristics of skin disease morphology in skin of colour particularly for inflammatory dermatoses. Not only is the colour of lesions different, but in many instances the pattern of distribution may differ markedly from what is observed in white skin. Wherever possible we have updated and expanded our image library to capture these changes and have started to phase out outdated terms such as erythema. We recognise that this is a process, but we have at least begun the change. As previously, watermarked Rook figures and tables are downloadable as PowerPoint slides for educational purposes.

The spirit of Rook lives on as exemplified by our predecessors, the editors of the first edition, Arthur Rook, Darrell Wilkinson and John Ebling. Even in the modern age of instantly accessible facts and shortened attention spans, the comprehensive, thoughtful textbook nature of Rook still has a place in our armamentarium of dermatological knowledge.

Our thanks go as always to the team at Wiley and to the team of freelancers with special mention of the indefatigable Nik Prowse.

Chris Griffiths
Jonathan Barker
Tanya Bleiker
Walayat Hussain
Rosalind Simpson

Preface to the First Edition

No comprehensive reference book on dermatology has been published in the English language for ten years and none in England for over a quarter of a century. The recent literature of dermatology is rich in shorter texts and in specialist monographs but the English-speaking dermatologist has long felt the need for a substantial text for regular reference and as a guide to the immense monographic and periodical literature. The editors have therefore planned the present volume primarily for the dermatologist in practice or in training, but have also considered the requirements of the specialist in other fields of medicine and of the many research workers interested in the skin in relation to toxicology or cosmetic science.

An attempt has been made throughout the book to integrate our growing knowledge of the biology of skin and of fundamental pathological processes with practical clinical problems. Often the gap is still very wide but the trends of basic research at least indicate how it may eventually be bridged. In a clinical textbook the space devoted to the basic sciences must necessarily be restricted but a special effort has been made to ensure that the short accounts which open many chapters are easily understood by the physician whose interests and experience are exclusively clinical.

For the benefit of the student we have encouraged our contributors to make each chapter readable as an independent entity, and have accepted that this must involve the repetition of some material.

The classification employed is conventional and pragmatic. Until our knowledge of the mechanisms of disease is more profound no truly scientific classification is possible. In so many clinical syndromes multiple aetiological factors are implicated. To emphasize one at the expense of others is often misleading. Most diseases are to some extent influenced by genetic factors and a large proportion of common skin reactions are modified by the emotional state of the patient. Our knowledge is in no way advanced by classifying hundreds of diseases as genodermatoses and dozens as psychosomatic.

The true prevalence of a disease may throw light on its aetiology but reported incidence figures are often unreliable and incorrectly interpreted. The scientific approach to the evaluation of racial and environmental factors has therefore been considered in some detail.

The effectiveness of any physician in practice must ultimately depend on his ability to make an accurate clinical diagnosis. Clinical descriptions are detailed and differential diagnosis is fully discussed. Histopathology is here considered mainly as an aid to diagnosis but references to fuller accounts are provided.

The approach to treatment is critical but practical. Many empirical measures are of proven value and should not be abandoned merely because their efficacy cannot yet be scientifically explained. However, many familiar remedies old and new have been omitted either because properly controlled clinical trials have shown them to be of no value or because they have been supplanted by more effective and safer preparations.

There are over nine hundred photographs but no attempt has been made to provide an illustration of every disease. To have done so would have increased the bulk and price of the book without increasing proportionately its practical value. The conditions selected for illustrations are those in which a photograph significantly enhances the verbal description. There are a few conditions we wished to illustrate, but of which we could not obtain unpublished photographs of satisfactory quality.

The lists of references have been selected to provide a guide to the literature. Important articles now of largely historical interest have usually been omitted, except where a knowledge of the history of a disease simplifies the understanding of present concepts and terminology. Books and articles provided with a substantial bibliography are marked with an asterisk.

Many of the chapters have been read and criticized by several members of the team and by other colleagues. Professor Wilson Jones, Dr R.S. Wells and Dr W.E. Parish have given valuable assistance with histopathological, genetic and immunological problems respectively. Many advisers, whose services are acknowledged in the following pages, have helped us with individual chapters. Any errors which have not been eliminated are, however, the responsibility of the editors and authors.

The editors hope that this book will prove of value to all those who are interested in the skin either as physicians or as research workers. They will welcome readers' criticisms and suggestions which may help them to make the second edition the book they hope to produce.

Arthur Rook, Darrell Wilkinson and John Ebling

About the Companion Website

Rook's Textbook of Dermatology, Tenth Edition is accompanied by a companion website:

https://www.wiley.com/rooksdermatology10e

The website includes:

– Full list of references
– Videos

PART 1
Foundations of Dermatology

CHAPTER 1

History of Dermatology

Nick J. Levell

Norwich Medical School, Norfolk and Norwich University Hospital, Norwich, UK

Introduction: when did dermatology history begin?, 1.1
Ancient dermatology writings, 1.1
The first medical texts, 1.1
Ancient Egypt, 1.2
Mesopotamia, 1.2
Ancient Greece, 1.2
Ancient India, 1.2
Growth of rational medicine, 1.2
The Silk Road: the pathway of rational medicine, 1.2
China, 1.2
South Indian early Buddhism, 1.2
The Holy Bible, 1.3
Greeks: the rational age, 1.3
Roman Empire, 1.3

Dermatology after the fall of Rome, 1.3
Early Islamic medicine and dermatology, 1.3
Italy during the European Renaissance, 1.3
European Enlightenment, 1.3
Growth of scientific dermatology, 1.4
Willan and Bateman: definition of skin diseases, 1.4
L'Hôpital St Louis, Paris: the first skin hospital, 1.4
Natural Sciences Hebra and the German-speaking Europeans, 1.5
Britain in the late 19th century, 1.6
United States in the 19th century, 1.7
Development of dermatology as a global specialty in the 20th century, 1.7
Skin infections, 1.7

Inflammatory disease and immunomodulatory treatments, 1.8
Dermatology surgery, 1.8
Medical dermatology, 1.8
Contact dermatitis and allergy, 1.8
Phototherapy, 1.8
Genital dermatology, 1.8
Psychodermatology and social medicine, 1.8
Cosmetic dermatology, 1.9
Paediatric dermatology and genetics, 1.9
Overcoming prejudice in dermatology, both from outside and within, 1.9
Images, technology and teledermatology, 1.9
Key references, 1.10

Introduction: when did dermatology history begin?

Dermatology history is the story of humanity. For all species, good skin care improves survival. Primates groom each other to reduce infestation. Many animals lick wounds. For most living beings, including humans, healthy, well-functioning skin is more likely to facilitate reproduction and hence survival of genes. Caring for the skin and hair improves the appeal to a potential mate. Genital skin disorders can prevent reproduction. Since earliest times, poor wound care or untreated inflammation would increase the risk of skin infections and reduce chances of survival.

Before the development of agriculture around 12 000 years ago, humans lived in small hunter gatherer groups so had little to fear from epidemic infectious diseases. Those who know how to keep skin healthy are more able to nuture, feed and support children and so pass on knowledge of skin care to future generations. The genes and habits of those with good dermatological care in ancient times, as now, were more likely to survive. Dermatology activity, removing parasites, applying grease to dry skin and cleaning and dressing wounds and burns, must have been important roles for the Shamans and Wise Women in primitive hominid tribal groups.

With the onset of agriculture came more sedentary group living and so diseases changed. Pandemics began and have plagued humanity to this day. Bioarchaeologists provide evidence of disease and early medical activity from times before the invention of writing. Palaeodermatologists have identified changes compatible with smallpox, lice and basal cell naevus syndrome in ancient Egyptian mummies [1,2] (Figure 1.1). Possible metastatic melanoma was found in 2400-year-old pre-Colombian Inca mummies [3]. More recently, tuberculosis, leprosy and syphilis leave changes on skeletons.

Writing became essential as humans built the first cities in Africa (Egypt *c*.3100 BC), the Middle East (Mesopotamia *c*.3000 BC), India (Indus valley *c*.2500 BC), Europe (Crete *c*.1800 BC) and China (Shang *c*.1400 BC). Early texts were mainly for administrative or religious purposes, but medical writings soon appeared. Many of these related to skin disorders.

Ancient dermatology writings

The first medical texts

Medical writings between *c*.3000 BC and 400 BC in most cultures had a theoretical basis founded on religious beliefs with pragmatic practical tips. Historians have often stated that there was an initial age of medicine dominated by magic, followed by the growth of rational medicine led by Hippocrates around 400 BC. However, evidence and logic suggest that the reality was not so clear-cut. Experience makes it obvious that doctors who relied solely on magic and religion would not have cured many patients and would have been rejected by people seeking out health care that worked.

Rook's Textbook of Dermatology, Tenth Edition. Edited by Christopher Griffiths, Jonathan Barker, Tanya Bleiker, Walayat Hussain and Rosalind Simpson.
© 2024 John Wiley & Sons Ltd. Published 2024 by John Wiley & Sons Ltd.

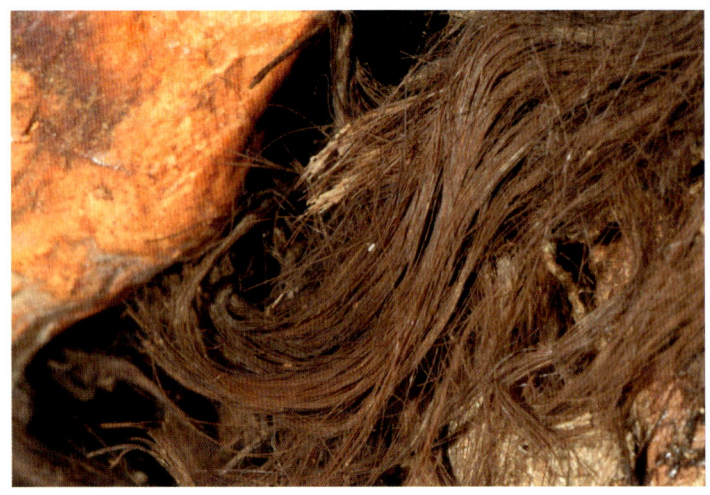

Figure 1.1 Suspected head lice eggs on female mummified body in British Museum from Gebelein area of Egypt pre-dynastic period (4400–3000 BC). Reproduced from Leslie and Levell 2006 [2], with permission of John Wiley & Sons.

A pharmacopoeia, written by an unknown Sumerian (Mesopotamia in the Middle East) in the third millennium BC may be the earliest medical writing [1]. It is on a clay tablet and describes a selection of external salves comprising cedar oil, wine and botanical, mineral and animal materials. Other preparations include clay mixed with honey, water and oil.

Medical writing moved from clay tablets, to papyrus to paper and now technology has moved medical textbooks such as *Rook's Textbook of Dermatology* back to tablets of a different type.

Ancient Egypt

Imhotep, the Chief Vizier to the Pharaoh Zoser (2700 BC), was renowned as a physician and was deified by the Egyptians. Egyptian medical writings date from a millennium later. The Edwin Smith Papyrus (*c*.1600 BC) known as the 'Book of Wounds' mentions wound dressings using fresh meat and then honey, grease and lint. However, the most important medical text is the Ebers Papyrus (1550 BC) written on over 20 metres of papyrus [2]. This describes 700 magical formulae and 800 formulae to treat 15 diseases of the abdomen, 29 of the eyes and 18 of the skin. Although dermatologists today use topical mixtures called 'Specials', the ancient ingredients differ from modern formulae. The text includes a baldness cure: a drink made from black ass testicles, or vulval and penis extracts from a black lizard. The Ebers Papyrus also describes an effective treatment for the Guinea worm: wrap the emerging end of the worm around a stick and slowly pull it out.

Mesopotamia

Over 1000 clay tablets that refer to medicine, of which 40 comprise a medical diagnostic handbook, and written *c*.1000 BC, are attributed to Esagil-kin-apli, a Babylonian physician. The writings on skin disease demonstrate the interplay of magic and empiricism [3]:
- Tablet 9, line 48: 'If his face is covered in white boils: Hand of the Sun God Ama, he will survive …'.
- Tablet 9, line 49: 'If his face is covered in black boils: Hand of the God I tar, he will die …'.
- Table 14, line 128: 'If his testicles are black he will die …' (possibly the first description of Fournier gangrene).

Ancient Greece

Asclepius is thought to have practised about 1000 BC in Greece. The reality of his work is lost in stories around his deification. Greek legend confuses him with the Egyptian God/physician Imhotep and also describes him as a son of the God Apollo (the healer) and the Goddess Panacea. Asclepius is said to have been executed by the gods for taking gold to raise the dead, a lesson for modern clinicians tempted by greed or arrogance to behave unethically. Temples to Asclepius included healing dogs to lick wounds. His followers in Greece persisted for centuries and included Hippocrates and Aristotle.

Ancient India

Early Brahmana (hereditary priests) guarded the Sanskrit religious teachings, the Veda (knowledge), from 1500 BC. Much of the medicine revolved around a magico-religious approach that paralleled that of Mesopotamia and Egypt. Early Vedic rites involved animal sacrifice, but writings included information on practical dermatology such as the use of cautery for haemostasis.

Growth of rational medicine

The Silk Road: the pathway of rational medicine

The trading route known as the Silk Road linked China, India, the Middle East and eastern Europe *c*.400 BC. At around this time, a growth of rational medicine appeared in Europe along with similar ideas in south India and China, so it seems likely that a two-way flow of medical ideas took place in parallel with the trade items. It can be debated whether knowledge flowed mainly from East to West or from West to East. The 'Diagnostic Handbook' from Mesopotamia, from 1000 BC, remained in print but between 600 and 400 BC changed radically in nature to show that disease was subject to the forces of nature and originated from the body rather than being of a divine nature.

China

Existing texts date back to at least 200 BC, but they may have originated over 2000 years before. Some original formulae are thought to be still in use today. Although there is little relationship to what western medicine considers to be an anatomical- or physiological-based system, the underlying concepts were not based on religion or spirits. Disease is seen to be based on a loss of harmony of the yin/yang system upsetting the qi (energy) and the meridians [1]. This is a generalist approach: skin disorders are considered to be manifestations of an internal problem. Sections on skin disease exist in classic works from 652 BC. Urticaria or 'wind type concealed rash' was considered to be due to excess lesser yin causing fluid obstruction in the skin. The 'Yellow Emperor's Inner Canon' describes urticaria and eczema.

South Indian early Buddhism

The Pali scripts date back to around 400 BC and describe the work of the Buddha [2]. The *Girimananda Sutra* described dermatology nursing, psychodermatology, occlusion therapy for foot eczema and possible early descriptions of skin diseases including leprosy, boils/abscesses, scrofula, ringworm, scabies, pustular eruptions, plethora, fistula and sexually transmitted diseases.

The Holy Bible
The Book of Leviticus written c.450 BC gave an account of how to diagnose 'leprosy' – although the descriptions of skin disease in this text could include many chronic cutaneous infections including tinea infection, impetigo and infected eczema. Practical tips on the management of contagious cutaneous disease include burning clothes and isolation of those afflicted.

Greeks: the rational age
Hippocrates (c.400 BC) was known to his contemporaries as Hippocrates the Great – an accolade indeed in the age of Plato and Socrates. He was an Asclepian physician and teacher on the island of Cos. Some great ideas attributed to him may have been written by his pupils at his school over later generations, who built up a body of medical knowledge. Hippocrates' school moved away from the magical and religious approach to medicine and adopted a method based on logic and reason. His approach was, like the Chinese, to see disease in the context of the whole patient and to see people as physical entities subject to the same laws of nature as the world. He used diet and exercise as therapies and adopted an expectant approach, not rushing to intervene. His writings on leg ulcers are relevant now: 'In the case of an ulcer, it is not expedient to stand; more especially if the ulcer be situated in the leg; but neither, also, is it proper to sit or walk. But quiet and rest are particularly expedient …'.

Roman Empire
Galen was born in Pergamon, Turkey in 120 AD and travelled to Egypt to learn about African and Indian medicine prior to settling in Rome. He studied anatomy through the dissection of animals (not humans), but then set Hippocratic ideas into an incorrect anatomical and physiological framework. This was based on four humours that might lead to fever if in excess: yellow bile, black bile, phlegm and blood. This led to an enthusiasm for blood-letting in his followers, aiming to restore balance in those with fever or if the physician wished to prevent fever.

Galen had a powerful intellect, an overbearing personality and a gift for self-publicity and was a prolific writer. Consequently, perhaps, this theoretical basis for medicine became entrenched in Europe and the Middle East. A period of relative intellectual stagnation regarding underlying disease processes persisted for over 1500 years. This may have been partly due to religious and cultural bans on human dissection until Renaissance times.

For 500 years after Galen, a series of Greek and Roman writers defined diseases within this flawed model of basic science. Therapeutic advances were made with various herbal and mineral remedies for skin disorders. Wood tars and coal tars were described for inflammatory skin disorders, presumably eczema and psoriasis [3]. The last of the series of Greco-Roman authors was Paul of Aegina (around 700 AD) who wrote a medical encyclopaedia in seven books of which book IV concerns skin disease [4]. This may be considered the earliest dermatology textbook.

Dermatology after the fall of Rome

Early Islamic medicine and dermatology
With the failure of the Roman Empire and the onset of the Dark Ages in Europe, the baton of medical knowledge in the West was passed back to the Middle East. Much would have been lost were it not for translations into Arabic by Christian and Islamic scholars at the Bayt al Hikma centre set up in 832 in Baghdad, the capital of the Islamic Empire. Hundreds of Greek, Latin and Sanskrit texts were translated, making Islamic culture the centre for learning. A series of medical compendia were produced, the first being the 'Paradise of Wisdom' (*Firdaws al-bikma*) by Ali ibn Rabban al-Tabari (c. 850 AD).

The great Persian physician, Muhammad ibn Zakariya al-Razi (865–925; known as 'Rhazes' in the West) studied in Rayy near Tehran, before settling in Baghdad. He wrote over 200 texts and initially challenged many of Galen's precepts – although ultimately describing himself as a Galen's disciple. He wrote *al-Jadari wa'l-hasba* ('Smallpox and Measles') in which he was the first to distinguish between febrile exanthemas: 'The rash of measles usually appears at once, but the rash of smallpox spot after spot'. Al-Razi's work was renowned in the Arabic world and was translated into Latin, still being reprinted in the West in 1542, over 600 years after his death.

The Persian writers, al-Majusi (Haly Abbas: 10th century), Ibn Sina (Avicenna: 980–1037) and al-Zahrawi (Albucasis: 936–1013), all wrote influential medical texts.

Italy during the European Renaissance
In the mid-16th century Europe was slowly struggling out of the religious superstition that characterised the Dark Ages and Middle Ages. A group of brilliant doctors in Padua, including Vesalius and Mercurialis (Geronimo Mercuriale), set up a system of learning and wrote medical texts that revitalised medicine in Europe. Mercurialis wrote *De Morbis Cutaneis* in 1572: this summarised work of earlier writers and had a focus on hair disorders, but still represents the first dermatology textbook in the West since the time of Paul of Aegina, 800 years before.

European Enlightenment
A series of dermatology textbooks written in the 18th century pulled dermatology through to the beginning of the modern age.

Daniel Turner (Figure 1.2) wrote the first English language dermatology textbook in 1712 [1] (Figure 1.3). This was a series of case reports which gives much insight into how skin disease was diagnosed and treated. The book was popular, running to four editions over 20 years. Turner was an English surgeon, who aspired to be a physician, and he dedicated his book to the President of the London Royal College of Physicians, perhaps hoping for acceptance. He was awarded association to the Royal College only as a 'Licentiate', as a medical degree (then only available in England from Oxford or Cambridge) was required to be a full member. Turner then endowed a medical library at Yale University in America and was given the first medical degree ever awarded in America, but, even with this distinction, he still failed to achieve his London Royal College membership.

Dermatology was linked with venereology in many European countries, and Jean Astruc, physician to the Parisian Court, wrote

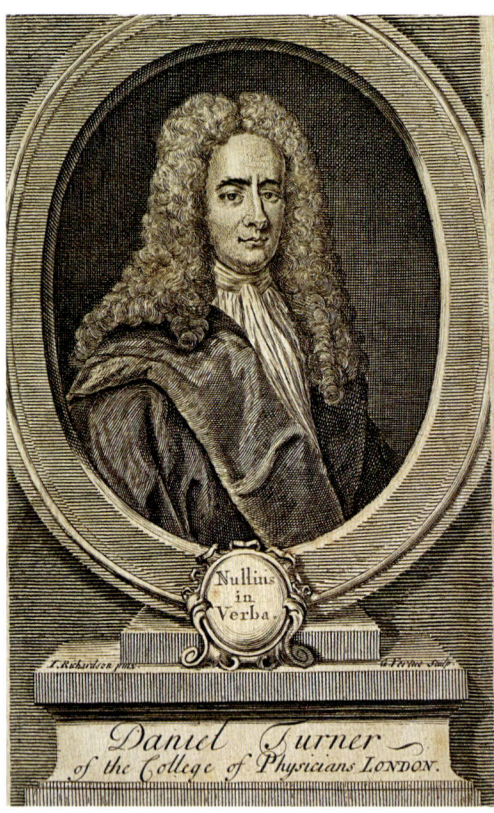

Figure 1.2 Daniel Turner. Writer of first English language dermatology textbook, who received the first medical degree from North America. Courtesy of Nick J. Levell.

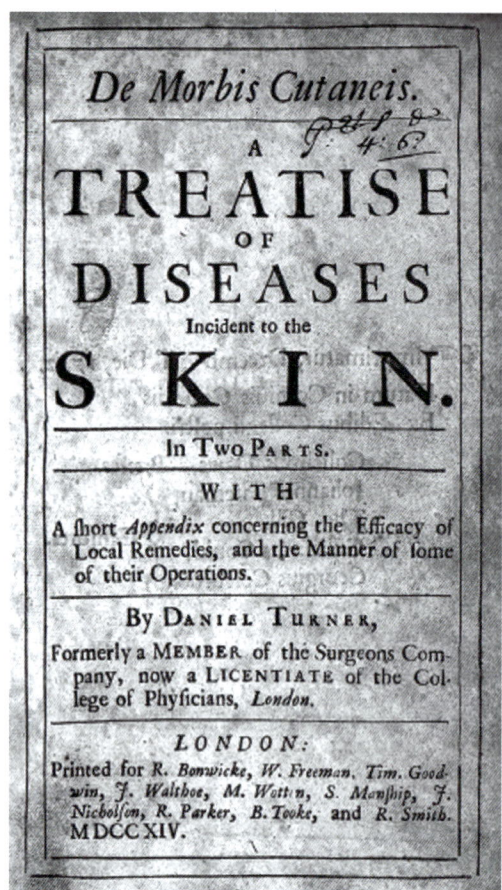

Figure 1.3 The first English language dermatology textbook by Turner. Reproduced from Wellcome Library/CC BY 4.0.

a definitive text summarising all knowledge on syphilis. He described the anatomy of the skin and linked cutaneous diseases to the sebaceous glands.

In Italy, Bernadino Ramazzini wrote a textbook on industrial disease in 1700, which classified occupational dermatoses ranging from varicose veins in priests to syphilis in midwives and wet nurses [2].

Classification was in the air: following Linnaeus, clinicians across Europe strove to classify cutaneous disease. Joseph Jacob Plenck, a Viennese-born professor in Buda, wrote a classification of skin disease in 1776 that divided skin disease into 14 categories [3]. This was a landmark for dermatology, being the first serious attempt to classify skin diseases. The following year, Antoine Charles Lorry in France wrote a text that considered the pathology, physiology and aetiology of skin diseases [4].

Growth of scientific dermatology

Willan and Bateman: definition of skin diseases

Prior to Robert Willan, terms were used loosely to describe skin diseases. Two doctors might use the same descriptive term to mean different appearances. Attempts to describe disease characteristics in classifications were ambiguous. Textbooks had no useful images, so there was no way to standardise terminology. Willan (Figure 1.4) defined precisely the terms used to describe skin disease. He wrote a classification based on these definitions, clearly illustrating these, first published in Breslau from 1798 onwards [1] (Figure 1.5). He died before finishing his work, but it was completed by his friend and student, Thomas Bateman in 1813. Bateman's *A Practical Synopsis of Cutaneous Disease* was translated into the main European languages and it was reprinted in America. This remained the standard textbook across much of the world until the 1830s [2].

Willan produced images of skin diseases in his textbook (Figure 1.6), the first dermatology atlas, that was completed in a larger atlas by Bateman in 1817 [3]. This atlas went through many editions after Bateman's death and was still in print in 1877.

Willan and Bateman changed the way dermatology was practised, with followers all around Europe: Biett and Cazenave in France, Chiarugi in Florence, Alfaro in Spain and Klaatch and Schreiver in Germany.

L'Hôpital St Louis, Paris: the first skin hospital

The time of war in Napoleonic Europe not only produced a great step forward in England, but also led to the encouragement of science in France. In 1801 the L'Hôpital St Louis became a dermatology hospital under the leadership of Jean-Louis Alibert (Figure 1.7). He had a flamboyant personality, wrote prolifically with elegant descriptions and produced several atlases. He introduced the famous 'arbre des dermatoses' classification (Figures 1.8 and 1.9) which had considerable artistic and also a little clinical merit. He was balanced by the scholarly Laurent Biett, his student, who studied under Bateman in 1816 and brought Willanism to France.

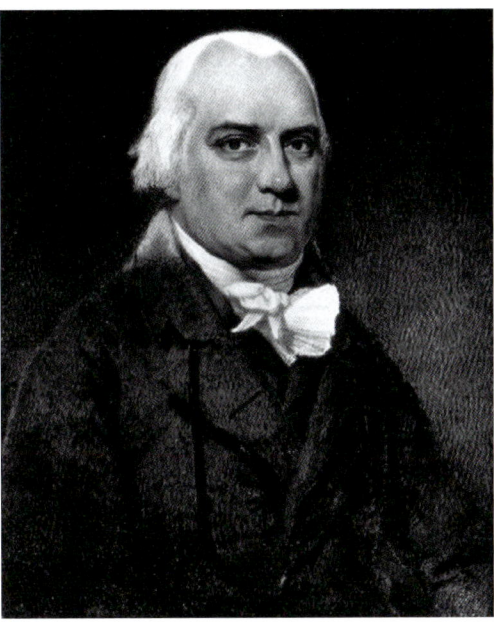

Figure 1.4 Robert Willan. Reproduced from A.C. Cooper/Wikimedia Commons/Public domain.

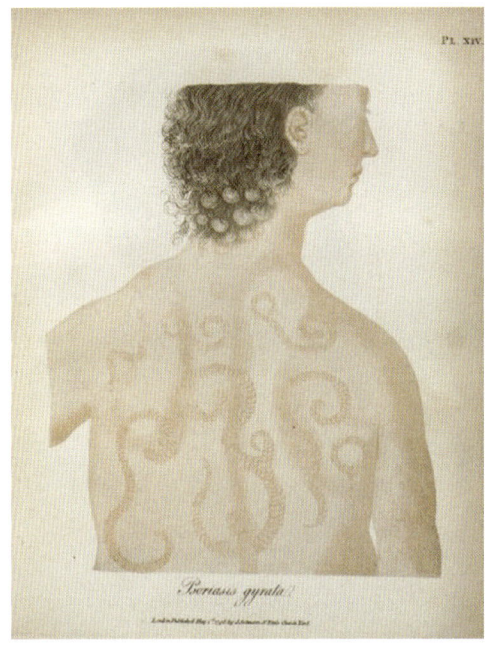

Figure 1.6 Psoriasis gyrata in Willan's textbook. Reproduced from Wellcome Library/CC BY 4.0.

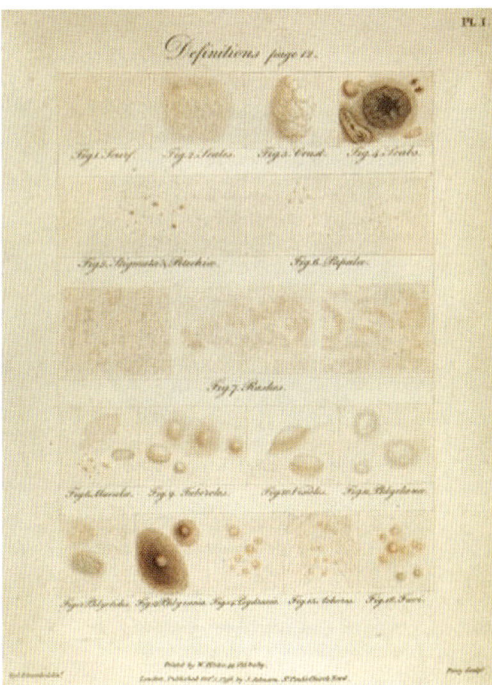

Figure 1.5 Willan's definitions. Reproduced from Wellcome Library/CC BY 4.0.

Biett then further developed and refined this work with Cazenave, Rayer and Bazin, making France and L'Hôpital St Louis the leading centre for dermatology in the early 19th century.

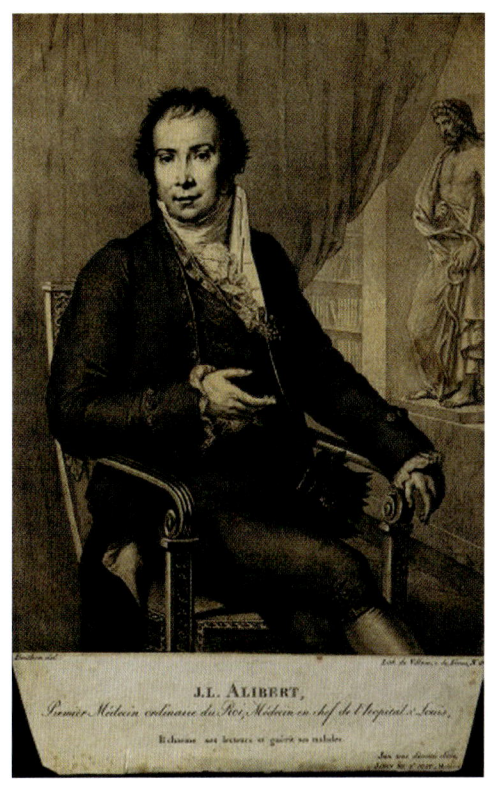

Figure 1.7 Jean Louis Alibert. Reproduced from Berthon/Wikimedia Commoms/Public domain.

Natural Sciences Hebra and the German-speaking Europeans

The integration between hospitals and universities was pioneered by German-speaking countries in central Europe in the second half of the 19th century. The new sciences of bacteriology and histopathology led to the understanding of underlying disease processes in dermatology. This greater understanding of underlying mechanisms ended Galen's ancient teachings and, together with the work on disease classification, marked the origin of modern scientific dermatology.

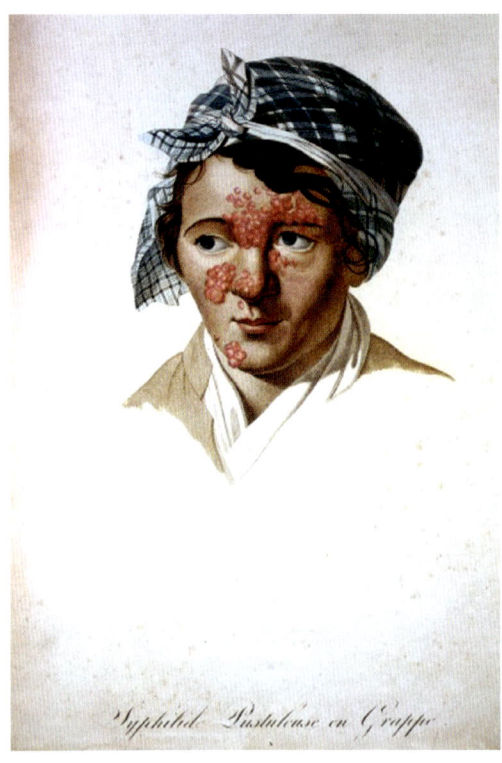

Figure 1.8 Alibert's syphilide pustuleuse en grappe. Reproduced from Wellcome Library/CC BY 4.0.

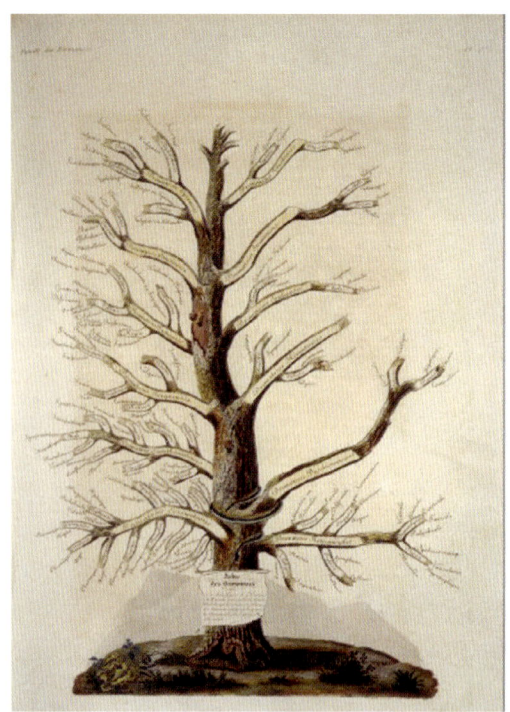

Figure 1.9 Alibert's arbre des dermatoses. Reproduced from Wellcome Library/CC BY 4.0.

In Vienna, Austria, the Allgemeines Krankenhaus became the world centre for medical teaching. From a group of brilliant clinicians, Ferdinand von Hebra (Figure 1.10) arose to introduce the new science of pathology into dermatology. He reclassified skin diseases using an anatomical and pathological framework, defined cutaneous fungal infections, and made great contributions to the definitions of many inflammatory disorders including eczema. Many great dermatologists studied under von Hebra and took his methods across the world. These included Filip Pick to Prague and Schwimmer to Budapest [4]. Moriz Kaposi and various English writers helped complete a popular five-volume English translation of von Hebra's work.

Heinrich Köbner, and then Oscar Simon and Albert Neisser in Breslau (now Wrocław), developed the Allgemeines Krankenhaus as the centre for German and Polish dermatology. Köbner moved to Berlin in 1872 to set up the Berlin Dermatology Society. Neisser utilised his knowledge of histopathology, microbiology, immunology, X-rays and ultraviolet and by the age of 25 had discovered the gonococcus and worked with Hansen to stain the lepra bacillus. He became the pre-eminent figure in European dermatology making advances in many areas, including work with Wassermann in syphilis [5].

Britain in the late 19th century

Sir Erasmus Wilson (Figure 1.11) was a famous Victorian dermatologist. A wealthy and charismatic surgeon and anatomist, he founded a dermatology chair for himself at the London Royal College of Surgeons, paid for Cleopatra's needle to be transported from Egypt to London, and founded and edited the first English dermatology journal in 1867. His evidence at an inquest led to the abolition of

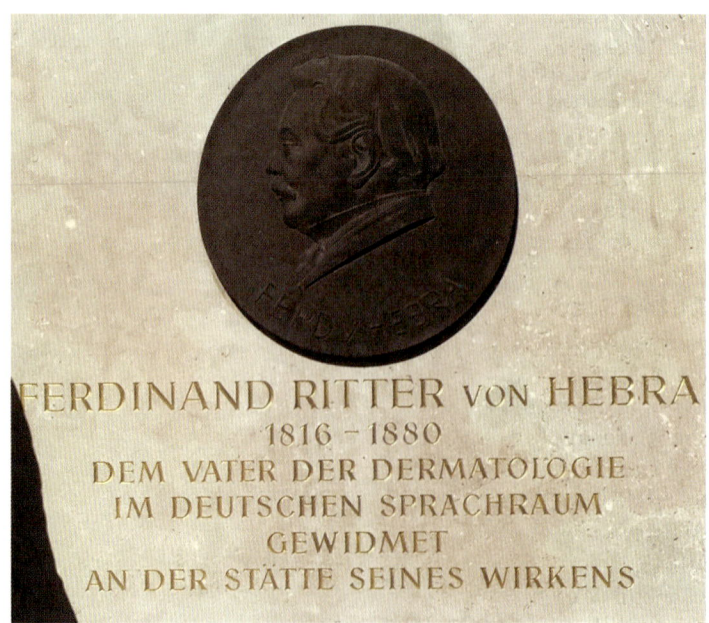

Figure 1.10 Ferdinand Ritter von Hebra, 1816–1880; father of dermatology in the German-speaking world. Courtesy of Nick J. Levell.

flogging in the British Army. He co-founded the controversial St John's Hospital for dermatology in London, with John Laws Milton. Another co-founder, William Tilbury Fox, became the first British university hospital consultant, defined impetigo and wrote an early text describing skin disease in India.

Sir Jonathan Hutchinson was a polymath surgeon, ophthalmologist, neurologist and dermatologist who described signs in syphilis and a host of other dermatology conditions. He often renamed these,

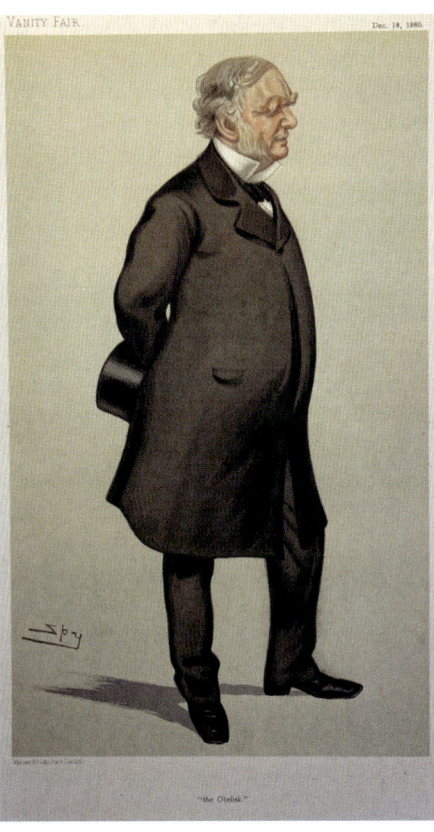

Figure 1.11 Erasmus Wilson: a cartoon from *Vanity Fair*. He was named 'the Obelisk' in humour because he had organised the transportation of Cleopatra's Needle from Egypt to London. The obelisk was a gift to the English by the Egyptian nation after the Battle of the Nile. Courtesy of Nick J. Levell.

causing confusion when diseases had previously been named by others, for example the recurrent summer eruption of Hutchinson, previously described by Bazin as hydroa vacciniforme.

United States in the 19th century

Henry D. Bulkley studied under Cazenave and Biett in France, and then returned to New York City. He set up the Broome Street Infirmary for Diseases of the Skin in 1837 with John Watson. He translated Cazenave into English and was the first President of the New York Dermatology Society in 1869 – the first dermatology society in the world. Noah Worcester was influenced by Willan and Bateman to write *Diseases of the Skin*, the first American dermatology textbook in 1845.

Faneuil Weisse studied under Sir Erasmus Wilson in Britain, and then helped establish the New York Dermatology Society when working as lecturer on skin disease at the University of New York City from 1865. In 1871 James White, a student of von Hebra, was appointed to the new chair of dermatology at Harvard, after lecturing for 8 years at the medical school, then practising at Massachusetts General. White was a strong force in developing American dermatology and medical education at Harvard and was president of the Massachusetts Medical Society.

Louis Duhring (Figure 1.12), another student of von Hebra, occupied the first chair of dermatology at the University of Pennsylvania from 1875 for 35 years. He had also studied in Paris and London, influencing his vision of dermatology as a part of general medicine.

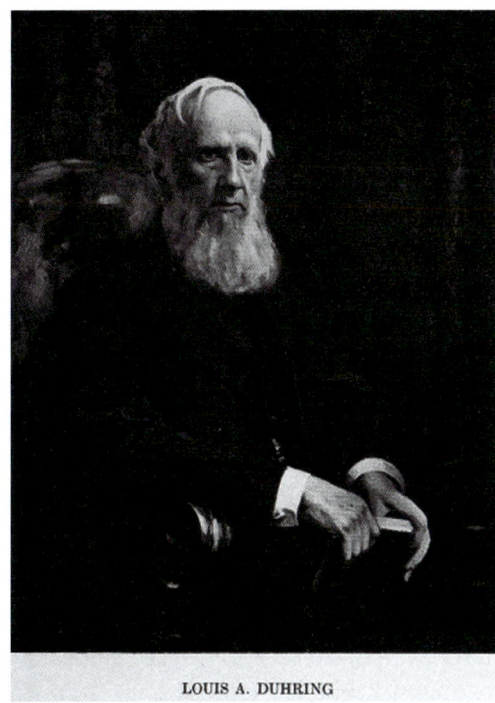

Figure 1.12 Louis Duhring. Reproduced from Hugh H. Breckenridge/Wellcome Collection/CC BY 4.0.

Duhring's book, *A Practical Treatise on Diseases of the Skin*, and work on dermatitis herpetiformis, together with his great wealth and benefactions to the specialty, helped establish dermatology in the United States.

Development of dermatology as a global specialty in the 20th century

At the beginning of the 20th century, dermatology was developing in most European and North American countries with fledgling dermatology societies and dermatology journals. The work often crossed national boundaries as international travel became easier. From this point on we can consider the development of dermatology as a global specialty. This coincided with the growth of subspecialty dermatology and science. The early 20th century saw treatments for infections that had ravaged humanity for centuries and the development of effective treatments for inflammatory diseases. These, together with public health initiatives, led to great increases in longevity. The later 20th century saw skin surgery develop to deal with the skin cancers that arose in an ageing population. The discovery of DNA in Cambridge, UK brought about the birth of molecular genetics that promises an even greater revolution in redefining diseases and predicting responses to treatment in a future era of personalised medicine.

Skin infections

Paul Ehrlich from Germany and Sarachiro Sata from Japan, working with Paul Uhlenhuth in Frankfurt, developed arsphenamine in 1910, Ehrlich's silver bullet, which offered effective chemotherapy for syphilis. This remained a mainstay of treatment until Alexander

Fleming, in London, UK, by serendipity discovered penicillin in 1928. This was produced commercially after its first synthesis by Florey, Heatley and Chain in Oxford and provided a cure for syphilis and many other cutaneous infections in the 1940s.

Leprosy has been a misdiagnosed, stigmatising and confused condition since ancient times. It is likely that many cases who were excluded from society in all ages of mankind actually suffered from other skin diseases. Norwegian Gerhard Hansen, together with Neisser in Breslau, described the bacterium between 1873 and 1880. Promin, a sulfone drug, was introduced in 1941; R. G. Cochrane then introduced dapsone in 1950 following research in Carville, Louisiana, USA. Research in Malta resulted in multidrug therapy in the 1970s, which was then adopted by the World Health Organization in 1981 and since has led to the reduction or eradication of the disease in many countries.

The Covid-19 pandemic, from 2020 onwards, reminded us that infections will evolve and adapt to be successful in the evolutionary race and will likely continue to challenge us. Each new infection brings new cutaneous presentations, keeping dermatologists as diagnosticians in the forefront of acute medicine. The stress imposed by pandemics on health care systems forces innovation in practice and delivery of care: Covid-19 has accelerated the adoption of new digital technology by dermatologists.

Inflammatory disease and immunomodulatory treatments

The discovery of corticosteroids revolutionised dermatology in the middle of the 20th century [1]. Further drugs that modified the immune system and that were introduced later in the century, such as azathioprine, methotrexate and ciclosporin, enabled the control of serious inflammatory diseases that had scourged humankind. Management of these disorders changed from episodic long-term hospital admissions to outpatient management using potentially toxic systemic agents requiring close monitoring. Increasing knowledge of the molecular basis for diseases has led to more targeted and personalised treatment, using less toxic biological agents and new small molecules, as dermatology moves through the 21st century.

Dermatology surgery

The practice of dermatology changed in the last three decades of the 20th century in Europe and North America due to the great increase in skin cancer presenting mainly in white-skinned people. This was thought to be due to an ageing population, greater international travel and improved awareness and recognition. This paralleled the growth of dermatology surgery. Dermatologists developed the technique of Mohs micrographic surgery and adopted plastic surgery procedures such as flap and graft repairs [2]. Many innovations in skin surgery were introduced by dermatologists as the number of practitioners increased. Advances in the understanding of cellular mechanisms heralded new drugs offering medical treatments for previously untreatable advanced skin cancers. With increased complexity of cancer management came the multidisciplinary team involving many specialties in skin cancer and a blurring of boundaries between specialties.

The adoption of skin surgical techniques by dermatologists, consumer demand and financial rewards have led to the growth of cosmetic dermatology in affluent societies since the end of the 20th century. Hair dyes, tattooing and other cosmetic procedures have been found in mummies from ancient Egypt. However, the growth and spending on cosmetic products to adorn and preserve the skin has paralleled economic growth. The spending on fillers, muscle relaxants, cosmetic surgery and hair transplantation has provided a change in direction for some dermatologists.

Medical dermatology

In the early 21st century, the growth of subspecialisation in dermatology and the increasing complexity of diagnosis and management of serious illness, using new treatments including biological agents, led to the need for a term for those providing education and courses in this area. Medical dermatology quickly became established as an important and popular area for subspecialisation, with clinicians establishing multidisciplinary clinics managing diseases such as lupus, psoriasis and vasculitis.

Contact dermatitis and allergy

Industrial skin disease has been present since antiquity but patch testing for allergic contact eczema was developed by Jadassohn in Breslau in 1895 [3]. Bloch in Basel and Zurich, Bonnevie in Copenhagen and Sulzberger in New York developed the technique and led its introduction across the world. In 1967 Niels Hjorth founded the International Contact Dermatitis Research Group, a group of clinicians from Europe and the United States (including Darrell Wilkinson, an original editor of this book), which standardised patch testing technique across the world.

Phototherapy

Niels Finsen's academic studies from 1894 to 1897 on the value of ultraviolet light as a treatment for tuberculosis put phototherapy on a scientific basis [4]. However, the use of topical and oral plant extracts combined with sunlight was used over 3000 years ago in India and Egypt. Broad-band UVB was used until the development of psoralen and UVA (PUVA) in 1974. The initial enthusiasm for this treatment was tempered by caution when the first patients who were on maintenance treatment began to develop skin cancers. Intermittent phototherapy was introduced and the use of PUVA further declined when narrow-band UVB equipment became available from 1990. Extracorporeal photophoresis for cutaneous T-cell lymphoma was introduced in 1987 and in the 1990s photodynamic therapy was developed.

Genital dermatology

In much of the world, dermatology and genito-urinary medicine developed as the same specialty, but in the USA and UK they have been separate specialties since the mid-20th century. In these countries, male and female genital dermatology developed as a subspecialty with the increasing awareness of the morbidity caused by genital disorders.

Psychodermatology and social medicine

Medicine and dermatology changed its focus in the latter half of the 20th century. The paradigm moved from being a process applied by doctors to generally passive patients to correct disease. It became an engagement with active patients encouraged to express their needs and wishes, which the medical teams aimed to fulfil. With this change came an awareness of the impact and morbidity that all disease has on activities of daily living and on mental health. There was a change in perception of the definition of success in medicine. Disease outcome measures focused on the experience of individuals undergoing investigation and treatment and the effect of disease and treatment on the patient's ability to function in their normal activities and the patients' perception of their own wellbeing. Terminology changed as patients asked instead to be described as people with a disease.

With greater consideration of psychological issues, some beginnings in the reduction of stigma and better awareness of the prevalence of mental illness, the subspecialty of psychodermatology developed in the late 20th century and early 21st century, closely linked with psychiatrists and psychologists.

Cosmetic dermatology

Dermatology textbooks from the 16th century included treatments for male pattern alopecia. Henna was used as a dye in ancient Egypt. Skin disease and skin surgery often has an impact on appearance and so cosmetic dermatology is integrated into all parts of dermatology. With greater affluence of society and individuals, the demand increases for interventions to reduce the self-perception of flawed appearance. Dermatology skills are helpful in this, so cosmetic dermatology as a subspecialty grew through the 20th and early 21st century, adopting interventions such as lasers, surgery, botulinum toxin and fillers.

Paediatric dermatology and genetics

A greater understanding of molecular genetics is revolutionising the relatively new subspecialty of paediatric dermatology. Diseases that were originally described by their appearance, then by phenotype, are now being defined by their genetic abnormalities. This understanding is allowing a reclassification of dermatology based on genetic abnormality, which will progress to a new understanding of more complex inflammatory diseases and cancers associated with multiple genetic abnormalities. This will result in splitting up diseases and enabling personalised treatment, maximising benefit and reducing the risks from new drugs targeting the precise molecular abnormality.

Overcoming prejudice in dermatology, both from outside and within

Dermatologists and those with skin disease are familiar with prejudice: through history there has been stigma against those with skin diseases, often made worse by confusion in terminology. Hansen disease and psoriasis were given similar names in older textbooks. This prejudice was deeply integrated so that evil characters in popular films or literature were often given skin diseases.

Many historical figures described in this chapter were white and most are male. Most images of skin disease in textbooks and in educational lectures were in white skin. Photographs of European medical meetings and universities before the mid-20th century illustrate the institutionalised discrimination in societies and in medical organisations that had reduced opportunities in education and promotion for those with protected characteristics.

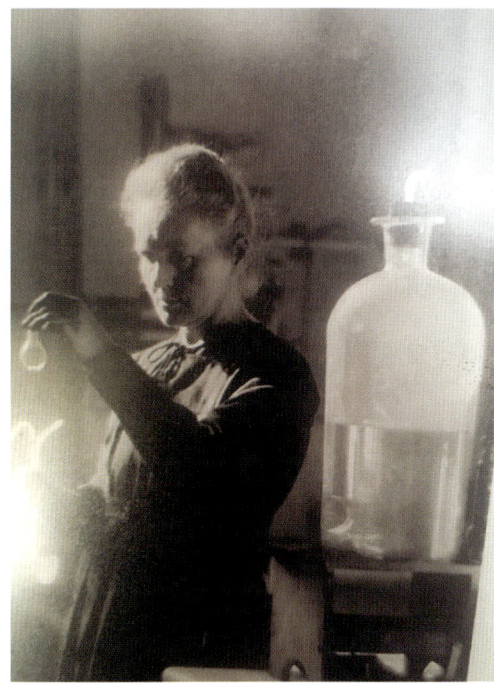

Figure 1.13 Marie Curie: photograph taken of image at the Marie Curie Museum, Paris. Courtesy of Nick J. Levell.

However, some exceptional women worked on science relating to skin disease, such as Marie Curie (Figure 1.13) from Poland, the first female Professor at the University of Paris, who discovered radioactivity and its use in cancer. Curie won the Nobel Prize for Physics in 1903 (in the same year, rules meant that a male had to read out her paper at the London Academy of Sciences) and the Nobel Prize for Chemistry in 1912.

As dermatology develops as a global specialty in the 21st century, there is growing recognition, particularly in younger generations, that any organisation is weakened if it limits opportunity due to factors other than competency, skills, ability and hard work. Those who offer opportunities to the best, irrespective of ethnicity, skin colour, gender, background, sexuality and belief, become stronger.

Images, technology and teledermatology

A good clinical history is essential in dermatology. However, clear images of skin disease facilitate education, diagnosis and management of skin disease. Illustrated textbooks allowed skin disease classification in the early 19th century. Dermatologists adopted photography in textbooks and produced large collections of wax models (moulages) to aid medical school teaching (Figure 1.14). The widespread use of computers in the workplace and digital photography began in the 1990s. This led to digitised images in research to measure disease severity, in education and in clinics to manage those who were unable to travel to hospital. However, change was resisted by some and the management of patients using digital technology, teledermatology, progressed slowly for 25 years [5]. Then, in 2020, the Covid-19 pandemic forced a revolution in the use of digital technology as social distancing minimised travel to hospital. Dermatology management by email, telephone and video consultation progressed further in a year than it had in the previous quarter of a century.

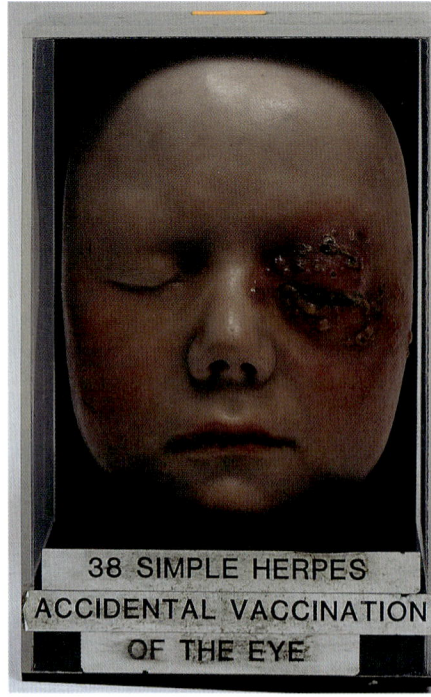

Figure 1.14 Herpes infection of the eye: moulages at the Gordon museum, Guy's Hospital, London, UK are still used today to teach dermatology A clear clinical image with relevant history can allow a diagnosis to be made and useful management advice to be given for many people with skin diseases. Courtesy of Nick J. Levell.

We live in a time of great changes in science and society. Dermatology has never been at a more exciting time in its history. Read on.

Key references

The full list of references can be found in the online version at https://www.wiley.com/rooksdermatology10e

Ancient dermatology writings
2 Ebbell B, translator. *The Papyrus Ebers: The Greatest Egyptian Medical Document*. Copenhagen: Levin and Munksgaard, 1937.

Growth of rational medicine
2 Elangasinghe V, Lee KYC, Levell N. An historical account of dermatology from Buddhist Sri Lankan literature. *Int J Dermatol* 2014;53:390–2.

Dermatology after the fall of Rome
1 Turner D. *De Morbis Cutaneis*. London: Bonwicke, Walthor, Wilkin, Ward and Tooke, 1712.
3 Plenck JJ. *Doctrina De Morbis Cutaneis*. Vienna: Graeffer, 1776.

Growth of scientific dermatology
1 Willan R. *On Cutaneous Diseases*. London: Johnson, 1808.
2 Bateman T. *A Practical Synopsis of Cutaneous Disease*. London: Longman, Rees, Orme, Brown and Green, 1813.
4 Pusey WMA. *The History of Dermatology*. Baltimore: Charles C Thomas, 1933.
5 Bilianicki-Birula R. The 100th anniversary of the Wasserman–Neisser–Bruck reaction. *Clin Dermatol* 2008;26:79–81.

Development of dermatology as a global specialty in the 20th century
3 Adams R. Profiles of greats in contact dermatitis. Josef Jaddasohn (1863–1936). *Am J Contact Dermatitis* 1993;4:58–9.
4 Honigsmann H. History of phototherapy in dermatology. *Photochem Photobiol Sci* 2013;12:16–21.

CHAPTER 2

Structure and Function of the Skin

John A. McGrath[1] and Jouni Uitto[2]

[1] St John's Institute of Dermatology, King's College London, London, UK
[2] Department of Dermatology and Cutaneous Biology, Thomas Jefferson University, Philadelphia, PA, USA

Components of normal human skin, 2.1	Desmosomes, 2.18	Collagen cross-linking, 2.31
Skin development, 2.3	Adherens junctions, 2.19	Collagen degradation, 2.31
Epidermal and adnexal structures, 2.5	Gap junctions, 2.20	Elastic fibres, 2.32
Keratinocytes, 2.7	Tight junctions, 2.20	Elastin, 2.33
Eccrine and apocrine glands, 2.8	Dermal–epidermal basement membrane, 2.21	Elastin-associated microfibrils, 2.35
Pilosebaceous unit, 2.9	Basement membrane collagen, 2.22	Proteoglycan/glycosaminoglycans, 2.36
Nails, 2.10	Laminins, 2.23	Fibroblasts, 2.39
Merkel cells, 2.11	Hemidesmosomes, 2.25	Blood vessels and lymphatics, 2.40
Skin immune ecosystem, 2.12	Focal adhesions, 2.26	Subcutaneous fat, 2.42
Skin microbiome, 2.13	Anchoring fibrils, 2.26	Physiological functions of skin, 2.42
Langerhans cells, 2.13	Extracellular matrix, 2.27	Skin homeostasis, 2.43
Immune surveillance, 2.15	Collagens, 2.28	Skin ageing, 2.45
Mast cells, 2.15	Collagen biosynthesis, 2.29	Key references, 2.47
Melanocytes, 2.17	Collagen biology, 2.29	

Components of normal human skin

Skin is the largest organ in the body. In a 70 kg individual, the skin weighs over 5 kg and covers a surface area approaching 2 m^2. Human skin consists of a stratified, cellular epidermis and an underlying dermis of connective tissue, separated by a dermal–epidermal basement membrane (Figure 2.1). Beneath the dermis is a layer of subcutaneous fat, which is separated from the rest of the body by a vestigial layer of striated muscle.

The epidermis is mainly composed of keratinocytes and, for the living cell layers, is typically 0.05–0.1 mm in thickness. It is formed by the division of cells in the basal layer, which give rise to the spinous layer. This layer contains cells that move outwards and progressively differentiate, forming the granular layer and the stratum corneum. The cellular progression from the basal layer to the skin surface takes about 30 days but is accelerated in diseases such as psoriasis. The 'brick-like' shape of keratinocytes is provided by a cytoskeleton made of keratin intermediate filaments. As the epidermis differentiates, the keratinocytes become flattened. This process involves the filament-aggregating protein filaggrin, a protein component of keratohyalin granules. Indeed, keratin and filaggrin comprise 80–90% of the mass of the epidermis.

The outermost layer of the epidermis is the stratum corneum, where cells (now called corneocytes) have lost the nuclei and cytoplasmic organelles. The corneocyte has a highly insoluble, cornified envelope within the plasma membrane, formed by cross-linking of soluble protein precursors, including involucrin and loricrin, the latter contributing 70–85% to the mass of the cornified cell envelope. It also contains several lipids (fatty acids, sterols and ceramides) released from lamellar bodies within the upper, living epidermis. The stratum corneum can be divided into three distinct biochemical and functional zones – an outer absorber of solutes, a middle absorber of water for hydration and an inner mechanical defence barrier.

Other cells in the epidermis are the melanocytes, Langerhans cells and Merkel cells. Melanocytes are dendritic cells that distribute packages of melanin pigment in melanosomes to the surrounding keratinocytes to give skin its colour. The number of melanocytes does not differ much between skin types. Rather it is the nature of the melanin and the size of the melanosomes that account for the different appearances. The Langerhans cells are also dendritic in nature, although these are of mesenchymal origin and originate from bone marrow. Langerhans cells are antigen-presenting cells, process antigens encountered by the skin to local lymph nodes and

---

Rook's Textbook of Dermatology, Tenth Edition. Edited by Christopher Griffiths, Jonathan Barker, Tanya Bleiker, Walayat Hussain and Rosalind Simpson.
© 2024 John Wiley & Sons Ltd. Published 2024 by John Wiley & Sons Ltd.

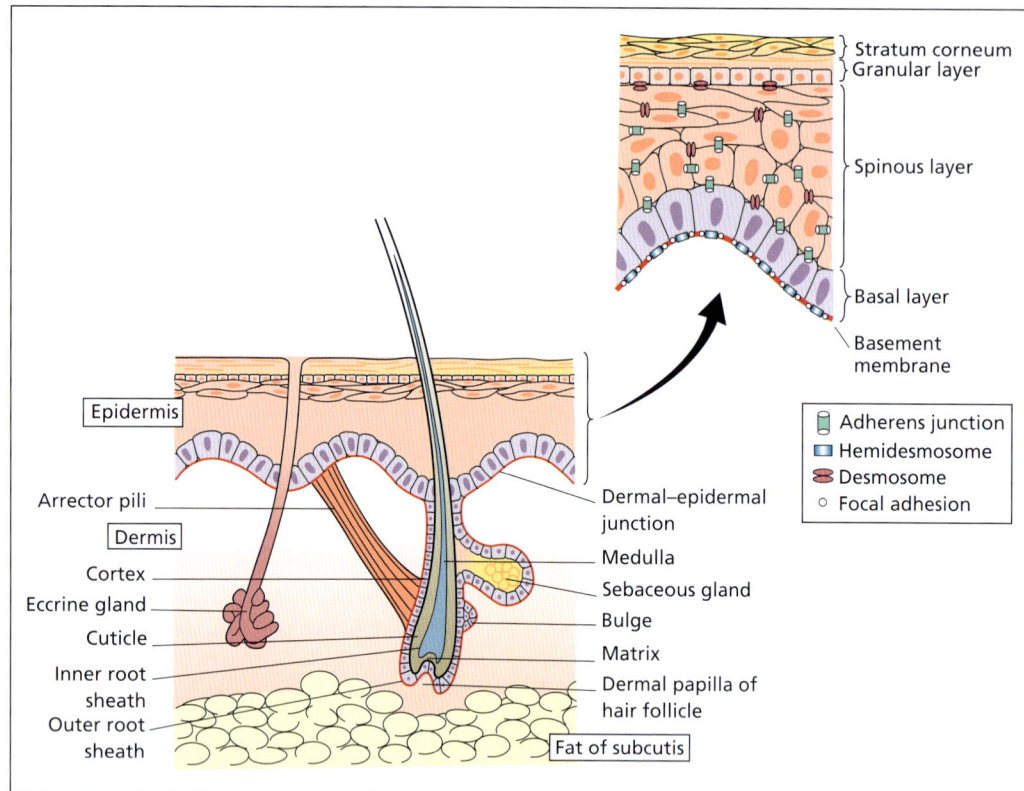

Figure 2.1 The skin and its appendages.

thus have a key role in adaptive immune responses in the skin. Merkel cells are probably derived from keratinocytes. They have a role as mechanosensory receptors in response to touch.

Human skin contains pilosebaceous follicles and sweat glands. The hair follicles comprise pockets of epithelium that are continuous with the superficial epidermis, but which also envelop a small papilla of dermis at their base. A bundle of smooth muscle, the arrector pili, extends at an angle between the surface of the dermis and a point in the follicle wall. Above the insertion, there are holocrine sebaceous glands which open into the pilary canal. In some sites, such as the axillae, the follicles may be associated with apocrine glands. Also derived from the epidermis and opening directly to the skin surface are the eccrine sweat glands.

The epidermis is attached to the dermis via a complex network of proteins and glycoproteins that extend from inside basal keratinocytes into the superficial dermis. Besides adhesion, the dermal–epidermal junction components also contribute to cell migration (for example during wound healing) as well as epithelial–mesenchymal signalling events. Over 30 different macromolecules (collagens, laminins and integrins) interact within a basement membrane zone that is less than 200 μm across.

The dermis consists of a supporting matrix in which polysaccharides and proteins are enmeshed to a network that provides resilience to the skin and has a remarkable capacity for retaining water. The thickness of the dermis varies from less than 0.5 mm to more than 5 mm depending on the skin site. There are two principal types of protein fibre: collagen and elastic tissue.

Collagen is the major extracellular matrix protein, comprising 80–85% of the dry weight of the dermis. Twenty-nine different collagens have been identified in vertebrate tissue (depicted by Roman numerals in the order of their discovery, from I to XXIX), of which at least 12 are expressed in skin. The main interstitial dermal collagens are types I and III, whereas the principal basement membrane collagen (at the dermal–epidermal junction and around dermal blood vessels, nerves and appendages) is type IV collagen. Triple-helical collagen monomers polymerise into fibrils and fibres, which then become stabilised by the complex formation of both intra- and intermolecular cross-links. Collagen fibres are extremely resilient and provide skin with its tensile strength.

In sun-protected adult skin, elastic fibres account for no more than 2–4% of the extracellular matrix in the dermis and consist of two components, elastin and elastin-associated microfibrils, which together give skin its elasticity and resilience. Elastic microfibrils are composed of several proteins, including fibrillin, which surround the elastin, and which can extend throughout the dermis in a web-like configuration to the junction between the dermis and the epidermis. The dermis also contains several non-collagenous glycoproteins, including fibronectins, fibulins and integrins. These extracellular matrix components facilitate cell adhesion and cell motility.

Between the dermal collagen and elastic tissue is the ground substance made up of glycosaminoglycan/proteoglycan macromolecules. These contribute only 0.1–0.3% of the total dry weight of the dermis but provide a vital role by maintaining hydration, mostly due to the high water-binding capacity of hyaluronic acid. About 60% of the total weight of the dermis is water.

The dermis has a very rich blood supply, although no vessels pass through the dermal–epidermal junction. There is a superficial and a deep vascular plexus. The motor innervation of the skin is autonomic and includes a cholinergic component to the eccrine

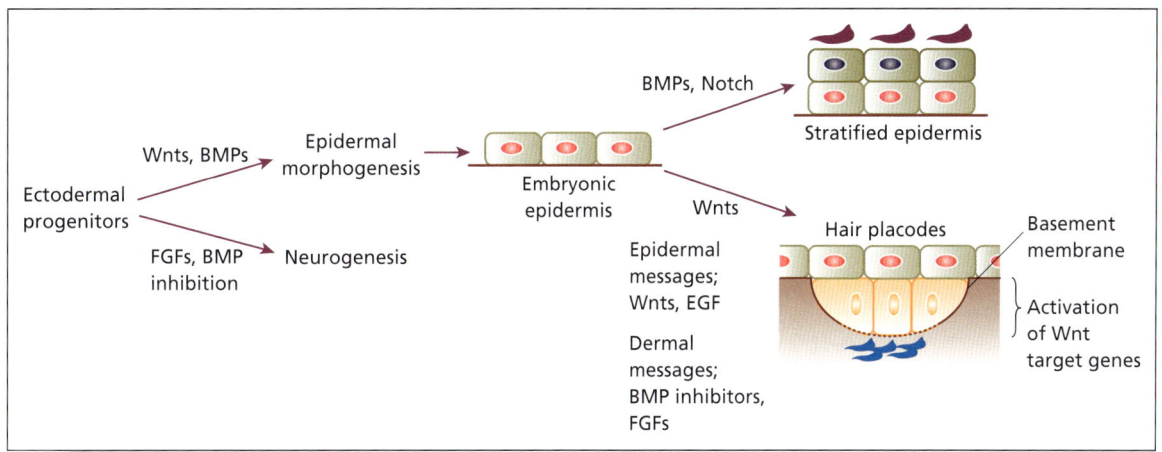

Figure 2.2 Embryonic development of the skin depends on specific signalling molecules. Relative stimulation or inhibition by these signalling molecules also determines whether embryonic epidermis progresses to a stratified epidermis or whether formation of skin appendages is induced. BMP, bone morphogenic protein; EGF, epidermal growth factor; FGF, fibroblast growth factor; Wnts, wingless and Int-1 signalling.

sweat glands and adrenergic components to both the eccrine and apocrine glands, to the smooth muscle and the arterioles and to the arrector pili muscle. The sensory nerve endings are of several kinds; some are free, some terminate in hair follicles and others have expanded tips.

Skin development

The skin arises by the juxtaposition of two major embryological elements: the prospective epidermis that originates from a surface area of the early gastrula, and the prospective mesoderm that contacts the inner surface of the epidermis during gastrulation. The mesoderm not only provides the dermis but is essential for inducing differentiation of the epidermal structures, such as the hair follicle. The melanocytes are derived from the neural crest.

After gastrulation, there is a single layer of neuroectoderm on the embryo surface; this layer will go on to form the nervous system or the skin epithelium depending on the molecular signals it receives (Figure 2.2). Activation of Wnt signalling will block the ability of the ectoderm to respond to fibroblast growth factors (FGFs). Without FGFs the cells express bone morphogenic proteins (BMPs) and progress to an epidermal lineage. Conversely, lack of Wnt signalling promotes a neural fate [1]. One key transcription factor in skin development is p63, which contributes to epidermal lineage commitment, epidermal differentiation, cell adhesion and basement membrane formation [2]. The embryonic epidermis consists of a single layer of multipotent epithelial cells, which is covered by a special layer known as periderm that is unique to mammals (Figure 2.3). Periderm provides some protection to the newly forming skin as well as exchange of material with the amniotic fluid.

During the first trimester, the embryonic dermis is very cellular, and includes several immune cells or their precursors (Figure 2.4). These cells become less numerous and are modified during the second trimester, although precise functions for many of these immunocytes remain to be fully characterised [3]. From weeks 14 to 21, fibroblasts are numerous and active, and perineural cells, pericytes, melanoblasts and Merkel cells can be individually identified. Two distinct lineages of fibroblasts are present: one that

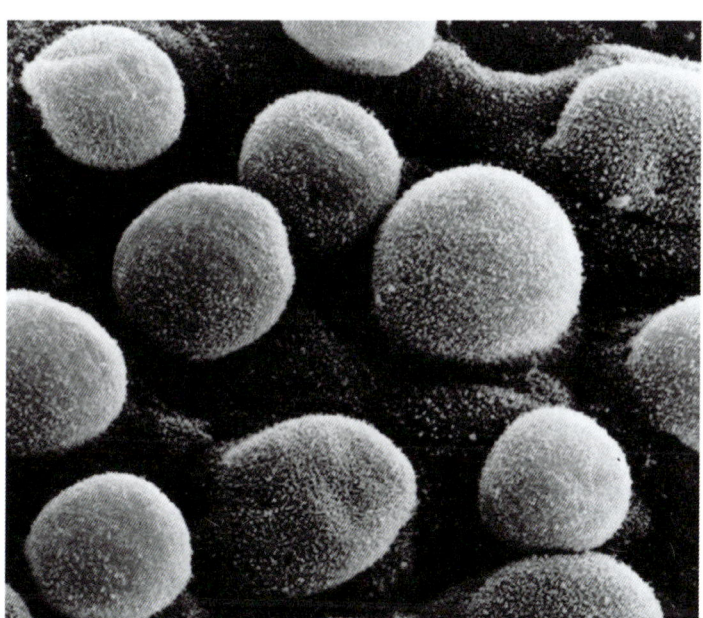

Figure 2.3 Scanning electron micrograph of an 85–110 day (estimated gestation age) human embryo. Single globular blebs project from the periderm cells. Courtesy of Professor K. A. Holbrook.

gives rise to the upper papillary dermis and hair follicle formation, and another that helps generate the deep reticular dermis and subcutaneous fat [4].

The various structural components of the skin that can be recognised postnatally start to appear at different embryonic time points, for example hair follicles and nails (9 weeks), sweat glands (9 weeks for the palms and soles, 15 weeks for other sites) and sebaceous glands (15 weeks). Touch pads become recognisable on the fingers and toes by week 6 and reach their greatest development at week 15. After this, they flatten and become indistinct. It is these areas that determine the pattern of dermatoglyphics that take their place.

The mesoderm not only provides the dermis but is essential for inducing differentiation of the epidermal structures, such as the hair follicle in mammals [5]. The earliest development of the hair

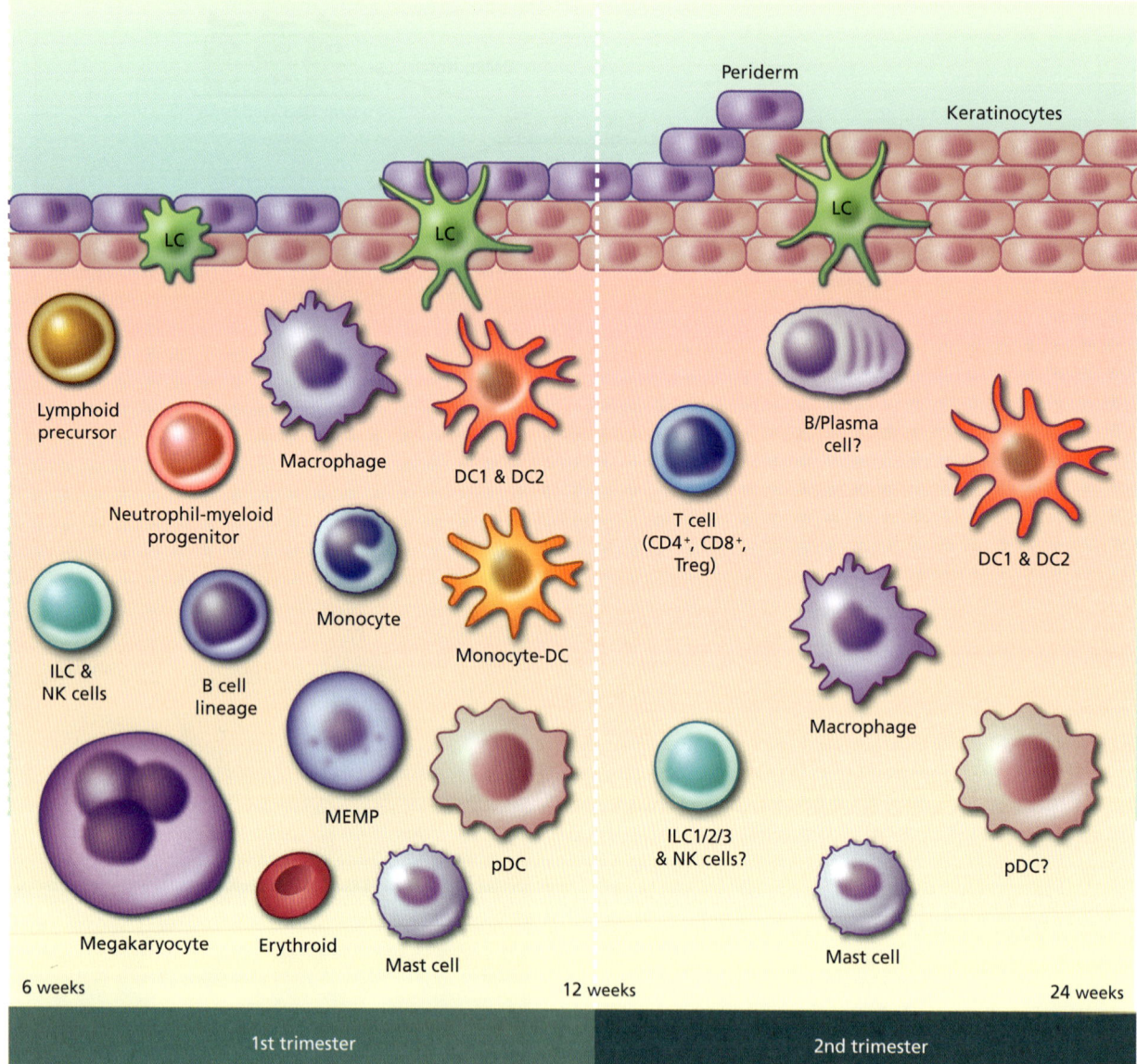

Figure 2.4 Overview of the immune cells present in first- and second-trimester human skin. ?, unknown; DC, dendritic cell; ILC, innate lymphoid cell; LC, Langerhans cell; MEMP, megakaryocyte-erythroid-mast cell progenitor; Monocyte-DC, monocyte-DC hybrid; NK, natural killer. Adapted from Botting and Haniffa 2020 [3] with permission from Wiley.

rudiments occurs at about 9 weeks in the regions of the eyebrow, upper lip and chin (Figure 2.5). Mesenchymal cells, derived from the dermomyotome, populate the skin and interact with the overlying epidermis to induce the formation of hair placodes [6]. Key components of the mesenchymal signals to produce hair follicles include FGFs and BMP-inhibitory factors such as Noggin; excessive BMP stimulation can reduce hair follicle density. The epidermal response to form the hair placode is generated by Wnt signals such as Wnt10b and sonic hedgehog (Shh), which also has a key role in the formation of the dermal papilla [7]. After it is formed, the dermal papilla sends further signals to transform the placode into a hair follicle. At the centre of the signalling cross-talk is the bipartite transcription factor composed of lymphoid enhancer-binding factor 1 (LEF-1) and stabilised β-catenin, which is essential for hair follicle formation. Hair follicle development is also influenced by Smads, a group of signalling mediators and antagonists of the transforming growth factor β (TGF-β) superfamily. Smad-4 affects hair follicle differentiation by mediating BMP signalling; Smad-7 affects hair follicle development and differentiation by blocking TGF-β/activin/BMP pathways [8]. Skin development is governed by complex, balanced waves of gene activation and silencing; cross-talk between small non-coding micro-RNAs and messenger RNAs is very important for the coordination of signal transduction and transcriptional activation [9].

Signalling responses differ between follicular and interfollicular epidermis: BMP signalling is active in the interfollicular epidermis and is both an epidermis-promoting signal as well as a follicle-inhibiting signal; epidermal growth factor receptor (EGFR) signalling may have a similar role in governing follicle density. As hair follicles mature to form inner and outer root sheaths, several signalling pathways are involved, including Wnt, Notch and BMP receptors. There are also marked changes in certain cell adhesion proteins, notably E-cadherin and P-cadherin. The hair follicles

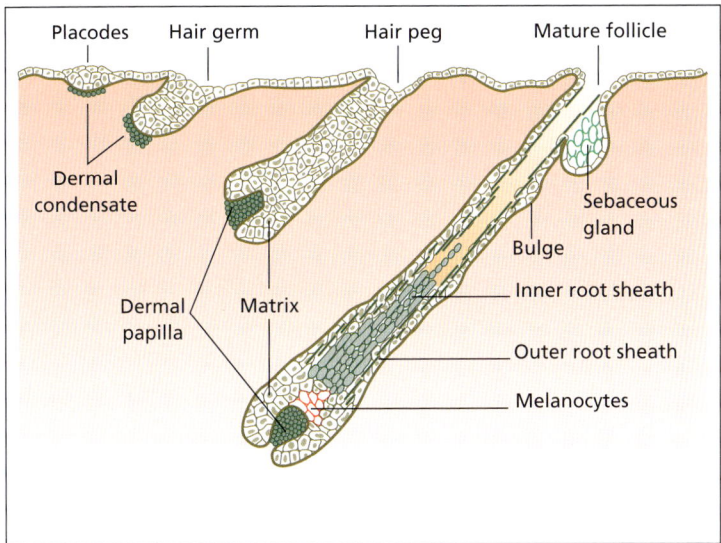

Figure 2.5 Embryonic stages of hair follicle morphogenesis.

are arranged in patterns, usually in groups of three. It appears that the first follicles develop over the surface at fixed intervals of between 274 and 350 μm. As the skin grows, these first hair germs become separated, and new rudiments develop between them when a critical distance, dependent on the region of the body, has been reached. There is no large-scale destruction of follicles during postnatal development, only a decrease in actual density as the body surface increases; nor do any new follicles develop in adult skin. In interfollicular epidermis, the undersurface of the epidermis is smooth, but during the fourth month, at the same time as the hair follicle starts to develop, it becomes irregular.

Sebaceous glands first appear as hemispherical protuberances on the posterior surfaces of the hair pegs. The cells contain moderate amounts of glycogen, but soon the cells in the centre lose this, and become larger and accumulate droplets of lipid. The sebaceous glands become differentiated at 13–15 weeks and are then large and functional. The sebum forms part of the vernix caseosa. At the end of fetal life, sebaceous glands are well developed and generally large. After birth, the size is rapidly reduced, and they enlarge to become functional again only after puberty. The molecular signals that induce sebaceous gland differentiation involve the c-Myc transcription factor as well as the adipogenic transcription factor peroxisome proliferator-activated receptor γ (PPAR-γ) [10].

Eccrine glands start to develop on the palms and soles at about 3 months, but not over the rest of the body until the fifth month [11]. In embryos of 12 weeks, the rudiments of eccrine sweat glands are first identifiable as regularly spaced undulations of the developing epidermis. Cells that go on to form the eccrine sweat glands are oblong, palisading and lie closely together, but otherwise they do not differ from the rest of the developing basal epidermis. By 14–15 weeks, the tips of the eccrine sweat gland rudiments have penetrated deeply into the dermis and have begun to form the coils. In the overlying epidermis, columns of cells that are destined to form the intraepidermal sweat ducts are recognisable. Each column is composed of two distinct cylindrical layers, comprising two inner cells that are elongated and curved so that they embrace the inner cylinder. The intraepidermal duct appears to form by the coalescence of groups of intracytoplasmic cavities formed within two adjacent inner cells. In the intradermal segment, the lumen forms by dissolution of the desmosomal attachment plaques between the cells that compose the inner core of the eccrine duct germ.

Nails begin to develop in the third month. Key signalling events in nail development involve the R-spondin family of transcription factors [12]. In fetuses at 16–18 weeks (crown to rump length 120–150 mm), keratinising cells from both dorsal and ventral matrices can be distinguished. Melanocytes take their origin from the neural crest. This can be identified in early human embryos, but the elements arising from it soon lose themselves in the mesenchyme, and pigmented melanocytes cannot be identified, even in darker skin fetuses, before 4–6 months of gestation. However, dopa-positive melanocytes can be demonstrated earlier. Langerhans cells are derived from the monocyte–macrophage–histiocyte lineage and enter the epidermis at about 12 weeks. Merkel cells appear in the glabrous skin of the fingertips, lips, gingiva and nail bed, and in several other regions, around 16 weeks.

Although some cells of the dermis may migrate from the dermatome (ventrolateral part of the somite) and take part in the formation of the skin, most of the dermis is formed by mesenchymal cells that migrate from other mesodermal areas [13]. These mesenchymal cells give rise to the whole range of blood and connective tissue cells, including the fibroblasts and mast cells of the dermis and the fat cells of the subcutis. In the second month, the dermis and subcutis are not distinguishable from each other but distinct collagen fibres are evident in the dermis by the end of the third month. Later, the papillary and reticular layers become distinct and, at the fifth month, the connective tissue sheaths are formed around the hair follicles. Elastic fibres are first detectable at 22 weeks.

Epidermal and adnexal structures

The normal epidermis is a terminally differentiated, stratified, squamous epithelium. The major cell type, making up 95% of the total, is the *keratinocyte*, which moves progressively from attachment to the epidermal basement membrane towards the skin surface, forming several well-defined layers during its transit [1]. Thus, on simple morphological grounds, the epidermis can be divided into four distinct layers: *stratum basale* or *stratum germinativum*, *stratum spinosum*, *stratum granulosum* and *stratum corneum*. The term *Malpighian layer* includes both the basal and spinous cells. Other constitutive cells within the epidermis include melanocytes, Langerhans cells and Merkel cells (Figure 2.6).

The stratum basale is a continuous layer that is generally only one cell thick. The basal cells are small and cuboidal (10–14 μm in diameter) and have large, dark-staining nuclei and dense cytoplasm that contains many ribosomes and dense tonofilament bundles. Immediately above the basal cell layer, the epibasal keratinocytes enlarge to form the spinous/prickle cell layer or stratum spinosum (Figure 2.7).

The stratum spinosum is succeeded by the stratum granulosum or granular layer, which contains intracellular granules of keratohyalin. At high magnification, the dense mass of keratohyalin

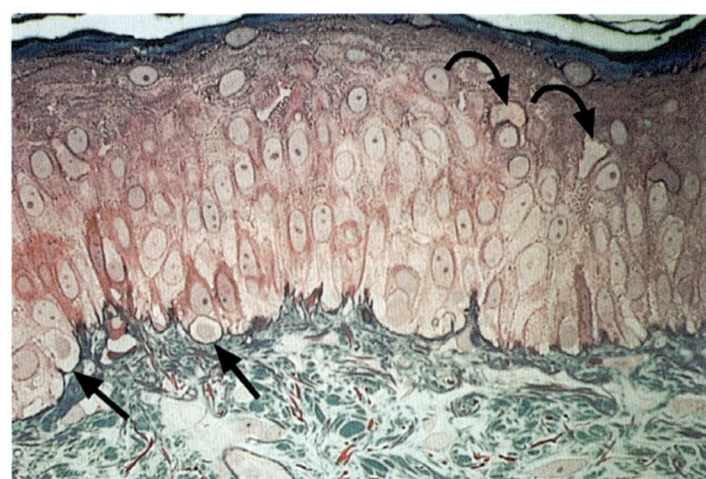

Figure 2.6 Photomicrograph of a 1 μm-thick plastic section of normal human skin. The tissue was fixed with half-strength Karnovsky medium and embedded in Epon. This technique allows the cellular components of the epidermis, including keratinocytes, melanocytes (straight arrows) and probable Langerhans cells (curved arrows), to be clearly resolved. Magnification 400× (basic fuchsin and methylene blue).

granules from human epidermis has a particulate substructure, with particles of irregular shape, on average 2 nm in length, and occurring randomly in rows or lattices. The cytoplasm of cells of the upper, spinous layer and granular cell layer also contains smaller lamellated granules averaging 100–300 nm in size. These are known as lamellar granules or bodies, membrane-coating granules or Odland bodies. They are numerous within the uppermost cells of the spinous layer and migrate towards the periphery of the cells as they enter the granular cell layer (Figure 2.8). They discharge their lipid components into the intercellular space, playing important roles in barrier function and intercellular cohesion within the stratum corneum (Figure 2.9) [2,3].

The outermost layer of epidermis is the stratum corneum where cells, now known as corneocytes, have lost the nuclei and cytoplasmic organelles. The cells become flattened and the keratin filaments align into disulphide cross-linked macrofibres, under the

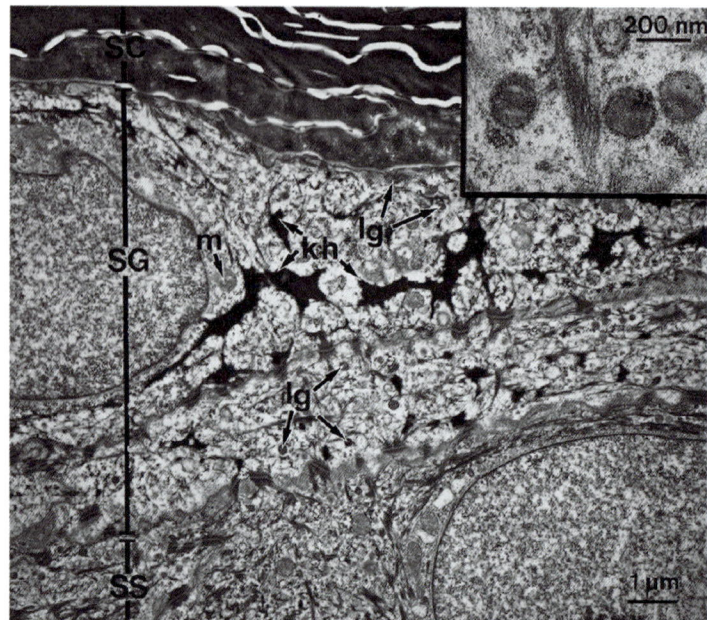

Figure 2.8 Electron micrograph showing details of the upper part of the epidermis including the stratum corneum (SC), stratum granulosum (SG) and most superficial cell layer of stratum spinosum (SS). Note the irregularly shaped keratohyalin granules (kh) and the small, round, lamellar granules (lg). The latter are present in both SS and SG and are smaller than mitochondria (m). The inset shows details of lamellar granules.

influence of *filaggrin*, the protein component of the keratohyalin granule. Filaggrin is responsible for keratin filament aggregation and is subsequently broken down into individual hygroscopic amino acids that form the basis of the natural moisturising factor within corneocytes. The key role of filaggrin in skin biology has been demonstrated by the discovery of common loss-of-function mutations in the filaggrin gene as the cause of the genetic disorder ichthyosis vulgaris and as a major risk factor for the development of atopic eczema, atopic asthma and systemic allergies [4]. The corneocyte has a highly insoluble, cornified envelope within the plasma membrane, formed by cross-linking of the soluble protein

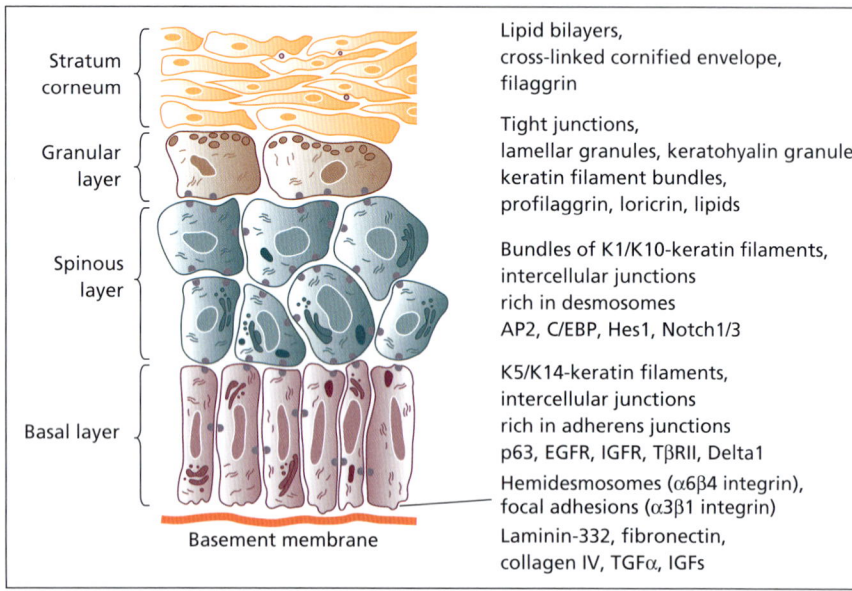

Figure 2.7 The process of epidermal differentiation is associated with the expression of different structures, macromolecules, transcription factors and other signalling molecules and their receptors in the different keratinocyte layers. EGFR, epidermal growth factor receptor; IGF, insulin-like growth factor; IGFR, IGF receptor; TGF, transforming growth factor.

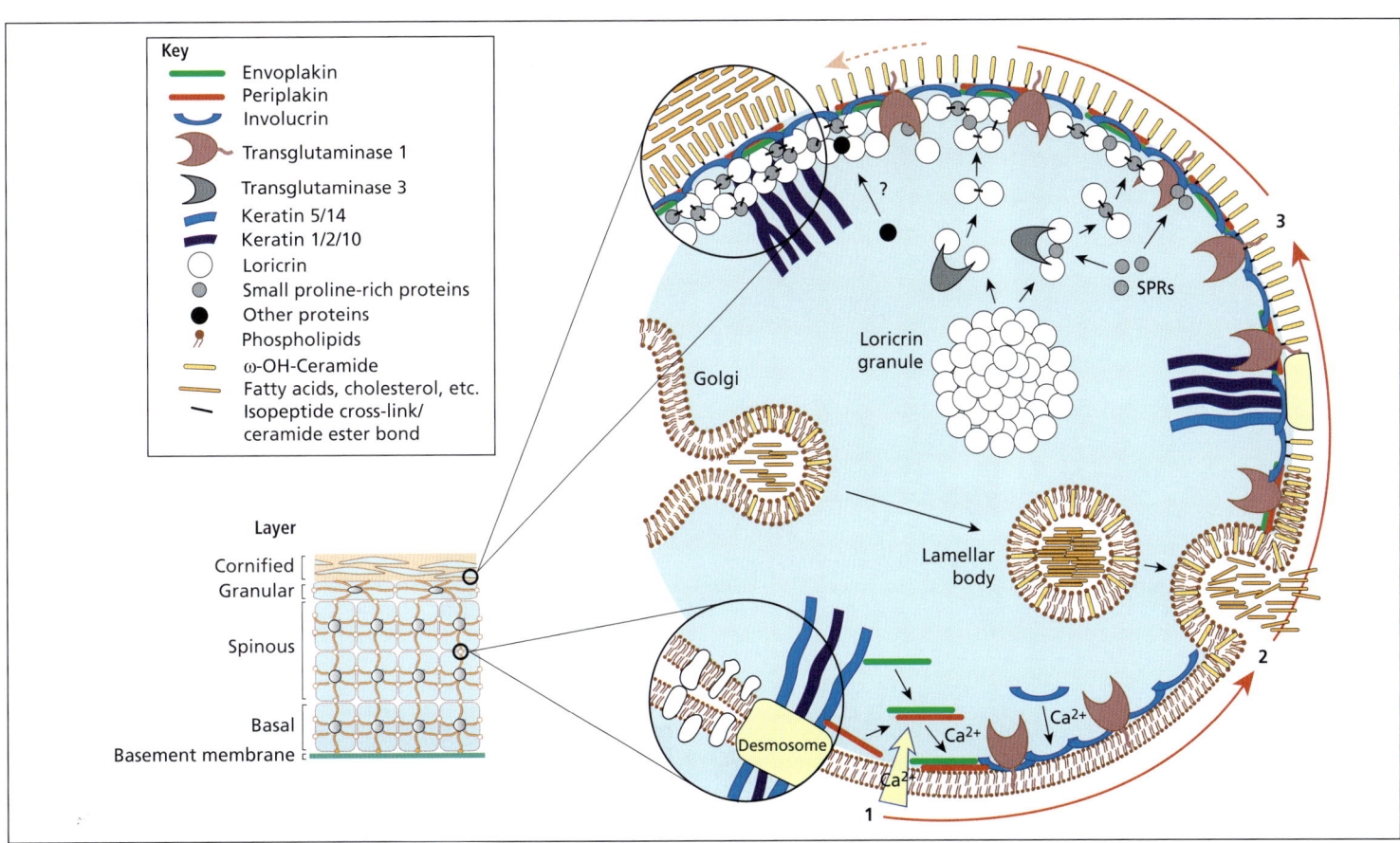

Figure 2.9 Assembly of the epidermal cornified cell envelope. In response to increasing intracellular calcium, an internal scaffold of desmosomal proteins is made along the plasma membrane. The contents of lamellar bodies (ceramides and other fatty acids, cholesterol and cholesterol esters) are released into the extracellular milieu to form a lipid membrane. The developing envelope is then added to and reinforced by the recruitment of various proteins, including loricrin, small proline-rich proteins (SPRs), other desmosomal remnants and attached keratin filaments. The resulting cornified cell envelope is durable and flexible and provides important mechanical and barrier functions.

precursor *involucrin*, following the action of a specific epidermal transglutaminase also synthesised in the high stratum spinosum (Figure 2.10). Many of the proteins involved in terminal differentiation are derived from a cluster of about 25 genes located within a *c.*2 Mb region on the long arm of chromosome 1. Termed the epidermal differentiation complex (EDC), these coding elements are derived from at least three families of structurally, functionally and evolutionarily related genes. Together, the EDC proteins have roles in structural integrity, signal transduction and cell cycle progression and may be primarily or secondarily disrupted in several inflammatory or neoplastic disorders.

The process of desquamation involves degradation of the lamellated lipid in the intercellular spaces and loss of the residual intercellular desmosomal interconnections [5]. In palmoplantar skin there is an additional zone, also electron-lucent, the *stratum lucidum*, between the granulosum and corneum. These cells are still nucleated and may be referred to as 'transitional' cells.

Keratinocytes

The filamentous cytoskeleton of all mammalian cells, including epidermal keratinocytes, is composed of actin-containing microfilaments approximately 7 nm in diameter; tubulin-containing microtubules 20–25 nm in diameter; and filaments of intermediate size, 7–10 nm in diameter, known as intermediate filaments. There are six types of intermediate filaments: keratins in epithelial cells; vimentin within mesenchymal cells; glial filament acidic protein (GFAP) in glial cells; neurofilaments in neurons; desmin in muscle cells; and peripherin in peripheral nerves. The nuclear matrix proteins, nuclear lamins A, B and C, are also intermediate filaments. The polypeptide building blocks of all intermediate filaments have a similar backbone structure of a classic α-helical region with heptad repeats, having four separate helical zones with interhelical linker sequences, and non-helical carboxy- and amino-terminals. There are 70 intermediate filament genes (including those encoding keratins, desmins and lamins), which are now known to be associated with numerous human diseases, including skin blistering, muscular dystrophy, cardiomyopathy, premature ageing syndromes, neurodegenerative disorders and cataract [1,2].

The human genome possesses 54 functional keratin genes located in two compact gene clusters, as well as many non-functional pseudogenes scattered around the genome [3]. Keratin genes are very specific in their expression patterns. Each one of the many highly specialised epithelial tissues has its own profile of keratin gene expression. Hair and nails express modified keratins, containing large amounts of cysteine which forms numerous chemical cross-links to further strengthen the cytoskeleton. The

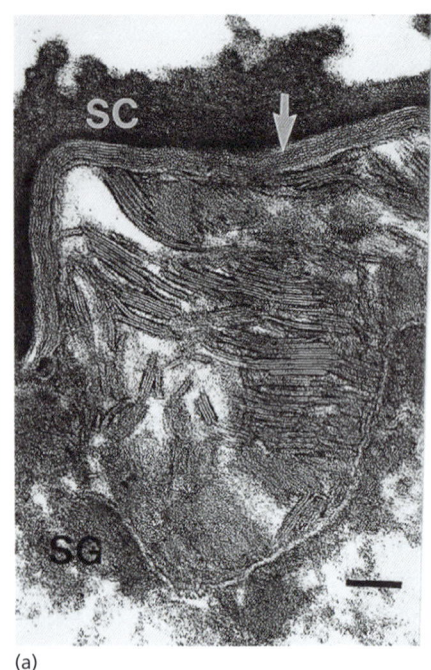
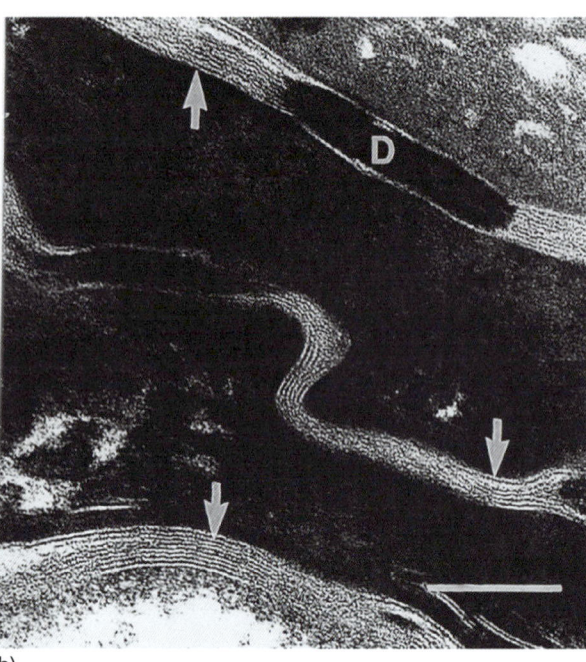

Figure 2.10 Electron micrograph showing the location of epidermal lipids by ruthenium oxide staining. (a) Extrusion of lamellar body lipids or sheets can be seen at the interface between the stratum granulosum (SG) and stratum corneum (SC). Scale bar 0.1 μm. (b) Sheets of lipid bilayers (arrowed) are present in the intercellular spaces of the SC. Some regions show a repetitive pattern of staining. D, desmosome. Scale bar 0.1 μm. Courtesy of Dr M. Fartasch, Department of Dermatology, University of Erlangen, Germany.

genes encoding individual keratins fall into two families: type I (acidic) and type II (basic). Mapping the tissue distribution of keratins shows coexpression of partner acidic–basic pairs in a cell- and tissue-specific manner. Heterodimers are assembled into higher-order protofibrils and protofilaments by an antiparallel stagger of some complexity.

Simple epithelia are characterised by the keratin pair K8/K18, and the stratified squamous epithelia by K5/K14 (Figure 2.11). In addition, stratified squamous epithelia express up to four other keratin pairs during epithelial differentiation. In skin, suprabasal keratins K1/K10 are characteristic of epidermal differentiation. In the stratum granulosum, release of filaggrin from the keratohyalin granules forms macrofibres. Retinoid levels, growth factors and hormones may regulate keratin gene expression. Mesenchymal signals may also direct or permit intrinsic patterns of keratinocyte differentiation. K15 is expressed in basal keratinocytes of the hair follicle bulge region at the site of pluripotential stem cells. K9 and K2 expression is site restricted in skin: K9 to the palmoplantar epidermis and K2 to the superficial interfollicular epidermis. Apart from their structural properties, keratins may also have direct roles in cell signalling, the stress response and apoptosis [1,4]. In epidermal hyperproliferation, as in wound healing and psoriasis, the expression of suprabasal keratins K6/K16/K17 is rapidly induced.

Currently, at least 21 of the 54 known keratins (28 type I and 26 type II) have been linked to monogenic genetic disorders, and some have been implicated in more complex traits such as idiopathic liver disease or inflammatory bowel disease [5]. The first genetic disorder of keratin to be described was epidermolysis bullosa simplex, which involves mutations in the genes encoding K5 or K14. About half of the 54 keratin genes are expressed in the hair follicle (trichocyte 'hard' keratins), although only a minority of these have been linked to human genetic disorders (monilethrix, hair–nail ectodermal dysplasias, pseudofolliculitis barbae and woolly hair) [6].

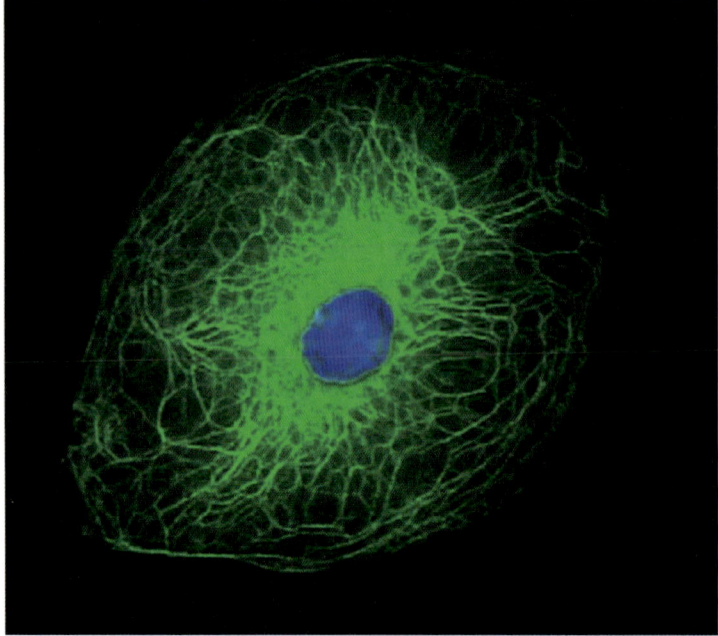

Figure 2.11 Structural organisation of the keratin filament network within a keratinocyte. Courtesy of Professor W. H. I. McLean, University of Dundee, UK.

Eccrine and apocrine glands

Human sweat glands are generally divided into two types: apocrine and eccrine [1]. The eccrine gland is the primary gland responsible for thermoregulatory sweating in humans. Eccrine sweat glands are distributed over nearly the entire body surface. Sweat glands become identifiable in the palms and soles in the 16th fetal week, and in the rest of the body from the 22nd week onwards. The number of sweat glands in humans varies greatly, ranging from 1.6 million to 4.0 million. The structure of the eccrine sweat gland consists of a bulbous secretory coil leading to a duct. The secretory coil is sited in the lower dermis, and the duct extends through the dermis and opens directly onto the skin surface. The active sweat glands are present most densely on the sole, forehead and palm, somewhat less on the back of the hand, still less on the lumbar region and the lateral and extensor surfaces of the extremities, and least on the trunk and the flexor and medial surfaces of the extremities. The uncoiled dimension of the secretory portion of the gland is approximately 30–50 μm in diameter and 2–5 mm in length. The size of the adult secretory coil ranges from 1 to 8×10^{-3} mm^3.

Human perspiration is classified into two types: insensible perspiration and active sweating. Insensible perspiration involves water loss from the respiratory passages and the skin. In the skin, the epidermis is supplied with water originating from blood in the skin microcirculation and interstitial spaces so that water can evaporate from its dry surface. Thus, the evaporation of water from the skin may depend on several environmental factors such as ambient temperature and ambient humidity. Heat, mental stimuli and muscular exercise can all induce active sweating in human beings. Active sweating may be classified into two types: thermal and mental/emotional. Thermal sweating plays an important role in keeping the body's temperature constant and involves the whole of the body's surface [2]. Mental or emotional sweating usually appears on the palms and soles. The physiological features of mental sweating differ considerably from those of thermal sweating. Mental sweating has a shorter latent period for its onset and immediately attains a certain rate of secretion that corresponds to the intensity of stimulation, remaining for the duration of the stimulation and subsiding quickly after it ends [3]. Eccrine glands contribute to both types of sweating.

The secretory nerve fibres innervated in human sweat glands are sympathetic and seem to be cholinergic in character as sweating is produced by pilocarpine and stopped by atropine [4]. Vasoactive intestinal peptide (VIP) coexisting in the cholinergic nerve fibres may act as a candidate neurotransmitter to control the blood circulation of the sweat glands. The sudorific nervous system is also separated into parts for thermal and emotional sweating, each being controlled by its own regulatory centre in the brain that is associated with the sweat glands in its respective region of the skin. The exact neurological pathways responsible for sweating are not entirely understood.

Sympathetic nerve terminals cluster mainly around the secretory coil of the sweat gland, but a few projections extend to the sweat duct. Acetylcholine is the primary neurotransmitter released from cholinergic sudomotor nerves and binds to muscarinic receptors on the eccrine sweat gland, although sweating can also occur via exogenous administration of α- or β-adrenergic agonists. Released acetylcholine is rapidly hydrolysed by acetylcholinesterase, and this response may be one of several mechanisms by which the rate of sweating is regulated.

When acetylcholine binds to muscarinic receptors on the sweat gland, intracellular Ca^{2+} concentrations increase. This results in an increase in the permeability of K$^+$ and Cl$^-$ channels, which initiates the release of an isotonic precursor fluid from the secretory cells [5]. This precursor fluid is similar to plasma but is devoid of proteins. As the fluid travels up the duct towards the surface of the skin, sodium and chloride are reabsorbed, resulting in sweat on the surface being hypotonic relative to plasma. When the rate of sweat production increases, however, for example during exercise or heat stress, ion reabsorption mechanisms can be overwhelmed due to the large quantity of sweat secreted into the duct, resulting in higher ion losses. The sodium content in sweat on the skin's surface, therefore, is greatly influenced by sweat rate.

Apart from eccrine glands, the skin also contains apocrine sweat glands [6]. Eccrine glands do not show cytological changes during secretion, whereas apocrine glands are characterised by decapitation secretion, in which part of the cell is pinched off and released into the lumen. Apocrine glands are located only in genital, axillary and mammary areas, where they are always connected to a hair follicle. Apocrine glands have a low secretory output and hence no significant role in thermoregulation. They are composed of a coiled secretory portion and an excretory duct. The inner layer of the secretory portion contains a single columnar secretory cell type with numerous, large, dense granules located at the apical aspect, which contribute to the lipid-rich secretion produced. The inner layer is also surrounded by a fenestrated layer of myoepithelial cells, but the lumen is generally larger in diameter than that present in eccrine tissue. The apocrine excretory duct does not have any known reabsorptive function and consists of a double layer of cuboidal cells that merge distally with the epithelium of the hair follicle, resulting in emptying of the secretion into the hair follicle. The exact role of apocrine glands in humans is unknown. A third type of intermediate sweat glands, the apoeccrine glands, has also been described in axillary skin but their existence is not universally accepted.

Pilosebaceous unit

The pilosebaceous units develop from epidermal downgrowths under the influence of specific mesenchymal cell condensations between the 10th and 14th weeks of estimated gestational age. They have complex groups of specialised cell layers with distinctive pathways of differentiation. There are four classes of pilosebaceous unit: terminal on the scalp and beard; apopilosebaceous in the axilla and groin; vellus on most skin; and sebaceous on the chest, back and face. The dermal papilla is located at the base of the hair follicle with a rich extracellular matrix. Around the papilla are germinative (matrix) cells that have a very high rate of division and give rise to spindle-shaped central cortex cells of the hair fibre, and the single outer layer of flattened, overlapping cuticle cells. A central medulla is seen in some hairs, with regularly stacked, condensed cells interspersed with air spaces or low-density cores. The cortical cells are filled with keratin intermediate filaments orientated along the long axis of the cell, interspersed with a dense interfilamentous protein matrix.

Terminal differentiation of cortical cells is associated with the appearance of a contiguous, laminated, intercellular layer, which appears critical for filament integrity. The cuticular cells are morphologically distinct; these are flattened, outward-facing cells, with three layers inside the cuticle of condensed, flattened protein granules: endocuticle, exocuticle and 'a' layer [1]. Around the cuticle is the inner root sheath (IRS), which is composed of three

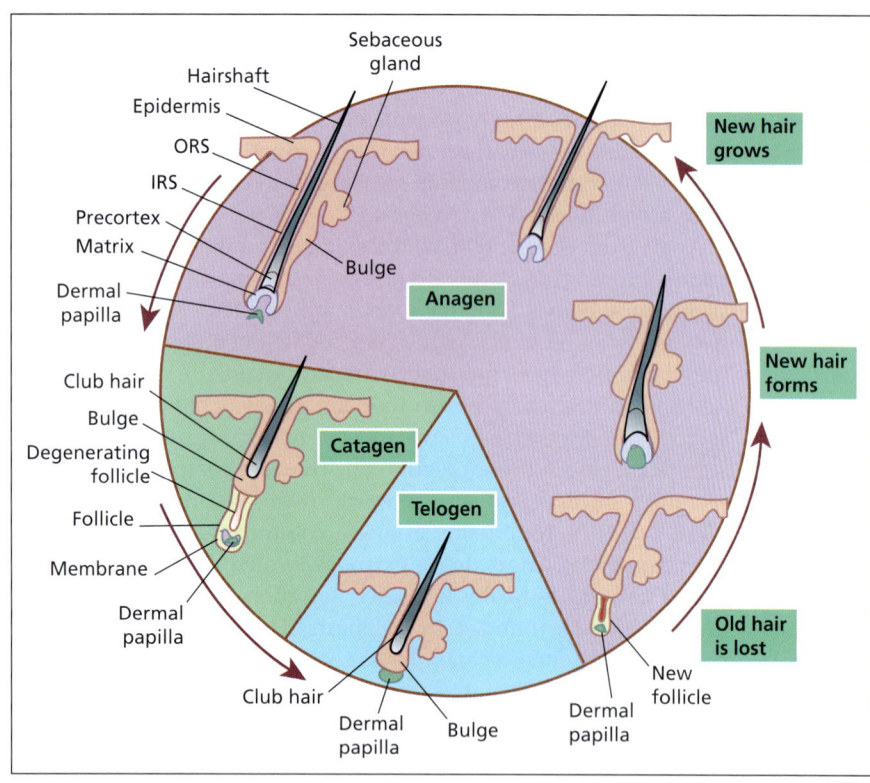

Figure 2.12 There are three components to the hair cycle: anagen (where new hair forms and grows), followed by catagen (regressing phase) and telogen (resting phase), and then loss of old hair. The hair cycle is associated with discrete changes in hair follicle anatomy, both in the shape of the follicle and in the subjacent dermal papilla. IRS, inner root sheath; ORS, outer root sheath.

distinct layers of cells that undergo keratinisation: the IRS cuticle, the Huxley layer and the outermost Henle layer [2]. Differentiation in the IRS involves the development of trichohyalin granules, with 8–10 nm filaments orientated in the direction of hair growth. The IRS moves up the follicle, forming a support for the hair fibre, and degenerates above the sebaceous gland. The outermost layer is the outer root sheath (ORS), which is continuous with the epidermis and expresses epithelial keratins K5/K14, K1/K10 and K6/K16 in the upper ORS and K5/K14/K17 in the deeper ORS.

Normal growth of the hair fibre is 300–400 μm/day, generated by the high rate of proliferation of progenitor cells in the follicle bulb. Compartmentalisation within the bulb gives rise to the different layers within the follicle, with most bulb cells forming the IRS. There are three phases of cyclical hair growth: anagen, when growth occurs; catagen, a regressing phase; and telogen, a resting phase (Figure 2.12). The follicle re-enters anagen, and the old hair is replaced by a new one.

Immediately above the basal layer in the hair bulb, cells undergo a secondary pathway of 'trichocyte' or hair differentiation, and express a further complex group of keratins, the hard keratins [3]. Two families of hair keratins, types I and II, are present in mammals, which have distinctive amino- and carboxy-terminals with high levels of cysteine residues, but lack the extended glycine residues of epidermal keratins. The proteins differ from epithelial keratins in their positions on two-dimensional gels, but they can be grouped into acidic and basic families; there are four major proteins in each of these families and several minor proteins, Ha 1–4 and Hb 1–4. Cloning of the hair keratin genes, which cluster on chromosomes 12 and 17, has shown a greater number of hair keratin genes, *HaKRT1–6* (including 3.1 and 3.2) and *HbKRT1–6*. Mutations in hair keratin genes have been found to be causative for autosomal dominant forms of the human disease monilethrix. In addition, keratin 17 null mice also demonstrate varying degrees of alopecia, depending on the age and strain of the mice.

Over the last two decades, several naturally occurring, inherited human disorders of hair have provided fascinating insight into hair development and growth. These include key signalling molecules such as ectodysplasin, as well as transcription factors, including hairless, WNT10A and the vitamin D receptor, structural hair keratins, desmosomal proteins, a G protein-coupled receptor, a serine protease and a copper transporter [4]. More common hair variants, such as curly hair, may be explained by dynamic changes during hair growth [5]. Curvature of curly hair is programmed from the very basal area of the follicle and the bending process is linked to a lack of axial symmetry in the lower part of the bulb, affecting the connective tissue sheath, ORS, IRS and hair shaft cuticle.

Nails

The main purposes of the nail apparatus are to provide protection to the digit tips, enhance sensory discrimination, help increase dexterity, facilitate scratching or grooming and, in some individuals, to function as a cosmetic accessory [1]. The earliest signs of finer nail development occur at 8–9 weeks' gestation: there is an invagination of the primitive epidermis to form an uninterrupted groove delineating a flattened surface at the end of each digit, known as the nail field. A key transcription factor in nail initiation is R-spondin 4, mutations in which underlie congenital anonychia [2]. A group of cells from the proximal part of the nail fold then grows proximally into the digit, stopping approximately 1 mm from the phalanx and giving rise to the matrix primordium. This site will eventually contribute to the epithelium of the proximal nail fold as well as the distal and intermediate matrix epithelium. From the distal part of the nail fold, a visible mound of cells emerges on the dorsum of the distal tip of each digit, which is known as the distal ridge [3]. At 13 weeks' gestation, the proximal nail fold is formed, and the first signs of nail plate growth are observed from the lunula. At this stage, the stratum corneum and the stratum granulosum start to materialise from the nail field epithelium, beginning distally and advancing towards the proximal nail fold. At 18 weeks' gestation, the granular layer recedes, and the nail bed epithelium takes on a postnatal appearance. Likewise, at 20 weeks' gestation, the process of cellular differentiation and maturation within the matrix is like that seen in adult nails. By 32 weeks' gestation, virtually all the components of the nail can be recognised. Toenail development is similar to that of fingernails but the stages occur about 4 weeks later.

The nail unit is composed of the nail plate and four epithelial structures: the proximal nail fold, the matrix, the nail bed and the hyponychium (Figure 2.13) [4]. The nail plate is a rectangular, translucent and relatively inflexible structure, and contains calcium, phosphate, iron, zinc, manganese and copper, but it is mainly the sulphur within the nail matrix that is responsible for the nail plate's physical qualities. The nail plate arises from beneath the proximal nail fold and is bordered on both sides by the lateral nail folds. The proximal aspect may contain white semicircular areas called lunulae, which are the visible portions of the distal matrix [5]. The dorsal surface of the nail unit appears pink in colour because of the enhanced vasculature of the underlying nail bed. The proximal nail fold has a dorsal and a ventral epithelial surface. It is a continuation of the skin of each digit (the dorsal surface) that folds underneath itself, resting above the nail matrix (the ventral surface). The dorsal proximal nail fold is devoid of hair follicles, sebaceous glands and dermatoglyphic markings and the ventral proximal nail fold also lacks rete ridges. At the junction between the dorsal and ventral surfaces is the eponychium (cuticle) which protects the matrix from damage. The lateral nail folds are extensions of the skin surface of the sides of the digits and join the nail bed medially.

The nail matrix forms the nail plate and is divided into three regions: the dorsal section of the matrix contributes to the most superficial layers of the nail plate, whereas the intermediate region of the matrix forms the deeper layers. The ventral subdivision is the most distal part of the nail matrix. The nail bed is the area underneath the nail plate (between the lunula and the hyponychium). It has a role in forming the deeper layers of the nail plate, as its thin epidermal layer represents the ventral portion of the nail matrix. The hyponychium is located underneath the free edge of the nail plate and denotes the transition of the nail bed to the normal epidermis of the fingers and toes. There is also part of the hyponychium, known as the onychodermal band, that reflects onto the ventral surface of the nail plate to protect the nail parenchyma from trauma.

The epithelium of the matrix is composed of at least two to three actively dividing, basal keratinocyte layers. These cuboidal cells have their vertical axes aligned in a diagonal manner, which allows the nail plate to develop in an upward and outward direction. As these cells differentiate and migrate, they become flatter, losing their nuclei and becoming integrated into the developing nail plate as onychocytes, or nail plate cells. This process of cellular

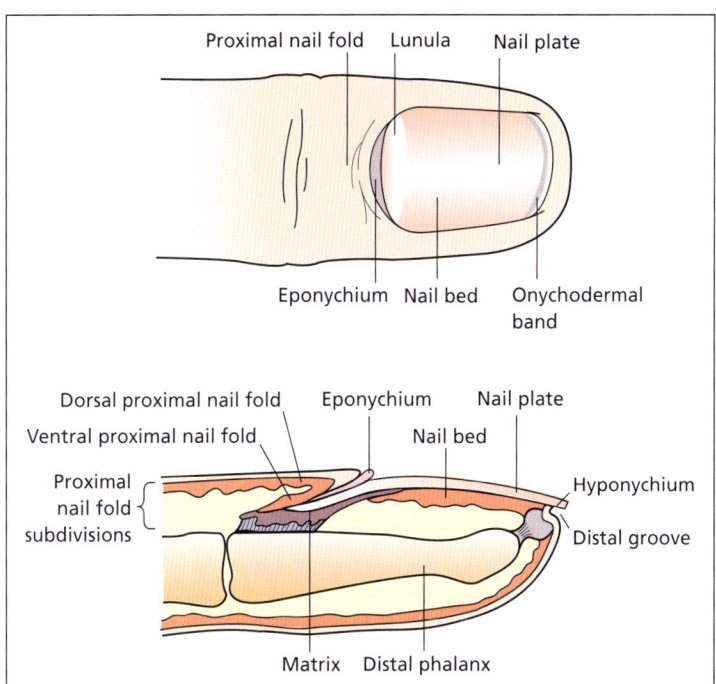

Figure 2.13 Anatomy and structure of the human nail.

maturation is akin to stratum corneum formation within the epidermis but does not require keratohyalin. The matrix also contains melanocytes, which pigment the surrounding keratinocytes and manifest as longitudinal bands across the nail plate; this may be a common racial variant in darker-skinned individuals. The nail bed is composed of a thin epidermal layer and a dermal layer, but there is no subcutaneous fat. As the epidermis is thin, the differentiation of keratinocytes to onychocytes occurs within one to two cell layers. The epidermis of the nail bed also contains parallel longitudinal ridges from the lunula to the hyponychium. These ridges interlock to provide strong binding between the nail bed and the nail plate. The dermal layer of the nail bed contains blood vessels to supply the nail unit, as well as lymphatics. Trauma to these vessels results in splinter haemorrhages.

Merkel cells

Merkel first gave the name *tastzellen* to certain cells that he found near the base of the rete peg in the snout skin of the mole. As there were intraepidermal neurites with expanded tips (Merkel discs) adjacent to them, he believed them to be transducers of physical stimuli. Merkel cells are postmitotic cells scattered throughout the epidermis of vertebrates and constitute 0.2–5% of epidermal cells [1]. They are located amongst basal keratinocytes and are mainly found in hairy skin, tactile areas of glabrous skin, taste buds, anal canal, labial epithelium and eccrine sweat glands, all regions of high tactile acuity (Figure 2.14).

Sun-exposed skin may contain twice as many Merkel cells as non-sun-exposed skin. They form close connections with sensory nerve endings and secrete or express a number of peptides. Human Merkel cells express immunoreactivity for various neuropeptides including met-enkephalin and vasoactive intestinal polypeptide,

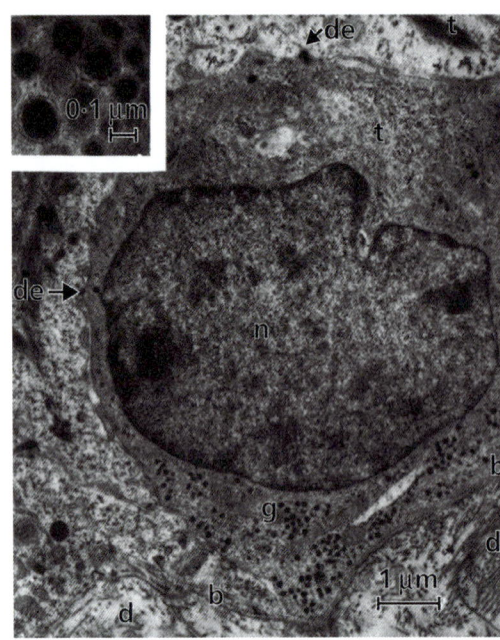

Figure 2.14 Merkel cell in human epidermis. The dermis (d) with collagen fibres is seen in the lower part of the picture. b, Basement membrane; de, desmosomes making connections with adjacent basal keratinocyte; g, spherical granules (see inset); n, nucleus of Merkel cell; t, tonofilaments. Courtesy of Professor A. S. Breathnach.

in addition to neuron-specific enolase and synaptophysin-like and pancreastatin-like material. They also contain chromogranin A [2].

Merkel cells are easily identifiable on transmission electron microscopy. They are oval with a long axis of approximately 15 μm, orientated parallel to the basement membrane. They also have a large bilobed nucleus and clear cytoplasm, which reflects a relative scarcity of intracellular organelles. Merkel cells contain numerous neurosecretory granules, each 50–160 nm across; these are found opposing the junctions with the sensory nerve endings. The close contact between Merkel cells and nerve fibres represents a Merkel cell–neurite complex. Indeed, Merkel cells actively participate in touch reception, displaying fast, touch-evoked mechanotransduction currents, and provide evidence for a direct, functional, excitatory connection between epidermal cells and sensory neurons [3,4].

Human skin contains an extensive neural network that consists of cholinergic and adrenergic nerves and myelinated and unmyelinated sensory fibres. The skin also contains several transducers involved in the perception of touch, pressure and vibration, including Ruffini organs surrounding hair follicles, Meissner corpuscles, Vater–Pacini corpuscles located in the deep layer of the dermis, and nerve endings that pass through the epidermal basement membrane. Some of these contain Merkel cells, which form the Merkel cell–neurite complex, while others are free nerve endings. The cell bodies for all these neurons reside in the dorsal root ganglion. The Merkel cell–neurite complexes are thought to serve as mechanoreceptors and to be responsible for the sensation of touch.

In glabrous skin, the density of Merkel cells is approximately 50 per mm^2. They are clustered near unmyelinated sensory nerve endings, where they group and form 'touch spots' at the bottom of rete ridges. These complexes are also known as hair discs, touch domes, touch corpuscles or Iggo discs. The complex is innervated by a single, slowly adapting type 1 nerve fibre. In hairy skin, Merkel cells also cluster in the rete ridges and in the outer root sheath of the hair follicle where the arrector pili muscles attach. The function of Merkel cells in hair follicles is unclear, although they may be involved in the induction of new anagen cycles.

There are two hypotheses for the origin of Merkel cells: one possibility is that they differentiate from epidermal keratinocyte-like cells and the other is that they arise from stem cells of neural crest origin that migrated during embryogenesis, in a similar fashion to melanocytes. A unifying view, however, could be that there is very early migration of the Merkel cells from the neural crest and population of the epidermis during the sixth or seventh embryonic week in humans and that these cells subsequently only undergo further differentiation once in the epidermis.

Circulating autoantibodies against Merkel cells have been described in pemphigus and graft-versus-host disease. Merkel cells are absent in vitiligo lesions, in keeping with an autoimmune destruction or neural involvement. Merkel cell hyperplasia is a common histological finding and may accompany keratinocyte hyperproliferation as well as being frequently seen in adnexal tumours such as naevus sebaceus, trichoblastomas, trichoepitheliomas and nodular hidradenomas [5]. Merkel cell hyperplasia is associated with hyperplasia of nerve endings that occurs in neurofibromas, neurilemmomas, nodular prurigo or neurodermatitis. Merkel cell carcinoma is a highly aggressive neuroendocrine carcinoma, the incidence of which appears to be increasing; most cases are associated with the Merkel cell polyomavirus, although the precise disease pathophysiology remains to be elucidated [6].

Skin immune ecosystem

The skin continuously encounters microbial pathogens, and to prevent infection, cells within the epidermis, dermis and fat have evolved several innate strategies. Immune surveillance and homeostatic regulation of skin function are governed by complex interactions between resident lymphoid and myeloid cells and their communications with the surrounding epithelial cells, fibroblasts, adipocytes and neurons to ensure barrier homeostasis. These parenchymal cells help to regulate the tissue residency, recruitment and activation of immune cells, while the immune cells produce effector cytokines as well as growth and regulatory factors to maintain and promote barrier function. In addition, the skin also harbours a community of resident microbes that have symbiotic relationships with host immune cells. The tissue-resident immune cells are highly varied and comprise αβ and γδ T cells, dendritic cells (DCs) and macrophages, as well as a population of an innate immune subset of lymphoid lineage cells, referred to as innate lymphoid cells (ILCs) [1]. ILCs produce effector cytokines similarly to T helper (Th) cells and have been considered as the innate counterpart of adaptive T lymphocytes. In contrast to T-cell activation, which requires T-cell receptor–major histocompatibility complex (MHC) class interactions, ILCs are activated by sensing epithelial cell-, stromal cell- or myeloid cell-derived signals such as alarmins, cytokines and other inflammatory mediators, which enable rapid responses to environmental cues [2]. There are three

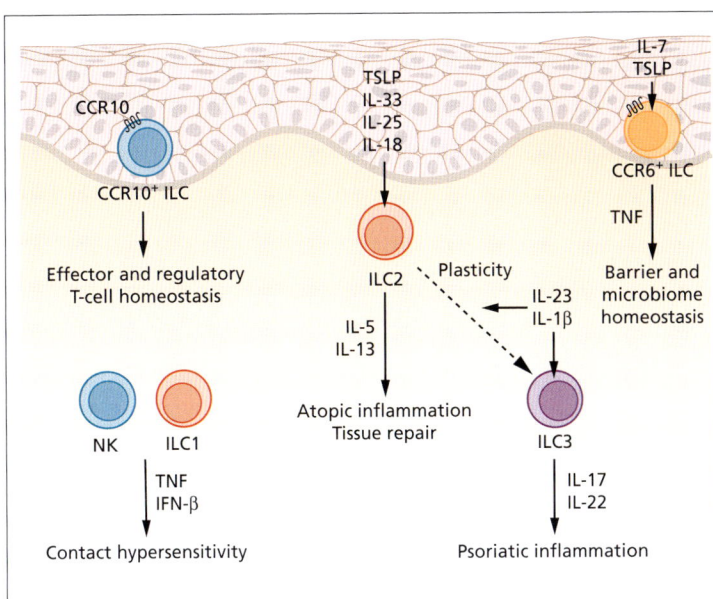

Figure 2.15 Heterogeneous populations of innate lymphoid cells (ILCs) with distinct functions reside in the skin. Skin-resident CCR6+ ILCs maintain the microbiota by regulating sebaceous gland function. CCR10+ ILCs maintain adaptive lymphocyte homeostasis. Natural killer (NK) cells and ILC1s play a role in contact hypersensitivity. ILC2s, which are activated by thymic stromal lymphopoietin (TSLP), interleukin (IL)-33, IL-25, and/or IL-18, contribute to atopic inflammation by production of type 2 cytokines. ILC2s also promote tissue repair. ILC3s produce IL-17 and IL-22, which mediate psoriatic inflammation. IFN, interferon; TNF, tumour necrosis factor. Reproduced from Kobayashi et al. 2020 [1] with permission of Elsevier.

main groups of ILCs which respond to different types of organisms and intracellular and extracellular or other triggers (Figure 2.15).

Some ILCs traffic between the circulation and lymph nodes whereas others are resident within skin, with sites of residency governed by cross-talk between parenchymal and immune cells as well as their patterns of chemokine receptor expression. It is also evident that ILCs contribute to the pathogenesis of several skin diseases, including contact hypersensitivity, atopic inflammation [3] and psoriasis, as well as physiological processes such as wound healing. Still to be determined is how skin ILCs are activated and regulated under different contexts and how they communicate with microorganisms and other tissue-resident immune cells, as well as with the surrounding stroma. A specific immune surveillance complex restricted to epidermis consists of the Ever1-Ever2-CIB1 complex which provides immunity to human papillary viruses (HPVs). As a result of genetic mutations inactivating any of the three proteins in this complex, skin becomes susceptible to HPV infections, a disease known as epidermodysplasia verruciformis.

Skin microbiome

Present on the skin are thriving complex communities of bacteria, fungi and viruses, with approximately 1 million bacteria (involving hundreds of distinct species) inhabiting each square centimetre of skin [1]. The bacteria mostly comprise Actinobacteria, Firmicutes, Bacteroidetes and Proteobacteria, with numerous subspecies thereof. Actinobacteria represents the largest phylum and includes Propionibacteria and Corynebacteria; Firmicutes includes Clostridia and Bacilli, the latter including the class *Staphylococcus*. The precise composition of these organisms depends on sebaceous gland concentration, moisture content and temperature, as well as on host genetics and exogenous environmental factors, but may be very diverse (Figure 2.16). For example, a survey of the palm microbiome found 4742 distinct species in 51 healthy subjects, with an average of 158 species coexisting on a single palm [2]. It has also become clear that these organisms are not just commensals but play a much bigger role in immune modulation and epithelial health than previously expected. There is cross-talk between the skin microbiome and organisms in other tissues, such as the gut [3]. Understanding microbe–host interactions and discovering the factors that drive microbial colonisation are likely to provide greater insight into the pathogenesis of skin diseases, such as the role of staphylococci in atopic eczema, and the development of new promicrobial and antimicrobial therapeutics [4].

Langerhans cells

Dendritic cells resembling melanocytes, but free from pigment and dopa-negative, were first described by Langerhans, who demonstrated their existence in human epidermis by staining with gold chloride. Subsequently, the dynamic behaviour of epidermal Langerhans cells has been investigated by combining time-lapse, intravital, confocal imaging technology and I-Aβ-enhanced green fluorescent protein (EGFP) knock-in mice in which Langerhans cells can be identified by EGFP-associated fluorescence. Without stimulation, some Langerhans cells exhibit a unique motion, which has been termed *dendrite surveillance extension and retraction cycling habitude* (dSEARCH) and which is characterised by rhythmic extension and retraction of dendritic processes between intercellular spaces. The topical application of an antigen such as dinitro-fluorobenzene leads to greater dSEARCH motion, and also triggers direct cell-to-cell contact formation between adjacent Langerhans cells. It appears that, *in vivo*, dSEARCH motion allows for a more efficient antigen sampling through scanning of a wide area. It is also evident that, under pathological stimulation, adjacent Langerhans cells may exchange antigens between cells (Figure 2.17) [1].

Langerhans cells, in combination with macrophages and dermal dendrocytes, represent the skin's mononuclear phagocyte system [2]. Langerhans cells are capable of phagocytosis, antigen processing, antigen presentation and interactions with lymphocytes (Figure 2.18). They highly express the lipid CD1a which orchestrates a complex interaction between Langerhans cells, a subset of T cells, the skin microbiome and other lipid moieties in skin physiology and antigen presentation [3]. Langerhans cells are intraepidermal macrophages whose dendrites trap antigens among keratinocytes. The cells then leave the epidermis and migrate via lymphatics to a regional lymph node. In the paracortical region of lymph nodes, the Langerhans cell (or 'interdigitating reticulum cell' as it is then known) expresses protein on its surface to present to a T lymphocyte that can then undergo clonal proliferation. There may be some selectivity in whether certain antigens are presented to lymph nodes by Langerhans cells or by dermal dendrocytes. The timing of antigen presentation may also vary, with the possibility

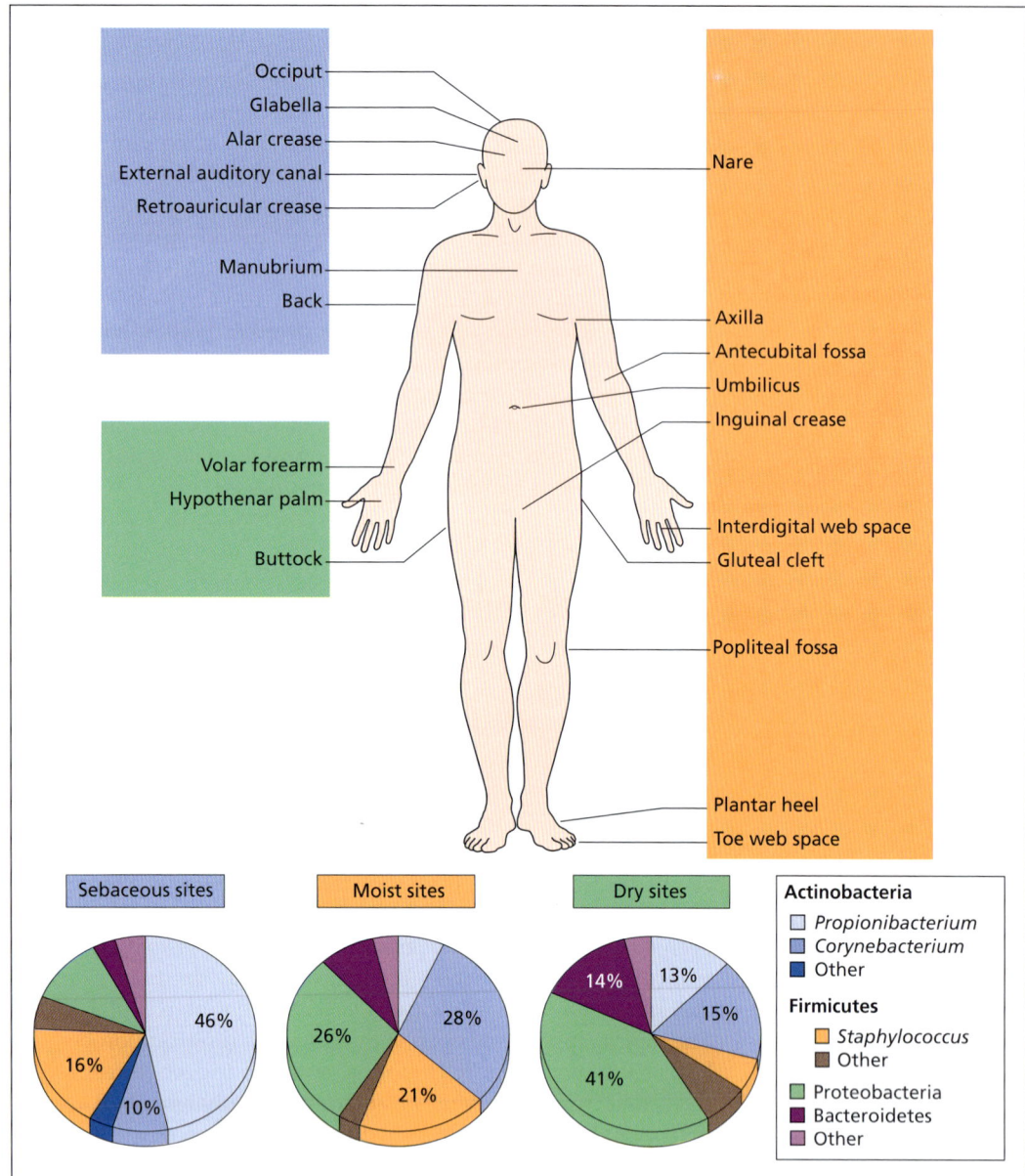

Figure 2.16 The skin microbiome contains numerous bacteria that are variably present in different body regions. Adapted from Chen and Tsao 2013 [4].

that sequential presentation of skin-acquired antigens may regulate cell-mediated immunity.

Langerhans cells may contribute to several skin pathologies including infections, inflammation and cancer, and they play a pivotal role in regulating the balance between immunity and peripheral tolerance [4]. Langerhans cells appear, however, to have characteristics distinct from other dendritic cells in that they are more likely to induce Th2 responses than the Th1 responses that are usually necessary for cellular immune responses against pathogens. It has also been shown that Langerhans cells are dispensable for contact hypersensitivity and that dermal dendrocytes can serve as antigen-presenting cells in the absence of Langerhans cells. Indeed, Langerhans cell-deficient mice appear to have enhanced contact hypersensitivity. With regard to a specific function, Langerhans cells, or a subset thereof, may have regulatory properties that counteract the pro-inflammatory activity of surrounding keratinocytes. It is plausible that under non-inflammatory steady-state conditions, Langerhans cells carry skin-specific components to draining lymph nodes to prevent immunisation and to induce peripheral tolerance against epidermal self-determinants [5]. It also appears that Langerhans cells may indeed consist of distinct subsets, since Langerhans cells that repopulate the skin after inflammation have been shown to derive from monocyte precursors.

Under the electron microscope, Langerhans cells share with melanocytes a lobulated nucleus, a relatively clear cytoplasm and well-developed endoplasmic reticulum, Golgi complex and lysosomes (Figure 2.19). They differ in lacking melanosomes or premelanosomes, and in possessing a characteristic granule that is either rod or racquet shaped. These 'Birbeck' granules have been shown to represent subdomains of the endosomal recycling compartment and form at sites where the protein langerin accumulates. Using ultrastructural evidence of the presence of the characteristic granules, Langerhans cells have been identified in the outer root sheath of the human hair and the secretory duct of the sebaceous

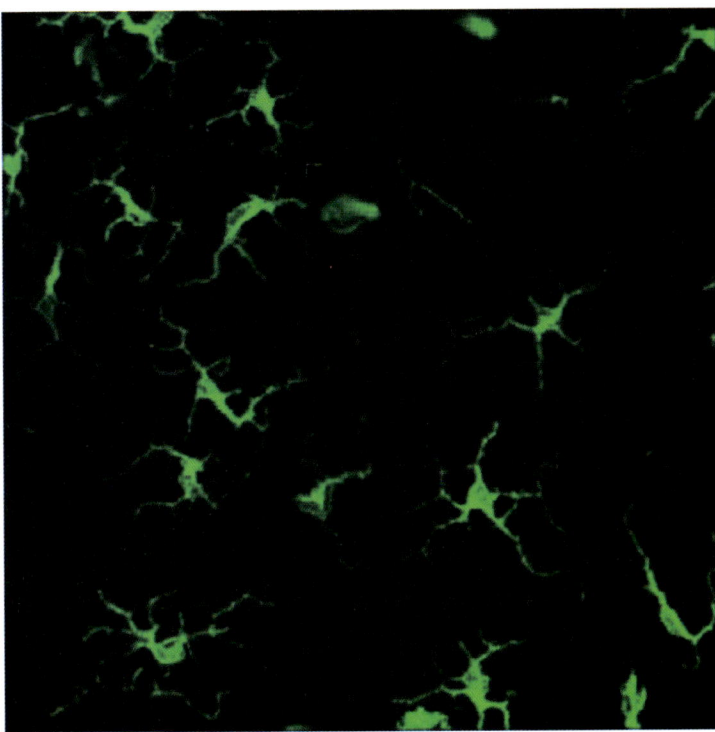

Figure 2.17 Dendritic appearance of epidermal Langerhans cells. Exposure to antigen provokes an increased movement of Langerhans cells as well as direct cell–cell contact between Langerhans cells. Courtesy of Dr R. Mohr, University of Toledo, Ohio, USA.

gland and in the epithelium of the crypts of the human tonsil. The discovery of similar granules in cells in the dermis in histiocytosis X resulted in the renaming of this condition as Langerhans cell histiocytosis.

Immune surveillance

Besides the antigen detection and processing role of epidermal Langerhans cells, cutaneous immune surveillance is also carried out in the dermis by an array of tissue-resident T cells, macrophages and dendritic cells (Figure 2.20) [1]. These immune sentinel and effector cells can provide rapid and efficient immunological backup to restore tissue homeostasis should the epidermis be breached. Resident memory T cells act as alarm-sensor cells or cytotoxic cells, often persisting in the skin for a long time, and can be reactivated upon reinfection with the same antigen. The dermis contains a very large number of resident T cells; remarkably, there are approximately 2×10^{10} skin-resident T cells, which is twice the total number of T cells in the circulating blood [2,3]. There are several distinct populations of dermal dendritic cells; some have potent antigen-presenting capacities, others have low antigen-presenting capacity but the potential to develop into CD1a+ and langerin-positive Langerhans cells, while some are pro-inflammatory.

The cellular diversity of dermal immune sentinels is reflected in some flexibility or plasticity in function. For example, immature dendritic cells, including dermal dendritic cells, can be phagocytic, which is a cellular function usually attributed to macrophages [4]. Alternatively, macrophages, which normally are phagocytic cells, can also be potent antigen-presenting cells for CD8+ T cells. This means that tissue-resident mononuclear sentinels of the dermis are likely to exist in a pluripotent state. Depending on microenvironmental factors and cues, they may acquire an antigen-presenting mode, a migratory mode or a tissue-resident phagocytic mode.

Mast cells

Mast cells were first described by Ehrlich in 1877, who distinguished them from other connective tissue cells by their ability to stain metachromatically with basic aniline dyes. Mast cells are larger than eosinophils and basophils. They occur in most tissues, but are particularly numerous in the skin, bronchus, nasal mucosa and gut. In the skin, mast cells are distributed close to blood vessels, nerves and appendages, and are most numerous in the subpapillary dermis, in the region of the superficial dermal vascular plexus. There are about 7000 mast cells/mm^3 in normal skin.

Dermal mast cells are ovoid or spindle shaped, mononuclear or occasionally binuclear, and only rarely show signs of mitosis in normal skin. Their major distinguishing feature is the presence of numerous, round, cytoplasmic granules (Figures 2.21 and 2.22). Mast cells are heterogeneous and fall into two main types – connective tissue and mucosal – which can be differentiated by their morphology, tissue distribution, histochemical characteristics and responses to degranulating agents. Solubility of the granules in formaldehyde and the content of neutral proteinase, namely tryptase and chymase (chymotryptic proteinase), will vary according to the type of cell. For example, human foreskin mast cells contain both proteinases, whereas mast cells in intestinal mucosa and the lung contain mainly tryptase [1].

Human mast cells arise from CD34+ pluripotent stem cells in the bone marrow. They then circulate in the blood as precursors and home to tissues where they mature under the influence of stem cell factor (SCF) and local cytokines and other factors. Mast cell growth and differentiation are also influenced by several other cytokines, including interleukin 3 (IL-3), -4, -6, -9, -10 and nerve growth factor. Mast cells are long lived and may proliferate in association with immunoglobulin E (IgE)-dependent activation and in the presence of IL-4 [2].

Kit (CD117), expressed on haematopoietic stem cells and progenitor cells, is the tyrosine kinase transmembrane receptor for SCF that is involved in the differentiation of both myeloid and lymphoid lineages. While Kit is downregulated on other bone marrow-derived cells during their differentiation, Kit remains highly expressed on mast cells and is critical for many mast cell functions such as survival, differentiation, chemotaxis and enhancement of signalling events during mast cell activation. The importance of Kit is shown by the finding of activating mutations in the *KIT* gene in patients with urticaria pigmentosa [3].

Upon activation of mast cells via cross-linking of the high-affinity IgE receptor (FcεRI) or non-IgE-mediated activation through complement receptors or Toll-like receptor (TLR) activation, mast cells can release histamine, serotonin and proteases as well as newly synthesised leukotrienes, prostaglandins, cytokines and chemokines. In addition to IgE-mediated activation, human mast cells exposed to interferon γ (IFN-γ) can be activated following IgG-mediated aggregation of FcγRI to release similar mediators.

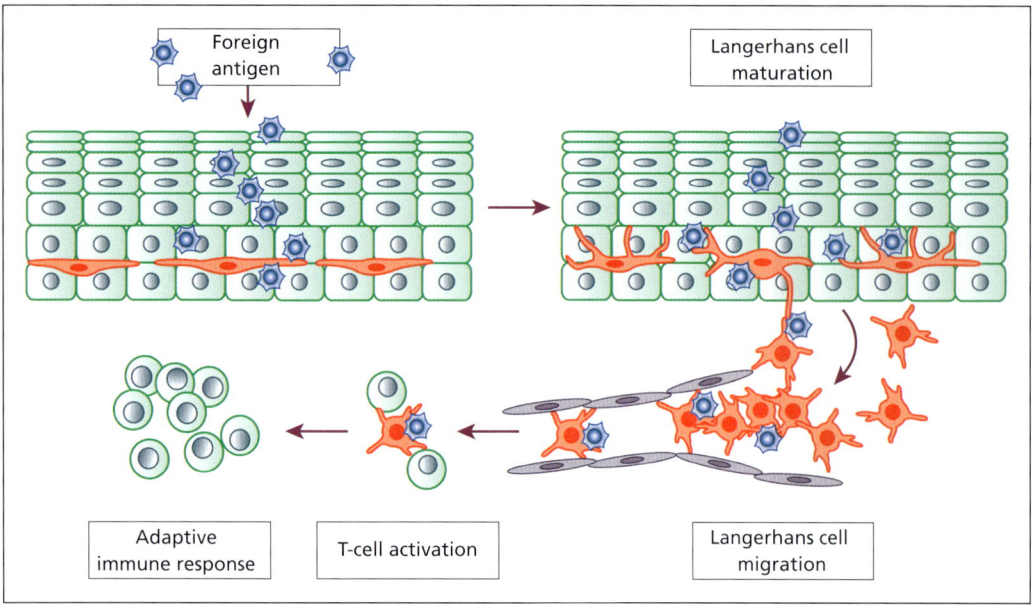

Figure 2.18 When exposed to foreign antigen, the activity of resting Langerhans cells increases, and the cells mature. Antigen is then processed and transported to the lymph nodes. T cells are then activated, and an immune response is triggered.

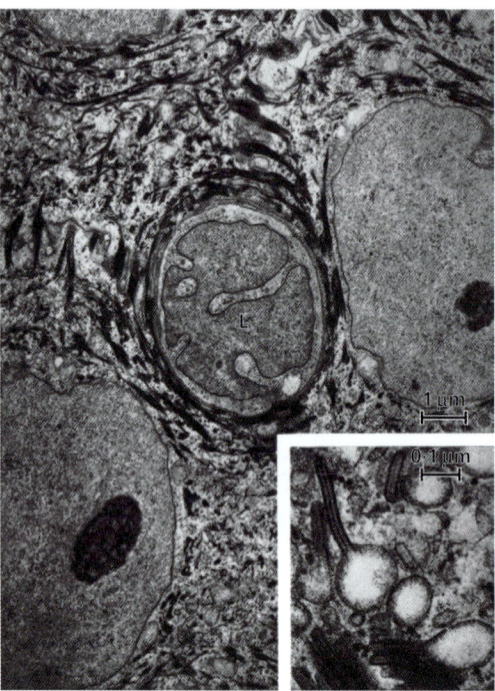

Figure 2.19 Langerhans cell (L) with its characteristically indented nucleus, situated between keratinocytes. The inset shows Langerhans cell granules with racquet-shaped profiles. Courtesy of Professor A. S. Breathnach.

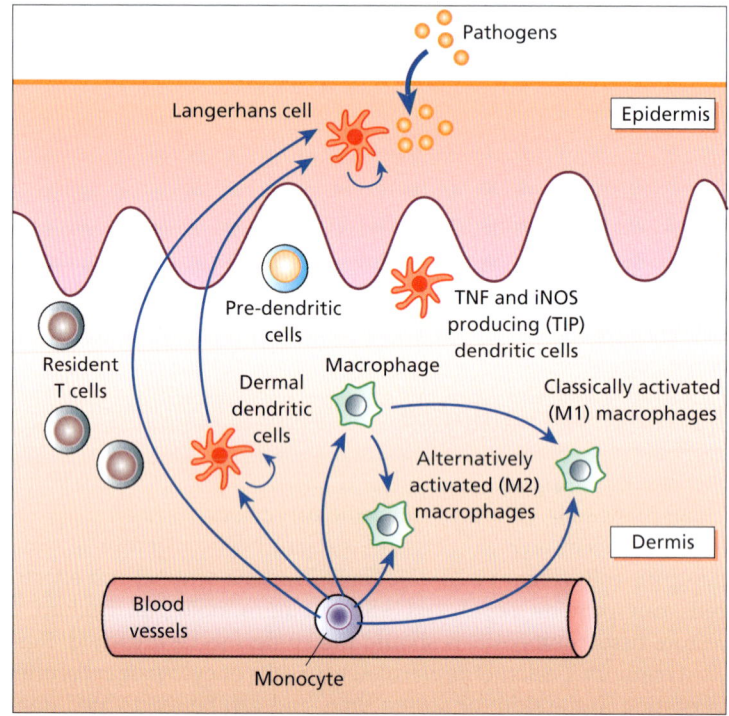

Figure 2.20 Immune surveillance in normal skin is carried out by an array of skin-based dendritic cells, macrophages and resident T cells. iNOS, inducible nitric oxide synthase; TNF, tumour necrosis factor.

Additional IgE-independent mast cell triggers have been described, including SCF, complement (C3a and C5a), neuropeptides (substance P), adenosine, TLR and scavenger receptors.

Mast cell products may both induce an immediate reaction and contribute to a late phase reaction. The immediate phase reaction occurs within minutes of FcεRI cross-linking and its consequences are referred to as an immediate hypersensitivity reaction. Late phase reactions peak 6–12 h following antigen challenge and are associated with cytokines and chemokines from eosinophils, neutrophils and basophils that have been secondarily recruited.

Mast cell activation results in increased vascular permeability and smooth muscle contraction, as well as fibroblast deposition of collagen, induction of B cells to class switch to synthesise IgE, basophil histamine release, recruitment of neutrophils and eosinophils, and promotion of T cells to a Th2 phenotype.

Mast cells play an important role in both adaptive and innate immunity and contribute to the skin pathology seen in contact dermatitis, atopic eczema (AE), immunobullous disease, scleroderma and chronic graft-versus-host disease; they also have a

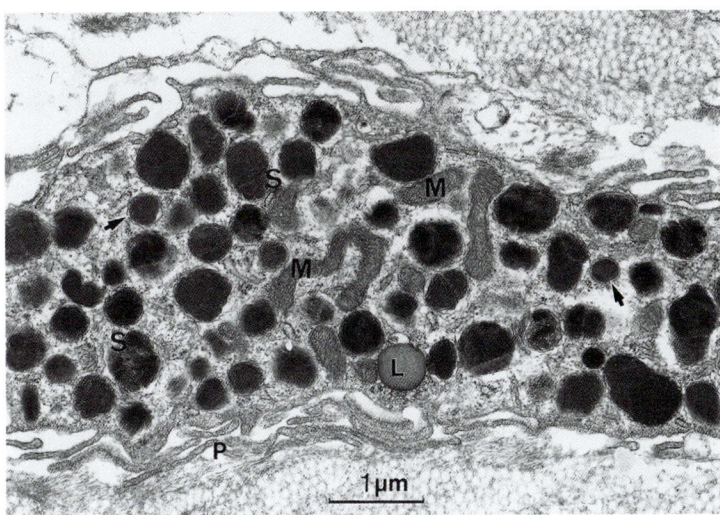

Figure 2.21 Part of a human skin mast cell showing characteristic granules, some with scroll-like profiles (S). Arrows indicate perigranular membrane; L, lipid droplet; M, mitochondria; P, peripheral processes. Courtesy of Professor R. A. J. Eady, St John's Institute of Dermatology, King's College London, UK.

Melanocytes

Melanocytes are pigment-producing cells located in the skin, inner ear, choroid and iris of the eye. In skin, melanocytes are dendritic in shape, are mainly located at the dermal–epidermal junction, and connect to the basement membrane by a dense plate structure that shares similarities with hemidesmosomes. Melanocytes in adult skin and hair develop from embryonically derived melanocyte precursors called melanoblasts [1]. During development, melanoblasts emerge from a subset of neural crest cells and migrate to the interfollicular skin and to developing hair follicles (Figure 2.23). In the hair follicle, melanocytes are divided into two distinct populations: differentiated melanocytes, located in the hair bulb where they provide melanin to the growing hair matrix, and melanocyte stem cells, located at the hair bulge. Melanocyte stem cells are typically quiescent but undergo cyclical proliferation, differentiation and migration. Melanocytes maintain their polarity similarly to neuronal cells, driving cellular asymmetry to control, for example, protrusion and spine formation, organelle transport and metastasis. Polarity regulators may be relevant to melanocyte architecture, function and quiescence and dysregulation therein may be implicated in both hypopigmentation and malignant melanoma. The life cycles of the follicular melanocytes and melanocyte stem cells are closely related to the cyclical nature of the hair follicle, and during anagen new melanocytes are generated from the pool of slow-proliferating melanocyte stem cells [2].

Melanin is synthesised and accumulates within the melanosome, an organelle within the melanocyte. In the skin and hair, two forms of melanin pigment are produced: brown/black eumelanin and yellow/red phaeomelanin (Figure 2.24). Eumelanin has photoprotective qualities via its ability to absorb and scatter ultraviolet (UV) radiation and scavenge reactive oxygen species. In contrast, phaeomelanin is photosensitising and produces reactive oxygen species when exposed to UVA. After melanin is synthesised, pigment-containing melanosomes are transported to keratinocytes, internalised and trafficked to perinuclear locations where they can absorb UV light and protect keratinocyte nuclei from UV-associated radiation damage [3]. One of the critical transcription factors

role in immune regulation [4]. In AE, there is an increase in mast cell numbers in lesional skin. Mast cells reside in the papillary dermis and undergo migration through the basal lamina into the epidermis. Although overall levels of histamine are not increased in AE, tryptase and activation of proteinase-activated receptor-2 (PAR-2) may contribute to the pruritus seen in AE, as tryptase is reported to be increased up to fourfold in AE patients and PAR-2 expression is markedly enhanced on primary afferent nerve fibres in skin biopsies from patients with AE. Chymase may play a role in eliciting and maintaining chronic inflammation in AE by increasing spongiosis and compromising the skin barrier. Mast cell–nerve interactions may also play a role in promoting inflammation in AE. There is an increased number of contacts between mast cells and nerves in both lesional and non-lesional skin, which may lead to inflammation mediated by neuropeptides such as substance P, calcitonin gene-related peptide, vasoactive intestinal peptide and nerve growth factor.

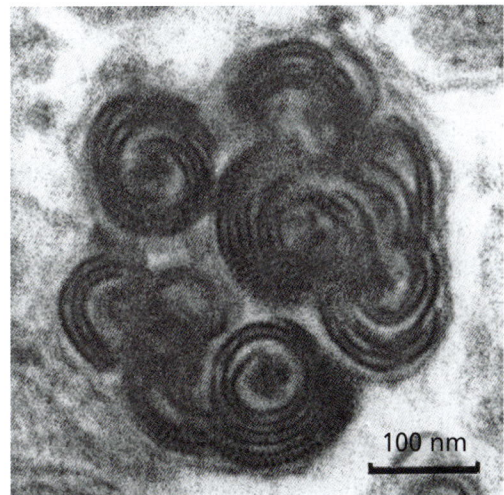
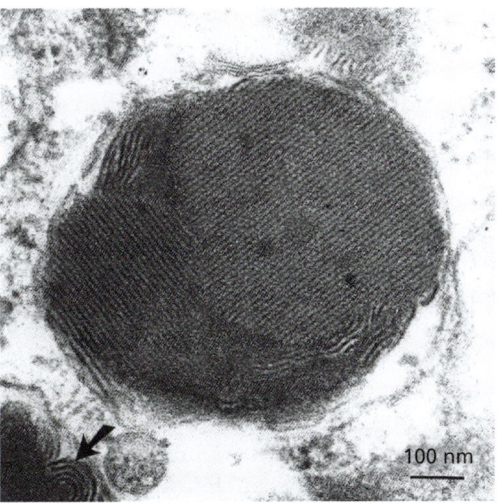

Figure 2.22 High-magnification views of dermal mast cell granules. (a) Typical scroll-like configuration of lamellae, some of which show a cross-banding of regular periodicity. (b) The substructure of this granule is a highly organised lattice (arrow). Courtesy of Professor R. A. J. Eady, St John's Institute of Dermatology, King's College London, UK.

(a)   (b)

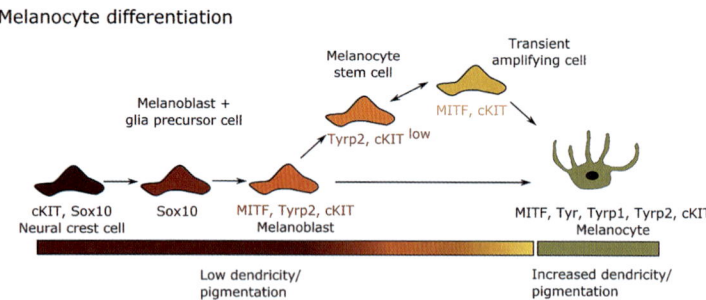

Figure 2.23 Melanocyte differentiation. During murine embryonic development, neural crest cells mostly specify via melanoblast/glial bipotent progenitors to melanoblasts. These then either directly differentiate to interfollicular and follicular melanocytes (marked by expression of MITF, Tyr, Tyrp1, Tyrp2 and a high level of cKIT) or become melanocyte stem cells residing in the hair follicle bulge (marked by expression of Tyrp2 and a low level of cKIT).

modulating melanogenesis, melanocyte survival and proliferation is the melanocyte-specific microphthalmia-associated transcription factor (m-MITF).

Variation in skin pigmentation and tanning ability between individuals mainly reflects differences in melanogenesis and melanin distribution rather than differences in the number of melanocytes. Across all races, ethnicities and skin phenotypes there are broad similarities in the number of melanocytes. In contrast, darkly pigmented skin has higher constitutive activation of MITF and melanosome maturation. Red-haired individuals do not typically experience skin darkening after UV exposure, with just a slight increase in melanocyte number following chronic UV exposure. The red-haired phenotype is mainly the result of polymorphic variants in the melanocortin 1 receptor (MC1R) on melanocytes. Loss-of-function variants in *MC1R* lead to diminished production of eumelanin and phaeomelanin predominance [4].

Desmosomes

Desmosomes are the major adhesion complex in the epidermis, anchoring keratin intermediate filaments to the cell membrane, bridging adjacent keratinocytes and allowing cells to withstand trauma. Desmosomes are also found in the myocardium, meninges, gastrointestinal mucosa, bladder and cortex of lymph nodes. The desmosome has a characteristic ultrastructural appearance, in which the cell membrane of two adjacent cells forms a symmetrical junction with a central intercellular space of 30 nm containing a dense line (Figure 2.25). Plaques of electron-dense material run along the cytoplasm parallel to the junctional region, in which three ultrastructural bands can be distinguished: an electron-dense band next to the plasma membrane, a less dense band and then a fibrillar area [1].

The main components of desmosomes in the epidermis consist of the products of three gene superfamilies: the desmosomal cadherins, the armadillo family of nuclear and junctional proteins, and the plakins [2]. The transmembranous cadherins comprise mostly heterophilic associations of desmogleins and desmocollins. There are four main epidermis-specific desmogleins (Dsg1–4) and three desmocollins (Dsc1–3), all of which show

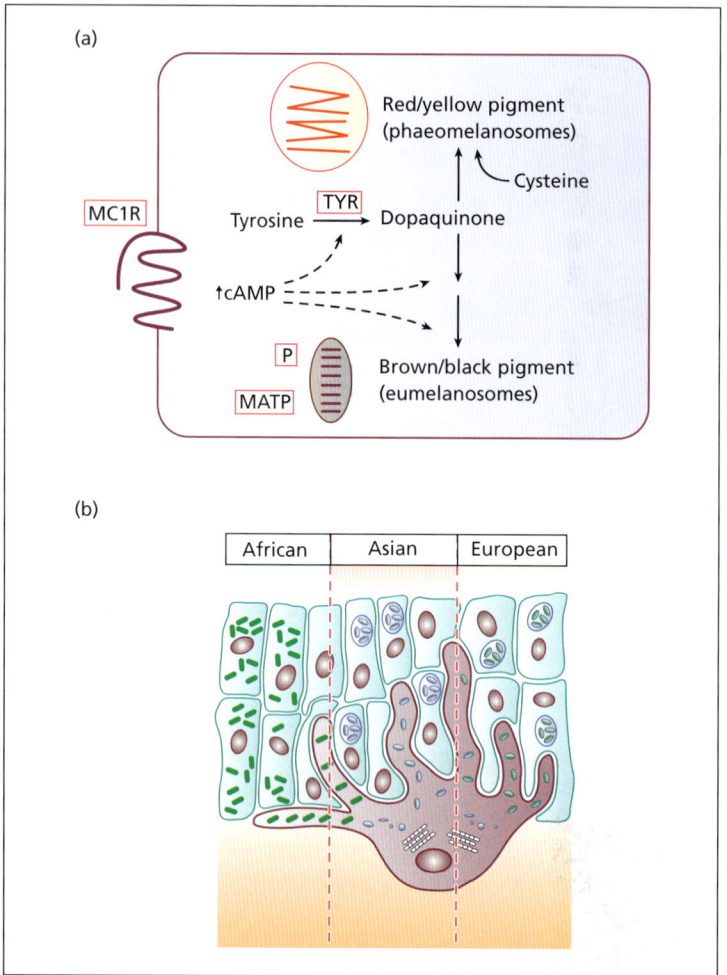

Figure 2.24 (a) Activation of the melanocortin 1 receptor (MC1R) promotes the synthesis of eumelanin at the expense of phaeomelanin. Oxidation of tyrosine by tyrosinase (TYR), however, is required for the synthesis of both pigment types. Melanosomal membrane components, including the membrane-associated transport protein (MATP) and the pink-eyed dilution protein (P), play a role in determining the amount of pigment synthesis within melanosomes. (b) In the skin of individuals of African, Asian and European ancestry there is a gradient of melanosome size and number; in addition, melanosomes in African skin are more widely dispersed.

differentiation-specific expression. For example, Dsg1 and Dsc1 are preferentially expressed in the superficial layers of the epidermis, whereas Dsg3 and Dsc3 show greater expression in basal keratinocytes. The intracellular parts of these glycoproteins are attached to the keratin filament network via desmoplakin, plakoglobin and other macromolecules, including the armadillo protein plakophilin 1, an important stabiliser of keratinocyte adhesion in differentiated keratinocytes, as well as other site-specific plakin cell envelope proteins, such as envoplakin and periplakin [3]. The network of the major interactive desmosomal proteins is depicted in Figure 2.26.

Further clues to the biological function and *in vivo* contribution to keratinocyte adhesion of these desmosomal components have arisen from various mouse models and human diseases, both inherited and acquired [4,5], and desmosome proteins may also serve as autoantigens in several immunobullous blistering skin diseases [6]. Antibodies to multiple desmosomal proteins may

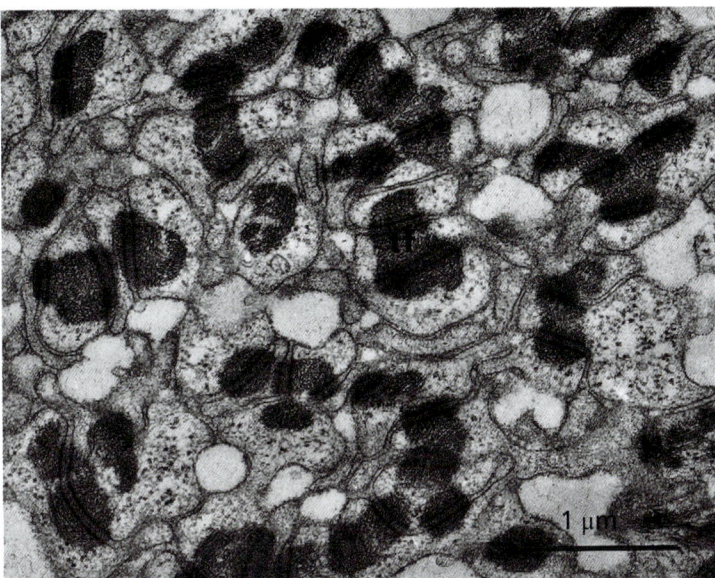

Figure 2.25 Electron micrograph of desmosomes in the spinous layer. These intercellular junctions are closely associated with tonofilaments (tf), many of which, in this view, are cross-sectioned. Courtesy of Professor R. A. J. Eady, St John's Institute of Dermatology, King's College London, UK.

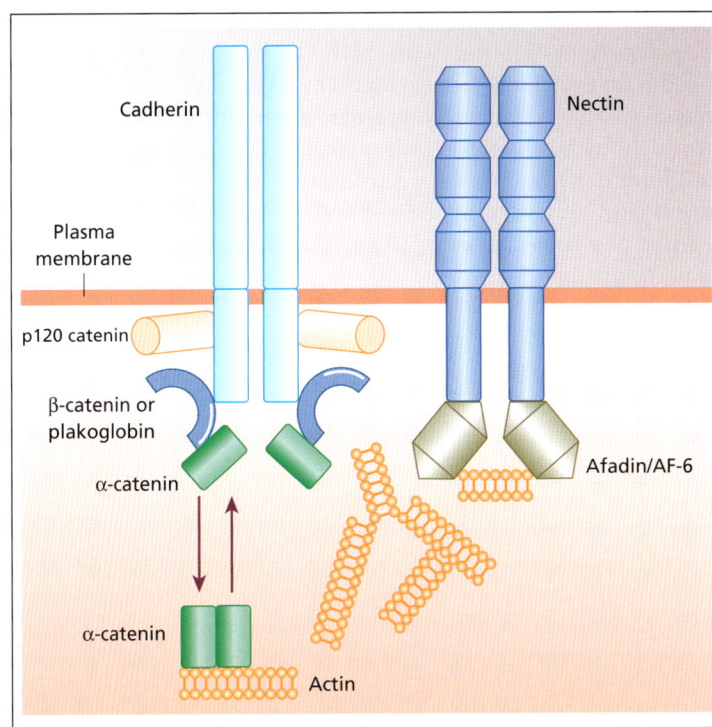

Figure 2.27 Macromolecular composition of an adherens junction in keratinocytes. There are two main components, nectin–afadin and the classic cadherin–catenin complex, which can both attach to the actin cytoskeleton.

Adherens junctions

Adherens junctions are electron-dense, transmembrane structures that engage with the actin skeleton [1]. They can associate with tight junctions and desmosomes or exist separately from these junction complexes. Adherens junctions contribute to epithelial assembly, adhesion, barrier formation, cell motility and changes in cell shape. They are characterised by two opposing membranes separated by approximately 20 nm and are 0.2–0.5 μm in diameter. Adherens junctions may also spatially coordinate signalling molecules and polarity cues as well as serving as docking sites for vesicle release. They comprise two basic adhesive units: the nectin–afadin complex and the classic cadherin–catenin complex (Figure 2.27) [2,3].

There are several different nectins and cadherins and these may be variably incorporated into adherens junctions; the precise composition will impact on the adhesive specificity and other functions of the junction. The nectins form a structural link to the actin cytoskeleton via afadin (also known as AF-6) and may be important in the initial formation of adherens junctions. The cadherins form a complex with the catenins (α-, β- and p120 catenin) and help mediate adhesion and signalling. Cell signalling via β-catenin can activate several Wnt pathways, which implicates adherens junctions in coordinating morphogenetic movements with cell fate determination. Adherens junctions are also associated with a variety of actin-binding molecules, suggesting multiple dynamic interactions with the cytoskeleton.

The first human gene mutation reported in a component of adherens junctions was in plakoglobin, also a component of desmosomes, in individuals with Naxos disease [4]. However, mutations have subsequently been reported in the *CDH3* gene,

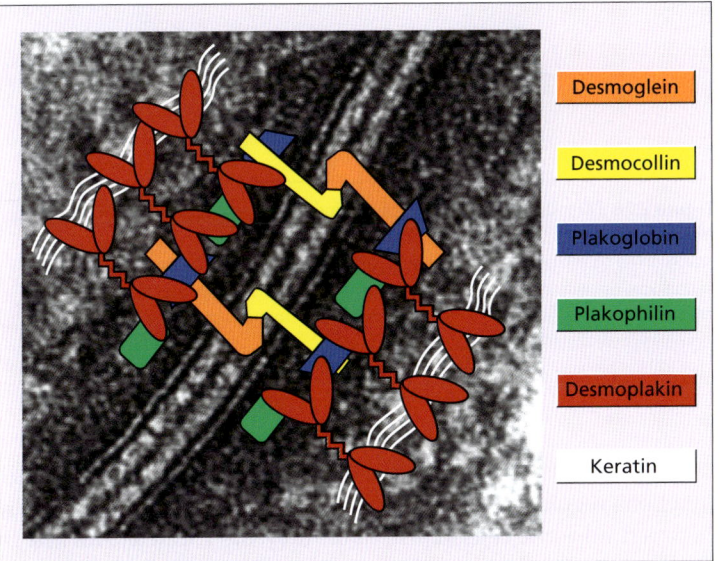

Figure 2.26 Macromolecular composition of desmosomes linking adjacent keratinocytes. Cells are connected via transmembranous cadherin glycoproteins (desmogleins and desmocollins). Attachment of these molecules to the keratin filament cytoskeleton occurs via a network of desmosomal plaque proteins (desmoplakin, plakoglobin and plakophilin). The background to this figure is a transmission electron micrograph of a desmosome to highlight how the molecules function as an adhesive complex.

develop in diseases such as paraneoplastic pemphigus, possibly through the phenomenon of epitope spreading [7]. Disruption of the extracellular domain of Dsg1 has also been demonstrated as the basis of staphylococcal scalded skin syndrome and bullous impetigo, in which this desmosomal cadherin is cleaved by the bacterial toxin [8].

which encodes P-cadherin; these mutations result in autosomal recessive hypotrichosis with juvenile macular dystrophy [5]. P-cadherin mutations are also found in a different disorder, ectodermal dysplasia–ectrodactyly–macular dystrophy (EEM) syndrome, in which there is hypotrichosis, macular degeneration, hypodontia and limb defects, including ectrodactyly, syndactyly and camptodactyly [6]. Mutations in nectin-1 and -4 have also been reported in a group of ectodermal dysplasia syndromes, sometimes referred to as nectinopathies [7].

Gap junctions

Gap junctions comprise clusters of intercellular channels, known as connexons, which directly form connections between the cytoplasm of adjacent keratinocytes (and other cells) [1]. Thirteen different human connexins have been described. Connexons originate following the assembly of six connexin subunits within the Golgi network that are then transported to the plasma membrane. The connexins are divided into three groups (α, β and γ) according to their gene structure, overall gene homology and specific sequence motifs [2]. At the plasma membrane, connexons associate with other connexons in the adjacent cell to form a gap junction (Figure 2.28).

Homotypic or heterotypic connexins (formed from one or more than one type of connexin, respectively) can be identified, and the formation and stability of gap junctions can be regulated by protein kinase C, Src kinase, calcium concentration, calmodulin, cyclic adenosine 3′,5′-monophosphate (cAMP) and local pH [3]. Apart from the connexins, vertebrates also contain another class of gap junction proteins, the pannexins, which are related to the innexins found in non-chordate animals [4]. The function of gap junctions is to permit the sharing of low-molecular-mass metabolites (<1000 Da) and ion exchange between neighbouring cells, thus allowing intercellular coordination and uniformity to maintain tissue/organ homeostasis in multicellular organisms [3]. Gap junction communication is essential for cell synchronisation, cell differentiation, cell growth and metabolic coordination of avascular organs, including epidermis.

Inherited abnormalities in genes encoding four different connexins (Cx26, Cx30, Cx30.3 and Cx31) have been detected in several forms of keratoderma and/or hearing loss, but non-dermatological disorders can also arise from mutations in the higher-molecular-weight connexins (Cx32, Cx40, Cx43, Cx46 and Cx50). Gap junction proteins can regulate immune responses, cell proliferation, migration and apoptosis [5]. Thus, alterations in gap junction profile and expression levels are also observed in hyperproliferative skin disorders, fibrotic disorders, wound healing, lymphatic vessel diseases, inflammatory lung diseases, liver injury and neoplastic disorders. Modulating the function or expression of connexins, such as with the use of synthetic mimetic peptides and small interfering RNA (siRNA) technology, may have therapeutic value.

Tight junctions

Tight junctions are the major regulators of permeability in simple epithelia, but they are also present in the skin, with a key role

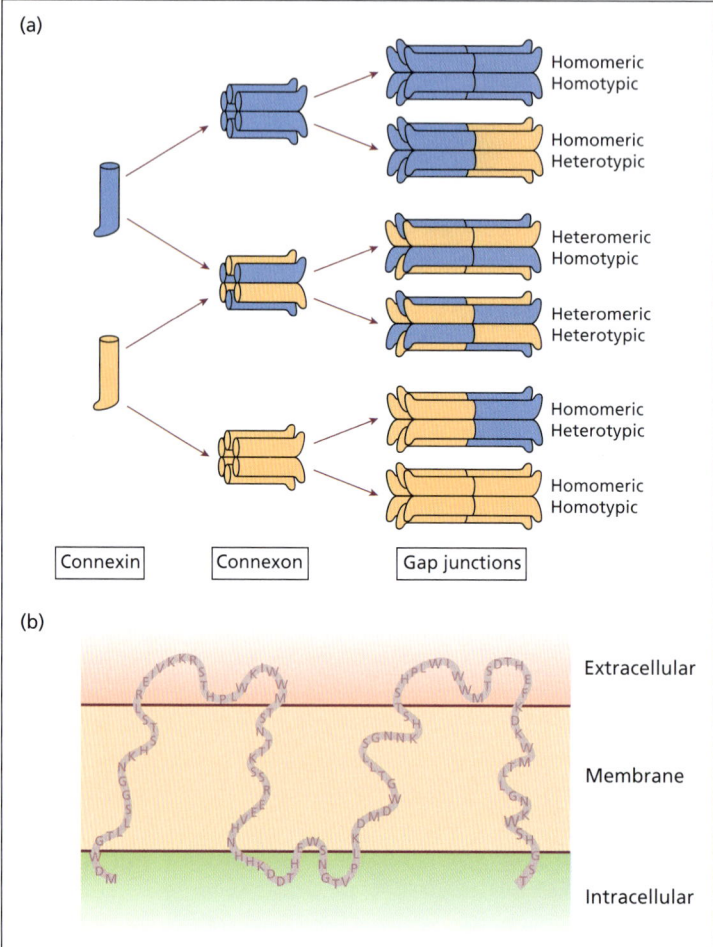

Figure 2.28 Formation and structure of gap junctions in human skin. (a) In the Golgi network six connexin subunits assemble to form a connexon. The connexon is then transported to the plasma membrane. Other connexons then co-aggregate to form homotypic or heterotypic gap junctions. (b) The gap junction protein is a transmembranous molecule with intracellular, transmembranous and extracellular domains (here illustrated for Cx26).

in skin barrier integrity and maintaining cell polarity [1]. Tight junctions regulate the paracellular flux of water-soluble molecules between adjacent cells [2]. In skin, they are located between the first and second layers of the granular cell layer. Tight junctions are highly dynamic structures: spatiotemporal regulation of dynamic tight junction replacement from cell to cell maintains skin barrier homeostasis, despite continuous cellular turnover [2].

The principal structural proteins of tight junctions are the claudins, of which there are approximately 24 subtypes. The other component transmembranous proteins are the IgG-like family of junctional adhesion molecules (JAMs) and the occludin group of proteins. Seven claudins are expressed in human epidermis, although the main claudins are 1 and 4. These transmembranous proteins do not bind to one another, but the claudins and occludins can bind to the intracellular zonula occudens proteins ZO-1, ZO-2 and ZO-3. These proteins can also interact with actin, thus providing a direct link with the cytoskeleton [1,3]. The structural organisation of a tight junction is shown in Figure 2.29.

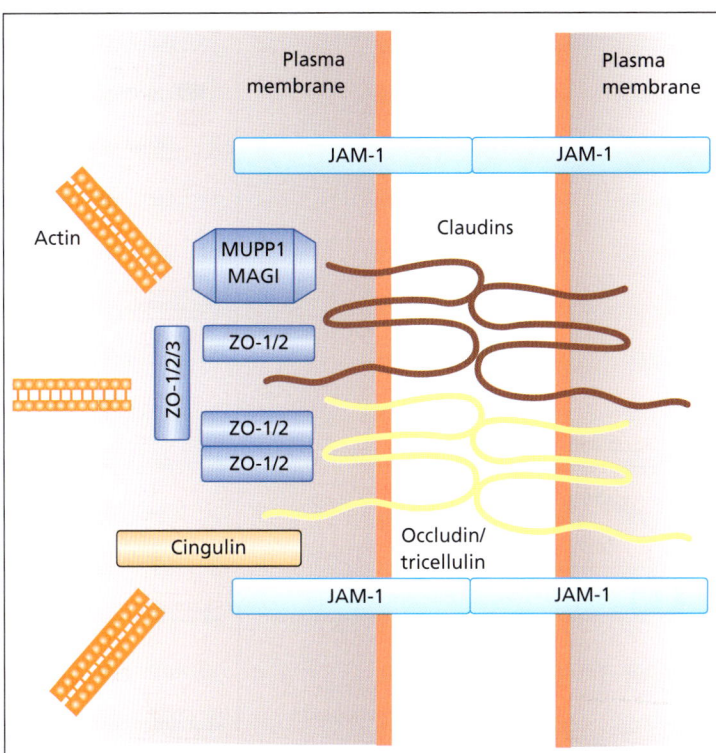

Figure 2.29 Structural composition of a tight junction in human skin. There are three transmembranous families of proteins, the junctional adhesion molecules (JAMs), the claudins and the occludins, of which the latter two bind to zonula occludens proteins (ZOs) and then directly to actin. MUPP1, multiple PDZ domain protein; MAGI, membrane-associated guanyl kinase inverted protein.

Mutations in claudin 16 (also known as paracellin-1) result in familial hypomagnesaemia with hypercalciuria and nephrocalcinosis; mutations in claudin 14 underlie the autosomal recessive deafness disorder DFNB29 leading to cochlear hair cell degeneration; mutations in claudin 19 result in renal and ocular disease [4]. In addition, the gene encoding the ZO-2 protein may be mutated in some cases of familial hypercholanaemia. With respect to skin, mutations in claudin 1 have been demonstrated in a few individuals with neonatal ichthyosis sclerosing cholangitis (NISCH) syndrome [5]. Collectively, these human genetic disorders, all of which are autosomal recessive in nature, demonstrate the key role tight junctions play in the skin, kidney, ear, eye and liver.

Dermal–epidermal basement membrane

The interface between the lower part of the epidermis and the top layer of the dermis comprises the dermal–epidermal basement membrane zone (BMZ), which consists of a number of extracellular matrix macromolecules (Box 2.1; Figure 2.30) [1]. Many of these components are glycoproteins, and the BMZ can be recognised histologically by positive labelling with periodic acid–Schiff (PAS) stain. Ultrastructural examination of the BMZ by transmission electron microscopy shows the presence of two distinct layers with different optical densities (Figure 2.31) [2].

Box 2.1 Molecular components of the epidermal basement membrane zone

Intermediate filament (IF) components
- Keratin 5
- Keratin 14

Hemidesmosomal plaque components
- 230 kDa bullous pemphigoid antigen (BP230/BPAG1/epithelial dystonin)
- Plectin

Focal adhesion components
- Actin
- Talin
- Kindlin-1 (fermitin family homologue-1)
- Vinculin

Transmembrane components
- $\alpha 6\beta 4$ integrin
- CD151 tetraspanin
- Type XVII collagen (180 kDa bullous pemphigoid antigen/BPAG2)
- $\alpha 3\beta 1$ integrin
- Type XIII collagen
- Syndecans 1 and 4

Lamina lucida/lamina densa components
- Laminin 332 (laminin 5)
- Laminin 311 (laminin 6)
- Laminin 511 (laminin 10)

Lamina densa components
- Type IV collagen
- Laminin 111 (laminin 1)
- Nidogen
- BM-40/SPARC
- Perlecan

Anchoring fibril components
- Type VII collagen
- GDA-J/F3 antigen

The upper layer, the lamina lucida, is a less electron-dense region and directly abuts the plasma membranes of the basal keratinocytes. Below the lamina lucida is the lamina densa, an electron-dense region that at the lower part interacts with the mesenchymal matrix of the upper dermis. The major biochemical components of the BMZ are type IV collagen and a number of non-collagenous glycoproteins, including laminin 322. Associated with the cutaneous BMZ are ultrastructurally recognisable attachment structures that form a contiguous network extending from the intracellular milieu of basal keratinocytes through the plasma membrane of basal cells, traversing the dermal–epidermal basement membrane and extending to the upper papillary dermis (Figure 2.30). The components of this network are the hemidesmosomes, anchoring filaments and anchoring fibrils. The biochemical components of the BMZ are synthesised by basal keratinocytes and dermal fibroblasts, which both contribute to the development and repair of the basement membrane. Focal adhesions at the dermal–epidermal junction anchor the actin microfilaments but are not visible by transmission electron microscopy.

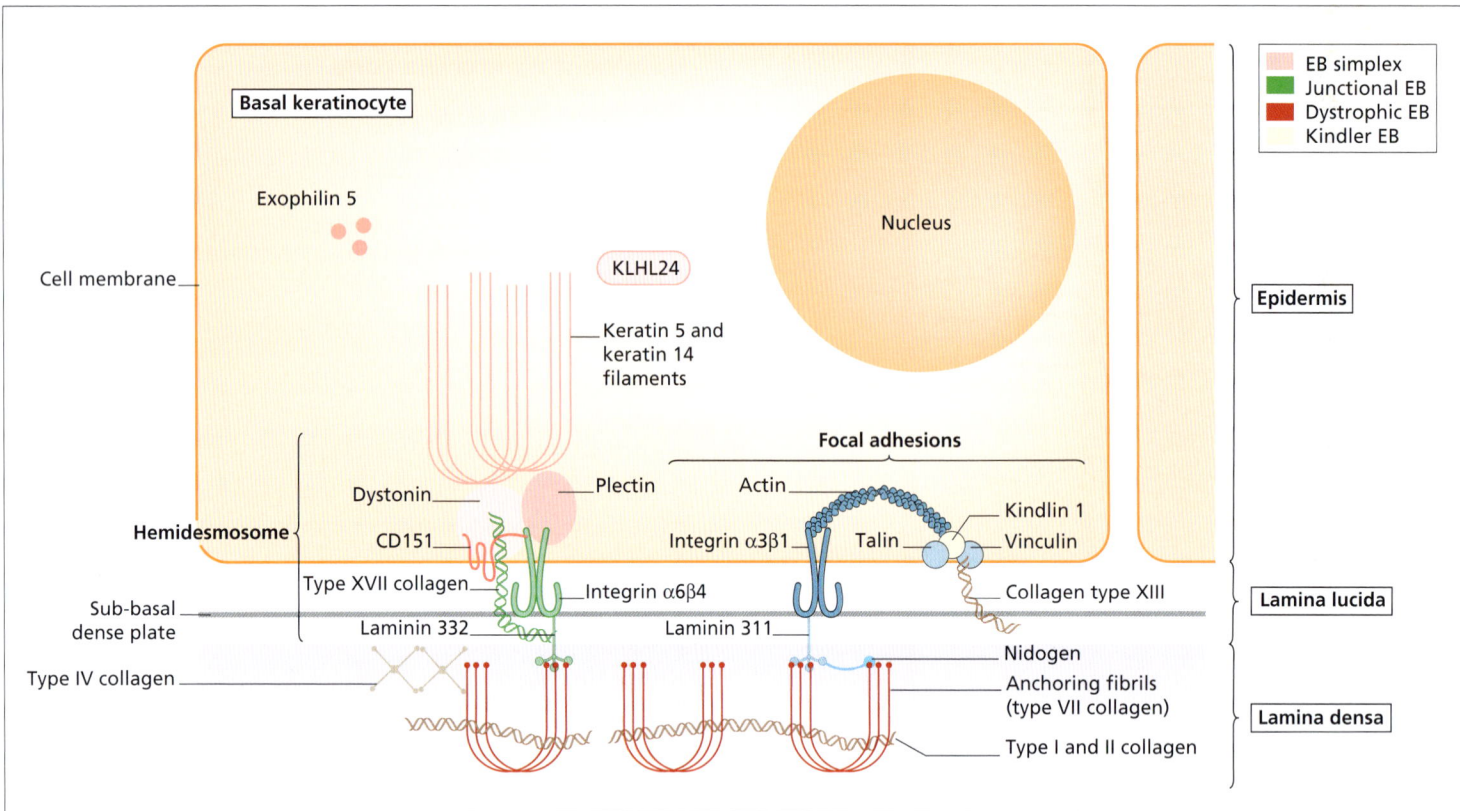

Figure 2.30 Structural components at or close to the dermal–epidermal junction that have physiological or disease relevance to maintaining adhesion at the dermal–epidermal junction and signalling between the epidermis and dermis. The colours denote the component involved in the pathobiology of the different forms of the inherited blistering skin disease epidermolysis bullosa (EB). Adapted from Bardhan et al. 2020 [1].

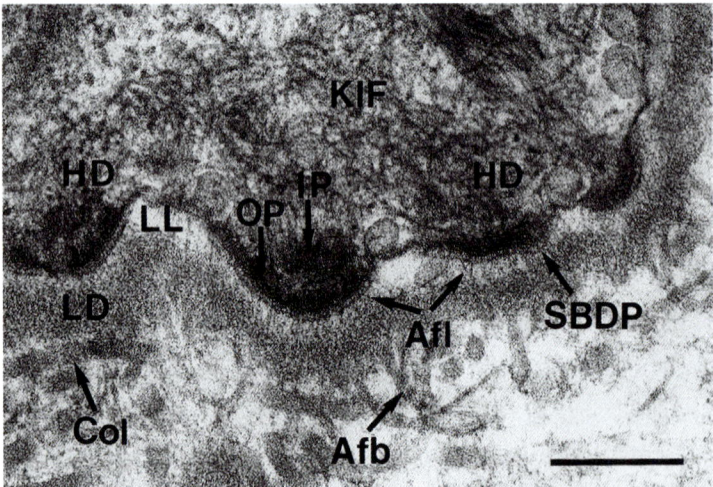

Figure 2.31 Transmission electron microscopy of the dermal–epidermal junction in human skin recognising hemidesmosomes (HD), anchoring filaments (Afl) and anchoring fibrils (Afb). The HD consists of an intracellular inner plaque (IP) and outer plaque (OP) as well as a sub-basal dense plate (SBDP) in the upper lamina lucida (LL). The anchoring filaments traverse the LL, appearing as thread-like structures that concentrate under the HDs and merge with the lamina densa (LD). Anchoring fibrils extend from the lower part of the LD to the upper papillary dermis where they closely associate with interstitial collagen fibres (Col). Keratin intermediate filaments (KIFs) associate with intracellular components of the HDs. Scale bar 0.25 μm. Courtesy of Professor R. A. J. Eady, St John's Institute of Dermatology, King's College London, UK.

The critical importance of this network structure in securing the adherence of the epidermis to the underlying dermis is reflected in the group of diseases, epidermolysis bullosa, in which components of the hemidesmosomes, anchoring filaments or anchoring fibrils are genetically altered or missing. As a result, fragility at the dermal–epidermal junction ensues, clinically manifesting as erosions and blisters following minor trauma [3,4].

Basement membrane collagen

The major component of the dermal–epidermal basement membrane is type IV collagen, a heterogeneous group of macromolecules that are present in diverse combinations in various basement membranes (Figure 2.32) [1]. Like all collagens, each type IV collagen molecule consists of three polypeptide subunits, known as α-chains. Some collagen molecules are homopolymers, that is the three α-chains are genetically identical, as in the case of type II, III and VII collagens. Others are heteropolymers so that there are two or even three different kinds of polypeptides, as for example in type I and type VI collagens. For type IV collagen, there are six genetically distinct but structurally related α-chains, and the precise composition of the α-chains varies with the tissue location of the basement membranes. In the case of the cutaneous BMZ, the major type IV collagen consists of α1 and α2 chains, with the chain composition $[\alpha 1(IV)]_2 \alpha 2(IV)$, although other type IV collagen

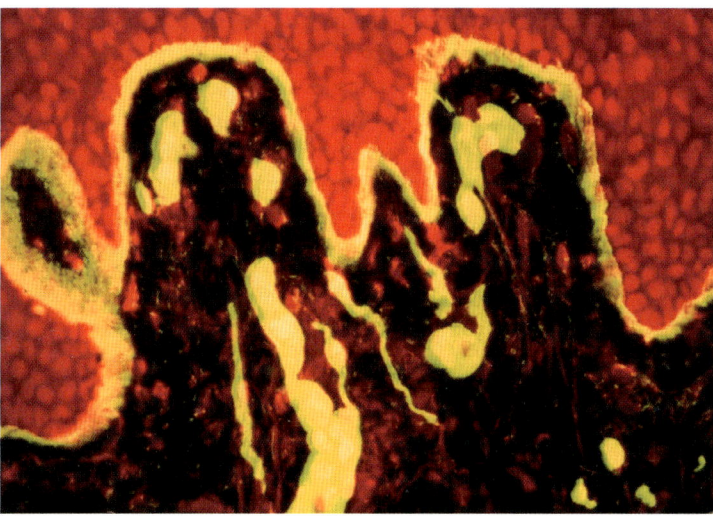

Figure 2.32 Immunofluorescence staining of the dermis and cutaneous basement membrane zone with an antibody for type IV collagen. Note positive staining at the dermal–epidermal basement membrane and around the dermal blood vessels. Original magnification 250×.

subunit polypeptides are also present in lower quantities. The α3 chain of type IV collagen has been shown to be the antigen recognised by circulating autoantibodies characteristic of Goodpasture syndrome, while structural aberrations in the α5 chain of type IV collagen are associated with Alport syndrome [2,3]. Autoantibodies against α5 and α6 chain epitopes have also been reported in patients with glomerulonephritis and subepidermal blistering [4].

The characteristic fibre structure of interstitial collagens, as exemplified by type I collagen, results from the lateral aggregation of individual molecules in a quarter stagger array; this gives rise to a 640 Å cross-striation pattern when examined by transmission electron microscopy (Figure 2.33). In the case of type IV collagen, the non-collagenous globular domains at both the amino and carboxyl ends of the individual collagen molecules interact to form dimers and tetramers which then assemble into

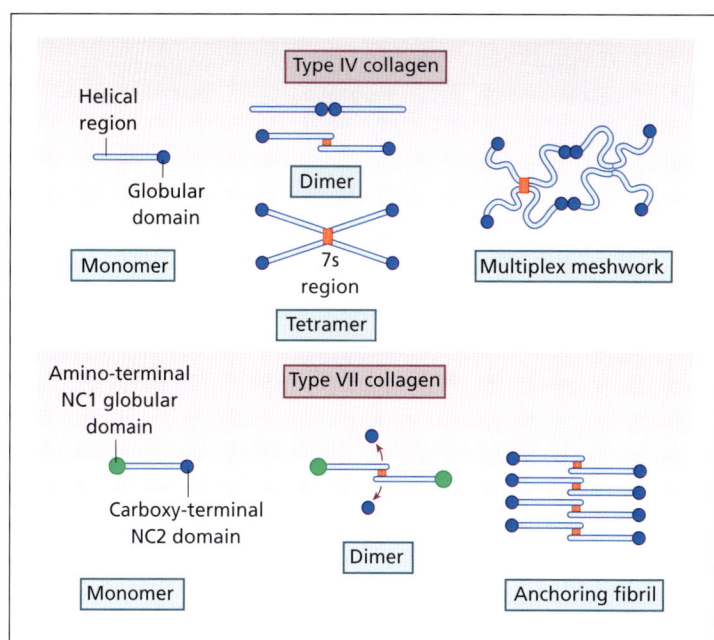

Figure 2.34 Assembly of type IV and type VII collagen molecules into supramolecular structures. The red rectangles represent intermolecular disulphide bonds.

lattice-like structures and associate laterally in a complex hexagonal arrangement (Figure 2.34). This arrangement allows the basement membrane structure to be highly flexible and makes interactions with other collagenous and non-collagenous basement membrane components possible [1].

Laminins

Other components that contribute to the cutaneous BMZ include members of the laminin family of multidomain proteins. As many as 16 different laminins have been identified thus far and at least four of

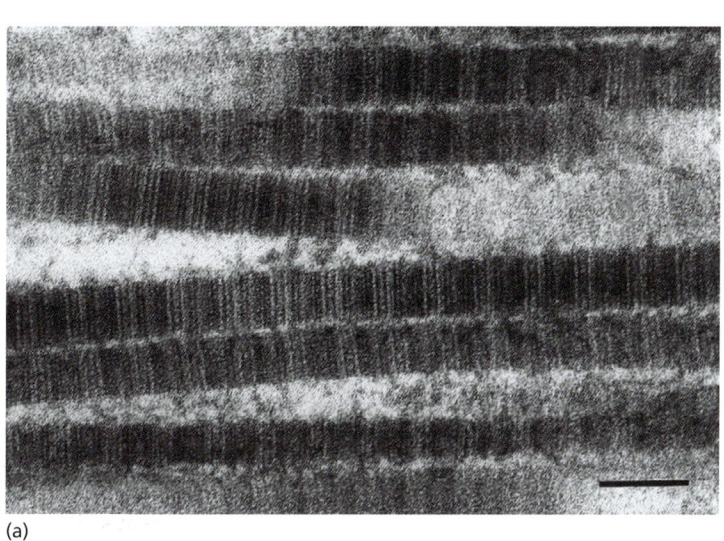

(a)

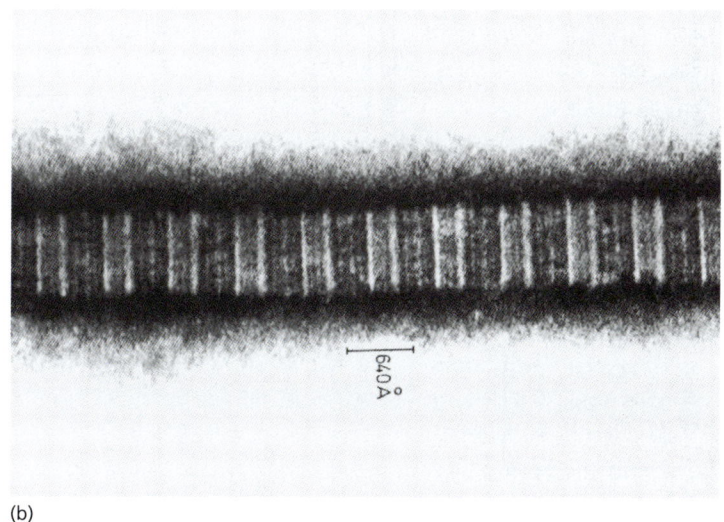

(b)

Figure 2.33 Demonstration of periodicity in collagen fibres of 640 Å. (a) Collagen fibrils in the reticular dermis show a characteristic banding pattern after standard processing and staining with uranyl acetate and lead citrate for transmission electron microscopy. Scale bar 0.1 μm. (b) Transmission electron micrograph of a shadowed replica of unfixed, freeze-frozen and surface-sublimated rat-tail tendon collagen showing the step-like banding of the fibres. Original magnification 40 500×. Courtesy of G. A. Meek.

2.24 Chapter 2: Structure and Function of the Skin

Table 2.1 Chain composition of the major laminins in the skin.

Type	Chain composition	Old designation	Distribution in basement membranes
111	α1β1γ1	1	Blood vessels, LD
332	α3β3γ2	5	LL/LD
311	α3β1γ1	6	LL/LD
511	α5β1γ1	10	LL/LD

LD, lamina densa; LL, lamina lucida.

them are physiologically present in the skin in significant quantities (Table 2.1) [1,2]. Each laminin molecule consists of three polypeptide subunits, α-, β- and γ-chains, which form a cruciform structure with three short arms and one long arm when visualised by rotary shadowing electron microscopy (Figure 2.35).

The short arms represent the N-terminal segments of the α-, β- and γ-chains. The long arm consists of an extended rod-like structure of the triple-stranded, coiled-coil domain of all three chains. This domain serves as the site of chain assembly of the three subunit polypeptides. The α-chain contains an additional C-terminal segment that has five globular segments located at the tip of the long arm, known as the G domain. The major laminin within the cutaneous BMZ is laminin 332, previously known as laminin 5 (Figure 2.36). In addition, laminin 311 and laminin 511 are integral components of the cutaneous BMZ, while laminin 111 is also present in basement membranes of the blood vessels in human dermis [3].

The cell binding of laminins is mediated by integrins, a family of cellular receptors, each consisting of two subunit polypeptides (Figure 2.37). Integrins also mediate outside-in signal transduction elicited by laminins and regulate cell migration, proliferation, differentiation and adhesion [4]. The principal integrin in the cutaneous BMZ is the α6β4 integrin, which is critical for the adhesion of basal cells to the underlying BMZ.

The cruciform structure of laminins contains both globular and rod-like segments that have been individually implicated in various functions, including interactions with other extracellular matrix

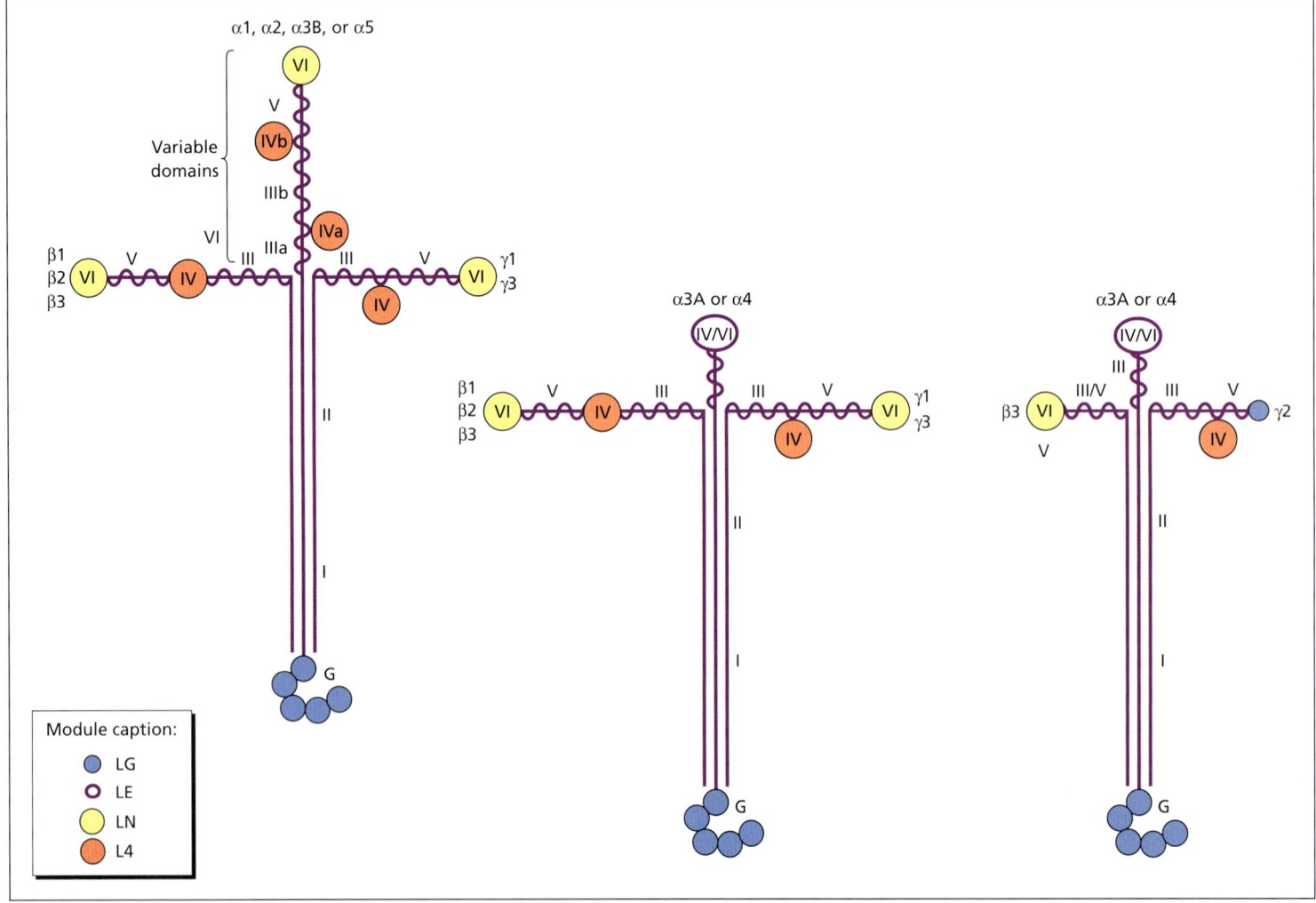

Figure 2.35 Different isoforms and domain organisations of laminin, each consisting of three distinct subunit polypeptides, α-, β- and γ-chains. The LE modules are formed by approximately 60 residues each and have homology to epidermal growth factor. The LN and L4 modules are folded into globular structures located between the LE modules (domain IV) or at the amino terminus of each chain (domain VI). The coiled-coil central region, comprising all three polypeptides, is represented as vertical straight lines. Note the presence of a G domain consisting of five globular segments (LG) at the carboxy terminus of the α-chains. Adapted from Aumailley and Rousselle 1999 [8] with permission of Elsevier.

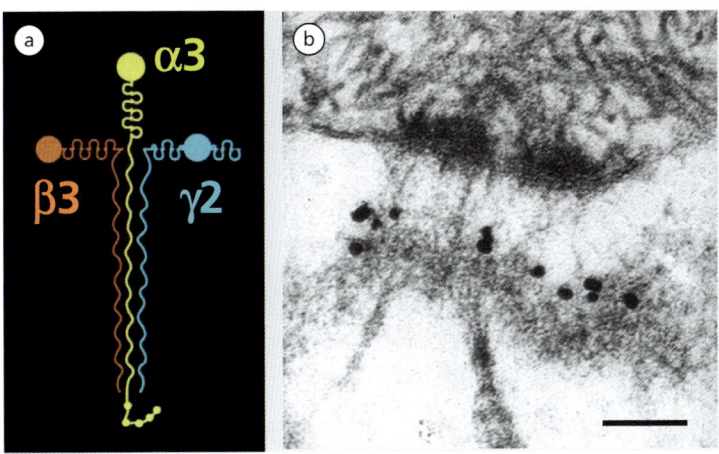

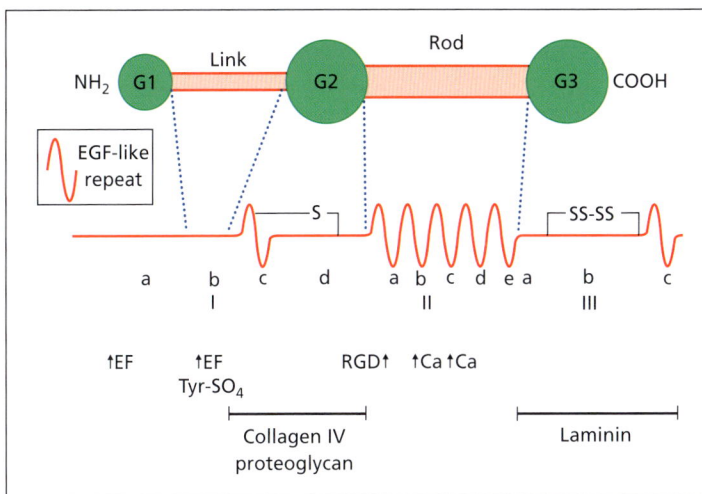

Figure 2.36 (a) Laminin 332 expressed in the cutaneous basement membrane zone. (b) Immunogold electron microscopy using an antibody to the γ2 chain of laminin 332 showing labelling at the lamina lucida–lamina densa interface below a hemidesmosome. Scale bar 50 nm.

Figure 2.38 Model of nidogen, containing subdomains with predicted binding activities to type IV collagen, proteoglycans and laminin 1. EF and Ca refer to putative calcium-binding sites; RGD is a putative cell-binding sequence. EGF, epidermal growth factor. Adapted from Niessen et al. 1994 [9] with permission of Elsevier.

molecules, such as the hemidesmosomal components and type VII collagen, as well as in cell attachment and spreading, neurite outgrowth and cellular differentiation. Collectively, the laminins play vital roles in the development and maintenance of the supramolecular organisation of the basement membrane [5]. The critical role of laminin 332 in providing integrity to the cutaneous BMZ is evident by observations that genetic mutations in any of the three polypeptide subunits – that is the *LAMA3*, *LAMB3* or *LAMC2* genes which encode the α3, β3 and γ2 chains, respectively – can result in junctional forms of epidermolysis bullosa (EB) with profound fragility of the skin. Furthermore, mutations in the *ITGA6* and *ITGB4* genes – encoding the α6 and β4 subunit polypeptides of integrin, respectively – cause a form of junctional EB frequently associated with pyloric atresia [6].

Other BMZ components at the dermal–epidermal junction include a glycoprotein known as nidogen (previously called entactin) that interacts with type IV collagen either alone or as a laminin–nidogen complex (Figure 2.38) [7]. Nidogens are a family of highly conserved, sulphated glycoproteins within a spectrum of binding proteins. Although nidogens are an abundant component of various basement membranes, genetic analyses have shown that they are not required for the overall architecture of the basement membrane. Instead, nidogens appear to play a critical role in the development of basement membranes in tissues undergoing rapid growth or turnover.

Another class of integral basement membrane component is that of the heparan sulphate proteoglycans (HSPGs). These molecules consist of a core protein with different numbers of covalently associated heparan and sulphate chains that make these molecules highly negatively charged and hydrophilic. These proteoglycans can interact with several other basement membrane components and are likely to contribute to the overall architecture of the basement membrane. Specific cell surface HSPGs are found also on the surface of epithelial cells and possibly mediate cell–matrix interactions.

Hemidesmosomes

The dermal–epidermal junction of skin is characterised by the presence of specific structures that are critical for the functional integrity

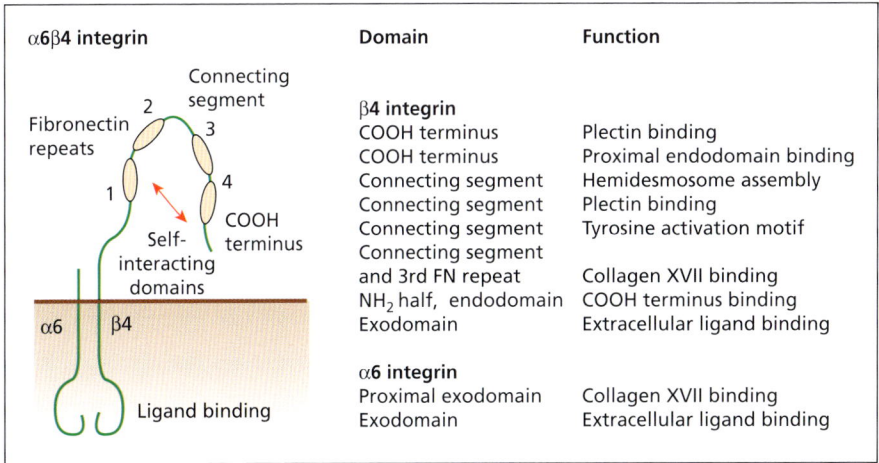

Figure 2.37 Molecular composition, domain organisation and functions of the α6β4 integrin, the main keratinocyte integrin in hemidesmosomes. This integrin is important in hemidesmosome assembly and protein–protein interactions. FN, fibronectin.

of the skin. These ultrastructurally recognisable components include hemidesmosomes, anchoring filaments and anchoring fibrils. The molecular composition and the specific domain organisations of the component macromolecules have been largely characterised (see Figures 2.30 and 2.31).

The hemidesmosomes are seen ultrastructurally as electron-dense attachment complexes, which extend from the intracellular compartment of the basal keratinocytes to the lamina lucida in the upper portion of the dermal–epidermal basement membrane [1]. The intracellular domains of hemidesmosomes within the basal keratinocytes attach to the keratin intermediate filament network, while in the extracellular space within the lamina lucida the hemidesmosomes are contiguous with anchoring filaments; this unit is termed the hemidesmosome–anchoring filament complex.

The inner plaques of hemidesmosomes contain plectin, a large intracytoplasmic adhesion molecule, and the 230 kDa bullous pemphigoid antigen, a non-collagenous protein of the plakin family. The 180 kDa bullous pemphigoid antigen, a transmembrane collagenous protein, also known as type XVII collagen, interacts with $\alpha6\beta4$ integrin and extends from the intracellular compartment of basal cells to the extracellular space, thus stabilising the association of basal keratinocytes to the underlying basement membrane.

Attesting to the critical importance of the hemidesmosomes in providing stability to the association of basal keratinocytes with the underlying BMZ is the finding that mutations in the genes encoding hemidesmosomal proteins have been shown to result in different forms of EB (see Figure 2.31) [2]. The causative nature of the mutations in these hemidesmosomal genes has been verified by the development of targeted mutant (knock-out) mouse models, which frequently recapitulate the clinical, genetic, histological and ultrastructural features encountered in patients with EB [3].

The hemidesmosomes are complexed with anchoring filaments, which are thread-like structures that tend to coalesce below the hemidesmosomal outer plaques (see Figure 2.31). Electron microscopy and immunohistochemical analyses have suggested that laminin 332 may be the major component of the anchoring filaments, although the presence of additional molecules has also been suggested. As indicated, laminin 332 is a disulphide-bonded complex of $\alpha3$, $\beta3$ and $\gamma2$ chains that associate into a trimeric, cruciform structure. After the initial assembly, the $\alpha3$ and $\gamma2$ chains are proteolytically processed, and many of the conformational epitopes are recognised by specific antibodies. Complete absence of any of the three subunit polypeptides of laminin 332, due to loss-of-function mutations in both alleles of the corresponding gene, results in severe generalised junctional EB [1]. Since laminin 332 binds to $\alpha6\beta4$ integrin in the hemidesmosomes and to type VII collagen in the anchoring fibrils, the severity of skin fragility in this form of EB apparently reflects the loss of its ability to bridge the hemidesmosomes and the anchoring fibrils. This results in a separation of the epidermis from the dermis within the lamina lucida as a result of minor trauma to the skin.

Focal adhesions

Focal adhesions, also known as focal contacts, are large multiprotein cell matrix adhesion complexes, which regulate multiple cellular functions, such as adhesion and migration [1]. They also transmit mechanical forces and regulatory signals between the extracellular matrix and an interacting cell. Found at the dermal–epidermal junction in skin, they are also present in cell matrix interactions in other tissues, such as kidney and lung. Two key proteins within focal adhesions are talin and vinculin, which connect integrin (mainly the $\alpha3\beta1$ integrin complex) to actomyosin networks in the cell. Both proteins bind to F-actin and each other, providing a foundation for network formation within the focal adhesion complex. The biological significance of focal adhesions in skin and other organs is underscored by two genetic disorders, Kindler epidermolysis bullosa and the interstitial lung disease, nephrotic syndrome and epidermolysis bullosa (ILNEB) syndrome, in which mutations affect focal adhesion proteins, fermitin-1 (kindlin-1) and the integrin $\alpha3$ subunit, respectively [2].

Anchoring fibrils

Anchoring fibrils are ultrastructurally recognisable, U-shaped structures that extend from the lower part of the lamina densa to the upper reticular dermis (Figure 2.39). Type VII collagen is the major, if not the exclusive, component of anchoring fibrils [1]. Individual collagen molecules are approximately 450 nm long, consisting of a central, triple helical segment flanked by non-helical globular domains at each end of the triple helix: NC1 at the amino terminus and NC2 at the carboxy terminus of the molecule (see Figure 2.34). In addition, the triple helical segment of type VII collagen contains imperfections in the triple helix, including a central 39 amino acid non-collagenous segment. These interruptions in the glycine-X-Y sequence are thought to provide flexibility to the type VII collagen molecules.

The gene encoding type VII collagen (*COL7A1*) is extremely complex, consisting of 118 exons on the short arm of human chromosome 3 [2]. Type VII collagen is synthesised by both dermal fibroblasts and epidermal keratinocytes, although the basal cell appears to be the major source of type VII collagen during the early prenatal development of skin. Upon secretion to the extracellular

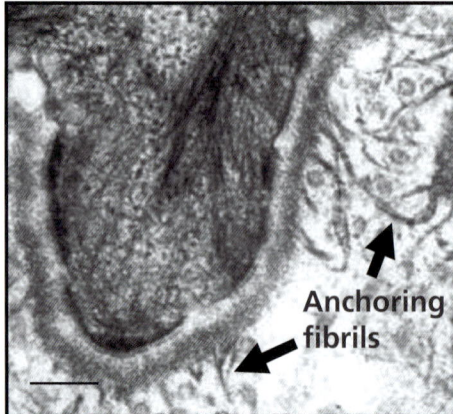

Figure 2.39 Transmission electron microscopy of the dermal–epidermal junction revealing wheatsheaf-shaped anchoring fibrils beneath the lamina densa. These fibrils help secure adhesion between the epidermal basement membrane and interstitial collagens within the dermis. Scale bar = 100 nm.

space, two type VII collagen molecules align into an antiparallel dimer with overlapping NC2 domains, and after partial proteolysis of the NC2 domain, the dimer is stabilised by intermolecular disulphide bonds. Subsequently, several type VII molecules laterally aggregate to form anchoring fibrils in which the NC1 domains at both ends attach to the basement membrane. The U-shaped loops then entrap, and possibly interact with, large interstitial collagen fibres consisting of type I, III and V collagens [3]. In addition to type VII collagen, anchoring fibrils have been suggested to have a component recognised by a monoclonal antibody GDA-J/F3 which was initially raised against sperm cells. While this epitope has not been well characterised, it has been suggested to be a type VII collagen-associated protein whose expression is altered in recessive dystrophic epidermolysis bullosa.

The critical importance of the anchoring fibrils in securing the adhesion of the dermal–epidermal basement membrane to the underlying dermis as well as in wound healing is illustrated by the dystrophic forms of EB [4]. Specifically, a complete absence of type VII collagen results in severe forms of recessive dystrophic EB with fragility of the skin and mucous membranes, leading to mutilating scarring of the hands and feet. Missense mutations, particularly glycine substitution mutations, can result in somewhat milder, dominantly inherited dystrophic EB [5].

Extracellular matrix

The major component of human skin is the dermis, demarcated on the top by the lamina densa in the lower border of the dermal–epidermal basement membrane and at the bottom by the subcutis. In contrast to the epidermis, the dermis is largely acellular and consists primarily of the extracellular matrix of connective tissue, a complex meshwork of various macromolecules. There are four major classes of extracellular matrix components: (i) collagen fibres, which provide tensile strength to allow the skin to serve as a protective organ against external trauma; (ii) elastic structures, which provide elasticity and resilience to normal human skin; (iii) non-collagenous glycoproteins, such as fibrillins, fibulins and integrins, which often serve as organisers of the matrix and facilitate cell–matrix interactions; and (iv) proteoglycan/glycosaminoglycan macromolecules, which provide hydration to the skin [1]. The maintenance of proper quantities and appropriate interactions between the extracellular matrix components is a prerequisite for the physiological homeostasis of the dermis.

The major extracellular matrix component in the dermis is collagen, which comprises a family of closely related yet genetically distinct proteins [1–4]. The major collagen fibres in the dermis provide tensile strength to the skin to serve as a protective organ against external trauma (Figure 2.40). A characteristic feature of all collagens is the triple helical conformation, which is predicated upon the primary amino acid sequence of the subunit polypeptides, α-chains, depicting a repeating glycine-X-Y sequence. The collagens also demonstrate non-collagenous flanking segments at the ends of the individual molecules. Currently, 29 distinct collagens have been identified in vertebrate tissues, and have been characterised to the extent that they are referred to by Roman numeral designation (I–XXIX) in the order of their discovery, many of them being present in the skin (Table 2.2).

All collagen molecules consist of three subunit polypeptides, which can either be identical as homotrimers or can consist of two or even three genetically different polypeptides in heterotrimeric molecules. Since the different subunits are all distinct gene products, there are over 40 different genes in the human genome that

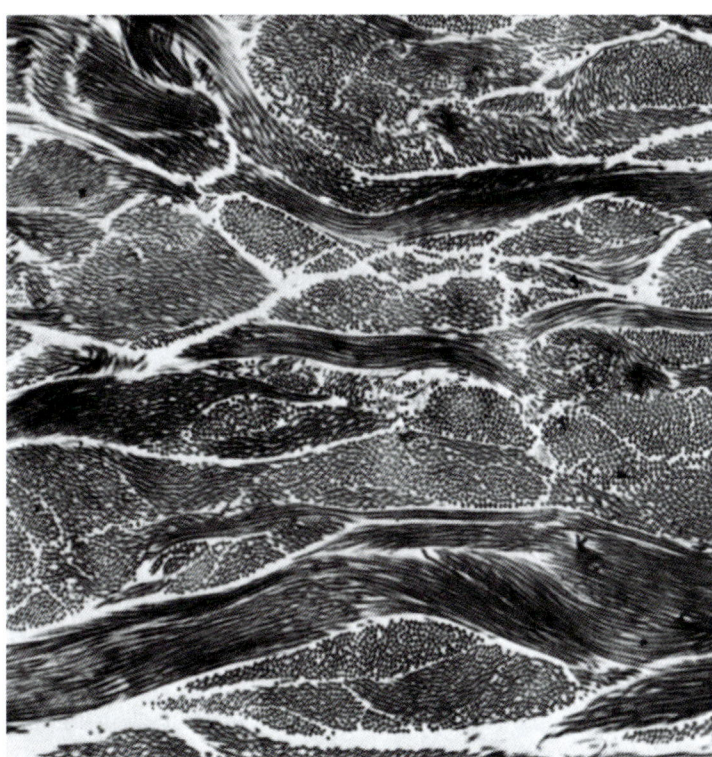

Figure 2.40 Transmission electron micrograph of a section of dermis from the human forearm showing bundles of collagen fibres, in both transverse and longitudinal sections. Original magnification 4900×. Courtesy of Professor A. S. Breathnach.

Table 2.2 Genetic heterogeneity of collagens.

Collagen type	Chain composition	Supramolecular assembly	Tissue distribution[a]
I	$[\alpha1(I)]_2\alpha2(I)$	Fibrillar	Dermis, bone, tendons
III	$[\alpha1(III)]_3$	Fibrillar	Blood vessels, GI tract
IV	$[\alpha1(IV)]_2\alpha2(IV)$[b]	Basement membrane	Ubiquitous
V	$[\alpha1(V)]_2\alpha2(V)$[b]	Fibrillar	Ubiquitous
VI	$[\alpha1(VI)\alpha2(VI)\alpha3(VI)]$[b]	Microfibrils	Ubiquitous
VII	$[\alpha1(VII)]_3$	Anchoring fibrils	Epithelial basement membranes
VIII	$[\alpha1(VIII)]_3$	Network forming	Endothelia
XIII	$[\alpha1(XIII)]_3$	Transmembrane	Ubiquitous, including epidermis
XIV	$[\alpha1(XIV)]_3$	FACIT	Skin, cornea
XV	$[\alpha1(XV)]_3$	Basement membrane	Ubiquitous
XVII	$[\alpha1(XVII)]_3$	Transmembrane	Hemidesmosomes
XXIX	Unknown	Unknown	Epidermis

[a] Distribution in the skin and other major tissues is indicated; lesser amounts may be present in other tissues.
[b] Additional α-chains have been identified.
FACIT, fibril-associated collagens with interrupted triple helices; GI, gastrointestinal.

encode the different subunit polypeptides, the α-chains, of these distinct collagens.

Collagens

On the basis of their fibre architecture in tissues, the genetically distinct collagens can be divided into different classes [1]. Types I, II, III, V and IX align into large fibrils and are designated as fibril-forming collagens. Type IV is arranged in an interlacing network within the basement membranes, while type VI is a distinct microfibril-forming collagen, and type VII collagen forms anchoring fibrils. FACIT collagens (fibril-associated collagens with interrupted triple helices) include types IX, XII, XIV, XIX, XX and XXI. Many of the latter collagens associate with larger collagen fibres and serve as molecular bridges, stabilising the organisation of the extracellular matrices [2]. The major collagens significantly contributing to skin physiology and pathology are presented in Table 2.2. Other collagen types, including types II, IX, X, XI, XIX, XX and XXI, are not discussed in detail because they are not present in the skin to a significant extent or their participation in maintaining skin physiology is unclear.

Type I collagen, the most abundant form, is the predominant collagen in human dermis, accounting for approximately 80% of the total collagen. Type I collagen contains two different kinds of α-chain with an $[α1(I)]_2α2(I)$ stoichiometry. A collagen consisting of three identical α1(I) chains has also been identified (so-called α1(I) trimer), but it appears to be only a minor component of connective tissue in the skin. Type I collagen associates with type III collagen to form broad, extracellular fibres in the human dermis. Mutations in type I and III collagens, or in their processing enzymes, can result in connective tissue abnormalities in the different forms of Ehlers–Danlos syndrome, and mutations in the type I collagen gene are responsible for the fragility of bones in osteogenesis imperfecta [3].

Type III collagen accounts for about 10% of the total bulk of collagen found in adult human dermis. It was originally shown to predominate in human skin during embryonic development, but during the early postnatal period type I collagen synthesis accelerates, resulting in the ratio of type I to type III collagen in the adult human skin being approximately 8 : 1. Type III collagen is most prominent in vascular connective tissues, the gastrointestinal tract and the uterus. It consists of three identical α-chains, α1(III), and mutations in the type III collagen gene can cause the vascular type of the Ehlers–Danlos syndrome [4].

Type IV collagen is a basement membrane collagen present within the dermal–epidermal junction as well as in the vascular basement membranes. The predominant form of type IV collagen in human skin is a heterotrimer of $[α1(IV)]_2α2(IV)$, although occasional homopolymers from these two chains may be assembled. The type IV collagen molecule is characterised by the presence of non-collagenous interruptions within the triple helical domains, thus conferring flexibility to the molecule. In addition to α1(IV) and α2(IV) chains, four other polypeptides of type IV collagen have been identified [5]. Type IV collagen molecules containing these polypeptides are present primarily in the glomerular basement membranes, and their importance for renal physiology is attested by the fact that mutations in the gene encoding the α5(IV) polypeptide result in Alport syndrome. The α3(IV) chain harbours the epitopes recognised by antibodies in Goodpasture syndrome, and the α5 chain of type IV collagen has been shown to be a target of circulating autoantibodies in a novel autoimmune disease with subepidermal blisters and renal insufficiency.

Type V collagen consists of interrelated collagens containing four different types of α-chains. Type V collagen is present in most connective tissues, including the dermis, where it represents less than 5% of the total collagen. Type V collagen is located on the surface of large collagen fibres in the dermis, and its function is to regulate the lateral growth of these fibres. Thus, in the absence of type V collagen, the collagen fibre diameter is variable and the contour of the individual fibres can appear irregular, some of them having 'flower-like' morphology in cross-section. The importance of type V collagen in contributing to connective tissue stability is attested by the fact that mutations in the type V collagen gene underlie most patients with classic, autosomal dominant forms of Ehlers–Danlos syndrome [6].

Type VI collagen, as originally discovered, consists of three distinct α-chains, α1(VI), α2(VI) and α3(VI), which fold into a relatively short, triple helical domain and contain large globular domains at both ends. More recently, three additional α-chains have been suggested to belong to the type VI family of collagens. Type VI collagen is a relatively minor collagen in human dermis, where it assembles into thin microfibrils independent of the broad collagen fibres, which consist primarily of type I and type III collagens. The microfibrillar network has an anchoring function, stabilising the assembly of collagen fibres as well as basement membranes. Mutations in the three type VI collagen genes can lead to different forms of muscular dystrophy with little effect on the physiology of skin [7].

Type VII collagen, the major if not the exclusive component of anchoring fibrils, consists only of one type of α1 chain, α1(VII). This polypeptide has a characteristic modular structure, with the central collagenous domain being flanked by amino-terminal (NC1) and carboxy-terminal (NC2) collagenous domains with homology to known protein sequences. Type VII collagen molecules become organised into anchoring fibrils through the formation of antiparallel dimers linked through their carboxy-terminal ends (see Figure 2.34). The large amino-terminal, non-collagenous NC1 domains interact with type IV collagen and laminin 332 at the dermal–epidermal basement membrane, forming U-shaped loops that entrap larger fibres in a manner that stabilises the association of the lower part of the lamina densa to the upper papillary dermis (see Figure 2.39). Consequently, altered primary structure, reduced level of expression or changes in the molecular interactions of type VII collagen with other basement membrane components can result in skin fragility, as exemplified by the dystrophic forms of EB [8]. In addition to the heritable forms of EB, type VII collagen serves as an autoantigen in the autoimmune blistering skin disease EB acquisita, with the majority of the antigenic epitopes residing within the NC1 domain [9].

Type XVII collagen was initially identified as the 180 kDa bullous pemphigoid antigen (BPAG2) recognised by circulating autoantibodies in the sera of patients with bullous pemphigoid or herpes gestationis. Subsequent characterisation of the protein and the

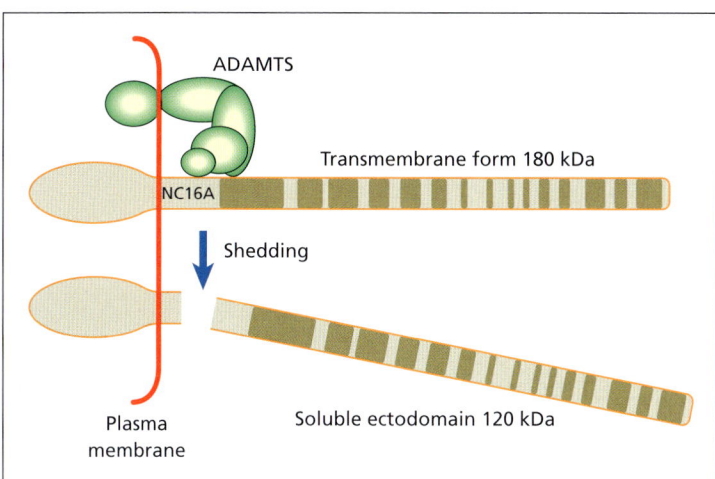

Figure 2.41 Type XVII collagen, a transmembrane protein in type 2 orientation. Note that the ectodomain traversing the lamina lucida contains 15 distinct triple helical collagenous segments (COL1–15). The non-collagenous segment between COL15 and the transmembrane domain, NC16A, harbours the major epitopes recognised by autoantibodies in bullous pemphigoid. ADAMTS, a disintegrin and metalloproteinase with thrombospondin motifs family of proteases, cleaves the protein at a sequence in the NC16A, resulting in release of the ectodomain. Adapted from Powell et al. 2005 [12].

corresponding gene has indicated that BPAG2 is, in fact, a collagenous molecule consisting of 15 collagenous domains with characteristic Gly-X-Y repeat sequences which form triple helices (Figure 2.41) [10]. Type XVII collagen is a transmembrane protein in type 2 topography, that is the amino-terminal segment of the molecule is intracellular while the carboxy-terminal ectodomain, containing the collagenous segments, is in the extracellular space. In the extracellular space, just adjacent to the plasma membrane is a non-collagenous peptide domain, NC16A, which serves as a site of proteolytic cleavage leading to release of the soluble ectodomain (Figure 2.41). This cleavage results in the generation of neoepitopes which will be recognised by circulating autoantibodies in bullous pemphigoid. The importance of type XVII collagen to the stability of the dermal–epidermal junction is attested to by the fact that mutations in the corresponding gene (COL17A1) result in an intermediate variant of junctional EB. Type XVII collagen is also implicated in skin ageing and hair greying [11].

Collagen biosynthesis

The genetically distinct collagens demonstrate considerable tissue specificity and, accordingly, they are synthesised by a number of different cell types, including dermal fibroblasts, epidermal keratinocytes, vascular endothelial cells and smooth muscle cells. The individual α-chains are initially synthesised as precursor molecules, pro-α-chains, with non-collagenous extensions at the ends of the collagenous domain (Figure 2.42).

While in the rough endoplasmic reticulum, three individual pro-α-chains assemble into a trimeric molecule through interactions of the non-collagenous sequences at the carboxy-terminal end. Upon completion of the prolyl hydroxylation reactions, the collagenous domains of the α-chains fold into a triple helical conformation, and the collagen molecules are then secreted through Golgi vesicles into the extracellular milieu. In the extracellular space, in the pericellular milieu, parts of the non-collagenous peptide extensions are cleaved by specific proteases. Specifically, the amino-terminal propeptides are cleaved by procollagen N-proteinases, including ADAMTS2, -3 and -14, while the carboxy-terminal propeptide is removed by C-proteinases of the tolloid family. This procollagen to collagen conversion allows the collagen molecules then to assemble into their tissue-specific supramolecular organisation. For example, the fibrillar collagens align into a characteristic quarter-stagger arrangement and form fibres, the growth occurring at the tip of the growing fibre. The coarse collagen fibres in the mid-dermis consist primarily of type I and III collagens, and type V collagen associates with them on the surface of the fibre so as to regulate the diameter of the growing fibre. Type VII collagen assembles into centrosymmetrical anchoring fibrils within the dermal–epidermal BMZ, and type XVII collagen assumes a transmembrane type 2 orientation as a component of the hemidesmosomes. A characteristic feature of collagen is the presence of hydroxyproline and hydroxylysine residues, two amino acids that are post-translationally synthesised by hydroxylation of proline and lysine residues, respectively (Figure 2.43) [1].

These hydroxylation reactions are catalysed in the rough endoplasmic reticulum by prolyl and lysyl hydroxylases, respectively, enzymes that require ascorbic acid, molecular oxygen and ferrous iron as cofactors. The hydroxylation of prolyl residues is necessary for the stabilisation of the triple helical conformation at physiological temperatures, and hydroxylysyl residues are required for the formation of stable covalent cross-links. Thus, for example, as a result of ascorbic acid deficiency in scurvy, the hydroxylation reactions are suboptimal, the newly synthesised collagen is poorly functional, and clinically scurvy manifests with connective tissue weakness. Similarly, low oxygen tension in chronic ulcers and wounds due to poor circulation may impair collagen production, resulting in poor healing. Finally, deficiency in lysyl hydroxylation due to non-functional lysyl hydroxylase results in the kyphoscoliotic type of Ehlers–Danlos syndrome.

Hydroxylation of the lysyl residues is followed by O-glycosylation, catalysed first by galactosyltransferase, which adds a galactosyl residue to the hydroxyl group of hydroxylysine, followed by a glucosyltransferase reaction to form glucosyl-galactosyl-hydroxylysine in O-glycosidic linkage. Additional glycosylation in N-glycosidic linkage will take place on the non-collagenous extensions at the end of the triple helical molecule, but the functional significance of these glycosylation reactions is currently unclear.

Collagen biology

The regulation of collagen gene expression must be tightly controlled to maintain normal amounts and ratios of genetically distinct collagens under physiological conditions. At the same time, regulatory mechanisms need to be responsive to rapid collagen synthesis in repair processes, such as wound healing. On the other hand, uncontrolled collagen synthesis can lead to excessive accumulation of collagen in fibrotic diseases, as exemplified by systemic sclerosis, keloids and hypertrophic scars [1].

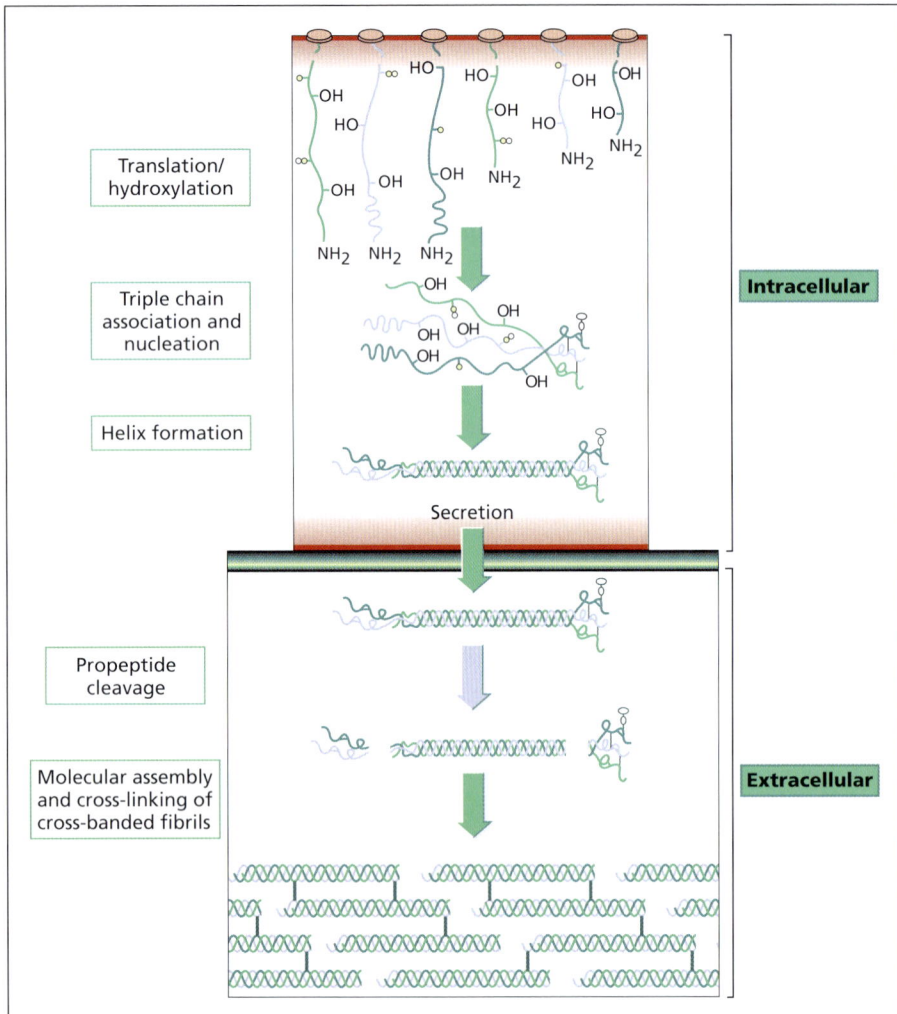

Figure 2.42 Steps in the intracellular biosynthesis of triple helical type I procollagen, its secretion into the extracellular space, and assembly and cross-linking of mature collagen fibres in the extracellular space.

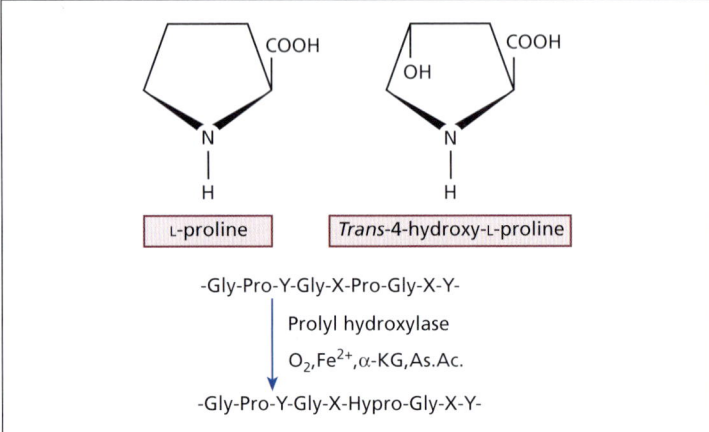

Figure 2.43 Enzymatic hydroxylation of prolyl residues in the Y-position of the repeating Gly-X-Y amino acid sequence to form hydroxyproline, an amino acid characteristic of collagen. Note that the reaction requires molecular oxygen, ferrous iron, α-ketoglutarate (α-KG) and ascorbic acid (As.Ac.) as cofactors.

An important control mechanism is at the level of collagen mRNA formation through regulation of the transcriptional activity of the corresponding genes. In general, there is a good correlation between the rate of collagen biosynthesis and the corresponding procollagen mRNA levels, as demonstrated in several *in vitro* models, including cultured fibroblasts. The transcriptional regulation of collagen gene expression involves both *cis*-acting elements and *trans*-acting factors. The *cis*-acting elements, representing nucleotide sequences within the regulatory regions of the gene that serve as binding sites for *trans*-acting regulatory proteins, have been identified in most collagen gene regulatory regions. Such factors can either upregulate or suppress the transcriptional promoter activity. An example of such *trans*-acting factors are the retinoic acid nuclear receptors (RAR and RXR) that form a complex with the ligand (a retinoid), which then binds to the retinoic acid-responsive elements (RARE) in the target gene. Retinoids, such as all-*trans*-retinoic acid, have been shown to modulate collagen gene expression both *in vitro* and *in vivo*, and quiescent non-proliferating cells can be stimulated by retinoic acid to activate type I collagen synthesis. These observations may have relevance to the elevated rate of collagen synthesis observed in photo-damaged dermis treated by the topical application of retinoids [2]. All-*trans*-retinoic acid has also been demonstrated to increase the density of anchoring fibrils along the cutaneous BMZ in adult human skin, suggesting that retinoids are capable of upregulating type VII collagen gene expression.

Collagen gene expression can also be modulated by several cytokines and growth factors, and one of the most powerful modulators of connective tissue gene expression is TGF-β [3]. In general, TGF-β is profibrotic and it has been shown to upregulate the expression of several extracellular matrix protein genes, including those encoding collagen types I, III, IV, VI and VII. Elevated levels of TGF-β have also been demonstrated in various fibrotic lesions, including the skin in systemic sclerosis and keloids. The upregulatory activity of TGF-β can be counteracted by other cytokines, including tumour necrosis factor α and interferon γ, which antagonise the TGF-β action. These cytokines have been tested for their efficacy for the treatment of keloids and other fibrotic diseases, with variable results.

A number of hormones clearly regulate collagen gene expression, as certain endocrine disorders dramatically change the amount of collagen found in connective tissues, including the skin. Glucocorticosteroids also affect collagen biosynthesis; inhibition is much more pronounced with fluorinated steroids compared with hydrocortisone. The glucocorticosteroid inhibition of collagen biosynthesis occurs in lower concentrations at the transcriptional level through inhibition of promoter activity. In higher concentrations and with more potent glucocorticosteroids, inhibition of prolyl hydroxylase activity also is evident, leading to deficient hydroxylation of collagen polypeptides and subsequently to reduced amounts of newly synthesised collagen. These mechanisms would explain the connective tissue side effects, such as dermal atrophy, associated with intralesional or prolonged topical application of fluorinated glucocorticosteroids.

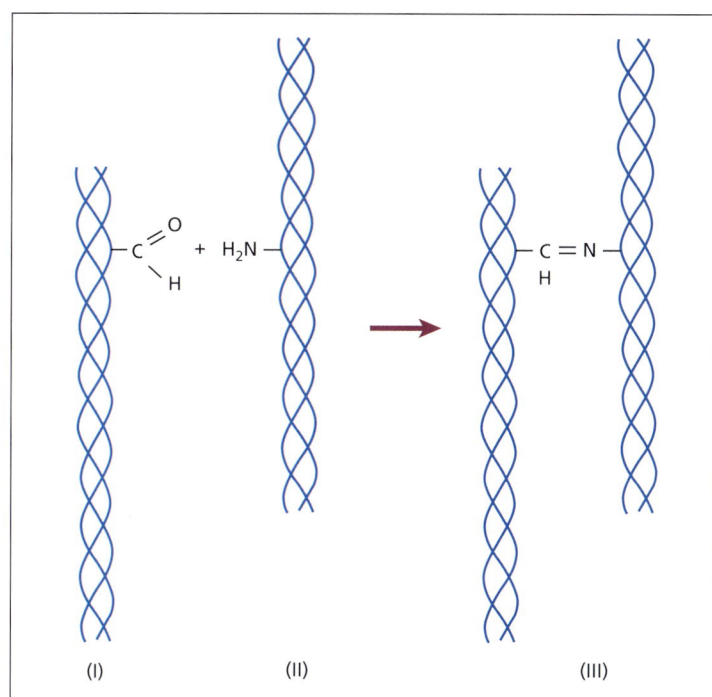

Figure 2.44 Formation of intermolecular cross-links between individual collagen molecules. The cross-linking is initiated by the conversion of lysine or a hydroxylysine residue that contains an ε-amino group to a corresponding aldehyde (I). The aldehyde then reacts with an unmodified ε-amino group in an adjacent collagen molecule (II) to form a Schiff base-type covalent cross-link (III).

Collagen cross-linking

The alignment of collagen molecules into their specific supramolecular organisation occurs spontaneously, but these fibre structures do not attain the necessary tensile strength until the molecules have been covalently linked together by specific intra- and intermolecular cross-links [1]. The most common forms of cross-link in type I collagen are derived from lysine and hydroxylysine residues, and in some collagens there are also cysteine-derived disulphide bonds. The first step in the cross-linking process is enzymatic synthesis of aldehyde residues from lysyl and hydroxylysyl residues by removal of the ε-amino group of these amino acids (Figure 2.44). This oxidative deamination reaction is catalysed by the lysyl oxidases, a group of enzymes that require copper as a cofactor. These enzymes act primarily upon native collagen fibrils and poorly, if at all, on denatured collagen (gelatin) or isolated α-chains. A similar deamination reaction catalysed by lysyl oxidase occurs also in elastin.

In addition to the classic human lysyl oxidase, four additional lysyl oxidase-like (LOXL1–4) genes/proteins have been identified [2]. These lysyl oxidase-like enzymes have been postulated to play a role in a number of disease processes, including susceptibility to exfoliation glaucoma, cancer biology and age-related changes in the cardiovascular system [2].

Collagen degradation

Collagen fibres, once fully matured by the cross-linking processes, are relatively stable and can exist in tissues under normal physiological conditions for long periods. However, there is continuous, yet slow, degradation and turnover of collagen in normal situations, as attested by continuous urinary excretion of hydroxyproline as a marker of collagen degradation. In addition, in certain physiological situations, as exemplified by reabsorption of the postpartum uterus, and in pathological conditions, such as tissue invasion and tumour metastases, degradation of connective tissues and particularly collagen is accelerated. There are several enzymes that comprise the family of matrix metalloproteinases (MMPs), enzymes capable of degrading the extracellular matrix components. These proteinase families include the collagenases, gelatinases, stromelysins, matrilysins and membrane-type MMPs (Figure 2.45) [1,2].

Native collagen is resistant to non-specific proteolytic degradation in physiological situations because the triple helical conformation is not readily degradable by general proteases. However, collagenases can degrade collagen triple helix at physiological pH and temperature. The vertebrate collagenase was initially isolated from tadpole tails which, when cultured upon reconstituted type I native collagen substrate, exercise proteolytic activity. Similar techniques were subsequently employed to demonstrate the presence of collagenase in human skin. Interstitial collagenase (MMP1) was initially shown to be synthesised as a proenzyme by cultured fibroblasts, and later different cell types, including epidermal keratinocytes, were shown to express a similar or identical enzyme. The ability of interstitial collagenase to digest the type I collagen triple helix is based on its ability to specifically cleave the α1(I) chain at a particular glycine–isoleucine peptide bond, or the α2(I) chain at a glycine–leucine peptide bond. This initial cleavage results in

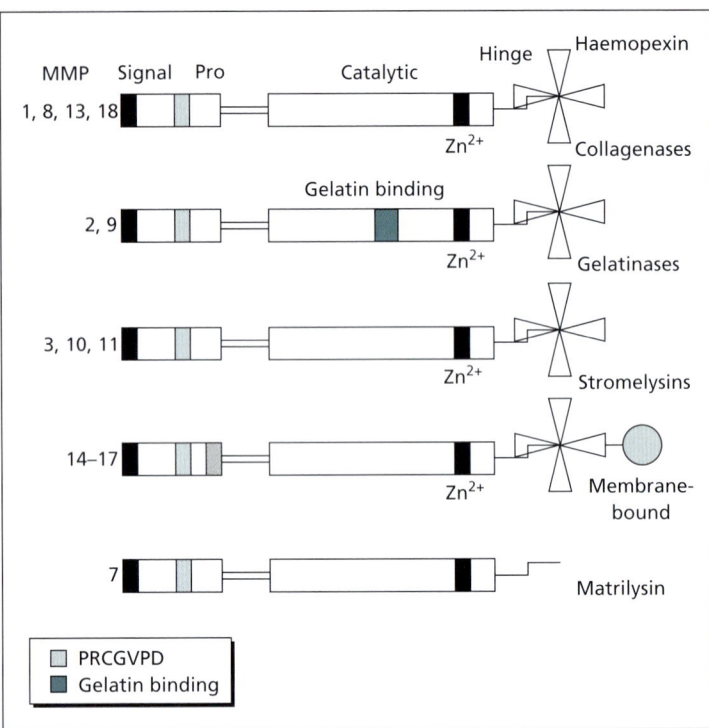

Figure 2.45 Structural organisation of various matrix metalloproteinases (MMPs) divided into different subclasses. The signal peptide, propeptide, active catalytic hinge and haemopexin regions are indicated. Note that MMP7 lacks the haemopexin region, while MMP14–17 harbour membrane-binding sequences at the carboxy-terminal end.

two degradation products, three-quarters and one-quarter of the size of the original collagen molecule. These shortened triple helical fragments have a lower helix-to-coil transition temperature (T_m) than the full-length molecule. Subsequently, at a body temperature of 37°C the triple helix unravels, rendering the individual polypeptides susceptible to general proteolytic degradation. It should be noted that type I collagen has several additional glycine–isoleucine and glycine–leucine sequences, but these are not susceptible to collagenase degradation in this collagen when in the native triple helical conformation. A similar enzyme (MMP8) has been identified in human neutrophils with comparable degrading characteristics. The neutrophil collagenase is stored in neutrophil granules and released upon stimulation. MMP1 and MMP8 can, in addition to type I collagen, degrade several other collagens, including types III and VII.

Another group of extracellular proteolytic enzymes is that of the gelatinases, which can degrade denatured collagen (gelatin) but can also cleave certain native collagens, such as types IV, V and VII, with certain interruptions or imperfections in their collagenous triple helices, thus allowing the proteolytic cleavage at these sites. Basement membrane collagen IV can also be degraded by MMP3 (stromelysin-1) and MMP10 (stromelysin-2).

In general, MMPs are synthesised and secreted as inactive proenzymes, which become activated proteolytically by removal of the propeptide. The MMPs are zinc metalloenzymes and require calcium for their activity. Consequently, the enzymes can be inhibited by chelators of divalent cations and, pharmacologically, tetracyclines have been suggested to inhibit MMP proteolytic activity due to their ability to bind calcium. The MMPs also have specific, small-molecular-weight peptide inhibitors, so-called tissue inhibitors of metalloproteinases (TIMPs). These proteins complex stoichiometrically with MMPs to prevent the degradative events.

In normal human skin, several MMPs are synthesised and secreted by fibroblasts and keratinocytes. The expression of these enzymes is activated in various pathological situations, including the invasion and metastasis of cutaneous malignancies, as well as during dermal wound healing and epidermal regeneration [3]. Finally, proteolytic enzymes play a pathophysiological role in tissue separation in a number of blistering diseases, such as bullous pemphigoid, dermatitis herpetiformis and epidermolysis bullosa acquisita.

Another metalloproteinase family has been designated as ADAMTS (a disintegrin and metalloproteinase with thrombospondin motifs family of proteases) [4]. The prototype, *ADAMTS-1* gene can be induced by IL-1 *in vitro* or by lipopolysaccharide injection in mice and, thus, this metalloproteinase was initially associated with inflammatory processes. Subsequently, several ADAMTS genes have been identified with similar domain organisations, consisting of a signal sequence, a propeptide, a metalloproteinase domain, a disintegrin-like domain, a cysteine-rich region and a variable number of thrombospondin type 1 molecules (Figure 2.46). These molecules are zinc-dependent proteases with a high level of expression in fetal tissues. ADAMTS proteases also have high levels of expression in tumour cells and tissues, including melanoma and colon carcinoma. Of particular interest in the context of collagen processing is ADAMTS2, which serves as a procollagen I/II amino-propeptide-processing enzyme.

Regulation of extracellular matrix turnover and collagen degradation during postpartum involution of the uterus has been attributed to relaxin, a hormone initially implicated in pregnancy-related conditions. More recently, it has become clear that many tissues, including skin, can serve as targets of relaxin. These tissues contain a relaxin family peptide receptor 1 (RFPR1) that mediates the relaxin effects on connective tissue metabolism, contributing to the maintenance of tissue homeostasis. The critical role of relaxin and its receptor has been illustrated by targeted mutant mice in which the absence of relaxin leads to collagen accumulation in several tissues, similar to systemic sclerosis.

Elastic fibres

An integral component of the dermal connective tissue is the elastic fibre network, which provides resilience and elasticity to the skin [1,2]. Elastic fibres are a relatively minor component in normal sun-protected adult skin, being less than 2–4% of the total dry weight of the dermis. The elastic fibre system in the reticular dermis consists of horizontally orientated fibres that interconnect to provide a network structure. Extending from these horizontal fibres is a network of vertical extensions of relatively fine fibrils, which consist either of bundles of microfibrils (oxytalan fibres) or of small amounts of cross-linked elastin (elaunin fibres) (Figure 2.47).

Elastic fibres have two principal components: (i) elastin, a well-characterised connective tissue protein that forms the core of the mature fibres; and (ii) the elastin-associated microfibrils

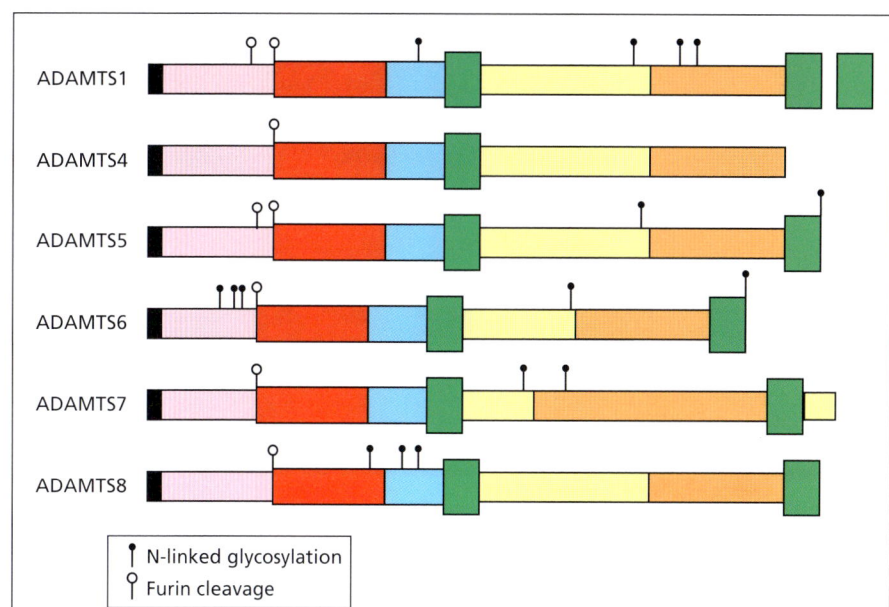

Figure 2.46 Main organisation of various ADAMTS family metalloproteinases. The catalytic domain is shown in red, while other domains include the thrombospondin type I repeat sequences (green), disintegrin-like domain (blue) and cysteine domain (yellow). The signal peptide is shown in black, the propeptide sequence is coloured pink and the spacer domain is in orange. ADAMTS, a disintegrin and metalloproteinase with thrombospondin motifs family of proteases.

which consist of a family of proteins, some of them less defined. Examination of mature elastic fibres by transmission electron microscopy reveals an electron-pale core that consists of elastin (Figure 2.48). Surrounding the elastin core are distinct microfibrillar structures, which appear electron dense under routine electron microscopy staining. While elastin is the major component and the microfibrils are less conspicuous in fully mature elastic fibres, the relative proportion of these two components varies during the embryonic development of elastic fibres and/or connective tissue repair. The first elements of elastic fibres that form consist of bundles of microfibrils, which can be visualised by electron microscopy during the first trimester of gestation. These microfibrils form a scaffold, allowing alignment of the elastin molecules in parallel array which guides the growth of fibres with relatively uniform diameters. During the second trimester of fetal development, the elastic fibres remain immature, but with increasing fetal age maturation of the fibres occurs and the elastin component becomes more prominent. In fully developed elastic fibres, well over 90% of the total content is elastin with relatively few microfibrillar components, mostly confined to the outer surface of the fibres.

Elastin

Elastin is initially synthesised as a precursor polypeptide, 'tropoelastin', which consists of approximately 700 amino acids with a molecular mass of approximately 70 kDa [1]. The amino acid composition of tropoelastin is similar to collagen in that about one-third of the total amino residues consists of glycine. However, glycine is not evenly distributed in elastin in every third position as it is in a typical collagenous sequence. Instead, the tropoelastin primary sequence shows domains rich in glycine, valine and proline, alternating with lysine- and alanine-rich sequences. A characteristic sequence motif in the latter setting is the presence of two lysine residues separated by two or three alanine residues (Figure 2.49).

The lysine residues in tropoelastin are critical for the formation of covalent cross-links, desmosine and its isomer, isodesmosine, which are unique to elastin. The first step in the formation of these elastin-specific cross-links is oxidative deamination of three lysine residues to form corresponding aldehydes, so-called allysines. Three of these resulting aldehydes, together with a fourth lysine residue containing the intact unmodified ε-amino group, spontaneously fuse to form a stable desmosine compound that covalently links two of the tropoelastin polypeptides. The addition of desmosines to other parts of the molecule progressively converts tropoelastin molecules into an insoluble fibrous structure which can be stretched, but upon release the fibres recoil, providing resilience and elasticity to the skin (Figure 2.50). The content of desmosine in various elastin preparations is almost constant, with approximately 1.5 residues per 1000 amino acids, and desmosine or isodesmosine can therefore provide a quantitative measure of the insoluble elastin content in tissues.

The human elastin gene spans approximately 45 kb of genomic DNA on chromosome 7 and consists of 34 exons corresponding to 3.5 kb of human elastin mRNA sequences. Examination of the gene structure reveals that the alternating cross-link domains, characterised by the presence of lysyl residues separated by two or three alanines, and the hydrophobic domains are encoded by individual exons. The elastin mRNAs are synthesised in several cell types present in elastin-rich tissues, as for example the vascular smooth muscle cells in arterial connective tissues. In the skin, the primary cell type responsible for elastin production appears to be the fibroblast which, under tissue culture conditions, expresses the elastin gene. Keratinocytes have also been suggested to express the elastin gene, but the level of expression is very low in comparison with dermal fibroblasts and the potential significance of elastin in the epidermis remains unclear.

Primary mutations in the elastin gene have been demonstrated in cutis laxa, a group of diseases that manifest with loss or fragmentation of elastic fibres [2]. It should be noted, however, that

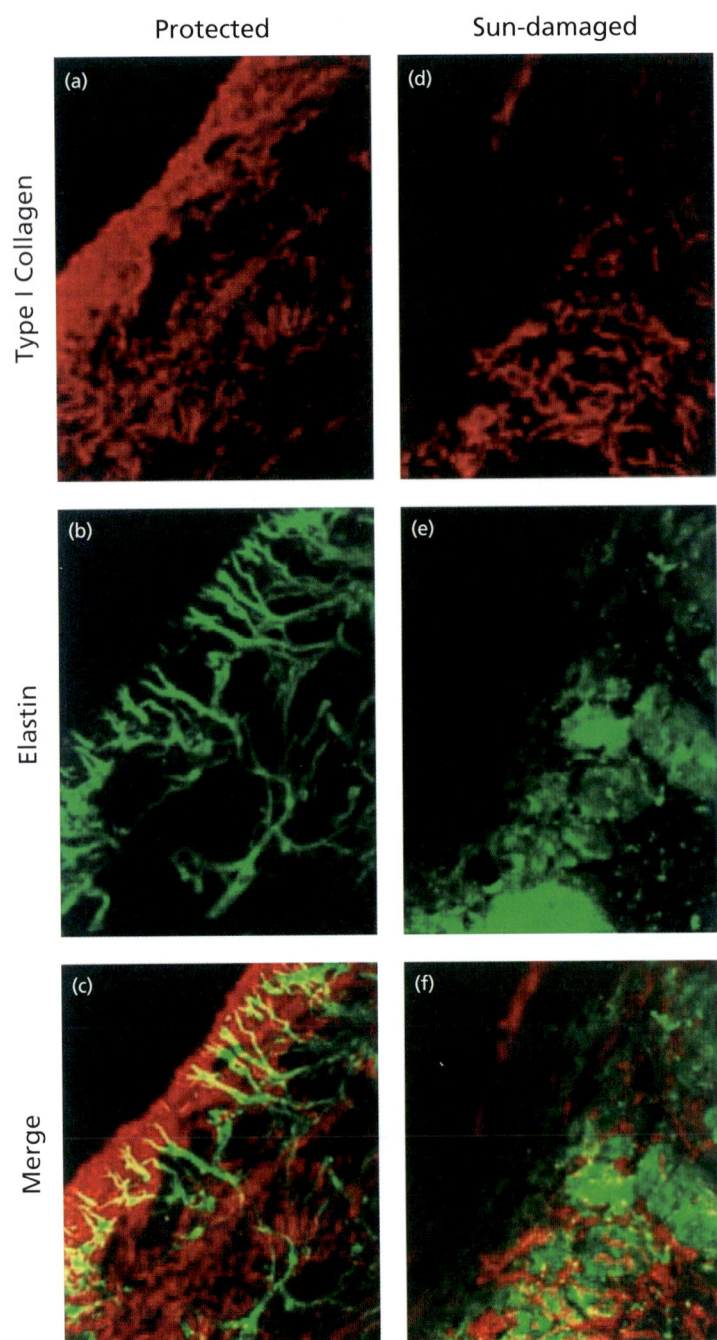

Figure 2.47 Immunofluorescence staining of type I collagen (a, d) and the elastic fibre network (b, e) in the dermis of human skin visualised by confocal laser scanning microscopy. Merging of the images (c, f) reveals that the elastic fibres assume a horizontal orientation in the mid-dermis while vertical extensions (oxytalan and elaunin fibres) reach the upper dermis, terminating just below the dermal–epidermal junction in normal, sun-protected areas of skin. In sun-damaged skin there is a dramatic decrease and disorganisation of both collagen and elastic fibres in comparison with sun-protected skin. Adapted from Uitto and Bernstein 1998 [3] with permission of Elsevier.

this group of heritable diseases is highly heterogeneous, and mutations in the fibulin-4 and fibulin-5 genes have also been observed. Williams syndrome is a contiguous gene deletion syndrome that also involves the elastin gene, with clinical manifestations predominantly in the cardiovascular system [3]. Finally, cutis laxa can

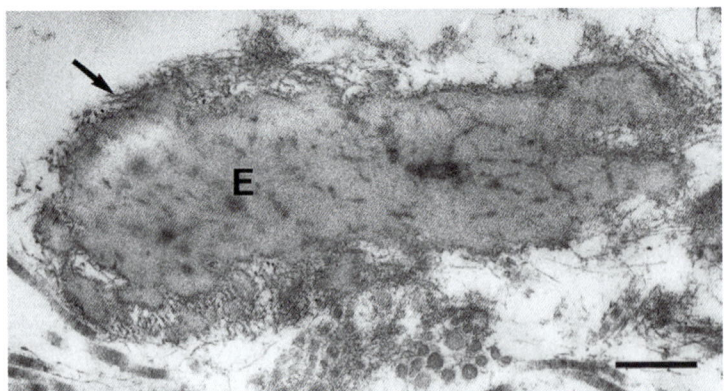

Figure 2.48 Transmission electron microscopy of an elastic fibre in the reticular dermis. The central electron-pale core consists of elastin (E), while the electron-dense areas represent the elastin-associated microfibrillar proteins which are particularly evident at the periphery of the fibre (arrow). Scale bar 0.5 μm. Courtesy of Professor R. A. J. Eady, St John's Institute of Dermatology, King's College London, UK.

develop as a postinflammatory condition, probably mediated by proteolytic enzymes released from the inflammatory cells.

An interesting observation during the processing of elastin mRNA precursor molecules is that they undergo extensive alternative splicing, leading to the formation of elastin molecules of varying primary sequences. In fact, at least six exons in the human elastin gene have been reported to be subject to alternative splicing, and this mechanism can provide significant variation in the primary sequence composition of elastin polypeptides, leading to different types of elastic fibres in different tissues. However, the physiological significance of the alternative splicing has not been established.

The oxidative deamination of lysyl residues to corresponding aldehydes is catalysed by a group of enzymes, lysyl oxidases, which require copper for their activity. Thus, copper deficiency can lead to reduced lysyl oxidase activity and the synthesis of elastic fibres that are not stabilised by enough desmosines. In such a situation, the individual tropoelastin polypeptides remain soluble and susceptible to non-specific proteolysis, and the elastin-rich tissues are fragile. Clinical manifestations of copper deficiency can vary depending on the level of copper and its circulating transport protein, caeruloplasmin, as manifested by Menkes syndrome and the occipital horn syndrome, two allelic conditions due to mutations in the copper transporter protein gene *ATP7A* [4]. Copper deficiency can also occur in patients undergoing long-term treatment with high doses of D-penicillamine, a copper chelating agent, which can result in abnormalities in the elastic structures in the skin and other tissues.

The metabolic turnover of elastin is slow, but a portion of elastin in the body is continuously degraded, as reflected by the continuous presence of desmosines in the urine. Thus, there may be ongoing turnover and repair of elastic fibres in normal tissues. In addition, there are some pathological states in which degradation of elastin is the histopathological hallmark, such as in some forms of cutis laxa and cutaneous ageing. Elastic fibres are degraded by elastases, a group of elastolytic enzymes in different tissues and with different cleavage specificities. The classic elastases, such as those originally

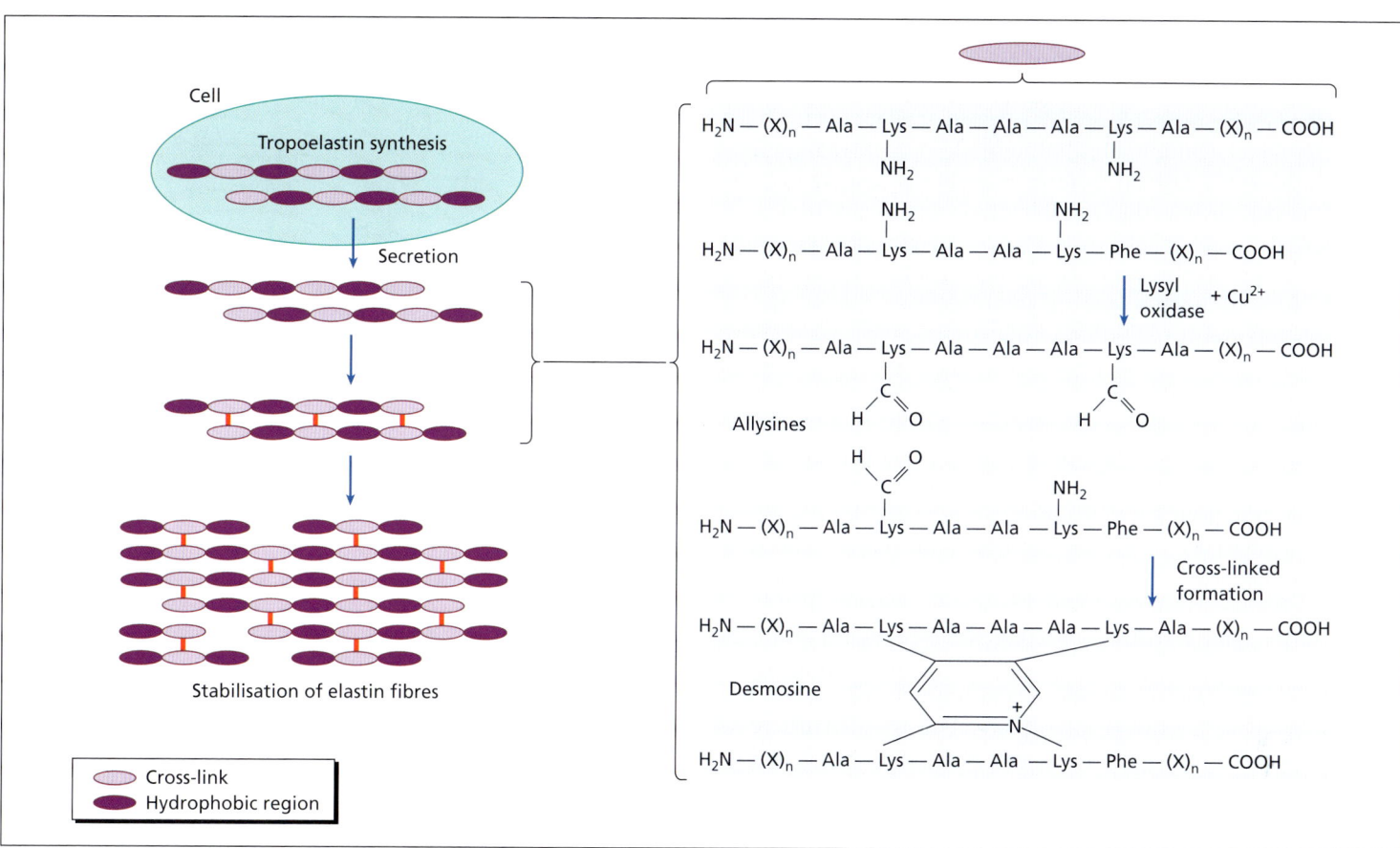

Figure 2.49 Assembly and cross-linking of elastic fibres. Newly synthesised elastin precursor polypeptides, tropoelastins, with alternating hydrophobic and cross-link regions are secreted into the extracellular milieu. Lysine residues in characteristic lys-ala-ala-lys or lys-ala-ala-ala-lys sequences in the cross-link region undergo oxidative deamination of the ε-amino groups catalysed by lysyl oxidase, an enzyme requiring copper as a co-factor. Three resulting allysine residues fuse with an unmodified lysine residue to form desmosines, elastin-specific cross-link molecules. Adapted from Mahoney et al. 2009 [5].

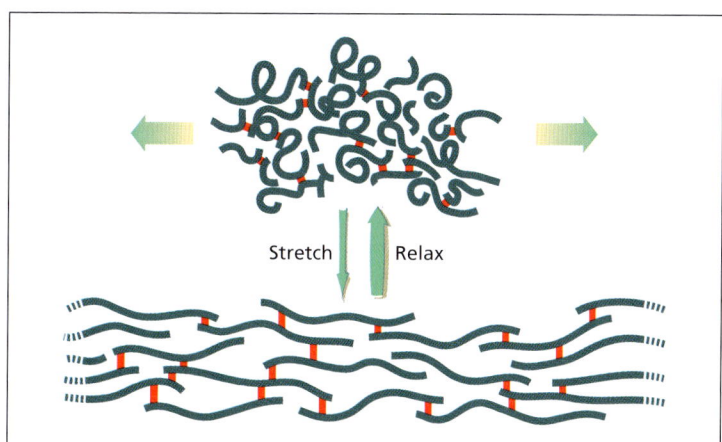

Figure 2.50 Elastic fibres cross-linked by desmosines (red). In the relaxed state, the fibres assume coiled-coil conformations. When the fibres are stretched and then released, they return to a relaxed state, the contraction providing elasticity and resilience to the skin.

isolated from the pancreas, are serine-proteases, and their activity can be inhibited by serum factors such as α_1-antitrypsin and α_2-macroglobulin. In addition to these classic serine-elastases, there are several metalloenzymes that are capable of degrading elastic structures, particularly the microfibrillar components. These metalloelastases are present in the skin and originate from fibroblasts and monocyte–macrophages.

Elastin-associated microfibrils

Elastin-associated microfibrils consist of tubular structures approximately 10–12 nm in diameter. Both ultrastructural evidence and biochemical analyses have confirmed that the microfibrils differ from elastin, and they may also be found in several tissues as individual microfibrillar structures without direct association with elastin. It is now known that elastin-associated microfibrils consist of a number of proteins, which can be divided into several different categories based on their molecular characteristics. Many of them form gene families with closely related structure and function, but clearly differ from other groups in their structural features.

One of the microfibrillar protein families is that of the fibrillins, which are a critical part of the microfibrillar structure [1]. Two distinct, yet closely homologous, human genes encode fibrillin 1 (FBN1) and fibrillin 2 (FBN2), proteins characterised by multiple repeats of sequence motifs previously observed in the epidermal growth factor (EGF) precursor molecule, with each motif having six conserved cysteine residues. Electron microscopy has established that monomeric fibrillin molecules synthesised by fibroblasts show an extended flexible molecule, which is approximately 148 nm long and 2.2 nm wide. Multiple fibrillin molecules can then align in a parallel, head-to-tail fashion to form microfibrils associated with elastin in tissues, such as skin and the arterial connective tissues. It should be noted that fibrillin is also a major component of microfibrils in tissues such as the ocular ciliary zonule and the periodontal ligament, without microscopic or immunoreactive evidence of elastin. The importance of fibrillin 1 is illustrated by the fact that the mutations in the corresponding gene (*FBN1*) underlie Marfan syndrome, manifesting with skeletal abnormalities, aortic dilatations, subluxation of the lens and cutaneous laxity [2]. Fibrillin 2 (*FBN2*) mutations cause congenital contractural arachnodactyly with some similarities, but also differences, to Marfan syndrome.

The latent TGF-β binding family of proteins (LTBP) has some structural similarities with the fibrillins, including repeating EGF-like domains [3]. TGF-β, a profibrotic cytokine, is secreted as a latent complex bound to LTBP. There are at least four distinct proteins in the family, with a molecular weight ranging from 125 to 310 kD. One of the putative functions of LTBP is to facilitate the secretion of TGF-β or binding of the inactive complex to the cell surface where activation takes place. However, LTBPs have also been found as free proteins associated with components of the extracellular matrix. LTBP1, a prototype of this subfamily of elastin-associated microfibrillar proteins, is clearly a component of the elastic fibres in human skin, and its levels are altered in solar elastosis.

Another family of the elastin-associated microfibrillar proteins consists of fibulins, extracellular matrix glycoproteins with characteristic calcium-binding EGF-like domains. Eight distinct fibulins have been characterised (fibulins 1–8; FBLN-1–8), and at least four of them have been located within the elastic fibres in different tissues [4]. In addition, FBLN-5 has been shown to bind both muscle cells and elastin, thus apparently facilitating cell–matrix interactions. The importance of FBLN-4 and FBLN-5 in skin physiology is attested by the demonstration of mutations in the corresponding genes in patients with cutis laxa, manifesting with loose and sagging skin and loss of recoil [5].

In addition to fibrillins, LTBPs and fibulins, other proteins have been shown to be associated with elastic fibres in the microfibrillar network. Several of these proteins belong to the families of microfibril-associated glycoproteins (MAGPs) or microfibril-associated proteins (MFAPs), highly acidic, relatively small molecules, some of which have been characterised in detail. Finally, interface proteins, so-called emilins, as well as lysyl oxidases critical for the cross-linking and stabilisation of elastic fibre structures, have been shown to be associated with elastic fibres [6].

Proteoglycan/glycosaminoglycans

Proteoglycans comprise several subfamilies defined by a core protein to which polymers of unbranched disaccharide units, glycosaminoglycans (GAGs), are linked by an *O*-linkage to serine residues (Figure 2.51). There are a number of distinct core proteins,

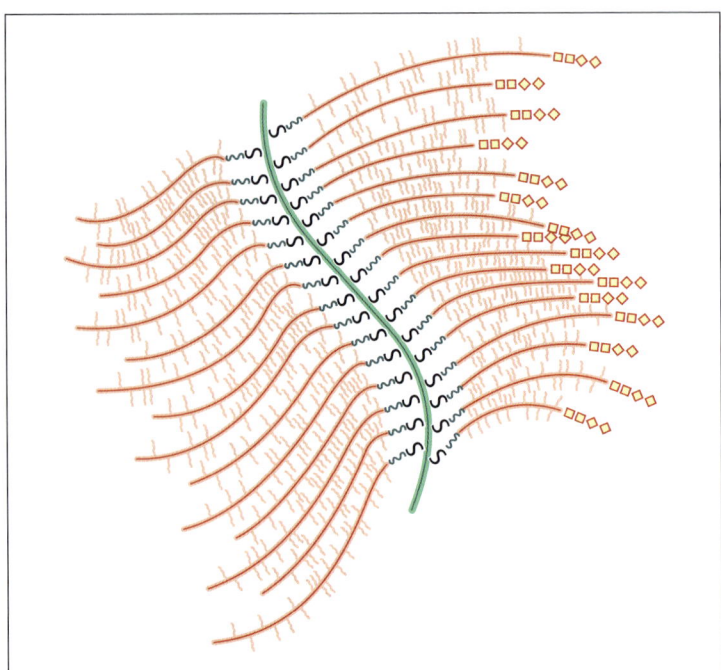

Figure 2.51 Prototypic proteoglycan in which the central core (green) is hyaluronic and the link proteins are represented by S-shapes, joining the protein side chains and carbohydrate polymers. Adapted from Stryer 1995 [6].

the number of attached disaccharides varies and the molecular mass of GAGs is highly variable. Commensurate with variability in structure, different proteoglycans are of different functional importance as critical components of cell membranes and the extracellular matrix of the skin during development, homeostasis and disease [1].

GAGs are highly charged polyanionic molecules that attach to the core protein. The characteristic feature of GAGs is their primary structure, consisting of alternating pairs of different monosaccharides, glucose or galactose, joined in 1–3 or 1–4 linkage (Figure 2.52). After the initial synthesis of GAGs, the polymers undergo complex post-assembly modifications catalysed by specific enzymes. Sulphatases catalyse replacement of *N*-acetyl by *N*-sulphate and epimerases convert D-glucuronic to L-iduronic acid. The linear GAG chains, consisting of linked disaccharide units, are highly variable in size, ranging from just a few to several thousands. Consequently, the molecular mass of naturally occurring GAGs can range from 5×10^3 to 5×10^7 Da.

The degree of post-assembly modifications is highly variable, and the control of this reaction depends on the specific characteristics of the GAGs, the associated core protein as well as the cell type and tissue environment (Figure 2.53). The simplest GAG, hyaluronic acid, is not sulphated, while other GAGs show sulphation of varying degrees. Within the individual GAG chains there are regions that show either a low or high degree of sulphation, a feature that may facilitate interactions of proteoglycans and GAGs with their numerous binding partners.

The core proteins of proteoglycans have been increasingly characterised through cloning and sequencing of the corresponding genes. These genes are expressed in a number of different types of cells, including dermal fibroblasts which are the principal cell

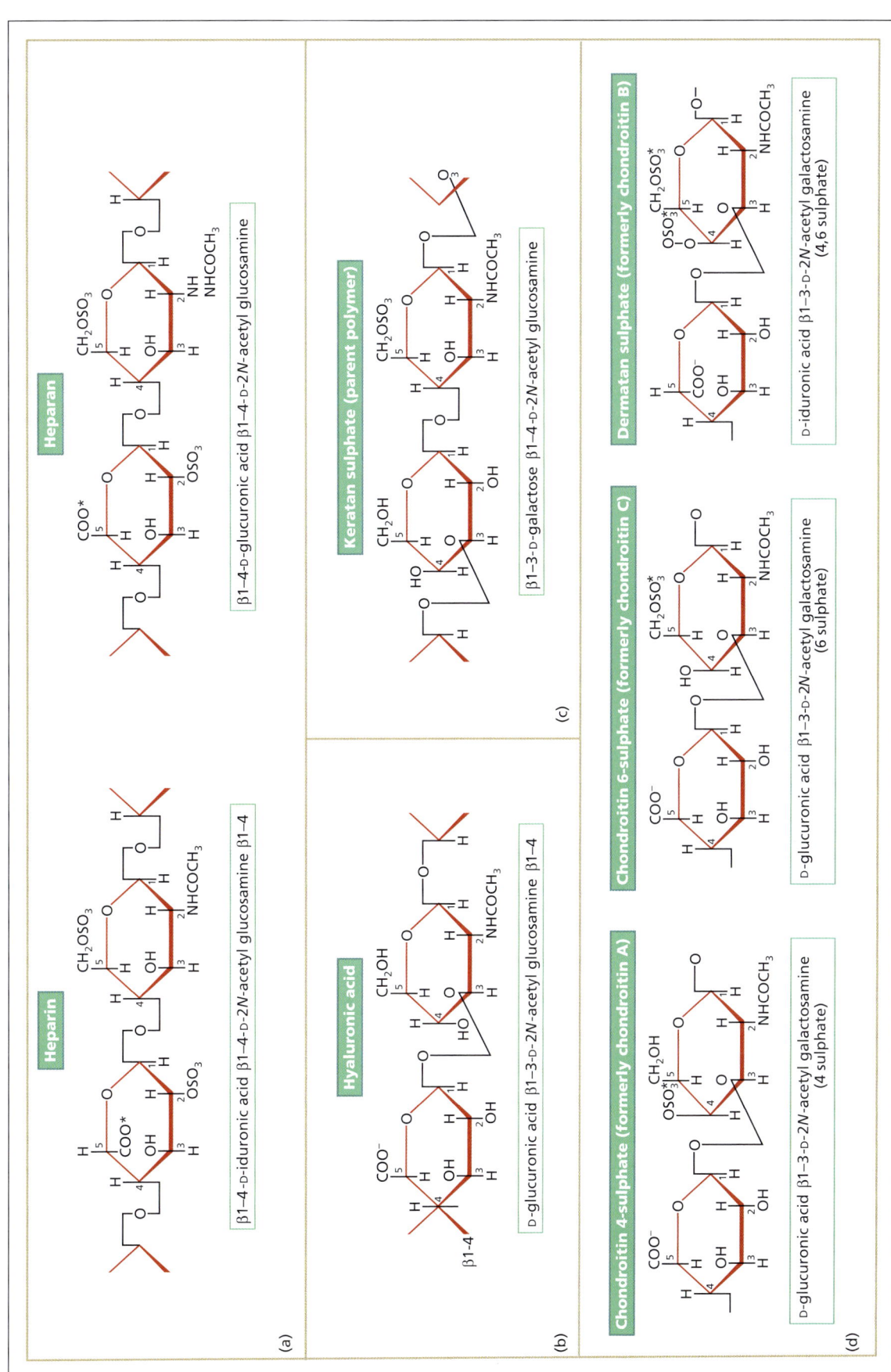

Figure 2.52 Glycosaminoglycan molecules that comprise the carbohydrate polymer side chains of proteoglycan molecules, including (a) heparin and heparan, (b) hyaluronic acid, (c) keratan sulphate and (d) various chondroitin sulphates. Note the variants that include O-sulphation at the 6 position of both glucosamine and galactose.

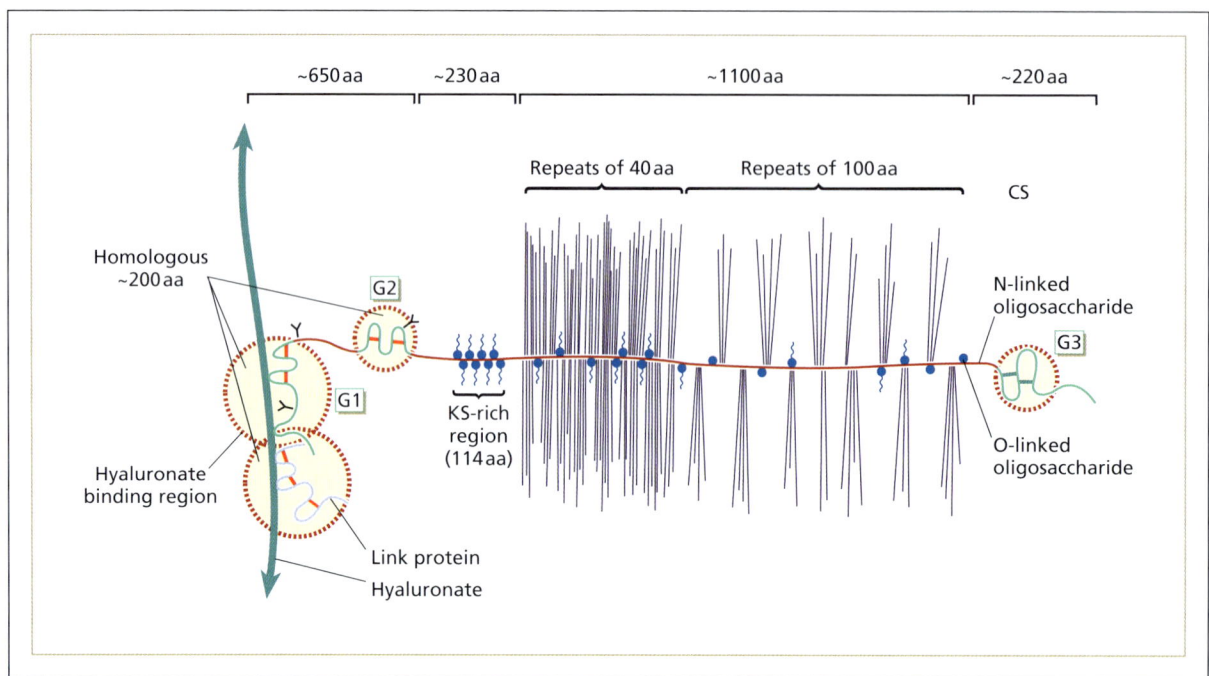

Figure 2.53 Core protein aggrecan is joined by link proteins to hyaluronate, with keratan sulphate (KS, blue) and chondroitin sulphate (CS, purple) side chains. aa, amino acids. Adapted from Heinegard and Oldberg 1993 [7].

type for proteoglycan synthesis in the dermis. Newly synthesised core protein polypeptides are transferred to Golgi vesicles where the attachment of GAG chains occurs. The final product, consisting of a core protein with attached GAG chains, allows classification of the proteoglycans. It should be noted that hyaluronic acid is a GAG produced without synthesis of a core protein; instead, this macromolecule is synthesised by a complex of enzymes at the plasma membrane, with subsequent extrusion into the extracellular space.

Known core proteins with their predominant tissue distribution and associated GAG components are listed in Table 2.3. The core proteins can be intracellular, reside on the cell surface or be part of the extracellular matrix. For example, serglycin shows an intracellular core protein present in the secretory granules of haematopoietic cells, such as mast cells and eosinophils, associated with either heparan sulphate or chondroitin sulphate GAGs. This proteoglycan is found in the skin in areas infiltrated by mast cells or eosinophils, and, on subsequent release, serglycin is a major form of highly sulphated heparan sulphate GAG in the skin.

There are several cell surface proteoglycans that function at the interface between the plasma membranes and the extracellular matrix. The mode of attachment to the cell surface is variable. For example, the glypican family of proteoglycans is attached to the cell surface by a phospholipid anchor, while the syndecans have membrane-spanning core proteins. Syndecans and glypicans are present in many cells and tissues, including abundant expression in the skin. Syndecan expression varies during the development and maturation of tissues and, for example, syndecan-1 is particularly abundant in keratinocytes. The nature of the attached GAG chains, however, changes as keratinocytes differentiate. Syndecans-1 and -4 are also induced in the dermis and granulation tissue, and it has been shown that deletion of syndecan-4 from mice greatly decreases the rate of wound repair. Furthermore, there are alterations in syndecan-1 expression because of malignant transformation.

The extracellular matrix contains different proteoglycans as an integral component of the connective tissue meshwork. In the dermis, fibroblasts produce large proteoglycans, as exemplified by versican, consisting of a core protein with attachment sites for 12–15 GAG side chains (Figure 2.54). The GAGs in versican are primarily chondroitin sulphate or dermatan sulphate, but versican can also bind hyaluronic acid, resulting in the formation of large aggregates. In the skin, versican has been identified in the dermis and epidermis as a product of fibroblasts and keratinocytes, respectively.

Extracellular matrix contains many small proteoglycans, exemplified by the family of leucine-rich repeat motifs. The prototype of this family is decorin, abundantly present in the skin. The decorin core protein is relatively small in size and has a single dermatan sulphate side chain covalently bound to a serine residue at the amino acid position 4 of the core protein. This proteoglycan was designated 'decorin' due to the observation that it associates with collagen and 'decorates' the fibres *in vivo*. This binding is attributed to the availability of decorin core protein to bind type I collagen, but the single GAG chain of decorin also binds to tenascin X, another extracellular component with affinity for collagen fibrils. Consequently, these interactions contribute to the connective tissue organisation and architecture with functional consequences for normal skin physiology [2].

Proteoglycan–GAG complexes have a multitude of functions. For example, the proteoglycans containing heparan sulphate and dermatan sulphate can bind extracellular matrix components, including various collagens. In addition, these proteoglycans bind several growth factors, cytokines, cell adhesion molecules and growth factor-binding proteins and they can serve as antiproteases. In addition to binding to various extracellular molecules, proteoglycans also play a role in the adhesion of cells to the extracellular

Table 2.3 Molecular characteristics and tissue distribution of selected proteoglycans (PGs).

PG	Protein (kDa)	Glycosaminoglycan(s)	Gene location	Tissue distribution
Decorin	36	CS/DS	12q21–23	Connective tissue
Biglycan	38	CS/DS	Xq28	Cell surface
Fibromodulin	42	KS	1q32	Collagen matrix
Lumican	38	KS	12q21–22	Cornea, bowel, cartilage, muscle
Epiglycan	36	CS/DS		Epiphyseal cartilage
Versican	260–370	CS/DS (10–30)	5q13	Skin, blood vessel, cartilage, brain
Aggrecan	220	CS (100)	15q26	Cartilage, blood vessel, brain
Perlecan	400–470	HS/CS	1p36	Cartilage, bone, marrow
Agrin	210	HS (3–6)	1q32	Cell membranes, kidneys, neuromuscular
Neurican	136	CS (3–7)		Brain
Brevican	100	CS (1–3)		Brain
Testican	44	HS/CS	21	Testis

CS, chondroitin sulphate; DS, dermatan sulphate; HS, heparan sulphate; KS, keratan sulphate.

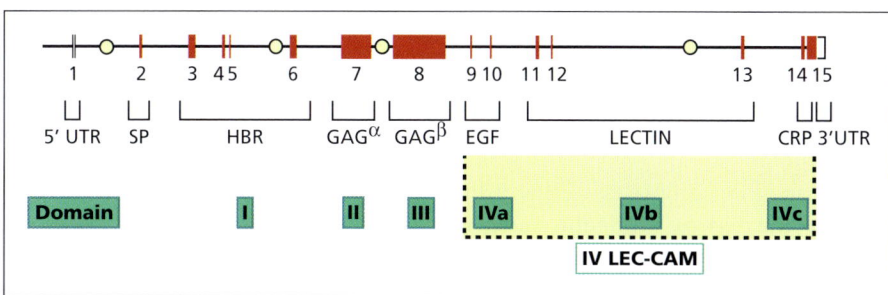

Figure 2.54 Human versican gene: intron–exon organisation (top) and deduced functional domains of the encoded protein. CRP, complement regulatory protein; EGF, epidermal growth factor; GAG, glycosaminoglycan; HBR, hyaluronan-binding region; SP, signal peptide; UTR, untranslated region. Adapted from Dours-Zimmerman and Zimmerman 1994 [8].

matrix. For example, syndecan-4, which is selectively enriched in dermal fibroblasts, facilitates the adherence of the cells in conjunction with other extracellular matrix-binding molecules, such as the integrins. Furthermore, the formation of focal adhesions requires heparan sulphate and subsequent activation of protein kinase C by a domain in the syndecan-4 core protein cytoplasmic tail [3].

Proteoglycans also interact with other extracellular matrix molecules besides collagen. In addition to decorin, which is known to associate primarily with type I collagen, chondroitin sulphate and dermatan sulphate bind fibronectin and laminin. The largest extracellular GAG, hyaluronic acid, plays an important role in providing physicochemical properties to the skin, mediated at least in part by its hydrophilicity and viscosity in dilute solutions. Most notably, hyaluronic acid has an expansive water-binding capacity, providing hydration to normal skin. The expression of hyaluronan is developmentally regulated in the skin, and the gene required for its synthesis, hyaluronan synthase, has been characterised. During wound healing, the physicochemical properties of hyaluronan may serve to expand the matrix and thus aid cell movement. The relatively high content of hyaluronan may also explain the finding that wounds in fetal skin heal without scarring. Other properties attributed to large proteoglycan complexes, such as those formed with versican or basement membrane proteoglycans, include their ability to serve as ionic filters, to regulate salt and water balance and to provide an elastic cushion [4].

Quantitative changes in the deposition of tissue proteoglycans have been encountered in various pathological processes. These include elevated hyaluronic acid synthesis in keloids and other fibrotic processes, as well as in pretibial myxoedema. In other skin conditions, including lichen myxoedematosus, systemic scleroderma and pseudoxanthoma elasticum, the lesional areas of skin have been reported to display abnormal amounts of proteoglycans. In most of these cases, the changes in proteoglycan/GAG content are secondary to an unrelated primary event. Finally, during innate cutaneous ageing in sun-protected areas of skin, the content of hyaluronic acid diminishes, possibly explaining the reduced turgor in aged skin [5].

Fibroblasts

The principal cell type responsible for the synthesis of connective tissue in the dermis is the fibroblast, which is of mesenchymal origin. The term fibroblast refers to a fully differentiated, biosynthetically active cell, while the term fibrocyte refers to an inactive cell. Biosynthetically active fibroblasts, as detected in developing or regenerating tissues, have an abundant cytoplasm, well-developed rough endoplasmic reticulum and prominent ribosomes attached to the membrane surfaces – features characteristic of cells engaged in active synthesis and secretion of extracellular matrix macromolecules (Figure 2.55). As indicated in the case of collagen, the newly synthesised polypeptides are first assembled in the cisternae of the rough endoplasmic reticulum, and the precursor polypeptides subsequently undergo extensive post-translational modifications. The polypeptides are then transferred to the Golgi vesicles and secreted into the extracellular milieu. Fibroblasts synthesise the extracellular matrix of connective tissue and play an essential role in maintaining the structural integrity of most tissues.

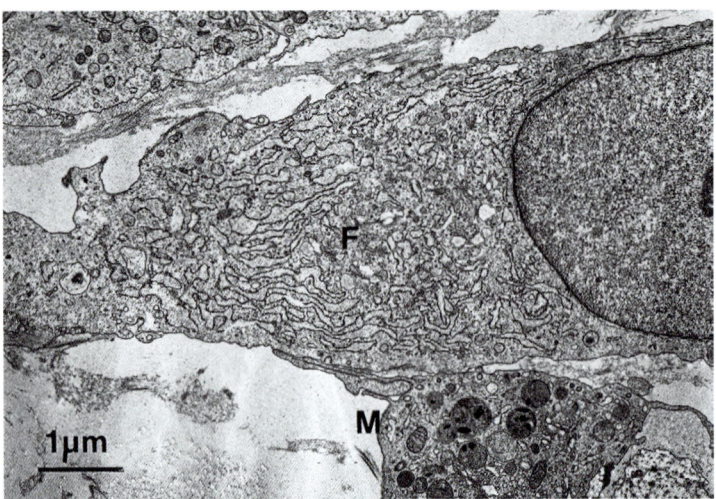

Figure 2.55 Transmission electron microscopy of an activated dermal fibroblast (F) in a healing wound. Note the prominent rough endoplasmic reticulum in the cytoplasm of this cell. There is an adjacent macrophage (M) with characteristic phagolysosomes, some of which contain ingested melanosomes. Courtesy of Professor R. A. J. Eady, St John's Institute of Dermatology, King's College London, UK.

Human skin fibroblasts are the principal cells synthesising collagen in the dermis. While the source of elastic fibres in the skin is less clear, fibroblasts clearly have the capacity to synthesise elastic tissues *in vitro*, and they probably are the primary source of elastin within the dermis as well. Finally, fibroblasts are the primary, if not the exclusive, cellular source of proteoglycan/glycosaminoglycan macromolecules. There is, however, considerable heterogeneity within fibroblast populations [1].

The multiple functions of the stroma of vertebrate animals are dependent on the architecture of the extracellular matrix, which contains mesenchymal cells and provides a structural scaffold for blood and lymphatic vessels and nerves. Reciprocal interactions between the mesenchymal and epithelial cells are known to play a critical role in the development and morphogenesis of tissues, such as skin. More recently, the specific gene expression patterns in cultured fibroblasts derived from fetal and adult human skin at different anatomical sites have been explored [2,3]. Fibroblasts from different sites were shown to display distinct and characteristic transcriptional patterns, and groups of differentially expressed genes include some involved in extracellular matrix synthesis, lipid metabolism and cell signalling pathways that control proliferation, cell migration and fate determination. Large differences in the gene expression programmes were also related to anterior–posterior, proximal–distal and dermal versus non-dermal anatomical divisions.

In human skin, fibroblasts from within the papillary or reticular dermis show differences in rates of cell division, contraction and the expression of various collagens and proteoglycans. Observations in mouse skin have also shown that papillary fibroblasts are required for new hair follicle formation following wounding, whereas reticular fibroblasts mediate the early events in wound repair and express so-called fibroblast activation markers such as α-smooth muscle actin (αSMA) [2]. In hair follicles, there are two separate populations of fibroblasts: hair follicle dermal papilla fibroblasts and dermal sheath fibroblasts. The former play a central role in the development of hair and the coordination of the hair cycle. The latter encapsulate the hair shaft external to epithelial components of the hair follicle. Additional populations of fibroblasts in the dermis include pericytes, preadipocytes and myofibroblasts. Pericytes are associated with and encircle vascular channels; preadipocytes are fibroblasts with the capacity to differentiate to adipocytes; myofibroblasts contribute to wound healing and may also transdifferentiate to adipocytes. Cellular identity is determined both by intrinsic mechanisms, including transcriptional regulatory networks and epigenetic processes, and by extrinsic factors, including cell–cell signalling, soluble signalling mediators or extracellular matrix components. Key signalling pathways include Wnt, bone morphogenic protein, β-catenin, Notch and TGF-β signalling [3]. Fibroblasts play a critical role in maintaining the structural integrity of the dermis and can adapt and respond to mechanical stress. Implicated in these responses are Hippo and focal adhesion kinase signalling [4].

Fibroblasts can be induced to become pluripotent stem cells, essentially indistinguishable from embryonic stem cells [5,6]. Specifically, the transduction of cultured fibroblasts with four transcription factors, *Oct4*, *Sox2*, *Klf4* and *cMyc*, generated inducible pluripotent stem cells, which may be used for disease modelling, drug and small molecule screening assays and potential cell therapy purposes.

Blood vessels and lymphatics

The arteries entering the skin form a deep plexus, the 'fascial' network, from which individual vessels rise to the border between the subcutaneous adipose tissue and the dermis to form a 'cutaneous' vessel network. These vessels then branch out towards various cutaneous appendages and provide ascending arterioles to generate a subpapillary plexus, which forms capillary loops entering the papillary dermis between the rete ridges. From these capillaries the blood is drained by venules which form intermediate plexuses. Thus, the cutaneous vasculature is rather elaborate and limited to the dermis, while the epidermis has no blood vessels (Figures 2.56 and 2.57) [1].

In addition to providing nutrients and oxygen to the skin, the vasculature plays a major role in regulating the body temperature. This is accomplished by controlling the blood flow through the capillaries in the upper dermis so that opening blood vessels allows dissipation of excess heat while constriction of blood vessels slows the blood flow to the skin and conserves the core energy. The amount of blood flowing through the superficial layers of the dermis can also be controlled by arterial–venous anastomoses, which act as shunts to short-circuit the flow.

The innermost component of the blood vessels is the endothelium, consisting of adjoining endothelial cells that surround the lumen. Arterioles are characterised by a subendothelial layer of elastic tissue (Figure 2.58), while venules generally do not have elastic tissue in their walls (Figure 2.59). The endothelium of capillaries and small arterioles and venules is surrounded by pericytes, which appear to share certain characteristics with both endothelial and smooth muscle cells. Capillaries contain a single, discontinuous layer of pericytes, whereas venules may include more than one pericyte layer in their periendothelial investment. Smooth muscle cells are found chiefly in the walls of ascending arterioles but also within

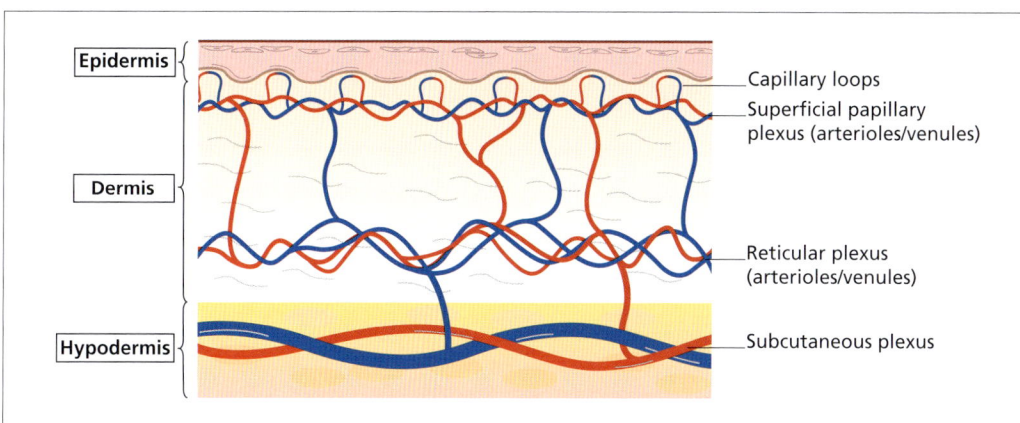

Figure 2.56 The vasculature of human skin is composed of capillary loops, the superficial papillary plexus, the reticular plexus and the subcutaneous plexus. Reproduced from Deegan *et al.* 2019 [1] with permission of IOP Publishing.

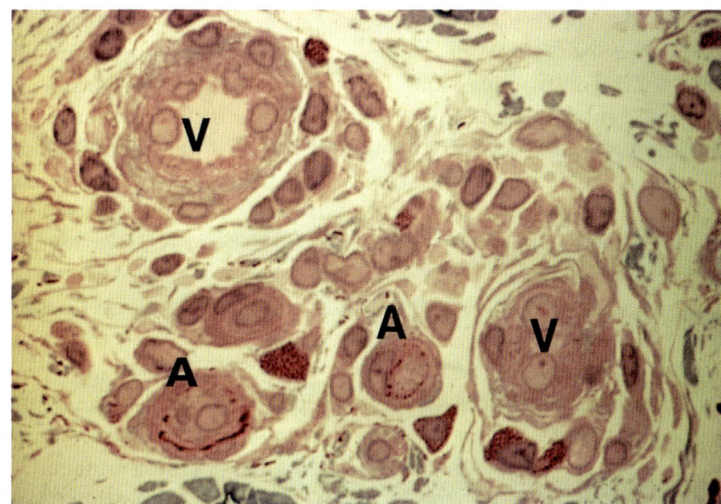

Figure 2.57 Histology of microvessels in the reticular dermis. Arterioles (A) can be distinguished from venules (V) by the presence of elastic lamina, which stains dark red. Surrounding mast cells can be distinguished by their prominent red/blue cytoplasmic granules. Original magnification 400× (basic fuchsin and methylene blue stain). Courtesy of Professor R. A. J. Eady, St John's Institute of Dermatology, King's College London, UK.

the arterioles of the superficial and deep plexus and in collecting venules. Smooth muscle cells and pericytes are surrounded by a basement membrane, which also encompasses the outer surface of endothelial cells. Veil cells are long, thin cells with an attenuated cytoplasm, and they more closely resemble fibroblasts than pericytes. They do not have a basement membrane investment and are located outside the vessel wall.

At the ultrastructural level, endothelial cells possess many of the common cellular organelles, including rough and smooth endoplasmic reticula, mitochondria and lysosomes; micropinocytotic vesicles are also evident. Intermediate filaments containing vimentin are present and have been reported to be more abundant on the venous than on the arterial site. Dense bodies associated with actin-like filaments of 5–6 nm diameter are found in the endothelial cells of the larger arterioles, and they may have a role in endothelial contraction.

Weibel–Palade bodies are endothelium-specific inclusions that occur more frequently in the venous side of the microvasculature (Figure 2.60). They are not found in dermal lymphatics but have been reported in larger lymph vessels. Weibel–Palade bodies contain

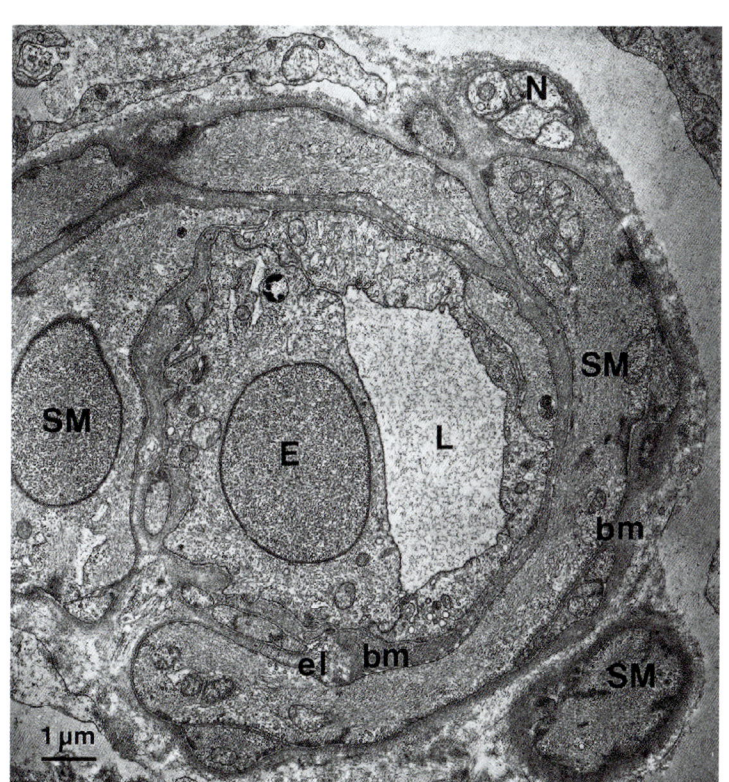

Figure 2.58 Transmission electron microscopy of a cross-section through a small arteriole in the skin. Note the relatively smooth surface of the endothelial cell (E) surrounding the lumen (L) and the presence of smooth muscle (SM) with an associated nerve (N). There is a small amount of elastic tissue (el) adjacent to the endothelial basement membrane (bm). Courtesy of Professor R. A. J. Eady, St John's Institute of Dermatology, King's College London, UK.

factor XIII-related antigen, von Willebrand factor and GMP-140, a protein that was first described in platelet α-granules.

A major feature distinguishing arterial from venous microvessels is the ultrastructural appearance of the basement membrane. Venules and venous capillaries have a multilaminated basement membrane, whereas arterioles possess a more homogeneous matrix, lacking the electron-dense strands. Vascular basement membrane contains laminin 111, type IV collagen, fibronectin and heparan sulphate proteoglycans. It does not contain, however, bullous pemphigoid antigens, type VII collagen or laminin 332, components of the epidermal BMZ.

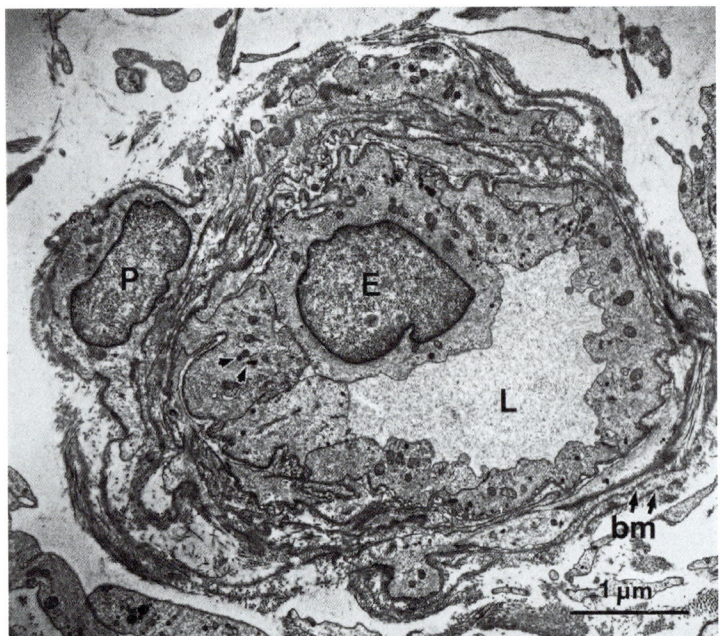

Figure 2.59 Transmission electron microscopy of a transverse section through a venule in the skin. The surface of the endothelial cells (E) in the lumen (L) is more convoluted than in its arteriolar counterpart (see Figure 2.58). The endothelial cells are surrounded by pericytes (P) and not smooth muscle cells, and the basement membrane (bm) contains dense strands (small arrows). The arrowheads indicate Weibel–Palade bodies. Courtesy of Professor R. A. J. Eady, St John's Institute of Dermatology, King's College London, UK.

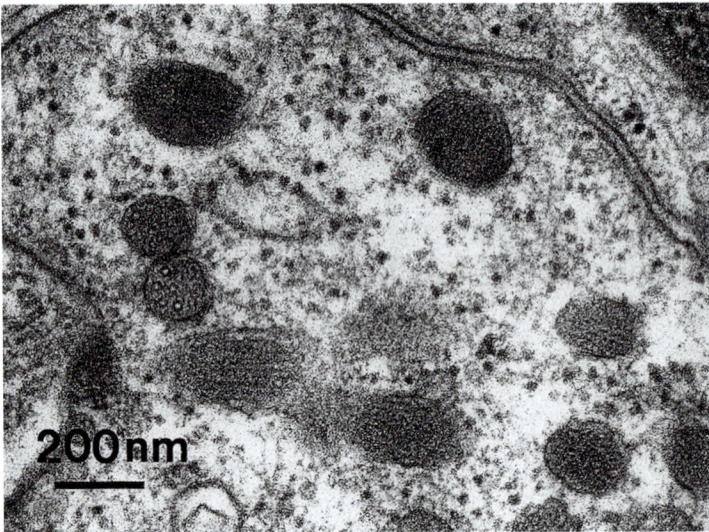

Figure 2.60 High-magnification view of Weibel–Palade bodies revealing tubular profiles in cross-section. Courtesy of Professor R. A. J. Eady, St John's Institute of Dermatology, King's College London, UK.

A number of endothelium-specific antigens have been recognised, and they may have a special value in studies of cutaneous pathology. Endothelial cells are the major source of angiotensin-converting enzyme as well as various cytokines and adhesion molecules. The microvasculature is also a rich source of enzymes that may be involved in cellular processes, such as endocytosis and vesicular transport. Acid phosphatase has been localised to lysosome-like structures in the endothelium, and alkaline phosphatase reactivity has been used extensively to map the distribution and arborisation of the arterial network in the upper dermis.

The lymphatic network in the skin serves to transport particulate and liquid materials, such as proteins, from the extravascular compartment of the dermis. Interconnecting lymphatic spaces arise from terminal bulbs in the papillary layer and ultimately form the system that drains into the lymph nodes. The vessels have a broad lumen surrounded by a single endothelial layer, which is discontinuous in the terminal components and rests on an often discontinuous basal lamina. These processes are critical for the normal function of skin, as altered function and development of lymphatics can lead to diseases, including primary and secondary lymphoedemas [2].

Subcutaneous fat

Fat is a major component of the human body and approximately 80% of fat is in the subcutis; the rest surrounds internal organs. In non-obese males, 10–12% of body weight is fat, while in females the figure is 15–20%. Fat comprises white and brown adipose tissue. Brown fat is more common in infants and children and is characterised by different mitochondrial properties and increased heat production [1]. The function of fat is to provide insulation, mechanical cushioning and an energy store. In addition, fat may have an endocrine function, communicating with the hypothalamus via secreted molecules such as leptin to alter energy turnover in the body and to regulate appetite [2]. Adipocytes also have important signalling roles in osteogenesis and angiogenesis, and additional physical functions such as phagocytosis. Multipotent stem cells have been identified in human fat, which are capable of developing into adipocytes, osteoblasts, myoblasts and chondroblasts. Molecular biological insights into genes, proteins, hormones and other molecules that influence fat deposition and distribution are gradually being realised, from both research on rare inherited disorders (such as the lipodystrophies or obesity syndromes) as well as population studies on more common forms of obesity [3].

Physiological functions of skin

A key role of skin is to provide a mechanical barrier against the external environment [1]. The cornified cell envelope and the stratum corneum restrict water loss from the skin, while keratinocyte-derived endogenous antibiotics (defensins and cathelicidins) provide an innate immune defence against bacteria, viruses and fungi [2]. The epidermis also contains a network of about 2×10^9 Langerhans cells, which serve as sentinel cells whose prime function is to survey the epidermal environment and to initiate an immune response against microbial threats, although they may also contribute to immune tolerance in the skin. Melanin, which is mostly found in basal keratinocytes, also provides some protection against DNA damage from UV radiation.

An important function of skin is thermoregulation. Vasodilatation or vasoconstriction of the blood vessels in the deep or superficial plexuses helps regulate heat loss. Eccrine sweat glands are found at all skin sites and are present in densities of 100–600/cm^2; they play a role in heat control and produce approximately 1 litre of sweat per hour during moderate exercise. Secretions from apocrine sweat glands contribute to body odour (pheromones). Skin lubrication and waterproofing are provided by sebum secreted from sebaceous glands [3].

Subcutaneous fat has important roles in cushioning trauma as well as providing insulation and a calorie reserve. In non-obese subjects, about 80% of the body's total fat is found in subcutaneous tissue. Fat also has an endocrine function, releasing the hormone leptin, which acts on the hypothalamus to regulate hunger and energy metabolism. Other functions of fat cells include tissue remodelling and phagocytosis.

Nails provide protection to the ends of the fingers and toes as well as being important in pinching and prising objects. Hair may have important social and psychological value, reflecting the notion that the appearances of human skin and its associated structures have a major impact on interpersonal relationships and personal well-being. Skin also has a key function in synthesising various metabolic products, such as vitamin D.

There are two main kinds of human skin: glabrous skin (non-hairy skin) and hair-bearing skin. Glabrous skin is found on the palms and soles and has a grooved surface with alternating ridges and sulci giving rise to the dermatoglyphics (fingerprints). Glabrous skin has a compact stratum corneum which may be up to 10 times thicker compared with other body sites such as the flexures, where the epidermis is at its thinnest. Glabrous skin also contains encapsulated sense organs within the dermis, as well as a lack of hair follicles and sebaceous glands. In contrast, hair-bearing skin has both hair follicles and sebaceous glands but lacks encapsulated sense organs. Hair follicle size, structure and density vary between different body sites; the scalp has large hair follicles that may extend into the subcutaneous fat whereas the forehead has only small, vellus hair-producing follicles, although sebaceous glands are large [4]. The number of hair follicles remains unchanged until middle life, but there is a changing balance between vellus and terminal hairs throughout life. In certain hair-bearing sites, such as the axilla, there are apocrine glands in addition to the eccrine sweat glands. Sebaceous glands are actively functioning in the newborn and from puberty onwards, and the relative activity modifies the composition of the skin surface lipids. The structure of the dermal–epidermal junction also shows regional variations in the number of hemidesmosomal-anchoring filament complexes that exist (more in the leg than the arm). In the dermis, the arrangement and size of elastic fibres vary from very large fibres in perianal skin to almost no fibres in the scrotum. Marked variation in the cutaneous blood supply is found between areas of distensible skin such as the eyelid and more rigid areas such as the fingertips. There are also regional differences in biomechanical properties which can affect percutaneous absorption of creams and ointments.

Skin homeostasis

To maintain skin homeostasis, regenerate skin appendages and repair itself after injury, the skin contains stem cells that reside in the bulge area of hair follicles, the basal layer of interfollicular epidermis and the base of sebaceous glands (Figure 2.61) [1]. These stem cells generate a proliferative progeny that can undergo

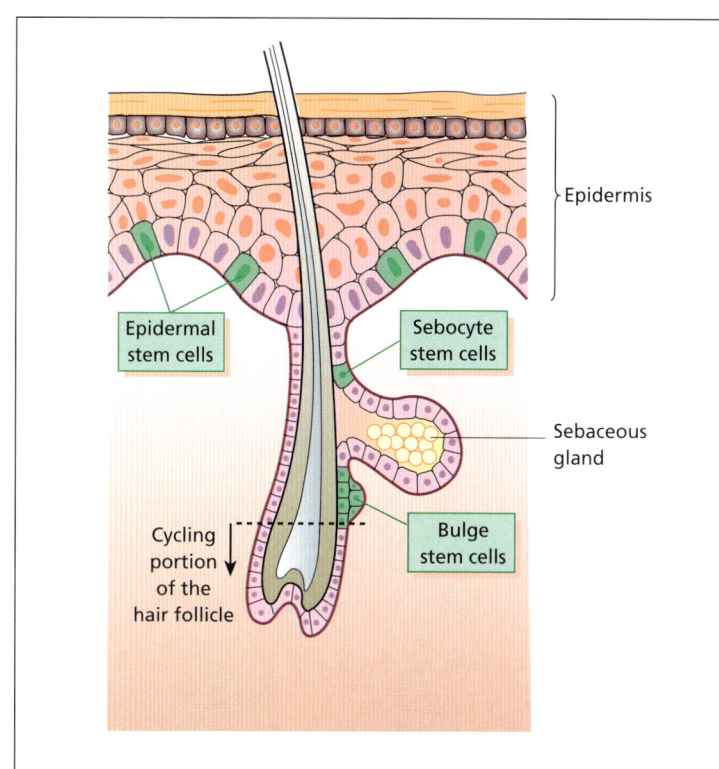

Figure 2.61 Epithelial stem cells are found within the interfollicular epidermis, the base of sebaceous glands and the bulge area of hair follicles.

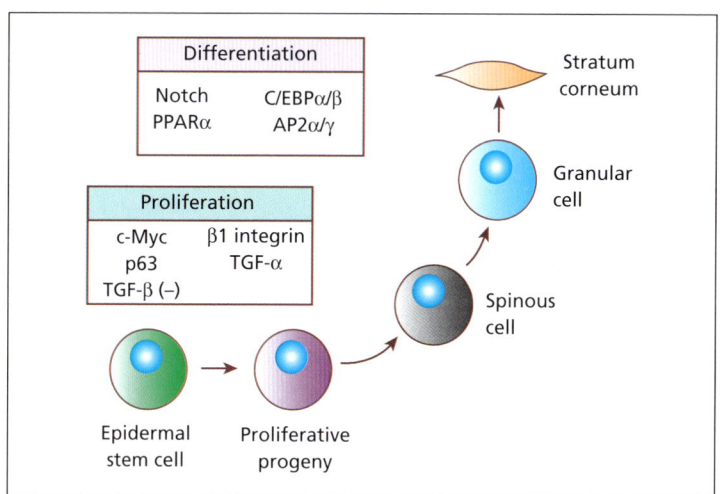

Figure 2.62 Epidermal stem cell proliferation is regulated positively by β1 integrin and transforming growth factor α (TGF-α) and negatively (−) by TGF-β signalling. The transcription factors c-Myc and p63 also promote epidermal proliferation. Notch signalling and the transcription factors peroxisome proliferator-activated receptor α (PPARα), AP2α/γ and C/EBPα/β control the differentiation of epidermal cells.

differentiation. The molecular signals involved in regulating epidermal stem cell proliferation and differentiation are illustrated in Figure 2.62.

Stem cells are able to self-renew as well as give rise to differentiating cells [2]. In the epidermis, some basal cells can periodically withdraw from the cell cycle and commit to terminal differentiation. It is still not clear, however, what proportion of cells in the basal layer can function as a stem cell. One long-established theory divides basal keratinocytes into epidermal proliferation units, which comprise one self-renewing stem cell and about ten tightly packed, transient, amplifying cells (each capable of dividing several times and then exiting the basal layer to undergo terminal differentiation) [3]. This unit gives rise to a column of larger and flatter cells that culminates in a single hexagonal surface. Stem cells within epidermal proliferation units are associated with a profile of particular chemical, molecular and biological characteristics. For example, stem cells retain labelling with injected ^{3}H-thymidine or 5-bromo-2-deoxyuridine after repeated cell division. In culture, actively growing clones present after serial passaging are considered to indicate an origin from stem cells. Potential markers of interfollicular epidermal stem cells are α6 and β1 integrin as well as p63, whereas sebocyte stem cells express Blimp1. Markers of hair follicle bulge stem cells include CD34, NFATc1, vitamin D receptor, TCF3, Sox9 and Lhx2, although considerably more markers exist in this and other parts of the hair follicle, highlighting the protean nature of the stem cell population in being able to respond to the requirements of tissue homeostasis, injury or growth spurts [4].

In the epidermal proliferation unit concept of stem cell behaviour, the division of basal cells has been viewed as a symmetrical process in which equal daughter cells are generated; the basal cells progressively reduce their adhesiveness to the underlying epidermal basement membrane, delaminate and commit to terminal differentiation (Figure 2.63). However, data also suggest that basal cells can undergo asymmetrical cell division, shifting their spindle orientation from lateral to perpendicular [5]. Asymmetrical cell divisions provide a natural means of maintaining a proliferative daughter cell that retains the cell markers associated with stem cells, while the other daughter cell has reduced markers such as β1 integrin and increased expression of Notch signals, and is committed to terminal differentiation. Asymmetrical cell divisions, therefore, can bypass the need for transient amplifying cells.

The structural and biological composition of the dermal–epidermal junction also influences the proliferative properties of basal keratinocytes. Laminin 332 promotes anchorage as a ligand via α6β4 integrins in hemidesmosomes and signalling/migration via its association with α3β1 in focal adhesions. Signalling via α3β1 integrin stimulates the mitogen-activated protein kinase (MAPK) pathway, turnover of focal adhesions and epidermal migration. The basement membrane is also a reservoir for growth factors that can promote epidermal proliferation (e.g. TGF-α, EGFs, insulin growth factors) or restrict it (e.g. TGF-β). EGFR signalling also enhances proliferation and migration in the epidermis, possibly by phosphorylating β4 integrin and promoting hemidesmosome disassembly. Thus, the control of basal keratinocyte stem cell activity in maintaining homeostasis and responding to injury is through the regulation of at least two opposing tyrosine kinase pathways and two integrin structures.

A key transcription factor in regulating the self-renewal and long-term proliferative capacity of the stem cell is p63, a member of the p53 family of proto-oncogenes [6]. However, the precise role of p63 is not clear; it may have a direct effect on stem cell renewal or lineage commitment, and/or an effect on switching from proliferation to terminal differentiation. Notch signalling also appears to have an important gatekeeper function in the transition from basal to suprabasal cells; there is basal expression of Notch ligands such as Delta1 and suprabasal expression of Notch receptors and Notch downstream targets such as Hes1.

Stem cells in hair follicles are located in the lowest permanent part of the follicle, within the outer root sheath. These cells cycle more slowly than other cells and have the capacity to migrate (e.g. to the base of the hair follicle in follicular regeneration), as well as to differentiate into diverse lineages (e.g. outer root sheath, inner root sheath, hair shaft, sebocytes, interfollicular epidermis). Despite this multipotency, however, the follicle stem cells only

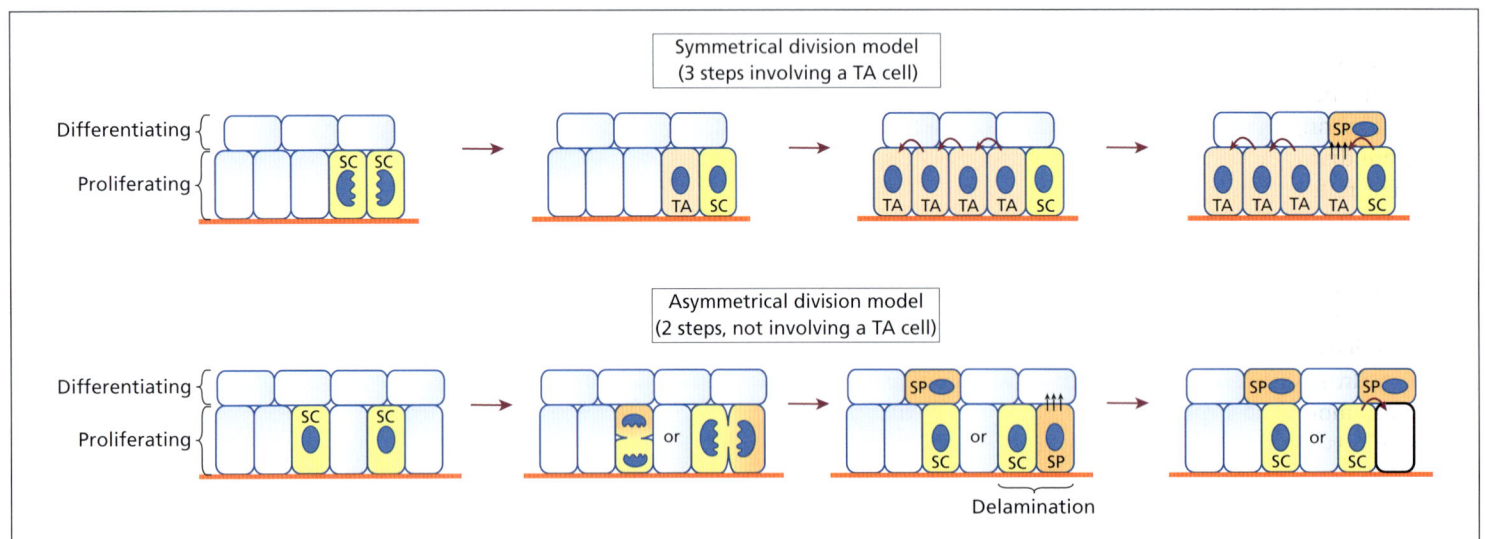

Figure 2.63 Possible mechanisms for the proliferative potential of stem cells (SC) in the basal keratinocyte layer. In the symmetrical division model, two stem cells are produced. Some of these cells in contact with the epidermal basement membrane are transient-amplifying cells (TA). These cells are capable of dividing four to five times before leaving the basal layer (delamination, small black arrows) to become a spinous layer cell (SP) and entering terminal differentiation. In the asymmetrical division model, there is preferential partitioning of proliferation-associated factors into the stem cell daughter cell and, conversely, preferential partitioning of differentiation-inducing components into the daughter cell that is destined to become an SP. Depending on the orientation of the cell spindle, the daughter cell destined for differentiation can either become an SP directly or delaminate from the basal layer to enter terminal differentiation. *In vivo*, both mechanisms may exist.

function in pilosebaceous unit homeostasis and do not contribute to interfolliclular epidermis unless the skin is wounded.

Hair follicles undergo cycles of degeneration and regeneration throughout life. During the growth phase (anagen), which requires activation of hair follicle stem cells, matrix cells proliferate rapidly but then undergo sudden apoptosis (catagen). The hair bulb and root shrivel to form an epithelial strand which forces the dermal papilla to rest at the base of the non-cycling part of the hair follicle [7]. The hairs then enter a resting phase (telogen). At a molecular level, inhibition of BMP signalling and activation of Wnt signalling converge to regulate stem cell activation. From microarray studies, *Sox9*, *Tcf3* and *Lhx2* appear to be markers of follicular stem cells whether they are quiescent or proliferative.

Apart from stem cells in the hair follicles and interfollicular epidermis, other cells in the dermis and subcutis may have stem cell properties. These include cells that have been termed skin-derived precursors, which can differentiate into both neural and mesodermal progeny. In addition, a subset of dermal fibroblasts can have adipogenic, osteogenic, chondrogenic, neurogenic and hepatogenic differentiation potential. Moreover, dermal fibroblasts can be reprogrammed into cells bearing an embryonic stem cell (pluripotent) phenotype by the insertion of just four key transcription factors, *Oct4*, *Sox2*, *Klf4* and *Myc* [8].

Skin ageing

Skin ageing represents an inevitable physiological consequence of getting older, but the impact on personal health and well-being can be significant. Considerable efforts have therefore been made to understand the biology and pathophysiology of skin ageing to try to identify new targets that might offer therapeutic intervention and prevention.

For many years, attempts have been made to define and characterise the physiological and pathological changes that occur in skin ageing, which is often subdivided into intrinsic (chronological) skin ageing and photoageing (sun-exposed sites). However, it is clear that this distinction is somewhat arbitrary, with light microscopy typically showing overlapping features of loss of collagen fibres, elastic fibre disruption, irregular pigmentation, a reduced number of thin hair follicles with grey hairs and altered inflammatory cells in the dermis, as well as shared age-associated physical changes such as reduced epidermal water-retaining capacity and reduced skin surface acidification (Figure 2.64) [1]. The often lax appearance to aged skin, however, does not reflect changes in skin water content. Indeed, the amount of water may not alter in intrinsically aged skin. In skin ageing, there is an increase in the number of mast cells, mononuclear cells and neutrophils. In photoageing, the fibroblasts show a stellate phenotype and, ultrastructurally, a highly activated endoplasmic reticulum, reflecting increased biosynthetic activity. With age, there are increasing levels of circulating pro-inflammatory cytokines and a shift towards cellular senescence, sometimes referred to as 'inflammaging' [2].

Age often decreases sensory perception and increases the threshold for pain. Aged skin displays a progressive disorganisation or loss of some sense organs; for example, the density of Meissner corpuscles in terminal digit skin falls from over 30/mm² in young adults

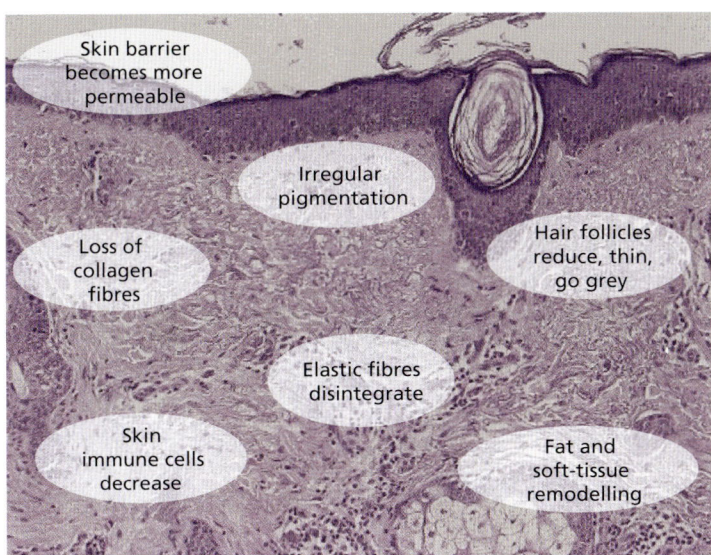

Figure 2.64 Structural and functional changes associated with skin ageing.

to approximately 12/mm² by the age of 70 years. Langerhans cells become considerably reduced in number in elderly people, even in sun-protected areas. There is a reduction in the number of epidermal Langerhans cells with age, coupled with a reduced ability to migrate from the epidermis in response to tumour necrosis factor α, although exogenous IL-1β can improve the impaired Langerhans cell migration in aged skin.

Peripheral immune function is altered in the elderly [3]. The responses of both T and B cells to specific mitogens change in elderly skin, despite the fact that the absolute numbers of T and B cells do not alter significantly. Nevertheless, a decreased intensity in delayed hypersensitivity reactions, an increased risk of photocarcinogenesis [4] and a greater susceptibility to chronic skin infections are all consequences of the ageing of the (skin) immune system. Additional contributors to ageing may include endocrine factors, nutritional or calorie intake, mechanical stress/tissue tension or inflammation and electromagnetic radiation.

Understanding why and precisely how these changes in the skin occur is a major challenge and one that is pivotal in trying to develop new and effective therapeutic agents that can delay or prevent the ageing skin phenotype [5]. One approach in trying to address this has involved the comparison of young and old skin, using various chemical, physical, biological and molecular techniques, and over the last 60 years several theories have been proposed to explain ageing (in general and in the skin). In the 1950s, oxidative damage, with an accumulation of free oxygen radicals capable of damaging cell proteins, lipids and nucleic acids, was considered to be an aetiological factor. Further cellular changes that promoted ageing were suggested to include the accumulation of nuclear DNA damage, misfolded proteins and increased frequency of mitochondrial DNA deletions, as well as alteration in the regulation of cell polarity [6]. These are not mutually exclusive contributors and indeed chronic inflammation, both immune and non-immune mediated, has been identified as another factor that can promote ageing, in a manner linked to oxidative damage.

Apart from cellular damage, other factors may include telomere shortening, as ageing cells fail to express sufficient telomerase to maintain the telomere ends that prevent replicative senescence [7]. Overall, it is plausible that different types of damage occur at different rates in a population of individuals, with a variable impact (timing and extent of ageing) as thresholds for toxicity are reached. Indeed, studies on fibroblast cell senescence in culture have identified the contribution of cell stress, the accumulation of intracellular damage and the secretion of factors that can affect the behaviour of other cells in their vicinity. Thus, the surrounding microenvironment that bathes cells may have a direct impact on cellular ageing, tissue integrity and the ageing phenotype.

One other investigative approach in skin ageing has been to focus on differences in the severity and time course of skin ageing between different individuals. This has been done predominantly using genomics platforms facilitated by improvements in the annotation of the human genome as well as new technical advances for functional studies. The concept has been that key events in ageing might be gleaned from the analysis of cohorts of individuals who demonstrate traits such as shorter or longer than average lifespans, as well as those with phenotypically accelerated forms of ageing such as the progeria syndromes [8]. Such studies do not relate exclusively to skin ageing but, as an expression of the ageing process, skin provides a useful model to observe the downstream functional consequences of specific variations in the genome that might be implicated in ageing.

From a reductionist point of view, rare genetic diseases, in which the pathology associated with normal ageing seems to accumulate at an accelerated rate, also have the potential to improve our understanding of the pathophysiology of normal skin ageing. These conditions include diseases such as the Werner syndrome, Hutchinson–Gilford progeria syndrome, Cockayne syndrome and trichothiodystrophy. Collectively, molecular characterisation of these diseases has identified particular abnormalities in enhanced DNA damage, defective DNA repair, genomic instability, susceptibility to genotoxic stress and impaired epigenetic homeostasis – processes which, when studied in specific individual disease models, demonstrate some overlap with ageing-related events. For example, fibroblasts from individuals with Hutchinson–Gilford progeria syndrome show similar changes to normally aged fibroblasts with regard to increased reactive oxygen species accumulation, increased basal DNA damage, reduced proliferation and early senescence. It is plausible, although not yet proven, that more common coding or non-coding variants in the genes that cause these rare monogenic syndromes (i.e. less disruptive changes than the disease-associated mutations) may confer some increased or decreased susceptibility to ageing via similar processes that occur on a grander scale in the rare genetic diseases.

With regard to photoageing, studies on the pathological changes following UV exposure have provided other insights into skin ageing mechanisms. For example, it is known that UV radiation can induce the synthesis of various destructive enzymes, specifically the MMPs [9]. Notably, there is increased expression of MMP1, MMP3 and MMP9. The MMP1 enzyme can cleave the major interstitial collagens type I and type III and these fragments can be further degraded by MMP3 and MMP9. It has also been shown that different individuals can have variable activity in the MMP1 enzyme and that some of this variability may be due to functional polymorphisms within the promoter of the MMP1 gene. Of note, at the −1607 position, there is a common polymorphic variant that either gives a single G nucleotide or a GG sequence. This GG sequence creates a binding site for ETS (E26 transformation-specific) transcription factors that leads to increased activity of MMP1 and a greater breakdown in dermal collagen.

It is possible that this single nucleotide polymorphism in MMP1 (or others with similar functionality) might provide some insight into differential rates of skin ageing: those with the GG genotype might be prone to accelerated or more marked visible changes of skin ageing. For now, however, this possibility is merely speculative. Nevertheless, the GG genotype in the MMP1 promoter has been shown to have a marked effect on contrasting skin phenotypes, for example in the severity of scarring in the inherited blistering skin disorder recessive dystrophic epidermolysis bullosa. MMP1 activity has also been shown to be greater in the skin of smokers (sun-exposed and sun-protected), a finding that may partially explain why many smokers display greater signs of skin ageing compared with age-matched non-smokers [10]. Nevertheless, MMP1 is just one of $c.20\,000$ genes and it is clear that the analysis of single genes in isolation is not the optimal approach in trying to dissect out what contributes to a skin ageing phenotype in the general population.

With regard to the extracellular matrix gene expression patterns, there is typically a markedly increased expression of elastic fibre components in photoaged skin, with reduced expression of some dermal collagens during skin ageing (particularly in intrinsically aged skin), although a paradoxical increase in some collagens can occur in both photoageing and intrinsic ageing [11]. Aside from different changes in extracellular matrix patterns of gene expression, some similarities occur for markers of stress in aged skin that are indicative of oxidative stress. Of note, all aged skin shows a decreased capacity to detoxify hydrogen peroxide and other free radicals along with reduced antioxidant defences.

Overall, it is evident that intrinsic ageing and photoageing clearly affect many of the same biological processes. Themes common to both types of skin ageing include abnormalities in lipid biosynthesis, epidermal differentiation and oxidative stress. Contrasting differences between photoaged and intrinsically aged skin mainly involve extracellular matrix composition. Transcriptomic analysis also provides clues to biomarkers of aged skin, particularly involving abnormalities of proteases, matrix proteins and inflammation as well as structural protein pathology in both the epidermis and dermis. The challenge will be to see whether these types of data will generate new targets for intervention and a rationale for developing new agents that delay or prevent some of the pathophysiological changes noted at both an individual gene/protein level as well as in the analysis of integrated or interactive biological pathways. An -omics approach to dissecting the pathophysiology of skin ageing is insightful at a basic science level, and at least provides a platform for further anti-ageing research and therapies, particularly to counter the visible effects of skin ageing.

Key references

The full list of references can be found in the online version at https://www.wiley.com/rooksdermatology10e

Skin development
3 Botting RA, Haniffa M. The developing immune network in human skin. *Immunology* 2020;160:149–56.

Keratinocytes
1 Redmond CJ, Coulombe PA. Intermediate filaments as effectors of differentiation. *Curr Opin Cell Biol* 2021;68:155–62.

Skin immune ecosystem
2 Kabashima K, Honda T, Ginhoux F, Egawa G. The immunological anatomy of the skin. *Nat Rev Immunol* 2019;19:19–30.

Skin microbiome
1 Ederveen THA, Smits JPH, Boekhorst J, Schalkwijk J, van den Bogaard EH, Zeeuwen PLJM. Skin microbiota in health and disease: from sequencing to biology. *J Dermatol* 2020;47:1110–18.

Mast cells
4 Olivera A, Rivera J. Paradigm shifts in mast cell and basophil biology and function: an emerging view of immune regulation in health and disease. *Methods Mol Biol* 2020;2163:3–31.

Tight junctions
2 Yokouchi M, Kubo A. Maintenance of tight junction barrier integrity in cell turnover and skin diseases. *Exp Dermatol* 2018;27:876–83.

Laminins
1 Nyström A, Bruckner-Tuderman L. Matrix molecules and skin biology. *Semin Cell Dev Biol* 2019;89:136–46.

Fibroblasts
1 Shaw TJ, Rognoni E. Dissecting fibroblast heterogeneity in health and fibrotic disease. *Curr Rheumatol Rep* 2020;22:33.

Physiological functions of skin
4 Li KN, Tumbar T, Li KN et al. Hair follicle stem cells as a skin-organizing signaling center during adult homeostasis. *EMBO J* 2021;40:e107135.

Skin homeostasis
2 Dekoninck S, Blanpain C. Stem cell dynamics, migration and plasticity during wound healing. *Nat Cell Biol* 2019;21:18–24.

CHAPTER 3

Histopathology of the Skin: General Principles

Eduardo Calonje and John Mee

St John's Institute of Dermatology, Guy's and St Thomas' NHS Foundation Trust, London, UK

Introduction, 3.1
Biopsy of the skin, 3.2
Techniques of skin biopsy, 3.3
Information to be provided with the specimen, 3.4
Care of the specimen, 3.4
Laboratory methods, 3.5
Specimen preparation, 3.5
Routine tissue processing, 3.7
Routine staining techniques, including histochemistry, 3.7
Immunopathology, 3.10

Immunofluorescence methods, 3.10
Immunoenzyme methods, 3.14
Applications of immunopathology techniques, 3.16
Other diagnostic methods, 3.29
Cytodiagnosis and Tzanck smears, 3.29
Electron microscopy, 3.30
Viral disease techniques, 3.31
Immunogenotyping, 3.31
Artefacts, 3.31
Digital pathology, 3.32

Approach to microscopic examination of tissue sections, 3.32
Preparing for microscopy, 3.32
Microscopic interpretation, 3.33
How to produce a histopathology skin report, 3.38
Commonly used descriptive terms in dermatopathology and their diagnostic significance, 3.38
Histological sections that reveal little or no abnormality, 3.44
Conclusions, 3.45
Key references, 3.45

Introduction

As well as clinical examination, microscopic examination of skin tissue is probably the single most important diagnostic ancillary technique used by dermatologists in the management of patients with skin disorders. The correlation of clinical appearances with the dermatopathological findings is not only of direct benefit to individual patients, but has also led to the recognition of many new skin disorders and increased our understanding of the mechanisms of skin disease. The science and art of dermatopathology had its beginnings in early 19th century Europe with the writings of pioneers such as Simon, von Baerensprung and Gans. It is interesting that these individuals were dermatologists, and this tradition of dermatologists writing about histopathological aspects of skin disease was carried on by researchers such as P. Unna, F. Pinkus, A. Civatte, J. Darier, H. Montgomery, H. Pinkus and W. Lever, and in the last half of the 20th century by R.K. Winkelmann, E. Wilson-Jones and A.B. Ackermann. During the last 20 years, the definition of numerous new disease entities and great advances in histopathological and related techniques have led to a wealth of publications on the histopathology of skin disease. Many major reference texts are now available [1–3,4].

Close cooperation between the clinician and the diagnostic dermatopathologist is not only desirable, but also essential. The spectrum of skin disease, including rare genetic disorders, infectious diseases, neoplasms and a wide range of inflammatory disorders, is huge, and although in many conditions the histological features are relatively distinctive of a particular skin disorder, in others the changes may be fairly non-specific. Only by close liaison between the disciplines of clinical dermatology and histopathology can the usefulness and limitations of skin biopsy examination be appreciated. The clinician who reviews the histology of his or her own biopsies appreciates the problems of interpretation of an inadequate biopsy, a biopsy from an inappropriate or unrepresentative lesion, and the effects of artefact caused by undue trauma at the time of biopsy. The pathologist in turn can learn, for instance, that epidermal spongiosis, exocytosis of lymphocytes and mild dermal inflammatory changes are the hallmark of a spongiotic process and that a wide variety of clinical entities may show a similar histological picture. Using the term 'chronic non-specific dermatitis' to denote this picture is unhelpful and misleading. What the pathologist should do is to closely correlate the clinical picture with the histological findings and try to reach a more specific diagnosis. Even if this is not possible, the clinician often finds it very useful if a number of differential diagnoses are ruled out.

Dermatopathology as a medical specialty continues to be an expanding discipline, as witnessed by the plethora of publications (including original papers and books), the development of many national societies for dermatopathology and the many international meetings. In the UK for more than three decades, the Diploma in Dermatopathology of the Royal College of Pathologists has assessed proficiency in dermatopathology for both pathologists and dermatologists. In Europe, a similar exam has been established by the European Union of Medical Specialists/Sections of Dermatovenereology and of Pathology [5]. This initiative has been received enthusiastically by physicians in both specialties not only throughout Europe but also worldwide. The exam has been so successful that it also takes place in Latin America and Asia under the auspices of the Ibero-Latin American and Asian Societies of Dermatopathology.

Biopsy of the skin

A thorough understanding of both the indications for skin biopsy and the various biopsy techniques and their limitations is essential if the histopathologist is to provide the maximum useful information from the study of biopsy sections [6–8]. In addition to light microscopic examination of paraffin-embedded tissue, material obtained from skin biopsy may be used for a variety of investigative procedures. These include ultrastructural examination (only very seldom used nowadays), immunofluorescence studies, antigen mapping in congenital bullous disorders, immunohistochemistry, microbiological studies, tissue culture and molecular biological methods such as *in situ* hybridisation (including FISH: fluorescent *in situ* hybridisation), polymerase chain reaction (PCR), mainly for immunoglobulin, T-cell-receptor gene rearrangement studies and infectious diseases, comparative genomic hybridisation, SNP (single nucleotide polymorphism) arrays and next generation sequencing. Molecular techniques will not be discussed in the chapter. The various investigative techniques often require specific specimens and transport conditions. The individual undertaking skin biopsy should have a clear idea, before carrying out the procedure, of the studies that are to be performed on the specimen obtained. It should be borne in mind that division of the specimen into many small portions for various techniques such as culture, direct immunofluorescence studies and light microscopy may lead to specimens being too small, too unrepresentative or too traumatised to provide useful results. It is often better to perform two biopsies or more to guarantee enough tissue to maximise the amount of information from the samples obtained.

Of the various indications for skin biopsy (Box 3.1), a diagnostic skin biopsy is frequently used to confirm a clinical diagnosis or to aid in the establishment of a diagnosis where a clinical diagnosis is not apparent. An excisional biopsy is the method of choice in treatment of skin lesions, particularly malignant neoplasms. It is less often used to remove lesions for cosmetic reasons.

> **Box 3.1 Indications for skin biopsy**
> - Excision of epidermal or dermal neoplasm, whether benign or malignant. Clear margins are required in a malignant neoplasm
> - An incisional biopsy (shave or punch biopsy) for confirmation of diagnosis of a lesion too big for removal, which will be treated by alternative methods, e.g. more complex surgery (wide excision, Mohs), radiotherapy or cryotherapy. Most useful for basal cell carcinoma or *in situ* squamous cell carcinoma (Bowen disease); avoid in melanocytic lesions, particularly lesions suspected of melanoma
> - An incisional biopsy of a hard-to-categorise skin eruption. Most will be inflammatory and a punch biopsy is often performed; sometimes cutaneous T-cell lymphoma is suspected and more than one biopsy may be necessary
> - Fresh-tissue incisional skin biopsies for immunopathological study, especially immunofluorescence, in suspected autoimmune dermatoses, e.g. blistering disorders (perilesional skin) or lupus erythematosus (lesional skin)
> - Simultaneous processing of contiguous incisional biopsies for pathology and for culture of fresh, unfixed tissue when infection is suspected. The tissue can be cultured for various organisms including mycobacteria and deep fungi or examined for protozoa or filarial worms

The type of biopsy, the selection of the site to be biopsied and the type of lesion to be biopsied, where there is a widespread eruption, are of utmost importance. Ideally, the lesion biopsied should be an early and untreated lesion and representative of the skin disorder as a whole. Avoiding secondary changes is crucial to obtain adequate information. Excoriated lesions and areas where secondary changes may obscure the primary features should be avoided. If lesions are present at all stages of evolution, such as may be seen in pityriasis lichenoides, it may be appropriate to biopsy more than one lesion. Multiple biopsies are also often helpful in conditions such as early cutaneous T-cell lymphoma (mycosis fungoides), where definite histopathological diagnosis is often difficult. Normal skin should be included with a diagnostic biopsy wherever possible, and the inclusion of perilesional skin is essential when submitting biopsies for direct immunofluorescence studies. In certain conditions, such as connective tissue naevi, the changes may be subtle and comparison with normal neighbouring skin may be very helpful. When this is done the clinician should mark the area of normal skin with a stitch to facilitate comparison. It is equally important to ensure that the biopsy is deep enough. It is frustrating for the pathologist and clinician alike to receive a specimen with a request form suggesting a diagnosis of panniculitis where sections from the biopsy show only a portion of epidermis and superficial dermis. The general tendency in cases suspected of panniculitis is to perform a punch biopsy. However, not infrequently, the information obtained from this type of biopsy in the setting of panniculitis is minimal and, ideally, a large, deep incisional biopsy should be performed to obtain maximum yield. If lesions are widespread and there is a choice of biopsy sites, it is sensible to avoid areas liable to heal badly, such as areas over bony prominences and the lower limbs, and to avoid cosmetically important areas. Secondary changes in some areas of the body, such as changes of venous stasis in biopsies from the lower legs of older people, may be confusing to the inexperienced diagnostic dermatopathologist, and such sites are also best avoided.

Prior to skin biopsy, written informed consent is normally obtained from the patient, and in all but the smallest biopsies, local anaesthetic – usually 1% or 2% lidocaine (lignocaine) with or without epinephrine (adrenaline) – is injected around the biopsy site. Superficial blebs resulting from injecting local anaesthetic into the skin itself should be avoided. Injection of too much local anaesthetic into one area of the skin can cause a prominent distortion artefact in sections that are prepared from biopsy tissue. The effect of epinephrine on dermal blood vessels and mast cells has probably been overemphasised in the past. However, when performing biopsies for conditions such as urticaria pigmentosa, it may be prudent either to avoid the biopsy site itself and inject the anaesthetic in a circle around it or to use an anaesthetic not containing epinephrine. Epinephrine and other vasoconstrictors should not be used in biopsies taken from the fingers or toes, as occasional intense vasospasm can result in tissue necrosis. Topical anaesthetic creams or gels are available as an alternative to injections for removal of superficial skin lesions. These topical anaesthetics are particularly helpful for biopsies performed in children and for biopsies obtained from genital skin. The main topical anaesthetic used is a combination of lignocaine and prilocaine (EMLA: eutectic mixture of local anaesthetics). Although this topical preparation is extremely useful, it is important to know that it may cause secondary histological changes that may alter the interpretation of the biopsy. This is due to an irritant contact dermatitis and seems to be associated with the time of exposure to the medication and is more common in samples taken from patients with inflammatory dermatoses [9,10]. The histological changes consist of vacuolar change of keratinocytes in the upper layers of the epidermis, clefting at the dermal–epidermal junction with pallor of the superficial layers of the epidermis, lysis of keratinocytes and granular basophilic material, papillary dermal oedema and congestion of small superficial blood vessels.

Techniques of skin biopsy (Table 3.1)

Elliptical surgical biopsy [8]

This is one of the most commonly used diagnostic skin biopsy techniques. The equipment required includes scalpel, fine-toothed forceps, needle holder, scissors and eyeless needle with suture (Figure 3.1). The use of a skin hook greatly facilitates manipulation of the biopsy specimen and avoids undue trauma. A reasonable size for an elliptical biopsy is about 5 mm, but smaller specimens may be adequate where indicated for cosmetic reasons. Small lesions may be totally excised, but a biopsy of a larger lesion should be at right angles through the margin to include adjacent normal skin. The long axis of the wound should, where possible, follow the natural crease lines of the skin. For suspicious melanocytic lesions, a simple excision with narrow margins is performed and this is followed by a wider excision on confirmation of the diagnosis. A full discussion of surgical techniques and suture materials is beyond the scope of this chapter, but there are several excellent reviews [7,8] and issues relating to dermatological surgery are discussed in Chapter 20.

Punch biopsy [11]

The biopsy punch is a metal cylinder of variable diameter with a sharp cutting edge at one end, usually attached to a plastic handle (Figure 3.2). The punch is pushed into the skin with a downward twisting movement, and then removed. The tissue specimen is lifted and separated from the underlying tissue, and removed from the biopsy punch. The wound may be left to heal without suturing, the base of the wound being cauterised by electrocautery or some other haemostatic agent. Many operators, however, prefer to insert one or two sutures to secure haemostasis.

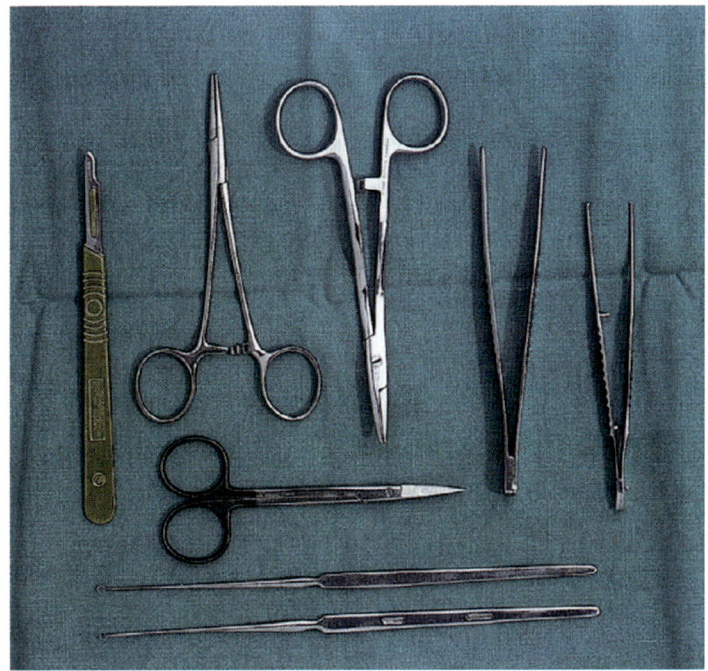

Figure 3.1 Instruments for skin biopsy, including scalpel, scissors, needle holder and skin hooks.

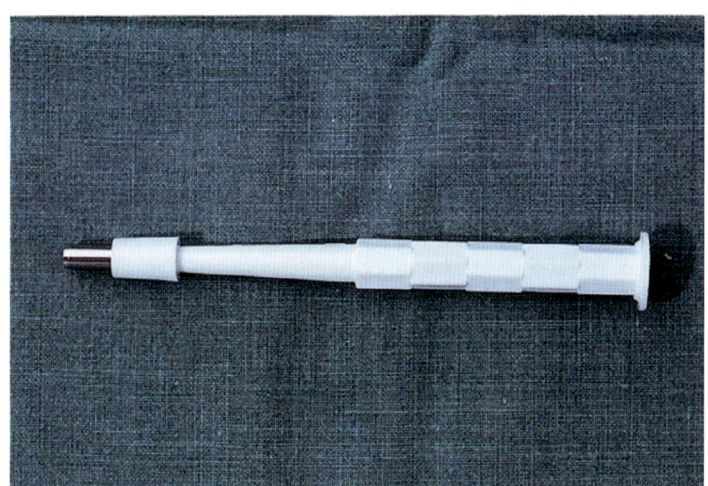

Figure 3.2 Disposable punch for cutaneous biopsy.

Punch biopsies are convenient and quick to use, but it is preferable to use at least a 3 mm punch to obtain a satisfactory specimen. A problem with small punch biopsies is that the specimen is often difficult to orientate, and most pathologists greatly prefer elliptical excision biopsies for diagnostic interpretation. Nevertheless, punch biopsies play an important role in busy out-patient departments and office practices, particularly for the diagnosis and management of small cutaneous lesions and in the diagnosis of inflammatory processes.

Curettage [12,13]

The technique of curettage with a sharp-edged Volkmann spoon or disposable curette followed by cautery is often used for the treatment of small benign and malignant skin lesions, such as viral warts, solar and seborrhoeic keratoses, and basal cell carcinomas.

Table 3.1 Skin biopsy techniques [6–8].

Technique	Application
Excision	For removal of a single lesion; an elliptical or fusiform-shaped area of skin is removed
Incision biopsy ('wedge')	Similar to excision, but narrower; to include fat in suspected panniculitis; some normal perilesional skin is included for comparison
Punch biopsy (3–6 mm)	Useful if tissue available is limited, but accurate sampling is essential; a rapid procedure, sometimes useful in children
Curettage	For hyperkeratotic lesions, e.g. seborrhoeic keratoses, viral warts, basal cell carcinomas; usually accompanied by cautery
Shave biopsy	For facial protuberant lesions, e.g. benign intradermal naevi
Snip	For skin tags; skin snips also for onchocerciasis

The resulting specimen is fragmented, and it is often impossible to comment on adequacy of removal. A combination of curettage and shave excision has been proposed to overcome this problem. Curettage alone is more useful as a therapeutic procedure than as a technique for providing ideal specimens for histopathological diagnosis. It must be emphasised that all specimens should be submitted for histopathological examination. Haemostasis may be achieved by electrocautery, alginate dressings or using aluminium chloride hexahydrate solution on a cotton bud rolled over the wound. It is important to mention a further haemostatic agent, Monsel solution (ferric subsulphate) that is no longer widely used but may cause problems in the histological interpretation of re-excision specimens. The pigment coats the collagen bundles and induces a histiocytic reaction with numerous siderophages [14]. This may make the interpretation of biopsies very difficult, particularly in the setting of melanocytic lesions.

Shave biopsy

Certain superficial, benign papular or nodular lesions may be treated by shaving off the lesion flush with the surface of the surrounding skin. Many sorts of superficial skin lesion may be treated in this way, in particular melanocytic naevi. Although often a useful cosmetic result may be obtained, this technique has several drawbacks. The whole lesion is rarely removed, and recurrence of the lesion is sometimes a problem. In the case of melanocytic naevi, lesions that recur following partial excision often demonstrate atypical histopathological features, sometimes leading to an erroneous diagnosis of a malignant lesion (pseudomelanoma phenomenon) [15]. This technique is also used to confirm the diagnosis of non-melanoma skin cancers, namely, basal cell carcinoma and squamous cell carcinoma. However, its use should be discouraged in the latter as it is often very difficult or impossible to distinguish between an *in situ* squamous cell carcinoma and an invasive neoplasm due to the superficial nature of the sample or to problems with orientation. As with the techniques of curettage and punch biopsy, the wounds resulting from the procedure of shave biopsy normally require some form of cauterisation or use of aluminium chloride hexahydrate to achieve haemostasis.

Other biopsy techniques

Various other ways of obtaining portions of skin tissue for diagnostic purposes have been described, including needle biopsy, similar to that used for tissue diagnosis of liver disease and lymph node pathology (see section on cytodiagnosis and Tzank smears). The results from such a technique are generally unsatisfactory for skin lesions, and in no way compare with those achieved using more conventional surgical procedures. Techniques for slit-skin smears for leprosy and skin snips for onchocerchiasis are discussed in Chapters 28 and 33, respectively.

Information to be provided with the specimen

For the clinician to obtain the optimum help from the pathologist, it is essential that full clinical details be provided. A fully completed histopathology request form should include the following details for each specimen. The patient should be identified by name, sex, age and usually a hospital reference number, or some other identification record number. It is useful to know the patient's racial group, as prominent epidermal basal layer melanin pigmentation may be pathological in some situations but represents normal skin for other individuals. A brief clinical history of the duration of the skin condition should be provided, together with details of any treatment including topical and systemic therapy. Ideally, a clinical differential diagnosis should be provided. The site of each biopsy taken should be clearly identified on the request form, and accompanied by specimens in separate, individually labelled containers. Unfortunately, it is not uncommon to receive several biopsies from what are thought to be trivial lesions from the same patient in one container. Sometimes it turns out that one of these lesions is histologically malignant and the others are benign and, in these circumstances, it may be impossible to determine the site of the malignant tumour.

Details of previous biopsies, and where possible the histopathology report reference numbers, should always be included on a request form, and finally a suggested clinical diagnosis or list of differential diagnoses is helpful. Where possible, abbreviations should be avoided. It may be that many pathologists will recognise the letters PLC as standing for pityriasis lichenoides chronica, but perhaps there would be fewer who would immediately recognise the letters TMEP as representing a form of urticaria pigmentosa.

Finally, but most importantly, the dermatologist or surgeon sending the biopsy material to the pathologist should give some clear indication on the request form from whom the biopsy is being sent, or to whom the report should be forwarded. If some of the simple advice above were more often heeded by clinicians performing biopsies, it would make the life of a dermatopathologist very much easier.

Care of the specimen

Care is required throughout the biopsy procedure to avoid trauma to the specimen with forceps or any of the other instruments used during biopsy. The use of skin hooks in manipulating the specimen during biopsy is helpful in this respect [16] and, in order to avoid trauma artefact, the division of small specimens into multiple smaller portions of tissue for different diagnostic purposes should be avoided. If a specimen is needed for four separate studies – such as paraffin embedding, direct immunofluorescence studies, electron microscopy and microbiological culture – it is often better to take two separate specimens and divide each of these into two portions than to attempt to divide one specimen into quarters. Biopsies taken for ultrastructural studies should be small (of the order of 1–2 mm cubes) to allow for adequate fixation. Skin samples for electron microscopy should be placed into fixative first, i.e. before other skin samples are put into their respective fixatives for other pathology studies.

For routine diagnostic microscopy of paraffin-embedded material, 10% neutral buffered formalin is still the most widely used fixative and is satisfactory for most purposes [17]. Many other fixatives and transport media such as Michel medium (Table 3.2) [17] are available, and these are indicated for either the study of specific diseases or tissue components, or for the application of specific diagnostic techniques such as immunofluorescence [18]. The use of Michel medium allows the preservation of antigens for immunofluorescence studies for up to 6 months [19]. By using Michel medium, specimens may be sent safely without the need for immediate freezing. This medium is also useful for fixation of samples used in

Table 3.2 Michel transport medium for fresh cutaneous tissue.

Component of medium	Reagents
Ammonium sulphate Buffer	55 g in 100 mL buffer 1 mol/L potassium citrate (pH 7), 2.5 mL 0.1 mol/L magnesium sulphate, 5 mL 0.1 mol/L ethyl maleimide, 5 mL Distilled water, 87.5 mL Mix 1 : 2 with 1 mol/L potassium hydroxide to pH 7.0

immunoelectron microscopy studies [20], seems to preserve the antigens relevant for the investigation of genetic blistering skin diseases [21] and may be used for short-term preservation of DNA in samples submitted for DNA analysis [22]. The specimen has to be washed thoroughly on receipt before freezing it to avoid artefacts. Sodium chloride 0.9% has been proposed as an alternative transport medium to Michel medium [23]. However, preservation of antigens only lasts for 24 h and frequent artefacts, including hydropic degeneration of keratinocytes and splitting of the dermal–epidermal junction, are seen. Furthermore, this method is not suitable for samples obtained for immunoelectron microscopy or antigen mapping. Table 3.3 gives some details of the more important fixatives and transport media. Honey has also been advocated as a transport medium for direct immunofluorescence samples and antigen mapping, but its efficacy is much less than that of Michel medium after 4 weeks [24].

Laboratory methods

Specimen preparation

Frozen sections are not used routinely in dermatopathology, except for Mohs micrographic surgery (described in Chapter 20) and immunofluorescence. Most antibodies used in diagnostic dermatopathology work adequately in samples fixed in formalin and, except in the context of research, frozen sections are therefore not used on a regular basis for immunohistochemical studies. Frozen sections are used for the diagnosis of autoimmune blistering disorders and also for the diagnosis of blistering genetic skin diseases (antigen mapping, see Chapter 50). Although it has been advocated that autoimmune blistering disorders may be diagnosed with immunohistochemistry performed on samples fixed in formalin, the results are often of inferior quality and interpretation is difficult, leading to false negative and false positive results. This method is therefore not recommended.

Careful identification and preparation of tissue specimens prior to processing is most important. The first requirement is that the biopsy specimen be placed immediately into a fixative solution. Various routine fixatives are employed; most contain 10% formalin. Because a stock solution of formalin consists of 40% formaldehyde, 10% formalin is really 4% formaldehyde. A minimum of 12 h fixation is recommended for most specimens, but small specimens may only need 6 h, and larger specimens a longer period of fixation, to produce optimal results. After fixation, the biopsy tissue is removed from its container, double-checking that the specimen corresponds with details given on the request form, and the pathologist produces a macroscopic description together with details of 'the cut up'.

Special care should be taken where multiple fragments of tissue are present, for example in specimens obtained by curettage. It may be necessary to pass the contents of the biopsy container through a filter paper to ensure that all relevant portions of tissue are processed and examined. After orientating the specimen, a description should be made of the size and shape of the specimen, and a note made of whether subcutaneous or other tissue is included. A careful description of surface changes is then made, with particular reference to changes of colour and surface texture, such as erosion or ulceration. Any obvious clinical lesion present on the gross specimen should be described. In some surgical specimens, an identification label, such as a skin suture, is left in place in the biopsy specimen by the surgeon to enable precise orientation of the specimen. This is particularly important when dealing with neoplastic lesions, where clearance of tumour in the margins of the biopsy specimen needs to be assessed.

Prior to sectioning a gross specimen, especially excised tumours, it is good practice to paint the margins of the biopsy specimen with

Table 3.3 Fixatives and transport media for skin biopsy specimens.

Investigative technique	Fixative/transport medium	Comments
Most routine diagnostic studies on paraffin-processed material	10% neutral buffered formalin solution (pH 7) 10% aqueous formalin (unbuffered) Carnoy solution (pH 2.8)	Most useful fixative for general use H&E staining generally better than with buffered preparation Formalin pigment a nuisance Good preservation of nuclear chromatin Haemolyses red blood cells; use small specimens
Where rapid fixation required	Place specimen in the oven in alcohol	Microwave fixation
Transmission electron microscopy and some electron immunocytochemistry	Karnofsky solution or 2.5% buffered glutaraldehyde solution Post fixation with osmium tetroxide	Small specimens required, normally no more than 1 mm cube
Immunofluorescence and immunoenzyme techniques	Various; periodate lysine paraformaldehyde fixation and cold processing useful for some endothelial cell markers	Various fixatives suitable depending on technique and antigen/substance to be identified Frozen tissue may be required
Transport of specimens for immunofluorescence studies	Michel medium	Specimen must be thoroughly washed in phosphate-buffered saline before immersion in Michel medium
Microbiological studies, studies on fat tissue and some immunohistological investigations	Fresh or frozen tissue	Specimens for microbiological examination should be placed in sterile containers and transported to the laboratory as soon as possible

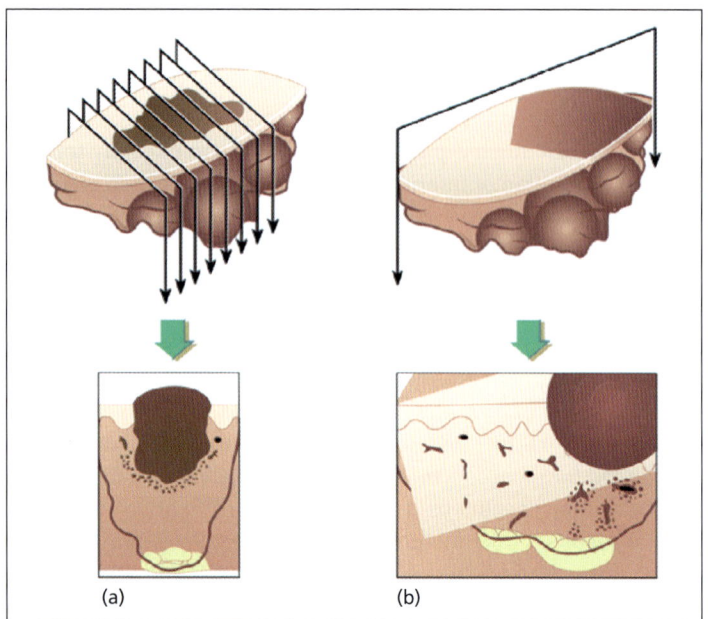

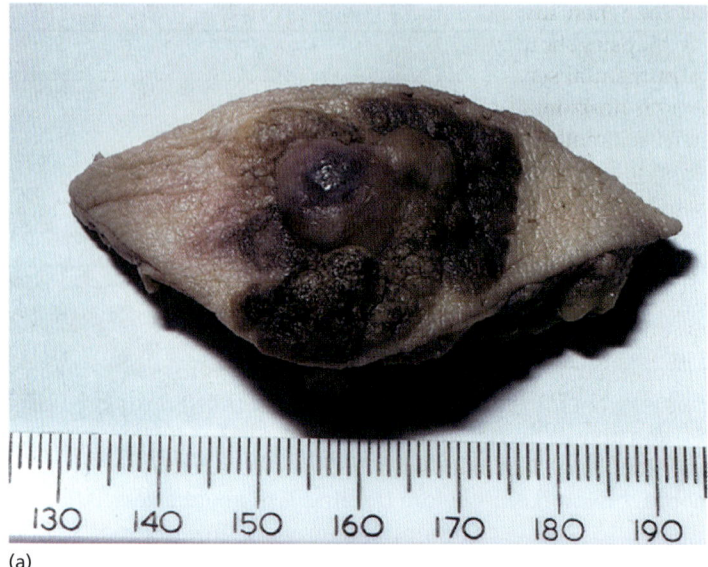

Figure 3.3 Blocking of elliptical skin biopsy specimens. (a) Neoplastic lesions. Multiple transverse blocks through the whole lesion allow for histopathological examination of the tumour at all levels and assessment of the narrowest excision margins. (b) Incisional biopsy of inflammatory lesion. Longitudinal blocking is recommended; this allows optimal visualisation of the affected and adjacent normal skin.

coloured dyes that are resistant to tissue processing. Various commercial preparations are available, and one or several colours may be used. If the dye is visible on the final tissue section examined by the pathologist, this implies that no tissue has been lost in processing, and that the edge of the section corresponds to the genuine margin of the biopsy. After painting the biopsy margins, the gross specimen is then sectioned prior to the preparation of histological blocks. There are various techniques for cutting up a standard elliptical skin biopsy. The ideal method depends to some extent on the nature of the suspected diagnosis. A specimen from an excision biopsy of a benign or malignant skin tumour is better handled by taking transverse blocks through the specimen, so that the narrowest excision margins may be examined. For malignant lesions, particularly for suspected melanoma, ideally transverse blocks should be taken at 2 mm intervals throughout the whole length of the lesion (Figure 3.3a) [1]. An elliptical biopsy taken, for instance, from the margin of a patch of an inflammatory dermatosis, is best sectioned longitudinally, so that both normal and abnormal skin can be visualised (Figure 3.3b). With larger specimens, examination of a selection of transverse blocks made from various portions of the tumour may be adequate for diagnostic purposes. Any biopsy tissue not processed should be labelled and returned to the fixative in the container and stored. Laboratories have different policies regarding the retention of fixed tissue specimens. Ideally, all specimens should be retained, but limitations of space often mean that most routine specimens can be discarded after a period of a few weeks after the histopathological report has been approved and signed.

In addition to a written description of the gross specimen, and how it has been prepared for blocking, a rough diagram of the specimen is very useful, particularly with larger specimens. This enables clear identification of the portion of the specimen from

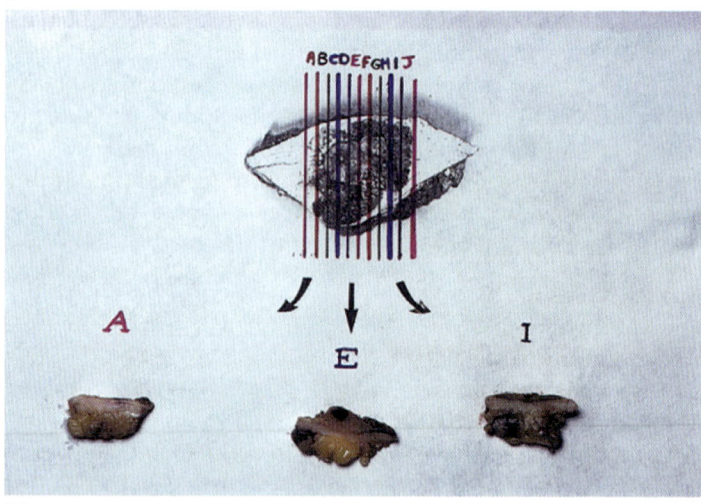

Figure 3.4 Photocopy procedure for recording the preparation of blocks. (a) The appearance of a macroscopic specimen of melanoma. (b) Transverse blocks are taken from the specimen, and their exact position is recorded on a photocopy made from the surface of the gross specimen.

which various blocks have been taken. An alternative approach for larger specimens, especially when dealing with neoplastic lesions, is either to photograph the specimen or to wrap the specimen in clear cling-wrap film and take a photocopy of the surface. This produces an image the same size as the gross specimen, and details of the blocks taken can be recorded directly on the photocopy image (Figure 3.4).

Very small specimens may be blocked in their entirety after trimming. Other blocking techniques may be used for specific purposes. An example is the blocking of transverse sections of cylindrical punch biopsies (at least 4 mm in diameter) of scalp disorders [2,3–5]. This technique is particularly useful in the assessment of various forms of inflammatory alopecia, and facilitates the quantitative morphometric analysis of pilosebaceous follicles and the hair itself. The technique also provides a useful method of studying the morphological details of the normal transverse anatomy of follicular structure, including the various phases of the normal hair cycle.

Ideally, when investigating a condition presenting with alopecia, two biopsies should be provided: one for vertical sectioning and one for horizontal sectioning. It has been shown that the interpretation of both horizontal and vertical sections in scalp biopsies is better than each method on its own to obtain a high diagnostic yield [4]. If immunofluorescence studies are required, the specimen for vertical sectioning can be divided into two portions.

The use of *ex vivo* dermoscopy-guided histological sectioning of melanocytic lesions has been demonstrated to improve accuracy in diagnosis and clinicopathological correlation of these challenging tumours. More recently, *ex vivo* dermoscopy with added derm dotting and adapted sectioning has been advocated as a technique allowing better clinicopathological correlation and more accurate diagnosis in the evaluation not only of melanocytic lesions but also of non-melanoma skin cancers [6–9,**10**]. This technique also allows better evaluation of excision margins and improvement in turnaround reporting times.

Routine tissue processing

Although the skin biopsy specimen may be examined with various techniques, at least a portion of most skin biopsies is routinely processed for light microscopic evaluation of sections from paraffin-embedded tissue. The tissue processing is carried out using automated machines. Two main types of automated tissue-processing machine are in use: the traditional carousel type and the enclosed pumped fluid type. Both types of machine have the facility for multiple separate stages in processing. After completion of fixation the same basic steps of dehydration, clearing and embedding are involved. The process of dehydration removes aqueous fixative and any tissue water. Clearing refers to the use of a substance such as xylene, which is totally miscible with both the dehydrating agent that precedes it and the embedding agent that follows it.

For embedding, paraffin wax at 56°C remains by far the most popular material. It is cheap, large numbers of tissue blocks may be processed in comparatively short times, and later sectioning and staining are straightforward. The use of vacuum impregnation in modern and automated tissue-processing machines considerably reduces the overall processing time. At the end of the embedding procedure, paraffin blocks are cut and stained and are then ready for microscopic examination. The dermatopathologist should be aware of relatively common potential artefacts that can cause confusion and misinterpretation [11]. When urgent preparation of tissue specimens is required, various processing steps can be shortened. The use of very thin portions of tissue, increasing the temperature of the fixative, microwave-fixation techniques [12,13] and shortening the time used for clearing can all facilitate rapid processing. Alternatively, cryostat sections can be examined.

Routine staining techniques, including histochemistry

By far the most widely used stain for sections from skin biopsies used in histopathology laboratories is haematoxylin and eosin (H&E). This staining technique gives good definition of many cellular and tissue structures in the skin, and is sufficient for the diagnosis of most skin diseases. This stain, however, does not clearly demonstrate certain tissue components, such as elastic fibres (Figure 3.5), and does not allow differentiation between melanin, haemosiderin and other skin pigments. Special stains are required for these purposes, and also for confirming the nature of abnormal dermal deposits, such as calcium, mucin and amyloid. Another important indication for special staining techniques is the demonstration of microorganisms. Full details of the techniques and applications of special stains used in diagnostic dermatopathology are given in standard reference texts [14,15,16]. Examples of commonly used staining techniques that are useful in the diagnosis of specific conditions are given below and in Table 3.4.

The periodic acid–Schiff (PAS) stain demonstrates the presence of carbohydrates, particularly some polysaccharides such as glycogen, and mucoproteins containing neutral mucopolysaccharides. These substances are stained reddish purple by the PAS reaction. Because the cell walls of fungi and yeasts contain neutral polysaccharides, they also stain positively with the PAS reaction (Figure 3.6). This is a cheap and reliable diagnostic method, and it has been advocated that a PAS stain should be routinely used in all biopsies of inflammatory dermatoses [17]. The reasoning for this proposal is based on the clinical and histological appearances of tinea often being non-specific. The technique is also useful in demonstrating blood vessel walls, basement membrane (Figure 3.7), fibrin deposition and the presence of glycogen deposits, for instance in certain sweat gland and follicular tumours, such as clear cell hidradenoma, trichilemmoma and some epithelial lesions of uncertain histogenesis, such as the clear cell acanthoma. The identification of glycogen can be further confirmed by removal by enzyme digestion with diastase in 1% aqueous solution at 37°C for 30 min. Positive staining after the use of diastase indicates the presence of neutral mucopolysaccharides.

Table 3.4 Some tinctorial stains used in dermatology.

Special stains	Tissue constituent	Appearance
Periodic acid–Schiff (PAS)	Glycogen	Magenta red (diastase sensitive)
	Mucopolysaccharides	Red (fungal wall red)
Van Gieson	Collagen	Red
	Muscle, nerve	Yellow
Congo red	Amyloid	Red with green birefringence
Acid orcein–Giemsa	Elastic fibre	Dark brown
	Collagen	Pink
	Melanin	Black
	Haemosiderin	Green/yellow
	Amyloid	Light blue
	Mast cell granules	Purple
Masson trichrome	Collagen	Green
	Muscle + fibrin	Red
Aldehyde fuchsin	Elastic fibres	Purple
Gomori	Reticulin	Black
Alcian blue (pH 4.5, 0.5)	Acid mucopolysaccharides	Blue
Toluidine blue	Acid mucopolysaccharides	Metachromatic purple including mast cells
Perls Prussian blue	Iron (haemosiderin)	Blue
Masson Fontana	Melanin	Black
Von Kossa	Calcium salts	Brown/black
Grocott	Fungus wall	Black
Methenamine silver	Bacteria	
	Gram positive	Blue/violet
	Gram negative	Red/pink
Ziehl–Neelsen/Wade–Fite	Acid-fast bacilli	Red

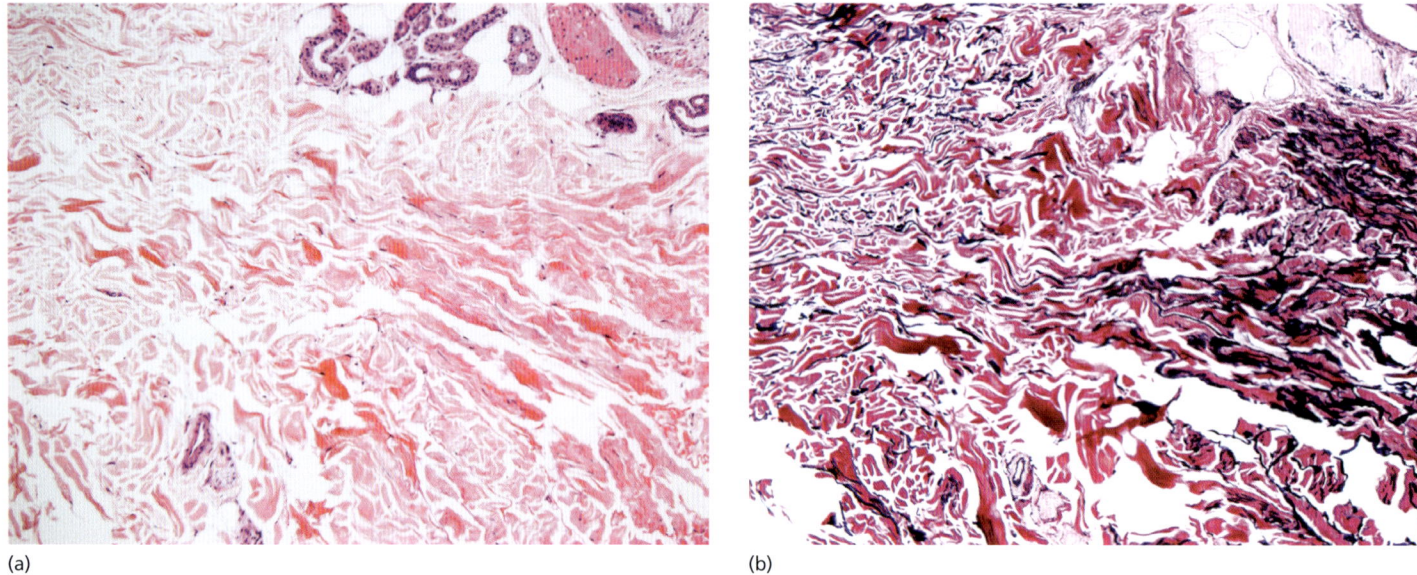

Figure 3.5 (a) Connective tissue naevus. The section stained with H&E only shows focal condensation of the collagen. (b) An elastic van Gieson stain shows marked focal increase in the number of elastic fibres.

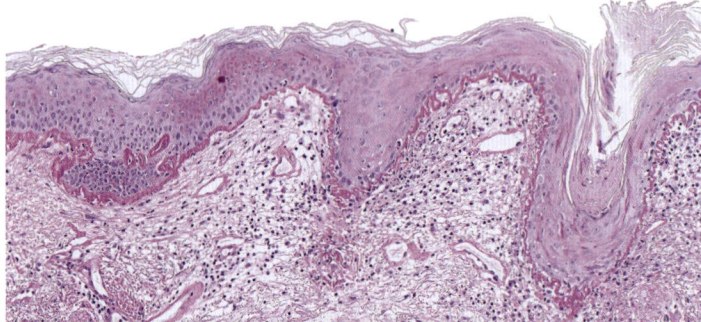

Figure 3.7 Periodic acid–Schiff stain showing thickening of the basement membrane zone in cutaneous lupus erythematosus.

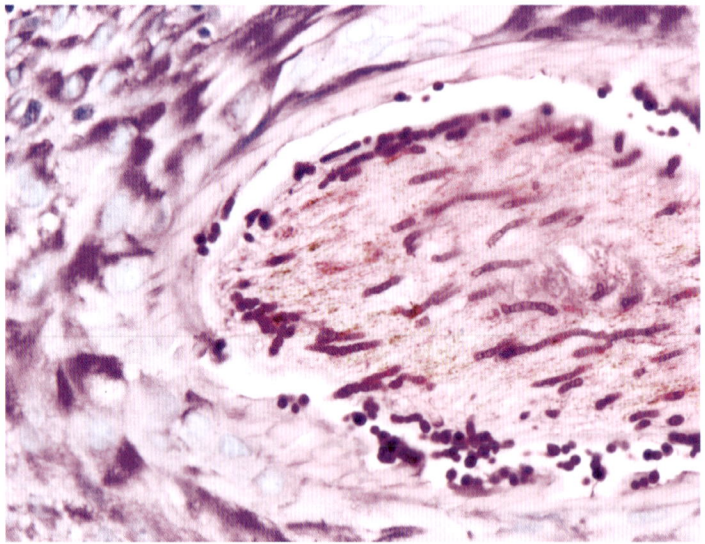

Figure 3.6 Periodic acid–Schiff stain showing numerous hyphae within the hair shaft in an endothrix infection.

The Alcian blue reaction produces a blue coloration in the presence of acid mucopolysaccharides. In addition to demonstrating the presence of mucin in cutaneous mucinoses, the technique is also of value in some cases of extramammary Paget disease, and occasionally in the demonstration of goblet cells in metastatic carcinoma of the gut. There are small amounts of acid mucopolysaccharide present in the ground substance of normal dermis, and the Alcian blue reaction is very pH dependent. Care should therefore be exercised in the interpretation of a positive result.

Acid orcein and Giemsa stain was popularised by Pinkus and Mehregan who recommend its use as a second routine stain [18]. It is a valuable technique that demonstrates, in addition to structures normally visible with H&E stain, the presence of mast cells, eosinophils, metachromatic substances and elastic fibres. The routine use of the orcein–Giemsa stain often avoids the recutting of blocks for other special stains. Orcein itself is a constituent in other staining methods, particularly those used to demonstrate elastic fibres.

Special staining techniques are often essential to differentiate between epidermal and dermal deposits of melanin, haemosiderin and other substances. The Masson ammoniacal silver nitrate technique produces a densely black reaction product with melanin. Melanin deposits appear greenish black with the acid orcein–Giemsa stain. Iron, which in the context of skin biopsy material normally means haemosiderin pigment, is demonstrated by the Perls Prussian blue reaction, which yields a deep blue reaction product in the presence of ferric and ferrous iron (Figure 3.8).

Trichrome stains can demonstrate various elements of connective tissue. Common examples are the van Gieson stain, in which collagen appears red and muscle and nerves yellow, and the Masson trichrome stain, in which collagen is green and muscle red. The latter stain is seldom used nowadays.

Certain types of cells present within the skin may be difficult to recognise on conventional H&E-stained material. Mast cells are best demonstrated either by using a metachromatic staining technique, such as toluidine blue, or with one of the few enzyme histochemical

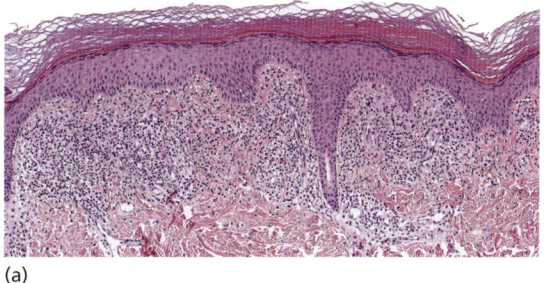
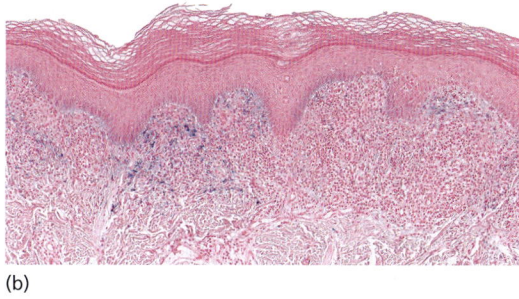

Figure 3.8 (a) A prominent lymphocytic infiltrate which is focally lichenoid and is associated with extravasation of red blood cells in a case of lichen aureus (H&E). (b) Perls stain highlighting numerous haemosiderin-containing macrophages, a useful technique to confirm the diagnosis of lichen aureus.

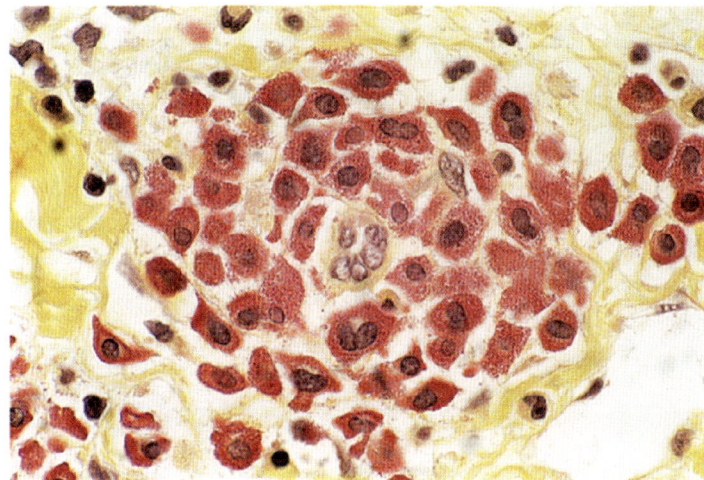

Figure 3.9 Chloroacetate esterase stain. Mast cells appear red with this technique.

methods that may be carried out on paraffin-embedded tissue, such as the chloroacetate esterase reaction. The use of this technique applied to formalin-fixed paraffin sections was described by Leder [19], and mast cells and myeloid white cells are easily identified by their bright pinkish red staining (Figure 3.9). Other histiocytic and dendritic cells that are difficult to visualise on routinely stained material are best visualised with immunohistochemical methods.

Cutaneous deposits of various naturally occurring and foreign substances often require special staining techniques for their demonstration. The von Kossa method produces a black coloration in the presence of calcium salts, and amyloid deposits may be demonstrated using crystal violet or Congo red. With this latter technique, amyloid deposits stain pinkish red, and under polariscopic examination there is a green birefringence. Another technique useful for the demonstration of amyloid deposits is the thioflavine T method, yielding green fluorescence on examination with a fluorescence microscope. Unfortunately, several of the staining techniques recommended for the demonstration of amyloid are technically unreliable, and none is totally specific for amyloidosis. Some cotton dyes other than Congo red, such as pagoda red, have been claimed to be as sensitive as Congo red while being more specific [20]. It is recommended that more than one special stain be used if amyloid is suspected. Occasionally, even with the use of several special stains, amyloid cannot be demonstrated and then electron microscopy is necessary for this purpose.

A wide range of techniques is employed for the demonstration of microorganisms in the skin. Reference has already been made to the usefulness of the PAS stain in the demonstration of yeasts and fungi. The silver staining technique of Grocott is also very helpful in the identification of fungal hyphae and yeast bodies. These structures stain black on a pale green background. Other silver techniques, including the Warthin–Starry technique, are useful in demonstrating spirochaetes and *Bartonella henselae* (the organism that causes bacillary angiomatosis). *Bartonella* may also be demonstrated using a Giemsa stain. The traditional Gram stain demonstrates coccal and bacillary organisms in the skin. Several techniques are available for the demonstration of acid-fast bacilli. The Ziehl–Neelsen method is widely used for the demonstration of mycobacteria, particularly *Mycobacterium tuberculosis*. It is based on the capacity of the lipid-rich cell wall of mycobacteria to take up strong phenol dye solutions. This dye is retained after differentiation in acid or alcohol. Mycobacteria stain magenta and the background is blue. Auramine–rhodamine stain is also a sensitive method for demonstrating mycobacteria in tissue sections. Its main drawback is that it requires the use of a fluorescence microscope for interpretation [21]. The Ziehl–Neelsen method should not be used for the demonstration of leprosy bacilli. The use of this technique often leads to a false negative result. The reason for this is that the leprosy bacilli are less acid- and alcohol-fast. The Wade–Fite stain, or a modification of this technique, is more appropriate for identification of leprosy bacilli and atypical mycobacteria because it uses minimal treatment with alcohol and acid. In fact, in cases with very few organisms, if Ziehl–Neelsen is used instead of Wade–Fite, the diagnosis may be missed.

Even with the above techniques, sensitivity remains very low and the demonstration of small numbers of microorganisms in the skin may be very difficult and may require the examination of many sections. Thankfully, increasing numbers of newer tests for the detection of microorganisms in paraffin-embedded tissue have become available, simplifying the task of pathologists and dermatopathologists. These techniques include *in situ* hybridisation, PCR and immunohistochemistry and are used for the detection of a wide variety of microorganisms, including bacteria, fungi, mycobacteria, viruses, rickettsia and leishmania [22–25,**26**,27–31,**32**,33–36]. Although PCR is a valuable diagnostic tool in infections such as those caused by leishmania, bartonella and rickettsia, this technique has important limitations in the diagnosis of fungal, mycobacterial and RNA viral infections due to the large number of false positive and negative results. PCR is useful in cases with suspicious histology in which special stains have been negative and in which fresh tissue is not available for culture. It is important to highlight that mycobacterial DNA has been found in cutaneous lesions of nodular vasculitis and papulonecrotic tuberculid [37,38]. While this confirms the relationship between these two entities and tuberculosis, it does not necessarily mean that the finding may be interpreted as evidence of tuberculous infection in the affected sites. A polyclonal antibody for BCG is very useful as a screening technique for the presence of fungi and bacteria in tissues and this is based on the presence of wide cross-reactivity of this antibody between different species [39–41]. The antibody is, however, not useful in detecting viruses, leishmania or spirochaetes. A monoclonal antibody to *Treponema pallidum* is very useful and much more sensitive than the silver technique to demonstrate organisms in tissue sections [42]. *Borrelia burgdorferi* can be identified in tissue sections by an immunohistochemical method using focus floating microscopy [28].

Immunopathology

There are some situations where even after careful biopsy of an appropriate lesion, expert tissue processing and sectioning and the use of several special staining techniques, a specific histological diagnosis is still not possible. The use of immunological methods permits the identification of antigens, antibodies and various other cell and tissue components and has greatly facilitated our ability to achieve a specific diagnosis. Hybridoma monoclonal antibody technology paved the way for the development of numerous antibodies to cell and tissue structures (Box 3.2).

Immunofluorescence methods

John Mee

Immunofluorescence techniques were pioneered in the 1940s and have been widely used subsequently, both in research and clinical diagnostics. Applications include the evaluation of cells in suspension, cultured cells, tissue, beads and microarrays for the detection of specific protein(s). In this technique, antibodies are chemically conjugated to fluorescent dyes such as fluorescein

---

Box 3.2 Immunocytochemistry panels of cell markers

Undifferentiated malignancy panel
- MNF 116 (keratin)
- AE1/AE3 (keratin)
- CAM 5.2 (low-molecular-weight keratin)
- Epithelial membrane antigen (EMA)
- Leukocyte common antigen (LCA)
- S-100 protein
- SOX10
- CD31
- ERG

Spindle cell panel
As in Undifferentiated malignancy panel plus:
- Desmin
- H-caldesmon
- Calponin
- Smooth muscle actin
- Q bend 10 (CD34)

Melanocyte panel
- S-100 protein
- HMB45
- Mart-1 (Melan-A)
- MIFT-1
- Tyrosinase
- Melanoma cocktail
- SOX10

Small blue cell panel
- Chromogranin
- Synaptophysin
- NSE (neuron-specific enolase)
- Cam 5.2
- EMA
- CEA
- S-100 protein
- Cytokeratin 20
- Human polyomavirus
- Neurofilament
- CD99

- FLI-1
- Desmin
- Myogenin
- MYOD1
- Muscle-specific actin
- Smooth muscle actin

Lymphoma panel
- LCA (CD45)
- CD20, CD79a (pan B-cell markers)
- CD2, CD3, CD5, CD7, CD43 (pan T-cell markers)
- CD4 (T-helper/inducer lymphocytes)
- CD8 (T-cytotoxic/suppressor lymphocytes)
- UCHL (CD45Ro) (pan T-cell marker)
- βF1 (anti-T-cell-receptor B chain antibody)
- TCR δ-chain
- Ber-H2 (CD30)
- κ light chain λ light chain (now also done by *in situ* hybridisation)
- ALK-1
- Bcl-2
- CD10 (marker of follicle-centre cells)
- Bcl-6 (marker of follicle-centre cells)
- Ki-67 (proliferation marker)
- CD56 (natural killer cell marker)
- TIA-1 (marker of cytotoxic granules)
- Granzyme (marker of cytotoxic granules)
- Perforin (marker of cytotoxic granules)
- MUM 1
- FPOX-1
- PD1 (marker of follicular T helper cells)
- ICOS (marker of follicular T helper cells)
- CXCL13 (marker of follicular T helper cells)
- Immunoglobulins: IgG, IgM, IgD, IgM, IgG4

Leukaemia panel
- LCA
- Lysozyme

- Myeloperoxidase
- CD33
- HLA-DR
- MT1 (CD43)
- KP1
- PGM1
- CD163
- TDT
- CD34
- CD4
- CD56

Langerhans cell panel
- S100 protein
- CD1a
- Langerin (CD207)

Vascular panel
- ERG
- CD31
- Q bend 10 (CD34)
- FLI-1
- Podoplanin (D2–40) (lymphatic endothelial cell marker)
- HHV8

Mast cell markers
- CD117
- Tryptase
- Microphthalmia transcription factor

Immunofluorescence labelling (frozen sections)
- IgM
- IgG
- IgA
- Complement-3 (C3)
- Fibrinogen

isothiocyanate (FITC) or tetramethyl rhodamine isothiocyanate (TRITC). These labelled antibodies bind (directly or indirectly) to the antigen(s) of interest in cells or tissue sections, which can be visualised by fluorescence or confocal microscopy and quantified by flow cytometry, array scanner or automated imaging instrument.

In clinical immunodermatology, there are two basic types of immunofluorescence detection methods: (i) direct immunofluorescence, in which the primary antibody is labelled with a fluorescent dye (Figure 3.10a); and (ii) indirect immunofluorescence, where a secondary antibody labelled with a fluorochrome is used to recognise a primary (circulating) antibody (Figure 3.10b). These techniques are both reliable and reproducible and have allowed major advances in the diagnosis of autoimmune blistering diseases.

Accuracy in the diagnosis of bullous diseases is important, as some of these disorders can be life threatening. Although some bullous diseases can have definitive clinical and histological features, a positive diagnosis is typically confirmed using immunofluorescence techniques, which are regarded as the 'gold standard' in the investigation and management of immunobullous diseases. In other conditions, such as connective tissue diseases and vasculitis, they are not diagnostic but can be helpful.

Photobleaching or fading is a technical limitation of immunofluorescence. Prolonged or repeated examination reduces the intensity of emission, which also diminishes if preparations are exposed to sunlight. This fading can be reduced through storage of immunofluorescence slides in the dark and the use of commercial mountant solutions containing an antifade reagent.

Findings from immunofluorescence techniques have enabled dermatologists to classify blistering diseases and to develop new assays utilising techniques such as immunoblotting, immunoelectron microscopy and enzyme-linked immunosorbent assays. Using these techniques, the principal antigens recognised by antibodies in autoimmune blistering diseases have been identified and characterised. Their respective genes have been cloned and used to produce recombinant proteins, which can be used to study the functional aspects of these molecules. The collective information obtained from the findings of these techniques is extremely valuable to dermatologists.

It is important to understand that immunofluorescence is not a substitute for histopathology but is, in fact, complementary to it. Maximum diagnostic accuracy is achieved by considering the clinical, histological and immunofluorescence findings together. The values of positive or negative immunofluorescence findings are dependent on the experience and skill of the laboratory staff in performing these techniques but also on the knowledge and experience of the reporter. Coordination with the clinician, to ensure the selection of appropriate lesions for biopsy, is also highly desirable. Weaknesses in any of these areas may result in the immunofluorescence findings being unhelpful or misleading.

Direct immunofluorescence

Direct immunofluorescence (DIF) is a single step procedure used to identify antibodies bound to target cutaneous or mucosal antigens *in situ* and other proteins of relevance to immunobullous diseases. The most commonly used panel of fluorescently conjugated antibodies detect tissue-bound IgM, IgG, IgA, the C3c subunit of complement and fibrinogen. The sensitivity of DIF is superior to that of indirect immunofluorescence, hence it is the preferred method for establishing a diagnosis. However, DIF provides only limited information on quantities of antibodies present and no information at all on the antigenic targets of the autoantibodies detected. Therefore, for maximal diagnostic utility, simultaneous submission of biopsy and serum specimens should be considered, to facilitate both direct and indirect immunofluorescence analysis.

Specimen preparation

Clinically, it is important to collect a biopsy for DIF analysis from an appropriate site(s) for the type of autoimmune bullous disease under investigation. Ideally, the biopsy should be taken from an area where blisters or lesions have recently occurred. Biopsies close to older blisters and inflamed sites should be avoided because immune deposits at these sites may be degraded and changes such as degeneration or secondary infection may occur. These changes, in turn, make the microscopy interpretation particularly challenging. Two further key considerations in determining the optimal biopsy site for meaningful DIF analysis are the suspected underlying disease and proximity to a blister. A biopsy of normal-appearing skin adjacent to a lesion should be taken where immunobullous blistering conditions are suspected. However, lesional tissue is required for positive immunofluorescence in other conditions including lichen planus, connective tissue diseases, vasculitides, porphyria and amyloidosis (Table 3.5). For patients with suspected systemic lupus erythematosus, two separate biopsies should be taken if the lesional site is sun-exposed, because connective tissue disorder-like immunofluorescence findings can sometimes be detected in normal sun-exposed skin.

Because intact epithelial tissue is required for optimal DIF interpretation, biopsies from suspected immunobullous patients should always be taken at least 1 cm from an active bulla or lesion. This location differs from lesional areas that are typically biopsied for standard histopathological analysis (Figure 3.11). Additionally, attempting to bisect a biopsy, submitting half for histopathology and the other half for DIF analysis, should be avoided, because the shearing forces required to divide a biopsy can result in epithelial separation (especially in mucosal tissue) and damage to the specimen which, again, make DIF interpretation difficult.

Table 3.5 Specimen selection for direct immunofluorescence by disease.

Disease	No. of biopsies	Biopsy site
Pemphigus (all forms)	1	Perilesional uninvolved
Pemphigoid (all forms)	1	Perilesional uninvolved
Epidermolysis bullosa acquisita	1	Perilesional uninvolved
Linear IgA bullous dermatosis	1	Perilesional uninvolved
Dermatitis herpetiformis	1	Perilesional uninvolved
Discoid lupus erythematosus	1	Lesional
Systemic lupus erythematosus	2	Lesional *and* uninvolved (non-sun-exposed)
Lichen planus	1	Lesional
Porphyria	1	Lesional
Vasculitis	1	Lesional
Amyloidosis	1	Lesional

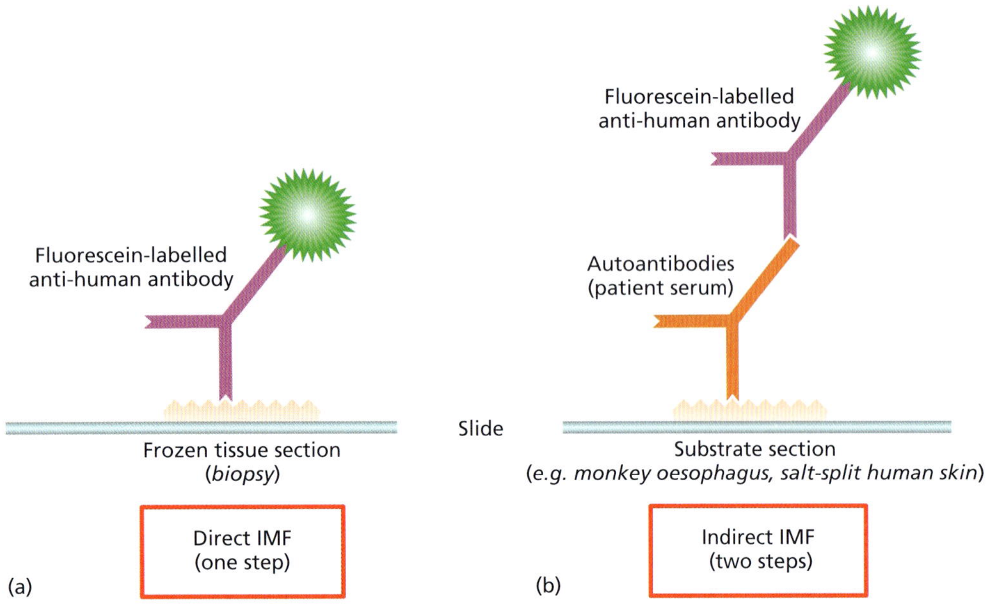

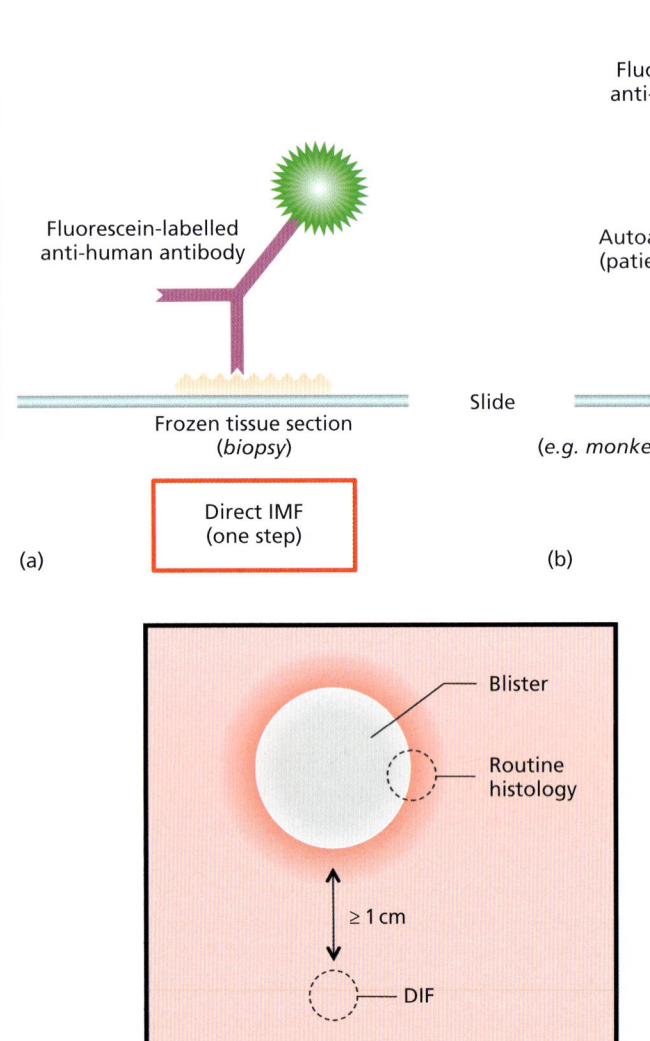

Figure 3.10 Different immunofluorescence (IMF) techniques in clinical immunodermatology: (a) direct and (b) indirect.

Figure 3.11 Biopsy site requirements for direct immunofluorescence (DIF) and routine histology studies of autoimmune blistering diseases.

Ideally, a biopsy for DIF examination should be rinsed in saline, embedded in a freezing medium such as optimum cutting temperature (OCT) compound and snap-frozen immediately after collection. In most cases, however, facilities for DIF are not available in clinical areas and tissue specimens will need to be transported to a laboratory. In this situation, biopsies should be rinsed in distilled water or normal saline and placed in Michel medium, which is widely available commercially or can be prepared locally (Table 3.3). This medium comprises a buffered, saturated ammonium sulphate solution with a proteolytic enzyme inhibitor, which prevents autolysis of tissue structures and immunoreactants. Washing of the tissue removes blood proteins and ensures maintenance of a neutral pH in the medium. This will facilitate immunoreactant preservation at ambient temperatures for up to 6 months for standard immunofluorescence [1]. Specimens in Michel medium can be posted to a laboratory. Unused Michel medium containers may be stored at room temperature for 1 year without any deterioration.

In the laboratory, tissue specimens received in Michel medium are washed extensively in phosphate buffered saline (PBS) to remove ammonium salts and any residual blood proteins and are then snap-frozen. Typically, a small amount of OCT embedding compound is placed on a piece of cork or plastic and briefly immersed in a liquid nitrogen-cooled heptane bath until the peripheral OCT is frozen. The skin biopsy is then appropriately orientated in the central fluid portion, covered with further OCT and briefly returned to the bath. The frozen skin biopsy is then transferred either to a cryostat for sectioning or to a freezer at −20°C or lower, for storage prior to cryotomy.

Specimen processing

A series of frozen tissue sections of 4–6 μm thickness are cut using a cryostat and placed on microscope slides. These are subsequently dried to increase adherence and then washed in PBS, to remove residual OCT compound. Sections are dried again, prior to incubation at 37°C with one of a panel of FITC-conjugated antihuman antibodies. Sensitivity and specificity of fluorescence is maximised following the determination of an optimal dilution of the labelled antibodies. Following incubation, slides are washed in PBS to remove unbound antibodies, then dried, mounted in buffered glycerol and either examined immediately by fluorescence microscopy or stored in the dark at −20°C or lower, prior to reporting.

Indirect immunofluorescence

Indirect immunofluorescence (IIF) is a two-step procedure used to identify circulating autoantibodies to cutaneous or mucosal antigens in patient serum. These antibodies are most commonly of IgG or IgA isotypes. Although serological antibody concentrations are usually lower than those found in tissues of patients with immunobullous diseases, IIF is a useful tool, both for confirming diagnoses made using DIF and for facilitating further characterisation of the antibody profile in patients, including titration of antibody levels, which can be useful in treatment monitoring. This technique can also be used to establish diagnosis in patients where a tissue biopsy is not possible or considered inappropriate. In recent years, IIF techniques have been performed alongside ELISA methodologies on patient sera, to improve detection sensitivity and provide further data on autoantibody specificity.

Specimen preparation

Serum samples are required for the detection of circulating autoantibodies by IIF procedures. Although blister fluid specimens can also yield successful results using this technique, serum is preferable, due to the superior consistency of results. Blood should be collected in a serum separator tube (often with a gold-coloured top) or similar, containing a clot activator and no anticoagulant, and delivered to a diagnostic laboratory within 7 days of collection. It is not necessary to refrigerate sera during storage or transit. Serum is separated by centrifugation, transferred to sterile containers and can be stored at 4°C for up to 1 month, prior to analysis. Longer-term storage requires freezing of sera at −20°C or lower. Care should be taken to avoid haemolysis of serum samples, which can result in autoantibody deterioration, and clotted blood is unsuitable for IIF analysis, for similar reasons. Plasma samples can be used for IIF if no serum is available. However, they are suboptimal, due to potential interference to antibody binding from clotting proteins.

Substrates for IIF

To detect circulating autoantibodies, tissues containing the corresponding antigens must be used as a substrate. Two principal tissue types are used for the routine detection of autoantibodies in immunobullous disorders by IIF. Monkey proximal oesophageal tissue provides a rich source of desmoglein proteins, particularly desmoglein-3 and is therefore the substrate of choice for the detection of pemphigus antibodies. Microscope slides containing thin 4–6 μm sections of monkey oesophagus prepared from frozen blocks of freshly prepared tissue are available from a number of commercial suppliers, are widely used in diagnostic laboratories and can be stored at 4°C for several months, prior to use.

Normal human skin, ideally prepared from surgically obtained tissue excised from the breast or abdomen and processed into frozen tissue blocks within 48 h, is the second most commonly used tissue for IIF studies. Skin from the scalp, face, sun-damaged sites and neonatal foreskin should not be used as these substrates produce a high rate of false positive results.

While both tissues can be used to screen for and titrate out circulating antibodies in most immunobullous diseases, normal human skin offers several advantages, including greater sensitivity (with the exception of antibodies associated with pemphigus vulgaris) and antigenic localisation options unavailable when using monkey oesophagus. It is recommended to use a combination of monkey oesophagus and normal human skin substrate for IIF screening in pemphigus. The use of these two substrates enhances diagnostic sensitivity and is also helpful for disease monitoring, compared with the use of a single substrate.

There are two key limitations to the use of monkey oesophagus substrate for IIF detection in immunobullous diseases. Firstly, this substrate is known to exhibit non-specific intercellular fluorescence of epithelial tissue in sera from a subpopulation of individuals with no underlying immunobullous disease, potentially resulting in false positive diagnoses of pemphigus. Pre-adsorption of test sera with soluble A/B blood group antigens, as a blocking step, may reduce this non-specificity [2]. Secondly, monkey oesophagus expresses very low levels of BP180 protein, the most common antigen targeted in bullous pemphigoid and, therefore, false negative diagnosis of this disease is possible if monkey oesophagus is the sole substrate used in IIF analysis [3]. Combined use of multiple substrates, particularly human salt-split skin, will reduce this possibility.

A third substrate that is used much less frequently for IIF studies is rat (or monkey) urinary bladder or similar tissues that contain transitional epithelium. Unlike the stratified squamous epithelium found in skin, transitional epithelium does not produce desmoglein-1 or desmoglein-3, the predominant antigens in pemphigus, but expresses high levels of desmosomal plakin family proteins, especially envoplakin, periplakin and desmoplakins. Antibodies against these proteins are found in the serum of most patients with paraneoplastic pemphigus and intercellular IgG fluorescence on this substrate is regarded as a diagnostic indicator of this disease, although it is not seen in 100% of these patients [4].

Split-skin indirect technique

The split-skin technique is valuable in the study of most subepidermal blistering disorders, enabling localisation of the antibody binding sites to be visualised. Circulating antibasement membrane zone antibodies are characteristic features of subepidermal immunobullous diseases. Immunoelectron microscopy divides them into two groups based on their ultrastructural binding sites. In bullous pemphigoid and pemphigoid gestationis, antibodies target proteins in the hemidesmosomes of the upper lamina lucida and are termed epidermal binding. In epidermolysis bullous acquisita, they target antigens in the sublamina densa and are termed dermal binding. Distinguishing between these diseases is important, especially in those cases where clinical and histological diagnostic features may overlap.

The split-skin method is a relatively simple and reliable technique for distinguishing between epidermal and dermal-binding autoantibodies. The method relies on splitting human skin through the lamina lucida, such that bullous pemphigoid antigens localise to the epidermal side (often referred to as the 'roof' of the split) whereas components of the lamina densa, including laminin proteins and the epidermolysis bullous acquisita antigen, type VII collagen, localise to the dermal side (often referred to as the 'base' or 'floor' of the split).

Various methods exist to split skin through the lamina lucida, the most frequently used being incubation of skin in 1 M normal saline for 24–48 h at 4°C [5]. Similar results can be achieved more quickly, with a consequent reduction in trauma to the tissue, using 20 mM di-sodium ethylenediaminetetraacetic acid (EDTA) for 18–24 h at 4°C. Following incubation, the epidermis can be gently teased apart from the underlying dermis using a fine pair of forceps. In addition to creating a substrate for IIF screening, this technique can also be used to split biopsies in DIF studies to assess basement membrane zone antibody distribution.

Specimen processing

To detect the presence of circulating autoantibodies in a patient with a suspected autoimmune bullous disease, microscope slides containing several 4–6 μm sections of appropriate tissue substrates are required. Ideally, these should include monkey oesophagus and human skin (split and unsplit). Slides should be thoroughly washed in PBS and dried immediately prior to use. Serial dilutions of patient serum in PBS are added to the sections and incubated at 37°C for optimal antibody binding. After incubation, slides are washed in PBS to remove unbound antibodies, dried and incubated again with diluted, fluorescently labelled antihuman IgG or IgA conjugates at 37°C. They are then washed extensively again in PBS and briefly in distilled water, then dried prior to mounting in buffered glycerol and subsequent fluorescence microscopy. Results are typically reported either qualitatively (positive or negative for intercellular or basement membrane zone fluorescence) or semi-quantitatively (by end-point titre where fluorescence remains visible) for both IgG and IgA conjugates.

Every series of IIF studies must include known negative and positive controls. For the negative controls, sections are primarily incubated with serum from individuals with no known underlying immunobullous disease and positive control sera for key immunobullous diseases are typically selected from previous known cases. These controls provide information about any non-specific binding of the immunglobulins to the tissue substrates and provide quality assurance around preparation of the fluorescent conjugates and all associated processing steps.

Calcium enhancement indirect technique
Calcium-containing buffers can enhance the sensitivity of IIF in some patients by two or more doubling dilutions. This is observed on both monkey oesophagus and human skin substrates. In cases where an increase in sensitivity occurs, it is likely to be seen in the detection of desmoglein (DSG) autoantibodies, which bind to calcium-sensitive conformational epitopes. Both DSG1 and DSG3 are members of the cadherin family of calcium-dependent adhesion molecules and previous studies have shown that conformational epitopes on DSG1 and DSG3 are calcium dependent. This technique will not enhance the detection of antibasement membrane zone antibodies in subepithelial blistering diseases [6].

Immunoenzyme methods
The immunoenzyme (immunoperoxidase) methods have several advantages over immunofluorescence (Box 3.3) [1,**2**,3].

> **Box 3.3 Advantages of immunoenzyme (immunoperoxidase) methods over immunofluorescence**
> - Standard microscopes and illumination are used
> - The preparations are permanent and the reaction products do not usually fade on repeated examination
> - Counterstains enable cells containing antigen to be identified with more certainty than using immunofluorescence with dark-ground illumination
> - Examination is less tiring for the microscopist
> - The preparations may be examined by electron microscopy

Technical limitations
Inflammatory lesions may contain endogenous peroxidase activity and such sections have to be pre-treated to remove it [3]. Furthermore, it is possible for the antigen to be modified by the pre-treatment, with the result that it is more difficult to detect. This mainly applies to examination of lesions. Normal tissues, for example those used as a substrate to detect antibodies in a patient's serum, rarely require pre-treatment. The problem with endogenous peroxidase is analogous to the disadvantage of autofluorescence in the immunofluorescence preparations.

There is less contrast with immunoperoxidase methods than in slides treated by the immunofluorescence technique and fine stippling or cytoskeletal structures seen by immunofluorescence are not quite so easily detected by immunoperoxidase. Although immunofluorescence may be more discriminating in detecting small amounts of antigen in cryostat-cut sections, the immunoperoxidase methods, used on paraffin-embedded tissues for antigens that are stable during preparation, provide more definite resolution of the tissue and sites of antigen.

Immunoperoxidase methods have another advantage in being the preferred method to re-examine tissues stored in paraffin blocks after routine histology, provided that the antigens are stable in the fixative and dehydrating agents. Recent improvements in immunoenzyme techniques have resulted in their application to many investigations. The reagent antibody is conjugated with an enzyme, usually horseradish peroxidase, and the antibody conjugate combines with the antigen in the test preparation. The site of binding is detected by adding a substrate for the enzyme: the degradation of many molecules of substrate leaves a deposit confined to the site of binding. Sites of peroxidase activity appear as dark brown granular deposits that are seen distinctly in contrast to suitable counterstains, for example methyl green or Mayer haemalum.

Although the application described here is for the detection of antigen in tissue sections and cell suspensions or monolayers, the principle of the method is the same as that of ELISA.

Chemical conjugation of peroxidase to antibody
Antiglobulins conjugated with peroxidase, and peroxidase–antiperoxidase (PAP) complexes, described here, are available commercially.

Use of conjugates
The horseradish peroxidase, conjugated to antibody or to globulin, may be applied to sections to detect antigen by procedures similar to those used for immunofluorescence. There are, however, modifications that increase the sensitivity of the method so that it is equal to, or possibly more sensitive than, IIF.

The diagrammatic representation of the procedures seen in Figure 3.12 shows the different forms of conjugate. Antibody against the antigen to be detected may be conjugated directly with the enzyme (Figure 3.12a). This is not a very discriminating procedure. The indirect or two-stage procedure, whereby the unlabelled antibody bound to the antigen is detected by antiglobulin conjugated to enzyme (Figure 3.12b), increases sensitivity by increasing the number of conjugated antibodies binding to the site, and is more versatile, because one conjugated antiglobulin can detect any antibody of that species.

Two other procedures increase the sensitivity of the technique. The antibody bound to the antigen is treated with unconjugated antiglobulin, which in turn is treated with normal globulin of the same species as the first antibody (Figure 3.12c): for example, a sequence of rabbit antibody, goat antirabbit globulin and then

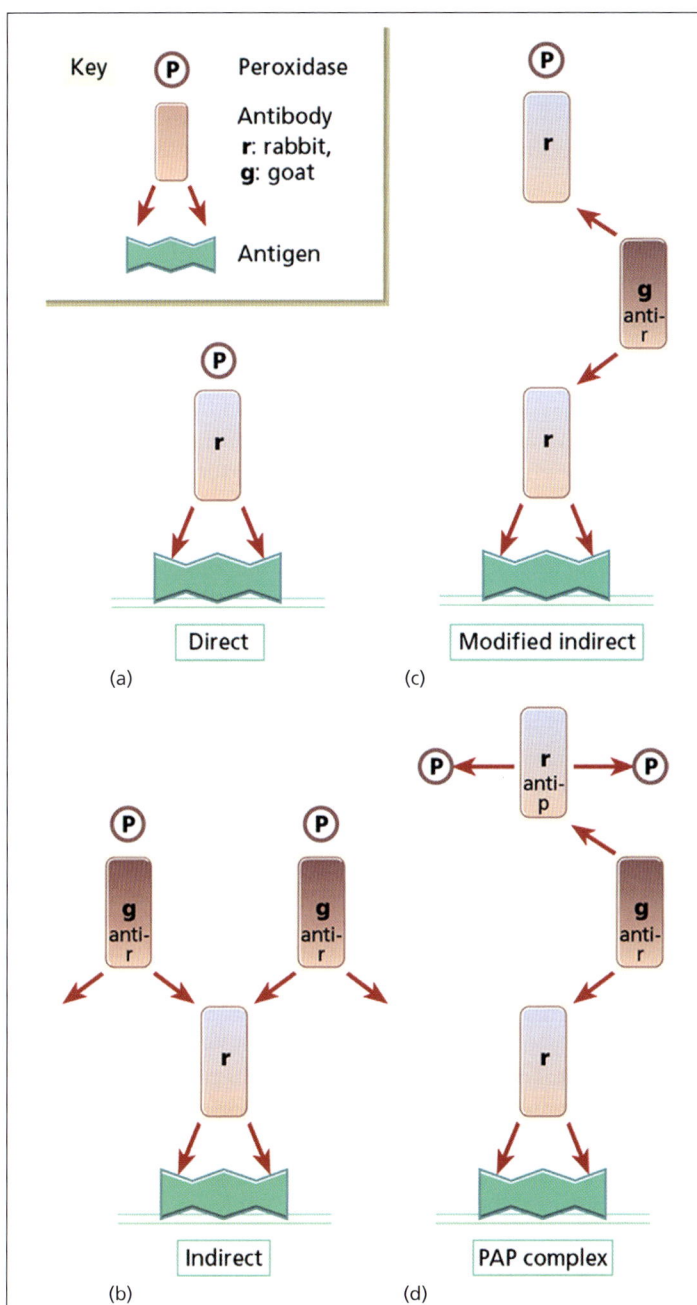

Figure 3.12 Different immunoperoxidase techniques: (a) direct, (b) indirect, (c) modified indirect and (d) with peroxidase–antiperoxidase (PAP) complex.

antibodies on the same tissue or cells to detect different antigens and to examine the relationship of one antigen to another (i.e. double staining). A further enzyme may be used to obtain a more permanent red product that is preferable in cases where interpretation of the results may be hampered by the presence of pigment (haemosiderin and, particularly, melanin). This is 3-amino-9-ethylcarbazole [4].

Examination of fixed frozen sections

There are three stages in the procedure:
1 Preparation of the tissue sections.
2 Treatment of the sections with the peroxidase-labelled antibody.
3 Chemical reaction to detect the peroxidase in the tissue.

Preparation and fixation of sections. Sections may be prepared from routine cryostat-cut samples or paraffin-embedded material and may be treated for antigen retrieval as previously described. Some improvement in cryostat prepared sections may be achieved by short-term fixation in dilute formalin.

Treatment of the sections with antibody. Control for antibody specificity as described for immunofluorescence. Sections may be treated by the methods described above (Figure 3.12). The indirect method is probably the most suitable for general use, applying unlabelled antibody, followed by labelled antiglobulin.

Detection of the peroxidase reaction product by staining. The substrate is a carcinogen and should be handled in small quantities with appropriate precautions.

Controls

It is necessary to confirm that the reaction observed reflects antibody-conjugated peroxidase and not endogenous peroxidase and that the antibody binding is specific for the antigen. One section should be stained with DAB only; another section with DAB–methanol–H_2O_2, to confirm the absence of endogenous peroxidase.

Paraffin sections

If the antigens to be detected are stable in the fixatives and dehydrating agents, the immunoperoxidase methods may be applied to sections from paraffin-embedded tissue. The paraffin is removed from the sections with xylol and alcohols; the sections are subsequently treated as for frozen sections. The identity of the cells and tissues containing the antigen is much more easily determined by this method than by cryostat-cut sections or by immunofluorescence. Immunoglobulins and hormones may be readily detected, but some antigens, such as those of bacteria in vasculitic lesions, tend to be extracted during processing.

Conjugates involving avidin–biotin coupling of antibody and enzyme

Instead of chemical covalent binding of antibody to enzyme to prepare conjugates, the two reagents may be linked non-covalently by the very strong affinity between biotin (a vitamin widely distributed in mammalian tissues) and avidin (a glycoprotein of egg white).

rabbit normal globulin conjugated with peroxidase. In the second modification, instead of using globulin conjugated chemically with enzyme in the third stage, a PAP complex is added (Figure 3.12d): for example, rabbit antibody to peroxidase, which gives a more discrete, intense reaction product than chemically prepared conjugates of normal globulin–peroxidase. This is possibly because chemical treatment tends to alter the antigenic determinants of the normal globulin, and to polymerise the peroxidase.

The enzyme most frequently used is horseradish peroxidase, which forms a dark brown product from its substrate. Alkaline phosphatase may also be used and the reaction product with its substrate is red. The two enzymes may be used with appropriate

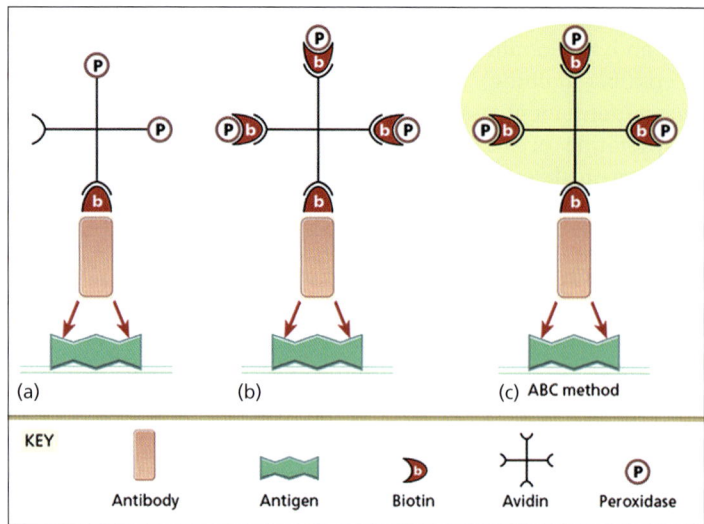

Figure 3.13 Avidin–biotin staining methods. (a) Antibody coupled with biotin binds with the antigen in the tissue. Avidin coupled with peroxidase binds to the biotin on the antibody. Treatment with enzyme substrate reveals the bound peroxidase and therefore the site of antigen. (b) Antibody coupled with biotin binds with the antigen in the tissue. Avidin will bind the biotin–antibody complex. Biotin coupled with peroxidase will then bind to the free avidin-combining sites. Finally, treatment with enzyme substrate reveals the bound peroxidase. (c) Complexes (shown within yellow circle) are formed of biotin, coupled with peroxidase, incubated with a moderate excess of avidin (ensuring some free avidin-combining sites). Antibody coupled with biotin binds to antigen in the tissue. The complexes are added to the tissue and the free avidin sites bind to the biotin on the antibody. Finally, treatment with enzyme substrate reveals the bound peroxidase.

Biotin is coupled to the reagent antibody through the formation of an intermediate biotin derivative and the avidin is coupled to the selected enzyme by glutaraldehyde [5]. Each biotin molecule has one combining site for avidin, and avidin has four sites for biotin, although not all of these would combine in a test system, and there are two main applications [5]:

1. The antibody–biotin conjugate is incubated with and combines with antigen in the test section or cell. This is followed by the addition of peroxidase conjugated with avidin. The avidin binds the peroxidase to any biotin, and subsequent treatment with the substrate for the enzyme reveals the antigen sites (Figure 3.13a).
2. The antibody–biotin conjugate is used as above to bind to any antigen. Avidin is then added, which becomes strongly linked to the biotin. Then biotin-labelled enzyme is added and the avidin bridges the biotin molecules. As the avidin has a potential four valencies for biotin, there is an enhancement or amplification of the enzyme binding, and therefore greater discrimination of the sites of antigen (Figure 3.13b).

A further modification is the avidin–biotin–peroxidase complex (ABC) method (Figure 3.13c), similar to the PAP method already described. A prepared ABC follows the use of biotin-labelled antiglobulin (to detect unlabelled reagent antibody or tissue-bound antibody in the tissue). The complex binds through the avidin bridge to biotin on the antiglobulin. The method results in a greater intensity of staining.

As in the other immunodetection techniques, it is necessary to ensure that there is no autologous tissue background activity that will cause confusion when interpreting results. In the avidin–biotin methods, it is necessary to eliminate the possibility of endogenous peroxidase activity as in any peroxidase method. It is also necessary to inactivate endogenous biotin present in tissues that would bind the avidin-labelled reagents. However, overcoming any endogenous activity is a complex multistep activity and is not necessary if the appropriate controls (e.g. tissue treated with the avidin conjugates) show no binding.

Enzyme-linked immunosorbent assay (ELISA)

In addition to IIF techniques, circulating antibodies in serum from patients with autoimmune bullous diseases can be detected using enzyme-linked immunosorbent assay (ELISA) methodologies. Unlike IIF, ELISA methodologies are specific for known autoantigens and offer higher sensitivity and a greater degree of quantitation, which can be particularly useful for treatment monitoring of patients. They are routinely performed using 96-well microtitre plates that have been pre-coated with recombinant antigenic peptides. Diluted serum is added to a well and any specific antibodies in the serum will bind to the immobilised antigen. Following washing to remove unbound antibodies, a secondary antibody raised against human immunoglobulin and conjugated with an enzyme that catalyses a colorimetric reaction is added. After further incubation and washing steps, a substrate for the enzyme conjugated to the secondary antibody is added and a colour change occurs which is directly proportional to the quantity of specific antibody present in the patient serum sample. This colour change is quantified using spectrophotometry and compared with that produced from known standards in other wells on the plate to generate quantitative data.

These assays are normally performed using commercial kits to assess the most commonly occurring autoantibodies seen in immunobullous diseases, i.e. DSG1 and DSG3 antibodies in pemphigus [6], BP180 and BP230 antibodies in pemphigoid diseases [7,8] and collagen VII antibodies in epidermolysis bullosa acquisita [9]. A limitation of these assays is that not all epitopes of a particular antigen will be represented in a specific ELISA, depending on the source and production protocol of the coating peptide used. In addition, ELISA systems only detect antibodies against specific, known antigens and are, therefore, of limited value in assessing patient sera that contain antibodies to other, less common antigens seen in autoimmune bullous disorders. This technique is, therefore, most useful when used in combination with IIF methodologies or for monitoring levels of antibodies in patients with known, previously characterised positivity, undergoing continued treatment.

Applications of immunopathology techniques

John Mee

The immunopathological methods described previously revolutionised diagnostic histopathology and have helped us to recognise, classify and understand the pathogenesis of a wide variety of cutaneous disorders [1,2,3,4]. Although there are some antigens of diagnostic value that are not stable following formalin fixation and paraffin embedding of tissue, there is a wide range of antigens that are stable. A few of the more important areas of diagnostic dermatopathology that highlight the usefulness of immunopathological techniques are described.

Direct immunofluorescence

Immunopathological techniques for the diagnosis of autoimmune blistering diseases rely on the use of immunofluorescence methods [3,4]. Although some have suggested that immunoperoxidase methods are equally reliable in this setting, formalin fixation results in poor preservation of the antigens of interest and false negative results are frequent [5]. The histological diagnosis of the various cutaneous autoimmune blistering diseases should always be confirmed with DIF studies. Although in many non-autoimmune bullous diseases a diagnosis can be made based on light microscopic features in biopsies from formalin-fixed tissue, in immunological diseases, a specific diagnosis is often not possible. In these circumstances, immunofluorescence studies are essential.

The results of DIF studies on skin biopsies vary considerably, depending on the disease being investigated and the site of biopsy. The distribution and type of immunoreactant deposition is recorded. The class of immunoglobulin and the presence or absence of C3 and fibrinogen is noted. Immunoreactants are deposited in two main patterns: in the epidermal intercellular space and at the basement membrane zone (BMZ). Intercellular immunoreactants may be observed throughout the epithelium or restricted to certain layers. BMZ deposits may be smooth and linear, granular and discontinuous or a combination of the two [6].

A key skill in DIF reporting is differentiating specific immunofluorescence from artefactual deposits which commonly arise. In addition, autofluorescence of proteins such as keratin and elastic fibres can be a significant problem and high background fluorescence is sometimes seen, particularly in sections exposed to anti-IgG conjugates, which can partially occlude specific fluorescence patterns present in the tissue.

A summary of DIF findings for the main cutaneous diseases in which this technique can be diagnostically informative is presented in Table 3.6.

Serration pattern analysis

Careful microscopic examination of linear IgG fluorescence at the dermo-epidermal junction can help to differentiate between different subepithelial autoimmune bullous disorders through identification of two distinct serration patterns, termed n-serration and u-serration, within the deposits [7]. Linear fluorescence exhibiting n-serration feature a series of small arches which are closed at the top, resembling the letter 'n', whereas u-serrated linear IgG fluorescence contains regions with fine, epithelial-facing protrusions resembling growing grass, with inverted closed arches, analogous to the letter 'u'. A u-serration pattern is specific to antibody binding to type VII collagen, as seen in epidermolysis bullosa acquisita, whereas n-serration is associated with all other pemphigoid diseases. Distinct serration patterns are often focal in nature and require sufficiently thin sections (typically 4–6 µm), at least 400-fold overall magnification (without oil) and prior training for optimal identification.

Pemphigus

Direct immunofluorescence findings in pemphigus exhibit a sharp, 'chicken-wire' pattern, representing intercellular deposition of IgG antibodies and/or C3 within the epithelium (Figure 3.14). IgA may also be seen with a similar distribution in a small percentage of cases. Although there are differences in the expression of DSG1 and DSG3 between cutaneous and mucosal epithelial tissues, pemphigus vulgaris and pemphigus foliaceus cannot be reliably differentiated by DIF studies and serum is required to achieve this. Presence of linear IgG and/or C3 deposition at the BMZ, in addition to epithelial intercellular IgG raises the possibility of paraneoplastic pemphigus, which also requires serological follow-up for accurate diagnosis.

Pemphigoid

In contrast to the intra-epithelial fluorescence observed in pemphigus, diseases of the pemphigoid family show a linear deposition of IgG and/or C3 at the BMZ by DIF, due to the hemidesmosomal location of the antigens targeted in these diseases. IgA linear BMZ fluorescence is also seen in some pemphigoid patients, particularly those with mucous membrane pemphigoid (MMP). Salt-splitting of biopsies from the majority of patients with bullous pemphigoid and subsequent repeated processing for DIF reveals localisation

Table 3.6 Direct immunofluorescence findings in cutaneous diseases.

Disease	Direct immunofluorescence findings
Pemphigus (all forms)	Epithelial intercellular deposition of IgG and/or C3 (IgA in IgA pemphigus)
Bullous pemphigoid	Linear deposition of IgG and/or C3 at the basement membrane zone, most commonly localising to the epithelial side, following salt-splitting of the biopsy
Mucous membrane pemphigoid	Linear deposition of IgG and/or IgA and/or C3 at the basement membrane zone, most commonly localising to the epithelial side, following salt-splitting of the biopsy
Pemphigoid gestationis	Linear deposition of C3 (+ occasionally IgG) at the basement membrane zone
Linear IgA disease	Linear deposition of IgA and/or C3 (+ occasionally IgG) at the basement membrane zone
Epidermolysis bullosa acquisita	Linear deposition of IgG and/or C3 at the basement membrane zone, localising to the subepithelial side, following salt-splitting of the biopsy
Dermatitis herpetiformis	Focal, granular (occasionally fibrillary) deposition of IgA in dermal papillae
Lupus erythematosus	Granular deposition of (most commonly) IgM +/− IgG, IgA, complement-3 and fibrinogen at the dermo-epidermal junction
Lichen planus	Coarse, ragged deposition of fibrinogen at the dermo-epidermal junction
Amyloidosis	Fluorescence of dermal amyloid deposits with thioflavin-T dye
Porphyria	Hyaline mantle formation around dermal blood vessels
Vasculitis	Peri- or intravascular deposition of C3 and/or fibrinogen (occasionally IgA) in dermal blood vessels (non-diagnostic)

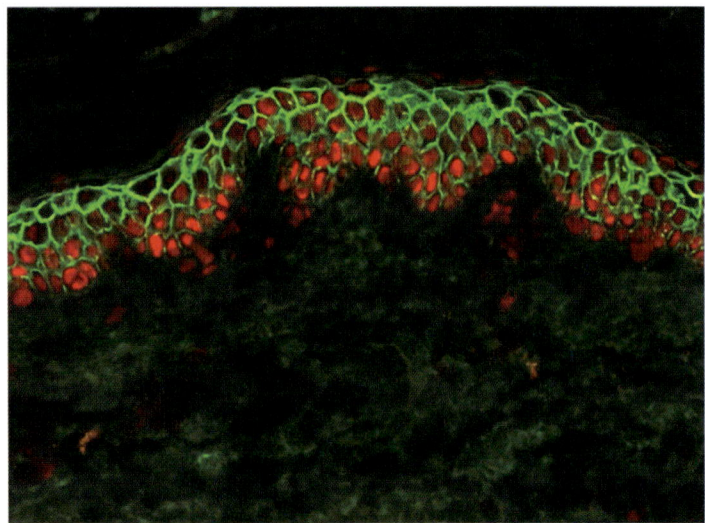

Figure 3.14 Direct immunofluorescence of pemphigus showing deposition of intercellular IgG in the epidermis.

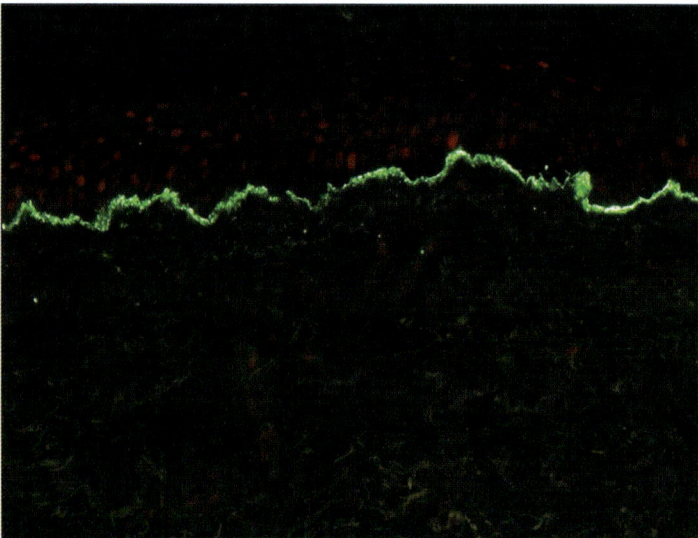

Figure 3.16 Direct immunofluorescence of linear IgA bullous dermatosis showing linear basement membrane zone deposition of IgA.

fluorescence intensities of the IgG and IgA deposits can be useful in differentiating linear IgA disease from MMP, when this is unclear from the clinical or histological presentations.

Epidermolysis bullosa acquisita

Direct immunofluorescence studies in epidermolysis bullosa acquisita (EBA) also result in linear deposition of IgG ± C3 at the BMZ, which can be easily mistaken for pemphigoid. However, careful microscopic examination may indicate a slightly thicker band than that seen in BP, with a u-serrated, rather than the n-serrated pattern seen at higher magnifications. Salt-splitting of the biopsy and repeated DIF assay always results in localisation of the linear deposition to the dermal side/base of the split, due to targeting of autoantibodies to collagen VII (Figure 3.17). Serum is required to differentiate EBA from dermal-binding pemphigoid, through the detection of specific anticollagen VII antibodies by ELISA analysis in EBA patients.

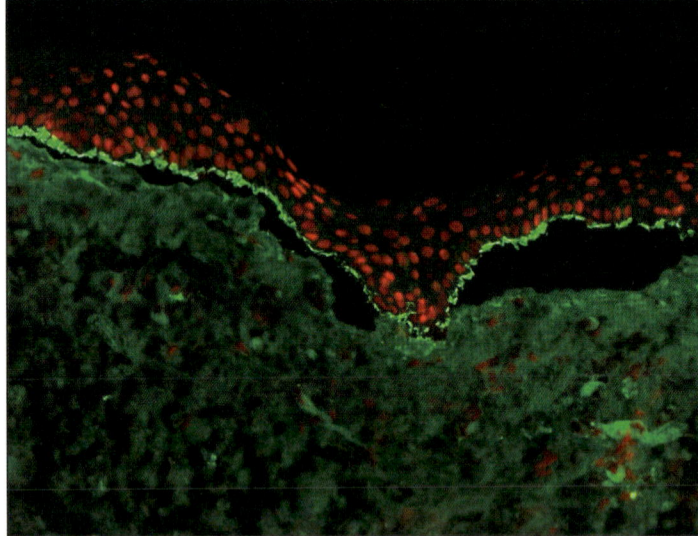

Figure 3.15 Direct immunofluorescence of bullous pemphigoid showing linear basement membrane zone deposition of IgG.

of the linear fluorescence pattern to the epidermal side/roof of the split, representing targeting of antibodies to epitopes within BP180 and/or BP230 proteins (Figure 3.15). Localisation of linear fluorescence to the dermal side/base of salt-split skin is indicative of a dermal-binding pemphigoid, including those that target chains of laminin proteins (e.g. laminin-332 and γ-1 laminin/p200 pemphigoid) which have a higher association with malignancy and are less responsive to immunosuppressive treatment.

Linear IgA bullous dermatosis

Similar to pemphigoid, patients with linear IgA disease, or the childhood variant, chronic bullous dermatosis of childhood (CBDC), present a bright, linear deposition of IgA along the BMZ with DIF analysis (Figure 3.16). In addition, there may be weak linear IgG and/or C3 BMZ fluorescence in some patients. The relative

Dermatitis herpetiformis

Patients with dermatitis herpetiformis, the predominant cutaneous manifestation of coeliac disease, exhibit a characteristic pattern of granular (sometimes fibrillar) deposition of IgA, either just beneath the basement membrane zone, in dermal papillae (Figure 3.18) or, occasionally, at the BMZ. Deposits may be subtle and easily missed and serology using standard IIF substrates is uninformative, because the target antigen in DH (epidermal transglutaminase) is not retained during substrate preparation.

Lichen planus

A thick, 'ragged' fibrinogen deposition is seen at the BMZ in exclusively lesional areas of cutaneous or mucosal tissue in lichen planus (Figure 3.19). In addition, an extensive lymphocytic infiltrate is often seen in the papillary dermis and colloid bodies (degenerating keratinocytes), which often fluoresce brightly with IgM, are also associated with this DIF pattern.

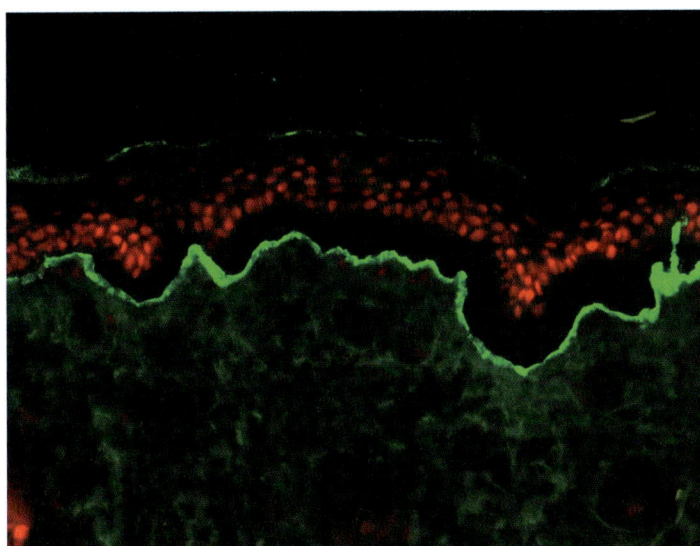

Figure 3.17 Direct immunofluorescence of epidermolysis bullosa acquisita showing thick linear basement membrane zone deposition of IgG, localising to the base of natural clefts.

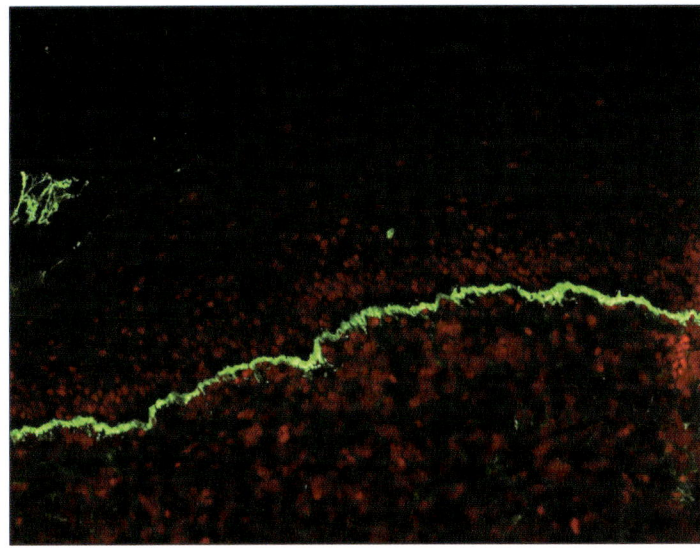

Figure 3.19 Direct immunofluorescence of lichen planus showing ragged basement membrane zone deposition of fibrinogen.

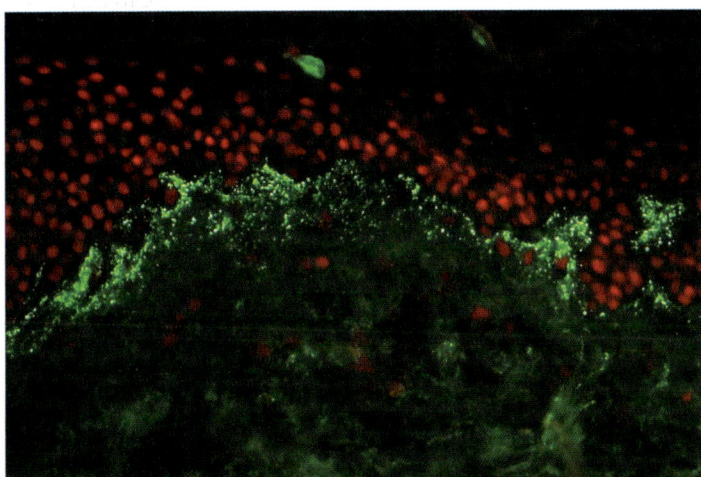

Figure 3.18 Direct immunofluorescence of dermatitis herpetiformis showing granular deposition of IgA in dermal papillae.

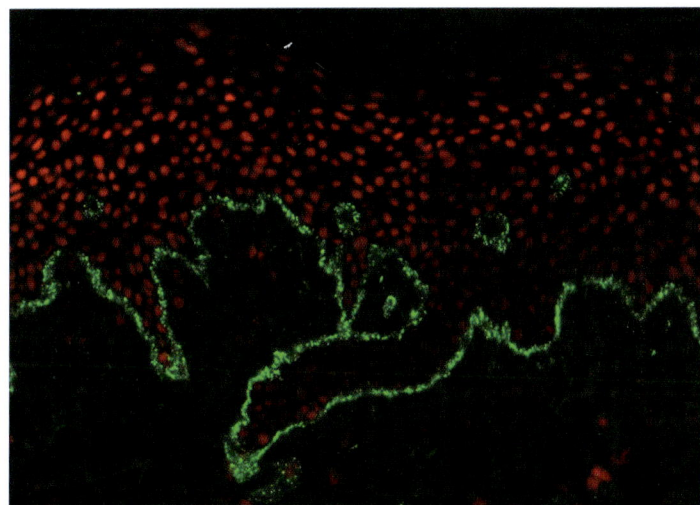

Figure 3.20 Direct immunofluorescence of lupus erythematosus showing granular basement membrane zone deposition of IgM.

Connective tissue diseases

Although non-diagnostic, connective tissue diseases can present with positive immunofluorescence when examined by DIF. In particular, continuous fine or coarse granular deposition of IgM at the BMZ, sometimes referred to as a lupus band, is observed in approximately 60% of patients with lupus erythematosus (Figure 3.20). A similar pattern may be observed with additional conjugates in different subtypes of lupus. A positive lupus band is usually seen in involved skin in cutaneous lupus erythematosus, but false positive results may be seen in sun-exposed skin from patients who do not have lupus [8]. Additionally, antinuclear antibody fluorescence within epithelial keratinocytes, typically of IgG isotype, may be seen in patients with a connective tissue disease during DIF analysis. However, this is also non-diagnostic and is observed in patients with no history of an underlying connective tissue disorder.

Indirect immunofluorescence

The combined utility of monkey oesophagus, normal human skin and split human skin tissue as substrates for the detection of circulating antibodies in patients with autoimmune blistering diseases using IIF methodologies constitutes an important tool in diagnosis (either through confirmation of DIF findings or, in the absence of a tissue biopsy, as a primary indicator) and monitoring of disease activity. In addition, use of these techniques, in combination with quantitative ELISA studies for specific immunobullous antigens, facilitates disease subtyping that is not possible with DIF techniques and which has important therapeutic and prognostic implications [9].

Monkey oesophagus is the most sensitive and widely used substrate for detection of desmosomal binding antibodies in pemphigus patients. Similar to DIF analysis, a 'chicken wire' pattern is seen on this tissue with an IgG detection antibody and fluorescence may be particularly bright with serum from patients with pemphigus vulgaris. Pemphigus foliaceus sera show a similar pattern on monkey oesophagus, although often at a lower intensity. Conversely, circulating antibodies from pemphigus foliaceus patients fluoresce more strongly on normal human skin than those from pemphigus vulgaris. In addition, the fluorescence seen is in suprabasal epidermal layers, compared with sera from pemphigus vulgaris, where fluorescence is concentrated in basal layers, as a result of the relative distributions of DSG1 and DSG3 within the epidermis.

Rat transitional epithelium can be used to detect antibodies against plakin proteins, most commonly envoplakin and periplakin, in patients with the uncommon, malignancy-mediated disease, paraneoplastic pemphigus. Sera from these patients typically exhibit positive intercellular immunofluorescence for IgG on both monkey oesophagus and transitional epithelium substrates.

By contrast, salt-split human skin is the substrate of choice for characterising subepithelial blistering diseases. The IgG linear BMZ depositions observed with DIF in these diseases can be subdivided into those localising to the 'roof' or the 'base' of the split-skin substrate. Most commonly, this is used to differentiate bullous pemphigoid, in which the linear fluorescence localises to the roof in most patients, from epidermolysis bullosa acquisita, where fluorescence always localises to the base of the split, reflecting the different antigens targeted in these two diseases. It is important to note that a base-binding linear IgG deposition does not diagnose epidermolysis bullosa acquisita, because a subset of pemphigoid patients produce antibodies targeting other antigens that localise to the base of split-skin substrate, in particular laminin proteins (eg. γ-1 laminin chains and laminin 332). Use of a collagen VII antibody ELISA can be helpful in distinguishing dermal-binding pemphigoid from epidermolysis bullosa acquisita (Figure 3.21).

IIF can also be used to detect IgA antibodies, in addition to IgG, in patients with linear IgA bullous dermatosis, mucous membrane pemphigoid and IgA pemphigus, although IgA levels are typically much lower than IgG antibodies targeting the same antigens and in the case of mucous membrane pemphigoid, only approximately 50% of cases can be detected with this method.

In addition to detection, IIF can provide semiquantitative data on circulating autoantibody levels by serially diluting aliquots of patient serum and assessing fluorescence intensity, to determine the lowest titre at which visible fluorescence is still observed. This is a rather subjective assessment with a large number of variables and is less accurate and sensitive than ELISA. However, unlike ELISA methodologies, serum titration is not limited to antibodies of known specificity and provides a method to assess total tissue-binding autoantibodies in a serum sample under investigation, irrespective of known antigenic specificity.

ELISA

ELISA assessment of sera from patients with immunobullous diseases can be used alone or, more usefully, in addition to IIF techniques to confirm diagnosis, establish disease subtypes and provide quantitative data on specific autoantibody levels (Figure 3.21).

In patients with pemphigus, ELISA analysis of DSG1 and DSG3 antibodies can be used to subtype the disease into either pemphigus vulgaris (DSG3 ± DSG1 antibodies) or pemphigus foliaceus (DSG1 antibodies alone) (Figure 3.22) and can also be used to monitor disease activity. In pemphigus vulgaris patients with both DSG1 and DSG3 antibodies, DSG1 antibody levels are typically more responsive than those targeting DSG3 following successful treatment. This finding also facilitates early detection of possible disease flares, if patients are being treated with tapering immunosuppression therapies.

Antibodies against BP180 (also known as BPAG2/collagen XVII) and/or BP230 (also known as BPAG1/dystonin) provide diagnostic confirmation in most cases of bullous pemphigoid and can also be used to monitor disease activity, although the correlation between ELISA values of these two autoantibodies and disease severity is

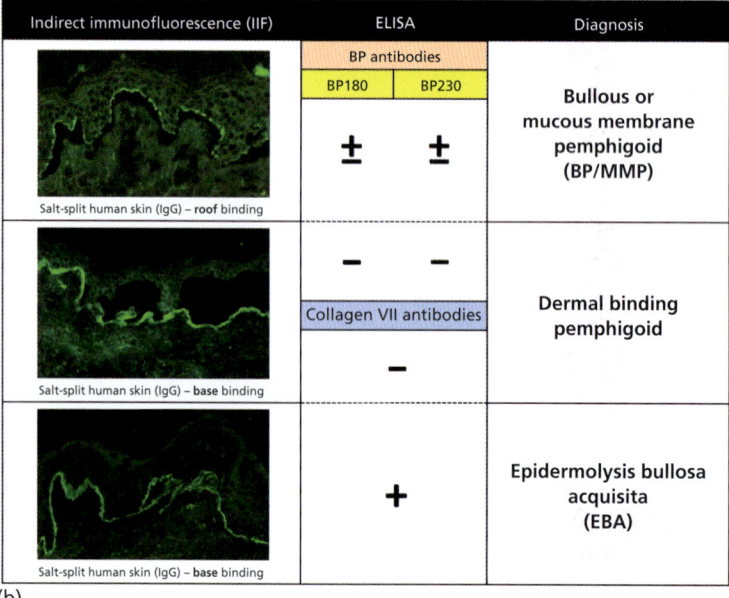

Figure 3.21 Serological diagnosis of (a) intraepithelial and (b) subepithelial immunobullous disorders using indirect immunofluorescence and ELISA techniques.

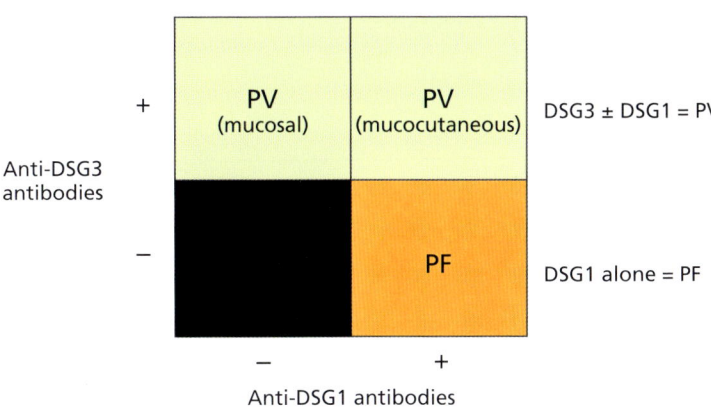

Figure 3.22 Pemphigus subtyping by desmoglein antibody profile. DSG1: desmoglein-1; DSG3: desmoglein-3; PV: pemphigus vulgaris; PF: pemphigus foliaceus.

lower than that seen between DSG antibodies and pemphigus disease activity. BP180 ELISA provides a highly sensitive and specific test for the diagnosis of pemphigoid gestationis, which commonly presents with low IgG antibody levels and in patients with mucous membrane pemphigoid, ELISA utilising these two antibodies provides a more sensitive assay than IIF.

ELISA analysis for anticollagen VII antibodies in sera with linear, base-binding IgG on human split-skin substrate by IIF analysis can be used to differentiate EBA from base-binding pemphigoids, because collagen VII is the sole target antigen in EBA. Quantification of anticollagen VII antibodies also facilitates disease activity monitoring in this disease.

Cutaneous neoplasms [10,11,12,13]

One of the most useful applications of immunopathology is in helping to determine the line of differentiation of poorly differentiated benign and malignant neoplasms that may arise from the various cellular components within the skin and related tissues. All the antibodies discussed below work well in formalin-fixed paraffin embedded material.

Keratins and other epithelial markers

Cytokeratins represent a group of intermediate filaments, known as tonofilaments, of variable molecular weight that may be demonstrated in keratinising and non-keratinising epithelia [14,15]. They represent the main structural component of the cytoskeleton of epithelial cells. More than 50 different keratins have been demonstrated in humans. Their molecular weight ranges from 40 to 68 kDa. Keratins are divided according to molecular weight and their charge properties into acidic (type I) and neutral-basic (type II) [15]. They associate as pairs of one acidic and one basic keratin polypeptide molecule with each epithelial cell containing at least one keratin pair.

The antibodies against keratins most frequently used in dermatopathology include AE1/AE3, MNF116 (Figure 3.23) and CAM 5.2. They are all cocktails containing several monoclonal antibodies of different molecular weight. CAM 5.2 is a low-molecular-weight keratin antibody, which labels most epithelia, with the exception of stratified squamous epithelia [16]. CAM 5.2 is usually negative in squamous cell carcinoma. It should therefore not be used in the diagnosis of poorly differentiated squamous cell carcinoma, as a negative result is the norm. The main use of CAM 5.2 in dermatopathology is in the diagnosis of Merkel cell carcinoma (primary cutaneous neuroendocrine carcinoma), as tumour cells in this lesion display a typical perinuclear dot-like positivity for this antibody.

Cytokeratin 20 (CK-20), a low-molecular-weight cytokeratin expressed usually only in urothelium, gastrointestinal epithelium and Merkel cells, is also very useful in the diagnosis of Merkel cell carcinoma [17,18]. The staining pattern is identical to that of CAM 5.2 (perinuclear dot-like; Figure 3.24), and a positive result strongly

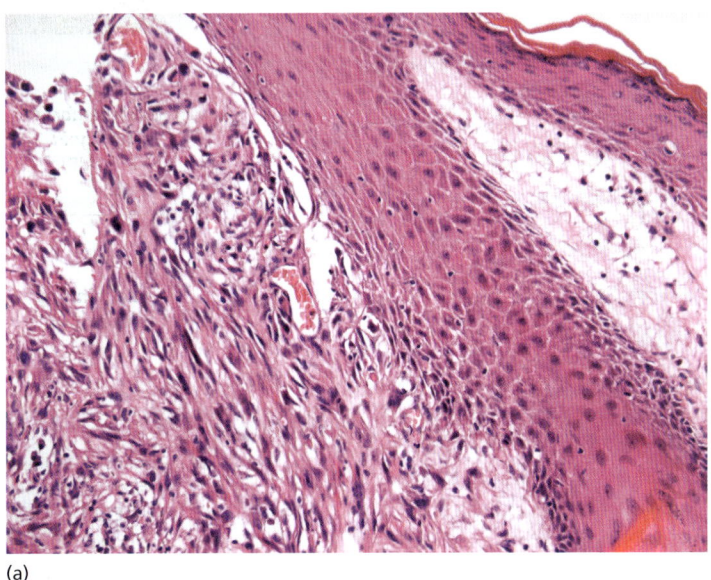
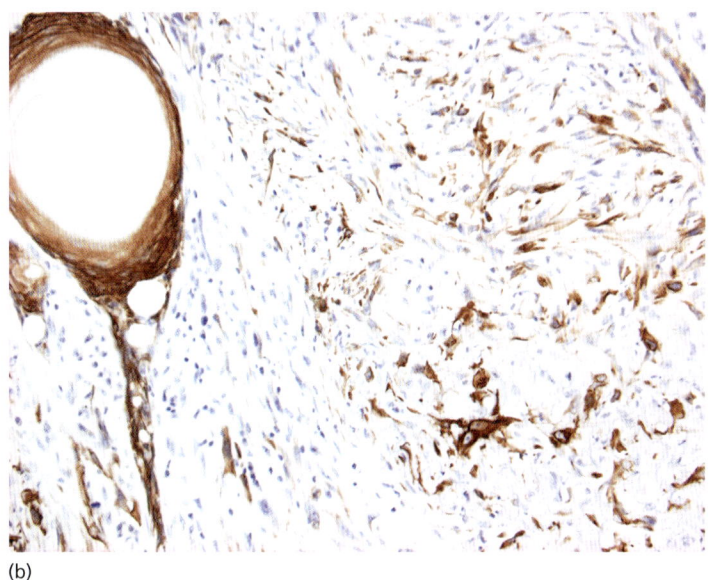

(a) (b)

Figure 3.23 (a) Poorly differentiated tumour composed of pleomorphic spindle-shaped cells in the dermis (H&E). (b) Diffuse positivity of tumour cells for the pan-keratin marker MNF116, confirming that the tumour is a sarcomatoid squamous cell carcinoma.

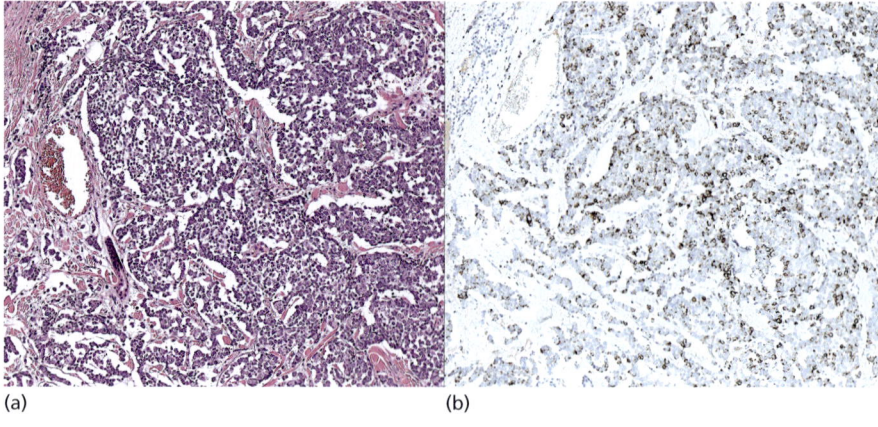

(a)   (b)

Figure 3.24 (a) Typical example of a Merkel cell carcinoma consisting of hyperchromatic cells with scanty cytoplasm. (b) Immunostaining with cytokeratin 20 highlighting the typical perinuclear dot-like positivity of tumour cells.

suggests a primary cutaneous origin rather than a metastatic neuroendocrine carcinoma originating in another organ. Only Merkel cell carcinoma and salivary gland small cell carcinoma tend to be positive for this marker, while neuroendocrine tumours from other organs are consistently negative.

CK-7 is a very useful antibody for confirmation of the diagnosis of mammary and extramammary Paget disease (Figure 3.25) [19,20]. Tumour cells in the latter stain consistently for this antibody while the surrounding epidermis is negative. However, staining for keratin 7 is not specific for mammary and extramammary Paget disease as positivity has been described in clonal Bowen disease and in rare cases of actinic keratoses [21,22]. It is important to remember that keratin and also epithelial membrane antigen (EMA) expression is commonly seen in various sarcomas, including epithelioid sarcoma, synovial sarcoma, epithelioid angiosarcoma and more rarely in other tumours such as leiomyosarcoma and rhabdomyosarcoma [23–26].

EMAs [27] are derived from human milk fat globulin membrane and consist of high-molecular-weight glycoproteins. Antibodies to EMA and related labels react with a range of normal and neoplastic epithelia, and positivity may be found in squamous and ductal epithelia as well as eccrine, apocrine and sebaceous glands. EMA tends to be at least focally positive in squamous cell carcinoma, sebaceous carcinoma, perineurioma and a wide variety of adnexal carcinomas. It is also positive in plasma cells, in epithelioid sarcoma, synovial sarcoma, epithelioid angiosarcoma, epithelioid fibrous histiocytoma and in systemic and, less commonly, primary cutaneous CD30+ large-cell anaplastic lymphoma [28].

Carcinoembryonic antigen is a protein that is normally found in the goblet cells of the small and large intestine. It is found in many adnexal carcinomas, particularly tumours displaying ductal differentiation [29]. It is also expressed in many glandular carcinomas arising in other organs. Its main use in dermatopathology is to highlight ductal differentiation in adnexal tumours.

An antibody against adipophilin, a lipid droplet-specific marker, is used as an aid in the differential diagnosis of tumours with sebaceous differentiation [30]. The pattern of staining in the latter tumours is membranous vesicular, while non-sebaceous tumours that are positive for this marker tend to show granular staining. Tumour cells in squamous and basal cell carcinomas are usually negative for this marker but metastatic renal cell carcinoma may be positive.

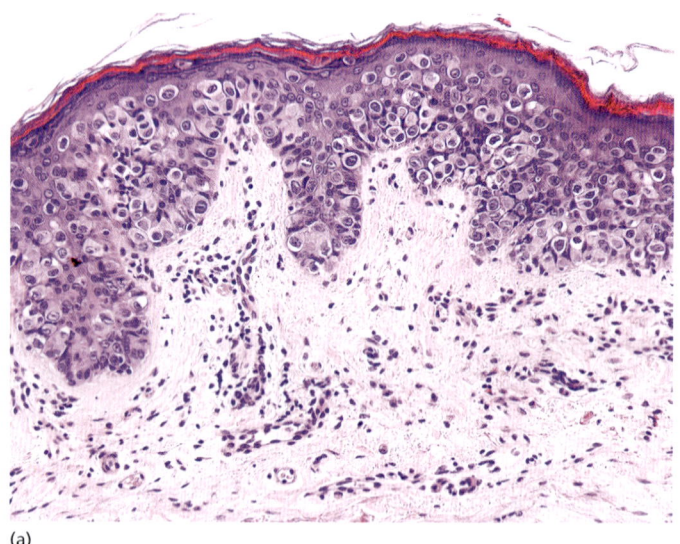

(a)

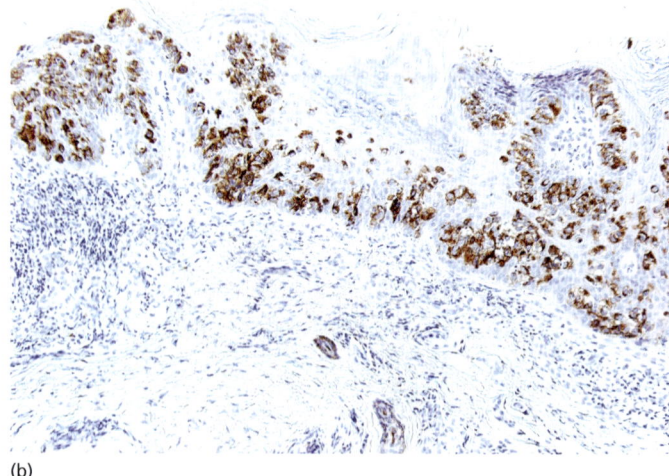

(b)

Figure 3.25 (a) Extramammary Paget disease showing prominent colonisation of the epidermis by numerous, atypical, rounded cells with pink cytoplasm. (b) Tumour cells stain diffusely for cytokeratin 7.

BerEP4 is a monoclonal antibody that detects the EpCam antigen, a transmembrane epithelial glycoprotein cell adhesion molecule present in epithelial progenitor cells and in a number of carcinomas arising in different organs. This protein is expressed consistently in basal cell carcinomas and it is negative in squamous cell carcinoma.

Expression in adnexal neoplasms is variable and it is therefore not useful in the differential diagnosis between the latter and basal cell carcinoma [31].

Neuroendocrine markers

Besides CK-20, whose use in the diagnosis of Merkel cell carcinoma has been described, markers of neuroendocrine differentiation include neuron-specific enolase, chromogranin and synaptophysin. Neuron-specific enolase is an enzyme described in the brain but also found in neuroendocrine cells [32]. Its use in diagnostic pathology is very limited because of the lack of specificity. Chromogranin A is part of a family of calcium-binding proteins present in the secretory granules of neuroendocrine cells. This protein is very specific but poorly sensitive for neuroendocrine differentiation [33]. Synaptophysin is a transmembrane glycoprotein with a molecular weight of 38 kDa and is a specific marker of neuroendocrine differentiation [34]. CD56 (neural cell adhesion molecule) is expressed in neural tissues, natural killer cells and a subset of T cells, among other tissues [35]. Neurofilament is consistently expressed in tumour cells in Merkel cell carcinoma in a paranuclear dot pattern, a feature that is not seen in neuroendocrine carcinomas arising in other organs [36]. This protein is often expressed in tumours with neuroendocrine differentiation and is sometimes included in the immunohistochemical panel used to diagnose Merkel cell carcinoma. This marker is particularly useful in the setting of CK20 negative Merkel cell carcinoma. Other useful more recently described markers include SATB2 (special AT-rich sequence-binding protein 2) and Merkel cell polyomavirus-large T antigen [37].

Melanocytic markers and antibodies used in the diagnosis and classification of melanocytic neoplasms and in monitoring response to treatment in melanoma

Over the years, a wide array of markers for melanocytes has been described including S-100 protein, HMB45, Melan-A, Mel-5, tyrosinase, MIFT-1 (microphthalmia transcription factor 1) and SOX-10. It is important to emphasise that no marker allows distinction between benign and melanocytes and that the sensitivity and specificity of different markers is variable. S-100 protein is very sensitive but much less specific than other markers including HMB45, Melan-A and MIFT-1. Melanocytic markers are particularly useful as part of a panel in the differential diagnosis of poorly differentiated malignant tumours. Desmoplastic melanomas are usually positive for S-100 protein but negative for melanocytic markers such as Melan-A, HMB45 and MIFT-1.

S-100 protein is an acidic protein, originally derived from ox brain, and named because of its solubility in 100% ammonium sulphate. It is a sensitive marker of melanocytes (Figure 3.26) [38–40]. Antibodies to S-100 protein, however, also react with Schwann cells, glial cells, adipocytes, chondrocytes, myoepithelial cells, Langerhans cells and cells of the eccrine sweat coil, and therefore tumours from these cells. S-100 protein also stains the cells in Rosai–Dorfman disease. S-100 protein is particularly useful in the study of suspected melanoma, as the great majority of, but by no means all, melanomas are positive for this marker [41]. In this context, the technique is particularly valuable in the differentiation of melanoma from other spindle cell neoplasms, and in identifying small deposits of melanoma that may be present in deep dermal tissues, as in the

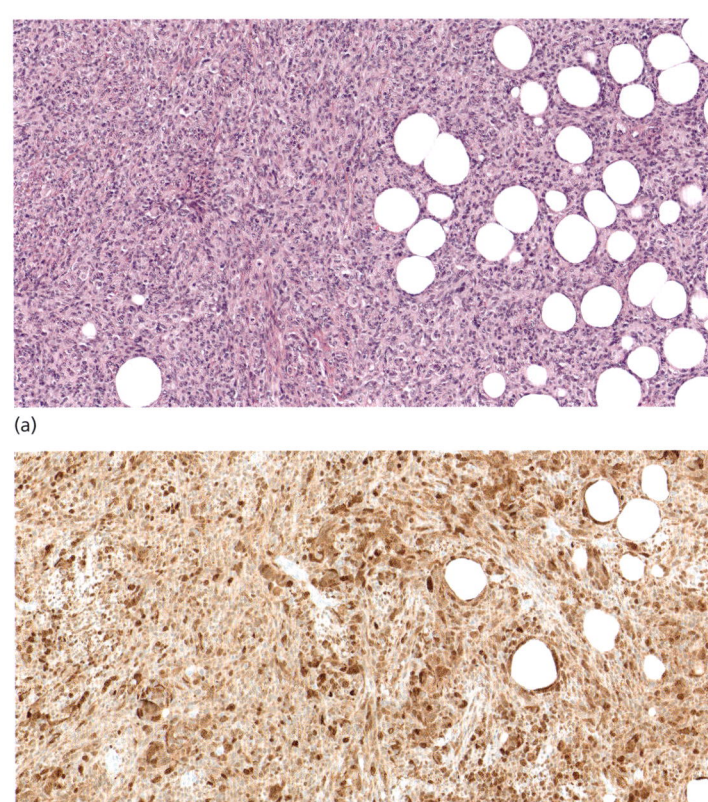

Figure 3.26 (a) Cellular blue naevus. Bland spindle-shaped cells with poor pigmentation and vesicular nuclei. (b) Diffuse cytoplasmic and nuclear staining for S100 protein.

determination of accurate Breslow thickness and/or intravascular spread, or the evaluation of spread to sentinel lymph nodes. S-100 protein is less reliable when used to delineate the epidermal component of a melanocytic lesion. The reason for this is that it also stains Langerhans cells. More specific markers of melanocytes such as Melan-A should be used for this purpose. S-100 protein is also often focally positive in a number of soft-tissue tumours and should therefore be used as part of a panel of markers in the diagnosis of poorly differentiated tumours.

HMB-45 (gp100) [42–44] recognises a 10 kDa antigen localised in premelanosomal vesicles. The antibody was developed from an extract of a lymph node metastasis of melanoma. This antibody does not stain normal adult melanocytes or intradermal naevi. It is a very specific antibody and is usually negative in desmoplastic melanoma. Around 90% of primary and metastatic melanomas are positive for this marker.

Melan-A (MART-1) [45,46] is a melanocyte marker that recognises an antigen present in melanoma cells and is recognised by CD8+ cytotoxic T lymphocytes. It is a fairly specific marker of melanocytes. Melan-A stains naevi and melanomas, but it tends to be negative in desmoplastic melanoma, spindle cell melanoma and neurotised naevi. Although Melan-A is a useful melanocytic marker, its usefulness in distinction between *in situ* melanoma arising in sun-exposed skin and pigmented actinic keratosis has been challenged [47]. The reason for this is that Melan-A may also occasionally stain melanocytes, probably as a result of transference of the protein from melanocytes to keratinocytes.

Mel-5 is a monoclonal antibody developed against a 75 kDa glycoprotein present in melanocytes, naevus cells and melanoma cells [48]. As for Melan-A, it does not tend to be expressed in desmoplastic melanoma, spindle cell melanoma and neurotised naevi.

MIFT-1 is a nuclear protein involved in the development of melanocytes and in the regulation of melanin synthesis [49]. It stains naevi and melanomas but is usually negative in desmoplastic melanomas. Although it was initially regarded as fairly specific, it has been found to be expressed in macrophages, mast cells, fibroblasts, lymphocytes, Schwann cells and even smooth muscle cells [50]. Its utility as part of a panel for the diagnosis of difficult tumours has proven to be limited due to its lack of specificity.

SOX-10 is a transcription factor that has a crucial role in the development of Schwann cells and melanocytes. The pattern of staining is nuclear and it is useful in the differential diagnosis between desmoplastic melanoma and tumours that are histologically confused with it, including sarcomatoid carcinoma, atypical fibroxanthoma and various sarcomas. Malignant peripheral nerve sheath tumours display positivity for this marker but these tend to be focally positive only, whereas in desmoplastic melanoma tumour cells are diffusely positive for this marker [51]. Because of its nuclear staining, SOX-10 is very useful in the evaluation of the intraepithelial component of melanocytic proliferations (Figure 3.27).

Cocktails consisting of a mixture of different monoclonal antibodies against melanocytes have been developed and advocated as being effective, particularly in the detection of low-volume melanoma cells in sentinel lymph node biopsies. One of the main cocktails used consists of a mixture of Mart-1, Melan-A and tyrosine (MCW) [52].

CDKN2A, a tumour suppressor gene located on chromosome 9p21, is a member of the INK4 class of cell cycle inhibitors. Its product, a cyclin-dependent kinase inhibitor 2A or protein p16 plays a role in the regulation of the cell cycle. The expression of this marker has been proposed as a discriminant between benign and malignant melanocytic proliferations. However, although melanomas often show loss of expression of the marker in contrast with naevi which display diffuse positivity, there are too many exceptions for it to be reliably used on its own as a diagnostic tool [53,54]. Loss of staining in a melanocytic tumour cannot be equated with malignancy and loss of heterozygosity should be confirmed by molecular tests.

Proliferation markers are useful not only in the evaluation of melanocytic tumours but also in other skin neoplasms including lymphoproliferative disorders. Antigen KI-67 is a non-histone nuclear protein expressed during the G1, S, G2 and M phases of the cell cycle and it is the main cell proliferation marker used in dermatopathology. The antibodies used are MIB1, a monoclonal antibody and anti-Ki67, a polyclonal antibody. A further less used proliferation marker is an antibody against phosphorylated histone H3 (pHH3). Histone H3 becomes phosphorylated between late anaphase and telophase and is a reliable marker of mitoses. Proliferation markers can be used with a cytoplasmic melanocytic marker as a counterstain to accurately evaluate proliferating cells of melanocytic lineage [55,56].

BRAF encodes a cytoplasmic serine/threonine kinase in the MAPK pathway upstream of ERK/MEK. Mutations in *BRAF* are not only found in melanoma (mainly those arising in non-chronically sun-exposed skin) but also in naevi. One of the most frequent mutations found in melanoma is BRAF V600E and although this is usually demonstrated by molecular testing, there is a sensitive and specific monoclonal antibody that can be used in paraffin embedded sections [57].

In the recent two decades, the understanding of the molecular mechanisms underlying an increasing number of melanocytic tumours has allowed a more logical classification of these challenging neoplasms, mainly but not only restricted to Spitz lesions. A number of genetic abnormalities and gene fusions have been described and these can not only be confirmed by molecular testing but also by the use of immunohistochemistry. These fusions are usually mutually exclusive not only within the group of protein kinases but also in relation to other driver mutations. Antibodies available for testing include *ALK*, *BRAF*, *NTRK1* and *ROS1* [58].

Germline mutations in BRAC1-associated protein (BAP-1) result in loss of expression of the protein, BRAF mutations and are associated with distinctive epithelioid Spitz-like neoplasms that can be multiple in a hereditary setting and associated with uveal melanoma and other internal cancers or more commonly, sporadic and with no known associations [59,60]. The loss of BAP-1 can be demonstrated by immunohistochemistry. Nuclear expression of ß-catenin is very useful in distinguishing between deep penetrating naevi/melanocytoma from other melanocytic neoplasms [61].

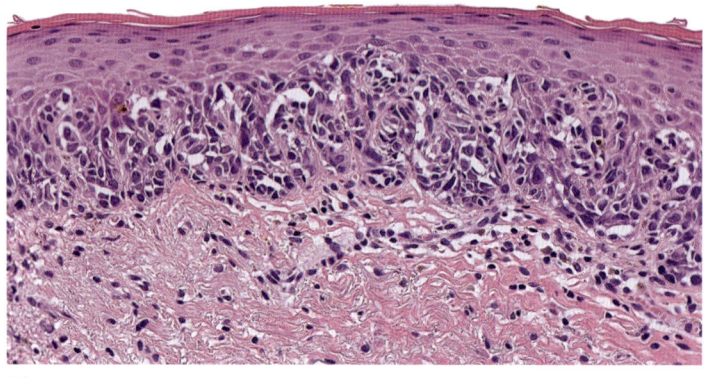

(a)

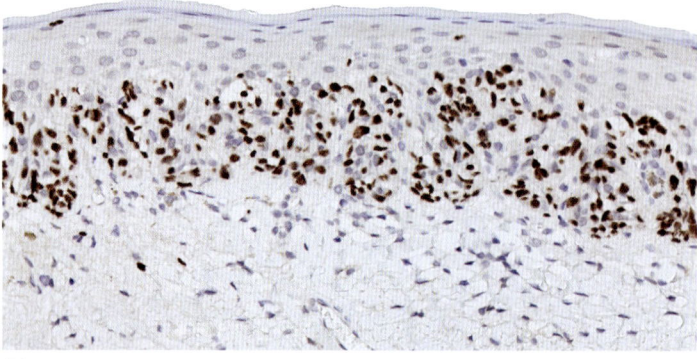

(b)

Figure 3.27 (a) Melanoma *in situ*. Atypical melanocytes in the epidermis with focal nest formation. (b) SOX10 highlights the nuclei of melanocytes.

Antibodies to CTLA-4 (cytotoxic T lymphocyte antigen-4), PD-1 (programmed cell death) and PD-L1 (programmed cell death ligand) have been used in the immunohistochemical evaluation of melanomas and other cancers to predict response to immunotherapy. The main problem with this approach, however, has been the standardisation and reproducibility of the results. Furthermore, a percentage of patients that are negative for these markers show good response [62,63].

PRAME (PReferentially expressed Antigen in Melanoma) is a melanoma-associated antigen and its expression can be assessed in melanocyte tumours by a monoclonal antibody. This protein is usually diffusely expressed in melanomas (except the desmoplastic variant) and tends to be negative or minimally expressed in naevi and it can be used with caution, as an aid in differential diagnosis of melanocytic lesions [64]. It is also particularly useful in the evaluation of excision margins in melanoma *in situ*.

Mesenchymal markers

There are many markers of mesenchymal differentiation that are useful in the differential diagnosis of neoplasms, particularly those that are poorly differentiated. As with many of the other antibodies discussed so far, the specificity and sensitivity of each of these markers is very variable. What this means is that they should always be used as part of a wider panel of markers. Commonly used markers include vimentin, S-100 protein, desmin, smooth muscle actin, muscle-specific actin, calponin, h-caldesmon, CD34, CD10, CD31 and Fli-1.

Vimentin has a molecular weight of 57 kDa and it is found in all mesenchymal cells and their tumours. It has a very low specificity and can be found in melanomas, lymphomas and even carcinomas. Its value is therefore very limited [65].

S-100 protein has already been described above. It is a very useful marker for neurofibroma and schwannoma. While the latter tumour tends to be uniformly positive for S-100 protein, the percentage of tumour cells positive for this marker varies in neurofibroma.

Desmin is a polypeptide with a molecular weight of 53 kDa, and is characteristic of smooth, skeletal and cardiac muscle [66,67]. In skeletal muscle, desmin filaments are found in association with the Z-discs of the sarcomeres and the sarcolemmal attachment plaques. In smooth muscle cells, desmin filaments interconnect the fusiform dense bodies with the plasmalemmal dense bodies. Desmin is very specific for muscular differentiation and is a useful marker as it is only occasionally reported in other tumours such as cellular fibrous histiocytoma, schwannoma and epithelioid sarcoma [68,69].

Actin represents a family of intermediate filaments present in the cytoskeleton of eukaryotic cells. They are contractile proteins involved in the control of the motility of muscle cells and non-muscle cells. Actin proteins are classified according to their amino acid sequences and six major isoforms have been described. Of the monoclonal antibodies used in diagnostic pathology the most useful ones are HHF35 (muscle-specific actin) and 1A4 (alpha smooth muscle actin) [70–72]. The former reacts with skeletal and smooth muscle and the latter only reacts with smooth muscle. Both types of antibody stain myofibroblasts, pericytes, glomus cells (Figure 3.28) and myoepithelial cells [73].

Calponin is a basic troponin T-like protein that modulates the interaction between actin and myosin. It is a good marker of smooth

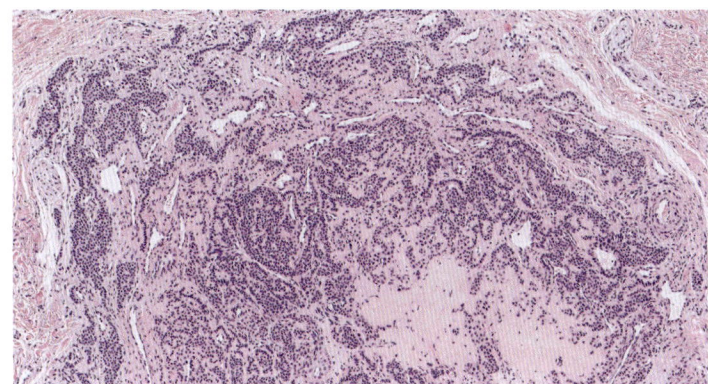

(a)

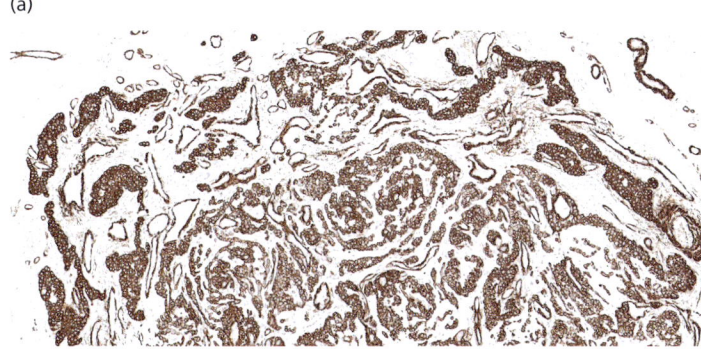

(b)

Figure 3.28 (a) Glomus tumour composed of uniform, round cells with pale cytoplasm and well-defined cytoplasmic membrane. (b) Strong cytoplasmic staining for smooth muscle actin in a case of glomus tumour.

muscle and myofibroblastic differentiation [73]. It is seldom used due to its lack of specificity.

H-caldesmon is a protein combined with actin and tropomyosin that regulates cell contraction. It is fairly specific for smooth-muscle differentiation and less often stains myofibroblasts [74,75].

CD34 is a glycosylated transmembrane protein with a molecular weight of 110 kDa. It is normally present on haematopoietic progenitor cells and vascular endothelial cells [76,77]. This marker, however, is fairly non-specific and it is expressed in a wide number of soft-tissue tumours including dermatofibrosarcoma protuberans (DFSP) (Figure 3.29), neurofibroma and spindle cell lipoma. Its main use in dermatopathology is as an endothelial cell marker and in the differential diagnosis between DFSP and fibrous histiocytoma and its variants, particularly cellular fibrous histiocytoma. CD34 tends to be diffusely positive in the former and negative or only focally positive, mainly in the periphery of the tumour, in the latter [78,79].

One large group of soft-tissue tumours where useful markers are badly needed is the group of fibrohistiocytic tumours. These tumours, despite their name, do not show true histiocytic differentiation. Factor XIIIa, a polyclonal antibody produced against the blood coagulation transglutaminase, seems to be a cell marker for a particular subpopulation of dermal dendritic mononuclear macrophage cells termed dermal dendrocytes [80]. A number of positive cells may be identified in very many different types of soft-tissue tumours. However, combined with other markers, factor XIIIa is useful in the differential diagnosis between benign fibrous histiocytoma (dermatofibroma) and DFSP. The former is normally rich in factor XIIIa-positive cells particularly at the periphery, in

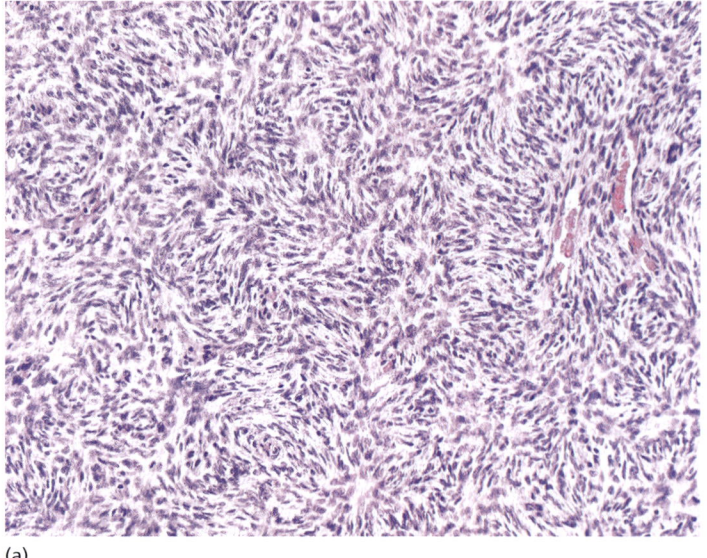

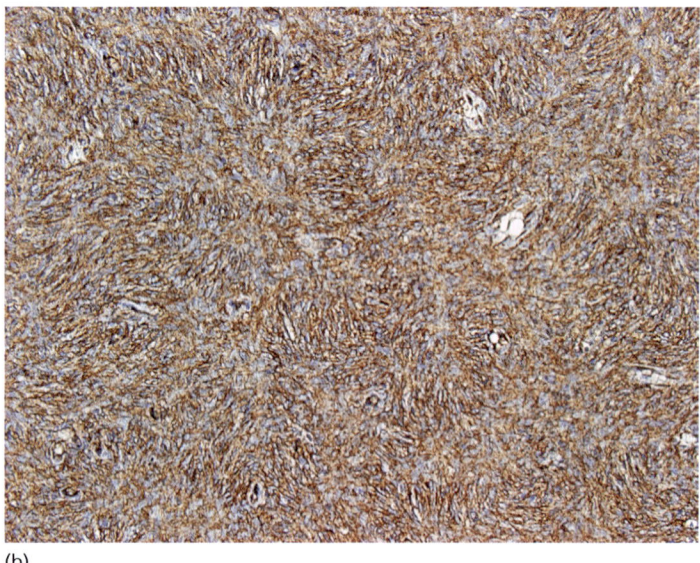

Figure 3.29 (a) Typical dermatofibrosarcoma protuberans composed of monotonous, spindle-shaped cells with hyperchromatic nuclei arranged in a prominent storiform pattern (H&E). (b) Diffuse staining of tumour cells for CD34.

A wide range of endothelial markers now available are useful in the histological diagnosis of vascular tumours. The most useful of these markers are CD31, CD34, Fli-1 and more recently ERG (Ets-related gene). There is also an expanding range of markers of lymphatic endothelium, the most commonly used being podoplanin (D2-40).

CD31 refers to a glycoprotein that belongs to the immunoglobulin supergene family and has a molecular weight of 130 kDa. It is also known as platelet–endothelial cell adhesion molecule type 1 (PECAM-1) and it stains endothelial cells and some haematopoietic cells. CD31 is a sensitive but not very specific marker of endothelial cells [83–85]. Interpretation should be cautious as CD31 also stains macrophages [86].

Fli-1 (friend leukaemia virus integration 1) is a DNA-binding transcription factor member of the ETS gene family. Most cases of Ewing sarcoma (90%) show a translocation t(11;22) (q24;q12) indicating fusion of EWS with Fli-1. Fli-1 is also expressed in endothelial cells and is a useful and fairly specific marker of endothelial cell differentiation [87]. The positive product displays nuclear staining.

ERG, an ETS family regulatory transcription factor, is now regarded as the most specific and sensitive marker of endothelial cells [88]. The pattern of staining is nuclear. This marker is also positive in a percentage of prostatic cancers and may be expressed by epithelioid sarcomas [89].

None of these endothelial cell markers allow distinction between lymphatic and vascular endothelium. In recent years, a number of antibodies have been described with claims as to their specificity for lymphatic endothelium. These antibodies include vascular endothelial growth factor receptor 3 (VEGFR-3), podoplanin, LYVE-1 (lymphatic vessel–endothelial hyaluronan receptor) and Prox-1 (a nuclear transcription factor important in lymphangiogenesis) [90–96]. Some of these markers are not very specific in lymphatic differentiation, particularly VEGFR-3.

INI 1 (hSNF5/SMARCB1) is a putative tumour-suppressor gene located on chromosome 22q11.2. Immunohistochemistry for INI 1 is consistently negative in epithelioid sarcomas and this is a very useful diagnostic tool as other tumours confused with the former tend to be positive for this marker [97].

Metastatic cutaneous tumours

It is important to remember that all tumours that are present in the skin are not necessarily of cutaneous origin. Reference has already been made to several epithelial markers, many of which may be useful in diagnosing metastatic adenocarcinoma. Immunohistochemistry, however, does not usually allow determination of the site of the primary tumour except in a few instances. The latter include prostate-specific antigen in prostatic carcinoma and thyroglobulin in thyroid carcinoma. Markers for oestrogen and progesterone receptors are not useful in the diagnosis of metastatic breast carcinoma, because adnexal carcinomas may also be positive for one or both markers. A combination of a number of markers may often be useful, however, in determining whether a tumour is primary or metastatic. Immunohistochemical markers that are not entirely specific but which may be used in a panel include among others, GATA-3 and mammaglobin (breast, but often positive in cutaneous adnexal neoplasms), CDX2 (colonic adenocarcinoma), RCC and PAX8 (renal cell carcinoma) and calretinin (mesothelioma).

contrast to DFSP which is negative. A number of fibrous histiocytomas, particularly variants such as cellular fibrous histiocytoma (cellular dermatofibroma), display variable expression of SMA in a population of cells that are likely to be of myofibroblastic lineage. D2-40 (podoplanin) identifies a 40 kDa O-linked sialoglycoprotein present in lymphatic endothelium and has been reported to be expressed consistently in fibrous histiocytomas and not in dermatofibrosarcoma protuberans [81].

CD10, a cell membrane metallopeptidase that is present in many haematopoeitic neoplasms – mainly those of B cell lineage – is also widely expressed in mesenchymal neopasms. Its use has been advocated in the differential diagnosis between atypical fibroxanthoma and sarcomatoid squamous cell carcinoma and spindle cell melanoma [82]. However, the latter two can also be positive for this marker, although usually in a more focal pattern.

Thyroid transcription factor 1 (TTF-1) is a 38 kDa nuclear protein expressed in epithelial cells of lung and thyroid. TTF-1 is therefore a useful marker in the diagnosis of cutaneous metastatic tumours [98]. p63, a homologue of the *p53* gene, has been demonstrated to be useful in the differential diagnosis between primary and metastatic adenocarcinomas in the skin. Metastatic adenocarcinomas to the skin are usually negative for p63 while primary adnexal adenocarcinomas tend to be positive for this marker [99,100]. Similar findings are obtained in adnexal carcinomas metastatic to other organs. The same finding has been recently reported with podoplanin as metastatic adenocarcinomas to the skin tend to be negative in tumour cells, while tumour cells in primary adnexal carcinomas are positive for this marker. ERG is useful in the diagnosis of metastatic prostatic carcinoma [101].

Histiocytic markers
CD68 (KP1) has been for many years the main marker used to demonstrate histiocytic differentiation in paraffin-embedded material [102,103]. It is an antibody raised against a 110 kDa glycoprotein present in pulmonary macrophages. This antibody stains normal histiocytes, granulocyte precursors, tumour cells in myelomonocytic neoplasms and true histiocytic lymphomas. KP1, however, is not specific for histiocytic differentiation, and expression may be seen in many tumours, including carcinomas, melanomas, granular cell tumours and a variety of sarcomas [104–106]. A more specific marker of histiocytic differentiation is PG-M1, a member of the CD68 group of proteins, which is present only in macrophages and not in myeloid cells [107,108]. CD163 is a glycoprotein of the scavenger receptor cysteine-rich superfamily that is more specific than CD68 as a marker of histiocytes [109] (Figure 3.30).

Langerhans cell markers
The main markers of Langerhans cells are S-100 protein and CD1a. More recently, langerin (CD207, a Langerhans cell-specific lectin) has been introduced as a sensitive and specific marker of Langerhans cells, as is CD1a [110,111]. S-100 protein is very sensitive but poorly specific, particularly as it stains melanocytes. Both the latter and Langerhans cells are present in healthy and abnormal epidermis. Often in inflammatory conditions there is hyperplasia of the Langerhans cells within the epidermis and they are often arranged in nests. This may lead to an erroneous diagnosis of mycosis fungoides as the nests of cells are confused with Pautrier microabscesses. In this setting, immunohistochemistry for Langerhans cells (Figure 3.31) and other histological parameters are useful to make the distinction.

Lymphoid markers
One of the most difficult areas in diagnostic dermatopathology is the interpretation of heavy lymphoid infiltrates in cutaneous biopsies. The wide range of conditions that may produce a histological picture simulating lymphoma ranges from insect bites and viral infections, through syphilis, to reactive lymphoid hyperplasia, where an aetiological factor cannot be demonstrated. Furthermore, recognition of the number of different varieties of malignant lymphoproliferative disorders that may be encountered in the skin continues to increase. Very many different markers for lymphocytes and their subsets are now available and are particularly useful when

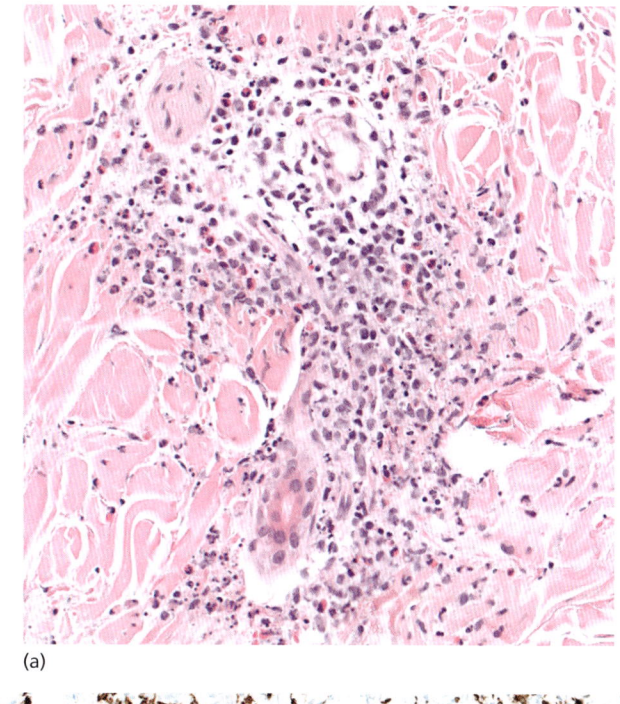

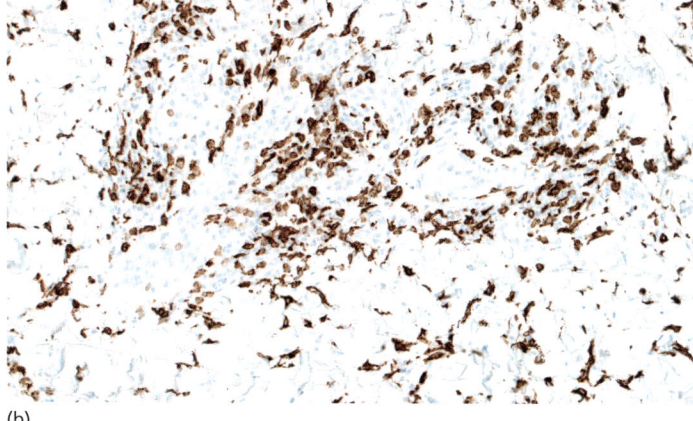

Figure 3.30 (a) Histiocytic-rich infiltrate with eosinophils in the background. (b) CD163 is a fairly specific marker of histiocytes.

used as a battery. It should be remembered that histological and antibody-labelling patterns of cutaneous lymphomas do not necessarily mirror their nodal counterparts, and that very few markers are absolutely specific for the cells of one lineage. Furthermore, it must be realised that in the course of a disease process, many lymphoid cell types may lose their antigenic determinants and may label in an anomalous fashion. This is particularly common in some forms of advanced cutaneous lymphoma. Nevertheless, with careful interpretation and the use of antibody panels, considerable information can be derived from the use of monoclonal antibodies.

The rationalisation of nomenclature in relation to human leukocyte antigens, the CD (or cluster of differentiation) nomenclature, has been a great advance, enabling useful comparisons of numerous different monoclonal antibodies developed in different laboratories, and facilitating their classification [2,112,113]. As in other areas of immunopathology, a further bonus for the diagnostic dermatopathologist is the possibility of using many of these leukocyte

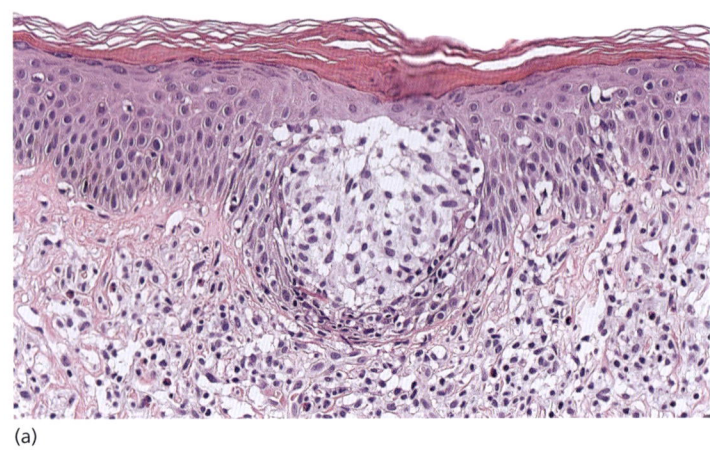

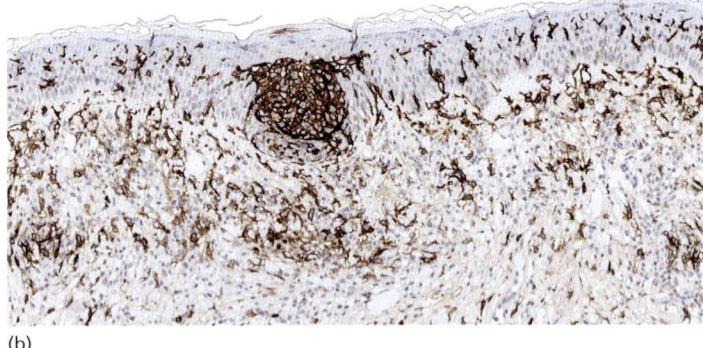

Figure 3.31 (a) Subacute spongiotic process (eczema) with hyperplasia of Langerhans cells presenting in a large nest within the epidermis mimicking a Pautrier microabscess (H&E). (b) Staining for CD1a highlighting the nature of the nested cells within the epidermis.

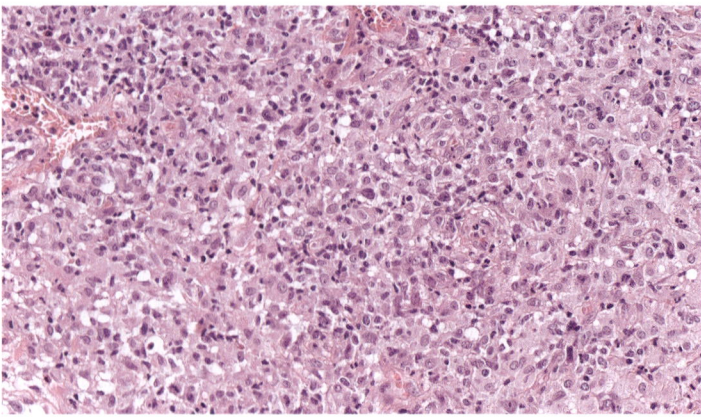

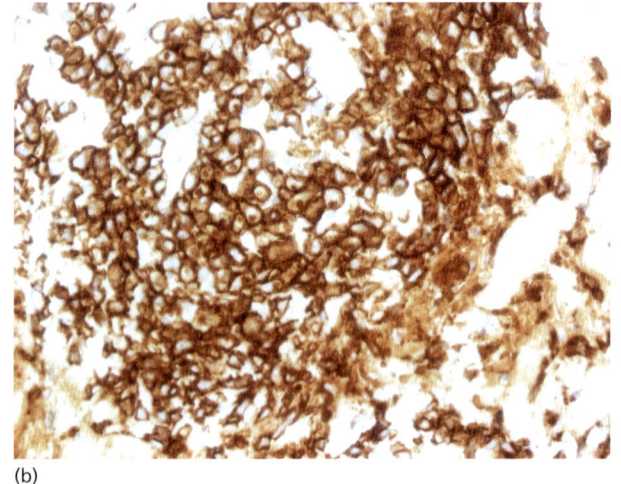

Figure 3.32 (a) Sheets of large, atypical lymphoid cells with pleomorphic nuclei and pink cytoplasm. (b) Positive staining of atypical cells in a case of CD30-positive, anaplastic, large T-cell lymphoma. Note the typical strong cytoplasmic membrane positivity and dot-like perinuclear staining.

antigen markers in paraffin-embedded tissue [114,115]. A full discussion of the applications of immunopathology to the recognition of subsets of lymphocytes in skin biopsies is beyond the scope of this chapter. Useful antibodies available for use on routinely processed material include CD45 (leukocyte common antigen), pan B-cell markers such as CD20 (L26), Pax5 and CD79a, and pan T-cell markers such as CD3, CD2, CD5 and CD7 [116,117]. The determination of the subset of T cells in paraffin-embedded skin biopsies is also possible as there are commercially available antibodies to CD4 (helper T cells) and CD8 (cytotoxic T cells) T cells [2,118,119]. Immunohistochemistry is also very useful in the determination of clonality, particularly in B-cell infiltrates. Antibodies against κ and λ light chains can be used in paraffin-embedded material to demonstrate clonality [2,120,121]. More recently, however, *in situ* hybridisation for κ and λ light chains has replaced immunohistochemistry as the method of choice as the results with this procedure are much easier to interpret [122]. Monotypic immunoglobulin light chain expression is very suggestive of a B-cell lymphoma.

Other markers of interest include determinants closely associated with T-cell activation, such as the CD30 antigen. An example of an antibody to the CD30 epitope is Ber-H2, which identifies activated T cells, B cells and Reed–Sternberg cells. In cutaneous biopsies it is commonly present in examples of CD30-positive lymphoproliferative disorders, including lymphomatoid papulosis and CD30-positive anaplastic large cell lymphoma (Figure 3.32) [123–125]. It is also frequently and variably expressed in cutaneous T-cell lymphoma (mycosis fungoides) in transformation.

Anaplastic lymphoma kinase (ALK) is a marker of the protein that results from translocation 2;5 between the ALK and nucleophosmin. Its usefulness resides in the fact that this protein is expressed in systemic large-cell anaplastic lymphoma, but it is usually not expressed in primary cutaneous large-cell anaplastic CD30+ lymphomas [126,127].

CD4, BCL-6, PD1, ICOS, CD10 and CXCL13 are markers of follicular helper T cells and are now used in the diagnosis of cutaneous lymphoproliferative disorders of these cells including CD4+ small/medium-sized pleomorphic T-cell lymphoproliferative disorder and cutaneous follicular helper T-cell lymphoma [128,129].

CD56 (neural cell adhesion molecule) is expressed in the central and peripheral nervous system, and is also a marker of natural killer (NK) cells. Its main use in dermatopathology is in the diagnosis of cutaneous NK/T-cell lymphoma [130,131]. Some subcutaneous panniculitis-like T-cell lymphomas may also express this marker [132].

TIA-1, granzyme and perforin are cytotoxic proteins present in the cytoplasmic granules of NK and cytotoxic T cells. Expression of these proteins can be demonstrated in paraffin-embedded material and this is useful in the diagnosis of NK or cytotoxic lymphomas [133,134].

CD123 is the α-subunit of the human interleukin 3 receptor and is a fairly specific marker of plasmacytoid dendritic cells. It is useful in the diagnosis of plasmacytoid dendritic cell leukaemia/lymphoma (previously known as CD4+/CD56+ haematodermic neoplasm) [135].

Markers of B follicle-centre cells such as CD10 and bcl-6, although not entirely specific, are useful in demonstrating the presence of these cells in the skin. Positive staining does not indicate that the cells are neoplastic but that they are of follicle-centre origin [136–138]. Reactive cutaneous germinal centres are positive for these markers. On the other hand, an infiltrate with follicle-centre cells that are positive for bcl-2 is very suggestive of a follicle-centre cell lymphoma, and usually indicates the presence of a 14;18 chromosomal translocation [139]. Many primary cutaneous follicle-centre cell lymphomas, however, do not stain for this marker and the t(14;18) chromosomal translocation is often absent [140]. It is worth remembering that normal reactive T lymphocytes are usually bcl-2 positive and these tend to be prominent in B-cell infiltrates. Normal mantle B cells are also bcl-2 positive.

Further markers of B-cell differentiation are also used including MUM-1/ITRF4 (multiple myeloma 1/interferon regulatory factor 4) and FOXP-1. MUM-1 is a protein expressed by late centrocytes and post-germinal centre B cells and FOXP-1 is an essential transcriptional regulator of B-cell development [119]. Cutaneous follicle-centre cell lymphomas do not tend to express either MUM-1 or FOXP-1, while diffuse large B-cell lymphoma leg type tend to be diffusely positive for both markers [141]. In cutaneous marginal zone lymphoma, MUM-1 is only expressed by the plasma cells. This pattern of staining, coupled with the other commonly used immunohistochemical markers, is helpful in differential diagnosis [142].

The field of immunopathology in general, and in relation to the study of lymphoid proliferations in particular, continues to grow apace. In addition to the techniques discussed here, it is likely that within the next few years further information of use to the diagnostic pathologist will be gained from studies of cytokines, adhesion molecules and similar substances. The correlation of immunophenotypic studies with immunogenotyping using the latest molecular biological techniques is likely to contribute further to our understanding of cutaneous and systemic lymphomas.

Other diagnostic methods

Cytodiagnosis and Tzanck smears

Cytodiagnosis in dermatopathology should not be regarded as a substitute for formal biopsy. The technique has been used as an aid to the rapid diagnosis of numerous skin conditions, including epithelial tumours, Paget disease, melanoma, cutaneous lymphomas and skin metastases. In most of these conditions, a diagnostic surgical biopsy rather than fine needle biopsy is always preferable. The examination of cytological specimens from skin lesions is of most value in bullous disorders, vesicular virus eruptions and basal cell epithelioma.

In blistering disorders, a small, early, uninfected lesion should ideally be selected. The roof of the blister is removed with scissors, and the base of the blister gently scraped with a blunt scalpel so as not to produce bleeding. The material obtained is spread thinly on a glass slide. This is called a Tzanck smear. However, herpes simplex infections cannot be differentiated from herpes zoster infections using such a simple technique. For the cytodiagnosis of suspected basal cell epitheliomas, any surface crust should be removed from ulcerated tumours, and non-ulcerated tumours should be incised with a sharp, pointed scalpel. The incision should be superficial enough to avoid undue bleeding. A sample of tumour is then obtained with either a blunt scalpel or a small curette, and the tissue obtained is pressed between two glass slides. Smears from blisters and basal cell epitheliomas should be fixed immediately for 2 min in absolute alcohol, and stained with H&E. Following rinsing and drying, the smears are cover slipped for microscopic examination.

Microscopic appearances
Bullous disorders

Cytodiagnosis is of most value in pemphigus in its various forms, and in Hailey–Hailey disease, because of the presence of numerous acantholytic keratinocytes. In pemphigus vulgaris, pemphigus vegetans and Hailey–Hailey disease, the cells obtained in the skin smear are usually rounded and more or less uniform in size, with a relatively large nuclear : cytoplasmic ratio. There may be a perinuclear pale halo, with the peripheral part of the cell staining more darkly. In the more superficial forms of pemphigus, including pemphigus foliaceus and Senear–Usher pemphigus, the keratinocytes tend to be more cuboidal in shape, with a small nucleus and more prominent cytoplasm. The cells may contain keratohyalin granules and show evidence of keratinisation. Occasional giant cells may be seen, but are quite unlike virus giant cells, which show ballooning degeneration. In addition to the acantholytic disorders mentioned previously, occasional acantholytic cells may be obtained in Darier disease, where dyskeratosis may also be present, and in bullous impetigo. In this latter condition, normally in addition to acantholytic cells, there are numerous neutrophil polymorphs and bacteria. The usefulness of cytodiagnosis in subepidermal bullous eruptions is limited; the smear in most instances contains only inflammatory cells. Eosinophils are commonly found in bullous pemphigoid but may also occur in dermatitis herpetiformis.

Viral disorders

The cytology of herpes simplex, herpes zoster and varicella is often diagnostic because of the presence of characteristic multinucleated giant cells. Keratinocytes of varying size are seen, and as the cell enlarges the nucleus shows some blurring of chromatin pattern and loss of staining. Some of the cells may show condensation of chromatin of the nuclear membrane. The multinucleate giant cells often contain eight or more nuclei, and these nuclei show great variation in size and shape (Figure 3.33).

Eosinophilic inclusion bodies are very occasionally identified in the herpesvirus group of disorders, but commonly the examination of many smears may fail to reveal any evidence of this change. Typical ballooning degeneration and giant cell formation as described above does not normally occur in vaccinia or cowpox, but occasionally somewhat enlarged acantholytic cells may be found,

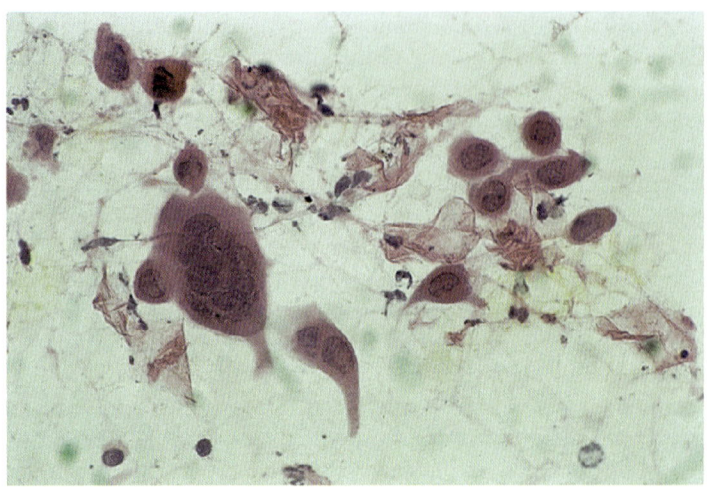

Figure 3.33 An H&E-stained smear from a lesion of herpes simplex showing multinucleate giant cells and degenerative nuclear changes.

and sometimes eosinophilic intracytoplasmic inclusion bodies may be detected. In molluscum contagiosum, characteristic molluscum bodies are easily identified. These are large, rounded, eosinophilic bodies, and may be identified without H&E stain in a potassium hydroxide preparation.

Basal cell carcinoma

In smears obtained from basal cell carcinoma, clumps of closely set, oval or round, deeply basophilic cells are found. The cytoplasm is usually very scanty and, in some cases, may not be detectable. The nuclei are finely granular with poorly defined nucleoli, and the cells in the smear are very regular in size and shape. In the presence of significant cytological atypia, an alternative diagnosis, such as squamous cell carcinoma or Bowen disease, should be considered.

Electron microscopy

Electron microscopic examination of cutaneous tissues is performed much less often than light microscopy and is nowadays rarely used in diagnostic dermatopathology. Electron microscopy has been replaced by antigen mapping using immunohistochemistry in the diagnosis of many genetic disorders, particularly those in the epidermolysis bullosa group. This technique and its applications are described in Chapter 69. Transmission and scanning electron microscopy have greatly increased our understanding, not only of the microanatomy of normal skin, but also of many disease processes. The use of newer embedding material has enabled ultrastructural examination to be carried out on single blocks of tissue prepared primarily for light microscopy. With care, even routinely fixed and paraffin-embedded material may produce electron micrographs that provide useful diagnostic information. In recent years, the combination of electron microscopy with immunopathological techniques, autoradiography and cytochemical methods has greatly enhanced our knowledge of tissue and cell pathophysiology. The contribution of ultrastructural studies to our understanding of the normal microanatomy of skin structures and their variants has been referred to in Chapter 2. Below are listed some of the cutaneous disorders where electron microscopy may be of diagnostic help.

Bullous disorders

The classification and subdivision of bullous disorders has been dramatically advanced by electron microscopy and immunoelectron microscopy. With the electron microscope it is much easier to separate the varieties of epidermolysis bullosa. In epidermolysis bullosa simplex, the plane of cleavage is within the basal cells. Additionally, tonofilament clumping may be seen. Junctional epidermolysis bullosa has various clinical forms, and, although with the electron microscope there is separation in the lamina lucida zone, junctional epidermolysis bullosa is probably a heterogeneous group of disorders. In some forms of this condition, hemidesmosomes are reduced in number, and this may represent a primary defect. In other forms of junctional epidermolysis bullosa, however, hemidesmosomes may be apparently normal. In dystrophic epidermolysis bullosa, again, various abnormalities are observed, but in this case the split is below the lamina densa. Immunoelectron microscopic techniques provide further information in epidermolysis bullosa, and also in some of the other idiopathic blistering disorders. In cicatricial pemphigoid, for instance, immunoreactants may be identified at a lower level in the lamina lucida than in classic bullous pemphigoid. In linear IgA disease, immunoreactants may be found either in the lamina lucida or below it. Sublamina densa deposits of immunoreactants are also seen in epidermolysis bullosa acquisita.

Pigmentary disorders

The quantitative and qualitative evaluation of melanocytes and melanosomes at ultrastructural level can be of great value in the examination of disorders of hyper- and hypopigmentation. In albinism, normal numbers of melanocytes are present, although melanosomes are immature. In vitiligo, a biopsy from affected skin shows either a complete absence or greatly diminished population of melanocytes. In early stages of vitiligo, some vacuolar degeneration of epidermal melanocytes may be identified.

Cellular identification

In addition to the demonstration of melanocytes, various other cells, both in inflammatory and neoplastic disorders, can be identified clearly with the aid of the electron microscope. The shape of the convoluted nucleus in the peripheral blood from patients with Sézary syndrome is diagnostic. Annulate lamellae, large, dense granules and decapitation secretion are all found ultrastructurally in apocrine secretory cells. Other cellular substructures that may be of diagnostic value are the identification of desmosomes in various epithelia, myofilaments in tumours of muscular origin, the Birbeck granule characteristic of Langerhans cells, and the Weibel–Palade body found in the endothelial cells of blood vessels.

Identification of dermal deposits

Ultrastructural examination of various forms of amyloidosis shows characteristic deposits of straight, non-branching, non-anastomosing filaments of approximately 6–7 nm in diameter. The apparent increased electron density at their periphery produces a superficial appearance of hollow cylinders. Colloid milia of both the adult and juvenile type may on occasion be confused with amyloid deposition at the light microscopic level. Ultrastructurally, however, the fibres of colloid milia are of a different thickness from those seen in amyloidosis and are wavy rather than straight. Other conditions where amorphous hyaline deposits may be seen with the light microscope, such as forms of porphyria and lipoid proteinosis, also have characteristic electron microscopic appearances.

Viral disease techniques

Many of the conventional techniques for confirmation of a diagnosis of virus infection, such as virus isolation and culture and the various serological tests, are slow and the patient has often recovered by the time the diagnosis is established with certainty. Conventional histology either from biopsy or from the scraping of the base of blisters, for instance in herpes simplex or zoster infections, can be useful in experienced hands, but there is quite a high rate of false negative results. Molecular biological techniques including PCR are more specific, especially for the identification of human papillomavirus infection, but are not widely available. Direct visualisation of virus particles with the electron microscope, using a negative staining technique, can give a positive result within half an hour of a lesion being sampled. This technique has become invaluable for the confirmation of diagnosis in disorders caused by many of the main families of viruses, particularly lesions such as herpes simplex and zoster, and hand, foot and mouth disease. Immunohistochemical stains are widely available for various viruses including herpesvirus 1 and 2, varicella zoster and also for cytomegalovirus, and are quite useful in establishing a diagnosis in paraffin-embedded sections. Human herpesvirus 8 is a type of herpesvirus that can be detected in all tumours in patients with Kaposi sarcoma [1]. A monoclonal antibody raised against the nuclear latent antigen of the virus is very sensitive and specific. A monoclonal antibody against the HIV-1 p24 Gag protein is a useful diagnostic tool in the setting of HIV infection [2]. *In situ* hybridisation for the Epstein–Barr encoding region (EBER) has been established as the method of choice for the detection of Epstein–Barr virus in paraffin-embedded tissue [3]. *In situ* hybridisation (on paraffin-embedded sections) and immunohistochemistry may be used for the detection of human papillomavirus [4]. SARS-CoV-2 can be demonstrated by immunohistochemistry in the chilblains-like lesions in patients with the virus [5]. SARS-CoV-2 has also been demonstrated by PCR in the macular eruption associated with the virus [6].

Immunogenotyping

In most inflammatory disorders, the lymphocyte population in the skin tissue is normally polyclonal, containing progeny of many different parent lymphocytes. In contrast, most lymphomas are monoclonal, with cells being derived from the same parent cell. With the development of DNA probes to detect rearrangements of genes encoding for immunoglobulin and T-cell receptor molecules, it is now a routine technique to assess clonality of T- and B-cell populations by immunogenotyping [1,2–4]. Refinements in technique mean that significant results can now be obtained from relatively small portions of tissue. The PCR technique is now widely used for the study of clonality in cutaneous lymphoid infiltrates. This subject is discussed in detail in Chapter 139.

Artefacts

The microscopic appearance of the end-product produced by processing a tissue specimen is in many ways an artificial representation of what is going on in a complex organ at one point in time. The procedures of biopsy fixation and tissue processing produce significant alterations in size, shape and structure of tissue constituents. We tend to think of fat cells as large, round, empty cells with peripheral nuclei, because this is how we are used to visualising them microscopically. Cysts that normally contain lipid-rich substances, such as those of steatocystoma multiplex, appear relatively empty when sections from paraffin-embedded material are viewed. The clear halo often seen around melanocytes in the lower layers of the epidermis is at least in part an artefactual change. Some routinely observed tissue artefacts are useful for diagnostic purposes. The so-called separation artefact, where dermal connective tissue separates away from islands of basal cell carcinoma, aids us, for instance, in differentiating a basal cell carcinoma from a trichoepithelioma. In addition to these everyday artefacts, there are a wide range of other changes that may be induced accidentally or by poor processing technique (Box 3.4). These changes may in some instances mislead the diagnostic pathologist.

> **Box 3.4 Potential dermatopathological artefacts**
> - Poor orientation: cross-sectioning makes it difficult to evaluate the epidermis and dermis; sometimes this results in complete loss of the epidermis
> - Formaldehyde fixation: vacuolation of epidermis
> - Fixation in non-buffered formaldehyde: pigment deposition
> - Freezing artefact: prominent intracytoplasmic vacuoles in keratinocytes
> - Scratch marks across tissue due to nick in microtome knife
> - Tissue carry-over from microtome knife
> - Foreign bodies, e.g. formaldehyde pigments, suture, *Alternaria*, spores, starch
> - Polarisation of cell nuclear material by electric current in curetted specimen
> - Clumped mitoses in podophyllin-treated warts
> - Pyknotic prickle cells from methotrexate- or hydroxyurea-treated patients

Artefacts due to poor biopsy technique

Undue squeezing of the specimen with forceps can produce a marked artefact, causing the connective tissue to become amorphous and basophilic. Considerable distortion of cellular infiltrates is also seen. Toothed forceps can produce a hole within the tissue specimen, which, although rarely causing diagnostic confusion, is aesthetically unpleasing. When a small tissue specimen is cut up into even smaller pieces, the pressure produced by the knife at the edge of the smaller biopsy portions may lead to connective tissue and cell distortion. It is far better to carry out several small separate biopsies from the same area, perhaps with a punch, than to try and divide a single specimen after it has been removed from the patient.

Various techniques of cautery used to secure haemostasis following either a shave biopsy or curettage can lead to unusual histological appearances. Diathermy produces a bizarre alteration of cellular and nuclear morphology, as well as producing a stringy eosinophilic and homogenised appearance to connective tissue. The haemostatic agent, Monsel solution (20% aqueous ferric subsulphate), can occasionally produce extensive ferrugination of fibrin, dermal collagen and even striated muscle in skin biopsies [1]. The iron pigment deposition can be very confusing and simulate melanin. Particular problems are encountered where this technique is used following shave biopsy of melanocytic naevi. The deposition of this pigment could lead to an erroneous diagnosis of a melanoma [2]. Artefacts may occasionally be induced by local anaesthetic. The epinephrine contained in some local anaesthetics may result in some degranulation of mast cells and have minor effects on dermal blood vessels, but these are not normally important problems. A large quantity of local anaesthetic, particularly when injected directly into a lesion or superficially in the dermis, can cause appearances simulating marked tissue oedema, or in the case of a cellular naevus, disruption of the normal architecture of the tumour.

Artefacts related to fixation media

It has already been stressed that an adequate fixation of skin tissue biopsy specimens is needed for optimum histological interpretation. Specimens that have been fixed for an insufficient time show a poor definition of cell structure and connective tissue. Cells may appear swollen and staining of such poorly fixed specimens often produces a rather smudged appearance. Similar results may be seen when the specimen has not been placed in the correct fixative, but rather in some inappropriate solution such as normal saline. Formalin pigment may be precipitated out into the tissues in some skin biopsies, particularly where the biopsies have been fixed in a formalin-containing fixative with an acid pH. Formalin pigment artefact is particularly common in biopsies from tissue containing large amounts of haemorrhage or tissues heavily congested with blood. Even in neutral buffered formal saline, a long fixation may increase the tendency to produce formalin pigment. There are some fixatives, such as Zenker fluid and Heidenhain Susa, that contain mercuric chloride. Tissues fixed in these media may develop a granular, brownish black deposit. This deposit can be removed, normally by treatment in Lugol iodine followed by sodium thiosulphate.

Artefacts due to blocking and sectioning

One of the most commonly encountered problems is with the orientation of the specimen. Oblique blocking can give a very misleading picture – for example, suggesting that there is pseudoepitheliomatous hyperplasia of the epidermis or psoriasis, when one is in fact dealing with normal skin. Correct and accurate vertical sectioning and blocking is particularly important where measurements are to be made, such as in the assessment of Breslow thickness and the Clark level of melanoma. Occasionally, fragments of a biopsy adhere to the microtome blade and 'knife carry' may occur, with the result that, for instance, a fragment of basal cell carcinoma may be seen just above the epidermis in a section from a histiocytoma. Normally this artefact is easy to spot, but occasionally it can give rise to confusion. Partial blunting of the microtome knife causes uneven thickness of the histological section. This can give a false impression, both of the density of cellular infiltrates and of the qualities of the connective tissue. Irregularities in the microtome knife's edge can cause an unaesthetic artefact known as shatter marks. In the presence of very hard or dense foreign material in the tissues, such as calcium, the foreign material may be drawn through the tissue, forming a tear in the resulting sections.

Artefacts due to staining techniques

It should be remembered that the various staining solutions have a very short shelf-life once made up, and that staining solutions that are old produce a very unsatisfactory end result. It is also quite common for staining solutions to be contaminated with various foreign materials, such as plant hairs [3] or microorganisms, which may appear to be present within the biopsied tissue when viewed in the finished mounted preparation.

Digital pathology

With the use of whole slide imaging (WSI), digital pathology was introduced in 1999. Its introduction has been slow but steady and has revolutionised the world of pathology in the last few years [1,2,3,4,5,6,7]. The technique allows the conversion of tissue sections on a glass slide into high resolution virtual slides. Initial problems with its introduction consisted of high costs, technical problems with the application and use of the technique and reluctance of many pathologists to adapt to a new and unproven technology. Since then, however, the technology has been refined and simplified; and, although the costs of introducing and maintaining a good digital system remain high, the long-term benefits outweigh these shortcomings. As opposed to traditional systems of slide evaluation, the benefits of the system are countless. Digital images are easily accessed everywhere on the internet, there is no need for physical storage space and the images do not deteriorate and can be kept and accessed indefinitely. The system can be used for diagnostic routine use after validation, for teaching, to generate data for research and for quality assurance programmes. Describing the technique in detail is beyond the scope of this chapter, but excellent articles on the subject have been published [1,2,3,4,5,6,7].

Approach to microscopic examination of tissue sections

Some understanding of the basic principles of microscopy and careful microscope maintenance are essential for optimal visualisation of tissue sections, and ultimately therefore for achieving a correct histopathological diagnosis. Knowledge of the techniques and applications of fluorescence microscopy, interference microscopy and polarised light microscopy is also recommended.

Preparing for microscopy

Before using the microscope, some attention should be given to various practical points. Are all the optical surfaces clean? Greasy fingerprints and dust may seriously impair the quality of the image, and before using the microscope all lens surfaces should be cleaned. This may be done with an optical lens tissue. Petroleum spirit is recommended by some manufacturers. The cleaning of objectives with a concave shape can be difficult. A recommended method is to use a small, freshly broken-up piece of expanded polystyrene. It is important that there is no trace of xylene or other organic solvent on an objective treated in this way, or there is a risk of a film of dissolved plastic being left behind.

The microscope light source should be centred, and on most modern microscopes this is easily achieved by a pair of centring screws acting against a spring, or by loosening a screw column and orientating the lamp holder. The condenser is then adjusted. The aperture diaphragm in the base of the microscope should be closed, and the condenser height adjusted, until the image of the field diaphragm is in focus. The diaphragm should then be centred with the adjusting screws. After centring, the field diaphragm should be opened until it just disappears from view. The aperture (substage iris diaphragm) is then adjusted. With experience, this can be done while viewing the image on the slide. Alternatively, an eyepiece can be removed, and while looking down the eyepiece tube the diaphragm is opened until it occupies approximately one-third of the field of view. In this position, the numerical aperture of the condenser is approximately that of the objective in use and optimum resolution is achieved.

The slide to be examined should then be viewed with the naked eye. Is the specimen a section of solid tissue, or uniformly spread across the slide, like a tissue or cell smear? The size and shape of sections on the slide should be noted, and it may be possible with naked eye examination to identify several tissues. It is important to note the number of sections mounted on one slide and whether these are likely to represent sections from the same block or different blocks mounted together. Finally, before putting the slide on the microscope stage, the name or identification number carried by the slide should be correlated with the details on the clinical request form. When inserting the slide into the microscope, make sure that it is the right way up, otherwise it may be impossible to focus the image with higher power objectives.

Microscopic interpretation
Examination of sections
The normal and recommended procedure is to start with lower power examination of the sections and gradually move up to higher power, detailed examination. Low-power scanning examination with a ×2.5 or ×4 objective provides a wealth of information. Identification of tissues is made, orientation of the specimen is possible and the main site of any pathological changes is often identified. The basic nature of the pathological changes may also be recognised – for example, whether the main pathology represents a neoplastic or inflammatory process. Low-power scanning of all the material on the slide makes it clear whether all sections are from the same block or whether they represent different portions of tissue. Low-power examination of biopsy material is the first step in the problem-solving exercise and is the key to good diagnostic dermatopathology. During low-power examination, the site of biopsy and whether this correlates with the clinical information should be evaluated and, secondly, some attempt at pattern diagnosis should be made.

When a foreign body is suspected it is very useful to examine the section under polarised light. This is a quick method of confirming the presence of foreign material within the tissue. However, it is important to emphasise that some endogenous substances polarise and that not all external particles polarise.

Site of biopsy and normal histological variation
Without a working knowledge of the differences in skin microanatomy in the different regions of the body, it is very easy to come to a wrong diagnostic conclusion. For instance, the prominent sebaceous glands seen on facial skin, particularly the nose, may lead to a diagnosis of sebaceous hyperplasia, and the normally thick stratum corneum present on the palms and soles may be interpreted as hyperkeratosis. The following notes describe some of the more typical features seen in skin biopsies from specific sites.

Skin from the palms and soles. In biopsies from these sites, there is a fairly thick Malpighian layer with a thickened basket-weave stratum corneum and a very prominent epidermal rete ridge pattern. Occasionally, specialised nerve endings (Meissner corpuscles) may be seen in the dermal papillae. Eccrine sweat glands are fairly numerous, but no pilosebaceous follicles are identified. Vater–Pacini corpuscles are characteristically found in the subcutis. They are large, specialised nerve endings and have an ovoid or round shape with a typical onion ring appearance.

Skin from the areola of the nipple and the scrotum. In these sites, papillomatosis is a common finding, and in the upper dermis there are often numerous small fascicles and fibres of smooth muscle. In biopsies from the areola and nipple, occasional lactiferous ducts may be identified.

Mucous membranes. Histology of mucosal surfaces often shows fairly thick epithelium lacking well-defined keratinisation. Focal mild parakeratosis is often seen. The rete ridge pattern normally associated with glabrous skin is not marked, and the cells of the Malpighian layer are large, pale and typically vacuolated.

Axillary skin. In skin from the axillae, papillomatosis of the skin surface is often marked. Abundant hair follicles are present, as are numerous apocrine glands, which are seen in addition to eccrine glands commonly present in other sites.

Scalp skin. Biopsies from the scalp are normally readily identified by the presence of numerous, large hairs (terminal hair follicles) with the hair bulbs frequently in the subcutaneous fat.

Facial skin. Facial skin is characterised by the presence of smaller hair follicles than in the scalp and, particularly in the central facial area, large numbers of mature sebaceous glands. The epidermis is very thin and melanocytes are numerous. The rete ridge pattern at the dermal–epidermal junction is often very poorly developed, which makes a distinction between papillary and reticular dermis often difficult to assess. *Demodex* organisms may be seen in the ostia of hair follicles and deeper within the sebaceous glands. Muscle may be identified relatively close to the epidermis in certain areas of the face, such as round the eyes or mouth.

Truncal skin. Skin from the trunk shows no very specific histological hallmarks. However, it is normally quite thick, with the distance between the epidermis and the subcutaneous fat being much greater than in biopsies from other sites. Eccrine sweat glands are normally identified at the junction between the dermis and the subcutaneous fat, and may, in skin from the trunk, appear within the reticular dermis itself. The skin from the back contains a very thick dermis with thick collagen bundles in which the ground substance is minimal. This normal pattern is often confused with evidence of a sclerosing dermal process such as morphoea.

Low-magnification histological pattern diagnosis

Having attempted to recognise the site of the biopsy, and having correlated this with the clinical information, the next task is to interpret any abnormal findings and attempt to come to some diagnostic conclusions. Sometimes, the site of the abnormality in the section is immediately obvious on scanning magnification. This then leads one to examine the appropriate area in more detail. When there is no obvious pathology in the section, a useful approach is to examine each identifiable cutaneous structure in turn. For instance, starting outwards with the stratum corneum and working inwards, is it increased or decreased in thickness? Is parakeratosis present? Is the pattern of keratinisation normal, producing a basket-weave pattern, or is the stratum corneum compacted? Examination of the epidermis may reveal atrophy or acanthosis, spongiosis or cell atypicality, and may also reveal colonisation of the epidermis by inflammatory or other abnormal cells. Various forms of epidermal degeneration may be noted. Some variants of these are described below. A vesicle or bulla may be present within the epidermis or below it.

Moving on to the dermis, is the arrangement of connective tissue fibres in the papillary and reticular dermis normal, or are the collagen fibres thickened and hyalinised? Is there an increase in interstitial oedema fluid, or is there evidence of increased amounts of mucin separating the collagen bundles? Is the elastic pattern normal? Careful examination of all adnexal structures should be made, and then, finally, any dermal infiltrate should be assessed. The density of the infiltrate, the pattern of the infiltrate (diffuse and interstitial and/or focal and localised) and the composition of the infiltrate are important. The position of the infiltrate in the dermis, whether it is predominantly deep or predominantly involves the epidermis, is also worth noting, as is the relationship of the infiltrate to adnexal structures and blood vessels. The blood vessels themselves should also be examined carefully for evidence, for example, of any vasculitic change or dilatation, increased tortuosity or thickening. A search should be made for any abnormal deposits or pigments such as amyloid, calcium or tattoo pigment. When one has some experience in assessing the different structures in a skin biopsy, one soon learns to recognise certain patterns of neoplastic change and inflammation. Ackerman established a method of pattern diagnosis appropriate for the study of inflammatory diseases [1]. He suggests recognition of nine major patterns of inflammatory change in the skin, ranging from superficial perivascular dermatitis to panniculitis. Having classified the appearances in the section according to one of these patterns, closer examination enables one to come to a more precise diagnosis. Other authors have described similar schemes of microscopy. The system of pattern analysis can be recommended to those new to dermatopathology. More experienced pathologists have almost always developed their own pattern analysis system.

High-magnification microscopic examination

By the time a histological section has been examined with a ×2.5 objective, a ×4 to ×8 objective depending on personal preference, and a ×10 objective, one should have some idea in most cases of a differential diagnosis. High-magnification examination with a ×25, ×40 or ×50 and sometimes with a ×100 oil-immersion lens provides an opportunity to confirm the initial impressions.

Under high-magnification examination, cells and other structures in the skin should be carefully examined in various specific ways. When dealing with neoplastic disorders, the cytology of individual tumour cells should be studied, with particular reference to nuclear detail and the variation in size and shape between cells of the same population. The number of mitotic figures and the number of abnormal mitoses are noted. The pattern of relationship of tumour cells to each other is also an important feature. Loss of polarity of keratinocytes in squamous epithelium is a characteristic feature associated with premalignant epithelial dysplasias, such as Bowen disease and actinic keratoses, although it can of course also occur in invasive epithelial tumours. The relationship of tumour cells to neurovascular bundles is also important and the pattern of neoplastic cells in relation to dermal connective tissue should also be evaluated. The so-called Indian filing pattern of tumour cells lining up one behind another, sandwiched between collagen bundles, is in some contexts suggestive of malignant disease.

In inflammatory conditions under high magnification, there is an opportunity to try and categorise the different types of cells in the infiltrate. It is important to look over the whole section, as in some areas the infiltrate may be composed of one cell type and in other areas another cell type may predominate. Some infiltrates are composed of almost pure populations of, for example, lymphocytes, and are described as monomorphic, whereas other infiltrates are composed of plasma cells, histiocytes, lymphocytes and eosinophils, and are described as polymorphic. It is only with experience that one becomes confident in recognising the cytology of cutaneous infiltrates and one must remember that in some biopsy material, cells may be seen that are impossible to classify by conventional criteria. The following notes describe the more typical appearances of commonly seen inflammatory and related cells, and describe some of the situations where they may be encountered.

Lymphocytes

Lymphocytes originate in the bone marrow and mature through a series of stages both in the bone marrow and the thymus gland, before being released into the peripheral blood and body tissues. The family of lymphocytes is a very heterogeneous one, with many subtypes of lymphocytes. T lymphocytes and B lymphocytes are indistinguishable by normal light microscopy, although on scanning electron microscopy *in vitro* B lymphocytes appear to have rather rougher surfaces than T lymphocytes and show villous projections. On light-microscopic examination of sections stained with H&E, lymphocytes are roughly 7–12 µm in diameter and possess small, round, deeply basophilic nuclei, surrounded by a thin rim of cytoplasm, which is usually very difficult to visualise (Figure 3.34). Numerous immunohistochemical methods are available that readily distinguish T and B lymphocytes, and most of these methods can be carried out using paraffin-embedded sections. In the majority of inflammatory conditions affecting the skin where a significant dermal infiltrate is seen, T cells outnumber B cells. Mature T and B cells are, of course, not the only lymphoid cells that may be found in the skin. In addition to plasma cells, various follicular centre cells and T and B immunoblasts may be seen under certain conditions.

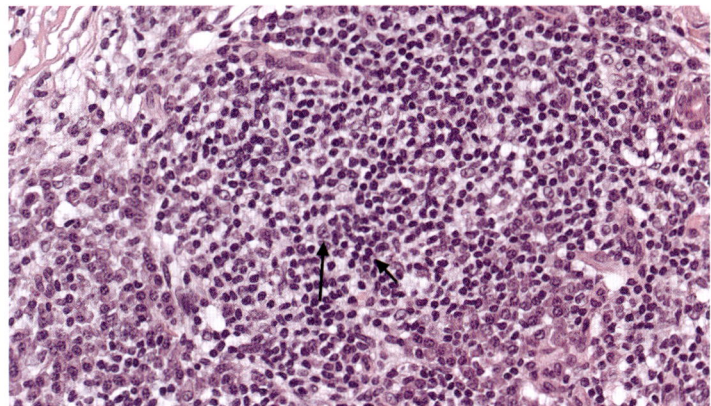

Figure 3.34 Inflammatory cell infiltrate composed of numerous lymphocytes and histiocytes. Lymphocytes have scanty non-visible cytoplasm and a small dark round homogeneous nucleus (short arrow). In contrast, histiocytes are larger with ill-defined cytoplasm, bean-shaped vesicular nucleus and a single small nucleolus (long arrow).

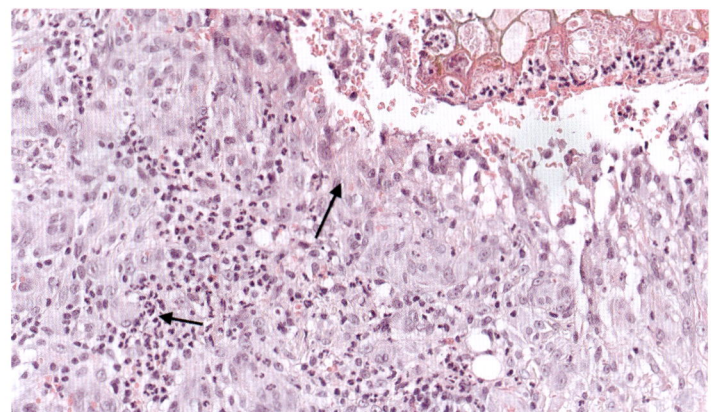

Figure 3.36 Neutrophils. Note ill-defined non-visible cytoplasm and nuclei with three lobules (short arrow). In addition, palisading histiocytes with pink cytoplasm, vesicular nuclei and a single nucleolus (long arrow) are seen surrounding a foreign body.

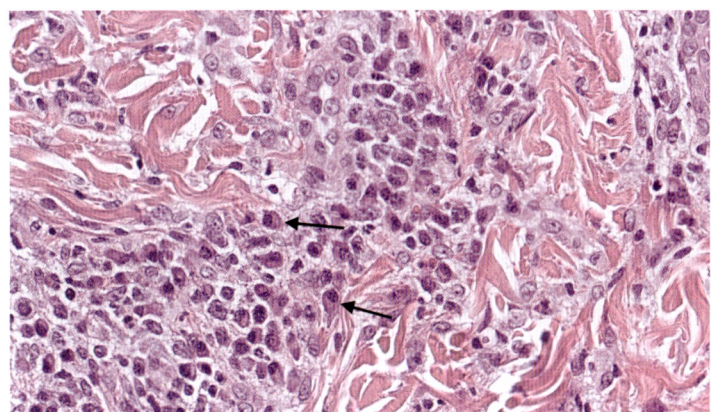

Figure 3.35 Numerous plasma cells with eccentric nuclei, clock face arrangement of the chromatin and abundant cytoplasm (arrows).

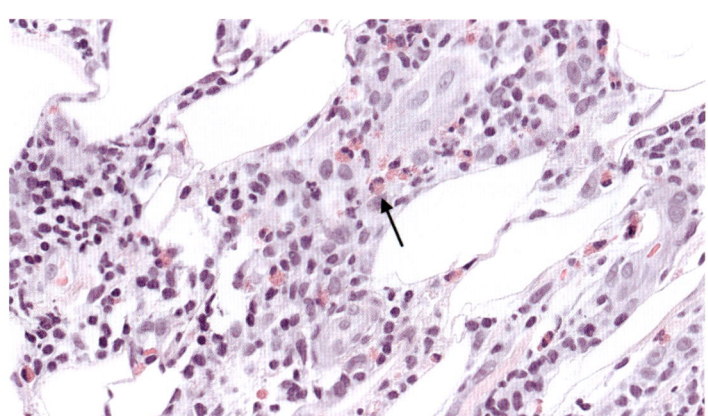

Figure 3.37 Eosinophils. Note cytoplasm with abundant red granules and bilobed nucleus (arrow).

Plasma cells

Plasma cells are responsible for immunoglobulin production. They are a variety of B lymphocyte, approximately 10 μm in diameter, that have a distinct appearance in H&E-stained sections. They have abundant basophilic cytoplasm with a round, eccentrically placed nucleus (Figure 3.35). The nuclear chromatin is scattered in coarse clumps at the periphery of the nucleus, giving it a 'clock face' appearance. Closely adjacent to the nucleus there is a zone of pallor in the cytoplasm, sometimes called the perinuclear hof. This area corresponds to the site where the Golgi apparatus is located. Older plasma cells often contain homogeneous eosinophilic globules of varying size within their cytoplasm, known as Russell bodies. Plasma cells are seen in many situations in the skin, particularly in inflammatory conditions affecting hairy areas, near mucous membranes and in the late stages of some granulomas.

Neutrophils

Neutrophils are the most numerous of the circulating white blood cells, comprising in normal individuals 50–70% of the blood leukocytes. They have a multilobed nucleus (three to four), with the lobes connected by narrow bridges of nucleoplasm (Figure 3.36). The slightly basophilic cytoplasm contains many smallish granules, many of which ultrastructurally correspond to membrane-bound lysosomes. Neutrophils function primarily as phagocytes, and are directed by chemotactic factors, including the complement cascade to noxious materials present in tissue. Such foreign materials include bacteria, fungi and tissues that have been injured. Collections of neutrophils may be seen in the skin in various infectious conditions (such as impetigo and staphylococcal folliculitis), in various inflammatory disorders of unknown cause (such as pyoderma gangrenosum and Sweet syndrome) and in various vasculitic disorders, including leukocytoclastic vasculitis, granuloma faciale and erythema elevatum diutinum.

Eosinophils

Eosinophils, like neutrophils, originate in the bone marrow, but are rather larger than neutrophils, being 12–17 μm across. The nucleus of the eosinophil is usually bilobed, and the cytoplasm is filled with eosinophilic granules that are larger than the granules found in neutrophil leukocytes (Figure 3.37). Eosinophils are highly phagocytic, are capable of ingesting various bacteria, fungi, immune complexes and inert particles and, like neutrophils, they contain hydrolytic and proteolytic enzymes within membrane-bound granules. Eosinophils are seen in skin biopsies in certain infections, in reactions to insect bites and other foreign bodies, in some drug

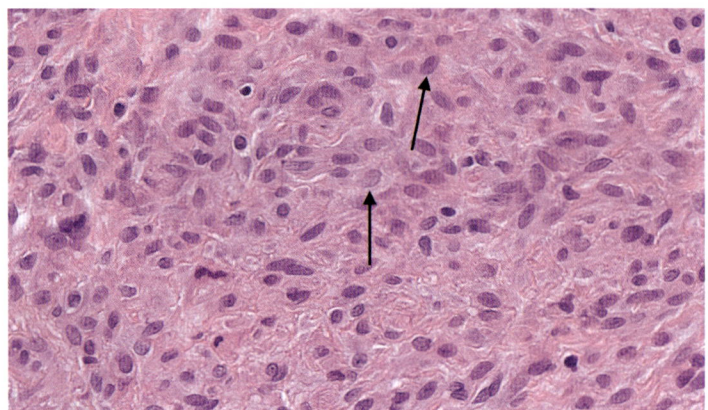

Figure 3.38 Numerous histiocytes (arrows) as described in Figure 3.34.

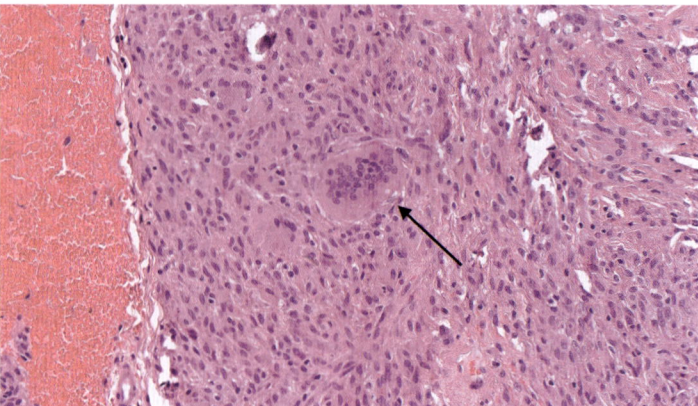

Figure 3.39 Foreign body giant cell. Large multinucleated cell with pink cytoplasm and crowding of the nuclei (arrow).

reactions, and in bullous eruptions such as bullous pemphigoid and some forms of pemphigus. They are of major importance in the condition known as eosinophilic cellulitis and may also occur in association with proliferations of cells of the lymphoid series in certain cutaneous T-cell lymphomas.

Histiocytes/monocytes/tissue macrophages

The term histiocyte is used by different authors to mean different things and is an unsatisfactory term. Monocytes circulating in the blood may be attracted into the skin for the purposes of phagocytosis. They are then called histiocytes or tissue macrophages. However, many other mesenchymal cells and cells of the granulocyte series are also capable of phagocytosis. The appearances of a histiocyte vary considerably. Many of the cells are fairly large with a lightly staining, sometimes vesicular, elongated nucleus. The cytoplasm is usually pale and cell margins may be indistinct (Figure 3.38). The cells may be dendritic, spindle shaped or epithelioid, taking on the latter form particularly in epithelioid cell granulomas. Epithelioid histiocytes frequently display a palisading arrangement (Figure 3.36). The size of histiocytes is also very variable, ranging from 15 to 25 μm. Compared with some of the cells described earlier, they are less easy to identify in skin biopsies, particularly for the novice, and immunohistological methods are often necessary to demonstrate histiocyte subsets. Several factor XIIIa-positive dendritic phagocytes (dermal dendrocytes) are seen in close proximity to the superficial microvascular plexus. These cells, together with other immune cells, mast cells and endothelial cells, probably collaborate to coordinate antigen presentation, induction of cellular inflammation, wound healing and haemostasis in this microenvironment. Various histiocytes are found in a wide range of inflammatory and neoplastic disorders but are particularly important in the production of granulomatous inflammation, both in conditions such as granuloma annulare and in response to cutaneous infection such as mycobacteria.

Giant cells

Many types of giant cell may be recognised in skin tissues. The three best known are the Langhans giant cell, the foreign body giant cell (Figure 3.39) and the Touton giant cell (Figure 3.40). All these giant cells are derived from tissue macrophages, and

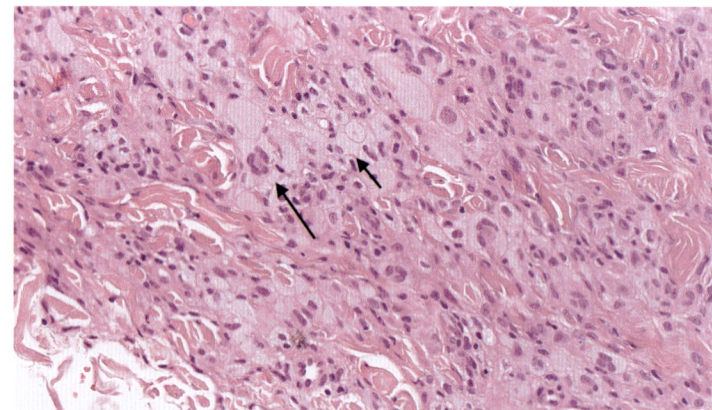

Figure 3.40 Touton giant cell. Note a foamy peripheral cytoplasm and a central, multiple nuclei with a wreath-like distribution of the nuclei (long arrow). Histiocytes with foamy cytoplasm and a single nucleus are also seen (short arrow).

forms intermediate between the different characteristic types are sometimes seen. The size of these cells varies greatly but is usually of the order of between 40 and 120 μm. Langhans giant cells show a characteristic horseshoe distribution of the nuclei arranged at the cell periphery. They are most characteristically seen in sarcoidosis and tuberculosis. Foreign body giant cells contain a haphazard arrangement of nuclei scattered throughout the cell cytoplasm and may also contain foreign material. Although typically seen in foreign body granulomas, they are common in other forms of granulomatous inflammation and in situations where there is disruption of pilosebaceous follicular structures with keratin release into the dermal connective tissue. Touton giant cells have a central ring of nuclei enclosing a layer of ground-glass cytoplasm, with a peripheral zone of clearer cytoplasm. They are typically seen in some xanthomas and juvenile xanthogranuloma. It should be noted that many other forms of giant cell are also seen, such as the fairly typical giant cell with scattered nuclei, prominent nucleoli and PAS-positive cytoplasm in multicentric reticulohistiocytosis. Not all giant cells are derived from cells of the macrophage series. Multinucleate cells derived from infected keratinocytes may be seen in various virus infections such as herpes and poxvirus infections, and multinucleate cells derived from melanocytes are quite typical of epithelioid and spindle cell (Spitz) naevi (Figure 3.41).

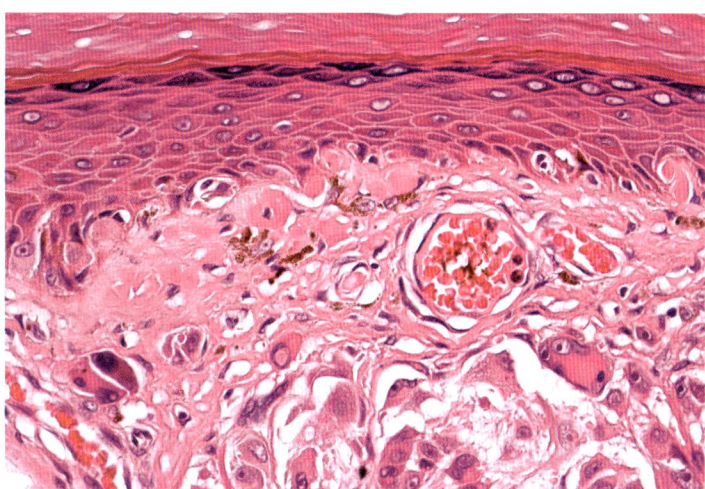

Figure 3.41 Bizarre multinucleated giant cells from a Spitz naevus.

Mast cells

Mast cells, unlike the white blood cells and some histiocytes, all of which probably originate from the bone marrow, are likely to arise from undifferentiated mesenchymal cells. In normal skin, they are present around small blood vessels in the dermis. They are approximately 9–16 μm in diameter and they possess a central round to ovoid, dark-staining nucleus (Figure 3.42). The cytoplasm contains small granules that stain metachromatically with such stains as toluidine blue. The granules contain vasoactive substances such as heparin, histamine, and eosinophilic and neutrophilic chemotactic factors of anaphylaxis. Mast cell activation may be triggered by neuropeptides derived from unmyelinated axons that surround perivascular mast cells. This in turn triggers adhesive events between leukocytes and endothelial cells, resulting in angiocentric inflammation.

Although in normal skin the cells tend to have a dendritic morphology, in various pathological conditions, including some forms of urticaria pigmentosa, the cells are larger and polygonal with a central, rounded nucleus. In addition to being found in increased numbers in the mastocytoses, they are also commonly seen in various benign and malignant nerve tumours, and in association with some melanocytic naevi.

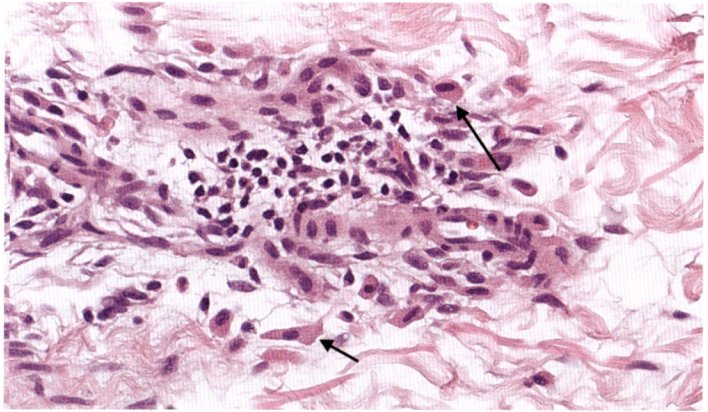

Figure 3.42 Mast cells. Typical 'fried-egg' appearance (long arrow). Another mast cell with a more elongated appearance is seen (short arrow).

Fibroblasts

Fibroblasts are often difficult to identify on routine light microscopy. Their nuclei tend to be oval or spindle shaped and with moderate basophilic staining. They are usually found between collagen bundles and may be prominent in conditions where there is an increase in the production of dermal connective tissue or ground substance, such as morphoea and scleromyxoedema. They may also contribute to the histogenesis of the wide range of so-called fibrocytic tumours that may occur in the skin.

Myofibroblasts

These cells are mainly defined by their electron microscopic appearances and display features intermediate between those of fibroblasts and smooth muscle cells. They are mainly seen in reactive reparative processes and in neoplasms. Histologically, they have an indistinct cytoplasmic margin, pink pale cytoplasm and vesicular tapering nuclei with a single inconspicuous nucleolus. Myofibroblasts can only be identified with certainty by electron microscopy.

Smooth muscle cells

Smooth muscle cells occur normally in the skin in the arrector pili muscles, in the tunica dartos of the external genitalia, in the areola of the nipple and in the walls of blood vessels. They are easy to identify by recognising the normal structures in which they occur and also by their cytomorphology, which consists of abundant, bright, eosinophilic cytoplasm and vesicular nuclei with a single inconspicuous nucleolus.

Rhabdomyocyte (striated muscle cell)

Skeletal muscle occurs in the skin of the neck and of the face. The constituent cells are arranged in bundles and have characteristic cross-striations and abundant, bright pink cytoplasm.

Schwann cells

Schwann cells are the main constituent cells of nerves. They envelop the neuroaxons and are characterised by a slender, hyperchromatic, thin nucleus and inconspicuous cytoplasm.

Endothelial cells

A single layer of endothelial cells lines all types of vascular channels in the skin. These cells usually appear flat with inconspicuous cytoplasm and small histiocyte-like vesicular nuclei. However, in most pathological processes, they become more prominent and may appear somewhat hyperchromatic. This, coupled with an increase in mitotic activity, may lead to confusion with malignant cells, particularly in cross-section, where the normal architecture of the vascular channel is often not apparent.

Pericytes

Pericytes occur as a single layer of indistinct cells around small dermal blood vessels. They are recognised by their location and by positive staining for actin.

Miscellaneous

In addition to closely examining cytology under the high-power objective, the opportunity should also be taken to look carefully for organisms, foreign bodies or deposits of foreign material such as amyloid. Special staining techniques will often be needed to confirm suspicions, and with these stains bacterial, fungal and protozoal organisms may be identified as well as various forms of parasite. The presence of viral organisms can also be inferred by the presence of characteristic cytopathic changes such as occur for instance with herpesvirus infections and infections with cytomegalovirus. Close examination of nerves and blood vessels should be carried out, particularly in relation to the presence of any organisms or tumour deposits. After examining adnexal structures and the subcutaneous tissues, it is useful to return to low-power examination and attempt to be certain one has not missed any pathology. It is not uncommon to discover more than one abnormality in a tissue section. Patients who develop solar keratoses may also have seborrhoeic warts, naevi and basal cell epitheliomas. Biopsies from patients with AIDS often have multiple pathologies, and one may, for example, see a biopsy of perianal tissue in which there is evidence of cytomegalovirus infection in the endothelial cells, human papillomavirus infection of the overlying epithelium and the presence of Kaposi sarcoma.

The importance of carefully assessing both the low-power pattern of changes in a skin section, as well as a more detailed examination of the cytology of the pathological changes, cannot be too strongly emphasised.

How to produce a histopathology skin report

After carefully carrying out the recommended procedure for low scanning power and high-power examination of a skin biopsy slide, the pathologist will either need more information, or will be in a position to provide a microscopic histopathological report to supplement the report on the gross pathological appearance of the biopsy specimen before processing. If there is very little obvious abnormality, it may be appropriate to cut deeper levels from the tissue block, or even consider blocking any remaining wet tissue that is in storage. If the specimen has been blocked obliquely or, for instance, the epidermis is missing, reblocking will be necessary. Serial sections may be required to determine pathological features that are only focal, such as changes affecting pilosebaceous follicles in a biopsy from the scalp. Special stains may be required for the evaluation of abnormal dermal deposits, to detect the presence of organisms or to elucidate the nature of various pigments in the biopsy material. Immunohistochemical studies may also be requested in, for example, cases of cutaneous lymphoma or malignant spindle cell tumours. If there is going to be undue delay in these various extra investigations, a preliminary report should always be issued.

Although reporting of histopathology is to some extent a subjective art, and every pathologist will have his or her own idea of what is an appropriate report, a description of the objective histological changes, and either a suggested diagnosis or a differential diagnosis, are always desirable. In a description of the pathology, it is important that features that are not present are never described, even though they may be consistent with the correct diagnosis. The differential diagnosis suggested by the pathologist should fully take into account the clinical information supplied by the clinician. If the clinician suggests on the request form chronic superficial scaly dermatitis, it would be churlish to sign out the report as subacute eczema without further qualification. In addition to a description of the objective pathological changes and a diagnostic suggestion, it is quite legitimate to add a further comment in certain situations. If the clinician suggests a tumour has been excised, then a comment on the adequacy of excision is obviously useful. Conversely, if the clinician states that this is a diagnostic/incisional or superficial biopsy, it is irritating for the clinician to receive a report stating that tumour extends to one margin of excision.

In some situations where the various histopathological parameters need to be recorded repeatedly in biopsies from specific skin disorders, for example melanoma, especially designed forms facilitate both the recording of information and subsequent computer analysis.

There is some degree of disagreement as to whether it is the role of the histopathologist under any circumstances to make recommendations for treatment, and no general rule can be given on this. If one knows one's clinical colleagues well, it is quite appropriate under certain circumstances to recommend a modest re-excision of the biopsy site, for instance in early superficial spreading melanoma. Some pathologists prefer to make such comments in a separate covering note. With some rarer conditions, particularly if they have serious implications for the patient, a telephone call to the clinician, or again a covering note, may be a reasonable approach. An offer from the pathologist to discuss any interesting case in more detail is often a good idea and is usually taken up. It is always in the best interests of the patient for there to be a close working relationship between the histopathologist and the clinician.

Finally, it is most important always to appreciate one's own limits of ability. One should never be afraid of asking for a second opinion from a colleague. It has been said that sections from skin biopsies fall into three groups. Firstly, there are those sections where the histological appearances are easy for anyone to interpret and diagnose. Secondly, there are sections from biopsies – for instance of a very poorly differentiated spindle cell tumour – where one does not know what the diagnosis is and that it is likely that no one else will either. Thirdly, there are sections where one does not know how to interpret the histological appearances oneself but that it is likely that someone else will! Once one is able to divide histological material into one of these three groups, one is already on the way to becoming an accomplished diagnostic dermatopathologist.

Commonly used descriptive terms in dermatopathology and their diagnostic significance

Acantholysis

Acantholysis is the term used to describe a loss of cohesion between keratinocytes due to the breakdown of intercellular bridges. It results in the formation of intraepidermal clefts, vesicles and bullae. It appears to be the primary pathological change in a group of diseases including pemphigus and its variants, Darier disease (Figure 3.43), transient and persistent acantholytic dermatosis and warty dyskeratoma. The site of acantholysis in these disorders is important. In pemphigus foliaceus and pemphigus erythematosus, acantholysis is usually confined to the upper portion of the epidermis, whereas in pemphigus vulgaris the split is formed at a lower level in the epidermis. In benign familial pemphigus (Hailey–Hailey disease), although acantholysis is often focal or incomplete, where it does occur it tends to affect the full thickness of the epidermis.

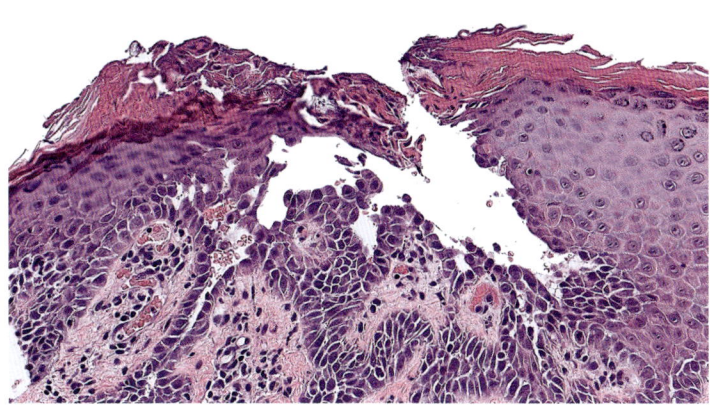

Figure 3.43 Biopsy from a case of Darier disease showing the histological features of parakeratosis, dyskeratosis and acantholysis and the formation of villi.

Acantholysis may also be seen secondary to some other pathological change, where there is alteration or damage to epidermal cells. It may occur, for example, in bullous impetigo, viral disorders, solar keratoses and some forms of squamous cell carcinoma. When acantholysis occurs in these disorders, the term secondary acantholysis is often used to distinguish the process from primary acantholysis, which occurs in pemphigus and related diseases.

Acanthosis

This term is used to describe an increase in number of cells in the Malpighian or prickle cell layer of the epidermis (from the Greek for prickle or thorn). Sometimes, a distinction is made between an increased thickness of the epidermis due to enlarged keratinocytes (pseudoacanthosis) and true acanthosis due to increased numbers of keratinocytes. In practice, acanthosis is commonly used to cover both senses. Increased thickness of the epidermis may result from an increased length of rete ridges, as in a psoriasiform tissue reaction, or may affect the whole epidermis, such as in lichenification. Acanthosis is commonly accompanied by other histological changes such as hypergranulosis, hyperkeratosis and papillomatosis.

When reactive epidermal proliferation is marked, the process may simulate an epithelial carcinoma and in this situation is referred to as pseudoepitheliomatous hyperplasia. Acanthosis may be seen in a wide variety of inflammatory and neoplastic disorders. Some of the common situations where this feature may be seen include the following:

1. Naevoid conditions and localised benign epidermal tumours – for example keratodermas, epidermal naevi and seborrhoeic keratosis.
2. Virally induced papillomas – for example viral warts and molluscum contagiosum.
3. Secondary to inflammatory conditions affecting the epidermis, particularly where chronic – for example persistent friction, lichenification, prurigo and chronic eczema, psoriasis and lichen planus.
4. Secondary to conditions associated with loss of keratinocyte adhesion – for example the pemphigus group of disorders and Darier disease.
5. Secondary to conditions associated with the presence of foreign cells within the epidermis – for example melanoma, Paget disease, mycosis fungoides and Langerhans cell histiocytosis.
6. Acanthosis is commonly seen overlying a variety of abnormalities in the dermis:
   - Dermal tumours such as fibrous histiocytoma and granular cell tumour.
   - Certain forms of cutaneous infection such as lupus vulgaris and blastomycosis.
   - Overlying dermal deposits of substances such as amyloid, abnormal elastic tissue or in association with foreign bodies.
   - In association with chronic oedema, such as chronic lymphoedema of the lower limb and myxoedema.

Anaplasia

This is a term used to describe variations in nuclear size, dense and clumped heterochromatin, and nuclear contour angulation typical of malignant cells, as in metastatic melanoma.

Apoptosis

This is a morphologically distinct type of cell degeneration and death, usually applied to keratinocytes that become homogeneous and eosinophilic and are extruded into the underlying upper dermis. These eosinophilic bodies (known as Civatte or colloid bodies), and the process of apoptosis, occur characteristically in lichenoid tissue reactions. A similar process may be observed in many other processes, for example following UV light exposure, in graft-versus-host disease and in cutaneous lupus erythematosus.

Basal lamina (see Chapter 2)

This structure, also known as the basement membrane, is a submicroscopic structure approximately 40 nm in thickness, which extends along the undersurface of the epidermal basal cells. It is not visible with light microscopy. The term basement membrane zone is sometimes applied to the area that may be visualised with the PAS-staining technique (Figure 3.7). The basement membrane is a very complex structure composed of large numbers of proteins with important functions in maintaining the structure of the skin. Many of these proteins are of great importance in genetic (epidermolysis bullosa) and acquired diseases (autoimmune blistering diseases).

Bullae

Bullae represent fluid-containing cavities occurring within or below the epidermis. Small bullae are known as vesicles. Determination of the site of bulla formation is most important in histological assessment of skin biopsies. Intraepidermal bullae may arise as the result of spongiosis, as in acute eczema, from reticular and ballooning degeneration seen in association with viral disorders or from acantholysis or epidermal cell necrosis. Subepidermal blisters usually result either from: (i) a defect in the basement membrane region, such as occurs in some forms of epidermolysis bullosa and porphyria; (ii) from a disruption of the basement membrane from intense liquefaction degeneration or necrosis of the basal cell layer, such as may occur in bullous lichen planus or bullous lupus erythematosus; or (iii) as a result of dermal inflammatory processes involving the upper dermal connective tissue and basement membrane region. In some conditions, such as erythema multiforme, both subepidermal and intraepidermal factors seem to be involved in bullae formation.

Colloid body
This term, usually regarded as synonymous with the Civatte body, describes the homogeneous, eosinophilic, rounded body resulting from degeneration and death of keratinocytes, particularly in the lower layers of the epidermis. This structure is found in various lichenoid tissue reactions and is involved in the process of apoptosis.

Crust
This term is used to describe collections of inflammatory cells, red blood cells, plasma and fibrin in the superficial portion of the epidermis. A crust may also contain microorganisms, and often replaces a partial or total loss of the epidermis itself.

Curlicue (storiform) pattern
This descriptive term refers to the twisting and curving of dermal fibrohistiocytic cells around collagen bundles, often at the margins of a dermal tumour. The pattern is mainly observed in dermatofibrosarcoma protuberans. The pattern described by this term is the same as that referred to by the term storiform (Figure 3.29a).

Degenerations
Dermal
Colloid degeneration. Colloid degeneration refers to the deposition of extracellular, homogeneous, gelatinous material of variable composition. It is typically seen in colloid milium but may also be found in certain epithelial tumours.

Elastotic degeneration. This describes the degenerative changes that develop with increasing age, particularly in the upper part of the dermis in sun-exposed skin. Early changes include an increase in the number and size of connective tissue fibres staining with elastic stains. In advanced stages of the condition there are masses of disorganised elastotic fibres occurring particularly in the upper third of the dermis and appearing to replace the normal collagen. This elastotic degeneration is normally separated from the epidermis by a narrow band of normal-staining connective tissue. In sections stained with H&E, the elastotic material is basophilic.

Fibrinoid degeneration. This term describes the deposition in tissue of eosinophilic, granular or fibrillary material resembling fibrin. The composition of the eosinophilic amorphous material may vary in different situations, but fibrinogen, plasma proteins, immunoglobulins and dermal ground substance may be components of the material. It is most typically seen in forms of necrotising vasculitis and is also found in disorders such as lupus erythematosus and the collagen diseases.

Hyaline degeneration. This term refers to the presence of homogeneous, eosinophilic, degenerative material in dermal connective tissue or in relation to blood vessels. The material has a glassy and refractile appearance. Hyaline degeneration occurs in forms of porphyria, lipoid proteinosis and sometimes in lichenoid tissue reactions. Epithelial structures may also show a similar type of change, for instance the tumour cells of cylindroma frequently undergo hyaline change.

Myxoid degeneration. This indicates the deposition or replacement of dermal connective tissue by amorphous, stringy, basophilic material. This pattern of degeneration is seen in localised myxoedema, papular mucinosis, scleroedema and dermatomyositis, as well as being seen in various neural, epithelial and adnexal neoplasms.

Epidermal
Ballooning degeneration. This form of degeneration of keratinocytes is associated with marked swelling and pallor of individual cells, with loss of intercellular bridges. A blister forms as a result of the consequent acantholysis. Ballooning degeneration along with reticular degeneration is characteristic of virus disorders affecting epithelia, such as herpesvirus infections.

Hydropic degeneration. This is also known as liquefaction degeneration and refers to a vacuolar change that affects the basal cell layer of the epidermis. Small droplets and vacuoles develop within and in-between basal cells. The process is commonly associated with pigmentary incontinence and when marked may lead to subepidermal blister formation. It occurs typically in the whole range of lichenoid tissue reactions, including lupus erythematosus, lichen planus, dermatomyositis, poikiloderma atrophicans vasculare and lichen sclerosus (Figure 3.44).

Reticular degeneration. This indicates the development of large, multiple, intraepidermal vesicles, where there remains a ragged network of epidermal cell remnants. As mentioned before, reticular degeneration often occurs in association with ballooning degeneration in acute virus infections of the herpesvirus and poxvirus

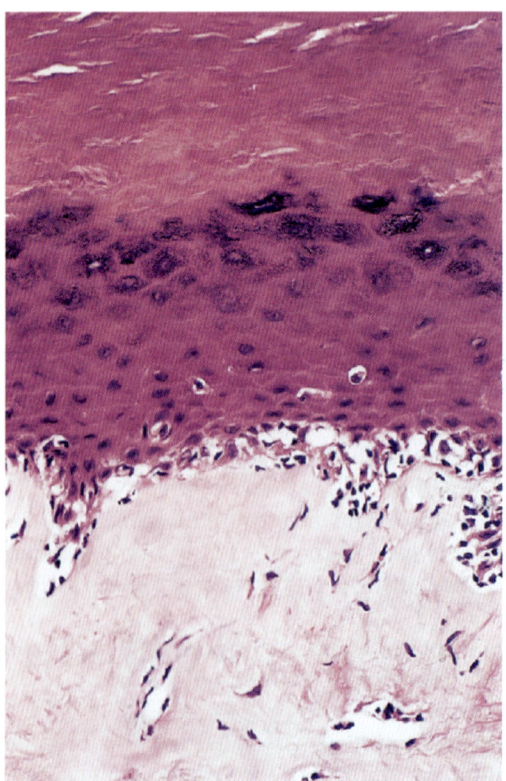

Figure 3.44 Prominent liquefaction degeneration from a case of lichen sclerosus.

groups. This pattern of epidermal degeneration may also sometimes be seen in the acute bullous reaction of contact dermatitis.

Desmoplasia

This term describes a pattern of fibrosis or sclerosis of dermal connective tissue, usually in association with an epithelial or melanocytic proliferative lesion. Examples of the use of this term are in desmoplastic trichoepithelioma and desmoplastic melanoma.

Dyskeratosis

This term relates to some abnormality in the process of epidermal cell keratinisation. The changes usually consist of nuclear pyknosis and bright pink condensation of the cytoplasm of keratinocytes. The process occurs in two main contexts: firstly, in malignant and premalignant epithelial lesions, such as squamous cell carcinoma, Bowen disease and solar keratosis; secondly, in various forms of acantholytic disorder such as Darier disease. In this latter condition, specific types of dyskeratotic cell include corps ronds and grains (Figure 3.43).

Dysplasia

This term is a confusing one, especially when used to describe atypical melanocytic naevi, because if communication with the clinician is inadequate it may be interpreted to mean different things. Its use normally reflects some abnormality in cell maturation, cytomorphology or the relationship between cells in epithelial structures. It has the connotation of possible progression to neoplastic disease.

Exocytosis

This term describes the migration of inflammatory cells from the blood vessels of the dermis into the overlying epidermis. The process may be associated with spongiosis, as in eczema, or may occur in the absence of spongiosis, such as may be seen in mycosis fungoides. In the latter setting, the word epidermotropism is usually preferred.

Granuloma

A granuloma describes circumscribed foci of inflammation containing monocytes, macrophages, lymphocytes and epithelioid cells. Multinucleated giant cells of foreign body, Langhans or Touton type may also be observed. Varying degrees of epidermal hyperplasia, capillary proliferation and dermal fibrosis are common accompanying changes. Granulomatous inflammation occurs in a wide variety of infectious and non-infectious conditions. Many different types of organism, ranging from viruses through bacteria to fungi, can produce a tissue granuloma. The presence of granulomas in a skin biopsy may indicate a systemic disease, such as sarcoidosis or a localised dermatosis of unknown cause, such as granuloma annulare or acne agminata. The precise histological appearance of a dermal granuloma depends not only on the underlying cause, but on the period over which the disease has been active and the immune status of the host.

Grenz zone

This comes from the German word for border and in dermatopathology is applied to a narrow zone of normal dermis between the epidermis and pathological changes in the underlying dermis.

Hypergranulosis

This refers to an increase in thickness of the granular layer of the epidermis and is commonly accompanied by hyperkeratosis and acanthosis. It is often seen in chronic lichenification and lichen planus and related disorders.

Hyperkeratosis

Hyperkeratosis refers to increased thickness of the stratum corneum and may be associated with acanthosis of the Malpighian layer. Hyperkeratosis may occur in various disorders of keratinisation, such as the keratodermas and some ichthyotic disorders, and relative hyperkeratosis is quite common in chronic discoid lupus erythematosus. In certain conditions, such as in Flegel disease, in addition to an increased thickness of the stratum corneum there is a change from the normal basket-weave pattern to a compact arrangement of the stratum corneum cells. When assessing the thickness of the stratum corneum, it is important to correlate the histological appearances with the site of the biopsy. The stratum corneum is normally thick on the palms and soles, and very thin, or even absent, around the eyelids and near mucous membrane junctions.

Epidermolytic hyperkeratosis

This particular change, also sometimes referred to as granular degeneration, is a peculiar and characteristic change seen in a number of skin disorders. There is an increase in the thickness of the granular layer, where keratinocytes appear to contain an increased number of keratohyalin granules. Perinuclear vacuolisation occurs in this area, and the cell boundaries may be indistinct. The vacuolisation may be marked, in some cases appearing to lead to intraepidermal vesicle formation. Although this change is best known as the characteristic histopathological feature of bullous ichthyosiform erythroderma (Figure 3.45), it also occurs in many other inherited and acquired conditions, including a form of palmoplantar keratoderma, so-called epidermolytic acanthoma and some forms of linear epidermal naevus. It is also occasionally seen as an incidental finding, either in normal skin or in association with a lesion, such as a naevus, a viral wart or a seborrhoeic keratosis.

Follicular hyperkeratosis

This describes varying degrees of hyperkeratosis and plugging of the ostia of hair follicles, and this change may be associated with the

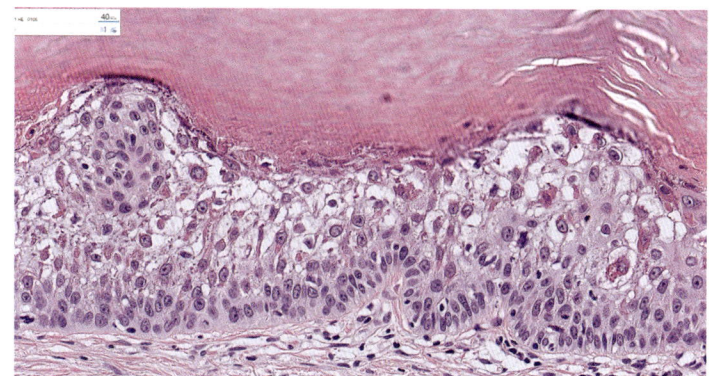

Figure 3.45 Epidermolytic hyperkeratosis seen in a biopsy from a patient with congenital bullous ichthyosiform erythroderma.

rupture of the follicular wall. It occurs in many conditions, including pityriasis rubra pilaris, lupus erythematosus, lichen planopilaris and lichen sclerosus.

Kamino bodies (eosinophilic globules)
This term describes the eosinophilic globules seen in the epidermis or in the region of the dermal–epidermal junction in spindle and epithelioid cell (Spitz) naevi. They are almost always found in Spitz naevi but may also be seen in some cases of melanoma.

Karyorrhexis
This refers to the fragmentation of cell nuclei and the process may be seen in various forms of neutrophilic dermatoses and cutaneous pyoderma. It is commonly seen in necrotising vasculitic processes. The term leukocytoclasis specifically refers to the fragmentation of nuclei of neutrophil polymorphonuclear leukocytes. However, the latter term is sometimes used to refer to fragmentation of other inflammatory cells such as lymphocytes.

Lichenoid tissue reaction
This is a pattern of changes occurring both in the epidermis and especially the dermis, seen in a wide variety of conditions, ranging from lichen planus itself to lupus erythematosus, lichen sclerosus and the poikilodermas. Lichenoid changes may also be seen in some examples of cutaneous drug eruptions. In the upper dermis, there is a band-like infiltrate consisting predominantly of mononuclear cells. This is closely related to the dermal–epidermal junction, which itself may have a saw-toothed pattern. Liquefaction degeneration of the basal cell layer is seen and colloid body formation may be present. There is often an increase in thickness of the overlying epidermis, affecting both the Malpighian layer and the stratum corneum (Figure 3.46).

Metaplasia
This term is used to indicate an alteration of one type of tissue into another, such as the formation of bone in certain epithelial tumours, for example pilomatricoma.

Necrobiosis
Necrobiosis is an unsatisfactory term derived from words for life and death. It is applied to certain granulomatous disorders where the dermal connective tissue becomes homogenised and loses its normal staining characteristics, resulting in mucinous, fibrinoid or sclerotic alteration. The outlines of the normal architecture are usually still present, and the amount of inflammation varies. Changes of necrobiosis are normally surrounded by a palisading histiocytic granuloma. The condition is seen in association with granuloma annulare, necrobiosis lipoidica, rheumatoid nodule and acne agminata.

Necrolysis
This is used to describe the separation of tissue constituents as a consequence of cell death. Epidermal changes of necrolysis are seen in various inflammatory reactions such as erythema multiforme, toxic epidermal necrolysis and necrolytic migratory erythema seen in association with the glucagonoma syndrome.

Necrosis
This term describes the death of cells or tissue.

Papilloma
This term indicates a tumour or tumour-like proliferation exhibiting both papillomatosis and hyperkeratosis. Acanthosis is also present. Examples of skin papillomas include viral warts, seborrhoeic keratoses and some epidermal naevi.

Papillomatosis
This change is characterised by elongation upwards of the dermal papillae, giving an accentuated and sometimes irregular, undulating configuration to the dermal–epidermal junction. The feature is commonly seen in psoriasis, and a wide variety of other inflammatory and neoplastic cutaneous disorders.

Parakeratosis
Parakeratosis can be defined as the retention of keratinocyte nuclei within the horny cell layer. It represents a disturbance of keratinisation and is normally associated with an absence or reduction in thickness of the granular cell layer. The histological feature of parakeratosis is commonly seen in many different forms of inflammatory dermatosis and is closely associated either with increased epidermal cell turnover or with inflammatory changes in the epidermis itself. It is commonly seen in psoriasis and subacute eczematous reactions, and in conditions such as pityriasis lichenoides where the change reflects an earlier disturbance in the underlying epidermis. In chronic inflammatory conditions where epidermal turnover is unaffected, such as in lichenoid reactions, parakeratosis is rarely seen. Dysplastic epithelial changes, such as those occurring in actinic keratoses and Bowen disease, are normally accompanied by parakeratosis.

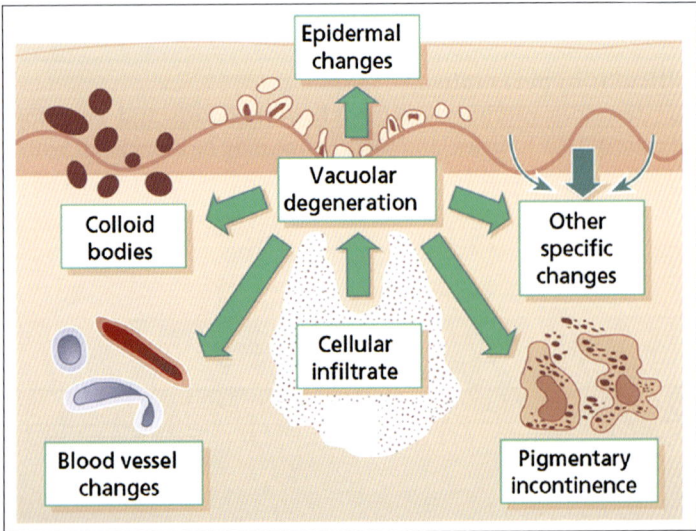

Figure 3.46 Lichenoid tissue reaction. Various histopathological consequences follow damage to the dermal–epidermal junction. These histopathological changes are seen in a wide variety of lichenoid reactions, ranging from lichen planus to lupus erythematosus, poikiloderma atrophicans vasculare, lichen sclerosus and lichenoid drug eruptions.

Pigmentary incontinence

This refers to the loss of melanin from cells of the basal layer of the epidermis, and the accumulation of melanin, both free and within dendritic macrophages, in the underlying dermis. It is associated with damage to keratinocytes of the lower epidermis and is commonly seen in lichenoid tissue reactions. Small amounts of melanin may be seen in the upper dermis in normal pigmented skin.

Pleomorphism

This describes variability in the appearance of cells and in particular the nuclei of cells of the same type. Although it may be seen in malignant and premalignant conditions, pleomorphism may also be seen in benign lesions such as pleomorphic fibroma.

Polymorphism

Conventionally this is used to describe a variation in types of cells in a cutaneous lesion. This term is not the same as pleomorphism.

Pustules and abscesses

These terms are used to describe cavities within the epidermis or dermis formed by collections of neutrophil or eosinophil polymorphonuclear cells. Occasionally, the term is used to describe collections of other leukocytes, as in the term Pautrier microabscesses. Cutaneous pustules may be sterile or associated with an infectious microorganism. Certain specific types of microabscess and pustule are of diagnostic value in dermatopathology.

Kogoj spongiform pustule. This describes the multilocular micropustules that form in the superficial portions of the epidermis in pustular psoriasis. They form in a similar manner to Munro microabscesses but the process is more extensive.

Munro microabscesses. These lesions are small collections of neutrophil polymorphs usually found within the stratum corneum. They are normally seen in lesions of chronic established psoriasis and the other histological features of the psoriatic reaction, such as irregular epidermal thickening and parakeratosis, are normally present.

Papillary tip microabscesses. These are small focal collections of neutrophil polymorphs, or occasionally eosinophils, in the tips of dermal papillae. Although they are characteristic of dermatitis herpetiformis, they may occur in other bullous eruptions such as epidermolysis bullosa acquisita and the bullous form of lupus erythematosus.

Pautrier microabscesses. These small, intraepidermal collections of lymphoid cells in the absence of marked spongiosis are characteristic of mycosis fungoides. The cells within the epidermis may show some degree of nuclear hyperchromatism or atypia. Single cell colonisation of the epidermis is more commonly seen than true Pautrier microabscess formation in many cases of early mycosis fungoides.

Subcorneal pustules. Large, subcorneal collections of neutrophil polymorphs usually represent either impetigo or subcorneal pustular dermatosis. Sometimes, the distinction of either of these two conditions from pustular psoriasis may be difficult.

Pyknosis

This term is used to refer to hyperchromatism and shrinkage of the cell nucleus. It is normally associated with cell death and may be seen in a wide variety of conditions, including epithelial dysplasias, drug reactions and reactions to UV light.

Saw-toothing

This refers to an alteration in the pattern of the dermal–epidermal junction where dermal papillae are expanded and the tips of the rete pegs are pointed. The resulting pattern bears a superficial resemblance to the teeth of a saw and the change is seen in lichen planus and other lichenoid reactions.

Spongiosis

Spongiosis is also known as intercellular oedema and describes the widening of intercellular spaces between keratinocytes due to fluid accumulation. Spongiosis is the characteristic histopathological change seen in acute and subacute eczematous reactions, but is also seen in a wide variety of other conditions; when spongiosis is marked it leads to intraepidermal vesiculation. Spongiosis of follicular epithelium may be associated with increased mucin deposition in the histopathological reaction pattern known as follicular mucinosis.

Storiform patterning

This is a pattern of proliferation commonly seen in various dermal and soft-tissue tumours, where strands of spindle-shaped tumour cells or even collagen bundles are arranged so as to resemble the pattern seen in woven cloth. The term is also sometimes applied to the presence of strands of spindle-shaped tumour cells or connective tissue cells that appear to extend radially from a central hub, similar to the spokes of a wheel. Cartwheel patterning is probably a better term to describe this particular appearance. Storiform and cartwheel patterning, although commonly referred to in DFSP, are by no means specifically diagnostic (Figure 3.29a).

Theque

This term is derived from French and Greek words for a box (*thèque*, θηκη) and is conventionally used in dermatopathology to describe small aggregates or nests of cells, particularly the collections of naevus cells at, and in the region of, the dermal–epidermal junction.

Villi

This term refers to elongated dermal papillae covered usually with a single layer of epidermal cells, which form the base of a blister cavity that has resulted from the process of suprabasal acantholysis. Villi are seen in the various forms of pemphigus and Darier disease (Figure 3.32), warty dyskeratoma and transient and persistent acantholytic dermatosis.

Histological sections that reveal little or no abnormality

It is not uncommon for the diagnostic dermatopathologist to come across histological sections where at first sight the appearances resemble normal skin. It may be that the pathological changes have been missed. This can be the fault of the clinician who has perhaps taken too superficial a biopsy from a lesion of suspected panniculitis, or it can be the fault of the pathologist who has inappropriately blocked the biopsy specimen or taken too few sections from the material. The importance of studying numerous serial sections in this situation cannot be overemphasised. There are a number of conditions, however, where subtle pathological abnormalities are present, but where a high index of suspicion is needed to make a correct diagnosis. The following list includes some of the more important of these.

Epidermal lesions

Actinic keratoses. Some flat actinic keratoses may show very little evidence of keratinocyte atypia, and unless a reasonable amount of normal skin is included the biopsy material may be signed out as non-diagnostic.

Fungal infections. In the presence of patchy epidermal spongiosis and focal overlying parakeratosis, it is always important to exclude the presence of a fungal infection with a PAS stain. Occasionally, a few neutrophil polymorphs may be seen in the upper Malpighian layer of the stratum corneum and this may provide a clue to the correct diagnosis. Pityriasis versicolor may be present in the absence of spongiosis and is frequently missed.

Ichthyotic disorders. The dominant form of ichthyosis vulgaris is usually characterised by some degree of compact hyperkeratosis and an absent or attenuated granular layer. If the hyperkeratosis is not significant, the diagnosis may be overlooked. When assessing the stratum corneum, it is always important to look at not only the thickness but also the quality of the corneocytes. An alteration from the normal basket-weave pattern to a compact cornified layer usually indicates some pathological abnormality.

Porokeratosis. The epidermal changes, usually of atrophy, in the various forms of porokeratosis are often not striking, and the diagnostic cornoid lamella may not be seen on the first sections cut from the block. In diagnostic biopsies, the cornoid lamella may not be present or may be missed if the orientation is not correct. All forms of porokeratosis may be misdiagnosed, but the disseminated actinic form of the disorder is the most commonly overlooked.

Pigmentary disorders

Various disorders of epidermal pigmentation may be difficult to diagnose with certainty, particularly if one is not certain of the skin colour of the patient from whom the biopsy has been taken. The loss of pigment in established vitiligo is normally associated with the absence or reduction in number of melanocytes. However, in café-au-lait spots and ephelides, melanocytes are normal in number. A melanin stain may reveal a difference between lesional and adjacent skin. In post-inflammatory hypo- or hyperpigmentation, the number of melanocytes remains normal with an increase or decrease in melanin in basal cells. Often, melanophages are seen in the papillary dermis, particularly in postinflammatory hyperpigmentation.

Dermal deposits

The small amounts of amyloid seen in macular amyloidosis are often difficult to visualise with H&E stain. Special stains are indicated, but the presence of slightly expanded dermal papillae, together with a hint of lichenoid tissue reaction, may alert the pathologist to this possibility. A further useful clue is the presence of scattered apoptotic keratinocytes. The presence of iron pigment in small quantities in the dermis is easily missed, either in common conditions such as bruising or in rare situations such as idiopathic haemochromatosis. A Perls stain usually highlights iron deposits that have not been detected in slides stained with H&E. The deposits of silver in argyria are often best seen around the basement membrane zone of dermal sweat ducts.

Connective tissue diseases

Scleroderma, particularly in the late stages, often shows little histopathological abnormality. The coarsening and hyalinisation of collagen bundles, with a reduction in the space between them, is often not prominent, particularly in the superficial form of morphoea. In the early stages of the condition, there is normally some increase in cellularity around the dermal blood vessels. It is always important to try and assess normal skin if there is some present in the biopsy. Similar problems may be encountered with various forms of connective tissue naevi and abnormalities of elastic tissue such as anetoderma. In atrophoderma, the elastic pattern is more or less normal, but there is a reduction in total thickness of the dermis, which may be difficult to evaluate. A solution to this problem is to obtain an ellipse of skin in which half of the specimen represents clinically normal skin. To indicate the clinically normal skin, the clinician marks the specimen with a stitch.

Dermal infiltrates

Blue naevus and related disorders. The dendritic melanocytes seen in the dermal melanocytoses, particularly Mongolian spots, are often difficult to recognise without the use of a melanocytic marker such as melan-A or SOX10. S-100 protein, a very sensitive melanocytic marker, may be negative in some of these lesions. The main problem resides in the distinction between melanophages and melanocytes, as most dermal melanocytoses excluding blue naevus contain only a few scattered dermal pigmented melanocytes. The use of an immunohistochemical marker for melanocytes is useful, but the product obtained in the detection of the final peroxidase product is usually brown and this is very similar to melanin. This problem can be overcome by bleaching the slide before immunohistochemistry or by changing the diaminobenzidine for amino-ethyl carbazole, which results in a red product.

Granuloma annulare. In the majority of cases this diagnosis is straightforward, with evidence of a dermal palisading granuloma with necrobiosis. However, in the disseminated form of the condition the changes are often very slight and may be represented by just a few mononuclear cells dissecting bundles of collagen.

Mast cell disorders. The adult form of urticaria pigmentosa, and particularly its variant telangiectasia macularis eruptiva perstans, frequently shows only a relatively slight increase in numbers of mast cells within the dermis. In these forms of urticaria pigmentosa, the mast cells tend to be rather dendritic or short spindle shaped. Their granules may not be obvious and they may resemble normal connective tissue cells such as fibroblasts. In mastocytoma and some juvenile forms of mastocytosis, the mast cells are larger, rounded cells with central nuclei and are easier to recognise.

Urticaria. In biopsies from urticarial lesions there may be very little more than slight dermal oedema, which is often difficult to evaluate on processed tissue, together with a slight increase in inflammatory cells around the upper dermal blood vessels. It should be remembered that, in normal skin, a few mononuclear cells, fibroblasts and other cells are present in the dermis. A clue to the diagnosis of urticaria is the presence of at least a few eosinophils.

Scalp disorders

Unless an adequate biopsy is available for examination, many disorders of the scalp may be difficult to evaluate. Conditions such as telogen effluvium and longstanding alopecia areata show very little sign of inflammation, and a diagnosis may have to be made purely on the number of pilosebaceous structures and the relative number of follicles in different phases of the hair cycle. The study of horizontally sectioned biopsies is the ideal method to study hair follicles with regard to their cycle, pathological alterations and numbers (Chapter 87).

Conclusions

As mentioned at the start of this chapter, histopathological examination of a skin biopsy taken from an appropriate lesion is a great help in assisting the clinician to come to a correct diagnosis and therefore to come to a decision regarding management of the patient. Light microscopic examination of sections from skin biopsy tissue fixed in formalin and embedded in paraffin is likely to remain the single most useful diagnostic technique for the foreseeable future. The wide range of tissue and cytological changes that may be encountered within normal skin and inflammatory and neoplastic conditions mean that considerable experience is required for the dermatopathologist to contribute helpfully to patient management. Many excellent texts are now available on the histopathology of the skin, but there can be no substitute for personal study on a day-to-day basis of as much material as possible under the supervision of an experienced guide. Feedback and communication between the clinician and pathologist is essential, and has been perhaps one of the most important factors in the advances in dermatopathology in the last decade. The light microscopist already has a very wide range of additional techniques available to assist in diagnosis and to study the anatomy and physiology of normal and diseased tissues, some of which are outlined in this chapter. The numerous new areas of investigation that have developed over the last decades, including molecular biological techniques, such as PCR, *in situ* hybridisation, comparative genomic hybridisation, SNP arrays and studies on biological response modifiers, cytokines and adhesion molecules, continue to further major advances in our understanding of skin in health and disease.

Key references

The full list of references can be found in the online version at https://www.wiley.com/rooksdermatology10e

Introduction, Biopsy of the skin
1 Calonje E, Brenn T, Lazar A, Billings S. *McKee's Pathology of the Skin with Clinical Correlations*, 5th edn. New York: Elsevier Mosby, 2019.
2 Patterson JW. *Weedon's Skin Pathology*, 5th edn. New York: Elsevier, 2019.
3 Ackerman AB, Boer A, Bennin B, Gottlieb GG. *Histologic Diagnosis of Inflammatory Skin Diseases*, 3rd edn. New York: Ardor Scribendi, 2004.

Laboratory methods
Specimen preparation, Routine tissue processing, Routine staining techniques, including histochemistry
2 Du X, Li Z, Xu W et al. Diagnostic value of horizontal versus vertical sections for scarring and non-scarring alopecia: a systematic review and meta-analysis. *Eur J Dermatol* 2016;26:361–9.
10 Haspeslagh M, Hoorens I, Degryse N et al. Pathologic evaluation of skin tumors with ex vivo dermoscopy with derm dotting. *JAMA Dermatol* 2017;153:154–61.
14 Suvarna KS, Layton C, Bancroft JD, eds. *Bancroft's Theory and Practice of Histological Techniques*, 8th edn. Edinburgh: Churchill Livingstone, 2018.
26 Sunderkötter C, Becker K, Kutzner H et al. Molecular diagnosis of skin infections using paraffin-embedded tissue – review and interdisciplinary consensus. *J Dtsch Dermatol Ges* 2018;16:139–47.
32 Müller N, Hentrich B, Frey CF et al. Quantitative PCR for the diagnosis of cutaneous leishmaniasis from formalin-fixed paraffin-embedded skin sections. *Mol Cell Probes* 2015;29:507–10.

Immunopathology
Immunofluorescence methods
3 Emtenani S, Yuan H, Lin C et al. Normal human skin is superior to monkey oesophagus substrate for detection of circulating BP180-NC16A-specific IgG antibodies in bullous pemphigoid. *Br J Dermatol* 2019;180:1099–106.
5 Gammon WR, Briggaman RA, Inman AO, Queen LL, Wheeler CE. Differentiating anti-lamina lucida and anti-sublamina densa anti-BMZ antibodies by indirect immunofluorescence on 1.0 M sodium chloride-separated skin. *J Invest Dermatol* 1984;82:139–44.

Immunoenzyme methods
2 Schach CP, Smoller BR, Hudson AR et al. Immunohistochemical stains in dermatopathology. *J Am Acad Dermatol* 2000;43:1094–100.
9 Komorowski L, Müller R, Vorobyev A et al. Sensitive and specific assays for routine serological diagnosis of epidermolysis bullosa acquisita. *J Am Acad Dermatol* 2013;68:e89–95.

Applications of immunopathology techniques
2 Oh KS, Mahalingam M. Immunohistochemistry as a genetic surrogate in dermatopathology: pearls and pitfalls. *Adv Anat Pathol* 2019;26:390–420.
6 Witte M, Zillikens D, Schmidt E. Diagnosis of autoimmune blistering diseases. *Front Med (Lausanne)* 2018;5:296.
9 Saschenbrecker S, Karl I, Komorowski L et al. Serological diagnosis of autoimmune bullous skin diseases. *Front Immunol* 2019;10:1974.
11 Compton LA, Murphy GF, Lian CG. Diagnostic immunohistochemistry in cutaneous neoplasia: an update. *Dermatopathology (Basel)* 2015;2:15–42.
37 Kervarrec T, Tallet A, Miquelestorena-Standley E et al. Diagnostic accuracy of a panel of immunohistochemical and molecular markers to distinguish Merkel cell carcinoma from other neuroendocrine markers. *Mod Pathol* 2018;32:499–510.
55 Nielsen PS, Riber-Hansen R, Jensen TO et al. Proliferation indices of phosphohistone H3 and Ki67: strong prognostic markers in a consecutive cohort with stage I/II melanoma. *Mod Pathol* 2013;26:404–13.

58 Quan VL, Panah E, Zhang B et al. The role of gene fusions in melanocytic neoplasms. *J Cutan Pathol* 2019;46:878–87.
60 Murali R, Wiesner T, Scolyer RA. Tumors associated with BAP1 mutations. *Pathology* 2013;45:116–26.

Other diagnostic methods
Viral disease techniques
5 Colmenero I, Santonja C, Alonso-Riaño M et al. SARS-CoV-2 endothelial infection causes COVID-19 chilblains: histopathological, immunohistochemical and ultrastructural study of seven paediatric cases. *Br J Dermatol* 2020;183:729–37.

Immunogenotyping
1 Mahe E, Pugh T, Kamel-Reid S. T cell clonality assessment: past, present and future. *J Clin Pathol* 2018;71:195–200.

Digital pathology
3 Kumar N, Gupta R, Gupta S. Whole slide imaging (WSI) in pathology: current perspectives and future directions. *J Digit Imaging* 2020;33:1034–40.
6 Kent MN, Olsen TG, Feeser TA et al. Diagnostic accuracy of virtual pathology vs traditional microscopy in a large dermatopathology study. *JAMA Dermatol* 2017;153:1285–91.

Approach to microscopic examination of tissue sections
1 Ackerman AB, Boer A, Bennin B, Gottlieb GG. *Histologic Diagnosis of Inflammatory Skin Diseases*, 3rd edn. New York: Ardor Scribendi, 2004.

CHAPTER 4

Diagnosis of Skin Disease

Ian H. Coulson[1], Emma C. Benton[2] and Stephanie Ogden[3]

[1]Burnley General Hospital, East Lancashire NHS Trust, Burnley, UK
[2]St John's Institute of Dermatology, Guy's and St Thomas' NHS Foundation Trust, London, UK
[3]Salford Royal Hospital, Greater Manchester, UK

Fundamentals of diagnosis, 4.1	Palpation of the skin, 4.16	**Skin testing (prick and scratch, intradermal and patch testing), 4.23**
Disease definition, 4.1	Additional simple clinical examination, 4.17	Techniques for skin testing, 4.23
The history, 4.2	Additional clinical investigations, 4.17	Immediate-weal tests, 4.24
The presenting complaint, 4.2	**Clinical microscopy, dermoscopy and other imaging systems, 4.19**	Delayed (4–8 h) tests, 4.24
Quality of life in dermatology patients, 4.5	Dermoscopy, 4.19	Intradermal tests for the detection of delayed sensitivity to bacterial, fungal and viral antigens, 4.24
Examination of the skin, 4.5	Other imaging systems for localised lesions, 4.21	**Teledermatology, 4.25**
Description of skin lesions, 4.5	Other simple microscopy procedures, 4.22	**Mobile smartphone applications, 4.26**
Examination of skin of colour, 4.5	**Fine-needle aspiration of lymph nodes, 4.22**	**Artificial intelligence and dermatology, 4.26**
Sites involved and their distribution, 4.5	**Radiological and imaging examinations, 4.22**	**Key references, 4.27**
Individual lesions – nomenclature, 4.10		
Distribution of lesions, 4.14		

Fundamentals of diagnosis

Accurate and precise diagnosis of any disease is paramount in guiding prognosis, prevention and effective therapy. Skin diseases are usually but not always visible, and there is a preconception both among patients and other physicians that inspection is all that is required to make a diagnosis.

As in almost all other branches of medicine, arrival at a dermatological diagnosis depends upon, at times, an almost forensic approach to history taking, inspection of the entirety of the integument including the scalp, flexures, palms and soles, nails and mucous membranes, supplemented by appropriate special investigations, including 'low-tech' techniques such as inspection with a dermoscope, Wood's light, skin biopsy, microbiology, through to 'high-tech' investigations such as genetic testing and *in vivo* confocal microscopy. Ultimately, some patients will need intimate amalgamation of clinical and investigatory information to arrive at the best clinicopathological diagnosis [1]. Re-evaluation of all of these factors, and being open to a different and even novel diagnosis, is part of developing dermatological maturity.

Increasingly, self-taken digital images are proffered by patients to aid diagnosis, and are often helpful in assessing changing, recurrent or evanescent eruptions (e.g. urticaria, erythema multiforme or herpes simplex).

The history, particularly the past medical and drug exposure history, may need to be supplemented by interrogation of all the available medical and general practitioner notes. Senses other than visual can aid diagnosis. Palpation will identify induration (such as in panniculitis and morphoea), quality of crusting and scaling, hardness (as in calcinosis) and temperature [2]. Smell can be helpful in the diagnosis of some disorders (such as trimethylaminuria).

Disease definition

Many skin diseases do not yet have an identifiable cause, so their definition is based on a constellation of symptoms, signs and histopathological features (e.g. rosacea). Additional information (e.g. genetic and immunopathological) may be used to refine a diagnosis further (e.g. linear immunoglobulin A (IgA) bullous dermatosis). Even when a cause for a condition is known, the same cause can produce a variety of reaction patterns (e.g. *Borrelia burgdorferi* can induce erythema chronicum migrans, acrodermatitis atrophicans and lymphocytoma cutis). Even with common diseases like psoriasis, there are no strict diagnostic criteria, and with the advent of new genetic information, different morphological types of psoriasis may be genetically distinct, justifying subclassification rather than 'lumping' [1].

For everyday clinical use, rather loose disease definition may be pragmatically acceptable, but in epidemiological studies and therapeutic trials, strict criteria may be required for complete uniformity of enrolment. Such criteria exist for a number of disorders, such as

Rook's Textbook of Dermatology, Tenth Edition. Edited by Christopher Griffiths, Jonathan Barker, Tanya Bleiker, Walayat Hussain and Rosalind Simpson.
© 2024 John Wiley & Sons Ltd. Published 2024 by John Wiley & Sons Ltd.

the American Rheumatism Association criteria for the diagnosis of systemic lupus erythematosus, where major and minor criteria may be used to define both the disease and the specificity and sensitivity for the diagnosis in a given individual [2]. Diagnostic criteria exist for several other diseases of dermatological importance, such as Behçet disease [3], atopic eczema [4], hidradenitis suppurativa and Sweet syndrome. Such criteria must not be fixed, but should take into account new scientific discoveries as they arise (e.g. fillagrin mutation in atopic disease, and the inclusion of drug-induced Sweet syndrome). To compound problems, for some conditions, more than one set of diagnostic criteria exist (e.g. the Hanifin and Rajka criteria and the Williams–Pembroke criteria for atopic eczema [5]).

Molecular and genetic techniques are revolutionising the definition of genodermatoses and diseases will become increasingly defined by their precise molecular aberration as well as their clinical phenotype.

Collation of diagnostic data is driven by a variety of motives. It is useful for the assessment of the health needs of populations, and therefore the allocation of funding by both state financed and insurance reimbursement-based health economies. The value of such information is dependent upon the validity of the data and concerns about the accuracy of coding, costing and case mix. Some of the diagnostic coding systems, such as the World Health Organization's International Classification of Diseases (ICD) system, have been felt to be too general for clinical and epidemiological use in dermatology, and national bodies have created their own diagnostic indexing systems (e.g. the British Association of Dermatologists Dermatological Diagnostic Index System). Collection of severe drug reaction diagnostic information is invaluable in the identification of evolving culprit drugs, but the voluntary nature of collection may skew their interpretation, with new drugs and more severe reactions being more likely to be reported.

The history

A careful, thorough and at times directed history is of paramount importance to making an accurate diagnosis in dermatology (Box 4.1). It is likely to be relatively quick in the assessment of some skin tumours (e.g. a dermatofibroma), and time consuming in inflammatory dermatoses and occupational diseases (where the relationship to work, work practice, the nature of agents that the patient has been exposed to, the involvement of other employees, the nature of personal protection and treatment used can be complex). History taking must remain an ongoing practice in patients where there is diagnostic uncertainty, or an unexpectedly slow or suboptimal response to therapy. Open questioning such as 'Do you have any ideas what may be causing this?' may lead to fruitful avenues of investigation, or a valuable chance to allay unnecessary fears. Detailed questioning about concordance, particularly with topical therapy, may identify why there has been a disappointing response. Many disease guidelines and guidelines for the introduction of systemic therapies now prescribe what should exist in the history section of minimum datasets [1–5].

Box 4.1 Essential points in history taking

Essential points in the history – rashes
- Location – where did the rash start, where did it spread to?
- Temporal – when did it start, does it come and go, if so, how long does it last?
- Exacerbating factors – what made it worse (e.g. physical factors, menstrual cycle, diet, topical and oral treatments, stress, medication)?
- Drugs and co-morbidities – was the rash there before or after drug (or herbal) medication was introduced?
- Alleviating factors – physical factors, diet, treatment?
- What are the predominant symptoms – itch, sleep disturbance, pain, disfigurement?
- Occupational factors – does it get worse at work, does it improve away from work, is it affecting work, are others at work similarly affected?
- Open questions – do you have any thoughts as to what has caused this? What do you fear most about this problem?

Essential points in the history – lesions
- Where is the lesion? Have others arisen since the first?
- Was there anything there before this developed?
- Was there any type of injury before it arose?
- Temporal – how long has it taken to develop to this size? Is it still growing or is it resolving?
- Symptoms – is it sore, tender or painful? What makes any pain worse?
- Past history – have you had anything similar before?
- Family history
- Sun exposure – have you had considerable sun exposure in your past?

The presenting complaint

The following areas are likely to form part of the dermatological history, especially for the diagnosis of inflammatory dermatoses. Generic questions relevant to skin tumours and preoperative history taking are specified below.

Symptoms

Itch

This is the cardinal dermatological symptom. Itch may be generalised or localised to a particular area and may be associated with or without visible rash. Scabies, for example, may cause intense generalised itch particularly when an individual is warm, with at first minimal visible rash, and prior to the pathognomonic burrow and scabies nodules becoming apparent. Itch may be localised to where an inflammatory eruption exists (such as an area of tinea corporis or discoid eczema). Generalised itch is characteristic of atopic eczema, and is likely to be worse at night and result in sleep disturbance. Lichen planus is usually intensely itchy though rubbing of lesions rather than scratching may be noted. Pityriasis rosea and versicolor and seborrhoeic eczema may be less itchy than atopic eczema of similar extent.

Intense itch localised to the lower scapular area with initially normal appearing skin is characteristic of notalgia paraesthetica. Ultimately, scratching results in lichenification, pigmentary change and even localised amyloid.

Pain

Some dermatoses and lesions may be painful or tender on palpation.

Herpes simplex and zoster and bacterial cellulitis are often preceded by pain before the eruption develops. Chondrodermatitis nodularis helicis is painful particularly at night when the lesion is subjected to pressure when lain upon. Tumours such as glomangiomas may be exquisitely painful when pressure is applied to them, particularly those under the nail. Angiolipomas, blue rubber bleb naevi and eccrine spiradenomas are painful. Leiomyomas may be tender when they are subject to cold stimuli. Pain in patients with multiple keratosis after organ transplantation is an early clue to lesional change and progression to squamous cell carcinoma.

Urticaria, when developing on the palms and soles, and especially pressure urticaria, can be painful rather than itchy. Erythema nodosum is often tender. Ischaemic ulcers caused by large vessel disease, vasculitis and drugs (e.g. nicorandil and hydroxycarbamide) are painful. Acute eruptions associated with pain may indicate the more serious onset of skin necrosis (such as in necrotising vasculitis, calciphylaxis and necrotising fasciitis).

Disfigurement

Sometimes an eruption is itch and pain free, and the physical appearance of an eruption or lesion is the principal concern (such as with vitiligo or post-inflammatory hyperpigmentation). Fear of cancer and infection or infestation may require specific questioning and reassurance if these are not considerations. Disfigurement is the source of considerable psychosocial upset.

Duration

The onset of a lesion or an eruption is usually apparent to the patient, but basal cell carcinomas may have actually been present for months or even years but only when it begins to weep or bleed is it evident to the sufferer. Keratoacanthomas arise rapidly over weeks and spontaneously resolve by 6 months. Lesions of urticaria characteristically arise and resolve within 24 h although the duration of the eruption may continue over months or years in chronic disease. Longer lasting lesions are likely to be those of urticarial vasculitis. Lesions of erythema annulare centrifugum spread out over a few weeks. Larva migrans tracks extend over a matter of days whereas the tracks of larva currens due to *Strongyloides* will elongate over minutes. Lesions that 'go black overnight' do so usually because of intralesional haemorrhage rather than becoming malignant.

Evolution

The patient's description of the evolution of an eruption can be diagnostically helpful. Typical distal subungual onychomycosis starts at the free edge of the nail and spreads proximally, whereas the nail dystrophy of chronic candidal paronychia starts with bolstering of the proximal nail fold, and the subsequent nail dystrophy spreads distally. Classical pityriasis rubra pilaris often starts in the scalp and spreads caudally. Cellulitis of the lower leg usually starts in the toe web and the erythema spreads proximally. Pityriasis rosea may demonstrate the characteristic herald patch preceding the widespread rash by days to weeks. A contact dermatitis can spread beyond the confines of where an allergen has been applied to the skin, so elucidating where the eruption first started can help in culprit allergen identification.

Periodicity

The behaviour of lesions or eruptions that recur over time in a stereotypic fashion may have diagnostic significance. Herpes simplex infections may be preceded by pain before the typical vesicles appear in the same location at each recurrence. Similarly, a fixed drug eruption will recur in exactly the same location often within hours of re-exposure to the culprit drug trigger. A relationship to the menstrual cycle, with an eruption resolving during the first half of the menstrual cycle, and recurring shortly after ovulation and reaching a crescendo just before menstruation may indicate an autoimmune progesterone dermatitis. Cutaneous deposits of endometriosis (often umbilical) fluctuate in synchrony with the menses.

Eruptions that only occur during vacations may be due to light exposure (e.g. polymorphic light eruption), but can be due to allergy to personal care products kept in the holiday wash bag, but not used when at home. Degradation products of some perfumes may be allergenic, whereas fresh undegraded products are tolerated, so that an identical product used frequently at home causes no problem, whereas the same product that has spent time opened in a holiday home or travel bag may be reactive.

General history

General medical conditions may have cutaneous features, and should be noted, especially in patients with rashes or generalised skin symptoms. Recent illnesses, even if apparently resolved, deserve special attention, as conditions such as urticaria, vasculitis, guttate psoriasis and erythema multiforme can be triggered by viral or bacterial infections in the weeks preceding the onset of the rash.

Medication

Any recent or current systemic medication should be noted, including regular or intermittent self-medication or that received from relatives or friends, both as a possible cause of drug eruptions and to avoid interactions with treatment prescribed for the skin complaint. It can sometimes be useful to ask an individual to describe the contents of their medicine box or cabinet to jog their memory. A new problem is that patients can easily forget that they are receiving a potent injection therapy perhaps only once every few months (such as ustekinumab or infliximab); such therapies are often not included on their medication list.

The timing of the introduction of a drug, and the effect of stopping and restarting medication, is paramount in the consideration of drug eruptions. Topical therapies should also be considered, both in terms of their efficacy (or lack of), as well as because they may conceal or even cause a dermatosis. Allergies to medicaments or other agents (including local anaesthetics and skin cleaners used preoperatively) may be important, as are drugs that might interact with anaesthetics and vasoconstrictors (e.g. β-blockers and epinephrine) or cause surgical bleeding (e.g. aspirin, warfarin and clopidogrel). The presence of medical implants (e.g. pacemakers, defibrillators, dental and joint prostheses) may have implications for imaging, the use of haemostatics such as the hyfrecator, and may occasionally be responsible for specific dermatoses.

Diet
Dietary history may be important in some individuals, especially those with intermittent urticaria or anaphylaxis, and in infants with atopic eczema. A food diary listing foods ingested and the timing of suspect symptoms can be helpful. However, diet is often erroneously blamed for skin eruptions.

Family history
This may be important if a genodermatosis is suspected, in disorders with more complex inheritance (e.g. atopic eczema, psoriasis), and in some non-inherited disorders in which family contact is important (e.g. scabies, chickenpox).

Occupational factors
An occupational contact dermatitis may improve when the sufferer has a holiday only to recur on return to work. Hand eczema is the most frequent manifestation, and a painstaking history is needed to determine the exact work practice, and to determine potential irritants or allergens. Perusal of the health and safety data sheets will be required, as well as noting the personal protective equipment that has been used (e.g. gloves, barrier creams and after work creams may help but can also occasionally hinder). Specific dermatological problems related to different occupations are outlined in Table 4.1.

Leisure factors
Certain dermatoses are related to leisure and sporting activities (e.g. jogger's nipples, jogger's toenails, cyclist's perineum, fiddler's neck). DIY can lead to exacerbations of atopic eczema due to solvent and dust exposure. Acrylate and epoxy adhesives can be problematic in some hobbies, producing localised and an airborne pattern of contact eczema. Gardening can expose the skin to a variety of irritant, allergen, phototoxic, arthropod and actinic insults, with often a seasonal periodicity.

Geographical factors
Both recent and distant travel can extend the differential diagnosis of both lesions and eruptions, and should be documented. Even short stopovers can result in a return with an unwanted exotic souvenir.

Ethnicity and cultural factors
Several disorders have a predilection for specific racial groups, for example sarcoidosis in black people [6] and prurigo pigmentosa in Japanese people [7]. Some disorders are of greater severity in some racial groups, such as atopic eczema in Afro-Caribbean and Chinese people [8,9].

The custom of cousin marriage can increase the frequency of recessive genetic disorders such as some types of epidermolysis bullosa. Religious rituals can produce distinctive lesions such as prayer nodules on the feet and forehead, and turban wearers may develop chondrodermatitis on the lower pinna from garment pressure. Alternative medical treatments popular in some areas and ethnic groups can produce unexpected appearances (e.g. marks from acupuncture and cupping) and should be sought in the history. Unregulated products may be imported and distributed illegally producing a variety of skin problems (e.g. super-potent topical steroids sold as skin lighteners, high concentration hydroquinone creams that can induce ochronosis, and unlabelled hair dyes or 'henna' containing paraphenylene diamine). Patients may also not always volunteer that they have had cosmetic procedures (such as filler insertion) and may not realise that delayed reactions can occur several years afterwards unless they are specifically questioned about it.

Social and psychological factors
The living conditions including bathing facilities, economic status and the standard of nutrition of the patient and access to transport may be relevant both as a guide to diagnosis and to ensure compliance with the treatment advised. The availability of a spouse or carer, and proximity to health care professionals or facilities are important

Table 4.1 Some dermatoses occurring in occupational groups.

Activity	Examples of dermatological conditions that may occur
Agricultural	Irritant dermatitis (e.g. to disinfectants, physical 'wear and tear')
	Contact allergy (e.g. rubber chemicals in gloves or footwear)
	Hazards from animals (e.g. tinea)
	Hazards from plants (e.g. lichen allergy in forestry)
	Actinic damage
	Cold damage – chilblains and chondrodermatitis
Gardening	Irritant or contact allergic dermatitis related to many plants
	Contact allergy to gloves
	Bites and stings; harvest mites, etc.
Building trade and DIY	Irritant dermatitis from cement (also causes chemical burns), plaster, solvents, preservatives, fibreglass
	Contact allergic dermatitis, especially from chromate in cement, epoxy resins, formaldehyde resins, colophony in soldering flux
	Mechanical – frictional palmar dermatitis from tools; vibration white finger related to use of some tools
Cars (trade or home)	Irritant dermatitis from solvents, paints, hand cleansers
	Contact allergic dermatitis from paints, resins, metals, rubber (gloves, tyres, tubing)
	Chemical leukoderma from rubber chemicals in tyre manufacture
Cooking (work or home)	Irritant dermatitis (detergents/hand washing, juices of meat, fruit and vegetables)
	Contact allergic dermatitis (or urticaria in some cases) from fruits, garlic, spices, meat, fish, gloves
	Physical – cuts, burns
Cleaning (work or home)	Irritant dermatitis from detergents
	Contact allergic dermatitis to fragrances or antimicrobials in detergents, polishes, etc., or to gloves
Health workers	Irritant dermatitis from cleaning agents/hand washing
	Contact allergies – latex allergy (urticaria or dermatitis), medicament allergies (dentists – allergy to balsam flavourings, mercury, resins)
	Contact urticaria and anaphylaxis from latex
	Infections and infestations, e.g. scabies, especially nursing homes
Hairdressers	Irritant dermatitis from shampoos, bleaches, etc.
	Contact allergic dermatitis from perfumes, dyes, bleaches, lanolin, antimicrobials; contact urticaria due to henna
Textiles (work or hobby)	Irritant dermatitis from solvents, bleaches, detergents/hand washing
	Contact allergic dermatitis – dyes, formaldehyde resins (finishes), mordants
Travel	Physical – photodermatoses, prickly heat
	Animals – bites, stings, seabather's eruption, swimmer's eruption, other marine invertebrate hazards
	Infections – cutaneous larva migrans, tungiasis, leishmaniasis, tropical viral exanthems
	Contact allergy – exotic plants, phytophotodermatitis

in determining the likelihood of therapy (particularly topical or phototherapy) being practical or possible.

Specific examples of important social factors include the strong association between cigarette smoking and palmoplantar pustulosis, and the multiple influences of excessive alcohol intake on the severity and therapeutic options in psoriasis.

A sexual history is also required in some instances, particularly where there may be a suspicion that an eruption may be due to a specific sexually transmitted disease such as syphilis or HIV.

It is unlikely that many skin eruptions are due entirely to 'nerves', but psychological factors can clearly be of importance in aggravating or perpetuating symptoms (most notably psoriasis) but may be the primary abnormality in some instances (see Chapter 84).

Quality of life in dermatology patients

The effects of skin problems on lifestyle, relationships, recreational activities, costs to the patient and costs to the community from work days lost are important, and it is helpful to know the patient's main concerns. This applies particularly to chronic skin eruptions. Quality of life tools are readily available, generic (e.g. the Dermatology Life Quality Index (DLQI)), disease specific (e.g. the Assessment of Psychological and Social Effects of Acne, Severity Assessment for Hidradenitis Suppuritiva) and age specific (Children's DLQI), take only minutes for patients to complete, and can give important information that they may not have readily volunteered [1,2,3]. They are valuable adjuncts to disease assessment or severity tools (e.g. the Psoriasis Area Severity Index) in determining aspects of therapy efficacy. Indeed they are required by funding bodies prior to qualification for expensive biological interventions in psoriasis in many countries. However, they may not be exhaustive in their scope (the DLQI does not include sleep disturbance), and can be discriminatory to some groups (e.g. the effects on sport, work and sexual relations may be less relevant to the elderly), but nonetheless, essential data to be collected during history taking.

Examination of the skin

Many patients referred to the dermatologist have objective changes in the appearance or consistency of the skin. Even those who describe itch without rash often have dry skin or other features that can be elicited, such as dermographism. With the availability of camera phones and tablet computers, patients are increasingly able to bring photographs of their lesions or eruptions, which, provided they are of sufficient quality and well illuminated, can be a helpful adjunct to direct examination, particularly when a rash is evanescent. Most lesions and eruptions can either be diagnosed fully, or at least assigned to a diagnostic category, by clinical examination; indeed, clinical diagnosis is more precise than laboratory tests in many disorders. The ability to elicit and interpret cutaneous physical signs is therefore of fundamental importance in dermatological training.

The patient should always be examined in a good light, preferably daylight, and with magnification of lesions if necessary. Artificial light can alter the appreciation of colour, and lesions like lichen planus can have a less easily recognised red hue. A mobile light on an articulated stand can be helpful in illuminating areas that are often in the shade from overhead lights such as the natal cleft, perianal and vulval areas and the mouth.

Ideally, the entire skin should be examined in every patient, particularly if the diagnosis is not initially obvious, as this may reveal lesions that are more easily identifiable and have not been modified by secondary changes. Adolescents and elderly people will often deny the existence of lesions other than those presented for examination, the former because they are unwilling to undress and the latter because they have not seen them.

In the examination of the skin, it is helpful to consider the morphology of individual lesions, their overall pattern and spatial relationship to each other, and their body site distribution. Each of these aspects is discussed more fully below. Specific attention to hair, nails and the mucous membranes is required. Careful description and use of nomenclature aids the monitoring of changes during follow-up, and any discussion with colleagues.

Touching the skin is important in most instances, and is discussed in more detail below. Gloves should be worn for examination of the mouth, genital/perineal region, or in the case of infective or infected dermatoses.

Additional simple aids to clinical examination include use of Wood's light, diascopy, dermoscopy, starch iodine testing to identify sweat duct orifices and hair microscopy.

Description of skin lesions

It is essential to elucidate the following features in describing skin lesions or eruptions as they constitute the features that, with the aid of features of the history, are paramount in the formulation of a diagnosis.

Examination of skin of colour

Examination of pigmented skin requires a degree of practice, as the physical signs may be modified. Erythema is often subtle or is seen as a dark area, macular or diffuse. Dermal oedema lightens the skin and weals appear pale. Papules may be pale or dark according to the degree of oedema or the presence of acanthosis or hyperkeratosis, which mask pigment. Purpura may be difficult to detect, but may appear jet-black in lighter pigmented skin. Post-inflammatory depigmentation and hyperpigmentation are exaggerated compared with paler skin – for example, after herpes zoster, syphilis, leprosy, lichen simplex and many other conditions. Normal pigmentary variation between body sites is also more apparent in darker skin, and may cause confusion (e.g. dark crease lines on the relatively pale palms); pigmentary demarcation lines may also be visible (Futcher and Voigt lines) [1] (See Figure 4.1).

Sites involved and their distribution

Both dermatoses and tumours can show a predilection for affecting certain sites; frequently there is no known explanation for this characteristic. Their distribution may be symmetrical or asymmetrical, or determined by 'special' factors, such as following Blaschko lines, or confined to major or minor flexures.

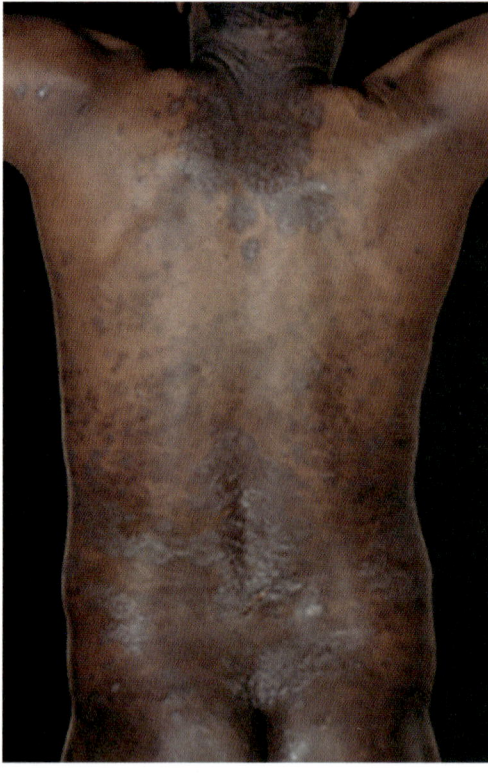

Figure 4.1 The back of a patient with pigmented skin showing variation in clinical features of psoriasis.

Known factors that determine distribution include the following.

Anatomical factors
- Blood supply, e.g. venous eczema, livedo reticularis.
- Skin appendages, e.g. acne, hidradenitis.
- Type of skin, e.g. eruptions may be localised to the glabrous skin of palms and soles.
- Neural, e.g. herpes zoster.
- Developmental or embryological, e.g. disorders which follow lines of Blaschko (see Chapter 8), dermoid cysts.
- Regional variation in the skin surface microenvironment, e.g. erythrasma is usually localised to flexures.
- Others, e.g. polychondritis is restricted to sites where there is cartilage, affecting ears, nose, joints (and extracutaneous areas like trachea).

External factors
- Solar exposure, e.g. photosensitivity disorders, squamous cell carcinoma.
- Chemical exposure, e.g. contact dermatitis.
- Infective, e.g. orf.

Distribution
- Symmetrical distribution – classical psoriasis affects the elbows and knees symmetrically, as does dermatitis herpetiformis. Atopic eczema has a symmetrical predilection for the minor flexures of the antecubital and popliteal fossae. Syringomas are commonly symmetrically distributed on the lower lids.
- Asymmetrical – cutaneous T-cell lymphoma and dermatophyte infection, impetigo and contact dermatitis often have an asymmetrical distribution.

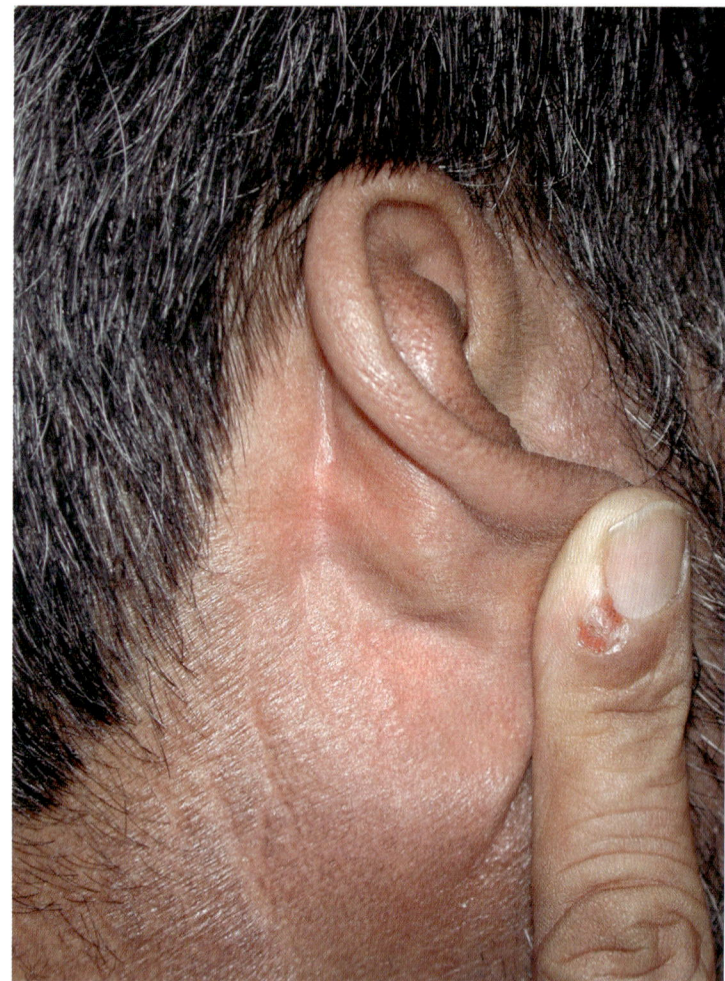

Figure 4.2 Sparing underneath the concha of the ear in chronic actinic dermatitis – sometimes called Wilkinson triangle after the late Dr D. S. Wilkinson, one of the first editors of *Rook's Textbook of Dermatology*.

- Flexural – flexural psoriasis and benign familial pemphigus characteristically affect the major flexural sites of the axillae and groins.
- Photo-distributed – dermatoses caused by light such as chronic actinic dermatitis affect the face, bald scalp, 'V' area of the chest and the backs of the hands with a cut-off at the point where sleeves cover the skin. Light-spared sites within this area include the upper lids, immediately behind and below the ears (Wilkinson triangle), under the chin, in the finger webs and below watch straps (Figures 4.2 and 4.3).
- Airborne distribution – this includes the face and hands, similar to photo distribution but the light-shaded sites of the upper lid, Wilkinson triangle and finger webs are affected, as airborne allergens can reach these sites. Allergens include plants, epoxy resins, phosphorus sesquisulfide (the red tip match allergen) and wood dusts.

Pattern and arrangement
The arrangement of individual lesions may create a characteristic pattern (Figure 4.4), such as the grouping of vesicles in herpes simplex – this pattern is so striking that it is applied to other lesions which do not share the same aetiology (e.g. herpetiform mouth ulcers, dermatitis herpetiformis).

Description of skin lesions 4.7

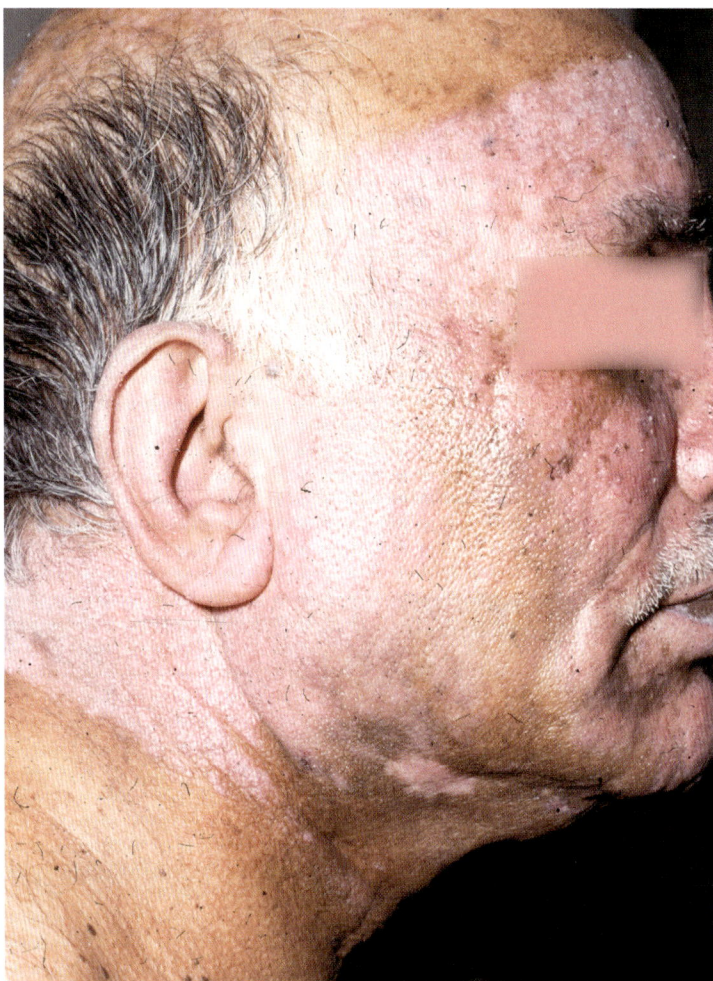

Figure 4.3 Sparing of the head and neck by garments in quinine-induced photo-lichenoid eruption.

skin disease such as psoriasis, atopic or seborrhoeic eczema, drug induced, congenital (such as in the ichthyosiform erythrodermas), due to T-cell lymphoma of the skin or idiopathic.

Linear, sporotrichoid, annular, arcuate, polycyclic, livedoid and discoid lesions

The shape of each lesion and the pattern in which neighbouring lesions are arranged in relation to each other is often of great significance and may provide an easily recognisable clue to a rapid visual diagnosis (Figures 4.5–4.9 and 4.10). The main shapes, with examples, are listed in Table 4.2. The mechanism or anatomical factor dictating the shape can sometimes be inferred, as in the case of many linear lesions (see Table 4.2) or the vascular patterning leading to livedo (Figure 4.9); in other instances, such as many annular lesions (Box 4.2) and reticulate lesions, the explanation for the pattern is less clear.

Box 4.2 Examples of lesions that are characteristically annular or often include annular morphology

Infections
- 'Ringworm' dermatophyte infections
- Impetigo
- Erythema chronicum migrans
- Syphilis (secondary, tertiary)
- Leprosy

Inflammatory
- Psoriasis
- Seborrhoeic dermatitis
- Atopic eczema (some)
- Halo eczema (Meyerson phenomenon)
- Subacute cutaneous lupus erythematosus
- Lichen planus
- Sarcoidosis
- Granuloma annulare
- Actinic granuloma
- Erythema multiforme
- Urticaria
- Serum sickness and serum sickness-like eruption
- Linear immunoglobulin A (IgA) disease/chronic bullous dermatosis of childhood
- Bullous pemphigoid
- Subcorneal pustular dermatosis
- Erythema annulare centrifugum
- Jessner lymphocytic infiltrate
- Erythema marginatum rheumaticum
- Pityriasis rosea (herald patch)

Vascular
- Purpura annularis telangiectoides

Neoplastic
- Superficial basal cell carcinoma
- Mycosis fungoides
- Other cutaneous lymphomas

Keratinisation disorders
- Porokeratosis

Useful terminology to describe patterns includes the following.
- *Agminate* – clustered; used to describe lesions such as acne agminata, where granulomatous lesions cluster around the lids, or agminate naevi, an unusual clustering of melanocytic naevi.
- *Grouped or clustered* – characteristic of some infections (e.g. herpetic vesicles, molluscum contagiosum, plane warts), flea bites, as well as of endogenous lesions such as lichen planus, leiomyomas, lymphangioma circumscriptum.
- *Satellite* – a cluster of lesions around a larger central lesion. May occur due to local lymphatic spread of neoplasm such as melanoma; may occur in chronic bullous disease of childhood/linear IgA disease.
- *Confluent* – lesions merging together, locally or widespread, e.g. pityriasis versicolor.
- *Scattered, disseminated and exanthematous* – for example, many drug eruptions, viral exanthems, as well as some extrinsic causes.
- *Spared* – patterns of sparing may also be diagnostically important, e.g. islands of sparing occur within the otherwise often confluent orange–red colour of pityriasis rubra pilaris, sparing within skin folds in papuloerythroderma of Ofuji, or areas shielded by clothing or a wristwatch may be overtly spared in photosensitivity.
- *Erythroderma* – this is defined as generalised redness often with scaling, affecting 90% of the skin surface. It may be a primary

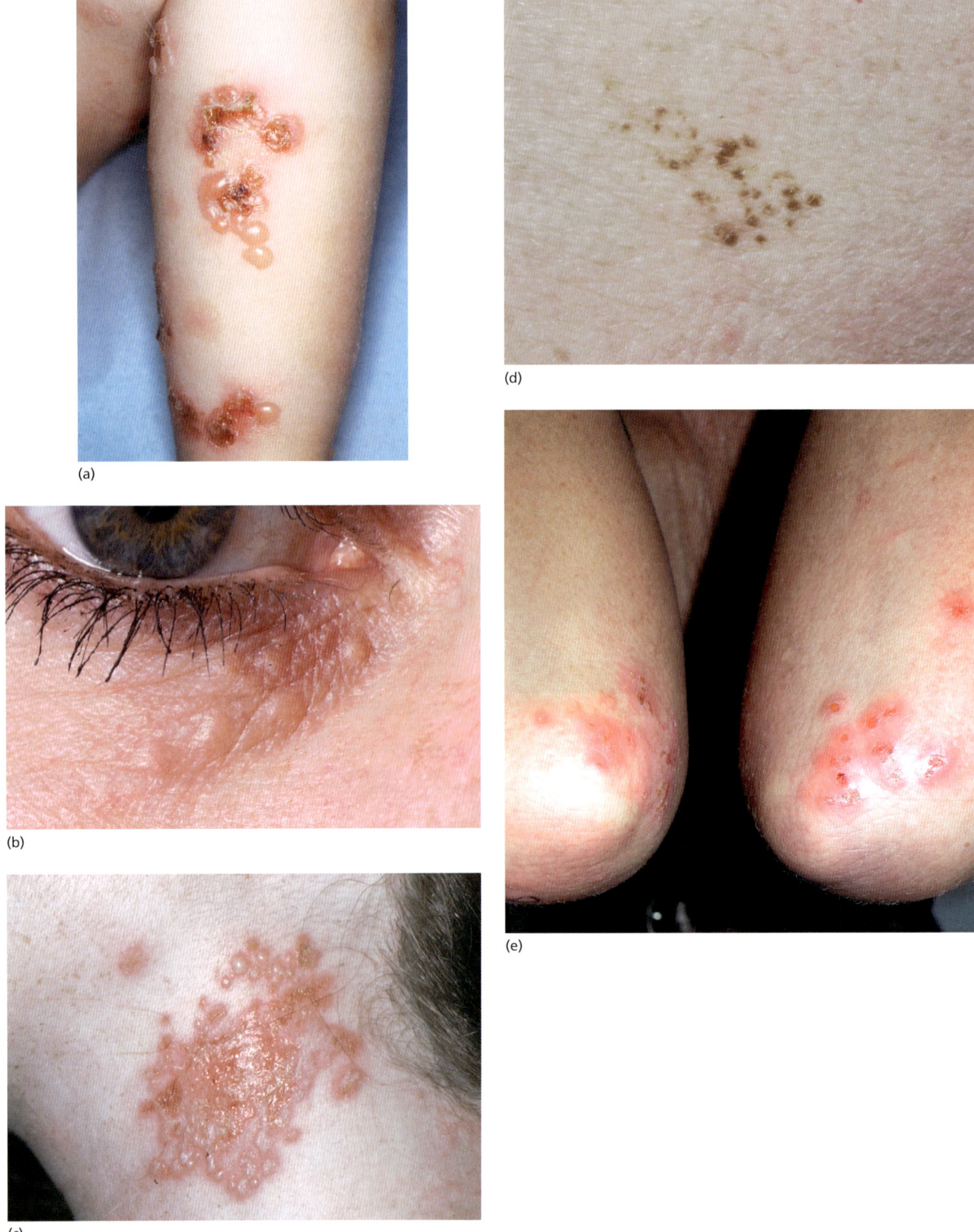

Figure 4.4 Characteristic grouping of lesions: (a) blisters in a ring like a 'string of pearls' in linear immunoglobulin A (IgA) bullous dermatosis; (b) grouped papules on the lower lid in syringomas; (c) grouped vesicopustules in herpes simplex on the neck; (d) pigmented papules in naevus spilus; (e) clustered lesions on the elbows in dermatitis herpetiformis.

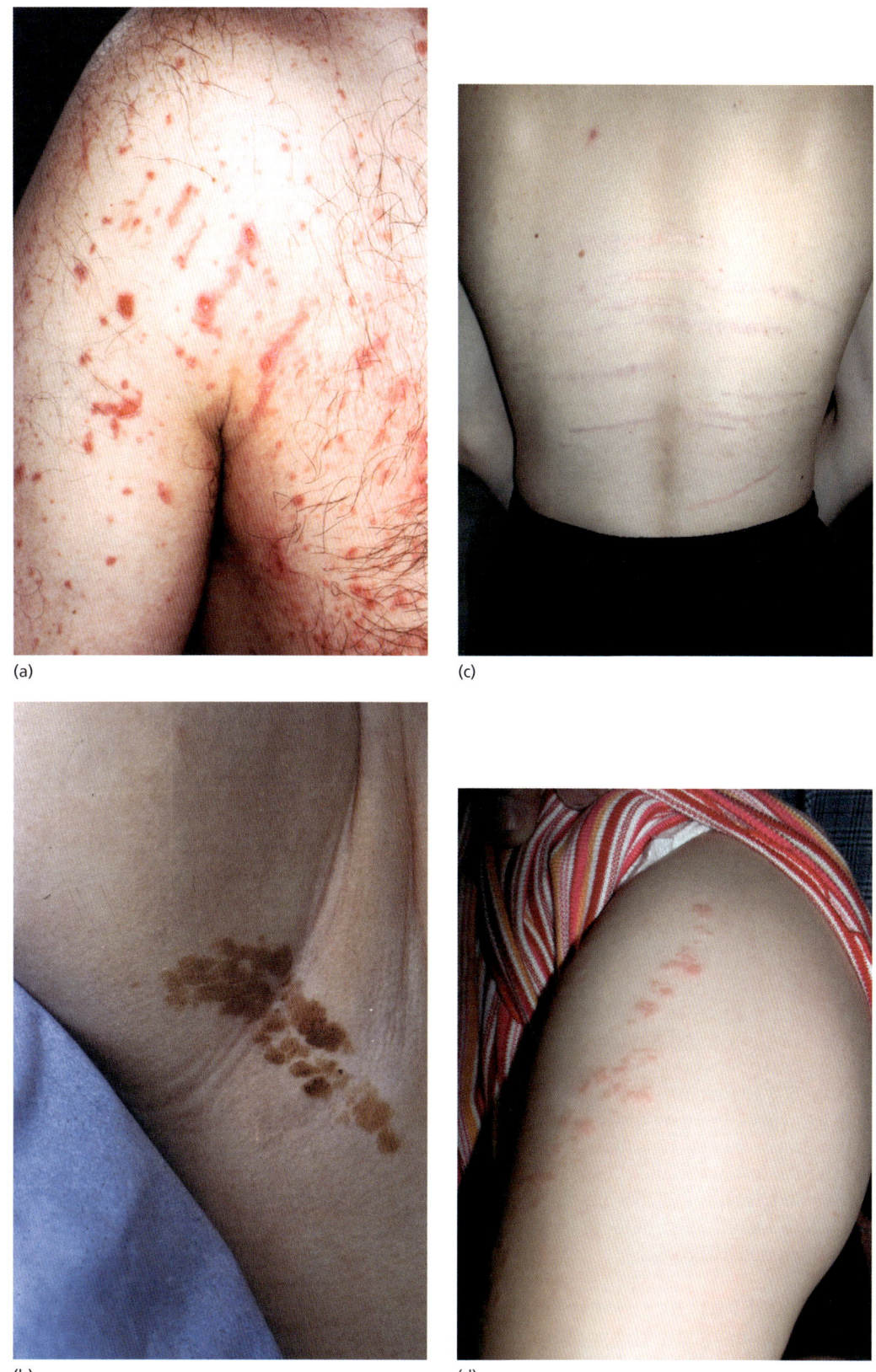

Figure 4.5 Examples of linear lesions: (a) 'strimmer' phytophotodermatosis; (b) linear epidermal naevus; (c) growth striae; and (d) lichen striatus.

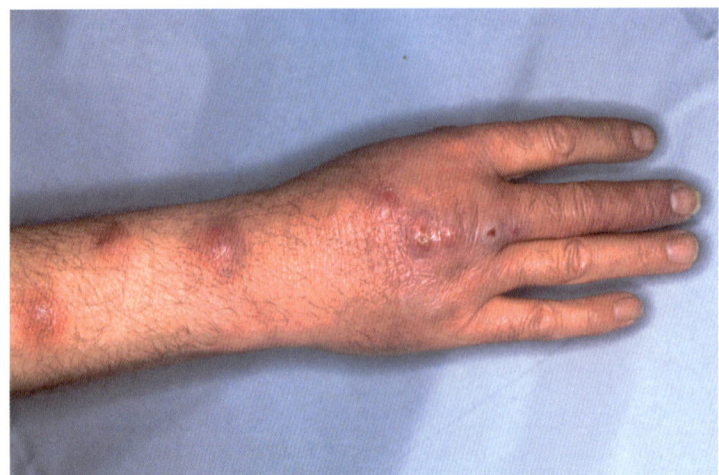

Figure 4.6 Grouping in a linear distribution ascending the distal limb – so-called sporotrichoid distribution of a *Mycobacterium marinum* infection.

A specific cause of a linear lesion is the Koebner or isomorphic phenomenon [2]. This term is applied when localised non-specific trauma provokes lesions of a dermatosis which is usually spontaneously present elsewhere, and usually in a relatively 'active' or eruptive phase. It is particularly characteristic of psoriasis (see Chapter 35) and lichen planus, but occurs in several other dermatoses (Table 4.3). The trauma may be mild, and is usually a scratch or similar, although light or heat may do the same. Occasionally, one disease may be responsible for the localisation of another, such as granuloma annulare developing at sites of herpes zoster, or psoriasis developing at sites of contact dermatitis; this has been termed the isotopic response [3]. Development of lesions of pyoderma gangrenosum or Behçet disease at sites of injection of serum or saline (or even just pinprick or venepuncture) is known as pathergy.

Some annular shapes result from centrifugal extension of an infection from the point of inoculation (e.g. tinea corporis with dermatophyte fungi or erythema chronicum migrans in *Borrelia burgdorferi* infection). In others, a spreading neoplastic or inflammatory process leaves central scarring or ulceration, for example superficial basal cell carcinoma and discoid lupus erythematosus. In eruptions in which an allergic process is probably involved, the annular configuration is attributed to the refractory state of the central area. In some conditions, annular shapes can be related to the vascular network. Some involve an iatrogenic component, for example warts recurring at the margin of a blistered cryotherapy site. However, in many diseases, such as lichen planus, sarcoidosis or psoriasis, there is no satisfactory explanation for the occurrence of annular lesions. In the clinical evaluation of annular lesions, it is particularly helpful to consider surface features such as scaling as an aid to identifying epidermal involvement and thus narrowing the differential diagnosis.

Individual lesions – nomenclature

The more common descriptive terms applying to cutaneous lesions are listed below. These definitions are broadly in agreement with those recommended by the Nomenclature Committee of the International League of Dermatological Societies [2]. However, it is important to note that some of these definitions have been

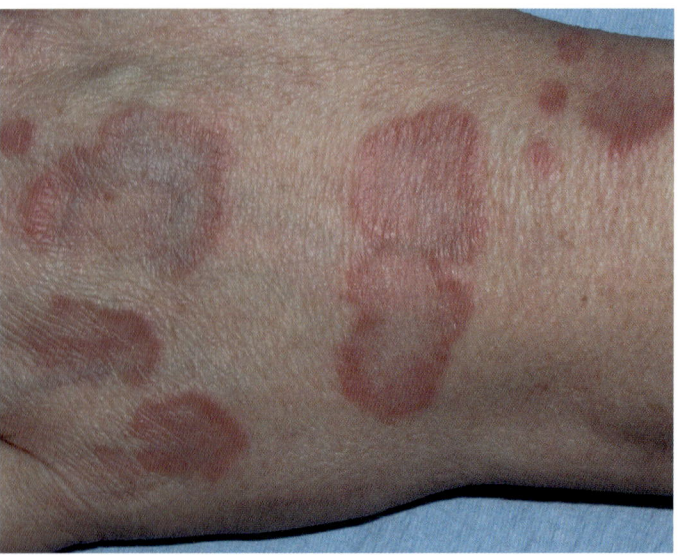

(a)

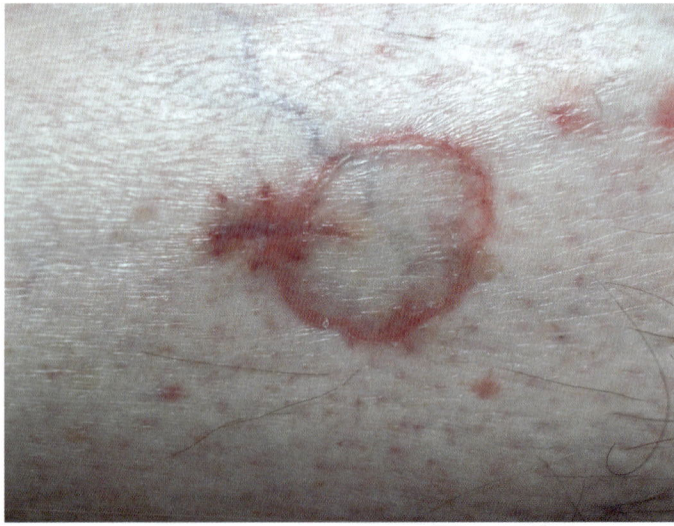

(b)

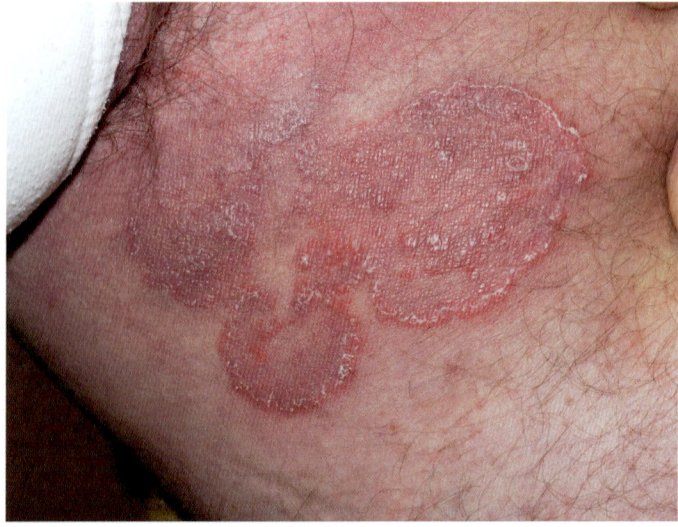

(c)

Figure 4.7 Examples of annular lesions: (a) granuloma annulare; (b) porokeratosis; and (c) tinea corporis.

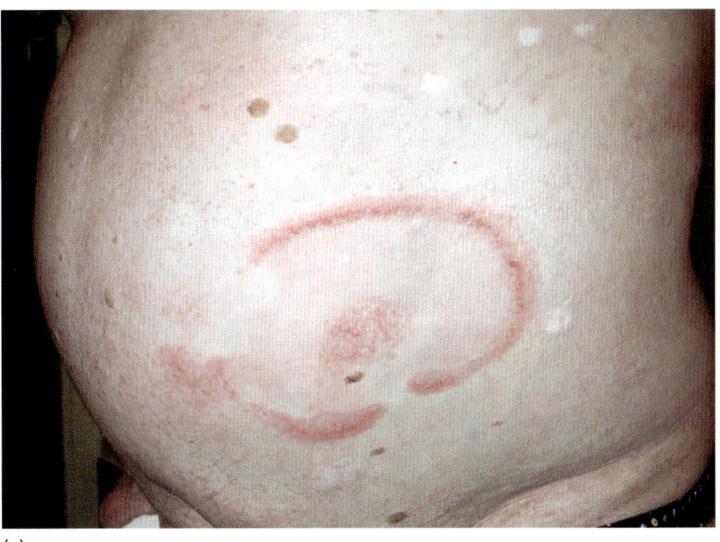

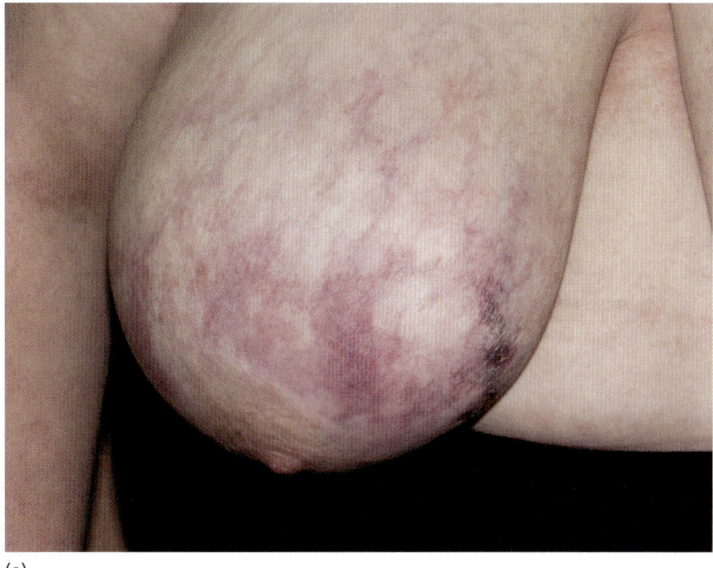

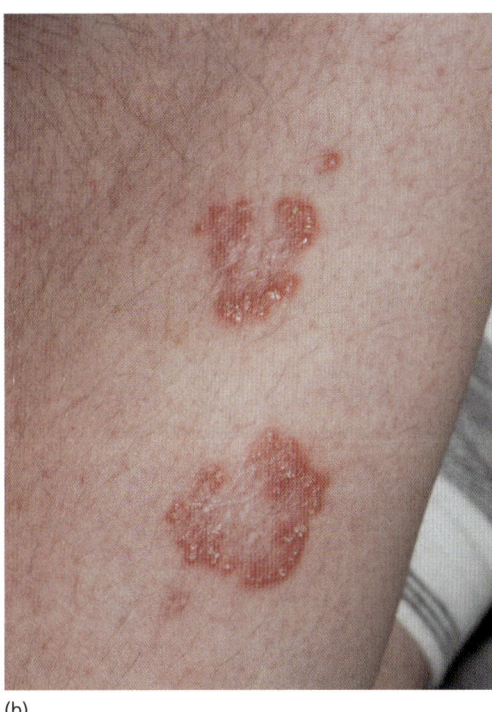

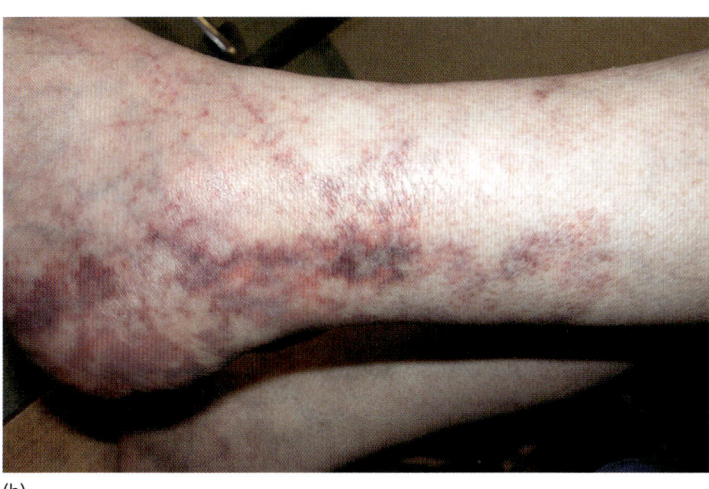

Figure 4.8 Examples of arcuate and polycyclic lesions: (a) erythema annulare centrifugum; (b) elastosis perforans serpiginosum – note the abnormal elastic tissue that is undergoing transepidermal elimination.

Figure 4.9 Livedoid lesions: (a) diffuse dermal angiomatosis of the breast; (b) broken livedo reticularis in cutaneous polyarteritis nodosum.

challenged subsequently [3–7]. A particular problem that many authors have glossed over is the dynamic aspects of skin disease. For example, some papules (<0.5 or 1 cm, depending on the source of the definition) are destined to grow larger and become nodules, whereas others (such as syringomas) rarely do so. Additionally, some eruptions may have essentially similar lesions but whose size may include both papules and nodules. Recording of actual size of lesions, or the range of sizes, is often a more useful clinical record.

Glossary

Alopecia	Absence of hair from a normally hairy area.
Aphtha	A small ulcer of the mucosa.
Atrophy	A loss of tissue from one or more of the epidermis, dermis or subcutaneous tissues. There may be fine wrinkling and increased translucency if the process is superficial.
Burrow	A small tunnel in the skin that houses a parasite, such as the scabies acarus.
Callus	A localised hyperplasia of the stratum corneum.
Cellulitis	An inflammation of cellular tissue, particularly purulent inflammation of the deep dermis and subcutaneous tissue.
Comedo (pl. comedones)	A plug of keratin and sebum in a dilated pilosebaceous orifice.
Crusts (scabs)	Crusts consist of dried serum and other exudates.
Cyst	Any closed cavity or sac (normal or abnormal) with an epithelial, endothelial or membranous lining and containing fluid or semi-solid material.
Ecchymosis (bruise)	A macular area of haemorrhage more than 2 mm in diameter.

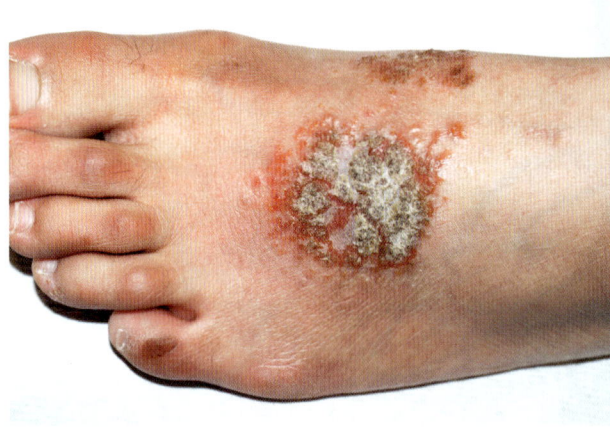

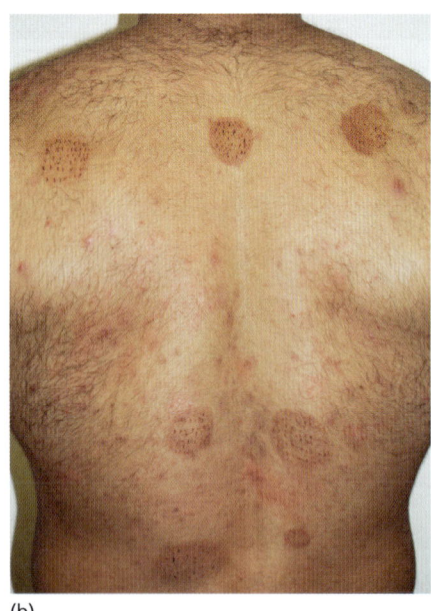

Figure 4.10 Discoid lesions: (a) discoid eczema; (b) discoid hyperpigmentation and unusual haemorrhagic lesions due to the practice of cupping.

Table 4.2 Main shapes of skin lesions.

Shape	Description	Examples
Discoid (nummular)	A filled circle	Discoid eczema, psoriasis
Petaloid	Discoid lesions which have merged together	Seborrhoeic dermatitis on the trunk
Arcuate	Incomplete circles	Urticaria
Annular	Open circles with different central skin compared with the rim	Tinea corporis, granuloma annulare
Polycyclic	Circles which have merged together	Psoriasis
Livedo	Chicken-wire criss-cross pattern	Erythema ab igne, polyarteritis nodosa, microvascular occlusion disorders
Reticulate	Fine lace-like pattern	Oral lichen planus
Target	Multiple concentric rings	Erythema multiforme
Stellate	Star-shaped	Lesions of meningococcal septicaemia
Digitate	Finger-shaped	Chronic superficial dermatosis
Linear	Straight line	Koebner reaction to a scratch in lichen planus or psoriasis
Serpiginous	Snake-like	Cutaneous larva migrans
Whorled	Swirling pattern	Epidermal naevi, late-stage incontinentia pigmenti

Adapted from Lawrence and Cox 2000 [7]. Reproduced with permission from Elsevier.

En cocarde (or 'cockade')	A rosette pattern of concentric rings, usually applied to naevi.
Erosion	A loss of epidermis, which heals without scarring. It commonly follows a blister.
Erythema	Redness of the skin produced by vascular congestion or increased perfusion.
Excoriation	Loss of skin substance, specifically produced by scratching.
Exfoliation	The splitting off of the epidermal keratin in scales or sheets.
Fibrosis	The formation of excessive fibrous tissue.
Fissure	Any linear gap or slit in the skin surface.
Fistula	An abnormal passage from a deep structure, such as a hollow viscus, to the skin surface or between two structures. It is often lined with squamous epithelium.
Gangrene	Death of tissue, usually due to loss of blood supply.
Guttate lesions	Small round or oval lesions distributed as a 'shower' of droplets. Usually applied to a form of psoriasis.
Haematoma	A localised tumour-like collection of blood.
Keratoderma	A horny thickening of the skin.
Lichenification	Thickening of the epidermis (and to some extent also of the dermis) in response to prolonged rubbing.
Macule	A flat circumscribed non-palpable lesion that differs in colour from the surrounding skin. It can be of any colour or shape. In North America, a macule is less than 1 cm in diameter, larger lesions are a patch.
Maculopapular	Rash consisting of both macules and papules.
Milium	A tiny white cyst containing lamellated keratin.
Nodule	A solid palpable lesion in the dermis or subcutis, which can be observed as an elevation or can be palpated. It is more than 0.5 cm in diameter; some would define it as being greater than 1 cm. It may consist of fluid, other extracellular material (e.g. amyloid), inflammatory or neoplastic cells.
Papilloma	A nipple-like mass projecting from the surface of the skin.
Papule	An elevated solid lesion that is less than 1 cm in diameter. The only distinction between a papule and a nodule is the size, and this is artificial; some lesions characteristically occur at the smaller size of a papule, whereas others typically enlarge from a papule to become a nodule. Recording a finite size, its topography, border and colour is useful.

Table 4.3 Anatomical and causative factors in linear lesions.

Determinant of pattern	Examples
Blood vessels	Thrombophlebitis, Mondor disease (linear thrombophlebitis on the trunk)
	Eczema related to varicose veins
	Temporal arteritis
Lymphatics	Lymphangitis
	Sporotrichosis, fish tank granulomas
Dermatome	Herpes zoster, zosteriform naevus, zosteriform Darier disease, zosteriform metastases
Nerve trunks	Leprosy (thickened cutaneous nerves)
Developmental, Blaschko lines	Pigmentary demarcation line, linea nigra
	Epidermal naevi, incontinentia pigmenti, hypomelanosis of Ito
	Linear psoriasis, linear lichen planus, lichen striatus
Skin stretching	Striae due to growth spurt (on lower back)
Infestation	Scabies, larva migrans (both usually serpiginous)
External factors	
Plants	Phytophotodermatitis
Allergens	Elastoplast, nail varnish (neck), necklace, waistbands, etc.
Chemical	Caustics, e.g. phenol
Thermal	Burns
Physical	*Trauma to previously normal skin*
	Keloid scar, bruising, dermatitis artefacta, amniotic constriction bands
	Trauma to skin with a pre-existing dermatosis
	Purpura (cryoglobulinaemia, amyloid, vasculitis)
	Blisters (epidermolysis bullosa, porphyrias)
	Koebner phenomenon
	Psoriasis, lichen planus, lichen nitidus, vitiligo, lichen sclerosus, pityriasis rubra pilaris
	Inoculation
	Warts, molluscum contagiosum
	Other mechanism
	Scar sarcoid
Other determinants	Linear scleroderma (limb, central forehead)
	Senear–Caro ridge (on hands in psoriasis)
	Dermatomyositis (dorsum of fingers; Gottron sign)
	Interstitial granulomatous dermatitis (rope or cord sign)
	Flagellate pigmentation due to cytotoxic drugs (e.g. bleomycin)

Adapted from Lawrence and Cox 2002 [7]. Reproduced with permission from Elsevier.

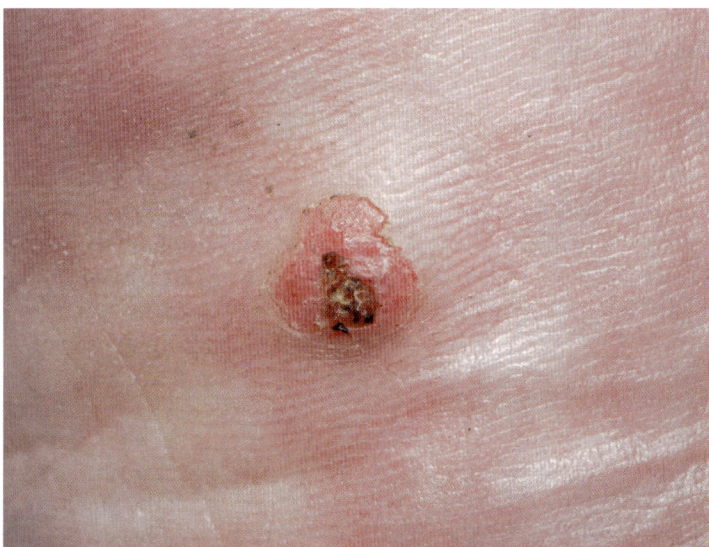

Figure 4.11 A collarette scale surrounding an eccrine poroma.

Petechia (pl. petechiae) — A punctate haemorrhagic spot, approximately 1–2 mm in diameter.

Plaque — An elevated circumscribed lesion greater than 1 cm diameter; its surface is usually flat. Plaques may form from coalesced papules.

Poikiloderma — The association of cutaneous pigmentation, atrophy and telangiectasia.

Pustule — A circumscribed lesion that contains purulent material. It may occur within a pilosebaceous follicle or a sweat duct or, less often, on glabrous skin. Most commonly due to infections, but some eruptions typically cause sterile pustules.

Pyoderma — Any purulent skin disease.

Scale — A flat plate or flake of stratum corneum. A *collarette* scale is a fine, peripherally attached and centrally detached scale at the edge of an inflammatory lesion (Figure 4.11). Annular scaling is also seen in porokeratosis. *Furfuraceous or pityriasiform* scales are fine and loose. *Ichthyotic* scales are large and polygonal. Scaling may accompany or follow many inflammatory disorders. Silvery scales are characteristic of processes involving parakeratosis, especially psoriasis. The silvery colour is due to reflection of light at the many air–keratin interfaces and can be altered by wetting the skin.

Scar — Replacement by fibrous tissue of another tissue that has been destroyed by injury or disease. An *atrophic* scar is thin and wrinkled. A *hypertrophic* scar is elevated, with excessive growth of fibrous tissue. A *cribriform* scar is perforated with multiple small pits.

Sclerosis — Diffuse or circumscribed induration of the subcutaneous tissues. It may also involve the dermis, when the overlying epidermis may be atrophic. It is characteristically seen in scleroderma, but may occur as a sequel to or in association with many different processes.

Sinus — A cavity or track with a blind ending.

Target lesions — These are less than 3 cm in diameter and have three or more zones, usually a central area of dusky redness or purpura, a middle paler zone of oedema, and an outer ring of redness with a well-defined edge.

Tumour — Literally a swelling. The term is used to imply enlargement of the tissues by normal or pathological material, or cells that form a mass. It may be inflammatory or non-inflammatory, benign or malignant. The term should be used with care, as many patients believe it implies a malignancy with a poor prognosis.

Ulcer (of skin) — A loss of dermis and epidermis, often with loss of the underlying tissues.

Vegetation — A growth of pathological tissue consisting of multiple closely set papillary masses.

Vesicles and bullae	A vesicle is a circumscribed elevation less than 1 cm in diameter that contains fluid (clear, serous or haemorrhagic) and often grouped. Bullae are more than 1 cm in diameter, and should be subdivided as multilocular (due to coalesced vesicles, typically in eczema) or unilocular.
Weal	A transient elevation of the skin due to dermal and hypodermal oedema, often pale centrally with a red rim. It is the characteristic lesion of urticaria.

Erythema

Erythema is defined as redness that blanches on pressure, due to dilated capillaries. Pressure empties the capillaries, making the lesion or eruption temporarily paler. It should be distinguished from purpura, which does not fade with pressure, and telangiectasia where the redness is due to visible dilated blood vessels.

Surface features

Lesions or rashes may be smooth, uneven (due to scale), or rough (often appreciated by touch as well as inspection), due to the presence of crusts or keratin. Where crusting is present, its gentle removal may reveal important diagnostic features (such as telangiectasia in a basal cell carcinoma, or pigment in an ulcerated malignant melanoma).

Colour

Normal skin colour is due to melanin, phaeomelanin, haemoglobin, oxyhaemoglobin and carotenoids (Figure 4.12). The colour of the skin is greatly modified by the scatter of light, which is responsible, for example, for the whiteness of scale and the blueness of any melanin deep in the dermis, although colour contrast with surrounding skin also alters perception of the colour of skin and subcutaneous structures [8].

The range of colours that may be seen in individual skin lesions is enormous (Table 4.4). Although many red, scaly rashes tend to resemble each other, many dermatoses have their own distinctive colour, which aids recognition – for example, the orange and yellow-orange palms of pityriasis rubra pilaris and carotenaemia, respectively. Some colours can be logically explained – for example, the purple of lichen planus is due to the redness of inflammation combined with the blue-brown of melanin within the dermis.

Unusual colours can occur due to the effect of drug accumulation in the skin (such as with minocycline and hydroxychloroquine), and adherence of exogenous pigments to the skin.

Border

Tumours or inflammatory lesions may show clearly defined well-circumscribed borders. Such lesions can confidently be drawn around with a clear distinction between affected and non-affected skin. Bowen disease and superficial basal cell carcinomas have distinct edges, as does psoriasis. Poorly defined lesions have borders that merge indistinctly into normal skin (such as eczema). Some lesions have active edges, with both increased erythema and scale at the periphery, and relative central clearing, such as dermatophyte infections.

Shape

Lesion shape can be a vital diagnostic sign. Round and oval lesions are frequently a feature of benignity. Irregularity can be an indicator of malignancy (e.g. superficial spreading malignant melanoma, Bowen disease). Vascular patterning may indicate and explain the morphology of livedo reticularis.

Linear lesions may occur for inexplicable reasons (such as lichen striatus), but they may be the result of the Koebner phenomenon, when often minor physical, thermal and surgical trauma may provoke the onset of new lesions at the sites of these assaults. Koebner lesions tend to occur during active phases of inflammatory disorders, and are seen characteristically in psoriasis, lichen planus and vitiligo. Some conditions have a predilection for arising in scars (such as scar sarcoidosis and scar pigmentation with drugs, notably minocycline), and therefore may have a linear distribution. Lesions of pyoderma gangrenosum and Behçet disease may arise in areas of recent physical skin trauma in a phenomenon known as pathergy.

Annular lesions may result from centrifugal extension of an infection (as in tinea corporis with dermatophyte infection or erythema chronicum migrans with *Borrelia burgdorferi*). In neoplastic conditions such as basal cell carcinoma, central regression can result in annular lesions. Annular lesions in discoid lupus erythematosus are the result of scarring occurring within the centre of a lesion, and progression peripherally. Annular warts can occur with viral warts overenthusiastically treated with cryotherapy, and warts seeding into the cryotherapy-induced peripheral blisters. In many instances, why some lesions are characteristically (e.g. subacute lupus erythematosus and granuloma annulare) or occasionally annular (e.g. sarcoid and psoriasis) is unexplained. Concentric circles of erythema give a bull's eye or target-like appearance to the lesions of erythema multiforme (Figure 4.13). Irregular sigmoid lesions give an appearance like that of a snake (or serpiginous), as in cutaneous larva migrans (Figure 4.14). A net-like morphology (reticulate; Figure 4.15) is characteristic of some dermatoses (buccal lichen planus, confluent and reticulate papillomatosis). Finger-like elongated lesions may be appreciated in digitate dermatosis (Figure 4.16).

Distribution of lesions

The overall distribution of lesions in many common dermatoses may be so characteristic that it is of great assistance in clinical diagnosis, even though the mechanism in most instances is not understood. Examples of body site predilection of dermatoses are provided in Table 4.5. Some of these are explained by anatomy, sites of contact, and so on, but even some demarcations that presumably have an anatomical basis are not fully understood, for example Wallace line on the foot or the equivalent on the hand. Some, for example those at flexural sites (Table 4.6), are often modified in appearance by moist occlusion. Important factors in determining the distribution of dermatoses include the following.

Anatomical factors

- Blood supply, e.g. venous eczema.
- Skin appendages, e.g. acne, hidradenitis.
- Type of skin, e.g. eruptions may be localised to the glabrous skin of palms and soles.

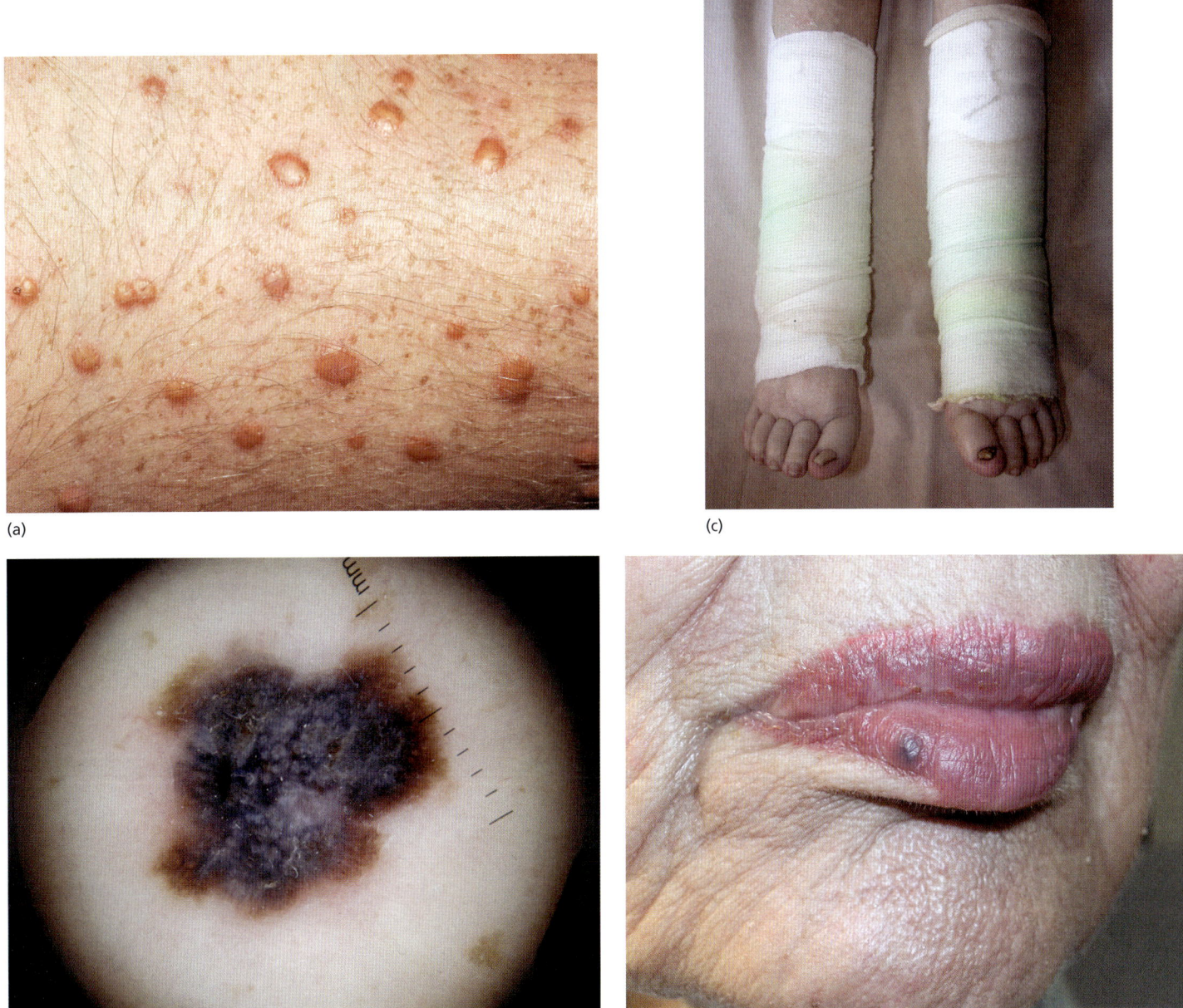

Figure 4.12 Colour and its variability can be diagnostically invaluable: (a) the yellow colour of xanthomas; (b) black, blue, grey and white in a malignant melanoma; (c) green discoloration of dressings with *Pseudomonas* colonisation of a wound; and (d) blue-purple colour of a venous lake on the lip.

- Neural, e.g. herpes zoster.
- Developmental, e.g. disorders which follow the lines of Blaschko.
- Regional variation in the skin surface microenvironment, e.g. erythrasma is usually localised to flexures.
- Others, e.g. polychondritis, is restricted to sites where there is cartilage, affecting ears, nose, joints (and trachea).

External factors
- Solar exposure, e.g. photosensitivity disorders, squamous cell carcinoma.
- Chemical exposure, e.g. contact dermatitis.
- Infective, e.g. orf.

Dermatomal distribution
Some eruptions can arise in a distribution that follows the distribution of the sensory neurological dermatomes. This can occur as an example of an isomorphic response for example pyoderma gangrenosum arising in lesions initially shingles, or for less apparent reasons such as zosteriform lichen planus.

Blaschkoid distribution
Blaschko recognised in the 1900s that some naevoid (e.g. hypomelanosis of Ito, incontinentia pigmenti and the atrophoderma of Conradi–Hunnerman disease) and inflammatory conditions (such as lichen planus) followed a series of lines that did not conform to

Table 4.4 Colours of skin lesions.

Colour	Examples
Black	Melanin, e.g. some naevi, melanoma
	Exogenous pigments, e.g. tattoos, pencil/ink
	Exogenous chemicals, e.g. silver nitrate, gold salts
	Deeply situated blood or melanin, e.g. angiomas, blue naevus
Blue-grey	Inflammatory diseases, e.g. orf
	Drug-induced pigmentation, e.g. phenothiazines, minocycline
Dark brown	Melanin near the skin surface, e.g. most melanocytic naevi
	Exogenous pigments, e.g. dithranol (anthralin) staining
Pale brown	Melanin near the skin surface, e.g. lentigo, freckles
Muddy brown	Melanin in the superficial dermis, e.g. post-inflammatory pigmentation
Purple	Vascular lesions, e.g. angiomas
	Other disorders where telangiectasia is a prominent feature, e.g. lupus pernio (chronic sarcoidosis), dermatomyositis
Dusky blue	Reduced amounts of oxygenated haemoglobin, e.g. poor arterial supply, central causes of cyanosis, methaemoglobinaemia
Violaceous and lilac	Lichen planus, edge of plaques of morphoea, connective tissue disorders, e.g. dermatomyositis
Pink-red	Many exanthems and common disorders, such as psoriasis
Red-brown	Inflammatory dermatoses, e.g. seborrhoeic eczema, secondary syphilis
	Haemosiderin, e.g. pigmented purpuric dermatoses
Scarlet red	Lesions with a strong arterial supply, e.g. pyogenic granuloma, spider naevus
	Altered haemoglobin, e.g. carbon monoxide poisoning
Orange	Haemosiderin, e.g. lichen aureus
	Inflammatory disorders, e.g. pityriasis rubra pilaris
Yellow-white/ yellow-pink	Xanthomatous disorders
Yellow-orange	Carotenaemia (ingested carotene, myxoedema)
Yellow-green	Jaundice
Green	Exogenous pigment, e.g. copper salts
White-ivory	Lichen sclerosus et atrophicus, morphoea
White (or pale pink, depending on vascularity)	Vitiligo, naevus anaemicus, arterial insufficiency, chemical depigmentation on vascularity

Adapted from Lawrence and Cox 2002 [7]. Reproduced with permission from Elsevier.

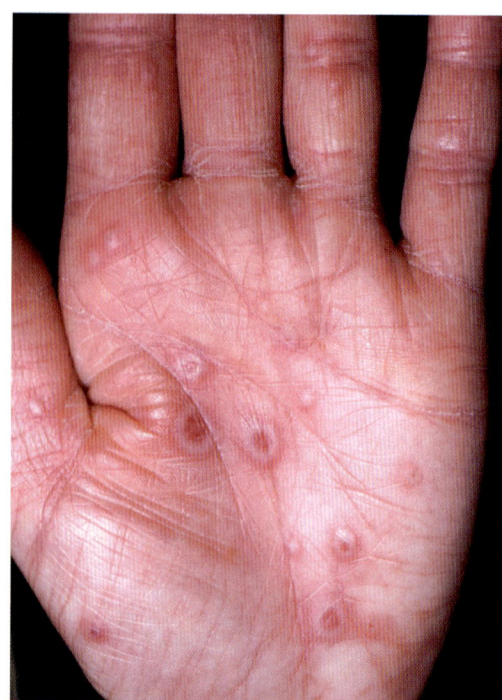

Figure 4.13 Target lesions in erythema multiforme.

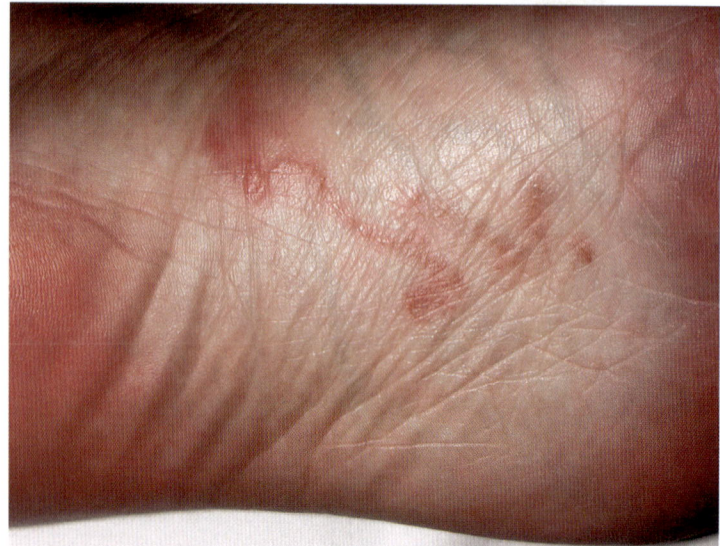

Figure 4.14 Serpiginous lesions on the foot in cutaneous larva migrans.

the distribution of any recognisable structure, such as a nerve, blood vessel or lymphatic (Figure 4.17). Most are regarded as a manifestation of a condition that is demonstrating genetic mosaicism.

Palpation of the skin

Palpation of rashes or localised lesions imparts additional information about texture, consistency, thickness, tenderness and temperature (Figure 4.18) [9]. It has been shown, using a trained 'blinded' observer, that the scaling of psoriasis and eczema can be distinguished by palpation alone [10]. Gentle scratching or rubbing alters the visibility of scaling and may elicit dermographism. The main 'touch' modalities in examining the skin are as follows.

- *Simple palpation* – to determine texture, etc., as above.
- *Blunt pressure* – e.g. to detect oedema, assess capillary refill, identify the dermal defect that occurs in anetoderma.
- *Linear or shearing pressure* – to elicit dermographism, or Nikolsky sign in pemphigus.
- *Squeezing or pinching* – to determine localisation and consistency of lesions, e.g. a pinch of skin can be lifted up over a subcutaneous nodule, whereas squeezing a tethered intradermal process such as a dermatofibroma produces dimpling.
- *Stretching* – may produce blanching of vascular lesions, and helps in visualising lesions such as 'submarine' comedones, the elastomas of Buschke–Ollendorf syndrome and the glassy edge of a superficial basal cell carcinoma.
- *Rubbing* – may cause release of chemicals, e.g. rubbing a mastocytoma causes urtication and a flare due to histamine release (Darier sign), rubbing a neuroblastoma causes surrounding pallor due to catecholamine release.
- *Scratching and picking* – scratching scales in psoriasis makes the scale appear more silver in colour by introducing air–keratin interfaces; more vigorous scratching or picking off the scale

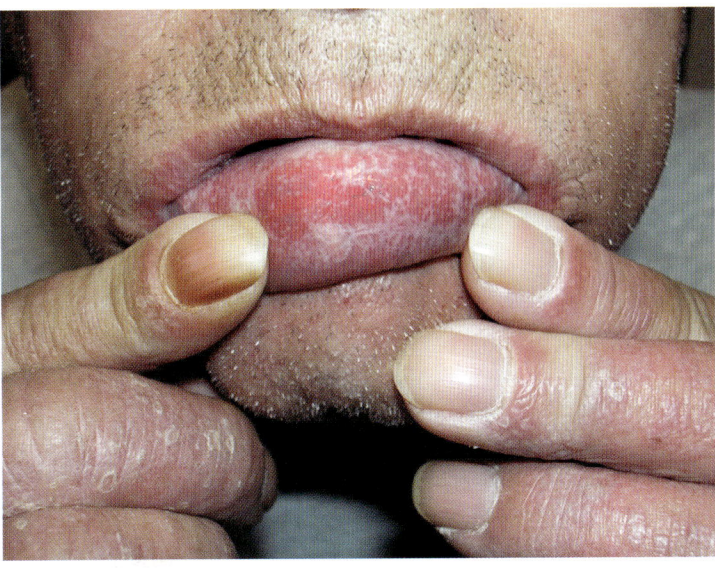

(a)

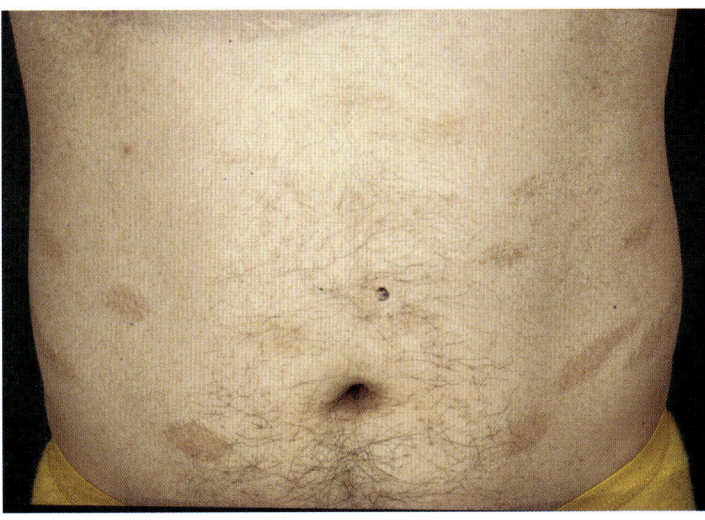

Figure 4.16 Digitate lesions in chronic superficial scaly dermatosis.

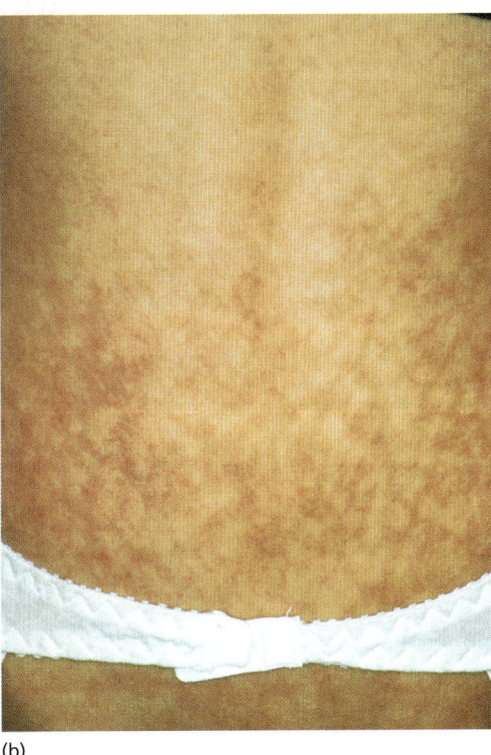

(b)

Figure 4.15 Reticulate lesions: (a) reticulate lichen planus on the lower lip – note also florid lichen planus on the fingers; and (b) erythema ab igne from resting against a radiator.

produces small bleeding points (Auspitz sign). Neither of these is specific to psoriasis. Removal of crusts overlying nodules may demonstrate the extent of the lesion, and additional diagnostic features, more accurately.

Additional simple clinical examination

- *Wetting the skin* with water or mineral oil (which lasts longer) fills air spaces in scale and allows underlying features to become more visible. In some instances, this just enhances underlying redness, for example, in psoriasis. In other instances, diagnostic features may become apparent to the naked eye (such as Wickham striae in lichen planus) or with the aid of additional magnification (e.g. use of a dermoscope to examine pigmented lesions). Soaking of the skin may make the lesions of pitted keratolysis more apparent.
- *Application of heat or cold* may identify specific physical urticarias. Whole-body warming may confirm cholinergic urticaria. Even whole-body cooling has been used to identify dysarthria as being due to Raynaud phenomenon of the tongue.
- *Pinprick sensation* may be lost in leprosy, and decreased *light touch sensation* (using specific graded monofilaments) can predict diabetes-related neuropathic ulceration.
- *Paring the skin* allows distinction between a wart and a corn, or may confirm the presence of old blood in talon noir or a haematoma.
- *Smell* may be useful – for example, in suspecting anaerobic wound infection, or in the diagnosis of rarities such as trimethylaminuria.
- *Simple microscopy* may be diagnostic for hair shaft abnormalities and for distinguishing between hair casts and head lice egg cases (nits), and is used to detect cutaneous fungal disease. Dermoscopy, an *in vivo* form of magnification, is discussed in Chapter 145.

Additional clinical investigations
Photography
Most patients or a family member own a smartphone equipped with a high quality camera, and many now come to consultations with photographs outlining the pictorial history of their eruption. They can be helpful and diagnostic in evanescent eruptions which have resolved by the time of examination. The progression of conditions such as erythema annulare centrifugum, Jessner lymphocytic infiltrate and uticarial vasculitis can be appreciated by the physician and help diagnostically. The skin and mucosal lesions in Behçet disease are recurrent and transient, and image capture at their zenith by patients is invaluable in diagnosis.

Diascopy
Pressing a glass slide or (more safely) a stiff, clear, colourless piece of plastic onto the skin compresses blood out of small vessels, to allow evaluation of other colours. Diascopy is of particular value in

Table 4.5 Some examples of disorders that have a predilection for specific body sites.

Body site	Type of disorder	Examples
Scalp	Hair disorders/alopecia	Alopecia areata, androgenetic alopecia
	Inflammatory dermatoses	Psoriasis, seborrhoeic dermatitis, lichen simplex
	Localised lesions	Pilar cysts, organoid naevus, squamous cell carcinoma, atypical fibroxanthoma, cutaneous metastases
Eyelids	Inflammatory dermatoses	Atopic eczema, contact allergy (cosmetics, nickel), seborrhoeic blepharitis, angio-oedema, dermatomyositis
	Localised lesions	Basal cell carcinoma, xanthelasma
Ears	Inflammatory dermatoses	Seborrhoeic dermatitis, psoriasis, atopic eczema, relapsing polychondritis
	Infection	Pseudomonas ('malignant') otitis externa
	Localised lesions	Actinic keratosis, squamous cell carcinoma, chondrodermatitis nodularis, atypical fibroxanthoma, angiolymphoid hyperplasia with eosinophilia, gouty tophi
Face	Inflammatory dermatoses	Acne, atopic eczema, seborrhoeic dermatitis, rosacea, lupus erythematosus, lupus pernio, photosensitivity
	Infections	Herpes zoster, erysipelas, impetigo
	Localised lesions	Naevi and freckles, actinic keratoses, basal and squamous cell carcinomas, keratoacanthoma, lentigo maligna
Lips	Inflammatory dermatoses	Dermatitis (atopic, contact), cheilitis (angular, actinic), angio-oedema, contact urticaria, erythema multiforme
	Infections	Herpes simplex, viral warts
	Localised lesions	Vascular lesions (venous lake, pyogenic granuloma), squamous cell carcinoma
Hands	Inflammatory and other dermatoses	Dermatitis (dyshidrotic, pompholyx, contact), psoriasis and palmoplantar pustulosis, keratodermas, erythema multiforme, photosensitivity (dorsal hand), collagen vascular disorders and vasculitis, granuloma annulare
	Infections	Paronychias, onychomycosis, scabies (especially finger webs), viral warts
	Localised lesions	Actinic keratoses, squamous cell carcinoma, subungual melanoma
	Nail disorders	Koilonychia, pachyonychia congenita, many others
Limbs	Inflammatory and other dermatoses	Psoriasis (elbows, knees), atopic eczema (limb flexures), discoid eczema, venous eczema and ulceration (lower leg), asteatotic eczema (lower leg), lichen simplex (lower leg), lichen planus (flexor forearms, shins), dermatitis herpetiformis (knee, elbow), granuloma annulare (elbows), erythema nodosum (legs), vasculitis (legs), papular urticaria/flea bites (lower leg)
	Localised lesions	Bowen disease (lower leg), dermatofibroma
Feet	Inflammatory and other dermatoses	Dermatitis (pompholyx, contact, juvenile plantar), psoriasis and palmoplantar pustulosis, vasculitis and arterial disease, callosities/corns
	Infections	Dermatophyte fungal infection (skin and nails), pitted keratolysis, verrucae
	Localised lesions	Eccrine poroma, subungual exostosis
Axillae (see also Table 4.6)	Inflammatory dermatoses	Psoriasis, contact dermatitis, hidradenitis suppurativa, acanthosis nigricans, fibroepithelial polyps, freckles in neurofibromatosis (Crowe sign)
	Infections	Staphylococcal boils, erythrasma
	Localised lesions	Apocrine hidrocystoma
Genital	Inflammatory and other dermatoses	Psoriasis/reactive arthritis, lichen planus and lichen nitidus (penis), lichen sclerosus (penis, vulva), lichen simplex (scrotum, vulva), fixed drug eruption (penis), Zoon balanitis (glans penis), plasma cell vulvitis, other vulval dermatoses
	Infections	Sexually transmitted diseases, genital warts, molluscum contagiosum
	Localised lesions	Epidermoid cysts (scrotal), squamous cell carcinoma (penis, vulva)

detecting granulomatous nodules, which have a translucent brownish colour known as 'apple jelly' nodules (e.g. in lupus vulgaris). In naevus anaemicus, a localised area of vasoconstriction, other pigments are unaltered – diascopy of adjacent skin therefore reveals an identical colour to that of the 'depigmented' area. By contrast, diascopy of skin adjacent to vitiligo, in which there is loss of melanin, demonstrates that the vitiligo remains paler. Application of medium pressure to a spider naevus can compress radiating arterioles and allow visualisation of pulsatile flow in the feeding vessel.

Wood's light

This is a source of ultraviolet light from which virtually all visible rays have been excluded by a Wood's (nickel oxide) filter. Applications of Wood's light are listed in Table 4.7 [1,2].

Variations in epidermal pigmentation are more apparent under Wood's lamp than under visible light, whereas variations in dermal pigment are less apparent [3]. Thus, for example, it can be used to distinguish vitiligo from naevus anaemicus. Vitiligo is due to loss of epidermal melanin, and the depigmented areas are greatly exaggerated under Wood's light; naevus anaemicus is due to localised dermal vasoconstriction with normal overlying epidermal pigmentation, and the pallor completely disappears under Wood's light. The ash leaf macules of tuberous sclerosis are much more prominent under Wood's lamp [3].

Many organisms produce chemicals that fluoresce under Wood's light [4,5] including *Propionibacterium acnes* [6], and *Corynebacterium minutissimum*, the bacterium responsible for erythrasma (Figure 4.19), and conversion of aminolaevulinic acid to protoporphyrin occurs in several tumours and other skin lesions, leading to the technique of photodynamic diagnosis [7] as well as photodynamic therapy. Fluorescein can be added to topical agents in studies of their use – for example, to detect areas that are missed during sunscreen application [8]. Wood's light can also be used to view *ex vivo* specimens, such as blood or urine in porphyrias [9], or even inanimate objects, such as clothing from patients with chromhidrosis [10]. The light has been advocated for confirming the diagnosis of suspected dermatitis artefacta – skin adjacent to the artefact has a tetracycline containing cream applied, and then occluded. The presence of fluorescence on the fingers under Wood's light is evidence that the dressings have been tampered with [11]. Postmenopausal vaginal atrophy results in a pale green fluorescence under Wood's light absent in the normal premenopausal individual.

Table 4.6 Some disorders that have a predilection for flexural sites.

Type of disorder	Disorder	Comment (all refer to major flexures unless specified)
Inflammatory dermatoses	Psoriasis	Common in flexures, typically red and shiny rather than the usual white scale; may be termed the 'inverse pattern' if mainly flexural distribution
	Seborrhoeic dermatitis	Usually with lesions elsewhere also; central face, scalp, etc.
	Contact dermatitis	Irritant or allergic; may affect the vault of the axilla (e.g. deodorants) or axillary folds (e.g. clothing dermatitis)
	Intertrigo	Especially inframammary; may be due to simple maceration, but also secondary infection may occur (staphylococcal, streptococcal, candidal)
	Napkin rash	Many causes, the commonest are irritant and candidal
	Lichen planus	Not often mainly flexural, but may cause confusion as flexural and genital lesions are often brown in colour and/or annular in morphology, rather than the usual purplish plaques, and may lack the anticipated pruritus
	Hidradenitis suppurativa	Affects axillae, groin, inframammary area
	Crohn disease	Cutaneous lesions affect especially the perineum
	Atopic eczema	Affects elbow and knee flexures, uncommonly the major flexures other than in infants when the process may be generalised
Bullous diseases	Pemphigus vegetans	Rare, mainly flexural
	Hailey–Hailey disease	Inherited, variable
Infections	Dermatophytes	Especially male groin; usually associated with tinea pedis
	Erythrasma	Brownish colour, fluoresces under Wood's light
	Trichomycosis axillaris	Coated hair shafts
	Candidosis	Especially in napkin rash or bedbound elderly adults, commoner in diabetes; satellite pustules are characteristic
	Bacterial	Various types – follicular infections (furuncles), perianal abscesses, secondary infection of intertrigo, Gram-negative toe-web infections, etc.
	Scabies	Multiple itchy flexural nodules are highly suggestive of the relatively chronic nodular variant – penile lesions are also common in this pattern
	Parvovirus B19	Often acral, but the laterothoracic type may include axillary involvement, and a bathing trunk pattern involves groin flexures; often purpuric
Localised lesions	Fibroepithelial polyps (skin tags)	A common normal variant
	Neurofibromatosis	Axillary freckling is seen (Crowe sign)
	Fox–Fordyce disease	An apocrine occlusion dermatosis
	Pseudoxanthoma elasticum	Inherited defect of elastic tissue, most apparent on the neck and axillae
Miscellaneous	Hyperhidrosis and other sweat apparatus disorders	Mainly axillae
	Acanthosis nigricans	May be endocrine-related or paraneoplastic
	Acrodermatitis enteropathica/zinc deficiency	Severe napkin rash and perioral rash in an infant; acquired version in adults; necrolytic migratory erythema of glucagonoma syndrome may have the same pattern
	Langerhans cell histiocytosis	May present as severe napkin rash
	Mycosis fungoides	Often affects shielded sites, may be limited to main flexures ± buttocks
	Granular parakeratosis	Rare – hyperkeratotic, mainly adult female axilla
	'Inverse' pattern of drug eruption	

Adapted from White and Cox 2000 [7]. Reproduced with permission from Elsevier.

There are pitfalls of using Wood's light:
- It is useful to diagnose tinea capitis acquired from cats or dogs, but most fungi do not fluoresce, so a negative test does not exclude the diagnosis.
- There is some reflection of light from any scaly dermatosis, which may be confused with the relatively subtle colour change of pityriasis versicolor.
- Optical brighteners in detergents fluoresce strongly – white shirts and coats may be a considerable distraction.
- Erythrasma fluoresces pink due to porphyrins – it is a reasonably frequent finding that the expected fluorescence is negative if the affected skin has been washed prior to a clinic appointment.

Clinical microscopy, dermoscopy and other imaging systems

Microscopy is an important laboratory technique, discussed briefly below. However, microscopy in a clinical setting also has several uses.

Dermoscopy

This technique, also known as dermatoscopy or epiluminescence microscopy, is an extension of the use of simple magnification. Dermoscopes have built-in illumination and are applied to the skin surface with a film of oil on the lesion to enhance the visibility of subcorneal structures. The technique is mainly used in the diagnosis of doubtful pigmented lesions (Chapter 145). The images may be viewed directly, photographed or recorded digitally for subsequent or sequential analysis. A structured system of analysing the colours and appearances of the structural elements (e.g. pigment network, globules and dots, horn cysts and pseudofollicular openings and the vascular patterns visualised) may increase the accuracy of diagnosing malignant melanoma [1,2]. Scoring systems such as the ABCD dermoscopy score (assessing *a*symmetry, *b*order, *c*olour and *d*ermoscopic structures) [3] and a 'seven-point check list' have been devised. Non-specialists may be trained to triage suspect pigmented lesions to aid triage for biopsy [4]. Computerised image analysis is being developed to aid in distinguishing benign melanocytic lesions from melanoma [5]. Dermoscopes can

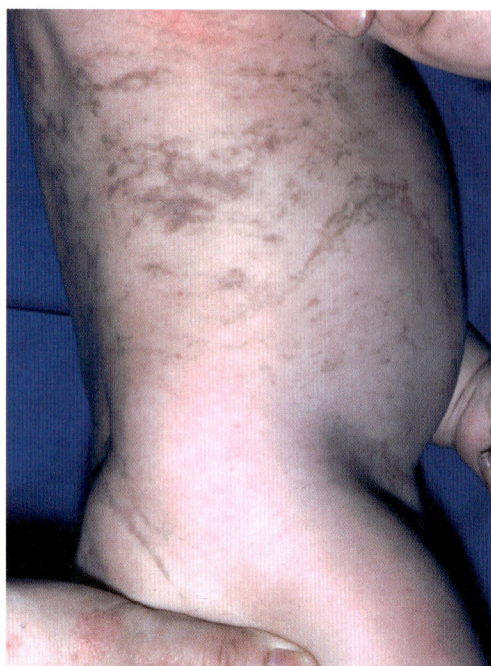

Figure 4.17 Blaschkoid lesions in incontinentia pigmenti.

also be useful in distinguishing haemangiomas, angiokeratomas, pigmented basal cell carcinomas and seborrhoeic keratoses from melanocytic lesions. Inflammatory papulosquamous disorders that dermoscopy may help differentiate include sarcoidosis, cutaneous leishmaniasis, lupus vulgaris, granuloma faciale and demodicidosis, acquired keratodermas (chronic hand eczema, palmar psoriasis, keratoderma due to mycosis fungoides, keratoderma resulting from pityriasis rubra pilaris, tinea manuum, palmar lichen planus and aquagenic palmar keratoderma), sclero-atrophic dermatoses (necrobiosis lipoidica, morphea and cutaneous lichen sclerosus), hypopigmented macular diseases (extragenital guttate lichen sclerosus, achromic pityriasis versicolor, guttate vitiligo, idiopathic guttate hypomelanosis, progressive macular hypomelanosis and postinflammatory hypopigmentations), hyperpigmented maculopapular diseases (pityriasis versicolor, lichen planus pigmentosus, Gougerot–Carteaud syndrome, Dowling–Degos disease, erythema ab igne, macular amyloidosis, lichen amyloidosus, friction melanosis, terra firma-forme dermatosis, urticaria pigmentosa and telangiectasia macularis eruptiva perstans), itchy papulonodular dermatoses (hypertrophic lichen planus, prurigo nodularis, nodular scabies and acquired perforating dermatosis), erythrodermas (due to psoriasis, atopic dermatitis, mycosis fungoides, pityriasis rubra pilaris and scabies), non-infectious balanitis (Zoon plasma cell balanitis, psoriatic balanitis, seborrheic dermatitis and non-specific balanitis) erythroplasia of Queyrat and assess nail fold capillaries in scleroderma [6].

Trichoscopy [7] (use of the dermoscope for hair and scalp lesions) aids diagnostic accuracy, and is helpful in the diagnosis of inflammatory cicatricial alopecias (scalp discoid lupus erythematosus, lichen planopilaris, frontal fibrosing alopecia and folliculitis decalvans), non-scarring alopecias (alopecia areata, trichotillomania, androgenetic alopecia and telogen effluvium) and scaling disorders of the scalp (tinea capitis, scalp psoriasis).

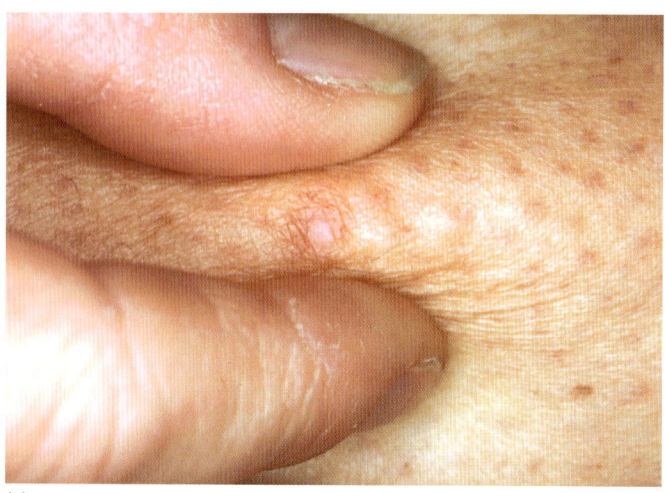

(a)

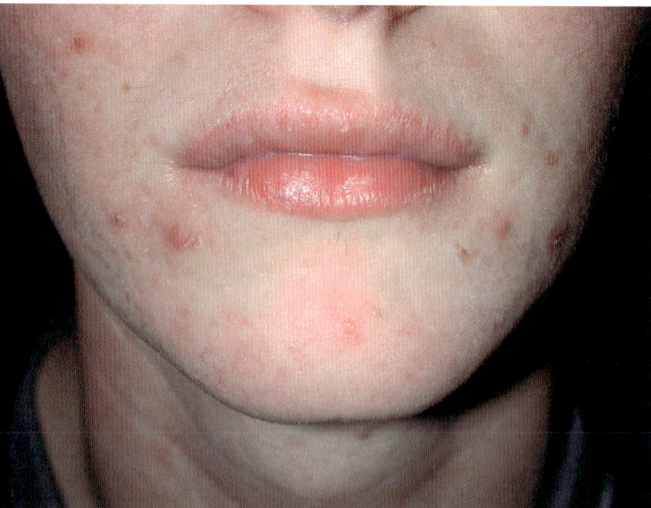

(b)

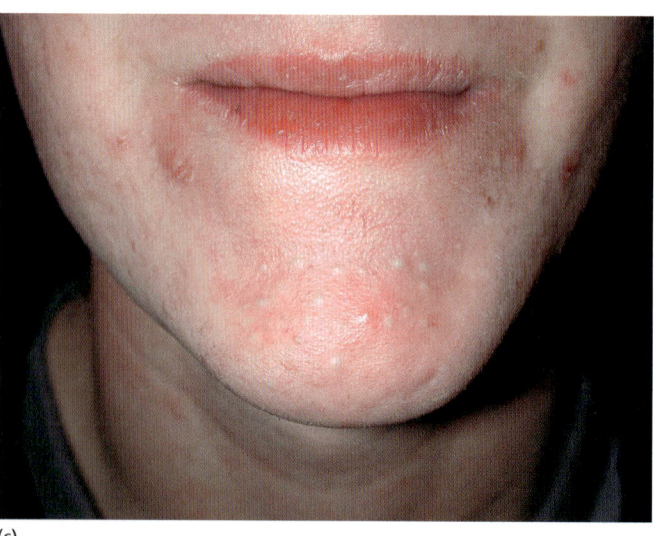

(c)

Figure 4.18 Pinching and stretching of the skin can elicit diagnostic features in some lesions: (a) pinching a dermatofibroma between the fingers causes it to dip deeper into the dermis eliciting the 'pinch sign'; (b,c) tensing the skin on the chin by grimacing makes 'submarine' comedones in acne become more evident.

Table 4.7 Uses of Wood's light.

Fungal infection	Tinea capitis – green fluorescence associated with *Microspora* species and favus (see also Chapter 32)
	Pityriasis versicolor – yellow
Bacterial infections	Erythrasma, acne – coral pink (porphyrins)
	Pseudomonas pyocyanea – yellowish green (pyocyanin)
Infestations	Scabies – fluorescein solution fills the burrows and can be viewed with Wood's light
Porphyrias (see also Chapter 58)	Urine, faeces and occasionally blister fluid fluoresce in porphyria cutanea tarda; teeth in erythropoietic porphyria; blood in protoporphyria
Pigmentary disorders	Vitiligo is accentuated, dermal pigment becomes less apparent
	Detection of ash leaf macules in tuberous sclerosis
Drugs and chemicals	Detection in tissues, e.g. staining of teeth or sebum from tetracyclines and of the nails from mepacrine
	Detection of fluorescent contact or photosensitisers on the skin, or in cosmetics and industrial agents, e.g. ballpoint pen ink, eosin, furocoumarins, halogenated salicylanilides, pitch ingredients
	Fluorescein can be added to topical medications to investigate sites of application or of manipulation (e.g. in the investigation of dermatitis artefacta)
Tumours	Red fluorescence can occur in some malignant tumours and other lesions of the skin, especially squamous cell carcinomas
	Conversion of aminolaevulinic acid to protoporphyrin IX occurs within tumours as the first step in photodynamic therapy and can be detected with Wood's light
Miscellaneous	Lipofuscins in sweat from patients with chromhidrosis can be identified by Wood's light examination of stained clothing
	Research use of fluorescent 'markers' for the investigation of cutaneous penetration and epidermal turnover
	Detection of mineral oil on the skin in the assessment of barrier creams

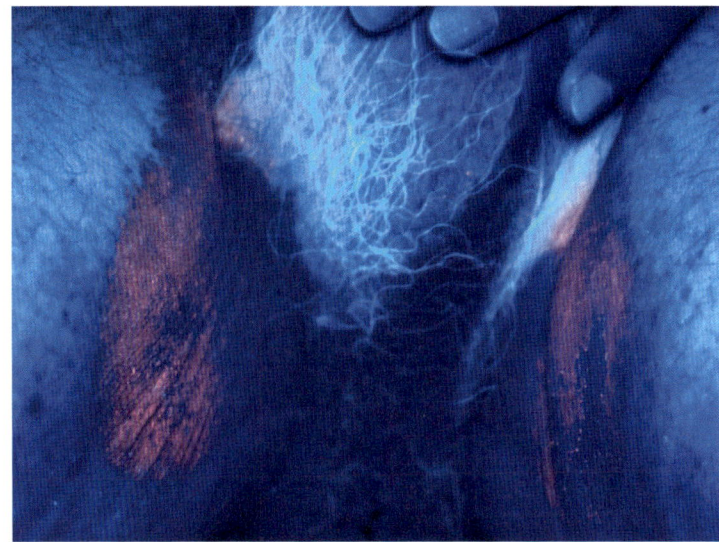

Figure 4.19 Wood's light illumination of erythrasma of the groins – the fluorescence is coral pink.

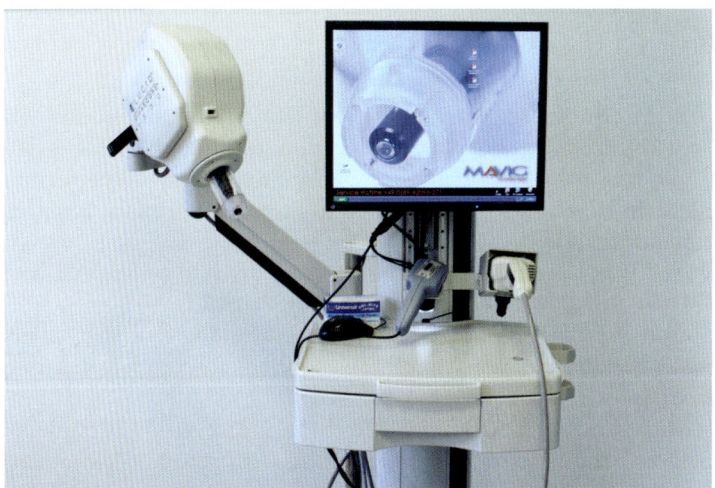

Figure 4.20 A reflectance confocal microscope.

Other imaging systems for localised lesions

Spectrophotometric image analysis of pigmented lesions (SIAo-scopy) allows the assessment of eight narrow-band spectrally filtered images of the skin over an area of 24 × 24 mm with radiation ranging from 400 to 1000 nm. The value of this technique as an adjunct to clinical examination and dermoscopy has produced differing opinions [1,2,3]; it has also been used in the diagnosis of non-melanoma skin cancers [4] and used with an algorithmic approach to diagnosis [5].

Reflectance confocal microscopy (RCM) allows for non-invasive imaging of the epidermis and superficial dermis to a depth of approximately 250 μm (Figures 4.20 and 4.21). Images are taken *en face* and there is visualisation of the skin at the cellular level. These images may provide an alternative to histopathology for diagnosis. The device uses a laser diode with a near infrared wavelength of 830 nm which penetrates into the skin illuminating a small point inside the tissue; this light is reflected back through a small pinhole to reach the detector. Only reflected light from the focal point is detected, hence the name, confocal. The detected images are on a greyscale and the contrast relies on the differences in reflectivity of the tissue. Structures with a high refractive index such as melanin appear bright. The examination is fast, pain free and the result immediate. An 8 × 8 mm glass and metal ring is placed on the skin over the lesion and the objective lens is then attached to this magnetically. Images are then obtained in the horizontal plane and fed back to the monitor. The use of RCM in dermatology is increasing dramatically. In skin cancer screening clinics, it is used as a screening tool for both melanocytic and non-melanocytic lesions in place of biopsy for equivocal lesions [6,7]. It can be used for the diagnosis of basal cell carcinoma pre-Mohs micrographic surgery or radiotherapy. It is particularly useful for margin assessment and determination of treatment in lentigo maligna and basal cell carcinoma [8]. It can be used in place of a biopsy in hair clinics, for inflammatory diseases and monitoring of mucosal disease. RCM can also be used on *ex vivo* tissue. When combined with fluorescence this is termed fluorescence confocal microscopy. This is particularly useful for the rapid assessment of excised tissue such as in Mohs micrographic surgery [8]. In this situation, the Mohs surgeon removes the tissue in the usual manner, acridine orange is applied to the excised tissue and the objective lens is placed onto the tissue. The images are detected within 3 min and, if tumour remains, the Mohs surgeon can continue to the second stage. The advantage of this over traditional Mohs is the speed at which sections can be read [9].

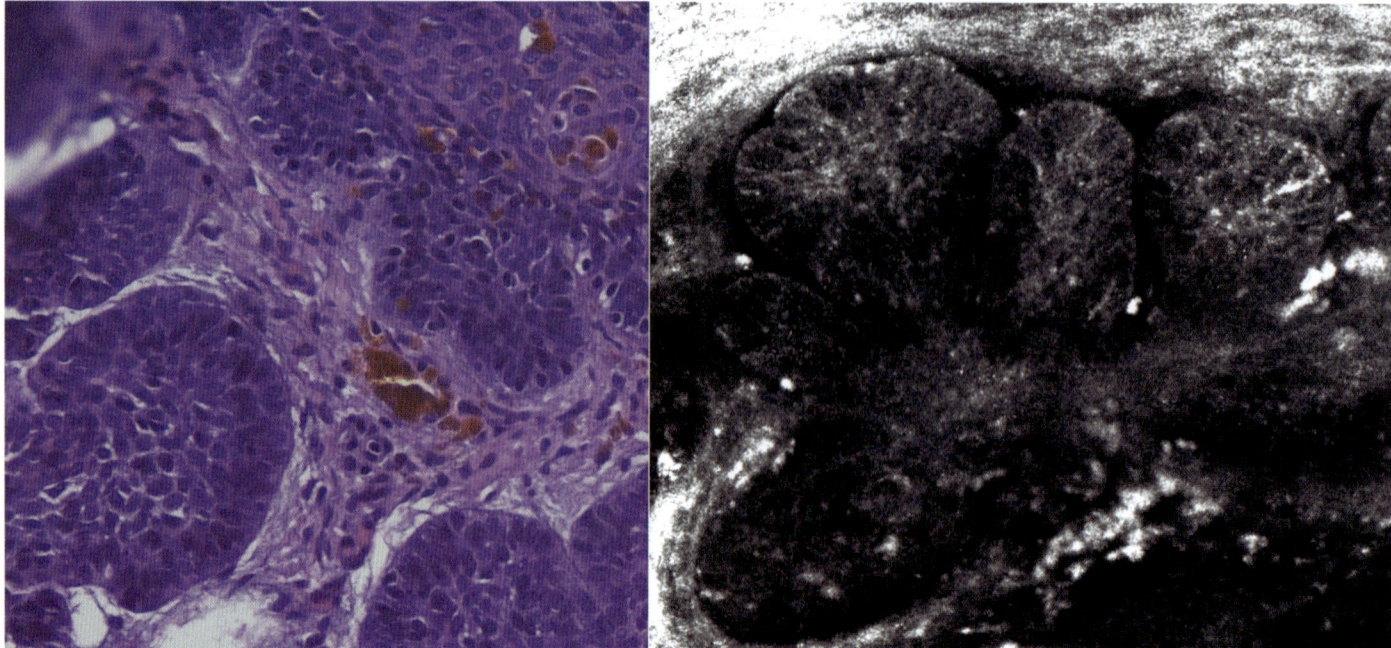

Figure 4.21 Basal cell carcinoma. A comparison of standard H&E histology and reflectance confocal microscopical appearances.

RCM can be used in combination with telecommunication with an expert reader at a distant location reading the images [10]. There has been some criticism, with punch biopsy outperforming RCM in diagnosing and subtyping suspected primary basal cell carcinomas [11].

Other simple microscopy procedures

Simple light microscopy is helpful in evaluating hair shaft abnormalities (this, and more complex electron microscopy, are discussed in Chapter 87).

Microscopy of skin scrapings for fungi is discussed in Chapter 32. Scraping the base of a herpetic vesicle with simple Giemsa staining may reveal giant cells (Tzanck smear); molluscum contagiosum can be identified in a similar fashion. Examination of skin pustule smears after fixation and H&E staining may be useful in the rapid diagnosis and confirmation of infantile eosinophilic folliculitis and incontinentia pigmenti; in both conditions, the pustules are filled with eosinophils.

Microscopy can be invaluable for confirmation of infestations of crab, body and head lice and their empty egg cases (nits), and for the examination of specimens brought by those suffering from delusional parasitosis.

Skin surface biopsies using tape-stripping or adhesive microscope slides pressed onto the skin allow observation of cells of the stratum corneum and of bacteria, fungi such as *Pityrosporon* species, and *Demodex* mites [1–3]. Plastic polymer (Silflo®) skin surface impressions may be useful for the study of eccrine gland pore size and numbers.

Scabies mites can be extracted from the end of a burrow using a needle, with microscopy to confirm the diagnosis. The technique can be useful to convince sceptical sufferers of their infestation. Alternatively, application of mineral oil [4] or 5% potassium hydroxide to an affected interdigital space, followed by light scalpel scraping, reveals the acarus or its eggs. The faecal pellets (scybala) of the mite are also diagnostic, but are dissolved by potassium hydroxide; they remain intact in oil. Burrows can also be removed by a very superficial shave technique and can be made more apparent by application to the skin of either black ink, or fluorescein with Wood's light visualisation. Dermoscopy (see previously) can also be used – the mite appears as a dark triangle shape – or higher-resolution microscopy with a standard light microscope [5]. Outwith the scope of this section, scabies can also be identified using polymerase chain reaction to detect mite antigens [6].

Fine-needle aspiration of lymph nodes

Aspiration of lymph node tissue using a 25- or 27-gauge needle allows cytological assessment of lymph nodes and is useful in the staging of metastatic malignant melanoma and squamous cell carcinoma of the skin. In melanoma patients with palpable and even impalpable but ultrasonically abnormal lymph nodes, the technique has been shown to have high specificity and sensitivity [1,2]. Combining the technique with flow cytometry can help in the differentiation of lymphoma from reactive and dermatopathic lymphadenopathy [3].

Radiological and imaging examinations

These have an important role in dermatology, but less than in many other specialties, because the skin can so readily be seen and felt. Ultrasound [1,2], magnetic resonance imaging (MRI) [3–5], radioisotope scans and even positron emission tomography [6,7,8], are all used in clinical dermatological practice, mainly in relation to the detection of lymphadenopathy or other metastatic skin cancer, and in the identification of occult malignancy in paraneoplastic conditions such as dermatomyositis. High-resolution ultrasound is increasingly important in the documentation of nodal enlargement and tumour infiltration, and can be used to guide biopsies, and in some countries is recommended in national guidelines for routine follow-up in melanoma with a Breslow thickness more than 1 mm. Combining ultrasound and colour Doppler scanning may provide additional help in assessing metastatic lymphadenopathy. It can also be used to measure tumour thickness and delineate margins particularly of larger non-melanoma skin cancers. It may be useful in the preoperative assessment of cysts and lipomata, particularly on the forehead where they are often located subfacially. Other uses of ultrasound in dermatology include, for example, for the accurate assessment of the thickness of lesions in scleroderma, the extent of infection in severe forms of cellulitis (and distinction, using MRI, from necrotising fasciitis) and assessing the extent of cystic lesions of hidradenitis suppurativa. Various imaging techniques are also important in the management of diseases such as neurofibromatosis and tuberous sclerosis, where there may be central nervous system involvement, or in the assessment of muscle change in dermatomyositis and the identification of inflammatory changes in eosinophilic fasciitis. With the advent of small high-resolution coils, MRI can be used to image digits, and may be useful in the diagnosis of myxoid cysts and other periungal pathology. MRI is invaluable in the assessment of disorders of fat (such as lipoatrophy and lipoedema). Lymphoscintigraphy may be a useful functional assessment of the lymphatic system of the swollen lower limb (Chapter 103). Doppler assessment of the peripheral lower limb arteries is an essential bedside technique prior to the use of high-compression bandaging in the management of venous leg ulcers (see Chapter 102); the use of standard electronic sphygmomanometer systolic pressure measurements is not accurate in the measurement of peripheral arterial pressures [9].

Skin testing (prick and scratch, intradermal and patch testing)

Substances may be introduced into the skin by a variety of techniques to study pharmacological and immunological reactions under controlled conditions [1]. Such tests are extremely valuable, but details of the type of test and the time at which it is read must correspond to the pathological process under consideration. Interpretation of the relevance of tests, either positive or negative, must always be correlated with the clinical picture. All too often, evidence adduced from tests is either meaningless or misleading.

Absorption of many substances through the intact skin is poor and variable, but direct application to the surface of the skin is used for patch testing. The epidermal barrier may be overcome either by removing it or by introducing the material directly into the dermis. The following techniques for skin testing are most commonly used.

Techniques for skin testing
Epicutaneous tests – patch tests
Patch tests are usually used to detect contact allergy of the delayed hypersensitivity type. They are usually read at 48–72 h and again up to 1 week, but can also be read at 15–30 min to detect contact urticaria. At times, patch testing may usefully be combined with scratch testing. Details of these techniques are discussed in Chapter 126.

Intradermal injection
The injection is made into the superficial layer of the dermis through a fine-bore (26- or 27-gauge) needle with its bevel pointing upwards. The quantity that may conveniently be injected varies from 0.01 to 0.1 mL. Precise measurement of smaller quantities is difficult and requires syringes with especially well-fitting plungers and a micrometer screw gauge. For routine clinical purposes, an approximation is sufficient – either 0.05 mL or the amount that just causes a visible weal (0.01–0.02 mL).

The optimal time for reading the reaction naturally varies with the pharmacological agent or the type of immunological reaction. Most such tests are read at either 15–20 min or at 48 h, but it may be important to read the tests at other times, for example at 4–12 h or after 4 days. The response to be observed at 15 min (e.g. after an injection of histamine or after immediate-weal allergy tests) is a weal with a surrounding flare. The weal is a more accurate measure than the flare. When the test is read at 48 h (e.g. in the tuberculin reaction), the sizes of the indurated papule and of the erythematous reaction should be observed.

The site of the test is of some importance [2,3]. In general, the whole skin surface is capable of responding to skin tests, but there are regional variations. The back and the flexor aspects of the forearms are most conveniently used. The skin on the ulnar aspect of the forearm is more sensitive than the radial, and the proximal more sensitive than the distal. These differences are not of sufficient magnitude to affect routine testing, but must be taken into account by using symmetrical areas for controls in any accurate quantitative testing.

A test solution must always be compared with a control solution injected in a comparable site at the same time. A positive test may be taken as one that is significantly different from the control. Assessment of what is significant is difficult and varies with the enthusiasm of the tester. If a difference of less than 5 mm is accepted, reproducible results may not be obtained on retesting [4].

The measurement of a weal is usually made by diameter, although more sophisticated methods, such as volume measurements and Doppler flow, have been used [5]. If the weal is not circular, an approximation may be made by averaging maximum/minimum diameters, or more accurately the area may be calculated by the formula $D_1 \times D_2 \times \pi/4$, where D_1 and D_2 are the maximum and minimum diameters [6]. For irregular weals, a tracing may be made on squared paper. Pseudopodia should be noted, but for measurement of diameter they are ignored. Attempts to assess the volume of a weal are less satisfactory for routine use.

The size of the weal is not directly proportional to the dose of the active agent, but varies also with the total volume of fluid injected. An approximation of a linear relationship may best be achieved, often only over a narrow range, by plotting the response against the log dose. For accurate quantitative observations, weal diameters below 4 mm or above 15 mm cannot be relied upon.

Antihistamines may greatly inhibit the immediate-weal tests. In the case of very long-acting agents, this effect may last as long as 3 weeks. They have no appreciable effect on delayed hypersensitivity patch tests. Moderate to large doses of corticosteroids, in

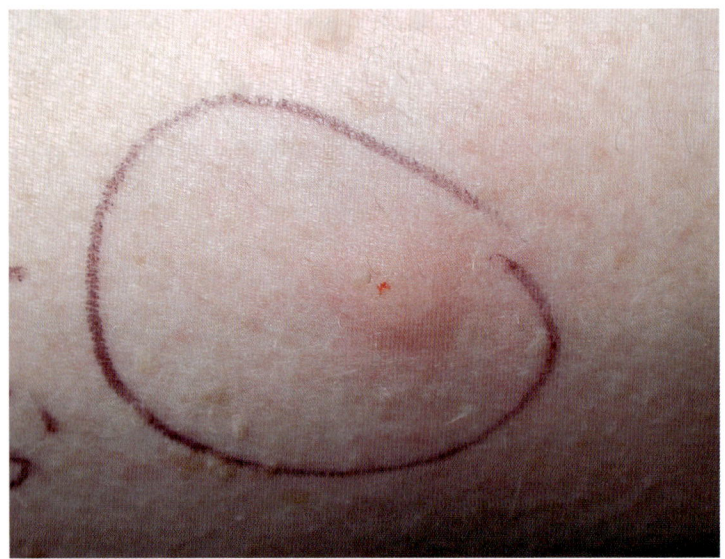

Figure 4.22 A positive prick test to latex.

contrast, may somewhat inhibit patch tests, although smaller doses (e.g. prednisolone 10 mg daily) are not necessarily a contraindication to testing. Steroids do not greatly inhibit the immediate-weal tests. When a patient feels faint, any immediate-weal test may be completely inhibited.

Prick test

This is a modification of the intradermal injection. A small quantity of the test solution is placed on the skin and a prick is made through it with a sharp needle. This should be superficial and not sufficient to draw blood. The quantity has been estimated as 3×10^{-6} mL [3]. The size of the weal and flare are measured after 15 min (Figure 4.22). This test gives reproducible results and is convenient for much routine allergy testing. Because of the discrepancy in the quantities injected, the testing solutions are made up at different strengths for prick testing and intradermal testing. The intradermal injection of prick-test solutions may be dangerous.

Scratch test

The scratch test resembles the prick test. A linear scratch about 1 cm long, but not sufficient to draw blood, is made through the epidermis. This test gives less reproducible results than the prick test.

Modified prick test

Here, a drop of the test solution is placed on the skin. A needle is then inserted very superficially and almost horizontally into the skin and lifted to raise a tiny tent of epidermis. This test is slightly more sensitive than the ordinary prick test, but gives no more reproducible results.

Skin-window technique

The surface of the skin over an area a few millimetres square is scratched off with a scalpel, the test solution applied and the area covered with a coverslip [7,8]. This is removed at various intervals (e.g. 3 h, 6 h, 12 h, 24 h and 48 h) and immediately replaced by another coverslip. The cells on the coverslip are stained with ordinary haematological stains. The cellular response at varying time intervals can be assessed.

Immediate-weal tests

These tests are used for detecting immunoglobulin E (IgE) antibodies. The passive transfer test has been used to detect circulating IgE, but is now deemed hazardous and unethical because of the risk of serum hepatitis or HIV. These antibodies play a role in hay fever, asthma, atopic eczema and anaphylactic reactions. They occur especially, but not exclusively, in patients with a personal or family background of atopy. Positive skin tests to a wide variety of antigens are extremely frequent in these patients and must always be correlated with the history. They are principally used in the assessment of hay fever and asthma and have a limited place in the management of atopic eczema. They are disappointing in the diagnosis of urticaria. False positive and false negative reactions are common.

Severe systemic reactions and, very rarely, fatalities may occur after correct use of standard testing solutions, and epinephrine and hydrocortisone injections should always be at hand when skin tests are performed [9,10].

Alternative methods of detecting and measuring circulating antibodies are the radioallergosorbent assay (RAST) and the enzyme-linked immunosorbent assay. RAST correlates well with skin testing [11,**12**]. It is particularly useful (i) in testing very young children; and (ii) with allergens associated with risk on prick testing (e.g. drugs).

The autologous serum test is a technique used in the investigation of chronic idiopathic urticaria whereby the patient's own serum is injected intradermally. It is regarded as being positive if at 30 min there is a weal 1.5 mm larger than at the saline control injection site. Positive reactions are indicative of functional autoantibodies against the high-affinity IgE receptor FcεRI, or against IgE [**13**] (Chapter 42).

Delayed (4–8 h) tests

The clinical interpretation of tests that are positive at 4–8 h can be difficult. Sometimes, these represent an Arthus reaction, but ideally this should be confirmed histologically. Other such tests represent a delayed variant of the immediate-weal (15 min) test.

Intradermal tests for the detection of delayed sensitivity to bacterial, fungal and viral antigens

Tuberculin test

Testing for evidence of tuberculosis has achieved new importance in dermatology, in part because of an increasing incidence of tuberculosis associated with HIV infection, and also because screening is a necessary part of the work-up before the use of antitumour necrosis factor biological drugs (e.g. in psoriasis). A positive result to the standard strength (10 tuberculin units, TU) is an indication of previous mycobacterial infection, but not necessarily by *Mycobacterium tuberculosis* (especially if the reaction is weak or doubtful). Reactions to 1 TU (1/100 dilution of purified protein derivative (PPD)) are, however, significant. In sarcoidosis, reactions may be wholly negative, or only positive to 100 TU. The minimum size of a positive reaction is taken as 5 mm. An intermediate (24 h) reaction sometimes occurs.

Comparable doses of PPD may vary according to their source. It is being replaced by interferon γ release assay (IRGA) tests such as the QuantiFERON-TB Gold In-Tube® test for the pre-evaluation for biological agents in inflammatory dermatoses. It is important to remember that after an immunomodulating drug, skin tuberculin tests may give false negative results. Tuberculin tests are discussed further in Chapter 27.

Heaf test
Used in mass testing and in children, this is roughly equivalent to, or perhaps slightly more sensitive than, a dilution of 1:100 old tuberculin [14].

Candida antigen
This is used in a similar manner to the tuberculin test. Depressed reactivity occurs in sarcoidosis and other immunosuppressed conditions. Negative reactions in normal subjects are, however, not uncommon and depend on age and locality.

Trichophytin
This detects past infection by *Trichophyton* species. Its value is limited.

Lepromin test
This is discussed in Chapter 28.

Histoplasmin, coccidioidin
These and similar antigenic tests are of most value in areas where these diseases are not endemic. The Frei test and cat scratch fever antigen are of some value in the UK, where the relevant diseases are comparatively rare. A positive reaction is then significant. Conversely, *Brucella* antigen and toxoplasmin are of limited use in dermatological practice.

Delayed-type bacterial antigen tests
Delayed-type bacterial antigen tests [15–17] are not widely used, partly because their specificity and interpretation are difficult to assess. They consist of standard preparations of bacterial extracts, each probably containing a mixture of antigenic components, which may produce an immediate, or delayed 48 h reaction, or an even later reaction. The normal 48 h response is a papule showing, histologically, a tuberculin-type reaction of lymphocytic type. Occasionally, however, especially in cases of vasculitis, an acute leukocytoclastic reaction occurs within 6–8 h [16] and is fully established at 24–48 h. Sometimes, the reaction is severe enough to produce a sterile abscess. It is tempting to believe that these reactions may be of some significance in conditions such as erythema multiforme, erythema nodosum (streptococcal), allergic vasculitis and, perhaps, pustular psoriasis. However, the antigens presently in use are relatively impure and the reactions may be non-specific. Further careful immunological studies are required.

Long-delayed (6-week) intradermal reactions
These comprise the Kveim test and the Mitsuda test. They are read at 6 weeks, but biopsy is essential with the Kveim test. Kveim test antigen is no longer available in the UK.

Pathergy and pathergy testing
This is a test that is used as part of the diagnostic criteria for the diagnosis of Behçet disease [18]. There is no standardised technique, but one frequently used is to puncture normal-appearing volar forearm

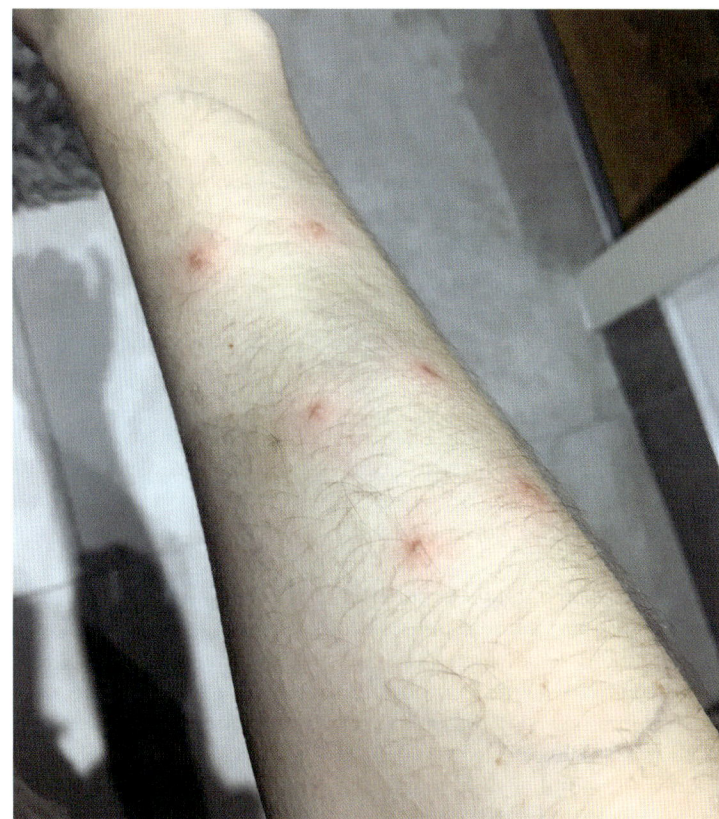

Figure 4.23 A positive pathergy test in Behçet disease at 48 h after skin puncture.

skin, which is examined 48 h later (Figure 4.23). Some feel it is important not to sterilise the skin with alcohol or an antiseptic before the puncture. The development of an inflammatory papule or pustule indicates a positive response. Recent studies have suggested that use of the patient's own saliva increases the sensitivity of the pathergy test in Behçet disease. Injury of the skin in some neutrophilic diseases such as pyoderma gangrenosum and Sweet syndrome can be followed by the development of the eruption in the injured site; this is an example of the pathergic response.

Teledermatology

Teledermatology has been used to improve patient access to dermatological care particularly in geographically remote areas or where there is a lack of local expertise and during enforced times of isolation as in the Covid-19 pandemic [1]. There are two principal forms of teledermatology: real-time teleconsultation and store-and-forward technology, where images and clinical information are sent electronically to be reviewed at a later time. There is evidence to suggest that store-and-forward teledermatology consultations are longer than traditional consultations for the primary care physician mainly due to the need to obtain images and complete electronic referral forms [2].

Diagnostic accuracy and reliability of teledermatology is reportedly similar to face-to-face consultation in selected referrals with an acceptable level of diagnostic concordance [3]. Management accuracy of teledermatology for non-skin cancer is also comparable to traditional consultation [4] and high levels of patient satisfaction [5,6]. However, clinic consultation has been shown to result in higher diagnostic accuracy in the assessment of malignant lesions, particularly malignant pigmented lesions [5,6]. Over recent years, teledermoscopy has been introduced in an attempt to improve accuracy in the diagnosis of both melanocytic and non-melanocytic skin lesions in store-and-forward teledermatology services [5] and patient satisfaction [7,8].

One major disadvantage of store-and-forward teledermatology is the inability to perform a full body skin examination. One study reported that over a third of melanomas detected in patients referred to secondary care with potential skin cancer were incidental findings on total skin examination; these may therefore have not been detected if a single image of the index lesion had been sent for teledermatology assessment [9,10]. The inability to palpate the skin in teledermatology consultations has also been cited as a drawback, for example in detecting small superficial actinic keratoses which are often more obvious on palpation [11].

In terms of economic considerations, store-and-forward consultation is cheaper than real-time teleconsultation; however, the former is more likely to result in a hospital consultation, particularly since supplementary clinical information and images cannot necessarily be obtained [11]. Store-and-forward teledermatology may be used to triage referrals from primary care and therefore potentially reduce the number of hospital consultations required [12] and for inpatient referrals [13]. When compared with traditional outpatient consultation, real-time teledermatology may not be cost-effective unless patients are travelling significant distances to attend [14–16]. Feedback from specialists reviewing teledermatology referrals may also have an educational value to the referring physician [17].

Mobile phones are increasingly being used to deliver telemedicine. Clinical and dermoscopic images of skin lesions or inflammatory dermatoses with relevant clinical information can be sent via mobile phone for review by a dermatologist at a distant location, which may be in a different country or continent [18]. Similar diagnostic accuracy and management concordance compared with traditional store-and-forward teledermatology has been reported, although interobserver concordance may be less with mobile teledermatology than with traditional face-to-face consultation. The process relies on having a mobile phone with a suitable camera and software and a method to ensure secure transmission of clinical information and and some degree of technical ability by the patient [19,20].

Mobile phone-based interventions may also be employed to educate and motivate patients with chronic skin conditions [20]. Text message reminders and educational tools have shown promise in improving adherence and outcomes in the short term in patients with psoriasis. Teledermatology has also been explored as a method of monitoring patients on systemic therapies for side effects and response to treatment, thus reducing the need for hospital appointments. Patients reported high levels of satisfaction, and it may be that if patients are required to submit data regularly through a teledermatology platform compliance would be improved, although there is limited data to support this.

General dermatologists may also use teledermatology to consult national experts in so-called 'tertiary teledermatology', and this may prevent the need for patients to travel long distances for tertiary review. It is important to note that although some patients may find teledermatology services convenient, a significant proportion of patients prefer face-to-face consultations and may even feel unable to speak freely about their condition if providing information for a teledermatology consultation [19]. However, teledermatology has been shown to be equivalent to traditional face-to-face consultation, in terms of skin-specific quality of life outcome measures, with comparable patient satisfaction and preferences.

Teledermatology is an expanding field that may be of particular use for triage and where there is limited access to local specialist care. Long-term data on the outcomes of patients managed by teledermatology are currently lacking and when available could determine the utility of more widespread use of teledermatology services.

Mobile smartphone applications

The internet has enabled patients to research medical conditions more easily, such that patients may present the clinician with information they have found online both about their diagnosis and treatment. Equally, clinicians often refer patients to appropriate sources of information and support on the internet. Smart phones are now also important patient resources. One recent study identified 229 dermatology-related mobile phone applications of which a significant number were aimed at patients [1]. The majority of applications were for general dermatology reference, followed by applications for self-diagnosis and monitoring. Some applications allowed patients to upload images of their skin and receive feedback from dermatologists. Educational applications were also available for both undergraduate students and dermatology trainees, including examination preparation aids. Clinicians may also use smart phones for teledermatology and education, and assessment tools such as Psoriasis Area Severity Index and DLQI calculators. However, it is important to note that applications are not necessarily well regulated and as yet there is little research on their safety and efficacy.

Artificial intelligence and dermatology

Artificial Intelligence (AI) is 'the ability of a computer or computer-controlled robot to perform tasks commonly associated with intelligent beings' (https://www.britannica.com/technology/artificial-intelligence, last accessed April 2022). In medicine AI may be used in diagnostics, monitoring and treatment protocol development. Visual pattern recognition is an important part of dermatology and there has been particular interest in the use of AI in analysis of images of skin conditions. In practice this may be used as a triage tool, to enhance face to face clinical assessment or in dermatopathology [1]. Convolutional neural networks are a form of deep learning architecture trained using multiple images and have been developed to classify skin conditions.

Most studies to date have focused on lesion assessment and commonly use binary classification (for example, benign versus malignant, or naevus versus melanoma) [2]. Studies have shown similar diagnostic accuracy to dermatologists, with dermatologists demonstrating improved outcomes with more clinical experience, clinical as well as dermoscopic images and accompanying clinical information [3]. Artificial intelligence-based mobile phone apps have also been developed to aid users in detecting melanoma, but concern has been raised regarding the accuracy of some such apps and further work is recommended [4]. There is more limited evidence to suggest deep learning systems can be used in the diagnosis of non-cancerous dermatoses, including inflammatory conditions, offering superior diagnostic accuracy to primary care physicians [5].

Future research should assess the real-world applicability of AI and ensure inclusion of diverse skin types. Technology should continue to be developed and used to improve patient pathways and access to services, and to support clinicians.

Key references

The full list of references can be found in the online version at https://www.wiley.com/rooksdermatology10e

Fundamentals of diagnosis

1 Lawrence CM, Cox NH. *Physical Signs in Dermatology*, 2nd edn. London: Mosby, 2002.

The history

8 Sladden MJ, Dure-Smith B, Berth-Jones J, Graham-Brown RAC. Ethnic differences in the pattern of skin disease seen in a dermatology department: atopic dermatitis is more common in Asian referrals in Leicestershire. *Clin Exp Dermatol* 1991;16:348–9.

Quality of life in dermatology patients

1 Finlay AY, Khan GK. Dermatology Life Quality Index (DLQI): A simple practical measure for routine clinical use. *Clin Exp Dermatol* 1994;19:210–16

Wood's light

2 Klatte JL, van der Beek N, Kemperman PM. 100 years of Wood's lamp revised. *J Eur Acad Dermatol Venereol* 2015;29:842–7.
7 Fritsch C, Lang K, Neuse W *et al*. Photodynamic diagnosis and therapy in dermatology. *Skin Pharmacol Appl Skin Physiol* 1998;11:358.

Dermoscopy

1 Stolz W, Braun-Falco O, Bilek P *et al*. *Color Atlas of Dermatoscopy*. Boston: Blackwell Scientific Publications, 1994.
4 Jones OT, Jurascheck LC, van Melle MA *et al*. Dermoscopy for melanoma detection and triage in primary care: a systematic review. *BMJ Open* 2019;9:e027529.
6 Errichetti E, Stinco G. Dermoscopy in general dermatology: a practical overview. *Dermatol Ther (Heidelb)* 2016;6:471–507.
7 Rudnicka L, Rakowska A, Olszewska M. Trichoscopy: how it may help the clinician. *Dermatol Clin* 2013;31:29–41.

Other imaging systems for localised lesions

1 Moncrieff M, Cotton S, Claridge E, Hall P. Spectrophotometric intracutaneous analysis: a new technique for imaging pigmented skin lesions. *Br J Dermatol* 2002;146:448–57.
2 Haniffa MA, Lloyd JJ, Lawrence CM. The use of a spectrophotometric intracutaneous analysis device in the real-time diagnosis of melanoma in the setting of a melanoma screening clinic. *Br J Dermatol* 2007;156:1350–2.
6 Gerger A, Koller S, Kern T *et al*. Diagnostic applicability of in vivo confocal laser scanning microscopy in melanocytic skin tumors. *J Invest Dermatol* 2005;124:493–8.
11 Woliner-van der Weg W, Peppelman M, Elshot YS *et al*. Biopsy outperforms reflectance confocal microscopy in diagnosing and subtyping basal cell carcinoma: results and experiences from a randomized controlled multicentre trial. *Br J Dermatol* 2021;184:663–71.

Radiological and imaging examinations

1 Kleinermann R, Whang T, Bard R, Marmur E. Ultrasound in dermatology: principles and applications. *J Am Acad Dermatol* 2012;67:478–87.
7 Böni R, Huch-Böni RA, Steinert H *et al*. Staging of metastatic melanoma by whole-body positron emission tomography using 2-fluorine-18-fluor-2-deoxy-D-glucose. *Br J Dermatol* 1995;132:556–62.
8 Selva-O'Callaghan A, Grau JM, Gámez-Cenzano C *et al*. Conventional cancer screening versus PET/CT in dermatomyositis/polymyositis. *Am J Med* 2010;123:558–62.

Skin testing (prick and scratch, intradermal and patch testing)

1 Pepys J. Skin tests. *Br J Hosp Med* 1984;32:120–4.
12 Seltzer JM. Correlation of allergy test results obtained by IgE RAST and prick-puncture methods. *Ann Allergy* 1985;54:25–30.
13 Sabroe RA, Grattan CE, Francis DM *et al*. The autologous serum skin test: a screening test for autoantibodies in chronic idiopathic urticaria. *Br J Dermatol* 1999;140:446–52.

Teledermatology

4 Andrees V, Klein TM, Augustin M, Otten M. Live interactive teledermatology compared to in-person care – a systematic review. *J Eur Acad Dermatol Venereol* 2020;34:733–45.
7 Chuchu N, Dinnes J, Takwoingi Y *et al*. Cochrane Skin Cancer Diagnostic Test Accuracy Group. *Teledermatology for diagnosing skin cancer in adults*. Cochrane Database Syst Rev 2018;12:CD013193.
9 Aldridge RB, Naysmith L, Ooi ET *et al*. The importance of a full clinical examination: assessment of index lesions referred to a skin cancer clinic without a total body skin examination would miss one in three melanomas. *Acta Derm Venereol* 2013;93:689–92

Mobile smartphone applications

1 Tongdee E, Markowitz O. Mobile app rankings in dermatology. *Cutis* 2018;102:252–6.

Artificial intelligence and dermatology

1 Young AT, Xiong M, Pfau J, Keiser MJ, Wei ML. Artificial intelligence in dermatology: a primer. *J Invest Dermatol* 2020;140:1504–12.

CHAPTER 5

Epidemiology of Skin Disease

Hywel C. Williams[1] and Sinéad M. Langan[2]

[1]Centre of Evidence-Based Dermatology, Population and Lifespan Sciences, School of Medicine, University of Nottingham, Nottingham; Nottingham University Hospitals NHS Trust, Nottingham, UK
[2]Department of Non-Communicable Disease Epidemiology, London School of Hygiene and Tropical Medicine, London, UK

What is epidemiology and why is it relevant to dermatology?, 5.1
Thinking in terms of populations rather than individuals, 5.2
Community diagnosis and control, 5.2
Skin diseases as 'entities' in the population, 5.2
Making comparisons and drawing inferences, 5.3
The prevention paradox, 5.3
More than one disease?, 5.4
How much of a public health problem is skin disease?, 5.4
The need for a clear disease definition in epidemiological studies, 5.4
Impairment, disability and handicap caused by skin disease, 5.5
Global Burden of Disease study, 5.6
What determines the frequency of skin disease in populations?, 5.7
Risk factors, association and causation, 5.7
Genetics, 5.10
Early environment, 5.10
Later environment, 5.10
Describing the natural history and associations of specific skin diseases, 5.11
Health services research in dermatology, 5.12
Needs assessments in dermatology, 5.12
Services available for people with skin diseases, 5.12
Relationship between need, supply and demand for dermatological care, 5.13
Conclusions, 5.14
Glossary of epidemiological terms, 5.14
Measures of disease frequency, 5.14
Measures of disease associations, 5.14
Interpreting results, 5.14
Validity and repeatability, 5.15
Types of epidemiological study, 5.15
Checklist for reading epidemiological studies in dermatology, 5.15
Recommended further reading and useful dermatoepidemiology resources, 5.15
General epidemiology, 5.15
Biostatistics, 5.15
Systematic reviews, 5.16
Dermatoepidemiology reports, 5.16
Dermatoepidemiology textbooks, 5.16
Epidemiology computer software, 5.16
Evidence-based dermatology, 5.16
Interest groups/societies, 5.16
Useful websites and online resources, 5.16
Key references, 5.16

What is epidemiology and why is it relevant to dermatology?

Epidemiology is the simplest and most direct method of studying the causes of diseases in humans and many contributions have been made by studies that have demanded nothing more than an ability to count, to think logically and to have an imaginative idea.

(Sir Richard Doll 1987 [1])

Many dermatologists still think of epidemiology as just describing the prevalence and age, sex and geographic characteristics of a particular skin disease. Whilst it is true that epidemiology is often used in this fashion to describe the *burden* of disease in human populations, as Sir Richard Doll pointed out above, epidemiology also offers one of the most powerful and direct methods of evaluating the *causes* of skin diseases in human populations. One definition of epidemiology is therefore 'the study of the distribution and causes of diseases in human populations'. In addition to describing the burden and causes of skin diseases in populations, *clinical epidemiology* is concerned with describing the natural history and prognosis of diseases and with evaluating interventions that seek to prevent or treat diseases [2]. The term *dermatoepidemiology* refers to the study of the epidemiology of dermatological disorders [3]. Because epidemiological studies are often concerned with making observations about highly complex natural experiments, methods for minimising bias or adjusting for confounding factors (see glossary at the end of this chapter) have had to be developed. Such methods, designed to ensure high scientific rigour when designing and interpreting epidemiological studies, are aspects from which all dermatological research can benefit. Epidemiology is therefore relevant to dermatology for the six reasons shown in Box 5.1.

Although epidemiology is still sometimes perceived as a novelty in dermatology, the first epidemiological discoveries in dermatology can be traced back to 1746, when James Lind [4] concluded that scurvy in sailors was related to dietary factors. He then showed, by means of a controlled study, that the disease readily responded to the addition of fresh oranges and lemons in the sailors' diet. The principles developed by Lind have resulted in the establishment of the virtual James Lind Library, documenting the history of development of fair tests in treatments in health care [5]. In 1914, Joseph Goldberger [6] observed that 8% of 418 patients admitted to the Georgia State Sanatorium developed pellagra, compared with

Box 5.1 The relevance of epidemiology to dermatology

- To quantify the burden of skin disease in the community
- To identify the causes or risk factors for skin diseases
- To describe the natural history, prognosis and disease associations of skin diseases
- To evaluate the effectiveness of prevention and treatment of skin disease and of the organisation of health care
- To provide a methodological framework for underpinning evidence-based practice in dermatology
- To provide appropriate methods for designing and interpreting clinical dermatological research

Table 5.1 Prevalence of scabies among 756 Kuna Indians on the island of Ticantiki, Panama.

Date	Community treatment status	Prevalence of scabies (%)
July 1986	Conventional treatment	33.0
October 1986	Community control and surveillance instituted	0.7
July 1987	Breakdown due to supply problem	3.6
December 1988	Programme running again	1.5
March 1990	US invasion of Panama	12.0

Adapted from Taplin et al. 1991 [3].

none of the 293 Sanatorium employees. He suggested that pellagra was due to an absence of 'essential vitamins', today recognised as nicotinic acid, and proceeded to test his suggestion in a community trial. Thus, dermatoepidemiology is not such a new subject, and with over 2000 skin disease reaction patterns described, the scope of the topic is vast. This chapter will therefore not deal with the epidemiology of specific skin diseases, which will be described where possible under the relevant disease sections. It will instead attempt to illustrate the relevance of modern epidemiology to dermatology by using specific examples. The principles of evidence-based dermatology, which relies heavily on methods developed from clinical epidemiology, are discussed in more detail in Chapter 17. A glossary of commonly used epidemiological terms and further reading sources are to be found at the end of this chapter.

Thinking in terms of populations rather than individuals

Community diagnosis and control

One of the first hurdles to overcome when considering the epidemiology of a skin disease is to think in terms of *populations* rather than *individuals*. Many physicians find this conceptual jump quite difficult as they are used to dealing with *individual* patients on a daily basis, whereas epidemiological studies refer to *groups* of individuals. Just as molecules, genes and individuals exhibit various aggregate characteristics, entire groups or populations exhibit their own unique characteristics and problems that enable a *community diagnosis* to be achieved [1].

Interesting patterns can occur when one explores the potential implications of treating an entire community (the public health approach) rather than sick individuals who present themselves to doctors (the high-risk approach). Rose [2], for example, showed that a 10 mm lowering of blood pressure distribution in an entire population (e.g. from reducing salt intake) would correspond to about a 30% reduction in the total attributable mortality, simply because of the shape of the change conferred on the distribution curve in relation to specific 'disease' cut-off points. In other words, a little bit of benefit spread across the entire population distribution may result in large population benefits in absolute terms.

During the scabies epidemics that occurred on the islands near Panama in the 1980s [3], it was found that even the best topical treatments when administered properly to individuals had no sustainable impact on the overall prevalence of scabies (which was very high in this population and was associated with considerable morbidity from secondary pyoderma). When a *population* approach was adopted, that is treating all individuals with a programme of continuing surveillance, the prevalence of scabies fell dramatically to less than 2%, as shown in Table 5.1, and was sustained at that level until the US invasion of Panama interrupted these efforts. Thus, just as individuals become 'diseased', entire populations can become sick [2]. In these situations, whether it be an infestation such as scabies or a disease of modern society such as obesity, tackling the problem based on a population diagnosis is usually beneficial, cost-effective and appropriate [4].

Population approaches are also critical to controlling infectious disease outbreaks. For example, there is little benefit in vaccinating a minority of enthusiastic or privileged individuals against SARS-CoV-2. High population coverage is needed in order to have a significant impact on disease transmission to produce herd immunity – a state whereby a large proportion of the community becomes immune to a disease making it difficult for the virus to spread [5]. Whilst not everyone, such as those with weak immune responses, is protected through vaccination, the group as a whole is protected as a result of making it difficult for the infectious agent to survive in enough people to spread – another example of why thinking in terms of populations rather than individuals is essential.

Skin diseases as 'entities' in the population

The concept of considering the health of entire populations also applies to the classification of skin diseases. Typically, dermatologists are preoccupied with deviants who present themselves to secondary and tertiary care because of troublesome symptoms associated with more severe or chronic disease and who are at the extreme end of the normal distribution curve of variations in skin health and disease. Such individuals usually have well-defined physical signs that prompt those studying them to declare them as discrete 'entities' [6,7]. Such distinctions often become blurred when community surveys are undertaken. In a community survey of atopic eczema, for instance [8], it was noticed that indeterminate or borderline cases who had limited areas of dry skin or a single patch of eczematous inflammation were quite common. In these circumstances, perhaps the more relevant question is not 'Has the person got eczema, yes/no?' but 'To what extent does this person have eczema?'

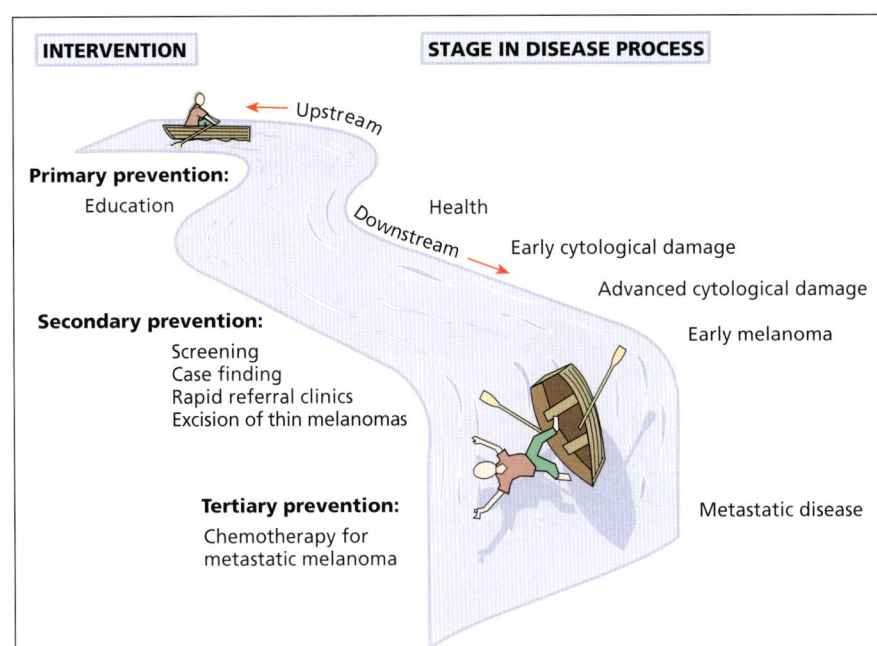

Figure 5.1 Disease prevention in a serious condition such as melanoma is much more sensible than treating sick individuals with expensive drugs at the end of a long chain of irreversible pathological events.

The concept of a continuum of skin disease or at least a distribution of disease severity at a population level may also be helpful in evaluating different treatment policies. For example, it has been estimated that a small change in the treatment threshold of isotretinoin from severe to moderate cases of acne could result in a 15-fold increase in prescriptions in absolute terms, simply because moderate cases outnumber severe cases by so much [9].

Making comparisons and drawing inferences

Epidemiological reasoning usually progresses in an ordered fashion, starting with a hypothesis that has been suggested by good clinical observations (e.g. palmoplantar psoriasis seems to be commoner in smokers) or descriptive studies of populations. The hypothesis (that smoking is a risk factor for palmoplantar psoriasis) is then tested in an epidemiological study, which gathers and analyses data in a systematic fashion in relation to an appropriate comparison group to see if a statistical association exists. Such a study was carried out, which confirmed a strong association between smoking prior to the onset of palmoplantar psoriasis [10]. *Analytical epidemiology* is therefore concerned with making comparisons. These comparisons rely upon the uneven distribution of disease and risk factors within and between populations to shed light on possible causes of ill health. Thus, previous case–control studies [11] showed that smoking was far more common in patients with lung cancer – a finding that led to more sophisticated studies to establish disease causality [12]. If everyone had smoked, it is unlikely that smoking would have been identified as a cause of lung cancer.

In the simplest form of epidemiological study, a count is made of the number of cases with a particular skin disease (the numerator) within a catchment population (the denominator). The probability or frequency of disease occurrence may then be compared in two or more populations – for example, one exposed to a putative causative agent compared with another that is not. Inferences are then drawn based on the magnitude of the differences of disease frequency between the populations considering possible alternative explanations such as chance, bias and confounding (see glossary). If such associations are genuine, further evidence is usually needed to determine whether they are causal in nature [13]. The whole process brings us one step nearer to the dermatoepidemiologist's ultimate goal – that of preventing skin disease, providing such causes are amenable to individual/public health manipulation. Prevention of skin disease, and hence any adverse consequences of having skin disease, is clearly a more desirable approach than treating a few diseased individuals who present to dermatologists after a long chain of pathological events (Figure 5.1).

When referring to an epidemiological study, it is important to make a distinction between the study population chosen for a particular study (e.g. those attending a hospital out-patient clinic) and the base population about whom one wishes to make inferences, as shown in Figure 5.2 [14].

The prevention paradox

Interventions that confer large population health gains may not confer much benefit as perceived by individuals. Thus, in the example of scabies in Panama [3], although the population's health as a whole benefited greatly, many apparently healthy individuals may have not appreciated being treated for scabies, as it was not known who would have developed scabies in the absence of the prevention programme. Similarly, it is difficult to say which child will benefit from being immunised for tuberculosis in a bacille Calmette–Guérin (BCG) immunisation programme, because events have not yet occurred. This conflict between large gains in the health of entire populations versus small gains in the health of individuals has been termed the 'prevention paradox' [4]. In the field of contact dermatitis, for example, eradication of a rare but potent contact sensitiser may have a great impact on affected individuals but little impact on the overall total burden of contact dermatitis in the general population. On the other hand, reduction in the amount of contact with formaldehyde, a less potent but far more common sensitiser in the general population, will result in a much larger

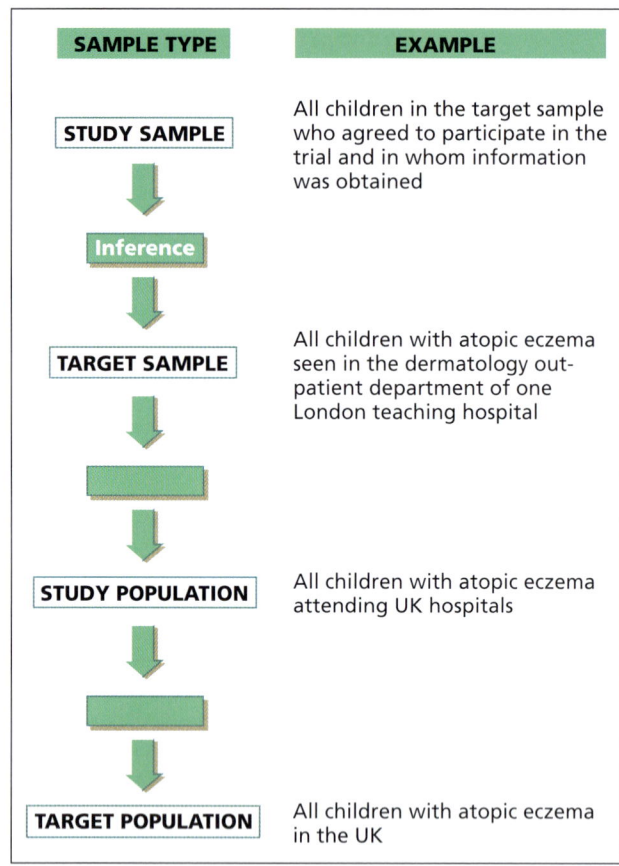

Figure 5.2 Generalising the results of a clinical trial of a new treatment for atopic eczema from a study of children attending one hospital department to all children with atopic eczema in the UK requires several jumps of inference.

Table 5.2 The prevention paradox: a little bit of harm affecting a lot of people can add up to more than a lot of harm affecting a few people.

	Eradication of exposure in:	
	The population	The individual
Rare: Exposure with high relative risk (e.g. contact sensitisation to diphencyprone)	Small benefit	Large benefit
Common: Exposure with low relative risk (e.g. smoking and psoriasis)	Large benefit	Small benefit

Reproduced from Williams 1996 [15] with permission of Karger.

reduction in the burden of contact dermatitis in that population, simply because far more people are exposed to formaldehyde [15]. As Table 5.2 illustrates, a little bit of harm affecting a lot of people can therefore add up to more than a lot of harm affecting a few people, in *population terms*. The first step when considering the epidemiology of skin disease is therefore to think about *populations* rather than *individuals*.

More than one disease?
Many of the conditions that are considered one disease today, such as atopic eczema and vitiligo, may turn out to be composed of several different diseases over time. Whilst it is easy to divide diseases into subtypes as a result of combinations of tests such as the division of atopic eczema into four subtypes on the basis of patch tests and immunoglobulin E (IgE) tests [16], the key issue when considering a change in nomenclature is that it should increase one's predictive ability – also known as progressive nosology. For example, the division of pemphigus, which formally referred to several diseases in which blistering was a feature, into pemphigus, pemphigoid, linear IgA disease and other variants on the basis of immunological discoveries, has been a key aspect to guiding the strength and duration of immunosuppressive therapy [17]. Techniques such as latent class analysis have been used with skin diseases such as hidradenitis suppurativa and atopic dermatitis that suggest that several main types may exist with different disease trajectories, which may require different treatment approaches [18,19]. The concept of stratified medicine based on exo-phenotypic features has been somewhat understudied and overshadowed by the concept of stratified or personalised medicine based on genetic or serological tests (the endo-phenotype).

How much of a public health problem is skin disease?

The need for a clear disease definition in epidemiological studies
A glance at the dermatological journals makes it clear that the subject matter of most current research is defined – wholly or in part – by diagnostic labels or criteria. But if these criteria are not explicitly stated, are prone to vary from one patient to the next in unpredictable ways, and vary systematically from place to place and in time, the usefulness of such research is gravely impaired. Although phrases such as 'diagnosed by experienced dermatologists' or 'all with typical symptoms' may be appropriate when dealing with individual patients, they are hopelessly inadequate when describing groups of individuals in epidemiological studies [1]. For instance, it has been shown that even experienced physicians are perfectly capable of disagreeing with each other over the classic signs of atopic eczema [2], and when two agree, a third is capable of disagreeing. What is regarded as 'typical' in London may be nothing of the sort in Lampeter, Lima, Lhasa or Lusaka.

Diagnostic criteria that work well in hospital studies may perform poorly in community studies because of the effect of low disease prevalence on positive predictive value (see glossary) and an increase in borderline cases. The properties of good diagnostic criteria for use in epidemiological studies are summarised in Box 5.2 [3].

Not only is it important to use diagnostic criteria of known validity and repeatability in epidemiological studies, but it is sometimes important to qualify cases identified by such criteria by some measure of disease severity (Box 5.3). For example, prevalence surveys of acne in the absence of severity measures are not very helpful in quantifying the disease problem, since physiological acne (non-inflammatory lesions) affects over 90% of adolescents [4]. Again, severity grading systems used in a hospital setting (which are usually non-linear and tend to favour severe and currently active disease) may not be so helpful in describing disease severity in milder community cases, where intermittent disease may be more common.

Box 5.2 Attributes of a good disease definition for use in epidemiological studies

- Validity: it measures what it purports to measure by including cases and excluding non-cases
- Repeatability: good replication of the definition between and within observers
- Acceptability to the study population in order to ensure high response rates
- Coherence with prevailing clinical concepts
- Easy to administer by field workers
- Reflects some degree of morbidity
- Comprehensiveness: applicable to a range of ages, ethnic groups and disease severities
- Comparability: they should contain elements that allow some comparison with previous studies

Reproduced from Williams 1997 [3] with permission of Taylor & Francis.

Box 5.3 Factors to consider when assessing skin disease severity at a population level

- Choose an instrument that is able to discern the whole range of severity from severe through to very mild disease
- Observers should be trained in the use of the severity examination methods and monitored against each other on a random selection of participants
- Consider pre-stating a cut-off point for defining 'significant' disease if measured in ordered categories or as a continuous score. For example, in acne, 'significant disease' could be defined as 'that associated with scarring'
- Consider the use of validated online or postal questionnaires; requiring a research nurse or doctor to examine thousands of cases is expensive and logistically difficult in population studies

Impairment, disability and handicap caused by skin disease

The burden of skin disease can refer to disease occurrence using terms such as prevalence or incidence (epidemiological burden), the effects of skin disease on a person's well-being (quality of life burden) or the direct and indirect costs associated with skin disease (economic burden). A working group affiliated to the US National Institute of Arthritis and Musculoskeletal and Skin Diseases (NIAMS) examined such conceptual frameworks in more detail, supplemented by thorough reviews of current data [5]. They concluded that further research is needed to reach consensus on how skin diseases and their associated burden should be defined.

In addition to the concept of burden, consideration of the three concepts of impairment, disability and handicap may be helpful in separating those effects that result from disordered function from those that are conferred on individuals by society. Impairment refers to the organic lesion produced by a disease, for example a broken limb; disability is the dysfunction that results from that impairment, for example not being able to walk; and handicap is the disadvantage that society confers upon the individual as a result of the impairment, for example unemployment. Handicap

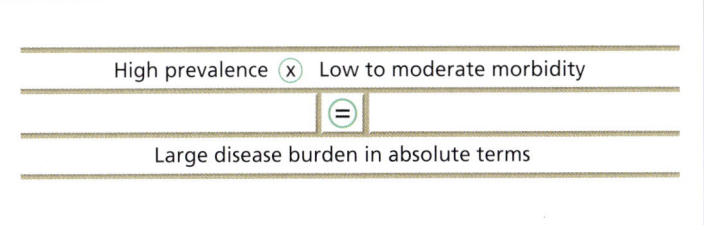

Figure 5.3 Skin disease is a major public health problem: in public health terms, a little bit of misery affecting a lot of people can add up to more than serious illnesses that affect only a few people.

in skin disease may not be as explicit as that associated with a broken limb, but the psychological consequences of skin disease, which include 'failure of display' [6,7], may be just as important. The concepts of stigma, discrimination and bias in relation to visible skin disease have been described for a wide range of skin diseases from psoriasis to neglected tropical diseases [8], but have received less specific research focus compared with quantitative aspects. Interestingly, it has been shown that relatively minor skin complaints often cause more anguish to people than other more 'serious' medical problems [6]. Also, because skin disease is so common, a little bit of morbidity affecting a lot of people can add up to far more in absolute terms at a population level than a lot of morbidity affecting only a few people. It is this product of high prevalence times moderate morbidity that makes skin disease very important from the public health point of view (Figure 5.3). Small changes in health policies for skin diseases such as changing the threshold for referring people to dermatologists with a pigmented lesion can have large financial implications and knock-on effects for other diseases, simply because they affect so many people.

One population-based, cross-sectional study conducted in the USA on a random sample of 20 479 people examined by dermatologists in 1971–74 [9] has pointed to the magnitude of disability and handicap from skin diseases: skin conditions were reported to limit activity in 10.5 per 1000 of the population aged 1–74 years, or 9% of those persons with such skin conditions. About 10% of those with skin complaints considered the condition to be a handicap to their employment or housework, and 1% considered themselves to be severely handicapped. About one-third of those persons with skin conditions indicated that the condition(s) were a handicap in their social relations. The dermatological examiners rated more than two-thirds of those with skin complaints as disfigured to some extent from the condition, and about one-fifth of those were rated moderately or severely disfigured. More than half of those with skin complaints reported some overall discomfort from the condition, such as itching or burning. An estimated 62.8 per 1000 US civilians (or 56% of those with skin complaints) indicated that the conditions were recurrent, with 49% active in the preceding 7–12 months.

The 1989 UK General Household Survey estimated that 16 per 1000 persons were affected by a longstanding skin disorder sufficiently severe to limit their activities [10]. Another survey of disability, amongst 14 000 adults conducted in the mid-1980s, found that 1% of complaints causing disability in private households and 2% in communal establishments were due to skin disease [11]. A survey of self-reported skin problems in 8000 adults in Uppland, Sweden, found that 20.5% reported skin problems [12]. Those reporting skin problems scored lower on all eight dimensions of the SF-36, a generic quality of life instrument.

In addition to disability and handicap, some chronic skin diseases such as atopic eczema also incur considerable additional direct costs to families, such as that needed to purchase moisturisers, special soaps, cotton clothing and bedding and extra laundry expenses. The Lothian Atopic Dermatitis Study estimated that the mean cost to the patient was £25.90 per 2 months, while the mean cost to the UK National Health Service was £16.20 in 1994 [13]. A systematic review of cost studies of atopic eczema in the USA found very wide-ranging estimates of 364 million to $3.8 billion per year, with very little information on indirect costs [14]. Another study estimated the direct cost of care for patients with psoriasis and psoriatic arthritis in the USA [15]. An ambitious project in the USA tried to estimate the direct and indirect costs of people with 22 of the commonest skin disease categories in 2004 and found that they accounted for around $29 billion in direct costs (medical care and products), $10 billion in lost productivity costs and a further $56 billion for loss of quality of life [16]. The recent expansion in use of high-cost biologic and small molecule drugs for severe skin diseases, such as psoriasis and eczema, and targeted therapies for cancer, e.g. melanoma, mean that focusing on economic aspects of skin diseases and their therapies is a key priority in terms of allocating resources. Cost-effectiveness thresholds may need to be applied, which are likely to be context-specific for specific geographies and settings. Quantifying skin disease burden in the elderly is particularly scant and requires more research in order to better serve the increasingly ageing population in many countries [17]. The same need for better data applies to people with skin of colour if they are to be served well by policy and clinical service developers [18].

Global Burden of Disease study

Estimating the global burden of skin disease in a standardised way remained elusive until the publication of the Global Burden of Disease 2010 (GBD 2010) study data [19]. Previous attempts at summarising world health in general had significant methodological shortcomings [20], many of which have been overcome by the GBD 2010 survey. The GBD 2010 survey (updated in various forms up to 2019 at the time of writing) covers all human disease and uses sophisticated Bayesian methods for estimating prevalence, incidence, mortality and disability for over 200 human diseases in 187 countries, broken down by age and sex, for the period 1990–2010. Data on disability-adjusted life years and years lived with disability for all diseases and injuries have been published elsewhere [21,22]. We illustrate the usefulness of GBD data by referring to GBD 2010 as it still contains the most comprehensive description of skin data that have been assembled as a result of an exhaustive search for relevant studies. Skin data for GBD 2010 include a description of disability caused by 16 common non-fatal skin groups: eczema, psoriasis, acne, alopecia areata, pruritus, pressure ulcers, urticaria, scabies, fungal skin diseases, impetigo, abscess and other bacterial skin diseases, cellulitis, viral warts, molluscum contagiosum/warts, non-melanoma skin cancer and other skin problems. These are described by country, age and sex in 187 countries. The key measures of disability used to describe the data include years lost due to disability (YLD) and the disability-adjusted life year (DALY). One DALY can be thought of as a year of lost healthy life, and is calculated by adding the sum of the years of life lost (YLL) due to premature mortality combined with the YLD for people living with the health condition or its consequences [23]. Assumptions used to calculate these estimates are described fully elsewhere [19].

Figure 5.4 shows the YLD due to the main 16 skin condition groupings by region in 2010 as a proportion of total YLD and as YLD per 100 000 of the population. Higher rates of disability due to infectious skin diseases are seen in regions such as Africa, whereas disorders such as pruritus and eczema are higher in Europe. Figure 5.5 shows YLD for skin disease according to age, and reveals a striking bimodal distribution with one peak in early life largely due to eczema and acne and a steady rise in a range of skin diseases in older life. Eczema as a group emerges as the commonest reason for YLD across the regions and over the different age groups. Figure 5.6 attempts to show the global distribution of DALYs for skin disease and illustrates the disproportionate burden of skin disease mainly in sub-Saharan Africa and lower rates across large parts of Russia, Mongolia and China.

When compared with other diseases, skin conditions in 2010 ranked as the fourth leading cause of non-fatal burden expressed as YLDs and as the 18th cause of DALYs. Three skin diseases (fungal infections, other skin and subcutaneous diseases, and acne) were amongst the 10 most common diseases globally, and another five (eczema, pruritus, molluscum/warts, impetigo and scabies) appeared in the top 50.

Karimkhani *et al.* have updated some aspects of GBD skin disease data up to 2013 [**24**], producing useful maps of DALYs for 15 common skin diseases according to age and 21 regions of the world (Figure 5.7). GBD 2013 showed that DALYs for skin and subcutaneous diseases ranked 18th globally and 4th for non-fatal disease burden. To provide some context, skin diseases ranked directly behind iron deficiency anaemia and tuberculosis. When mortality data are excluded, YLDs as a result of skin diseases (36.4 million) are greater than those for diabetes mellitus (29.5 million).

Others have interrogated the GBD data sets up to 2017 for quantifying the burden of specific skin diseases such as atopic dermatitis [25], psoriasis [26], leishmaniasis [27] and scabies [28], and have illustrated trends over time, co-morbidities and disparities according to age and geography. More detailed estimates of skin disease burden for specific countries such as Canada [29], Iran [30] and the USA [31] have also been produced that are helpful in health care planning. Skin disease data by gender and location can be interrogated freely from the GBD study using their Epi Visualization Hub [32].

Although the GBD data have limitations – such as missed studies and sparse data from some parts of the world – it is nevertheless the most comprehensive attempt to collate data and model missing data for disfigurement and other sequelae from skin diseases using a robust and explicit approach. The surveys provide essential data for health service planning and suggest that skin disease is a priority for most countries across the world. Some have already used the data, along with other sources, to come up with a World Health Organization list of essential medicines for skin disease [33].

It is important to point out that all of the above data refer to non-fatal skin disease, and that data on all diseases with significant impacts on mortality (including diseases treated by dermatologists such as melanoma and infectious diseases) up to 2019 have been

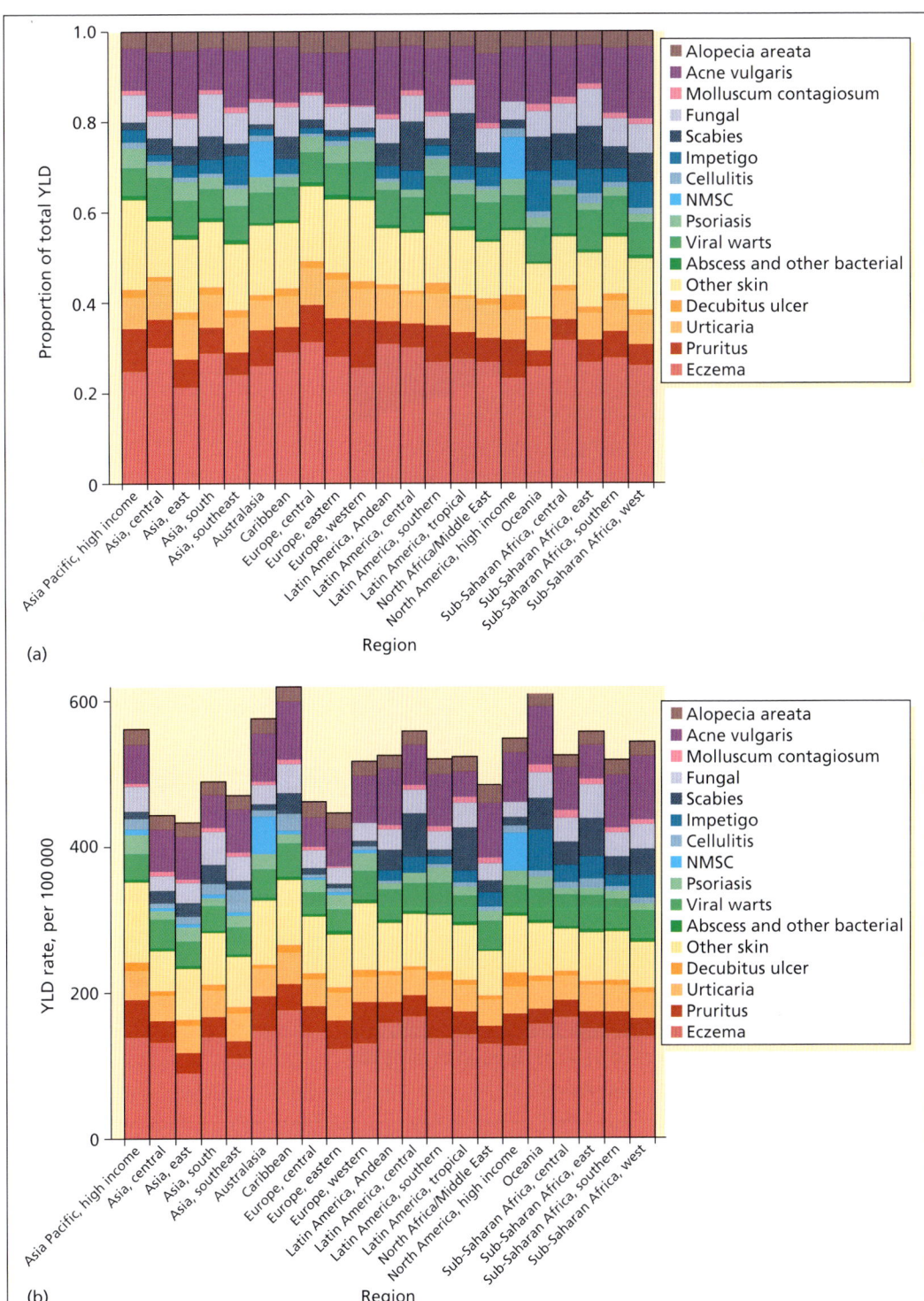

Figure 5.4 Years lost due to disability (YLD) for the main 16 skin condition groupings by world region in 2010 as a proportion of total YLD and as YLD per 100 000 of the population. NMSC, non-melanoma skin cancer. Reproduced from Hay et al. 2014 [19] with permission of Elsevier.

collated in other key publications [34]. Not surprisingly, infectious diseases such as dengue fever and measles appear as the top causes of mortality for skin disorders. Although the number of people diagnosed with melanoma increases steadily in older age, it is one of those cancers that seems to have a disproportionate mortality impact in younger, economically active people. Non-melanoma skin cancer, although rarely associated with mortality, shows mortality rates approaching melanoma, probably due to the much larger number of tumours (especially squamous cell carcinoma) involved.

What determines the frequency of skin disease in populations?

Risk factors, association and causation

In the first instance, epidemiological studies seek to establish *risk factors* for diseases, that is, factors that are *associated* with an increased frequency of disease. The term 'risk factors' can be used to describe factors that predict outcomes of interest (e.g. identifying who is at risk of a disease such as heart attack in a predictive statistical model)

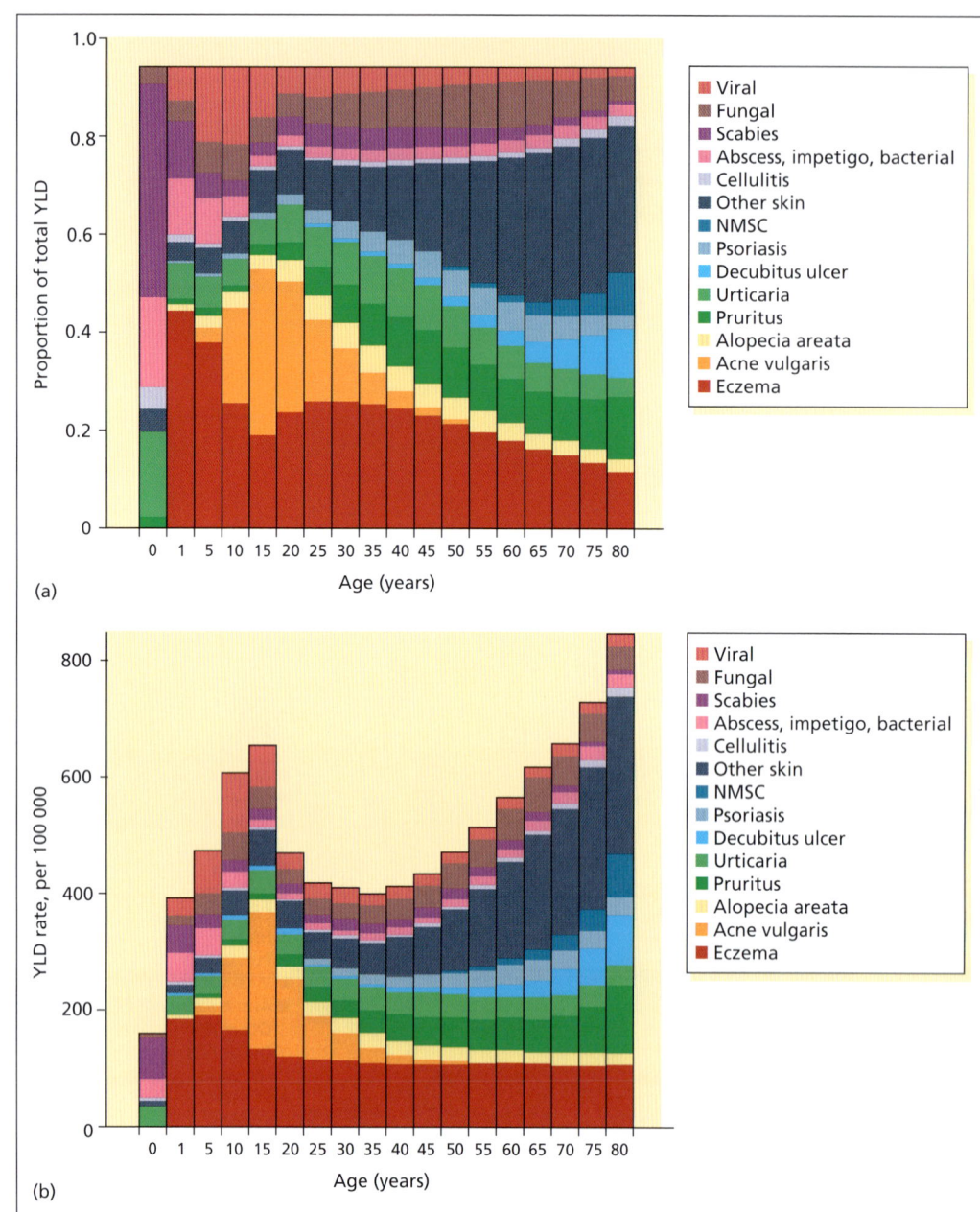

Figure 5.5 Years lost due to disability (YLD) for skin disease according to age from the 2010 Global Burden of Disease study showing a peak in younger life and a steady increase in burden in later life. NMSC, non-melanoma skin cancer. Reproduced from Hay *et al.* 2014 [19] with permission of Elsevier.

or explanatory factors that may help identify potential targets for intervention [1]. This chapter is using the term 'risk factors' to mean explanatory factors for skin diseases rather than predictors of who will develop skin disease.

When *associations* between skin diseases and risk factors are discovered (e.g. by demonstrating an increased risk of palmoplantar psoriasis in smokers [2]), it should be understood that such *associations* do not necessarily imply *causation*. The association between smoking and psoriasis may simply be a *chance* finding (around 1 in 20 studies with a *P* value of less than 0.05 in favour of rejecting the null hypothesis of no association will be wrong due to chance alone), or it could be due to *confounding* (i.e. a third factor such as alcohol or social class, which is independently associated with both smoking and psoriasis [3]). The association could be due to a *bias* – for example, people with psoriasis in hospital may be more likely to recall antecedent events or seek reasons for explaining their illness in comparison with healthy controls [4]. Further analyses or new studies are usually needed to establish whether risk factors are *causative* – for example, by evaluating the strength of the association, biological gradient, relationship in time, consistency between different studies, biological plausibility, coherence of evidence with external sources, experimental evidence and specificity of findings as suggested by the Bradford-Hill checklist for causality [5]. Recent studies also incorporate additional approaches such as Mendelian randomisation to help provide additional insights into causality; in this technique, genetic variants are used as natural experiments in an effort to reduce confounding. Such an approach has recently been used to demonstrate evidence for causality in associations between psoriasis and obesity [6].

The causes of some skin diseases are already established – for example, the herpes simplex virus causes cold sores – but for most

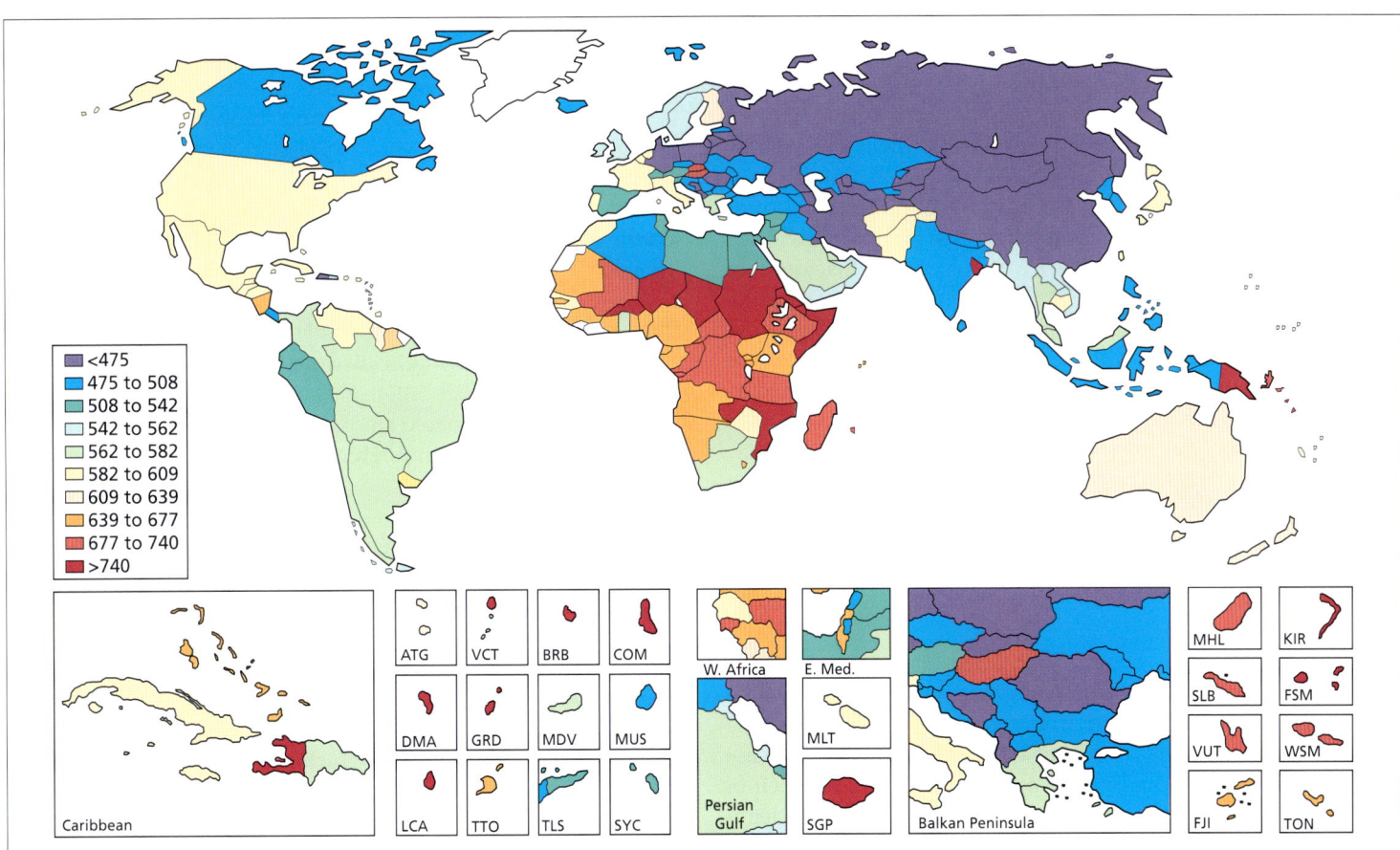

Figure 5.6 Global distribution of disability-adjusted life years (DALYs) for skin disease from the 2010 Global Burden of Disease study illustrating the disproportionate burden of skin disease in sub-Saharan Africa. Reproduced from Hay et al. 2014 [19] with permission of Elsevier.

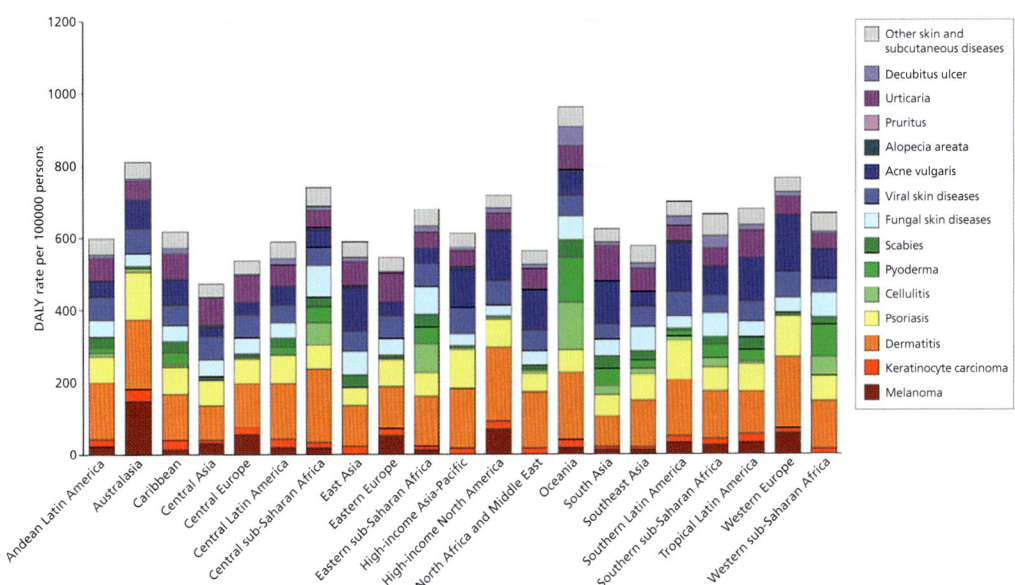

Figure 5.7 Regional distribution of skin and subcutaneous disease burden from the 2013 update of the Global Burden of Disease survey. This figure shows rate of disability-adjusted life years (DALY) per 100 000 persons from 15 skin disease categories throughout 21 world regions. Reproduced from Karimkhani et al. 2017 [24] with permission of American Medical Association/CC BY 4.0.

dermatological conditions the causes are unknown. Nevertheless, epidemiological research has established many *risk factors* for skin diseases which may help to serve as pointers to specific causes. Direct manipulation of these risk factors may help in preventing or reducing disease even before the specific cause is found. For example, in the London cholera epidemics of the 1850s, John Snow [7] postulated that the disease was spread by some 'morbid matter' in the water supply and proceeded to intervene by removing the pump handle in Broad Street. This resulted in a dramatic fall in incident cholera cases. All of this occurred some 20 years before germ theory had become established in Europe. Snow's work illustrates one of the beauties of epidemiological research, which is that knowledge of pathophysiology is not a prerequisite for determining aetiology.

Even when a causative agent is discovered, for example *Vibrio cholerae*, exposure to this agent does not necessarily imply disease. Of those exposed to cholera during an outbreak, some will die from the disease, some will be very ill, some will be slightly unwell, some will be apparently healthy (but still carry the organism) and some will not be affected at all. The absence of disease in some individuals following exposure is probably due to a whole range of factors such as chance, infecting dose, genetic heterogeneity and other constitutional and environmental factors that interact together to produce the final clinical picture. This phenomenon of apparent health in the presence of an established harmful exposure has been exploited by individuals in order to avoid modifying their behaviour. One often hears statements such as 'my grandfather smoked 40 cigarettes a day all his life and he did not get lung cancer' in order to justify their habits. In order to explain such phenomena, we return to the epidemiological concept of *groups* of people or *populations* and *probability* of disease [8]. On average, *groups* of people who smoke cigarettes are 10 times more likely to develop lung cancer when compared with those who do not smoke.

It is also important to separate risk factors associated with disease *incidence*, that is the number of new cases in a given population occurring over a defined period, from those that determine disease *chronicity*, that is the determinants of how long a particular disease will last once an individual has it, as the risk factors for each of these aspects may be different. Although many dermatoepidemiology surveys have measured the *prevalence* of skin disease when examining risk factors [9], prevalence is a function of incidence times chronicity. It is therefore often difficult to say in such studies whether these risk factors are important in people developing a disease for the first time, or if they lead to disease flares or maintain the disease once established. Measuring risk factors and disease in prevalence studies can also lead to the problem of reverse causality; for example, parents may remove pets from the household once eczema has developed in their child, resulting in a paradoxical protective effect of pet exposure and reduced eczema when measured at a single point in time [10].

Risk factors for skin disease may operate at many different levels. Some may predispose to disease (e.g. a parent with atopic eczema genetically predisposes their child to atopic eczema), some may precipitate disease (e.g. exposure to high levels of house-dust mite may precipitate atopic eczema for the first time) and some may be important in perpetuating that disease (e.g. failure to use prescribed treatments may worsen the course of atopic eczema). Some of the commonest risk factors for skin disease are discussed here.

Genetics

In addition to a few rare diseases such as epidermolysis bullosa, where specific chromosomal mutations have been closely correlated with different disease phenotypes, many genes may be important in many of the major inflammatory skin diseases. Thus, in atopic eczema, genes such as filaggrin mutations that play a key role in skin barrier function, as well as several other genes that code for inflammatory responses, may be important in explaining the variation in disease phenotype [11]. Genes such as those that predispose for melanoma may only express their beneficial or deleterious effects when individuals who carry them are additionally exposed to key environmental risk factors such as ultraviolet (UV) light [12]. Some genes may be responsible for disease predisposition and some may be responsible for disease severity and chronicity, as exemplified by molecular subsets in the gene expression signatures in the skin in scleroderma [13].

Early environment

There is evidence to suggest that the experience of the fetus *in utero* (e.g. in terms of nutrition) is critical in 'programming' adult diseases such as hypertension and diabetes [14]; *in utero* programming may well operate for many skin diseases such as atopic eczema [15]. Epigenetics is another interesting field whereby environmental exposures such as tobacco smoke or dietary factors may induce a persistent genetic state through gene transcription [16].

Later environment

Age and sex are often included in the descriptive epidemiology of many skin diseases and may point to further risk factors. The marked female preponderance of lichen sclerosus, for example, suggests that hormonal factors may be important in this disease.

Ethnic group may account for some variations in disease rates. Thus, it has been shown that atopic eczema is twice as common in black Caribbean children in comparison with similar white children in the UK [17]. Ethnic group, which refers to a way of life encompassing a whole range of dietary and cultural factors, must be distinguished from racial factors [18], which are often more difficult to define. Care also has to be taken in lumping many distinct ethnic groups together – for example, combining the diverse cultures of black Africans and black Caribbeans into people with black skin may be inappropriate, both in terms of respecting the identity of the separate cultures and because such lumping together may obscure important epidemiological associations [19]. The term 'race' should not be used in epidemiological studies as it has no scientific meaning [20]. Migration itself may be an important factor in determining skin diseases; for example, individuals who migrated from China (where atopic eczema is not very common) developed much higher rates of disease (similar to the rates in the local population) after migration to Hawaii [21]. Migrants may not be totally representative of their indigenous peoples, but they may nevertheless show the effect of the environment in determining the frequency of skin disease.

Secular factors may reflect changes in the natural history of skin disease or of transient environmental exposures. Thus, the epidemic of melanoma skin cancer has been attributed by some to increased exposure to sunlight over the last 50 years. However, recent epidemiological studies have suggested that some of this increase may relate to increased ascertainment as there is no associated increase in mortality rates [22,23]. There is now clear evidence from the International Study of Asthma and Allergies in Childhood that the prevalence of atopic eczema has increased in most countries across the world over a 10-year period with some evidence of plateauing in high-income, westernised countries, but the reasons for this change are less clear [24].

Socioeconomic factors may also be crucial in accounting for the distribution of skin disease. In many poorer countries where overcrowding and poor sanitation may occur, infectious or ectoparasitic skin diseases such as secondarily infected scabies or pediculosis are commoner [25,26]. In wealthier countries, where such infectious dermatoses are less common, new 'diseases' such as concern regarding the cosmetic appearance of sun-damaged skin or thread veins may preoccupy the population in their quest for a perfect skin. Some skin diseases, such as atopic eczema, also demonstrate a genuine positive social class trend: that is, higher prevalences in more wealthy groups [9]. Some of this increase in reported eczema may have been due to differences in reporting between socioeconomic groups, but other genuine environmental factors such as hygiene, carpets, central heating, family size or differences in treatment and other health-seeking behaviours also probably play a part.

Geography and climate are important considerations in describing the frequency of skin disease. Thus, consideration of the marked latitude gradient of melanoma in white-skinned peoples has supported the concept that exposure to sunlight is an important risk factor for this disease [27]. Paul [28] has drawn attention to the concepts of *macroclimate*, which in the ordinary geographic sense refers to temperature, rainfall and humidity, and *microclimate*, which refers to the immediate domestic and occupational environment a given individual finds themselves in. These are discussed further by Marshall [29] and Canizares [30]. The combination of temperature, rainfall and humidity may be crucial to sustain certain infectious disease vectors such as the *Simulium* fly in onchocerciasis, and may for example account for seasonal fluctuations in pyoderma secondary to scabies during the wet season in Lilongwe in Malawi [31]. An elegant study by Silverberg *et al.* merged data on the self-report of eczema from 91 642 children aged up to 17 years with national climatic data and reported a lower prevalence of eczema to be associated with higher outdoor humidity, high UV exposure and higher temperatures when analysed across the USA [32].

Occupational factors are occasionally a very important factor for skin disease. Thus, exposure to irritants and contact sensitisers in light and heavy industry accounts for a very large burden of hand dermatitis and lost revenue for both individuals and the state. Certain occupations, for example mining, where workers are constantly exposed to damp conditions, may predispose to fungal infections. Some diseases may occasionally occur in outbreaks from work-related substances, for example chloracne due to dioxins, vinyl chloride disease and hydroquinone-induced leukomelanoderma. The reader is referred to standard texts of occupational dermatoses and to Chapter 129 for further reading [33,34].

Infective agents may directly cause or be suspected to cause many skin diseases. Thus, for a long time it was suspected that fifth disease was caused by an infectious agent, but it was not until 1983 that human parvovirus B19 was identified as the causative organism [35]. Similarly, there is reasonable circumstantial evidence to suggest that diseases such as pityriasis rosea are caused by infectious agents, even though no specific agents have yet been consistently isolated [36,37]. Recent reports of skin manifestations related to SARS-CoV-2 infection in international registry and hospital-based settings provide clues to Covid-19 diagnosis in asymptomatic individuals [38], but would benefit from further assessment in a cohort study design with careful considerations of causality.

Dietary factors may be crucial in some skin diseases. As the examples of Lind and Goldberger in the opening section of this chapter illustrated, vitamin deficiency states may directly cause skin diseases. Other deficiency diseases with skin manifestations, such as acrodermatitis enteropathica, are completely reversible with the administration of the appropriate agent, in this case zinc. Some diseases, such as phenylketonuria and dermatitis herpetiformis, may be transformed by restricting substances that affected individuals cannot handle – for example, phenylalanine and gluten, respectively. Some skin diseases, such as atopic eczema and acute urticaria, may be modified by the avoidance of dietary allergens in a proportion of affected individuals. Leisure activities such as gardening or habits such as smoking cigarettes and drinking alcohol may be important risk factors for many skin diseases including contact dermatitis, psoriasis and porphyria cutanea tarda. Medicines, although intended to alleviate human disease, are a very common cause of cutaneous eruptions, some of which (e.g. toxic epidermal necrolysis) can be fatal. Recent evidence from a range of international epidemiological studies demonstrated strong associations between the use of antihypertensive drugs and increased skin cancer risks [39], resulting in new guidance from the Food and Drug Administration to increase awareness of this association amongst prescribers of these medicines [40].

Describing the natural history and associations of specific skin diseases

Patients with a skin disease often ask 'How long will it last?' and 'Will it come back again?', yet reliable answers to such questions are scarce. Special studies are required to answer these questions, which ideally involve following, over many years, individuals with typical and well-defined disease in terms of morphology and severity [1]. Such prospective studies are rare in dermatology [2]. Another approach is to identify people with a specific skin disease from old hospital records and then to trace them in order to find out what has happened to them since they were seen [3]. Studies on the natural history of disease are often difficult to interpret because of incomplete follow-up, the intermittent nature of many skin diseases, which can make the distinction between 'real' and 'apparent' clearance rates difficult [4], and because the treatment of many diseases can improve over time, rendering some with mild disease into the non-diseased category when they would previously have been classified as diseased. Guidelines regarding the attributes of what makes a good follow-up study are summarised elsewhere [**5**].

Disease associations of specific skin diseases may also give insight into possible causative factors. Thus, the high incidence of laryngeal carcinoma in psoriasis patients might be evidence for the possible role of cigarette smoking in psoriasis [6]. Many publications have emerged over the last 7 years linking psoriasis with the metabolic syndrome and cardiovascular events, suggesting that psoriasis is a systemic disease and that patients with psoriasis should be screened for cardiovascular risk factors [7,8]. Establishing disease co-occurrence, for example atopic eczema and psoriasis, may also shed light on shared or opposing immunopathological mechanisms [9–11]. Great care has to be exercised in interpreting disease associations generated from hospital sources because, in the absence of an appropriate denominator, many types of bias may occur [12].

Recent advances related to the increasing availability of international electronic health records and administrative data (collectively known as routinely collected health data) have transformed dermatoepidemiology research. These data sources are usually very large, often population-based, and may have key linked information on hospitalisation and demographic data, sometimes involving the whole population of a country, for example Denmark [13]. They provide unprecedented opportunities to answer questions that require very large sample sizes or where prolonged follow-up time is required, and they are an efficient method as data already exist; however, researchers have no opportunity to influence the collection of data, hence issues relating to misclassification and residual confounding are important to understand. Data linkage from large representative general practitioner databases has yielded valuable insights into disease associations such as an increased risk of stroke following chickenpox [14], a threefold increase in mortality for patients with pyoderma gangrenosum [15], a relative lack of association between atopic eczema and cancers except lymphomas [16] and increased risk of attention deficit hyperactivity disorder in children with atopic eczema [17].

Health services research in dermatology

Broadly defined, dermatological health services research is concerned with studying how dermatological health care is delivered with the ultimate aim of benefiting patients. Dermatological health services research thus covers a wide variety of service aspects, such as determinants of referrals to hospital departments, evaluation of cost-effectiveness of alternative treatment strategies, quantifying the dermatological needs of the community, evaluating the role of teledermatology and dermatological nurses and exploring economic aspects of screening and other prevention strategies. These diverse studies require a range of quantitative and qualitative research methods, such as focus groups, surveys, analysis of routinely collected referral and outcome data, before and after studies, comparative studies, interrupted time series, action research (studying the process and outcomes of change, often involving people who deliver care), randomised controlled trials, decision analysis and health economic modelling alongside evidence syntheses. Research establishes which treatments or services should be used, whereas audit seeks to establish whether health care providers perform these services to a required standard [1]. As in any other branch of epidemiology, health services research requires meticulous attention to be given to aspects of study design. A useful introduction to health services research in dermatology is given elsewhere [2].

Needs assessments in dermatology

When evaluating dermatological health services, certain steps need to be followed [3]:
1 Establish the size and nature of the dermatological need based on epidemiological data.
2 Summarise the currently available supply of services for that problem.
3 Appraise the evidence for effectiveness of those services.
4 Propose models of care that best fit the epidemiological data and evidence of effectiveness of care within current resources.
5 Propose outcome measures and targets that can be monitored after implementation.

Table 5.3 A guide to the number of persons per 100 000 per year using dermatology services in the UK.

Group	Number using service
Number with a skin complaint	25 000 (at least 25% of total population)
Number who will self-treat	7500 (30% of those with skin complaint)
Number who will seek advice from their GP	14 550[a] (15% of total population or 19% of all GP consultations)
Number referred to dermatologist	1162 (8% of those attending their GP for skin problems, or 1.2% of the total population)
Number admitted to hospital	24–31 (2–3% of all new dermatology referrals)
Number of deaths due to skin disease	5[b] (0.4% of all new dermatology referrals)

Reproduced from Williams 1997 [4] with permission of Radcliffe Group.
[a] Excludes skin neoplasms, viral warts, herpes simplex and scabies.
[b] Includes people dying from cellulitis, chronic ulcer of the skin and severe drug reactions who might not have been admitted under a dermatologist's care.

Such an assessment has been attempted for UK dermatological health services by this author [4], and a comprehensive update of the assessment was undertaken by Schofield *et al*. [5].

Services available for people with skin diseases

People with skin problems obtain help from various sources, including self-help, increasing use of social media, advice from pharmacists, and advice and treatment from the primary care team and specialist services. Little research has been conducted to clarify the relative health gain and appropriateness of the various health care settings for different subgroups of skin disease. The estimated number of people using current dermatology health services in the UK at various entry points, for a population of 100 000 over a 1-year period, is summarised in Table 5.3 [6–11].

Self-help

Although self-help/medication is not traditionally regarded as a health service, the range and availability of over-the-counter skin products are important elements in the equation of balancing need, supply and demand. Around 30% of those with a skin complaint decide to self-medicate, and this proportion is similar for trivial and for moderate to severe disease [6]. Many effective skin treatments are available over the counter in the UK, such as 1% hydrocortisone for mild eczema, topical aciclovir cream for cold sores, topical benzoyl peroxide for acne, and numerous antifungal preparations and wart removers. Pharmacists occupy a key role in advising the public on the use of these products, but whether this advice is beneficial or whether it simply delays appropriate medical consultation has not been studied adequately in the UK [12]. Self-help groups are often a useful source of advice and support for those with chronic skin diseases, with expanding recent use of social media for these purposes, but with much less oversight regarding the quality of that information, and emerging evidence that such guidance is frequently not coherent with standard guidance [13,14].

Primary care

The majority of those with a skin complaint who seek medical help in the UK and some other countries such as Canada and the Netherlands are treated by their family practitioner (general practitioner or GP). Skin conditions were the most frequent reason for people in England and Wales to consult their GP with a new problem in 2006, which equates to around 6.1% (0.8 million) of the population (12.9 million people). The most common reasons were skin infections and eczema [5]. In the USA, it has been estimated that around 36.5% of patients attending their family practitioner over a 2-year period had a skin complaint [15]. The range of skin disorders seen in general practice is similar to that in the general population, with relatively few subcategories accounting for the majority of consultations. As one would anticipate, proportionally more incident diseases such as skin infections (e.g. impetigo, herpes simplex and viral exanthems) are seen in general practice than in secondary care [8].

Secondary care

Although dermatology covers around 2000 disease–reaction patterns, over 70% of specialist activity is concerned with fewer than 10 main disease categories, as shown in Box 5.4 [4]. Age-specific attendance rates are more common in female patients and also rise with increasing age. Around 12% of referrals were considered inappropriate by dermatologists in one UK study [15]. There is considerable variation in referral rates to specialist care within the UK and there is some evidence to suggest that much of the regional variation in referral rates may be governed by established patterns of care and the number of available consultants, rather than by any objective dermatological need [4]. Roland and Morris [16] showed no relationship between referral rates for dermatology services and medical need as suggested by standardised mortality ratios or mean number of prescriptions issued by GPs (standardised regression coefficient of 0.1). It should be emphasised, though, that mortality ratios are not a suitable surrogate measure for dermatological need. A strong relationship between dermatology referral rates and the number of dermatology consultants per 100 000 population was present, however, in their study (standardised regression coefficient of 0.82, $P <0.001$).

> **Box 5.4 The nine categories of skin disease that account for over 70% of dermatological diagnoses in primary and secondary care**
>
> - Skin cancer (including melanoma)
> - Acne
> - Atopic eczema
> - Psoriasis
> - Viral warts
> - Other infective skin conditions
> - Benign tumours and vascular lesions
> - Leg ulceration
> - Contact dermatitis and other eczemas
>
> Reproduced from Williams 1997 [4] with permission of Radcliffe Group.

Digital transformations

Digital technologies and care pathways using teledermatology are likely to play an increasingly important part in the delivery of specialist care and the self-help/primary/secondary care interface in the future with tools for patients to assess their own disease severity [17]. Smartphone applications that may help skin diagnosis such as VisualDx and Derm Assist are already in existence, as are digital pathology technologies [18]. Digital technologies may not be a substitute for all aspects of dermatological care and some technologies may result in harm, for example algorithm-based smartphone apps missing cases of melanoma and delaying time-critical diagnosis [19]. It is also critical that digital technologies are developed and tested in the populations they are intended to be used in, using the entire spectrum of skin colours and not just predominantly white skin populations, if they are to achieve equality in the populations that they purport to serve [20].

Relationship between need, supply and demand for dermatological care

Unlike commerce, which aims to balance supply with demand, caring for sick human beings requires consideration of a third factor – that of medical need. Medical need may be defined as the ability to benefit from medical care; demand as that which people ask for; and supply as what the service does or could provide [3,4]. Not all dermatological need is demanded (e.g. a person may be unaware that they have an early melanoma), not all that is demanded is needed (e.g. cosmetic removal of all moles), although all that is supplied is usually needed or demanded. The division between what constitutes reasonable need (e.g. somebody worried that a mole may be cancerous) and demand (e.g. somebody requesting removal of an 'ugly' mole) is especially blurred in dermatology. Defining 'need' in dermatology is therefore quite difficult, and is a process that requires the participation of society so that appropriate policies can be set in the light of finite resources.

Two population surveys conducted in the 1970s have produced useful data on the relationship between the need, supply and demand for dermatological care. In a study of 2180 adults in the London borough of Lambeth who were examined for skin disease [7], it was shown that for those with moderate/severe skin disease, only 24% had made use of any medical service in the previous 6 months. A further 30% had used self-medication. Medical usage was still considerable for those with trivial skin disease, with 10% using medical services and 33% self-medicating.

In the US HANES-1 study [21], there was a considerable mismatch between what the dermatologists considered to represent medical need and what the population were concerned about. Only one-third (31%) of persons with significant skin pathology diagnosed by the dermatologists expressed concern about these specific skin conditions, whereas nearly 18% of those who complained about their skin conditions were not considered to have serious conditions by the dermatologists. Thus, both of these population studies suggest that, at any one time, around one-quarter to one-third of the population have a skin problem that could benefit from medical care, yet around 80% do not seek medical help.

The relationship between need, supply and demand for dermatology services in developing countries may be very different from that in developed countries. Many surveys have shown a high prevalence of need, mainly due to infectious dermatoses. There is marked maldistribution of care for people with skin diseases throughout the world, with meagre to absent dermatological services in many countries. Leprosy, onchocerciasis and leishmaniasis are probably the commonest skin diseases worldwide, but the epidemiological research afforded to these diseases is usually scanty. Groups such as the International Foundation for Dermatology work to remedy such inequalities, with the ultimate aim of a healthy skin for all [22]. Getting the right people to the right services is a major challenge. In the state of Guerrero in Mexico, for instance, skin complaints represent the second commonest reason for referral to rural clinics, resulting in a detrimental effect on other important activities such as vaccination programmes and antenatal care [23]. In addition to such opportunity costs, this study also showed how much family income is wasted on ineffective treatments for skin infections and scabies.

Conclusions

This chapter has demonstrated the fundamental importance of the discipline of epidemiology in understanding skin diseases in context, from the clinic to the population. Not only is epidemiology concerned with issues such as describing the incidence, prevalence and human and financial cost of skin disease, but it is also one of the most direct ways of finding out the causes of skin diseases. Finding out causes is important because it may lead to the prevention of skin disease on a massive scale. For example, it has been found through a number of epidemiological studies that atopic eczema is less common in large, less economically advantaged families [1,2]. This observation gave rise to the hygiene hypothesis, which postulated that increased exposure to microbes and infections in early life might protect against atopy [1,3]. The hygiene hypothesis led to a full-scale, randomised controlled trial of *Lactobacilli* cultures given to pregnant mothers and infants, a study that suggested that around 50% of atopic eczema could be prevented by such a measure in infants [4]. Even though this particular study had some potential flaws [5], it nevertheless demonstrates the potential power of prevention.

Epidemiological principles have been key to developing the principles of evidence-based medicine described in Chapter 17 and of health services research in relation to dermatology. Although traditional epidemiology may be superseded or enhanced by genetic epidemiology and other new hybrids as biomedical knowledge develops, there will always be a need for a thorough understanding of the principles of assessing risk and the roles that the 'big three' factors of chance, bias and confounding may play in any study. The same basic epidemiological principles apply to assessing digital transformations in the delivery of dermatological care such as the use of artificial intelligence systems to detect skin cancers [6]. Similarly, the principles of critically appraising published literature using a framework derived from epidemiology are as basic to dermatological clinical practice as diagnosing rashes [7]. Nijsten and Stern nicely summarise how modern epidemiology has led to better understanding of skin diseases and their treatments such as in Lyme disease, severe cutaneous reactions, long-term safety of PUVA (psoralen–UVA), co-morbidities in psoriasis and teratogenicity of isotretinoin [8]. The importance of clear reporting of the various types of epidemiological studies using the STROBE (STrengthening the Reporting of OBservational Studies in Epidemiology) guidance cannot be overemphasised [9,10].

Glossary of epidemiological terms

Measures of disease frequency
- *Prevalence*. The proportion of people with a disease at any one time. *Point prevalence* refers to prevalence at one point in time. *Period prevalence* refers to the proportion with a disease (existing and new cases) over a longer period, for example 1 year.
- *Incidence*. The rate of new cases developing over a specified time period, for example the incidence of melanoma in the USA in men in 1983–87 was 6.9 per 100 000 per year [1].

Measures of disease associations
- *Risk factor*. A factor that increases the risk of disease. This could be a specific exposure, for example asbestos giving rise to mesothelioma, or an attribute such as gender or social class which is indirectly associated with an increased frequency of disease.
- *Relative risk*. This is the *ratio* of the risk of disease occurring in those exposed to the agent under investigation divided by the risk of those not exposed. It is a measure of the strength of the risk factor.
- *Attributable risk*. This is the *difference* between the incidence rate in those exposed to a factor and the incidence rate in those unexposed. It is a measure of the absolute effect of the exposure.
- *Odds ratio*. An approximation of relative risk used in case–control studies. It is the ratio of the odds of exposure in cases to the odds of exposure in controls.
- *Hazard ratio*. This a special form of relative risk that is used in studies that examine survival to express the relative risk of an end point or 'hazard' occurring at any given time.

Interpreting results
- *Sampling error*. This refers to the variation in values that a given sample could be expected to show by chance alone.
- *P value*. When referring to the association of a disease with a particular exposure, a P value of <0.05 means that a value as extreme as that obtained by the study would be expected to be observed by chance in fewer than 1 in 20 such studies (or <5% of the time). It is convention at this level of significance to reject the null hypothesis of no difference between the compared groups.
- *Confidence intervals*. This refers to the range of plausible values for a main study finding. It is based on the size of the sample and the size of the difference between compared groups. For example, the 95% bounds of a relative risk of 2.0 for smoking in a sample of psoriasis sufferers was 1.5–2.5. If the association is a genuine one, this means that the reader can be 95% confident that the true population relative risk resides between the values of 1.5 and 2.5.
- *Bias*. Bias is a systematic error resulting in an incorrect conclusion about the association between an exposure and an outcome. Over 30 types of bias have been described [2], but they fall into two main groups: (i) *selection*, that is the two groups to be compared are not comparable in terms of factors in addition to the exposure of interest; and (ii) *information*, that is collection of information about the disease and exposure in a fashion that could bias response, for example those evaluating a new drug were aware of the treatment allocation when assessing patients' response to treatment. An excellent description of the main forms of bias in epidemiological research is to be found elsewhere [3].

- *Confounding.* This is where the association between an exposure and disease is mixed up with a third factor that is independently associated with both the exposure and the disease, for example the protective effect of prolonged breastfeeding (the exposure) on the development of atopic eczema (the disease) may be due to confounding by parental atopy. The risk of atopic eczema is increased in children born to atopic parents, and atopic parents are more likely to practise prolonged breastfeeding in their infants because they may be more aware of a possible protective effect of breastfeeding.
- *Association and causation.* Association between an exposure and disease does not necessarily imply causation. Other factors such as chance, bias and confounding may explain that association.

Validity and repeatability

- *Internal validity.* Internal validity, for example of a diagnostic test, refers to the extent to which the test measures what it is meant to measure. This is normally measured in terms of sensitivity (proportion of true cases correctly identified) and specificity (proportion of non-cases correctly identified).
- *External validity.* This refers to the extent to which findings from one particular study (the study population) can be generalised to the target population – for example, to what extent are the favourable results of a clinical trial to test a new oral agent for children with severe atopic eczema attending hospital applicable to children with milder eczema in the community?
- *Predictive value.* When comparing the performance of a test or diagnostic criterion with a gold standard (e.g. clinical diagnosis of melanoma against histological diagnosis), the positive predictive value refers to the probability that someone is a genuine case given a positive test result. Negative predictive value refers to the probability that a person does not have that disease given a negative test result. In addition to sensitivity and specificity, predictive value is dependent on the overall prevalence of the disease being studied [4].
- *Repeatability.* This refers to the extent to which two observations agree with each other. This may be between two observers (interobserver agreement) or between replicate measurements in one observer (within-observer agreement). Repeatability is measured by chance-corrected agreement measures such as the κ statistic [5], or by differences between two observers plotted against corresponding means of observations and *not* correlation coefficients [6].

Types of epidemiological study

- *Observational or descriptive studies.* These are studies where the frequency of a disorder is described in terms of its association with various background attributes such as age, sex and ethnicity.
- *Analytical studies.* These set out to test specific hypotheses on the relationship between a potential exposure and disease. These may be *cross-sectional* (e.g. 'Is atopic eczema more common in black Caribbean children in London compared with white children?'), *case–control* (e.g. 'Is a history of preceding infection more common in people with pityriasis rosea than in controls?') or *cohort* (e.g. 'Are people who are exposed to diesel fumes more likely to develop asthma than those who are not?').
- *Intervention studies.* These are studies in which groups of individuals are allocated to an experimental treatment prospectively. Clinical trials are the commonest examples. Occasionally, such trials are conducted at a community level, for example vaccine trials.
- *Screening.* This refers to the examination of healthy people who would not otherwise have sought medical help for the presence or absence of disease. Principles for evaluating the usefulness of screening are described elsewhere [7].

Checklist for reading epidemiological studies in dermatology

This checklist represents a general approach to exploring key elements that should have been included in an epidemiological study. For recommendations on what to include when reporting case–control, cohort and prevalence studies, please refer to the STROBE checklist at www.strobe-statement.org (last accessed January 2022).

1. Is there a clear objective(s)?
2. Is the study design appropriate and efficient for the question posed?
3. Have cases (numerators) been clearly defined?
4. Is there a population denominator?
5. Have the main hypotheses and outcome measures been stated *a priori*?
6. Is there a rationale for the study's sample size?
7. Have potential confounders been considered and measured?
8. Has the study attempted to minimise selection and information biases?
9. Have the data been analysed appropriately?
10. Are the main results clearly presented with confidence intervals?
11. Have subgroups or *post hoc* findings been treated appropriately?
12. Have the authors discussed alternative explanations such as chance, bias and confounding?
13. Are the study's conclusions supported by the main results?
14. Who sponsored the study? Could sponsorship have affected the choice of data and the way they were presented?

Recommended further reading and useful dermatoepidemiology resources

General epidemiology

Gordis L. *Epidemiology*, 3rd edn. Philadelphia: Elsevier Saunders, 2004.
Hennekens CH, Buring JE. *Epidemiology in Medicine*. Boston: Little, Brown, 1987.
Holmes L, Jr. *Concise Guide to Epidemiology and Biostatistics for Clinicians*. Boston: Jones and Bartlett Publishers, 2011.
Rothman KJ, Greenland S, Lash TL. *Modern Epidemiology*, 4th edn. London: Lippincott, Williams and Wilkins, 2021.
Sackett DL, Haynes RB, Guyatt GH, Tugwell P. *Clinical Epidemiology: A Basic Science for Clinical Medicine*, 2nd edn. Boston: Little, Brown, 1991.
Schlesselman JJ. *Case Control Studies: Design, Conduct, Analysis*. Oxford: Oxford University Press, 1982.

Biostatistics

Altman DG. *Practical Statistics for Medical Research*. London: Chapman and Hall, 1992.
Gilmore SJ. Evaluating statistics in clinical trials: making the unintelligible intelligible. *Aust J Dermatol* 2008;49:177–84; quiz 185–6.

Gore SM, Altman DG. *Statistics in Practice*. London: British Medical Association, 1991.
Kahn HA. *Statistical Methods in Epidemiology*. Oxford: Oxford University Press, 1989.
Kirkwood BR. *Essentials of Medical Statistics*. Oxford: Blackwell Scientific Publications, 1988.
Spiegelhalter D. *The Art of Statistics: Learning from Data*. London: Penguin Random House, 2020.

Systematic reviews

Chalmers I, Altman D. *Systematic Reviews*. London: British Medical Journal Publishing Group, 1995.
Cochrane Library: www.thecochranelibrary.com (last accessed January 2022).
Higgins JPT, Green S, eds. *Cochrane Handbook for Systematic Reviews of Interventions*, Version 5.1.0 (updated March 2011). Cochrane Collaboration, 2011. www.cochrane-handbook.org (last accessed January 2022).
Reddi A, Prescott L, Doney E et al. The Cochrane Skin Group: a vanguard for developing and promoting evidence-based dermatology. *J Evid Based Med* 2013;6:236–42.

Dermatoepidemiology reports

Barzilai DA, Mikkilineni R, Davis BR, Stevens SR, Mostow EN. Implementation of dermato-epidemiology curriculum at Case Western Reserve University dermatology program. *Dermatol Online J* 2004;10:1.
Chuang TY. Dermatoepidemiology. 1: Epidemiologic methods. *Int J Dermatol* 1993;32:251–6.
Grobb JJ, MacKie RM, Stern R, Weinstock MA. *Epidemiology, Causes and Prevention of Skin Diseases*. Oxford: Blackwell Science, 1997.
Langan SM, Bouwes Bavinck JN, Coenraads PJ et al.; European Dermato-Epidemiology Network. Update on the activities of the European Dermato-Epidemiology Network (EDEN). *Dermatology* 2006;213:1–2.
Marks R. Dermatoepidemiology: wherefore art thou in this perilous time of need? *Int J Dermatol* 2001;40:167–8.
Nijsten T, Stern RS. How epidemiology has contributed to a better understanding of skin disease. *J Invest Dermatol* 2012;132:994–1002.
VanBeek M, Beach S, Braslow L et al. Highlights from the report of the working group on 'Core measures of the burden of skin diseases'. *J Invest Dermatol* 2007;127:2701–6.
Weinstock MA. Dermatoepidemiology. *Dermatol Clin* 1995;13:505–716.
Williams H, Svensson A, Diepgen T et al.; European Dermato-Epidemiology Network (EDEN). Epidemiology of skin diseases in Europe. *Eur J Dermatol* 2006;16:212–18.

Dermatoepidemiology textbooks

Williams HC. *Atopic Dermatitis*. Cambridge: Cambridge University Press, 2000. (A textbook dedicated to the epidemiology of atopic eczema.)
Williams HC, Strachan DP. *The Challenge of Dermato-epidemiology*. Boca Raton, FL: CRC Press, 1997. (This contains a comprehensive 'toolbox' section at the start of the book, followed by a summary of the epidemiology of specific skin diseases.)

Epidemiology computer software

Centers for Disease Control. *Epi Info™*, Version 7.2. Atlanta, GA: Centers for Disease Control, 2008. Available as a free download from http://www.cdc.gov/epiinfo/ (last accessed January 2022).
Gardner MJ, Gardner SB, Winter PD. *Confidence Interval Analysis (CIA)*, Version 1.2. London: British Medical Journal Publishing Group, 1991.

Evidence-based dermatology

Bigby M. Evidence-based medicine in a nutshell: a guide to finding and using the best evidence in caring for patients. *Arch Dermatol* 1998;134:1609–18.
Bigby M. Snake oil for the 21st century. *Arch Dermatol* 1998;134:1512–14.
Rees J. Evidence-based medicine: the epistemology that isn't. *J Am Acad Dermatol* 2000;43:727–9.
Williams H. Dowling Oration 2001. Evidence-based dermatology – a bridge too far? *Clin Exp Dermatol* 2001;26:714–24.
Williams HC. Why is the center of evidence-based dermatology relevant to Indian dermatology? *Indian J Dermatol* 2009:54:118–23.
Williams HC, Bigby M, Herheimer A et al. *Evidence-Based Dermatology*, 3rd edn. London: BMJ Books/Wiley Blackwell, 2014.
Williams HC, Dellavalle RP. The growth of clinical trials and systematic reviews in informing dermatological patient care. *J Invest Dermatol* 2012;132:1008–17.

Interest groups/societies

American Dermato-Epidemiology Network (ADEN) and American Academy of Dermatology DermatoEpidemiology Expert Resource Group (DERM EPI-ERG): http://adenet.us/.
European Dermato-Epidemiology Network (EDEN): https://www.dermepi.eu/dermepi.eu. (Website containing details of current epidemiological projects and meetings.)
(Both last accessed January 2022.)

Useful websites and online resources

Centre for Evidence-Based Medicine (CEBM): www.cebm.net/. (The CEBM is based at Oxford, UK. The website contains a list of useful teaching resources for evidence-based medicine, along with a glossary of terms and resources.)
Centre of Evidence Based Dermatology (CEBD): http://www.nottingham.ac.uk/dermatology/. (Includes the Cochrane Skin Group and the UK Dermatology Clinical Trials Network. The website has a large resource section that includes databases of all randomised controlled trials for eczema, the UK Diagnostic Criteria for Atopic Dermatitis manual, annual evidence updates for common skin diseases and details about the international Harmonising Outcomes for Eczema (HOME) project. It also runs annual courses in better evaluation of evidence and statistics in dermatology.)
Cochrane Library: http://www.thecochranelibrary.com. (Widely acknowledged as the most reliable source of evidence, it contains the largest collection of systematic reviews and clinical trials in the world. It is free to any user in the UK with an IP address, and also in many other countries such as India, Finland, Ireland and Norway.)
Cochrane Skin – Core Outcomes Set Initiative (CS-COUSIN): http://cs-cousin.org/. (A collaboration between Cochrane Skin and various international groups developing core outcome sets for skin diseases. CS-COUSIN has recently joined with the Consortium for Harmonizing Outcomes Research in Dermatology (CHORD) to form one organisation dealing with core outcomes for the whole of dermatology called Chord COUSIN Collaboration (C3).)
Equator network (Enhancing the QUAlity and Transparency Of health Research): www.equator-network.org/. (Guidelines on reporting various study designs such as epidemiological studies, randomised controlled clinical trials, diagnostic test studies, etc. are all to be found on this website.)
International DermatoEpidemiology Association (IDEA): http://www.nottingham.ac.uk/~muzidea/aadcurric.htm. (Trainees' curriculum for dermatoepidemiology. A list of guided reading and questions developed by dermatoepidemiologists from IDEA in conjunction with the American Academy of Dermatology (AAD).)
ProQolid (Patient-Reported Outcome and Quality of Life Instruments Database): www.qolid.org/.
(All last accessed January 2022.)

Key references

The full list of references can be found in the online version at https://www.wiley.com/rooksdermatology10e

What is epidemiology and why is it relevant to dermatology?

6 Goldberger J. The etiology of pellagra. *Public Health Rep* 1914;29:1683–6.

Thinking in terms of populations rather than individuals

3 Taplin D, Porcelain SL, Meinking TL et al. Community control of scabies: a model based on the use of permethrin cream. *Lancet* 1991;337:1016–18.

How much of a public health problem is skin disease?

3 Williams HC. Defining cases. In: Williams HC, Strachan DP, eds. *The Challenge of Dermato-Epidemiology*. Boca Raton, FL: CRC Press, 1997:13–23.
24 Karimkhani C, Dellavalle RP, Coffeng LE et al. Global skin disease morbidity and mortality: an update from the Global Burden of Disease Study 2013. *JAMA Dermatol* 2017;153:406–12.

What determines the frequency of skin disease in populations?

6 Budu-Aggrey A, Brumpton B, Tyrrell J et al. Evidence of a causal relationship between body mass index and psoriasis: a mendelian randomization study. *PLoS Med* 2019;16:e1002739.

Describing the natural history and associations of specific skin diseases

5 Williams HC, Wuthrich B. The natural history of atopic dermatitis. In: Williams HC, ed. *Atopic Dermatitis: the Epidemiology, Causes and Prevention of Eczema*. Cambridge: Cambridge University Press, 2000:41–59.

15 Langan SM, Groves RW, Card TR, Gulliford MC. Incidence, mortality, and disease associations of pyoderma gangrenosum in the United Kingdom: a retrospective cohort study. *J Invest Dermatol* 2012;132:2166–70.

Health services research in dermatology

5 Schofield J, Grindlay D, Williams H. *Skin Conditions in the UK: a Health Care Needs Assessment*. Nottingham: Centre of Evidence-Based Dermatology, University of Nottingham, 2009.

23 Hay RJ, Hernandez HA, Lopez GC et al. Wastage of family income on skin disease in Mexico. *BMJ* 1994;309:848.

Conclusions

8 Nijsten T, Stern RS. How epidemiology has contributed to a better understanding of skin disease. *J Invest Dermatol* 2012;132:994–1002.

9 Langan S, Schmitt J, Coenraads PJ, Svensson A, von Elm E, Williams H; European Dermato-Epidemiology Network (EDEN). The reporting of observational research studies in dermatology journals: a literature-based study. *Arch Dermatol* 2010;146:534–41.

CHAPTER 6

Health Economics and Skin Disease

Matthias Augustin

Institute for Health Services Research in Dermatology and Nursing, University Medical Center Hamburg-Eppendorf, Hamburg, Germany

---

Background, 6.1
Introduction to methods and approaches in health economics, 6.1
Perspectives of health economic evaluations, 6.2
Types of health economic evaluation, 6.2
Implementation of health economic findings in decision making, 6.5

Economic burden of disease in dermatology, 6.5
Skin cancer, 6.5
Psoriasis, 6.8
Atopic dermatitis, 6.10
Cost comparisons of atopic dermatitis and psoriasis, 6.10

Critical reflection of studies on disease burden, 6.10
Impact for decision making in dermatology practice, 6.10

Key references, 6.11

Background

Economic burden is defined as the total amount of direct, indirect and intangible costs of defined diseases. Health economic evaluation of treatments and procedures to optimise resource allocation are necessitated by increasing life expectancy, continuous innovations in medicine and health care, changes in national and international health policies as well as limited financial resources. In dermatology, the past decade has been characterised by an increasing incidence and prevalence of many diseases leading to a rising need for health care and resource consumption. In several fields, such as skin cancer and allergies, this increase exceeds the expected rise due to the general ageing of the population. For example, in Australia, skin cancer has steadily increased in number, proportion and burden to society; today, it poses the greatest economic impact among all cancers [1]. In European countries, the incidence is also rising [2–5]. For instance, in the UK, the incidence of basal cell carcinoma (BCC) increased by 12% from 134/100 000 in 1996 to 162/100 000 in 2003 [6]. In Slovakia, the incidence of non-melanoma skin cancer (NMSC) has risen by 59.1% in males and 58.5% in females between 1978 and 1995, and in Denmark from 46.2/100 000 to 121.2/100 000 between 1987 and 2007 [7,8]. The overall increase in Germany between 2003 and 2010 was about 80% both for NMSC and for melanoma [9], meaning an average annual increase of about 8–10%.

Trends of increasing prevalence are also evident for allergic diseases and atopic eczema (AE). For example, in England, an increase of AE prevalence from 9.6% in 2001 to 13.6% in 2005 in the general population was observed. In Denmark, it increased from 17.3% in 1986 to 27.3% in 2001 in children [10,11]. Contrarily, also in Danish children, a stable incidence was found between 1993 and 1998 [12]. Likewise, no reliable conclusion can be drawn from a Swiss study which showed an increase in patient-reported symptoms for AE from 4.6% in 1992 to 7.6% in 2001 but a stable incidence in doctor-diagnosed diseases [13]. An example of an ageing population being responsible for an increasing burden of skin diseases is chronic wounds. These often occur in elderly people. For instance, the incidence is about 0.76/1000 in men and 1.42/1000 in women aged 65 years or older in the UK [14]. In 1997, it was estimated that about 1% of the population in European countries was affected by chronic leg ulcers [15]. Since society is steadily ageing, one can expect this prevalence to be even higher and to rise in the future, which leads to an increase in costs and in the economic burden of disease.

Changing epidemiology combined with the continuous development of innovations and limited financial resources create the need for health economic decisions based on fair resource allocation. Here, health economic analysis can provide some support and guidance for decision makers in health policy, hospitals, the pharmaceutical industry and other areas of the health care sector. Moreover, dermatologists are key specialists in the proper use of medical resources for the management of skin diseases.

This chapter gives an overview of health economics in general and its use in determining the burden of disease in dermatology.

Introduction to methods and approaches in health economics

Health economics analyses the economic aspects of health care [16]. It is an empirical, theoretical and interdisciplinary science, which focuses on the production and allocation of health services and their economic consequences in the health sector. It especially concerns the balanced use and distribution of resources such as personal capacity, drugs, hospital density and utilisation, supply of diagnostic and therapeutic procedures as well as the associated efficacy, effectiveness, quality and equity regarding access to health services. Therefore, areas of responsibility for health economists include the acquisition, assessment and comparison of the costs, benefits, efficacy and effectiveness of different types of health care. The scope and methods of health economics vary depending on the underlying perspective and professional background of authors and target groups, including social policy, finance, actuarial science, governance or microeconomics.

Health economic evaluation is the general term for different types of analyses that use economic methods to examine and assess medical procedures [17]. Different approaches to benefit and cost estimation can be chosen for the analysis, depending on the question, the perspective and the aim of the study. The description, evaluation, allocation and appropriate distribution of the available resources are the fundamental tasks of health economics. Therefore health economic evaluation can be designed to assess the costs and cost–benefit ratios of particular interventions, health structures and procedures across indications or the impact of conditions of health care systems on the stakeholders concerned [18]. In any case, its results serve as the basis to optimise the health outcome, given a restricted budget for health services.

Perspectives of health economic evaluations

Before data on costs and benefits can be assessed, the perspective of the health economic evaluation has to be chosen (Figure 6.1). This defines the point of view from which information is assessed. The *societal* perspective contains various costs, irrespective of who bears them. Besides direct medical costs for treatments, drugs and medical devices, this perspective also includes direct non-medical costs, for example the costs for travelling, care or child care and indirect costs like the loss of productivity that results from health impairment. From the perspective of *third-party payers* (e.g. health insurers) costs within their budget responsibility in particular are taken into account. Potential savings in other sectors, for example due to prevention of premature retirement, are either not considered or, if they are, are considered to be less relevant. The physician responsible for the patient's care is mainly concerned with the direct costs arising from treatment with drugs or medical devices. Subsequent costs that are relevant for society and health insurers are not included. Like individual physicians, hospital managers are also concerned with costs arising from treatment, but they also have to take account of a wider range of direct costs, such as staff, accommodation and catering. Unlike the perspectives already described, the *patient's* perspective focuses on out-of-pocket payments and patient benefits of treatment. Health economic evaluations from the patient's perspective are commonly not conducted independently, but are usually made complementary to other evaluations. As shown, inputs included in evaluations vary depending on the perspective.

Types of recommended perspectives likewise vary between countries. For instance, in Sweden a holistic perspective is used including medical, humanitarian and socioeconomic aspects; and in the UK the perspective derives from the National Health Service (NHS) and patients [19,20]. In Germany, researchers can choose between the perspective of statutory health insurance and the societal perspective; while, in Spain, both the societal and the third-party payer perspective are required [21,22]. In France, the perspective depends on the aim of the study [23]. This is one reason why the results of health economic analyses from different perspectives should only be compared with caution.

Types of health economic evaluation

In the next step of an economic appraisal, the source of data has to be defined. If retrospective data are to be analysed, secondary research can be conducted. In this case, already existing data are used. Examples of secondary research are meta-analysis and modelling methods such as decision trees, Markov models or discrete event

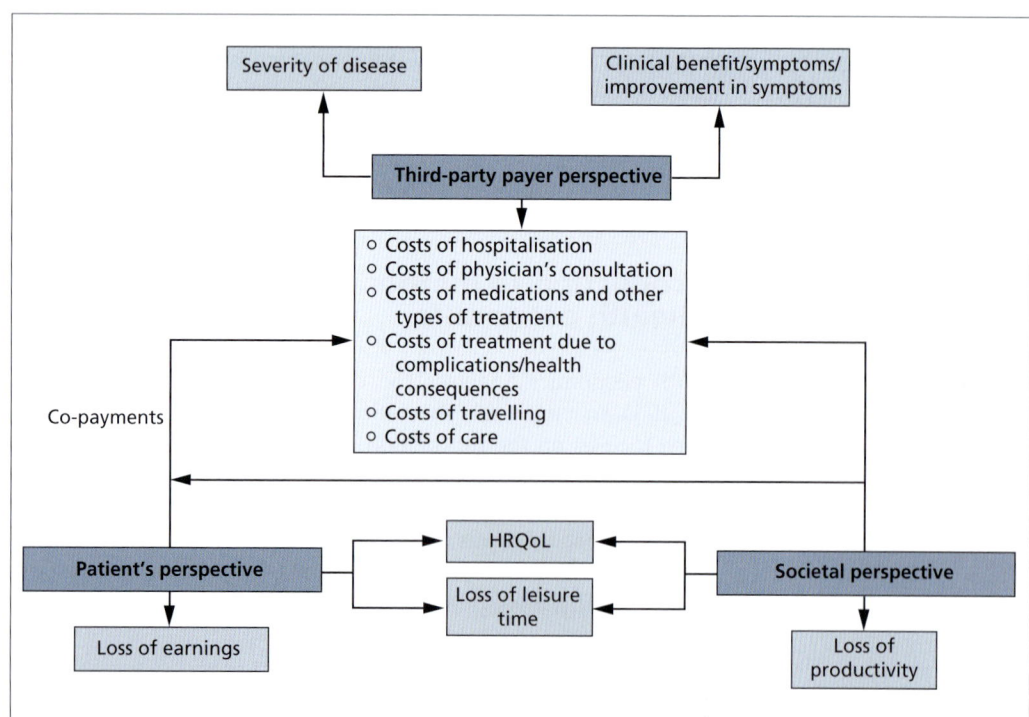

Figure 6.1 Perspectives of health economic analysis. HRQoL, health-related quality of life.

simulations. Another kind of study design is based on field research, where data are explicitly recorded for the given research question. Data gained from field research are highly acceptable because of their increased levels of accuracy and timeliness, and therefore they are of greater value in health economic evaluations. Here, retrospective or prospective analysis can be performed. Examples of field research include Delphi surveys and clinical or observational studies. Furthermore, a distinction is made between the bottom-up and top-down approach. The bottom-up approach means the collection of epidemiological, medical and economic data on an individual level. Using this method, input and output can be traced back to a specific person. It is mainly used in field research. The advantage lies in the possibility of conducting analysis on an individual level, in subgroups or on a superordinate level. In contrast, the top-down approach uses aggregated data from bottom-up studies. Therefore it is mainly used in secondary research, for example by including secondary data from official statistics. The major advantages of this approach are the low cost and the easier availability of data. However, a disadvantage is the fact that data were collected for a different objective than health economic evaluation. Data can only be used for analysis with restrictions due to the varying quality and completeness of the information.

As shown, health economic evaluations have different study designs using different sources of data on different levels with variable quality. But there is also a distinction between the types of studies depending on the costs and benefits data included. In the first step, it begins to matter whether a *non-comparative* or a *comparative* study should be conducted (Figure 6.2).

Conducting a non-comparative study is the simplest way to carry out a health economic analysis. It can either be designed as a *cost analysis* or as a *cost-of-illness study* in which direct, indirect and intangible costs are determined.

Indirect costs are the costs of those resources for which no payment is made, but for which there is an opportunity cost or foregone benefit. Typically, indirect costs are raised by disease-induced losses of productivity. Productivity costs include: (i) absenteeism; (ii) presenteeism; and (iii) unpaid labour. Both absenteeism (which is the costs due to time off work) and presenteeism (which is the costs due to time at work with impaired productivity related to disease) are important results of many skin diseases.

Indirect costs can be assessed in two different ways: either using the human capital or the friction cost approach. The human capital approach is the less conservative way to calculate productivity loss under the assumption of full employment for the rest of a life. However, the friction cost approach assumes some unemployment and thereby values lost productivity for the period of time it takes to find someone who replaces the person who has fallen ill. The calculation of indirect costs by the human capital approach results in higher costs if the disease leads to long-term absence from work. Given a short-term absence from work, the use of the human capital approach is also likely to overestimate indirect costs because either colleagues undertake the tasks or the person who has fallen sick is working again after convalescence [24,25]. Intangible costs reflect the impairment in quality of life (QoL) and can thus only be assessed on a single patient level. For the evaluation of health-related QoL, a large number of tools have been developed in dermatology [26,27]. The goal of cost-of-illness studies is to inform about the economic burden of a disease and to compare the impacts of different diseases. They are used by politicians and management service providers such as hospitals to support their

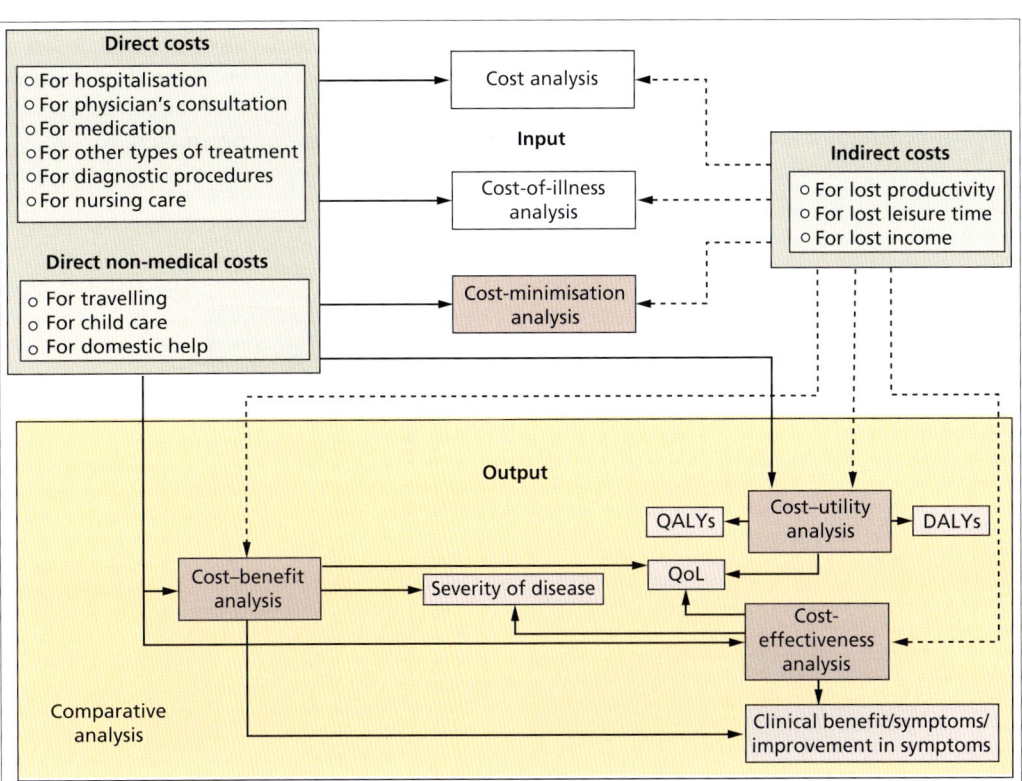

Figure 6.2 Types of health economic analysis. DALYs, disability-adjusted life-years; QALYs, quality-adjusted life-years; QoL, quality of life.

decision making. Costs can be analysed on an individual level for each patient, in subgroups for different stages of disease or for the entire population of a defined area. Furthermore, specific types of costs can be considered separately. These types of studies do not deal with the effects (output) of an intervention, but exclusively concentrate on its costs (input).

The objective of *comparative studies* is to assess costs and health outcomes of alternative therapies or diagnostic procedures. They include cost–benefit, cost–utility, cost-effectiveness and cost-minimisation analysis. *Cost-minimisation* studies deal with the same types of data as cost studies. The consequences are not analysed because the assumption is made that they were identical for all compared alternatives. One advantage of this study type lies in its feasibility. In *cost–benefit* analysis, in addition to the resources needed, the effect (output) is regarded which is assessed and expressed monetarily. The valuation is either based on the contribution of the effects of increasing human capital on the willingness to pay (WTP) or on conjoint analysis which reflects patient preferences [17]. The objective of this type of study is the net benefit defined as monetary value, which results from the difference of the cost and the benefit of two or more compared alternative treatments. Thereby, the advantage consists in the consideration of intangible benefit. Difficulties for this approach are the interdependence of WTP and human capital on one side and the net income of respondents on the other. A *cost-effectiveness* analysis is performed when every associate (player) in health care is given a fixed budget, of which the maximal beneficial effect for the patient and for society should be generated. The output is captured as clinical outcome, for example the skin area affected by psoriasis and its severity, the stage of melanoma or as QoL. QoL can be measured in four different ways [28]. The first is a survey using a general health profile questionnaire, for example the Short Form 36 Health Survey (SF-36) or the EuroQol (EQ-5D); and the second is a questionnaire to detect preferences, for example using conjoint analysis or discrete choice experiments [29,30]. Both result in values for general QoL. The last two methods assess the disease-specific and the condition-specific QoL. Dermatology-specific instruments, such as the dermatology life quality index (DLQI) or Skindex, can be used to compare the cost-effectiveness within a group of different skin diseases, but not to others; while QoL assessed with disease-specific instruments can only be compared within the same disease, for example the psoriasis disability index [31–33]. *Cost–utility* analysis can be classified as a subgroup of cost-effectiveness analysis which focuses on QoL as the outcome [17]. Here, utilities, precise preferences or values are determined by carrying out different types of survey [34]. It can be measured by a visual analogue scale (VAS), standard gamble, time trade-off (TTO) or questionnaires assessing QoL like EQ-5D or SF-36. VAS is a direct method and the simplest way to measure utility. Thereby, QoL is rated on a visual rating scale for defined diseases. Using standard gamble, people have to choose between two alternatives. The first is a defined state of health. The second is an uncertain condition with defined chances of living healthy or dying. Chances are varied until the person is indifferent between both alternatives. In contrast, TTO asks how much of the life time remaining people would give up to spend the rest of their life in health instead of suffering from a defined chronic disease. Under temporarily reduced health conditions people have to choose between intermediate reduced QoL for the duration of a disease and a worse QoL for a shorter period of time, both followed by perfect health. Duration of the worse QoL is varied until the person asked is indifferent between both the alternatives. These utilities can be used as weights for quality-adjusted life-years (QALYs) or disability-adjusted life-years (DALYs), considering not only life-years gained by a certain programme or therapy but also the QoL (Figure 6.3). A further advantage of this study design is the possibility of comparing interventions for different diseases, different outcomes and combinations of outcomes or the burden of different diseases.

Conclusions drawn from comparative studies of medical treatments or procedures fulfil the criteria for effectiveness if the costs incurred lead to an appropriate benefit. Thereby the benefit can be defined as a clinical (e.g. psoriasis area and severity Index), monetary (e.g. cost of illness) or intangible (e.g. QoL, well-being) parameter.

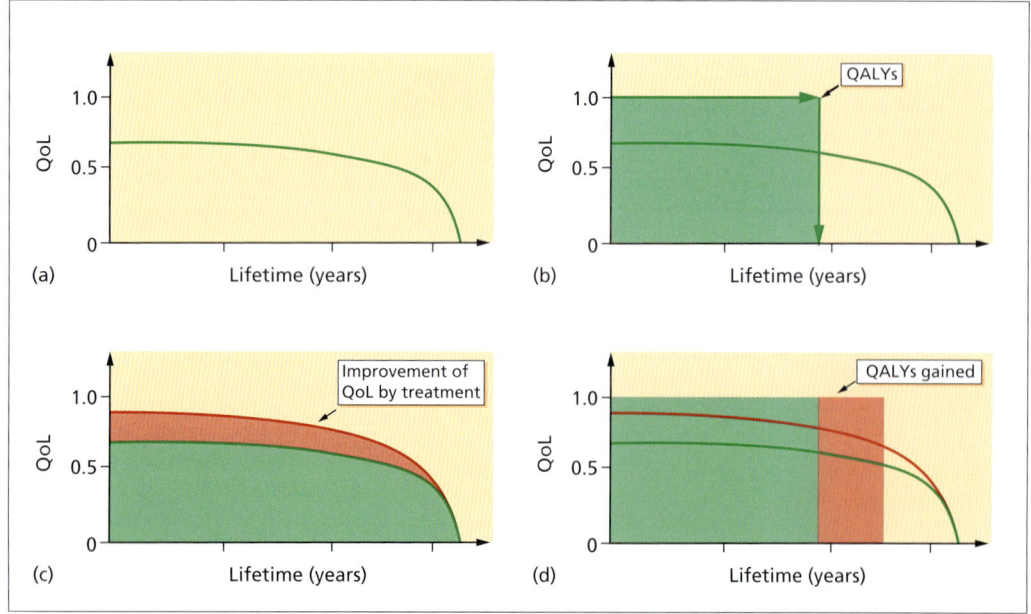

Figure 6.3 Quality of life (QoL) and quality-adjusted life-years (QALYs).

In health economic evaluation, it is thus of utmost importance to identify and include not only the therapy costs but also the therapeutic benefits in treatment decisions. In many cases, this means that a more expensive therapy is to be preferred if its benefit is relatively higher than that of a primarily cheaper therapy. There are numerous examples of such positive incremental cost–benefit ratios in innovative drugs for psoriasis, atopic dermatitis and other skin disorders.

Implementation of health economic findings in decision making

Results of these studies are used by decision makers to allocate resources and medical services. Therefore, consequences can be differentiated regarding their strength of regulation and restriction in prioritisation, rationalisation and scaling. *Prioritisation* stands for the development of an order of medical services according to their grade of medical necessity. Thereby a distinction is made between vertical and horizontal prioritisation [35]. While vertical prioritisation is made through treatments for the same indication, horizontal prioritisation happens between treatments for different diseases. Prioritisation can be used as the basis for scaling in a further step if the objective of this procedure is the limitation of medical services. *Scaling* means the withholding of necessary medical treatments or procedures because of limited resources. Therefore, it is the most radical instrument of cost containment. However, different degrees of scaling exist. While in its mildest form people are allowed to pay for services not covered by their health insurance out of their own pocket, it is not possible to use services not covered by health insurance when scaling occurs in its strictest form. In contrast to scaling, the purpose of *rationalisation* is to increase efficiency or productivity by cost reduction while the quality of supply remains stable. Furthermore, rationalisation is part of the economic principle that states that a defined goal should be achieved with minimal input or to achieve as much as possible with the given available means.

As shown, for health economic evaluations a wide range of different methods, approaches and study designs can be applied. In the following text, the burden of skin diseases and the relationship between costs and benefits are depicted closely. In the light of several thousand but individually small dermatological entities, health economics in dermatology can only be illustrated by a few frequent conditions.

Economic burden of disease in dermatology

The annual economic burden of disease was shown to be a relevant cost factor for society in the USA [36]. Bickers *et al.* analysed secondary data on direct, indirect and intangible costs. Total direct and indirect cost of the 22 dermatological indications considered summed up to US$39.3 billion, of which 3.5% ($1358 million) arose from psoriasis, 14.1% ($5555 million) from skin cancer and 30.4% ($11 951 million) from skin ulcers and wounds. In the following text, the national economic burden of three skin diseases with different clinical courses and cost structures are presented to provide an overview of costs arising from dermatological diseases, how health economic methods are used in practice and how this can lead to substantial differences in the results.

Skin cancer

Skin cancer is a life-threatening skin disease of major economic importance. Once a person is affected, it can lead to recurrence. This is more likely for NMSC than for melanoma. For instance, in Germany, 22/1815 (1.2%) melanomas diagnosed during a mass screening were recurrences while in NMSC they accounted for 1352/14 178 (9.5%) cases [37]. Another study conducted in the USA found recurrence in NMCS only appeared in 21/487 cases (4.3%). However, this is more than three times as high when comparing it with melanoma [38]. Because cost-of-illness studies possess the most appropriate study design for the determination of economic burden, this is the only type of study considered here.

The economic burden of melanoma was estimated for the US population aged 65 years and older ($n = 15 130$) in a cost study of Seidler *et al.* [39]. The authors extrapolated the cost of a Medicare cohort with 1858 melanoma patients to the US population. Direct costs of office visits and consultations, surgical and pathological treatment, radiological interventions, laboratory tests, emergency department visits, hospital stays and chemotherapy as well as external radiation were considered from the Medicare perspective solely. The annual expenses were differentiated by stage of disease instead of resources used and resulted in US$249 million for the entire population in 1996. They varied between $5247 and $23 285 per patient and year, depending on the stage of disease. The melanoma lifetime treatment costs which were calculated by using data from people who had died during the observation period of 5 years added up to $28 210.

Another retrospective cost evaluation from the USA dealing with economic costs concentrated on the productivity loss due to skin cancer mortality [40]. People aged 15 years and above were included. The average life expectancy was set as a cut-off for the calculation of potential life-years lost. The authors stated that, in 2006, 8437 deaths (5474 men and 2963 women) occurred as a result of melanoma in the USA with an average potential life loss of 20.4 years per person, which summed up to a total of 166 261 life-years lost. In order to determine the monetary value of productivity loss caused by mortality, the human capital approach was chosen by using the present value of further lifetime earnings. Average costs per death amounted to US$441 903 for men and $401 046 for women, thus giving a total of $3.5 billion.

The costs of skin cancer from a societal perspective in England in 2002 were taken from routine NHS data, using the top-down approach [41]. Costs resulting from GP consultation, out-patient attendance, in-patient treatment, absence from work and mortality were assessed. Continued payment of wages was considered if it was borne by the statutory sick pay system. Costs due to mortality were assessed by using the human capital approach. They were taken into account if death occurred before the age of 60 years for women or before the age of 65 for men according to the state retirement age in England at that time. Expenses for drugs were not included. Total costs borne by the NHS summed up to £101.6 million for the treatment of 67 571 newly diagnosed skin cancers, of which 6928 were malignant melanomas. They consisted of costs for 131 880 GP consultations (£2.6 million), 14 000 in-patient admissions (£24.9 million), 49 000 day cases (£13.5 million) and 907 000 out-patient attendances (£60.5 million). Out-of-pocket expenses for patients come to £19.3 million. They consist of costs for GP consultation (£0.9 million), in-patient admission (£0.06 million), day cases (£0.9 million) and out-patient attendance (£17.4 million). Productivity loss due to 218 000 working days missed lead to costs of £20.9 million. Additional costs caused by death occurring before reaching retirement age came to £98.2 million. Therefore, the total cost caused by illness in the UK in 2002 was £240 million.

Tinghög et al. analysed the cost of illness in Sweden in 2005 from the societal perspective [42]. They used a top-down approach for in-patient care and a bottom-up approach for out-patient and primary care. In this case, expenses for suspected diagnoses were also taken into account. Direct medical costs for 3125 in-patient episodes of €13.1 million, for 100 982 out-patient attendances of €60 million and for 42 135 episodes of primary care of €6.5 million added up to €79.6 million. Neither drug costs nor direct non-medical costs were included. Indirect costs due to mortality and morbidity were included for persons aged 25–64 years to take account of periods of education and the legal retirement age. In total, 181.5 working years were lost due to sick leave and 87.75 due to early retirement. This production loss resulted in indirect costs of €9.5 million. An additional cost was the production loss caused by the premature deaths of 454 patients. These led to 1816 working years lost and the cost of €53.3 million. In total, the societal costs for skin cancer in Sweden amounted to €142 million in 2005.

Chevalier et al. evaluated the economic burden of melanoma in France in a hospital setting from the health care perspective [43]. Data were obtained retrospectively from the national database of the Ministry of Health for 2004. A total of 42 911 hospital stays were recorded because of melanoma or melanoma in situ leading to costs of €58.95 million. The majority of patients ($n = 32 989$) received out-patient treatment, which was defined as a hospital stay of less than 48 h. The average duration of stay varied between 1 and 14.4 days depending on diagnosis and led to average costs between €161 for radiotherapy and €913 for surgery per day. Treatment of 26 735 (62.3%) patients without metastasis caused costs of €32.2 million (54.6%) while treatment of 16 176 (37.7%) patients with metastasis caused costs of €26.7 million (45.4%).

Fransen et al. analysed the incidence and treatment costs for NMSC in Australia from a societal perspective [1]. Data from Medicare Australia were evaluated for the time period between 1997 and 2010 retrospectively and extrapolated until 2015. Costs for in-patient and out-patient (GP and specialist) treatment, drugs prescribed and pathology testing were included but not analysed separately. In 1997, 412 493 services were performed for the diagnosis and treatment of NMSC. Until 2010, total services rose by 86% to 767 347 with discounted total costs including private co-payments of AU$511 million. Extrapolating from these data, a further increase is predicted for 2023.

Stang et al. evaluated the economic burden of NMSC and melanoma in 2003 in Germany from the perspective of statutory health insurance [44]. Cost analysis for hospitalisation was performed retrospectively by multiplying the number of cases treated for each diagnosis with diagnosis-related group (DRG) fees. In order to estimate the costs for out-patient treatment, data on ambulatory services were derived from 35 dermatologists and extrapolated to the entire population. In total, 159 083 days were spent in hospital due to melanoma or melanoma in situ causing costs of €61.6 million. A total of 332 500 days were spent in hospitals due to NMSC. This led to costs of €136.9 million. In out-patient care, 372 850 services were used for the diagnosis and treatment of melanoma and 711 350 for NMSC. Costs for out-patient care were not calculated.

Comparing the results of these studies, consultations are the medical service most often used in skin cancer (Table 6.1). It accounts for 94.2% of services in England and 99.2% in Germany, causing 66.9% and 83.5% of expenses for medical services, respectively. This is in accordance with earlier findings that found consultations leading to about three-quarters of all direct medical costs for the treatment of skin cancer (Table 6.2) [36]. In studies that analysed direct and indirect medical costs, direct costs resulted in a slightly greater proportion of total costs: they amounted to 55.9% in Sweden and 50.1% in England. Additionally, studies have been published focusing on the cost-effectiveness of prevention programmes. For some of these programmes, the potential to reduce mortality and the economic burden of skin cancer is discussed [45,46].

Krensel et al. investigated the costs for skin cancer based on a meta-analysis at a European level (Table 6.3; Figure 6.4) [47,48]. As expected, there was a wide range of costs for melanoma depending on the country observed and the methodology used. Adjustment by purchasing power and discounting led to fairly comparable

Table 6.1 Resources used and persons affected by skin cancer.

Reference	Country	Perspective	Number of:					
			Consultations	Hospitalisations	Medications	Population	Persons	LYL
Seidler et al. [39]	USA	Medicare	Yes	Yes	Yes	–	1858	–
Ekwueme et al. [40]	USA	Society	–	–	–	–	8437	166 261
Morris et al. [41]	England	NHS patients	1 038 800	63 000	–	–	67 571	–
Tinghög et al. [42]	Sweden	Society	143 117	3125	–	–	–	–
Chevalier et al. [43]	France	Hospital	–	42 911	–	–	–	–
Fransen et al. [1]	Australia	Society:						
		1997	412 493	–	–	18 514 741	–	–
		2010	767 347	–	–	21 911 011	–	–
		2015	938 991	–	–	23 626 109	–	–
Stang et al. [44]	Germany	SHI	1 084 200	64 622	–	82 500 000	–	–

SHI, statutory health insurance; LYL, life-years lost.

Table 6.2 Cost of illness of skin cancer in selected countries.

Reference	Country	Perspective	Direct medical costs in millions			Indirect costs in millions	Total costs in millions
			Consultations	Hospitalisations	Medications	Productivity lost	
Seidler et al. [39]	USA	Medicare	Yes	Yes	Yes	–	US$249
Ekwueme et al. [40]	USA	Society	–	–	–	US$3500	US$3500
Morris et al. [41]	England	NHS	£63.1	£39.3	–	£119.1	£240.8
		Patients	£18.3	£1.0	–	–	
Tinghög et al. [42]	Sweden	Society	€66.5	€13.1	–	€62.8	€142.4
Chevalier et al. [43]	France	Hospital	–	€58.95	–	–	€58.95
Fransen et al. [1]	Australia	Society:					
		1997	Yes	Yes	Yes	–	
		2010	Yes	Yes	Yes	–	US$511.0
		2015	Yes	Yes	Yes	–	US$703.0
Stang et al. [44]	Germany	SHI	–	€198.5	–	–	€198.5

SHI, statutory health insurance.

Table 6.3 Cost-of-illness meta-analysis of malignant melanoma on a European level, converted to Euros and adjusted for reference year 2012 and for purchasing power parity.

Country	Stage	Cost/case	Cost/patient	Number of:								
				Hospital	Hospice	Out-patient	GP	Day cases	Drugs	Patient	Morbidity	Mortality
UK	III–IV	–	€6272	3259	2419	593	–	–	–	–	–	–
Italy	III–IV	–	€2972	2736	204	32	–	–	–	–	–	–
France	III–IV	–	€6388	6072	289	27	–	–	–	–	–	–
Italy	III–IV	–	€5548	4703	203	31	–	–	–	–	–	–
Sweden	III–IV	–	€17 408	x	–	x	x	–	–	–	–	–
Sweden	I–IV	–	€4106	x	–	x	x	–	–	–	–	–
England	I–IV	–	€3261	1339	–	1401	158	363	–	–	–	–
England	I–IV	–	€3321	x	–	x	x	x	–	–	–	–
Sweden	I–IV	–	–	x	–	x	x	–	–	–	x	x
France	I–IV	€1425	–	x	–	–	–	–	–	–	–	–
England	I–IV	–	€28 940	1423	–	2427	99	315	–	830	4550	20 408
Germany	I–IV	€3365	–	x	–	–	–	–	–	–	–	–
Denmark	I–IV	–	€10 460	7111	–	2370	–	269	78	–	658	–
Sweden	I–IV	–	€4316	417	–	440	16	–	50	–	103	3511

Reproduced from Krensel et al. 2019 [48] with permission of John Wiley & Sons.
GP, general practitioner; x, cost category was assessed but not described separately.

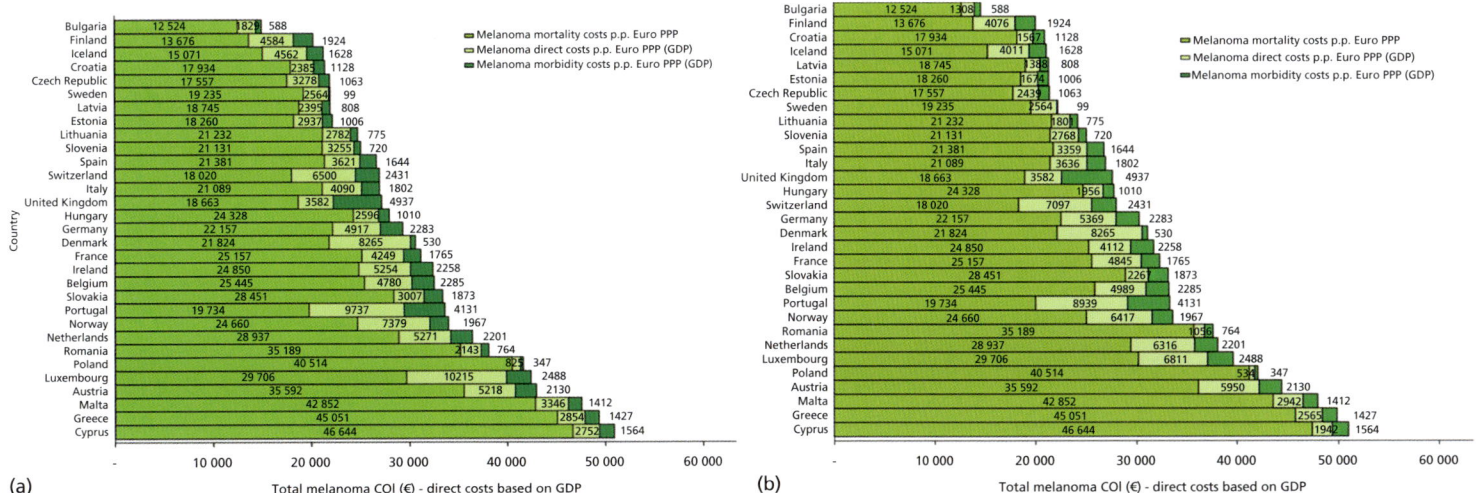

Figure 6.4 Direct, mortality and morbidity costs of melanoma per patient (p.p.). (a) Direct costs derived from gross domestic product (GDP). (b) Direct costs derived from national health expenditure (HE). COI, cost of illness; PPP, purchasing power parity. Reproduced from Krensel et al. 2019 [47] with permission of John Wiley & Sons.

Psoriasis

Psoriasis is a chronic skin disease which affects about 1.5% of the UK population [50], 2.5% in Germany [51] and 1.17–1.43% in Spain [52]. Worldwide 0.2–4.8% of all people suffer from this disease [53] (Chapter 35). Prevalence in children has been 0.7% in Germany [54]. Its economic burden is not only attributable to the high prevalence but also to the high prices of innovative pharmaceutical products like biological agents. Moreover, indirect costs due to absenteeism and presenteeism can be considerable. In a recent study from the USA, 49% of psoriasis patients missed work days regularly due to psoriasis [55]. In the following text, studies investigating the economic burden of psoriasis are discussed (Table 6.4).

The costs of illness due to moderate to severe plaque psoriasis in Canada were evaluated by Levy et al. from a societal perspective [56]. Expenses due to physician consultations, drug prescriptions, over-the-counter drugs, phototherapy sessions, hospitalisation, laboratory tests and procedures, lost productivity at work and losses in leisure activity were included. Therefore, direct medical costs as well as indirect cost were included. The DLQI was also assessed, but not analysed with respect to costs. For analysis, the bottom-up approach was used; data were collected from 90 patients in three clinics and extrapolated to the entire population of Canada. The mean annual direct medical cost for the treatment of psoriasis was CDN$4557 per patient. Costs caused by lost productivity due to psoriasis were $2953. In this analysis, lost productivity costs not attributed directly to psoriasis were considered as well, which amounted to an additional $489. Transferring these expenses onto the entire population of Canada with approximately 212 500 persons affected by moderate to severe psoriasis, annual direct medical costs added up to $1 billion for direct lost productivity and $0.7 billion for lost productivity not directly attributed to psoriasis.

The cost of illness of psoriasis in Switzerland was estimated by Navarini et al. for the year 2005 using mixed methods [57]. To determine out-of-pocket expenses, health-related QoL and lost productivity, severity of disease, prescribed drugs, and consumption of diagnostic and therapeutic procedures, a patient and physician survey was conducted using the bottom-up approach. Utilisation of in-patient treatment, average length of stay per case, number of cases and the number of cases per patient were derived from the Federal Statistic Offices using the top-down approach. A total of 383 patients returned their questionnaires and stated their annual out-of-pocket expenses to be CHF1185. Physicians returned 170 questionnaires concerning their patients. Of these, average treatment costs resulted in CHF1100 for mild, CHF2500 for moderate and CHF9900 for severe psoriasis. Additional expenses of CHF2 154 547 arose from the treatment of severe psoriasis with biologics. Regarding in-patient care, in total 3578 cases and 3043 patients were treated in 2004 in Swiss hospitals with an average length of stay of 18.3 days. Multiplied with the average day fee of CHF1070, costs for in-patient treatment due to psoriasis added up to CHF19 581 per patient and CHF59 584 983 for the entire population. Consultations and medications resulted in expenses of CHF929 and CHF3780, respectively. Extrapolated to the Swiss population with 86 170 persons affected, total direct medical costs rose to CHF458 million in 2005 with the assumption that 38% suffered from mild, 43% from moderate and 19% from severe psoriasis. The annual costs per person affected for medication (CHF2658), consultations (CHF779), hospitalisation (CHF691) and out-of-pocket expenses (CHF1193) added up to CHF5321. Health-related QoL and lost productivity were not considered in this analysis although these items were part of the questionnaire.

One study evaluating the economic burden of psoriasis from a societal perspective in Germany retrospectively included direct medical and non-medical costs as well as indirect costs borne by patients, insurers, employers and the sickness fund [58]. Data from 184 patients was collected by handing out questionnaires to patients and physicians. Fifty-two patients had 63 hospital admissions in total with an average length of stay of 29.8 days causing costs of €2299 per patient. Annual out-of-pocket expenses for patients were €794. Productivity loss was estimated using the friction cost approach by multiplying the average daily gross income of employed person with days of sick leave ($n = 57$), being out of work ($n = 6$) or having a 'reduction in earning capacity' ($n = 44$) due to

Table 6.4 Cost of illness of psoriasis in selected countries.

| Reference | Country | n | Perspective | Direct medical costs per patient and year | | | Indirect costs | Total costs |
				Consultations	Hospitalisations	Medications	Productivity lost	
Levy et al. [56]	Canada	90	Society	–	CDN$4557[b]	–	CDN$2953	CDN$7510
Navarini et al. [57]	Switzerland	170	Physicians	CHF779	CHF691	CHF2658	–	CHF5321
		383	Patients	–	CHF1193	–	–	
Sohn et al. [58]	Germany	184	SHI Patients	€204	€2299	€2014	€1310	€6621
				€794[b]	–	–	–	
Berger et al. [59]	Germany	192	SHI Patients	€350[c]	–	€513	€1441	€2866
				€562[c]	–	–	–	
Yu et al. [60][a]	USA	56 528	Hospital	US$720	US$111	US$847	–	US$1976
Carrascosa et al. [61]	Spain	797	Society	€352	€36	€503	€189	€1079
Colombo et al. [62][a]	Italy	150	Society	€158	€2510	€1092	€2682	€8371

Adapted from Gutknecht et al. 2016 [63].
[a] Costs for other procedures are also included in total costs.
[b] Total direct medical costs (consultations + hospitalisations + medications).
[c] Direct medical costs for consultations + hospitalisations.
SHI, statutory health insurance.

psoriasis for the first 3 months of absence. Indirect costs resulted in €1310 per patient and year. Average out-patient and medication costs were €204 and €2014 per year. Thus, total average costs added up to €6709 per patient. Classifying patients into three groups regarding their type of therapy (those receiving therapy other than systematic therapy, those receiving conventional systemic therapy and those with inadequately controlled disease), out-of-pocket expenditures, productivity loss and risk for hospitalisation, as well as length of stay and therefore costs for in-patient treatment, increased their (unmet) medical needs from €609 to €1002, €1048 to €1635 and €1187 to €3887, respectively. In contrast, in the ambulatory setting, costs for physician consultations and medication were highest in the group treated with conventional systemic therapies (€224 and €3089, respectively). Nevertheless, total costs were highest (€6709) for patients with inadequately controlled psoriasis. These findings were not extrapolated to the entire population to estimate the national economic impact.

Another multicentre study evaluating cost of illness in patients with moderate to severe psoriasis in Germany from a societal perspective included direct and indirect costs [59]. Data were obtained from 192 patients by survey retrospectively, prospectively and by patients' records; 106 patients suffered from moderate and 82 from severe psoriasis. Services included 7.2 physician consultations and 0.4 days of hospitalisation leading to annual costs on average of €350.85 per patient. Medication was prescribed to 91.7% of the patients generating costs of €513.50. Therefore, direct medical costs for the third-party payer added up to €864.35. From the patient's perspective, co-payments and expenses for non-reimbursable therapies and devices amounted to an additional €561.68. Annual indirect costs were calculated using the human capital approach including work days lost because of sick leave, early retirement, unemployment or inability to work due to psoriasis and this resulted in a €1440.20 cost per patient. Total annual costs for psoriasis treatment in Germany amounted to €2866.23 per patient. Differentiated by the severity of disease no significant differences were found, but total costs for patients receiving systemic therapy were significantly higher (€4985) than costs for patients receiving other therapies (€1173). Here, findings were not extrapolated to the entire population to estimate the national economic impact.

Yu *et al.* evaluated the annual direct costs of psoriasis in the USA retrospectively from the third-party payer perspective using information obtained from a national database [60]. They chose another study design comparing total expenses for health services for any cause of 56 528 patients suffering from psoriasis with a matched healthy cohort. Occurrence of co-morbidities, health care utilisation and health care costs were significantly higher in patients with psoriasis. Allocating the incremental economic burden of US$1976.3 per patient, annual costs for out-patient treatment amounted to $719.5, for in-patient treatment $111.4 and for drugs $846.8. Patients receiving systemic therapy were rated to have moderate to severe psoriasis. About 9.3% of all patients received systemic medication. The treatment of patients who did not receive any systemic therapies generated costs of $5010.9. For patients with systemic medication, expenses were $10 592.5. Their drug prescription as well as in-patient and out-patient utilisation was significantly higher compared with patients with other types of therapy or without therapy, resulting in adjusted direct health care costs higher by $3886.4, $166.5 and $1747.7, respectively. Thus incremental costs for patients treated with systemic therapies compared with the patients without were $7517. An extrapolation to the entire population was not carried out. Because of the chosen perspective, neither out-of-pocket expenses nor indirect costs were considered.

In Spain, a prospective observational study was conducted considering direct and indirect costs of psoriasis from the societal perspective using the bottom-up approach [61]. A total of 797 patients were included and asked to keep a diary on health resource consumption which was then priced monetarily by the authors. Direct costs included expenses for prescribed drugs, over-the-counter drugs, diagnostic procedures, physicians' consultations (e.g. routine visits, private dermatologists, out-patient hospital department visits) and in-patient treatment. They accounted for €890.5 (82.5%) annually on average, of which €502.9 (46.6%) was for drugs, €36.4 for hospitalisation and €351.4 for consultations. Patients had to bear the costs of €154.9 for over-the-counter drugs on average. Indirect costs were defined as lost productivity because of sick leave due to psoriasis and amounted to €188.5. Total costs added up to €1079. Classified by severity of disease, treatment of severe psoriasis (€2169.3) caused significantly higher costs than treatment of moderate psoriasis (€1265.4) or mild psoriasis (€893.3). Extrapolating these findings onto the population of Spain, the economic burden of psoriasis is approximately €532 million annually.

Colombo *et al.* evaluated the costs of moderate to severe psoriasis in a multicentre prospective study in Italy from a societal perspective [62]. The study was carried out as a survey of 150 patients and their physicians using the bottom-up approach. Direct costs included expenses for hospitalisation, day-hospital admission, medical examinations, laboratory tests, phototherapy and medication. These costs amounted to €5690.10 of which 44% were caused by hospitalisation and 19% by medication only. No patient was treated with biologics. Indirect costs were defined as lost productivity because of leaving work earlier, sick leave and lost leisure time due to psoriasis. They were calculated by the human capital approach multiplying lost productivity with the average national gross income and resulted in a cost of €2681.51 per patient. Total annual costs for psoriasis added up to €8371.61. Expenses for patients with severe psoriasis were €11 434.4 on average and significantly higher compared with expenses for patients with moderate psoriasis (€5226.04). Extrapolating these results on the population of Italy, national costs are approximately €2403 million per year. Out-of-pocket expenses were not included in this analysis.

Besides data on the cost and budget impact of antipsoriatic drugs, comparative data on the cost-effectiveness of treatments are needed. In particular, given the high annual costs of biologics, it needs to be investigated whether such costs are balanced by higher benefits from treatment. Such cost-effectiveness studies have been started in many countries. Since resource utilisation and prices are very specific for each health system, no general conclusions from the data can be drawn. Nevertheless, several studies have shown that more expensive drugs can be the most cost-effective choices when the overall outcomes (e.g. proportion of responders with a lower psoriasis area and severity index (PASI) score, gains in QoL) are relatively higher compared with cheaper drugs. For example, it has been shown that more recent innovations like interleukin 17 (IL-17) and IL-23 blockers are superior in efficiency when used as first line biologics compared with tumour necrosis factor-inhibitors [64,65].

Atopic dermatitis

Atopic dermatitis (AD) is an equally important, very common skin condition which leads to substantial disease burden and has a large impact on the patient, family and social contacts and society [66]. Compared with psoriasis, pharmacological innovations have been delayed and thus there has been less pressure and resources to generate epidemiological and health economic data. However, given the introduction of highly effective biologic drugs (in particular dupilumab and tralokinumab) and small molecules (the first being baricitinib, upadacitinib and abrocitinib), there is now an increased requirement for health economic data in AD. Thus several publications indicate relevant cost burden from AD in different countries [67]. In a recent review, 84 articles were identified depicting costs of illness in AD; 30 assessed direct costs and health care resource use, nine assessed patient/family out-of-pocket costs, 17 assessed indirect costs due to work productivity impairment and 47 assessed humanistic burden [66]. Direct medical costs of up to €6993 per patient per year (PPPY) were observed for adults with uncontrolled moderate to severe disease, with further patient out-of-pocket costs of up to €927 PPPY. Work absenteeism losses were also high and reached €10 040 PPPY in patients with moderate to severe AD in the Netherlands. In Italy, work productivity losses of €2604 PPPY were observed which comprised 60.8% of the total costs for patients with moderate to severe disease. The human costs associated with AD such as sleep disruption, depression, anxiety and impact on education adds further weight to the indirect cost burden.

In conclusion, the burden of AD on patients, their families and society is extensive and complex, with effects continuing throughout patients' lives. When all aspects of costs are considered, it is evident that AD is associated with substantial burden in most countries, amounting to estimated annual direct costs of €10 billion and indirect costs of up to €8 billion in Europe [66].

Cost comparisons of atopic dermatitis and psoriasis

Although the overall disease burden is substantially high in AD, the overall average costs of illness per capita have been shown to be higher in psoriasis in more recent years (Figure 6.5). For example, in Germany the average costs for psoriasis in 2014 were about €5500 [68] compared with about €3500 in atopic dermatitis in 2019 [69]. The reason for this is the much wider use of innovative drugs in psoriasis. Interestingly, once innovations are available, there is a shift in costs for psoriasis from the hospital sector to drug costs [68]. Further, in parallel to higher use and resource utilisation for drugs, the indirect costs were reduced, thus better balancing cost and benefit.

Critical reflection of studies on disease burden

For health economic evaluations a broad range of approaches and study designs exist. Even if the analysis only covers the cost of illness, publications show a large variation of underlying assumptions and methods used which results in limited comparability of findings even within countries. These inconsistencies correspond to the findings of a systematic review of methods used to determine cost of illness of several diseases [70]. For instance, 78% of the articles analysed costs for in-patient care, 64% expenses for medications and 45% for lost productivity only. Further differences between the studies were found in the study designs (e.g. top-down versus bottom-up approach and total versus incremental costs). The assessment of indirect costs varied even if only one indication was considered: in some cases the friction approach was used, in others the human capital. When the human capital approach was used, a further differentiation in absenteeism and presenteeism was found.

The cost structures of these two high-expense diseases differ significantly [36]. First, direct costs account for the largest proportion of expenses in psoriasis (91.6%), while in skin cancer it accounts for 31.4% only. Second, the more detailed examination also showed a huge difference in the composition of direct costs. While the largest proportion of expenses was medication in psoriasis (84.6%), it was office visits in skin cancer (75.0%). Intangible costs, which take loss in QoL into account, were an additional US$56 244.

Thus, any data on disease burden need to be critically checked for the methods applied, the quality of data collection, the time of study conduction and the framework of the health system.

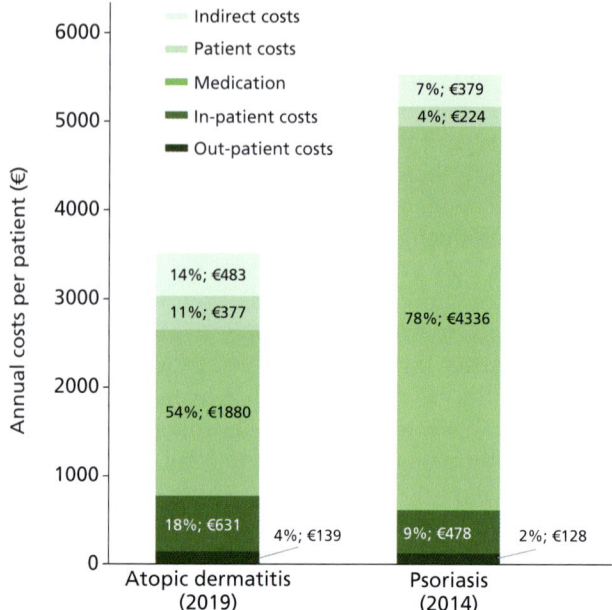

Figure 6.5 Comparison of costs of illness between psoriasis and atopic dermatitis in Germany, showing typical differences in the course of psoriasis care and between psoriasis and atopic dermatitis.

Impact for decision making in dermatology practice

The economic burden of skin diseases includes the costs to the payers and patients, indirect costs to society and intangible costs to the patient and relatives. These overall costs are difficult to determine for an individual patient in practice. However, in routine care, the evaluation of the patient's perspective, in particular their health-related QoL, is essential. Economically, it is the patient's disease burden that justifies the expenses for medical measures such as diagnostics and drug treatment. In practice, the explicit treatment goals for an individual patient should be used to define the cost-effectiveness of the treatment. Following health economic rules, the dermatologist provides the most efficient treatment if the treatment goals (i.e. patient benefits) are achieved with the least costs. Consequently, if the least costly treatment fails, a more expensive therapy is justified. Hence, among several treatment options having the same chances of success, the cheapest should be chosen. All costs following the treatment decision need to be included, not just medication costs. Furthermore, a long-term perspective needs to be used since 'early investment' may lead to a return of the disease in the long run. Within the national frameworks of social laws and ethics, individual decision making should favour patient benefits to costs.

Key references

The full list of references can be found in the online version at https://www.wiley.com/rooksdermatology10e

17 Drummond MF, Sculpher MJ, Torrance GW, O'Brien BJ, Stoddart GL. *Basic Types of Economic Evaluation of Health Care Programmes*, 3rd edn. Oxford: Oxford University Press, 2005.

18 Icks A, Chernyak N, Bestehorn K *et al*. Methods of health economic evaluation for health services research. *Gesundheitswesen* 2010;72:917–33.

25 Evans C, Mertzanis P, Abetz L. Measurement strategies for indirect costs in economic evaluations. *Expert Rev Pharmacoecon Outcomes Res* 2003;3:703–16.

27 Augustin M, Langenbruch A, Gutknecht M, Radtke MA, Blome C. Quality of life measures for dermatology: definition, evaluation, and interpretation. *Curr Derm Rep* 2012;1:148–59.

28 Both H, Essink-Bot M, Busschbach J, Nijsten T. Critical review of generic and dermatology-specific health-related quality of life instruments. *J Invest Dermatol* 2007;127:2726–39.

36 Bickers DR, Lim HW, Margolis D *et al*. The burden of skin diseases: 2004, a joint project of the American Academy of Dermatology Association and the Society for Investigative Dermatology. *J Am Acad Dermatol* 2006;55:490–500.

39 Seidler AM, Pennie ML, Veledar E, Culler SD, Chen SC. Economic burden of melanoma in the elderly population: population-based analysis of the Surveillance, Epidemiology, and End Results (SEER) – Medicare data. *Arch Dermatol* 2010;146:249–56.

56 Levy AR, Davie AM, Brazier NC *et al*. Economic burden of moderate to severe plaque psoriasis in Canada. *Int J Dermatol* 2012;51:1432–40.

58 Sohn S, Schoeffski O, Prinz J *et al*. Cost of moderate to severe plaque psoriasis in Germany: a multicenter cost-of-illness study. *Dermatology (Basel)* 2006;212:137–44.

70 Akobundu E, Ju J, Blatt L, Mullins CD. Cost-of-illness studies: a review of current methods. *Pharmacoeconomics* 2006;24:869–90.

CHAPTER 7

Global Health Dermatology

L. Claire Fuller
Chelsea and Westminster NHS Foundation Trust, London, UK

What is global health?, 7.1	Neglected Tropical Disease Non-Governmental Organisation Network (NNN), 7.6	Community dermatology, 7.7
History of global health, 7.1		WHO NTD RoadMap, 7.7
Global health today, 7.1	The Skin Related NTDs Cross Cutting Group (NNN Skin NTD CCG), 7.6	**Improving global skin health, 7.7**
Global burden of disease – dermatology, 7.2		Developing capacity in global health dermatology, 7.7
Dermatology in the global health context, 7.2	GLODERM – International Alliance for Global Health Dermatology, 7.6	Initiatives to improve access – equity of access to dermatological expertise, 7.8
Climate change and the skin, 7.3	Centers for Disease Control and Prevention (CDC), 7.6	Building educational capacity for dermatology, 7.11
Key stakeholders in global health dermatology, 7.4	American Society of Tropical Medicine and Hygiene (ASTMH), 7.6	Building academic capacity for global health, 7.12
United Nations (UN), 7.4		Simple needs assessments, 7.12
World Health Organization (WHO), 7.5	Royal Society of Tropical Medicine and Hygiene (RSTMH), 7.6	Migrant health dermatology, 7.13
International League of Dermatological Societies (ILDS), 7.5		Getting involved, 7.13
International Foundation for Dermatology (IFD), 7.6	**Terms used in global health dermatology, 7.6**	**Conclusion, 7.14**
	Sustainable Development Goals, 7.6	**Key references, 7.15**

What is global health?

Global health describes an evolving concept, an approach or discipline that aims to improve people's health worldwide through better health care and access to it. It embraces a focus on both individual, patient-based clinical care as well as intervention at the population level, understood as 'public health'.

Achieving this requires a broad range of potential areas of engagement including research, teaching and clinical practice. It requires addressing social and political determinants of health, and finding solutions while working across political boundaries.

History of global health

The term global health first started appearing in the English literature in the 1990s taking over from the previous prevailing term 'International Health'. However, its origins can be considered to have developed from various predecessors such as 'colonial' and 'tropical' medicine. These terms emerged during the 19th century and focused on infectious disease control, in the main driven by national security priorities.

Global health continues to be seen in the context of foreign policy and connected to international security. However, over time, proponents of the global health concept have acknowledged the opportunities of recognising the benefits of including national security and foreign policy considerations within their advocacy framework. This assists in achieving alignment with the Sustainable Development Goals (SDGs) drafted in 2015. The SDGs were agreed by 193 countries at the United Nations (UN). They aim to rid the world of poverty and hunger and be safe from the worst effects of climate change by 2030. The 17 goals and 163 targets built on momentum established by the Millennium Development Goals (MGDs) that report achieving a 50% reduction in extreme poverty over 15 years.

The SDGs, which include specific global health targets, consider health and well-being a general human right. They necessitate engagement from a range of potential contributors including international agencies, governments, charities and individual philanthropists.

Global health today

National public health departments and health protection agencies work together for global health security conforming to the international health regulations specifically committing countries to ensure they have the capacity and capability to detect, assess and report global health threats. While current global events highlight the dangers of infectious disease, exemplified dramatically by the Covid-19 global pandemic, other hazards such as chemical, radiation, nuclear and biological threats can also impact on health.

Several universities now have departments of global health with many of them collaborating through networks and consortia to

Rook's Textbook of Dermatology, Tenth Edition. Edited by Christopher Griffiths, Jonathan Barker, Tanya Bleiker, Walayat Hussain and Rosalind Simpson.
© 2024 John Wiley & Sons Ltd. Published 2024 by John Wiley & Sons Ltd.

promote sharing of good practice, rapid communication of activities and results and pooling of resources. As yet there are only a very few specifically with dermatological global health departments within them.

The global heath 'approach' may involve three themes:
1 Equitable partnerships – incorporating principles of respect and trust, planned together, and carried out together with measurable outputs.
2 Expanding capability – supporting the strengthening of health systems in low- and middle-income countries (LMIC).
3 Sustainability – ensuring that skills and capacity generated remains and continues once a partnership arrangement has reached its conclusion.

Global burden of disease – dermatology

Disease burden as a concept was first devised in the 1990s to collate the impact of effect from death and health loss due to disease and injuries as well as other health hazards across all regions of the world. Harvard School of Public Health working with the World Bank and World Health Organization (WHO) used disability adjusted life years (DALYs) as the unit of measurement which collates the time lost because of premature death with the time spent in a health limited situation state. This combined calculation of the numbers of years lost due to premature mortality or disability generate the DALYs for specific diseases. The approach of calculated disease burden cannot comprehensively be limited to DALYs as this misses the impact of stigma as well as involvement of robust heath economic evaluations becoming increasingly relevant when considering finite resources available for health care. The Global Burden of Diseases Study 2013 identifies skin diseases as the fourth most common cause of all human disease, affecting nearly one third of the world's population and the 18th leading cause of DALYs [1].

Dermatology in the global health context

The impact of skin ill health can be felt throughout life in a variety of ways that were illustrated in an editorial review from the International League of Dermatological Societies, titled Global Challenge for Skin Health in 2015 [2]. They noted the rising incidence of atopic dermatitis (AD) that is affecting 165 million children worldwide. AD results in intrusive itching that interrupts sleep and scratching that can lead to secondary infection. In LMIC, infestation with scabies mite is widespread, affecting more than 160 million children globally. In addition to causing intractable itching, it is the commonest cause of bacterial pyoderma. Long-term sequela of pyoderma through glomerulonephritis contributes to the worldwide epidemic of lifelong hypertension [3]. Occupational skin diseases including hand dermatitis are reported to cost €5 billion each year when addressing treatment, loss of productivity and compensation costs [4]. Skin cancer can occur throughout life but is more common in the elderly. Loss of pigment caused by the genetic disorder oculocutaneous albinism is a major determinant of life-threatening skin cancer in the resource-poor

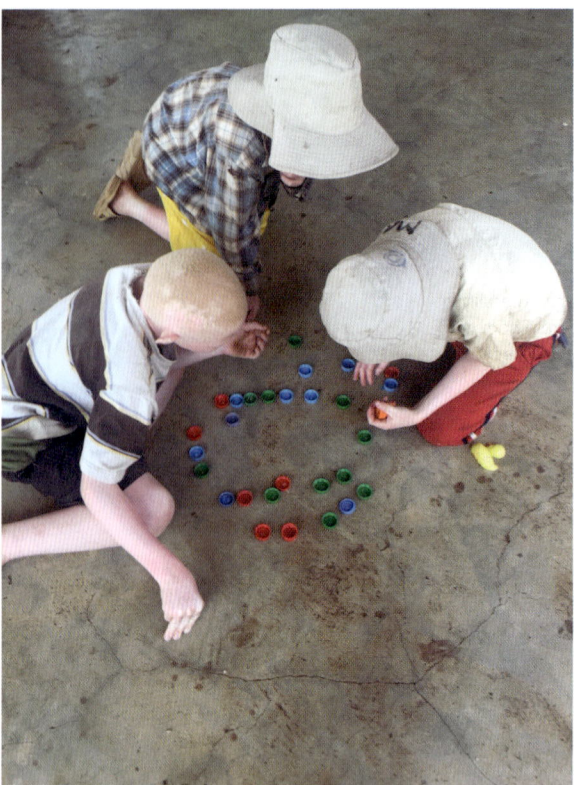

Figure 7.1 Children with albinism playing at a workshop.

tropics. Not only is access to prevention and treatment limited, but persons with albinism (PWA) are also at risk of persecution, including violent attack and ritual murder (Figure 7.1). These represent just a few examples of challenges to global skin health.

As can be seen in Table 7.1, in addition to the widespread prevalence of common skin diseases, there is further burden from the so-called 'neglected tropical diseases' (NTDs), many of which have cutaneous manifestations and are known as the skin NTDs. Skin NTDs include those NTDs that have recognised skin manifestations that are either primary manifestations of the disease such as Buruli ulcer, leprosy, scabies and mycetoma or an associated clinical feature such as the urticarial rash that can occur in schistosomiasis, soil-transmitted helminths and foodborne trematodiases, or lymphoedema that occurs with podoconiosis (Figure 7.2), lymphatic filariasis and leprosy.

NTDs are a diverse group of diseases most common in tropical and subtropical conditions that affect more than a billion people. They account for 62.3 million DALYs according to the 2017 Global Burden of Disease study [1]. In addition to their impact on health, NTDs, often, through their highly visible cutaneous manifestations, contribute to stigma, disability and exacerbate poverty of those affected. The WHO hosts a list of priority NTDs that include conditions that disproportionally affect populations living in poverty and cause significant morbidity and mortality, and primarily affect communities living in tropical and subtropical areas. They include conditions that are generally amenable to control, elimination or eradication and have been relatively neglected by research.

Table 7.1 The impact of common skin diseases. Reproduced from Hay, Augustin, Griffiths and Sterry 2015 [2].

Skin condition	Global distribution	Impact
Atopic eczema	RPS/AE	Predominantly affects children. Itching leading to sleep loss, inattention and disruption of family life
Psoriasis	RPS/AE	Mainly adults. In addition to skin disability, risk of arthritis and cardiovascular disease
Scabies	RPS	All ages but particularly children. High prevalence, e.g. >50% in some areas. Risk of nephritis and rheumatic fever
Pyoderma	RPS	Associated with scabies. Risk of secondary complications (see Scabies)
Skin ulcers, especially leg ulcers and decubitus ulcers	RPS/AE Elderly	Associated secondary infection and major loss of mobility
Pruritus, from both dermatological and non-dermatological diseases	RPS/AE	Loss of sleep, particularly in elderly; depression and mental illness
Genetic disorders such as epidermolysis bullosa and albinism	RPS/AE	Risks range from severe disability and death, e.g. in epidermolysis bullosa, to aggressive skin cancer in albinos in Sub-Saharan Africa
Skin cancers: both melanoma and non-melanoma	Mainly AE but both for non-melanoma skin cancer	Rising mortality with melanomas in younger adults. Very high prevalence of SCC in the elderly (>70–80 years)
Diseases of an ageing population: leg ulceration, pruritus	RPS/AE	See previously
The skin as initial indicator of serious medical conditions such as NTDs (RPS), e.g. leprosy, yaws, onchocerciasis etc., or autoimmune damage, e.g. SLE (RPS/AE)	RPS/AE	Risk of mortality or severe morbidity. Early recognition leads to early treatment and prevention of major sequelae. Failure to recognise signs of NTDs may compromise control programmes

RPS, resource-poor settings; AE, advanced economies; SCC, squamous cell carcinoma; NTD, neglected tropical disease; SLE, systemic lupus erythematosus.

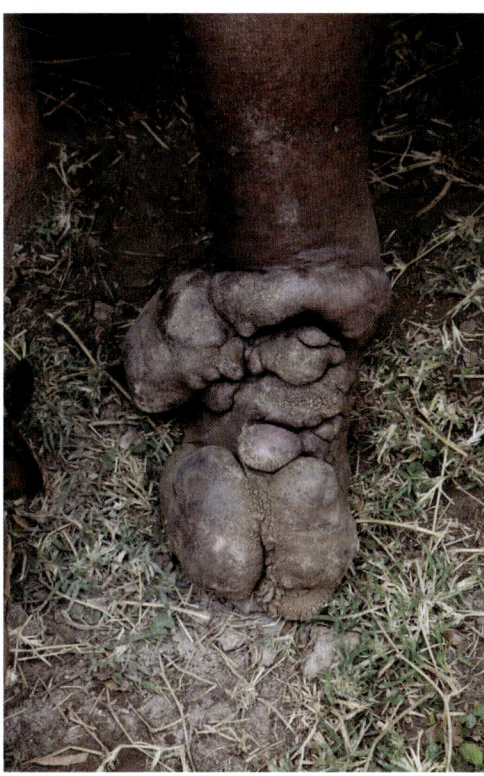

Figure 7.2 Podoconiosis – a typical foot with nodular variant of non-filarial elephantiasis.

While dealing with these challenges needs a multifaceted approach, recognition and management of common skin diseases as well as neglected diseases can be enhanced by access to dermatological expertise. It has been previously widely acknowledged that there is a gap in the provision of specialist dermatology expertise in many settings including high income countries such as the UK [5]. However, this gap is vast in the context of LMIC. Formal maps detailing the availability of dermatologists across the world are limited. However, a recent review estimating the density of dermatologists across Sub-Saharan Africa presented in numbers of consultants per million of the population demonstrates that in contrast to the USA where there are an estimated 20 000 dermatologists to 328 million population, Lesotho and The Gambia have no dermatologists and Eritrea and Liberia just one for the whole country [6]. Updated details are shown in Figure 7.3.

Efforts required to progress the global skin health initiative can be divided into four key areas:
1 Research.
2 Education.
3 Clinical intervention programme application through translation.
4 Advocacy and funding.

Dermatologists have long been involved in global health. For example, Castellani followed a career in tropical and infectious diseases predominantly affecting those in resource-limited settings and eventually founded the International Society of Dermatology, originally known as the International Society of Tropical Dermatology [7]. Samuel Plumbe acknowledged the global dimensions of skin diseases including sections on leprosy, lymphatic filariasis and even the Aleppo boil (leishmaniasis) in his texts in the 1830s [8]. However, the formal involvement of dermatologists within global health agencies, academic departments or ministries of health is scanty.

Climate change and the skin

Climate change affects the social and environmental determinants of health such as clean air, safe drinking water, sufficient food and secure shelter. Over the next 30 years climate change is anticipated to cause around 250 000 additional deaths per year from malnutrition, malaria, diarrhoea and heat stress. The direct costs to health are estimated to be $2–4 billion/year by 2030. Countries with fragile health systems, mainly LMIC, are the least able to cope without assistance to prepare and respond (Figure 7.4).

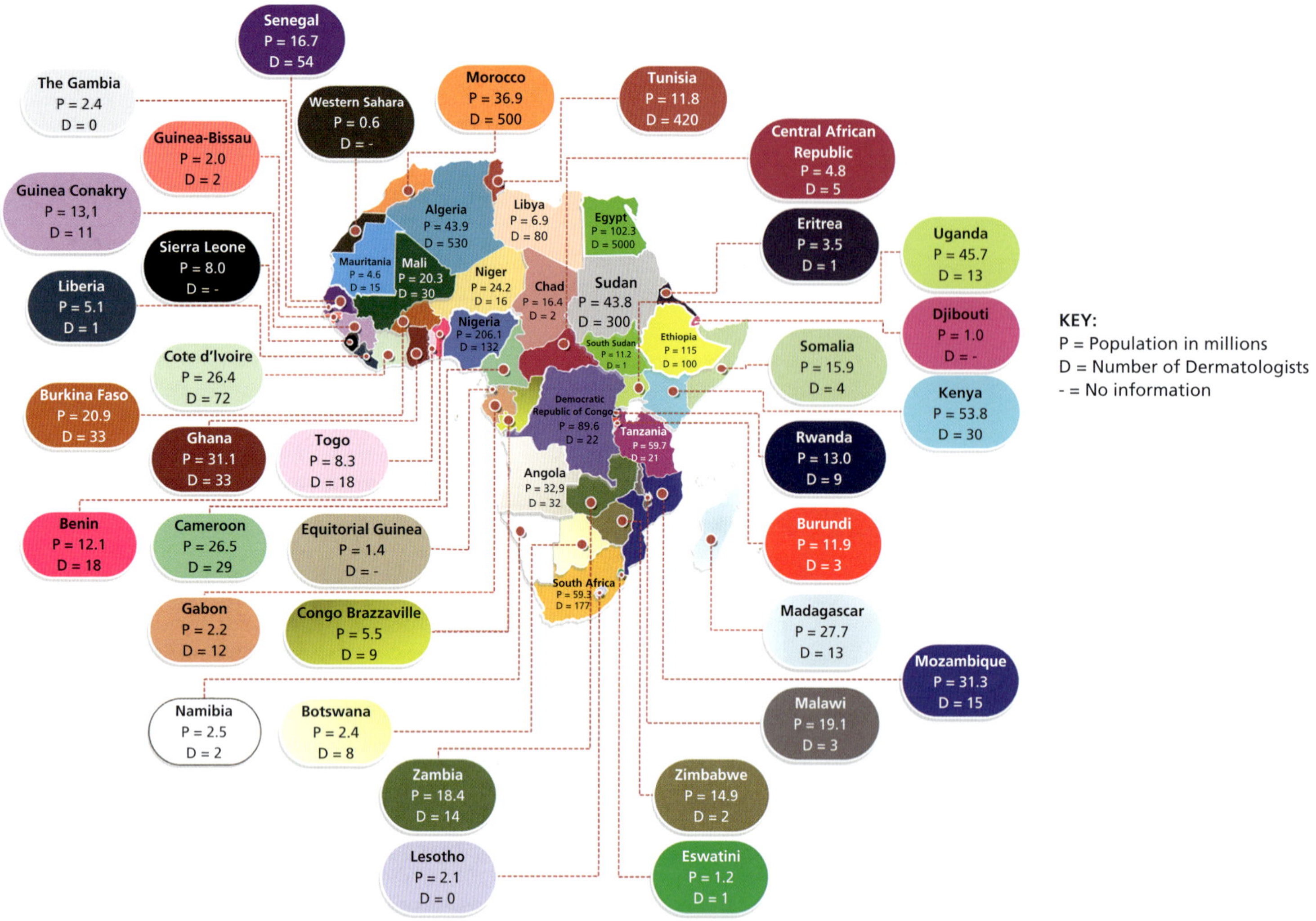

Figure 7.3 Map of Africa showing population of countries and number of dermatologists.

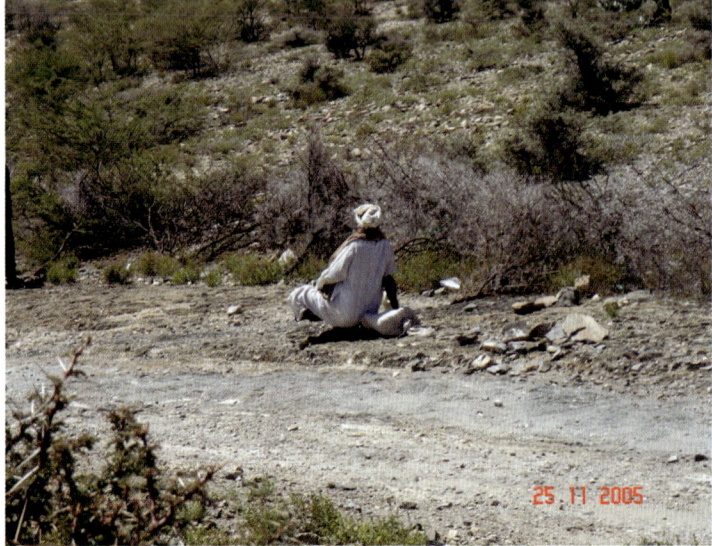

Figure 7.4 Waiting for a lift, Somaliland 2005. Courtesy of Professor Anisa Mosam.

A survey of a group of 158 dermatologists in 2019 reported that the vast majority believed that climate change will alter their work as dermatologists, modifying the incidence of skin diseases in general as well as more specifically in fungal, vector-borne and water-borne diseases. One third reported unusual skin conditions noted already within their communities that they attributed to climate change including common and atypical infections, ultraviolet or heat-related diseases such as skin cancers, and inflammatory dermatoses [9]. A detailed review of the impact of climate change on skin health in Africa produced by the International Society of Dermatology's Climate Change Committee classifies the effects and concludes that the continent, with its delicate health infrastructure, is the most susceptible to the negative influences of climate change and threatens to undermine many of the public health accomplishments made in recent years [10].

Key stakeholders in global health dermatology

United Nations (UN)

The UN is an international organisation founded in 1945. It is currently made up of 193 member states. Its founding charter guides the mission and work and bestows power to enable the UN to take action on issues confronting humanity. These include peace and security, climate change, sustainable development, human rights, disarmament, terrorism, humanitarian and health emergencies, gender equality, governance and food production.

World Health Organization (WHO)

The WHO is a specialised agency of the UN headquartered in Geneva, Switzerland, responsible for international public health. It was established in 1948 and works with 194 member states across six regions and from more than 150 offices. The commitment of the WHO is to achieve 'better health for everyone everywhere'. Their General Programme of Work sets the framework for the financial resources and expenditure every 5 years. They aim to direct and coordinate international health work through collaboration. The WHO partners with countries within the UN system, international organisations, civil society, foundations, and academic and research institutions. In order to protect its work from potential risks such as conflict of interest, reputational risks and undue influence the WHO has adopted the WHO Framework of Engagement with Non-State Actors [11].

The WHO headquarters is organised into a number of departments, many of which include potential for skin health to be specifically considered (Figure 7.5).

International League of Dermatological Societies (ILDS)

The ILDS has been promoting skin health around the world for more than 80 years. The ILDS represents dermatology at the highest level with over 180 Member Societies from more than 80 countries, acting for at least 200 000 dermatologists worldwide. The ILDS is the only dermatology non-state actor in official relations with the WHO. It aims to increase awareness, cooperation and communication within the global dermatology community to promote high quality education, clinical care, research and innovation that will improve skin health globally. It engages with the WHO to encourage consideration of skin health and dermatological issues at several relevant and strategic points. These include:
- Occupational disease, e.g. skin cancer in PWA in the tropics, working outside and occupational contact allergies.
- NTDs.

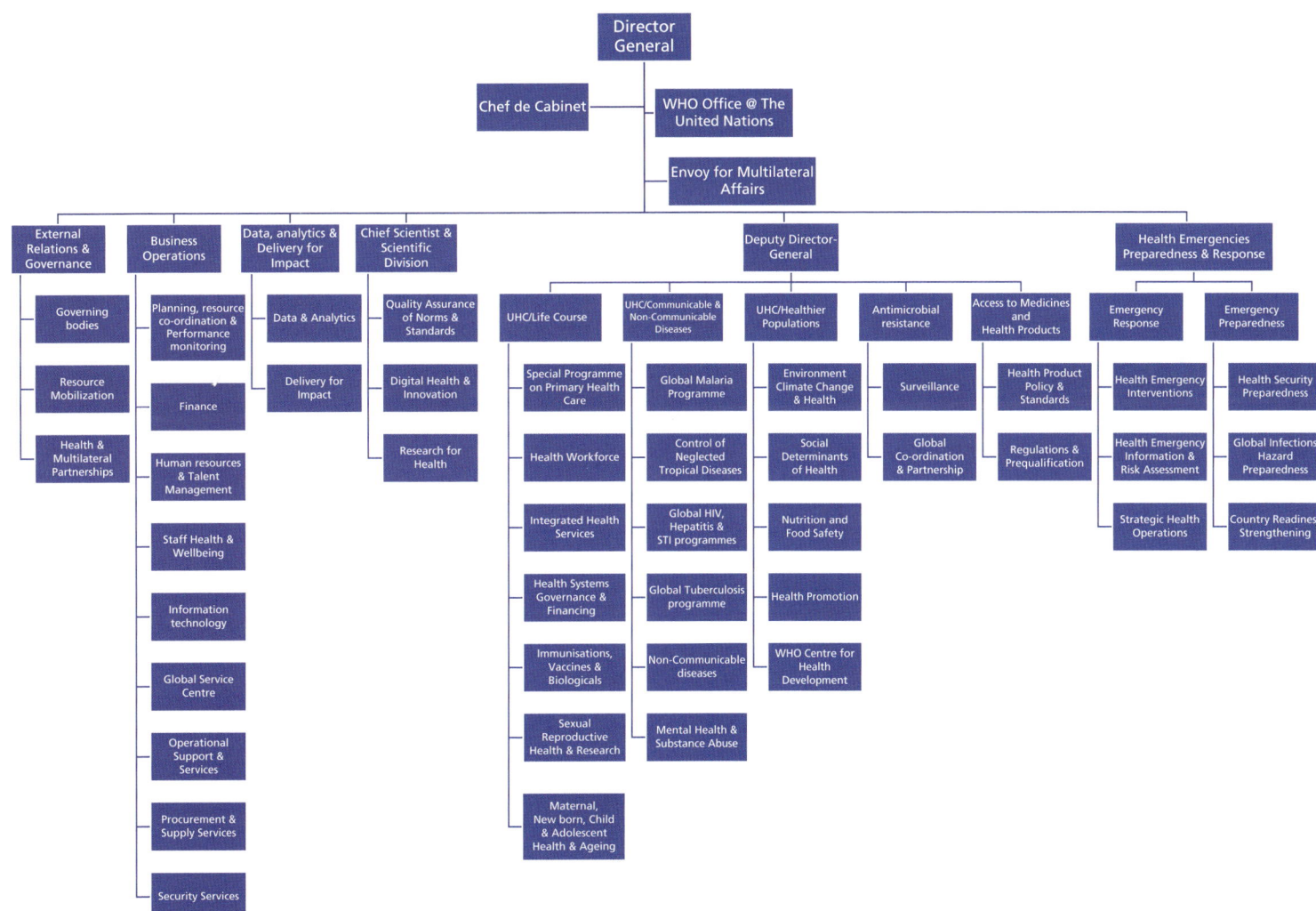

Figure 7.5 Organogram of the World Health Organization as of 10 May 2021 (available from WHO website).

- Essential Medicines List.
- International Classification of Diseases and Related Health Problems (ICD).

International Foundation for Dermatology (IFD)

The IFD is a section of ILDS that specifically focuses on the needs of underresourced areas to enhance awareness of skin health and improve accessibility to dermatological care. Established in 1987 by ILDS, the IFD works to ensure skin health services in areas of low resource are available, accessible and effective for all patients, regardless of ethnicity, disability or social background. It works by supporting partners in underserved parts of the world to improve the provision of, access to and understanding of skin health and skin health services. It achieves this working in three main ways:
1. Education, training and knowledge sharing.
2. Global health partnerships and networks.
3. Policy influencing.

Neglected Tropical Disease Non-Governmental Organisation Network (NNN)

This is a forum for partners working together to improve health for the world's poorest populations. It has over 80 non-governmental organisations (NGOs) as members. It works in support of WHO and governments of endemic countries as an innovative platform for shared learning and programming to generate and disseminate evidenced-based practices. Working across diseases, between cross cutting issues and with governments, the NNN has developed the 'BEST framework' encouraging embedding cross-sectoral approaches and systems in all programmes. BEST is an anagram for the components in the framework and includes: Behaviours, Environment, Social Inclusion and Treatment/care elements. Moving away from the previously traditional methods of vertical, single disease programmes for managing NTDs towards integrated approaches, NNN has fostered identifying common themes and cross cutting approaches and shifts towards integration, coordination and health system strengthening. This shift has been supported by funders and the WHO and reflected in emerging international policies.

The Skin Related NTDs Cross Cutting Group (NNN Skin NTD CCG)

This is one of several NNN cross cutting groups. It works by promoting and supporting the integrated approach to skin-related NTDs detailed previously, recognising the opportunities integrated approaches offer around raising community awareness, conducting epidemiological surveillance and diseases mapping, training for health workers and community health workers, and programme monitoring and evaluation initiatives directed at managing NTDs.

GLODERM – International Alliance for Global Health Dermatology

GLODERM (www.gloderm.org) is a community of health professionals focused on global health dermatology that provides expertise to international health agencies, shares best practice, pools technical know-how and supports trainees wishing to pursue a career in global health dermatology. It undertakes to advance the discipline of population-based medicine and public health in the practice of dermatology.

Global health dermatology is rapidly expanding in the areas of medical education, telehealth, capacity building, task shifting, research, and academic career development. In order to develop a central organisation in which to train in best practice and seek out collaborations and mentorship, the alliance was launched at the American Academy of Dermatology with help from the IFD and the International Society of Dermatology as a novel entity to unite dermatologists, allied health professionals and trainees. It is now supported by the IFD. It has established a trainee committee hosting monthly educational webinars free to registered dermatologists from anywhere in the world and is working towards developing a mentorship scheme to guide trainees in this new dermatology specialty.

Centers for Disease Control and Prevention (CDC)

The US Centers for Disease Control and Prevention is the national public health agency of the USA. It is a US federal agency, under the Department of Health and Human Services, and is headquartered in Atlanta, Georgia. Its role is to protect America from health safety and security threats both foreign and in the USA. It achieves this through conducting strategic scientific investigations and provides health information to protect the USA against health threats and respond when they arise.

American Society of Tropical Medicine and Hygiene (ASTMH)

The ASTMH, founded in 1903, is a large international scientific organisation of experts dedicated to reducing the worldwide burden of tropical infectious diseases and improving global health.

Royal Society of Tropical Medicine and Hygiene (RSTMH)

The RSTMH is a charity and member society based in London striving to save lives and improve health around the world through increased access to and greater equity in global health care.

Terms used in global health dermatology

Sustainable Development Goals

The 2030 Agenda for Sustainable Development was adopted by all UN member states in 2015 and provides a future-proofed scheme for peace and prosperity for people and the planet. It consists of 17 SDGs which represent a call to all countries for action in a global partnership. The SDGs acknowledge that ending poverty and other deprivations must operate in tandem with strategies that improve health and education, reduce inequality, and spur economic growth while tackling climate change and working to preserve our natural environment.

Sustainable Development Goal 3 of the 2030 Agenda for Sustainable Development is to *'ensure healthy lives and promoting well-being for all at all ages'*. The associated targets aim to: reduce the global maternal mortality ratio; end preventable deaths of newborns and children; end the epidemics of AIDS, tuberculosis, malaria and other communicable diseases; reduce mortality from non-communicable diseases; strengthen the prevention and treatment of substance abuse; halve the number of deaths and injuries from road traffic accidents; ensure universal access to sexual and reproductive health care services; achieve universal health coverage; and reduce the number of deaths and illnesses from hazardous chemicals and pollution.

Universal health coverage means that all people have access to the health services they need, when and where they need them, without financial hardship. It includes the full range of essential health services, from health promotion to prevention, treatment, rehabilitation and palliative care. Currently, at least half of the people in the world do not receive the health services they need. About 100 million people are pushed into extreme poverty each year because of out-of-pocket spending on health. This goal is embedded in SDG 3 – Ensure Healthy Lives and Promote Well-being.

Community dermatology

Community dermatology is a term conceived to describe activities or interventions where the dermatologist's role extends beyond the individual to the community as a whole. The approach of community dermatology models adopted initially in Mexico and Argentina (see below) aims to increase access to dermatology experts through education aimed at rural communities currently cut off from dermatology expertise either geographically or socioeconomically, or both.

WHO NTD RoadMap

The WHO has launched a road map for NTDs for 2021–30 'ending the neglect to attain the sustainable development goals'. This sets out global targets and milestones to prevent, control, eliminate and eradicate a diverse set of 20 diseases. Generated through extensive international consultation including IFD, NNN Skin NTD CCG and GLODERM, and endorsed by the World Health Assembly in November 2020, this new roadmap concentrates on integrated approaches needed to achieve the published targets that intersect multiple diseases though cross cutting actions. There are three pillars described to support the global efforts for control and elimination:

1 Accelerate programmatic action.
2 Intensify cross cutting approaches.
3 Change operating models and culture to facilitate country ownership [12].

Improving global skin health

Developing capacity in global health dermatology

We have seen the scarcity of dermatologists within Sub-Saharan Africa. Initiatives to address this include establishing dermatology training centres in resource limited settings both within Sub-Saharan Africa and in other resource limited settings.

Regional Dermatology Training Centre, Moshi, Tanzania (RDTC)

The RDTC (Figure 7.6), situated on the slopes of Mount Kilimanjaro in Tanzania, was established in 1992 through a collaboration between the Government of Tanzania Ministry of Health, the IFD and the Good Samaritan Foundation (NGO responsible for the

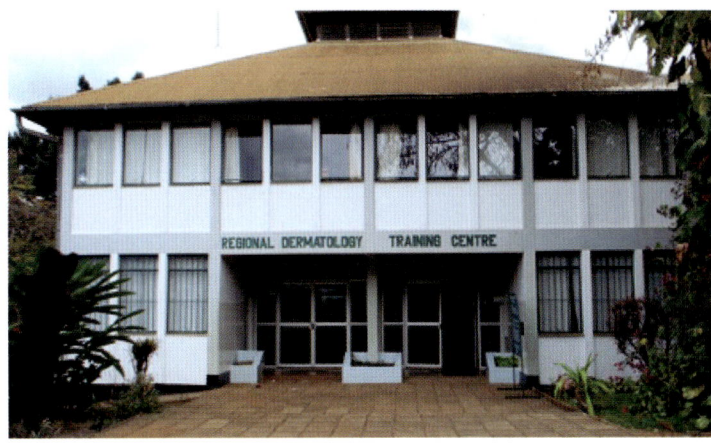

Figure 7.6 Regional Dermatology Training Centre, Moshi, Tanzania.

Kilimanjaro Christian Medical Centre (KCMC)). The centre is integrated within KCMC and provides dermatological services for this teaching hospital as well as being a dedicated training institution. The broad objective for the centre to prevent, treat and rehabilitate patients with skin diseases, leprosy and sexually transmitted infections in Sub-Saharan Africa was initially achieved through training of appropriate cadres of health care workers. The first programme, an Advanced Diploma of Dermato-venereology, directed at clinical officers, has now trained more than 300 dermatology officers and returned them to start dermatology services in 17 African countries. Subsequently a 4-year residency programme has begun and trained 42 dermato-venereology consultants for eight African countries. Moves towards financial sustainability include encouraging the sending countries ministries to demonstrate financial support for their candidates through robust and regular representation to the ECSA-HC (East, Central and Southern African Health Community).

Botswana–UPENN Partnership

This initiative represents a partnership between the Perelman School of Medicine Centre for Global Health, Botswana Ministry of Health and the University of Botswana to build health care and research capacity in Botswana. It was established in 2001. With about 120 full-time staff in Botswana supported by the programme, this initiative takes an interdisciplinary approach emphasising a focus on internal medicine and its subspecialties. The initial drive was to improve the treatment of HIV and its complications. It has developed postgraduate training programmes within the University of Botswana, supports global health experience for Perelman trainees and has developed a joint research agenda guided by the needs of the citizens of Botswana. There is specific and successful dermatology involvement with this programme, focusing on local dermatology capacity building and teledermatology.

Cambodia – rebuilding dermatology services after the Kymyer Rouge era: clinical officers training

With support of overseas, mainly German and French donors and lecturers, dermato-venereology services have been strengthened in Cambodia through the establishment of a dermatology diploma course. Working with the only internationally fully certified dermatologist (fully trained in Germany) a 20-week course consisting of 2-week modules and bolstered by 320 hours of internship in

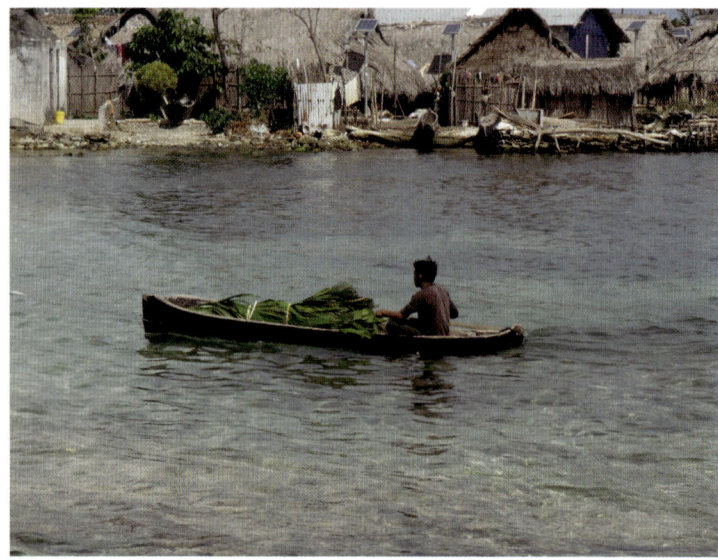

Figure 7.7 Local transport solutions in Cambodia.

hospitals and laboratories was delivered. Classes of 10 students completed basic dermatology diagnostics and therapeutics training to enable identification and management of the common dermatoses seen in Cambodia. Between 2005 and 2013, five courses were completed, with roughly 50 clinicians graduating with a diploma in basic dermatology. Following this, full specialisation training commenced in 2013 that is conducted partly in Cambodia and partly in overseas placements. International collaboration continues to play a significant role in supporting dermatology specialty development within Cambodia [13] (Figure 7.7).

UK Ethiopia Residents Programme – moving towards sustainability

Ethiopian medical education has escalated significantly since 2006, when there were three Ethiopian medical schools from which 122 doctors graduated each year. All 22 dermatologists in the country of about 80 million individuals had trained abroad. After rapid expansion there are now about 30 medical schools training 2700 doctors each year. Developing the teaching faculty as well as the service providers to support this increase has been testing.

In 2006, the Tropical Health and Education Trust (THET) approached a UK dermatologist with experience of working in Ethiopia to assist with teaching medical students in Gondar, Northern Ethiopia. From this initial contact, the UK connection blossomed and a residents training programme for dermatology was born, initially enrolling six trainees. The curriculum was devised locally by the Ethiopian dermatologists at the ALERT Institute in Addis Ababa with UK collaboration. Delivery was assisted by a team of volunteer UK dermatologists acting as visiting lecturers and examiners. This partnership has continued and there are now over 100 trained dermatology consultants serving a population of about 100 million and three new dermatology training centres. With this first phase of establishing a dermatology specialty within Ethiopia now complete, delivering the training of residents is now undertaken by the Ethiopian consultants. However, visiting dermatology specialists to support ongoing training remain welcome as does offering overseas placements for the developing Ethiopian dermatologists. An Association of Ethiopian Dermatology and Venereology has been formed and the development of a robust programme of continuing professional development is in progress within the country.

Community dermatology in Mexico and Argentina

This model involves a regional dermatology team delivering short periods of training over two working days (known as 'journadas') held in various rural areas using volunteer dermatologists, residents and medical students. The journadas include short, targeted dermatology classroom-based courses for the local health care workers (LHCW) followed by massive, free of charge dermatology clinics seeing large numbers of patients but also teaching the LHCW, embedding the theoretical training with 'hands on' experience.

As well as improving dermatology education, training of the LHCW and delivering dermatology clinics for the local community these events enable a number of other objectives to be addressed:
- Surveying the dermatology pathologies prevalent in the rural populations that can then be analysed and shared to stimulate research activities as well as tailoring subsequent teaching to focus on the common diseases seen.
- Initiate activities aimed at preventing common dermatoses.

Training the community to prevent common dermatoses

In Argentina the community teams noted sun-related dermatoses such as actinic prurigo accounted for a significant number of dermatoses seen in rural communities, particularly among the Mapuche living in the Andes. In addition to targeting training of the health care workers on the predominant pathologies seen, the Community Dermatology Argentina has developed an innovative approach, educating young school children under 8 years old on photoprotection using the input of theatre, humour and student participation [14].

One day training programmes – Mali

Noting that skin disease training for health workers is frequently neglected in many settings including those of low resource, a short training programme for general health care workers on the management of common skin diseases was trialled in Bamako, Mali. The benefit was assessed on the basis of evaluating diagnostic and treatment selection accuracy before and immediately after the training. Diagnostic accuracy increased from 42% before training to 81% afterwards. Prescription costs fell by 25% following training. These improvements in knowledge and practice were recorded to persist for at least 18 months after the training [15].

Initiatives to improve access – equity of access to dermatological expertise
Teledermatology in global health

This is now a well-established subspecialty in the medical field of dermatology in general and arguably the most advanced example of applications of telemedicine and e-health. Telecommunication technologies are used to exchange medical information over distance using a combination of audio, visual and data transfer. Many dermatological services from high income countries (HIC) to LMIC are embracing the opportunities offered by this technology. Although different challenges apply across the world, the overarching driver is to improve timely access of dermatological care to patients.

Models exist to support education and development of clinical staff in virtual situations, supporting clinicians in isolated localities to diagnose and manage dermatology patients, as well as consulting with patients in remote settings [16].

Teledermatology training in Mexico

After 25 years of undertaking training in person within the inaccessible rural communities (see the journadas section), faced with challenges of funding and other resources, the Dermatologica Communitaria team from Guerrero state began to shift this teaching to a teledermatology course in Chilpancingo Guerrero, Mexico. Since 2010, with the support of the Guerrero State Health Secretary and Telemedicine Guerrero, they now deliver four basic dermatology courses per year reaching 22 health centres with telemedicine systems and have contact with 11 198 health personnel. These take the form of lectures and short videos accompanied by a simple hard copy manual that is distributed to embed the learning. They also support the referral and management of complex patients using this network.

Africa Teledermatology Project (ATP)

A store-and-forward teledermatology consultation network was established in 2007 in order to assist in providing dermatology care to 12 countries (Botswana, Eritrea, Kenya, Lesotho, Liberia, Malawi, Mozambique, Nigeria, South Africa, Swaziland, Tanzania and Uganda). Since its inception, the project connected clinicians via a secure, password-protected website. This virtual collaboration is between African partners, the USA and Austria. Using cameras and laptop personal computers to capture and send images of patients to specialists in other African countries, Austria and the USA, it provides diagnostic and treatment support to local physicians, dermatologists and health care workers in hospitals and clinics in underserved areas [17].

Teledermatology in Kenya

Colleagues from AMPATH (see later) have led the establishment of a teledermatology service in rural Kenya. The system allows clinicians at remote clinics to utilise an iPad to photograph patients with skin issues that are then transmitted by a secure platform and reviewed by a local Kenyan dermatologist. The team estimates that 65% of patients can be treated by their primary care providers without having to make a long and potentially expensive journey to see a specialist in person. Eventually, the goal is that artificial intelligence could be developed to make the diagnosis based on the photos that are loaded into the system.

Advocating for appropriate attention for skin diseases

International Alliance for the Control of Scabies (IACS)

IACS (www.controlscabies) is a global network committed to the control of human scabies and the promotion of health and well-being of all those living in affected communities. It is a multiprofessional group which partners with government and non-government organisations including the WHO. It is involved in producing global control measures, focusing on advocacy, global burden of scabies monitoring, generation of diagnostic and management guidelines and prioritising the research gaps to achieve control.

Why is scabies important? This parasitic skin infection affects people in every country in the world. Young children and the elderly are particularly vulnerable; secondary infection is common and may lead to severe complications such as sepsis, renal damage and possibly rheumatic heart disease.

Since its launch in 2012, IACS has held annual global scabies control meetings, published strategic position statements and succeeded in presenting the case of scabies to be included as a neglected tropical disease by the WHO in 2017. Through coordinated research efforts evidence has emerged to suggest that scabies is amendable to population level control particularly through mass drug administration. In order to develop a global control programme, key operational research questions need to be resolved. Approaches to diagnosis and disease burden mapping require standardised approaches. Safety of treatments with ivermectin and moxidectin for younger children require investigation. Studies to support the design of optimum implementation of mass treatment including the threshold prevalence for intervention, as well as dosing and frequency, are also needed [18].

As a result of the success of IACS activities, an area of unmet health need has been exposed, and significant financial support has been forthcoming to initiate the World Scabies Programme. This organisation, an initiative of the Murdoch Children's Research Institute in Australia, aims to work with government and partners to translate innovative research in scabies control and establish public health programmes that will reduce the burden of scabies and its complications.

It will work to:
- Translate research on scabies control strategies into practice.
- Increase global awareness on the impact of scabies.
- Support governments to put scabies control on the national health agenda.
- Establish country programmes to implement community-wide control strategies.
- Partner with communities to reduce the impact on families and livelihoods.
- Strengthen health systems to manage and monitor disease.

Footwork: the International Podoconiosis Initiative (www.podo.org)

Podoconiosis, a type of elephantiasis found in subsistence farming communities in the tropics, is an abnormal reaction to irritant mineral particles found in soils of volcanic origins. This poorly understood and neglected disorder is estimated to affect 4 million people in highland tropical Africa with endemicity suggested in more than 15 countries worldwide. Although the disease is both preventable (by avoiding contact with irritant soils) (Figure 7.8) and treatable (through simple inexpensive foot hygiene and protection methods) government-backed assistance programmes have been lacking. Individuals with podoconiosis suffer debilitating physical effects including acute attacks, common to all lymphoedemas, and they are often ostracised from their communities because of myths and misconceptions about the cause of their disease. Footwork was established to coordinate a cross cutting programme of work to achieve the vision of a world free of podoconiosis within our lifetime. By bringing together public and private partners to support

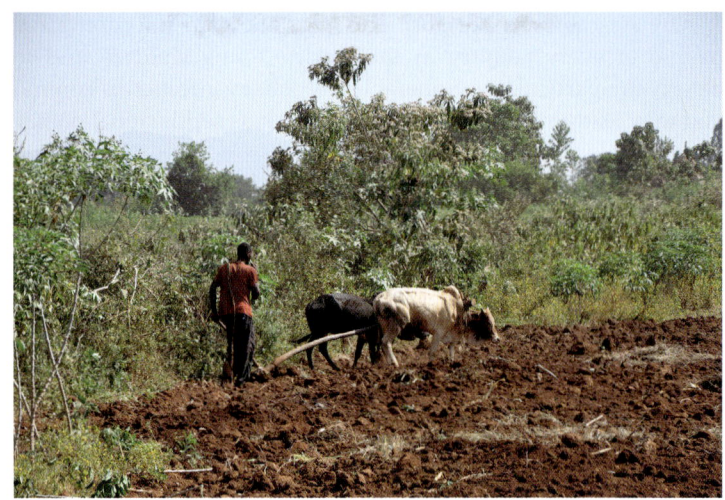

Figure 7.8 Ploughing barefoot in highland Ethiopia, which increases the risk of podoconiosis.

prevention and treatment of and advocacy for podoconiosis Footwork grouped its work in three areas of advocacy and awareness, research and data collection and intervention.

Increasing advocacy for podoconiosis to be included in global health and NTD agendas encourages endemic countries to include the condition within the master plans for health. This has been achieved in Ethiopia. Raising awareness as to the causes and impact of podoconiosis within affected communities and the relative simplicity of disease prevention and treatment reduces stigma and the ostracisation of affected individuals. Advocating for shoes as 'the next bednets' against foot-related conditions including basic wounds, parasitic worms, tetanus, madura foot, tungiasis and snake bite has the ability to prevent disease, reduce morbidity, and increase quality of life and economic opportunities.

Establishing the research priorities enable targeted data collection to clarify the global picture of podoconiosis. Accelerating the collection of scientific data will assist in further establishing the cause of podoconiosis, the most effective treatments and the means of preventing the disease. Supporting mapping of podoconiosis distribution in countries identified as having the appropriate geology, topography and climate has already been undertaken enabling care and support programmes for those affected to be rapidly organised.

Footwork has succeeded in supporting the integration of podoconiosis intervention programmes into primary health care programmes. Additionally, in Ethiopia it has established a method of capturing, propagating and continually updating best practice in diagnosis, prevention and treatment of podoconiosis for use in national guidelines and health professional criteria through the Ethiopian National Podoconiosis Action network.

Global Alliance to Eradicate Lymphatic Filariasis (GAELF)

GAELF connects a diverse collection of public–private partners to support the global programme to eliminate lymphatic filariasis. Acting together, they are able to be more effective in mobilising political, financial and technical resources to achieve a future free of lymphatic filariasis.

International Federation of Anti-Leprosy Associations (ILEP)

A consortium of international NGOs with a common purpose of a world free from leprosy. Through its 13 members working across 62 countries, they support 1028 project locations fighting against leprosy.

Intervention to support and improve skin health

Skin cancer prevention and management in PWA in the tropics: Comprehensive Care Programme with Persons with Albinism (CCPWA)

Occulo-cutaneous albinism, a genetic disorder affecting 1 in 18 000 people worldwide. It is much more common in Sub-Saharan Africa, affecting approximately 10 times more people (1 in 1400). Occulo-cutaneous albinism limits the production and process of melanin distribution in the body, leading to a reduction or absence of it in the skin, eyes and hair. This results in a complex visual impairment, altering retinal development and neural connections, and eliminates natural sun protection leading, in the tropics, to skin cancer development early in life. However, with careful yet simple interventions supporting visual development and introducing sun protection practices and skin surveillance early in life, these health challenges can be mitigated, significantly improving life quality in PWAs.

Starting as an initiative from the RDTC in Moshi, Tanzania with the aim to assist the many PWA in Tanzania with the prevention of cancer and treatment of complications, CCPWA has developed a number of key strands to its programme.
- Skin cancer prevention and treatment.
- Eye assessment and visual improvement.
- Improving access to education.
- Improving independence of PWA.
- General public awareness of issues for PWA.
    - Stigmatisation.
    - Persecution.

Skin cancer prevention through manufacture and provision of free, bespoke sunscreen accompanied by education on sun avoidance and appropriate clothing to minimise sun damage and reduce the development of skin cancer is provided. The educational programmes are directed not only to the PWA beneficiaries but also to community leaders, health care workers, teachers and care givers to support the message, reduce myths and reduce stigmatisation (Figure 7.9).

Skin cancer treatment is delivered through regular outreach clinics screening the PWA and identifying skin cancers or lesions that need cryotherapy, biopsy or excision. A key success for this model is partnering with others. RDTC works with Standing Voice, an international NGO based in Tanzania, Malawi and the UK committed to defending the rights of PWA in Africa. Standing Voice supports the delivery of health, education, advocacy and community programmes not only with the RDTC but also in Malawi. They provide infrastructure capacity for the outreach clinics and work with the RDTC to develop financial and practically sustainable services. Standing Voice has coordinated the development of a skin cancer prevention workshop programme for dermatology officers incorporating classroom components, practical surgical teaching, how to conduct patient education workshops and sun protection education sessions. This is supported with a Manual of Best Practice Skin

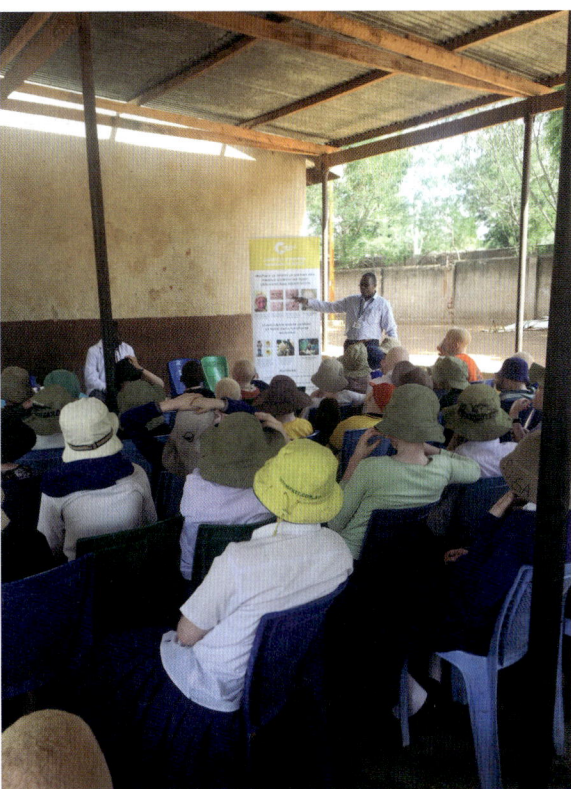

Figure 7.9 Health education workshop for persons with albinism in Tanzania.

Cancer Prevention and Management for Persons with Albinism in Sub-Saharan Africa which is downloadable for free from the ILDS website.

Additional specialist support is provided by annual weeklong practical dermatology surgical workshops led by members of the Academia Espanola de Dermatologica y Venereologia. These hone the surgical skills of those dermatology officers involved in PWA care enabling them to care for those affected locally and minimise the need for the patients to travel long distances for specialist surgical care.

Encouraged and inspired by the Tanzania model, other PWA projects have been established in Fiji and Panama.

Additional projects caring for PWAs have been established in Botswana and Malawi led by local dermatologists and supported by colleagues at the Perelman School of Medicine at the University of Pennsylvania and Tumaini, Austria (a charitable NGO) and Primary Care Dermatology Society, Ireland respectively.

Burma Skincare Initiative (BSI)

Founded in 2018, BSI, a charitable incorporated organisation registered in the UK, aims to improve access to skincare in Myanmar in a sustainable manner working with the country's dermatological and health care communities across the three domains of education, research and clinical services.

Building educational capacity for dermatology
Community Skin Health Journal (CSH)

CSH is the official journal of the IFD and is a resource for health care workers in underserved areas. It provides up-to-date, practical information for the diagnosis and management of skin disease

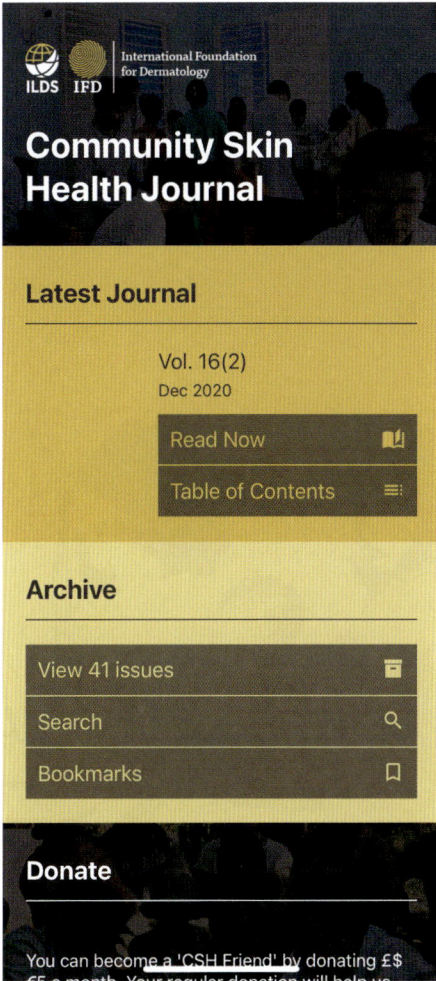

Figure 7.10 *Community Skin Health Journal* app.

appropriate to resource limited settings targeted towards the needs of general community health care workers. There are two editions published each year and these are available free of charge in hard copy with 10 000 copies sent to contacts in more than 180 countries. It is also available electronically as a downloadable PDF from the ILDS resource centre (https://ilds.org/resource-centre/tags/cdj/) as well as via a fully subject searchable app on android or iOS. It is available in English, French, Spanish and Chinese with plans to widen the languages covered (Figure 7.10).

Community dermatology teaching materials

A manual produced by the Communitaria Dermatologia team in Mexico is available in hard copy for participants in the Mexican teledermatological training events. It is also available digitally and provides dermatological teaching material appropriate for community health workers in resource limited settings.

Recognising NTDs through changes on the skin – a training guide for frontline health workers

This manual was published in 2018 as a freely downloadable resource from the WHO NTD department. It has recently been supplemented by the launch of an interactive app, 'the Skin NTDs Guide App' available in four languages and focuses, as does the

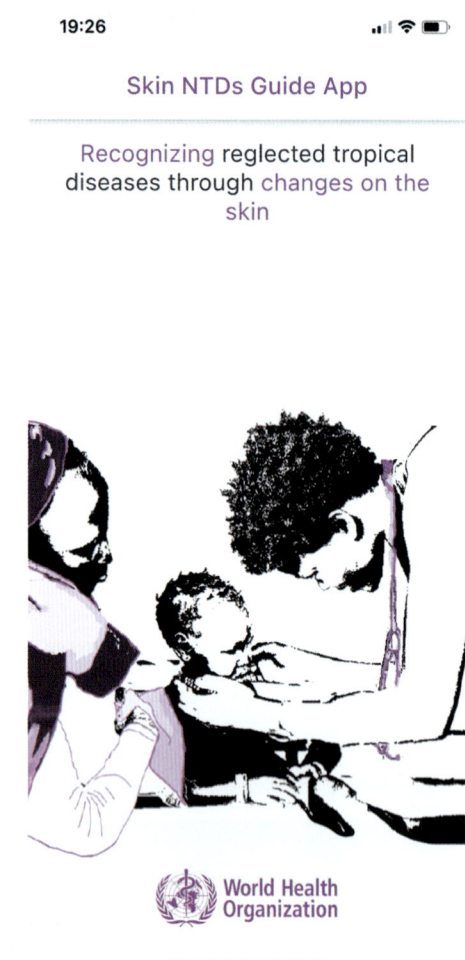

Figure 7.11 WHO Neglected Tropical Diseases Guide app.

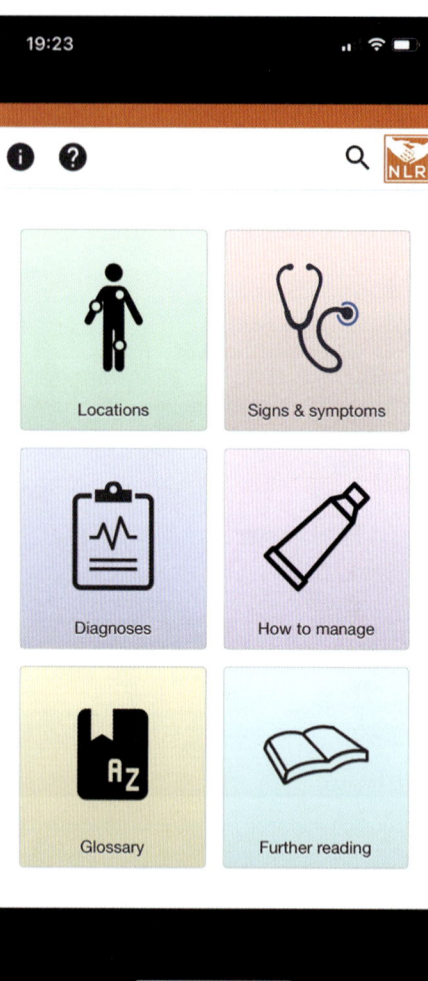

Figure 7.12 SkinApp from NLR – until No Leprosy Remains.

manual, on grouping the disorders around their skin signs, e.g. lumps, ulcers, swollen limbs and patches [19] (Figure 7.11).

NLR SkinApp
This is a tool to help identify common, NTD and HIV-related skin diseases with which patients present at the peripheral health level. It is designed to support diagnosis and as a source of information on signs, symptoms and therapies for common dermatoses [20] (Figure 7.12).

Manual of Best Practice – Skin Cancer Prevention and Management for Persons with Albinism in Sub-Saharan Africa
This is an internationally recognised resource developed by Standing Voice in collaboration with the IFD in 2019. It is directed at clinicians to assist them in delivering effective quality care to PWA across the African continent and beyond. It aims to consolidate previous learning and drive improvements in clinical practice for professionals working to promote the dermatological health of PWA. It is accessible from the ILDS website (Figure 7.13).

Tropical Dermatology: A Syndrome-Based Approach
This is an online course presented by the University of Minnesota aimed at primary care clinicians working in resource-limited settings and/or with mobile human populations, dermatology trainees including residents and fellows planning rotations abroad, and dermatologists planning to work in resource-limited settings. It is organised by presenting complaint and is designed to reflect how we as clinicians evaluate patients by the clinical presentation rather than the cause of the disease.

Building academic capacity for global health
AMPATH (Academic Model Providing Access to Healthcare) is a partnership between Moi University, Moi Teaching and Referral Hospital in Kenya and the AMPATH Consortium of North America Universities led by Indiana University. It was launched officially in 2001. The Indiana Centre for Global Health coordinates the involvement from North America, holds the institutional relationships with the Kenyan partners and facilitates several full-time faculty from Indiana University to be present in Eldoret, Kenya year round.

Simple needs assessments
Understanding need is an important way to gain objective information on the impact of diseases in large communities. This is especially important prior to allocating scarce resources. Establishing prevalence, impact and obstacles to management prior to planning intervention were the objectives behind a simple needs

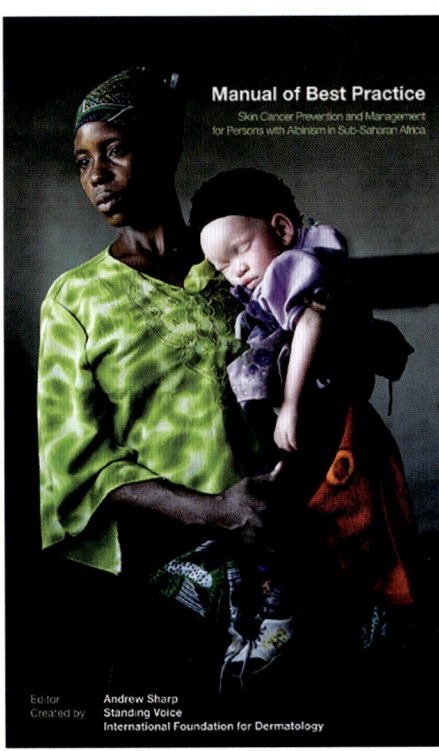

Figure 7.13 Cover image of *Manual of Best Practice for Skin Cancer Prevention and Management for Person with Albinism in Sub Saharan Africa*. Courtesy of Standing Voice and International Foundation for Dermatology.

assessment undertaken in Cambodia. Patients from both rural and urban settings completed and administered questionnaires and were then examined and their diseases recorded. The survey showed that 10 diseases accounted for nearly 60% of the cases seen: acne, eczema and scabies were the top three. The majority of the participants had mild to moderate disease for a median duration of 12 months. More than half the patients had previously spent an average of $10 USD on treating their skin disease unsuccessfully. The survey concluded that educating community health workers and their patients about simple management of common skin diseases with locally available treatment could significantly reduce the impact of dermatoses for the patient and community. Such an approach is a pragmatic adjunct to accompany the more formal capacity building of specialist dermatology units and may well serve to amplify access to dermatology care at an earlier stage of specialist service development [21].

Migrant health dermatology

There are nearly 80 million refugees and internally displaced people. Skin diseases are highly prevalent amongst migrants, and access to specialised health care services is often limited. This situation has been further exacerbated by the Covid-19 pandemic. Diagnosing and managing skin diseases and understanding the context in which they present will contribute to alleviating and addressing the burden of ill health due to the skin and also contribute to the overall well-being of the migrant community. Skin health is global health. The burden of sexually transmitted infections (STIs) and HIV in migrant populations varies according to the prevalence in the country of origin, due to sexual abuse during the transit phase, social inequalities associated with migration, human trafficking, HIV-related stigma and discrimination, and changes in sexual behaviour after migration. In response to this IFD established a Migrant Health Dermatology Working group to coordinate responses to these challenges. Initiatives to develop improvements in skin and sexual health care for refugees, migrants and internally displaced people are underway. These include:

1 Establishing a curriculum to prepare health workers in displaced persons camps (DPCs) with relevant dermatological expertise.
2 Developing a dermatological formulary for DPCs.
3 Launching locally supported teledermatological services for DPCs and their surrounding communities.

Following a field visit in December 2019, The IFD Migrant Health Working Group has enabled the AMPATH teledermatology model (see previously) to be rolled out in Bangladesh. This was achieved following support by OBAT Helpers (USA based) and The Refugee Crisis Foundation (UK based) NGOs. The IFD Migrant Health Working Group team also worked closely with the dermatologists at the University of Chittagong and together they have launched a sustainable system of teledermatology support to link the health care workers in the refugee camps with the dermatologists in Chittagong to provide dermatological care for the 800 000 Rohingya refugees residing in the Kutupalong refugee camp. Identifying the common dermatoses in the camp is also facilitating the development of targeted training [22] (Table 7.2).

Getting involved

Many of the actors in global health dermatology conduct this work outside their remunerated job plans. In time it is hoped that formal, funded global health dermatology positions will develop. Until then, dermatologists continue to volunteer their time and expertise.

Short-term field trips – medical volunteerism opportunities and potential hazards

While short-term international medical service work has the potential to advance global health by promoting patient care, education and health infrastructure in underserved communities, it also has the power to work against health equity and empowerment of the local health community. How is this so? Brief and intermittent visits often fail to facilitate appropriate patient follow-up to evaluate the safety and usefulness of the interventions. Volunteers, in particular trainees, may be tempted to practise beyond their scope of competency. Even if the volunteer covers their own travel and accommodation expenses, volunteer visits often consume host community resources in terms of time, logistical support and culturally mandated hospitality. The observation of ethical principles developed by Stoff *et al.*, adapted from DeCamp, provide useful guidance for the short-term medical volunteer [23] (Table 7.3).

Particular care should be paid when considering the donation of medicines. The WHO stipulate that 'medicine donations are neither a long-term solution to the underfunded health systems nor a solution to the lack of access to medicines in poor countries – especially for diseases that require lifelong treatment or large numbers of treatments' [24].

Table 7.2 Summary of skin diseases diagnosed in the Kutupalong Refugee Camp in December 2019.

ICD-10 category	Patients (n)
Infections and infestations	
Viral skin infections	3
Fungal skin infections	
Dermatophytosis	215
Other superficial mycoses	3
Candidiasis	5
Chromomycosis	1
Bacterial skin infections	
Impetigo	11
Cellulitis	39
Ecthyma	1
Ectoparasite skin infections	
Scabies	16
Inflammatory diseases	
Dermatitis and eczema	
Atopic dermatitis	1
Seborrhoeic dermatitis	9
Unspecified contact dermatitis	9
Exfoliative dermatitis	1
Lichen simplex chronicus	14
Prurigo nodularis	4
Other dermatitis	36
Erythema intertrigo	2
Pityriasis alba	5
Papulosquamous disorders	
Psoriasis	4
Lichen planus	5
Oral lichen planus	1
Gianotti Crosti	1
Other	
Urticaria and erythema	1
Disorders of skin appendages	
Acne	6
Alopecia totalis	1
Other disorders of skin appendages	2
Congenital disorders[a]	
Congenital ichthyosis	1
Striate keratoderma	1
Pachyonychia	1
Hyperhidrosis	1
Fissured nipples	2
Insect bite	1
Benign neoplasms	1
Diseases of the digestive tract	
Aphthous stomatitis/ulcer	1
Angular cheilitis	3
Glossitis	1
Other disorders[b]	
Vitiligo	12
Asteatotic eczema	14
Other/not classified	22
Total	457

Adapted from Khan *et al.* 2020 [22].
[a] Congenital malformations, deformations and chromosomal abnormalities.
[b] Other disorders of skin and subcutaneous tissue/not classified. ICD-10, WHO International Classification of Diseases version 10.

Sustainable educational and health care partnerships

Tropical Health and Education Trust (THET)

With a vision of a world where everyone has access to quality health care, THET works to achieve this by training and educating health workers in Africa and Asia. It has partnered with over 130 UK National Health Service (NHS) trusts, royal colleges and academic institutions. In addition, THET has worked closely with the British Government and is in official relations with the WHO. The partnerships deliver health worker training programmes based on the needs of the overseas partner institutions. At the centre of the effort has been the UK NHS. Over the past 4 years over 100 NHS institutions and 2000 NHS staff have provided more than 95 000 days of their time to work with colleagues overseas. In addition to bringing benefit to health systems in LMIC, there is benefit to the NHS. Staff return home with increased knowledge, improved leadership skills and a greater understanding of how to innovate in delivering health care with limited resources. This vision of co-development and bilateral innovation fosters the sustainable relationship and mutual advantage.

American Academy of Dermatology Resident International Grant Scheme

This funds 12 US and Canadian residents each year to participate in international electives spending between 4 and 6 weeks at one of four partner sites. The competitive submission process, requiring support from the residents' educational supervisors, includes a detailed application form. Comprehensive information is provided from each elective site and careful monitoring and evaluation processes are in place to support the trainees and the host organisations.

British Association of Dermatologists (BAD) – global health activities

Many UK dermatologists have been involved in supporting global health activities, from providing volunteer teaching assistance for the RDTC in Moshi to supporting the Ethiopian Dermatology training programme to name just two. The Roger Harman Fellowship provides financial support for Association members to undertake global health dermatology activities. Recently the BAD has established an annual Global Health Dermatology meeting and a global health session within the BAD annual meeting. It has also committed to setting up a global health dermatology subcommittee to facilitate a strategic focus on the place of British dermatology within the international health arena.

Conclusion

Global health dermatology is a rich and varied field of medicine with emerging prospects to influence the improvement in health and well-being of many currently neglected individuals around the world. With the recently articulated emphasis on the role of understanding skin disease for improving universal health coverage and achieving control of neglected tropical disease, dermatologists have a significant opportunity to provide international leadership and expertise, making a difference for the many and not just our individual patients.

Table 7.3 Ethical principles to guide global short-term medical volunteer trips. Adapted from DeCamp 2011. Taken from Toff and McMichael (2014) [23] with permission of Elsevier.

Guideline	Example
Create a statement of common purpose	Promotion of global health equity through an expression of mutual caring and the relief of suffering
Establish a collaborative partnership	Formulate goals for the trip through open, mutual input from volunteers and representatives of host site well in advance of the trip
Ensure fairness in site selection	Make transparent the rationale for a project at a given site and include ethically relevant features, including perceived medical need, efficiency of resource impact, and safety for volunteers and patients
Commit to benefits of social value	Allow representatives of the local community to determine the desirability and feasibility of the service work to be performed
Engage in bidirectional educational initiatives targeting the local community and team members	In collaboration with local health care providers, create a series of interactive lectures and other educational materials targeting local health care providers and covering commonly encountered diseases in their community
Build the capacity of and work within the limits of local health care infrastructure	Donate resources to establish a high-speed internet connection and telemedicine capacity at the host site
Evaluate programme outcomes	For an educational goal, measure durable gains in knowledge; for a patient care goal, measure long-term responses to treatment
Engage in frequent ethical review	After working with local health care leaders to define guiding principles and benchmarks, periodically seek external, independent review (e.g. from a member of a different volunteer organisation) of goals and deliverables for adherence to these principles

Key references

The full list of references can be found in the online version at https://www.wiley.com/rooksdermatology10e

2 Hay RJ, Augustin M, Griffiths CEM, Sterry W. The global challenge for skin health. *Br J Dermatol* 2015;172:1469–72.

10 Coates SJ, Enbiale W, Davis MDP, Anderson LK. The effects of climate change on human health in Africa, a dermatologic perspective: a report from the International Society of Dermatology Climate Change Committee. *Int J Dermatol* 2020; 59:265–78.

11 Framework for Engagement with Non-State Actors. May 2016. WHA 69.10 https://apps.who.int/gb/ebwha/pdf_files/wha69/a69_r10-en.pdf (last accessed January 2022).

14 Casas IM. Community dermatology in Argentina. *Dermatol Clin* 2021;39:43–55.

15 Mahe A, Faye O, N'Diaye HT *et al.* Integration of basic dermatological care into primary health care services in Mali. *Bull World Health Organ* 2005; 83:935–41.

19 Recognizing Neglected Tropical Diseases Through Changes on the Skin. A Training Guide for Front-Line Health Workers. WHO Department of Control of Neglected Tropical Diseases. https://apps.who.int/iris/bitstream/handle/10665/272723/9789241513531-eng.pdf?sequence=1&isAllowed=y (last accessed January 2022).

21 Mey S, Fuller LC, Bendick C. Impact of skin disease on patients in Cambodia – a survey and simple needs assessment. *Comm Dermatol J* 2015;11:13–28.

23 Stoff BK, McMichael JR. Short term international volunteerism in dermatology; ethical considerations. *J Am Acad Dermatol* 2014;71:822–5.

24 World Health Organization. Guidelines for medicine donations – revised 2010. Available at: https://apps.who.int/iris/bitstream/handle/10665/44647/9789241501989_eng.pdf?sequence=1&isAllowed=y (accessed January 2022).

CHAPTER 8

Genetics and the Skin

John A. McGrath
St John's Institute of Dermatology, King's College London, London, UK

Advances in genetics, 8.1
Nosology and principles of medical genetics, 8.2
Mutations and disease, 8.5
Mosaicism, Lyonisation and the lines of Blaschko, 8.7
Genome sequence and analysis of inherited disorders, 8.8
Prenatal diagnosis, 8.9
Key references, 8.11

Advances in genetics

Progress in the field of genetics in medicine continues rapidly. Most of the known single-gene inherited skin disorders have at least been mapped to particular chromosomal regions and the causal genes have been identified in ever increasing numbers [1,2]. Moreover, the introduction of next generation sequencing technologies (whole genome and whole exome sequencing) has led to several skin disease gene discoveries and provided new insights into skin disease pathophysiology as well as novel diagnostic approaches for inherited skin diseases [3].

The molecular genetic basis of the more common complex skin disorders (e.g. psoriasis and atopic eczema) is also advancing. The identification of the impact of certain genes or gene variants on disease susceptibility, clinical manifestations, optimal therapy and prognosis is gradually and selectively becoming realised. One ambition is to progress towards personalised, precision or P4 (predictive, personalised, preventative, participatory) medicine. For example, recent studies on pustular psoriasis have identified that at least seven genes may influence disease biology [4], with evidence that interleukin-36 may be a common target for both pathobiology and therapy. These data, when combined with pharmacogenomics and other factors, then start to provide a basis for improved individual case management in dermatological practice.

One key issue for dermatologists is trying to work out how relevant genetics might be to the patient with a skin condition in their clinic. Clearly for the Mendelian genodermatoses the role of genetics is very evident, but what about for an inflammatory skin condition or another individual with a similar disorder? One relatively new entity addressing this issue is the polygenic risk score (PRS). A PRS, also known as a polygenic score, genetic risk score or genome-wide score, is a number that summarises the estimated effect of many genetic variants on an individual's phenotype, typically calculated as a weighted sum of trait-associated alleles. In other words, a PRS estimates how likely an individual is to have a given trait based only on genetics, without taking environmental factors into account.

Over the next few years, PRS data are expected to become more clinically relevant in health and disease prediction.

Another important point for dermatologists is to be aware that genetics is still a science very much in its infancy, particularly regarding understanding the nuances of a patient's skin disease. We are still very much in an era of information gathering to try to improve the interpretation of genetics. Gathering skin, blood and saliva from dermatology patients and control subjects is vital in advancing the relevance of genetics. Biobanking refers to the process by which samples of bodily fluid or tissue (and other information) are collected for research use to improve our understanding of health and disease. Samples may be kept for years so that long-term research may be carried out, and researchers may track the health of the participants by looking at their past and future medical records, if people have given them permission to do so. Projects such as the UK Biobank recruit large groups of healthy people from across the population, and then use the samples over time to see if it can be established why some people go on to develop certain illnesses or conditions while others do not.

The Human Genome Project, launched in 1990 and completed in 2003, was an international effort to describe the entire human genetic sequence. The project has led to rich catalogues of human genomic variants, an improved understanding of the functional complexities of the human genome and the capacity to determine the genomic basis of thousands of human diseases. The project has also heralded the era of genomic medicine, converting research successes into health care benefits, including somatic genome analysis for cancer (and hence targeted therapies), genomics-based tests for a myriad of paediatric conditions and rare disorders, and the option of non-invasive prenatal genetic screening [5]. To date, however, much of genomic medicine has involved merely describing and comparing genomic sequences. More challenging is to begin to understand more about function. One project that has been comprehensively annotating all the functional sequences in the human genome is the Encyclopedia of DNA Elements (ENCODE) Project [6]. This project, begun in 2003, offers data pertinent to a

Rook's Textbook of Dermatology, Tenth Edition. Edited by Christopher Griffiths, Jonathan Barker, Tanya Bleiker, Walayat Hussain and Rosalind Simpson.
© 2024 John Wiley & Sons Ltd. Published 2024 by John Wiley & Sons Ltd.

broad range of genomic analyses, facilitating insights into specific phenotypes as well as genome-wide properties and principles. Given the relative ease of phenotyping skin disorders compared with some other diseased organs, dermatologists may be in an enviable position of being able to match new data from the genome to specific changes in patients' skin. This will allow the creation of much more refined genotype–phenotype correlations that provide far greater insight into genetic skin diseases and how to improve clinical care of patients.

Another recent advance has been the advent of single-cell genomics which enables high-resolution analysis of human tissues, including skin. Deconstructing skin into single cells and assessing their gene expression has provided data on novel cell states and biological pathways underpinning human development, tissue homeostasis and disease. The Human Cell Atlas project is attempting to identify the molecular properties of each cell that forms a healthy human [7]. With regard to disease, the ambition is to understand how individual cells interact with one another and to translate such knowledge into precision medicine [8].

Online access to genetic information, databases and tools provides a vital support link for both clinicians and researchers. The internet provides useful updates on several aspects of genetic research and data, and several informative sites are listed below:

- Medical Research Council (MRC) Human Genetics Unit, Institute of Genetics and Molecular Medicine: www.hgu.mrc.ac.uk. This link provides access to a wide range of databases and resources for genetic studies.
- National Center for Biotechnology Information (NCBI): www.ncbi.nlm.nih.gov/guide/. This site offers a main entry point for information about the Human Genome Project.
- Human Gene Mutation Database, Institute of Medical Genetics in Cardiff: www.hgmd.cf.ac.uk/ac/index.php. This site provides valuable updated information about mutations that have been identified in various inherited disorders.
- Leiden Open Variation Database: www.databases.lovd.nl/shared/genes. This site provides a comprehensive database of variants in genes associated with disease.
- University of California Santa Cruz (UCSC) Genomics Institute: www.genome.ucsc.edu/. This site contains the reference sequence and working draft assemblies for a large collection of genomes. It also provides portals to several other useful genomics projects.
- Genome Aggregation Database (gnomAD): https://gnomad.broadinstitute.org. This is an international resource that aggregates and harmonises both exome and genome sequencing data from various large-scale sequencing projects.
- Human Cell Atlas (HCA): www.humancellatlas.org. This site outlines the comprehensive reference maps for all human cells to provide a basis for understanding human health and diagnosing, monitoring and treating disease.
- ENCODE Project: www.encodeproject.org. This site offers access to the latest information on functional elements within the genome being generated by the ENCODE Project.
- UK Biobank: www.ukbiobank.ac.uk/. This is a large-scale biomedical database and research resource, containing in-depth genetic and health information from half a million UK participants. The database is regularly augmented with additional data and is globally accessible to approved researchers undertaking vital research into the most common and life-threatening diseases.
- Online Mendelian Inheritance in Man (OMIM): www.ncbi.nlm.nih.gov/omim/. OMIM is a catalogue of over 12 000 known human Mendelian characters, and was created by the late Dr Victor McKusick of Johns Hopkins Hospital, Baltimore, USA. OMIM is an excellent starting point for acquiring up-to-date information on human Mendelian characters or *phenotypes*. Each character is given a six-digit MIM number, which is widely used to identify inherited disorders in the medical literature. The first digit of the MIM number indicates the mode of inheritance (historical): 1, autosomal dominant; 2, autosomal recessive; 3, X loci or phenotype; 4, Y loci or phenotype; 5, mitochondrial loci; and 6, autosomal loci or phenotypes added after 1994.

(All last accessed January 2022.)

Nosology and principles of medical genetics

The terms 'familial', 'inherited' and 'congenital' are frequently misunderstood and misused. *Familial* refers to the clustering of a disorder, with more close relatives affected than predicted by the population prevalence of the condition. *Inherited* disorders require the transmission of genetic variants from one generation to the next. The term *congenital* simply means that the character was present at or detectable before birth; such abnormalities may not be genetically determined and include developmental defects due to environmental infectious agents (e.g. rubella) and malformations arising from physical injuries (e.g. amniotic bands). Only a proportion of inherited disorders reveal themselves at birth (i.e. are congenital), with many having their onset in later life. Such age dependence may result from a wide number of factors, including the maturation of cells or tissue-specific functions, exposure to exogenous agents or accumulation of a noxious substance.

A further and important example of adult age of onset is provided by hereditary cancer syndromes, such as neurofibromatosis (NF) type 2, in which a second mutation impacting upon the normal allele of a *tumour suppressor gene* is required to induce tumour formation. Such a mutation occurs as a 'somatic' change.

Of the inherited skin abnormalities, the largest group is that of the single-gene disorders, which require an alteration in the function of a gene and are known commonly as the genodermatoses [1]. There are four inheritance patterns for classic genodermatoses: autosomal dominant (Figure 8.1), autosomal recessive (Figure 8.2), X-linked recessive (Figure 8.3) and X-linked dominant (Figure 8.4). Predisposition to the more common skin disorders, including atopic eczema and psoriasis, is determined by the action of more than one gene (sometimes involving gene–gene interactions, known as *epistasis*), with significant evidence for further modulation by environmental factors. Such disorders display complex patterns of clustering in families and are referred to as *multifactorial*. Chromosomal abnormalities, either in number (*aneuploidy*) or form (*translocation*, *complex rearrangements* or *microdeletions*) are important to the clinician, particularly if the patient presents a range of abnormalities including developmental delay. However, chromosomal anomalies rarely present solely with dermatological problems.

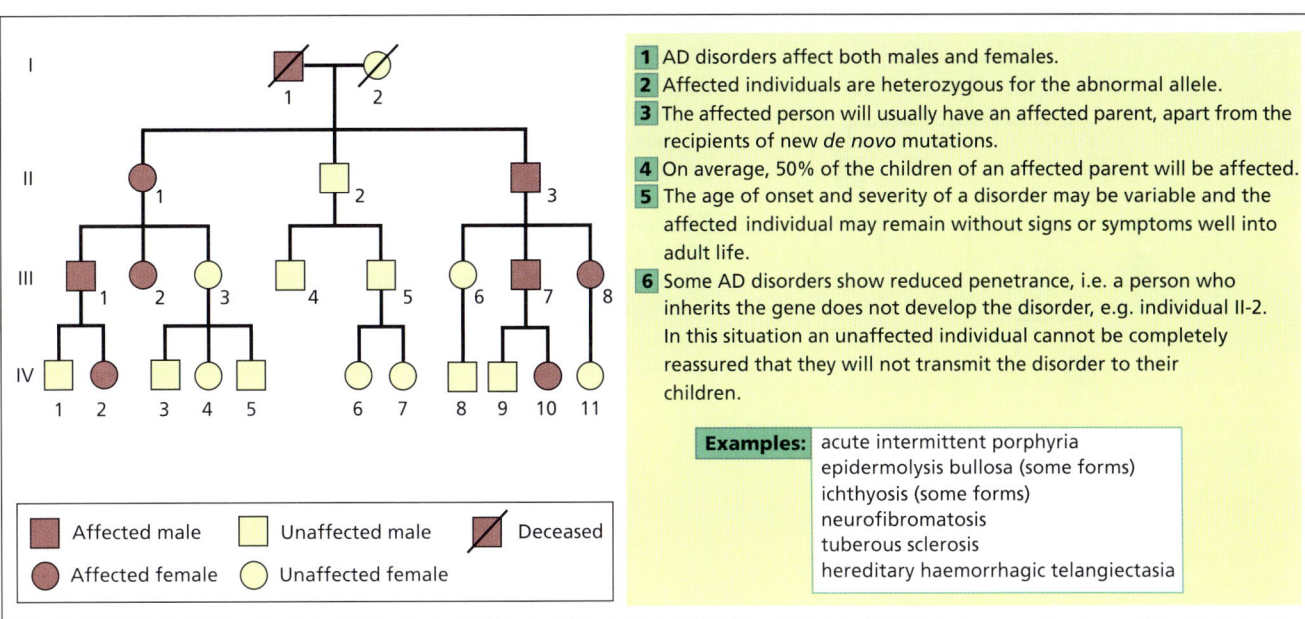

Figure 8.1 Autosomal dominant (AD) inheritance.

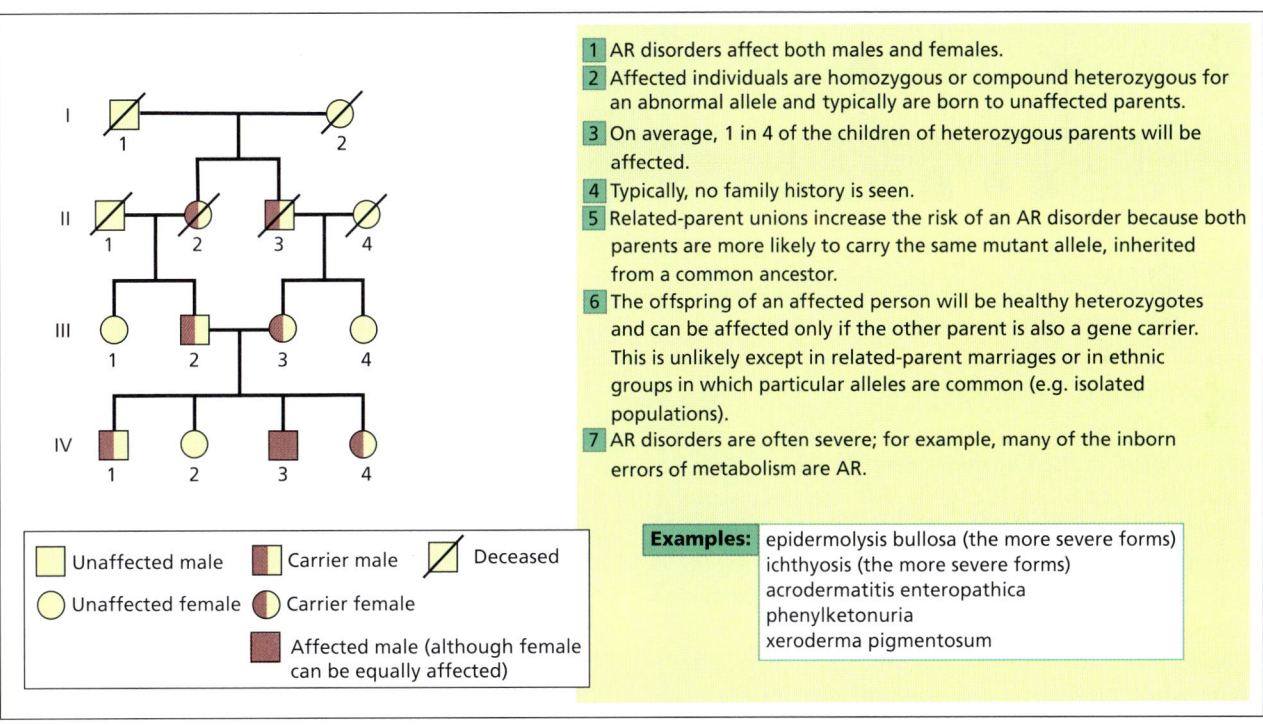

Figure 8.2 Autosomal recessive (AR) inheritance.

Inherited characteristics are transmitted from one generation to the next by chromosomes, composed of double helix strands of DNA. A *gene* is a sequence of bases in the DNA encoding a polypeptide. The precise position of the gene on a genetic map is known as its *locus*. In females, the 46 chromosomes found in most somatic cells present in homologous pairs; hence two copies of every gene exist, one maternal and the other paternal in origin. In males, the Y chromosome only pairs with the X chromosome at the pseudo-autosomal region. *Meiosis* is the process of cell division by which male and female gametes (germ cells) are produced. Alternative genes at a single locus are called *alleles*. An individual with two different alleles at a particular locus is *heterozygous*; where both alleles are identical, the individual is described as *homozygous* at that locus. As with all complex mammalian genomes, the human sequence is made up of considerable amounts of repetitive DNA (Figure 8.5). The total number of genes is now estimated to be c.20 000, with an average size, including introns, of between 10 and 15 kb. The genome may contain multiple copies of genes, known

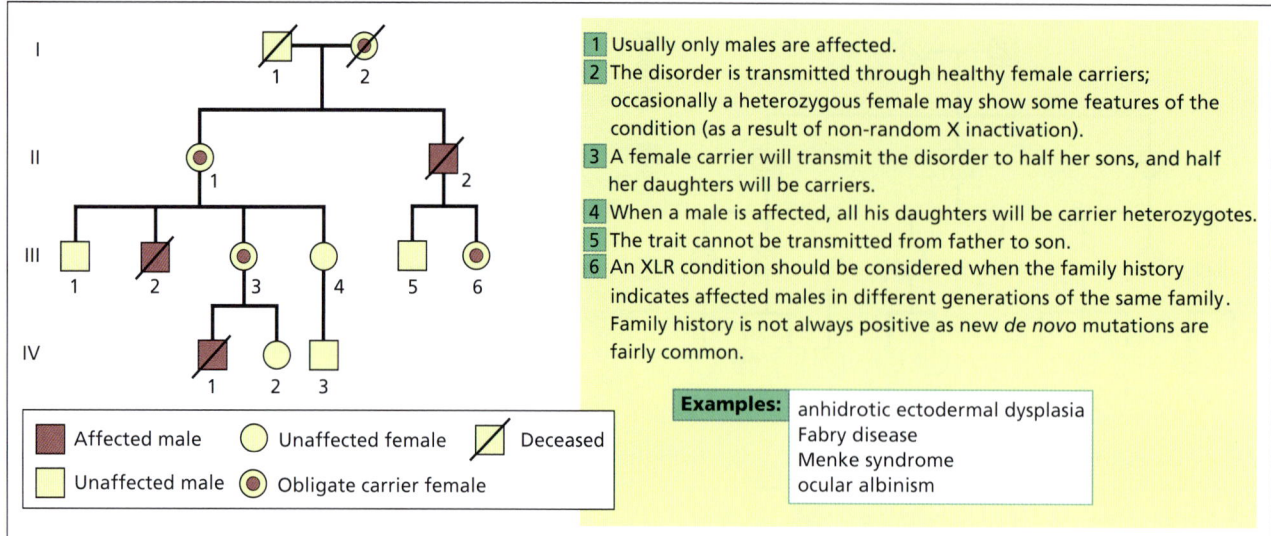

Figure 8.3 X-linked recessive (XLR) inheritance.

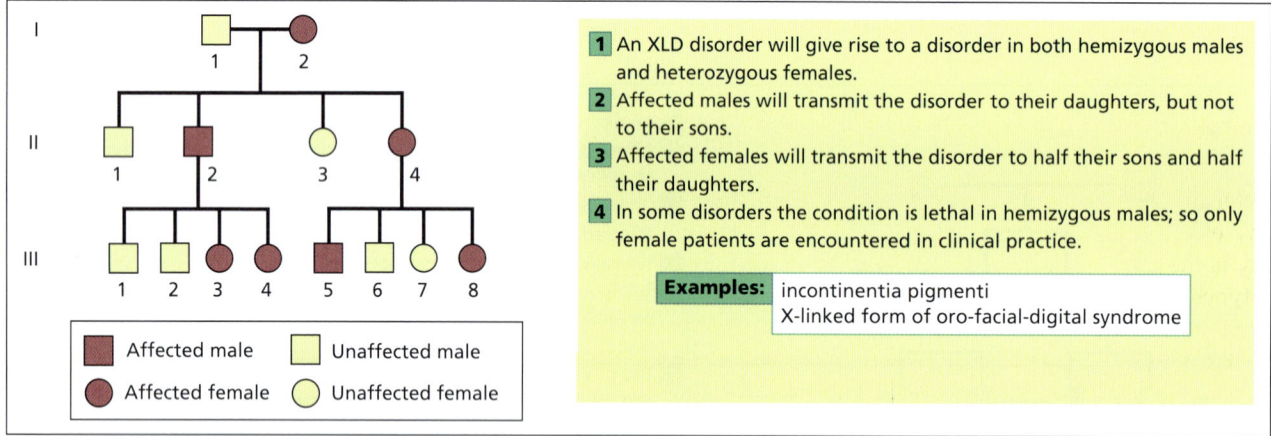

Figure 8.4 X-linked dominant (XLD) inheritance.

as *copy number variation*. Individual genes may also show *intragenic copy number variation*, such as the *FLG* gene that encodes a variable number (either 10, 11 or 12) of filaggrin repeat units [2]. The clinical significance of this intragenic copy number variation in *FLG* is variability in skin dryness (10 repeats is associated with a drier skin phenotype).

An allele is regarded as *dominant* (Figure 8.1) if it manifests as a phenotype when present on only one member of the chromosome pair (heterozygous state) and as *recessive* (Figure 8.2) if it must be present at both corresponding loci (homozygous or compound heterozygous state) before it can exert its full effect. *Semidominant* refers to the consequences of inheriting one or two mutant alleles resulting in a phenotype, usually the two alleles having more substantive clinical manifestations. An autosomal dominant trait may occur in more than one sibling, even though both parents are apparently unaffected. This phenomenon may be explained by gonadal mosaicism, due to the presence of a mutation in the germline but not somatic cells [3]. It is important to note that the terms 'dominance' and 'recessivity' refer to a phenotypic characteristic rather than a gene.

Genes borne on chromosomes other than the sex chromosomes (X and Y) are known as *autosomal*. Characters controlled by genes borne on the X or Y chromosomes are termed *sex-linked* (Figures 8.3 and 8.4). The Y chromosome is much smaller than the X chromosome. The great majority of sex-linked genes are exclusive to the X chromosome, having no active counterpart on the Y chromosome. For these traits the term 'recessive' applies to males who carry only one (mutant) allele. Genes on the X chromosome are not one of a pair in males and when such a gene is abnormal in a male, the term *hemizygous* is used. Females who carry X-linked mutations are typically heterozygous and, with rare exceptions, including markedly skewed X inactivation, display no clinical abnormalities. A region of homology sufficient for pairing between the X and Y chromosomes exists on the end of the short arm of the X chromosome, known as the *pseudo-autosomal region*, enabling sex-linked transmission comparable to autosomal traits. Genes that are Y-linked are primarily involved in male sex determination (e.g. the *SRY* gene controlling the testis determining factor) or spermatogenesis.

The effects of a mutant allele are not necessarily constant. The degree to which the effects are variable is a measure of the *expression*

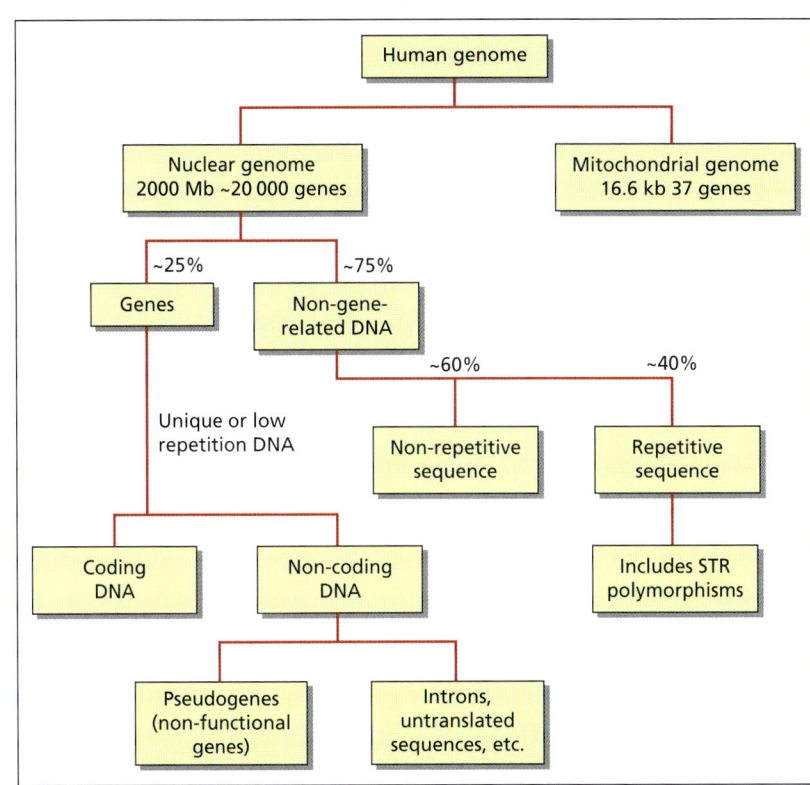

Figure 8.5 Human genome organisation. STR, short tandem repeat.

of the character in question, and the frequency with which a gene produces any effect at all is a measure of its *penetrance*. Genetic heterogeneity is the term used to describe clinically similar disorders (phenotypes) that result from different genetic defects. The concept of genetic heterogeneity is important for several reasons: (i) disorders that appear the same can be due to entirely different molecular defects, with a different natural history and requiring different treatment; (ii) for accurate genetic counselling as defects may have different inheritance patterns; and (iii) because genetic heterogeneity plays a significant role in common complex disease states. Different alleles at the same locus (allelic) and genes at different loci (non-allelic) can give rise to similar phenotypes. The term *genomic imprinting* is used to describe the phenomenon whereby a DNA sequence derived from one parent acts in a different way compared with that derived from the other parent [4]. Imprinting (coding or non-coding) carries a signal or imprint that indicates to nuclear transcription machinery the parent of origin for that sequence. For the majority of the human genome, no distinction is made between paternal and maternal copies, with the exclusion of polymorphic variation. The molecular basis of imprinting is thought to be *methylation*, the process whereby a methyl group (CH_3) is added to DNA nucleotides (typically cytosine). Methylation is usually associated with reduced levels of expression of a gene, and for certain genes is applied exclusively to either the paternal or maternal copies [5].

In addition to nuclear DNA, which accounts for 99.995% of the total genetic pool, mitochondria contain a circular chromosome comprising 14 protein-coding regions. The mitochondrial DNA mostly encodes for enzymes involved in the respiratory chain and oxidative phosphorylation [6]. Mitochondrial disorders are predominantly muscular, neurological and ophthalmological diseases and transmission is almost exclusively from the mother. Alteration in the mitochondrial genome may also be implicated in aspects of ageing [7].

Mutations and disease

Most mutations are spontaneous and unexplained; however, certain factors such as mutagenic chemicals and ionising radiation can increase the rate. In the absence of such agents, the mutation rate is of the order of 1 base pair (bp) substitution for every 10^9–10^{10} bp replicated. If a mutation occurs in a somatic cell (*somatic mutation*), only the descendants of that cell are affected and there will be no transmission of the abnormality to further generations. Only mutations occurring in the gametes or their precursors can be transmitted to offspring. Normally, the replication of DNA is accurate, but mutations can occur, either induced by exposure to mutagenic agents or spontaneously through errors in the process of DNA replication and repair during meiosis. Chromosomal disorders may be due to abnormalities of chromosome number or structure and may involve autosomes or sex chromosomes [1]. Somatic cells are *diploid*, with a complement of 46 chromosomes, whereas gametes (ova and sperm) are *haploid*, with only 23 chromosomes following reduction division in meiosis. Numerical abnormalities that involve the gain or loss of one or more chromosomes are known as *aneuploidies*. Structural chromosome rearrangements result from chromosome breakage with subsequent reunion in a different configuration. They may be balanced or unbalanced, depending on whether or not gain (or loss) of genetic material occurs. Approximately 7.5% of all conceptions have a chromosomal disorder, but most of these are spontaneously aborted, so the birth frequency is 0.6%. Among early spontaneous abortions, the frequency of chromosomal disorders is 60%, whereas in late spontaneous abortions and stillbirths the frequency is 5%. Chromosomal abnormalities generally cause multiple congenital malformations. Children with more than one physical abnormality, particularly if there is developmental delay, should undergo chromosomal analysis as part of their investigation. Chromosomal disorders are incurable but can be reliably detected by prenatal diagnostic techniques.

Mutations that impinge on the function of a gene most commonly occur within the coding regions (*exons*) and may alter the amino acid sequence and hence structure and function of the protein (Figure 8.6). In addition to gross structural chromosomal changes, submicroscopic alterations including *substitutions* (replacement of a single nucleotide by another), *deletions* (loss of one or more nucleotides) and *insertions* (addition of one or more nucleotides) may occur. Single-base substitutions, often referred to as *point mutations*, have been most extensively characterised. These mutations alter the DNA sequence so that either a different amino acid is encoded (*missense*), or a *codon* (the code of three nucleotides specifying an amino acid) is altered to code for a *stop codon*, leading to premature termination of the protein (*nonsense*). Deletions and insertions, other than in multiples of three, will lead to disruption of the reading frame for RNA translation, resulting in a frameshift mutation and premature termination (Figure 8.6). Point mutations may also affect *splicing*, the process by which mature messenger RNA (mRNA) is produced from RNA that has been transcribed directly from the gene. Large genome deletions may involve several neighbouring genes leading to contiguous gene defects. Mutations exert their effects by leading to a loss or gain of function of the gene's protein product. In general, loss-of-function mutations lead to either reduced activity or complete loss of the protein. Gain-of-function mutations result in either increased levels of expression or the acquisition of a new function of a protein. The term 'mutation' has traditionally been applied to genetic variation causative of a Mendelian disorder. As further studies are undertaken to unravel the genetic contribution of common and complex disorders, understanding the subtle functional consequences of all genetic variation, including *polymorphisms*, will be increasingly important. Polymorphisms are alterations in the DNA sequence that are present in unrelated individuals (some are common (50%), some are rare (<1%)) that usually do not cause disease although they may modify disease expression or contribute to some phenotypic manifestations [2]. Polymorphisms occur in both non-coding and coding DNA; in the latter they may be silent or lead to an amino acid change.

The phenotypic features of a disease often reflect the result of the interaction between a particular genotype and the environment, but sometimes variation can be attributed to neither, as might occur in monozygotic twins. These differences are referred to as epigenetic phenomena as they occur due to additional influences at the biochemical, cellular, tissue and organism levels. Epigenetic effects involve chemical modifications to DNA that do not alter the DNA sequence but do alter the probability of gene transcription, for example by DNA methylation [3]. DNA hypermethylation contributes to gene silencing by preventing the binding of activating transcription factors and by attracting repressor complexes that induce the formation of inactive chromatin structures. The DNA methylation machinery in mammals is made up of two components: (i) DNA methyltransferases, which establish and maintain genome-wide DNA methylation patterns; and (ii) the methyl-CpG-binding proteins, which are involved in scanning and interpreting the methylation patterns. The analysis of any changes in these processes is known as *epigenomics*. Such changes may affect DNA accessibility to local transcriptional complexes, thus providing a link between genome structure and regulation of transcription. Epigenome analysis is now the focus of considerable attention to identify genome-wide methylation patterns and the profiles of all human genes. Over the course of any individual's lifespan, epigenetic mutations will occur more frequently than DNA mutations, and appreciating the role of epigenetic phenomena in influencing phenotypic variation is a key area of future research activity.

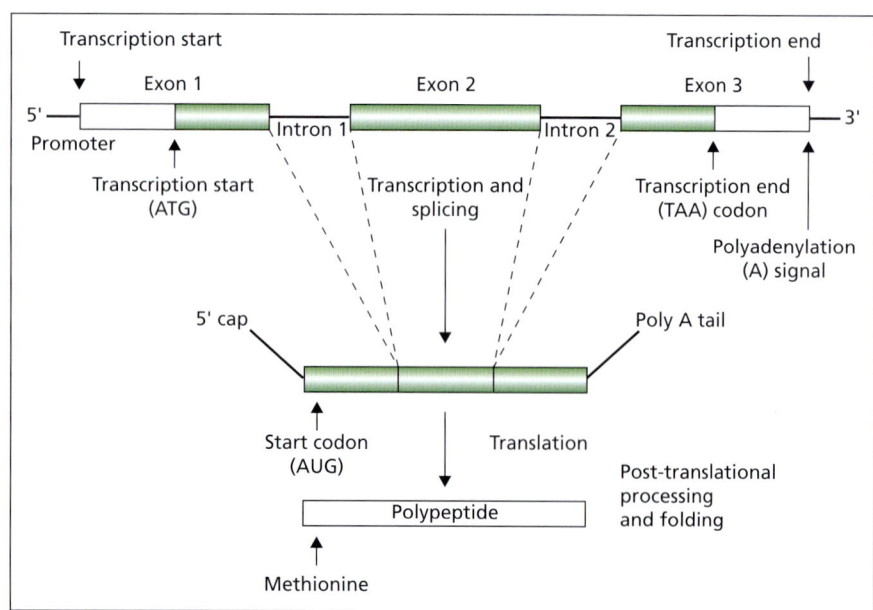

Figure 8.6 Features of a typical human gene.

One topic that has absorbed geneticists over the years has been the association between human leukocyte antigens (HLAs) and various diseases, including multifactorial disorders in dermatology, as well as drug metabolism or hypersensitivity [4]. HLAs are glycoproteins on the cell surface of most nucleated human cells. These differ in subtle ways from person to person and uniquely fingerprint each person's cells. These fingerprints allow an individual's immune system to recognise if a given cell is its own. The importance of the HLA system has been highlighted by the need to match donors and recipients in the transplantation of human tissues. The HLA region is located on the short arm of chromosome 6, referred to as the major histocompatibility complex (MHC). A person inherits HLAs as a set, one set (haplotype) from each parent. There are at least four or five genetic loci that produce HLAs, termed A, B, C, D and DR (in order of their discovery not their location), and their gene products are called HLA-A, HLA-B, HLA-C, HLA-D and HLA-DR. Each locus has multiple allelic determinants (polymorphism). Previous methods to define HLA subtypes by the serotyping of cellular assays have now been replaced by DNA sequence approaches to determine sequence feature variant types. Each allele at each locus controls an antigen, which is identified by a number placed after the letter of that series, for example HLA-A1 or HLA-B5. The letter 'w' in front of a number indicates that its specificity was studied in an international workshop, and it continues to undergo further definition. HLAs that code at the A, B and C loci are determined by serological cytotoxicity methods, whereas those occurring at the D locus are detected by the mixed lymphocyte reaction. The HLA-DR antigens are serologically determined and are similar, if not identical, to the D locus antigens. DNA-based methods for typing at all HLA loci are now available.

The association of an HLA with a given disease means that there is a higher incidence of that antigen in a group of patients with the disease than in a group of people without the disease. There are various ways in which the presence of a particular HLA might be involved in the pathogenesis of a disease:

1 *Molecular mimicry*. An infective agent may have a similar configuration to the HLA, so that the agent is then not attacked by the body's defence system. Alternatively, the agent might differ only slightly from the HLA, so that antibodies are produced that attack both the infective agent and the cells containing the HLA, thus inducing autoimmune damage.
2 *Receptor effects*. Many chemicals, including drugs and toxins, bind to the cell surface before they are taken into the cytoplasm. As HLAs are present on the cell surface, they could modify the binding of these potentially toxic substances, and the specificity for such binding may be determined, at least in part, by DNA variation for HLA molecules.
3 *Genetic linkage*. The HLA may be close to another gene on the same chromosome that produces a disease, either directly (e.g. due to an enzyme deficiency) or indirectly due to an effect on the immune response, which may be abnormally enhanced, leading to autoimmunity, or abnormally decreased, leading to infection.

The association between an HLA and a particular disease is rarely absolute. There are many possible explanations for this, including the role of environmental factors or triggers (such as chemicals or infective agents) in disease causation. Non-HLA-linked genes are probably also important, including some that may confer resistance to disease. The relative risk is the numerical answer to the question 'How many times is a person with a given HLA phenotype more likely to develop a given disease than a person without that HLA phenotype?'

In dermatological practice, HLA testing is particularly relevant to drug prescribing and the enhanced risk of drug hypersensitivity in certain populations. For example, individuals carrying the HLA-B*1502 allele are 100-fold more likely to develop toxic epidermal necrolysis following treatment with the anticonvulsant drug carbamazepine. This allele is common in South-East Asian countries and pre-prescribing screening for HLA-B*1502 led to a decreased incidence of this adverse drug reaction [5].

Mosaicism, Lyonisation and the lines of Blaschko

The term *mosaicism* can be used to describe an individual with two or more cell lines of different genotypes derived from the same zygote [1]. Indeed, any tissue that contains a mixed population of cells with different genetic or chromosomal contents leading to phenotypic diversity can be referred to as *mosaic*. The actual type of mosaicism may vary and includes single-gene (somatic), chromosomal, functional and revertant mosaicism [2]. *Somatic mosaicism* indicates a mutational event occurring after fertilisation. The earlier this occurs during development, the more downstream cells will be affected and the more likely it is to affect the clinical expression of a disease. *Gonosomal mosaicism* refers to involvement of both gonads and somatic tissue, but if the mosaicism occurs exclusively in gonadal tissue, this is called *gonadal mosaicism*. Segmental mosaicism for autosomal dominant disorders can occur in one of two ways, referred to as type I or type II. In *type I segmental mosaicism* either there is a postzygotic mutation in the segment with the skin or outside the segment, with normal genomic DNA. In *type II segmental mosaicism* there is a heterozygous genomic mutation in all cells that is then exacerbated by loss of heterozygosity or a second mutation within a segment or along the lines of Blaschko. Blaschko lines were first described in 1901 and originally described as a 'system of lines on the human skin which the linear naevi and dermatoses follow' (Figure 8.7) [3]. Many naevoid skin lesions display an arrangement following these lines. The lines do not correspond to any known nervous, vascular or lymphatic structures, but represent the developmental growth pattern within the skin [4]. Mosaicism following the Blaschko lines is also seen in chromosomal mosaicism and functional mosaicism (random X chromosome inactivation through Lyonisation). Chromosomal mosaicism results from non-disjunction events that occur after fertilisation. Functional mosaicism relates to genes on the X chromosome because during embryonic development in females, one of the X chromosomes, either the maternal or the paternal one, is inactivated. In health, all females exhibit functional mosaicism with regard to their X chromosomes. One of the two X chromosomes in the cells of normal females undergoes inactivation at an early stage of embryonic development (12–16 days after fertilisation), a process known as *Lyonisation* [5]. The inactive X remains condensed as a densely stained mass of chromatin known as the *Barr body*. For each somatic cell it is random whether the paternal X or the maternal X is inactivated,

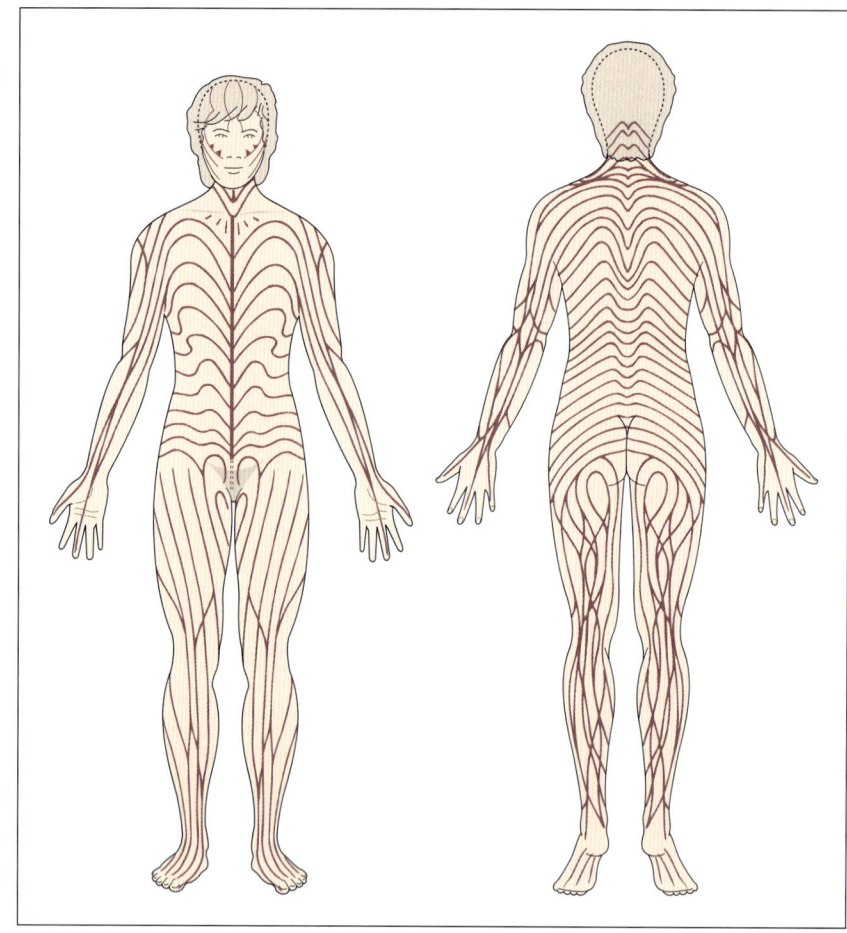

Figure 8.7 The lines of Blaschko as illustrated in his 1901 article 'A system of lines on the surface of the human body which the linear naevi and dermatoses follow'. Reproduced from Blaschko 1901 [3] with permission of W. Braumüller/Public Domain.

but the choice is fixed for all subsequent descendants of that cell. Thus, a female has a mixture of two populations of cells, some of which have an active paternal X chromosome and some of which have an active maternal X chromosome. The relative proportions vary from female to female (even in identical twins) due to the randomness of the inactivation process. As a result of Lyonisation, the heterozygous state of various X-linked gene defects may give rise to a mosaic pattern of cutaneous lesions, which conforms to the lines of Blaschko.

Revertant mosaicism, also known as *natural gene therapy*, refers to genetic correction of an abnormality by multiple different phenomena including back mutations, intragenic crossovers, mitotic gene conversion and second site mutations [6]. Indeed, multiple different correcting events can occur in the same patient. The clinical relevance of the reversion process depends on several factors, including the number of cells involved, how much reversal occurs and at what stage in life the reversion occurs. The phenomenon of revertant mosaicism has translational potential for treating genetic skin disease and has been tested in patients using punch grafting or by culturing and grafting revertant keratinocytes to unreverted areas [7]. Revertant keratinocytes have also been used to generate inducible pluripotent stem cells for future clinical applications. These reverted cells can thereby generate a bank of cells for regenerative medicine that does not require further genomic editing of the disease causing the mutation(s) (Figure 8.8).

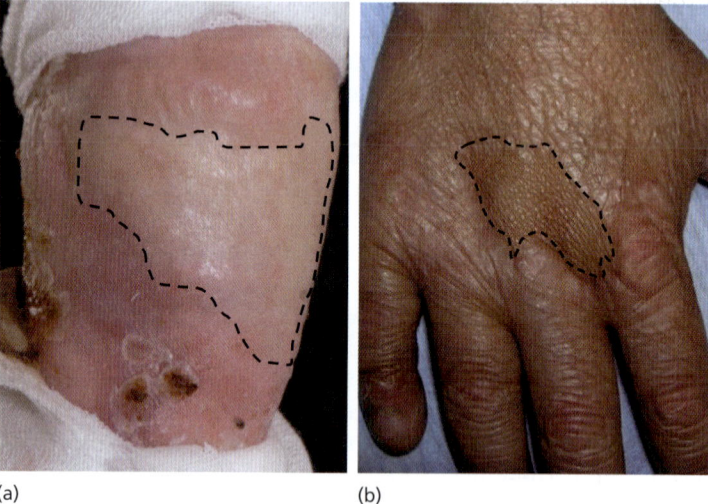

(a) (b)

Figure 8.8 Revertant mosaicism in (a) recessive dystrophic epidermolysis bullosa and (b) Kindler epidermolysis bullosa. In both cases, the area within the dashed line has undergone spontaneous improvement with a partial functional and biochemical correction due to additional somatic genetic events.

Genome sequence and analysis of inherited disorders

Completion of the human genome sequencing effort has led to phenomenal progress in gene mapping techniques, with thousands of DNA markers now available, each defined and covering all chromosomes. These markers have greatly facilitated linkage studies within families with Mendelian disorders. Linkage analysis questions whether each DNA marker co-inherits with the disease more often than expected by chance. The statistical test of linkage is the *lod* (logarithm of the odds) score. A lod score of 3 or greater is accepted as significant evidence of linkage, whereas a score of −2 excludes linkage at that location. Most genetic markers are now detected rapidly by polymerase chain reaction (PCR)-based methods of analysis, exploiting an abundant class of DNA sequence variation known as simple tandem repeats or single nucleotide polymorphisms. *Gene tracking* is the term given to the use of a known linkage between a marker and a disease locus to predict the genotype at the disease locus in a particular family member, such as in asymptomatic carrier testing or prenatal diagnosis. Early linkage studies relied on use of a few scattered markers, often widely spaced throughout the genome and therefore of limited practical value. With the advent of human genome sequence data, however, many more polymorphic markers have been identified and collectively used in genome-wide association studies, providing more detailed links between genes (or groups of genes) and specific diseases. Examples of recent genome-wide association studies include those in acne vulgaris and frontal fibrosing alopecia [1,2].

Alleles at gene loci residing close to each other on the same chromosome remain linked in transmission so long as the chromosome remains intact. However, during reduction division (meiosis), such linkages may be disrupted if *crossing over* occurs. The closer two gene loci are situated on a chromosome, the less likely they are to be separated by crossing over and the more likely they are to be inherited together. Two such gene loci are said to be linked and it is possible to demonstrate genetic linkage in a family using appropriate genetic markers. When two alleles occur together more frequently, or less frequently, in a population than would have been expected from the individual allele frequencies, they are said to be in *linkage disequilibrium*. This may arise because of a recent mutation or for a particular combination of DNA sequences, which may have, for example, a selective advantage and hence achieve disequilibrium by natural selection [3]. Linkage disequilibrium is one important cause of disease association. Genetic linkage is a phenomenon demonstrable within families. In contrast, association due to linkage disequilibrium is a phenomenon demonstrated by comparing a population of affected individuals with a control population.

Although DNA markers have been used for decades to track and identify disease traits and relevant genes, much of the elegant detective work has been superseded by advances in DNA sequence technologies. These technologies have introduced rapid and comprehensive direct sequencing of the entire genome (*whole genome sequencing*) or the coding region (*whole exome sequencing*) [4]. Thus, even genome-wide association studies have now evolved to add in, or be replaced by, one of these next generation sequencing approaches, which offer a universal tool for the diagnosis and discovery of genetic disorders or genetic contribution to disease. As access to accurate and efficient next generation genetic diagnosis improves, the need for expensive and invasive hospital investigations for inherited skin diseases is likely to decrease in the future. Given that over a 20-year period the cost of DNA sequencing technologies has come down 100 000-fold, this is expected to continue falling until it becomes affordable to most institutions. As this technology continues to evolve, an appreciation of its ethical implications is essential. Every whole genome or whole exome data set generated will reveal sequence alterations in several genes, and although the potential effect on health is currently unknown for most of these alterations, they will likely be well understood in the future. Therefore, the most pertinent ethical issues centre around the use of the genetic information generated. This plethora of emerging information raises several ethical issues, such as how much of the data should be disclosed to patients? Should consent from individuals be sought to allow for both diagnosis and prognosis? What implications will the data have on family planning? Can terminations of pregnancy be justified from the global data? Or in a broader context, will insurance companies determine premiums based on a patient's genetic profile? Despite these ethical and social challenges, however, the technical advances in next generation sequencing and implications for clinical activity in dermatology are set to continue.

In addition to genomic data, research tools that generate other -omic data sets such as transcriptomics, proteomics, metabolomics, lipidomics, etc. are also being incorporated into multi-omic analyses to help characterise disease pathobiology, discover biomarkers of disease activity, and help drive targeted therapies for stratified or personalised medicine. New technologies that assess disease processes at single-cell levels are also emerging that will provide fundamental new insights into disease aetiology, classification and management [5].

The availability of swathes of new multi-omic data highlights the importance of accurate genetic counselling in many areas of clinical genetics. Genetic counselling is defined as 'the process of helping people understand and adapt to the medical, psychological and familial implications of genetic contributions to disease'. Such counselling should include (i) an interpretation of family and medical histories to assess the chance of disease occurrence or recurrence; (ii) education about inheritance, testing, management, prevention, resources and research; (iii) counselling to promote informed choice and adaptation to the risk or condition; and (iv) information exchange on the implications or limitations of personal genetic data. Genetic counselling must be based on an understanding of the genetic principles and usual behaviour of hereditary and congenital abnormalities. It is also important to be aware of the spectrum of clinical severity for a particular condition, the availability of treatment (if any) of specialist centres and the options for molecular investigations and prenatal testing in subsequent pregnancies at risk for recurrence. These principles are straightforward to apply to monogenic diseases, but counselling for multifactorial disorders such as psoriasis or atopic eczema is more difficult.

Prenatal diagnosis

In most countries, sustained improvements in obstetric and perinatal care have meant that more children with congenital malformations survive so that congenital malformations, single-gene defects and chromosomal abnormalities are increasing in their relative importance as causes of infant mortality and morbidity. Up to 5% of live-born infants may be affected by congenital defects or hereditary disease, and approximately 20% of all infant deaths today are the result of such disorders. Congenital defects and hereditary diseases can have a huge impact on individual sufferers and families at risk of genetic disease as well as creating substantial health, economic and financial burdens for health care providers and society in general.

The purpose of prenatal diagnosis is the detection or exclusion of a hereditary disease or congenital defect *in utero*. The option of an elective abortion of affected pregnancies can help parents at risk of having affected children to produce normal offspring. A consequence of early prenatal diagnosis is that many pregnancies can proceed to term with the delivery of a normal child, instead of being terminated on the basis of a high risk.

Over the last 40 years there has been considerable progress in developing prenatal testing for severe inherited skin disorders. In the late 1970s, fetal skin was examined by transmission electron microscopy in a limited number of conditions, including severe (Herlitz) junctional epidermolysis bullosa (EB) and epidermolytic ichthyosis (bullous congenital ichthyosiform erythroderma). The tests were reliant on being able to demonstrate clear structural differences in the fetus compared with age- and site-matched control skin [1].

The early fetal skin biopsy sampling procedures were performed using a rigid fetoscope to directly visualise the fetus. Later samplings were obtained using finer, more flexible devices under ultrasound guidance. The fetal skin biopsy samples obtained during the early 1980s could be examined only by light microscopy and transmission electron microscopy [2]. In the mid-1980s, however, the availability of a number of monoclonal and polyclonal antibodies to certain basement membrane components led to the development of immunohistochemical tests to complement ultrastructural analysis in establishing accurate diagnoses. For example, in severe recessive dystrophic EB, transmission electron microscopy may reveal structural abnormalities in the anchoring fibrils and cleavage below the lamina densa, but reduced immunolabelling for type VII collagen at the dermal–epidermal junction by immunohistochemistry can provide valuable diagnostic support, especially if no clear evidence of blistering was noted in the fetal skin [3]. Fetal skin biopsies for disorders such as EB are usually obtained at 16–17 weeks' gestation, although for some forms of ichthyosis, such as harlequin ichthyosis, the diagnostic skin abnormalities may not be present until 20–22 weeks' development. Fetal skin biopsies for oculocutaneous albinism often necessitated biopsying hair-bearing sites, such as the eyebrows, or subjecting the skin to an immunohistochemical analysis of tyrosinase enzyme activity.

Nevertheless, since the early 1990s, as the molecular basis of an increasing number of inherited skin diseases has been discovered, fetal skin biopsies have gradually been superseded by DNA-based diagnostic screening using fetal DNA from chorionic villi or amniotic fluid cells [4]. Chorionic villi are usually sampled at 10–12 weeks' gestation (i.e. at the end of the first trimester), whereas amniocentesis is often performed early in the mid-trimester. Chorionic villi can be obtained before 10 weeks, but sampling is usually deferred until later because of a possible risk of inducing fetal limb abnormalities. The chorionic villi can be obtained through the cervix or through the mother's abdomen, depending on gestation and location of the placenta (Figure 8.9).

Knowing the molecular basis of an inherited skin disease has made it feasible to test a much broader range of genodermatoses

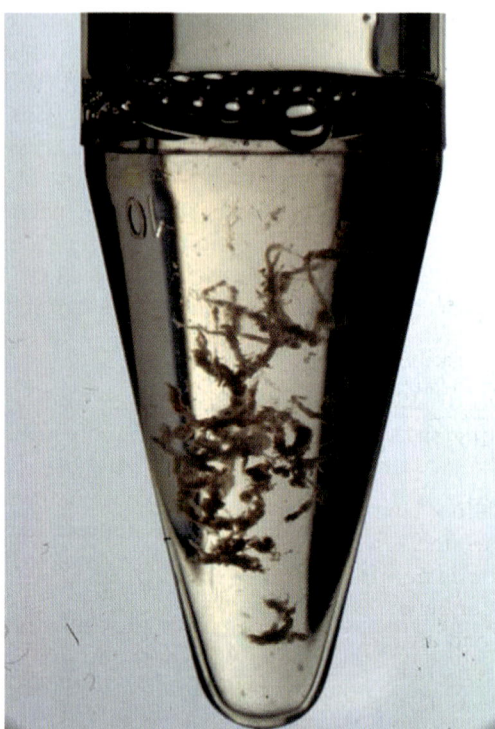

Figure 8.9 Chorionic villi for DNA-based prenatal diagnosis.

by fetal DNA analysis, provided that the molecular basis of the disease has been fully characterised. This information should include knowledge of the mutation in the previously affected child as well as the carrier status in both parents. Having this information available can exclude compounding factors, such as the occurrence of *de novo* mutations (i.e. mutations occurring for the first time in parental gametes), uniparental isodisomy (i.e. the previously affected child having inherited two copies of a gene abnormality from one parent only) or the finding of non-paternity [4,5].

More recently, advances with *in vitro* fertilisation and embryo micromanipulation have led to the feasibility of even earlier DNA-based assessment through preimplantation genetic diagnosis (PGD) (Figure 8.10) [6], an approach that has been successfully applied to inherited skin diseases [7]. Improvements in DNA markers have also refined the approaches used for PGD such that

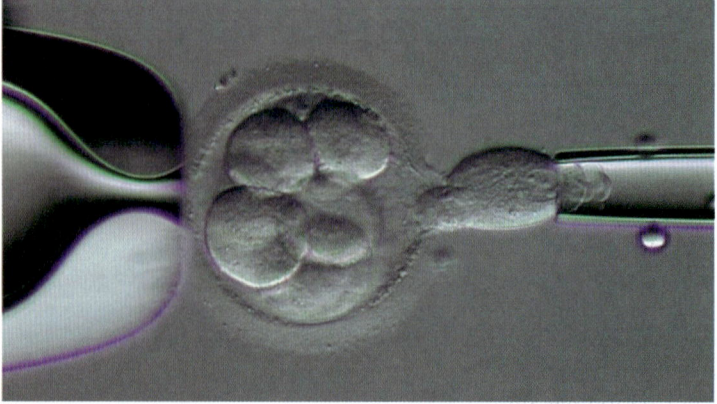

Figure 8.10 Biopsy of a single cell from a blastocyst (3-day-old embryo) for preimplantation diagnosis or haplotyping. Courtesy of Assisted Conception Unit, Guy's Hospital, London, UK.

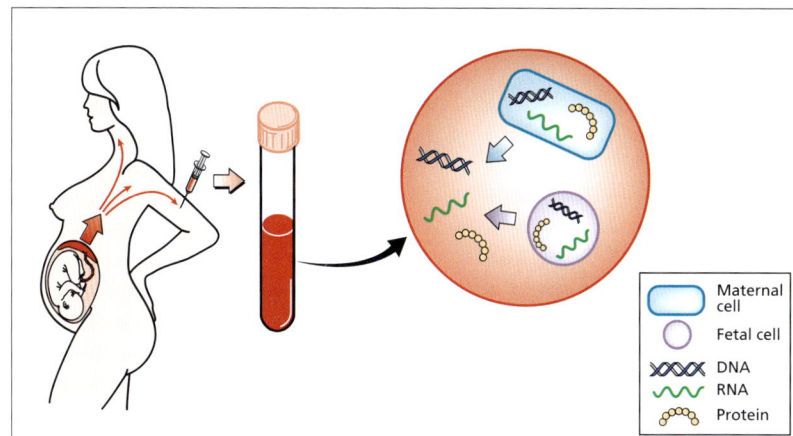

Figure 8.11 The blood of a pregnant woman contains maternal and placental cells along with cell-free fetal elements (DNA, RNA and proteins) which have the potential to be used as biomarkers for prenatal testing and diagnosis. Adapted from Pös et al. 2019 [9].

preimplantation genetic haplotyping (PGH) is now performed in many centres, including for genodermatoses [8]. PGH technology means that it is not necessary to screen for the precise mutations in a particular gene; rather a selection of polymorphic informative markers in and around that gene locus will suffice. The advantage of PGH means that more couples can be screened more quickly and PGH tests for conditions such as severe junctional EB have been approved, licensed and used clinically. Ethically, this approach may be more acceptable for some couples.

For some inherited skin disorders, alternative, less invasive methods of testing are now also being developed, given that fetal cells, DNA, RNA and proteins may be detected in the maternal circulation in early pregnancy (Figure 8.11) [9].

Free fetal DNA is present in the maternal circulation from 6 weeks' gestation and is rapidly cleared from the circulation after delivery [10]. The challenge in diagnosing monogenic diseases, however, is the presence of maternal DNA. Although non-invasive prenatal testing has not become established for inherited skin diseases, combining targeted haplotyping of both parents with targeted sequencing of cell-free DNA extracted during pregnancy offers one technical way forward to clinical realisation. Likewise, isolating fetal cells or defining fetal epigenetic markers may also improve diagnostic options. Considerable ethical, legal and social issues, however, remain to be addressed over the introduction and adoption of non-invasive prenatal testing [11]. Some inherited skin disorders, such as harlequin ichthyosis, can also be screened for by three-dimensional ultrasound [12]. Given that at present there is no cure for any inherited skin disease, prenatal diagnosis offers couples at risk of having affected children options for family planning, although genetic counselling should also be offered as part of patient and family management.

In a clinical setting, the topic of prenatal diagnosis usually becomes relevant to dermatologists only when a mother of a child with a genodermatosis wishes to discuss risk in future pregnancies. Less commonly, she may consult once she is already pregnant and at risk for another affected child. The first objective for the dermatologist is to establish an accurate diagnosis and pattern of inheritance. The next task is to see what laboratory diagnostic information has previously been identified in the family, or if none is available, the challenge is to find a diagnostic laboratory that can undertake the necessary testing. It is important to establish how quickly such information might be made available – if it is going to take several weeks, then this may be too late for the current pregnancy. Then a centre that can perform the prenatal diagnostic test needs to be contacted so that a specific type of test can be planned, and arrangements made for counselling and follow-up. In most cases, the detailed planning can be referred on to the clinical genetics services or, in some countries, tertiary referral centres that diagnose and care for patients with inherited skin diseases.

Key references

The full list of references can be found in the online version at https://www.wiley.com/rooksdermatology10e

Advances in genetics

2 Chiu FP, Doolan BJ, McGrath JA, Onoufriadis A. A decade of next-generation sequencing in genodermatoses: the impact on gene discovery and clinical diagnostics. *Br J Dermatol* 2021;182:606–16.
5 Green ED, Gunter C, Biesecker LG et al. Strategic vision for improving human health at The Forefront of Genomics. *Nature* 2020;586:683–92.
7 Regev A, Teichmann SA, Lander ES et al. The Human Cell Atlas. *Elife* 2017;6:e27041.
8 Dubois A, Gopee N, Olabi B, Haniffa M. Defining the skin cellular community using single-cell genomics to advance precision medicine. *J Invest Dermatol* 2021;141:255–64.

Nosology and principles of medical genetics

5 Cheng JB, Cho RJ. Genetics and epigenetics of the skin meet deep sequence. *J Invest Dermatol* 2012;132:923–32.

Mosaicism, Lyonisation and the lines of Blaschko

1 Cheraghlou S, Lim Y, Choate KA. Mosaicism in genodermatoses. *Clin Dermatol* 2020;38:408–20.
2 Kinsler VA, Boccara O, Fraitag S, Torrelo A, Vabres P, Diociaiuti A. Mosaic abnormalities of the skin: review and guidelines from the European Reference Network for rare skin diseases. *Br J Dermatol* 2020;182:552–63.

Genome sequence and analysis of inherited disorders

4 Kanzi AM, San JE, Chimukangara B et al. Next generation sequencing and bioinformatics analysis of family genetic inheritance. *Front Genet* 2020;11:544162.

Prenatal diagnosis

4 Fassihi H, Eady RA, Mellerio JE et al. Prenatal diagnosis for severe inherited skin disorders: 25 years' experience. *Br J Dermatol* 2006;154:106–13.
11 Zaami S, Orrico A, Signore F, Cavaliere AF, Mazzi M, Marinelli E. Ethical, legal and social issues (ELSI) associated with non-invasive prenatal testing: reflections on the evolution of prenatal diagnosis and procreative choices. *Genes (Basel)* 2021;12:204.

CHAPTER 9

Inflammation, Immunology and Allergy

Muzlifah Haniffa

[1]Wellcome Sanger Institute, Cambridge, USA
[2]Department of Dermatology and NIHR Newcastle Biomedical Research Centre, Newcastle Hospitals NHS Foundation Trust, Newcastle upon Tyne, UK
[3]Biosciences Institute, Newcastle University, Newcastle upon Tyne, UK

Introduction, 9.1	Skin microbiota and the immune system, 9.7	Mast cell and IgE-related type I skin hypersensitivity, 9.9
Immunology, 9.2	**Inflammation, 9.8**	Allergic contact dermatitis, 9.10
Immune cells in human skin, 9.2	Pathological skin inflammation, 9.8	**Summary, 9.10**
Resetting skin homeostasis: healing and repair, 9.6	Inflammatory memory, 9.9	**Acknowledgements, 9.10**
Skin immune network in humans and mice, 9.7	**Allergy, 9.9**	**Key references, 9.10**

Introduction

The skin is the largest human organ, measuring about 1.5–2 m^2 in adults and representing about 15% of body weight [1]. It forms a mechanical, biochemical and immunological barrier with the external environment, including the microbiota, and is contiguous with the oral and anal epithelial lining of the human body. Creating an exchange interface between the internal and external environment, the skin is vital to the maintenance of homeostasis, notably through regulating body temperature and water loss.

The basic structure of the human skin comprises a stratified epithelial layer followed by the basement membrane and the dermis, moving from superficial to deep (Figure 9.1) [1]. The avascular epidermal layer comprises keratinocytes including stem cells in the basal layer, which give rise to basal keratinocytes that undergo progressive differentiation through the sublayers of the epidermis into the stratum corneum located at the most superficial epithelial layer. Keratinocyte differentiation is a dynamic process that forms the sublayers of the epidermis and is characterised by the production of keratin and intercellular connections called desmosomes (spinous layer) followed by accumulation of keratohyalin granules (granular epithelial layer) and cellular compaction with loss of nuclei (stratum corneum) before the corneal layer desquamates (sloughs off). Terminally differentiated keratinocytes, known as corneocytes, are embedded in a hydrophobic lipid matrix of ceramides, fatty acids and cholesterol which act as a waterproof barrier to maintain skin integrity. Each of these sublayers of the epidermis can be identified by the unique expression pattern of key epidermal proteins such as keratins. For example, K5 and K14 in the basal layer, K10 in the spinous layer and filaggrin and loricrin in the stratum corneum [2,3]. In addition to keratinocytes, the basal epidermis also contains melanocytes producing the pigment melanin, Merkel cells for mechanosensing and immune cells. Therefore, the epidermis undergoes a continuous renewal process supported by both immune and non-immune cells, vital to the maintenance of a homeostatic state. The complex network of epidermal cells and immune cells provides protection against ultraviolet (UV) radiation, chemicals, injury and pathogens.

Separated from the epidermis by the dermal–epidermal junction, the dermis is a collagen-rich extracellular matrix (ECM) structure populated by fibroblasts, endothelial cells lining blood and lymphatic vessels, pericytes, neuronal cells, Schwann cells and immune cells [4]. The dermis provides mechanical resilience of the skin and has a key role in thermoregulation due to the cell populations present. A simple analogy of the dermis is that of jelly (the ECM) with fruit pieces (the cells) embedded in it. There are two broad dermal regions: the papillary and reticular dermis. The papillary dermis has invaginations (rete ridges) from the epidermis that also lines appendageal structures such as eccrine sweat glands and the pilo-sebaceous unit, the latter comprising the hair follicle and hair shaft, sebaceous glands and arrector pili muscles. On a cross-section view of the skin, the papillary dermis has vertically orientated, densely packed collagen bundles, in contrast to the reticular dermis where the collagen fibres are horizontally orientated and more sparsely organised. The papillary dermis has capillary loops and the superficial blunt-ended lymphatic vessels and is rich in immune cells in comparison to the reticular dermis, which contain arterioles, venules and draining lymphatics. Immune cells such as antigen-presenting cells and T cells form cords around the dermal papillary vessels and are best appreciated on *en face* rather than cross-section view [4]. The subcutis deeper to the dermis is rich in adipocytes and will not be discussed in detail in this chapter.

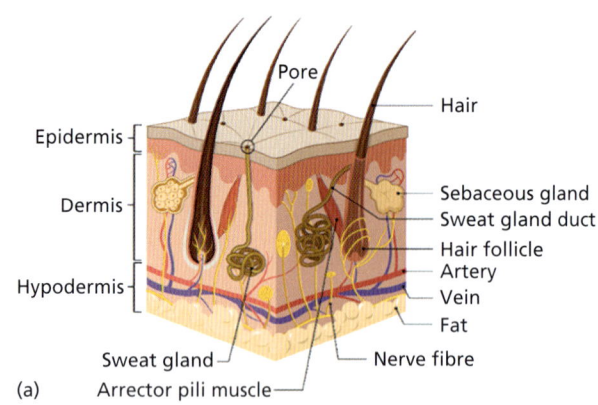
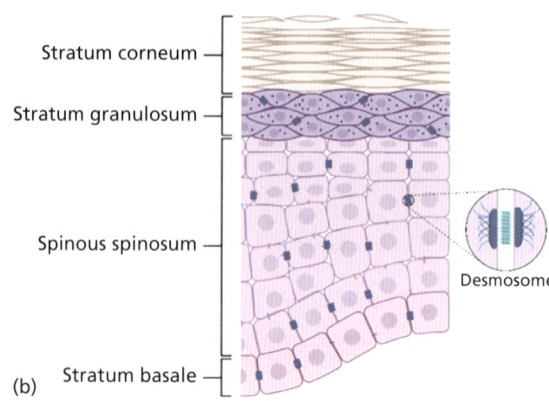

Figure 9.1 Anatomy of (a) the skin and (b) the epidermis.

Immunology

The skin is one of the major non-lymphoid barrier tissues that are interconnected with all organs primarily via the vascular and lymphatic systems. Immune cells constantly traffic into and out of the skin and are in dynamic equilibrium with the rest of the tissue compartments in the human body during health. This harmonious relationship allows the immune system to signal via the different cell types in the major organs and, therefore, when challenged can mediate the necessary immune response. Perturbations to the equilibrium occur upon exposure and response to a stimulus, which can result in resolving or pathological inflammation mediated by various immune cells and molecules. The first section of this chapter describes the components of the human skin immune network during health. The second half will focus on the consequences to human skin when the immune network equilibrium is perturbed.

Immune cells in human skin

The identity of immune cells in the human skin were initially described based on morphology, protein and gene expression. All cells contain DNA, which confers individual identity. The respective segments of DNA transcribed by each cell into RNA is variable and confers cellular identity (e.g. keratinocytes, lymphocytes). Some of these RNAs encode proteins which are translated, determining cellular functions. Non-protein-coding RNAs also contribute to cellular function, but these have received little attention compared with protein-coding RNAs and proteins, which are widely used to assign cell identity.

The earliest descriptions of immune cells in the skin were based on chemical staining, for example gold chloride for Langerhans cells or haematoxylin and eosin (H&E) staining performed on skin sections usually cut at cross-section [1]. Further advances occurred following the discovery of antibodies that could be used to label specific antigens (components of proteins) expressed by immune cells and visualised using chemical- or fluorescence-based imaging, which are currently used in clinical pathology [2,3]. While these approaches allow the visualisation of cells *in situ*, they are limited by the number of antigens that can be measured simultaneously.

Alternative approaches to *in situ* imaging involved culturing skin explants *ex vivo* or dissociating skin to release cells into a suspension for further analysis. It was observed that immune cells such as antigen-presenting cells and lymphocytes migrated out of skin explants over 24–60 h of culture and was originally thought to recapitulate lymphatic migration to the lymph node [4,5]. However, recent studies have shown that cells were not necessarily entering lymphatics during *ex vivo* migration from skin explants [5]. Both *ex vivo* migration from skin explants and skin dissociation (mechanical, enzymatic or both) enable cells to be collected in a suspension and can be analysed using technologies such as flow cytometry and fluorescence activated cell sorting (FACS), frequently used to study peripheral blood cells [5,6]. The advantage of this method is the greater multiplexity of antigens that can be simultaneously measured. However, those analyses lack precious *in situ* spatial information, impairing our understanding of how the cells' microenvironment influences their fate and functions.

Advances in single-cell RNA sequencing (scRNA-seq), single-nuclei RNA sequencing (snRNA-seq) and spatial genomics (e.g. spatial transcriptomics, *in situ* hybridisation and sequencing) technologies leveraging next generation sequencing have provided unprecedented resolution in depth and breadth of analysis of human tissues in recent years [7]. These methods enable whole cell (nuclei and cytoplasm) or nuclei RNA/transcriptome profiling of single cells in suspension as well as near single-cell resolution *in situ* RNA profiling [8]. They can be performed at high throughput and applied to the analysis of small skin biopsies of 4–6 mm in diameter [7]. These recent studies are beginning to highlight the heterogeneity of cell types and cell states in healthy human skin based on each cell's RNA expression, enabling a reference atlas of human skin to be assembled for comparisons with skin upon perturbation and in disease. scRNA-seq can be combined with surface protein profiling and snRNA-seq can be combined with regulatory DNA analysis (e.g. open chromatin and methylation) [8]. This allows different properties of a cell to be analysed simultaneously, providing a multifaceted view of cell identity.

ScRNA or snRNA sequencing requires cells to be dissociated from tissue into suspension, so there is loss of spatial information of the cells within the tissue as well as incurring potential effects of dissociation during data analysis. Nevertheless, as snRNA-seq profiles nuclear RNA extracted from frozen tissues, this overcomes tissue digestion effects but does not include cytoplasmic RNA profiling. *In situ* spatial genomics technologies do not require tissue dissociation and can be performed on frozen or chemically fixed skin tissues, and therefore retain spatial information of the cells and their neighbours. Spatial transcriptomics provides data on cells' localisation relative to their cellular and tissue microanatomical structure, thus allowing a finer level of understanding of the different cues and interactions that cells are exposed to, and therefore giving a better comprehension of what can influence their functions and fate.

On top of providing a physical and mechanical barrier, the skin acts as an active immune organ, shielding the internal environment from any pathogen or noxious breach. As such, immune cells are a vital component of skin homeostasis when in a resting state but are also recruited during tissue repair, inflammation and allergy mechanisms in activated skin.

Innate immune cells are of particular interest as they are generated in a relatively pathogen-free embryonic environment at a time when organogenesis and tissue morphogenesis occur [9]. Whether this is to protect against maternal–fetal transmission of pathogens, to prepare for perinatal challenges or immune cells having an undervalued non-canonical role in skin morphogenesis is still to be determined. Several mouse studies have described a role for immune cells, particularly macrophages, in murine skin development, wound healing and tissue repair. Although *in vivo* mechanistic studies of human skin morphogenesis are logistically challenging, recent advances in skin organoid culture from human inducible pluripotent stem (iPS) and embryonic stem (ES) cells are beginning to facilitate these investigations [10].

The skin-resident immune cells are the first line of defence against any noxious breach of the barrier and have a sentinel function where they continuously sample their environment in search of non-self-antigens [11]. Upon activation by harmful antigens, some skin immune cells can migrate to the lymph nodes to induce a targeted immune response against specific antigens [12]. In steady state, the skin-resident immune cells are also largely involved in the maintenance of homeostasis and tolerance, preventing an overactivation of immune cells or autoimmune responses. This fine balance between an immunogenic and tolerogenic environment is crucial to support skin homeostasis and to ensure an appropriate immune response.

Epidermal immune cells

In healthy skin, the epidermal immune environment is composed of T cells and antigen-presenting cells called Langerhans cells (LCs) (Figure 9.2). The mechanical and immunological functions of the epidermis cannot be exclusively attributed to non-immune and immune cells, respectively, but are the collective function of all epidermal cells acting in synergy. Innate immune sensing and acute inflammatory responses mediated by keratinocytes have been demonstrated by recent studies, along with their capacity to promote immune tolerance via self-antigen presentation to T cells [13]. These elements further highlight the importance of the cross-talk between immune and non-immune cells for adequate surveillance of the epidermal microenvironment and maintenance of barrier integrity.

Langerhans cells

Langerhans cells are unique skin-resident immune cells that are thought to originate from macrophage precursors early during prenatal development [14]. LCs, characterised by the expression of CD207, major histocompatibility complex (MHC) class II and high CD1a molecules, are found in the basal layer but extend their dendrites all the way to the granular layer to constantly survey and probe their local environment [12]. Recent studies based on scRNA-seq and mass spectrometry refined the classification of epidermal LCs and dendritic cells (DCs) by identifying two main populations: LC1, excelling at antigen presentation and innate immune responses and LC2, specialised in adaptive responses and related to dermal DCs [15,16]. There are 300 LCs per 1 mm^2 area of skin [17] that form an interdigitating cellular network providing an immunological barrier that complements the mechanical barrier of the keratinocytes interdigitating via desmosomes in the spinous layer.

LCs sample antigens in the epidermis and migrate into the dermis where they enter lymphatic vessels, enabling them to travel to skin-draining lymph nodes to present the antigens to T cells. LC migration occurs during homeostasis to maintain healthy skin integrity and also on antigen challenge, such as from pathogen/exogenous molecules, to initiate protective immune responses. This is done by activating CD8+ T-cell differentiation into cytotoxic T cells and by supporting CD4+ T-cell differentiation into primarily T helper 2 (Th2) cells. LCs are also largely involved in the maintenance of a tolerogenic environment during homeostasis. While sampling the environment, non-activated LCs internalise self-antigens (mainly from apoptotic keratinocytes) without triggering autoimmune responses but rather promoting the secretion of anti-inflammatory cytokines, such as interleukin 10 (IL-10) and transforming growth factor β (TGF- β), and the induction of regulatory T-cell (Treg) survival and differentiation [12,17]. Therefore, LCs present both tolerogenic and immunogenic phenotypes and their promotion is tightly orchestrated by the antigen origin and environment cues they receive. LCs are also studied as a potential candidate for vaccination strategies to induce antitumour immune responses in various skin cancers [18].

T cells

T cells are broadly categorised as CD8+ cytotoxic T cells, CD4+ T helper cells and Tregs. T cells that have yet to encounter antigen are called naïve T cells and after activation by cognate antigen in the lymph node, naïve T cells proliferate and differentiate into memory T cells [19]. Human skin is populated primarily by memory T cells that enter the skin from the blood circulation [18,19,20,21]. Some memory T cells gain long-term residency in the skin (resident memory T cells) and others can recirculate (circulating memory T cells). Epidermal T cells are skin-resident memory T lymphocytes, primarily cytotoxic CD8+ T cells (with some CD4+ T cells), expressing CD103. They are derived from circulating T cells that enter the dermis through endothelial vessels and subsequently differentiate into skin-resident T cells, similar to other tissue-resident memory T cells. These cells provide a rapid immune response to previously encountered antigen challenges in the skin, such as protective immunity to viruses (e.g. herpes simplex virus) that can cause cutaneous infection. Their activation can also lead to hypersensitivity reactions, an unwanted immune response to allergen, such as drug molecules. LCs can directly present antigens to memory T cells in the skin, promoting their proliferation and activation and allowing for a thorough screening of the environment for harmful substances. T-cell functions are also influenced by their interactions

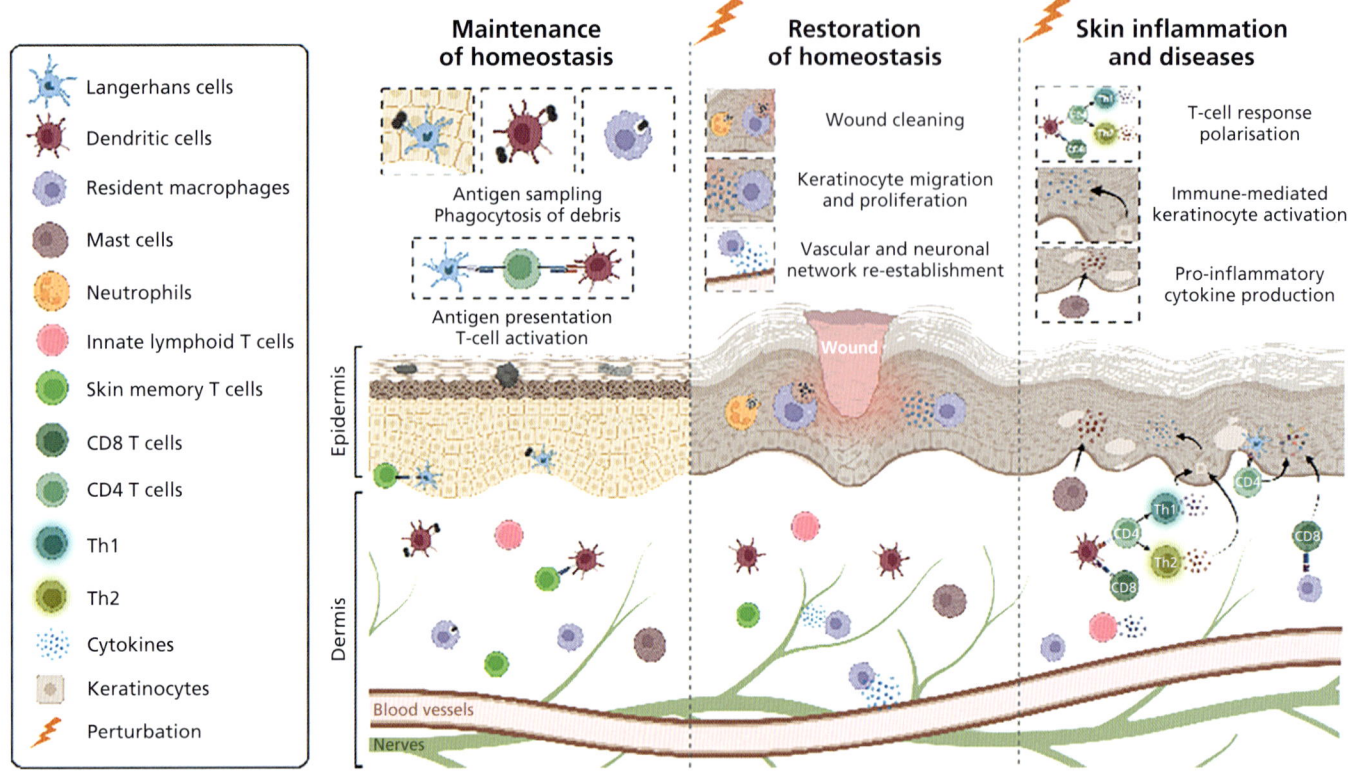

Figure 9.2 Immune cells in skin homeostasis and disease.

with keratinocytes. Besides cell–cell interactions, keratinocytes can communicate via cytokine secretion, such as IL-1α and TNF-α, promoting the initial step of the inflammatory response along with immune tissue infiltration. These elements reinforce the vital role of immune/non-immune interactions to regulate skin homeostasis.

Dermal immune cells

The healthy dermis has a variety of immune cells, including dermal antigen-presenting cells (DCs, macrophages and monocyte-derived cells), T cells expressing the lymphocyte antigen receptor/T-cell receptor comprising αβ chains (αβ T cells) and γδ chains (αβ T cells), innate lymphoid cells (natural killer (NK) cells and innate lymphoid cells (ILCs)), mast cells and plasma cells (Figure 9.2). Notably, neutrophils and B cells are absent in healthy skin but can be observed during inflammation and disease.

Myeloid lineage cells

Antigen presenting cells. Dendritic cells are divided into two broad subtypes: conventional DCs and plasmacytoid DCs. The classification of DC populations is constantly evolving based on phenotype and ontogeny studies [12]. Each DC subpopulation is unique and distinct from one another through their transcriptome and phenotype. All DC populations appear to originate from a common DC progenitor via the action of the growth factor FLT3-L, although plasmacytoid DCs may arise from lymphoid progenitors. The dermis is composed of several subsets of conventional DCs, such as DC1, DC2 and DC3. Plasmacytoid DCs are very rare/absent in healthy skin. Similar to the LCs in the epidermis, DCs are potent antigen-presenting cells at the interface between innate and adaptive immunity by sensing and integrating environmental cues to polarise T-cell responses appropriately. Immature DCs are effective at antigen capture and processing as well as environment screening through the pattern recognition receptors on their surface. When patrolling, DCs can sense danger through pathogen-associated molecular pattern signals leading to the release of cytokines (type I and III interferon (INF) and TNF-α) and to direct cytotoxicity (via TRAIL (TNF-related apoptosis-inducing ligand) and Fas ligand interactions). Immature DCs can also internalise antigen and migrate into the skin lymphatics to the skin draining lymph nodes while maturing on their way. Once activated or mature, DCs are less effective at antigen capture but are potent activators of T cells.

In the skin draining lymph nodes, DCs prime and activate T lymphocytes by presenting exogenous antigens bound to MHC II to CD4+ T cells and endogenous antigens (derived from the cell's protein synthesis endoplasmic reticulum compartment) bound to MHC I to CD8+ T cells. All cells express MHC I molecules and as such can present endogenously derived antigens to CD8+ T cells. MHC II presentation is restricted to antigen-presenting cells such as DCs, but MHC II can be upregulated during inflammation by epithelial and stromal cells such as keratinocytes, fibroblasts and endothelial cells. However, DCs are unique in their ability to migrate to skin draining lymph nodes to activate T cells and coexpress many co-stimulatory molecules such as CD80, CD83 and CD86 to efficiently activate T cells.

DC subsets are functionally specialised [22]. For example, although CD8+ T-cell activation via MHC I machinery relies on endogenously derived antigens, there is a DC subset that can sample exogenous antigen and shuttle it to MHC I molecules for efficient presentation to CD8+ T cells. This process, called cross-presentation, is efficiently performed by skin CD141+CLEC9A+XCR1+ DC1, enabling CD8+ T-cell activation to phagocytosed skin cancer antigens and viral antigens without the DCs becoming infected by the virus. CD1c-expressing DC2 and DC3 specialise in exogenous antigen presentation on MHC II to activate CD4+ T cells [23]. DCs are generally short-lived and are continuously replenished by DCs and DC precursors in the peripheral blood and bone marrow haematopoietic stem cells (HSCs) via a lineage distinct from monocytes. Like their epidermal counterpart, DCs can either promote an immunogenic or a tolerogenic environment giving them a key role in skin homeostasis regulation.

Dermal dendrocytes, which express FXIIIa, are skin-resident macrophages and not DCs [24]. Macrophages have a broad range of functions that differ depending on the tissue they are found in, for example microglia in the brain and Kupffer cells in the liver, but are essentially critical for tissue maintenance, homeostasis and local immunity. Dermal macrophages engulf melanin granules and were historically also called melanophages. Macrophages are one of the earliest immune cells to seed the developing skin where they likely contribute to skin morphogenesis. Tissue-resident macrophages arise from several sources including prenatal yolk sac progenitors and HSCs in the fetal liver and bone marrow [22]. There is increasing evidence for tissue-resident macrophages contributing to tissue morphogenesis in several organs in murine models, and their role in human prenatal skin morphogenesis remains to be explored. Dermal-resident macrophages are long-lived, can self-renew and persist locally in homeostasis but can also be reconstituted by bone marrow-derived HSCs if required [22,24].

Monocytes are made in the bone marrow from HSCs and released into the circulation where they seed peripheral non-lymphoid tissues such as the skin, where they rapidly undergo differentiation into cells with properties of DCs or macrophages based on local tissue requirements. Monocytes form a pool of cells in the bone marrow and peripheral blood that can be rapidly mobilised to replenish tissue DCs and macrophages in times of need (e.g. inflammation and infection). Monocyte-derived DCs can subsequently acquire lymph node migratory capacity like conventional DCs. Following inflammation, circulating monocytes replenish the dermal macrophage population but the longevity of monocyte-derived macrophages is unclear.

Mast cells. Mast cells are tissue-resident cells that are packed with mast cell mediators such as histamine, tryptase, prostaglandins and cytokines [25]. Mast cells reside in all vascularised tissues in the body but are particularly abundant in tissues that are in frequent contact with the external environment such as the skin. This ensures that the mast cells are in a prime position to regulate inflammatory mediators upon infection or disease. Mast cell mediators are rapidly released following activation of the high affinity receptor FcER1, on the surface of mast cells, that recognises the Fc region of immunoglobulin E (IgE) molecules. IgEs are a subtype of antibody that are made in response to allergens. Interestingly, mast cells are also generated in the yolk sac and, similar to the other innate cells such as macrophages, NK cells and ILCs, seed the developing skin very early in the first trimester [9]. The role of mast cells in allergic responses is well characterised but additional homeostatic roles have been reported, such as angiogenesis, and remain to be better characterised.

Lymphoid lineage cells

Innate lymphoid cells. Innate lymphoid cells, such as NK cells and ILCs, do not express a lymphocyte antigen receptor and as such lack antigen-specific memory capacity [26,27]. These cells are able to respond rapidly via cytokine and/or cytoplasmic granule secretion upon stimulation in the skin. NK cells are innate counterparts of CD8+ T cells and recognise cells that lack self MHC I for destruction through granzyme and perforin release. ILCs are the innate counterparts of CD4+ Th cells with similar cytokine-producing subsets including ILC1 (IFN-γ), ILC2 (IL-4/IL-13) and ILC3 (IL-17). NK cells and ILCs are generated in the yolk sac and fetal liver prior to the formation of the thymus and are also found in the fetal bone marrow. These cells seed the human skin very early in the first trimester but can be replenished by bone marrow-derived progenitors in postnatal life.

Mucosal associated invariant T (MAIT) cells. MAIT cells are evolutionary conserved, innate-like T cells that present a semi-invariant T receptor restricted to MHC class I molecules [28]. They specifically recognise riboflavin metabolites of bacterial origin presented on MR1 (MHC class I related) and therefore defend the body in the event of a microbial insult. These cells are especially enriched in the blood and liver but they are also found to populate tissues in contact with the external environment. In the skin, MAIT cells are mainly located in the basal membrane where they interact with the microbiota and actively participate in the maintenance of barrier integrity. Skin-resident MAIT cells show an effector memory phenotype and can be activated either in a T-cell receptor (TCR)-dependent or -independent manner through cytokines such as IL-7 and IL-12. Upon stimulation, MAIT cells produce a variety of cytokines depending on their polarisation. In mice, skin-resident MAIT cells seem to be skewed towards a Th17 profile, supporting epithelial survival. Recently, studies of MAIT cells' genome revealed their involvement in tissue repair in addition to canonical immune functions.

T lymphocytes. T cells form the adaptive arm of the immune response and have the capacity for immune memory through their lymphocyte antigen receptor/T-cell receptor. αβ T cells are CD4+ or CD8+ and conventionally recognise exogenous peptides presented by MHC II (usually on antigen-presenting cells) or endogenous peptides on MHC I (any cells), respectively [29]. The vast majority of T cells in the skin are memory T cells that are recruited via dermal capillaries into the skin following cognate antigen presentation by DCs in skin-draining lymph nodes [19,20]. Central memory T cells retain the capacity to recirculate but effector memory T cells are generally skin-resident. Differentiation of memory T cells into long-lived skin-resident memory T cells (characterised by the expression of CD69, CD103 and CD49a) is thought to be antigen-specific and locally mediated [20].

CD4+ T cells in the skin can be IFN-γ-producing T helper (Th1), IL-4/IL-13-producing T helper (Th2) and IL-17-producing T helper (Th17) cells. In addition, human skin also contains CD4+ Tregs, which have been shown to confer an immune privilege in the hair follicle bulge where they protect stem cells. During the hair follicle anagen phase, Tregs support an immune permissive environment allowing high levels of proliferation and differentiation to promote hair follicle regeneration. Bulge immune privilege is also achieved through the downregulation of MHC I-mediated antigen processing and presentation. γδ T cells are also found in the dermis but their precise role in homeostasis and disease is still unclear. Recent studies have demonstrated the presence of unconventional αβ T cells in human blood and tissues, including in the skin, that recognise lipids presented by CD1a on antigen-presenting cells such as LCs and dermal DCs. In addition, some αβ T cells may not express CD4 or CD8 and recognise glycolipids presented by CD1d. Both CD1a and MR1 (presents riboflavin metabolite to MAIT cells) are also expressed by LCs and dermal DCs. In humans, adaptive T cells begin to seed human skin at the start of the second trimester following their differentiation in the thymus.

Plasma cells and B cells. B cells also have a similar innate and adaptive cellular equivalent to ILCs and T cells. Innate-like B cells (B1 cells) spontaneously secrete IgM but the adaptive B cells undergo antigen-specific somatic hypermutation and differentiation into memory B cells and long-lived plasma cells specialised in antibody secretion and antibody class switching (IgM, IgG). B1 cells have been described in mouse tissues but their presence in human tissues has been debated. Recently, putative human B1 cells were described in prenatal tissues but not in adult tissues [30]. Plasma cells reside in the healthy dermis, but B cells are rare [31]. Skin-associated B lineage cells are a heterogeneous population, different from the lymph node-associated B lineage cells, and are able to recirculate through the healthy dermis via CCR6–CCL20 interaction [31]. Their precise role in health and disease is still unclear but B cells are also known to be involved in autoimmune-mediated skin disorders (e.g. pemphigus vulgaris), infection (e.g. leprosy) and skin cancers (e.g. cutaneous B-cell lymphoma).

Immune surveillance: peripheral blood and skin draining lymph node

The skin vascular and lymphatic vessels as well as nervous system facilitates the coordination of local and body-wide homeostasis and responses when required. Immune cells are mobile and can travel around the body mediating homeostatic equilibrium and physiological and pathological responses. Immune cells differentiate from HSCs in the bone marrow in postnatal life and egress from the bone marrow to enter the peripheral blood circulation where they can travel to various tissues in the human body. Cells destined to peripheral tissues often express specific surface adhesion proteins that act as tissue-homing receptors, for instance T cells expressing cutaneous lymphocyte adhesions, addressins that can act as postcodes for traffic to the various tissues including skin during both homeostasis and inflammation or disease.

Immune cells seed the human skin as early as the first trimester of gestation [9]. The earliest cells found in prenatal skin are innate cells including macrophages, mast cells and ILCs. T and B lymphocytes are seeded in the skin from the onset of the second trimester of gestation (about 12 postconception weeks) following the development of the thymus, where T cells differentiate, and the onset of bone marrow haematopoiesis, when B-cell differentiation scales up.

There is one major travel route for immune cells into the skin via blood vessels but two exit routes from the skin via the blood and lymphatic vessels. Myeloid and lymphoid cells enter the skin through vascular endothelial cells, primarily through post-capillary high endothelial venule-like structures in the papillary dermis. Lymphocytes (e.g. central or effector memory T cells) can re-enter the peripheral blood through these postcapillary vessels and circulate around the body. Some lymphocytes that enter the skin differentiate into skin-resident T cells (characterised by the expression of CD103 and CD62L) and are primarily found in the epidermis.

DCs and monocytes enter the skin through the circulation. Monocytes can differentiate into tissue DCs or macrophages. Macrophages are resident in the skin and are often long-lived [24]. DCs in the skin and other peripheral non-lymphoid tissues express the chemokine receptor CCR7 which enables their traffic from the skin to skin-draining lymph nodes via lymphatic vessels, the second exit route from skin.

Resetting skin homeostasis: healing and repair

Skin homeostasis can be altered in many ways following physical, environmental and microbial stimulation or perturbation [32]. Homeostasis needs to be reset following perturbation and a classic response is following skin wounding resulting in repair. Wound healing has been extensively studied in murine skin and is a tightly regulated multifactorial programme of phases that involves haemostasis, inflammation, proliferation and remodelling at the injured site. The different phases of wound healing are overlapping and occur in a synchronised fashion throughout the process. Wound healing in the skin relies on many different cells working together such as the resident hair follicles and dermal fibroblasts, along with epithelial–mesenchymal cross-talk signals, for cell migration and epidermal regeneration to take place [33]. The role of macrophages in regulating repair has been described and is in keeping with observations of poor wound healing in an immunodeficiency context and with immunosuppressive treatments, which are used in organ transplant and skin inflammation. This highlights the crucial role of immune cells as orchestrators of the wound healing and tissue repair processes.

Haemostasis is the first step of the wound healing process and starts rapidly after the injury. Transient vascular constriction is induced and the extravascular collagen produced by the injury activates platelets and ensures their recruitment to initiate fibrin clot formation at the site of injury, preventing further blood loss. The fibrin clot acts as a provisional matrix supporting the wound healing process and is replaced by a definitive matrix in the following phases. During haemostasis, the clots and the surrounding cells secrete pro-inflammatory cytokines and chemokines such as TGF-β, platelet-derived growth factor and epidermal growth factor to promote vascular dilatation and therefore allow immune cell recruitment and extravasation. The products of the injury also act as chemoattractants for immune cells.

The inflammatory stage starts as soon as the immune cells are recruited at the injured site. Neutrophils are the first to arrive and their main role is to decontaminate the wound by phagocytosing any microbial particles and cellular debris. They also release elastase and collagenase to eliminate the components of the skin that were damaged by the injury. Once the site of injury is thoroughly cleaned, neutrophils die by apoptosis. About 24 h after the injury, monocytes migrate to the relevant site and differentiate to macrophages in response to the chemokines secreted by the cells surrounding the site of injury and the products of the injury themselves (i.e. degraded collagen). Once at the site of injury, macrophages secrete cytokines to support the wound healing process. Macrophages likely play a role in re-establishing vascular and neuronal networks as well as keratinocyte migration during wound healing and repair.

The proliferative phase mainly consists of epithelial cell migration to the injured site and proliferation, a process called re-epithelisation. The fibroblasts in the injury bed secret collagen and other ECM components to help rebuild the wounded tissue. This high level of cell activity implies a high demand in oxygen, which triggers angiogenesis via the secretion of TGF-α, basic fibroblast growth factor (bFGF) and vascular endothelial growth factor (VEGF) by endothelial cells activated during haemostasis. The remodelling phase is the final step of the wound healing process and usually starts 21 days after the initial injury. It is characterised by the full closure of the wound and ECM remodelling. The initial ECM laid out by fibroblasts during the proliferation phase is disorganised and weak.

Wound healing is accompanied by fibroblasts that secrete collagen and ECM that is organised in an abnormal lattice network forming scar tissue. Immune cells such as macrophages also contribute to scar tissue formation. The destruction of hair follicles and their stem cells in the injured skin results in hair loss within the scar tissue. Interestingly, human prenatal first trimester skin heals without scar formation. The precise differences between prenatal and postnatal human skin that results in scarless healing during development remains unclear and are likely mediated by multiple factors involving cross-talk between immune and non-immune cells.

Skin immune network in humans and mice

Murine models are widely used to study skin and have contributed to furthering our understanding of cutaneous biology. Therefore, it is important to understand the shared and distinct properties of the immune network in human and mouse skin to fully appreciate the lessons learned from animal models and how these findings can be extrapolated into clinical settings [22]. The extrapolation of findings in mouse studies to human biological relevance needs to consider three key factors. The first is the difference between the often-studied young mice and adult human skin, leading to comparisons between two different corresponding biological ages between species. The second is the general use of a specific pathogen-free environment to house mice for experimental studies that contrasts with the natural environment human skin is exposed to immediately after birth. The third is the hair-bearing nature of mice skin and although studies are often done on mouse ear skin that lacks hair, its architecture is very different from human trunk and limb skin. Nevertheless, animal models do provide the advantage of undertaking perturbational mechanistic studies that are often not possible to perform in humans *in vivo*, but careful consideration of their implications to human biology is required.

The composition of skin immune cells in both species are broadly similar but with the notable absence of dendritic epidermal T cells (DETCs) in the human epidermis [34]. DETCs are from the family of intraepithelial lymphocytes that are also seen in other epithelial tissues such as the gut. DETCs express γδ TCR and are abundant in the mouse epidermis, forming a similar interconnected network to epidermal LCs in mouse and human skin. In mice, DETCs have been shown to be vital for tissue repair. It has been proposed that DETCs are linked to the presence of hair follicles in murine skin tissue after wounding, which are absent in human scar tissue.

The role of macrophages in tissue homeostasis and regeneration has been well described in mice, including in cardiac repair following injury, iron recycling and the regulation of body heat and peristalsis. Notably, Csf1op/op mice and humans with homozygous CSF1R deficiency lacking macrophage populations suffer developmental abnormalities including defects of tissue patterning, branching morphogenesis and embryonic HSC differentiation [35]. Human maternal NK cells regulate angiogenesis and fetal trophoblast invasion and mouse Tregs promote hair follicle growth and lung tissue repair [35–37]. Also, although the cellular composition of the skin immune network is similar between humans and mice, there are differences in the abundance and molecular features of these cells across species. For example, dendritic epidermal T cells prominent in the murine epidermis are not present in human skin. In healthy murine skin, antibody-secreting B cells are seen after 8 weeks of age and constitutively secrete IgM in the absence of antigen challenge, showing a role in skin homeostasis and defence. Furthermore, inflammation positively influences antibody-secreting cells leading to their accumulation in the skin.

Skin microbiota and the immune system

In addition to human skin cells, a rich community of microorganisms colonise the human skin that through host–microbiota interactions contribute to homeostasis and barrier integrity and tune immune responses to pathogens and perturbations and in disease [38,39]. The use of 16s ribosomal RNA sequencing or shotgun metagenomic sequencing has enabled the identification of a diverse species of microbiota beyond traditional culture-dependent methods. Commonly found healthy skin microbiota include *Staphylococcus*, *Corynebacterium* and *Cutibacterium* (predominates in the pilosebaceous unit) bacterial species, eukaryotic viruses in low numbers, the fungal *Malassezia* species and the arachnid genus *Demodex* that resides in the hair follicles. There are many external factors that can influence the composition of the skin microbiota including local (e.g. electrolytes, sebum) and systemic (age, hormones) host factors, and environmental (e.g. UV radiation, pollution) and lifestyle (e.g. skin products) factors.

Recent research has illustrated the influence of skin microbiota particularly *Staphylococcus epidermidis*, a common commensal, on local tissue and systemic immune responses [11]. These studies have primarily been done on mice housed in germ-free facilities with regulated introduction of microbiota at birth. The host–microbiota interactions involve direct and indirect interactions with skin immune cells such as *S. epidermidis* triggering Treg influx in infant mouse skin and antimicrobial and immunomodulatory molecule production by keratinocytes. In short, mice that do not encounter skin microbiota have impaired local immune responses to pathogenic bacterial strains and are more vulnerable to infection and inflammation. The skin host–microbiota interactions can also affect distant organs (e.g. gut microbiota) affecting skin immunity, or mediate a systemic response (e.g. toxin activating a systemic pain response). Skin microbiota has also been shown to promote the expression of host-specific endogenous retroviruses as a means of communication between host and exogenous microbiota to control homeostasis and inflammation.

The composition of skin microbiota is altered in skin disease suggesting a role for microbiota in their pathogenesis. However, research in this field has struggled with the 'chicken or egg' conundrum of whether the change in microbiota drives disease or is a consequence of disease. The microbiota in atopic dermatitis (AD) is enriched for *Staphylococcus* species, which is known to exacerbate AD, but there is little change to the microbiota in psoriasis skin. Although it is hard to know if skin microbiota alterations cause or are a consequence of skin disease, there is evidence in mice that skin inflammation can be dampened by modulating the skin microbiota. Further studies are required to better understand how complex skin microbial colonies modulate regional immunity and how to harness these functions for clinical therapy.

Inflammation

Inflammation is a cellular and molecular response that was conventionally characterised by tissue redness (Latin *rubor*), swelling (*tumor*), heat (*calor*) and pain (*dolor*). These signs and symptoms of inflammation, mediated by immune infiltration and tissue oedema, are generally viewed as a pathological tissue response in contrast to steady-state tissue homeostasis. Inflammation is mediated by different types of immune infiltrates into the skin including lymphohistiocytic (primarily lymphocytes and mononuclear phagocytes) and granulocytic (e.g. neutrophilic and eosinophilic), and are accompanied by extravascular fluid extravasation. Inflammation can be triggered by many causes such as pathogens, UV radiation and mechanical injury.

However, there is increasing evidence that the cellular and molecular processes involved in inflammation are also shared by a range of other non-pathological biological processes including tissue remodelling and morphogenesis [1]. This has been observed during wound healing and in early human development. As such, some researchers have proposed a reinterpretation of the conventional viewpoint of inflammation as purely reflecting a response mediating disease.

A recent perspective put forward is of inflammation as a molecular response that arises from loss of tissue structure, cell loss or loss of homeostatic control mediated by a diverse range of triggers. The corollary would also support inflammation as a process critical for tissue development and homeostasis which occurs during embryogenesis and regeneration. This perspective is helpful in contextualising inflammation as a process that has enormous benefits in normal physiology as well as potentially causing damage or pathology to the organism.

In this context, the human skin, as an accessible organ that regularly undergoes tissue structure changes, wounds, repairs and heals, is an ideal tissue to interrogate the cellular and molecular mechanisms of inflammation. The same shared molecular processes are also implicated in a range of skin diseases that are described in other chapters of this textbook.

Pathological skin inflammation

Inflammation that does not result in re-establishing homeostasis can result in a range of skin diseases, including inflammatory skin disease, chronic ulceration and neoplasia. Inflammatory skin disease is common and affects all age groups [2]. Common inflammatory skin diseases include AD, psoriasis, hidradenitis suppurativa and lichenoid disorders. These skin disorders cause a huge burden on the quality of life in patients and traditionally treatment focused on controlling symptoms rather than necessarily addressing the cause of the inflammatory response. Inflammatory skin disorders such as psoriasis and AD are often characterised by visible erythematous (red) skin eruptions during disease flares which can subside during remission. The red skin rash accompanies the infiltration of immune cells into the skin, including T cells and myeloid cells that induce epidermal hyperplasia/hyperproliferation, and the secretion of cytokines that creates the characteristic well-defined scaly plaques of psoriasis and ill-defined reddish papules and plaques of AD [3].

These two common inflammatory skin disorders are characterised by a preponderance of unique cytokines secreted by primarily immune cells in the local skin milieu. In psoriasis, there is activation of the IL-23/IL-17 axis whereby IL-23-induced stimulation of IL-17+ T cells leads to phosphorylation in the JAK (Janus kinase)/STAT (signal transducers and activators of transcription) pathway, which then induces the expression of IL-17 [4]. IL-17+ T cells target the epidermal keratinocytes which secrete chemokines such as CCL20 and CXCL8, subsequently attracting infiltration of more T cells and neutrophils, resulting in psoriatic skin and inducing further disease activity. LCs and dermal myeloid cells are sources of IL-23 in psoriasis. Psoriasis-like skin in murine models can be induced by topical application of imiquimod (a Toll-like receptor 7 agonist). Reducing LC secretion of IL-23 reduces T-cell interactions and IL-17 secretion, which improves psoriasis-like symptoms in these murine models. Notably, overexpression of CD1a in murine LCs aggravates psoriasis. In humans, anti-CD1a antibodies have been shown to reduce the amount of cytokines in the skin such as TNF, IL-1 and IL-17 and to alleviate inflammation.

AD has a multifactorial pathogenesis that incorporates barrier defects, bacterial overload and Th2-biased immune responses. The enhanced colonisation of skin with *S. aureus* is shown to further exaggerate the Th2 microenvironment, exacerbating disease. Mutation and aberrant expression of filaggrin, a major protein of the cornified layer in the epidermis, was described as a major predisposing genetic factor. However, more recently, dysregulation of the Th2 immune response, an imbalance in the skin commensals of the microbiome and increased colonisation of skin with *S. aureus* have been shown to underpin AD. It is thought that the dysregulated Th2 response is further exacerbated by a defective epidermal barrier integrity, increased secretion of factors such as thymic stromal lymphopoietin and IL-33 by keratinocytes and *S. aureus* colonisation. Activation of Th2 cells to release IL-4 and IL-13 further induces B cells to produce IgE, resulting in a vicious loop of Th2 cytokine-mediated inflammation.

The cytokines and inflammatory mediators in both psoriasis and AD also mediate cross-talk between immune cells and neurons in the skin. These interactions mediate itch and pain as well as modulating skin inflammation. As such, therapies targeting psoriasis- and AD-associated cytokines using biologics (e.g. anti-TNF, anti-IL-17 for psoriasis and anti-IL-4/IL-13) and reducing *S. aureus* burden in the context of AD have proven to be highly effective in dampening inflammation, improving symptoms such as itch and enhancing the quality of life of patients [5].

Inflammatory memory

Immune memory is the ability of cells to respond more effectively and efficiently upon reinfection or re-exposure to an inflammatory stimulus. Conventionally this has been attributed to adaptive T and B lymphocytes and mediated by the selection of highly specific TCR and B-cell receptor (BCR) for the specific immune response causing the inflammatory process. However, it is becoming a more widely accepted concept that immunological/inflammatory memory can also be retained by long-lived innate immune cells such as macrophages and non-immune cells such as epithelial stem cells [6]. Inflammatory memory can contribute to the tissue-wide immune response and exert its effect well after the initial inflammatory process.

Researchers studying the epithelial barrier, tissues that are more routinely exposed to injury or pathogenic infection, noted that the response to injury is enhanced with repeated episodes of trauma. Investigation into the IL-17-mediated inflammatory response such as psoriasis demonstrated that the same area of lesional skin can undergo re-epithelialisation more quickly. The mechanism of inflammatory memory in epithelial stem cells is thought to be epigenetically encoded. Epithelial stem cells retain memory of wound healing through altered chromatin accessibility, which remains open long after the inflammatory resolution, and is then recalled following a secondary insult resulting in a rapid reactivation of relevant gene expression and a quicker molecular response. In addition to this, an interesting discovery is that epithelial stem cells can also retain memory of their previous microenvironments and cellular functions. This was elegantly demonstrated in stem cells responsible for regenerating hair follicles to retain memory of their origin and the capacity to make hair even after moving out of the hair follicle niche into a new environment, which aided epithelial barrier repair following trauma.

The mechanism of inflammatory memory lies in the specific epigenetic landmarks left after injury or infection. In response to inflammation, cells undergo histone and chromatin accessibility modifications to activate transcription of genes associated with inflammation or the stress response. Usually, these genes are returned to baseline after a period of resolution but epithelial stem cells can remain poised in a primed state for rapid gene expression upon further insult. Recent studies have begun to provide some answers to this. One layer to this is the idea of inflammation-sensing transcription factors that are activated upon cytokine or microbial exposure such as the activation of STAT3 in skin during the IL-17 cytokine response which is essential for establishing epigenetic memory in epithelial stem cells. However, other researchers have highlighted that these transcription factors, such as STATs, alone are not enough. In addition to a stimulus-specific factor, establishing memory requires the general stress-responsive transcription factor FOS and one of its associated factors, such as JUN, to gain chromatin access for remodelling. This then allows for prolonged binding of transcription factors long after the inflammation or stress is removed and allows reactivation of inflammatory memory via various cellular stresses that trigger FOS. Despite the recent advances in understanding the mechanisms of inflammatory memory, some questions remain unanswered: how does a cell decide whether to retain epigenetic memory of inflammation, how is memory retained during normal cellular processes such as cell division and differentiation and whether there is variation in the way different cell lineages acquire and retain inflammatory memory.

Inflammatory memory is an exciting conceptual development in skin biology and has the potential to better understand skin diseases, including cancers, where immune memory can be hijacked or exploited mediating disease. Precise manipulation of inflammatory memory, well beyond the active skin flare during disease, promises to open exciting new therapeutic avenues and also to potentially facilitate therapeutic cure of common inflammatory skin diseases.

Allergy

Allergy is a type of abnormal inflammatory response triggered by sensitivity to an otherwise harmless substance such as food, pollen or animal fur. Skin allergies can be classified more specifically by the type of hypersensitive reaction triggered. Skin allergies manifest due to type I hypersensitivity, characterised by hives in acute or chronic urticaria, or type IV hypersensitivity reactions, such as contact allergic dermatitis following contact with allergen. A type I hypersensitivity reaction is immediate (within *c*.24 h) and is mediated by an IgE response to the allergen causing mast cell degranulation. This releases histamine, prostaglandin and other vasoactive molecules resulting in oedema, itch and redness. In contrast, a type IV hypersensitivity reaction occurs *c*.48–72 h later and is T-cell mediated. Allergen-specific T cells are activated by DCs in the skin draining lymph nodes.

Mast cell and IgE-related type I skin hypersensitivity

One of the main players in the skin allergic-type response is the mast cells. Mast cells are an important immune cell type that produce mediators that can actively enhance inflammation and promote wound healing through re-epithelialisation and scarring. In terms of allergy, mast cells are vital to skin immunity as they reside in the tissue available to rapidly mediate regulatory response to any infection or disease. Mature mast cells contain various mediators, cytokines and proteoglycans that are released upon activation of mast cell surface receptors. IgE binding to FcER1 on mast cells triggers the release of histamine and other mediators in defence against potentially harmful molecules. However, in certain individuals, the inappropriate activation of mast cells to allergens results in urticaria [1]. Urticaria, characterised by the appearance of wheals/hives on the skin, can be triggered by a range of stimuli and is named depending on the inducible factor, such as solar urticaria caused by sensitivity to UV light and cold urticaria caused by exposure to cold. When the trigger is unknown, the rash is labelled spontaneous urticaria. Histamine and other mediators released by degranulating mast cells are associated with the pathogenesis of urticaria, and mast cell degranulation can be observed at the sites of wheals in the skin. The first evidence of the immunological mechanisms underlying chronic spontaneous urticaria demonstrated that IgG antibodies against the patient's own IgE were instrumental in causing wheal formation. It has also been shown that in patients with chronic spontaneous urticaria, there were more than 200 IgE autoantigens in the serum that are not observed in healthy controls, suggesting that IgE-dependent mechanisms underlie forms of urticaria. Therefore, the development of novel anti-IgE therapies such as omalizumab changed the landscape for many urticaria patients [2]. However, there is now an appreciation of an alternative pathogenesis of chronic spontaneous urticaria that is IgE independent, where some patients do not respond [3].

Allergic contact dermatitis

Allergic contact dermatitis is a common T-cell-mediated, delayed-type hypersensitivity response to often relatively mild sensitising antigens that come into contact with the skin [4]. Clinically, it presents as an eczematous red rash with itch within 72 h. It has recently been shown that different allergens have unique molecular patterns, for example nickel-induced contact dermatitis promotes a Th1/Th17 axis whereas fragrance demonstrates a Th2/Th22 response. This was missed in previous work in mouse models using strong sensitisers that suggested a more consistent response despite the different allergens.

Contact allergy response involves both innate and adaptive immune pathways in three stages. Initially, sensitisation takes place in which exposure to the allergen is taken up by LCs and dermal DCs, which are activated by the cytokine secretion of epidermal keratinocytes [4,5]. DCs then migrate and present the antigen to naïve T cells which are activated and generate effector T cells. The effector stage is antigen non-specific and then antigen-specific. With antigen non-specific inflammation, the antigen stimulates keratinocytes to secrete pro-inflammatory cytokines such as IL-1β and TNF-α and mast cells to release histamines. Together this activates the endothelial cells to guide T cells in the blood to migrate and increase vascular permeability, triggering the neutrophils and CD8+ T cells to infiltrate, respectively. Antigen-specific inflammation then begins once T cells have migrated and are activated by the production of IFN-γ and IL-17. This leads to further T-cell recruitment and intensifies the response. The response in the effector stage can be elicited following antigen re-exposure and the recruitment of primed T cells, which is visible as inflamed redness and pruritus. Finally, resolution begins in which residing regulatory T cells control the expansion of cytotoxic T cells and dampen the immune response through the release of anti-inflammatory cytokines (IL-10) and deactivation of effector cells via cell-to-cell contact in the skin. Regulatory T cells can also impart suppressor activity by affecting the functions of antigen-presenting cells and negatively regulating mast cell degranulation in the allergy response. It has been shown that regulatory T cells, especially those expressing high FOXP3, are instrumental in maintaining cutaneous memory and self-tolerance [3,**6**,7].

Some researchers have begun to demonstrate an appreciation that AD is actually a risk factor for developing irritant or allergic contact dermatitis. This is in part due to the recruitment of eosinophils into the skin, defective barrier integrity and increased production of IL-4 and IL-13, which promote IgE and increase the susceptibility to IgE-mediated allergic reactions and more broadly other autoimmune responses. In AD, this again becomes a loop of disease activity.

It is now appreciated that in AD the defective barrier is a secondary response to Th2 and Th22 signalling; these epidermal changes are perpetuated by epicutaneous antigen exposure that in turn prolongs inflammation and immune-related changes to the epidermal barrier, in a similar mechanism to that in AD. One such example of this is the propensity for chemical sensitisation of non-lesional AD skin regardless of filaggrin (*FLG*) mutation status compared with healthy individuals. Interestingly, it has been noted that although there is a heightened sensitivity to allergic responses in AD patients, these immune responses are resolved in these patients compared with healthy controls. This is potentially due to the skin and residing immune cells being readily active at the site of disease.

Summary

The skin is a rich immune organ where complex interactions between immune and non-immune cells maintain homeostasis in health. Skin immune cells are in dynamic equilibrium with peripheral blood, the lymphatic system including skin draining lymph nodes and the skin microbiota. In this chapter we also discussed the observation of many cellular and molecular responses characteristic of inflammation in a variety of physiological and pathological processes, which can leave epigenetic memory in immune and non-immune cells. Allergic inflammation is one form of inflammation that results from the response to allergen and can trigger two different types of skin hypersensitivity reactions. An in-depth understanding of the skin immune system in health and disease will facilitate a greater understanding of skin diseases and new avenues for therapeutic strategies for patient benefit.

Acknowledgements

The author is grateful to April Foster and Chloe Admane for co-writing this chapter, Chloe Admane for the illustrations and Bayanne Olabi for critical reading of the chapter.

The author is funded by the Wellcome Trust (WT107931/Z/15/Z and WT206194).

Key references

The full list of references can be found in the online version at https://www.wiley.com/rooksdermatology10e

Introduction

1 Gallo RL. Human skin is the largest epithelial surface for interaction with microbes. *J Invest Dermatol* 2017;137:1213–14.
4 Kashem SW, Haniffa M, Kaplan DH. Antigen-presenting cells in the skin. *Annu Rev Immunol* 2017;35:469–99.

Immunology

6 Wang XN, McGovern N, Gunawan M *et al.* A three-dimensional atlas of human dermal leukocytes, lymphatics, and blood vessels. *J Invest Dermatol* 2014;134:965–74.
8 Stephenson E, Webb S, Haniffa M. Multiomics uncovers developing immunological lineages in human. *Eur J Immunol* 2021;51:764–72.
10 Lee J, Rabbani CC, Gao H *et al.* Hair-bearing human skin generated entirely from pluripotent stem cells. *Nature* 2020;582:399–404.

11. Belkaid Y, Naik S. Compartmentalized and systemic control of tissue immunity by commensals. *Nat Immunol* 2013;14:646–53.
12. Kashem SW, Haniffa M, Kaplan DH. Antigen-presenting cells in the skin. *Annu Rev Immunol* 2017;35:469–99.
20. Strobl J, Haniffa M. Functional heterogeneity of human skin-resident memory T cells in health and disease. *Immunol Rev* 2023;316:104–19.
32. Medzhitov R. The spectrum of inflammatory responses. *Science* 2021;374:1070–5.
38. Byrd AL, Belkaid Y, Segre JA. The human skin microbiome. *Nat Rev Microbiol* 2018;16:143–55.

Inflammation

1. Medzhitov R. The spectrum of inflammatory responses. *Science* 2021;374:1070–5.
2. Kabashima K. *Immunology of the Skin: Basic and Clinical Sciences in Skin Immune Responses*. Berlin: Springer, 2016.
4. Hawkes JE, Chan TC, Krueger JG. Psoriasis pathogenesis and the development of novel targeted immune therapies. *J Allergy Clin Immunol* 2017;140:645–53.
6. Naik S, Fuchs E. Inflammatory memory and tissue adaptation in sickness and in health. *Nature* 2022;607:249–55.

Allergy

4. Strobl J, Haniffa M. Functional heterogeneity of human skin-resident memory T cells in health and disease. *Immunol Rev* 2023;316:104–19.
5. Kabashima K. *Immunology of the Skin: Basic and Clinical Sciences in Skin Immune Responses*. Berlin: Springer, 2016.
6. Guttman-Yassky E, Zhou L, Krueger JG. The skin as an immune organ: tolerance versus effector responses and applications to food allergy and hypersensitivity reactions. *J Allergy Clin Immunol* 2019;144:362–74.

CHAPTER 10

Photobiology

Antony R. Young
St John's Institute of Dermatology, School of Basic and Medical Biosciences, Faculty of Life Sciences and Medicine, King's College London, London, UK

Basic principles, 10.1	Action spectroscopy, 10.4	Clothing and shade, 10.12
UVR and its production and sources, 10.1	**Normal effects of UVR on the skin, 10.5**	**Personal and population exposure to UVR, 10.12**
Measurement of UVR, 10.2	Molecular and cellular effects, 10.5	The sun, 10.12
Terrestrial UVR, 10.2	Clinical effects of UVR, 10.7	UV index, 10.13
Artificial sources of UVR, 10.2	**Photoprotection, 10.11**	Non-solar sources with emphasis on sunbeds, 10.13
Interaction of UVR with the skin (physicochemical aspects), 10.3	Melanin, 10.11	Risks versus benefits of population UVR exposure, 10.13
	Sunscreens, 10.11	**Key references, 10.14**

Basic principles

Photobiology is the study of the effects of ultraviolet (UV) and visible radiation on life but may also include the effects of infrared radiation (IR). This chapter focuses on UV photobiology of normal skin. This is important because the skin is the body's interface with the environment, and solar ultraviolet radiation (UVR) is probably our most important natural environmental hazard. Many people also expose themselves to artificially generated UVR for cosmetic tanning. Solar UVR exposure has many detrimental effects on skin that can be minimised by photoprotection strategies. However, solar UVR is also necessary for vitamin D production, and there is increasing evidence of other beneficial effects [1] such as a reduction of blood pressure. UV and visible radiation may be exploited in photo(chemo)therapy and photodynamic therapy for the treatment of skin disorders (Chapters 21 and 22), and indeed for internal diseases. Furthermore, many people have disorders that render their skins abnormally sensitive to UV and visible radiation. These aspects of photodermatology are discussed in Chapter 126.

UVR and its production and sources

Ultraviolet and visible radiation, which comprises a very small part of the electromagnetic radiation spectrum (Figure 10.1), is energy released during the transition of a molecular electron from a higher-energy outer molecular orbital to a less energetic inner one. Each such emission, known as a photon, is a discrete oscillating electromagnetic pulse of energy E (joules, J), wavelength λ (nanometres, nm, 10^{-9} m) and velocity through space c (3×10^8 m/s), such that $E = h\nu = hc/\lambda$, where $h = 6.63 \times 10^{-34}$ J/s (Planck's constant) and ν = photon frequency (Figure 10.2). Thus, a 300 nm photon has energy of 6.63×10^{-19} J, where 1 J is defined as the work required to accelerate 1 kg over 1 m in 1 s to a velocity of 1 m/s in a frictionless

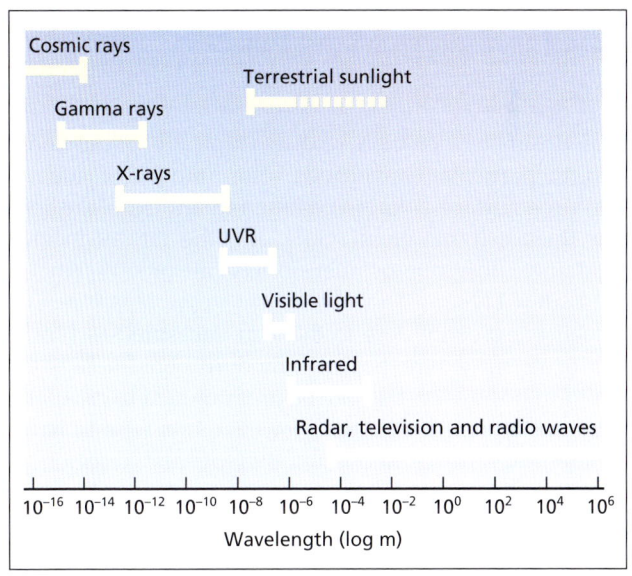

Figure 10.1 The electromagnetic spectrum.

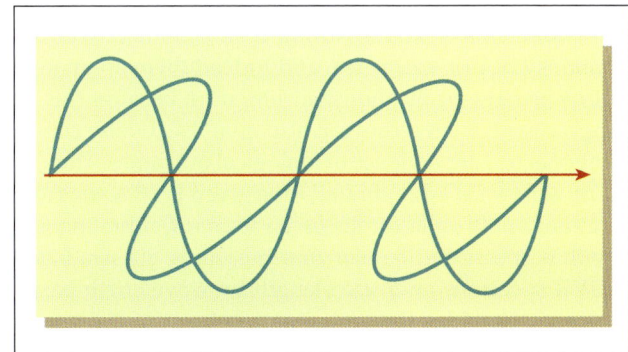

Figure 10.2 Schematic representation of an electromagnetic wave.

environment. Repeated molecular emissions from a point source lead to multiple spherical radiation wave fronts, each of total energy equal to the sum of the individual photon energies, but diverging with gradually diminishing intensity per unit surface area. UVR can be defined in terms of photons (i.e. particles) or waveform.

Ultraviolet radiation is, by convention, divided into three subcategories officially designated by the Commission Internationale de l'Eclairage (CIE):
- UVC (200–280 nm).
- UVB (280–315 nm).
- UVA (315–400 nm).

However, a UVB/UVA boundary of 320 nm is very widely used in photodermatology. Furthermore, UVA is often subdivided into UVA1/I (340–400 nm) and UVA2/II (315/320–340 nm). This subdivision of UVA is based on different molecular mechanisms within the UVA spectral region. In general, UVA2/II is thought to act more like UVB in the ways that it exerts its molecular and biological effects.

Measurement of UVR

Accurate measurement of UVR is important for all aspects of photobiology. Such measurement is called dosimetry, which can be approached physically [2] or biologically.

Physical dosimetry

Physical dosimeters contain sensors, typically photodiodes that respond to particular wavebands. The amount of such energy incident on a surface is known as the radiant exposure, exposure dose or fluence (J/m^2 or mJ/cm^2), and the rate of incidence as the irradiance, dose rate or intensity (W/m^2 or mW/cm^2), where $1 W = 1 Watt = 1 J/s$.

In practice, exposure dose to the skin, measured as J/m^2, is the product of $W/m^2 \times$ time (s). Most modern phototherapy cabinets have built-in dosimeters that can be programmed to calculate exposure time for a prescribed dose. However, it is wise to have these independently verified, and phototherapy and research departments will benefit considerably from close links to physicists with expertise in UVR measurement.

The spectral responsivities of different photodiodes in hand-held dosimeters vary considerably and typically have a bell shape. This means, for example, that a designated UVB sensor may also have some sensitivity in the UVA region or vice versa. This can result in false measurements when measuring UVB irradiance with a source that contains UVA or vice versa, and indeed there are many errors of UVR measurement in published literature because this has not been appreciated. Such errors can also give rise to false conclusions about the spectral dependence of biological outcomes. Thus, a given UVR dosimeter *must* be calibrated for a given UVR source and such a calibration is only valid for the given source. Calibration is widely done with a spectroradiometer that measures the irradiance of a given UVR spectrum on a wavelength by wavelength basis. Such measurement provides the emission spectrum of a given source. A good spectroradiometer will have a dynamic range of about six orders of magnitude. This is very important because even low levels (<1.0%) of a given waveband (usually UVB) may have very important biological effects. Spectroradiometers are themselves calibrated against national standard lamps.

Biological dosimetry

In biological dosimetry, the skin is the sensor and the most widely used measurement outcome is the minimal erythema dose (MED), which is typically assessed *c*.24 h after UVR exposure. The MED is determined by exposing small areas of skin (e.g. 1 cm^2) to a geometrically increasing series (e.g. × 1.25 or × $\sqrt{2}$) of UVR doses and determining the lowest dose that results in either just perceptible redness or redness with definite borders. The MED is widely used as a measure of exposure in experimental photobiology and phototherapy. It is also used in the diagnosis of photodermatoses (Chapter 126). A threshold assessment by eye, such as the MED, is subjective but is reproducible and reliable if performed carefully [2] with standardised lighting. The MED is a measure of individual sensitivity to UVR of a given spectrum, but it should be noted that it varies with body site [3], especially when comparing regions that are habitually sun exposed with those that are normally sun protected. There is increasing use of the standard erythema dose (SED) [4], especially in research and epidemiology, which is a mathematical construct. One SED is equivalent to an erythemally effective radiant exposure of 100 J/m^2. This is obtained by weighting a spectroradiometric measurement with the CIE action spectrum for erythema (see the section on action spectroscopy later in this chapter). One great advantage of the SED is that, in contrast to the MED, it is independent of personal UVR sensitivity and the emission spectrum of the UVR source.

Terrestrial UVR

The spectrum of terrestrial solar UVR is modified by several factors including the absorption of UVC and UVB by oxygen (O_2) and stratospheric ozone (O_3). Thus, the stratospheric ozone layer absorbs all UVC and attenuates UVB but has very little effect on UVA. The UVR spectral profile of terrestrial sunlight is strongly influenced by the height of the sun, which is dependent on latitude, season and time of day. Particulate and gaseous (e.g. O_3, NO_2, SO_2) pollution in the troposphere (0–10 km above sea level) can also influence the UVR spectrum. UVB is at its most intense when the sun is directly overhead, for example at solar noon on the equator. This is because the pathway through the stratosphere is shorter (i.e. less attenuation of UVB) than when the sun is low in the sky (Figure 10.3). This means that the ratio of UVB to UVA varies with the height of the sun (e.g. time of day and time of year) [5], especially at higher latitudes, because there is more seasonal fluctuation of UVB irradiance compared with UVA. However, even when the sun is directly above (e.g. on the equator at noon at sea level) the vast majority of solar UVR is UVA (>90%). Examples of solar spectra are given in Figure 10.4, in which UVB content is about 5% when the sun is high in the sky. Thus, it can be said that the sun is primarily a UVA source, especially UVA1 (>70%). It should be noted that solar irradiance increases with altitude, for instance on mountains. For example, in an Alpine region in summer, total UVR and UVA irradiance increases by about 8–9%/1000 m. When total irradiance is erythemally weighted (see the section on action spectroscopy later in this chapter) this increases to 18%/1000 m [6].

Artificial sources of UVR

There are many man-made sources of UVR, but the most common is the fluorescent tube, which is widely used in photo(chemo)therapy

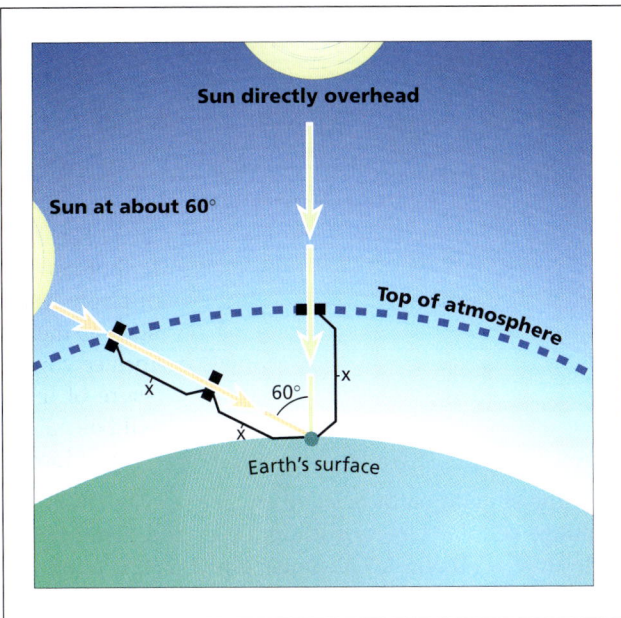

Figure 10.3 Ultraviolet radiation path lengths for differing solar elevations.

and by the tanning industry. This is a sealed glass tube that contains mercury and an inert gas, typically argon. The inner lining of the tube is coated with a phosphor powder. The mercury is excited when an electric current is passed though the tube and releases UVR photons, which interact with the phosphor. UV and visible radiation are released by this interaction, the emission spectra of which can be tailored by the composition of the phosphor. The tubes widely used in phototherapy typically emit narrow-band, more or less monochromatic, UVB (c.313 nm), broad-band UVB and UVA. Cosmetic tanning tubes generally contain primarily UVA1 with a small amount of UVA2 and UVB. See examples of phototherapy tube emission spectra in Figure 10.4.

Some UVR sources are based on the xenon (Xe) arc, which emits a very broad UV and visible spectrum that can be modified by suitable optics. Solar simulating radiation (SSR) (Figure 10.4) can be generated with suitable glass filters, and is used in research, clinical phototesting and the assessment of sunscreens. The Xe arc can also be coupled with a monochromator to generate 'monochromatic' radiation that is required to determine action spectra (see later section). However, it should be noted that in reality this is narrow-band polychromatic radiation with a bell shape. Such monochromatic spectra are characterised by their spectral bandwidth at full width at half maximum (FWHM), which is defined as the width of the spectral band at 50% of the peak maximum. For example, monochromatic radiation at 300 nm might have a FWHM of 5 nm.

Metal halide lamps are used to generate high-output UVA1 that is used in high-dose UVA1 phototherapy in which exposures are more than 60 J/cm^2. A more recent development with promise in phototherapy and photobiology is the light-emitting diode (LED) [7].

Interaction of UVR with the skin (physicochemical aspects)

Radiation incident on a surface is either reflected, or transmitted and scattered within the medium beneath, particularly at short wavelengths (Figure 10.5). It then eventually exits, unless it first collides with and is absorbed by an appropriately structured molecular moiety, known as a chromophore. In the skin these include DNA, *trans*-urocanic acid (tUCA), proteins with aromatic amino acids, melanins, metabolites of melanogenesis, flavins and porphyrins [8]. A broad range of contiguous wavelengths may be absorbed, with slightly differing probabilities, resulting in a highly characteristic absorption spectrum (Figure 10.6) for a given chromophore; for example, naked DNA has an absorption maximum at c.260 nm. This results in electronic excitation to an outer higher-energy molecular orbital (Figure 10.7), enabling chemical reactions to occur which can lead to molecular, cellular and clinical outcomes. Thus, the basis of all skin photobiology, whether acute or long term, is photochemistry.

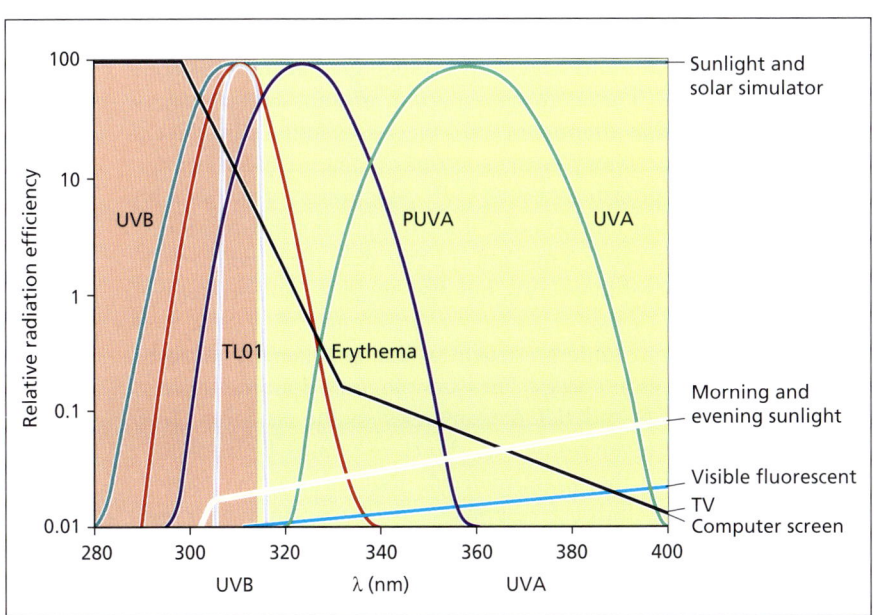

Figure 10.4 Approximate emission spectra of typical sources encountered in dermatological photobiology and elsewhere, with the action spectrum for human cutaneous erythema for comparison. PUVA, psoralen and UVA; UV, ultraviolet.

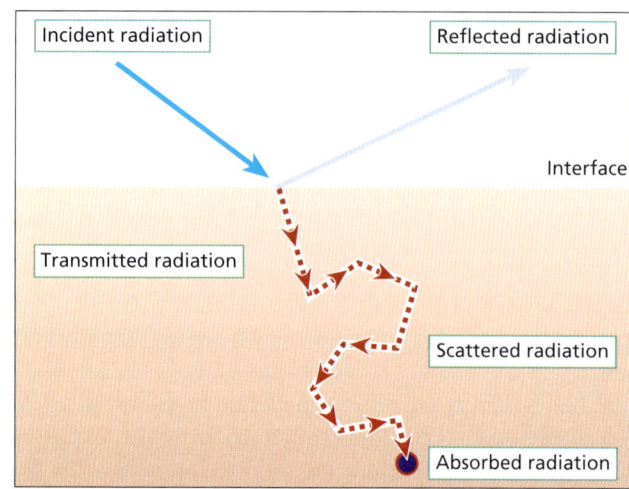

Figure 10.5 Interaction of ultraviolet radiation with physical matter.

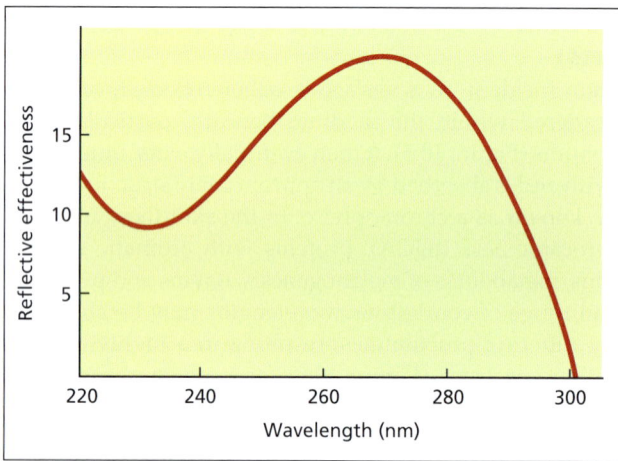

Figure 10.6 Typical appearance of wavelength probability curve for excitation of orbiting electron to outer electronic orbital (absorption spectrum).

The penetration (transmission) of UVR through the skin is a major determinant of the location of photobiological outcome. Transmission studies of UVR have usually been done on isolated mouse and human epidermis and have shown much greater transmission of UVA than UVB. This is to be expected as some of the major chromophores in skin attenuate UVB as it passes to the basal layer and the dermis. For example, the stratum corneum is very rich in tUCA. Another approach to assess UVR penetration of the skin is to measure molecular markers of photodamage after *in vivo* irradiation. Such studies, using a marker of DNA damage, confirm that UVA penetrates better than UVB, but also suggest more scattering of UVA [9,10].

Chromophores may undergo structural change when they absorb UV or visible radiation energy. For example, dipyrimidine lesions are formed in DNA and tUCA isomerises to the *cis* form. The above examples are referred to as direct responses because the chromophore is also the target molecule that initiates the photobiological response. Indirect responses also occur, in which the chromophore is not the molecule that causes the photobiological response *per se*. For example, a chromophore may absorb UV or visible radiation energy and transfer this energy to oxygen, which

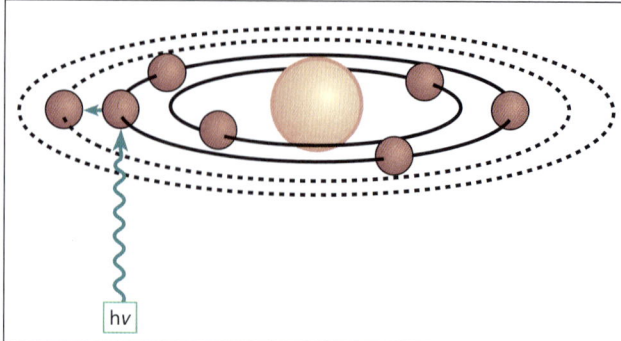

Figure 10.7 Schematic representation of photon absorption, leading to excitation of an orbiting electron to outer electronic orbital. The green arrow, hv, is the energy of a photon.

results in the generation of reactive oxygen species (ROS) that can then damage cellular targets such as DNA and membranes. As a rule of thumb, UVB and UVA2 cause direct effects in normal skin whereas UVA1 causes indirect effects, but there are many exceptions. It should be noted that this rule of thumb is largely based on *in vitro* work.

Action spectroscopy

An action spectrum (wavelength dependence) determines the relationship between wavelength (λ) and photobiological outcome, usually expressed on a logarithmic scale because of the very large differences between different spectral regions for many biological outcomes. Figure 10.8 shows the CIE action spectrum for erythema in normal human skin and demonstrates that UVB is orders of magnitude more erythemogenic than UVA for a given UVR dose (J/m^2). The relative difference between UVB and UVA for erythema will depend on the exact wavelengths being compared, but a rule of thumb for broad UVB and UVA spectra is that the former is about 1000 times more erythemogenic than the latter.

Action spectroscopy has two main purposes. The first is the identification of the chromophore that is responsible for the biological response, and this is critical for the understanding of a given

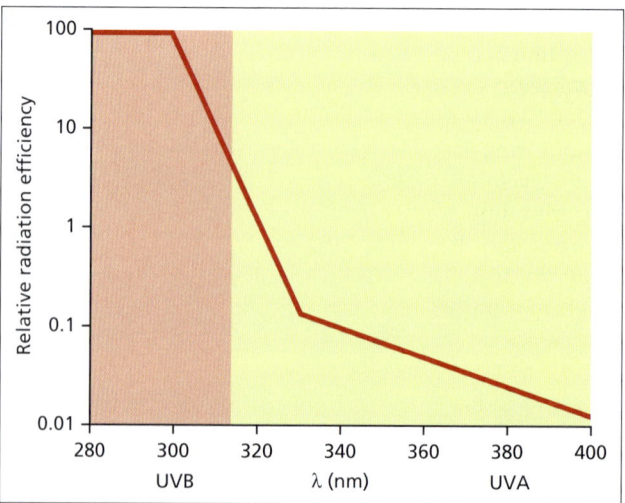

Figure 10.8 Action spectrum for the induction of erythema in human skin. UV, ultraviolet.

photobiological mechanism. Under ideal conditions, an action spectrum of a given biological response can be superimposed on the absorption spectrum of the chromophore that initiates the response. A good non-dermatological example is similarity of the action spectrum for photosynthesis and the absorption spectrum of chlorophyll. However, in more complex structures like human skin, such a match is much less likely because of competing chromophores and the scattering of UVR that modify skin optics. The second and more important practical purpose of action spectra is their use as biological weighting functions for given UVR emission spectra. Biological weighting is the process whereby a given emission spectrum (e.g. solar UVR) is multiplied, wavelength by wavelength, by a given action spectrum to generate a third curve to define biologically effective energy. As described in the section on terrestrial UVR, the sun is primarily a UVA1 source; however, it is the small UVB (typically <5%) content that is primarily (>80%) responsible for sunburn. One practical consequence of this is that sunscreens would be ineffective without good UVB filtering. Biological weighting with action spectra can often give surprising results, such that <1% of a given emission spectrum may be responsible for the vast majority of a given biological or clinical response [11]. The determination of good action spectra for human skin is technically demanding and very time consuming. Reliable biological weighting requires very high-quality spectroradiometric measurements. The action spectrum for normal erythema can be altered by the administration of an exogenous chromophore. For example, the addition of 8-methoxypsoralen (8-MOP) to the skin, orally or topically, will result in an erythema action spectrum with a peak in the UVA region of about 330–340 nm [12].

Normal effects of UVR on the skin

Molecular and cellular effects

The epidermis is rich in UVR-absorbing chromophores [8] and is therefore very vulnerable to photobiological effects. A summary of the main molecular and cellular effects is given in Table 10.1. The most important chromophore is probably nuclear DNA that, upon absorption of UVR, can give rise to varying DNA photolesions [13]. Pyrimidine dimers (also known as dipyrimidine lesions) form after the absorption of photon energy that splits the C5=C6 double bonds of two adjacent pyrimidine bases and forms new covalent bonds linking the two pyrimidines at the C5 and C6 positions. A 4-carbon cyclobutane ring is produced, giving the dimer its characteristic name – the cyclobutane pyrimidine dimer (CPD). Another lesion is the 6-4 pyrimidine-pyrimidone (6-4PP), in which the C5=C6 double bonds break and the surplus energy results in the rotation of one of the pyrimidine rings, which offers its C4 to form a new bond with the C6 of the adjacent pyrimidine. In this case, only one new covalent bond is formed. CPD and 6-4PP can be readily detected in skin *in vivo* after suberythemal exposure of UVB and SSR. The 6-4PP is also induced by UVB but not by UVA1 [9]. The CPD is the most important DNA photolesion. Immunostaining of CPD and 6-4PP by UVB (300 nm) and UVA1 in human skin is shown in Figure 10.9. A new phenomenon of delayed or dark CPD (dCPD) has been described in human skin after long-wave UVA radiation (385 nm) [14] and in black and white skin after exposure to SSR [15].

Table 10.1 Summary of the main normal effects of ultraviolet radiation on the skin.

Molecular/cellular	Clinical	
	Acute	Chronic
DNA photodamage (and its repair) and mutation	Erythema	Skin cancer
Melanogenesis	Delayed tanning	Photoageing
Inflammatory infiltrate, hyperplasia and stratum corneum thickening	Immediate pigment darkening	
Reactive oxygen species that damage DNA and cell membranes	Persistent pigment darkening	
Apoptosis (sunburn cells)	Suppression of acquired immunity	
Langerhans cell depletion	Enhancement of innate immunity	
Gene and protein expression		
Vitamin D photosynthesis	Reduction of blood pressure	

Conventional CPDs are formed within pico (10^{-12}) seconds, during the UVR exposure, whereas dCPDs occur hours after exposure by photosensitising mechanisms [16,17]. The biological significance of these lesions is not known.

Oxidative stress (a state in which the cellular antioxidant system is overwhelmed by ROS) induces modification of cellular biomolecules such as lipids, proteins and DNA. Deoxyguanine (dG) has a low threshold for oxidation, and many different types of potentially mutagenic oxidatively induced DNA damage occur, such as 8-oxo-7,8-dihydroguanine (8oxoGua) [18] and 8-oxo-7,8-dihydro-2′-deoxyguanosine (8oxodG) [19]. These can be induced by UVA and UVB, although it is widely reported that UVA produces relatively more oxidative damage than UVB.

Repair of DNA damage

DNA photodamage is ubiquitous in life and most organisms have elaborate DNA repair mechanisms. The basic principle of DNA repair in skin is the recognition of the photolesion to be removed and replaced with a new base(s) followed by ligation to give intact DNA. Faithful DNA repair is critical for genomic integrity. The insertion of an incorrect base in proliferating epidermal cells may result in mutations that give rise to skin cancer.

Nucleotide excision repair

The most important repair process in human skin is nucleotide excision repair (NER). This process is dependent on a large group of enzymes with specific roles in the recognition and excision of DNA photolesions, and their repair using the opposite strand as a template. NER is triggered by the activation of p53 protein which occurs in response to cellular stress including DNA damage, oncogenic stimulation and hypoxia. This triggers a G1/S cell cycle arrest and transcriptional activation of NER genes. NER is also called unscheduled DNA synthesis (UDS), as opposed to the scheduled DNA synthesis that is observed in cells undergoing mitosis. Failure to repair DNA through the lack of one or more repair proteins may have catastrophic consequences, as exemplified by patients with xeroderma pigmentosum (XP) who are extremely prone to skin cancer [20,21] (Chapter 76). Studies on cell cultures from XP patients have greatly increased our understanding of DNA repair and indeed many of the DNA repair proteins are described by the XP prefix.

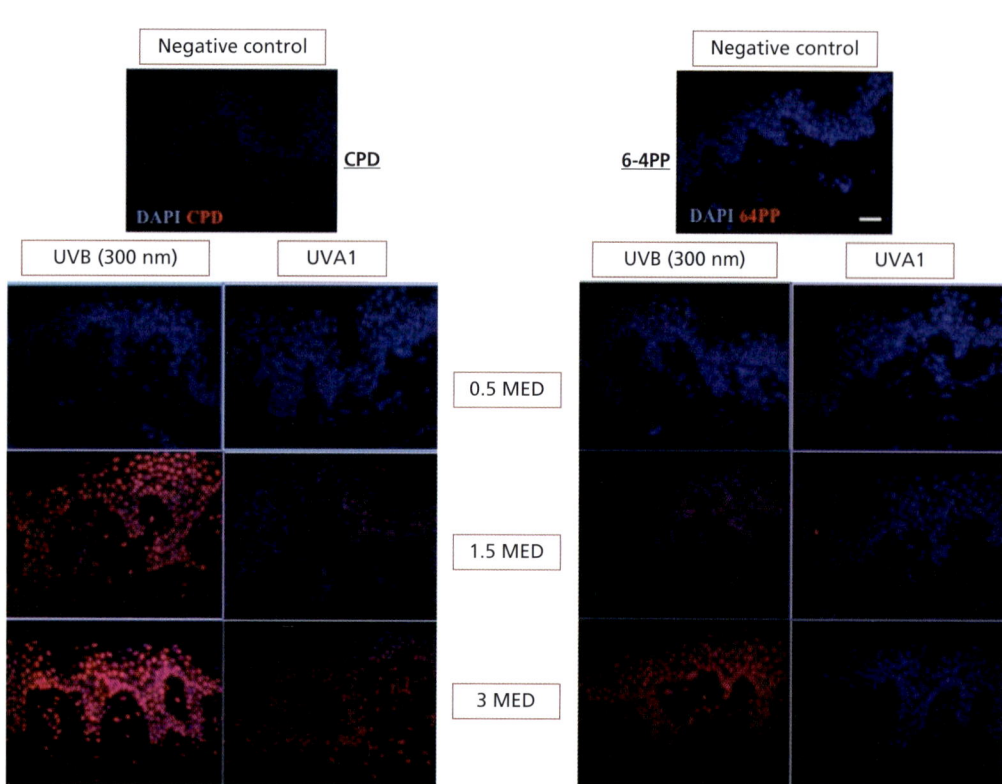

Figure 10.9 Cyclobutane pyrimidine dimer (CPD) and 6-4 pyrimidine-pyrimidone (6-4PP) in skin immediately after ultraviolet B (UVB) (300 nm) and UVA1 exposure. Note the UVR dose response, damage to dermal cells and lack of 6-4PP with UVA1. This damage is potentially mutagenic and is removed by nucleotide excision repair. DAPI (4′,6-diamidino-2-phenylindole) stain identifies the nuclei. MED, minimal erythema dose. DNA damage images courtesy of Dr Angela Tewari, with permission.

NER has two subpathways: global genome repair (GGR) and transcription coupled repair (TCR) in which repair is selectively directed at the actively transcribing strand [22]. In GGR damage is recognised by XPE and/or XPC, whilst in TCR the photoproducts cause RNA polymerase II to stall and damage recognition is done by Cockayne syndrome protein A (CSA) and CSB. Thereafter, both processes follow a common pathway that requires multiple proteins in human cells. Assessment of GGR in human epidermis *in vivo* shows that the repair of 6-4PP is relatively rapid and typically complete within 6 h. In contrast, the half-life for the removal of the CPD is about 30 h [23]. This difference may be because the 6-4PP causes a more significant distortion in the double helix than the CPD, which may result in more rapid recognition and repair.

It should be noted that there is *in vitro* evidence that UVA inhibits NER, possibly due to the oxidation of NER proteins which results in loss of function [24,25].

Base excision repair

Base excision repair (BER) mends damage to non-distorting single base modifications caused by oxidation [19], for example 8oxodG, 2,6-diamino-4-hydroxy-5-formamidopyrimidine (FapyG), 4,6-diamino-5-formamidopyrimidine (FapyA), alkylation (3-methyladenine, 7-methylguanine), hydrolysis or deamination (hypoxanthine from deaminated adenine or xanthine from deaminated guanine). BER is initiated by DNA glycosylases that recognise and remove specific damaged or inappropriate bases. This leaves an apurinic/apyrimidic site or naked sugar phosphate backbone commonly referred to as an AP site. Once cleaved by an AP endonuclease, the resulting single-strand break can then be processed by either short-patch BER (where a single nucleotide is replaced) or long-patch BER (where between 2 and 10 new nucleotides are synthesised). One of the most well-described glycosylases is human 8-oxoguanine glycosylase (hOGG1) which repairs 8oxodG and is poorly expressed in the basal layer [26]. Consequently, UVA-induced 8oxodG is repaired more slowly in the basal layer than upper layers of the human epidermis in which lesions can be repaired within 2 h of UVA exposure [27].

Cellular effects

Ultraviolet radiation exposure of the skin results in a wide range of cellular effects. One of the most striking is the formation of epidermal sunburn cells (SBCs) with pycnotic nuclei and eosinophilic cytoplasm [28]. SBCs are apoptotic keratinocytes that are readily induced by SSR and UVB but not by UVA1. Their formation is regulated by p53 which can be readily demonstrated by immunostaining. The role of p53 in UVR-induced apoptosis is clear from mouse studies [**29**,30] in which UVR irradiation of p53 wild-type mice induced the formation of SBCs, whilst p53-null mice were resistant to such apoptosis and accumulated CPD and skin cancers. Multiple factors lead to SBC formation in which p53 upregulates intrinsic and extrinsic apoptotic signalling that initiates keratinocyte death through a caspase-associated pathway. Thus, potentially carcinogenic cells, with high levels of DNA damage, are eliminated.

The loss of Langerhans cell dendricity and number is also seen. These changes may be accompanied by epidermal spongiosis along with dermal vasodilatation and neutrophil and CD3+ lymphocyte infiltration. Skin hyperplasia develops over hours to days after UVB or SSR (but generally not UVA) exposure, and results from a marked increase in cell mitosis, DNA, RNA and protein synthesis rates, after some hours of early inactivity. This is followed by a thickening of the epidermis, particularly the stratum corneum. This thickening, along with pigmentation, may play a role in photoadaptation [31,32].

Table 10.2 Summary of skin types based on the Fitzpatrick classification. There is a relationship between the acute and carcinogenic effects of ultraviolet radiation, the basis of which is poorly understood.

Fitzpatrick skin type	Skin colour on sun-protected site (constitutive pigmentation)	Sunburn risk	Approximate SED for 1 MED on sun-protected site	Tanning ability (facultative pigmentation)	Skin cancer risk
I	White	++++	2–3	±	High
II	White	+++	2–3	+	High
III	White	++	4–6	++	Moderate
IV	Olive	+	4–6	+++	Moderate
V	Brown	±	6–20[a]	++++	Low
VI	Black/dark brown	±	6–20[a]	++++	Low

[a] Data on skin types V/VI are less reliable because melanin masks sunburn.
MED, minimal erythema dose, SED, standard erythema dose.

Clinical effects of UVR

It has been generally assumed that the effects of UVR on human health are mediated through the skin, and indeed exposure of human skin *in vivo* to UVR upregulates a large number of genes [33], but studies also show that UVR can have a direct effect on the blood transcriptome [34]; UVR has considerable impact on immune cells in human blood [35]. The acute and chronic effects of UVR depend on skin type, which is usually a phenotypic assessment of skin colour (melanin pigmentation) coupled with self-reported acute responses to solar UVR [36]. A summary of skin type, known as Fitzpatrick skin type (FST), and associated risks is shown in Table 10.2. Fair-skinned FST I and II are at greatest risk from the acute and long-term effects of solar UVR. In general, MED on previously unexposed buttock skin increases with FST [37], but there is considerable overlap and MED cannot be used to predict skin type or vice versa. The genetic basis of human pigmentation is increasingly understood [38].

Acute effects

The acute clinical effects of UVR are those that occur within seconds to weeks after a single UVR exposure.

Erythema

The most obvious acute clinical effect is erythema, which is UVR-induced skin inflammation. Typically, with SSR/UVB, this is apparent after about 6 h and peaks at about 24 h and gradually resolves over a few days. Erythema may be associated with pain, warmth and oedema (blanching) in severe cases. It is also associated with increased sensitivity to pain from mechanical and thermal stimuli, resulting in the skin feeling tender after sunburn [39]. Repeated daily suberythemal (0.65 MED) exposure in skin type FST II has a cumulative effect resulting in frank erythema after a few days, which is not the case in skin type IV [40], even though the latter received twice the physical dose because of its higher MED. This suggests that those with fair skin resolve erythema less well than those who tan readily.

Erythema action spectra have been studied for over 90 years and a library of such spectra has been compiled [41]. A standard CIE action spectrum for erythema [42] is shown in Figure 10.8. Typically, the MED is around 500 J/m^2 for the UVC–UVB boundary (280 nm), 250 J/m^2 for UVB (300 nm) and 320 kJ/m^2 for UVA (360 nm). The CIE erythema action spectrum is similar to that for CPD induction in human skin *in vivo* in the solar UVB and UVA range and provides indirect evidence that the CPD initiates the erythemal response [43]: wavelengths around 300 nm are the most DNA damaging and erythemogenic. A role for DNA in erythema is also supported by some animal studies. However, it is likely that other unknown non-DNA chromophores/mechanisms contribute to erythema, especially in the UVA1 region. For example, a human erythema action spectrum determined with lasers showed a main UVB peak at 298.5 nm and a smaller peak at 362 nm [44], suggesting a UVA1-absorbing chromophore. Furthermore, it has been shown that UVA erythema is oxygen dependent which is not the case for UVB [45]. This is supported by studies that show a lack of correlation between UVB and UVA1 MED in the same individuals, suggesting different independent mechanisms [9]. The pharmacology of UVR-induced erythema is incompletely understood but there is evidence that it occurs via mediators [46] such as prostaglandins and nitric oxide [47].

Pigmentation and tanning

Skin colour is largely dependent on the quantity and quality of melanin. Constitutive pigmentation is indicative of pigmentation in typically non-habitually UVR-exposed body sites such as the buttock; skin types V and VI have high levels of constitutive pigmentation. Irrespective of skin type, there is a melanin gradient in the epidermis with the highest concentration in the basal layer. Facultative pigmentation (i.e. tanning) is the response to exposure to UVR. There are three types with different action spectra [41]:
- Immediate pigment darkening.
- Persistent pigment darkening.
- Melanogenesis or delayed tanning.

Immediate and persistent pigment darkening. Immediate pigment darkening (IPD) presents as a transient grey colour which is thought to be due to immediate photo-oxidation of existing colourless melanin precursors after exposure to UVA (action spectrum peak at 340 nm) and visible (400–500 nm) radiation. IPD, which fades within 15 min, is induced at low UVA doses (1–4 J/cm^2). It is almost undetectable in fair-skinned individuals but is easily observed in skin type IV or darker. IPD is not protective against sunburn and its biological significance is unclear, although it has been suggested that its oxidised products absorb in the visible wavebands and thus prevent photodamage by visible radiation to other important molecules such as folate (5-methyltetrahydrofolate (5MTHF)) in the blood [48]. 5MTHF deficiency may increase the risk of cardiovascular diseases, colorectal carcinoma, megaloblastic anaemia, depression and dementia. Interestingly, serum folate shows seasonal variation with lower concentrations in summer [49].

Persistent pigment darkening (PPD) is a brown colour in response to higher UVA doses (>10 J/cm^2) peaking 2 h post-irradiation and lasting for up to 20 days in a range of FSTs [50]. IPD and PPD are not thought to be due to new melanin synthesis but rather to a more persistent oxidation of melanin precursors. PPD is an end point that is used to assess UVA protection of sunscreens.

Melanogenesis. Delayed tanning (DT) is due to stimulation of new melanin synthesis by basal epidermal melanocytes, which is then transported via dendrites to adjacent keratinocytes and redistributed towards the surface of the skin [51]. The ability to tan depends on skin type as described in Table 10.2. The density of melanin varies with body site and declines with age. Melanin is synthesised either as dark-coloured brown-black insoluble eumelanin or light-coloured red-yellow, alkali-soluble, sulphur-containing phaeomelanin. Eumelanin is thought to be the major factor in the photoprotective properties of melanin, which when induced in white skin types results in a protection factor of about 2–4 against DNA photodamage and sunburn as well as a visible tan [31]. There is *in vitro* and animal evidence that products relating to melanogenesis, particularly phaeomelanin, may have photosensitising properties contributing to the skin cancer susceptibility of people with red hair. New melanin is redistributed with the transit of keratinocytes through the epidermis and is typically evident c.3 days post-irradiation. The tan fades when the stratum corneum is shed over several weeks.

UVR-induced DT results from an increase in tyrosinase activity stimulating the oxidation of tyrosine to dopaquinone (DQ) which is the rate-limiting step. Other precursors for eumelanin derived from DQ include 5,6-dihydroxyindole (DHI) and 5,6-dihydroxyindole-2-carboxylic acid (DHICA). DQ is also the starting point for phaeomelanin that is synthesised via a different cysteine-dependent pathway.

Tyrosinase activity can be stimulated directly by UVR on melanocytes and by indirect activation by keratinocytes, whereby UVR induces the release of membrane-associated diacylglycerol (DAG) from plasma membranes, which activates protein kinase C-β and in turn activates tyrosinase. A study of gene expression after multiple UVR doses *in vivo* in humans showed that UVB is a strong stimulator of various pigment-related genes, such as the tyrosinase (*TYR*) gene, tyrosinase-related protein 1 (TRP1) and dopachrome tautomerase (DCT), as well as the transcription factor microphthalmia-associated transcription factor (MITF) [52]. SSR is more effective in eliciting these effects than UVB, suggesting a synergistic effect on melanogenesis when UVA and UVB are combined. UVA alone did not induce such upregulation of pigment cell-specific genes, suggesting UVA-induced pigmentation likely occurs via a distinct mechanism [53]. Melanogenesis is also mediated via DNA photodamage, which is indicated by its action spectrum. *In vitro* experiments show that the topical DNA repair enzyme (T4N5) treatment of murine S91 melanoma cells and human melanocytes exposed to SSR demonstrated greater melanogenesis than when treated with heat-inactivated enzyme [54] and that accelerated and/or more extensive excision of CPD enhances tanning.

The release of single-stranded DNA fragments during CPD repair may stimulate melanogenesis by increasing tyrosinase activity, leading to an increase in tyrosinase protein and downstream new melanin formation [55].

UVR-induced DNA damage activates p53 protein [56,57], which is also a mediator of melanogenesis. It causes an upregulation of pro-opiomelanocortin (POMC), which is then processed to adrenocorticotrophic hormone (ACTH) and α-melanocyte stimulating hormone (α-MSH). Secreted α-MSH binds to the melanocortin 1 receptor (MC1R) on melanocytes and via an increase in cyclic adenosine monophosphate (cAMP) increases the activity of tyrosinase.

Recent studies suggest that pigmentation may also be activated via skin opsins that belong to the photosensitive G protein-coupled receptor (GPCR) super family, which are expressed in human keratinocytes and melanocytes [58]. One study has reported that blue light induces pigmentation in melanocytes via opsin-3 [59]. Another study shows a role for opsin-5 when melanogenesis is induced by broad spectrum UVR [60].

Immunomodulation

The skin is an important arm of the innate and acquired immune system (Chapter 9) and the epidermis is rich in antigen-presenting Langerhans cells. UVR has profound effects on skin immunity [61,**62**] and, for example, readily depletes the epidermis of Langerhans cells. Classic experiments in the 1970s showed that UVR-induced immunosuppression in the mouse played a major role in the development of UVR-induced squamous cell carcinoma (SCC). A similar role is likely to occur for humans, although this is impossible to test experimentally. An intact immune system is important for skin cancer surveillance and tumour rejection because organ transplant patients, maintained on immunosuppressive drugs, have a high incidence of all types of skin cancer, especially on sun-exposed sites. A major difference between drug-induced immunosuppression and photoimmunosuppression is that the latter is antigen specific. This can be demonstrated using the contact hypersensitivity (CHS) model of acquired immunity in mice and humans. This model is widely used to represent the photoimmunological events in skin cancer. Skin can be sensitised to a universal sensitiser such as dinitrochlorobenzene (DNCB) and shows a typical CHS response when subsequently challenged on a distal site with DNCB. However, the CHS response to DNCB is reduced or inhibited if the sensitisation site is pre-exposed to UVR. Such animals could not be subsequently resensitised with DNCB but could be sensitised with another antigen. Mechanistic studies in mouse skin show that suppression of the CHS response is mediated by the generation of antigen-specific T-regs which results in 'immunotolerance'.

Suppression of the CHS response can readily occur in humans with suberythemal exposure [63]. There is good evidence that DNA [64] and tUCA [65] are chromophores for CHS suppression. It is likely that antigen-specific photoimmunosuppression evolved to prevent chronic allergic reactions to new antigens that arise from UVR-induced alterations to skin molecules that result in the generation of photoantigens. There is some evidence to suggest that polymorphic light eruption (PLE) is a consequence of the failure to suppress the CHS response to unspecified photoantigens [66–68]. The downside of the suppression of photoimmunosuppression is the failure of the immune system to reject potentially carcinogenic clones of keratinocytes and melanocytes. Selection pressure is likely to have preferred the prevention of allergic reactions, given that skin cancer typically occurs well past the age of reproduction and child rearing. Interestingly, there is evidence to suggest that PLE patients are less prone to skin cancer [69].

Mouse studies have shown that UVR can suppress acquired immunity to a range of pathogens and this has raised concerns about a possible role of UVR in human vaccination programmes. However, to date, there is some circumstantial but no definitive evidence that supports these concerns [70].

This discussion has focused on the effects of UVR on the sensitisation (primary) arm of the CHS response. However, UVR can also suppress the elicitation (memory) arm of the CHS response, which can be demonstrated by irradiating skin prior to challenge with recall antigens. The significance of this is not known.

UVR suppresses acquired and recall immunity, but studies have also shown that it enhances innate immunity through the induction of antimicrobial peptides such as β-defensin, especially in the upper layers of the epidermis [61].

In summary, UVR inhibits acquired immunity with antigen specificity. This has probably evolved to prevent CHS reactions to photochemically induced antigens in the skin. However, its long-term consequences are increased susceptibility to skin cancer. In contrast, it appears that innate immunity is enhanced by UVR, which may give better protection against microbial infection.

Vitamin D

The production of vitamin D is an established benefit of solar UVR exposure. Vitamin D has long been known to be important for skeletal health, but there is considerable and often controversial evidence that vitamin D is important for a wide range of health outcomes [71,72]. The skin (mostly epidermal) chromophore for vitamin D synthesis is 7-dehydrocholesterol (7DHC), also known as provitamin D. It is converted to previtamin D by solar UVB, with an action spectrum that is like that for erythema in the UVB region. There is no evidence that UVA is involved in vitamin D production, but there is evidence that it may induce photodegradation. Previtamin D is converted to the final biologically active vitamin D (in fact a hormone) by thermal and enzymatic steps. Vitamin D status is usually assessed by measuring serum 25-hydroxy vitamin D (25(OH)D). Several studies have estimated that the sun is the most important source of vitamin D for most people, mainly because relatively few components of typical diets are rich in vitamin D (found, for example, in oily fish). In temperate climates, vitamin D status is seasonal.

Studies have shown that people with darker skin types have poorer vitamin D status at a given latitude [73], and such observations have been often attributed to photoprotection by melanin. Indeed, it has been argued that melanin as humans migrated from Africa was due to selection pressure to maintain vitamin D status [74], but some authors have proposed other explanations [75]. The role of melanin in vitamin D synthesis has been addressed in a few laboratory studies with conflicting results. A recent study has demonstrated that skin pigment has a very modest effect on vitamin D status [76]. This may be because 7DHC is in sufficient quantity above the heavily melanised basal layer.

Cardiovascular disease

Several studies have postulated a relationship between blood pressure and cardiovascular disease and solar UVR exposure. This has been attributed to vitamin D (i.e. a UVB effect) but has not been supported by intervention studies. A vitamin D effect was also eliminated in a study in which a single suberythemal dose (2 SED) of UVA (320–400 nm) lowered blood pressure via the release of nitric oxide from the skin into the systemic circulation [77]. A 3-year study of 342 459 haemodialysis patients showed an inverse relationship between systolic blood pressure and UVB and UVA radiation [78]. These findings are important with implications for other diseases that have latitude gradients. It will be important to confirm and expand on these data because they have very significant public health implications and may also impact on photoprotection strategies.

Chronic effects

Subject to ethical approval, it is relatively easy to study the acute effects of UVR on human skin in the laboratory. However, this cannot be done for chronic effects for which an epidemiological approach is necessary. There has been extensive epidemiological research on skin cancer, including molecular epidemiology, that has been supported by animal and *in vitro* studies. In contrast, there has been very little epidemiological work on photoageing, almost certainly because it has been traditionally viewed as a cosmetic rather than a health problem. Most of our understanding of photoageing has come from chronic animal studies and the use of acute molecular surrogates in human skin.

Skin cancer

Epidemiological data and body site studies have long supported an association between solar radiation exposure and skin cancer, including basal cell carcinoma (BCC) (Chapter 140) and SCC (Chapter 141), which are keratinocyte cancers, and malignant melanoma (MM) (Chapters 142–144), which is a cancer of the melanocyte. Solar UVR exposure is also associated with actinic keratoses that are indicative of SCC risk. The risk of skin cancer is very dependent on skin type (see Table 10.2). For example, the risk factors for MM include self-reported higher levels of sunburn, and genetically determined phenotypic characteristics associated with greater sensitivity to UVR, including fair skin, light hair and eye colour, poor ability to tan, freckling and multiple naevi. The following text summarises some important trends from two recent reviews [79,80].

The incidence of MM has steadily increased in many countries from 1982 to 2015 although there has been some evidence of a decline in New Zealand and Denmark. A study based on 18 European cancer registries over 1995–2012 showed an average annual percent (AAPC), increase in invasive melanoma of 4.0% and 3.0% for men and women, respectively. In the USA, MM incidence increased in all ethnicities in those aged 40 or older between 2001 and 2015 with an AAPC change of 1.8%. However, there was a decline in AAPC in younger populations. It is likely that public health sun protection campaigns, beginning in the 1980s, have contributed to the decrease in new cases in younger age groups. It is estimated that MM represents only about 4% of cases of skin cancer. However, it accounts for about 80% of skin cancer deaths.

Data spanning 1985–2015 from 31 countries taken from the World Health Organization Mortality Database showed an overall increase in mortality in men, but stable rates or a decline in women.

There is considerable evidence that the incidence of keratinocyte cancers is increasing, even though it is very difficult to obtain accurate incidence rates for a variety of reasons including the widespread lack of mandatory reporting of keratinocyte cancers to cancer registries, and because population-based studies are rare. Data from South Australia show a 59% increase in age-standardised incidence rates of keratinocyte cancers between 2000 and 2015. A study in Iceland based on registry data showed that from 1981 to 2017, there were 2.3- and 3.7-fold increases in BCC incidence in men and women, respectively. Given low levels of ambient UVR in Iceland, it is probable that these increases reflect more sun holidays and/or greater use of tanning beds.

Table 10.3 Summary of the main histological features of chronological ageing and photoageing.

Location	Chronological ageing	Photoageing
Epidermis	Flattened dermal–epidermal junction Variable keratinocyte size and epidermal thickness Loss of melanocytes	Flattened dermal–epidermal junction Epidermal thickening and atrophy Variable keratinocyte size, with increase in melanocytes (often atypical) and melanin content
Dermis	Atrophy with reduction of collagen, elastic fibres and proteoglycans Loss of vascularity	Elastosis (elastin degradation) and collagen degeneration Increased proteoglycans Low-grade perivascular inflammation Thickening of vascular walls

Adapted from Herschenfeld and Gilchrest 1999 [93].

Experimental evidence for UVR as a carcinogen. The association between skin cancer and solar range UVR (c.295–400 nm) component has been extensively confirmed with animal studies, especially with hairless mice that readily develop SCC with chronic UVR exposure, including SSR. Murine models have also shown a relationship between UVR and MM [81–83]. Mouse studies have generated an action spectrum for SCC, which has been used to produce an action spectrum for human SCC after correcting for differences in the UVR transmission optics in human and mouse skin [84]. This shows that UVB is the main cause of SCC. The human SCC action spectrum is comparable with those for human erythema and epidermal CPD, which implicates DNA as a chromophore. This has been supported by a direct molecular link with UVR in actinic keratoses, BCC and SCC. UVR results in specific 'fingerprint' mutations (T $\rightarrow$ C and TT $\rightarrow$ CC transitions) that have been found at high frequencies in these lesions. For example, the *TP53* gene shows UVR fingerprint mutations in up to 90% of SCC, and over 60% of BCC *TP53* UVR mutations were at nine hotspots [85]. UVR-induced C $\rightarrow$ T mutations have been found in 80% of *TP53* mutations in actinic keratoses [86] and 63% of *TP53* mutations in Bowen disease [87]. An analysis of mutations in SCC and BCC combined in XP patients showed that 90% were G:C to A:T [88,89]. Mutations in *TP53* inhibit cellular arrest and DNA repair, which results in their incorporation into daughter cells. UVR fingerprint mutations in *TP53* have been reported in melanoma, but also in other genes that are known drivers of melanomagenesis such as *CDKN2A*, *BRAF* and *NRAS* [90].

Effect of different patterns of UVR exposure on skin cancer. Patterns of UVR exposure seem to be important in the genesis of skin cancer [91]. SCC is associated with low-dose chronic exposure whereas MM and probably BCC are associated with intermittent high-dose sunburning exposure [92]. Studies show that childhood sun exposure may be particularly important, with studies showing that migration from countries of low insolation (e.g. Scotland) to those of high insolation (e.g. Australia) after the age of 10 years is associated with a markedly lower risk of MM development in later life compared with migration before the age of 10 years. Interestingly, a mouse model for MM will only develop lesions if exposure is done within a few days of birth [83].

Photoageing

Skin ageing occurs as two distinct phenomena: intrinsic chronological ageing (Chapter 156) in which changes are attributable to the passage of time, and photoageing that is the superimposition of structural and functional changes caused by chronic UVR exposure. This may be seen as a deterministic (i.e. inevitable) process in contrast to skin cancer which is stochastic. The main clinical features of photoageing are fine and course wrinkling, dryness, coarseness, telangiectasia, yellowness and irregular patchy pigmentation. Skin also loses its mechanical properties. Table 10.3 summarises the main histological differences between photoageing and chronological skin ageing. The mechanical and elastic properties of the skin derive from the extracellular matrix (ECM) of the dermis of which the major proteins are collagen, and elastin to a lesser extent. The degradation of elastin, known as elastosis, is a typical histological feature of skin that has been chronically exposed to solar UVR. Elastosis is often observed close to SSC, which is associated with chronic low-level UVR exposure.

Collagen and elastin degradation. Collagens and elastin are subject to degradation by matrix metalloproteinases (MMP) that have low levels of expression in sun-protected skin. MMP are a large family of proteases that share common structural and functional elements. They contain a zinc-containing binding site that is found in their catalytic domain. MMP are released as proenzymes where a blocking cysteine residue must be removed to activate enzyme activity. This is largely in order to ensure MMP activity is focused on target sites. Their main physiological function is ascribed to the modulation and regulation of ECM turnover by direct proteolytic degradation of dermal ECM proteins and non-matrix proteins, as well as the liberation of biologically active cytokine growth factors and chemokines from their membrane anchored preforms. MMP upregulation forms part of normal physiological processes such as wound healing and angiogenesis. However, MMP also play an important role in cancer invasion.

Both UVB and UVA1 have been shown to induce a range of MMP at the gene, protein and protein activity level [94,95]. Most studies have focused on MMP1, which is a collagenase. Tissue inhibitors of MMP (TIMP), the expression of which is much less responsive to UVR exposure, regulate MMP activity [96]. Thus, photoageing appears to be the consequence of an imbalance between MMP and TIMP activity and possibly the consequence of imperfect repair when new extracellular proteins are synthesised in response to MMP-induced degradation [97]. Most laboratory studies on UVR induction of MMP protein and its activity have shown much greater expression/activity of MMP in the epidermis [98] than the dermis. This conundrum has yet to be explained, but it has been suggested that MMP may migrate from the epidermis to the dermis. It should also be noted that laboratory studies are typically acute and that photoageing is a long-term process.

Several studies have indicated that ROS initiate MMP production. Research has also shown that UVR can have a direct non-enzymatic effect on ECM and that this may be mediated by ROS [99]. Furthermore, UVR-damaged ECM may be more susceptible to MMP degradation. However, there are data to suggest that the CPD may be a trigger, at least for the induction of MMP1 [100]. A recent study of UVA exposure to cultured human dermal fibroblasts showed that opsin 3 upregulates several MMP via the calcium-dependent G protein-coupled signalling pathway [101]. Overall, the data suggest that MMP can be induced via multiple pathways.

Role of damage to mitochondria. Genetic damage and instability outside the nuclear genome have been suggested to contribute to photoageing [102]. Cellular mitochondria generate energy (adenosine triphosphate) via a series of redox reactions mediated through the electron transport chain and antioxidants (nicotinamide adenine dinucleotide, flavin adenine dinucleotide 2 and coenzyme Q). Despite these constitutive enzymes and mitochondrial base excision repair, mitochondrial DNA (mtDNA) is sensitive to ROS-induced damage, and the mutation incidence for mtDNA is much greater than for nuclear DNA. Photodamaged skin has a higher mtDNA mutation frequency when compared with sun-protected skin, which also correlates with higher MMP1 levels [103]. It has been suggested that mitochondrial dysregulation may lead to increased oxidative stress which in turn activates MMP production.

Spectral dependence. It is often stated that UVA is the main cause of photoageing on the basis that it penetrates deeper into the dermis. Furthermore, there have been a few case reports of photoageing on one side of the face that has been habitually exposed to solar UVR through glass (which attenuates UVB). However, an action spectrum for elastosis in the hairless mouse is very similar to that for human erythema [104], which supports UVB as the major cause. Other mouse studies for different photoageing end points also reported UVB as the major cause apart from skin sagging [105], which was primarily a UVA effect. Erythemal responses to different spectra, including UVA1, have been shown to predict the expression of MMP1 mRNA in human skin [106], also implicating UVB. However, it seems likely that many MMP play a role in photoageing and that different MMP may have different spectral dependencies [94]. Overall, the data suggest that in a solar environmental context, UVB is the major cause of photoageing, but UVA certainly plays a role.

Relationship between photoageing and skin cancer. Finally, it should be noted that photocarcinogenesis and photoageing have usually been treated as separate phenomena, when it is very likely that they are closely related. This has been demonstrated in hairless mouse studies in which a neutrophil elastase-deficient strain was resistant to UVR-induced SCC [107] and photoageing [108].

Photoprotection

Photoprotection reduces the molecular and clinical damage caused by solar UVR. This may occur by constitutive or facultative pigmentation or by behavioural strategies such as the use of sunscreens and clothing. A good rule of thumb is that behavioural photoprotection is necessary when your shadow is shorter than you, because this is indicative of high levels of UVB. This is especially important for FST I and II but, depending on circumstances, it may also be advisable for more sun-resistant skin types.

Melanin

Tanning in skin types II–IV offers some protection against sunburn and DNA damage, but the level of protection is modest [109]. Melanin in black skin is more protective. Studies comparing black and white skins show that melanin affords a protection factor of about 7 for sunburn [110]. The protection factor for DNA damage varies with epidermal location but is about 60 in the melanin-rich basal layer (containing keratinocyte stem cells and melanocytes) [111]. This may explain the large difference in skin cancer incidence in black and white skins.

Sunscreens

Sunscreens are topical formulations that contain agents that filter and/or scatter UVR [112]. In effect, UVR-absorbing molecules are exogenous chromophores applied to the skin. A typical product contains a mix of organic filters with different absorption spectra as well as micropigments that may be physical (e.g. titanium dioxide) or organic. In Europe sunscreens are regulated as cosmetics, but they are regarded as drugs in the USA. Sunscreens are designed and tested to prevent sunburn and their main index of protection is the sun protection factor (SPF). The SPF is calculated by the formula SPF = [24 h MED on protected skin]/[24 h MED on unprotected skin], according to strict protocols prescribed by regulatory bodies. Included in these protocols is a sunscreen application density of 2 mg/cm^2 on skin and the use of well-defined SSR. In theory, an SPF of 15 if used correctly will reduce erythemal exposure to 1/15th of that which would otherwise have been received for a given time in the sun. However, there have been recent concerns that SSR overestimates protection compared with solar UVR [113].

The action spectrum for erythema in Figure 10.8 shows that no sunscreen could be effective without good UVB protection, but there has been an increasing trend for better UVA protection resulting in broad spectrum coverage, and this is now required by regulatory bodies [114] although the indices of UVA protection may vary with regulatory body. These indices may be based on the ability to prevent PPD (of unknown biological significance) or the UVR transmission properties of the sunscreen. Labelling of sunscreens within the European Union (EU) is divided into low (SPF 6–10), medium (SPF 15–25), high (SPF 30–50) and very high (SPF 50+) protection, with the level of UVA protection at least one-third of the SPF.

One *de facto* consequence of better UVA protection for a *given SPF* is reduced UVB protection. However, the UVA protection index must be regarded as secondary to the prevention of sunburn as indicated by the SPF. The long-term benefits of improved UVA protection have yet to be determined.

Assuming beach use, a typical person should use about 100 mL/day, assuming three whole-body applications, to achieve the labelled SPF. In practice, people apply sunscreen much less thickly than SPF test conditions [115,116] which results in much less protection than indicated by the labelled SPF. This means that people may overestimate their degree of protection. Thus, the typical use of a labelled SPF 15 product may result in a considerably lower SPF. However, if sunscreens are used optimally, they offer excellent protection against sunburn, even under very high UV index conditions [117]. Overall, people are probably getting much less photoprotection than they think from sunscreens, especially with intentional solar exposure. This is a public health issue that must be addressed either by encouraging people to use more sunscreen or to use a higher SPF to compensate for inadequate application.

Effects of sunscreens on non-erythema end points

Protection against sunburn does not necessarily mean protection against other types of photodamage that may occur with suberythemal exposure. For example, suppression of the induction phase of the CHS reaction in skin types I/II occurs with doses of <0.5 MED [63]. There are few data on the ability of sunscreens to prevent molecular damage to the skin that may result in skin cancer or photoageing, but there is evidence that sunscreens are effective in the prevention of SSR-induced CPD in human skin *in vivo* [118,119]. Intervention studies suggest that regular sunscreen use may be beneficial in the inhibition of actinic keratoses [120,121] and SSC but not BCC [122]. However, a large population-based study in Norwegian woman found no difference in SCC when comparing use of SPF ≤15 versus SPF ≥15 sunscreens [123]. There are sunscreen intervention data for a beneficial effect against melanoma [124] and the population-based study in Norway, just referred to, reported that SPF ≥15 versus SPF ≤15 reduced melanoma incidence by 18% [125]. The role of sunscreens in skin cancer prevention is controversial with authors of recent reviews reaching opposite conclusions [126,127]. There are also studies that indicate that regular sunscreen use may inhibit photoageing [128].

Concerns about the possible adverse effect of sunscreen use on vitamin D synthesis have been addressed by two reviews that concluded that such use has little or no impact on vitamin D status [129,130], possibly because of inadequate application. However, an intervention study in which sunscreens (SPF = 15) were used optimally during a sun holiday has also shown excellent vitamin synthesis in the absence of sunburn [131]. The most likely explanation for this observation is that the threshold dose for vitamin D synthesis is much lower than that for sunburn. It should be noted that we lack data on the effect of high SPF sunscreens on vitamin D status [132,133].

Traditional topical sunscreens depend on the filtering or scattering of UVR and may be described as 'passive' photoprotection. There has, however, been a trend for 'active' photoprotection at a topical and systemic level. These include topical products with natural antioxidants, and liposome-containing DNA repair enzymes [134,135]. Another approach is the delivery of α-MSH analogues and other strategies that stimulate melanogenesis [136].

Clothing and shade

It should be remembered that sunscreen use is not the only option for photoprotection. Clothing reduces the skin surface area exposed to solar UVR. It offers good protection against sunburn that is dependent on fabric properties such as colour, weave, wetness, etc. Some clothing is designed and tested for photoprotection, and the level of protection is expressed by the UV protection factor (UVP) [137] that can be seen as equivalent to the SPF of a sunscreen. Clothing can be very effective as witnessed by the poor vitamin D status that is common in the Middle East and North Africa, especially in women [138]. Vitamin D supplementation is necessary when the body is typically fully clothed, even in sunny countries.

Shade seeking is a well-recognised and very effective way of reducing solar UVR exposure, especially when the sun is high. The construction of shaded areas [139] should be explored as a means of reducing UVR burden.

Personal and population exposure to UVR

The sun

The sun is the most important source of UVR exposure for most people and the degree of exposure is primarily dependent on behaviour. In people with indoor jobs, exposure may be adventitious (e.g. taking a lunch break) or from deliberate sun seeking, as with sunbathing and beach holidays. Occupational exposure will occur in those with outdoor work such as farmers. There are different ways to assess personal exposure, but the most reliable is with personal dosimetry, in which people wear the dosimeter on a specified part of the body. There are two basic types of personal dosimeter. The first is an integrating device, such as the polysulphone film badge, which records total exposure over a fixed period. The second is a time-stamped electronic device that records the exposure in real time. The latter are much more expensive and technically demanding but provide important information on behaviour. Such data are very important because behavioural knowledge provides a better basis for informed public health interventions. For example, one study with time-stamped dosimeters showed that Danes on holiday in Tenerife received most of their UVR round about noon (88% of time outdoors was between 12.00 and 15.00) [140], despite widespread advice to an educated population to avoid this period. Time-stamped dosimeters can also show how solar UVR exposure varies on different parts of the body with orientation and movement [141].

Several studies have been done in which personal UVR exposure has been measured over extended periods in different populations in spring/summer in Copenhagen, Denmark (56°N), using time-stamped personal electronic dosimeters. In people working indoors without 'risk, or sun-seeking, behaviour' the median daily dose was 0.3 SED (range 0–3.9) on working days and 0.6 SED (range 0.1–3.5) on days off [142]. It has been estimated that indoor workers in northern Europe receive about 150–200 SED/year, which is approximately 5% of the total available ambient UVR. Outdoor workers are exposed to more UVR, perhaps up to 400–600

SED/year. Children spend more time outdoors and it has been previously estimated that those in the UK receive an annual dose of about 300 SED [143]; however, this may be less now because of increasing levels of indoor activity. A very high proportion of annual exposure may be received during holidays. It has been estimated that about a third of annual UVR exposure to the face in northern Europe is received during a 2-week summer vacation at home [144]. A study of Danish holidaymakers showed that they obtained 43% of their annual sunburning UVR exposure in just 6 days in Tenerife in March [140]. This was associated with high levels of sunburn, despite the use of sunscreens.

Unsurprisingly, higher daily exposures have been measured, using polysulphone badges, in Queensland, Australia, with for example Brisbane (27.4°S) home workers having weekday shoulder exposure medians of 2.0–8.00 SED depending on the time of year [145]. Outdoor workers at the same latitude showed values of 3.0–10.0 SED. It has been estimated that an average American is exposed to about 250 SED per working year, mostly in the spring and summer [146]. This can be increased by 78 SED (i.e. about 30%) with a 3-week vacation (i.e. by 3.7 SED/day) when sunscreens are more likely to be worn. Behaviour is a major determinant of UVR exposure, such that it is possible for children in the UK to have higher solar exposure levels than in Queensland, Australia [147].

Personal UVR measurements are only possible with limited participants and duration of study, however modelling is possible to estimate UVR exposure given to larger well-defined populations and specific body sites [148,149].

UV index

The UV index (UVI) is increasingly used to inform the public about ambient sunburning UVR at a given location [150]. Such information can help guide sun exposure behaviour and the need for photoprotection. The UVI is readily available and is often presented in weather forecasts and can be easily found online for a particular geographical location. In reporting the UVI, most emphasis is placed on the maximum UVR level on a given day, which is at solar noon ± 2 h. The UVI ranges from 1 to 11+, the latter being classed as extreme. Photoprotection for fair-skinned people is recommended once the UVI reaches 3 [151].

It could be argued that there is a need for cheap, reliable, personal, user-friendly dosimeters so that people can measure their own UVR exposure based on UVI that would allow them to modify their UVR exposure. In addition, there are smartphone applications for this purpose. One possible disadvantage of these devices is that they would encourage maximal exposure, especially in cases where typically there is inadequate sunscreen application.

Non-solar sources with emphasis on sunbeds

People may be exposed to UVR from a range of artificial sources: some indoor workers are significantly irradiated by, for example, arc welding devices and, possibly, from hospital phototherapy equipment if due care is not taken. Office workers and home dwellers may be at risk from low-intensity UVR from fluorescent or, more importantly, quartz halogen lamps used for indoor lighting. The increased use of LED lighting decreases this risk. The most common artificial source of UVR exposure is sunbed use. A study in 30 European countries showed variation in prevalence of sunbed use ranging from 0.5% in Malta to 26.5% in Belgium [152]. There was a significant correlation with latitude and a negative correlation with hours of local sunshine.

Sunbeds are designed to induce tanning (melanogenesis), the action spectrum of which is similar to that for erythema, with a peak in the UVB region at about 300 nm in the solar UVR range [**41**]. Generally, the emission spectra of tanning devices are primarily in the UVA1 region (c.80%), with a small amount of UVB (2–3%). This UVB will be responsible for most of the tanning based on the action spectrum for melanogenesis. The EU standard is that the erythemally weighted irradiance of sunbeds should not exceed 0.3 W/m^2, and that levels above that are unsafe. A survey in England showed that more than 90% of more than 400 sunbeds studied exceeded this limit [153] with an average erythemally weighted irradiance of almost twice the EU limit. When the emission spectra of these sources were weighted with an action spectrum for keratinocyte cancer, the average irradiance was over twice that of Mediterranean noon sun. That is, the average carcinogenic risk per minute of exposure was 2.3 times greater than intense solar exposure. These data show that small errors in sunbed dosimetry/timing of exposure can easily result in sunburn and give cause for concern, especially as sunbed operators are unlikely to have much technical knowledge. They also show that regulations are not being enforced.

There is considerable evidence that sunbed use increases the risk of melanoma and BCC and that this risk is greater when sunbed use started at an early age [154]. Sunbed use has also been shown to increase the risk factors associated with melanoma such as atypical naevi [155]. Some authors consider that the relationship between sunbed use and melanoma has been unequivocally established [156] while others disagree [157]. Many national and international organisations have issued guidelines/laws to restrict sunbed use, especially in those under 18 years of age. Some countries have banned sunbed use.

Risks versus benefits of population UVR exposure

The long-term risks of UVR exposure are well established with damage to epidermal DNA leading to mutation and skin cancer. Chronic UVR exposure also results in photoageing. In the context of terrestrial UVR (with no UVC), most action spectrum studies, whether *in vitro*, or in animal or human skin *in vivo*, have shown that these effects are primarily caused by UVB. The only universally accepted benefit of solar UVR exposure is vitamin D production, which is also caused by UVB, but other benefits, of yet unknown wavelength dependence, are being investigated. Field studies have shown that vitamin D production and DNA damage are related to the product of skin area exposed and solar UVB dose over a wide dose range [158]. Thus, benefit is always associated with some risk, which will be influenced by skin type. More recently, it has been argued that exposure to solar UVA and UVB is beneficial because it reduces blood pressure, and this would have major health benefits at a population level [**78**,159]. Any proposal to increase solar exposure would be controversial, especially in the dermatology community. Until recently, most emphasis on the immunological effects of UVR on the skin has been focused on its suppression of acquired immunity, but it is recognised that UVR can enhance innate immunity. At present, we lack the information to prescribe solar UVR exposure to obtain the best risk–benefit outcome for health. As such, it is probably best to advise that daily exposure be restricted to suberythemal doses (e.g., about 2 SED for light-skinned individuals), whether through sunscreen or not, which are sufficient for vitamin D synthesis. There is, however, no case for additional UVR exposure from tanning beds, which significantly adds to MM risk. Sunbed use, popular with the young, is often unregulated and the non-cosmetic beneficial effects can be readily obtained from the sun or vitamin D supplementation.

Key references

The full list of references can be found in the online version at https://www.wiley.com/rooksdermatology10e

1. Alfredsson L, Armstrong BK, Butterfield DA et al. Insufficient sun exposure has become a real public health problem. *Int J Environ Res Public Health* 2020;17:5014.
8. Young AR. Chromophores in human skin. *Phys Med Biol* 1997;42:789–802.
9. Tewari A, Sarkany RP, Young AR. UVA1 induces cyclobutane pyrimidine dimers but not 6-4 photoproducts in human skin in vivo. *J Invest Dermatol* 2012;132:394–400.
13. Cadet J, Douki T. Formation of UV-induced DNA damage contributing to skin cancer development. *Photochem Photobiol Sci* 2018;17:1816–41.
29. Ziegler A, Jonason AS, Leffell DJ et al. Sunburn and p53 in the onset of skin cancer. *Nature* 1994;372:773–6.
33. Bustamante M, Hernandez-Ferrer C, Tewari A et al. Dose and time effects of solar-simulated ultraviolet radiation on the in vivo human skin transcriptome. *Br J Dermatol* 2020;182:1458–68.
41. Schmalwieser AW, Wallisch S, Diffey B. A library of action spectra for erythema and pigmentation. *Photochem Photobiol Sci* 2012;11:251–68.
62. Hart PH, Norval M. Ultraviolet radiation-induced immunosuppression and its relevance for skin carcinogenesis. *Photochem Photobiol Sci* 2018;17:1872–84.
78. Weller RB, Wang Y, He J et al. Does incident solar ultraviolet radiation lower blood pressure? *J Am Heart Assoc* 2020;9:e013837.
79. Neale RE, Barnes PW, Robson TM et al. Environmental effects of stratospheric ozone depletion, UV radiation, and interactions with climate change: UNEP Environmental Effects Assessment Panel, Update 2020. *Photochem Photobiol Sci* 2021;20:1–67.

CHAPTER 11

Cutaneous Response to Injury and Wound Healing

Edel A. O'Toole

Centre for Cell Biology and Cutaneous Research, Blizard Institute, Queen Mary University of London, UK

Introduction, 11.1	Fibroblast recruitment, matrix synthesis and scarring, 11.7	Physiological basis of the treatment of wounds, 11.10
Inflammation and the immune response, 11.2	Abnormal wound healing and scarring, 11.8	Novel therapies for wound healing, 11.11
Neutrophils and platelets, 11.2	Chronic wounds, 11.8	Growth factors to augment wound healing, 11.11
Macrophages, 11.3	Diabetes, 11.9	Stem cell therapy, 11.11
Lymphocytes, 11.3	Hypertrophic and keloid scarring, 11.9	Tissue engineering, 11.11
Re-epithelialisation, 11.4	Age-related changes in wound healing, 11.10	
Angiogenesis, 11.5		Key references, 11.13

Introduction

Skin, the largest organ in the body, is vital for humans and animals to protect against dehydration, bleeding and environmental microorganisms. Humans and animals have evolved a sophisticated mechanism of wound healing to plug any gap in skin integrity quickly, re-epithelialise over the defect and rapidly replace the lost dermis with new matrix. The final product is not normal skin, for adult human skin does not regenerate, but rather is a repair in the form of a scar, which is visible on the skin surface.

Adult wound repair consists of a series of overlapping stages [1], beginning with aggregation and degranulation of platelets, blood clotting and the formation of a fibrin plug (eschar), which initially fills the wound (Figure 11.1). This is followed by the inflammatory phase, where initially polymorphonuclear leukocytes appear, which stimulate the recruitment of monocytes, macrophages and lymphocytes that kill microorganisms and secrete a wide variety of growth factors and cytokines, which modulate the remaining wound healing response. These immune cells invade the fibrin-filled wound space and, together with fibroblasts and blood vessels from the deep fascia and surrounding dermis, begin to lay down a temporary matrix of granulation tissue consisting initially of a proteoglycan- and fibronectin-rich tissue, which serves as a guiding substratum for the migrating and proliferating cells. Cellular behaviour and coordination of the wound response is controlled during this granulation phase by a wide range of growth factors, extracellular matrix molecules and their receptors. There are extensive cell–cell and cell–matrix interactions. Epidermal cells proliferate and move down the edge of the wound until they reach the new granulation tissue, where they dissect between the overlying fibrinous eschar and the underlying granulation tissue to close the wound. At the same time, the wound contracts predominantly by forces exerted by contractile elements contained within the myofibroblasts. The transitory granulation tissue phase ends as immune cells, fibroblasts and endothelial cells undergo apoptosis, while the remaining fibroblasts lay down collagen (mostly types I and III), a process that continues for several months In the final remodelling stage of wound healing, the matrix is remodelled with a decrease in the relative levels of fibronectin, proteoglycans and type III collagen and an increase in the levels of predominantly type I collagen, which is organised into thick bundles and extensively cross-linked to form the mature scar.

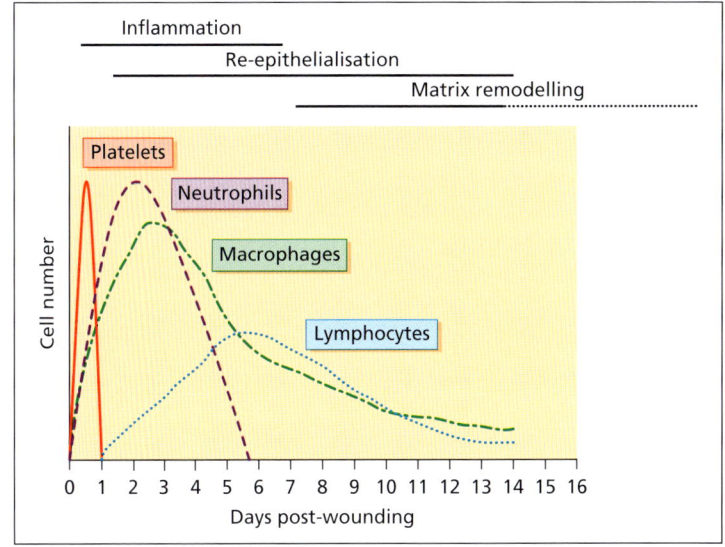

Figure 11.1 Wound inflammatory cells during the first 2 weeks of wound healing showing the stages of acute wound healing and the inflammatory infiltrate present in the wound bed.

Rook's Textbook of Dermatology, Tenth Edition. Edited by Christopher Griffiths, Jonathan Barker, Tanya Bleiker, Walayat Hussain and Rosalind Simpson.
© 2024 John Wiley & Sons Ltd. Published 2024 by John Wiley & Sons Ltd.

Acute wound healing proceeds quickly and with few problems in the vast majority of cases. Clearly, the speed of wound healing depends upon many factors, including the size of the wound (incisional or excisional), blood supply to the area, presence of foreign bodies and microorganisms, age and health of the patient, nutritional status of the patient, drugs that the patient may be taking and a variety of systemic diseases. Oxygen plays a critical part in wound healing [2,3], as does nitric oxide [4]. Leptin may be another regulator of wound healing [5]. Wound healing is subject to regulation by a large number of different cytokines and growth factors [6,7]. Oestrogens promote wound healing, while androgens inhibit it [8–11]. Opioid peptides may also favour wound healing [12]. Circadian timekeeping can also influence wound healing via regulation of the actin cytoskeleton resulting in better healing of daytime wounds [13].

Sometimes, the wound healing process does not proceed normally and chronic wounds result. The most common forms of chronic wounds in humans include venous ulcers, diabetic ulcers and pressure sores. In each of these cases there is normally an underlying pathology, such as venous insufficiency in the case of venous ulcers, or abnormal microvasculature and high blood sugar levels in diabetic ulcers. These underlying pathologies create a situation where the wound healing response is impaired. Thus, for example, in the case of venous stasis ulcers, there is often a chronic ischaemia–reperfusion injury resulting in high levels of local cytokines, complex cuffs forming around the blood vessels and increased levels of wound proteases, particularly matrix metalloproteinase 8 (MMP-8), MMP-26 and elastase, and decreased levels of protease inhibitors such as tissue inhibitor of matrix metalloproteinase 2 (TIMP-2) [14,15]. In the case of diabetic ulcers, there are often extensive abnormalities in the microcirculation, thickening of the blood vessel wall, thrombi and areas of focal necrosis [16]. In such chronic wounds, it is necessary to treat the underlying pathology if long-term non-recurrent healing of the ulcer is to be achieved. Understanding the molecular pathogenesis of these chronic wound healing states can lead to novel therapeutic targets for pharmacological intervention (e.g. the application of dressings containing protease inhibitors or 'smart matrix'). MicroRNA regulation of wound healing is a growing area of interest [17]. The wound healing response can also be disrupted by excessive healing (adverse scarring), which is represented at the extremes by hypertrophic scars or keloids. These excessive wound healing states result from the abnormal deposition of connective tissue within the healing wound, such that the scar is elevated and may extend beyond the boundaries of the original wound. Excessive scarring shows a clear genetic basis with racial tendencies (e.g. it is more common in Black and Oriental people than it is in White people).

Finally, the acute wound healing response varies with the age of the individual. Wounds made on very early embryos heal by complete regeneration, while wounds made on later embryos or early fetuses (in the middle trimester of pregnancy) display scar-free healing but the absence of regeneration of dermal appendages. Embryonic wounds exhibit a markedly reduced inflammatory response and alterations in cellular mediators, cytokines, growth factors, extracellular matrix modulators, tyrosine phosphorylation patterns and homeobox gene expression [18]. Wounds in children and young adults often heal quickly with excessive scarring, while elderly patients show specific disruptions in the wound healing cascade, such as elevated levels of proteases, altered ratios of growth factors and their receptors and a slower rate of healing but often with enhanced quality (reduced scarring). Age-related changes in the inflammatory response to wounding have been reported [19]. Wound healing is impaired by stress, possibly due to increased serum cortisol [20].

Despite the fact that the various phases of wound healing overlap, it is convenient to consider the principal cellular and molecular mechanisms regulating the basic biology of wound healing in three phases: inflammation and the immune response, re-epithelialisation and matrix remodelling.

Inflammation and the immune response

Following wounding, there is an almost immediate release of inflammatory mediators from damaged cells, degranulating platelets or resident tissue macrophages and mast cells. Furthermore, wounding causes a transient permeabilisation of cells near the wound margin, with the rapid exchange of extracellular and intracellular ions, resulting in the switching on of early response genes in such cells within seconds following wounding. These mediators initially cause arteriole dilatation, resulting in an increased blood flow into the wound area. This process is further aided by growth factors such as vascular endothelial growth factor (VEGF), which causes hyperpermeability of endothelial cells [1]. This results in an influx of fluid and plasma components into the wound space, while inflammatory cells adhere to the vascular endothelium and migrate through the vascular wall into the wound.

Neutrophils and platelets

Neutrophils are the predominant, initial inflammatory cells recruited to the wound, which together with platelets release a complex mixture of cytokines and growth factors. These amplify the inflammatory response, resulting in an influx of monocytes and lymphocytes, the proliferation of monocyte precursors within the wound and their differentiation into mature macrophages [2]. The use of knock-out mouse models to dissect the contribution of individual cytokines to wound repair revealed important roles for tumour necrosis factor α (TNF-α), interleukin 1 (IL-1) signalling, chemokine (C-X-C motif) receptor 2 (CXCR2), chemokine (C-X-C motif) ligand 10 (CXCL10), IP-10, Smad3 and secretory leukocyte protease inhibitor in inflammatory cell recruitment in acute wound healing [2,3]. Stress-induced catecholamines can increase neutrophil recruitment resulting in delayed wound healing [4].

Platelets respond very quickly, and when they reach the wound they adhere through selectin and integrin receptors [5], degranulate and release a variety of factors, including thromboxanes, prostaglandins, 12-lipoxygenase products, serotonin, adhesive glycoproteins (including fibrinogen, Von Willebrand factor, fibronectin and thrombospondin) and growth factors (including platelet-derived growth factor (PDGF), epidermal growth factor (EGF) and transforming growth factor β1 (TGF-β1)). These factors contribute to the initial fibrin plug that closes the wound and also modulate subsequent cellular behaviour, including attachment, migration, proliferation and matrix deposition. However, wound closure, angiogenesis and collagen synthesis are not significantly impaired in thrombocytopenic mice [6].

These signals from the wound site, together with changes in vascular permeability, cause leukocytes to pavement in the blood vessels, and undergo rolling and attachment to activated endothelial P- and E-selectins and integrins, for example heterodimers of CD18 (β2 integrin) and variable α subunits [7]. Neutrophils, recruited early in wound healing, are responsible for destroying invading bacteria by phagocytosis and the release of reactive oxygen species, eicosanoids and proteolytic enzymes (elastase, cathepsin G, urokinase-type plasminogen activator), which may cause further tissue damage and inflammation. Once in the wound, neutrophils may be activated by cytokines such as granulocyte–macrophage colony-stimulating factor (GM-CSF) and TNF-α, complement, or proteases such as thrombin. Unless stimuli for neutrophil recruitment persist, after a few days neutrophils are eliminated by macrophage phagocytosis or apoptotic cell death.

Macrophages

Monocytes and macrophages are recruited in large numbers to the healing wound as neutrophil numbers begin to decline. Classic studies by Leibovich and Ross [8] demonstrated the importance of these cells in wound healing; experimental depletion of wound macrophages resulted in prolonged inflammation and delays in fibroblast proliferation, matrix deposition and subsequent wound closure. The transition from a resting to an active state in monocytes and macrophages is controlled by cytokines including TNF-α and interferon γ (IFN-γ), as well as bacterial products such as lipopolysaccharide. Monocytes and macrophages produce a range of cytokines in response to pro-inflammatory signals, including TGF-β and TGF-α, basic fibroblast growth factor, VEGF and PDGF. The interactions between these growth factors and monocyte/macrophage differentiation/activation are complex and often self-regulatory. Thus, TGF-β1 acts as a pro-inflammatory cytokine early in the wound healing phase, as it is chemotactic to immature monocytes, which are recruited to the wound site and synthesise and secrete more TGF-β1, due to a self-inducing response element in the TGF-β1 promoter. However, TGF-β1 is anti-inflammatory to mature or activated monocytes/macrophages, because it inhibits their activation and modulates receptor expression. Although wound healing is initially normal in the TGF-β1 knock-out mouse, the accumulation of inflammatory cells and reduction in angiogenesis and collagen deposition lead to delayed epithelial closure [9].

In addition to the production of cytokines, wound macrophages also produce a range of extracellular matrix molecules, which – together with fibrinogen and fibrin from the blood clot, matrix molecules from degranulating platelets, recruited fibroblasts and endothelial cells – form the granulation tissue or provisional matrix. This provisional matrix is rich in molecules, such as fibronectin, vitronectin, thrombospondin, SPARC (secreted protein, acidic, cysteine-rich; also known as osteonectin), tenascin and proteoglycans such as dermatan, chondroitin and heparan sulphate. It acts as an early scaffold for the re-establishment of the dermis and for the migration of epidermis as it promotes both cell migration and proliferation. Regulation of this provisional matrix is complex and achieved partially through control at the transcriptional level, for example with alternative splicing of the primary transcript for fibronectin resulting in embryonic-like cellular fibronectins being deposited within the wound space, which better facilitate cell migration and proliferation [10].

Lymphocytes

Pro-inflammatory cytokines such as TNF-α and IFN-γ can stimulate the production of chemokines by endothelial cells [11]. Endothelial and macrophage chemokines (e.g. IL-8, CXCL10, platelet factor 4 (PF-4), chemokine (C-C motif) ligand 3 (CCL3), CCL4, CCL5 and CCL2) attract lymphocytes to the wound area, and may have a role in the progression of healing to fibrosis [3]. These lymphocytes include both B and T lymphocytes, and there is growing evidence that the particular type of T-lymphocyte response (Th1 or Th2), each characterised by a different profile of cytokine secretion, may be one of the factors underlying abnormal fibrosis and scarring [12]. Early life exposure to microbes induces development of mucosal-associated invariant T (MAIT) cells. In adults, cutaneous MAIT cells are a dominant population of interleukin-17A-producing lymphocytes, which display a distinct transcriptional signature and respond to skin commensals and promote wound repair [13]. Interleukin-33, a member of the IL-1 family, facilitates the development of alternatively activated macrophages (M2) with the resolution of inflammation, increased fibronectin and type III collagen deposition and improved wound repair [14].

Human γ/δ T lymphocytes express and synthesise connective tissue growth factor (CTGF), known to regulate fibrogenesis and wound healing, as well as fibroblast growth factor 7 (FGF-7), FGF-10 and insulin-like growth factor 1 (IGF-1) regulating keratinocyte differentiation and proliferation and FGF-9 linked to hair follicle neogenesis [15,16]. In addition, this T-cell subgroup regulates keratinocyte hyaluronic acid deposition in the provisional matrix, and subsequent macrophage infiltration into the wound [17]. The type of T-lymphocyte response itself may be determined by the profile of growth factors in the early wound. Thus, for example, natural killer (NK) cell migration out of blood vessels is promoted by VEGF but inhibited by FGF-2 [18]. IL-6 also has a crucial role in wound healing, probably by regulating early leukocyte infiltration and tissue remodelling in the later stages of wound repair [19]. Recent *in vivo* functional studies reveal the roles of different transcriptional regulators in wound repair. Mice deficient for PU.1 transcription factor, that lack macrophages and functional neutrophils, surprisingly showed normal scar-free healing of incisional wounds [20]. Mice deficient in Nrf2, a leucine zipper transcription factor involved in the detoxification of reactive oxygen species, have increased and prolonged macrophage infiltration in wounds, suggesting that Nrf2 regulates the resolution of inflammation [21]. Components of the innate immune system, such as Toll-like receptor 4, are also important regulators of wound inflammation [22].

These early inflammatory responses clear the wound of foreign antigens such as bacteria and supply combinations of growth factors (Table 11.1) and extracellular matrix molecules, which orchestrate the subsequent healing of the provisional matrix by providing the signals and scaffold for fibroblast, endothelial and keratinocyte influx. Inflammatory cells such as monocytes and macrophages decrease towards the end of the inflammatory phase, largely through apoptosis resulting from a reduction in the levels of survival factors (e.g. specific cytokines and matrix molecules).

Table 11.1 Main source of growth factors/cytokines during wound healing.

	Platelet	Macrophage	Lymphocyte	Keratinocyte	Fibroblast	Endothelial cells
PDGF	X	X		X	X	X
VEGF	X	X		X	X	X
EGF	X	X				
FGF-1/2		X	X			X
FGF-7					X	
CTGF					X	X
IGF-1	X				X	
HGF		X			X	
TNF-α		X	X	X		X
TGF-α	X	X		X		
TGF-β	X	X		X	X	X
GM-CSF		X				
IFN-γ			X	X		
IL-1β		X	X	X		
IL-2		X	X	X		
IL-6		X	X	X		
IL-8		X	X	X		

CTGF, connective tissue growth factor; EGF, epidermal growth factor; FGF, fibroblast growth factor; GM-CSF, granulocyte–macrophage colony-stimulating factor; HGF, hepatocyte growth factor; IFN, interferon; IGF, insulin-like growth factor; IL, interleukin; PDGF, platelet-derived growth factor; TGF, transforming growth factor; TNF, tumour necrosis factor; VEGF, vascular endothelial growth factor.

Re-epithelialisation

The process of re-epithelialisation commences about 24 h after wounding when keratinocytes migrate from the wound edge or hair follicles, across the provisional wound matrix to invade the wound bed, where they proliferate to form new epidermis [1]. Keratinocyte injury alters the ratio of magnesium and calcium ions, which induces keratinocytes to adopt a migratory phenotype [2]. The migrating keratinocyte flattens and elongates with the formation of lamellipodia to aid cell movement, loss of cell–cell (desmosomes) and cell–matrix contacts and rearrangement of the actin filament network. The K1 and K10 suprabasal cytokeratin filaments are replaced by the flexible cytokeratins K6 and K16, whose expression is regulated by growth factors such as EGF, TGF-α and TGF-β present at high levels within the provisional matrix, as well as the rhomboid protease, iRhom2 [3].

Following wounding, signals from the matrix and growth factors induce phosphorylation of numerous keratinocyte proteins, including focal adhesion kinase, c-Met, the small guanine triphosphatase, Rac, extracellular signal-regulated kinases 1/2, phosphatidylinositol-3-kinase, mitogen-activated protein kinases (MAPKs), and the AP-1, Stat3 and Tcf3 families of transcription factors. These transcription factors regulate many of the genes involved in keratinocyte migration, for example integrins, MMPs and growth factors [4–10]. TNF-α stimulates transcription of the PPARβ/δ (peroxisome-proliferator-activated receptor β/δ) gene, also via an AP-1 site in its promoter, with subsequent upregulation of the expression of integrin-linked kinase and 3-phosphoinositide-dependent kinase 1, which activates the anti-apoptotic protein, Akt [11]. Keratinocytes in the basal layer some 300–400 cell diameters away from the wound margin proliferate extensively; such proliferation peaks within 1–2 days post-wounding and then falls back again to reach basal levels about 14 days post-wounding. The transcription factor, c-Myc, is a potent regulator of keratinocyte proliferation during wound healing [12]. Suprabasal cells derived from this extensive proliferation roll over the attached basal cells to form new basal cells at the wound margin, a process repeated by successive basal cells until re-epithelialisation is complete.

To reach the wound bed, migrating keratinocytes express MMPs (enzymes that degrade basement membrane components and interstitial collagens) (Figure 11.2) and urokinase-type plasminogen activator, an enzyme that activates plasmin for fibrinolysis of fibrin [13,14]. Upregulation of MMP-9 and urokinase plasminogen activator, induced by hypoxia, results in increased keratinocyte migration [15,16]. This upregulation is mirrored by the concurrent upregulation of plasminogen-activator inhibitors (Figure 11.3), which control the extent of plasminogen activation [16]. This suggests a key role for the plasmin–plasminogen system in wound healing, an assertion given experimental weight by wound healing studies on mice with targeted disruption of the plasminogen gene [17]. These mice showed substantial delays in wound re-epithelialisation and the aberrant persistence of fibrin within the wound matrix, demonstrating the importance of the plasminogen–plasmin system for fibrin removal during wound healing. Syndecan-1 is a cell-surface proteoglycan that enhances keratinocyte proliferation and re-epithelialisation [18].

During wound healing, the migrating keratinocytes come into contact with dermal collagens and the fibrin clot constituents fibrin, fibronectin and vitronectin. Thus, α5, β1, αV and β5 integrin subunits, the primary keratinocyte receptors for fibronectin and vitronectin, are upregulated in migrating keratinocytes during re-epithelialisation (Figure 11.3) [19]. Expression of these integrins may be induced by TGF-β1 [20]. Once re-epithelialisation is complete, the keratinocytes switch from the vitronectin/fibronectin receptor (αVβ5) to the tenascin/fibronectin receptor (αVβ6). This switch may be involved in the redifferentiation of the epidermis as the β6 integrin subunit has been associated with epithelial remodelling during development and tumorigenesis [21]. Because

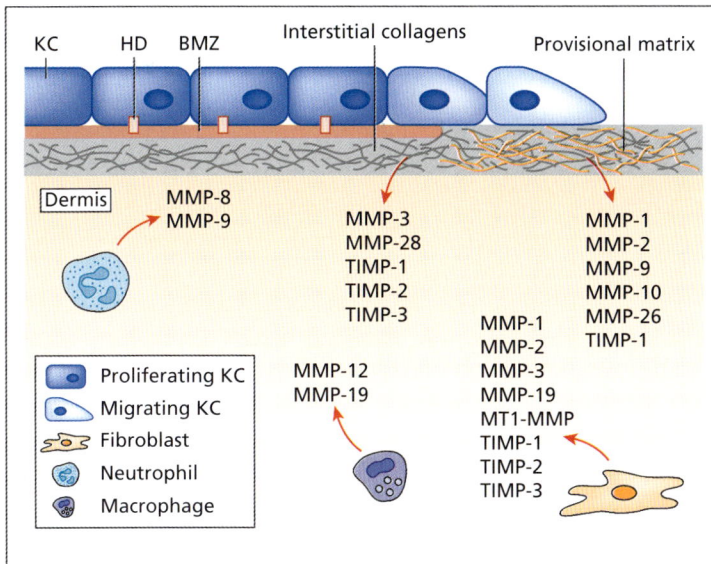

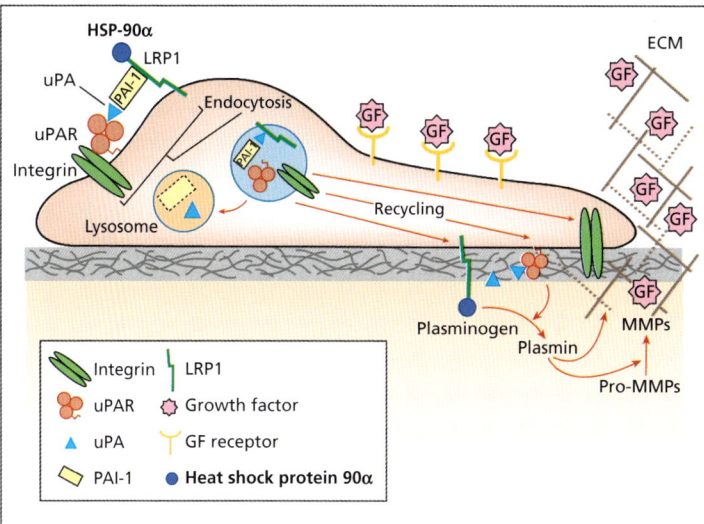

Figure 11.2 Matrix metalloproteinases (MMPs) and tissue inhibitor of matrix metalloproteinases (TIMPs) in wound healing showing the expression and cellular source of MMPs and TIMPs in cutaneous wound healing. Keratinocytes (KC) change their phenotype as they lose their hemidesmosomes (HD), which attach them to the underlying basement membrane zone (BMZ), thus coming in contact with a provisional wound matrix made of fibronectin and fibrin (in orange). Below the basement membrane lies the interstitial matrix composed mainly of type I collagen (in grey). A differential pattern of expression of MMPs and their inhibitors seems to be critical for wound healing, with some MMPs being expressed by migrating keratinocytes at the leading edge of the wound, while others are only expressed by the proliferating population of keratinocytes adjacent to the wound edge. MMPs expressed by fibroblasts and inflammatory cells such as neutrophils and macrophages also contribute to regulating the wound healing process. Reproduced from [35] with permission from Springer Nature.

Figure 11.3 Mechanisms involved in matrix degradation during keratinocyte migration. Physiological control of pericellular proteolysis occurs primarily through the regulation of plasminogen activation at the cell surface, which in turn contributes to downstream matrix metalloproteinase (MMP) activity. Focal proteolysis disrupts extracellular matrix (ECM) architecture, breaking cell–matrix interactions with receptors, such as integrins, and releasing bioactive fragments of ECM molecules, as well as growth factors that stimulate migratory behaviour. Plasminogen activator inhibitor type 1 (PAI-1), through its ability to inhibit urokinase-type plasminogen activator (uPA) dependent activation of plasmin, titres this process maintaining the scaffolding necessary to facilitate cell migration. uPAR, uPA receptor; GF, growth factor; LRP1, low-density lipoprotein receptor-related protein 1; HSP90α, heat shock protein 90α (ligand for LRP1 and a potent regulator of keratinocyte migration). Reproduced from [36]/Hindawi/CC by 3.0.

keratinocytes do not express the fibrin-specific integrin αVβ3, instead of invading the fibrin clot, the migrating cells dissect the fibrin clot from the wound bed [22].

A number of growth factors secreted by keratinocytes, fibroblasts or inflammatory cells promote keratinocyte proliferation and migration (see Tables 11.1 and 11.2 and [23–26]). Fibroblast growth factor 7 (FGF-7/KGF) stimulates hyaluronan synthesis, which also promotes keratinocyte migration [27]. The anti-microbial peptides, human β-defensins, stimulate epidermal keratinocyte migration, proliferation and production of pro-inflammatory cytokines [28]. Secreted heat shock protein 90α induced by TGF-α, promotes both epidermal and dermal cell migration [29]. Keratinocytes can stimulate FGF-7 production by underlying dermal cells, which then acts specifically on the overlying epidermal cells expressing the FGF-7 receptor [30]. During wounding, cells come into contact with human serum, which promotes keratinocyte motility via p38 MAPK and the induction of epidermal MMP expression [31].

In normal skin, the basement membrane separates the epidermis from the dermis. Following wounding, this dermal–epidermal junction must be reconstituted as part of the re-epithelialisation process. Basement membrane components are synthesised and deposited into the dermal–epidermal junction by both the fibroblasts and the keratinocytes, and a scanty basement membrane is usually present by 7–9 days after wounding [32,33]. Maturation of anchoring fibrils may take up to 3 years [34].

Table 11.2 Function of cytokines/growth factors in acute wounds.

	Leukocyte chemotaxis	Re-epithelialisation	Angiogenesis	Wound remodelling
PDGF	+	++	++	++
VEGF			+	
EGF	+	+++	+	+
FGF-1/2		+	+++	+
FGF-7		+++		+
HGF	+	+++	++	+
IGF-1			++	
TNF-α	++			
TGF-α		++	++	
TGF-β		+	+	
GM-CSF	+			
IFN-γ	+			
IL-1β	+++	+		++
IL-6				+
IL-8	++	++	++	

EGF, epidermal growth factor; FGF, fibroblast growth; GM-CSF, granulocyte–macrophage colony-stimulating factor; HGF, hepatocyte growth factor; IGF, insulin-like growth factor; PDGF, platelet-derived growth factor; TGF, transforming growth factor; TNF, tumour necrosis factor; VEGF, vascular endothelial growth factor.

Angiogenesis

Formation of new blood vessels within the provisional matrix is stimulated by day 2 of the inflammatory stage of wound healing. Immediately following injury, angiogenic factors including VEGF,

PDGF, FGFs, TGF-β and complement 1q (C1q) are secreted by platelets, fibroblasts, wounded keratinocytes and macrophages [1,2]. VEGF induces endothelial cell proliferation and migration through three receptors, VEGFR-1/Flt1, VEGFR-2 and neuropilin-1 [3,4]. Periostin, a known inducer of VEGFR-2 expression which plays a role in regulating vascular smooth muscle cell migration, is up to 100-fold upregulated in wound vessels compared with normal blood vessels [5]. The sprouting endothelial cells participate in granulation tissue formation (the capillary loops within the provisional matrix give granulation tissue its red granular appearance). Hypoxia and reactive oxygen species also regulate VEGF expression via the activation of hypoxia-inducible factor 1α, which is strongly expressed by keratinocytes at the wound edge, and the Sp1 transcription factor, respectively [6,7]. Endothelial cells from nearby blood vessels and, in larger wounds, endothelial progenitor cells from bone marrow, activated by VEGF and mobilised by the CXCR4 ligand, stromal cell-derived factor 1 (SDF-1), move to the wound bed [8]. Macrophages also positively influence wound angiogenesis by reducing antiangiogenic wound neutrophils and secreting VEGF to drive vessel sprouting [9]. Subsequently, macrophages also play a role in blood vessel regression during the resolution phase of wound repair, and their absence, or shifted activation state, impairs appropriate vessel clearance.

Laminin 411 (previously laminin 8) and laminin 511 (previously laminin 10) are the major laminin isoforms in the basement membrane of dermal microvascular endothelial cells [10]. Laminin 411 promotes endothelial cell attachment, migration and tubule formation. Endothelial cells use both β1-containing and αVβ3 integrins in their interactions with the G1-3 domains of the α4 chain of laminin 441 [11]. Proteolytic enzymes, for example MMPs, are released at the growing tips of capillaries, degrading the extracellular matrix for forward movement [12]. Ephrin ligand–receptor interactions guide the patterning of vascular loops and tubes [13].

Adequate revascularisation of the wound is essential for healing (Figure 11.4); ineffective angiogenesis results in impaired wound healing [14]. At the end of the provisional matrix phase, the numbers of blood vessels within the healing wound decrease by a process of apoptosis, probably induced by the depletion of vascular survival factors, such as VEGF, and the appearance of pro-apoptotic factors such as TGF-β [15].

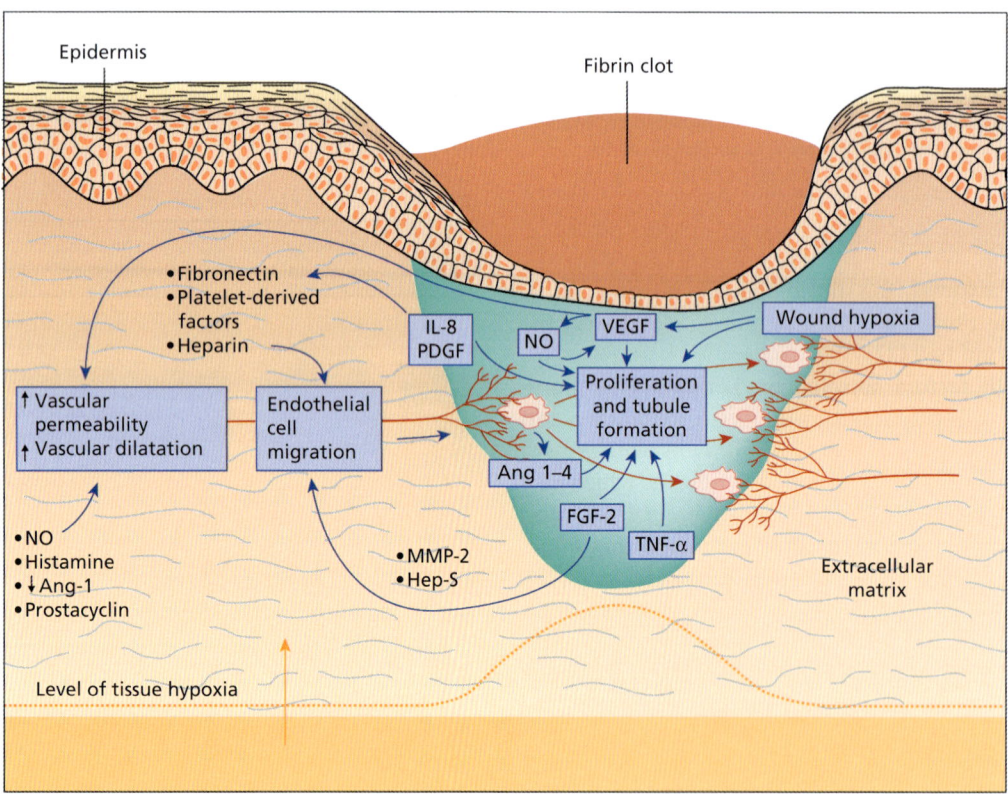

Figure 11.4 Molecular and cellular factors required for angiogenesis in order to promote endothelial cell migration, proliferation and tubule formation. After wounding, angiogenesis functions to re-establish normoxia and nutrient delivery to damaged and regenerating tissue. Existing capillaries in the wound margin become dilated with increased permeability secondary to the influence of inflammatory mediators including nitric oxide (NO), histamine, angiopoietin 1 (Ang-1), prostacyclin and vascular endothelial growth factor (VEGF). This facilitates endothelial cell extravasation and migration into the perivascular space. The process is further encouraged by platelet-derived factors, extracellular matrix components (heparan sulphate (HEP-S) and fibronectin), platelet-derived growth factor (PDGF), interleukin 8 (IL-8) and fibroblast growth factor 2 (FGF-2), which may be fibrin or fibrinogen bound. FGF-2-induced integrin expression facilitates matrix metalloproteinase 2 (MMP-2) localisation, resulting in collagen degradation and thereby facilitating endothelial cell migration. Once present in the wound bed, endothelial cells proliferate and form new capillary tubules contributing to granulation tissue formation and restoration of circulatory integrity. VEGF replaces FGF-2 as the predominant stimulant of this process after 7 days and is secreted by a range of cellular mediators including macrophages, neutrophils, endothelial cells, keratinocytes and fibroblasts. Other important proliferative factors include tissue hypoxia, NO, tumour necrosis factor α (TNF-α) and Ang-1–4. Reproduced from [3], with permission from Elsevier.

Fibroblast recruitment, matrix synthesis and scarring

The fibroblasts migrate into, and proliferate within, the provisional wound matrix, depositing additional extracellular matrix molecules. Most wound fibroblasts are derived from proliferation of fibroblast progenitor cells in the lower dermis and the septae of the underlying fat; in mouse models adipocytes are necessary for fibroblast recruitment during wound healing [1]. Fibroblast precursors in the upper dermis of murine wounds form new hair follicles, stimulated by epidermal β-catenin signalling, explaining why re-epithelialising wounds lack hair follicles initially [2]. Single cell transcriptomic profiling of human dermis has revealed there are at least four subpopulations of fibroblasts with different functions including skin regeneration [3]. Like the keratinocytes, fibroblasts alter their integrin profile, expressing receptors for fibronectin, fibrin and vitronectin and downregulating receptors for collagen during the early phases of migration. During the early stages of provisional matrix deposition, collagen synthesis in the surrounding unwounded skin is suppressed, while fibronectin synthesis is enhanced [4]. Fibroblasts within the provisional matrix secrete and assemble a complex extracellular matrix. Initially, this consists predominantly of fibronectin and proteoglycans, but later consists of mature type I collagen bundles. The ratio of collagen types during wound healing varies, the early wound being characterised by elevated levels of type III collagen, whereas later in wound healing type I collagen predominates. Minor collagens, such as types XII and XIV, as well as proteoglycans such as decorin, are also present in the early healing wound and play a key part in collagen fibril organisation. The degree of collagenous cross-linking also varies with time after wounding: the early wound has fewer and more immature cross-links compared with the later wound, which has extensive mature cross-links, resulting in a more insoluble collagenous matrix.

Both mesenchymal and epidermal secreted factors stimulate fibroblast proliferation and migration and extracellular matrix synthesis in a paracrine and autocrine fashion, including the TGF-β family, IGF-1, PDGF, CTGF and hypoxia-induced heat shock protein 90 [5,6]. There is extensive cross-talk between the extracellular matrix-derived signals and growth factor signalling in this process. Thus, for example, clustering of integrin receptors on the fibroblast leading edge leads to associated clustering of growth factor receptors, which then interact with the growth factors bound to the matrix.

The early granulation tissue is characterised by transformed wound fibroblasts called myofibroblasts, which show elevated levels of α-smooth muscle actin and are morphologically and functionally intermediate between fibroblasts and smooth muscle cells. Differentiation into myofibroblasts is induced by growth factors such as TGF-β1 and IL-6, coagulation protease factor (F)Xa, extracellular matrix proteins such as the fibronectin splice variant EDA FN (extra domain A fibronectin) and tenascin, and the mechanical microenvironment [7,8]. Myofibroblasts may contribute to the contractile forces involved in wound contraction (Figure 11.5). In murine models, in early wound healing myofibroblasts can be reprogrammed into adipocytes aiding tissue regeneration [9]. They are preferentially eliminated during the apoptotic phase of wound healing, which may be induced by wound relaxation [7]. The Smad family of proteins mediates signal transduction of the TGF-β superfamily including the induction of CTGF expression and the synthesis of collagens and TIMP-1, and TGF-β induces the fibroblast contraction necessary for efficient wound healing [10]. Turnover of the extracellular matrix is facilitated by a range of proteases and protease inhibitors, including plasmin, MMPs, hyaluronidase and elastase [11]. Levels of these active proteases are carefully and focally controlled both by growth factors, for example IL-6, and by proteolytic inhibitors such as TIMP and syndecans [12,13]. IL-10

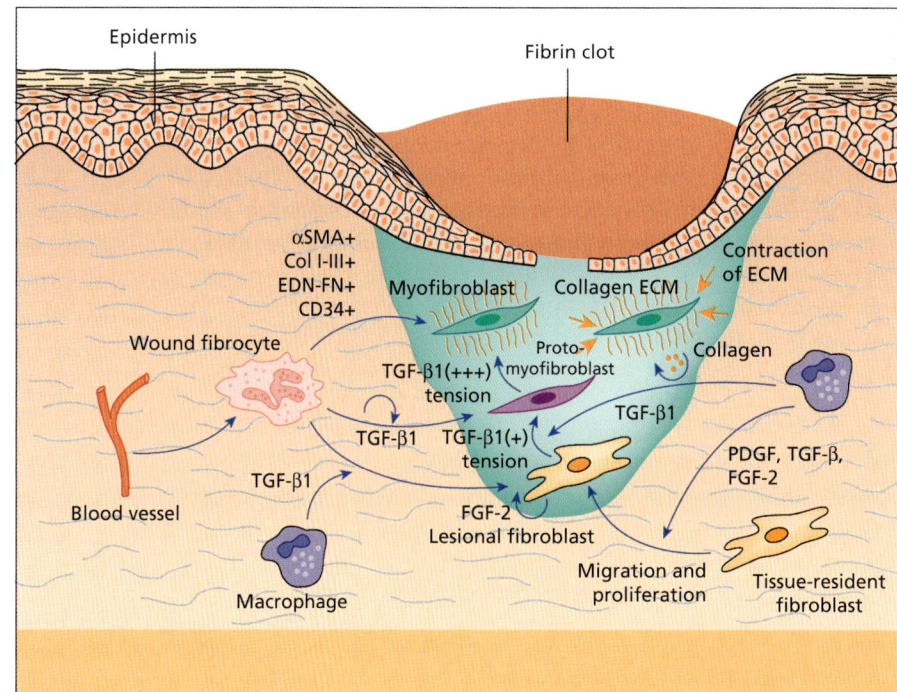

Figure 11.5 Wound contraction to initiate scarring. Macrophage-derived platelet-derived growth factor (PDGF), transforming growth factor-β (TGF-β) and fibroblast growth factor 2 (FGF-2) result in the migration of fibroblasts from surrounding healthy tissue to the wound site where they begin the process of fibroplasia. TGF-β1 can also induce bone-marrow-derived fibrocyte differentiation into fibroblasts, proto-myofibroblasts and myofibroblasts. Later in the proliferative phase fibroblasts convert to proto-myofibroblasts in response to increased tissue tension and TGF-β. A positive feedback loop is created where tension facilitates further TGF-β release and final maturation into myofibroblasts, which generate the majority of contractile forces in the wound. Myofibroblasts are recognised by increased expression of α-smooth muscle actin (αSMA), collagen I and III, extra domain A fibronectin (EDA-FN) and CD34+ cells. ECM, extracellular matrix. Reproduced from [31], with permission from Elsevier.

and FGF-2 both regulate remodelling of the extracellular matrix during wound healing [14,15].

As healing proceeds, the numbers of fibroblasts and endothelial and inflammatory cells decrease, and the predominantly collagenous matrix becomes organised into thicker, more heavily cross-linked bundles. This marks the establishment of the mature scar. Scars continue to remodel for a long time after wounding and cannot be considered to be in a steady state condition until at least 2 years postwounding. Cutaneous scarring is defined as a macroscopic disturbance of the normal structure and function of the skin architecture, resulting from the end-product of a healed wound [16]. Scarring may manifest itself as an elevated or depressed site, with an alteration of skin texture (e.g. hard), colour (e.g. hyperpigmentation or redness), vascularity, nerve supply, reflectance and biomechanical properties (e.g. elasticity). Histologically, dermal scars are characterised by thickened epidermis with a flattened dermal–epidermal junction, and an abnormal organisation of the dermal matrix into parallel bundles of scar tissue collagen, as opposed to the normal basket-weave appearance of dermal collagen. The scar collagen fibres are usually smaller and more densely packed and often have higher proportions of type III collagen and fibronectin compared with the surrounding normal skin. Elastin appears early in the wound healing process but then disappears (presumably because of the activity of elastase) to reappear again later in the scar [17]. However, the elastin is abnormally organised into fragmented and chaotic structures, as opposed to the normal elastin fibre arcades that characterise normal dermis [17]. Epidermal appendages such as hair follicles and sebaceous glands do not regenerate in scars, although the experimental addition of dermal papilla fibroblasts to a wound can induce hair follicle formation [18]. In a mouse model, wounding in association with Wnt signalling can induce hair follicles from epidermal progenitor cells [19]. Proliferative scarring or chronic wounds may result from overexpression or dysregulated activity of the fibrogenic isoforms of TGF-β (1 and 2) [20]. All three isoforms of TGF-β, and its receptors, are strongly expressed in adult wounds but not in fetal wounds, which do not scar [21]. Activin-A, a member of the TGF-β family, also contributes to fibrosis [22].

The severity of scarring can be assessed clinically using visual analogue scales and the severity of macroscopic scarring correlates with histological abnormalities predominantly in the epidermis and papillary dermis [23]. Scar redness lasts on average for about 7 months after excisional wounding [24]. The initial inflammatory phase of wounding is thought to be critical to the morphology and severity of scarring. The application of antiscarring therapies, such as neutralising antibodies to the profibrotic TGF-β isoforms, TGF-β1 or TGF-β2, or exogenous TGF-β3, which is elevated in non-scarring fetal epidermis, is necessary at the time of, or shortly after, wounding to achieve maximum antiscarring effect [25]. Smad3 is a key mediator of the TGF-β pathway and the Smad3 null mouse exhibits impaired wound healing, suggesting that inhibition of TGF-β may not always have beneficial effects [26]. Translating preclinical studies into human wound healing clinical trials will require further knowledge of the biology of this complex pathway in skin [27].

Gap junctions – intercellular communication channels composed of connexin isoforms – are present in epidermis. The application of connexin 43 (Cx43) antisense oligonucleotides reduced the inflammatory cell infiltrate with accelerated healing in murine wounds and reduced scarring after cutaneous thermal injury [28,29]. Short bioengineered peptides derived from the Cx43 carboxyl terminus accelerated wound healing and reduced scarring [30]. Scarring of skin is a major clinical problem resulting in adverse cosmesis, loss of function (particularly if over joints) and interference with growth in children. Strategies to reduce scarring in the skin may also be beneficial in the eye, the central nervous system and other organs where cytokine secretion or gap junction communication play a role in fibrosis.

Abnormal wound healing and scarring

Chronic wounds

The series of biological events that close any defect in the skin may be impaired by factors interfering with inflammation, angiogenesis, re-epithelialisation and wound remodelling. Most wounds will have a tendency to heal, however longstanding, but this process may be very slow. Recurrent injury over a previous scar, as in a leg ulcer or pressure sore, and recurrent breakdown following healing, can give rise to chronic skin wounds or ulcers that appear to have lost the capacity to heal (see Chapter 102). Although the mechanisms of skin ulceration are understood, the biological profile of the chronic wound is still not fully understood.

The chronic wound environment may be deficient in the stimulatory growth factors, growth factor receptors or proteolytic enzymes required for growth factor activation or may be overproducing any of these factors [1,2]. A mouse model lacking TNF superfamily member 4 has many features of chronic wounds including excessive production of chemokines, defective basement membrane and granulation tissue with high levels of type III collagen [3]. Resolution of inflammation is important for wound closure. Continued wound inflammation from inflammatory macrophages (M1) results in tissue damage and impaired wound healing [4]. Chronic wound fluid has been shown to decrease the proliferation of fibroblasts, endothelial cells and keratinocytes, in part mediated through Ras- and MAPK-signalling pathways [5–8]. In contrast, acute wound fluid stimulates growth of these cells [9]. Fibrin accumulates in chronic wounds (unlike acute wounds) and forms complexes that may bind or inactivate other molecules such as growth factors. A proteomic study showed increased levels of the γ- and β-chains of fibrinogen as well as vitronectin, fibronectin, lumican and α2-HS-glycoprotein in non-healing wound exudates. Olfactomedin-4, a matrix protein possibly important in developmental biology, was found exclusively in non-healing wounds [10].

The MMPs are proenzymes requiring activation [11]. Three classes of MMPs are collagenases, gelatinases and stromelysins (Table 11.3) – single-chain proteins, the production of which is stimulated by soluble factors and matrix proteins and inhibited by TIMP [12]. Chronic wounds have excess proteases, including

Table 11.3 Metalloproteinases (MMPs) involved in wound repair.

Enzyme	Substrate
MMP-1 (collagenase 1)	Collagens I, II, III, VII and X, aggrecan, serpins
MMP-8 (collagenase 2)	Collagens I, II and III, aggrecan, serpins
MMP-13 (collagenase 3)	Collagens I, II, III, IV, IX, X and XIV, gelatin, fibronectin, laminin, tenascin
MMP-2 (gelatinase A)	Gelatin, collagens I, IV, V, VII and X, laminin, aggrecan, fibronectin, tenascin
MMP-9 (gelatinase B)	Gelatin, collagens I, III, IV, V and VII, aggrecan, elastin, fibrillin
MMP-3 (stromelysin 1)	Collagens IV, V, IX and X, fibronectin, elastin, gelatin, aggrecan, nidogen, fibrillin
MMP-10 (stromelysin 2)	Collagens IV, V, IX and X, fibronectin, elastin, gelatin, laminin
MMP-11 (stromelysin 3)	Serine protease inhibitors
MMP-7 (matrilysin)	Elastin, fibronectin, laminin, nidogen, collagen IV, tenascin, versican
MMP-12 (metalloelastase)	Collagen IV, gelatin, fibronectin, laminin, vitronectin, elastin, fibrillin
MMP-14 (MT1-MMP)	Collagens I, II and III, gelatin, fibronectin, laminin, vitronectin, aggrecan, tenascin, nidogen, perlecan, fibrillin

Table 11.4 Differences between hypertrophic and keloid scars.

	Hypertrophic scar	Keloid scar
Site of injury	Localised to injury site	Grows beyond injury site
Progression	Stabilises	Increases in size
Sites of excessive wound tension	Yes	Yes
Genetic predisposition	No	Yes
Ethnic predisposition	No	Increased in type V and VI skin

MMP-1, MMP-8 and MMP-9 [10–13]. Keratinocytes in chronic wounds fail to migrate across a wound bed despite a hyperplastic epithelium and may lack specific matrix proteins in the wound bed to permit cell movement. Keratinocytes migrate most effectively on fibronectin, usually present in the wound bed, and on type I and IV collagens, but not on laminin [14]. Keratinocyte mesenchymal interactions therefore require a vascularised appropriate matrix and this is impaired in chronic persistent wounds. Microbial colonisation of wounds also impairs chronic wound healing by causing excessive inflammation and amplifying the innate immune response [15]. Mast cells seem to be critical in regulating bacterial load and healing of infected wounds [16].

Diabetes (Chapter 150)

Peripheral neuropathy and micro- or macrovascular disease, causing tissue ischaemia and hypoxia, render the diabetic foot more susceptible to skin wounding and ulceration, particularly in vulnerable areas like the lower limbs. Hyperglycaemia also has a negative effect on wound healing through the production of advanced glycation end-products that induce inflammation and impair collagen turnover [17]. High glucose levels also affect keratinocyte differentiation and proliferation. Changes in growth factors, elevated levels of MMPs and reduced levels of TIMPs and increased cell death also contribute to chronic wounding in diabetes [18]. Diabetic wounds have increased chronic inflammation, which is detrimental to wound repair with an increase in the ratio of pro-inflammatory (M1) to anti-inflammatory (M2) macrophages and decreased neutrophil recruitment, mediated by the transcription factor, FOXM1 [19]. Hyperglycaemia and chronic inflammation cause impaired endothelial progenitor cell recruitment from the bone marrow in diabetes resulting in defective angiogenesis [20]. Dysregulated neuropeptide signalling may also play a role as peripheral nerve fibres of the skin are stimulated immediately after injury [21]. A fragment of secreted heat shock protein 90α, called F5, promotes diabetic wound healing by stimulating keratinocytes, fibroblasts and endothelial cells [22]. Laminin heparin-binding peptides bind to growth factors and also improve murine diabetic wound healing [23].

Hypertrophic and keloid scarring (Chapter 94)

Keloids and hypertrophic scars are abnormal fibrous reactions to trauma, inflammation, surgery or burns in predisposed individuals, particularly in Afro-Caribbean skin, and most occur between the ages of 10 and 30 years. Hypertrophic scars remain restricted to the original wound, but keloids extend beyond the original wound and rarely regress. Most keloids commence within a year of trauma in areas of highest skin tension: on the upper back, shoulders, anterior chest and upper arms. Reducing wound tension by orientating the wound along lines of relaxed tension may reduce scar formation. A genetic predisposition to keloid formation is suggested by reports of dominant and rarely recessive inheritance. Linkage and genome-wide association studies have identified susceptibility loci for keloids on chromosomes 1–3, 7 and 15 in Japanese families with autosomal dominant inheritance and a case–control study, respectively [24,25].

Hypertrophic scars are distinguished from keloids by growth, course and outcome (Table 11.4). They occur soon after the trauma or inflammation, are limited to the site of the wound and regress in months to years, but may be difficult to distinguish from keloids in their early actively growing phase. Pathological distinction is not easy. Normal healing involves fibroplasia following the inflammatory phase. In keloids, this is progressive and forms nodular vascular proliferations surrounded by fibroblasts. These nodules transform into avascular collagenous bundles with persistent swirls of fibroblasts; myofibroblasts are prevalent in active keloids. The collagen bundles are randomly aligned and not orientated to the skin surface, whereas in normal scars the bundles lie parallel to the epithelial surface. There are suggestions from *in vitro* studies with keloid fibroblasts that abnormal collagen cross-linking, degradation or regulation by TGF-β may be involved in the pathogenesis [26,27]. Other cellular changes identified include alterations in α1β1 integrin collagen receptor expression [28] and in the regulation of fibroblast apoptosis [29]. *In vitro* studies suggest that keloid keratinocytes influence keloid fibroblasts (and normal fibroblasts) to increase procollagen I and III gene and protein expression [30]. Gene expression arrays demonstrate that keloid keratinocytes exhibit an elevated expression of genes involved in wound healing, cell motility and angiogenesis, including VEGF [31]. Keloid tissue has increased M2 macrophages, mast cells and 'keloid-associated lymphoid tissue', suggesting that chronic inflammation perpetuates keloid growth [32].

Age-related changes in wound healing

Wounds even of a very substantial size created in certain lower vertebrates (e.g. amphibians) heal by complete regeneration. Similarly, wounds made in early (first trimester) embryos also heal by complete regeneration [1]. However, for wounds to heal in this way they tend to be made before the skin has established even a simple differentiated structure. During the second trimester, experimental studies in numerous animals have shown that late embryonic and early fetal dermal wounds heal with the absence of scarring, but without the regeneration of dermal appendages such as hair follicles or sebaceous glands [2]. This scar-free embryonic wound healing then gradually turns into a scarring healing phenotype during the last trimester and after birth. Scar-free embryonic wounds lack fibrin clots and platelet degranulation, have altered matrix components (including increased tenascin C and hyaluronic acid) and have a sparse, poorly differentiated inflammatory response with less dermal mast cells [3,4]. Consequently, the growth factor profile at the embryonic wound site is different, with reduced levels, for example, of TGF-β1 and TGF-β2, but increased levels of TGF-β3 [5]. These observations of scar-free fetal healing have led to experimental studies to manipulate TGF-β isoforms to try and mimic the fetal situation with good results [6]. A highly conserved RNA-binding protein, Lin26, which is expressed during embryogenesis, has been shown to promote the tissue repair of adult tissue by reprogramming cellular metabolism [7].

Interestingly, ageing during adult life also brings alterations to the wound healing process [8]. Many studies of human age-related changes in the wound healing profile are methodologically flawed because of failure to control for concurrent morbidity and disease. However, experimental investigations on health status in defined human subjects of varying ages have shown profound alterations in the wound healing process with age [8]. Wounds in elderly subjects heal more slowly, with a reduced inflammatory response, an altered cytokine profile and an increased level of active proteases [8–10]. Of major interest is the observation that, in normal ageing skin, the levels of proteases such as MMPs and elastase increase, while the levels of proteolytic inhibitors (e.g. TIMP) decrease, tipping the balance towards proteolytic digestion of the dermis [11]. This may account for some of the age-related changes seen in normal skin structure. It may also predispose certain individuals to ulcer formation, as chronic venous ulcers are characterised by an excessive proteolytic profile. By contrast, the quality of wound healing in elderly subjects is markedly improved with reduced scarring. In part, this correlates with the altered inflammatory and growth factor response, which to some extent mimics that seen in embryonic skin [8]. These ageing studies have also shown marked differences between how males and females heal their wounds, and between the healing of pre- and postmenopausal females [12,13]. In general, postmenopausal women heal more slowly but with a better scar quality than premenopausal women. The exogenous therapeutic addition of topical oestrogen to the healing wounds of postmenopausal women causes a marked acceleration of wound healing and reverses the age-related changes in speed and quality [14]. Selective oestrogen receptor modulators, such as tamoxifen, appear to act as oestrogen receptor agonists in the skin, accelerating cutaneous wound healing in a murine model [15]. Inhibition of microRNA-7 reverses an age-associated loss of EGF receptor and hyaluronan-dependent differentiation in fibroblasts [16]. These results have significant implications for the treatment of wounds in older individuals.

Physiological basis of the treatment of wounds

Healing by primary intention refers to wounds where the edges have been brought into apposition by sutures, which is possible when there is a good blood supply and no contamination or necrotic debris. Optimal healing requires the wound edges to be everted, carefully aligned and free from tension. Epidermis will cross the gap by 24 h, but by 5 days the tensile strength is only about 5% that of normal skin [1]. Thus, sutures help to take some tension off the wound. Buried absorbable sutures are helpful in reducing dead space and supporting the wound for longer, as the tensile strength is still only about 20% that of normal skin at 3 weeks. Staples or clips may be used for primary wound closure, especially postoperatively, and have the advantage of producing a good cosmetic result. Tissue adhesives and sterile skin closure strips may also be used, particularly for traumatic lacerations where sutures would increase tissue tension and threaten viability, and have the advantage of not requiring suture removal. See Chapter 20 for further detail about skin surgery.

Healing by secondary intention occurs when a wound is allowed to heal from the edge without surgical closure, so re-epithelialisation is a crucial process. This technique is often used when there is wound contamination and a risk of infection. The depth of the wound is critical to the manner of healing. In a partial-thickness wound, not only will part of the dermis remain intact, but retention of critical regions of hair follicles and other skin appendages will also provide a rapid source of epidermal regeneration. The density of skin appendages therefore influences the rate of healing. In contrast, full-thickness wounds will have lost dermal and appendageal components and can only be healed from the wound edge, requiring a stimulation of granulation tissue – a mixture of proliferating microvasculature, fibroblasts and the deposition of matrix components. Recent lineage studies demonstrated that there are two distinct mesenchymal fibroblast precursors in the skin during wound healing: the lower dermal lineage forming the reticular dermal fibroblasts, fibrillar matrix and adipocytes, and the upper dermal lineage forming the hair follicle, stimulated by epidermal β-catenin [2]. Wound contraction occurs after 1–2 weeks via activated fibroblasts or myofibroblasts, which decreases the surface area to be closed. Different body sites vary in the results of secondary intention healing, concave surfaces being better than convex, and the face being better than extremities. Tertiary intention healing refers to wounds that are closed to allow primary intention healing, but wound dehiscence occurs and the wound then heals by secondary intention.

In open wounds, the normal water-retaining properties of the skin are lost, and the inflammatory exudate on the surface dries to form a crust or scab. This acts as a barrier to external infection, but it prevents epidermal migration across the surface of the wound. A wound that is kept moist by an appropriate dressing will epithelialise faster than a wound that has been allowed to form a crust.

Accelerated epithelial healing under an occlusive, non-permeable dressing is associated with a gelatinous coagulum containing fibrin and fibronectin, which provides a suitable matrix for epidermal cell migration [3].

Chronic wounds are often caused by systemic diseases, including vascular disorders (e.g. congestive cardiac failure, hypertension, atherosclerosis, venous insufficiency or lymphoedema), as well as metabolic disorders (e.g. chronic renal failure, chronic liver disease or diabetes). Poor nutritional status, infection, mechanical pressure and drugs may also play a detrimental role in wound healing. Many of these factors are more likely to be present in the elderly.

Novel therapies for wound healing

Growth factors to augment wound healing

All cells involved in the wound healing process (inflammatory cells, epidermal keratinocytes and mesenchymal cells) can synthesise a wide range of membrane-bound and free growth factors, whose effects are mediated by specific growth factor receptors for each family of growth factor. Growth factors are multifunctional and have differing effects on different cell types, and can induce expression of other cytokines and their receptors in an autocrine and paracrine fashion. Growth factor activity can also be regulated via extracellular matrix components and proteolytic activation. The addition of exogenous growth factors in pharmacological amounts may have measurable effects in wound healing models but can be disappointing in the clinical arena [1–3]. Furthermore, elevated MMPs and bacterial superinfection of wounds may completely obliterate any possibility of a useful therapeutic response from exogenous growth factors because of rapid degradation of the recombinant protein [4]. Bioengineering of protease-resistant growth factors is a possible solution to this problem [5].

In animal models, a number of growth factors have positive effects on granulation tissue formation and angiogenesis, including PDGF, FGFs and TGF-β [6,7]. EGF family members appear to enhance re-epithelialisation, as well as having mesenchymal effects [8–10]. Repifermin, a truncated form of recombinant KGF-2 (FGF-10), showed promise in a phase IIA randomised clinical trial on venous ulcers, but in a subsequent trial failed to meet its primary end-point [11]. PDGF-BB (becaplermin gel) is currently the only licensed recombinant growth factor for treating recalcitrant wounds and its usefulness in the management of chronic neuropathic diabetic ulcers has been demonstrated in clinical trials [12]. However, use of becaplermin is limited by cost and the requirement for daily application, and controversy about an increased risk of cancer. A recent matched cohort study showed no evidence of increased cancer mortality in patients using becaplermin gel compared with matched controls [13]. A 115 amino acid fragment, F5, of the secreted heat shock protein 90α has a greater effect than becaplermin gel on re-epithelialisation of wounds in the db/db mouse model of diabetes through its effect on keratinocytes, fibroblasts and endothelial cells suggesting this may be a promising drug for wound healing (Figure 11.6) [14].

Stem cell therapy

Recent advances in stem cell biology provide promise for new therapeutic strategies for wound healing. Several types of stem

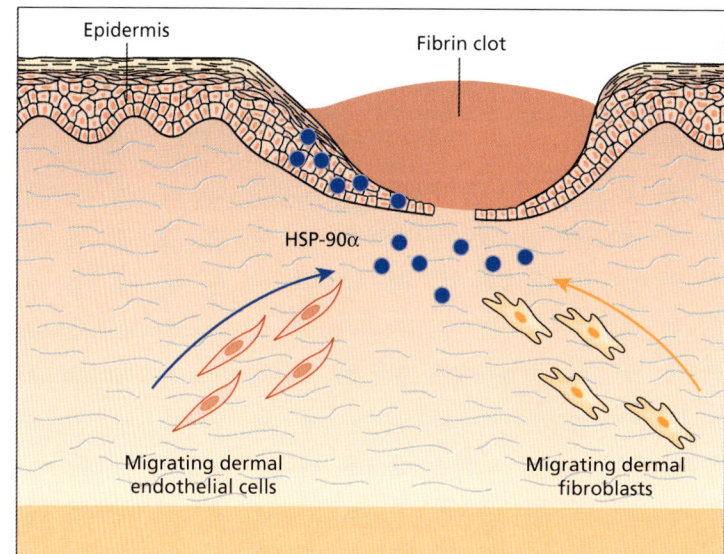

Figure 11.6 Model of how secreted heat shock protein 90α (HSP-90α) promotes wound repair. Injury to the skin triggers the release of transforming growth factor β (TGF-β) from several sources, and keratinocytes become more motile and release conventional growth factors. However, the growth factors will not be able to recruit the dermal cells at the wound edge to the wound bed due to the presence of TGF-β. When the keratinocytes are migrating, they release/secrete HSP-90α. When the secreted HSP-90α reaches a concentration of >0.1 μmol/L, it will drive migration of fibroblasts and endothelial cells into the wound.

cells have been studied in preclinical and clinical settings including bone-marrow-derived stem cells, adipose tissue-derived stem cells, endothelial progenitor cells and keratinocyte and fibroblast stem cells [1,2]. Strategies to mobilise bone marrow stem cells (such as high mobility group box 1 (HMGB1)) as well as direct topical application are the subject of intense preclinical research [3]. Bone marrow transplantation improved wound healing dramatically in the rare skin disease recessive dystrophic epidermolysis bullosa, most likely due to bone marrow stem cells [4]. A single topical application of a direct antagonist of C-X-C chemokine receptor type 4, AMD3100, has been shown to increase wound healing in diabetic mice. This was associated with increased numbers of bone marrow endothelial precursor cells, increased cytokine production and increased activity of fibroblasts and macrophages [5]. Combining AMD3100 with low-dose topical tacrolimus had a synergistic effect resulting in more rapid wound repair of full-thickness wounds (Figure 11.7) [6,7].

Tissue engineering

For pinch grafts, small (2–3 mm²) pieces of partial-thickness skin can be removed under local anaesthetic, as an out-patient procedure or by a specialist nurse within the home, and planted across the wound bed to form islands for re-epithelialisation with greatly increased healing. The time-consuming nature of the procedure is the major problem, but repeated grafts can be performed, and the donor sites heal very rapidly. The approach may benefit both arterial and venous leg ulcers and its suitability for primary care settings has been demonstrated [1]. For split-thickness skin grafts, a large sheet of partial-thickness skin is removed using a dermatome. The plane of cleavage may be variable, either within the papillary or reticular dermis. The graft is usually meshed before application as this tends to reduce the chances of the graft subsequently detaching as a result

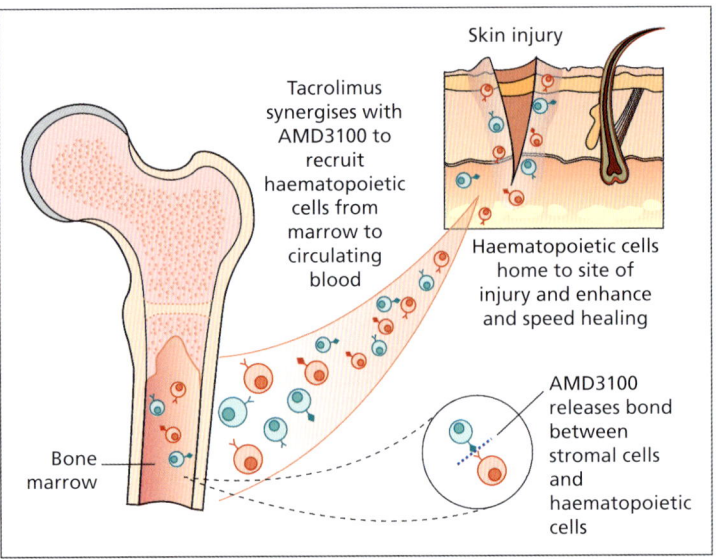

Figure 11.7 Better and faster skin wound healing is achieved by the combined action of AMD3100 and tacrolimus. AMD3100 interferes with the interaction of the CXC chemokine receptor 4 (CXCR4) and its ligand CXC motif chemokine 12 (CXCL12) and releases bone marrow cells into the peripheral blood. Tacrolimus inhibits calcium-dependent T-cell activation and expansion. This novel approach for boosting innate healing potential, in which blood cells are mobilised and engaged in productive skin repair, is further evidence of systemically administered bone marrow cells migrating to injured skin and contributing to its repair. Adapted from Tolar and McGrath 2014 [7].

of the wound exudate. Split-thickness skin graft donor sites are often painful.

The feasibility of growing human keratinocytes in culture was first established in 1975 [2] and the possibility of expanding a small donor site up to 10 000-fold led to the application of cultured keratinocytes for grafting [3]. Use of Rho kinase inhibitors can allow further expansion of keratinocyte cultures [4]. Grafts established from the patient's own skin (autografts) or from allogeneic donors (allografts) have subsequently been formulated for clinical use.

The earliest clinical use was to treat major burns patients, and the translucent sheets became a permanent stable epidermis, visible after 12–14 days [5]. The resulting graft remained fragile and remodelling of the dermis occurred slowly [6]. Without a well-vascularised dermis, cultured keratinocytes alone are of limited use, and provision of a dermal equivalent in the graft on the wound bed appears to enhance graft take [7]. Cultured epidermal autografts have also been used to treat epidermolysis bullosa wounds [8], wound beds of congenital naevi [9] and chronic leg ulcers [10], where repeated grafting from passaged cultures is a major advantage. Preparation of a cultured keratinocyte sheet can take 2–3 weeks (Figure 11.8). Keratinocytes can also be suspended in fibrin and sprayed onto wounds or delivered on polymer carrier systems, such as hyaluronate membranes, allowing earlier grafting than previously possible [11,12]. Allografts of cultured keratinocytes do not survive long term [13,14], but have been shown to have a wound healing effect in chronic leg ulcers [15], probably because of the production of appropriate growth factors and extracellular matrix proteins.

The field of tissue engineering to generate skin in the laboratory using keratinocytes, fibroblasts, growth factors and biomaterials has advanced considerably [16]. Available products can be categorised into three groups: (i) epidermal substitutes; (ii) dermal substitutes; and (iii) combined epidermal and dermal substitutes (Figure 11.9). Full-thickness wounds require the replacement of both the epidermis and dermis. Current skin substitutes lack a vascular plexus or appendageal structures. Pluripotent stem cells, such as mesenchymal cells from bone marrow and adipose tissue, are recruited into the dermis during wound healing [17,18]. Gene-corrected autologous keratinocyte skin grafts were used to successfully restore large areas of skin in junctional epidermolysis bullosa and are stable at 5 year follow-up [19]. Human pluripotent stem cells can now be manipulated to produce a skin organoid containing hair follicles and nerves, producing hope for complete skin regeneration in the future [20].

Topical application of the basement membrane component, type VII collagen, increases re-epithelialisation in mouse wounds [21]. The development of synthetic polymers with incorporated matrix and cells should be possible in the future. Micropatterning

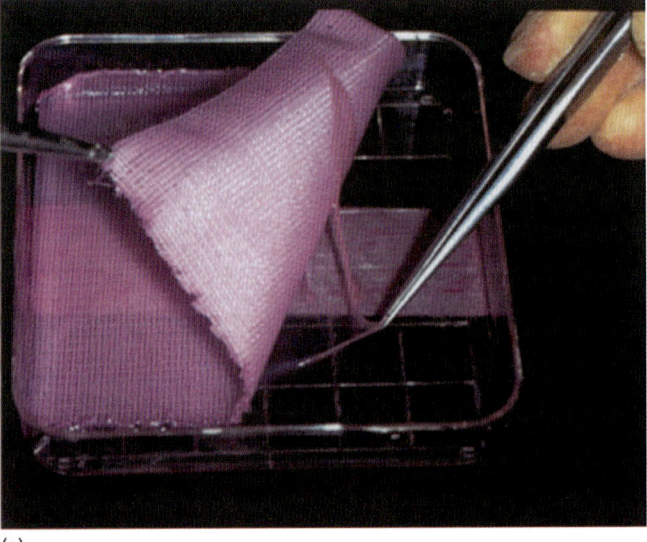

(a)

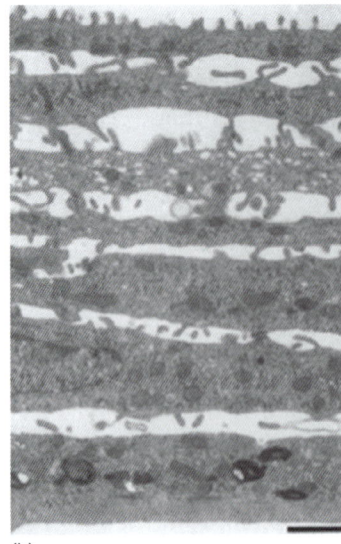

(b)

Figure 11.8 Keratinocyte grafting. (a) Sheet of cultured keratinocytes for grafting (b) Ultrastructure of keratinocyte graft. Scale bar 1 µm. Courtesy of Professor John McGrath, King's College London, UK.

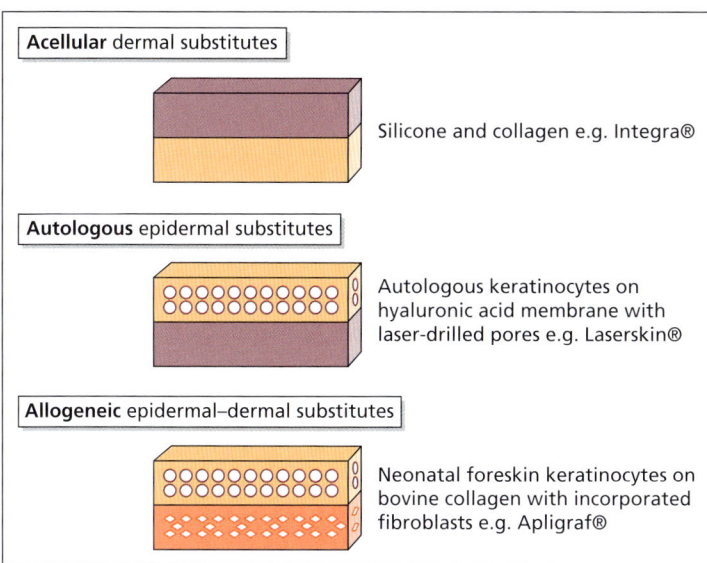

Figure 11.9 Examples of biological skin substitutes.

of polymers may also enhance re-epithelialisation by enhancing regeneration from stem cells and promoting keratinocyte and fibroblast migration [22].

Key references

The full list of references can be found in the online version at https://www.wiley.com/rooksdermatology10e

Introduction
13 Hoyle NP, Seinkmane E *et al*. Circadian actin dynamics drive rhythmic fibroblast mobilization during wound healing. *Sci Transl Med* 2017;9(415):eaal2774.

Inflammation and the immune response
13 Constantinides MG, Link VM, Tamoutounour S *et al*. MAIT cells are imprinted by the microbiota in early life and promote tissue repair. *Science* 2019;366(6464):eaax6624.

Re-epithelialisation
3 Maruthappu T, Chikh A, Fell B *et al*. Rhomboid family member 2 regulates cytoskeletal stress associated Keratin 16. *Nat Commun* 2017;8:14174.

Angiogenesis
9 Gurevich DB, Severn CE, Twomey C *et al*. Live imaging of wound angiogenesis reveals macrophage orchestrated vessel sprouting and regression. *EMBO J* 2018;37:e97786.

Fibroblast recruitment, matrix synthesis and scarring
3 Philippeos C, Telerman SB, Oulès B *et al*. Spatial and single-cell transcriptional profiling identifies functionally distinct human dermal fibroblast subpopulations. *J Invest Dermatol* 2018;138:811–25.
11 Martins VL, Caley M, O'Toole EA. Matrix metalloproteinases and epidermal wound repair. *Cell Tissue Res* 2013;351:255–68.

Abnormal wound healing and scarring
4 Willenborg S, Eming SA. Macrophages – sensors and effectors coordinating skin damage and repair. *J Dtsch Dermatol Ges* 2014;12:214–21.
19 Sawaya AP, Stone RC, Brooks SR *et al*. Deregulated immune cell recruitment orchestrated by FOXM1 impairs human diabetic wound healing. *Nat Commun* 2020;11:4678.

Novel therapies for wound healing
Tissue engineering
19 Lee J, Rabbani CC, Gao H *et al*. Hair-bearing human skin generated entirely from pluripotent stem cells. *Nature* 2020;582(7812):399–404.
20 Kueckelhaus M, Rothoeft T, De Rosa L *et al*. Transgenic epidermal cultures for junctional epidermolysis bullosa – 5-year outcomes. *N Engl J Med* 2021;385:2264–70.

CHAPTER 12

Topical Drug Delivery

Richard H. Guy[1] and Adrian F. Davis[2]

[1]Department of Pharmacy and Pharmacology, University of Bath, Bath, UK
[2]Limeway Pharma Design Ltd, Dorking, UK

Introduction: skin barrier function, 12.1	Efficiency of topical drug delivery – what fraction of the 'dose' is absorbed?, 12.4	Assessment of topical drug bioavailability and bioequivalence between formulations, 12.7
Penetration pathways: mechanisms of percutaneous absorption, 12.1	Patient-centred optimisation of topical dermatological products, 12.4	*In vitro* methods, 12.7
The relationship between drug structure/properties and skin permeation, 12.2	Formulation design and choosing the right dose, 12.5	*In vivo* approaches, 12.7
Topical drug formulations used to treat dermatological disease, 12.3	Optimisation of dermatological drug delivery – options available, 12.5	Conclusion, 12.8
		Key references, 12.9

Introduction: skin barrier function

The delivery of drugs to dermatological targets in the skin is in large part controlled, and indeed limited, by the barrier function of the stratum corneum (SC). The ability of a topical drug formulation designed to alleviate skin disease is therefore directly dependent on the composition and structural organisation of the SC and the physical chemical mechanisms involved in the uptake of the active compound from the vehicle and its subsequent diffusion to the site(s) of action.

The SC impedes molecular transport either from the 'inside–out', as in the case of water, or from the 'outside–in' with respect to topically contacting drugs or other foreign substances. Microscopically, the SC is often compared with a 'brick wall', with the corneocytes representing the bricks and the intercellular lipids the cement (Figure 12.1) [1,2,3]. Corneo-desmosomes act as bridges holding corneocytes together until their controlled enzymatic degradation towards the SC surface provokes (the roughly daily) desquamation of the outer cell layer. The effectiveness of the SC to limit transepidermal water loss (TEWL) is demonstrated easily by measuring the rate of water 'escape' across the skin as the outer layers of corneocytes are progressively removed by adhesive tape stripping, with TEWL increasing by about an order of magnitude once the barrier has been fully deranged [4].

Similar tape stripping experiments have also shown that the SC presents the principal barrier to drug penetration following topical application. Exceptions to this general rule are limited to very lipophilic compounds which, although taken up into the SC quite easily, are then limited in their entry into the underlying, viable epidermal tissue by their unfavourable partitioning and very low solubility in this predominantly aqueous environment.

Penetration pathways: mechanisms of percutaneous absorption

The 'brick and mortar' model of the SC offers two obvious, potential pathways for penetration across the barrier (Figure 12.1) [5,6]: (a) transcellularly, involving the most direct route and multiple transfers of the permeant between corneocytes and interstitial lipids, and (b) intercellularly, a tortuous route constraining transport uniquely to the lipid 'cement' between the bricks. In addition, the opportunity for topically contacting chemicals to access apparent 'shunt' paths, involving the skin appendages (and, in particular, the follicles), represents a further alternative.

As no active transport mechanism across the SC has been identified, and accepting therefore that percutaneous absorption involves passive diffusion, molecules must follow the path of least resistance across the barrier. At face value, the transcellular route appears most likely: it has the largest surface area and volume available for transport and the path length is short (*c*.0.01 mm). In contrast, the intercellular lipid domains comprise only about 15% of the SC volume and, given the flattened corneocyte dimensions, the path length around the cells is closer to 0.5 mm (i.e. 50 times longer than transcellularly).

However, a combination of elegant analytical chemistry, electron microscopy and biophysical research in the 1980s and early 1990s has led to a consensus that the intercellular route is, in fact, the dominant pathway. Unravelling the composition and arrangement of the SC intercellular lipids was a key first step in reaching this conclusion [1,2,3]. The absence of phospholipids and the presence of an array of ceramides were important and noteworthy features and their precise organisation, with the approximately equimolar quantities of fatty acids and cholesterol, into two distinct lamellar

---

Rook's Textbook of Dermatology, Tenth Edition. Edited by Christopher Griffiths, Jonathan Barker, Tanya Bleiker, Walayat Hussain and Rosalind Simpson.
© 2024 John Wiley & Sons Ltd. Published 2024 by John Wiley & Sons Ltd.

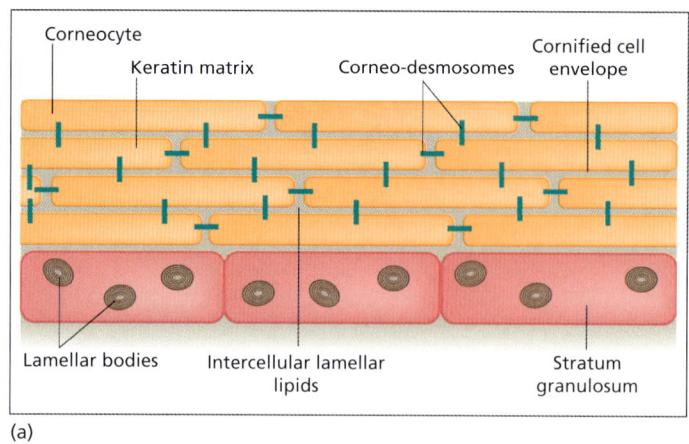
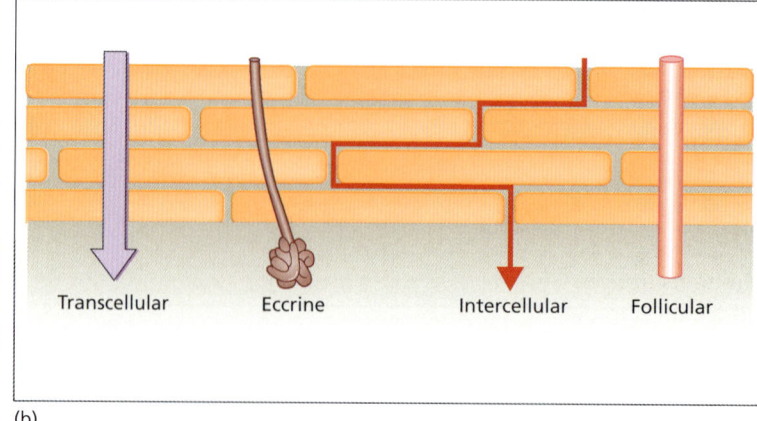

Figure 12.1 (a) A schematic representation of the stratum corneum (SC) as a brick wall. (b) Potential penetration pathways across the SC. Adapted from [5,6].

phases immediately suggested a more important role for these domains than that of a simple 'filler' in between the bricks. It was then noted, in an attempt to visualise chemical penetration across the SC *in situ*, that the permeating molecules were indeed localised to the intercellular spaces, reinforcing the impression that transport might be constrained to these lipid-rich regions. This led to a defining and confirmatory study that demonstrated that water permeability through the SC was highly correlated with the conformational order of the intercellular lipid domains: as the lipids became progressively disordered by increasing temperature, the permeation of water increased concomitantly. In addition, even as the lipids went through a phase transition (and became markedly more disordered), the permeation of water was enhanced in a correspondingly discontinuous way (Figure 12.2) [7,8]. The inescapable conclusion from these data was that the path of diffusion for water through the SC was via the intercellular lipids. This deduction was reinforced in a further series of experiments that independently assessed the path length of transport to be more than 50-fold greater than the SC thickness.

In terms of appendageal transport, a variety of experimental data point to two common features: (i) the hair follicles, in particular, appear to offer more rapid, 'shunt' pathways circumventing the SC barrier; and (ii) the capacity of the pathway is limited by the low density of follicles on most body sites. As a result, although the first molecules reaching the viable skin layers after the application of a topical drug formulation, for example, may well have diffused via the available hair follicles [1,2,3], the overall contribution to delivery at a 'steady state' (when transport across the SC will have caught up, so to speak) is small.

The relationship between drug structure/properties and skin permeation

The absorption of a chemical into the skin depends upon its physicochemical properties, its presentation to the skin (i.e. the 'vehicle' in which it is applied), the skin 'environment' (i.e. skin condition, disease state, etc.) and the duration of exposure.

The permeation of a specific molecule may be expressed in terms of its flux (J) across the SC [9], defined as:

$$J = k_p \times C_v = (D \times K_{sc/v}/h) \times C_v \qquad \text{(eqn 12.1)}$$

where C_v is the concentration of the compound in the vehicle in which it is applied, and k_p is its permeability coefficient across the skin when it is applied in that vehicle. The units of J are amount per unit area per unit time (e.g. µg/cm^2/h). k_p has units of velocity (e.g. cm/h) and depends on the chemical's diffusivity (D) across the SC, its partition coefficient between the SC lipids and the vehicle in which it is applied ($K_{sc/v}$) and its path length of diffusion across the SC (h). If the vehicle does not interact with the skin in any way (for example, to alter its structure or composition), and does not change the drug's solubility in the SC, then the maximum flux of the compound (J_{max}) is achieved when it is applied at a concentration equal to its saturation solubility in the formulation ($C_{v,sat}$):

$$J_{max} = k_p \times C_{v,sat} \qquad \text{(eqn 12.2)}$$

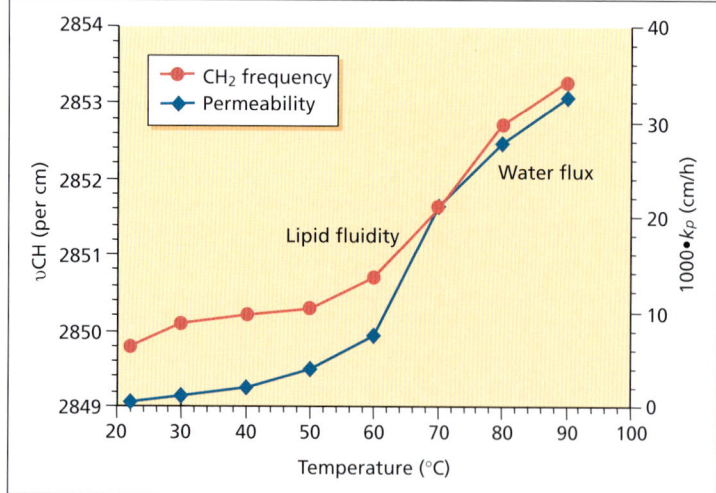

Figure 12.2 Correlation between the permeability coefficient (k_p) of water across the stratum corneum (SC) with the conformational order of the SC intercellular lipid domains (as measured by the frequency of the asymmetrical methylene group vibration (υCH_2)) as a function of increasing temperature. Adapted from [7,8].

The permeability coefficients of a large number of drugs and other chemicals from water have been determined experimentally and this has permitted a simple algorithm to estimate k_p (in units of cm/h) from water to be derived [9] and validated:

$$\log k_p = -2.7 + 0.71 \times \log P - 0.0061 \times MW \quad \text{(eqn 12.3)}$$

where P is the octanol–water partition coefficient of the chemical and MW is its molecular weight (in Daltons). The log P and MW are readily available physicochemical parameters of the permeant, the first defining its lipophilicity (a very commonly used metric in pharmaceutical development to assess a molecule's ability to be absorbed across lipid barriers), the second describing its size, and hence the rate at which it is able to diffuse.

Equation 12.3 assumes (as is typically the case) that the SC is the rate-determining barrier for percutaneous absorption. However, as noted earlier, for very lipophilic compounds penetration is controlled by their ability to partition/dissolve into the viable skin layers. In this case, the value of k_p predicted by equation 12.3 must be corrected [9]:

$$k_{p,corr} = k_p / (1 + (k_p \times MW^{1/2})/2.6) \quad \text{(eqn 12.4)}$$

An estimate of J_{max} for a chemical is now possible using equation 12.2, with $k_{p,corr}$ determined from equations 12.3 and 12.4 and its water solubility (i.e. $C_{water,sat}$). The latter is frequently determined in the course of drug development, or (like log P, in fact) can be calculated using any one of a number of available algorithms.

Estimated J_{max} values for the 91 drugs currently approved for topical and transdermal administration, in either Europe or the USA (or both), are presented in Figure 12.3 as a function of MW. As anticipated by equation 12.3, drug flux is inversely dependent upon MW; furthermore, within a group of compounds of approximately similar MW, J_{max} increases with increasing lipophilicity (log P). Notably, the majority of topical and transdermal drugs manifest rather modest maximum flux rates across the skin (the dotted horizontal line in Figure 12.3 signifying a J_{max} of only 1 µg cm^{-2} h^{-1}), and attest to the considerable pharmacological potency of these compounds.

Topical drug formulations used to treat dermatological disease

Broadly speaking, current topical formulations can be categorised as follows [10,11]:

1 *Hydrocarbon-based formulations.* For chronic skin disease, these formulations are preferred for their occlusive and protective properties. However, while useful as emollients, the value of these vehicles as topical release systems is limited by poor drug solubility. The latter can be enhanced by using a formulation with hydrocarbon-miscible solvents such as isopropyl myristate or propylene glycol. For example, high potency 0.05% clobetasol propionate ointment contains the partition coefficient enhancer propylene glycol dispersed in a liquid paraffin base. These anhydrous formulations are usually rather inelegant, sticky, greasy, white or off-white ointments, providing high occlusion of the skin. They are typically used to treat psoriasis, chronic eczema and mycosis, involving small areas of application to dry or very dry skin.

2 *Polar gel formulations.* These are more elegant single-phase systems. They are usually water- and/or alcohol-based (hydrogel, hydro-alcoholic gel) with low or no lipid content. Fluocinolone acetonide gel, 0.025%, contains the active ingredient dissolved in a propylene glycol/ethanol/water co-solvent system gelled with a carbomer carboxy-vinyl polymer. Physically, the gels are transparent to opaque semi-solid gels, rapidly absorbed, non-greasy, non-occlusive and may elicit a skin 'cooling' effect upon application. These gels are used to treat acne, acute eczema, rosacea and allergic skin conditions (but are not favoured for psoriasis and chronic eczema) and are applied to small areas of oily or inflamed skin (e.g. on the face). There is a variety of gelling agents available (such as cellulose derivatives, polysaccharide gums and acrylate polymers, such as carbomers) allowing the creation of diverse formulations. Variations of this vehicle class include hydrogels containing a dispersed lipid phase, a so-called emulsion gel or emulgel, and suspensions of water-insoluble drugs in hydrogels (suspension gel).

3 *Creams.* Creams are dispersed systems – that is, emulsions – and represent the majority of aqueous-based topical formulations. Cream formulations of corticosteroids include those containing clobetasol propionate, betamethasone valerate, fluocinolone acetonide, fluticasone propionate and mometasone furoate. The readily adjustable properties of these vehicles have led to their wide application in dermatological therapy. Creams require 'emulsifiers' (i.e. surfactants) to stabilise the mixture of oil and water phases; the dispersion of oil droplets in water or water droplets in oil is complicated and the arrangement of emulsifier films at the oil–water interface determines the internal structure (crystalline or liquid–crystalline regions, hexagonal or lamellar structures, etc.) of these formulations. Water acts as either the outer, continuous phase (oil-in-water, o/w emulsion) or the inner, discontinuous phase (water-in-oil, w/o emulsion). The latter blends easily with SC lipids, improving the bioavailability

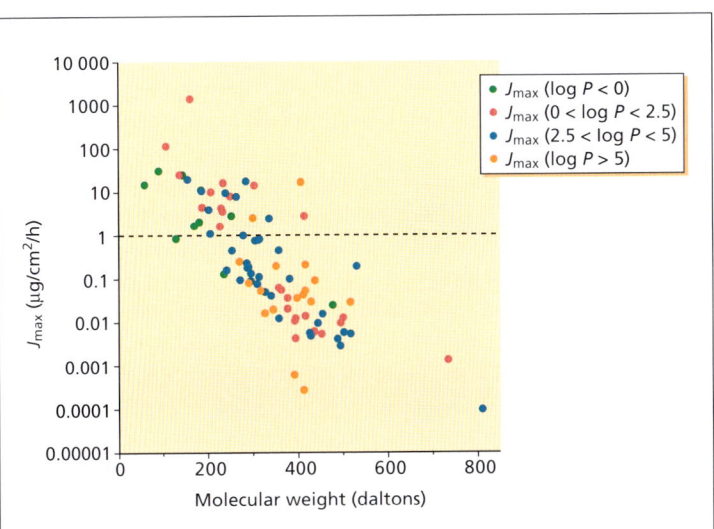

Figure 12.3 Estimated maximum flux (J_{max}) values for approved topical and transdermal drugs as a function of their size (molecular weight).

of lipid-soluble drugs and moisturising the skin via a modest occlusive effect. The continuous lipid phase typically comprises triglycerides or waxes. These white to off-white emulsions have a high lipid-replenishing effect and are applied to broad areas of normal to dry skin, treating diseases such as psoriasis, chronic eczema and mycosis. The former (o/w emulsions) are more cosmetically appealing (less sticky and greasy) as the lipids therein are finely dispersed and contact of the outer aqueous phase with the skin increases water evaporation, producing a cooling effect after application (however, it should also be noted that the surfactant-like emulsifiers in o/w emulsions can withdraw moisture from the skin and facilitate both SC lipid extraction and perturbation). These formulations are hydrating, milky white, spreadable emulsions, suitable for application to large skin areas (both normal, slightly dry and inflamed) affected by acne and acute and subacute eczema.

4 *Other dispersed systems for specific applications*. These more complex formulations include (i) those that are created with vesicular structures, such as liposomes or niosomes, based on phospholipids and non-ionic surfactants, respectively; (ii) multiple, nano- and microemulsions, which require relatively high levels of surfactant to maintain their stability; and (iii) sprays, foams and lacquers, the latter being most typically used in treating diseases of the nail.

Efficiency of topical drug delivery – what fraction of the 'dose' is absorbed?

The amount of drug in a topical dermatological product is usually described as the percentage concentration of the active ingredient in the formulation. As formulations are applied, typically, in milligram amounts per cm^2 of skin, a 1% hydrocortisone cream might be better described from a clinical perspective as containing 0.01 mg of drug per mg of the formulation. Of course, the dose applied is both a function of the concentration of drug in the formulation and of the amount of formulation applied per unit area of skin. Application of 5% acyclovir cream at 2.5 mg of cream per cm^2 of skin therefore equates to a drug dose of 0.125 mg/cm^2 of skin (= 0.05 mg/mg × 2.5 mg/cm^2).

As discussed previously, drug delivery across the skin is quantified in terms of flux, which is measured, for example, in units of $\mu g\ cm^{-2}\ h^{-1}$. It follows that a more transparent assessment of topical bioavailability is made on the basis of both the dose applied and the dose absorbed over time. In the case of aciclovir permeating human skin after application of several 5% creams, fluxes in the range of 0.01–0.05 $\mu g\ cm^{-2}\ h^{-1}$ have been reported [12]. Assuming that such fluxes were sustained over 12 h, then the drug absorbed following administration of 2.5 mg of a 5% cream per cm^2 of skin would be 0.12–0.60 $\mu g\ cm^{-2}$; that is, only about 0.1–0.6% of the applied dose. This observation is at the lower end of reported absolute bioavailabilities, which are typically 1–2% and rarely much higher. As a result, most of the applied drug is 'wasted' [13] and often the amount absorbed is poorly correlated with that applied. To make matters worse, dosing intervals are typically based on consumer habits/convenience and derived from oral drug usage and, generally, have little or no basis in science.

Although, as described in the next section, formulation can have significant effects in clinical practice, the skin, and not the formulation, controls the dose absorbed for the majority of topical formulations. This lack of formulation control means that skin site and skin condition are the major factors which determine the potential risk of local and systemic adverse effects. For example, the use of topical corticosteroids on the face and anogenital regions is contraindicated because local adverse effects are much more common at these permeable skin sites. Similarly, topical corticosteroid application in children with extensive, severe eczema, where the skin barrier is damaged, can lead to systemic adverse effects on adrenal function [14].

The poor efficiency of topical drug delivery is a far from novel observation, of course. It has been recognised for some time that, as the amount of drug applied is increased – by increasing either drug concentration or the amount of formulation applied – it is common for the amount of drug absorbed to remain relatively constant. As a result, dose titration, which is essential to optimise clinical response when there is large variation between subjects in skin pharmacodynamics and/or skin pharmacokinetics, may be difficult or impossible. The need to address this issue (and driven by the recognised side effects of topical steroids highlighted previously) was recognised over 50 years ago and there have been repeated calls for dosing rationalisation to stipulate suitable therapeutic regimens involving minimally effective doses at the skin target without local and/or systemic adverse effects. A telling observation from 1974 was that 'concentrations of active substances in practically all topicals are in the range 1 to 3% suggesting the influence of fashion rather than of a rigorous appraisal' [15]. More recently, it has been argued that [16] 'The arbitrary and empirical selection of antimicrobial concentration would be unacceptable for systemically administered drugs and should also be so for topical therapies'. Yet, still today, irrational dosing is the norm and clinical performance is adversely affected.

Patient-centred optimisation of topical dermatological products

Adherence to the use of topical dermatological products is disappointingly low [17] and is the result of a number of factors, namely:

- Those relating to the patient (social, economic, psychological).
- Those associated with the health care system and with interactions between the patient and health care professionals.
- Disease-related factors.
- Those pertaining to formulation design, specifically dissatisfaction with efficacy or onset of efficacy, local and systemic adverse effects (or fear of these), posology and consumer experience in use.

With respect to formulation design, the first three factors relate to drug delivery and biopharmaceuticals, areas that are underpinned by design skills in the pharmaceutical industry; the fourth represents essentially the domain of cosmetic sciences and emphasises its crucial role, when integrated with 'medicines design', in the improvement of patient adherence to topical dosing regimens.

Formulation design and choosing the right dose

Assume, for clinical efficacy, that the concentration of drug at the target site in the viable skin must reach a threshold, effective level of C^*. This may be equal, for example, to an IC_{50} or IC_{90} concentration determined in preclinical development. If the drug product is formulated correctly and dosed repeatedly to the skin, then it should be possible to deliver a fairly steady average flux (J^*) that satisfies the relationship

$$J^* = P_D \times C^* \qquad \text{(eqn 12.5)}$$

where P_D is a measure of the 'clearance' of drug from its site of action and can be equated to the ratio of its diffusivity in the viable skin (D_D) to the distance (h_D) it must travel before encountering, and being removed by, the dermal microcirculation [18].

This concept has been validated [18] using aciclovir and extended to a wide range of drug classes and to different targets in the skin [19]. For antiviral activity, the required J^* for aciclovir has been estimated to be about $1.25\,\mu g\,cm^{-2}\,h^{-1}$ (or $30\,\mu g\,cm^{-2}\,day^{-1}$) but typical, measured fluxes of the drug across human skin from various 5% creams are at best only $0.01–0.05\,\mu g\,cm^{-2}\,h^{-1}$ [12], a result consistent with observed (poor) clinical outcomes. Equally pertinent is the simple calculation from the required J^* that the twice-daily application of aciclovir should deliver $15\,\mu g\,cm^{-2}$. Assuming that this is achieved by the normal application of 2.5 mg of cream, then it is simple to calculate the minimum dose of aciclovir required in the cream to sustain C^* at the target level, i.e. $(0.015\,mg/2.5\,mg) \times 100\% = 0.6\%$, indicating – as is well-known – that a substantial amount of drug in existing formulations is completely wasted (and unnecessary).

Optimisation of dermatological drug delivery – options available

To optimise the use of dermatological medicines (i.e. drug plus delivery system) [10,11], a useful starting point is to revisit the earlier discussion of a drug's flux (J) across the skin. Equation 12.1 shows that J is directly dependent upon the product of the compound's SC/vehicle partition coefficient ($K_{sc/v}$) and its concentration in the vehicle (C_v). The partition coefficient, of course, is a measure of the drug's relative affinity for the SC as compared with that for the vehicle and, as such, can be expressed as the ratio of its solubilities in these two phases, that is:

$$K_{sc/v} = C_{sc,sat}/C_{v,sat} \qquad \text{(eqn 12.6)}$$

Substitution of equation 12.6 into equation 12.1 and re-arranging yields:

$$J = DS \times C_{sc,sat} \times (D/h) \qquad \text{(eqn 12.7)}$$

where $DS = C_v/C_{v,sat}$, the degree of saturation of the drug in the vehicle. The form of equation 12.7 reveals three formulation options for improving drug delivery into the skin:
- Increase DS to as close to 1 as possible (i.e. aim to make $C_v = C_{v,sat}$).
- Introduce an excipient, which itself partitions into the SC, and permits $C_{sc,sat}$ to be increased.
- Add a penetration enhancer that increases drug diffusivity (D) across the SC.

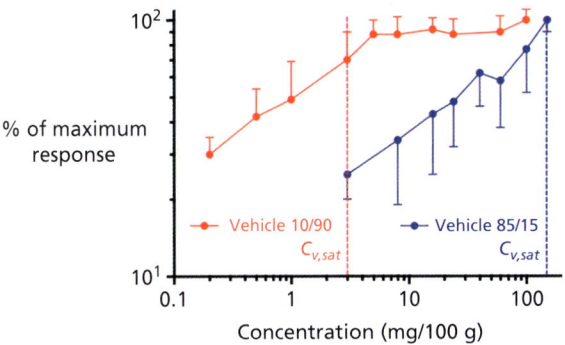

Figure 12.4 Dose–vasoconstriction response profiles for betamethasone 17-benzoate following application in vehicles comprising 10:90 (red) and 85:15 (blue) v/v mixtures of neutral oil and mineral oil. Data redrawn from [21].

Option 1 – use of simple saturated solutions

From a thermodynamic, drug delivery point of view, this strategy is straightforward in concept. However, to sustain a target flux is impossible when $C_{v,sat}$ is very small. To solve this problem, combinations of solvents, in one of which the drug is significantly more soluble than the other, have been used [20] and the approach has been particularly applied to the formulation of corticosteroids. Figure 12.4 illustrates the idea and shows the vasoconstriction response to betamethasone 17-benzoate as a function of the drug concentration in two formulations comprising neutral oil and mineral oil in ratios (v/v) of either 10:90 or 85:15, respectively [21]. The drug's solubility in the 10:90 vehicle is $2.8\,mg/100\,g$; that in the 85:15 mixture is $150\,mg/100\,g$.

When the drug concentrations are below the solubilities in the two vehicles (i.e. to the left of the dashed vertical lines in Figure 12.4), there is an evident and essentially linear dose–response behaviour. However, for the 10:90 formulation, as the drug concentration is increased beyond the saturation solubility, there is no significant further change in vasoconstriction response to the six suspensions containing $5–100\,mg/100\,mg$. This makes sense, of course, because – as indicated in equation 12.7 – the degree of saturation (DS) of the drug is the same (and equal to 1) in all suspensions; the presence of excess solid makes no significant contribution to drug delivery. It follows that understanding dose–response is an imperative for optimal dermatological therapy.

A further teaching of equation 12.7, at least in theory, is that formulations in which $C_v/C_{v,sat}$ (= DS) is greater than 1 would enable drug delivery rates in excess of J_{max}. Such so-called supersaturated systems can be prepared under controlled conditions and (as discussed later) can be formed extemporaneously during application of a formulation but suffer from inherent instability. Approaches by which DS may be maintained above 1 for more than a transient period have been, and continue to be, explored.

Option 2 – use of saturated solutions containing partitioning enhancers

Propylene glycol (PG) is a co-solvent excipient that is frequently present in topical formulations at quite high levels. When the vehicle is applied, the co-solvent not only influences the drug's solubility and its partitioning into the SC, it also transfers itself from the administered delivery system into the skin. The physicochemical properties of co-solvents are such that they are typically

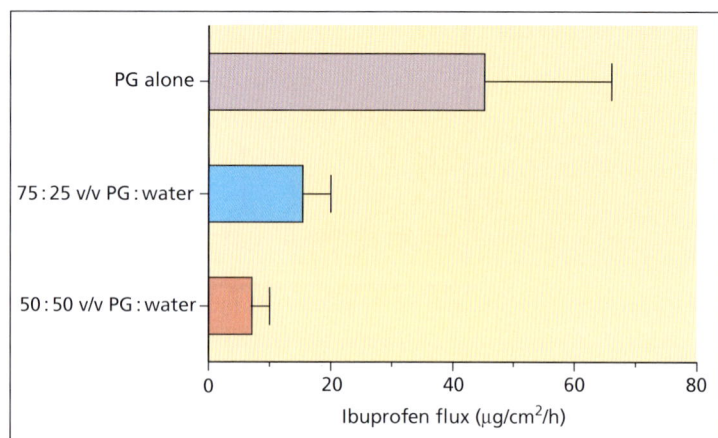

Figure 12.5 Flux of ibuprofen into human stratum corneum *in vivo* from three formulations in which the drug was present at its saturation concentration. PG, propylene glycol. Adapted from [22].

well absorbed into the SC. Having done so, they are then capable of changing the drug's solubility in this outer layer of the skin [22]; that is, one key principle, upon which equation 12.7 was derived (i.e. the assumption that the vehicle has no impact on the drug's solubility in the SC), is violated and drug delivery can therefore be increased. Figure 12.5 illustrates this point for the delivery of ibuprofen into human SC *in vivo* from three formulations in which the drug was saturated: 50:50 v/v PG:water, 75:25 v/v PG:water and PG alone [22]. The ideal analysis developed mathematically earlier predicts that drug flux from the three vehicles should have been identical. In fact, with increasing PG, ibuprofen availability increased, relative to the 50:50 PG:water formulation, by about 2- and 6.5-fold, respectively, for 75:25 PG:water and PG alone.

Option 3 – use of saturated solutions containing partitioning and diffusion enhancers

The other assumption inherent in the derivation of equation 12.7 is that the formulation composition has no effect on drug diffusivity (D) across the SC. However, the transfer of co-solvent(s) (such as PG) into the SC will also facilitate the uptake of other excipients, e.g. surfactants or emulsifiers, from the vehicle. These compounds, and others, have been shown capable of structurally perturbing and/or extracting SC intercellular lipids and thereby compromising barrier function to some extent. Such penetration enhancers may therefore impact upon both the SC/vehicle partition coefficient of the drug and its diffusivity across the skin. This combined partitioning and diffusion enhancement strategy is already used in marketed, topical drug products, including Elidel® (pimecrolimus) cream and Voltarol™ 12-hour Emulgel (diclofenac), which both contain PG and oleyl alcohol, and Xerese™ (aciclovir and hydrocortisone combination) cream, with PG and isopropyl myristate.

Formulation 'metamorphosis' and design of the non-volatile residual phase

The discussion so far has been silent on the fact that the majority of dermatological formulations contain volatile solvents (water, ethanol, isopropyl alcohol). The incorporation of a volatile solvent is a useful means by which to solubilise a poorly soluble drug in the vehicle (i.e. the volatile excipient is also acting as a co-solvent). Upon administration, such a solvent will itself rapidly partition into the SC and assist in transferring the drug quickly from the formulation into the barrier. In parallel, the solvent will be evaporating, causing the drug, which has been up to this point solubilised – at least in part – by the solvent's presence, to concentrate in the vehicle and hence increase the driving force for its diffusion across the SC. From a thermodynamic point of view, the loss (by evaporation and SC uptake) of the volatile will eventually reach the point at which the amount of drug remaining at the skin surface may no longer be fully solubilised and its precipitation might occur – a step which will significantly impede any further transfer into the SC. However, as mentioned previously, because this change in the formulation can occur quite quickly, it is possible that there will be a transient, supersaturation [23] of drug in the vehicle providing a period during which the active compound may be delivered into the skin at a rate greater than J_{max}. The duration of supersaturation may be prolonged by (for example) certain polymers, such as those used to gel the vehicle or to adjust its viscosity.

This 'metamorphosis' of the formulation [23] has attracted the attention of regulatory bodies with a particular interest in understanding how the loss of volatile vehicle components affects the solubility and partitioning of the drug and functional excipients (e.g. penetration enhancers) into the skin that, in turn, potentially impacts upon therapeutic outcome. Equally, developers of topical drug products are increasingly focused on not only the form of the manufactured product but also on that of the non-volatile residual phase that remains postapplication and transformation of the original formulation.

As a result, a quality-by-design process is now being followed to optimise the non-volatile residual phase [19]. The procedure begins by first estimating the required drug concentration in the formulation and then determining the ratio of the volatile phase to that of the non-volatile residual phase. Using aciclovir as an example, it was previously shown that a sensible minimum dose is approximately 0.6% w/w; it follows that if the ratio of volatile to non-volatile components of the formation is 1:1, then the drug's solubility in the non-volatile residual phase should be ~1.2% w/w.

The further design requirements mirror those identified previously but are now specifically applied to the *non-volatile residual phase*: (i) the drug should be in solution, approximately at or above saturation; (ii) an effective amount of a partitioning enhancer should be present (recognising that an additional, miscible co-solvent may be needed to satisfy criterion (i)); and (iii) an effective amount of a diffusion, or penetration, enhancer should be present and, like the drug, approximately at or above saturation.

In this way, for example, gels may be formulated by the addition of volatile solvents (typically, ethanol and water) and acrylate or cellulose polymers to the non-volatile residual phase. Upon application to the skin as a thin film, the volatiles are lost by evaporation and the optimised residual phase is formed. When the objective is to formulate a cream, a particular challenge is incorporation of a diffusion enhancer at or above saturation in the residual phase. This is because the hydrocarbon ester emollients often used in creams are exceptionally good solvents for typical diffusion enhancers, very large (and unfeasible) concentrations of which are therefore needed to achieve saturation. The problem can be circumvented by borrowing technology from the cosmetic industry and using silicone-based volatile fluids, emollients and elastomers. The result is efficient drug delivery and an exceptional consumer experience in use.

Assessment of topical drug bioavailability and bioequivalence between formulations

Bioavailability (BA) may be defined as the 'rate and extent to which the drug is absorbed from the formulation and becomes available at the site of action'. Bioequivalence (BE) is 'the absence of a significant difference in the rate and extent to which the active ingredient or active moiety in pharmaceutical equivalents or pharmaceutical alternatives become available at the site of drug action when administered at the same molar dose under similar conditions in an appropriately designed study'. For new chemical entities, their approval as drug products requires the successful demonstration of safety and efficacy in a series of increasingly detailed clinical trials. With respect to the commercialisation of bioequivalent, generic drug products for oral delivery, the accepted approach is relatively straightforward and is principally based on matching blood level profiles (rate and extent of absorption). For topical drug products, in contrast, other than the corticosteroids, a clinical trial has been and remains the primary route for the approval of a generic product or for the replacement of an already approved dermatological product that has appreciable compositional changes. Comparative clinical trials are relatively insensitive, time consuming and costly; to gain the adequate statistical power needed to clearly evaluate bioequivalence can require a very large number (i.e. hundreds or more) of subjects.

Methods for the determination of topical BA and BE are summarised in Figure 12.6 and separated into *in vitro* and *in vivo* approaches [24]. The methods in *italics* have not yet been accepted as independent means with which to evaluate topical BA/BE; the others have each, to some extent, been employed to compare different topical drug products.

In vitro methods

The US Food and Drug Administration (FDA) has described a method to assure consistent release kinetics of the active component(s) from semi-solid formulations typical of those found in topical products [25]. The technique measures the delivery of the active pharmaceutical ingredient (API) from the product across an artificial (e.g. polymeric) porous membrane and serves as a valuable quality control measurement of a number of important product characteristics, such as solubility and particle size of the API and its rheological properties. Thus, in many cases, the *in vitro* release rate is a useful test to assess product sameness when minor formulation changes are made. However, the *in vitro* release test for semi-solid dosage forms is *not* a surrogate test for *in vivo* BA or BE (as is often the case for the *in vitro* dissolution of solid oral dosage forms).

The use of *ex vivo* human skin to study the process of percutaneous absorption is widespread and has applications within multiple areas of the drug development process as well as in the field of toxicology [24]. Though substantial literature has emerged utilising this model system, the degree to which it mimics the living state and, therefore, the extent to which the data can be extrapolated with confidence must be critically examined. While not a perfect model, perhaps, the weight of evidence accumulated over more than 40 years suggests that, when a consistent and robust protocol is employed, the data are reliable and correlated with those obtained from living subjects. Despite having carefully examined the principles and practice of *in vitro* percutaneous absorption studies, and their relevance to BA/BE, the regulatory authorities have yet to formally embrace this approach. In the interim, however, it is clear that *in vitro* skin penetration studies are in routine use in manifold applications, including the screening and optimisation of transdermal, topical, cosmetic and personal care formulations, and in the assessment of risk associated with dermal exposure to potentially harmful chemicals in the home, workplace and environment.

In vivo approaches
Clinical end point studies

A number of important issues have been identified with respect to the use of this approach for the assessment of topical BA/BE, including (i) when the reference listed drug (RLD) has low efficacy it is difficult to demonstrate that the test product and RLD are active, and that the study is sufficiently sensitive to detect differences between products; (ii) when the RLD is indicated for a relatively small patient population; (iii) the typically high variability of clinical end points means that BE can only be proven when the products are tested in very large patient populations – given the costs of clinical trials, this makes evaluation prohibitively expensive; and (iv) the creation of a potential barrier to postapproval changes to improve quality.

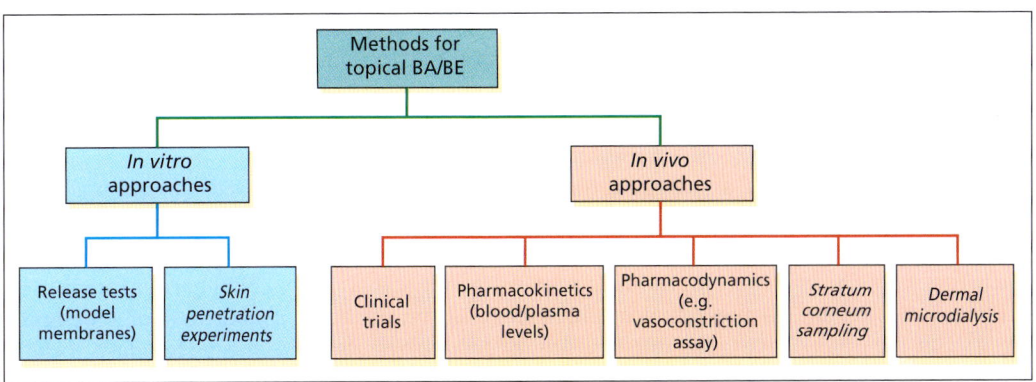

Figure 12.6 Methods, both accepted and under consideration by the regulatory authorities (see text for details), for the determination of topical bioavailability (BA) and bioequivalence (BE). Mathematical modelling and simulation and spectroscopic/imaging methods represent complementary tools under evaluation and development.

'Classic' pharmacokinetic approach

Measurement of blood or plasma levels of drug as a function of time postapplication for the evaluation of topical BA/BE has been largely ignored because, in general, the amount of API that can be found in the blood is small and difficult to quantify, and the levels present are typically considered (but rarely, if ever, proven) to be irrelevant to therapeutic activity at the site of action within the skin. Two key facts, however, are worthy of consideration. First, for a large fraction of *all* topically applied drugs (and this includes those used in dermatology, drugs to treat local, subcutaneous pain and inflammation, and transdermal drugs for systemic effect), the principal barrier to their absorption to the site of action – whether within the skin, beneath the skin at the application site, or in the central compartment – is the SC. Once the SC is breached, transport within the viable skin and uptake by the microcirculation proceed relatively quickly, such that it is reasonable to hypothesise that drug levels in the sub-SC compartments (epidermis/dermis, subcutaneous tissue, blood/plasma) will be proportional to one another, albeit progressively smaller with increasing distance from the skin surface. If true, then a conventional plasma concentration (C_p) versus time profile may well reflect the fluctuation of drug levels at the target site in the skin, and a comparison of classic pharmacokinetic metrics for two topical drug products would then allow an assessment of *local* BE to be performed. Second, the recent and rapid development and evolution of coupled liquid chromatography and mass spectrometry (LC-MS) technology means that the very low levels of API in the blood postadministration of conventional topical dosage forms are now quantifiable with an accuracy and precision sufficient to allow pharmacokinetic studies to be performed. Of course, there are potential exceptions to the use of this approach, for which it makes little sense (e.g. for the evaluation of a topical antifungal, or for a drug with a specific action within a hair follicle). In contrast, for drugs acting in subcutaneous compartments, such as non-steroidal anti-inflammatory drugs in muscle, joints, etc., a sensitive comparison of C_p–time profiles may offer a far more sensitive approach to local BE assessment than currently available alternatives.

The vasoconstriction assay

Corticosteroids, after permeation through the epidermal barrier, exert a quantifiable blanching effect on the skin, caused by vasoconstriction of the dermal microvasculature. This pharmacodynamic effect has been adopted as an acceptable method for assessing the BA/BE of topical corticosteroids [26]. While the approach is non-invasive and much less onerous than a clinical trial, refining the rather complicated protocol of subject selection, assessment of blanching (visual versus chromameter) and the determination of dose duration has not reduced the significant variability associated with the assay. As a surrogate tool for comparing topical dosage forms, therefore, the vasoconstriction assay is of limited value: on the one hand, being applicable only to the steroids that elicit the requisite pharmacological response (which, it should be added, is not related to the actual mechanism of action of these drugs); on the other, leaving the relevant skin pharmacokinetics as a black box.

Stratum corneum sampling by tape stripping

This so-called dermato-pharmacokinetic (DPK) method to assess the BE of topical products for application to the skin has been examined carefully over the past 20 years. A draft FDA Guidance, which was subsequently withdrawn, required quantification of the amount of drug in the SC as a function of time, akin to the typical C_p–time profiles of traditional pharmacokinetic studies using blood sampling. However, the inconsistent results of a pivotal study, which compared tretinoin gel formulations, prompted concern about both the reproducibility and the adequacy of this method to assess drugs whose target site is beyond the SC. Considerable subsequent effort has been directed at the identification of problems/limitations of the original DPK protocol and the development of an improved procedure to generate data of much higher quality and reproducibility. The end product of this research is a relatively straightforward method that examines only one uptake and one elimination time per formulation [27]. The total amount of drug in the SC is measured for each site, and the ratios of these quantities for RLD and test formulations can then be compared to assess (in)equivalence. The method has been successively applied retrospectively to the comparison of retinoid gels and prospectively to the analysis of DPK data obtained for econazole creams consistent with clinical outcome.

Microdialysis

This technique samples free drug concentrations in the subcutaneous or intradermal extracellular fluid [24]. A thin dialysis membrane tube is inserted into the skin and perfused with a site-compatible physiological solution. Molecules of interest diffuse across the membrane, allowing the percutaneously absorbed drug content of the extracellular fluid of the dermis to be continuously sampled and measured over a period of hours. The successful monitoring of the skin penetration of several drugs has been reported. However, the technically demanding procedure remains a research tool, with challenges related to tissue reactions as the probe is inserted, the need for highly sensitive analytical tools to detect very low amounts of the permeating drug (especially those that do not cross the SC rapidly) and the length of time (c.6 h) that subjects can be comfortably immobilised with dialysis probes in place. Inter- and intraindividual variability is relatively large, with coefficients of variation as large as 100%.

In sum, it is evident that topical BA/BE can be assessed using appropriately selected *in vitro* and/or *in vivo* surrogate tests. All surrogate tests have some, but different, limitations, meaning that results from distinct approaches can be complementary and increase confidence in the outcome of (in)equivalence deduced. The adoption of alternative methodologies to facilitate the approval of topical drug products can be anticipated in the not-too-distant future.

Conclusion

Skin barrier function is principally determined by the SC, a remarkable feat of bioengineering that provides an extremely efficient means to retard water loss from the 'inside–out' and to the penetration of xenobiotics from the 'outside–in'. While there are multiple potential pathways for drug diffusion across the SC, it appears that most compounds are constrained to transport via the lipid-filled intercellular domain of the barrier, significantly extending the distance that must be travelled from one side of the barrier to the other (and hence substantially lowering the permeability of the membrane).

Analysis of the substantial percutaneous absorption literature reveals unequivocally that molecular penetration of the barrier depends upon the drug's lipophilicity (consistent with the principal permeation pathway), its size and its solubility properties. Key physicochemical parameters that ultimately determine a drug's maximum flux across the SC are hence its octanol–water partition coefficient (P), molecular weight (MW) and aqueous solubility ($C_{water,sat}$); compounds with extreme values of lipophilicity (e.g. log $P > 5$), MW of $>400–500$ and low $C_{water,sat}$ (less than about 1 mg/mL) are unlikely to penetrate the skin well.

A variety of topical drug formulations has been developed to treat dermatological disease and many potent drugs are successfully used to resolve diverse skin problems. The efficiency of most drug products approved for therapeutic use is, however, rather poor. Typically, only a few per cent of the applied drug dose actually becomes available at the site of action. Because of this disappointing performance, it is not surprising that drug treatment of skin disease is associated with large variability and that the demonstration of safety and efficacy (and indeed the bioequivalence between formulations of the same drug) currently requires clinical trials with very large patient numbers.

To improve the quality of topical dermatological therapy, two substantial challenges, which have been addressed in some detail in this chapter, must be overcome. First, it is essential to create better formulations that contain lower drug loads, but which deliver a greater proportion of that load. At present, a substantial fraction of the applied drug is probably 'stranded' on the skin surface in the solid state following the loss of co-solvent excipients (by volatilisation and skin permeation) during the application process (i.e. massage of the formulation into the skin). Greater attention needs to be paid to the nature of the residual formulation after this metamorphosis of the vehicle to ensure that the drug remains in a molecularly absorbable form from the residual film. Second, additional research is required to evolve validated, surrogate tests with which to objectively, rapidly and economically evaluate DPKs – that is, the bioavailability of topically applied drugs and the bioequivalence between different formulations containing the same drug that are designed to achieve the same clinical end point.

Key references

The full list of references can be found in the online version at https://www.wiley.com/rooksdermatology10e

1 Menon GK, Cleary GW, Lane ME. The structure and function of the stratum corneum. *Int J Pharm* 2012;435:3–9.
5 Scheuplein RJ. Mechanism of percutaneous adsorption. I. Routes of penetration and the influence of solubility. *J Invest Dermatol* 1965;45:334–46.
7 Potts RO, Francoeur ML. Lipid biophysics of water loss through the skin. *Proc Natl Acad Sci USA* 1990;87:3871–3.
10 Barry BW. *Dermatological Formulations: Percutaneous Absorption*. New York: Dekker, 1983.
23 Surber C, Davis AF. Bioavailability and bioequivalence of dermatological formulations. In: Walters KA, ed. *Dermatological and Transdermal Formulations*. New York: Informa Healthcare, 2002:401–98.

CHAPTER 13

Clinical Pharmacology

Richard T. Woolf and Catherine H. Smith

St John's Institute of Dermatology, Guy's and St Thomas' Hospitals NHS Foundation Trust and King's College London, London, UK

Introduction, 13.1
Types of drugs and terminology, 13.1
Pharmacokinetics, 13.1
Absorption, 13.2
Distribution, 13.3
Metabolism, 13.3
Elimination, 13.3
Pharmacodynamics, 13.4

Molecular mechanisms underlying drug action, 13.5
Drug toxicity and adverse effects, 13.6
Factors that affect therapeutic outcome, 13.7
Drug choice and medical decision making, 13.7
Clinical factors that affect drug pharmacokinetics and pharmacodynamics, 13.7
Drug interactions, 13.9
Patient adherence to treatment, 13.9

Medication errors, 13.9
Personalised medicine and pharmacogenomics, 13.11
Drug development and licensing procedures, 13.11
Preclinical drug identification, 13.11
Drug development, 13.12
Ethics and trial reporting, 13.13

Key references, 13.13

Introduction

Drug therapy offers a real opportunity to dramatically improve the lives of people suffering from skin disease. In dermatology, there has been a transformative change over the last 20 years in terms of treatment options available. An abiding principle in medicine is 'to help, or at least to do no harm' (Hippocrates) and it is a sobering fact that an estimated 3–6% of hospital admissions are due to adverse drug reactions [1,2] and, of these, over half could have potentially been avoided [3,4]. Clinical pharmacology deals with the actions, mechanisms of action, uses, adverse effects and fate of drugs in humans, and underpins all aspects of drug therapy from novel drug development through to safe, effective prescribing.

Types of drugs and terminology

Traditional pharmaceutical agents are typically small (<500 kDa), organic molecules (small-molecule drugs) and have, until recently, dominated medicine. With the advent of recombinant DNA technology and advances in biotechnology manufacturing, the design and large-scale production of proteins became possible and consequently brought in the era of biological medicines (in this context 'large-molecule' drugs) [1]. The nomenclature around this group of medicines is somewhat confusing in the literature, with biological products, biotherapeutics, biopharmaceuticals and biological medicinal products all being used interchangeably. From a regulatory perspective the European Medicines Agency (EMA) describes a biological medicine as a 'medicine whose active substance is made by a living organism' and can be used to describe therapeutic agents that are produced by or extracted from a biological source [2]. In the broadest sense, these include recombinant proteins, monoclonal antibodies, fusion proteins, blood products, immunological medicinal products such as sera and vaccines, allergens and advanced technology medicinal products such as gene and cell therapies. In practice (and in this chapter unless otherwise stated), the term biologics (or biologicals) usually references monoclonal antibodies and related protein-based therapeutics which are very widely used, powerful agents that have revolutionised the management of skin disease. The principles of clinical pharmacology apply to all types of intervention, but due to the size and complexity of biologics, the pharmacokinetics and pharmacodynamics often differ from small-molecule drugs, as does the ethical and regulatory framework around their development and licensing.

Pharmacokinetics

Pharmacokinetics describes the processes involved in drug absorption, distribution, metabolism (biotransformation) and elimination, and is often referred to by the acronym ADME (i.e. what the body does to the drug) (Table 13.1) [1]. Understanding these principles is fundamental to safe, effective prescribing as it dictates how, and when, a drug will be delivered to the main site(s) of action. *Clinical pharmacokinetics* aims to describe and quantify the relationship between a given dose of drug and the pharmacological effect, be it therapeutic, toxic or 'off target' (i.e. unrelated to the known therapeutic efficacy or toxicity), and assumes that the concentration of drug measured in the central compartment (usually blood or plasma) can be related to the concentration at the site of pharmacological action. In general, for most small-molecule drugs administered within the therapeutic dose range, this relationship is linear (first order kinetics) because the systems in place for drug elimination such as metabolising enzymes and transporters are not saturated. In contrast, biologics are generally characterised by non-linear pharmacokinetics due to saturation of binding,

---

Rook's Textbook of Dermatology, Tenth Edition. Edited by Christopher Griffiths, Jonathan Barker, Tanya Bleiker, Walayat Hussain and Rosalind Simpson.
© 2024 John Wiley & Sons Ltd. Published 2024 by John Wiley & Sons Ltd.

Table 13.1 Common terms used in clinical pharmacology.

Term	Meaning
Pharmacokinetics	The rates of process related to drug absorption, distribution, metabolism (biotransformation) and elimination
Pharmacodynamics	The study of the biochemical and physiological effects of drugs and their mechanisms of actions (i.e. what the drug does to the body)
Drug disposition	A collective term to describe the absorption, distribution, metabolism and elimination of a drug
Bioavailability	The fraction of a drug absorbed into the systemic circulation (where intravenous administration describes 100% bioavailability)
Volume of distribution	A measure of the *apparent* space in the body available to contain a drug calculated according to the amount of drug given, and the concentration found in the systemic circulation (a proportionality constant that reflects the degree to which a drug is distributed in body tissue relative to the plasma)
Clearance	A measure of the body's efficiency in eliminating a drug from the systemic circulation (the volume of blood or plasma from which a given drug is completely removed per unit of time)
Elimination half-life	A measure of the rate of removal of a drug from the systemic circulation (the amount of time required for 50% of the drug to be removed from the blood (plasma))
Equilibrium dissociation constant (K_D)	A measure of drug/receptor binding affinity (a drug with high affinity binding will have a low K_D)
Half maximally effective concentration (EC_{50})	A measure of drug potency (concentration of a drug required to induce 50% of the therapeutic effect)
Median effective dose (MD_{50})	Dose of drug required to produce a specified effect in 50% of the population
Lethal effective dose (LD_{50})	Dose of drug required to cause death in 50% of experimental animals (preclinical)
Therapeutic window	Range of steady-state drug concentration required to produce the desired clinical effect with minimal toxicity

Adapted from Buxton 2018 [1].

distribution and/or elimination pathways as well as the development of antidrug antibodies [2,3]. *Target-mediated drug disposition*, which refers to the situation where a significant proportion of a drug (relative to dose) is bound with high affinity to a pharmacological target, such that this interaction is reflected in the pharmacokinetic properties of the drug, is commonly reported with therapeutic monoclonal antibodies. Complex, multiple compartment pharmacokinetic modelling is frequently required to adequately describe biologic drug disposition and is an area of ongoing development and challenge [2]. Even so, for many biologic drugs, the central premise that drug level concentration in the central compartment is related to the therapeutic effect remains true.

Absorption

Absorption describes the movement of a drug from its site of administration to the central compartment, and is critically dependent on the route of administration used.

Topical. In skin disease, a topical approach to treatment (Chapter 12) is often preferred as it allows direct application of the drug to the site of pathology (skin disease), potentially limiting 'off target' effects and systemic exposure. The active agent (drug) can be applied to the skin in a variety of vehicles, including creams, foams, gels, lotions and ointments. Many vehicles are lipid based to facilitate drug penetration of the stratum corneum of the epidermis. Not all drugs can be effectively delivered in a topical form. The decision as to whether a topical or systemic approach is required will depend on the nature, extent, site and severity of disease, practicability and patient choice. Where topical therapy alone is insufficient, a combined topical and systemic approach may minimise the dose requirement of potentially more toxic systemic drug therapy.

Oral. Oral drug administration is convenient for patients, but bioavailability is highly variable and dependent on drug characteristics (e.g. lipophilicity, pH), patient characteristics (e.g. variation in molecular/transmembrane transporter mechanisms, rate of gastric emptying) and concomitant food intake (e.g. chelation of tetracyclines by calcium in milk). Drug formulation is also important [1]. Enteric-coated preparations are useful for drugs that cause significant gastric irritation, such as prednisolone, but may be incompletely dissolved and absorbed. Similarly, controlled release preparations have relevance where the half-life of the drug is short (<4 h) but are associated with wide interpatient variation and risk of 'dose dumping' when the dosage form fails.

Parenteral administration. Parenteral administration (intravenous, intramuscular, subcutaneous) circumvents the gastrointestinal tract with consequent improved drug bioavailability. Therapeutic proteins (biologics) have very limited oral bioavailability due to intestinal enzymes and poor permeability across the intestinal mucosal membrane barrier, and are almost exclusively administered via parenteral routes, either as an intravenous infusion (e.g. rituximab or infliximab) or, more conveniently, subcutaneously (the route used for most biologics used to treat skin disease). Following subcutaneous administration, a drug is absorbed via the lymphatic and/or capillary networks into the systemic circulation at varying rates that are determined, at least in part, by molecular size, with most molecules larger than 20 kDa absorbed completely by lymphatics [4]. For example, the maximum systemic concentration (T_{max}) occurs 3–7 h after subcutaneous administration of anakinra (molecular weight 17.3 kDa) as compared with 5 days for the monoclonal antibody adalimumab (molecular weight 148 kDa). Factors operating to influence absorption, and consequent drug bioavailability following subcutaneous administration, include patient characteristics (e.g. age), local factors at the injection site (e.g. subcutaneous blood flow, local adiposity) and injection technique, drug-specific factors (e.g. formulation, volume, dose, concentration, presence of an Fc receptor, degree of glycosylation) and degree of presystemic elimination (influenced in turn by multiple factors; see 'Elimination' later in this chapter) [4]. The reported range of bioavailabilities for different biologics thus ranges from 25% to 95%, with significant interpatient variation for any single agent.

Novel methods of drug delivery aim to limit systemic drug exposure (and therefore potential toxicity) and/or optimise bioavailability, particularly for large-molecule drugs (including DNA and proteins). These include facilitating access to the systemic circulation through traditional routes (skin, lung, gut) or harnessing the specificity of the immune system to target drug action once inside the body. Advances in transdermal drug delivery systems [5,6] include the use of chemical enhancers, iontophoresis, electroporation (where short, high-voltage pulses disrupt the lipid bilayer of the skin), cavitational ultrasound (already approved for optimising the delivery of topical lignocaine), microneedles (painless, spontaneous dissolution), laser-assisted drug delivery (ablative fractional lasers such as carbon dioxide or erbium:yttrium-aluminium-garnet (Er:YAG) lasers, which perforate the epidermis) and thermal ablation. Inhalation also offers potential for rapid systemic delivery of small-molecule drugs and can confer better bioavailability than oral ingestion given the much lower concentrations of drug-metabolising enzymes in the lungs compared with the gastrointestinal tract. Oral drug delivery systems for oral peptides include permeation enhancers, gut enzyme inhibitors and co-formulating therapeutic peptides with mucolytic or cell penetrating functions [7]. Antibody–drug conjugates comprise a monoclonal antibody tethered to a cytoxic drug (known as the payload). These antibody–drug conjugates offer the possibility of delivering a toxic payload directly to cancer cells, while minimising off target exposure. As an example, brentuximab vedotin, the anti-CD30 (cluster of differentiation 30) antibody has been covalently linked to monomethyl auristatin E (cytoxic) and is approved for the treatment of CD30+ lymphoproliferative disorders [8].

Distribution

The volume of distribution of a drug is mainly determined by its physicochemical properties (such as charge and lipophilicity), protein-binding capacity and the degree to which it is subject to active transport mechanisms. Small-molecule drugs are distributed into interstitial and intracellular fluids with well-perfused organs such as the liver, kidney and brain receiving most of the drug initially, and skin and fat levels accumulating more slowly. The degree to which a drug is bound to plasma proteins and tissues determines blood–tissue partitioning, which in turn can be affected by disease states. Preferential accumulation of drugs in certain tissues may also be of clinical relevance. For example, retinoids tend to preferentially accumulate in adipose tissue so that dosing may need alteration in obese patients. Albumin is a major carrier for acidic drugs, which when reduced by liver, renal or malnutritional disease can lead to elevated levels of unbound drug and increased clearance. On the other hand, α_1-acid glycoprotein binds basic drugs and so if it is increased in acute inflammatory states, unbound drug levels may be correspondingly reduced.

For most therapeutic proteins, in contrast to small-molecule drugs, distribution is limited by their large mass and hydrophilic properties, so that the measured volume of distribution is close to the plasma volume and increases with increasing body size (weight) [2]. Measured drug concentrations in tissue are generally a fraction of those present in plasma. The specific, high-affinity binding properties of therapeutic proteins mean that these very low concentrations of drug are still able to effect marked pharmacological action within the target tissue. The distribution of a drug may also be influenced by the distribution and concentration of the target antigen, as exemplified by monoclonal antibodies, which in turn may be affected by disease activity. This phenomenon is also referred to as 'antigen sink' (part of target-mediated disposition) and can further contribute to non-linear pharmacokinetics [2].

Metabolism

Drug metabolism is traditionally described as occurring in two phases [1]. Phase I reactions are catalysed by cytochrome P450s (CYPs), flavin-containing mono-oxygenases and epoxide hydrolases, and lead to oxidation, reduction or hydrolysis of the drug. Usually this results in a loss of drug function, but for some drugs (so-called prodrugs), it results in drug activation (e.g. mycophenolate mofetil is an ester prodrug, which is hydrolysed to biologically active mycophenolic acid by plasma esterases). Of the large CYP superfamily, subfamilies CYP2C, CYP2D and CYP3A account for the majority of drug-metabolising activity, and CYP3A4, specifically, metabolises over half of all small-molecule drugs in clinical use. These CYPs demonstrate significant overlapping substrate specificity and can also metabolise a single compound at different positions, which explains their significant role in the context of drug interactions (see later in this chapter).

Phase II reactions catalyse conjugation of the phase I product with a second molecule (sulphate, glucuronic acid, glutathione, acetyl group, methyl group). This inactivates potentially toxic phase I metabolites, and also facilitates drug elimination as a consequence of improved water solubility and increased molecular weight. Drug-metabolising enzymes are found in most tissues in the body, including the skin, but are found in the greatest quantity in the gastrointestinal tract (liver, small and large intestine). Thus when a drug is given orally, substantial metabolism and clearance may occur before it reaches the systemic circulation, firstly by metabolising enzymes within the gastrointestinal epithelium, and subsequently following absorption into the portal vein, within the liver (so-called *first pass effect*). Liver disease (as well as bowel disease or resection) may therefore have a clinically relevant impact on drug metabolism and subsequent drug concentration in the systemic circulation; however, the degree to which this occurs is unpredictable and standard measures of liver function are not especially helpful.

Elimination

Drugs are eliminated (excreted) from the body either unchanged or as drug metabolites. The most important excretory organs are the kidney and liver, with drugs eliminated in urine or bile, respectively; however, drugs can also be excreted in sweat, saliva, tears and milk. Within the kidney, drug and drug metabolite elimination depends on glomerular filtration, active tubular secretion and passive tubular absorption. Renal function is therefore a critical factor in determining drug bioavailability and potential toxicity, and when reduced due to age, kidney disease or concomitant therapy (e.g. non-steroidal anti-inflammatory drugs (NSAIDs), diuretics) becomes a very common source of adverse drug reactions.

Therapeutic proteins are eliminated (commonly described as cleared) from the circulation and interstitial tissue fluids in a variety of ways, including: (i) target-mediated clearance, where a drug is taken up intracellularly following antigen binding; (ii) non-specific endocytosis; and (iii) formation of circulating immune complexes [2,9]. Once inside cells, whether prior to systemic absorption (following subcutaneous administration), in the circulation or target tissue, proteins are broken down into peptide fragments and/or amino acids. These protein degradation products, as well as biologics of low molecular weight (<30 kDa, for example anakinra), are then cleared by renal excretion. How, and to what extent, these various elimination mechanisms operate for any particular drug, and in different diseases, is only partially understood. Target-mediated clearance depends on antigen mass – so that high tumour burden or inflammatory disease activity can correspondingly lead to increased clearance. Molecules with an Fc domain such as monoclonal antibodies and fusion proteins are actively protected from this intracellular proteolytic degradation via the FcRn present in endothelial cell endosomes. This FcRn/Fc complex is then transported back to the cell surface where it dissociates, releasing the active drug back into the circulation. This is why albumin levels are inversely correlated with monoclonal antibody clearance since both are recycled via FcRn (i.e. high albumin corresponds to low antibody clearance). At low levels of albumin, factors other than FcRn may influence this inverse relationship, since (for example) low albumin can be driven by high inflammatory disease burden and increased target-mediated elimination. This FcRn-mediated salvage pathway, which presumably evolved to maintain levels of endogenous immunoglobulin G (IgG) for health reasons, results in a therapeutically helpful long half-life (around 4 weeks) for most monoclonal antibodies. This is also relevant when using these agents during pregnancy as antibodies cross the placenta via FcRn-mediated mechanisms (see 'Conception, pregnancy and lactation' later in this chapter). The development of antidrug antibodies is most commonly reported in association with tumour necrosis factor (TNF) inhibitor monoclonal antibodies, and can lead to enhanced drug clearance (and correspondingly reduced drug exposure) through the development of antidrug antibody–drug complexes.

Pharmacodynamics

Pharmacodynamics is the study of the biochemical and physiological effects of drugs and their mechanisms of actions (i.e. what the drug does to the body) [1]. The term encompasses desired therapeutic effects as well as unwanted toxic effects. Most drugs work by interacting with a specific cellular macromolecule (drug target or drug receptor). This drug–receptor interaction is the initiating event in a multistep process that ultimately alters tissue function and depends on two key principles: (i) the affinity and specificity of drug/receptor binding; and (ii) the intrinsic activity of a receptor-bound drug to activate the receptor. The intrinsic activity of a drug describes whether binding to a receptor completely mimics the effect of the endogenous ligand (an *agonist*), prevents or blocks this response (an *antagonist*) or is somewhere in between (*partial agonists*). Many receptors exhibit constitutive activity in the absence of endogenous ligand binding; *inverse agonists* inhibit this activity by binding to and stabilising the receptor in an inactive form. Drugs may bind to the same recognition site as the endogenous ligand (*syntopic* binding) or to a different region (*allosteric* or *allotopic* binding), and this may be reversible or irreversible, competitive or non-competitive. All of these variables ultimately determine the potency of the drug (Table 13.2).

Table 13.2 Major mechanisms underlying drug actions.

Structural family	Functional family	Physiological ligands	Effectors and transducers	Example drugs
Transmembrane transduction mechanisms				
G-protein-coupled receptors	Muscarinic cholinergic receptors	ACh	G_i and G_q; adenyl cyclase, ion channels, phospholipase	Botulinum toxin
	Eicosanoid receptors	Prostaglandins, leukotrienes, thromboxanes	G_s, G_i and G_q proteins	Montelukast
	Histamine receptors (1–4)	Histamine	$G_{q/11}$, G_s, $G_{i/10}$	Fexofenadine, ranitidine
Ion channels	Ligand gated	ACh, GABA, 5-HT	Na^+, Ca^{2+}, K^+, Cl^-	Nicotine, gabapentin
	Voltage gated	None (activated by membrane polarisation)	Na^+, Ca^{2+}, K^+, other ions	Lignocaine
Transmembrane enzymes	Receptor tyrosine kinases	Insulin, PDGF, EGF, VEGF, growth factors	SH2 and phosphotyrosine-binding domain containing proteins	Herceptin, imatinib, vemurafenib
Transmembrane non-enzymes	Cytokine receptors	Interleukins and other cytokines	JAK/STAT, soluble tyrosine kinases	Janus kinase inhibitors
	Toll-like receptors	LPS, bacterial products	NFκB, MyD88, IRAKs	Imiquimod
Intracellular transduction mechanisms				
Nuclear receptors	Steroid receptors (includes retinoic acid receptors, retinoid X receptors)	Oestrogen, testosterone	Co-activators	Corticosteroids, alitretinoin, bexarotene
	PAR-ϒ	PAR-ϒ		Thiazolidinediones, clofibrate
Intracellular enzymes	Cyclic phosphodiesterases	Cyclic GMP, cAMP	Protein kinase A, exchange proteins activated by cAMP, cAMP responsive element binding protein	Vasodilators, anti-inflammatory agents (apremilast, roflumilast)

Adapted from Blumenthal and Garrison 2018 [1].
ACh, acetylcholine; cAMP, cyclic adenosine monophosphate; EGF, epidermal growth factor; GABA, γ-aminobutyric acid; GMP, guanosine monophosphate; 5-HT, 5-hydroxytryptamine; IRAKs, interleukin-associated kinases; JAK, Janus kinase; LPS, lipopolysaccharide; MyD88, myeloid differentiation primary response 88; NFκB, nuclear factor κB; PAR-ϒ, proteinase activated receptor ϒ; PDGF, platelet-derived growth factor; SH2, Src homology 2; STAT, signal transducers and activators of transcription; VEGF, vascular endothelial growth factor.

Molecular mechanisms underlying drug action

Initial drug/receptor coupling may result in a direct effect on the cellular function, or convey a message to intermediary cellular signalling molecules (transducers). The receptor, its cellular target and any intermediary molecules are termed the *receptor–effector system* or *signal transduction pathway*. Often, the transducer proteins mediate the actual physiological effect via generating, moving or degrading small molecules known as second messengers (e.g. nitric oxide or cyclic adenosine monophosphate (cAMP)). This system allows the cell to coordinate, and to amplify, signals from multiple ligands, and explains how tiny amounts of drug at a particular receptor result in a significant biological effect. This complexity can also underpin unintended or unexpected 'off target' drug effects. The site of drug/receptor coupling and associated underlying mechanism can be outside the cell, at the cell membrane or within the cell. In dermatology, as in other areas of medicine, for many established drugs in clinical use the site of drug action is unknown, having been introduced either by serendipity, trial and error, or following traditional drug development where drugs were selected for development based on their effects at a whole organism rather than molecular level. However, this is changing as we have a greater understanding of molecular and cellular biology in both health and disease, and particularly the identification of 'druggable' pathways/processes that are dysregulated in disease. This increased understanding has, in great part, been achieved through the elucidation of genetic determinants of disease; indeed, drug targets with genetic support are more likely to be therapeutically valid [2,3].

Extracellular mechanisms

A number of drugs act outside the cell to affect cellular function, typically in one of two ways. The first is to alter the activity of extracellular enzymes involved in the synthesis or degradation of endogenous signalling molecules (e.g. angiotensin-converting enzyme (ACE) inhibitors). The second is by directly interacting with the endogenous ligand to prevent binding to its site of action (e.g. monoclonal antibodies, such as TNF antagonists adalimumab or infliximab).

Transmembrane mechanisms

Hydrophilic drugs (and their physiological counterparts) cannot easily access the cell and so rely on membrane-bound receptors to exert their action (see Table 13.2 for further details and examples of drugs that exploit these receptors). These fall into five broad categories.

1 *G-protein-coupled receptors* (GPCRs) couple to a family of heterotrimeric guanosine triphosphate (GTP) binding regulatory G proteins. Following ligand binding, G proteins signal to various effector proteins including enzymes such as adenyl cyclase phospholipase C and cyclic guanosine monophosphate (cGMP), which then leads to a cascade of intracellular events via second messenger systems and ultimately a drug effect. G proteins exist in as many as 23 isoforms coupled to different signalling paths and it is the type(s) of G protein coupled to the receptor that determines the response to receptor activation.
2 *Receptors linked to intracellular enzymes* have an extracellular binding domain directly coupled in some way to enzymatic activity within the cell so that, on ligand binding, the consequent enzymatic activity initiates and amplifies the intracellular signals and feedback responses by changing the phosphorylation status of the cellular proteins. The types of receptor described include: (i) receptor tyrosine kinases (RTKs), where the tyrosine kinase is part of the transmembrane receptor; (ii) transmembrane receptors that recruit cytoplasmic tyrosine Janus kinases (JAKs), which then phosphorylate STAT (signal transducers and activators of transcription) proteins that translocate to the nucleus and regulate transcription; and (iii) receptor serine/threonine kinases, analogous to the RTKs except they have a serine/threonine cytoplasmic domain.
3 *Transmembrane receptors without enzyme-linked activity* include Toll-like receptors, fundamental components of innate immune signalling, which on ligand binding ultimately recruit interleukin-associated kinases and downstream pathway signalling via the nuclear factor κB (NFκB) pathway. TNF-α receptor signalling operates in a very similar way to that of Toll-like receptors in that it has a transmembrane domain with a non-enzymatic cytoplasmic domain (death domain) that on ligand binding triggers a cascade of intracellular events.
4 *Ion channels* facilitate the flux of cations and anions across the impermeable plasma cell membrane to maintain electrochemical gradients critical to excitable cells such as nerves and muscles as well as non-excitable cells, to trigger biochemical and secretory cell function. These channels may be open, closed or inactive and drugs may affect their function by directly opening or closing the channel (ligand-gated channels), by influencing the voltage-dependent characteristics of the channels (voltage-gated channels) and by the amount of time the channel spends in a given state, or by generating second messengers that subsequently open or close the channel (second messenger gated).
5 *Membrane-bound transporters* play a key role in drug pharmacokinetics as they determine drug entry to and elimination from cells, but are also drug targets, particularly those used in neuropsychiatric disorders (e.g. the transporter SERT (SLC6A4) is responsible for the uptake and clearance of serotonin in the brain, and the target for selective serotonin reuptake inhibitors).

Intracellular mechanisms

Some small-molecule drugs diffuse or are actively transported into the cell to access intracellular drug targets. There are two main types.

1 *Nuclear hormone receptors* comprise a superfamily of receptors that act as ligand-activated transcription factors able to interact with specific DNA sequences and directly regulate gene expression following ligand binding. Classic family members are hormonal ligands, including sex hormones, cortisol, thyroid hormones and vitamin D receptors.
2 *Intracellular enzymes* may be targeted directly by drugs. Identifying such enzymes that are relevant to processes dysregulated in disease is an area of active drug development. For example, cyclic nucleotide phosphodiesterases (PDEs) are a major family of cytoplasmic enzymes important in cell signalling as they hydrolyse cAMP and cGMP. The specificity of PDEs varies, with some able to hydrolyse cAMP, cGMP or both. Inhibitors of PDE3 are drug targets for the treatment of asthma and cardiovascular

disease, while the PDE4 inhibitors (e.g. apremilast, crisaborole) have been developed for the treatment of psoriasis and atopic dermatitis. Other examples of dermatological drugs that target intracellular enzymes are calcineurin inhibitors, such as ciclosporin, tacrolimus and pimecrolimus, which act as antagonists of calcineurin, a cytoplasmic phosphatase enzyme. This prevents dephosphorylation of the cytoplasmic nuclear factor of activated T cells (NFAT) and its translocation to the nucleus.

Drug toxicity and adverse effects

An ideal drug would only mediate a desired therapeutic effect. However, few drugs are sufficiently specific, so unwanted effects are part of therapeutics. Drug toxicities can be classified in five, somewhat overlapping, broad categories based on the underlying mechanism.

1 *On target drug toxicity* can be defined as drug toxicity following modulation of the primary, pharmacological target (e.g. receptor or enzyme). This may arise due to altered drug exposure at the target site, leading to an exaggerated pharmacological response. Sources of this type of event include deliberate or accidental dosing error, alterations in the pharmacokinetics of the drug (e.g. due to liver or kidney disease or to interactions with other drugs) or changes in the pharmacodynamics of the drug–receptor interaction that alter the pharmacological response (e.g. changes in receptor number). Activation of the drug target in an unintended tissue is another example of on target toxicity (e.g. osteoporosis secondary to corticosteroid use, myositis with statin therapy).

2 *Off target toxicity* results from the interaction of a drug with targets other than the intended therapeutic targets, for example the H_1-receptor antagonist terfenadine also inhibits a cardiac potassium channel (Kv11.1 encoded by the gene *hERG*) which led to fatal cardiac arrhythmias and ultimately drug withdrawal.

3 *Biological activation of drugs* to toxic metabolites capable of binding to proteins, DNA and small molecules such as glutathione (GSH) is an increasingly recognised mechanism of drug toxicity. Paracetamol-induced hepatic necrosis is a classic example of this, due to GSH binding (and depletion) by the active intermediate metabolite *N*-acetyl-*p*-benzoquineimine.

4 *Allergic reactions (hypersensitivity)* to drugs are due to an enhanced immunological or inflammatory response to the medication and extend from type I to type IV reactions. These are not dose related and are generally unpredictable.

5 *Idiosyncratic drug reactions* are very rare (e.g. toxic epidermal necrolysis), and typically no obvious mechanism is apparent. Pharmacogenetics offers an opportunity to interrogate the molecular mechanisms underlying many of these reactions. For example, severe, life-threatening fluoropyrimidine toxicity (which can include hand–foot syndrome) is now known to be mediated by genetic variants in the gene encoding dihydropyrimidine dehydrogenase, with homozygotes having a complete absence of the enzyme. Such reactions are thus no longer 'idiosyncratic' but, instead, predictable – and avoidable with genetic screening [4].

Assessing the potential for a drug to produce adverse effects begins at the earliest stage of drug development right through to postmarketing surveillance mechanisms (Table 13.3). In general, clinical trials are powered for efficacy rather than safety and are performed in patient populations that are not necessarily generalisable to those in whom the drug will be used in clinical practice. So although common adverse effects are likely to be picked up prior to drug marketing, rare (<1 : 10 000) idiosyncratic events (e.g. cases of progressive multifocal leukoencephalopathy observed with efalizumab), events with a long latency period (e.g. skin cancer secondary to psoralen and ultraviolet A) or problems using a drug in the context of other morbidities, may take many years to establish. This is particularly relevant to drugs that may be used over very prolonged periods for chronic conditions. Pharmacovigilance registries are critical to evaluate these longer term safety issues, especially those with a longer latency period.

Table 13.3 Methods used to identify drug-related adverse events and their respective roles within the lifetime of a drug, from drug development through to post-licensing pharmacovigilance.

Method	Benefits	Problems
Preclinical studies (*in vitro* or *in vivo* (animal))	Controlled Can establish potential therapeutic and toxic dose ranges Identifies new/unexpected adverse events and drug–drug interactions before human exposure to drug Can study high-risk situations, such as drug effect on pregnancy/fetal development	May not be able to directly extrapolate to human responses to drug Short-term exposure Ethical considerations
Clinical trials (phase I–IV)	Controlled Rigorous collection of high-quality data Will identify common, short-term side effects	Short term Powered for efficacy not safety Data may not be relevant to clinical practice Will miss effects with long latency period
Spontaneous reporting	Identifies new/rare/unexpected adverse events and drug–drug interactions	Relies on voluntary reporting May overestimate the risk (no denominator) May miss common/less severe morbidity
Registries/electronic health records	Reflects real-life clinical practice Population based May allow relative risk–benefit analysis Allows collection of adverse effects with longer latency period	Incomplete data sets Observational; multiple confounders May lack control group

Factors that affect therapeutic outcome

Drug choice and medical decision making

Before initiating any therapy, a comprehensive and holistic assessment of the patient is essential, considering the diagnosis, the natural history of the condition if not treated, available treatment options, the wider context of the whole patient, the patient's attitudes and beliefs and shared treatment goals. The evidence base for a therapeutic intervention enables the clinician to define and communicate the probability of certain outcomes, such as disease remission or an adverse effect. When starting an intervention in an individual patient it can also be considered a trial (of $n = 1$) for that patient requiring appropriately defined 'outcome measures' and timelines for judging success or failure. This is perhaps especially important in dermatological practice. The rarity of many skin diseases and historic lack of investment in drug development means that robust evidence to guide treatment choice and optimise drug use is often unavailable. In addition, many drugs are used for unlicensed dermatological indications so clear documentation of benefit (or harm) is also important. Continuing an ineffective or insufficiently effective treatment exposes patients to the ongoing risk of adverse events and suboptimal management of their skin disease.

Multiple factors determine the relationship between the dose of any particular drug and outcome (Figure 13.1). Therapy needs to be carefully and precisely tailored to the needs and clinical circumstance of each patient. This can be a highly complex, dynamic process that requires constant re-evaluation and refinement during the course of treatment.

Clinical factors that affect drug pharmacokinetics and pharmacodynamics

Age

Drug pharmacokinetics and pharmacodynamics are altered in the very young and in older people, and available drug-specific information is often limited as these groups are often excluded from clinical trials. There are also age-specific considerations that are pertinent to medical errors, adherence to treatment and co-therapy.

Growth and development during childhood is associated with marked physiological change, especially during infancy and puberty, with consequent non-linear changes in drug disposition such that dose adaptation is required for most drugs [1,2]. Specific (additional) considerations are relevant in preterm neonates. Systemic exposure to topically applied therapies is more likely in infants and children compared with adults. During infancy, this relates in part to the presence of a thinner stratum corneum and, during childhood, to increased cutaneous perfusion and hydration of the epidermis compared with adults. The ratio of total body surface area to body mass in infants and young children also far exceeds that in adults. With maturation, increases in weight, drug-binding proteins such as albumin (during the first 1–3 years) and fraction of fat mass (and corresponding fall in total body water) all influence drug distribution. The impact on drug metabolism is highest in the first few years of life. Most hepatic drug-metabolising enzymes are expressed at very low levels at birth, increasing to adult levels during the first few months of life. For many metabolised drugs, clearance is increased in infants and toddlers with consequent reduction in drug exposure due to an overall increase in metabolic capacity due to the large size of the liver at this age. The glomerular

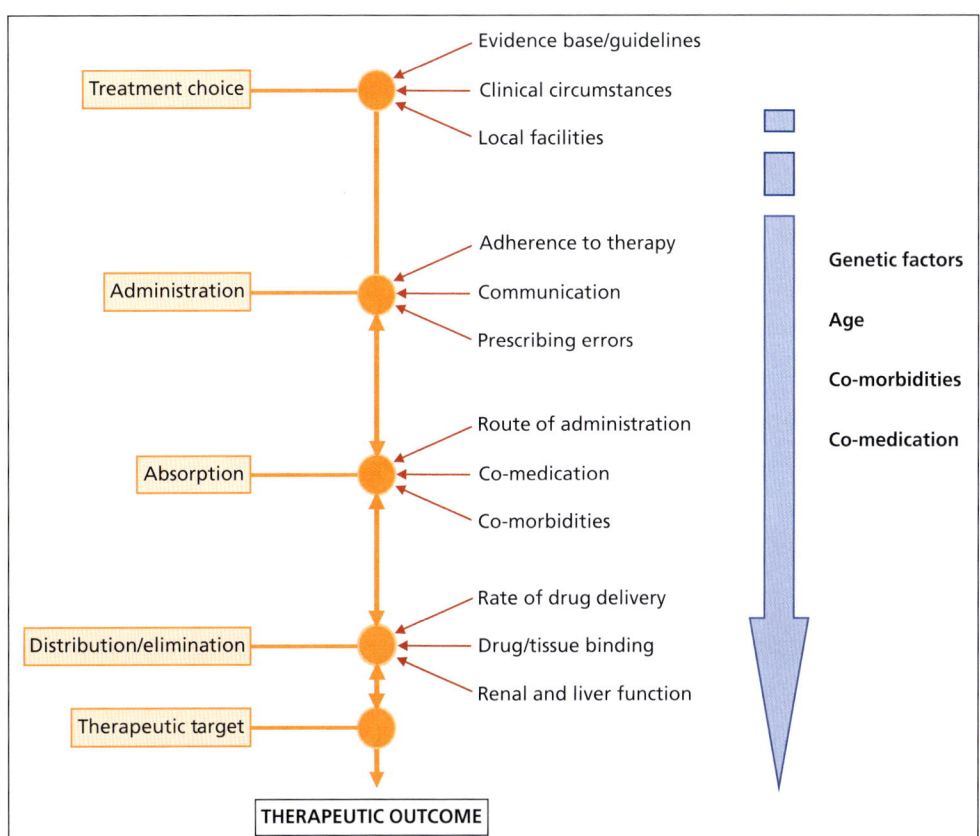

Figure 13.1 An overview of the relationship between the dose of any particular drug and therapeutic outcome. Multiple, often interdependent, factors impact at critical points (orange circles) along the pharmacological pathway, some of which are relevant throughout (blue arrow).

filtration rate increases rapidly to achieve full maturity before 2 years; less is known about tubular function but tubules appear to mature more slowly [2]. With respect to biologics, in general, the elimination of monoclonals seems to be faster in children compared with adults although the precise mechanisms are unclear [3].

Ageing is associated with a number of progressive physiological changes including cutaneous atrophy, reduction in lean body mass, 40% reduction in hepatic blood flow, reduced activity of hepatic enzyme activity (especially CYP phase I) and reduced renal function. The decline in glomerular filtration rate has been estimated to be around 1 mL/min/year (or less) after middle age and is a critical determinant of disposition for many drugs. The high prevalence of co-morbidities such as hypertension, diabetes and ischaemic heart disease, together with widespread use of nephrotoxic therapies such as diuretics and NSAIDs, contribute to this decline. In completely healthy older people, renal function may not necessarily be reduced significantly. Collectively, physiological and pathological changes in older people tend to increase drug bioavailability and reduce drug metabolism and elimination (for a comprehensive review see [4]), so accounting for the general advice to start drug therapy at the lowest possible dose and increase the dose slowly. Pharmacodynamic responses to drugs may also change with age – the increased effect of drugs that depress the central nervous system is a good example – and the pathophysiology of the disease itself may be different from that in younger people, as in the case of psoriasis where genetic susceptibility loci are distinct in late-onset disease.

Polypharmacy is common with 20–40% of older people taking five or more medications, with consequent impact on medicine adherence and risk of drug interactions. All these factors lead to increased variability in drug response with age. Adverse drug reactions are also more common, and tend to be more severe and less likely to be recognised or reported by the patient [5,6]. The elderly also have both increased risk of and severity of infections, in part due to the prevalence of co-morbidities, variation in drug responses and immunosenescence (dysregulated immune function) with ageing. This should be a consideration when starting certain drugs that affect (reduce) the immune system, such as systemic immunosuppression to treat inflammatory skin disease.

Conception, pregnancy and lactation

Any drug exposure prior to, during or after conception can result in an adverse fetal outcome or risk to the mother. This risk, which is closely related to drug dose and duration, should always be considered when prescribing in women of child-bearing potential and the patient should be fully informed of the potential hazard. The pre-implantation period (fertilisation to implantation) is considered the 'all or nothing' period since injury will result either in embryonic loss or, if only a small number of cells are affected, embryo survival, as the remaining cells are not yet committed to a particular path of development and can therefore compensate for the loss. Drug exposure during the embryonic period (week 2 to week 9) carries the greatest risk of fetal malformation as this is when organogenesis occurs. Nevertheless, maternal drug exposure at any period may be associated with longer term functional or developmental changes that are not immediately apparent. For example, in a cohort of 31 children born to mothers exposed to isotretinoin, nearly half had evidence of developmental delay, regardless of whether the children had structural malformations at birth [7]. Drugs given just before term or during labour can have adverse effects on labour or the neonate (e.g. sedative antihistamines) as well as the mother (e.g. risk of postpartum infection with certain types of immunosuppression); ongoing maternal drug use post-pregnancy may be secreted in breast milk.

Thalidomide, acitretin and isotretinoin are notable examples of drugs with specific, known risks of teratogenicity, and all of these are used in dermatology with rigorous pregnancy prevention plans attached. Additional drugs are also commonly used in dermatology with known risk of teratogenicity, such as methotrexate and mycophenolate mofetil. However, for the majority of drugs, there is insufficient evidence to properly categorise the level of risk and so in general, where possible, drug exposure is avoided or minimised in women planning conception or who are pregnant. Nevertheless, very many women with skin disease will require treatment, and often the benefit of any intervention – the health and well-being of the woman – will outweigh poorly described or uncertain risks. Referencing up-to-date information on risks (for example the summary of product characteristics) and regular review (to ensure effectiveness and/or continuing need for treatment) will contribute to optimal treatment selection and outcome. Topical therapy is generally considered the safest route of drug use for skin disease during pregnancy since systemic, and therefore fetal, exposure is minimised. Large volumes applied to extensive, inflammatory skin disease may still result in systemic drug exposure so risk is not completely avoided. For example, there is some evidence suggesting an increased risk of low birth weight with the use of very significant amounts of potent or very potent corticosteroids during pregnancy [8] but even here, depending on the clinical circumstances, such risks may be less than that associated with other interventions – for example oral corticosteroids – or leaving disease untreated.

Drug disposition can alter significantly during pregnancy [9] with most of the changes beginning during the first trimester and peaking during the second trimester. Overall these physiological changes tend to increase the volume of drug distribution, reduce the amount of albumin-bound drug, and increase hepatic and renal clearance, with consequent variable effects on drug concentration depending on the drug. The use of therapeutic monoclonal antibodies and therapeutic peptides during pregnancy requires particular care since maternal antibodies are actively transported across the placenta from around the 14th week of pregnancy, via the Fc receptor expressed on trophoblasts, rapidly increasing over the second and third trimesters. Data on the use of anti-TNF monoclonal antibodies during pregnancy suggest that therapeutic antibodies are handled in the same way as naturally occurring antibodies, with drug levels of infliximab and adalimumab in infants at birth being at least equivalent to those of the mother. Interestingly, transplacental transfer of certolizumab pegol, a pegylated humanised antibody Fab' fragment against TNF, appears to be very low or absent because it lacks an Fc receptor. Maternal immunoglobulins (predominantly IgA) are present in breast milk, so therapeutic antibodies might also be predicted in breast milk. Limited human data indicate that drug levels in breast milk are only a fraction of those in the mother, with infant drug levels falling over time despite continuation of breast feeding. This suggests that the infant intestinal mucosal barrier and enzymatic digestion limit the bioavailability of any drug present in breast milk.

In men, drugs may affect fertility and/or spermatogenesis, although reliable information on absolute risk is scarce. Drugs that directly interact with DNA (e.g. methotrexate, azathioprine, cytotoxics) theoretically carry particular risk although recent studies are reassuring [10,11].

Drug interactions

A drug's effect may be significantly altered by the co-administration of another drug with a consequent impact on efficacy and/or induction of toxicity. The principal mechanisms underlying most drug interactions relate to drug-metabolising enzymes and transporters.

Whereas all major drug-metabolising enzymes have been associated with drug–drug interactions, cytochrome P40 enzymes are the major contributors to clinically relevant drug interactions, with CYP1A2, CYP2B6, CYP2C8, CYP2C9, CYP2C19, CYP2D6 and CYP3A being commonly implicated. For example, ciclosporin is extensively metabolised by CYP3A isoforms. Co-therapy with erythromycin or itraconazole, both potent inhibitors of CYP3A, can therefore lead to significantly increased levels of ciclosporin, whereas phenytoin, a potent inducer of CYP3A, may reduce ciclosporin levels. Alternative remedies are also relevant here. St John's wort contains a potent inducer of CYP3A (hyperforin), for example, and has been reported in association with reduced levels of ciclosporin, while echinacea variously inhibits intestinal CYP1A2 and CYP3A and induces hepatic CYP3A activities.

Drug–transporter interactions arise either due to a change in activity (increased or decreased) or competition at the transporter site. For example, the activity of the efflux transporter P-glycoprotein, which normally acts to reduce gastrointestinal absorption and increase biliary excretion of drugs, is inhibited by intraconazole and ciclosporin, with a resultant increase in relevant drug substrate levels (e.g. fexofenadine).

Aside from these pharmacokinetic mechanisms, drugs may interact at a pharmacodynamic level. This may be used to therapeutic advantage – prednisolone is often combined with azathioprine or mycophenolate mofetil in order to achieve the same level of immunosuppressant effect, while reducing the toxicity of higher dose steroid monotherapy, for example.

From a pharmacokinetic perspective, in contrast to small molecules, there are few clinically relevant drug interactions reported in relation to protein-based therapeutics, specifically monoclonal antibodies. For individuals who are receiving *two* therapeutic monoclonal antibodies, competition for the FcRn-mediated salvage pathway can potentially influence bioavailability.

Patient adherence to treatment

The extent to which patients follow the instructions they are given for a prescribed medication (i.e. adherence) varies enormously, from missing an occasional dose to completely stopping treatment. The corresponding impact on treatment outcome is therefore variable. The science of quantifying the three measurable phases of adherence – initiation, implementation and persistence/discontinuation – and their respective contribution to drug outcome is known as *pharmionics* [12]. Non-adherence is very common and the underpinning reasons are multiple and complex. The COM-B framework (that is, capability, opportunity and motivation), which is a conceptual framework widely used to understand behaviours and, crucially, influence change, has recently been advocated as a better framework for investigating and managing adherence than the two-category *unintentional* and *intentional* approach. Here, *capability* relates to psychological (e.g. memory, poor comprehension or recall of the details of the prescribed therapeutic regimen) and/or physical (e.g. dexterity, difficulty applying topicals/injecting treatments) factors. *Motivation* relates to any brain processes that energise and direct behaviour whether reflective (such as beliefs about treatment) or automatic (e.g. mood, anticipatory nausea with methotrexate). *Opportunity* encompasses anything that lies outside the individual, whether these are physical factors (such as ability to pay, lack of access, complexity of the treatment schedule) or the social/cultural environment (e.g. stigma around skin disease, religious beliefs). Helpfully, this framework explicitly acknowledges interactions between the three themes, for example poor adherence being explained by low mood (motivation) which also influences ability to plan (psychological) [13]. Few patients will voluntarily declare non-adherence to health care professionals and assessment is best approached in a non-judgemental way. In general, patients wish to minimise drug exposure and/or the number of medicines they take, and where multiple treatments have been recommended may prioritise one over the other. They will evaluate for themselves the side effects and effectiveness of any given treatment – and, of course, the effectiveness of treatment in skin disease is manifestly obvious. Some may stop therapy to see the outcome. Overall, adherence to prescribed therapy, especially for chronic conditions, is poor, with no major change in rates over the last 50 years.

Strategies to improve adherence need to take into account these multiple and complex drivers to non-adherence, and inevitably evidence for benefit is inconsistent [14]. Adherence rates may improve when patients are empowered with knowledge, skills and confidence to manage their own health [15]. Key practical aspects to this ambition include clear written and verbal communication about how, why and when the treatment needs to be taken, always prescribing the simplest dosing schedule possible and using a route of administration that is acceptable and practical. Techniques to remind and support patients in different situations (e.g. telephone reminders, dosette boxes) are part of this [14]. Dermatology nurse specialists and pharmacists also play a role with education and support, practical demonstration of where and how to apply topical treatments and, in some instances, application of treatments in formal out-patient settings.

Medication errors

Some drug-related adverse events are accepted risks of treatment as characterised at different stages of drug development and pharmacovigilance (Table 13.3) [16]. Although these may be minimised with careful prescribing and medicine use, some are unavoidable. In contrast, medication errors and any associated harm are avoidable, and have been described as any preventable event that may cause or lead to inappropriate medication use or patient harm while the medication is in the control of the health care professional, patient or consumer [17]. The steps involved between writing a

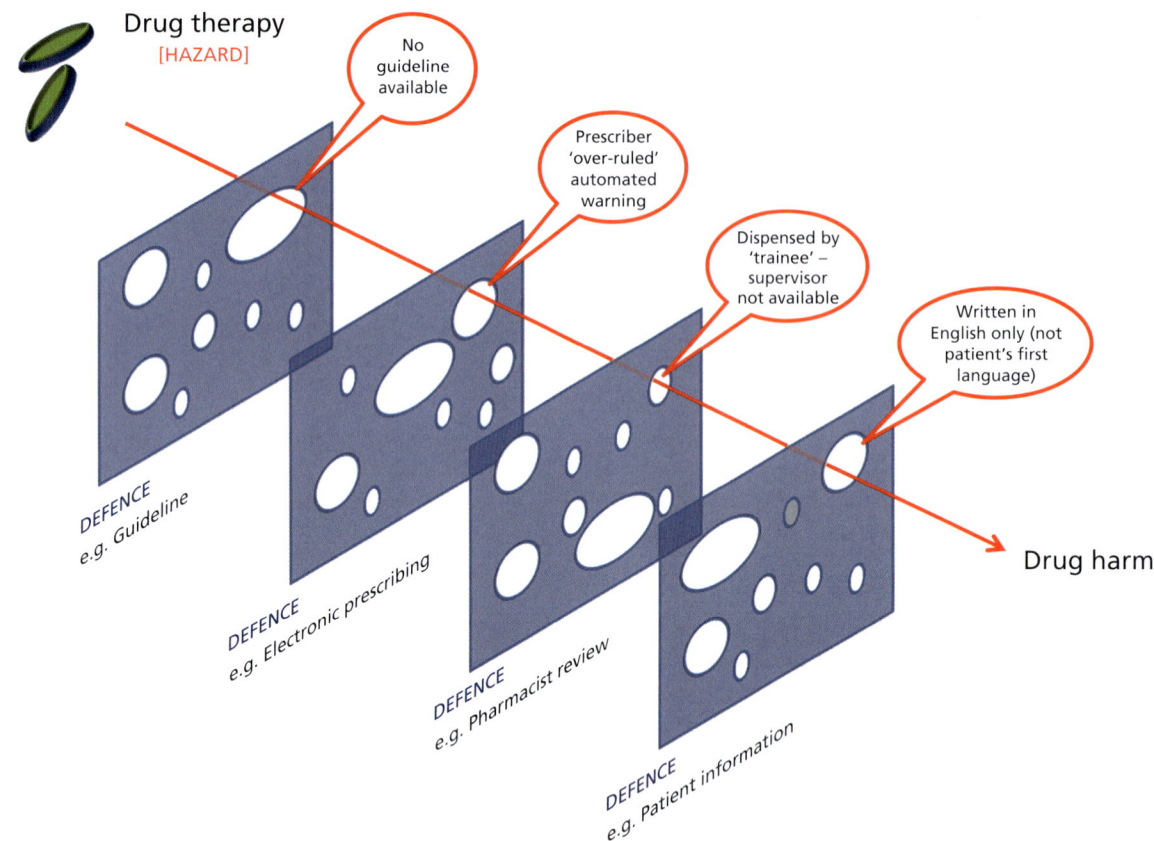

Figure 13.2 Swiss cheese model to illustrate the cumulative effect of multiple failures (holes) in defence mechanisms that ultimately translate drug hazard into actual, drug-related patient harm. The 'holes' in the defence may be latent such as organisational flaws (e.g. no supervisor being present) or active (e.g. the prescriber actively overruling an automated alert). Understanding the origin of near misses and/or actual drug-related adverse events is a crucial step towards safer prescribing and the avoidance of preventable drug harm.

prescription and the patient receiving the medicine are multiple, and each is subject to potential error. Medication errors that lead to serious or fatal adverse events invariably occur due to a series of events, and reflect human error (active failure) arising in the context of certain predisposing environmental or system factors (latent failures), the so-called 'Swiss cheese model' (Figure 13.2).

Reasons are multiple, and include inadequate knowledge of the patient (for example their clinical condition, drug history and known allergies) or the drug being prescribed, drug dose calculation errors, errors relating to communication such as illegible handwriting, confusing drug names and/or product labelling, errors in dispensing and administration, and failure to monitor adequately and thus minimise the impact of adverse reactions (for example interrupting methotrexate therapy if bone marrow depression occurs) [16,18].

One of the commonest sources of error is in the prescription itself. In hospital, often the most junior member of the team with the least knowledge and experience is tasked with prescribing; this in itself is a risk, but also fails to create a culture where prescribing is perceived to be important [19]. Additional factors that predispose to errors include repeated interruptions when writing a prescription and depression in the prescriber.

Poor communication among clinicians, particularly where care crosses or is transferred from one clinical setting (e.g. hospital) to another (e.g. primary care), is also a significant source of error. This is both in relation to the dose and type of medication to be used, and also, as importantly, review and monitoring of the treatment. In this situation, a disconnect can arise between the prescriber who initiated the treatment and the clinician responsible for ongoing care, so the necessary adjustments in drug therapy and monitoring fail to occur and/or drug errors remain unchecked for prolonged periods of time, with sometimes catastrophic results. This was specifically identified as a major contributory factor in a review of 137 adverse events arising in relation to methotrexate, which included 25 deaths and 26 serious incidents requiring hospital admission in the UK. It was also the commonest reason in ambulatory care for adverse drug reactions leading to hospital admission.

Certain types of medication are subject to frequent medication errors: (i) drugs with a narrow therapeutic index and/or where the therapeutic dose is close to the toxic dose (e.g. chemotherapeutic agents, anticoagulants, narcotics); (ii) drugs with an unusual dosing schedule that patients may easily confuse (e.g. once-weekly methotrexate); or (iii) drugs requiring intravenous administration where the speed of infusion or extravasation of drug into tissue can lead to problems (e.g. rapid immunoglobulin infusion and the risk of thromboembolic events, cytotoxic drugs). The drug groups most frequently associated with preventable, drug-related hospital admissions are anticoagulants, antiplatelet agents, diuretics and NSAIDs, with around a third due to problems with prescribing, a third due to adherence issues and a third due to inadequate monitoring [20–22]. Patient groups vulnerable to medication error include infants and children, where complex dose calculations are required using drugs that may not be licensed for use in children, and older patients due to communication difficulties, multimorbidity, and related to this, polypharmacy.

While something is known about the cause and prevalence of medication errors, there is relatively little good evidence to indicate which interventions effectively reduce error [23,24]. Prescribing is no longer the sole remit of doctors and extends to nurses, pharmacists and physiotherapists, all of whom need to take professional responsibility for their prescribing practice. Prescribers need to be supported by appropriate training in clinical pharmacology and the practicalities of prescribing with ready access to clear guidelines and protocols on the use of drugs. Clearly defined 'care pathways' can also provide clarity over where responsibility lies for prescribing and monitoring, as has been implemented as part of the National Patient Safety Agency alert on methotrexate in the UK. However, all humans are subject to errors and lapses so additional, multiple checks need to be in place. Pharmacists play a critical role in cross-checking prescriptions (although paradoxically knowing that this safeguard is in place has been identified as a source of inaccurate prescription writing in clinical practice). Numerous and varied information technology initiatives focusing on all aspects of the prescribing pathway have been developed, although not all are necessarily associated with a reduction in error risk. For example, electronic prescribing has been shown to reduce the incidence of illegible scripts and adverse drug reactions [25] but automated alerts about potential drug interactions and dose errors may overwhelm the prescriber or be ignored. Electronic prescribing also has the benefit of standardising the use of medicines and can be used to align drug choices to local formularies or guidelines. It seems likely, though, that further refinement of existing systems and new developments in this area will yield substantial benefit.

Legislation from the UK Medicines and Healthcare Products Regulatory Agency on standards for product labelling should help to reduce confusion and thus minimise dispensing errors. Perhaps most important of all, ensuring the patient is fully informed about the treatment plan can allow patients themselves to understand the intervention and potentially identify and/or correct mistakes.

Personalised medicine and pharmacogenomics

Personalised medicine aims to provide the right drug to the right patient at the right time [26]. Pharmacogenomics describes the intersection between genomic medicine and pharmacology, focusing on the identification of genome variants that influence drug effects via alterations in a drug's pharmacokinetics or via modulation of a drug's pharmacodynamics [27,**28**]. Genome variations of clinical relevance are primarily in the germline DNA; however, in cancer therapeutics, important somatically acquired mutations also influence response, and for infectious disease genomic variation in the infecting vector itself may alter their sensitivity to antimicrobial agents.

Historically, work to identify genetic determinants of variation in response has largely focused on drug pharmacokinetics. The well-described phenotypic subtypes fast and slow 'acetylators' and 'slow metabolisers' for example, have been found to originate from specific genetic polymorphisms in *NAT2* and *CYP2D6*, respectively. Deficiencies in enzymes metabolising azathioprine and 6-mercaptopurine are also established pharmacokinetic phenotypes determined by genetic variation, and account for at least some of the rare but severe drug-related myelotoxicity. Specifically, thiopurine *S*-methyltransferase deficiency is caused by homozygous or compound heterozygotes in *TPMT*3C*, *TPMT*3A TPMT*2* and nudix hydrolase deficiency, caused by *NUDT15* polymorphisms especially in Asian populations where the frequency of TMPT deficiency is low [29]. More recently, with the advent of the Human Genome Project, genome-wide investigation of genetic variation and the falling cost of sequencing, pharmacogenetic discovery has accelerated. More than 80 actionable germline gene–drug relationships have been identified – in other words where genetic information should be used to change prescribing of the affected drug. However, with the exception of azathioprine and mercaptopurine, these are not for interventions routinely used in dermatology [30]. In cancer, targeting certain somatically acquired gene mutations has driven both drug development and precision medicine. This is exemplified in melanoma, where the identification of activating mutations in *BRAF* (encoding protein kinase B-raf) led to the rapid development of highly specific oral BRAF inhibitors such as vemurafenib and improved progression-free survival in patients with advanced melanoma.

Bringing findings into practice is, however, challenging. Genetic (or other biomarker) assessment of treatment outcome may fail to move into the clinic because when evaluated in real life they fail to demonstrate added value over and above more traditional 'clinical' indicators of treatment response. This may be for a variety of reasons, including ethnic diversity, and the fact that other influences are in play (such as adherence). The transition from a research environment into clinical practice also requires capacity: clinical research capacity to validate and test, capacity for clinicians to take up new investigative tools and understand their meaning in the context of the patient in front of them, the capacity of laboratories to process new tests, and financial capacity within health care systems [**28**,29].

Drug development and licensing procedures

The process of developing a drug that meets statutory efficacy and safety requirements for use in patients is long, complex and expensive (Figure 13.3). Very substantial investment in drug research and development over the past few decades across medicine and specifically within dermatology, together with the genomics era and technological advances, have brought many new and 'game changing' interventions.

Preclinical drug identification

The two principal approaches used to identify potential candidate drugs are *phenotypic screening* and *target-based screening*. Phenotypic screening investigates the effects, or phenotypes, that a compound induces in cells, tissues or whole organisms and historically was the primary method of new drug identification. However, phenotypic screens have been largely replaced with a target-based approach due to huge developments in medicine (including technology and computing) and our increased understanding of disease mechanism through molecular biology and genomics. The identification of a candidate target requires a detailed understanding of the molecular basis of a particular disease or pathogenic pathway and such data

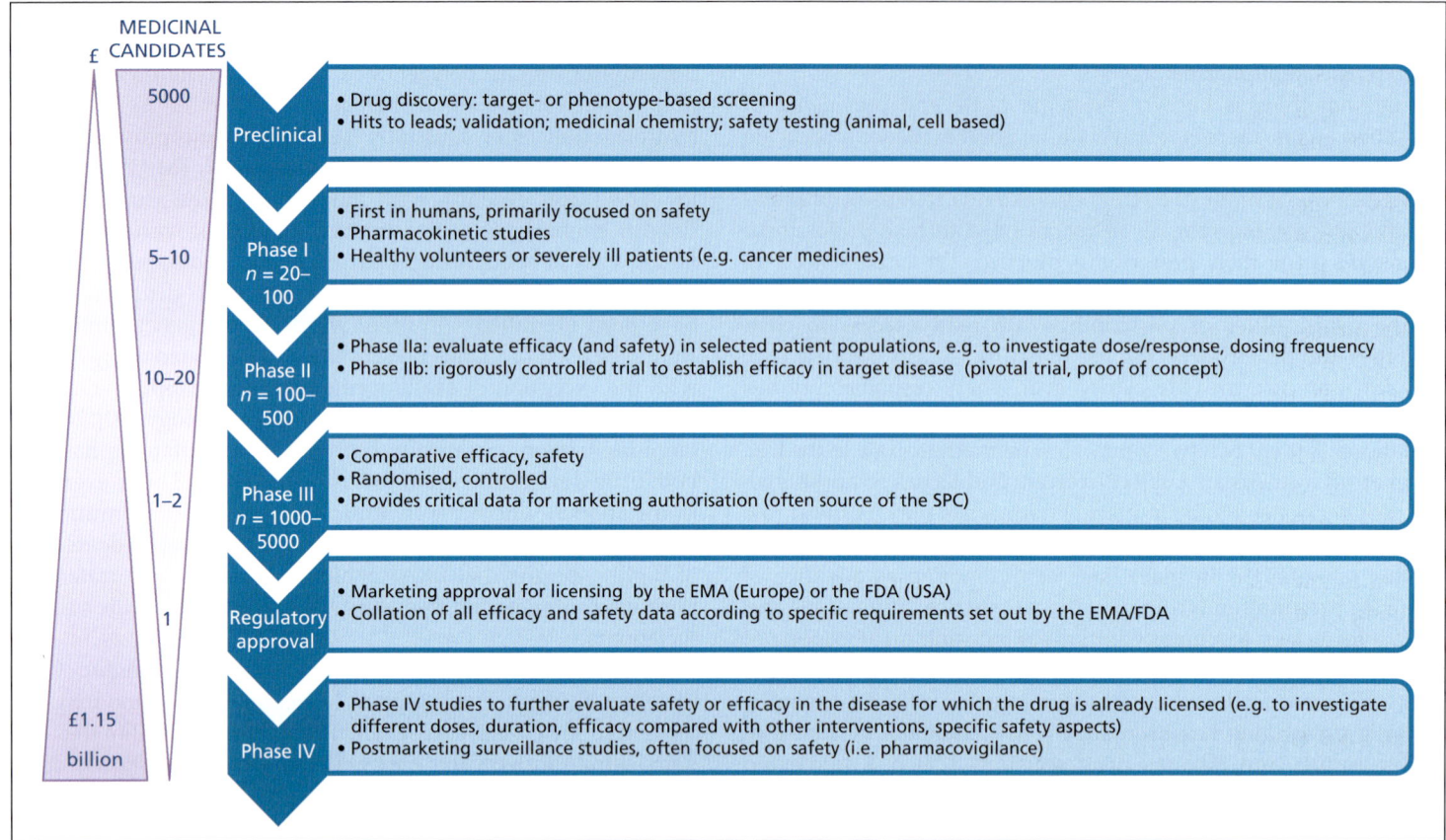

Figure 13.3 An overview of the phases of drug development from discovery through to licensing and postmarketing surveillance (phase IV). Toxicity, failed efficacy and commercial reasons contribute to the slow attrition in numbers of promising candidate drugs that successfully progress along this pathway. The parallel, almost exponential, increase in the cost of delivering each phase of drug development means that for each drug that reaches the market, the investment is substantial. EMA, European Medicines Agency; FDA, US Food and Drug Administration; SPC, summary of product characteristics.

can come from a variety of sources, including academic and clinical research and from the commercial (pharmaceutical) sector. Potential candidate medicines are then screened for their ability to alter a specific biologically critical target within that pathway (usually a protein). Structure-based techniques, which are increasingly done using computational modelling (*in silico*), enable precise delineation of the target. Libraries of 'small-molecule' compounds that interact with these targets can be rapidly screened using high throughput technology (*in silico* and/or *in vitro*), and subsequently tailored to optimise target binding (reiterative redirected compound synthesis). The development of biological therapy similarly employs a target-based approach, with the design and development of large-molecule protein-based drugs (often monoclonal antibodies) that aim to modulate endogenous pathways known to be pathogenically relevant.

These two approaches can be very effectively combined, capitalising on the benefit of knowing that candidate molecules identified in a phenotypic screen show pharmacological activity in a complex, biologically relevant system, and then using all the -omics technology to identify the underlying molecular mechanism of action and tailor the drug accordingly.

Drug development

Once candidate drugs are identified, further optimisation, pharmacokinetic and pharmacodynamics studies and preclinical testing are completed in a variety of *in silico*, *in vitro* (including cellular or organotypic assays) and animal models. The technology and platform depend on the therapeutic target. Animal testing is kept to an absolute minimum (as mandated by the recent European '3 Rs' directive: reduce, replace and refine) but remains an essential component of drug development prior to the first human trials in order to establish drug pharmacokinetics and to give an indication of early safety (e.g. genotoxicity, mutagenicity, unexpected toxicity). Phase I trials investigate the use of the drug in humans for the first time (Figure 13.3). These studies usually involve a small number of healthy volunteers but may, particularly in cancer medicine, involve patients with advanced disease and poor prognosis or limited treatment options. Because the drug effects can be unpredictable and, rarely, catastrophic, these studies are always completed in a highly supervised, clinical research environment [1]. Phase I studies intensively assess safety and pharmacokinetics, often in a staggered programme of drug exposure that starts with minimal drug exposure, up-titrating to a modelled or predicted therapeutic dose range, with the trial only progressing through each stage of escalated dosing if all safety parameters are met. If the phase I studies reveal no untoward findings and are consistent with the known pharmacology of the drug, phase II trials proceed in the target disease with the aim of establishing drug efficacy. Phase III trials follow, with at least two independent, large, randomised, comparative trials generally required for regulatory approval.

Throughout the phase II and phase III trial programme the comparative control populations are exposed to a placebo and/or another medical intervention (often current standard care).

New drug applications for regulatory approval are made to national or regional agencies such as the Medicines and Healthcare products Regulatory Agency (MHRA) (UK), the European Medicines Agency (EMA) (European Union) and the Food and Drug Administration (FDA) (USA) on submission of a detailed dossier of requisite information. This includes all preclinical testing, data from the phase I–III trials, technical information on drug manufacturing processes, proposed labelling, directions for use, safety updates, overdose information, additional studies outside of the regulatory region, patent information and plans for postmarketing pharmacoviligance (see 'Drug toxicity and adverse effects' earlier in this chapter). Drugs can be assigned 'orphan' status when indicated for rare diseases ('orphan' diseases) where the feasibility of large-scale trials as well as cost (in terms of likely market return) will probably be prohibitive. Here regulatory requirements are adjusted to encourage industry investment (e.g. early access and marketing of drugs prior to the completion of formal approval) in order to maintain focus and investment on what are often very high-need groups.

Ethics and trial reporting

The International Conference on Harmonisation Good Clinical Practice (ICH-GCP) guideline has established an internationally agreed ethical and scientific quality standard for the design, conduct, recording and reporting of drug intervention trials involving human subjects.. This aims to: (i) ensure that the rights, safety and well-being of trial subjects are protected, consistent with principles that have their origin in the Declaration of Helsinki; (ii) ensure that the clinical trial data are credible; and (iii) facilitate mutual acceptance of clinical data by the different regulatory authorities. All trials conducted on human subjects are mandated to adhere to ICH-GCP standards.

The reporting of trials and trial results has been subject to much debate, with concern over lack of transparency and significant reporting bias with large tracts of trial data remaining with either regulators or unpublished. Collectively, this all contributes to clinicians having an incomplete picture of a drug's efficacy and safety, and thus limits their ability to achieve optimal outcomes. A number of strategies have been put in place to improve this situation with some evidence for benefit [2]. First, investigators are strongly encouraged to register trials on publicly available databases such as ClinicalTrials.gov with protocol details, recruitment progress and eventually the trial results. This strategy has been strongly endorsed by the International Committee of Medical Journal Editors who agreed to make this a requirement for journal publication. Second, standards have been developed to improve the quality of trial reporting by the EQUATOR Network and many journals subscribe to adherence to these standards for trial reports submitted for publication. Third, within the biopharmaceutical industry, the European Federation of Pharmaceutical Industries and Associations (EFPIA) and the Pharmaceutical Research and Manufacturers of America (PhRMA), have developed joint 'Principles for responsible clinical trial data sharing'. The EMA, as well as a number of large pharmaceutical companies, have also agreed to the release of previously unpublished data.

Resources

Further information

EQUATOR (Enhancing the QUAlity and Transparency Of health Research) Network: http://www.equator-network.org/ (last accessed April 2023).

Key references

The full list of references can be found in the online version at https://www.wiley.com/rooksdermatology10e

Pharmacokinetics

1 Buxton I. Pharmacokinetics: the dynamics of drug absorption, distribution, metabolism, and elimination. In: Brunton LL, Hilal-Danden R, Knollmann BC, eds. *Goodman and Gilman's: The Pharmacological Basis of Therapeutics*, 13th edn. New York: McGraw Hill Medical, 2018.
2 Bensalem A, Ternant D. Pharmacokinetic variability of therapeutic antibodies in humans: a comprehensive review of population pharmacokinetic modeling publications. *Clin Pharmacokinet* 2020;59:857–74.

Pharmacodynamics

1 Blumenthal DK. Pharmacodynamics: molecular mechanisms of drug action. In: Brunton LL, Hilal-Danden R, Knollmann BC, eds. *Goodman and Gilman's: The Pharmacological Basis of Therapeutics*, 13th edn. New York: McGraw Hill Medical; 2018.

Factors that affect therapeutic outcome

1 Kearns GL, Abdel-Rahman SM, Alander SW, Blowey DL, Leeder JS, Kauffman RE. Developmental pharmacology – drug disposition, action, and therapy in infants and children. *N Engl J Med* 2003;349:1157–67.
4 Klotz U. Pharmacokinetics and drug metabolism in the elderly. *Drug Metab Rev* 2009;41:67–76.
12 Vrijens B, De Geest S, Hughes DA *et al*. A new taxonomy for describing and defining adherence to medications. *Br J Clin Pharmacol* 2012;73:691–70.
16 Neberker JR, Barach P, Samore MH. Clarifying adverse drug events: a clinician's guide to terminology, documentation, and reporting. *Ann Intern Med* 2004;140:795–801.
23 Ciapponi A, Fernandez Nievas SE *et al*. Reducing medication errors for adults in hospital settings. *Cochrane Database Syst Rev* 2021;Issue 11: CD009985.
28 Relling MV, Evans WE. Pharmacogenomics in the clinic. *Nature* 2015;526:343–50.

Drug development and licensing procedures

2 Baronikova S, Purvis J, Southam E, Beeso J, Panayi A, Winchester C. Commitments by the biopharmaceutical industry to clinical trial transparency: the evolving environment. *BMJ Evid Based Med* 2019;24:177–84.

CHAPTER 14

Adverse Immunological Reactions to Drugs

Michael R. Ardern-Jones

Faculty of Medicine, University of Southampton, Southampton General Hospital, Southampton, UK

Introduction, 14.1	Drug reaction with eosinophilia and systemic symptoms, 14.3	Pharmacological interaction (p-i) model, 14.6
IgE-mediated drug hypersensitivity, 14.1		Altered peptide repertoire model, 14.6
Pseudoallergic reactions, 14.2	Other types of drug hypersensitivity, 14.4	Understanding the clinical phenotype, 14.6
T-cell-mediated drug hypersensitivity, 14.3	T-cell recognition of drugs, 14.4	Conclusions, 14.7
Stevens–Johnson syndrome and toxic epidermal necrolysis, 14.3	Hapten/pro-hapten model, 14.5	Key references, 14.7

Introduction

Many drugs are designed carefully to avoid interaction with the immune system. However, some such as imiquimod are designed to induce 'on-target' immunological effects through direct induction of immune responses via binding of immunostimulatory receptors such as TLR7 [1]. 'Off-target' induction of an immune system-mediated reaction is an adverse immunological reaction. A hypersensitivity reaction is an adverse immunological reaction that involves antigen-specific recognition but does not include induction of inflammatory responses via activatory receptors. Consequently, hypersensitivity reactions are mediated by antibodies and T cells and demonstrate immunological memory. The cellular machinery of the immune system that may be involved in a drug hypersensitivity reaction is the same as that involved in immune-mediated host defence against infection. Consequently, many overlapping clinical, biochemical, molecular and immunological features exist between drug hypersensitivity and infection. One important difference between the two states is that drug hypersensitivity reactions frequently only involve the skin, although the precise reasons for cutaneous restriction of inflammation secondary to a drug that has wide bioavailability remain unclear. However, drug hypersensitivity-mediated multiorgan involvement must be considered in all reactions.

The four main types of immune reaction were originally defined by Coombs and Gell (Table 14.1) [2] and modified by Pichler (Table 14.2) [3]. Hypersensitivity reactions types 1–3 are antibody mediated while type 4 processes are mediated by T cells, but there are many different overlapping clinical syndromes that can be produced.

IgE-mediated drug hypersensitivity

Antibodies recognise antigen in the soluble form and do not require antigenic processing. Thus, the recognition/binding repertoire of antibodies is significantly greater than that of T cells. The role of immunoglobulin E (IgE) is convincing and has been demonstrated in organ transplants from allergic donors to non-allergic recipients, with subsequent confirmation of transfer of drug-specific IgE producing B cells and clinical drug allergy [4]. IgE-mediated drug reactions including urticaria, angioedema and anaphylaxis are type 1 hypersensitivity reactions and involve drug-specific IgE bound to the high-affinity IgE receptor (FcεR1) on the surface of mast cells and basophils. IgE binding to a multivalent allergen (drug) induces receptor aggregation and leads to cellular activation, followed by degranulation and release of inflammatory mediators including histamine. The mediators are divided into three groups: (i) those that are preformed on granules; (ii) newly synthesised lipid mediators; and (iii) cytokines and chemokines. In the skin, the release of histamine, leukotriene C4 (LTC4), prostaglandin D2 (PGD2) and proteases contributes to early vasodilatation and increased vascular permeability, which induce redness and oedema associated with weal and flare (urticaria and sometimes angioedema). The effects of histamine and mast cell chymase on smooth muscle in the lungs or gastrointestinal tract result in bronchoconstriction (asthma) or intestinal cramps and diarrhoea [5]. LTC4 and cytokine release induces an eosinophil (interleukin 5 (IL-5)) and neutrophil (IL-8 and tumour necrosis factor α (TNF-α)) influx which contributes towards a late phase reaction [5]. If the vasodilatory effect is sufficient to cause hypotension, anaphylactic shock can follow with cardiac decompensation and ultimately death if untreated.

Whilst histamine can induce all the features of anaphylaxis, it is likely that other factors are involved. Good evidence points to an early role for platelet-activating factor (PAF) in disease pathogenesis [6,7]. PAF is a phospholipid synthesised and secreted by mast cells as well as monocytes and macrophages. Its role has been supported by injection into humans causing grade 1 anaphylaxis symptoms [8], and levels correlate better with severity of anaphylaxis [7].

Although drug-specific IgE is identifiable in most cases of drug-induced anaphylaxis, it is not detectable in all. These latter are

Rook's Textbook of Dermatology, Tenth Edition. Edited by Christopher Griffiths, Jonathan Barker, Tanya Bleiker, Walayat Hussain and Rosalind Simpson.
© 2024 John Wiley & Sons Ltd. Published 2024 by John Wiley & Sons Ltd.

Table 14.1 Types of hypersensitivity reaction, mechanisms and clinical correlations.

Type of hypersensitivity	Immune effector mechanisms	Clinical manifestations relevant to drug hypersensitivity
Type 1: immediate or anaphylactic	IgE is bound to the surface of mast cells or basophils. Antigen binding causes mast cell degranulation and the release of histamine and other mediators	Urticaria, asthma, anaphylaxis
Type 2: cytotoxic	Antigenic determinants on cell surfaces are targets for antibodies – may be IgG or IgM. The antibodies damage cells/tissues by activating complement, or by binding to cells through Fcγ receptors they activate cytotoxic killing, e.g. by NK cells	Pemphigus Blood cell penias: haemolytic anaemia, neutropenia, thrombocytopenia
Type 3: immune complex	Circulating immune complexes are deposited in vascular beds or on tissue surfaces. Complement is activated, neutrophils are attracted and their products damage tissues	Vasculitis – hypersensitivity vasculitis, Henoch–Schönlein purpura
Type 4: delayed type, T-cell mediated	Effector T lymphocytes, which may be CD4+ or CD8+, produce different patterns of cytokines and/or cytotoxic factors	There are many clinical patterns that are subcategorised in Table 14.2

Adapted from Coombs and Gell 1968 [2].
NK, natural killer.

Table 14.2 Types of type 4 hypersensitivity reaction, mechanisms and clinical correlations.

	Immune mediators	Inflammation characterised by	Clinical pattern
Type 4a	Th1/Tc1 cells: IFN-γ, TNF-α	T cells, macrophages	Contact dermatitis, tuberculin reaction
Type 4b	Th2 cells: IL-4/-13, IL-5	Eosinophils	Maculopapular rash, exanthemata with eosinophilia
Type 4c	Cytotoxic T/NK/NKT cells: granulysin perforin, granzyme B	T cells Keratinocyte apoptosis	Contact dermatitis, maculopapular rash, drug-induced exanthemata, bullous eruptions (SJS/TEN)
Type 4d	T cells: IL-8, CXCL8, GM-CSF	Neutrophils	Acute generalised exanthematous pustulosis

Adapted from Pichler 2007 [3].
GM-CSF, granulocyte–macrophage colony-stimulating factor; IFN, interferon; IL, interleukin; NK, natural killer; SJS, Stevens–Johnson syndrome; TEN, toxic epidermal necrolysis; TNF, tumour necrosis factor.

termed idiopathic anaphylaxis or anaphylactoid reactions. In such cases, drug-specific IgG has been identified in numerous cases [9] and it has been proposed that activation of neutrophils and other FcγR-bearing cells may be implicated in disease pathogenesis, and that these cells contribute to the expression of PAF [10]. The role of PAF has been proposed for many years, while supporting evidence has increased and the mechanism has become more widely acknowledged; this understanding has increased the interest in PAF inhibitors as therapeutic targets.

The current understanding of the genetic factors driving individual susceptibility to type 1 hypersensitivity drug allergy is less well understood than that for type 4. The regulation of B-cell IgE production is dependent upon antigen-specific Th2 signalling in the lymph node and therefore, to some degree, the two systems are linked. Thus despite the disparate clinical phenotypes, the activation of drug-specific T cells is critical for type 1 hypersensitivity. In view of this, the reported associations between type 1 hypersensitivities and human leukocyte antigen (HLA) alleles are surprisingly weak.

Previous work has associated the risk of IgE-mediated penicillin allergy with atopy, IL-13, IL-18, IL-10 promoter, IL-4Rα and FcεR1 polymorphisms [11–16]. Similarly, STAT6 polymorphisms have been reported to specifically predispose to penicillin allergy but not atopy [17]. Interesting work has recently identified polymorphisms in FcεR1 associated with non-steroidal anti-inflammatory drug (NSAID) hypersensitivity [18]. Although mostly of weak predictive value, the association between penicillin allergy and IL-4Rα polymorphisms has been shown to be the most replicated of the genetic associations.

Further insights into the relationship between environmental exposures and subsequent IgE allergic responses have been gained from studies of populations at risk of tick bites in North America. Ticks of the genus *Amblyomma* are recognised to mainly interact with animals but bite humans incidentally. Individuals who have suffered a tick bite have shown increased risk of inducing a specific IgE against a mammalian epitope (galactose-α-1,3-galactose or alpha-gal) which is a blood group substance of non-primate mammals. This specific IgE is associated with clinical allergy to non-primate meat including beef, pork and lamb, presumably through recognition of the animal blood group antigen. However, interestingly, the alpha-gal-specific IgE also recognises a structurally similar glycosylation site on the anticancer monoclonal antibody cetuximab produced in murine cells. This explains why individuals who have suffered a tick bite are at increased risk of immediate anaphylactic reactions at first exposure to cetuximab [19]. Thus environmental sensitisations can be relevant to subsequent allergic reactions to drugs.

Pseudoallergic reactions

Activation of immune cells independent of unique antigen recognition, for example by direct binding of drug to a cell surface receptor, is termed 'pseudoallergic', although this term is most commonly applied to non-specific activation of mast cells. In these cases, the drug directly induces mast cell degranulation or release of inflammatory mediators such as leukotrienes which produce clinical syndromes such as urticaria, asthma or anaphylaxis that can be indistinguishable from true immunological hypersensitivities. Until recently, these reactions were thought to be largely idiosyncratic. However, recent work identifying the Mas-related G protein-coupled receptor member X2 (MRGPRX2) [20] has shone a light on previously unexplainable reactions. MRGPRX2 is expressed on human skin mast cells and binds many different drugs including morphine, contrast agents, anaesthetic agents and ciprofloxacin, which induces mast cell degranulation and causes anaphylaxis. Other areas of interest include other cascades such as those triggered by factor XII (FXII) associated with penicillin allergy [21].

T-cell-mediated drug hypersensitivity

Drug reactions including acute generalised exanthematous pustulosis (AGEP), Stevens–Johnson syndrome (SJS), toxic epidermal necrolysis (TEN) and drug reaction with eosinophilia and systemic symptoms (DRESS) are severe cutaneous adverse reactions to drugs which are quite heterogeneous in their presentation [22]. These are acknowledged to be dominantly T-cell mediated [23]. This is shown by the detection of activated cytotoxic T cells in the skin of people with acute reactions and drug-specific T cells *in vitro* [24,25]. T-cell or type IV hypersensitivity reactions are classically referred to as 'delayed type' because they develop over many hours. However, the clinical phenotype is likely to correspond to differences in immuno-phenotype, as recently expanded with relevance to drug hypersensitivity by Pichler (see Table 14.2) [3].

Stevens–Johnson syndrome and toxic epidermal necrolysis

Stevens–Johnson syndrome and TEN form a clinical spectrum characterised by widespread skin and mucous membrane blistering in association with histological evidence of full-thickness epidermal necrosis (keratinocyte apoptosis and/or necroptosis). In most cases a drug cause is identified although some cases have been identified in association with infection, especially with *Mycoplasma pneumoniae*. Evidence that drug-specific T cells are evident in blisters of TEN [26] favours a critical role for a T-cell-mediated pathogenesis. This is supported by evidence of immunological memory responses (TEN onset is faster on accidental re-exposure to the causative drug [27]) and genetic associations with molecular structures critical to T-cell activation (strong drug-specific association between certain HLA class I alleles and risk of TEN [24]). In addition to classic T cells, natural killer (NK) T cells and NK cells have also been implicated in SJS/TEN [28]. However, the precise mechanism for keratinocyte apoptosis is still not completely understood.

Fas is a death receptor and its activation initiates an apoptotic signalling cascade resulting in cell death. Keratinocytes constitutively express Fas receptors and apoptosis can be induced by contact with another cell bearing the ligand FasL. Therefore, much attention has been given to the observation that keratinocytes themselves upregulate surface FasL during TEN [29]. FasL is thought to be maintained intracellular in keratinocytes in non-inflammatory conditions, to prevent initiation of apoptosis. Following exposure to drug-activated T-cell cytokines TNF-α and interferon γ (IFN-γ), keratinocytes induce nitric oxide expression which then signals the increased expression of FasL at the surface [30]. FasL can also be released in soluble form (sFasL) and high levels have been found in blister fluid [31], but sFasL is thought to be unable to trigger apoptosis and so is unlikely to be the primary mediator. Subsequently, higher levels of FasL expression on TEN keratinocytes have not been detected by all groups, therefore it remains unclear how important this pathway is [32–35]. Furthermore, the initial demonstration that intravenous immunoglobulin (IVIg) contained blocking anti-Fas antibodies led to the widespread introduction of this treatment in TEN [29], but its effectiveness in TEN has since been questioned and remains controversial.

The induction of keratinocyte apoptosis by blister lymphocytes from cases of TEN but not controls, and apoptosis mediated by blister fluid alone, suggests a key role for a lymphocyte-released soluble mediator. Molecular and immunohistochemical evidence of lymphocyte (including CD8+, NK and NKT cells) production of granulysin is significantly upregulated in TEN [36]. Granulysin can initiate cell death by triggering cytolysis and a cascade of signalling which dysregulates membrane ion channels, damages mitochondria and ultimately initiates apoptosis. Thus, a strong case for the role of granulysin has been made in the initiation of TEN. Injection of this molecule into the skin induced widespread epidermal necrosis in a mouse model [37]. Interestingly, a similar clinical and immunological phenotype is recognised in severe cases of cutaneous graft-versus-host disease [37]. However, granulysin is important beyond TEN because it plays an important role in host defence against a variety of cancers [38] and microbes including skin infections such as leprosy [39], which could potentially account for infection-triggered SJS/TEN. Therefore, further work to understand the regulation expression of granulysin in the skin is of central importance to further understanding of this disease.

Others pathways and altered drug metabolism [40] have also been implicated in TEN pathogenesis including CD40/CD40L activation [41,42]. Studies of CD8+ cytotoxicity have suggested a role for perforin and granzyme in cytotoxic killing of keratinocytes in TEN which was inhibited *in vitro* by inhibition of perforin/granzyme but not by anti-Fas antibodies [26,43]. TNF-α has also been found at higher levels in TEN blister fluid and skin as compared with blistering burns [31,44] and activates apoptotic pathways through the death receptor TNF-R1. The only randomised controlled trial in the management of TEN was conducted on the basis of TNF-α inhibition with thalidomide, but had to be stopped early because of increased mortality in the treatment arm [45]. Some authors have concluded that this supported a bystander role for TNF-α [31], but, of note, levels of the cytokine were not reduced in blisters of thalidomide-treated patients. Furthermore, a number of case reports have suggested a benefit from monoclonal antibody TNF inhibitor therapy in TEN [46–49].

Drug reaction with eosinophilia and systemic symptoms

Synonyms of DRESS include drug-induced hypersensitivity syndrome (DIHS) and hypersensitivity syndrome (HSS). In contrast to SJS/TEN, both CD4+ and CD8+ T cells are implicated in DRESS pathogenesis. In addition, as implied in the name, eosinophil infiltrations in affected organs contribute to inflammation [50] and are recruited by IL-5 from Th2 polarised CD4+ cells [51]. However, the other Th2 cytokines, including IL-4 and IL-13, are also important in mediating tissue inflammation [52,53]. Recruitment of Th2 cells to tissues is mediated by chemokines including CCL17 (thymus and activation-regulated chemokine or TARC), and TARC levels in DRESS have been found to be higher than in other drug hypersensitivity reactions affecting the skin such as SJS/TEN or exanthems [54]. As a consequence of this understanding, anti-Th2 therapies including mepolizumab (anti-IL-5) [55] and Janus-activating kinase (JAK) inhibition have been proposed [53] as therapeutic options.

The cardinal features of DRESS include the rash (an exanthem-like eruption often with oedema) and systemic inflammation (including fever, organ dysfunction, haematological abnormalities and lymphadenopathy), which are reflected in diagnostic criteria from Europe [56] and Japan [57]. The similarity to viral infection is well recognised and sometimes difficult to distinguish. The pathogenesis of DRESS is thought to be the prototypical T-cell-mediated hypersensitivity reaction as suggested by *in vitro* demonstration of drug-specific T cells [58–60].

The association between human herpesvirus (HHV) and drug exanthems has been recognised for many years, most commonly in the association of an ampicillin-induced exanthem arising in 80% of those with acute Epstein–Barr virus (EBV) infection versus approximately 5% of controls. However, in DRESS, the finding that reactivation of long-lived viruses occurs in approximately 75% of cases suggests a more complicated pathogenesis than drug-specific T cells alone.

Reactivation of herpesviruses, especially EBV, HHV-6 and HHV-7, is a common finding and proposed as an explanation for flares in disease despite withdrawal of the culprit drug [61–65]. Indeed some authors have suggested that the detection of viral reactivation is a useful diagnostic marker of DRESS [66].

Although no clear consensus has emerged, several hypotheses have been suggested to explain the association between drug and virus reactivation. One suggestion is that the Th2 environment during DRESS may predispose towards induction of regulatory T cells. This impairs host virus control and results in viral reactivation followed by a surge in anti-viral CD8+ T cells, which cause a secondary flare in the skin eruption [67,68]. An alternative hypothesis has been derived from work showing that in DRESS a large proportion of proliferating CD8+ T cells from the skin, blood or other organs are virus-specific, and that causative drugs specifically enhanced viral replication and production in patients' B cells. This suggests that the induction of virus replication rather than drug-specific immune responses may be the principal pathogenic feature of this condition [65]. In accordance with this, T-cell receptor (TCR) sequencing has demonstrated a diverse TCR usage in DRESS T cells and that HHV-6b DNA was detected at higher levels in these cells [53]. Interestingly, *in vitro* studies of drug-induced T-cell activation from a patient with sulfamethoxazole-induced DRESS showed evidence that anti-HHV-6 therapies block drug-induced proliferation [53], thus suggesting a direct role of viral reactivation in DRESS pathogenesis.

Other types of drug hypersensitivity

Acute generalised exanthematous pustulosis is a rare type of drug hypersensitivity that has not been well characterised at an immunological level. As with other delayed drug hypersensitivity reactions, drug-specific CD4 and CD8 T cells have been implicated [69–72] and the neutrophil chemoattractant IL-8 is thought to be central to manifesting the pustulosis [72]. Although drug-specific T-cell production of IL-8 has largely been considered to be the source of the cytokine, recent work has suggested that increased frequencies of Th17 cells in AGEP and consequent high levels of circulating IL-22 may be central to disease pathogenesis by causing upregulation of keratinocyte IL-8 production [73].

Fixed drug eruptions (FDEs) are incompletely understood, but show immunophenotypic similarity to SJS/TEN, with a demonstration that effector memory CD8 T cells predominate early in skin lesions [74] and these cells show cytolytic activity against keratinocytes [75]. An interesting phenomenon is the finding that patch test elicitation of an FDE is most likely to be positive in lesional skin and not in unaffected skin. Resident memory cells in the skin reside in tissue and are non-recirculating and the best characterised show a phenotype of CD8+, CD103+ and CD69+ [76,77]. The finding that in FDEs T cells share this phenotype neatly explains the reason for repeated inflammation at precisely the same skin site in an FDE, and also why patch test investigation needs to be undertaken at the affected site.

A variant of FDEs named generalised bullous fixed drug eruption (GBFDE) causes widespread epidermal detachment but is reported not to progress to TEN [78,79]. GBFDE tends to affect an older population but shows a better prognosis than SJS or TEN [80]. Individuals with GBFDE tend to show fewer systemic features of inflammation with minimal evidence of fever. Additionally, the involvement of mucosal surfaces is less. Ocular surfaces are generally not affected, but oral and genital surfaces may be affected.

Type 2 hypersensitivity reactions are mediated by cell surface antigens (modified by drugs) which are recognised by antibodies (usually IgG). A variety of cell types are recognised targets of such hypersensitivity reactions including platelets in drug-induced thrombocytopenia; although skin cells can be involved, these are less common cutaneous reactions. In some drug-induced type 2 hypersensitivities the drug is part of the antigen [81], whereas in others, such as pemphigus foliaceous, autoantibodies target self-proteins and the precise role of the drug is unclear. Type 3 hypersensitivity reactions result in IgG–antigen complexes in the circulation. Whilst they are relatively low-affinity interactions, adherence to endothelial surfaces results in complement fixation and accumulation and activation of neutrophils. This causes damage to the endothelium sufficient to allow extravasation of erythrocytes and the clinical syndrome of allergic or hypersensitivity vasculitis with purpuric lesions in skin.

T-cell recognition of drugs

Activation of the T cell via its receptor (TCR) is constrained by the requirement for antigen recognition in the context of the major histocompatibility complex (MHC) molecule. Therefore, drugs in solution do not activate T cells. Instead, it is necessary for drug-specific T-cell activation to arise because of drug modification of the MHC–peptide–TCR interaction. Three non-mutually exclusive models for T-cell interaction with drugs have been proposed (Figure 14.1).

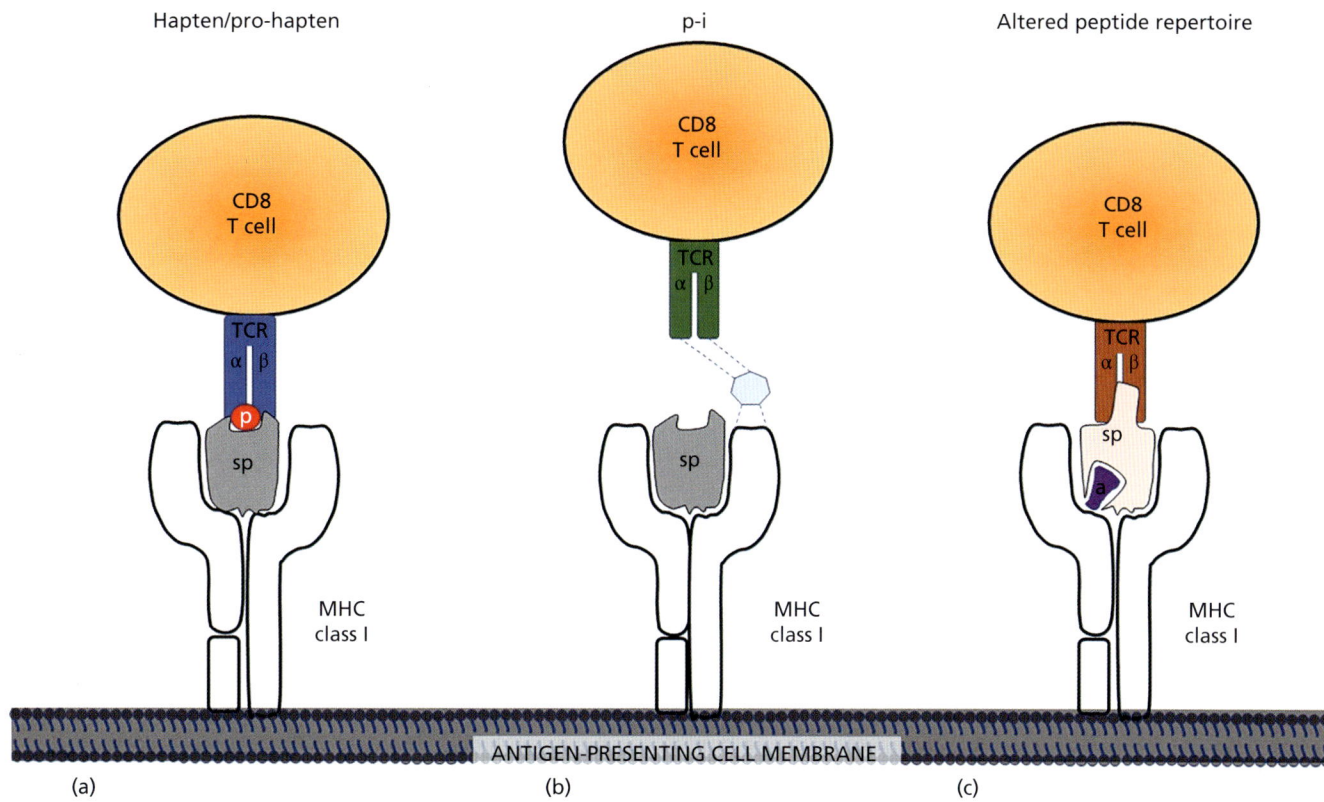

Figure 14.1 Three proposed models of T-cell recognition of drugs. (a) The hapten/pro-hapten model suggests that drugs or metabolite directly bind self-peptides (sp) in the intracellular antigen-processing pathway and result in presentation of the drug–peptide complex at the cell surface in the antigenic groove of the major histocompatibility complex (MHC) molecule. The example shown is that of penicillin haptenated to a self-peptide for presentation. (b) The p-i model suggests that the drug can act to stabilise T-cell receptor (TCR)–MHC interactions by providing weak non-covalent binding in an antigen-independent manner. (c) Direct binding of the drug in the antigenic groove of the MHC results in conformational changes in the groove to facilitate the binding of self-peptides which would ordinarily not be presented by that particular MHC and are therefore recognised as non-self. The example shown is that of abacavir (a) binding into the HLA-B*5701 molecule.

Hapten/pro-hapten model

The precise reason for a drug hypersensitivity reaction in any individual is the product of drug factors and individual factors. Drugs with a low molecular weight which would ordinarily be too small for direct immune recognition (less than 1000 Da) may become 'haptens' by binding to a self-protein carrier (haptenation). Such haptenated self-proteins are then processed as normal by antigen-presenting cells and the hapten-modified carrier protein is degraded to peptides that are individually loaded into the molecular groove of an MHC molecule in the classic way. Evidence for this model has been shown recently using a mass spectrometry peptidomics approach to analyse every MHC-presented peptide on the cell surface after keratinocyte exposure to a contact allergen. This work confirmed the presence of drug-altered peptides at the cell surface and demonstrated T-cell-specific immune responses in allergic patients targeting these antigens [82]. The hapten–peptide–MHC complex is then displayed on the cell surface and may be recognised by T cells as non-self. The intrinsic capacity of drugs to bind self-proteins depends on the formation of molecular bonds. Whilst multiple interactions with low-energy bonds such as hydrogen bonds may possibly be sufficiently stable to survive the antigen-processing pathway, it is thought that stable high-energy covalent bonds are most likely to determine the potential for neoantigen formation through haptenation. Many native drug molecules are not intrinsically protein-reactive, although some, including penicillins, cephalosporins and captopril, can bind directly to serum or cellular proteins [83,84]. Once the drug–peptide complex is presented in the context of MHC class I or II, the limiting factor is the presence of T cells expressing a T-cell receptor with sufficient functional avidity to induce T-cell activation. The random somatic recombination critical in defining the TCR repertoire in humans has been predicted to provide 10^{15} potential receptors of different specificities, yet adult humans are thought to have only 10^7 of these in circulation [85,86]. Therefore, it is entirely possible that drug sensitivity may also be reflected by whether certain individuals possess T cells with specific receptors for that drug. Pre-clinical drug development pathways are now very efficient at screening for protein-reactive drugs and these generally do not make it through to clinical testing.

However, inert drugs that are unable to bind self-proteins directly may become reactive following metabolism during biodegradation and detoxification. For example, after phase 1 metabolism by the cytochrome P450 superfamily of enzymes, the potentially reactive intermediates are not fully detoxified by phase 2 metabolism. Such reactive intermediates are then capable of binding 'self' cellular proteins which can be processed through the classic antigen-presenting cell pathways leading to display of the metabolite–protein–MHC complex to T cells. Such drugs are therefore known as 'pro-haptens'. Investigators have attempted to identify carrier proteins in this process without much success. However, some studies have implicated CYP450 enzymes, such as drug-induced hepatitis from halothane, where the metabolite of halothane, trifluoroacetyl halide, becomes bound to the cytochrome P450 enzyme (CYP2E1). This is thought to inhibit the enzyme function and result in drug metabolite/CYP2E1 proteolytic degradation and antigen formation that can be recognised by antibodies [87,88]. Similarly, antibodies targeting CYP450 enzymes have been reported in anticonvulsant hypersensitivity reactions [89]. Susceptibility to drug hypersensitivity reactions through such a pro-hapten concept may be dependent upon altered metabolic pathways as a consequence of enzymatic polymorphisms and mutations. However, efforts to demonstrate inadequate or defective phase 2 metabolism in drug-allergic individuals have been generally unsuccessful.

As the immune system is intrinsically unable to differentiate between a foreign protein from a benign source and one from a pathogen, a system to sense 'danger' has evolved [90]. This signalling is critical to host defence against infection. It has been suggested that innate immune activation as a danger signal may be critical for the initiation of immune responses against drugs. This may provide an explanation for the role of the environment in drug hypersensitivity reactions that could explain individual susceptibility. Bacterial, viral and fungal molecules provide classic danger signals that are sensed by pattern recognition receptors resulting in enhanced antigen-presenting cell priming of T-cell responses. A possible mechanism for the initiation of drug immune responses may be coexistent infection-related danger signals, which are inevitably associated during exposure to antibiotics and may explain why this class of drugs most frequently cause hypersensitivity reactions [91].

Interestingly, some drugs have been reported to deliver danger signals themselves. One of the likely mechanisms for this is the oxidative stress that occurs during drug metabolism. The generation of reactive oxygen species depletes intracellular antioxidant defences and induces activation of transcription factors including activator protein 1 (AP-1) [92], nuclear factor κB (NF-κB) [93,94] and nuclear factor erythroid 2-related factor 2 (NRF2) [95,96]. These in turn induce innate immune responses resulting in the release of cytokines and chemokines. It seems likely that endogenous antioxidant reserves and defences may be crucial in determining whether a particular drug generates danger signals in an individual that can result in an active immune response.

Pharmacological interaction (p-i) model

Despite the extensive data to support the hapten and pro-hapten concepts, evidence suggests that some drugs are antigenic in their native, non-reactive state; some do not require antigen processing; and some involve reversible rather than covalent binding for antigen presentation. These observations are considered to support the concept that drugs may facilitate T cell–MHC interaction by externally binding the MHC, stabilisation of low-affinity interactions or direct TCR binding. The concept that drugs may activate immune responses without forming a hapten yet in an HLA-dependent manner is known as the 'pharmacological interaction with immune receptors' (p-i) concept [97]. The p-i concept is therefore also processing and metabolism independent. It has been suggested that the T cells involved in p-i reactions may arise from the circulating memory T-cell pool [98].

Table 14.3 HLA associations with severe cutaneous adverse reactions caused by drugs.

Drug	HLA allele	Studied populations	Phenotype	OR
Abacavir	B*5701	Australian, European, African	DRESS	960
Allopurinol	B*5801	Han Chinese, Thai, Japanese, Koreans	SJS/TEN/DIHS/DRESS/MPE	>800
Carbamazepine	A*3101	Europeans, Japanese, Koreans, Han Chinese	DRESS	9.5
Carbamazepine	B*1502	Han Chinese, Indians, Thai	SJS/TEN	>1000
Carbamazepine	B*1511	Japanese, Koreans	SJS/TEN	16–18
Dapsone	B*1301	Chinese, Papuans, Aboriginals, Japanese	DRESS	20
Lamotrigine	B*1502	Chinese	SJS/TEN	
Nivirapine	C*0401	Thai	DRESS	3–7
Vancomycin	A*3201	North American	DRESS	

Adapted from Redwood et al. 2018 [24] and Kaniwar and Saito 2013 [107]. DIHS, drug-induced hypersensitivity syndrome; DRESS, drug reaction with eosinophilia and systemic symptoms; HLA, human leukocyte antigen; MPE, maculopapular exanthem; OR, odds ratio; SJS, Stevens–Johnson syndrome; TEN, toxic epidermal necrolysis.

Altered peptide repertoire model

The association of drug-induced adverse reactions with particular HLA phenotypes is increasingly well recognised (Table 14.3). For example, in some cohorts, abacavir induces a hypersensitivity reaction in HLA-B*5701 individuals with an odds ratio (OR) of 1945 (95% confidence interval (CI) 110 to 34 352) [99], allopurinol in HLA-B*5801 individuals up to OR 580 (95%CI 34 to 9780) [100] and in Han Chinese populations carbamazepine hypersensitivity is predicted by HLA-B*1502 (OR 1357; 95%CI 193 to 8838) [101]. As a result of the discovery of such strong HLA associations, most regulatory agencies including those in the USA and UK suggest pre-screening for at-risk HLA alleles prior to the initiation of abacavir and for carbamazepine use in individuals with Chinese or Thai ancestry.

The nature of the interaction between these drug molecules and the MHC-associated peptides has recently been further characterised. Studies using X-ray crystallography data confirmed that abacavir non-covalently binds directly into the MHC peptide binding cleft of HLA-B*5701 during its synthesis [102,103]. The abacavir-altered MHC allele is then capable of presenting a different repertoire of self-peptides as compared with untreated HLA-B*5701. Thus, in the context of abacavir/HLA-B*5701, the non-classic self-peptides in this allele represent neoantigens and result in a polyclonal T-cell response. It is as yet unclear how many other drug–HLA associations reflect a similar mechanism.

Understanding the clinical phenotype

Despite the detailed understanding of molecular mechanisms involved in adverse immunological reactions to drugs as outlined earlier, the link between drug and individual and hypersensitivity phenotype is still poorly understood. A major clue to the complexity of these pathways is derived from understanding hypersensitivity reactions to drugs that are very strongly associated with risk HLA alleles. However, despite great interest in this area, strong associations between HLA alleles and drug-induced severe cutaneous adverse reactions are so far limited to a small number of drugs (see Table 14.3) and it remains unclear what proportion of hypersensitivity reactions will eventually be deemed truly HLA dependent.

The strongest association and best described of these is that of abacavir and HLA-B*5701. In those exposed to abacavir, 5% suffer clinically diagnosed adverse drug reactions. Of these, approximately 50% are HLA-B*5701-positive individuals. Interestingly, as has been shown in multiple studies, following a hypersensitivity reaction, positive abacavir patch tests arise only in HLA-B*5701-positive individuals [104]. Ninety-four per cent of all abacavir reactions arise within 6 weeks (median 10–11 days) and have been reported up to 318 days after initiation of therapy [105], and death can result on rechallenge [106]. Typically, the abacavir hypersensitivity reaction begins with fever followed by organ involvement including the skin. Whilst abacavir hypersensitivity syndrome is considered an exemplar of systemic drug hypersensitivity paralleling DRESS, there are some important differences. In contrast to classic DRESS, the rash arises in only 66% of cases and is generally mild or moderate in severity (urticarial or maculopapular) [105,106]. Gastrointestinal symptoms of nausea, vomiting and diarrhoea are the next most frequent (approximately 38%) followed by respiratory involvement [105]; hypotension is a common finding. Investigations show that eosinophilia is not common and deranged liver biochemistry, renal function and haematological abnormalities arise in 5–9% [105]. Thus, there are clear and important differences between abacavir hypersensitivity and our current understanding of DRESS, which suggests that the dominant skin phenotype of DRESS may be a distinct subset of T-cell-mediated drug hypersensitivity reactions. Furthermore, of HLA-B*5701 positive individuals, only 61% demonstrated hypersensitivity reactions on exposure to the drug for 6 weeks [104] and some individuals tolerant of abacavir are HLA-B*5701 positive. These observations suggest that there is an additional layer of complexity to the induction of classic drug hypersensitivity phenotypes beyond HLA-restricted immunological responses.

Carbamazepine hypersensitivity has also been closely studied and as described previously shows a strong association to HLA-B*1502 in Han Chinese populations. However, despite the well-recognised potential for carbamazepine induction of other types of hypersensitivity reaction, in the context of HLA-B*1502 association is only seen with SJS/TEN and not with exanthems or DRESS [101]. This could suggest that HLA associations are determinant of the T-cell phenotype and thus clinical reaction pattern. However, this theory is challenged by the simultaneous association of HLA-A*3101 with carbamazepine-induced SJS/TEN, DRESS and drug exanthems [107]. Similarly allopurinol-associated HLA-B*5801 is associated with both SJS/TEN and DRESS [107]. Furthermore, aligning the strong HLA genetic associations against the data to suggest a role for viral reactivation in DRESS makes a confusing and incompletely understood picture. Thus it seems that although in some circumstances the exposure of an individual with a specific HLA allele to a drug is necessary to induce a restricted clinical phenotype, this is not sufficient by itself to determine the type of clinical reaction in many cases. It is possible that as yet undefined haploinsufficiencies with the HLA alleles could explain the phenotype. Indeed, although not yet replicated, an early report of the association between abacavir and HLA-B*5701 showed co-segregation with a heat shock protein (Hsp70-Hom) variant, suggesting a role for Hsp70 in mediating the hypersensitivity response [108].

Conclusions

In conclusion, hypersensitivity reactions to drugs are common and the clinical presentations are diverse. Although the hapten hypothesis has dominated understanding of T-cell-mediated hypersensitivity pathogenesis over the last 20 years, recent work identifying direct interaction between the drug and host immune receptors suggests the exciting possibility that it will be possible to predict many adverse cutaneous immunological reactions to drugs based upon HLA testing.

Key references

The full list of references can be found in the online version at https://www.wiley.com/rooksdermatology10e

1 Hemmi H, Kaisho T, Takeuchi O *et al*. Small anti-viral compounds activate immune cells via the TLR7 MyD88-dependent signaling pathway. *Nat Immunol* 2002;3(2):196–200.

5 Bischoff SC. Role of mast cells in allergic and non-allergic immune responses: comparison of human and murine data. *Nat Rev Immunol* 2007;7:93–104.

20 McNeil BD, Pundir P, Meeker S *et al*. Identification of a mast-cell-specific receptor crucial for pseudo-allergic drug reactions. *Nature* 2015;519:237–41.

37 Chung WH, Hung SI, Yang JY *et al*. Granulysin is a key mediator for disseminated keratinocyte death in Stevens-Johnson syndrome and toxic epidermal necrolysis. *Nat Med* 2008;14:1343–50.

53 Kim D, Kobayashi T, Voisin B *et al*. Targeted therapy guided by single-cell transcriptomic analysis in drug-induced hypersensitivity syndrome: a case report. *Nat Med* 2020;26:236–43.

77 Jiang X, Clark RA, Liu L, Wagers AJ, Fuhlbrigge RC, Kupper TS. Skin infection generates non-migratory memory CD8+ T(RM) cells providing global skin immunity. *Nature* 2012;483:227–31.

102 Illing PT, Vivian JP, Dudek NL *et al*. Immune self-reactivity triggered by drug-modified HLA-peptide repertoire. *Nature* 2012;486:554–8.

PART 2
Management

CHAPTER 15

Psychological and Social Impact of Long-Term Conditions and Principles of Holistic Management

Sandy R. McBride and Alexandra Mizara
Royal Free Hospital, London, UK

Introduction, 15.1	Cumulative life course impairment, 15.3	Social considerations, 15.5
The psychological and social impact of long-term dermatological conditions, 15.1	Psychological factors relevant to specific skin conditions, 15.3	Spiritual considerations, 15.5
Appearance and society, 15.1	Principles of holistic management of skin disease, 15.4	Effective communication, 15.6
Body image, self-esteem and social inclusion, 15.1		Key practical skills for use in busy clinics, 15.6
The relationship between emotion, behaviour and beliefs, 15.1	Physical considerations, 15.4	Conclusion, 15.7
	Psychological considerations, 15.5	Key references, 15.7

Introduction

Psychological factors such as stress, coping and personality play a pivotal role in health and illness. Living with a long-term skin condition can be life altering or even life ruining [1]. Skin conditions cause visible difference and can lead to stigmatisation [2–4], low self-esteem, negative body image [5–7], distress [8,9] and adoption of unhelpful coping behaviours [10,11]. Stress and distress may affect treatment outcomes [12], trigger flares of skin disease [12,13] and affect adherence [14], suggesting a need to address the psychological as well as physical needs of patients. Clinicians working in dermatology are well placed to identify patients in need of psychological support [15]. Recognising the individual needs and beliefs of patients enables a holistic approach to care. In this chapter we aim to provide an overview of challenges posed by living with a long-term skin condition, discuss the need for a holistic approach to care and describe some key consultation skills useful in busy clinics.

The psychological and social impact of long-term dermatological conditions

Appearance and society
The appearance of skin is fundamental to the evaluation of attractiveness. Smooth, unblemished skin is associated with youth, health and fertility – attributes likely to confer an evolutionary advantage and valued across cultures for centuries [16]. Today, social media and the use of 'beauty filters' on photographs add to pressure to conform to a narrow, unrealistic image of beauty.

Beauty is commonly (and wrongly) associated with positive character traits such as honesty, kindness and intelligence. This bias, termed the 'halo effect', leads to attractive people being treated favourably, receiving greater rewards and less punishment than less attractive people [17]. Conversely, visibly different faces trigger decreased activity in areas of the brain associated with empathy and understanding [18] and increased activity in areas associated with disgust [19]. Filmmakers exploit this phenomenon by using visible difference, often in the form of a skin condition, to dehumanise villains [20], adding to prejudice associated with skin conditions.

Body image, self-esteem and social inclusion
Body image is a key concept in dermatology. Body image refers to an internalised view of appearance, it refers to how we think others perceive us [16] and is developed through seeing our own image and from feedback from others. Negative body image is an obstacle to forming and sustaining relationships and can lead to low self-esteem.

Self-esteem represents a sense of worth and value. Low self-esteem is associated with feelings of shame, inferiority and worthlessness, leading to self-disgust, avoidance behaviours and social isolation.

Social inclusion is a fundamental evolutionary need, generating a powerful drive for acceptance and inclusion. The experience of being socially excluded causes considerable hurt [21,22], leading dermatology patients to conceal their skin disease and avoid situations that may result in rejection.

The relationship between emotion, behaviour and beliefs
Aaron T. Beck pioneered cognitive behavioural therapy (CBT). His 'cognitive model' [23] describes beliefs, behaviours, and emotions as being linked. For example, if someone *believes* a medication will not be effective or side effects to be dangerous they might *feel*

Rook's Textbook of Dermatology, Tenth Edition. Edited by Christopher Griffiths, Jonathan Barker, Tanya Bleiker, Walayat Hussain and Rosalind Simpson.
© 2024 John Wiley & Sons Ltd. Published 2024 by John Wiley & Sons Ltd.

anxious or fearful of taking the medication and the resulting *behaviour* may be non-adherence.

Beck's cognitive model is relevant to understanding and managing patients with skin conditions. Observing beliefs, behaviours and emotional reactions gives an indication of possible underlying issues of coping and adjustment. Importantly, behaviours or emotions are all amenable to change. Professionals working in dermatology have a unique opportunity to enable their patients to develop constructive attitudes and beliefs about their skin condition. Education and therapeutic recommendations can change unproductive coping strategies and reduce emotional distress.

Emotions

Long-term skin conditions are associated with high rates of distress [9]. Psychological distress is defined as a state of emotional discomfort connected with burdens and demands that are difficult to cope with. In dermatology patients, distress is typically manifested by the emotions of stress, anxiety, depression and/or anger.

Anxiety is the feeling when worried, tense or afraid, particularly about future events, and is characterised by persistent, excessive worries that do not go away even without an external trigger. Anxiety evolved from a need to escape danger – the 'flight, fright, freeze' response and becomes a mental health problem when it impacts on the ability to live life fully.

Depression is a mood disorder characterised by a persistent feeling of sadness and loss of interest. A key symptom is anhedonia – an inability to feel pleasure in normally pleasurable activities.

Anger is an intense emotional state associated with poor psychological adjustment [24] and feelings of rejection [25] and can be a sign of underlying anxiety or depression [26]. Evolutionarily, anger is an empowering emotion providing energy and drive for change, so in a clinic situation understanding the grounds for anger can be enlightening and benefit both patient and clinician.

Shame is a strong, all encompassing, self-conscious emotion associated with powerful feelings of humiliation and worthlessness. It is a consequence of negative evaluation (either by oneself or others) in relation to what is perceived as normal or expected in society. Shame plays a major role in psychological problems or disorders such as anxiety, depression, obsessive-compulsive and eating disorders, risky behaviours and addictions [27].

Psychological stress occurs when events exceed an individual's perceived ability to cope [28] and has been linked to the development or evolution of several long-term skin conditions including acne [29], vitiligo [30], alopecia areata [31], chronic urticaria [32] and psoriasis [33]. Symptoms can be psychological and physical including irritability, anger, fatigue and difficulty sleeping. Stress and anxiety have similar symptoms but stress resolves with the absence of a trigger.

The *physiological response to stress* acts via three main pathways: (i) the release of nerve-related factors from peripheral sensory nerves, (ii) the hypothalamic–pituitary–adrenal (HPA) axis and (iii) the sympathetic nervous system (SNS) [34].

The *'brain–skin axis'* is a concept used to describe the interaction between the psyche, the immune system and cutaneous inflammation [12]. The brain and the skin share an embryological origin and are intrinsically linked; the skin has a fully functional peripheral HPA axis equivalent to the brain stress axis [35] and most immune cells in the skin express receptors for stress-related mediators [36]. Hence, the skin responds to psychological stress [37,38] and the relationship appears bidirectional with peripheral inflammation associated with changes in the brain observed with depression [39] and stress [40].

Skin function is affected by stress. Delayed wound healing is observed in people in hostile relationships [41] and during exam stress [42], but can be improved with positive lifestyle behaviours such as regular exercise [43]. Skin barrier function is disrupted during periods of stress [44] and enhanced by having a positive affect (optimistic personality) [45].

Behaviour

Behaviour is an individual's activity in response to external or internal stimuli. Behaviours are linked with (or guided by) emotions and beliefs and provide insight into patients' thoughts and/or feelings. Recognition of unhelpful behaviours facilitates introduction of helpful coping and adjustment strategies.

People living with long-term skin conditions may develop complex avoidant strategies. Social avoidance, abstaining from activities that expose the skin, concealment of skin with clothing, excessive alcohol/drug intake etc. are all methods to protect from rejection or humiliation [2,46]. Forming relationships, seeking intimacy and sexual interactions are avoided due to insecurities about appearance and desirability. Compensatory behaviours, to manage distress, may involve overeating [46], obsessive skin checking, hair-pulling and elaborate personal hygiene regimens.

In an ideal world all patients would take their medications as they are prescribed, but patients' behaviour varies. *Medication adherence* is defined as the 'extent to which the patients' behaviour matches agreed recommendations from the prescriber' [47]. Non-adherence is an avoidable cause of treatment failure, increased use of healthcare services and unnecessary escalation of treatment.

Intentional non-adherence describes a deliberate decision not to take or alter the regimen of their prescribed medication. Patients' beliefs about their condition, their need for medication and potential side effects [48] are common drivers of intentional non-adherence. Beliefs, however, are modifiable [49] and exploration of patients' medication beliefs [50] can improve intentional non-adherence.

Unintentional non-adherence, such as forgetting a medication, is influenced by strength of routine or habit [50] and low mood [14] in long-term conditions. Habit-based interventions can be effective.

General strategies to improve treatment adherence are using shared decision-making skills [51] (as recommended by NICE [52] and the GMC [53]), simplifying treatment regimens, empowering patients to take responsibility for their treatment, raising awareness of poor adherence and helping patients build a solid medication-taking habit [54,55].

Beliefs

Beliefs are fundamentally linked to emotions and behaviour [23] and provide an insight and explanation for patients' feelings and behaviours. Beliefs concerning the causes of a skin condition, exacerbating factors and treatments are particularly relevant to adherence.

Beliefs, behaviours and emotions are all influenced by personality. *Personality traits* develop early and persist over a lifetime [56]. Personality is a substantial factor in explaining the variability in psychological and emotional response (adjustment) to living with a skin condition. Adjustment is predicted by individual perception and interpretation of experiences, rather than disease severity. For example, an individual's response to rejection depends on the interpretation of motives behind the rejection. Two key personality traits are optimism and alexithymia.

Optimism is crucial in adjustment to long-term health conditions including psoriasis [57] and vitiligo [58]. Optimism confers resilience, protects against mental health issues and is associated with better socioeconomic status and social integration [59]. Optimism can be developed using CBT techniques [59], which have been used in long-term skin conditions [60].

Alexithymia is a personality trait associated with difficulty in identifying, describing and communicating emotions. A high prevalence of alexithymia has been identified in patients with hidradenitis suppurativa [61], urticaria [62] psoriasis [63], alopecia areata [64], and vitiligo [65]. Alexithymia is related to unhelpful coping strategies such as unhealthy eating and alcohol/drug use and anxiety and depression in dermatology patients [66]. People with alexithymia have fewer close relationships, fewer social skills and less social support, with consequent adverse impact on health and well-being [67]. In a clinic situation, patients with alexithymia will have difficulty answering the question 'How do you feel?' yet can recount trivial life events in detail.

Identifying people with alexithymia is important, as their distress is often not readily apparent, yet they may benefit most from effective treatment. Sampogna *et al.* [68] found effective treatment of psoriasis also reduced levels of alexithymia. Participants who were alexithymic at baseline experienced the largest improvement in anxiety, depression and Dermatology Life Quality Index (DLQI) and (perhaps) consequent reduction in alcohol consumption.

Cumulative life course impairment

Cumulative life course impairment (CLCI) describes the impact of a long-term health condition over time. This contrasts with the cross-sectional analysis provided by the DLQI. The lifetime consequences (life course impairment) of living with a long-term skin condition can be physical, psychological, social and/or economic [69]. A key concept in life course impairment is accumulation of risk – over time the risk of significant life impairment increases with ongoing or repeated episodes of skin disease. Identifying people at risk early in the course of their skin condition may prevent life impairment.

Life impairment is not only dependent on the nature and severity of a skin condition – protective factors such as resilience, personality, social support and positive coping skills play a role [69]. Other considerations are stigmatisation, mood, coexistent health conditions and age.

Childhood and adolescence

During early *infancy* until 3 years of age, self-image is shaped by attachment with caregivers [70]. Attachment is, in turn, affected by the emotions of carers towards their child. Relationships with peers become important from *2 to 10 years of age* [70] and, by 7 years, children recognise visual differences between themselves and peers, which can influence self-esteem and bullying may be encountered.

Entering *teenage years*, children generally have lower self-esteem and are more pessimistic and self-critical, which can affect motivation, confidence and resilience. Adolescents become more self-conscious and experience pressure to fit in [16] and visible difference can be an easy target for bullies. Skin conditions can lead to missing out on sporting and social activities and education.

Adolescence is a time when young people formulate ambitions and make key decisions about their future. Given the right support, they can build resilience and helpful coping strategies to enable them to achieve their aspirations. It is, however, also a time when unhelpful coping strategies and lifelong mental health burdens may develop. Early psychological intervention in children can prevent escalation of problems and have major societal benefits [71].

Having a child with a skin condition presents a considerable burden to families [72]. Treatments take up time and detract from other family members, loss of sleep can affect the whole family, differing opinions as to how the condition should be managed may lead to conflict and the skin condition may restrict family activities [73].

Adulthood

Early adulthood is a period of completing education, starting careers and forming relationships. There is a relatively short period, particularly for women, when childbearing is possible and optimal. Compatibility of treatment strategies with family planning needs to be considered and discussed with both men and women. Planning ahead, regularly discussing family planning and responding to changing needs is key to management during this period.

Middle age brings challenges and opportunities. Medications can be changed if childbearing is no longer an issue. Attendance at hospital may be easier after retirement or other health issues may start to be a problem. It is a time of change, which can be reflected in management plans.

Older age brings medical and physical complexity. For some individuals there may be a change of importance, with less concern about appearance and more emphasis on safety and independence. For others this may not be the case. Beliefs are individual and require individual exploration.

Psychological factors relevant to specific skin conditions

Not only does each individual patient have a unique experience of, and response to, living with a skin condition, individual skin conditions present a varied array of challenges to patients.

Acne

Although acne is often seen as a teenage issue, it can have a protracted course and be resistant to treatment [74]. Acne is associated with low attachment to friends, not thriving at school, never having romantic relationships and never having sexual intercourse [75,76]. Acne itself appears to be a risk factor for suicide, with attempted suicide progressively escalating in the years prior to isotretinoin medication [76]. There have also been suggested links between isotretinoin and mental health issues [77–79]. Scarring, as a consequence of untreated acne, can also have an enduring psychological and social impact. Ultimately both acne and depression require effective treatment.

Atopic dermatitis
Childhood eczema has a considerable impact on both the child and their family [3,80,81]. The impairment in quality of life for children with eczema is equivalent to that found in children with cystic fibrosis and renal disease [82] and the effect on education and socialisation can lead to difficulties in adulthood [83].

Atopic dermatitis in adulthood is associated with anxiety, depression, sleep disorders, work absenteeism, activity impairment [84] and significantly higher levels of suicidal ideation [85]. It can be triggered or exacerbated by stress [86] and also causes considerable stress [87]. Career choice is important in patients with atopic dermatitis, further influencing life course [88,89].

Atopic eczema is a risk factor for hand eczema. Severe occupational hand eczema can lead to job loss and in one study almost a quarter of people with severe hand eczema had lost their job within the last year [90] and in another hand eczema was mostly within service occupations such as hairdressing [91].

Urticaria
There are multiple reports of a relationship between stress and urticaria and adrenergic urticaria invariably follows acute stressful events [92]. An additional difficult factor for patients with chronic urticaria is that for 80–90% a specific trigger cannot be identified, which can lead to extensive lifestyle restrictions [93]. Pruritus causes sleep deprivation, negatively affecting work, social life and mood [94].

Hidradenitis suppurativa
Hidradenitis suppurativa (HS) has profound consequences for patients [95] with symptoms including pain, fatigue, malodour, exudate and scarring and affects body sites important in intimate and sexual relationships. Diagnosis is often delayed by many years, treatments are incompletely effective and the course of the disease is unpredictable and protracted. Unsurprisingly the condition has a profound effect on the emotional, social, working and economic lives of patients and is associated with significant psychological morbidity [96] and a greater than twice the risk of completed suicide [97].

Psoriasis
Many studies have described the potentially life-ruining impact of psoriasis, including social, emotional, economic and sexual aspects [**69**]. Much has been written about the link between stress and psoriasis, with emotional stressors preceding the onset of psoriasis [33] and triggering flares [98,99]. Yet, despite the availability of effective treatment for many patients, there is considerable delay to receiving effective treatment [100], high treatment dissatisfaction and 'doctor shopping' remains. Patients feel others (including clinicians) do not understand their lived experience and the 'incurable' nature of psoriasis is frequently interpreted as there are no effective treatments [101]. Psychological and social interventions have been shown to improve outcomes for patients living with psoriasis [102–104] but are not readily available.

Vitiligo
Stressful events have been associated with the onset of vitiligo [105], but this is not consistent [106]. Vitiligo is associated with high levels of alexithymia and lower social support and higher attachment-related problems than controls [58]. Depending on the background skin colour, it can be very visible and frequently affects high impact sites such as the hands and face. In some communities, vitiligo can carry considerable stigmatisation and attract discrimination, being associated with leprosy and a reason for divorce [107]. The psychological burden of vitiligo [108] is exacerbated by a lack of effective treatment, unpredictable prognosis and individual perception of disease severity [109]. CBT benefits coping with the condition and may have a beneficial effect on disease progression [110].

Hair loss
Hair possesses great psychological and social importance. Consequently, hair loss is a major source of distress. The psychological and social effects of hair loss are more profound than the biological significance of losing hair [111]. Stress has been linked causally with some forms of hair loss – telogen effluvium [112], alopecia areata [113] and female and male pattern alopecia [114,115] are all reported to be caused or exacerbated by stress. Alopecia areata is associated with higher rates of psychiatric disorder [116,117]. A corollary of this is that psychological intervention and coping strategies may be helpful in the management of people with hair loss, particularly as medical interventions tend to be incompletely effective.

Skin cancer
Cancer, including skin cancer, is increasingly becoming a long-term condition. Although most skin cancers have a low mortality risk, almost all patients with skin cancer experience some worry [118] and the potential for recurrence or further spread can cause distress [119]. Protective factors for melanoma-associated worry are being male with a partner (as opposed to female with a partner), increasing age, lower stage of melanoma (IB-IIC), being in employment and receiving emotional support from health care workers [119]. A mindfulness-based intervention [120] reduced fear of melanoma recurrence and a telephone administered psycho-educational intervention was 'beneficial' [121]. Understanding patients' concerns about skin cancer is key to alleviating unnecessary worry and providing support where appropriate.

Principles of holistic management of skin disease

Holistic care is an approach in which the whole person (physical, psychological, social and spiritual) is considered in management decisions, as opposed to focusing on diagnosis and treatment.

Physical considerations
Accurate diagnosis and effective treatment (if possible) are clearly fundamental to the management of patients with skin conditions. In the treatment of psoriasis, achieving completely clear or almost clear skin (Psoriasis Area and Severity Index (PASI) 90–100) is associated with a significantly greater proportion of patients reporting

Table 15.1 Psychological care: a stepped approach. See end of chapter for online resources.

	Level of care	Facilitators	Access	Examples
Level 0	Self-help	Patient Dermatology clinicians	Signposting Self access Self-referral	Patient support websites Patient organisations Professional associations
Level 1	Primary care	Psychological well-being practitioners Psychologists	Self-referral Referral by GP	Community mental health services Online mental health services
Level 2	Secondary care	Dermatology clinicians Psychologist Liaison Psychiatrist	Referral by dermatology clinician	Multidisciplinary meetings with dermatology clinicians, psychologists and psychiatrists
Level 3	Tertiary care	Specialist Dermatologist, Dermatology and/or Psychiatric Nurse Specialist Psychiatrist Specialist Psychologist	Referral to (usually) regional clinic by dermatology clinician	Dedicated psychodermatology clinic

their quality of life not being affected (DLQI 0/1) by psoriasis, than those with a 75% (PASI 75–89) improvement [122].

Lifestyle interventions, such as weight reduction, can be beneficial in long-term conditions such as hidradenitis suppurativa and psoriasis, which are associated with obesity, smoking and/or excessive alcohol [123,124].

Maintaining a healthy weight, a healthy diet and regular exercise will clearly have a beneficial impact on health and well-being for all patients. Addressing unhelpful coping strategies such as smoking and alcohol excess offers potential benefit.

A pragmatic, time sensitive and responsible approach to lifestyle issues is to identify patients at need of intervention and to sensitively signpost towards available support from allied services. Motivational interview techniques can be readily learned and practised by clinicians [125].

Psychological considerations

Most psychological difficulties affecting dermatology patients relate to the impact of living with a long-term condition that is often incurable, unpredictable, appearance-altering and stigmatising [126]. Stress, either resulting from the skin condition or as an exacerbating factor, is an issue for many.

Identifying patients in need of psychological support is the first step to improving mental health. Dermatology clinicians are often the only health care professionals who regularly see patients with long-term skin conditions and are therefore ideally placed to identify those who may benefit from psychological input.

Questionnaires such as the Hospital Anxiety Depression Scale (HADS) [127], Generalised Anxiety Disorder Assessment (GAD-7) [128] and Patient Health Questionnaire (PHQ-9) [129] are useful screening tools for anxiety and depression.

A 'yes' response to one of the two questions below has high specificity but low sensitivity for depression [130].

1 'During the past month have you often been bothered by feeling down, depressed, or hopeless?'
2 'During the past month have you often been bothered by little interest or pleasure in doing things?'

The DLQI [131] is a measure of quality of life, not distress.

Questionnaires should be used in conjunction with careful questioning and insightful observation of behaviour as a means of identifying patients in need of support.

The importance of identifying patients experiencing stress and/or distress is that mood directly affects effective management of the skin condition. Examples include:

- Worry is a major determinant of outcome for people with psoriasis treated with photochemotherapy [**12**].
- Depression affects adherence [**14**].
- Stress is a trigger or exacerbating factor of several long-term skin conditions [29–33,132].

Psychological and educational interventions as an adjunct to standard medical treatment are shown to improve both physical and psychological well-being in dermatology patients [**60**].

A stepped approach for psychological care of people with skin conditions is recommended [133] [**1**] (Table 15.1) and is manageable for all dermatology clinicians. Simple skills, such as active listening, demonstrating professional curiosity, optimism and effective signposting, can fulfil the needs of most patients.

Where there is a moderately severe psychiatric disorder it may be necessary to refer the patient to allied services such as psychology, psychiatry or their family practitioner for further support.

Social considerations

People living with skin conditions frequently experience discrimination, stigmatisation and social isolation [134,135]. Social relationships are robust predictors of physical health outcomes. Social support is linked to better adjustment to conditions including psoriasis [136] and vitiligo [106] and lower levels of inflammation [137]. Belonging to a social network and perceptions of support are protective for mental health, well-being and adjustment to health conditions that affect appearance [138] and a reduction in mortality rate comparable to not smoking and undertaking physical activity.

Being aware of an individual patient's support network is an important part of a holistic approach to care. Signposting to local patient groups (if available) and patient organisations and online support groups [139] can be beneficial.

Spiritual considerations

An individual's spirituality extends beyond religious or cultural beliefs – it refers to the essence of what is fundamentally important to a person. Individual beliefs and attitudes towards factors relating

Table 15.2 Key skills to use in busy clinics in order to facilitate patient-centred, holistic care.

Skill	What is this?	How to …	Tips
Active listening	Making a conscious effort to hear a patient and understand the complete message being communicated	Ask open questions Adopt behaviours that indicate listening and attention	Don't interrupt – most patients will speak for <2 minutes Paraphrase and reflect back to the patient your understanding of what has been said
Demonstrating interest	Showing professional curiosity, exploring further what the patient has said	'How', 'When', 'What', 'Where' are all good words to start 'demonstrating interest' questions	Be authentic and use a conversational style
Providing optimism	The importance of providing optimism cannot be overestimated Optimism gives cause to continue – the opposite of hopelessness	Focus on the possible, give hope and dispel unreasonable fears	Even when no treatment is available, hope of support and improved coping skills can be beneficial and appreciated
Demonstrating compassion	Feeling someone's distress and being motivated to relieve their pain	Showing empathy, acting appropriately to what has been heard Providing management aligned to the needs of the patient	Highly relevant to dermatology where levels of distress may not be linked to disease severity [1]
Signposting	Directing patients to sources of support and information Empowering patients to take ownership of their care and actively engage in shared decision-making processes	Education and support can be in several forms – directly from the clinician, or via sources of reliable information, patient organisations and patient decision aids if available [2]	Dermatology clinicians cannot, and need not, solve every problem presented. Signposting is often sufficient

to health are at the core of a holistic approach to care. For example, a Muslim patient may feel very strongly that they do not wish to take oral medication during Ramadan, when another may feel totally comfortable doing so.

Effective communication

Effective communication is key to the successful management of patients with long-term conditions [140]. Dermatology patients, however, report a lack of understanding of their experience, minimisation of their concerns and lack of timely individualised treatment. They want clinicians to demonstrate an appreciation of their suffering, provide hope of disease control, listen, show compassion and give patient-centred, individualised recommendations and information using simple to understand language [101,141,142]. There are some important principles that are fundamental to effective communication.

Preserving dignity is crucial for dermatology patients who frequently feel shame, embarrassment and anxiety, particularly around physical examination. Ensuring patients feel safe, asking permission to examine and explaining in advance what will happen are key to preserving dignity.

Privacy is essential for communication of private information. Patients may feel uncomfortable speaking openly in the presence of other people, such as students and visiting clinicians. Seeking permission for their attendance is usually routine.

Honesty is fundamental to effective communication. Mutual trust is needed for effective communication and honesty, and respect facilitates collaboration.

Clinicians will need to *make allowance for distress*. Demanding, challenging, unreasonable or difficult behaviours can result from patients being fearful, anxious, angry or ashamed of their skin condition. Curiosity regarding the origin of the behaviour is often a fruitful and pacifying endeavour.

Key practical skills for use in busy clinics

Active listening, demonstrating interest and compassion, providing optimism and signposting are all easily assimilated skills that are practical to use in busy clinics and essential to the provision of patient-centred, holistic care (Table 15.2).

Shared decision making is a move away from 'the doctor knows best' paradigm to clinicians working in partnership with patients to manage their health. It is 'a process in which clinicians and patients work together to select tests, treatments, management or support packages, based on clinical evidence and the patient's informed preferences' [143]. Shared decision making involves both provision of information and assessment of what patients need to make a decision.

The process of shared decision making involves three steps [144] (see Figure 15.1):

1 *Team talk* – information is shared between clinician and patient. *The patient* (the expert on themselves and their condition) provides information on their experience of their illness, social circumstances, attitude to risk, values and preferences. This process involves the clinician demonstrating active listening skills, professional curiosity and compassion. *The clinician* provides information on the diagnosis, disease aetiology, prognosis, treatment options and outcome probabilities. Effective signposting is key to this process.
2 *Option talk* – involves discussing treatment options available once patient factors and disease factors have been considered. This may involve discussing two or three options only, including not treating a condition. Discussion will include risk and potential outcomes. Decision aids can be helpful at this stage.
3 *Decision Talk* – making preference-based decisions with the patient including practicalities of implementation. Agreeing management goals, including those of self-care, is part of this process.

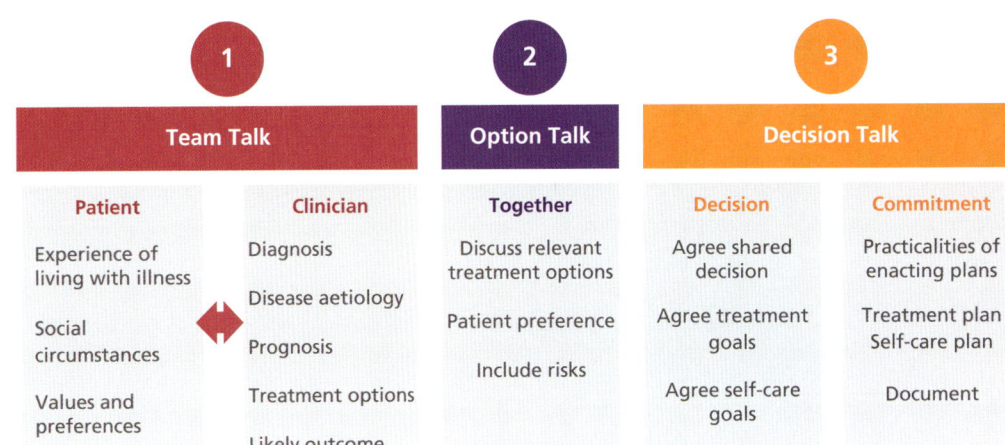

Figure 15.1 Shared decision making. Adapted from Elwyn *et al.* 2017 [144].

Conclusion

Living with a long-term skin condition can be life altering or even life ruining. No two patients with the same condition present in the same way or have the same experience. Skin conditions are typically visible to others, and patients often encounter stigma as part of their journey. Effective management of people living with long-term skin conditions involves a holistic approach. An approach that extends beyond diagnosis and treatment [15] and includes the physical, psychological, social and spiritual aspects of care. Understanding patients' beliefs and needs and empowering them to be active participants in their management through shared decision making leads to improved physical and psychological outcomes. Recognising and involving the person behind the skin condition is enriching and beneficial for both patients and clinicians.

Resources

Dermatology information sites

www.bad.org.uk. The British Association of Dermatologists website.
www.dermnetnz.org. This is a New Zealand-based website.
www.aad.org/dermatology-a-to-z. American Academy of Dermatology website

Patient support sites

The British Association of Dermatologists provides details of support groups for a wide range of skin conditions: https://www.bad.org.uk/patient-support-groups.
http://www.skinsupport.org.uk/ provides information to support people in psychological distress due to skin conditions (last accessed March 2022).

Key references

The full list of references can be found in the online version at https://www.wiley.com/rooksdermatology10e

1 Guterres S. *Mental Health and Skin Disease*. London: APPGS, 2020.
9 Dalgard FJ, Gieler U, Tomas-Aragones L *et al*. The psychological burden of skin diseases: a cross-sectional multicenter study among dermatological out-patients in 13 European countries. *J Invest Dermatol* 2015;135:984–91.
12 Fortune DG, Richards HL, Kirby B *et al*. Psychological distress impairs clearance of psoriasis in patients treated with photochemotherapy. *Arch Dermatol* 2003;139:752–6.
15 Gibbs S. Losing touch with the healing art: dermatology and the decline of pastoral doctoring. *J Am Acad Dermatol* 2000;43:875–8.
23 Beck AT. *Cognitive Therapy and the Emotional Disorders*. New York: International Universities Press, 1976.
37 Hunter HJA, Momen SE, Kleyn CE. The impact of psychosocial stress on healthy skin. *Clin Exp Dermatol* 2015;40:540.
60 Lavda AC, Webb TL, Thompson AR. A meta-analysis of the effectiveness of psychological interventions for adults with skin conditions. *Br J Dermatol* 2012;167:970–9.
68 Sampogna F, Puig L, Spuls P *et al*. Reversibility of alexithymia with effective treatment of moderate-to-severe psoriasis: longitudinal data from EPIDEPSO. *Br J Dermatol* 2019;180:397–403.
69 Kimball AB, Gieler U, Linder D, Sampogna F, Warren RB, Augustin M. Psoriasis: is the impairment to a patient's life cumulative? *J Eur Acad Dermatol Venereol* 2010;24:989–1004.
143 Coulter A, Collins A. *Making shared decision-making a reality: no decision about me, without me*. London: King's Fund, 2011. Available from: http://www.kingsfund.org.uk/document.rm?id=9190 (last accessed January 2022).

CHAPTER 16

Principles of Measurement and Assessment in Dermatology

Andrew Y. Finlay and Faraz M. Ali

Division of Infection and Immunity, Cardiff University School of Medicine, Cardiff, UK

Measurement of skin disease severity, 16.1
Why measure skin disease severity?, 16.1
What should be measured?, 16.1
Who should do the measuring?, 16.2
What can be measured?, 16.2
Electronic delivery of outcome measures, 16.2
Validation of measurement methods, 16.2
Core outcome measures, 16.3
Assessment tools, 16.3
Inflammatory disease, 16.3
Psoriasis, 16.3
Atopic eczema, 16.3
Acne, 16.4
Hidradenitis suppurativa, 16.4
Urticaria, 16.5

Symptoms, 16.5
Therapy benefit, 16.5
Objective methods for measuring skin properties, 16.5
Measurement of the impact of skin disease, 16.5
Quality of life assessment in patients with skin disease, 16.5
Quality of life measures used in dermatology, 16.6
General health measures, 16.6
Dermatology-specific measures, 16.6
Disease-specific quality of life measures, 16.7
Patient-specific and utility measures, 16.9
Measuring the impact of skin disease in children and adolescents, 16.9

Measuring the impact of skin disease on partners and the family, 16.10
Assessing life course impairment resulting from skin disease, 16.11
Practical clinical use of quality of life measures: a vital sign?, 16.11
Psychological impact measures, 16.11
Sexual functioning measures, 16.12
Work impact measures, 16.12
Occupational skin disease, 16.12
Work productivity, 16.12
Conclusion, 16.13
Declaration of interest, 16.13
Key references, 16.13

Measurement of skin disease severity

Why measure skin disease severity?

When general physicians manage chronic disease, they have long used reproducible measurements such as blood pressure, glycosylated haemoglobin or forced expiratory volume to follow their patients' progress. In contrast, dermatologists have only recently embraced methods of recording the course of their patients' chronic diseases. Skin disease is so visible that the drive to develop methods for assessing its activity has been slow [1]. Dermatologists still continue to record the success of their interventions using imprecise terms such as 'nearly clear', 'a bit better', 'slightly improved', 'stable', 'worse' or 'flaring'. If a new therapy has been started, they may be biased to record 'slightly better' rather than 'no change'. Wishful thinking of this kind is understandable but may lead to delays in changing to more effective therapy.

Even where dermatologists are able to keep patients requiring long-term review under their sole care, it is difficult to remember precisely how that patient's skin was 3 months earlier and the physician may have to rely on the patient's own assessment. If different doctors review a patient, it is even more difficult to make a valid assessment of change between patient visits without reproducible methods of recording disease activity or severity.

The introduction of powerful but expensive new therapies for inflammatory skin disease, and the need to demonstrate whether their cost can be justified by the benefit obtained, provided a spur to the development of methods to measure skin disease severity.

Assessment of skin disease severity has a major influence on clinical decision making and it is thus important to incorporate it into routine clinical practice. Formal assessment is, of course, an essential and well-established component of clinical research for comparing disease severity before and after intervention.

What should be measured?

There are many aspects of disease that can be measured but it is important to be sure that what is measured is relevant. The requirements for a proof-of-concept study of a novel pharmacological agent are completely different from those required in a routine clinic for monitoring a patient being treated for severe acne or psoriasis. Furthermore, there are objective measurements which can be made with some precision (e.g. transepidermal water loss or epidermal thickness) but they may have little relevance to a patient's perception of disease activity.

It is important to engage patients in discussions of what should be measured, as their concerns are frequently not fully appreciated by the professionals looking after them. What is easiest to measure

---

Rook's Textbook of Dermatology, Tenth Edition. Edited by Christopher Griffiths, Jonathan Barker, Tanya Bleiker, Walayat Hussain and Rosalind Simpson.
© 2024 John Wiley & Sons Ltd. Published 2024 by John Wiley & Sons Ltd.

is not always what patients feel is the aspect of their disease which has the greatest impact.

Fortunately, there is now a range of validated tools to measure the impact of skin disease. Some of these are specific to skin diseases in general and some are specific to a particular disease. Many of the 'objective' tools for assessing disease severity correlate poorly with patients' own perceptions of their disease. It is thus important to consider not only a disease itself but also its impact on the patients and their wider circle including family and employment.

Who should do the measuring?
Until recently, patients have not been engaged in making formal assessments of the state of their disease. In chronic disease, however, there are major advantages in involving patients. They are generally better able to judge how much a disease affects their daily lives than can an observer merely measuring visible signs. There is a place both for 'objective' assessments and for self-assessment by patients.

The move towards more patient engagement in assessing their progress is to be welcomed and a wide range of patient self-assessment tools has been developed. Many of these have been termed 'Patient-Reported Outcome Measures' (PROMs).

What can be measured?
The clinician considers key aspects of the patient's history, current symptoms, clinical signs and the impact of the disease that the patient is experiencing. All of these may be measured, either by subjective or by objective methods. The most widely used methods record clinical signs, using semi-objective approaches.

Before choosing or designing a specific method, it is essential to be clear about what aspect of disease requires measuring. For example, methods used in the long-term monitoring of individual patients may be different from those needed to compare patients in a short intervention study. A variety of measurement methods are required to assess different aspects of skin disease. The huge variety of clinical features of skin diseases calls for many diverse methods, but currently there are specific techniques available only for the most common skin conditions.

Electronic delivery of outcome measures
There is increasing preference to use computer-based assessments (CBAs) of measures of clinical severity and patient-reported outcomes rather than paper and pencil versions. This change in practice may be attributed to the inherent benefits of digital delivery of measures including reduced error rates, increased reliability of data, and better patient compliance [2,3]. There are some disadvantages of traditional paper-based completion including missing values and costs associated with storing large volumes of physical data. Research data are often manually transferred from paper to computers or electronic portals, which is time consuming and also has the capacity to introduce transcription errors [4,5], potentially reducing reliability of the data. These issues may be avoided by the use of CBAs of clinical outcome measures and PROMs. As a result, there is a concerted effort to validate measures electronically at the time of creating the measure, or alongside paper counterparts in order to benefit from reduced administrative costs and more efficient data analysis [6,7]. The International Society for Pharmacoeconomics and Outcomes Research (ISPOR) has issued recommendations for the migration of PROMs to electronic formats [8] and detailed reviews have been published on equivalence studies between paper and electronic formats [3,9].

However, CBAs also have limitations [10,11]. There may be a learning curve associated with the use of electronic applications, particularly in older users [12,13], with the requirement of considerable investment of resources. Although the degree of smartphone technology use amongst the elderly population remains unclear, it is likely that even this age group may embrace the new technology in the near future. Furthermore, the lack of consistent internet connectivity may pose challenges particularly where the infrastructure is not optimally supported [14]. In order to prevent cyber-attacks or exposure to computer viruses, data confidentiality and protection require much thought. Sensitive patient information may need regular backing up within a digital framework [15], and should always be collected in strict accordance with the principles of information governance and laws relating to data protection.

There is a technological revolution within medicine; more and more people are using smartphones in their daily lives [16]. User-controlled monitoring of health is a rapidly increasing market, with innovations such as 'wearable technology' becoming increasingly popular [17]. Within dermatology, for example, while the Psoriasis Area and Severity Index (PASI) has been electronically validated [18], computer-guided PASI measurements have been shown to have similar precision and better reproducibility compared with trained physicians [19]. Health care services will have to balance the challenges of financial constraints (e.g. purchasing 10 tablets versus 1000 printouts), but the capacity of such technology to improve health care in the near future remains considerable. Patients being able to record and monitor health-related data on a single device has the potential to develop into an integrated system that could streamline health care delivery.

Validation of measurement methods
Many methods for measuring skin disease have been introduced with little more than a description of the methodology. However, it is necessary to know whether a measurement method actually measures what it purports to measure, and how reliable it is. There are several aspects of validation that are considered desirable. These include:

- Internal consistency: this checks how well individual items in the measurement method that would be expected to correspond, do so. It is usually measured using the Cronbach α coefficient.
- Test–retest reliability: this measures the stability of a scale when used repeatedly under the same conditions.
- Construct validity: this explores how well an instrument measures what it is intended to measure. It is often checked by correlating with a similar existing instrument.
- Sensitivity to change: this examines whether an instrument detects change appropriately.

In the development of patient-reported assessment and outcome measures, both factor analysis and Rasch analysis are used to determine the most appropriate items to use. Application of these techniques ensures removal of redundant items that measure the same thing and tests whether it is appropriate for scores to be combined in an overall score.

The COnsensus-based Standards for the selection of health Measurement INstruments (COSMIN) checklist contains standards for evaluating the methodological quality of studies of health measurement instruments [20]. This checklist is a good starting point to learn more about measurement properties.

Core outcome measures

The ability to compare data and conclusions between studies is severely limited if different measurement methods are used. This has been a particular problem in acne and atopic dermatitis; in contrast, most studies in psoriasis use PASI and the DLQI. To address this, methodology to identify core outcome measures has been developed [21].

International groups, such as Harmonising Outcome Measures for Eczema (HOME) [22], International Dermatology Outcome Measures (IDEOM) [23], Acne Core Outcomes Research Network (ACORN) [24] and HIdradenitis SuppuraTiva cORe outcomes set International Collaboration (HISTORIC) [25] identify, develop and encourage use of core outcome measures in every clinical study of a particular condition, such as for eczema (Box 16.1). Additional measures can still be used as well as the core ones. If research groups internationally cooperate with these voluntary suggestions, within a few years data comparison and combination will be much enhanced, thereby enriching research quality.

> **Box 16.1 Core outcome measures for clinical studies of eczema, suggested by Harmonising Outcome Measures for Eczema (HOME) [22]**
>
> Core Outcome Set (COS) and core outcome instruments (for clinical trials)
> 1 Clinical signs: Eczema Area and Severity Index (EASI)
> 2 Patient-reported symptoms: Patient-Oriented Eczema Measure (POEM) and NRS-11 for peak itch over past 24 hours
> 3 Long-term control: Recap of Atopic Eczema (RECAP) or Atopic Dermatitis Control Test (ADCT)
> 4 Quality of life: DLQI (adults), CDLQI (children), IDQoL (infants)

Assessment tools

The following section discusses a number of tools available to assess common chronic inflammatory skin diseases.

Inflammatory disease

The *Dermatology Index of Disease Severity* (DIDS) [26] can be used across all inflammatory skin diseases and is responsive to change [27]. It assesses functional impairment and percentage of body surface area involvement, categorising each patient into one of five severity grades.

Psoriasis (Chapter 35)

Methods for psoriasis measurement are listed in Box 16.2. The PASI was introduced for a clinical trial [28] but with no supporting validation [29]. PASI requires the observer to give separate scores for erythema, infiltration and desquamation [28] for four body areas. The percentage area involvement in each area is estimated and a formula gives an overall score from 0 to 72. Most patients with psoriasis score less than 10. The scoring of PASI is equivalent, whether signs are recorded using an application (app) or on paper [18]. A patient-administered method, the *Self-Administered PASI* (SAPASI) [30], facilitates measurement in large surveys [31]. Modifications of PASI [32] have not gained widespread acceptance. The PASI system, although flawed because of problems measuring area, is used so widely that researchers seldom consider using alternative methods.

> **Box 16.2 Methods of psoriasis measurement**
>
> - Psoriasis Area and Severity Index (PASI) [28]
> - Self-Administered PASI [30]
> - Physician's Global Assessment [33]
> - Lattice System Global Assessment [35]
> - Simplified Psoriasis Index [38,39]
> - Photographs
> - Nail Assessment in Psoriasis and Psoriatic Arthritis [43]

The simplest scoring system is the *Physicians Global Assessment* (PGA) [33]; the PGA can be combined with body surface area [34]. The *Lattice System Global Assessment* [35] is an alternative better-validated measure [36]: body surface area and average plaque thickness, erythema and scale are combined to reach an overall descriptor [35]. Another proposal is the *Copenhagen Psoriasis Severity Index* [37] in which erythema, plaque thickness and scaling are each assessed at 10 sites, giving a score range of 0–90. The inherent inaccuracies of area assessment are avoided.

The *Simplified Psoriasis Index* (SPI) [38,39] includes three separate scores for clinical severity, psychological impact (a simple overall score) and the history of the psoriasis, including history of previous treatment. The SPI is well suited to describing, categorising and monitoring patients.

There are special considerations in sites such as the scalp, or presentations such as localised pustular psoriasis. The *Nail Psoriasis Severity Index* (NAPSI) [40] and a simpler variant [41] have been reviewed [42]. A three-component tool has been described, the *Nail Assessment in Psoriasis and Psoriatic Arthritis* (NAPPA) [43].

Up to 30% of patients with psoriasis may also suffer with psoriatic arthritis (PsA) [44], a progressive joint disease that may cause considerable chronic disability. Though several screening tools exist for the identification of clinical signs of PsA, the Psoriasis Epidemiology Screening (PEST) is a validated tool with high sensitivity and specificity [45] that is also recommended in psoriasis biological guidelines [46]. The PEST tool consists of five simple questions alongside a manikin to help the clinician immediately identify problematic joints. A score of 1 is allocated to each question answered in the affirmative, with a total score of 3 or more indicative of a potential diagnosis of PsA, warranting a rheumatology referral [45].

Atopic eczema (Chapter 41)

Core outcome domains for clinical use and trials should include symptoms, clinician-assessed signs and measurement of long-term flares [47]. Systematic reviews concluded that only *SCORAD* (SCORing Atopic Dermatitis) [48], *Eczema Area and Severity Index*

(EASI) and *Patient-Oriented Eczema Measure* (POEM) perform adequately [49] (Box 16.3) and that the EASI and SCORAD are the best instruments to assess the clinical signs of atopic eczema (atopic dermatitis) [50]. However, the original Rajka and Langeland system to grade AD severity [51] has been demonstrated to have good construct validity, reliability, internal consistency and responsiveness in adults and children [52]. Assessment methods have been reviewed as part of American Academy of Dermatology guidelines [53]. The minimal clinically important score difference for SCORAD is 8.7, objective SCORAD 8.2 and for POEM is 3.4 [54].

> **Box 16.3 Methods of atopic eczema measurement**
>
> - Rajka Langeland severity classification [66]
> - Nottingham Eczema Severity Score (NESS) [67]
> - SCORing Atopic Dermatitis (SCORAD) [**48**]
> - Eczema Area and Severity Index (EASI) [59]
> - Six Area Six Sign Atopic Dermatitis severity score (SASSAD) [68]
> - Patient-Orientated Eczema Measure (POEM) [69]
> - Three Item Severity Score (TIS) [70]
> - Objective Severity Assessment Atopic Dermatitis (OSAAD) [72]

SCORAD was created in 1993 [**48**], with guidelines [55] and further guidance [56,57]. SCORAD combines scores for clinical signs, disease extent and patient symptoms, including sleep. However, a modified objective SCORAD which omits pruritus and sleep may be more accurate [55]. 'SCORAD 75' has been defined as a 75% reduction in SCORAD following therapy [58].

The EASI is reliable in the clinical trial setting [59]: there is experience of its use in a large study [60]. A self-administered version of EASI has been validated [61].

The POEM [62], completed by patients, incorporates seven features: itchiness, sleep, bleeding, weeping or oozing clear fluid, cracked skin, flaking, dry or rough. The POEM score correlates well with quality of life (QoL) scores [62].

One aspect of measurement that has not been addressed previously in dermatology is the level of control of a chronic disease. In eczema there has been no consensus on what constitutes a 'flare' [63]. Recap of atopic eczema (RECAP) is a seven-item questionnaire to capture the experience of eczema control in all ages and eczema severities [64]. There are two versions: a self-reported version for adults and older children with eczema, and a caregiver-reported version for younger children with eczema. Another approach has been the Atopic Dermatitis Control Tool, consisting of six items with a seven-day recall period [65]. A method to differentiate between mild, moderate and severe atopic eczema [66] was refined as the *Nottingham Eczema Severity Score* (NESS) [67]. The *Six Area Six Sign Atopic Dermatitis* (SASSAD) severity score [68,69] has the advantage of not incorporating area estimation, as there is often no clear delineation between normal and abnormal skin. A very simple *Three Item Severity Score* [70], measuring excoriations, erythema and oedema/papulation may provide as much information as more detailed techniques [71].

Observer variation of scoring has spurred instrument-based and other objective approaches. The *Objective Severity Assessment of Atopic Dermatitis* (OSAAD) score incorporates measurements of stratum corneum barrier function and hydration with computer-assisted measurements of disease extent [72]. OSAAD scores correlate with SCORAD and with serum levels of interleukin-16 [73]. Interleukin-31 levels correlate with severity scoring [74].

Acne (Chapter 88)

Such a wide range of tools is used to assess acne severity that it is not possible to undertake secondary analysis of trial data [75]. Methods range from global assessments to lesion counting [76].

The revised *Leeds Acne Grading System* [77] involves direct counting of non-inflamed and inflamed lesions and includes grading systems for the back and chest and for the face. The original Leeds photographic grading technique [78] is rarely used as few patients now have persisting severe acne: a simpler photographic-based grading method with a 0–8 scale was used in several clinical trials [79]. Parallel-polarised and cross-polarised photography, video microscopy and fluorescence photography have also been described [80].

The *Echelle de Cotation des Lésions d'Acné* (ECLA) or 'Acne Lesion Score Scale' system has demonstrated good reliability [81] and may correlate with QoL scores [82,83].

Methods to measure post-acne scarring are needed: a global scarring grading system has been proposed with four grades of scarring described [84]. The *Echelle d'évaluation Clinique des Cicatrice d'Acné* (ECCA) [85] consists of recording the number of each of six types of acne scars: this has been used to assess laser therapy [86]. There are two other patient-reported outcome measures, both specific to facial atrophic acne scarring, the self-assessment of clinical acne-related scars (SCARS) and the facial acne scar quality of life (FASQoL) tools. These tools focus on symptoms (SCARS) and psychological and social well-being (FASQoL) [87].

Hidradenitis suppurativa (Chapter 90)

There is a lack of efficient and sensitive outcome measures for hidradenitis suppurativa (HS), with up to 30 instruments described in literature [88]. The *Hurley staging system*, based on the degree of sinus and scar formation, was the first severity assessment measure to be utilised by classifying patients into three categories: (i) mild, (ii) moderate and (iii) severe. However, as scarring is irreversible, this method of scoring is not entirely sensitive to change when monitoring treatment response [89]. The *HS Physician's Global Assessment* (HS-PGA) is relatively easy to use. It consists of a 6-point scale ranging from 'clear' (score = 0) to 'very severe' (score = 5), taking into account the number of inflammatory nodules, abscesses and draining fistulae. However, there is concern around the heterogeneity of patients at the severe end of the scale and its clinical discriminatory power [90].

The *Sartorius Score*, developed in 2003, incorporates lesion, region and inflammatory count as well as body surface area [91] and has subsequently been modified, resulting in the '*modified HS Score*', '*modified Sartorius Score*' (MSS) and '*HS lesion, area, and severity index*' (HS-LASI) [88,92]. These various versions have different items and despite some conceptual overlap, the scores cannot be directly compared.

Newer measures include the *Hidradenitis Suppurativa Clinical Response* (HiSCR) and the *Acne Inversa Severity Index* (AISI). The

HiSCR was created retrospectively from a randomised controlled trial and captures the acute phase of HS disease activity by incorporating total inflammatory lesion count (abscesses and inflammatory nodules) and is also responsive to treatment effects [90]. AISI is a composite instrument that incorporates a physician-rated assessment and a patient-rated visual analogue scale (VAS) pain and disability scale. The physician-rated element considers body sites as well as the nature of the type of lesions in its score calculation [93]. At present there are limited validation studies of HiSCR and AISI.

To address concerns around validation, the European Hidradenitis Suppurativa Foundation (EHSF) developed a novel validated tool: the 'International Hidradenitis Suppurativa Severity Score System' (IHS4), based on the number of nodules, abscesses and draining tunnels [94]. It correlates well with several other existing clinical and patient-reported measures and is therefore suitable for use in real-life as well as clinical trial settings. Similarly, the 'Severity and Area Score for Hidradenitis' (SASH) is a valid and reliable outcome measure that incorporates body surface area, induration, ulceration and inflammatory skin colour change (e.g. erythema) [95]. However, despite assessment of its psychometric properties, the instrument has only been designed to be utilised in a clinical trial setting and its responsiveness has yet to be formally established.

Urticaria (Chapter 42)

The current gold standard for measuring disease activity in chronic spontaneous urticaria (CSU) is the urticarial activity score (UAS) [96]. Due to the variable nature of urticaria, the UAS measure encourages patients to self-record disease activity over a 24-hour period for a total of 7 consecutive days, following which an aggregate score is calculated. There are two versions of this measure widely used in practice, UAS7 and UAS_{TD}. Both versions incorporate wheal count as well as itch severity with an overall weekly score range of 0–42. The main difference between these versions concerns the wheal score categories: whereas the UAS7 is scored once daily, the UAS_{TD} is scored twice daily. Though both tools produce comparable results [97], the UAS7 is the preferred tool in guidelines due to its simplicity of completion, discriminatory power and lower burden of completion for patients and physicians [98,99].

A separate measure has also been created to assess disease control in all forms of urticaria: the urticaria control test (UCT) [100]. This is a simple four-item questionnaire with a 4-week recall period, scoring disease activity from 'poorly controlled' to 'well-controlled'.

In a subset of patients who also experience symptoms of angioedema, the angioedema activity score (AAS) is a validated adjunct severity assessment tool [101].

Symptoms

Itch is usually measured using a single global question or VAS, either alone or as part of other standard tools such as SCORAD or DLQI. VAS should be combined with scratch activity scales [102] and QoL or patient-benefit scales [103]. The *Itch Severity Scale* records itch frequency and specific sensations during the day [104]. Efforts continue to improve itch assessment [105]. Psoriasis symptoms can be measured using the validated eight-item *Psoriasis Symptom Inventory* (PSI) [106,107].

Therapy benefit

The *Patient Benefit Index* (PBI) is the first validated measure to assess the patient's perspective of benefit from drugs and therapeutic procedures [108]. It has been used in lichen sclerosus, chronic wounds and psoriasis [109].

Objective methods for measuring skin properties

There are many objective ways to measure the physical properties of skin [110]. Few of them have, however, found their way into routine use either in the clinic or in clinical trials.

Ultrasound [111] can be used to measure psoriatic plaque thickness [112,113]. Stratum corneum hydration can be measured by assessing surface electrical properties [114,115], and barrier function of the skin is assessed *in vivo* by measuring transepidermal water loss (TEWL) [116]. Optical coherence tomography has been used to measure epidermal thickness [117].

There are guidelines for the standardisation of procedures to measure skin colour [118]. It is important to recognise that 'objective' properties may be influenced by factors such as ambient light conditions and the effect of melanin on erythema assessment and vice versa. Simple to use devices may aid clinical work [119]. A variety of techniques have been used to measure skin pigmentation [120], including diffuse reflectance spectroscopy [121].

Elasticity [122] and surface roughness and microcontours [123] can be measured, though not easily in the clinic.

Accurate measurement of skin disease extent is difficult. Photographs may be used to record psoriasis, but body contour distortion and difficulty in defining edges are problems in image analysis. Where an expert panel assesses photographs there is accurate global assessment [124]: enhanced imaging methods can improve PASI area estimation accuracy [125]. Computer-aided analysis of manual outlines of lesions on photographs [126] may enhance area estimation accuracy, but 'old-fashioned' point counting of photographs is still reliable in assessing vitiligo [127].

Artificial intelligence (AI) techniques [128] are likely to profoundly influence the ability to measure skin diseases accurately. They have been used to measure ulcers, using image recognition to measure precise wound boundaries [129,130]. In psoriasis AI has been used to measure and classify psoriatic plaques [131], and, in a window to the future of our specialty, giving predictions over response to biologic therapy from initial basic clinical criteria [132].

Measurement of the impact of skin disease
(Chapter 15)

Quality of life assessment in patients with skin disease

What does quality of life mean?

It is essential to assess the impact of skin disease in order to address the real needs of patients [133]. The importance of QoL in dermatology has been emphasised by the suggestion of a new word to describe quality of life impairment, 'quimp' [134]. However, defining QoL and the narrower concept of Health-Related Quality of

Life (HRQoL) is not easy [135–137]. Information about the absolute meaning of QoL scores is required, together with the interpretation of change in scores.

Why measure quality of life?

The most important use of QoL measurement is in the clinic, to inform clinical decisions, to improve clinician–patient communication, and to make clinicians more aware of skin disease burden [138]. QoL data may be useful to triage the urgency of referrals [139].

Measurement is also helpful for clinical therapeutic research, health service research, audit of effectiveness of services, use in patient registries [140] and research into psychological aspects of dermatology and patient behaviour. Skin disease burden data may strengthen arguments for appropriate funding of dermatology services and for education about skin diseases [141,142]. Generic HRQoL measures can be used to demonstrate the importance of skin disease in comparison to diseases of other organs [143,144].

Informing clinical decisions

The assumptions that clinicians make concerning the impact that diseases have on their patients' lives influence their clinical decisions, but these assumptions may not be accurate [145–147]. HRQoL measures with meaningful scores may give clinicians a more accurate assessment of disease impact, enabling them to make better judgements on the choice of therapy for the individual patient [148].

Current severe psoriasis can be defined by using a combination of physical and QoL descriptors [149]. The *Rule of Tens* is as follows:

current severe psoriasis = body surface area involved

> 10% *or* PASI > 10 *or* DLQI score > 10

If this is met, more active therapy should be considered [149]. The British Association of Dermatologists' guidelines [150] for the use of biologics use a variation on this concept, as do other national and international guidelines [151–153]. The International Psoriasis Council has suggested that patients with psoriasis should be classified as either candidates for topical therapy or candidates for systemic therapy; the latter are patients who meet at least one of the following criteria: body surface area >10%, disease involving special areas, and failure of topical therapy [154].

Methods of measuring quality of life in dermatology

There are at least 40 health status QoL measurement instruments for skin disease [155]: a European Academy of Dermatology and Venereology (EADV) Task Force has summarised the techniques available [156]. There is guidance over general principles concerning how to choose which to use [157,158]. A critical review recommended the use of a combination of the SF-36 and Skindex-29 for research studies [159]; however, in the busy clinical environment it is more practical to use a single simple short questionnaire.

There are comparisons of assessment of QoL in cutaneous disease [160] and in psoriasis [161], and there is advice about understanding QoL research [162] and QoL research methodology [163]. Minimum criteria to create and establish new instruments have been suggested [164] and there are techniques to address whether instruments are uni-dimensional [165,166]. Once QoL measures have been published, for them to become useful in the research or clinical arena, a long-term supportive framework is required to ensure continuing integrity of the measure, for example to validate and maintain quality of translations [167].

HRQoL measures usually assess the impact of skin disease 'at present' or over a fixed time (e.g. 'the last week'), allowing data comparison before and after intervention. However, the long-term impact on a patient's life may not be captured by these indices.

There are advantages in administering QoL measures electronically, which is now the preferred mode. As many QoL measures were designed and validated using paper, it is reassuring that equivalence has been confirmed between paper and electronic administration for the DLQI [168,169].

What do quality of life scores mean?

Descriptive bands to interpret scores, such as for the DLQI [170–172], can transform questionnaires to be useful in routine clinical practice. There also needs to be information about the minimal clinically important difference (MCID) of score that is of relevance to patients. It may be that other standard differences, such as the concept of 2MCID [173], could be calculated to provide more understanding of the meaning of change.

Where HRQoL measures are used in international studies, culturally validated translations should be used. However, psoriasis patients from different countries respond differently to items from both the DLQI and Skindex, despite having the same underlying HRQoL impairment [174].

Quality of life measures used in dermatology

General health measures

General health measures can be used across a wide range of diseases and are needed to compare the impact of skin diseases with diseases of other systems. Examples include the *UK Sickness Impact Profile* [143,175–177], the *SF-36* [178–180] and *WHOQOL-26* and *-100* [181,182]. For the *Patient-Generated Index*, a subject identifies key ways in which their life is affected, and ranks and assigns importance to each aspect [183]. This method gains insight into individual patients' problems, but is unsuitable for large surveys. The *EuroQol EQ-5D* [184] is used by European drug licensing authorities as a basis for utility analysis [185,186]. There is growing experience of its use in dermatology [187,188], and a mapping study now allows DLQI data to be converted to EQ5D data [189].

The *General Health Questionnaire* is designed to detect psychiatric disorder and is reliable in dermatology patients [190]. Depression can be detected using the *Mini International Neuropsychiatric Interview* questionnaire [191]. Psychiatric co-morbidity and QoL impairment are closely related [192].

Dermatology-specific measures

Dermatology-specific measures are used to compare the impact of different skin diseases, and to measure change before or after intervention. Having a single simple measure for use across all skin disease is of great practical advantage. The *DLQI* [193] and

Skindex [194] are the most widely used. Other measures include the *Dermatology Quality of Life Scales* [195], the *Dermatology-specific Quality of Life instrument* [196], the German *DIELH* [197], the French *VQ-Dermatol* [198] and a Turkish measure [199]. The *Freiburg Life Quality Assessment* (FLQA) questionnaires combine a common core module with a disease-specific module [200]. The *Pictorial Representation of Illness and Self Measure* (PRISM) is a pictorial QoL instrument [201].

The DLQI and Skindex measure mainly physical, psychological and social functioning. A broader instrument, the *Impact of Chronic Skin Disease on Daily Life* (ISDL) [202], has five categories, good reliability and validity, but has over 72 items and takes 20 min to complete.

The Dermatology Life Quality Index

The DLQI has 10 questions (Box 16.4), each is answered by a simple tick-box method and scored 0–3 [193]. DLQI completion takes on average 2 min [203].

Box 16.4 The Dermatology Life Quality Index

The aim of this questionnaire is to measure how much your skin problem has affected your life OVER THE LAST WEEK. Please tick one box for each question.

1. Over the last week, how **itchy, sore, painful** or **stinging** has your skin been?
2. Over the last week, how **embarrassed** or **self-conscious** have you been because of your skin?
3. Over the last week, how much has your skin interfered with you going **shopping** or looking after your **home** or **garden**?
4. Over the last week, how much has your skin influenced the **clothes** you wear?
5. Over the last week, how much has your skin affected any **social** or **leisure** activities?
6. Over the last week, how much has your skin made it difficult for you to do any **sport**?
7. Over the last week, has your skin prevented you from **working** or **studying**?
   If 'no', over the last week how much has your skin been a problem at **work** or **studying**?
8. Over the last week, how much has your skin created problems with your **partner** or any of your **close friends** or **relatives**?
9. Over the last week, how much has your skin caused any **sexual difficulties**?
10. Over the last week, how much of a problem has the **treatment** for your skin been, for example by making your home messy, or by taking up time?

Please check you have answered every question. Thank you.

Each question is answered either 'Very much' (score 3), 'A lot' (score 2), 'A little' (score 1) or 'Not at all' (score 0). Questions 3–10 also have the option 'Not relevant' (score 0). The first part of question 7 has the choices 'Yes' (score 3),'No', or 'Not relevant'. The second part of question 7 has the choices 'A lot', 'A little' or 'Not at all'. The maximum score (indicating highest possible impairment of quality of life) is 30 and the minimum 0. For further information [205] see https://www.cardiff.ac.uk/medicine/resources/quality-of-life-questionnaires/dermatology-life-quality-index (last accessed January 2022).

Reproduced from Finlay and Khan 1994 [193]. © A.Y. Finlay and G.K. Khan April 1992.

By 2021, there were over 1500 articles describing the use of the DLQI in over 120 translations [204,205]. The DLQI is now used in guidelines and national disease registries in over 45 countries [206]. Validation studies have been carried out in the UK, in secondary [193] and primary [207] care, and in over 32 countries [208–218]. When illustrations are added, the questionnaire is completed more rapidly but answers are influenced [203]. Descriptive score bandings for the DLQI are given in Box 16.5. In psoriasis [219] and urticaria [220], a score change of at least 3 is needed for a patient to experience a minimum clinically important change in HRQoL. A score change of at least 4 (the MCID) is required to indicate an equivalent change in HRQoL if the DLQI is used to assess patients with a diverse range of inflammatory skin diseases rather than a specific dermatosis [221]. Although criticised [222], the DLQI has contributed to a paradigm shift to patient-centred outcomes [223]. A mapping technique now allows EQ-5D population data to be calculated from DLQI scores [189].

Box 16.5 Descriptive score bandings for the Dermatology Life Quality Index

Score	Meaning
0–1	No effect on patient's life
2–5	Small effect on patient's life
6–10	Moderate effect on patient's life
11–20	Very large effect on patient's life
21–30	Extremely large effect on patient's life

Adapted from Hongbo *et al.* 2005 [170].

Although the DLQI is copyright, clinicians may freely use the DLQI in routine clinical practice without seeking permission and without charge [205].

Skindex

Skindex has been developed and extensively validated in four versions with 61 [194], 29 [224], 16 [225] or 17 [226] questions. Further validation studies have been carried out in several countries [227–234]. There is extensive experience of the use of this measure in a wide range of languages, countries and dermatological diseases. The appropriateness of using Skindex in psoriasis along with the generic SF-29 has been emphasised [161]. *Skindex-29* scores have been categorised into four levels to aid interpretation of scores [171,172].

Disease-specific quality of life measures

Disease-specific measures may be the most sensitive to change and are suitable for comparing outcomes of patients with the same disease. However, most skin conditions affect patients' lives in broadly similar ways, so dermatology-specific measures can also be used. From a practical clinical perspective there is no need for a disease-specific measure for every skin disease.

Psoriasis

A systematic review of QoL assessment of psoriasis identified 21 questionnaires [235]. Psoriasis-specific measures have been described [236] and critically reviewed [237]. A systematic review of the use of QoL instruments in RCTs in psoriasis found that the DLQI was the most commonly used QoL instrument (83% of studies), followed by the SF-36 (31%), EQ-5D (15%) and the PDI (14%) [238].

The 15-item *Psoriasis Disability Index* (PDI) [239,240] was the first dermatology disease-specific QoL measure. It has been extensively used [241–243] in over 23 languages [**204**]. Some aspects of its validation have been criticised [244].

The stigmatising effects of psoriasis can be recorded using a 33-item questionnaire [245]. A technique for measuring stigma across all dermatology patients, the *Questionnaire on Experience with Skin complaints* (QES) [246], has been used in psoriasis [247]. Stress caused by psoriasis can be measured using the 15-item version of the *Psoriasis Life Stress Inventory* [248,249].

The 11-item version *Impact of Psoriasis Questionnaire* (IPSO) [250,251] has good internal consistency [251]. The IPSO was used to assess changes in a cohort of psoriasis patients over 11 years [252].

The SPI (see earlier) consists of three independent scores describing *S*igns (disease activity), *P*sychosocial disability and history of *I*nterventions [**38**,39].

PSORIQoL is a 25-item questionnaire that assesses the impact of impairment and disability from psoriasis on the patient's perception of QoL [253]: a US version has been validated [254]. Another questionnaire, the 12-item *PQoL-12* [255], has been incorporated in a psoriasis severity assessment tool, the Koo–Menter Psoriasis Instrument [256]. *CALIPSO* is a 30-item psoriasis-specific QoL questionnaire, based on five other questionnaires [257].

Atopic eczema
The *Children's Dermatology Life Quality Index* (CDLQI) and the *Dermatology Life Quality Index* (DLQI) have been frequently used in the monitoring of patients with atopic eczema as well as several disease-specific QoL measures. Patient-assessed severity of atopic eczema was more closely correlated with the DLQI and CDLQI than provider-assessed severity [258]. Assessment of the burden of atopic eczema has been reviewed [259].

The *Psychosomatic Scale for Atopic Dermatitis* (PSS-AD) is a simple 12-item scale to measure the 'psychosomatic pathology' of adult atopic eczema [260]. It may help identify patients who would benefit from psychological intervention. In adults, perceived stigma and atopic eczema severity are both strong predictors of QoL impairment [261].

The 45-item *Childhood Atopic Dermatitis Impact Scale* (CADIS) assesses the impact on the QoL of affected young children and on their families [262], two separate concepts. CADIS scores correlate with SCORAD [263] and with *Infant's Dermatitis Quality of Life Index* (IDQoL), CDLQI and *Dermatitis Family Impact questionnaire* (DFI) [264].

The *Parents' Index of Quality of Life in Atopic Dermatitis* (PIQoL-AD) [265] measures the parent's assessment of the impact of the atopic eczema on the affected child (not the secondary impact on the parent). The minimum meaningful score difference is estimated to be 2 to 3 points [266]. In contrast, the DFI measures the impact of having a child with atopic eczema on the QoL of the family [267].

The lives of infants with atopic eczema may be severely disrupted: the IDQoL [268,269], completed by the parents, measures this impact on infants (see later).

Acne
QoL measures for use in acne have been reviewed [270]. The five-question *Cardiff Acne Disability Index* [271–273] has demonstrated reliability [274] and been validated in French [275], Persian [276] and Serbian [277]. The CADI and the CDLQI correlate well [278]. The *Assessments of the Psychological and Social Effects of Acne* (APSEA) questionnaire [279,280] has 15 questions, some of which relate to the overall impact and some to the recent past.

The *Acne Quality of Life Scale* (AQOL) [281] has nine questions that relate specifically to the social impact of acne. The *Acne-specific Quality of Life Questionnaire* (Acne-QoL) [282] was designed for use in clinical trials. A four-question condensed version of this, the Acne-Q4, is more practical to use [283,284]. The *Acne Symptom and Impact Scale* (ASIS) was developed for adults and adolescents specifically with facial acne [285].

Hidradenitis suppurativa
The DLQI is the most commonly used QoL measure in HS, followed by another dermatology-specific questionnaire, the Skindex-29 [286]. Only a few HS-specific QoL measures are described in the literature, though given the considerable impact of the disease, this is a fast-evolving area of interest.

A non-validated untitled measure was adapted from an instrument used for Crohn's disease with a focus on severe perianal disease, but has only had limited use in HS [287]. The Hidradenitis Suppurativa Quality of Life instrument (HS-QoL) is a 7-subscale measure consisting of 44 items that covers various QoL aspects as well as mental health and life satisfaction [288]. It has been shown to be reliable with strong evidence of validity [289]. Another measure, the Hidradenitis Suppurativa Burden of Disease (HSBOD), is based on interviews with dermatologists and patients and consists of 19 items that are self-administered using a visual analogue scale (0, no complaints, to 10, worst complaints) [290]. The instrument has two recall segments: '4 weeks' and 'total duration of HS disease', with various domains including 'symptoms and feelings', 'daily activities', 'leisure', 'work/school' and 'personal relationships'. The measure demonstrates internal reliability and correlates well with the DLQI.

The Hidradenitis Suppurativa Symptom Assessment (HSSA), consisting of 9 items, and the Hidradenitis Suppurativa Impact Assessment (HSIA), consisting of 17 items, were developed at the same time to assess HS symptoms and signs in a research setting. While both measures demonstrate construct validity, they do not have full psychometric evaluation [291].

To address the gaps in HS QoL measurement, the HIdradenitis SuppuraTiva cORe outcomes set International Collaboration (HISTORIC) [292,293] paved the way for another validated QoL tool for HS severity measurement in clinical trials: the Hidradenitis Suppurativa Quality of Life (HiSQOL) [294]. This is a 17-item questionnaire, with a 7-day recall period, and incorporates aspects such as odour and drainage. It correlates strongly with the DLQI and, unlike the majority of existing HS PROMs, has full psychometric evaluation.

Urticaria

Changes in clinical symptoms and signs correlate well with simultaneous impact on HRQoL for patients suffering with urticaria [295]. The *Chronic Urticaria Quality of Life Questionnaire* (CU-Q$_2$oL) is the first reliable and validated urticaria-specific measure to be developed [296] and is a recommended QoL measure for use in urticaria [297]. It has a recall period of 2 weeks and consists of 23 items across six domains: pruritus, impact on daily activities, sleep problems, limitations, look and swelling. The total score ranges from 0 to 100 (100 = worst HRQoL impairment) with a proposed MCID of 15 [298].

The HRQoL of patients with various types of angioedema may be assessed with the *Angioedema Quality of Life Questionnaire* (AE-QoL), a validated tool with a 4-week recall period. It consists of 17 items, categorised into four domains: functioning, fatigue/mood, fears/shame, and food [299]. It has an MCID of 6 [300] and has been widely used, demonstrating good evidence of reliability and validity [301].

Skin cancer

Skin cancer-specific questionnaires are more sensitive and responsive to HRQoL change than generic measures [302], such as the EQ-5D or SF-36 which are both commonly used [303]. However, the European TaskForce review also recommends the simultaneous use of dermatology-specific measures, such as DLQI or Skindex-29, to fully capture skin-related problems associated with skin cancer [303].

The *European Organisation for Research and Treatment of Cancer Core Questionnaire* (EORTC QLQ-C30) is a 30-item cancer-specific questionnaire with five functional scales: physical, role, cognitive, emotional and social functioning. It has been extensively validated [303,304] and has an 11-item melanoma module targeted at patients with advanced disease [305].

The *Functional Assessment of Cancer Therapy-Melanoma* (FACT-M) is a melanoma-specific measure with 51 items that also incorporates the impact of lymphoedema and surgical scarring. It consists of three QoL domains: physical well-being, emotional well-being and social well-being. It has been validated demonstrating internal consistency, reliability and responsiveness [306,307].

The *Skin Cancer Index* (SCI) is a 15-item skin cancer-specific measure with a focus on cervicofacial non-melanoma skin cancer and has three subscales: emotion, social and appearance [308]. The score ranges from 0 to 100 with higher scores reflecting a better QoL. It is clinically responsive and has also been extensively validated [309].

Patient-specific and utility measures

The *Patient Generated Index* [310] asks patients to identify five ways in which their lives are most affected and then assign them comparative values [311], providing insight into a specific patient's concerns.

Utility measures assess the hypothetical value placed by people on their health. The *Willingness To Pay* (WTP) method asks how much patients would be prepared to pay for a hypothetical cure, in acne [272], psoriasis [240,312,313] and atopic eczema [312,314]. WTP data showed strong test–retest reliability in an onychomycosis study [315].

In the *Time Trade-Off* (TTO) method, patients are asked how much time they would be prepared to give up for the sake of a cure. These 'trade-off' questions can be related to years of shortening of life, as in the *Quality-Adjusted Life Year* (QALY), or related to daily hours. The TTO method has been described in psoriasis [240,313], atopic eczema [314] and melasma [316]. Patients would choose a 40% shorter life expectancy in order to avoid uncontrolled eczema or psoriasis [317]. TTO questions have been used to calculate comparative mean utilities across a range of skin diseases [318], which can be compared with non-dermatological diseases.

Quality-adjusted and disability-adjusted life years (QALYs and DALYs)

Quality of life data, in particular EQ-5D score data, is used to calculate QALYs. The ability of new interventions to improve a skin condition can be expressed in terms of improvement in QALYs, and so the cost per QALY can be calculated. This information is used to compare the efficiency of different drugs and, by setting a cut-off level for cost per QALY gained, can assist health technology appraisers such as the National Institute for Health and Care Excellence (NICE) to decide whether or not to recommend drugs for use in health care systems.

The QALY method was first applied in dermatology in acne [319]. The advent of biologic drugs for psoriasis resulted in considerable attention being given to the concept [320]. The resulting QALY information has played a key role in influencing criteria for the use of these drugs. QALY calculations may use standard HRQoL information, such as EQ-5D or DLQI data, to compare the cost-effectiveness of different drug regimens [186,321].

Health state descriptors and the standard gamble technique have been combined for the calculation of QALYs [322] in atopic eczema. Such cost–utility and cost-effectiveness analyses, sometimes including QoL data [323,324], may demonstrate whether particular interventions can be economically justified.

More broadly, there have been huge challenges in meeting the need to measure the overall burden of skin disease [325,326]. The concept of disability-adjusted life year (DALY) has been used to provide comparative data. DALY data brings together the time spent with a skin condition that limits health, along with time lost because of early death. However, to appreciate the wider burden of skin disease, disease prevalence, QoL data and health care costs must also be taken into account [327], as well as the burden on partners and other family members and the wider societal impact.

Measuring the impact of skin disease in children and adolescents
Children

The assessment of QoL impairment in children is challenging because of communication, change in lifestyle with age and differing rates of maturing. General measures and disease-specific measures have been systematically reviewed [328,329].

The *CDLQI* [330] is for use from 4 to 16 years. Older children complete it unaided but parents can help younger children as necessary. Key question areas are given in Box 16.6. The illustrated cartoon version, using the same text, has been validated [331]. The CDLQI has been used in 28 countries in 102 clinical studies and is available in 44 languages, including six cultural adaptations [**332**]. It has been used in 14 skin conditions and in the assessment of 11 topical drugs, 9 systemic drugs, 13 therapeutic interventions and 2 epidemiological and other studies [333]. There is evidence of high internal consistency, test–retest reliability, responsiveness to change, and significant correlation with other subjective and objective measures.

> **Box 16.6 The Children's Dermatology Life Quality Index: aspects covered in 10 questions**
>
> 1. Symptoms
> 2. Embarrassment
> 3. Friendships
> 4. Clothes
> 5. Playing
> 6. Sports
> 7. School/holiday activities
> 8. Teasing
> 9. Sleep
> 10. Treatment
>
> Adapted from Lewis-Jones and Finlay 1995 [330].

The difficulties in measuring life quality changes in children are even greater in the very young. The *IDQoL* is completed by a parent and records the impact of atopic eczema on infants [268]. The IDQoL has been translated into 21 languages and used in 18 countries, including two multinational studies [287]. Thirty-one studies demonstrated its psychometric properties, such as test–retest reliability, internal consistency, validity, responsiveness to change and interpretability. Eight studies used the IDQoL to assess the effectiveness of therapeutic interventions such as education programmes, consultations and wet-wrap therapy, while seven studies described the use of IDQoL in topical interventions.

The *Infants and Toddlers Quality of Life* instrument (InToDermQoL) was created as a dermatology-specific proxy instrument for HRQoL assessment in children from birth to age 4 years [334]. Created across seven countries, there are three age-specific versions with 10, 12 and 15 items. An epidermolysis bullosa-specific module has been developed [335].

The *Pediatric Symptom Checklist* [336], which consists of 35 questions answered by the parent, has been used for psychosocial screening in paediatric dermatology clinics.

Adolescents

Skin disease may profoundly affect adolescents in several ways, including psychological, social, lifestyle, education and employment [337]. Although the CDLQI and the DLQI are widely used in teenagers, and there is some overlap [338], there are special aspects of life quality impairment experienced by adolescents that may be captured by specific teenage measures. *Skindex-Teen* [339] is a 21-item questionnaire assessing physical symptoms and psychosocial functioning: the questions originated from experts but were validated on patients. The questions of the *Teenagers' Quality of Life Index* (T-QoL©) [340] were based on the results of a qualitative study of teenage patients with skin disease [337]. T-QoL has 18 questions covering three domains: 'self image', 'physical well-being and future aspirations' and 'psychological impact and relationships'. T-QoL has been used to assess the benefit of a specialised teenage and young adult dermatology clinic [341].

Measuring the impact of skin disease on partners and the family

'The Greater Patient'

The concept of 'the Greater Patient' describes the wider family unit, including the partner or close relatives. The lives of all of these may be affected by an individual within the family unit having skin disease [342]. The variety of methods used to measure the family impact of skin disease using dermatology-specific instruments have been reviewed [343].

This impact on the family has been assessed in atopic eczema, for example in causing parental sleep disturbance [344]. Two disease-specific methods [267,345] measure this secondary impact, and another questionnaire records the impact both on an affected child and on the parents [262]. The *Dermatitis Family Impact* questionnaire (DFI) [267,346] has been used in 50 studies in 16 countries to assess the impact of therapy and of different care interventions, and to demonstrate the relationship of childhood dermatitis severity to family life quality [347]. Support groups for children with atopic eczema and their families [348] may help to address some of these Greater Patient issues. The families of adults with atopic eczema also experience a secondary impact: for example, the sex life of 36% of partners of adult patients with atopic eczema was affected, as measured by a questionnaire designed to assess sexual functioning [349].

The 10-item *Family Dermatology Life Quality Index* (FDLQI) can be used across all skin diseases [350,351]. Key areas affected and enquired about are shown in Box 16.7. The FDLQI allows comparison between the family impact of different skin diseases and it has been used in psoriasis, atopic eczema, acne, chronic wounds, hidradenitis suppurativa, vitiligo, pemphigus and epidermolysis bullosa. It can also be used to demonstrate change in family QoL after therapeutic intervention, such as following biologic therapy for psoriasis [352].

> **Box 16.7 The Family Dermatology Life Quality Index: aspects covered in 10 questions**
>
> 1. Emotional distress
> 2. Physical well-being
> 3. Personal relationships
> 4. Other people's reactions
> 5. Social life
> 6. Recreation/leisure activities
> 7. Time assisting therapy
> 8. Housework
> 9. Work/study
> 10. Expenditure
>
> Adapted from Basra, Sue-Ho and Finlay 2007 [350].

It is important to understand the attitudes and beliefs held by patients with psoriasis and their partners [353]. The *Psoriasis Family Impact* [354,355] and *FamilyPso* [356] questionnaires can assess the psoriasis-specific issues.

New ways are needed to develop interventions to address these impacts on family members and to assess outcomes [357].

The *Family Reported Outcome Measure* (FROM-16) is a 16-item questionnaire that can be used across all of medicine to measure the impact of disease on the partner or the family members of patients [358]. It was based on interviews with over 130 family members of patients from 26 specialties [359]. It is primarily an assessment tool that enables comparison of the secondary impact caused by skin disease with that caused by other diseases. It could, however, also be used to explore whether an intervention with a beneficial outcome for the patient has a corresponding beneficial effect on the patient's partner and family. FROM-16 has been used to measure the family impact of cancer, urinary stones, myalgic encephalitis [360] and Covid-19 [361], as well as a variety of systemic diseases: its use in dermatology [362] will therefore allow comparisons with the impact of non-dermatological disease.

Assessing life course impairment resulting from skin disease

One of the three key dimensions [363] of burden of skin disease (the others are impact now and impact on the family) is life course impairment [364]. Skin diseases influence many major life-changing decisions, such as career choice or choice of partner [365,366]. The magnitude of this influence can be recorded using the *Major Life Changing Decision Profile* (MLCDP) [367]. Having psoriasis leads to long-term cumulative life changes [364]. It has been postulated that the impact of psoriasis on life course is likely to be more significant during young adulthood because it is a sensitive and critical period in a patient's life [368]. Life course impairment has also been assessed in vitiligo [369], skin cancer [370], alopecia [371] and several other skin diseases [372,373].

The cumulative and ongoing burden of disease may result in the failure of patients to reach 'full life potential', a process that has been termed 'cumulative life course impairment' (CLCI) [364]. This impairment may also be assessed by examining milestones, such as in psychosocial and psychosexual development [374]. The *Course of Life Questionnaire* (CoLQ) was designed to measure such domains in young adults who have grown up with chronic disease [375].

While it may be argued that some aspects of CLCI are irreversible, formal assessment of life course impairment may assist clinicians to identify risk factors at an earlier stage, allowing more tailored and individualised intervention [376].

Practical clinical use of quality of life measures: a vital sign?

Clinicians use a subjective view of the QoL of their patients to inform many decisions. A better understanding of this impact has led to a focus on 'patient-centred care' [377] or 'patient-based medicine' [378]. In psoriasis, there is a relationship between the type of management decision taken and patient-rated HRQoL [379]. However, there is a lack of HRQoL discussion during dermatology out-patient consultations [380]. Where DLQI information was routinely available in a general dermatology clinic, treatment decisions were influenced in 9% of consultations, mainly in patients in whom there was high HRQoL impairment [381].

Patient-generated information, as assessed by HRQoL outcome measures, is essential for understanding the impact of skin disease on the individual patient and thus for influencing management decisions [382]. Challenges remain in the capturing and use of HRQoL data: QoL assessment adds to but cannot replace effective patient–physician communication [383]. A further challenge to dermatologists is to identify the full range of interventions, beyond drugs, that may be of benefit in improving impaired QoL [384].

Psychological impact measures (Chapter 15)

The psychological impact of skin disease is considerable and patients may experience depression, anxiety and suicidal ideation [385–387]. Psychiatric morbidity can range from 25% to 40% in dermatological patients, with higher rates in pruritic conditions, skin infections and alopecia [388,389]. A multicentre European review of psychological burden of skin disease highlights chronic leg ulcers as the leading cause of depression, often due to feelings of isolation [385], and is supported by previous findings [390]. Certain subsets of eczema have a higher incidence of depression [385,391], while anxiety is more common in conditions such as psoriasis and acne [385]. Nevertheless, psoriasis is also strongly associated with depression and suicidal ideation [392]. Psychological stress may depend on attachment styles of dermatological patients and may consequently play a further role in exacerbating chronic skin diseases [393,394]. However, dermatologists often underdiagnose mood disorders and further clinical training may be necessary to address these concerns [395]. Though routine QoL assessment may capture elements of depression [396], the formal identification and assessment of psychological disorders associated with dermatological conditions are crucial to ameliorate patient health care. The involvement of a psychodermatology team is important when managing patients with psychocutaneous disease [393].

Two psychiatric measures commonly used alongside QoL assessment include the *Hospital Anxiety and Depression Scale* (HADS) and *Beck Depression Inventory* (BDI) [396].

The HADS scale, developed in 1983 [397], is a screening tool composed of 14 items, with a score range 0–21. The questions are categorised into two domains: anxiety (HADS-A) and depression (HADS-D). Each domain has seven questions with a four-level response scale. Total scores are banded from 0 to 7 ('normal'), 8 to 10 ('borderline abnormal') and 11 to 21 ('abnormal'), which would warrant further investigation or management. HADS has good psychometric properties and is a well-validated instrument [397–399] with good correlation with other outcome measures [396,400].

The BDI was originally published in 1961 [401]. It is a 21-item patient-reported outcome measure with a score range 0–63 and is routinely used to assess the severity of depression in clinical studies [248,396,402]. The BDI covers various aspects of mental health, as well as physical and behavioural manifestations of ill health.

The *Brief Symptom Inventory* (BSI) is a 53-item instrument that measures psychological symptoms across nine subscales: somatisation, compulsive symptoms, interpersonal sensibility, depression, anxiety, hostility, phobia, paranoia and psychoticism (a personality pattern typified by aggressiveness and interpersonal hostility) [403].

Another measure often used for screening psychiatric conditions is the 12-item *General Health Questionnaire* (GHQ-12) [404]. This is a self-administered questionnaire which is scored either by a binary method or by using a Likert method, which has been shown to be a valid way to assess psychological distress in dermatological patients

[405]. However, it does not specifically measure anxiety and depression [385].

Though several other measures exist, further studies are required for identifying the optimal way to measure psychiatric morbidity in patients with skin disease.

Sexual functioning measures

The sexual life of patients suffering from skin disease is an important consideration when assessing their overall psychological, emotional and physical well-being. Patients' sexual life may be affected due to localised genital involvement [406,407] or due to chronic generalised conditions including hidradenitis suppurativa, psoriasis, eczema, urticaria and blistering disorders [408]. Sexual impairment may manifest as decreased sexual functioning [409], decreased sexual desire [410], difficulties with achieving arousal or orgasm [411] or physical discomfort. Given the sensitive nature of these issues, they are usually ignored and not discussed or addressed in up to 96% of patients [412]. They may be associated with anxiety, depression or suicidal ideation [408]. Therefore, the use of specific self-assessment questionnaires as well as certain aspects of QoL measures may be valuable in allowing these concerns to be addressed.

There are numerous sexual functioning-specific questionnaires that cover a wide range of relevant domains including satisfaction, interest, frequency, importance, performance, desire, worry, arousal, current behaviour, orgasmic capacity, libido, urological problems and feelings of femininity and masculinity. At least 45 sexual-specific questionnaires have been described, though not all are validated for different sexual orientations [413]. Ermertcan [414] evaluated sexual dysfunction in dermatological diseases and identified several measures suitable for assessing sexual dysfunction according to gender, systemic disease or dermatological condition. The *Female Sexual Function Index* (FSFI) for females and *International Index of Erectile Dysfunction* (IIEF) for males were recommended for use in skin disease.

The FSFI is a 19-item questionnaire assessing six domains of female sexuality: sexual desire, arousal, lubrication, orgasm, satisfaction and pain. The score range is 2–36, with scores less than or equal to 26.6 indicating sexual dysfunction [415].

The IIEF is a 15-item measure that incorporates five domains of male sexuality: erectile function, orgasmic function, sexual desire, intercourse and overall satisfaction. The score range is 5–75 with higher scores indicative of better sexual function [416]. Sexual dysfunction is indicated with erectile function domain scores less than, or equal to, 25 [417].

Cuenca-Barrales *et al.* [418] have identified several sexual-function measures utilised in hidradenitis suppurativa studies including the *Arizona Sexual Experience Scale* (ASEX) [419], *Sexual Quality of Life Questionnaire for Use in Men* (SQoLM) [420], *Frankfurt Self-Concept Scale for Sexuality* (FKKS SEX) [421] and the original and revised version of the *Female Sexual Distress Scale* (FSDS and FSDS-R, respectively) [422,423].

Generic, dermatology and disease-specific outcome measures may also capture elements of sexual impairment. For example, item 9 of the DLQI asks about 'sexual difficulties'. The Skindex-29, PDI and Impact of Psoriasis on Quality of Life Questionnaire measures have also been utilised to assess impact on sexual life in psoriasis sufferers [424].

Work impact measures

Occupational skin disease

Within Europe, work-related skin problems may represent up to 40% of recognised occupational health diseases [425]. Allergic contact dermatitis (ACD) accounts for a majority of occupational skin diseases, with a prevalence range of 70–90% [426], followed by irritant contact dermatitis (ICD). Both ACD and ICD may impact a wide range of professions from health care workers, aestheticians and hairdressers to construction workers. Increasingly, skin cancer is also being recognised as an occupational hazard leading to compensation claims and an increased drive for secondary targeted insurance schemes [427,428]. Preventative measures at an early stage are crucial to avoid occupational skin diseases from becoming chronic, which may consequently have significant implications for future employment and disability [429,430]. The consequences of occupational skin disease may not be limited to the workplace, but potentially have a wider effect on patient QoL. Although clinical outcome measures are useful tools, it is equally important to consider work-specific outcome measures to fully assess the impact of changes in occupation on patient well-being.

A European review of QoL measurement of occupational skin disease highlights the DLQI as the most commonly used measure, followed by the generic SF-36 and *The Life Quality Index Occupational Dermatoses* (LIOD) [431]. Skindex-16, Skindex-29 and PDI have also been utilised, though less frequently and in some cases as modified versions [427].

The LIOD has been designed specifically for occupational skin diseases, but due to a 3-month recall period, there are concerns around recall bias, routine use and applicability in clinical trials [427].

The DLQI has one item regarding the impact of skin disease on work and, along with the SF-36 and Skindex measures, is a well-validated tool. However, it is recommended that non-validated modified versions of QoL instruments should be avoided [432–434].

Work productivity

Chronic skin disease may have a considerable impact on work productivity but is often overlooked by policy makers and the general public due to the perception that skin disease is usually non-life-threatening. However, skin disease burden may be comparable to other chronic medical conditions [435]. Psoriasis and eczema are examples of chronic skin conditions whereby the psychological, physical and social burden of disease may contribute to decreased work productivity. This may manifest as absenteeism (physically too disabled to work) or presenteeism (compromised work productivity). For example, 30% of patients not in work attribute their employment status to their psoriasis [240], whereas patients suffering with atopic dermatitis experience an increased number of sick days [436]. Furthermore, parents may need to take time off work to care for children with atopic dermatitis [437].

Measures already listed in this chapter, such as the DLQI, capture elements of work impairment. Clinical outcome measures such as the PASI correlate moderately at best with DLQI scores, suggesting the influence of other factors impacting patient well-being [438,439]. It is therefore important to consider work-productivity measurement as part of routine patient assessment.

The *Work Productivity and Activity Impairment: General Health* (WPAI:GH), developed in 1993, is a six-item instrument to evaluate the impact of health problems on the subject's productivity, and *'Specific Health Problem'* (SHP) versions also exist for use in particular conditions [440]. It has a 7-day recall period. The instrument screens for impairment in both unpaid and paid work by yielding four scores: (i) absenteeism, (ii) presenteeism, (iii) total work productivity impairment (TWPI) (% overall work impairment, including absenteeism/presenteeism) and (iv) total activity impairment (TAI) (% total impairment in non-work daily activities, e.g. housework).

The *WPAI:SHP* version has been used to assess work impairment in hidradenitis suppurativa [441]. The *WPAI–Psoriasis* version is sensitive to change and has been utilised in comparing intervention efficacy on work impairment in psoriatic patients [442,443]. The *WPAI* has also been used in the relevant specific form for studies in atopic dermatitis [444], chronic hand dermatitis [445] and urticaria [446].

The combination of clinical outcome, HRQoL and work impairment measures can help provide physicians and health authorities with important information about the clinical course of disease and overall disease burden as well as financial and real-life impact of a chronic skin condition.

Conclusion

Although dermatology has taken longer than some other specialties to focus on the importance of measurement of disease, there is now a major interest in the creation of new measurement methods for use across all of the common skin diseases. However, the recent profusion of new techniques leaves unanswered the question as to how many of these newly proposed methods will improve the standard of care of patients, in contrast to their more immediately obvious use in clinical research. The challenge for researchers is to demonstrate the specific scenarios where measurement can be of value, and to develop validated methods that can be translated for clinical use, to enhance the quality of dermatology care. In the meantime, dermatologists can take advantage of those few methods where such validation has been established.

Declaration of interest

AYF is joint copyright holder of the following questionnaires described here: ADI, CADI, CDLQI, DFI, DLQI, FDLQI, FROM-16, IDQoL, MLCDP, PDI, PFI and T-QoL. FMA is employed by Cardiff University, who own several of the quality of life measures described in this chapter.

Key references

The full list of references can be found in the online version at https://www.wiley.com/rooksdermatology10e

28 Fredriksson T, Pettersson U. Severe psoriasis – oral therapy with a new retinoid. *Dermatologica* 1978;157:238–44.
38 Chularojanamontri L, Griffiths CEM, Chalmers RJG. The Simplified Psoriasis Index (SPI): a practical tool for assessing psoriasis. *J Invest Dermatol* 2013;133:1956–62.
48 European Task Force. Severity scoring of atopic dermatitis: the SCORAD index. Consensus report of the European Task force on atopic dermatitis. *Dermatology* 1993;186:23–31.
138 Finlay AY, Salek MS, Abeni D *et al*. Why quality of life measurement is important in dermatology clinical practice. An expert-based Opinion Statement by the EADV Task Force on Quality of Life. *J Eur Acad Dermatol Venereol* 2017;31:424–31.
193 Finlay AY, Khan GK. Dermatology Life Quality Index (DLQI): a simple practical measure for routine clinical use. *Clin Exp Dermatol* 1994;19:210–16.
204 Basra MK, Fenech R, Gatt RM *et al*. The Dermatology Life Quality Index 1994–2007: a comprehensive review of validation data and clinical results. *Br J Dermatol* 2008;159:997–1035.
205 Quality of Life Questionnaires: School of Medicine, Cardiff University. https://www.cardiff.ac.uk/medicine/resources/quality-of-life-questionnaires (last accessed January 2022).
226 Nijsten TEC, Sampogna F, Chren M-M, Abeni DD. Testing and reducing Skindex-29 using Rasch analysis: Skindex-17. *J Invest Dermatol* 2006;126:1244–50.
332 Salek MS, Jung S, Brincat-Ruffini LA *et al*. Clinical experience and psychometric properties of the Children's Dermatology Life Quality Index (CDLQI), 1995–2012. *Br J Dermatol* 2013;169:734–59.
343 Sampogna F, Finlay AY, Salek SS *et al*. Measuring the impact of dermatological conditions on family and caregivers: a review of dermatology-specific instruments. *J Eur Acad Dermatol Venereol* 2017;31:1429–39.
358 Golics CJ, Basra MK, Finlay AY, Salek S. The development and validation of the Family Reported Outcome Measure (FROM-16)© to assess the impact of disease on the partner or family member. *Qual Life Res* 2014;23:317–26.

CHAPTER 17

Principles of Evidence-based Dermatology

Michael Bigby[1] *and Hywel C. Williams*[2]

[1] Harvard Medical School and Beth Israel Deaconess Medical Center, Boston, MA, USA
[2] Centre of Evidence-Based Dermatology, Nottingham University Hospitals NHS Trust, Nottingham, UK

Evidence-based medicine, 17.1	**Critically appraising evidence and applying it to individual patients, 17.8**	Conclusions, 17.18
What is evidence-based medicine?, 17.1		**Evaluating the data in clinical research papers and a shortcut method for reading clinical research papers, 17.18**
The need for evidence-based medicine, 17.1	Critically appraising the evidence, 17.8	
Practising evidence-based medicine, 17.2	Critically appraising systematic reviews, 17.8	
Limitations of evidence-based medicine, 17.2	Critically appraising individual clinical trials, 17.12	Evaluating the data in clinical research papers, 17.18
Threats to evidence-based medicine, 17.3	Critically appraising a study about a diagnostic test, 17.15	Statistical methods, 17.20
Formulating questions and finding evidence, 17.3		Shortcut method for appraising clinical research papers, 17.24
Formulating well-built clinical questions, 17.3	Critically appraising a study about adverse events (case–control and cohort studies), 17.17	
What is the 'best evidence'?, 17.4		**Key references, 17.25**
Finding the best evidence, 17.6	Applying the evidence to individual patients, 17.18	

Evidence-based medicine

What is evidence-based medicine?

Evidence-based medicine (EBM) is the integration of best research evidence *with* clinical expertise *and* patient values. [1]

The need for evidence-based medicine
Distinguishing effective treatments from those that are ineffective or harmful

Distinguishing effective treatments from those that are ineffective or harmful has been a problem facing medical practitioners since medicine has been practised [2]. Prior to the 1940s, determination of treatment efficacy was based on expert opinion, trial and error, uncontrolled observation and small case series. The only treatments that could be distinguished as effective were those that produced dramatic increases in survival such as streptomycin for tuberculous meningitis [2]. The publication of the randomised controlled clinical trial (RCT) that demonstrated that streptomycin was effective in the treatment of pulmonary tuberculosis was a landmark event in determining treatment efficacy [3]. Since then, the RCT has become the gold standard for determining the efficacy of therapeutic interventions. Hundreds of RCTs were conducted between 1950 and 1980. However, their results were not catalogued or used systematically to inform medical decision making.

Evidence-based medicine is a framework designed to help practitioners distinguish interventions that are effective from those that are ineffective or harmful. The origin of evidence-based medicine is most often traced to Pierre Charles Alexander Louis who introduced the teaching of statistical methods into the study of medicine in post-revolutionary France. However, a strong case can be made that its modern originator was Archie Cochrane, a British epidemiologist and physician, who in 1971 published his response to being asked to evaluate the effectiveness of the British National Health Service in delivering health care to the population of the UK. In his analysis he concluded that medical science was poor at distinguishing interventions that were effective from those that were not and that physicians were not using available evidence from clinical research to inform their decision making [2,4].

Like-minded epidemiologists and physicians responded to Archie Cochrane's challenge by examining the methods by which medical decisions and conclusions were reached and proposed an alternative method of summarising evidence based on finding, appraising and utilising available data from clinical research performed on patients. In 1985 Sackett, Haynes, Guyatt and Tugwell published a landmark book entitled *Clinical Epidemiology: A Basic Science for Clinical Medicine* that detailed the rationale and techniques of this evidence-based approach [5]. These authors and others reduced the rules of evidence to a small subset of principles that were easier to teach and to understand and reintroduced the concept in 1992. They named this technique 'evidence-based medicine'. It was defined as 'the conscientious, explicit and judicious use of the best current evidence in making decisions about the care of individual patients' [6]. The definition was expanded to include the integration of independent clinical expertise, best available external clinical evidence from systematic research, and patients' values and expectations [7]. Others like Iain Chalmers were instrumental in setting

Rook's Textbook of Dermatology, Tenth Edition. Edited by Christopher Griffiths, Jonathan Barker, Tanya Bleiker, Walayat Hussain and Rosalind Simpson.
© 2024 John Wiley & Sons Ltd. Published 2024 by John Wiley & Sons Ltd.

up the Cochrane Collaboration, a global network of mainly volunteers tasked with preparing and maintaining unbiased systematic reviews of all RCTs, organised according to specialty [8]. Whereas making a decision about therapy has been the primary focus of EBM, its principles have been extended to diagnosis, prognosis, harmful effects of interventions and economic analyses [2].

It has been estimated that physicians need evidence (e.g. about the accuracy of diagnostic tests, the power of prognostic markers, the comparative efficacy and safety of interventions) about twice for every three out-patients seen (and five times for every in-patient). They get less than a third of this evidence because they do not look for it, cannot find it or it does not exist [2,9,10].

Keeping up with the literature

The best external evidence that informs patient care comes from clinical research involving patients. It has a short doubling-time (10 years) and replaces currently accepted diagnostic tests and treatments with new ones that are more powerful, more accurate, more efficacious and safer [2].

In the field of medicine the amount of data published far exceeds our ability to read it. Keeping up by reading the literature is an impossible task for most practising physicians. It would require reading around 19 articles a day, 365 days a year. The average practising physician spends 30 min per week reading the medical literature related to the patients he or she sees (Figure 17.1) [2,7,9]. The burden of literature for dermatologists is no less daunting since there are now more than 300 journals devoted to dermatology worldwide [2,11,12]. Such expansion in the biomedical literature has been one of the main reasons for developing secondary research synthesis summaries (systematic reviews) of all available evidence, so that the busy physician can go to just one place for an up-to-date summary.

The expansion of the biomedical literature and the increases in demand on physicians' time (e.g. for seeing more patients and interacting with electronic health records) fuelled the development, proliferation and use of point-of-service products. These products provide frequently updated reviews and recommendations for most diseases written by chosen authors many of whom may be recognised as experts in their respective fields. The products vary in cost, features, editorial quality, evidence-based methodology and breadth of coverage [13].

Even if he or she had the time, the best clinical evidence published in journals is often inaccessible to the average practising physician. Most are not adequately trained in clinical decision making, clinical research, epidemiology or statistics to read many articles published in the primary medical literature. Commonly used techniques and concepts such as odds ratio, confidence interval, Bayesian credibility intervals, utility, Yates correction or fixed effects model, as examples, are inadequately understood. EBM provides a systematic method to evaluate the medical literature that allows the average practising physician to understand the medical literature and to apply it to the care of individual patients.

Practising evidence-based medicine

Practising EBM consists of five steps (Box 17.1) that are explained in detail in the following sections of this chapter. Once learned, the techniques of EBM can be performed rapidly and efficiently to use available external evidence from the medical literature with clinical experience and patient preferences to make clinical decisions.

Box 17.1 The five steps of practising evidence-based medicine

1 Formulating a well-built clinical question generated from a patient encounter
2 Searching for valid external evidence
3 Critically appraising that evidence for relevance and validity
4 Applying the results of that appraisal of evidence back to the patient
5 Recording the information for future use

Limitations of evidence-based medicine

Practising EBM is limited by several inherent weaknesses predominately resulting from having to rely on evidence published in the medical literature (Box 17.2). Publication bias results from allowing factors other than quality of the research to influence its acceptability for publication (e.g. sample size, statistical significance or investigators' or editors' perception of whether the results are 'interesting') [2,14]. There is a strong bias favouring studies with positive results even if they have methodological weaknesses and small sample size. Negative studies with small sample size are much less likely to be published. Even studies with large sample sizes and negative results may go unpublished: for example two RCTs that demonstrated that topical imiquimod was ineffective in the treatment of molluscum contagiosum have not yet been published [15].

Box 17.2 Limitations of evidence-based medicine

- Publication bias
- Poor quality of many trials
- Lack of evidence in some areas
- Use of summary statistics in reporting results

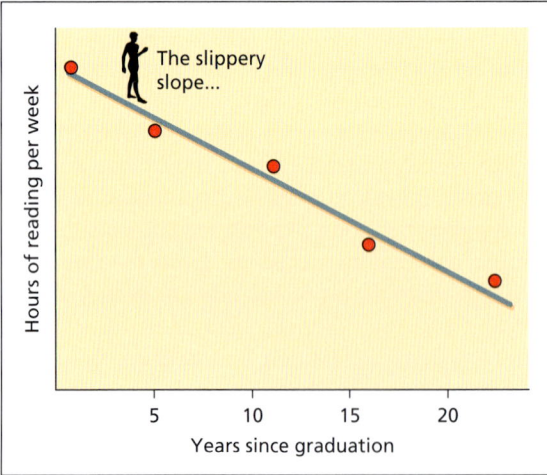

Figure 17.1 Relationship between reading and years from graduation from medical school. Adapted from Sackett 1997 [26]. Reproduced with permission of Elsevier.

As a result of publication bias, easy to locate studies are more likely to show 'positive' effects [2,14]. In many areas, the primary studies published are dominated by company-sponsored trials of new, expensive treatments. Treatment is often only compared with placebo in these studies, making it difficult for practising clinicians to decide how the new treatment compares with existing therapies.

Many trials published in the dermatological literature (and in the medical literature generally) are of poor methodological quality. Surveys of clinical trials published in the dermatological literature list the features of trials most important in limiting the risk of bias (e.g. adequate randomisation, concealed allocation, intention-to-treat analysis and masking). These features were reported less than 50% of the time [16,17]. Reporting has improved over time. In a study of quality of reporting of controlled trials in dermatology published in 2018, method of randomisation and concealed allocation were reported 70% and 58% respectively [18].

Sufficient evidence is lacking in many areas in dermatology (and in medicine in general). An analysis of systematic reviews of dermatological topics found insufficient evidence to inform practice in 60% (63/105) [19]. Many dermatological diseases are very uncommon and have not been studied in controlled clinical trials. Case series, case reports and expert opinion based on experience are still legitimate evidence for rare skin diseases where no clinical trials or systematic reviews are available.

'All or none' clinical observations such as the use of streptomycin for tuberculous meningitis and insulin for diabetes provide strong evidence of treatment efficacy and obviate the need for expensive and time-consuming clinical trials [20]. The use of dapsone for dermatitis herpetiformis and pulsed tunable dye laser for vascular malformations may serve as examples of 'all or none' clinical observations in dermatology.

Results in published clinical trials are almost always expressed in summary statistics that refer to the groups treated in the study. Summary statistics refer to groups not individuals (e.g. PASI-75 (psoriasis area and severity index) or proportions who cleared). Some participants may respond a lot and others very little, whereas only the average response is reported. Ideally, in addition to group data, the raw data of individual treatment responses should be presented or made available to determine whether it is possible to identify factors that make it more or less likely that a patient will respond to treatment. These data are rarely provided. Unfortunately in dermatology, most trials are relatively small and of short duration. As a result, they are underpowered to identify predictors of response that could help to identify those groups of people who might respond better or worse to a particular treatment. Small studies are also at risk of falsely concluding no treatment benefit when in fact the study was underpowered to detect even moderate benefits [21].

Threats to evidence-based medicine

The practice of EBM faces threats from several entities that seek to exploit it for gain (Box 17.3). Some authors approach systematic reviews and meta-analyses as a quick way to get published. A common practice is to look into the literature for areas in which many trials have been published and write a data-driven systematic review. These reviews tend to include many company-sponsored trials of new and expensive treatments compared with placebo that do not necessarily address important clinical questions raised in clinical practice.

> **Box 17.3 Threats to evidence-based medicine**
>
> - Data-driven systematic reviews
> - Sponsored systematic reviews
> - Selective outcome reporting bias
> - Failure to publish trials with negative results
> - Spinning of trial results
> - Ghost writing of research papers and reviews
> - Expansion of drug indications through selective reporting of trials with positive results

Many published therapeutic trials are company-sponsored trials of new treatments. These trials are more likely to have results favourable to the sponsor [22]. Compared with trials funded by other sources, company-sponsored trials that are pre-registered with government registration sites (e.g. https://clinicaltrials.gov/ and https://www.clinicaltrialsregister.eu/; both last accessed February 2022) are less likely to be published, perhaps indicating that trials with negative results are intentionally not finished or published [22].

Trials with negative results for the primary outcome are often 'spun' to give the appearance that the treatment is effective [23]. This objective is accomplished by de-emphasising the primary outcome and selectively reporting or emphasising results in secondary outcomes, subgroup analyses, within-group analyses or post hoc analyses. In a representative sample of RCTs published in 2006 with statistically non-significant primary outcomes, the reporting and interpretation of findings was frequently inconsistent with the results [24]. Selective outcome reporting bias can be partially overcome by systematic reviews stipulating the preferred clinically important outcomes and by those conducting clinical trials to register their protocol and to state their primary outcome measures of success in publicly accessible trial registers before recruitment starts [25].

Formulating questions and finding evidence

Formulating well-built clinical questions

Practising EBM centres on trying to find answers to clinically relevant questions that arise in caring for individual patients. Asking *well-built clinical questions* may be the most important step in practising EBM [1]. A well-built clinical question has four elements: a patient or problem, an intervention, a comparison intervention (if necessary) and an outcome. One easy way of remembering these key components is the acronym PICO (patient, intervention, comparator and outcome). A fifth element, time frame (i.e. the time it takes for the intervention to achieve the outcome or how long participants in a study are observed), has been suggested as an additional component for the well-built clinical question yielding the acronym PICOT (Figure 17.2) [2,3].

Well-built clinical questions about individual patients can be grouped into several categories: aetiology, diagnosis, therapy,

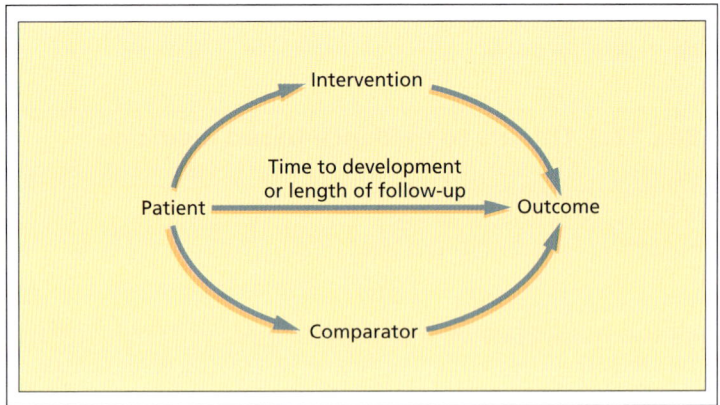

Figure 17.2 The PICOT format.

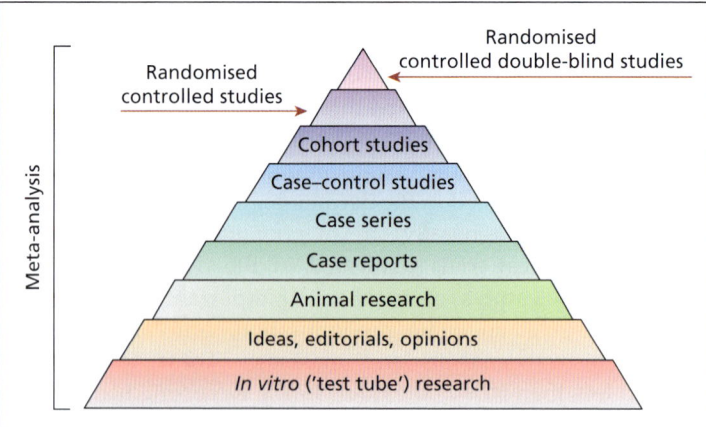

Figure 17.3 The hierarchy of evidence.

prevention, prognosis and harm. An example of a well-built question about diagnosis is 'In patients with dystrophic toenails due to onychomycosis [P], would a fungal culture [I] or a periodic acid–Schiff stain (PAS) of a nail clipping [C] be more likely to establish a diagnosis of onychomycosis [O]?' An example of a well-built question about therapy is 'In immunocompetent children with cutaneous warts [P], would treatment with imiquimod [I] or vehicle [C] result in clearance of all lesions [O] after 2 months of treatment [T]?' An example of a well-built question about harm is 'What is the likelihood that a patient with severe nodular acne [P] treated with isotretinoin [I] or not exposed to isotretinoin [C] will develop ulcerative colitis [O] within 12 months after completing a course of treatment [T]?'

A well-formed clinical question has two strong advantages. Firstly, a major benefit of careful and thoughtful question forming is that it makes the search for, and the critical appraisal of, the evidence easier. The well-formed question makes it relatively straightforward to elicit and combine the appropriate terms needed to tailor the search strategies for the database(s) you choose (e.g. MEDLINE, EMBASE, Cochrane Library). Secondly, having to formulate well-built clinical questions will also train you to define your patient clearly, be specific about the interventions used and choose carefully the outcomes that would make a difference to your patient and you.

What is the 'best evidence'?

Practising EBM is predicated on finding and utilising the best evidence [4]. Potential sources of evidence include empirical reasoning based on the aetiology and pathophysiology of disease, personal experience, colleagues or experts, textbooks, articles published in journals, and systematic reviews and guidelines. An important principle of EBM is that the quality (strength) of evidence is based on a *hierarchy of evidence* (Figure 17.3). The order of the hierarchy of evidence is dependent on the type of question being asked (Table 17.1). The hierarchy of evidence for evidence of treatment benefits typically starts with the combined results of well-designed experimental studies such as RCTs (especially if the studies have results of similar magnitude and direction, and if there is homogeneity among studies), results of observational studies such as case series, expert opinion and personal experience, in descending order. The hierarchy was created to encourage the use of the evidence that is most likely to be true and useful in clinical decision making. The ordering of this hierarchy has been widely discussed, actively debated and sometimes hotly contested [5]. It is important to consider study quality when referring to the evidence hierarchy. For example, a well-designed cohort study may provide more reliable evidence than a small, poorly conducted RCT (even though the RCT hypothetically offers a stronger design for minimising bias).

A systematic review is an overview of available evidence that answers a specific clinical question, contains a thorough, unbiased search of the relevant literature, explicit criteria for assessing studies and structured presentation of the results. When there are similar studies in a systematic review (i.e. RCTs using the same interventions and outcomes), the authors of a systematic review may use a statistical technique called meta-analysis to combine quantitative data from several studies in order to provide a more precise and informative overall estimate of treatment effects.

Meta-analysis is credited with allowing recognition of important treatment effects by combining the results of small trials that individually lacked the power to demonstrate differences among treatments. For example, the benefits of intravenous streptokinase in acute myocardial infarction were recognised by the results of a cumulative meta-analysis of smaller trials at least a decade before it was recommended by experts and before it was demonstrated to be efficacious in large clinical trials [6]. Meta-analysis has been criticised for the discrepancies between the results of meta-analysis and the results of large clinical trials [7]. For example, results of a meta-analysis of 14 small studies of calcium to treat pre-eclampsia showed benefit of treatment but a large trial failed to show a treatment effect [8]. The frequency of discrepancies ranges from 10% to 23% [8]. Discrepancies can often be explained by differences in treatment protocols, heterogeneity of study populations or changes that occur over time [8]. Unfortunately, with the exception of Cochrane systematic reviews and a few notable others, the quality of dermatology systematic reviews is generally poor, with around 90% assessed as being low quality in a recent study [9]. Systematic reviews have become a very popular publication type in the dermatological literature, yet they are subject to abuse such as addressing topics of limited interest, salami publication, selective reporting of 'interesting' outcomes, duplicate publication and errors such as including the same primary study more than once in a meta-analysis [10].

Table 17.1 Levels of evidence.

Level of evidence	Therapy/harm	Diagnosis
1a	Multiple randomised controlled trials (RCTs) with homogeneity[a]	Multiple level 1b (see 1b entry) diagnostic studies with homogeneity; or clinical decision rules[b] with 1b studies from different clinical centres
1b	Individual RCT (with narrow confidence intervals)	Independent blind comparison of an appropriate spectrum of consecutive patients, all of who have undergone both the diagnostic test and the reference standard
1c	All or none[c]	Very high sensitivity or specificity[d]
2a	Cohort studies with homogeneity	Multiple level ≥2 (see entries below) diagnostic studies with homogeneity
2b	Individual cohort study (including low-quality RCT; e.g. <80% follow-up)	Independent blind comparison but either in non-consecutive patients, or confined to a narrow spectrum of study individuals (or both), all of whom have undergone both the diagnostic test and the reference standard; or a diagnostic clinical decision rule (CDR) not validated in a test set
2c	'Outcomes' research[e]	
3a	Case–control studies with homogeneity	Multiple level 3b and better studies (see below) with homogeneity.
3b	Individual case–control study	Independent blind comparison of an appropriate spectrum, but the reference standard was not applied to all study patients
4	Case series (and poor quality cohort and case–control studies)	Reference standard was not applied independently or not applied blindly
5	Expert opinion without explicit critical appraisal, or based on physiology, bench research or logical deduction	

Adapted from NHS R&D Centre for Evidence-Based Medicine (https://www.cebm.ox.ac.uk/resources/levels-of-evidence/oxford-centre-for-evidence-based-medicine-levels-of-evidence-march-2009, last accessed February 2022).
[a] Homogeneity means lacking variation in the direction and magnitude of results of individual studies.
[b] Clinical decision rules are algorithms or scoring systems that lead to a prognostic estimation or a diagnostic category.
[c] All or none – these are interventions that produced dramatic increases in survival or outcome such as streptomycin for tuberculous meningitis.
[d] A diagnostic finding whose specificity is so high that a positive result rules in the diagnosis or a diagnostic finding whose sensitivity is so high that a negative result rules out the diagnosis.
[e] Outcomes research includes cost–benefit, cost–effectiveness and cost–utility analysis.

Network meta-analyses are being increasing published and utilised to compare treatments in situations where direct head-to-head trials are few or lacking. Network meta-analysis (NMA) is a technique for comparing multiple treatments in a single analysis by combining direct evidence (from head-to-head trials) and indirect evidence (from trials of different treatments against placebo or a third treatment) in a network of RCTs. NMA allows for comparing treatment effects between any pair of interventions. It also allows for ranking of the effectiveness of the included interventions. To be valid, there should be no systematic differences between the comparisons included in a NMA other than the treatments being considered [11]. Despite their appeal, NMA are also prone to some of the same problems as those associated with conventional systematic review such as duplicate publications, e.g. there are over 21 NMAs of systemic treatments for psoriasis at the time of writing. Living systematic reviews denote that reviews that are updated frequently as new evidence become available in real time, and individual patient data (IPD) meta-analysis refers to the use of IPD from each contributing trial as opposed to aggregate summary data. An example of a living IPD review in the prevention of atopic dermatitis can be found here [12].

The type of question being asked determines the type of clinical study that constitutes the best evidence. Questions about therapy and interventions for disease prevention are best addressed by RCTs. Questions about diagnosis are best addressed by cohort studies. RCTs are usually a good source of evidence for the harmful effects of interventions for adverse events that occur frequently, but not for rare but potentially important adverse events. For adverse effects that occur infrequently, cohort studies, case–control studies, postmarketing surveillance, pharmacovigilance and large database studies are best. Case reports are often the first line of evidence for very rare adverse events and sometimes they are the only evidence.

Over 1.7 million RCTs have been conducted in medicine. Studies have demonstrated that failure to use randomisation or adequate concealment of allocation results in larger estimates of treatment effects, predominantly caused by a poorer prognosis in non-randomly selected control groups compared with randomly selected control groups [13]. However, studies comparing RCTs and non-RCTs of the same interventions have reached disparate and controversial results [14,15]. Some found that observational studies find stronger treatment effects than RCTs [13]. Others found that the results of well-designed observational studies (with either a cohort or case–control design) do not systematically overestimate the magnitude of the effects of treatment as compared with RCTs on the same topic [14,15]. Sifting through the controversy leads to the following limited conclusions: trials using historical controls result in larger estimates of treatment effects compared with RCTs. Large, inclusive, fully masked controlled trials that generate and conceal the randomisation sequence properly and include all those who are originally allocated to the treatment groups (intention-to-treat analysis) are likely to provide the best evidence about effectiveness [5]. RCTs and systematic reviews of well-designed clinical studies have informed the care of dermatological patients [16].

Whereas personal experience is an invaluable part of becoming a competent physician, the pitfalls of relying too heavily on personal experience have been widely documented. Nisbett and Ross extensively reviewed people's ability to draw inferences from personal experience and document several pitfalls [17]. They include:
- Overemphasis on vivid, anecdotal occurrences and underemphasis on significant statistically strong evidence.

- Bias in recognising, remembering and recalling evidence that supports pre-existing knowledge structures (e.g. ideas about disease aetiology and pathogenesis) and parallel failure to recognise, remember and recall evidence that is more valid.
- Failure to characterise population data accurately because of ignorance of statistical principles including sample size, sample selection bias and regression to the mean.
- Inability to detect and distinguish statistical association and causality.
- Persistence of beliefs in spite of overwhelming contrary evidence.

Nisbett and Ross provide numerous examples of problems associated with recall from controlled clinical research. Physicians may remember patients who improved, often assume that patients who did not return for follow-up improved and conveniently forget the patients who did not improve. A patient treated with a given medication may develop a severe life-threatening reaction. On the basis of this single undesirable experience, the physician may avoid using that medication for many future patients, even though, *on average*, it may be more efficacious and less toxic than the alternative treatments that the physician chooses.

Few physicians keep adequate, easily retrievable records to codify results of treatments with a particular agent or of a particular disease; and even fewer actually carry out analyses. Similarly, few physicians make provisions for tracking those patients who are lost to follow-up. Therefore, statements made about a physician's 'clinical experience' may be biased. Finally, for many conditions, a single physician sees far too few patients to enable reasonably firm conclusions to be drawn about the response to treatments. For example, suppose a physician treated 20 patients with lichen planus with tretinoin and found that 12 (60%) had an excellent response. The confidence interval for this response rate (i.e. the true response rate for this treatment in the larger population from which this physician's sample was obtained) ranges from 36% to 81% (http://statpages.org/confint.html; last accessed February 2022). Thus the true overall response rate might well be substantially less (or more) than the physician concludes from personal experience.

Expert opinion can be valuable, particularly for rare conditions in which the expert has the most experience, or when other forms of evidence are not available. However, several studies have demonstrated that expert opinion often lags significantly behind conclusive evidence. Experts may rely too heavily on bench research, pathophysiology and treatments based on logical deduction from pathophysiology, and from the same pitfalls noted for relying on personal experience.

It is widely believed that clinical decisions can be made on the basis of understanding the aetiology and pathophysiology of disease and logic [18]. This paradigm is problematic since the accepted hypothesis for the aetiology and pathogenesis of disease changes over time. For example, in the last 20 years, hypotheses about the aetiology of psoriasis have shifted from a disorder of keratinocyte proliferation and homeostasis, to abnormal signalling of cyclic adenosine monophosphate, to aberrant arachidonic acid metabolism, to aberrant vitamin D metabolism, to the current favourite, a T-cell-mediated autoimmune disease. Each of these hypotheses spawned logically deduced treatments. The efficacy of many of these treatments has been substantiated by rigorous controlled clinical trials, whereas others are used even in the absence of systematically collected observations. Therefore, many options are available for treating patients with severe psoriasis (e.g. UVB, narrow-band UVB, the Goeckerman regimen, psoralen–UVA (PUVA), methotrexate, ciclosporin, tumour necrosis factor (TNF) inhibitors, IL-12/23 or IL-17 inhibitors) and mild to moderate psoriasis (e.g. anthralin, topical corticosteroids, calcipotriol and tazarotene). However, a clear sense of what is best, in what order they should be used, or in what combinations, is still lacking.

Treatments based on logical deduction from pathophysiology may have unexpected consequences. For example, it was postulated that thalidomide might be a useful treatment for toxic epidermal necrolysis, based on the observation that thalidomide showed anti-TNF-α properties. However, an RCT of thalidomide was stopped early because it was found that mortality was significantly higher in the thalidomide group than in the placebo group [19].

Textbooks can be valuable, particularly for rare conditions and for conditions for which the evidence does not change rapidly over time. However, textbooks have several well-documented shortcomings. They tend to reflect the biases and shortcomings of the authors who write them. By virtue of how they are written, produced and distributed, most are at least 2 years out of date *at* the time of publication. Most textbook chapters are narrative reviews that do not systematically search for all available evidence and appraise the quality of the evidence reported.

Finding the best evidence

The ability to find the best evidence to answer clinical questions is crucial for practising EBM [2]. Finding evidence requires access to electronic searching, searching skills and available resources. Evidence about therapy is the easiest to find. The best sources for finding the best evidence about treatment include:
- The Cochrane Library.
- Searching the Medline and EMBASE databases.
- Point-of-service products.
- Primary journals.
- Secondary sources that summarise important new research.
- Evidence-based dermatology and EBM books.
- The National Guideline Clearinghouse (https://www.ahrq.gov/gam/index.html; last accessed February 2022).
- The National Institute for Health and Care Excellence (NICE) (www.nice.org.uk; last accessed February 2022).

The Cochrane Collaboration formed in response to Archie Cochrane's challenge to organise a critical summary, by specialty or subspecialty, adapted periodically, of all relevant RCTs. The Cochrane Library contains the Cochrane Database of Systematic Reviews, the Cochrane Central Register of Controlled Trials (Central) and the Health Systems Evidence (HSE) database. The Cochrane Library is the most complete and well-indexed database of systematic reviews of therapy, RCTs and controlled clinical trials and is the best and most efficient place to find evidence about therapy.

The Cochrane Database of Systematic Reviews is the most comprehensive collection of high-quality systematic reviews available. Volunteers, according to strict guidelines developed by the Cochrane Collaboration, write the systematic reviews in the Cochrane Library. Systematic reviews conducted within the Cochrane Collaboration are rated among the best [20]. The last issue of the Cochrane Library (2021, Issue 3, accessed March 2021) contained 8546 completed systematic reviews. The number of reviews identified as skin disorders is 255.

CENTRAL is a database of over 1.76 million controlled clinical trials (https://www.cochranelibrary.com/central/about-central; last accessed February 2022). It is compiled by searching several databases including Medline, EMBASE and Literatura Latino Americana em Ciências da Saúde (LILACS), and hand-searching many journals. Hand-searching journals to identify controlled clinical trials and RCTs was undertaken because members of the Cochrane Collaboration noticed that many published trials were incorrectly classified in the Medline database. As an example, Adetugbo et al. hand-searched the Archives of Dermatology from 1990 through 1998 and identified 99 controlled clinical trials. Nineteen of the trials were not classified as controlled clinical trials in Medline and 11 trials that were not controlled clinical trials were misclassified as controlled clinical trials in Medline [21].

HSE consists of completed and ongoing health systems assessments (studies of the medical, social, ethical and economic implications of health care interventions) from around the world. The aim of the database is to improve the quality and cost-effectiveness of health care. The latest issue of the Cochrane Library contained 14 354 HSE reviews (2021, Issue 3, last accessed March 2021).

The Cochrane Library is the best source for evidence about treatment. It can be easily searched using simple Boolean combinations of search terms and by more sophisticated search strategies. The Cochrane Database of Systematic Reviews, CENTRAL and HSE can be searched simultaneously. The Cochrane Library is available on a personal or institutional subscription basis on the World Wide Web from the Cochrane Collaboration (https://www.cochranelibrary.com/help/how-to-order; last accessed February 2022). The Cochrane Library is offered free of charge in many countries such as the UK by national provision, and to faculty and students by many medical schools in the USA. It is also available free to those in developing countries through a programme called Health InterNetwork Access to Research Initiative (HINARI). Daily pay-per-view access is also available.

Epistemonikos has emerged as a useful source to identify systematic reviews that are relevant to health care decision making, with 10 databases (including the Cochrane Library) searched and updated regularly (https://www.epistemonikos.org/en/; last accessed February 2022). Epistemonikos is free and has retrieved 1 613 996 references from different databases and other sources, which in turn have been sorted by human screeners and a machine learning algorithm, leading to a total of 371 499 systematic reviews at the time of writing.

DARE is a database of abstracts of systematic reviews published in the medical literature (https://www.crd.york.ac.uk/CRDWeb/HomePage.asp; last accessed February 2022). It contains abstracts and bibliographic details on over 35 000 published systematic reviews. DARE is the only database to contain abstracts of systematic reviews that have been quality assessed.

The second best method for finding evidence about treatment and the best source for finding most other types of best evidence in dermatology is by searching the Medline or EMBASE databases by computer. MEDLINE is the National Library of Medicine's bibliographic database covering the fields of medicine, nursing, dentistry, veterinary medicine, the health care system and the preclinical sciences. The MEDLINE file contains bibliographic citations and author abstracts from approximately 5200 current biomedical journals published in the USA and 80 other countries. The file contains approximately 32 million records dating back to 1948. The new PubMed interface was introduced in September 2019. It has enhancements for searches. Users would benefit from examining the Users Guide and FAQs (https://pubmed.ncbi.nlm.nih.gov/help/; last accessed February 2022).

Medline searches have inherent limitations that make their reliability less than ideal [4]. For example, Spuls et al. conducted a systematic review of systemic treatments of psoriasis [22]. Treatments analysed included UVB, PUVA, methotrexate, ciclosporin and retinoids. The authors used an exhaustive strategy to find relevant references including Medline searches, contacting pharmaceutical companies, polling leading authorities, reviewing abstract books of symposia and congresses, and reviewing textbooks, reviews, editorials, guideline articles and the reference lists of all papers identified. Of 665 studies found, 356 (54%) were identified by Medline search (range 30–70% for different treatment modalities). The 17 of 23 authorities who responded provided no references beyond those identified by Medline searching.

Specific search strategies, 'filters', have been developed to help find relevant references and exclude irrelevant references for systematic reviews, and for the best evidence about aetiology, diagnosis, therapy and prevention, prognosis and clinical prediction guides (https://pubmed.ncbi.nlm.nih.gov/clinical/, last accessed February 2022). PubMed Clinical Queries is the preferred method for searching the Medline database for the best, clinically relevant evidence. It can be freely used by anyone with Internet access.

EMBASE is Elsevier's database covering drugs, pharmacology and biomedical specialties. EMBASE contains bibliographic citations and author abstracts from approximately 8500 current biomedical journals published in 95 countries, with a focus on drugs and pharmacology, medical devices, clinical medicine and basic science relevant to clinical medicine. The file contains over 32 million records dating back to 1947. EMBASE has a better coverage of European and non-English language sources and may be more up to date than Medline [23]. EMBASE includes all records indexed by Medline. EMBASE is available online (https://www.embase.com; last accessed February 2022). Personal and institutional subscriptions are available. EMBASE performs simultaneous searches of EMBASE and Medline databases and eliminates duplicate records. EMBASE has special search features such as PICO searches for systematic reviews and searches for adverse drug reactions, medical devices, drugs and diseases.

Clinicians are increasingly using general Internet search engines such as Google and Google Scholar to search for medical evidence. In a comparison of searches in three areas in respiratory medicine, PubMed Clinical Queries had better precision (positive predictive value) than Google Scholar for both overall search results (13% versus 0.07%, $P < 0.001$) and full-text results (8% versus 0.05%, $P < 0.001$). PubMed Clinical Queries and Google Scholar had similar recall (sensitivity) for both overall search results (71% versus 69%) and full-text results (43% versus 51%) [24]. In contrast to Clinical Queries searches, general searches of Medline are not consistently better than Google Scholar searches and are considerably worse in some studies [25,26]. SumSearch (http://sumsearch.org; last accessed February 2022) is a free search tool for searching the medical literature for clinically relevant evidence. It was the strategy that had the highest precision defined as the proportion of relevant, high quality citations among the first 50 citations retrieved when compared with PubMed Clinical Queries narrow and Google Scholar. It was also the most likely to find at least one high quality citation (73% of searches; 95% CI 68%–78%) [27].

The UK NICE produces guidance on public health, health technologies and clinical practice based on the best available evidence. It is accessible online at https://www.nice.org.uk (last accessed February 2022) and, for example, includes guidance for treating atopic eczema in children, the use of calcineurin inhibitors for atopic eczema, the use of biologicals for psoriasis and alitretinoin for hand eczema, and a full set of guidelines for skin cancers including melanoma.

The Centre of Evidence Based Dermatology (http://www.nottingham.ac.uk/research/groups/cebd/resources/index.aspx; last accessed February 2022), includes clinical tools, outcome measure and collections of evidence specifically relevant to skin diseases.

Critically appraising evidence and applying it to individual patients

Critically appraising the evidence

After finding evidence, the next step in practising EBM involves *critically appraising the evidence* [1,2]. Key questions that can be used to critically appraise systematic reviews and papers about treatment, diagnostic tests and harmful effects of exposures are described in Boxes 17.4, 17.5, 17.6 and 17.7. Papers that meet these criteria are more likely to provide information that is true and useful in the care of patients. Detailed explanation of each criterion and examples using a patient with a dermatological complaint are available [1].

Critically appraising evidence consists of three steps to determine whether the results are:
1 *Valid* (i.e. as unbiased as possible).
2 *Clinically important.*
3 *Applicable to the specific patient being seen.*

Determining the validity of evidence centres on ascertaining whether the evidence was produced in a manner most likely to eliminate and avoid bias. Clinical importance is determined by looking at the magnitude of the effect of the intervention (e.g. response difference and number needed to treat for therapy, likelihood ratio for diagnostic studies and relative risk, odds ratios or number needed to harm for studies of harm) and its corresponding precision (usually expressed as the 95% confidence interval). To determine whether the evidence is applicable to a specific patient requires physician expertise, knowledge of the patient's preferences and an evaluation of the availability, risks and benefits of the intervention.

Critically appraising systematic reviews

Not all systematic reviews and meta-analyses are equal. A systematic review should be conducted in a manner that will include all of the relevant trials, minimise the introduction of bias, and synthesise the results to be as truthful and useful to clinicians as possible [1,2]. Criteria for reporting systematic reviews were developed by a consensus panel first published as Quality of Reporting of Meta-analyses (QUOROM) and later refined as Preferred Reporting Items for Systematic Reviews and Meta-analyses (PRISMA) (http://www.prisma-statement.org/; last accessed February 2022). This detailed, 27-item checklist contains the items that should be included and reported in high-quality systematic reviews and meta-analyses [3]. Several PRISMA extensions for special types of systematic reviews such as network meta-analyses and IPD meta-analyses are also available and should be used when reporting such studies.

All systematic reviews should follow a planned protocol that should be published in the public domain before the review is carried out in order to avoid duplication of effort and in order to minimise selective outcome reporting bias (i.e. emphasising the outcomes that turn out to be statistically significant). The international Prospective Register of Systematic Reviews (PROSPERO) now exists for this purpose (http://www.crd.york.ac.uk/PROSPERO/; last accessed February 2022).

Are the results of the systematic review valid?

The items that strengthen the validity of a systematic review include having clear objectives, explicit criteria for study selection, an explicit and thorough search of the literature, an assessment of the quality of included studies, criteria for which studies can be combined, and appropriate analysis and presentation of results (Box 17.4). Meta-analysis is only appropriate if the included studies are conceptually similar. Meta-analyses should be conducted only within the context of a systematic review [1,4].

Box 17.4 Critical appraisal of a systematic review

Are the results of this systematic review valid?
- Did the review address a focused clinical question?[a]
- Were the criteria used to select articles for inclusion appropriate?[a]
- Is it unlikely that important, relevant studies were missed?[b]
- Was the validity of the included studies appraised?[b]
- Were assessments of studies reproducible?[b]
- Were the results similar from study to study?[b]

Are the valid results of this systematic review important?
- What are the overall results of the review?
- How precise were the results?

Can you apply this valid, important evidence in caring for your patient?
- Can the results be applied to your patient's care?
- Were all clinically important outcomes considered?
- Are the benefits worth the harms and costs?

Adapted from
https://www.cebm.ox.ac.uk/resources/ebm-tools/critical-appraisal-tools?o=1157 (last accessed February 2022).
[a] Primary guides.
[b] Secondary guides.

Table 17.2 Other sources for data on adverse reactions to drugs.

Resource	Source	Comments
Side Effects of Drugs Annuals	https://www.elsevier.com/search-results?labels=books&book-series=Side%20Effects%20of%20Drugs%20Annual	Data 1–2 years old
Reactions Weekly	https://www.springer.com/journal/40278	Requires registration and fee
Drug Safety Update	https://www.gov.uk/drug-safety-update	Drug safety bulletin of the Medicines and Healthcare Products Regulatory Agency (MHRA); issues freely searchable
Medicines Safety Update	https://www.tga.gov.au/publication/medicines-safety-update#.Ur3Yx2RDt0o	Back issues and free email subscription available
MedWatch	http://www.fdable.com/	Searchable database of spontaneous reports of adverse reactions to drugs maintained by the US Food and Drug Administration

All websites last accessed February 2022.

A systematic review should have clear, focused clinical objectives. Like the well-built clinical question for individual studies, a focused clinical question for a systematic review should contain four elements: (i) a patient, group of patients or problem; (ii) an intervention; (iii) comparison intervention(s); and (iv) specific outcomes. The patient populations should be similar to patients seen in the population to which one wishes to apply the results of the systematic review. The interventions studied should be those commonly available in practice. Outcomes reported should be those that are most relevant to physicians and patients.

A sound systematic review can be performed only if most or all of the available data are examined. An explicit and thorough search of the literature should be performed. It should include searching several electronic bibliographic databases including the Cochrane Controlled Trials Registry (CCTR), Medline, EMBASE and LILACS. Bibliographies of retrieved studies, review articles and textbooks should be examined further for studies fitting the inclusion criteria. There should be no language restrictions. Additional sources of data include scrutiny of citation lists in retrieved articles, hand-searching for conference reports, prospective trial registers (e.g. http://clinicaltrials.gov for the USA and www.clinicaltrialsregister.eu for the European Union; both last accessed February 2022) and contacting key researchers, authors and drug companies [1,5]. Regulatory agencies such as the EMA and FDA are also important sources for additional data that may not appear in trial reports [6].

The overwhelming majority of systematic reviews involve therapy. Because of their ability to minimise bias, RCTs should be used as the preferred study design for inclusion in systematic reviews of therapy if they are available. The criteria commonly used to assess the quality of included trials are described in the Cochrane Collaboration risk of bias tool and include: concealed, random allocation, groups similar in terms of known prognostic factors, equal treatment of groups, masked (also known as blinded) evaluation of treatment outcomes and accounting for all patients entered into the trial in analysing results (intention-to-treat design) [7,8].

Systematic reviews of treatment efficacy should always include a thorough assessment of common and serious adverse events as well as efficacy in order to come to an informed and balanced decision about the utility of a treatment. A thorough assessment of adverse events should include data from RCTs, case–control and postmarketing surveillance studies and some of the other sources shown in Table 17.2.

Publication bias (i.e. the tendency that studies that are easy to locate are more likely to show 'positive' effects) is an important concern for systematic reviews [9]. It results from allowing factors other than the quality of the study to influence its acceptability for publication. Several studies have shown that factors such as sample size, direction and statistical significance of findings, or investigators' perception of whether the findings are 'interesting', are related to the likelihood of publication [10].

Language bias may also be a problem, that is, the tendency for studies that are 'positive' to be published in an English language journal and also more quickly than inconclusive or 'negative' studies. A thorough systematic review should therefore include a search for high-quality, unpublished trials and not be restricted to journals written in English.

Studies are less likely to be published if they have negative results, especially if they have small sample size. By emphasising only those studies that are positive, this type of publication bias jeopardises one of the main goals of meta-analysis (i.e. an increase in power when pooling the results of small studies). The creation of study registers (e.g. http://clinicaltrials.gov/, https://www.clinicaltrialsregister.eu or http://www.anzctr.org.au; all last accessed February 2022) and advance publication of research designs have been proposed as ways to prevent publication bias.

For many diseases, published clinical trials are dominated by drug company-sponsored trials of new, expensive treatments, and in the absence of legislation that mandates publication of all clinical trials, many trials remain unpublished [11,12]. This bias in publication can result in data-driven systematic reviews that draw more attention to those medicines. This problem underlies the need to develop and publish a protocol for a systematic review before the data are explored, as is the current practice with Cochrane reviews and those systematic reviews that are registered with PROSPERO. Question-driven systematic reviews answer the clinical questions of most concern to practitioners. In many cases, studies that are of most relevance to doctors and patients have not been done in the field of dermatology due to inadequate sources of independent funding.

Systematic reviews that have been sponsored directly or indirectly by industry are prone to bias by the overinclusion of unpublished positive studies that are kept 'on file' by that company and the exclusion of negative trials that are not published [11,13]. Until it becomes mandatory to register all clinical trials conducted on human beings in a central register and to make all of the results available in the public domain, distortions may occur due to selective withholding or release of data.

Generally, reviews that have been conducted by volunteers in the Cochrane Collaboration are of better quality than non-Cochrane reviews [14]. However, potentially serious errors have even been noted in up to a third of Cochrane reviews [15].

In general, the studies included in systematic reviews are analysed by at least two individuals. Data, such as numbers of people entered into studies, numbers lost to follow-up, effect sizes and quality criteria, are recorded on pre-designed data abstraction forms. Any differences between reviewers are usually settled by consensus or by an arbitrator. A systematic review in which there are large areas of disagreement among reviewers should lead the reader to question the validity of the review.

Various frameworks for assessing the quality of systematic reviews are available, the most notable of which is the AMSTAR2 tool [16]. It contains 16 items, is easy to use and can be applied to systematic reviews that contain non-randomised studies as well as RCTs.

Are the results of the systematic review important?

Results in the individual clinical trials that make up a systematic review may be similar in magnitude and direction (e.g. they may all indicate that a treatment is superior to its comparator by a similar magnitude). Assuming that publication bias can be excluded, systematic reviews with studies that have results that are similar in magnitude and direction provide results that are most likely to be true and useful. It may be impossible to draw firm conclusions from systematic reviews in which studies have results of widely different magnitude and direction.

The key principle when considering combining results from several studies is that they should have conceptual homogeneity. Results of several different studies should not be combined if it does not make sense to combine them (e.g. if the patient groups or interventions studied are not sufficiently similar to each other). The trials should involve similar patient populations, have used similar treatments and have measured results in a similar fashion at a similar point in time. Although what constitutes 'sufficiently similar' is a matter of judgement, the important thing is to be explicit about one's decision to combine or not combine different studies and to consider conducting sensitivity analyses by excluding studies with certain features to see how the effect estimate alters.

There are two main statistical methods by which results are combined: random-effects models (e.g. DerSimonian and Laird) and fixed-effects models (e.g. Peto or Manzel-Haenszel) [17]. Random-effects models assume that the results of different studies may come from different populations with varying responses to treatment. Fixed-effects models assume that each trial represents a random sample of a single population with a single response to treatment (Figure 17.4). In general, random-effects models are more conservative (i.e. random-effects models are less likely to show statistically significant results than fixed-effects models). When the

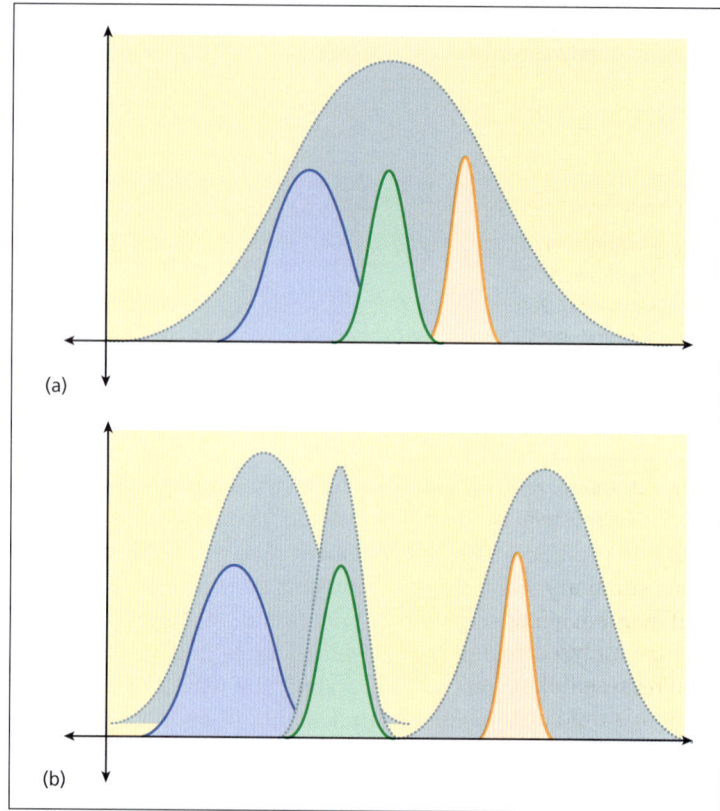

Figure 17.4 (a) Fixed-effects models assume that each trial represents a random sample (coloured curves) of a single population with a single response to treatment. (b) Random-effects models assume that the results of different trials (coloured curves) may come from different populations with varying responses to treatment.

combined studies have statistical homogeneity (i.e. when the studies are reasonably similar in direction, magnitude and variability), random-effects and fixed-effects models give similar results.

The point estimates and confidence intervals of the individual trials and the synthesis of all trials in a meta-analysis are typically displayed graphically in a forest plot [18] (Figure 17.5). Results are most commonly expressed as the odds ratio of the treatment effect (i.e. the odds of achieving a good outcome in the treated group divided by the odds of achieving a good result in the control group), but can be expressed as risk differences (i.e. difference in response rate) or relative risk or risk ratio (probability of achieving a good outcome in the treated group divided by the probability in the control group). An odds ratio of 1 (null) indicates no difference between treatment and control and is usually represented by a vertical line passing through 1 on the x-axis. An odds ratio of greater or less than 1 implies that the treatment is superior or inferior to the control respectively. Risk ratios rather than odds ratios should be used for summarising systematic reviews of common events because of the tendency of odds ratio to overestimate true risk in such conditions [19].

The point estimate of individual trials is indicated by a square whose size is proportional to the size of the trial (i.e. number of patients analysed). The precision of the trial is represented by the 95% confidence interval that appears in forest plots as the brackets surrounding the point estimate. If the 95% confidence interval (brackets) does not cross null (odds ratio of 1), then the individual trial is statistically significant at the level of $P = 0.05$.

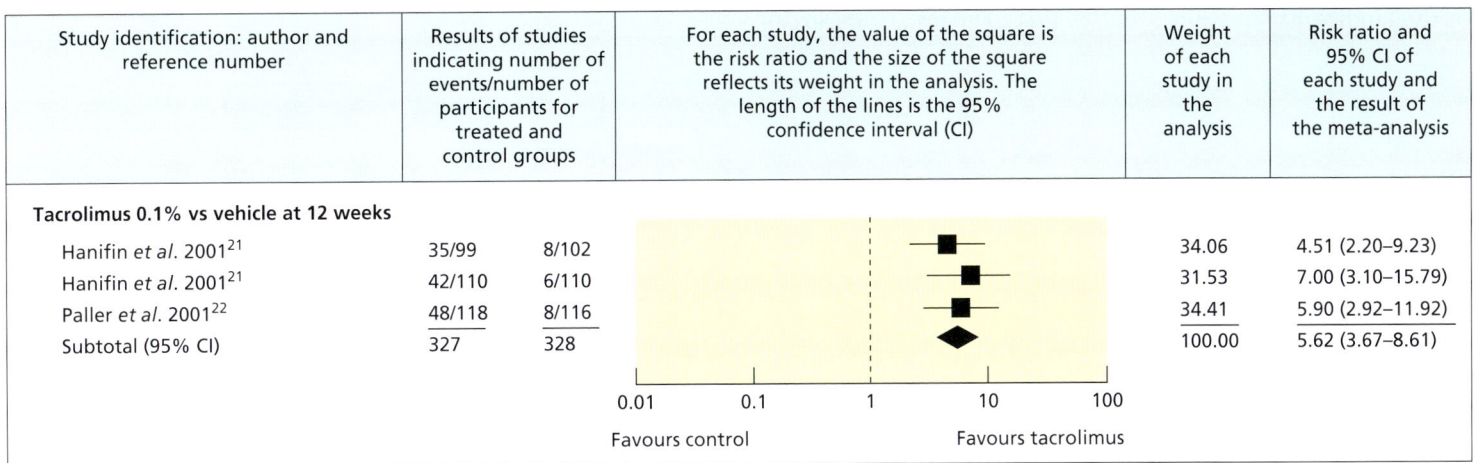

Figure 17.5 Typical forest plot showing the results of a meta-analysis of trials of tacrolimus 0.1% ointment versus vehicle in the management of moderate to severe atopic eczema. The x-axis represents the rate ratio of the investigator global assessment of response. Adapted from Ashcroft et al. 2005 [47].

The summary value for all trials is shown graphically as a parallelogram whose size is proportional to the total number of patients analysed from all trials. The lateral tips of the parallelogram represent the 95% confidence interval and if they do not cross null (odds ratio of 1), then the summary value of the meta-analysis is statistically significant at the $P = 0.05$ level. Odds ratios can be converted to risk differences and the number needed to treat (NNT) if the event rate in the control group is known (Table 17.3) [20].

The most easily understood measures of the magnitude of the treatment effect are the difference in response rate and its reciprocal, the NNT [1,2,21]. The NNT represents the number of patients one would need to treat on average to achieve one additional cure. Whereas the interpretation of NNT might be straightforward within one trial, the interpretation of NNT requires some caution within a systematic review as this statistic is highly sensitive to baseline event rates. For example, if treatment A is 30% more effective than treatment B for clearing psoriasis, and 50% of people on treatment B are cleared with therapy, then 65% will clear with treatment A. These results correspond to a rate difference of 15% (65 – 50) and an NNT of 7 (1/0.15). This difference sounds quite worthwhile clinically. However, if the baseline clearance rate for treatment B in another trial or setting is only 30%, the rate difference will be only 9% and the NNT now becomes 11; and if the baseline clearance rate is 10%, then the NNT for treatment A will be 33, which is perhaps less worthwhile. In other words, it does not make sense to provide one NNT summary measure within a systematic review if 'control' or baseline events rates differ considerably between studies. Instead, a range of NNTs for a range of plausible control event rates that occur in different clinical settings should be given, along with their 95% confidence intervals.

The data used in a meta-analysis can be tested for statistical heterogeneity by methods including the χ^2 and I^2 [2,13,22]. When there is evidence of statistical heterogeneity, reasons for heterogeneity between studies – such as different disease subgroups, intervention dosage or study quality – should be sought [13]. Detecting the source of heterogeneity generally requires subgroup analysis that is only possible when data from many or large trials are available [1,2]. Tests for statistical heterogeneity are typically of low power, so that failure to detect statistical heterogeneity does not ensure homogeneity.

Publication bias can be detected by using a simple graphic test (funnel plot), by calculating the 'fail-safe' N, or using the Begg rank correlation method, Egger regression method and others [23]. These techniques are of limited value when fewer than 10 RCTs are included. Testing for publication bias is almost never possible in systematic reviews of skin diseases because of the limited number and sizes of trials.

Sometimes, the robustness of an overall meta-analysis is tested further by means of a sensitivity analysis. In a sensitivity analysis the data are re-analysed excluding those studies that are suspect because of quality or patient factors, to see whether their exclusion makes a substantial difference in the direction or magnitude of the main original results. In some systematic reviews in which a large number of trials have been included, it is possible to evaluate whether certain subgroups (e.g. children versus adults) are more likely to benefit than others. Subgroup analysis is rarely possible in dermatology because few trials are available.

The conclusions in the discussion section of a systematic review should closely reflect the data that have been presented within that review. The authors should make it clear which of the treatment recommendations are based on the review data and which reflect their own judgements. The approach developed by the Grading of Recommendations, Assessment, Development and Evaluations (GRADE) working group (https://gradepro.org/last accessed February 2022) links the quality of evidence to clinical recommendations by means of summary of findings tables that are used in Cochrane reviews. The GRADE approach assesses methodological flaws of included studies, the consistency of study results, how generalisable the results are to a broader group of patients, and the magnitude of effect of treatment.

Many reviews in dermatology find little evidence to address the questions posed. The review may still be of value, especially if the question addressed is an important one [1,24]. For example, the systematic review may provide the authors with the opportunity to call for primary research in an area, and to make recommendations on study design and outcomes that might help future researchers [25].

Table 17.3 Deriving numbers needed to treat (NNTs) from a treatment's odds ratio (OR)[a] and the observed or expected event rates of the control group.

		\multicolumn{9}{c}{Odds ratio}								
		1.5	2	2.5	3	3.5	4	4.5	5	10
						Number needed to treat				
	0.05	43	22	15	12	9	8	7	6	3
	0.1	23	12	9	7	6	5	4	4	2
CER or PEER	0.2	14	8	5	4	4	3	3	3	2
	0.3	11	6	5	4	3	3	3	3	2
	0.4	10	6	4	4	3	3	3	3	2
	0.5	10	6	5	4	4	3	3	3	2
	0.7	13	8	7	6	5	5	5	5	4
	0.9	32	21	17	16	14	14	13	13	11

Data from https://www.cebm.ox.ac.uk/resources/ebm-tools/number-needed-to-treat-nnt (last accessed February 2022).
[a] The formula for converting ORs to NNTs is:
$$NNT = [\{PEER*(OR - 1)\} + 1] / [PEER*(OR - 1)*(1 - PEER)]$$
CER, control event rate (the rate of good events or outcomes in the control group); PEER, patient expected event rate (the rate of good events or outcomes in your patient or the population in which you are interested).

Can the results of the systematic review be applied to your specific patient?

Applying external evidence to the patient in front of you is one of the most difficult steps of EBM. Having identified some relevant and valid information from a systematic review in relation to a clinical question generated by a patient encounter, three questions now need to be asked in order to guide the application of such information to that patient (Box 17.4).

Firstly, physicians should ask themselves whether there are any compelling reasons that the results should *not* be applied to the patient, rather than expecting a perfect match of the study participants and patient. Only if the answer is 'yes' are the study's results not applicable to the patient. Participants in clinical trials may be different from the patient who originally prompted you to ask an evidence-based question in obvious biological ways such as age, sex and clinical disease type, but in most circumstances these differences do not prevent you from making some useful generalisations from the literature. Perhaps one of the most frequent problems encountered is that of having to generalise trials of adult therapy to children, in whom RCTs are rarely performed. Yet children can suffer almost all of the 'adult' skin diseases, and practitioners frequently have no choice but to use adult-based data as a means of informing treatment decisions.

Secondly, the outcomes desired by the patient should have been included in or be deducible from the outcomes of the systematic review. Finally, the benefits of the intervention should outweigh the risks and the intervention should be available and affordable.

Critically appraising individual clinical trials
[1,2,26,27]

Are the results of the trial valid?
To determine whether an individual clinical trial is valid, pay particular attention to the features that strengthen clinical trials and help validate their conclusions (Box 17.5). The 'big three' that should always be assessed are:
1 Is the method of generating the randomisation sequence and subsequent concealment of allocation of participants clearly described and appropriate?
2 Were participants and study assessors masked to the intervention?
3 Were all those who originally entered the study accounted for in the results and analysis (i.e. was an intention-to-treat analysis performed)?

Box 17.5 Critical appraisal of a paper about therapy

Are the results of this single preventative or therapeutic trial valid?
- Was the assignment of patients to treatments randomised? And was the randomisation list concealed?
- Were all patients who entered the trial accounted for at its conclusion? And were they analysed in the groups to which they were randomised?
- Were patients and clinicians kept 'blind' to which treatment was being received?
- Aside from the experimental treatment, were the groups treated equally?
- Were the groups similar at the start of the trial?

Are the valid results of this trial important?
- Calculations:

Intervention response rate	IRR
Comparison (intervention) response rate	CRR
Difference in response rates DRR	(IRR − CRR)
Number needed to treat	NNT (1/DRR)

- What is the 95% confidence interval of the difference in response rates (DRR)?[a]
- What is the 95% confidence interval of the NNT?[b]

Can you apply this valid, important evidence in caring for your patient?
- Do these results apply to your patient?
  - Is your patient so different from those in the trial that its results cannot help you?
  - How great would the potential benefit of therapy actually be for your individual patient?

- Does the regimen and its consequences satisfy your patient's values and preferences?
    - Do your patient and you have a clear assessment of your values and preferences?
    - Do this regimen and its consequences meet them?

Adapted from https://www.cebm.ox.ac.uk/files/ebm-tools/rct.pdf (last accessed February 2022).

[a] The 95% confidence interval of the difference in response rates (DRR) is from:

$$DRR - 1.96 \times SE \text{ to } DRR + 1.96 \times SE \text{ where } SE$$
$$= \sqrt{\frac{IRR(1 - IRR)}{\text{No.intervention patients}} + \frac{CRR(1 - CRR)}{\text{No.comparison patients}}}$$

[b] The 95% confidence interval of the NNT = 1/limits on the confidence interval of its DRR.

Ideally, patients should be randomly assigned to treatment groups to avoid the introduction of biases and to distribute intrinsic prognostic factors equally among treatment groups. Randomisation controls patient selection and evaluation bias by physicians and study personnel. Non-randomised studies have limited value in distinguishing useful from useless or even harmful therapy. When compared with RCTs, studies in which patients are not allocated randomly more commonly show larger effects, many of which are false positive. For example, the belief that azathioprine reduces the dose of corticosteroids necessary to treat bullous pemphigoid was suggested by several uncontrolled or non-randomised studies. However, a randomised trial of the effects of azathioprine on corticosteroid dose in patients with bullous pemphigoid and a systematic review of interventions for bullous pemphigoid indicated that azathioprine had no or negligible effect on remission or corticosteroid doses [28,29].

Randomisation has the disadvantage of depending on chance for an equal statistical distribution of prognostic factors among groups. Therefore, it is always important to identify known prognostic factors such as disease severity and compare their distribution among treatment groups at baseline. The common practice of assigning *P* values to differences in characteristics at baseline is inappropriate. Demographic and known prognostic factors may not be equally distributed among treatment groups when patients are randomly assigned to them. However, the impact of the unequal distribution of prognostic factors on treatment results should be assessed by performing adjusted statistical analyses. Inequality of groups is a more significant problem in studies with few patients.

When patients are assigned randomly, the method used to randomise should be reported. The most widely accepted and unbiased methods are to use sealed random numbers obtained from tables or random numbers generated by computers. In this method, patients are assigned a random number after they are admitted to a trial. That number has been previously assigned to a treatment group and the assignment is unknown to the patient and the investigator. Randomisation or concealment of assignment is often not done in published studies, and the methods of randomisation are often not reported adequately. Many commonly encountered methods of randomisation (e.g. on the basis of the admitting team, alternative assignment, odd or even days of entry, birth dates, social security numbers or day of the week) can lead to significant introduction of selection bias. For example, a physician who would like a new treatment to be shown to be superior in efficacy to an older treatment may be able to enter patients most likely to respond to treatment on even days and patients least likely to respond on odd days, if he or she can foretell the allocation sequence according to odd or even days.

Concealment of treatment allocation refers to the steps taken by the trialists to conceal the allocation of participants to the intervention groups from those recruiting trial participants, and is a crucial step in the construct of an RCT. Concealing the sequence from recruiters is adequate if investigators and patients cannot foresee the assignment to intervention groups (e.g. numbered and coded identical sealed boxes prepared by a central pharmacy or sealed opaque envelopes). It is inadequate if the allocation schedule is open for the recruiting physician to view beforehand (e.g. unsealed envelopes).

The randomisation list should be kept away from enrolment sites (e.g. by a central clinical trials office or pharmacy). Internet randomisation by a third party, whereby details of a new, potentially eligible trial participant are entered irrevocably onto a trial database before an allocation code is offered, is another very secure way of concealing allocation.

It is important to make the evaluation of the outcome of a trial as masked as possible to avoid the introduction of information/detection bias. Masking can refer to at least four groups of people: those recruiting patients, the study participants themselves, those assessing the outcomes in study participants, and those analysing the results, so it is important that trials report who is masked rather than just using the phrase 'double-blind'. The masking of physicians and patients is especially important when subjective outcomes such as pain are being measured. The masking of patients and evaluators also ensures that ancillary therapies and outcome evaluations are applied equally, thus minimising performance bias. A patient who is known to be receiving a new treatment may be observed more closely, may receive better ancillary care and may have different expectations than a control patient. Changes in disease status may receive greater (or lesser) emphasis and adverse events may similarly receive more (or less) attention. Masking is less of an issue for some studies that use very objective outcomes such as death, since the risk of detection bias is low for such an outcome.

Sometimes masking is not possible. Many treatments produce skin changes that make it apparent what treatment is being used. For example, the drying effects of topical and systemic retinoids and the tanning effects of UVB therapy make the recipients of those therapies readily apparent. An unmasked study may still be valid, but the designers of an unmasked study must make allowances for the possibility that bias may have been introduced and should increase the statistical rigour for demonstrating differences and consider objective outcome measures measured by masked third parties.

The whole purpose of randomisation is to create two or more groups that are as similar to each other as possible, the only difference being the intervention under study. In this way, the additional effects of the intervention can be assessed. A potentially serious violation of this principle is the failure to take into account all those who were randomised when conducting the final main analysis, for example participants who deviate from the study protocol, those who do not adhere to the interventions and those who subsequently drop out for other reasons. People who drop out of trials tend to differ from those who remain in them in several ways. People may drop out because they encounter adverse events, get worse (or no better) or simply because the proposed regimen is too complicated for them to follow. They may also drop out because the treatment is working so well. Ignoring participants who have dropped out in the analysis is not acceptable as their very reason for dropping out is likely to be related in some direct or indirect way to the study intervention. Excluding participants who drop out after randomisation potentially biases the results. One way to reduce bias is to perform an intention to treat (ITT) analysis, in which all those initially randomised are included in the final analysis.

Unless one has detailed information on why participants dropped out of a study, it cannot be assumed that analyses of those remaining in the study to the end are representative of those randomised to the groups at the beginning. Failure to perform an ITT analysis may inflate or deflate estimates of treatment effect. Performing an ITT analysis is regarded as a major criterion by which the quality of an RCT is assessed.

It may be entirely appropriate to conduct an analysis of all those who remained at the end of a study (a 'per protocol' analysis) alongside the ITT analysis, especially in early efficacy studies and in equivalence or non-inferiority studies. Discrepancies between results of ITT and per protocol analyses may indicate the potential benefit of the intervention under ideal compliance conditions and the need to explore ways of reformulating the intervention so that fewer participants drop out of the trial. Discrepancies may also indicate serious flaws in the study design [30].

A considerable degree of detail needs to be provided in the methodology section of a published clinical trial. This need has led to the development of reporting guidelines, for example the Consolidated Standards of Reporting Trials (CONSORT) and its various extensions (http://www.consort-statement.org/; last accessed February 2022). Most of the top dermatology journals now insist that all RCT submissions are reported according to the CONSORT checklist.

Other features that strengthen the validity of trials
[1,2,3,22,23]

In evaluating a clinical trial in dermatology, look for clinical outcome measures that are clear cut and clinically meaningful to you and your patients. For example, in a study of a systemic treatment for warts, the complete disappearance of warts is a meaningful outcome, whereas a decrease in the volume of warts is not. Historically, three principal methods are used to determine patient outcomes in dermatological clinical trials. The first involves examining patients before, during and at the conclusion of treatment, and reporting how the patients appear at the various time points. The second involves determining the degree of improvement during treatment [31]. A third method, determining the impact of therapy on the quality of the patient's life, is being increasingly used in dermatological trials.

An example of the first method is commonly encountered in therapeutic trials of psoriasis. A common practice is to assign numerical values to the amount of redness, scaling and degree of infiltration, to determine the area of the body surface involved, and to formulate an 'index' by calculating a derivative of some product of these four numbers. The overall condition of the patient can then be represented by this index. A common example is the psoriasis area and severity index (PASI) that ranges from 0 to 72 [32].

The major problem with indices is that they confound area of involvement with severity of disease. For example, a patient with thick plaque-type psoriasis of the knees, elbows and scalp may have the same index as a patient with diffuse but minimal psoriasis of the trunk and arms. Whereas the former patient is notoriously difficult to treat, the latter will generally respond rapidly and easily to many forms of therapy. The second problem with indices is that they lend an air of spurious precision to the analysis and presentation of data that is not warranted. For example, Tiling-Grosse and Rees demonstrated that physicians and medical students were poor at estimating the area of skin disease, and, therefore, some of the components that make up indices may be inaccurate [33]. Finally, calculating the means, differences in means and percentages of change in indices in response to treatment often do not convey an accurate clinical picture of the changes that have occurred.

The second method of assessment groups patients according to their degree of improvement such as investigator global improvement. Treatments are then compared by their ability to move patients to higher degrees of improvement. There are two major problems with this form of assessment. The first is that the categories of improvement are often not well defined. The second problem is that the categories are not additive. That is, 60–80% improvement is often assumed to be twice as good as 20–40%, although no such numerical relationship exists between these subjectively defined categories.

To be most useful, the outcome variables to measure must be clearly defined, be as objective as possible, and have clinical and biological significance. The best indices and scales are those that accurately reflect the state of the disease and the patient's view of treatment and quality of life. The development of scales and indices for cutaneous diseases, and testing their validity, reproducibility and responsiveness has been inadequate. Therefore, a lack of clearly defined and useful outcome variables remains a major problem in interpreting dermatological clinical trials.

Several groups in medicine are now developing the concept of core outcome measures, a set of which should always be included in clinical trials (http://www.comet-initiative.org/; last accessed February 2022). The measures are designed to ensure that the key features or domains of a disease are included and that the best instrument for measuring that domain is used. The best known core outcome sets are for arthritis. Similar groups, such as the Harmonising Outcome Measures for Eczema (HOME) (http://www.homeforeczema.org/index.aspx; last accessed February 2022), have developed a complete core outcome set for atopic dermatitis. The HOME initiative led to the development of the Cochrane Skin Core Outcomes Initiative (CS-COUSIN) (http://cs-cousin.org/; last accessed February 2022) and at least 12 other groups in dermatology are now developing core outcome sets for common skin diseases such as acne and skin cancer [34].

Until better scales and more core outcome sets are developed, trials with the simplest and most objective outcome variables are the best. They lead to the least amount of confusion and have the strongest conclusions. Thus, trials in which a comparison is made between death and survival, patients with recurrence of disease and those without recurrence, or patients who are cured and those who are not cured are studies whose outcome variables are easily understood and verified. For trials in which the outcomes are less clear-cut and more subjective in nature, a simple ordinal scale is probably the best choice. The best ordinal scales involve a minimum of human judgement, have a precision that is much smaller than the differences being sought and are sufficiently standardised that they can be used by others and produce similar results.

In addition to being clearly defined, outcome variables should have clinical and biological significance. For example, in a therapeutic trial of patients with severe acne, treatment was associated with a decrease in lesion count from a mean of 400 to a mean of 350. This numerical difference may be of statistical significance, but it does not convey the clinical significance. This aggregate nature of the result may mean that some patients with severe acne cleared completely whereas other patients remained the same or got worse. It could also mean that most patients got slightly better. Furthermore, does an individual patient look better when their lesion number has been reduced from 400 to 350? Are scarring and complications less?

To strengthen clinical trials and help validate their conclusions, the outcome variables should be few in number and should be chosen before initiation of the study. Having many outcome variables increases the likelihood that spurious, chance differences will be detected that may be highlighted in the abstract. Such selective reporting outcome bias can be overcome by prospectively registering clinical trials in clinical trial registers such as https://clinicaltrials.gov/. An ineffective treatment may be claimed to be efficacious when tested using poorly designed outcome assessment tools. Conversely, an effective therapy may be found ineffective by an insensitive scale.

Special precautions are recommended when dealing with 'substitute or surrogate end points', especially when no differences are detected in clinically important outcomes. Examples of such end points include CD4:CD8 ratios instead of survival in studies of treatments of AIDS; antinuclear antibody levels or sedimentation rates instead of clinical measures of disease activity in lupus erythematosus; and transepidermal water loss for atopic dermatitis instead of proportion of patients cleared. Carefully chosen and validated surrogate end points often allow studies to provide answers to questions that would typically require much larger or longer trials if the targeted clinical end points were utilised. For example, a well-designed, short clinical trial may be sufficient to demonstrate that a new drug effectively lowers serum cholesterol or that another drug is effective in controlling hypertension. In both cases much longer and larger studies would be required to demonstrate that the cholesterol-lowering drug and the antihypertensive drug reduced morbidity and mortality from atherosclerotic and hypertensive cardiovascular diseases, respectively. Surrogate end points must, however, correlate with clinical outcomes and their validity must be demonstrable in prior studies.

Are the results of the clinical trial important? [1,2,22,23]

Once sound, clinically relevant outcome measures are chosen, the magnitude of the difference between the treatment groups in achieving these meaningful outcomes, the NNT and the precision of these estimates should be determined.

Examples of the application of the concepts of NNT and confidence intervals are found in a trial comparing placebo, aciclovir, prednisolone and aciclovir–prednisolone in the treatment of herpes zoster [35]. At day 30 of the trial, 48 of 52 patients treated with aciclovir were totally healed compared with 22 of 52 patients who received placebo. The response rates for aciclovir and placebo were 0.92 and 0.42, respectively, and the difference in response rates was 0.5. The NNT was 2 (1/0.5). This result means that for every two patients treated with aciclovir instead of placebo, one additional patient would be totally healed by day 30. The 95% confidence interval for the difference in response rates is from 0.35 to 0.65, and the 95% confidence interval for the NNT is from 2 to 3.

Misinterpreting trials that fail to show statistically significant differences among treatments is a common error of interpretation in clinical trials in dermatology. It is important to remember that 'not statistically significant' means that a difference has a reasonably high probability of having been due to chance; it does not mean that there is no difference or that treatment is necessarily ineffective. Significant differences in treatment effects in comparison trials may be missed if the number of study participants is small. For example, in a 1978 survey of 71 published trials with negative results, Freiman *et al.* found that a 25% or 50% improvement in outcome might have been missed in 57 (80%) and 34 (48%) of the studies, respectively [36]. A follow-up study conducted by Moher *et al.* in 1994 indicated that 25% or 50% improvements in outcome might have been missed in 84% and 64% of 102 negative studies, respectively [37]. The sample sizes of many dermatological trials are often inadequate to detect clinically important differences. For example, 58 clinical trials with negative conclusions, published in three British dermatological journals over 4 years, were reviewed to determine the risk of their having missed an effective treatment. All but one of the 44 evaluable trials had a greater than one in 10 risk of missing a 25% relative treatment difference (median risk 81%), and 31 of the trials (70%) were so small that they had a greater than one in 10 risk of missing a 50% relative treatment difference (median risk 42%) [38].

Can the results of the trial be applied to your specific patient?

Applying evidence from a clinical trial to specific patients is similar to the process used to apply the results of a systematic review to specific patients (see previous section). Four questions now need to be asked in order to guide the application of such information to that patient (see Box 17.5).

Critically appraising a study about a diagnostic test [1,2,3]

Are the results valid?

To be valid, studies about diagnostic tests should include masked comparison with a criterion ('gold') standard, evaluation in an appropriate spectrum of patients and consistent application of the criterion standard (Box 17.6). Few studies in dermatology meet this standard [39,40] when judged against the QUADAS-2 quality assessment instrument for diagnostic test accuracy studies.

> **Box 17.6 Critical appraisal of a paper about a diagnostic test**
>
> **Are the results of this diagnostic study valid?**
> - Was there an independent, blind comparison with a reference ('gold') standard of diagnosis?
> - Was the diagnostic test evaluated in an appropriate spectrum of patients (like those in whom it would be used in practice)?
> - Was the reference standard applied regardless of the diagnostic test result?
>
> **Are the valid results of this diagnostic study important**
> - Calculations:
>
> | | | Target disorder | |
> |---|---|---|---|
> | | | Present | Absent |
> | Diagnostic test result | Positive | a | b |
> | | Negative | c | d |
>
> Sensitivity $= a/(a+c)$
> Specificity $= d/(b+d)$
> Likelihood ratio for a positive test result $= [a/(a+c)]/[b/(b+d)] =$ sensitivity$/(1-$specificity$)$
> Likelihood ratio for a negative test result $= [c/(a+c)]/[d/(b+d)] = (1-$sensitivity$)/$specificity
>
> **Can you apply this valid, important evidence about a diagnostic test in caring for your patient?**
> - Is the diagnostic test available, affordable, accurate and precise in your setting?
> - Can you generate a clinically sensible estimate of your patient's pre-test probability (from practice data, from personal experience, from the report itself or from clinical speculation)?
> - Will the resulting post-test probabilities affect your management and help your patient? (Could it move you across a test treatment threshold? Would your patient be a willing partner in carrying it out?)
> - Would the consequences of the test help your patient?
>
> Adapted from https://www.cebm.ox.ac.uk/files/ebm-tools/diagnostic-accuracy-studies.pdf (last accessed February 2022).

Are the results important?

Important terms and concepts that must be understood to determine whether the results of a paper about a diagnostic test are clinically important include the likelihood ratio, pre-test probability, post-test probability and threshold for action. The *likelihood ratio* is the percentage of people with the disease who have a positive test divided by the percentage of people who do not have the disease who have a positive test. The likelihood ratio is traditionally taught as being the sensitivity divided by 1 minus the specificity: it provides an estimation of how much higher the likelihood of the disease is, given a positive test (post-test probability), compared with the probability before the test is done (pre-test probability). An ideal test is one that will almost always be positive when the disease is present and negative when the disease is absent, i.e. a test with a high sensitivity and specificity. Such a test would have a very high likelihood ratio.

In order for the likelihood ratio to be useful, one has to have an idea of how likely the disease is to be present before the test is done (i.e. the pre-test probability) and a sense of how certain one needs to be to conclude that the patient has the disease and to act on it (i.e. the threshold for action) [41]. The *pre-test probability* is determined from available published data or based on physician experience and judgement. Once the pre-test probability is known or estimated and the likelihood ratio determined, a nomogram can be used to estimate the *post-test probability* (Figure 17.6).

If the nomogram is not available, the calculations can be done manually after conversion of probabilities to odds. The odds of disease is defined as the probability of disease divided by 1 minus the probability (odds = probability/1 − probability). For a defined group of individuals or patients, it can also be calculated as the ratio of the number of those with disease to those without disease. Thus, if the probability of (proportion with) a disease is 0.20 (20%), the odds of that disease are 0.20/1 − 0.20, or 0.20/0.80, or 1:4. This result means that for every person with the disease, there are four people without the disease. The post-test odds are equal to the pre-test odds times the likelihood ratio (post-test odds = pre-test odds × LR). The formula (probability = odds/odds + 1) is used to convert odds back to probability.

For example, suppose that, based on clinical judgement, the estimated probability that a patient with a cluster of vesicles on his cheek has herpes zoster is 0.6 (60%), then his odds of having herpes zoster are 1.5:1 (0.6/1 − 0.6). Assume, for this example, that the sensitivity and specificity of a direct fluorescent antibody (DFA) test for herpes zoster are 80% and 96%, respectively. Therefore, the likelihood ratio for a positive DFA is 20 (0.80/1 − 0.96). If this patient's DFA test is positive, his post-test odds are 30 (1.5 × 20) and the post-test probability of herpes zoster is 0.97 (97%) (30/30 + 1). This probability is certainly high enough to act upon.

Whether formally or informally, physicians develop thresholds of certainty at or above which they are comfortable with establishing a diagnosis and acting on the diagnoses. Action may take the form of communicating the diagnosis or prognosis to the patient, prescribing treatment or referring the patient. When historical and physical evidence leads a clinician to suspect a diagnosis, but the degree of certainty does not exceed the threshold for establishing a diagnosis, a test is done to increase the probability that the disease is present above the clinician's *threshold for action* [34]. Diagnostic studies should always be interpreted in the context of specific clinical encounters so that the diagnostic value of the test can be assessed [42,43]. Studies reporting diagnostic tests in dermatology should adhere to established international reporting standards [44].

adequate follow-up. The effects of selection bias when choosing cases and controls need particular consideration in the absence of randomisation. In addition, the results should make clinical and biological sense (Box 17.7).

> **Box 17.7 Critical appraisal of a paper about harm**
>
> **Are the results of this harm study valid?**
> - Were there clearly defined groups of patients, similar in all important ways other than exposure to the treatment or other cause?
> - Were treatment exposures and clinical outcomes measured the same ways in both groups (e.g. was the assessment of outcomes either objective (e.g. death) or blinded to exposure)?
> - Was the follow-up of study patients complete and long enough?
> - Do the results satisfy some 'diagnostic tests for causation'?
> - Is it clear that the exposure preceded the onset of the outcome?
> - Is there a dose–response gradient?
> - Is there positive evidence from a 'de-challenge–re-challenge' study?
> - Is the association consistent from study to study?
> - Does the association make biological sense?
>
> **Are the valid results from this harm study important?**
> - Calculations:
>
> | | | Adverse outcome | |
> |---|---|---|---|
> | | | Present (case) | Absent (control) |
> | Exposed to treatment | Yes (cohort) | a | b |
> | | No (cohort) | c | d |
>
> In a randomised trial or cohort study:
>
> relative risk = $[a/(a+b)]/[c/(c+d)]$
>
> In a case–control study: odds ratio (or relative odds) = ad/bc
>
> **Should these valid, potentially important results of a critical appraisal about a harmful treatment change the treatment of your patient?**
> - Can the study results be extrapolated to your patient?
> - What are your patient's risks of the adverse outcome?
> - What are your patient's preferences, concerns and expectations from this treatment?
> - What alternative treatments are available?
>
> From Sackett et al. 1996 [48]. Reproduced with permission of Elsevier.

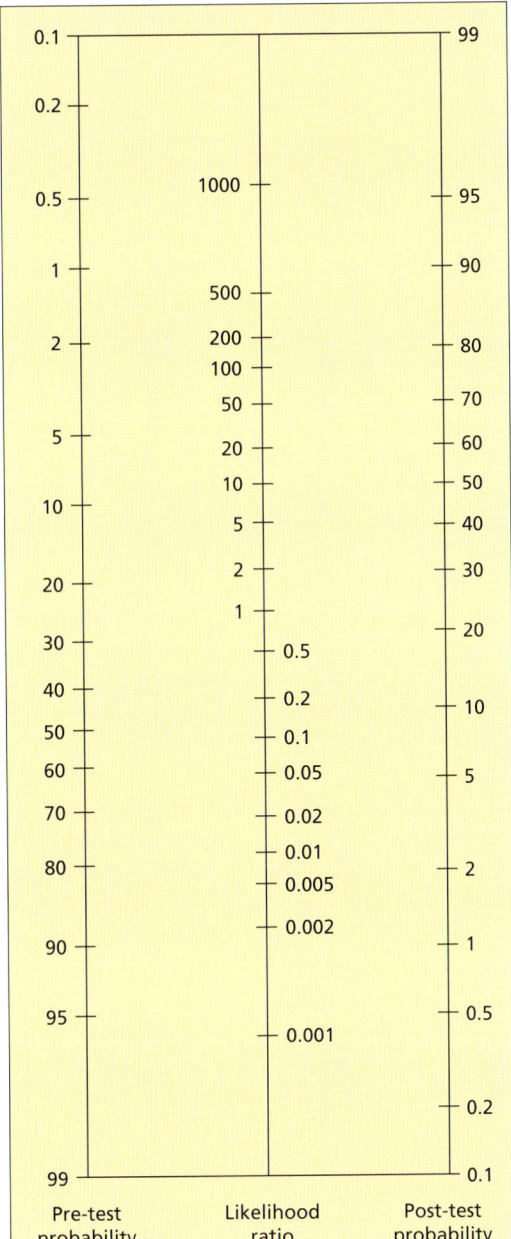

Figure 17.6 Nomogram for determining the post-test probability. To determine the post-test probability, draw a straight line through the pre-test probability and the likelihood ratio and read the post-test probability on the right.

Can the results of the diagnostic study be applied to your specific patient?

The key questions to ask to determine whether the results of a diagnostic study can be applied to a specific patient are shown in Box 17.6.

Critically appraising a study about adverse events (case–control and cohort studies) [1,2]

Are the results valid?

To be valid, studies about the harmful effects of exposures should include cohorts with comparable groups of exposed and unexposed individuals, or cases and controls, objective outcome measures and

Are the results important? [1,2,3,34]

Important terms and concepts that must be understood to determine whether the results of a paper about harmful effects of exposures are clinically important include case–control and cohort studies, relative risk and odds ratios. In a *cohort study* a group of individuals who are exposed to an agent is compared with an appropriately selected unexposed control group and both groups are followed until an event of interest occurs or for a pre-specified length of time. The association of exposure to the harmful outcome is expressed as the relative risk (Box 17.7). A relative risk of 1 implies no association. If the relative risk is greater than 1, then the result implies a positive association between exposure and the harmful outcome. If it is less than 1, then the implication is of an inverse association. However, in order to infer a causal association reflected by either an increase in risk (relative risk of more than 1) or a protective effect (relative risk less than 1), it is important to evaluate the validity and precision of the relative risk estimate. The precision can be readily assessed by means of the 95% confidence interval. A confidence interval that does not include 1.0 denotes a statistically significant association. Because the most likely result of a study is the point estimate (i.e. the reported result), the observed association (expressed by the point estimate) may be causal, even if the confidence interval includes 1.0 as a result of a small sample size. Other criteria such as dose–response effect, consistency, biological plausibility and specificity need to be considered when inferring causality from observational data [45].

Case–control studies can be used when the undesirable outcome (e.g. lymphoma) is recognised and the causative agent not yet discovered. They are also used when there is a very long time lag between exposure and outcome or when the frequency of adverse events is very small. In a case–control study, patients with a disease of interest are compared with appropriately selected controls. The odds of exposure to suspected aetiological agents are ascertained in the cases and controls (Box 17.7). The odds of an event are the ratio of the number of events to the number of non-events. Events are exposures to potentially harmful risk factors in case–control studies. The odds of exposure of cases are divided by the odds of exposure among controls to derive the *odds ratio*, which is a good estimate of the relative risk when the outcome (e.g. disease, death) is relatively rare (i.e. when it is less than 5% in exposed subjects). An odds ratio of 1 implies no association. If the odds ratio is greater than 1, then the result implies a positive association between exposure and the harmful outcome. If the odds ratio is less than 1, then the result implies a protective effect of the exposure. As noted above, it is important to evaluate the validity and precision of the odds ratio estimate by examining the 95% confidence interval.

For example, suppose a case–control study was performed to study the relationship between limb deformity and exposure to thalidomide. The results of the study indicated that patients with limb deformities were more likely than controls to have been exposed to thalidomide *in utero*. The odds ratio for thalidomide exposure was 3.5 and the confidence interval was from 1.8 to 6.6. Thus the odds that patients with limb deformities were exposed to thalidomide *in utero* were 3.5 times the odds of thalidomide exposure in controls. Since the odds ratio is greater than 1, and its 95% confidence interval does not include 1, the result implies the positive association between thalidomide use and limb deformities was not likely to have been due to chance. These results (an odds ratio of 3.5 and confidence interval of 1.8–6.6) were actually the results of a study by Wolf *et al.* who studied the relationship between sunscreen use and melanoma in a case–control study in Austria [46]. Their results indicated that patients with melanoma were more likely than controls to report having used sunscreen often. In order to infer causality it is important to assess whether the data could have resulted from confounding (i.e. the association between exposure and outcome can be explained by other factors such as age, sex or bias (e.g. people with melanoma may be more likely to recall sun protective behaviour)) and that the results are biologically plausible.

To add confusion to an already difficult area, clinical researchers will often report results of meta-analyses, cohort studies and RCTs using odds ratios. Odds ratios are used because they have stronger statistical properties than other measures [34]. For example, odds ratios can take any value between zero and infinity, are symmetrical in a log scale and can be used to make adjustments for confounding factors using multiple regression. Unfortunately, they are the measure of association least intuitively understood. If a meta-analysis, controlled trial or cohort study is reported using odds ratios, the relative risk, difference in response rates or NNT can often be calculated if the primary data are provided. Alternatively, these more readily understandable measures can be derived if the number of subjects in each group, odds ratio and overall event rate are provided (https://www.cebm.ox.ac.uk/resources/ebm-tools/number-needed-to-treat-nnt; last accessed April 2021).

Applying the evidence to individual patients
Can the results be applied to your specific patient?
The key questions to ask to determine whether the results of a study of adverse events (usually a case–control or cohort study) can be applied to a specific patient are shown in Box 17.7.

Conclusions
EBM is the use of the best current evidence in making decisions about the care of individual patients. It is predicated on asking structured clinical questions, finding the best evidence to answer the questions, critically appraising the evidence, applying the evidence to specific patients and saving the critically appraised evidence. The EBM approach is most appropriate for common, frequently encountered conditions.

Results from well-designed clinical studies on patients are near the top of the hierarchy of evidence used to practise EBM. Recommendations about treatment, diagnosis and harm made in this textbook and in other sources should take into account the validity, magnitude, precision and applicability of the evidence upon which it is based.

Evaluating the data in clinical research papers and a shortcut method for reading clinical research papers

Evaluating the data in clinical research papers [1]
Are the data adequately reported?
The authors of a study should present their results in sufficient detail to allow the reader to perform his or her own preferred analysis of the data. At a minimum, the presentation of interval data (i.e. discrete or continuous data such as lesion counts or area of involvement) should include a summary measure of the centre of the data for each group and a measure of the variability of the data. The mean and median are most commonly used to indicate the centre of the data. The mean is simply calculated as the sum of the data points divided by the total number of data points. The mean is the most appropriate choice for normally distributed data (i.e. data that are distributed in the shape of

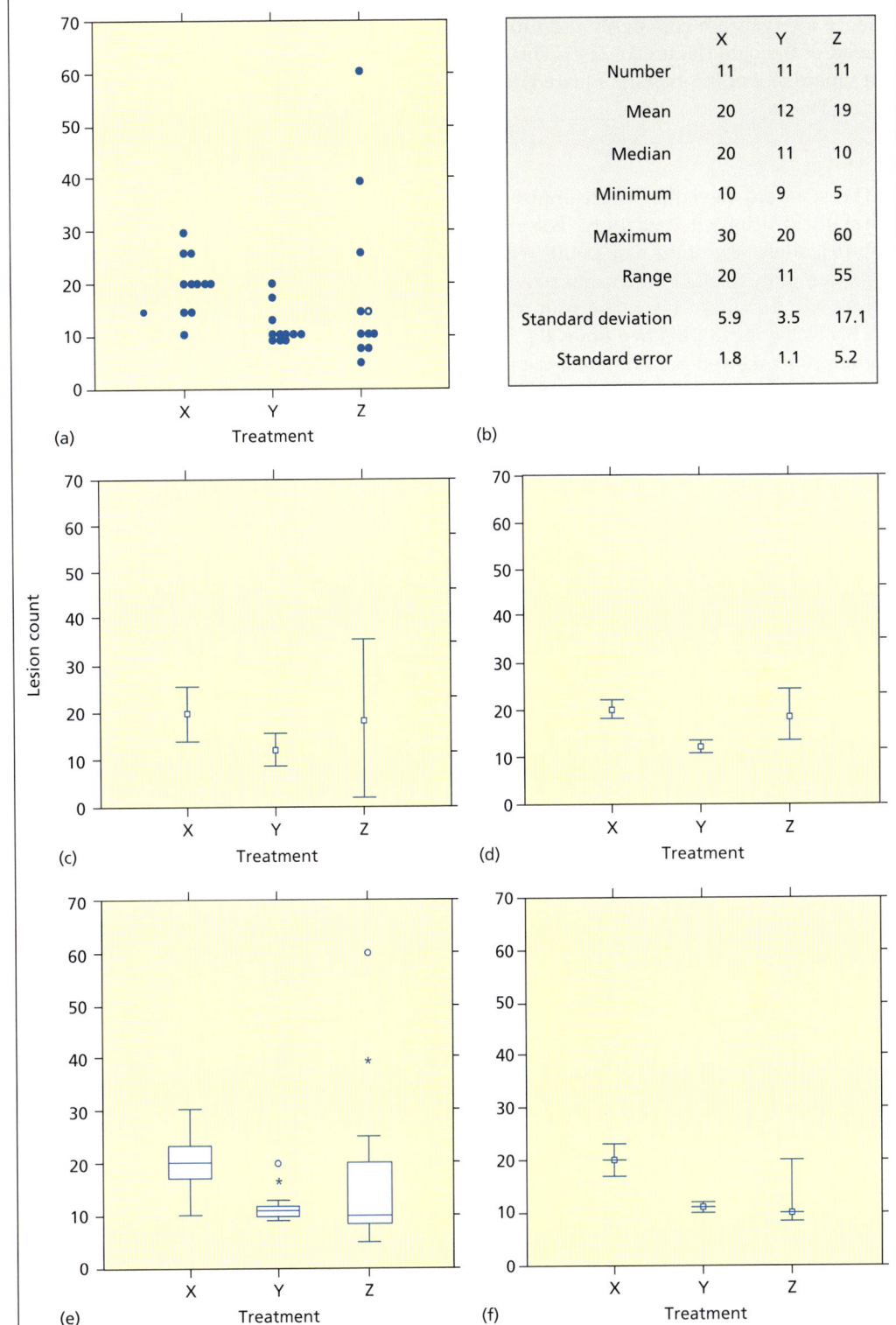

Figure 17.7 Hypothetical final lesion counts in a clinical trial of treatments X, Y and Z. The same data are displayed or summarised in each panel. A graphical display of all of the data points (a) gives an accurate description of the magnitude and distribution of the results. Commonly used summary statistics (b). The mean with error bars consisting of 1 SD (c) or 1 SE (d) provide little useful information even for the normally distributed response to treatment X and are totally misleading for treatment Y, which is skewed, and treatment Z, which has outliers. A box plot of the data (e) shows the median (line within the box), the interquartile range (top and bottom of the box) and adequately represents skewed data (note the asymmetry of the median within the box in the Y plot) and the presence of outliers (note the asymmetry of the median within the box in the Z plot and the outliers indicated by an asterisk and open circle). The 95% confidence interval about the median (f) adequately represents skewed data and the presence of outliers. If the 95% confidence intervals around two means or medians do not overlap, you can be confident at about the 95% level that the two population means or medians are different.

the bell curve). The median is a better choice for data that are skewed or contain outliers (Figure 17.7a, b). The median for an odd number of data points is the value in the middle when the data are ordered from lowest to highest. The median for an even number of data points is determined by taking the mean of the two numbers in the middle when the data points are ordered from lowest to highest. Half the data points fall above and half fall below the median. The magnitude of the difference between the mean and the median is a crude indicator of the degree of skewing. If the difference is none or small, the data are or approach normal (i.e. are symmetrical); if the difference is large the data are skewed.

The standard deviation, range, interquartile range and 95% confidence intervals are commonly used to indicate the variability or spread of the data (Figure 17.7c–f). The standard deviation (SD) is the square root of the average squared deviation of values from the mean. That is:

$$SD = \sqrt{\Sigma(X - \overline{X})^2/(n - 1)}$$

The standard deviation is an important summary statistic for normally distributed data only. For normally distributed data, approximately 68% of the data points will lie within the range from the mean minus 1 SD to the mean plus 1 SD; and 95% of the data points will lie within the range from the mean minus two times the SD to the mean plus two times the SD. These relationships do not apply to skewed data or small data sets that contain outliers. Note in Figure 17.7c that the mean and standard deviation do not adequately describe the centre of the data or its distribution for skewed data or data with outliers (treatments Y and Z).

The range is the interval from the highest to the lowest data points. The range may be a good indicator of variability for data that are tightly arranged around the mean and for small data sets. The range is greatly influenced by outliers and may not give an adequate indication of skewed data. Therefore the range is not a good descriptive statistic for skewed data sets or for data with outliers (Figure 17.7a, b).

The interquartile range is the interval that contains the middle 50% of the data points. It excludes the highest 25% of the data points and the lowest 25%. The interquartile range is a reasonable descriptive statistic to describe skewed data and data with outliers (Figure 17.7e).

Confidence intervals are the best way to present the degree of uncertainty of normally distributed data as well as skewed data or data with outliers (see discussion of confidence intervals later). The 95% confidence interval around the mean can be calculated for normally distributed data using the sample mean, standard error and the t distribution. For skewed data, the confidence interval around the median should be used (Figure 17.7f).

The standard error (SE) is the standard deviation divided by the square root of the number of data points ($SE = SD/\sqrt{n}$). Unfortunately, the standard error is commonly but incorrectly used to summarise the variability of data. This choice is made because of tradition and because the SE is always smaller than the SD and 95% confidence interval and, therefore, looks better (Figure 17.7c, d, f). The standard error is correctly used to analyse normally distributed data in inferential statistics (see discussion of the t-test later). The common practice of reporting the mean ± SE is firmly ingrained in the medical and scientific literature but is often misleading and inappropriate, and should be discouraged. The standard error is an important and useful statistic only for normally distributed data sets. It is used to make predictions or inferences about the population from which the sample is chosen. That is, for large, normally distributed data sets, the chance that the true or population mean (from which the sample was drawn) will lie outside the range from the sample mean minus two times the SE to the sample mean plus two times the SE is only 5%. The relationship between the sample mean, the population mean and the standard error does not apply to skewed data or small data sets that contain outliers.

Descriptive statistics are at best incomplete summaries of the data; considerably more information may be conveyed by graphic displays (Figure 17.7) [2]. Figures that show individual observations are an excellent tool for presenting small data sets, and data that are skewed or have outliers (Figure 17.7a) [2]. Unfortunately, such diagrams are underutilised in the scientific and medical literature. Graphic displays of data using 'error bars' showing 1 SD or 1 SE depict at best 68% of the sample or 68% confidence intervals, respectively, and are therefore misleading and should be avoided or approached with scepticism (Figure 17.7c, d).

Categorical data are preferably presented in tables in which the treatments and outcomes are represented in rows and columns. Examples of categorical outcomes include cured and not cured, survived and died, and minimal, moderate and marked improvement. Categorical outcomes should be clearly defined, limited in number, clinically important and declared before the trial is begun.

Are the data subjected to statistical testing and are the tests used correctly?

Observed differences in outcome in clinical trials may be due to chance alone. It is therefore imperative that statistical analyses be performed to verify that the results are from treatment and not from chance. This admonition is especially true for trials containing few patients, as is the case for many published dermatological trials.

Statistical methods
Understanding *P*

Understanding the meaning of P is fundamental to understanding and interpreting statistical testing. In the simplest terms, all clinical trials begin with the null hypothesis – that the effects of each treatment are the same. If the results of the trial indicate that the outcomes of treatment are different, then a statistical test is performed to determine the probability that a difference as large or larger than the observed difference could be observed if the treatment effects were the same. If the probability is sufficiently small, the null hypothesis that the outcomes of each treatment are the same is rejected.

The error of believing that a difference in treatment outcomes exists, when in fact there is no difference is referred to as a Type I or α error. The statement that 'the difference was statistically significant ($P = 0.05$)' means that the probability that a difference as large as the observed difference might arise if the treatment effects were the same is one in 20 and that the author will accept this degree of chance as being sufficiently unlikely that the null hypothesis (that the treatment outcomes are the same) can be rejected. Conversely, the statement that 'the difference was not statistically significant ($P = 0.10$)' means that the probability that a difference as large as the observed difference might arise if the treatment effects were the same was one in 10 and that the author will not accept this degree of chance as being sufficiently unlikely that the null hypothesis (that the treatment outcomes are the same) can be rejected. It is important to remember that 'not significant' means that a difference is not proven; it does not mean that there is no difference.

The acceptance of a significance level of 0.05 as the cut-off for rejecting the null hypothesis is a tradition based on the history of hypothesis testing and is not an absolute truth [3]. In 2016 the American Statistical Association issued a statement decrying the use of P less than 0.05 as the gatekeeper for determining the significance and worthiness for publication of scientific research. Their statement's six principles are shown in Box 17.8.

> **Box 17.8 Interpreting P-values**
>
> From the ASA statement of P-values: Context, Process, and Purpose:
> 1 P-values can indicate how incompatible the data are with a specified statistical model
> 2 P-values do not measure the probability that the studied hypothesis is true or the probability that the data were produced by random chance alone
> 3 Scientific conclusions and business or policy decisions should not be based only on whether a P-value passes a specific threshold
> 4 Proper inference requires full reporting and transparency
> 5 A P-value, or statistical significance, does not measure the size of an effect or the importance of a result.
> 6 By itself, a P-value does not provide a good measure of evidence regarding a model or hypothesis

Tests that do not meet the $P=0.05$ standard sometimes may be significant. For example, a trial of a new chemotherapeutic agent involving 30 randomised patients with metastatic melanoma produced a 5-year survival of seven of 15 patients treated with the new agent, and three out of 15 in control patients treated with conventional surgery, chemotherapy and radiation. Whereas the result does not achieve statistical significance when compared by χ^2 testing (see later section) (Yates corrected $\chi^2 = 1.35$; $P = 0.25$), the result is, nonetheless, potentially significant. If the therapy is beneficial and the estimated difference in response rates is the true difference in response rates, it may result in the saving of 2528 lives annually in the USA (based on 9480 deaths from melanoma annually and the improvement in survival in this hypothetical example). Because of the biological and clinical importance of the results suggested by the study, the treatment should be subjected to study in a larger patient population with more power to detect a difference, if one exists (see discussion of power later). Others might argue that the adherence to the 95% standard ($P=0.05$) should be relaxed in cases like this one. The potential benefit of the treatment may be revealed by the use of confidence intervals (see discussion of confidence intervals later).

Investigators should indicate what statistical procedures were utilised to compare results. Simply stating that the difference was statistically significant ($P<0.05$) does not constitute an adequate description of the statistics used. The exact procedure used (e.g. t-test or χ^2) and the results obtained must be specified. The t-test and the analysis of contingency tables (e.g. χ^2 and Fisher exact test) are the most commonly employed procedures and should be understood by all physicians.

The t-test

The t-test is the most commonly used statistical test in the biomedical literature. It is used to determine whether the difference in the means of two samples is from chance (sampling variation) alone. It should be emphasised that the t-test at a significance level of 0.05 is designed to compare the difference in the means of only two samples or populations. The t-test has additional important restrictions. It should be used to compare the means of interval data that are normally distributed. The data analysed by the t-test should be sufficiently large, should not contain outliers, should be statistically independent and the variability of the two treatment groups should be similar. In most instances a two-sided t-test is appropriate. When a one-sided t-test is performed the reasons should be specified. A two-sided test should be used when either treatment may be superior. A one-sided test is used when the authors are only interested in whether one treatment is better than the comparator [4].

The unpaired t-test should be used to analyse two different groups (e.g. patients receiving alternative treatments). The paired t-test should be used to analyse the effects of two different treatments on the same patients (e.g. in a cross-over or left–right comparison study).

Statistical analysis using the t-test can be illustrated using data from a study comparing calcipotriol and betamethasone ointments in the treatment of stable plaque psoriasis [5]. In this multicentre RCT, 201 and 200 patients were randomised to treatment with calcipotriol and betamethasone, respectively. Outcomes were measured by changes in PASI scores. At the end of 6 weeks of treatment the improvement (decrease) in PASI scores were 5.50 and 5.32 for calcipotriol and betamethasone, respectively. The statistical significance of the small difference in the change in PASI scores was evaluated using an unpaired t-test. The t value and corresponding significance level can be determined using computer programs or calculated using a t distribution table and the formula. Not surprisingly, the result indicated that the difference was not statistically significant ($P=0.76$). Thus, the trial failed to demonstrate a difference between the two treatments.

Misuse of the t-test was one of the most commonly encountered errors in the use of statistics found by Gore *et al.* in their review of the use of statistical methods in the *British Medical Journal* [6]. They found that 52% (32/62) of analytical reports that utilised statistical analyses contained at least one error in the use of statistics. Eleven of the errors were misuse of the t-test. The errors included using the t-test to analyse data that were not normally distributed or had different variability, and using an unpaired t-test to analyse paired data. Another commonly encountered error in the use of the t-test is its use to compare the means of more than two samples. This error in the use of the t-test occurred in 61% and 44%, respectively, of articles that used statistical analyses published in *Circulation Research* and *Circulation* in 1977 [7].

The t-test should not be used to analyse data that are skewed, or data in which the variability (standard deviation) is very different between treatment groups. Nor should it be used to analyse small data sets because it is impossible to verify that small data sets are normally distributed. In these situations, the Mann–Whitney U test, the distribution-free equivalent of the t-test, may be used for unpaired data, and the Wilcoxon test can be used for paired data. The t-test also should not be used to compare more than two groups because it ignores possible associations among groups and it increases the likelihood that spurious results will be obtained. Testing of the means of more than two groups can be performed with different forms of analysis of variance.

Table 17.4 Format of a four-fold contingency table.

	Good response	No or poor response	Total
Treatment A	a	b	H1
Treatment B	c	d	H2
Total	V1	V2	N

The χ^2 for unpaired data is calculated using the formulae:

$$\chi^2 \text{ (uncorrected)} = \frac{|a*d - b*c|^2 N}{H1*H2*V1*V2}$$

$$\chi^2 \text{ (Yates corrected)} = \frac{(|a*d - b*c| - 0.5*N)^2 N}{H1*H2*V1*V2}$$

in which $|a*d - b*c|$ indicates the absolute value of $a*d - b*c$.

Contingency tables

Chi-square is the most commonly used test to determine whether the categorical data in contingency tables differ because of chance alone. The format of a typical four-fold (2 × 2) contingency table is shown in Table 17.4. The numbers in the table (indicated by a, b, c and d) are the numbers of patients in each treatment group that fall into each outcome category. The assumption made to formulate the null hypothesis that the treatment outcomes are the same is that the overall response rate (i.e. the total number of patients with good responses divided by the total number of patients; V1/N in Table 17.4) is the same for both treatments. Chi-square is then used to determine how likely it is that the actual numbers observed could be obtained by chance or sampling variation if the response rate for the two treatments were the same. A continuity correction in the χ^2 is recommended to analyse smaller data sets (20–40 patients). This correction is used to account for the use of continuous curves to approximate the discrete frequencies in contingency tables. The Yates correction is most commonly used (Table 17.4). Chi-square should not be used to analyse small trials (trials with fewer than 20 patients) or when the predicted number of patients in any cell (positions a, b, c or d in Table 17.4) is fewer than five. In those circumstances, the Fisher exact test should be performed. Chi-square is used to analyse unpaired data and the McNemar test is used to analyse paired contingency table data. Contingency table analyses can be easily modified and used to compare more than two treatments and more than two outcomes.

Like the t-test, the χ^2 test is frequently used incorrectly in published clinical trials. In their analysis of the use of statistics in medical papers published in the *British Medical Journal*, Gore et al. found that χ^2 was used incorrectly in 12 of 62 published papers [6]. The errors included omission of the continuity correction for studies with few patients, omission of clearly stated hypotheses to be tested, lack of consideration of degrees of freedom and misuse of the test to study paired data.

Confidence intervals

Standard statistical hypothesis testing generally results in a determination of a P value that is the probability that a difference as large as the observed difference might arise by chance. If this probability is equal to or less than a predetermined 'critical value' (usually 0.05), the null hypothesis is rejected and the difference is considered statistically significant. If the P value exceeds the predetermined value, the null hypothesis is not rejected and the difference is considered not statistically significant. This dichotomous treatment of the results of clinical trials as being significant or not significant sometimes may be misleading and may hide meaningful estimates in the differences between the treatments. What matters most in a therapeutic trial is whether investigators have been able to detect a medically significant difference in treatments and how large the difference is likely to be. The conventional significance levels are useful guides to the interpretation of trial results but they should not be considered strict rules. The absurdity of the dichotomous significance testing approach is best appreciated by considering two trials, one of which has a P value of 0.05 and the other a P value of 0.06. The difference in the level of significance is very small, yet the former is considered statistically significant and the latter is not.

Reporting results with confidence intervals is an alternative or complementary way to present the results of clinical trials. Many believe it is far preferable. In simple terms, the reported result provides the best estimate of the treatment effect and the confidence interval provides a range of values in which the 'population' or true response to treatment lies. If the trial is repeated many times, 95% of the confidence intervals produced will contain the true or population mean response to treatment. The population or true mean has only a one in 20 chance of falling outside the 95% confidence interval. The true response rate will most probably lie near the middle of the confidence interval and will rarely be found at or near the ends of the interval. If the 95% confidence intervals around two means or medians do not overlap, you can be confident at the 95% level that the two population means or medians, from which the samples were drawn, are different.

The confidence interval provides a direct, numerical measurement of the imprecision of the estimate of the response to treatment that is due to sampling variability. The width of the confidence interval is determined by the sample size (the larger the sample, the narrower the interval), the variability of the response being measured (the larger the variability, the wider the interval) and the degree of confidence desired (the higher the confidence desired, the wider the interval) (Figure 17.8). Confidence intervals can be determined for means and their differences, and for proportions and their differences by looking them up in tables, by calculating them with formulae or by using computer software. In comparative studies, confidence intervals should be reported for the differences between groups, not for the results of each group separately.

There is a close relationship between the results of a test of a hypothesis and the associated confidence interval; if the difference between treatments is significant at the 5% level, then the associated 95% confidence interval excludes the zero difference. The advantage of using confidence intervals instead of, or in addition to, P values is that confidence intervals provide an indication of the size of the differences in treatments and give numerical measurements of the inexactness in our knowledge of the real differences in treatments.

Confidence intervals can be valuable in interpreting data from trials in which the difference is not statistically significant (i.e. the P value is greater than 0.05). To determine whether a treatment effect may have been missed in a study reporting negative results one should look at the upper boundary of the 95% confidence interval. If this value would be clinically important if it were the

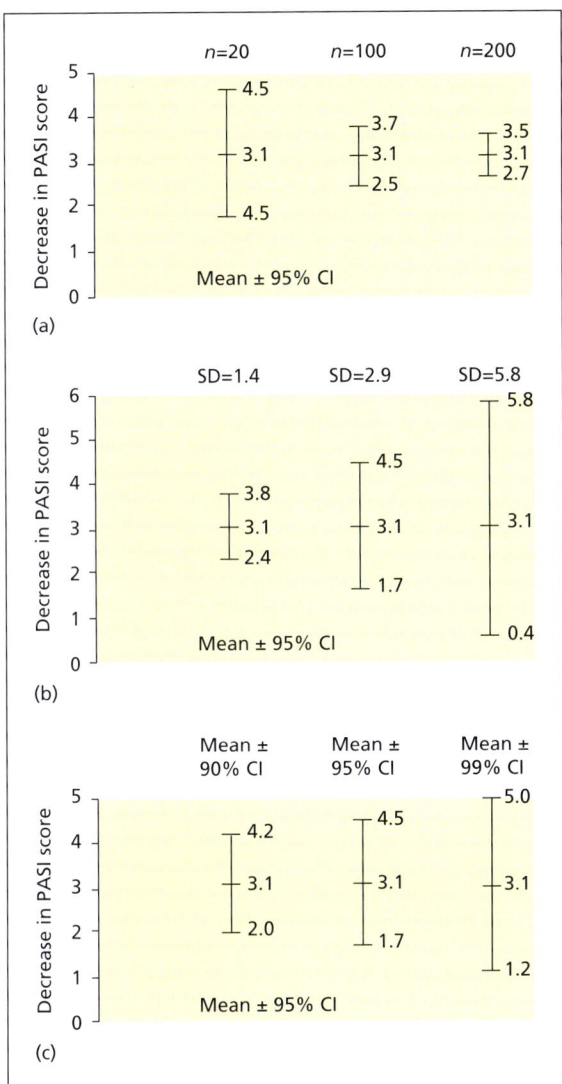

Figure 17.8 The effects of (a) sample size, (b) variability and (c) desired confidence level on confidence intervals (CIs). (a) The mean change in psoriasis area and severity index (PASI) score was 3.1 with a standard deviation (SD) of 2.9. The 95% CI is shown and narrows as the number of patients studied increases from 20 to 200. (b) The mean change in the PASI score of 20 patients was 3.1. The 95% CI is shown and widens as the sample variability (SD) increases. (c) The mean change in the PASI score of 20 patients was 3.1 with an SD of 2.9. The CI widens as the degree of confidence desired increases from 90% to 99%.

true response, then an important treatment effect may have been missed in the study. In the calcipotriol and betamethasone trial as an example, the upper boundary of the difference in PASI scores was 0.78. This difference in PASI scores would be unlikely to have much clinical significance and therefore it is unlikely that a significant treatment advantage for calcipotriol was missed in this study.

In contrast, consider our hypothetical new treatment for metastatic melanoma that had a cure rate of 7/15 versus 3/15 for conventional treatment. The cure rate for the new treatment and conventional treatment were 47% and 20% respectively, and the difference between them was 27%. The 95% interval for the difference in proportions was –10% to 51%. The upper boundary of the difference in cure rates was 51%. This difference would clearly have a significant impact on the treatment of patients with metastatic melanoma and, therefore, a significant treatment advance may have been missed in this study. Also note that the 95% confidence interval of the difference in proportions does not exclude the zero difference; therefore, we cannot be 95% certain that the response rates of the two treatments are different.

Confidence intervals may also be useful in interpreting the response to a single treatment. Ninety-five per cent confidence intervals for the response rate of a single treatment can be determined using formulae, tables, nomograms and computer programs. For example, suppose a physician treated 20 patients with lichen planus with metronidazole and found that 12 (60%) had an excellent response. The confidence interval for this response rate ranges from 36% to 81%. Thus the true overall response rate might well be substantially less (or more) than the physician concludes from personal experience. An important point can be made from determining the confidence interval of a single proportion. There is a degree of uncertainty in reported response rates that can be expressed in exact numerical terms by determining the confidence interval.

Confidence intervals may also be useful in interpreting the rate of side effects observed in a clinical trial. For example, in the calcipotriol study 40 out of 201 patients (20%) treated with calcipotriol developed lesional or perilesional irritation. The 95% confidence interval for this adverse reaction would be 14–26%. Thus a high rate of local irritation can be anticipated with calcipotriol and the rate may be as high as 26%. If no untoward reactions occur in a study, it is still possible to determine the 95% confidence interval of adverse reactions. Accurate upper 95% limits of the reaction rate can be obtained by referring to available tables. If the number exposed is at least 30, a reasonable approximation of the 95% confidence limit of the rate of adverse reactions can be obtained by dividing three by the number of patients that were exposed to the studied treatment. For example if no events occur in 100 exposed patients, the upper 95% confidence interval is 3/100 or 0.03 [8].

Power

Significant differences in treatment effects in comparison trials may be missed if the number of subjects tested is small. For example, in a 1978 survey of 71 published trials with negative results, Freiman et al. found that a 25% or 50% improvement in outcome might have been missed in 57 (80%) and 34 (48%) of the studies, respectively [9]. The importance of this observation and the importance of determining the power of studies to detect clinically significant differences in treatments are illustrated by the fact that this study has been cited more than 700 times. In spite of the recognition of the importance of power, a follow-up study conducted by Moher et al. in 1994 indicated that 25% or 50% improvements in outcome might have been missed in 84% and 64% of 102 negative studies, respectively [10].

Power is an expression of the ability of a trial to detect a difference in treatments if one exists. The investigators in a well-designed clinical trial should have an estimate or prediction of the anticipated differences between treatments, and a knowledge of the magnitude of differences that would be clinically important. The trial should then be designed to enrol a sufficient number of patients to ensure with reasonable certainty that a statistically significant difference would be obtained if the anticipated or clinically important differences between the treatments existed. The error of believing that there are no differences between treatments, when in fact there are differences, is a Type II or β error.

The power of a trial to detect a significant difference is determined by the response rates of the treatments, the significance level desired by the investigators and the number of patients treated. The power of a trial to detect differences between treatments can be calculated using formulae, nomograms, programmable calculators or computer software. Conventionally, a power of 80% with a significance level of 0.05 is considered adequate. The choice of a power of 80% means that, if the anticipated or clinically important difference in treatments really exists, four of five trials with the specified number of patients in the treatment groups will show a statistically significant difference. However, a higher power sometimes may be desirable. For example, increasing the power to 90% means that nine out of 10 trials would detect a statistically significant difference between treatments if the difference really exists. The power of a study design to detect clinically significant differences in treatments is best considered before the trial is initiated. However, studies that fail to demonstrate statistically significant differences among treatments should always include a discussion of power.

The sample size needed to detect a difference is small when the difference in treatments is large. Conversely, the sample size needed to detect differences is large when the difference in treatments is small or when the response rate of the comparison treatment is high.

As noted by Moher *et al.* [10]

If a trial with negative results has a sufficient sample size to detect a clinically important effect, then the negative results are interpretable – the treatment did not have an effect at least as large as the effect considered to be clinically relevant. If a trial with negative results has insufficient power, a clinically important but statistically insignificant effect is usually ignored or, worse, is taken to mean that the treatment under study made no difference. Thus, there are important scientific reasons to report sample size and/or power calculations.

The importance of statistical analyses must be kept in proper perspective. Statistics are a tool for trying to ensure that results of clinical trials are not due to chance or sampling variation alone. The combination of hypothesis testing and the use of confidence intervals give a measure of the likelihood that results of a trial are due to chance and the precision of the estimated difference in treatments, respectively. Statistical analyses cannot tell you the medical significance of differences in treatments. In other words, statistically significant should not, and cannot, be equated with medically significant. Conversely, a trial whose results indicate that the difference in treatments was not statistically significant does not necessarily mean that there is not a medically important difference between treatments. It may simply mean that too few patients were used to detect the difference that does exist.

Shortcut method for appraising clinical research papers

The EBM criteria for appraising evidence represent subsets of other schemes for appraising the quality of clinical research [1]. These methods include reporting guidelines and their extensions such as CONSORT for clinical trials [11], PRISMA for systematic reviews, STARD for diagnostic test accuracy studies and STROBE for observational studies all of which are available and updated

Table 17.5 Shortcut method for evaluating clinical research papers.

Step	Comments
Read title	If interesting, continue
Read abstract	If still worthy of your time, continue
Look at the figures and tables	Find the most important data. Are the data adequately reported? Is there a control group? Are the outcomes clinically important? Are the data subjected to statistical testing and are the tests used correctly? If still worthy of your time, continue
Read the results	Are complications reported? Are compliance and lost patients considered? Ask yourself 'If everything the authors say is true, is it important for my patients, my practice or for the field of dermatology?' If 'no', stop reading; if 'yes or possibly', continue
Read the methods	How were the patients chosen and allocated? Are the outcomes clearly defined and assessed blindly? Are the conclusions valid? If yes, continue
Record the citation	Note the authors, citation and conclusions of the study for easy retrieval later
Read the discussion	If you have time
Read the introduction	The last sentence in the introduction should contain a clear statement on why the study was needed

on the EQUATOR (Enhancing the QUAlity and Transparency Of health Research website (https://www.equator-network.org/; last accessed February 2022). Other specific tools for assessing study quality such as AMSTAR for systematic reviews and QUADAS for diagnostic test accuracy studies have already been mentioned. What is common to all of these methods is that they require the entire paper to be read, especially the methods section. Doing so is often not possible for busy clinicians trying to find answers to specific problems. Nor is it the most efficient use of his or her time. Instead, a shortcut method for evaluating the literature is available (Table 17.5). A shortcut method to evaluate clinical trials will enable you to use your time efficiently. It allows you to decide not to read the majority of poorly conceived, designed, executed or reported trials and those trials with insignificant results. After each step you should re-ask the questions, 'Am I still interested in this trial?' and 'Is it worth spending my valuable time on it?'

First read the title. If the title holds interest for you, read the abstract. If after reading the abstract you still feel that the article is worthy of your time, look at the figures and tables. Authors generally display their best or most convincing data in these. In a well-written study, you should be able see the important results in summary figures and tables. Try to pick out the one or two figures or tables that hold the most important data. Look at the data to see whether they are summarised and displayed correctly. Determine whether there is an appropriate control group, whether the outcomes are clinically and biologically important, whether the data are subjected to statistical analysis and whether the correct statistical methods were used. *It is important that you examine and assess the data yourself.* If you are still convinced that the article is worthy of your time, read the results. Determine whether complications are reported, and whether compliance and lost patients were considered. After reading the results, ask yourself the question, 'If everything the authors say is true, is it important for my patients, for my practice or for dermatology as a whole?' If the answer is an emphatic 'no', stop reading; if 'yes or possibly', continue to the methods.

While reading the methods pay particular attention to the features that strengthen clinical trials and help validate their conclusions. In particular, determine the eligibility criteria, whether patients were randomly allocated and whether the outcome is clearly defined and assessed masked. Make an effort to find out who paid for the study and whether all possible conflicts of interest were declared [12]. If your conclusion is that the trial was conducted in a reasonable manner and the conclusions are valid, then make some notation of who the authors are and the conclusions of the study. Several software packages for cataloguing and managing references are available for most computer platforms (e.g. EndNote® and Reference Manager®). Finally, if you still have time and interest, read the discussion and introduction, in that order.

Key references

The full list of references can be found in the online version at https://www.wiley.com/rooksdermatology10e

Evidence-based medicine

2 Bigby M, Corona R, Szklo M. Evidence-based medicine. In: Goldsmith LA, Katz SI, Gilchrest BA, Paller A, Leffell DJ, Wolff K, eds. *Fitzpatrick's Dermatology in General Medicine*, 8th edn. Columbus, OH: McGraw-Hill, 2012:9–15.

4 Cochrane A. *Effectiveness and Efficiency. Random Reflections on Health Services*. London: Nuffield Provincial Hospital Trust, 1972.

5 Sackett DL, Haynes RB, Guyatt GH, Tugwell P. *Clinical Epidemiology: A Basic Science for Clinical Medicine*. Boston: Little, Brown and Company, 1991.

7 Sackett DL, Rosenberg WM, Gray JA, Haynes RB, Richardson WS. Evidence based medicine: what it is and what it isn't. *BMJ* 1996;312:71–2.

12 Williams HC. Dowling Oration 2001. Evidence-based dermatology – a bridge too far? *Clin Exp Dermatol* 2001;26:714–24.

16 Bigby M, Stern RS, Bigby J. An evaluation of method reporting and use in clinical trials in dermatology. *Arch Dermatol* 1985;121:1394–9.

22 Lexchin J, Bero LA, Djulbegovic B, Clark O. Pharmaceutical industry sponsorship and research outcome and quality: systematic review. *BMJ* 2003;326:1167–70.

Formulating questions and finding evidence

1 Bigby M, Rzany B. Formulating well built clinical questions. In: Williams HC, Bigby M, Herxheimer A *et al.*, eds. *Evidence-based Dermatology*, 3rd edn. London: Wiley-Blackwell and BMJ Books, 2014:25–7.

2 Guyatt G, Drummond R, Meade M, Cook D. *The Evidence Based Medicine Working Group Users' Guides to the Medical Literature*, 2nd edn. Chicago: McGraw-Hill, 2008:17–28.

4 Bigby M, Corona R, Szklo M. Evidence-based medicine. In: Goldsmith LA, Katz SI, Gilchrest BA, Paller A, Leffell DJ, Wolff K, eds. *Fitzpatrick's Dermatology in General Medicine*, 8th edn. Columbus, OH: McGraw-Hill, 2012:9–15.

8 Lau J, Ionnidis JPA, Schmid CH. Summing up evidence: one answer is not always enough. *Lancet* 1998;351:123–7.

13 Kunz R, Oxman AD. The unpredictability paradox: review of empirical comparisons of randomised and non-randomised clinical trials. *BMJ* 1998;317:1185–90.

14 Benson K, Hartz AJ. A comparison of observational studies and randomized, controlled trials. *N Engl J Med* 2000;342:1878–86.

16 Williams HC, Dellavalle RP. The growth of clinical trials and systematic reviews in informing dermatological patient care. *J Invest Dermatol* 2012;132:1008–17.

23 Greenhalgh T. *How to Read a Paper: The Basics of Evidence Based Medicine*, 5th edn. London: BMJ Publishing Group, 1997.

Critically appraising evidence and applying it to individual patients

1 Bigby M, Corona R, Szklo M. Evidence-based medicine. In: Goldsmith LA, Katz SI, Gilchrest BA, Paller A, Leffell DJ, Wolff K, eds. *Fitzpatrick's Dermatology in General Medicine*, 8th edn. Columbus, OH: McGraw-Hill, 2012:9–15.

2 Bigby M. Understanding and evaluating systematic reviews. *Indian J Dermatol* 2014;59:134–9.

4 Egger M, Smith GD, Sterne JA. Uses and abuses of meta-analysis. *Clin Med* 2001;1:478–84.

18 Schriger DL, Altman DG, Vetter JA, Heafner T, Moher D. Forest plots in reports of systematic reviews: a cross-sectional study reviewing current practice. *Int J Epidemiol* 2010;39:421–9.

26 Bigby M, Gadenne A-S. Understanding and evaluating clinical trials. *J Am Acad Dermatol* 1996;34:555–90.

27 Williams HC. How to critically appraise a randomized controlled trial. In: Williams HC, Bigby M, Herxheimer A *et al.*, eds. *Evidence-based Dermatology*, 3rd edn. London: Wiley-Blackwell and BMJ Books, 2014:39–45.

30 Fergusson D, Aaron SD, Guyatt G, Hebert P. Post-randomisation exclusions: the intention to treat principle and excluding patients from analysis. *BMJ* 2002;325:652–4.

36 Freiman JA, Chalmers TC, Smith JH, Kuebler RR. The importance of beta, the type II error and sample size in the design and interpretation of the randomized control trial. *N Eng J Med* 1978;299:690–4.

37 Moher D, Dulberg CS, Wells GA. Statistical power, sample size, and their reporting in randomized controlled trials. *JAMA* 1994;272:122–4.

Evaluating the data in clinical research papers and a shortcut method for reading clinical research papers

1 Bigby M, Gadenne A-S. Understanding and evaluating clinical trials. *J Am Acad Dermatol* 1996;34:555–90.

2 Moher D, Liberati A, Tetzlaff J, Altman DG, PRISMA Group. *Preferred Reporting Items for Systematic Reviews and Meta-Analyses: the PRISMA Statement. BMJ* 2009;339:b2535.

6 Gore SM, Jones IG, Rytter EC. Misuse of statistical methods: critical assessment of articles in BMJ from January to March 1976. *BMJ* 1977;1(6053):85–7.

7 Glantz SA. Current topics biostatistics: how to detect, correct and prevent errors in the medical literature. *Circulation* 1980;61:1–7.

9 Freiman JA, Chalmers TC, Smith J *et al.* The importance of beta, the Type II error and sample size in the design and interpretation of the randomized control trial. *N Eng J Med* 1978;299:690–4.

10 Moher D, Dulberg CS, Wells GA. Statistical power, sample size, and their reporting in randomized controlled trials. *JAMA* 1994;272:122–4.

11 Moher D, Hopewell S, Schulz KF *et al.* CONSORT 2010 explanation and elaboration: updated guidelines for reporting parallel group randomised trials. *BMJ* 2010;340:c869.

12 Williams HC, Naldi L, Paul C, Vahlquist A, Schroter S, Jobling R. Conflicts of interest in dermatology. *Acta Derm Venereol* 2006;86:485–97.

CHAPTER 18

Principles of Topical Therapy

Deirdre A. Buckley
Department of Dermatology, Sulis Hospital, Bath, UK

Introduction, 18.1	Preservatives, 18.8	Vitamin D analogues (deltanoids, secosteroids), 18.26
Prescribing topical treatment, 18.1	Antioxidants, 18.8	Cytotoxic and antineoplastic agents, 18.29
Drug concentration, 18.1	**Topical treatments used in the management of skin disease, 18.8**	Depigmenting agents, 18.31
Choice of vehicle, 18.2		Depilatories, 18.33
Quantity to be applied, 18.3	Emollients, 18.8	Sensitising agents, 18.33
Advice to patients, 18.4	Astringents, 18.9	Sunscreens, 18.34
Hazards associated with topical treatment, 18.4	Antiseptics, 18.9	Tars, 18.36
Formulation of topical medicaments, 18.5	Antibiotics, 18.10	Antiperspirants, 18.37
Lipids, 18.6	Antifungal agents, 18.12	Dyes, 18.38
Polyethylene glycols, 18.7	Antiviral agents, 18.13	Other traditional remedies, 18.38
Emulsifiers, 18.7	Antiparasitic agents, 18.13	Miscellaneous agents, 18.39
Humectants, 18.7	Topical glucocorticoids, 18.14	
Penetration enhancers, 18.7	Calcineurin inhibitors, 18.22	**Key references, 18.42**
Powders, 18.8	Retinoids, 18.23	

Introduction

Dermatologists have the good fortune to work on the most accessible organ of the body. This greatly facilitates not only the diagnosis but also the treatment of skin disease. Whilst systemic administration of drugs is often necessary in dermatology, many inflammatory and neoplastic conditions can be effectively managed using the wide range of locally applied physical or pharmacological modalities that are available. The latter are the subject of this chapter, which reviews the pharmacological treatments used topically, that is, by application to the surface of the skin. Some of these are time-honoured treatments that have been used for a century or more, whilst others belong to the ever-expanding range of newer and increasingly sophisticated agents constantly being developed and formulated for topical use.

Topical treatment offers the potential to achieve high concentrations of a drug in the skin with minimal exposure of other organs. This can greatly increase efficacy and also safety relative to systemic administration. When side effects do occur, they are most likely to take the form of localised reactions.

Prescribing topical treatment

Prescribing topical medication requires careful consideration of several factors if optimal results are to be achieved. The concentration of the drug, the vehicle and the frequency of application must be specified. In order to improve both compliance and efficacy, the patient requires advice on the quantity to be used, precisely where it should be applied and often further explanation about precise timing of application in relation to bathing and other treatments. The prescriber needs to be aware of the hazards associated with a topical treatment, particularly the likelihood of the medication inducing irritant or allergic reactions. It is also important to understand the factors that influence systemic absorption.

Drug concentration

The most used conventions for defining the concentration of a drug in a topical formulation are as follows:
- The concentration is usually written as a percentage representing the proportion of the formulation, by weight, that is the active constituent. A concentration of 1% indicates that 1 g of drug will be contained in 100 g of the formulation. For example, an over-the-counter treatment for plantar warts contains 50% salicylic acid, whereas calcitriol ointment is used at a concentration of 0.0003% in the treatment of psoriasis. A very low concentration such as this is more often written as 3 µg/g.
- A frequently used alternative, especially for liquid preparations, is to express the percentage of the drug as a proportion of the volume of the formulation, thus a 1% solution contains 1 g of drug in 100 mL of the formulation. The abbreviations w/w (weight in weight) and w/v (weight in volume) are often employed to indicate which convention is being used.

Rook's Textbook of Dermatology, Tenth Edition. Edited by Christopher Griffiths, Jonathan Barker, Tanya Bleiker, Walayat Hussain and Rosalind Simpson.
© 2024 John Wiley & Sons Ltd. Published 2024 by John Wiley & Sons Ltd.

- The concentration of a drug in solution is often denoted in 'parts', thus a 1 part in 10 000 solution of potassium permanganate contains 0.1 g in 1 L of solution, which could be expressed as 0.01% (w/v), equivalent to a 400 mg potassium permanganate tablet dissolved in 4 L of water, a treatment used frequently as a soak for malodorous leg ulcers.

The efficacy of a topically applied drug may not always be proportionate to the concentration, as the site of application, patient's age, skin thickness, volumes used, frequency of application, use of occlusion and the nature of the skin disease will all influence efficacy.

Choice of vehicle

Topical medication must be applied to the skin in a suitable vehicle. This term encompasses all the constituents of the formulation apart from the active pharmaceutical agent. The choice of vehicle depends on the anatomical site to be treated and the condition of the skin. As a rule, acutely inflamed skin is best treated with fairly bland preparations that are least likely to irritate. Moist or exudative eruptions are conventionally treated with 'wet' medications such as lotions or creams, whilst dry skin responds well to the occlusive action of ointments. Hair-bearing skin, especially the scalp, can be treated with medicaments formulated into shampoos, lotions, gels or mousses. The cosmetic properties of the vehicle assume particular importance when treating the face. Oily skin affected by acne is often best treated with lotions or gels, whilst the more sensitive skin affected by rosacea may benefit from the emollient effect of a cream. The physical properties of some types of vehicle are summarised here. Examples given are of non-proprietary preparations, but the principles discussed apply equally to proprietary products, to the formulation of which manufacturers will often devote considerable developmental effort.

Ointments. Ointments are semi-solid vehicles composed of lipid, such as white soft paraffin BP (petrolatum). They have useful occlusive and emollient properties. Some ointments contain emulsifying agents such as polyhydric alcohols (macrogols, polyethylene glycol) or cetostearyl (cetearyl) alcohol (e.g. emulsifying ointment BP). The latter have the advantage of being less greasy, with good solvent properties, and they are easily washed off. Ointments require fewer preservatives than other vehicles since they contain no water and do not sustain the growth of microorganisms.

Creams. These are semi-solid emulsions (i.e. suspensions), either of lipid droplets in water or water droplets in lipid. Aqueous creams, for example aqueous cream BP, are suspensions of lipid droplets in water. These are water miscible, cooling and soothing, and are well absorbed into the skin. Water-in-oil creams, for example oily cream BP, are suspensions of water droplets in lipid. These are immiscible with water and more difficult to wash off. They are emollient, lubricant and mildly occlusive (but less so than ointments).

Pastes. Pastes are semi-solid preparations containing a high proportion of finely powdered material such as zinc oxide or starch. Protective (fatty) pastes are greasy and therefore messy and water insoluble. They are difficult to apply and remove, but their stiffness permits accurate localisation of the paste and any constituent medication. They are occlusive, protective and hydrating. The consistency of these pastes can be 'softened' by adding oils or 'hardened' with hard paraffin. Dithranol is prepared in Lassar paste (zinc oxide 24%, salicylic acid 2%, starch 24%, white soft paraffin 50%) at specialist manufacturing pharmacy units at various concentrations to localise dithranol on plaques of psoriasis and avoid getting it on unaffected skin. Drying pastes, also called cooling pastes, are mixtures of powder with liquid. These are non-greasy, water miscible and easy to apply and remove. They are drying and soothing, and can be used in conjunction with dressings as paste bandages or as vehicles for active medicaments. Bandages impregnated with 10% zinc oxide paste mixed with glycerol, oil and water are commonly used on the limbs for the treatment of atopic prurigo and stasis dermatitis.

Lotions. These are liquid formulations that are usually simple suspensions or solutions of medication in water, alcohol or other liquids. Those containing alcohol often sting, especially when applied to broken skin. When left on the skin, the liquid will evaporate, leaving a film of medication on the surface. Lotions are a useful way of delivering topical steroid to scalp skin or to very hirsute skin on the trunk and limbs.

Gels. Gels can be regarded as thickened lotions. They are semi-solid preparations containing high-molecular-weight polymers, such as carboxypolymethylene (carbomer BP) or methylcellulose. Gels are also especially suitable for treating the scalp and other hairy areas of skin. Like lotions, gels tend to dry when left on the skin. Gels are particularly useful for frequent application during the working day in hand dermatitis, where compliance is greatly aided by their non-greasy texture.

Powders. Those applied directly to the skin are also known as *dusting powders*. They can reduce friction (talc) or excessive moisture (starch). They are occasionally used to deliver drugs such as antifungal agents applied to the feet.

Paints. Paints are liquid preparations, either aqueous, hydro-alcoholic or alcoholic (*tinctures*), which are usually applied with a brush to the skin or mucous membranes and then evaporate. Collodion preparations are also sometimes referred to as paints.

Collodions. Collodions, for example flexible collodion BP, are liquid preparations consisting of cellulose nitrate in organic solvent. They evaporate rapidly to leave a flexible film that can hold medicaments in contact with the skin. They are most frequently used to apply salicylic and lactic acids to warts. Another example is a topical preparation used for actinic keratoses containing 5 mg/g of fluorouracil and 100 mg/g of salicylic acid. Collodions may also be used as protectives to seal minor cuts and abrasions. They are easy to apply and water repellent, but inflammable.

Microsponges. These use porous beads, typically 10–25 μm in diameter, to form a reservoir loaded with the drug, enhancing drug penetration, sustaining its release, reducing irritation and prolonging shelf-life without requiring the use of preservatives. This approach has been used for cosmetics and sunscreens as well as topical medications such as benzoyl peroxide, imidazole antifungals, terbinafine, mupirocin, mometasone furoate, aciclovir and hydroquinone/retinoid combinations [1].

Liposomes. Liposomes are structures comprising an aqueous phase surrounded by a lipid capsule, ranging widely in diameter from several nanometers to several microns. They may contain several lipid layers so that the structure can be likened to that of an onion. Liposomes can be used to encapsulate a wide range of active pharmaceuticals. Used in this way, liposomes may be regarded as 'penetration-enhancing agents'. This technology is used in cosmetics more frequently than in dermatological treatment. However, liposomes can be useful for reducing irritation from topical use of agents including imidazole antifungals, can increase the penetration of topical steroids in atopic eczema and can improve delivery of topical minoxidil to scalp hair follicles [2].

Frequency of application. The frequency of application must be specified in order to maximise the response whilst avoiding side effects such as irritation. Excessive frequency of application may also result in unnecessary systemic exposure to the drug. Active preparations are usually applied just once or twice a day. As a general rule, twice-daily application of drugs such as corticosteroids is only marginally more effective than once-daily application, whilst requiring double the amount of medication and increasing both systemic exposure to the drug and cost. The pharmacological actions of a drug may persist long after it has left the surface of the skin. Thus the ability of a potent topical corticosteroid to inhibit flares of atopic eczema when applied just twice weekly [3] seems unlikely to be explained simply by the persistence of a reservoir of the drug. Increasing the interval between applications can be a useful method of gradually reducing the intensity of a treatment, especially when it is difficult to do so by using a lower concentration or less potent agent. Emollients should be applied frequently enough to maintain their physical effect. This may require several applications daily, something which must be clearly explained to patients. Patient use of emollients is often far less than recommended by the prescriber [4].

Quantity to be applied

The total quantity to be dispensed should be specified when prescribing, and it is helpful to inform the patient how long the prescribed quantity is expected to last. Patients routinely overinterpret the advice on the package inserts provided with their medication to apply topical steroids 'sparingly'. Minute quantities are rarely effective. Conversely, inappropriate use of active medicaments as emollients is not only wasteful but often hazardous. The potential for systemic absorption must be taken into account when prescribing, for example, topical corticosteroids or salicylic acid.

The quantity of cream or ointment required for 1 week of once-daily application to the whole body is approximately 140 g for males and 120 g for females, and for twice-daily application male and female patients require 280 g and 240 g per week, respectively.

Table 18.1 provides the approximate quantities required for single applications to specific anatomical regions. Table 18.2 provides a guide to total quantities required for a week of twice-daily total body treatment for children of various ages. All these guidelines can only be approximate and should be interpreted very flexibly. In addition to the obvious large differences between individuals of any age in body surface area, the condition of the skin may influence how far the medication will spread. Creams and ointments seem to cover a very similar area per unit of weight [5].

Simple, approximate, but practical guides to the quantity of a topical medication to apply are provided by the fingertip unit and the rule of hand:
- *Fingertip unit* [6]. An approximate but practical measure of topical medication is the quantity of ointment or cream, extruded from a tube with a nozzle of 5 mm diameter (note that nozzles do vary somewhat), extending from the distal crease of the forefinger to the ventral aspect of the fingertip (Figure 18.1). This unit weighs approximately 0.49 g in males and 0.43 g in females [7] and covers, on average, an area of approximately 300 cm^2. The number of units required for a single treatment of each anatomical region in adults and children of various ages is given in Table 18.3.
- The *rule of hand* states that an area of the size that can be covered by four adult hands (including the digits) can be treated by 1 g of ointment or 2 fingertip units [8].

The figures discussed are all based on the application of active medicaments. Emollients are applied for their physical properties

Table 18.1 Approximate quantities required for one topical application of cream or ointment medication to different anatomical regions.

	Quantity of medication (g)	
Region	Males	Females
Trunk (including buttocks)	6.6	5.8
One leg (groin to ankle)	2.9	2.5
One foot	0.9	0.7
One arm and forearm	1.7	1.3
One hand	0.6	0.5
Face, neck and ears	1.3	0.9
Whole body	20	17

Adapted from Long and Finlay 1991 [6] with permission of John Wiley & Sons.

Table 18.2 Quantities of medication required for twice-daily topical application of cream or ointment to the entire body at various ages in childhood.

	Age										
	3 months	6 months	12 months	18 months	2 years	3 years	4 years	5 years	7 years	10 years	12 years
Daily requirement (g)	8	10	12	13	14	16	19	20	25	30	37
Weekly requirement (g)	56	67	84	93	95	112	135	140	172	210	256

Adapted from Long et al. 1998 [9] with permission of John Wiley & Sons.

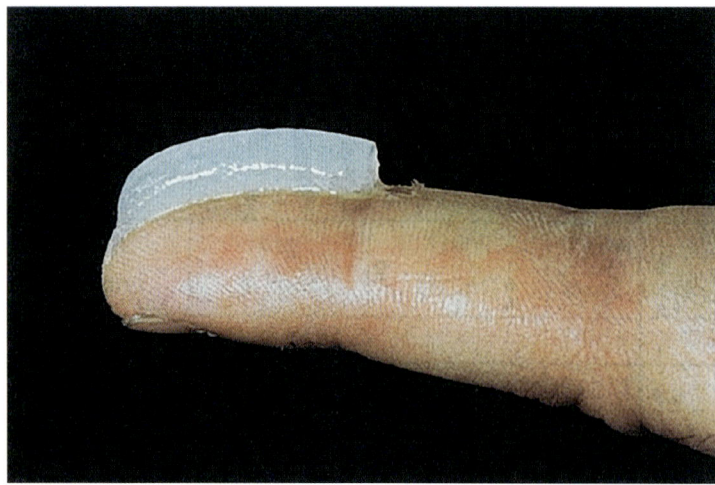

Figure 18.1 The fingertip unit.

rather than for the delivery of a drug, and are generally used much more liberally. Emollient treatment of the whole body may require 100 g daily when the skin is very dry.

Advice to patients

Detailed instructions are often required as to the timing of applications. In many cases it is most convenient to apply the medication immediately after bathing. If other topical treatments are in use it is important to explain how the applications should be timed relative to each other. For example, the application of an emollient immediately after the application of an active agent may dilute the active medication and might spread it over areas of skin where it is not required. In practice, for topical corticosteroids, this does not appear to cause any loss of efficacy. For medications with a tendency to induce irritation it is helpful to warn patients about this in advance.

If it is planned to use any form of occlusion, bandaging or other dressing with topically applied medication, detailed instruction is required and this should ideally take the form of a demonstration by a trained nurse, or by watching a training video. The simplest method of occlusion is the use of polythene gloves on the hands or plastic food-wrapping film (cling film) on the feet or limbs. Self-adhesive hydrocolloid dressings can be very useful for limited areas on the limbs or trunk. 'Wet wrap' bandaging is described in the treatment of atopic eczema (Chapter 41). Various additional types of bandaging (e.g. paste bandages) can be used to increase the penetration of topical medication and have the added benefit of protection from scratching.

When self-treatment fails, the efficacy of topical therapy can almost invariably be improved if the treatment can be applied by specialist nurses in an out-patient clinic. Many dermatology departments are able to provide this service for patients with severe skin disease who are able to attend on a daily basis. The response to treatment is improved even further by admission to hospital for a period of rest and regular, supervised treatment.

Hazards associated with topical treatment

The most frequent adverse effects associated with topical medication are localised irritant or allergic reactions. Irritant reactions, most commonly seen with antiacne preparations such as retinoids and benzoyl peroxide, can be minimised by applying treatment at the optimal concentration and treatment intervals and by selection of the correct vehicle. Irritation is frequent when topical emollient lotions containing antiseptics such as benzalkonium chloride and chlorhexidine are used as a leave-on product at flexural sites, particularly in elderly patients. Many photodamaged elderly patients develop irritant reactions to topical diclofenac gel used for actinic keratoses.

Table 18.3 Fingertip units required for a single treatment of various regions in children and adults. Note that the unit is measured using an adult finger.

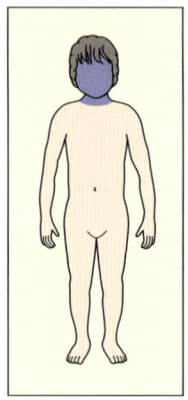 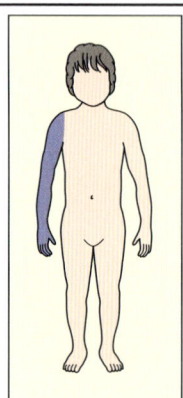 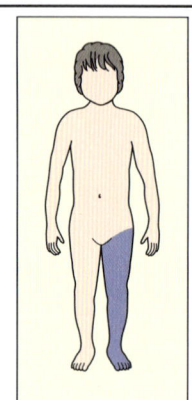 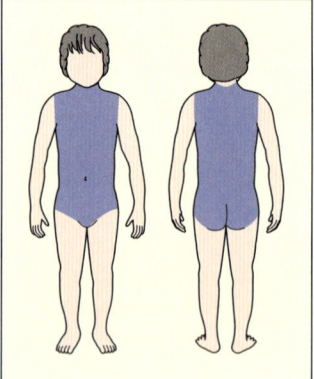 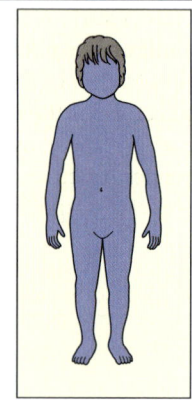

Age	Face and neck	One upper limb	One lower limb	Trunk (including buttocks)	Whole body
3–6 months	1	1	1.5	2.5	8.5
1–2 years	1.5	1.5	2	5	13.5
3–5 years	1.5	2	3	6.5	18
6–10 years	2	2.5	4.5	8.5	24.5
Adult	2.5	4.5	7.6	13.5	40

Adapted from Long and Finlay 1991 [6] and Long et al. 1998 [9] with permission of John Wiley & Sons.

Allergic sensitisation is more difficult to anticipate and to prevent. Contact allergy can develop not only to the active medicament (e.g. corticosteroid molecules or antibiotics) but also to preservatives, added fragrances or constituents of the vehicle. Almost any component may sensitise and notable examples include corticosteroids [1], antibiotics [2], topical anaesthetics [3], cetearyl alcohol [4], *Myroxylon pereirae* (balsam of Peru) [4], lanolin [4], colophonium [4], fragrances [5,6] and historically ethylenediamine (Tri-Adcortyl®/Mycolog® have now been withdrawn from the market in the UK/USA, respectively) [7] and isothiazolinones (now banned in leave-on preparations in the UK and the European Union) [8]. Patients with chronic otitis externa, ano-genital dermatoses, venous eczema or leg ulcers seem to be particularly susceptible [3,4,9–11]. The elderly appear to be more likely to develop multiple sensitivities [10]. Atopic dermatitis patients have higher rates of sensitisation to ingredients in their topical medicaments, relevance is established in most cases, and polysensitisation is frequent [12]. Sensitivity to topical medication is often overlooked as the symptoms tend to be attributed to the disease being treated.

Systemic side effects from topically applied medication are relatively rare. Nonetheless, all topically applied drugs are absorbed to some degree and on occasions unexpected systemic toxicity occurs. One of the best recognised risks is salicylism, resulting from excessive topical use of salicylic acid. It has been estimated that toxicity can occur with twice-daily application of 6% salicylic acid to 40% of the body surface, and at least four deaths have been attributed to topical salicylic acid [13]. Systemic effects from super-potent topical corticosteroids appear rare even with continuous use if amounts greater than 50 g per week are avoided [**14**].

Absorption varies very considerably depending on the region of skin being treated (Table 18.4) [15]. Occlusion greatly enhances drug penetration [16,17]. The mechanism of this effect is not fully understood but seems to be partly the result of retaining a reservoir of the medication on the surface of the skin, and partly the effect of increased hydration of the stratum corneum. Systemic exposure can be greater than expected in children due to their relatively high ratio of skin surface to body mass. Infants are particularly prone to systemic effects from topical steroids or salicylic acid [18]. In the elderly, penetration of drugs may be increased as a result of changes in the structure of the skin; this effect is most pronounced in those drugs that are most hydrophilic [19]. Inflammation of the skin impairs barrier function and significantly increases drug absorption. This is especially significant in the erythrodermic patient [20,21].

Table 18.4 Relative levels of absorption of hydrocortisone applied at various sites.

Site	Relative absorption
Forearm	1
Sole	0.1
Ankle	0.4
Palm	0.8
Back	1.7
Scalp	3.5
Axilla	3.6
Forehead	6
Scrotum	42

Adapted from Feldmann and Maibach 1967 [15].

Formulation of topical medicaments

The formulation of the vehicle in which a drug is delivered topically to the skin is critical in obtaining effective and consistent results. The vehicle plays many roles. It must provide rapid delivery of the drug to the stratum corneum and into the viable layers of the skin, be soothing and comfortable to use, cosmetically acceptable, and provide a chemical environment in which the drug remains sufficiently stable prior to use to have a practical shelf-life. The simplest role of a vehicle is dilution of an active drug to the desired concentration. Agents such as beeswax, liquid paraffin, polyethylene glycol and powders are often added for their physical properties to adjust the thickness or texture of the medication. In addition to this, various constituents act as emollients, emulsifiers, humectants, penetration enhancers, preservatives, antioxidants, solvents or fragrances. Some of the constituents most often employed are listed in Box 18.1 and some are discussed further here. A single constituent often serves more than one function.

Box 18.1 Frequently employed constituents of vehicles

Lipids (emollients)
- Beeswax (cera alba)
- Castor oil
- Cetyl alcohol
- Cocoa butter
- Isopropyl myristate
- Isopropyl palmitate
- Lanolin
- Liquid paraffin
- Stearic acid
- Stearyl alcohol
- White soft paraffin (petrolatum)

Emulsifiers
- Alkyl sulphates and sulphonates
- Glyceryl monostearate
- Lanolin and derivatives
- Phosphoric acid esters
- Polyethylene glycols
- Polyvalent metallic soaps
- Propylene glycol fatty acid esters
- Quaternary ammonium cationic compounds
- Sorbitan monolaurate, monopalmitate and mono-oleate
- Triethanolamine oleate

Humectants
- Gelatin
- Glycerin
- Propylene glycol
- Pyrrolidone carboxylic acid
- Sorbitol
- Urea

Penetration enhancers
- Azone
- Dimethyl sulfoxide
- Propylene glycol
- Salicylic acid
- Urea

Preservatives
- Benzyl alcohol (also acts as a fragrance)
- Chlorocresol
- Edetic acid/disodium edetate
- Hydroxybenzoates (parabens)
- Propylene glycol
- Sodium metabisulphite
- Sorbic acid/sorbates
- Phenoxyethanol

Antioxidants
- Butylated hydroxyanisole
- Butylated hydroxytoluene
- Octyl gallate
- Dodecyl gallate
- Propyl gallate
- Vitamin E (tocopherol)
- Vitamin C

Solvents
- Acetone
- Chloroform
- Ethanol
- Ether
- Glycerin
- Isopropyl alcohol
- Methanol
- Propylene glycol
- Water

Most topical medicaments are now commercially formulated in vehicles that have been carefully designed for optimal results. An understanding of the roles played by the various constituents of vehicles is important [1]. Only the most frequently used components are reviewed here. Extemporaneous or personalised formulations of medicaments (known as 'specials') had been widely used in dermatological practice, with enormous benefit to patients. Stricter financial, legislative and safety controls in recent years have made many pharmacists reluctant to prepare or dispense them. In the UK, a limited range of specials is recommended by the British Association of Dermatologists (BAD) [2].

Lipids

Lipids incorporated into vehicles can act as diluents and solvents but are especially valuable as emollients, that is they have the ability to form a coating on the surface of the stratum corneum that inhibits the evaporation of water, thus providing a softening and moisturising effect. Generally speaking, the greater the proportion of lipid in the formulation, the greater will be the emollient action. Ointments are therefore more emollient than oily creams, which are more so than aqueous creams, whilst most lotions have no emollient effect. Lipids from a variety of sources are incorporated into topical treatments for skin disease.

Vegetable oils

Oils can be obtained from numerous vegetable sources by pressing or by solvent extraction. Vegetable oils are largely composed of triglycerides which tend to contain high proportions of unsaturated fatty acids such as oleic acid and linoleic acid. These are vulnerable to oxidation, with resulting rancidity manifesting as an unpleasant odour, hence the use of antioxidants to delay the process.

Arachis oil, derived from the ground nut (peanut), has been the subject of some concern over possible contamination with allergens that could cause hypersensitivity reactions in peanut-sensitive individuals, including primary sensitisation to peanuts in infants with impaired skin barrier function who have never eaten peanut [3]. Cocoa butter, also known as theobroma oil, is a product of the cocoa bean and consists chiefly of the triglycerides of palmitic, stearic and oleic acids. It also contains antioxidants, which make it remarkably stable for a vegetable oil and it can even help to preserve other constituents with which it is compounded. It is brittle at room temperature but melts at between 30 and 35°C. Castor oil, obtained from the castor bean *Ricinus communis*, is composed almost entirely of triglycerides of the 18-carbon long-chain fatty acid ricinoleic acid. Olive oil contains a large proportion of oleic acid. Shea butter is extracted from the fruit of the shea tree, *Vitellaria paradoxa*. This is a useful emollient, containing somewhat variable proportions of palmitic, stearic, oleic and other fatty acids as well as cinnamates. The latter constituent can provide a modest degree of photoprotection.

Mineral oils and greases

Vaseline® was first patented in the USA in 1872 and extracts of crude oil (petroleum) have been widely used since then for the treatment of skin disease.

Emollient products extracted from crude oil can be produced as fluids, semi-solids or solids and include liquid paraffin BP, mineral oil USP, yellow and white soft paraffin BP, petrolatum USP, etc. The extraction process involves treatments to remove elements other than hydrogen and carbon. Aromatic and unsaturated compounds are also eliminated, leaving a diverse range of hydrocarbon molecules, some straight chained, some branched and some polycyclic [4]. As a result of their fully saturated nature, these hydrocarbons are far more stable than the constituents of vegetable oils. They are remarkably inert and not vulnerable to oxidation or rancidity. For this reason, mineral oils are favoured as the lipids used in emollients and topical treatments. The inert nature of petrolatum makes it the ideal diluent for the majority of patch test materials.

Lanolin

The use of wool extracts for cosmetic and medicinal purposes dates back at least as far as ancient Greece. Lanolin (wool fat) is extracted from wool and is essentially the product of the sheep sebaceous gland. It is available in abundance and, since its natural purpose is to protect the skin and wool of the sheep, it is perhaps an obvious choice of lipid material for use as an emollient. There are occasional patients who may wish to avoid lanolin for cultural reasons, e.g. vegans.

Lanolin comprises a complex mixture of higher fatty acids esterified with mono and dihydric alcohols, including aliphatic alcohols and cholesterol and related sterols. Its precise composition varies qualitatively and quantitatively with humidity, temperature and method of collection. It is prone to auto-oxidation and is therefore often formulated with the antioxidant butylated hydroxytoluene. Lanolin is miscible with water and is a useful emulsifying agent when mixed with other lipids.

Lanolin has gained a largely undeserved reputation as a frequent contact sensitiser, but sensitisation still occurs and is slightly more frequent in those with atopic dermatitis [5]. Irritant patch test reactions to lanolin are often incorrectly interpreted as a positive patch test, and patients themselves may confuse the irritant effect of fibres in a woollen garment touching atopic skin with lanolin allergy.

Partly because of its reputation as a sensitiser, numerous lanolin extracts and derivatives are often used instead of the natural material. These are produced by a range of processes including hydrolysis to yield the constituent acids and alcohols, acetylation, ethoxylation and solvent fractionation. Wool alcohols BP is the wool alcohol fraction of wool fat, and contains cholesterol and isocholesterol. It is mixed with liquid, soft and hard paraffin to form ointment of wool alcohols BP, which, on the addition of water, produces hydrous ointment BP, a vehicle for many water-in-oil creams (see the section on emulsifiers later in this chapter).

Fatty acids and alcohols

Long-chain fatty acids (e.g. palmitic and stearic acids and their alcohols, cetyl alcohol and stearyl alcohol) are very frequently used as emollients and also serve as emulsifiers for cream preparations. Cetostearyl (cetearyl) alcohol is a frequently used mixture of cetyl and stearyl alcohols. These can be obtained by hydrolysis of triglycerides from many different animal and vegetable fats and oils.

Waxes

Beeswax is secreted by worker bees to make the cell walls of the honeycomb. It has a melting point of around 60°C and is composed mainly of free cerotic acid and myricyl palmitate. It is used as a thickening agent for creams, ointments and lip salves. Occasional cases of sensitisation occur, due either to components of the wax or contamination with plant-derived materials such as propolis [6].

Emulsifying wax comprises cetostearyl (cetearyl) alcohol, sodium lauryl sulphate and water. This is a constituent of emulsifying ointment BP.

Polyethylene glycols

Polyethylene glycols, also known as PEGs or macrogols, are dihydric alcohols. They are polymers of ethylene glycol linked by ether bonds with the general formula $H(O\text{-}CH_2\text{-}CH_2)_n\text{-}OH$ in which n may range from 2 to 90 000. PEGs can be designated by a number indicating the average molecular weight. At low molecular weights, up to 2000, they are hygroscopic. They variously serve as emollients, emulsifiers or thickeners and can also be used to impart a pleasant feel or texture to a formulation. Rarely, they can cause immediate (type 1) hypersensitivity reactions; a suggestive history would be immediate allergic reactions to a wide range of systemic drugs, some vaccines and to cosmetics and topical medicaments.

Cetomacrogols are cetyl ethers of PEGs, for example cetomacrogol 1000 is the monocetyl ether of PEGs with an average molecular weight of 1000. It is useful as a non-ionic emulsifying agent.

Emulsifiers

An emulsion is a two-phase system consisting of two immiscible components, one (the dispersed or inner phase) being suspended in the other (the continuous or outer phase) as small droplets. One phase is aqueous, the other oily. Stable emulsions remain in this form; unstable emulsions, with a large droplet size, tend to separate as cream does from milk. The production of a stable emulsion requires the presence of an emulsifier, which is a large molecule with both strongly polar (i.e. water soluble) and non-polar (i.e. oil soluble) groups allowing it to bridge the gap between polar and non-polar substances. A large and chemically diverse range of compounds can be used for this purpose and some examples are given in Box 18.1.

Water in oil (abbreviated by pharmacists to W/O) systems result from the dispersion of an aqueous phase in an oily phase, as in oily cream BP. Oil in water (O/W) systems have a less greasy texture and are formed when oil is the dispersed phase and water the continuous phase, as in aqueous cream BP. It is sometimes possible to produce both types of emulsion in the same system [7]: these are called ambiphilic creams.

Humectants

These are compounds with a high affinity for water (hygroscopicity). They draw water into the stratum corneum and therefore have an emollient effect on dry skin. However, most of the water is drawn out from within the skin, and in dry atmospheric conditions water loss from the skin surface may be increased by the presence of humectants. Some patients, for religious or cultural reasons, may wish to avoid the humectant gelatin because of its bovine or porcine origin. Commonly used humectants are listed in Box 18.1.

Penetration enhancers

Agents that have been shown to enhance the penetration of drugs through the skin include propylene glycol [8], azone [9], urea [10] and dimethyl sulfoxide (DMSO) [11]. Mechanisms for this effect include hydration of the stratum corneum and keratolytic actions. The effect of salicylic acid as a penetration-enhancing agent seems to be variable. *In vitro* studies have suggested that the penetration of drugs is enhanced but this effect was not observed during *in vivo* studies of steroid penetration through normal skin [12,13]. However, in treatment of psoriasis, the addition of salicylic acid does seem to improve the response to topical corticosteroids [14].

DMSO is a highly polar, stable substance with exceptional solvent properties. It releases histamine *in vivo* and may induce weals when applied topically. It reacts with water, liberating heat. The stratum corneum retains significant amounts of DMSO and, as most drugs are more soluble in DMSO than water, this tends to promote percutaneous absorption. Toxicological considerations have precluded its more widespread use, but 50% DMSO cream is sometimes prescribed for complex regional pain syndrome.

The use of liposomes incorporated into topical formulations such as creams and gels to enhance penetration is a subject of much ongoing research [15]. A wide range of large and small molecules can be encapsulated in liposomes. Under certain conditions liposomes can release their contents close to a target cell, fuse with the cell membrane or be endocytosed by the cell. Liposomes do not appear to penetrate intact into the intracellular compartment of the epidermis, although an *in vitro* study using reconstructed human skin has suggested that liposomal lipids can be incorporated into the intercellular lipids of the stratum corneum and cell membranes in the uppermost viable layers of the epidermis [16]. Numerous drugs including topical minoxidil have been shown to have increased penetration in a liposomal formulation [17].

Transferosomes and ethosomes are liposome variants with more flexible structures that may further enhance penetration of the skin [15].

Powders

Inorganic powders are an important component of many dermatological treatments and include zinc oxide, titanium dioxide, talc, bentonite and calamine. Organic powders include various starches and zinc stearate.

Zinc oxide is widely used as a component of many dusting powders, shake lotions and pastes. It has covering and protective properties, gives consistency to creams and pastes, and is said to have cooling and slightly astringent properties.

Titanium dioxide is chemically very inert and for this reason it can be used instead of zinc oxide in pastes containing salicylic acid. Like zinc oxide, it has useful ultraviolet (UV)-reflecting properties, and is an alternative sunscreen ingredient in patients sensitised to chemical UV blockers.

Talc is inert magnesium polysilicate, with a very low specific gravity. It contributes 'slip' and has a cooling effect.

Calamine may be either zinc carbonate or zinc oxide, coloured with a little ferric oxide, and has bland, soothing and antipruritic properties.

Starch is more absorbent than inorganic powders, but tends to deteriorate and is prone to microbiological decomposition. Some powders, for example bentonite (colloidal hydrated aluminium silicate), aluminium magnesium silicate, tragacanth, methylcellulose and carbomer, are used in gels or as stabilisers in shake lotions.

Preservatives

Ointments and creams with oil as the continuous phase do not usually require preservatives. Lotions, oil-in-water creams and gels, however, because they contain accessible water, are easily contaminated by moulds or bacteria. The ideal preservative should be non-toxic, non-irritant, non-sensitising, odourless, colourless and effective even at very low concentrations and under conditions of normal usage. In addition, it must be chemically compatible with both the vehicle and the active ingredients.

Hydroxybenzoates (parabens), esters of parahydroxybenzoic acid, are effective and widely used preservatives. Commonly used esters are methyl, ethyl and propyl (respectively methylparaben, ethylparaben and propylparaben). Because, individually, they are only sparingly water soluble, and as their effects are additive, mixtures are usually preferred. This also increases their spectrum of activity and lowers the risk of sensitisation, as lower concentrations can be used. Despite public concern about parabens in cosmetics, and their widespread use, their sensitising potential appears to be low.

Chlorocresol is a preservative used especially in the UK. It is more effective in acid than in alkaline solution. It has a low sensitising potential and is used in several corticosteroid and emollient creams.

Sorbic acid (2,4-hexadienoic acid) is also a good preservative, which maintains its activity in the presence of non-ionic detergents. It also has a low sensitisation index. It can only be used, however, in preparations with a pH of less than 6.5 and can cause non-immunological contact urticaria.

Propylene glycol can inhibit the growth of moulds and fungi, and can therefore be used as a preservative, as well as a humectant and a penetration enhancer.

Organic mercurials such as thimerosal are now rarely used as preservatives, but historically were present in some ophthalmic preparations, vaccines and prick test solutions; they are occasionally incorporated into topical skin preparations. Thiomersal was removed from UK vaccines by 2005, but was included in the swine flu vaccine used between 2009 and 2011 [18]. Ethylenediaminetetraacetate is a widely used preservative in ear, nose and eye drops.

Isothiazolinones are significant contact allergens and were widely used as antimicrobial preservatives in cosmetics, but have been banned in leave-on cosmetic products in the European Union. They are generally not present in topical medicaments, but occasionally may be found in medical products such as ultrasound gel [19].

Antioxidants

Animal and vegetable oils, unless protected from oxidation, tend to become rancid and malodorous. Antioxidants such as butylhydroxyanisole, butylhydroxytoluene, vitamin E (tocopherol), vitamin C, and octyl, propyl and dodecyl gallate are used to prevent rancidity in oily and fatty preparations.

Topical treatments used in the management of skin disease

Emollients

These agents form a fundamental component of dermatological therapy in any condition where discomfort is caused by the skin feeling dry.

The word emollient is derived from the Latin verb *mollire*, to soften, and reflects the use of these agents to soften and moisturise the surface of the skin via their protecting, lubricating and moisturising effects. Emollients include creams, ointments, gels, bath oils and soap substitutes. These are largely formulated using the various materials described as 'constituents of vehicles', especially lipids. The efficacy of an emollient is not related to its cost, but efficacy is closely related to compliance with its use. Cosmetic acceptability aids compliance; while the most effective emollient is probably white soft paraffin (petrolatum), many patients find this unacceptable to use on extensive areas of the skin because of its messiness. A compromise that may be more acceptable is to use a cream or gel formulation in the morning and an ointment at night. Recent evidence suggests that where adults and children are *prescribed* emollients in primary care, there is an accompanying reduction in the use of topical steroids and antimicrobials, and in the frequency of general practitioner (GP, family doctor, primary care physician) visits. This study suggested an overall reduction in health care costs. Savings were most marked in those prescribed a cosmetically acceptable colloidal oatmeal preparation *ab initio* rather than at a delayed stage [1].

Bath oils have been widely used in the UK. Most contain lipids such as liquid paraffin, which probably helps reduce the drying effect of bathing by protecting the stratum corneum with a layer of lipid. Some also contain antiseptics and antipruritic compounds. Recently, questions have arisen about the additional benefit of using bath emollients to treat atopic eczema in children versus using their leave-on emollient additionally as a soap substitute [2].

The use of soaps on inflamed skin, especially in atopic eczema, is generally considered harmful and likely to exacerbate damage to the stratum corneum [3]. Compounds used as soap substitutes are lipid materials containing emulsifiers; most emollients can be used in this way, including aqueous cream BP, ointments and gels. These can effectively remove lipid-soluble dirt and contamination from the skin surface whilst reducing damage done to the stratum corneum by surfactants. Patients with dry skin conditions generally report that soap substitutes improve the condition of the skin [4]. Aqueous cream has fallen out of favour as a leave-on emollient due to a high frequency of irritant reactions (burning, stinging, etc.). In experimental studies it caused a significant increase in transepidermal water loss [5,6].

Attempts at primary prevention of atopic eczema in high-risk infants treated for the first year of life with daily emollient have been unsuccessful to date [7].

Emollient-soaked clothing can present a fire hazard, particularly with emollients with a high paraffin content in the presence of oxygen and a naked flame or cigarette [8]; the Medicines and Health care products Regulatory Authority issued an alert in the UK in 2016 to this effect. Bath oils may be hazardous for elderly patients as they tend to make the bath slippery.

Astringents

Astringents are compounds used to reduce exudation by precipitation of protein. Those most frequently employed are aqueous solutions of potassium permanganate, aluminium acetate and silver nitrate.

Potassium permanganate ($KMnO_4$)

This is an oxidising agent with antiseptic and fungicidal activity which is invaluable in the treatment of very acute exudative eczematous dermatoses. It is highly effective for removing malodour in leg ulcers and drying up weeping skin lesions. It is most commonly used at concentrations of 1 : 10 000 to 1 : 12 000; the solution may be diluted further, to achieve a pale pink colour. It can be applied as a wet dressing on gauze (for example to weeping flexures), a soak (for example to malodorous leg ulcers) or a bath (for widespread weeping or blistering eruptions). A bucketful of $KMnO_4$ 1 : 10 000 may be prepared by adding 1 × 400 mg tablet to 4 L water, and a bath containing $KMnO_4$ 1 : 25 000 by adding 2 g (5 × 400 mg tablets) to each 50 L of water. Potassium permanganate stains with a brownish colour the skin, toenails and fingernails, bucket, bath, sink, towels and other materials. Fingernails and toenails may be protected with petroleum jelly prior to soaking to prevent staining. It is important to ensure that $KMnO_4$ tablets are fully dissolved before the patient (or patient's leg) is immersed in the solution.

Aluminium acetate

Also known as Burow solution, this astringent is mildly antiseptic and has the advantage of not causing the staining associated with potassium permanganate. The solution contains 5% aluminium acetate and is diluted 1 : 10 to 1 : 40 in water for use in soaks, rinses or wet dressings. Aluminium acetate 8% ear drops are used for weeping otitis externa.

Aluminium chloride hexahydrate

Aluminium chloride hexahydrate 20% solution is an astringent used for hyperhidrosis of the axillae, hands and feet. It is highly irritant in the axillae. It may be used as a chemical cauterising agent after shave or curette excision of benign skin lesions.

Silver nitrate

In concentrations of 0.1–0.5% silver nitrate is an effective astringent and antiseptic used in the management of leg ulcers and burns. Higher concentrations may cause pain. Silver nitrate causes staining of the skin and most other materials. Silver nitrate sticks may be used to cauterise bleeding granulation tissue, for example hypergranulation around a stoma, or a recurrent histigically confirmed pyogenic granuloma.

Antiseptics

This term is used for a very wide variety of topical agents applied to the skin for cleansing and treatment of infection, as opposed to the term 'disinfectants', used to describe agents employed to clean and sterilise inanimate materials, surfaces, instruments, etc. Some antiseptics are also astringents. Antiseptics, by their nature, exhibit broad spectrum antimicrobial efficacy, but some organisms tend to be more sensitive than others. Gram-positive bacteria such as *Staphylococcus aureus* tend to be more sensitive than Gram-negative bacteria. *Pseudomonas aeruginosa* is one of the most resistant Gram-negative organisms. Bacterial spores (e.g. those of *Clostridium difficile*) are relatively protected from antiseptics, explaining the importance of handwashing with soap and water in outbreaks of *C. difficile* infection, which is more effective than the use of alcohol-based hand gel alone. Viruses, fungi and mycobacteria often require higher concentrations of antiseptics, and prions are extremely resistant to them.

Alcohols

Isopropyl alcohol, ethanol and *n*-propanol are widely used for skin cleansing. These are rapidly acting agents with a broad spectrum of antimicrobial activity that denature cell membranes and proteins, hence the use of high-concentration alcohols in hand gels used to prevent the spread of the SARS-CoV-2 virus during the global pandemic which began in late 2019.

Aldehydes
Formaldehyde and glutaraldehyde are broad spectrum antimicrobials used more often for sterilising equipment than for treatment of the skin as they are potential contact sensitisers. Soaks with 3% formaldehyde may be used for pitted keratolysis associated with plantar hyperhidrosis.

Cetrimide and benzalkonium chloride
These are quaternary ammonium, cationic surfactants with a wide spectrum of activity against bacteria and fungi. They have many applications, including use in proprietary antiseptic creams and as a constituent of shampoos for treating seborrhoeic dermatitis.

Chlorhexidine
This is one of the most frequently used antiseptics, especially in antiseptic creams, hand cleansing products and as a skin cleanser prior to surgery. The ability of chlorhexidine to persist and remain active in the skin makes it especially useful for these purposes. It is most active at a neutral or alkaline pH. It exhibits a wide spectrum of antibacterial activity by multiple mechanisms including disruption of membrane structure and function. Activity against mycobacteria and viruses is rather limited. Allergy to chlorhexidine may cause both eczematous and anaphylactic reactions [1]. Irritant reactions readily occur when combined emollient preparations containing chlorhexidine and benzalkonium chloride are used as leave-on products, particularly in the flexures [2].

Chlorine-releasing agents
Sodium hypochlorite (domestic bleach) has a broad spectrum of action but is used mainly as a disinfectant. Dilute bleach baths or a bleach wash may reduce skin colonisation by *Staphylococcus aureus* in children with atopic eczema [3] (Chapter 41).

Chloroxylenol
Chloroxylenol (4-chloro-3,5-dimethylphenol) is a bactericidal compound that has been used as a domestic antiseptic and disinfectant for many years. It is not effective against *Pseudomonas aeruginosa*.

Hydrogen peroxide
Hydrogen peroxide (H_2O_2) is a colourless liquid available in various concentrations, also sold as a 1% antiseptic cream over the counter in the UK. H_2O_2 demonstrates broad spectrum efficacy against bacteria, viruses and yeasts, with somewhat greater activity against Gram-positive than Gram-negative bacteria. H_2O_2 acts as an oxidant by producing hydroxyl free radicals (•OH) that damage various cell components, including lipids, proteins and DNA.

Iodine
Iodine and iodine-releasing agents are rapidly acting, broad spectrum antimicrobial agents demonstrating cidal activity against Gram-positive and Gram-negative bacteria, mycobacteria, viruses, fungi and yeasts. Iodine is available in a range of aqueous and alcoholic solutions (tinctures). Free molecular iodine (I_2) is the most potent and rapidly acting microbicide. To reduce the irritancy, staining and risk of toxicity, formulations containing 'iodine-releasing' compounds (iodophores) have been developed, which are widely used (such as povidone iodine, cadexomer iodine and poloxamer iodine), but are less potent antimicrobials.

Iodine toxicity seems to be unusual when iodine-releasing compounds are used, but hypothyroidism, hyperthyroidism, renal failure and metabolic acidosis have occasionally been reported with use of topical povidone iodine [4]. Systemic exposure is related to the area treated, so patients with extensive burns are at particular risk. Iodine is excreted largely by the kidneys and the risk of accumulation is higher in the presence of renal impairment. Prolonged treatment is not recommended for patients with thyroid dysfunction, including endemic goitre. Hypersensitivity reactions, irritant reactions and allergic contact dermatitis can also occur.

Proflavine
Proflavine is most frequently used for inflammatory conditions of the skin of the external ear where *Pseudomonas* infection is suspected. It stains the skin and clothing yellow.

Triclosan, triclocarban and hexachlorophene (hexachlorophane)
These are bisphenol compounds widely used in personal hygiene products such as deodorants and toothpastes. They are most active against Gram-positive bacteria and probably act mainly by impairing the cytoplasmic membrane.

Antibiotics
Topical antibiotics are most frequently used in the treatment of superficial infections such as impetigo, superficially infected surgical wounds, infected leg ulcers and infected eczema. They are also widely used for acne and rosacea. In view of the increasing concerns over the global spread of antibiotic resistance, it is important to limit topical use of those antibiotics that are important for treating systemic infections. When treating infected skin the option of using an antiseptic rather than, or in addition to, a topical antibiotic should therefore always be considered; an additional advantage is that antiseptics cover a wider spectrum of organisms.

The value of antibiotics such as neomycin, framycetin and clioquinol is limited by their tendency to sensitise when used topically. Erythromycin and clindamycin are the antibiotics most used for acne and topical metronidazole for rosacea. Because of concerns over antibiotic resistance there is a trend away from the use of topical antibiotics for these disorders [1].

Bacitracin
This is an antibiotic that is too toxic for systemic use. Its antibacterial action is principally against Gram-positive organisms, so it is generally used topically in combination with other antibiotics such as neomycin or polymyxin B. In leg ulcer patients it was reported to be the most potent sensitiser of all the topical antibiotics tested [2], and products containing it are no longer marketed in the UK.

Clindamycin
This has been used for many years as a topical treatment for acne vulgaris but, in common with other topical antibiotics, has become less popular as monotherapy due to the emergence of antibiotic-resistant strains of *Propionobacterium acnes*. The risk of resistance may be lessened by combining it with benzoyl peroxide or tretinoin.

Dapsone

Dapsone 7.5% gel is an effective treatment for mild to moderate acne, particularly in females [3], but is not licensed for use in all countries. There are also isolated reports of the successful use of topical dapsone in cases of pyoderma gangrenosum [4], erosive pustular dermatosis of the scalp [5], erythema elevatum diutinum [6], granuloma faciale [7], subcorneal pustular dermatosis [8], leukocytoclastic vasculitis [9], granuloma annulare [10] and, in combination with topical tacrolimus, circinate balanitis [11]. Excessive use, for example in widespread facial and truncal acne, can lead to methaemoglobinaemia [12].

Erythromycin

Lipid-soluble forms of erythromycin, for example the base, propionate or stearate, have been widely used in topical preparations for acne vulgaris. As with clindamycin, combination with benzoyl peroxide may reduce the risk of antibiotic resistance (Chapter 88). In the UK, topical erythromycin is available as combination preparations containing zinc or tretinoin.

Fusidic acid

Derived from the fungus *Fusidium coccineum*, fusidic acid is active against staphylococcal infections and effective in erythrasma [13] and pitted keratolysis [14]. It is available in combination with topical corticosteroids for the treatment of infected eczema.

Sensitisation may complicate its use [15,16]; bacterial resistance following topical use in atopic dermatitis is common [17]. This is of potential public health relevance because of the value of systemic fusidic acid for the treatment of meticillin-resistant *Staphylococcus aureus* (MRSA) infection.

Gentamicin

The particular dermatological value of gentamicin lies in its broad spectrum of activity, including against *Pseudomonas aeruginosa*. Contact allergy is fairly frequent in patients with chronic otitis externa [18] and, compared with other agents, it remains a common sensitiser [19]. Cross-sensitivity can develop with other aminoglycosides [20].

Metronidazole

Metronidazole 0.75–1% has been shown to be a safe and effective treatment for rosacea (Chapter 89) [21]. Topical metronidazole has also been used with some success in patients with stasis and pressure ulcers, rapidly eliminating malodour [22].

Mupirocin

This topical antibiotic is derived from *Pseudomonas fluorescens* [23] and is chemically unrelated to other antibiotics. It acts by arresting bacterial protein synthesis and is active against a wide range of Gram-positive and some Gram-negative organisms. Naturally, it is not active against *Pseudomonas* and may allow overgrowth of this organism. It can be highly effective for cutaneous bacterial infections [24,25]. It has also proved useful in the elimination of nasal carriage of staphylococci [26], including multiply resistant organisms, but strains resistant to mupirocin are now an increasing problem [27]. It is available as a 2% cream or ointment in the UK.

Neomycin and framycetin

These are highly effective aminoglycoside antibiotics with a broad spectrum of action against Gram-positive and Gram-negative organisms. Both are considered too toxic for systemic use. Many preparations containing one or other of these are available, although less commonly used than in the past because of the risk of sensitisation. Contact dermatitis is particularly associated with use under occlusion, around leg ulcers, or in patients with chronic otitis externa, pruritus ani/vulvae or recurrent eye infections [28]. Simultaneous contact allergy to neomycin, bacitracin and polymyxin has been reported [29]. There has been a reduction in sensitisation to neomycin in recent years [30], likely related to a reduction in its use, but it is still present in ear drops, eye drops, creams and ointments, combined with topical steroids and other antimicrobial agents.

Ozenoxacin

Ozenoxacin 1% cream is an effective treatment for impetigo in adults and children from the age of 2 months. It has a low probability of selecting spontaneous resistant mutants in quinolone-susceptible or quinolone-resistant bacterial strains and has shown to be active against MRSA isolates [31,**32**].

Polymyxin B

This antibiotic is a cyclic peptide derived from a Gram-positive bacterium (*Bacillus polymyxa*) and has valuable activity against Gram-negative organisms including *Pseudomonas aeruginosa*. It is used in several proprietary topical formulations for application to the skin, eyes and ears, usually combined with other antibiotics. In the UK is it still present in licensed ear drops and eye drops, combined with topical corticosteroids and other antimicrobial agents.

Retapamulin

This is a member of a novel class of antibiotics known as pleuromutilins, derived from *Clitophilus scyphoides*, an edible mushroom, which exert antimicrobial activity by the inhibition of bacterial protein synthesis following interaction with the peptidyltransferase centre of the 50S subunit of bacterial ribosomes [33]. Retapamulin was licensed in the USA in 2007 and is available as a 1% ointment for the treatment of impetigo from the age of 9 months. Retapamulin is effective *in vitro* against *Staphylococcus aureus* (including meticillin-resistant strains) and *Streptococcus pyogenes* (including macrolide-resistant strains) [34], and against a diverse range of anaerobic organisms including *Clostridium* species, anaerobic cocci and *Propionibacterium acnes* [35,36]. In clinical trials, retapamulin has shown efficacy comparable with topical fusidic acid in the treatment of impetigo and appeared effective in treating infections caused by strains of *S. aureus* resistant to other antibiotics [37,38]. Efficacy was comparable with oral cephalexin in the treatment of infected wounds [39] and infected dermatitis [40]. Resistance to retapamulin has been reported [41,**42**]. It is not licensed in the UK.

Silver sulfadiazine

First introduced in the 1970s [43], silver sulfadiazine 1% cream has become established as a safe and convenient preparation for burns, although a recent systematic review suggested that healing may be faster with alternative dressings [44]. Bacterial resistance can occur. Even when applied over wide areas, systemic absorption is minimal and the risk of renal damage is thought to be slight [45]. However, caution should still be exercised when applied over very large areas due to the risk, albeit low, of systemic argyria. In the management of leg ulcers it provides good prophylaxis against *S. aureus* and some Gram-negative organisms. It is frequently used as a topical treatment for blisters including those in autoimmune bullous diseases.

Tetracyclines

Tetracyclines were discovered in the 1940s and have a wide range of activity against Gram-positive and Gram-negative bacteria, chlamydia, mycoplasma, rickettsiae and protozoan parasites. In the USA, 3% tetracycline hydrochloride ointment is available without prescription for minor skin lesions. In the UK, topical oxytetracycline is prescribable in mild and moderate potency topical corticosteroid/antimicrobial combination preparations. Bacterial resistance is common, especially in *S. aureus* infections. Tetracyclines also tend to stain skin and clothing yellow.

Antifungal agents

Topical application of antifungal agents is used by dermatologists mainly for the treatment of mild dermatophyte and yeast infections. Infections of the hair and nails and severe and extensive infections are usually treated systemically. The most frequently prescribed topical antifungal agents are the allylamines, imidazoles, morpholines and polyenes. Older compounds such as tolnaftate and undecenoic acid are sold mainly over the counter. A Cochrane review of topical therapies for dermatophytosis provides support for the use of allylamines and imidazoles in tinea pedis [1].

Allylamines

These inhibit the fungal synthesis of ergosterol, an essential component of fungal cell membranes, by inhibiting squalene epoxidase with a resultant toxic accumulation of the fungicidal hydrocarbon squalene within the organism. This class includes naftifine, butenafine and terbinafine. The fungicidal nature of these compounds results in a rapid response of dermatophyte infection to topical application [1]. Naftifine and butenafine also possess anti-inflammatory activity. Terbinafine is also active topically against *Malassezia* yeasts and is effective in treating pityriasis versicolor. *Trichophyton* clinical isolates resistant to terbinafine have been reported in about 1% of samples [2]. Topical terbinafine is also licensed for the treatment of cutaneous candidiasis.

Ciclopirox olamine

This hydroxypyridone compound has a different mode of action to most other antifungal agents and does not directly inhibit sterol synthesis [3]. It binds with high affinity to trivalent cations such as Fe^{3+} that are essential for the functioning of numerous enzymes including cytochromes. Several metabolic pathways are likely to be disrupted by this process including mitochondrial electron transport. It demonstrates activity against a broad spectrum of dermatophytes, yeasts and moulds including *Scytalidium* and *Scopulariopsis* species and is also effective against Gram-positive and Gram-negative bacteria, including MRSA. Ciclopirox is commercially formulated in a variety of creams, lotions, powders, nail lacquers and shampoos, available over the counter in the UK.

Imidazoles

This is a large group of compounds that includes bifonazole, clotrimazole, econazole, fenticonazole, isoconazole, ketoconazole, miconazole, oxiconazole, sertaconazole, sulconazole, terconazole, tioconazole and others. These have largely similar properties and act by inhibiting the synthesis of ergosterol. They are fungistatic. They are active against a wide range of fungal organisms including *Candida* and *Malassezia* yeasts as well as dermatophytes. The range of available formulations includes creams, powders, sprays, shampoos, suspensions and nail lacquer. Many are available without prescription. In the treatment of seborrhoeic dermatitis, ketoconazole is as effective as topical corticosteroid with fewer side effects [4].

There are also combined formulations available that contain imidazoles and corticosteroids. The precise role of these combined formulations is controversial. They can occasionally be useful to accelerate the resolution of symptoms when infected skin is very inflamed and pruritic, for example in skin flexures. However, it is also possible that they may impair the response to the antifungal agent [5] and the familiar hazards of topical corticosteroids include the potential to mask a persisting infection.

Morpholines

Amorolfine inhibits two separate stages in the synthesis of ergosterol and is fungicidal. It is marketed as a nail lacquer containing 5% amorolfine for treatment of onychomycosis, and is available without prescription. It may need to be applied for 12 months or more and is of value only for limited nail infections [1]. An advantage of amorolfine in this application is that, in addition to efficacy against dermatophytes, it is also active against other filamentous fungi that cause onychomycosis, such as *Neoscytalidium* species and *Scopulariopsis* species (Chapter 32).

Polyenes

The important member of this group is nystatin – one of the earliest antifungal agents developed. Nystatin is a fungal metabolite with activity against *Candida albicans* and several other *Candida* species. It damages the fungal cell membrane by binding irreversibly to ergosterol, an action that is fungistatic at low concentrations and fungicidal at high concentrations. It is not effective against dermatophytes. It is a safe and well-tolerated compound which is not significantly absorbed when taken orally or when used topically on skin and mucous membranes. Nystatin is available in a range of formulations including cream, ointment, oral suspension, lozenges and pessaries. There is also a range of creams and ointments containing combinations of nystatin with antiseptics such as chlorhexidine, antibiotics and various potencies of corticosteroids.

Tolnaftate

This compound is available in a variety of formulations (creams, lotions, powder) generally sold over the counter for topical treatment of dermatophyte infections. It is a thiocarbamate derivative, chemically unrelated to other antifungal drugs, and an inhibitor of squalene epoxidase. It is considered less effective than more recently developed agents but is superior to placebo [6].

Undecenoic acid
Undecenoic acid, a monounsaturated fatty acid, is largely used as an over-the-counter topical treatment for tinea pedis. In addition to its fungistatic activity it has antiseptic and antiviral properties. Various formulations are produced including cream, ointment, paint, spray and powder. It is probably less effective than terbinafine [7]. Occasional cases of sensitisation are reported.

Other topical antifungal agents
Whitfield ointment, a combination of 6% benzoic acid and 3% salicylic acid in a petrolatum base, is effective in the treatment of superficial dermatophyte infections. Studies in the tropics suggest that cure rates are quite acceptable when very low cost is a priority [8]. However this formulation is not very cosmetically acceptable. In some countries it has to be prepared as a 'special' (extemporaneously prepared unlicensed) product, making it a potentially expensive treatment.

The antiseptic properties of benzoyl peroxide have been put to use in the treatment of dermatophyte infection and pityriasis versicolor; it is, however, irritant and bleaches clothing, so some caution is required [9].

Zinc pyrithione 1% and selenium sulphide 2.5% are used in shampoos to treat dandruff and seborrhoeic dermatitis. Both compounds have also been shown in placebo-controlled trials to be effective in the treatment of pityriasis versicolor at these concentrations [10]. Zinc pyrithione shampoo can be lathered over the affected skin for 5 min and then rinsed off, every day for 2 weeks. Selenium sulphide has been shown to be effective, used in the same way, but applied for 10 min daily for 7 days. Some irritation may develop.

Griseofulvin 1% spray is available over the counter for the treatment of tinea pedis.

Resorcinol (1,3-dihydroxybenzene) is an antiseptic agent and preservative that is also added to some shampoos to suppress dandruff by inhibition of *Malassezia* yeasts.

Azelaic acid demonstrates antifungal properties and is discussed in the section on depigmenting agents later in this chapter.

Antiviral agents
There are few topical agents available with specific antiviral activity although many antiseptics, especially povidone iodine [1], are known to inactivate viruses. Although their action is not specific to viruses, alcohol gels have been a cornerstone in hand disinfection during the SARS-CoV-2 pandemic by disrupting the envelope of the coronavirus [2]. The use of imiquimod, 5-fluorouracil and podophyllin in the treatment of viral warts is discussed elsewhere in this chapter. Aciclovir, penciclovir and idoxuridine are used topically in the management of herpes simplex and the latter is also used for herpes zoster.

Aciclovir and penciclovir
Topical aciclovir is used in the treatment of primary and recurrent herpes simplex types I and II [3]. The drug is a nucleoside analogue and is phosphorylated by a viral thymidine kinase to an active form that inhibits effective replication of viral DNA. A recommended regimen is the application of 5% aciclovir cream every 4 h for 5–10 days. Both labial and genital lesions may respond. Severe episodes are best treated systemically. Unlike oral aciclovir, regular prophylactic application of aciclovir cream has little effect in the prevention of recurrent herpes labialis [4]. Penciclovir is applied as a 1% cream every 2 h for 4 days and has a similar mechanism of action to aciclovir. Both of these agents should be applied as early as possible in the course of the episode of infection.

Idoxuridine
Idoxuridine was the first agent to become available for topical treatment of herpes infections. It is a thymidine analogue that inhibits viral DNA replication. Topical idoxuridine is now only rarely used for cutaneous herpes simplex and zoster infection. In the USA, idoxuridine eye ointment is used for herpes simplex keratitis; however aciclovir 3% ointment has been shown to be more effective [5].

Podophyllin and podophyllotoxin
Podophyllin (podophyllum) is a plant extract traditionally used to treat genital warts [6]. Podophyllotoxin, the most active constituent, is an antimitotic agent that arrests cells in metaphase by binding to tubulin and is available in standardised formulations free of the unwanted constituents of the extracted resin. Podophyllin is known to be highly mutagenic, and although podophyllotoxin may be less hazardous, both of these treatments should be avoided in pregnancy. Podophyllotoxin is available as a 0.15% cream and a 0.5% ethanolic solution. It is recommended for soft non-keratinised external ano-genital warts, applied twice daily for 3 days, with weekly repeat courses for 4–8 weeks. Irritant reactions are common and severe necrosis may rarely occur. Podophyllotoxin 0.5% solution is twice as effective as 5% imiquimod cream in the clearance of external genital warts, but has a higher rate of adverse events [6]. No added benefit was found when podophyllotoxin cream was combined with weekly liquid nitrogen cryotherapy [7].

Other antiviral agents
Agents with broader ranges of indications, including bleomycin, fluorouracil, imiquimod and retinoids, which can be used for human papillomavirus infections, are discussed elsewhere in this chapter.

Cidofovir is a nucleotide analogue of deoxycytidine monophosphate, with broad spectrum anti-DNA virus activity. Although it is not commercially marketed in a topical application, there are interesting reports of the use of variously formulated creams, gels and lotions containing 1–3% cidofovir. Responses have been reported in refractory molluscum contagiosum [8], viral warts [8–10], genital warts [6] and herpes simplex [11].

Antiparasitic agents
The principles of treatment of lice infestations and scabies are discussed in Chapter 34. Insecticide resistance has emerged as a significant problem in the treatment of head lice [1] and may necessitate treatment with a second agent or the use of non-pharmacological approaches.

Pyrethroids

Pyrethroids are highly effective [2] and are now probably the most widely used agents. They are insecticides that are neurotoxic to parasites. Permethrin 5% cream is a first line treatment for scabies [3] and for pubic lice. It is licensed for use in scabies from the age of 2 months. Permethrin 5% is also available as a creme rinse for treating head lice. It is important to use the correct formulation according to the type of infestation [3,4]. Phenothrin is another pyrethroid available for eradicating head and pubic louse infestations.

Malathion

Malathion is an organophosphorus cholinesterase inhibitor that paralyses parasites. It is used for scabies [3], head lice and pubic lice, commonly as a 0.5% solution, and is licensed for use from the age of 6 months.

Dimeticone

Dimeticone is licensed for the treatment of head lice from the age of 6 months, available as a 4% lotion or spray [5]. Two applications a week apart are recommended. Dimeticone is silicone based and coats lice, possibly killing them by preventing them from excreting excess water. It has little activity against the eggs (nits), hence the need for a second treatment. As it is not an insecticidal chemical, resistance should not be a problem.

Ivermectin

This is an important agent that has been used systemically in the treatment of filariases, notably onchocerciasis, for over 30 years [6]. Both topical and oral ivermectin have been successfully used for scabies and head lice [2,3,6]. A 1% solution in propylene glycol applied twice with a 1-week interval has proved highly effective in scabies [6] as has a 0.5% lotion for head lice [7]. Its activity against *Demodex* mites has made it an important and effective new topical treatment for rosacea [8], including ocular disease [9], and superior to topical metronidazole [10,11] (Chapter 89).

Other antiparasitic agents

Benzyl benzoate is believed to be neurotoxic to parasites. It can be used as a scabicide in a 25% lotion applied daily for 3 days but is somewhat irritant, and is no longer available as a licensed preparation in the UK. It is recommended as a first line treatment in European guidelines [3] and a recent toxicological assessment found it to be safe in the concentrations used [12]. Carbaryl is another organophosphorus insecticide that can be used for head and pubic lice. It is available as 1% aqueous and 0.5% alcoholic lotions which are usually left on the skin for 12 h. A single application may be effective, but a second application after 7 days is often recommended. Resistance to carbaryl means that it is not recommended as a first line treatment [13]. Gamma benzene hexachloride (lindane), used as a 1% lotion, is an effective scabicide but was withdrawn in the UK as a result of concern over systemic absorption and possible neurotoxicity [14]. The risks are relatively greater in infants and young children, and if multiple applications are used. Permethrin is more effective [15]. Crotamiton has weak scabicidal activity and is an antipruritic. It is often used in a cream preparation as a follow-up to other therapies.

Topical glucocorticoids

Topical glucocorticoids, more commonly known by dermatologists and generally referred to in this book as topical corticosteroids, have been in use for treating skin disease since the introduction of 'compound F' or hydrocortisone (cortisol) in 1952 [1]. Their impact has been immense. In addition to becoming the mainstay of treatment in eczematous dermatoses, they are used either regularly or occasionally in the management of most inflammatory skin diseases.

All other topical corticosteroid molecules are derived from hydrocortisone. The basic structure of the steroid moiety is shown in Figure 18.2. Modifications to both the ring structure and the side chains have increased the specificity of action, increased penetration, dramatically increased potency and, to some degree, reduced side effects.

Hydrocortisone's considerable mineralocorticoid activity can be reduced by methylation or hydroxylation at position 16; its lipid solubility and stratum corneum penetration increased by esterification at positions 16, 17 and 21 (e.g. betamethasone dipropionate and triamcinolone acetonide). Its glucocorticoid activity is enhanced by fluorination of the 9α position, the introduction of an unsaturated bond between the first two carbon atoms and changes in the nature of the side chains, particularly in the 21 position [2]. Fluticasone propionate, available as a 0.5% cream and ointment, a nasal spray for allergic rhinitis and an inhaler for asthma, has a fluoride thioester carbothiate at C21, a propionate ester at C17 and a methyl group at C16; this molecule is inactivated rapidly on first passage through the liver, conferring greater systemic safety. Similar properties are demonstrated by methylprednisolone aceponate and mometasone furoate, whilst systemic exposure to prednicarbate is minimised by metabolism within the skin.

In view of the great differences in potency between different corticosteroids it is essential for the dermatologist to be able to rank or classify them by potency in order to predict the response and possible adverse effects. This classification ideally needs to take account not only of the relative potency of the molecules, but also factors such as the concentration and nature of the vehicle, which can significantly alter penetration.

Many different approaches have therefore been developed to compare potencies of topical corticosteroids. The most widely used approach has been the vasoconstrictor assay in human healthy volunteers, assessing pallor of the skin from corticosteroid-induced

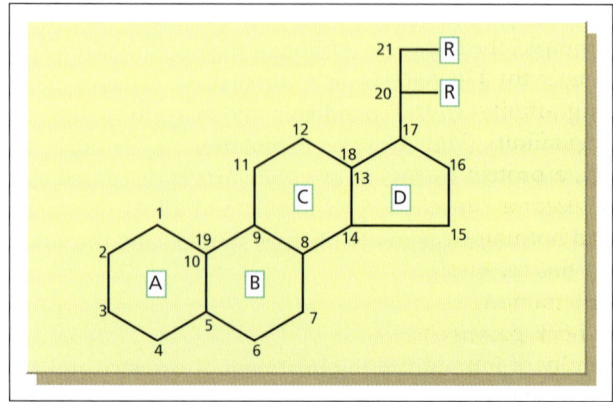

Figure 18.2 Configuration of the basic corticosteroid structure.

vasoconstriction visually, or measuring it instrumentally. This evaluates not only the intrinsic potency of the molecule but also its ability to penetrate the stratum corneum from a specific vehicle and even takes into account certain aspects of the removal and metabolism of the drug. The degree of pallor produced following the application of a compound to the skin seems to correlate fairly well with clinical potency and with the potential for side effects such as atrophy. Typically, pallor reaches a peak at around 9–12 h after application and then falls, initially fairly rapidly over the next 10 h, then more slowly [3]. The total duration of action varies considerably between different compounds.

The various classifications adopted to provide a guide to the relative potencies of different compounds are substantially based on the vasoconstrictor assay but also take into account other evidence such as comparative clinical trials. The British National Formulary (BNF) employs a four-category scale: mild, moderate, potent and very potent. In the USA, topical corticosteroids are ranked using a scale ranging from class 1 (super potent) to class 7 (mild). There is some discordance between international classifications of topical corticosteroid potency. For example, the American Society of Health System Pharmacists (ASHP) classifies betamethasone dipropionate 0.05% as 'moderate' potency if prescribed as a lotion and 'ultra-high' potency if prescribed as a cream or ointment in an optimised vehicle. The World Health Organization (WHO) and the BNF classify both betamethasone dipropionate 0.05% cream and ointment as 'high' potency or 'potent' (Table 18.5) [4].

Indications

The anti-inflammatory, immunosuppressant and antiproliferative properties of corticosteroids find numerous applications in dermatology, which are considered in more detail in the relevant sections of this text. Table 18.6 lists some of these applications together with the potencies of compounds that are most often used and the level of evidence available to support their efficacy [5].

Mechanism of action

Corticosteroids diffuse through the stratum corneum barrier and through cell membranes to reach the cytoplasm of keratinocytes and other cells present in the epidermis and dermis. Diffusion through the stratum corneum is generally considered to be the rate-limiting step in delivery of the drug. In the cytoplasm they bind to a specific receptor, glucocorticoid receptor α (GRα). Clinical potency of corticosteroids seems to be strongly related to receptor-binding affinity, which is very sensitive to certain structural changes in the steroid. For example, the introduction of a double bond in the A ring, esterification in the 17α position and fluorination at position 9α increase binding affinity, whereas esterification in the 21 position reduces binding affinity (Figure 18.2).

GRα, a protein of molecular weight 330 kD, is a member of the same receptor superfamily as receptors for other classes of steroid, thyroid hormone, calcitriol, etc. When not associated with a steroid ligand this receptor is found in the cytoplasm, as a component of a heterotetrameric structure containing two molecules of the 90 kD heat shock protein hsp90, and a 59 kD protein p59 (a member of the family of immunophilins that interact with other immunosuppressant drugs). The binding of the receptor to its ligand results in its activation and dissociation from the other components of the tetrameric complex [6]. The ligand-bound receptor then enters the nuclear compartment and interacts with specific response elements on the genome, glucocorticoid response elements (GREs). This modulates transcription of numerous genes. In addition, the ligand-bound receptor can inhibit, directly or indirectly, the activity of other transcription factors including nuclear factor κB (NF-κB), AP-1 and nuclear factor of activated T cells (NFAT) [7]. These interactions lead to changes in the expression of a wide range of genes, resulting in diverse cellular effects that include suppression of the production of inflammatory cytokines, inhibition of T-cell activation, changes in the function of endothelial cells, granulocytes, mast cells and fibroblasts, and inhibition of proliferation. Part of the anti-inflammatory activity of corticosteroids may be explained by their ability to induce the synthesis of lipocortin [8], a family of glycoproteins that regulates the activity of phospholipase A_2. This enzyme effects the production of arachidonic acid, the precursor for leukotrienes and prostaglandins.

The transcriptional activity of the steroid receptor seems likely to be regulated by an alternative isoform of the receptor known as glucocorticoid receptor β (GRβ), formed by alternative splicing. GRβ is an endogenous inhibitor of glucocorticoid action that does not bind steroid ligands but competes with ligand-bound receptor for binding to GREs [9]. Staphylococcal superantigen can upregulate expression of GRβ [10], providing a potential mechanism by which these bacteria might induce corticosteroid resistance.

Side effects

The potential side effects of topical corticosteroids are significant but must be kept in proportion. When these compounds are prescribed appropriately they can be of enormous benefit and clinically significant side effects are rare, especially in the short term (over a few days or weeks) (Table 18.7). Pharmacists, general practitioners and the public are very aware of (and frequently overestimate) the hazards. Patients are routinely encountered whose dermatosis requires potent corticosteroids but who are denied effective treatment by the inappropriate prescription of hydrocortisone or simple emollients. Others apply the medication so 'sparingly' that it is completely ineffective, or stop the treatment almost immediately, leading to rapid relapse. The fear of using topical corticosteroids can be quite out of proportion to the likelihood of side effects developing. Among patients with atopic dermatitis and their carers, a systematic review showed 21–83.7% to have 'steroid phobia', which was strongly linked to non-adherence to treatment [11].

With the exception of structural changes introduced to minimise systemic exposure to topical corticosteroids, it has proved difficult to separate the various unwanted actions of these compounds from those that are so desirable. The side effects of topical steroids are directly related to their potencies, as well as to the patient's age, body site treated and the quantity and duration of use. It is often appropriate to use more than one compound simultaneously, so that mild or moderate steroids are used on areas such as the face and flexures, whilst the more potent preparations are used only where they are required, such as the trunk and limbs.

Local effects

The most common side effects are localised to application sites. Cutaneous atrophy, skin fragility and purpura may be seen in

Table 18.5 Comparison of different classifications of topical corticosteroid potency.

WHO model prescribing information classification [4]	WHO anatomical therapeutic chemical classification [4]	ASHP classification [4]	BNF scale
Class VII Low Dexamethasone sodium phosphate 0.1% cream Hydrocortisone acetate 1% cream Methylprednisolone acetate 0.25% cream *Class VI Low* Betamethasone valerate 0.05% lotion Desonide 0.05% cream Fluocinolone acetonide 0.01% solution	*Group I Weak* Methylprednisolone Hydrocortisone Prednisolone	*Class VI Low* Alclometasone dipropionate 0.05% cream or ointment Desonide 0.05% cream Fluocinolone acetonide 0.01% solution	*Mild* Hydrocortisone 0.1–2.5% cream or ointment Fluocinolone acetonide 0.0025% cream
Class V Moderate Betamethasone dipropionate 0.02% lotion Betamethasone valerate 0.1% cream Fluocinolone acetonide 0.025% cream Fludroxycortide 0.05% cream Hydrocortisone butyrate 0.1% cream Hydrocortisone valerate 0.2% cream Triamcinolone acetonide 0.1% lotion	*Group II Moderate* Clobetasone Hydrocortisone butyrate Flumetasone Fluocortin Fluperolone Fluoromethalone Fluprednidene Desonide Triamcinolone Alclometasone Hydrocortisone buteprate Dexamethasone Clocortolone Combinations of corticosteroids	*Class V Medium* Betamethasone benzoate 0.025% cream Betamethasone dipropionate 0.05% lotion Betamethasone valerate 0.1% cream and lotion Fluocinolone acetonide 0.025% cream Flurandrenolide 0.05% cream Hydrocortisone butyrate 0.1% cream Hydrocortisone valerate 0.2% cream Prednicarbate 0.1% cream Triamcinolone acetonide 0.1% cream and lotion	*Moderate* Alclometasone dipropionate 0.05% cream Betamethasone valerate 0.025% cream and ointment Clobetasone butyrate 0.05% cream and ointment Fludroxycortide 0.0125% cream and ointment Fluocinolone acetonide 0.00625% cream and ointment
Class IV Moderate Desoximetasone 0.05% cream Fluocinolone acetonide 0.025% ointment Fludroxycortide 0.05% ointment Hydrocortisone valerate 0.2% ointment Triamcinolone acetonide 0.1% cream *Class III High* Betamethasone dipropionate 0.05% cream Betamethasone valerate 0.1% ointment Diflorasone diacetate 0.05% cream Triamcinolone acetonide 0.1% ointment		*Class IV Medium* Desoximetasone 0.05% cream Fluocinolone acetonide 0.2% cream or 0.025% ointment Flurandrenolide 0.05% ointment Triamcinolone acetonide 0.1% ointment *Class III Medium to high* Betamethasone benzoate 0.025% gel Betamethasone dipropionate 0.05% cream Betamethasone valerate 0.1% ointment Diflorasone diacetate 0.05% cream Mometasone furoate 0.1% ointment Triamcinolone acetonide 0.5% cream	
Class II High Amcinonide 0.1% ointment Betamethasone dipropionate 0.05% ointment Desoximetasone 0.025% cream or ointment Fluocinolide 0.05% cream, ointment or gel Halcinonide 0.1% cream	*Group III Potent* Betamethasone Fluclorolone Desoximetasone Fluocinolone acetonide Fluocortolone Diflucortolone Fludroxycortide Fluocinonide Budesonide Diflorasone Amcinonide Halometasone Mometasone Methylprednisolone aceponate Beclometasone Hydrocortisone aceponate Fluticasone Prednicarbate Difluprednate Ulobetasol	*Class II High* Amcinonide 0.1% ointment Betamethasone dipropionate 0.05% ointment Desoximetasone 0.25% cream or ointment and 0.05% gel Diflorasone diacetate 0.05% ointment Fluocinonide 0.05% cream, gel or ointment Halcinonide 0.1% cream	*Potent* Beclometasone dipropionate 0.025% cream and ointment Betamethasone valerate 0.1% cream, ointment, foam, scalp application and lotion Betamethasone dipropionate 0.05% cream, ointment and lotion Diflucortolone valerate 0.1% cream and ointment Fluocinolone acetonide 0.025% cream, ointment and gel Fluocinonide 0.05% cream and ointment Fluticasone propionate 0.05% cream and 0.005% ointment Hydrocortisone butyrate 0.1% cream, ointment and lotion Mometasone furoate 0.1% cream, ointment and scalp lotion
Class I Ultra-high Clobetasol propionate 0.05% cream Diflorasone diacetate 0.05% ointment	*Class IV Very potent* Clobetasol Halcinonide	*Class I Ultra-high* Betamethasone dipropionate optimised vehicle 0.05% cream or ointment Clobetasol propionate 0.05% in any vehicle Diflorasone diacetate optimised vehicle 0.05% ointment	*Very potent* Clobetasol propionate 0.05% cream, ointment, foam, scalp application and shampoo Diflucortolone valerate 0.3% cream and ointment

ASHP, American Society of Health System Pharmacists; BNF, British National Formulary; WHO, World Health Organization.

Table 18.6 Indications for topical corticosteroids, potency of preparations generally employed and level of evidence available for efficacy [5]. Occlusion and intralesional injection indicate that these approaches have been reported to be useful in selected cases.

Indication	Potency[a]	Evidence grade[b]	Occlusion and intralesional use
Actinic prurigo	P, VP	C	
Allergic contact dermatitis	Mod, P	B	
Alopecia areata	P, VP	B	Ocl, I/L
Aphthous stomatitis	P	A	
Atopic eczema	M, Mod, P	A	
Bullous pemphigoid	P, VP	B	
Chronic actinic dermatitis	Mod, P	C	
Cutaneous T-cell lymphoma	Mod, P	B	
Discoid eczema	P, VP	C	
Discoid lupus erythematosus	P, VP	B	I/L
Geographic tongue	P	C	
Granuloma annulare	P, VP	E	Ocl, I/L
Granuloma faciale	Mod, P	E	Ocl, I/L
Grover disease	P	D	
Hailey–Hailey disease	M, Mod, P	C	
Infantile haemangioma	VP	D	I/L
Irritant contact dermatitis	M, Mod, P, VP	C	
Juvenile plantar dermatosis	Mod, P	C	
Lichen nitidus	P	E	
Lichen planopilaris	P, VP	D	I/L
Lichen planus	P, VP	C	Ocl, I/L
Lichen sclerosus	P, VP	A	
Lichen simplex	P, VP	A	Ocl, I/L
Lymphocytoma cutis	P	E	I/L
Lymphomatoid papulosis	P, VP	E	
Morphoea	P	E	I/L
Mucous membrane pemphigoid	P, VP	C	
Necrobiosis lipoidica	P	D	Ocl, I/L
Nodular prurigo	P, VP	D	Ocl, IL
Pemphigoid gestationis	P, VP	C	
Pityriasis rosea	Mod, P	E	
Pompholyx	P, VP	A	Ocl
Polymorphic eruption of pregnancy	P	B	
Pretibial myxoedema	P	C	Ocl
Pruritus ani	M, Mod	A	I/L
Pruritus vulvae	Mod, P	B	I/L
Psoriasis	M, Mod, P, VP	A	Ocl
Pyoderma gangrenosum	P, VP	D	
Sarcoidosis	P, VP	C	Ocl, I/L
Scleromyxoedema	P	E	Ocl, I/L
Seborrhoeic eczema	M, Mod	A	
Subacute cutaneous lupus erythematosus	Mod, P	E	
Subcorneal pustular dermatosis	Mod, P	D	
Sweet syndrome	P	C	I/L
Urticaria pigmentosa	P, VP	C	Ocl
Vitiligo	P, VP	A	

[a] Potency: M, mild; Mod, moderate; P, potent; VP, very potent.
[b] Evidence grade: A, double-blind trial; B, clinical trial; C, small trial or >20 cases reported; D, at least 5 cases reported to respond; E, fewer than 5 cases reported.

Table 18.7 Side effects of topical corticosteroids.

Local side effects	Systemic side effects (rare)
Cutaneous atrophy	Adrenal suppression
Skin fragility	Cushingoid features
Purpura	Hypertension
Striae	Hyperglycaemia
Telangiectasia (vasodilatation)	Low birth weight (with super-potent topical corticosteroids)
Perioral/periocular dermatitis	
Acneiform/rosaceiform eruptions	
Tachyphylaxis	
Rebound	
Contact allergy	
Promotion of infection (herpes simplex, dermatophyte, candida)	
Cataracts	
Glaucoma	
Impaired wound healing	
Hypertrichosis	
Pigment alteration	

elderly patients using large quantities of potent or super-potent topical corticosteroid on the dorsal forearms, where the ageing photodamaged skin is already atrophic. Striae are most frequent on the inner arms (Figure 18.3) and inner thighs. Perioral/periorbital dermatitis, and acneiform or rosaceiform eruptions of the face, may occur with regular use of moderately potent or potent topical corticosteroids. Other problems include the development of contact allergy (uncommon, but difficult to detect as the anti-inflammatory effect of the topical corticosteroid can mute the delayed hypersensitivity response) and the risk of promoting infection, such as fungal infection.

Atrophic changes affect both the epidermis and the dermis. The epidermis becomes thinner. This is initially due to a diminution in the size of epidermal cells, which reflects a reduction in metabolic activity [12]. After intense or prolonged steroid exposure the number of cell layers is reduced, the stratum granulosum disappears and the stratum corneum is thinned [13–16]. There is suppression of many aspects of cell metabolism, including the synthesis of stratum corneum lipids, the synthesis of keratohyalin granules and the formation of corneodesmosomes required for structural integrity of the stratum corneum [17]. Inhibition of melanocyte function may develop, giving rise to localised hypopigmentation. This complication is most likely to occur with steroids applied under occlusion or with intracutaneous steroid injections [18,19].

In the dermis, topical corticosteroids induce resorption of mucopolysaccharide ground substance. This is likely to explain the rapid development of skin thinning which amounts to an approximately 15% reduction in thickness after 3 weeks of treatment under occlusion with 0.1% betamethasone valerate [20]. Collagen synthesis is suppressed within 3 days of treatment with betamethasone valerate [21]. Even mild corticosteroids such as hydrocortisone have been shown to inhibit collagen synthesis [22,23]. In a study in which betamethasone valerate was applied for 3 days only, there was still significant inhibition of collagen synthesis 2 weeks after treatment was discontinued [24].

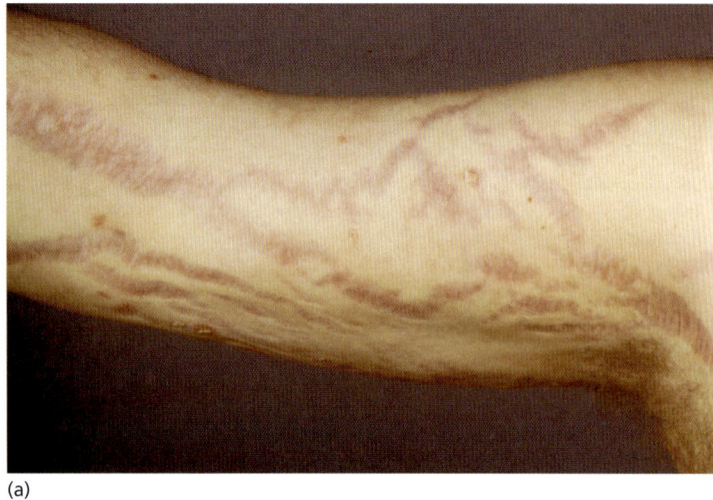 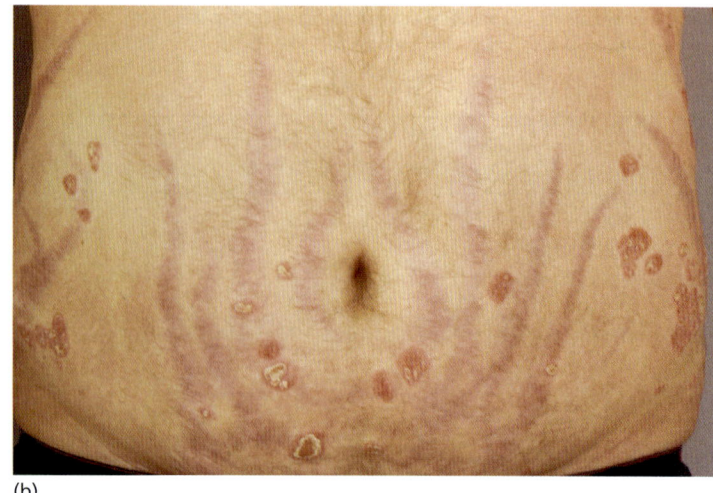

Figure 18.3 (a, b) Permanent striae induced by repeated use of clobetasol propionate for psoriasis.

When steroid exposure is prolonged, thinning becomes clinically evident and fragility and striae may develop. The loss of connective tissue support for the dermal vasculature results in redness, telangiectasia and purpura. With long-term use of potent preparations these atrophic changes can become irreversible. The areas most vulnerable to developing atrophy are those where the skin is already relatively thin, including the flexures and especially the face. In general, potent steroids should be used on the face only when treating recalcitrant dermatoses such as chronic discoid lupus erythematosus.

Contact allergy to corticosteroids is probably often missed, as symptoms may be attributed to the disease being treated. Sensitivity to hydrocortisone was first reported in 1959 but was initially considered a rare problem [25]. Rates of sensitivity to topical corticosteroids of 0.2–5.0% of patch tested patients are reported [26]. Tixocortol pivalate and budesonide are considered the best patch test reagents for screening, with rates of 1.2% and 1.6% respectively in consecutively patch tested patients [27], and are used in baseline (screening) patch test series internationally. Cross-reactions between topical corticosteroids are common. Chemical groupings have been identified within which, it has been proposed, cross-reactivity is most likely to occur, and these groupings have been updated and rationalised from four to three (Box 18.2) [26] (Chapter 127), replacing previous classifications [28,29]. Two patterns of cross-reactivity occur: either within group 1 only, or a patient being potentially allergic to all corticosteroid molecules with cross-reactivity to group 2 and/or group 3 molecules [26]. Air-borne exposure to inhaled corticosteroids, including those used nearby by others, can sensitise, as can exposure to mucosal surfaces such as the nasal, conjunctival or respiratory mucosa [26]. Systemic exposure is unlikely to induce cutaneous sensitisation. Reactivation of allergic contact dermatitis at previously affected cutaneous sites after inhalation of a corticosteroid may occur [30], and generalised eruptions following systemic administration of corticosteroids have been reported (systemic allergic contact dermatitis) [26]. Immediate hypersensitivity reactions are not a concern in patients sensitised by topical application of corticosteroids, although type 1 hypersensitivity can (rarely) occur as an independent phenomenon, most frequently with intravenous hydrocortisone and methylprednisolone [26].

> **Box 18.2 Groups of topical corticosteroids within which cross-sensitisation is most likely to occur**
>
> **Group 1**
> - Budesonide (S-isomer)
> - Cloprednol
> - Cortisone
> - Cortisone acetate
> - Fludrocortisone acetate
> - Fluoromethalone
> - Hydrocortisone
> - Hydrocortisone acetate
> - Hydrocortisone-17-butyrate
> - Methylprednisolone acetate
> - Prednisolone
> - Prednisolone acetate
> - Tixocortol pivalate
> - Triamcinolone
>
> **Group 2**
> - Amcinonide
> - Budesonide (R-isomer)
> - Desonide
> - Flunisolide
> - Fluocinolone acetonide
> - Fluocinonide
> - Halcinonide
> - Triamcinolone acetonide
> - Triamcinolone diacetate
>
> **Group 3**
> - Alclometasone dipropionate
> - Beclomethasone dipropionate
> - Betamethasone
> - Betamethasone dipropionate
> - Betamethasone sodium phosphate
> - Betamethasone-17-valerate
> - Clobetasol-17-propionate
> - Clobetasone-17-butyrate
> - Dexamethasone
> - Dexamethasone sodium phosphate
> - Diflucortolone valerate
> - Diflorasone diacetate
> - Flumethasone pivalate
> - Fluocortolone
> - Fluocortolone caprylate
> - Fluocortolone pivalate
> - Fluprednidene acetate
> - Fluticasone propionate
> - Mometasone furoate
>
> Adapted from Baeck and Goossens 2012 [26].

Infections may be exacerbated by topical corticosteroids. Obvious bacterial superinfection of eczema is usually treated specifically with topical or oral antimicrobial agents, concurrently with the use of topical corticosteroids. There is evidence that colonisation with *Staphylococcus aureus* is reduced if the condition of the skin can be improved by use of potent or very potent topical corticosteroids [31,32]. It is traditionally advised that the use of topical corticosteroids should be avoided, whenever possible, in the presence of active viral infection including herpes simplex, viral warts or molluscum contagiosum. However, evidence for this approach is lacking; a recent systematic review of randomised clinical trials comparing topical corticosteroid combined with a topical antiviral agent in the treatment of recurrent herpes simplex labialis versus topical antiviral alone or placebo found increased efficacy when the combined preparation was used, with a reduced rate of recurrence [33]. When dermatophyte infections are not recognised and are inappropriately treated with a potent topical corticosteroid, the symptoms and signs may transiently improve but the infection continues to spread, a phenomenon known as tinea incognita (unrecognised tinea) (Figure 18.4). Scabies presents a similar trap, as the pruritus can be improved by topical corticosteroids whilst the infestation persists unless a scabicidal treatment is also applied. Topical corticosteroids are, however, invaluable for treating the eczema associated with scabies, between applications of scabicidal treatments. Nodular granulomatous candidiasis of the napkin area (infantile gluteal granuloma) (Chapter 32) is found only in infants who wear nappies (diapers) and is often associated with the use of topical corticosteroids. Impairment of the immune response to *Candida* by the steroids has been suggested as the cause [34]. It has become much less common in recent decades.

The use of topical corticosteroids on the face can result in the development or exacerbation of rosacea and perioral dermatitis (Chapter 89). A similar eruption of inflammatory papules which may develop from using corticosteroids around the eyes has been termed periocular dermatitis (Figure 18.5) [35]. The term periorificial dermatitis has been proposed as a unifying term. In other individuals acne may be triggered, with the development of comedones, inflammatory papules and pustules on treated areas of skin, usually on the face or upper trunk. Comedones have also been induced in perianal skin by the application of potent corticosteroids [36]. The mechanisms involved in these eruptions are not well understood.

It is possible that the use of topical corticosteroids on the eyelids and periorbital skin may result in some exposure of the eye to the steroid. The use of corticosteroid eye drops is known to raise intraocular pressure, increase the risk of cataract formation and aggravate infections, especially herpes simplex. There have been only occasional reports of such ocular complications arising from the use of topical steroids applied around the eyes to treat skin disease [37–39]. Glaucoma has also been reported in a patient regularly treating hand eczema with betamethasone valerate at night with the presumption that inadvertent contamination of the eyes with the steroid was responsible [40]. These few reports, mainly historical, should be offset against the benefit of treating periocular skin disease, especially atopic eczema, which is associated with keratoconus, probably as a result of frequent rubbing around the eyes [41].

Wound healing and re-epithelialisation have been shown to be impaired by locally applied corticosteroids in a variety of animal and human models [42–44].

Vascular effects of corticosteroids include prompt vasoconstriction of the superficial small vessels, followed by a phase of rebound vasodilatation. After prolonged treatment the vasodilatation may become fixed and more conspicuous as a result of dermal and epidermal atrophy [45].

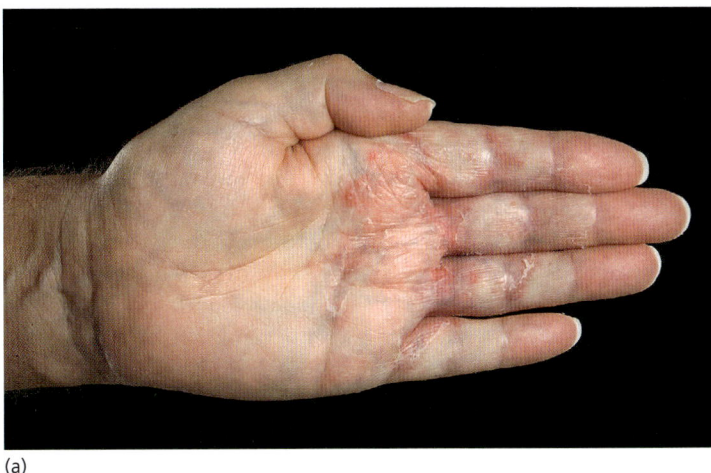

(a)

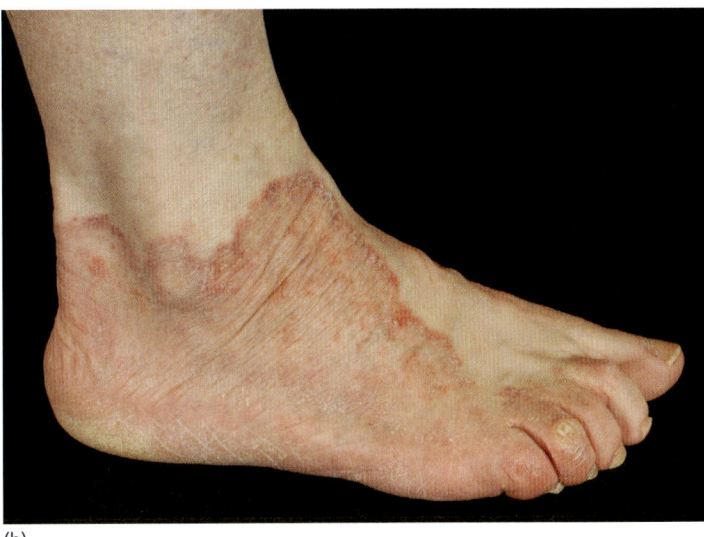

(b)

Figure 18.4 Tinea incognita. (a) Signs of tinea manuum are partly suppressed by treatment with a potent topical steroid. (b) Rash on a foot extending progressively for 5 months whilst applying clobetasol propionate cream (note the characteristic well-defined raised edge of the eruption with papulopustules and minimal scale).

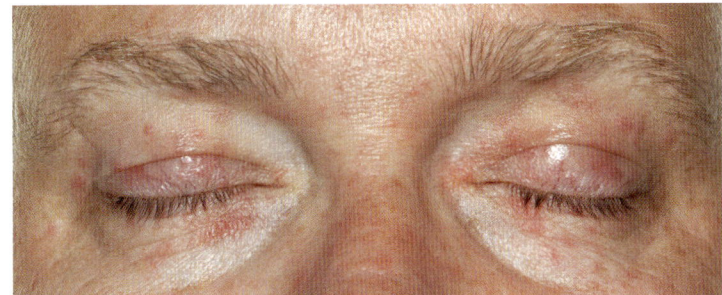

Figure 18.5 Periocular dermatitis.

Systemic effects

Inhibition of the pituitary–adrenal axis by excessive application of moderately potent topical steroids or by relatively modest use of stronger steroids is well documented [46]. Eight of 40 subjects developed temporary reversible adrenal suppression after applying 98 g of a super-potent corticosteroid preparation over

2 weeks [47]; similar results were seen in two further studies [48,49]. Significant suppression was reported in three patients using less than 50 g/week [50]. It is recommended that patients should use no more than 50 g of a super-potent steroid or 100 g of a potent steroid preparation per week and that prolonged usage at this high rate should be avoided. Children and babies have a high ratio of surface area to body volume and are more vulnerable to pituitary–adrenal suppression as a result of systemic absorption. Even hydrocortisone applied topically may (rarely) suppress the adrenocortical response in some children [51]. Cushingoid features may be seen in inappropriately treated infants and children [52,53]. Severe clinical problems are fortunately rare, even in the presence of abnormal biochemical parameters.

Excessive concern about adverse effects of topical steroids has caused a trend amongst patients to seek 'alternative' therapies such as topical and oral Chinese herbal treatments, which are perceived to be safer. In many cases such 'herbal' creams may be adulterated with super-potent topical steroids, and 'herbal' teas adulterated with oral steroids, leading to predictable cutaneous and systemic side effects including striae and Cushing syndrome [54–57]. A herbal 'Good Night Tea' containing *Glycyrrhiza glabra* (a potent inhibitor of the CYP3A4 cascade, hence inhibiting the metabolism of topical corticosteroids) triggered Cushing syndrome in a patient with atopic eczema using modest amounts of medium to high potency topical corticosteroids, although the tea itself did not contain corticosteroids [58]. Potent topical corticosteroids may be concealed in cosmetics sold openly, but illegally, on the high street and in markets, such as a product being used on the face of a 2-year-old girl and her mother, purchased in the UK in a Nigerian hair and beauty shop (Figure 18.6).

The use of very potent topical corticosteroids in pregnancy may be associated with a low birth weight, but there is no association with congenital abnormality, preterm delivery or stillbirth [59].

Tachyphylaxis and rebound phenomena

The question of whether tachyphylaxis develops during continued treatment with corticosteroids remains controversial. It is very common for patients to report that a topical corticosteroid which was highly effective during the first few days of application has subsequently lost efficacy. On occasions, withdrawal of corticosteroids is followed by a flare of disease. The hypothesis that these phenomena are due to tachyphylaxis is supported by data from vasoconstrictor assays showing that successive applications of topical corticosteroids are associated with a decreasing response [60]. Furthermore, inhibitory effects on epidermal cell proliferation decreased during repeated administration of topical corticosteroids to hairless mice [61]. However, tachyphylaxis has not been shown to occur in clinical trials of corticosteroids in treatment of atopic eczema or psoriasis.

It has been proposed that patients report that the effect of the corticosteroid is diminishing when the underlying disease activity is increasing. Physicians observing patients intermittently may mistake stable disease activity for a failure to improve, even when there has been improvement from baseline, and may interpret this as tachyphylaxis. In a survey of dermatologists with 70 respondents, 57% believed that tachyphylaxis occurred within 8 weeks of initiating treatment of chronic plaque psoriasis with a potent corticosteroid. When this was put to the test in a clinical trial of 12 weeks' treatment duration, tachyphylaxis was not observed [62]. Some patients with eczema believe that they are suffering from 'steroid withdrawal syndrome' if they abruptly stop treatment and their disease predictably flares up due to the absence of anti-inflammatory treatment. There has been confusion between the predictable effects of long-term excessive use of potent topical steroids on facial or genital sites, resulting in burning, stinging and redness on withdrawal, and a poorly defined entity labelled as 'steroid withdrawal syndrome' or 'steroid addiction' [63].

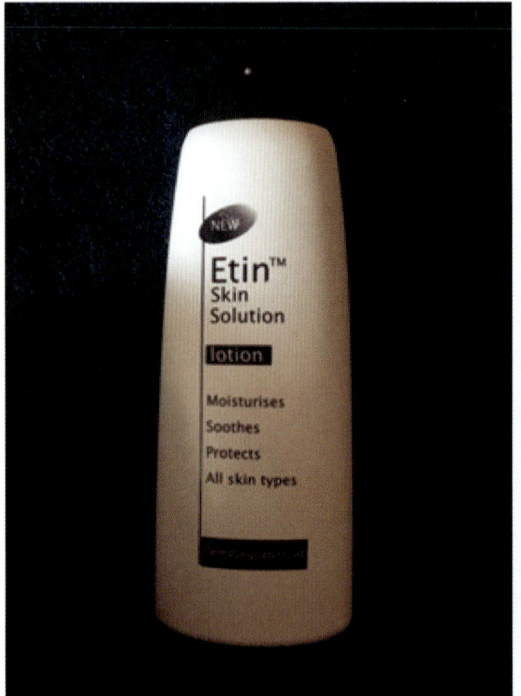
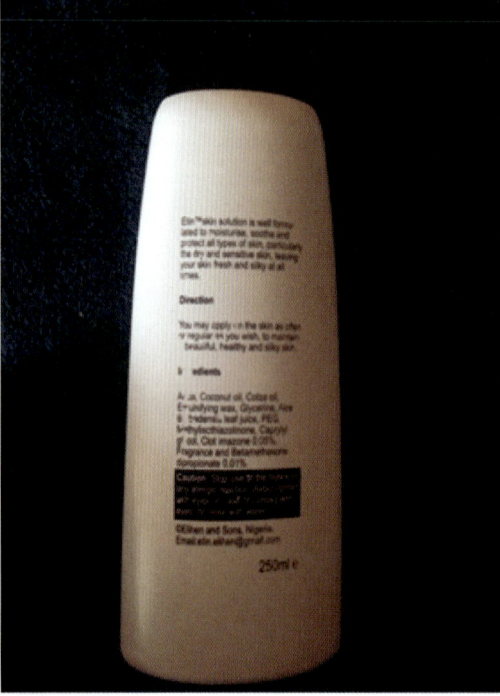

Figure 18.6 Cosmetic lotion containing potent topical corticosteroid purchased for use on the face of a toddler. Courtesy of Heulwen Wyatt, paediatric clinical nurse specialist, Newport, Gwent, UK.

Rebound phenomena when topical corticosteroids are withdrawn have principally been of concern in the management of psoriasis. In several cases, withdrawal of treatment with potent or very potent corticosteroids has been followed by the eruption of severe generalised pustular psoriasis. This seems to have been especially likely to happen after potent or very potent corticosteroids have been used in large quantities or applied under occlusion [64]. In these cases, it is likely that significant systemic exposure to the steroid was occurring and this was consequently withdrawn at the same time. The risk of this happening when unoccluded treatment with topical corticosteroids is used for chronic plaque psoriasis of moderate severity and disease extent is clearly very small as this treatment has been so widely used, especially in the USA, and generalised pustular psoriasis remains rare. There has been a general reluctance of dermatologists in the UK to rely on topical steroids for the treatment of psoriasis vulgaris, which has had the undoubted benefit of sparing patients other side effects such as cutaneous atrophy. Potent topical corticosteroids should only be used for the treatment of psoriasis when they are really necessary and/or there is no alternative, and only in the short term, except at thick skin sites such as the palms and soles. The advent of combined calcipotriol/betamethasone dipropionate preparations, which are now very widely prescribed globally for psoriasis, has been associated with cutaneous atrophy, rebound and tachyphylaxis in long-term users [65].

Vehicles and formulations

There is a large range of topical formulations of corticosteroids on the market. At first glance this may seem more than necessary, but it is undoubtedly helpful to have a variety of compounds available in a range of formulations. It is clearly important to be able to adjust the potency of the steroid being used so that the least potent compound that is effective can be employed at each site and at each stage in the course of the dermatosis. Generic formulations of a licensed topical corticosteroid may have different relative potencies and cosmetic features to the branded alternative, often remarked upon by patients [4]. It is necessary to be able to avoid corticosteroids to which patients are known or suspected to be sensitised. It is also helpful to have a range of formulations for each compound. Ointments are helpful when eczema is dry, whilst creams are more effective if the eruption is moist or exudative. Lotions, gels, mousses, foams and shampoos are useful for the scalp. The concentration (and hence the potency) of topical corticosteroid in a foam increases as the volatile ingredients evaporate on the skin [4]. When the distribution of the dermatosis is limited, as is often the case in lichen simplex chronicus or prurigo, the use of a steroid-impregnated tape will simultaneously prevent scratching and increase drug penetration by effective occlusion [66].

Several antimicrobial agents are commercially formulated in combination with topical steroids including clioquinol, clotrimazole, fusidic acid, miconazole, neomycin and nystatin. These compound formulations are the subject of some controversy. They can be helpful when there is a clear indication for each constituent, but are probably used more often when the diagnosis is unclear in the hope of 'covering all possibilities'. The latter approach is not recommended. Disadvantages include the risks of obscuring the diagnosis, promoting development of microbial resistance to antibiotics and sensitisation of patients to antimicrobial agents which may then be impossible to use topically or systemically in future. The aminoglycosides, including neomycin, carry a significant risk of sensitisation [67].

Some cases of atopic eczema are exacerbated by the presence of *Staphylococcus aureus* on the skin. Superantigen production by *S. aureus* may play a role in the exacerbation of atopic eczema [68] and may also have the effect of reducing sensitivity to corticosteroids [10]. The use of topical steroid/antibiotic combinations in both clinically infected and uninfected eczema may be slightly more effective than topical corticosteroids alone, but the level of evidence remains poor [69]. The case for the use of combination preparations is much stronger in the treatment of eczema with clear clinical or microbiological evidence of secondary infection, although many dermatologists still prefer to give an antibiotic systemically.

There are also commercially developed formulations combining corticosteroids with other active constituents. Mixtures containing tar, salicylic acid or calcipotriol can be useful in the treatment of psoriasis, although the range of licensed tar-containing products has dramatically lessened due to a combination of a reduction in prescribing and global shortages of raw ingredients.

Traditionally, many dermatologists found it useful to create their own formulations by dilution of proprietary steroid products or addition of other medicaments such as tar and salicylic acid. In the modern era, the use of such unlicensed preparations is often discouraged, and it can be difficult to persuade small pharmacies to manufacture them, even when no licensed alternative exists. The stability of a steroid in a novel formulation is unpredictable [4,70], and changes in the vehicle may also alter levels of steroid penetration into the skin and systemic absorption [71]. In the UK, the British Association of Dermatologists publishes a regularly updated recommended list of a restricted number of extemporaneously prepared topical treatments ('specials'), in an attempt to standardise the manufacture of such unlicensed topical agents [72].

Occlusion and topical steroids

The penetration of a topical corticosteroid can be greatly increased by occlusion using polythene film or gloves, or by using hydrocolloid dressings [73]. Polythene gloves are most easily used overnight, although they are uncomfortable, especially in warm weather. Wet cotton gloves worn over a potent or super-potent topical corticosteroid and an emollient, for a 30 min period twice daily, are an effective treatment for severe, acute weeping hand dermatitis. A similar occlusive effect is obtained when a steroid is covered by paste bandages and by the use of wet wrap bandaging in the treatment of atopic eczema. Using corticosteroids in this way can undoubtedly increase adverse as well as beneficial effects. However, judicious use of occlusion can be an invaluable strategy in the management of pompholyx, of a refractory plaque of psoriasis on the leg, or a patch of lichen simplex. The incorporation of a corticosteroid such as fludroxycortide (flurandrenolone) into the adhesive of a plastic tape provides another effective method of using occlusion. Whole body occlusion of corticosteroids was formerly used, but adverse effects were common, so this has fallen out of favour.

Intralesional steroids

Recalcitrant dermatoses (e.g. alopecia areata, keloid scars, lichen simplex, nodular prurigo) may respond to injection of steroid into the lesions. Triamcinolone acetonide 2.5–40 mg/mL is often used; dermal atrophy and leukoderma may occur at higher concentrations, so diluted strengths are often used for alopecia areata, especially of the eyebrows.

Calcineurin inhibitors

Topical formulations of tacrolimus and pimecrolimus (first licensed in the USA in 1994 and 2001, respectively) were developed for topical treatment of atopic eczema, and have found numerous additional applications. Their mechanism of action is similar to that of ciclosporin. Lymphocyte activation is suppressed by inhibition of the cytoplasmic enzyme calcineurin, a calcium- and calmodulin-dependent serine/threonine phosphatase, which activates NFAT, a transcription factor regulating numerous lymphokines in both Th1 and Th2 lymphocyte subsets, and which constitutes an important link in signal transduction from the T-cell receptor to the nucleus [1]. Similar mechanisms operating in other cell types, including mast cells [2,3], antigen-presenting cells [4] and keratinocytes [5], may provide additional targets for these drugs. In contrast to ciclosporin, tacrolimus and pimecrolimus have sufficiently low molecular weight to penetrate the stratum corneum, at least when barrier function is impaired, as is the case in atopic eczema. They are therefore active when applied topically. A notable advantage of these agents is that they do not induce cutaneous atrophy [6,7], even with long-term regular application [8,9,**10**,11]. It is therefore possible to apply them to facial and flexural areas where prolonged use of topical corticosteroids would cause concern. Theoretically, the local immunosuppression related to these compounds could increase the risks of infections and neoplasia. In practice, these risks have not proved problematic, and the initial hypothetical concerns about risk of neoplasia have shown no justification after more than two decades of use [11].

Tacrolimus

Tacrolimus (an abbreviation of *t*sukuba *m*acrolide *im*munosuppressant, also known as FK-506), is a macrolide lactam antibiotic (macrolactam) discovered in Japan, where it was first isolated from a soil fungus *Streptomyces tsukubaensis*. It has been used systemically in transplantation since 1994 and is known to be an effective systemic treatment for psoriasis [12]. It has a molecular weight of 822 Da and a complex structure (Figure 18.7).

The efficacy of 0.1% topical tacrolimus in atopic eczema has been demonstrated in several placebo-controlled trials in both adults [13,14] and children [15,16] and found to be comparable in efficacy to potent topical corticosteroids [16–19] (Chapter 41). A lower concentration of 0.03% tacrolimus has been shown to be nearly as effective as 0.1% in children [15,16] but this does not apply for adults [17,20].

The most frequently encountered side effect is a burning sensation lasting for a few minutes after application. This appears to be related to the ability of tacrolimus to induce substance P release and cause phosphorylation of TRPV1 (transient receptor potential subtype vanilloid 1), which plays a role in the induction of pain [21]. The burning tends to resolve after a few days and is rarely of sufficient severity to require withdrawal of the treatment. Systemic exposure is low and drug levels in the blood are usually too low to measure [11,15,22]. Using data obtained from the application of 0.3% tacrolimus ointment, systemic bioavailability has been estimated at 0.5% of that obtained by intravenous administration [22]. It is therefore unlikely that topical application of tacrolimus will have systemic activity. Percutaneous absorption appears to fall further as eczema improves and barrier function is restored [23]. Rarely, a rosacea-like eruption has been reported [24].

Additional indications for topical tacrolimus have to date been less formally investigated. It should be noted, in particular, that extensive safety data relating to systemic exposure are available only for atopic eczema. The use of topical tacrolimus in Netherton syndrome (ichthyosis linearis circumflexa) has been reported to result in clinically significant systemic exposure to the drug [25], indicating that some care is required.

Tacrolimus does not appear to penetrate sufficiently to be effective in chronic plaque psoriasis but is of value for facial and intertriginous psoriasis [26]. There are many reports of the successful use of topical tacrolimus in a wide range of other inflammatory skin diseases (Table 18.8), with high-quality evidence for its use in seborrhoeic dermatitis and oral lichen planus [27,28].

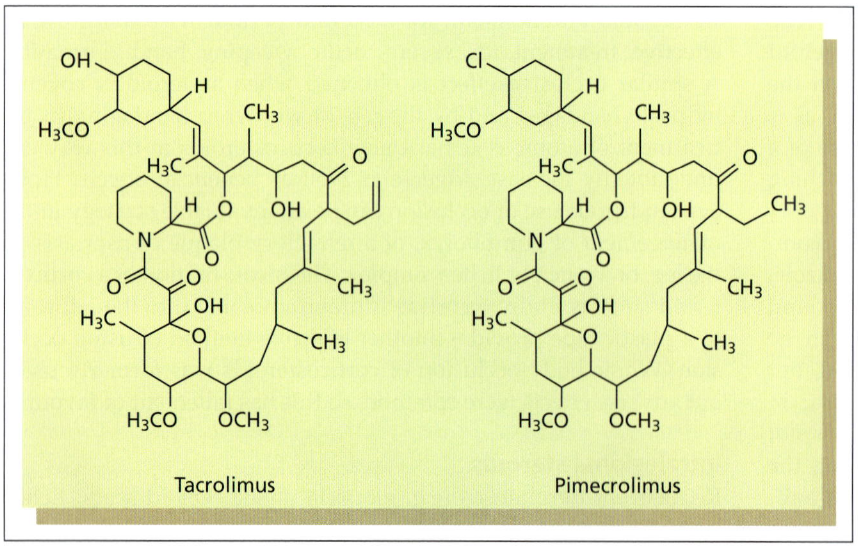

Figure 18.7 Structures of tacrolimus and pimecrolimus.

Table 18.8 Summary of the reported use of tacrolimus and pimecrolimus in unlicensed indications and levels of evidence for efficacy [25,37–51].

Dermatoses	Tacrolimus	Pimecrolimus
Eczematous dermatoses		
Allergic contact dermatitis	B	B
Chronic actinic dermatitis	B	E
Eyelid dermatitis	C	
Lichen simplex	E	C
Pompholyx	C	C
Prurigo nodularis	E	
Seborrhoeic dermatitis	A	A
Other dermatoses		
Amyloidosis	E	
Angiolymphoid hyperplasia with eosinophilia	E	
Balanitis	B	A
Behçet disease (genital ulceration)		A
Crohn disease (oral and perineal lesions)	D	
Darier disease	E	
Dermatomyositis	D	
Discoid lupus erythematosus	B	B
Eosinophilic pustular folliculitis	E	E
Epithelioid haemangioma (angiolymphoid hyperplasia with eosinophilia)	E	
Erosive pustular dermatosis of the legs	E	
Erosive pustular dermatosis of the scalp	E	
Erythema annulare centrifugum	E	
Follicular mucinosis	E	E
Folliculitis decalvans	E	
Fox–Fordyce disease		D
Geographic tongue	E	
Graft-versus-host disease	D	
Granuloma annulare (generalised)	E	E
Granuloma faciale	E	E
Hailey–Hailey disease	E	E
Jellyfish stings	E	E
Jessner's lymphocytic infiltrate	E	E
Juvenile plantar dermatosis	C	
Keratosis pilaris	C	
Leprosy (type 1 reversal reaction)	E	
Lichen myxoedematosus	E	E
Lichen nitidus	E	E
Lichen planus	E	E
Lichen planus (oral)	A	A
Lichen sclerosus	B	A
Lupus erythematosus (cutaneous)	B	B
Lymphocytoma cutis	E	
Mastocytosis		E
Morphoea	C (occluded)	
Mucous membrane pemphigoid	E	
Necrobiosis lipoidica	E	
Netherton syndrome	E	E
Paronychia	C	
Perioral dermatitis		A
Pityriasis lichenoides chronica	E	
Pruritus ani	A	
Pruritus vulvae		C
Psoriasis (facial and flexural)	A	A
Pyoderma gangrenosum	C	E
Rheumatoid leg ulceration	E	
Rosacea	C	D
Sarcoidosis	E	
Steroid-induced rosacea	C	B
Uraemic pruritus	E	
Vitiligo	B	B
Wells syndrome	E	

[a] Evidence grade: A, double-blind trial; B, clinical trial; C, small trial or >20 cases reported; D, at least 5 cases reported to respond; E, fewer than 5 cases reported.

Pimecrolimus

Pimecrolimus (SDZ ASM 981) is a macrolactam similar in molecular structure to tacrolimus (Figure 18.7), compared with which it is more lipophilic but less potent. Most of the initial clinical research on this compound was in atopic eczema. Placebo-controlled trials of a 1% cream demonstrated efficacy and safety in adults [29–31] and children from age 3 months upwards [32,33], although it is less effective than betamethasone valerate 0.1% cream [30]. Used in long-term studies, pimecrolimus has effectively inhibited flares of the disease and reduced the requirement for topical corticosteroids [11,31,33]. Systemic exposure to pimecrolimus has been found to be low and usually undetectable [34]. Pimecrolimus cream is usually well tolerated but may initially produce a burning sensation, which typically resolves after a few days. Infections have not been increased and there has been no evidence of increased neoplasia [35]. Paradoxical rosacea is a rare side effect [36]. As with tacrolimus, topical pimecrolimus has been reported to be effective in a diverse range of off-licence indications (Table 18.8).

Ciclosporin

The high molecular weight of ciclosporin (1202 Da) and its consequent poor penetration through the stratum corneum probably explain why topical preparations have not been found to be effective for skin disease. Early reports of efficacy in oral lichen planus were encouraging, but controlled studies using triamcinolone as comparator have been disappointing and generally found no difference between the treatments [52,53].

Ophthalmic formulations of ciclosporin have been used successfully for a range of indications, including ocular rosacea [54] and atopic keratoconjunctivitis [55]. Recent reviews have found it effective for Sjögren syndrome but not for dry eye syndrome [56,57]. Topical ciclosporin drops are irritant.

Retinoids

The retinoids can be defined either as compounds related structurally to retinol (vitamin A) (e.g. tretinoin (retinoic acid) and isotretinoin (13-*cis* retinoic acid)), or as compounds that are able to interact with retinoid receptors (e.g. the synthetic retinoids adapalene, tazarotene and bexarotene) (Figure 18.8). All three synthetic retinoids are effectively absorbed into the epidermis when applied topically [1].

Retinol (the alcohol, also known as vitamin A) and retinoic acid (the acid, also known as tretinoin) are both produced from retinal (the aldehyde) in most cells, including keratinocytes. Retinal, a chromophore which binds to the protein opsins and is the chemical basis of animal vision, is ingested directly from meat or produced from

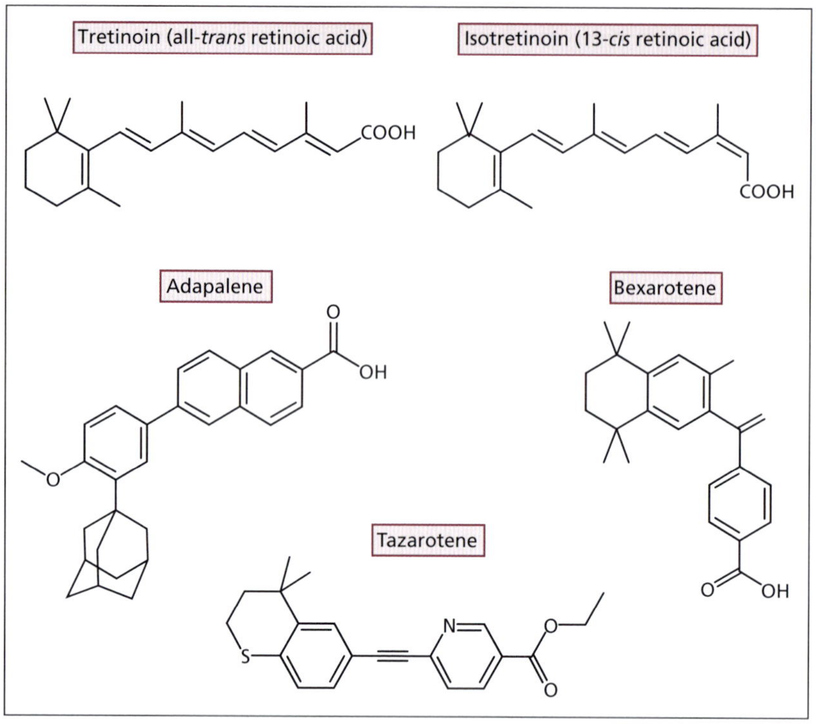

Figure 18.8 Structures of retinoid molecules used topically.

dietary plant carotenoids and xanthophylls. Retinoic acid can isomerise to 13-cis and 9-cis retinoic acid, a process that occurs readily in the presence of visible light. The level of free retinoic acid is tightly controlled. Topical retinoic acid (tretinoin) has been used in the treatment of acne vulgaris for over three decades. Retinoids are now used for many indications including psoriasis, photoageing and numerous disorders of keratinisation, as well as for the suppression of dysplasia and malignancy.

Endogenous retinoids regulate cell differentiation and proliferation, and their activity within the cell is regulated by binding proteins known as cellular retinol-binding proteins (CRBP-I and -II) and cellular retinoic acid-binding proteins (CRABP-I and -II). These proteins are widely distributed throughout the body in many cell types. CRABP-II predominates in skin, and is found in keratinocytes and fibroblasts [2]. This protein is upregulated by tretinoin [3] and other compounds demonstrating retinoid activity, and is believed to play a role in regulating the availability of free tretinoin within the cell.

Within the nucleus, retinoids bind to specific receptors, retinoic acid receptors (RAR-α, -β and -γ) and retinoid X receptors (RXR-α, -β and -γ). Alternative splicing of each of these receptors generates further diversity (the subtypes being known as RAR-α1, RAR-α2, etc.) [4]. All-trans retinoic acid is the endogenous ligand for the RARs whilst 9-cis retinoic acid is the endogenous ligand for the RXRs. The receptors most abundantly expressed in the epidermis are RAR-γ and RXR-α. They bind to 'response elements', specific regions of DNA within the regulatory regions of numerous genes, increasing or decreasing transcription of the gene. RXRs can dimerise with several other similar receptors such as the vitamin D receptor, the thyroid receptor and orphan receptors (which have no established endogenous ligand). This range of different receptors and their dimers, the various possible states of binding with different ligands, and the wide range of different response elements allow for the highly diverse and complex signalling required to regulate cellular metabolism, and the ability of retinoids to normalise keratinocyte differentiation in diverse circumstances where this is disturbed.

Metabolism of retinoids can take place within keratinocytes. The initial step is usually 4-hydroxylation by cytochrome P450 enzyme systems, such as CYP2S1 and CYP26, which can be induced by their substrate and may show considerable interindividual variation [5]. This variation may explain some of the variability between individuals in responses to topical retinoids.

Systemic retinoids are known to be highly teratogenic. Systemic exposure to retinoids applied topically seems to be minimal [6,7], but it is recommended that topical use of retinoids should be avoided during pregnancy to avoid any hypothetical risk of teratogenicity.

The retinoids currently used in the topical treatment of skin disease are retinol, retinal, retinoic acid (tretinoin), isotretinoin and the synthetic retinoids adapalene, bexarotene and tazarotene.

Retinol

Retinol is widely used in cosmetics. Retinal appears to be more irritant than retinol and is marketed as a faster way to reduce wrinkling [1]. Topical retinol exhibits many of the pharmacological properties of tretinoin, increasing levels of retinyl esters within the epidermis [8]; these long-chain fatty acids constitute an intracellular reservoir of inactive vitamin A, an autoregulatory mechanism that inhibits excess synthesis of retinoic acid [8]. In addition, topically applied retinol induces 4-hydroxylase activity, increasing metabolism and inactivation of tretinoin [9]; higher levels of CRABP-II and CRBP are also induced by the topical application of retinol [7]. Tretinoin is also much more irritating than retinol, although both increase epidermal thickness in a similar manner [7,10].

Retinol 10% gel has been used as a component of a depigmenting regimen with results considered comparable to those obtained from tretinoin. However, this high concentration of retinol was irritant [11].

Retinoic acid (tretinoin)

Retinoic acid is also known as tretinoin, all-*trans* retinoic acid and vitamin A acid. It is well absorbed into the skin when applied topically, exerts potent local effects on cellular metabolism, and is the endogenous ligand for the retinoic acid receptors. Isomerisation of tretinoin (accelerated in visible light) results in formation of 13-*cis* and 9-*cis* retinoic acid [12], the latter being the naturally occurring ligand for the RXRs.

Tretinoin is used in the treatment of acne vulgaris, particularly comedonal acne (Chapter 88). It is normally applied once or twice daily at a concentration of 0.01–0.025% in a lotion, cream or gel, and often used as a combination treatment with 1% clindamycin or 4% erythromycin [13,14], although erythromycin may be more effective if combined with benzoyl peroxide. It is most frequently applied as a nighttime treatment. Tolerance of irritancy can be improved by initially using it on alternate nights.

Topical tretinoin improves several features of photoageing including fine and coarse wrinkling and dyspigmentation [15] (Chapter 156).

Tretinoin has both a therapeutic and prophylactic effect on chemically induced skin tumours. Clinically, it exhibits an antineoplastic effect, and may be used to treat small actinic keratoses either alone [16] or in combination with 5% 5-fluorouracil cream [17] (Chapter 141). It also has a 'normalising' effect on the histological appearance of dysplastic naevi [18].

Tretinoin can help to reduce various forms of hyperpigmentation (see the section on depigmenting agents in this chapter).

Tretinoin has been shown to accelerate wound healing if it is applied for several weeks before wounding [19] and has been claimed to improve results after chemical peeling [20] and dermabrasion [21]. Its usefulness in this context is limited by its irritancy, a major drawback of topical tretinoin. A new lotion formulation of tretinoin is less irritant than the gel [22].

Topical tretinoin has been advocated for a wide range of other conditions including senile comedones [23], comedo naevus, verrucous epidermal naevus, plane warts, reactive perforating collagenosis, localised mild Darier disease [24], keratosis pilaris [25], lamellar ichthyosis, ichthyosis vulgaris [26], oral lichen planus [27], geographic tongue [28], Fox–Fordyce disease (apocrine miliaria) [29,30] and hypertrophic scars and keloids [31,32]. It has not found a role in the treatment of psoriasis.

Although sensitisation to tretinoin has been reported this seems to be a rare event [33].

Isotretinoin

Isotretinoin (13-*cis* retinoic acid) is readily isomerised to tretinoin and vice versa. It therefore exhibits a similar receptor specificity to tretinoin, interacting with RARs. Isotretinoin is used both topically and systemically for the treatment of acne vulgaris (Chapter 88). When used topically it is considered somewhat less irritant than tretinoin but may be more irritant than adapalene [34]. Topical isotretinoin is believed to work mainly by inhibiting comedogenesis, although it is also known to penetrate into sebaceous glands [35] and may reduce sebum secretion [36]. A combination preparation with erythromycin is also available.

Like tretinoin, it has been advocated for the treatment of photoageing [37,38] and actinic keratoses [39]. Benefit has been claimed in isolated reports for dissecting cellulitis [40], oral leukoplakia [41], squamous cell hyperplasia of the vulva (leukoplakia) [42], oral lichen planus [43], hyperkeratosis of the nipple [44], actinic granuloma [45] and limited Darier disease [46,47].

Alitretinoin

A 0.1% gel preparation of alitretinoin (9-*cis* retinoic acid), which is used systemically for chronic hand dermatitis, has been approved by the US Food and Drug Administration (FDA) in 1999 as a twice- to four-times daily treatment for human immunodeficiency virus (HIV) related Kaposi sarcoma [48,49] and has also shown promise in the treatment of photodamage, seborrhoeic keratoses, actinic keratoses and pyogenic granuloma [49].

Adapalene

Adapalene is a synthetic retinoid used for the treatment of acne vulgaris. In randomised comparative trials, adapalene gel 0.1% has proved at least as effective as, but less irritant than, retinoic acid gel 0.025% [34] and isotretinoin gel 0.05% [50,51]. Adapalene appears to retain comedolytic activity whilst showing less potential for irritancy than other topical retinoids, and improved tolerance with similar efficacy [52]. It exhibits specificity for RAR-β and -γ receptors with low affinity for RAR-α relative to retinoic acid [53]. It is highly lipophilic, a property likely to enhance efficacy by increasing penetration into the hair follicle. In addition, adapalene has anti-inflammatory properties that may improve both efficacy and tolerability [53]. Formulations available are cream, aqueous gel, lotion and single use pledgets, all containing 0.1% adapalene. A combination treatment containing 0.1% adapalene and 2.5% benzoyl peroxide in gel form is effective for acne in patients 12 years and over, is more effective than either constituent used alone and has a more rapid onset of efficacy [54]. A higher concentration of 0.3% adapalene with 2.5% benzoyl peroxide may help prevent and reduce atrophic acne scars [55]. Adapalene has no benefit in the prophylaxis of the acne-like rash induced by anti-epidermal growth factor receptor agents [56].

Bexarotene

Bexarotene is a novel synthetic retinoid with specificity for RXRs (rexinoids). In addition to its systemic use for cutaneous T-cell lymphoma, it is approved by the FDA as a 1% gel for early (plaque stage) mycosis fungoides [57,58], with a complete or partial response observed in 21% and 42% of patients, respectively [57].

Tazarotene

Tazarotene is a synthetic retinoid prodrug that is rapidly hydrolysed to its active form, tazarotenic acid. The molecule has a rigid structure that can undergo conformational changes, in contrast to that of tretinoin. Tazarotene exhibits a degree of receptor specificity, interacting with RARs α, β and γ. The latter receptor is likely to be most important in the epidermis. Tazarotene does not bind to RXRs and, unlike tretinoin, it is not susceptible to isomerisation into a conformation which might do so [59]. It was developed mainly for the treatment of psoriasis and acne vulgaris and is available in gel and cream formulations at concentrations of 0.1% and 0.05%. The higher concentration appears more effective in psoriasis, but also more irritant. In the treatment of acne, the higher concentration is used most frequently. It is also known to be active in the treatment of psoriasis when administered orally.

A 0.1% gel formulation of tazarotene is marketed for psoriasis. Although psoriasis has been shown to respond, with 65% of patients showing 50% or greater improvement at 12 weeks [60], its value is limited by irritancy. Tazarotene lotion appears to be less irritant than cream [22]. Improvement of nail psoriasis was reported in a small controlled trial [61]. There are isolated reports of severe genital ulceration [62] and pyogenic granuloma, a well-recognised side effect of systemic retinoid therapy, developing during topical treatment of psoriasis with tazarotene [63].

Tazarotene 0.1% gel has also been advocated for acne vulgaris [64–66], photoageing [67], oral lichen planus [68], lamellar ichthyosis [69,70], X-linked ichthyosis and ichthyosis vulgaris [71], confluent and reticulate papillomatosis [72], elastosis perforans serpiginosa [73], Darier disease [74,75], warty dyskeratoma [76], benign acanthosis nigricans [77], spiny keratoderma [78], keratoderma blenorrhagicum [79] and discoid lupus erythematosus [80]. As an O/W emulsion, 0.01% tazarotene has also been claimed to be beneficial for keratosis pilaris [81]. Ectropion in ichthyosis has been reported to respond to tazarotene [82]. Its usefulness in the treatment of onychomycosis has been reported [83], but tazarotene has no benefit in the prevention of basal cell carcinomas in basal cell naevus (Gorlin) syndrome [84].

Trifarotene

Trifarotene, a fourth-generation tretinoin, has selective agonist activity for RAR-γ and has increased stability in keratinocytes, whilst being rapidly metabolised in hepatic microsomes, indicating a potentially more favourable safety profile when compared with first- and third-generation tretinoins. It was developed to reduce the incidence of common retinoid-associated side effects such as burning, redness and peeling, but to date there have been no head-to-head investigations comparing trifarotene with existing topical retinoids [22,85,86].

Vitamin D analogues (deltanoids, secosteroids)

The term vitamin D refers to a group of fat-soluble secosteroids (compounds with a break in the steroid nucleus) which increase intestinal absorption of calcium, magnesium and phosphate. The most important members of this group in humans are cholecalciferol (vitamin D_3) and ergocalciferol (vitamin D_2). The therapeutic potential of vitamin D in psoriasis has been recognised for many years. The doses required for it to be effective as a systemic agent risk the development of hypervitaminosis D and hypercalcaemia. Topical use, however, permits considerable efficacy with a wide safety margin. Calcipotriol was the first vitamin D analogue to be developed and evaluated for treating psoriasis; since then calcitriol, tacalcitol and maxacalcitol have been developed (Figure 18.9).

Vitamin D is not strictly a vitamin, because an exogenous source is not essential. Photochemical cleavage of 7-dehydrocholesterol (the physiological precursor located in the membranes of basal and spinous layer keratinocytes) by UVB reaching the skin is required to form the hormonally inactive precursor of vitamin D, cholecalciferol. Fairly limited exposure to UVB is sufficient to permit physiological quantities of cholecalciferol to be synthesised.

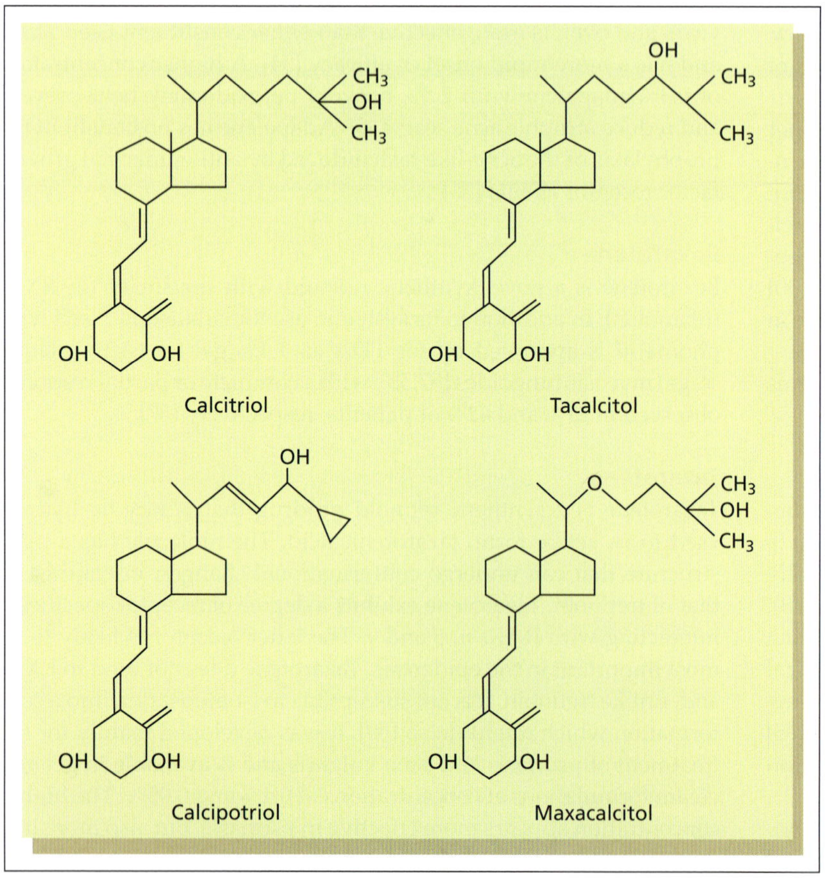

Figure 18.9 Structures of calcitriol, tacalcitol, calcipotriol and maxacalcitol.

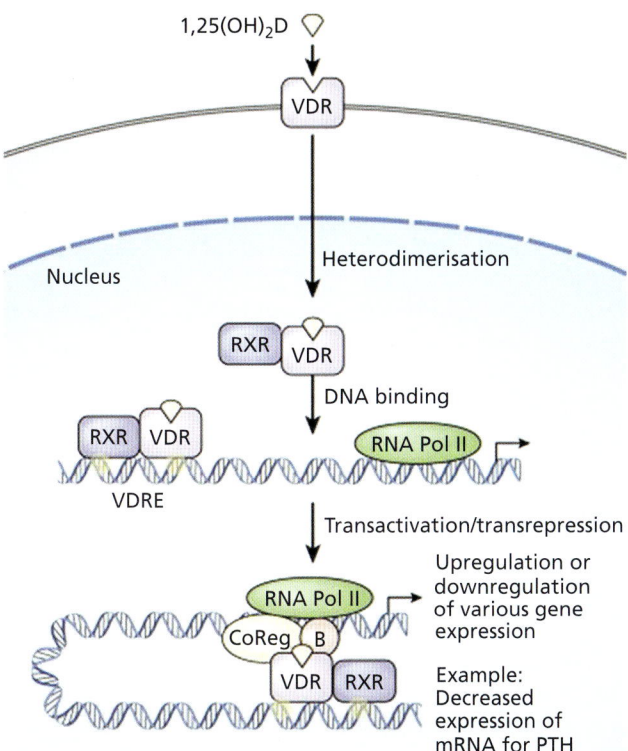

Figure 18.10 The vitamin D_3 receptor (VDR) is present in the cytoplasm and nucleus of most cells. $1,25(OH)_2D$ binds to the VDR and facilitates the interaction of VDR with the retinoic acid receptor/retinoid X receptor (RXR). This heterodimer of VDR:RXR with bound vitamin D translocates to the nucleus. The $1,25(OH)_2D$–VDR–RXR complex interacts with specific vitamin D response elements (VDREs) in vitamin D-responsive genes. Various coregulating proteins may also be recruited to this site. VDREs may be within the promoter region, within introns or far distal from the transcription start site. VDR activation upregulates some genes and downregulates others. For example, parathyroid hormone (PTH) mRNA is downregulated by activation of VDR. Reproduced from DiMeglio and Imel 2014 [84] with permission of Elsevier.

Cholecalciferol requires two hydroxylations for activation. The first step is 25-hydroxylation, to produce 25-hydroxycholecalciferol, which occurs mainly in the liver and is not tightly controlled [1]. 25-Hydroxycholecalciferol is the main storage form of vitamin D within the body. This is converted to the hormonally active form, 1α-25-dihydroxycholecalciferol, by a very tightly regulated hydroxylation, which takes place mainly in the kidney [2,3]. 1α-25-Dihydroxycholecalciferol has three hydroxyl groups and is also known as calcitriol (Figure 18.9). It regulates calcium absorption from the gut.

The receptor for calcitriol (the vitamin D receptor complex) is expressed in virtually all types of cell, and is of fundamental importance in the regulation of differentiation and proliferation. It is a phosphopeptide with molecular weight of around 60 kD that is able to move freely between the cytoplasm and the nucleus. The complex is a member of the steroid receptor superfamily, being similar in structure to the retinoid receptors, the thyroid hormone (T3) receptor and receptors for other classes of steroid hormone. It is active mainly as a heterodimer in combination with the retinoid X receptor (RXR) [4]. It regulates transcription of numerous genes by binding to regulatory regions of DNA, vitamin D response elements (VDREs), specific but heterogeneous regions of DNA that are generally situated upstream of regulated genes (Figure 18.10) [4].

Calcitriol and its receptor regulate the differentiation and proliferation of keratinocytes, the balance of the cutaneous immune system and the process of apoptosis. Proliferation of keratinocytes is reduced, upregulation of S100A7 levels in psoriatic skin induced by interleukin 22 (IL-22) is reduced, and the synthesis of keratins (K1 and K10), involucrin, transglutaminase, loricrin and filaggrin in the stratum spinosum is increased [1]. The synthesis of glycosylceramides required for barrier integrity and permeability in the stratum corneum is also regulated. Induction of the calcium receptor and the phospholipase C enzymes by calcitriol regulate intracellular calcium level. Conversely, a deficiency in calcitriol, or a loss of function of its receptor, has been shown to disrupt the differentiation of the epidermis, with reduced levels of involucrin and loricrin and the loss of keratohyalin granules, resulting in hyperproliferation of the basal layer [1].

The increase in calcium absorption from the bowel stimulated by vitamin D, especially in activated (1α-hydroxylated) forms, is normally compensated for by increased calcium excretion in urine, but with high levels of exposure serum calcium rises. All the analogues currently used in the treatment of psoriasis are 1α-hydroxylated compounds, which effectively bypass the regulatory step of 1α-hydroxylation and can thus potentially cause hypercalcaemia in overdose, although vitamin D analogues are otherwise very safe. The goal of secosteroid research is to develop an analogue that would normalise proliferation and differentiation without influencing calcium metabolism.

In comparison with traditional treatments for psoriasis, vitamin D analogues have many advantages. They are more cosmetically acceptable than tar or dithranol, are odourless, do not stain skin or clothing and (when used as monotherapy) do not cause cutaneous atrophy, so are ideal preparations to use as monotherapy for a lifelong disease. However, they can all cause irritant reactions, which are concentration dependent [5]. Sensitisation can also occur but seems to be rare [6]. A characteristic pattern of circumlesional scaling appears around psoriatic lesions treated with vitamin D analogues (Figure 18.11), which gives a guide to compliance almost as reliable as the staining produced by dithranol [7]. It is

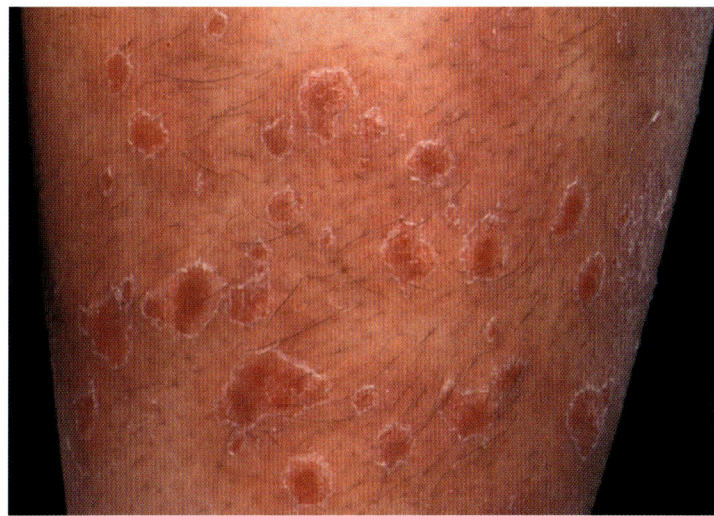

Figure 18.11 Circumlesional scaling characteristic of psoriasis lesions treated with vitamin D analogues.

Tacalcitol

Tacalcitol (1,24-dihydroxycholecalciferol) has been used for topical treatment of psoriasis for many years in Japan [8]. In Europe tacalcitol is normally used once daily at a concentration of 4 µg/g. Efficacy of this regimen has been demonstrated in placebo-controlled and dose-ranging studies [9,10]. Once-daily application of tacalcitol 4 µg/g is less effective than twice-daily calcipotriol at 50 µg/g [11] but is less irritant. It is therefore useful for treating facial or flexural psoriasis [12]. A long-term trial has indicated that in patients who have responded well the benefit can be maintained for up to 18 months, although only 64 of 299 subjects continued treatment for the full duration of this trial [13]. Tacalcitol has been used in conjunction with both UVB [14] and psoralen and UVA (PUVA) [15] and accelerates the response to these treatments, potentially reducing the UV exposure required.

Currently, the recommended maximum dose of tacalcitol 4 µg/g is 10 g daily. However, no significant increase in serum or urine calcium was observed with daily doses of 15–20 g for up to 26 days [16]. It also appears safe to use tacalcitol at the higher concentration of 20 µg/g [8]. Hypercalcaemia has not yet been reported but sensitisation may rarely occur [6]. Other indications for which topical tacalcitol has been employed with reported success include Nekam disease [17], confluent and reticulate papillomatosis [18], Grover disease [19], subcorneal pustular dermatosis [20], Hailey–Hailey disease [21], disseminated superficial actinic porokeratosis [22], prurigo [23], acquired perforating collagenosis [24] and generalised pustular psoriasis [25].

Calcitriol

Calcitriol (1α-25-dihydroxycholecalciferol) is the naturally occurring form of activated vitamin D, which is known to be active both topically and systemically in the treatment of psoriasis [26,27]. It is not used systemically because of the need to monitor serum calcium to exclude any risk of hypercalcaemia.

Calcitriol has been used topically at various concentrations ranging from 0.3 to 15 µg/g [28,29]. At the higher end of this range, changes are seen in urine and/or serum calcium levels, especially when large areas of skin are treated. At the lower end, efficacy is very limited. When applied twice daily at a concentration of 3 µg/g, controlled trials have demonstrated that a degree of efficacy can be maintained with minimal risk of effects on calcium homeostasis [30]. Calcitriol ointment 3 µg/g seems to have very little potential for irritancy or sensitisation [31], and has the significant advantage that it can be used for facial psoriasis.

Calcipotriol

Calcipotriol (calcipotriene) has been more intensively investigated than any other secosteroid for the treatment of psoriasis. The molecule has a cyclopropane group at the end of the side chain, which facilitates rapid metabolism (see Figure 18.9). It is therefore ideal for topical administration and can be safely used in higher concentrations than calcitriol or tacalcitol [32]. Placebo-controlled and dose-ranging trials demonstrated maximal response at the concentration of 50 µg/g [33,34] and this is the concentration used in clinical practice.

Efficacy and safety of calcipotriol in childhood psoriasis have been confirmed in trials on children aged from 2 years upwards [35,36] and satisfactory response in an infant has been reported [37]. Although topical calcipotriol may benefit generalised pustular psoriasis [38] and erythrodermic psoriasis [39,40], absorption of the drug may be significantly increased and for severe generalised psoriasis systemic therapy is generally preferred. Generalised pustular psoriasis was thought to have been precipitated by calcipotriol in one reported case [41]. Some patients with acropustulosis of Hallopeau [42] or nail psoriasis [43,44] have been reported to respond, although the results are not consistent.

In comparative studies calcipotriol 50 µg/g generally compares well against other topical treatments for psoriasis, being at least as effective as coal tar and short-contact dithranol, although with more irritant potential than potent topical corticosteroids [**45**]. It has shown efficacy similar to potent topical corticosteroids such as betamethasone-17-valerate and to tacalcitol 4 µg/g [11] and calcitriol 3 µg/g [30]. The response has been relatively well sustained over time in long-term trials [46,47]. Continuous long-term treatment is generally required. New formulations with improved efficacy are being developed [48].

Calcipotriol has also been investigated in a wide range of combinations with other antipsoriatic medication. Combination with a moderately potent or potent topical corticosteroid preparation may increase efficacy and reduce irritation. When each preparation is applied once daily, the combination reduces irritation and, in the case of a potent corticosteroid, increases efficacy relative to twice-daily calcipotriol alone [49]. A combined formulation containing betamethasone dipropionate 0.05% and calcipotriol 50 µg/g has proved more effective and less irritant than twice-daily application of calcipotriol alone, and is now widely used worldwide in primary care as a first line treatment for chronic plaque psoriasis [50]. The continuous long-term use of calcipotriol with potent steroids carries the risk of skin atrophy (Figure 18.12), which does not apply to the use of calcipotriol alone. Despite publications suggesting that calcipotriol counteracts the betamethasone-induced decrease in extracellular matrix component related to skin atrophy [51], in practice long-term use is associated with atrophy and the other side effects that potent topical corticosteroids are well known to induce [52]. New foam preparations are even more potent in efficacy and the induction of steroid-induced vasoconstriction [53,54]. It is important that all those prescribed a combination of calcipotriol with betamethasone dipropionate recognise that it does contain a potent corticosteroid.

There is increasing evidence for the use of calcipotriol in combination with 5-fluorouracil both in the treatment of actinic keratoses and the prevention of cutaneous squamous cell carcinoma [**55**,56]. The combination has also been used for palliative treatment of refractory extramammary Paget disease [57].

Calcipotriol not uncommonly induces irritant reactions, especially when applied to the face. Sensitisation can also rarely occur [58–60]. In one case propylene glycol in the base was responsible for the reaction [61].

The maximum recommended dose is 100 g of ointment per week. Exceeding this can induce hypercalcaemia, although serious harm

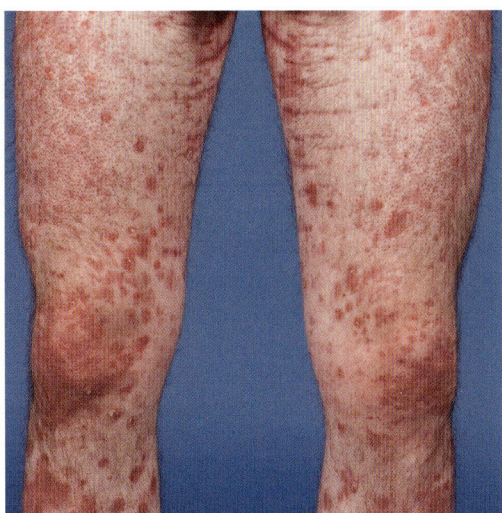

Figure 18.12 Cutaneous atrophy and striae in a 21-year-old man from the unsupervised use of calcipotriol and betamethasone ointment 60 g weekly for 2 years.

appears to be unlikely if serum calcium concentration and urinary calcium excretion are monitored. Efficacy in psoriasis can, however, be improved by using higher doses [62] and in this situation, or when calcipotriol is used for indications other than psoriasis vulgaris, monitoring is advisable, especially if large areas of skin are treated. Obtaining serum calcium levels presents little difficulty but measurement of urine calcium excretion depends on obtaining accurate 24 h urine collections.

There is now a wide range of dermatoses in addition to psoriasis that have been reported to respond to calcipotriol, although the evidence is largely anecdotal. These include confluent and reticulate papillomatosis [63], disseminated superficial actinic porokeratosis [64], erythema annulare centrifugum [65], extragenital lichen sclerosus [66], Flegel disease [67], Grover disease [68,69], inflammatory linear verrucous epidermal naevus [70], keratosis lichenoides chronica [71], lichen amyloidosus [72], lichen planus [73], nodular prurigo [74], naevoid hyperkeratosis of the nipple [75], morphoea [76], pityriasis rubra pilaris [64], Reiter syndrome [64], ichthyoses [77,78], vitiligo [79], epidermolytic palmoplantar keratoderma [80] and alopecia areata [81].

Calcipotriol has not proved beneficial in trials for Darier disease [77], hereditary palmoplantar keratoderma [77], keratosis pilaris [77] or seborrhoeic dermatitis [82].

Maxacalcitol

Maxacalcitol (22-oxa-calcitriol) is another analogue with efficacy in psoriasis similar to calcipotriol [83]. It is used in Japan and elsewhere but is not marketed in the UK.

Cytotoxic and antineoplastic agents
5-Fluorouracil

This pyrimidine analogue is an antimetabolite that inhibits pyrimidine metabolism and DNA synthesis.

5-Fluorouracil (5-FU) 5% cream is a very effective treatment for actinic keratoses [1] and for selected patients with Bowen disease or superficial basal cell carcinoma. Its use for these indications is fully described in Chapter 141. Lesions on the scalp and face respond more readily than lesions on the limbs. A commonly used regimen is twice-daily application for 2 weeks, but there are many variations on this which are used to improve tolerability: examples include once-daily application for 4 weeks, twice-daily application for a week on alternate weeks for 4 weeks, or twice-daily application 5 days a week for 4 weeks. A brisk inflammatory response should occur within the keratoses, otherwise clearing is likely to be incomplete; some patients require longer periods of treatment or polythene film occlusion to achieve clearance. Severe ulcerative reactions may occur but will heal within a few weeks once treatment is discontinued; the therapeutic outcome is generally good after a significant inflammatory response. Allergic contact dermatitis to excipients in the cream may be mistaken for a severe inflammatory response [2]. Combination with a potent topical corticosteroid has been shown to limit the intensity of the inflammatory response without reducing efficacy [3]. Seborrhoeic dermatitis-like eruptions can rarely occur at sites distant to the sites of application [4]. Combination with oral isotretinoin 20 mg daily proved to be highly effective in a series of cases with disseminated actinic keratoses [5]. Actinic cheilitis and labial keratoses may also respond [6]. When applied as a 5% cream to the head and neck twice daily for 2–4 weeks, the risk of squamous cell carcinoma is significantly reduced for at least 12 months [7]. It may be marginally more effective than imiquimod in the prevention of keratinocyte carcinoma [1]. It produces no reduction in the signs of photoageing, such as wrinkling [8]. In the treatment of actinic keratoses, the combination of 5-FU 5% cream and calcipotriol applied twice daily for 4 days can greatly shorten treatment duration while preserving efficacy [9]. This combination has also been shown to reduce the incidence of progression of actinic keratoses to squamous cell carcinoma [10] and may be effective in the palliative treatment of extramammary Paget disease [11].

5-FU as monotherapy has also been used for a range of other indications including genital warts in females [12] and males [13] and, applied under adhesive plasters, for common warts [14], extramammary Paget disease [15], naevoid keratotic disorders including Darier disease [16], disseminated superficial actinic porokeratosis [17] and erythroplasia of Queyrat [18]. It has not found a standard place in the therapy of any of these conditions. In combination with imiquimod and tretinoin it has been recently used as a treatment for melanoma *in situ*, when excision was not possible [19].

Dihydropyrimidine dehydrogenase is the most important enzymatic pathway for metabolism and inactivation of 5-FU. Genetic variation in the activity of this enzyme seems likely to account for some of the variability in inflammatory responses observed when this treatment is used topically. Systemic toxicity, including abdominal pain, fever, diarrhoea, mucositis and myelosuppression, has been reported from topical application of 5-FU in a patient with very low activity of this enzyme [20].

Bleomycin

Bleomycin is a cytotoxic agent with antitumour, antibacterial and antiviral activity. It binds to DNA, causing strand scission and elimination of pyrimidine and purine bases. It has been used intralesionally for the treatment of recalcitrant viral warts for over three decades [21]. The mechanism of action in warts is not known. The results from two large, double-blind, placebo-controlled trials were similar and showed that 75–95% of warts on the hands and 60% of plantar warts cleared following one to three injections of 0.1% bleomycin. This compared with 10% and 0% clearance in controls [22,23]. Pre-treatment of recalcitrant warts under local anaesthesia with a pulsed dye laser to induce haemorrhagic blistering before the injection of bleomycin has been reported to produce 60% and 15% complete and partial response rates, respectively, at a mean of 24 months after treatment [24].

The small volumes used do not cause systemic toxicity but local pain at the time of injection is very significant. Treatment of a periungual wart has resulted in permanent nail dystrophy [25]. The injection pain may be better tolerated by patients who have previously received many unsuccessful treatments. Bleomycin must be handled with care, and in some countries it is no longer commonly used due to concerns about handling and disposal issues.

Bleomycin has also been used in the treatment of oral leukoplakia: a 1% solution of bleomycin in dimethyl sulfoxide applied for 5 min daily for 14 consecutive days was reported to reduce lesion size and histological dysplasia [26].

Diclofenac

This compound is a non-steroidal anti-inflammatory drug that has been developed in a gel formulation containing 3% diclofenac and 2.5% hyaluronic acid for the treatment of actinic keratosis. The mechanism of action remains uncertain, although it has been proposed that inhibition of cyclo-oxygenase may be involved [27]. In an open-label study in which the gel was applied twice daily until patients were clinically clear, for up to 180 days, 22 of 27 patients who completed the study and were assessed 30 days after treatment was discontinued were judged to have had a complete response and another 4 (15%) showed marked improvement [28]. These results have been supported by double-blind trials in which 3% diclofenac gel has been applied twice daily for 30–90 days and proved superior to vehicle in clearing solar keratoses [27,29,30]. Consistently, the largest and most statistically significant difference between diclofenac and vehicle has been observed at follow-up 30 days after treatment has been discontinued. This has occurred even when the difference has not been significant at the end of treatment [30]. As assessed at this follow-up visit, the proportions of patients completely cleared were approximately 16% when treatment duration was 30 days, 31% when this was 60 days, 38% for 12 weeks and 47% for 90 days; hence the clearance rate may continue to increase with increasing treatment duration [30].

The treatment seems to be well tolerated, although pruritus is a potential side effect, severe irritant dermatitis is not infrequent and allergic contact dermatitis to topical diclofenac may occur [31].

Imiquimod

Imiquimod is an imidazoquinolone that interacts with the Toll-like receptor 7 (TLR-7), a cell surface receptor found on cells of monocyte lineage [32]. The naturally occurring ligands for Toll-like receptors are evolutionally highly conserved microbial molecules. Interaction of TLR-7 with these ligands stimulates the innate immune response by activating a signalling pathway that results in the release of large amounts of interferon-α, IL-12, tumour necrosis factor α and other potent cytokines, which in turn promote the development of antigen-specific, cell-mediated immune responses.

The first clinical application in which imiquimod proved useful was for treatment of genital warts. In large placebo-controlled [33] and open-label [34] trials, imiquimod 5% cream applied three times weekly for 16 weeks produced complete clearance in 35–75% of treated patients [33–35], although with recorded relapse rates by 3 and 6 months of 13% [33] and 23% [34], respectively. Long-lasting or therapy-resistant common warts [36–38] and stucco keratoses [39] have also been reported to respond. Clearance rates of warts in children [37] may be higher than those in adults [36], though how imiquimod compares with rates of natural resolution has not been adequately studied. In the treatment of molluscum contagiosum, imiquimod appears to be no more effective than placebo [40].

Imiquimod is also effective in the treatment of actinic keratoses and *in situ* malignancy. In a placebo-controlled trial, actinic keratoses cleared in 84% of patients who applied imiquimod three times weekly for up to 12 weeks, but in none applying the vehicle control [41]. Fourteen of 15 patients with Bowen disease had no residual lesion after daily application for up to 16 weeks [42]. Local skin reactions were common, but these are thought to reflect the immune response to the tumour. In a series of similar size, actinic cheilitis responded well to imiquimod applied three times weekly for up to 6 weeks [43]. Partial and complete responses have been observed in the treatment of cervical, vaginal, vulval and penile intraepithelial neoplasia and Bowenoid papulosis, although results have not been consistent [44–46].

Trials on superficial basal cell carcinoma (BCC) have demonstrated unequivocal efficacy in dose-ranging and placebo-controlled studies. In superficial BCCs, resolution occurred in 81–88% of lesions treated daily, or treated on 5 days per week, for 6 or 12 weeks [47,48] with no obvious advantage of continuing to 12 weeks. Applying imiquimod for 6 weeks on only 3 days per week produced cure rates of 76%, or 87% when occluded [49]. Cure rates for nodular BCCs are lower, even with occlusion, and imiquimod is generally not recommended for them [49,50], although it can be useful for periocular nodular BCC where excision (the gold standard treatment) is not possible [51].

Response to imiquimod has also been reported in extramammary [52] and vulval [53] Paget disease and in one case of porokeratosis of Mibelli [54]. Apparent complete clinical resolution of lentigo maligna has been reported [55] with a low recurrence rate [56], but the subsequent development of nodular melanoma has also been observed [57], so imiquimod is best considered as a potential palliative treatment for the frail or elderly, or where surgery is impracticable [19]; long-term monitoring is required in such cases. Complete [58] and partial [59,60] responses have been observed in cutaneous metastatic melanoma, although this does not, of course, prevent metastases developing elsewhere [61]. Imiquimod has also been reported helpful, in isolated case reports and in case series, in the suppression of recurrent keloids following surgery [62] and in discoid lupus erythematosus [63].

Ingenol mebutate

This compound, a plant extract from *Euphorbia peplus*, is effective in the treatment of actinic keratoses, with the advantage of a short duration of treatment. The proposed mechanism of action includes prompt induction of cell necrosis, disruption of mitochondria, brisk neutrophil infiltration and a tumour-specific immune response [64,65].

Ingenol mebutate was permanently withdrawn from the world market in 2020 due to concerns about the potential development of cutaneous squamous cell carcinoma during its use [66].

Mechlorethamine

Mechlorethamine (mustine, nitrogen mustard) is a cytotoxic drug that is highly active when applied topically. It is an alkylating agent and acts by binding covalently to DNA and thus inhibiting replication. Its use is constrained by its marked tendency to induce contact allergic dermatitis, and by concerns in some countries' health systems about safe disposal following topical use. Immediate hypersensitivity reactions can occur but are uncommon. It is also potentially carcinogenic, although the precise level of risk is difficult to establish, as many groups of treated patients have received additional carcinogenic treatments. Mechlorethamine has a number of dermatological applications.

The most frequent use is in the treatment of cutaneous T-cell lymphoma, once daily at concentrations of 0.01–0.02% [67]. Aqueous solutions and ointment formulations are highly effective. The latter seem to carry a lower risk of sensitisation, although irritant reactions still occur. In a large series, 137 patients with stage T1 or T2 disease were treated with topical mechlorethamine alone for a median period of 5 years. Complete remission was achieved in the majority and only four progressed to a more advanced stage [67]. A new gel formulation appears to reduce the rate of allergic contact dermatitis, but increases irritancy and is less effective [68]. Topical carmustine is used in some centres.

Topical mechlorethamine 0.02% can be highly effective and seems to be well tolerated in children with Langerhans cell histiocytosis [69]. In this series treatment was initially applied daily to affected areas of skin and the children were bathed to remove excess medication 10 min after the application was completed. The frequency of application was later reduced to every second or third day as the skin improved. Only 2 out of 20 children treated developed an irritant dermatitis [70].

Topical mechlorethamine has been recognised as an effective treatment for psoriasis since a placebo-controlled trial was published in 1970, but its use is now largely historical [71]. Ulcerating lesions of chronic granulocytic leukaemia have been reported to respond to topical mechlorethamine [72].

Methotrexate

Topical methotrexate has been used in psoriasis, but it is unlikely to become a licensed treatment and, although generally well tolerated and superior to placebo, results have been inconsistent [73–76].

Depigmenting agents

Depigmenting agents are most frequently used by dermatologists in the treatment of disorders of hyperpigmentation such as melasma (Chapter 86). Conversely, in skin diseases associated with extensive depigmentation, such agents can improve the appearance of the skin by removing the residual patches of normal pigmentation. There is also high demand among populations with darker skin types for agents to reduce the intensity of pigmentation for cosmetic purposes. In parts of Africa, treatments marketed for this purpose include very potent topical corticosteroids, mercury compounds and high concentrations of hydroquinone, up to 18%, sometimes labelled as dioxybenzene [1–3].

For melasma, hydroquinone is widely used, usually at a 2–5% concentration, and often combined with tretinoin 0.025–0.1%, and a weak topical corticosteroid such as 1% hydrocortisone, the combination being significantly more effective at lightening melasma than hydroquinone alone [4].

Hydroquinone

Hydroquinone (1,4-dihydroxybenzene) is widely used as a depigmenting agent in both clinical and cosmetic contexts. It is sold globally over the counter in skin lightening creams at a concentration of 2%. It probably reduces pigmentation at least partly as a result of inhibition of melanin synthesis, since it is known to inhibit tyrosinase. It has also been proposed that its action may be partly mediated by the release of free radicals. In animal models, the effect of the drug is potentiated by the use of buthionine sulphoximine or cystamine to inhibit synthesis of the protective free radical scavenger glutathione [5]. Its use is discussed in detail in Chapter 86.

Epidemiological studies indicate that a very large proportion of the African population (perhaps the majority of women), a significant number in India and a much smaller number in China have used hydroquinone cosmetically as a skin lightening agent [1–3,**4**,6]. This practice, often not disclosed to the clinician, has been strongly associated with the development of exogenous ochronosis [1–3,6–8].

The pigment in exogenous ochronosis strongly resembles that in the endogenous form and may result from the inhibition of homogentisic acid oxidase by hydroquinone. Milder cases show only macular 'sooty' pigmentation, whilst more advanced cases develop irregular stippling, papulation and pigmented colloid milia [8,9]. These features tend to be most prominent over the areas of skin most intensely exposed to the sun. Histologically, deposits of pigment are observed in the papillary and reticular dermis and probably represent accumulations of the pigment in association with degenerated collagen [9,10]. Characteristic dermoscopic findings of distinctive blue-grey dots and globules, obliterating follicular openings, are reported [6].

In many countries, the concentration of hydroquinone in cosmetic products has been legally restricted to 2%, with the aim of reducing the risk of ochronosis. However, it is not established that this risk is dependent on the concentration, and prolonged use, even of a 2% concentration, may be equally relevant [6,11]. Use of hydroquinone should be limited to 6 months to minimise the risk of ochronosis, and concomitant photoprotection is important. Higher concentrations of hydroquinone may cause more irritancy [**4**]. Hydroquinone should be avoided in pregnancy, although over-the-counter products are often not labelled to advise avoidance of use during pregnancy [12].

In striking contrast to Africa, exogenous ochronosis seems to be rare in the USA, even though hydroquinone-containing compounds are widely used there [13–15]. Possible explanations put forward for this paradox in the USA include concomitant use of sunscreens, relatively cautious use of these compounds and underreporting, and in Africa the use of different formulations (especially hydro-alcoholic solutions), combined use with other compounds and intense solar irradiation.

Exogenous ochronosis occurs mainly in black skin, although occasional cases have occurred in Hispanics, Chinese and people with white skin [6,15]. The relatively high levels of enzyme activity associated with melanin synthesis in black skin, and additional stimulation of these pathways by intense sun exposure, seem to be required for ochronosis to develop.

Ochronosis is very difficult to treat, but Q-switched lasers with long wavelength may be helpful [16].

Kligman cream
This formulation comprises 5% hydroquinone, 0.1% tretinoin and 0.1% dexamethasone in hydrophilic ointment [17]. It has been widely used as a depigmenting treatment, especially for melasma. Variations on this preparation are widely used globally; when a potent topical steroid such as mometasone furoate 0.1% is substituted, predictable corticosteroid side effects occur [4].

Monobenzyl ether of hydroquinone
Skin bleaching with 20% monobenzyl ether of hydroquinone (monobenzone) is generally reserved for the treatment of carefully selected cases of vitiligo. The resulting depigmentation may be permanent, so this treatment is only suitable for those with extensive disease, in whom the appearance of the skin would be improved by removing the residual pigment. Patients should be warned that results are unpredictable. Treatment may need to be prolonged and is not always successful [18]. Depigmentation may occur at sites other than those being treated. Spontaneous repigmentation may occur unexpectedly after cessation of the treatment, slowly or rapidly, at both treated and untreated sites [19]. Contact dermatitis can develop [18,20]. It has also been reported that this treatment may cause corneal and conjunctival pigmentation [21].

The addition of monobenzyl ether of hydroquinone to cosmetic skin lightening preparations caused an epidemic of leukomelanoderma in South Africa during the early 1970s [9].

Additional phenol derivatives
Mequinol (4-hydroxyanisole, 4-methoxyphenol) is another phenol derivative with depigmenting properties. It is a constituent of a commercially formulated solution containing 2% mequinol and 0.01% tretinoin, marketed for the treatment of solar lentiginosis. In trials with a treatment duration of 24 weeks, this combination appeared to be more effective than either of the constituents used alone, or than placebo [22]. Mequinol has also been used with benefit in the treatment of melasma, but there is insufficient evidence to date to recommend its use [4]. Mequinol 20% cream has been successfully used to remove residual pigmentation in severe vitiligo, with efficacy considered comparable with monobenzyl ether of hydroquinone [23].

Retinoic acid
Retinoic acid (tretinoin) has been successfully used to reduce pigmentation in a variety of disorders including melasma [24], actinic lentiginosis [25,26] and post-inflammatory hyperpigmentation [27]. In most trials, tretinoin 0.1% cream has been used for 40 weeks. Retinoid dermatitis is a common side effect and may result in postinflammatory hyperpigmentation. Some mild reduction of pigment may occur in normal skin surrounding the treated areas. The mechanism of action is not fully understood, but may be at least partly explained by a reduction in melanogenesis consequent upon reduction of tyrosinase activity [28].

Attempts have been made to use other retinoids for this purpose, with variable results; 10% all-*trans* retinol gel proved effective, although irritant, in a Japanese study [29]. A study on the use of topical 0.05% isotretinoin in melasma showed no difference from placebo after 40 weeks [30].

Azelaic acid
This non-phenolic dicarboxylic acid is a relatively safe, although mildly irritant, agent with several roles to play in dermatology. As a depigmenting agent, azelaic acid is moderately effective in the treatment of melasma. The proposed mechanism is direct or indirect inhibition of tyrosinase [31]. Azelaic acid 20% cream proved more effective than 2% hydroquinone cream after 24 weeks of treatment [32]. In two other studies with the same treatment duration, 20% azelaic acid proved equivalent in efficacy to 4% hydroquinone cream [33,34]. Another study on facial hyperpigmentation in darker skinned individuals compared a combination of azelaic acid 20% cream and glycolic acid 15% or 20% lotion, with 4% hydroquinone cream; similar efficacy was observed from the two regimens [35]. Azelaic acid has also proved effective in the treatment of Kitamura reticulate acropigmentation [36].

Azelaic acid has antineoplastic properties, inhibiting mitochondrial enzymes and DNA synthesis [4,37], and has been used as a palliative treatment for lentigo maligna and melanoma [38,39], although some cases of lentigo maligna have progressed to invasive melanoma whilst using this treatment [39].

Azelaic acid 20% cream is effective in the treatment of acne and rosacea [40,41]. This is likely to be due to a combination of antimicrobial and anti-inflammatory properties. It inhibits the growth of *Propionobacterium acnes* and *Staphylococcus epidermidis*, the production of free radicals by polymorphonuclear leukocytes [42], and the growth of dermatophytes [43] and antibiotic-resistant *Staphylococcus aureus* [44].

Kojic acid
This is a fungal metabolite known to inhibit tyrosinase by chelating copper at the active site of the enzyme [4,45]. Used at 1–4%, it is a constituent of over-the-counter depigmenting creams sold globally. In the treatment of melasma, 1% kojic acid proved of equal efficacy to 2% hydroquinone when each was used in combination with glycolic acid [46,47], but it is less effective when used as monotherapy [4].

Liquiritin
This compound, which can be extracted from liquorice (*Glycyrrhiza glabra*) and other herbal sources, has been reported to be effective in reducing the pigmentation of melasma in a double-blind trial [48].

Arbutin
Arbutin is a derivative of D-glucopyranoside that competitively inhibits tyrosinase and is cytotoxic to melanocytes [4,49]. A 3% preparation in combination with 4% nicotinamide and 1% bisabolol and 0.05% retinal has resulted in improvement in melasma and it has also been used successfully in combination with the neodymium:yttrium-aluminium-garnet (Nd:YAG) laser [4].

Ascorbic acid (vitamin C)
Ascorbic acid acts as a reducing agent at various oxidative steps in melanin synthesis, but preparations can be unstable due to rapid oxidation. Ascorbic acid 5% has less adverse effects than 4% hydroquinone, but is less effective [4].

Niacinamide
Niacinamide, the active amide of vitamin B_3, inhibits the transfer of melanosomes to keratinocytes. A 4% cream is better tolerated than 4% hydroquinone, but is slightly less effective [4].

Resveratrol
Resveratrol, a polyphenol found in many edible plants, including grape skin, inhibits tyrosinase and has potent antioxidant effects. It is unstable in cosmetics and is acetylated to resveratryl triacetate to improve stability. At a concentration of 0.8% it reduces skin pigmentation in human volunteers exposed to UV light, and resveratryl triacetate 0.4% in combination with glycolic acid reduces UV-induced tanning in human volunteers [50].

Other agents
Topical tranexamic acid, 4-*n*-butyl resorcinol, flutamide 1% cream and glycolic acid 5–10% (used as an exfoliator to brighten the skin) are other agents that may be effective in lightening skin pigmentation [4,51–53].

Depilatories
Depilation can be defined as temporary removal of hair, whilst epilation denotes permanent destruction of the follicle. Epilation requires physical methods of destruction of the follicle such as electrolysis, lasers and intense pulsed light (IPL). Depilation can be achieved by shaving, waxing, plucking, threading and by use of topical depilatory creams. Systemic androgen antagonists have a role to play in some cases; only topical treatments are discussed here.

Traditional depilatory creams depend upon breaking the disulphide bonds in hair. Three main classes are used. The oldest are various sulphides (e.g. 20% strontium or barium sulphide), which have a powerful effect but may irritate, and in the presence of water generate malodorous hydrogen sulphide. They are effective on terminal hair in the axillae. Thioglycolates are being used more frequently, but they are slower to work than sulphides. Concentrations of 2.5–4% produce an effect in 5–15 min. Substituted mercaptans (thioalcohols) are those most widely used. They work slowly, but are suitable for use on the face. The hair shafts are only removed down to skin surface level, so the reduction in hair is of short duration. Irritant dermatitis may occur.

Eflornithine hydrochloride is an irreversible inhibitor of ornithine decarboxylase, an enzyme required for hair growth. This is marketed as an 11.5% cream, applied twice daily, that can slow the growth of facial hair, and was approved by the US FDA for topical treatment of hirsutism in 2000. A response takes 4–8 weeks to develop and the effect wears off over a similar period when the treatment is discontinued, so treatment needs to be ongoing [1]. The benefit seems to be rather modest in many cases, with only 32% of patients reporting marked improvement [1–3]. Some irritation may occur, but contact sensitisation is rare. In a prospective randomised clinical trial, the combination of IPL and eflornithine was much more effective than IPL alone [4].

Sensitising agents
These chemicals are known as universal sensitisers. The principal ones used clinically have been dinitrochlorobenzene (DNCB), squaric acid dibutyl ester (SADBE) and diphencyprone (diphenylcyclopropenone, DCP). Almost every individual will develop allergic dermatitis after repeated skin contact with these substances, usually after the first exposure. Animals are also readily sensitised.

For many years dermatologists have tried to utilise the induction of contact sensitisation, using these and other allergens to manipulate immune responses to advantage in a wide variety of benign and malignant skin diseases [1]. Numerous attempts have been made, with some reported success, to use sensitisers to stimulate an immune response to malignancies including melanoma [1,2]; for example, there are isolated reports showing benefit in cutaneous melanoma metastases not responding to immune checkpoint inhibitor treatment alone [3]. Currently, topical sensitisers have found two main roles in dermatology: for alopecia areata and for viral warts [1].

The sensitisers that have been most intensively investigated are DNCB, SADBE and DCP. The earliest of these to be used was DNCB, which was subsequently found to be mutagenic, and is no longer routinely used in clinical practice. The use of SADBE or DCP avoids this hazard, and DCP has the advantage of a practical shelf-life. The latter has therefore become the most widely used sensitiser for the treatment of alopecia areata and warts. DCP does not cross-sensitise patients to any other household or medicinal substances. An additional advantage is that it is photochemically unstable and degrades in the presence of visible light. Accidental spills will therefore not result in longlasting environmental contamination. Because of this property, DCP must be stored in the dark, and is dispensed in dark brown bottles.

The precise mechanisms by which induction of contact allergy can induce hair regrowth in alopecia areata have not been established. It seems likely that regulatory mechanisms activated to modulate the contact allergic reaction also downregulate the autoimmune reaction responsible for the alopecia. Increased production of IL-10 may explain this effect [4]. DNCB [5], SADBE [6] and DCP [7] have all been shown to stimulate hair regrowth on treated areas of the scalp in studies using untreated areas as a control. The same effect has been achieved, in sensitised individuals, by use of *Primula* leaves [8] and nickel patch test reagent [9].

Hair regrowth on one side of the scalp that has been treated with allergen, whilst there is none on the other side, has been clearly demonstrated in innumerable studies, and constitutes part of the treatment regimen in many protocols. Sensitisation can usually be achieved by the application of 2% concentration of DCP to the skin of a small area of the scalp or upper arm, repeated after 1–2 weeks if there is no reaction. Subsequent treatment can begin with a 0.01% solution and usually continues on a weekly basis, adjusting the concentration as required to maintain mild dermatitis. Attempts have been made to achieve the same effect by the use of a simple inflammatory response induced by contact irritants. Phenolics, cantharides, camphor and other irritants have been used for many years, mostly without controlled trials [10]. Trials using croton oil and retinoic acid have not confirmed a response to these irritants [10,11]. With the possible exception of dithranol [12], it has proved difficult to establish the efficacy of irritants.

The effect of contact sensitisation in alopecia areata is of value to patients who are particularly distressed by the condition. In a meta-analysis, complete regrowth was observed in 24.9% of patients with alopecia totalis/universalis. However, recurrence rates are high, occurring in 38.3% of patients receiving maintenance treatment and 49.0% of those not receiving maintenance treatment. Disease extent of 50% or greater, atopic history and nail involvement were associated with poorer therapeutic outcomes [13]. In children with alopecia areata, the efficacy of satisfactory hair regrowth has been reported to range from 11% to 33% [14].

In the treatment of warts with topical sensitisers, most published efficacy data are retrospective, and published controlled trials have been small and inconclusive [1,15]. A Cochrane review found two controlled trials showing that DNCB was more than twice as effective as placebo [16]. Uncontrolled data are convincing but inconsistent, perhaps because treatment regimens have also been variable [1]. The best results with DCP have been obtained by first sensitising patients at a site remote from the warts and then applying DCP 0.01–6% to the lesions at intervals of 1–4 weeks. Complete clearance was reported in 70–85% of patients with this method [17,18]. Again, the mechanism of action has not been fully clarified but it is likely that the induction of an inflammatory reaction within the wart induces an influx of immunocompetent cells, which can then promote an appropriate immune response to the infecting human papillomavirus. The reaction is non-specific, and allergic contact dermatitis to alkyl bromide has also resulted in the contemporaneous clearance of longstanding viral warts [19]. A combination of DCP and acitretin may improve efficacy in resistant viral warts [20]. DCP can clear recalcitrant viral warts in immunosuppressed patients, including patients on biologic treatment, but with a lower rate of efficacy than in the immunocompetent, with a requirement for more prolonged treatment [21].

Topical contact sensitisers have been used with success in the treatment of ano-genital warts in children [22], molluscum contagiosum [23], including recalcitrant molluscum contagiosum in the context of HIV infection where antiretroviral treatment alone was ineffective [24], and in the prevention of recurrent herpes simplex labialis [25,26].

Adverse effects of topical contact sensitisers include hypopigmentation and/or hyperpigmentation at the sensitisation and/or treatment sites in darker skin types, regional lymphadenopathy during treatment (particularly in the treatment of alopecia areata), persistent dermatitis, bullous reactions, (rarely) urticaria and (very rarely) anaphylaxis [1,27].

Sunscreens

It is likely that in the early evolution of *Homo sapiens*, pigmentation of the skin developed primarily as protection from the risk of sunburn. Subsequent migration away from our equatorial origins reduced the risk of sunburn, and skin pigmentation was lost in order to facilitate adequate penetration of UVB into the skin for photochemical synthesis of vitamin D. Unlike vitamin D deficiency, the adverse consequences of this loss of endogenous sunscreen may not have reduced genetic fitness, since they tend to occur mainly in later life. However, individuals with white skin are clearly at greater risk from melanoma and non-melanoma skin cancer as well as photoageing.

Sunscreens, if applied correctly, reduce UV penetration into the skin. This may enable those with fair skin, who would normally burn with any significant sun exposure, to expose themselves to intense sunlight for prolonged periods, thus achieving a significantly greater cumulative UV irradiation than would otherwise have been possible. This is especially likely to happen if sunscreens with low protection against UVA are used. The ideal sunscreen should block completely the transmission of both UVB (280–320 nm) and UVA (320–400 nm), whilst at the same time be cosmetically acceptable (for example, not stain clothing) and pleasant to use. Additional desirable properties are durability on the surface of the skin, including photostability and water resistance. The latter is especially important if the sunscreen is to be used when swimming. Sunscreens are generally more effective in blocking UVB than UVA but effective filtration of UVA is as important. Recent studies have shown that, although UVB causes much more DNA damage than UVA to cells near the epidermal surface, the epidermal basal layer is particularly sensitive to UVA, which is able to penetrate easily through the epidermis to inflict DNA damage (as measured by cyclobutane pyrimidine dimer formation) at the level at which both melanocytes and basal keratinocytes are located [1,2]. It is now thought that UVA exposure is a signicant contributor to carcinogenesis [3–5] as well as to photoageing [6,7]. UVA has also been shown to induce local immunosuppression [8,9], can play a central role in photodermatoses such as polymorphic light eruption [10] and drug-induced photosensitivity [11], and penetrates window glass.

No single compound can achieve all the desired aims, so most commercial formulations contain a mixture of active constituents. These fall into two broad categories: physical sunscreens that act by reflecting and scattering UV light, and chemical agents that absorb UV light [7,12–14]. Frequently used compounds are listed in Table 18.9.

Physical agents such as titanium dioxide and zinc oxide can block a broad spectrum of UVB, UVA and visible light; the latter property may be important in some photodermatoses in which there is sensitivity to visible light. Their efficacy against UVA and visible light depends on particle size. Larger particle size results in superior efficacy but reduced cosmetic acceptability due to the increased whitening of the skin (which is, of course, reflection of visible light). There has been some concern over the potential for UV light to interact with zinc and titanium oxides and release free radicals [15]. Fortunately, the oxide particles do not seem to penetrate the stratum corneum and the risk would appear to be very limited [16]. The US FDA deems physical sunscreens to be very safe [17].

Chemical agents vary in their absorption of UV radiation, with some blocking predominantly UVB whilst others absorb UVA. Relatively few absorb longwave UVA (UVA1: 340–400 nm), exceptions being butylmethoxydibenzoylmethane, which has an absorption spectrum of 320–400 nm, and terephthalylidene dicamphor sulfonic acid, with an absorption spectrum of 290–400 nm. Some, such as butylmethoxydibenzoyl methane, become unstable when exposed to UV light, and hence potentially less effective in products exposed to UV over time, but this can be counteracted by combining it with other sunscreens such as benzophenone-3 [7]. Chemical UV blockers may cause irritant, allergic, phototoxic or photoallergic reactions. Benzophenones are probably the commonest sensitisers, whilst dibenzoylmethanes, *para*-aminobenzoic acid (PABA) and

Table 18.9 Compounds used as active constituents of sunscreens.

	Type of UV light protected against
Physical agents	
Titanium dioxide	UVA, UVB, visible
Zinc oxide	UVA, UVB, visible
Ferrous (iron) oxide	UVA, UVB, visible
Mica (talc)	UVA, UVB
Calamine	UVA, UVB
Ichthammol	UVA, UVB
Kaolin	UVA, UVB
Chemical agents	
Anthranilates (e.g. methyl anthranilate)	UVA
Methoxybenzenes (e.g. bis-ethylhexyloxyphenol methoxyphenyl triazine/bemotrizinol/Tinosorb® S)	UVA, UVB
Camphor derivatives (e.g. terephthalylidene dicamphor sulfonic acid/ecamsule/Mexoryl® SX and 3,4-methylbenzylidene camphor/enzacamene/Eusolex® 6300)	UVA, UVB
Benzophenones (e.g. benzophenone-3/oxybenzone)	UVA, UVB
Benzotriazoles (e.g. methylene bis-benzotriazolyl tetramethylbutylphenol/ bisoctrizole/Tinosorb M and drometrizole trisiloxane/silatriazole/Mexoryl XL)	UVA, UVB
Cinnamates (e.g. octyl methoxy cinnamate/octinoxate)	UVB
Dibenzoylmethanes (e.g. butylmethoxydibenzoyl methane/avobenzone/Parsol® 1789 and 4-isopropyl-dibenzoylmethane)	UVA
Octocrylene	UVB
Para-aminobenzoic acid (PABA) and derivatives (e.g. ethylhexyl dimethyl PABA/padimate O)	UVB
Phenylbenzimidazole sulfonic acid	UVB
Salicylates (e.g. benzyl salicylate, ethyl hexyl salicylate/octisalate and homomenthyl salicylate/homosalate)	UVB

cinnamates may cause photoallergic dermatitis [18,19]. Allergy may also be due to other constituents such as fragrances and stabilisers.

Sunscreens are frequently added to cosmetics; 60% of leave-on haircare products contain sunscreens [20]. Benzyl salicylate, a chemical sunscreen, has been linked with the development of frontal fibrosing alopecia in males and females, either by induction of allergic contact dermatitis or through endocrine or enzymatic pathways [20,21]. It is present in 46% of leave-on hair products, 61% of fine fragrances, 26% of cosmetic and hygiene products sold in supermarkets, and in 8% of domestic cleaning products [21].

Sun protection factor (SPF) labelling was introduced to help consumers evaluate the level of protection from UVB and the risk of sunburn. Unfortunately, different systems of assay are used in different countries, making direct comparisons very misleading. However, all depend on deriving a ratio of the time or the amount of energy to reach a given end point (such as minimal redness) when using the sunscreen, to that required without using the sunscreen:

$$\text{SPF} = \frac{\text{Dose of UVB radiation producing minimal erythema with sunscreen}}{\text{Dose of UVB radiation producing minimal erythema without sunscreen}}$$

It should be noted that the SPF is based on the presumption that sunscreen is applied in a sufficient quantity to produce a specified thickness on the skin, usually 2 mg/cm^2. This is more than is used by most people. In a prospective study measuring actual usage of sunscreen by young adults on holiday, the median thickness of sunscreen applied was calculated to be less than 0.4 mg/cm^2 [22]. It is generally accepted that the thickness of sunscreen application on which SPF calculation is normally based is far greater than that which is generally used – which is usually taken as around 0.5 mg/cm^2 [23]. There is an exponential reduction in SPF with decreasing thickness of application so that sunscreens declared to provide SPFs of 4, 8 and 16 would in fact result in SPFs of only 1.4, 1.7 and 2.0 with such typical usage [23]. Nowadays many higher SPF sunscreens (SPF ≥50) are available and should provide an SPF of 15 or more in typical conditions [24]. The UV radiation dose reaching the skin is doubled between SPF 60 and 30 (1.7% versus 3.3%) and again between SPF 30 and 15 (3.3% versus 6.7%) [25]. There has been some debate as to whether increasing SPF beyond 50 provides any additional benefit. This has, however, been demonstrated *in vivo* in a blinded study in which there was a significantly greater protection from sunburn provided by an SPF 85 sunscreen compared with an SPF 50 preparation [24].

It is important that a sunscreen also provides adequate protection from UVA. A star system from 1 to 5 is often used in the assessment of protection against UVA [7]. Most modern sunscreens provide protection against UVA as well as UVB. Measurement of resistance to water has also not been standardised and can be assessed by several methods [26].

Whilst it would seem likely that correct use of sunscreens reduces the risk of malignancy, this has not been easy to confirm, especially in retrospective studies. Part of the difficulty is the presumed association between the use of a sunblock and a desire for sun exposure. Sunscreens have been shown to reduce UV-induced immunosuppression, which is considered to play a role in cutaneous carcinogenesis. Both the sensitisation [27] and elicitation [8] phases of immune responses can be preserved by the use of sunscreens. In a hairless mouse model, sunscreen combinations that block both UVA and UVB prevent cutaneous keratinocyte carcinogenesis, but individual sunscreen components that claim to block both UVA and UVB will not always prevent carcinogenesis [28].

In a placebo-controlled trial in a high-risk population, appropriate-strength sunscreens were shown to be effective in reducing the incidence of actinic keratoses [29]. In an Australian prospective controlled study, regular use of sunscreen reduced the incidence of new squamous cell but not basal cell carcinomas [30], although a Cochrane review found the evidence in this trial to be of low quality [31]. A study of BCCs indicated that there were fewer p53 mutations in those that developed in patients who had used sunscreen. This might be indicative of effective protection against UV-induced DNA mutations [32], but these are not the only factors involved in the development of BCCs. Another important population who require protection with sunscreens are patients who are immunosuppressed such as organ transplant recipients, patients taking azathioprine, ciclosporin or biologic agents, and patients with haematological disease. The use of sunscreen in transplant patients is increased by an intense educational programme, although the use of protective clothing increases more [33]. A recent reduction in the incidence of keratinocyte cancer in transplant patients may be related to changes in immunosuppressive regimens as well as sun protective behaviour [34].

Whether the risk of melanoma is reduced by the use of sunscreens is also a difficult question to answer. Two case–control studies have linked sunscreen usage to an increased incidence of melanoma, especially if sunscreens with an SPF below 10 are used [35,36]. These findings may possibly be explained in part by the probability that the subjects studied had previously used sunscreens that provided protection against UVB radiation alone, and were thus able to expose themselves to higher doses of solar radiation than those who did not use sunscreen. A randomised controlled trial showed a significant decrease in the development of invasive melanomas with regular use of sunscreen, but did not show a statistically significant decrease in the total number of melanomas [37]. Other studies have examined the development of naevi as a marker for risk of melanoma. A retrospective epidemiological study from Israel found that use of sunscreen was associated with a higher number of naevi [38]. Conversely, a prospective controlled trial from Vancouver demonstrated a reduced rate of development of naevi over a 3-year period in children provided with sunblock and instructed on its use. The effect was especially evident in those children who were freckled [39].

In addition to the protection of healthy skin, sunscreens have an important role in the management of patients with photodermatoses. The commonest of these, polymorphic light eruption, often seems to show rather limited benefit from sunscreens but may respond well to formulations that block a broad spectrum of UVA including longer wavelengths [40]. Sunscreens effective in blocking the offending wavelengths of UV light can also be helpful in the management of less common photodermatoses including actinic prurigo, chronic actinic dermatitis, hydroa vacciniforme, lupus erythematosus [41], porphyrias and solar urticaria (Chapter 126).

Whether sunscreens are applied to prevent solar damage to healthy skin or to manage a photodermatosis, it is important that these should not be regarded as the only means of limiting sun exposure. Staying indoors during the hours of peak sunlight intensity, and covering the skin with suitable clothing and headwear when outdoors, constitute more effective strategies than using sunscreens.

Tars

Tars are distillation products of organic material. Tars derived from wood have been used in the topical treatment of skin disease for millennia, including by the ancient Greeks; tars derived from shale, and especially coal, more recently [1]. By their nature, these products contain vast numbers of chemical constituents, and are difficult to standardise.

Wood tars

Oils of cade (juniper), pine, beech and birch are used for treating eczema and psoriasis. Oil of cade is particularly used in scalp preparations or when tar preparations are needed on the face. Wood tars are normally applied in 1–10% strength in various formulations including ointments, pastes, paints and shampoos. Pine tar has antipruritic, anti-inflammatory, antibacterial and antifungal effects. It is thought to reduce DNA synthesis and mitotic activity, which promotes a return to normal keratinisation. Bathing in pine tar improves atopic dermatitis in children, whereas bathing in tea does not [2]. Pine tar and topical triamcinolone have a similar suppressive effect on inflammation [1]. Irritation from wood tars is uncommon, especially with pine tar, but may occur when treating unstable, facial or flexural psoriasis. Wash-off pine tar products may be better tolerated [1]. Folliculitis occurs occasionally. Wood tars do not photosensitise and have an excellent safety profile, but may occasionally induce allergic sensitisation, for example pine tar contains terpenes related to colophonium, turpentine and linalool.

Shale tars (bitumen)

Ichthammol (ichthyol) is shale tar. It contains a very high proportion of organic sulphur. Shale tars have antiseptic and anti-inflammatory properties that can be useful in the management of eczematous dermatoses, but they are generally less effective than coal tars. They are not photosensitisers. Ichthammol is often used in paste bandages for treating atopic eczema.

Coal tar

Coal tar is a black, viscous fluid with a potent characteristic smell, a product of various distillates of heated coal. The precise chemical composition of the tar depends on the source of the coal and the temperature of the distillation, as well as any subsequent processing.

Coal tar has been used for decades to treat psoriasis and other inflammatory skin diseases. It is still used in the treatment of psoriasis, either alone or in combination with UVB, and is the basis of the Goeckerman regimen combining tar and UVB [3] (Chapter 35). This regimen is still used in many countries, including the USA. Crude coal tar (black tar) 2–10% or liquor picis detergens 20% preparations are used, in combination with broad- or narrow-band UVB. The Goeckerman regimen has the advantage of an excellent safety profile, including in pregnancy, and can induce remission periods of more than a year. An adapted version may also be used to treat atopic eczema [4]. The time commitment of 4–5 hours' treatment per day at a hospital out-patient unit, 5 days per week for 6 weeks, is a potential disincentive for patients. Purified coal tar 3% with salicylic acid 6% once daily for 12 weeks applied to chronic plaque psoriasis is as effective as calcipotriol/betamethasone dipropionate ointment, although the onset of efficacy is slightly slower [5]. Coal tar is superior in efficacy to vehicle [6] and 5% is superior to 1% crude coal tar [7].

Randomised controlled trials support the use of coal tar products in terms of efficacy, cost and their low side effect profile in the treatment of both psoriasis and atopic dermatitis [8]. Prior to the advent of topical corticosteroids, coal tar was widely used in the treatment

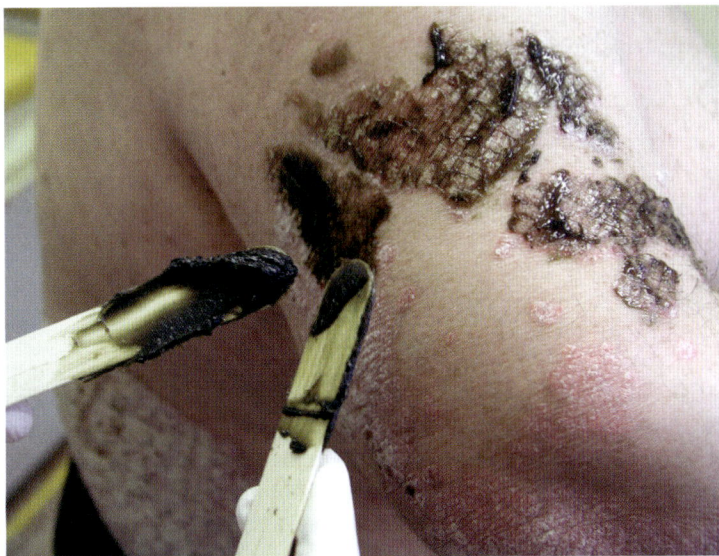

Figure 18.13 Crude coal tar in white soft paraffin being applied to chronic plaque psoriasis.

of eczematous dermatoses and it remains useful as an alternative to steroids, as a steroid-sparing agent and as an antipruritic. Coal tar can be added to paste bandages, although ichthammol is often preferred.

The disadvantages of coal tar include the smell, messiness (Figure 18.13), staining of clothing, potential for irritancy, phototoxicity (from both UVA and visible light) and rarely allergic sensitisation [9]. There may be cross-sensitisation with wood tars [10]. Prolonged contact is usually required for good results. Over the years, a wide range of more 'acceptable' formulations of tar have been developed, as creams, ointments, pastes, bath additives and shampoos, with a view to improving acceptability. None of these completely removes the odour or the risk of staining clothing. A study comparing 5% liquor carbonis detergens (an alcoholic solution of crude coal tar) with calcipotriol 0.005% cream found significantly better results with coal tar, with less relapse on withdrawal [11]. Many dermatologists believe that the more 'acceptable' tar extracts have tended to be less effective than crude coal tar, but only extracts are now commercially available. The range of proprietary products has also diminished in recent years, due to reduced uptake by patients, a reduction in the provision of nurse day treatment and in-patient beds, deskilling of doctors and nurses in the use of tar, shortages of raw ingredient materials for manufacturing tar preparations, concerns over possible carcinogenicity and, in particular, increased use of systemic immunosuppressants and monoclonal antibody treatments.

The active constituents, and the mechanisms by which tar exerts its effects, remain uncertain. Tar plus UV light reduces epidermal DNA synthesis [12,13]. This may be related to the formation of cross-links between opposite strands on the DNA double helix [14]. A cytostatic effect of crude coal tar has also been postulated [15], following the finding that prolonged application to normal skin produces epidermal thinning associated with retention hyperkeratosis. In the treatment of atopic eczema, coal tar may promote restoration of skin barrier function, upregulating the expression of key barrier proteins such as filaggrin, and exert anti-inflammatory activity through interaction with the aryl hydrocarbon receptor, increasing epidermal differentiation and suppressing the Th2 cytokine response [16].

The well-established carcinogenicity of pitch and heavy tar fractions, which contain large quantities of polycyclic aromatic hydrocarbons, has given rise to concerns about potential carcinogenicity of tar preparations intended for use on human skin [17,18]. Reports of malignant tumours in humans in relation to tar therapy are historical and rare. Rook *et al.* reported five cases [19] and Greither *et al.* 13 cases [20]; most had genital or groin involvement, but these are nowadays unlikely sites for tar application. Several large, long-term, follow-up studies have shown no increase in the incidence of skin or bladder tumours [**21**,22–25].

Antihistamines

Topical antihistamines (e.g. diphenhydramine, mepyramine maleate, promethazine) are widely employed in non-prescription preparations as antipruritic agents. The efficacy of such preparations is questionable. Limited efficacy, combined with the marked potential for many antihistamines to sensitise when applied topically, has tended to deter dermatologists from advocating them.

Topical application of doxepin, a potent H_1- and H_2-receptor antagonist and anticholinergic agent, reduced the pruritus associated with atopic eczema [1] and other eczematous dermatoses such as lichen simplex [2], in placebo-controlled trials. Doxepin mouthwash reduces pain from radiation-induced mucositis significantly more than placebo [3]. Like other topical antihistamines, this compound may sensitise [4,5]. Systemic absorption may be significant, especially in children, and may give rise to sedation [1,2,6].

Antiperspirants

Most antiperspirants marketed for cosmetic purposes contain aluminium chloride hexahydrate. In contemporary products, refined formulations of aluminium chlorohydrates (or aluminium zirconium complexes) are often used to maximise precipitation of aluminium hydroxide within the sweat duct [1]. Cosmetic antiperspirants are often combined with antimicrobial agents that reduce axillary odour by inhibiting the action of bacterial metabolism on various components of apocrine sweat. Fragrances are often added to mask or adjust the odour in various ways, around eight individual fragrances being labelled in the average product [2], and 91% of products containing fragrances [3]. Hence sensitisation may occur; axillary dermatitis is a frequent presenting symptom of fragrance allergy. The management of hyperhidrosis is discussed in Chapter 92.

In treatment of hyperhidrosis of the axillae, palms and soles, higher concentrations of aluminium chloride hexahydrate (e.g. 20–25% in ethanol) are generally used as first line treatment. These are more effective, more irritant and more likely to damage clothing than cosmetic formulations. Blockage of the sweat duct is regarded as the principal mechanism of action [1,4], although secondary degeneration of the secretory cells may develop after long-term use, as a result of the increased pressure in the duct [5]. For maximal efficacy the treatment should be applied when the skin is dry and sweating is minimal. Drying the axilla with a hairdryer on a low heat before application may be beneficial. Application at night is often recommended and this also helps minimise damage to clothing. Polythene occlusion may enhance efficacy and irritancy. Irritation often limits the use of this treatment but may settle with reduced frequency of application and the use of a mild or moderately potent topical steroid.

Traditional remedies that have fallen out of favour include the aldehydes. These are believed to work by a similar mechanism to aluminium salts. Aqueous glutaraldehyde solution (up to 10%) can be applied on a swab to the soles of the feet [6,7]. The keratin stains orange-brown when higher concentrations are used. Formaldehyde solution BP (1–3%) used as a twice-daily soak also helps mild cases. Both compounds are potential sensitisers and are therefore not ideal for prolonged use.

Anticholinergic agents inhibit the anomalous sympathetic (cholinergic) innervation of the sweat glands and can be applied topically to minimise the side effects associated with systemic administration. Topical glycopyrronium swabs have been recently licensed in the USA for the treatment of primary axillary hyperhidrosis in adults and in children from the age of 9 years [8,9]. Glycopyrrolate 2% cream or lotion has been used with success in patients suffering from severe facial hyperhidrosis or gustatory sweating following parotidectomy [10,11]. Glycopyrronium bromide can also be very effective when administered by iontophoresis [12]. Dry mouth is common and visual accommodation may be disturbed for 24–48 h following treatment. Iontophoresis with tap water is also effective, by an unknown mechanism [13,14], and avoids these side effects.

Surgical treatments and injection of botulinum toxin are considered in Chapter 92.

Dyes
Gentian (crystal) violet
This is a triphenylmethane dye that has antiseptic properties against bacteria (e.g. *Staphylococcus* and *Streptococcus*) and yeasts (e.g. *Candida albicans*). Gentian violet (hexamethyl pararosaniline) irreversibly fixes Gram-positive bacteria, leading to the development of the Gram stain by Hans Gram in 1884, using gentian violet. It is effective in the treatment of *Staphylococcus aureus*-colonised atopic eczema and eradicates MRSA from infected leg ulcers [1]. Employed for many years as a topical treatment for bacterial and fungal skin infections in the pre-antibiotic and antifungal era, its use was greatly reduced after experimental studies demonstrated that it interacted with the DNA of living cells [2]. Long-term high oral doses in animals have been associated with tumours of internal organs, but no malignancies have been seen with over a century of external use in humans. The main adverse effect is reversible skin staining, and permanent staining of clothing. If applied to ulcers, it can cause permanent tattooing of the skin. It is available over the counter in many countries as a 1% and 2% solution for application to unbroken skin. It has the advantages of being cheap, easy to prepare, is chemically stable at room temperature for years and does not have the risk of antimicrobial resistance.

Brilliant green
This is also a triphenylmethane dye and has properties similar to gentian violet. It was often used in combination with the latter but does not seem to increase the spectrum of activity [3]. It has suffered similar restrictions in usage, as have other members of the group, such as malachite green.

Magenta (basic fuchsin)
An active component of Castellani paint (also containing acetone, boric acid, ethanol, phenol, resorcinol and water), magenta is known to have activity against Gram-positive bacteria and fungi, but is no longer used because of potential carcinogenicity. Colourless Castellani paint (the same formula without the magenta) has been used to reduce secondary bacterial contamination in onycholysis and in chronic paronychia.

Eosin
Eosin is a red dye that has astringent and antiseptic properties. A 2% solution is used for ulcerative, erosive or weeping wounds, or inflammatory skin disease, including around stomas, applied when the dressing or device is changed. In the past it was used in some centres to reduce inflammation in severe inflammatory dermatoses, in particular erythrodermic psoriasis.

Other traditional remedies
Camphor
Camphor is an extract from the camphor laurel *Cinnamonum camphora*, best known as a moth repellent. It is sometimes added to lotions for its antipruritic and cooling effects. It is widely used in proprietary chilblain preparations.

Honey
Honey inhibits bacterial growth and has been in use since ancient times for dressing wounds. Potential indications include decubitus ulcers, venous ulcers, surgical wounds, anal fissures, seborrhoeic dermatitis and tinea pedis [1]. A range of commercially formulated products is available. Manuka honey, made from nectar collected from the manuka bush (a native shrub of New Zealand), has been popular recently, and has a higher content of the therapeutically active components methylglyoxal and hydrogen peroxide [1]. The use of honey on surgical wounds can result in a finer scar than standard wound dressings [2] and published results of manuka honey in the treatment of venous ulcers appear to be satisfactory [3].

Menthol
Menthol is still extracted mainly from the Japanese mint (*Mentha arvensis*), although synthetic sources are now available. It is added to calamine and other lotions and creams to induce a cooling sensation and relieve pruritus. At concentrations of 0.5–5% (usually 1%) in aqueous cream BP, it is a very useful and safe treatment for severe pruritus, particularly in the elderly.

Thymol
This compound is found in plants of the genus *Thymus* and contributes much of the characteristic flavour to thyme (*Thymus vulgaris*). It is a traditional and potent antibacterial and antifungal agent. It has limited solubility in water and is therefore most often used as a solution in chloroform or absolute alcohol. A traditional formulation is 4% thymol in chloroform. This has been used for paronychia and fungal nail infections and should be applied two or three times daily.

Miscellaneous agents

Becaplermin
Becaplermin (recombinant human platelet-derived growth factor (PDGF) BB) is a dimeric glycoprotein. Whilst PDGF occurs naturally as homodimers or heterodimers of A and B chains, becaplermin comprises only the BB homodimer. Amongst other properties, this cytokine is known to stimulate fibroblast proliferation and angiogenesis.

A gel containing becaplermin 0.01% has been demonstrated to accelerate healing of deep diabetic ulcers [1]. Pressure ulcers have also been reported to respond [2] and there are isolated case reports of its use as adjunctive treatment in severe ulceration due to pyoderma gangrenosum and calciphylaxis [3]. The gel is applied directly to the wound for 12 h daily.

There has been concern that the properties of this cytokine may promote the growth of a pre-existing malignancy. A post-marketing survey of a cohort of 1622 patients who had used three or more tubes of becaplermin revealed increased cancer mortality relative to controls [4], although the incidence of malignancy was not increased. A black box warning has been issued by the US FDA. This product is not currently marketed in Europe, but it is licensed in the USA.

Bimatoprost
This drug is a prostaglandin analogue and an agonist of the prostamide α-F_2 receptor, used in the treatment of glaucoma. It was incidentally observed to induce eyelash hypertrichosis, and licensed in the USA in 2008 as a 0.03% preparation to treat eyelash hypotrichosis. It also stimulates eyebrow growth [1] and in a randomised study was more effective, and better tolerated, than mometasone furoate in the treatment of patchy alopecia areata [2]. When used intraocularly in the treatment of glaucoma, it can cause iris hyperpigmentation, periorbital hyperpigmentation and loss of periorbital fat [1]; when used in the treatment of eyelash hypotrichosis, iris hyperpigmentation and loss of periorbital fat do not occur.

Brimonidine
This drug, related to clonidine, is an α_2-adrenoceptor agonist widely used in the topical treatment of glaucoma. It was observed that the eye drops caused cutaneous vasoconstriction when they contaminated facial skin. Brimonidine tartrate gel 0.5% was developed specifically for the treatment of rosacea and licensed in 2014. It proved significantly effective in vehicle-controlled trials in the treatment of moderate to severe redness in rosacea [1]. Onset of effect is rapid, within 30 min, and duration of action is at least 12 h. Marked rebound redness and worsening of rosacea may occur [2]; systemic side effects such as bradycardia, hypotension and dizziness may uncommonly occur after topical application. Sensitisation has been reported [3].

Caffeine
Caffeine is a relatively small molecule with the potential for adequate penetration when applied topically. It is a phosphodiesterase inhibitor with potential anti-inflammatory activity mediated by changes in cyclic adenosine monophosphate levels in the epidermis.

In mice, caffeine has been shown to enhance UVB-induced apoptosis and to inhibit UVB-induced carcinogenesis [1].

In a study using *ex vivo* cultured human hair follicles, caffeine increased the rate of hair growth [2] and counteracted testosterone-related reduction in hair growth. An open randomised study showed 0.2% caffeine solution to be non-inferior to 5% minoxidil in the treatment of androgenetic alopecia in males [3]. Shampoos and hair tonics have been developed incorporating caffeine as a putative method of retarding androgenetic alopecia.

Capsaicin
Capsaicin is a remarkably potent compound extracted from chilli peppers and is responsible for the gustatory discomfort they induce. It is a very stable alkaloid, probably produced by these plants to prevent the seeds being eaten by animals (but not by birds, which lack the receptor required for its effects). Capsaicin stimulates the release of substance P, which is subsequently depleted in sensory neurons [1]. It also activates transient receptor potential vanilloid 1 (TRPV1), a Ca^{2+}-permeable ion channel in nociceptors [2], causing reversible ablation of nociceptor terminals and temporary hypoalgesia.

The first application established for this drug was in the treatment of postherpetic neuralgia [3]. However, an increasing range of conditions has been reported to benefit including diabetic neuropathy [4], burning mouth syndrome [5], nodular prurigo [6], notalgia paraesthetica [7], pruritus ani [8], pruritus caused by pityriasis rubra pilaris [9], psoriasis [10,11], PUVA itch [12] and uraemic pruritus [13].

Cromoglicate
Sodium cromoglicate is a member of the chromone group of drugs that also contains nedocromil sodium. These remarkably safe compounds inhibit the release of inflammatory mediators from mast cells and may also inhibit sensory nerve activation in response to histamine [1]. They are used topically in the treatment of asthma, rhinitis and conjunctivitis; systemic absorption is minimal. Oral cromoglicate is used for mast cell disorders.

The results from trials of topical sodium cromoglicate in the treatment of atopic eczema have been inconsistent, but a 4% lotion appears to have a modest effect on disease severity and a steroid-sparing action [2,3]. A 4% emulsion has been successfully used in combination with oral sodium cromoglicate in an infant with diffuse cutaneous mastocytosis [4].

Dihydroxyacetone
Dihydroxyacetone (DHA) reacts with amino acids in the stratum corneum to form a brown pigment, hence its widespread use in self-tanning creams, lotions and sprays. It is also incorporated into sunscreen products; the 'tan' itself offers little photoprotection. Some sufferers from vitiligo and other disorders of hypopigmentation find the use of DHA helpful as a cosmetic camouflage [1]. The hands must be washed after application to other body sites, or temporary staining of the palms and flexor aspect of the fingers will result. DHA appears to be remarkably safe.

Dithranol
Dithranol (anthralin, dihydroxyanthranol) is a time-honoured topical treatment for psoriasis [1], similar in its irritating and staining properties to chrysarobin, which it supplanted in the early 20th century, but more effective. It has been used in ointments, pastes and creams and as a pomade for use on the scalp. Historically, it was used

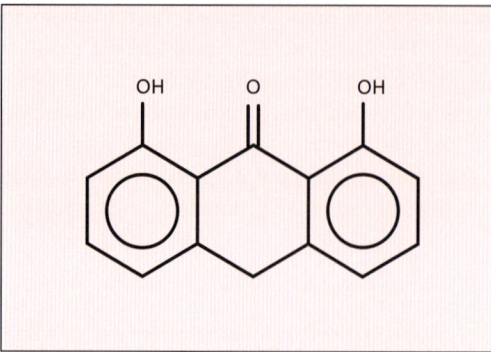

Figure 18.14 Structure of dithranol.

for chronic plaque psoriasis as part of the Ingram regime, where gradually increasing concentrations of dithranol were applied to the plaques in an in-patient setting in combination with UVB irradiation, resulting in prolonged psoriasis remission times. Its structure is shown in Figure 18.14.

The mechanism of action of dithranol is still uncertain. In the early response to dithranol in human psoriatic skin, the genes for keratinocyte and epidermal differentiation pathways and IL-1 family members (i.e. *IL36RN*) are differentially expressed, but elements of the IL-17/IL-23 axis are not. There is a rapid decrease in expression of keratinocyte differentiation regulators (e.g. involucrin), antimicrobial peptides (e.g. ß-defensins and S100 proteins) and chemotactic factors for neutrophils (e.g. *CXCL5*, *CXCL8*). Initial neutrophilic infiltration is later followed by a reduction in T-cell infiltration [2]. In healthy mouse skin, topical dithranol leads to a strong increase in mRNA expression of antimicrobial peptides, keratinocyte differentiation markers and inflammatory cytokines [3]. Dithranol induces a marked antiproliferative effect [4].

The use of dithranol has proved remarkably safe, although staining of skin, clothing and baths is a drawback (Figure 18.15a). Local reactions are common and temporary irritation of normal skin accidentally contaminated with dithranol can be severe (Figure 18.15b). Any irritation can be readily resolved by interrupting treatment for a couple of days and (if necessary) applying a moderate strength topical corticosteroid. There is no evidence of systemic toxicity with dithranol and it is not considered to be carcinogenic.

Dithranol, especially when incorporated in zinc oxide, is slowly oxidised by alkaline impurities to an inactive pink anthrone [5]. The effect of salicylic acid in preventing this has been known for a long time [6]. Salicylic acid neutralises hydroxyl ions in an alkaline medium, and perhaps reacts with free zinc ions to form an inactive zinc–dithranol complex. The combination of tar with dithranol is said to reduce dithranol irritancy without inhibiting its therapeutic effect [7]. The use of a water-soluble antioxidant, ascorbic acid, has allowed the production of stable dithranol cream preparations [5]. These are not as therapeutically potent as equivalent strengths of pastes or ointments but show much greater patient acceptability for home usage [8]. The development of a lipid-encapsulated cream formulation may increase acceptability by further reducing staining and irritation [9], but traditional preparations in zinc oxide paste appear more effective.

The introduction of new systemic therapies such as biologic agents, and the concomitant reduction in the availability of in-patient and out-patient facilities for intensive dermatology treatment, have greatly reduced the use of dithranol for extensive psoriasis. In recent years, it has become difficult for manufacturers to source dithranol as a raw ingredient, leading to a reduction in availability of both licensed and unlicensed preparations containing it. Dithranol still has a useful place in the treatment of more limited stable chronic plaque psoriasis, with the advantages of a potential induction of disease remission, often lasting many months, and no toxicity with long-term regular or intermittent use. Short-contact applications of strong dithranol pastes or creams are known to be almost as effective as prolonged contact use and facilitate treatment on an out-patient basis and self-treatment at home [10].

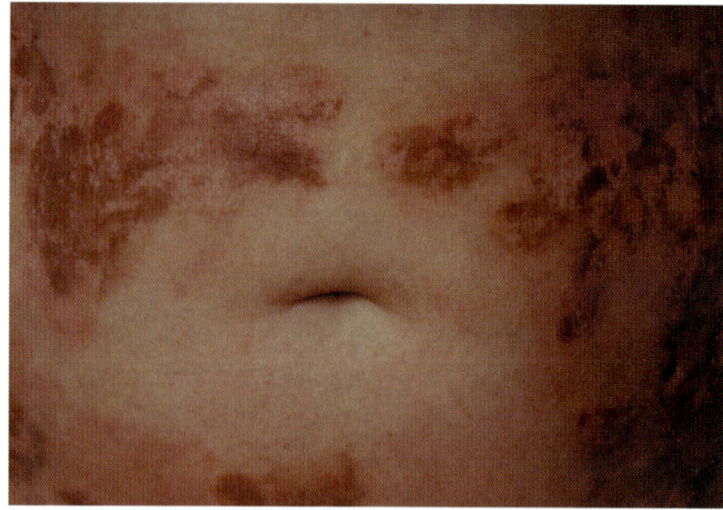

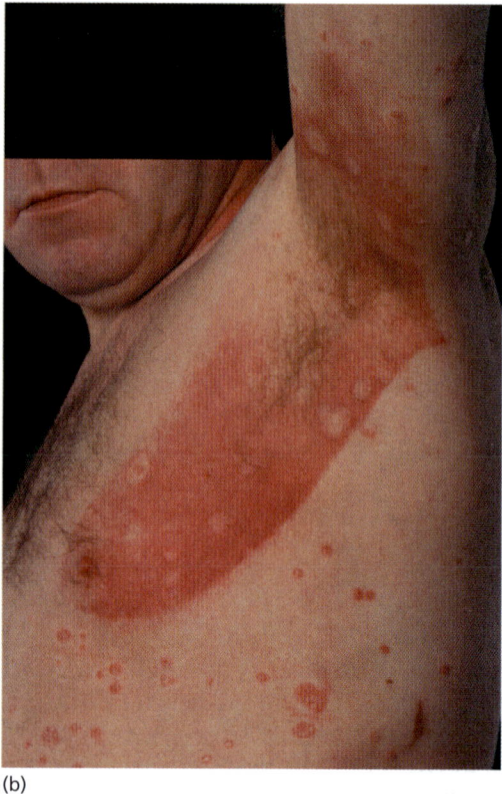

Figure 18.15 (a) Staining of the skin due to dithranol treatment. (b) An irritant reaction following accidental contamination of normal skin with dithranol.

Dithranol has also been used to stimulate an inflammatory response and regrowth of hair in patients with alopecia areata [11], and for the treatment of warts [12].

Glycyrrhetinic acid
Glycyrrhetinic acid is extracted from the root of the liquorice plant *Glycyrrhiza glabra*. This compound has anti-inflammatory properties that may be partly related to inhibition of cortisol metabolism by 11β-hydroxysteroid hydrogenase. It has been incorporated into topical preparations for the treatment of atopic eczema, being more effective than its vehicle in controlled trials in children and adults [1,2]. A Cochrane review showed moderate evidence for improved disease severity, a reduction in itch, lower eczema area and severity index (EASI) scores, fewer flares and increased patient satisfaction versus vehicle. However, the effects reported by patients were more prominent than those noted by investigators [3].

Minoxidil
This vasodilating agent was initially introduced as a systemic treatment for hypertension and was found to cause hypertrichosis [1]. A 2% minoxidil solution was marketed in 1986 and a 5% solution in 1993; these concentrations are approved by the US FDA for the treatment of androgenetic alopecia. The 2% solution is preferred in female-pattern baldness due to the risk of hypertrichosis [1,2]. Treatment results are usually modest [3]. Minoxidil can also accelerate hair regrowth after chemotherapy [4] or irradiation [5], and there is possibly some modest benefit in patients with alopecia areata and other types of alopecia [1]. Contact sensitisation to topical minoxidil, or to its propylene glycol excipient, may occur [6]. The use of minoxidil is discussed in detail in Chapter 87.

Morphine
Topical administration of opioids is potentially advantageous as a means of avoiding the central nervous system side effects associated with systemic administration of these drugs.

Alleviation of pain by using varied formulations of topically applied morphine has been reported in a range of conditions including pressure ulcers [1], sickle cell ulceration [2] and ulcerated scleroderma [3]. Results from small controlled trials in patients with leg ulcers of varied aetiology have yielded less consistent results [4,5], perhaps reflecting the size and other limitations of these trials. In oncology patients with ulcerated skin and mucosal lesions, 0.2% morphine ointment and gel, respectively, had very significant and sustained effects in relieving pain when used as a palliative treatment [6].

Nicotinamide and nicotinic acid
The marked anti-inflammatory properties of nicotinamide, the amide derivative of vitamin B_3 (niacin, nicotinic acid), have been used in the topical treatment of acne vulgaris. In a multicentre trial, a 4% alcoholic gel used for 8 weeks gave a global reduction in acne of 82%, compared with 68% for 1% clindamycin gel [1]. A Cochrane review found low-quality evidence that nicotinamide compared with clindamycin or erythromycin had similar withdrawal rates, but patient global assessment was not measured [2]. A potential advantage of nicotinamide is that the risk of antibiotic resistance is avoided.

Unlike nicotinamide, topical nicotinic acid causes vasodilatation, and it has been used to increase the diameter of cutaneous capillaries to facilitate the treatment of flushing and telangiectasia with lasers or intense pulsed light [3].

Nitrite, nitric oxide and glyceryl trinitrate
Nitric oxide (NO) is a short-lived gaseous free radical. Its synthesis by endothelial cells regulates vascular smooth muscle contraction. Macrophages and neutrophils also synthesise NO, which exerts potent antimicrobial activity against a wide range of organisms.

Acidification allows the gas NO to be applied to the skin as sodium nitrite in a cream, together with ascorbic or acetic acid. The mixture generates NO at the site of application, which can permeate the stratum corneum and nails. NO-releasing preparations are being investigated as potential topical agents to accelerate wound healing via vasodilatation [1]. The antimicrobial properties of NO generated from acidified nitrite have been exploited to treat dermatophyte infections of skin and nails [2], and an NO-releasing gel SB206 (berdazimer 12%) shows a modest effect in the treatment of molluscum contagiosum [3].

Glyceryl trinitrate (GTN) is another source of NO. Topical application of GTN increases blood flow in normal skin, and is used as a 0.1–0.4% ointment for the treatment of anal fissure [4]. It induces relaxation of the anal sphincter, increases blood flow and appears to be as effective as botulinum toxin [4]. Diltiazem 2% (as gel, cream or ointment) is used as an alternative for this purpose, and is less likely to cause headache as a side effect [5]. Allergic contact dermatitis to topical GTN may occur [6].

Salbutamol
Salbutamol acts on the $β_2$-adrenoceptor, which is present on immunocytes including CD4 lymphocytes and Langerhans cells. Salbutamol therefore has potential as a topical immunosuppressant and anti-inflammatory agent.

An uncontrolled trial suggested that both discoid and subacute lupus erythematosus may respond to salbutamol 0.5% cream [1]. A placebo-controlled trial in 37 patients with discoid lupus using R-salbutamol 0.5% cream twice daily for 8 weeks showed a significant improvement in symptoms (itching and pain), signs and patients' global assessments compared with placebo [2,3].

Silicone
A range of silicone gels and sheet dressings is marketed for the prevention and treatment of hypertrophic and keloid scars; they appear to be safe and well tolerated. The most likely mechanism of action is the effect of occlusion on keratinocyte hydration, which could alter epidermal cytokine signalling directed to dermal fibroblasts [1]. There is weak evidence of the benefit of silicone gel sheeting in the prevention of abnormal scarring in high-risk individuals, but the poor quality of research means a great deal of uncertainty prevails [2]. Trials evaluating silicone gel sheeting as a treatment for hypertrophic and keloid scarring showed improvements in scar thickness and scar colour, but are of poor quality and highly susceptible to bias [2].

In high-risk intensive care patients, silicone dressings applied to the sacrum and heels reduce the incidence of pressure ulcers [3].

Key references

The full list of references can be found in the online version at https://www.wiley.com/rooksdermatology10e

Prescribing topical treatment
6 Long CC, Finlay AY. The finger-tip unit: a new practical measure. *Clin Exp Dermatol* 1991;16:444–7.

Hazards associated with topical treatment
14 Nakamura M, Abrouk M, Zhu H *et al.* Update on the systemic risks of superpotent topical steroids. *J Drugs Dermatol* 2017;16:643–8.

Topical treatments used in the management of skin disease
Emollients
2 Santer M, Rumsby K, Ridd MJ *et al.* Adding emollient bath additives to standard eczema management for children with eczema: the BATHE RCT. *Health Technol Assess* 2018;22:1–116.

7 Chalmers JL, Harris RH, Bradshaw LE *et al.* Daily emollient during infancy for prevention of eczema: the BEEP randomized controlled trial. *Lancet* 2020;395:962–72.

Antiseptics
3 Majewski S, Bhattacharya T, Asztalos M *et al.* Sodium hypochlorite body wash in the management of Staphylococcus aureus-colonized moderate-to-severe atopic dermatitis in infants, children, and adolescents. *Pediatr Dermatol* 2019;36:442–7.

Antibiotics
1 Dessinioti C, Katsambas A. Propionibacterium acnes and antimicrobial resistance in acne. *Clin Dermatol* 2017;35:163–7.

32 Torrelo A, Grimalt R, Masramon X *et al.* Ozenoxacin, a new effective and safe topical treatment for impetigo in children and adolescents. *Dermatology* 2020;236:199–207.

42 Chen W, He C, Yang H *et al.* Prevalence and molecular characterization of methicillin-resistant *Staphylococcus aureus* with mupirocin, fusidic acid and/or retapamulin resistance. *BMC Microbiol* 2020;20:183.

Antifungal agents
4 Okokon EO, Verbeek JH, Ruotsalainen JH *et al.* Topical antifungals for seborrhoeic dermatitis. *Cochrane Database Syst Rev* 2015;Issue 5:CD008138.

Antiviral agents
2 Leslie RA, Zhou SS, Macinga DR. Inactivation of SARS-CoV-2 by commercially available alcohol-based hand sanitizers. *Am J Infect Control* 2021;49:401–2.

Antiparasitic agents
11 Taieb A, Ortonne JP, Ruzicka T *et al.* Superiority of ivermectin 1% cream over metronidazole 0.75% cream in treating inflammatory lesions of rosacea: a randomized, investigator-blinded trial. *Br J Dermatol* 2015;172:1103–10.

Topical glucocorticoids
4 Oakley R, Arent BWM, Lawton S *et al.* Topical corticosteroid vehicle composition and implications for clinical practice. *Clin Exp Dermatol* 2021;46:259–69.

65 Hunter A, Keith D, Buckley DA. Side-effects resulting from long-term use of topical calcipotriol and betamethasone in patients with psoriasis. *Br J Dermatol* 2017;177(Suppl. 1):68–9.

Calcineurin inhibitors
10 Ohtsuki M, Morimoto H, Nakagawa H. Tacrolimus ointment for the treatment of adult and pediatric atopic dermatitis: review on safety and benefits. *J Dermatol* 2018;45:936–92.

35 Siegfried EC, Jaworski JC, Kaiser JD, Hebert AA. Systematic review of published trials: long-term safety of topical corticosteroids and topical calcineurin inhibitors in pediatric patients with atopic dermatitis. *BMC Pediatr* 2016;16:75.

Retinoids
6 Chen C, Jensen BK, Mistry G *et al.* Negligible systemic absorption of topical isotretinoin cream: implications for teratogenicity. *J Clin Pharmacol* 1997;37:279–84.

52 Kolli SS, Pecone D, Pona A *et al.* Topical retinoids in acne vulgaris: a systematic review. *Am J Clin Dermatol* 2019;20:345–65.

Vitamin D analogues (deltanoids, secosteroids)
45 Ashcroft DM, Po AL, Williams HC, Griffiths CE. Systematic review of comparative efficacy and tolerability of calcipotriol in treating chronic plaque psoriasis. *BMJ* 2000;320:963–7.

55 Cunningham TJ, Tabacchi M, Eliane J-P *et al.* Randomized trial of calcipotriol combined with 5-fluorouracil for skin cancer precursor immunotherapy. *J Clin Invest* 2017;127:106–16.

Cytotoxic and antineoplastic agents
7 Weinstock MA, Thwin. SS, Siegel JA *et al.* Chemoprevention of basal and squamous cell carcinoma with a single course of fluorouracil 5% cream. A randomized clinical trial. *JAMA Dermatol* 2018;154:167–74.

Depigmenting agents
4 Sarkar R, Gokhale N, Godse K *et al.* Medical management of melasma: a review with consensus recommendations by Indian Pigmentary Expert Group. *Indian J Dermatol* 2017;62:558–77.

Sensitising agents
21 Audrain H, Siddiqui H, Buckley DA. Diphencyprone immunotherapy for viral warts in immunosuppressed patients. *Br J Dermatol* 2013;168:1138–9.

Sunscreens
21 Pastor-Nieto MA, Gatica-Ortega ME, Sanchez-Herreros C *et al.* Sensitization to benzyl salicylate and other allergens in patients with frontal fibrosing alopecia. *Contact Dermatitis* 2021;84:423–30.

Tars
21 Roelofzen JH, Aben KK, Oldenhof UT *et al.* No increased risk of cancer after coal tar treatment in patients with psoriasis or eczema. *J Invest Dermatol* 2010;130:953–61.

CHAPTER 19

Principles of Systemic Therapy

Andrew E. Pink, Richard T. Woolf and Catherine H. Smith
St John's Institute of Dermatology, Guy's and St Thomas' NHS Foundation Trust, London, UK

Introduction, 19.1
General aspects, 19.1
Risk reduction, 19.1
Anti-inflammatory and immunomodulatory drugs, 19.2
Antihistamines, 19.3
Antimalarial agents, 19.4
Apremilast, 19.7
Azathioprine, 19.8
Ciclosporin, 19.10

Colchicine, 19.12
Dapsone, 19.13
Fumarates, 19.15
Systemic glucocorticoids, 19.17
Hydroxycarbamide, 19.21
Janus kinase inhibitors, 19.22
Methotrexate, 19.24
Mycophenolate mofetil, 19.28
Potassium iodide, 19.30
Biologic therapies (protein therapeutics), 19.31

Intravenous immunoglobulin therapy, 19.40
Systemic retinoids, 19.41
Thalidomide, 19.44
Antimicrobial therapies, 19.46
Systemic antibiotics, 19.46
Anti-inflammatory effects of antibiotics, 19.48
Antifungal drugs, 19.48
Antiviral drugs, 19.49

Key references, 19.49

Introduction

General aspects

Drugs can target the skin by either topical, intralesional (for certain localised conditions) or systemic routes. The topical route is often the default approach in skin disease since it allows direct application of the drug to the site of pathology and potentially limits 'off target' effects and systemic exposure. When the bioavailability of topically applied drugs is insufficient, impractical to achieve and/or associated with unacceptable risks of local toxicity, systemic drug delivery is indicated. Drugs may also be used systemically if a topical formulation is not available. Systemic therapy is commonly combined with topical therapy to improve overall disease management and/or to minimise systemic drug exposure where this is a concern.

Risk reduction

As is the case when starting any therapeutic intervention (Chapter 13, and see section on patient education later in this chapter), it is important that the clinician ensures that the patient is fully informed about the benefits and harms of the proposed option, reasonable alternatives and the option to take no action. This includes use of a drug outside the licensed indication either for a disease not specified or at an unlicensed dose. It is the responsibility of the clinician prescribing a medication to maintain the safety of the individual patient on that drug, as well as to report any adverse events through relevant pharmacovigilance channels such as the UK Yellow Card Scheme (https://yellowcard.mhra.gov.uk/; last accessed August 2023) (Chapter 13 has further detail).

Standards of care

A wide range of clinical guidelines and patient pathways exist to help standardise clinical care with the overall aim of maintaining good clinical outcomes and patient safety. Specific guideline methodology provides a transparent framework for summarising evidence through to a systematised, unbiased, approach to recommendations [1]. Example organisations that develop guidelines for use in dermatology include the National Institute for Health and Care Excellence (NICE), the British Association of Dermatologists, the European Academy of Dermatology and Venereology and the American Academy of Dermatology. In addition, for specific medications with well-characterised risk(s) there may be specific processes to maintain patient safety, such as the pregnancy prevention plan and iPLEDGE for oral isotretinoin.

Patient selection

In the context of inflammatory skin disease, systemic therapy is offered to those individuals with more extensive body surface involvement, where topical approaches are ineffective or impractical. Less extensive disease that has failed to respond to topical therapy may also justify systemic therapy if there is associated significant functional impairment and/or high levels of distress, for example involvement of high-impact body sites, such as the face or hands/feet. Disease pathology may be deep in the dermis/subcutis or 'systemic', also necessitating systemic therapies, for example lupus profundus, panniculitis and vasculitides. Validated quality-of-life assessments and tools to measure/score clinical severity can be helpful in making therapeutic decisions. As with any shared clinical decision making that requires patient consent for an intervention, the treatment approach to a skin condition is tailored to the needs and clinical circumstance of each patient. In this context, the decision as to whether a topical or systemic approach is required will depend on disease factors (such as the nature, extent, site and severity), patient factors (such as age, co-morbidities, views on administration route and likelihood of adherence to treatment) and drug factors (such as efficacy, side effect profile, cautions/contraindications, potential drug interactions, monitoring requirements and cost).

Patient education

Active participation of the patient (the 'therapeutic partnership') in the decision-making process of treatment choice (shared decision making) is important as a means of enabling informed consent, empowering the patient to manage their own condition and reducing the risk of dissatisfaction with the outcome. This may include relatives and/or the patient's primary care doctor. Being transparent about the goal of therapy, from both the patient's and clincian's perspectives, and the likelihood of this being achieved, is a crucial component of this process. With many newer systemic treatments for common skin conditions, high-quality clinical trial and real-world data have been translated into decision aids [2] and online tools [3] to support these discussions. Organisations such as the British Association of Dermatologists provide publicly available patient-facing resources, such as information leaflets about skin conditions and treatments, which are specifically designed for a lay audience (https://www.bad.org.uk/patient-information-leaflets/; last accessed August 2023). Drug-specific information will also be provided by the manufacturer or other patient groups. In educating patients about their condition/treatment it is important to also allow them adequate time to consider such information in making an informed decision. This may vary from patient to patient, and for a chronic low-acuity medical issue there may not be an immediate need to start an intervention.

Once a decision on treatment has been made, patients should again be instructed about the practicalities in how and when to take the medication, potential relevant severe side effects and the importance of any required monitoring tests. They should be instructed how to seek medical advice if there is a query or problem associated with the treatment. If a patient is on a systemic medication that may have an impact on other medical care, such as an immunosuppressive medication, it is important that the patient is made aware of this and the importance of telling other care providers of their treatment. Mechanisms of doing this include the provision of a steroid card for someone on long-term systemic corticosteroid therapy to reduce the risk of adrenal insufficiency caused by medication being stopped abruptly. Patients may also consider wearing a MedicAlert® bracelet or necklace with their medical information inscribed.

Pre-treatment screening and monitoring tests

To minimise predictable risks of systemic drug therapy, certain clinical and investigational assessments may be indicated prior to and during therapy. These may be part of the licensed use of a drug – for example full blood count (FBC) monitoring during methotrexate use – or, more commonly, have evolved as part of the standard of care. Assessment requirements will need to be adapted to the individual needs of each patient, according to their clinical characteristics and risk profile including age, underlying disease, coexisting morbidities and co-therapies.

Drug interactions

Clinicians are strongly advised, when they recommend a systemic treatment, to check potential interactions with the patient's existing medications and to highlight common drugs that may interact with the new drug. In this context, the hospital pharmacist, utilising the local drug information service, also becomes part of the therapeutic partnership. Drug interactions listed in this chapter are not exhaustive.

Record keeping

Good clinical documentation is essential for risk management. When systemic medications are started by a specialist in secondary care it is important that the patient's primary care provider is informed. The discussion with the patient regarding the decision to start a systemic treatment, including potential benefits and harms of the intervention, should be documented. Copy letters sent to the patient can improve this communication and empower the patient regarding certain aspects of their care, such as the need for certain monitoring investigations.

Prescribing and monitoring practice

Every effort has been made in this chapter to provide the clinician with sufficient knowledge of the pharmacology, potential adverse effects, interactions and monitoring requirements for a comprehensive list of systemic treatments used in dermatology outside cancer. Nevertheless, clinicians are strongly advised to also reference local practices, national guidelines and the summary of product characteristics (SmPC) to optimise benefit and minimise harm. The authors make no claim to complete comprehensiveness. Furthermore, in recognising that practices may vary between individual dermatologists depending on personal experience, local factors and international differences, our suggestions for drug usage should not be considered prescriptive.

This chapter focuses on therapeutics for cutaneous inflammation and infection, the systemic therapies most commonly prescribed by dermatologists. For an update on novel therapeutics in other specialist areas, for example melanoma and cutaneous lymphoma, please see the respective chapters in this book.

Anti-inflammatory and immunomodulatory drugs

The terminology around drugs that affect the immune system – referred to in this chapter as immunomodulatory drugs – is evolving [1]. Therapeutic immunosuppression was originally used in the context of transplantation, where drugs such as tacrolimus, mycophenolate and sometimes corticosteroids are used to suppress organ rejection. This strategy comes with an important risk of infection and cancer because each of these drugs influences multiple immune pathways and they are generally used in combination and over long periods of time. Thus, the overall burden of immunosuppression is high and broad-based. When used to manage immune-mediated skin conditions, the prescribing pattern and thus associated risk are different: standard (also referred to as conventional) immunosuppressants are generally (but not always) used as monotherapy and/or at low doses. The advent of targeted therapies with selected action on specific immune pathways may further modify drug-related risks, although this depends on the drug. Words matter. The term immunosuppressant carries negative attributions for both prescribers and patients and the term immunomodulatory (defined by the European Medicines Agency (EMA) as a substance that changes the activity of the body's defences [2]) is increasingly used especially in the context of targeted therapies. The risks associated with drugs that affect the immune system will be determined by the drug's mechanism of action, how the drug is being prescribed (dose, duration, concomitant therapies) and the risk profile of the individual being treated (for example, older age and co-morbidity burden increase the risk of serious infection with tumour necrosis factor (TNF) antagonists). Broad areas to consider are listed in Box 19.1, with close reference to the relevant guidelines, and the SmPC (see also Chapter 13 for important principles underpinning safe, effective prescribing).

> **Box 19.1 Suggested checklist to consider before and during the use of immunomodulatory drugs**
>
> - Drug-specific risks and overall likely burden of therapeutic immunosuppression:
>   - Guidelines
>   - Summary of product characteristics (SmPC)
> - Individual susceptibility to or pre-existing factors:
>   - Infection
>   - Bone marrow suppression
>   - Malignancy including skin cancer
> - Risk mitigation:
>   - Vaccination status including travel plans
>   - Concordance with routine cancer screening programmes
>   - Conception-related risk
>   - Monitoring schedule (clinical review, investigations)
> - Patient communication and education:
>   - Drug information leaflet
>   - How and when to seek advice
>   - Risk reduction strategies (e.g. sun protection)
>   See individual sections for further drug-specific considerations.

The use of immunomodulatory therapy can lead to reactivation of asymptomatic or 'dormant' infection which, in some cases, can be associated with serious morbidity and mortality. The clinical presentation of infections in this setting may be atypical. Some risks are drug-specific – for example reactivation of latent tuberculosis is particularly associated with TNF antagonists and Janus kinase (JAK) inhibitors. Screening for latent blood-borne viruses such as hepatitis B and C and human immunodeficiency virus (HIV), checking vaccination schedules are up to date, and advice to have flu, Covid-19 and pneumoccoal vaccines have become routine practice. This screening and vaccination strategy needs to be optimised in line with the individual's likely exposure to infections (e.g. working in high-risk environments for tuberculosis, absent history of chickenpox and need to consider screening for varicella immune status) and the local and/or national public health vaccination policies.

Antihistamines

Histamine is synthesised by and stored in mast cells and basophils, together with a variety of other pro-inflammatory mediators, and its release results in inflammation, which contributes to a variety of cutaneous disorders, particularly urticaria. Histamine receptors are expressed in skin on endothelial cells, neurons and T lymphocytes. Specifically, histamine-induced itch, vasodilatation and increased vascular permeability are mediated by H_1 receptors; H_2 receptors do not participate in the aetiology of itch [1], but contribute to vasodilatation and vascular permeability. The role of H_3 and H_4 receptors in cutaneous inflammation remains to be fully defined. In theory, supressing the inflammatory actions of histamine may result from inhibiting its synthesis in mast cells, reducing its release (e.g. with ketotifen, a mast cell stabiliser) and accelerating its degradation in tissues, but in clinical practice the only effective way of minimising histamine-mediated inflammation is by the use of antihistamines, primarily those that act on H_1 receptors [1].

The first generation of antihistamines (represented by alimemazine, chlorphenamine, clemastine, cyproheptadine, hydroxyzine and promethazine) are able easily to cross the blood–brain barrier, interfering with the neurotransmitter function of histamine, thus causing sedation and impairing cognitive function. The second-generation antihistamines (such as acrivastine, bilastine, cetirizine, levocetirizine, loratadine, desloratadine, fexofenadine, mizolastine and rupatadine) are, in contrast, minimally sedating.

Dermatological uses (Chapters 42, 44 and 46)

H_1 antihistamines are the mainstay of treatment for chronic urticaria and angioedema, and may be symptomatically beneficial in the physical urticarias [2], urticarial vasculitis, cutaneous mastocytosis, insect bite reactions, anaphylaxis and allergic reactions to drugs. H_1 antihistamines have a very limited role in atopic eczema, although short-term intermittent use of sedating H_1 antihistamines may be useful in the setting of sleep loss secondary to itch [3]. The combination of H_1 and H_2 antihistamines (off-licence) has been advocated for the treatment of urticaria, although the quality of evidence is low and generally superseded by other strategies such as the use of omalizumab [2]. The H_2 antihistamine ranitidine was taken off the market in 2019 due to the presence of low levels of an impurity called N-nitrosodimethylamine (NDMA), a probable human carcinogen. An alternative, famotidine, is now available.

Pharmacological properties
Formula and structure

H_1 antihistamines differ markedly in structure, with six structural classes: alkylamines, ethanolamines, ethylenediamines, phenothiazines, piperidines and piperazines. The first generation of antihistamines have representatives in each structural group, but the majority of second-generation antihistamines are piperidines and piperazines. Doxepin is a tricyclic antidepressant with antihistamine activity.

Pharmacokinetics

Just as H_1 antihistamines differ in structure so they differ in their pharmacokinetic characteristics. In general, they are readily absorbed from the gastrointestinal tract, reaching peak plasma levels within 2–3 h, and are substantially protein bound [1]. The lipophilicity of the first-generation antihistamines determines their ability to cross the blood–brain barrier, in contrast to the second-generation antihistamines. The first-generation drugs are metabolised by the hepatic cytochrome P450 system, usually followed by predominantly renal excretion. A number of the second-generation antihistamines, some of which are derived from a prodrug or are active metabolites of other antihistamines, may be excreted unchanged into the gut (fexofenadine) or urine (cetirizine and levocetirizine).

Pharmacodynamics

Traditionally, antihistamines have been thought of as reversible competitive inhibitors of histamine. However, molecular characterisation has suggested that histamine receptors have an intrinsic level of activity, and that H_1 and H_2 antihistamines are now best regarded as inverse agonists, not just blocking the interaction of histamine with its receptors but inducing an opposite pharmacological response by decreasing the constitutive activity of the receptors [1].

Additionally, it is thought possible that H_1 antihistamines, especially the second-generation compounds, may have H_1 receptor-independent anti-inflammatory effects, including inhibiting the release of histamine from mast cells and basophils, inhibiting the tissue activation and accumulation of inflammatory cells such as eosinophils, and directly inhibiting pro-inflammatory mediators such as bradykinin [4]. However, the experimental data are inconclusive and the potential clinical relevance is questionable [4].

The first-generation antihistamines, in contrast to the highly specific actions of the second generation, generally tend to have a high affinity for muscarinic cholinergic receptors, thereby inducing anticholinergic side effects [1].

Potential adverse effects

The first-generation antihistamines tend to cause sedation, impaired cognitive function, paradoxical excitability (especially in children and the elderly when given in high doses), anticholinergic effects (blurred vision, dry mouth, micturition difficulties and constipation) and weight gain. The second-generation antihistamines are relatively free from such adverse effects and have a high therapeutic index. Rarely, antihistamines may cause headaches, hypotension, palpitations, arrhythmias, sleep disturbances, dizziness, confusion, extrapyramidal effects, tremor, convulsions, depression and hypersensitivity reactions (see relevant SmPC). The potentially cardiotoxic antihistamines terfenadine and astemizole are not available in most countries and should no longer be prescribed.

Contraindications

Antihistamines are contraindicated in those rare instances of hypersensitivity to them [5].

Cautions

Although the available data do not suggest that H_1 antihistamines pose a significant risk to fetal well-being, it is generally recommended that they be avoided during pregnancy and lactation unless there is a clearly favourable risk–benefit ratio (see relevant SmPC for individual drug information). Avoid sedating antihistamines near term due to risk of sedation in the infant post-delivery.

The first-generation antihistamines in particular, because of their sedating and anticholinergic actions, should be used with caution in patients with epilepsy, glaucoma and prostatic hypertrophy [6]. Advice should be given regarding concurrent alcohol consumption, driving and operating dangerous machinery in view of the possibility of impaired judgement or dexterity [6].

In general, caution should be exercised if there is severe hepatic or renal impairment, severe hypertension, respiratory problems, porphyria or a predisposition to cardiac arrhythmias [6].

Drug–drug interactions

See Box 19.2.

> **Box 19.2 Antihistamines: drug–drug interactions**
>
> - CYP3A4 inhibitors, such as macrolide antibiotics, azole antifungal agents, HIV-1 protease inhibitors and grapefruit juice, may inhibit the metabolism and increase the serum levels of those antihistamines that are metabolised in the liver and may cause an increase in adverse events
> - Alcohol, anxiolytic and hypnotic drugs may exacerbate the sedative effects of first-generation antihistamines
> - Antacids reduce the absorption of fexofenadine
> - Antidepressant drugs (tricyclics and monoamine oxidase inhibitors (MAOIs)) may increase the sedative and antimuscarinic effects of antihistamines

Dose and regimens

In the context of urticaria, if the recommended dose of individual antihistamines [6] is not clinically effective, it is common clinical practice to prescribe second-generation antihistamines up to four times the licensed doses, although there is a limited evidence base for the efficacy and safety of this [1,2,7].

Antimalarial agents

Quinine, a natural anti-inflammatory alkaloid derived from the bark of the South American *Cinchona* tree, has medicinal properties that have been utilised since the 17th century. It was the treatment of choice for malaria until synthetic derivatives with fewer side effects were developed in the 1930s and 1940s. Of these, mepacrine (known in the USA as quinacrine), chloroquine and hydroxychloroquine have been employed as anti-inflammatory agents in various clinical settings, primarily dermatological and rheumatological. Mepacrine is now relatively little used, and in the UK is available only from 'special order' manufacturers or specialist importing companies [1], but both chloroquine and the more commonly prescribed hydroxychloroquine have product licences in the UK for chronic cutaneous (discoid) and systemic lupus erythematosus as well as for rheumatoid arthritis. Additionally, the product licence for hydroxychloroquine extends to dermatological conditions caused or aggravated by sunlight [1]. Hydroxychloroquine appears less toxic but also less effective than chloroquine [2,3].

Dermatological uses (Chapters 51, 58, 95, 96, 97 and 126)

The dermatological licensed indications include cutaneous forms of lupus erythematosus and photodermatoses (including polymorphic light eruption, solar urticaria and porphyria cutanea tarda), but, off-label, antimalarials are used in granulomatous dermatoses (cutaneous sarcoidosis and granuloma annulare), panniculitides (lupus panniculitis, chronic erythema nodosum, idiopathic panniculitis) and a miscellany of other conditions (including Jessner lymphocytic infiltrate, oral lichen planus, urticarial vasculitis and reticular erythematous mucinosis) [3].

Pharmacological properties
Formula and structure
Hydroxychloroquine (empirical formula: $C_{18}H_{26}ClN_3O$; systematic name: (RS)-2-[{4-[(7-chloroquinolin-4-yl)amino]pentyl}(ethyl)amino] ethanol) is a substituted 4-aminoquinoline, differing from chloroquine only by the presence of a hydroxyl group in a β position at the end of the ethyl side chain.

Mepacrine (empirical formula: $C_{23}H_{30}ClN_3O$; systematic name: (RS)-N′-(6-chloro-2-methoxy-acridin-9-yl)-N,N-diethyl-pentane-1,4-diamine) differs from the 4-aminoquinolines in having a third benzene ring.

Administration
Hydroxychloroquine sulphate, chloroquine phosphate or sulphate and mepacrine hydrochloride are administered orally, in tablet form [1].

Pharmacokinetics
The pharmacokinetic characteristics of the antimalarials are complex, and there is great variability between individuals. Hydroxychloroquine and chloroquine are water soluble and readily absorbed from the gastrointestinal tract, with peak plasma concentration within 8–12 h and approximately 60% binding to plasma proteins [3]. They are widely distributed to the tissues, and accumulate in the liver, spleen, kidney, lung, leukocytes and within melanin-containing cells of the skin and retina [3]. The 4-aminoquinolines are metabolised in the liver by enzymes of the cytochrome P450 (CYP) group (CYP2D6, -2C8, -3A4 and -3A5) to active metabolites, hydroxychloroquine into N-desethylhydroxychloroquine, and chloroquine into desethylchloroquine and bisdesethylchloroquine [3]. Excretion is largely in the urine, but also in the bile, sweat and saliva. Elimination is slow, because of tissue accumulation, with a terminal half-life of 30–60 days [3], and maximum clinical efficacy may take up to 3–6 months.

The pharmacokinetics of mepacrine is similar to the 4-aminoquinolines [3].

Pharmacodynamics
Despite recent advances, the mechanisms underlying the anti-inflammatory properties of the antimalarials are still incompletely understood. The traditional explanation centres on antimalarials, which are lipophilic weak bases, being 'lysosomotropic', penetrating cellular membranes and preferentially accumulating in lysosomes [3]. The resultant rise in lysosomal pH results in the inhibition of proteases and consequent dysfunctional protein processing. In immunologically competent cells, this causes disruption of protein secretion, receptor recycling and reduced production of pro-inflammatory cytokines and other immunological mediators (such as TNF-α, interleukin 6 (IL-6) and interferon γ (IFN-γ)). The effects of this include reduced antibody production and cell-mediated cytotoxicity by lymphocytes, reduced natural killer (NK) cell activity, impaired antigen presentation by monocytes, macrophages and dendritic cells to CD4 T cells, and decreased chemotaxis, phagocytosis and superoxide production by neutrophils [3,4], thereby downregulating immune responsiveness.

More recently, the 4-aminoquinolines have been demonstrated to have a potent and important inhibitory effect on intracellular Toll-like receptor (TLR) signalling, which may be their principal mode of action [3]. The lysosomotropic nature of antimalarials appears to prevent the proper functioning of endosomal TLRs, particularly TLR9, primarily within antigen-presenting cells, thereby inhibiting the activation of the innate immune system that would otherwise result from the recognition by TLRs of self nucleic acid components, including immune complexes, found in connective tissue disorders [4].

Antimalarials also exert other complex immunological and anti-inflammatory effects, including inhibition of phospholipase A2, thereby reducing prostaglandin formation, and photoprotection by virtue of being able to absorb ultraviolet (UV) light [3].

Furthermore, antimalarials have anticoagulant, lipid-lowering and hypoglycaemic properties [3]. Hydroxychloroquine has been demonstrated to restore the binding of annexin A5 (a potent natural antithrombotic agent) to intravascular surfaces in the presence of antiphospholipid antibodies [5], thus reducing thrombotic events in the antiphospholipid antibody syndrome. Antimalarials have a beneficial effect on cholesterol, triglyceride and low-density lipoprotein (LDL) levels [3,6], and thus on the development of atherosclerosis via effects on cholesterol synthesis and inhibition of a TLR9-mediated accumulation of lipids in macrophages [7]. Antimalarials also influence glucose metabolism, decreasing insulin degradation [3] and reducing the risk of diabetes [4], possibly also involving blockade of TLR9 [8]. The relevance, if any, of these interesting antimalarial properties to cutaneous disorders is as yet unclear.

Pharmacogenetics
The majority of patients respond to hydroxychloroquine and chloroquine, although a significant proportion do not or cannot tolerate them. Haemolysis has been reported in glucose-6-phosphate dehydrogenase (G6PD)-deficient individuals with malaria treated with chloroquine; recently this has been attributed to the underlying disease rather than the drug [9,10].

Potential adverse effects
Pharmacological
Myelotoxicity. Although very uncommon, all the antimalarials (but particularly chloroquine and mepacrine) can suppress bone marrow function [3] and leukopenia is thus a risk; agranulocytosis and aplastic anaemia have been recorded. Antimalarials may cause haemolysis in G6PD-deficient individuals [3].

Cutaneous toxicity. It is generally considered that antimalarials, especially chloroquine and mepacrine, may result in exacerbation of psoriasis, and it is reasonable to warn patients regarding this, although a systematic review has concluded that the evidence for this is equivocal [11]. Mepacrine can give the skin a yellow colour and the 4-aminoquinolines may impart a blue-grey discoloration [12]. Antimalarials have also been associated with bleaching of hair and transverse bands affecting the nails [3]. A miscellany of adverse cutaneous reactions has been reported with antimalarials, including pruritus, erythroderma, urticaria, lichenoid eruptions, photosensitivity and alopecia [13].

Idiosyncratic

Oculotoxicity. Antimalarial-induced retinopathy is an important vision-threatening side effect with hydroxychloroquine and chloroquine [14], but is not associated with mepacrine [15]. This manifests with damaged photoreceptors, degeneration of the retinal pigment epithelium and insidious 'bull's eye maculopathy'. The subsequent loss of central vision commonly presents with difficulty reading [16]. If allowed to progress, the typical 'bull's eye' macular changes become visible on fundoscopy. Once developed, the maculopathy may be permanent and may even progress despite stopping therapy [16,17]; there is no effective treatment. Prevalence estimates vary but increase with time, with the risk of toxicity up to 5 years under 1% and increasing to almost 20% by 20 years. Additional risk factors include those on more than 5 mg/kg/day, taking concomitant tamoxifen and with renal impairment. Hydroxychloroquine is also deposited in the cornea: it is usually asymptomatic, but may cause visual haloes. These corneal deposits are reversible on stopping the drug, are not related to retinal toxicity and are not a contraindication to continuing treatment.

Given that there is no treatment for established retinopathy, early detection at a reversible stage before there are changes in the retinal pigment epithelium is critical. Recently issued guidelines (2020) from the UK Royal College of Ophthalmologists in collaboration with the British Association of Dermatologists recommend annual monitoring with both spectral domain optical coherence tomography and, ideally, wide-field fundus autofluorescence imaging. The risk of retinopathy is greater with chloroquine than hydroxychloroquine, so screening with these tests is recommended after 1 year of therapy for everyone taking chloroquine, and after 5 years for those on hydroxychloroquine. The exception to this is for those on high-dose hydroxychloroquine, tamoxifen or with renal impairment when screening should start after 1 year. Updated US guidelines (2016) provide comparable recommendations, emphasising the importance of looking beyond the macula in people of Asian heritage where early damage can occur with a peripheral pattern [18].

Neuromuscular toxicity. Rarely, antimalarials can induce myalgia, fatigue and myopathy [19] and they have been associated with headaches, dizziness, tinnitus, hearing loss, nightmares, irritability, seizures and psychosis [21].

Cardiotoxicity. Both hydroxychloroquine and chloroquine are rarely reported as being associated with corrected QT interval (QTc) prolongation by directly affecting cardiac repolarisation, and in the long term with cardiomyopathy and heart failure [21]. A pre-treatment electrocardiogram (ECG) has been recommended to exclude pre-existing QTc prolongation or other conduction defects [13].

Gastrointestinal toxicity. Hydroxychloroquine is the least likely of the antimalarials to cause gastrointestinal symptoms which include nausea, vomiting, diarrhoea, anorexia and heartburn. Abnormal liver function tests are uncommon and routine monitoring is not generally recommended [13], although chloroquine and hydroxychloroquine should be used with caution in moderate to severe hepatic impairment [22].

Contraindications

Hypersensitivity reactions to antimalarials are a contraindication to their use. The 4-aminoquinolines and mepacrine do not cross-react, and so an adverse reaction to one does not preclude the use of the other [3].

Should a patient develop retinopathy on a 4-aminoquinoline, its continued use is contraindicated.

Cautions

The 4-aminoquinolines readily cross the placenta and are also excreted into breast milk. Data concerning 4-aminoquinolines during pregnancy and lactation are limited (see relevant SmPC) and the licence states these drugs should be avoided [22]. Nevertheless, recent European rheumatology guidelines found no evidence for congenital malformations with either hydroxychloroquine or chloroquine, and the group reached broad consensus that where clinically required these drugs could be continued during pregnancy and lactation [23]. Mepacrine, on the other hand, should be avoided.

Antimalarials should be used with caution in patients with a neuromuscular disease or a psychotic condition. Antimalarials should be given in low dosage when used to treat porphyria cutanea tarda (PCT) in view of the risk of causing hepatitis.

Drug–drug interactions

See Box 19.3.

Box 19.3 Antimalarial agents: drug–drug interactions

The most clinically important interactions involving antimalarials include the following:
- Antacids and kaolin may impair absorption of antimalarials (a 4 h interval between the drugs should be allowed)
- Cimetidine may increase serum antimalarial levels
- 4-Aminoquinolines may increase plasma digoxin levels
- Antimalarials may enhance the effects of hypoglycaemic therapy
- Risk of ventricular arrhythmias may increase with amiodarone, droperidol and moxifloxacin
- Aminoglycoside antibiotics may exacerbate neuromuscular adverse effects
- Possible risk of convulsions when given with antiepileptics
- 4-Aminoquinolines may increase plasma concentrations of ciclosporin
- May diminish effect of neostigmine and pyridostigmine
- Concomitant administration of antimalarials may prevent successful immunisation with oral typhoid vaccine [1] and human diploid cell rabies vaccine [22]

Pre-treatment screening
Pre-treatment checks include an FBC and liver and renal function tests; consider G6PD testing depending on the country and label [24].

Counsel patients about the risk of visual damage and the importance of screening, alongside written information.

Dose and regimens
The standard dose of hydroxychloroquine for adults is 200–400 mg daily, and of chloroquine is 2.5 mg daily. Dose according to real, rather than ideal, body weight and avoid doses >5 mg/kg to minimise the risks of eye toxicity. Mepacrine doses may be effective on as little as 50 mg three times each week and up to 100 mg three times daily [25].

Although there is only limited published evidence, combination therapy of hydroxychloroquine or chloroquine with mepacrine (quinacrine) may result in an enhanced therapeutic response [26,27].

Monitoring
Consider checking the FBC and liver function tests every 3 months during the first year, and then every 4–6 months while on treatment [3]. Patients should undergo ophthalmology assessment as stated in the ocular toxicity section.

Apremilast
Apremilast is an immunomodulatory small-molecule inhibitor of phosphodiesterase 4 (PDE4).

Dermatological uses
Apremilast is widely approved for the treatment of psoriasis, psoriatic arthritis and Beçhet disease in adults.

Pharmacological properties
Formula and structure
Apremilast (empirical formula: $C_{22}H_{24}N_2O_7S$; systematic name: N-[2-[(1S)-1-(3-ethoxy-4-methoxyphenyl)-2-methylsulfonylethyl]-1,3-dioxoisoindol-4-yl]acetamide) is a small-molecule inhibitor of PDE4.

Administration
Apremilast is available as oral tablets (10, 20 and 30 mg).

Pharmacokinetics
Apremilast is readily absorbed from the gastrointestinal tract with an oral bioavailability of 73% [1]. The peak plasma concentration occurs 2.5 h after an oral dose, with a terminal elimination half-life of 9 h. Apremilast is extensively metabolised by both CYP- and non-CYP-mediated pathways with only a fraction of the parent compound eliminated unchanged by the kidneys and gastrointestinal tract. Strong inducers of CYP3A4 such as rifampycin may reduce apremilast efficacy.

Pharmacodynamics
Phosphodiesterase 4 is the dominant PDE in inflammatory cells. Inhibition of PDE4 by apremilast increases intracellular cyclic adenosine monophosphate (cAMP), which downregulates the inflammatory response by modulating the expression of pro-inflammatory signals such as TNF-α, IL-23 and IL-17 and anti-inflammatory cytokines such as IL-10.

Potential adverse effects
Pharmacological [1]
Gastrointestinal. Tolerability issues with apremilast are common and often relate to gastrointestinal disturbance. These include upper abdominal pain, dyspepsia, nausea, vomiting, diarrhea and reduced appetite. These are often more prominent at initiation and can improve with time.

Headache. Headache or tension headache is common.

Weight loss. Apremilast can be associated with weight loss, which can be helpful in the context of psoriasis.

Infections. Upper respiratory tract infection, bronchitis and nasopharyngitis were reported in patients on trial but serious infection is rare in practice.

Depression and suicide. Depression and suicidal ideation have been reported, irrespective of a background of low mood. These problems are prevalent in the psoriasis population. The label states that suicidal ideation is rare and the exposure-adjusted incidence rate over the first 3 years of exposure has been reported as 0.1/100 patient-years [1].

Other side effects. Other reported side effects include cough, insomnia and fatigue. Hypersensitivity, angioedema and urticaria are uncommon.

Contraindications
Apremilast is contraindicated in individuals with hypersensitivity to the medicine or any of its ingredients as well as in pregnancy and breastfeeding.

Cautions
Severe renal impairment. The dose should be halved (30 mg once daily as opposed to twice daily).

Psychiatric disorders. Given reports of low mood and suicidal ideation on apremilast it is important to risk-assess patients and discuss this with them prior to initiating therapy. Patients and caregivers should be notified to inform prescribers of any change in mood or suicidal ideation and stop treatment.

Lactose intolerance. Apremilast should be avoided in patients with total lactase deficiency, galactose intolerance or glucose-galactose malabsorption.

Pre-treatment screening
No routine screening is stipulated as part of the licence, however European guidelines recommend a pre-treatment check of FBC, serum creatinine and liver function [2].

Dose and regimens
Apremilast is taken as oral tablets, 30 mg twice daily, ideally 12 h apart, with or without food. Gradual uptitration of dose is recommended over the first 6 days increasing by 10 mg each day. A final dose of 30 mg once daily is advised for those with renal impairment.

Monitoring
Routine monitoring is not required as part of the licence; depending on the patient characteristics, symptoms and signs, additional monitoring with FBC and renal and liver function may be indicated every 4–6 months.

Azathioprine
Azathioprine (AZA) is a potent immunosuppressive, anti-inflammatory and antiproliferative drug that has been used over the last six decades to prevent graft rejection and to treat haematological malignancies and a variety of rheumatological, gastrointestinal, neurological and dermatological inflammatory disorders.

Dermatological uses (Chapters 30, 41, 51, 52 and 126)
AZA is licensed in Europe for the treatment of systemic lupus erythematosus, dermatomyositis, Behçet disease, pemphigus vulgaris and bullous pemphigoid. It has been used off-label for a range of skin conditions, notably atopic eczema, chronic actinic dermatitis, lichen planus, leukocytoclastic vasculitis and pyoderma gangrenosum. It is often used as an adjunct to other immunosuppressive agents such as prednisolone and may exert a steroid-sparing effect, thereby minimising the adverse effects associated with the prolonged high-dose use of systemic corticosteroids. The now well-established link between the use of AZA and increased risk of keratinocyte malignancy means that where possible alternative agents are used [1].

Pharmacological properties
Formula and structure
Azathioprine (empirical formula: $C_9H_7N_7O_2S$; systematic name: 6-[(1-methyl-4-nitro-1H-imidazol-5-yl)sulfanyl]-7H-purine) is a thiopurine with a molecular structure consisting of imidazole and mercaptopurine moieties.

Administration
AZA is commonly available as oral (25 and 50 mg tablets) and intravenous preparations.

Pharmacokinetics
AZA is readily absorbed from the gastrointestinal tract, the peak plasma concentration occurring 1–2 h after an oral dose, and it is distributed rapidly throughout the body. The plasma half-life is 3–5 h with up to 30% bound to plasma proteins [2,3].

AZA is a prodrug that is rapidly transformed *in vivo* into 6-mercaptopurine (6-MP) by non-enzymatic cleavage of the imidazole ring, facilitated by glutathione. Further metabolism of 6-MP continues by three metabolic pathways: (i) methylation of 6-MP to 6-methyl-mercaptopurine (6-MMP), which is biologically inactive, catalysed by thiopurine methyl transferase (TPMT); (ii) oxidation of 6-MP to thiouric acid, also biologically inactive, catalysed by xanthine oxidase (XO); and (iii) conversion of 6-MP by a number of enzymatic steps, via 6-thioinosine monophosphate (6-TIMP) and 6-thioguanine monophosphate (6-TGMP) to a variety of 6-thioguanine nucleotides (6-TGNs), which are considered to be the active metabolites (Figure 19.1).

AZA and its metabolites are excreted via the kidneys and gastrointestinal tract. There is no enterohepatic circulation. A lowered dose in cases of reduced renal function may be necessary [3].

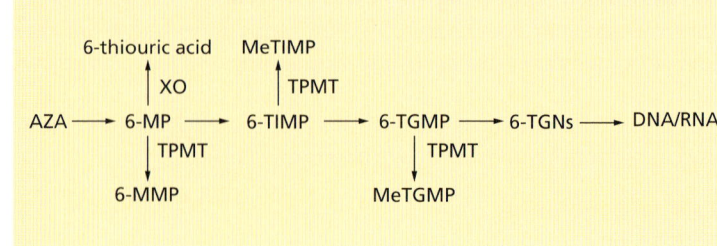

Figure 19.1 A simplified diagram of thiopurine metabolism (see text for abbreviations).

Despite the rapid absorption, metabolism and excretion of AZA, its active metabolites only slowly accumulate in tissues, and thus the therapeutic immunosuppressive effects of AZA may take 6–12 weeks to develop.

Pharmacodynamics
Despite over five decades of clinical use, the precise mechanism of action of AZA remains uncertain. AZA is a purine analogue and the accepted theory has been that its antiproliferative, anti-inflammatory and immunosuppressant properties are the result of the incorporation of 6-TGNs into DNA, thus interfering with its replication [4], and are perhaps also due to the suppression of purine synthesis, as methylthioinosine monophosphate (MeTIMP) is an *in vitro* inhibitor of *de novo* endogenous purine synthesis [5]. The relative specificity of its action on lymphocytes, with the consequence of altered T-cell and B-cell function, can be explained by the lack of a purine salvage pathway in lymphocytes [9]. However, it appears that AZA may additionally induce lymphocyte apoptosis and T-cell anergy, possibly by the modification of CD28 signalling [6], and thus the immunosuppressive effect of AZA may be due to a combination of antimetabolic and pro-apoptotic actions [7].

Pharmacogenetics
There are a number of allelic variants of *TPMT* and this polymorphism results in clinically important phenotypes in Europeans. Approximately 90% of individuals have normal TPMT activity (homozygous for the wild-type allele), 10% intermediate (heterozygous) and less than 1% low (homozygous or compound heterozygous for a mutant allele) TPMT activity [7]. TPMT is an important enzyme in the metabolic pathway of AZA. Not only does it catalyse the conversion of 6-MP to inactive 6-MMP, but it also inactivates 6-TIMP and 6-thioguanine by methylation. Therefore, in those individuals with inherited TPMT deficiency, the metabolism of AZA is shunted in the direction of excessive production and toxic accumulation of 6-TGNs (Figure 19.1); standard dosages of AZA in such individuals risk causing severe bone marrow suppression and consequent pancytopenia. In South and East Asians, Hispanic and American Indian populations, variants in *NUDT15* are more commonly responsible for thiopurine toxicity. *NUDT15* encodes the nucleoside diphosphatase nudix hydrolase 15, and deficiency of this protein leads to the excessive incorporation of toxic thiopurine nucleotides into DNA [8]. Pre-treatment testing for *TPMT* variants and additionally *NUDT15* variants (particularly in Asian populations) with appropriate dose adjustment (or in the

case of absent TMPT, complete avoidance) is now recommended [9]. For indeterminate genotypes, TPMT activity can also be measured in erythrocytes to support dosing strategies.

Potential adverse effects
Pharmacological
Myelosuppression. Bone marrow suppression is more likely with intermediate TPMT levels, and increasingly likely in individuals with low TPMT activity. However, a normal TPMT level with low 6-TGN production does not negate the possibility of myelotoxicity. Haematological monitoring is therefore required throughout the duration of treatment with AZA, independent of the TPMT status [2]. Leukopenia is the most common haematological side effect, but anaemia, thrombocytopenia and pancytopenia can occur. Patients should be warned to report infection, bruising, mouth ulcers and sore throat, which might be indicative of myelotoxicity.

Carcinogenesis. There is strong epidemiological evidence for an association between AZA use and an increased risk of cutaneous squamous cell carcinoma that increases with age, cumulative dose and duration of AZA use. Recently, whole exome sequencing has identified a novel, AZA 'mutational footprint' (designated signature 32) providing mechanistic evidence that this association is causal [10]. Replacement of DNA guanine with the AZA metabolite 6-thioguanine causes UVA photosensitivity, and this alongside increased UVB mutagenicity through the impaired DNA repair is likely to drive skin cancer risk [11].

Rarely, myeloid malignancies (myelodysplastic syndrome and amyeloid leukaemia) and lymphoma have also been associated with the use of AZA in autoimmune diseases [12].

These risks, although real, are rare and in the case of skin cancer can be mitigated, and need to be balanced with likely therapeutic benefit alongside the benefits and risks of alternative strategies.

Infection. AZA therapy is associated with an increased risk of infection, in particular by disseminated herpes simplex, varicellazoster virus and human papillomavirus [2]. However, true opportunistic infections are uncommon in patients treated with AZA for dermatological conditions.

Gastrointestinal. Nausea, vomiting and diarrhoea are common side effects of AZA and can be minimised by dose reduction, dose division and taking AZA with food [2]. Pancreatitis has been reported with AZA therapy [2].

Hepatic. Although generally well tolerated, mild derangement of liver function tests is not uncommon and may not require alteration of dosage [13]. However, AZA can rarely cause severe, occasionally life-threatening hepatitis. The mechanism is uncertain but may involve oxidative stress [14]. Furthermore, AZA, in the context of treating inflammatory bowel disease, has been associated with nodular regenerative hyperplasia of the liver [15] with resultant portal hypertension presenting with thrombocytopenia and splenomegaly. Liver function should be monitored throughout treatment with AZA [2].

Idiosyncratic
Hypersensitivity syndrome. AZA hypersensitivity syndrome is a rare but potentially fatal adverse effect. It occurs in approximately 2% of patients treated with AZA and typically develops early in the course of treatment, usually within the first month. It may be easily overlooked as it can mimic infection or disease exacerbation [16–19]. The syndrome is characterised by fever, malaise, arthralgia, myalgia, nausea, vomiting and diarrhoea, with occasional renal and liver dysfunction, pancreatitis, hypotension, cardiogenic shock and leukocytosis [16,18]. In about 50% of cases it has a cutaneous component, which may assist in its recognition [16,17]. In the majority of cases in which rash is a feature, the clinical and histological features are of a neutrophilic dermatosis and, although the eruption can be non-specific in appearance, it may resemble Sweet syndrome, erythema nodosum, acute generalised exanthematous pustulosis or leukocytoclastic vasculitis [16]. The symptoms and signs of hypersensitivity syndrome settle within days of discontinuing AZA; rechallenge with AZA should not be undertaken for fear of causing a life-threatening shock reaction [16,17].

Contraindications
Azathioprine is contraindicated (i) in those with high pharmacogenomic risk (homozygous, compound heterozygous or heterozygous diplotypes with any two variants of *TPMT*3A*, *-3C* or *-*2* or *NUDT15*2*, *-*3* or *-*9*); (ii) if there is a history of hypersensitivity to AZA; (iii) in the presence of severe infection, severely impaired hepatic or bone marrow function or pancreatitis; and with concomitant administration of live attenuated vaccines; and (iv) in women who are pregnant or considering conception (unless the benefits to the patient outweigh the potential risks) [13].

Cautions
Lactation and conception. Available data do not demonstrate that AZA exposure during early pregnancy increases the risk of congenital malformation, preterm delivery or adversely affects fetal growth. Data on longer-term outcomes are sparse. AZA is thus not recommended in men or women planning conception, or during pregnancy without careful evaluation of the risks and the need for treatment [3,13,20]. Recent European rheumatology guidelines indicate that where needed to maintain the health of the mother, AZA may be used [21].

Drug–drug interactions
See Box 19.4.

Box 19.4 Azathioprine: drug–drug interactions

- Allopurinol and febuxostat, by inhibiting XO and thus shunting the metabolism of AZA to increased production of 6-TGNs (Figure 19.1), enhance the effect and increase the toxicity of AZA
- Angiotensin-converting enzyme inhibitors (such as captopril and enalapril) increase the risk of myelosuppression with AZA
- AZA possibly reduces the anticoagulant effect of coumarins
- Both sulfamethoxazole and trimethoprim may increase the myelotoxicity of AZA
- Aminosalicylates may also increase the myelotoxicity of AZA
- Ribovirin, an antiviral guanosine analogue, may enhance the myelosuppressive effect of AZA

Pre-treatment screening [13]

As AZA has significant immunosuppressive activity, pre-treatment screening should incorporate all the aspects of Box 19.1. An FBC, including white cell differential, kidney function and liver function, should be determined at baseline. Renal impairment may require a dose reduction [22], and hepatic dysfunction will necessitate close supervision of haematological and liver parameters.

The pre-treatment assessment of *TPMT* (and *NUDT15*) genotypic or phenotypic status is recommended in order to minimise the risk of potentially life-threatening myelosuppression [9].

Dose and regimens

For individuals with low pharmacogenomic risk and/or normal TPMT activity use the standard daily dose of AZA of 2–3 mg/kg [8]. For those with some risk of myelotoxicity (e.g. heterozygous or with any one variant of *TPMT*3A, -*3C* or *-*2* or *NUDT15*2, -*3* or *-*9*) and/or measureable TPMT activity in the intermediate range consider giving 50% of the recommended daily dose, 1–1.5 mg/kg [8]. Avoid AZA with very high-risk pharmacogenomic variants and/or low/absent TPMT activity [8].

Monitoring

Patients taking AZA should be monitored regularly irrespective of genotypic status/TMPT activity for signs of toxicity, in particular hepatotoxicity and myelosuppression. Liver function tests and FBC should be checked weekly for 4–8 weeks after initiating therapy and after any dose increment, and, once the dose is stable, at least 2–3-monthly thereafter. Macrocytosis is a common unremarkable feature of AZA therapy.

It is not yet routine clinical practice to measure levels of 6-TGNs and other AZA metabolites (such as 6-MMP), but such monitoring may prove to assist in the determination of the dose required to optimise efficacy and minimise adverse effects.

Ciclosporin

Ciclosporin is a highly effective and rapidly acting potent inhibitor of T-cell function [1]. It has remained of central importance in the management of severe inflammatory skin disease since the early 1990s.

Dermatological uses (Chapters 35, 41, 42 and 47)

Ciclosporin is licensed for use in psoriasis (plaque type) and atopic eczema. Common off-label uses include chronic urticaria, pyoderma gangrenosum, hand eczema and palmoplantar pustulosis. It is also used sporadically for a variety of other inflammatory conditions including Behçet disease, lichen planus, prurigo nodularis, chronic actinic dermatitis and toxic epidermal necrolysis.

Pharmacological properties
Formula and structure

Ciclosporin (originally named cyclosporine A) is a neutral, strongly hydrophobic, cyclic undecapeptide (hence the prefix 'cyclo' or 'ciclo') of 11 amino acids that was first detected in the early 1970s in the spores (hence the suffix 'sporin') of the fungus *Tolypocladium inflatum* Gams. A hydrophilic, microemulsion formulation was developed to circumvent problems with variable bioavailability, and there are a number of different generic formulations now available.

Administration

Ciclosporin is given orally, in the dose range 2.5–5 mg/kg daily, in two divided daily doses.

Pharmacokinetics [1,2]

The absorption of ciclosporin from the gastrointestinal tract is incomplete and variable, and depends on the individual patient, the patient population and the formulation. The absolute bioavailability is poor (around 25% of the total administered dose) due to extensive first-pass metabolism as well as active transport of absorbed drug back into the intestinal lumen by the efflux transporter P-glycoprotein (encoded for by the *ABCB1* gene), which is present at high concentrations in the villus tip of enterocytes of the small intestine. If taken with a high-fat meal, bioavailability may be further reduced. There may be differences in bioavailability between different formulations of ciclosporin (including generics which are licensed on the basis of bioequivalence) that may be clinically important in certain circumstances and so, in general, when switching from one formulation to another, additional monitoring and careful review are advised, specifying which particular brand of ciclosporin is to be dispensed.

Ciclosporin is highly lipophilic, readily absorbed through cell membranes and distributed widely throughout the body. The average apparent distribution volume is 3.5 L/kg. It is highly protein bound in circulating blood.

Ciclosporin undergoes extensive metabolism, mainly in the liver via CYP3A4, which gives rise to a number of important drug interactions. The main pathways of metabolism consist of mono- and dihydroxylation and *N*-demethylation at various positions in the molecule. All metabolites (up to 25) identified so far retain the intact peptide structure of the parent compound; some possess weak immunosuppressive activity (up to one-tenth that of the unchanged drug).

Excretion is primarily biliary; of the total oral dose, only around 6% is detected in the urine (a fraction of which is unchanged). Renal impairment thus has only minimal impact on the pharmacokinetics of ciclosporin. There is a high variability in the data reported on the terminal half-life of ciclosporin depending on the assay applied and on the target population, ranging from 6.3 h in healthy volunteers to 20.4 h in patients with severe liver disease.

Pharmacodynamics

Ciclosporin is a prodrug that becomes active only after forming a complex with an intracytoplasmic immunophilin (protein) known as cycliphilin. This ciclosporin–cycliphilin complex inhibits calcineurin phosphatase, an enzyme catalysing dephosphorylation of the cytoplasmic protein nuclear factor of activated T cells (NF-ATc). Ordinarily, dephosphorylation of NF-ATc allows it to translocate to the nucleus, where it enables transcription of a number of pro-inflammatory cytokines including IL-2, IL-4, IFN-γ, transforming growth factor β and upregulation of receptors such as IL-2R (CD25). Inhibition of calcineurin phosphatase, and possibly also the JNK (MAPK8) and p38 (MAPK14) pathways, thus suppresses production of IL-2 and IL-2 receptor expression, key regulators of T-cell activation. Additional actions of therapeutic relevance include reduced histamine release and downregulation of high-affinity immunoglobulin E (IgE) receptors on mast cells and basophils.

Pharmacogenetics

CYP3A4, *CYP3A5* and *ABCB1* genes code for enzymes and transporters that play a central role in ciclosporin disposition. All three genes are highly polymorphic, with marked differences in population prevalence depending on ethnicity. These genetic variants are likely to be major contributors to the wide interpatient variation in drug pharmacokinetics and have been subject to intensive investigation, predominantly in the transplant field. For example, in one large renal cohort, variation in liver CYP3A4 and enterocyte P-glycoprotein activity explained up to 75% of the variation in ciclosporin clearance. The clinical utility of these genetic variants (as well as others) to individualise ciclosporin dosing remains to be established [3].

Potential adverse effects

There are a large number of potential adverse effects reported with ciclosporin [1,2], with hypertension, nephrotoxicity, hyperlipidaemia, myalgia and headache being the most common. Others include gingival hyperplasia, fatigue, gastrointestinal disturbances, tremor and paraesthesiae in the hands and feet, and a variety of metabolic abnormalities (hyperbilirubinaemia, hypercalcaemia, hypomagnesaemia, hyperuricaemia).

Most are dose related and respond rapidly to dose reduction or, if necessary, treatment cessation. In general, though, ciclosporin is a very well-tolerated drug when used in the short term (6–12 months), whereas longer-term use carries significant, predictable risk, particularly of nephrotoxicity, and is generally not recommended if other interventions can be used.

Nephrotoxicity

Acute nephrotoxicity can occur within weeks of treatment initiation, is reversible and arises due to dose-dependent vascular dysfunction involving afferent arteriolar constriction, which results in increased vascular resistance and a decrease in glomerular filtration rate. Tubular dysfunction may also occur and is characterised by decreased magnesium reabsorption, decreased uric acid excretion, decreased potassium and hydrogen ion secretion and distal tubular acidosis. Chronic nephrotoxicity [4,5] is largely irreversible and is characterised by progressive arteriolar hyalinosis, interstitial fibrosis, tubular atrophy and glomerular sclerosis. Chronic nephrotoxicity is more likely to occur with higher daily doses, larger cumulative doses and long-term therapy (more than 1–2 years); particular risk factors include age over 50 years, pre-existing hypertension and/or renal impairment and concomitant treatment with non-steroidal anti-inflammatory drugs (NSAIDs) and other nephrotoxic drugs. Intermittent rather than continuous therapy is widely cited as a sensible, dose-minimising strategy. However, with each treatment course, the time taken for creatinine levels to rise tends to become shorter. Change in serum creatinine from baseline is the single most important indicator of nephrotoxicity and thus is a critical component of monitoring.

Hyperlipidaemia

Triglycerides and, less commonly, cholesterol levels may become elevated within 2 weeks of treatment initiation, usually returning to normal on withdrawal of therapy. If hyperlipidaemia does require active intervention, management requires care due to an increased risk of statin-induced myopathy; fibrates may be a preferred treatment option (see drug–drug interactions).

Malignancy

Long-term use of immunosuppressants, such as ciclosporin, is associated with a potential increase in the risk for developing certain types of malignancy, particularly cancers of the skin and lymphoid system. This risk has been identified in organ transplant populations where the burden of immunosuppression and duration of therapy are likely to be greater than in those being treated for skin disease. Data from psoriasis cohorts indicate that the incidence of non-melanoma skin cancer (principally squamous cell carcinoma) is significantly increased with use of ciclosporin [6,7], predominantly in those who have previously received psoralen and ultraviolet A (PUVA), for whom the increased risk of squamous cell carcinoma following exposure to ciclosporin approaches that associated with 200 PUVA treatments [6]. The absolute risk of systemic malignancy is unclear, with the studies that do exist often being underpowered and/or not controlling for important confounders and any background disease-associated cancer risk, such as is the case in psoriasis [7].

Contraindications

Ciclosporin is contraindicated in uncontrolled hypertension, renal disease, serious infections and in those with a previous history of malignancy (excluding basal cell carcinoma) or a high cumulative dose of PUVA.

Cautions

In women planning conception and during pregnancy, ciclosporin has a relatively favourable risk–benefit profile, and in contrast to agents such as methotrexate (MTX) and retinoids is not teratogenic. However, data from use in the transplant population indicate an increased risk of pregnancy-associated complications such as pre-eclampsia and low birth weight and so it should only be used where the benefits of use outweigh risk to the fetus. Small amounts of ciclosporin are excreted in breast milk; most formulations also contain ethanol and the licence indicates that breastfeeding should be avoided (or the drug stopped). However, limited data report no side effects for breastfed children exposed to ciclosporin and recent guidance for the rheumatology community suggests maternal ciclosporin may be 'compatible' with breastfeeding [8].

Drug–drug interactions

Ciclosporin interacts with multiple drugs, many of which have important clinical implications. First, drugs may inhibit or induce enzymes involved in the metabolism of ciclosporin, in particular CYP3A4. For example, co-therapy with rifampicin or St John's wort, both potent CYP3A4 inducers, increases ciclosporin metabolism and so reduces efficacy; conversely, erythromycin inhibits CYP3A4 and thus increases ciclosporin levels by up to sevenfold with consequent risk of toxicity [2]. Second, ciclosporin itself is an inhibitor of CYP3A4, the multidrug efflux transporter P-glycoprotein and organic anion transporter proteins, and may therefore increase plasma levels of co-medications that are substrates of this enzyme and/or transporters. Statins, for example, are oxidised via CYP3A4, and so ciclosporin-mediated inhibition of statin metabolism is the likely mechanism underlying the risk of rhabdomyolysis associated with concomitant ciclosporin therapy. Certain statins (rosuvastatin and simvastatin) should be avoided completely whereas others may be used but at a reduced dose (e.g. a maximum dose of atorvastatin 10 mg or fluvastatin 20 mg) with monitoring of creatine kinase. Grapefruit juice increases ciclosporin bioavailability via inhibition of intestinal CYP3A4 [9].

Pre-treatment screening
Routine recommended clinical and investigational assessments aim to identify those at risk of the principal adverse effects (nephrotoxicity, hypertension), altered pharmacokinetics (liver disease, drug–drug interactions) and to minimise the risks of immunosuppression. Prior to commencing ciclosporin, screening as outlined in Box 19.1 should be undertaken.

A full history and examination should focus on past or current infection, malignancy (including a full skin check and counselling to ensure patients are up to date with national screening programmes), renal disease, liver disease, excess alcohol intake and previous phototherapy, especially PUVA.

Investigations include FBC, fasting lipids, alanine aminotransferase (ALT), aspartate aminotransferase (AST), γ-glutamyl transferase (γ-GT) and bilirubin as well as a comprehensive renal assessment (urinalysis, urine protein : creatinine ratio, baseline creatinine ideally calculated from the mean of two serum creatinine measurements, urea and electrolytes, including potassium and magnesium, and a urate level). In patients over 60 years, in those with suspected renal impairment or where therapy is likely to be required long term, an accurate assessment of renal capacity can be helpful (ethylenediaminetetraacetic acid (EDTA) clearance).

As with all immunosuppressive agents, ciclosporin may enhance the adverse and toxic effect of live attenuated vaccines (i.e. vaccinal infections), and in addition may diminish the therapeutic effects of vaccines, so that appropriate counselling about avoidance of live vaccination and a review of planned travel are important [10].

Dose and regimens
Generally, patients start treatment in the lower dose range (2.5 mg/kg/day), escalating to higher doses (up to 5 mg/kg/day) after a month of therapy in the event of a poor response. In circumstances where disease is acute, severe and/or unstable, treatment may be started at 5 mg/kg/day, but this carries an increased risk of side effects. The lowest possible therapeutic dose should be used to maintain remission and, ideally, a treatment course should last no more than 1 year. In obese patients, dosing per actual body weight may lead to toxicity as, although highly lipophilic, observations suggest that distribution of the drug is limited primarily to lean body mass.

Monitoring
In transplant medicine, in view of the narrow therapeutic index, requirement for long-term (lifelong) treatment and the critical importance of maintaining adequate immunosuppression to ensure organ viability, therapeutic drug monitoring with either serum trough and/or 2 h post-dose measurement of ciclosporin is part of routine practice. In dermatology, routine measurement of drug levels offers no specific advantage in terms of optimising efficacy, although the measurement of trough levels to predict risk of nephrotoxicity may be helpful in patients who cannot avoid long-term treatment. Blood pressure, FBC, liver function tests and renal function are generally checked every 2 weeks for 3 months after initiation and after any subsequent dose increase; once established on therapy, they should be checked at 8–12-weekly intervals, although fasting lipids may be monitored less frequently. If the creatinine level rises by more than 30% above baseline, the dose should be reduced; if it fails to normalise, the drug should be stopped.

Drug-induced hypertension should be managed as for ordinary hypertension; calcium-channel blockers are often the preferred first line agents due to their vasodilatory effect on the afferent renal arteriole, which is thought to protect against nephropathy. All drugs of this class are associated with gum hypertrophy (in common with ciclosporin). However, amlodipine has no impact on ciclosporin drug levels, in contrast to nifedipine and diltiazem, and so is often considered the preferred agent.

Angiotensin-converting enzyme inhibitors may be used although they lead to a rise in serum creatinine that, although not pathological, may be difficult to distinguish from changes attributable to ciclosporin. Potassium-sparing diuretics should be avoided since ciclosporin tends to increase serum potassium levels, and, where psoriasis is the indication for use, β-blockers should also be avoided.

Summary
Ciclosporin remains an extremely useful, predictably effective and generally well-tolerated drug for short-term use. Long-term use is complicated by nephrotoxicity, as well as risks associated with ongoing potent immunosuppression.

Colchicine
Colchicine is an ancient drug, originally derived from the roots and seeds of plants of the genus *Colchicum*, particularly *C. autumnale* (the autumn crocus). In the UK, it is licensed only for the treatment of acute gout, but it has recognised benefit in familial Mediterranean fever, Behçet disease and recurrent pericarditis [1].

Dermatological uses (Chapters 35, 49, 50, 52, 54, 100 and 108)
Colchicine has been used off-label for a wide variety of dermatological conditions, particularly those characterised by a neutrophilic inflammatory infiltrate, including neutrophilic dermatoses (Sweet syndrome, recurrent aphthous stomatitis), cutaneous vasculitis, autoimmune bullous disorders (dermatitis herpetiformis, epidermolysis bullosa acquisita, linear IgA disease), autoimmune connective tissue diseases (Behçet disease, dermatomyositis, scleroderma) and papulosquamous disorders (psoriasis), with variable efficacy [2].

Pharmacological properties
Formula and structure
Colchicine (empirical formula: $C_{22}H_{25}NO_6$; systematic name: N-[(7S)-1,2,3,10-tetramethoxy-9-oxo-5,6,7,9-tetrahydrobenzo[a]heptalen-7-yl] acetamide) is a tricyclic alkaloid consisting of two seven-member and one six-member carbon rings, with nitrogen in the side chain (a protoalkaloid).

Administration
Colchicine is administered orally; parenteral use has given rise to serious safety concerns [1].

Pharmacokinetics
Colchicine is lipophilic and is absorbed in the small intestine. There is a wide interindividual variation in bioavailability. The peak plasma concentration after oral administration is reached at 30–90 min, with a second peak at approximately 6 h [1]. Protein binding is between 10% and 30% and the terminal half-life is about 10 h. It is metabolised in the liver, with deacetylation via the CYP3A4 system, and excretion is predominantly into bile, with 10–20% eliminated unchanged in urine [2]. Colchicine is widely distributed in tissues but accumulates preferentially in neutrophils, where the concentration may exceed 16 times the peak plasma concentration [1].

Pharmacodynamics
Colchicine is both antimitotic and anti-inflammatory, but its precise mechanism of action is uncertain. By binding to β-tubulin it appears to interfere with the assembly of microtubules, thereby causing mitotic arrest in metaphase and inhibiting cellular chemotaxis. Its anti-inflammatory action results from the modulation of pro-inflammatory molecule production and the reduction of neutrophil degranulation, chemotaxis and phagocytosis [1,3].

Potential adverse effects
Gastrointestinal
Colchicine commonly causes watery diarrhoea, vomiting, abdominal pain, bloatedness and hyperperistalsis [1,2].

Toxicity and poisoning
Acute overdosage with colchicine commences within hours with burning sensations in the mouth and throat, and severe gastroenteritis-like symptoms. After 24–72 h, signs of multiorgan dysfunction and sepsis may develop: bone marrow failure, renal and hepatic damage, respiratory distress, muscle weakness, central nervous system toxicity, myocardial damage, disseminated intravascular coagulation, metabolic acidosis, electrolyte disturbances and hypovolaemic shock may supervene, and are potentially fatal consequences [1,4].

Contraindications
Colchicine is contraindicated if there is known hypersensitivity to it, and in the presence of blood dyscrasias [2].

Cautions
Colchicine should be used with caution if there is renal or hepatic dysfunction, and should be avoided during pregnancy [5].

Drug–drug interactions
Drugs that inhibit the CYP3A4 and P-glycoprotein systems may increase colchicine levels and toxicity: they include ciclosporin, erythromycin, clarithromycin, ketoconazole, itraconazole, antiviral drugs and verapamil; grapefruit juice has a similar action [1,4,5]. Co-administration with statins may increase the risk of myopathy [1,4,5].

Pre-treatment screening
Full blood count, renal and hepatic biochemistry, urinalysis and, if appropriate, a pregnancy test should be undertaken.

Dose and regimens
A starting dose of 0.5 mg/day, increasing to 0.5 mg twice or three times daily over several weeks, may enhance tolerability [2]. The dose can be subsequently tapered as disease activity allows [2].

Monitoring
Full blood count, renal and hepatic biochemistry and urinalysis should be checked monthly for several months, then 3-monthly thereafter [2].

Summary
Oral colchicine is a safe drug in the long term when used appropriately [1], but it has a narrow therapeutic range [1,3], and care should be taken to avoid overdosage.

Dapsone
The synthesis of dapsone in 1908 developed out of research on azo dyes and it was subsequently discovered in the 1930s to have beneficial anti-infective properties like other sulphones [1,2]. It still retains important roles in the treatment of leprosy and the prophylaxis of malaria and pneumocystis pneumonia, and has recently been shown to have antiepileptic activity [3]. It was, however, the realisation in the 1950s that dapsone is a potent anti-inflammatory agent that paved the way for its use in a wide variety of primarily dermatological inflammatory disorders. The related drugs, sulfapyridine and sulfamethoxypyridazine, have been used in the treatment of dermatological disorders, but are now only rarely prescribed.

Dermatological uses (Chapters 49, 50 and 100)
In the UK, dapsone is licensed for the treatment of dermatitis herpetiformis and the rapidity of its action (usually between 1 and 3 days) has been used as a diagnostic test for this condition. Dapsone is also predictably beneficial for the treatment of linear IgA disease, chronic bullous disease of childhood, bullous lupus erythematosus, erythema elevatum diutinum, IgA pemphigus and subcorneal pustular dermatosis. It has been widely used off-licence in many other inflammatory dermatoses, although its efficacy tends to be unpredictable. These dermatoses include:
- Autoimmune blistering disorders (bullous and cicatricial pemphigoid, pemphigus and epidermolysis bullosa acquisita).
- Vasculitis (leukocytoclastic vasculitis, urticarial vasculitis, granuloma faciale and Behçet disease).
- Neutrophilic dermatoses (Sweet syndrome and pyoderma gangrenosum).
- Miscellaneous other conditions (lupus erythematosus, panniculitis, acne vulgaris, hidradenitis suppurativa, pustular psoriasis, delayed pressure urticaria and relapsing polychondritis) [1,5].

Pharmacological properties
Formula and structure
Dapsone (4,4'-diaminodiphenylsulphone) is a sulphone with a simple structure consisting of an atom of sulphur linking two aromatic amine rings.

Administration
Dapsone is taken orally in tablet form: 50 and 100 mg tablets are available in the UK. A topical preparation, dapsone 5% gel, is available in the USA and Canada as a treatment for acne.

Pharmacokinetics [1,5]
Dapsone is lipid soluble and water insoluble. Orally, it is absorbed very efficiently from the gastrointestinal tract and appears to have a significant enterohepatic circulation. The peak plasma concentration occurs 2–6 h after ingestion and in the circulation it is approximately 70% protein bound. It is widely distributed, crossing the placenta and passing into breast milk. Dapsone is metabolised in the liver along two pathways: acetylation (by an N-acetyltransferase) and hydroxylation (by an N-hydroxylase). Acetylation results in the non-toxic metabolites monoacetyl dapsone and diacetyl dapsone. Hydroxylation yields the potentially toxic dapsone hydroxylamine. Metabolites are subsequently glucuronidated and excreted in the urine, and a small percentage is excreted in bile. Dapsone has a relatively long elimination half-life of 1–2 days, with wide individual variation.

Pharmacodynamics
Dapsone affects the folic acid metabolic pathway, an important process in DNA synthesis. It is selectively toxic to bacterial cells as it inhibits bacterial synthesis of dihydrofolate (DHF) by competing with para-aminobenzoic acid for the catalytic activity of dihydropteroate synthetase [5]. While this explains its antibiotic activity, the mechanisms underpinning the anti-inflammatory effects of dapsone are still poorly understood. The fact that dapsone seems to be particularly effective in inflammatory reactions characterised by a polymorph response has resulted in mechanistic theories centred on neutrophil function. Dapsone has inhibitory actions on neutrophil and eosinophil myeloperoxidase: the former, as part of the neutrophil 'respiratory burst', is an important element in tissue damage. It also inhibits neutrophil chemotaxis by inhibiting IL-8 release and function [6]. Further actions include stabilisation of neutrophil lysosomes, inhibition of neutrophil lysosomal enzymes and suppression of integrin-mediated neutrophil adhesion and neutrophil recruitment [1,5].

Pharmacogenetics
Dapsone hydroxylamine has strong oxidising properties, with the potential to induce a state of oxidative stress sufficient to cause severe haemolysis and methaemoglobinaemia in individuals with G6PD deficiency, the result of a number of polymorphisms of the G6PD gene on the X chromosome. G6PD is the rate-limiting enzyme in the pentose phosphate metabolic pathway, one of the main functions of which is the generation of nicotinamide adenine dinucleotide phosphate (NADPH), which is integral in maintaining the intracellular supply of reduced glutathione that prevents accumulation of free radicals that would otherwise cause oxidative damage to proteins. The pentose phosphate pathway is the only source of reduced glutathione in red blood cells, which are therefore at particular risk of damage to their cell membranes and haemoglobin by a variety of oxidants, including dapsone hydroxylamine, if G6PD is deficient. If this defence against oxidative stress is overwhelmed, consequent damage to the erythrocyte plasma membrane results in haemolysis or phagocytosis, and the ferrous ion of the haemoglobin molecule is oxidised to the ferric state (methaemoglobin), with a decreased oxygen-carrying capacity. Therefore, it is prudent to screen for functional G6PD deficiency prior to commencing dapsone therapy [1].

Potential adverse effects
Pharmacological
Haemolysis and methaemoglobinaemia. Haemolytic anaemia and methaemoglobinaemia are dose-dependent side effects, occurring to some degree in all dapsone-treated patients, but showing great individual variability [4]. Methaemoglobinaemia is manifest by lethargy and headache, and a cyanotic hue to the skin and mucous membranes. The decreased oxygen-carrying capacity of the blood consequent on haemolysis or methaemoglobinaemia may exacerbate pre-existing cardiac and pulmonary insufficiency. Mild or moderate degrees of methaemoglobinaemia may be treated with cimetidine (400 mg three times daily), which reduces dapsone hydroxylamine formation by inhibiting the cytochrome P450 system of enzymes [7], although this effect declines after several months, possibly because of cytochrome P450 enzyme induction [8]. Vitamin E and ascorbic acid (vitamin C) have also been used to counter methaemoglobinaemia [1], and lipoic acid, as a dietary supplement, may prove to be a useful adjunct to cimetidine in improving patient tolerance of dapsone [9].

Idiosyncratic
Agranulocytosis. Agranulocytosis is a rare unpredictable idiosyncratic adverse effect of dapsone that is potentially life threatening and for which the mechanism is unknown. Dapsone-induced agranulocytosis is more common in older individuals (>60 years) and those of non-white descent, and represents a particular risk in the treatment of dermatitis herpetiformis (compared with a negligible risk when used in leprosy and as prophylaxis for malaria) [10]. Agranulocytosis may present with fever, sore throat and signs of infection and usually manifests within 3 weeks to 3 months of treatment being commenced. Recovery of the neutrophil count tends to occur within 7–14 days of withdrawing the drug, although there is a mortality rate of 14–33% [4].

Peripheral neuropathy. Rarely, dapsone may cause peripheral neuropathy, which is more commonly motor than sensory [4]. The onset of distal neuropathy is often subtle and slowly progressive. Symptoms may persist long after dapsone therapy is terminated (sometimes as long as 1–3 years) [11,12], although recovery usually occurs eventually. It typically presents with weakness of the hands or legs, loss of fine motor skills, gait disturbance, foot drop, glove and stocking loss of sensation and wasting of the hand muscles [11]. Typically dapsone-induced peripheral neuropathy develops after several years of treatment, although it may occur as quickly as within 6 weeks [11,12]. Electrophysiological studies have demonstrated axonal degeneration, although the mechanism is unknown [4,11].

Ocular. Dapsone therapy may also very rarely be associated with ophthalmic side effects including optic neuritis, optic atrophy and macular infarction, potentially resulting in severe visual impairment. Diabetes, hypertension, hypercholesterolaemia and coagulopathy are contributory risk factors [13].

Dapsone hypersensitivity syndrome. Dapsone hypersensitivity syndrome is an idiosyncratic adverse reaction of unknown mechanism, usually occurring in the first 3–5 weeks of commencement of dapsone. It comprises at least two of four signs: fever, lymphadenopathy, generalised rash and hepatitis [14]; it resembles DRESS syndrome (drug rash with eosinophilia and systemic symptoms) [15]. The prevalence is 1.4% and the fatality rate 9.9% [14], with liver failure the most frequent cause of death. Mucosal involvement, rash (which ranges from a maculopapular eruption to toxic epidermal necrolysis [4]) and delayed cessation of dapsone therapy are associated with an increased risk of a fatal outcome [14]. Nausea and vomiting are common, as are eosinophilia and leukocytosis. Other internal organs (kidneys, heart, lungs, pancreas) may be affected.

The presence of HLA-B*13:01 has been shown to be associated with the development of dapsone hypersensitivity syndrome [6].

Systemic glucocorticoid (GC) therapy appears to be beneficial when there is internal organ or mucosal involvement: it should be tapered over 1 month [14]. The cautious reintroduction of dapsone without recurrence of dapsone hypersensitivity syndrome has been reported [17,18].

Other side effects. Dapsone is generally well tolerated at the doses normally used for dermatological conditions. However, it may cause gastrointestinal upset and anorexia, hepatitis, hypoalbuminaemia, headache, insomnia, rashes (varying from a morbilliform eruption and exfoliation to erythroderma and toxic epidermal necrolysis) and, rarely, acute psychosis or photosensitivity [4].

Contraindications
Dapsone is contraindicated for patients with known hypersensitivity to it, and is relatively contraindicated in severe G6PD deficiency and in advanced cardiovascular or pulmonary disease that may be exacerbated by dapsone-induced haemolytic anaemia and methaemoglobinaemia [4].

Cautions
When its use during pregnancy is unavoidable, it is generally considered that dapsone is moderately safe [4,19], although haemolysis and methaemoglobinaemia may develop *in utero* and breastfeeding infants, especially if the child is G6PD deficient [4,20]. Folic acid (5 mg daily) for the mother is advised during pregnancy [7,19].

Dapsone should be used with caution when there is G6PD deficiency, significant cardiopulmonary disease, severe hepatic and renal impairment and pre-existing peripheral neuropathy [4].

Drug–drug interactions
Drug interactions are relatively uncommon with dapsone [4], although the plasma concentration of dapsone may be reduced by rifamycins, carbamazepine, phenytoin, griseofulvin, proton pump inhibitors, calcium and H_2 antihistamines, and be increased by probenecid. MTX, sulphonamides, trimethoprim and hydroxychloroquine may increase the risk from the haematological side effects of dapsone.

Pre-treatment screening
It is important to establish whether the patient has pre-existing conditions that may increase the risk of toxicity from dapsone, such as cardiopulmonary, renal, hepatic or neurological disease. There should be a baseline clinical examination of peripheral motor and sensory function. An FBC and liver and renal function tests should be undertaken, and the G6PD level determined.

Dose and regimens
It is usual to commence dapsone in a single daily dose of 50–100 mg, depending on the pre-treatment screening, subsequently increasing to 100–200 mg/day. Once adequate disease control has been attained, the dose should be gradually tapered to the lowest effective level in order to minimise dapsone toxicity.

Monitoring
An FBC with differential white cell count should be checked every week for the first 4 weeks, and then fortnightly for the next 8 weeks, to monitor for agranulocytosis. Patients should, of course, also be warned to discontinue the medication immediately in the event of fever, chills and sore throat occurring within 3 months of commencing dapsone.

An FBC with reticulocytes should be checked 3–4 monthly: signs of haemolysis (such as raised reticulocytes and bilirubin) should prompt requests for a blood film (Heinz bodies within red blood cells in G6PD-induced haemolysis), lactate dehydrogenase (elevated in haemolysis) and a haptoglobin level (decreased in haemolysis). Methaemoglobin levels should be checked if there are signs or symptoms to suggest methaemoglobinaemia. It is prudent to check the liver function tests fortnightly for the first 3 months; thereafter liver and renal function tests should be performed with the FBC every 3-4 months.

At each follow-up appointment, the peripheral motor and sensory nervous system should be assessed.

Fumarates
Common fumitory (*Fumaria officinalis*) is a plant rich in fumaric acid that is known to have been in use for the treatment of skin complaints, including leprosy, as early as the 17th century when Nicholas Culpeper claimed it to be 'very effectual for … clarifying the blood from saltish, choleric humours which cause leprosy, scabs, tetters, and itches, and such like breakings-out of the skin' [1]. Its use at this time may represent an early example of systemic therapy for psoriasis, as it was not until the 19th century that psoriasis was clearly differentiated from leprosy. The beneficial properties of fumaric acid in psoriasis were first reported by Schweckendiek in 1959: both a chemist and a psoriasis sufferer, he found through self-experimentation a combination of esters of fumaric acid that was both tolerable and effective in improving his psoriasis. Recently, there has been renewed interest in fumarates with the development and licensing of dimethyl fumarate for the treatment of psoriasis and multiple sclerosis.

Dermatological uses
Dimethylfumarate is licensed in Europe, and a mixture of fumarates (under the brand name Fumaderm®) is licensed (only) in Germany, for moderate to severe plaque psoriasis.

Pharmacological properties

Formula and structure
Dimethylfumarate (DMF) is an α,β-unsaturated carboxylic acid ester. Fumaderm also contains three monoethyl hydrogen fumarates (calcium, magnesium and zinc salts).

Administration
Fumarates are taken orally in three divided doses each day, ideally before meals.

Pharmacokinetics
Following oral ingestion, DMF is absorbed from the small intestine in the preportal circulation and rapidly hydrolysed by ubiquitous esterases to the active metabolite, monomethylfumarate. Only monomethylfumarate is detectable in serum, reaching maximum levels by around 4 h [2]. Food intake may significantly delay or reduce absorption, and fumarates should therefore be taken before meals [2]. There is no evidence for a CYP-dependent metabolism in the liver. The half-life of monomethylfumarate is approximately 2 h [3–5].

Pharmacodynamics
Fumarates, and specifically monomethylfumarate, appear to modulate T-helper cell differentiation away from Th1/Th17 development in favour of Th2, which may explain therapeutic efficacy in Th1-mediated disease and the eosinophilia and elevated IgE that can occur with therapy. The molecular mechanisms underlying this are incompletely understood, but data from studies on FAEs in the dermatology literature and data on experimental animal models of multiple sclerosis indicate that both DMF and monomethylfumarate modulate oxidative stress response pathways by binding both to glutathione [6,7] and to KEAP-1 (kelch-like ECH-associated protein 1) [8]. Glutathione is the most important intracellular scavenger of reactive oxygen species and leads to impaired IL-12 and IL-23 production with consequent induction of type II dentritic cells [9]. KEAP-1 is an inhibitor of NFE2L2 (nuclear factor erythroid 2-like 2 or Nrf2), which promotes the synthesis of antioxidant proteins protective against oxidative tissue injury [8].

Potential adverse effects
Two-thirds of patients experience gastrointestinal symptoms, such as nausea, cramps and diarrhoea, and one-third report episodic flushing lasting minutes to hours, with or without headache. These symptoms may settle with time and/or dose reduction but often lead to treatment discontinuation. Transient eosinophilia occurs between weeks 4 and 10, and lasts 1–2 months. A fall in lymphocyte count seen in nearly all patients is not usually of any clinical significance and may correlate with treatment response; in about 10% of patients, the fall is greater than a 50% reduction below baseline values. Rare cases of confirmed progressive multifocal leukoencephalopathy [10,11,**12**] have been reported in patients taking fumarates, all of which were associated with profound lengthy lymphopenia, as well as with other potentially relevant factors (cancer and other immunosuppressive therapies); this highlights the importance of monitoring for and avoiding lymphocyte counts below 0.7×10^9/L. With long-term use, proteinuria with associated renal impairment may rarely develop, with a risk of acute renal failure [4].

Contraindications
Toxicology studies have shown that fumarates have neither teratogenic nor mutagenic potential; nonetheless, conception (for men and women), pregnancy and breastfeeding are contraindicated. Severe hepatic or renal disease, severe gastrointestinal disease (such as untreated peptic ulceration) and significant leukopenia are also contraindications.

Cautions
Recent guidelines suggest caution when fumarates are used with MTX, retinoids, psoralens, ciclosporin, immunosuppressants, cytostatics and any drugs with known nephrotoxicity [**13**]. Live vaccines or live attenuated vaccines should be avoided during fumarate therapy.

Drug–drug interactions
There are no reported interactions of fumarate with other drugs; limited data are available so a high index of suspicion should remain for potential drug interactions.

Pre-treatment screening
Routine baseline blood tests (FBC, liver function tests, renal function), lipids and accurate assessment of urinary protein, ideally with measurement of the albumin to creatine ratio, are needed [**13**,14,15].

Dose and regimens
Fumarates are available as DMF tablets (30 and 60 mg) and as fumarate mixture low strength (Fumaderm initial®; 30 mg DMF, 67 mg monoethylfumarate calcium salt, 5 mg monoethylfumarate magnesium salt, 3 mg monoethylfumarate zinc salt) and high strength (Fumaderm®; 120 mg DMF, 87 mg monoethylfumarate calcium salt, 5 mg monoethylfumarate magnesium salt, 3 mg monoethylfumarate zinc salt). Typically, treatment is initiated with one tablet (equivalent to 30 mg DMF), increasing each week, as tolerated, over 9 weeks (Table 19.1) up to the maximum dose of six tablets of high-strength (equivalent to a daily dose of 720 mg of DMF). Treatment at this dose can be continued as long as there is a clinical need and provided monitoring is satisfactory.

Monitoring
Full blood counts, renal and liver function tests and albumin to creatinine ratios should be checked at monthly intervals during

Table 19.1 Dosage of fumarates (number of tablets).

Week	Morning	Noon	Evening	Fumarate formulation (dose of dimethylfumarate)
1	1	–	–	Low strength (30 mg)
2	1	–	1	Low strength (30 mg)
3	1	1	1	Low strength (30 mg)
4	1	–	–	High strength (120 mg)
5	1	–	1	High strength (120 mg)
6	1	1	1	High strength (120 mg)
7	2	1	1	High strength (120 mg)
8	2	1	2	High strength (120 mg)
9	2	2	2	High strength (120 mg)

dose escalation and then every 3 months once a therapeutic dose is established. If the lymphocyte count falls below $1.0 \times 10^9/L$ but is $\geq 0.7 \times 10^9/L$, blood monitoring should be performed monthly until levels return to $1.0 \times 10^9/L$ or higher for two consecutive blood tests at which point monitoring can again be performed every 3 months. If the lymphocyte count falls below $0.7 \times 10^9/L$, the blood test must be repeated and if the levels are confirmed to be below $0.7 \times 10^9/L$, then treatment must be stopped immediately.

Summary

For those patients who tolerate fumarates, the therapy is straightforward to manage. Licensing of DMF for psoriasis and multiple sclerosis has improved availability and will provide important additional safety data, particularly in relation to rare serious adverse effects.

Systemic glucocorticoids

The glucocorticoids (GCs) are a family of steroid hormones that have vital immunomodulatory and metabolic functions and are the most frequently used and consistently effective anti-inflammatory agents for dermatological conditions. The term *glucocorticoid* is often used synonymously with *corticosteroid*, although, strictly, the latter includes both GCs and mineralocorticoids, both produced within the adrenal cortex. The principal naturally occurring GC is cortisol (hydrocortisone), possessing modest GC potency; there are also a number of synthetic systemic GCs with intermediate (prednisolone, methylprednisolone, triamcinolone) and high (betamethasone, dexamethasone) GC potency.

Dermatological uses: licensed indications and off-label usage (Chapters 35, 36, 37, 39, 40, 41, 42, 49–55, 96 and 100)

Glucocorticoids are used in a very wide variety of dermatological inflammatory conditions [1], including bullous dermatoses, connective tissue diseases, vasculitides, neutrophilic dermatoses, eczematous and papulosquamous disorders and miscellaneous conditions such as severe urticaria and sarcoidosis. Low-dose dexamethasone has also been used in androgen excess syndromes [1].

Pharmacological properties

Formula and structure

The basic ring structure of all GCs is the cyclopentanoperhydrophenanthrene nucleus, consisting of three hexane rings and one pentane ring. GCs with increased anti-inflammatory potency are formed by modifications of the hydrocortisone molecule: introducing a 1,2 double bond (prednisolone); a 1,2 double bond and a 6-methyl group (methylprednisolone); a 1,2 double bond and fluorine at the 9α position, with a 16α hydroxyl group (triamcinolone); a 16α methyl group (dexamethasone); or a 16β methyl group (betamethasone).

Administration

Although GCs are usually administered orally, there are occasional indications for intramuscular, intravenous and intralesional administration.

Oral GCs are ideally given in the early morning to conform to the natural circadian rhythm of endogenous GC production. Traditionally, prednisolone (the biologically active metabolite of prednisone) is the favoured oral GC for dermatological use in the UK, although betamethasone, deflazacort, dexamethasone, hydrocortisone and methylprednisolone can be given orally [2].

Intramuscular administration of GCs has the advantages of guaranteeing that a possibly unreliable patient receives treatment and also avoids the potential gastrointestinal side effects of oral GCs. However, intramuscular GCs may cause fat atrophy and occasional abscess formation at the injection site, as well as being more likely than oral GCs to induce menstrual irregularities in women [1], possibly because the intramuscular route results in constant levels of circulating GCs without diurnal variation, thereby suppressing gonadotropin release. Traditionally, triamcinolone acetonide has been favoured for intramuscular use [3].

Intravenous administration of GCs, usually given in 'pulses' on an in-patient basis, is generally only used in situations where it is desirable to bring very serious steroid-responsive conditions under rapid control. Methylprednisolone is the usual intravenous GC of choice. The risks particularly associated with intravenous pulsed GCs include sudden death of presumed cardiac origin secondary to acute electrolyte shifts, cardiac arrhythmias, potentially life-threatening anaphylaxis, gastric erosions and sepsis [1]. Serious cardiovascular adverse effects are rare, tending to occur in patients with heart or kidney disease [4], and pulsed intravenous GC therapy is considered to have an acceptable risk–benefit profile, in the appropriate clinical context [5].

Formerly, corticotropin (adrenocorticotropic hormone) and its analogue, tetracosactide, were used as an alternative to GCs but had the disadvantages of variable and unpredictable therapeutic responses and a gradual waning of effect [2].

Pharmacokinetics

The synthetic GCs are readily absorbed from the small bowel after oral administration and peak plasma concentrations occur after 1–2 h. They are significantly protein bound in the circulation to cortisol-binding globulin (transcortin) and corticosteroid-binding albumin, become widely distributed in body tissues and also cross the placenta.

They are metabolised predominantly in the liver and the metabolites are then conjugated with sulphate or glucuronic acid to make them water soluble, before being excreted in the urine. Inactivation is mainly by reduction of both the 3-keto group (by 3α-hydroxysteroid dehydrogenase) and the 4,5 double bond in the steroid A ring (by 5α-reductase and 5β-reductase).

The biological half-life of GCs varies from 8 to 12 h for the short-acting GCs (hydrocortisone, cortisone), 24–36 h for the intermediate-acting GCs (prednisolone, methylprednisolone, triamcinolone) and 36–54 h for the long-acting GCs (betamethasone, dexamethasone) [1].

Pharmacodynamics

Endogenous GC (cortisol) plays vital physiological roles in anti-inflammatory homeostasis and in certain metabolic processes, including gluconeogenesis and fluid/electrolyte regulation. The synthetic GCs have been developed primarily as anti-inflammatory agents for the treatment of conditions unresponsive to natural anti-inflammatory processes.

The intracellular mechanisms of action of GCs are complex and still incompletely understood [6]. They are known to act within the nucleus at a genomic level but also to have non-genomic effects [7]. Being lipophilic, GCs cross plasma membranes into the cytoplasm of cells with ease, where they bind to cytosolic GC receptor (cGCR) encoded by the NR3C1 (nuclear receptor subfamily 3, group C, member 1) gene.

Unactivated cGCR, which is ubiquitous in vertebrate cells, is a 94 kDa protein present in the cytoplasm as a complex with various other proteins (chaperones), including heat-shock proteins and several kinases of the mitogen-activated protein kinase (MAPK) signalling system that are thought to be important in maintaining the conformational state of the cGCR to enable high-affinity binding with GCs. It has a complex structure that includes specific domains for binding GCs and DNA and for undertaking transcription functions. On binding to GC (endogenous or synthetic), the cGCR rapidly dissociates from its protein chaperones, enabling the GC/cGCR complex to pass into the nucleus. There, the GC/cGCR complex binds to specific DNA binding sites (GC response elements) within the promoter regions of GC-inducible genes, from where it modifies the transcription of those genes. Depending on the target gene, transcription is either activated ('transactivation') or inhibited [7,8]. Numerous genes are targeted by the GC/cGCR complex, many of which produce proteins that regulate the inflammatory process and apoptosis and others which regulate metabolic functions: it is estimated that GCs influence the expression of approximately 1% of the entire genome [7].

In addition to their DNA binding effects on transcription, GC/cGCR complexes also prevent the binding to their target genes of a variety of natural transcription factors (such as activator protein 1, NF-ATc and nuclear factor κB (NFκB)), resulting in the reduced expression of many immunoregulatory and pro-inflammatory proteins ('transrepression') [7,8]. Furthermore, GCs also seem to have post-transcriptional and post-translational effects [7].

GCs have several non-genomically mediated actions still to be precisely defined. These include the release of the protein chaperones when the GC/cGCR complex is formed, which may have important signalling effects, such as those involving the T-cell receptor (TCR). Via this mechanism, GCs impair TCR signalling and consequently T-cell cytokine production, proliferation and differentiation [9]. There may also be an important non-specific non-genomic mechanism of GC action involving intercalation of GC molecules in cell plasma membranes, resulting in altered cation transport, which in the case of immune-competent cells is considered to contribute to immunosuppressive and anti-inflammatory actions [7]. Finally, GCs may also cause specific non-genomic actions, mediated through a cell surface membrane-bound GCR known to be present on the cell surfaces of human monocytes and B lymphocytes [7].

This is a very simplified summary of the complex mechanisms that in combination are thought to regulate GC-induced immune modulation and apoptosis of immune-competent cells. In addition to these desirable anti-inflammatory properties in the context of treating disease states, the enhanced effect compared with that of endogenous cortisol of the synthetic GCs on gene transcription results in a number of undesirable metabolic consequences. These include important effects on gluconeogenesis, causing increased carbohydrate production by the enhanced metabolism of endogenous protein (from bone, muscle, skin and blood vessels) and on fat metabolism with associated peripheral insulin resistance; the less potent GCs also have important mineralocorticoid actions. It has long been assumed that the unwanted effects of prolonged treatment with GCs are largely the result of transactivation, while the beneficial anti-inflammatory effects are the result of transrepression [7,8], but doubt has been cast on this hypothesis [10,11].

Pharmacogenetics

The pharmacogenetic factors of clinical relevance to dermatologists are still to be established. However, GCR polymorphisms may explain in part the wide individual variation in response to GCs [12–14] and may influence GC-induced bone mineral density [13] and metabolic [15] changes. GCR polymorphisms have also been associated with depression and bipolar disorder [16–18] and may therefore possibly be relevant to the mood disturbances that may complicate GC therapy.

Potential adverse effects

Glucocorticoids have the potential for a wide variety of side effects, particularly when used in high (supraphysiological) doses and in long-term regimens (Figure 19.2). Short courses (2–3 weeks) of GCs are generally relatively safe [1].

Hydrocortisone has a significant mineralocorticoid action, but with increasing potency the mineralocorticoid effect of GCs diminishes: GCs of intermediate potency (prednisolone, methylprednisolone, triamcinolone) have some mineralocorticoid action and the high-potency GCs (betamethasone, dexamethasone) negligible action [2].

Malignancy

The development of immunosuppression-related malignancies, such as lymphoma, squamous cell carcinoma and Kaposi sarcoma, is very uncommon when GCs are used in isolation [1].

Steroid withdrawal syndrome

The withdrawal of GCs may be occasionally and apparently idiosyncratically associated with signs and symptoms of variable degree resembling adrenal insufficiency [19]. Steroid withdrawal syndrome may occur when the dose of GC is still supraphysiological or even after complete withdrawal without biochemical evidence of subnormal hypothalamopituitary–adrenal (HPA) axis integrity. Symptoms include fever, anorexia, nausea, vomiting, lethargy, fatigue, weakness, malaise, emotional lability, depression, myalgia, arthralgia, headache, abdominal pain, skin peeling, influenza-like symptoms and weight loss. Signs include postural hypotension, hyponatraemia and hyperkalaemia [19].

The precise mechanism underlying the steroid withdrawal syndrome is unknown, although it is possible that the symptoms are mediated by increased circulatory levels of pro-inflammatory cytokines such as IL-6, TNF-α and IL-1β consequent on the reduction of GCs [20]. Its treatment is to reinstitute or increase GC therapy, followed by more gradual tapering of the dose [20].

Contraindications

Glucocorticoids are relatively contraindicated if there is systemic infection unless specific therapy is being given [2]. Vaccination with live virus should be avoided in patients taking GCs.

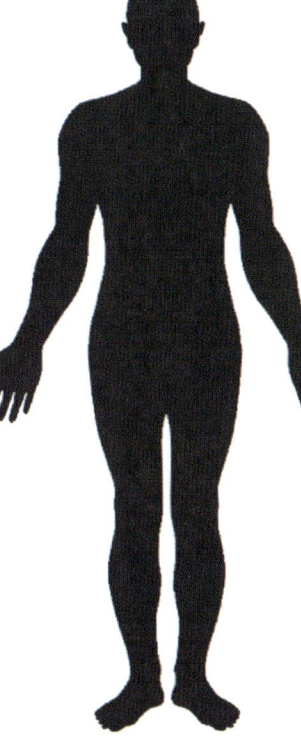

 OCULAR
- Ocular hypertension and glaucoma
- Cataracts – posterior subcapsular
- Central serous chorioretinopathy
- Ocular infections, including herpes simplex

 INFECTION
- Tuberculosis reactivation
- Opportunistic infections

 MINERALOCORTICOID
- Hypernatraemia and water retention
- Hypertension and weight gain
- Hypokalaemia, hypocalcaemia

 GLUCOCORTICOID
- Hyperglycaemia, development of diabetes
- Deterioration of diabetic control
- Dyslipidaemia – hypertriglyceridaemia, hypercholesterolaemia
- Increased appetite, weight gain
- Menstrual irregularities
- Cushingoid features (lipodystrophy) – moon face, 'buffalo hump', central obesity (thin limbs, plump trunk)

 BONE
- Osteoporosis
- Osteonecrosis (avascular necrosis)
- Growth impairment in children

 PSYCHIATRIC
- Psychosis
- Euphoria, depression, agitation
- Suicidal ideation
- Insomnia, nightmares
- Irritability, mood lability

 CUTANEOUS
- Purpura, bruising, striae, dermal and epidermal atrophy, telangiectasia
- 'Steroid acne', rosacea-like syndrome
- Impaired wound healing
- Hirsutism
- Fat atrophy with injected GCs
- Cutaneous infections – staphylococcal and herpetic
- Hyperhidrosis

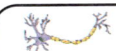 **GASTROINTESTINAL**
- Peptic ulceration
- Bowel perforation (particular risk with active diverticulitis and recent bowel anastomosis)
- Pancreatitis
- Fatty liver
- Gastro-oesophageal reflux
- Candidiasis

 NEUROMUSCULAR
- Muscle weakness (proximal myopathy)
- Intracranial hypertension (pseudotumor cerebri)
- Spinal epidural lipomatosis

Figure 19.2 Potential side effects of glucocorticoids.

Cautions

Adrenal suppression

Endogenous cortisol production in the physiological state is regulated by a negative feedback homeostatic mechanism on corticotropin-releasing factor secretion from the hypothalamus and adrenocorticotropic hormone release from the pituitary – the HPA axis. Synthetic GCs also suppress the hypothalamopituitary drive of the adrenal glands and will abolish endogenous cortisol production by the adrenals if the dose and duration of treatment are sufficient, resulting in the potential, albeit rare, for acute adrenal insufficiency (Addisonian crisis) if the GC is stopped abruptly. It can take very many months for the normal adrenocortical response to fully recover, and vulnerability to stress may last for a year or more [1].

There is significant individual variation in susceptibility to GC-induced adrenal suppression [1]. GCs given in divided doses or at times other than the morning are more likely to induce HPA axis suppression. Alternate day GC therapy reduces the risk of HPA axis suppression [1].

The early morning cortisol level and 24 h urinary cortisol level both provide a measure of basal HPA axis function for a patient on GCs, and the short synacthen stimulation test is a measure of the stress responsiveness of the adrenal: these are an option for assessing adrenal reserve towards the end of long-term GC therapy.

GCs taken in a daily dose of more than 40 mg for more than 1 week (or a lesser dose for more than 3 weeks) should be tapered gradually [2]. Intercurrent illness, infection, surgical procedure or trauma requires a temporary increase in GC dose or, if a prolonged GC course has recently been completed, a temporary reintroduction of GC to compensate for a diminished adrenal response. Anaesthetists must know if their patient is taking or has been taking a GC within 3 months of surgery [2]. Patients on long-term GC therapy should carry a steroid treatment card with them at all times.

Acquired resistance (tachyphylaxis)

The therapeutic response to GCs in chronic inflammatory disorders may be compromised by the development of an acquired resistance or insensitivity to GCs [21,22]. The precise mechanisms for this phenomenon are not fully elucidated but are thought to include down-regulation of GCR expression and inhibition of GCR translocation by pro-inflammatory cytokines, oxidative stress and hypoxia in the cellular microenvironment occurring over time [22]. The consequent higher doses of GCs that are necessary to maintain disease control increase the risk of adverse effects.

Infections

Prolonged courses of GCs increase susceptibility to infection and may modify and perhaps mask signs of infection, especially septicaemia and tuberculosis [2]. GCs predispose to severe chickenpox and measles if the patient is not already immune to these infections: exposure to them requires passive immunisation. Fungal or viral ocular infections may be exacerbated, as may amoebiasis and strongyloidiasis [2].

Bone protection
Glucocorticoid-induced osteoporotic fractures are a real risk with long-term therapy, even in low dosage, and monitoring with bone mineral density measurements (dual-energy X-ray absorptiometry (DEXA) scans) is advisable in patients on long-term GC therapy. Preventative measures, such as calcium/vitamin D supplements and biphosphonate therapy, together with lifestyle advice including weight-bearing exercise, smoking cessation and avoiding excessive alcohol intake, should be considered early when initiating long-term GC therapy to limit the likelihood of osteoporosis.

Gastrointestinal protection
Although controversial, the prophylactic administration of a proton pump inhibitor or an H_2 antagonist should be considered in high-dose GC therapy, particularly for high-risk groups (e.g. anticoagulation therapy or a history of peptic ulcer disease) [1].

Psychiatric reactions
Glucocorticoids should be prescribed with caution for patients with a personal or family history of psychiatric disorders.

Pregnancy
Glucocorticoids may increase the risks of spontaneous abortion and stillbirth, and the possibility of fetal HPA axis suppression should be considered when GCs are given to the mother close to delivery [1].

General cautions
Care should be taken when prescribing GCs for children, the elderly, pregnant women or patients with diabetes, hypertension, osteoporosis, raised intraocular pressure, a history of peptic ulceration, diverticulitis, recent bowel anastomosis or tuberculosis, or if there is hepatic or renal impairment.

Contraindications
Glucocorticoids are relatively contraindicated if there is systemic infection unless specific therapy is being given [2]. Vaccination with live virus should be avoided in patients taking GCs.

Drug–drug interactions
There are a large number of potential interactions between systemic GCs and other drugs (see *British National Formulary* for complete list), although only a small number are potentially serious, with only very few of these involving prednisolone (Box 19.5) [1].

Pre-treatment screening
If a short course (up to 3 weeks) of GC therapy is envisaged, it is reasonable to establish whether there are coexisting conditions that might be influenced by GCs (such as diabetes, psychosis, glaucoma, infections, peptic ulcer disease, active diverticulitis and recent surgery), to enquire about medications that might influence or be influenced by GCs and to monitor for rising blood pressure and glycosuria.

If extended treatment is anticipated, baseline assessment of blood pressure, weight, height (in children), serum electrolytes, fasting glucose and fasting lipids should be undertaken. Consideration should be given to screening for active and latent tuberculosis, especially in those considered to be at particular risk, by means of a Mantoux test followed if positive by an IFN-γ test and chest X-ray [23]. Baseline ophthalmic examination for cataracts and ocular hypertension should also be considered.

Prior to initiating GC therapy, the patient and family members should receive appropriate education, in particular about the potential adverse effects and the monitoring details. A steroid treatment card should be provided and the information on it kept up to date.

> **Box 19.5 Glucocorticoids: drug–drug interactions**
> - Glucocorticoids (GCs) antagonise the hypotensive effects of angiotensin-converting enzyme inhibitors, α-blockers, angiotensin-II receptor antagonists, β-blockers, calcium-channel blockers and clonidine
> - GCs increase the risk of gastrointestinal bleeding when given synchronously with non-steroidal anti-inflammatory drugs
> - Anticonvulsants reduce plasma levels of GCs
> - GCs have a variable effect on the anticoagulant action of coumarins
> - GCs antagonise the oral hypoglycaemics
> - GCs antagonise diuretics and increase risk of hypokalaemia
> - Oestrogen-containing oral contraceptives increase plasma concentrations of GCs
> - GCs may impair immune response to vaccines

Dose and regimens
Oral administration
Depending on the clinical diagnosis, its severity and the presence or otherwise of cautionary factors, it is reasonable to consider commencing prednisolone at a starting dose of up to 1 mg/kg body weight daily, ideally given as a single dose in the morning. A single daily dose is less likely than a divided dose to cause adverse effects, and a morning dose less likely to result in HPA axis suppression than when given at other times of day [1]. In some circumstances, higher doses may be considered [1].

Intramuscular administration
A typical regimen for intramuscular triamcinolone is 80 mg two or three times a year [1].

Pulsed intravenous administration
A typical regimen for in-patient-based pulsed intravenous methylprednisolone is 500–1000 mg (approximately 10–15 mg/kg) daily, given over at least 60 min, for 3–5 consecutive days, with continuous cardiac monitoring and daily measurement of electrolytes and glucose levels recommended [1]. Thereafter, oral prednisolone and/or a non-steroidal immunosuppressive may be required to maintain the therapeutic effect of pulsed intravenous therapy.

Tapering steroid dose
Generally, as soon as there is adequate disease control, consideration should be given to tapering long-term GCs to the minimal effective dose in order to minimise the risk of side effects, although, despite their use over many decades, the optimal regimen has yet to be determined. The rate of dose reduction is determined by disease activity, assessed by clinical features and laboratory parameters. When withdrawing GCs, it is reasonable to attempt to reduce the dose rapidly to a physiological level (7.5 mg prednisolone daily or equivalent [2]), followed thereafter by a more gradual reduction. If a patient has been on steroids for more than 3 weeks or on >40 mg for more than 1 week then it is advisable to check a 9 am cortisol (and short synacthen test if low) prior to reducing below 7.5 mg. Endocrine advice should be sought prior to further weaning if there is evidence of HPA axis suppression. If supraphysiological doses of GCs are required in the long term, adjusting to an alternating day regimen may ultimately allow recovery of the HPA axis and cause less metabolic disruption than continuing to give GCs in a daily dose [1].

Monitoring
A reasonable follow-up frequency for patients on oral GC treatment is at 1 month and then every 2–3 months [1]. At each visit specific enquiries should be made for side effects, blood pressure and weight (and height in children) should be recorded, and serum electrolytes, fasting glucose and lipids measured [1]. An ophthalmic examination every 6–12 months is recommended [1].

A neutrophilia frequently occurs with GC therapy. This should not be assumed to be necessarily the result of infection as it is often innocent, resulting from a shift of neutrophils from the marginated to the circulating pool, with a minor contribution from an increased release from bone marrow [24].

Depending on therapeutic response and the likely duration of therapy with GCs, active consideration should be given to steroid-sparing strategies.

Summary
Glucocorticoids have a very important place in the dermatological therapeutic armamentarium and their prudent use and monitoring will minimise, although not obviate, adverse effects. For the future, enhancement of the risk–benefit ratio of GCs may be possible by the targeted delivery of GCs (long-circulating liposomal GCs), by combining GCs with synergistic anti-inflammatory moieties (such as nitric oxide) or by the modified release of GC to conform to circadian rhythms (chronotherapy) [25]. Novel non-steroidal drugs such as SEGRAs (selective GCR agonists) and SGRMs (selective GCR modulators) may have the anti-inflammatory properties of conventional GCs with fewer side effects [25].

Hydroxycarbamide
Hydroxycarbamide (formerly known as hydroxyurea) is an antimetabolite cytotoxic drug that is used primarily in the treatment of chronic myeloid leukaemia and certain solid malignancies, for conditions with a high risk of thromboembolic complications (including polycythaemia rubra vera and essential thrombocythaemia) and for reducing the crises of sickle cell disease [1].

Dermatological uses
Off-label, the primary dermatological indication for hydroxycarbamide has been for the treatment of recalcitrant chronic plaque psoriasis [2]. The advent of novel targeted therapies means that where these are available, hydroxycarbamide is rarely used. It has also been used for the treatment of Sweet syndrome, erythromelalgia and hypereosinophilic syndrome [3].

Pharmacological properties
Formula and structure
Hydroxycarbamide (empirical formula: $CH_4N_2O_2$; systematic name: hydroxyurea) is a simple organic molecule consisting of a carbonyl functional group attached to single amine and hydroxylamine functional groups. It was first synthesised in 1869.

Administration
Hydroxycarbamide is administered orally and is available in the UK as 100, 500 and 1000 mg tablets [1].

Pharmacokinetics
Hydroxycarbamide has excellent oral bioavailability, with maximum plasma concentrations reached between 0.5 and 2 h [1,4]. Despite therapeutic use over many years, there is still only a limited understanding of hydroxycarbamide absorption, distribution, metabolism and clearance [4]. The metabolic pathways include saturable hepatic metabolism and also degradation by urease-producing intestinal bacteria [1]. It is cleared relatively rapidly, mainly via the kidneys, with a plasma half-life of 2–4 h [1].

Pharmacodynamics
Hydroxycarbamide is thought to act by inhibiting the ribonucleotide reductase system, thus blocking the formation of deoxyribonucleotides and thereby inhibiting DNA synthesis [1].

Potential adverse effects
Myelosuppression
Dose-related bone marrow toxicity, causing anaemia, leukopenia or thrombocytopenia, is the most common adverse effect of hydroxycarbamide, although clinically significant complications are rare provided that there is close haematological monitoring [2]. Mild megaloblastic changes, which are common and of little significance [3], are unrelated to vitamin B_{12} or folate deficiency [1] and are a good indicator of adherence [2].

Gastrointestinal
Diarrhoea, constipation, nausea, vomiting and stomatitis may occur [1]. Upper gastrointestinal symptoms may be reduced by administration of hydroxycarbamide with food, milk or antacids [3].

Cutaneous
Hydroxycarbamide is associated with a number of cutaneous side effects including painful leg ulceration [5], a dermatomyositis-like eruption [6–8], a lichen planus-like rash [9], alopecia [3], lupus erythematosus [10], photosensitivity [3], radiation recall [3] and hyperpigmentation of the skin and nails [11–13].

The mutagenic potential of hydroxycarbamide and its impairment of DNA repair mechanisms may increase the long-term risk of non-melanoma cutaneous malignancy [14–17], particularly in patients being treated for myeloproliferative disorders. Although it is prudent to offer standard advice regarding sun protection, the risk to patients being treated for dermatological conditions appears to be low [2,3,18]. Similarly, although hydroxycarbamide has been associated with the development of leukaemic change when used in myeloproliferative disorders, myelodysplasia has not been established as a long-term concern in dermatological usage [2,5].

Other side effects
Rarely, hydroxycarbamide has been associated with acute pulmonary inflammation, abnormal liver function, neurological symptoms, pyrexia, hypersensitivity and hallucinations.

Contraindications
Hydroxycarbamide is contraindicated if there is significant pre-existing bone marrow dysfunction, or if there is known sensitivity to the drug.

Cautions
Hydroxycarbamide should be avoided during pregnancy and breastfeeding, and men should be advised to avoid conception during treatment and for 3 months after its discontinuation [1].

Drug–drug interactions
Hydroxycarbamide is associated with few drug interactions likely to be of clinical relevance when used for dermatological indications [2]. Other myelosuppressive and antineoplastic drugs should be avoided. Hydroxycarbamide may enhance the potential side effects of nucleoside reverse transcriptase inhibitors such as didanosine and stavudine.

Pre-treatment screening
Prior to commencing hydroxycarbamide, screening as outlined in Box 19.1 should be undertaken.

Dose and regimens
When used for cutaneous disorders, an initial dose of 1 g once daily is recommended [2]. Depending on clinical response and haematological parameters, this can be gradually increased to 2 g daily in a divided dose. In the elderly and those with renal impairment, consider a starting dose of 500 mg daily [2].

Monitoring
It is reasonable for the FBC to be checked weekly for the first month, then fortnightly for the next 3 months, monthly for a further 3 months, then quarterly thereafter [3]. Dose adjustment or temporary cessation of therapy should be considered if significant myelosuppression occurs [2]. Monthly electrolyte, creatinine and liver function tests, reducing to every 3–6 months if stable, are also reasonable [3].

Janus kinase inhibitors
Janus kinase inhibitors (JAKi) are small-molecule inhibitors of intracellular JAK activity. JAKs are a family of intracellular tyrosine kinases that transduce cytokine-mediated signals via the JAK/STAT (signal transducers and activators of transcription) pathway, comprising four members, JAK1, JAK2, JAK3 and TYK2. These recently introduced immunomodulatory agents are effective at treating multiple inflammatory conditions. There are multiple JAKi in use/development, all of which target specific members of the JAK family to different extents. JAKi licensed for dermatological indications currently comprise abrocitinib and upadacitinib, both more specific to JAK1, and baricitinib, more specific to JAK1 and JAK2 [1–3].

Dermatological uses
Abrocitinib, baricitinib and upadacitinib are all licensed for the treatment of moderate to severe atopic dermatitis in adults [1–3]. Trials have shown additional promising effect of JAK inhibition in autoimmune hair loss, vitiligo and psoriasis (TYK2 targeting agents specifically). Outside of dermatology, other inflammatory indications include psoriatic arthritis (tofacitinib and upadacitinib), rheumatoid arthritis (tofacitinib and upadacitinib), ulcerative colitis (tofacitinib) and ankylosing spondylitis (upadacitinib).

Pharmacological properties
Formula and structure
- Abrocitinib: empirical formula: $C_{14}H_{21}N_5O_2S$; systematic name: N-[3-[methyl(7H-pyrrolo[2,3-d]pyrimidin-4-yl)amino]cyclobutyl]propane-1-sulfonamide.
- Baricitinib: empirical formula: $C_{16}H_{17}N_7O_2S$; systematic name: 2-[1-ethylsulfonyl-3-[4-(7H-pyrrolo[2,3-d]pyrimidin-4-yl)pyrazol-1-yl]azetidin-3-yl]acetonitrile.
- Upadacitinib: empirical formula: $C_{17}H_{19}F_3N_6O_2$; systematic name: (3S,4R)-3-ethyl-4-(1,5,7,10-tetrazatricyclo[7.3.0.0^{2,6}]dodeca-2(6),3,7,9,11-pentaen-12-yl)-N-(2,2,2-trifluoroethyl)pyrrolidine-1-carboxamide.

Administration
Abrocitinib, baricitinib and upadacitinib are available in the UK as oral tablets (100/200 mg tablets, 2/4 mg tablets, 15/30 mg tablets, respectively).

Pharmacokinetics
Abrocitinib, baricitinib and upadactinib are well absorbed with absolute oral bioavailabilities of between 60% and 79%. Peak plasma concentrations are achieved within 1–4 h. Abrocitinib is metabolised by CYP2C19, CYP2C9 and CYP3A4. Baricitinib and upadactinib are primarily metabolised by CYP3A4. Abrocitinib and baricitinib are primarily renally excreted, while upadacitinib is excreted via urine and faeces. The half-lives of abrocitinib, baricitinib and upadacitinib are 5, 12.5 and 8–14 h, respectively.

Pharmacodynamics
Cytokines are extracellular and once they associate with their receptors many exert their downstream intracellular effects via JAK-STAT signalling (Figure 19.3). When these cytokines (including key inflammatory cytokines such as IL-4, IL-13 and IL-31 relevant to atopic dermatitis, and IL-12 and IL-23 relevant to psoriasis) bind to their receptor, the two arms of the receptor come together. Attached to each arm is a JAKi, and every cytokine receptor has a specific combination of JAKi attached to each arm. These can be

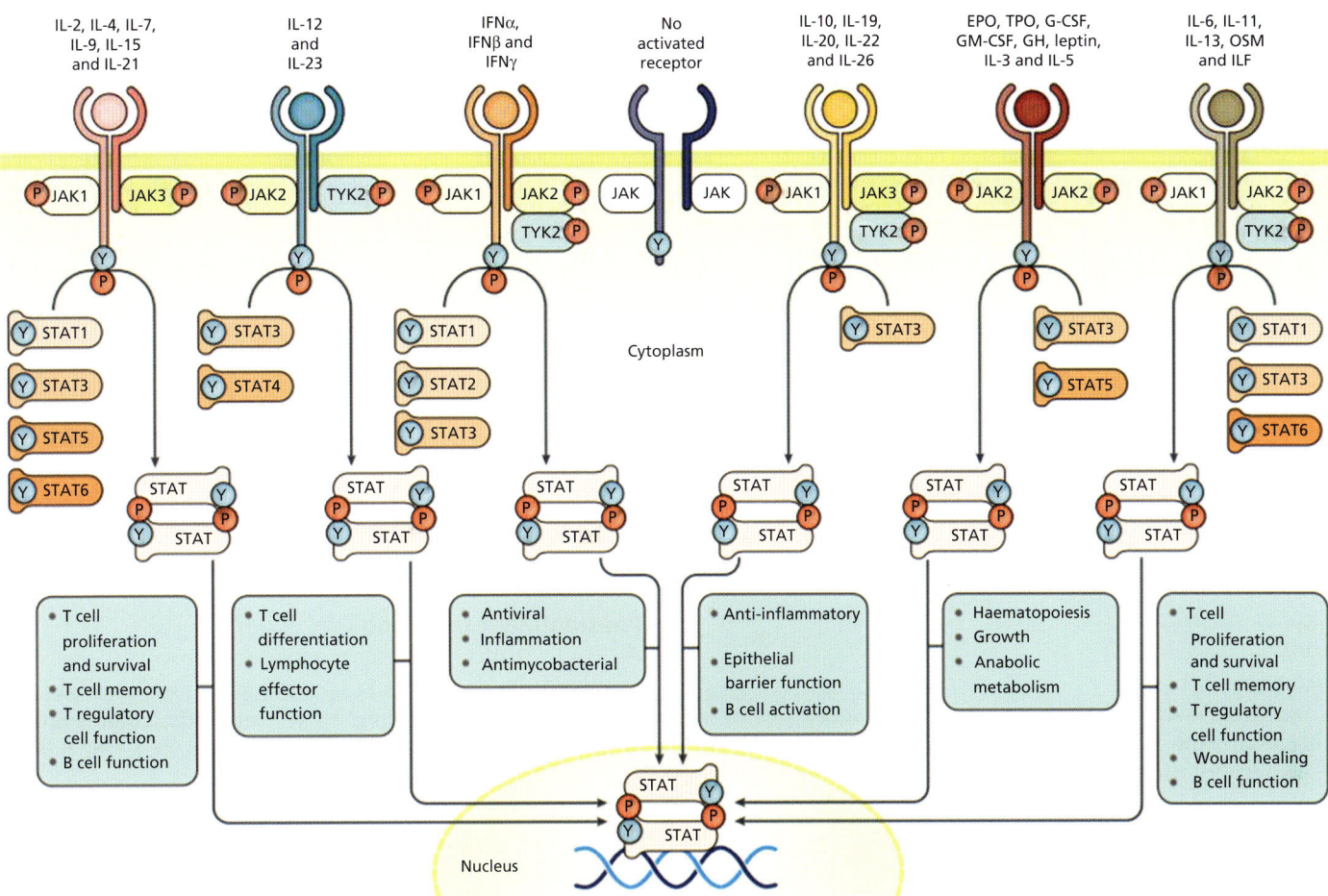

Figure 19.3 Extracellular signals involving the JAK/STAT pathway and their respective downstream functions. JAKs (Janus kinases) are intracellular tyrosine kinases that transduce cytokine-mediated signals. The combination of JAKs required on the respective arms of a receptor varies depending on the signal, for example IL-4 requires both JAK1 and JAK2 function. On stimulation, JAKs phosphorylate STATs (signal transducers and activators of transcription) which results in dimerisation and translocation of STATs to the nucleus to modulate target gene expression and downstream effects. GM-CSF, granulocyte–macrophage colony-stimulating factor; EPO, erythropoietin; G-CSF, granulocyte colony-stimulating factor; GH, growth hormone; IFN, interferon; IL, interleukin; LIF, leukemia inhibitory factor; OSM, oncostatin; P autophosphorylation and/or transphosphorylation; TPO, thrombopoietin; Y, tyrosine residues. Reproduced from Salas et al. 2020 [10].

homodimers (e.g. JAK1 on both arms, JAKI1/JAK1) or heterodimers (e.g. JAK1/JAK2, JAK1/JAK3, JAK1/TYK2, etc.). Specific examples include IL-4 which requires JAK1 and JAK3, and IL-23 which requires JAK1 and TYK2. When the two arms come together the JAKs cross-phosphorylate one another and then phosphorylate the tyrosine residues on the arms themselves in turn facilitating STAT binding, phosphorylation detachment and downstream activity on gene transcription in the nucleus.

Cytokines that are integral to atopic dermatitis, such as IL-4, IL-13 and IL-31, all require JAK1 (Figure 19.3). Relative JAK1 inhibition via abrocitinib, baricitinib and upadacitinib can therefore modulate the effects of these signals and has proven effective at improving the severity of atopic dermatitis [4–6]. JAKi have a very rapid onset of action in atopic dermatitis with itch improvement noticed within a week and clinical improvement within 4 weeks. Cytokines integral to psoriasis, such as IL-23, requiring TYK2 and TYK2 inhibition can therefore modify that signal, and there is emerging evidence to support TYK2 inhibition in that context [7].

In addition to this, JAK signalling is an important component for multiple other signalling pathways including interferons, EPO, TPO, G-CSF, GM-CSF, GH and leptin (Figure 19.3, with abbreviations in full). Inhibiting JAK function can therefore impact on wide-ranging biological pathways including haematopoiesis, lipid metabolism, growth and defence against infection. The relative specificity of JAKi is therefore important in terms of the tolerability of the individual agents.

Potential adverse effects

There are broad tolerability issues relevant to all three JAKi [1–3]. Common side effects include infection (including herpes simplex and herpes zoster), gastrointestinal upset (nausea, vomiting, abdominal pain), acne, headache and a rise in creatinine kinase. There is variability in the relative frequency of these side effects across the agents with, for example, nausea and vomiting more common on abrocitinib and acne more common on upadactinib. Uncommon side effects include hyperlipidaemia and venous thrombotic events, including pulmonary embolism and deep vein thrombosis. Drug-specific effects include thrombocytopenia (abrocitinib), thrombocytosis (baricitinib), anaemia (upadacitinib), neutropenia (baricitinib and upadacitinib), diverticulitis (baricitinib and upadacitinib) and transaminitis (baricitinib and upadacitinib).

A safety trial comparing tofacitinib and anti-TNF therapy for rheumatoid arthritis in a trial population enriched for cardiovascular risk showed risks of major adverse cardiovascular events and cancers were higher in the tofacitinib arm [8]. This has led the US Food and Drug Administration (FDA) to issue a warning for all medicines in this class (pending further information) about an increased risk of serious heart-related events, cancer, blood clots and death [9]. The UK Medicines and Healthcare products Regulatory Agency (MHRA) has issued similar guidance.

Contraindications

Abrocitinib and upadacitinib are contraindicated in people with a hypersensitivity to the active substance or excipients, active tuberculosis or serious infection, severe hepatic impairment, pregnancy or breastfeeding. Baricitinib is contraindicated in people with a hypersensitivity to the active substance or excipients and pregnancy.

Live vaccination should be avoided within 2 weeks of initiation, while on therapy and for 6 months (or longer dependent on local guidance) post-treatment cessation.

Cautions
Infection

Risks and benefits should be considered in the context of recurrent infection, exposure to tuberculosis (or risk thereof), history of serious or opportunistic infection or underlying conditions that may predispose to infection.

Viral reactivation is reported with these agents; consideration should be given to risk from herpes simplex virus (HSV), varicella-zoster virus (VZV) and the potential merits of vaccination where available/recommended.

Thrombotic events

Janus kinase inhibitors should be used with caution in those with risk factors for deep-vein thrombosis or pulmonary embolism. These might include older age, obesity, previous history, prothrombotic disorder, combined oral contraceptives, hormone replacement therapy, planned major surgery or immobility.

Malignancy

The risks and benefits of JAKi therapy should be carefully considered in patients with a history of previous or current malignancy. There are no long-term data available for abrocitinib and upadacitinib but the incidence of cancer for patients on baricitinib for rheumatoid arthritis was 0.9/100 patient-years (excluding non-melanoma skin cancer).

Haematological abnormalities

Janus kinase inhibitors should not be commenced if platelets are $<150 \times 10^3/mm^3$, lymphocyte count $<.5 \times 10^3/mm^3$, neutrophil count $<1 \times 10^3/mm^3$ and haemoglobin <8 g/dL.

Renal impairment

A dose reduction is required for those with a creatinine clearance of 30–60 mL/min and treatment is contraindicated in those with a creatinine clearance of <30 mL/min.

Table 19.2 Dosage for Janus kinase inhibitors.

Drug	Lower dose	Upper dose
Abrocitinib	100 mg (50 mg available)	200 mg
Baricitinib	2 mg	4 mg
Upadacitinib	15 mg	30 mg

Hepatic impairment

No dose reduction is required with mild to moderate hepatic impairment, and treatment is not recommended with severe hepatic impairment.

Age

A greater proportion of older people (>65 years) in trials discontinued therapy, experienced serious adverse events, developed haematological abnormalities or experienced HSV/VZV. Lower-dose therapy is recommended for older people.

Pre-treatment screening

As JAKi have significant immunosuppressant activity, pre-treatment screening should incorporate all the aspects of Box 19.1. Check the FBC, including white cell differential, kidney function, liver function and lipids, and screen for latent tuberculosis, hepatitis B and C and HIV.

Dose and regimens

The doses for abrocitinib, baricitinib and upadacitinib are 100–200 mg once daily, 2–4 mg once daily or 15–30 mg once daily, respectively (Table 19.2). The lower dose is recommended for those with a creatinine clearance between 30 and 60 mL/min (treatment is not recommended for those with a creatinine clearance of <30 mL/min) and for the elderly (>65 years).

Monitoring

Only abrocitinib and baricitinib require blood monitoring as per licence; abrocitinib requires 4-week blood counts and lipids, and baricitinib requires 12-week lipids. While these requirements were derived from trial data (thromobocytopenia on abrocitinib and lipid derangement on abrocitinib and baricitinib), given the potential side effects of all three agents, one might consider monitoring a blood count and then renal and hepatic function at 4 weeks, 4 months and then 4–6 monthly thereafter on all of them.

Methotrexate

Methotrexate is an antimetabolite that has been used as a chemotherapeutic agent since the early 1950s. It also has immunosuppressive and anti-inflammatory effects and is used therapeutically in a variety of rheumatological, gastrointestinal, neurological and dermatological inflammatory disorders. It has been used as an abortifacient.

Dermatological uses (Chapters 35, 41, 42, 49, 50, 52, 53, 54, 55, 95, 100 and 139)

In the UK, MTX is licensed for and effective in the treatment of severe psoriasis. Off-label MTX is used (often as a steroid-sparing measure) to treat multiple inflammatory dermatoses, including:

- Atopic dermatitis.
- Connective tissue diseases (dermatomyositis, lupus erythematosus and scleroderma).
- Vasculitides.
- Immunobullous disorders (pemphigus, bullous pemphigoid, cicatricial pemphigoid and epidermolysis bullosa acquisita).
- Neutrophilic dermatoses (pyoderma gangrenosum and Sweet syndrome).
- Lymphoproliferative cutaneous disorders (lymphomatoid papulosis, mycosis fungoides and Sézary syndrome).
- Miscellaneous other inflammatory dermatoses (such as sarcoidosis, cutaneous Crohn disease, chronic spontaneous urticaria, pityriasis lichenoides and pityriasis rubra pilaris) [1].

Pharmacological properties
Formula and structure
Methotrexate (empirical formula: $C_{20}H_{22}N_8O_5$; systematic name: (2S)-2-[(4-{[(2,4-diaminopteridin-6-yl)methyl](methyl)amino}benzoyl) amino]pentanedioic acid, abbreviated to 4-amino-N^{10}-methyl folic acid) is a weak organic acid with a very similar structure to folic acid (pteroylglutamic acid).

Administration
In dermatological usage, MTX is usually taken orally in weekly (not daily) doses. Prescribing 2.5 mg tablets (only) is strongly encouraged to avoid confusion with the also available 10 mg tablets. It can also be administered by subcutaneous or intramuscular routes. Intravenous administration is only for oncology indicatations (i.e. not in skin disease).

Pharmacokinetics
MTX is absorbed from the gastrointestinal tract rapidly and efficiently, actively transported by a carrier-mediated uptake system, reduced folate carrier 1 (RFC1). RFC1 is a saturable protein transporter and therefore the bioavailability of oral MTX (which demonstrates considerable interindividual variation) declines with higher doses [2]. Bioavailability can be improved with parenteral administration.

MTX is widely distributed in body tissues, although penetration of the blood–brain barrier is poor. In the circulation it is approximately 50% protein bound and, if displaced from protein by other drugs (such as aspirin, NSAIDs or sulphonamides), the increase in the level of active (non-bound) MTX will increase the risk of significant side effects, such as pancytopenia. Furthermore, alterations in circulating albumin levels (e.g. as the result of severe liver or kidney disease) may necessitate an adjustment of dosage.

MTX is actively transported into cells by RFC1. Contrary to the historical perception that it is not metabolised to a significant degree, approximately 10% of MTX is converted to 7-hydroxymethotrexate in the liver and in all cells a proportion of MTX and 7-hydroxymethotrexate is transformed by γ-glutamyl hydrolase to pharmacologically active polyglutamate derivatives [2]; this process may delay cellular clearance and contribute to MTX toxicity [3].

MTX and 7-hydroxymethotrexate are excreted mainly through the kidneys via glomerular filtration and active transport, although a small proportion is excreted into the bile. If renal function is compromised, a reduced dosage may be necessary to prevent accumulation and minimise adverse effects. Other weak acids, such as salicylates, probenecid and sulphonamides, may interact with MTX at this level.

The serum half-life of MTX is approximately 6–8 h and the drug is undetectable in the serum after 24 h, although intracellular accumulation is of long duration.

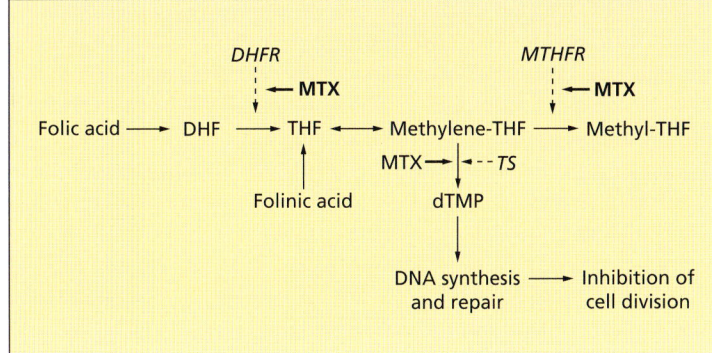

Figure 19.4 Methotrexate interaction with the folate metabolic pathway (see text for abbreviations).

Pharmacodynamics
The mechanisms of action of MTX are complex. It inhibits a number of key enzyme systems. By virtue of it being a structural analogue of folic acid, MTX blocks the metabolism of folic acid through competitive inhibition of dihydrofolate reductase (DHFR), which catalyses the conversion of DHF to tetrahydrofolate (THF), a single-carbon transfer source essential to the generation of purine and pyrimidine nucleotides and therefore for nucleic acid and protein synthesis (Figure 19.4). It also inhibits thymidylate synthase (TS), which converts deoxyuridine monophosphate by methylation to the nucleotide thymidine monophosphate (dTMP), which is essential for normal DNA replication. Additionally, MTX inhibits the enzyme methylenetetrahydrofolate reductase (MTHFR), reducing the conversion of methylenetetrahydrofolate (methylene-THF) to methyltetrahydrofolate (methyl-THF), which is the methyl donor for the recycling of homocysteine to methionine. By inhibiting this recycling, MTX may prevent the accumulation of polyamines that contribute to inflammatory injury [4]. MTX also inhibits the enzyme 5-aminoimidazole-4-carboxamide ribonucleotide (AICAR) transformylase (ATIC), which plays important roles in *de novo* purine metabolism (by catalysing the reversible conversion of 10-formyl THF to THF) and inflammatory regulation.

While the suppression of transmethylation reactions and the reduction of purine and pyrimidine synthesis by the inhibition of folate-dependent enzymes may play important roles in the antiproliferative and immunosuppressive properties of MTX, particularly in relation to lymphocytes which are dependent on *de novo* synthesis of nucleotides, there is a growing body of evidence supporting adenosine as a key mediator of the anti-inflammatory action of MTX through the potent inhibition of ATIC [5]. Inhibition of ATIC by MTX and hydroxymethotrexate results in an intracellular accumulation of AICAR which inhibits adenosine monophosphate (AMP) deaminase. This in turn causes the release of intracellular adenine nucleotides into the extracellular space, where they are dephosphorylated to adenosine, an endogenous purine nucleoside and an important signalling molecule mediating cytokine secretion and expression of adhesion molecules in immunologically competent cells. In the peripheral circulation and in inflammatory exudates, adenosine binds to specific cell surface receptors (belonging to the family of G-protein-coupled receptors), where it modulates a wide variety of physiological functions: these include the regulation of acute and chronic inflammatory processes [5]. *In vitro* and *in vivo* models also demonstrate MTX modulating JAK/STAT, NFκB and p38 MAPK intrasignalling pathways (recently comprehensively detailed in [6]).

Pharmacogenetics
There are multiple functionally relevant polymorphisms in genes relevant to MTX pharmacology which might be expected to contribute to the observed interindividual variation in MTX effectiveness and safety. Many, including those encoding elements of the folate metabolic pathway including *MTHR*, *SLC19A1*, *SLCO1B1*, *ABCB1* and *ABCC2*, have been very extensively investigated but studies are small and/or conflicting. To date none of the pharmacogenomic variants associated with safety or effectiveness has been validated for clinical use [7].

Potential adverse effects
Myelotoxicity
Most cases of dose-dependent MTX-induced bone marrow suppression occur during the first 2 months of treatment, although this can occur at any time during therapy and may result in pancytopenia or any combination of anaemia, leukopenia or thrombocytopenia, with potentially lethal consequences. Folate supplementation provides some protection. Particular risk factors include poor kidney function, older age, displacement of MTX from protein-binding sites (particularly by NSAIDs or sulphonamides) and hypoalbuminaemia. Inadvertent daily (rather than weekly) MTX dosing greatly increases the risk of pancytopenia. Should significant myelosuppression occur during MTX therapy, prompt folinic acid rescue should be considered [1,5].

Hepatotoxicity
Methotrexate may be associated with an acute transaminitis or, in the long term, liver fibrosis [8]. Co-morbidities, such as obesity, diabetes, high alcohol intake and previous hepatic problems, may be significant aggravating or confounding factors. The extent to which MTX is causally related to the liver fibrosis reported in many (predominantly psoriasis) cohorts has been unclear, given that other drivers to liver fibrosis, particularly fatty liver disease and metabolic syndrome, are also prevalent in these populations [9]. However, a (secondary) analysis of a large randomised controlled trial (RCT) in a population with known cardiovascular disease and diabetes or metabolic syndrome suggests that MTX itself confers risk of fibrosis [10].

Gastrointestinal toxicity
Methotrexate commonly causes nausea and anorexia: vomiting, diarrhoea and stomatitis are occasionally encountered. Folate supplementation and/or administration of MTX parenterally can reduce gastrointestinal side effects.

Nephrotoxicity
Although high-dose MTX as used in the treatment of malignant conditions may cause renal damage from precipitation in the renal tubules, this is an unlikely consequence of low-dose therapy.

Reproductive toxicity
Methotrexate is teratogenic and an abortifacient. MTX has also been reported to cause oligospermia, menstrual dysfunction and amenorrhoea in humans, during and for a short period after cessation of therapy, and to cause impaired fertility, affecting spermatogenesis and oogenesis during the period of its administration – effects that appear to be reversible on discontinuing therapy. It is thus crucial that women avoid MTX during conception and pregnancy. Recent data on pregnancy outcomes following paternal MTX exposure within 3 months of conception are nevertheless reassuring [11,12], with no increase in congenital abnormalities, preterm birth and small for gestational age, or (in the longer term) no increase in autism, schizophrenia or attention deficit disorder. Updated guidance from the EMA nevertheless recommends both men and women avoid MTX for 6 months before conception, as well as throughout pregnancy. It is excreted in breast milk and should thus be avoided by breastfeeding women [13].

Pulmonary toxicity
Methotrexate-induced pulmonary toxicity, although well recognised in rheumatoid arthritis, is uncommon in psoriatic patients. However, pneumonitis or pulmonary fibrosis can occur with low doses of MTX and is a serious, unpredictable and potentially fatal adverse reaction. It may develop shortly after initiating MTX [14,15] or after many years [16]. The development of cough and dyspnoea should prompt immediate cessation of MTX and appropriate investigation and treatment.

Malignancy
Lymphoma, and other lymphoproliferative disorders, in some cases associated with Epstein–Barr virus, have been reported in patients on MTX. MTX may also be associated with an increased risk of keratinocyte cancer [17]. As with immunosuppressants more generally, risks are likely to relate to MTX duration and dose as well as the context in which it is being used.

Other side effects
Other adverse effects of MTX include fatigue, headaches, dizziness, alopecia, phototoxicity, 'recall' reactions at sites of sunburn or radiotherapy, anaphylaxis, acral redness, vasculitis and cutaneous ulceration [1].

Contraindications
MTX is contraindicated in the treatment of pregnant or breastfeeding women and if there is known MTX hypersensitivity. Significant impairment of hepatic and renal function, pre-existing blood dyscrasias, immunodeficiency and latent infection (such as tuberculosis, viral hepatitis B and C) are relative contraindications, as are excess alcohol consumption and concern regarding the reliability of the patient to conform to necessary monitoring procedures [1].

Cautions
Where, as in the UK, there are two strengths of tablet (2.5 and 10 mg) available, confusion regarding dosage can easily occur. It is recommended that only one strength, usually 2.5 mg, is prescribed.

Drug–drug interactions
See Box 19.6.

> ### Box 19.6 Methotrexate: drug–drug interactions
>
> The interaction of methotrexate (MTX) with other drugs can occur via a number of mechanisms:
> - Reduced absorption from gut: digoxin (absorption reduced by MTX), neomycin
> - Displacement from plasma proteins: non-steroidal anti-inflammatory drugs (NSAIDs) (aspirin, diclofenac, ibuprofen, indometacin, ketoprofen, meloxicam, naproxen), sulphonamides
> - Added antifolate effect: nitrous oxide, trimethoprim, sulphonamides, dapsone, phenytoin, pyrimethamine
> - Diminished renal excretion: ciprofloxacin, NSAIDs, omeprazole, penicillins, probenecid, sulphonamides
> - Increased renal excretion: acetazolamide
> - Cumulative toxicity: tetracyclines, acitretin, clozapine, ciclosporin, cisplatin, leflunomide, alcohol
> - Other: theophylline (plasma levels increased by MTX)

Folate supplementation
Low-dose MTX is generally well tolerated. However, a number of toxic adverse reactions that appear to result from the inhibitory effect of MTX on purine and pyrimidine synthesis, such as myelotoxicity, hepatotoxicity and stomatitis, may limit its long-term use. Folate supplementation, which has as its rationale that folic acid competes with MTX for DHFR, has been shown in a number of principally rheumatological studies to reduce the adverse reactions to MTX, particularly those related to the gastrointestinal tract, liver and bone marrow, thus enabling MTX to be better tolerated without impairing its clinical efficacy [4,18]. Two recent dermatological studies, however, have suggested a detrimental effect of folate supplementation on MTX efficacy [19,20] and so the issue remains contentious. However, the balance of evidence favours supplementation [18], although the optimal dosage regimen remains uncertain.

Folinic acid (leucovorin, N^5-formyl-THF) is as effective as folic acid in reducing MTX toxicity [18]. By direct conversion to THF it bypasses the step catalysed by DHFR, thus allowing some purine and pyrimidine synthesis despite DHFR inhibition by MTX. Additionally, folinic acid competes with MTX for RFC1 intracellular transportation. Folinic acid is particularly useful in the 'rescue' of bone marrow and gastrointestinal cells from MTX toxicity and acute MTX overdose. To avoid impairing intracellular uptake of MTX, folinic acid should not be taken within 12 h of the weekly MTX dose.

Furthermore, both folic acid and folinic acid reduce plasma homocysteine levels during MTX therapy and therefore theoretically may benefit those patients at risk of cardiovascular disease [18].

Pre-treatment screening
Potential recipients of MTX should be counselled about the risks of immunosuppressive therapy, provided with written details of the medication and warned about drug–drug interactions. Prior to commencing MTX, screening as outlined in Box 19.1 should be undertaken.

Pregnancy should be excluded before initiating treatment and contraception (ideally employing two methods) carefully discussed. A pre-treatment chest X-ray is probably not necessary unless the patient is at increased risk of tuberculosis, as in some ethnic communities or immigrants from countries with a high prevalence of tuberculosis.

Dose and regimens
For the treatment of dermatological conditions, the administration of MTX once weekly is standard practice. While splitting the dose over the week (e.g. twice or three times weekly) to improve tolerability has been historically advocated, recently updated EMA guidance strongly recommends against this, given the risks of dosing error and toxicity. MTX is now widely available in a self-administered subcutaneous formulation, and this can be useful where bioavailability is poor or where gastrointestinal side effects are a problem.

For most individuals, MTX can be initiated at 10 or 15 mg weekly. Individuals at greater risk of MTX toxicity (e.g. older people, those with renal impairment or underlying bone marrow disease) or where there is concern about potential tolerability issues, a lower starting dose may be prudent. Common practice involves checking an FBC and liver function tests 1 week later, and then an FBC weekly until the dose (and monitoring results) have stabilised. The dose can be gradually increased by 2.5–5 mg/week until there is a satisfactory response without significant toxicity. Ordinarily, the dose should not exceed 25 mg weekly and, in view of the reduced bioavailability of oral MTX at higher doses, consideration should be given to switching to a subcutaneous route of administration if response remains poor. Once an optimal response has been achieved, the dose of MTX can be tapered by 2.5 mg each week to determine the lowest dose necessary to maintain clinical benefit.

It is also standard practice to administer oral folic acid, an example regimen being 5 mg once weekly, usually on the day following MTX, although the timing is not crucial [21].

Oral folinic acid, three doses of 5 mg at 12 h intervals commencing 24 h after the weekly MTX dose, should be considered if folic acid is not improving gastrointestinal symptoms or correcting abnormalities of the liver enzymes or macrocytosis.

Monitoring
Close monitoring is required until MTX dosage has been stabilised, particularly for elderly patients and those with renal impairment. Initially, the FBC, liver function tests and creatinine should be checked every 1–2 weeks for 4–8 weeks following the last dose escalation; thereafter the frequency of blood tests can be gradually reduced to 2–3 monthly. Deterioration in blood parameters or an intercurrent illness requires resumption of closer monitoring and consideration of dose reduction. Macrocytic red blood cell indices are common during MTX therapy.

During the early months of treatment, the opportunity should be taken at clinic attendances to reinforce warnings regarding symptoms of bone marrow suppression (bruising, sore throat, mouth ulcers), the importance of contraception and the avoidance of drugs that might interact with MTX.

The development of abnormal liver function tests can be a sign of MTX damage, but liver enzyme levels may be normal despite the presence of significant hepatic fibrosis. Elevation of liver transaminases to double the upper limit of the normal range necessitates discontinuation or dose reduction of MTX. Routine liver biopsy for the histological assessment of hepatic structure was for many years considered an integral part of MTX usage to identify liver fibrosis but is no longer justified given the attendant risks of the procedure and the low absolute risk of significant fibrosis. Recent advances in non-invasive assessment for liver fibrosis (whatever the cause) include scoring systems combining clinical and conventional laboratory parameters for use as screening tools, direct serum biomarkers of fibrogenesis and tissue elastography using both ultrasound (FibroScan®) and magnetic resonance (reviewed in [22]). These can be useful adjuncts to monitoring for MTX-associated liver fibrosis, and selection of those needing onward referral for consideration of liver biopsy, ideally in close collaboration with hepatology colleagues.

Mycophenolate mofetil

Mycophenolate mofetil (MMF) is a potent immunosuppressant prodrug of mycophenolic acid (MPA), used primarily to prevent solid-organ graft rejection, but it is used off-label in the treatment of a variety of immunologically mediated dermatological conditions as a single agent or as a steroid-sparing drug.

Dermatological uses

Mycophenolate mofetil has a predictably beneficial effect in the treatment of immunobullous disorders (in particular pemphigus and pemphigoid), and a less consistent effect in psoriasis, atopic eczema, connective tissue disorders and vasculitides [1,2,3,4].

Pharmacological properties
Formula and structure
Mycophenolate mofetil (empirical formula: $C_{23}H_{31}NO_7$; systematic name: 2- morpholinoethyl (E)-6-(1,3-dihydro-4-hydroxy-6-methoxy-7-methyl-3-oxo-5-isobenzofuranyl)-4-methyl-4-hexenoate) is the 2-morpholinoethyl ester of MPA.

Administration
When given for dermatological reasons, MMF is usually administered orally, although there is an intravenous preparation. An enteric-coated form of MPA is also available (720 mg of enteric-coated MPA is therapeutically equivalent to 1000 mg of MMF).

Pharmacokinetics [1,5]
Mycophenolate mofetil is absorbed efficiently and completely from the gastrointestinal tract and is rapidly converted to its active metabolite, MPA, which is 97% bound to plasma albumin. The half-life of MPA is approximately 16 h. The peak plasma level occurs at about 1 h, followed by a second peak at 6–12 h that is the result of enterohepatic recirculation.

MPA is metabolised predominantly in the liver by uridine diphosphate glucuronosyl transferase to its phenolic glucuronide (MPAG), which is pharmacologically inactive but which can be converted back to MPA by β-glucuronidase, especially in the epidermis and gastrointestinal tract.

Biliary excretion of MPA/MPAG involves several transporters including organic anion transporting polypeptides and multidrug-resistant protein 2 (MRP-2). More than 90% of the administered dose of MMF is excreted in the urine, mainly as MPAG (and involving, at least in part, MRP-2), with the remainder eliminated in the faeces.

The pharmacokinetics of MPA are complex and there is substantial intersubject variation [6].

Pharmacodynamics
Like AZA, the mechanism underlying the immunosuppressive action of MMF involves purine biosynthesis. Purine nucleotides are either formed by a complex *de novo* pathway or are recycled by a salvage pathway (in which bases and nucleosides released in the breakdown of nucleic acids are recovered and converted back into nucleotides).

Adenine and guanine, the purine nucleobases, are both derived from the nucleotide inosine-5′-monophosphate (IMP), which is the first compound in the *de novo* pathway of purine synthesis to have a completely formed purine ring. MPA interferes with this process by inhibiting the action of IMP dehydrogenase (IMPDH) in catalysing the conversion of IMP to xanthine monophosphate, the rate-limiting step to the *de novo* formation of guanine nucleotides (guanosine mono-, di- and triphosphates), which have important roles in a variety of biological processes including the synthesis of DNA and RNA.

This effect of MMF is specifically targeted towards T and B lymphocytes as, in contrast to other nucleated cells, they lack the ability to produce purines via a salvage mechanism and are thus critically dependent for their DNA/RNA synthesis, growth and proliferation on the *de novo* synthesis of purines. Interruption of the *de novo* pathway by MMF therefore results in a relatively selective immunosuppressive effect on lymphocytes which, among other immunological effects, includes the suppression of cell-mediated immune responses and the inhibition of antibody production by activated lymphocytes.

Additionally, humans have two *IMPDH* genes, encoding hIMPDH1 and hIMPDH2 isoenzymes, which have similar structural and kinetic properties [7]. MPA has a fivefold greater inhibitory effect on the type 2 isoform of IMPDH, which is expressed in activated lymphocytes, than the type 1 isoform, which is expressed preferentially in other cell types, thereby exerting a more potent cytostatic effect on lymphocytes than other cell types [8].

Furthermore, several other factors may contribute to the anti-inflammatory effects of MPA. MPA can induce apoptosis of activated T lymphocytes; it can inhibit the presentation of antigen to T lymphocytes by dendritic cells; by depleting guanosine nucleotides, it can suppress glycosylation and the expression of certain adhesion molecules, thereby decreasing lymphocyte and monocyte recruitment in sites of inflammation; and also, by depleting guanosine nucleotides, MPA depletes tetrahydrobiopterin, thus suppressing the production of nitric oxide by the inducible form of nitric oxide synthase and consequent tissue damage mediated by peroxynitrite [8–11].

Clinical response to MMF is slow and typically takes 6–8 weeks [1].

Potential adverse effects
Gastrointestinal toxicity
The most common side effects of MMF are gastrointestinal and dose dependent [2]. Nausea, vomiting, abdominal pain, diarrhoea and constipation occur in up to 20% of patients [2]. These are usually mild and tend to improve with time. Administration with food and the use of enteric-coated MPA may help to ameliorate these adverse effects [1]. MMF is not considered to be hepatotoxic [1]. Gastrointestinal ulceration and cytomegalovirus-associated colitis may rarely occur [1].

Haematological toxicity
Anaemia, neutropenia and thrombocytopenia are not uncommon, and are usually mild, dose related and reversible with discontinuation of therapy or dose reduction [2]. MMF has also been associated with pseudo-Pelger–Huët anomaly, a form of neutrophil dysplasia in which the nuclei tend to be bilobed rather than hypersegmented [13].

Infections
Mycophenolate mofetil, by dampening the normal immune response, appears to increase susceptibility to opportunistic infections, particularly in organ transplant recipients and specifically to cytomegalovirus and BK virus [14], although other herpesvirus infections (varicella-zoster and herpes simplex), bacterial sepsis, atypical mycobacterial and fungal infections have been reported in the dermatological literature [1]. Systemic immunosuppression carries with it the risk of reactivation of other latent virus infections, such as hepatitis B, hepatitis C and JC virus (associated with progressive multifocal leukoencephalopathy), as well as reactivation of dormant tuberculosis [1]. Conversely, MMF has antimicrobial activity *against* certain pathogens, including hepatitis C, HIV and *Pneumocystis jirovecii* [14]. Mucocutaneous candidosis, urinary tract infections and pneumonia are commonly associated with MMF therapy [5].

Carcinogenicity
The magnitude of the potential for MMF specifically to cause lymphoproliferative malignancy is uncertain, and much of the available evidence relates to the transplant population receiving combinations of immunosuppressive agents [5]. However, the development of Epstein–Barr virus-related B-cell lymphoma involving the central nervous system has been recorded with MMF used to treat autoimmune conditions [1,15].

There is no clear evidence base for an association between MMF and non-melanoma cutaneous malignancy [1], but it would appear prudent to offer sun protection advice [5].

Teratogenicity
Mycophenolate mofetil appears to be teratogenic when given in early pregnancy, being particularly associated with early miscarriage and with cranio-facial and cardiac malformations [16–19]. Appropriate measures should be taken to minimise the risk of pregnancy in women of child-bearing potential [20]. There is limited clinical evidence relating to paternal exposure so men are advised to use reliable contraception while on treatment and for 3 months post-cessation [21].

Other side effects
Genito-urinary symptoms, including frequency, dysuria, urgency, haematuria and sterile pyuria, may occur during the first year of treatment [2]. Tremor, dizziness, anxiety, depression, confusional states, dysgeusia, headache, electrolyte abnormalities, hypercholesterolaemia, rashes (urticaria, hand dermatitis, alopecia), hypo- and hypertension, dyspnoea, cough, interstitial lung disease, pulmonary fibrosis, arthralgia and pyrexia are also recorded [5].

Drug–drug interactions
See Box 19.7.

> **Box 19.7 Mycophenolate mofetil: drug–drug interactions**
>
> - Antacids and proton pump inhibitors reduce absorption of mycophenolate mofetil (MMF)
> - Iron and calcium supplementation reduces the absorption of MMF [1]
> - Antibiotics: certain antibiotics, including metronidazole, cephalosporins, penicillins, sulphonamides and macrolides, may reduce serum levels of mycophenolic acid (MPA) by a reduction in enterohepatic circulation [1]
> - Lipid-regulating drugs: cholestyramine also reduces enterohepatic circulation of MPA, and therefore the efficacy of MMF
> - Antivirals: the serum levels of aciclovir and ganciclovir are increased by MMF
> - Salicylates, phenytoin and xanthine bronchodilators may increase the free fraction of circulating MPA by displacement from plasma-binding proteins
> - Probenecid may increase the serum levels of MPA by interfering with its renal tubular secretion

Contraindications
Mycophenolate mofetil is contraindicated in pregnancy, breastfeeding women and in those with a history of hypersensitivity to it [5].

Cautions
Mycophenolate mofetil should be used with caution in patients with active gastrointestinal disease, and live attenuated vaccines should be avoided.

Pre-treatment screening
Before commencing treatment with MMF, the items listed in Box 19.1 should be addressed. MMF is teratogenic so prescribing clinicians must ensure women are adequately counselled on this risk, alongside access to relevant pregnancy prevention strategies. Pregnancy testing is advised prior to and 1 week after treatment initiation. Although there is no evidence to date of malformations or miscarriage following paternal conception, nevertheless, in line with the licence, men should be advised to avoid conception during and for 3 months after stopping MMF.

Dose and regimens
Twice-daily dosing is recommended, and a reasonable starting dose for dermatological indications is 250 mg twice daily for the first week, then 500 mg twice daily, increasing thereafter if tolerated by 500 mg daily or twice daily every 4 weeks until a maximum of 1.5 g twice daily is reached. Dosage should be tailored to individual tolerance and response. Patents should be reminded that the clinical response is slow.

Monitoring
The FBC should be monitored regularly during initiation, for example checked weekly for the first month, then fortnightly for 2 months [22]. This can then be monitored less frequently (e.g. every 3 months) once established on therapy. Electrolytes, creatinine and liver function tests should be monitored every 2–4 weeks following dose escalation, then every 2–3 months [1].

Potassium iodide
Medicinally, potassium iodide is used principally as an emergency treatment for hyperthyroidism, and for thyroid protection during treatment with radiopharmaceuticals and following exposure to nuclear radiation.

Dermatological uses (Chapters 32, 47, 48 and 97)
Potassium iodide is a traditional and inexpensive off-label option advocated historically in a variety of cutaneous disorders, including cutaneous sporotrichosis, erythema nodosum, subacute nodular migratory panniculitis, nodular vasculitis, Sweet syndrome, Behçet syndrome, pyoderma gangrenosum and erythema multiforme [1,2,3]. With the advent of newer therapies, the use of potassium iodide has substantially reduced or stopped.

Pharmacological properties
Formula and structure
Potassium iodide is an inorganic ionic compound, with chemical formula K^+I^-.

Administration
Potassium iodide can be given as drops of a saturated solution of potassium iodide, but in the management of dermatological conditions it is most conveniently given in tablet form.

Pharmacokinetics
Potassium iodide is well absorbed orally, and is distributed to the thyroid and, to a lesser extent, to the salivary glands, breasts, choroid plexus and gastric mucosa [2]. It crosses the placenta and is found in breast milk [2]. It is excreted predominantly in urine, with small amounts excreted in sweat and faeces [2].

Pharmacodynamics
The mechanism by which potassium iodide exerts its anti-inflammatory effects is unknown, although there is evidence that it has a detrimental effect on neutrophil chemotaxis and the generation by neutrophils of pro-inflammatory oxygen intermediates [1,2,3].

Potential adverse effects
Wolff–Chaikoff effect
Potassium iodide can induce the Wolff–Chaikoff effect, which is the inhibition of organic binding of iodide in the normal thyroid gland by excess iodide. This is a protective mechanism, blocking thyroid hormone synthesis, and predisposing to temporary hypothyroidism [4,5]. Resolution usually occurs within several weeks, although thyroid replacement therapy may need to be considered [1].

Jod–Basedow phenomenon
There is a risk that the therapeutic administration of potassium iodide to a person with thyroid dysfunction lacking pituitary control, such as Graves disease or a multinodular goitre, may cause a significant exacerbation of hyperthyroidism [2,5].

Potassium toxicity
Rarely, potassium iodide may cause symptoms of hyperkalaemia, including fatigue, confusion, palpitations, muscle weakness and numbness and tingling of the extremities.

Other adverse effects (iodism)
- Sialadenitis (in particular parotid and submaxillary glands).
- Hypersalivation.
- Metallic taste, halitosis, burning sensation in the mouth.
- Coryzal symptoms, headache.
- Gastric irritation, diarrhoea, nausea.
- Urticaria/angioedema, acneform pustulation, iododerma.

Contraindications
Potassium iodide is contraindicated in pregnancy and if there is known hypersensitivity to iodine. It has been associated with fetal malformations [6] and may cause hypothyroidism in the fetus [1].

Cautions
Potassium iodide should be used with caution in patients with thyroid and cardiac disorders, with conditions associated with hyperkalaemia, or with active tuberculosis [3]. It may exacerbate dermatitis herpetiformis, pustular psoriasis [1] and hypocomplementaemic vasculitis [3].

Drug–drug interactions
Potassium iodide may interact with antithyroid drugs, lithium, amiodarone and sulphonamides to cause hypothyroidism, and with potassium-sparing diuretics and angiotensin-converting enzyme inhibitors to cause hyperkalaemia [2].

Pre-treatment screening
Specific enquiries should be made regarding a history of thyroid disease and the use of medications that might interfere with thyroid function. Suspicion of thyroid disease should prompt the checking of thyroid function (T_4, thyroid-stimulating hormone (TSH) and circulating thyroid antibody). A baseline check of electrolyte and urea levels should be undertaken.

Dose and regimens
For dermatological conditions, a reasonable initial dose is 300 mg daily, increasing to 900 mg daily depending on disease activity and tolerability.

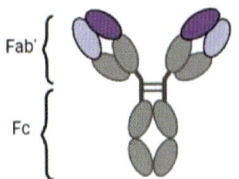 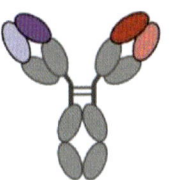 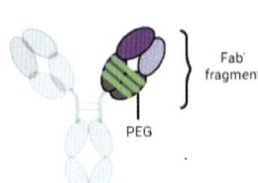 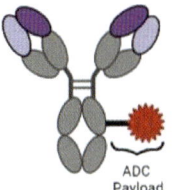 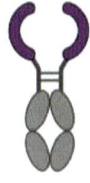

Monospecific (conventional) monoclonal Ab. Both fragment antigen-binding (Fab') domains recognise the same antigen (e.g. adalimumab targeting tumour necrosis factor)

Bispecific monoclonal Ab with two different fragment antigen-binding domains (e.g. mosunetuzumab)

Fragment antigen-binding domain conjugated with polyethylene glycol (PEGylation) to delay systemic elimination (e.g. certolizumab)

ADC. Monoclonal Ab tethered to a cytotoxic drug (ADC payload) (e.g. brentuximab vedotin)

Fusion protein. Fc fragment fused to receptor (e.g. etanercept)

Figure 19.5 Example structures of therapeutic proteins (biologics). Developments in bioengineering have enabled the production of therapeutic proteins with divergent structures and enhanced function. To date, bispecific antibodies (Abs) and antibody–drug conjugates (ADCs) are predominantly in development or licensed for use in cancer. Created with BioRender.com.

Monitoring

The TSH level should be checked 1 month after initiation of therapy to exclude iodide-induced hypothyroidism [2] and, if abnormal, it would be prudent to monitor thyroid function thereafter. It is reasonable to monitor potassium levels.

Biologic therapies (protein therapeutics)

Biologic therapy (also known as protein therapeutics) is a term that encompasses, in its broadest sense, a group of pharmacologically active protein (or peptide)-based molecules produced by living organisms that are designed to alleviate disease by inhibiting or imitating the actions of naturally occurring proteins in the body. Insulin could be considered the very first 'biologic' therapy, purified from bovine and porcine pancreas in 1922 to treat diabetes, while pooled intravenous immunoglobulins (IVIgs), introduced in the 1980s, remain an important intervention for a number of dermatological diseases. However, the advent of recombinant DNA technology, which allows the large-scale production of recombinant proteins with highly specific structure and function, together with a better understanding of the complex role of endogenous proteins in health and disease (including enzymes, receptors, membrane channels and molecule 'transporters'), has led to an exponential increase in drug development in the field of biologic therapy. Biologic therapies include those that are identical to an endogenous protein and function either to replenish or to enhance an endogenous supply (e.g. interferons, pooled immunoglobulins; and those proteins that target a specific pathway) or those that use the specificity of the antigen-recognition site of immunoglobulins or the receptor-binding domains of native protein ligands to guide the immune system to destroy the relevant molecule or cell.

Monoclonal antibodies (mAbs) are the largest class of biologic products in clinical use. They comprise a large variety of different structures, from small fragments to intact, modified or unmodified immunoglobulins, all of which contain an antigen-binding domain (Figure 19.5). Until recently, all mAb-based drugs were recognised by the suffix -mab, preceded by a source infix such as -xi- (chimeric), -zu- (humanised) or -u- (human) designating the species from which the antibody was derived. In 2021, the World Health Organization (WHO) International Nonproprietary Names (INN) Programme issued a revised naming system to better reflect the diversity of therapeutic antibodies and to provide capacity to meet the demand for distinct names (Table 19.3). In this new scheme, as before, the naming system infers both the structure and function. This comprises (i) a prefix, which is random, and is only required to give the molecule a distinctive name; (ii) an infix, which indicates the proposed mode of action/target (e.g. -ki cytokine or cytokine receptor; -ta tumour); and (iii) a suffix, groups 1–4, depending on the structure. Immunoglobulin fusions are only included in the mAb nomenclature scheme if both domains have immunoglobulin-derived variable domains (e.g. mAb fused with a cytokine is under the -fusp nomenclature scheme). The stem -mab has been dropped and four new groups have been assigned to mAb with a variable domain. Already licensed agents will retain their original name.

This therapeutic field confers many potential advantages over small-molecule pharmacology. A high degree of functional specificity and extracellular binding should result in fewer 'off-target' actions compared with small molecules, which often have direct intracellular effects with consequent hepatotoxicity and other toxic effects. However, this does not necessarily translate to safer drugs, since the complexities of biological systems are such that interruption of a particular pathway may nevertheless result in undesired pharmacodynamic effects. Reactivation of latent tuberculosis with TNF antagonist therapy for psoriasis is one such example, as was the catastrophic trial of the CD28 agonist which invoked a 'cytokine storm' in the six volunteers involved [1]. Further disadvantages include the fact that, since these drugs are proteins, all those currently available for dermatological conditions (and, at present, also for the majority of other indications) have to be given parenterally, and also that immunogenicity remains a significant problem, even

Table 19.3 World Health Organization International Nonproprietary Names scheme for all substances that contain an immunoglobulin variable domain.[a]

	Group 1	Group 2	Group 3	Group 4
Suffix	-tug unmodified immunoglobulin	-bart antibody artificial	-mig multi-immunoglobulin	-ment fragment
Structure	Monospecific full length and Fc unmodified immunoglobulins of any class. Molecules which might occur as such in the immune system	Monospecific full length immunoglobulins with engineered constant domains (CH1/2/3)	Bi- and multispecific immunoglobulins regardless of the format, type or shape (full length, full length plus, fragments)	All monospecific domains, fragments of any kind, derived from an immunoglobulin variable domain (all monospecific constructs that do not contain an Fc domain)

[a] Antibody–drug conjugates (ADCs) also follow this new monoclonal antibody (mAb) nomenclature scheme.

in the context of 'fully human' monoclonal antibodies such as adalimumab.

The number of biologic therapies available for use is rapidly increasing and the disease indications are constantly changing; drug acquisition costs are high, and so use is generally limited to severe recalcitrant disease. Access may however improve with the recent introduction of 'biosimilars' (a biologic medicine that is similar to another biologic medicine that has already been authorised for use, without any meaningful differences in terms of quality, safety or efficacy). Treatment with biologic therapies should always be supervised by clinicians who are experienced in their use, and, because these are (generally) novel treatments, participation in long-term pharmacovigilance registries is actively encouraged. Brief detail is provided here on a number of biologic therapies with a focus on those agents that are licensed for use in skin disease; however, the list is not comprehensive and additional information is available in the relevant disease chapters.

Biologic therapies directed against cytokines

Cytokines are potent regulators of inflammation, and their neutralisation by antibodies or receptor antagonists can be an extremely effective therapeutic strategy as well as a major contributor to understanding the underlying disease pathogenesis.

Tumour necrosis factor antagonists

Tumour necrosis factor is a pro-inflammatory cytokine produced by a wide variety of cell types including keratinocytes. It plays a complex role in innate immunity and host defence, particularly against mycobacterial infection, and can both enhance and suppress adaptive immunity. Over the last 20 years, it has been shown to play a central role in the pathogenesis of a number of chronic inflammatory disease states, evidenced in large part by the striking clinical efficacy of TNF antagonists in disorders such as psoriasis, rheumatoid arthritis and Crohn disease. There are currently two types of biologic agents that target TNF: the first binds directly to TNF and is represented by the monoclonal antibodies adalimumab, certolizumab, golimumab and infliximab; the second, represented by the fusion protein etanercept, a soluble TNF receptor, competitively inhibits the binding of TNF to TNF receptors so inhibiting the biological activity of TNF.

Dermatological uses

Licensed indications (Chapters 35 and 90). Adalimumab, certolizumab, etanercept and infliximab have all been shown to be very effective in psoriasis in large-scale RCTs. These interventions now form a standard part of the treatment approach for severe psoriasis (and also psoriatic arthritis). Golimumab is only licensed for psoriatic arthritis. Adalimumab is also licensed for use in hidradenitis suppuritiva (infliximab is extensively used off-licence for this indication too).

Off-label uses (Chapters 47, 48, 90 and 96). TNF antagonists are used in a wide spectrum of inflammatory skin conditions, largely based on observational data and/or small trials. These include skin diseases associated with inflammatory bowel disease and rheumatoid arthritis where TNF antagonists are of proven efficacy. Examples include pyoderma gangrenosum, Sweet syndrome and Behçet disease. Severe treatment-resistant cutaneous sarcoidosis has also been reported to benefit from infliximab and adalimumab [2,3], whereas etanercept is of no benefit (and possibly harmful). Case reports of positive treatment responses to TNF antagonists (mainly infliximab) exist for an even wider spectrum of diseases [4], but require further study. Proper assessment of the risk–benefit ratio in all these 'off-label' indications is hampered by a lack of controlled trial data, poorly defined treatment outcomes and limited follow-up.

Pharmacological properties

Formula and structure. Infliximab is a chimeric human–murine mAB (c.25% mouse-derived protein), whereas golimumab and adalimumab are fully human IgG1 antibodies. Etanercept is a fusion protein composed of a dimer of the extracellular portions of human TNFR2 (p75) fused to the Fc domain of human IgG1. Certolizumab pegol is a humanised anti-TNF Fab' fragment conjugated to a polyethylene glycol that increases the half-life of the attached molecule.

Administration. All TNF antagonists are given parenterally and, with the exception of infliximab, can be self-administered subcutaneously (Table 19.4).

Pharmacokinetics. Following subcutaneous administration the drugs are slowly absorbed, probably predominantly via lymphatics, to reach peak plasma concentrations after 2–4 days. The disposition of TNF antagonists, as with other mAbs and protein-based molecules, is complex and incompletely understood (Chapter 13) [5]. It is affected by multiple interrelated factors including body weight

Table 19.4 Dose and regimens of some tumour necrosis factor antagonists.

	Infliximab[a]	Adalimumab[a]	Certolizumab	Etanercept[a]
Route	IV, over 2 h	SC	SC	SC
Dose[b]	5 mg/kg week 0, 2, 6 and then 8 weekly	80 mg (week 0), 40 mg week 1 and then 40 mg every other week	400 mg (week 0, 2 and 4) and then 200 or 400 mg every other week	50 mg weekly
Bioavailability	[100%]	64%	80%	76%

[a] Biosimilar available.
[b] For psoriasis, licensed indication.

(which is associated with more rapid clearance of adalimumab), the degree of drug binding to TNF within target tissues such as the skin and synovium (so-called target-mediated drug disposition) and drug immunogenicity (see later). Circulating drug levels do, however, correlate with treatment efficacy and explain some of the variability in treatment response. In contrast to small molecules, renal filtration and biliary secretion are not relevant to drug elimination, so dose adjustment is not required in the event of impaired renal or hepatic function.

Drug immunogenicity. In common with biologic agents in general, all TNF antagonists can generate an immune response with consequent development of antidrug antibodies [6,7]. These are increasingly recognised as an important mechanism underlying treatment failure either by competing with endogenous ligand (TNF) and preventing the neutralising effect of the TNF antagonist or through formation of drug/antidrug antibody complexes and accelerated drug clearance. These mechanisms may coexist and may also contribute to the adverse event profile. While the majority of patients develop antidrug antibodies, typically within the first 6 months of therapy, not all lose treatment efficacy, as antibodies may be transient or at a low level. This interindividual variability in development and amplification (or tolerance) of immune response appears to relate to multiple factors, including route and dosing schedule (e.g. an initial high dose and continuous dosing may confer a reduced risk), route of administration, patient factors (e.g. genetic factors, level of disease activity) as well as drug-specific considerations. Notably, methotrexate [6,8] (and possibly other immunosuppressants) significantly reduces the risk of development of antidrug antibodies and is often co-prescribed with TNF antagonists. The clinical utility of drug and antidrug antibody level evaluation to optimise drug dosing and strategies to minimise or avoid antibody formation is subject to ongoing research [9–11].

Pharmacodynamics. TNF is released from a wide variety of cells including keratinocytes as a soluble cytokine (sTNF) following cleavage from its cell surface-bound precursor (tmTNF). Both sTNF and tmTNF are biologically active and bind to either of two distinct receptors [9]: TNF receptor 1 (TNFR1, p55) and TNF receptor 2 (TNFR2, p75). This leads to NFκB activation (which promotes inflammation) and/or cell apoptosis. In addition, tmTNF can itself act as a ligand via a process of reverse signalling to induce cell activation, cytokine suppression or apoptosis of the tmTNF-bearing cell.

All TNF antagonist biologic agents specifically bind both soluble and transmembrane forms of TNF and act by (i) blocking TNFR-mediated mechanisms; and (ii) inducing tmTNF (reverse-signalling) events. Etanercept also binds members of the lymphotoxin family (LTα3 (also known as TNF-β) and LTα2β1), whereas certolizumab, because it lacks an Fc' portion, cannot bind complement or cause antibody-dependent cell-mediated cytotoxicity (in vitro). Whether these differences in function account for differences in overall efficacy and/or safety in clinical practice is unclear.

Potential adverse effects. Principal side effects include injection site reactions, infusion reactions (infliximab) and infection. Reactivation of tuberculosis is a particular risk, given the role of TNF in host defence against mycobacterial infection and granuloma formation, and frequently presents with extrapulmonary or other atypical site involvement. Heart failure (both new onset and worsening of pre-existing heart disease) and demyelinating disorders have also been reported. Paradoxically, new-onset psoriasis (including palmoplantar pustulosis) and sarcoidosis have developed in patients on TNF antagonists, particularly when given for rheumatological indications or Crohn disease, illustrating that the impact of TNF blockade on what is a highly complex cytokine network is not always predictable. Idiosyncratic hepatitis reactions, autoimmune hepatitis, cytopenias, pancytopenias and serious opportunistic infections are also rarely reported. Historically, there has been concern that TNF antagonists may confer an increased risk of malignancy, particularly in relation to lymphoma and skin cancer. However, to date, data are reassuring [1,13].

Contraindications. Contraindications include the presence of severe cardiac failure (New York Heart Association class III/IV), a personal history of demyelinating disease, active infection or untreated latent tuberculosis. Live and live attenuated vaccinations may potentially lead to severe or fatal infections and must be avoided during therapy. Check for up-to-date vaccine-specific advice in the relevant SmPC and in national guidelines, for example in the UK the so-called 'Green Book' [14]. A current or recent past history of malignancy (unless the malignancy has been diagnosed and treated more than 5 years previously, and /or where the likelihood of cure is high, e.g. adequately treated non-melanoma skin cancer) is also generally considered a contraindication although there may be instances where the treatment may be used due to the severity of the underlying disease and/or the absence of alternative therapeutic options. In these circumstances, prescribers are strongly encouraged to consult with the relevant multidisciplinary team members.

Cautions. Patients with multiple co-morbidities, who are older or have a history of cancer may be at increased risk of serious adverse events and should be carefully reviewed and monitored [15]. Caution is also required when considering use in patients with chronic viral infections including hepatitis B and C and HIV due to risks of reactivation and/or progression and lack of information on safety. IgG is actively transported from mother to fetus via the neonatal Fc receptor (FcRN) from around 14 weeks, so that all the TNF antagonists with the exception of certolizumab, which lacks an Fc portion, would be expected to cross the placenta during the second and third trimesters. Measurable drug levels in infants born to mothers on infliximab and etanercept have been reported [16]. Use during pregnancy, especially in the second and third trimesters, thus needs careful consideration. Live vaccinations must be avoided in infants (up to 6 months of age) whose mothers have received biologic therapy beyond 16 weeks' gestation [17]. Maternal use of TNF antagonists is compatible with breastfeeding since although TNF antagonists are excreted in breast milk, the concentrations are very low and bioavailability in the infant is poor due to intestinal proteolysis [18]. Surgery while on TNF therapy is associated with an increased risk of postoperative infection. In all these instances, specialist advice and consideration on a case-by-case basis with reference to relevant clinical guidelines are strongly recommended.

Drug–drug interactions. There are no clinically important interactions between TNF antagonists and small-molecule drugs. With the exception of methotrexate, co-administration with other immunomodulatory agents including biologic therapies is, in general, avoided due to the potential for increased risk of infection.

Pre-treatment screening. All patients should have a comprehensive history taken and a thorough clinical examination and appropriate investigations performed to identify contraindications to or cautions for therapy, with particular focus on the presence or risks of infection, including active tuberculosis, demyelination or cancer. Planned conception, pregnancy and travel, given the risk of tuberculosis and possible vaccination requirements, should be discussed. Screening for latent tuberculosis should include a chest X-ray and a tuberculin skin test. In instances where this is unreliable, however, as in bacille Calmette–Guérin-vaccinated individuals or those on immunosuppressants, an *in vitro* IFN-γ release assay (IGRA) test (QuantiFERON®-TB Gold In-Tube, Cellestis, Australia, and T-Spot®.TB, Oxford Immunotec, UK) should be performed [19]. In patients with investigations supportive of a diagnosis of latent tuberculosis, treatment with antituberculous therapy may be indicated, although it is worth noting that this only reduces the risk of reactivation of latent tuberculosis during subsequent TNF antagonist therapy by 50%, so a high index of suspicion should remain during therapy. Relevant national guidelines [20] are helpful since specific details on recommended pre-treatment screening and treatment for latent tuberculosis [19] will vary depending on population and individual patient risk profiles. Where available, patients should be encouraged to participate in national long-term safety registries.

Monitoring. Careful clinical review and advice to patients to seek early medical review in the event of new symptomatology, as well as routine blood investigations (FBC, renal and liver function tests), are part of the routine monitoring of patients on TNF therapy.

Annual IGRA testing (for those who are negative at treatment outset) may be useful in those at especially high risk of tuberculosis (e.g. people who work or live in high-risk settings, or who travel to high-prevalence countries).

Other cytokine antagonists

IL-23/IL-17 antagonists. Drugs that target IL-23 and IL-17 include the anti-p40 mAb ustekinumab, anti-IL-23 mAbs guselkumab, risankizumab and tildrakizumab [17] and the IL-17 antagonists bimekizumab, brodalumab, ixekizumab and secukinumab. The striking efficacy of all of these agents in psoriasis [21] underpins the critical importance of the IL-23/Th17 axis in the disease pathogenesis; in time, their clinical utility may well extend to other immune-mediated skin diseases.

Preassessment screening, cautions, contraindications and monitoring recommendations are broadly in line with those discussed in relation to the TNF antagonists. Class- and/or drug-specific recommendations are detailed here.

Ustekinumab. Ustekinumab is licensed for use in plaque psoriasis (and also psoriatic arthritis). There have also been recent reports of its value for treating pityriasis rubra pilaris but formal studies have yet to be undertaken (Chapter 36).
- **Pharmacological properties**:
  - *Formula and structure.* Ustekinumab is a fully human IgG1κ monoclonal antibody that binds with specificity to the shared p40 protein subunit of human cytokines IL-12 and IL-23.
  - *Administration.* It is given by self-administered subcutaneous injection.
  - *Pharmacokinetics.* The estimated bioavailability of ustekinumab is 57% following a single subcutaneous injection, with a median half-life of approximately 3 weeks (range 15–32 days). Enhanced drug clearance occurs with increasing body weight and the presence of ustekinumab antidrug antibodies [22].
  - *Pharmacodynamics.* IL-12 and IL-23 are heterodimeric cytokines secreted by activated antigen-presenting cells and share a common protein subunit, p40. IL-12 activates CD4 and NK cells to induce expression of type 1 cytokines (TNF and IFN-γ), while IL-23 stimulates survival and proliferation of a subset of T cells that produce IL-17 (Th17 cells). Ustekinumab binds specifically to the p40 protein subunit thereby preventing IL-12 and IL-23 from binding to the IL-12Rβ1 receptor protein expressed on the surface of T cells, NK cells and antigen-presenting cells. The marked efficacy of ustekinumab in psoriasis is likely to be mainly attributable to the inhibition of IL-23, given the central role for the IL-23/IL-17 pathway in the pathogenesis of psoriasis.
- **Potential adverse effects.** Ustekinumab is generally well tolerated, with nasopharyngitis, headache, upper respiratory tract infection and injection site reactions being the most commonly reported adverse effects in clinical trials. Rarely, serious infections may also occur. IL-12 and IL-23 have been implicated in atherogenesis, and there has been a reported possible excess of major adverse cardiovascular events in RCTs involving the use of ustekinumab and another mAb, briakinumab, with specificity for the p40 subunit. The latter was subsequently withdrawn from clinical development [23].

- **Contraindications.** These are as for TNF antagonists and include active infection or untreated latent tuberculosis, a current or recent past history of malignancy (unless the malignancy has been diagnosed and treated more than 5 years previously and/or where the likelihood of cure is high, e.g. adequately treated non-melanoma skin cancer) and live vaccination within 2 weeks preceding the first injection or within 15 weeks after the last injection. Ustekinumab has an Fc portion, and so will cross the placenta via the FcRN from 16 weeks, and will be excreted in breast milk. Advice to women planning conception or who are pregnant is as for the TNF antagonists.
- **Drug–drug interactions.** There are no known specific drug interactions. Co-therapy with other immunosuppressant drugs should generally be avoided due to the risk of excess immunosuppression and limited data on the safety of such combinations.
- **Pre-treatment screening.** The recommended pre-treatment assessment for ustekinumab is comparable to that for TNF antagonists [17,24].
- **Dose and regimens.** The standard licensed dosing regimen is as a fixed dose according to body weight (<100 kg, 45 mg; >100 kg, 90 mg) at weeks 0 and 4 and then at 12-weekly intervals thereafter. Off-label use of escalated dosing schedules is occasionally used in poor responders, for example increasing the dose from 45 to 90 mg (in those who are <100 kg) or increasing the frequency of injections (45 or 90 mg) to 8 weekly.
- **Monitoring.** This is as for TNF antagonists [17,24].

IL-23 antagonists. Guselkumab, risankizumab and tildrakizumab are all licensed for use in plaque psoriasis. (Mirikizumab although established as effective for psoriasis is only being developed for regulatory approval in inflammatory bowel disease.)
- **Pharmacological properties**:
  - *Formula and structure.* All three agents selectively bind with high affinity to the p19 subunit of human IL-23. Guselkumab is a human IgG1λ mAb; risankizumab and tildrakizumab are humanised IgG1 mAbs.
  - *Administration.* This is given as a self-administered subcutaneous injection, with differing loading schedules. Maintenance injections are given at 8-weekly (guselkumab) or 12-weekly (risankizumab, tildrakizumab) intervals.
  - *Pharmacokinetics.* The estimated bioavailability ranges from 49% (guselkumab) to 89% (risankizumab). Enhanced drug clearance occurs with increasing body weight; antidrug antibodies (including neutralising antibodies) to all three agents have been detected. While making cross-drug comparisons is difficult given different assays, in general the p19 monoclonal antibodies are less immunogenic than TNF antagonists.
  - *Pharmacodynamics.* All three agents prevent IL-23 from interacting wih the IL-23 receptor complex and thus inhibit IL-23-dependent cell signalling and the release of pro-inflammatory cytokines. In particular, IL-23 plays a key role driving pathogenic Th17, γδT and group 3 innate lymphoid cells to produce high levels of IL-17, hence accounting for the marked efficacy of IL-23 blockade in psoriasis.
- **Potential adverse effects.** These agents are generally well tolerated, with upper respiratory infection, headaches and arthralgia being the most commonly reported problems in trials. Serious adverse events are rare (estimated at <0.02% in a recent meta-analysis in psoriasis) [21].
- **Contraindications.** These include active infection or untreated latent tuberculosis, a current or recent past history of malignancy (unless the malignancy has been diagnosed and treated more than 5 years previously, and/or where the likelihood of cure is high, e.g. adequately treated non-melanoma skin cancer) and live vaccination within 4 weeks preceding the first injection or 12–21 weeks (depending on the drug) after the last injection. All IL-23 antagonist mAbs have an Fc portion, and so will cross the placenta via the FcRN from 16 weeks and be excreted in breast milk. Advice to women planning conception or who are pregnant is as for the TNF antagonists.
- **Drug–drug interactions.** There are no known specific drug interactions. Co-therapy with other immunosuppressant drugs should generally be avoided due to the risk of excess immunosuppression and limited data on the safety of such combinations.
- **Pre-treatment screening.** The recommended pre-treatment assessment for IL-23 antagonists is comparable to that for TNF antagonists [17,24].
- **Monitoring.** This is as for TNF antagonists [17,24].

IL-17 antagonists. Bimekizumab, brodalumab, ixekizumab and secukinumab are all licensed for use in plaque psoriasis [25].
- **Pharmacological properties**:
  - *Formula and structure.* Bimekizumab is a humanised IgG1/κ mAb with divalent specificity for both IL-17A and IL-17F. Brodalumab is a human IgG2 mAb that binds to the IL-17 receptor. Secukinumab is a human IgG1/κ mAb that binds to IL-17A. Ixekizumab is a humanised IgG4 mAb, also binding to IL-17A.
  - *Administration.* This is given as a self-administered subcutaneous injection, with differing loading schedules. Maintenance injections are given at 2-weekly (brodalumab), 4-weekly (ixekizumab, secukinumab) or 8-weekly (bimekizumab) intervals.
  - *Pharmacokinetics.* The estimated bioavailability ranges from 55% (brodalumab) to 90% (ixekizumab) depending on the drug and study. Enhanced drug clearance occurs with increasing body weight; antidrug antibodies (including neutralising antibodies) to all IL-17 antagonists have been reported. While making cross-drug comparisons is difficult given different assays, in general the IL-17 monoclonal antibodies are less immunogenic than TNF antagonists.
  - *Pharmacodynamics.* IL-17A and IL-17F are Th17 cell 'signature' cytokines, as well as being produced by innate immune cells resident in the skin, gut and lung, playing key roles in immune responses to fungal and bacterial infections at the mucosal and skin barrier, and in driving inflammation in diseases such as psoriasis, psoriatic arthritis and rheumatoid arthritis. Secukinumab and ixekizumab both bind IL-17A, whereas brodalumab, through binding of the IL-17A receptor, disrupts signalling of IL-17A, IL-17C, IL-17F and IL-17A/F heterodimers. Bimekizumab exerts bivalent specificity for both IL-17A and IL-17F.
- **Potential adverse effects.** These agents are generally well tolerated. Nasopharyngitis, upper respiratory infections, transient

neutropenia and injection site reactions are common. Mucocutaneous candidiasis is a problem specific to Il-17 blockade, is usually mild or moderate and is estimated to affect around 4% of patients. IL-17 antagonists may trigger or worsen pre-existing inflammatory bowel disease. Serious adverse events are rare (estimated at <0.03% in a recent meta-analysis in psoriasis) [21].

- **Contraindications.** These include active infection or untreated latent tuberculosis, inflammatory bowel disease, recurrent candidiasis, live vaccination within 4 weeks preceding the first injection or 6–12 months (depending on the drug) after the last injection. All IL-23 antagonist mAbs have an Fc portion, and so will cross the placenta via the FcRN from 16 weeks and be excreted in breast milk. Advice to women planning conception or who are pregnant is as for the TNF antagonists.
- **Drug–drug interactions.** There are no known specific drug interactions. Co-therapy with other immunosuppressant drugs should generally be avoided due to risk of excess immunosuppression and limited data on the safety of such combinations.
- **Pre-treatment screening.** The recommended pre-treatment assessment for IL-17 antagonists is comparable to that for TNF antagonists [17]. In addition, take a focused history and, if indicated, investigate to rule out inflammatory bowel disease and/or significant candidiasis.
- **Monitoring.** This is as for TNF antagonists [17,24].

IL-4/IL-13 antagonists. Drugs that target IL-4 and IL-13 include the anti-IL-4 receptor α mAb dupilumab and the anti-IL-13 mAb tralokinumab. Lebrikizumab is a further anti-IL-13 mAb in the late stages of clinical development. All of them have proven effective in treating atopic dermatitis [26–28]. Dupilumab confers additional benefit in other atopic diseases including asthma, allergic rhinitis and nasal polyps.

Dupilumab. Dupilumab is licensed for use in adults with moderate to severe atopic dermatitis, severe asthma with type 2 inflammation and severe chronic rhinosinusitis with nasal polyps. It is licensed for use in children >5 years of age for atopic dermatitis and adolescents >11 years of age for asthma.
- **Pharmacological properties**:
  - *Formula and structure.* Dupilumab is a fully human IgG mAb. Dupilumab binds with specificity to the shared IL-4 receptor α subunit of the IL-4 and IL-13 cytokine receptors.
  - *Administration.* This is given by a self-administered subcutaneous injection.
  - *Pharmacokinetics.* The estimated bioavailability of dupilumab is 61–64% following a single subcutaneous injection [29]. Drug elimination is mediated by parallel linear and non-linear pathways. After the last steady-state dose, the median time for drug levels to reduce below the lower limit of detection is 10–11 weeks on a 300 mg every 2 weeks regimen. Enhanced drug clearance occurs with increasing body weight. Approximately 5% of patients on trials developed antidrug antibodies, 2% of which were neutralising.
  - *Pharmacodynamics.* IL-4 and IL-13 are major drivers of human type 2 inflammatory disease including atopic dermatitis and asthma. IL-4 induces differentiation of naïve helper T cells to Th2 cells, which in turn produce further IL-4 to create a positive feedback loop. Th2 cells also produce IL-13 which is a mediator of allergic inflammation affecting the skin barrier, pathogen defence, fibrosis and neuronal sensitisation within the skin [30]. They share a common receptor subunit, IL-4 receptor α. By binding to that subunit, dupilumab inhibits IL-4 signalling through the type I receptor (IL-4Ra/yc) and IL-4 and IL-13 signalling through the type II receptor (IL4Ra/IL-13Ra).
- **Potential adverse effects.** Dupilumab is generally well tolerated. Conjunctivitis (termed dupilumab-induced ocular surface disease in some reports) is the most common side effect, affecting up to 20% of participants in trials and up to 60% of patients in real-world practice [31,32]. This generally arises in the first 4 months of therapy and is managed topically [32]. Some patients require specialist ophthalmology care and strong topical treatment including tacrolimus ointment, ciclosporin eye drops or steroid eye drops. Few patients have to stop dupilumab because of eye symptoms. Other side effects include eosinophilia, which is usually transient and improves over the first 4 months, oral herpes and injection site reactions. Rarer side effects include blepharitis, keratitis, athralgia (including arthritis and enthesitis), psoriasiform skin rashes, facial eczema flares, anaphylaxis, angioedema, serum sickness reactions and serum sickness-like reactions.
- **Contraindications.** These include previous hypersensitivity to the drug or constituents or live vaccination within 2 weeks preceding the first injection. Live vaccination should be avoided while on treatment and for at least 6 months (following relevant national guidance) post-treatment cessation. It is recommended that active helminth infections are treated prior to initiation of therapy (due to the role of IL-4/IL-13 in helminth defence).
- **Drug–drug interactions.** There are no known specific drug interactions. Co-therapy with other immunosuppressant drugs should generally be avoided due to the risk of excess immunosuppression and limited data on the safety of such combinations.
- **Pre-treatment screening.** No routine blood tests are recommended but clinicians may consider a blood count, renal and hepatic function.
- **Dose and regimens.** The standard licensed dosing regimen for adults with atopic dermatitis is 600 mg loading followed by 300 mg every other week. Children aged between 12 and 17 years with a body weight of <60 kg should receive 400 mg loading and then 200 mg on alternate weeks; those >60 kg should receive the standard dose. Children aged 6–11 years weighing 15–60 kg should receive 300 mg loading, 300 mg 2 weeks later and then 300 mg every 4 weeks; those >60 kg should receive the standard dose.
- **Monitoring.** No routine blood monitoring is recommended but clinicians may consider a blood count and renal and liver function at 1 month, 4 months and then annually as they deem appropriate.

Tralokinumab. Tralokinumab is licensed for use in adults with moderate to severe atopic dermatitis [33].
- **Pharmacological properties**:
  - *Formula and structure.* Tralokinumab is a fully human IgG4 mAb that binds to type 2 cytokine IL-13.
  - *Administration.* It is given by self-administered subcutaneous injection.

- *Pharmacokinetics.* The estimated bioavailability of tralokinumab is 76% following a single subcutaneous injection with a half-life of 22 days. Enhanced drug clearance occurs with increasing body weight.
- *Pharmacodynamics.* IL-13 is a driver of human type 2 inflammatory disease including atopic dermatitis. IL-13 is a mediator of allergic inflammation directly affecting the functional integrity of the skin barrier, pathogen defence, fibrosis and neuronal sensitisation within the skin. By binding to IL-13, tralokinumab prevents binding to IL-13 receptors.
- **Potential adverse effects.** Tralokinumab is generally well tolerated. Conjunctivitis (termed dupilumab-induced ocular surface disease in some reports), eosinophilia, upper respiratory tract infections and injection site reactions are common; keratitis is rare. The real-world frequency and severity of conjunctivitis are yet to be established but cases reported in trials were generally mild and did not require treatment cessation [34].
- **Contraindications.** These include previous hypersensitivity to the drug or constituents or live vaccination within 2 weeks preceding the first injection. Live vaccination should be avoided while on treatment and for at least 6 months (following relevant national guidance) post-treatment cessation. It is recommended that active helminth infections are treated prior to initiation of therapy (due to the role of IL-13 in helminth defence).
- **Drug–drug interactions.** There are no known specific drug interactions. Co-therapy with other immunosuppressant drugs should generally be avoided due to the risk of excess immunosuppression and limited data on the safety of such combinations.
- **Pre-treatment screening.** No routine blood tests are recommended but clinicians may consider a blood count and renal and hepatic function.
- **Dose and regimens.** The standard licensed dosing regimen for adults with atopic dermatitis is 600 mg loading followed by 300 mg every other week.
- **Monitoring.** No routine blood monitoring is recommended but clinicians may consider a blood count and renal and liver function at 1 month, 4 months and then annually as they deem appropriate.

IL-1 antagonists. IL-1 plays a central role in a wide range of inflammatory conditions, and there are a number of novel biologic agents targeting IL-1, both approved and in development, that may be of potential therapeutic benefit in pustular skin diseases such as autoinflammatory disorders, Behçet syndrome and SAPHO syndrome (synovitis, acne, pustulosis, hyperostosis and osteitis) [35–37]. All three agents detailed here are licensed for use in the 'orphan indication' cryopyrin-associated autoinflammatory syndromes that include familial cold autoinflammatory syndrome (FCAS) and Muckle–Wells syndrome.

Anakinra is a recombinant IL-1 receptor antagonist and acts to competitively inhibit both IL-1α and IL-1β binding to the IL-1 receptor. It is administered as a single daily self-administered subcutaneous injection (100 mg/day in adults or 1–2 mg/kg/day). Bioavailability is 95%, with rapid renal clearance (median half-life 4–6 h). Adverse effects include injection site reactions (very common), allergic reactions, anaphylaxis (rare), infection including serious infections, neutropenia and raised liver enzymes [38,39].

Canakinumab is a human IgG1κκ anti-IL-1β mAb that acts by binding to endogenous IL-1β and thus prevents interaction with IL-1 receptors. It is administered as a single dose (initially 150 mg or 2 mg/kg escalating as indicated by clinical response) with maintenance therapy at 8-weekly intervals [40]. The bioavailability is 66% with a mean half-life of 26 days (comparable with other therapeutic mAbs). The adverse event profile is similar to anakinra [41].

Rilonacept (IL-1 trap) is a dimeric fusion protein that contains in a single chain the extracellular domains of IL-receptor type 1 and IL-1 receptor accessory protein fused to the human Fc portion of IgG. It acts as a soluble decoy receptor to block primarily IL-1β signalling and, to a lesser extent, IL-1α and endogenous IL-1 receptor antagonist (IL-1ra) signalling. It is available only in the USA.

B-cell directed biologic therapies

Available B-cell directed therapy has until recently been limited to rituximab, a potent B-cell-depleting anti-CD20 mAb that was originally developed for the treatment of a wide range of B-cell malignancies including cutaneous B-cell lymphoma. However, belimumab, now licensed for use in systemic lupus erythematosus, is one of a number of new recombinant antibodies targeting surface-bound proteins on B cells [42,43] that may have clinical utility in autoimmune/inflammatory skin disease (Figure 19.6).

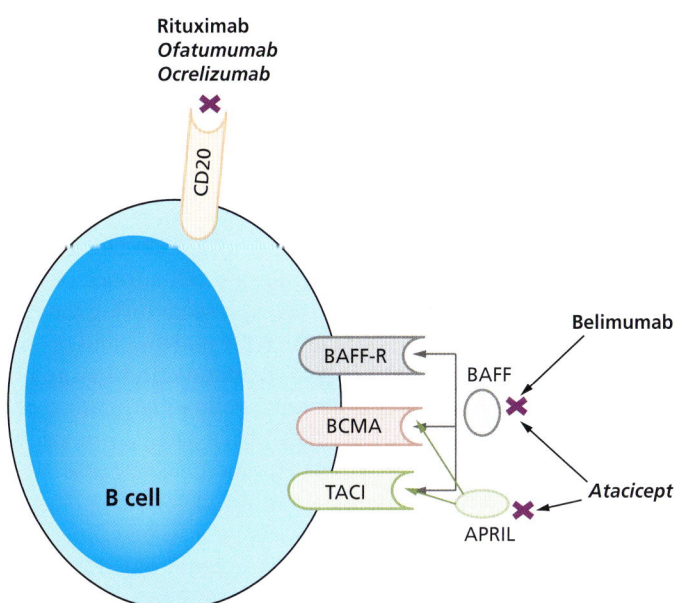

Figure 19.6 B-cell directed biologic therapies. In common with rituximab, ofatumumab and ocrelizumab both target CD20 but with enhanced complement- and antibody-dependent cell-mediated cytoxicity [43]. Belimumab binds to B-cell activating factor of the tumour necrosis factor (TNF) family (BAFF; also known as B-lymphocyte stimulator (BLyS), a crucial soluble B-cell survival factor, to prevent activation of TNF receptor superfamily member 13C (BAFF receptor (BAFF-R) or BLyS receptor 3 (BR3)), TNF receptor superfamily member 17 (B-cell maturation antigen (BCMA)) and TNF receptor superfamily member 13B (transmembrane activator and cyclophilin ligand interactor (TACI)). Atacicept is a fusion protein containing the extracellular, ligand-binding portion of TACI and the modified Fc portion of human immunoglobulin G (IgG): it binds and neutralises both BAFF and a second soluble B-cell activating factor known as a proliferation-inducing ligand (APRIL). Both belimumab and atacicept show efficacy in systemic lupus erythematosus and have potential applications in autoimmune skin disease [43,47,48]. Drugs given in italics are in clinical development. Adapted from Faurschou and Jayne 2014 [43] and Vincent et al. 2014 [47].

Rituximab

Dermatological uses (Chapters 50–53 and 100). Rituximab is licensed for use, in combination with GCs, for the induction of remission in adults with antineutrophil cytoplasmic antibody (ANCA)-associated vasculitis (granulomatosis with polyangiitis and microscopic polyangiitis) [43,44]. It is used off-label in a wide spectrum of severe autoimmune and chronic inflammatory diseases including vasculitis, pemphigus, systemic lupus erythematosus, dermatomyositis and primary Sjögren syndrome, usually in combination with other immunomodulatory agents [43,45].

Pharmacological properties

Formula and structure. Rituximab is an IgG1, chimaeric mouse/human anti-CD20 mAb.

Administration. Rituximab is given as a slow intravenous infusion. Premedication with an analgesic/antipyretic (e.g. paracetamol), an antihistaminic drug (e.g. chlorphenamine) and a GC (e.g. methylprednisolone) is given to reduce or avoid infusion reactions.

Pharmacokinetics. In non-malignant conditions, the mean terminal half-life following IV infusion is around 20 days (range 9–35 days depending also to some extent on the dose), with metabolism and elimination as for IgG in general (Chapter 13). Population pharmacokinetic modelling indicates that body surface area and sex (men have a larger volume of distribution and clearance) are the most significant covariates to explain interindividual variability in pharmacokinetic parameters, although sex differences are not considered clinically relevant.

Pharmacodynamics. CD20 is a four-transmembrane phosphoprotein that is specifically expressed on the cell surface of B cells and is regulated by differentiation. It is expressed during the transition from pre-B to immature cell in the bone marrow, and on naïve, activated and memory B cells in the circulation and tissue, but is lost on differentiation into plasma cells. Following binding of the rituximab Fab fragment to CD20, B-cell lysis occurs, primarily via antibody-dependent cellular cytotoxicity mediated by one or more of the Fcγ receptors on the surface of granulocytes, macrophages and NK cells, although other mechanisms have also been implicated. Naïve B cells disappear rapidly from peripheral blood circulation and also, to a more variable extent, from tissues, depending on the pathology and setting. Circulating B-cell populations recover to normal over the ensuing 3–6 months. Since the CD20 antigen is not expressed by pro- or pre-B cells or by terminally differentiated plasma cells, rituximab does not prevent regeneration of CD20+ B cells from precursor cells and does not directly interfere with the production of immunoglobulins. Demonstration of efficacy in diseases where autoantibodies *per se* have not historically been considered to be of direct pathogenic significance (e.g. rheumatoid arthritis, dermatomyositis and systemic sclerosis) reflects the increasingly recognised, highly diverse nature of B-cell function including antigen presentation, cytokine production, lymphoid organ remodelling and immune cell regulation (by regulatory B cells) [46].

Potential adverse effects. Infusion reactions are common and occur in up to 25% of patients following the first infusion; most are mild to moderate in degree and decrease in severity with subsequent infusions. There is a predisposition to infection, including serious and opportunistic infections, herpes zoster and candidosis (rate of clinically significant infection in rheumatoid arthritis trials 0.05 per patient-year). Progressive multifocal leukoencephalopathy has been reported in patients treated for lymphoproliferative disease and, very rarely, for systemic lupus erythematosus [47,48]. Cytopenias including neutropenia may occur months after treatment. The cohort of patients receiving rituximab tend to have severe recalcitrant disease and have therefore necessarily received significant, often very long-term immunosuppression prior to treatment, which probably further increases the risks of infection. Human antichimaeric antibodies develop in about 25% of patients treated and can be associated with worsening of infusion or allergic reactions and failure to deplete B cells, although not predictably so.

Contraindications. These include those with active infection; severely immunocompromised patients (e.g. with hypogammaglobulinaemia or where levels of CD4 or CD8 are very low); uncontrolled heart disease or heart failure (New York Heart Association grade IV); and live vaccination within 4 weeks of infusion and/or while B-cell depleted.

Cautions. Patients with pre-existing heart disease should be closely monitored as a variety of cardiac events have been reported during infusions (e.g. angina, cardiac arrhythmias) and infusion reactions may be poorly tolerated. Caution should be exercised when considering the use of rituximab in patients with a history of recurring or chronic infections or with underlying conditions that may further predispose patients to serious infection [49].

Drug–drug interactions. There are no known specific drug interactions.

Pre-treatment screening. To minimise risk, rituximab should be instigated only by clinicians experienced in its use, in a multidisciplinary environment and where a comprehensive pre-treatment history, clinical and investigation protocol is in place. Screening prior to rituximab should aim to identify in particular those with cardiac disease and any current or past infection at risk of progression or reactivation. This includes a past history of tuberculosis, risk factors for or presence of active infection, together with relevant screening tests for latent tuberculosis and blood-borne viral infections (HIV, hepatitis B and C) [49,50]. Fulminant hepatic failure following hepatitis B reactivation is well documented in the oncology literature, although rituximab may not be absolutely contraindicated in the presence of positive hepatitis B or C serology, given appropriate antiviral prophylaxis (for hepatitis B) and relevant expert hepatology advice [49]. Vaccination status against *Pneumococcus* and influenza as well as any travel plans likely to require live vaccination should be checked. The importance of avoidance of pregnancy during and for 12 months post-infusion should be emphasised. Commonly recommended additional investigations include FBC, renal and liver function, serum immunoglobulins and lymphocyte subsets.

Dose and regimens. Dosing schedules have varied in different clinical trials and according to the disease being treated. For most dermatological conditions, a single cycle of treatment is given (usually 375 mg/m^2 or 1 g total dose, weekly for 2–4 weeks) in the context of concomitant immunosuppressant agents such as corticosteroids. Subsequent cycles may be given on disease relapse if necessary, but not usually until 6 months have elapsed.

Monitoring. Ongoing monitoring is necessary for signs of infection and neurological disturbance. Routine blood investigations (FBC and renal and liver function tests) should be carried out at regular intervals (e.g. monthly) or more frequently in the event of abnormalities. Immunoglobulins and lymphocyte subsets should be checked prior to any subsequent infusions.

Miscellaneous biologic therapies
Omalizumab
Omalizumab was first licensed for use in severe allergic (IgE-mediated) asthma and is effective in treating chronic urticaria. Further mAbs, such as ligelizumab (also targeting IgE), are in late-stage development.

Dermatological uses. It is licensed for use as an add-on therapy for the treatment of chronic spontaneous urticaria in adults and adolescents (12 years and above) with inadequate response to H$_1$ antihistamine treatment. Off-label, it is used in other forms of urticaria [51] and treatment-resistant atopic eczema, although with variable outcomes [52,53].

Pharmacological properties
Formula and structure. Omalizumab is a recombinant humanised mAb (IgG1κ) against the Cε3 domain of IgE.

Administration. It is given by subcutaneous injection.

Pharmacokinetics. Following injection, the absolute bioavailability is 62%, reaching peak serum concentrations after an average of 6–8 days. Metabolism and elimination are as for IgG in general (Chapter 13) via the reticuloendothelial system and by targeted binding (omalizumab–IgE complex formation), with a mean elimination half-life of 24 days.

Pharmacodynamics. Omalizumab binds specifically to free IgE only, since Cε3, the IgE antigenic determinant recognised by omalizumab, constitutes part of the high-affinity IgE receptor (FcεR) binding site. This results in lower serum levels of free IgE, prevention of IgE binding to FcεRI and subsequent downregulation of FcεRI expression on basophils, mast cells and dendritic cells. Omalizumab–IgE immune complexes may also sequester allergens/autoantigens and, through downregulation of IgE-expressing B lymphoblasts and memory B cells, reduce the number of IgE-secreting plasma cells. These mechanisms clearly play a key role in the treatment effect where urticaria is caused by autoreactive IgG antibodies against FcεRI and/or IgE or autoreactive IgE antibodies against autoallergens. In other forms of urticaria the precise mechanism of action is unclear, although its effectiveness points to the IgE–mast cell axis being central to all forms of urticaria.

Potential adverse effects. The most common adverse effects include headache, sinusitis, joint pain, upper respiratory tract infection and injection site reactions. Reported adverse events that will require longer-term, larger-scale pharmacovigilance studies that properly control for confounders to evaluate true risk include arterial thromboembolic events (such as stroke, transient ischaemic attack, myocardial infarction), anaphylaxis, theoretical concerns around immune complex-mediated pathology and abnormal immune responses to parasitic infections [54].

Contraindications. These include hypersensivity reactions to omalizumab or injection excipients.

Cautions. Type 1 allergic reactions including anaphylaxis have been reported following omalizumab, usually within 2 h of injection but occasionally up to 24 h post-injection. Patients should be warned about this possibility and injections always given under medical supervision (see monitoring). Omalizumab may present particular risk to patients with a susceptibility to helminthic/other parasitic infections in endemic areas.

Drug–drug interactions. No specific drug interactions have been reported.

Pre-treatment screening. This should include routine history, clinical assessment and blood tests (FBC, liver and renal function tests). Dosing for asthma (only) is based on serum IgE.

Dose and regimens. The licensed dosing for chronic urticaria is 300 mg subcutaneously every 4 weeks. Injections should be given under supervision with post-treatment monitoring for allergic reactions for 1–2 h.

Monitoring. Routine bloods investigations should be undertaken, in particular to exclude thrombocytopenia [52].

C1-esterase inhibitor replacement therapy
Three forms of C1-esterase inhibitor (C1INH) replacement therapy are approved for use in hereditary angioedema (type 1 and 2): Cinryze® and Berinert®, both of which are derived from human plasma, pasteurised and nanofiltered to reduce the risk of infection transmission; and Rhucin®, which is a recombinant human C1INH concentrate purified from rabbit breast milk [55,56]. CINH replacement therapy is given as an intravenous infusion, either as short-term prophylaxis prior to procedures at high risk of triggering an attack (e.g. surgery, extensive dental work) or as an emergency intervention during an acute attack. Cinryze is also licensed for the 'routine' prevention of recurrent hereditary angioedema (e.g. 1000 IU every 3–4 days). Acute anaphylaxis (rarely) and the theoretical transmission of as yet unidentified infectious agents are the principal adverse effects.

Intravenous immunoglobulin therapy

Intravenous immunoglobulin refers to the intravenous infusion of high doses of human IgG pooled from the plasma of thousands of healthy donors. As well as its use as replacement therapy in primary and secondary immunodeficiency syndromes with impaired antibody production, IVIg has immunomodulatory actions and is licensed in the UK for use in primary immune thrombocytopenia, Guillain–Barré syndrome and Kawasaki disease [1].

Dermatological uses (Chapters 38, 42, 50–54 and 57)

Off-label, IVIg, either as monotherapy or in combination with other immunomodulating drugs, has been utilised in a variety of autoimmune and inflammatory dermatoses including autoimmune bullous disorders (pemphigus, pemphigoid, epidermolysis bullosa acquisita, linear IgA disease), autoimmune connective tissue disorders (dermatomyositis, systemic sclerosis, systemic lupus erythematosus) and miscellaneous other conditions including chronic autoimmune urticaria, graft-versus-host disease, scleromyxoedema and Stevens–Johnson syndrome/toxic epidermal necrolysis [2].

Pharmacological properties

Formula and structure

The IgG antibodies present in IVIg preparations reflect those present in the normal population, with the proportions of its four subclasses approximating to the *in vivo* state [1].

Administration

It is given intravenously and should be administered in accord with the infusion rate recommended for the particular brand being used. Adequate hydration of the patient should be established prior to use [1].

Pharmacokinetics

Following infusion, IVIg is distributed relatively rapidly between intra- and extravascular compartments, with equilibrium after 3–5 days [1]. IVIg crosses the placenta and may be excreted into breast milk [2]. The half-life of the immunoglobulins, which are gradually degraded by cells of the reticuloendothelial system, is approximately 4 weeks [1].

Pharmacodynamics

The mechanisms underlying the immunomodulatory actions of IVIg remain poorly understood, and in particular the apparent contradiction between the well-established pro-inflammatory properties of IgG antibodies and the anti-inflammatory activity of high-dose pooled IgG has yet to be reconciled. Suffice to say that IVIg has complex effects on both the innate and adaptive components of the immune system that act in the direction of immune homeostasis. These include (i) the blockade of Fc receptors on B lymphocytes by 'natural' antibodies, resulting in a reduction of pathogenic autoantibody and cytokine production, and B-cell apoptosis; (ii) blocking of Fc receptors on macrophages (particularly by IgG in IVIg with sialylated Fc, thereby inhibiting the secretion of pro-inflammatory cytokines) and on granulocytes, thus inhibiting degranulation; (iii) saturation of Fc receptors leading to increased clearance of pathogenic antibodies; (iv) anti-idiotypic antibodies in IVIg neutralising the effect of pathogenic antibodies; (v) inhibition by natural antibodies of complement-mediated cellular damage, including interference with the formation of the membrane attack complex; (vi) inhibition by natural antibodies of certain cytokines (including TNF-α and IFN-γ); (vii) inhibition of the maturation and function of dendritic cells, imposing on them a tolerogenic phenotype; and (viii) expansion of the population of regulatory T cells (T-regs) and enhancement of their suppressive functions [3–13]. However, the precise mechanistic process for the anti-inflammatory action of IVIg remains to be definitively established.

Pharmacogenetics

Little is known about the pharmacogenetic aspects of IVIg therapy, although there is some evidence that genetic factors may influence clinical response to IVIg in Kawasaki syndrome [14].

Potential adverse effects

In general IVIg is considered to have a good safety profile, with side effects tending to be mild and transient and with a low incidence of serious adverse effects [15–18]. However, older patients tend to be at greater risk of acute renal failure and venous and arterial thrombosis [18].

General infusion-related effects

Symptoms, usually mild, may occur during the course of the infusion of IVIg and include fatigue, malaise, shivering, raised temperature, flushing, headache, myalgia, arthralgia, back pain, chest tightness, dyspnoea, nausea, vomiting, diarrhoea, rashes, blood pressure variation and tachycardia [1,15]. These side effects usually settle if the infusion rate is slowed or temporarily discontinued and may be pre-empted in susceptible individuals by pre-treatment with analgesia, antihistamines, NSAIDs or low-dose intravenous corticosteroid [2].

Acute kidney injury

Rarely, IVIg may cause renal dysfunction by inducing osmotic nephrosis, in which cells of the proximal renal tubules are damaged [19–22]. Risk factors for osmotic nephrosis include age (>65 years), diabetes, pre-existing renal impairment, dehydration, concomitant administration of other nephrotoxic drugs [21] and the use of a sucrose-stabilised brand of IVIg [20,21]. Circulating rheumatoid factor and cryoglobulins may also be risk factors [2]. Gradual recovery of renal function is the rule [21], although there is a risk of fatal outcome [19]. If any risk factors are present, diuretics should be avoided for the period around the transfusion, hydration of the patient should be monitored and the infusion rate should be reduced [21].

Haemolysis

Haemolytic transfusion reactions with IVIg are uncommon, although non-O blood group recipients with an underlying inflammatory disorder appear at particular risk [23]. They have been linked to the presence of anti-A and anti-B haemagglutinins in the IVIg preparation and may be both IgG and complement mediated [23]. Haemolysis is manifest by a drop in haemoglobin following IVIg transfusion, elevated unconjugated bilirubin, elevated lactate dehydrogenase, a positive direct antiglobulin (Coombs) test and evidence of spherocytes and polychromasia on a peripheral blood film [23].

The immediate management of IVIg-related haemolysis is to stop the transfusion and, if red cell replacement is required, group O cells should be given [23]. To minimise the risk of further haemolytic transfusion reaction for a particular individual, a different IVIg product containing a lower titre of ABO haemagglutinins may be considered, together with cross-matching between the IVIg preparation and the recipient [23].

Thrombotic events
By increasing blood viscosity and thereby altering the rheological properties of the blood and decreasing its flow, IVIg is associated with an increased risk of venous and arterial thrombosis and subsequent embolic complications, including deep-vein thrombosis, pulmonary embolism, myocardial infarction and cerebrovascular accidents [24–28]. In 50% of cases such thrombotic events may be manifest during the IVIg infusion, although detection may not occur until later [29], with arterial thrombosis tending to be evident before venous thrombosis [24]. IVIg-related thrombosis, especially arterial, is associated with significant mortality, with the risk factors being older age, arterial hypertension, atherosclerosis, obesity, immobility, dehydration, diabetes, history of thrombosis, hyperviscosity syndromes and hypercholesterolaemia [1,24,25]. The risk of thrombotic events may be reduced in those considered to be particularly vulnerable by administering IVIg at a slow rate, giving a lower dose and using prophylactic aspirin or low-molecular-weight heparin [26].

IgA-mediated anaphylaxis and hypersensitivity reactions
The presence of trace amounts of IgA in IVIg preparations may induce allergic reactions and even anaphylaxis in otherwise symptomless IgA-deficient recipients with circulating anti-IgA antibodies of IgG or IgE class [29]. However, such IgA-dependent transfusion reactions are rare. Strategies have been developed to prevent IgA-related anaphylaxis in patients with a history of hypersensitivity [29].

Aseptic meningitis
Aseptic meningitis, presenting with headache, fever, photophobia, neck stiffness and vomiting, is a rare adverse reaction to IVIg, tending to occur within 48 h of the infusion [30]. Patients with pre-existing migraine may be more susceptible [30]. Examination and culture of cerebrospinal fluid are usually necessary to exclude bacterial meningitis. The prognosis for aseptic meningitis is good, and usually symptomatic treatment is all that is required. Ensuring adequate pre-treatment hydration, pre-medication analgesia or antihistamine and using a slow rate of infusion may enable continuation of IVIg therapy in patients who have experienced aseptic meningitis [30].

Infection risk
As a biological product derived from pooled human plasma, IVIg carries the potential risk of transmission of pathogens, which is minimised by the use of donor selection, screening of donations and plasma pools for specific markers of infection, scrupulous preparation hygiene and validated techniques for the removal or inactivation of infectious agents [1,31]. Nonetheless, the possibility of transmitting infection with known and unknown organisms cannot be totally excluded [1] and for medicolegal reasons it has been suggested that a pre-treatment serum sample from the recipient be stored [2], although this does not appear to be a general view.

Contraindications
Severe anaphylaxis resulting from a previous infusion is a contraindication to further use. The presence of risk factors for acute kidney injury and thrombosis are relative contraindications.

Cautions
The recommended infusion rate should not be exceeded. IVIg administration may impair the efficacy of live attenuated virus vaccines for up to 3 months (1 year in the case of measles) [1].

Drug–drug interactions
For the period immediately before and after IVIg infusions, the administration of loop diuretics should be avoided [1].

Pre-treatment screening
When assessing the risk–benefit ratio of a course of IVIg, factors predisposing that individual to acute kidney injury and thrombosis should be assessed. It is reasonable to consider measuring serum IgA and undertaking a thrombophilia screen.

Before each cycle of IVIg, an FBC, creatinine level and liver function tests should be checked. The hydration of the patient should be optimised, especially for the older person [18].

Dose and regimens
The standard regimen for high-dose IVIg for the treatment of dermatological conditions is 2 g/kg/cycle, based on the ideal weight of the patient, in divided doses over 2–5 days [1]. The rate of infusion should not exceed that recommended by the supplier. Cycles are repeated at approximately monthly intervals until effective disease control is obtained, after which the interval between cycles is gradually increased empirically up to 16 weeks, when IVIg can be discontinued if remission continues [2].

Fluid intake should be encouraged during and after the infusion. Consider paracetamol, with or without codeine, an NSAID or an antihistamine as a pre-medication if infusion-related symptoms have previously occurred. In those patients considered susceptible to thrombosis, aspirin or low-molecular-weight heparin are prophylactic options [26].

Monitoring
During and immediately after IVIg infusions, the vital signs, hydration status (to exclude both fluid overload and dehydration) and urine output should be monitored. Post-transfusion, an FBC with film and bilirubin level will screen for the possibility of haemolysis. Mobility should be encouraged in all patients to minimise the risk of thrombosis.

Systemic retinoids
The synthetic retinoids are a class of organic molecules derived from and with similar biological activity to the naturally occurring vitamin A group of retinoids, which includes retinol, retinal and retinoic acid.

While the naturally occurring retinoids are involved in the regulation of diverse and important biological processes, not least cell signalling in embryogenesis, the synthetic retinoids exert their medicinal properties principally via their specific effects at the genome level on epidermal cell proliferation, differentiation and apoptosis, tumour suppressor gene expression and immune function [1–4,5]. Their development over the last seven decades was initially prompted by the observed cutaneous effects of vitamin A deficiency, although their medical significance has subsequently extended far beyond the dermatological sphere. They are showing great potential in a number of different fields, including chemotherapeutic and chemoprotective use in a variety of haematological and solid malignancies; in metabolic diseases, as regulators of adipogenesis and as antidiabetic agents; in the prevention or treatment of neurodegenerative conditions; in certain renal disorders; and in stem cell-based regenerative medicine [6].

This section concerns those synthetic retinoids administered systemically for dermatological conditions, rather than the topical retinoid preparations. There are three generations of dermatologically useful systemic retinoids: first, the non-aromatic retinoids, represented by isotretinoin (13-*cis* retinoic acid) and alitretinoin (9-*cis* retinoic acid); second, the monoaromatic retinoids, including acitretin, a metabolite of etretinate, which it has now replaced; and third, the polyaromatic group, which includes bexarotene.

Dermatological uses (Chapters 88, 89 and 90)

Isotretinoin is licensed for the treatment of severe acne resistant to adequate courses of standard therapy, although off-label it has been used in rosacea, hidradenitis suppurativa and dissecting cellulitis of the scalp.

Alitretinoin has a product licence to treat severe chronic hand eczema (and has also been approved by the US FDA for the topical treatment of the cutaneous lesions of Kaposi sarcoma).

Acitretin is licensed in the UK for the treatment of severe psoriasis resistant to standard therapies, palmoplantar pustulosis, inherited ichthyoses and Darier disease. Off-licence, it has been used as chemoprophylaxis to reduce the risk of actinically induced non-melanoma cutaneous malignancy [5,7].

Bexarotene is indicated for the treatment of the cutaneous manifestations of advanced cutaneous T-cell lymphoma [8].

Retinoids have also been used off-licence to treat pityriasis rubra pilaris, lupus erythematosus and lichen planus.

Pharmacological properties

Formula and structure

The basic structure of a retinoid has three parts: a hydrophobic trimethylated cyclohexene ring; a conjugated polyene linker side chain; and a hydrophilic polar moiety [6].

Isotretinoin (systematic name: 13-*cis* retinoic acid), acitretin (systematic name: (2E,4E,6E,8E)-9-(4-methoxy-2,3,6-trimethyl-phenyl)-3,7-dimethylnona-2,4,6,8-tetraenoic acid), alitretinoin (systematic name: (2E,4E,6Z,8E)-3,7-dimethyl-9-(2,6,6-trimethyl-1-cyclohexenyl) nona-2,4,6,8-tetraenoic acid) and bexarotene (systematic name: 4-[1-(3,5,5,8,8-pentamethyltetralin-2-yl)ethenyl] benzoic acid) are the four principal retinoids currently used in dermatological therapy.

Administration

All the systemic retinoids are administered orally.

Pharmacokinetics

The pharmacokinetics of retinoids are complex. The broad principles are absorption from the gut into intestinal mucosal cells, chylomicron-borne passage to the liver, intracellular processing by hepatocytes, secretion into blood (where they are bound to albumin) and finally uptake by and transport to the nucleus of the target cells [6]. This involves a sequence of intracellular transporter proteins that include cellular retinol-binding proteins, plasma retinol-binding proteins and cellular retinoic acid-binding proteins [6].

Being taken with food or milk enhances their bioavailability. In the circulation, they are bound to albumin, and are widely distributed; they cross the placenta and are secreted into breast milk.

Retinoids are metabolised via isomerisation and oxidation by enzymes of the CYP system, followed by glucuronidation into inactive water-soluble forms [5,8] and biliary or renal elimination.

The elimination half-lives of the retinoids vary, with that of alitretinoin up to 10 h, isotretinoin approximately 20 h and acitretin 50–60 h. Isotretinoin and alitretinoin are endogenous retinoids and after cessation of treatment normal physiological levels are reached within 2 weeks for isotretinoin and a few days for alitretinoin [8]. Bexarotene has a clearance profile similar to isotretinoin [5].

Acitretin is cleared from the body within 1 month of stopping therapy [5]. However, because alcohol ingestion by patients on acitretin results in re-esterification to etretinate, which has a comparatively long half-life of 80–160 days, adequate contraceptive precautions are necessary for 2 years [5,8].

Pharmacodynamics

In the target cells, retinoids enter the nucleus to regulate the transcription of a variety of target genes. The complex process of retinoid signalling involves two families of retinoid nuclear receptor, the retinoic acid receptors (RARs) and the retinoid X receptors (RXRs) [9]. Each family has three isotypes (α, β and γ) and each isotype several isoforms [4,6]. Each receptor has a DNA-binding domain and a ligand-binding domain. In order to regulate the expression of target genes, the receptors form dimers, each containing an obligatory RXR and either a second RXR (RXR-RXR) or an RAR (RAR-RXR). The receptor dimers bind to specific sequences of DNA (retinoic acid response elements) within the promoter regions of the target genes, and it is the conformational change in the receptor consequent to binding of the ligand that promotes the transcription process, resulting in mRNA and then protein formation. Isotretinoin and acitretin act as ligands for RAR, bexarotene is a ligand for RXR, and alitretinoin is a panagonist, binding to both RAR and RXR [4].

Details regarding the genes targeted by retinoids and the mechanistic processes by which their protein products influence epidermal cell and immune cell function remain to be fully elucidated.

In addition to this genomic action, retinoids also have non-genomic effects, in particular retinoylation, a post-translational modification of certain proteins, including cytokeratins [6].

Potential adverse effects

Teratogenicity
Natural retinoids, in particular retinoic acid, play a fundamental role in embryonic patterning, growth and organogenesis, and perplexingly excess retinoid activity results in many of the same embryonic developmental defects as vitamin A deficiency [6]. Fetal exposure to retinoids in early pregnancy puts at risk normal neurological, ocular, cardiovascular and renal development, as well as that of the pulmonary system, skeleton, pancreas and limbs [6]. Administration of retinoids to women during the first trimester of pregnancy may cause cranio-facial deformities (including cleft palate and external ear malformations), central nervous system abnormalities (such as hydrocephalus, microcephaly and cerebellar malformation), heart defects (tetralogy of Fallot, transposition of the great vessels and septal defects) and abnormalities of the thymus and parathyroid glands in up to 50% of pregnancies, with increased numbers of early and late stillbirths [5,6].

There appears to be negligible risk of retinoid-induced embryopathy in fetuses fathered by men taking systemic retinoids [5].

Psychiatric
The SmPC for all licensed retinoids carries a warning about a potential relationship between psychiatric disorders and systemic retinoids. These drugs are often prescribed for conditions where psychiatric problems such as depression and anxiety are prevalent, causing concern to both prescribers and patients. Retinoids cross the blood–brain barrier, and there are biologically plausible mechanisms by which they may influence mood. Much of the evidence relates to isotreinoin where findings are mixed and often inconclusive. Recently published, large, population-based studies are however reassuring, and do not suggest that isotretinoin is independently associated with adverse psychiatric adverse events at a population level [10,11]. Nevertheless, it would seem prudent to advise patients and members of their families to be watchful for signs and symptoms of depression and to make specific enquiries relating to mood and suicidal thoughts [12] at each review consultation. Severe or frequent headaches may be a warning of retinoid-induced depression [13]. It is not clear whether patients with a pre-existing history of psychiatric problems are at increased risk [5,14], but oral isotretinoin therapy should not automatically be refused to such individuals [12,15,16]. Rather joint management with a psychiatric colleague should be undertaken, with measures in place to ensure that any deterioration in mental state is recognised at an early stage (including the use of a validated rating scale for anxiety and depression).

Ocular
Dry irritated eyes caused by blepharoconjunctivitis, occasionally complicated by bacterial infection, result from retinoid-induced alterations in conjunctival epithelium [17] and decreased meibomium gland secretion [18]. These problems can be alleviated by artificial tears, and affected individuals should be advised to temporarily discontinue contact lens use.

Asymptomatic corneal opacities may occur with retinoid therapy but these do not adversely affect vision [5].

Retinal toxicity causing impaired night vision is a potential adverse effect of retinoids which may persist for a number of years [19,20]. The possibility of this may justify electrophysiological screening in those individuals who have occupations that are dependent on satisfactory night vision.

Gastrointestinal
Of the retinoids, isotretinoin in particular has been implicated as a cause of inflammatory bowel disease, both ulcerative colitis and Crohn disease [5]. However, the evidence is conflicting [21] and, if indeed isotretinoin does predispose to inflammatory bowel disease, the overall risk is likely to be very low [21]. Patients with inflammatory bowel disease that require isotretinoin should be managed jointly with their gastroenterologist. Mild gastrointestinal upset is relatively common.

Musculoskeletal
Vitamin A toxicity may result in hyperostosis (in particular diffuse interstitial skeletal hyperostosis), premature epiphyseal closure, calcification of tendons and ligaments and lowered bone mineral density [5]. However, under the clinical conditions that retinoids are normally used in the treatment of acne and keratinisation disorders, there appears to be only a very low risk of these complications [5,22–24]. The possibility, albeit rare, of premature epiphyseal closure should be considered in preadolescent children.

Myalgia is a common side effect, particularly in physically active patients on isotretinoin, and may be accompanied by elevated creatine phosphokinase levels [5].

Mucocutaneous
Dryness of the skin (particularly in atopic patients) and mucous membranes (especially the nasal lining, vermilion of the lips and conjunctivae) is very common and dose related. It may be associated with pruritus, facial redness, impetiginisation, asteatotic eczema and skin fragility. Epistaxis can be troublesome. Patients on acitretin occasionally complain of 'sticky skin'. Emollient therapy is usually effective: a non-comedogenic preparation is recommended for acne-prone areas.

A temporary deterioration in acne frequently occurs when isotretinoin therapy is initiated but this does not normally require dose adjustment; very rarely, acne fulminans may develop [25]. Telogen effluvium, nail fragility, onycholysis and photosensitivity are occasional complications [5]. Isotretinoin-induced pyogenic granuloma-like lesions can arise in association with acne lesions and over nail folds: they tend to resolve on discontinuation of treatment [26]. There are rare postmarketing reports of severe skin reactions (Stevens–Johnson syndrome and toxic epidermal necrolysis) associated with isotretinoin therapy [27].

Neurological
Transient headaches are a common side effect, but very occasionally oral retinoids may cause benign intracranial hypertension (pseudotumor cerebri) with associated nausea, vomiting and visual disturbances, potentially with loss of vision [28], especially when isotretinoin is used concomitantly with an oral tetracycline.

Hyperlipidaemia
Dyslipidaemia, especially hypertriglyceridaemia but also hypercholesterolaemia, is a common consequence of retinoid therapy, particularly with bexarotene, and requires monitoring during

retinoid therapy. The management of modest dyslipidaemia involves dietary modification, increased physical activity and weight control to reduce cardiovascular risk, with more severe impairment of lipid levels necessitating pharmacological intervention to minimise the risk of pancreatitis [29]. Retinoid-induced hyperlipidaemia is reversible on discontinuation of treatment [5].

Hepatotoxicity
Retinoid-induced elevations of liver transaminases are common, and, although usually of little clinical significance, require monitoring [5]. Severe hepatitis is rare and probably idiosyncratic.

Haematological
Neutropenia is a common laboratory observation with isotretinoin and bexarotene, and isotretinoin may result in platelet abnormalities and anaemia [8].

Endocrinological
Bexarotene [30] and alitretinoin [8] may both cause central hypothyroidism, and monitoring for this adverse effect is necessary.

Contraindications
The oral retinoids are contraindicated in (i) women who are pregnant or breastfeeding; (ii) women of child-bearing potential unless all the conditions of a retinoid pregnancy prevention plan are met; (iii) patients who are receiving concomitant treatment with a tetracycline; and (iv) patients who are hypersensitive to the retinoid or an excipient (in particular soya and peanuts). Relative contraindications include renal and hepatic insufficiency and severe hyperlipidaemia.

Cautions
Patients should not donate blood during treatment or for at least 1 month thereafter in the case of isotretinoin and alitretinoin, and 6 months thereafter for acitretin, because of the potential risk to the fetus of a pregnant transfusion recipient [8]. Exposure to intense sunlight should be avoided and sun-protection measures used. Wax depilation should be discouraged for 6 months following retinoid treatment for fear of epidermal stripping, and dermabrasion or laser resurfacing should be postponed for at least 6 months because of the risk of hypertrophic scarring and dyspigmentation [8]. Retinoids may affect blood glucose control in diabetics.

Drug–drug interactions
See Box 19.8 [31].

Box 19.8 Systemic retinoids: drug–drug interactions

- Tetracyclines increase the risk of benign intracranial hypertension
- Alcohol induces acitretin re-esterification to etretinate
- Effects of coumarin anticoagulants and simvastatin are possibly reduced by acitretin
- Carbamazepine plasma concentrations are possibly reduced by isotretinoin
- Ketoconazole increases plasma concentrations of alitretinoin
- Possible methotrexate toxicity with acitretin
- Gemfibrozil increase bexarotene plasma levels
- Concomitant vitamin A may induce hypervitaminosis A

Pre-treatment screening
Women of child-bearing potential should receive explicit counselling on the teratogenicity of retinoids and prescribing clinicians must ensure women have access to relevant pregnancy prevention strategies. Pregnancy should be excluded prior to commencing retinoid therapy, and pregnancy avoided for the duration of therapy and for an appropriate time thereafter (1 month for isotretinoin, alitretinoin and bexarotene, and 2 years for acitretin). Pregnancy prevention plans in place for isotretinoin can be adapted for the other retinoids.

Pre-treatment laboratory tests should include an FBC, liver function tests, renal function tests and a full fasting lipid profile. Alitretinoin and bexarotene treatments necessitate monitoring of thyroid function.

Dose and regimens
There are standard dosage regimens for each of the retinoids [8,31,32,**33**,34].

Monitoring
A reasonable follow-up regimen is monthly clinical evaluation and blood tests (liver function tests and fasting lipid profile, with occasional renal function tests and FBC) for 3–6 months, then 3-monthly reviews with blood tests [5]. Thyroid function should be monitored in patients receiving alitretinoin and bexarotene.

Serum or urinary pregnancy tests are required monthly for women of child-bearing potential, and again 5 weeks after the drug is discontinued.

Specifically enquire about adverse effects, particularly those relating to mood and vision. Asymptomatic patients do not require routine monitoring for skeletal toxicity or osteoporosis [5] but if a patient reports restricted mobility and bone pain consideration they should be given to relevant radiological examination.

Thalidomide
Thalidomide acquired pharmacological notoriety in the early 1960s when it became clear that its use as a sedative and antiemetic for pregnant women could cause limb defects (phocomelia) and internal deformities in their children. Its subsequent reinvention as a useful therapeutic agent with potent immunomodulatory, anti-inflammatory, antiangiogenic and antineoplastic properties has seen it licensed as a component of first line treatment for myeloma and, in the USA, for erythema nodosum leprosum.

Dermatological uses (Chapters 31, 48, 51, 81, 126 and 135)
Thalidomide has also been used off-licence in a wide variety of dermatoses, including nodular prurigo, actinic prurigo, cutaneous lupus erythematosus, aphthous stomatitis, Behçet disease, sarcoidosis, graft-versus-host disease, Langerhans cell histiocytosis, cutaneous manifestations of advanced HIV infection and Kaposi sarcoma [**1**,2–10].

Pharmacological properties
Formula and structure
Thalidomide (empirical formula: $C_{13}H_{10}N_2O_4$; systematic name: (RS)-2-(2,6-dioxopiperidin-3-yl)-1H-isoindole-1,3(2H)-dione) is a

piperidinyl isoindole, consisting of a phthaloyl ring and a glutarimide ring. It has a chiral centre and exists as a racemic mixture of left- and right-handed enantiomers [2].

Administration
Thalidomide Celgene® is available in the UK as capsules containing 50 mg of thalidomide [11].

Pharmacokinetics
Absorption following oral administration is slow with peak plasma levels being reached within 1–5 h [12]. It appears to be degraded by non-enzymatic hydrolysis, with liver or kidney impairment having no appreciable impact on thalidomide pharmacokinetics. The mean elimination half-life after a single oral dose is 5.5–7.3 h, with a linear relationship between body weight and thalidomide clearance. It readily crosses the placenta.

Pharmacodynamics
In vitro and *in vivo*, thalidomide exerts a wide range of anti-inflammatory, immune-modulatory and antineoplastic activities. Cereblon has been identified as a key molecular target for thalidomide. This receptor forms part of the cullin-ring ligase 4 E3 ubiquitin ligase complex, binding substrates for ubiquitination and proteasomal degradation. On binding to cereblon, thalidomide causes an allosteric modification of this complex, with downstream effects dependent on the proteins that are subsequently ubiquinated. These include cytoxic, antiapoptic and teratogenic effects [13].

Potential adverse effects
Teratogenicity
In addition to phocomelia, thalidomide has been associated with congenital heart disease, ocular and aural malformations, urological abnormalities, autism and intellectual disability [14]. The critical exposure period during which it appears to exert its devastating embryopathic effects is between 20 and 36 days after conception [14–16].

Peripheral neuropathy
Peripheral neuropathy is a very significant adverse effect of thalidomide, and the predominant factor limiting its use. It occurs in 20–55% of patients, with women and the elderly at greatest risk. The peak incidence is in the first year of treatment [17,18]. The precise neurotoxic mechanism is not known but it seems likely that affected individuals may have a genetic susceptibility [19]. This results in a symmetrical, mainly sensory, length-dependent axonal polyneuropathy, with reduced sensory nerve action potential (SNAP) amplitudes and relative conservation of nerve conduction velocities [20–22]. It presents clinically as symmetrical painful parasthesiae of the hands and feet, sensory loss and, occasionally, muscle weakness or cramps, signs of pyramidal tract involvement and carpal tunnel syndrome [2]. Recovery tends to be slow and often incomplete, and neurotoxicity may even be progressive after thalidomide therapy is withdrawn [2].

Other adverse effects
See Box 19.9.

> **Box 19.9 Other adverse effects of thalidomide** [2,11]
> - Venous and arterial thrombosis
> - Endocrine effects – hypothyroidism, hypo- and hyperglycaemia, hypocalcaemia
> - Anaemia, neutropenia, lymphopenia, thrombocytopenia
> - Erythroderma, Stevens–Johnson syndrome/toxic epidermal necrolysis
> - Hypersensitivity reaction
> - Drowsiness, dizziness, depression, confusion, anxiety, agitation, anorexia
> - Intestinal obstruction and perforation
> - Dry mouth, constipation, nausea
> - Bradycardia, peripheral oedema, dyspnoea, cardiac failure
> - Decreased libido
> - Xerosis, pruritus

Contraindications
Thalidomide is absolutely contraindicated during pregnancy and for those individuals with a known sensitivity to it [1]. It should be avoided in breastfeeding mothers [11].

Cautions
Women of child-bearing potential receiving thalidomide must practise strict contraception. Men with sexual partners who are women of child-bearing potential are advised to use condoms as thalidomide is found in seminal fluid at concentrations comparable to those in the plasma.

Thalidomide is relatively contraindicated in patients with an existing peripheral neuropathy or other neurological disorder, or if there is significant renal or hepatic impairment, congestive heart failure, hypertension, hypothyroidism, gastrointestinal disease or increased risk of thrombosis [1,11].

When used in the treatment of myeloma, anticoagulation as prophylaxis for thrombosis is recommended for at least the first 5 months of treatment, particularly if there are specific risk factors such as smoking, hypertension or hyperlipidaemia [11].

Drug–drug interactions
Thalidomide may potentiate the effects of drugs that cause sedation, bradycardia or peripheral neuropathy. In women of child-bearing potential requiring oral contraception because of thalidomide therapy, the possibility of drug interactions involving the contraceptive preparation should be considered [1]. Furthermore, the combined oral contraceptive is not recommended because of the possible increased risk of thrombosis with thalidomide.

Pre-treatment screening
Thalidomide is licensed by the EMA [23] and FDA [24] and can only be prescribed and dispensed following formal registration with the aligned pregnancy prevention plan by the physician, pharmacist and patient, and fully informed consent from the patient.

Careful counselling and education of patients are necessary, alongside detailed written information.

Patients should be assessed regarding risk of thrombosis and, if considered necessary, anticoagulation commenced. A clinical neurological examination should be undertaken and baseline electrophysiological testing (measurement of SNAP amplitudes) should be considered.

In women of child-bearing potential, two reliable methods of contraception must be employed, commencing at least 1 month before therapy is started, throughout treatment and for 1 month after stopping. Pregnancy must be excluded before initiating treatment.

An FBC and renal and liver function tests should be checked.

Dose and regimens
The dose range for dermatological conditions is 50–300 mg/day, taken as a single dose at bedtime to reduce the impact of sedation.

Monitoring
Peripheral neuropathy
It is recommended that patients are examined at monthly intervals for the first 3 months of thalidomide therapy and periodically (1–6 monthly as indicated [1]) thereafter for signs or symptoms of peripheral neuropathy. Electrophysiological testing should be considered every 6 months to detect subclinical neuropathy.

Laboratory tests
Pregnancy testing should be performed monthly for women of child-bearing age, and again 4 weeks following cessation of treatment. An FBC and liver function tests should be performed monthly until the dose of thalidomide is stable, then every 2–3 months.

Antimicrobial therapies

Systemic antibiotics and antiviral, antifungal and antiparasitic drugs constitute a very significant proportion of medications prescribed by dermatologists. While the majority of antimicrobial agents are for infectious conditions, certain antibiotics, such as the tetracycline and macrolide groups, are also utilised for their anti-inflammatory properties, particularly in the treatment of acne vulgaris, rosacea, immunobullous disorders, pyoderma gangrenosum, palmoplantar pustulosis and sarcoidosis [1].

Constraints of space prevent detailed descriptions of individual antimicrobial drugs, and the reader is referred to excellent overviews [1–4].

Systemic antibiotics
There is a wide variety of orally administered antibiotics that are effective in the treatment of skin and soft-tissue infections, including penicillins, cephalosporins, macrolides, tetracyclines, fluoroquinolones, glycopeptide and lipopeptide antibiotics, rifamycins, folate synthesis inhibitors, lincosamides and oxazolidinones [5].

Penicillins
Penicillins are β-lactam antibiotics, with a β-lactam ring attached to a thiazolidine ring. They prevent stable bacterial cell wall formation by inhibiting the enzyme DD-transpeptidase, which normally catalyses peptidoglycan cross-linkage, thus weakening the structural integrity of the cell wall and resulting in cell death.

The natural first-generation penicillins were benzylpenicillin (penicillin G) and phenoxymethylpenicillin (penicillin V), active against Gram-positive cocci and bacilli, Gram-negative cocci and anaerobes. These were followed by a variety of semi-synthetic penicillins: (i) penicillinase (β-lactamase)-resistant penicillins, including flucloxacillin and dicloxacillin, active against penicillinase-producing staphylococci, and temocillin, active against Gram-negative bacteria (but not *Pseudomonas aeruginosa* or *Acinetobacter* spp.); (ii) broad spectrum penicillins, such as ampicillin and amoxicillin, which extend the activity spectrum to include Gram-negative bacilli but which are inactivated by penicillinases; (iii) extended spectrum penicillins, such as pivmecillinam, active against many Gram-negative bacteria, including *Escherichia coli* and *Klebsiella*, *Enterobacter* and *Salmonella* spp.; and (iv) antipseudomonal penicillins, including piperacillin and ticarcillin, both having a broad spectrum of activity against a range of Gram-positive and Gram-negative bacteria and anaerobes, and both available in the UK only in combination with a β-lactamase inhibitor [1,5].

Hypersensitivity is the most important adverse effect of the penicillins. Allergic reactions occur in 1–10% of exposed individuals, with anaphylaxis occurring in less than 0.05% [5]. Penicillin-allergic patients may also react to cephalosporins and other β-lactam antibiotics [5]. An ampicillin-induced pruritic maculopapular eruption in patients with infectious mononucleosis, lymphocytic leukaemia or receiving allopurinol is not truly allergic and is not a contraindication to future treatment with penicillins [1].

Cephalosporins
Cephalosporins are also β-lactam antibiotics and have the same mode of antibacterial action as the penicillins. The fusion of the β-lactam ring with a dihydrothiazine ring in cephalosporins confers a relative protection against penicillinases. There are currently five generations of cephalosporins, with the first generation having most activity against Gram-positive cocci, and subsequent generations having greater action against Gram-negative organisms and lesser action against Gram-positive bacteria.

The orally active first-generation (cefalexin, cefradine, cefadroxil), second-generation (cefaclor, cefuroxime axetil) and third-generation (cefpodoxime proxetil) cephalosporins are licensed for the treatment of skin and soft-tissue infections [5,6].

Hypersensitivity reactions are the principal adverse effect of cephalosporins [5,6]. About 0.5–6.5% of penicillin-allergic individuals will also be allergic to cephalosporins [6] and cephalosporins should be avoided if possible in patients with a history of penicillin allergy.

Carbapenems
Carbapenems are also β-lactam antibiotics, sharing the mode of action of penicillins. Like cephalosporins, they too can remain stable in the presence of penicillinases, but additionally in the presence of cephalosporinase. They therefore have a broad spectrum of activity against aerobic, anaerobic, Gram-positive and Gram-negative bacteria (including *Pseudomonas aeruginosia* and *Enterococcus*). They are often used to treat multidrug-resistant bacterial infections, however the evolution of carbapenemases has resulted in developing resistance. Carbapenems include imipenem, meropenem, ertapenem, doripenem, panipenem, biapenem and tebipenem. Cross-reactivity rates in those with penicillin allergy are high so, where possible, they should be avoided in those with a known penicillin allergy.

Macrolides

The macrolide group of antibiotics (with the azalide and ketolide subclasses) includes erythromycin, clarithromycin, azithromycin and telithromycin, with a structure that includes a macrocyclic lactone ring. They exert a bacteriostatic action by binding reversibly to the 50S subunit of the bacterial ribosome, thus inhibiting bacterial protein synthesis [1]. Macrolides also have anti-inflammatory properties unrelated to their antibiotic action. They have an antibacterial spectrum that is similar to penicillin, and so erythromycin has traditionally been an alternative in penicillin-allergic patients [5]. The emergence of resistant strains of *Staphylococcus aureus* and streptococci (as well as *Propionibacterium acnes*), together with its gastrointestinal side effects and CYP inhibition (resulting in a number of potential drug interactions), has limited the clinical usefulness of erythromycin [1,5]. QT interval prolongation and cardiac arrhythmias are rare adverse effects.

Tetracyclines

The tetracycline class of antibiotics is broad spectrum and bacteriostatic, and includes tetracycline, oxytetracycline, doxycycline, lymecycline, minocycline and demeclocycline. They have a basic four-hydrocarbon ring structure and inhibit bacterial protein synthesis by binding to the 30S ribosomal subunit [1]. Their clinical usefulness has lessened with increasing bacterial resistance [5], but they are the most common antibiotics prescribed by dermatologists [1], usually for their anti-inflammatory properties but also for the treatment of Lyme disease and atypical mycobacterial infections. Modified-release (subantimicrobial) preparations of doxycycline and minocycline appear to minimise the development of antibiotic resistance without loss of anti-inflammatory effect [1]. They are contraindicated in children and in pregnant or breastfeeding women as they are incorporated in growing bones and teeth. With the exception of doxycycline and minocycline, tetracyclines may exacerbate renal impairment [5]. Photosensitivity, hypersensitivity reactions, dyspigmentation and benign intracranial hypertension are potential side effects [5]. Minocycline may induce a lupus-like syndrome and vasculitis.

Tigecycline is a glycylcycline, structurally similar to the tetracyclines with a similar mechanism of action, used in the treatment of complicated skin and soft-tissue infections [5].

Fluoroquinolones

The quinolones are a family of synthetic broad spectrum antibiotics, with a structure based on a quinoline ring system. Their antibiotic effect results from the inhibition of topoisomerases, which prevents bacterial DNA from unwinding and replicating. Ciprofloxacin, levofloxacin, moxifloxacin and ofloxacin are licensed for the treatment of skin and soft-tissue infections, although staphylococcal resistance to the quinolones is common [5]; their use should be avoided in meticillin-resistant *Staphylococcus aureus* (MRSA) infections. They are effective against most Gram-negative organisms, including *Pseudomonas aeruginosa*, and are also active against mycobacteria and in anthrax [1]. Tendon damage may occur with quinoline therapy [5].

Glycopeptides

Vancomycin and teicoplanin are glycopeptide antibiotics that work by inhibiting synthesis and cross-binding of peptides in the cell wall of Gram-positive bacteria via a mechanism different to the β-lactams. They have bactericidal activity against Gram-positive bacteria, including multiresistant staphylococci (such as MRSA) and *Clostridium difficile*. Because of poor gastrointestinal absorption, vancomycin and teicoplanin are administered parenterally but can be given orally in the treatment of *C. difficile*. Monitoring of the plasma concentrations of vancomycin (and teicoplanin, in certain circumstances) is required [5].

Daptomycin

Daptomycin is a lipopeptide antibiotic with a spectrum of activity similar to vancomycin. Its mechanism of action involves depolarisation of bacterial cell membranes, which results in inhibition of protein and nucleic acid synthesis and subsequent cell death. It is given intravenously and should be reserved for complicated skin and soft-tissue infections caused by resistant Gram-positive bacteria, including MRSA [5,6].

Rifamycins

The rifamycins include rifampicin and rifabutin. Their antibacterial action is the result of binding to bacterial RNA polymerase, causing 'steric occlusion' which prevents RNA transcription. Rifampicin has a broad spectrum of activity including mycobacteria, staphylococci and *Neisseria* and is the rifamycin most commonly used by dermatologists worldwide, mainly for the treatment of cutaneous tuberculosis, atypical mycobacterial infection, leprosy, leishmaniasis and *S. aureus* infections [1]. In combination with clindamycin it is frequently used to treat such chronic inflammatory dermatoses as hidradenitis suppurativa, folliculitis decalvans and dissecting cellulitis. The rapid development of bacterial resistance to the rifamycins is the reason why they are usually used in combination with other antibiotics, rather than as monotherapy. Rifampicin is a potent inducer of the CYP system and this may result in reduced blood concentrations of a wide range of concomitantly administered drugs.

Folate synthesis inhibitors

Sulfonamides inhibit dihydropteroate synthetase and trimethoprim inhibits DHFR. In combination, sulfamethoxazole and trimethoprim (co-trimoxazole) act synergistically to inhibit production of tetrahydrofolic acid, an essential component of thymidine synthesis, lack of which interferes with bacterial DNA formation. Folate synthesis inhibitors are bacteriostatic against a variety of Gram-positive aerobic cocci and certain Gram-negative organisms and protozoa [1]. Co-trimoxazole, as well as having significant antibiotic uses, is also an unlicensed alternative treatment for acne (as is trimethoprim alone) and hidradenitis suppurativa [1]. The major side effects are Stevens–Johnson syndrome and blood dyscrasias.

Lincosamides

Clindamycin is a semi-synthetic derivative of lincomycin, with a similar mechanism of action to the macrolides. It is bacteriostatic to Gram-positive cocci and against many anaerobes [5], including *P. acnes*. It is an alternative to the macrolides in the treatment of erysipelas or cellulitis in penicillin-allergic patients [5]. Clindamycin can also be useful in MRSA infections so long as lincosamide resistance has not developed. Potentially fatal antibiotic-associated colitis is perhaps the most concerning side effect, and treatment with clindamycin should be stopped immediately should diarrhoea develop.

Oxazolidinones
Linezolid has an oxazolidinone core and is a protein synthesis inhibitor, consequent to binding to the 23S portion of the 50S bacterial ribosomal subunit [1]. It is active against Gram-positive bacteria including MRSA and vancomycin-resistant enterococci [5]. Haematopoietic disorders and severe optic neuropathy are the main adverse effects [5].

Anti-inflammatory effects of antibiotics
The mechanisms by which the tetracyclines and erythromycin exert anti-inflammatory effects are incompletely understood. However, their beneficial effects in acne may be based on inhibition of the fibroblast growth factor receptor 2 (FGFR2) signalling cascade, which is thought to play a role in sebaceous gland function and follicular hyperkeratinisation in that condition [7]. Tetracyclines may inhibit FGFR2b-mediated overexpression of matrix metalloproteinases, and erythromycin may attenuate FGFR2 signalling via an inhibitory effect on CYP and consequent interference of endogenous retinoid catabolism and amplification of endogenous retinoid signalling [7,8]. Furthermore, decreased nuclear levels of the transcription factor Fox01 and increased activity of the protein synthesis regulator mTORC1 have been implicated in the pathogenesis of acne [9,10]: it has been shown that tetracyclines and erythromycin may enhance nuclear Fox01 activity and inhibit mTORC1 [10,11].

Antifungal drugs
The medically important systemic antifungal drugs can be broadly classified by their mechanistic properties into those that act on the fungal wall or cell membrane and those that act intracellularly.

The fungal wall/cell membrane agents are subdivided into those that inhibit ergosterol (a molecule unique to fungi and an integral part of the fungal cell membrane) function and those that inhibit β-glucan synthase.

The ergosterol inhibitors are categorised into the azoles (inhibitors of lanosterol 14α demethylase, essential for the synthesis of ergosterol), allylamines (inhibitors of squalene epoxidase, also essential in ergosterol synthesis, such as *terbinafine*) and polyene antifungals (such as *nystatin* and *amphotericin*, which bind to ergosterol and thereby interfere with the integrity of the fungal cell membrane).

The systemically active azoles are further subdivided into the imidazoles (based on a five-membered aromatic ring with two nitrogen and three carbon atoms, and including *ketoconazole*) and triazoles (based on a five-membered ring with three nitrogen and two carbon atoms, and including *fluconazole, itraconazole, posaconazole* and *voriconazole*). Lanosterol 14α demethylase is CYP dependent and the imidazoles and triazoles have different inhibitory effects on CYP.

The β-glucan synthase inhibitors interfere with the synthesis of glucan, an important component of the fungal cell wall, and are represented by the echinocandin antifungals (*anidulafungin, caspofungin* and *micafungin*).

The antifungal drugs that have intracellular mechanisms of action include *flucytosine*, a pyrimidine analogue that inhibits fungal DNA and RNA synthesis, and *griseofulvin*, a spiro-benzo[b] furan [2] that inhibits fungal mitosis by binding to tubulin and thereby disrupting microtubule function.

Dermatological uses
Triazole antifungals
Fluconazole is well absorbed orally, and its dermatological uses include dermatophyte infections (tinea), pityriasis versicolor and mucocutaneous candidosis [5]. It should be used with caution in those at risk of cardiac arrythmias [2].

Itraconazole is indicated for dermatophytosis, onychomycosis, pityriasis versicolor, mucosal candidosis, aspergillosis, histoplasmosis and cryptococcosis. Rarely it may cause severe hepatotoxicity, and liver function should be monitored if it is used for longer than 1 month [5]. It has been associated with heart failure and cardiac arrhythmias in those at risk [5]. Itraconazole can be used to treat onychomycosis in a 'pulsed' fashion (treatment for 1 week, repeated after an interval of 3 weeks; two courses for fingernails and three courses for toenails) [5].

Posaconazole and voriconazole are rarely used for dermatological reasons.

Imidazole antifungals
Oral ketoconazole has a place as second line treatment for dermatophytoses, mucocutaneous candidosis and *Malassezia* (pityrosporum) folliculitis when the oral triazoles and terbinafine are ineffective or poorly tolerated. Potentially life-threatening hepatotoxicity can rarely occur and liver function should be monitored [5].

Allylamine antifungals
Oral terbinafine is indicated for dermatophyte infections of the skin and nails. Although it is not licensed for use in children, it has been widely used off-label in this group of patients. Hepatotoxicity and a lupus erythematosus-like condition have been reported.

Polyene antifungals
Neither nystatin nor amphotericin is absorbed from the gastrointestinal tract. Nystatin is effective against *Candida*, and can be used orally to treat oesophageal and genital *Candida* infections and to prevent fungal infections in immunocompromised patients.

Amphotericin is active against most fungi and yeasts and can be given parenterally for severe systemic and deep mycoses [5].

Echinocandin antifungals
The echinocandin antifungals are active only against *Aspergillus* spp. and *Candida* spp., and are rarely used for dermatological indications [5].

Flucytosine
Flucytosine is used intravenously for systemic fungal (including yeast) infections, such as cryptococcal meningitis and severe systemic candidosis, but not for cutaneous disorders [5].

Griseofulvin
Griseofulvin is indicated for dermatophyte infections of the skin and nails, although it has been largely superseded by the newer azole and allylamine antifungals [2,5]. In contrast to terbinafine it has a product licence for use in children. It can be hepatotoxic and may exacerbate lupus erythematosus and the acute porphyrias [5].

Antiviral drugs
Dermatological uses
The systemic antiviral drugs of most relevance to dermatological practice are those used to treat herpesvirus infections, in particular HSV and VZV.

Guanosine analogues
The three main drugs are aciclovir, valaciclovir (a prodrug of aciclovir) and famciclovir (a prodrug of penciclovir). Foscarnet is indicated for mucocutaneous HSV infection unresponsive to aciclovir in immunocompromised individuals. Inosine pranobex is also licensed for herpes simplex infections, although it is not widely used [12].

Aciclovir (chemical name: acycloguanosine) is a guanosine analogue. It is phosphorylated by viral thymidine kinase to aciclovir monophosphate and then enzymes in the host cell convert it to aciclovir triphosphate, which inactivates viral DNA polymerase, preventing viral DNA synthesis and thus replication [3]. Valaciclovir, an ester of aciclovir, has a much greater oral bioavailability than aciclovir; it is de-esterified *in vivo* to aciclovir. Famciclovir is converted to penciclovir which, after phosphorylation to penciclovir triphosphate, inhibits viral DNA polymerase in the same way as aciclovir, although penciclovir triphosphate has a much longer intracellular half-life in herpesvirus-infected cells than aciclovir triphosphate [3].

These drugs are indicated in the treatment of severe herpes simplex infections, suppression of recurrent herpes simplex infections, herpes zoster, herpes simplex and varicella-zoster in immunocompromised patients, eczema herpeticum and recurrent erythema multiforme.

Key references

The full list of references can be found in the online version at https://www.wiley.com/rooksdermatology10e

Introduction
1 BMJ Best Practice. *What is GRADE?* https://bestpractice.bmj.com/info/toolkit/learn-ebm/what-is-grade/ (last accessed August 2023).

Anti-inflammatory and immunomodulatory drugs
Antimalarial agents
18 Marmor MF, Kellner U, Lai TY, Melles RB, Mieler WF. Recommendations on screening for chloroquine and hydroxychloroquine retinopathy – 2016. *Ophthalmology* 2016;123:1386–94.
24 Callen JP, Camisa C. Antimalarial agents. In: Wolverton SE, Wu JJ, eds. *Comprehensive Dermatologic Drug Therapy*, 4th edn. London: Elsevier, 2021:234–44.

Azathioprine
13 Meggitt SJ, Anstey AV, Mohd Mustapa MF et al. British Association of Dermatologists' guidelines for the safe and effective prescribing of azathioprine 2011. *Br J Dermatol* 2011;165:711–34.

Ciclosporin
1 Berth-Jones J, Exton LS, Ladoyanni E et al. British Association of Dermatologists guidelines for the safe and effective prescribing of oral ciclosporin in dermatology 2018. *Br J Dermatol* 2019;180:1312–38.
5 Maza A, Montaudié H, Sbidian E et al. Oral cyclosporin in psoriasis: a systematic review on treatment modalities, risk of kidney toxicity and evidence for use in non-plaque psoriasis. *J Eur Acad Dermatol Venereol* 2011;25:19–27.

Colchicine
2 Davis LS, LeBlanc KG, Knable AL, Owen CE. Miscellaneous systemic drugs: colchicine. In: Wolverton SE, Wu JJ, eds. *Comprehensive Dermatologic Drug Therapy*, 4th edn. London: Elsevier, 2021:445–64.

Fumarates
12 Ermis U, Weis J, Schulz JB. PML in a patient treated with fumaric acid. *N Engl J Med* 2013;368:1657–8.
13 Nast A, Boehncke W-H, Mrowietz U et al. S3 – Guidelines on the treatment of psoriasis vulgaris (English version). Update. *J Deutsch Dermatol Gesellsch* 2012;10:S1–95.

Systemic glucocorticoids
1 Wolverton SE, Rancour EA. Systemic corticosteroids. In: Wolverton SE, Wu JJ, eds. *Comprehensive Dermatologic Drug Therapy*, 4th edn. London: Elsevier, 2021:133–55.

Hydroxycarbamide
2 Smith CH. Use of hydroxyurea in psoriasis. *Clin Exp Dermatol* 1999;24:2–6.
3 High WA. Cytotoxic agents. In: Wolverton SE, Wu JJ, eds. *Comprehensive Dermatologic Drug Therapy*, 4th edn. London: Elsevier, 2021:209–21.

Methotrexate
1 Callen JP, Kulp-Shorten CL. Methotrexate. In: Wolverton SE, Wu JJ, eds. *Comprehensive Dermatologic Drug Therapy*, 4th edn. London: Elsevier, 2021:156–68.
10 Solomon DH, Glynn RJ, Karlson EW et al. Adverse effects of low-dose methotrexate: a randomized trial. *Ann Intern Med* 2020;172:369–80.

Mycophenolate mofetil
1 Schadt CR, Zwerner JP. Mycophenolate mofetil and mycophenolic acid. In: Wolverton SE, Wu JJ, eds. *Comprehensive Dermatologic Drug Therapy*, 4th edn. London: Elsevier, 2021:178–86.
2 Orvis AK, Wesson SK, Breza TS, Jr, Church AA, Mitchell CL, Watkins SW. Mycophenolate mofetil in dermatology. *J Am Acad Dermatol* 2009;60:183–99.

Potassium iodide
1 Davis LS, LeBlanc KG, Knable AL, Owen CE. Miscellaneous systemic drugs: potassium iodide. In: Wolverton SE, Wu JJ, eds. *Comprehensive Dermatologic Drug Therapy*, 4th edn. London: Elsevier, 2021:445–64.

Biologic therapies (protein therapeutics)
13 Waljee AK, Higgins PDR, Jensen CB et al. Anti-tumour necrosis factor-α therapy and recurrent or new primary cancers in patients with inflammatory bowel disease, rheumatoid arthritis, or psoriasis and previous cancer in Denmark: a nationwide, population-based cohort study. *Lancet Gastroenterol Hepatol* 2020;5:276–84.
21 Sbidian E, Chaimani A, Garcia-Doval I et al. Systemic pharmacological treatments for chronic plaque psoriasis: a network meta-analysis. *Cochrane Database Syst Rev* 2021;Issue 4:CD011535.
45 Ntatsaki E, Carruthers D, Chakravarty K et al. BSR and BHPR guideline for the management of adults with ANCA-associated vasculitis. *Rheumatology* 2014;53:2306–9.

Intravenous immunoglobulin therapy
2 Goerge T, Luger TA. Intravenous immunoglobulin therapy. In: Wolverton SE, Wu JJ, eds. *Comprehensive Dermatologic Drug Therapy*, 4th edn. London: Elsevier, 2021:397–404.

Systemic retinoids
5 Patton TJ, Ferris LK. Systemic retinoids. In: Wolverton SE, Wu JJ, eds. *Comprehensive Dermatologic Drug Therapy*, 4th edn. London: Elsevier, 2021:245–62.
33 Ormerod AD, Campalani E, Goodfield MJ. British Association of Dermatologists guidelines on the efficacy and use of acitretin in dermatology. *Br J Dermatol* 2010;162:952–63.

Thalidomide

1 Davis LS, LeBlanc KG, Knable AL, Owen CE. Miscellaneous systemic drugs: thalidomide. In: Wolverton SE, Wu JJ, eds. *Comprehensive Dermatologic Drug Therapy*, 4th edn. London: Elsevier, 2021:445–64.

Antimicrobial therapies

1 Kim S, Brent DM, Kim GK, Del Rosso JQ. Systemic antibacterial agents. In: Wolverton SE, Wu JJ, eds. *Comprehensive Dermatologic Drug Therapy*, 4th edn. London: Elsevier, 2021:69–98.

2 Gupta AK. Systemic antifungal agents. In: Wolverton SE, Wu JJ, eds. *Comprehensive Dermatologic Drug Therapy*, 4th edn. London: Elsevier, 2021:99–113.

3 Magel GD, Haitz KA, Lapolla WJ *et al*. Systemic antiviral agents. In: Wolverton SE, Wu JJ, eds. *Comprehensive Dermatologic Drug Therapy*, 4th edn. London: Elsevier, 2021:114–25.

4 Elston D. Systemic antiparasitic agents. In: Wolverton SE, Wu JJ, eds. *Comprehensive Dermatologic Drug Therapy*, 4th edn. London: Elsevier, 2021:126–32.

CHAPTER 20
Principles of Skin Surgery

S. Walayat Hussain[1], Christopher J. Miller[2] and Timothy S. Wang[3]

[1]Leeds Centre for Dermatology, Chapel Allerton Hospital, Leeds Teaching Hospitals NHS Trust, Leeds, UK
[2]Penn Dermatology Oncology Center, Hospital of the University of Pennsylvania, Philadelphia, PA, USA
[3]Cutaneous Surgery Unit and Micrographic Surgery and Dermatologic Oncology (Mohs) Fellowship Program, Johns Hopkins Health System, Baltimore, MD, USA

Introduction, 20.1
Critical anatomical considerations, 20.1
Head and neck, 20.1
Limbs, 20.4
Ideal tissue planes for excising and undermining, 20.4
Presurgical equipment, local anaesthetic and biopsy techniques, 20.4
Equipment and sterilisation, 20.4
Safety aspects, 20.6
Local anaesthetics, 20.7
Biopsy techniques, 20.8
Preoperative preparation, 20.11
Surgical procedures and techniques, 20.11
Simple excision, suture technique and wound closure, 20.11
Reconstruction, 20.19
Mohs micrographic surgery, 20.30
Dressings and postoperative care, 20.37
Complications, 20.40

Electrocautery and electrosurgery, 20.42
Electrocautery, 20.42
Electrosurgery, 20.43
Cryosurgery, 20.46
Clinical methods, 20.46
Clinical uses, 20.46
Side effects, 20.46
Caustics, 20.47
Intralesional corticosteroid therapy, 20.47
Surgical indications, 20.47
Intralesional therapies for skin malignancies, 20.47
Miscellaneous surgical procedures and techniques, 20.48
Curettage, 20.48
Haemostasis for open wounds, 20.48
Snip excision, 20.48
Management of specific conditions, 20.49
Epidermoid cysts, 20.49
Lipomas, 20.49

Hidradenitis suppurativa, 20.49
Chondrodermatitis nodularis, 20.49
Digital myxoid cysts, 20.49
Axillary and palmar hyperhidrosis, 20.49
Hypertrophic scars and keloids, 20.49
Lesions on the shoulder, upper back and sternum, 20.49
Benign naevi, 20.49
Non-melanoma skin cancer: basal cell and squamous cell carcinomas, 20.49
Lesions of the mucous membranes, 20.49
Keratoacanthoma, 20.50
Pigmented lesions, 20.50
Minor skin lesions: mollusca, milia and comedones, 20.50
Acknowledgement, 20.50
Video legends, 20.50
Key references, 20.50

Introduction

The acquisition of dermatological surgery skills is an integral component of dermatological training. Indeed, the increasing burden of skin cancer has resulted in competence in dermatological surgery being a mandatory requirement for all dermatologists. This chapter provides an overview of the fundamental basics of skin surgery and provides an introduction to more advanced surgical techniques, including Mohs micrographic surgery (MMS). For more in-depth coverage a selection of introductory [1,2,3] and intermediate textbooks [4,5,6] are be recommended.

Critical anatomical considerations

A knowledge of critical anatomy is essential for efficient and safe surgery [1,2–7,8,9]. This section outlines critical anatomic structures and relationships.

Head and neck
Blood vessels of the face

The external carotid artery and its branches supply most of the soft tissue of the head and neck. The two major branches of the external carotid artery are the superficial temporal and facial arteries (Figure 20.1). The veins of the face generally accompany the arteries. A notable exception is the angular vein, which runs laterally and independently to the angular artery.

The superficial temporal artery, the terminal branch of the external carotid artery, supplies the soft tissue of the lateral cheek, temple, forehead and scalp. Its pulse can first be palpated as it emerges anterior to the tragus between the condyle of the mandible and the external auditory meatus. The superficial temporal artery travels superiorly anterior to the ear then divides into the temporal and parietal branches approximately 2 cm superior to the zygomatic arch. The temporal branch of the superficial temporal artery is often visible through the skin immediately anterior to the temporal hairline. It anastomoses at the lateral forehead with branches of the

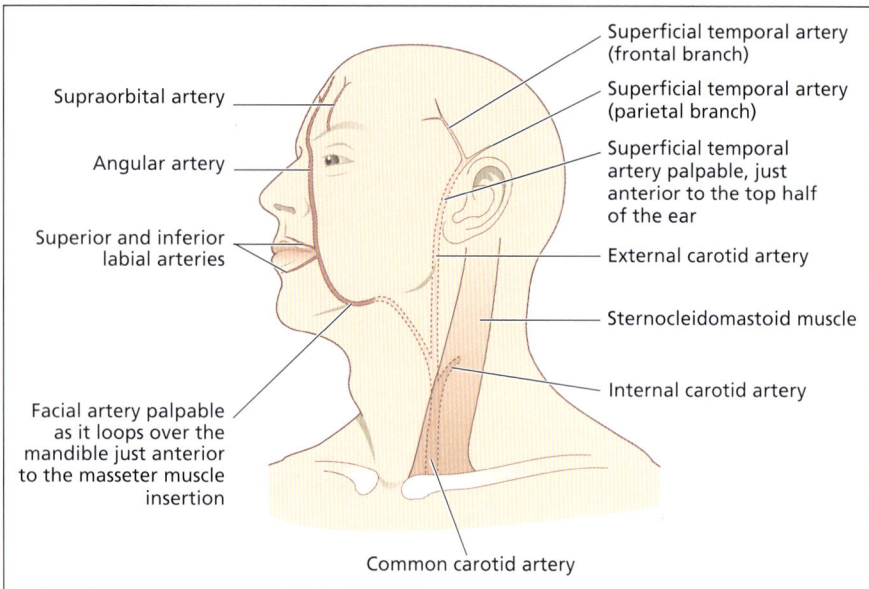

Figure 20.1 Arteries of the head and neck encountered in skin surgery. The labial artery lies on the inside (mucosal) surface of the lip approximately 5 mm from the visible vermilion border. (---) Arteries that are rarely encountered are indicated with dashed lines and arteries that are frequently identified during superficial skin surgery on the face are given as solid red lines.

ipsilateral supraorbital artery from the internal carotid system. The parietal branch may be palpated along its course over the temporal and parietal scalp. The superficial temporal artery and its branches run in the deep subcutaneous fat immediately superficial to the superficial fascia (superficial temporal fascia on the temple; galea aponeurotica on the scalp). Local anaesthesia may be injected to hydrodissect the fat from the superficial fascia, making it easier to preserve the arteries during excision and reconstruction.

The facial artery (Figure 20.1) supplies blood to the soft tissues of the medial cheek, lips, chin and lateral nose. Its pulse can first be palpated along the margin of the mandible immediately anterior to the masseter muscle. As it travels superomedially along the naso-labial fold, it sends named branches to the chin, lips, and nose. It continues in the naso-facial sulcus as the angular artery and anastomoses with the internal carotid system at the medial canthus.

The internal carotid artery supplies blood to a mask-like region of the central face, including the central forehead and upper two-thirds of the central nose. The central forehead is supplied by the supraorbital and supratrochlear arteries after they emerge from the orbit. The upper two-thirds of the central nose is supplied by the external nasal artery. Inadvertent injection of filler into the branches of the internal carotid artery can cause blindness if filler travels retrograde to occlude the central artery of the retina.

Lymphatics of the face

The lymphatic system produces lymphocytes, drains fluid from the extracellular space back into the bloodstream and defends the body from infection and cancer. Cancer spreads to lymph nodes along routes of lymphatic drainage, therefore surgeons must know which parts of the body drain to which lymph node basins. Lymphatics of the face generally follow the venous drainage and course inferiorly and posteriorly. Midfacial lymphatics drain into the facial, submental and submandibular lymph nodes. The lateral face and frontotemporal scalp lymphatics drain into the parotid lymph nodes. The parietal scalp drains to the parotid lymph nodes anteriorly and the retroauricular (mastoid) nodes posteriorly. The occipital scalp drains posteriorly into the occipital lymph nodes.

Sensory nerves of the face

Sensation to the face is supplied by the trigeminal cranial nerve (CN V). Since the target organ of the sensory nerves is the skin, skin surgery may transect nerve branches and cause temporary or permanent anaesthesia. If the proximal nerve has not been transected, sensation may gradually return over approximately 12 months. During preoperative consent, patients should be advised of the possibility of sensory damage.

CN V has three divisions: the ophthalmic (V1), maxillary (V2) and mandibular (V3). For precise injections of anaesthesia, it is important to know the distribution of each division and the location of the main nerve branches (Figure 20.2).

The ophthalmic division supplies sensation to the forehead, anterior scalp and nasal dorsum. Its largest branches are the supratrochlear and supraorbital nerves. The maxillary division supplies sensation to the cheek, the conjunctiva and skin of the lower eyelid, the side of the nose and the nasal vestibule, and the skin of the upper lip. Its largest cutaneous branch is the infraorbital nerve. The mandibular division supplies sensation to the chin, lower lip, beard distribution of the cheek and the upper third of the auricle. Its most accessible cutaneous branches are the mental and auriculotemporal nerves.

The supraorbital, infraorbital and mental nerves emerge from the skull via the palpable foramina, and all lie in the same plane, just medial to a mid-pupillary vertical line [10]. Targeted nerve blocks at the foramina block the skin supplied by each branch.

Sensation to the neck and posterior scalp is supplied by the cervical nerves CN II–IV. Large areas of the posterior scalp, neck and lower ear can be anaesthetised by injecting local anaesthesia along the posterior border of the middle third of the sternocleidomastoid muscle approximately 10–20 mm above and below the Erb point, where the great auricular, transverse cervical and lesser occipital nerves emerge [11]. The Erb point is located where a plumb line from the midpoint of a line drawn between the mastoid process and the angle of the jaw intersects with the posterior border of the sternocleidomastoid muscle. The spinal accessory nerve (CN XI) also emerges from behind the sternocleidomastoid muscle

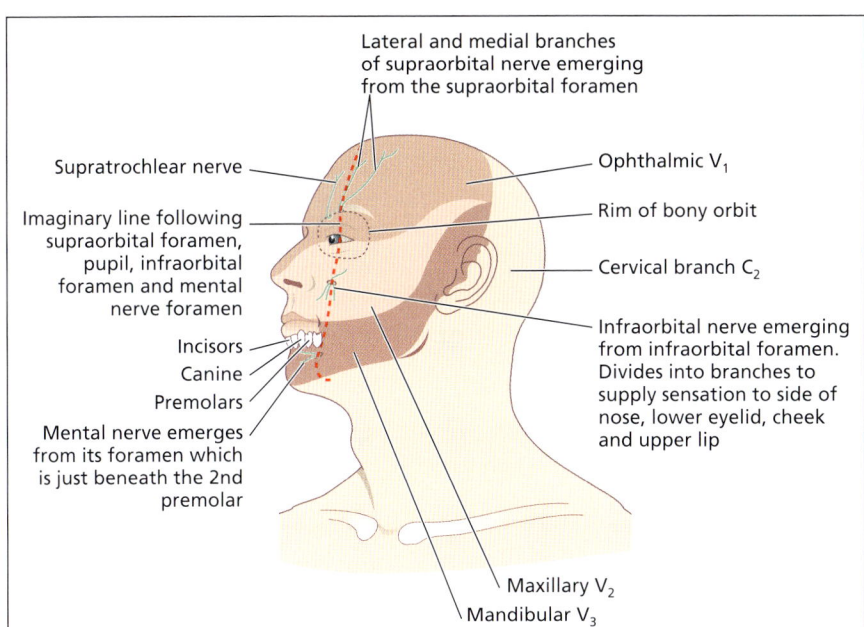

Figure 20.2 Sensory nerves on the face used in nerve block anaesthesia. Sensation on the face is served by the three main divisions of the trigeminal nerve: the ophthalmic, maxillary and mandibular divisions. Three important branches of these nerves – the supraorbital, infraorbital and mental nerves – emerge in the same plane along a vertical line running through the pupil.

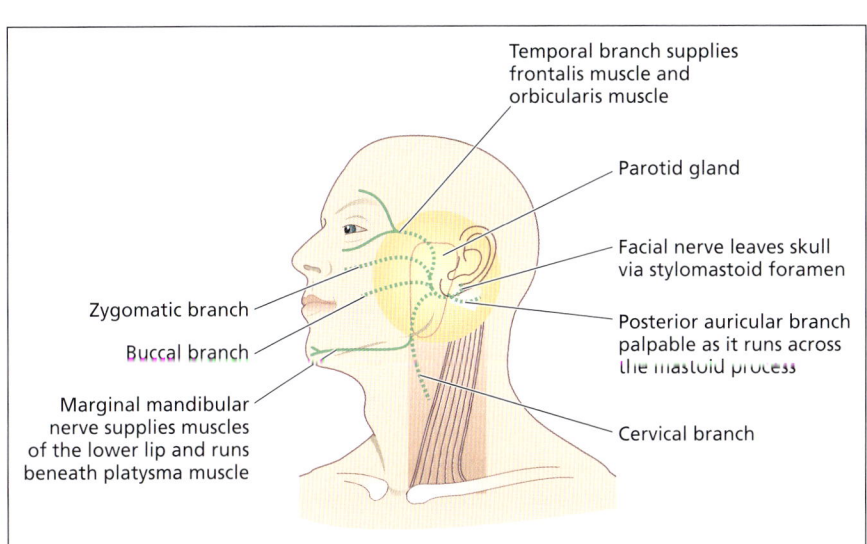

Figure 20.3 Motor branches of the facial nerve vulnerable in skin surgery. (---) Nerves that are rarely encountered are indicated with dashed lines and nerves at risk during superficial skin surgery on the face are given as solid green lines.

near the Erb point, but this motor nerve is rarely affected by the local anaesthesia, as it lies deep to the superficial layer of the deep cervical fascia [12].

Motor nerves of the head and neck

The facial nerve (CN VII) provides motor innervation to the muscles of facial expression. The main trunk of the facial nerve exits the stylomastoid foramen approximately 6–8 mm medial (deep) to the trypanomastoid suture line. The main trunk immediately enters the parotid gland before dividing into its five main branches: temporal, zygomatic, buccal, marginal mandibular and cervical. The branches emerge from the parotid and innervate the muscles of facial expression from their lateral undersurface, except for three deep muscles (buccinator, levator anguli oris and mentalis), which are innervated at their superficial surface.

The temporal and marginal mandibular nerves are the branches at greatest risk for injury during skin surgery (Figure 20.3).

The temporal branch of the facial nerve innervates the frontalis, corrugator supercilii and superior portion of the orbicularis oculi muscles. After exiting the parotid gland, it runs deep to the superficial fascia approximately along a line connecting a point 0.5 cm inferior to the tragus and a point 1.5 cm superior to the lateral eyebrow. Transecting the nerve makes the patient unable to wrinkle the ipsilateral forehead or raise the ipsilateral brow (Figure 20.4).

The marginal mandibular nerve innervates the lip depressors. The marginal mandibular branch of the facial nerve exits from the anteroinferior portion of parotid gland near the angle of the mandible. The nerve travels medially toward the chin either slightly above or up to 3 cm inferior to the lower border of the mandible. When the nerve crosses over the facial artery (its pulse may be palpated at the anterior border of the masseter muscle along the margin of the mandible), it courses superior to the border of the mandible before entering the lateral undersurface of the lip depressors. The nerve is always deep to the platysma muscle. Transecting

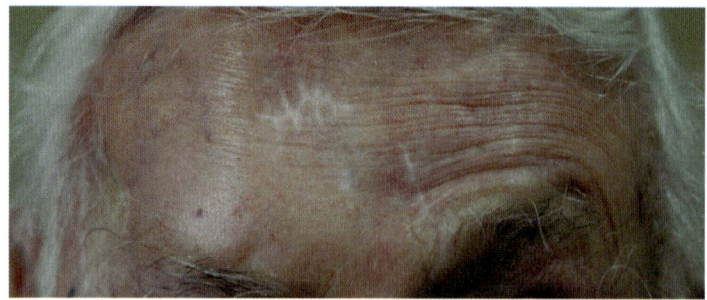

Figure 20.4 Nerve damage: transection of the temporal branch of the facial nerve resulting in ipsilateral paralysis of the frontalis muscle.

the nerve renders the patient unable to depress the ipsilateral lower lip, resulting in drooling and asymmetry of the mouth when smiling or grimacing.

The spinal accessory nerve (CN XI) provides motor innervation to the sternocleidomastoid and trapezius muscles. The nerve is vulnerable to transection in the posterior triangle of the neck, where it runs immediately deep to the superficial layer of the deep cervical fascia (Figure 20.5). To approximate the course of the nerve in the posterior triangle, divide the sternocleidomastoid muscle into thirds. CN XI enters the posterior triangle at the posterior border of the sternocleidomastoid muscle near the junction of its upper and middle thirds. It courses posteroinferiorly until it enters the trapezius at a horizontal angle from the junction of the middle and inferior thirds of the sternocleidomastoid muscle. Transecting CN XI causes weakness and wasting of the ipsilateral trapezius, resulting in drooping and chronic aching of the ipsilateral shoulder as well as difficulty abducting the arm superior to horizontal. Lateral winging of the scapula may be elicited on examination by asking the patient to push against a wall with their arms horizontally extended.

Limbs

The only superficial motor nerve on the limbs is on the lateral aspect of the knee, where the common peroneal nerve (lateral popliteal) can be palpated against the bone as it winds round the neck of the fibula. Injury to the nerve at this site will produce a foot drop resulting from paralysis of the foot dorsiflexors and elevators.

The sensory innervation of the hand is supplied by branches of the radial, ulnar and median nerves. Digital sensory nerves and arteries run together in a neurovascular bundle along the lateral aspects of the fingers. Care should be taken when obtaining haemostasis on the lateral finger to avoid damage to the associated nerve. Loss of sensation can occur distal to the site of injury.

Postoperative lymphatic leakage sometimes occurs after lower limb or axillary excision. This resolves spontaneously with conservative management.

Ideal tissue planes for excising and undermining

When excising or undermining tissue, the preferred anatomical plane should protect the motor nerves and minimise bleeding (Table 20.1).

Presurgical equipment, local anaesthetic and biopsy techniques

Equipment and sterilisation

Although most dermatological surgical procedures can be safely performed in well-lit, dedicated out-patient units using relatively simple equipment and surgical instruments [1,2,3], the absence of a need for either expensive equipment or a completely sterile environment does not justify the use of inadequate facilities or inappropriate equipment.

Dermatological surgery ranges from superficial tissue destruction and removal to complex surgical excision and repair. A range of basic surgical instruments for commonly performed procedures should be available to all dermatologists. The basic equipment, with optional items that should be available for those who undertake more specialised procedures, is shown in Box 20.1. Advanced skin surgery (e.g. excision with or without margin control and complex repair for extensive tumours) requires both dedicated facilities and specialised surgical instruments to achieve the best results.

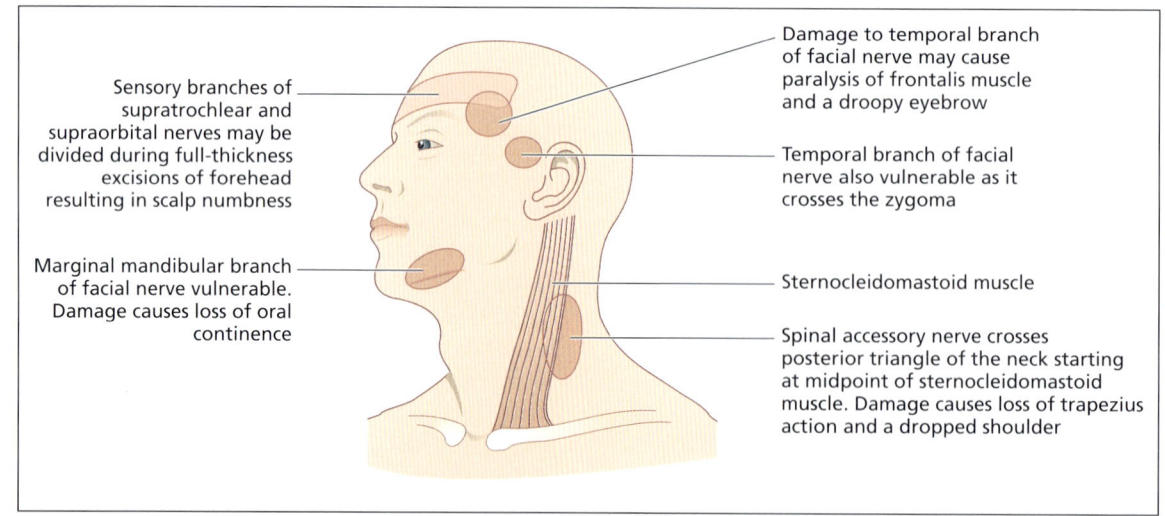

Figure 20.5 Potential surgical hazard sites to nerves during skin surgery on the head. Reproduced from Lawrence 2002 [13] with permission of Elsevier.

Table 20.1 Undermining levels in surgical procedures.

Anatomical location	Preferred anatomic plane	Comments and critical structures to consider
Trunk and extremities	Junction of subcutaneous fat and deep fascia	In areas on the trunk and proximal extremities, with a thicker layer of subcutaneous fat, the ideal surgical plane is the junction between the tightly organised, compact, columnar fat lobules adherent to the underside of the dermis and the underlying, looser, larger and more disorganised fat lobules that invest and obscure the fascia
Lateral face and neck	Junction of subcutaneous fat and superficial fascia	The motor branches from the facial nerve always lie deep to the superficial fascia. Excision at the junction of the subcutaneous fat and superficial fascia will always protect the motor nerves
Central third of face and scalp	Junction of subcutaneous fat and superficial fascia *or* Deep to the muscles of superficial fascia or galea (on scalp)	Because the branches of the facial nerve have arborised before reaching the central third of the face, excision deep to the muscles of facial expression in the central face is less likely to cause motor deficits (e.g. excision of the midline and paramedian frontalis muscle does not leave a motor deficit on the forehead). On the midline nose, forehead and scalp, undermining deep to the superficial fascia is frequently desirable

Box 20.1 Essential surgical equipment

Equipment
- Examination couch accessible from both sides with adjustable backrest
- Stool for surgeon
- Good-quality manoeuvrable lighting source
- Electrosurgical unit (e.g. hyfrecator):
  - Handpieces for both monopolar and bipolar electrosurgery (or electrocautery)
- Electrocautery device (pen or unit)
- Sharps container
- Autoclave or other mechanism for instrument sterilisation and related packaging
- Cryosurgery gun
- Optional:
  - Operating theatre table, adjustable back-, head-, arm- and footrest
  - Overhead theatre lights
  - Additional seating
  - Hand mirrors

Disposables

General
- Clean, non-sterile disposable examination gloves (latex-free preferred)
- Alcohol-based hand sanitiser
- Alcohol prep pads
- Non-sterile clean examination gloves
- Skin markers
- Eye and face protection
- Cotton-tipped applicators/gauze swabs

Haemostasis
- 30–50% aluminium chloride in alcohol
- Silver nitrate sticks or Monsel (ferric subsulphate) solution

Dressings
- Sterile skin closure strips (e.g. steri-strips)
- Transparent waterproof film dressing (e.g. Opsite®)
- Compound benzoin tincture (Friar balsam)
- Gauzepads
- Bandages:
  - Adhesive (e.g. Elastoplast®)
  - Gauze (e.g. Kerlix®)
  - Surgical tape (e.g. Transpore® and Micropore®)
  - Non-woven fabric sheet (e.g. Hypafix®)
  - Self-adherent elastic (e.g. Coban®)
  - Paraffin gauze dressing (e.g. Jelonet®, Xeroform®)

Histopathology
- Specimen pots
- Fixatives:
  - 10% buffered formalin (standard processing)
  - Michel medium (immunofluorescence staining)
- Tissue culture pots and swabs

Cryosurgery
- Supply of liquid nitrogen

Preoperative
- Surgical hand scrub
- Sterile disposable surgical gloves (latex-free preferred)
- Skin preparation solution:
  - Chlorhexidine gluconate, iodophors or alcohol-containing products
- Sterile draping towels:
  - Autoclavable cloth or disposable paper drapes or autoclavable cloth drapes

Anaesthesia
- Disposable syringes 1 or 2 mL and 5 mL (Luer lock if available)
- Needles (18 and 25, 27 or 30 gauge)
- Lidocaine (lignocaine) at 1:100 000 or 1:200 000 dilutions:
  - 1% and/or 2% plain
  - 1% and/or 2% with epinephrine (adrenaline)
- Optional:
  - Longer acting local anaesthetic (e.g. bupivacaine)
  - Methylparaben-free plain lidocaine

Instruments
- Scalpel handles – autoclavable or disposable
- Scalpel blades:
  - No. 15, 10
  - Optional: no. 11, 22
- Forceps:
  - Fine-toothed or 1 × 2:
    - Large (e.g. Adson or Adson–Brown)
    - Small (e.g. Bishop–Harmon)
  - Non-toothed and/or serrated
- Skin hook(s)
- Scissors:
  - Tissue, undermining, suture and bandage-cutting

- Needle-holders:
  - Small for smaller needles
  - Medium for larger needles
- Haemostats:
  - Straight and curved
- Sutures with attached needles:
  - Absorbable (2/0–5/0)
  - Non-absorbable (3/0–6/0)
- Punch biopsies – disposable or autoclavable (3–6 mm)
- Ring curettes – disposable or autoclavable (2–10 mm)
- Nail surgery:
  - Periosteal elevator
  - English anvil nail splitter

Wound infection, an uncommon complication of dermatological surgery, is more commonly related to poor surgical technique than inadequate instrument sterilisation or intraoperative cleanliness. However, correct hand-washing techniques are vital to the prevention of cross-infection [4]. The tradition of protracted 'scrubbing up' is not essential prior to most dermatological surgical procedures – two washes in warm running water using 4% chlorhexidine or 10% povidine–iodine solution are sufficient.

Hand hygiene in UK National Health Service (NHS) hospitals has been the subject of much publicity and concern. The routine use of alcohol-based hand rubs [5] has been recommended to help prevent the spread of hospital-acquired infections, particularly meticillin-resistant *Staphylococcus aureus* (MRSA). Hand disinfection using such alcohol-based hand rubs is associated with less skin irritation [6] and less skin barrier disruption [7] than hand washing using soap or detergent-based products.

During surgery, the use of either clean non-sterile or sterile surgical gloves is mandatory, and the wearing of eye protection and a face mask is strongly recommended [8].

The sterilisation of non-disposable medical and surgical instruments is an important factor in reducing the risk of infection. Many surgical departments are now utilising single-use instruments to avoid the need for robust sterilisation. For reuseable instruments, individual manufacturers often provide specific information and requirements for sterilisation of their equipment. Three levels of importance have been described in this area [9]: (i) non-critical items (e.g. dermatoscopes, which normally come into contact with intact skin) require only simple disinfection between patients; (ii) semi-critical items (e.g. endoscopes, which contact mucous membranes) require high-level disinfection between patients; and (iii) critical items (e.g. surgical instruments, which come into contact with sterile tissues) require sterilisation between patients. Both high-level disinfection and sterilisation should be preceded by manual or ultrasonic cleaning in order to remove any dried tissue, pus or blood [9,10,11]. Older methods of sterilisation, for example boiling in water at atmospheric pressure and the use of various chemical agents (e.g. glutaraldehyde, phenolic agents) are no longer recommended [3]. The new variant Creutzfeldt–Jakob disease (vCJD) prion cannot be destroyed by sterilisation, and equipment suspected of being contaminated must be quarantined. If contact is confirmed, the equipment must be destroyed.

Safety aspects

Certain basic safety measures and protocols are essential within a dermatological surgery unit in order to minimise the risks of infection and accidental injury to both patients and staff [1].

The routine use of aseptic technique minimises the risk of bacterial colonisation at the operation site, and prevents contamination from adjacent sites. Antisepsis and equipment sterilisation are discussed earlier in this chapter. Control of blood-borne infections, especially human immunodeficiency virus (HIV) and hepatitis viruses, should focus on the prevention of transmission from patient to patient and protection of the surgical team. It is now mandatory for all British medical and nursing staff to be adequately vaccinated against hepatitis B, and for hospitals to have both dedicated infection control staff and protocols to ensure instrument sterility. One approach suggested by the US Centers for Disease Control and Prevention (CDC) is to treat all patients as if they were infected with HIV, hepatitis B or other blood-borne pathogens and to adopt 'universal precautions' [1,2].

Needle-stick injuries and other sharp instrument cuts are particularly important, and all members of the surgical team should take extreme care with the use and disposal of sharps. It is extremely dangerous either to leave uncapped needles on the instrument tray or to attempt needle recapping by the two-handed method. Ideally, the surgeon should make a habit of both disposing of used needles and syringes immediately after use and removing all sharp disposable instruments (e.g. needles, scalpel blades) from the tray after the operation, placing these directly into a sharps disposal box. All relatives and those theatre personnel not directly concerned with the procedure should be excluded from the operating room. Clothing should be specific for surgery – apart from potentially introducing a variety of organisms to the procedure room, clothes may become contaminated [3].

At the preoperative consultation, a careful history may identify certain potential problems (e.g. diabetes, epilepsy) or the presence of cardiac pacemakers, implantable defibrillators and cochlear implants [4,5]. A full drug history including any potential allergies (both prescribed and over the counter) is important – aspirin, clopidogrel, ticlopidine, anticoagulants (both coumarin and non-coumarin) and herbal preparations and supplements such as St John's wort, ginseng, glucosamine and *Gingko biloba* promote bleeding. Non-selective β-blockers (e.g. propranolol) may rarely interact with epinephrine (adrenaline) in local anaesthetics, resulting in malignant hypertension. On direct questioning, some people may admit to a tendency to faint very easily, and some patients with epilepsy may have a history of fits triggered by surgery or dental procedures. As there is always a risk of patient collapse in operating rooms, there must be adequate space available for an emergency resuscitation to be performed. Resuscitation drugs and equipment, together with both suction and an oxygen supply, should be readily available. All theatre personnel should ideally be trained in basic life support and resuscitation techniques. A modern computerised portable automated external defibrillator (AED) should be locally available and its location known to all staff within the department.

Covid-19 and skin surgery

The SARS-CoV-2 global pandemic focused the minds of all practitioners regarding the potential risk posed by the virus in the context of dermatological surgery. Many institutions still require patients to wear face masks where feasible during a procedure as well as subjecting patients to appropriate screening measures prior to any intervention. Additionally, although local anaesthetic procedures are not aerosol generating, dermatologists and allied health professionals frequently perform procedures using electrosurgical and ablative laser devices, generating surgical smoke (plume), which may pose harm to both patients and staff. Although no reported cases of Covid-19 transmission via surgical plumes have been reported, the small size of the coronavirus virions makes the possibility of the virus existing in inhaled surgical plumes plausible [6,7]. Appropriate safety measures for surgical plumes including masks, eyewear, smoke evacuation, ventilation and suction are therefore highly recommended.

Local anaesthetics
Principles and types
Local anaesthetics work by blocking the conduction of nerve impulses within the peripheral nerves. They do so by reversibly binding sodium-specific ion channels, inhibiting the influx of sodium and thus preventing the action potential necessary for signal conduction. Based on chemical structure, there are two classes of local anaesthetics: amide type and ester type.

An ideal local anaesthetic agent would be non-toxic, painless on injection, rapid in onset, highly effective and carry a low risk of sensitisation. The best compromise is found in 0.5–2% lidocaine hydrochloride (lignocaine), an amide-type local anaesthetic, which is the agent of choice for most dermatological surgery. Other amide-type local anaesthetic agents include mepivacaine, bupivacaine and ropivacaine, which have a slower onset but more sustained duration of action than lidocaine [1]. Local anaesthetics in 'multiuse' bottles generally contain parabens preservative, but those supplied in glass ampoules are often preservative-free. Special care should be taken when using multidose bottles of lidocaine. It is all too easy to inadvertently contaminate the contents of a bottle by extracting lidocaine using a needle that has already been used for a patient. Subsequent users of the bottle may be unaware that the contents are contaminated. The only safe way to use multidose bottles of lidocaine is for their contents to be completely extracted into one or several syringes as soon as the seal is removed. It is not acceptable practice to take lidocaine from a previously opened multidose bottle. Multidose vials are prohibited in some countries because of the risk of cross-contamination when used between patients.

Ester-type local anaesthetics, for example procaine (ester of *p*-aminobenzoic acid (PABA)), are seldom used by dermatologists.

Epinephrine 1 : 80 000 to 1 : 200 000, when added to local anaesthetic solutions, prolongs the duration of anaesthesia and produces local vasoconstriction, thereby reducing bleeding into the operative field. By reducing absorption, it may also reduce the risk of systemic lidocaine toxicity. Buffering the pH of the lidocaine solution with sodium bicarbonate can reduce the pain associated with infiltration and increase its duration of action. The pH of plain lidocaine is about 6.3–6.4, but the addition of sodium bicarbonate converts about 50% of the drug to the free base, at a pH of about 8.0. This increases the rate of penetration of the anaesthetic into nerve cells, decreases the burning sensation of infiltration and speeds up the onset of anaesthesia.

Tumescent anaesthesia describes the practice of injecting a very dilute solution of local anaesthetic combined with epinephrine (and sodium bicarbonate) into tissue until it becomes firm and tense (tumescent). Although initially described in the field of liposuction it is now widely used in both hospital- and office-based environments and enables dermatological surgeons to perform large flaps and excisions entirely under local anaesthesia in an out-patient setting.

Other anaesthetic agents include the following:
1 Ethyl chloride (which is highly flammable) and liquid nitrogen spray give short-lived periods of anaesthesia by skin refrigeration. This may be sufficient for quick, superficial procedures such as the incision of small cysts and milia, abscesses, removal of skin tags or the curettage of multiple small warts. In many departments, machines that produce a variable flow of cold air are now used in preference for simple topical cryoanaesthesia.
2 The anaesthetic effect of antihistamines (e.g. 1% diphenhydramine hydrochloride solution) can be used when hypersensitivity to other agents is present or strongly suspected.
3 The intradermal injection of normal saline produces a brief anaesthetic effect [2].
4 Hypnosis and acupuncture may be useful when performed by an experienced practitioner and in a suitable subject.
5 General anaesthesia is rarely used in dermatological surgery. Patients requiring a general anaesthetic (e.g. children requiring treatment of large facial birthmarks) are best admitted to hospital either as a day case or overnight.

Toxic reactions
Toxic reactions to lidocaine are rare, and more likely to occur with the use of high volumes of high-concentration solutions or if accidental intravascular injection occurs. Lidocaine toxicity usually presents as a sensation of numbness or tingling. Systemic reactions include vasodilatation, cardiac or respiratory depression, or central nervous system manifestations such as dizziness, drowsiness, tinnitus, slurring of speech, muscle twitching and seizures. These side effects are, to some extent, reversible with diazepam but full resuscitation measures may be required.

Ester-type local anaesthetics should be used with caution in patients with renal impairment. They also cross-react with a number of drugs of the PABA ester type (e.g. sulphonamides, paraphenylenediamine) [3,4]. Amide-type anaesthetics should be used with care in patients with hepatic impairment.

The maximum recommended dosage for lidocaine with epinephrine is 7 mg/kg or approximately 50 mL of a 1% lidocaine solution for an average adult. In practice, most dermatological procedures require substantially lower anaesthetic doses. In order to minimise the risk of accidental intravascular injection, it is a wise precaution either to aspirate prior to infiltration or, if using very fine (e.g. 30 gauge) needles which will not aspirate blood, to keep moving the needle about in the skin while slowly infiltrating small volumes.

Systemic absorption of epinephrine may be associated with mild tachycardia and an excited state. More serious reactions are rare but, as with lidocaine toxicity, are more likely to occur with the use of high-volume high-concentration solutions or following accidental intravascular injection. The use of epinephrine in local anaesthetics should be avoided, or it should be used with caution, during pregnancy, in combination with inhalation anaesthesia or in patients suffering from severe narrow-angle glaucoma [5]. Interaction with non-selective β-blockers (e.g. propranolol) may rarely cause malignant hypertension [2], but this is not a risk with 'cardioselective' β-blockers (e.g. atenolol).

Patients should always be asked if they have had any untoward reactions to local anaesthetics (e.g. in dental procedures). These may have been nothing more than fainting, as vasovagal attacks are commonly associated with local anaesthesia, and should not be confused with serious toxic reactions. In cases of serious doubt, alternative methods of anaesthesia are necessary.

True immunoglobulin E (IgE) mediated reactions to local anaesthetics are exceedingly rare. They occur more commonly with ester-type local anaesthetics as their break-down products include PABA. Metabolism of amide-type local anaesthetics does not produce PABA. However, methyl paraben, which is often added to multidose vials of local anaesthetics, is structurally similar to PABA and could cross-react.

When a patient reports an 'allergy' to a local anaesthetic it is important to elicit a history regarding the nature of the reaction. If true allergy is suspected, using an alternative anaesthetic in the other class and also using a methyl paraben-free (MFP) formulation should be considered. Referral for specialist evaluation can also be valuable for future procedures.

Injection techniques

To minimise discomfort when injecting a local anaesthetic, consideration should be given to using a fine needle, injecting slowly and using both verbal and tactile distraction techniques. Injecting into the subcutaneous fat is less painful than intradermal infiltration, although it does take longer for the skin surface to become anaesthetised. Whenever possible, anaesthetic solutions should be at room temperature. Pain on injection is less when lidocaine solutions are buffered with sodium bicarbonate immediately prior to use [6]. Plain 0.5% lidocaine without epinephrine is an ideal agent to initiate local anaesthesia in children and very nervous patients [7]. It causes no discomfort but the duration of action is brief and so it is usually necessary to top up with a second injection of lidocaine with epinephrine. For most dermatological procedures, lidocaine with epinephrine is beneficial.

Topical anaesthetics include lidocaine cream (LMX4®), tetracaine (amethocaine) cream (Ametop®) or a eutectic lidocaine–prilocaine cream (EMLA®) [4]. LMX4 can be simply applied to the skin; EMLA and Ametop are applied under occlusion before the procedure. The duration of application required varies according to the product used. Ametop is the fastest acting, working within 20 min, but if left for significantly longer periods may cause urticaria and even superficial blistering of the skin. LMX4 generally achieves satisfactory anaesthesia in 30 min. It usually takes at least 60 min for adequate anaesthesia to be achieved with EMLA: the depth of anaesthesia can be increased by leaving the cream in place for longer. The treated skin is vasoconstricted following EMLA application.

Conjunctival anaesthesia is best achieved using proxymetacaine eye drops, which sting much less than tetracaine. The lower eyelid should be gently retracted and 2–3 drops of local anaesthetic placed in the inferior fornix. Reflex tear formation washes away some of the anaesthetic and so further drops should be instilled after a minute or so. Tetracaine is useful for more prolonged and intensive anaesthesia and may be instilled after proxymetacaine.

Other methods of anaesthesia include field block and nerve block anaesthesia [3,5], which produce temporary blockade of sensory nerve function in a given area. Field block involves infiltration of local anaesthetic at several points around surgical sites such as the nose and ear [2], and nerve block anaesthesia involves blockade of one or more major sensory nerves. The most useful nerve blocks on the face in dermatological surgery involve branches of the trigeminal cranial nerve (CN V) (see Figure 20.2) – the supraorbital (forehead), supratrochlear (glabella), infraorbital (lower eyelid, nasal side wall, upper lip) and mental (lower lip) nerves [4,5]. The choice of local anaesthetic method depends upon a number of factors, including the procedure itself, the anatomical site and expected duration of the operation.

Historically, there was controversy surrounding the use of epinephrine in digital nerve block ('ring block') anaesthesia because of a real or perceived theoretical risk of digital ischaemia. Some believe it is absolutely contraindicated [8], whereas others describe routine use without incident [9,10]. Careful review of the literature and current experience has shown that the combination of lidocaine and epinephrine is safe both for ring block anaesthesia and for direct infiltration into the digits (where the addition of epinephrine will reduce bleeding and prolong anaesthesia). The use of epinephrine-containing local anaesthetics should not therefore be considered contraindicated in anaesthetising the digits, penis, nose or ears (as is often mistakenly promulgated).

Biopsy techniques
Incisional and excisional elliptical biopsy

The elliptical excision biopsy is used for the removal of tumours or suspect moles and is the 'workhorse' surgical procedure performed by dermatologists (Figure 20.6). An incisional biopsy is used to take diagnostic biopsies of rashes and tumours before treatment is started. The technique has the advantage that the entire thickness of skin down to the fat is excised, which provides the dermatopathologist with an optimal amount of tissue to provide accurate histological assessment. An appropriate margin can be selected if required and the incision line placed in the optimal direction [1].

Planning the biopsy

For lesions on the face, orientate the ellipse so that the scar runs parallel to or within an existing skin crease (wrinkle), or follows a boundary line between two adjacent cosmetic units (Figure 20.7). Excision direction is best assessed with the patient standing or seated upright rather than lying flat, to allow for the effect of gravity on the skin crease lines. Wrinkle or smile lines can be exaggerated by asking the patient to grimace or smile, or by manipulating the skin [2]. In an excisional biopsy, measure the margin to be excised and mark the optimal line of closure before injecting the anaesthetic. When drawing on the skin, use a recognised skin marker pen as other inks may permanently tattoo the skin when performing the excision or repair. The length of the wound should be at least three times its breadth (the angles at the ends of the ellipse should ideally not exceed 30° to minimise the size of any 'dog ears' at the

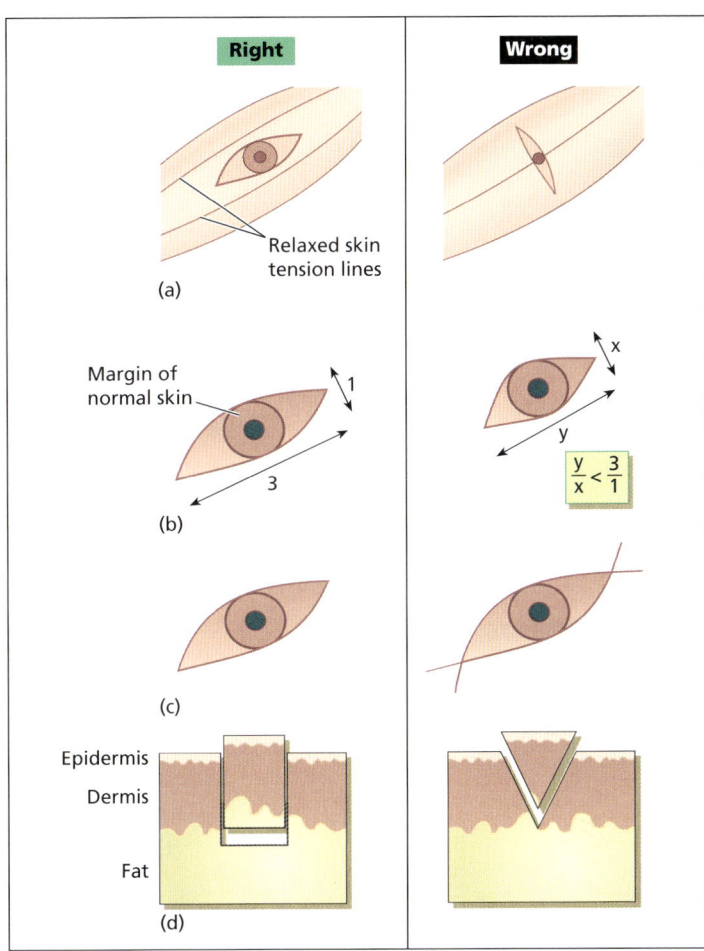

Figure 20.6 Principles of elliptical excision. The ellipse is designed to follow skin-crease lines (a), and should be approximately three times as long as it is wide (b). (b) Ensure that an appropriate margin of normal skin is also excised. (c) At the ends of the ellipse, hold the blade vertically so that the incision lines do not cross over. The blade should be held at 90° to the skin when cutting the ellipse so that the wound has vertical sides down to fat. (d) Do not bevel the blade towards the specimen as this makes the wound more difficult to close and may cut into the dermal component of the lesion. Reproduced from Lawrence 2020 [3] with permission of Elsevier.

apices), taking care not to allow the incisions to cross each other ('fishtailing') at either end [3]. A larger angle may be acceptable at some sites or in older people [4].

Performing the biopsy

The incision should be made as a smooth, single, continuous movement rather than a series of small nicks. The scalpel blade should be aligned at 90° to the skin, not angled inwards, so that the ellipse sides are vertical [5]. The incision lines should meet neatly without crossing over at the tip by starting and finishing each sweep with the blade held vertically. Incisions should be down to the fat. When the ellipse sides and tips have been completely separated from the surrounding skin, the ellipse should be sitting on a bed of fat. The fat under the ellipse should be separated using sharp and blunt dissection using curved tissue dissection scissors, while the ellipse is gently pulled away from the skin using a skin hook or fine-toothed forceps [6]. Undermining of the edges at the appropriate level is required to enable tension-free wound closure and allow optimal wound edge eversion. The wound should be

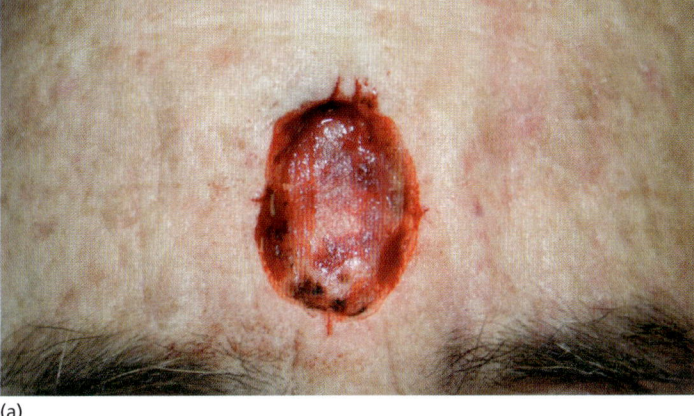
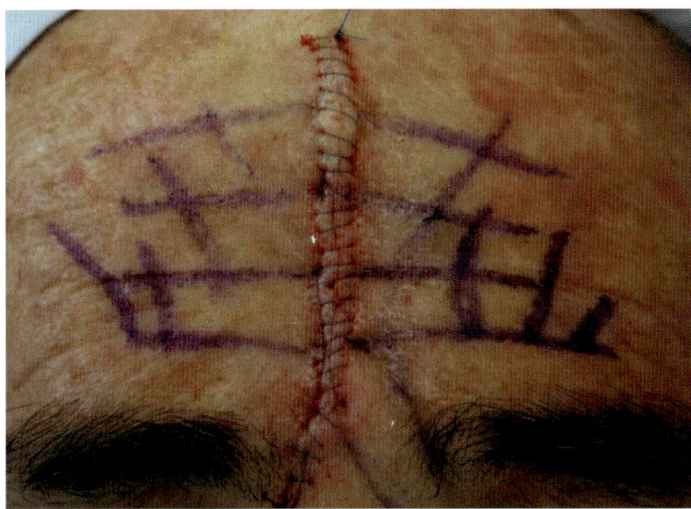
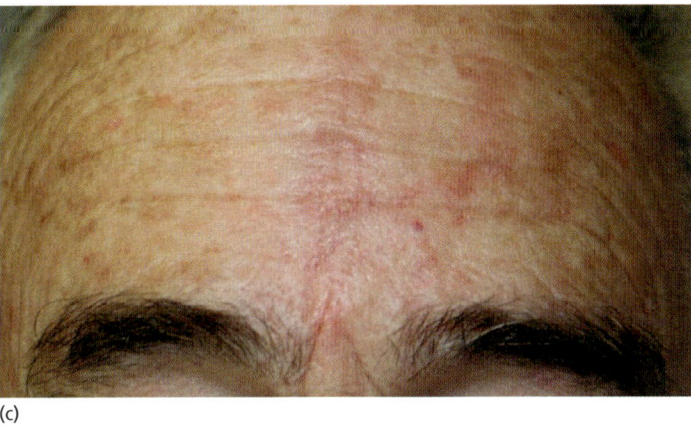

Figure 20.7 Scar orientation. (a) A surgical defect on the central forehead. (b) Having marked out the forehead skin rhytids, the defect is closed primarily ensuring the rhytids are aligned on wound approximation. (c) The result, even at 4-week review, is pleasing.

closed in a layered fashion utilising both subcutaneous and surface sutures if necessary, using the correct suture technique to maximise wound edge eversion.

Punch biopsy

A punch biopsy produces a core of skin down to the fat. It is quick and easy to perform, and leaves only a small wound. The disadvantages include: (i) the potential for sampling error; (ii) with skin tumours there is a risk associated with breaching the dermis and the potential for tumour implantation; (iii) depth control in critical sites in less experienced hands; and (iv) the difficulty in stopping bleeding if a small arteriole is punctured at the base of the wound – although in practice, given the small wound size, firm constant pressure for 10–15 min will deal with this. Punch biopsies can also be used to excise naevi on the trunk. Punch biopsy wounds may sometimes be allowed to heal by second intention, with acceptable cosmetic results [7]. Subcutaneous tissue lesions can be sampled using a punch biopsy by pinching up a fold of skin to include the subcutaneous tissue before the biopsy is taken [8].

Disposable and reusable 2–8 mm diameter punches are available. When the skin is numb, the circular punch biopsy blade should be 'drilled' down to the fat with gentle downward pressure and a rotating/twisting motion [5]. To minimise the scar size, stretching the skin at right angles to the relaxed skin tension lines (RSTLs) while taking the biopsy creates an oval rather than a round wound, with its long axis parallel to the RSTL [6]. The skin core may pop up when the surrounding skin is pressed down, or it may be hooked out using a needle. Cutting through the fat at the base with scissors releases the specimen, which should then be carefully removed to avoid crush artefact during tissue processing. The wound can be sutured or allowed to granulate; the latter produces an acceptable small round or oval scar. If the wound is to be allowed to heal by second intention, stopping bleeding using a collagen matrix dressing results in a better cosmetic result than using Monsel solution (ferric subsulphate), which may tattoo the skin [9].

Shave biopsy

Shave excision is a simple, rapid and effective method for removing benign superficial lesions and obtaining tissue samples from protuberant nodular skin tumours. Shave biopsy of dermatoses affecting the epidermis or high dermis provides adequate tissue for diagnosis, and the subsequent re-epithelialisation from follicular epithelium produces a good cosmetic result. The use of card upon which to place the specimen prevents it curling up during histopathological processing, thus allowing adequacy of margins to be assessed [10].

Shave biopsy of a solid tumour is faster and easier than an incisional biopsy, which needs to be sutured. A fragment can be shaved off to confirm the diagnosis prior to definitive treatment. This biopsy technique is unsuitable if histological examination of the deep margin or edge of a tumour is required to confirm the diagnosis. If melanoma is therefore suspected clinically, a full-thickness excisional biopsy is preferred. Bleeding can be stopped using silver nitrate stick coagulation, as the cosmetic outcome will be determined by the subsequent treatment.

Benign naevi may be shave excised using a number 15 blade held horizontally or using a flexible safety razor blade or commercial equivalent (Dermablade®) [11]. This allows the naevus to be shaved off flush with the skin. Haemostasis should be obtained using cautery, electrodesiccation or a chemical haemostatic agent. Any remaining wound edge tissue fragments may be destroyed using cautery or electrodesiccation. On average, such wounds take 2–3 weeks to heal. In approximately 45% of head and neck and 30% of truncal naevi, no visible scar remains (Figure 20.8). In the remainder, the scar is smaller than the original naevus on the head,

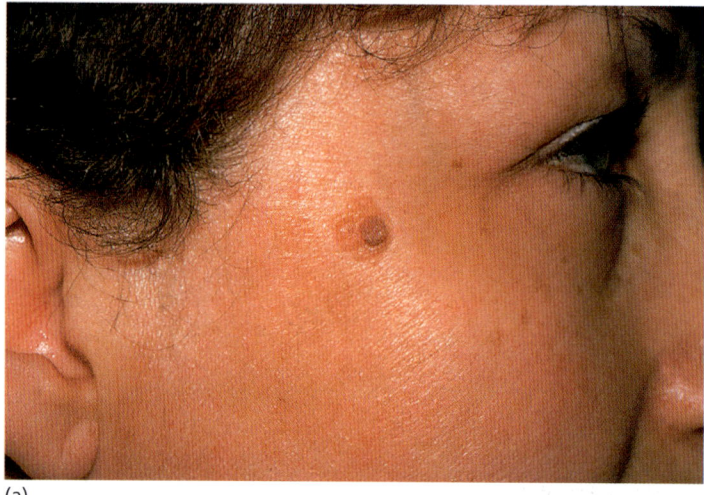
(a)

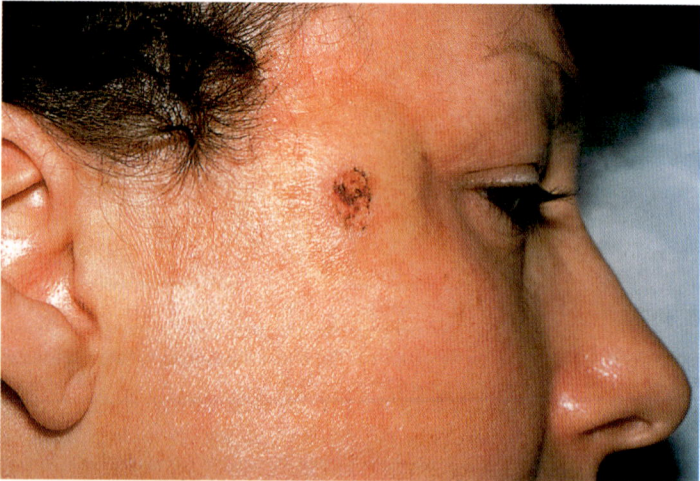
(b)

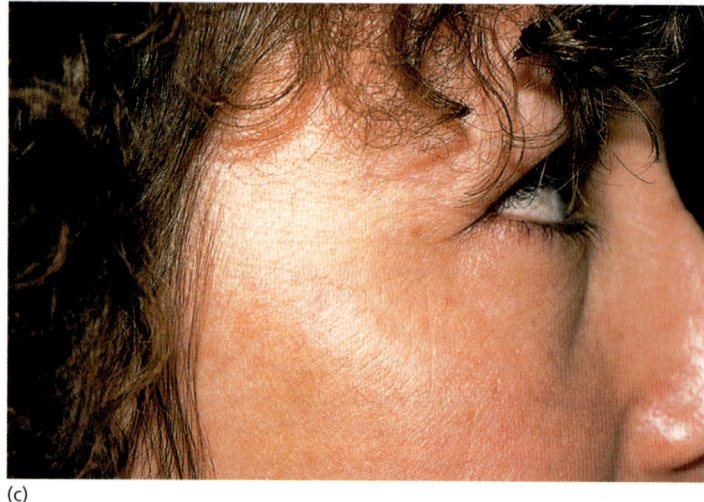
(c)

Figure 20.8 Shave biopsy of benign papular naevi. (a) This patient had a benign tan-coloured naevus on the face that was removed by shave excision followed by cautery (b), resulting in a good cosmetic result 6 months later (c).

neck and limb sites and a little larger than the naevus on truncal sites. Pigmentation at the scar edge or centre remains in approximately 25% of initially pigmented naevi after shave excision – it is therefore important to forewarn patients about this possibility; non-pigmented naevi rarely, if ever, leave a pigmented scar [12]. Persistent pigmentation is even more common when aluminium chloride haemostasis is used rather than cautery [13]. Recurrent or retained pigment does not need to be excised. If a further specimen is sent, the pathologist must be given the full history in order that the changes may be correctly interpreted. Hairs remain in 25% of initially hairy naevi; these can be destroyed by electrolysis if necessary.

Preoperative preparation
Surgeon preparation
Dermatologists should be confident that they are competent to perform the proposed procedure and to manage any possible complications. If not, they should ask for a second opinion. The surgeon should be fully immunised against hepatitis B, and should observe safe practices with regard to handling sharps and tissue specimens. Surgical gloves should always be worn and face and eye protection is strongly recommended.

Patient preparation and consent
Patients should be fully aware of the significant risks, benefits and possible complications associated with the planned procedure. Informed consent [1] should be obtained, both verbally and in writing, for all invasive procedures. In the UK, the regulatory body (General Medical Council) has recently updated its guidance on 'shared decision making and consent'. This information is readily available on its website (www.gmc-uk.org; last accessed August 2023). Usually, consent should be obtained from the parent or guardian in the case of minors, although some adolescents may be fully capable of both giving and withholding consent. Most patients about to undergo surgery are anxious and usually respond positively to appropriate reassurance as well as a calm and professional manner displayed by all members of the surgical team.

The use of a surgical checklist is helpful in minimising risks during skin surgery. Such checklists confirm the patient's identity, highlight relevant medication (e.g. warfarin) and raise awareness of implanted devices (e.g. pacemakers) and allow all members of the team to ensure the correct patient is attending to have the correct lesion treated by an agreed surgical modality. Wrong site surgery is an increasing cause of litigation in dermatological surgery and various strategies have been suggested to minimise the risk of its occurrence [2,3].

Preoperative planning and preparation
It is important to consider which method of biopsy or skin lesion removal is most appropriate in each individual circumstance. Often techniques other than elliptical excision are preferable, many of which (e.g. curettage, shave biopsy) do not result in a linear scar. Consequently, the decision on which surgical technique to use should balance the possible cosmetic advantages of these other techniques (e.g. epidermal lesions and benign facial naevi) against the need to provide a full-thickness tissue specimen for histological examination (e.g. possible melanoma) by performing a formal surgical excision.

Examination and palpation of skin lesions will help to estimate their extent, depth and proximity to large blood vessels, nerves or other important structures. Langer lines of skin tension [4] were previously used as a guide to incision, but the best cosmetic results are usually obtained by following the RSTL [5,6], which on the face tend to lie perpendicular to the major underlying muscles. Langer lines and RSTLs often coincide, as on the neck. When they do not, as on the limbs, the choice depends on other factors. Excisions on the lower leg, for instance, close more easily along the long axis of the limb, rather than transversely. Testing for skin laxity by manipulating the skin usually clarifies the best direction in which to plan an excision. The size and type of excision made will also depend upon many factors, including the site and nature of the lesion to be excised and the nature of the planned skin closure.

The skin surface should be cleaned prior to operation with a detergent–antibacterial combination, most commonly containing either chlorhexidine [7] or povidone–iodine [8]. This helps to reduce the risk of wound infection by removing pathogens and reducing the resident cutaneous bacterial flora [9].

Surgical procedures and techniques

Simple excision, suture technique and wound closure
Elliptical excision: general technique [1–3]
It is recommended that the planned excision lines are marked prior to cleansing the skin surface and infiltrating local anaesthetic. A reasonable period of time should be allowed for the anaesthetic and epinephrine, if used, to take full effect (ideally a minimum of 5 min).

A number 15 blade is most commonly used to make two hemielliptical incisions perpendicularly through the skin into the subcutaneous tissues (see Figure 20.6). Once incised, the ellipse of tissue is held firmly but gently with either fine-toothed Adson forceps or a skin hook, and separated from its base ideally using sharp and blunt dissection with curved tissue scissors. For both histological purposes and to facilitate wound closure, the excised specimen should contain subcutaneous fat.

For standard histological processing, the specimen should be placed in a formaldehyde–saline specimen bottle, clearly labelled with the patient's details. As with a shave excision specimen, to prevent curling of small biopsy or excision samples, these may be placed on small squares of filter paper and floated into the formalin solution. With any potentially malignant skin lesion, a marker suture (e.g. at the 12 o'clock position) should be placed to enable specimen orientation during histopathological processing. Blunting of one end of the specimen, away from the main lesion, will also allow orientation without the need for a marker suture [4]. For immunofluorescence studies, specimens are placed in Michel medium, a tissue transport medium that preserves tissue well for up to 5 days at room temperature.

Intraoperative bleeding is controlled by a combination of pressure, electrosurgery, clamping and ligation of vessels. Bleeding from superficial wounds may be controlled with topical agents such as aluminium chloride.

Depending upon the size of the defect and the body site, a variable degree of undermining of the wound edges will be necessary to facilitate the placing of subcutaneous absorbable sutures and to reduce wound tension. Finally, non-absorbable or absorbable surface sutures are used to neatly appose and evert the wound edges [1,2].

The timing of suture removal depends upon the site and the amount of tension across the wound. With appropriate surgical technique and use of buried vertical mattress sutures all cutaneous sutures may be removed at 7 days. Where there is a history of skin reactivity, sutures on the face may be removed after 4–5 days. When the wound is expected to heal slowly (e.g. on the lower leg), is under greater than usual tension due to its size or location, occurs at a site difficult for the patient to immobilise or lacks the support of buried sutures, then it is sensible to leave the surface sutures in place for 10–14 days or even up to 21 days. Note that after 14 days, the wound may only possess approximately 15% of its final wound strength. Postoperative instructions should include decreased activity and recommend a gradual increase after sutures are removed.

Surgical needles and suture materials

An ideal suture material would have high tensile strength, handle easily, provide good knot security and cause no tissue reaction. Skin sutures are of two main types: absorbable, which are generally used beneath the skin, and non-absorbable, which are generally used in the skin surface. The gauges normally used for skin surgery range from 3/0 (strong) to 6/0 (fine), with suture selection depending on the wound size, anatomical site and surgeon preference.

Monofilament sutures are less likely to become bacterially contaminated but are harder to knot and stiff to work with compared with braided sutures. Absorbable sutures such as Vicryl®, which is braided (Vicryl polyglactin 910), and polydioxanone (PDS), which is a monofilament (PDS II® polydioxanone), are designed to be used as buried sutures. They lose their strength and are resorbed over several weeks (PDS lasts longer than Vicryl and is stronger and better for large wounds, especially on the trunk). Fine-gauge Vicryl can be used as a surface suture for eyelids and mucosal surfaces when a soft flexible suture is required. It has been previously believed that it should not normally be used as a surface suture as it carries a higher risk of creating suture marks on the skin although clinical practice and evidence from scar evaluation studies suggests this may not in fact be the case.

Non-absorbable sutures are of monofilament construction and may be of polyamide 6 (e.g. Ethilon®) or polypropylene (e.g, Prolene®).

Both types of suture are suitable for surface use, but polypropylene is completely non-reactive and suitable for use as a permanent buried suture when this is required.

Most skin sutures use a 3/8th curved needle, which is generally the most useful shape, although a compound bicurved needle can be easier to use when placing buried sutures in small wounds. Many are 'prime' quality – these maintain their sharpness for longer – which is important when multiple needle punctures are being made with the suture. Most needles have a 'cutting' edge – without this it would be very difficult to penetrate the

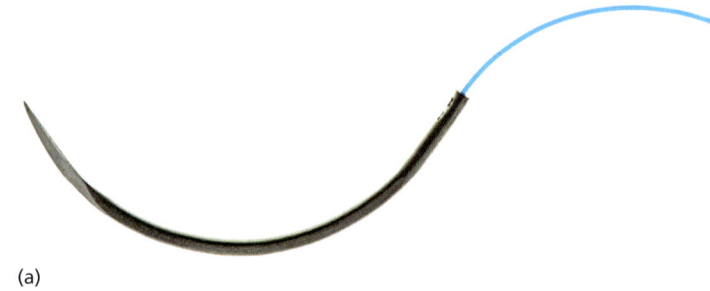

(a)

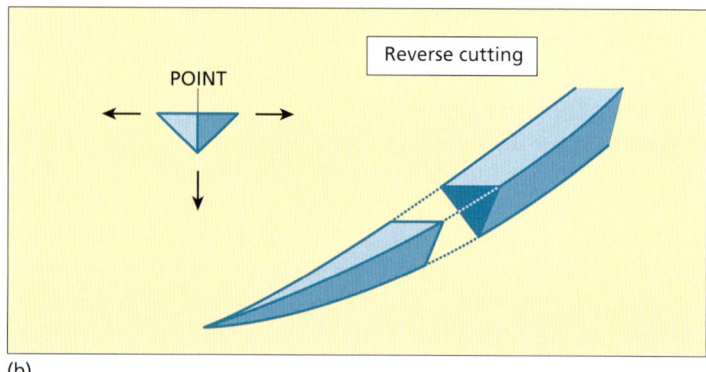

(b)

Figure 20.9 (a) Reverse cutting needle. (b) Cross-section of the reverse cutting needle.

skin – and many are 'reverse cutting' which means the triangular shape of the needle is orientated with the base of the triangle to the inside of the curve and the sharp apex on the outside (Figure 20.9). The reverse cutting needle is less likely to 'cut out' of the skin edge if any tension is applied when the needle is inserted into the skin and the suture is less likely to pull through if tension is applied to the sutured wound. It is better for tougher, more difficult to penetrate tissues. The conventional cutting needle has the sharp edge in the inside of the curve and there is a risk that slight tension applied with the needle in the skin will result in an extended cut through the skin surface. In addition, tension on the sutured wound may pull the suture through the hole more easily.

The front two-thirds of the needle is hardened metal with a sharp triangular tip with a more squared or flattened body. The final third or swage is soft metal into which the suture is crimped. Quality and durability of the needle depend on the alloy of metal, geometry and coating which in turn affect cost. The needle should be gripped in the tip of the needle-holder at the junction between the middle and end thirds, not on the swage which is easily bent. Needle-holders should be fine enough not to distort the needle but should hold it firmly. The suture material should not be gripped in its working length with the needle-holder as the jaws may damage the material and lead to premature rupture.

Suture and needle size generally relate to the tension across the wound, for example low tension closures may require a small needle and a fine suture, and vice versa. A small 'bite' taken with a large diameter suture may under tension result in the suture simply pulling through the dermis.

Surgical knots

The ideal surgical knot should allow precise adjustment of tension on the wound and then tie securely without risk of slipping.

No single knot will be ideal in all circumstances and it is helpful to be familiar with the principles of creating a knot and several variations of it. Knots are usually tied using the needle-holder, which is the most efficient method and saves time and suture material, but there are occasions where tying the knots by hand is preferable.

Modern suture materials require careful handling and knot creation, and incorrectly tied knots are all too common. It is simple to test the security of a knot by stretching the tied suture until it breaks or, if the knot is poor, the knot slips.

A tied suture has several components:
- The loop of suture material that holds the tissue together.
- The knot that is composed of a number of throws snuggled against each other.
- The suture ends or 'ears'.

A throw is a wrapping of one strand around another. When two throws in opposite directions are pulled to form a knot, depending on the direction of 'twist' of the throws, the ends may emerge parallel to each other on one side of the loop – a 'square' knot – or on opposite sides – a 'granny' knot. The granny knot is less secure and more easily comes undone.

The ideal surgical knot should hold its initial position after the first throws while still being adjustable by the surgeon who makes sure the tissues are correctly apposed and completes the knot with further throws to make it secure and resistant to slipping. The ends of the suture should be about 3 mm long to allow for a little stretching of the suture material without the knot coming undone. With buried knots, the ends may be cut short and security obtained by putting an additional throw on the knot.

Tying knots with the needle-holder

For simplicity, we have assumed the surgeon is right-handed and places the suture through the tissues of the wound with a forehand movement – from right to left. The short end of suture material will be on the surgeon's right and the long end, with the needle attached, on the left.

In the first move, the surgeon places the needle-holder between the short and long ends, wraps the long end twice around the tips of the needle-holder in a clockwise direction, creating two full loops of suture around the needle-holder. The short end of the suture is then grasped in the tips of the needle-holder and pulled back towards the left side, while the left hand still holding the main length of suture is taken over to the right side. This creates a simple, double wrap throw, which has greater friction and less slippage than a single throw. In many cases, the edges of the wound can be apposed with this first throw (Figure 20.10). It is important to pull in a direction perpendicular to the wound edge and in the plane of the skin.

The next step is to secure the knot by applying a square knot on top of the initial double throw. The needle-holder is again placed between the long and short ends of the suture and the long end of the suture is wrapped once around the needle-holder in the opposite direction (anticlockwise as viewed from the handle of the needle-holder). The short end is once again grasped with the needle-holder and pulled to the opposite (right) side, while the left hand takes the long end of the suture to the left side. The knot should be pulled perpendicular to the wound edge and flat, in the plane of the skin. At this stage, the knot is called a surgeon's friction knot (Figure 20.11) – but it is insufficiently secure for modern suture

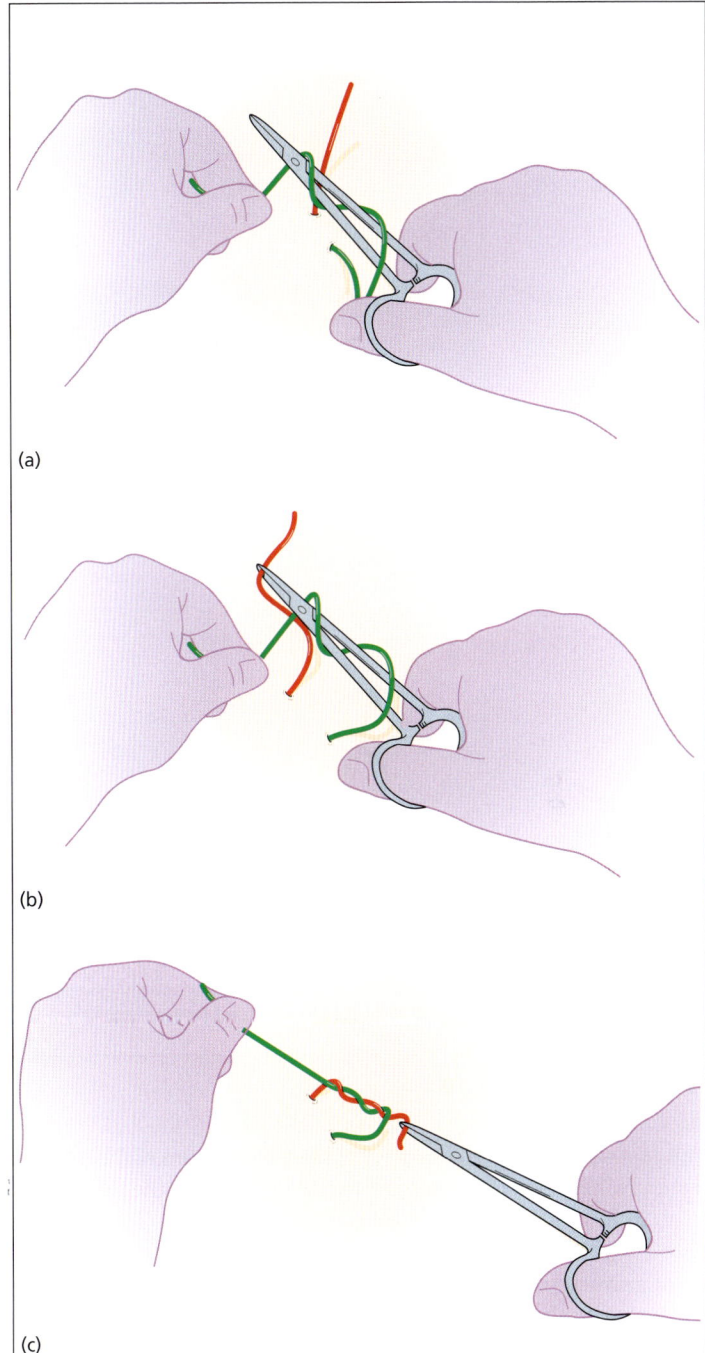

Figure 20.10 (a–c) Tying knots with the needle-holder.

material at this point. Taking one final throw, the needle-holder is positioned between the long and short ends, the long end is wrapped clockwise around the needle-holder, the short end is grasped and the ends are pulled to opposite sides of the wound (Figure 20.12). The knot is then placed on one side of the wound (usually placing the knot on the side which is marginally more depressed to correct any minor depression). It is essential that the suture ends are pulled in opposite directions after each throw and the final throw is pulled tightly to secure the knot.

Sometimes the elasticity of the skin pulls the first double wrap of the knot apart and the edges are not held in apposition. A simple

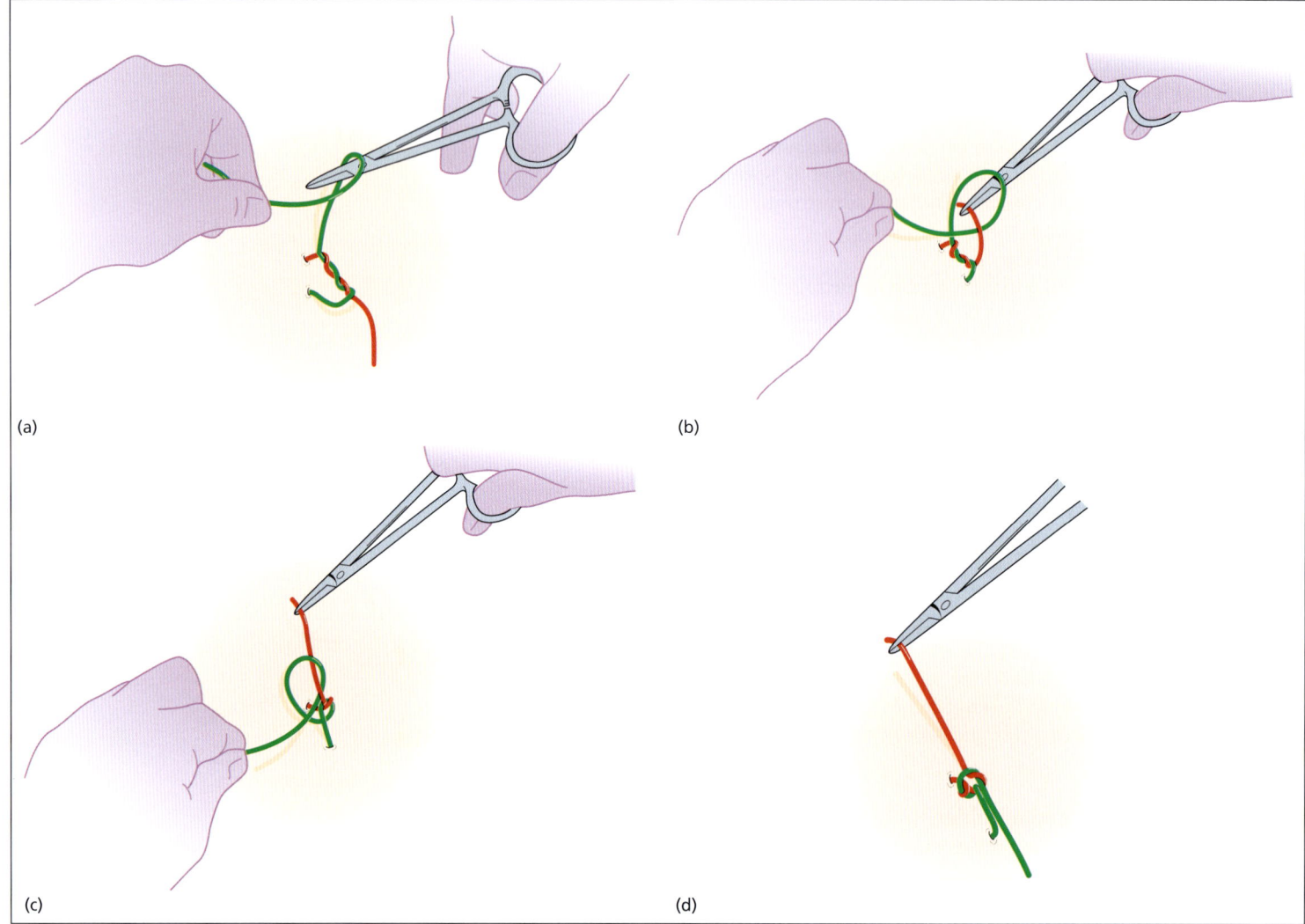

Figure 20.11 Surgeon's friction knot.

way of reducing slippage is to pull the short suture end back to the original side, prior to the second throw, converting the intertwining throw into two loops around the short suture end. The two loops have a tightening action on the suture and hold it in place, but if the alignment of the suture ends is disturbed it will loosen its grip. The knot can then be secured with a conventional square knot. An alternative is to use a triple wrap on the first throw.

If this manoeuvre is not sufficient, it can be helpful to create a more powerful 'slipping' knot. This can be done using two conventional alternate throws, but instead of pulling the suture ends in alternate directions, the short end of the suture is kept on its original side. This creates a series of loops around the short suture end. The short end is then grasped with the needle-holder and gently pulled, while gently 'easing down' the knot of loops. When the desired apposition has been achieved, the 'slipping' knot is secured with a conventional square knot on top. This slipping knot is particularly useful for buried dermal sutures but also clearly demonstrates the importance of pulling the suture ends in opposite directions to create a secure knot and the ease with which this becomes a slipping knot if the directions of pull are not reversed between throws.

It is also helpful to be familiar with tying knots by hand – particularly for buried sutures. Although hand tying is more wasteful of suture material, the tension on the suture ends is more evenly distributed and makes it easier to create a knot where the suture is under tension.

One of the problems with instrument-tied knots is that the tension of the throws is unevenly distributed, which may generate sufficient frictional heat to break the suture as it is tightened.

Suture technique

The ability to employ several different suture techniques is one of the skills needed in order to become proficient in dermatological surgery. The dermatological surgeon should be proficient at techniques for both superficial and deep or buried sutures [1,2–4].

The simple interrupted suture is the mainstay of superficial skin closure. They are normally 4/0–6/0 gauge, and are placed close to the skin edge for fine approximation. Useful superficial stitches to be familiar with include: simple interrupted, simple running, horizontal and vertical mattress, tip and running interlocking stitches.

The horizontal mattress suture (with or without bolsters) is useful for wounds under tension and can also be used to approximate long

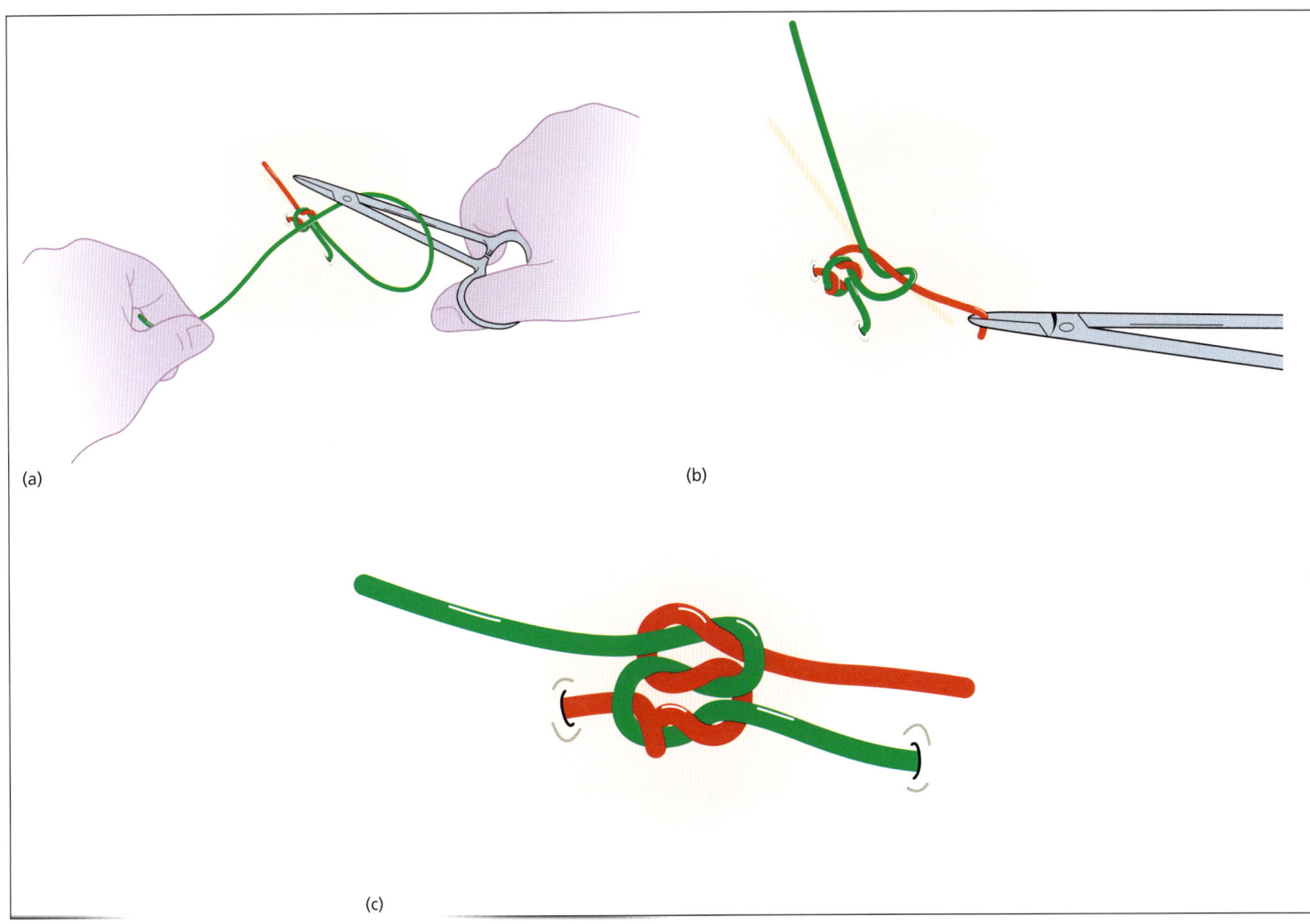

Figure 20.12 Final throw.

wounds. Vertical mattress sutures are useful for wound eversion, the tip stitch, also termed the half-buried mattress, is useful as a corner stitch when insetting the tips of flaps and the running interlocking stitch is useful for haemostasis at the wound edge.

Deep or buried sutures are used to close off 'dead space' in a deep wound and to relieve tension across the wound. They are typically performed using dissolving sutures and optimally placed as a heart shape to give the wound eversion and to take advantage of the tensile strength of the dermis by following a longer course within the dermis.

Prior to closure, wound tension can be decreased by undermining. Meticulous haemostasis prior to closure and good surgical technique can minimise the risk of complications.

Excess tension on superficial stitches will increase the risks of infection and wound dehiscence, and often leaves permanent unsightly, papular or linear suture marks known as 'train tracks'.

To minimise tension across the wound, tape closure materials such as sterile adhesive tapes can be used in conjunction. The running intradermal (subcuticular) suture, although difficult to learn, is an elegant suture technique, and it can be left in place for long periods, leaving only two suture marks. Cyanoacrylate glue (Dermabond®) can also be used for superficial wound closure for wounds that are well approximated and under little tension.

Simple interrupted suture

The simple interrupted suture penetrates the skin surface on one side of the wound, passes under the dermis of both sides and exits on the other side and is tied securely with a surgical knot. It is important that the tension within the suture is sufficient to hold the wound edges together but not so tight as to impair the microcirculation in the area; allowance should be made for postoperative swelling that may increase tension in the suture. The edges of a wound naturally contract and invert, this tendency should be countered by careful insertion of the needle through the skin in a way that creates a stitch with a wider base; this encourages wound eversion (Figure 20.13). The skin sutures should puncture the skin typically 1–3 mm from the edge, depending on skin thickness; the distance from the edge should match the thickness of the skin. Greater distances can lead to a loss of control of the skin edges with a risk of overlapping. The sutures should be placed at intervals equal to the span of the suture, creating a 'square' or 'cuboidal' relationship between the track of the suture and the thickness of the skin. In general, the distance from the

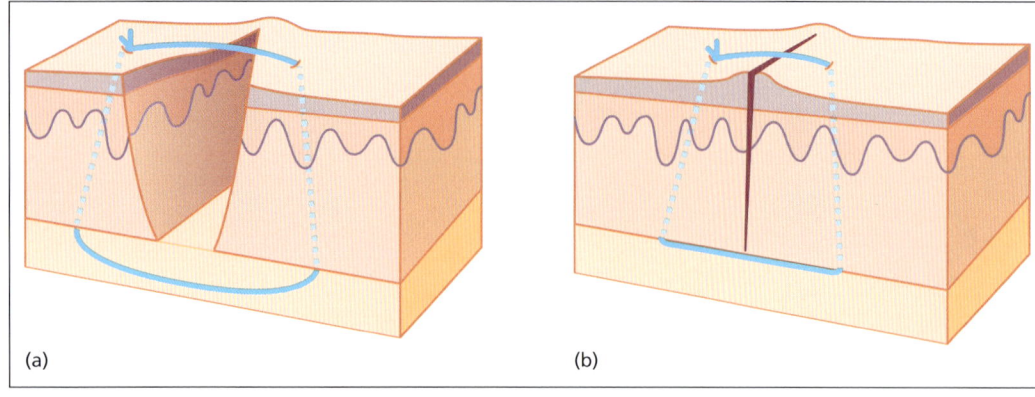

Figure 20.13 (a, b) Simple interrupted suture.

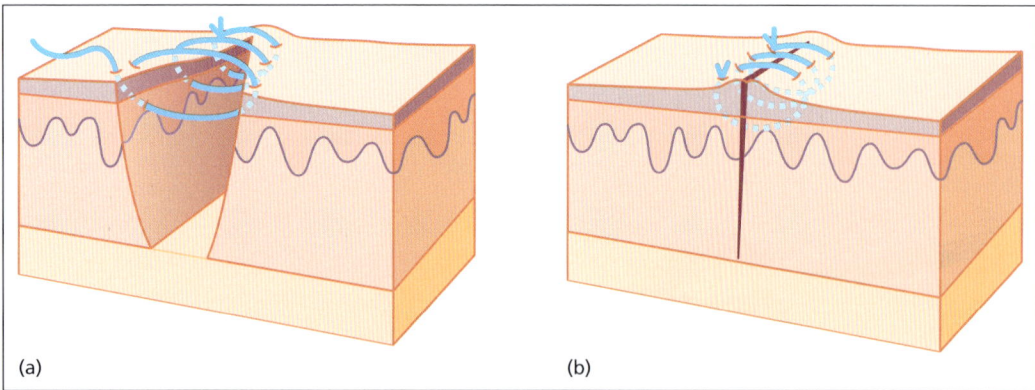

Figure 20.14 (a, b) Simple running sutures.

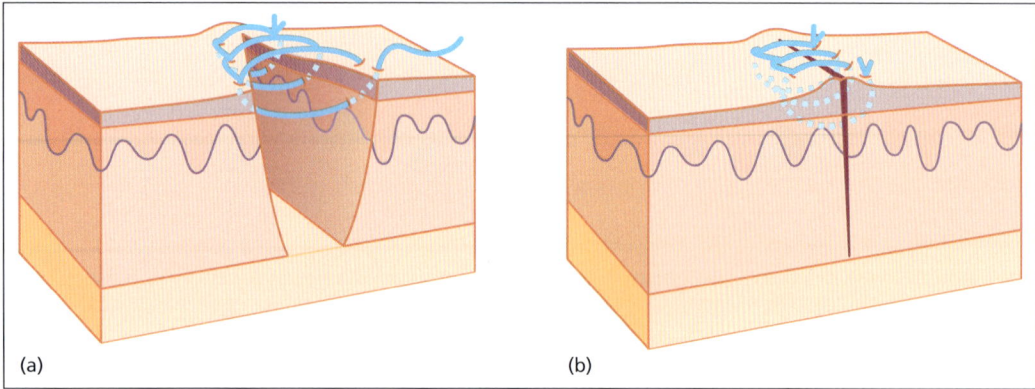

Figure 20.15 (a, b) Running locked sutures.

wound edge should be proportional to the depth of the stitch below the surface.

A number of simple interrupted sutures may be used as superficial closure. With experience, running simple or running locked sutures are often preferred for speed and economy of suture material (Figures 20.14 and 20.15).

In general, buried dermal sutures promote healing and improve scarring. Their primary roles are to reduce tension and to aid in alignment and eversion of the wound edges but they also reduce dead space and assist in haemostasis via tamponade. Most skin wounds will benefit if one or more buried dermal sutures are used. The buried dermal suture enters the dermis from below, courses within the dermis and exits. It then passes across the wound, enters the opposite side and its course is mirrored. The entire length of the suture and knot are buried beneath the skin surface (Figure 20.16).

Slowly absorbable suture is typically used, providing support for the wound for several weeks while the wound regains its strength.

When the buried stitch is tied, the vertical cut edges of the wound should be in direct, gentle but firm apposition (without strangulation) and the epidermis aligned with slight eversion and no stepping. Direct contact between the cut vertical edges facilitates dermal healing. Good alignment of the epidermis assists in superficial healing and top sutures are often used for final fine alignment.

In an ideal stitch, the needle enters and exits in a single vertical plane within the vertical cut edge of the incision and follows a heart-shaped course. When tightened, tension 'ovalises' the suture's course, the wound everts and the knot is tied. Tissue within the loop is directly apposed and neighboring tissue is stabilised. The dermis provides the majority of tensile strength, and therefore the more dermis contained within the loop, the more tension that

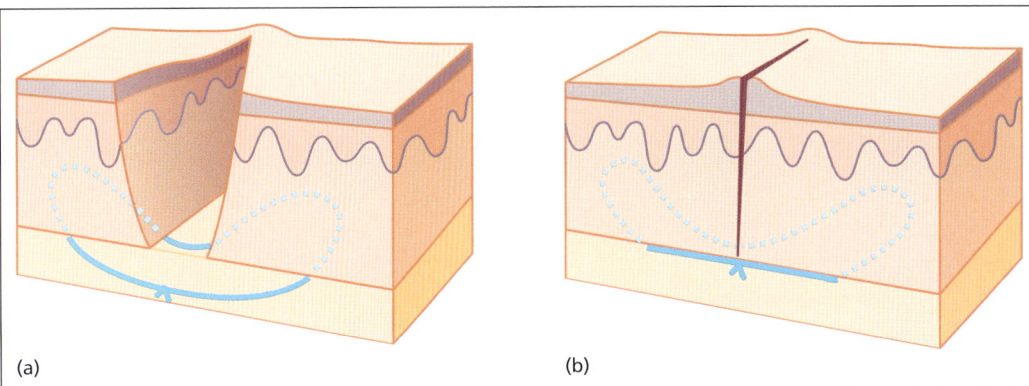

Figure 20.16 (a, b) Buried dermal (vertical mattress) suture.

can be applied to close the defect. In areas of thick dermis or in closures that require higher tension, a larger needle resulting in a larger bite and/or stronger suture may be helpful. To facilitate the heart-shaped course, one may visualise the needle pointing slightly downward as it exits the dermis and pointing slightly upward as it enters the dermis on the opposite side.

Optimally, in the first part of the buried stitch, the needle enters and exits in a single vertical plane within the vertical cut edge of the incision. In practice, however, the needle may need to enter on the underside of the flap a short distance back, away from the vertical cut edge. This is usually inconsequential, however, when the entrance and exit points occur in different (horizontal and vertical) planes (and are mirrored on the other side), tightening leads to greater pressure at the corners where the planes meet; they are more compressed within the loop. If the bite size is held constant, the further back from the vertical cut edge the needle enters, the greater the compression at the corners and the greater eversion but less apposition of the vertical cut edges. If both entrance and exit points occur in the underside of the flap, tension will bring the undersides of the wound together, exaggerating eversion but giving little direct apposition of the vertical cut edges. The compressed corners may even act as a fulcrum, separating the epidermal edges.

The surgeon should carefully assess the entrance and exit points of buried sutures in regard to distance 'back' from the vertical cut edge and distance 'up' the vertical cut edge. Factors involved include depth of undermining, thickness of dermis, elasticity of skin, size of bite, tension required, bevel, etc.

The first buried suture is usually placed in the middle of the wound. Subsequent buried sutures are placed at the midpoint of the resulting two segments and so on – the so-called rule of halves. If the wound is under high tension and closure in the middle of the wound is difficult, the following may help.

1. *Evaluate the undermining*. Attachment to underlying tissues limits movement. However, undermining can only help so much and increased undermining increases the risk of bleeding.
2. *Consider repositioning the patient*. This is especially helpful for patients undergoing surgery on the back as they tend to raise their arms above their head, increasing tension across and/or distorting some wounds. For wounds near the pretibia, raising and supporting the knee can help off-load forces on the calf and wound. Forearm sites can be affected by supination and pronation, etc.
3. *Lengthen the incision*. This tends to distribute the tension along a greater distance.
4. *Use a temporary top stitch in the middle of the defect to close the wound initially and then proceed with deep suture placement*. A simple interrupted suture may suffice but, if more force is needed, consider a horizontal mattress, a pulley or even a tandem pulley stitch. After multiple deep sutures have been placed, remove the temporary top suture and close as normal.
5. *Use a force multiplying deep stitch as an initial suture*.
6. *Use a plicating suture*. These buried sutures are placed in deep tissues below the undermined plane and partially close the defect prior to more superficial deep sutures.
7. If all else fails, *most wounds can be at least be partially closed* with large top stitches only. If closure is performed without buried deep sutures, consider leaving them in place longer than usual. Partial closure requires some healing by second intention.

Although perfectly regularly spaced and placed sutures look attractive, there is a disadvantage to being too uniform in suture placement, particularly with running sutures. If all the sutures have the same line of entry and the skin can move on one axis, it is possible that the wound edges may 'slip' relative to one another allowing overlap to occur. This can be avoided by slight variation in the width and depth of the suture placement along the wound.

Vertical mattress suture

The vertical mattress suture (Figure 20.17) is particularly useful in everting the wound edges and in areas where the skin has to be closed under some tension, or where it is very thin and fragile and a greater amount of tissue is necessary to hold the needle without tearing through (if a large bite were taken as a simple suture the outer edges would tend to invert).

Horizontal mattress suture

The horizontal mattress suture is the most everting suture of all. It is useful in areas requiring high tension as the force of the stitch is distributed across two transverse stitches and the tissue included between them. The needle is inserted through the skin on one side of the wound at a distance from the edge, it passes underneath to the opposite side, emerges and is reinserted a little further laterally and passes back, under the wound to emerge on the opposite side. This suture takes a wide bite of skin, but passes entirely under the wound, thus preventing any tendency to invert the edges and

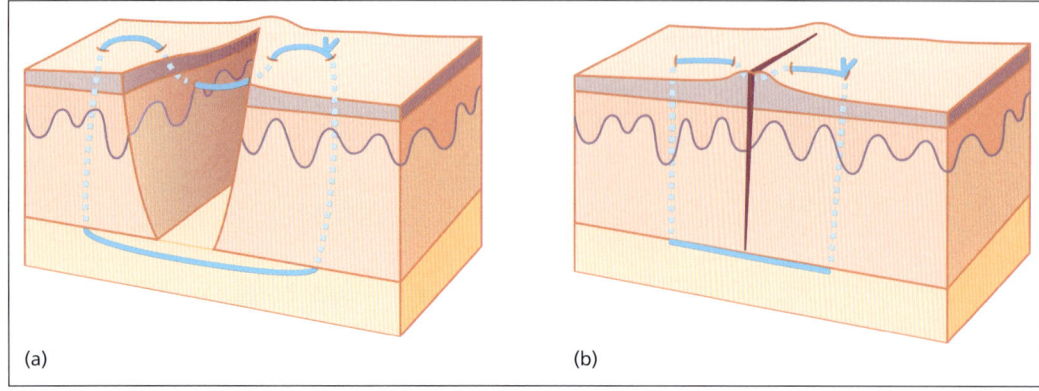

Figure 20.17 (a, b) Vertical mattress suture.

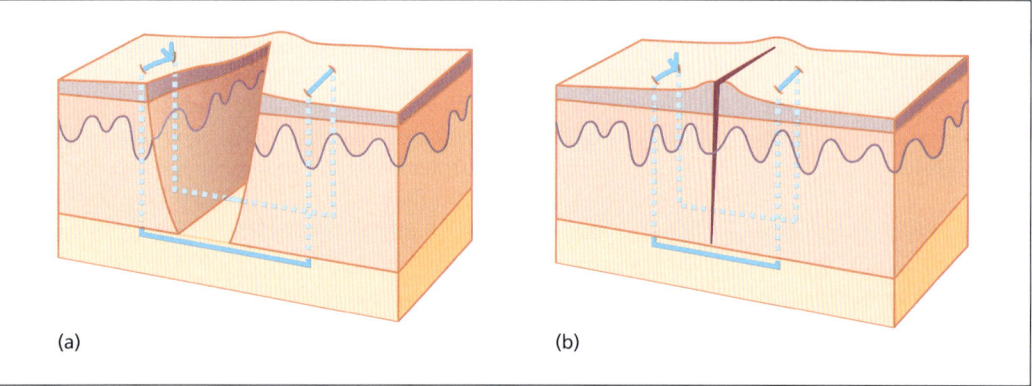

Figure 20.18 (a, b) Horizontal mattress suture.

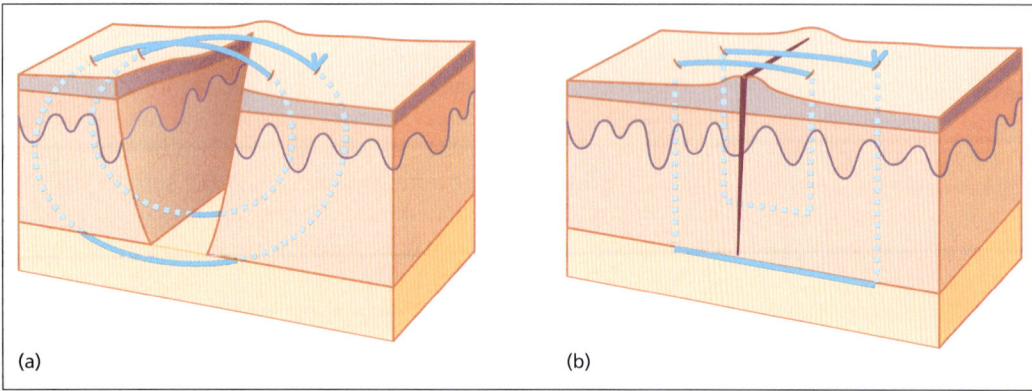

Figure 20.19 (a, b) Pulley suture.

ensuring maximum eversion. It is usually used in combination with simple or running sutures at the wound edge (Figure 20.18).

Pulley suture

There are times in closing a wound under tension when it is clear from moving the skin with finger pressure that the edges could come together but attempts to persuade this to happen with a simple suture fail – either because the suture breaks, or the tension results in it cutting through the skin. Under these circumstances, a pulley suture is most useful and perhaps most often used on scalp wounds. In the simple pulley suture, the needle takes a large bite from the skin of one side of the wound, passes to take a small bite from the opposite side, returns to take a small bite from the original side and then passes to take a large bite from the opposite side before being tied (far, near – near, far). This creates a powerful suture that has twice as many points of contact in the skin and twice as many suture strands as a simple suture. The double loop creates a pulley action that will pull the edges together and may be used in a tandem fashion so as to combine a pulley stitch and a horizontal mattress. Pulley stitches are perhaps best used to initially take tension off a wound allowing easier placement of buried sutures and then removed prior to final closure (Figure 20.19).

There is a slight risk of compromising the vascular circulation if the pulley loops overlap, this can be countered by slightly staggering the loops along the wound. This suture should not be used when a wound does not close with reasonable finger pressure – if excessive pressure is used to close a wound it will become avascular and necrosis will result. If the wound edges are white when the edges are closed, the wound is too tight. Pulley stitches can be used to initially take tension off a wound allowing easier placement of buried sutures and then removed prior to final closure.

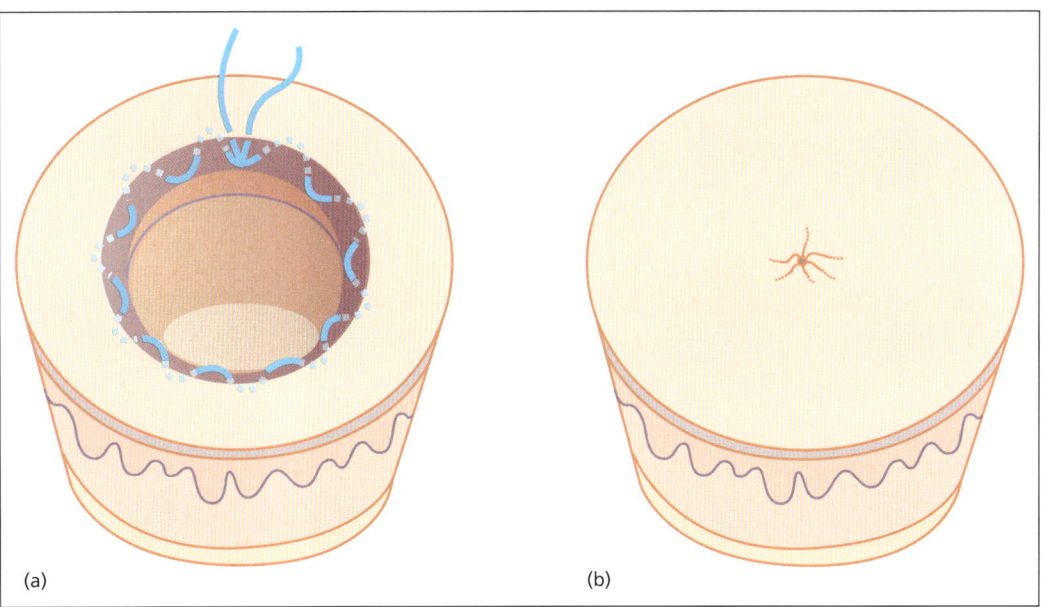

Figure 20.20 (a, b) Purse string suture.

Purse string suture
This is a very useful way of reducing the size of a wound, which will then heal by second intention. It is particularly useful for large tumours that are necrotic or infected or where the exact nature of the tumour or the adequacy of excision is in question. Having excised the lesion with a suitable margin, a running monofilament absorbable PDS intradermal suture is then run around the margin, taking bites into the edge of the dermis. The suture is tightened drawing the edges together. This causes some distortion of the skin surface but the distortion disappears as the wound heals. The suture should be left in place for at least 6 weeks or until the wound has healed. Absorbable sutures do not need to be removed unless they are causing irritation (Figure 20.20).

Running intradermal (subcuticular) suture
This suture technique may be employed where sutures are to remain in the skin for prolonged periods of time and when it is desirable to avoid visible sutures or the necessity for their removal. It is quite commonly employed to close incisional wounds in various branches of surgery and when used in combination with a soluble monofilament suture such as polydioxanone can obviate the need for suture removal, although the placement of the running suture is often combined with external placement of the ends of the suture at either end of the wound.

The subcuticular suture is confined to the dermis and passes from one side of the wound to the opposite side like the rungs of a ladder. Before placing a subcuticular suture, the wound should be apposed with buried dermal sutures. Care should be taken to ensure that needle insertion is of equal depth on both sides of the wound and the needle should cross the wound perpendicularly. It may be preferable to start by placing a buried dermal suture at what will become the final end of the wound, leaving a free suture end to secure to the end of the subcuticular suture. The subcuticular suture then starts at the opposite end of the wound with a buried suture and proceeds in a ladder-like manner, along the length of the wound before being finally secured to the first-placed buried suture at that end. It is the authors' preference to use monofilament soluble sutures such as polydioxanone which do not require removal. This suture technique is commonly employed following wide local excision of lesions on areas of mobility such as the limbs or the back where wound stretch often occurs.

Reconstruction
Reliable outcomes after surgery depend on adhering to fundamental principles of reconstruction and understanding tissue biomechanics. Disregarding these fundamental principles leads to inconsistent outcomes or noticeable scars. This section reviews basic principles for designing reconstructions, and then highlights the key features of secondary intention healing, linear closures, flaps and grafts.

Principles of surgical design
In descending order of importance, the fundamental principles of reconstructive design are: (i) to preserve and restore free margins and contour; (ii) to hide scars in cosmetic subunit junctions and relaxed skin tension lines; and (iii) to optimise colour and texture match with imported tissue.

Free margins. The eyelids, distal nose, lips and helical rim are 'free margins' because they are unsupported on one side. Preserving and restoring the free margins of the eyelids, distal nose, lips and helical rim is a top priority in maintaining symmetry during reconstructive surgery (Figure 20.21). Tension from reconstructive surgery or subsequent contraction from resulting scars can change the position of these delicate structures and create noticeable changes in contour and symmetry. Strategies to preserve free margin position include: orientating tension vectors parallel to the free margins; transferring tension to tissue reservoirs remote from the free margins; or tacking tissue to immobile deep structures so that dermal sutures near the free margins are tension-free.

Contour. Contour determines how light reflects off our faces. Concavities (alar groove, medial canthus, philtrum) cast shadows;

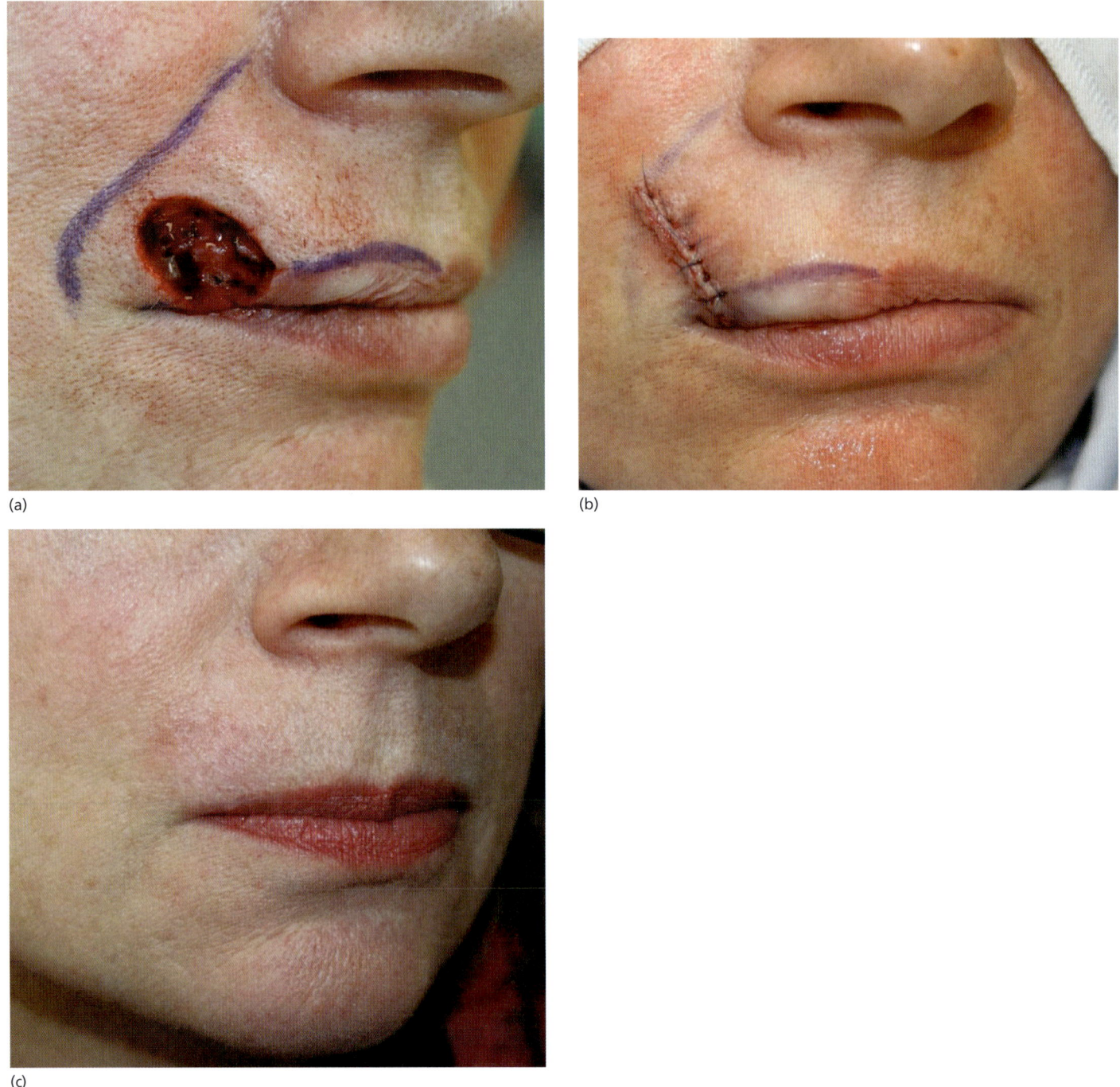

Figure 20.21 Free margin approximation. (a) The vermilion border and melo-labial crease have been marked prior to closure of the Mohs surgical defect. (b) The surgical defect is closed in a linear fashion ensuring the vermilion border is meticulously aligned to prevent unsightly asymmetry and notching. (c) Eight week outcome showing a pleasing alignment of the vermilion border with no distortion of this free margin.

convexities (zygoma, tip of nose) reflect shiny light; and planar surfaces (cheek, forehead) reflect a subtle, even light. Unnatural contours draw attention by interrupting the expected shadows and reflections. A top priority of reconstructive surgery is to recreate scars with natural contours.

Cosmetic subunit junction lines. Cosmetic subunit junction lines create natural shadows and reflections at transitions between facial structures. For example, around the mouth, the vermilion cutaneous junction divides the shiny red vermilion from the textured skin of the cutaneous lip, and the naso-labial fold separates the lip from the cheek. Scars are less noticeable when they fall in cosmetic subunit boundaries. Crossing such boundaries may lead to suboptimal aesthetic outcomes (Figure 20.22).

Relaxed skin tension lines. Relaxed skin tension lines are natural lines of tension on the skin. In general, wounds that are parallel to RSTLs close with less tension. On the face, these lines are obvious,

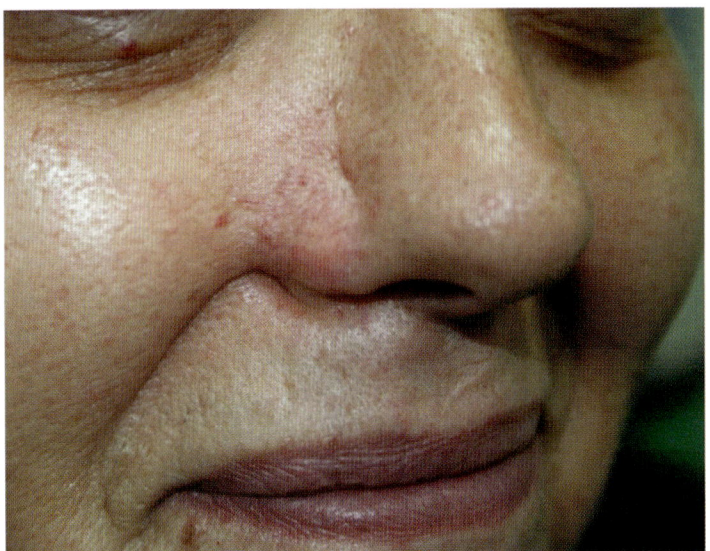

Figure 20.22 Cosmetic unit bridging. A poorly designed and executed transposition flap has effaced the aesthetically important alar–cheek sulcus and also blunted the apical triangle of the upper cutaneous lip.

because they are accentuated with animation of the muscles of facial expression, such as crow's feet lines while squinting the eyes. On the trunk and extremities, these lines can be accentuated by pinching the skin. As a rule, the lines of tension should be determined with the patient upright with the arms by the side and the hands facing forward. Placing scars in relaxed skin tension lines should not violate higher priority reconstruction principles. For example, if a horizontal closure on the forehead would cause an asymmetrical lift of the eyebrow, it is better to perform a vertical closure that crosses RSTLs but preserves brow position.

Colour and texture. Mismatches in colour and texture can make scars more noticeable. Reconstructive surgery ideally creates thin scars surrounded by skin of similar colour and texture. When it is impossible to reconstruct with skin of similar colour and texture, conforming to higher priority reconstruction principles (free margins, contour, cosmetic subunit junction lines, RSTLs) often makes these differences acceptable.

Secondary intention healing

Cutaneous wounds may be left to heal by secondary intention (Figures 20.23 and 20.24) [1,6–8]. Second intention scars contract and have a shiny texture. The shiny scars from secondary intention healing are less noticeable in naturally shiny skin, such as a bald scalp, upper forehead, ear and nasal dorsum or proximal sidewall. Since secondary intention wounds contract, they can pull on nearby free margins and cause webbing of adjacent, loose skin, such as the eyelid. The ideal defect to minimise distortion from second intention healing is shallow and is surrounded by stiff skin. Occipital scalp wounds after excision of acne keloidalis nuchae [7] or axillary and inguinal wounds after excision of hidradenitis suppurativa [8] may heal by secondary intention with excellent results.

Linear closure

Linear closure is the side-to-side approximation of the edges of a fusiform wound. Tension lies along a single vector running perpendicular to the long axis of the fusiform wound and is greatest at the centre of the wound. To avoid standing cones and to maintain normal contour, the ideal angles at the apices of a fusiform excision are <30°, which requires a length:width ratio of 3 : 1 or greater.

Primary linear closure is the most common reconstruction and ideally aligns with cosmetic subunit junctions or RSTLs (see Figure 20.7), unless the orientation must be modified to preserve free margin position.

M-plasty [1,2]

M-plasty is a useful technique to shorten an elliptical excision and avoid crossing an important anatomical or cosmetic line (Figure 20.25). The angle at the apex of a fusiform excision is divided into two adjacent 30° apical angles that are half the length of a single apex. The appearance of these neighbouring triangles mimics the letter 'M'.

S-plasty

Elliptical excision over convex surfaces may cause an inverted scar. To avoid inversion of scars from fusiform excisions over convex surfaces, a straight fusiform design may be converted to a 'lazy-S' shape. As the scar contracts, the 'lazy-S' shape usually straightens, but the extra length gained from the curved design reduces the risk of scar inversion. The 'lazy-S' design is most common over the

Figure 20.23 (a) Defect on the scalp after Mohs surgery for an undifferentiated pleomorphic sarcoma and adjacent squamous cell cancers. The wound was left to heal by secondary intention. (b) At 4 months after surgery, the central wound has filled with healthy granulation tissue and the periphery of the wound has begun to re-epithelialise with healthy epidermis. (c) By 6 months after surgery, the wound has re-epithelialised except for small crusts in the centre of the scar. The re-epithelialised skin of large secondary intention scars is more fragile than native skin, and scabbing from trauma is common.

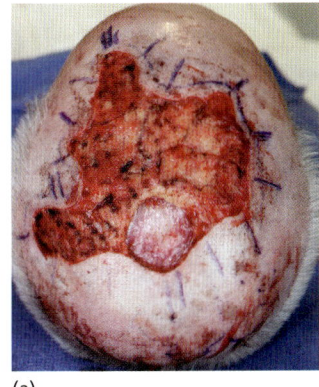 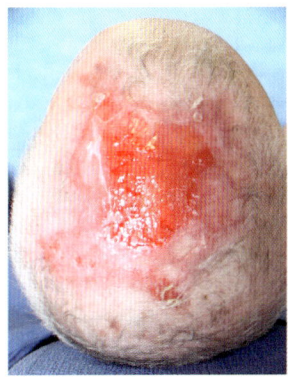 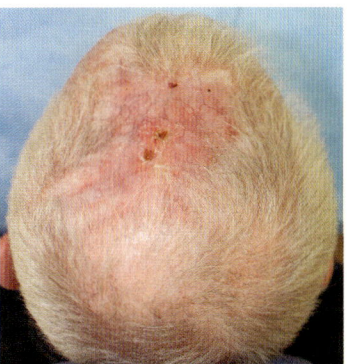

(a) (b) (c)

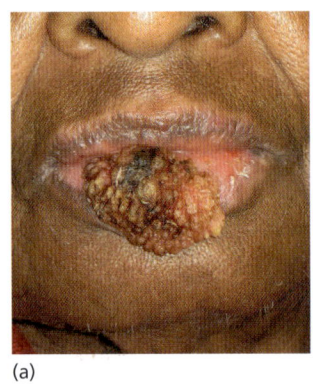
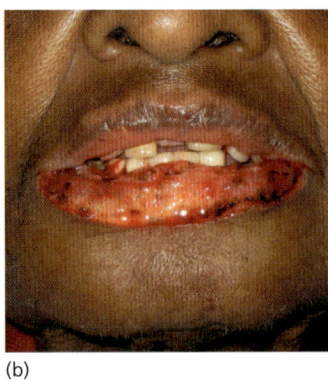
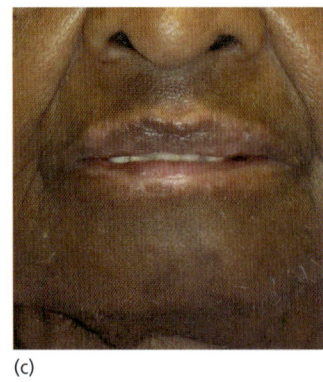

Figure 20.24 (a) Exophytic squamous cell cancer of the lower vermilion lip. (b) Superficial defect of the lower lip after obtaining clear microscopic margins with Mohs surgery. The wound was left to heal by secondary intention. (c) Appearance of the scar 8 months after surgery.

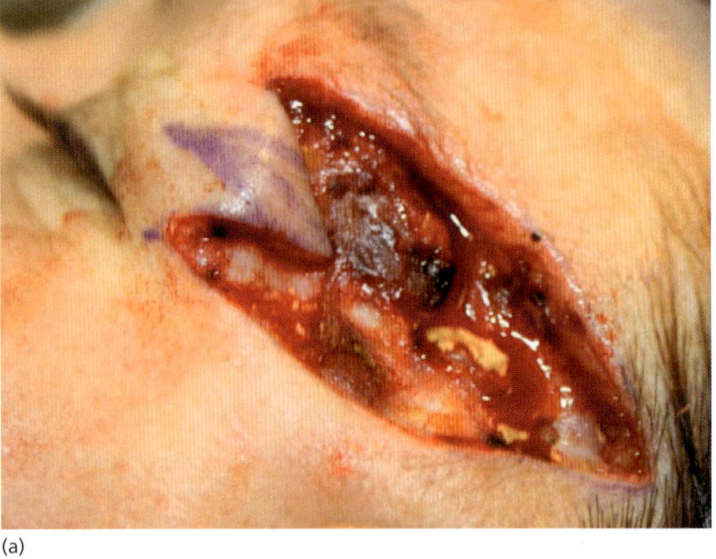
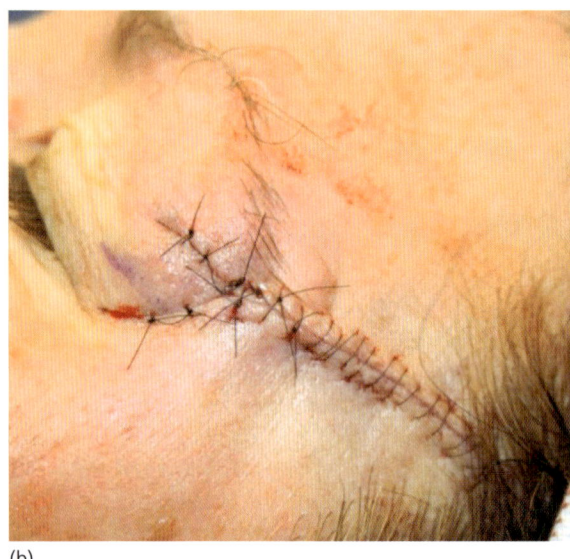

Figure 20.25 (a, b) An M-plasty design in this case prevents the scar extending onto the eyelid skin.

convexities of the premaxillary cheek, chin and dorsal forearms and hands (Figure 20.26).

Wedge excision: lip, eyelid and ear

Defects on the eyelid, lip and ear can be closed by removing a wedge of tissue, and then suturing the different layers of the defect in a straight line. Wedge closures are easiest on the relatively elastic lip and eyelid. However, the unyielding ear cartilage can buckle during a wedge repair [3].

'Dog ear' repair

There are several synonyms of the 'dog ear' repair: tricone repair, standing cutaneous deformity repair and standing cone [4]. 'Dog ears' tend to occur when the length to width ratio of an excision is insufficient to prevent the skin at the apices from bulging outwards when the opposing skin edges are brought together. 'Dog ears' form most commonly when fusiform excisions are designed with apical angles >30°. 'Pseudo-dog ears' may form if the excision plane of a fusiform excision is shallower at the apices compared with the centre of the wound.

There are several ways to correct a 'dog ear' [5]:
1 The excision can be extended and the redundant overlapping skin excised.
2 One side of the pucker can be cut back flush with the skin and the excess skin from the other side identified by drawing it across the wound; this can then be cut off (Figure 20.27).
3 The excess skin of the 'dog ear' can be removed by converting it into a T-plasty or an M-plasty. This is a useful technique when the length of the wound cannot be extended [6].

Vermilionectomy and mucosal advancement flap

A mucosal advancement may be used to repair defects after vermilionectomy, usually of the lower lip [1–3]. The labial mucosa may be pulled outward and sutured to the skin edge to recreate a vermilion–cutaneous junction. The exposed mucosa often scales and has a bright red colour.

Flaps (Table 20.2)

A flap is defined as skin, fascia or muscle that is moved from one area of the body to cover a tissue defect [1]. The most common types of flaps performed by dermatological surgeons are 'local' flaps, which are loosely defined by donor tissue that lies close to the tissue defect. A local flap is comprised of elevated tissue (skin with or without fascia or muscle) with a pedicle that remains attached to a blood supply at the flap's base. The pedicle may have either a random pattern blood supply from subdermal and subcutaneous plexuses or

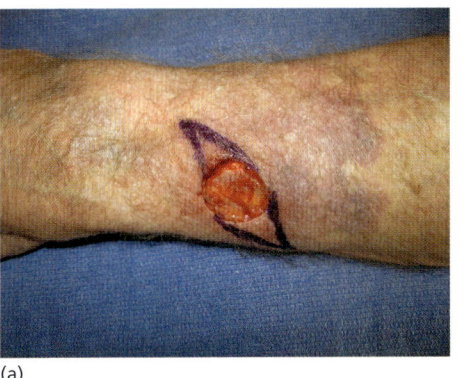
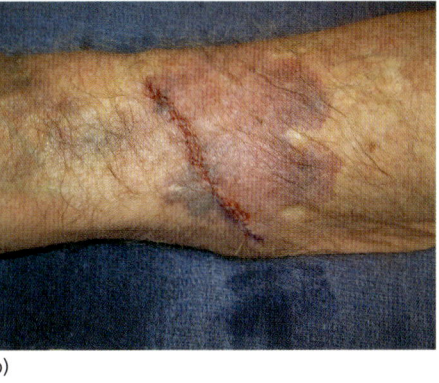

Figure 20.26 (a) An S-plasty is designed to repair this wound on the ulnar aspect of the dorsal forearm. (b) Appearance immediately after surgery. The S-shaped curve of the scar can prevent inversion as the wound contracts.

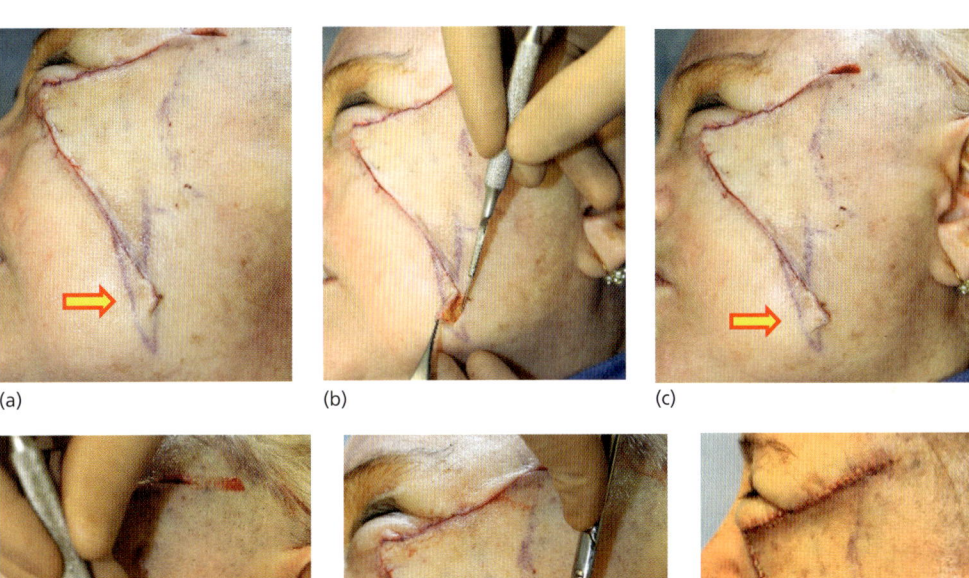

Figure 20.27 (a) A standing cone, or 'dog ear' (arrow), has formed at the inferior apex of this rotation flap. (b) The leading edge at the base of the standing cone is incised, and the skin is undermined. (c) The undermined skin now drapes flat against the cheek (arrow). (d) The trailing edge of the standing cone is incised to match the incision along the leading edge. (e) The standing cone is cut, and the skin edges now align with good contour. (f) Appearance after layered closure of the standing cone.

an axial pattern blood supply from a named artery (e.g. the supratrochlear artery for a paramedian forehead flap).

Local flaps may be further classified based on various characteristics, such as vascular supply (e.g. random pattern versus axial) or primary motion (e.g. advancement versus rotation versus transposition). However, overlapping features of these classifications can cause confusion. For simplicity, this chapter classifies flaps as either sliding or lifting.

Sliding flaps move adjacent tissue directly into a defect without 'jumping' over interposed tissue. The greatest point of tension is at the primary defect. Sliding flaps include advancement, rotation and island pedicle flaps.

Lifting flaps move tissue into a defect by 'jumping' over interposed tissue. Lifting flaps transfer the greatest tension away from the primary defect to the donor site. Lifting flaps include transposition (e.g. rhombic, bilobed, trilobed) and interpolation flaps (e.g. forehead flap).

Sliding flaps

Advancement flaps. Advancement flaps are useful for wounds that could be closed with a fusiform excision, except one of the standing cones would encroach on a free margin (e.g. eyelid, lip, distal nose, helical rim) or cosmetic subunit junction (e.g. eyebrow, vermilion–cutaneous junction, alar groove). Like fusiform closures, advancement flaps maintain tension along a single vector, but they displace one or both of the standing cones to preserve a free margin or hide the scar in a cosmetic subunit junction line or RSTL (Video 20.1).

Common locations for advancement flaps are near free margins on the face, such as the upper and lower cutaneous lip, the nasal sidewall, the infraorbital cheek and lower eyelid, the forehead and

Table 20.2 Common flap type and uses [1,2–7,8,9–13,14,15,16,17,18,19,20–26,27–31,32,33].

Flap type	Random pattern flap (synonym/s)	Uses	Comments
Advancement [1]	Crescentic advancement flap	Cheek/nose Cheek/apical lip	In effect a side-to-side closure with special attention to cosmetic boundaries; a useful technique
Unilateral	Single advancement (U-plasty)	Cheek Temple Forehead Upper lip	May employ a degree of rotation. A Burow unilateral advancement often produces superior aesthetic results
Bilateral (H-plasty)	Double (bilateral) advancement (H-plasty)	Forehead Eyebrow	Propagated in all surgical texts but the H-shaped scar is aesthetically suboptimal
	O-T plasty (A-T plasty, V-T plasty)	Upper lip Supra-eyebrow forehead Glabellar/nasal root Temple	Unless the defect is centrally located, the majority of flap movement is in a unilateral direction
	Single advancement (unilateral Burow wedge flap)	Upper lip Temple/forehead Preauricular cheek Helical rim	Workhorse flap for temple, preauricular, upper cutaneous lip and helical rim defects. Enables excellent concealment of incision lines
Island pedicle	V to Y (island pedicle flap)	Upper lip Cheek Lower cutaneous eyelid Medial canthus Nasal sidewall	Efficient flap in terms of tissue dissection. May be elevated in a number of ways to facilitate movement. Triangular-shaped scar however is often very noticeable
V-to-Y / Rotating island–pedicle	Rotating/lenticular island pedicle flap	Temple Cheek Lower cutaneous eyelid Naso-jugal fold	Combines motions of advancement and rotation. Provides favourable aesthetic results as it enables scar lines to run parallel with relaxed skin tension lines
Rotation Single	Single rotation (nasal sidewall rotation, Tenzel rotation, Mustardé flap)	Nasal tip Lower eyelid Naso-jugal fold/lower eyelid	Larger flaps necessitate meticulous dissection and haemostasis. Utilised around free margins and if executed correctly produce favourable aesthetic and functional results
Double (O-to-Z)	Single rotation with a back-cut (hatchet flap)	Apical lip Nasal root Medial canthus	Useful for small defects and enables principle of cosmetic subunit repair to be respected
	Single rotation with advancement (AIRNS flap, Rieger flap)	Nasal tip Lower nasal dorsum	Subnasalis tissue dissection provides a robust vascular supply for these flaps. Utilise secondary tissue movement of the cheek and glabella to enable tension-free closure
	Double rotation (O to Z plasty)	Scalp Chin	Best results produced in scalp repair. Requires significant subgaleal tissue dissection
	Double rotation (O to W plasty – Peng flap)	Nasal tip and dorsum	Has a pinch effect on nasal contour: useful when a slight reduction in nasal width is desirable
Transposition	Standard (Limberg) transposition	Cheek Temple Medial canthus Nose	Most commonly used flap in cutaneous facial reconstruction. Frequently designed as a 'square peg to fit a round hole'. A Z-plasty modification enhances flap mobility

(continued)

Table 20.2 (continued)

Flap type		Random pattern flap (synonym/s)	Uses	Comments
Single (Limberg) Double (bilobed)				Naso-labial transposition is frequently performed to resurface alar and nasal sidewall defects. However, without meticulous planning and execution it may blunt the alar crease and tent across the apical triangle of the upper lip
		Webster 30° variant	Nasal dorsum Lateral canthus	Versatile flap. May be bilateral
		Dufourmental variant	Cheek Temple Medial canthus Nose	Alteration in flap design allows scars to be concealed at junction of cosmetic units
		Bilobed flap	Nasal tip, sidewall and ala Temple Cheek Medial canthus	Two transposition flaps in continuity. The most frequent flap in distal nose reconstruction but requires careful planning and execution
		Trilobed flap	Nasal tip	Three transposition flaps in continuity
		Median or paramedian forehead flap	Nasal dorsum Nasal tip Full-thickness defects of lower third of nose including ala	Two or three staged procedure. Reliable flap based on the supratrochlear artery
		Cheek interpolation flap	Nasal tip Nasal ala	Care should be taken in males to ensure hair is not transposed from the cheek onto the nose
		Auricular interpolation flap	Ear, especially helical rim defects	Allows height of ear to be maintained

temple (Figure 20.28), the preauricular cheek (Figure 20.29) and the helical rim. For defects of the midline face, the primary tissue motion of advancement flaps is usually lateral to medial so the tension vector parallels the free margins of the eyelids, nose and lips. For defects of the lateral face, the primary motion is usually inferior to superior.

Variations of advancement flaps include the Burow advancement flap, U-plasty, H-plasty and O-T flap.

Rotation flaps. The hallmark of a rotation flap is the arciform incision used to mobilise the surrounding skin (Figure 20.30). Rotating the flap into the primary defect creates a secondary defect along the arciform incision. The secondary defect enlarges as the arc of rotation increases, and surgeons must plan for closure of both the primary and secondary defects. In contrast to the single tension vector of advancement flaps, rotation flaps distribute tension across multiple vectors along both the primary and secondary defects.

A simple test to choose between a rotation and advancement flap is to push the wound edges together. If there is a clearly preferred tension vector at the primary wound but the standing cone of a linear closure would impinge on adjacent free margins, then an advancement flap will work. If there is no clearly dominant tension vector, but the wound edges nearly approximate by pushing in multiple directions, then a rotation flap may be ideal to distribute tension across multiple vectors at the primary defect. The scalp is a classic location for rotation flaps to repair wounds that do not have a preferred tension vector (Figure 20.31).

Rotation flaps on the face are most commonly used to repair medial cheek defects (Video 20.2) that recruit skin from the lateral cheek and neck; lateral forehead defects that recruit from the temple; and nasal tip defects that recruit skin from the nasal sidewall and glabella (Figure 20.32).

Island pedicle flaps. Island pedicle advancement flaps differ from the other sliding flaps (i.e. advancement and rotation) in that their entire blood supply comes from a pedicle on the flap's undersurface. Island pedicle flaps can have numerous shapes, such as a triangular V to Y flap or a rhomboid-shaped keystone flap. Regardless of the shape, the island pedicle flap is defined by incising through the skin around its periphery, creating the 'island' that gives the flap its name (Video 20.3). A key suture advances the leading edge of the flap toward the primary defect, where the greatest amount of tension resides. A secondary defect must be closed at the trailing edges of the flap.

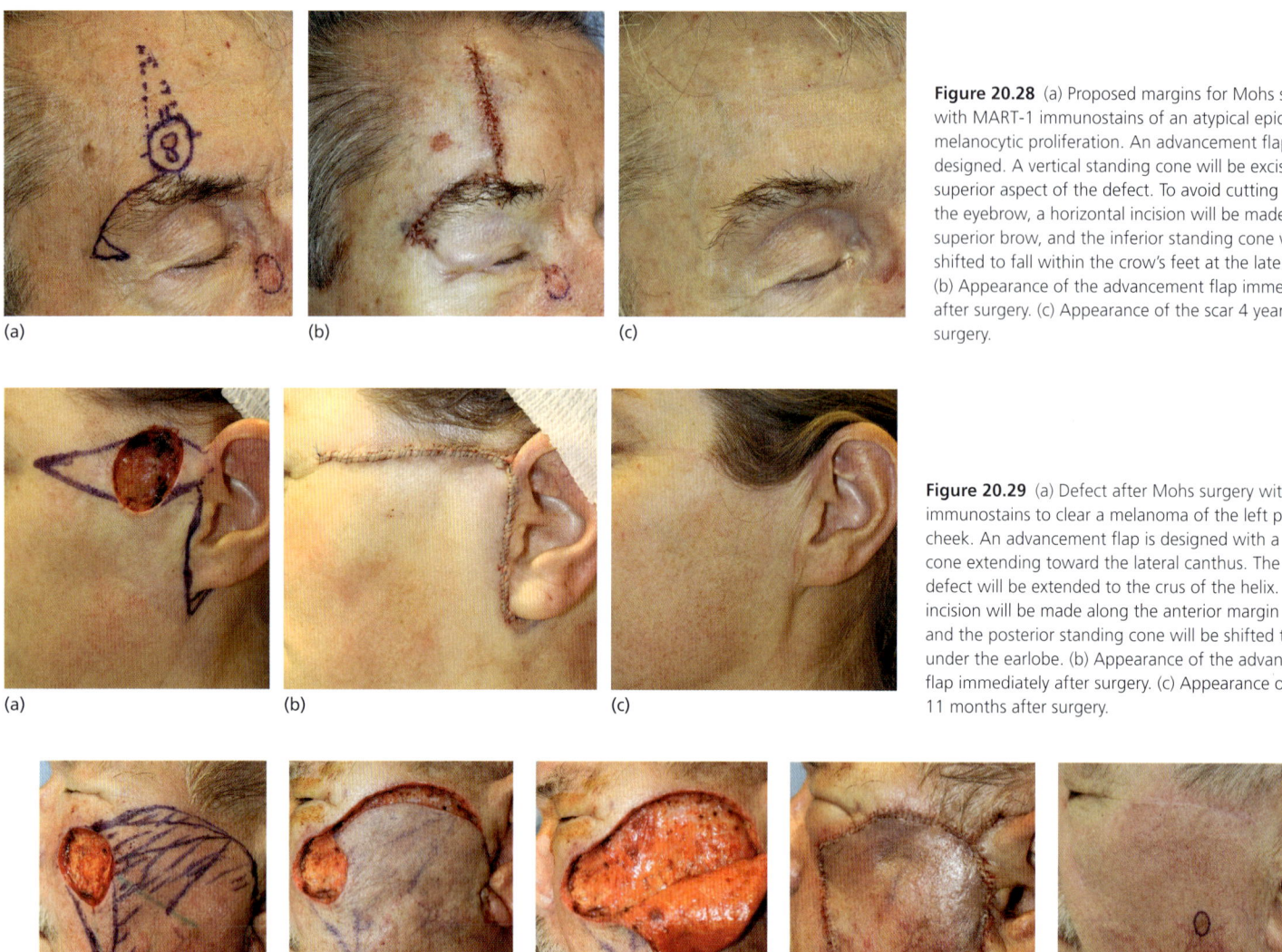

Figure 20.28 (a) Proposed margins for Mohs surgery with MART-1 immunostains of an atypical epidermal melanocytic proliferation. An advancement flap is designed. A vertical standing cone will be excised at the superior aspect of the defect. To avoid cutting through the eyebrow, a horizontal incision will be made along the superior brow, and the inferior standing cone will be shifted to fall within the crow's feet at the lateral brow. (b) Appearance of the advancement flap immediately after surgery. (c) Appearance of the scar 4 years after surgery.

Figure 20.29 (a) Defect after Mohs surgery with MART-1 immunostains to clear a melanoma of the left preauricular cheek. An advancement flap is designed with a standing cone extending toward the lateral canthus. The posterior defect will be extended to the crus of the helix. A vertical incision will be made along the anterior margin of the ear, and the posterior standing cone will be shifted to hide under the earlobe. (b) Appearance of the advancement flap immediately after surgery. (c) Appearance of the scar 11 months after surgery.

Figure 20.30 (a) Defect after Mohs surgery for an infiltrative basal cell carcinoma of the zygomatic cheek. A rotation flap is designed. The shaded areas on the flap represent the anticipated extent of undermining. (b) Intraoperative photo with the arcs of the rotation flap incised on the superficial fascia. Note the secondary defect along the arc of the rotation flap. (c) Intraoperative photo with the flap elevated in the immediately superficial to superficial fascia. (d) Appearance of the rotation flap immediately after surgery. A standing cone was excised at the preauricular cheek along the outer edge of the arch of the rotation flap. (e) Appearance of the scar several months after surgery. The circled lesion indicates the site for a biopsy of an unrelated lesion.

A common example of an island pedicle flap is a V-Y advancement flap for lateral upper cutaneous lip defects (Figure 20.33).

Lifting flaps

Transposition flaps. As opposed to sliding flaps, which have the greatest tension at the primary defect, transposition flaps displace the greatest tension to the final donor site (i.e. secondary defect of a rhombic flap; tertiary defect of a bilobed flap; and quaternary defect of a trilobed flap). Closing the terminal donor site allows rotation of the flap into the primary defect with minimal tension. Transposition flaps are useful to transfer tension away from the primary defect to a more generous tissue reservoir. Three common transposition flaps include the (single-lobed) rhombic flap (Figures 20.34 and 20.35) (Video 20.4), bilobed flap (Figures 20.36 and 20.37) and trilobed flap (Figures 20.38 and 20.39) (Video 20.5). Adding lobes to transposition flaps recruits tissue from reservoirs increasingly remote from the primary defect and displaces tension to more favourable vectors.

Because they transfer key tension vectors away from the primary defect, transposition flaps are especially useful to repair facial defects near the free margins of the nose, eyelids and lips.

Z-plasty. A Z-plasty is a double transposition flap used to reorientate the scar direction or to lengthen a webbed scar over a concavity [2]. The central limb of the Z-plasty has a greater increase in length

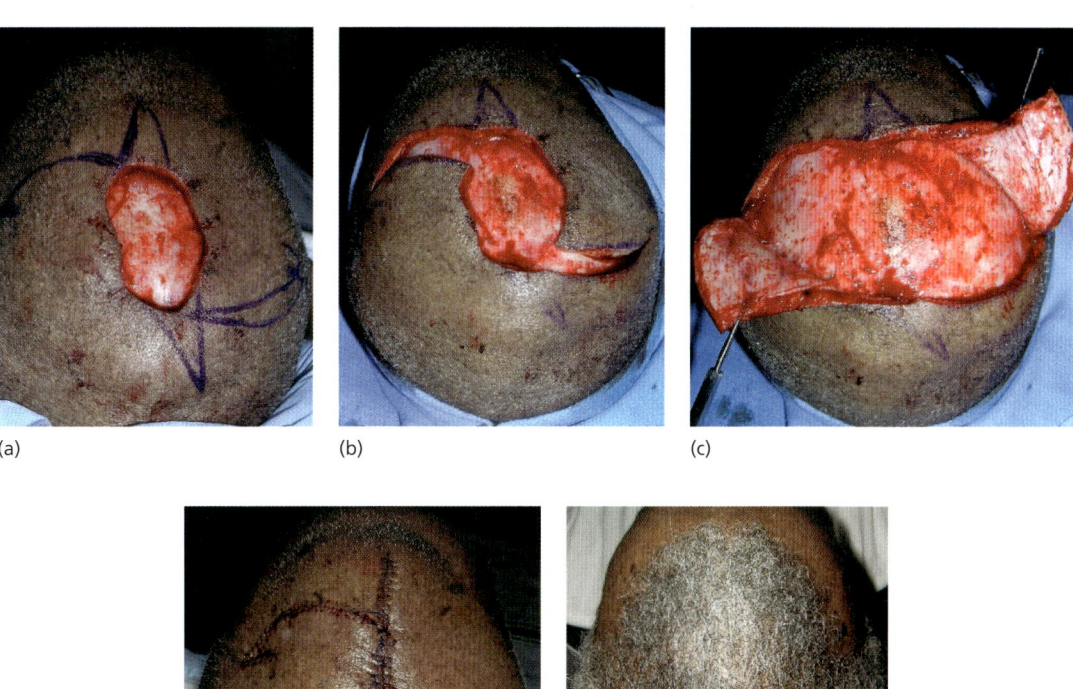

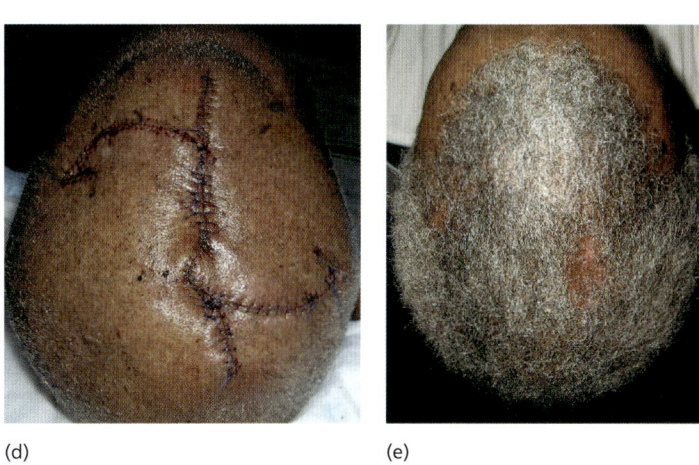

Figure 20.31 (a) Defect after Mohs surgery for a squamous cell cancer of the vertex of the scalp. Bilateral rotation flaps (O to Z) are designed. (b) Intraoperative photo with the arcs of each rotation flap incised through the galea aponeurotica. Note the secondary defects along the arcs of each rotation flap. (c) Intraoperative photo with the flaps elevated in the loose areolar connective tissue deep to the galea aponeurotica. The arteries on the scalp run superficial to the galea aponeurotica. (d) Appearance of the rotation flaps immediately after surgery. Standing cones were excised in the midline along the arc for each rotation flap. (e) Appearance of the scar 5 months after surgery.

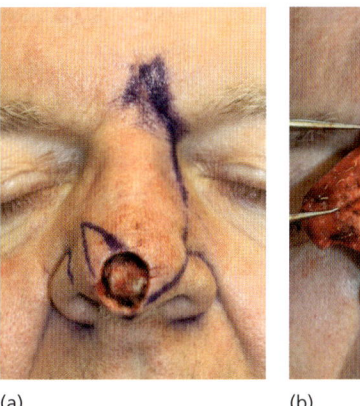
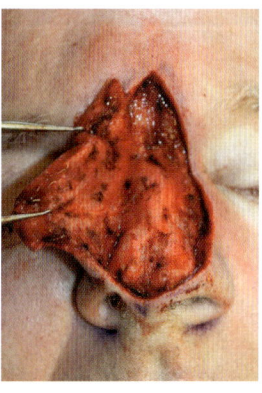
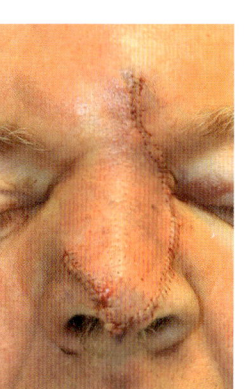
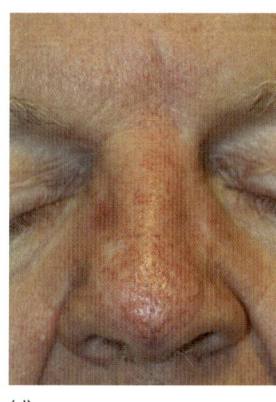

Figure 20.32 (a) Defect after Mohs surgery for a basal cell carcinoma of the nasal tip. A dorsal nasal rotation flap is designed. (b) Intraoperative photo with the flap elevated at the perichondrial plane, deep to the nasalis muscle. The blood supply to the flap pedicle comes from the right dorsal nasal artery, which runs superficial to the nasalis muscle. (c) Appearance of the rotation flap immediately after surgery. (d) Appearance of the scar 4 years after surgery.

as the angles at the apices of each flap widen (Figures 20.40, 20.41 and 20.42).

Interpolation flaps. Interpolation flaps transfer skin from remote reservoirs with a pedicle that bridges an isthmus of skin between the primary defect and the donor site. After approximately 3–4 weeks, the flap integrates with the blood vessels at the recipient site and the pedicle is divided in a second surgical procedure. The pedicle of interpolation flaps may or may not contain a named artery. For example, the pedicle of a paramedian forehead flap includes the supratrochlear artery, but the pedicle of the naso-labial interpolation flap relies on perforators from the angular artery.

Interpolation flaps are ideal for defects at or near free margins of the face. The paramedian forehead flap (Figure 20.43) (Videos 20.6 and 20.7) and naso-labial interpolation flap (Figure 20.44) repair distal nasal defects; the retroauricular interpolation flap repairs helical rim defects (Figure 20.45) (Video 20.8); the Abbe flap repairs large defects of the lip margin (Video 20.9); and the Hughes and Cutler–Beard flaps repair defects of the eyelid margin. All of these flaps transfer tension away from the primary defect and help to preserve and restore free margins.

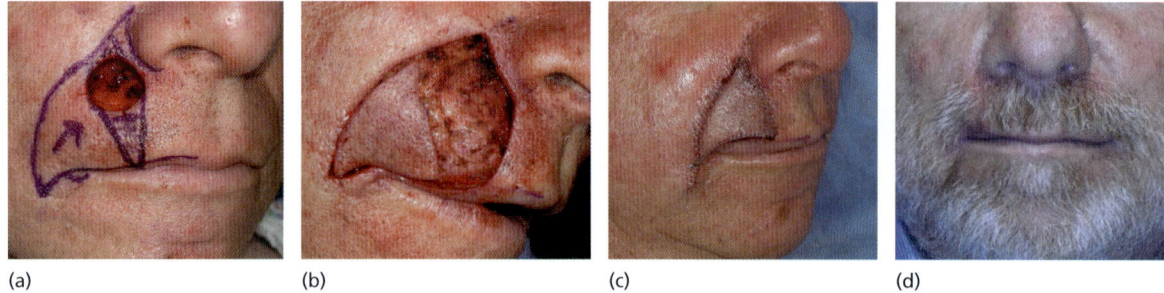

Figure 20.33 (a) Defect after Mohs surgery for a basal cell carcinoma of the right upper cutaneous lip. A V–Y island pedicle flap is designed. (b) Intraoperative photo with the defect enlarged to form a column from the vermilion cutaneous junction to the naso-labial fold. The lateral incisions of the triangular flap hide in the cosmetic subunit junctions of the vermilion–cutaneous junction and naso-labial fold. (c) Appearance of the island pedicle flap immediately after surgery. (d) Appearance of the scar 2 months after surgery.

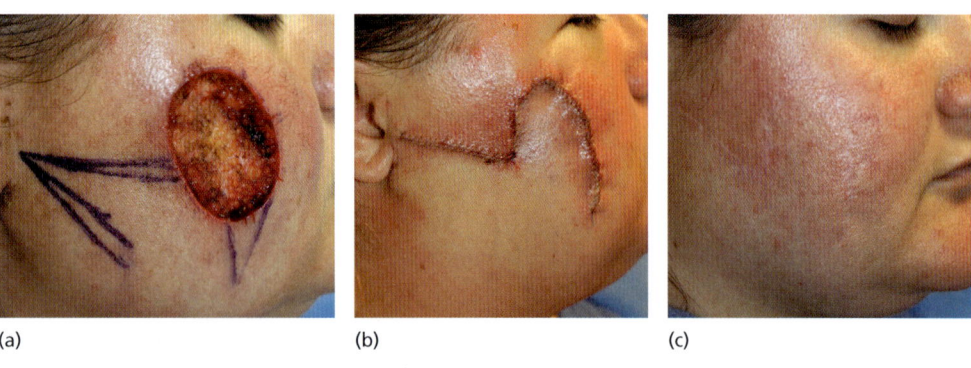

Figure 20.34 (a) Defect after Mohs surgery with MART-1 immunostains for a melanoma of the right preauricular cheek. A rhombic flap (single-lobed transposition flap) is designed to recruit skin from the preauricular cheek. The inverted triangle at the inferior border of the defect represents the anticipated standing cone after transposing the flap into the primary defect. (b) Appearance of the rhombic flap immediately after surgery. (c) Appearance of the scar 10 months after surgery.

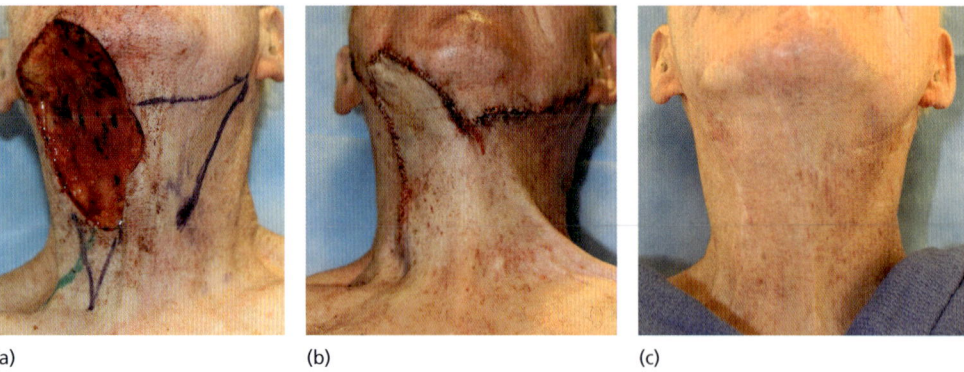

Figure 20.35 (a) Defect after Mohs surgery with MART-1 immunostains for a melanoma *in situ* of the right mandibular cheek and neck. A rhombic flap (single-lobed transposition flap) is designed to recruit skin from the contralateral neck. The inverted triangle at the inferior border of the defect represents the anticipated standing cone after transposing the flap into the primary defect. (b) Appearance of the rhombic flap immediately after surgery. (c) Appearance of the scar 13 months after surgery.

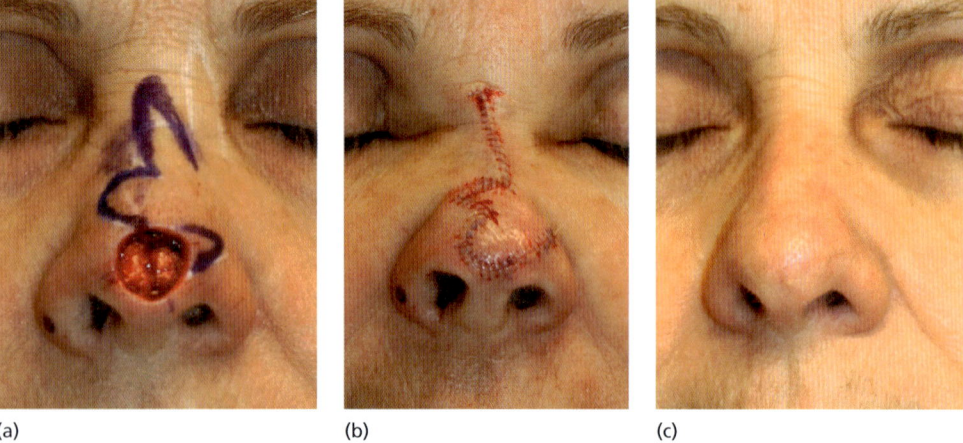

Figure 20.36 (a) Defect after Mohs surgery for a basal cell carcinoma of the nasal tip. A bilobed flap is designed to recruit skin from the dorsum of the nose. (b) Appearance of the bilobed flap immediately after surgery. (c) Appearance of the scar 8 months after surgery.

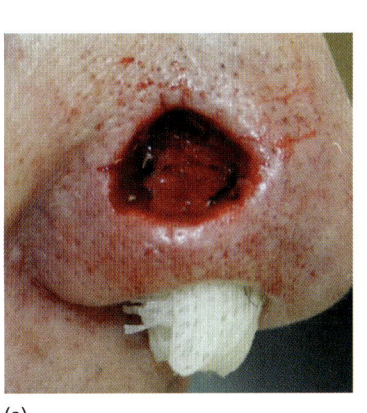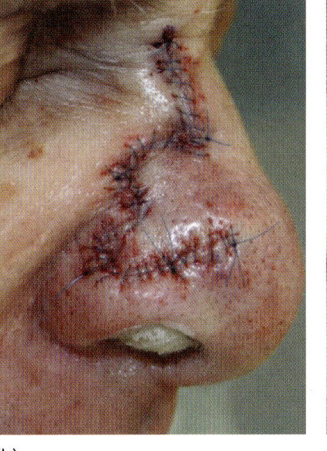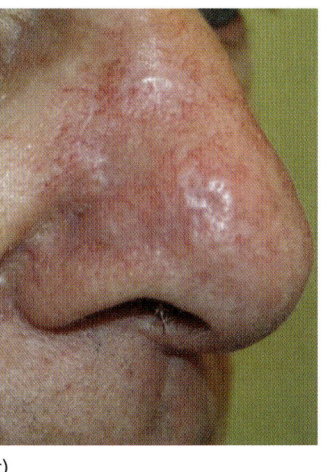

Figure 20.37 Bilobed flap repair on the nose. (a) A Mohs surgical defect of the right lower nasal sidewall and alar. To prevent effacement of the aesthetically critical alar–cheek sulcus, a medially based flap was designed. (b) Immediately at closure. (c) A satisfactory outcome at the 3-month review.

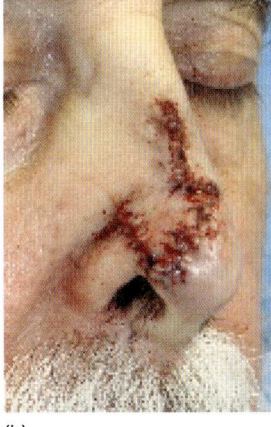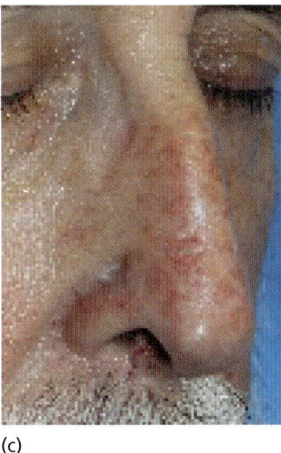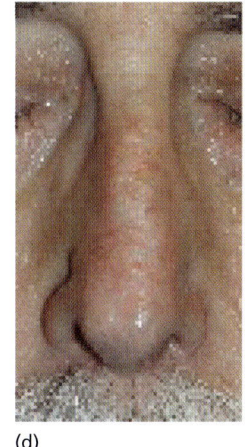

Figure 20.38 (a) Defect after Mohs surgery for basal cell carcinoma of the distal lateral nasal tip. The third lobe of the trilobed flap was necessary to recruit skin from the dorsum of the nose. (b) Appearance of the trilobed flap immediately after surgery. (c, d) Appearance of the scar 18 months after surgery.

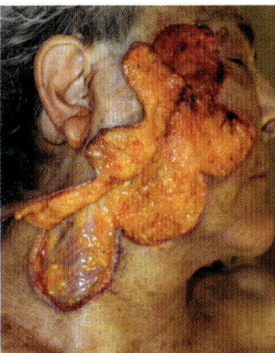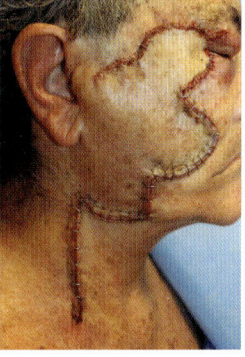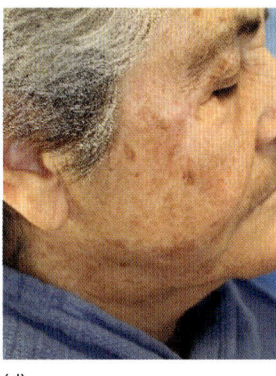

Figure 20.39 (a) Defect after Mohs surgery with MART-1 immunostains for a melanoma of the temple and lateral canthus. A trilobed flap is designed to recruit skin from the lateral neck. (b) Intraoperative photo with the flap elevated immediately superficial to the superficial fascia. (c) Appearance of the trilobed flap immediately after surgery. (d) Appearance of the scar 11 months after surgery.

Flap complications

Complications from flap reconstruction may include necrosis (Figure 20.46) or distortion of the free margins. Both complications can be avoided with careful flap design and selection. Flap necrosis can be prevented by minimising tension along the flap's leading edge and by ensuring adequate blood supply at the flap's pedicle. Stopping cigarette smoking 2 days before and 7 days after surgery may also decrease the risk for flap necrosis [3]. Free margin distortion can be avoided by keeping tension vectors parallel to the free margins or by using lifting flaps that transfer tension away from primary defects near the margins of the eyelids, nose, lips and ears. Scar revisions or staged reconstruction may be necessary to address unaesthetic scarring from necrosis or free margin distortion [4].

Grafts

Grafts are comprised of tissue that has been completely separated from its blood supply, and their survival depends on developing new attachments to the blood vessels at the recipient site [1,2,3]. While grafts are useful to repair defects that are too large for local flaps, they may be conspicuous if the colour, texture or thickness differs between the donor and recipient sites.

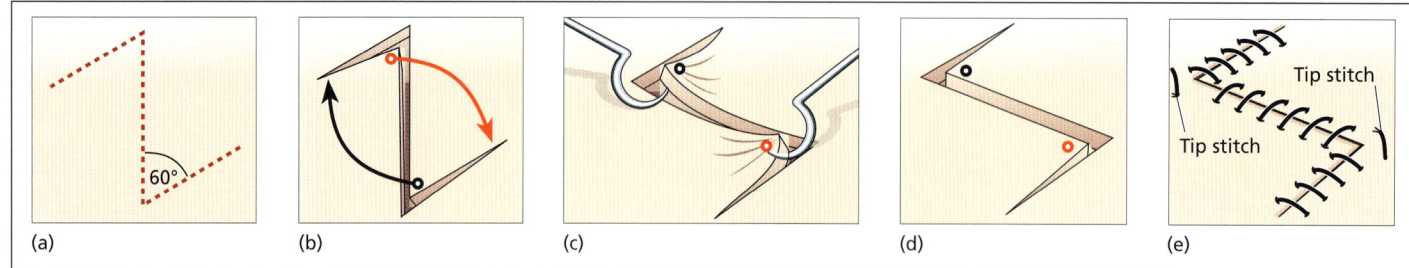

Figure 20.40 Technique of Z-plasty. Reproduced from Eedy *et al.* 1996 [30] with permission of John Wiley & Sons.

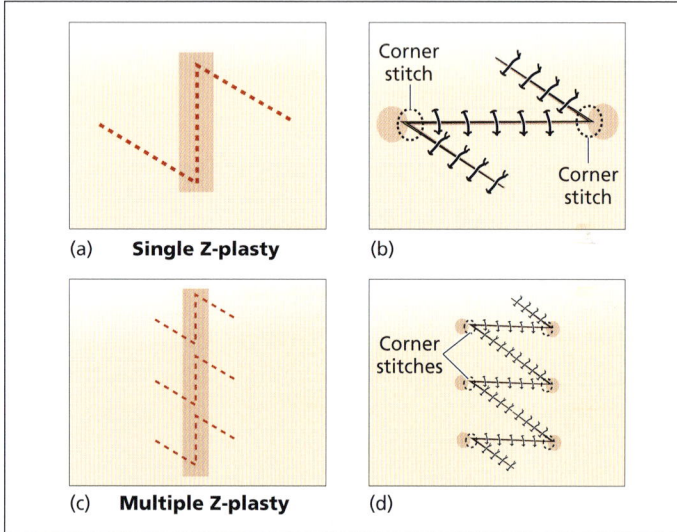

Figure 20.41 Single and multiple Z-plasty. (a, b) Single Z-plasty. (c, d) Multiple Z-plasty. Note breaking up of the zone of lateral tension (shaded areas) with multiple Z-plasty. Reproduced from Eedy *et al.* 1996 [30] with permission of John Wiley & Sons.

Grafts are classified by what tissue they contain. Split-thickness skin grafts contain the epidermis and a 'split' superficial portion of the dermis. Full-thickness skin grafts contain the epidermis and the 'full' dermis. Composite grafts contain skin and deeper tissues, usually cartilage for a dermatological surgery. Thicker grafts have increased metabolic demand and increased risk for necrosis.

Split-thickness skin grafts

Split-thickness skin grafts are useful to cover large defects (Figure 20.47). They are usually harvested from the thigh or buttock with a hand-held knife or mechanical dermatome (Figure 20.48). Split-thickness skin grafts may include variable amounts of dermis, but they generally lack adnexal structures and therefore do not grow hair or produce sweat or sebum. Thicker grafts may worsen scarring at the donor site, which is left to heal by second intention. If a split-thickness skin graft is smaller than the recipient site, it can be enlarged by meshing, or cutting multiple parallel slits that allow the graft to stretch like a fishnet stocking (Figure 20.49). The meshes also allow serous fluid (e.g. on the leg) to drain without collecting under the graft.

While split-thickness skin grafts are quick to harvest and cover large surface areas, the colour, texture or thickness often contrasts with the recipient site. They are also more fragile and prone to shearing from trauma, especially on the scalp [4].

Full-thickness skin grafts

A full-thickness skin graft (Video 20.10) is used when a donor reservoir is generous enough to suture the defect after harvesting the graft. The donor site may be selected based on the size of the graft. For smaller grafts for facial defects, common donor sites include the periauricular skin, naso-labial fold and upper preseptal eyelid. For larger grafts, common donor sites include the upper inner arm, periclavicular skin or lower abdomen. Full-thickness grafts include adnexa so they retain hair follicles and sweat glands. Ideally, the donor and recipient sites have similar colour, thickness and density of sebaceous glands and hair follicles. The donor site is usually closed with layered sutures, but hidden donor sites (e.g. postauricular sulcus) may be left to heal by second intention.

The graft is harvested by using a scalpel to separate the dermis from the subdermal fat. Residual fat on the graft may be trimmed with sharp tissue scissors. The graft is secured to the recipient site with a combination of peripheral and quilting sutures. The quilting sutures secure the graft to the base of the primary defect and close dead space to prevent the collection of blood or serous fluid (Figure 20.50). A bolster dressing is usually tied over the graft to push it against the base of the wound and to prevent shearing. The bolster dressing is usually removed 1 week after surgery.

Grafts are more likely to survive when the base of the primary defect has a good blood supply. Necrosis and infection are more likely if the recipient site has a poor blood supply, such as exposed bone or cartilage, or if the recipient site develops oedema, such as on the lower leg. If the primary defect is deep or has a poor blood supply, grafting may be delayed until granulation tissue fills the wound bed to allow increased survival and improved contour [5].

Composite grafts

Composite grafts contain skin and deeper tissue, usually cartilage. Composite grafts are typically harvested from the ear [6] to repair small full-thickness defects of the alar rim or from the contralateral eyelid to repair eyelid margin defects. Large or thick composite grafts have an increased risk for necrosis, so composite grafts are ideally small (<1 cm) and should approximate as much surface area of the primary defects as possible.

Mohs micrographic surgery
Definition
Mohs micrographic surgery (MMS) is a specialised treatment for skin cancer that offers extremely high cure rates and maximal preservation of healthy tissue. Intraoperative microscopic

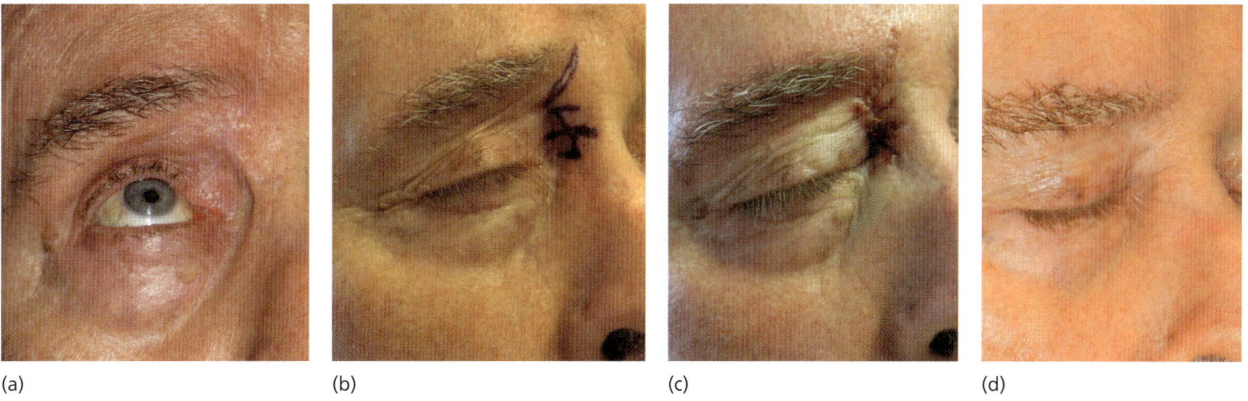

Figure 20.42 (a) Webbed scar of the skin of the medial canthus. The webbed scar is more noticeable with the eyebrow raised. (b) A double Z-plasty is designed to lengthen the webbed scar so it conforms to the concavity. The inverted scar at the medial brow will also be excised and resutured. (c) Appearance of the double Z-plasty immediately after surgery. (d) Appearance of the scar 4 years after surgery.

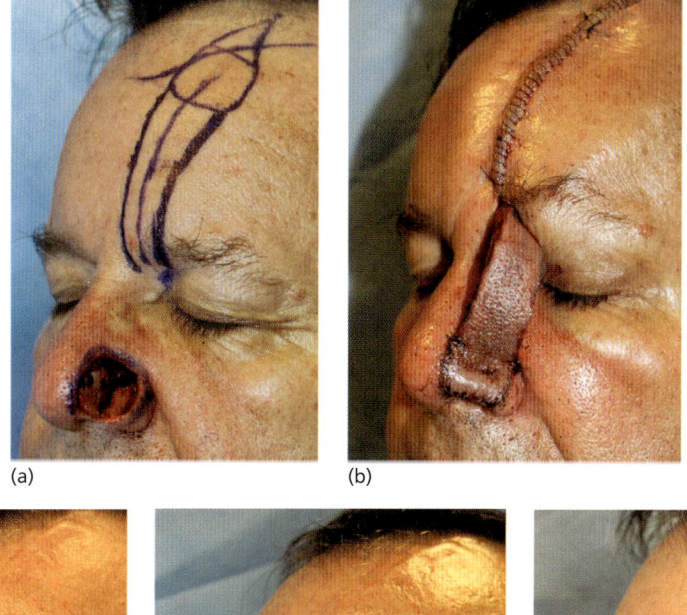

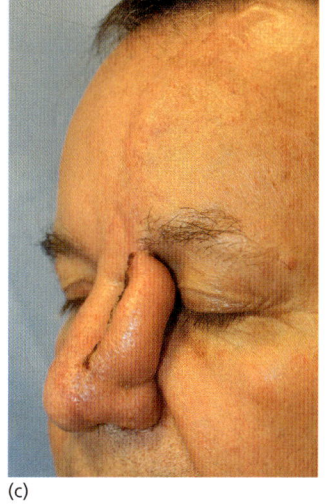
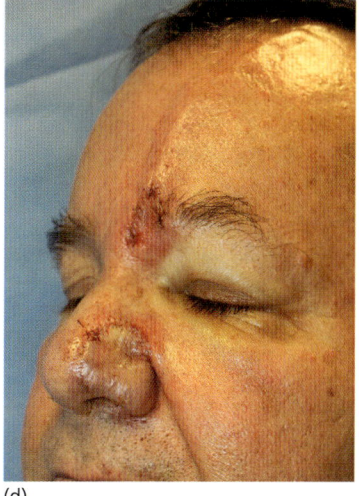
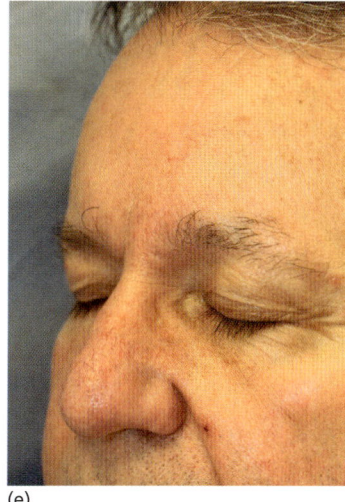

Figure 20.43 (a) Defect after Mohs surgery with MART-1 immunostains for a *melanoma in situ* of the left ala. A template of the defect was transferred to the upper forehead, immediately inferior to the hairline (delineated with a tangential line on the upper forehead). The path of the supratrochlear artery was mapped with a Doppler and is represented by the vertical line in the centre of the flap. (b) Appearance of the flap immediately after the first stage of surgery. The templated portion of the flap has been secured to the ala with layered sutures, and the donor site along the forehead has been closed linearly with layered sutures. (c) The patient returns for division and inset of the pedicle 3–4 weeks after the first stage. The templated portion of the flap has integrated into the blood supply on the ala. (d) Appearance immediately after division and inset. (e) Appearance 4 months after division and inset.

examination of the entire surgical margin by the surgeon allows accurate and dependable identification and removal of all residual invasive tumour while preserving adjacent uninvolved skin. MMS is most often used to treat the most challenging forms of facial basal and cutaneous squamous cell carcinoma, where it is rightly considered the gold standard. There is, however, a growing body of literature supporting its use in non-facial sites for recurrent disease and/or particularly large or aggressive tumours.

History

The technique evolved from the pioneering work of Frederic E. Mohs while working as a cancer research assistant at the University

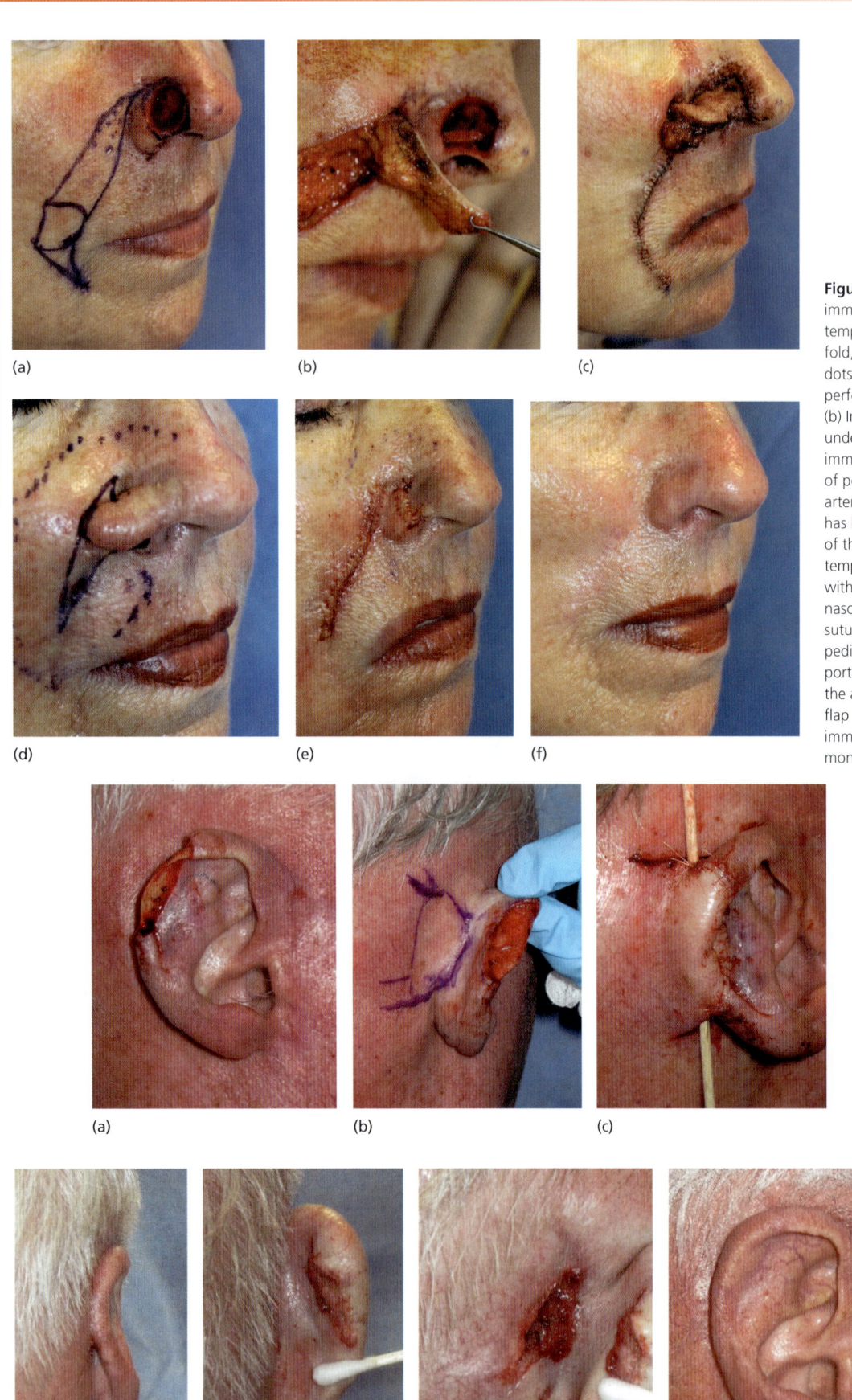

Figure 20.44 (a) Defect after Mohs surgery with MART-1 immunostains for a melanoma *in situ* of the right ala. A template of the defect was transferred to the naso-labial fold, and a naso-labial interpolation flap is designed. The dots at the base of the flap pedicle represent angular artery perforators, which were mapped with a Doppler device. (b) Intraoperative photo showing the planes of undermining. The templated portion of the flap is elevated immediately superficial to the naso-labial fat pad. The base of pedicle includes the naso-labial fat pad and the angular artery perforators. An auricular free cartilage batten graft has been placed to secure the alar margin. (c) Appearance of the flap immediately after the first stage of surgery. The templated portion of the flap has been secured to the ala with layered sutures, and the donor site along the naso-labial fold has been closed linearly with layered sutures. (d) The patient returns for division and inset of the pedicle 3–4 weeks after the first stage. The templated portion of the flap has integrated into the blood supply on the ala. An elliptical excision is planned at the base of the flap pedicle at the naso-labial fold. (e) Appearance immediately after division and inset. (f) Appearance 9 months after division and inset.

Figure 20.45 (a) Defect after Mohs surgery with MART-1 immunostains for a melanoma *in situ* of the right helical rim. (b) A staged retroauricular interpolation flap is designed. (c) Appearance of the retroauricular interpolation flap immediately after surgery. The cotton-tipped applicator is placed in the space between the flap pedicle and the mastoid scalp. (d) The patient returns 3–4 weeks after surgery for division and inset. The template portion of the flap has integrated with the blood vessels on the helical rim. (e) Appearance of the ear immediately after division and inset. (f) The donor site of the flap is left to heal by secondary intention. (g) Appearance of the ear 1 month after division and inset.

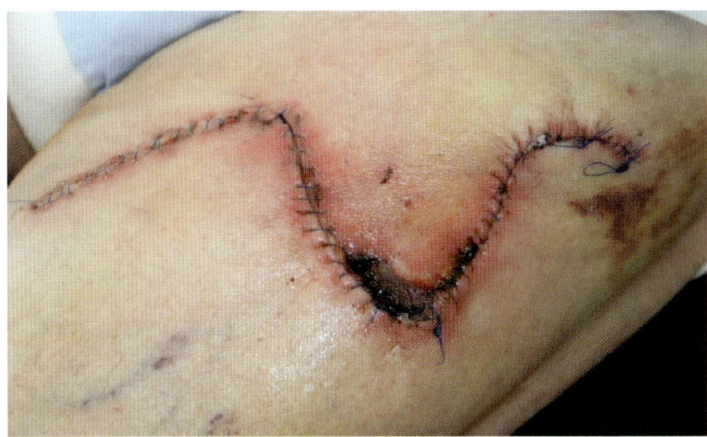

Figure 20.46 Flap complications: necrosis. A large modified rhombic transposition flap on the left anterior thigh of a heavy smoker that has undergone a degree of tip necrosis. This area will subsequently healed by secondary intention.

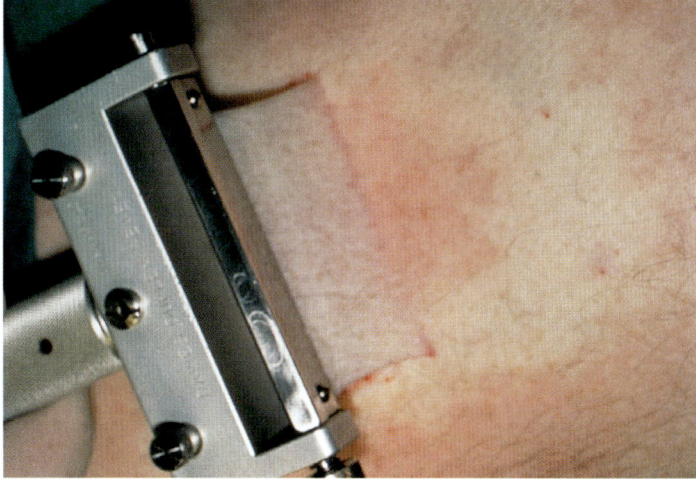

Figure 20.48 A split-skin graft can be harvested from the thigh skin using a power dermatome.

of Wisconsin, USA, in the early 1930s. Initially called chemosurgery, the original technique involved the overnight application of zinc chloride paste, with subsequent excision of the devitalised preserved tissues, and microscopic examination of histological tissue sections. Consequently, the wounds created had to be allowed to heal by secondary intention. Mohs introduced three features that remain fundamental to the success of the modern technique:

1. Tissues were sectioned and examined in a horizontal plane.
2. Excised specimens were marked and colour coded using a novel technique.
3. A mapping process was used to accurately identify the location of any residual tumour that could then be excised with further cycles of treatment.

As experience with the technique grew, the combination of consistently high cure rates for large and extremely destructive tumours, and the surprisingly acceptable results of wound healing by secondary intention [1], resulted in a gradual acceptance of the technique by the medical community.

Mohs first published his results in the general surgical literature [2], but as the main interest in his work was among dermatologists he subsequently began to publish in the dermatological literature [3]. Practical use of chemosurgery spread slowly among dermatologists, and nearly 30 years passed before there were enough 'chemo-surgeons' to form a society; the original 23 members of the American College of Chemosurgery (ACC) first met in 1967 [4].

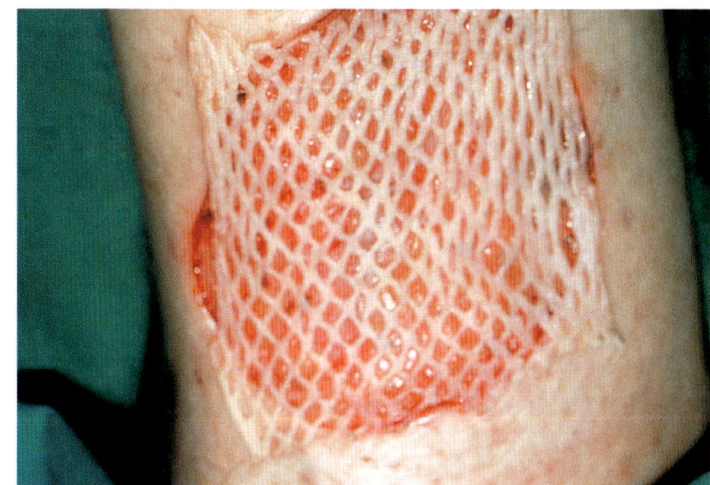

Figure 20.49 In a split-skin graft the harvested skin is meshed on a mesher, and the meshed graft applied to the defect.

Figure 20.47 (a) Large defect after Mohs surgery with MART-1 immunostains for a melanoma of the forehead and temple. (b) Appearance immediately after covering the wound with split-thickness skin grafts. A mechanical dermatome was used to harvest the split-thickness skin grafts from the thigh. (c) Appearance of the of the split-thickness skin grafts 14 months after surgery. (d) Defect on the thigh immediately after harvesting the split-thickness skin grafts with a dermatome.

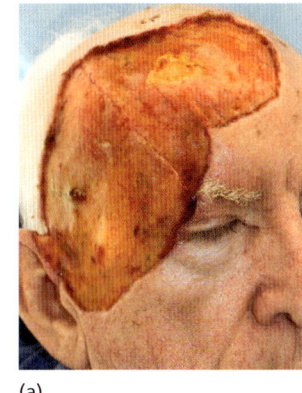 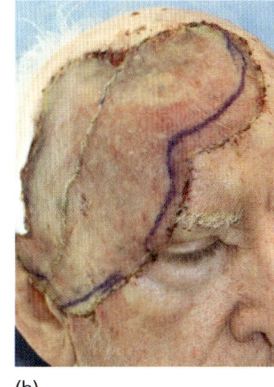 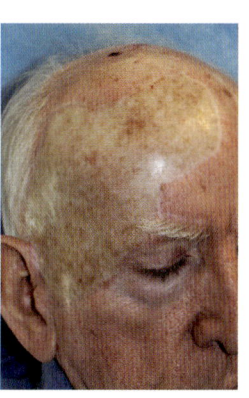 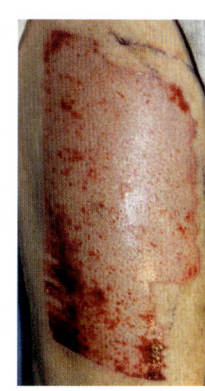

(a)   (b)   (c)   (d)

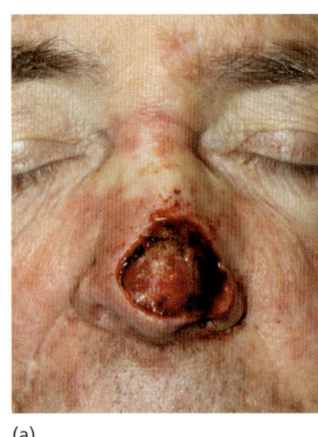 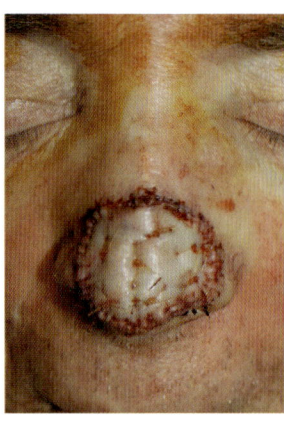 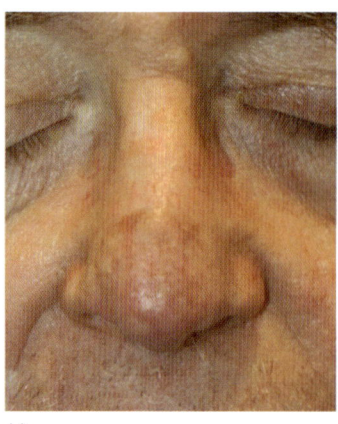

(a) (b) (c)

Figure 20.50 (a) Superficial defect after Mohs surgery for a basal cell cancer of the nasal tip. The defect was enlarged to include the entire nasal tip cosmetic subunit, and a full-thickness skin graft was harvested from the clavicle. (b) Appearance of the full-thickness skin graft immediately after surgery. Quilting sutures were placed to affix the graft to the base of the wound and a bolster dressing was placed for 1 week. (c) Appearance of the scar 8 months after surgery.

The evolution of chemosurgery into the technique that is now widely practised worldwide began at the 1970 meeting of the ACC when Tromovitch reported no recurrences in 99 (97%) of 102 patients following excision of basal cell carcinomas using the Mohs technique but omitting the use of zinc chloride paste and simply excising living tissue under a local anaesthetic [5,6]. This 'fresh tissue' technique had first been used by Mohs himself in 1953 and had become his preferred technique for the removal of periorbital tumours, a site where the use of zinc chloride paste led to particularly severe inflammation, swelling and morbidity [7].

As confidence in chemosurgery grew, it became increasingly clear that the success of the procedure was fundamentally linked to the comprehensive microscopic control of resection margins, rather than *in situ* tissue fixation. Consequently, there began a gradual move away from the use of chemosurgery and an increased adoption of the fresh tissue technique of Mohs surgery, most commonly using rapidly prepared frozen tissue sections. As a result, a painful prolonged technique, producing sloughy granulating wounds, was replaced by a procedure that could be performed comfortably under local anaesthesia, lasting hours rather than days, and resulting in defects that could be immediately reconstructed when necessary [8].

Treatment of skin cancer

Skin cancer can be treated with a variety of techniques including topical therapy, destructive procedures, surgical excision and radiotherapy. However, only surgical excision and MMS provide tissue suitable for histological examination of the surgical margins. The following are the fundamental differences between traditional surgical excision and MMS:

- Traditional surgical excision involves removing a predetermined margin of clinically normal skin from around and underneath the cancer; generally, wider and deeper margins are recommended for more advanced, difficult and recurrent tumours. MMS does not rely upon clinical estimation as the true extent of the cancer is revealed as the technique proceeds through the number of stages required to clear the tumour (Figure 20.51).
- Traditional surgical excision is generally followed by immediate reconstruction of the wound, with histological examination of the surgical margins occurring days later. MMS uses intraoperative histological examination to establish complete tumour

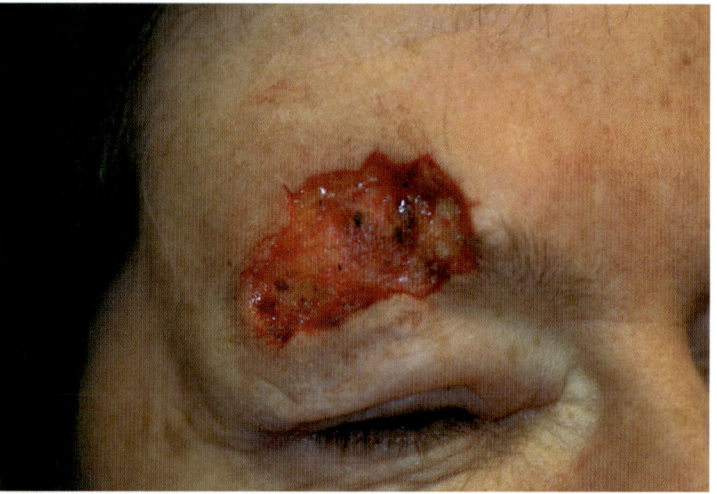

Figure 20.51 Defects following Mohs micrographic surgery (MMS) for 'high risk' facial basal cell carcinoma (BCC) illustrating significant tumour extension beyond the apparent clinical margins medially into the eyebrow.

removal on the day of surgery. Consequently, traditional surgery may result in incomplete excision of the cancer, and difficult management decisions as the wound has already been repaired. In contrast, MMS confirms complete tumour resection prior to wound reconstruction.
- Traditional surgical excision generally relies upon histological evaluation of the surgical margins using vertically orientated tissue sections ('bread-loafing'), which has been estimated to have a sensitivity no greater than 44% [9] as it involves assessment of <1% of the entire surgical margin. In contrast, the horizontally orientated tissue sections used in MMS are designed to allow microscopic examination of theoretically nearly 100% of the true surgical margin.
- Traditional surgical excision involves the surgeon, pathologist and possibly an anaesthetist. MMS is performed by the Mohs surgeon who also acts as anaesthetist, pathologist and in the vast majority of cases as the reconstructive surgeon.

Procedure

The practical aspects of modern fresh tissue MMS have been well described [8,10]. The technique involves sequential cycles of local anaesthetic surgery and pathological investigation. The visible skin cancer is initially excised as a flat layer with bevelled edges, which is accurately orientated, colour coded, mapped, horizontally sectioned and examined microscopically (Figure 20.52).

Any residual tumour identified at any part of the surgical margin is marked on the Mohs map, which accurately guides the Mohs surgeon in the re-excision of all residual tumour-involved areas (Figure 20.53). This meticulous and extremely methodical use of highly accurate, staged excisions underpins the very high cure rates associated with the technique. In contrast, those areas of the wound that do not contain tumour are not excised further, thus providing the maximal tissue preservation associated with the technique. Each tissue layer is examined microscopically and, if there is still residual cancer, the process continues, layer by layer, until the cancer has been completely removed. Frozen section histology is the preferred option for most experienced Mohs surgeons excising basal and squamous cell carcinoma [11], but permanent section histology is used by some, and this means that the wounds cannot

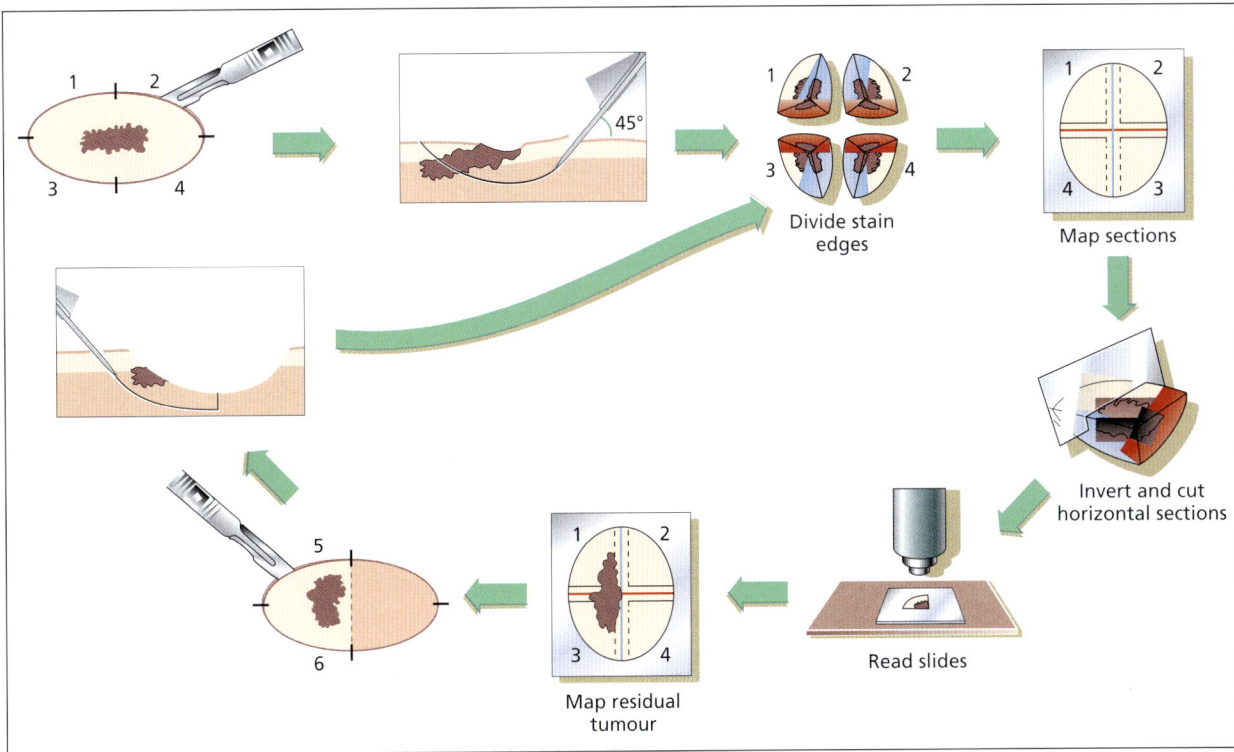

Figure 20.52 The stages of Mohs micrographic surgery.

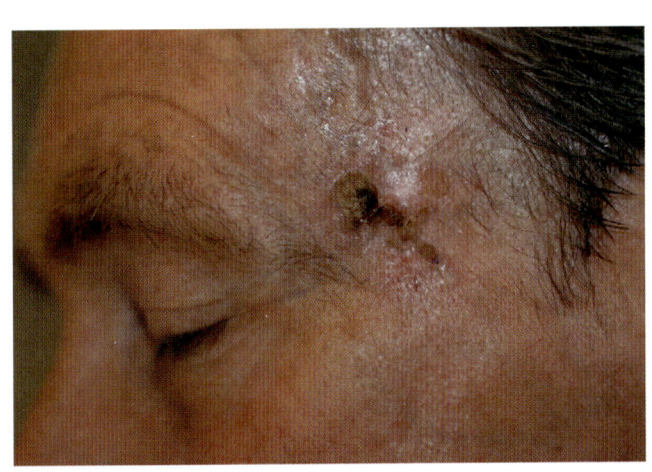
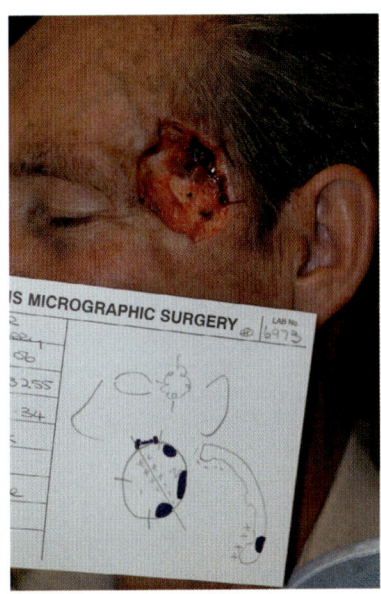

Figure 20.53 Intraoperative picture during Mohs micrographic surgery illustrating the role of the Mohs map in identifying the location of residual tumour. (a) Poorly defined basal cell carcinoma of the left temple, recurrent following excision. (b) Intraoperative picture showing correlation between residual tumour (blue areas on Mohs map) and the Mohs defect.

(a) (b)

be repaired on the same day [12]. Mohs surgeons who routinely use frozen section histology may occasionally use permanent section histology when treating highly infiltrative or uncommon tumours such as dermatofibrosarcoma protuberans [13,14].

In a feature unique to MMS, the final decision on the exact mode of wound repair is made only after the cancer has been completely removed, although likely wound repair options in a particular anatomical area can be discussed in advance. All wounds resulting from the old chemosurgical technique had to heal by secondary intention, but wounds following MMS are suitable for immediate reconstruction or secondary intention healing, whichever is most likely to result in the best cosmetic and functional outcome. In selected cases, other surgical specialists may perform reconstruction of the Mohs defect as part of a multidisciplinary approach to the management of aggressive facial skin cancer. In many major Mohs units, Mohs surgery is frequently performed in collaboration with plastic [15], maxillofacial, otorhinolaryngeal [16] or oculoplastic [17] colleagues.

Results

With MMS, a 98–99% 5-year cure rate for basal cell carcinoma and a 94.4% 5-year cure rate for squamous cell carcinomas was reported by Mohs himself [18]. There is considerable evidence supporting the use of MMS to treat the most difficult cases of basal cell carcinoma. A review of studies published since the mid-1940s suggested an overall 5-year cure rate of 99% following MMS for primary basal cell carcinoma [19] and 94.4% for recurrent disease [20]. Two prospective studies have been reported from Australia; in one, 5-year cure rates of 100% and 92.2% for primary and recurrent tumours were reported in 819 patients with periocular basal cell carcinoma [21]. In another study of 3370 basal cell carcinomas on the head and neck treated with MMS there were 5-year cure rates of 98.6% for primary basal cell carcinoma and 96% for recurrent disease [22]. A retrospective review of 620 patients with 720 lesions gave estimated 5-year cure rates of 98.8% for primary basal cell carcinoma and 93.3% for recurrent disease (Box 20.2 and Table 20.3) [23,24].

> **Box 20.2 Types of basal cell carcinoma (BCC) that should not be treated by curettage**
>
> - Large tumours (≥2 cm diameter)
> - Tumours at sites where the appearance of the scar produced by curettage is cosmetically unacceptable to the patient or where recurrence of the tumour has an unacceptable risk of further morbidity
> - Morphoeic, infiltrating or basosquamous BCCs
> - Recurrent tumours
> - Ill-defined tumours
> - Tumours penetrating muscle, fat, bone, etc.

Cutaneous squamous cell carcinoma can also be successfully treated by MMS [18,25,**26**]. In an Australian multicentre study of 1263 cases (38.9% were recurrent lesions) treated over a 10-year period, there was an overall 5-year cure rate of 96.1% (97.4% for primary and 94.1% for recurrent disease) [27].

Table 20.3 Sites to avoid curettage and cautery of basal cell carcinomas.

Sites with a high recurrence rate after all treatment modalities	Sites where curettage is technically difficult	Sites associated with poor cosmesis after curettage
Nose	Lips	Vermilion border
Naso-labial fold	Eyelid	Alar rim
Around the eye	Hair-bearing scalp	Nose tip
Around the ear		Chin
Scalp		

MMS with melanocytic immunohistochemical stains treats specialty site and recurrent primary melanomas *in situ* and invasive melanomas with a <1% local recurrence rate [28–30]. Melanocytic immunohistochemical stains have proven to be accurate to detect the presence or absence of melanoma on frozen sections [31]. By comparison, conventional wide local excision of specialty site melanomas has local recurrence rates of approximately 10% [32]. As a result of the improved outcomes, MMS in the USA has grown 304% from 2001 (2.6% of melanomas) to 2016 (7.9% of melanomas) [33]. In its latest guidelines for cutaneous melanoma, the National Comprehensive Cancer Network indicates that comprehensive histological assessment of margins with MMS or staged excision should be considered 'for large and/or poorly defined' *in situ* or minimally invasive melanomas (<0.8 mm) associated with high cumulative sun damage [34].

The cost of MMS has been compared with traditional management [**24**,35–37]. The procedure (to produce tumour-free margins) has a similar cost to traditional excision [35] but is less expensive than excision using intraoperative frozen section control [36]. A study from the Netherlands found MMS was more expensive than traditional surgery [37], but as MMS is likely to produce higher cure rates than standard excision in selected cases it remains intuitively cost-effective compared with the resources required to treat difficult recurrent disease. The only study to date that tried to compare cure rates following standard excision and MMS [38] appeared to show little difference between the two treatment modalities. However, a failure to adhere to the study design (with 24 of 301 patients randomised to have standard surgical excision being moved into the MMS treatment group) raises concerns about the conclusions of this study [39].

Practical aspects and indications

Mohs micrographic surgery is a remarkably safe procedure when performed under local anaesthesia on a day-case basis [40–42]. The complete surgical margin control achieved by MMS lends itself ideally to the excision of tumours that grow in a contiguous fashion (all parts of the tumour are directly connected to all other parts), and whereas the two most common tumours treated by MMS are basal cell carcinoma and squamous cell carcinoma, many less common cutaneous tumours can be excised by experienced clinicians working in a multidisciplinary fashion and using either standard or modified forms of MMS (Box 20.3).

The success of MMS has led to the development of other surgical/pathological techniques offering more comprehensive surgical margin control than is available using standard histology techniques.

Techniques such as 'peripheral in-continuity tissue examination' [43] and 'three-dimensional histology' [44] all have their merits, but none has gained widespread popularity.

> **Box 20.3 Tumours treated by Mohs micrographic surgery**
>
> **Common**
> - Basal cell carcinoma and squamous cell carcinoma
>
> **Less common**
> - Melanoma, melanoma *in situ*/lentigo maligna [47]
> - Dermatofibromasarcoma protuberans [25,48]
> - Microcystic adnexal carcinoma [25,49]
> - Sebaceous carcinoma [25]
> - Extramammary Paget disease [25]

Basal cell carcinoma and squamous cell carcinoma can often be adequately managed without the use of MMS, and the technique is generally reserved for 'high-risk lesions' (Figure 20.54) [45,46], which can be defined by various criteria, including those listed in Box 20.4.

> **Box 20.4 Criteria for high-risk lesions that preferably should be managed with the use of Mohs micrographic surgery**
>
> - Size (especially larger (>2 cm) lesions) (Figure 20.54a)
> - Site (especially the perioral, periorbital, perinasal and periauricular areas where a combination of a high cure rate and maximal preservation of normal tissues and structures is vital) (Figure 20.54c)
> - Lesions with very poorly defined clinical borders (where it is difficult to accurately identify appropriate surgical resection margins)
> - Failure of previous treatment (recurrent disease) (Figure 20.54b)
> - Histologically incompletely excised lesions
> - Histological features (aggressive growth patterns, perineural spread)

As the use of MMS became widespread, the ACC first changed its name to the American College of Mohs Micrographic Surgery and Cutaneous Oncology (ACMMSCO), and is now the American College of Mohs Surgery (ACMS), with over 2000 members worldwide. For many years, the college and its members have undertaken a long-term policy of improvement of the specialty, through scientific and technical development and through the formalisation of training for new Mohs surgeons with minimum 12-month, college-approved fellowships. Successful graduates from fellowship training, and others trained outside the college training schemes, should not only be proficient in the technique, but also be expert in cutaneous oncology and highly competent reconstructive surgeons. The continuing success and development of MMS as a recognised specialty is dependent upon a consistent demonstration of high cure rates, maximal tissue conservation and good aesthetic outcomes of the technique, which can only result from appropriate training and experience.

In the UK, the British Society for Dermatological Surgery has also created training standards for MMS with postgraduate fellowship training programmes, which have been ratified by the relevant postgraduate training authorities. In the USA, many of the criteria for postgraduate training have been adopted by the Accreditation Council for Graduate Medical Education (ACGME) under the recently renamed Fellowship in Micrographic Surgery and Dermatologic Oncology. In addition to training in MMS and skin oncology, this fellowship includes training in aesthetic procedures including lasers and injectables such as fillers and Botox®.

Dressings and postoperative care

Although perhaps not strictly necessary, a dressing following a cutaneous surgical procedure is likely to produce a better final result and, furthermore, conform to the expectations of most patients.

An ideal dressing should have the following characteristics:
- It should soak up excess exudate from the wound surface, thereby reducing the risk of bacterial penetration.
- It should maintain a moist wound–dressing interface to encourage migration of epidermal cells over the granulating tissue. Partial-thickness wounds heal faster if they are covered than if they are left to dry [1]. A scab is a poor barrier against loss of moisture from the dermal surface because it allows the surface to dry out, thus forcing the epidermis to grow under the dry wound surface. As the epidermal cells migrate, they secrete a proteolytic enzyme which dissolves the base of the scab; migration ceases when cell–cell contact occurs [2].
- It should not contain organisms or fibres that may contaminate the wound. Cellulose-derived dressings may shed fibre fragments into the wound [3], causing a foreign-body reaction and leading to increased risk of infection.
- It should be impermeable to bacteria.
- It should cause minimal injury to healing tissue when removed.

It is often claimed that a dressing that permits increased oxygen permeability aids wound healing. Such dressings do aid healing in partial-thickness wounds [4]. However, in full-thickness wounds, the same synthetic wound dressings create hypoxic conditions at the healing surface [5]. Paradoxically, tissue hypoxia in full-thickness wounds appears to stimulate rather than retard granulation tissue formation [6].

Basic dressings

This includes contact, absorbent and outer layers [7]. The layer in contact with the wound is non-adherent, either because it contains a greasy ointment (e.g. paraffin gauze) or because it is made from a specially designed, low-adherence material (e.g. polyethylene) [8]. The absorbent layer soaks up the excess wound exudate and cushions the wound. The outer layer (e.g. tubular bandage, elasticated tape) holds the other two layers in place and applies slight pressure. The basic dressing may be left in place until suture removal, but should be changed if it becomes wet or is saturated with exudate, as this greatly increases bacterial penetration. Many proprietary dressings combine two or all three components (e.g. Melolin® contains a polyethylene non-adherent layer attached to an absorbent cellulose component).

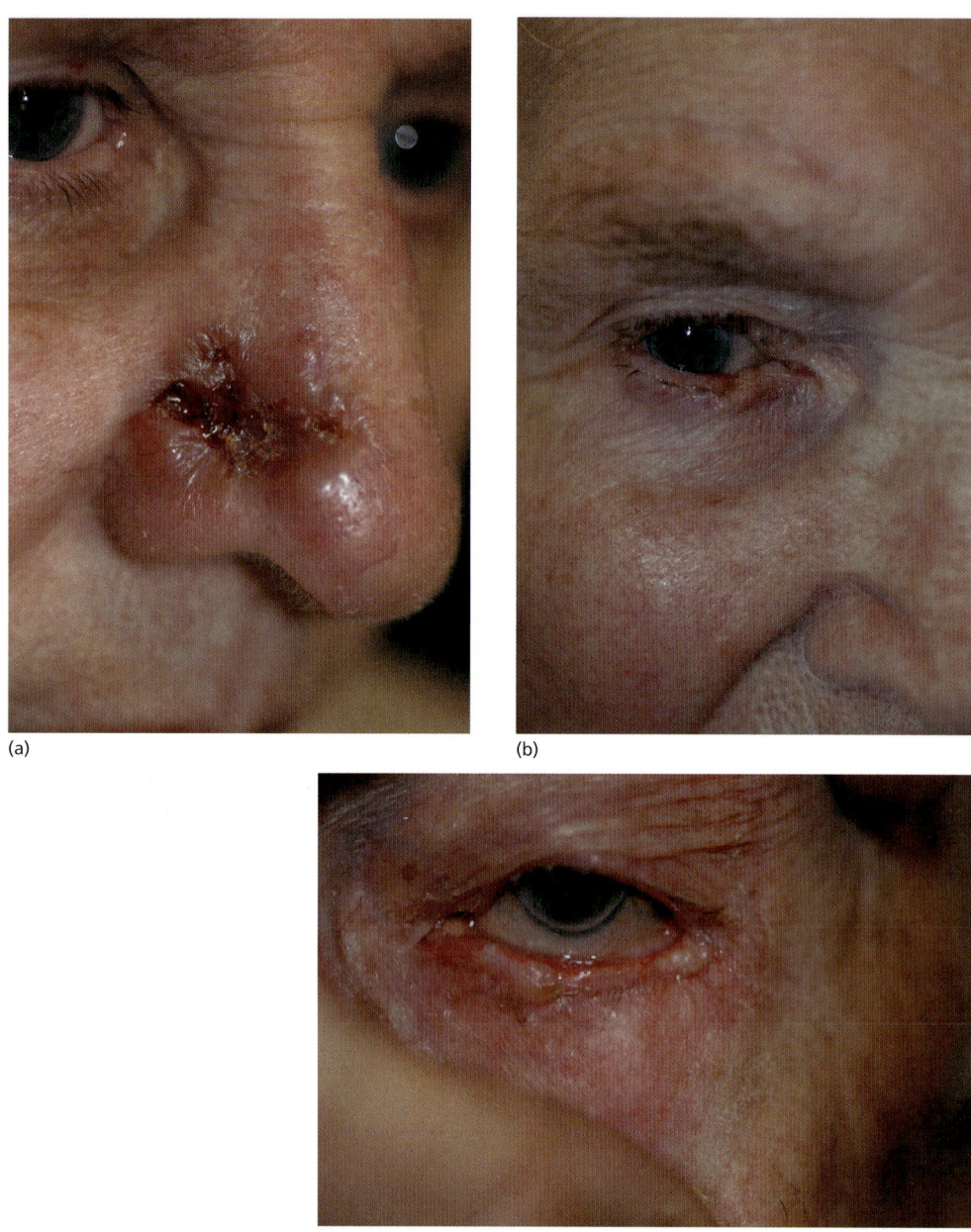

Figure 20.54 'High-risk' facial basal cell carcinoma (BCC) suitable for Mohs micrographic surgery (MMS). (a) Extensive nasal BCC. (b) Extensive lower eyelid BCC, recurrent following radiotherapy. (c) Infiltrative medial canthal BCC involving medial portions of both eyelids.

Pressure dressings

These are typically placed over the basic dressing and are useful in the immediate postoperative period to assist with haemostasis. Most commonly, and on suitable sites, a piece of compressible padded dressing (e.g. cotton-wool, dental roll, sponge, eye pad) is pressed down onto the wound with an elasticated or crepe bandage for 24–48 h. Where bandage application is difficult, adhesive tape can be used. A tie-over pressure dressing is commonly applied over skin grafts, but can be used on any wound. Paired sutures are placed around the wound and tied together to hold down a three-layered contact, absorbent and compression dressing, so that the graft is held down onto the recipient site to stabilise the graft and prevent a haematoma forming beneath it; alternatively skin staples may be used in this setting. Aquaplast®, a conforming thermoplastic material, may also be used to tie over skin grafts [9].

Postoperative care of granulating wounds

After surgery, an initial contact dressing is applied, and covered by a pressure dressing for 24–48 h. Thereafter, the dressing can be changed at 2–4-day intervals, depending on the amount of exudate. At each dressing change, the wound is cleaned to remove crust or debris and a greasy ointment (e.g. petrolatum jelly) and non-adherent dressing are applied [10]. On average, a 25 mm diameter head and neck wound takes approximately 35 days to heal [5]. These wounds are pain-free during the healing process. Bacterial contamination may occur, but tissue infection is rare. The patient should be made aware of the predicted time course for healing and that even a successfully healing wound will develop a somewhat reddened, elevated margin. A yellow exudate is common in the first few days. Before granulation tissue appears, a yellowish fibrin clot covers the wound. Exposed

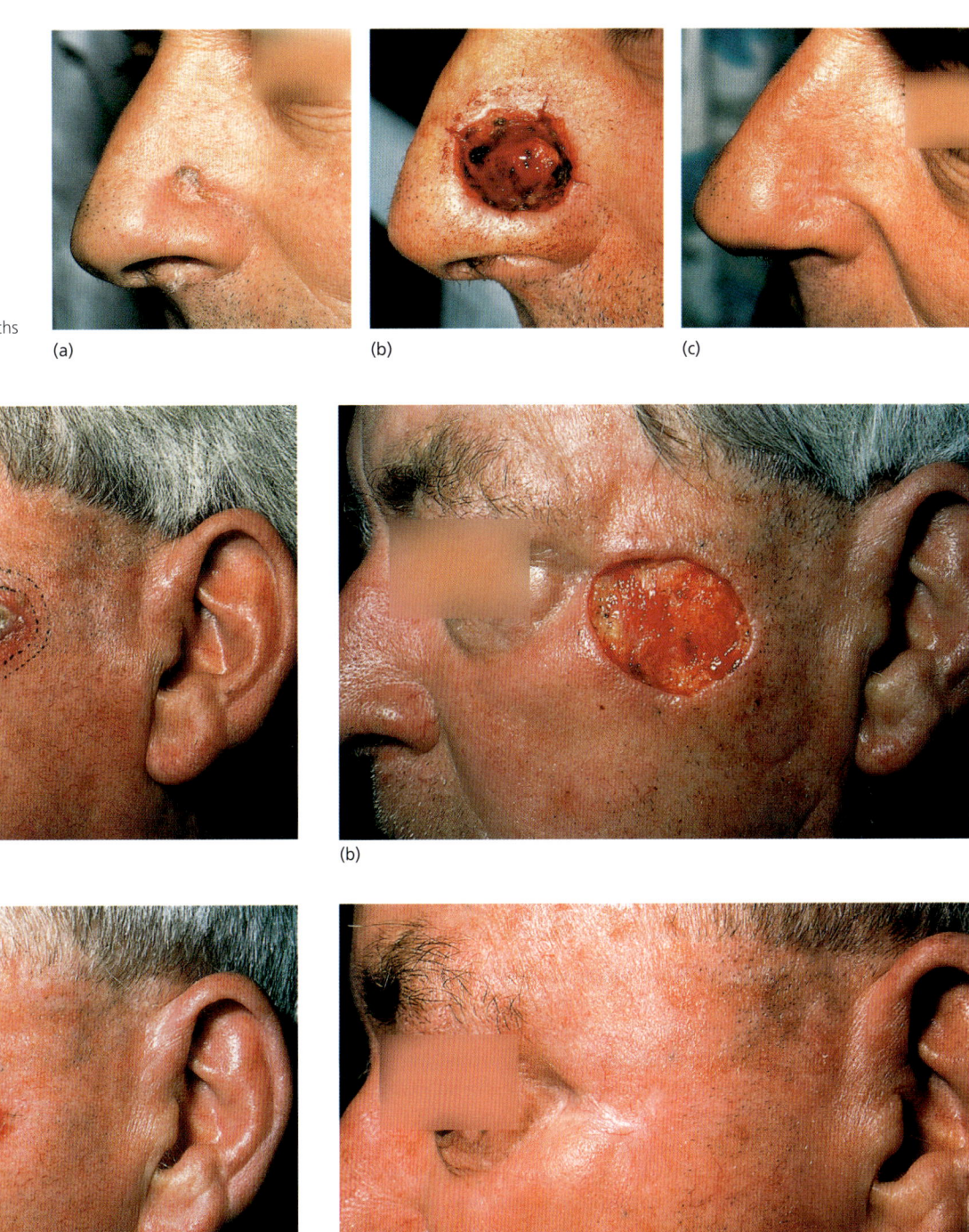

Figure 20.55 (a) This man had a basal cell carcinoma on the side of the nose; (b) this was excised and the wound was allowed to heal by second intention. (c) The cosmetic result 4 months later was good.

Figure 20.56 (a) This man had a basal cell carcinoma on the temple which was excised (b). (c) Three months later, the wound had healed but the scar was thick and red; (d) 15 months later this scar had become considerably less conspicuous.

periosteum and perichondrium must be kept moist and viable by using petrolatum jelly plus a moistened alginate dressing. This encourages granulation tissue to migrate over the exposed area and also reduces the risk of bone or cartilage desiccation and necrosis [6]. If the periosteum has been stripped off, the exposed bone can be fenestrated or abraded to encourage the formation of granulation tissue and hence enhance re-epithelialisation [7]. When the wound first heals, the scar often contains large looped vessels, which slowly disappear as the scar thickens. A slightly elevated red hypertrophic scar is then present, and the cosmetic result is not optimal until approximately 1 year (Figures 20.55 and 20.56).

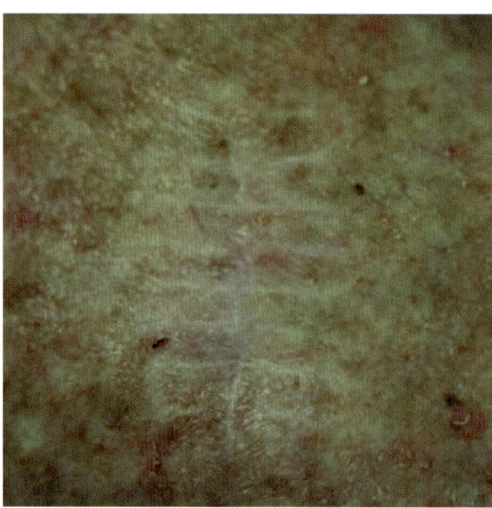

Figure 20.57 'Railroad' track marks arising as a consequence of skin sutures being left in place under tension and for too long.

Removal of sutures

The timing of removal of surface sutures varies according to the anatomical site of the surgery, wound tension and the surgeon's preference. In general, facial skin sutures may be removed on days 4 to 7; on the trunk and limbs between 7 and 10 days. The longer surface sutures remain in place, the greater the risk of cosmetically unsatisfactory surface 'track marks' occurring (Figure 20.57).

Complications

All dermatological surgical procedures may result in complications [1], most commonly bleeding, infection and poor wound healing (Table 20.4). Although complications inevitably occur, most may be prevented by a combination of thorough preoperative preparation and good surgical technique.

The incidence of complications following general dermatological surgery and MMS is in the main very low. In a prospective, multicentre study published in 2005, 84 French dermatologists performed 3788 out-patient dermatological surgical procedures under local anaesthesia. These included excision of benign and malignant tumours (excluding 'sebaceous' cysts and pyodermas) [2]. There were 236 recorded complications occurring in 213 (6%) procedures. Excessive bleeding (3%), vasovagal syncope (1.4%) and wound infection (2%) were the main complications. Infection was superficial in 92% of cases, with only one case of systemic infection. Antibiotic therapy or further surgery was required in 1%; haemorrhagic complications appeared to be independently associated with the risk of wound infection. In 2007, the same authors reported an almost identical study (73 dermatologists performed 3491 procedures) [3]. Overall, 67 (1.9%) patients developed wound infections, with a higher rate (4.3%) of infection following complex wound repair. Again, haemorrhagic complications were independently associated with the risk of development of wound infection.

MMS is also a safe procedure associated with a low risk of complications. An overall infection rate of 2.3% was reported following 530 Mohs procedures and 517 non-Mohs excisions performed on out-patients [4]. One US Mohs unit reported its complication rate to be equal to or lower than the published complication rates from specialists in other surgical disciplines [5]. The common practice of using clean but non-sterile gloves during Mohs tumour excision stages appears to be both safe and cost-effective. A retrospective case note review of 1239 Mohs patients (1400 Mohs procedures) revealed 25 cases of wound infection, with no significant difference in infection rates seen between those treated with either sterile or non-sterile gloves in the Mohs excision stages [6]. A more recent prospective study from Perth, Western Australia looked at 2370 dermatological surgery procedures including 934 Mohs surgery cases. The rate of complications of bleeding and infection were extremely low: 0.2% and 0.5%, respectively [7].

Bleeding (Figure 20.58)

Warfarin and other novel oral anticoagulant agents such as rivaroxaban pose a significant risk of postoperative bleeding complications. In a prospective study of 102 patients undergoing minor plastic surgery (37 regularly taking aspirin, 21 taking warfarin and 44 on neither drug), 57% of the patients taking warfarin developed complications, significantly more than the control and aspirin-taking groups [8].

Similarly, antiplatelet drugs (e.g. aspirin, clopidogrel, ticlopidine) potentially increase the risks of bleeding complications. In one study of patients undergoing minor plastic surgery, no significant difference in bleeding complication rates was seen between aspirin-taking and control groups [8]. However, other reports have found a link between aspirin therapy and a small but significant increased risk of postoperative bleeding following excision of cutaneous head and neck lesions [9], the risk being particularly pronounced in patients undergoing local flap wound repair. Current opinion favours continuing anticoagulation therapy in all its forms for patients undergoing dermatological surgery procedures. The increased risks of bleeding should be explained to the patient, and the surgeon should take measures to accommodate this – these include meticulous haemostasis, minimising tissue undermining, using pressure dressings, perforating grafts and even using small suction drains where indicated. It is important to make sure that patients taking warfarin do not have an excessively prolonged international normalised ratio (INR) and it is reasonable to check this prior to surgery, especially if they have a history of widely fluctuating INR readings. The preoperative evaluation is thus critical in identifying whether the patient has a history of a bleeding disorder or possible platelet dysfunction such as thrombocytopenia. Individual surgical units and hospital departments will have guidance and protocols pertaining to surgery and anticoagulation medication. It is recommended to be familiar with such guidance. National organisations such as the British Society for Dermatological Surgery have published their recommendations and guidance on antithrombotics and skin surgery on their websites (e.g. www.bsds.org.uk, last accessed October 2023).

New oral anticoagulants such as dabigatran, rivaroxaban and apixaban target key coagulation factors rather than vitamin K. Compared with warfarin, they have more rapid onset of action, stable pharmacokinetic properties and lack significant drug interactions. They do not require coagulation monitoring. Like warfarin, their use can result in postoperative complications. Perioperative management of new oral anticoagulants should balance the risk of bleeding with the risk of thrombosis. Comprehensive reviews on the topic have been published [10,11].

Table 20.4 Complications in wound healing.

Complications	Predisposing factors	Prevention
Infection (Figure 20.59)	Infected lesions	Careful preoperative and operative techniques
	Poor sterility	Sutureless closure
	Steroids	Antibiotic sprays
	Adjacent infectious source	Prophylactic antibiotics for infected or potentially infected wounds
	Occlusive dressings	
	Poor blood supply	
	Fat, haematoma and foreign material	
	Sutures	
	Poor technique	
	Excessive devitalised tissue from careless handling or electrocoagulation	
Delay in closure	Poor blood supply	Layered closure
	Excess movement	Gentle tissue handling
	Infection	Minimise devitalisation of tissues
	Tension	Care in decision to operate
	Steroids	Warmth
	Debilitated patient	Careful postoperative dressings
	Poor nutritional status	
'Gaping scar'	Inadequate apposition	Careful apposition
	Dermal instability	Subcutaneous or subcuticular sutures
	Excess movement	Adequate postoperative support (e.g. antitension dressings)
	Infection	
	Tension	
Painful scars	Feet and fingers especially	Avoid pressure sites if possible
		Dressings to reduce subsequent pressure and/or movement
		Careful apposition
Hypertrophic scars	Site	Avoid 'cape' area if possible
	Tension	Good surgical technique including undermining of edges where necessary
	Reaction to embedded material	
	Trauma	
	Individual susceptibility	
Keloids	Previous history	Avoid surgery where possible
	Fitzpatrick skin types V and VI	Antitension measures for 3 weeks
	Upper half of body	Watch and prepare to treat
	Tension	
'Railroad tracks' (Figure 20.58)	Skin sutures under too much tension	Good suture technique
		Use of 'non-reactive' suture material
Stitch marks 'abscess'	Sutures left in too long	Early suture removal
Wound edge inversion	Poor technique	Good surgical technique
		Occlusive or semiocclusive dressings
Bleeding and/or haematoma formation (Figure 20.58)	Bleeding tendency	Preoperative screening
	Aspirin	Good haemostasis
	Clopidogrel	Use of epinephrine (adrenaline) in local anaesthetic
	Ticlopidine	
	Eptifibatide	
	Tirofiban	
	Coumarin	
	Dabigatran	
	Rivaroxaban	
	Apixaban	
	Edoxaban	

The use of epinephrine-containing local anaesthetics results in vasoconstriction and prolongs the duration of anaesthesia. Intraoperatively, bleeding can be controlled by a combination of electrosurgery, pressure and ligation. Postoperatively, the use of appropriate wound dressings is important, ranging from simple dressings for superficial wounds to layered dressings with pressure pads for larger wounds where there is a significant risk of haematoma formation (e.g. following cyst or lipoma excision, or with widely undermined wounds). This is largely a matter of personal surgical preference with no data showing the 'superiority' of one type of dressing over another. All patients should be given verbal and written information regarding wound care and how to contact the surgical unit if problems arise. Haematoma formation may occur at various times after surgery and usually results in acute pain and swelling. The clinical appearances, together with the age and size of the haematoma, will dictate whether to open the wound,

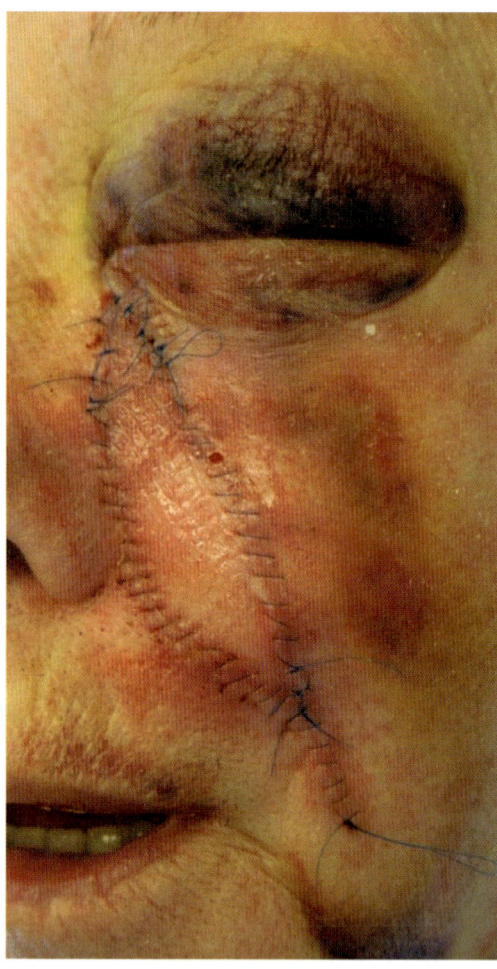

Figure 20.58 Postoperative swelling and haematoma formation.

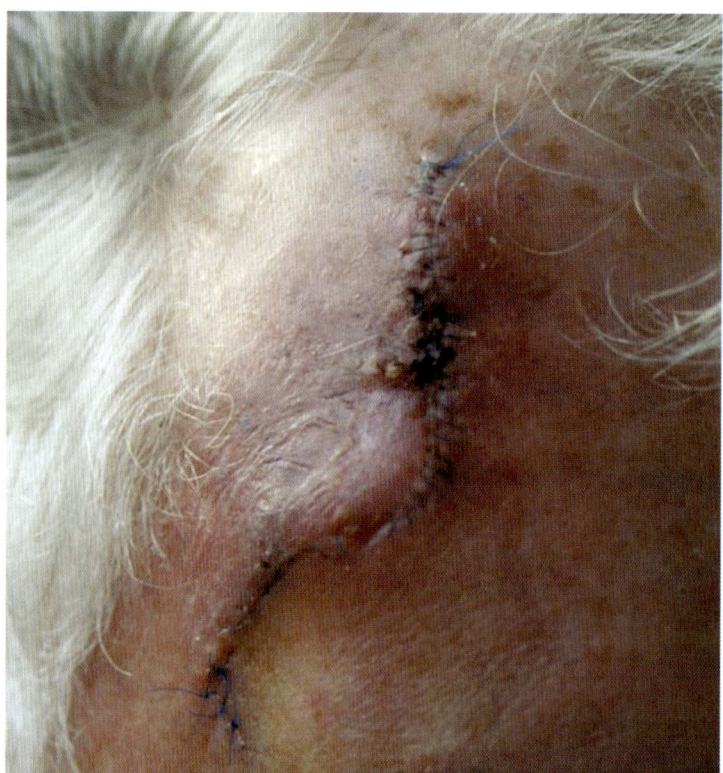

Figure 20.59 Postoperative infection characterised by redness, crusting and wound swelling and tenderness.

evacuate the haematoma and obtain haemostasis, or to manage the complication conservatively.

Infection (Figure 20.59)

Wound infection is a major concern, but is fortunately relatively uncommon following skin surgery of all types [2,3,4]. Antibiotic therapy may be appropriate for operations on ulcerated skin tumours: these are commonly colonised with *Staphylococcus aureus*, which considerably increases the risk of postoperative wound infection. Antibiotics may also be used prophylactically for wounds that are repaired with skin flaps or skin grafts or for wounds in the groin or on the lower leg. If the risk of infection is higher than normal (e.g. following excision of an ulcerated tumour from a flexural site), prophylactic antibiotic therapy may be appropriate. Postoperative infection usually presents as redness, pain and swelling in and around the wound, 4–8 days after the procedure. Depending upon the clinical appearances, management will range from wound care, topical and systemic antibiotics, through to incision and drainage of a frank wound abscess.

Unsatisfactory outcomes

Other significant problems relate both to the adequacy of excisional surgery and to the cosmetic and functional outcome.

Incomplete excision

Incomplete excision of malignant and benign skin lesions may occur either because of poor technique or, even with judicious clinical assessment of margins, due to subclinical tumour extension. Patients should be forewarned about these risks and the potential need for further surgery.

Unsatisfactory scars

The risk of abnormal or greater than predicted scarring must be carefully explained prior to surgery, with special attention to the possibility of distortion of free margins and unsightly hypertrophic scars in high-risk body sites (e.g. upper arm, shoulders, chest). Altered pigmentation in and around the wound is an additional cosmetic risk in those with Fitzpatrick darker skin types V and VI.

Nerve damage

Nerve damage is a significant concern, as both sensory and motor nerves may be damaged during dermatological surgery, particularly at certain 'high-risk' anatomical sites (see Figures 20.2 and 20.3).

Electrocautery and electrosurgery

Electrocautery

Cautery is the application of heat to living tissue. Heat causes tissue coagulation but if excessive can lead to unsightly scarring. In electrocautery, a thin metal element is heated by resistance to the flow of electricity and applied to the skin. No electricity passes through the patient so it is safe in patients with implanted cardiac or other electrical devices. However, due to the high temperature of the heated element, electrocautery may ignite inflammable liquids, vapours and gases and even dry cotton gauze so care must be taken to exclude these from the operative field [1–4].

Electrocautery units vary in size from small disposable pen size units that are popular for eyelid surgery to portable battery and mains-powered units. The more powerful units tend to have more rugged elements that last longer. It is common to heat the element until red-hot to sterilise the tip before use, but the tip should be allowed to cool before applying to the skin and only the lowest temperature for the shortest time should be used to achieve the desired effect.

Electrocautery may be used on its own or in combination with curettage to destroy a wide range of superficial skin lesions such as seborrhoeic keratoses or sebaceous hyperplasia. It can also be used for haemostasis after simple shave excisions. The most effective technique is to apply the element to the skin surface and move it around in a rotating motion while triggering the current and watching carefully for the first indication of tissue coagulation.

While heating the element may sterilise the tip, the body of the element remains cooler and may carry a risk of cross-contamination from patient to patient. It is therefore desirable to use a newly sterilised or sterile disposable element for each new patient.

Electrosurgery
Characteristics
Electrosurgery, also known as radiosurgery, radiofrequency surgery or surgical diathermy, uses high-frequency alternating current to heat the tissue. The frequencies used (0.3–5.0 MHz) fall within the radiofrequency band of electromagnetic radiation. Electrosurgical units (ESUs) and their output is seen on an oscilloscope as a continuous sine wave.

Low-frequency alternating currents such as the 230 volt 50 Hz or 110 volt 60 Hz currents as in domestic mains are hazardous to health because they stimulate muscle tissue and can cause cardiac ventricular fibrillation. The higher frequencies used in electrosurgery do not stimulate muscle and fibrillation does not occur.

In the most commonly used forms of electrosurgery, the surgeon holds a single active electrode (pole) to apply the energy to the patient. For current to flow, there must be a ground or sink to accept the electrons. At low energy levels, the patient's capacitance is sufficient to act as a ground and the current can flow without the use of a return pad. At higher energy levels, current cannot flow to the patient unless a return pad is used. The return allows current to flow back to the ESU and then to ground. In this case, charge enters from the active pole, travels through the patient, collects at the return pad, flows to the ESU and to ground. The return pad is also called a dispersive, collector, grounding pad/plate or passive electrode.

In both cases, energy flows through the patient and care should be taken in those with implanted electrical devices.

Terminology
Most commonly, the surgeon holds a single active electrode (pole) to apply the radiofrequency energy to the patient. This is termed *monopolar* electrosurgery. Conversely, if the surgeon holds both the active and passive electrodes in their hand, this is termed *bipolar* electrosurgery.

When energy is returned to the ESU (such as via a grounding pad or specialised forceps), the ESU is labelled as *biterminal*. When energy is not returned to the ESU, the unit is *monoterminal*.

The hyfrecator is a low-power unit and does not require a return of energy to the ESU. Thus, the hyfrecator as typically used is a monopolar, monoterminal device. Higher energy ESUs require a return (grounding pad) and as typically used are monopolar, biterminal devices.

Return or no return, electricity does pass to the patient during monopolar electrosurgery and due to possible interference, care should be taken in those with implanted electrical devices.

In contrast, current does not pass through the patient in bipolar electrosurgery. Bipolar electrosurgery appears similar to monopolar surgery as the surgeon holds only a single instrument. However, instead of holding only the single, active electrode, the surgeon holds both the active and passive electrodes in the form of electrically isolated forceps. Current travels to the patient down one (active) blade of the forceps and returns in the other (passive) blade. Only the tissue held between the two blades is affected and no charge enters the patient. Bipolar electrosurgery can therefore be used without regard to implanted electrical devices. As there is a return of energy to the ESU, bipolar electrosurgery is biterminal.

Electrosurgical units
Hyfrecator
Most dermatologists today primarily use a hyfrecator (named as a portmanteau of 'high frequency eradicator') in monopolar mode. The hyfrecator does not require an electrical return. However, if an alternate ground is present, for example if the surgeon touches the patient or if the patient touches metal on the surgical table, an electrical shock can be felt. Hyfrecators are only safe to use in conscious patients able to alert staff to inadvertent alternate site grounding.

With the hyfrecator, current enters the patient's body and care should be taken in those with implanted electrical devices such as pacemakers, deep brain stimulators and cochlear implants. As with any electrosurgical device, sparking can ignite inflammable liquids, vapours and gases and care must be taken to exclude these from the operative field. Supplemental oxygen should be discontinued during use if tolerated.

Most hyfrecators are configurable to be used in either mono- or bipolar modes.

Higher power electrosurgical units
Higher power ESUs require a return (dispersive) pad and are therefore biterminal. With these units, current will not travel to the patient unless connected to a return. As with the hyfrecator, the surgeon typically manipulates a single active electrode in a monopolar manner. Current enters the patient's body and care should be taken in patients with implanted electrical devices.

These units often have cutting, coagulating and blended settings. In 'cut', a continuous sine wave of energy is produced (similar to the hyfrecator but at higher power). In 'coag', the sinusoidal waveform is not altered but is only 'on' approximately 5% of the time. This results in slower heating – coagulating and desiccating the tissue rather than vapourising and cutting it. In blended settings, the on/off percentages are modified but the sinusoidal waveform remains. To maintain set power levels, the amplitude of the waveform (voltage) is automatically increased in these discontinuous or intermittent modes.

Return pads may be conductive (placed in direct contact with the skin) or capacitive (placed next to the skin). Conductive pads must make good electrical contact with the patient. Capacitive pads work through capacitive coupling and do not need to make direct electrical contact with the skin. Capacitive pads are less safe than conductive pads but are more convenient in the clinical setting on conscious patients. Many ESUs will alarm if contact between the patient and the return pad is broken.

Most high-power ESUs are also configurable to be used in either mono- or bipolar modes.

Electrosurgical effects

Monopolar electrosurgery can be used to produce a spectrum of effects with cutting at one end and coagulation/desiccation at the other. The ultimate result is influenced by the power setting, the tip of the electrode, the type of tissue and the surgeon's technique. Focused, high-energy results in rapid heating and vapourisation which cuts the tissue. More broadly distributed, low energy, over a greater area, results in slower gentler heating which coagulates blood and desiccates tissue. Both effects can be obtained by adjusting technique only.

In monopolar electrosurgery, radiofrequency energy is delivered to the patient at the tip of the electrode. When the tip is held above the skin, the charge 'jumps' and is dispersed to patient in a conical shape. This results in more superficial heating and charring. As the tip moves closer to the skin, the area of distribution (base of the cone) becomes smaller and smaller until the tip touches the skin. When the tip is held in direct contact with the skin, the charge density is greater and the tissue is heated more deeply.

Electrocoagulation (haemostasis)

Electrosurgery is extremely useful for haemostasis during dermatological surgery. For best results, place the electrode tip on or very near to the bleeding vessel. Use the lowest effective power setting and accurately place the tip as close as possible to the opening of the bleeding vessel. Frank blood should be removed prior to haemostasis to maximise energy transfer to the open vessel and to minimise energy wasted by simply charring and boiling the blood.

Electrodesiccation

Electrodesiccation refers to the technique where the tip of the monopolar electrode is in direct contact with the skin (Figure 20.60). It also describes the use of electrosurgery to coagulate and dehydrate (desiccate) the tissue. Tissues are fixed rather than vapourised. Lower power settings, intermittent waveforms and broader tips can result in more desiccation than cutting of tissue.

Electrofulguration

The term fulguration ('fulgur' = lightning) refers to the technique where the tip of a monopolar electrode is held above the skin and a train of sparks strikes the surface (Figure 20.61). This results in superficial heating and a blackened, non-conductive char. Due to the area of its conical base and shallow effect, fulguration is used for superficial haemostasis over a larger area such as after shave excisions and curettage.

Electrosection (cutting)

Focused high energy is used to cut the tissue. Optimally, a fine tip is utilised and the tip is held very near if not in direct contact with the tissue. Some tension on the tissue helps to separate the two sides. Much has been made of the possibility of cutting tissue without causing bleeding, but this is only possible if a degree of

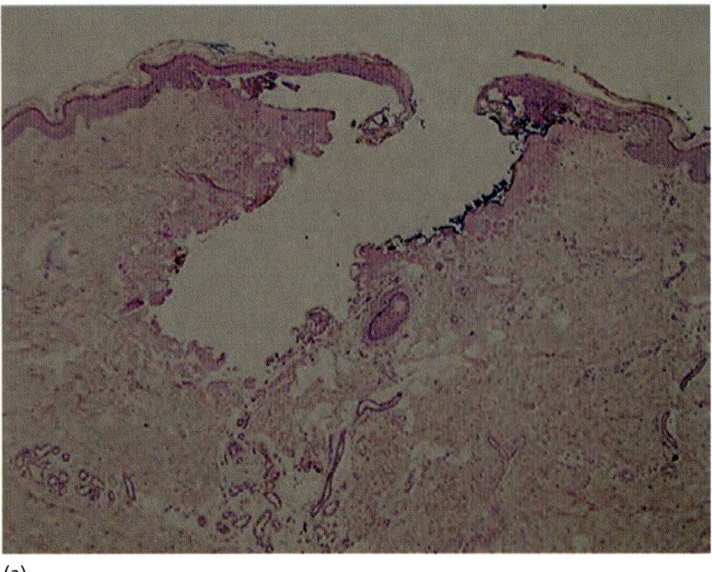
(a)

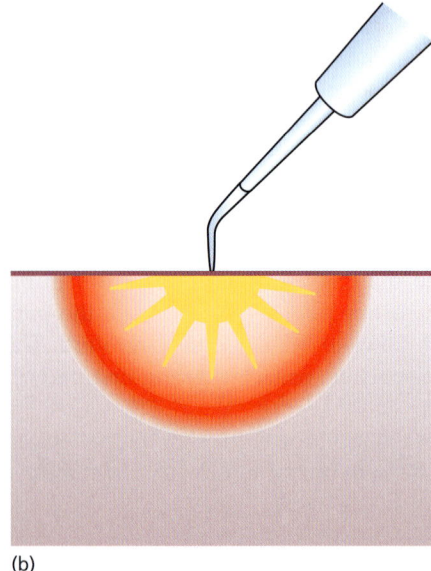
(b)

Figure 20.60 (a, b) Electrodesiccation. Focused coagulation, for example of bleeding points, can be achieved with a monopolar unit using a fine-tipped needle to deliver more concentrated energy to a focal point.

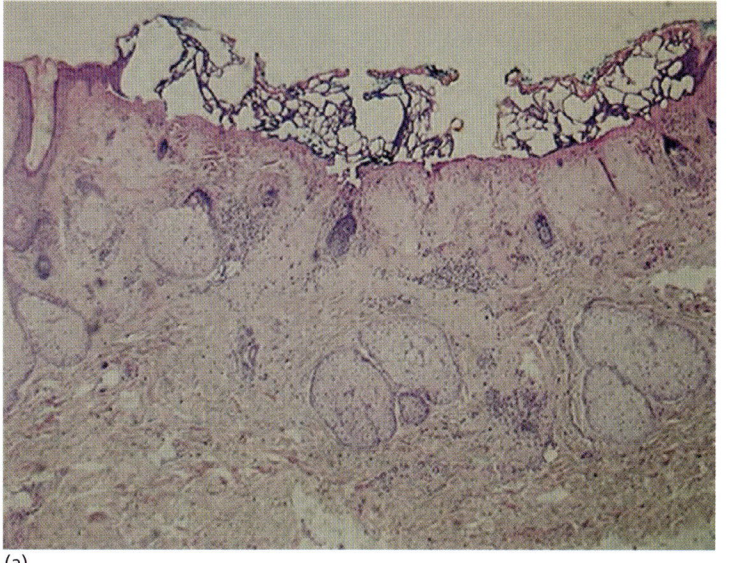
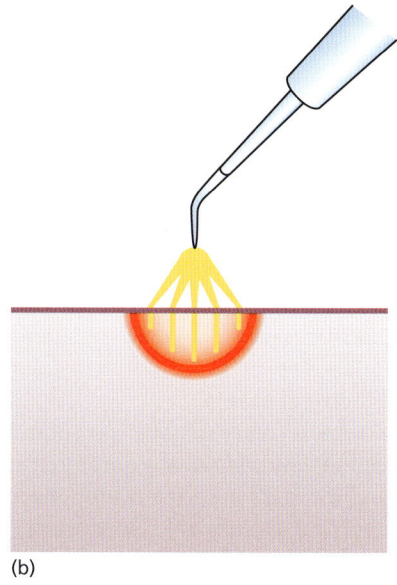

Figure 20.61 (a, b) Electrofulguration. Diffuse superficial coagulation can be achieved by passing the electrode of a monopolar electrosurgical unit over the skin without touching it. Energy is dispersed over a wide area by the spark which jumps from the needle to the skin.

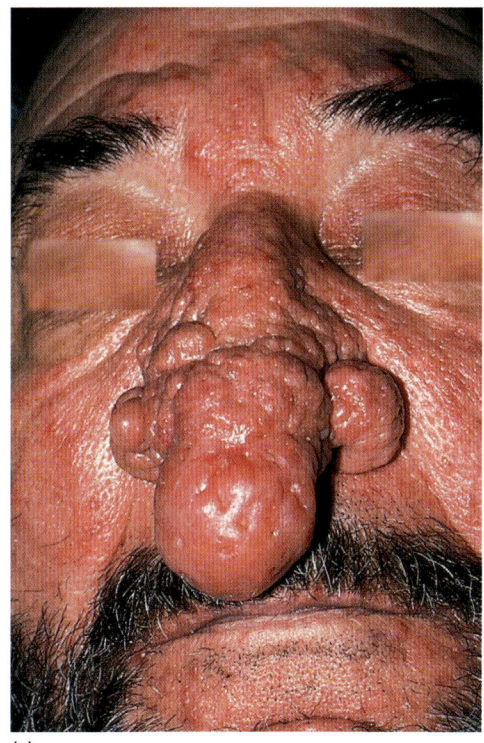
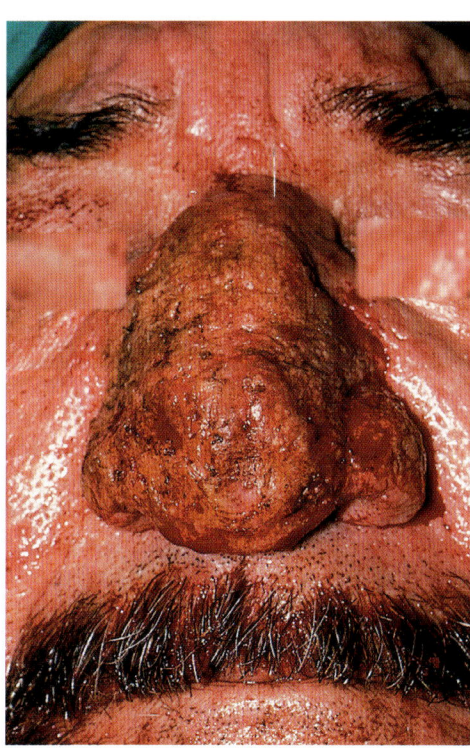
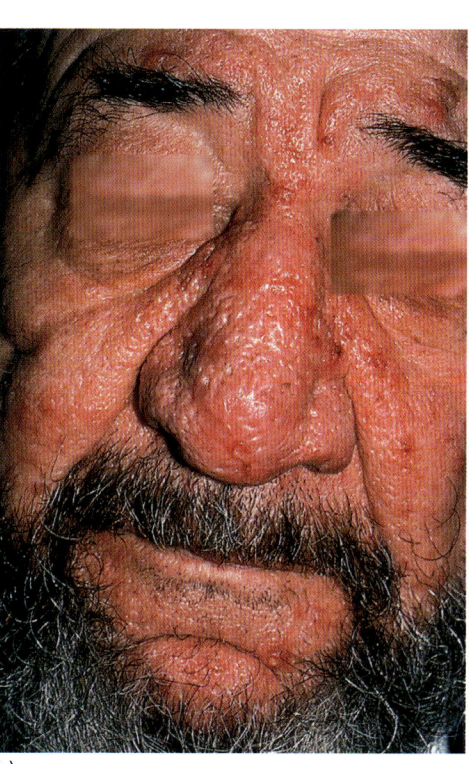

Figure 20.62 Shave excision and electrosurgery of a rhinophyma. (a) This disfiguring rhinophyma was reduced in size, and (b) the nose shape recreated by shave excision and electrodesiccation of the bleeding surface under local anaesthetic, (c) resulting in an acceptable cosmetic result at 4 months.

lateral tissue coagulation occurs. With the hyfrecator, electrosection can be used to undermine. In higher power ESUs, electrosection can be used with a loop tip to remove excess tissue in rhinophyma (Figure 20.62) although some coagulation also occurs. When using electrosurgery to treat rhinophyma especially, smoke and tissue fluid splatter will occur and a suitable smoke evacuator should be used; appropriate surgical masks and eye protection should also be worn by medical staff.

Hazards and risks of electrosurgery
Surgical smoke
Electrosurgical procedures result in a plume of smoke and steam that can contain particulates, formaldehyde, toluene, acetaldehyde and a variety of trace toxic gases. These substances can produce upper respiratory irritation and have *in vitro* mutagenic potential. The potential for generating infectious viral fragments, particularly following the treatment of verrucae, may exist. An effective smoke

evacuation or ventilation system should be considered to prevent the inhalation of noxious smoke and vapours produced during electrosurgical operations.

Fire
Electrosurgery may ignite inflammable liquids, vapours and gases. Particular care should be taken with alcoholic skin cleansers which may pool in anatomical recesses such as the conchal bowl or umbilicus and create a fire risk. Supplemental oxygen can also accumulate and removing or shutting off the supply during electrosurgery should be considered.

Electrical safety
Electrical safety may be considered from two perspectives: the safe use of any electrical equipment in the operating room, and the specific risks associated with electrosurgical current. As with any electrical equipment, electrosurgical equipment should be tested regularly and handled carefully; in particular, there should be no liquids in proximity to the equipment. Many electrosurgical machines have in-built safety features and will not work unless correctly set up and with a patient return electrode attached to the patient when this is required. It is important to be familiar with the individual machine.

Current passes from the active electrode to the patient return electrode and so the position of the patient return electrode, relative to the operative site, will determine the direction of current flow. This should generally be positioned to avoid any metal prosthetic joints and to avoid the chest in patients with implanted cardiac devices.

In general, most implanted cardiac devices will resist interference from electrosurgery but it is sensible to seek advice from the cardiac electrophysiologist responsible for the device if there are concerns or doubts.

Cryosurgery

Various methods of freezing skin lesions have been described [1]. Liquid nitrogen is the most effective and most studied cryogen and the only one that will be considered in further detail here. Nitrous oxide may be used with a cryotherapy gun – particularly for treating genital warts. Volatile (and highly flammable) ether and propane mixture sprays are sold in pharmacies for home treatment of warts. Neither of these achieve the same depth of freeze as liquid nitrogen, but can be effective for treating viral warts and benign skin lesions.

Cryotherapy is believed to cause cell death in four ways:
1. Ice crystals formed in the cell damage cellular components [2].
2. Uneven intracellular ice formation during freezing leads to osmotic differences arising during thawing, which in turn causes cell disruption.
3. Cold injury to small blood vessels results in ischaemic damage.
4. Immunological stimulation produced by the release of antigenic components results in cell damage.

The extent of injury is determined by the rate of freezing, the coldest temperature reached, freeze time and rate of thawing. Maximum damage is produced by rapid freezing and slow thawing. Repeating the freeze–thaw cycle produces much greater tissue damage than a single freeze because the greater conductivity of the previously frozen skin and the already impaired circulation both allow a greater and faster depth of cold penetration. It is suggested that a temperature of −30°C is required to produce cell death. In practice, tissue temperatures achieved during cryotherapy do not need to be measured because clinical studies have determined the duration of liquid nitrogen spray freeze times for common skin conditions.

Clinical methods
Liquid nitrogen is best stored in a pressurised container to reduce evaporative loss and the canister kept in a secure ventilated outside area. One litre of liquid nitrogen held in an unsealed vacuum flask will last approximately 6 h. Liquid nitrogen can be applied using cotton-wool swabs dipped into the liquid. However, a liquid nitrogen spray can is easier to direct accurately, faster and more convenient.

Clinical uses
Liquid nitrogen cryotherapy has been used to treat a wide range of skin lesions [3]. The simplicity and speed of cryosurgery treatment is both a strength and a weakness. Cryotherapy can easily be done incorrectly and ineffectively. The correct technique and freeze times are required to produce results similar to those described in published studies. It is important to recognise fundamental differences in the descriptions of cryotherapy techniques between British literature, which describes 'freeze' times, and American literature, where 'thaw' times are recorded. The development of post-cryotherapy complications also remains one of the most frequent sources of litigation for dermatologists [4].

Cryosurgical treatment of basal cell carcinomas gives cure rates that compare favourably with other modes of therapy [5–7] provided the correct technique is used and the treatment limited to small (<20 mm), well-defined, previously untreated tumours, avoiding basal cell carcinomas on the inner canthus of the eye, naso-labial and retroauricular folds and the hair-bearing scalp. The temperature reached and the number of freeze–thaw cycles are also critical. Debulking the tumour using curettage or electrosurgery prior to cryotherapy is advocated by some authors [8,9] although this is not routinely performed.

Side effects
Cryotherapy pain is significant but usually transient, and tissue swelling is common [1]. Inflammation can be reduced with potent topical corticosteroid applications [10]. Haemorrhagic blisters may occur but blister formation is not necessary for the cure of lesions such as viral warts. Sun-damaged and senile atrophic skin, and areas previously treated with topical steroids or radiotherapy, are more likely to blister or become necrotic after freezing. Skin necrosis is a desirable part of the treatment of neoplastic and many pre-neoplastic lesions, and several weeks may elapse before healing is complete. Hypopigmentation is common after liquid nitrogen cryosurgery, is particularly noticeable in dark-skinned patients and may be permanent [2,11]. Temporary postinflammatory hyperpigmentation is to be expected following less intense freezing. Nerve damage resulting in paraesthesiae, distal anaesthesia and motor paralysis occasionally occur [12]. Similarly, deep freezing

over the lacrimal ducts may, very rarely, lead to permanent ductal obstruction [1].

Caustics

In experienced hands, caustics provide a simple and readily available means of destroying many superficial skin lesions. The operator should be well acquainted with the action and degree of penetration of individual caustics, and the toxic effects that may result from absorption, especially if they are to be used on large areas and particularly when applied to the face [1–3]. In treating individual lesions, caustics are usually applied by means of a cotton-bud applicator or a wool-tipped orange stick, pointed if necessary.

Aluminium chloride hexahydrate. A 20% solution (Driclor®, Anhydrol Forte®), usually applied on a cotton-bud, is a very useful styptic for superficial wounds such as those following shave excision. Ferric subsulphate (Monsel solution) is widely used but may leave a pigmented scar.

Silver nitrate [4]. This is used in the form of a pencil or as a strong solution to suppress exuberant granulation. It is haemostatic and may be used to arrest bleeding after curettage. Repeated use tends to lead to unsightly staining of the skin.

Trichloroacetic acid. This is an effective haemostatic caustic with many uses. The 30–50% concentration can be used as a styptic, and may be employed in conjunction with superficial curettage in the treatment of solar keratoses, seborrhoeic warts, etc.

The supersaturated solution can also be used on its own to treat many benign and dysplastic skin lesions. Trichloracetic acid 35% is used for its destructive effect on the epidermis and may be a useful treatment for xanthelasmas and actinic lentigines. It must be applied with great care, however, especially around the eyes. Its action is rapid, and a white 'frosting' occurs within a few seconds of application. The caustic action can be partially neutralised by applying alcohol, water or sodium bicarbonate-soaked gauze, but this is unlikely to have any effect once the acid has penetrated the skin.

Excess sebum should first be removed using detergent or isopropyl alcohol. Trichloroacetic acid should then be applied with an 'almost dry' cotton applicator. The concentration to be used will vary according to the site, the condition to be treated and whether the trichloroacetic acid is being used as a styptic or a superficial skin caustic. Weaker solutions of trichloroacetic acid are sometimes used. Xanthelasma can also be treated using the blunt end of an orange stick, dampened with trichloroacetic acid and dabbed onto the affected area.

Intralesional corticosteroid therapy [1]

Aqueous suspensions of triamcinolone acetonide (10 mg/mL (Adcortyl®) and 40 mg/mL (Kenalog®)) are available and can be diluted with saline or lidocaine. Intralesional hydrocortisone acetate (25 mg/mL) can also be used. Triamcinolone acetonide 10 mg/mL is sufficient for all conditions except keloids, for which the more potent preparation is required in order to achieve the desired degree of collagen resorption.

The amount injected normally ranges from 0.1 to 0.5 mL of 10 mg/mL solution, depending on the size and nature of the lesion. The injection should be given using a 27–30 gauge needle deep in the dermis when possible to minimise the risk of collagen atrophy. The manufacturers recommend that no more than 30 mg of triamcinolone acetonide should be given in one session, with a maximum of 5 mg at any one site. (Steroid equivalence: 5 mg prednisolone = 4 mg triamcinolone = 20 mg hydrocortisone.)

It is important to note that triamcinolone acetonide is particulate in nature and serious adverse effects may result from inadvertent intravascular injection. The avoidance of intravascular injection is especially important when injecting lesions around the forehead – where accidental intra-arterial injection and retrograde flow of a bolus of particles may result in retinal artery occlusion and blindness. In this location, counter pressure should be applied around the injection site at the time of injection to avoid this disastrous complication.

Plasma cortisol levels are suppressed for a few days by 20 mg of intralesional triamcinolone acetonide given into various sites; higher doses suppress cortisol levels for longer [2]. Cushing syndrome has occurred in a child 2–3 weeks after a single treatment with 40 mg triamcinolone acetonide injected into keloids [3]. Local side effects include collagen atrophy with localised indentation of the skin [4], hypopigmentation [5], skin necrosis [5], perilymphatic linear depigmented and atrophic streaks [6,7] and telangiectasia [8].

Surgical indications
Intralesional triamcinolone therapy may be used for keloid scars, acne and pilar cysts, chondrodermatitis nodularis helicis, alopecia areata and many other steroid-responsive conditions [9].

Intralesional therapies for skin malignancies

Surgical excision is the treatment of choice for skin malignancy, but in *exceptional* circumstances, on a case-by-case basis, intralesional chemo- or immunotherapy may be considered. The agents that have been used most frequently are methotrexate, 5-fluorouracil, bleomycin and various forms of interferon. High cure rates have been reported, but most of the published literature consists of case reports and lacks long-term follow-up.

Intralesional therapy has been mainly used for keratoacanthomas and it is easy to appreciate the desire to control this rapidly growing but spontaneously resolving tumour by non-surgical means. Intralesional methotrexate or fluorouracil have been used most commonly. Bleomycin and interferon cost about 10 times as much as methotrexate and fluorouracil. Intralesional injections of methotrexate and interferon are painless, whereas bleomycin and fluorouracil cause severe pain and require concurrent use of local anaesthesia. A useful practical review of intralesional chemotherapy has been published [1].

In addition to keratoacanthomas, intralesional therapies have been used for basal and squamous cell carcinomas and for bowenoid papulosis.

Intralesional bleomycin followed by electrical stimulation (electrochemotherapy) has been used for a range of skin tumours and has a place in the management of multiple cutaneous metastases [2,3].

Miscellaneous surgical procedures and techniques

Curettage

Curettage can be used to treat benign lesions as well as small, lower risk squamous cell carcinoma *in situ* (Bowen disease), basal cell carcinoma (Figure 20.63a) and small, low-risk, well-defined squamous cell carcinoma. The technique relies on the principle that the curetted material is more fragile than normal skin (e.g. basal cell carcinoma) or there is a natural cleavage plane between the lesion and the surrounding skin (e.g. seborrhoeic wart). Disposable ring curettes are now the most commonly employed in practice. They come in ring sizes ranging from 2 to 7 mm and contain a sharp (cutting) edge on one side enabling a clean plane of cleavage.

On mobile or fragile skin areas, a starting point for curettage can be made by fulgurating the rim of the lesion using an electrosurgery machine or scoring the skin with a size 15 blade or the sharp side of a disposable curette. Haemostasis is achieved using either a chemical haemostatic agent (e.g. aluminium chloride 20% in isopropyl alcohol), cautery or electrosurgery (Figure 20.63b). Alcohol-based skin-cleansing solutions should not be used for the latter because of the fire risk. The resulting partial-thickness wound heals by re-epithelialisation from the retained adnexal epithelium.

Performing the curettage in a direction away from the operator ensures the creation of a shallow, superficial wound that usually heals excellently by secondary intention (Figure 20.63c) [1].

Haemostasis for open wounds

Bleeding from open wounds can be stopped readily using an absorbable haemostatic dressing such as Surgicel® (glucosic copolymer) although the mechanism of action is poorly understood. These materials may behave like a foreign body while dissolving in the wound and thus increase the risk of infection; large pieces should be removed before wound closure.

Chemical haemostatic agents [1,2] are effective on oozing skin wounds, for example after curettage and shave excision, but are ineffective in the presence of arterial or arteriolar bleeding and should not be used in sutured wounds as they cause cell death, which predisposes to infection. Application should be followed by pressure on the wound for 2–3 min to allow haemostasis to occur without the chemical being washed away. Ferric subsulphate (Monsel solution) solution carries the risk of iron tattooing [3]. Silver nitrate sticks are effective but caustic and may leave scars. Aluminium chloride 20% is effective: occasionally, and causes histiocytic reactions in treated skin [4].

Snip excision

Small tags can be snipped off with a pair of sharp scissors without the need for local anaesthetic. The tag should be pulled away from the skin with dissecting forceps and snipped off at its base: bleeding, if any, usually stops spontaneously. Haemostasis may be a problem with larger polyps with a well-developed blood supply; hence, an anaesthetic will be required. The wounds can be left to heal by second intention, with excellent cosmetic results.

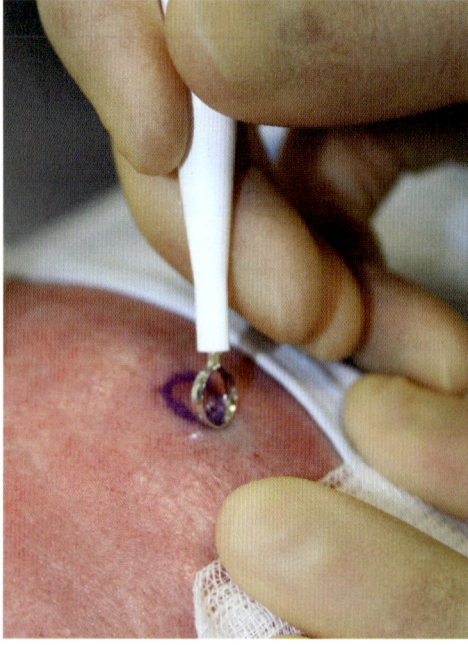
(a)

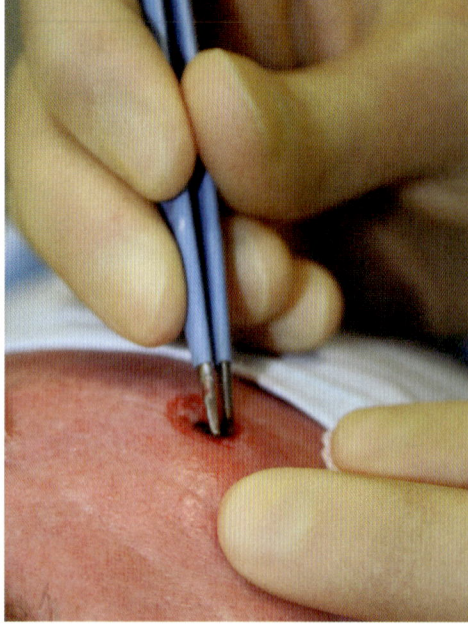
(b)

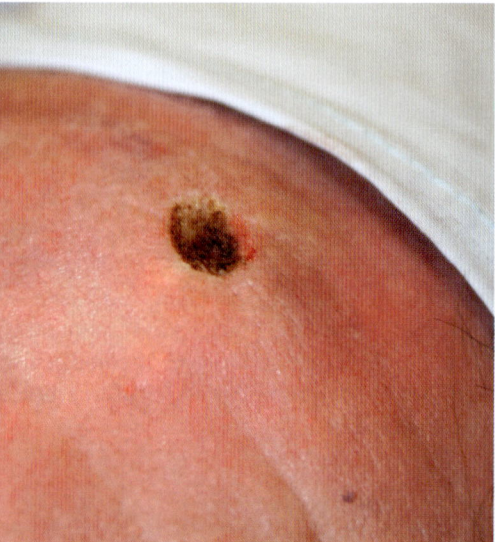
(c)

Figure 20.63 Ring curette. (a) Curettage of a small nodular basal cell carcinoma (BCC) on the forehead using a ring curette. (b) Haemostasis with bipolar diathermy. (c) Wound bed post treatment.

Management of specific conditions

Epidermoid cysts (Chapter 133)

Epidermoid cysts (erroneously called sebaceous cysts) are lined by a keratinising epithelium, which produces the cheesy keratinous contents. Patients may request excision if they are disfiguring, cause discomfort or are repeatedly infected.

The inflamed tissue around an infected epidermoid cyst is friable, making it difficult to excise without fragmenting the cyst wall. An infected cyst should therefore be drained, and the patient treated with an appropriate antibiotic. When the inflammation settles, the cyst can be excised. Cysts inflamed as a result of a foreign-body giant cell reaction to released keratin are best treated by triamcinolone injection followed by subsequent removal.

Freely mobile cysts can be easily shelled out through the smooth tissue plane that separates the very thin cyst wall from the surrounding tissue, although at this plane the cyst wall is easily punctured and must be handled gently. In all cases, the entire cyst wall and punctum should be removed, the latter at the centre of a small skin ellipse, which can also be used to manipulate the cyst during removal. If the cyst ruptures during extraction (a not infrequent occurrence), every effort should be made to remove residual wall fragments to prevent recurrence. Irrigation of the wound prior to closure will help remove residual cyst contents which might otherwise cause a granulomatous tissue reaction.

To avoid long scars, very large cysts can be decompressed via a 4 mm punch biopsy before excision. The wound is either left to heal for 4–6 weeks before definitive removal of the shrunken cyst or an attempt can be made to pull the cyst inside out through the circular wound using artery forceps. Immobile cysts are surrounded by extensive scar tissue and usually have to be excised with the surrounding fibrotic tissue and overlying skin. Excision of large skin cysts leaves subcutaneous dead space, which must be obliterated with deep sutures to minimise the risks of haematoma formation, infection and wound dehiscence.

Lipomas (Chapter 136)

Simple skin incision and lipoma excision ensures complete removal but produces a large scar. Scar size can be minimised by breaking up the lipoma into smaller fragments using blunt-ended forceps or a needle-holder inserted via a 4–6 mm punch biopsy wound made over the centre of the lipoma. The fragmented contents can then be squeezed out through the small wound. The fat can also be removed using liposuction. A subfrontalis lipoma (Figure 20.64) must be distinguished from a forehead epidermoid cyst. The former can be particularly difficult to remove because of its site beneath the frontalis muscle of the forehead, and care must be taken to divide the frontalis muscle vertically to minimise the risk of damage to the sensory nerves that lie on its surface or, more laterally, to the temporal branch of the facial nerve (damage to which will cause ipsilateral paralysis of the frontalis muscle).

Hidradenitis suppurativa

The surgical management of hidradenitis suppurativa is fully discussed in Chapter 90.

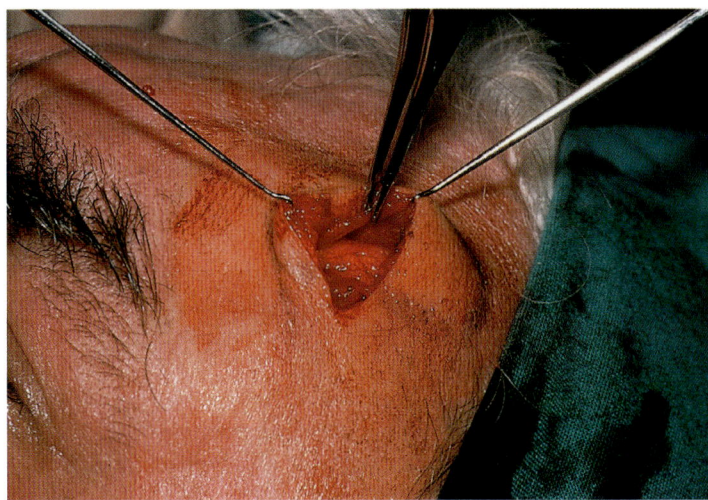

Figure 20.64 Subfrontalis lipoma. This lipoma lies beneath the frontalis muscle. The muscle has been split vertically and is held back with forceps to reveal the lipoma.

Chondrodermatitis nodularis

The surgical management of hidradenitis suppurativa is fully discussed in Chapter 106.

Digital myxoid cysts

The surgical management of digital myxoid cysts is fully discussed in Chapter 93.

Axillary and palmar hyperhidrosis

The use of surgical techniques for hyperhidrosis, including injection of botulinum toxin and sympathectomy, is fully discussed in Chapter 92.

Hypertrophic scars and keloids

The topic is fully discussed in Chapter 94.

Lesions on the shoulder, upper back and sternum

Surgical excision on the shoulders, upper back and sternum frequently produce poor cosmetic results, with the formation of stretched and frequently hypertrophic scars. Although meticulous surgical technique, appropriate undermining and careful suture technique may minimise these problems, patients should be carefully counselled and only offered surgical excision in these areas when it is absolutely necessary.

Benign naevi

Surgical excision, even by experts, leaves scars and consequently benign naevi are best either left alone or removed by shave excision when possible. See also Chapter 130.

Non-melanoma skin cancer: basal cell and squamous cell carcinomas

The management of these is fully discussed in Chapters 140 and 141.

Lesions of the mucous membranes

For management see Chapters 108, 109 and 110.

Keratoacanthoma

This is often difficult to differentiate, both clinically and histologically, from a well-differentiated squamous cell carcinoma. Management is fully discussed in Chapter 141. In general, it is best to remove these lesions surgically without delay.

Pigmented lesions (Chapters 131, 142–145)

The diagnosis and management of pigmented lesions is a key component of clinical dermatology and forms an important part of the multidisciplinary treatment of malignant melanoma, which also involves pathology, plastic surgery, clinical oncology, radiology and specialist skin cancer nurses.

Common and blue melanocytic naevi, pigmented basal cell carcinomas, seborrhoeic keratoses and dermatofibromas are usually easily recognisable to the trained eye, although diagnostic difficulties occasionally occur. Dermoscopy can provide a valuable non-invasive diagnostic adjunct (Chapter 145). When diagnostic doubt persists, and especially when malignancy is suspected, the lesion should be excised and submitted for histopathological examination.

When the lesion is too large to excise and repair directly, an incisional biopsy may be indicated (e.g. possible malignant change in a large congenital naevus or facial lentigo). In these cases, if malignant melanoma is proven on biopsy, a second procedure, possibly involving complex wound reconstruction, will often be necessary. The determination of key prognostic features (e.g. growth phase, depth of invasion, mitotic count, presence of vascular invasion) can only be made accurately from examination of the full excision specimen. For this reason, excision rather than biopsy of a pigmented lesion is recommended whenever possible.

Minor skin lesions: mollusca, milia and comedones

An orange stick can be used to apply small quantities of a caustic agent precisely to a skin lesion. When 90% liquid phenol is used to treat mollusca contagiosa or small cysts, the orange stick tip may need to be sharpened so that it just fits the cavity being treated.

Mollusca can be squeezed to express the cellular debris from the centre of the lesion before phenol application. The tip of the orange stick is dipped into the phenol, any excess wiped off and the stick is then placed in the centre of the lesion and gently twisted. The solution does not need to be neutralised. After initial whitening, the molluscum becomes inflamed and then resolves 7–10 days later. Treatment is painful and not usually tolerated by small children. The use of hydrogen peroxide cream has also been reported to clear molluscum.

Multiple small facial epidermoid or acne cysts can be treated using the blunt end of an orange stick, dampened with trichloroacetic acid or phenol. The cyst is incised, the contents expressed and trichloroacetic acid or phenol carefully applied to the cyst lining using an orange stick. No dressing is required, but a local anaesthetic is necessary. The same technique may be employed without the need for a specific caustic agent.

Milia are tiny, keratin-filled, epithelial-lined cysts with no connection to the overlying skin. They can be removed via a small skin incision made with a sterile venesection needle. No anaesthetic is required. Prick the needle tip into the skin and, by pulling the cutting edge upwards, incise the skin overlying the milium. Hook or squeeze out the cyst through the skin incision.

Comedones may be emptied using a comedo expressor, a metal instrument with a small cup-shaped end in the centre of which is a small hole.

Acknowledgement

The authors express their immense gratitude to Leela Raj (medical student) at the Sidney Kimmel Medical College Philadelphia, USA for her contribution towards the chapter's reconstructive videos.

Video legends

Videos for this chapter are available on the companion website (https://www.wiley.com/rooksdermatology10e).

Video 20.1 O-to-T advancement flap for a forehead, brow and eyelid defect.

Video 20.2 Rotation flap for a cheek defect.

Video 20.3 Two-staged 'pacman' island pedicle advancement for large cheek, nose and eyelid defect.

Video 20.4 Rhombic transposition flap for a cheek defect.

Video 20.5 Trilobed transposition flap for a cheek defect.

Video 20.6 Paramedian forehead flap for a large defect of the nose.

Video 20.7 Paramedian forehead flap: pedicle division and inset.

Video 20.8 Retroauricular interpolation flap for a helical rim defect.

Video 20.9 Abbe flap for a lower lip defect.

Video 20.10 Full-thickness skin graft for a helical rim defect.

Key references

The full list of references can be found in the online version at https://www.wiley.com/rooksdermatology10e

Introduction

3 Lawrence CM. *An Introduction to Dermatological Surgery*, 2nd edn. St Louis: Mosby, 2002.
6 Rohrer TE, Cook JL, Kaufman AJ. *Flaps and Grafts in Dermatologic Surgery*, 2nd edn. Philadelphia: Elsevier, 2017.

Critical anatomical considerations

1 Salasche SJ, Bernstein G, Senkarik M. *Surgical Anatomy of the Skin*. Norwalk: Appleton and Lange, 1988.
8 Romanes GJ. *Cunningham's Manual of Practical Anatomy. Vol. 3 Head and Neck and Brain*, 15th edn. Oxford: Oxford University Press, 1986.

Presurgical equipment, local anaesthetic and biopsy techniques
Equipment and sterilisation

3 Diwan R. Instruments for dermatologic surgery. In: Lask GP, Moy RL, eds. *Principles and Techniques of Cutaneous Surgery*. New York: McGraw-Hill, 1996:85–100.

10 Sebben JE. Survey of sterile technique in dermatological surgeons. *J Am Acad Dermatol* 1988;18:1107–14.

Safety aspects

1 Centers for Disease Control and Prevention (CDC). Recommendations for preventing transmission of human immunodeficiency virus and hepatitis B virus to patients during exposure-prone invasive procedures. *Morb Mortal Wkly Rep* 1991;40:1–9
2 Centers for Disease Control and Prevention (CDC). Perspectives in disease prevention and health promotion update: universal precautions for prevention of transmission of human immunodeficiency virus, hepatitis B virus, and other bloodborne pathogens in health-care settings. *Morb Mortal Wkly Rep* 1988;37:377–88.
6 Searle T, Ali FR, Al-Niaimi F. Surgical plume in dermatology: an insidious and often overlooked hazard. *Clin Exp Dermatol* 2020;45:841–7.

Local anaesthetics

1 Auletta MJ, Grekin RC. *Local Anesthesia for Dermatologic Surgery*. New York: Churchill-Livingstone, 1991.
6 Matarasso SL, Glogau RS. Local anaesthesia. In: Lask GP, Moy RL, eds. *Principles and Techniques of Cutaneous Surgery*. New York: McGraw-Hill, 1996:63–75.
7 Charalambides M, Yannoulias B, Gnanappiragasam D et al. Local anaesthetics in dermatological surgery: a review of adjuncts and pain reduction techniques. *Clin Exp Dermatol* 2022;47:1781–93.

Biopsy techniques

3 Lawrence CM. *An Introduction to Dermatological Surgery*, 2nd edn. St Louis: Mosby, 2002.
5 Zachary CB. *Basic Cutaneous Surgery: a Primer in Technique*. New York: Churchill Livingstone, 1991.

Preoperative preparation

6 Lawrence CM. *An Introduction to Dermatological Surgery*, 2nd edn. St Louis: Mosby, 2002.
8 Zachary CB. *Basic Cutaneous Surgery: a Primer in Technique*. New York: Churchill Livingstone, 1991.

Surgical procedures and techniques
Simple excision, suture technique and wound closure
Elliptical excision: general technique

1 Epstein E, Epstein E, Jr, eds. *Skin Surgery*, 5th edn. Springfield: Thomas, 1982.
2 Stegman SJ. *Basics of Dermatologic Surgery*. Chicago: Year Book Medical, 1982.
3 Miller CJ, Antunes MB, Sobanko JF. Surgical techniques for optimal outcomes, Part 1. Cutting tissue: incising, excising and undermining. *J Am Acad Dermatol* 2015;72:377–87.

Suture technique

2 Stegman SJ. Suturing techniques for dermatologic surgery. *J Dermatol Surg Oncol* 1978;4:63–8.
3 Stegman SJ, Tromovitch TA, Glogau RG. *Basics of Dermatologic Surgery*. Chicago: Year Book Medical, 1982.
4 Miller CJ, Antunes MB, Sobanko JF. Surgical techniques for optimal outcomes, Part 2. Repairing tissue: suturing. *J Am Acad Dermatol* 2015;72:389–402.

Reconstruction
Secondary intention healing

1 Zitelli JA. Wound healing by secondary intention. *J Am Acad Dermatol* 1983;9:407–15.

Linear closure

2 Wisco OJ, Wentzell JM. When an M is a V: vector analysis calls for redesign of the M-plasty. *Dermatol Surg* 2009;35:1271–6.

Flaps

1 Rohrer TE, Cook JL, Kaufman AJ. *Flaps and Grafts in Dermatologic Surgery*, 2nd edn. Philadelphia: Elsevier, 2017.

8 Hussain W, Tan E, Salmon PJ. Inferiorly based crescentic "sliding" cheek flaps for the reconstruction of paranasal surgical defects. *Dermatol Surg* 2012;38:249–55.
14 Salmon PJ, Klaassen MF. The rotating island pedicle flap: an aesthetic and functional improvement on the subcutaneous island pedicle flap. *Dermatol Surg* 2004;30:1223–8.
16 Tan E, Mortimer NJ, Hussain W et al. The nasal sidewall rotation flap: a workhorse flap for small defects of the distal nose. *Dermatol Surg* 2010;36:1563–7.
19 Hafiji J, Salmon P, Hussain W. The AIRNS flap: an alternative to the bilobed flap for the repair of defects of the distal nose. *J Am Acad Dermatol* 2012;67:712–16.
27 Zitelli JA. The bilobed flap for nasal reconstruction. *Arch Dermatol* 1989;125:957–9.
28 Cook JL. Reconstructive utility of the bilobed flap: lessons from flap successes and failures. *Dermatol Surg* 2005;31:1024–33.
29 Ricks M, Cook J. Extranasal applications of the bilobed flap. *Dermatol Surg* 2005;31:941–8.
30 Albertini JG, Hansen JP. Trilobed flap reconstruction for distal nasal skin defects. *Dermatol Surg* 2010;36:1726–35.
31 Jellinek NJ, Nguyen TH, Albertini JG. Paramedian forehead flap: advances, procedural nuances, and variations in technique. *Dermatol Surg* 2014;40(Suppl. 9):S30–42.

Mohs micrographic surgery

4 Brodland DG, Amonette R, Hanke CW, Robins P. The history and evolution of Mohs micrographic surgery. *Dermatol Surg* 2000;26:303–7.
10 Telfer NR. Mohs micrographic surgery for nonmelanoma skin cancer. *Clin Dermatol* 1995;13:593–600.
14 Charalambides M, Yannoulias B, Malik N et al. A review of Mohs micrographic surgery or skin cancer. Part 1: Melanoma and rare skin cancers. *Clin Exp Dermatol* 2022;47:833–49.
24 Brown AC, Brindley L, Hunt WTN et al. A review of the evidence for Mohs micrographic surgery. Part 2: basal cell carcinoma. *Clin Exp Dermatol* 2022;47:1794–804.
26 Hunt WT, Earp E, Brown AC et al. A review of Mohs micrographic surgery for skin cancer. Part 3: squamous cell carcinoma. *Clin Exp Dermatol* 2022;47:1765–73.

Dressings and postoperative care

2 Harris DR. Healing of the surgical wound. I. Basic considerations. *J Am Acad Dermatol* 1979;1:197–207.
7 Telfer NR, Moy RL. Wound care after office procedures. *J Dermatol Surg Oncol* 1993;19:722–31.
10 Axibal E, Brown M. Surgical dressings and novel skin substitutes. *Dermatol Clin* 2019;37:349–66.

Complications

1 Stasko T. Complications of cutaneous procedures. In: Roenigk RK, Roenigk HH, eds. *Dermatologic Surgery*, 2nd edn. New York: Marcel Dekker, 1996:149–75.
2 Amici JM, Rogues AM, Lasheras A et al. A prospective study of the incidence of complications associated with dermatological surgery. *Br J Dermatol* 2005;153:967–71.

Electrocautery and electrosurgery

1 Boughton RS, Spencer SK. Electrosurgical fundamentals. *J Am Acad Dermatol* 1987;16:862–7.
2 Taheri A, Mansoori P, Sandoval LF et al. Electrosurgery: part I. Basics and principles. *J Am Acad Dermatol* 2014;70:591.e1–14.
3 Taheri A, Mansoori P, Sandoval LF et al. Electrosurgery: part II. Technology, applications, and safety of electrosurgical devices. *J Am Acad Dermatol* 2014;70:607.e1–12.
4 Bigony L. Risks associated with exposure to surgical smoke plume: a review of the literature. *AORN J* 2007;86:1013–24.

Cryosurgery

3 Kuflik EG. Cryosurgery updated. *J Am Acad Dermatol* 1994;31:925–44.
11 Graham GF, Deltas RL, Garrett AB et al. Guidelines of care for cryosurgery. *J Am Acad Dermatol* 1994;31:648–53.

Caustics

3 O'Connor AA, Lowe PM, Shumack S, Lim AC. Chemical peels: a review of current practice. *Australas J Dermatol* 2018;59:171–81.

Intralesional corticosteroid therapy

1 Callen JP. Intralesional corticosteroids. *J Am Acad Dermatol* 1981;4:149–51.
9 Lebwohl M, Heymann WR, Coulson I, Murrell DF, eds. *Treatment of Skin Disease – Comprehensive Therapeutic Strategies*, 6th edn. London: Elsevier, 2022.

Intralesional therapies for skin malignancies

3 Good LM, Miller MD, High WA. Intralesional agents in the management of cutaneous malignancy: a review. *J Am Acad Dermatol* 2011;64:413–22.

Miscellaneous surgical procedures and techniques
Curettage

1 Kapadia A, Hussain W. Optimizing curettage with a 'backhand'. *J Eur Acad Dermatol Venereol* 2013;27:e139.

Haemostasis for open wounds

1 Larson PO. Topical haemostatic agents for dermatologic surgery. *J Dermatol Surg Oncol* 1988;14:623–32.
2 Palm MD, Altman JS. Topical hemostatic agents: a review. *Dermatol Surg* 2008;34:431–45.

CHAPTER 21

Principles of Phototherapy

Kevin McKenna[1] and Sally Ibbotson[2]

[1] Dermatology Department, Belfast Trust, Belfast, UK
[2] Photobiology Unit, University of Dundee, Ninewells Hospital and Medical School, Dundee, UK

Introduction, 21.1	Extracorporeal photochemotherapy, 21.7	**Patient selection, assessment and education, 21.15**
History and background, 21.2	**Administration of different therapies, 21.7**	Patient selection and assessment, 21.15
Ultraviolet radiation, 21.2	UVB phototherapy, 21.7	Patient education, 21.16
What is ultraviolet radiation?, 21.2	Psoralen and UVA, 21.9	**Patient and staff safety, 21.16**
Artificial sources, 21.2	Combination therapy, 21.10	Patient follow-up: skin cancer surveillance, 21.16
Equipment for the delivery of phototherapy, 21.2	UVA-1 phototherapy, 21.10	**Clinical governance, 21.17**
Ultraviolet calibration and dosimetry, 21.3	Extracorporeal photochemotherapy, 21.11	Documentation, 21.17
Indications for phototherapy, 21.3	**Adverse effects, 21.11**	Risk management, 21.17
UVB phototherapy and PUVA, 21.3	UVB phototherapy, 21.11	Audit, 21.17
Choice of phototherapy modality: UVB versus PUVA, 21.5	PUVA, 21.13	**How to set up a phototherapy unit, 21.17**
	UVA-1 phototherapy, 21.15	**What's new: developments, 21.18**
UVA-1 phototherapy, 21.6	Extracorporeal photochemotherapy, 21.15	**Key references, 21.18**

Introduction

Phototherapy (or 'light therapy') is a form of treatment for skin conditions involving the controlled administration of non-ionising radiation (most commonly within the ultraviolet (UV) part of the electromagnetic spectrum). A wide variety of dermatoses are responsive to phototherapy, which is used most commonly for psoriasis and eczema. Photodynamic therapy and laser therapies are distinct types of visible light-based treatments, which are discussed elsewhere (Chapters 22 and 23). Extracorporeal photochemotherapy (ECP), in which the target is white blood cells rather than skin, is, however, included in this chapter as it involves UV irradiation.

The UVB part of the spectrum is usually defined as that between 280 and 320 nm (although the International Commission on Illumination (CIE) has set the upper limit of the range at 315 nm). It can be delivered with the 'full spectrum' (broad-band UVB (BB-UVB) lamps 270–350 nm, which also include shorter UVA wavelengths) or with just a narrow part of the UVB spectrum (narrow-band UVB (NB-UVB) lamps 311–313 nm) (Figure 21.1). Since the 1980s, NB-UVB has largely replaced the use of BB-UVB [1,2,**3**].

The UVA spectrum is commonly defined as that between 320 and 400 nm and is typically used in combination with a psoralen photosensitiser, either orally or topically. This UVA activation of psoralen is known as photochemotherapy (PUVA) [4,5,**6**]. Skin diseases responsive to PUVA are similar to those responsive to UVB phototherapy, particularly psoriasis and eczema. ECP (photopheresis) involves the addition of psoralen to the patient's white blood cells after they have been separated from whole blood *ex vivo*. The photoactivated white blood cells are then irradiated with UVA and reinfused back into the patient. Photopheresis is used to treat the erythrodermic stage of cutaneous T-cell lymphoma, graft-versus-host disease (GVHD) and other conditions [7,**8**,9]. The longer wavelengths of UVA are known as UVA-1 (340–400 nm) and these have been shown to be beneficial in a number of chronic dermatoses including atopic eczema and sclerosing skin disorders [10,11,**12**,13].

UVB phototherapy has anti-inflammatory, immunosuppressive and cytotoxic properties. The mechanisms of its action are unclear, but include the induction of *cis*-urocanic acid, Langerhans cell depletion, altered antigen presentation, decreased activity of natural killer (NK) cells, increased activation of regulatory T cells and apoptosis of T lymphocytes and keratinocytes [14–17].

The mechanisms of action of PUVA include the cross-linking of DNA by psoralen photoadducts, the inhibition of DNA replication, Langerhans cell depletion, immunosuppressive effects on T-lymphocyte function and migration and the restoration of Th17/regulatory T-cell imbalance in psoriasis [18–20]. Photopheresis results in dendritic cells acquiring antigen from apoptotic

---

Rook's Textbook of Dermatology, Tenth Edition. Edited by Christopher Griffiths, Jonathan Barker, Tanya Bleiker, Walayat Hussain and Rosalind Simpson.
© 2024 John Wiley & Sons Ltd. Published 2024 by John Wiley & Sons Ltd.

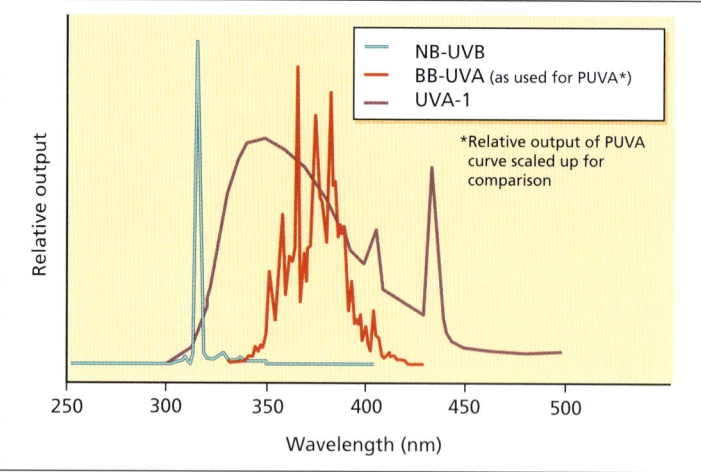

Figure 21.1 Spectra of narrow-band ultraviolet B (NB-UVB), broad-band UVA (BB-UVA) and UVA-1. PUVA, psoralen and UVA.

lymphocytes, which elicit a specific immune response without causing systemic immunosuppression [21–23]. UVA-1 phototherapy penetrates deeper into the dermis and induces interstitial collagenase and several cytokines, resulting in a softening of sclerotic skin [24,25]. In addition, UVA-1 phototherapy causes a reduction in tumour necrosis factor α (TNF-α) in the skin, among other mediator effects; it is also cytotoxic with T-cell apoptosis being a prominent feature [26].

History and background

The beneficial effects of sunlight or heliotherapy on the skin have been known since antiquity. The treatment of vitiligo with psoralen extract from seeds in combination with sunlight is recorded in ancient Egyptian, Indian and Chinese manuscripts [4,27,28]. The primary therapeutic component of sunlight, ultraviolet radiation (UVR), would not be discovered until 1801 by Johann Ritter [29]. The lethality of UVR to bacteria was demonstrated by Downes and Blunt in 1877. The father of modern phototherapy, Niels Finsen, demonstrated the effectiveness of UV therapy for lupus vulgaris at the end of the 19th century [30,31]. Finsen went on to be awarded the Nobel Prize for his work in 1903.

It was suggested by Alderson in 1923 that a mercury quartz lamp be used to treat psoriasis [32]. The combination of tar and UVB therapy for psoriasis was promoted by Goeckerman in the USA in 1925, and the combination of UVB and dithranol (anthralin) for the same by Ingram in England in 1953 [33,34]. A broad-band fluorescent UVB system for the treatment of psoriasis was developed by Wiskemann in the 1960s. These lamps had a much higher output than the mercury quartz lamp. The action spectrum for the clearance of psoriasis with a peak at 313 nm was defined in 1976 by Parrish and Jaenicke in the USA [35]. This work paved the way for the development of the more specific and efficient narrow-band UVB phototherapy for psoriasis in the 1980s [36,37].

Photochemotherapy was revived in 1947 with the isolation of 8-methoxypsoralen and 5-methoxypsoralen from plant extracts [38,39]. El Mofty *et al.* demonstrated the clinical benefit of these psoralens with natural sunlight or with UV lamps for the treatment of vitiligo [40]. Photochemotherapy or PUVA was revolutionised by Parrish *et al.* in 1974 with the introduction of a high-intensity fluorescent UVA tube for the treatment of psoriasis [41]. A decade later, ECP or photopheresis was introduced by Edelson for the treatment of cutaneous T-cell lymphoma (CTCL) [7]. ECP is recommended as first line treatment for erythrodermic CTCL. In 1981, Mutzhas and colleagues first reported the development of an irradiation device that emitted long-wave UV radiation (UVA-1; 340–400 nm) [42]. It was noted that it readily provoked pigmentation and polymorphic light eruption (PLE). It was thus initially used for PLE provocation testing. The therapeutic potential of UVA-1 was not to be recognised until the early 1990s when it was reported to be beneficial for atopic eczema [10].

Ultraviolet radiation

What is ultraviolet radiation?

Ultraviolet radiation is that part of the solar electromagnetic spectrum that lies between X-rays and visible light. UVR is normally defined as UVA (320–400 nm), UVB (280–320 nm) and UVC (<280 nm), although the International Commission on Illumination uses 315 nm rather than 320 nm as the boundary between UVA and UVB [43,44].

UVC radiation is absorbed by the earth's atmosphere before it reaches the surface of the earth. UVB radiation is significantly more effective (100–1000 times more potent) than UVA at producing erythema, cellular effects and DNA damage. UVA radiation is less energetic but penetrates more deeply into the skin, particularly the longer UVA-1 wavelengths, and as such has been implicated in chronic skin photoageing [45].

Artificial sources

The most common means of producing UVR artificially is by the passage of an electric current through mercury vapour enclosed in a fluorescent tube. The excited electrons of the mercury are absorbed by a phosphor coating on the inside of the tube, which results in re-emission of radiation of longer wavelengths by the process of fluorescence (Figure 21.2). By changing the phosphors used, a variety of different spectra in the UVA or UVB regions can be produced [46]. Tubes commonly used for PUVA lamps include NB-UVB: TL-01 (Waldmann/Cosmedico/Hybec/Lumenis); BB-UVB: TL-12 (Philips) or the more selective UV-6 (Sylvania); and UVA: TL-09 (Philips). UVA-1 can be produced either by low output fluorescent tubes, such as the TL-10 (Philips), or by the higher output metal halide UVA-1 sources (Sellamed, Dr Hönle, Dermalight), which require significant cooling [12].

Equipment for the delivery of phototherapy

A wide variety of NB-UVB (TL-01) units are available, including whole body cabins, whole body panels, small panel irradiators and point sources (Figure 21.3) [1,3]. Whole body cabins contain 1800 mm long fluorescent tubes that line the walls in front of reflective metal surfaces which enable greater dose uniformity and greater treatment efficiency to be achieved. Whole body panels

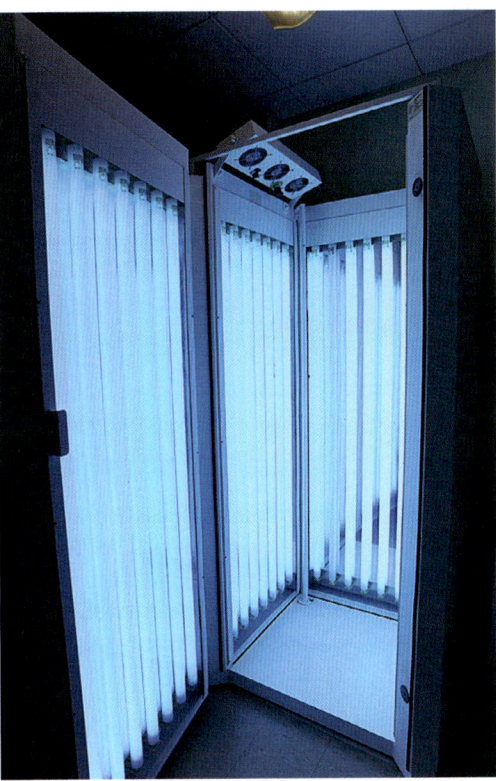

Figure 21.2 Whole body narrow-band UVB cabinet.

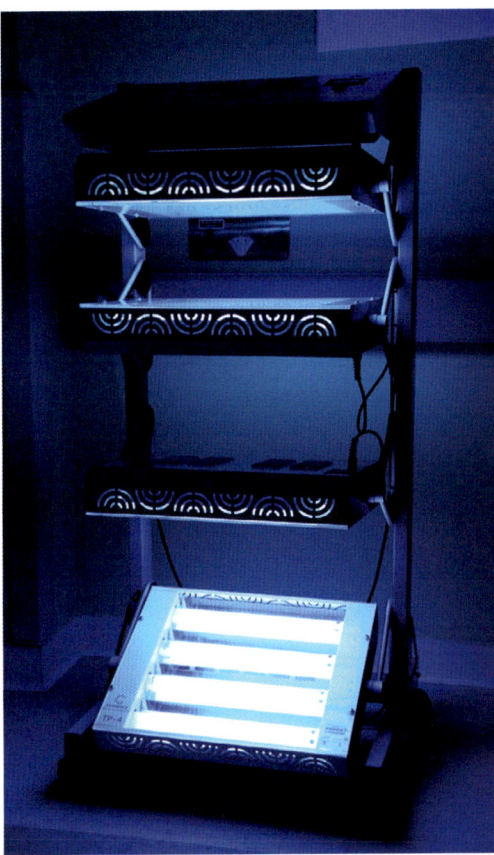

Figure 21.3 Narrow-band UVB unit for the treatment of hands and feet.

necessitate rotation of the patient to provide uniform irradiation: careful attention to position and posture is required to avoid under- or overdosing. Furthermore, these units are a significant UV hazard to others, who must avoid passing in front of the panel. They may, however, be useful for home phototherapy. Small panel irradiators are used for the treatment of palmar and plantar skin. Point source devices avoid unnecessary irradiation of unaffected skin but care is needed to avoid under- or overdosing at overlap areas.

PUVA units are either whole body cabins or small panel irradiators for the treatment of the hands and feet or other localised areas of the body, such as the lower legs or scalp [43,44].

Space and expense may be saved by using a cabin with a combination of UVB and UVA tubes. However, as only half the number of tubes of each type can be accommodated, longer treatment times are required. They also pose a significant hazard if the wrong tubes are selected and so in general are not recommended.

Ultraviolet calibration and dosimetry

To provide consistency and repeatability of treatment doses it is essential that the irradiance of the UV unit being used is determined at regular intervals. The dose is calculated from the formula:

$$\text{Dose (mJ/cm}^2) = \text{irradiance (mW/cm}^2) \times \text{time (seconds)}$$

It is important that this is performed using calibrated radiometers that are traceable back to a national reference. This ensures that treatment delivered at one phototherapy centre is the same as that given at any other phototherapy centre. Some whole body cabins have built-in radiometers, but these are unreliable. They may give inaccurate readings when the tubes are changed if the radiometer is not cleaned or if shielding occurs with very obese patients.

To determine the mean UV irradiance to which a patient will be exposed in a whole body cabin, a *designated patient irradiance* (DPI) is determined [43,44]. This is for a subject of average height and build at chest, waist and knee levels. The irradiance should be measured at the anterior, posterior and both lateral positions, that is, at 12 body sites. This can be determined in one of two ways, the direct or the indirect methods. In the direct method the irradiance at the specified sites must be measured while the investigator (usually from the nearest medical physics department) is standing in the unit. The skin and eyes must be protected with suitable protective clothing and goggles. In the indirect method the irradiance is measured while the unit is unoccupied. This can be done with the radiometer clamped to a stand whose position can be adjusted up or down (Figure 21.4). The mean value of the DPI is multiplied by a correction factor (typically 0.8–0.9) to take into account the occupancy effect of the patient in the cabin.

Indications for phototherapy

UVB phototherapy and PUVA
Psoriasis
Psoriasis is the most frequent indication for both UVB and PUVA [2,6,47,48,49]. NB-UVA (TL-01) can be used to treat all variants except generalised pustular and erythrodermic psoriasis, for which PUVA can, however, be considered [50]. NB-UVB is more effective

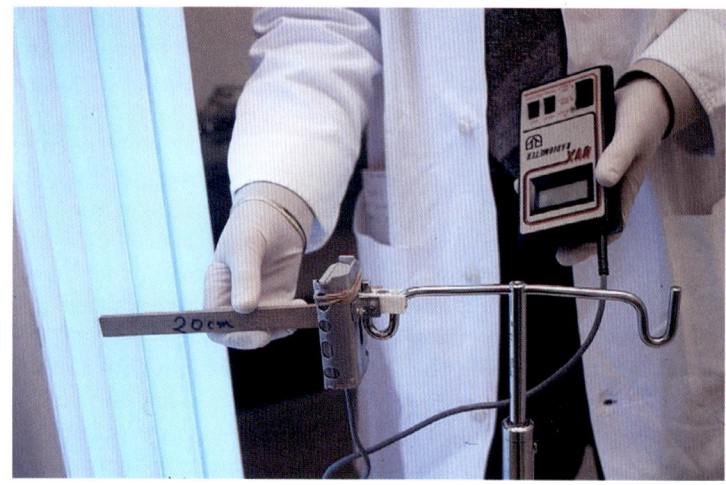

Figure 21.4 Irradiance of UV tubes being measured by a radiometer clamped in position at a fixed distance.

than BB-UVB and is on average of similar efficacy to PUVA for the treatment of psoriasis (Figure 21.5). Thin plaques as seen in guttate and seborrhoeic psoriasis respond readily to UVB therapy. NB-UVB has been shown to be a cost-effective treatment modality for psoriasis [51,52]. UVB is generally used in preference to PUVA: it has a lesser skin cancer risk than PUVA, is easier to administer and, with its shorter exposure times, facilitates a greater throughput of patients. PUVA should be considered in those patients who have failed to respond to UVB or whose duration of remission following UVB is consistently of short duration.

Atopic eczema

Atopic eczema has been treated effectively with BB-UVB [53], combined UVB and UVA [54], UVA-1 [10], NB-UVB (Figure 21.6) [1,3,55] and PUVA [56,57]. It is commonly stated that it is preferable that UVA-1, if available, should be used for acute flares and NB-UVB should be used for chronic disease, although there is no evidence to support this. Recent evidence confirms the efficacy of NB-UVB for atopic eczema, with 70% of patients requiring less topical steroid prescribing for at least a year after phototherapy [58]. A flare of disease is often seen in the early stages of phototherapy, usually due to the heat generated in the cabinets. Lower dose increments and more prolonged treatment courses than used for psoriasis are often required [59]. The clinical impression is that relapse also tends to be more frequent than in psoriasis, although there is no firm objective evidence for this. PUVA may be effective if UVB has failed.

Cutaneous T-cell lymphoma

Narrow-band UVB and PUVA have been used effectively for the treatment of CTCL (mycosis fungoides) [60–62]. UVB is particularly useful for patch stage CTCL, but PUVA is preferable for the plaque stage. Increased inflammation may be seen in the early stages of treatment but this usually settles without stopping therapy. 'Sanctuary sites' such as the flexures, which are less accessible to phototherapy, may be areas where disease persists. The use of maintenance therapy PUVA after initial clearance of mycosis fungoides remains unproven and controversial [9,63]. It has been suggested that maintenance therapy may be considered to prevent relapse in rapidly recurrent disease [6].

Vitiligo

Vitiligo may respond both to NB-UVB and to PUVA [64–66]. NB-UVB is more effective than PUVA but response is variable and treatment usually has to be prolonged, often over many months to a year or more. Affected areas that tend to be more photoresponsive include those on the face and those of recent onset, of limited extent, containing pigmented hairs or involving non-acral sites [67,68]. Acral areas typically respond less well but are often the sites that bother the patient most. Tanning of normal skin, which exaggerates the contrast with vitiliginous skin, is more obvious in patients with darker skin types. Patients of skin types I and II are more at risk of burning. Patients should be carefully selected and the risks and benefits clearly discussed.

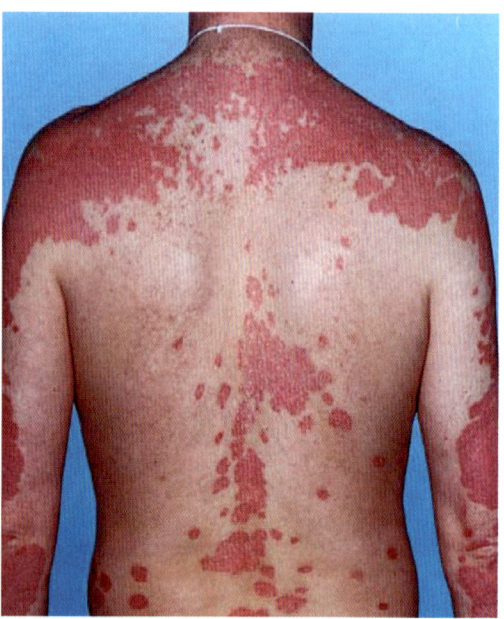
(a)

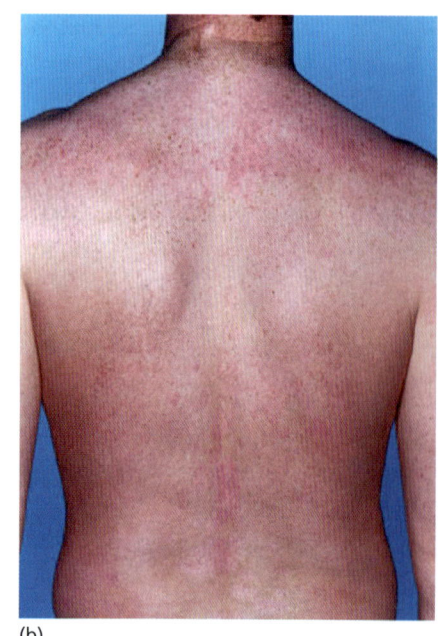
(b)

Figure 21.5 Psoriasis affecting a patient's back (a) before and (b) after narrow-band UVB (TL-01) therapy, showing the effectiveness of the treatment. Reproduced with permission of British Dermatological Nursing Group.

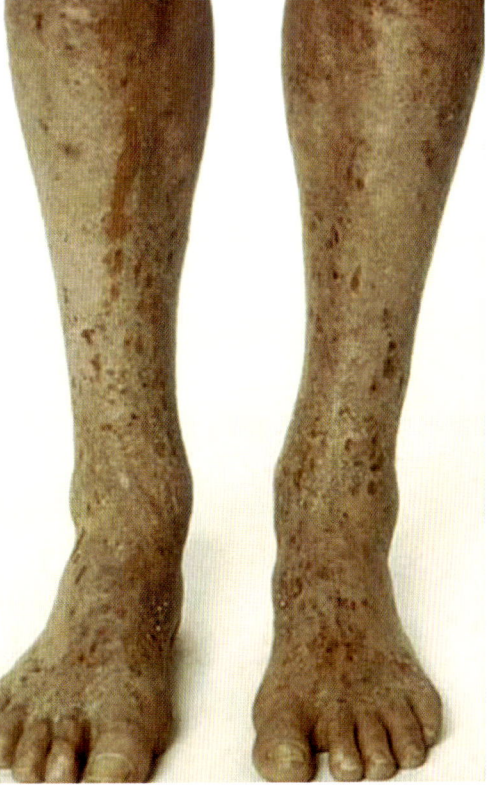
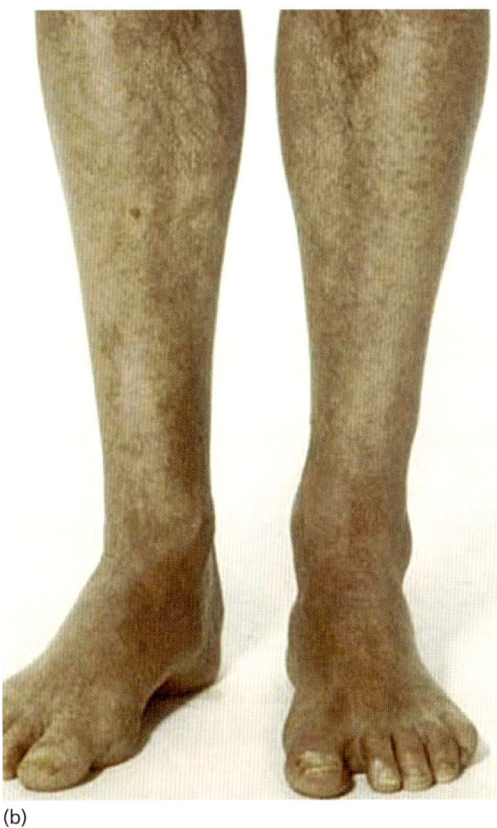

Figure 21.6 Atopic eczema affecting a patient's legs (a) before and (b) after narrow-band UVB therapy.

(a)   (b)

Polymorphic light eruption

Narrow-band UVB and PUVA are equally effective for the desensitisation of PLE but the former is used more frequently nowadays as it has a better side effect profile [69,70]. It is usually administered in spring time or before travel to sunny locations. Provocation of the rash, which occurs in approximately 50% of patients, can be managed with topical corticosteroid creams and reduction of dose. Patients are typically given 15 treatments (three times per week for 5 weeks) for three consecutive years prior to a year without treatment to assess whether there is any change in disease expression. Evidence as to the optimal regimen to use is lacking.

Other conditions

Many other skin conditions have been treated with UVB and PUVA therapy with variable efficacy. Representative examples of such conditions are listed in Table 21.1.

Choice of phototherapy modality: UVB versus PUVA

Narrow-band UVB therapy is much more widely used than PUVA. This is primarily due to the well-documented cumulative risk of skin cancer associated with PUVA [99,100]. In addition, many studies have shown the efficacy of NB-UVB for psoriasis and other dermatoses to be comparable with that of PUVA [1,3]. It should not be forgotten that PUVA penetrates more deeply into the skin than UVB radiation and is thus better suited for thick plaque disease and for treating the palms and soles (Box 21.1). The relapse rate of psoriasis following PUVA therapy is less than that of NB-UVB therapy. PUVA can also be highly effective for generalised pustular or erythrodermic psoriasis [6].

Table 21.1 Other conditions that may respond to ultraviolet B (UVB) phototherapy or psoralen and UVA (PUVA).

Condition (and reference)	Comment
Alopecia areata [71,72]	Efficacy of PUVA is not clearly established; relapse is common
Graft-versus-host disease [73,74]	PUVA is helpful in extensive lichenoid disease
Granuloma annulare [75]	Can be beneficial
Lichen planus [76,77]	Response is variable; PUVA is useful for palmar disease
Necrobiosis lipoidica [78]	PUVA can be beneficial – in ulcer healing and camouflage effect
Nodular prurigo [79,80]	Can be beneficial; relapse is common
Other photodermatoses (actinic prurigo, chronic actinic dermatitis, erythropoietic protoporphyria, solar urticaria) [81–83]	Can be effective but close supervision is required; consider referral to a centre with special interest
Palmoplantar pustulosis [84]	PUVA is more effective
Pityriasis lichenoides chronica [85]	Can be beneficial
Pityriasis rosea [86]	Rarely needed; used in severe symptomatic disease
Pityriasis rubra pilaris [87,88]	PUVA only
Pompholyx eczema [89,90]	PUVA is more effective
Pruritus [91,92]	Can be beneficial; UVB is effective for itch of renal failure or liver disease
Seborrhoeic dermatitis [93]	Responsive to UVB but rapid relapse is common
Subcorneal pustular dermatosis [94,95]	Can be beneficial
Systemic sclerosis/morphoea [96]	PUVA is beneficial
Urticaria [97]	Good evidence to support a role for UVB
Urticaria pigmentosa [98]	Can be beneficial; relapse is common

> **Box 21.1 Ultraviolet B (UVB) and psoralen and UVA (PUVA) compared**
>
> **Factors favouring the use of UVB**
> - Convenience – there is no need for oral medication or protective eyewear before/after therapy
> - Thin plaque/macular disease
> - Pregnancy
> - Skin type I/II is at a higher risk of PUVA-induced skin cancer
> - Photosensitivity to UVA but not to UVB
> - Liver or gastrointestinal disease
> - Poor patient cooperation/compliance
> - Age <18 years
>
> **Factors favouring the use of PUVA**
> - Failure to respond to UVB or rapid relapse following UVB
> - Thick plaques
> - Palmoplantar disease
> - Nail disease
> - Photosensitivity to UVB
> - Erythrodermic or generalised pustular psoriasis
> - Pityriasis rubra pilaris – which usually flares with UVB but can respond well to PUVA

> **Box 21.2 Contraindications to ultraviolet B (UVB) and psoralen and UVA (PUVA)**
>
> **Absolute contraindications**
> - Dysplastic naevus syndrome
> - Systemic lupus erythematosus
> - Dermatomyositis
> - Genetic skin cancer syndromes (xeroderma pigmentosum, Gorlin syndrome)
> - Bloom syndrome, Cockayne syndrome
> - Concomitant specific oral immunosuppressive medication: azathioprine, ciclosporin, mycophenolate mofetil and tacrolimus
> - Patients unwilling or unable to comply with safety procedures
> - Patients who are medically unfit and unable to stand, e.g. severe cardiovascular or respiratory disease
>
> **Relative contraindications**
> - Age <16 years
> - Previous or current non-melanoma skin cancer
> - Previous melanoma
> - Previous exposure to arsenic or ionising radiation
> - Current premalignant skin lesions
> - Previous or concomitant oral immunosuppressive therapy
> - Photo-induced epilepsy
> - Pregnancy[a]
> - Bullous pemphigoid/pemphigus
> - Cataracts[a]
> - Significant liver dysfunction[a]
>
> [a] Contraindication to oral PUVA only.

Contraindications to UVB and PUVA

Patients should be assessed for their suitability for either UVB or PUVA therapy prior to starting therapy (Box 21.2). Individual risk and benefit must always be assessed. Being on a photosensitising medication is not a contraindication to phototherapy but a note of caution is needed to ensure good drug record keeping and to reinforce the importance of baseline minimal erythema dose (MED)/minimal phototoxic dose (MPD) and that a lower incremental dose regimen may be appropriate in some settings.

UVA-1 phototherapy

The evidence base for using UVA-1 relates mainly to its use in atopic eczema, the sclerosing skin conditions, in particular morphoea and scleroderma, and various subtypes of lupus erythematosus. The application of UVA-1 has also been investigated for several other skin diseases (e.g. urticaria pigmentosa, disseminated granuloma annulare, CTCL and psoriasis in patients infected with human immunodeficiency virus (HIV)), although the evidence base is largely restricted to case series and case reports [12,101]. In general, UVA-1 is probably most useful as an option to be considered for some of the rarer skin diseases where other treatment options are limited. It is not usually first line phototherapy and its availability at present is limited to specialist centres.

Atopic eczema

Ultraviolet A-1 phototherapy can be of benefit, particularly for atopic prurigo, and, if it is available, should be considered for the patient who has failed to respond to NB-UVB or PUVA [10,102,103]. Studies have shown that high- and medium-dose UVA-1 are of equivalent efficacy although medium-dose treatment is more effective than low-dose. Recently high-dose UVA-1 has been shown to be more effective than medium-dose in individuals of higher skin phototype with atopic eczema [104]. UVA-1 has been shown to be superior to potent topical corticosteroid and broadband UVA/B. UVA-1 is of equivalent efficacy or possibly slightly less effective than NB-UVB and is less effective than PUVA.

Sclerosing skin conditions

There is evidence of the utility of UVA-1 for the treatment of cutaneous sclerosis in morphoea and systemic sclerosis, particularly if the disease is progressive, symptomatic and/or restricting movement [105]. Recently, the utility of high-frequency ultrasonographic response of morphoea to UVA-1 has been reported [106]. There is also limited evidence to support its use in the treatment of cutaneous GVHD [107], nephrogenic fibrosing dermopathy [108] and both extragenital and genital lichen sclerosus [109,110]. UVA-1 at medium dose has been shown to be superior to NB-UVB and even low-dose treatment can be effective, although prolonged treatment courses may be needed.

Lupus erythematosus

Paradoxically there is good evidence for the use of very low-dose UVA-1 (about 6 J/cm^2 per individual dose) for systemic lupus erythematosus (LE) with demonstrable reduction in systemic disease activity [111,112]. UVA-1 has also been used successfully for subacute cutaneous LE, tumid LE and, although generally less responsive, for chronic cutaneous (discoid) LE.

Mycosis fungoides

There are limited reports of UVA-1 phototherapy in the treatment of mycosis fungoides and most are case reports or short series of cases [113]. In a study of 19 patients with early mycosis fungoides (stage IA–IIA), complete responses were achieved in 12 (63%) and partial responses in 7 (37%) after UVA-1 treatment [114]. In addition, the deeper penetration of UVA-1 into the skin may provide a role of such therapy for more refractory forms of mycosis fungoides such as the folliculotrophic variant. Of 12 patients with early-stage folliculotrophic mycosis fungoides treated with UVA-1, 11 experienced >80% improvement (8 complete remission and 3 partial remission) [115].

Extracorporeal photochemotherapy

Extracorporeal photochemotherapy, or photopheresis, has evidence of benefit for the treatment of erythrodermic CTCL [7,8,9,116–118] and for GVHD [119–121]. It has also been used for a wide range of skin diseases such as systemic sclerosis [122,123], some immunobullous disorders [124,125], psoriasis [126], atopic eczema [127,128], lichen planus [129,130], LE [131], scleroedema [132] and dermatomyositis [133]. Evidence of benefit for any of these conditions is generally weak. It is of interest that the best evidence for the efficacy of ECP is in the prophylaxis of cardiac transplant rejection [134].

Cutaneous T-cell lymphoma

Extracorporeal photochemotherapy is licensed for the treatment of CTCL, particularly in patients with erythrodermic disease, including those with Sézary syndrome [135,136]. Patients who respond best have a disease of shorter duration, have near normal CD8+ cell counts [137], are immunocompetent [138], have circulating Sézary cells [139,140] and have an absence of bulky lymphadenopathy or major organ involvement [136]. Evidence for ECP for the treatment of non-erythrodermic mycosis fungoides is poor [141–143]. A more recent report found an overall response rate of only 42% in patients with early-stage mycosis fungoides treated with ECP [144]. Added benefit has been claimed when ECP is combined with interferon [139,145], bexarotene [146] or electron beam therapy [147]. Response rates have been reported to be highest, reaching levels >80%, with combinations of interferon and bexarotene [148].

Graft-versus-host disease

Graft-versus-host disease complicating allogeneic bone marrow transplantation can be subdivided into acute and chronic phases. There is evidence that ECP is of benefit for both the acute and chronic phases [135,136,149]. A systematic review of studies of ECP for the treatment of GVHD found an overall response rate for acute phase disease to be 69%. The highest response rates were 84% for cutaneous involvement, followed by 65% for gastrointestinal and 55% for hepatic manifestations [150]. A review of the literature of ECP treatment for chronic GVHD reported a mean response for cutaneous disease of 74%, for mucosal of 62%, for hepatic of 62%, and of 46% for both gastrointestinal and pulmonary manifestations [135]. Treatment of GVHD with ECP has also demonstrated a significant steroid-sparing effect.

Administration of different therapies

UVB phototherapy

Phototherapy is most frequently referred to as UVB therapy and historically was delivered either as broad-band or narrow-band UVB. However, NB-UVB is more effective than BB-UVB for psoriasis and is now the standard form of UVB used. BB-UVB is now rarely used in modern phototherapy. It is recommended that the starting dose of UVB is based on the MED in order to reduce the risks of burning on the one hand or undertreatment on the other, and to detect unsuspected photosensitivity [1].

Minimal erythema dose

The MED is defined in the UK as the dose of radiation that produces minimal, just perceptible, erythema at 24 h post-irradiation (in other countries it is defined as the dose that produces well-defined erythema) [151]. There is a poor correlation between MED and skin type (as determined by physician estimate based on information provided by standard questioning of patients) [152]. The UVB MED gives an objective measure of a patient's threshold cutaneous sensitivity to UVB.

The MED can be determined by the use of a homemade template, or nowadays the usual practice is the use of automatic or semi-automatic hand-held UV exposure devices. If using a homemade template, any UV-opaque material with a number of apertures (typically eight) can be used, through which different doses of UVB can be delivered to the skin. A geometric series of doses are selected, based on skin phototype [153], such as 25, 50, 70, 100, 140, 200, 280, 390, 550, 650 and 770 mJ/cm^2 for NB-UVB (Figure 21.7). The usual site for testing with the template is on the mid-back, avoiding the midline. The UVB testing source uses a bank of UVB tubes identical to those used in the irradiation cabinet and whose irradiance is regularly monitored. In some units the actual irradiation cabinet is

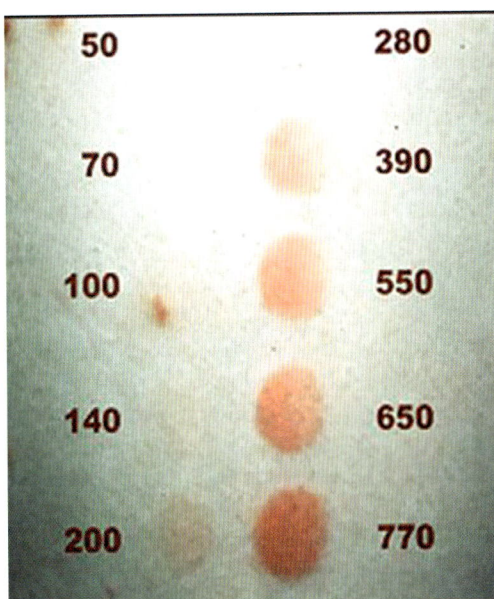

Figure 21.7 Narrow-band UVB minimal erythema dose (MED) reading 24 h after the irradiation of phototest sites. Doses are in mJ/cm^2.

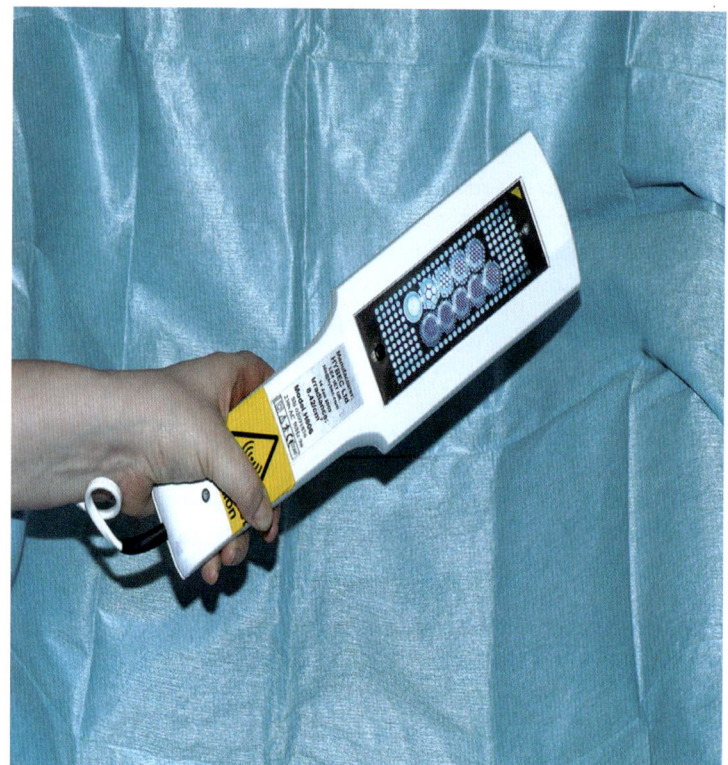

Figure 21.8 Hand-held Hybec 'Durham' phototesting unit.

used with the patient standing or sitting within it, but this requires careful covering of the patient to avoid unnecessary erythema and to some patients this can be very claustrophobic. In addition to being time consuming it also means that this cabinet is not available for treatment while the procedure is undertaken. Alternatively, a hand-held semiautomated UV device can be used and is placed directly on the skin being tested. The plate in contact with the skin is perforated with a number of apertures fitted with UV-attenuating mesh foil. Essentially, the finer the mesh, the more UV it blocks. One such device delivers 10 doses with an attenuation factor of 1.26 between apertures allowing a sequence of doses to be delivered (Figure 21.8) [154].

Regimen variables

Starting dose. The evidence for optimal dose regimens mainly relates to psoriasis. The action spectrum for the clearance of psoriasis peaks in the UVB region around 311–313 nm and it was with this in mind that NB-UVB lamps were designed by Philips. To achieve clearance of psoriasis it is not necessary to use erythemogenic dose regimens. The starting dose is commonly initiated at a percentage of the MED (usually 70% or 50%) to minimise the risk of developing significant erythema. Interestingly, one study showed increased erythemal episodes with a 50% MED starting dose regimen when compared with 70% MED or arbitrary skin phototype-based starting dose regimens, and showed no difference in efficacy between any of the three regimens [155]. However, undertaking a MED or a small area test dose is important to detect unsuspected abnormal photosensitivity.

Increments. As the skin acclimatises to UVB therapy by epidermal thickening and pigmentation, it is necessary to increase the dose incrementally. Comparison of a low-increment regimen (20%) with a high-increment regimen (40%) showed the former to result in 50% fewer episodes of erythema requiring postponement of treatment [156]. A low-dose regimen is advocated with a reduction to 10% increments if significant erythema develops.

Frequency. Treatment three times a week is preferred to a five times per week schedule for patients of skin phototypes I–III. This is because the advantage of a marginally more rapid clearance of psoriasis with the latter regimen is outweighed by the inconvenience to the patient of a higher frequency of treatment, and the higher cumulative UVB dose received [157]. Both twice and three times a week regimens are effective for psoriasis, although three times a week treatment results in faster clearance.

Number of exposures. Clearance of psoriasis can usually be achieved with 20–25 treatments, although more prolonged courses may be needed, particularly with stubborn disease. Atopic eczema also usually requires more prolonged treatment courses than those used for achieving clearance in psoriasis. A course of 15 treatments is usually used for PLE desensitisation, although optimal treatment parameters have not been established.

Ways to deliver phototherapy

Ultraviolet B phototherapy is most commonly delivered in a cabinet in which the patient is surrounded by TL-01 fluorescent tubes (Figure 21.9). Hand and foot units can also be used for localised hand and foot disease.

Involved psoriatic skin has a much higher tolerance of UVB than the surrounding uninvolved skin. With UVB devices that can be targeted directly at individual psoriatic plaques, higher doses of UVB can therefore be used [158,159]. Treatment with 2–6 multiples of MED can clear localised plaques of psoriasis after five or six treatments. Coherent UVB in the form of the 308 nm excimer laser can also be used for stubborn localised psoriatic plaques, although availability is limited [160].

Home phototherapy has been particularly advocated for patients who cannot attend hospital because of geographical, work, economic or other reasons [161,162]. Such treatment has raised concerns of suboptimal therapy, greater risks and medicolegal implications, which have not been confirmed [163]. However, a study from the Netherlands, in which home phototherapy for psoriasis was compared with out-patient UVB, found that the treatments had similar efficacy and that the cumulative doses and rates of short-term side effects were comparable [164]. Cost analysis of home phototherapy for psoriasis versus hospital UVB therapy in Scotland concluded that home phototherapy was cost-effective and that the development of this means of treatment delivery should be encouraged [162,165,166]. Despite evidence of non-inferiority for the efficacy and safety of home phototherapy compared with hospital-based phototherapy, the uptake of the former is poor in UK National Health Service departments [167]. Recent studies have also recommended the utility of home phototherapy for the treatment of vitiligo [168–170].

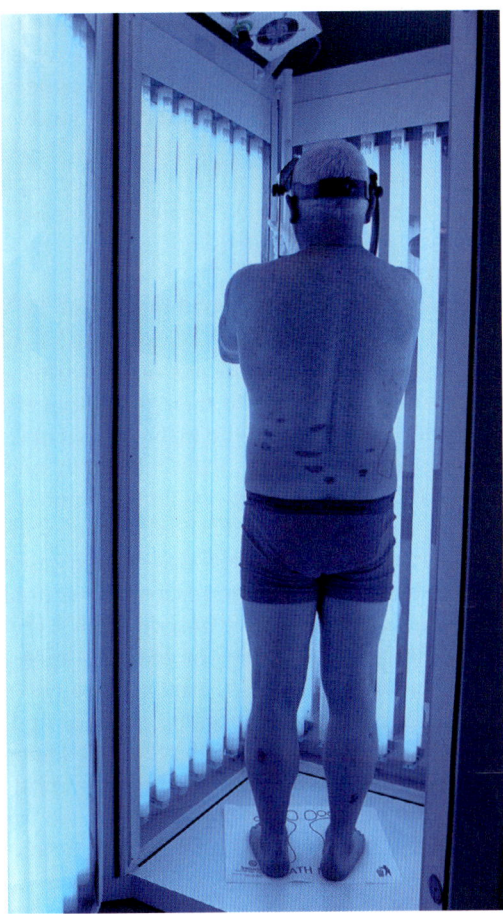

Figure 21.9 Patient with psoriasis receiving narrow-band UVB in a whole body cabinet.

Psoralen and UVA

Psoralens

The most frequently used psoralens for oral use are 8-methoxypsoralen (8-MOP) and 5-methoxypsoralen (5-MOP) [4,6,59,171]. The former is used preferentially as it is considered to be more effective and is less expensive. Nausea is a common side effect of 8-MOP and, if troublesome, switching to 5-MOP is helpful. The dose of psoralen used is most commonly determined on the basis of body weight: 0.6 mg/kg for 8-MOP and 1.2 mg/kg for 5-MOP. Some authorities advocate calculating the dose according to body surface area: 25 mg/m^2 for 8-MOP and 50 mg/m^2 for 5-MOP [172]. The latter method of dosing has been shown to improve the therapeutic effect of PUVA in psoriasis.

Oral 8-MOP is taken 2 h before treatment with a light meal and 5-MOP should be taken 2–2.5 h before treatment.

Topical psoralens have been used for centuries for the treatment of vitiligo. Psoralens currently used for topical therapy include 8-MOP and trimethylpsoralen (TMP) [173]. In equivalent concentrations TMP is up to 30 times more phototoxic than 8-MOP, although it is now rarely used [174]. Psoralen can be applied topically in a variety of ways: a bath solution for whole body treatment and soak, paint, cream or gel for hands and feet, scalp and other localised areas.

Topical therapy is preferable to oral therapy in patients with hepatic dysfunction, gastrointestinal disease, cataracts, poor compliance with eye protection and risk of drug interactions (e.g. warfarin), and to allow shorter irradiation times (e.g. for children, the elderly or those with claustrophobia).

A frequently used bath PUVA regimen in the UK involves dissolving 30 mL of a 1.2% 8-MOP lotion in 140 L of water (final concentration 2.6 mg/L) [173]. The patient bathes in this for 15 min, followed by immediate exposure to UVA. When treating the hands and feet with topical PUVA there should be a 30 min delay prior to irradiation to allow psoralen absorption into palmar and plantar skin [175].

Minimal phototoxic dose

The MPD is determined in a similar way to MED except that the UVA geometric doses series is undertaken in psoralen-sensitised skin, 2 h after oral ingestion of a standard dose of 8-MOP (or 2.5 h for 5-MOP). Typical UVA test doses used include 0.5, 0.7, 1.0, 1.4, 2.0, 2.8, 3.7, 5.5, 7.7 and 10.8 J/cm^2 but may vary between centres. The test sites are read after 72–96 h [176].

MPD testing allows the determination of the optimal starting dose, allows identification of underdosage due to poor psoralen absorption and may identify patients with abnormal photosensitivity.

Regimen variables

Starting dose. The starting dose should ideally be based on the patient's MPD, and between 40% (topical PUVA) and 70% (oral PUVA) of the MPD is recommended [177,178]. If MPD testing is unavailable or the patient's skin is too extensively involved to measure the MPD, the starting dose is based on skin phototype: I, 0.5 J/cm^2; II, 1.0 J/cm^2; III, 1.5 J/cm^2; and IV, 2.0 J/cm^2. The starting dose of bath PUVA should always be based on MPD testing because of the risk of severe photosensitivity.

Increments. Doses are normally increased in 20–40% increments; lower increments may be indicated if significant erythema develops. If barely perceptible asymptomatic erythema develops, the dose can be kept the same until the erythema settles.

Frequency. PUVA therapy is usually administered twice weekly as PUVA erythema is delayed [179]. It had been assumed that topical PUVA erythema was maximal at 72 h but more recent studies have shown the peak to occur at between 96 and 144 h [180,181]. Some centres still use PUVA three times per week, but this regimen can result in an increased incidence of burning and is therefore not advised, particularly given the cumulative carcinogenic risk of PUVA.

Number of exposures. A typical twice weekly course of PUVA for psoriasis may last for 6–8 weeks, with the number of exposures required being similar to or less than that of NB-UVB, given that the latter is generally used three times per week. As there is a significantly increased risk of skin cancer with increasing cumulative exposure to PUVA, the number of treatments should be kept to a minimum and maintenance therapy avoided.

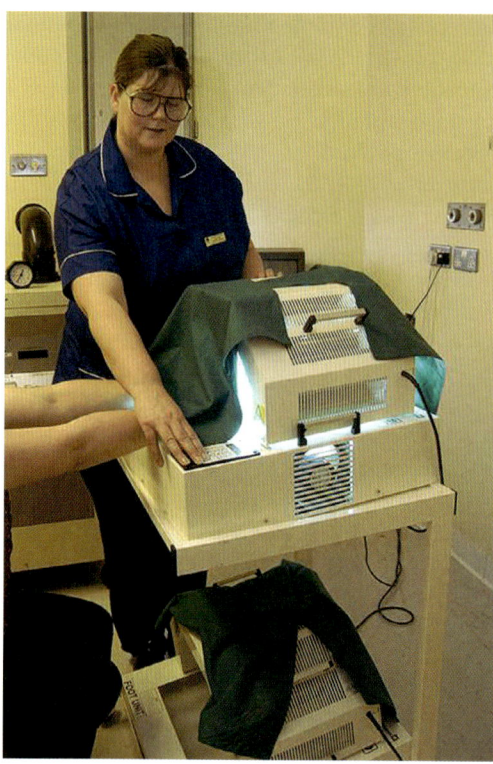

Figure 21.10 Patient's hands being irradiated with UVA following a topical psoralen soak.

Ways to deliver PUVA
As with UVB phototherapy, PUVA is usually delivered in a cabin with fluorescent tubes that surround the patient. PUVA can also be delivered locally with units that can be used to irradiate the hands and feet (Figure 21.10). Bath PUVA and localised PUVA are also available for patients when systemic PUVA is not recommended or is less appropriate.

Eye protection
Following the ingestion of psoralen tablets, patients are required to wear UVA-absorbing glasses before therapy and for at least 12 h after therapy (24 h for children and patients with pre-existing cataracts or atopic eczema) [6,59]. During therapy UV-blocking goggles must be worn. Eye protection with bath PUVA is only necessary in patients with very extensive disease when the risk of systemic absorption becomes significant.

Combination therapy
Combination therapy (i.e. UVB or PUVA combined with topical or systemic therapy) is used to increase the clinical response of psoriasis and to decrease the number of phototherapy exposures and thus the cumulative dose.

Topical agents
A variety of topical agents, including emollients [182], tar [183], dithranol (anthralin) [184], tazarotene [185] and vitamin D analogues such as calcipotriol [186,187], have been used in combination with phototherapy. Evidence for significant adjuvant or UV-sparing effects is limited. Studies of both calcipotriol and tazarotene have shown faster clearance of psoriasis with significantly lower median cumulative UV exposure. Vitamin D analogues are best used after UV exposure as they are unstable if exposed to UV radiation [188]. Topical immunomodulatory agents such as tacrolimus and pimecrolimus should be avoided. A multicentre study showed significant benefit when patients were treated with TL-01 UVB in the presence of Dead Sea salt solution [189]. In practice, if phototherapy is used optimally, the role of adjunctive therapies is less clear.

Systemic agents
There is good evidence that the combination of PUVA or UVB with an oral retinoid (so-called Re-PUVA or Re-UVB, respectively) increases efficacy and has a significant dose-sparing effect [190]. Retinoids are also beneficial due to their protective effects against skin cancer development [191]. In the management of CTCL, PUVA has been combined successfully with interferon and also with bexarotene [192,193]. Concomitant systemic immunosuppressive agents should in general be avoided in combination with phototherapy in order to avoid an augmented risk of skin cancer. Eruptive skin cancers have been reported when ciclosporin is used in patients who have received high cumulative doses of PUVA [194]. NB-UVB enhances the efficacy of a variety of biologic agents including alefacept [195], etanercept [196,197], adalimumab [198] and ustekinumab [199]. There have been recent reports of apremilast and fumaric acid esters in combination with NB-UVB demonstrating an enhanced treatment response [200,201]. However, most studies did not include a phototherapy-alone control group, so it is not feasible to conclude that any increased effect was due to combination therapy as opposed to the effect of NB-UVB alone. The potential for enhanced skin carcinogenesis is a significant concern with such combinations and they should, in general, be avoided. However TL-01 therapy could be considered in combination with selected systemic agents (not ciclosporin) as a short-term rescue therapy to control flares.

UVA-1 phototherapy
Ultraviolet A-1 phototherapy uses long-wavelength UVA radiation (340–400 nm), filtering out the erythemogenic UVA-2 and UVB wavelengths (280–340 nm). UVA-1 phototherapy has been used at a wide variety of doses, typically described as high (>60 J/cm^2), medium (30–60 J/cm^2), low (10–20 J/cm^2) and very low (<10 J/cm^2). There is very little evidence to define what the optimal UVA-1 treatment regimen should be, although common practice is stated here [**12**,101].

Minimal erythema dose
This is determined using a range of doses which reflect whether a low, medium or very high dose schedule is being used.

Regimen variables

Starting dose. The starting dose is based on the MED and is usually 50% of the latter.

Increments. Increments of 10–20% can be used at each treatment depending on whether or not erythema develops.

Frequency. Treatment is administered 3–6 times per week.

Number of exposures. In general, a trial of a minimum of 15 treatments would be recommended before deciding on whether to continue treatment or not.

Ways to deliver UVA-1
Ultraviolet A-1 can be delivered either via low-irradiance lamps (such as Philips TL-10) or from metal halide portable or whole body UVA-1 units. The latter provide a much higher irradiance thus allowing increased dose delivery.

Extracorporeal photochemotherapy
The photopheresis procedure takes place in three stages: leukapheresis, photoactivation and reinfusion [116,202]. Whole blood is removed from the patient and then centrifuged to separate the red blood cells (RBCs) from the white blood cells (WBCs). The WBCs (along with some plasma and RBCs) form the buffy coat. The latter is then mixed with saline and 8-MOP (UVADEX®) and photoactivated by being passed through a plastic film which is irradiated by UVA lamps (Figure 21.11). The irradiated buffy coat is then reinfused into the patient.

Phototesting
Minimal phototoxicity dose testing is not necessary as irradiation occurs outside the body in a machine.

Regimen variables

Standard dose. The dose of UVA delivered to the patient's lymphocytes is 1–2 J/cm^2.

Increments. None, the standard dose is used for each treatment.

Frequency. It is administered on 2–3 consecutive days once per month (for GVHD every 2–3 weeks). The frequency of treatment can be increased in non-responders.

Number of treatments. Treatment is generally continued for 6 months before declaring treatment failure if there is a lack of response. In patients who respond to therapy this can be continued at a decreased frequency to provide maintenance control if necessary.

Ways to deliver extracorporeal photochemotherapy
Extracorporeal photochemotherapy has been most commonly delivered using the UVAR XTS^R system (Therakos). The CELLEX (Therakos) system has recently replaced the latter system and is used in all UK sites [135]. The CELLEX system shortens treatment times using double needle access and allows patients of lower body weight to be treated [136]. Although 8-MOP may be given orally to administer ECP, plasma levels can be erratic, side effects such as nausea, vomiting and diarrhoea may be troublesome, and there is a risk of burning from exposure to ambient UV [203,204].

Adverse effects

UVB phototherapy
Acute effects
Erythema
Erythema and burning are the most common side effects of treatment. Erythema peaks at 12–24 h and can be associated with pain, swelling and blistering (Figure 21.12) [1,205,206]. Burning is

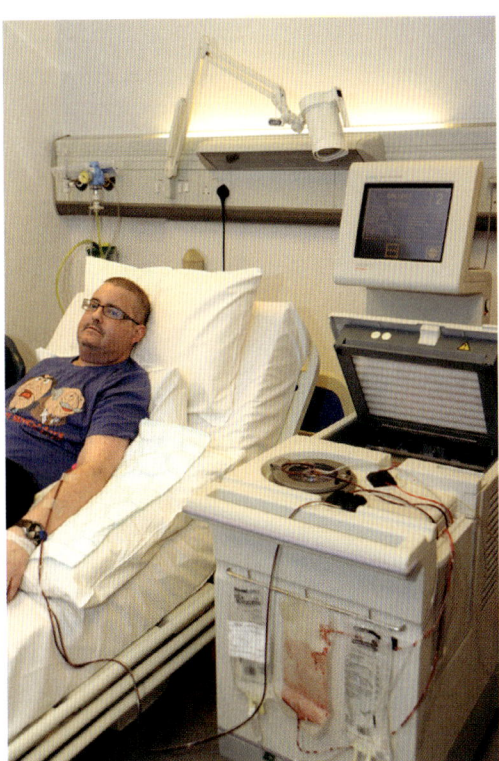
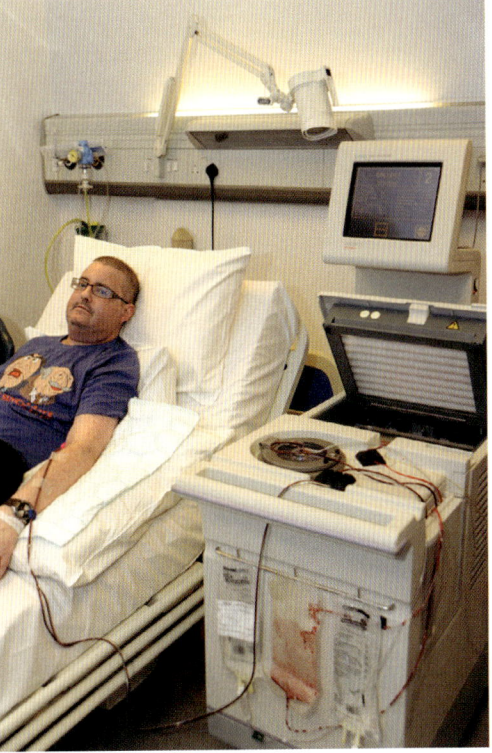

Figure 21.11 (a) Patient receiving extracorporeal photopheresis. (b) Close-up of the upper part of the photopheresis equipment showing the patient's buffy coat containing white blood cells being circulated between UVA tubes.

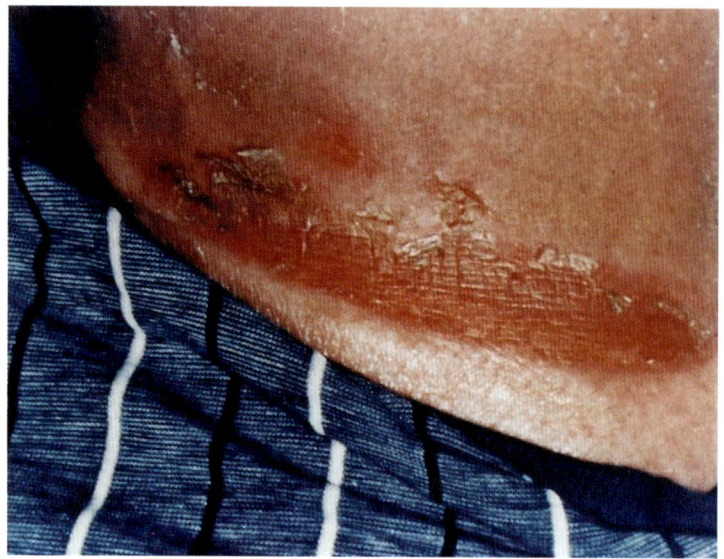

Figure 21.12 Burn sustained to the lower trunk during narrow-band UVB therapy due to slipping of the patient's underpants.

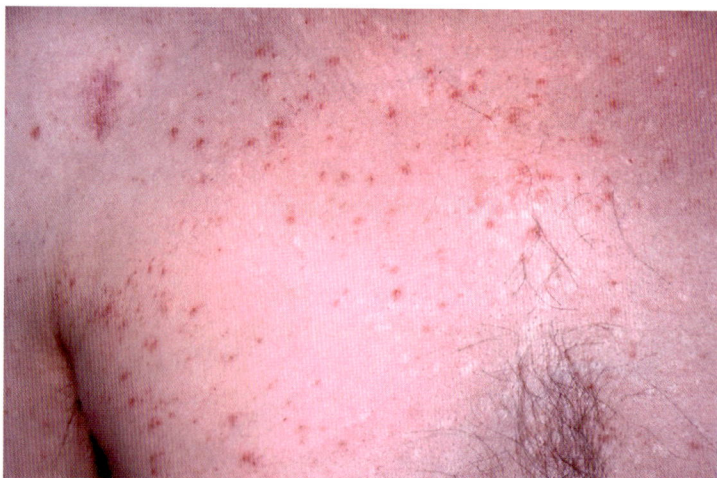

Figure 21.13 Flare of polymorphic light eruption on the chest induced by UVB therapy.

more likely in patients who are of skin phototype I/II, are obese, have inadvertent exposure of previously covered skin (e.g. after a haircut), are taking phototoxic drugs or herbal medication or have unknown photosensitivity (e.g. lupus erythematosus) [207]. Burning may also be due to operator error in programming the cabinet timer or selecting the correct dose for the correct patient. Mild erythema is managed using topical corticosteroid creams and emollients. Further treatment is withheld until the erythema settles, after which a lower incremental dose regimen should be introduced. More severe reactions may require a short course of oral corticosteroids and/or non-steroidal anti-inflammatory drugs (NSAIDs).

Pruritus
This is usually due either to phototherapy-induced dryness of the skin or to the underlying disorder being treated. It can usually be controlled by emollients [208].

Herpes simplex virus reactivation
This most commonly affects the lip and occurs more frequently in those with a past history of such outbreaks [209]. The areas in question can be protected by a sunscreen or visor if necessary.

Lesional blistering
Blistering of psoriatic plaques is an uncommon side effect of TL-01 phototherapy and is usually asymptomatic [210]. It typically occurs mid-way through a treatment course and usually settles spontaneously or following dose reduction. It can occur in the absence of erythema or burning.

Flare of polymorphic light eruption
The precipitation of PLE is a not uncommon occurrence during phototherapy in those who are predisposed to it (Figure 21.13) [208]. This is managed by the use of topical corticosteroid creams and adjustment of the treatment regimen.

Idiopathic guttate hypomelanosis-like hypopigmented macules and lentigines
Idiopathic guttate hypomelanosis-like lesions have been reported in 7 of 87 patients with mycosis fungoides treated by NB-UVB or PUVA [211]. Four affected patients had received NB-UVB and three PUVA. Lentigines have also been reported to have occurred in 10 of 73 (13%) patients with mycosis fungoides who received NB-UVB treatment [212]. They were restricted to mycosis fungoides lesions in seven patients and both involved and uninvolved skin in three patients. Two of these patients also had concomitant idiopathic hypomelanosis lesions.

Folic acid depletion and phototherapy
Ultraviolet radiation is known to cause photodegration of folate *in vitro* and in human skin [213]. Studies of NB-UVB on serum folate levels are controversial. Some show no change [214–216] and others show a reduction [217,218]. El-Saie *et al.* reported after exposure to 18 and 36 treatment sessions that the decreases in folate were 19% and 27%, respectively [218]. The largest study to date has recently been reported in 1001 patients treated with NB-UVB [219]. This group found that a significant fall in folate occurred after 12 exposures, but no significant changes were observed between baseline and 24 or 36 exposures. It has been recommended that women of child-bearing age receiving phototherapy should take folate supplements [219,220].

Ophthalmological effects
Narrow-band UVB can induce both acute and chronic photodamage to the eye [221]. Acute exposure can result in photoconjunctivitis and photokeratitis. Chronic UVB exposure can result in corneal degeneration, cataract formation, ptergium and squamous cell carcinoma of the conjunctiva. In view of these risks protective goggles must be worn during treatment [221,222]. NB-UVB can be used to treat eyelid dermatoses without goggles as the eyelid blocks the majority of radiation to the eye [223]. The latter method can be considered in carefully selected patients who are compliant with keeping their eyes shut. If patients are poorly compliant or eyelid closure is incomplete, UV-blocking contact lenses can be used. Soft

contact lenses are preferable to gas permeable ones due to complete coverage of the cornea [222].

Chronic effects
Photoageing
Premature cutaneous ageing may be induced or exacerbated by UVB phototherapy. The skin develops a leathery appearance, xerosis, wrinkling, pigmentary changes, loss of elasticity and increased fragility [2].

Carcinogenesis
Broad-band UVB has a carcinogenic risk that is not well defined due to the many confounding variables; these include recreational sun exposure, exposure to sunbeds or PUVA, skin type and exposure to systemic immunosuppressive therapies. A meta-analysis of studies using BB-UVB estimated an excess risk of non-melanoma skin cancer of about 2% per year [224]. Stern's long-term follow-up study of PUVA recipients in the USA showed that the risk of developing genital squamous cell carcinoma was 4.6 times greater in men with psoriasis and a history of significant UVB exposure (>300 treatments) than in men with similar PUVA exposure but without UVB exposure [225]. Genital protection during phototherapy continues to be recommended to minimise this risk.

The carcinogenic risk of NB-UVB, which is being increasingly used for delivering phototherapy, is not fully defined in humans but is less than that of PUVA. Extrapolation from animal studies would suggest that NB-UVB is 2–3 times per MED more carcinogenic than BB-UVB [226]. It has been suggested that this risk is abrogated in clinical practice, as the number of MEDs to clear psoriasis with NB-UVB is less than a third that required with BB-UVB. Clinical studies to date have not identified a significant risk of skin cancer in patients treated with NB-UVB, but further long-term follow-up studies are required [227,229,**230**] and appropriate governance of phototherapy services and recording of treatment numbers are essential, with monitoring of those who have received high cumulative treatment numbers advisable.

PUVA
Acute effects
Acute phototoxicity
The erythema induced by PUVA is delayed, thus incurring a risk of cumulative injury if treatments are more frequent than twice per week. Peak erythema following the administration of oral and topical PUVA occurs between 72 and 120 h and between 96 and 144 h, respectively [231,232]. Acute PUVA phototoxicity can range from mild erythema to severe pain with oedema, blistering and systemic upset including malaise and fever. PUVA erythema not only appears later than UVB erythema but lasts longer. A rarer form of phototoxic reaction to PUVA is nail damage with photo-onycholysis [233] or subungual haemorrhage [234]. Episodes of burning are more common with topical PUVA than with oral PUVA due to greater epidermal concentrations of psoralen and uneven absorption into the skin. The smaller risk of burning from oral PUVA can be lessened further by using 5-MOP rather than 8-MOP [235]. Predisposing factors for the development of erythema are similar to those discussed for UVB-induced erythema.

The management of phototoxic reactions depends on their severity and can range from dose increment adjustments to withdrawal of treatment. Mild to moderate erythema can be managed with moderate to potent topical corticosteroid creams and emollients. Severe reactions with blistering may require a potent topical corticosteroid such as clobetasol propionate supplemented by a short course of systemic corticosteroids.

Pruritus and pain
Pruritus occurs in up to 25% of patients and is associated with dryness of the skin [234,236]. This can usually be controlled with emollients. A rare but severe idiosyncratic side effect is PUVA pain that can last for weeks or months and does not appear to correlate with PUVA phototoxicity [237,238]. PUVA pain is important to identify as management is difficult. Low-frequency electrotherapy [239], topical capsaicin [240] and oral gabapentin [241] or phenytoin [242] have all been advocated. The continuation of PUVA or further courses in the future are contraindicated as recurrence of pain is common.

Nausea
Nausea is a common side effect in patients treated with oral 8-MOP PUVA. This can be lessened by taking the psoralen with a light meal or by using an antiemetic. Alternatively switching to 5-MOP or topical PUVA may help [59].

Blistering
Subepidermal bullae have been reported to be induced by PUVA [4,243]. Phototoxic reactions to PUVA can result in bullae that occur most commonly in an acral distribution. Induction of bullous pemphigoid or a flaring of this in a patient with pre-existing disease is recognised.

Provocation of photodermatoses
Polymorphic light eruption can be precipitated by PUVA, as can undiagnosed lupus erythematosus [208].

Herpes simplex reactivation
As with UVB phototherapy, outbreaks of herpes can be precipitated by PUVA [244]. Management is no different.

Other side effects
Less commonly observed side effects include transient nail pigmentation, a facial dermatitis resembling seborrhoeic dermatitis, folliculitis, facial hypertrichosis [208,234], disseminated superficial actinic porokeratosis [245], lichenoid eruptions [246], headaches, insomnia [247] and allergic reactions to 8-MOP [248,249].

Chronic effects
Photoageing
PUVA induces features resembling photoageing (dermatoheliosis) except that the changes are not confined to sun-exposed sites. The clinical features are similar to those described for UVB therapy but pigmentary changes and xerosis are more prominent. These changes are cumulative and dose related [208,**250**].

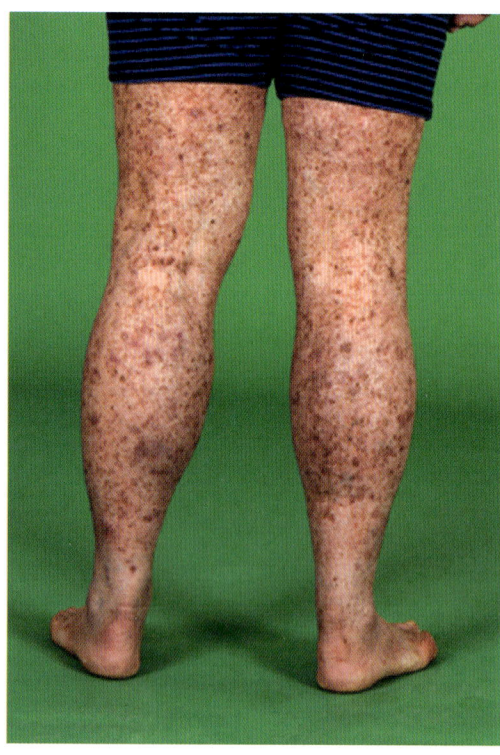

Figure 21.14 PUVA lentigines affecting a patient's legs.

PUVA keratoses
These manifest as multiple hyperkeratotic papules, most commonly located on non-sun-exposed sites, for example the legs, trunk and sides of the hands, feet and digits [251]. They occur most frequently in those patients exposed to high cumulative doses and are associated with an increased risk of non-melanoma skin cancer.

PUVA lentigines
These are large, irregular, stellate, darkly pigmented macular lesions (Figure 21.14) that histopathologically consist of large and atypical melanocytes. They occur most frequently in patients of skin type I/II who have received high numbers of PUVA treatments [252,253]. There is no proven link between PUVA lentigines and the development of melanoma. Interestingly, however, a recent study has found that the T1799A *BRAF* mutation is commonly found in PUVA lentigines, suggesting premalignant potential [254].

Non-melanoma skin cancer
There is now substantial evidence for the carcinogenic risk of PUVA therapy in large cohorts of patients followed up for prolonged periods of time, particularly from the USA and Sweden [255–261]. There is a marked and dose-dependent increased risk of squamous cell carcinoma (SCC): in the most recent report from the American cohort, the risk of developing one or more SCCs in a year was strongly associated with the total number of PUVA treatments (350–450 versus <50 treatments; incidence rate ratio (IRR) of 6.01) [262]. The overall excess risk of SCC in the high exposure group was significantly greater than this (IRR of 20.92). A 16-fold increase in incidence of genital SCC was observed in males from the same cohort whose exposure to PUVA was high (>240 treatments) rather than low (<140 treatments) [225]. It is recommended that lifetime exposure should be limited to 150–200 treatment sessions or a cumulative dose of 1000–1500 J/cm^2. Maintenance therapy should be avoided [6,59].

Important risk factors for PUVA-induced skin cancer include skin types I/II, a previous history of skin cancer, previous exposure to radiotherapy or arsenic [263–266], immunosuppressive therapy, especially ciclosporin [194,258,267,268] or UVB therapy [269], and the presence of PUVA keratosis [251] or lentigines [253].

PUVA is mutagenic [270,271], immunosuppressive [272–274] and carcinogenic [275,276]. p53 mutations have been detected in 65% of PUVA-induced SCCs. The mutational pattern consists not only of PUVA-specific mutations (T to A transversions) but also 'fingerprint' mutations, as seen following solar exposure and UVB therapy (i.e. C to T or CC to TT mutations) [277–279]. PUVA has various effects on the immune system including decreasing the number of CD3+, CD4+ and CD8+ T lymphocytes in both the epidermis and dermis and affecting Langerhans cell immune expression [272,273]. In addition, PUVA has also been reported to reduce a variety of circulating lymphocyte subsets [274]. Decreased immune surveillance may contribute to the carcinogenic effects of PUVA. To date there is no evidence to support an increased risk of skin cancer occurring in patients who have received bath or topical PUVA [280].

Melanoma
Psoralen and UVA can stimulate the growth of melanoma cells and induce melanocytic tumours in animal experiments [281,282]. A fivefold increase over the expected incidence of melanoma 15 years after first treatment was reported from a US 16-centre PUVA cohort [283]. Follow-up of the same cohort (an average of 2.25 years later) has showed a further increase to nine times the expected incidence [284]. The melanomas were more common in patients of skin type I/II and in those who had received at least 250 PUVA exposures. European study groups, on the other hand, have not found an increased risk of melanoma with PUVA [261,265,285,286]. In particular, the study of 4799 Swedish patients treated with PUVA with an average follow-up of 16 years did not detect an increased incidence of melanoma [261]. Due to the long latent period of melanoma, further follow-up of these cohorts will be required to clarify melanoma risk in patients treated by PUVA.

Internal malignancy
It is known that patients with psoriasis have a threefold increased risk of lymphoma compared with the general population [287]. As PUVA alters immune function and surveillance there is a concern that the risk of internal malignancy, particularly of lymphoproliferative neoplasms, may be increased. To date studies have not demonstrated a significant association of PUVA with the development of lymphoma [288], nor a consistent relationship with other internal malignancies [259,261,289].

Ophthalmological effects
Psoralens can penetrate the ocular lens, where 8-MOP has been detected in humans at 12 h and in rats at 12–24 h after systemic administration [290,291]. Following exposure to UVA, psoralens can bind to proteins in the lens, where they can accumulate as a result of the lack of cell turnover [292].

Cataract development following PUVA has been reported in some animal experiments [4]. Several studies of patients who have received PUVA have not shown an association between PUVA and cataract development [293–295]. A study of 82 patients who refused to wear protective sunglasses after PUVA did not observe any lens abnormalities. Decreased lacrimation and conjunctival hyperaemia occurred in some cases, however [296]. It is recommended that protective eyewear be worn for 12 h after the ingestion of psoralen and for 24 h in individuals with pre-existing cataracts or who may be at increased risk of cataract (e.g. children and patients with atopic eczema). A survey of protective eyewear used for PUVA showed that all sunglasses tested were suitable and the UV400 label was proven to indicate appropriate protection [222].

UVA-1 phototherapy

Acute effects

Ultraviolet A-1 is generally well tolerated. Expected acute adverse effects include erythema, pigmentation, induction of PLE and recrudescence of herpes simplex virus infection [**12**]. Erythema induced by UVA-1 has a biphasic time course, with an early peak at 15–60 min and a delayed peak that may be maximal as early as 8 h after exposure, although this latter peak may be broad and plateau between 8 and 24 h [297].

Chronic effects

Ultraviolet A-1 phototherapy, in common with NB-UVB and PUVA, is photogenotoxic, photomutagenic and carcinogenic in a mouse model. There is no evidence as yet of increased risk of skin cancer in humans [298]. There are, however, concerns about its potential carcinogenic risk as it has been shown to induce cyclobutane pyrimidine dimers, particularly thymine dimers, and the basal layer is particularly vulnerable [299]. Oxidative DNA damage occurs at both genomic and nucleotide levels and there is also altered calcineurin signalling, which may impair tumour suppression [300].

Extracorporeal photochemotherapy

Adverse events occurring with ECP are uncommon providing psoralen is added to the treatment bag and not given orally [301]. Side effects reported include transient hypotension, low-grade pyrexia, an increase in erythema of the skin, anaemia with long-term use and thrombocytopenia [136,202,302].

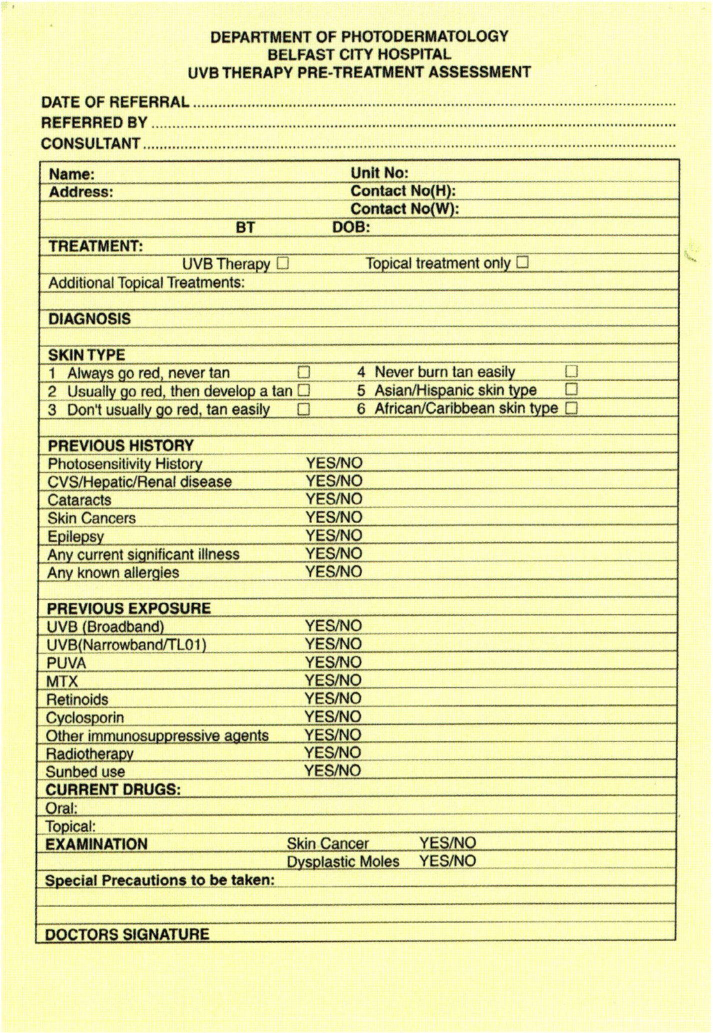

DEPARTMENT OF PHOTODERMATOLOGY
BELFAST CITY HOSPITAL
UVB THERAPY PRE-TREATMENT ASSESSMENT

DATE OF REFERRAL ....
REFERRED BY ....
CONSULTANT ....

Name:	**Unit No:**	
Address:	**Contact No(H):**	
	Contact No(W):	
BT	**DOB:**	
TREATMENT:		
UVB Therapy ☐	Topical treatment only ☐	
Additional Topical Treatments:		
DIAGNOSIS		
SKIN TYPE		
1 Always go red, never tan ☐	4 Never burn tan easily ☐	
2 Usually go red, then develop a tan ☐	5 Asian/Hispanic skin type ☐	
3 Don't usually go red, tan easily ☐	6 African/Caribbean skin type ☐	
PREVIOUS HISTORY		
Photosensitivity History	YES/NO	
CVS/Hepatic/Renal disease	YES/NO	
Cataracts	YES/NO	
Skin Cancers	YES/NO	
Epilepsy	YES/NO	
Any current significant illness	YES/NO	
Any known allergies	YES/NO	
PREVIOUS EXPOSURE		
UVB (Broadband)	YES/NO	
UVB(Narrowband/TL01)	YES/NO	
PUVA	YES/NO	
MTX	YES/NO	
Retinoids	YES/NO	
Cyclosporin	YES/NO	
Other immunosuppressive agents	YES/NO	
Radiotherapy	YES/NO	
Sunbed use	YES/NO	
CURRENT DRUGS:		
Oral:		
Topical:		
EXAMINATION	Skin Cancer	YES/NO
	Dysplastic Moles	YES/NO
Special Precautions to be taken:		
DOCTORS SIGNATURE		

Figure 21.15 Ultraviolet B referral form.

Patient selection, assessment and education

Patient selection and assessment

Patients requiring phototherapy should be appraised for factors relating to skin cancer risk (see Box 21.2) [**3**,**6**]. A referral form completed in the clinic should document the patient's risk factor profile and should include documentation of skin type, previous natural sunlight/UVB/PUVA/sunbed use, previous skin cancer or precursors, previous systemic immunosuppressive drug therapy and exposure to radiotherapy (Figure 21.15). In addition, a full skin examination should be performed to assess solar damage and to look for the presence of multiple freckles/moles, premalignant skin lesions and skin cancers.

It is also important to document all medication, especially any oral photoactive drug or herbal product being taken such as a thiazide diuretic or St John's wort (*Hypericum perforatum*). Most photoactive drugs absorb maximally in the UVA region and only some (including thiazides and quinine) have an extension of their action spectrum into the UVB region. In one study, patients taking NSAIDs, calcium channel antagonists and phenothiazines were reported to have a lower NB-UVB MED, a factor which may need to be taken into consideration in patients being assessed for phototherapy [303]. Furthermore, photosensitising drugs may increase the risk of erythemal episodes during a course of NB-UVB phototherapy, even if the baseline MED was normal [207].

Photosensitivity with UVA-1 phototherapy is more likely in patients taking photoactive drugs [**12**]. With PUVA, the overwhelming photosensitisation by psoralen usually means that other photoactive drugs are unlikely to cause any additional clinically important photosensitisation.

Patient selection is particularly important for home phototherapy. Candidates for such therapy include those living some distance from the local phototherapy unit, who have poor transport links, have disability or mobility problems or have work/childcare or other caring responsibilities. Suitable candidates should also be required to have a good understanding of how to perform such therapy after appropriate training and monitoring [167].

Topical therapies should also be assessed. Consideration should be given to discontinuation of topical calcineurin inhibitors, such as tacrolimus [304]. Patients with epilepsy should be asked whether seizures can be induced by light exposure. As PUVA therapy is mutagenic this treatment should be avoided in pregnancy. Oral PUVA should be used with caution if the patient has significant liver dysfunction.

Patient education

Patients who are commencing phototherapy or PUVA should be counselled regarding both the acute and chronic potential side effects of treatment. This should be reinforced by providing a patient information leaflet. Patients should be advised regarding the appropriate use of emollients. The importance of reporting any new medication and of avoiding fragrance-containing products, sunbathing and sunbeds during the course of treatment should be emphasised. Also, it is important to advise patients to maintain a consistent hairstyle and to explain the rationale for this advice. Males should be advised of the need to protect the genitalia. The importance of wearing protective eyewear should be stressed. The treatment cabin should be shown to the patient and the protocol explained, stressing the importance of regular attendance. A consent form should be signed by the patient before treatment is commenced. A recent report assessed educational benefits for patients using a computer tablet education session compared with traditional education before phototherapy. The tablet-based sessions led to higher levels of patient phototherapy safety knowledge [305].

Patient and staff safety

Both patient and staff safety should be ensured. For patient safety, see Box 21.3.

Individuals who may be exposed to UV radiation include nurses and nursing assistants, medical physicists, doctors or, less commonly, physiotherapists. The most important risk to staff is exposure to UVB. Staff who conduct dosimetry should wear goggles, face shields, appropriate clothing and a sunscreen (sun protection factor >30) if they have to enter the cabinet with the lamps on. When UV cabinets are being used, the lamps should be switched off before opening or entering the cabinet.

Patient follow-up: skin cancer surveillance

It is well recognised that systemic PUVA therapy is associated with a dose-related increased risk of non-melanoma skin cancer, particularly SCC. It has been recommended that the maximum lifetime dose should not exceed 1000–1500 J/cm^2 or 150–200 exposures [6,59]. The increased carcinogenic risk seen with systemic PUVA has not been seen with bath PUVA. Bath PUVA involves lower UVA doses but results in a much higher epidermal psoralen concentration than oral PUVA. Thus the potential for induction of mutagenic DNA lesions remains and ongoing vigilance in these patients is required. It is important to take into account total UVA dose in addition to treatment numbers when considering the carcinogenic risk of PUVA. The British Association of Dermatologists (BAD) *Service Guidance and Standards for Phototherapy Units* has recommended a threshold of >500 UVB exposures for skin cancer screening review [306]. It is recommended that patients who exceed these maximum thresholds of exposure should have an annual skin examination carried out to detect premalignant and malignant skin lesions. This is particularly important for those patients with other risk factors, such as those of skin type I/II.

Box 21.3 Patient safety during ultraviolet (UV) phototherapy or psoralen and UVA (PUVA)

Eye protection
- Patients must wear UV-blocking goggles while receiving treatment
- Individuals receiving oral PUVA must wear UVA-blocking glasses for 12 h following the ingestion of psoralen (longer if risk factors for cataract development are present)
- Patients should be provided with a list of approved UV protective eyewear and have their own glasses checked [307–309]

Prevention of burning
- Minimal erythema dose/minimal phototoxic dose testing: this allows more accurate determination of starting dose than that based on skin type
- Accurate dosimetry: the irradiance of cabinets should be regularly checked by a medical physicist using an appropriately calibrated radiometer. In-built radiometers in cabinets have been found to be unreliable. Exposure times for the full range of doses used should be precisely calculated for each individual cabinet. It is helpful if these can be displayed in tabular form with the corresponding doses according to the measured irradiance
- Patient education: factors that can lead to inadvertent burning should be discussed with each patient
- Obese patients may require a modified treatment protocol, i.e. a lower starting dose, as areas such as the breasts, buttocks and abdomen are closer to the lamps
- Use of correct UV source: in cabinets that have combined UVB and UVA lamps it is essential that the correct tubes are selected for treatment
- Lamp maintenance: cabins should be kept clean and lamps should be inspected regularly. Tubes should be replaced when their output falls to a predetermined threshold as agreed with the local medical physicist. If a number of tubes need to be changed at the same time, the new tubes should be spaced out and not replaced side by side to minimise the risk of burning due to uneven irradiance from the cabinet. The irradiance should be rechecked once lamp replacement has been completed
- Psoralen dosage: it is important to ensure that the patient has taken the correct number of tablets at the correct time prior to skin irradiation

Reducing skin cancer risk
- Male patients should wear appropriate clothing to protect the genitalia [310]
- The face (if not involved by the dermatosis being treated) should be shielded with a visor to avoid unnecessary UV exposure
- For some indications, whole body treatment may not be required (e.g. for polymorphic light eruption desensitisation, treatment limited to the photoexposed skin may be sufficient). Treatment planning should take such factors into account to reduce overall UV exposure load

Assimilation of long-term follow-up data for NB-UVB is ongoing, although the preliminary data have not, however, suggested a significant increase in skin cancer risk from NB-UVB [227–229].

Mathematical models have been created in attempts to quantify the risk of skin cancer resulting from NB-UVB but the methodologies used are very variable. One group, on the premise that an increased risk of non-melanoma skin cancer of no more than 50% is 'acceptable', has recommended limiting lifetime exposure to 450 treatments [311]. However, there are concerns about defining a ceiling number of treatments in the absence of robust clinical data to support this and, more importantly, without assessing risk/benefit on an individual basis.

Clinical governance

Skin burning secondary to phototherapy is a leading cause of negligence legal claims in dermatology [312,313]. To reduce the risk of this adverse event and to ensure maintainance of safety, good clinical governance practice is essential. A phototherapy service should have a designated responsible person or lead clinician (usually a consultant dermatologist). This individual should ensure that high quality standards are maintained. Guidelines and protocols should be maintained and updated. Staff should be suitably trained and their knowledge should be updated through formal clinical professional development (CPD). The service should be delivered by a multidisciplinary team which should consist of the lead clinician, lead phototherapy nurse, medical physicist and other relevant assistant staff. Areas that require being audited regularly include patient outcomes, documentation, adverse events, equipment maintenance and risk management. Governance may be overseen through managed clinical networks, such as in Scotland where phototherapy is standardised and governed through the oversight of Photonet, the Scottish Managed Clinical Network for Phototherapy.

Documentation

In most of Europe and North America there is a legal requirement for documentation that should include patient records, dosimetry and equipment maintenance, adverse events and summary records of departmental activity.

Patient records
Referral forms for phototherapy or PUVA must be completed by a dermatologist or authorised dermatology practitioner. The content of this form should include patient identity, the disease being treated, type of phototherapy requested, current systemic medications, previous phototherapy and details about the absence or presence of any contraindications or risk factors for phototherapy. A record of informed consent must be obtained and patients must receive a patient information leaflet. A formal nursing assessment should be recorded. Phototest results, treatment type (including details of psoralen dose), incremental regimen prescribed, all treatment visits, UV doses administered, response to treatment and adverse incidents must all be systematically documented.

Dosimetry and equipment maintenance
The UV equipment used must be 'CE' marked as a medical device and be appropriately maintained by an approved engineer or medical physicist. Assessment of the electrical safety and inspection of the integrity of all UV units should form part of a regular maintenance schedule, careful records of which must be kept.

Records must be kept of all UV calibration readings, which must be carried out by an approved medical physicist. Any radiometer used must be calibrated with traceability to the UK National Physics Laboratory or equivalent authority elsewhere [44]. A policy for the replacement of low-output or failed UV lamps should be in place.

Adverse incidents
All adverse incidents should be recorded. The circumstances should be clearly described with the action taken. These incidents should be discussed at department meetings to minimise the risk of recurrence of such events.

Performance indicators
These reflect the workload of the department and should include the total number of patients treated, total number of treatment sessions with a breakdown by treatment modality, number of patients on the waiting list and average waiting time from referral to treatment.

Risk management
A formal risk assessment of potential hazards in the phototherapy department, especially from inadvertent exposure to UV radiation, should be undertaken at least annually. Employee exposure to UV radiation should not exceed exposure limit values (ELVs) as required by control measures of the Artificial Optical Radiation Directive (AORD) [314]. The waiting areas must be separate from treatment areas. Warning signs should be displayed on entering areas where UV is being used. An infection control and hygiene policy should be established, particularly with regard to cleaning the phototherapy equipment.

Audit
The phototherapy service should be regularly audited to ensure it is maintaining standards and adhering to guidelines [1,3,6]. Many aspects of the service can be audited, including quality of phototherapy records; clinical outcome including adverse events; workload and activity statistics; waiting list management and access to the service; and discharge and follow-up procedures.

How to set up a phototherapy unit

The setting up of a phototherapy service involves the participation of different groups – including medical and nursing staff, the medical physics service, local health service management and hospital engineers (with regard to both electrical supply and safety) [1,6]. The involvement of patient organisations may help persuade administrators and funders of the desirability of providing such a service.

It is vital that adequate space is provided. For a modest district-based service serving a population of 200 000 people there should be sufficient room to accommodate one NB-UVB cabinet, one PUVA cabinet, a set of UV units for the local treatment of hands and feet and UV units for phototesting. If topical bath PUVA is to be offered, bathing facilities are necessary. In addition to the treatment area, which requires adequate ventilation to cope with heat emitted by the UV equipment, space is also required for a waiting area with access to toilet facilities and for reception and nursing administration areas with appropriate IT facilities and document storage space.

Policies need to be established for ongoing UV cabinet maintenance, lamp replacement and radiometry [44]. Staff should have a background of experience and training in dermatology and should have attended a core phototherapy course followed by a period of supervised practice in a unit where UV therapy is already provided. Protocols and evidence-based guidelines must be in place and staff training completed before the service is opened.

The introduction of a home phototherapy service also requires a multidisciplinary team approach. Patient selection and appropriate training and supervision by staff are essential. Standardised treatment protocols need to be adhered to and the supervising nurse should contact the patient regularly during treatment to assess progress and any problems [167,315,316].

What's new: developments

Phototherapy is a highly effective and safe treatment option for many skin diseases and continued awareness of the availability of this form of treatment is important.

One of the factors limiting further therapeutic advances in phototherapy sources has been our relative lack of understanding of the action spectra for the clearance of diseases other than psoriasis. Most of the developmental work relating to optimising phototherapy regimens has been with psoriasis in mind. Future work to define the optimal wavelengths for the treatment of diseases such as eczema, mycosis fungoides and vitiligo is required in order to promote the development of light sources and treatment regimens that are disease-specific.

Advances in technology are enabling the development of compact, portable, efficient and inexpensive UV and visible light-emitting diode (LED) light sources. Taken together with modern methods of instant communication, these may facilitate the development of patient self-administered home phototherapy services with ready access to expert supervision and assistance coordinated from a central phototherapy department. Clinical governance is essential and the development of national networks to centralise this is ongoing. The future of phototherapy is encouraging. As new insights into skin biology are gained, there will be opportunities to refine treatment further to improve its already good efficacy/risk profile.

Key references

The full list of references can be found in the online version at https://www.wiley.com/rooksdermatology10e

3 Goulden V, Ling TC, Babakinejad P et al. British Association of Dermatologists and British Photodermatology Group guidelines for narrowband ultraviolet B phototherapy (NB-UVB) 2021. *Br J Dermatol* 2022;187:295–308.

6 Ling TC, Clayton TH, Crawley J et al. British Association of Dermatologists and British Photodermatology Group guidelines for the safe and effective use of psoralen-ultraviolet A therapy 2015. *Br J Dermatol* 2016;174:24–55.

8 Scarisbrick JJ, Taylor P, Holtick U et al. UK consensus statement on the use of extracorporeal photopheresis for the treatment of cutaneous T-cell lymphoma and chronic graft-versus-host disease. *Br J Dermatol* 2008;158:1365–2133.

12 Kerr AC, Ferguson J, Attili SK et al. Ultraviolet A1 phototherapy: a British Photodermatology Group workshop report. *Clin Exp Dermatol* 2012;37:219–26.

27 Roelandts R. The history of phototherapy: something new under the sun? *J Am Acad Dermatol* 2002;46:926–30.

36 Van Weelden H, Baart de La Faille H, Young E, van der Leun JC. A new development in UVB phototherapy of psoriasis. *Br J Dermatol* 1988;119:11–19.

47 Dawe RS. A quantitative review of studies comparing the efficacy of narrow-band and broad-band ultraviolet B for psoriasis. *Br J Dermatol* 2003;149:669–72.

171 Stern RS. Psoralen and ultraviolet light therapy for psoriasis. *N Engl J Med* 2007;357:682–90.

230 Archier E, Devaux S, Castela E et al. Carcinogenic risks of psoralen UV-A therapy and narrowband UV-B therapy in chronic plaque psoriasis: a systematic literature review. *J Eur Acad Dermatol Venereol* 2012;26(Suppl. 3):22–31.

250 Matz H. Phototherapy for psoriasis: what to choose and how to use: facts and controversies. *Clin Dermatol* 2010;28:73–80.

CHAPTER 22

Principles of Photodynamic Therapy

Sally Ibbotson[1] and Kevin McKenna[2]

[1] Photobiology Unit, University of Dundee, Ninewells Hospital and Medical School, Dundee, UK
[2] Dermatology Department, Belfast Trust, Belfast, UK

What is photodynamic therapy?, 22.1	Basal cell carcinoma, 22.6	Treatment schedules, aftercare and follow-up, 22.12
History and background, 22.1	Other indications, 22.7	**Adverse effects**, 22.12
Photosensitisers used for photodynamic therapy in dermatology, 22.2	**Contraindications**, 22.8	Acute effects, 22.12
	Methodology and regimens, 22.8	Chronic effects, 22.14
Light sources, 22.3	Diagnosis and patient selection, 22.8	**Clinical governance**, 22.15
Indications, 22.4	Conventional PDT, 22.9	How to set up a PDT service, 22.15
Actinic keratosis, 22.4	Ambulatory photodynamic therapy, 22.11	**What's new?**, 22.15
Bowen disease, 22.6	Daylight photodynamic therapy, 22.11	**Key references**, 22.15

What is photodynamic therapy?

The aim of all dermatology treatments is to clear diseased tissue, while sparing normal healthy skin. Photodynamic therapy (PDT) has three key components: tissue-localised photosensitiser, photochemical activation by light of appropriate wavelength(s) and oxygen, which together result in oxidative stress, inflammation and cell death [1,2]. Treatment for diseased tissue alone is achieved by photosensitiser localisation and targeted light delivery, and it is this relative selectivity that has led to considerable interest in the clinical application of PDT. Systemic or topical photosensitisation can be used but as most dermatological PDT is topical, this will be the focus of this chapter.

Interestingly, although many studies have investigated the mechanisms of effect of PDT *in vitro*, there is little known about what happens following topical PDT to human skin *in vivo*. The effects of PDT depend on the subcellular localisation and concentration of photosensitiser, accessibility of light of the appropriate wavelength and oxygen availability, which will in turn be influenced by the treatment parameters used.

During PDT, the photosensitiser absorbs light, is photochemically activated and is converted to a higher energy singlet state; when it returns to the ground state, fluorescence occurs. Alternatively, the singlet state may transfer to the more stable triplet state. Both type I and type II photo-oxidative reactions occur: type I involves direct hydrogen and electron transfer from the triplet state of the photosensitiser to a substrate; type II occurs when electrons or energy are transferred to molecular oxygen in the ground state and singlet oxygen is generated. The generation of reactive oxygen species, in particular singlet oxygen, is thought to be important in terms of causing nuclear, mitochondrial and membrane damage and in initiating signalling pathways with subsequent gene transcription, pro-inflammatory changes, cell cycle arrest, apoptosis and necrosis [3,4].

In vivo studies have shown that prostaglandin E_2, histamine and nitric oxide are released following topical PDT [5,6]. Activation of the tumour suppressor gene, *p53*, is thought to be less important following PDT than following UV irradiation [7]. Topical PDT is immunosuppressive in humans and reduces epidermal Langerhans cell numbers after exposure; paradoxically, despite its immunosuppressive effects, it is widely and effectively used for the treatment of skin malignancies and dysplasia and may have both direct antitumour effects and immunogenic cell toxicity [4,8–11]. Effects on the vasculature, including endothelial cell damage, vasoconstriction and vessel occlusion, are considered important for systemic PDT, where photosensitiser delivery is principally via the intravenous route, but is thought to be less important for topical PDT, where there is local cutaneous uptake and metabolism of photosensitiser prodrugs. The effects of PDT are considered to be mainly membrane-mediated, but DNA damage, strand breaks and mutagenesis can occur [4,12]. To date, however, there is no evidence for a carcinogenic effect. Interestingly, topical cutaneous PDT may have an important role in delaying the development of actinic keratosis and invasive squamous cell carcinoma in organ transplant recipients.

History and background

The term 'photodynamic reaction' was first coined at the beginning of the 20th century following a series of experiments by a medical student, Oscar Raab, who was working for Hermann von Tappeiner in Munich. He observed amplification of the cytotoxic effects of acridine orange on protozoa in the presence of daylight. In 1903, the therapeutic effects of this photodynamic reaction were explored by Jesionek and von Tappeiner and they demonstrated the beneficial effects of topical eosin and sunlight or arc lamp exposure for a range of skin diseases, including skin cancers and lupus vulgaris [13].

The effects of systemic photosensitisers were investigated by Friedrich Meyer-Betz in 1912. He injected himself with haematoporphyrin and, when subsequently exposed to daylight during a tram journey, he experienced an extreme cutaneous phototoxic reaction. Subsequent clinical studies using intramuscular haematoporphyrin and UV exposure showed some therapeutic effect in psoriasis. However, it was not until Dougherty and colleagues undertook key early clinical studies in the 1970s using purified haematoporphyrin derivative for PDT in patients with a range of skin tumours that the potential of PDT, with its selective phototoxic effects, was recognised as suitable for development as an anticancer treatment [14]. A purified haematoporphyrin preparation is now approved for use in systemic PDT for several internal malignancies, although not for skin cancers [2].

An ideal photosensitiser needs to accumulate in the target tissue, absorb light at clinically relevant wavelengths, be photochemically activated efficiently and have rapid clearance and minimal dark toxicity. Several chemicals have been investigated for their potential in systemic PDT: these include porphyrins, chlorins, porphines, phthalocyanines and texapyrins. The most widely used systemic photosensitisers for PDT have been porfimer-sodium (Photofrin®), particularly for lung and oesophageal cancer and temoporfin (tetrakis (hydroxymethyl) phosphonium chloride; Foscan®) for head and neck squamous cell carcinoma [15]. Both are associated with prolonged photosensitivity to visible light over several weeks and there is also a risk of phototoxicity occurring at sites of injection if extravasation occurs. The benzoporphyrin derivative BPD-MA (Verteporfin®), has also been used for systemic PDT for wet macular degeneration. Other systemic photosensitisers are in development but not in routine clinical use [16].

Systemic PDT is rarely required in dermatology, other than in the occasional setting of treating Gorlin naevoid basal cell carcinoma (BCC) syndrome, when multiple lesions may be treated simultaneously, and if treating larger less accessible areas, for example in extensive vulval intraepithelial neoplasia [17,18].

The accessibility of skin led to further investigation of the use of topical photosensitisation for PDT. In 1990, Kennedy reported the successful use of topical 5-aminolaevulinic acid (ALA) as a prodrug for PDT for malignant and pre-cancerous skin lesions [19,20]. Topical 'porphyrin' PDT is now widely incorporated into dermatology services such that dermatologists involved in the management of patients with skin cancer and pre-cancers should have access to a PDT service [21–27,**28**,29–34].

Photosensitisers used for photodynamic therapy in dermatology

Topical 'porphyrin' PDT employs the principles of the haem cycle (Figure 22.1). A non-photosensitising prodrug is used. The licensed prodrugs in current use are ALA (Levulan® Kerastick®, Ameluz® and Alacare®) and the methyl ester of ALA, methyl aminolaevulinate (MAL) (Metvix®/Metvixia®), which penetrate the epidermis due to their low molecular weight. Following the application of prodrugs to a skin lesion (usually a superficial non-melanoma skin cancer or dysplastic lesion) and uptake, the rate-limited step of ALA synthase is bypassed and, due to a second rate-limited step at ferrochelatase, protoporphyrin IX (PpIX) accumulates in the target tissue. PpIX is a potent photosensitiser expressed in all mammalian nucleated cells at very low sub-photosensitising levels. When it is present in increased amounts, however, it is a potent and efficient photosensitiser, which can be activated by light of the appropriate wavelengths. It has a short half-life and is cleared within 24–48 h.

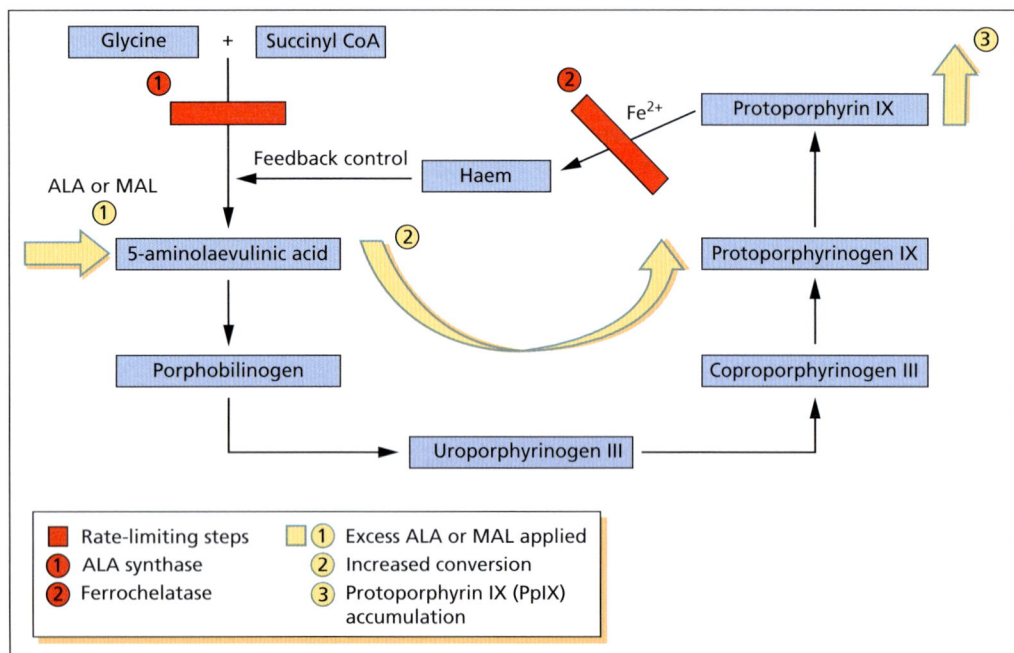

Figure 22.1 'Porphyrin' photodynamic therapy uses the haem cycle. ALA, 5-aminolaevulinic acid; CoA, co-enzyme A; MAL, methyl aminolaevulinate.

PpIX has a characteristic crimson red fluorescence when exposed to UVA (Wood's light), a phenomenon that can be used diagnostically, for example in the delineation of skin tumour margins (Figure 22.2) [27,35,36], or, when ALA is administered systemically, for the diagnosis of gastrointestinal malignancies or dysplasia or delineation of brain tumours. When ALA and MAL are applied topically the processes involved in the preferential uptake of PpIX by diseased skin are poorly understood. Surface measurements 6 h after topical ALA application show that PpIX fluorescence in non-melanoma skin cancer is up to 15 times more intense than in adjacent normal skin. Although this does not necessarily fully reflect deep accumulation of the photosensitiser, PpIX does in general reach higher concentrations in tumour tissue than in the surrounding skin (Figure 22.2) [37]. It is likely that altered permeability of the stratum corneum overlying a skin cancer or pre-cancer facilitates the uptake and conversion of these small molecules. Whereas ALA is hydrophilic, MAL is lipophilic and was introduced with the aim of increasing uptake and specificity for diseased skin. Esterases are, however, required to remove the methyl chain from MAL prior to conversion to PpIX. The vehicle may also play an important role in uptake, as for example with the ALA preparation in nanocolloid emulsion (Ameluz®). In clinical studies in humans, both ALA PDT and MAL PDT are highly effective when used in the appropriate clinical setting [28]. There may be other factors involved in determining the relative specificity of PpIX accumulation in diseased skin. *In vitro* studies have led investigators to propose that relative iron deficiency, altered haem cycle enzyme expression, change in pH and state of cell differentiation in diseased tissue may each influence this, although the actual mechanisms *in vivo* are unknown and, importantly, are not specific to tumour cells. This is demonstrated by relative PpIX accumulation after prodrug application in benign hyperproliferative conditions, such as psoriasis and viral warts.

Many of the earlier published studies of topical PDT used non-licensed proprietary preparations of ALA. However, approved licensed preparations of both ALA and MAL are now available. MAL is available as Metvix/Metvixia (16%, Galderma) for PDT and is used for actinic keratoses (AK) on the face and scalp in both conventional and daylight PDT, Bowen disease and superficial BCC (and also for nodular BCC when other available treatments are considered less suitable). The use of MAL for these indications has been approved by the licensing authorities of most European countries and a significant number of countries elsewhere (e.g. Australia, South Africa, Canada, Brazil).

A preparation of ALA in solution (Levulan Kerastick; 20%, DUSA Pharmaceuticals) is approved by the US Food and Drug Administration (FDA) for PDT of mild to moderate AK on the face and scalp [38]. ALA in a nanocolloid emulsion (Ameluz; 8%, Biofrontera) is also approved for clinical use: this has been shown to result in an increased depth of PpIX accumulation after prodrug application when compared with MAL in a porcine skin model *ex vivo* [39]. Ameluz PDT is licensed for use in thin to moderately thick AK of the face and scalp both in conventional and daylight PDT and for superficial and thin nodular BCC [40–42]. In addition, an ALA patch (Alacare; 8 mg, 2 mg/cm^2, Spirig HC) is licensed for use in several European countries for PDT for thin AK on the face and scalp [43–45]. Other developments in the formulations for prodrug delivery include the use of penetration enhancers or iron chelators, such as dimethyl sulfoxide (DMSO), ethylenediaminetetraacetic acid (EDTA), desferrioxamine or the hydroxypyridinone, CP94 [46–48]. These have the potential to improve PDT outcomes but are not in routine clinical use and are mainly still at the experimental stage [49–53]. Physical methods to improve prodrug uptake are also under investigation and include laser pre-treatment, microdermabrasion or microneedling [54–60].

Light sources

The majority of photosensitisers used in PDT absorb maximally in the visible waveband. The absorption of porphyrins is broad, with peak absorption in the Soret band around 410 nm and several other smaller peaks between 500 and 650 nm (Figure 22.3). For PDT to be effective the photosensitiser needs to be activated within the target tissue. Although short wavelengths in the blue/violet range of the visible spectrum are the most potent at activating PpIX *in vitro*, tissue penetration *in vivo* is limited to 1–2 mm. Photochemical activation of PpIX by red light at 630–635 nm is, however, still significant and red light has the advantage of penetrating tissue to a depth of 6–7 mm. For this reason these longer wavelengths are the ones most commonly used in conventional PpIX-based PDT. The exception to this is the approved regimen for PDT for AK in the USA using Levulan Kerastick and a blue light-emitting diode (LED) light source (BLU-U®). This provides sufficient efficacy for these superficial lesions but would be unlikely to offer adequate depth of effect for superficial BCC or Bowen disease [38]. Furthermore, advances in the use of daylight PDT employ the visible component of daylight exposure, with relative emphasis on the blue light part of the spectrum [61].

Historically, either filtered photographic slide projectors or lasers were used as light sources. In the limited studies that have been undertaken, there is no evidence that the efficacy of topical PDT

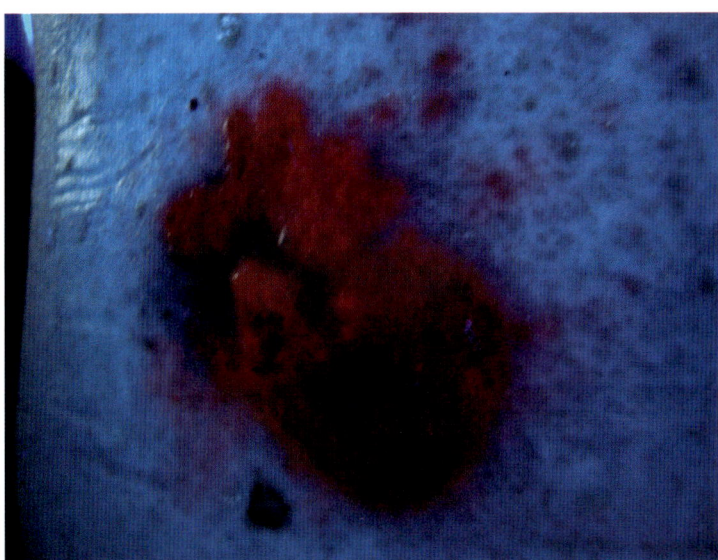

Figure 22.2 Crimson red protoporphyrin IX fluorescence in a superficial basal cell carcinoma 3 h after methyl aminolaevulinate application, showing the tumour specificity and adjacent tumour islands that need to be included in the irradiation field.

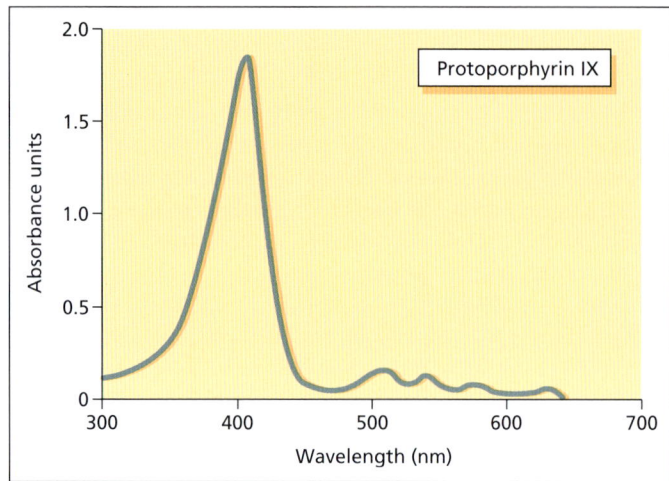

Figure 22.3 Absorption spectrum of protoporphyrin IX.

is superior if a monochromatic rather than a polychromatic light source is used [52,54–56,62]. Indeed, there are theoretical grounds for supposing that polychromatic sources might be more effective given that there are additional PpIX photoproducts that have absorption peaks around 670 nm.

A range of polychromatic light sources has been used in PDT, including filtered tungsten filament, metal halide and short arc xenon sources with peak emission in the 630–635 nm waveband [63–65]. The field size, irradiance, uniformity of irradiation and treatment times vary considerably between the different types of devices. Laser sources, including dye lasers and the compact and cheaper diode lasers, again using the 630–635 nm wavelengths, have also been employed. Intense pulsed light sources may also be successfully used for PDT [66].

The increasing developments in LEDs for PDT has resulted in the availability of portable, efficient, cheap and easy to maintain sources of relatively uniform irradiance, which can be used to treat field diameters of up to approximately 20 cm. These LED sources have more therapeutically weighted emission spectra that are narrower than other polychromatic sources and thus deliver light more efficiently. There is evidence from *ex vivo* studies that low irradiance light delivery may improve PDT efficiency. The efficiency of different light sources for PDT can be considered in the concept of total effective fluence, which takes into account incident spectral irradiance, optical transmission through tissue and photosensitiser absorption [67].

It is difficult to compare the results of published studies as there is wide variation in the treatment parameters used in PDT: these include variables in light delivery, such as the light source, irradiance and dose used [68]. Although high irradiance light delivery reduces treatment times, this may reduce PDT efficiency as a result of rapid oxygen depletion. On the other hand, fractionation of light delivery as an alternative to low irradiance light delivery might also be therapeutically beneficial [69–73]. The timing of light delivery to coincide with peak photosensitiser accumulation is also important and, for topical PDT, most regimens typically include irradiation 3–6 h after prodrug application. Blue or green light may be effective for AKs but the depth of effect will limit its use for most other conditions. Regular calibration of light sources is essential for light delivery during PDT, as lack of uniformity of irradiation may lead to inaccuracy in dose delivery and consequently suboptimal treatment.

Developments in light delivery include the use of daylight. Daylight PDT is now widely used as a convenient and effective treatment. The depth of the daylight PDT effect may be limited by the fact that most of the therapeutically effective wavelengths in daylight are in the blue light spectrum, thus mainly limiting its use to AK on exposed sites of the face and scalp. Other developments in light delivery include the use of very low irradiance portable LEDs and conformable light-emitting polymers and fabrics for lesions on curved body regions [74–78].

Indications

The main indications for topical PDT, with good supportive evidence, are in treating AK, Bowen disease and superficial basal cell carcinoma (sBCC); its role in other skin diseases is not as comprehensively established [17,21–23,26,**28**,**32**,**33**,79–88]. It is highly effective in selected cases and, because of its relative sparing of normal tissue, it can be used for multiple large 'field' areas and at sites of poor healing such as below the knee. Topical PDT is non-invasive, undertaken on an out-patient basis and treatment can be repeated without cumulative risk [21,**89**].

Actinic keratosis

Topical PDT is effective for thin- and moderate-thickness AK on the face and scalp using either MAL (Metvix/Metvixia) or ALA (Ameluz, Levulan Kerastick or non-licensed ALA preparations). PDT delivered either as conventional or daylight PDT is approved for this indication. Reported conventional PDT clearance rates (as assessed at 3 months after treatment) are in the region of 90% – while these are at least as good as those with liquid nitrogen cryotherapy or topical 5-fluorouracil, the cosmetic outcome is superior (Figure 22.4) [22,23,25,**32**,34,42,90,91]. There is, however, a relatively high recurrence rate of up to 19% at 1 year [92]. In meta-analyses, PDT was shown to be superior to cryotherapy and topical diclofenac in hyaluronan gel, in terms of efficacy, cosmetic outcome and patient satisfaction [93–95].

A head-to-head comparison of Ameluz, Metvix and placebo PDT for thin- to moderate-thickness facial and scalp AK showed superior efficacy of Ameluz PDT, particularly if a red light LED source was used, with sustained responses at 1 year [42,**96**]. Three months following completion of treatment with Ameluz or Metvix PDT, lesion clearance rates were 90% and 83% respectively, with sustained clearance of 53.1% and 40.8% at 1 year reported. There were no significant differences in adverse effects [**96**]. Follow-up at one year indicated lower recurrence rates with Ameluz PDT [**96**]. A meta-analysis of available published study evidence concluded that Ameluz PDT is more effective for thicker AK [97].

In an intra-subject comparison study, ALA PDT was more effective than imiquimod for moderate-thickness AK and was equivalent to imiquimod for thin AK on the upper limbs, although patient preference favoured PDT [98]. In a second similar study in patients with AK, in which patient tolerance and satisfaction with treatment were the main end points, both imiquimod and PDT were considered to be acceptable treatments for AK but patient satisfaction was

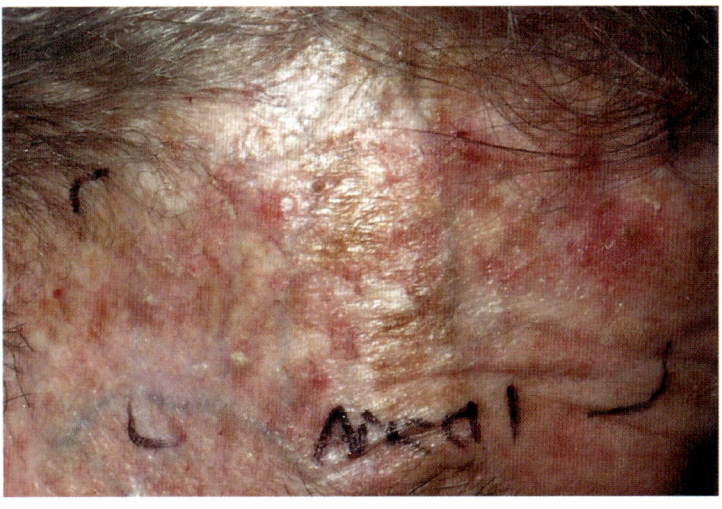 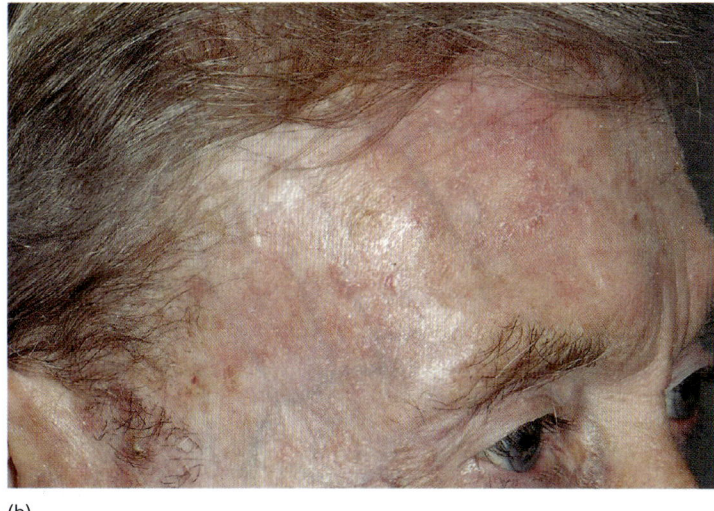

Figure 22.4 Field treatment of actinic keratoses on the forehead and temple (a) before and (b) 3 months after a single treatment of topical photodynamic therapy.

higher with PDT [99]. More recently, a small ($n = 9$) within subject pilot study compared PDT with 3.75% imiquimod for scalp AK, showing both treatments to be effective and with excellent cosmetic outcomes [100].

Patch ALA PDT (Alacare; Spirig HC) was shown to be superior to cryotherapy for mild AK of the face and scalp but is limited to a maximum of six individual AK and is not suitable for diffuse actinic damage ('field change') [43,45].

A single PDT treatment may be insufficient and repeat treatment has been shown to improve response rates, particularly for moderate-thickness AK [101]. The conventional topical PDT treatment regimen for AK thus involves a single treatment, and if this does not achieve clearance at 3 months then a double treatment cycle with treatments 1 week apart would be administered, although this is not usually required for thin AK [101]. It should be noted that the response to PDT of thick hyperkeratotic AK, particularly those on acral sites, is disappointing and may be less than 50%. With hyperkeratotic AK, if PDT is used, prior curettage is advisable. In one study, MAL PDT was less effective than cryotherapy for acral AK, although superior cosmetic outcome was reported for PDT [102]. However, pre-treatment with 5-fluorouracil prior to PDT may improve outcomes at acral sites [103].

While there is good evidence to recommend the use of topical 5-fluorouracil management of field change AK, patients typically require a rotational or even sequential approach to their chronic disease management and PDT is ideally suited for AK field treatment [**28,32**,104]. PDT enables large areas of subclinical disease to be treated and can be particularly advantageous at sites of poor healing, such as the lower leg, or where cosmetic outcome is a significant concern. Furthermore, PDT has an important role in the management of patients at high risk of invasive squamous cell carcinoma (SCC) – including those who are heavily photodamaged or have a history of multiple SCC – or patients who require immunosuppressive medication (e.g. organ transplant recipients) or who are otherwise immunosuppressed. In addition to clearing existing AK, PDT can reduce the rate of development of new AK; there may also be a reduction in the risk of developing non-melanoma skin cancers, although this needs further study [105–118]. PDT is more effective than 5-fluorouracil for treating AK in organ transplant recipients [119] and was also shown to be more effective at achieving clearance of AK in a within subject study in organ transplant recipients ($n = 35$) when compared with imiquimod [**120**]. Furthermore, longer term response rates (21 months) indicate equivalent efficacy of daylight PDT with cryotherapy for organ transplant recipients, but with patient preference for daylight PDT [121].

PDT has been used for actinic cheilitis and can be useful at this difficult treatment site, although recurrence is common: a combined approach using topical imiquimod in addition has been proposed for resistant cases [122–126]. PDT has a particular role for multiple, superficial lesions and for lesions occurring at sites of poor healing and should also be considered if other treatments have failed.

Topical PDT is thus ideal for widespread non-hyperkeratotic AK on the face and scalp. MAL (Metvix) and ALA (Ameluz) PDT are licensed in the UK for this indication (see Figure 22.4) and Ameluz PDT has now also been approved for use for AK on the trunk and extremities [127]. There are wide variations in the treatment protocols that have been used, although a 3–4 h interval between prodrug application and irradiation is most commonly advocated for conventional PDT. The Metvix/Metvixia and Ameluz PDT regimens specify a 3 h interval. The Alacare patch is applied for 4 h, with no surface preparation or additional occlusion required.

Red, blue and green light PDT may be effective for superficial AK. Blue light PDT using a topical solution of ALA (Levulan Kerastick) applied for 14–18 h without occlusion and a light dose of $10 J/cm^2$ is approved in the USA for the treatment of thin- to moderate-thickness AK [38]. However, ALA incubation times may in practice vary and may be as short as 1–2 h in some settings. However, most approved topical PDT regimens for AK using MAL or ALA employ red light at a dose of $37.5 J/cm^2$.

The use of daylight PDT for superficial non-hyperkeratotic AK on the face and scalp has rapidly developed worldwide, to the point where this is typically the PDT regimen of choice for patients with field change disease. Both MAL and ALA can be used, with daylight enabling continuous activation of PpIX [90,128,129]. Efficacy rates for daylight PDT are comparable with those of conventional PDT for AK, although daylight PDT is much better tolerated, with low pain scores and high levels of patient satisfaction reported for this convenient treatment approach [106,130–140,**141**,142–144,**145**,146]. In sunny climates daylight PDT can be undertaken all year, whereas in temperate climates it is best used between March/April to September/October [147–155]. Indoor surrogates of daylight exposure for potential application in PDT are also under investigation [156–159]. In an indirect analysis of published study data, MAL daylight PDT was shown to be more than four times as likely to achieve complete AK response as diclofenac in hyaluronic acid gel (Solaraze) [160].

Bowen disease

Topical MAL (Metvix/Metvixia) PDT using red light LED irradiation at 37.5 J/cm^2 is licensed for Bowen disease with two treatments 1 week apart, repeated at 3 months if there is only partial response. Red light irradiation is required to achieve sufficient penetration of light for PDT: green light PDT has been shown to be of inferior efficacy for Bowen disease. Based on clearance assessed 3 months after the last treatment, response rates of 86–93% can be expected, with sustained remission of 68–71% at 2 years (Figure 22.5) [22–25,**28**,34]. Topical PDT has been shown in separate studies to be at least as effective for Bowen disease as cryotherapy and topical 5-fluorouracil but to be associated with fewer adverse effects and improved cosmetic outcome [86,161,162]. A systematic review and meta-analysis of published studies also concluded that PDT was more effective than 5-fluorouracil or cryotherapy for Bowen disease [87].

PDT is the treatment of choice for large or multiple areas of Bowen disease, particularly on poor healing sites such as the lower legs (Figure 22.5). It can also be used to treat other difficult sites such as the digits or genitalia. Response rates are reduced if there is evidence of microinvasive SCC or a high degree of cellular atypia. PDT is not indicated for invasive SCC because of the high risk of recurrence and the potential for metastasis.

Basal cell carcinoma

The same regimen of MAL PDT as used for Bowen disease is licensed for treating sBCC (and thin nodular BCC if not suitable for surgery), using a double treatment cycle of two treatments 1 week apart, with repeat treatment at 3 months if necessary (Figure 22.6) [22–24,**28**,32,34,**83**,163]. Clearance rates of 92–97% for sBCC treated with MAL PDT are reported at 3 months follow-up after one or two treatments [25,164,165]. Weighted clearance rates of 87% for sBCC and 53% for nodular BCC at follow-up intervals of up to 36 months following PDT were reported in one review of 12 studies [166].

In comparisons between cryotherapy and PDT, there were no differences in response rates for sBCC but the cosmetic outcome was superior with PDT [167]; similar 5-year recurrence rates of 22% for PDT and 20% for cryotherapy were observed in one study [164]. In another study comparing topical MAL PDT with 5-fluorouracil or imiquimod for sBCC ($n = 601$), PDT was inferior to imiquimod as assessed by tumour clearance at 12-month follow-up but equivalent in efficacy to topical 5-fluorouracil [165] and superiority of imiquimod was still seen at 5-year follow-up [169]. However, only patients who would be able to comply with the topical cream regimens were included and repeat PDT cycles were not allowed. More local adverse effects, including infected treatment sites, were seen with imiquimod and 5-fluorouracil. Thus, PDT remains a suitable treatment option for sBCC and each patient therefore needs to be evaluated on an individual basis in terms of what treatment approach is likely to suit best.

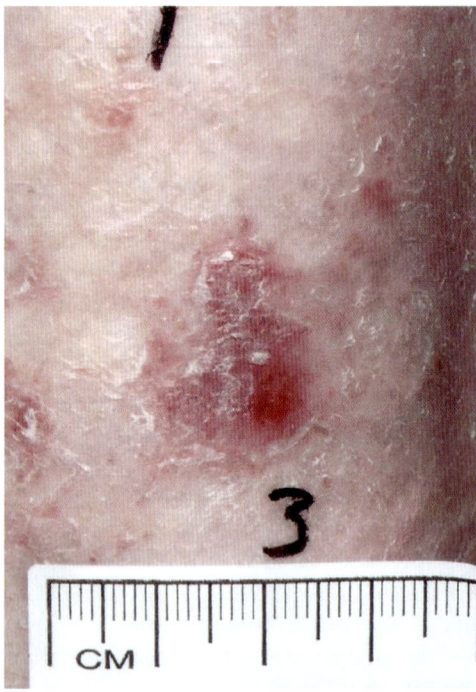
(a)

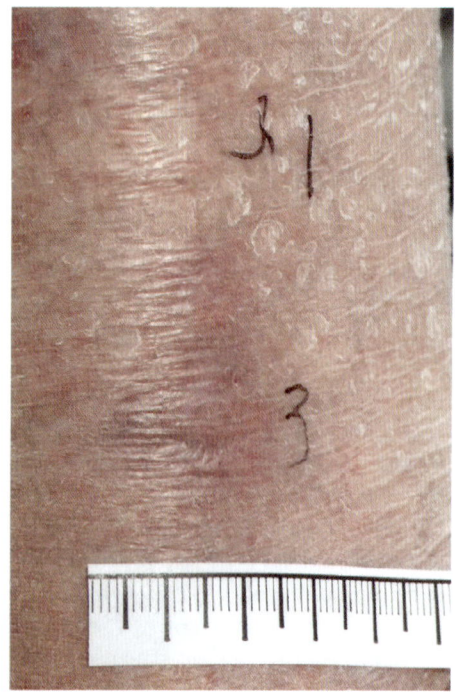
(b)

Figure 22.5 Bowen disease on the lower leg (a) before and (b) 1 year after photodynamic therapy (PDT). Stasis change, oedema and xerosis were prominent and although the risk of poor healing was significant, this patient had no problems after PDT.

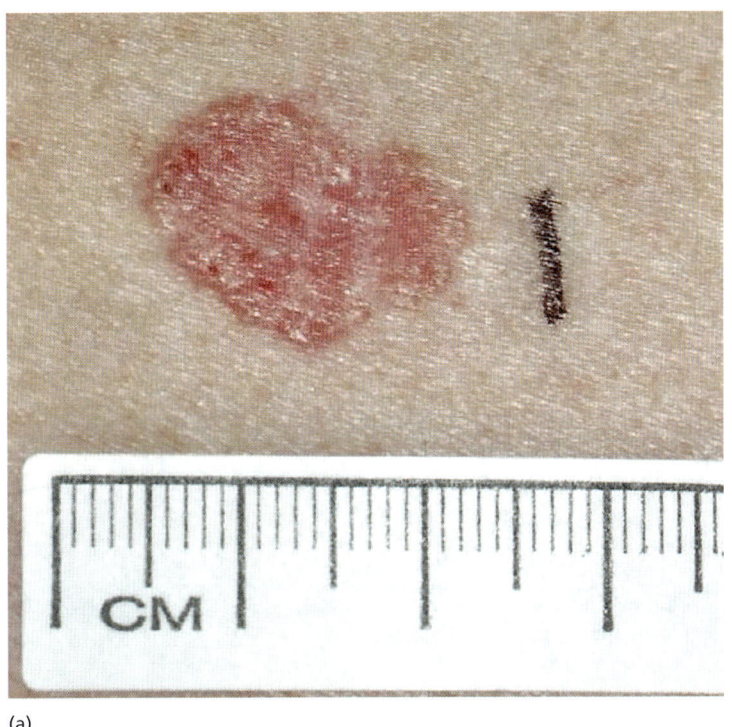 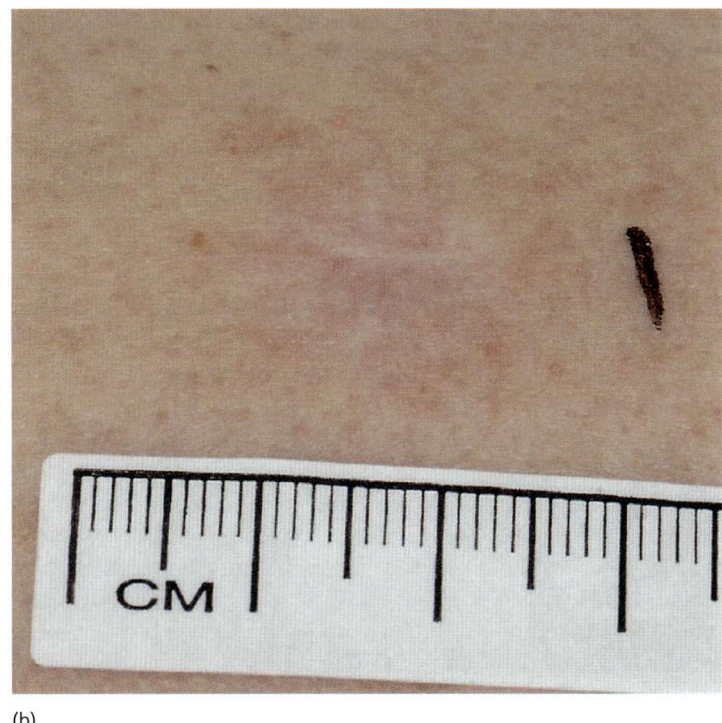

Figure 22.6 Superficial basal cell carcinoma on the back (a) before and (b) 1 year after photodynamic therapy. Note the excellent cosmetic outcome, with only the scar of the initial diagnostic biopsy evident.

Equivalent efficacy has been shown for PDT and surgery for sBCC at 1 year, although with improved cosmetic outcome with PDT [165,170]. Topical PDT is inferior to surgery for nodular BCC, with increased recurrence rates at 5-year follow-up [171–175]. This is likely to be due to a combination of inadequate PpIX accumulation in deeper tumour cells and poor light penetration. PDT should be reserved for thin BCCs with histological thickness <2 mm [176]. Only if surgery is contraindicated should PDT be considered for nodular BCC, as is reflected in the licensed approval for MAL (Metvix/Metvixia) PDT [177]. If topical PDT is used for nodular BCC, then prior debulking of the nodular component by curettage would be advised. Use of penetration enhancers, microneedling, laser pretreatment, iron chelators and fractionated regimens have been investigated in an attempt to improve efficacy, but there is no doubt that PDT is inferior to surgery for the treatment of nodular BCC.

A randomised controlled trial in 281 patients with sBCC and thin nodular BCC compared ALA (Ameluz) PDT with MAL (Metvix) PDT and showed high efficacy rates and low recurrence, with proven non-inferiority of Ameluz compared with Metvix [41] and thus both MAL and Ameluz are licensed for use in BCC in the UK.

Recent systematic reviews and study analyses indicate equivalent efficacy between PDT and either cryotherapy or surgery, with higher recurrence rates with PDT than surgery, but improved cosmetic outcome with PDT [83,84,85,178,179].

On a note of caution, morphoeic (sclerosing) infiltrative and thick nodular BCC should not be treated with topical PDT. Systemic PDT can be considered for high-risk patients such as those with the naevoid BCC (Gorlin) syndrome, although patients must be counselled about the associated prolonged visible light photosensitivity.

Topical PDT has also been recommended in Gorlin syndrome for superficial and thin (<2 mm) nodular BCC [180].

Other indications

Acne. Increasing evidence supports the value of topical PDT for inflammatory acne vulgaris in patients for whom more conventional therapies are ineffective or not possible [24,**28,33**,80,181–188]. Response rates of 54–68% reduction in inflammatory lesions may be expected but the adverse effects from treatment, including florid phototoxicity, sterile pustules and hyperpigmentation, can be significant. Non-inflammatory lesions may also respond to PDT but are less likely to do so. PDT is a treatment that should be kept in mind for patients who fail to respond to conventional acne therapies or if systemic retinoids are contraindicated. The optimal PDT treatment parameters to achieve efficacy and minimise adverse effects are not well established [189,190], but daylight PDT may also be effective [191,192].

Viral warts and HPV-related neoplasia. Topical PDT may also be effective for recalcitrant viral warts with response rates of approximately 50%, although treatment is often painful and can be difficult to tolerate [**28,33**,188,193]. Facial warts may also be responsive to PDT, with one study showing clearance rates of 65% at 3 month follow-up [194,195]. Daylight PDT may also be effective for facial warts and is well tolerated [196]. Modifications to drug and light delivery may facilitate improved outcomes, with minimised adverse effects as many variables exist in current PDT regimens [197,198]. Topical PDT has also been reported to be effective for genital warts [24,199–205], Bowenoid papulosis [206,207], vulval intraepithelial neoplasia [23,200,208–212] and penile intraepithelial neoplasia (erythroplasia of Queyrat) [23,213–219], although its role in these conditions has not been established [23,**28**,**33**,188].

Other forms of cutaneous neoplasia. There are individual case reports of response to PDT in extramammary Paget disease [220–226] and localised cutaneous T-cell [227–231] and B-cell lymphoma [232].

Aesthetic dermatology. PDT has been advocated for photorejuvenation, although further work is required to establish its place in this arena. Repeated daylight PDT is also being investigated for photorejuvenation and AK prevention [24,**28**,**33**,115,188,233,234].

Miscellaneous. There are also reports of efficacy of topical PDT in several other inflammatory and infective skin conditions including cutaneous leishmaniasis, onychomycosis, leg ulcers and wound healing, localised scleroderma, cutaneous sarcoid, lichen sclerosus, lichen planus, necrobiosis lipoidica, granuloma annulare, hidradenitis suppurativa and erosive pustular dermatosis (Box 22.1). Further studies are required to establish the role of PDT in these conditions [24,**28**,**33**,80,188,235–245], with the antimicrobial and wound healing effects of PDT being of particular interest [246–249]. On the other hand there is evidence to suggest that PDT is ineffective for psoriasis [**28**,**33**,188,250–254] and is unpredictable for porokeratosis [255,256].

> **Box 22.1 Topical photodynamic therapy (PDT) has been applied to a diverse range of conditions with varying levels of evidence to support its use**
>
> **Good evidence to support the use of PDT from randomised controlled trials**
> - Acne vulgaris
>
> **Fair evidence to support the use of PDT from randomised controlled trials**
> - Cutaneous leishmaniasis
> - Field change carcinogenesis
> - Genital warts (condyloma acuminata)
> - Organ transplant recipients – field change treatment and prevention
> - Photorejuvenation
> - Recalcitrant viral warts
>
> **Limited evidence, requiring further investigation**
> - Actinic cheilitis and leukoplakia
> - Alopecia areata
> - B-cell lymphoma
> - Breast metastases
> - Chondrodermatitis nodularis helicis
> - Chronic folliculitis
> - Cutaneous T- and B-cell lymphoma
> - Darier disease
> - Epidermodysplasia verruciformis
> - Erythroplasia of Queyrat
> - Erosive pustular dermatosis
> - Extramammary Paget disease
> - Granuloma annulare
> - Hailey–Hailey disease
> - Hidradenitis suppurativa
> - Hirsutism
> - Hypertrophic scar/keloid
> - Infected leg ulcers
> - Keratoacanthoma
> - Lichen planus
> - Lichen sclerosus
> - Melanoma
> - Molluscum contagiosum
> - Naevus sebaceous
> - Necrobiosis lipoidica
> - Perioral dermatitis
> - Porokeratosis
> - Psoriasis
> - Radiation dermatitis
> - Rosacea
> - Sarcoid
> - Scleroderma
> - Sebaceous hyperplasia
> - Superficial mycoses
> - Vulval intraepithelial neoplasia

Contraindications

Topical PDT is contraindicated for disease with metastatic potential such as invasive SCC or melanoma. Importantly, in highly pigmented lesions such as melanoma or heavily pigmented BCC, red light absorption by melanin may reduce efficacy of treatment. Topical PDT is not advisable for thick tumours such as thick nodular BCC or for morphoeic (sclerosing)/infiltrative BCC. Patients with porphyria should not be treated with PDT. Caution is required if considering PDT in xeroderma pigmentosum, although there are reports of its effective use in this condition [257–259]. Tumours at high-risk sites such as the mid-face should also not be considered for topical PDT unless a more conventional surgical approach is contraindicated. Under those circumstances, PDT may prove efficacious for those difficult-to-treat lesions, although it would not be the treatment of choice.

Methodology and regimens

Diagnosis and patient selection

A number of factors need to be taken into account when deciding whether to use PDT to treat a specific disorder in a particular patient. Hospital-based PDT may be preferred by elderly, frail patients who would not be able to self-treat with either topical preparations or daylight PDT. Others, however, may prefer to be involved in the administration of their own treatment with, for example, topical 5-fluorouracil, imiquimod or daylight PDT. PDT is a particularly good treatment choice for multiple and/or large low-risk (and therefore generally thin) lesions, diffuse field change at sites where healing may be problematic, such as the lower leg, or where cosmetic outcome is important (Figures 22.7 and 22.8). Thus, optimising efficacy of PDT depends on careful selection of patient and lesion(s).

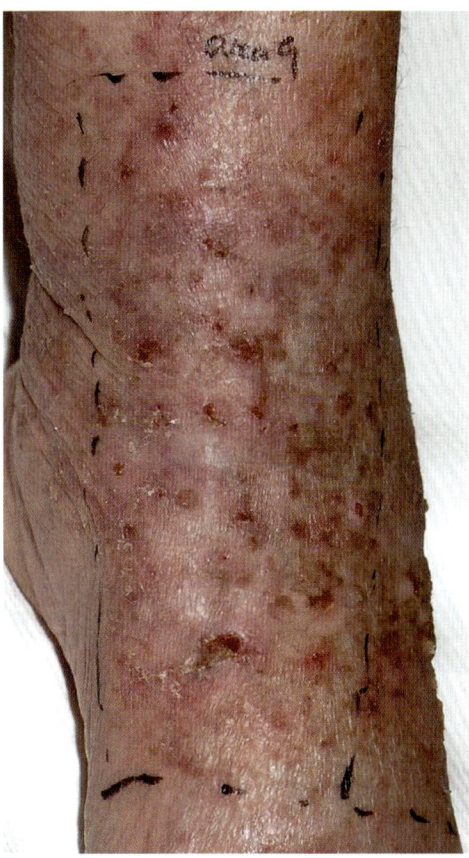

Figure 22.7 Photodynamic therapy (PDT) is ideal for multiple and/or large lesions and field change. This patient had extensive actinic keratosis, Bowen disease and field carcinogenesis following chronic sun exposure and was keen to obtain good healing and cosmetic outcome. She was therefore an ideal candidate for PDT.

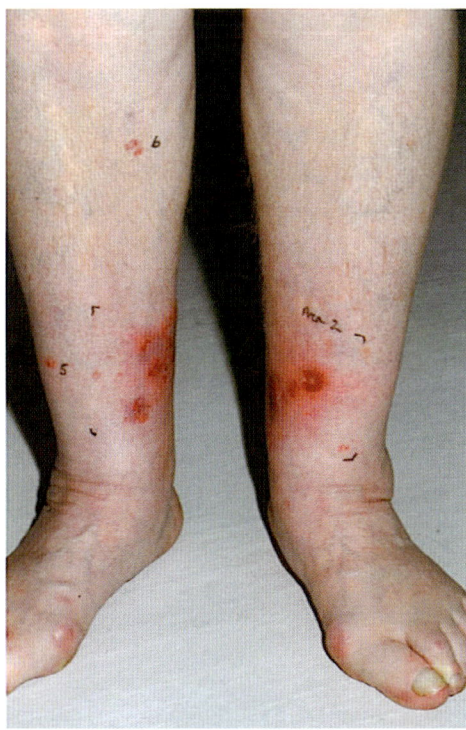

Figure 22.8 Photodynamic therapy (PDT) is ideal for lower leg sites as the risk of poor healing and ulceration is reduced. This patient has lower leg oedema, stasis changes and multiple areas of Bowen disease. PDT would be the treatment of choice.

Detailed history taking and clinical examination are required to establish patient co-morbidities that may be relevant: these include diabetes, immunosuppression, peripheral venous insufficiency and dependent oedema, all of which may impair healing following PDT. Immunosuppression may also increase the risk of recurrence. If there is significant dependent oedema, compression stockings may be advised in order to facilitate healing following PDT at lower leg sites.

A representative confirmatory biopsy is usually undertaken. If a BCC has a histological thickness of >2 mm, PDT is generally contraindicated. The site and size of the lesion should be assessed and baseline photography undertaken, as cosmetic outcome following clearance can be such that it may be difficult to identify where the lesion was.

The British Association of Dermatologists Service Standards are an important guide for anyone setting up and running a PDT service in the UK and provide guidance and structure with respect to clinical service delivery, governance, benchmarking, education and training [29]. It is important that patients are provided with verbal and written information about treatment and provide appropriate consent. Topical PDT generally takes place in dermatology departments and involves the patient in a half-day visit, although daylight PDT may be undertaken either entirely in the home setting or as a hybrid model. Conventional PDT is usually undertaken by a nurse or technician, who must be provided with adequate training [260].

Conventional PDT
Lesion preparation

Lesion preparation is important if there is marked hyperkeratosis or crusting. The experimental use of laser pre-treatment, microneedling and penetration enhancers such as DMSO and iron chelators has been investigated with the intention of improving prodrug uptake and PpIX accumulation. In practice, many centres simply advise the application of white soft paraffin (Vaseline®) to lesions for 1–3 days prior to treatment in order to soften hyperkeratosis and crusting and to facilitate subsequent lesion preparation immediately prior to PDT [28,32,49–52,54–56]. This involves using either a wooden spatula or a disposable ring curette to remove surface keratinous debris (Figure 22.9) and does not usually require local anaesthetic.

Prodrug application

The prodrug is applied after surface preparation, and in practice is usually MAL (Metvix 16%) or ALA (Ameluz 8%). In the US Levulan Kerastick (ALA HCL 20% solution) may also be applied as prodrug for use in AK with blue light (Figure 22.10). The prodrug is applied under plastic film occlusion (e.g. Tegaderm®) as a thin (c.1 mm thick) even application to the lesion including a rim of at least 5–10 mm of normal appearing skin (Figure 22.11). Metvix and Ameluz should be occluded for 3 h prior to irradiation; although this may vary, such as short incubation use in AK and acne [261–263].

If the lesion to be treated is on a light-exposed site, a UV and visible light opaque dressing (e.g. Mepore®) should be applied on top of the occlusive film dressing so that PpIX photobleaching and the PDT reaction do not commence prematurely. The ALA patch (Alacare, Spirig HC) PDT regimen does not require surface preparation or additional occlusion. PDT using Levulan Kerastick does not involve

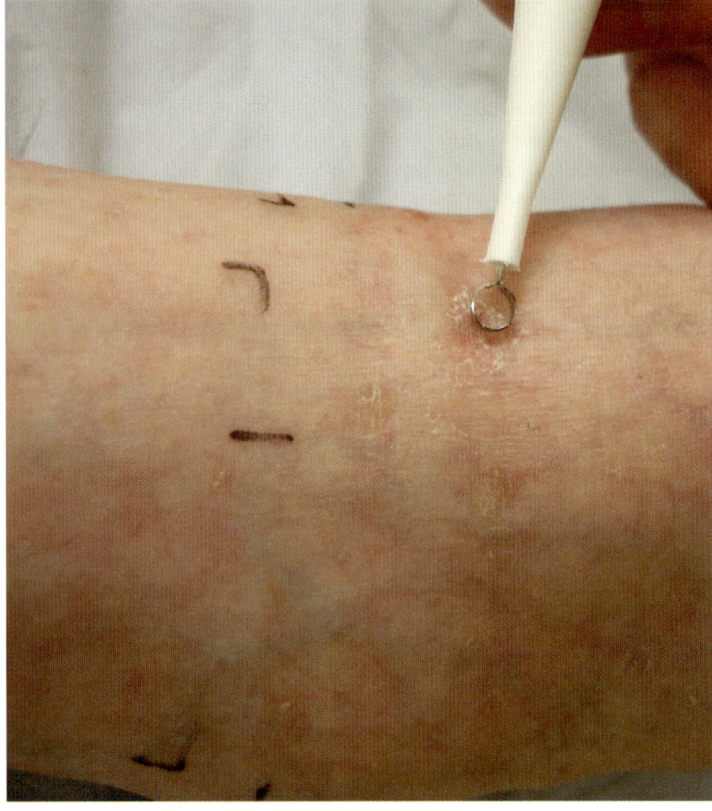

Figure 22.9 Lesion preparation using a disposable ring curette.

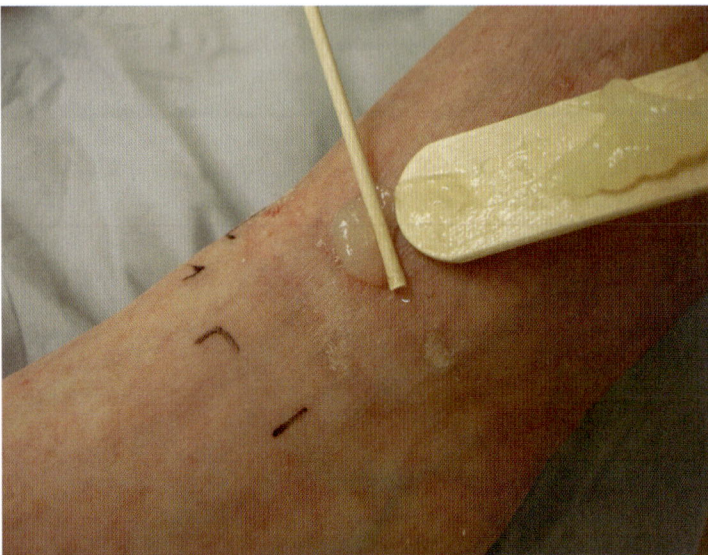

Figure 22.10 Prodrug application.

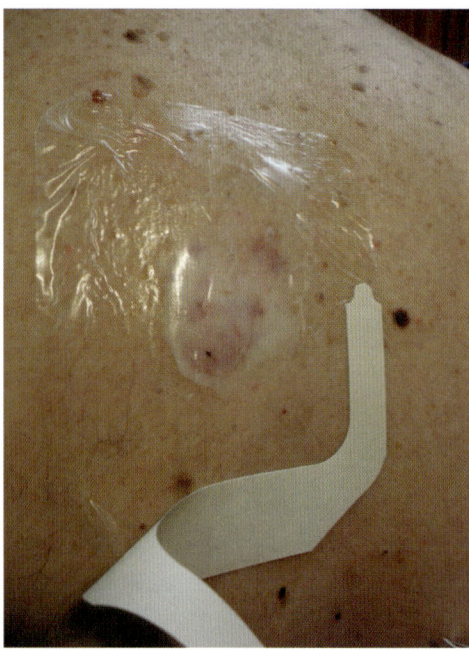

Figure 22.11 Prodrug occlusion under Tegaderm. An additional UV/visible light opaque dressing would also be applied if the lesion is on an exposed site.

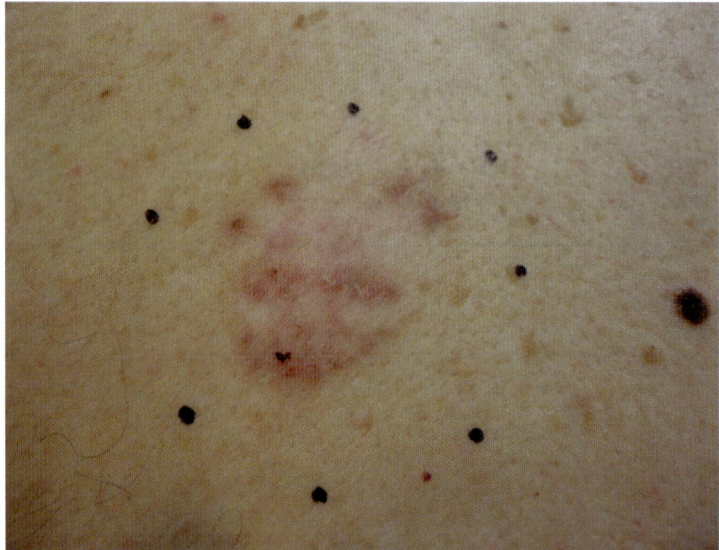

Figure 22.12 Mapping out the irradiation field to include a 5 mm rim of clinically uninvolved skin.

occlusion but the treatment site should be protected from sun and bright light.

Following the prodrug incubation period, the dressings should be removed and any residual cream wiped from the surface. Wood's light can be used to identify PpIX fluorescence, which is usually largely limited to the lesional site but can help reveal adjacent areas of subclinical disease that should then be included in the treatment field. A rim of 5 mm of clinically normal skin should be included in the irradiation field (Figure 22.12).

Irradiation

Irradiation may be performed using a variety of light sources, though the most commonly used are red light LED sources with peak emissions around 632–635 nm (e.g. Aktilite® or RhodoLED®) (Figure 22.13). The irradiance emitted by the source must be monitored and for LEDs this is usually approximately 80 mW/cm^2. The approved dose for use in MAL and ALA (Ameluz) PDT is 37.5 J/cm^2, although some centres use a higher dose (e.g. 75 J/cm^2), as there are experimental data to indicate that increased PpIX photobleaching may continue if higher doses are used.

Historically, when polychromatic or laser light sources were used, irradiation doses of 125–200 J/cm^2 or more were applied, although

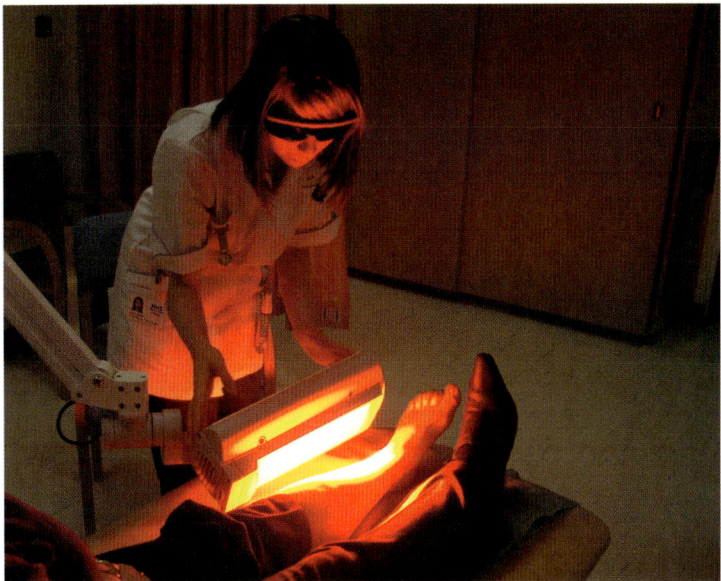

Figure 22.13 Photodynamic therapy to the lower leg using a red LED source.

it is important that irradiance is kept below 150 mW/cm² to avoid thermal effects. There is, however, no evidence that higher light doses are associated with improved outcomes. Likewise, as only low levels of PpIX accumulate in adjacent normal skin, red light toxicity to the surrounding skin is not a concern.

The time for irradiation using the LED sources is generally 8–17 min dependent on the dose and irradiance. A lesional field diameter of up to 20 cm² can be treated with standard PDT using either LED (e.g. Aktilite® or RhodoLED®) or metal halide sources (e.g. Waldmann 1200®).

Ambulatory photodynamic therapy

There is good evidence *ex vivo*, and increasing evidence *in vivo*, that light delivery at lower irradiance results in more efficient PDT and reduced pain during irradiation [264–267]. Ambulatory PDT employs this principle of very low irradiance light delivery over a prolonged time period [265,268–270]. One such method of light delivery is using a small lightweight portable red LED array, peak emission 633 nm (lower–upper full width at half maximum 624–639 nm), at very low irradiance (approximately 7 mW/cm²) (Ambulight®, Ambicare Health Ltd), which has been shown in a randomised controlled study of patients ($n = 50$) with BCC and Bowen disease to be very well tolerated and highly effective at one year follow-up, with non-inferiority to conventional hospital-based PDT and is thus an option for patients who prefer the convenience of home treatment (Figure 22.14) [270], although availability of these devices is currently limited. Another means of delivery of low irradiance PDT is using light-emitting fabric-based devices (Flexatheralight®, Fluxmedicare® and Phosistos® protocols), which have been shown in randomised controlled trials to be non-inferior to conventional PDT (using Aktilite®) for AK on the scalp and forehead and to be better tolerated [74–76].

Daylight photodynamic therapy

Daylight PDT is an alternative way to use low irradiance light delivery during PDT. This has the advantage of convenience for

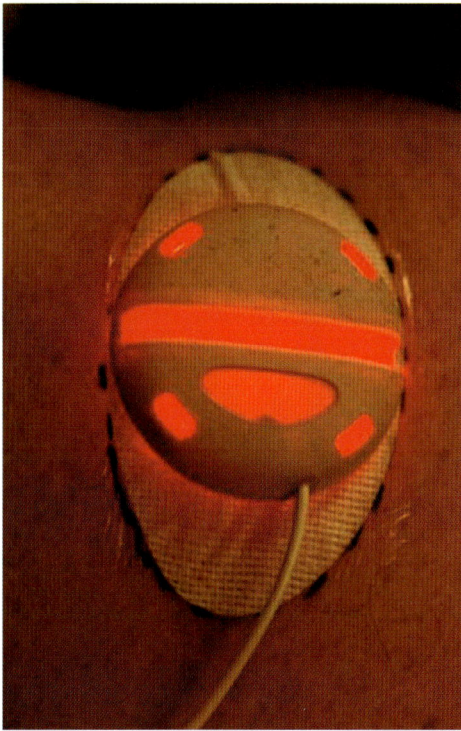

Figure 22.14 Ambulatory photodynamic therapy. Irradiation is underway, as indicated by the red light emission from the portable inorganic LED source (Ambulight®). The battery pack enables up to three lesions to be treated simultaneously. Lesions must be <2.4 cm diameter and not on highly curved surfaces, such as ears.

the patient and larger areas can be treated in one session and in the home setting (Figure 22.15) [153,271]. This has been extensively investigated for the treatment of AK on the face and scalp and is of equivalent efficacy to conventional PDT, but with much lower pain scores and higher levels of patient satisfaction and cosmetic outcome [**32**,**33**,**61**,136–140,**141**,142–144,149,156,272–279]. The therapeutically effective wavelengths of daylight are mainly in the blue light part of the spectrum and daylight PDT may not have sufficient depth of effect to treat lesions of Bowen disease or BCC. However, preliminary work has indicated that it may be possible to treat these with daylight PDT in selected patients, although it is likely to be less effective than conventional PDT [280,281]. Formal prospective studies are required to judge whether indeed this is the case.

In the daylight PDT regimen for facial and scalp AK, SPF50 absorbent sunscreen is applied to all sites, both the lesional areas to be treated and the unaffected normal skin that will be exposed to daylight, in order to prevent the development of UV redness (sunburn). Fifteen minutes after sunscreen application, the AK are prepared using a disposable ring curette. The photosensitiser prodrug (typically MAL or ALA) is then applied without occlusion to the areas to be treated and the patient is advised to expose the affected areas to continuous daylight for 2–2.5 h, preferably starting no later than half an hour after application of the photosensitiser prodrug. If it is impracticable to be out of doors because of inclement weather or patient frailty, then sitting indoors beside a window would be a reasonable alternative. In northern latitudes, treatment can be undertaken between April and September, whereas elsewhere, such as in Australia and Southern Europe, year-round treatment may be feasible [138,142,154,155]. In the UK, daylight

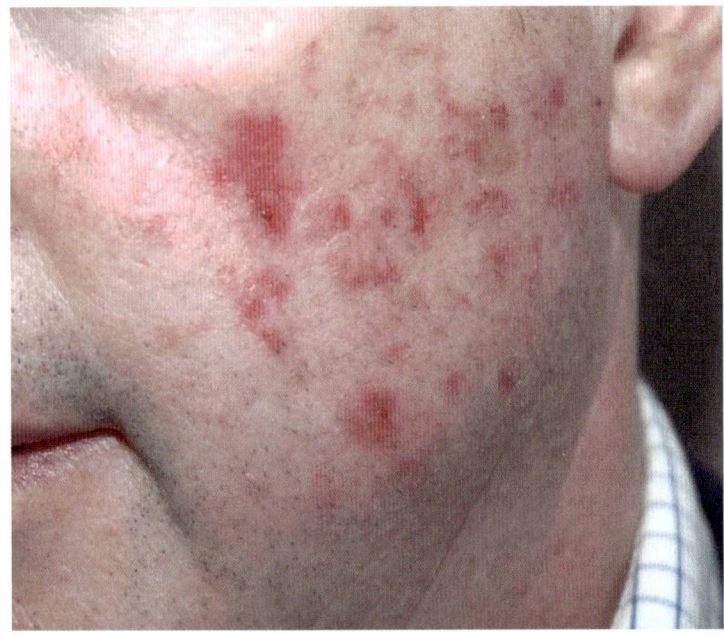

Figure 22.15 Daylight photodynamic therapy (PDT) allows field areas of superficial actinic keratosis on exposed sites to be treated in one session. This man had daylight PDT to the face and scalp and this shows the typical reaction 3 days after treatment with subclinical areas of disease becoming more apparent.

PDT can be performed on days with low UV index, but temperature may be the limiting factor for patient comfort [148–151].

Studies have shown that there is no difference in efficacy or adverse effects between a regimen involving 1.5 or 2.5 h of continuous daylight exposure, with no advantage to longer exposure times; 2 h continuous exposure is generally accepted as being sufficient [282]. It is the visible component of daylight that is important therapeutically and effective daylight PDT can be undertaken on any dry day, including cloudy days. No difference in the clearance rates of AK (c.75–79%) was seen between daylight or conventional PDT, but daylight PDT was associated with lower pain scores and higher patient satisfaction [**32,33,61**,106,136–140,**141**,142–144,**145**,149,156,273–279,282].

While formal measurememt of light exposure is not required during routine daylight PDT, real-time daylight exposure monitoring, such as via a smartphone app, is under evaluation and may help to increase patient engagement and practitioner confidence in daylight PDT [283].

Treatment schedules, aftercare and follow-up

Most topical PDT regimens involve a single PDT treatment for AK and two treatments a week apart for Bowen disease and sBCC. It is advisable to keep the areas out of direct sunlight for 24–48 h as photosensitivity can persist for this time period due to further PpIX accumulation following PDT [284]. The degree of phototoxic inflammation is of a similar degree after both conventional and daylight or ambulatory PDT.

Review should be undertaken at 3 months and if there is no, or only partial, clinical response then a second treatment cycle should be undertaken with two treatments a week apart, including for AK. Further review should be undertaken at 6 months and, given that Bowen disease and BCC recur in up to a quarter of patients at 5-year follow-up, this should be considered with respect to follow-up plans. The same principles of review times and treatment regimens also apply to ambulatory and daylight PDT. Careful treatment records and appropriate governance must be in place [29].

Adverse effects

Acute effects

The adverse effects of topical PDT (Box 22.2) include the expected acute phototoxic effects of pain, itch, discomfort, redness, oedema, exudation and crusting [**89**,285]. The degree of redness and phototoxicity is dependent on the size of the field treated and the degree of subclinical photodamage. Redness peaks about 1 h after PDT but persists for about 7–10 days. Exudation and crusting are common (Figures 22.16 and 22.17). Fair-skinned photodamaged patients are most at risk of extensive redness and phototoxicity (Figure 22.18). For this reason an initial test area of up to 5 × 5 cm may be advisable before more widespread treatment of patients with markedly photodamaged facial and scalp skin. Periocular oedema may occur and patients should be warned of this and advised that sleeping with an additional pillow for 48 h after treatment may minimise the problem. Urticaria occurs at the treatment site in the minority of patients during or immediately after PDT (Figure 22.19) [286]. Antihistamines have not been shown to be of benefit in reducing the acute effects of PDT [287]. However, topical corticosteroids may have a role in reducing inflammation induced by PDT, if applied before and after treatment, without compromising efficacy [288]. Furthermore, protection of the treatment site from light after PDT has also been shown to reduce the degree of inflammation [289].

Box 22.2 Adverse effects of topical photodynamic therapy

Acute/short-term effects
- Pain, itch, discomfort[a]
- Redness
- Oedema[a]
- Urticaria
- Exudation[a]
- Crusting[a]
- Infection, cellulitis
- Sterile pustules
- Bruising, purpura
- Dermatitis
- Erosive pustular dermatosis
- Bullous pemphigoid

Chronic/medium-term effects
- Scarring
- Milia
- Photo-onycholysis
- Pigmentary loss/gain
- Hair loss/gain

From Ibbotson 2011 [285]. Reproduced with permission of John Wiley & Sons.

[a] Common.

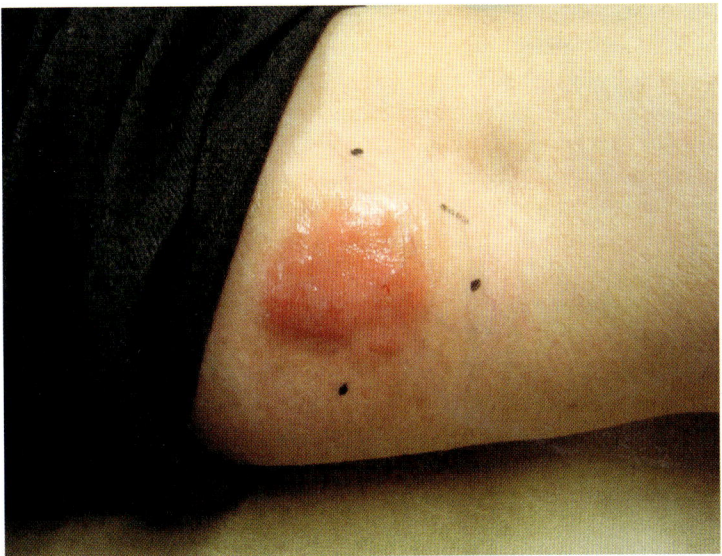

Figure 22.16 Redness and oedema immediately after photodynamic therapy.

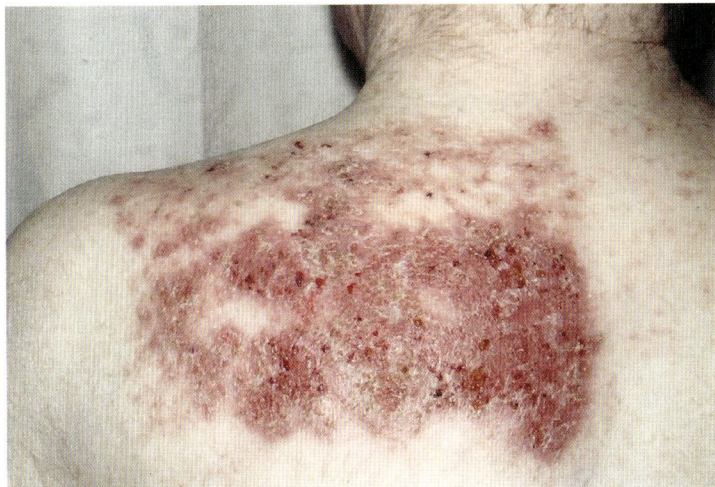

Figure 22.18 Severe phototoxic reaction persisting 1 week after photodynamic therapy in a fair-skinned subject with marked field change photodamage.

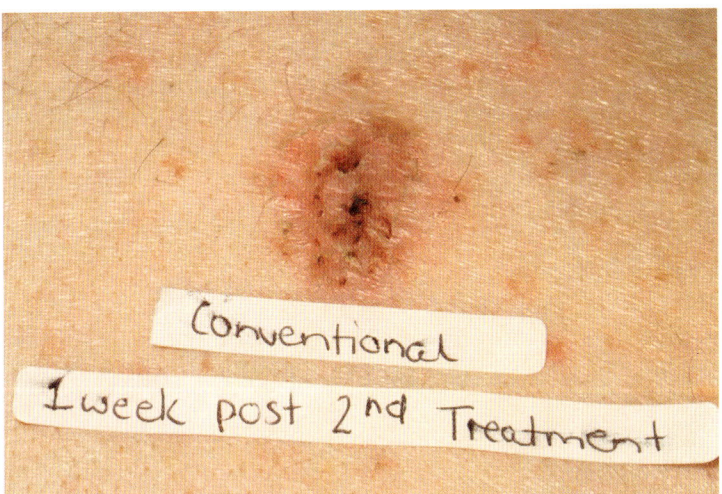

Figure 22.17 Expected residual redness and crusting 1 week after photodynamic therapy.

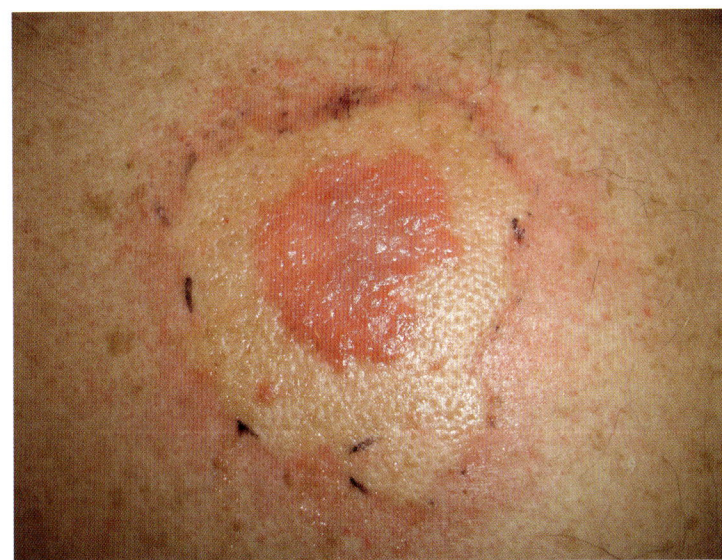

Figure 22.19 Urticaria at the treatment site immediately after photodynamic therapy.

Infection and cellulitis occur infrequently. Topical PDT has bactericidal and bacteriostatic effects and therefore infection occurs less commonly than, for example, with cryotherapy. The development of sterile pustules following PDT for acne vulgaris is common and patients should be warned of this adverse effect. Purpura and bruising are uncommon. Ulceration is more likely at lower leg sites, and if dependent oedema is present, the use of compression stockings throughout the PDT treatment course may assist with healing and reduce the risk of ulceration.

Dermatitis and allergy

Dermatitis may occur at the treatment site and may be secondary to phototoxicity or be irritant in nature. However, the possibility of allergic contact dermatitis to the prodrug needs to be considered. Patients who have had multiple treatments and treatments to large areas are particularly at risk (Figure 22.20) [290,293,**294**]. There may be cross-reaction between the prodrugs, although allergy to MAL does not necessarily imply allergy to ALA or vice versa. Patch testing should be organised if contact allergy is suspected (Figure 22.21), as further PDT in allergic patients may result in a generalised dermatitis or rarely systemic allergic contact dermatitis [295,296]. In addition, given that both MAL and Ameluz preparations contain arachis oil, PDT presents a potential, albeit unlikely, hazard for patients with extreme peanut allergy. Bullous pemphigoid has been reported in a single case localised to sites of PDT [252,297].

Pain

The main acute adverse effect of PDT is pain and most patients experience some discomfort, with severe pain in 16–20% [**89**,253,254,298,299]. The mechanism of PDT-induced pain is unknown although it occurs maximally in the first few minutes of treatment and is typically of a burning, prickling, stabbing nature. Pain usually rapidly subsides as soon as irradiation stops. It is not known if there are patient-dependent factors, such as genetic susceptibility, which influence pain. PDT treatment of

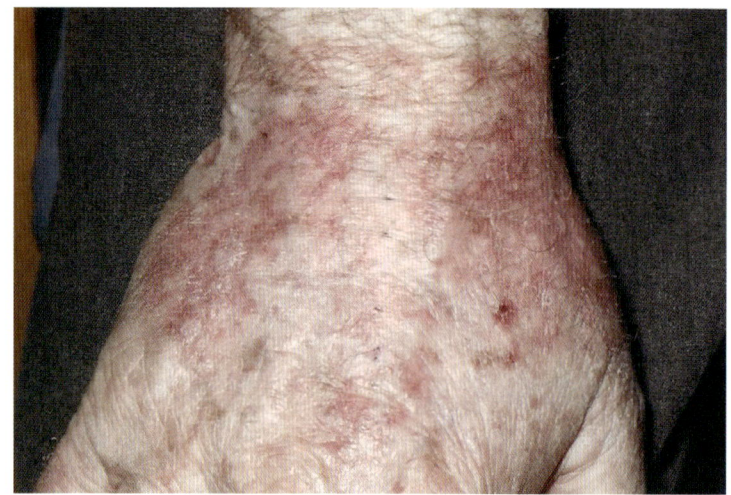

Figure 22.20 Dermatitis arising at the photodynamic therapy (PDT) treatment site in a patient who had received multiple treatments with topical PDT to field areas. This was confirmed to be contact allergic in nature by patch testing.

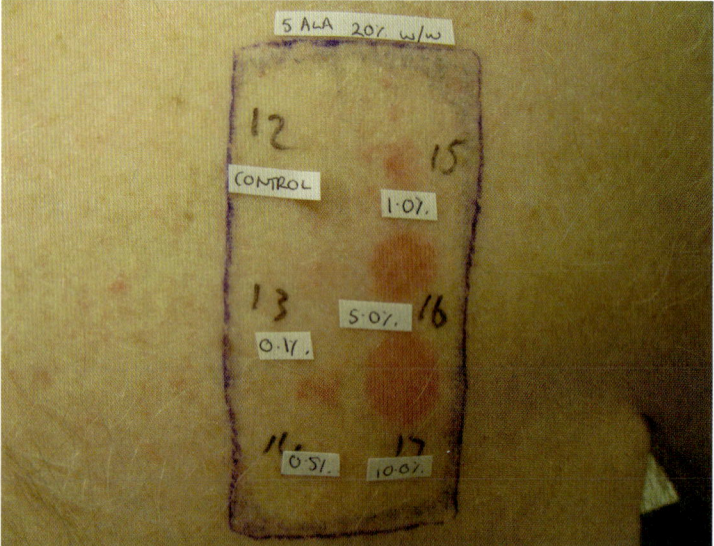

Figure 22.21 Positive patch tests confirming contact allergy to a proprietary preparation of 5-aminolaevulinic acid (ALA). Contact allergy to both ALA and methyl aminolaevulinate may uncommonly occur, particularly after multiple treatments, often to large areas.

large lesions and lesions on the head, neck and genital sites is more likely to be associated with significant pain. There is also some evidence that lesions with the strongest fluorescence may be associated with more severe pain [300–302]. PDT treatment of warts appears to be associated with particular discomfort during treatment.

In one study of 983 PDT treatments, 44% of patients required pain-reducing interventions [300]. However, methods of pain relief for PDT are generally not particularly effective. Cold water sprays and pausing irradiation may provide some relief, as may a fan or forced air cooling [303]. Distracting the patient and engaging in conversation is anecdotally of some help, although this has not been formally studied. However, given that one study reported a rise in blood pressure in eight of 36 (22%) patients after PDT, keeping the patient relaxed during treatment is advisable [304].

Pre-treatment with topical tetracaine gel, EMLA (eutectic mixture of local anaesthetics), capsaicin or morphine does not significantly alleviate pain [301,305–307]. The role of transepidermal nerve stimulation has been investigated but is of limited use and can only be applied to certain body sites [308]. Subcutaneous anaesthetic and nerve blockade can be used and the latter has been shown to be more effective than forced air cooling. These interventions are, however, invasive and are limited to use at certain sites [130,309,310].

It has been claimed that MAL PDT is of equivalent efficacy but less painful than ALA PDT, although in the studies in which this has been investigated there have been other variables such as time of application of the prodrugs which may have influenced the development of pain [131–134]. In one study comparing ALA (Ameluz) and MAL PDT for AK, no significant differences in pain experienced were detected [42].

Irradiation parameters influence the severity of PDT-induced pain. Variable pulse light delivery may be associated with less pain than LED sources. The latter appears to be comparable with broadband and laser sources in this regard [135]. Green light is associated with less pain than red light when used for PDT of AK but not in a study using PDT for Bowen disease; as green light has limited penetration into the skin it would not normally be recommended for treating Bowen disease [286,311]. The total light dose used during irradiation does not seem to influence pain but studies with low irradiance LEDs and daylight PDT indicate that reduced rate of light delivery (irradiance) is associated with reduced pain through continuous low-level PpIX activation [**89**,299,312].

Chronic effects

The risk of scarring following PDT is low (<1%) and when it does occur this is more likely to be atrophic than hypertrophic [26]. If the dermal–epidermal junction is disrupted, milia may appear, although this is rarely seen. Photo-onycholysis, hypo/hyperpigmentation and increased/reduced hair growth are also possible medium- to long-term risks of topical PDT, although again these are rare.

There is no evidence of long-term carcinogenic risk of PDT in humans. There have been anecdotal reports of, for example, an invasive SCC arising in an area of penile intraepithelial neoplasia following PDT and of melanoma occurring in actinically damaged skin previously treated with PDT. Whether such events are casually related is unproven [215,313–316] but there is some evidence to suggest that they are not. However, in one retrospective study of 357 patients with AK treated with PDT, 17 developed a SCC at the site of previous PDT. Those individuals who developed SCC were found to have more risk factors for non-melanoma skin cancer compared with those who did not develop SCC. This would suggest that factors other than PDT were dominant in the development of SCC, but the authors recommended more frequent follow-ups in individuals with multiple risk factors who are treated with PDT [317]. However, these patients are those who should be carefully reviewed anyway as they are at higher risk of skin cancer.

PDT has been shown in animal models to delay UV-induced carcinogenesis. There is also evidence that PDT may retard AK development and that repeated PDT field treatment might possibly reduce the risk of SCC in organ transplant recipients. Its potential preventative role is currently being explored.

Clinical governance

Despite the good evidence base for topical PDT in dermatology and the availability of British and European guidelines and NICE (National Institute for Health and Care Excellence) interventional procedures guidance, there have been significant areas where consensus on best practice was unclear and there was no clear governance in place [291]. However, the introduction of standards by the British Association of Dermatologists for the set up, delivery and governance of PDT services are particularly helpful in terms of provision of structured guidance with respect to how a PDT service should be established, organised, managed and audited. Standards have been set for services to benchmark against and in order to ensure that PDT services are available for patients, and that treatment is delivered appropriately, effectively and safely [29].

How to set up a PDT service

A business case to set up a new PDT service will need to explain in detail why the service is required, including an exposition of the advantages of PDT over existing therapies and the cost implications for using PDT rather than alternative treatment modalities. A full assessment of expected patient numbers, staffing requirements (including nurse and clinician time), drug costs and consumables, equipment and training should be undertaken. A dermatologist should be identified to oversee the service and clinician input is required as appropriate patient and lesion selection is essential. Furthermore, a PDT service should be accessible to all those involved in skin cancer management. Input from a medical physicist will also be needed for calibrating and measuring the irradiance of light sources. Adequate staff training is critical and protocols, guidelines and governance arrangements must be put in place [29].

What's new?

The place of topical PDT in the management of field change dysplasia and superficial non-melanoma skin cancer has been consolidated by the wealth of published studies, guidelines and standards that are available to support the use of this invaluable therapy. Further optimisation of PDT methodologies will help with the widespread acceptance of this treatment in routine dermatology practice. The explosion of studies and clinical use of daylight PDT is further proof that developing and refining techniques to improve patient tolerance and satisfaction while maintaining efficacy, reinforces the place of PDT. Further investigation into photosensitisers and prodrug delivery methods, along with refinement of light delivery methods, such as portable and conformable sources, continues to be a priority. In the post-Covid-19 recovery period, the need for home-based therapies is greater than ever and PDT, particularly daylight/portable PDT, lends itself to this, with patient engagement and confidence in treatment being essential. Fluorescence diagnostics and further investigation of the use of PDT in a wide range of dermatological conditions requires further study, as does the potential of PDT for preventative application in patients who are at high risk of skin cancer/pre-cancer, such as those who are immunosuppressed.

In conclusion, PDT has many advantages and few adverse effects. The continued development of improved mechanisms for drug delivery and irradiation will help refine the clinical practice of PDT. There is also great potential for the application of PDT in a diverse range of other cutaneous diseases, which requires further investigation.

Key references

The full list of references can be found in the online version at https://www.wiley.com/rooksdermatology10e

19 Kennedy JC, Pottier RH, Pross DC. Photodynamic therapy with endogenous protoporphyrin IX: basic principles and present clinical experience. *J Photochem Photobiol B* 1990;6:143–8.

28 Wong TH, Morton CA, Collier N et al. British Association of Dermatologists and British Photodermatology Group guidelines for topical photodynamic therapy (PDT) 2018. *Br J Dermatol* 2019;180:730–9.

32 Morton CA, Szeimies RM, Basset-Seguin N et al. European Dermatology Forum guidelines on topical photodynamic therapy 2019 Part 1: treatment delivery and established indications – actinic keratoses, Bowen's disease and basal cell carcinomas. *J Eur Acad Dermatol Venereol* 2019;33:2225–38.

33 Morton CA, Szeimies RM, Basset-Seguin N et al. European Dermatology Forum guidelines on topical photodynamic therapy 2019 Part 2: emerging indications – field cancerization, photorejuvenation and inflammatory/infective dermatoses. *J Eur Acad Dermatol Venereol* 2020;34:17–29.

61 Wiegell SR, Wulf HC, Szeimies RM et al. Daylight photodynamic therapy for actinic keratosis: an international consensus: International Society for Photodynamic Therapy in Dermatology. *J Eur Acad Dermatol Venereol* 2012;26:673–9.

83 Collier NJ, Haylett AK, Wong TH et al. Conventional and combination topical photodynamic therapy for basal cell carcinoma: systematic review and meta-analysis. *Br J Dermatol* 2018;179:1277–96.

89 Ibbotson SH, Wong TH, Morton CA et al. Adverse effects of topical photodynamic therapy: a consensus review and approach to management. *Br J Dermatol* 2019;180:715–29.

96 Dirschka T, Radny P, Dominicus R L et al. Long-term (6 and 12 months) follow-up of two prospective, randomized, controlled phase III trials of photodynamic therapy with BF-200 ALA and methyl aminolaevulinate for the treatment of actinic keratosis. *Br J Dermatol* 2013;168:825–36.

120 Togsverd-Bo K, Halldin C, Sandberg C et al. Photodynamic therapy is more effective than imiquimod for actinic keratosis in organ transplant recipients – a randomized intra-individual controlled trial. *Br J Dermatol* 2018;178:903–9.

141 Rubel DM, Spelman L, Murrell DF et al. Daylight photodynamic therapy with methyl aminolevulinate cream as a convenient, similarly effective, nearly painless alternative to conventional photodynamic therapy in actinic keratosis treatment: a randomized controlled trial. *Br J Dermatol* 2014;171:1164–71.

145 Lacour JP, Ulrich C, Gilaberte Y et al. Daylight photodynamic therapy with methyl aminolevulinate cream is effective and nearly painless in treating actinic keratoses: a randomised, investigator-blinded, controlled, phase III study throughout Europe. *J Eur Acad Dermatol Venereol* 2015;29:2342–8.

294 Pastor-Nieto MA, Jiménez-Blázquez E, Sánchez-Herreros C, Belmar-Flores P. Allergic contact dermatitis caused by methyl aminolevulinate. *Actas Dermosifiliogr* 2013;104:168–70.

CHAPTER 23

Principles of Cutaneous Laser Therapy

Vishal Madan[1] and Jill S. Waibel[2]

[1] Laser Division, Dermatology Centre, Salford Royal NHS Foundation Trust, Salford, UK
[2] Miami Dermatology and Laser Institute, Miami, FL, USA

Introduction, 23.1	Tissue cooling, 23.6	Photothermal ablation in the treatment of skin disorders, 23.20
Light and laser light characteristics, 23.1	**Clinical applications of lasers and flashlamps, 23.6**	Non-ablative and fractional modalities, 23.23
Lasers and laser beams, 23.2	General considerations, 23.6	Low-power lasers, 23.24
Tissue optics, 23.3	Vascular lesions and vascular lasers, 23.6	Laser-assisted lipolysis, 23.24
Light–tissue interaction, 23.4	Tattoos and pigmentary disorders, 23.12	**Key references, 23.24**
Selective photothermolysis, 23.5	Hair reduction, 23.17	

Introduction

Prior to the early years of the 20th century, light had been considered to exist as either particles or waves. In 1901, Planck resolved what had been an experimental contradiction with the prevailing wave theory by postulating that electromagnetic radiation (including light) consisted of discrete packets of energy or quanta. Einstein's subsequent study of the photoelectric effect ultimately formed the basis of the modern theory of light as a wave–particle duality [1]. 'Light' is a form of energy and falls within the electromagnetic spectrum which extends from X-rays to radio waves. Optical radiation refers to the specific range of energies as shown in Table 23.1.

In 1954, Charles Townes' experiments with the stimulation of ammonia molecules to emit extra energy as microwaves led to the term 'MASER' (*m*icrowave *a*mplification by the *s*timulated *e*mission of *r*adiation). The term 'LASER', which is also an acronym, seems to have been used first by Gould in a lecture entitled 'The LASER, light amplification by stimulated emission of radiation' in 1959. The first functional laser (ruby, 694 nm) was developed by Maiman in 1960 [3]. Its clinical applications were described 3 years later by Goldman [4] in the first dermatological paper on the subject. The theory of selective photothermolysis was postulated by Anderson and Parrish in 1983 [5], subsequent to which there has been an explosive development in the scientific study and application of this 'new technology' for skin disorders and cosmetic surgery. This chapter will largely restrict itself to the treatment of skin disorders. For a discussion of cosmetic applications of light and related technologies see Chapter 161.

Table 23.1 Divisions of the *optical region* of the electromagnetic spectrum.

Region of optical spectrum	Division	Wavelength (nm/mm)
Ultraviolet (UV) radiation – 'beyond' violet	UV-C	180–280 nm
	UV-B	280–315 nm
	UV-A	315–400 nm
Visible radiation (VIS) – 'light'	A sensation of violet coloured light through to red coloured light	400–780 nm
Infrared (IR) radiation – 'below red'	IR-A (near IR)	780–1400 nm
	IR-B (mid IR)	1400–3000 nm
	IR-C (far IR)	3000 nm–1 mm

Adapted from International Electrotechnical Commission [2].

Light and laser light characteristics

Atoms consist of a nucleus surrounded by electrons. In their resting state, electrons are usually at a low energy level and close to the nucleus. By absorbing energy in the form of a photon (i.e. a quantum of electromagnetic radiation or light), an electron will move to a higher energy orbit (Figure 23.1). The probability of absorption is proportional to the radiation intensity of the light, and also to the number of atoms in the resting state. In its excited and unstable state, the tendency of the electron is to drop back to the ground state. During this process, termed the *spontaneous emission* of radiation, a photon of energy is released.

Emission can also be stimulated, as in a laser. As stated previously, 'laser' is an acronym for '*l*ight *a*mplification by *s*timulated *e*mission of *r*adiation'. *Stimulated emission* occurs after an already excited

Rook's Textbook of Dermatology, Tenth Edition. Edited by Christopher Griffiths, Jonathan Barker, Tanya Bleiker, Walayat Hussain and Rosalind Simpson.
© 2024 John Wiley & Sons Ltd. Published 2024 by John Wiley & Sons Ltd.

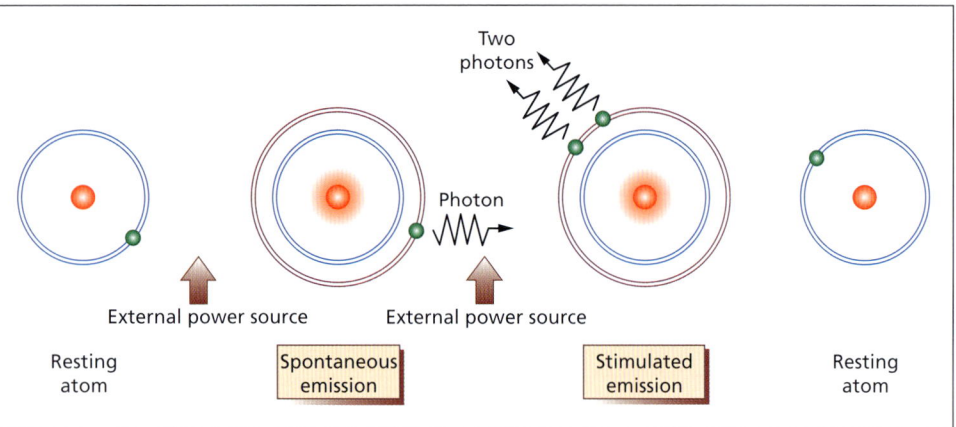

Figure 23.1 Excitation of an atom with (a) spontaneous and (b) stimulated emission of radiation.

atom is perturbed by a photon with a frequency (wavelength) corresponding to the energy gap between the excited and ground states. If this happens, the excited atom reverts to the resting state, releasing energy as a second photon of the same frequency as the incident photon. Because the incident photon is not absorbed, the atom emits two photons. Importantly, each of these has the same wavelength and phase, that is, they are coherent. It is this property which allows *light amplification* and the production of a laser system. During the operation of a laser, all three of these light–matter interactions take place simultaneously (namely, *energising* of atoms, *spontaneous emission* of photons and *stimulated emission* of photons). The energy that is required to excite the atoms in a laser is provided by an external power source in a process called *pumping*. When most of the atoms are in an excited (metastable) rather than in a lower energy state, they are described as having undergone *population inversion* (a condition in which stimulated emission is more likely).

Laser light differs from light emitted by a conventional light source in that it has the following characteristics:
1 *Monochromaticity*. The identity of the excited atom determines the wavelength of the radiation produced. In a laser this is, more precisely, a narrow band in a Gaussian distribution around a characteristic wavelength.
2 *Coherence*. Light can be likened to a sine wave. Laser light is both temporally and spatially coherent, that is, the waves are in phase in time and space.
3 *Collimation*. This is a consequence of coherence and refers to its non-divergent and energy conserving properties. It means that the diameter of the beam changes only minimally over distance, unless it is focused by a lens. Both forms may be useful, such as in CO_2 laser surgery where a focused beam can be used for excision or where a collimated beam can be scanned for resurfacing.

Lasers and laser beams

Lasers are usually named after the constituents of the *active* or *gain medium*, which may be a gas, liquid, solid or semiconductor. The active medium may take the form of:
1 A solid state material including crystals: ruby, alexandrite, Nd:YAG (neodymium:yttrium-aluminium-garnet), Er:YAG (erbium:yttrium-aluminium-garnet) or semiconductor diodes.
2 A liquid: organic dyes in a solvent, for example rhodamine.
3 A gas: carbon dioxide, argon, rare gas–halide mixtures and metal vapours.
4 Semiconductor materials, e.g. diodes and ceramics.

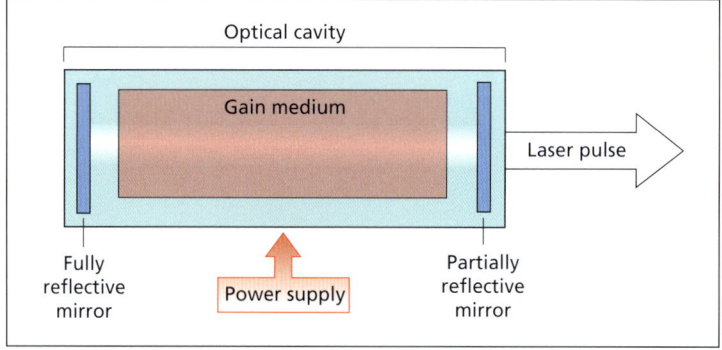

Figure 23.2 Diagram of a laser showing the external power source, the active medium within the optical cavity and a system of fully and partially reflective mirrors.

The active medium is contained within an *optical cavity* (Figure 23.2). In its simplest form the optical cavity consists of two opposing mirrors, one of which is fully (99%) reflective and the other, the *output coupler*, is partly transparent (1%). Photons moving parallel to the axis of the optical cavity are reflected between the two mirrors, in turn eliciting stimulated emission in the same axis, creating an *optical gain*.

When the beam first passes through the gain medium, it experiences gain. Losses occur as the beam is reflected back and forward through the gain medium. Steady-state operation is the point at which there is no change in the beam after one round trip, i.e. total gain and total losses are balanced. The feedback mechanism keeps the population inversion at this threshold level to maintain this balance.

The energy required for the process of light amplification is supplied by an external source such as an electric current (*electrical pumping* if the active medium is a gas) or by a light source (*optical pumping*, flash lamp or other laser, if the active medium is solid). This supply of energy amplifies the light until it is emitted through the output coupler. It then enters a delivery system that transmits it to the operator hand-piece.

Delivery systems may take the form of fibreoptic cables or articulated arms through which light is reflected by mirrors. Fibreoptic cables are lighter as well as easier to operate and maintain. However, they are also delicate and can break when bent or twisted beyond their tolerance. They are not sufficiently robust to transmit light emissions from systems such as CO_2, Er:YAG or the very short pulse nano- or picosecond Q-switched lasers, where articulated arms are required. Likewise, some wavelengths are absorbed by glass, limiting transmission through an optical fibre. Each delivery system ends in an operator hand-piece through which light can be focused by a lens or transmitted as a collimated beam. Either beam type can be scanned to limit exposure time. In contrast to lasers, the xenon flashlamp is mounted within the treatment hand-piece that produces a broad spectrum output beam. The beam is directed through a quartz or sapphire treatment block or tip. Internal cooling of the treatment block or tip provides a level of epidermal protection during treatment.

Lasers are sometimes classified according to the pulse characteristics of the beam, which may be continuous, pulsed or quality switched (Q-switched) (Figure 23.3). Continuous wave light consists of an uninterrupted beam of relatively low power, such as is emitted by the CO_2 laser. Light produced by lasers of this sort can be shuttered mechanically to interrupt the beam and may reduce the accumulation of unwanted heat. Another modification, *superpulsing*, was developed so that the laser emits a rapid train of higher peak power pulses of energy. One disadvantage of these so-called 'quasi-continuous' lasers is that the pulses are so close together that there is insufficient time for cooling. The tissue effect of this may therefore be very similar to a continuous wave laser beam. It was only with the development of high peak power lasers that clinically significant tissue effects could be achieved with single pulses. Examples include the pulsed dye laser and normal mode alexandrite and diode lasers as well as CO_2 lasers with pulse durations in the millisecond or high microsecond range.

Q-switching is a means of creating an ultrashort pulse (5–100 ns and picoseconds) together with an extremely high peak power. This is achieved by means of an *electro-optical switch* which consists of two polarisers. Depending on their alignment, these will either transmit or block light. Blocking the light will lead to the generation of peak powers which can then be transmitted to result in photomechanical/photoacoustic shattering of targets such as tattoo particles and melanosomes. The beam diameter is identical to the so-called spot size and is usually Gaussian in profile. This necessitates a degree of spot size overlap during treatment in order to irradiate tissue more uniformly. Q-switching is commonly used on solid-state lasers such as Nd:YAG, alexandrite and ruby lasers. Q-switching is described as *active* or *passive* according to the method used to achieve the pulsed output.

Tissue optics

The fate of incident light depends upon a number of important factors (Figure 23.4):

1 *Reflection*. Reflection occurs due to the difference in the refractive index between air ($n = 0$) and the stratum corneum ($n = 1.45$). About 4–6% of light is reflected at the skin surface. Reflection increases with increased angle of incidence – it is lowest when the beam is perpendicular.
2 *Absorption*. This is governed by Beer's law, which relates the absorption of light to the properties of the substance through which the light is travelling. In essence, the law states that there is a logarithmic dependence between the transmission of light through a substance and the concentration of that substance as well as between the transmission of light and its path length through the substance. Without absorption of light, there can be no effect on tissue. When a photon is absorbed by a target molecule or chromophore, all of its energy is transferred to that molecule. The basis for selective skin laser surgery is that light can be manipulated in terms of its wavelength, energy content and pulse duration so that a particular target chromophore absorbs light and is selectively damaged or destroyed. The endogenous chromophores of importance are melanin, haemoglobin,

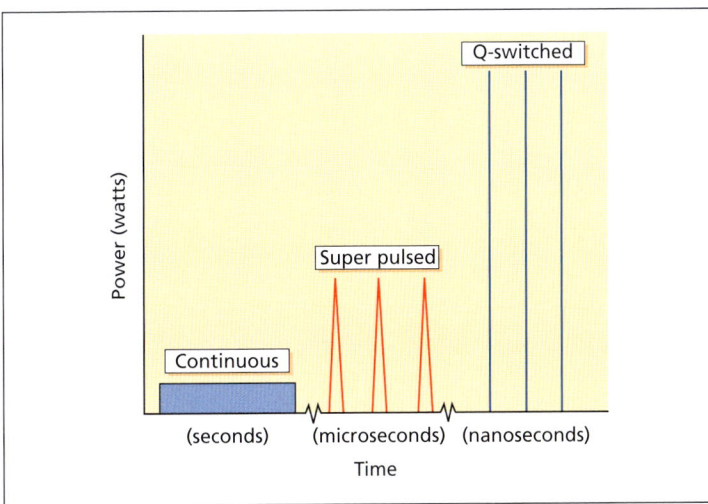

Figure 23.3 Simplified representation of the pulse types.

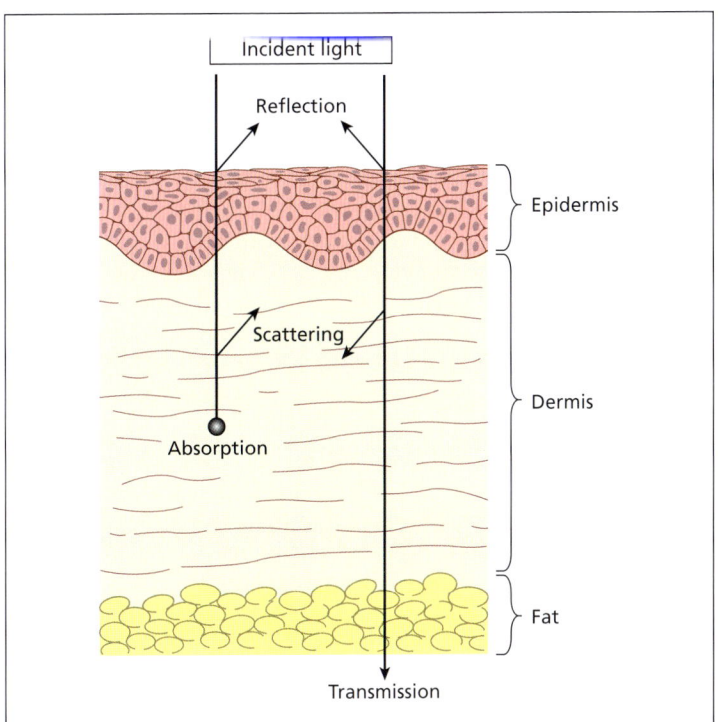

Figure 23.4 Fate of incident light on skin. Endogenous chromophores absorb in the visible and near infrared spectra, and water in the mid and far infrared regions. There are also exogenous chromophores, tattoo ink for example.

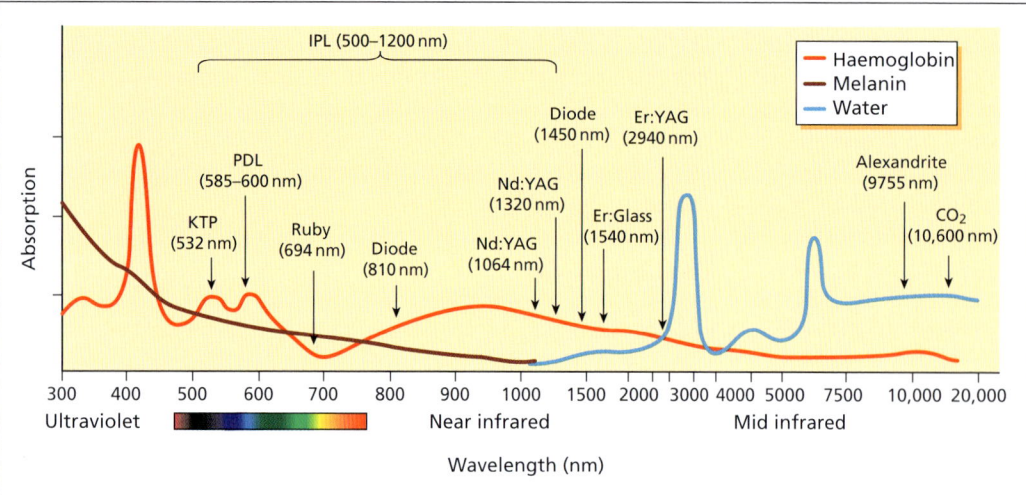

Figure 23.5 Absorption spectra of the principal tissue chromophores. Er:Glass, erbium:glass; Er:YAG, erbium:yttrium-aluminium-garnet; IPL, intense pulsed light; KTP, potassium titanyl phosphate; Nd:YAG, neodymium:yttrium-aluminium-garnet; PDL, pulsed dye laser.

water and collagen (Figure 23.5). Melanin is present in normal epidermis and hair follicles. Its principal function is to protect against sunlight and its absorption includes ultraviolet and visible light, with decreasing absorption into the near infrared spectrum. Haemoglobin has absorption peaks in the UVA, blue (400 nm), green (541 nm) and yellow (577 nm) wavelengths. Collagen absorbs in the visible and near infrared spectra, and water in the mid and far infrared regions. There are also exogenous chromophores, tattoo ink for example.

3 *Scattering*. This refers to the deviation of light by non-uniformities in the medium through which it passes. In skin, this is largely due to collagen in the dermis. Because the collagen molecule is similar in size to the wavelength of visible and near infrared light, scatter is mainly forward in direction. In certain situations, however, back scatter can be high enough to increase the energy density in the upper dermis to beyond that of the incident light. In relation to laser light, so-called coherent back scattering can be more than twice as much as would be the case if the incident light were incoherent.

Scattering in the skin is important in that it reduces the light energy available for absorption by the target chromophore and thereby decreases the clinical effect. Scattering diminishes with longer wavelengths, allowing these to reach deep dermal structures such as hair follicles. Light between 600 and 1200 nm has been described as an optical window into the skin because it is subject to low scattering in addition to being well absorbed by endogenous chromophores. Longer wavelength light is absorbed by water and does not penetrate deeply.

4 *Transmission*. Light that is not reflected, absorbed or scattered passes to deeper tissue. This is dependent on wavelength, shorter wavelengths (300–400 nm) being scattered and penetrating less than 0.1 mm. Wavelengths in the 600–1200 nm range penetrate more deeply because they are scattered less.

Light–tissue interaction

The wavelength of light determines its absorption by a tissue target or *chromophore*. In addition to being absorbed, light must have sufficient energy if it is to alter the target's structure. Energy is measured in joules (J) although it is usually more useful to consider its *fluence* or energy density (J/cm^2). *Power* is the rate at which energy is delivered and is measured in watts (i.e. W or J/s). The term *irradiance* refers to the power density (i.e. the rate at which energy is delivered per unit area) and is measured in W/cm^2. Fluence and irradiance are therefore inversely proportional to the square of the radius of the spot size. This means that for a fixed amount of energy, doubling the spot size decreases the fluence and the irradiance by a factor of 4. On the other hand, increasing the spot size (up to a maximum of about 12 mm) reduces scatter and allows more photons to be transmitted into the skin. In this way, more thermal energy is delivered than with a smaller spot size. The fluence should be accordingly reduced when using a larger spot size.

Pulse duration (the duration of each individual pulse of laser light) is the single most significant variable in light–tissue interaction (Table 23.2). Depending on these qualities, light may affect tissue as follows:

1 *Photostimulation/photobiomodulation*. It has been claimed that low-energy laser light expedites wound healing, although the evidence in support of this is equivocal and the mechanism by which it might do so is unclear.

2 *Photochemical change*. This forms the basis of photodynamic therapy (PDT) and usually involves the topical or systemic administration of a photosensitiser or precursor thereof. Subsequent irradiation with an appropriate light source elicits two types of photo-oxidative reaction and an immediate cytotoxic effect. PDT can also target endogenous chromophores (such as produced by *Pityrosporum acnes* and utilised in the blue light treatment of acne vulgaris). Direct photochemical interactions result from exposure to short wavelengths (high photon energy), specifically UV and blue light (200–400 nm), and is a cumulative process.

3 *Photothermal reactions*. The heat generated by the interaction of light (e.g. 595 nm) with the chromophore (e.g. oxyhaemoglobin) results in thermal disruption of the chromophore. An increase in local tissue temperature induced by longer wavelengths and continuous wave or long-pulsed exposures results in photothermal reaction/injury. Absorption of photon energy produces an increase in the vibrational energy and collisions between tissue molecules, part of which is seen as an increase in tissue temperature. The extent of injury to the tissue depends on the temperature reached and the duration held at that temperature [6]. In the absence of natural heat diffusion or epidermal cooling

Table 23.2 Interactions between light and tissue.

Pulse duration	Interaction	Typical application
Continuous wave or exposures >1 second	Photochemical interactions	Photodynamic therapy
Milliseconds to microseconds	Photothermal interactions	Hair reduction, vascular lesions
Microseconds to nanoseconds	Photoablation/ photomechanical	Pigmented lesions, ablative rejuvenation

Table 23.3 Comparison of lasers and flashlamps (intense pulsed light systems).

Lasers	Flashlamps
Single wavelength, e.g. pulsed dye laser (595 nm)	Multiple wavelengths tuned according to application, e.g. 590–950 nm for vascular indications
Small(er) circular or square spot sizes	Larger rectangular or square spot sizes or footprints
High(er) repetition rate (Hz)	Low repetition rate (Hz)
Smaller hand-piece	Bulkier hand-piece, which houses the lamp and lamp cooling device
Single pulses of variable or fixed duration for efficient heating of target	Multiple pulses with variable or fixed delay for slow heating of target and sparing of epidermis

significant tissue temperature increase can result in irreversible tissue damage. At the immediate impact site there may be a zone of vaporisation leading to zones of necrosis or carbonisation caused by thermal diffusion.

4 *Photomechanical interactions*. The interaction of nanosecond and picosecond domain high peak energy Q-switched laser pulses results in photomechanical or photoacoustic disruption of melanosomes or tattoo pigments.

5 *Photoablation* involves the direct breaking of molecular bonds by high-energy UV radiation causing selective removal of material with no peripheral thermal damage.

Selective photothermolysis

The theory of selective photothermolysis has been used to target structures containing haemoglobin, melanin and collagen. It postulates that light can be used to selectively damage or destroy a chromophore if (i) a wavelength is selected that offers as large a difference as possible between the absorption coefficient of the target and that of the surrounding tissue; (ii) its energy is high enough to damage the target; and (iii) its pulse duration is less than or equal to the thermal relaxation time. These are now considered in more detail.

1 *Wavelength*. Wavelength identifies a particular region of the electromagnetic spectrum, e.g. 635 nm (visible radiation) and the colour of the beam, e.g. 532 nm = green light. It also determines the fate of incident light on tissue (the light–tissue interaction), e.g. transmission or absorption by tissues, and helps determine the lens colour or material to be used in protective eyewear. The absorption spectra of important tissue chromophores are shown in Figure 23.5 in relation to the wavelengths of the lasers widely used in dermatology [5]. Haemoglobin has a number of different absorption peaks, whereas absorption by melanin gradually diminishes with longer wavelengths of incident light. The depth of the target structure must also be considered because scattering of light in the dermis is strongly influenced by wavelength. For this reason, long wavelength light that penetrates well but is poorly absorbed by a deep chromophore may be more damaging to it than a shorter wavelength with the opposite characteristics. In some situations, particularly in relation to melanin, a single wavelength may not be necessary. It may even be preferable to use flashlamps or intense pulsed lights (IPLs) because of their broad emission spectrum (500–1200 nm). These are cheaper to manufacture than lasers and can be used with light filters to allow a potentially wide range of applications. It is possible to vary their pulse durations from 0.5 to 88.5 ms and to introduce intervals between pulses of 1 and 300 ms. For example, a flashlamp hand-piece for hair reduction may irradiate at between 650 nm (red) and 110 nm (infrared), whereas an Nd:YAG laser used for the same purpose would irradiate with a single wavelength of 1064 nm. At present, flashlamps cannot substitute for lasers where focused, high-energy beams are required. The differences between lasers and IPL devices are listed in Table 23.3.

2 *Energy fluence*. The energy contained within light is expressed in joules (J) and its fluence or energy density per unit area in J/cm^2. For laser–chromophore interaction to be successful, the fluence should be high enough to cause destruction of the chromophore.

3 *Thermal relaxation time (TRT)*. The TRT is the time taken for the target to dissipate about 63% of the incident thermal energy. The TRT is related to the size of the target chromophore and varies from a few nanoseconds (tattoo particles) to several hundred milliseconds or more (leg venules). Estimated TRTs for typical chromophores are listed in Box 23.1.

Box 23.1 Estimated thermal relaxation time for typical chromophores

Epidermis	≈ 1–10 ms
Terminal hair (200–300 μm diameter)	≈ 40–100 ms
Blood vessels	≈ 1–50 ms
Melanosomes (1.0 μm diameter)	≈ 250–1000 ns
Cellular water	≈ 1000 ns

Some tissue targets, notably the hair follicle, are not uniform in their absorption of light, and it is possible that light-assisted hair removal is better explained by an 'extended theory of selective photothermolysis' [6]. This distinguishes between an 'absorber' chromophore (in which heat is generated) and a distant 'target', to which heat is transmitted and which is damaged as a result. This may also apply to hair removal, melanin in the hair shaft and matrix cells acting as the absorber, whereas the stem cells of the isthmus (and possibly blood vessels in the papilla) represent the distant target. The time to achieve selective damage of the target is the *thermal damage time* (TDT). This is how long it takes for the entire target, including the primary chromophore (e.g. melanin) and the surrounding target (e.g. a hair follicle), to cool by 63%. The TDT is longer than the TRT as it takes into account heat diffusion from the chromophore throughout the target.

A practical outcome of this theory has been termed 'thermokinetic selectivity' [7]. Because large structures cool more slowly than small structures, it has been proposed that, with appropriate manipulation of the light source, the former can be heated to higher and thus potentially more damaging temperatures. An example of this is light-assisted hair removal where a pulse is used that is longer than the TDT of the melanin-containing epidermis (1 ms) but not of the melanin-containing hair follicle (30–100 ms). Lasers or light sources with pulse durations of 5–50 ms can therefore enable sufficient thermal energy to be accumulated in the hair follicle to coagulate it. Even while the energy is being delivered, the epidermis is protected as it cools rapidly, so that its temperature is kept below its thermal coagulation threshold.

Tissue cooling

Light in the 500–1200 nm spectrum may be preferentially but not specifically absorbed by either haemoglobin or melanin, depending on the wavelengths employed. Epidermal melanin will therefore absorb both direct and back-scattered light from all such devices, whether or not it is the intended chromophore. Heat damage to the epidermis may result in blistering, dyspigmentation or scarring and is particularly likely in pigmented skin. To reduce this risk, the wavelength should be optimised with respect to the absorption characteristics and depth of the target chromophore. The use of long pulses [8] and cooling of the epidermis further reduce the risk of undesired damage to pigmented skin. The latter may be undertaken before, during or after the light pulse, or all three. Cooling may be achieved by three means:

1 *Cold air convection*. Air, chilled to temperatures as low as –30°C, is directed onto the area to be treated.
2 *Contact cooling*. This can involve simple application of icepacks or more sophisticated systems in which cold water flows between colourless and transparent plates (usually sapphire as it is a more efficient conductor than glass). Although this is a good method of cooling, the condensate that develops on the plates can obscure the skin and may require frequent removal.
3 *Cryogen spray (dynamic) cooling*. A frozen gas (e.g. tetrafluoroethane) is sprayed onto the skin immediately before the laser pulse. Evaporative cooling has a high heat transfer coefficient and this is therefore the most efficient way of pre-cooling. With timed, automated control this method is also relatively predictable and reproducible.

One important benefit of epidermal cooling has been to allow treatments at higher fluences than would otherwise be considered safe and in this way to reduce the number of treatments required. Cooling has also made it possible to safely treat patients with all except the most heavily pigmented skin types. Furthermore, cooling decreases the pain associated with treatment, thus reducing the need for topical or local anaesthetic. Cooling can itself cause cryogen injury if used inappropriately.

Clinical applications of lasers and flashlamps

General considerations

As the range of indications for lasers has steadily increased over the years, many treatments have become safer, more effective and better tolerated. From non-purpuric bleaching of port-wine stains to the eradication of signs of photoageing with minimal down time, laser treatments have become very acceptable and have gained tremendous popularity.

With the continuous evolution and popularisation of laser technology, it is understandable that patients may have a false perception of what lasers can achieve. Dermatologists should be able to explain to their patients that, despite the availability of a plethora of lasers, there still remain many dermatological conditions where lasers may have only a limited or no role to play. Even for established laser indications, it may not always be possible to predict the outcomes with any degree of certainty. Practitioners should refrain from making unattainable claims and should set realistic goals for treatment.

Patients with unrealistic expectations from laser treatments are invariably dissatisfied with the outcomes. Before offering laser treatment, therefore, it is important to have a fully informed patient who has realistic expectations of what can and cannot be achieved for them. During the initial assessment, the laser practitioner should also consider the possibility of dysmorphophobia, particularly in patients requesting treatment for barely perceptible clinical signs, as such patients are unlikely to benefit from any laser intervention and are likely to remain dissatisfied.

The main chromophores in the skin are oxyhaemoglobin, melanin (or exogenous pigment) and water, and interactions between laser light and these chromophores form the basis of dermatological laser treatments.

Vascular lesions and vascular lasers
Light–tissue interaction

The main absorption peaks of oxyhaemoglobin are at 418, 542 and 577 nm. Following the postulate of selective photothermolysis by Anderson and Parrish, a flashlamp-pumped dye laser was developed with a wavelength of 577 nm, a pulse duration of 0.3 ms and a fluence of 2 J/cm^2 [9]. The main limitation of 577 nm wavelength was limited depth of penetration into the skin. In subsequent treatment of port-wine stains (PWS), this wavelength was replaced with 585–600 nm light, which has the advantage of deeper dermal penetration (although with reduced oxyhaemoglobin absorption at the longer wavelengths) [10]. A slightly longer pulse duration (0.45 ms) was used in the first generation of pulsed dye lasers (PDLs) on the basis of a calculated TRT of <1 ms for vessel diameters of 10–50 μm. This may have been an underestimate and the TRT was measured in a subsequent *in vivo* study as 1–10 ms for vessel diameters of 30–150 μm [11]. PDLs are now manufactured with pulse durations of up to 40 ms, although the short pulse PDL is optimal for PWS in children because vessel diameters are relatively small [12]. Another laser useful for vascular anomalies (especially facial telangiectases) is the potassium titanyl phosphate (KTP) laser (532 nm); light from this laser does not penetrate beyond superficial vessels but is well absorbed. The alexandrite (755 nm) and Nd:YAG (1064 nm) lasers emit light with longer wavelengths and therefore relatively deep penetration. This is targeted at a low absorption peak at 900–1000 nm.

Devices for treating vascular lesions

There are a few devices commonly used to treat vascular lesions (Table 23.4):

- *KTP (532 nm) laser (frequency doubled Nd:YAG laser).* By passing the emission from an Nd:YAG (1064 nm) laser through a KTP crystal the emission frequency can be doubled with a halving of the wavelength from 1064 nm to 532 nm. The emissions may be flashlamp or diode pumped and are characterised by trains of short pulses that summate to give a wide, pulse-like or 'quasicontinuous' effect with a low risk of producing purpura. Light produced by KTP lasers is highly absorbed by haemoglobin (and melanin) but its wavelength penetrates only superficially. They are used, with or without cooling devices, to treat small facial vessels.
- *Pulsed dye lasers (585–600 nm) 0.45 and 1.5–40 ms.* These contain a rhodamine dye that is excited by a xenon flashlamp to produce light at 585–600 nm in pulses of 0.45–0.5 ms (short pulse PDL) or 1.5–40 ms (long pulse PDL) through spot sizes of up to 15 mm diameter. Light penetrates the dermis to a depth of 1.2 mm and photocoagulates vessels of up to 100 μm in diameter [13].
- *Alexandrite (75 nm) and Nd:YAG (1064 nm) lasers.* These emit light with longer wavelengths and therefore relatively deep dermal penetration. The wavelengths are absorbed by a small haemoglobin absorption peak at 900–1000 nm. Used with long pulses (up to several hundred milliseconds) and epidermal cooling systems, the Nd:YAG laser may have a role to play in treating relatively deep and large vessels, including those on the legs.
- *Flashlamps (500–1200 nm).* These emit non-coherent light over a broad spectrum. Filters are used to eliminate wavelengths shorter than selected thresholds. There is contact cooling and a large spot. Potential advantages are reduced likelihood of patterning, purpura or over-correction when treating fine facial telangiectases or diffuse facial redness.

Laser treatment of vascular lesions

Indications for vascular lasers are shown in Box 23.2. Note that their value is not restricted to primarily vascular conditions. For treating facial lesions in adults usually no anaesthesia is needed, but topical, local or regional anaesthesia may be required when treating children with vascular lasers. Cooling used with the vascular laser provides comfort and obviates the need for any topical anaesthetic in adults. Concerns regarding EMLA cream-induced vasoconstriction and reduced efficacy of PDL treatment of PWS have not been found to be true [18]. Bland emollients and analgesics relieve postoperative pain, swelling and redness. Ice packs may be used to alleviate the discomfort.

Table 23.4 Laser and light-based devices to treat vascular lesions.

Laser	Wavelength (nm)	Comment
Copper vapour	578	Good absorption spectrum for oxyhaemoglobin
		Limited by depth of penetration
KTP	532	Superficial penetration of wavelength
		High absorption by haemoglobin and melanin
		Higher risk of scarring
		Useful of smaller facial vessels
Pulsed dye	577, 585, 590, 595, 600	Favourable side-effect profile
		Purpuric and non-purpuric treatments possible.
		Different sized spots for flexible treatments
		Limited by depth of penetration so not useful for thicker lesions
Alexandrite	755	Good for deeper lesions
		Less purpura
		Not safe in darker skin types
Nd:YAG	1064	Safer in darker skin types
		Good for deeper lesions and thicker vascular lesions
		Greater range of pulse widths
		Less skin bruising
		Higher risk of scarring
Diode	800, 810, 930	Deeper penetration suitable for thicker lesions
		Poor absorption by oxyhaemoglobin
Flashlamp (not laser)	515–1200	Cost effective as multiple indications
		Effective for diffuse redness, e.g. in rosacea
		Lower efficacy than vascular lasers
		Use with caution in patients with darker skin

KTP, potassium titanyl phosphate; Nd:YAG, neodymium:yttrium-aluminium-garnet.

Box 23.2 Indications for vascular lasers

Primarily vascular conditions
- Haemangiomas
- Congenital capillary malformations (port-wine stains)
- Facial telangiectases and redness
- Angioma serpiginosum [14]
- Radiotherapy telangiectases [15] and telangiectases in CREST syndrome [16] and hereditary haemorrhagic telangiectasia [17]
- 'Spider' telangiectases
- Cherry angiomas
- Superficial leg veins and telangiectases
- Angiokeratomas
- Venous lakes
- Venous malformations

Other indications
- Angiofibromas
- Viral warts
- Red and hypertrophic scars
- Psoriasis
- Granuloma faciale
- Jessner's lymphocytic infiltrate
- Poikiloderma of Civatte
- Keratosis pilaris
- Ulerythema ophryogenes
  - Granuloma annulare
  - Sarcoidosis
  - Reticular red mucinosis
  - Lichen sclerosus
- Striae rubrae

Carefully performed test patches are helpful in gauging response to treatment and are a medicolegal requirement for most professional indemnity policies. They alert the patient to the degree of purpura that can be expected with treatment. Test shots can be

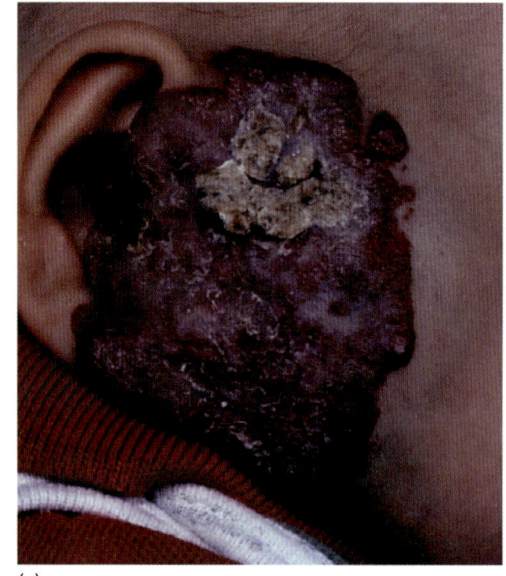
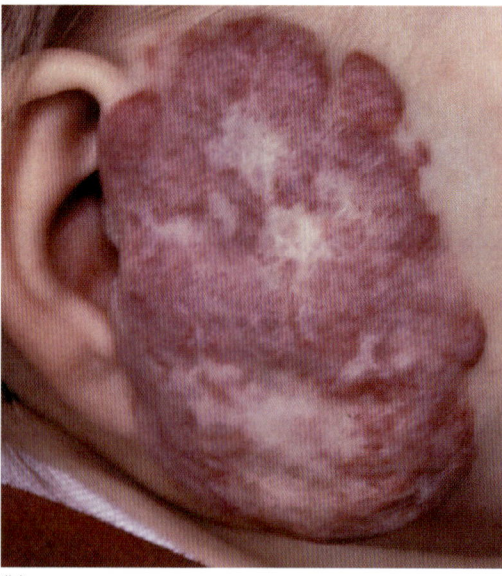

Figure 23.6 Ulcerated haemangioma (a) before and (b) after two pulsed dye laser treatments.

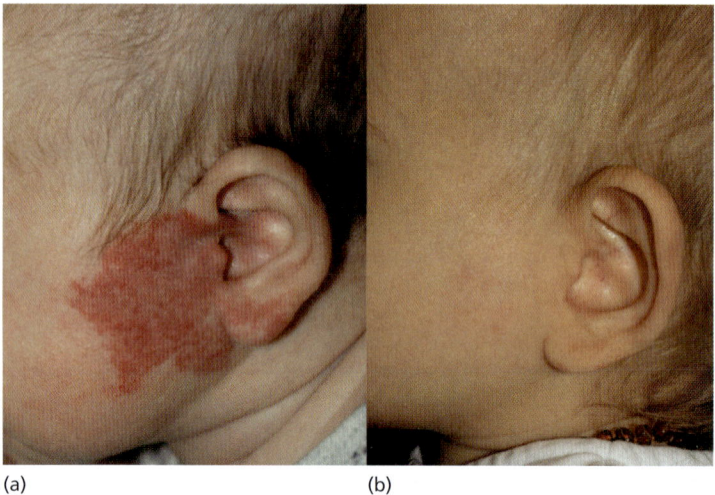

Figure 23.7 Changes in haemangioma associated with PHACES syndrome, baseline (a) versus following treatment with six sessions of PDL (b).

delivered on normal skin in children and on the lesional skin in adults. Assessments are usually undertaken in 2–4 weeks. The highest tolerable fluence resulting in a discernible improvement in the absence of post-laser hyperpigmentation or prolonged purpura should be used for the first session.

Infantile haemangiomas (capillary haemangiomas)

These appear within the first few weeks of life and are the commonest benign tumours of infancy. They are characterised by endothelial hyperplasia and may proliferate for months. It is possible that they originate in the maternal placenta, with which they share distinct tissue-specific markers [19]. The proliferative phase usually lasts for 6–9 months and is eventually followed by spontaneous but slow involution. Most regress, sometimes leaving redundant, atrophic skin or a telangiectatic patch or atrophic scar if there was ulceration. Intervention may be indicated if the site and/or size of the haemangioma is likely to cause functional impairment (e.g. periocular lesions), if the haemangioma is ulcerated and painful or if it is associated with abnormal psychological development. Non-selective β-blockade with topical timolol or systemic propranolol has become the treatment of choice for proliferative haemangiomas, especially complicated lesions on the face, near the eye or those with the potential of causing respiratory embarrassment [20]. As a consequence, the use of lasers in these situations is now rarely indicated.

Infantile haemangiomas have, however, been reported to show a reduction in both redness and size when treated with pulsed dye or Nd:YAG lasers [21]. Concurrent PDL and propranolol may have a role in treatment of haemangiomas. Laser treatment may sometimes be helpful in painful, ulcerated, involuting haemangiomas (Figure 23.6) [22], although ulceration is itself a rare complication of treatment [23]. Posthaemangioma involution, residual telangiectases also respond readily to vascular lasers [24] (Figure 23.7).

Port-wine stains (congenital superficial capillary malformations)

Vascular malformations may be arterial, venous, capillary or lymphatic and may include elements of more than one type. PWS are capillary malformations in which the vessels are characterised by flat endothelium with normal turnover. Sturge–Weber syndrome describes PWS involving skin in the distribution of the ophthalmic branch of the trigeminal nerve, together with involvement of the ocular choroid and leptomeninges. Patients with a periorbital PWS should also be tested for glaucoma.

PDL is the intervention of choice for uncomplicated lesions and 6–8 treatments spaced at 4–6-week intervals will achieve good results in as many as 60% (Figure 23.8) [25]. However, complete clearance is achieved in less than 10%, and roughly 20% of lesions fail to lighten at all [25]. It is generally accepted that laser treatment of PWS at a younger age improves prognosis [26].

Commencing treatment at 1–2 years of age may be the most appropriate clinical decision when weighing up the benefits of early laser treatment against the risks of multiple general anaesthetics in an infant. An alternative philosophy is to defer intervention until the child is self-advocating for treatment (typically of school age) as they

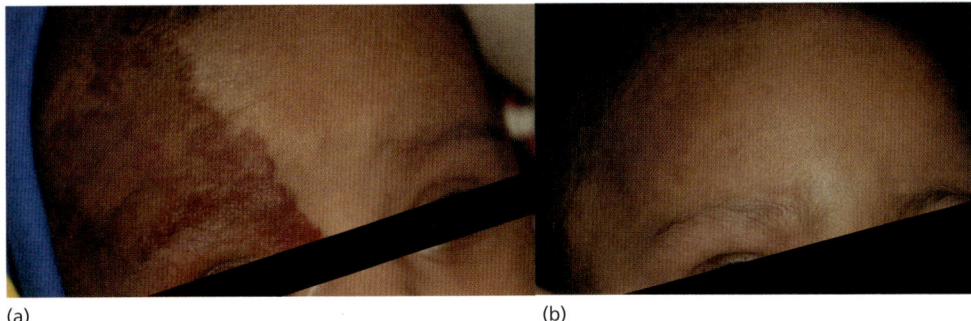

Figure 23.8 Changes in port-wine stain, baseline (a) and following 11 sessions of treatment (b).

may then be in a better position to tolerate treatment without the need for general anaesthesia.

In recent years, PDLs have been manufactured with longer wavelengths, larger spot sizes and longer pulses as well as with cooling devices that allow the use of higher fluences. The 585 nm short pulse PDL is probably optimal for treating PWS in infants, in whom vessel diameters are relatively small. More recently manufactured PDLs emit light with a wavelength of 595 nm, absorption of which by haemoglobin is fivefold lower than at 585 nm. Nevertheless, used in conjunction with a longer pulse, these may be most suitable for the deeper, larger vessels encountered in adult PWS [27]. The use of spray cooling and higher fluences with both short and long pulse (1.5–4.0 ms) PDLs has considerably shortened the duration of treatment for a PWS [28].

Lesions become purpuric if treated with both high fluences and pulse durations of 6 ms or less. Although reduced by both cooling and long pulsing, a degree of post-treatment purpura formation is thought to be necessary for effective treatment of lesions. Factors favouring a good response to PDL treatment are youth as well as flat and scarlet (as opposed to purple) PWS on the head and neck (excluding the cheeks or midline) (Figure 23.9) [29]. Proximal limb lesions do better than those sited more distally. Partial re-emergence (in up to 40% after 4 years) may occur after successful treatment [30]. Poor prognostic factors (Table 23.5) include age over 1 year, central facial location, size >40 cm², nodular or hypertrophic lesions, vessels >400 μm below the dermal–epidermal junction, vessel diameter >20 μm and more than five previous laser treatments [31,32].

PWS thicken diffusely over time with approximately two-thirds of patients developing hypertrophic or nodular lesions by age 50 years.

PDL-resistant and recurrent PWS represent a therapeutic challenge (Figure 23.10). The small-calibre deeper vessels are difficult to target with the available systems. Double-pass techniques or pulse stacking have been shown to further lighten some such resistant PWS, although the risks of blistering, scarring and hyperpigmentation are higher [32,33]. Longer wavelength, variable pulse width lasers such as the alexandrite, 810 nm diode and 1064 nm Nd:YAG lasers and IPL systems can be used to treat resistant or recurrent PWS [34]. Topical and intravenous PDT has been found to be at least as effective as PDL and may be useful for conventional laser-resistant PWS [35,36]. Topical antiangiogenic agents such as rapamycin and imiquimod applied after laser irradiation may improve treatment outcomes [37]. Treatment with sequential pulses of 595 and 1064 nm wavelengths has been shown to be of benefit for recalcitrant and hypertrophic PWS [38].

Table 23.5 Poor prognostic factors for PWS response to laser therapy [31].

Category	Poor prognostic factors
Port-wine stain characteristics	Central facial V2 area
	Distal limb area
	Darker colour at presentation
	Hypertrophic thickening at presentation
	Size >40 cm²
	Vessels >400 μm below the dermal–epidermal junction
	Vessel diameter >20 μm
Patient characteristics	Older age at presentation
	More than five previous treatments
Dermoscopy features	Subpapillary capillaries on dermoscopy, showing deep red linear vessels
	A bright red background
	Thick vessels
Reflectance confocal microscopy	Blood vessels with high blood flow, large diameter and located deeper in the skin
Video microscopy	Deeper vessels in the superficial horizontal plexus presenting as small fine capillary dots

Flashlamps (500–900 nm) have larger spot sizes and have also been used to treat resistant PWS, with supposedly good effect [39]. Other and more questionable options for treating resistant PWS include fractional ablative resurfacing, indocyanine green-augmented diode laser therapy and PDL therapy in conjunction with pneumatic skin flattening – a technique whereby vacuum-assisted compression of skin is claimed to improve outcomes while reducing the discomfort associated with laser treatment. Adult patients in whom progressive vascular ectasia has resulted in very exophytic lesions are probably best treated with longer wavelengths (Nd:YAG; 1064 nm) or CO_2 laser (Figure 23.11) [40].

Telangiectases and redness

Spider telangiectases consist of a central arteriole with a high filling pressure and are best treated with a PDL. The superficial telangiectases that are commonly found in a midfacial distribution in middle-aged and elderly fair-skinned patients and those associated with erythemotelangiectatic rosacea respond safely and well to a single treatment with a KTP laser. The same applies to telangiectases associated with autoimmune disease and following radiotherapy. KTP laser treatments do not produce purpura and hence are more acceptable to patients. More diffuse, finer telangiectases or diffuse redness associated with rosacea will respond to PDL

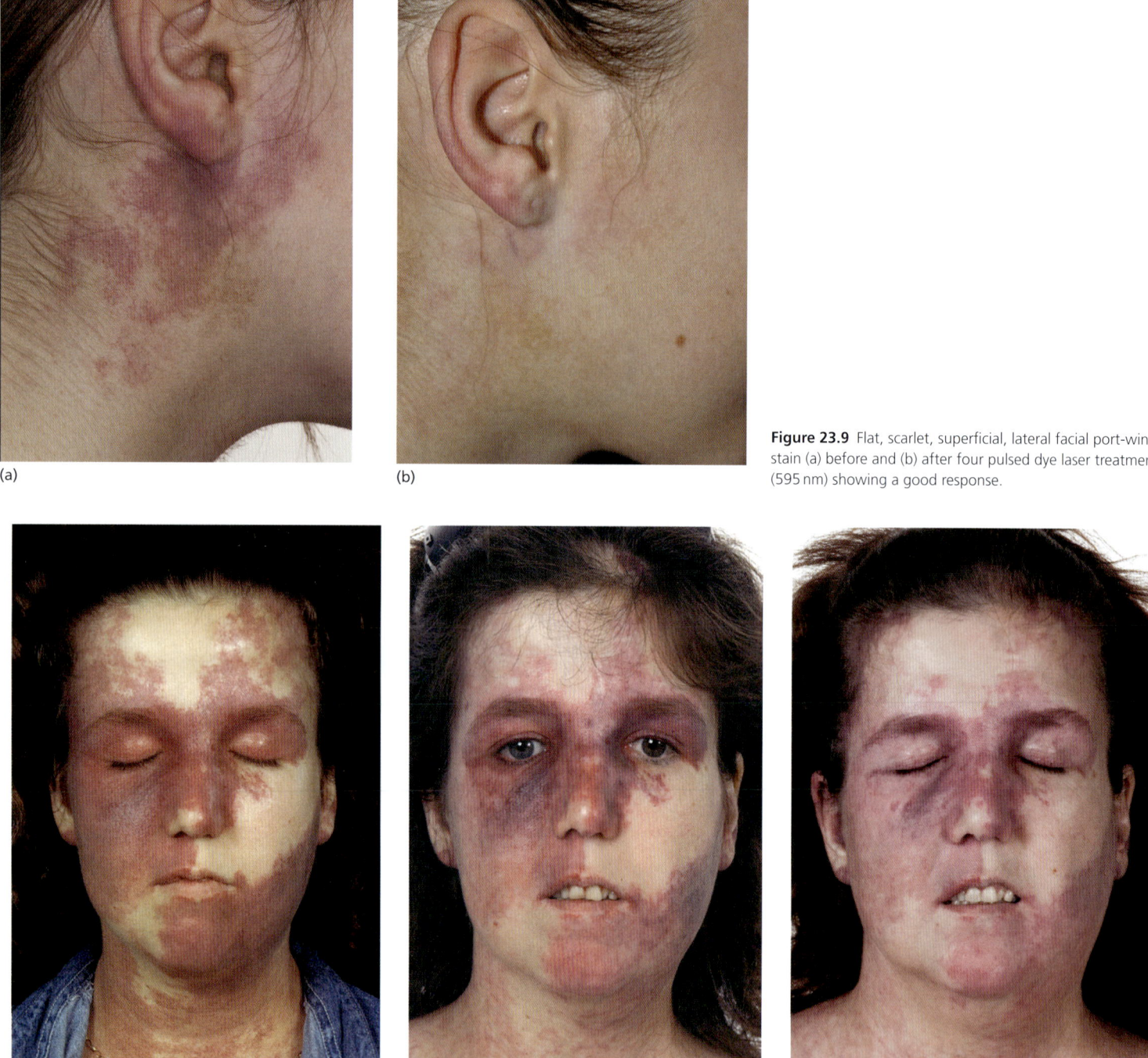

Figure 23.9 Flat, scarlet, superficial, lateral facial port-wine stain (a) before and (b) after four pulsed dye laser treatments (595 nm) showing a good response.

Figure 23.10 (a–c) Port-wine stain intermittently treated with the pulsed dye laser over a period of 12 years showing a relative lack of response in the mid-face port-wine stain.

treatment (Figure 23.12), not necessarily with associated purpura but with a risk of subsequent honeycomb patterning (Figure 23.13). Non-purpuric PDL treatments are popular but require more sessions to achieve comparable results to purpurogenic treatments. Treatments are repeated at 4–6-week intervals. Stubborn perinasal and nasal telangiectases respond to deeper penetrating Nd:YAG laser. However, this wavelength is associated with high risk of scarring and should be used with extreme caution on facial vessels. The flashlamp usually reduces redness more gradually than the PDL and is less likely to cause patterning (Figures 23.14 and 23.15). Nevertheless, the flashlamp may be more painful than laser treatment and several treatments may be required.

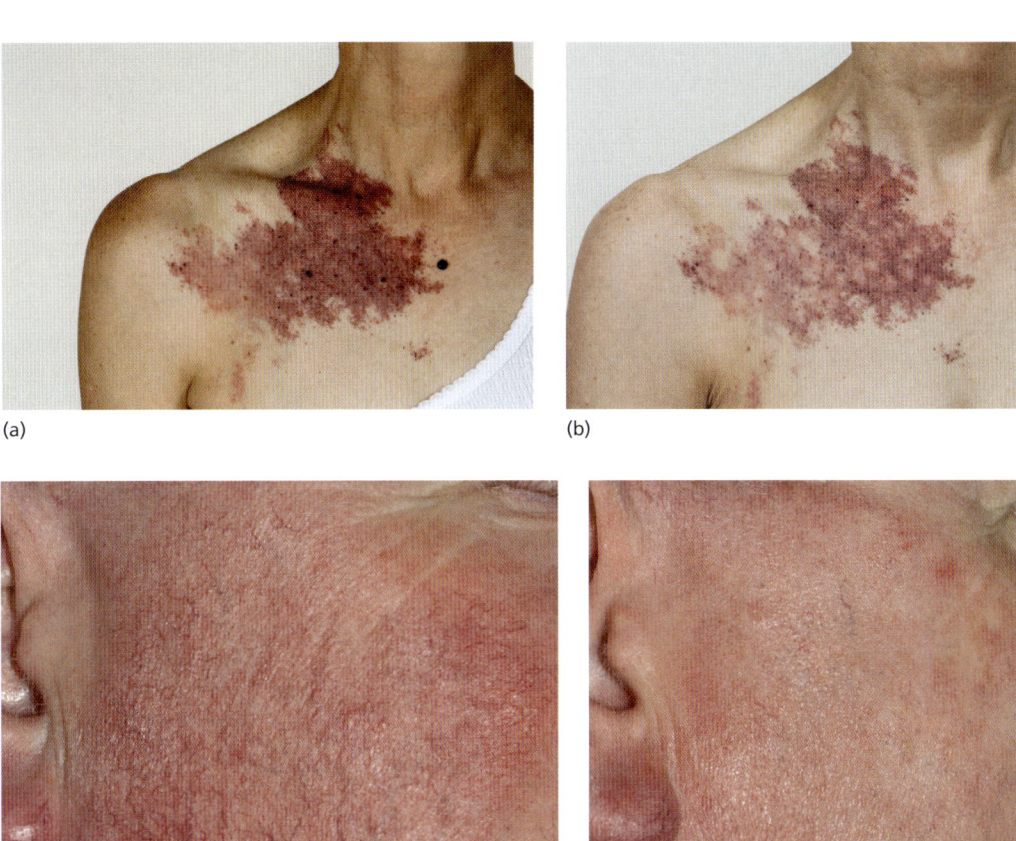

Figure 23.11 Carbon dioxide laser treatment of vascular ectasia in port-wine stain (a) before and (b) after treatment.

Figure 23.12 Facial telangiectasia (a) before and (b) after pulsed dye laser treatment.

Leg veins

These vary in terms of size, depth and flow characteristics. In the absence of deep venous insufficiency, superficial dilated venules are probably best treated by sclerotherapy using sclerosants such as aethoxysclerol, hypertonic saline or polidocanol. Nevertheless, some superficial small-calibre venules may respond to laser treatment [41]. Long pulsed (1.5–40.0 ms) PDLs with wavelengths in the 585–600 nm range and used with moderate fluences are sometimes useful for superficial vessels less than about 0.5 mm in diameter [42]. Longer wavelengths are used to target a different absorption peak of haemoglobin and achieve deeper penetration. The 3 ms alexandrite (755 nm) laser has been used with high fluences in treating leg venules of up to 2 mm in diameter [43] and the Nd:YAG (1064 nm) laser with fluences higher than 100 J/cm^2 and pulse durations of up to 1 s in treating even deeper and larger vessels [44]. Treatments may be repeated at 4–6-week intervals. Complications are relatively common and include ulceration, dyspigmentation and scarring [45]. There are few data on the flashlamp in this context but its emission spectrum and large applicator head would suggest a role only in treating widespread, fine telangiectases. Recently, indocyanine green-augmented diode laser therapy of telangiectatic leg veins has been shown to have better efficacy than long pulsed Nd:YAG lasers [46].

Miscellaneous vascular skin lesions

Other cutaneous vascular lesions that respond to laser treatment include *angiomas* and small *venous lakes*, for which PDL treatment is optimal. Larger venous lakes may respond to long pulsed Nd:YAG laser. Small, red *angiofibromas* may respond well in young patients with tuberous sclerosis in whom ablative treatments are inappropriate. These have recently been reported to respond to topical rapamycin which has been more acceptable to patients than vascular or ablative laser treatments [46]. *Angiokeratomas* are likely to recur unless treatment is sufficient to cause fibrosis, but smaller lesions respond well to treatment (Figure 23.16). *Pyogenic granulomas* should probably be treated by curettage rather than laser as obtaining histopathological confirmation of diagnosis should be considered. Medium-sized veins in the periorbital and temple area can be treated with long pulsed Nd:YAG (1064 nm) (Figure 23.17).

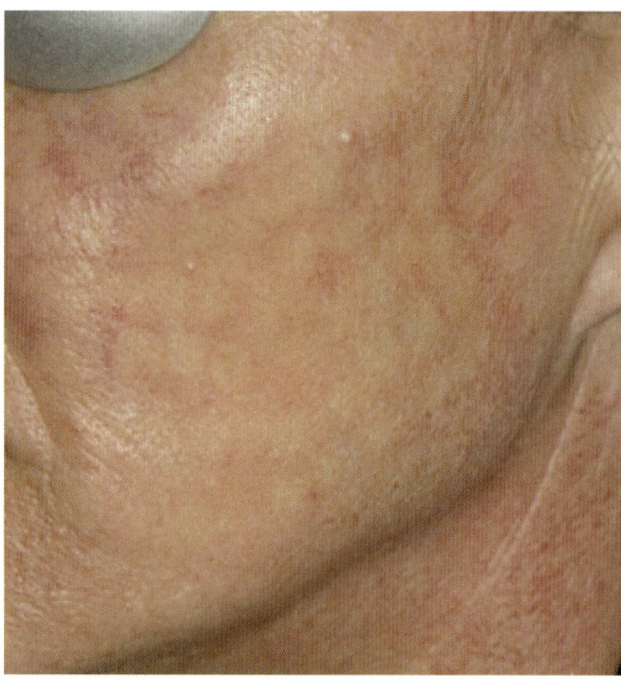

Figure 23.13 Honeycombing noted after pulsed dye laser treatment of facial erythema.

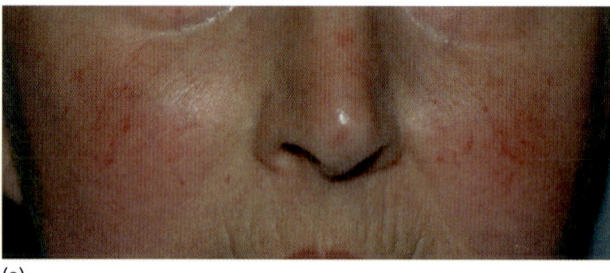
(a)

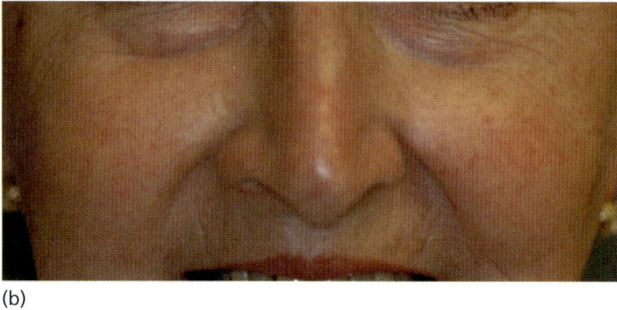
(b)

Figure 23.14 Changes in rosacea telangiectasia, baseline (a) versus following treatment (b).

Other applications of vascular lasers (Box 23.2)
Viral warts
Pulsed dye, CO_2 and Nd:YAG lasers have been used to treat viral warts [47], often at high fluences and without cooling (Figure 23.18). The rationale for this was originally that photocoagulation of the underlying dermal vessels compromised the viability of the abnormal epidermis. It seems more likely that it represents a non-specific thermal injury to the infected epidermis. Facial and perineal warts respond better than plantar warts [48]. PDL is equivalent to conventional therapies such as cryotherapy and cantharidin. Combination therapies with lasers and other agents including bleomycin, salicylic acid, and light-emitting diode have shown some success [49].

Hypertrophic scars
PDLs have been reported to improve the colour and contour of red and hypertrophic (but not keloid) scars in studies that have sometimes been supported with objective measurements such as reflectance spectrometry and silicone profilometry [50]. The mechanism of action is unknown, although it is also possible that the destruction of small vessels plays a part. In more elevated scars, lasers have been claimed to be most useful after the scars have first been substantially reduced in bulk by intralesional corticosteroids. Overall, evidence seems poor for laser treatment of scars (except the 595 nm PDL) [51].

Inflammatory cutaneous lesions
Some inflammatory skin conditions such as cutaneous and nail psoriasis, acne, granuloma faciale, granuloma annulare, lupus erythematosus, sarcoidosis, Jessner lymphocytic infiltrate, reticular erythematous mucinosis and lichen sclerosus may respond to PDL [52–54]. Whilst not fully understood, efficacy of PDL in these disorders appears to be mediated by antiangiogenesis and photodynamic effects. Currently, the role of lasers in these disorders is not well defined and lasers are only used for recalcitrant and localised lesions.

Complications of vascular lasers
The newer generation, long pulsed PDLs are safe and associated with a very low incidence of complications. Appropriate cooling prevents epidermal injury although excessive cooling must be avoided to prevent cryogen burns. Postinflammatory dyspigmentation, particularly hyperpigmentation, is the commonest side effect. Both atrophic and hypertrophic scarring can occur with vascular lasers. Redness, pallor, discomfort, vesiculation and crusting can follow KTP laser treatment. Likewise, atrophic scarring has been reported after the treatment of nasal telangiectases with KTP and Nd:YAG lasers. Non-purpuric PDL parameters may result in significant facial and periorbital oedema.

The efficacy of vascular lasers in the treatment of PWS and facial telangiectases is unquestionable. There are enough data and clinical experience supporting these claims. However, treatment of resistant PWS still poses a challenge to the laser clinician. Good-quality clinical research evaluating the role of vascular lasers in the treatment of other vascular indications is hampered by the large number of variables, which makes comparisons difficult.

Tattoos and pigmentary disorders
Light–tissue interaction
Melanin absorbs light in the wavelength range of 290–120 nm (Figure 23.5). At the shorter wavelengths, absorption is higher but penetration less deep than at the longer wavelengths. The 'therapeutic window' for treatment of pigmented lesions lies between 630 and 1100 nm, where absorption by melanin exceeds that by haemoglobin.

The Q-switch is an electro-optical device that is used to produce pulses of only a few nanoseconds. These are designed to be within the estimated TRT of melanosomes (0.5–1 µs) but longer

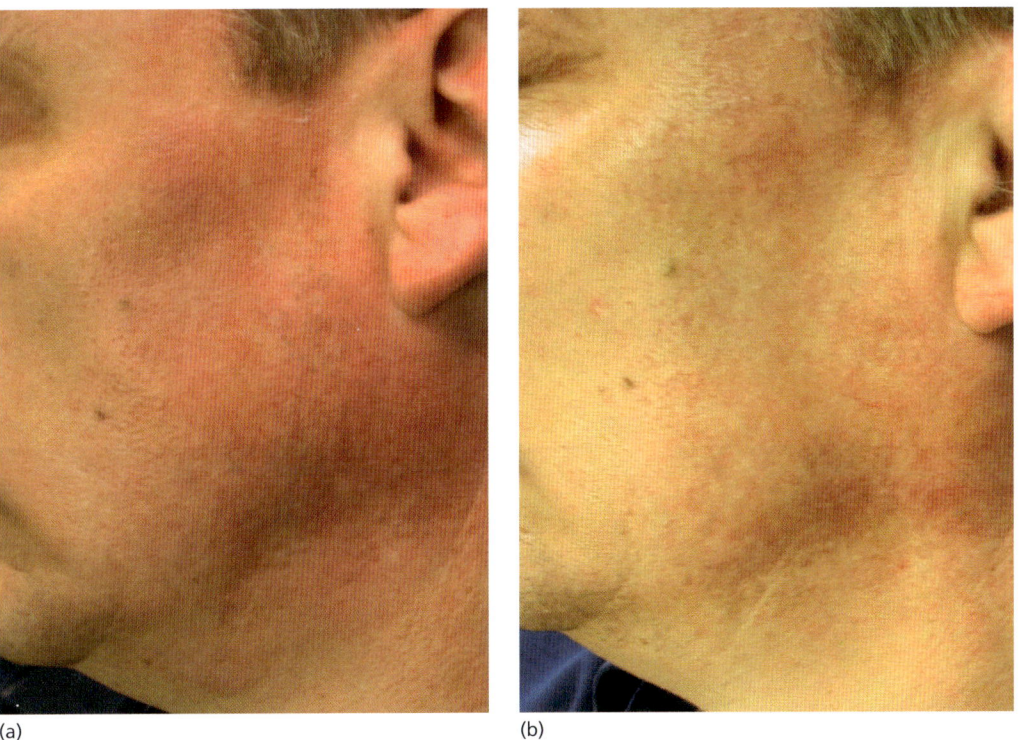

Figure 23.15 Facial redness (a) before and (b) after one treatment with a flashlamp, showing minimal patterning and a good clinical response.

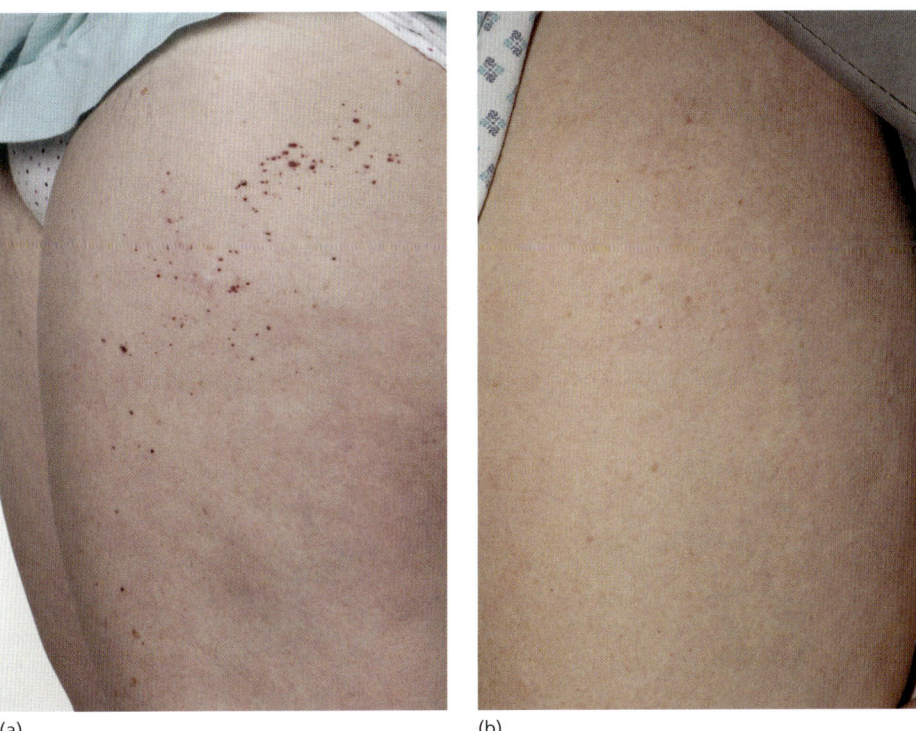

Figure 23.16 Angiokeratoma (a) before and (b) after pulsed dye laser treatment.

than that of tattoo particles, which are in the low nanosecond domain. Flashlamps can pulse within the millisecond range, which is relatively long in this context. Pulses in the nanosecond and subnanosecond range may fragment and disperse melanin and tattoo ink, thereby altering their optical properties. Laser tissue interaction produces intracellular steam and vacuole formation, which leads to immediate whitening. An audible popping sound is heard due to the photoacoustic effect. Most tattoo lightening is probably due to uptake and removal of the fragmented particles by activated macrophages through the lymphatic system. Some may also be removed by transepidermal elimination. Although nanosecond (10^{-9}) Q-switched lasers are 'gold standard' lasers for treating pigmentation and tattoos, picosecond (10^{-12}) lasers offer a greater than 10-fold reduction of pulse width allowing better

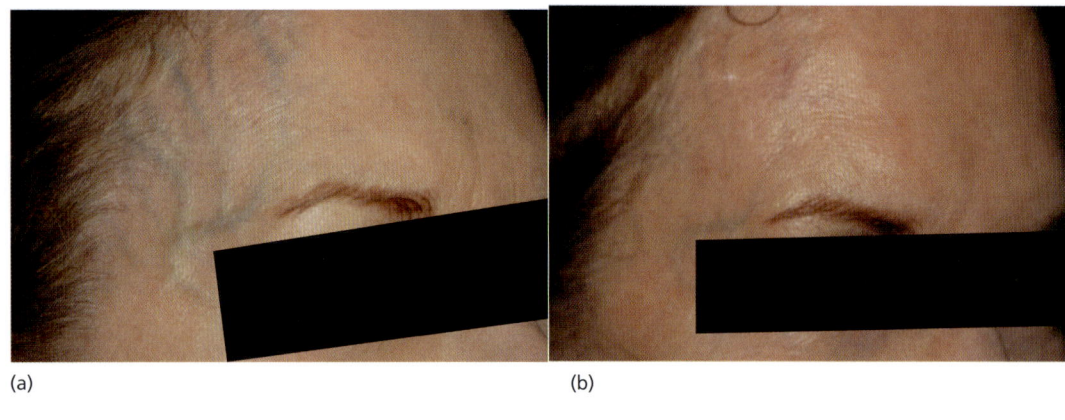

Figure 23.17 Changes in vein prominence on the right temple; baseline (a) versus following treatment (b).

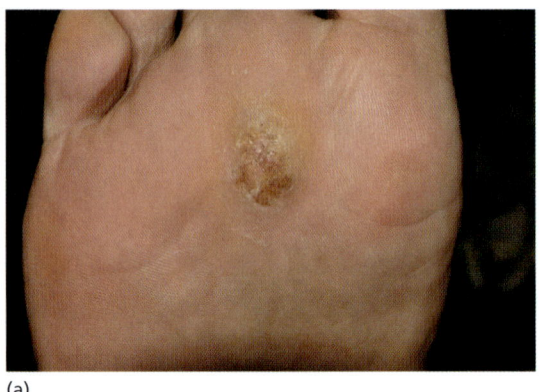
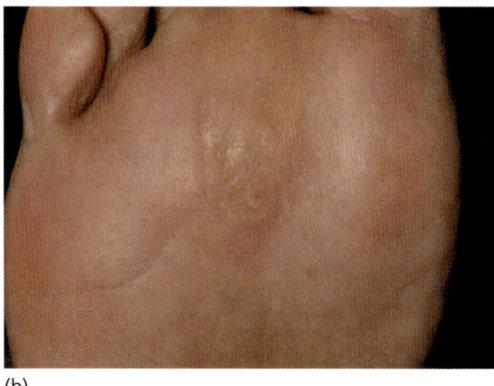

Figure 23.18 Improvement in plantar warts (a) before and (b) after four pulsed dye laser sessions.

targeting of the melanosomes and tattoo ink particles whose TRT is in the subnanosecond domain [55].

Devices for treating tattoos and pigmented lesions

1 *Q-switched Nd:YAG (106 nm) laser and Q-switched frequency doubled Nd:YAG (532 nm) laser.* The Q-switched Nd:YAG (1064 nm) laser emits light that penetrates 2–3 mm into the dermis and is therefore suitable for the removal of deeper dermal pigmentation. If the frequency is doubled (and the wavelength thus halved to 532 nm) by passing the laser beam through a KTP crystal as for the KTP laser, penetration is reduced. The Q-switched frequency doubled Nd:YAG (532 nm) laser is designed to have limited penetration into the dermis and is therefore more useful for the removal of epidermal pigment.
2 *Q-switched ruby (694 nm), alexandrite (755 nm) and diode (810 nm) lasers.* These also emit red light at intermediate wavelengths, allowing somewhat deeper dermal penetration although with some loss of absorption.
3 *Flashlamps (500–1200 nm).* These emit non-coherent light over a broad spectrum with potential advantages in terms of penetration and absorption. The relatively long pulse duration (0.5–88.5 ms) appears not to constitute a practical problem in treating pigment with TRTs in the nanosecond domain.

Anaesthesia pre-treatment considerations

Topical anaesthesia is usually satisfactory for treating pigmented lesions or tattoos. Topical anaesthetics may be appropriate for larger treatment areas but risk of systemic absorption should be borne in mind. Emollients and analgesics relieve postoperative pain, swelling and redness. Concomitant cooling of the epidermis is not required with Q-switched lasers. Periorbital treatments necessitate the need for intraocular metal shields to protect the globe.

Indications for laser treatment of tattoos and pigmented lesions

Indications for pigment-specific lasers are listed in Box 23.3.

Box 23.3 Indications for pigment-specific lasers

- Tattoos
- Epidermal lesions
  - Freckles
  - Lentigines
  - Labial melanotic macules
  - Flat and darkly pigmented seborrhoeic keratoses
  - Café-au-lait macules
- Dermal melanocytosis
  - Naevi of Ota and Ito
  - Hori naevus
  - Drug-induced pigmentation
  - Mongolian blue spot
  - Acquired dermal melanosis, e.g. lichen planus pigmentosus
- Mixed epidermal–dermal lesions
  - Postinflammatory hyperpigmentation
  - Melasma
  - Becker naevi
  - Riehl melanosis
  - Poikiloderma of Civatte

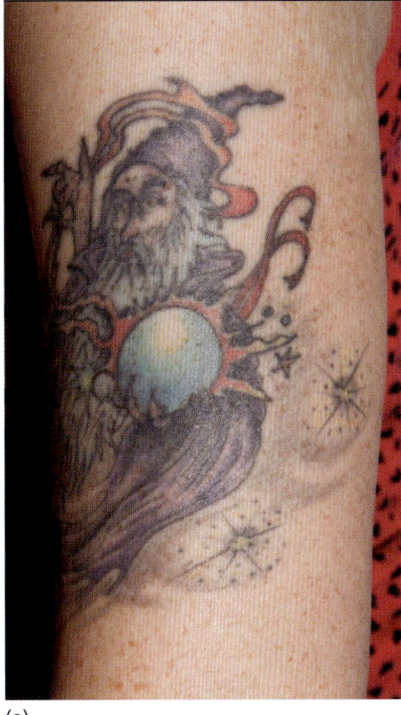
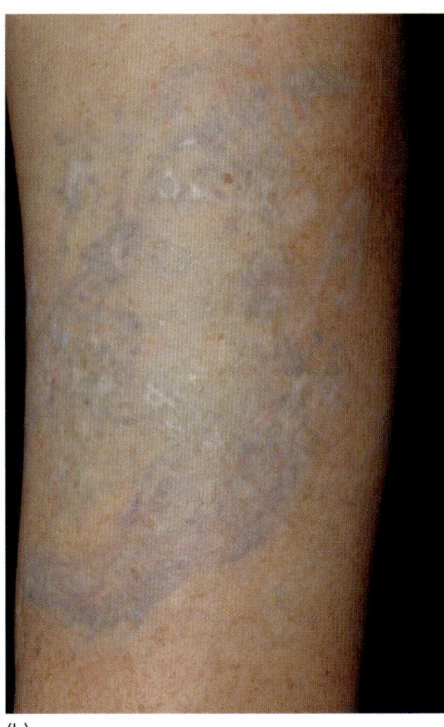

Figure 23.19 Professional tattoo (a) before and (b) after multiple Q-switched alexandrite (532 and 1064 nm) laser treatments. Note the hypopigmentation following the high fluence laser treatments. (a) (b)

Tattoos

Tattoos can be amateur, professional, cosmetic, traumatic or medical, e.g. radiotherapy. Q-switched treatment of tattoos is cosmetically superior to older destructive modalities. Black or blue amateur tattoo pigments absorb across a broad range of wavelengths in the visible and near infrared spectrum. Green inks respond optimally to the Q-switched ruby and Q-switched alexandrite lasers but often persist. Conversely, red pigments respond best to the green light emitted by the Q-switched frequency doubled Nd:YAG laser (532 nm). The Nd:YAG laser is effective for blue/black tattoos but is relatively poorly absorbed by green pigments. It has been used successfully to treat tattoos in pigmented skin. Lasers used for tattoo removal are listed in Table 23.6. Red, brown or flesh-toned inks may contain ferric oxide (Fe_2O_3), which can be reduced by laser treatment to ferrous oxide (FeO), which is black. Although test treatments are therefore important, this reaction is rare and usually responds to subsequent treatment with the appropriate wavelength. Yellow and pastel colours are difficult to treat and complete resolution is unusual.

Amateur tattoos usually require fewer treatments than professional tattoos. Q-switched lasers are also effective in clearing traumatic, cosmetic and radiotherapy tattoos.

Improving tattoo clearance with Q-switched lasers has been of much interest, especially as multicoloured professional tattoos may require more than 20 treatment sessions (Figure 23.19). Nanosecond domain pulses may be too long for certain tattoo particles, most of which vary in size from 40 to 300 nm *in vivo*. Picosecond pulse width lasers may therefore be more effective [56]. The intradermal injection of hyperosmotic substances such as glycerol in animal models reduces dermal scatter and improves tattoo clearance but can cause skin ulceration [57]. Other novel approaches include repeated exposures (R20) or combining Q-switched and fractional techniques [58,59].

Table 23.6 Q-switched lasers for the treatment of different tattoo inks.

	Brown	Black	Blue	Red	Green	Yellow	Orange
Nd:YAG (1064 nm)	+	+	+				
Nd:YAG (532 nm)	+	+		+		+	+
Alexandrite (755 nm)	+	+	+		+		
Ruby (694 nm)	+	+	+		+		

Nd:YAG, neodymium:yttrium–aluminium garnet.

Epidermal pigmentation

Ephelides (freckles) and *actinic (solar) lentigines* respond well to treatment with the Q-switched KTP laser (532 nm). Unlike the Q-switched ruby (694 nm) and Q-switched alexandrite lasers, this laser may cause bruising. Each lesion has to be treated individually, an often tedious exercise in photodamaged patients, who often present with mottled hyperpigmented lesions on a background of chronic 'bronzing' and guttate hypopigmentation.

Facial lentigines as well as labial lentigines associated with *Peutz–Jegher syndrome* have also been shown to improve with the Q-switched alexandrite laser [60].

Similarly, the Q-switched alexandrite laser can be very effective in the treatment of oral and *genital melanosis* (genital lentiginosis) (Figure 23.20). There are limited published data on the use of the flashlamp in this context as its pulse width is relatively long. However, its large beam diameter allows treatment of the entire affected area and not just the pigmented lesions themselves. Using a glass slide to compress the epidermis may allow the 595 nm PDL to treat superficial pigmented lesions by 'shifting' the competing chromophore haemoglobin.

Café-au-lait patches show a variable response to laser treatment and repigmentation occurs in 50% [61]. *Becker melanosis* consists of dermal melanophages as well as epidermal hyperpigmentation.

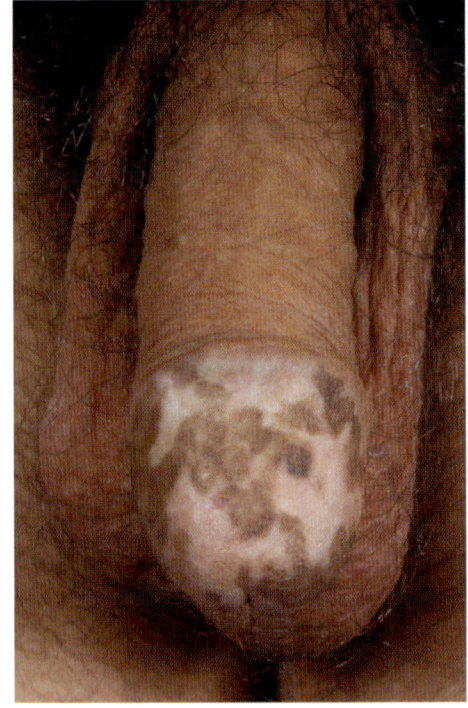
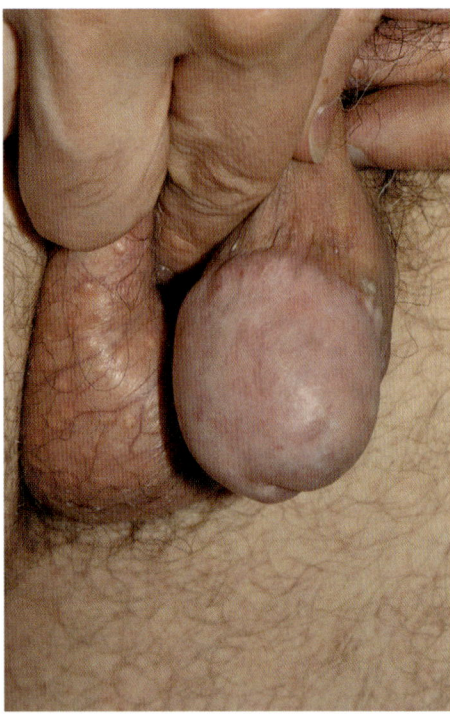

Figure 23.20 Penile lentiginosis (a) before and (b) after Q-switched alexandrite laser treatment.

Its response to Q-switched lasers or to flashlamps is unpredictable, particularly if there is hypertrichosis, and repigmentation may occur from the hair follicles. This has led some authors to suggest that ablative treatment with an Er:YAG laser may be preferable [62]. Despite early enthusiasm for fractional ablative lasers, treatment of Becker melanosis often results in postinflammatory hyperpigmentation and poor patient satisfaction [63].

Seborrhoeic keratoses, which resemble solar lentigines in being flat and brown, will respond well to laser treatment. However, lesions that are warty or poorly pigmented are likely to respond better to destructive treatment modalities.

Although lasers may lighten *lentigo maligna*, they may not eradicate amelanotic or deep perifollicular disease. Lentigo maligna and atypical naevi should not be treated with lasers [64].

Dermal pigmentation

Speckled and lentiginous naevus (naevus spilus) consists of a lentiginous patch speckled with compound naevi. A small, early study with both Q-switched ruby and Q-switched Nd:YAG (532 or 1064 nm) lasers suggested that the former was more effective. One of six patients developed dyspigmentation and another showed focal recurrence [65]. In a larger study of Japanese children, speckled and lentiginous naevi were noted to respond poorly to Q-switched alexandrite laser treatment [66]. The conclusions of this second study seem more plausible in view of generally disappointing experience with Q-switched laser treatment of both café-au-lait macules and compound naevi (Figure 23.21).

Naevus of Ota has been treated with the Q-switched ruby, alexandrite and Nd:YAG lasers (Figure 23.22) [67]. The relatively deep dermal pigmentation responds optimally and with fewer complications to treatment with the Q-switched Nd:YAG laser. Some patients re-pigment after treatment [68].

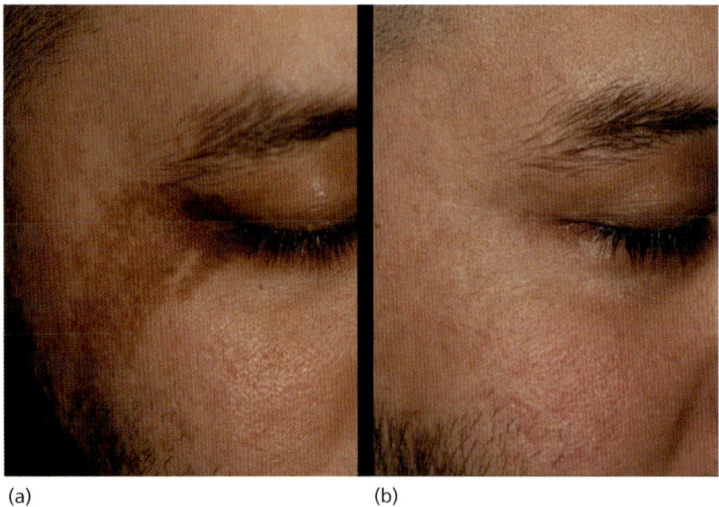

Figure 23.21 Changes in café-au-lait macule, baseline (a) and following 11 treatments (b).

Both *congenital and acquired melanocytic naevi* have been treated with Q-switched lasers [69], although this remains controversial. One reason is that the long-term effects of non-lethal laser irradiation of melanocytes are unknown. With the possible exception of flat, junctional naevi, melanocytic naevi tend to respond incompletely and many lesions re-pigment. In a study in which 31 congenital and acquired (including atypical) melanocytic naevi were treated with the Q-switched ruby laser, normal mode ruby laser or both, only 16 were visibly lighter 4 weeks after treatment [70].

Flat, medium-sized, congenital melanocytic naevi respond to pigment-specific lasers, but raised lesions only improve with ablative laser treatment, if at all. However, re-pigmentation can be seen

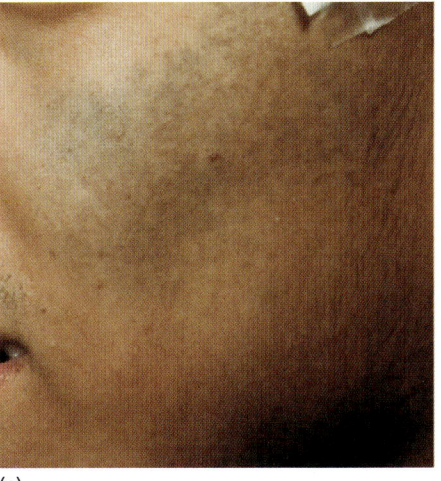
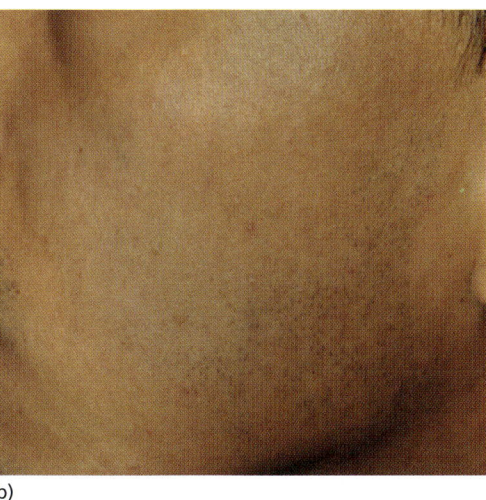

Figure 23.22 Naevus of Ota (a) before and (b) after seven treatments with a Q-switched Nd:YAG (1064 nm) laser, showing a reduction of abnormal pigment and minimal patterning.

in up to 50% of patients, perhaps because the laser light does not eliminate deep perifollicular melanocytes [71].

Melasma can be epidermal, dermal or mixed in type, and usually responds unsatisfactorily to Q-switched laser therapy [72]. More recently, the 'microthermal treatment zones' created by fractional non-ablative devices have been claimed to function as a 'pigment escalator'. Claims have also been made for successful treatment of melasma with the 1927 nm fractional thulium fibre laser (Figure 23.23) [73]. Likewise, there are advocates of low fluence 'skin toning' with the 1064 nm Q-switched Nd:YAG laser, but multiple treatments are usually required and long-term results are unpredictable [74].

As with melasma, the response of *postinflammatory hyperpigmentation* to lasers is unpredictable: there is a significant danger of increasing skin pigmentation (Figure 23.24). *Haemosiderin* seen in association with venous stasis will only occasionally respond to laser treatment. *Drug-induced hyperpigmentation* secondary to the administration of minocycline and amiodarone responds readily to treatment with the Q-switched ruby, alexandrite and Nd:YAG lasers. Riehl melanosis and lichen planus pigmentosus show diffuse grey to blue–grey and black facial hyperpigmentation. There are no good treatment approaches but multiple sessions of low fluence Q-switched Nd:YAG may lighten pigmentation in some patients [75].

Complications of pigment lasers

Whitening and subsequent redness or pin-point bleeding are common and expected end points. The most common complications are laser burns, dyspigmentation or scarring, which are more common in pigmented or tanned skin. It is preferable to defer laser treatment until the tan has faded. Undertaking test patches prior to full treatment may also be useful, not least medicolegally. Certain tattoo pigments can darken with laser treatments and care must be taken when treating traumatic tattoos, which may consist of combustible material. Treating allergic tattoo reactions with Q-switched lasers may result in a systemic allergic reaction.

Some pigmented lesions respond better to laser treatments than others. While epidermal pigmentation in freckles and solar lentigines responds readily to lasers, melasma and postinflammatory hyperpigmentation show a variable and unpredictable response.

Good-quality, long-term efficacy data supporting the use of lasers in the treatment of congenital melanocytic naevi are lacking but the high recurrence rate is a recognised problem despite early clearance seen with laser treatment.

Hair reduction

Hair reduction is the most commonly performed laser procedure in dermatology. Apart from their use in hirsutism, hair reduction laser devices are commonly employed to treat unwanted facial and extrafacial hair in women and men. The application of these devices extends to treatment of hypertrichosis associated with conditions such as hairy congenital melanocytic naevi and pilonidal sinuses.

Light–tissue interaction

The mechanism for light-assisted hair reduction remains incompletely understood. Light is probably absorbed by melanin in the hair shaft and matrix but it is likely that heat is then transferred to the true target structures, stem cells (mainly in the bulge area of the outer root sheath) and possibly blood vessels in the papilla. The TRT of a 200–300 μm follicle is about 25–50 ms, but much shorter pulse durations also seem to be effective. It has also been shown that considerably longer pulses (30–400 ms) are effective in damaging the stem cells and papillary vessels, neither of which contain melanin nor are in direct contact with the melanin-rich components of the follicle. This observation has been explained in terms of an 'extended theory of selective photothermolysis' [6]. Follicles in early anagen are thought to be most susceptible to laser treatment because they are more superficial than in other phases. Follicular disruption is an immediate effect and is followed by conversion from the anagen to the telogen phase, with subsequent miniaturisation of the hair follicle.

Devices for hair reduction

The normal mode (long-pulsed) ruby (694 nm), alexandrite (755 nm), diode (800 nm) and Nd:YAG (1064 nm) lasers have all been used for photoepilation, as have flashlamps. Cooling is required to protect the epidermis [76].

Laser-assisted hair removal

Laser hair removal is the most commonly performed laser procedure. Although extremely useful for the treatment of hirsutism,

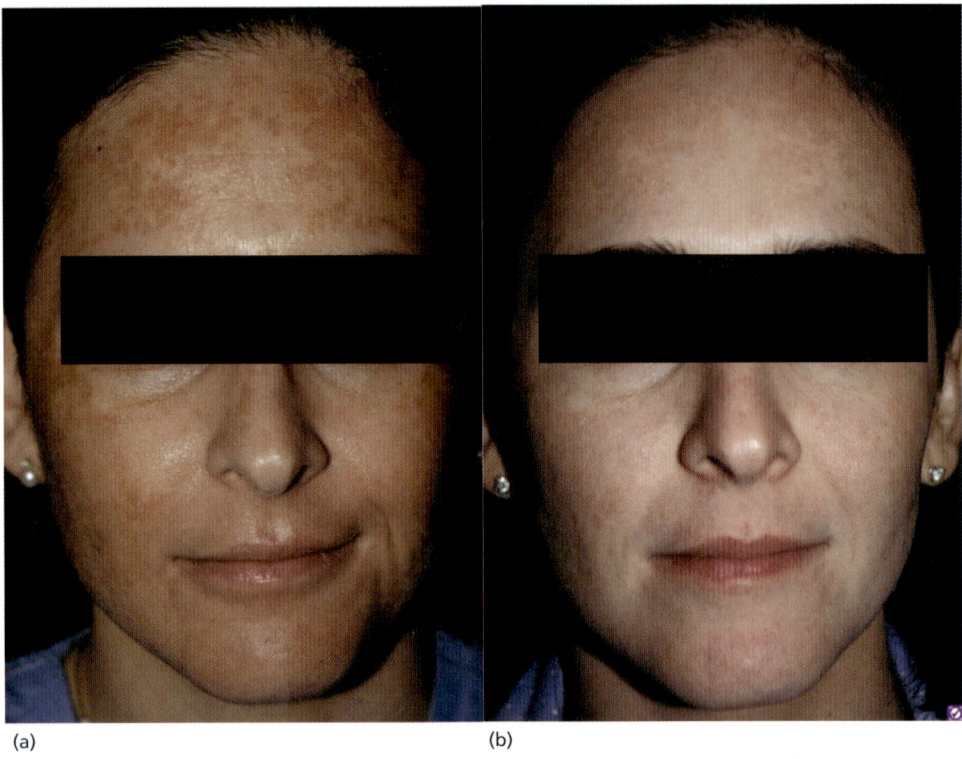

Figure 23.23 Melasma, baseline (a) and 4 months post-treatment (b).

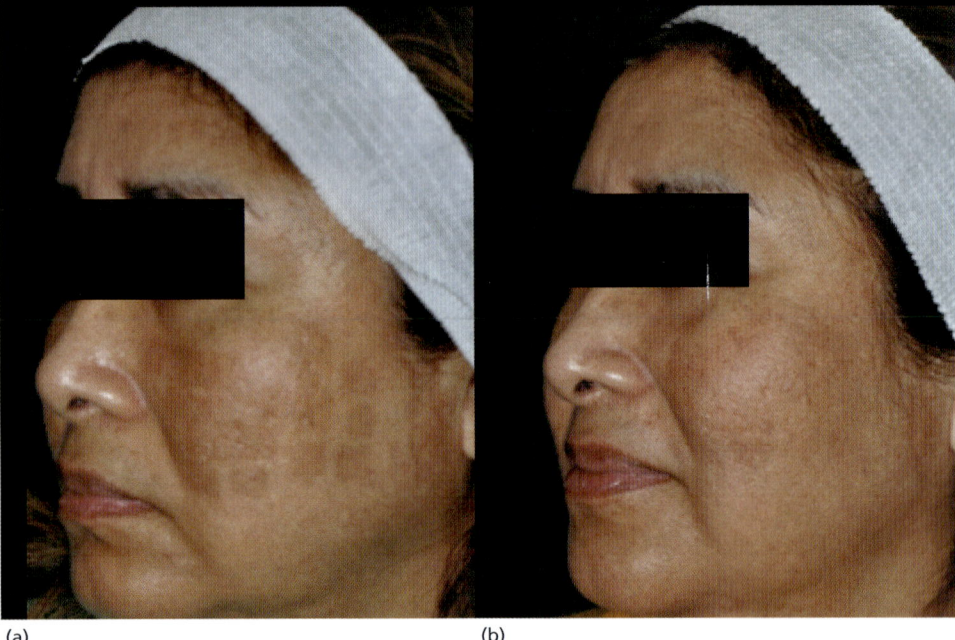

Figure 23.24 Postinflammatory hyperpigmentation, baseline (a) and following treatment (b).

many patients seek laser treatment for normal but unwanted body and facial hair (Figure 23.25), e.g. pre or post gender-confirming surgery. Patients with light skin colour and dark hair are best suited to laser hair removal. Patients should be informed that lasers may not work on light-coloured, red, grey or white hair nor on fine vellus hair.

A clinical end point of mild perifollicular redness and oedema is often recommended by manufacturers. Multiple treatments (three to six and often more) are necessary to achieve long-term reduction of hair growth. The term 'permanent hair reduction' has been loosely used in this context and is defined as a long-term, stable reduction in the number of hairs regrowing after a treatment course [77]. The number of hairs regrowing must be stable over a time period greater than the duration of the complete growth cycle of hair follicles, which varies from 4 to 12 months according to body location. Permanent hair reduction does not necessarily imply the elimination of all hairs in the treatment area [77]. Considerations such as repeated treatments as well as variable and temporary hair reduction should be included in patient selection and counselling.

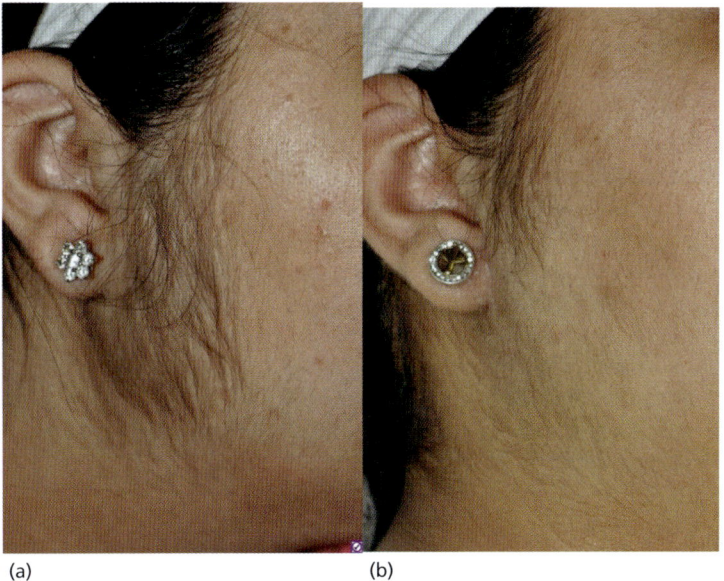

(a) (b)

Figure 23.25 Laser hair removal, baseline (a) and post-treatment (b).

Test patches are mandatory to determine the most effective treatment parameters for the patient's skin and hair type, and to judge how the skin will respond to treatment. The test patch should always be carried out in a small area, in or near the area for treatment, and if other body sites are to be treated subsequently, then a test patch must be carried out in the new treatment area.

Lasers with longer wavelengths are likely to be safer and more effective. A study of patients treated at least three times at 4–6-week intervals with the 3 ms alexandrite laser showed a mean long-term (12-month) hair reduction of 74% [78]. This was even higher in those patients with non-pigmented skin in whom higher fluences were used. Optimal results are obtained in patients with non-pigmented skin and with pigmented hair. The alexandrite laser may be best suited to treating skin phototypes I–III because of the paucity of competing epidermal melanin and, consequently, the relatively low risk of laser-induced dyspigmentation or burns. When treating darker skin phototypes, however, the 1064 nm Nd:YAG laser is preferred. Both the 810 nm diode and the Nd:YAG lasers are of comparable efficacy, but treatments with the low fluence diode laser are less painful [77]. Fair or white hair lacks melanin and is largely resistant to treatment. Flashlamps have been used to treat hypertrichosis and hirsutism, but it seems likely that subsequent blistering and dyspigmentation are more common than after laser treatment, especially in darker skin phototypes. Furthermore, when compared with the Nd:YAG laser, the flashlamp was found to be less effective in reducing axillary hair counts (54.4% versus 79.4%) [77].

Home use lasers and flashlamps are gaining popularity. They result in a hair reduction of about 30%, although there are safety concerns in the absence of clinical supervision.

Anaesthesia
Most patients require no anaesthesia, but topical anaesthetics may be needed. Preoperative analgesics may help in reducing operative discomfort. Emollients and analgesics relieve postoperative pain, swelling and redness. Sun avoidance and UV protection are advised. Concomitant cooling of the epidermis is essential.

Indications for laser hair removal
Skin and hair disorders in which laser-assisted hair removal may be beneficial are listed in Box 23.4.

Box 23.4 Medical indications for epilation lasers
[76,77,79]

- Hirsutism
- Hairy congenital naevi
- Faun tail and Becker naevi
- Hair-bearing skin grafts and flaps
- Folliculitis decalvans and dissecting folliculitis of the scalp
- Pseudofolliculitis barbae (Figure 23.26)
- Limb prosthesis in amputees
- Body odour reduction
- Pilonidal sinus
- Hidradenitis suppurativa
- Trichostasis spinulosa
- Gender-confirming laser hair removal including preoperative genital gender-confirming surgery
- Peristomal hair growth
- Hair restoration surgery to redesign frontal hairline in women

Complications of laser-assisted hair removal
There is a low incidence of usually self-limiting side effects, which depend on the laser used, the site treated and the skin type [80]. Pain, transient redness and perifollicular oedema and folliculitis

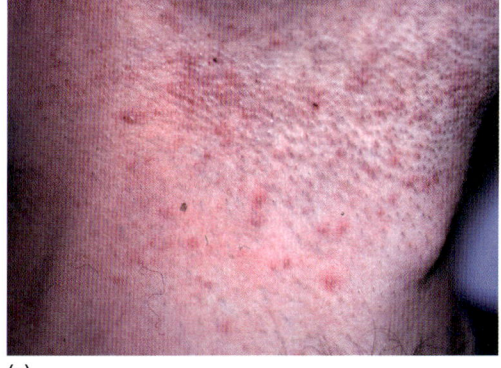 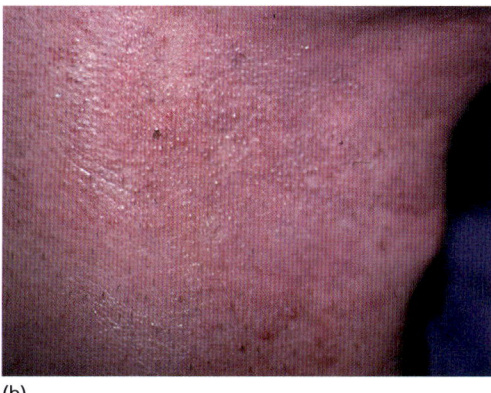

Figure 23.26 Pseudofolliculitis barbae (a) before and (b) after a treatment with a normal mode alexandrite (755 nm) laser. Residual hair is sparse and fine and there are no inflammatory lesions.

(a) (b)

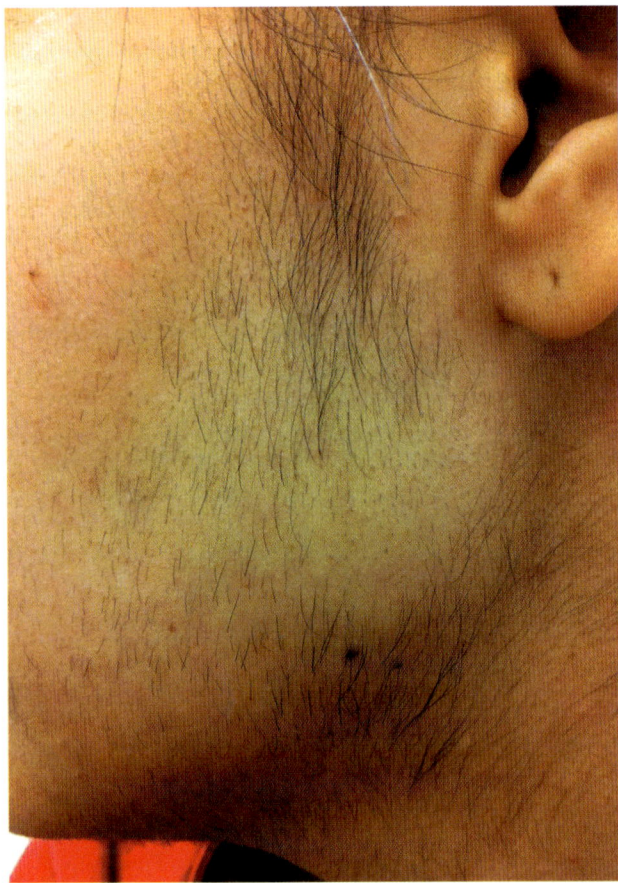

Figure 23.27 Paradoxical hypertrichosis on the neck seen after long pulsed Nd:YAG laser treatment.

are common and expected effects. Treating tanned skin, using inappropriate wavelengths for skin type and inadequate cooling of skin are some of the common causes of photoepilation laser side effects. Thermal burns resulting in blisters, hyperpigmentation or persistent hypopigmentation are uncommon and signify aggressive treatment or improper patient or laser selection. Permanent scarring is rare. Aggravation of pre-existing skin conditions, including acne, can occur.

The devices operate in the visible or near infrared region and there is therefore a risk of retinal injury. The risk of dyspigmentation is highest with the ruby laser and drops with longer wavelengths. Similarly, risk is higher in patients with pigmented skin although this can be reduced with use of the Nd:YAG laser (1064 nm). Paradoxical hypertrichosis, described as an increase in hair growth on or adjacent to the treatment site (Figure 23.27), is an uncommon side effect of treatment with all laser and IPL devices but more common in darker skin and patients with underlying hormonal imbalances, e.g. polycystic ovarian syndrome [81–83]. Subtherapeutic thermal injury induced terminal hair growth and thermally induced inflammatory response-induced activation of dormant hair follicles in untreated areas are plausible explanations [81].

Using higher laser fluences and actively cooling the neighbouring (non-treated) areas to prevent stimulation of the follicles by subtherapeutic light are recommended to treat paradoxical hair growth [83].

Photothermal ablation in the treatment of skin disorders

Light–tissue interaction

Ablation can be achieved by heating the water in the epidermis and dermis. The continuous wave carbon dioxide laser (CO_2 laser) in the far infrared region was the first laser to be used as an ablative laser. The abundance of water in the skin makes the ablative lasers tissue selective, but strictly speaking these devices do not follow the principles of selective photothermolysis. The absorption of water by the CO_2 laser makes it an ideal cutting (incising) and ablating laser.

There are two main types of applications:

1 *Incisional with haemostasis*. The CO_2 laser (10 600 nm) can be used as an incisional or resurfacing instrument. Tissue can be incised by using a high-power, focused beam that vaporises the tissue in its immediate path. The power, diameter and pulse characteristics of the beam determine the thickness of a surrounding cuff of thermal damage, which is also determined by scatter and temperature diffusion. The main advantage of thermal damage, in this context, is haemostasis.

2 *Ablative laser resurfacing*. This was performed initially with pulsed or scanned CO_2 lasers, the immediate effect of which is ablation (or vaporisation) of the epidermis and the superficial papillary dermis. In the healing period, re-epithelialisation occurs from the surrounding epidermis and from adnexal structures. There is also residual thermal damage to a band of underlying dermis, together with collagen denaturation, contraction and subsequently neo-collagenesis.

The CO_2 laser emits light that is relatively poorly absorbed by water and which therefore has a relatively high penetration (30 μm). Unless the irradiance is high, this elicits relatively little ablation compared with thermal damage (up to 300 μm) or less than was initially thought desirable. Furthermore, with each subsequent pass there is less and less ablation and more and more thermal damage as the water content drops from 80% in the epidermis to 60% in the underlying dermis. These considerations led to the development of the Er:YAG laser (2094 nm) because it emits a wavelength that is highly absorbed by water and therefore has a low penetration (3 μm). This in turn is associated with more ablation (2–4 μm per J/cm^2) and less thermal damage (10–15 μm). It soon became apparent, however, that a degree of thermal damage was necessary for haemostasis. In addition, the thermal damage that underlies CO_2 laser-treated sites may influence the thickness of subsequent fibrosis [84]. As a result, Er:YAG lasers were adapted to cause more rather than less thermal damage, in other words to make a wound more like a CO_2 laser. The differences between CO_2 and Er:YAG lasers are listed in Table 23.7. The 2790 nm erbium:yttrium-scandium-gallium-garnet (Er:YSGG) laser and plasma-emitting devices employ two further ablative modalities; the latter have gained popularity in the cosmetic sector.

Devices in common use

Carbon dioxide (10 600 nm) laser

The CO_2 laser produces light (10 600 nm) that is relatively poorly absorbed by the chromophore water, and which therefore penetrates relatively deeply (30 μm). Incisional surgery is achieved using a focused beam. For ablation, these lasers were originally operated in continuous wave, or the wave is pulsed using a rotating mirror

Table 23.7 Key differences between carbon dioxide and erbium:yttrium-aluminium-garnet (Er:YAG) lasers.

Laser	Carbon dioxide	Er:YAG
Affinity for water	High	Very high
Ablation per pass	20–60 μm	5–15 μm
Haemostasis	Yes	No
Ablation plateau	Yes	No
Residual thermal damage	150 μm	15 μm

or computerised pattern generator. Continuous wave CO_2 lasers resulted in unpredictable clinical results and scarring. Pulsed CO_2 lasers, on the other hand, deliver higher peak powers in pulsed durations which are shorter than the TRT and allow safer treatments. These systems effect ablation of up to 20–30 μm of skin per pass with a smaller residual thermal damage zone than continuous wave systems. These lasers have recently been modified to perform fractional ablative resurfacing (see the section on fractional modalities).

Er:YAG (2940 nm) laser

This laser emits light with a higher absorption coefficient for water and a lower optical penetration depth than the CO_2 laser. There is therefore limited ablation and reduced residual thermal damage. This results in efficient tissue ablation with lower recovery times and fewer side effects than seen with the CO_2 laser. Er:YAG lasers have been modified to effect the precise ablation capability of short pulse Er:YAG lasers with coagulative effects similar to those of CO_2 lasers.

Anaesthesia

Ablative treatments almost always require adequate anaesthesia. For the treatment of superficial benign lesions such as syringomas, topical anaesthesia may be adequate. For other deeper ablative or incisive procedures, local or general anaesthesia is preferred. Topical emollients are useful post procedure.

Indications for incisional and ablative laser surgery

Indications for photothermal ablation are listed in Box 23.5.

> **Box 23.5 Indications for photothermal ablation**
>
> **Malformations**
> - Epidermal naevi
> - Lymphangioma circumscriptum
>
> **Epidermal dysplasia and neoplasia**
> - Actinic keratoses and actinic cheilitis
> - Squamous cell carcinoma *in situ* (Bowen disease)
> - Porokeratosis
> - Melanoma metastases
>
> **Benign cutaneous tumours and proliferations**
> - Rhinophyma and sebaceous hyperplasia
> - Xanthelasma
> - Seborrhoeic keratoses
> - Dermatosis papulosa nigra
> - Syringomas
> - Angiofibromas
> - Familial trichoepitheliomas
> - Cylindromas
> - Hidrocystomas
> - Viral warts
> - Neurofibromas
>
> **Dermal infiltrates**
> - Xanthelasma
> - Granuloma faciale
> - Sarcoidosis
> - Amyloidosis
>
> **Miscellaneous**
> - Darier disease (keratosis follicularis)
> - Hailey–Hailey disease (familial benign chronic pemphigus)
> - Pemphigus vegetans
> - Colloid milium
>
> **Cosmetic**
> - Acne scarring
> - Rhytides

CO_2 laser incisional surgery may confer an advantage over conventional scalpel incisions on account of the associated haemostasis due to thermal damage around the beam. A potential disadvantage is that thermal damage of the apposed wound edges may result in slower healing and a more obvious scar. This technique may be most useful in making surgical wounds that are to heal by second intention. One example is the dissection of head and neck *keloids* below the hair follicles through the subcutaneous fat. Results have varied [85] but are probably better on the head than at other sites, particularly if augmented with intralesional corticosteroids before and after re-epithelialisation. A difficulty in doing or assessing studies on keloids is defining what is meant by cure, and when.

Ablative modalities remain the most effective means of resurfacing *wrinkles* and some *acne scars*, although with increased morbidity. This is explored in more detail in Chapter 161.

Epidermal dysplasia and neoplasia

CO_2 laser ablation may be a useful alternative option to topical therapies in treating *actinic cheilitis* as well as *Bowen disease* on the periungual folds and on the glans penis. Bowenoid papulosis has also been reported to respond well to ablative laser treatments [86]. *Superficial basal cell carcinomas (sBCC)* have also been managed with laser ablation, although this is unlikely to be the treatment of choice. Combined PDT and CO_2 laser treatment of small nodular and sBCC has been reported to be effective [87].

Benign cutaneous tumours and proliferations

Familial trichoepitheliomas and *angiofibromas* (Figure 23.28) can be flattened with lasers but lesions recur over time in some patients. Small angiofibromas associated with tuberous sclerosis may be better treated with PDL or topical sirolimus [88]. *Periorbital syringomas* (Figure 23.29) and *sebaceous hyperplasia* can be managed with any of a number of destructive modalities including CO_2 laser ablation. In periorbital skin, the dermis is thin and it may be difficult to ablate to a depth that does not lead to either recurrence of the lesions

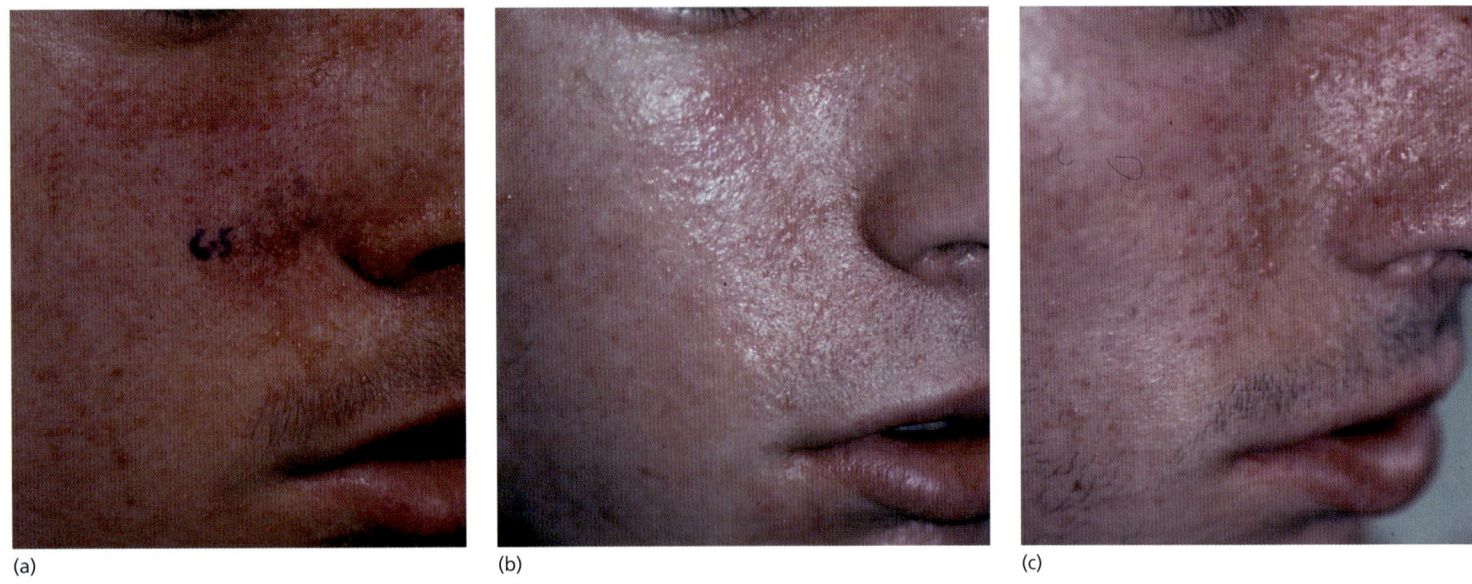

Figure 23.28 Angiofibromas (a) before, (b) 6 months after and (c) 24 months after CO_2 laser resurfacing, showing a gradual recurrence of lesions over time.

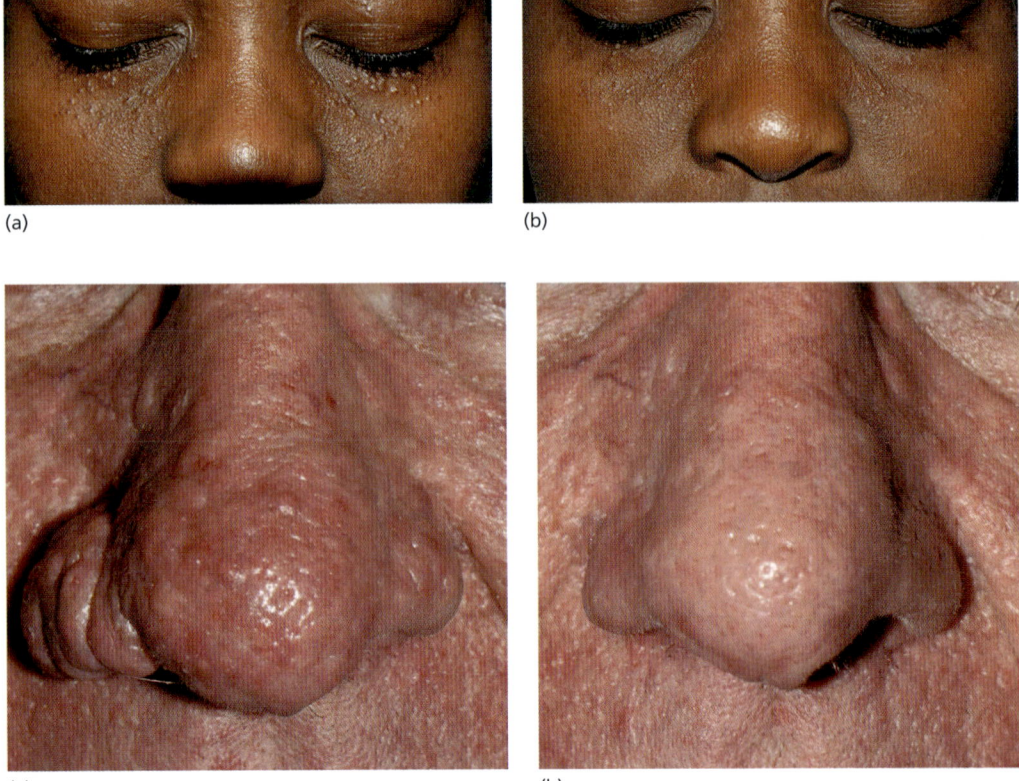

Figure 23.29 Periorbital syringomas in a patient with skin phototype VI (a) before and (b) after 3 months of treatment with a CO_2 laser.

Figure 23.30 Contouring of rhinophyma (a) before and (b) after treatment with a CO_2 laser usually produces excellent cosmetic outcomes.

or colour and texture change. *Rhinophyma* (Figure 23.30) can be recontoured for cosmetic purposes and in order to relieve nasal obstruction, when present; results are usually permanent [89].

Dermal inflammatory and other infiltrates

Granuloma faciale and facial *sarcoid* usually present with violaceous plaques and nodules. Both have been reported to respond to PDL treatment, although it seems likely that their colour owes more to the infiltrate than ectatic vessels. Plaques of granuloma faciale can be flattened with a CO_2 laser and will reform slowly, if at all [90]. Likewise, plaques and nodules of facial sarcoid can be usefully and often indefinitely debulked if the disease is stable [91]. Xanthelasmata respond well to a range of destructive techniques, including CO_2 laser surgery.

Miscellaneous

A number of other unrelated conditions have been treated with CO_2 laser ablation, of which the most relevant may be *periungual*

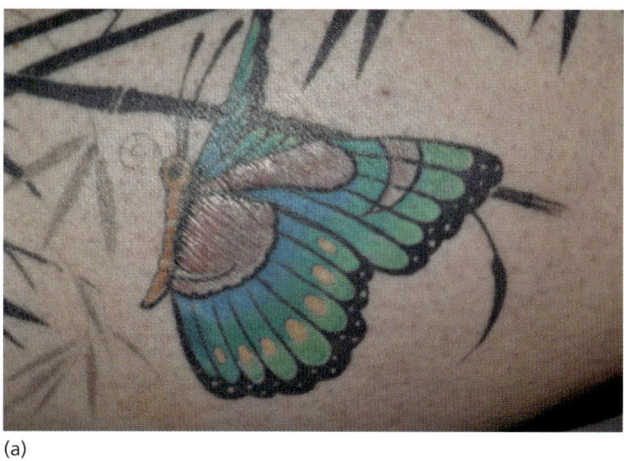
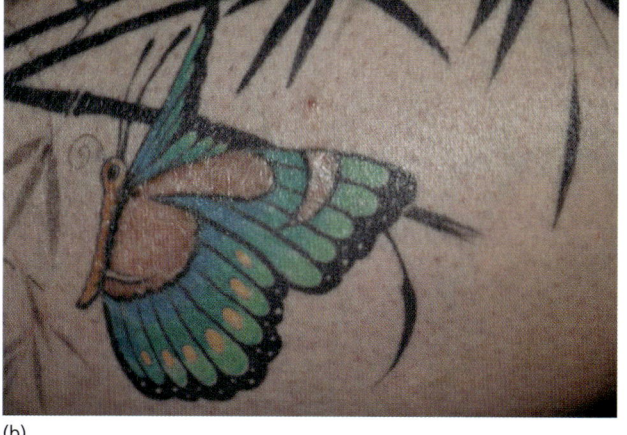

Figure 23.31 Tattoo granulomas in the centre of the tattoo (a) before and (b) after CO_2 laser ablation; they usually respond well.

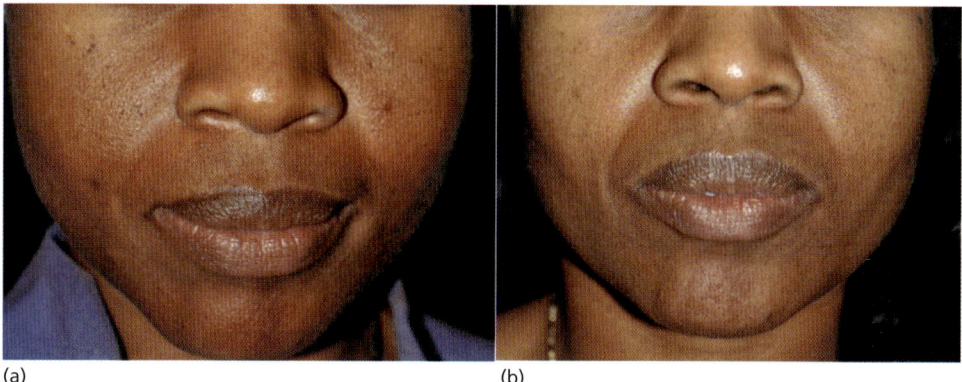

Figure 23.32 Non-ablative fractional resurfacing, baseline (a) versus following treatment (b).

and *plantar warts*, *Hailey–Hailey* and *Darier disease* and *vulval lymphangiectasia/lymphangioma* or *cysts* [92]. Non-infective, pruritic *tattoo granulomas* that have failed to respond to potent topical corticosteroids usually respond well when ablated with the CO_2 laser (Figure 23.31). Recurrent sinuses and nodules of *hidradenitis suppurativa* can be excised using the cutting mode of the CO_2 laser [93]. The dumb-bell tumours of *neurofibromatosis* can be excised using the CO_2 laser, leaving a flatter skin profile, albeit at the expense of hypopigmented scars [94].

Complications of photothermal ablation

The risk is dependent on the depth of photothermal ablation. Before re-epithelialisation, the major complication is infection, which occurs in about 4% of patients after full face resurfacing. This is usually due to staphylococci, although infections with *Candida* species and herpes simplex have also been implicated – all may cause scarring. Complications after the third week include acneform folliculitis and milia formation, contact reactions, dyspigmentation and scarring. Postoperative redness occurs in all patients and its duration is mainly a reflection of wound depth [95]. Hypopigmentation is not usually apparent until 6 months postoperatively and may be caused by loss of epidermal melanin or by underlying fibrosis. This is now quoted as one of the reasons for the swing from ablative to non-ablative resurfacing.

Most data on efficacy of ablative lasers come from case reports or case series, as conducting randomised controlled trials using ablative lasers is fraught with difficulties.

Non-ablative and fractional modalities

The prolonged healing times and side effects associated with ablative laser systems have led to the introduction of non-ablative and fractional non-ablative techniques [96]:

1 *Non-ablative resurfacing*. The aim of treatment is to selectively wound the upper dermis in order to induce dermal fibrosis (or collagen remodelling) (Figure 23.32). The epidermis is protected and retained to avoid the problems of the open wounds caused by ablative modalities. Prerequisites to this are therefore epidermal cooling systems and wavelengths that are sufficiently long to penetrate and injure the dermis. A variety of lasers (1064 and 1320 nm Nd:YAG, 1450 nm diode and 1540 nm erbium glass lasers) and flashlamps have been studied, including some originally developed for other purposes. Despite clear histological evidence of new collagen formation, clinical results with these systems are often modest. Radiofrequency and infrared devices designed to cause deep, volumetric heating and subsequent skin tightening have been used only for cosmetic purposes and are discussed in Chapter 161.

2 *Fractional non-ablative resurfacing*. This refers to the creation of microscopic treatment zones of coagulative damage to the epidermis and upper dermis. The diameter of these zones is about 100 µm and their depth and density determine the clinical response. They heal with microepidermal necrotic debris, which supposedly removes pigment, and with subsequent fibrosis [96]. The prototype was an erbium glass laser (1540 nm) that emits light through a fibre with an optical deflection and focusing

system. Other systems include 1540 and 1550 nm erbium fibre lasers, the 1320 and 1440 nm Nd:YAG lasers, the 825–1350 nm non-coherent infrared light source and the 1927 nm thulium fibre laser. Indications for fractional non-ablative systems include acne scarring, fine rhytides and, supposedly, melasma [97].

3 *Fractional ablative resurfacing*. This occupies a place between fractional non-ablative modalities on the one hand and ablative resurfacing on the other. Efficacy is greater than with non-ablative techniques but so are recovery times and complication rates. Both CO_2 and Er:YAG laser systems have been fractionated and are largely used for cosmetic indications, principally for acne scarring and wrinkles.

Apart from lasers, unipolar, bipolar and multipolar radiofrequency devices have been designed to effect non-ablative cosmetic skin tightening (see Chapter 160). *Sublative radiofrequency* refers to fractionated bipolar radiofrequency energy that is delivered in a manner that has the most impact on the dermis. Epidermal change is minimal, thus limiting the incidence of side effects such as hyperpigmentation [98].

Low-power lasers

There is anecdotal and conflicting evidence relating to the use of low-power lasers and light-emitting diodes for expediting wound healing and for treating aphthous ulcers. Increases in collagen synthesis and the stimulation of immune pathways have been proposed as mechanisms of action [99].

Laser-assisted lipolysis

Light, currently mainly at 1440 nm ('water selective') and 924/975 nm ('fat selective'), can be transmitted through optical fibres introduced directly into the subcutaneous fat to produce cellular damage to both the adipocyte and fibrous septa [100]. This may represent a safe and effective method of reducing small accumulations of body fat. As with conventional liposuction, larger volumes of laser-damaged fat can be aspirated. Advantages to laser-assisted lipolysis may be shorter procedures and concomitant tissue tightening. Devices employing ultrasound, radiofrequency, infrared light and cryolipolysis have been used to similar effect.

Key references

The full list of references can be found in the online version at https://www.wiley.com/rooksdermatology10e

5 Anderson RR, Parrish JA. Selective photothermolysis: precise microsurgery by selective absorption of pulsed radiation. *Science* 1983;220:524–7.
11 Dierickx CC, Casparian JM, Venugopalan V *et al*. Thermal relaxation of portwine stain vessels probed in vivo: the need for 1–10 millisecond laser pulse treatment. *J Invest Dermatol* 1995;105:709–14.
28 Chang C-J, Nelson JS. Cryogen spray cooling and higher fluence pulsed dye laser treatment improve port-wine stain clearance while minimizing epidermal damage. *Dermatol Surg* 1999;25:767–72.
34 Savas JA, Ledon JA, Franca K, Chacon A, Nouri K. Pulsed dye laser-resistant port-wine stains: mechanisms of resistance and implications for treatment. *Br J Dermatol* 2013;168:941–53.
51 Vrijman C, van Drooge AM, Limpens J *et al*. Laser and intense pulsed light therapy for the treatment of hypertrophic scars: a systematic review. *Br J Dermatol* 2011;165:934–42.
56 Saedi N, Metelitsa A, Petrell K, Arndt KA, Dover JS. Treatment of tattoos with a picosecond alexandrite laser: a prospective trial. *Arch Dermatol* 2012;148:1360–3.
81 Town G, Bjerring P. Is paradoxical hair growth caused by low-level radiant exposure by home-use laser and intense pulsed light devices? *J Cosmet Laser Ther* 2016;18:355–62.
88 Wataya-Kaneda M, Ohno Y, Fujita Y *et al*. Sirolimus gel treatment vs placebo for facial angiofibromas in patients with tuberous sclerosis complex: a randomized clinical trial. *JAMA Dermatol* 2018;154:781–8.
96 Manstein D, Herron GS, Sink RK *et al*. Fractional photothermolysis: a new concept for cutaneous remodelling using microscopic patterns of thermal injury. *Lasers Surg Med* 2004;34:426–38.

CHAPTER 24

Principles of Radiotherapy

Charles G. Kelly, John Frew and Najibah Mahtab
Northern Centre for Cancer Care, Freeman Hospital, Newcastle upon Tyne, UK

Introduction, 24.1
Ionising radiation in the treatment of skin cancer, 24.1
X-ray photon beams: megavoltage and kilovoltage X-ray therapy, 24.1
Electron beams, 24.1
Proton beam therapy for skin cancers, 24.2
Brachytherapy, moulds, applicators and implants, 24.3
Superficial radiotherapy treatment technique, 24.3
Megavoltage X-ray therapy technique, 24.3

Radiosensitivity, 24.4
Indications for radiotherapy, 24.4
Benign disease, 24.4
Keloids, 24.7
Malignant skin disease, 24.8
Radiotherapy for particular skin sites: basal cell and squamous cell carcinoma, 24.10
Radiotherapy for particular skin tumours, 24.12
Acute radiation reaction (acute radiodermatitis), 24.18

Management, 24.18
Late radiation reaction (chronic radiodermatitis), 24.18
Tumour recurrence after radiotherapy, 24.20
Radiation-induced tumours, 24.21
Management, 24.21
Rare tumours associated with previous irradiation, 24.21
Key references, 24.21

Introduction

The clinical effects of ionising radiation on the skin have been known since the discovery of X-rays in 1895 [1,2]. Initially, both benign and malignant skin conditions were irradiated and dose and clinical indications were chosen empirically with little knowledge of the late effects of radiation on skin and subcutaneous tissue. Indications for treating benign disease by irradiation have declined since the advent of topical steroids.

It is in the best interest of patients with skin tumours to be seen in a clinic where the expertise of specialists in radiotherapy and oncology, plastic surgery and Mohs micrographic surgery as well as dermatology is present, and this has been achieved with the mandatory development of multidisciplinary team meetings and clinics in the UK as described in improving outcomes guidance [3].

Ionising radiation in the treatment of skin cancer

X-ray photon beams: megavoltage and kilovoltage X-ray therapy

X-rays are part of the electromagnetic spectrum, of shorter wavelength and more energetic than ultraviolet (UV) light. The most commonly used form of therapeutic radiation is megavoltage radiotherapy using energies of greater than 1 million electron volts (>1 MeV), delivered by linear accelerators in the treatment of deep-seated tumours. Previously, these beams have usually not been suitable for the treatment of skin cancers because of their greater penetration and skin-sparing properties, but that has changed in the

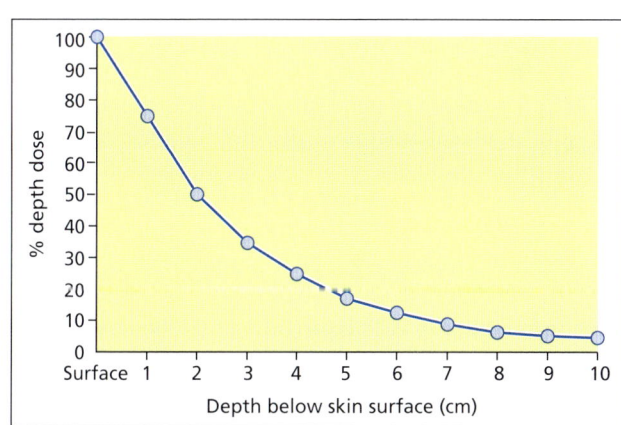

Figure 24.1 Approximate per cent depth dose values for 90 kV superficial X-ray beam.

last few years with advances in beam delivery technology, although megavoltage beams are still only used for a small minority of skin cancer patients and in particular clinical situations. X-rays in the kilovoltage range (50–140 kV) are very suitable for treating skin cancer as their maximum energy is deposited on the surface. Fall-off subsequently is exponential (Figure 24.1), and some radiation dose does reach underlying subcutaneous structures. Higher-kilovoltage beams can be used for thicker tumours.

Electron beams

Beta rays are electrons and can be derived from radioactive isotopes, such as strontium-90, or be produced by a linear accelerator. An electron beam differs from a superficial X-ray beam or other photon beams, as the energy does not fall off exponentially as the beam goes through tissue but builds up to a peak and then falls off rapidly

Rook's Textbook of Dermatology, Tenth Edition. Edited by Christopher Griffiths, Jonathan Barker, Tanya Bleiker, Walayat Hussain and Rosalind Simpson.
© 2024 John Wiley & Sons Ltd. Published 2024 by John Wiley & Sons Ltd.

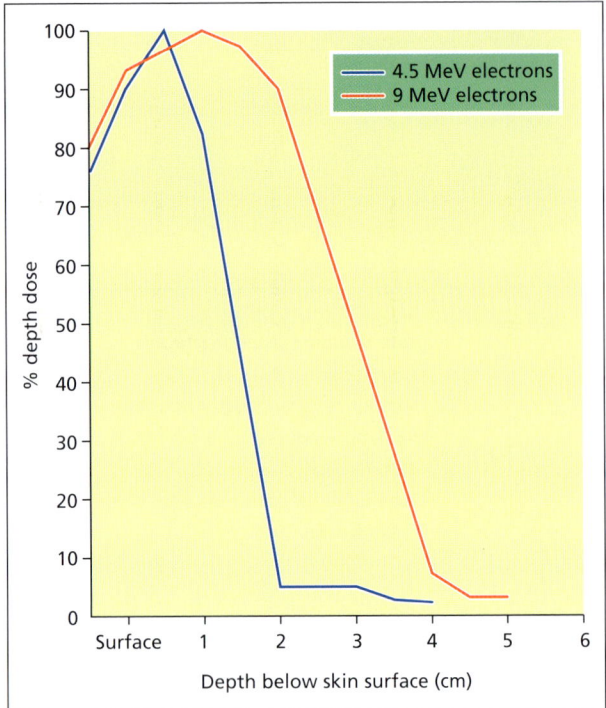

Figure 24.2 Approximate per cent depth dose curves for 4.5 and 9 MeV electron beams.

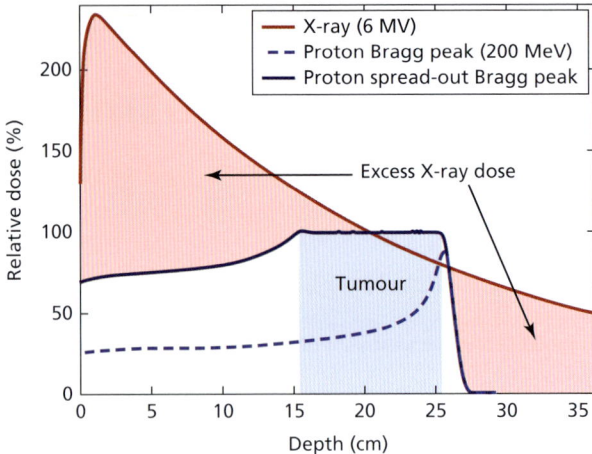

Figure 24.3 Proton depth–dose curve. Reproduced from [1] with permission from Nature Publishing Group.

(Figure 24.2). The depth of penetration is proportional to the energy of the beam. A useful treatment depth in centimetres is approximately one-third of the energy of the beam, so a 4.5 MeV electron beam will be useful for treating to a depth of 1.5 cm, and a 12 MeV beam to a depth of 4 cm. The width at the peak of the beam also increases with electron energy, giving more of the plateau at the peak at higher energies, as shown by the representation of the 9 MeV beam shape in Figure 24.2. This can be useful when trying to enclose all of a thick tumour within the highest-energy part of the beam. To avoid skin sparing, tissue equivalent material such as wax or paraffin gauze is applied over the tumour so that energy is deposited in this 'build-up' material, moving the beam peak left towards the skin surface in Figure 24.2.

Superficial X-ray therapy is indicated for the majority of skin cancer treatments. However, there is a theoretically slightly higher risk of late bone and cartilage necrosis with this modality (<5%), as X-rays are absorbed proportionally more in high-molecular-weight tissues than in soft tissue, but this is uncommon in clinical practice. Electrons are absorbed similarly in all tissues, and have the advantage of sparing sensitive underlying tissues. These may be the modality of choice for tumours on the pinna, scalp, dorsum of the hand and tibia. Superficial X-rays have been used successfully in the past in these sites [1], but electrons are now preferred [2].

Unfortunately, in practice, electrons have a limited use in the treatment of common skin cancers. As an electron beam is produced by a linear accelerator, which is much larger than a superficial X-ray machine, the treatment applicator is unwieldy and the minimum applicator size on the skin is 4 cm^2 for a reliable dose calculation. Air cavities can give unacceptable dose inhomogeneity with electrons, and eye shielding is not possible for the treatment of periorbital tumours. Setting up treatment fields with electrons is often more time consuming than with superficial X-ray therapy.

It is possible to irradiate the whole skin area with an electron beam [3–8]. The minimal depth dose characteristics that may be achieved avoid the irradiation of subcutaneous structures, which would occur if X-ray therapy that is absorbed exponentially was used. This technique is used in the treatment of mycosis fungoides [4]. Multiple radiation fields are combined to give a homogeneous dose to the whole skin down to a depth of approximately 1 cm.

Proton beam therapy for skin cancers

Proton beam therapy is a type of radiotherapy that uses protons (positively charged particles) rather than X-rays to treat cancer. The characteristic of the proton beam depth dose curve is unique in the sense that the dose peaks (also known as the Bragg peak) at a well-defined point of tissue, and allows for rapid fall-off in dose at the end of the energy deposition curve (Figure 24.3). This effectively allows the delivery of high radiation doses to tumour cells and very low or zero doses to the normal cells, protecting nearby critical structures such as the orbit, spinal cord and base of skull from radiotherapy collateral damage.

Non-melanoma skin cancers of the head and neck, in particular squamous cell carcinomas, can rarely present with extensive perineural infiltration with extension of disease involving the base of skull. These tumours benefit from adjuvant radiotherapy due to their high risk for local recurrence. However, radiotherapy planning poses a challenge as radical doses of up to 65 Gray (Gy), in 2 Gy per fraction, are normally recommended and the base of skull structures, optic nerves/chiasm and brainstem dose tolerance is a limiting factor in being able to encompass the target volume adequately. In this situation, the advantages of proton beam therapy may allow optimal conformity.

There is one reported study [2] that presents one centre's experience in treating this subset of patients with proton beam therapy. A total of 21 patients received treatment with both primary and postoperative proton beam therapy, and 71% also received concurrent systemic therapy; 5/21 patients recurred locally at a median of 0.6 years, 5/21 recurred regionally at 1.7 years. The 3-year overall survival was 50%. It was concluded that proton beam therapy may

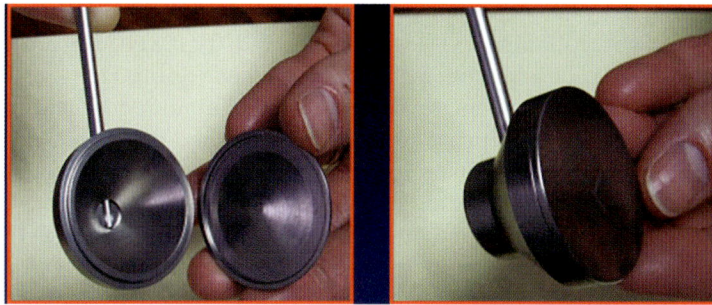

Figure 24.4 Brachytherapy applicator for skin cancer. When in use, a radioactive source is sent along the tube and a homogeneous radiation dose is then distributed through the flat end, which is applied directly to the skin tumour.

be an effective treatment option for this select group of patients, and the nerves at risk of lesion recurrence should be irradiated electively.

Proton beam therapy is available in a small number of cancer treatment centres worldwide, and should be considered as an alternative mode of therapy for head and neck skin cancers with infiltrative perineural invasion. Proton treatment, if available, is also used for uveal melanoma.

Brachytherapy, moulds, applicators and implants

Other treatment modalities available for the irradiation of skin cancer, but used less commonly, use a brachytherapy 'mould', which is a cast loaded with radioactive material applied to the surface of the tumour and secured in place for the required treatment time, or use interstitial brachytherapy as described later in this chapter for the treatment of keloids [1,2]. Brachytherapy or treatment at a 'short distance' is when a radioactive source is placed close to the area to be treated (Figure 24.4). The use of these techniques has seen a slight renaissance in some countries with the introduction of more modern applicators [3]. Cosmetic results are good but there is a need for hospital admission for radiation protection reasons and results depend on local expertise [4,5,6].

Superficial radiotherapy treatment technique

The superficial X-ray tube is manoeuvrable, and the patient can be made comfortable on a treatment couch with an applicator resting on the skin to be treated (Figure 24.5). The tumour and a margin of normal tissue are treated with a standard applicator. If the tumour is an irregular shape in two dimensions, a piece of lead shielding 1.5 mm thick can be 'cut out' in the shape of the skin to be treated, and the applicator rests on this (Figure 24.6). The individual surface area for treatment is measured and the treatment time adjusted by calculation, giving the number of machine units which have to be delivered for each treatment.

Once the applicator is in position, the radiographer leaves the treatment room. Treatments last for a few minutes on each occasion, and the patient is watched throughout using a remote camera system or special glass window.

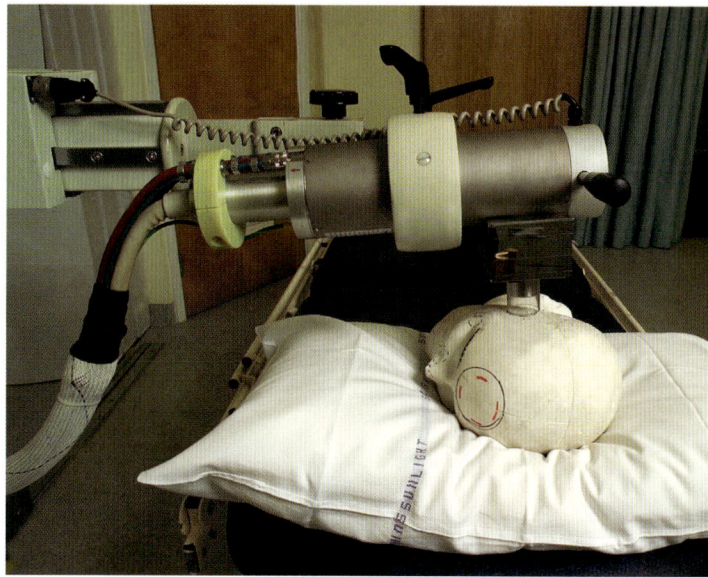

Figure 24.5 Superficial X-ray machine.

Megavoltage X-ray therapy technique

While kilovoltage beams remain the most common modality to treat skin tumours, developments in radiotherapy technology have increased interest in the use of megavoltage X-ray therapy in treating superficial skin lesions. The development of intensity modulated radiotherapy (IMRT) has enabled techniques where energy from megavoltage beams can be delivered separately and distinctly into individual, small tissue volumes, building up complex 3D photon distributions with different doses delivered to specific areas adjacent to each other and with no or very little dose being given to areas containing organs at risk (OAR).

These advances in technology have allowed developments such as a 'bathing cap' distribution, as seen in Figure 24.7, which allows homogeneous dose distribution across the skin of the scalp with rapid dose fall-off below the surface tissues, resulting in much less dose being delivered to the underlying brain.

Modern linear accelerators have machine heads that revolve around a patient with the beam being delivered as multiple small beamlets within the treatment beam, which can all be adjusted individually with regard to the radiation energy deposited. Using spiral or arc movements and varying beamlet deposition, widely differing dose distributions can be built up in separate, very small patient volumes or 'voxels' (similar in concept to children's building blocks). This allows the build-up of very complex 3D distribution patterns for individual patients.

These new megavoltage IMRT techniques are also useful whenever a relatively high homogeneous surface dose is required with sparing of underlying or neighbouring structures (OAR).

A further example of a 'stocking' distribution is shown in Figure 24.8a and b, where an appropriate dose can be delivered homogeneously to the foot and ankle of a patient with skin lymphoma, sparing underlying tissues. The benefit of using this method of treatment can be seen in Figure 24.8c and d before and

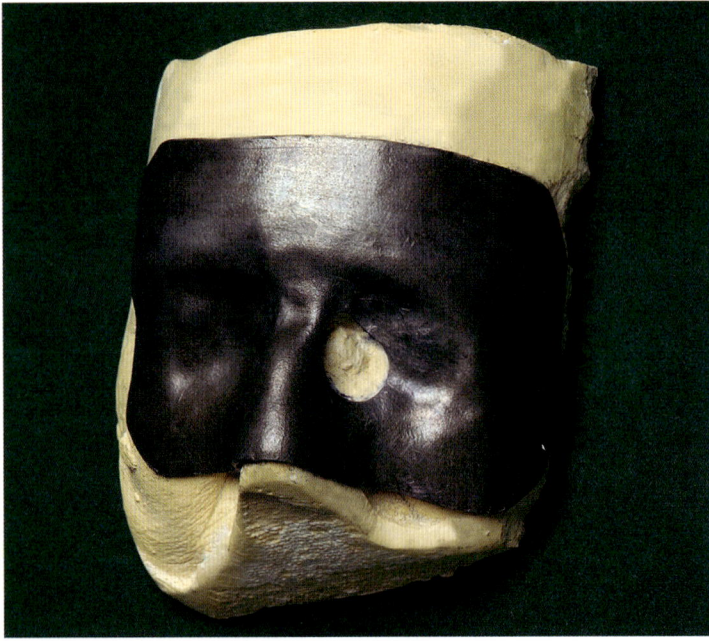

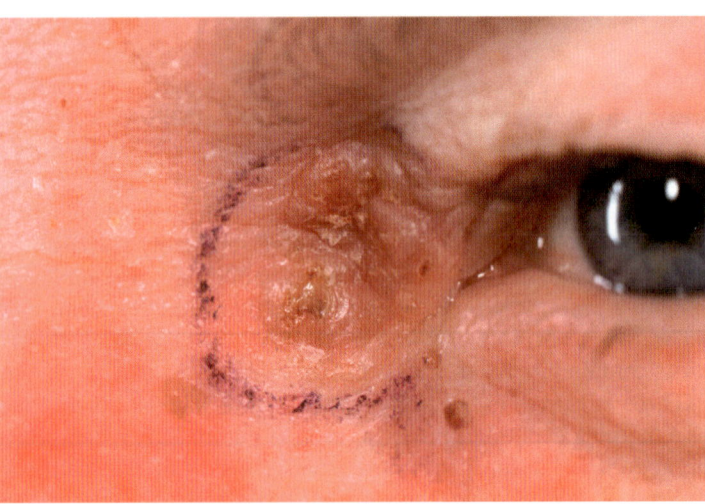

Figure 24.6 (a) Lead mask with area for treatment 'cut out'. (b) Basal cell carcinoma to be treated in this manner.

after treatment. The foot and lower leg were held in position for treatment using the immobilisation device in Figure 24.8e.

Radiosensitivity

All radiation is destructive. The basis of radiotherapy is that abnormal cells are more radio-responsive than differentiated cells. Radio-responsiveness and radio-curability are dissimilar and are functions of differences in cell population kinetics, so a rapidly resolving cancer may recur and a slowly resolving tumour may be completely cured. Radiotherapy is usually given as a fractionated course, as the intervals between doses allow for the recovery of normal cells. The effect of a dose of radiation is reduced by increasing the number of fractions in which it is given or by lengthening the total overall treatment time. The effect of irradiation can be modified by anoxia, infection, oedema, trauma and any inborn genetic susceptibility. The face tolerates irradiation well and radical dosages may be accompanied by good cosmetic results [1].

When irradiating benign conditions, the minimum dose and the lowest voltage appropriate to achieve the desired effect should be chosen. The threat of radiation carcinogenesis must clearly be seen in the context of the clinical indication for treatment. There is a threshold for somatic radiation changes that should not be breached in the treatment of benign conditions. The late radiation sequelae of treatment given many years ago are inexcusable with modern standards of dosimetry and equipment, and should not be seen in the treatment of benign diseases today [2,3].

Indications for radiotherapy

Benign disease

Some of the misconceptions about the role of radiotherapy have arisen because of its widespread use in the past for the treatment of benign conditions. X-ray production was discovered in 1895, and soon afterwards it was noted that the antiproliferative effect of low-energy X-rays was advantageous in the short term in a variety of visible tumours and benign dermatoses, and sometimes multiple re-treatments were offered. There was, however, no dose measurement apart from the biological effect of 'skin erythema', no radiation protection for workers or patients, and no appreciation of the late effects of radiodermatitis, leukaemia and other malignancies, and of skin cancer induction after a very long latent period.

Radiation epilation for tinea capitis, a treatment offered widely in Europe, effectively demonstrates the concept of radiation carcinogenesis. In Israel, between 1946 and 1960 over 20 000 immigrant children were treated with radiation soon after their arrival, by government order, with twice the subsequent incidence of cancer, usually of the brain, head and neck [1]. Skin cancers induced by this treatment have a very long latent period, often over 30 years, and cases treated in the 1930s and 1940s have been seen until recently in cancer treatment centres in the UK (Figure 24.9). For a fascinating and well-illustrated discussion of these early treatments and their consequences see Mould [2].

Radiotherapy is used much less now in the management of benign skin conditions than formerly and then usually only after other treatment modalities have failed or are contraindicated. Its use for benign conditions such as arthritis has been practised more in Europe than the UK. In some conditions, such as psoriasis and eczema, there is a response to radiotherapy but often the benefit is only temporary [3–8]. This coupled with the risk of late radiation-induced malignancy has led to the decline in its use in all but the most refractory of cases. It is also still used occasionally in the management of keratoacanthoma where the differentiation from squamous cell carcinoma (SCC) cannot be made with complete confidence [9,10]. Other rare uses are in Darier disease [7], familial benign chronic pemphigus [7] and acropustulosis of Hallopeau.

Recent UK National Institute for Health and Care Excellence (NICE) guidance on the use of Grenz rays, which are very low-kilovolt X-rays absorbed chiefly in the epidermis, advises that the evidence for their safety and efficiency is very limited, and that their use in inflammatory skin conditions be limited to

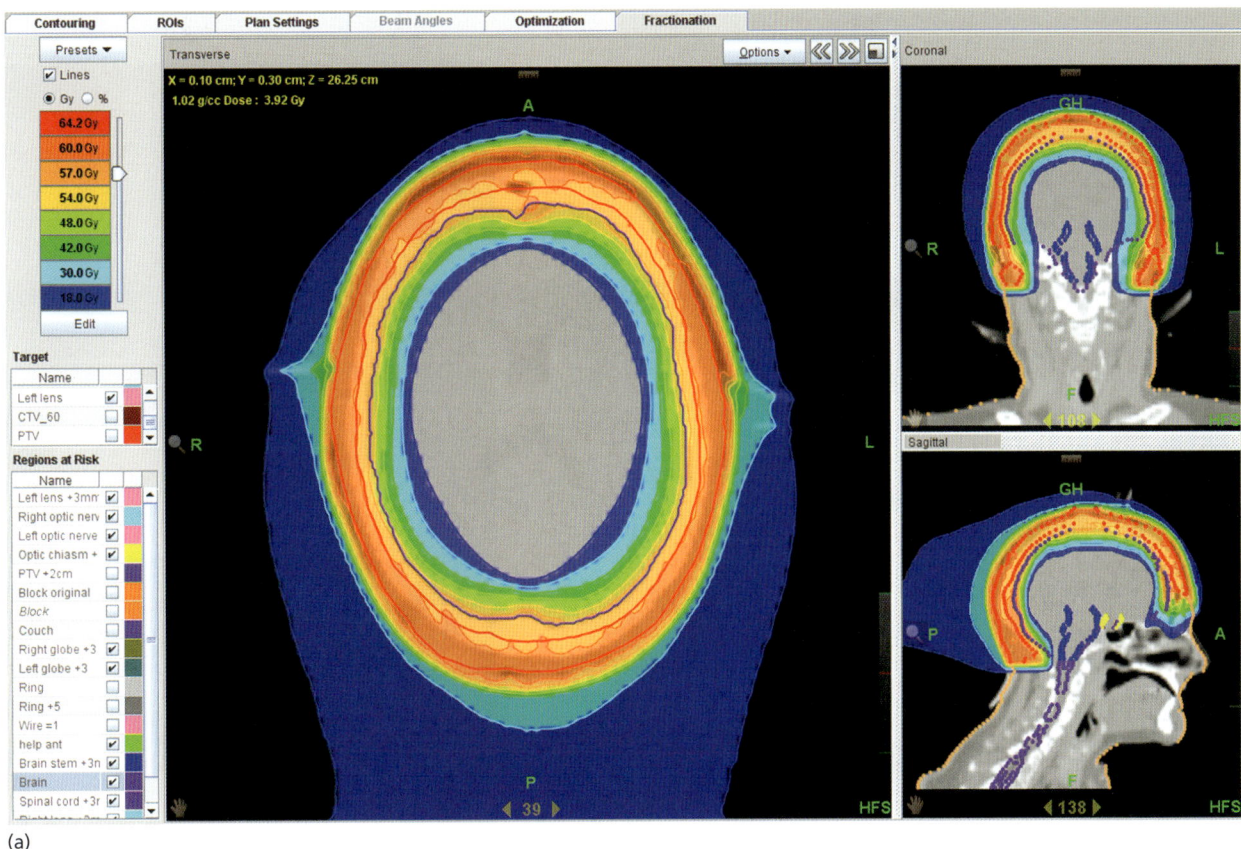

(a)

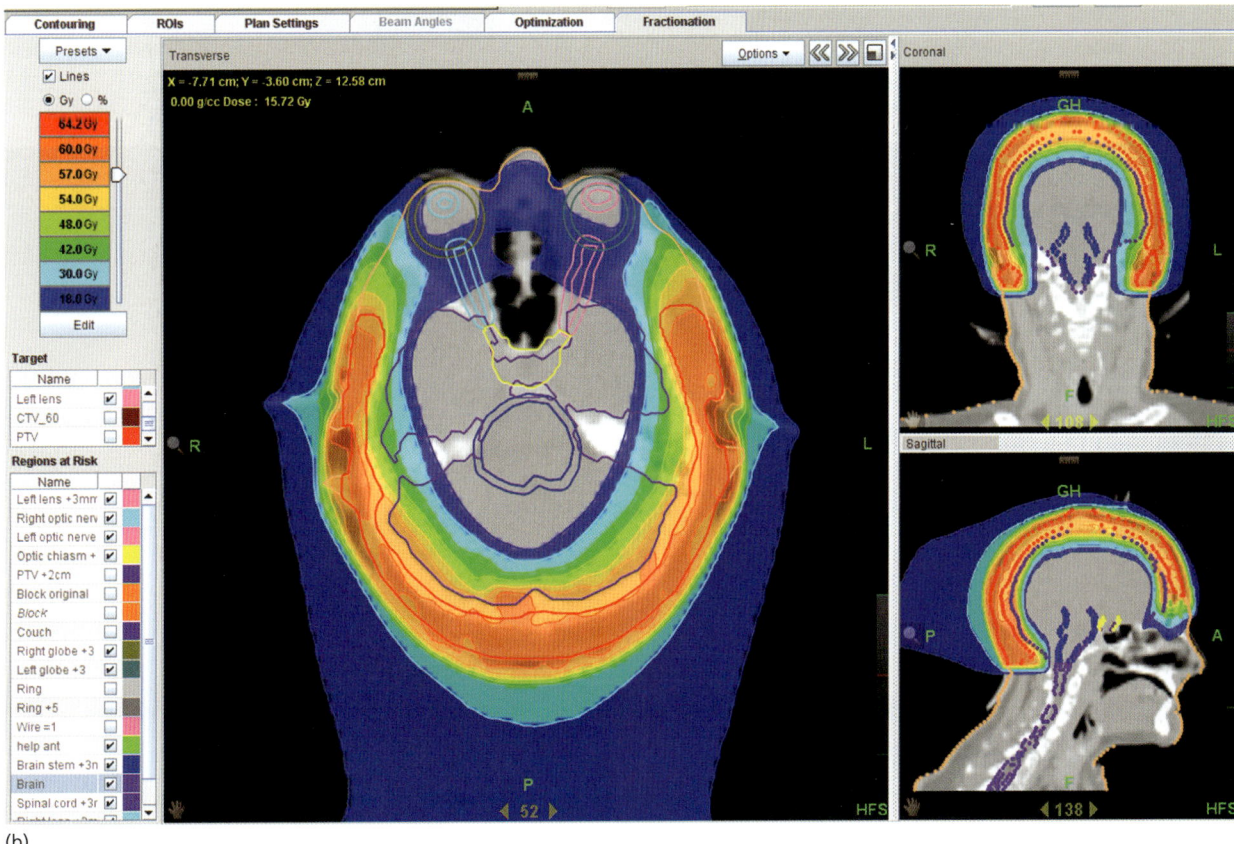

(b)

Figure 24.7 (a) 'Bathing cap' distribution showing minimal radiotherapy dose to the eyes, optic nerves and chiasm. (b) 'Bathing cap' showing high radiotherapy dose to the skin of the scalp and reducing dose to the brain.

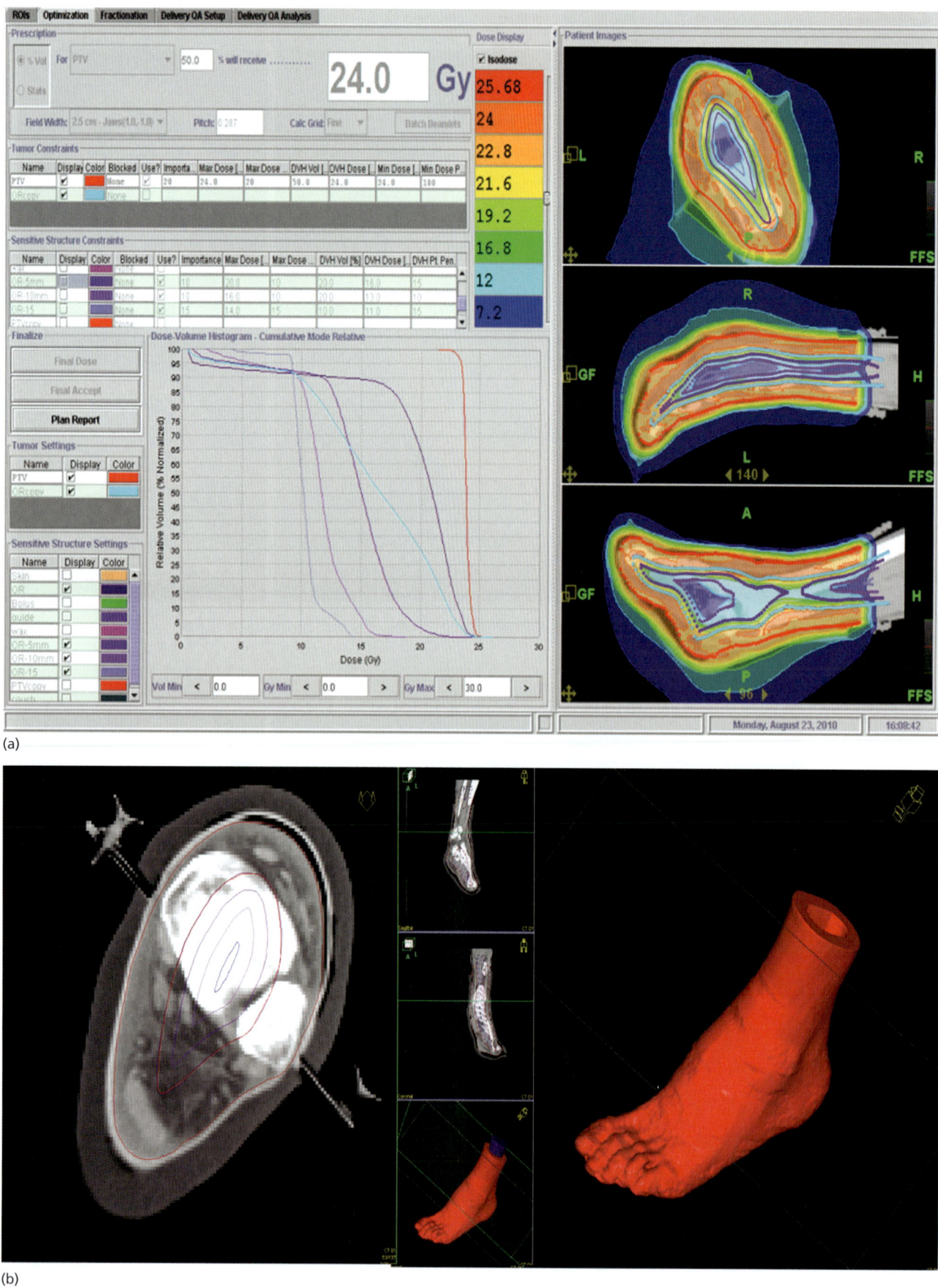

Figure 24.8 (a) Homogeneous dose distribution over the skin of the foot, ankle and lower leg using intensity modulated radiotherapy (IMRT). (b) Dose distribution for IMRT treatment of the foot, ankle and lower leg showing high-dose delivery to the skin with reducing dose to the centre of the limb. (c) Before and (d) after treatment for skin lymphoma lesions using IMRT. (e) Immobilisation device for set-up in (c) and (d) to enable very accurate dose to be given with no limb movement. © Newcastle upon Tyne Hospitals NHS Foundation Trust.

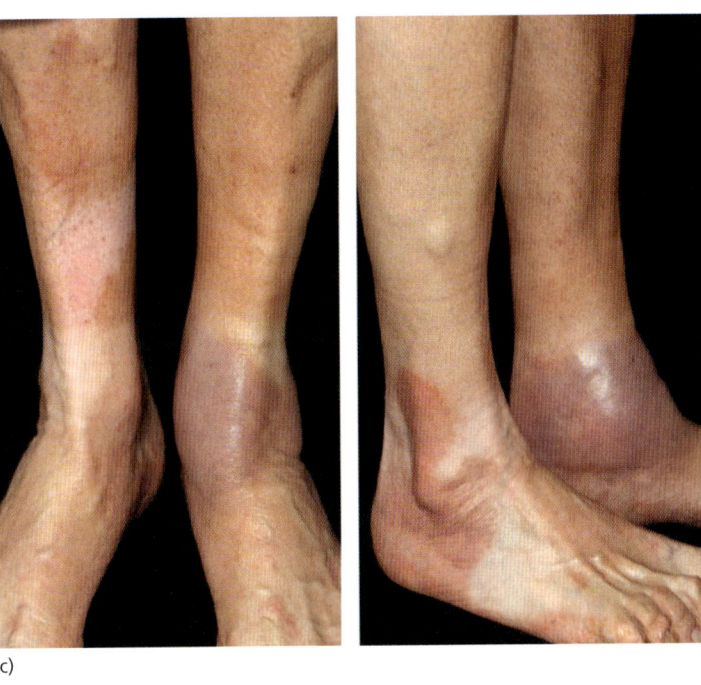
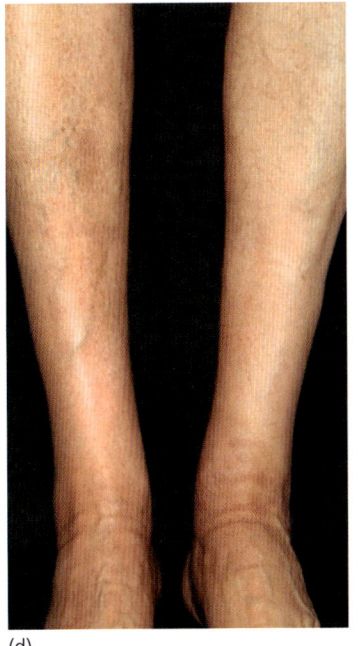
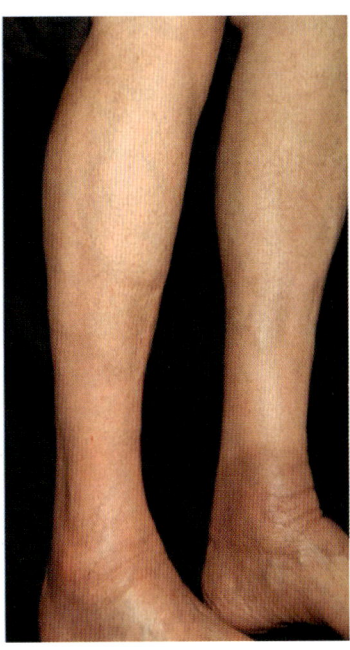
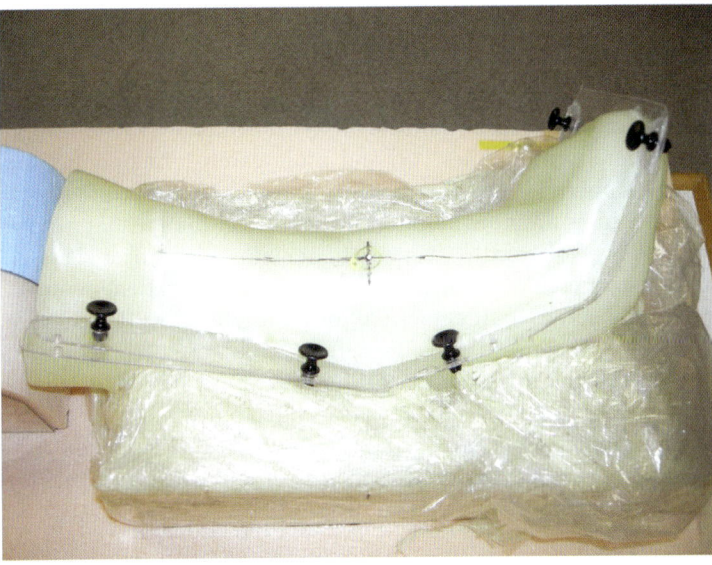

Figure 24.8 (*Continued*)

carefully selected patients who are refractory to other treatments, and preferably under trial conditions or at least with national data collection [3,7,11].

Keloids (Chapter 94)

These represent the most common benign condition now treated with radiotherapy. Intractable keloids resistant to intralesional steroids or other conventional treatment may respond well to radiation. Excision of the keloid with early irradiation of the scar is more successful, but in some sites, for example the tip of the shoulder or upper middle chest where surgery is inadvisable, good response of pain, itch and redness can be achieved with some regression of the keloid itself. Relatively high doses are necessary; these will cause temporary pigmentation, which will remain for many months in pigmented skin. Doornbos *et al.* [1] noted that 17 of 18 unexcised keloids that were less than a year old regressed with 1500 cGy given in three treatments over 6 days at 120 kV. Older keloids respond less well to irradiation. The most satisfactory management of keloids is postexcision irradiation where a dose–response relationship can be seen. Total doses less than 900 cGy, irrespective of fractionation and postsurgical interval, did not prevent recurrence. Three doses of 400 cGy were given by Kovalic and Perez [2] with a 73% success rate. Using the commonly employed dose of 900 cGy, Lo *et al.* [3] described an 85% success rate and Borok *et al.* [4] a 96% response rate. No late sequelae or carcinogenesis was described by any of the previously quoted authors with follow-up in excess of 30 years.

As well as using superficial X-rays or electron beam radiotherapy [5], treatment can be given using a radioactive iridium wire implant. With the latter technique, at the time of excision a small

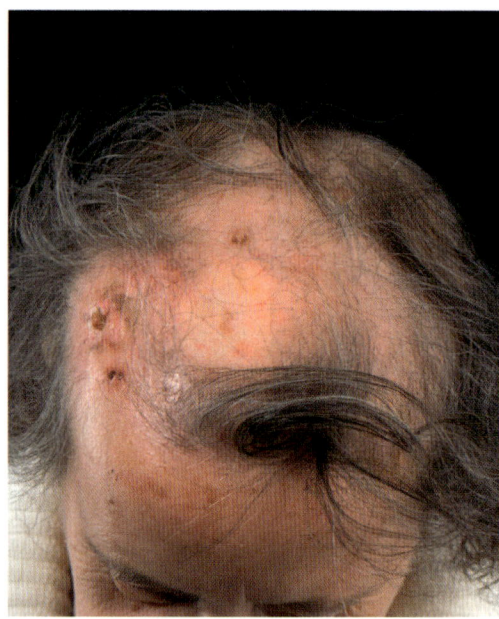

Figure 24.9 Late sequelae after radiation treatment for ringworm – atrophy, pigmentation change, alopecia, telangiectasia and multiple basal cell carcinomas.

plastic tube is inserted below the incision with both ends of the tube exposed. The patient is then transferred to the radiotherapy department within 24 h and the tube is loaded with iridium wire and the scar irradiated to a dose of 20 Gy at 2 mm from the wire over 2 days [6]. Escarmant *et al.* [7] described the results of treating 783 keloid scars in 544 patients with interstitial iridium implants. Skin applicators using either high-dose rate or low-dose rate brachytherapy have also been used [8].

Malignant skin disease

Basal cell carcinoma and squamous cell carcinoma of the skin (Chapters 140 and 141)

For most small basal cell carcinomas (BCC) or SCC without nodal involvement, surgical excision or radiotherapy will give excellent cure rates [1–4,**5**].

Superficial radiotherapy has a long history in the successful treatment of BCC and SCC. Nearly 1700 such patients received treatment in 1945 at the Queensland Radium Institute [6]. A number of mature series have been reported, dated from 1947 onwards [7], and have shown cure rates of 90% or over.

The incidence of both SCC and BCC is increasing rapidly but the number of patients referred with these tumours for radiotherapy does not reflect the increasing incidence, despite radiotherapy showing good treatment outcomes with low toxicity [8]. The American Society for Radiation Oncology has recently produced guidelines for the primary and adjuvant use of radiotherapy in patients with SCC or BCC from the evidence available [9].

Treatment of choice

If cure is the intention, then surgery and radiotherapy are the treatment options, although a variety of other modalities including cryotherapy, curettage, photodynamic therapy and topical therapies (e.g. imiquimod) may be appropriate for certain tumours [10,11,**12**,13–16].

The decision as to which is the most appropriate modality will depend on several factors. These include the size, depth and location of the tumour, any involvement of underlying tissues and the likely functional and cosmetic outcome. The majority of low-risk BCC can be managed satisfactorily by simple surgical techniques with good cosmesis and low recurrence rates. For larger BCC and SCC in critical sites, particularly around the eyes, ears and nose, Mohs micrographic surgery followed by appropriate surgical reconstruction is now widely used (Chapter 20). Radiotherapy should, however, still be considered as a valuable treatment option, and in some clinical situations as useful as surgery [17]. The patient's overall performance status and co-morbidities are as important as the complexity of any intervention under consideration. In reaching a decision, social factors such as accessibility of treatment centres, ability to cooperate with treatment and patient preference all need to be taken into account. The regular skin cancer multidisciplinary team meetings held throughout the UK are very helpful in guiding such decisions. Cure is not always a realistic proposition and radiotherapy can offer very worthwhile palliation (Figures 24.10 and 24.11) where it has been shown to improve quality of life [18].

Radiotherapy has a role to play in the treatment of almost all malignant skin conditions but, because there is considerable regional and national variation in access to radiotherapy and awareness of its value, its current use is patchy [10]. Although radiation damage with skin atrophy, telangiectasia, necrosis and ulceration occurred in the past, better dosimetry, a wider range of radiotherapy modalities [19] and more careful fractionation have considerably reduced this risk. In the UK, multidisciplinary skin cancer teams are now helping to ensure that the most appropriate modality is offered to every patient with skin cancer. This is in contrast to previous practice where only 2% of patients with BCC were referred to joint clinics [20] or a radiotherapeutic option was needlessly dismissed [21]. UK national guidance [22] recommends that all health professionals treating skin cancer should be members of such a team and should work to locally approved protocols based upon nationally accepted guidelines, such as those of the British Association of Dermatologists [23]. A similar approach has been recommended in American guidelines [24].

Surgery or radiotherapy

It is not disputed that surgery offers a better cosmetic result with the passage of time, nor that radiotherapy is able to preserve existing structure and function, although not of course able to replace tissue destroyed by tumour.

Few trials have compared surgery directly with radiotherapy. Avril *et al.* [25] showed that in 347 patients with facial tumours less than 4 cm in diameter, a surgical recurrence rate within 3–5 years was 1/174 in the surgery group compared with 11/173 for radiotherapy. The cosmetic result was better with surgery. However, the radiotherapy regimens were heterogeneous, and the surgical results exceptionally good, better even than for Mohs surgery, where one large series had a 30-month recurrence of 3/160 tumours, compared with 5/171 for conventional surgery [26]. Published studies of radiotherapy for skin cancer are, however, remarkably consistent in reporting high long-term control rates of well over 90% [27–30]. The advantages and disadvantages of each modality are summarised in Table 24.1.

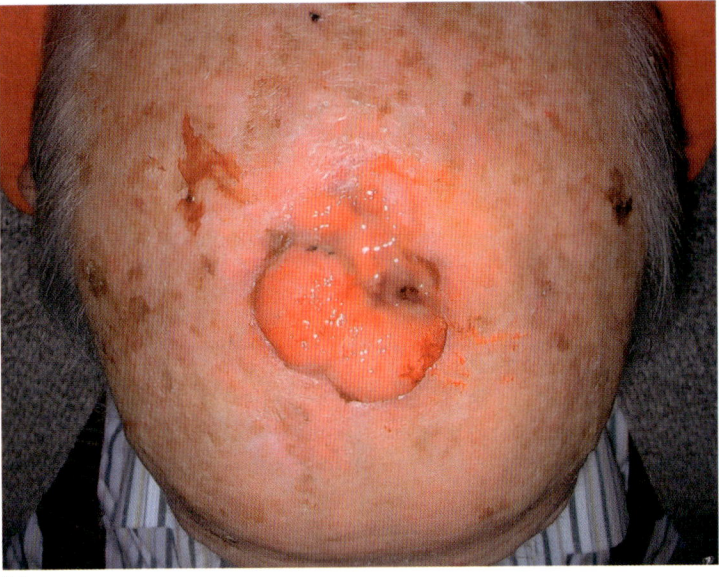

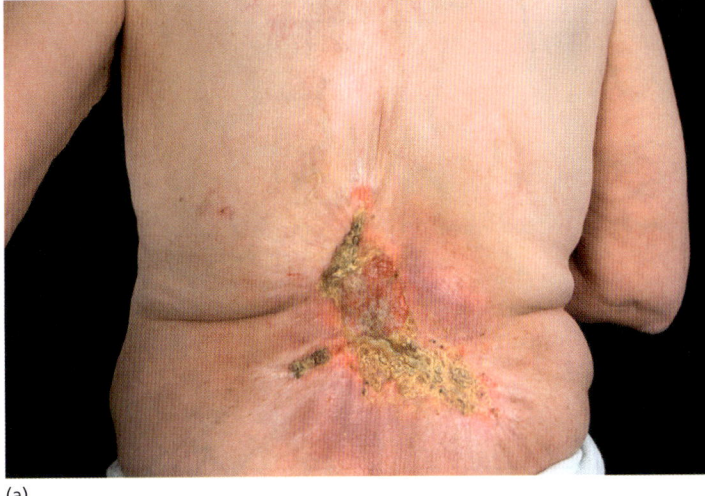

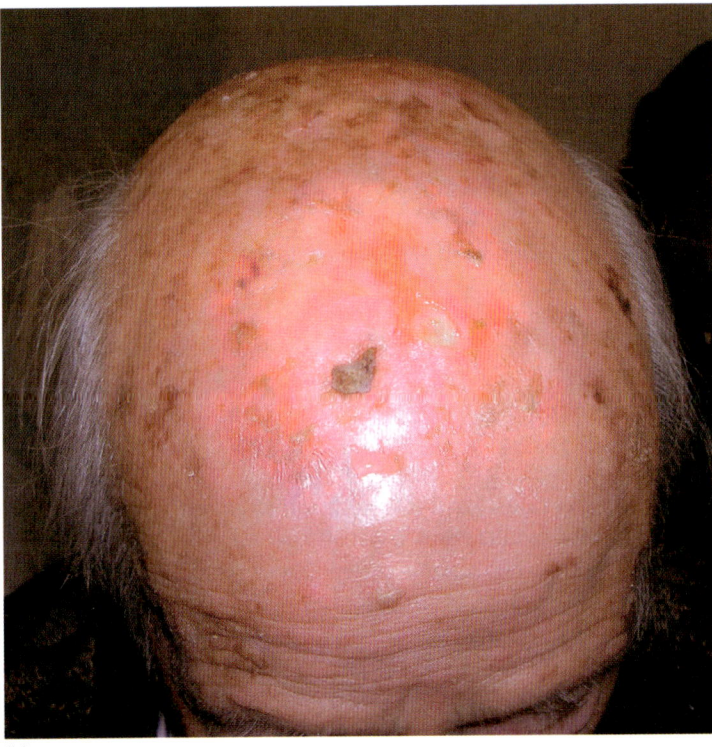

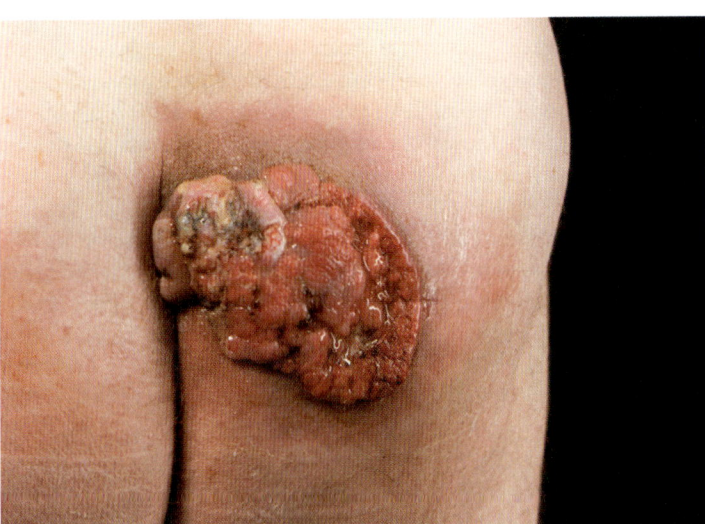

Figure 24.11 (a) Squamous cell carcinoma (SCC) on the back and (b) SCC on the buttock unsuitable for radiotherapy. These sites tolerate radiotherapy less well and are prone to painful acute reactions, infection and slow healing.

Figure 24.10 (a) Large squamous cell carcinoma on the frontal scalp. (b) Satisfactory clinical disease control at 6 months.

There is little difference in outcome between external beam radiotherapy using superficial X-rays or an electron beam [31,32]. Locally placed moulds or applicators have also been used for malignant skin tumours, placing a radioactive source over the tumour and leaving this in position for a predetermined period [19,20], or implanting radioactive wire into the tumour-bearing tissue. As described earlier, megavoltage radiotherapy using IMRT is now starting to be used for treating larger skin areas, often when surgery would not be possible, such as treating large areas of the scalp or peripheral limbs.

The areas which have traditionally been considered as not suitable for radiotherapy, such as over the nose, pinna, dorsum of the hand or anterior lower leg, can be treated if careful consideration is given to the volume treated, the total dose and the fractionation. It is also important to consider the general fitness of the patient and the condition and physiological reserve of the skin in the site to be treated [33–36].

There are some patients who, for practical reasons, cannot have radiotherapy. If patients are confused or unable to lie still because of confusion or neurological disease, then it can be impossible to deliver radiotherapy effectively and safely.

Adjuvant and salvage radiotherapy for skin cancer

Although ideally the patient should receive a single curative modality of treatment, sometimes patients are presented who have had a macroscopic excision of an SCC or a BCC but involved margins histopathologically.

Table 24.1 Patient factors influencing choice of skin cancer treatment.

Surgery generally preferred	Radiotherapy may be preferred
Younger patients	Older patients
Multiple tumours	If surgery would result in poor cosmetic result or loss of function, particularly if micrographic surgery not available (e.g. nasal tip, lips, periocular, ears) or there is refusal of surgery
Gorlin syndrome [22] where radiotherapy is usually contraindicated	
Infiltrative basal cell carcinomas	
Bulky tumours >6 cm	To avoid complex surgical reconstruction in the frail elderly
If there is erosion of bone or cartilage	
Tumours located on the trunk	To avoid general anaesthesia in patients who would not tolerate surgery under local anaesthesia
Ano-genital tumours	
Tumours below the knee [30]	
	To avoid general anaesthesia in patients who would otherwise require this for surgical management

Table 24.2 Commonly used superficial radiotherapy dosage regimens for definitive treatment of basal cell carcinomas and cutaneous squamous cell carcinomas. These fractionation regimens are only examples. Many centres will have other similar but locally derived dose fraction regimens.

Total dose (Gy)	No. of fractions	Fractionation interval
18	1	–
28	2	7 weeks apart
35	5	Daily (for tumours less than 4 cm in diameter)
45	10	Daily (for tumours more than 4 cm in diameter)

Adjuvant radiotherapy has been advocated by some authors [37–39]: (i) where there has been inadequate excision and further surgery is either not possible or not recommended; (ii) if the tumour shows prognostic indicators of poor outcome such as positive lymph nodes, especially with extracapsular spread; (iii) with a large primary SCC; or (iv) in higher-risk primary tumours of the head and neck. Adjuvant radiotherapy may improve outcome in SCC, especially if there is perineural invasion, when there is an increased risk of incomplete clearance even after Mohs surgery [38]; there is also some evidence that delaying radiotherapy may result in early tumour recurrence [40].

Because of the risk of nodal spread or perineural invasion from an incompletely excised SCC, if further surgery is not feasible it is sensible to offer postoperative radiotherapy to the scar and tumour bed using a full normal dose and fractionation regimen. With a well-healed scar or skin graft, the radiation reaction is often very mild.

A note of caution, in that the heterogenicity of studies, almost always performed retrospectively, even now does not give a definitive evidence base for the use of adjuvant radiotherapy [41]. However current guidelines do recommend adjuvant radiotherapy for BCC/SCC if perineural invasion is present.

The situation is different for BCC, where Lui et al. [42] reported a series of 186 incompletely excised BCC: 119 had immediate radiotherapy postoperatively, and 67 'wait and see' with radiotherapy for clinical recurrence. The predicted cure rates at 5 years were 91% versus 61%, respectively, but 10-year cure rates of 90–92% were observed for both immediate and delayed treatment. When surgical re-excision is inappropriate, it may thus be reasonable, particularly in the elderly, merely to observe and to offer adjuvant radiotherapy only for clinical recurrence.

Radiotherapy dose fractionation and treatment regimens

Radiotherapy regimens have evolved empirically over a long period of time and a wide range is in current use (Table 24.2). Generally, the greater the fractionation of the total dose (i.e. the smaller the individual dose administered at each session), the better the cosmetic outcome. This is very important to some patients, but others are content to accept a poorer cosmetic outcome in exchange for fewer hospital visits. There is renewed interest in using hypofractionated radiotherapy regimens, fewer fractions with higher dose/fraction and a shortened overall treatment time for frailer, poorer performance patients to reduce hospital visits particularly in the post Covid-19 era [43,44].

The SI unit of absorbed dose is called the Gray (Gy), and is 1 J/kg. This unit has replaced the rad. Note that 100 rad = 1 J/kg = 1 Gy and 1 rad = 1 cGy. The dose prescription is defined by the total dose given, the energy of the beam, the number of fractions given, the total number of days over which treatment is given and the volume or area treated. For example, a typical prescription for the treatment of a small BCC might be '35 Gy using 90 kV superficial X-ray beam given in five fractions over 5 days to a 3 cm diameter circular area'. This time–dose relationship is crucial to understanding the biological effect.

Dose and fractionation regimens are similar for BCC and SCC. There is a small therapeutic ratio between tumour cure and normal tissue necrosis, and even a slight alteration of dose or fractionation can be critical. In a retrospective study of 1005 BCC and SCC treated with superficial X-rays in 1976 at the Christie Hospital, Manchester, Chan et al. found that for a field size of 3 cm^2 or less, a single fraction of 20 Gy gave a 10-year disease-free rate of over 90%, with late necrosis rate of 6%. An increase of dose to 22.5 Gy did not improve tumour control rates, but did significantly increase late necrosis [45].

Fractionated radiotherapy is usually preferred for larger tumours, as cure rates are higher and better long-term cosmetic results are achieved [46–48].

Radiotherapy for particular skin sites: basal cell and squamous cell carcinoma

Eyelid

The upper eyelid, a rare site for skin cancer, is best treated surgically, as keratinisation of the tarsal conjunctiva may cause subsequent traumatic damage to the cornea. Tumours of the lower eyelid, however, are often suitable for treatment with superficial X-rays (Figure 24.12). A protective, metal, internal eyeshield is placed like a large contact lens over the globe of the eye after the application of local anaesthetic eye drops, with an applicator resting on this and on the lower lid tumour with an appropriate margin. The whole lower eyelid can be successfully treated in this manner if required.

Inner canthus

These tumours, close to the orbit, have a high cure rate if there is meticulous attention to dose calculation (Figure 24.13). An individual thin lead mask is made for the patient by mould technicians, with

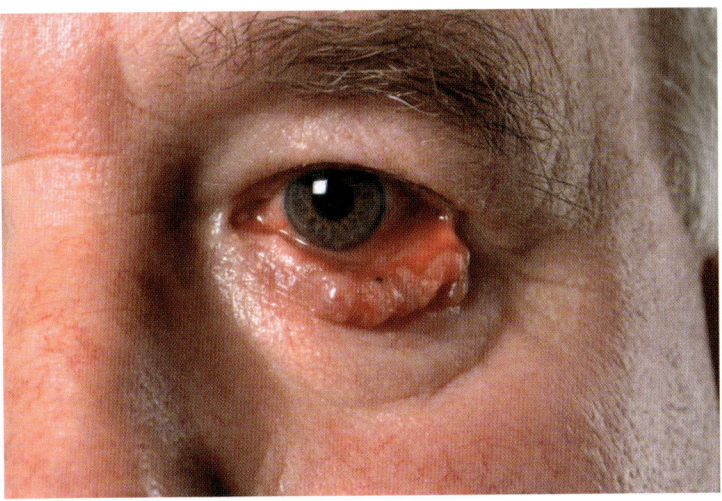

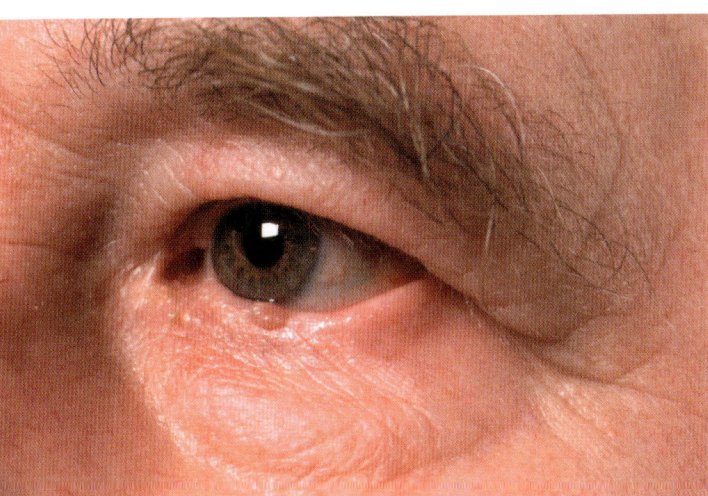

Figure 24.12 (a) Basal cell carcinoma of the lower eyelid. (b) The same patient 6 months after superficial X-ray treatment. There was no recurrence and the patient remained disease-free after radiotherapy.

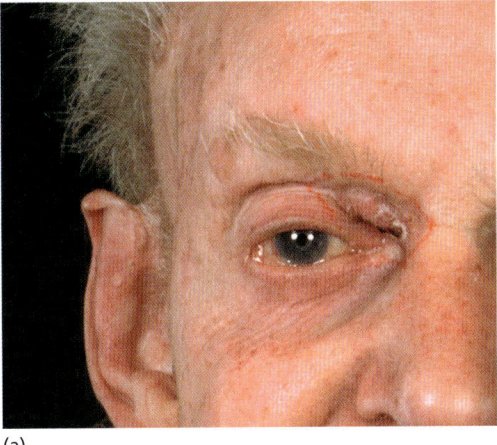

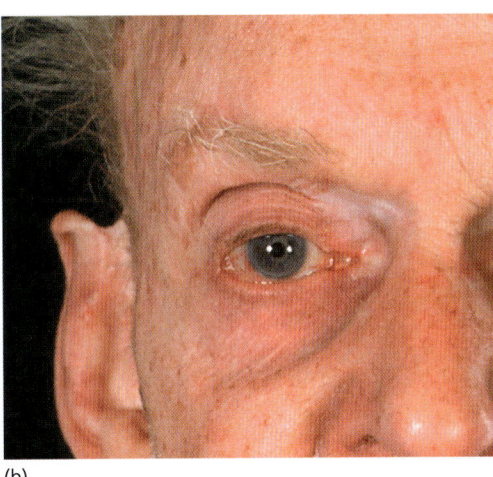

Figure 24.13 (a) Basal cell carcinoma of the upper inner canthus. (b) The same patient 5 years after superficial X-ray treatment.

the treatment area cut out. This provides a seating for the applicator, avoids the possibility of trauma on the treated side and protects the contralateral eye from the exit beam. If the naso-lacrimal duct has been damaged by the tumour and the patient has epiphora for this reason, then radiotherapy is not likely to reverse this symptom. However, it is uncommon for radiation *per se* to cause a new stenosis of the ductal system. Different authors advocate either radiotherapy or Mohs micrographic surgery depending on the size of the tumour, potential for disfigurement or loss of function [1,2].

Ear

Because tumours of the pinna and outer ear canal have close proximity to cartilage, electron beam techniques are preferred for treatment (Figures 24.14 and 24.15). In a study of 62 patients treated by orthovoltage techniques, local control was achieved in 97% of cases and only one of the six cases with clinically suspected cartilage necrosis failed to heal spontaneously [3]. In a large Canadian study, in which 93% of patients remained tumour-free at 10 years [4], persistent ulceration was observed in only 3%, and did not relate to beam energy but to dose and fractionation. However, electron treatment does give very good results for tumours covered by a 4 or 5 cm diameter applicator [5] and most departments will offer electrons unless for particular reasons the patient is unable to tolerate such procedures. The visible tumour is delineated, with a margin of at least 1 cm to account for the depth–dose characteristics of the electron beam, and the fact that the smallest reliable treatment applicator size is 4 cm diameter. The patient lies on the treatment couch with the ear for treatment uppermost, and wax or paraffin gauze is applied to make a level treatment surface, to fill in air gaps of sufficient thickness to avoid sparing the most superficial levels of skin, which can occur if a bolus is not used. If the tumour is on the posterior surface of the pinna, the ear itself can act as a build-up zone, with wax as a posterior filler to ensure an even dose. A lead shield behind this protects the scalp. Once this 'sandwich' is in place, the applicator is brought down firmly to rest on the surface, and treatment delivered using 5 or 6 MeV electrons.

Nose

Although skin cancers here are very closely applied to cartilage, in practice superficial X-rays give excellent control rates, and often a better cosmetic result than tumours irradiated at other sites. A lead plug is inserted inside the nostril to protect nasal mucosa from the

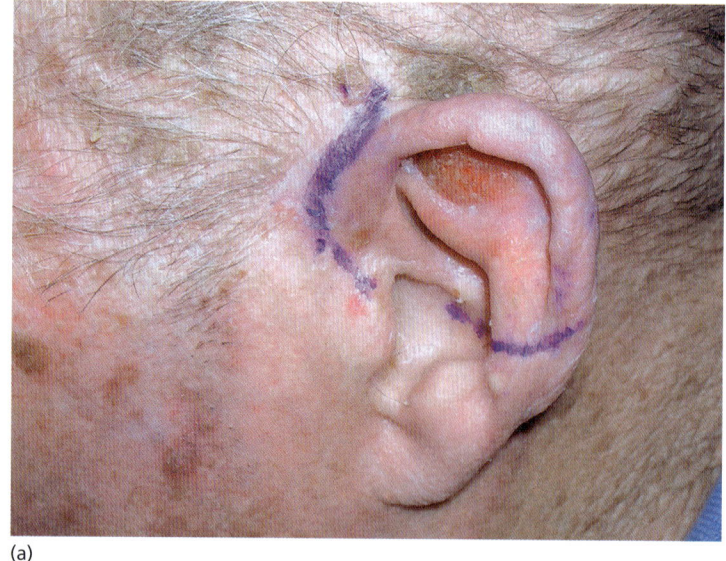

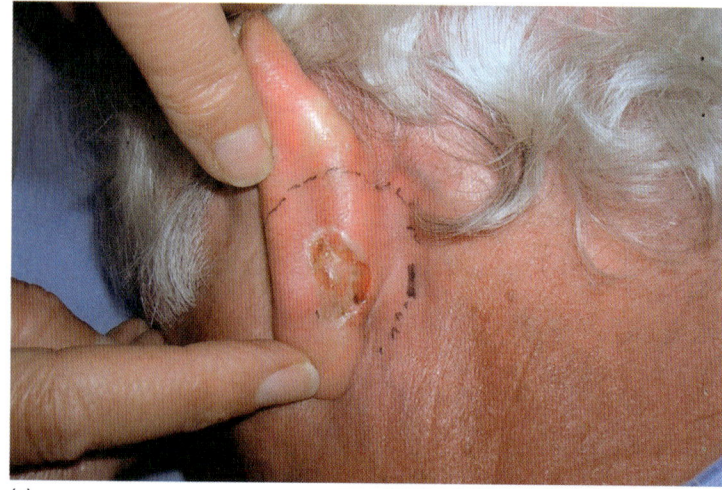

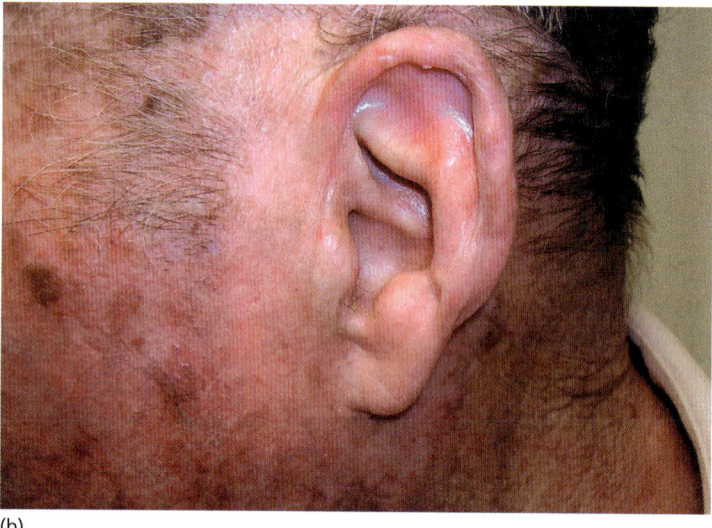

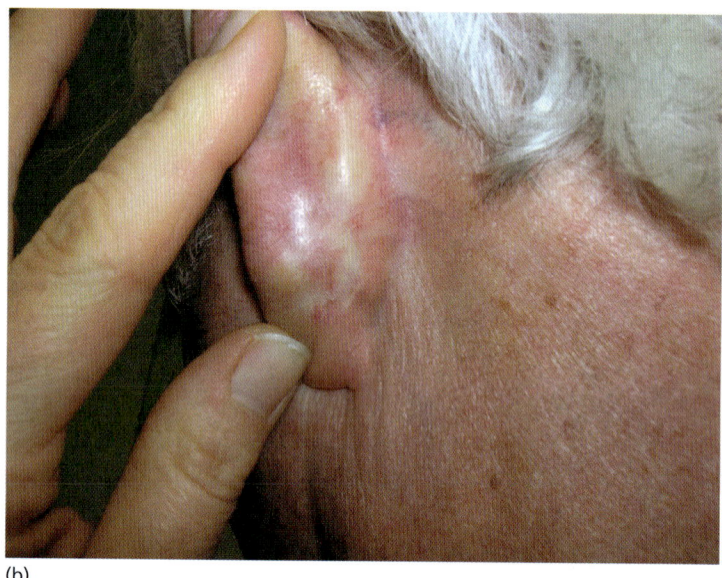

Figure 24.14 (a) Basal cell carcinoma of the scapha of the left ear. (b) The same patient 6 weeks after electron beam therapy.

Figure 24.15 (a) Basal cell carcinoma of the posterior aspect of the ear. (b) The same patient 6 months after electron beam treatment.

exit beam. At the naso-labial fold, the depth to be treated needs careful consideration.

Lip
Squamous cell carcinoma of the lip has a high local cure rate with radiotherapy using either electrons or kilovoltage X-rays (Figure 24.16a, b) [7]. Treatment margins should be generous because of the tendency for the tumours to spread mucosally, usually at least 1 cm of apparently normal tissue. The whole thickness of the lip is treated, choosing appropriate electron energy and build-up wax, or higher-energy kilovoltage X-rays (300 kV). A wax-coated lead gum shield protects the inner mouth from the exit beam, but a patch of mucositis within the mouth is inevitable, and will interfere with normal eating and drinking for a few days after treatment.

The patient is usually able to tolerate treatment to most of the upper or lower lip at one time, but not both areas simultaneously. The final cosmetic result is usually excellent (Figure 24.16c–e).

As well as electron treatment, local brachytherapy can also be used for non-melanoma skin cancer of the lip [8].

Other areas of the face
Even large BCC can do well with radiotherapy (Figure 24.17) [6].

Parotid and cervical lymph node involvement from cutaneous squamous cell carcinoma
A subset of patients who develop cutaneous SCC of the skin of the head and neck risk developing regional disease within the parotid or cervical nodes, with worse outcomes [9]. Several studies have now shown that combination treatment with surgery and adjuvant radiotherapy gives higher rates of local control of parotid and cervical node metastasis than either treatment given alone [9–13].

Radiotherapy for particular skin tumours
Basal cell carcinoma (Chapter 140)
Radiotherapy is useful for the primary treatment of small BCC or larger lesions where surgery may leave a poor functional or cosmetic

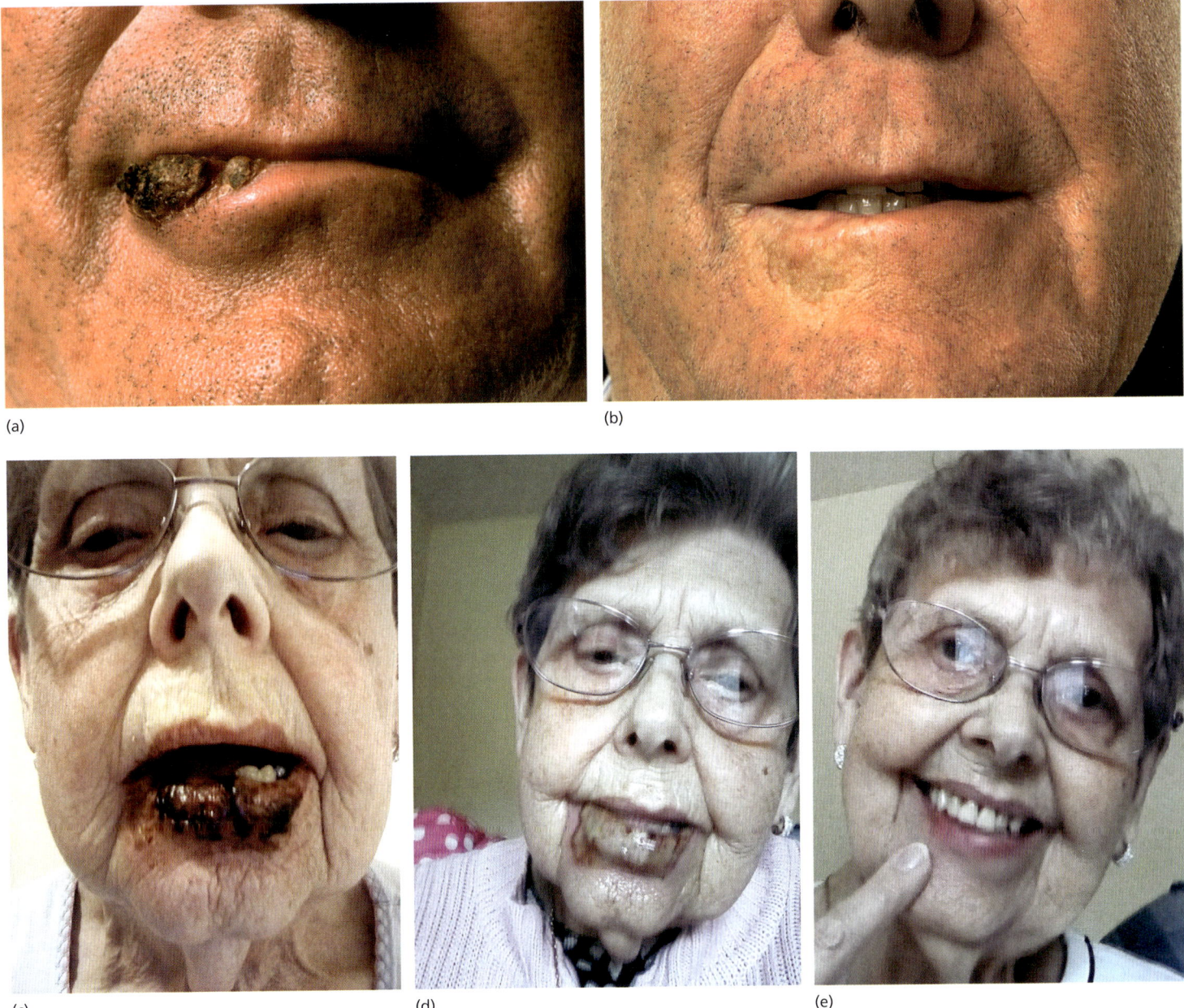

Figure 24.16 (a) Squamous cell carcinoma (SCC) of the lateral lower lip. (b) The same patient 8 years after higher-energy kilovoltage treatment. (c–e) Healing after radical radiotherapy to extensive SCC of the lower lip.

result (see earlier) [1,2,3]. Several European dermatology and oncology organisations have produced an 'easy to treat', 'more common' and 'difficult to treat' BCC classification [4].

Radiotherapy should not be used to re-treat BCC that have recurred after previous radiotherapy as they may then behave in a more aggressive manner [5]. The infiltrating (morphoeic) BCC subtype and the presence of underlying bone or cartilage involvement are relative contraindications to radiation treatment [6].

Squamous cell carcinoma of the skin (Chapter 141)

As with BCC, radiotherapy can be used as either the primary modality of treatment or as adjuvant treatment after surgery if there is a narrow surgical margin of clearance, the margin often being determined by the particular anatomical site of the tumour. The technique and dose are the same as those for treating a BCC, but a wider margin is taken around the tumour and the patient is subjected to a more frequent and longer follow-up, as suggested in the British Association of Dermatologists' guidelines [7]. If the SCC has developed on the face, it is mandatory to check for cervical lymphadenopathy. Radiotherapy may be especially useful for SCC on or around the nose where resection may be incomplete or the potential for reconstruction suboptimal [8].

The size of the SCC is also important, with one study showing radiotherapy giving local control in over 90% of SCC less than 1 cm, but in only 56% of tumours larger than 5 cm [9]. A large systemic review has also confirmed that local relapse after radiotherapy to the primary skin site increases with tumour stage [10].

Adjuvant radiotherapy may reduce the development of nodal disease in higher-risk cutaneous SCC as described by Veness [11], but

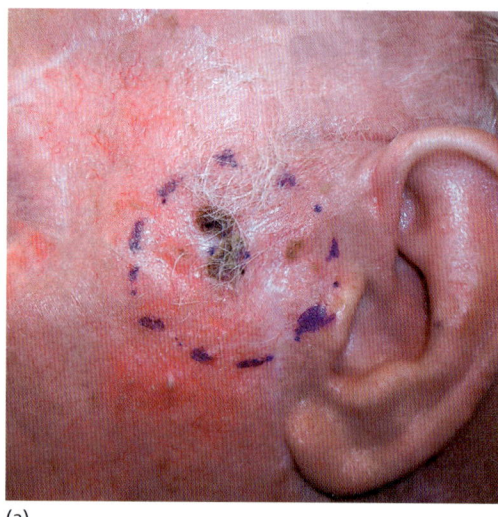

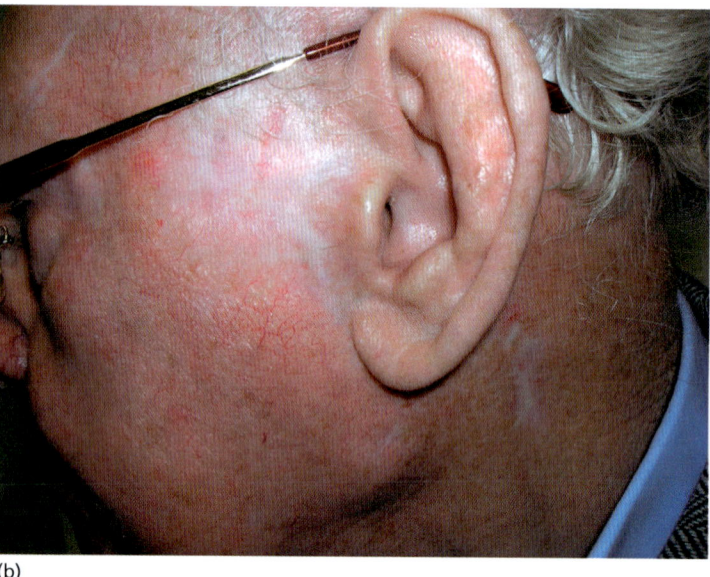

Figure 24.17 (a) Large pre-auricular basal cell carcinoma. (b) The same patient 6 months after superficial X-ray treatment.

whether adjuvant radiotherapy is required after excision with negative surgical margins has not been defined [12]. There may, however, be a benefit for higher-stage primary tumours and for tumours with risk factors such as perineural invasion, parotid involvement and in the immunosuppressed [13].

Porceddu *et al.* reported a Trans Tasman Radiation Oncology Group (TROG) prospective, randomised, phase III trial which showed no benefit in adding weekly chemotherapy to postoperative radiotherapy in patients with high-risk cutaneous SCC [14].

Radiotherapy can also be useful in palliation of advanced skin tumours and in some patients give long-term survival [15].

Bowen disease (Chapter 141)

Radiotherapy can be an effective treatment for Bowen disease [3], but it is not commonly used, particularly since the introduction of photodynamic therapy (Chapter 22). Lesions on the leg should be treated with caution [16,17] as there is a danger of ulceration and very slow healing if large areas are treated. A retrospective review of 44 cases by VanderSpek *et al.*, where radiotherapy was used as a primary treatment or for managing residual disease, showed a crude local control rate of 93% [18]. The British Association of Dermatologists has issued guidelines for the management of Bowen disease including the use of radiotherapy [19]. Complete responses are widely reported after radiotherapy but there can be impaired healing if used for lesions on the lower leg.

Melanoma (Chapters 142–145)

Melanoma cells are not insensitive to radiotherapy (Figure 24.18), as is sometimes stated, but they do require higher dose per fraction regimens to overcome their higher radio-resistance. Patients may thus be given larger individual doses in less frequent fractions ('hypofractionation') and there is increasing interest in using these hypofractionated regimens with stereotactic radiosurgery and stereotactic ablative radiotherapy (SABR) using smaller treatment margins than usual, especially for oligometastatic disease [20,21]. The main indication for the use of radiotherapy in melanoma is for palliation of cutaneous and visceral metastases [22]. There have been uncontrolled studies suggesting that adjuvant radiotherapy may improve local control [23,24]. The TROG trial reported that patients at risk of regional failure (as defined by having multiple nodes, large nodes or extracapsular spread) randomised to receive adjuvant radiotherapy had a decreased risk of such failure at a median follow-up of 6 years compared with those who were not. There was, however, a high (40%) incidence of severe lymphoedema in those receiving treatment of the groin and no relapse-free or overall survival benefit [25,26,**27**,28].

Adjuvant radiotherapy may improve outcome after wide local excision, specifically in early desmoplastic melanoma [29]. The European Society for Medical Oncology has produced consensus guidelines for melanoma including the management of loco-regional disease and local treatment strategies for localised metastatic melanoma [30].

An abscopal effect occurs where localised treatment results in a systemic antitumour response, for example giving radiotherapy to a single melanoma metastasis resulting in shrinkage of other distant metastases. The possible method of action is that cancer cells killed by radiotherapy break down, exposing a greater level of antigens which triggers a heightened immune reaction, attacking other metastases. It has been described in several cancers but research into this effect in melanoma has increased, especially using a combination of radiotherapy and immunotherapy, such as ipilimumab, looking for an improved summative efficacy with two agents working through differing mechanisms and with the hope of an added abscopal effect [31–34].

Lentigo maligna and lentigo maligna melanoma (Chapters 142–145)

Radiotherapy has been used successfully in both lentigo maligna (LM) and lentigo maligna melanoma (LMM). In one German study, there was no recurrence in any of 42 patients with LM, with a mean follow-up of 15 months, and only 2 of 22 patients with LMM showed local recurrence. Cosmetic results were also reported as good or excellent in the majority of patients [35]. Similar complete responses with good cosmetic outcomes have been reported from Australia [36] and Canada [37]. Further systematic reviews support the view

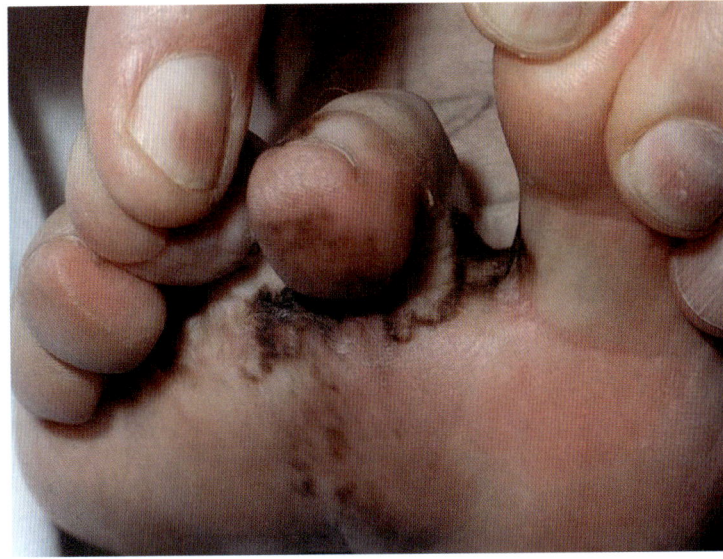

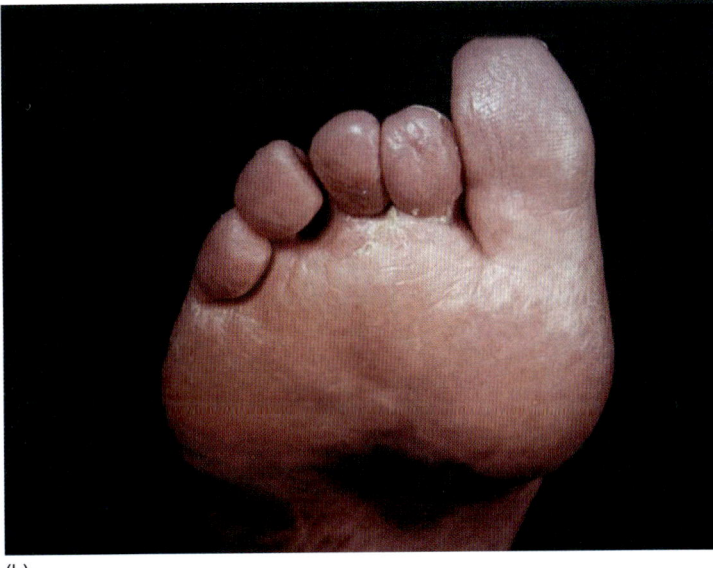

Figure 24.18 (a) Malignant melanoma, pre-radiotherapy. (b) Malignant melanoma, post-radiotherapy.

that superficial radiotherapy is a safe and effective treatment for LM and LMM with acceptable cosmetic outcomes [38,39].

Merkel cell carcinoma (Chapter 146)

These tumours of neuroendocrine origin are most common on the head and neck, but can occur elsewhere on the skin. They have a tendency to recur locally after conventional surgical removal and improved local control has now been shown in a large number of studies with a combination of wide excision and adjuvant postoperative radiotherapy to the primary tumour site and local nodal drainage [40–54]. There is no benefit in using adjuvant chemotherapy in Merkel cell carcinoma (MCC) [54], but there is some evidence that omitting radiotherapy even in patients with lower-risk MCC gives a significantly higher rate of recurrence [55]. Some studies have also shown improved survival [45]. Mohs surgery is now also used for removal of MCC in some centres, and, if complete excision is achieved, adjuvant radiotherapy may not add benefit in terms of improved local control or survival [52]. These are radiosensitive tumours and radiotherapy has been used as a primary treatment, with local control rates of over 75% [56–61]. Sentinel lymph node biopsy is being explored as to whether adjuvant radiotherapy or nodal dissection may improve outcomes [62].

Kaposi sarcoma (Chapter 136)

It is well known that these tumours are sensitive to low-dose radiotherapy, with a complete response rate of up to 84% [63]. Either superficial X-rays or electron beams can be used depending on the thickness of the lesion(s) and consequently the depth of treatment required. Treatment is used cautiously as patients are prone to develop severe local reactions and mucositis. Radiotherapy is also used to palliate systemic disease such as pulmonary masses [64,65].

Dermatofibrosarcoma protuberans (Chapter 136)

This low-grade sarcoma has a propensity to recur after surgery alone and local control is improved by giving adjuvant radiotherapy [66,67].

Carcinoma metastatic to the skin from other primaries

Radiotherapy can provide useful palliation for cutaneous metastases from visceral tumours such as breast, colon and lung (Chapter 148).

Squamous cell and basal cell carcinoma in transplant patients (Chapter 147)

Skin tumours developing after organ transplant are known to have more aggressive characteristics and carry a poorer prognosis [68]. These patients develop more SCC than BCC, reversing the normal ratio, and often develop multiple skin cancers at an earlier age. There is no contraindication to using radiotherapy if surgery is considered inappropriate and it may be used as adjuvant therapy for patients with more aggressive tumours [69].

Cutaneous lymphoma

Radiotherapy represents the single most effective treatment strategy for cutaneous lymphomas. In contrast to other skin cancers, lymphomas are extremely sensitive to radiotherapy with doses as low as 4 Gy sometimes sufficient for local control. Surgery is therefore rarely indicated unless there is a solitary nodule where excision biopsy can both be diagnostic and provide definitive local treatment. The low radiotherapy doses are almost always within the constraints of normal tissue tolerance and therefore radiotherapy can be safely delivered with minimal risk of long-term complications.

An overview of the classification and management of lymphomas is described in Chapter 139. The following summarises the technical aspects of radiotherapy with a focus on mycosis fungoides, which accounts for 50% of cutaneous lymphomas.

Mycosis fungoides

Mycosis fungoides evolves slowly with the majority of patients falling into a favourable prognostic group with a median survival of more than 35 years from presentation [70]. It is essential to involve specialist histopathologists, dermatologists, oncologists and haematologists in a multidisciplinary approach to management.

Individual patches, plaques and tumours. While mycosis fungoides is normally not isolated to one area, local radiotherapy is frequently utilised for troublesome lesions with a local control rate in excess of 90% [71]. The recurrence rates are dependent on the dose given, with a dose–response relationship observed up to doses of 30–40 Gy [72]. In practice, lower doses are preferred, as they still convey a high chance of local control, are more convenient for patients and permit overlap of adjacent fields or re-treatment if necessary [73]. The current recommended UK doses include 8 Gy in two fractions for patches and plaques, and 12 Gy in three fractions for tumours [74].

Radiotherapy can be delivered with X-rays (low-energy superficial or orthovoltage), or electrons as described earlier with a directly applied field. The target volume is the clinically defined lesion with a margin of at least 1 cm laterally. Patches and plaques are typically treated to a depth of 8–10 mm with careful assessment of tumour thickness to determine the appropriate beam energy and bolus requirement when using electrons.

More extensive tumours, particularly when extending around curved areas, require careful radiotherapy planning. Patient-specific immobilisation devices such as thermoplastic shells for the head and neck region are essential to ensure accurate delivery of the planned radiotherapy treatment. More complex techniques include matched field electrons and intensity-modulated radiotherapy plans as well as high-dose rate brachytherapy mould techniques (see Figures 24.7 and 24.8). When delivering radiotherapy to large tumours, treatment is normally fractionated with typical doses between 20 and 30 Gy in 10–15 fractions [74,75].

Total skin electron beam therapy. A significant number of patients with mycosis fungoides develop generalised skin involvement. Total skin electron beam therapy (TSEBT) can provide excellent palliation particularly when other skin-directed therapies including psoralen and ultraviolet A (PUVA) fail. The response rates and duration of response are dependent on the stage of the disease. A systematic review of TSEBT as monotherapy in 952 patients reported complete response rates of 96% in stage IA, IB and IIA disease. Despite this, the 5-year relapse-free survival rates were only 10–23% [76]. The standard dose for TSEBT is 30–36 Gy as endorsed by the European Organisation for Research and Treatment of Cancer (EORTC) and the American Association of Physicists in Medicine guidelines [77,78]. The conventional Stanford schedule is 36 Gy delivering 2 Gy fractions per 2-day cycle over 9 weeks to the whole skin, which has been modified in the UK to 30 Gy in 1.5 Gy fractions over 5 weeks.

In recognition of the palliative nature of TSEBT there has been growing interest in reduced dose schedules with favourable toxicity profiles. While doses as low as 4 Gy in four fractions have been investigated, the duration of remission is short [79]. However, doses between 10 and 30 Gy were found to have similar overall response rates (>50% improvement) and relapse-free survival rates to patients treated with conventional doses of 30–36 Gy [80]. A series of low-dose TSEBT (12 Gy in eight fractions over 2 weeks) in 103 patients has reported very high response rates, with a median duration of response of 18 months in patients with stage IB and 10 months in patients with stage IIB mycosis fungoides, with significantly less toxicity than standard-dose TSEBT [81].

The aim of TSEBT is to treat the entire target volume, which comprises the epidermis, adnexal structures and dermis, to a uniform dose. The EORTC recommendations are that the 80% isodose should be at least 4 mm deep to the surface of the skin, and that the dose at 20 mm depth should be less than 20% of the maximum dose at the skin surface [77]. A variety of techniques may be used to ensure total skin coverage including large-field electron-field techniques and rotational techniques. The modified Stanford technique has been most widely adopted and involves treating the patient with large electron fields standing in six positions holding onto a frame for stability (Figure 24.19). The distance between the linear accelerator and the patient needs to be at least 3 m. At this distance, the beams are angled approximately 20° above and below the central axis to deliver a reasonably uniform dose distribution. With this technique, the typical variation in dose at the skin surface is ±10%, dropping to ±5% at 3 mm depth [78].

The Stanford technique results in relative shielding of the scalp, perineum and soles of the feet which may require additional treatment. Conversely, some areas such as the wrists, ankles and ears may require shielding due to higher doses being received; shielding may also be required in previously treated areas. Sensitive areas that are spared from involvement with mycosis fungoides such as the nail beds and testicles can be shielded with lead fingernail shields and a cricket box, respectively. Custom-made lead-lined goggles are also used to shield the eyes which can be treated afterwards with superficial X-rays if there is involvement of the eyelids.

The side effects are related to the dose given, with an increased chance of toxicity with standard doses of 30–36 Gy. The most common acute complications of standard dose TSEBT are redness and moist desquamation which can be severe in patients with erythroderma. Temporary loss of fingernails and toenails also occurs if these are not shielded. Long-term side effects include xerosis and an inability to sweat properly for 6–12 months. Due to concern over possible skin atrophy and potential necrosis there is a reluctance to offer more than two conventional courses of TSEBT in a patient's lifetime, although lower dose schedules (e.g. 12 Gy in eight fractions) can be repeated on multiple occasions.

Other lymphomas

The technical approach to radiotherapy planning for other types of skin lymphoma is similar to that outlined earlier for individual patches, plaques and tumours of mycosis fungoides. A brief commentary on radiotherapy for specific histological subtypes is provided here.

Other cutaneous T-cell lymphomas

The approach to radiotherapy for primary cutaneous anaplastic large-cell lymphoma and subcutaneous panniculitis-like T-cell lymphoma is similar. Patients presenting with solitary or localised disease can be treated with radical radiotherapy with a recommended dose of 40 Gy in 20 fractions for subcutaneous panniculitis-like T-cell lymphoma and 24–30 Gy in 12–15 fractions for primary cutaneous anaplastic large-cell lymphoma [6]. Lower doses may be equally effective but there are no published data. Systemic therapies should be considered for patients with multiple lesions, although short palliative radiotherapy schedules can be useful. Primary cutaneous CD4+ small or medium-sized

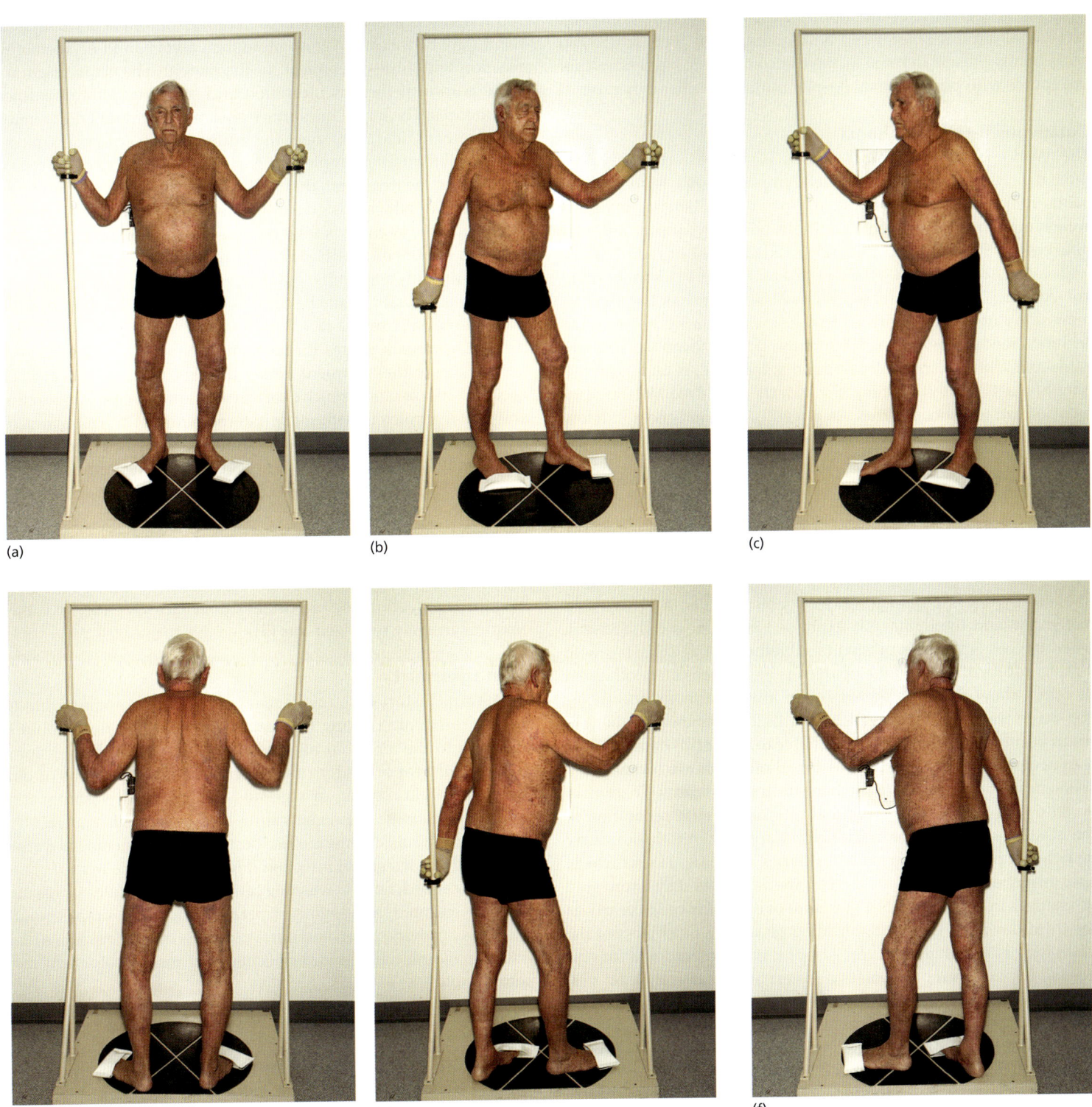

Figure 24.19 (a–f) The modified Stanford technique showing patient positions to optimise a uniform dose to all the skin when using total skin electron beam therapy.

pleomorphic T-cell lymphoproliferative disorder typically presents with a solitary nodule on the head and neck region which can be treated with surgery or radiotherapy [74].

Other cutaneous T-cell lymphomas including cutaneous γ-δ T-cell lymphoma, aggressive epidermotropic CD8+ T-cell lymphoma and extranodal natural killer T-cell lymphoma, nasal type, which can occasionally present in the skin, have in common an aggressive clinical course with poor survival despite multiagent chemotherapy.

Cutaneous B-cell lymphoma

The World Health Organization–EORTC classification describes three main types of cutaneous B-cell lymphoma [82]. Primary cutaneous follicle centre lymphoma and primary cutaneous marginal zone lymphoma are indolent conditions with 10-year survival rates in excess of 90%. The recommended radical dose of radiotherapy for localised disease is 24–30 Gy with a margin of 1–1.5 cm of uninvolved skin [74,75,82]. Palliative doses (2 Gy × 2) achieve a complete remission rate of 72%, with 30% of lesions requiring re-treatment within a median period of 6.3 months [73]. In contrast, primary cutaneous diffuse large-cell lymphoma, leg type, is an aggressive lymphoma typically affecting the elderly with frequent involvement of extracutaneous sites. As a result, systemic chemotherapy is indicated followed by radiotherapy to the lesion (36–40 Gy) with generous margins of 2–5 cm [74,75].

Acute radiation reaction (acute radiodermatitis)

Radiation works by damaging clonogenic cells, both benign and malignant, and the damage is expressed at the next cell division, when the cell either dies or repairs sublethal damage. Tissues with a rapid turnover such as the epidermis and mucosal endothelium therefore show radiation damage soon after treatment, and this is the 'acute reaction' (Figures 24.20 and 24.21). For the treatment to result in cure, the tumour must be unable to repair this damage [1,2].

In acute radiodermatitis, the histopathology shows oedema and sparseness of connective tissue beneath the epidermis. There may be flattening and loss of epidermal rete ridges with separation of the elastic tissue from the basal layer. Capillary endothelium may be hypertrophic and congested capillaries a feature. Haemorrhage and thrombosis are often observed. Special stains may show subtle changes in the DNA–RNA structure of epithelial cells as early as the third day [1,2]. During the healing phase, the patchiness of the pathology is a striking feature. Atrophy may be bordered by epidermal hyperplasia, pigmentation is very irregular and blood vessels are of variable size and shape; deeper vessels may be fibrosed [3]. Normal tissue repair occurs when normal clonogenic cells on the basement membrane, which have either not received damage or have repaired sublethal damage, repopulate the basement membrane and re-cover the epithelium [4].

In a commonly used regimen, where the patient attends at daily intervals for five doses of treatment, the irradiated skin starts to redden 5–7 days after the first treatment, because of increased vascularity and inflammation associated with cell damage. Subsequent doses add to the reaction, which proceeds through dry and sometimes moist desquamation and scabbing, usually reaching a height of discomfort at 3–4 weeks after treatment finishes. It then settles over the next 2–3 weeks with re-epithelialisation, which begins in the perifollicular areas and proceeds as cell colonies coalesce to cover the denuded surface.

If the skin is previously unbroken or the tumour is nodular, treatment may be followed by no more than a very mild erythematous reaction with little discomfort for the patient. The acute reaction is more painful if there is ulceration and scabbing before treatment commences. The larger the surface area of the tumour and therefore the treatment field, the longer the healing takes; even so, healing is commonly virtually complete by 6 weeks after the end of the course. The brisker the treatment, that is, the larger the dose and the shorter the time over which it is given, the more marked the acute reaction is likely to be, as there is less opportunity for normal tissue repair between treatments. Individual skin reactions vary, and those who burn in the sun tend to have a brisker reaction to X-ray treatment. Occasionally, healing may be complicated by secondary impetiginisation, especially on the face.

If the exit beam passes through mucosa, a patch of mucositis of similar size to the treatment field will ensue. This reaction usually occurs earlier and is of much shorter duration than the skin reaction, and heals completely without long-term sequelae. The nasal mucosa may swell and occasionally bleed, with the feeling of a blocked nose; in the mouth, a sore patch may make eating uncomfortable for a few days. Although protective lead can be used to protect structures beyond the inner mucosa, such as the gums and the nasal septum, the mucosa just beneath the cancer cannot be protected.

It is unusual to see acute radiation reactions with diagnostic imaging but it can occur with fluoroscopy. Both dose and length of the diagnostic procedure are important causal factors. Balter *et al.* have comprehensively reviewed this [5].

Management

The natural history of the acute reaction cannot be modified, but the patient can avoid making the reaction worse. The area should be left open to the air as far as possible and protected from trauma, extremes of heat or cold, irritation with medicated creams or ointments, physical rubbing or vigorous and repeated washing, all of which can damage the regenerating clonogenic cells and result in ulceration. Steroid creams are also best avoided. Patients are warned to seek advice if signs of infection develop. Once the treated area is dry and scabbed, normal washing can resume. The mucosal reaction must be endured, although soft paraffin and/or a simple mouthwash may provide relief, and if the patient is having excessive nasal crusting, simple saline nasal douches may make the patient more comfortable.

Late radiation reaction (chronic radiodermatitis)

Tissues with a slow rate of cell division such as subcutaneous fat, fibrous tissue and small blood vessels will not show radiation effects until months or years after treatment. At 6 months, treated skin is often slightly paler or pinker than adjacent untreated skin; with the passage of time, sequelae usually appear, with late appearances established at 5–10 years. The irradiated skin may show pallor

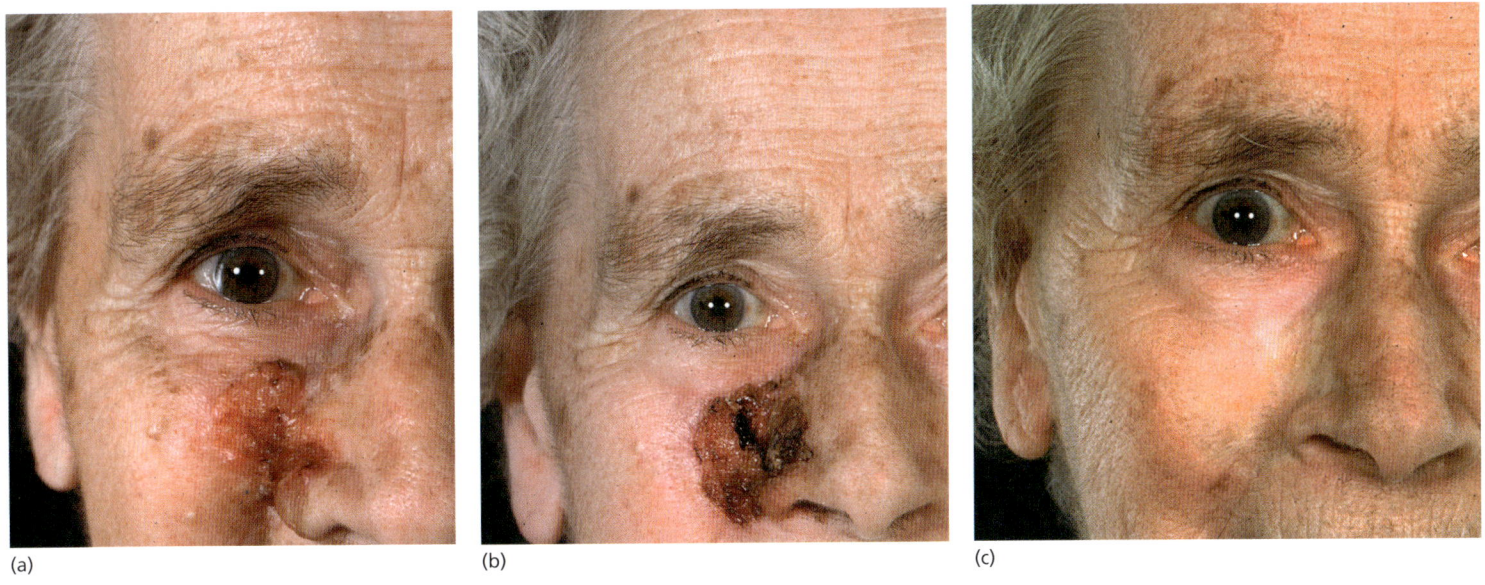

Figure 24.20 (a) Large basal cell carcinoma of the cheek. (b) The same patient showing acute radiation reaction 6 weeks after superficial X-ray treatment. (c) The same patient showing a settled reaction 6 months after superficial X-ray treatment.

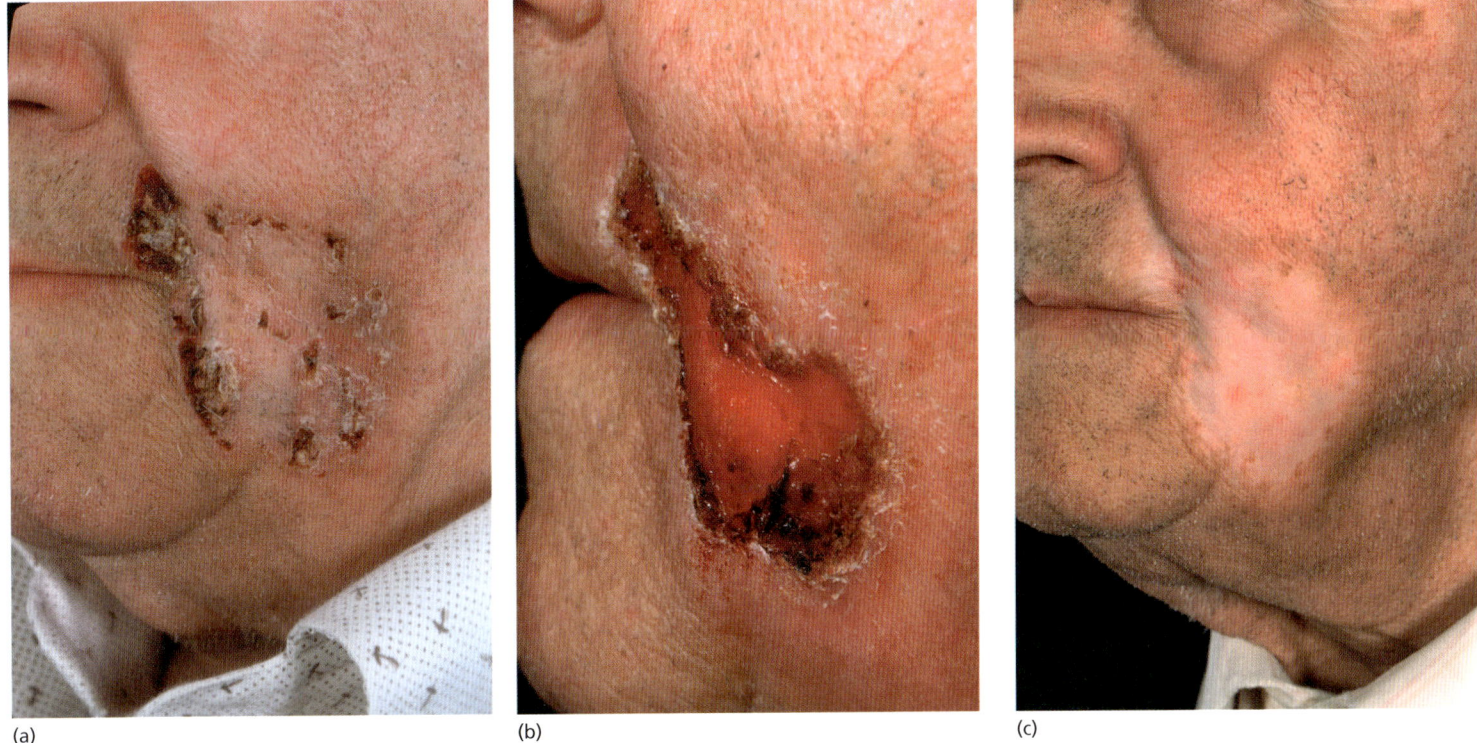

Figure 24.21 (a) Large basal cell carcinoma of the jaw. (b) The same patient showing acute radiation reaction 4 weeks after superficial X-ray treatment. (c) The same patient showing a settled reaction 6 months after superficial X-ray treatment.

or increased pigmentation, with variable atrophy, telangiectasia, fibrosis and loss of appendageal structures (Figures 24.22 and 24.23). With time, the blood supply of the treated area may become compromised, resulting in ulceration either spontaneously or after trauma; such ulcers often, however, heal spontaneously [1].

The fundamental histopathology of chronic radiodermatitis is fibrosis and occlusion of the cutaneous vasculature with varying degrees of homogenisation of the dermal connective tissue. Residual vessels may be enormously dilated. Bizarre, large, stellate fibroblasts may be seen in the dermis. Fibrosis of the deep dermis and subcutaneous tissue may occasionally occur after megavoltage radiotherapy [2]. The changes in the epidermis vary from simple atrophy to acanthosis and extreme dyskeratosis. There is usually loss of adnexa such as hair follicles.

The late cosmetic result varies and may reflect the underlying damage caused initially by the tumour as well as the patient's skin

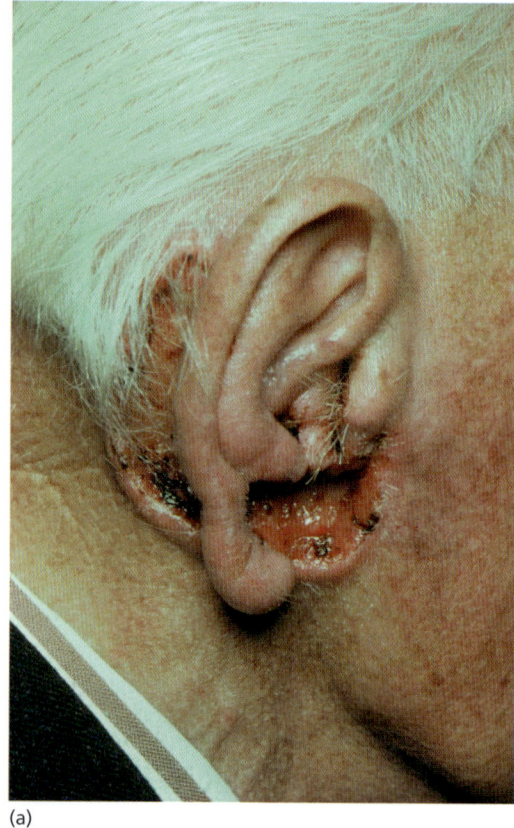
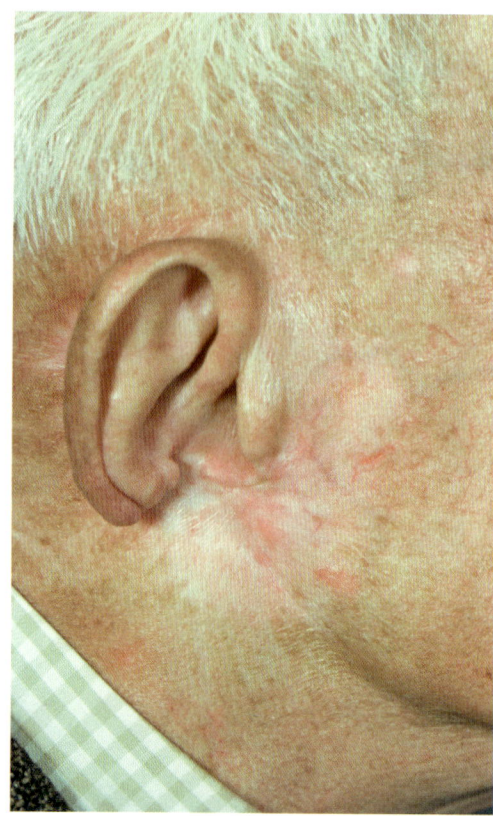

Figure 24.22 (a) Extensive erosive basal cell carcinoma of the ear. (b) The same patient 2 years after superficial X-ray treatment.

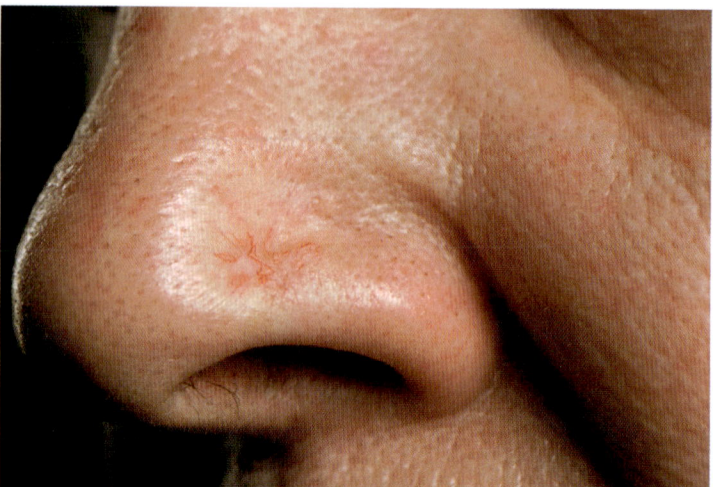

Figure 24.23 Telangiectasia after treatment for a small basal cell carcinoma of the nose.

type. In one study of 339 patients, telangiectasia, pigmentation and fibrosis were directly related to the increasing size of field needed for treatment rather than the treatment regimen used [3]. The late cosmetic result is also less good if the patient has had repeated cryotherapy to the area (authors' personal observation) or been left with a poor surgical scar. Chronic radiation change may sometimes be difficult to distinguish from tumour recurrence.

Ischaemic necrosis following radiotherapy should rarely be seen when modern techniques of dose fractionation are used. Radionecrosis typically occurs 1–2 years after treatment and is often precipitated by trauma or infection. Excision and grafting may provide the only satisfactory treatment of extensive radionecrosis, although small areas may slowly heal with conservative management [4].

The induction of skin tumours within irradiated fields is very rare indeed, as would be expected with the latency for this and the average age of the patient receiving radiotherapy for skin cancers.

Tumour recurrence after radiotherapy

Basal cell carcinoma and SCC are not always cured by radiotherapy [1–3], especially if the patient has had prior treatment with multiple modalities [4]. Ulceration lasting more than 6 months after therapy usually means persistent tumour. Some authorities suggest that one reason for avoiding primary radiotherapy is that surgical salvage is more difficult after treatment failure, but if the patient is referred on at an early stage, excision of the irradiated skin and grafting are usually possible. Mohs surgery may give the best results in these cases [4]. As with surgical treatment, radiotherapy for recurrent BCC has a higher relapse rate. Age, immunosuppression and treatment modality are also important as well as size of tumour for recurrence [5].

Re-treatment with radiation is not usually offered, because the primary is by definition relatively radioresistant. There is an increased risk of radionecrosis if normal tissues, which may have already received a 'tolerance dose', are exposed to further radiation. However, in practice, radiotherapy has been given successfully in these circumstances with acceptable cosmetic results, especially if there has been a sufficient time interval between the two radiotherapy treatments [6]. Occasionally, it is reasonable to offer treatment to persistent tumours at the edge of a previous radiotherapy field, when a small degree of overlap may be acceptable. Although the risk of a small area of necrosis will be higher, this strategy is often acceptable to the patient and is typically successful.

Radiation-induced tumours

There is evidence that the risk both of BCC and of SCC is increased in areas of skin previously irradiated for benign or malignant disease including Hodgkin disease, breast cancer, acne, ankylosing spondylitis and tinea capitis [1,2].

BCC of the scalp may not present until 50 years after X-ray epilation for ringworm. Such tumours are much more rarely seen since the virtual abandonment of radiotherapy for benign diseases, the development of more sophisticated radiotherapy machinery and advances in the understanding of radiobiology. It has not, however, been possible to demonstrate any precise quantitative relationship between the development of skin cancers and the amount of radiation received on the skin surface, nor is it known what total dose or fractionation regimen would be most carcinogenic.

Although a greater knowledge of the limitations and effectiveness of radiation should prevent the occurrence of late radiation damage including carcinogenicity, the long latent periods involved warn against early complacency [3–5].

As the number of childhood cancer survivors increases, there is some evidence for an increased incidence of BCC developing within irradiated skin sites [6], but this is not confirmed by all studies [7]. As most of these children will also have had treatment with chemotherapy, the aetiological factors causing their second malignancy cannot be easily disentangled.

Management

Most radiation-induced tumours should be excised. However, where there is no radiation damage evident on the skin, a subsequent radical dose of radiotherapy can normally be tolerated [8].

Rare tumours associated with previous irradiation

Atypical fibroxanthoma (see Chapter 136)

Atypical fibroxanthoma (syn. pseudosarcoma of the skin), seen particularly in fair-skinned males who have suffered actinic damage, may also follow radiation damage [1–3].

Radiation-induced sarcoma (Chapter 136)

Radiotherapy-induced sarcomas make up an estimated 5% of all sarcomas and occur in less than 0.2% of patients who have had radiotherapy [4,5]. Children are more susceptible to developing radiation-induced cancer [6]. There can be a long latent period with sarcomas appearing 5–15 years or even longer post-treatment [7,8].

Postirradiation sarcomas of both soft tissue and bone are characteristically high grade and include undifferentiated pleomorphic sarcoma (previously known as malignant fibrous histiocytoma), spindle cell sarcoma, osteosarcoma, leiomyosarcoma and angiosarcoma, the latter being especially associated with radiotherapy for breast cancer [7].

Development of sarcoma appears to be related to exposure to kilovoltage rather than megavoltage radiotherapy and to receiving higher doses of radiotherapy. It is also associated with a range of genetic syndromes which may predispose to cancer development such as Li–Fraumeni syndrome.

Diagnosis and investigation are as for primary sarcomas, including a carefully planned biopsy.

There is evidence that prognosis is worse for radiation-induced sarcomas compared with primary sarcomas [8]. Surgery and chemotherapy are the primary treatment modalities with re-irradiation usually avoided.

Key references

The full list of references can be found in the online version at https://www.wiley.com/rooksdermatology10e

Ionising radiation in the treatment of skin cancer
Brachytherapy, moulds, applicators and implants

3 Celada F, Rodriguez S, Botella R et al. Non-malignant skin cancer treated with HDR Valencia applicator: clinical outcomes. J Contemp Brachy 2014;6:167–72.
6 Tagliaferri L, Ciardo F, Fioda B et al. Non-melanoma skin cancer treated by contact high-dose-rate radiotherapy (brachytherapy): a mono-institutional series and literature review. In Vivo 2021;35:2313–19.

Indications for radiotherapy
Keloids

8 De Cicco L, Vischioni B, Vavassori A et al. Postoperative management of keloids: low-dose-rate and high-dose-rate brachytherapy. Brachytherapy 2014;13:508–13.

Malignant skin disease

5 Cho M, Gordon L, Rembielak A, Woo TC. Utility of radiotherapy for treatment of basal cell carcinoma: a review. Br J Dermatol 2014;171:968–73.
8 Visch M, Kreike B, Gerritsen M-J et al. Long-term experience with radiotherapy for the treatment of non-melanoma skin cancer. J Dermatolog Treat 2020;31:290–5.
9 Likacheva A, Awan M, Barker C et al. Definitive and postoperative radiation therapy for basal and squamous cell cancers of the skin: executive summary of the American Society for Radiation Oncology Clinical Practice Guideline. Pract Radiat Oncol 2020;10:8–20.
12 McPartlin AJ, Slevin NJ, Sykes AJ et al. Radiotherapy treatment of nonmelanoma skin cancer: a survey of current UK practice and commentary. Br J Radiol 2014;87:20140501.
17 Barrett-Lee P. Radiotherapy for skin cancer: as good as surgery? Br J Dermatol 2014;171:930.

Radiotherapy for particular skin sites: basal cell and squamous cell carcinoma

6 Matthiesen C, Thompson JS, Forest C et al. The role of radiotherapy for T4 non-melanoma skin carcinoma. J Med Imaging Rad Oncol 2011;55:407–16.
7 Sykes AJ, Allan E, Irwin C. Squamous cell carcinoma of the lip: the role of electron treatment. Clin Oncol 1996;8:384–6.
8 Guibert M, David I, Vergez S et al. Brachytherapy in lip carcinoma: long-term results. Int J Radiat Oncol Biol Phys 2011;81:e839–43.

Radiotherapy for particular skin tumours

2 Cho M, Gordon L, Rembielak A et al. Utility of radiotherapy for treatment of basal cell carcinoma: a review. Br J Dermatol 2014;171:968–73.
27 Henderson MA, Burmeister BH, Ainslie J et al. Adjuvant lymph-node field radiotherapy versus observation only in patients with melanoma at high risk of further

lymph-node field relapse after lymphadenectomy (ANZMTG 01.02/TROG 02.01): 6-year follow-up of a phase 3, randomised controlled trial. *Lancet Oncol* 2015;16:1049–60.

74 Gilson D, Whittaker S, Child FJ *et al.* British Association of Dermatologists and UK Cutaneous Lymphoma Group guidelines for the management of primary cutaneous lymphomas 2018. *Br J Dermatol* 2019;180:496–526.

77 Jones GW, Kacinski BM, Wilson LD *et al.* Total skin electron radiation in the management of mycosis fungoides: consensus of the European Organization for Research and Treatment of Cancer (EORTC) Cutaneous Lymphoma Project Group. *J Am Acad Dermatol* 2002;47:364–70.

PART 3
Infections and Infestations

CHAPTER 25

Viral Infections

Catherine A. Harwood[1] *and Jane C. Sterling*[2]

[1] Department of Dermatology, The Royal London Hospital, Barts Health NHS Trust, London, UK; Centre for Cell Biology and Cutaneous Research, Blizard Institute, Barts and the London School of Medicine and Dentistry, Queen Mary University of London, London, UK
[2] Department of Dermatology, Cambridge University Hospitals NHS Foundation Trust, Addenbrooke's Hospital, Cambridge, UK

Introduction, 25.2
General pathology of viral infections, 25.2

POXVIRUS INFECTIONS, 25.6
General description of disease domain, 25.6
Basic biology, 25.6
Smallpox, 25.6
Vaccinia, 25.7
Mpox (formerly monkeypox), 25.8
Cowpox, 25.12
Buffalopox, 25.13
Orf, 25.13
Milker's nodule, 25.15
Molluscum contagiosum, 25.15
Tanapox, 25.19

HERPESVIRUS INFECTIONS, 25.19
General description of disease domain, 25.19
Basic biology, 25.19
HERPES SIMPLEX VIRUS INFECTIONS, 25.19
General description of disease domain, 25.19
Primary infection, 25.19
Recurrent infection, 25.19
Subclinical viral shedding, 25.20
Basic biology, 25.20
Primary herpetic gingivostomatitis, 25.20
Recurrent oro-facial and cutaneous herpes, 25.22
Primary herpes genitalis, 25.24
Recurrent genital herpes, 25.26
Neonatal herpes, 25.27
Inoculation herpes simplex, 25.28
VARICELLA-ZOSTER VIRUS INFECTIONS, 25.28
General description of disease domain, 25.28
Basic biology, 25.28
Varicella, 25.28
Zoster, 25.32
EPSTEIN–BARR VIRUS INFECTIONS, 25.36
Introduction, 25.36
General description of disease domain, 25.36
Basic biology, 25.36
Infectious mononucleosis, 25.36
Oral hairy leukoplakia, 25.37

Chronic active Epstein–Barr virus infection, 25.38
Epstein–Barr virus-associated lymphoproliferative disorders and malignancy, 25.38
HUMAN HERPESVIRUS 6 AND 7 VIRUS INFECTIONS, 25.39
Definition, 25.39
Classification, 25.39
General description of disease domain, 25.39
Basic biology, 25.39
Roseola infantum, 25.39
Reactivation of herpesvirus 6 and 7, 25.40
OTHER HERPESVIRUS INFECTIONS, 25.41
Cytomegalovirus infection, 25.41
Human herpesvirus 8 infection, 25.42
Herpes B virus infection, 25.43
Eczema herpeticum, 25.43

POLYOMAVIRUS INFECTIONS, 25.46
Definition and general description of disease domain, 25.46
Merkel cell polyomavirus infection, 25.46
Trichodysplasia spinulosa, 25.48
Human polyomavirus 6 and 7 associated pruritic and dyskeratotic dermatoses (PDD), 25.48
Human polyomavirus-9 and hyperkeratotic skin lesions in organ transplant recipients, 25.49
Malawi polyomavirus; human polyomavirus-10, 25.49
Human polyomaviruses and keratinocyte skin cancers, 25.49

HUMAN PAPILLOMAVIRUS INFECTIONS, 25.49
Definition, 25.49
General description of disease domain, 25.49
Basic biology, 25.51
Subclinical and latent human papillomavirus infection, 25.51
Immunity to human papillomavirus, 25.52
Cutaneous warts, 25.52
Ano-genital warts, 25.61
Human papillomavirus-associated intraepithelial and invasive neoplasias of genitalia and mucosae, 25.64

Definition, 25.64
General description of disease domain, 25.64
Basic biology, 25.64
Cervical intraepithelial neoplasia and invasive carcinoma, 25.65
Cutaneous squamous cell carcinoma without immunosuppression, 25.65

IMMUNODEFICIENCY AND HPV INFECTION, 25.65
Overview, 25.65
Inborn errors of immunity and HPV infection, 25.65
Epidermodysplasia verruciformis, 25.65
Genetic EV (classic/typical and non-classic/atypical), 25.66
Other inborn errors of immunity and recalcitrant viral warts, 25.70
Human papillomavirus in acquired immunodeficiency, 25.71
HIV infection, 25.71
Haematological malignancies, 25.71
Immune-mediated inflammatory disorders (IMIDs), 25.71
Iatrogenic immunosuppression, 25.71
Acquired epidermodysplasia verruciformis (AEV), 25.71

HEPATITIS INFECTIONS, 25.73
Hepatitis B, 25.74
Hepatitis C, 25.75

PARVOVIRUS INFECTIONS, 25.77
General description of disease domain, 25.77
Erythema infectiosum, 25.77
Other parvoviruses, 25.78

HUMAN RETROVIRUS INFECTION, 25.78
General description of disease domain, 25.78
HUMAN T-CELL LYMPHOTROPIC VIRUSES, 25.79
General description of disease domain, 25.79
Epidemiology and transmission, 25.79
Basic biology, 25.79
Haematological and neurological disease associated with HTLV-1, 25.79
Infective dermatitis associated with HTLV-1, 25.79

Rook's Textbook of Dermatology, Tenth Edition. Edited by Christopher Griffiths, Jonathan Barker, Tanya Bleiker, Walayat Hussain and Rosalind Simpson.
© 2024 John Wiley & Sons Ltd. Published 2024 by John Wiley & Sons Ltd.

VIRAL INSECT-BORNE AND HAEMORRHAGIC FEVERS, 25.80	PICORNAVIRUS INFECTIONS (ENTEROVIRUSES), 25.93	Disease exacerbation by SARS-CoV-2 infection, 25.115
General description of disease domain, 25.80	General description of disease domain, 25.93	Covid-19 outcomes in patients with pre-existing mucocutaneous diseases, 25.115
Basic biology, 25.80	Basic biology, 25.93	Mucocutaneous manifestations of treatment for Covid-19 infection, 25.116
ARENAVIRUS INFECTIONS, 25.81	Foot and mouth disease, 25.93	
General description of disease domain, 25.81	Enterovirus infection, 25.93	MUCOCUTANEOUS REACTIONS TO SARS-COV-2 VACCINES, 25.117
Lassa fever, 25.81	Hand, foot and mouth disease, 25.94	
Lujo virus haemorrhagic fever, 25.82	Herpangina, 25.95	General description of disease domain, 25.117
Argentinian, Bolivian, Brazilian and Venezuelan haemorrhagic fevers, 25.82	Parechovirus infection, 25.96	COVID-19 vaccination and skin disease, 25.119
BUNYAVIRUS INFECTIONS, 25.83	Hepatitis A infection, 25.96	Skin disorders resulting from use of personal protective equipment (PPE), 25.119
General description of disease domain, 25.83	RHABDOVIRUS INFECTIONS, 25.97	Altered health care delivery during the Covid-19 pandemic on diagnosis and prognosis of skin cancer, 25.120
FILOVIRUS INFECTIONS, 25.84	Vesicular stomatitis virus infection, 25.97	
General description of disease domain, 25.84	PARAMYXOVIRUS INFECTIONS, 25.97	
Marburg and Ebola haemorrhagic fevers, 25.84	MEASLES AND RESPIRATORY SYNCYTIAL VIRUS, 25.97	OTHER CUTANEOUS PROBLEMS ASSOCIATED WITH VIRAL INFECTIONS, 25.120
FLAVIVIRUS INFECTIONS, 25.85	General description of disease domain, 25.97	
General description of disease domain, 25.85	Measles, 25.97	General description of disease domain, 25.120
Yellow fever, 25.85	Respiratory syncytial virus, 25.99	Papular-pruritic gloves and socks syndrome, 25.120
Dengue, 25.86	HUMAN CORONAVIRUS INFECTION, 25.100	TORCH syndrome, 25.121
Zika virus, 25.87	General description of disease domain, 25.100	Gianotti–Crosti syndrome, 25.121
TOGAVIRUS INFECTIONS, 25.87	Severe acute respiratory syndrome coronavirus-2 (SARS-CoV-2), 25.100	Asymmetrical periflexural exanthem of childhood, 25.123
General description of disease domain, 25.87	SARS-COV-2 IN SKIN HEALTH AND DISEASE: OVERVIEW, 25.102	Eruptive pseudoangiomatosis and eruptive hypomelanosis, 25.123
Basic biology, 25.88	Mucocutaneous manifestations of Covid-19 infection, 25.102	Pityriasis rosea, 25.123
Sindbis virus infection, 25.88	Covid-19 and skin disease in children, 25.113	
Chikungunya fever, 25.89	General description of disease domain, 25.113	Key references, 25.127
O'Nyong-Nyong fever, 25.89	Effects of SARS-CoV-2 infection on pre-existing mucocutaneous disease, 25.115	
Ross River virus, 25.90		
Barmah Forest virus, 25.90		
Mayaro virus infection, 25.91		
Rubella, 25.91		

Introduction

A virus particle, or virion, consists of a length of nucleic acid, either RNA or DNA, within a protein shell, the capsid. The genetic information is sufficient to encode proteins involved in viral replication and production of the protective coat, but requires host cell ribosomes for translation. This absolute dependence on the host is the distinguishing feature of viruses.

A simple classification of viruses that cause illness involving the skin in humans is given in Table 25.1 [1]. This classification is followed throughout this chapter. Other viral-associated skin diseases and pityriasis rosea, a condition of uncertain but possible viral aetiology, are also discussed.

General pathology of viral infections
Pathogenesis of viral disease

For a virus to produce infection, it must gain entry into a susceptible cell within an appropriate host. Many viruses, particularly those producing systemic infection, enter the body via mucous membranes after inhalation, ingestion or contact. The skin can act as a portal of entry, although this usually depends on some breach of the barrier function of the integument, for instance a scratch or fissure or by direct inoculation. Attachment to the cell surface by means of a receptor is followed by entry of the virion into the cell, by endocytosis or phagocytosis. Viruses differ in the range and type of cell which they can infect; host specificity and tissue tropism are hallmarks of viral infections. For example, poliovirus can infect neurons and is called a neurotropic virus, while human papillomaviruses (HPVs) have a tropism for epithelial cells. A cell in which a particular virus can replicate is described as permissive for that virus. After entry into the cell, pre-existing cell enzymes remove or damage the capsid sufficiently for the nucleic acid to emerge.

The next stage depends on the nature of the virus. In relatively simple ones, like enteroviruses, the RNA acts as a messenger, is infectious on its own and is immediately translatable by host ribosomes into viral proteins. More complex RNA viruses, such as influenza, have non-infectious RNA, called negative-strand RNA, which has to be transcribed into messenger RNA (mRNA) by a polymerase enzyme carried in the virus itself. RNA tumour viruses or retroviruses, such as human immunodeficiency virus, contain a reverse transcriptase enzyme which synthesises DNA from the viral RNA template. DNA viruses are generally more complex and are able to transcribe mRNA from their DNA using either cell polymerase (e.g. adenoviruses) or viral polymerase (e.g. vaccinia). At the same time, replication of the viral nucleic acid also occurs.

A variety of proteins – regulatory, enzymatic and structural – are produced and these, together with the products of cell damage,

Table 25.1 Classification of viruses causing human skin disease.

Nucleic acid	Family	Genus	Size (nm)	Species/disease
DNA-ds	Poxviridae	Orthopoxvirus	200 × 300	Variola
				Vaccinia
				Monkeypox (Mpox)
				Cowpox
				Buffalopox
		Parapoxvirus	150 × 200	Pseudocowpox
				Orf
		Yatapoxvirus		Tanapox
		Molluscipox virus		Molluscum contagiosum
	Orthoherpesviridae	Simplexvirus	180–250 enveloped (100 naked)	Herpes simplex 1 and 2 (human alphaherpesvirus 1 and 2)
				Cercopithacine herpesvirus (herpes B virus)
		Varicellovirus		Varicella-zoster
		Cytomelagovirus		Cytomegalovirus (human betaherpesvirus 5)
		Roseolovirus		Human betaherpesvirus 6A, 6B
				Human betaherpesvirus 7
		Lymphocryptovirus		Epstein–Barr virus (human gammaherpesvirus 4)
		Rhadinovirus		Human gammaherpesvirus 8
	Polyomaviridae	Polyomavirus	44 naked	Merkel cell carcinoma virus
				Human polyomavirus 6
				Human polyomavirus 7
				Human polyomavirus 10
	Papillomaviridae	α Papillomavirus	55 naked	Warts, mucosal intraepithelial neoplasia and squamous cell carcinoma
		β Papillomavirus		Epidermodysplasia verruciformis, skin cancer
		γ Papillomavirus		Cutaneous warts
		μ Papillomavirus		Palmar and plantar warts
		ν Papillomavirus		Cutaneous warts, skin cancer
DNA-ds*	Hepadnaviridae	Orthohepadnavirus	42 naked	Hepatitis B
DNA-ss	Parvoviridae	Erythroparvovirus	22 naked	Human parvovirus (B19)/erythroparvovirus
		Tetraparvovirus		Parvovirus 4
		Bocaparvovirus		HBoV-1, HBoV-2-4
RNA-ss (+)	Retroviridae	Deltaretrovirus	100 enveloped	HTLV-1, HTLV-2
		Lentivirus		HIV-1, HIV-2
	Matonaviridae	Rubivirus	42 enveloped	Rubella
	Togaviridae	Alphavirus		Ross River
				Sindbis
				Chikungunya
				O'Nyong-Nyong
				Mayaro
				Barmah Forest
	Flaviviridae	Hepacivirus	42 enveloped	Hepatitis C
		Orthoflavivirus		Dengue
				Yellow fever
				Kyasanur forest disease
				Omsk haemorrhagic fever
				Zika
	Hepeviridae	Pastahepevirus	33 naked	Hepatitis E
	Coronaviridae	Betacoronavirus	110 enveloped	SARS-CoV-2/Covid-19
	Picornaviridae	Aphthovirus	27 naked	Foot and mouth disease
		Enterovirus		Enterovirus A–L, rhinovirus A–C. Hand, foot and mouth disease, herpangina
		Hepatovirus		Hepatitis A
		Parechovirus		Human parechovirus
RNA-ss (−)	Rhabdoviridae	Lyssavirus	70 × 180 enveloped	Rabies
		Vesiculovirus		Vesicular stomatitis virus/Indiana vesiculovirus
	Filoviridae	Orthoebolavirus	Filamentous	Ebola disease
		Orthomarburgvirus		Marburg disease
	Paramyxoviridae	Morbillivirus	150 × 300 enveloped	Measles
		Respirovirus		Parainfluenza
		Orthorubulavirus		Mumps
		Metapneumovirus		Respiratory syncytial virus

(continued)

Table 25.1 (continued)

Nucleic acid	Family	Genus	Size (nm)	Species/disease
	Orthomyxoviridae	Influenzavirus A–D	>100 enveloped	Influenza
	Arenaviridae	Mammarenavirus	100 × 300 enveloped	Lassa fever
				Lujo virus haemorrhagic fever
				Junin virus
				Argentinian haemorrhagic fever
				Mapucho virus, Chapare virus
				Bolivian haemorrhagic fever
				Guanarito virus
				Venezuelan haemorrhagic fever
				Sabia virus, Latino virus
				Bolivian haemorrhagic fever
				Whitewater arroyo virus
	Hantaviridae	Orthohantavirus	100 enveloped	Hantaan virus
				Sin Nombre
	Nairoviridae	Orthonairovirus		Crimean–Congo haemorrhagic fever
	Peribunyaviridae	Orthobunyavirus		Bunyamwera
				Oropouche virus
	Pheniuviridae	Phlebovirus		Rift valley fever

ds, Double stranded; ds*, incomplete ds; ss, single stranded; ss (+), single stranded (plus strand); ss (−), single stranded (minus strand).

probably contribute to the local and general response to the infection. The time required for new virus production in acute infections is measured in hours and the number of new virions in thousands per cell. Newly produced virions can invade adjacent cells or be carried via the bloodstream and so the infection spreads. During this process the cell itself may be destroyed by a *lytic infection* (e.g. enterovirus and herpes simplex) or damaged transiently (e.g. myxovirus). With time, an immune response develops against the virus particles and processed viral proteins, which can lead to containment and clearance of the infection.

Not all virus infections end in this fashion. Some viruses infect cells that apparently remain normal and may multiply while virus replication continues within, that is *persistent infection*. When persistently infected cells produce no infectious virus because the replication cycle is arrested, the virus is said to be *latent*. From time to time, a latent virus can become active (*reactivation*), new virions are produced and other cells are infected. This process can result in clinical signs and symptoms as in the case of cold sores (reactivated herpes simplex) and shingles (reactivated varicella-zoster). Other viruses cause cell proliferation, for example poxviruses and HPVs. Viruses can also be implicated in the process of carcinogenesis, as in the development of cervical cancer and hepatoma.

Exanthems of viral infections

Widespread exanthems may be a manifestation of viral infections that cause a viraemia. An attempt to explain the different types of viral exanthem (Table 25.2) can be made by tracing the sequence of events following the arrival of blood-borne virus particles in the skin, where they lodge in dermal capillary loops. Some microorganisms (e.g. some togaviruses, poxviruses and rickettsiae) can replicate in capillary endothelium, causing damage directly or by a type III hypersensitivity reaction that results in infarcts and haemorrhages. The great majority of viruses, however, act as inert foreign particles, reacting with circulating antibodies and sensitised lymphocytes to produce inflammation. Circulating immune complexes of antibody and viral antigens also localise in dermal blood vessels and

Table 25.2 Viral exanthems.

Type of rash	Pathogen associated
Macular	Rubella
	Echovirus (esp. 2, 4, 6, 9, 11, 16, 18, 19, 23, 25, 32)
	Coxsackie A (esp. 4, 5, 6, 9, 10, 16) and B (esp. 5, 3)
	Epstein–Barr virus (infectious mononucleosis)
	Human herpesvirus 6 (roseola)
	Human herpesvirus 7
	SARS-CoV-2
Maculopapular	Togaviruses
	Echovirus (esp. 6, 9)
	Measles
	Human parvovirus (B19) (erythema infectiosum)
	SARS-CoV-2
Maculopapular-vesicular	Coxsackie A (occasional 5, 9, 10, 16)
	Echovirus (occasional 4, 9, 11)
	Ebola, Marburg
	SARS-CoV-2
Maculopapular-petechial	Togavirus (esp. chikungunya) and bunyavirus haemorrhagic fevers (including Lassa)
Urticarial	Coxsackie A9 (occasional)
	Hepatitis B (occasional)
	SARS-CoV-2
Vesicular	Herpes simplex virus
	Hand, foot and mouth disease (coxsackie 16, 4, 5)
	Vesicular stomatitis virus
	SARS-CoV-2
Vesiculopapular	Varicella-zoster
	SARS-CoV-2
Papulovesiculopustular	Vaccinia
	Variola
	Cowpox
Papulovesicular	Orf
	Milker's nodule
Papular	Molluscum contagiosum
	Warts
	Gianotti–Crosti syndrome
	SARS-CoV-2

are responsible for the rashes in many virus infections, for example human parvovirus. The complex cascade of inflammation in the dermis results in red macules and papules.

In the case of most RNA viruses where there is no replication, these are the only reactions and the intruding particle is removed (e.g. echoviruses, coxsackie A, most togaviruses and rubella). A few RNA viruses are, on occasion, able to enter actively metabolising epidermal cells and replicate for a limited time, with cytolysis and production of a vesicular lesion (e.g. the vesicular exanthem of coxsackie A and some rarer vesicular exanthems).

Replicative ability in epidermal cells is mainly a feature of the DNA viruses, which may explain why this group contains those viruses capable of replication after direct inoculation of the epidermis. Vesicles and pustules result from viral replication in the epidermis, where the focal necrosis is followed by an immune response and infiltration with leukocytes. Vesicular lesions are caused by poxviruses, herpes simplex, varicella-zoster and some coxsackievirus infections. The cell proliferation caused by HPVs and molluscum results in localised tumours.

The antibody production that produces local inflammatory lesions may serve to prevent further dispersal of infection by the bloodstream. However, the cell-mediated immune response is probably the major local inflammatory factor, the means of containment and healing of the infection. When it is not competent, as in immunosuppression or immunodeficiency, there may be serious spread of the lesions, as seen in vaccinia and varicella. The factors that influence the areas of distribution of the rash and the sequence of affected regions are imperfectly understood. Where there is an area of capillary trauma, caused for example by intermittent pressure or a pre-existing area of inflammation, viruses will localise, but the caudal progression in rubella and the centripetal distribution in varicella are unexplained.

Laboratory diagnosis [2,3,4,5]

The extent to which laboratory procedures are helpful depends on the nature of the infection and locally available resources. The general condition of the patient should always be considered and it is stressed that in early pregnancy any rash should be investigated to establish the possible risk to the fetus from rubella, parvovirus or other congenital infections. A considerable expansion of technical methods is taking place and clinicians are urged to discuss current local facilities with their microbiologists. Rapid methods are often feasible, using polymerase chain reaction (PCR) or fluorescence microscopy, so that laboratory confirmation may be possible on the day of receipt of specimens. Tissue culture can give an answer in 1–2 days.

Broadly, the following groups of tests are available:
1 Virus culture, usually done in cell cultures but occasionally in fertile eggs or laboratory animals.
2 Examination of histological specimens for features typical of a virus infection, for example inclusion bodies or koilocytes.
3 Visualisation of virus by electron microscopy.
4 Detection of viral antigens by immunological techniques, for example using fluorescent antibodies.
5 Detection of viral nucleic acid by molecular techniques such as PCR (for DNA viruses) or reverse transcription PCR (RT-PCR; for RNA viruses or for detection of viral transcripts).
6 Serological tests to detect seroconversion, rising antibody titres or specific antibodies (e.g. immunoglobulin M (IgM), low-avidity IgG).

Specimens for virus culture are most likely to be positive if taken early in the illness. After the onset, the amount of live virus declines, especially when accessible to circulating antibody. Specimens should be sent to the laboratory with the minimum of delay. Throat swabs should mop up the maximum nasopharyngeal material and the broken-off swab head should be immersed in a virus-transport medium and kept cool if in transit for more than 1 h. A swab of vesicle fluid transported in virus culture medium is also valuable. Small biopsies from proliferative skin lesions are best transported in medium or sterile normal saline. Crusts are sent dry in a sterile bottle. Cerebrospinal fluid should be transported rapidly, preferably chilled. Urine is of limited value; as a special transport medium may be needed, arrangements should be made with the laboratory. Faeces should be sent as a few grams in a sterile container.

Vesicle fluid for electron microscopy is best collected in a glass capillary, which can have one end sealed but not so as to heat the fluid. An alternative is to use a sterile disposable hypodermic needle and transport it in its plastic container.

The fraction of blood – white cells, plasma or serum – most suitable for PCR varies according to the viral nucleic acid to be detected. Blood for togavirus isolation must be chilled and reach the laboratory quickly. It is best processed without delay or rapidly frozen below −40°C because of inactivation of virus by antibody. PCR or RT-PCR can also be used for the detection of viral nucleic acid in vesicle fluid, skin exudate, skin biopsy, urine or cerebrospinal fluid.

If smallpox, Lassa fever, Marburg disease or other haemorrhagic fevers are suspected, consult both the laboratory director and the local community physician before any specimens are taken or transported and the patient should be kept in strict isolation.

Serological tests

Two specimens of clotted blood (5–10 mL each) should always be taken to achieve an unequivocal diagnosis in infections for which serology is available. The first must be taken as soon after the onset of symptoms as possible in order to have serum before appreciable antibody production has taken place. The second should be taken after a considered interval, depending on the type of infection. In general, 10 days is optimal, but when the antibody response immediately follows the rash, as in rubella, 5 days may suffice, provided the first blood was taken on the day of eruption of the rash.

A fourfold or greater rise in titre between acute and convalescent sera is taken as diagnostic. Because of technical variations it is customary to titrate both sera in parallel so that comparison of titres is accurate. Interpretation has to take into account possible anamnestic rises caused by organisms with some antigenic similarity.

Examination of a single serum may provide strong presumptive evidence of infection when it demonstrates a high relevant antibody titre, but this can be quite misleading at times as the particular antibody level may antedate the infection under consideration. The demonstration of specific IgM or IgA antibody in a single acute serum is also of diagnostic value in rubella and other infections. Unfortunately, in some infections such as HIV infections and in

Table 25.3 Human poxvirus infections.

Genus	Species	Abbreviation
Orthopoxvirus	Variola (smallpox)	VV, VARV
	Vaccinia	VACV
	Mpox (formerly monkeypox)	MPXV
	Cowpox	CPXV
	Buffalopox	BPXV
Parapoxvirus	Milker's nodule	–
	Pseudocowpox	PCPV
	Orf	–
Yatapoxvirus	Tanapox	TANV
Molluscipoxvirus	Molluscum contagiosum	MCV

severely immunodeficient or immunosuppressed people, serological responses to infection are unpredictable and cannot be relied upon for diagnosis.

POXVIRUS INFECTIONS

The poxviruses are the largest animal viruses, being only slightly smaller than the smallest bacteria, and they are just visible by light microscopy. Many species can infect both humans and other animals (Table 25.3).

General description of disease domain

Spread is mainly by direct-contact inoculation, with droplet spread in some, for example variola, which produce oropharyngeal and respiratory tract lesions. The skin lesions are inflamed vesicles or pustules in the ortho- and parapoxviruses. Yatapox and molluscipox produce small firm epidermal tumours.

Basic biology

These are complex double-stranded DNA viruses which replicate in the cytoplasm and are especially adapted to epidermal cells. Within the cytoplasm, they produce eosinophilic inclusion bodies (Guanieri bodies). They are generally resistant to physical damage; some, for example variola, have remarkable resistance to drying and can remain viable for months in crusts. Some grow readily in eggs and tissue culture, others not at all.

Smallpox

Synonyms and inclusions
- Variola virus (VARV)

Introduction and general description

Smallpox is an ancient human disease estimated to have caused 300–500 million deaths worldwide. It was the first human infectious disease to be successfully eliminated worldwide after a 10-year World Health Organization (WHO) vaccination programme and its eradication was certified at the World Health Assembly in 1980 [1]. The last case in an endemic area was in 1977 in Somalia. The last case in the UK was in Birmingham in 1978 and was the result of a laboratory accident. Routine vaccination against smallpox has now been discontinued, producing a decrease in herd immunity against the virus. However, concerns that the virus could be released as an agent of bioterrorism have led to an increase in the number of medical and military personnel receiving vaccinia vaccination, together with progress in smallpox laboratory diagnostics and antiviral medications, with an emphasis on heightened awareness of the clinical features of smallpox infection [2,3,4]. As a result of waning immunity to smallpox, there is also an increased risk of the emergence of other orthopoxviruses, as seen in the 2022 global outbreak of Mpox (see below).

Pathophysiology
Causative organisms

Variola is an orthopoxvirus which emerged 3000–4000 years ago in East Africa and is closely related to poxviruses in African gerbils and camels [3,4]. Stocks of smallpox virus still exist in government agencies in the USA (Center for Disease Control, Atlanta) and Russia (Vector Centre in Koltsovo, Siberia).

Clinical features
Predisposing factors

Human-to-human transmission occurs by inhalation of airborne droplets of saliva from an infected person. Transmission by contact with pustules/scabs can also occur but is much less infectious than respiratory secretions [2].

Presentation

There are four main clinical forms of smallpox: ordinary smallpox/variola major (accounting for 85% of cases in the smallpox era); modified type (occurring in previously vaccinated individuals); flat/malignant type (more frequent in children and causing intense toxaemia); and haemorrhagic (more common in adults and pregnant women).

The first features of ordinary smallpox are a prodrome of fever, headache, backache and malaise, appearing 10–14 days after infection. Within 1–4 days an eruptive phase develops as the fever subsides. A macular eruption evolves over about 3 days into a rash of tense vesicles which may umbilicate and evolve to pustules. This typically starts on the face and spreads caudally, usually affecting the extremities more than the trunk (Figure 25.1). The palms and soles are frequently affected. Lesions within an area are at the same stage. After about a week, the lesions dry, scab over and finally slough off 14 days after onset. Scarring due to virus-mediated necrosis and destruction of sebaceous glands is common following recovery. It can be marked and is still seen in areas of the world where the infection was last evident (Figure 25.2).

Disease course and prognosis

During the smallpox era, the mortality differed for the four clinical forms and overall was approximately 30% in unvaccinated individuals.

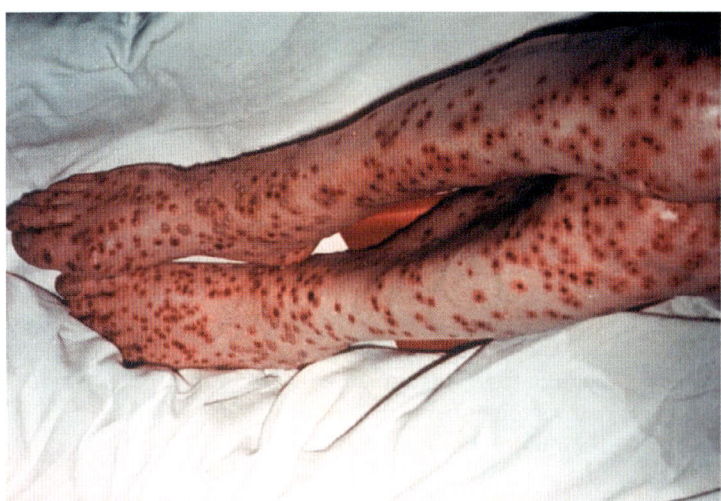

Figure 25.1 Smallpox. Papulovesicular lesions, some with haemorrhagic centres, concentrated on the extremities. Courtesy of Dr Colin Long, Cardiff and Vale NHS Trust, Wales, UK.

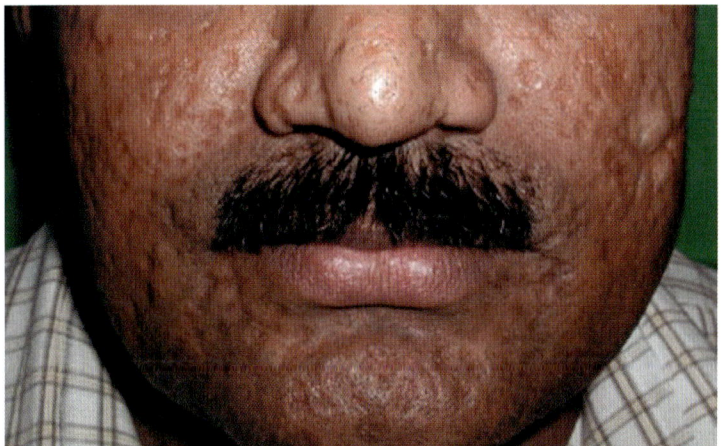

Figure 25.2 Scarring of face following smallpox infection. Courtesy of Dr S. B. Verma, Baroda Skin Clinic, Baroda, India.

Management

This generally involves supportive care. Vaccination with replication-competent smallpox vaccines can reduce disease severity if given within 2–3 days of exposure. As orthopoxvirus has a stable genome and highly conserved protein structure, smallpox vaccines provide cross-immunity with more than 80% efficacy for other orthopoxviruses such as mpox (formerly monkeypox) (see later) [3,4]. The Food and Drug Administration (FDA) approved the antiviral drugs tecovirimat and brincidofovir in 2018 and 2021, respectively, for treatment of smallpox [3].

Resources

Further information
World Health Organization: http://www.who.int/csr/disease/smallpox/en/
Centers for Disease Control and Prevention: https://www.cdc.gov/smallpox/
(Both last accessed August 2023.)

Vaccinia

Introduction and general description

Vaccinia virus (VAVC) was used in vaccination programmes against smallpox and human vaccinia disease is related to vaccination and its complications. Although routine vaccination was discontinued in the 1970s it continued for some years for laboratory workers using wild-type and recombinant vaccinia virus, but is now only performed for those in specific high-risk work. Vaccination has continued for military personnel and has increased over the last 10 years because of the potential risk that variola could be used in bioterrorism. Medical personnel who might potentially treat victims of biological attacks have also been vaccinated [3,4]. Since 1999, vaccinia-like virus has been found to be endemic in cattle in Brazil and more recently in monkeys, probably a result of infection spreading from vaccinated humans to animals [5,6,7]. Cases of human infection have been found in people working closely with animals [7,8]. In 2022, the global outbreak of mpox (formerly monkeypox) also led to increased levels of vaccination for exposed individuals (see later).

Pathophysiology
Causative organisms

Vaccinia virus is a distinct entity – poxvirus officinalis – and is unique in that it does not occur naturally but is the first stable virus to have resulted directly from human activity, that is, the serial propagation of cowpox orthopoxviruses originally used for human inoculation against smallpox. At the molecular level, it closely resembles cowpox and is postulated to have arisen as a mutant from cowpox [9]. Antigenically, it closely resembles variola and was used instead of cowpox in the 20th century in the WHO Smallpox Eradication Programme [3,4]. Vaccinia is also now being used in viral-vectored genetic vaccines against other infections (including coronavirus, tuberculosis, rabies and influenza) and in oncolytic virus-based therapies for malignancy [10].

Clinical features
Presentation

Following vaccination, a slightly itchy papule develops at the site of inoculation after 3–4 days. It develops into a pustule or blister, which may burst, before crusting and drying in about 2 weeks. The lesion heals by 3 weeks.

Clinical variants

A local or more generalised spread can occur, especially if the inoculation site is not adequately covered (Figure 25.3). Accidental infection can occur at sites distant to the inoculation site such as the eye or genitalia and autoinoculation in tattoos is also reported [11]. Spread to other individuals in close contact with a vaccinated person may occur, usually presenting 1–2 weeks after contact [12–14].

Complications and co-morbidities

In immunocompromised individuals, vaccinia infection can become persistent and locally progressive, with necrotic and fungating

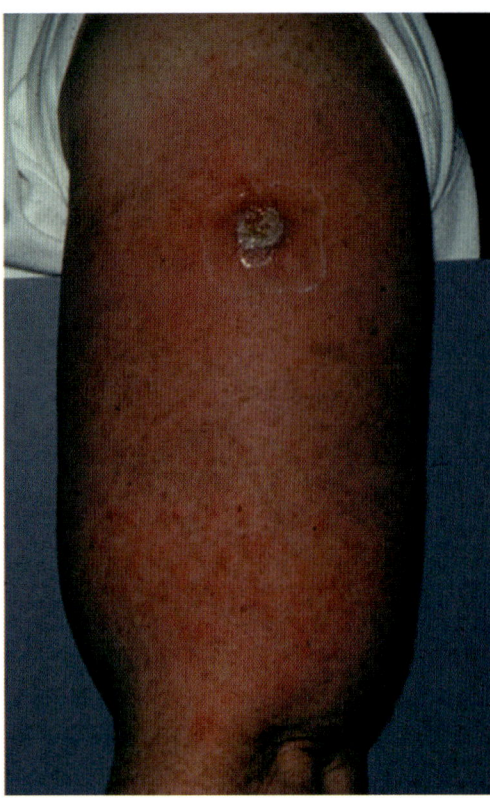

Figure 25.3 Vaccinia: vaccination site with generalised spread. Courtesy of Addenbrooke's Hospital, Cambridge, UK.

lesions, and may be fatal. Generalised vaccinia with disseminated vesicular or pustular lesions is also more common in immunocompromise [15,16]. In atopic individuals, vaccination can result in eczema vaccinatum in which localised or widespread infection occurs in eczematous skin [17]. Erythema multiforme/Stevens–Johnson syndrome may also complicate vaccinia infection.

Disease course and prognosis
The vaccination site usually scars and occasionally forms a hypertrophic scar. The scar may rarely be the site of development of a tumour such as a basal cell carcinoma [18].

Management
Care after vaccination should include adequate coverage of the vaccination site and avoidance of close contact with individuals who are immunosuppressed or atopic. Vaccinia immune globulin intravenous (VIGIV) is first line therapy for treatment of continued vaccinia virus replication after vaccination and antivirals may be considered as a secondary treatment.

Resources

Patient resources

http://www.who.int/csr/disease/smallpox/en/
https://www.cdc.gov/smallpox/
(Both last accessed August 2023.)

Mpox (formerly monkeypox)

Introduction and general description
Monkeypox virus (MPXV) infection was first described in 1958 in Denmark in research colonies of macaque monkeys transported from Africa and the first human case was described in 1970 in the Democratic Republic of Congo [19,20]. Despite being discovered in captive monkeys, it was subsequently documented in diverse mammals such as squirrels, rats, mice and prairie dogs; small forest mammals are thought to be the main reservoir driving zoonotic transmission, although this remains uncertain [20,21]. It produces a disease with a pustular rash and systemic symptoms that are similar to, but milder than, smallpox [19,21].

Epidemiology
Incidence and prevalence
The virus is endemic in 11 countries in Central and West Africa. The natural reservoir is uncertain, but is probably wild rodents [22]. Most outbreaks have been in the Congo Basin and West Africa, for example in Nigeria (2017–18) and Cameroon (2018), with occasional clusters of cases beyond the tropical rainforests [21,23–26]. There have been changes in the epidemiological characteristics of mpox, with increasing cases in West and Central Africa, particularly since 2010, and cases occurring in new geographic areas [19,21]. It is postulated that this re-emergence of mpox reflects waning of orthopoxvirus cross-protection resulting from cessation of smallpox vaccination after eradication of the disease in 1980, as this provides protection in 85% of cases [27,28]. There are also possible environmental factors affecting the interface between humans and the mpox animal reservoir, for example due to increased population density and displacement, climate change and deforestation, ease and rapidity of global travel, or possible new and widespread zoonotic reservoirs [21,22,25]. Outside endemic countries, an outbreak of 72 cases in the USA in 2003 followed illegal importation of infected rodents from Ghana which spread to native prairie dogs in a shared distribution centre [24]. Outbreaks were also reported in the USA and UK during the Covid-19 pandemic in 2021 [25,26]. However, prior to May 2022, transmission outside endemic areas and human-to-human transmission were uncommon [21,26,29].

In early May 2022 the first cases in a global outbreak of multiple clusters of mpox were reported, in countries across five WHO regions (Americas, African, European, Eastern Mediterranean and Western Pacific regions), but particularly in Europe. By July 2022 it was declared a Public Health Emergency of International Concern by the WHO. By October 2022, more than 75 000 cases had been confirmed in 109 countries, 102 of which had not historically reported mpox [30]. Multiple causes may have driven this outbreak, including a background of waning smallpox immunity globally [19] and relaxation of Covid-19 prevention measures with corresponding increases in international travel and sexual interactions in 2021. Transmission initially disproportionately affected gay, bisexual and men who have sex with men (GBMSM) communities and human-to-human transmission was particularly associated with close person-to-person or sexual contact not linked with travel from endemic countries [30,31,32]. The upsurge of subsequent interest in mpox resulting from the 2022 outbreaks in non-endemic high-income countries underscores its position as one of many neglected tropical diseases in endemic low-income countries [21].

Age

Most cases in endemic areas are in children. However, in the 2022 outbreak, cohort and other studies have reported a median age of around 38 years and particularly affecting males [**31**,32].

Pathophysiology

Causative organism

Mpox virus is a brick-shaped, enveloped, double-stranded DNA virus of the *Orthopoxvirus* genus (*Poxviridae* family), most closely related to vaccinia and smallpox [19]. Two genetic clades of the virus have been identified: clade 1 (Congo Basin/Central African clade – Democratic Republic of Congo, Republic of Congo, Gabon and Cameroon) and clade 2 (West African clade – Nigeria, Côte d'Ivoire, Sierra Leone, Liberia, Ghana) [33]. Clade 1 (Congo Basin) is associated with more severe disease in humans and a case fatality rate of 10%, with mortality rates of 15% in children [19,21]. Clade 2 (West African) is associated with milder disease and cases fatality rates of 1–4% [21,33,34]. In the May 2022 outbreak, molecular testing identified reported cases in the UK as due to clade 2 [35]. Factors determining differences in virulence between the clades are currently uncertain [21].

Transmission

In endemic regions, mpox is a zoonotic infection and is acquired via droplets from animal reservoirs: small forest animals are presumed to be responsible for most transmission to humans including squirrels, rats and monkeys. Mpox outbreaks typically occur in populations who hunt, kill, handle and consume bushmeat [19,21]. Mucocutaneous inoculation of a scratch or wound with animal secretions leads to more severe systemic symptoms and a shorter incubation period than if contact has been less close [36]. Human-to-human transmission is also through respiratory droplets during direct and prolonged face-to-face contact by large respiratory droplets, but also by close contact of skin lesions with infected bodily fluids, contaminated fomites and by vertical transmission. Possible sexual transmission was first proposed in the 2017 outbreak in Nigeria [37]. Mpox has a secondary attack rate of approximately 10% in contacts unvaccinated against smallpox [21]. The role of transmission from asymptomatic or pre-symptomatic carriers is unknown [30]. Possible human-to-animal transmission has also been reported [38]. In non-endemic countries, epidemiology may differ. In a multicentre study of the seven patients seen between 2018 and 2021 in the UK, four had acquired mpox from travel to Nigeria, but three acquired the infection in the UK: one was a health care worker involved in the care of an imported case and the other two were household contacts of a case imported from Nigeria (including an adult in whom a possible sexual transmission was also proposed, and a 2-year-old child) [29]. A notable longitudinal virological finding in these cases was prolonged (up to 3 weeks) viral DNA shedding from the upper respiratory tract after apparent skin lesion resolution [29].

In the 2022 global outbreak, most cases were not associated with recent travel to endemic areas, suggesting circulation within the GBMSM community [**31**,32,39–43,**44**,45]. Patients presented with lesions predominantly on the ano-genital area, indicating direct contact with body fluids and prolonged physical contact during sexual intercourse [**31**,32,40–43,**44**,45,46]. It is uncertain whether sexual transmission through seminal or vaginal fluids occurs [19,29,46]. No definitive explanation has been provided for this 2022 outbreak, although waning of cross-protective herd immunity for smallpox and potentially new mpox virus mutations have been proposed [45].

Clinical features

History

The incubation period is 5–21 days, but typically 7–17 days following exposure [**44**]. Patients are presumed to be infectious from the rash onset until desquamation of cutaneous lesions approximately 4 weeks later [19,**20**,21,**44**].

Presentation

A 1–4 day prodrome with fever (38.5–40.5°C), headache, fatigue, sore throat and myalgia may be accompanied by nausea, vomiting, dyspnoea and cough. A prodrome is not present in all patients [19,**20**,21,29,30,34,39,40,42,43,**44**]. Lymphadenopathy occurs around the time of fever onset and is a distinguishing feature from smallpox. About 1–2 days after the onset of the prodrome a rash appears with multiple lesions that can number as few as one or up to thousands. In endemic areas, the lesions are initially most common on the face and trunk, but spread centrifugally to the limbs, palms, soles and periungual areas as mpox 'whitlows' [19,**20**,29,40,**44**]. Pharyngeal, genital and conjunctival mucosae may also be involved. Individual lesions are initially macules and papules which evolve into whitish-yellow vesicles and pustules that may become umbilicated or crateriform, centrally eroded with a brownish crust, and may be complicated by superinfection [19,29,**44**]. Lesions last for approximately 1–3 days at each stage and usually progress simultaneously/synchronously, although lesions at multiple stages of evolution may coexist. In the pustular stage, a further fever may develop with complications such as pneumonia and encephalitis. After 2–4 weeks, the lesions dry and become crusted. Once the crust has fallen off and the wounds have healed the patient is no longer considered infectious. Lesions may leave atrophic or pitted scarring [19,**20**,29,39,40,42,**44**].

Presentation in the 2022 outbreak. In the 2022 global outbreak, clinical manifestations differed from those in countries where mpox is endemic in terms of patterns of transmission, prodromal symptoms and atypical cutaneous manifestations (Table 25.4). Transmission appears to be predominantly sexual, patients may develop fewer cutaneous lesions, which are often localised to the ano-genital region, and preceding systemic symptoms may be minimal [**20**,**44**]. Similar findings were reported in international case series [**31**], single-centre studies from the UK [32,43] and Italy [42], and multicentre cross-sectional and prospective observational cohort studies in Spain [39,40]. Registries established during the Covid-19 pandemic have also been extended to capture data on clinical aspects of the disease and its treatment [47].

In an international case series in 2022 of 528 patients attending 41 centres in 16 non-endemic countries from four WHO areas

Table 25.4 'Atypical' clinical features of monkeypox in the 2022 outbreak compared with endemic infection.

'Atypical' clinical features of monkeypox in the 2022 outbreak
More common in males, mid-30s, GBMSM, PLWH
Human-to-human transmission – mainly sexual contact
No association with travel to endemic areas
Mild or minimal systemic symptoms in prodrome
Ten or fewer lesions, usually initially at sites of ano-genital inoculation
Lesions localised to ano-genital area with no involvement at other sites
Anal pain and bleeding with no visible skin lesions; tonsillitis
Lesions at different stages of development (asynchronous)
Presence of other sexually transmitted diseases is common

GBMSM, Gay, bisexual, men who have sex with men; PLWH, people living with HIV.

(Europe, Americas, Western Pacific and Eastern Mediterranean), 98% of those with infection were GBMSM, 75% were white and 41% were living with HIV infection [31]. Prodromal symptoms of fever, lymphadenopathy and myalgia were observed in the majority, as in endemic monkeypox, although they may be less severe [20,40]. The ano-genital area was the most frequently involved anatomical site (73%), with trunk, arms or legs (55%), face (25%) and palms and soles (10%) less frequently involved. This pattern is likely to reflect primary inoculation sites related to sexual transmission with a later more generalised eruption of vesiculopustular lesions [40]. The localised initial lesions are more similar to the presentation of other orthopoxviruses (e.g. cowpox virus, camelpox virus, buffalopox virus) and parapoxviruses (e.g. orf virus) that also cause localised skin lesions in humans at sites of inoculation. It is also proposed in several studies that the primary lesions at inoculation sites are predominantly pseudopustules – firm papules with a central ulcerated/necrotic appearance and white periphery on a red base that simulate pustules, but from which it is impossible to de-roof and obtain pus, and which histologically are composed of inflammatory keratinocytic debris and not liquid [40,48] (Figure 25.4). This may help distinguish mpox from conditions such as varicella-zoster virus [40]. Most of those infected had fewer than 10 lesions each, and these are often painful, may group together in plaques or appear asynchronously [40]. A single lesion was present in 11% of patients in one series [40]; importantly, a single genital ulcer potentially increases the risk of misdiagnosis with other conditions causing penile and perianal ulcers such as herpes, primary syphilis, lymphogranuloma venereum, granuloma inguinale and chancroid [49,50]. Single whitlow-like lesions may also be misdiagnosed [40]. Mucosal involvement was observed in 41% [31], particularly ano-rectal involvement, which was associated with pain, proctitis and diarrhoea, and pharyngeal involvement causing tonsillitis and dysphagia [39,40]. Penile lymphoedema has also been reported in some [32,39,51] but not all [40] studies, possibly caused by marked inguinal lymphadenopathy [51]. Concomitant sexually transmitted infections were confirmed in 29% in this study [31] but up to 76% in other studies [40].

Complications and co-morbidities

Although usually a self-limiting disease in healthy adults [29], there is potentially increased severity in young children [34], those who are pregnant and in immunocompromised groups, including people living with HIV (PLWH) [20,21,30,52,53]. Local mucocutaneous complications include deep soft tissue abscesses [29], keratitis, corneal scarring (with possible loss of vision) and permanent pitted scarring often secondary to bacterial superinfection [21]. Systemic complications include encephalitis, bronchopneumonia, myositis and miscarriage [19,20].

Case fatality rates in African outbreaks with at least 50 cases have ranged from 0 to 10% in unvaccinated individuals [21]. Disease is milder in West African compared with Congo Basin clades, with fewer deaths and previously limited human-to-human transmission [21,34]. In the 2022 outbreak due to the West African clade, the illness generally appeared to be mild. In one series, 13% required hospital admission, usually to manage pain (particularly ano-rectal pain) and soft-tissue super infections [31]. Giant ulcerated lesions [42] and penile lymphoedema [51] are also described. Morbilliform eruptions are less common and appear later and an associated erythema multiforme is also reported [39,40]. Dissemination beyond the ano-rectal area was more common in association with HIV [53,54], although rare serious complications (myocarditis and epiglottitis) were also observed [31].

Overall mortality was low in the 2022 outbreak [30], but is significantly higher in people with advanced HIV [53]. An international case series reported clinical outcomes and mortality in 382 people with mpox and HIV with low CD4 count (<350 cells/mm^3) [53]. The series included 27 of the 60 people reported to have died of mpox between May 2022 and January 2023, all of whom had a CD4 cell count <200 cells/mm^3, with high HIV viral load an additional risk factor for death. Severe complications were also more common in those with CD4 cell count <100 cells/mm^3 and included necrotising skin lesions, lung involvement, secondary bacterial infections and sepsis [53].

Clinical variants

Atypical cases are recognised with, for example, few minimally symptomatic lesions, anal pain without skin lesions, absent prodromal period or minimal systemic symptoms [50]. Infection can occasionally cause illness without skin lesions, and this has been described in both endemic areas [21] and in non-endemic areas during the 2022 outbreak [50,55]. Severe skin infection in association with atopic dermatitis (eczema monkeypoxicum) is described [56] and asymptomatic virus-positive cases have also been reported [41,55].

Differential diagnosis

Mpox should be considered in the differential of vesicular and pustular rashes [20,55]. Varicella is the most common differential but is usually associated with less prominent fever, is not associated with lymphadenopathy, lesions are often itchy, frequently involving the scalp and mouth, and are more polymorphic in nature [44]. Secondary syphilis, herpes, molluscum contagiosum, scabies, varicella-zoster, disseminated vaccinia, hand, foot and mouth disease, orf, milker's nodule and pityriasis lichenoides et varioliformis acuta may all be considered with widespread disease [19,20]. With more localised disease reported in the 2022 outbreak, mpox should be considered in the differential diagnosis of other causes of ano-genital and oral ulceration as discussed earlier [20].

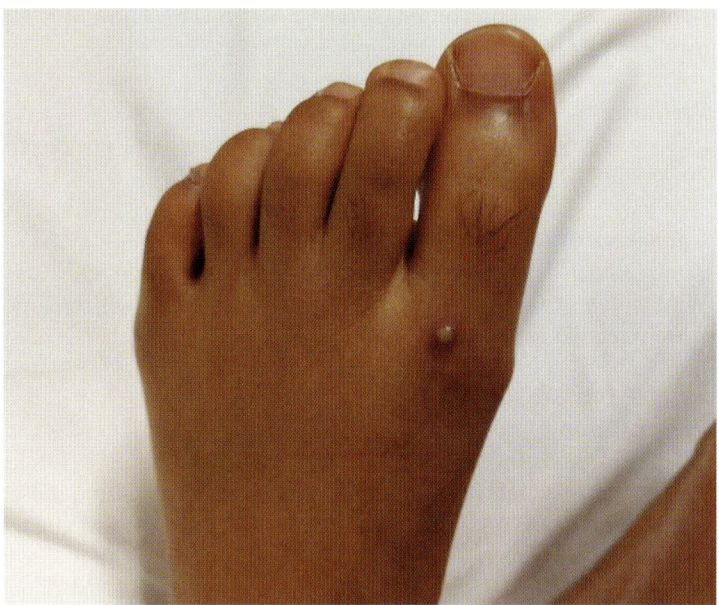
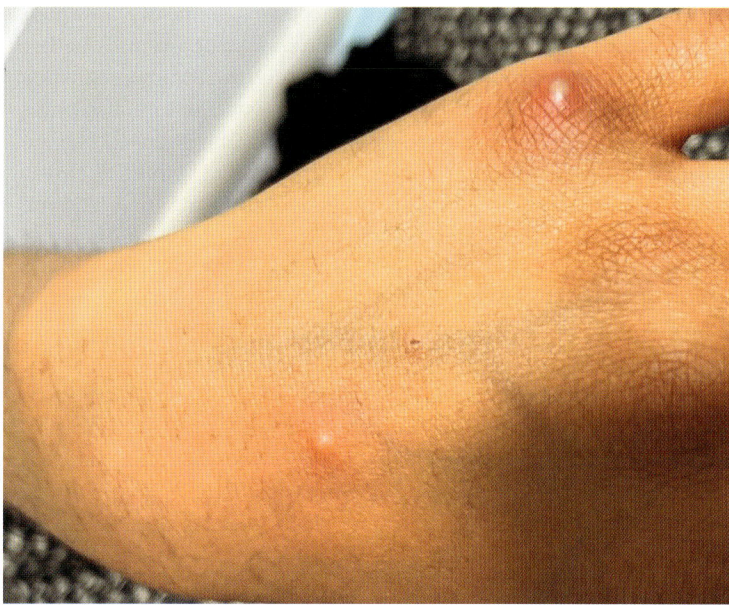

Figure 25.4 Pseudopustules associated with monkeypox infection. Courtesy of Professor Christopher Bunker, University College Hospitals, London, UK.

Investigations

Dermoscopy may provide diagnostic support: diffuse bright white structureless areas or bright white halos surrounded by a perilesional red rim are reported as a prominent finding in both vesicles and pustules [57]. Clinical suspicion can be confirmed by [20]:
- Demonstration of mpox virus DNA by real-time PCR analysis or next-generation sequencing of vesico pustular fluid and nasopharyngeal swabs.
- Isolation and culture of the virus from saliva, lesion exudate or crust specimens.
- Immunohistochemistry for viral antigen detection, including the point-of-care test Tetracore OrthopoxBioThreat®.
- ELISA for anti-orthopoxviruses IgM and IgG antibodies: there may be cross-reactivity to other orthopoxviruses [30,58].

However, most cases in remote endemic settings are clinically diagnosed.

Pathology

The epidermis shows degenerative changes with cell fusion, causing direct cytopathic changes including multinucleate cells and cytoplasmic inclusion bodies, and ground glass-like eosinophilic nuclei. Full-thickness epidermal necrosis and adjacent acanthosis may be present depending on the stage of the lesion [59,60]. A mixed inflammatory cell infiltrate of lymphocytes, neutrophils and eosinophils is found in the upper dermis in a perieccrine and perivascular distribution. With electron microscopy, the typical poxvirus brick-shaped enveloped particles are found in the cytoplasm [59,61].

Management

Supportive care. Mpox is usually self-limiting and treatment is primarily supportive and based on individual patient risk, underlying co-morbidities and complications. Hydration, anti pyretics, skin/mucosal care, analgesia and antibiotics for secondary infection may be required [20]. Those with confirmed infections should be isolated, with strict infection control [30,53,62]. There is evidence that viral DNA is present in 93% of surfaces and 20% of air samples in hospital isolation rooms [63]. Isolation of close contacts, contact tracing and surveillance are all essential to reducing transmission [30,53,62]. Avoidance of close contact with others, particularly children aged under 5 years and individuals who are pregnant or severely immunocompromised, should continue until all lesions have healed and crusted. There is some evidence that mpox DNA may be detected in semen after an acute infection [31]: it is unclear whether this is from seminal carriage, as the testes are immunologically protected sites, or from resolving meatal or urethral lesions. However, it has been recommended by the WHO UK that men who have had a confirmed or highly probable diagnosis of mpox should use condoms during sex for 12 weeks after complete recovery from mpox infection [64].

Direct-acting antiviral drugs. Brincidofovir and tecovirimat are broad spectrum direct-acting antivirals that have activity against orthopoxviruses. Tecovirimat inhibits p37 inhibitor, a protein involved in the release of enveloped virus and viral dissemination and virulence [65]. Efficacy has been demonstrated in animal models of mpox infection, it also has a favourable safety profile in healthy volunteers [66] and there are encouraging preliminary data from case reports/series [29,52,67,68]. It was approved by the European Medicines Agency (EMA) and Medicines and Healthcare products Regulatory Agency (MHRA) for use in more severe or complicated cases in the 2022 outbreak, but confirmatory randomised controlled trial (RCT) data for tecovirimat were awaited as of June 2023 [69; https://www.cdc.gov/poxvirus/mpox/clinicians/obtaining-tecovirimat.html#Summary-Recent-Changes]. Brincidofovir has also been used in case series but was associated with transaminitis in three cases where tecovirimat was better tolerated [29].

Vaccinia immunoglobulin. This may be considered in severe disease and in immunocompromised patients.

Vaccination. Although there are no vaccines specifically designed against mpox virus, the stable orthopoxvirus structure means that smallpox vaccines provide cross-immunity with efficacy of 80–85% [21,**28**,70]. Residual immunity from past vaccination also substantially reduces the severity of symptoms and signs [21]. The modified vaccinia Ankara (MVA-BN) (Imvanex, JYNNEOS, Imvamune) smallpox vaccine is a third-generation smallpox vaccine that contains a live but replication-defective virus and prevents lethal mpox in primate challenge models. In the USA, MVA-BN has been approved by the FDA and EMA for the prevention of both smallpox and mpox and can be used for immunosuppressed people such as PLWH and in atopic dermatitis or other dermatoses, although it has the disadvantage of requiring two vaccinations [**28**]. Although not specifically licensed for the prevention of mpox in Europe, MVA-BN vaccine has been used in response to the 2022 outbreak as postexposure prophylaxis with the aim of preventing infection and/or modifying disease severity [**28**,70]. This should ideally be administered within 4 days of exposure.

Resources

Further information

Centers for Disease Control and Prevention: https://www.cdc.gov/poxvirus/monkeypox/index.html
https://www.cdc.gov/poxvirus/mpox/clinicians/obtaining-tecovirimat.html#Summary-Recent-Changes
UK Health Security Agency:
https://www.gov.uk/government/collections/monkeypox-guidance
https://www.gov.uk/government/publications/monkeypox-outbreak-epidemiological-overview
World Health Organization:
https://www.who.int/news-room/questions-and-answers/item/monkeypox
European Centre for Disease Prevention and Control:
https://www.ecdc.europa.eu/en/news-events/monkeypox-situation-update
https://ecdc.europa.eu/en/mpox-monkeypox
(All last accessed August 2023.)

Cowpox

Introduction and general description

Cowpoxvirus (CPXV) infection causes inflammatory vesicular lesions which crust and heal with superficial scarring [71].

Epidemiology

Incidence and prevalence

Originally described in dairymaids in contact with the udders of infected cows, the natural reservoir of the virus is now wild rodents rather than cows, although cattle and zoo animals can also be infected [19]. Humans are more commonly infected by scratches and bites from domestic cats or pet rodents [19,71,72].

Pathophysiology

Predisposing factors

Contact with wild or domestic animals is almost always the route of infection [19]. Young people are those most frequently infected and smallpox vaccination confers some protection. Infection of laboratory workers has rarely been reported [73].

Pathology

In lesions, the epidermis is necrotic with prominent eosinophilic intracytoplasmic inclusions.

Causative organism

Cowpoxvirus is an orthopoxvirus, endemic in Europe and Russia. Viral isolates can be divided into two clades, one of which is more closely related to vaccinia virus [19].

Clinical features

Presentation

The skin lesion develops between 5 and 7 days (range 2–14) after contact with an infected animal. It starts as a painful papule and evolves rapidly to become vesicular, pustular or haemorrhagic with surrounding redness. The centre may show umbilication. In the second week, the lesion can erode and form a dark crust usually between 1 and 3 cm in diameter. There is often associated lymphangitis and lymphadenitis with general features of malaise, low-grade fever and myalgia. By 3–6 weeks the ulcerated lesion develops an eschar that heals, often with scarring, by 6–12 weeks [19].

Clinical variants

Lesions are most common on the hands, arms or face. One or a few lesions is the most common presentation, but sporotrichoid spread can occur [74]. Rarely, lesions present on mucosal surfaces such as the genitalia [75] or the eyes [76]. Scarring can be of greater significance if the lesions are near the eye, on the ear or if large with wider local necrosis.

Differential diagnosis

Differential diagnoses include orf, milker's nodule and mpox as well as herpes simplex, anthrax, sporotrichosis, primary tuberculosis, necrotising fasciitis and foreign-body granuloma. If lesions are widespread, chickenpox or other zoonotic orthopoxvirus infections should be considered [77].

Complications and co-morbidities

Secondary bacterial infection may occur and lesions on the face may be associated with conjunctivitis and a risk of conjunctival scarring. Although usually self-limiting in the immunocompetent, widespread cowpox infection has been reported in immunosuppressed patients including organ transplant recipients [78,79] and those with atopic eczema or Darier disease [80,81]. Fatality is rare, even in immunodeficiency [78,79,82].

Disease course and prognosis

The lesion usually heals with scarring in 6–12 weeks [19].

Investigations

Ultrastructural examination of vesicle fluid or crust will show orthopoxviruses. The viral DNA can be detected in blood as well as the lesions and PCR using a panel of primers for poxviruses will give precision regarding the causative virus [83,84]. Retrospectively, serology can confirm the infection.

Management
No specific treatment is usually required unless secondary bacterial infection occurs. Use of tecovirimat and vaccinia immune globulin has been described in severe cases [76,79].

Buffalopox

Epidemiology
Incidence and prevalence
Buffalopox is found as a resident in buffaloes but can infect cows, pigs and humans. Disease is usually confined to the Indian subcontinent and South-East Asia [19,85,86].

Pathophysiology
Predisposing factors
Infection is more common in those who have not received smallpox vaccination [19,86].

Causative organism
Buffalopoxvirus (BPXV) is an orthopoxvirus (Table 25.3).

Clinical features
History
Most infections occur in those working in close proximity to buffaloes, such as milkers and herdspersons. Laboratory-acquired infection is also described [87]. The incubation period is 1–2 weeks [19,85].

Presentation
The appearance of lesions is often accompanied by fever, malaise and painful local lymphadenopathy. Lesions are most common at sites of contact or contamination such as the fingers, hands and forearms rather than the face, although the mouth may be affected through contact with contaminated milk. They start as papules and evolve into blisters before then crusting and sometimes ulcerating. Healing, often with scarring, is complete in a month [85,88].

Complications and co-morbidities
Involvement near the eye can lead to corneal damage and scarring [88].

Investigations
Blister fluid or crusts can be examined ultrastructurally for poxvirus virions or used for molecular detection by PCR [19,85,88].

Management
Treatment is supportive.

Orf

Synonyms and inclusions
- Ecthyma contagiosum
- Contagious pustular dermatitis

Introduction and general description
Orf virus (ORFV) infection occurs worldwide and most commonly presents with a single lesion after contact with an infected animal [19,89].

Epidemiology
Incidence and prevalence
Infection is well recognised in individuals working with sheep and goats with the highest incidence during the breeding season. Although the virus is widespread in these animals, it is the young that most commonly show features of the disease, particularly around the lips, muzzle and mouth [19].

Pathophysiology
Predisposing factors
Contact with infected animals, usually domesticated sheep or goats, either directly or indirectly via contaminated fomites, precedes the human infection and occupational exposure is described in shepherds, slaughterhouse workers, butchers, animal skin and wool handlers and veterinarians [90]. The virus has also been acquired from wild rabbits, cats [91] or deer [92] and participants in religious ceremonies when animals are sacrificed [93]. Rarely, human-to-human transmission occurs [94] and progressive and/or multiple lesions are more common in the immunocompromised [95–98].

Pathology
The epidermis in an orf lesion shows ballooning degeneration of keratinocytes with eosinophilic cytoplasmic inclusions [99]. A dense cellular infiltrate in the dermis consists mainly of histiocytes and macrophages in the centre and of lymphocytes and plasma cells peripherally. There are very few polymorphonuclear leukocytes.

Causative organisms
Orf virus is a parapoxvirus (Table 25.3; Figure 25.5).

Environmental factors
Close contact between patients and health care workers within a hospital burns unit led to multiple cases and the first report of human-to-human transmission [94].

Clinical features
Presentation
The lesion develops 5–6 days (range 3–10 days) after contact with an infected animal or animal carcass. A small, firm, red or reddish-blue papule appears at the skin site of contact and enlarges into an uncomfortable, targetoid, haemorrhagic pustule or bulla (Figure 25.6). The size is usually 2–3 cm but may be as large as 5 cm. There is often lymphadenitis and lymphangitis and a mild fever [90].

Clinical variants
The most common sites of orf lesions are on the hands and forearms. Unusual sites relate to unusual contact and have been reported on the face and in the axillae and genital area [100,101].

Differential diagnosis
The clinical appearance of orf is similar to that of other orthopoxvirus and parapoxvirus infections. Giant orf can be similar to

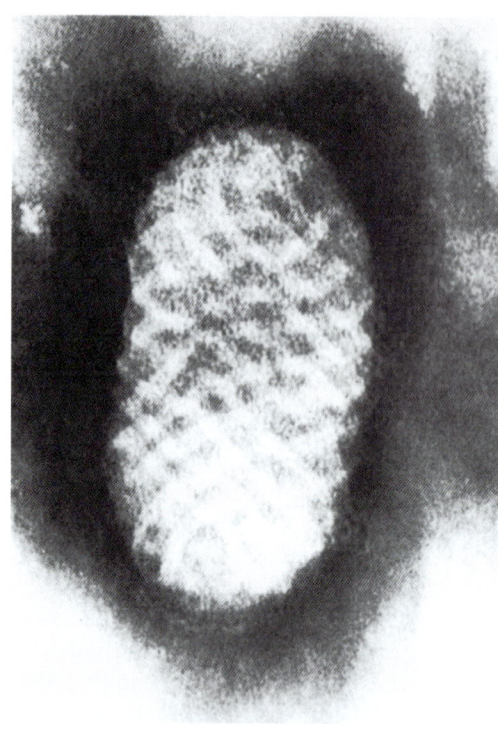

Figure 25.5 Orf virus. Phosphotungstate preparation (×230 000). Courtesy of Dr J. Nagington, Cambridge, UK.

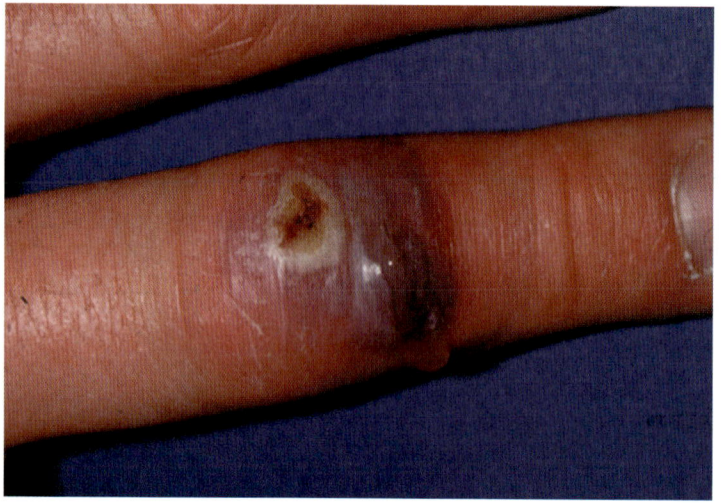

Figure 25.6 Orf. Courtesy of Addenbrooke's Hospital, Cambridge, UK.

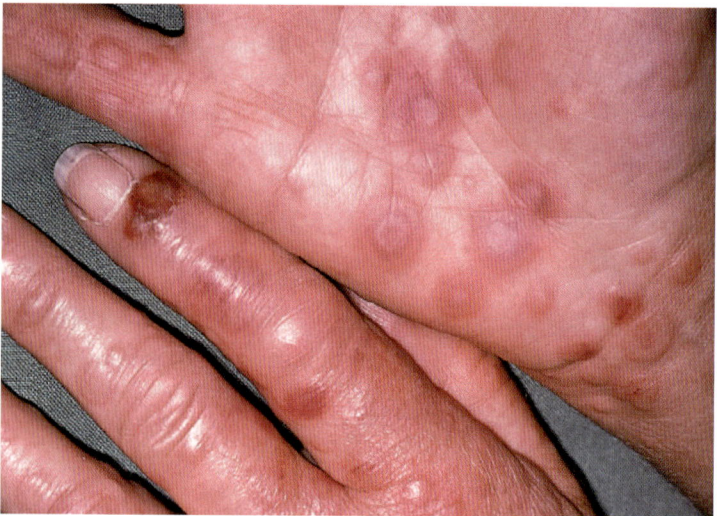

Figure 25.7 Orf with erythema multiforme. The orf lesion on the dorsum of the forefinger has been present for 14 days, the secondary erythema multiforme for 4 days. Courtesy of Dr A. S. Highet, York District Hospital, UK.

pyogenic granuloma and keratoacanthoma; widespread orf has similarities to chickenpox [90].

Complications and co-morbidities
Infection in the immunocompromised can result in giant orf [95] or widespread lesions that can be progressive, disfiguring, recurrent and recalcitrant to treatment and have been termed 'orf progressiva' [96,97]. Widespread lesions have also been observed in atopic eczema [102].

Erythema multiforme is a well-recognised complication of orf infection, presenting 2–3 weeks after the orf lesions in up to 10% of infections [103,104] (Figure 25.7).

The possibility of precipitation of an immunobullous disease with features of bullous pemphigoid about a month after orf has been raised in several anecdotal reports [105,106].

Disease course and prognosis
The lesions heal after 3–6 weeks. One infection is usually sufficient to confer immunity but second infections are not uncommon.

Investigations
The well-established methods of confirming a poxvirus infection are by electron microscopy of a skin biopsy or crust or culture on allantoic egg membrane. PCR of blister fluid, biopsy or crust is quicker and can distinguish orf from other poxviruses [107,108]. Serological confirmation can be made from about 1 week after the lesion appears.

Management
Treatment is not usually necessary. Secondary bacterial infection should be treated appropriately. Animals can be vaccinated against orf.

First line
Large exophytic lesions are best removed surgically.

Second line
Recurrent or persistent lesions, particularly in the immunocompromised, may clear with addition of cryotherapy [109], idoxuridine [110], imiquimod [111] or cidofovir cream [98,112], systemic acyclovir, and valaciclovir and interferon-α [97,113].

Resources

Further information
http://dermnetnz.org/viral/orf.html
(Last accessed August 2023).

Milker's nodule

Synonyms and inclusions
- Pseudocowpox
- Paravaccinia

Epidemiology
Incidence and prevalence
As its name suggests, this infection affects those in close contact with animals harbouring the virus, particularly around the teats and mouths of cows. It is distinct from cowpox, which more recently has been mainly acquired from cats and small rodents rather than cows. It is often an occupational infection of farmers, milkers and veterinary personnel. Those who handle raw beef may also become infected [114–116].

Associated diseases
One case of coinfection with pseudocowpox and vaccinia has been reported [117].

Pathophysiology
Causative organisms
Pseudocowpox virus (PCPV) or paravaccinia is a member of the *Parapoxvirus* genus (Table 25.3).

Clinical features
Presentation
Lesions may be single or multiple and are most common on the hands, forearms and occasionally face [115]. Following an incubation period of about 5 days to 2 weeks, six stages of milkers, nodule are described: (i) an initial red papule, which becomes (ii) targetoid with a red outer ring and paler inner ring; (iii) the nodule then ulcerates and (iv) becomes firmer, darker and crusted; (v) papillomas develop within the nodule and (vi) the nodule regresses without leaving a scar [114,115] (Figure 25.8). Secondary bacterial infection may occur.

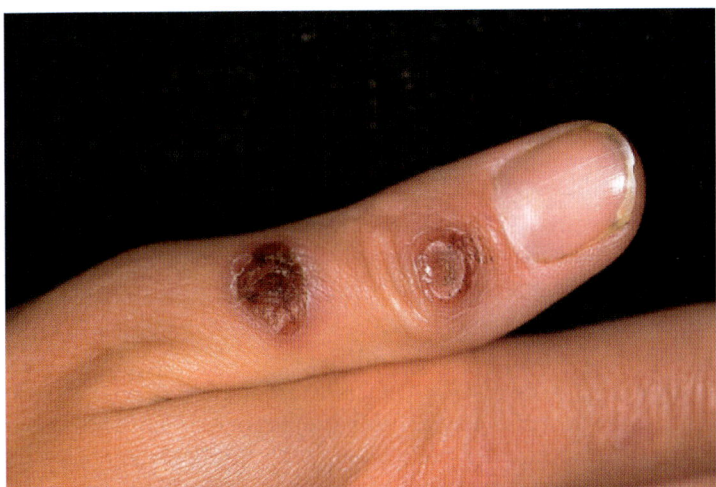

Figure 25.8 Milker's nodule. Courtesy of Dr J. B. Kurtz, Oxford, UK.

Differential diagnosis
The lesions are very similar to orf. Herpes simplex, cutaneous anthrax and pyogenic granuloma may also need to be considered, and in certain parts of the world, vaccinia, buffalopox and mpox are differential diagnoses [115].

Complications and co-morbidities
There is constitutional upset only rarely, but lymphangitis is not uncommon. Some patients develop erythema multiforme or a less distinct papular or papulovesicular eruption on the hands, forearms and arms, and sometimes on the legs and neck, 1–2 weeks after the appearance of the nodules which fades in 1–2 weeks [118].

Disease course and prognosis
The lesion crusts in the centre and heals without scarring in 4–6 weeks.

Investigations
Although electron microscopy of crusts can confirm the presence of a poxvirus, PCR is now the quickest and most reliable method to diagnose pseudocowpox infection [119,120]. Histological features include epidermal necrosis, spongiosis, inflammation and intracytoplasmic eosinophilic inclusions [121].

Management
No specific treatment is necessary other than treatment for any secondary bacterial infection.

Resources

Patient resources
https://dermnetnz.org/topics/milkers-nodule (last accessed August 2023).

Molluscum contagiosum

Epidemiology
Incidence and prevalence
Molluscum contagiosum (MC) infection is common [**122**,123], with an estimated prevalence of 5–11% [**122**]. The incidence appears to be increasing [124]. The molluscum contagiosum virus (MCV) occurs throughout the world, most commonly causing infection in childhood. Type 1 MCV (MCV-1) is responsible for most infections (76–97%) and there is some evidence to support a relatively higher incidence of MCV-2 infection in adults and PLWH [125]. There is no clear relationship between virus type and lesional morphology or anatomical distribution [126,127].

Viral DNA can be detected on the normal skin of people with molluscum and from objects in their environment, so it is assumed that infection follows contact with infected persons or contaminated objects [128]. It is not known if epidermal injury is important for establishing infection.

Age
Infection is rare under the age of 1 year, perhaps due to maternally transmitted immunity and a long incubation period. There

are rare reports of lesions detected in the first few days or weeks of life, suggesting that vertical transmission can occur [129]. In warmer climates where children are lightly dressed and in close contact with one another, spread within households is common and peak incidence is between 2 and 5 years [130,131]. In cooler climates, spread within households is less common and infection occurs at a later age and may be more closely correlated with use of swimming pools and shared bathing facilities [**122**,123,130,132,133]. A later incidence peak in young adults is attributable to sexual transmission, with lesions more common in the genital area.

Pathophysiology
Predisposing factors
Although MC appears to be more common in patients with atopic eczema [123,134], this is not consistently supported by cohort studies [135]. Use of topical steroids and topical calcineurin inhibitors are suspected as contributing factors [136,137].

MC is seen quite commonly on the genital, perineal and surrounding skin of children and although infection through sexual abuse is possible, abuse should not be regarded as likely unless there are other suspicious features.

Unusually widespread lesions have been reported in the context of immune compromise, including PLWH (Chapter 31), haematological malignancy [138], idiopathic CD4 lymphocytopenia [139], hyper-IgE syndrome [140], DOCK8 deficiency [141], thymoma [142] and in those receiving immunosuppressive therapy including methotrexate, anti-TNF therapy, JAK inhibitors, methotrexate and fingolimod [142–146]. Despite profound immunosuppression following organ transplantation, the incidence of MC infection is not greatly increased in this group and is much less common than other viral infections such as warts [147].

Pathology
The virus enters the basal epidermis where an early increase in cell division extends into the suprabasal layer [**122**,148]. The cellular proliferation produces lobulated epidermal growths which compress the papillae until they appear as fibrous septa between the lobules, which are pear shaped with the apex upwards. The basal layer remains intact. Cells at the centre of the lesion show the greatest distortion and are ultimately destroyed and appear as large hyaline bodies (molluscum bodies), 25 µm in diameter, containing cytoplasmic masses of virus material. These bodies are present in large numbers in the cavity which appears near the surface of the fully developed lesion. Inflammatory changes in the dermis are minimal, but in lesions of long duration there may be a chronic granulomatous infiltrate. It has been suggested that the inflammatory reaction may be induced by the discharge into the dermis of the contents of a papule [149] rather than by secondary infection. In spontaneous regression, the lesions are surrounded by an infiltrate of interferon-producing plasmacytoid dendritic cells [150].

Specific antibodies are present in 58–73% of patients with recognised MC and 6–16% of controls, but have not been demonstrated to play a role in clearance of infection [151].

Causative organisms
MCV belongs to the genus *Molluscipox virus* [152] (Table 25.3), which has features intermediate between orthopox and parapox. It cannot be grown in tissue culture or eggs. Although it seems to infect only humans and is not readily transmissible to laboratory animals, it produces typical changes in human skin cultured on immunodeficient mice [153]. Restriction endonuclease and PCR analyses of MCV DNA have identified two main types, MCV-1 and MCV-2, with two much rarer types, MCV-3 and MCV-4 [154,155].

Clinical features
Presentation
The incubation period is estimated at between 14 days to 6 months. Typical MC lesions appear as shiny, hemispherical papules with central umbilication (Figure 25.9a). Enlarging slowly, they may reach diameters of 5–10 mm in 6–12 weeks [**122**]. Rarely, and usually when one or very few are present, lesions may become considerably larger (giant MC). Plaques composed of many small lesions ('agminate' forms) may occur rarely. Lesions frequently spread and the large numbers of lesions may ultimately occur. After several months, spontaneous inflammatory changes result in suppuration, crusting and eventual destruction of the lesion, and this involution may be precipitated by trauma [**122**].

Clinical variants
The distribution of MC lesions is influenced by the mode of infection and by the type of clothing worn, and hence by the climate. In temperate regions, they are more commonly seen on the neck or on the trunk, particularly around the axillae. In the tropics, lesions are more common on the limbs in children. In teenagers and young adults for whom sexual transmission is a frequent mode of spread, lesions in the ano-genital area are most common. In otherwise healthy subjects, occasional facial lesions are seen, particularly on the eyelids. MC may affect the scalp and any other body surface [**122**].

Widespread and refractory MC on the face is commonly seen in PLWH [156] and iatrogenic immunosuppression [157] (Figure 25.9b). Lesions on the lips, tongue or buccal mucous membranes are rare, usually occur in immunosuppressed adults and may present in the absence of cutaneous lesions [158]. Giant or widespread MC infection is also more common in immunosuppression [159].

MC lesions may also occur in scars and tattoos [160]. Follicular MC has been reported, producing atypical, less exophytic pale papules [162].

Differential diagnosis
Solitary MC lesions may resemble pyogenic granuloma, basal cell carcinoma, sebaceous gland hyperplasia, keratoacanthoma or squamous cell carcinoma. Multiple small lesions can simulate plane warts [**122**]. In PLWH and other immunocompromised patients, cutaneous cryptococcosis and histoplasmosis should be considered (Chapter 31).

Complications and co-morbidities
In at least 10% of cases, particularly in atopic subjects, a patchy eczematous reaction may develop around one or more MC lesions a month or more after their onset [162]. Erythema annulare centrifugum and erythema multiforme have also been reported in association with MC infection [163–165]. Chronic conjunctivitis and

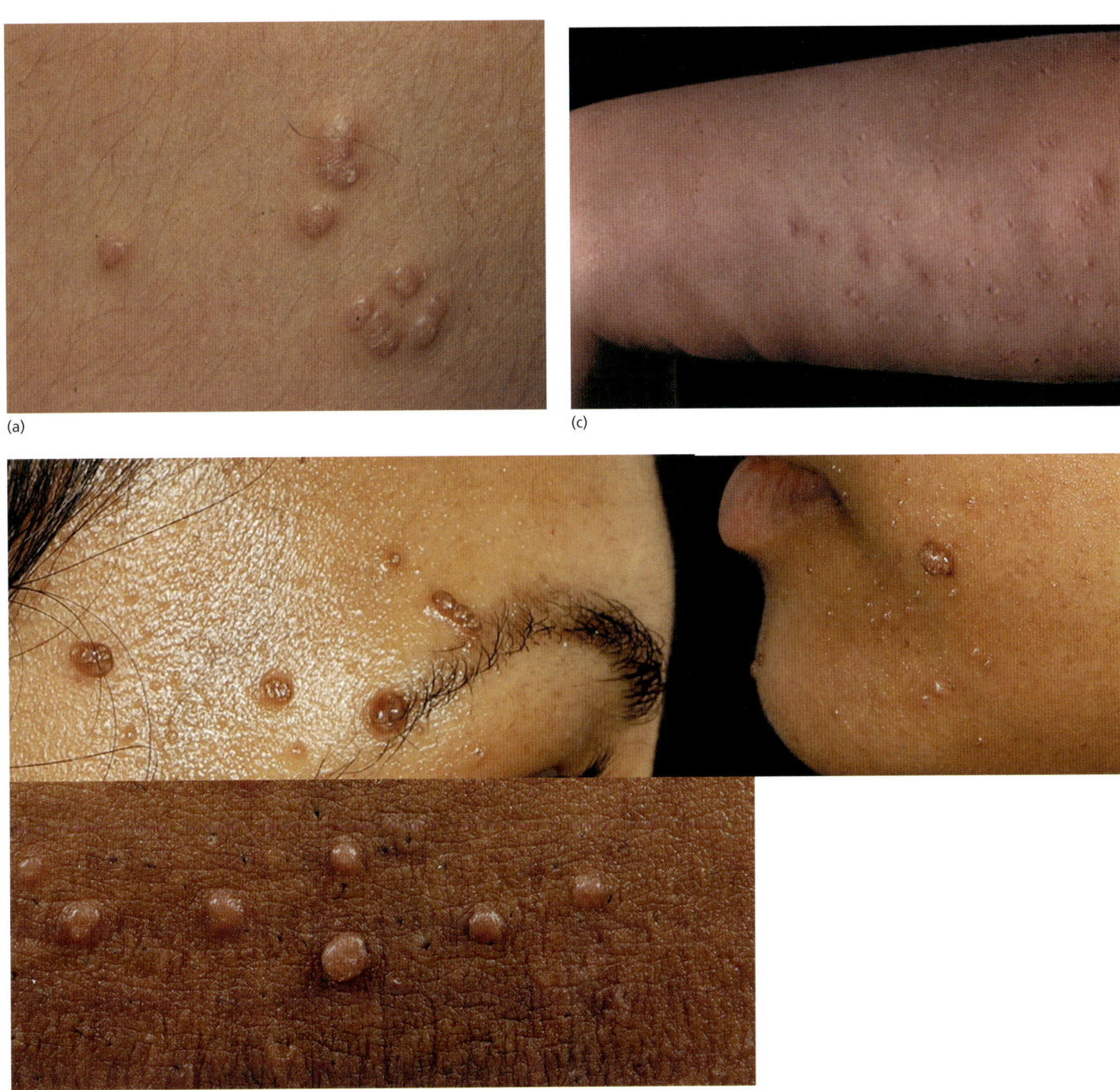

Figure 25.9 Molluscum contagiosum. (a) Typical umbilicated lesions. (b) Multiple lesions of varying sizes in a patient on fingolimod. (c) Depressed scars following infection. Courtesy of Addenbrooke's Hospital, Cambridge and Barts Health NHS Trust, London, UK.

superficial punctate keratitis may similarly complicate MC lesions on or near the eyelids [166]. Eczematous reactions and conjunctivitis tend to subside spontaneously when MC lesions resolve or are removed [166,167].

Disease course and prognosis

The duration of both individual lesions and of attacks is very variable. Although most cases are self-limiting and last 6–9 months, some may persist for 3 or 4 years [133]. Individual lesions are unlikely to persist for more than 2 months, but some lesions, particularly if solitary, may persist for up to 5 years [168].

Perilesional inflammatory responses may indicate that immunological resolution is likely to occur within a few months rather than the presence of bacterial superinfection: the so-called BOTE – 'beginning of the end' – sign [169]. A similar reaction has also been observed in association with Covid-19 vaccination [170].

Depressed scars or anetoderma-like lesions can remain when MC lesions clear [171,172] (Figure 25.9c).

Investigations

The diagnosis of MC is usually straightforward when typical umbilicated lesions at different stages of evolution are present. Typical dermoscopic features include yellow lobule-like structures around a central, amorphous white nodule with vascular patterns including crown, punctiform, radial and 'mixed flower' patterns [**122**,144,170,173]. Skin imaging techniques such as reflectance confocal microscopy and lone-field optical coherence tomography have also been proposed as providing an alternative non-invasive approach to diagnosis [174,175]. The diagnosis can be confirmed by direct or electron microscopy of the papule contents, histopathology and molecular analysis [**122**,176,177].

Management

In many instances, therapy is not necessary and spontaneous resolution can be awaited [**178**]. The risk of dissemination can be minimised by avoiding scratching, which spreads virus from mature papules. Associated eczema should be treated with emollients and a weak topical steroid may be considered. Transmission of infection to other individuals may be reduced by avoidance of shared towels, contact sports and communal bathing [131–133].

Treatment may be required if spontaneous clearance is slow, lesions are symptomatic or associated eczema is troublesome [179]. The choice of treatment will depend upon patient age, lesion numbers, severity and locations as well as patient (and caregivers) preferences. Treatments aim to destroy the infected epidermal cells, stimulate an immunological response and/or act directly against the virus. The most recent Cochrane systematic review evaluated 22 RCTs in 1650 participants without immune deficiency that had investigated 20 topical and 2 systemic treatments for non-genital MC; it concluded that no single intervention was convincingly effective in the treatment of MC and did not favour any one treatment [**178**]. A broadly similar approach is recommended for genital MC [180].

Most treatments cause stimulation of an antiviral immune response which may occur with:
1. Destructive or pro-inflammatory topical treatments
2. Immune-modulating treatments
3. Physical treatments
4. Antiviral treatments [**122**,**178**]

Destructive/pro-inflammatory topical treatments. Cantharidin is a topically applied vesicant and complete clearance of MC with a 0.7% w/v preparation applied every 3 weeks for a maximum of four applications using a specific application device was significantly higher compared with placebo in two phase III RCTs recruiting participants over the age of 2 years [181]. As with trichloroacetic acid and diluted liquefied phenol, cantharidin is a strong irritant which causes pain, blistering and scarring, but with careful application and appropriate dilution, all can increase lesion clearance [182–184].

Topical salicylic acid-based preparations [**178**,179], tretinoin [185], adapalene [167,186], 5–10% potassium hydroxide solution [187–189], benzoyl peroxide cream [189] and podophyllotoxin [190] all lead to an irritant reaction, but if the strength of preparation and the frequency of application are adjusted, individuals can tolerate repeated treatments until resolution occurs. Lemon myrtle oil [191] and tea tree oil [192] have been used, the former with apparent efficacy when compared with placebo.

Berdazimer gel, a nitric oxide-releasing agent, demonstrated greater complete lesion clearance compared with vehicle (32.4% vs 19.7%, $P < 0.01$) in a phase III RCT with 891 patients over 6 months old. The most commonly observed local skin reaction was mild to moderate redness and transient application-site pain was also observed [193–195].

Immune-modulating treatments. Immune-modulating treatments have been used with the explicit aim of enhancing the immune response, although trials are not always randomised or controlled. Efficacy has been reported with topical diphencyprone [196]. There is some evidence for the use of imiquimod cream from case series and case–control studies [197–199]. Compared with cryotherapy, lesions clear more slowly with imiquimod [200]. However, in two large but unpublished randomised trials, imiquimod was apparently of no benefit when compared with placebo and a systematic review of published RCTs indicates that 5% imiquimod cream is not more effective in clearing MC compared with placebo in children aged 2–12 years and caused more local adverse effects [**178**,179,201]. Intralesional or systemic interferon [139,202,203], systemic cimetidine [204] and intralesional immunotherapies including candida, combined measles, mumps, rubella vaccine, tuberculin purified protein derivative and streptococcal substrain OK-432 [203–206] have all been investigated, with variable evidence for effectiveness.

Physical treatments. Damage to the lesions by squeezing the contents or insertion of a pointed cocktail stick may stimulate inflammation and clearance. Cryotherapy is similarly effective and commonly used in older children and adults, but needs to be repeated at 3–4-weekly intervals. Carbon dioxide or pulsed dye lasers have produced useful effects [207,208] but can cause scars. Photodynamic therapy has also been used [209,210].

Surgical removal by curettage has been used for many years but the rate of successful clearance is reduced if there are multiple lesions [211]. Children usually need prior application of topical anaesthetic cream, with strict observance of the maximum safe dose [212].

Antiviral treatments. The antiviral agent cidofovir may effectively clear MC lesions when used topically as a 1–3% ointment or cream, intravenously or intralesionally [**122**,213–215]. It should be considered for extensive lesions in, for example, immunocompromised patients in whom lesions have proved recalcitrant to standard treatment regimens [216]. Although not specifically antiviral, successful use of intravenous paclitaxel has also been described for severe, recalcitrant MC in immunocompromised patients [217,218].

Resources

Further information

http://www.cdc.gov/ncidod/dvrd/molluscum/overview.htm
https://cks.nice.org.uk/topics/molluscum-contagiosum/

Patient resources

https://patient.info/childrens-health/viral-skin-infections-leaflet/molluscum-contagiosum

https://www.aad.org/public/diseases/a-z/molluscum-contagiosum-overview

(All last accessed August 2023.)

Tanapox

Introduction and general description

This is an acute febrile illness associated with localised nodular skin lesions which was first described in 1957 in the flood plain of the Tana River in Kenya [219,220].

Epidemiology

Incidence and prevalence

Sporadic cases and occasional outbreaks occur in equatorial Africa, especially in the Congo Basin [220]. Cases outside Africa are rare and described in contacts of laboratory animals in research facilities and in travellers returning from Africa [220].

Pathophysiology

Pathology

The epidermis shows degeneration and the keratinocytes have vacuolated cytoplasm with eosinophilic inclusions. Papillary dermal oedema and a mild inflammatory infiltrate are seen.

Causative organisms

The tanapox virus (TANV) belongs to the *Yatapoxvirus* genus and infects both monkeys and humans, but no other natural reservoir has been identified.

Clinical features

Presentation

A prodrome with a mild fever, myalgia and headache is followed within 2 days by the appearance of a skin papule, most commonly on the limbs. The general symptoms quickly subside, but the lesion grows to a maximum of 1–2 cm within 2 weeks and is usually tender, occasionally itchy and may ulcerate. There may be regional lymphadenopathy. The nodule clears within 6 weeks leaving a small scar [219,220].

Clinical variants

A solitary lesion is most common, but multiple lesions may occasionally be present.

Investigations

Electron microscopy of keratinocytes of the lesion will show the characteristic brick-shaped enveloped poxvirus [220]. PCR and sequencing can be used to identify tanapoxvirus DNA [221].

Management

The disease is self-limiting.

HERPESVIRUS INFECTIONS

The herpesvirus group consists of relatively large, enveloped DNA viruses. After primary infection, they can remain latent within the host.

General description of disease domain

Herpesviruses are subgrouped, according to genome similarities, into the α, β and γ herpesviruses (Table 25.5). Eight members of the group commonly infect humans. Herpes simplex virus (HSV) and varicella-zoster virus (VZV) predominantly cause cutaneous disease and viral exanthems can occur with β herpesvirus infections. The γ herpesviruses may cause skin disease during reactivation or latent infection.

Basic biology

The herpesviruses replicate within the nucleus and produce typical intranuclear inclusion bodies detectable in stained preparations.

A notable feature of infection by members of the herpesvirus group is the absence of virus elimination following clinical recovery. Virus persists throughout the person's life as a latent infection in the cells for which the strain is specific. Under certain conditions, especially immune suppression, the virus may become reactivated and produce an acute infective episode with cellular damage.

HERPES SIMPLEX VIRUS INFECTIONS

Herpes simplex infections are caused by HSV or human herpesvirus 1 (HHV-1), and are among the commonest infections of humans throughout the world. There are two major antigenic types: type 1, which is classically associated with facial infections; and type 2, which is typically genital, although there is considerable overlap in disease manifestations. After the initial infection, the virus becomes latent and may later reactivate.

General description of disease domain

Primary infection

This occurs in a previously seronegative individual and is often subclinical. When clinical lesions develop, the severity is generally greater than in recurrences. Genital primary disease is more commonly symptomatic than oral.

Recurrent infection

After the first infection, whether symptomatic or subclinical, there may be no further clinical manifestations throughout life. Recurrences occur in 30–50% of cases of oral herpes, but are more frequent after genital herpes infection, developing in 95% of those with type 2 HSV compared with 50% in individuals with type 1 infection [1,2].

Table 25.5 Herpesviruses causing disease in humans.

Subfamily	Genus		Virus	Abbreviation	Also called
Alphaherpesvirinae	α	Simplexvirus	Human simplex virus, type 1	HSV-1	Herpesvirus hominis 1, HHV-1
	α		Human simplex virus, type 2	HSV-2	Herpesvirus hominis 2, HHV-2
	α	Varicellovirus	Varicella-zoster virus	VZV	Herpesvirus varicellae, HHV-3
Betaherpesvirinae	β	Cytomegalovirus	Cytomegalovirus	CMV	HHV-5
	β	Roseolovirus	Human herpesvirus type 6	HHV-6	
	β		Human herpesvirus type 7	HHV-7	
Gammaherpesvirinae	γ	Lymphocryptovirus	Epstein–Barr virus	EBV	HHV-4
	γ	Rhadinovirus	Human herpesvirus type 8	HHV-8	Kaposi sarcoma-associated herpesvirus, KSHV

Recurrences may be triggered by minor trauma, or by infections including febrile illnesses but also trivial non-febrile upper respiratory tract infections, by ultraviolet radiation [3], by trigeminal neuralgia and especially after intracranial operations for that disease [4], by other neural surgery [5], by dental surgery [6], or by facial cosmetic procedures such as chemical peel [7], dermabrasion [8] or laser resurfacing [9]. Some women have more recurrences in the premenstrual period. Emotional stress is blamed in some cases, possibly related to the effect on immune function [10,11]. However, in many cases no reason for the eruption is evident.

Recurrent infections differ from primary infections in the smaller size of the vesicles and their close grouping, and in the usual absence of constitutional symptoms. In the immunocompetent, they do not as a rule affect the buccal mucosa.

Subclinical viral shedding

Asymptomatic shedding of HSV-2 is more frequent than of HSV-1 and correlates with the frequency of symptomatic recurrences. Inapparent oral shedding occurs in about 12% of the UK population. Genital shedding of HSV-2 is common in antibody-positive individuals. In those who have recurrent episodes, the virus is shed on approximately 20% of days, while asymptomatic individuals shed virus on 10% of days [12]. In the first year following acquisition of HSV-2, asymptomatic shedding is more common than in subsequent years.

Basic biology [1,13–16]

Both type 1 and type 2 HSV are acquired by direct contact with, or droplets from, infected secretions entering via skin or mucous membrane, where primary infection may become evident. The establishment of latent infection is common with the virus persisting in the ganglia of sensory nerves innervating the primary infection site. The virus produces no viral proteins while latent and can therefore remain undetected by host defence mechanisms. From this condition of latency, the virus may travel peripherally along the nerve fibre and, if it replicates in the skin or mucous membrane, may cause recurrent disease. The virus can be shed in saliva and genital secretions from asymptomatic individuals, especially in the months following the first episode of disease, although the amount shed from active lesions is 100–1000 times greater. Close contact with an infected individual, whether symptomatic or asymptomatic, can result in transmission of HSV and resultant disease.

Trauma facilitates transfer of the virus to fully keratinised skin. The virus can be inoculated into any body site to cause a new infection, whether or not there has been previous infection with either type. The source may be endogenous (autoinoculation), for example to the finger, especially in nail biters or thumb suckers. Examples of exogenous inoculation are lesions of the hand in health care workers (see later Figure 25.12) and others [17], facial lesions contracted during contact sports, and infection of a breastfeeding mother's nipples from the infected mouth of her baby [18].

Following primary infection, humoral and cell-mediated immune responses take place, the latter probably being more important [19]. They do not fully protect against reinfection or recurrent disease. The acquisition of HSV at a new site in a patient previously infected at a different site is referred to as a non-primary first-episode infection. Initial (non-primary) genital herpes tends to be less severe in patients who have had previous oral infection. Where immunity is deficient (either congenitally or due to disease or drugs), both primary and recurrent herpetic infections may be increased in incidence and severity, and may run a prolonged and atypical course. Examples include patients immunosuppressed following organ or marrow transplantation, patients receiving cytotoxic therapy for malignancy [20], including cutaneous T-cell lymphoma [21], and patients with HIV infection. Herpes simplex reactivation is not a major risk during treatment with biologics for psoriasis but may be increased with dupilumab therapy [22]. Topical immunomodulating treatment with corticosteroids or calcineurin inhibitors has also been implicated in herpetic eruptions [23–25].

Immunological abnormalities or variations, in addition to possible local cutaneous factors, may explain the increased incidence in atopic eczema of recurrent herpes simplex [26] and the evolution in some individuals of erythema multiforme, as well as the occasional more severe infections [27,28], including eczema herpeticum (see later).

Primary herpetic gingivostomatitis

Definition and nomenclature

Herpes simplex infection of the mouth and lips.

Synonyms and inclusions
- Herpes labialis
- Cold sore

Introduction and general description
This is the most common clinical manifestation of primary infection by type 1, although the sites infected by the two HSV types are not mutually exclusive. Primary type 1 infections occur mainly in infants and young children, when they are usually minimal and often subclinical. Primary infections may rarely produce a painful vesicular stomatitis [29].

Epidemiology
Incidence and prevalence
In crowded areas of the developing world, over 90% of children have antibody by the age of 5 years, but in more temperate areas and higher socioeconomic groups the incidence is lower in children, rising steadily with age [30]. For example, in western Europe and the USA, a quarter of children, a half to three-quarters of adolescents and young adults, and up to 90% of the elderly are HSV-1 antibody positive [31–33].

Age
Most cases of primary HSV gingivostomatitis occur in children between 1 and 5 years of age, but cases are well recognised in adults.

Pathophysiology
Pathology
In skin and mucosal lesions, the cytoplasm of the infected epithelial cells becomes oedematous and the cells swell, producing the so-called 'ballooning degeneration'. Intraepidermal vesicles are formed by the combination of intra- and intercellular oedema. The dermis, and later the epidermis, is infiltrated with polymorphonuclear leukocytes. Specific changes occur in the cell nuclei and different stages in the process of the development of the intranuclear inclusions can usually be seen in a single section. In addition, giant cells containing 2–15 or more nuclei are almost invariably present in cutaneous and corneal epithelium. The cytological changes are essentially the same in all organs, and foci of necrosis surrounded by a zone of inflammation are characteristically found in the brain and liver when these organs are involved.

Immunohistochemistry can be used to detect viral proteins in the virally infected cells. Viral particles can be identified ultrastructurally, mainly in the cell nucleus, and with detailed examination, HSV types 1 and 2 can be distinguished [34].

Causative organisms
Usually HSV-1, less frequently HSV-2.

Clinical features
History
The incubation period is approximately 5 days.

Presentation
The stomatitis begins with fever, which may be high, malaise, restlessness and excessive dribbling. Drinking and eating are very painful and the breath is foul smelling. The gums are swollen, inflamed and bleed easily. Vesicles presenting as white plaques are present on the tongue, pharynx, palate and buccal mucous membranes. The plaques develop into ulcers with a yellowish pseudomembrane. The regional lymph nodes are enlarged and tender.

Clinical variants
Recurrent disease due to reactivation (see later).

Differential diagnosis
Differential diagnoses of primary HSV infection include streptococcal infections, diphtheria, candidiasis, aphthosis, coxsackie infections including herpangina, Behçet syndrome and Stevens–Johnson syndrome.

Complications and co-morbidities
Eczema herpeticum is discussed later in this chapter.

Pharyngitis may accompany approximately 10% of primary orofacial herpes.

Disseminated or systemic infection may occur in the immunodeficient and in those neonates not protected by maternally acquired antibody, but rarely in otherwise healthy patients. Systemic infection may develop with or without widespread cutaneous lesions. At any age, encephalitis, untreated, has a high mortality and a high incidence of disability in survivors [35]; in neonates HSV-2 gave a worse prognosis than HSV-1, even with antiviral therapy [36]. HSV hepatitis is rare in adults, but when severe is often fatal [37,38]. Lower respiratory tract infection has occurred in immunosuppressed, burned or intubated patients [39], and in neonates [40].

Herpes simplex may occur in certain bullous disorders, complicating the presentation or disease manifestations of pemphigus [41,42], pemphigoid [43] and Hailey–Hailey disease [44], and occurring as severe infections in patients receiving immunosuppressive treatment.

Disease course and prognosis
After 3–5 days, the fever normally subsides and recovery is usually complete in 2 weeks.

Investigations
A swab taken from vesicle fluid, avoiding surface contamination, is the best sample for either virus culture or molecular analysis. PCR for HSV-1, HSV-2 and VZV is the quickest method and less likely than culture to be affected by surface organisms [45,46]. Primary infections can be distinguished by seroconversion or a rise in antibody titre. Recurrences tend to produce little change in antibody titre; measurement of antibody is therefore not helpful in the diagnosis of recurrent HSV, but type-specific antibodies will give some indication of the type causing reactivation episodes. A rapid diagnosis is also possible by detection of viral antigen by immunofluorescence in scrapings from lesions or the virus seen by electron microscopy in vesicle fluid. The detection of HSV DNA in the cerebrospinal fluid by PCR is the diagnostic method of choice for herpes encephalitis and aseptic meningitis [47] and can also be used to identify the virus and the type at other sites [48].

Management [49–51,52]
Mild uncomplicated eruptions of herpes simplex require no treatment.

Anaesthetic mouthwashes may help to relieve pain. The use of a topical antiseptic agent on affected skin may help to reduce the risk of secondary bacterial infection. In practice, antiviral therapy is usually justified to try to reduce the duration of symptoms.

First line
For less severe infections and when swallowing is not impaired, oral aciclovir treatment is adequate. The usual oral dose is 200 mg five times daily for 5 or more days, but 800 mg BD has been used with success [53]. In children, the oral suspension given at 15 mg/kg five times per day for 7 days reduces the duration of symptoms and virus shedding [54]. Valaciclovir 500 mg BD for 5 days or famciclovir 250 mg BD for 7 days is of similar efficacy to aciclovir [55].

Second line
Aciclovir systemically is the treatment of choice for severe or potentially severe primary herpes simplex infection, as in immune compromise, but there is no effect on establishment of virus latency and rates of recurrence after therapy. Treatment should be started as soon as possible. The usual dose is 5 mg/kg 8 hourly intravenously, though twice that dose has been used for neonatal herpes [53] and encephalitis [56]. As the drug is excreted via the kidneys, the dose must be scaled down in renal failure. Transient rises in blood urea and creatinine may occur with bolus injections; slow infusion over 1 h in an adequately hydrated patient is recommended.

Alternatives in this situation are valaciclovir 1 g BD for 10 days or famciclovir 500 g BD for 7 days.

Treatment ladder for primary herpetic gingivostomatitis

First line
- Aciclovir, PO, 200 mg five times daily, or 800 mg BD, for 5 days
- Valciclovir, PO, 500 mg BD for 5 days, or famciclovir 250 mg BD for 7 days

Second line
- Aciclovir, IV, 5 mg/kg 8 hourly
- Valaciclovir, PO, 1 g BD for 10 days, or famciclovir, PO, 500 mg BD for 7 days

---

Recurrent oro-facial and cutaneous herpes

Synonyms and inclusions
- Cold sore
- Herpes labialis

Introduction and general description
Reactivation of the latent virus can cause asymptomatic shedding or clinically evident recurrent disease.

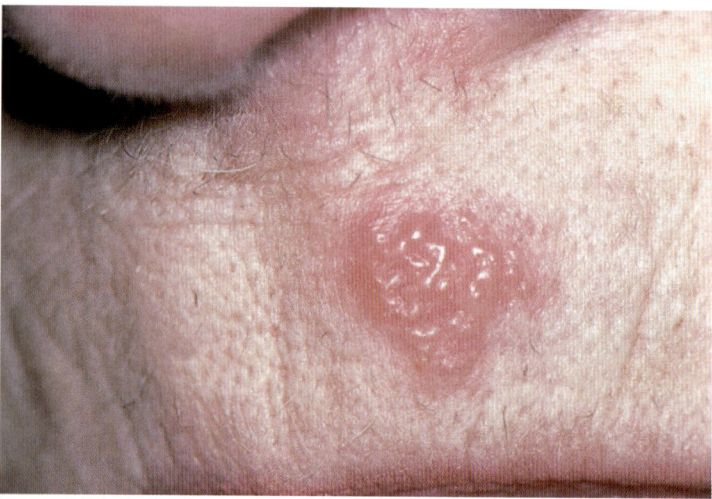

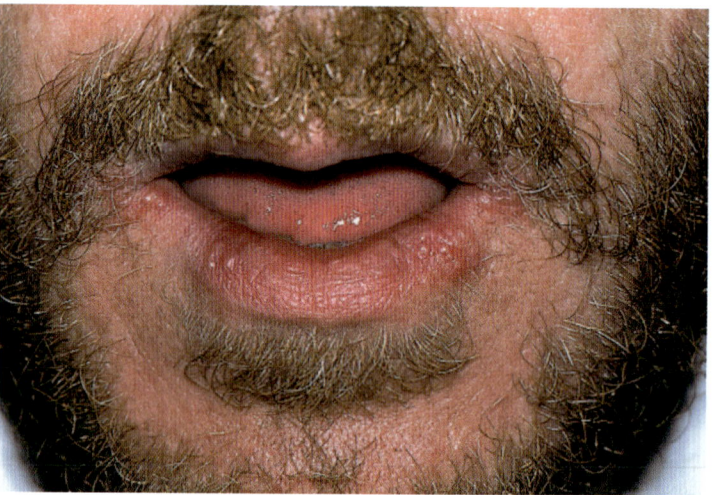

Figure 25.10 Herpes labialis. (a) Typical recurrent lesion on the upper lip. (b) More widespread recurrent lesions following streptococcal pyoderma with lymphangitis. Courtesy of Dr A. S. Highet, York District Hospital, UK.

Clinical features
Presentation
Itching or burning precedes by an hour or two the development of small closely grouped vesicles on an inflamed base. The eruption may be painful just at the onset or pain may last for a few days. Lesions occur most frequently on the face, particularly around the mouth (Figure 25.10), but can be situated anywhere on the body. Larger vesicles are not uncommon, especially in children. Recurrences tend to be in the same region, but not always on the identical site. Although the vesicles usually form an irregular cluster, they may be arranged in a line or in zosteriform distribution, particularly in the lower thoracic or lumbar region [57]. In such cases, there may be considerable deep pain and regional lymphadenopathy. Fever, pain and lymphangitis may also be associated with herpes of the hand or forearm and further complications of oedema and persistent pain may develop [58].

Recurrent herpetic lesions are most commonly vesicular and ulcerative, but occasionally they are atypical with the appearance, for example, of folliculitis, candidal fissures or minor 'frictional ulcers'. Laboratory confirmation is needed for the accurate diagnosis of atypical lesions.

Clinical variants
Although primary and recurrent herpes is most common in the oro-facial area, infections can occur at other sites such as the trunk and limbs (see Inoculation herpes later).

Complications and co-morbidities
In recurrent herpes of the face or lips, constitutional symptoms rarely occur but some individuals report temperature disturbance, tiredness and general malaise that often precedes the onset. In one child, fever and an organic psychosis accompanied each attack [59]. Cranial nerve palsies may occur [60], sometimes with each eruption. Rarely, neuralgic pain may precede each recurrence of herpes by 1 or 2 days, a syndrome often associated with the name of Mauriac [61], and trigeminal neuralgia can be associated with episodes of recurrence [62].

Eczema herpeticum can be associated with recurrent as well as primary HSV.

In the immunocompromised, persistent ulcerative or verruciform lesions may occur (Chapter 31). Although these chronic HSV lesions are seen most commonly in HIV infection, they may occur more rarely in haematological malignancy [63].

If recurrent herpes simplex involves the eye, keratoconjunctivitis, dendritic ulcers, disciform or hypopyon keratitis and iridocyclitis may occur. An ophthalmological opinion should be sought.

Lymphoedema has followed recurrent attacks on a limb [64]. Secondary leukoderma may develop in pigmented skin, and herpes has been recorded as appearing in scar tissue [65].

Erythema multiforme (herpes-associated erythema multiforme) [66] (Chapter 47). In 65% of adult patients with recurrent erythema multiforme, there is a history of herpes labialis, usually preceding the erythema multiforme by several days to 2 weeks, but occasionally seeming to coincide with it. Although virus cannot be seen by electron microscopy or isolated, HSV antigen gB has been detected in erythema multiforme skin lesions and HSV DNA has been demonstrated by PCR in lesions [67–69]. This evidence is not confined to cases with clinically apparent preceding herpetic lesions. Certain HLA types are associated with recurrent postherpetic erythema multiforme or with severity of site affected [70,71]. Erythema multiforme-like eruptions which are associated with HSV are not uncommon following stem cell transplantation [72]. Treatment of recurrent HSV-associated erythema multiforme, if started by the patient in the prodrome stage (with a 5-day course of aciclovir), will often prevent the development of erythema multiforme. If that is not effective and attacks are frequent, a 6-month course of prophylactic aciclovir should be tried even in patients in whom HSV is not obviously a precipitating factor [73]. Dapsone, azathioprine, ciclosporin or cimetidine has been reported to be effective in cases resistant to aciclovir or not associated with HSV [74–76].

Bell palsy. The suggestion that Bell palsy is due to viral reactivation (HSV or VZV) has been strengthened by the detection by PCR of the HSV-1 genome in saliva, facial nerve and muscle tissue in patients with this condition [77–79]. The use of an appropriate antiviral should therefore be considered in the early management of Bell palsy.

Recurrent lymphocytic meningitis. A benign form of aseptic meningitis that lasts 3–14 days and may recur at intervals of months or years is associated with HSV [80]. HSV is detectable by PCR in the cerebrospinal fluid. Prophylactic or pre-eruptive aciclovir has been reported to prevent recurrences.

Encephalitis. This severe disease can occur after the virus has established latent infection. Cases are recorded after the possible reactivating event of neurosurgery [81], or more commonly without a recognised trigger. Rapid diagnosis by PCR and treatment are essential to minimise the mortality and morbidity of the condition.

Disease course and prognosis
The initial vesicular lesions usually become pustular and crusted before healing in 7–10 days without scarring.

Management
Recurrent herpes labialis may need no treatment if attacks are mild or infrequent [82].

More troublesome recurrences merit antiviral treatment with aciclovir, valaciclovir or famciclovir.

Resistance of herpes simplex to aciclovir has not emerged as a significant problem in immunocompetent patients [83]. However, in the immunocompromised, resistant strains which cause intractable lesions have emerged following long-term or frequently repeated treatment. Resistance is usually due to a change in or loss of the viral thymidine kinase [84], or more rarely to alteration of the viral DNA polymerase [85]. The former strains may respond to antivirals that have a different mode of action (e.g. phosphonoformate, also known as foscarnet, or cidofovir).

Recurrences of herpes labialis may be prevented or reduced in intensity by the use of a topical sunscreen [86].

Prophylaxis against reactivation or spread of HSV may be useful before cosmetic laser treatment of the face, as widespread herpes has been reported following such procedures [87,88].

First line
Both emollient creams and a thin hydrocolloid dressing reduce discomfort [89] but may not alter healing rate. Similarly, there is no strong evidence that topical aciclovir applied five times daily influences the disease course in recurrent cutaneous HSV.

Topical penciclovir compares favourably with aciclovir [90] and reduces the duration of pain and the eruption in comparison with placebo [91].

Oral aciclovir started as soon as possible after onset of symptoms can shorten the duration and decrease the intensity of an episode [92]. Valaciclovir 2 g BD for one day or famciclovir (single 1500 mg dose or 750 mg BD for 1 day) also reduces time to healing [93,94].

A number of botanical extracts and also honey or propolis preparations have been reported to increase comfort and shorten the duration of blistering, but none is licensed for treatment.

Historically, topical idoxuridine has been used for the treatment of herpes but was superseded by the safer and more effective antiviral drugs. New formulations may enable its reconsideration as therapy [95]. Trifluorothymidine has also been used but its efficacy is uncertain [96].

Second line

If recurrences are frequent, long-term prophylactic aciclovir at a dose of 200–400 mg BD for 4–6 months may increase the time between episodes [51,**97**,98]. Valaciclovir 500 mg daily (if <10 episodes per year) or 1 g daily (if >10 episodes per year) given for 6–12 months is an alternative. There is some evidence that photodynamic therapy can reduce the frequency of recurrences of herpes labialis [99], but larger studies are needed to establish its utility.

Third line

In the immunocompromised patient, mucocutaneous herpes simplex responds well to intravenous aciclovir [100,101] or penciclovir [102]. Post-exposure, the infection can be prevented by intravenous [103] or oral [104] aciclovir, which should be started several days before the anticipated immunosuppression and continued throughout the period of greatest risk. Longer-term prophylaxis where indicated is also effective [105] (aciclovir 400–800 mg two or three times daily; oral valaciclovir 500 mg BD; famciclovir 500 mg BD for 7 days).

In the treatment of severe herpes simplex infection resistant to aciclovir, systemic phosphonoformate (foscarnet) may be considered [106]. An alternative antiviral is cidofovir, which acts to block DNA replication. This can be administered systemically but is also active topically. Small numbers of individuals with severe HSV resistant to conventional treatment are reported to have responded to topical or intravenous cidofovir [107,108].

Enhancement of the immune response to HSV could reduce recurrences. Imiquimod cream has been shown to reduce frequency of reactivation episodes [109]. Vaccines against the virus are under development but not yet in clinical use.

Treatment ladder for recurrent herpes labialis

First line for acute episode
- Aciclovir, topical, five times daily or more, for 5 days
- Hydrocolloid dressing
- Penciclovir, topical, every 2 hours for 4 days
- Aciclovir, PO, 200 mg five times daily for 5 days
- Valaciclovir, PO, 2 g BD for 1 day, or famciclovir, PO, 1500 g once

Second line for prophylaxis
- Aciclovir, long-term, prophylactic, 200–400 mg daily; higher dose if immune compromised
- Imiquimod, topical

Third line in immune compromise
- Aciclovir, IV, 5 mg/kg 8 hourly; PO, 800 mg every 8 hours
- Penciclovir, IV
- Phosphonoformate (foscarnet), IV
- Cidofovir, IV

Resources

Further information

cks.nice.org.uk/topics/herpes-simplex-oral/
https://www.who.int/news-room/fact-sheets/detail/herpes-simplex-virus

Patient resources

https://dermnetnz.org/topics/herpes-simplex
www.bad.org.uk/shared/get-file.ashx?id=208&itemtype=document
(All last accessed August 2023.)

Primary herpes genitalis [110]

Definition

Infection of the genital skin or mucosa with herpes simplex virus.

Introduction and general description

Both HSV-1 and HSV-2 can cause disease in the genital area. Primary HSV-2 infection is more commonly symptomatic than primary HSV-1 infection.

Epidemiology

Incidence and prevalence

Genital herpes is usually transmitted sexually. Seropositivity is low in children, but about a third of young adults are seropositive for type 2 and this rises to up to half the population by later life [111]. In one sample of women, overall transmission rates between couples, from infected to uninfected partner, averaged 4–30% annually [112]. In 2016, it was estimated that there were almost 24 million new cases of HSV-2 worldwide [113] with rates in women higher than those in men.

Age

Type 2 infections occur mainly after puberty. In children with genital herpes (HSV-1 or HSV-2), sexual abuse must be considered [114].

Pathophysiology

Causative organisms

HSV-2 has been the most common type in this area, although there is an increasing frequency of HSV-1 herpes genitalis, especially in young females, with some studies now reporting that type 1 is found more frequently than HSV-2 [111,115]. HSV-1 is most common in several European countries including the UK, North America and Australia, while HSV-2 remains the most common virus causing genital herpes in Africa [116–119]. Transmission occurs during reactivation episodes, but also frequently during asymptomatic periods, when shedding can occur in up to 10% of days [**120**].

Clinical features

Presentation

Primary infection is symptomatic in only about one-third of cases, with symptoms and lesions appearing after an incubation period of 2 days to 2 weeks. The most frequent presentation is of painful erosions, which may be preceded by a general malaise and fever and are often associated with oedema. In the male, the ulcers are most

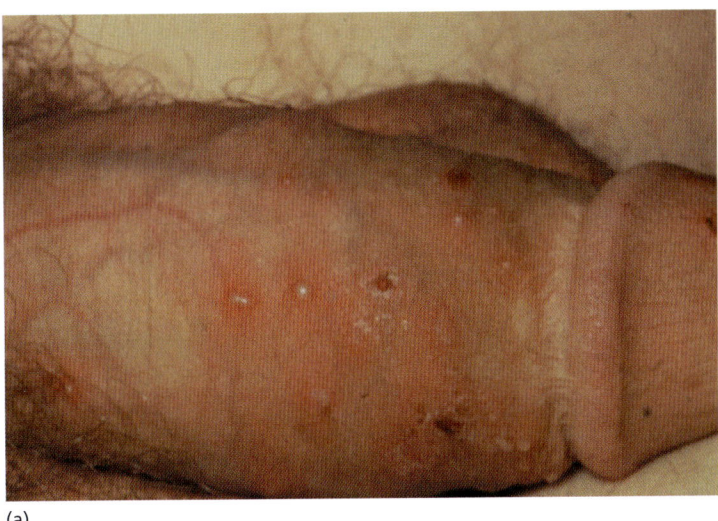
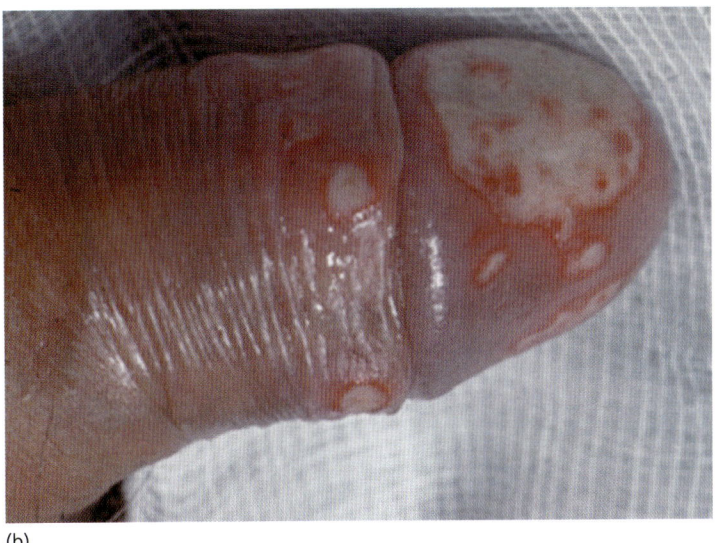

Figure 25.11 Herpes genitalis. (a) Scattered lesions on the penile shaft. (b) Confluent lesions resulting in large erosions. Courtesy of Addenbrooke's Hospital, Cambridge, UK.

frequent on the glans, prepuce and shaft of the penis (Figure 25.11). In the female, similar lesions occur on the external genitalia and mucosae of the vulva, vagina and cervix. In skin of colour, there may be marked postinflammatory hypopigmentation. In men who have sex with men, herpes simplex is common in the perianal area and may extend into the rectum. Infection of the cervix may progress to a severe ulcerative cervicitis. Dysuria is common in both sexes and there may be urethral discharge. Lymphadenitis occurs frequently.

Clinical variants
In HIV infection, ulceration of the primary infection may become chronic. It may become thickened and verrucous, causing diagnostic confusion with neoplasia.

Classification of severity
Where a person has had previous HSV-1 infection, this is likely to decrease the severity of a primary HSV-2 infection, shortening the clinical course and reducing systemic symptoms.

Complications and co-morbidities
Radiculoneuropathy is seen occasionally in primary ano-genital infection in women, and especially in perianal disease in homosexual men [121,122]. There may be sacral paraesthesia, urinary retention, constipation and, in men, impotence. Recovery takes a few days to a few weeks.

Headache and meningism affected 36% of women and 11% of men in a series of 268 patients with primary genital herpes simplex [121], with full recovery. In such patients, HSV DNA can be found by PCR in the cerebrospinal fluid. Encephalitis is a rare complication [123].

Disease course and prognosis
Genital lesions can last for 2–3 weeks if untreated. Recurrences are likely to be more frequent in HSV-2 disease.

Investigations
See Investigation of primary oro-facial herpes, earlier.

Management
Preventative strategies to avoid spread include the use of barrier contraception and, in the future, local microbicides [124]. Development of prophylactic vaccines is underway but not yet of proven efficacy [125]. For primary genital herpes in pregnancy, see Neonatal herpes.

First line
Initial eruptions of genital herpes [126] improve significantly with oral aciclovir [127], valaciclovir [55] or famciclovir. Pain control is usually needed.

Second line
In severe chronic verrucous herpes simplex, oral or intravenous aciclovir or valaciclovir may be ineffective. Combinations with cidofovir or imiquimod have proven useful in a few cases [128,129].

Treatment ladder for primary herpes genitalis

First line
- Aciclovir, PO, 200 mg five times per day or 400 mg TDS for 7–10 days
- Valaciclovir, PO, 1 g BD for 7–10 days
- Famciclovir, PO, 250 mg TDS for 7–10 days
- Pencilcovir, PO, 250 mg TDS for 5 days or longer; in immune compromise, 500 mg BD for 10 days

Second line
- Aciclovir, IV
- Cidofovir, IV

Recurrent genital herpes [130]

Epidemiology
Incidence and prevalence
Worldwide, it is estimated that one in eight adults is seropositive for HSV-2 with half a billion people having genital infection with HSV [113]. The prevalence is higher in women than in men and in Africa compared with Europe. Viral shedding is greatest at time of disease recurrence but also occurs at a low level between reactivation episodes [120].

Pathophysiology
Predisposing factors
Prior primary infection with establishment of latent infection.

Clinical features
Presentation
Recurrences are fairly common in HSV-2 infection, occurring two to six times per year, with clusters of small vesicles that produce non-indurated ulcers on the glans or shaft of the penis (Figure 25.11). Similar lesions may occur on the labia, vagina or cervix and can cause distressingly painful symptoms. In other individuals, the lesions can be unnoticed. Frequent recurrences are less likely in HSV-1 infection.

Clinical variants
In immune suppression, persistent HSV can cause verrucous lesions or chronic ulceration [131].

Complications and co-morbidities
Pharyngitis can occur in 1% of recurrent episodes of genital herpes. Episodic genital herpes increases the risk of HIV acquisition. Cases of chronic urticaria associated with recurrent genital herpes have been reported [132]. Genital ulceration can increase the risk of acquisition of other sexually transmitted infections.

Disease course and prognosis
Reactivation episodes of genital herpes are of shorter duration than the initial infection.

Management [126]
Soothing measures such as gentle bathing, petroleum jelly over ulcers and mild pain relief can all help during the acute episode. An infected individual may reduce the risk of spread to others by regular use of condoms and by avoiding sexual contact during a reactivation episode. Virus shedding and therefore spread of HSV can also be reduced but not prevented during treatment with aciclovir, valaciclovir and famciclovir, either for acute disease or as prophylactic therapy [133,134]. For recurrent genital herpes in pregnancy, see Neonatal herpes.

First line
In recurrent herpes genitalis, the effect of topical aciclovir is minimal and oral treatment is recommended [135,136].

Oral therapy for genital herpes is much more effective but can be ineffective unless initiated as early as possible and in adequate dose. Patients should have a supply of tablets in hand to be started on their own initiative [137–139]. Several dose regimes have been tested and the more recent trials of higher dose, shorter duration treatment give equivalent effects to the original treatment plans [140–142]. In immune compromise, dose and duration of the antiviral can both be increased, for example aciclovir 500 mg BD for 5–10 days.

Second line
Frequent recurrences, and also any associated erythema multiforme [143], can be suppressed by long-term treatment, but the efficacy is variable and does not necessarily reduce viral shedding between reactivation episodes [144]. Cessation of therapy, even after several years, may allow resumption of recurrences [145]. Prophylactic doses of aciclovir vary between 200 and 1000 mg daily; a typical regimen is 400 mg BD, gradually reduced to find the minimum effective dose for the individual patient. Valaciclovir, 250 mg BD or 1 g once daily or famciclovir 125 mg TDS or 250 mg BD [142,146,147], is also effective in suppression of recurrent episodes. The prophylaxis is continued for 6–12 months.

If immunosuppressed pencicovir 500 mg BD should be given.

Third line
Topical imiquimod and resiquimod, which cause local release of cytokines and enhancement of antigen presentation, showed initial promise but inadequate clinical effect in treatment of recurrent genital herpes [148,149]. Newer antiviral approaches to reduce virus shedding or reactivation are being trialled.

Treatment ladder for recurrent genital herpes

First line
- Aciclovir, 200 mg five times daily or 400 mg TDS or 800 mg BD for 5 days, or 800 mg TDS for 2 days

Second line
- Valaciclovir, 500 mg BD for 3 days or 1 g OD for 5 days
- Famciclovir, 1 g BD for 1 day or 125 mg BD for 5 days
- Aciclovir, long-term, prophylactic – see text

Resources

Further information
Patel R, Alderson S, Geretti A et al. IUSTI/WHO Europe. European guideline for the management of genital herpes, 2010. *Int J STD AIDS* 2011;22:1–10.
https://www.cdc.gov/std/treatment-guidelines/herpes.htm
https://www.ncbi.nlm.nih.gov/books/NBK554427/
https://cks.nice.org.uk/topics/herpes-simplex-genital/

Patient resources
www.herpes.org.uk
https://www.cdc.gov/std/Herpes/
(All last accessed August 2023.)

Neonatal herpes (Chapter 114) [150]

Definition
Herpes simplex infection of a baby within 28 days of birth is usually acquired vertically from the mother.

Introduction and general description
Primary genital herpes infection or active recurrent infection in the mother at the time of delivery risks transmission to the baby during vaginal delivery. Infection can occur *in utero* with premature membrane rupture, at the time of delivery or postnatally from the mother or other close contacts.

A maternal primary genital infection at the time of birth, before the maternal immune response has taken place, is transmitted to the infant in about 50% of cases and the neonatal infection may be severe and fatal [151]. Antiviral treatment and caesarean section delivery should be considered. Primary infection earlier in the third trimester may cause fetal growth retardation and prematurity. However, serious morbidity is rare if non-primary or recurrent genital infection occurs during pregnancy or at delivery, presumably due to protection by maternal antibody [152–154]. Primary oral herpes in late pregnancy does not carry such high risks for the baby [155].

Epidemiology
Incidence and prevalence
Worldwide, it is estimated that there are about 14 000 cases of neonatal herpes per year with 70% being caused by HSV-2 [156], which equates to about 10/100 000 births. Earlier estimates suggested 2/100 000 births in the UK and 8–60/100 000 in the USA [150], but there are several reports of increasing incidence in some countries in North America and Europe [157,158]. Overall, 70% of cases are caused by HSV-2, but in some countries HSV-1 has been found as the predominant cause [159].

Pathophysiology
Predisposing factors
Infection (primary, recurrent or asymptomatic viral shedding) of the mother during pregnancy or at the time of delivery is the main risk factor, but in most cases of neonatal herpes, there is no known history of maternal infection. The risk of infection of the baby is highest if the mother has a primary infection, when at least 40% of the babies are likely to develop infection [160]. With an active, recurrent herpes episode at the time of birth, the risk of acquisition is approximately 1–3% [153].

There is some evidence that severe infection may be related to subtle defects in the host immune system or variants in the herpes virus [161,162].

Clinical features
History
A history of genital herpes in the mother should alert the obstetrician to the possibility of infection in the neonate, although this risk is frequently missed prenatally and the mother may be unaware of her HSV infection. Vaginal discharge or fever in the mother in late pregnancy should initiate testing for HSV [163].

Presentation
Herpes infection acquired at delivery usually presents at 1–3 weeks of life. The effects on the baby range in severity and may be due to disseminated disease, affecting multiple organs but predominantly the central nervous system, or limited to the skin, eyes and mouth [163,164]. In the latter, which accounts for about 45% of neonatal herpes cases, there may be a vesicular eruption, or more subtle blistering or peeling of the skin. The mucosae are inflamed and may be ulcerated. If the infection is disseminated, as in 25% of cases, there is likely to be fever, lethargy, seizures, respiratory distress, hepatosplenomegaly with hepatitis and thrombocytopenia.

Disease course and prognosis
The potential mortality of untreated neonatal herpes is 60–80% and even when treated, mortality of disseminated disease can be 25–30% [165]. The disease can progress to haemophagocytic lymphohistiocytosis. The outcome is best for babies with skin and mucosal disease only who are treated promptly.

Even after treatment with aciclovir, relapse of skin and mucosal neonatal herpes is common [166], with outbreaks of infection during childhood.

Investigations
Swabs for PCR and confirmatory viral culture are taken from skin, eyes, mouth and rectum. Herpes simplex virus can be detected by PCR in the cerebrospinal fluid in encephalitis and often in blood in disseminated disease. Serology of the mother can aid in confirmation of the HSV type.

Management
If there is active primary herpes infection in the mother at the time of delivery or shortly before, the risk of infection to the baby is so great that caesarean section is indicated and prophylactic aciclovir should be considered for the neonate [165,167,**168**]. Primary genital herpes during pregnancy and especially in the third trimester warrants treatment of the acute episode with oral aciclovir. For women with a primary genital infection in the third trimester or known recurrent herpes genitalis, treatment with prophylactic aciclovir from 36 weeks of gestation until delivery is recommended, to reduce the chance of asymptomatic viral shedding. For a baby born to a mother with a previous history of genital herpes but no active lesions during pregnancy or at delivery, the baby is monitored and tested for the presence of herpes on the skin, since asymptomatic shedding may be a route for infection [169].

Once diagnosed or even strongly suspected, neonatal herpes must be treated urgently, even if confined to skin and mucosae, to reduce the risk of progressive spread of infection and mortality [170].

Neonatal herpes is treated with high-dose intravenous aciclovir (20 mg/kg TDS for 2–3 weeks) followed by oral aciclovir for 6 months [171,172].

Inoculation herpes simplex

Synonyms and inclusions
- Herpetic whitlow
- Paronychial herpes simplex

Introduction and general description

Accidental inoculation of herpes simplex into intact or damaged skin or mucosa via a contaminated instrument or trauma can result in a primary herpes simplex infection which may later be seen as reactivation episodes.

Clinical features
History
Skin lesions develop 5–7 days after inoculation.

Presentation
Indurated papules, irregularly scattered vesicles or large bullae may be seen at the site of injury (Figure 25.12). Inoculation of the fingertips results in a 'herpetic whitlow' in which painful deep vesicles coalesce to give a honeycombed appearance or to form a large bulla. The regional nodes are enlarged but fever and constitutional symptoms are usually mild.

Clinical variants
Multiple crops of vesicles and pustules on plaques or redness and oedema on the face, scalp and upper trunk, simulating impetigo and lasting some 10–12 days, have occurred in wrestlers (herpes gladiatorum) [173]. On the face of the adult male, the appearance of herpes may be deceptive; it may take the form of a folliculitis, but satellite umbilicated vesicles soon suggest the correct diagnosis. Facial contact during rugby is another recognised means of acquiring herpes simplex virus infection [174], commonly called 'scrumpox', and close combat in the military may be another means of spread [175].

The primary infection may be mild or subclinical. Reactivation episodes may be misdiagnosed as shingles, especially if the vesicular eruption appears to be limited to a possible dermatomal pattern (zosteriform herpes simplex).

Differential diagnosis
Herpetic whitlow may be confused with a pyogenic bacterial infection.

Complications and co-morbidities
Recurrences of herpetic whitlow may occur; the majority are reported to be due to HSV-2 and occur in women with recurrent genital herpes [176]. Recurrent episodes may be avoided by prophylactic treatment with oral aciclovir prior to precipitation sporting events.

VARICELLA-ZOSTER VIRUS INFECTIONS

Varicella-zoster virus (Figure 25.13) is the cause of both varicella (chickenpox) and zoster (shingles).

General description of disease domain

The primary infection of varicella includes viraemia and a widespread eruption, after which the virus persists in nerve ganglion cells, usually sensory. Zoster is the result of reactivation of this residual latent virus.

Basic biology

Varicella-zoster virus is an α herpesvirus. Genotyping has shown that there are at least seven clades, clades 1–6 and clade 9, distinguished according to molecular variation, which have geographic variation [177,178].

The virus is transmitted by droplet infection from the nasopharynx. A brief first viraemic stage, when the virus can disseminate to other organs, is followed by a second viraemia coinciding with the onset of the rash. Patients are infectious to others from about 2 days before to 5 days after the onset of the rash and 60–100% of non-immune individuals will contract the infection if exposed to someone in the infectious stage of chickenpox or zoster. Vesicle fluid in either disease contains a large amount of virus and may be a route of droplet infection. Completely dry scabs are not infectious.

Varicella

Definition and nomenclature
Primary infection with VZV [179].

Synonyms and inclusions
- Chickenpox

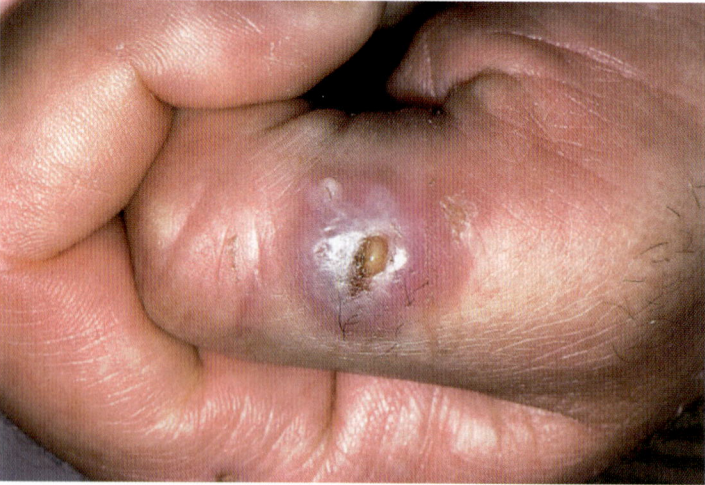

Figure 25.12 Herpes simplex. Inoculation lesion on the thumb of a dermatologist. Courtesy of Dr A. S. Highet, York District Hospital, UK.

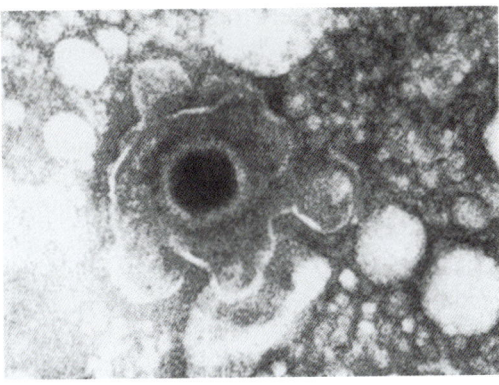

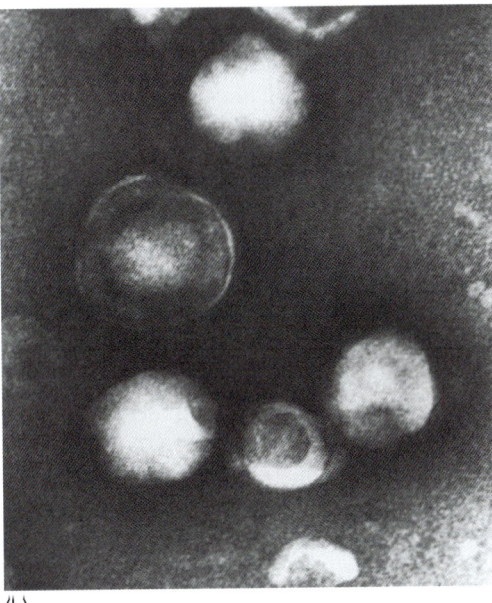

Figure 25.13 *Herpesvirus varicellae*. Phosphotungstate preparations from vesicle fluid. (a) The dark centre is due to penetration of the capsid by phosphotungstate (×72 000). (b) The envelope encloses the nucleocapsid and obscures detail (×116 250). Courtesy of Dr J. Nagington, Cambridge, UK.

Epidemiology

Incidence and prevalence
Varicella occurs throughout the world but infection occurs at a younger age in temperate zones compared with the tropics. Subclinical infections may occur. It is estimated that in non-immune populations, approximately 15 cases per 1000 people occur per year, leading to a seropositivity of about 95% of young adults with somewhat lower rates in tropical areas and in immigrants from tropical to temperate zones [**180**,181].

Age
Over half of primary infections occur before the age of 5 and 85% before puberty [182,183].

Pathophysiology

Pathology [184]
Following an initial period of replication in the oro-pharynx, a viraemia causes widespread dissemination. Within a few days, a second viraemia is detectable at the time when skin lesions become evident. In varicella skin lesions, cells of the Malpighian layer show ballooning of their cytoplasm by intracellular oedema and distinctive nuclear changes, comprising eosinophilic inclusions and marginated chromatin. Multinucleate giant cells with up to 15 nuclei, which are a characteristic feature of infections with HSV and VZV, are produced mainly by cell fusion. Intracellular oedema plus intercellular oedema and cellular necrosis produce the vesicle, the roof of which consists of the upper Malpighian and horny layers. A mild inflammatory reaction in the dermis later extends to the epidermis and the proportion of polymorphonuclear cells increases with ulceration.

In fatal cases of varicella, essentially similar cytological changes with areas of focal necrosis are found in the liver, kidney and other organs [185]. The lungs show interstitial pneumonia with focal consolidation and haemorrhage.

In varicella, IgG, IgM and IgA antibodies appear 2–5 days after the onset of the rash, and their levels peak during the second and third weeks. Thereafter, the titres gradually fall, although IgG persists at low levels. Antibodies seem to have an incomplete protective effect; maternal or administered antibody reduces the severity of infection, but does not prevent it and recurrent varicella has been reported [186].

Cell-mediated immunity is more important in both protection against and control of the infection. If the primary infection occurs when cell-mediated immunity is impaired, as in organ transplant patients, varicella may be severe and occasionally fatal.

Causative organisms
Varicella-zoster virus.

Environmental factors
In temperate climates, cases are more common in the cooler winter and spring months with a reduction in cases during the long school holidays [187]. In cities, epidemics occur at irregular intervals.

Clinical features

History
The incubation period is usually 14–17 days (range 9–23 days).

Presentation
After a day or two of fever and malaise, often slight or absent in children, an inconstant and fleeting scarlatiniform or morbilliform redness is followed by the development of papules which very rapidly become tense, clear, unilocular vesicles (Figure 25.14). Within a few hours, the contents become turbid and the pustules are surrounded by red areolae.

The vesicles appear in three to five crops over 2–4 days. They are most numerous on the trunk, then on the face and scalp and on the limbs. Their distribution is centripetal, and on the limbs the eruption is more profuse on the thighs and upper arms than on the lower legs and forearms. A characteristic feature is the presence of lesions at different stages in each site. The total number of lesions is very variable; they may be few or profuse. The distribution may be modified by pre-existing inflammatory changes at the sites of which lesions may appear in increased density [188]. The vesicles in such areas tend to be at the same stage and are often small, but may occasionally be bullous. In exceptional cases of normal distribution, the

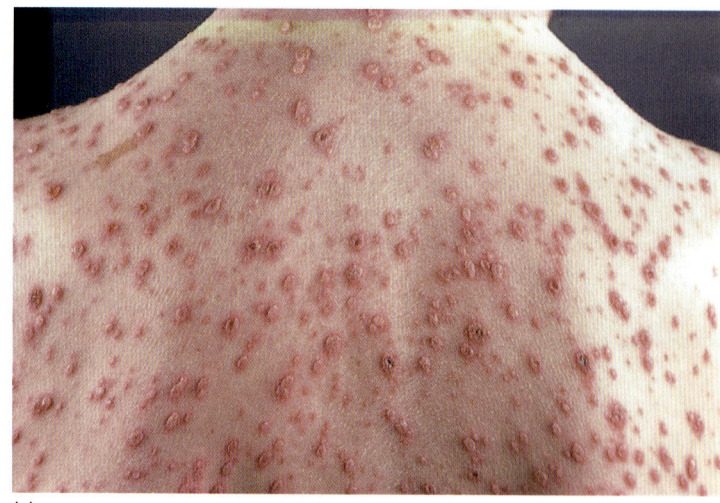

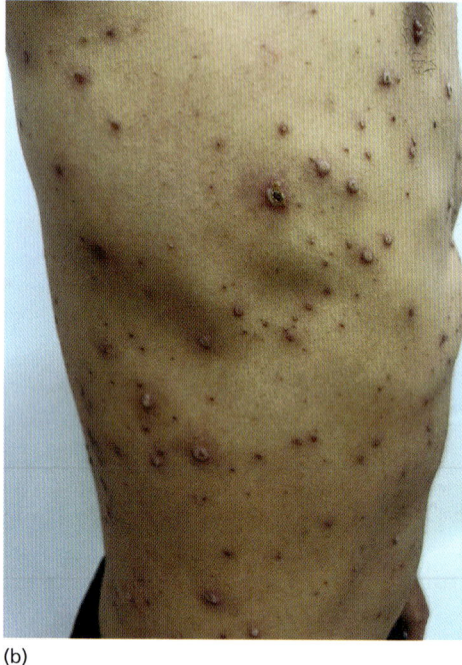

Figure 25.14 (a) Varicella in white skin. Courtesy of York District Hospital, UK. (b) Varicella in pigmented skin.

lesions are larger and umbilicated or varioloid. Vesicles are common in the mouth, especially on the palate, and are occasionally seen on other mucous membranes, including the conjunctiva and genitalia. On the anal mucosa, they may be followed by painful ulcers.

Fever is variable in severity and duration, and roughly parallels the extent of the eruption. It may be trivial or may reach 40°C or 41°C for 4 or 5 days. Constitutional symptoms tend to be proportionate to the fever. In some patients, pruritus is troublesome. When these features develop in an adult, a diagnosis of chickenpox may initially be overlooked.

Clinical variants

Haemorrhagic varicella, in which a very extensive eruption of haemorrhagic vesicles is accompanied by high fever and severe constitutional symptoms, is rare in the previously healthy patient. It is relatively more common in some tropical regions in which malnutrition may be a factor, but most cases now seen in temperate regions occur in immunocompromised patients.

Infection during pregnancy has extra risks for both mother and baby. Maternal infection may lead to pneumonitis in about 2.5% [189], with highest rates in the last trimester when there is a risk of maternal death due to respiratory failure. Infection in pregnancy, especially during the first and second trimesters, carries an approximate 2% risk of fetal damage, collectively called the congenital varicella syndrome. There may be skin scarring, multiple neurological problems including microcephaly, skin scarring and limb hypoplasia, with a 30% mortality within the first year of life [190].

Maternal primary infection at the time of delivery spreading to the immunologically unprotected neonate can result in very severe infection of the baby, with a mortality of about 30%. Chickenpox in a neonate when the mother is immune to VZV is usually mild, but infection later in the first year of life, once maternal antibodies in the baby have cleared, may be more severe [191].

A skin eruption may be seen after vaccination [192]. This may be localised or generalised, but is most commonly maculopapular and rarely vesicular.

Complications and co-morbidities

Complications are rare in otherwise healthy children, are less infrequent in neonates and adults, and are common in the immunosuppressed.

Encephalitis, often presenting with ataxia, in the otherwise healthy patient occurs in fewer than 1/1000 cases and complete recovery occurs in 80%. Other neurological complications, such as meningitis, transverse myelitis or ophthalmoplegia, are very rare. A vasculopathy with virus present within vessels can lead to infarction presenting as a stroke, but this is more common after zoster and is very rare in children after chickenpox [193]. The other main systemic complications are varicella pneumonia and hepatitis [194]. Varicella pneumonia is more common in adults than in children and can be more severe in pregnant women and smokers.

Secondary bacterial infection is seldom a serious problem in temperate climates, but under tropical conditions may be severe [195] and may be complicated by septicaemia. Cutaneous gangrene ('varicella gangrenosa') may follow secondary infection, but rarely extensive local gangrene may occur with or in the absence of proven bacterial involvement, and sometimes during a mild attack of varicella [196,197]. Thrombocytopenic purpura, beginning on the 5th to 10th day and usually recovering spontaneously after 3 or 4 months, occasionally follows otherwise benign varicella.

Other conditions rarely associated with varicella are rhabdomyolysis [198], Reye syndrome [199] and viral arthritis [200], although bacterial arthritis also occurs.

Stevens–Johnson syndrome occurring with varicella infection and after varicella vaccination has been reported [201,202], and should be considered if bullae develop in addition to the typical vesicles of chickenpox. Treatment with systemic corticosteroids, in addition to aciclovir, may be necessary. Erythema multiforme has been reported immediately prior to or coincidental with the eruption of chickenpox or zoster [203,204].

Varicella in immunocompromised people may be severe and progressive with a mortality of 7–10% [205]. Relatively short courses of oral steroid treatment in children and adults may permit the development of severe and potentially fatal chickenpox [206]. Features associated with a progressive varicella include haemorrhagic varicella, pneumonitis, hepatitis, encephalitis and acute retinal necrosis syndrome. Chronic varicella with persistent hyperkeratotic lesions [207] and repeated attacks of varicella have also been observed.

Disease course and prognosis
In 2–4 days, a dry crust forms and soon separates, to leave a shallow pink depression which, in the absence of secondary infection, heals without scarring.

After about 4 days, no new crops of lesions appear and existing vesicles dry and crust. It may be 1–2 weeks before the crusts separate and repair of lesion sites is complete. Hyper- or hypopigmentation may persist for weeks and small round depressed scars can occur in about 18% [208]. Rarely, hypertrophic scarring may develop [209].

Varicella confers lasting immunity and second attacks are uncommon, especially in immunologically healthy subjects, but clinical reinfection with a mild varicella-like illness occurs occasionally [210].

Investigations
In most cases, the diagnosis of varicella is clinical. The distinctive features of varicella are the centripetal distribution, the polymorphism in each affected site and the rapid progression of the individual lesion from vesicle to crust. In patients developing vaccinia eruption after vaccination, the eruption may be atypical and in these and other uncertain diagnoses, laboratory confirmation of the infection is desirable [211].

The quickest and most reliable way to confirm diagnosis is by PCR of vesicle fluid or a scraping taken from the base of a blister. Oral swabs can also be used, even when the eruption is fading [212]. PCR analysis is particularly useful in patients with suspected encephalomyelitis, in whom examination of the cerebrospinal fluid can lead to rapid diagnosis [213].

The virus is readily identified by electron microscopy of vesicle fluid and can be grown in tissue culture but this takes longer and is less reliable than for HSV. Detection of VZV antigen by direct fluorescent antibody staining of a smear from the base of a vesicle offers an alternative method. Titration of complement-fixing antibody in acute and convalescent sera may be a useful test in atypical infections.

In skin biopsies, the VZV proteins can be detected by immunohistochemistry [214], and the viral nucleic acid by *in situ* hybridisation [215] or PCR of extracted DNA [216].

Management
Prevention
This can be by pre-exposure vaccination, post-exposure immunoglobulin and antiviral prophylaxis.

Pre-exposure prophylaxis. A live attenuated vaccine developed from the Oka strain of VZV is effective in preventing varicella in healthy children [217]. The vaccine is given in two doses, 3 months apart, resulting in approximately 90% seroconversion with 75% of responding recipients maintaining detectable antibody for up to 10 years. The vaccine has been used routinely in the USA for 25 years and in many European countries for 15 years, but is not in routine use for children in the UK. Given in childhood, the vaccine does not appear to affect the incidence of zoster in adulthood [218]. The vaccine can also be used in children with HIV and a CD4+ count of at least 200 cells/μL [219] or children with leukaemia in remission, for whom it produces a seroconversion rate of over 80% and reduces the incidence and severity of varicella [220].

Before considering treatment with immunosuppressive agents, serotesting is advised and vaccination given to seronegative individuals [221] at least 2 weeks before starting therapy. If immunesuppressive therapy can be stopped, vaccination can be given at least 3 and preferably 6 months after discontinuation. In seronegative immunosuppressed adults, vaccination carries a risk of serious illness with vaccine-strain varicella [222] and is contraindicated.

Post-exposure prophylaxis. Specific varicella-zoster immune globulin (VZIG) administered within 10 days of contact reduces the severity of varicella but does not always prevent it [223]. It should be given to neonates whose mothers develop varicella within the period from 7 days before to 7 days after delivery [224,225,226]. Some advocate additional intravenous aciclovir, for the mother before delivery and the baby after delivery [227–229]. VZIG is also indicated for healthy neonates in contact with active chickenpox or zoster, and for immunocompromised children and adults, for example organ transplant recipients and patients who have taken oral steroids for at least 14 days within the previous 3 months who have not had previous chickenpox, if exposed to varicella or zoster [230]. It should also be given to exposed non-immune pregnant women, not only to reduce the severity of potential or actual chickenpox but also to reduce the risk of fetal transmission in those women who develop disease despite VZIG prophylaxis [226].

In children exposed to VZV, vaccination, if given within 3–5 days of exposure, will reduce the severity of chickenpox [225]. In the immunocompetent person, aciclovir given from about 9 days after exposure for 1 week appears to be effective in aborting or reducing the severity of chickenpox and allows immunity to develop. In the immunocompromised, such prophylaxis only delays the onset of the disease.

Antiviral prophylaxis. Long-term prophylaxis with aciclovir is effective in preventing zoster in the early months following bone marrow transplantation [231] and is also advocated for long-term prophylaxis at low dose [232]. Patients under treatment with short-term but high-dose immune suppression, such as prednisolone 40 mg daily for over a week or other long-term immunosuppressive drugs, benefit from prophylactic acyclovir, and this is strongly advised if immune status against the virus is low or absent.

First line
Varicella in the otherwise healthy child requires only symptomatic treatment. Soothing antiseptic applications may be helpful and secondary bacterial infection will require antibiotics.

Primary varicella infection during pregnancy should be treated with intravenous aciclovir to reduce the risk to the fetus. Infection of the mother in the 3 weeks before delivery or immediately after can result in neonatal varicella and treatment of the baby is essential [233].

Second line
The use of aciclovir in childhood chickenpox can reduce the severity and duration of the eruption [234]. It should be started within 24 h of the onset of the rash.

An antiviral is indicated for varicella in adults and for severe varicella or zoster infections at any age in the immunocompromised. Treatment should be started as early as possible, preferably within the first 1 or 2 days. The virus is less sensitive to aciclovir *in vitro* than HSV and higher doses are usually recommended, typically 10 mg/kg or 500 mg/m^2 8 hourly intravenously [235] or 4 g/day orally [236]. Courses of 5, 7 and 10 days have been used and some advocate a change from intravenous to oral drug after 48 h.

Third line
In chickenpox with immune suppression or in encephalitis, intravenous aciclovir should be started as soon as possible [237].

Treatment ladder for varicella

First line
- Antiseptic cream
- In pregnancy – acyclovir, IV, 10 mg/kg TDS

Second line
- Aciclovir, IV, 10 mg/kg TDS

Third line
- Aciclovir, IV, 10 mg/kg TDS

Resources

Further information
https://assets.publishing.service.gov.uk/government/uploads/system/uploads/attachment_data/file/1056198/Green_Book_Chapter_34_v3_0.pdf
https://cks.nice.org.uk/topics/chickenpox/
(Both last accessed August 2023).

Zoster

Definition and nomenclature
Zoster is a segmental eruption due to reactivation of latent VZV from dorsal root ganglia.

Synonyms and inclusions
- Herpes zoster
- Shingles

Introduction and general description [238]
Zoster (zoster = a girdle or belt, a reference to its segmental distribution) is a sporadic affliction of individuals who have previously had clinical or subclinical varicella. Zoster patients are infectious, both from virus in the lesions and, in some instances, the nasopharynx. In susceptible contacts of zoster, chickenpox can occur.

Epidemiology
Incidence and prevalence
The average annual incidence has been estimated at 2–4/1000 [239,240]. In one study in Australia, VZV infections were among the five most common dermatological causes of a visit to the emergency department [241].

Age
Zoster is not common in childhood and young adult life. Over the age of 50, the incidence rises and continues to rise in successive decades of life so that at age 80, the incidence is approximately 10 cases per 1000 patient-years. The mean age of zoster is about 60 years [242].

Sex
Zoster is slightly more common in females.

Pathophysiology
Predisposing factors
An earlier infection with varicella is essential before zoster can occur. Most commonly, chickenpox occurs in childhood and zoster in middle to older age. Zoster is more common in immunosuppression.

The factors determining the site of an eruption of zoster are often unclear, but it may be precipitated by pressure on or trauma to nerve roots, by neoplastic deposits, radiotherapy, surgery or other, often trivial, traumas [243].

Pathology
The skin lesions show similar features to those seen in chickenpox (see Chickenpox pathology earlier).

The posterior nerve roots and ganglia show inflammatory changes and sometimes these involve the anterior horn. Virus particles have been seen in ganglion cells and Schwann cells in the affected nerve bundles [244]. More extensive changes are sometimes reported: leptomeningitis, encephalitis with local demyelination, and myelitis. Disseminated lesions in other organs may occur as in varicella.

Zoster can cause some destruction of nerve fibres in the middle and lower dermis, detectable with silver impregnation techniques [245]. Partial denervation may persist for over a year and characteristically does so in patients with postherpetic neuralgia [246]. Corresponding fibres in the spinal cord degenerate and there may be scarring in the region of the ganglion.

In zoster, the levels of IgG antibody increase rapidly and reach a higher titre than during the primary infection.

Causative organisms
Reactivation of latent VZV.

Clinical features
Presentation [247]
The first manifestation of zoster is usually pain, which may be severe, and may be accompanied by fever, headache, malaise and

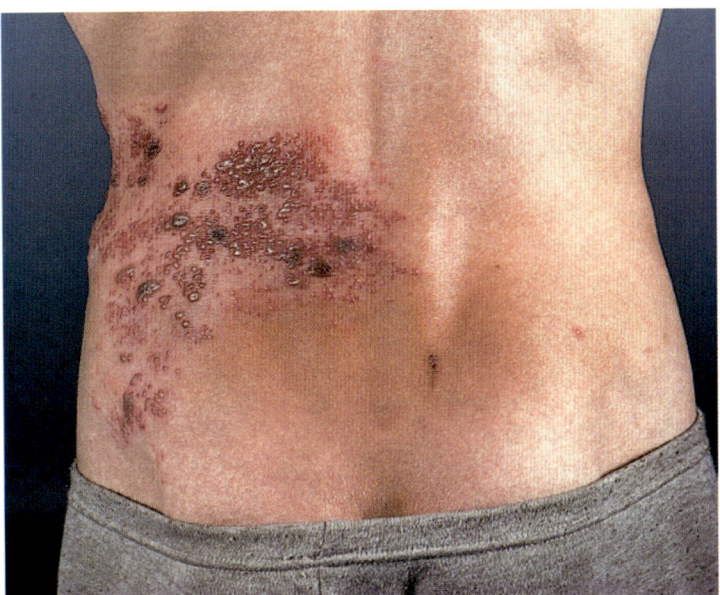

Figure 25.15 Zoster of the trunk. Courtesy of York District Hospital, UK.

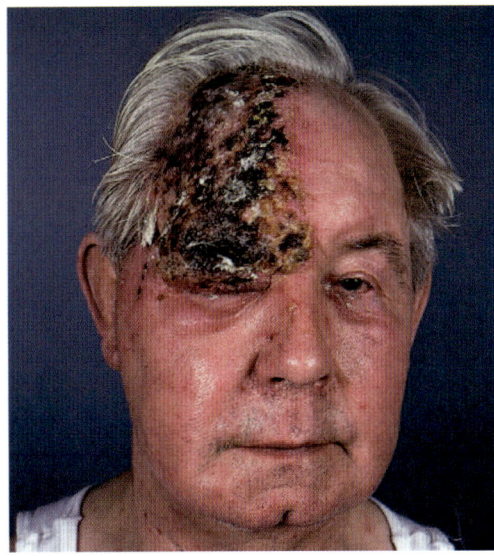

Figure 25.16 Ophthalmic zoster. Courtesy of York District Hospital, UK.

tenderness localised to areas of one or more dorsal roots. The pain may be sharply localised and unilateral, but may be more diffuse. Instead of or in addition to pain, occasionally pruritus may be an early feature of shingles. The time between the start of the pain and the onset of the eruption averages 1.4 days in trigeminal zoster and 3.2 days in thoracic disease. Closely grouped red papules, rapidly becoming vesicular and then pustular, develop in a continuous or interrupted band in the area of one, occasionally two and, rarely, more contiguous dermatomes. The striking feature is cut-off at the midline (Figure 25.15). Mucous membranes within the affected dermatomes are also involved. New vesicles continue to appear for several days. Often in children, and occasionally in adults, the eruption is the first indication of the attack. The lymph nodes draining the affected area are enlarged and tender.

Occasionally, the pain is not followed by the eruption ('zoster sine eruptione') [248].

The thoracic (53%), cervical (usually C2, 3, 4, 20%), trigeminal, including ophthalmic (15%), and lumbosacral (11%) dermatomes are most commonly involved at all ages, but the relative frequency of ophthalmic zoster increases in old age. Rarely, the eruption may be bilateral.

In some 16% of patients with zoster, vesicles develop beyond the dermatome involved within a few days of the local eruption. This is more common in the elderly, but in most cases only a few lesions appear and the course of the zoster is unchanged.

In the elderly and undernourished, the local eruption often becomes necrotic. Healing, which may require many weeks, may be followed by severe scarring. In the otherwise healthy child, zoster usually runs a benign course.

Variations in the zoster syndrome depend on which dorsal root is involved, on the intensity of its involvement and on the extension of the inflammatory changes into the motor root and anterior horn cells. Visceral involvement may be responsible for abdominal pain, pleural pain or temporary electrocardiographic abnormalities with or without precordial pain [249].

Clinical variants

Maternal zoster in pregnancy is not associated with intrauterine infection [250]. Zoster in infancy has followed maternal varicella, the baby's primary infection having occurred *in utero* [251].

In patients with lymphomas or who are otherwise immunocompromised, generalised varicella ('disseminated zoster') develops and may be haemorrhagic. Rarely in such cases the zoster may successively involve further dermatomes. Systemic involvement may follow and can be fatal.

Trigeminal nerve zoster. In ophthalmic nerve zoster (Figure 25.16), the eye is affected in two-thirds of cases, especially when vesicles on the side of the nose indicate involvement of the nasociliary nerve (Hutchinson sign). Ocular complications include uveitis, keratitis, conjunctivitis, conjunctival oedema (chemosis), ocular muscle palsies, proptosis, scleritis (which may be acute or delayed for 2–3 months), retinal vascular occlusion, and ulceration, scarring and even necrosis of the lid. Involvement of the ciliary ganglia may give rise to Argyll–Robertson pupil.

Zoster of the maxillary division of the trigeminal nerve produces vesicles on the uvula and tonsillar area, while with involvement of the mandibular division, the vesicles appear on the anterior part of the tongue, the floor of the mouth and the buccal mucous membrane. In oro-facial zoster, toothache may be the presenting symptom.

Herpes zoster oticus. The facial nerve, mainly a motor nerve, has vestigial sensory fibres supplying the external ear (including pinna and meatus) and the tonsillar fossa and adjacent soft palate. Classical sensory nerve zoster in these fibres causes pain and vesicles in part or all of that distribution, though the skin involvement may be minimal and limited to the external auditory meatus.

Herpes zoster oticus accounts for about 10% of cases of facial palsy (Figure 25.17). The paralysis is usually complete and full recovery occurs in only about 20% of untreated cases.

Complications and co-morbidities

Motor involvement [252]. This occurs overall in 5% of cases and is commoner in older patients and in those with malignancy, and

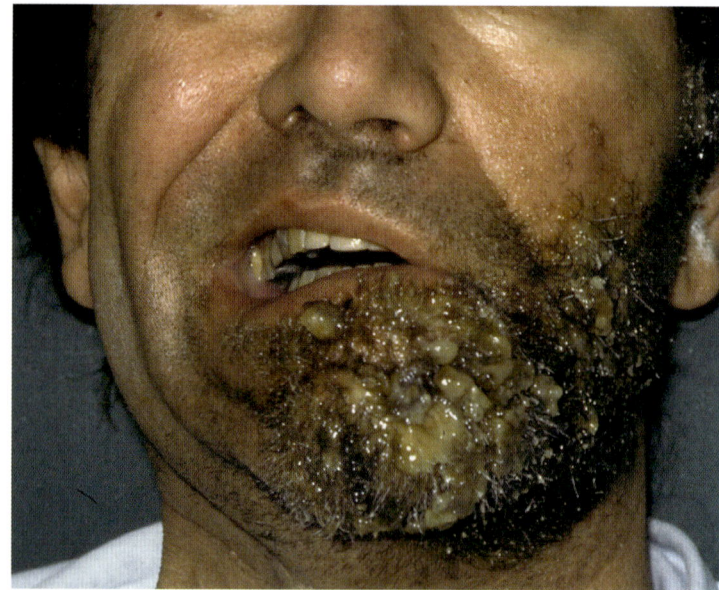

Figure 25.17 Herpes zoster oticus showing unilateral zoster with facial palsy (Ramsay Hunt syndrome).

in cranial compared with spinal nerve involvement. The motor weakness usually follows the pain and the eruption, by a few days to a few weeks, but occasionally precedes or accompanies them. The affected segment is usually but not always the same. Complete recovery is expected in 55% and significant improvement in a further 30%. Facial palsy in herpes zoster oticus is discussed earlier. In ophthalmic zoster, ocular or facial palsies may occur [253].

Zoster of the ano-genital area may be associated with autonomic effects including disturbances of defecation or urination [254]. In the abdominal area, this can present as a pseudohernia [255] or pseudo-obstruction (Ogilvie's syndrome) [256].

Post-herpetic neuralgia [257]. The commonest and most intractable sequel of zoster is postherpetic neuralgia, generally defined as persistence or recurrence of pain more than a month after the onset of zoster, but better considered after 3 months. It is unusual in childhood and increases in incidence and severity with age. It occurs in about 30% of patients over 40 and is most frequent when the trigeminal nerve is involved. It is more likely to develop if there was prolonged dermatomal pain prior to the eruption, if the acute pain of zoster was severe and if the zoster rash was prolonged [258]. The pain has two main forms, a continuous burning pain with hyperaesthesia, and a spasmodic shooting type, but a pruritic 'crawling' paraesthesia may also occur. Allodynia, pain caused by normally innocuous stimuli, is often the most distressing symptom and occurs in 90% of people with postherpetic neuralgia. The neuralgia varies in intensity from inconvenient to profoundly disabling.

Neurological symptoms can occur with VZV reactivation after or without a rash. The presentations include encephalitis, meningoencephalitis, cranial neuropathies, myelitis and stroke. Many of these effects can be grouped together as varicella vasculopathy, which may also include coronary artery disease and peripheral thrombotic vascular disease [259,260]. The risk of a neurological event remains raised in the 3 months post-zoster [261].

In patients with impaired immunity, both the incidence and severity of zoster are increased, and it is frequently complicated by disseminated cutaneous disease and systemic involvement, usually pneumonia, hepatitis or encephalitis. This is seen in malignancy, especially lymphomas, so that the incidence of zoster is at least 10% [262,263]. Also at risk are patients receiving cytotoxic or immunosuppressive therapy, especially the more profound suppression required for bone marrow transplantation; series suggest that 30–40% of patients may have varicella-zoster reactivation episodes during the first year post-transplant [264,265]. Anti-tumour necrosis factor (TNF)-α therapy is estimated to increase the risk of zoster threefold [266]. In patients infected with HIV, zoster is 10 times more common than in the normal population and may become disseminated and chronic.

Other complications

1 Erythema multiforme has been reported in association with the eruption of zoster [267].
2 Scar sarcoid [268], granuloma annulare [269] and fungal granulomas [270] have been reported in healed zoster scars. Other patterns of granulomatous inflammation, variously described as granulomatous dermatitis, giant cell lichenoid dermatitis, granulomatous folliculitis and granulomatous vasculitis, may occur after zoster [271]. These persistent lesions are more common in the immunosuppressed and may respond to prolonged antiviral treatment.
3 Bacterial infection of damaged skin, including necrotising fasciitis [272].
4 Acute retinal necrosis syndrome; this rare complication follows an attack of shingles affecting the ophthalmic nerve or an unrelated dermatome [273].
5 Guillain–Barré syndrome has also been noted occasionally following zoster.

Disease course and prognosis

The pain and the constitutional symptoms subside gradually as the eruption disappears. In uncomplicated cases recovery is complete in 2–3 weeks in children and young adults, and 3–4 weeks in older patients.

In immunosuppressed individuals, especially due to HIV infection, zoster may run a protracted course, with a small number of lesions developing into verrucous or crusted nodules.

Recurrent shingles can occur, either affecting the same dermatome (in 45% of cases) or at a different site [274]. Distinction from zosteriform HSV infection should be made.

Investigations

Diagnosis of typical zoster presents few difficulties once the eruption has developed and can be confused only with zosteriform herpes simplex. Where the diagnosis is uncertain, confirmation is made by PCR or culture as in chickenpox.

Detectable VZV DNA persists in saliva for days to months after a zoster infection [275] and this can be useful for diagnosis once the eruption has faded.

Management [276]

Shingles is a self-limiting infection but it is painful, and carries a risk of secondary infection and postherpetic neuralgia. Analgesia and measures to counteract the infection and facilitate healing are usually necessary.

Prevention
In later life, immunity against VZV wanes but may be boosted intermittently following contact with chickenpox [277]. Boosting by vaccination can help to reduce the occurrence or severity of zoster or the risk of postherpetic neuralgia [278,279]. The zoster attenuated virus vaccine (Zostervax®) is the same as the varicella vaccine but at a higher virus titre and is given as a single dose. In those for whom immunosuppressive treatment is being considered, for example pre-transplantation or for skin or rheumatic conditions, vaccination can be administered at least 2 weeks prior to commencing immunosuppression. The more recent development of the recombinant zoster vaccine (Shingrix®) now enables immunosuppressed individuals to receive antibody-boosting intervention without the risk of disseminated virus infection.

Vaccination is recommended where available (Shingrix for those over 50 years of age in the USA, where live vaccine use has been discontinued, and in the UK, where both vaccine types are still available in 2023, Shingrix for those turning 65 or Zostervax for those over the age of 70). In the immunosuppressed, the use of the live vaccine is contraindicated, and the recombinant vaccine can be used over the age of 50. In those for whom immunosuppressive treatment is being considered, for example pre-transplantation or for skin or rheumatic conditions, vaccination can be administered at least 2 weeks prior to commencing immunosuppression.

First line
Rest and analgesics are sufficient for mild attacks of zoster in the young. Higher-strength analgesia is often needed in older patients. Soothing topical preparations with dressings as blisters break can relieve discomfort.

An antiviral is indicated for painful zoster infections in adults and at any age in facial zoster and in the immunocompromised. Treatment should be started as early as possible, preferably within the first 1 or 2 days. The virus is less sensitive to aciclovir *in vitro* than HSV and higher doses are recommended. Oral treatment for zoster is with aciclovir 800 mg five times a day for 7–10 days or with valaciclovir 1 g or famciclovir 250 or 500 mg three times a day for 7 days [283]. Such treatment prevents progression of the eruption, reduces the systemic complications of varicella and zoster, and lessens zoster pain during treatment.

Studies of the benefits of corticosteroid therapy together with aciclovir in the treatment of shingles have given conflicting results. One study in immunologically normal patients found that, in conjunction with aciclovir, prednisolone 40 mg daily tailed off over the next 3 weeks hastened the return to normal activity, better sleep and reduced the time analgesia was required [284]. Another study [285] concluded that the addition of prednisolone conferred only a slight benefit on the rate of healing and reduction of acute pain, but at the expense of an increase in adverse effects. Without antiviral cover, serious dissemination of infection due to systemic steroids is a risk.

There is debate regarding the effect of antiviral treatment in reducing the risk of postherpetic neuralgia [286], but many believe that aciclovir or famciclovir, started early in shingles, can reduce both the chance and the duration of postherpetic neuralgia, especially in the older patient [287,288].

Second line
In immunosuppression, aciclovir may be given intravenously (10 mg/kg or 500 mg/m^2 8 hourly) or 4 g/day orally in five doses [276,289]. Courses of 5, 7 and 10 days have been used and some advocate a change from intravenous to oral drug after 48 h.

Third line
For postherpetic *neuralgia* the use of opiates should be avoided if possible but the disorder can be prolonged and debilitating [290]. A tricyclic antidepressant such as amitriptyline [291] or nortriptyline (or clomipramine or doxepin) is useful, especially for hyperaesthesia and constant burning pain, an effect independent of any antidepressant activity. For best results, it should be given early in a dose of 25 mg daily and continued for 3–6 months. These adrenergically active antidepressants may be most effective if antiviral treatment is given during the acute attack of shingles. For stabbing pain, sodium valproate (or other anticonvulsant, e.g. clonazepam or carbamazepine) is of value. Especially in the elderly, doses should be low initially and increased every few days as required. Gabapentin or pregabalin can be useful analgesics for the pain [291] but any benefits are variable [292]. Topical capsaicin 0.025%, a substance P depleter, may relieve pain in some patients, though its usefulness in some is limited by a burning sensation following application or an increased area of allodynia [293]. Topical anaesthetic applied as a cream or a patch can also give relief [294,295].

Treatment ladder for zoster

First line
- Aciclovir, PO, 800 mg five times a day for 8–10 days
- Valaciclovir, PO, 1 g TDS for 7 days
- Famciclovir, PO, 250–500 mg TDS for 7 days

Second line
- Aciclovir, IV, 10 mg/kg every 8 hours for 5–10 days

Third line
For postherpetic neuralgia, consider:
- Amitriptyline
- Nortriptyline
- Sodium valproate
- Gabapentin
- Pregabalin

Resources

Further information

Clinical Knowledge summaries: http://cks.nice.org.uk/shingles#!topicsummary
https://www.cdc.gov/shingles/resources-refs.html; https://www.cdc.gov/vaccines/vpd/shingles/public/shingrix/index.html
https://www.gov.uk/government/publications/shingles-herpes-zoster-the-green-book-chapter-28a

Chicken pox in adults – management: http://www.lhp.leedsth.nhs.uk/detail.aspx?id=1465
https://www.msdmanuals.com/en-gb/professional/infectious-diseases/herpesviruses/chickenpox
Werner RN, Nikkels AF, Marinović B *et al*. European consensus-based (S2k) Guideline on the management of Herpes Zoster – guided by the European Dermatology Forum (EDF) in cooperation with the European Academy of Dermatology and Venereology (EADV), Part 2: treatment. *J Eur Acad Dermatology Venereol* 2017;31:20–9.

Patient resources
NHS Choices: http://www.nhs.uk/conditions/shingles
https://www.nhs.uk/conditions/vaccinations/shingles-vaccination/
Centers for Disease Control and Prevention: (https://www.cdc.gov/shingles/; https://www.cdc.gov/vaccines/vpd/shingles/public/shingrix/index.html
(All last accessed August 2023.)

EPSTEIN–BARR VIRUS INFECTIONS

Introduction

Epstein–Barr virus (EBV) infection is very common and the great majority of adults in all populations are infected with EBV [296].

General description of disease domain

In early childhood, the virus is probably spread by contact with saliva on fingers or fomites. In more developed communities, early childhood infection is less frequent and primary infection occurs most commonly in early adult life, when kissing is the usual route of infection, though occasional droplet spread may occur. Most primary infection, especially in childhood, is asymptomatic or mild, but when it is delayed to adolescence or adulthood, clinically obvious infectious mononucleosis is more frequent, occurring in about two-thirds of those infected.

Basic biology

Epstein–Barr virus is a γ herpesvirus that usually infects oral epithelial cells and B lymphocytes of the tonsil and occasionally T lymphocytes or monocytes. In the oro-pharynx, liberation of virus into the saliva from localised differentiated B cells explains the spread of infection between individuals.

Primary infection, whether clinical or subclinical, is followed by lifelong persistence of the virus in a latent state in resting memory B cells. Although not actively replicating, the latent virus can produce some detectable proteins, including nuclear antigens [297]. Under certain conditions, especially in immune compromise, the virus may reactivate and then a range of viral and cellular proteins are expressed. No latent infection takes place in epithelial cells, although persistent infection with viral shedding may occur. Latent EBV is associated with nasopharyngeal carcinoma and with various B-lymphoproliferative lesions later in life.

Occasionally, the primary viral infection does not settle and a state of chronic active infection develops.

Infectious mononucleosis

Synonyms and inclusions
- Glandular fever

Introduction and general description

Infectious mononucleosis is an acute febrile illness with sore throat and cervical lymphadenopathy, presenting after an incubation period of about 6 weeks [298].

Epidemiology

Incidence and prevalence
An incidence of 500/100 000 per year is reported from the USA in 2010 [299] and there is an increasing incidence in the UK over the last decade [296]. Seropositivity is reported in over 95% of adults in the UK in 2020.

Clinical features

Presentation
Infectious mononucleosis is characterised by fever, sore throat with exudative pharyngotonsillitis and lymphadenopathy. There is a variable degree of malaise, fatigue and headache. Enlargement of the spleen or liver has been recorded in up to half of those acutely infected. Petechiae at the junction of the hard and soft palate are a distinctive feature of the disease and usually appear on the second or third day of fever.

An exanthem occurs in about 10% of cases, usually between the fourth and sixth days. Most common is a macular or maculopapular eruption of the trunk or upper arms, involving the face and forearms in some cases and the thighs and legs occasionally. Morbilliform and scarlatiniform eruptions are sometimes seen. Acute urticaria is occasionally a presenting feature [300] and periorbital oedema may be seen, more commonly in females. Skin lesions fade after a few days to a week. Rarely, the eruption may be vesicular or petechial [301].

If ampicillin or amoxicillin is taken during the course of the illness, an extensive maculopapular or morbilliform eruption develops in over 90% of cases, 7–10 days after the start of treatment. This eruption may be itchy, is most marked on extensor surfaces and pressure areas and can involve palms and soles. The eruption can last days to weeks and may be associated with arthralgia or gastrointestinal upset. A similar effect is occasionally seen with penicillin, tetracyclines and azithromycin [302].

Differential diagnosis
An acute mononucleosis-like disease can occur in infection with cytomegalovirus (CMV) (see later), HHV-6, primary HIV, hepatitis A, toxoplasma and SARS-CoV-19 [303].

Complications and co-morbidities

Cold agglutinins are common in infectious mononucleosis, usually without clinical manifestations, but they might explain occasional cases of transient cold urticaria [304], which may rarely be severe enough to result in ulceration [305]. EBV association is reported in several autoimmune diseases including rheumatoid arthritis, systemic lupus erythematosus, dermatomyositis, Sjögren syndrome and multiple sclerosis, although the causality is debated.

Thrombocytopenic purpura is common but counts below 100 000/μL are fortunately rare. Other complications include neutropenia, gammaglobulinaemia, pneumonia, myocarditis, nerve palsies, cerebellar ataxia and optic neuritis. Splenic rupture and encephalitis are life-threatening complications.

A number of other conditions affecting skin or mucosae have been reported with acute EBV infection, including airways obstruction due to enlarged tonsils, ulcerative pharyngitis and oesophagitis.

Gianotti–Crosti syndrome (see later). Epstein–Barr virus has been reported in association with this eruption, which is believed to be a reaction to viral infection in childhood [306,307].

Lipschütz ulcers (Chapter 110). These develop as acute painful genital ulceration, usually in adolescents without sexual contact [308]. Evidence of primary EBV infection [309] may be found but other infections are implicated [310]. The sloughy ulcers are often multiple and develop in association with malaise, fever and inguinal lymphadenopathy. They heal spontaneously but somewhat slowly.

Haemophagocytic lymphohistiocytosis (haemophagocytic syndrome). Acute EBV infection can rarely lead to this very severe disease with a high mortality. It was first described in genetic immunodeficiency syndromes such as X-linked lymphoproliferative disease [311], but also occurs in other causes of immune suppression or during immunosuppressive treatment or other severe infections [312,313]. The syndrome in immunocompetent individuals was originally described in Japanese patients, but other races can be affected [314] and has also been reported soon after Covid-19 immunisation [315]. It most commonly affects children and adolescents.

Infection of T lymphocytes or natural killer (NK) cells triggers T-cell proliferation and overactivity of NK cells with overproduction of cytokines, especially interferon-α and TNF-α. Investigations show a high viral EBV load in blood as well as elevated acute phase reaction proteins.

The presentation is usually with fever lasting several days, followed by the development of pancytopenia with coagulation defects and multiorgan failure. Lymphadenopathy, hepatosplenomegaly and haemorrhage into the lungs and bowel are common, and cerebral symptoms of meningitis or encephalitis may develop. The cutaneous findings may relate to coagulation defects, but reported features can include telangiectasia [316], a maculopapular rash with epidermal necrosis, panniculitis or nodules with granulomatous inflammation [317–319].

Treatment must include full supportive care, antiviral therapy and rapid commencement of immunosuppressive therapy, including biologics for refractory cases [320–323], but prognosis is often poor.

Kikuchi's histiocytic necrotising lymphadenitis. This has been rarely reported in association with EBV infection [324] (Chapter 149).

Other. There are reports of cases of EBV infection associated with a variety of reactive dermatoses: erythema multiforme [325], Stevens–Johnson syndrome, erythema nodosum [326], erythema annulare centrifugum [327], acute pityriasis lichenoides [328], chronic bullous disease of childhood [329], papular pruritic gloves and socks (see later), unilateral laterothoracic exanthem [330] and a predominantly facial eruption resembling inflammatory granuloma annulare [331].

Disease course and prognosis
The acute disease clears within a month but cervical lymphadenopathy may take 3 months to settle. There may be relapsing episodes of malaise, fatigue, fever and lymphadenopathy, but no recurrent skin eruption.

Reactivation of the latent infection is associated with the development of oral hairy leukoplakia in immune suppression and with drug hypersensitivity syndrome or drug reaction with eosinophilia and systemic symptoms (DRESS) [332].

Investigations
In acute disease, there is lymphocytosis with at least 10% atypical cells seen on blood film [333]. Abnormalities in liver function tests indicate hepatocellular damage which may lead to jaundice in about 4% of those infected.

Antibodies to viral antigens can be detected in early infection (early antigen, EA, and viral capsid antigen, VCA) and after acute infection (antibodies to the EBV nuclear antigen A, EBNA). Detection of these specific antibodies is used to distinguish acute, chronic active, reactivated and malignancy-associated latent EBV disease [334]. Anti-EA antibodies are detectable in 80% of individuals during acute infection and persist for several months. IgM class antibody against VCA persists for a few weeks after infection and IgG antibody for life. IgM is also detected in reactivation.

Tests for heterophile antibodies, which agglutinate sheep or horse red blood cells, become positive in 90% of patients after 1–2 weeks, so are not useful in the early stages of the infection. These tests (Paul–Bunnell and monospot) are less reliable in childhood, when false negative results are more common, and occasionally give false positives (for instance in several other infectious diseases and also lymphomas and leukaemias).

Viral DNA or RNA detection by PCR or RT-PCR in throat swabs, blood or tissue, or *in situ* hybridisation of tissue, are methods which can be applied in unusual cases [334,335].

Management
General measures include treatments for the symptoms of pyrexia and sore throat. Rest and recuperation are important aspects of management. Oral antiviral treatment has no effect on the acute disease [333]. Vaccines are under development.

If the skin eruption is symptomatic, an emollient and moderately potent topical steroid may be used, but clearance is usually within a week even when not treated.

Oral hairy leukoplakia (Chapter 108)

Introduction and general description
Oral hairy leukoplakia develops insidiously, presenting as white plaques on the sides of the tongue.

Pathophysiology
Predisposing factors
This disorder is due to reactivation of EBV infection and is seen most commonly in association with immunodeficiency due to HIV infection. It may develop in other immune-incompetent states such as haematological malignancy [336] or during immunosuppressive treatment [337,338] including biologics [339], and occasionally in immunocompetent individuals [340] such as with steroid inhaler use or in old age.

Pathology
Epstein–Barr virus replicates in maturing epithelial cells but is not present in basal and parabasal keratinocytes.

Clinical features
Presentation
White rippled plaques develop unilaterally or bilaterally on the sides of the tongue. They may appear to have hair-like projections. In more advanced disease, the plaques may extend over the tongue and into the oro-pharynx.

Differential diagnosis
Consider lichen planus, candidiasis, focal epithelial hyperplasia and squamous cell carcinoma.

Chronic active Epstein–Barr virus infection

Definition
Chronic or recurrent and relapsing disease following acute EBV infection and lasting for at least 3 months after primary infection.

Introduction and general description
The usual features are persistent or intermittent malaise, fever, lymphadenopathy, splenomegaly, hepatitis and arthritis. There may be evolution into haemophagocytic lymphohistiocytosis.

Epidemiology
The disorder is more common in children and young adults than in older adults. There are reported cases from Central and South America, but most are from East Asia.

Pathophysiology
Pathology
Investigations show high levels of EBV DNA in the blood with circulating IgG antibodies against VCA and EA-restricted proteins. An increasing defect of T and NK cell function can lead to immune suppression and opportunistic infection. Genetic defects relating to immune function have been identified in a number of patients with severe or chronic disease, but there is no clear predisposing abnormality [341].

Clinical features
Presentation
As well as the features already described, there may be leukocytoclastic vasculitis with cutaneous features similar to Henoch–Schoenlein purpura [342,343].

The course of the disease is variable, but lymphoma may develop in about 17% [344]. Patients with connective tissue disorders, especially systemic lupus erythematosus, are often found to have a viral load higher than in the healthy population. This may be due to a mild degree of immune compromise due to the disease and is likely to be exacerbated by immunosuppressive therapy [345].

Hydroa vacciniforme developing in children or adults as a UV-associated eruption is linked with high EBV viral loads [346,347]. Pruritic necrotic plaques as a presenting feature of lymphocytic variant hypereosinophilic syndrome have been ascribed to chronic active EBV infection [348].

Hypersensitivity to mosquito bites. This may indicate a primary persistent EBV infection, usually occurring in childhood. Most cases are reported from East Asia. Intense inflammation, often with purpura, bullae and necrosis, develops at the sites of mosquito bites [349]. There is usually regional lymphadenopathy and there may be systemic features such as pyrexia and hepatitis. These patients should be monitored for the possible development of NK/T-cell lymphoma.

Complications and co-morbidities
Natural killer/T-cell lymphoproliferative disease evolving to lymphoma associated with EBV can involve skin, rarely as a predominantly cutaneous disease [350]. Prolonged immunosuppression may be a predisposing factor. A notable presenting feature in some cases is hypersensitivity to mosquito bites and suggests chronic active EBV infection [351]. Papulonecrotic lesions, especially of the face, or severe hydroa vacciniforme-like lesions have been described as presenting features of NK/T-cell malignancies [352,353]. This clinical pattern, now described as hydroa vacciniforme-like lymphoproliferative disorder (HV-LLD), usually presents in childhood or adolescence. Nodular lesions and panniculitis are also reported [354]. Very rarely, the lymphoma may be intravascular, producing dusky plaques or nodules [355]. The skin lesions may be found to contain EBV RNA. These cases have been reported most commonly in Asia and in native Americans of Central and South America.

Epstein–Barr virus-associated lymphoproliferative disorders and malignancy

Introduction and general description
Epstein–Barr virus infection is implicated as a pathogenic factor in several proliferative and malignant disorders of the lymphoid system and also in gastric cancer. The global incidence of EBV-associated malignancies is over 250 000 per year with the highest rates in East Asia [356]:

1 *Burkitt lymphoma.* This occurs in equatorial Africa and New Guinea, presenting classically with huge cervical lymphadenopathy. It is most common in children but can occur in adults [357].
2 *EBV-associated lymphoproliferative disease.* B-cell tumours, histologically characterised as large-cell lymphomas, occur in

immunocompromised people and especially immunosuppressed transplant recipients. Systemic immunosuppressive agents associated with this include azathioprine and methotrexate [358]. In transplant recipients, EBV-associated post-transplant lymphoproliferative disease (PTLD) occurs in 0.5–1.5% of the recipients of solid organs, with 50–80% of PTLD cases progressing to abnormal lymphoid proliferative disease [359]. Skin involvement is not common, presenting with single or multiple papules or nodules, but in rare cases the skin is the primary site of disease [360]. Ulcers of the skin or mucosae may be classified as EBV-positive mucocutaneous ulcers [361].

3 *EBV-positive diffuse large B-cell lymphoma (DLBCL)*. This includes the previously named age-related EBV-associated B-cell lymphoma [362], occuring most commonly over the age of 50, in non-immunosuppressed individuals usually presenting with lymphadenopathy (80%). There may be extranodal involvement, particularly in the skin/mucosa (in 20%), gastrointestinal tract (in 15%) or lung (in 12%). Skin lesions are nodules and ulcers. It is an aggressive disease, usually proving fatal within 2–3 years.
4 *Nasopharyngeal carcinoma*, reported mainly in Asia, is often preceded by prolonged elevation of antibodies against EBV.
5 *Hodgkin lymphoma*.

HUMAN HERPESVIRUS 6 AND 7 VIRUS INFECTIONS [363,364]

Definition

Human herpesvirus 6 (HHV-6) is a worldwide virus infecting the majority of the population in early life. Primary infection is usually of little consequence, but later reactivation during immune suppression can produce more troublesome disease. Human herpesvirus 7 (HHV-7) produces very similar effects but has been less extensively studied.

Classification

HHV-6 was originally isolated in 1986 from circulating B cells of patients with HIV infection or lymphoproliferative disorders [365]. Two antigenically distinct varieties, HHV-6A and HHV-6B, were identified and these are now classified as separate viruses [366]. HHV-6B is almost always the cause of human disease, with HHV-6A rarely implicated [367,368]. HHV-6A and HHV-6B and the closely related HHV-7 (formally classified as human betaherpesviruses 6A, 6B and 7) are all in the genus *Roseolovirus* (see Tables 25.2 and 25.4).

HHV-7 infection is very similar to HHV-6. The virus was first isolated from human CD4+ T lymphocytes in 1990 [369].

General description of disease domain [370]

HHV-6 and HHV-7 cause roseola infantum (exanthem subitum) as a primary infection. Persistence or reactivation of HHV-6 can occur, especially in immune compromise; for example, it is estimated that about half of allogenetic haematopoetic stem cell transplant recipients experience HHV-6 reactivation [371]. This may be asymptomatic but has been associated with encephalitis, multiple sclerosis, Guillain–Barré syndrome, chronic fatigue syndrome, lymphoproliferative disorders, connective tissue disease [372] and Kikuchi–Fujimoto disease [373] (Chapter 149), although the importance of the associations is not clear. Reactivation of the viruses may underlie the development of pityriasis rosea, and two forms of drug rash: drug-induced hypersensitivity syndrome and DRESS (Chapter 12).

Basic biology

HHV-6 and HHV-7 are serologically and genomically distinct from other human herpesviruses but with some regions of the genome bearing similarities to the betaherpesvirus CMV. The cellular receptor for HHV-6 is CD46 [374] while CD4 on T lymphocytes is important for HHV-7. In culture, infected cells (B and especially T cells) are large and refractile and frequently contain intranuclear and/or intracytoplasmic inclusions.

In the acute stage of primary infection with HHV-6, there is a viraemia which is followed by the appearance of antibodies to the virus [375]. Seroprevalence studies have shown that by the age of 1 year, 75% of infants have antibodies to HHV-6 and 90–95% of adults are seropositive for HHV-6 and HHV-7 [376,377]. The main presentation of primary infection with either virus is roseola infantum, but most infections are subclinical [366,378–380], with estimates that only about one-third develop clinical disease. After the initial infection, the virus persists and can be detected in saliva from a high percentage of healthy subjects, the likely mode of spread [381].

HHV-6 can integrate into chromosomal DNA but still retain the ability to produce new virions [382]. As a latently integrated virus, it can be transmitted vertically [383] and it is estimated that approximately 1% of children are infected at birth and the virus is present in cells throughout the body of the newborn.

Roseola infantum [384,385]

Definition and nomenclature
Roseola infantum is an acute febrile illness with a maculopapular eruption.

Synonyms and inclusions
- Exanthema subitum
- Exanthem subitem
- Sixth disease

Epidemiology
Incidence and prevalence
Roseola infantum is the most common exanthematic fever in children under the age of 2 years, reported to account for 24% of acute febrile illness presenting at a paediatric emergency department [386].

Age
Peak incidence is between 6 and 9 months.

Pathophysiology
Causative organisms
- HHV-6
- HHV-7

Clinical features
History
The incubation period is from 10 to 15 days.

Presentation
The first sign of illness is abrupt onset of fever, sometimes ranging between 39.5°C and 40°C, which persists for 3–5 days and initially is usually accompanied by few or no symptoms. Irritability, inflamed tympanic membranes, ulcers at the posterior palate and uvula [387] and, occasionally, periorbital oedema and haematuria are early manifestations. As the temperature falls, an eruption of discrete rose-pink maculopapules develops on the neck and trunk; it may later spread to the arms, face and legs. The lesions may have surrounding pallor and rarely become vesicular [388]. The patient's cervical and occipital lymph nodes are usually enlarged.

Clinical variants
The eruption of primary HHV-6 infection is almost always restricted to the first 3 years of life. If primary infection occurs in adults, there may be a mononucleosis-like illness, with variable fever or rash and with mainly cervical lymphadenopathy, which may persist for up to 3 months; or an acute but self-limiting hepatitis [389,390].

Differential diagnosis
Measles, rubella.

Complications and co-morbidities
Febrile convulsions are not uncommon, occurring in 13% in one series [365].
Fatal encephalitis is rare, but has been reported in primary infection [391]. Other complications reported are thrombocytopenia [392], purpura fulminans [393] and haemophagocytic syndrome [394]. Primary HHV-6 infection has been rarely associated with papular purpuric gloves and socks syndrome [395], Gianotti–Crosti syndrome [396], Stevens–Johnson syndrome [397] and pityriasis rosea [398].

Disease course and prognosis
After 1 or 2 days the rash fades, leaving no scaling or pigmentation.
Reactivation of the latent virus may occur, especially in immune suppression (see later).

Investigations
The lack of symptoms during the febrile phase and the appearance of the eruption as the fever subsides should suggest the diagnosis, although clinical confusion with rubella or measles is not uncommon and the picture of roseola infantum can also be caused by HHV-7 infection. Confirmation is by demonstrating a seroconversion or rise in antibody titre to HHV-6, typically by indirect immunofluorescence using cells infected with HHV-6 as antigen. IgM antibody is usually present 5–7 days after the rash, maximal 2 weeks after infection, and persists for about 2 months. Current serological tests do not distinguish between HHV-6A and -6B. Molecular detection of viral RNA by RT-PCR or DNA by PCR is possible and distinguishes HHV-6A from -6B, but only quantitative PCR reliably distinguishes primary from latent infection [365,399]. HHV-6 DNA has been demonstrated in the cerebrospinal fluid of children with both primary HHV-6 infection and also at times of recurrent seizures following exanthem subitum, which suggests that HHV-6 is a direct cause of the associated encephalitides.

During the first 2 days there may be leukocytosis but as the rash develops, leukopenia with a relative lymphopenia is usual.

Management
First line
Only symptomatic measures are usually required.

Second line
Antiviral therapy with ganciclovir, valganciclovir, cidofovir or foscarnet would be appropriate in individuals with severe disease.

Reactivation of herpesvirus 6 and 7

In immunosuppression, latent HHV-6 and HHV-7 may reactivate and cause a variety of symptoms. Quantitative PCR detection is necessary to distinguish active primary or reactivated infection from past infection [399,400].

If it occurs, reactivation is most frequent in the first few weeks after transplantation and commencement of immune suppression. In one study, reactivation of HHV-6 occurred in just over 10% of transplant recipients [401]. The effects are usually subclinical, producing no recognisable disease, but in about 1%, HHV-6 reactivation and increase in blood virus titres are associated with presentations of fever, rash, hepatitis, gastroenteritis, encephalitis, pneumonitis and bone marrow suppression [399,402,403]. The eruption may be maculopapular or vesicular [404,405]. Antiviral therapy with gangciclovir or foscarnet, either alone or in combination, is indicated in severe disease. Reactivation of HHV-7 alone is unusual but it may accompany HHV-6 reactivation. Reactivation of the HHV-6 has been reported in graft-versus-host disease [399,406] and more recently in patients severely ill with SARS-CoV-2 [407].

In otherwise healthy individuals, reactivation of HHV-6 and HHV-7 is associated with pityriasis rosea. In recent years, a link between reactivation of these viruses and the development of reactions to certain drugs has been established. As with HHV-6, HHV-7 is possibly associated with pityriasis rosea [398] (see later) and it has also been proposed as a candidate trigger for lichen planus [408].

The viral evidence suggests that both drug-induced hypersensitivity syndrome and DRESS involve drug-triggered viral reactivation [409,410] and detection of the viral DNA in the blood is most likely in days 14–21 after the onset of the skin reaction.

OTHER HERPESVIRUS INFECTIONS

Cytomegalovirus infection

Synonyms and inclusions
- Cytomegalovirus (CMV) infection of the skin
- CMV infection, congenital

Introduction and general description
Cytomegalovirus infections are common throughout the world and are usually inapparent. Primary infection is followed by life-long carriage of the virus with intermittent shedding in various secretions. This may be increased by physiological stimuli such as pregnancy, and by immune suppression due to disease or therapy as in AIDS and transplant recipients, respectively.

Epidemiology
Incidence and prevalence
Depending on socioeconomic conditions, between 40 and 100% of adults in a community are infected as shown by seropositivity [411]. There are several ways of transmitting CMV, which are to some extent age dependent. Intrauterine transmission occurs in 0.1–1.0% of births. Perinatal and neonatal infections arise as a result of exposure to infectious cervical secretions in the birth canal, from infected breast milk or from close household contacts. Preschool children may acquire CMV from oral secretions or urine of other infected infants. At an older age, sexual transmission is important. CMV may be transmitted via blood transfusion and in transplanted organs from CMV seropositive donors.

Presentation [412,413]
Primary cytomegalovirus mononucleosis. In the otherwise healthy child or adult, infection is commonly symptomatic. When symptoms do appear, they resemble infectious mononucleosis with fever, lymphocytosis and mildly deranged liver function, although lymphadenopathy and splenomegaly are not usually striking. In up to a third of cases, there is a follicular, maculopapular or rubelliform eruption, often affecting the legs and lasting up to 2 days. Urticaria may occur [414].

As in EBV infectious mononucleosis, concomitant ampicillin commonly triggers a widespread eruption.

Vasculopathy presenting as cutaneous vasculitis or necrotic skin lesions has been reported [415,416] and Lipschütz ulcers, more commonly associated with EBV infection, have occurred with primary CMV infection [417].

Congenital CMV infection. Primary CMV infection in the first or second trimester of pregnancy can have multiple effects on the fetus. As both mother and baby at birth may be asymptomatic, diagnosis must be made by serological testing. In just over 10% of babies with congenital infection, there are signs including hepatosplenomegaly, jaundice and microcephaly. Skin signs include petechiae and purpura. Mortality can be high and survivors usually have severe neurological damage, especially deafness. There may be erythropoietic tissue in the dermis derived from undifferentiated dermal mesenchyme; this presents as purple or red papules or nodules lasting 4–6 weeks ('blueberry muffin' lesions) (Chapter 114). Vesicles occur very rarely in congenital CMV disease [418]. CMV can present as a congenital infection where there is underlying immune defect [419].

Clinical variants
Cytomegalovirus in the immunosuppressed. Cytomegalovirus infection in the immunocompromised may be due to primary infection or to reactivation of latent infection. It can be severe and even fatal, with pneumonitis, hepatitis, gastrointestinal ulceration, retinitis and superinfection with other opportunistic pathogens. Neurological complications include encephalitis, myelitis and especially myeloradiculitis when the peripheral nerve roots are infiltrated with lymphocytes in AIDS.

A wide variety of skin lesions may occur in disseminated CMV infection. A non-specific widespread maculopapular eruption may be seen that may become papular and purpuric, with vesiculobullous or pustular lesions and indurated pigmented nodules or plaques [420]. A characteristic histological feature of the eruption is the presence of cytomegalic ('owl-eye nucleus') cells in vascular endothelium. This may progress in some cases to vasculitis or a more diffuse vasculopathy [421]. Sharply demarcated ulceration may occur, mostly around the genitalia, perineum, buttocks and thighs [422,423], and there may be associated livedo reticularis [424]. Isolated nodules, keratotic or necrotic skin lesions and severe oral and skin ulceration have been reported [425–428], especially in AIDS.

Following a course of antiviral treatment for CMV in immunosuppressed or immunocompromised people, relapsing infection and progression of organ involvement may occur. Severe disease without known immunosuppression should prompt investigation for underlying disease or primary immune deficiency.

Other associations of cytomegalovirus infection. Cytomegalovirus has been suggested as the precipitating factor in scleredema, scleroderma, systemic sclerosis [429], sclerodermatous chronic graft-versus-host disease [430], vitiligo and alopecia areata, but these associations are unproven or contentious. One case of toxic epidermal necrolysis presenting with concomitant CMV viraemia has been reported [431].

Complications and co-morbidities
Gianotti–Crosti syndrome [432] (see later), papular purpuric 'gloves and socks' syndrome [433] (see later) and DRESS may occur together with CMV infection. Erythema multiforme and haemophagocytic lymphohistiocytosis have been reported as a consequence of CMV infection including congenital disease [434–437].

Investigations
Current diagnosis is with rapid and sensitive methods using viral DNA detection by PCR and detection of CMV antigenaemia. Primary infection can be diagnosed serologically by the appearance of CMV IgM and IgG antibodies. Congenital CMV can be detected by PCR analysis of saliva or urine neonatally and confirmed by virus isolation or the presence of CMV IgM antibody within 3 weeks of

birth [438]. Post-transplant, monitoring of CMV viral load can permit early diagnosis of reactivation.

Classically, the infection was diagnosed histologically by finding typical intranuclear inclusions surrounded by a clear halo in enlarged cells. This method is relatively insensitive, but with the addition of immunohistochemistry, cytomegalic inclusions are more readily demonstrable. Virus culture from throat washings, urine, bronchoalveolar lavage fluid, blood or biopsy material is carried out in human embryo fibroblast cells, but it takes 5–28 days to produce a cytopathic effect, seen as 'owl eye' nuclear inclusions. This can be accelerated by looking for CMV early antigen after 24–48 h culture.

Management
Most CMV infections do not require specific therapy, but in life-threatening situations or when CMV retinitis threatens sight, two antiviral agents – IV ganciclovir and foscarnet – have been used with some success [439]. Valganciclovir, a prodrug of ganciclovir, is used orally as prophylactic treatment in CMV antibody-negative transplant recipients receiving a solid organ from a CMV-positive donor [440] and has also been reported to be effective as treatment for acute or recurrent CMV disease [441].

Newer antivirals such as letermovir (also approved for prophylactic use in bone marrow transplant recipients) and maribavir are under assessment for use in wider prophylaxis and as active treatment.

When diagnosis of a primary infection or reactivation episode is made during pregnancy, treatment of the mother with the antiviral valaciclovir can reduce the risk of fetal infection [442]. Prompt treatment with valganciclovir when a diagnosis of congenital CMV infection is made may reduce the risk of progressive hearing loss.

Human herpesvirus 8 infection

Definition and nomenclature
Human herpes virus 8 (HHV-8) is found worldwide, but usually produces a subclinical primary infection. It leads to a risk of development of Kaposi sarcoma (KS), especially in immunosuppression.

Synonyms and inclusions
- Kaposi sarcoma-associated herpesvirus (KSHV)

Epidemiology
Incidence and prevalence
Antibody studies of healthy adults suggest that approximately 80% of the population have had infection with HHV-8 in African countries, with variation across the continent, but that less than 20% of the population is seropositive in western Europe [443,444]. Italy has a slightly higher rate of 35% in some areas of the country.

Pathophysiology
Pathology
Histology of the eruption of primary HHV-8 infection shows a perivascular upper dermal infiltrate which includes plasma cells [445] in which viral proteins may be detectable.

In KS, KSHV DNA has been detected in 98% of lesions and is present in the monocytes, endothelial cells and spindle cells. The mechanism by which KSHV produces tumours is different to most other malignancies. Many of the viral proteins expressed by the virus influence cell proliferation, angiogenesis and apoptosis and downregulate local immunity [446,447]. Early KS lesions are polyclonal although clonal growth may develop as a late event.

Causative organisms
Since it was recognised in association with HIV/AIDS, the epidemiology of KS suggested that it was caused by an infectious agent. In 1994, Chang *et al.* [448] identified novel DNA fragments in AIDS-associated KS tissue that had partial homology to other γ herpesviruses. Several genotypes are identified based on variation within specific areas of the genome.

As with other herpesviruses, latent infection persists after initial infection and later reactivation episodes may occur, especially with immunosuppression.

Clinical features
Presentation
Primary infection with HHV-8 may be subclinical or may occur with fever and maculopapular eruption. The red rash can affect all areas of the body but is usually most marked on the body and limbs. In countries with high seroprevalence, the primary infection may be seen in children [449].

Clinical variants
Primary infection with HHV-8 or reactivation in an HIV-positive individual can produce a severe disease with high-level viraemia, fever, wasting, anaemia and thrombocytopenia, and rapid development of KS. This has been called the KSHV-inflammatory cytokine syndrome (KICS) [450].

KS-associated herpesvirus, or HHV-8, has also been found in association with classic KS in immunocompetent people [451] and in post-transplantation KS (iatrogenic KS). Prolonged immunosuppression including with biologic therapy, and for reasons including pemphigus and psoriatic arthritis, has rarely been associated with HHV-8 in the skin and KS [452–454].

The virus is also found in multicentric Castleman disease, in which cutaneous involvement has been occasionally reported [455], in primary effusion lymphomas and in the related solid primary effusion lymphoma which may rarely present in the skin [456]. A multisystem disorder reported in Castleman disease (POEMS syndrome) is also associated with HHV-8 infection [457]. In POEMS syndrome (polyneuropathy, organomegaly, endocrinopathy, monoclonal gammopathy and skin changes) the cutaneous abnormalities include multiple haemangiomas, hyperpigmentation, hypertrichosis and thickened skin.

In a minority of cases, pityriasis rosea may be associated with HHV-8 [458].

Investigations
Quantitative PCR permits detection of the virus plus estimation of viral load, but is not yet in routine or widespread use [459,460]. In primary infection, the virus may be detected in saliva [449].

Management
Treatment of HHV-8 infection may be difficult as the primary infection is frequently subclinical or diagnosis may be made late.

First line
There is some evidence that antivirals (valaciclovir, famciclovir, valganciclovir) may reduce viral replication in primary or reactivation episodes [461,**462**].

Treatments for HHV-8-associated KS are multiple (Chapter 138). Regression of lesions frequently occurs in AIDS with antiretroviral treatment and post-transplant with reduction of immunosuppression or with change of immunosuppressive regime to include rapamycin or sirolimus [463]. Local treatments include cryotherapy, radiotherapy, photodynamic therapy, intralesional chemotherapy, intralesional interferon, topical 5% imiquimod cream [464] and topical beta-blocker [465].

Herpes B virus infection [466]

Definition and nomenclature
Herpes B virus is mainly an infection of primates, but can infect humans in close contact with animals.

> **Synonyms and inclusions**
> - Macacine herpesvirus 1
> - Previously named Cercopithecine herpesvirus 1 (CeHV-1)

Introduction and general description
Human infection with herpes B virus usually occurs via a bite from an infected macaque. The virus is highly pathogenic to humans, in whom it typically causes a fulminant encephalitis which is fatal in 80% of cases without treatment.

Pathophysiology
Predisposing factors
Human infections have occurred in attendants and research workers, most frequently following monkey bites, but occasionally in those who have handled monkeys or monkey tissues and have not been bitten. Person-to-person transmission is rare.

Causative organisms
Herpes B virus is genetically close to HSV-1 and -2 but is not naturally an infection of humans [467]. It causes a benign enzootic infection of Asiatic macaque monkeys (the *Macaca* genus) and readily spreads among other monkeys in captivity. The virus remains latent in infected monkeys and may reactivate spontaneously or at times of stress.

Clinical features
Presentation
Symptoms of infection are initially non-specific with fatigue, myalgia, fever and headache. Lesions resembling herpes simplex usually but not invariably develop after 5–21 days at the site of the bite or scratch. There may be symptoms of tingling, itching, numbness or pain before the vesicular eruption appears. The eruption may remain localised or show some extension with regional lymphangitis and lymphadenopathy.

Disease course and prognosis
Ascending myelitis and encephalitis, usually fatal, develops after 10–35 days in a high proportion of cases.

Investigations
There is usually a history of contact with monkeys or monkey tissue. Culture of the virus from vesicle fluid or brain biopsy material will confirm the diagnosis, but must be performed in a specialised laboratory and is slow. Specific primers for PCR are available for the direct detection of herpes B virus DNA in blood or tissue [468]. Serological tests of paired samples can also be helpful.

Management
Ideally, situations in which a monkey may bite should be avoided and there are guidelines to prevent herpes B virus infections in monkey handlers [469]. Steps should be taken to ensure that any captive colonies are pathogen free by testing for antibodies [470].

First line
Monkey-inflicted wounds should be vigorously cleaned with soap and water and followed by iodine or alcohol. Aciclovir used early may reduce the severity of the disease but may have little impact if used late [469]. Valaciclovir orally is now the recommended treatment given as soon as possible following exposure. The dose is 1 g TDS for 14 days.

Second line
Intravenous ganciclovir is more potent than aciclovir *in vitro* and has also been used clinically.

Third line
If neurological symptoms of herpes B virus disease develop, treatment is with intravenous aciclovir, 12.5–15 mg/kg TDS, or ganciclovir, 5 mg/kg BD [471], but if there are signs of encephalitis, ganciclovir is the treatment of choice. Even with treatment, mortality is high.

Resources

Further information
http://emedicine.medscape.com/article/235360-overview
http://www.cdc.gov/herpesbvirus/
https://rarediseases.org/rare-diseases/simian-b-virus-infection/
(All last accessed August 2023.)

Eczema herpeticum

Definition and nomenclature
A widespread cutaneous infection with a virus which normally causes localised or mild vesicular eruptions, occurring in a patient with pre-existing skin disease.

> **Synonyms and inclusions**
> - Kaposi varicelliform eruption

Introduction and general description
The great majority of cases are infections with HSV-1, and are now usually called eczema herpeticum rather than Kaposi varicelliform eruption. The more general eponymous title may be used to encompass similar widespread infections with other viruses including vaccinia, coxsackie and other herpesviruses.

Epidemiology
Incidence and prevalence
Most herpes simplex infections in patients with atopic eczema are not unusually severe or widespread. Approximately 3% of those with atopic dermatitis may develop eczema herpeticum [472]. There is no clear seasonal variation.

Age
Cases are seen at all ages, most commonly in the second and third decades [473,474].

Pathophysiology
Predisposing factors
Atopic eczema is by far the commonest predisposing condition. Eczema herpeticum can result from primary or recurrent infection [473].

Other susceptible dermatoses are listed in Table 25.6.

Extensive spread of herpetic infection has followed cosmetic procedures, such as dermabrasion [493], laser therapy [494], hair transplantation [495] and trauma, including burns [496,497] and skin grafting [498].

Eczema herpeticum only develops on skin with visible dermatitis. Eczema herpeticum may be worse in patients with severe, especially erythrodermic, atopic eczema, but frequently occurs in mild or quiescent cases [499]. In localised cases, local spread seems likely, but widespread dissemination is haematogenous.

Patients who develop eczema herpeticum are usually immunocompetent and have, or can develop, antibodies against the virus [500]. Several studies have identified possible risk factors for the development of eczema herpeticum in individuals with atopic eczema [501]. An early age of onset of atopic eczema, high IgE level [473], a tendency to other skin infections [502] and a low NK cell count [503] have all been found in eczema herpeticum patients. A further possible predisposing factor is a defect in the innate immune response as shown by a low skin level of the antimicrobial peptides LL-37 (cathelicidin) [504], human β-defensin [505] and keratinocyte-derived thymic stromal lymphopoietin (TSLP) [506]. Several abnormalities in the interferon signalling pathway have been described [507–510], suggesting that this aspect of viral defence may be of central importance to the susceptibility to eczema herpeticum.

An association with systemic or topical steroid treatment has not been consistently found [473,499]. Other topical and systemic immunosuppression has also been associated with eczema herpeticum, namely topical tacrolimus [511] or pimecrolimus [512], although this is not a significant risk factor. Dupilumab may reduce the incidence of eczema herpeticum, probably due to improved skin function during treatment [513]. It is possible that the predisposition to develop widespread herpes simplex is linked more with the severity of the eczema or a limited immune defect rather than with the type or quantity of treatment used.

Causative organisms
The usual causative virus is HSV-1. HSV-2 [514], VZV [515], coxsackie A6 and A16 (eczema coxsackium) [516] and vaccinia [517,518] (eczema vaccinatum) have all been associated with a similar eruption.

Clinical features
History
There may be a short history of a reactivation episode of herpes labialis, but this is frequently not seen. If there is known contact preceding the onset, the incubation period is about 10 days (range 5–19 days).

Presentation [499,501] (Figure 25.18)
Vesicles, which rapidly become pustular, erupt in massive crops. They may be confined to abnormal skin but are often widely disseminated and may generalise, simulating chickenpox or smallpox. They may be haemorrhagic and the face may become grossly oedematous. The skin is painful and generally red. The vesicles rupture quickly, leaving small round superficial erosions, usually 2–4 mm, which weep and crust (Figure 25.18c). New crops of vesicles may appear for 5–7 days. Fever, which may be high, commonly develops 2 or 3 days after the onset of the eruption and constitutional symptoms may be severe. The regional lymph nodes are enlarged.

Table 25.6 Skin disorders which may be affected by widespread herpes simplex.

Skin disorder	References
Atopic eczema	See text
Less common	
Darier disease	475
Pemphigus foliaceous	476
Benign familial pemphigus	477
Rarely	
Hailey–Hailey disease	478
Ichthyosis vulgaris	479
Congenital ichthyosiform erythroderma	480
Epidermolysis bullosa simplex	481
Grover disease	482
Allergic contact dermatitis	483
Irritant contact dermatitis	484
Psoriasis	485
Pityriasis rubra pilaris	486
Cutaneous T-cell lymphoma	487
Sézary syndrome	488
Rosacea	489
Drug eruption	490
Staphylococcal scalded skin syndrome	491
Sunburn	492

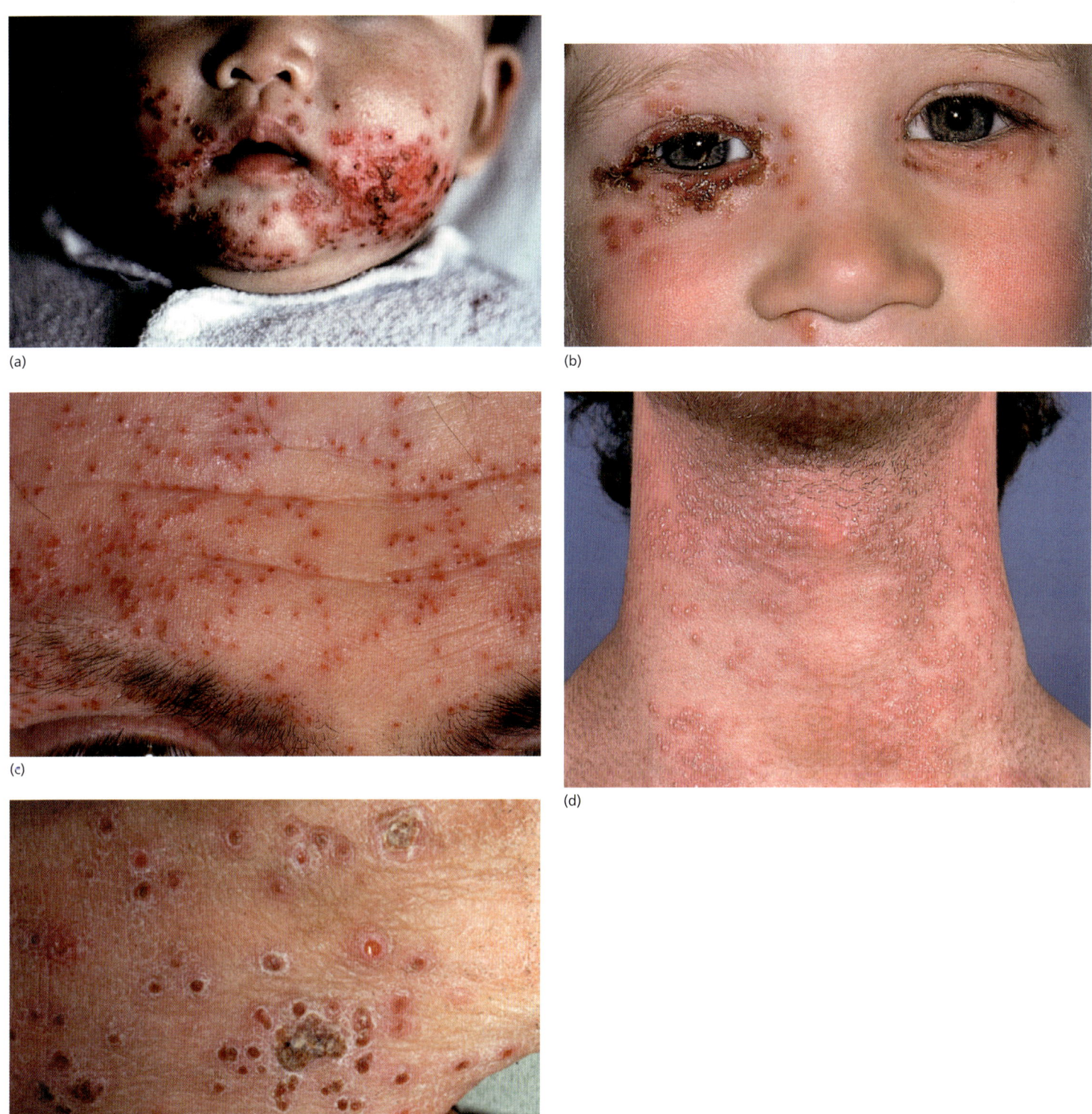

Figure 25.18 Eczema herpeticum. (a) Perioral. (b) Periocular. (c) Forehead. Courtesy of Addenbrooke's Hospital, Cambridge, UK. (d) Front of the neck of 20-year-old man. Courtesy of York District Hospital, UK. (e) Resolving lesions.

Clinical variants
When developing from a primary infection, there is more likely to be malaise, high fever and lymphopenia.

In immune compromise, whether iatrogenic or due to other disease, the presentation of eczema herpeticum may be atypical and the disease more severe.

Differential diagnosis
Chickenpox is the most important differential of a widespread blistering eruption evolving into punched-out erosions. In localised infections, the diagnosis may be confused by secondary bacterial infection [519] and by lesions in pre-existing blistering skin disorders. However, typical vesicles or subsequent erosions, generally

confined to eczematous or inflamed areas, should be sought, especially if there is a poor response to antibacterial therapy. These milder infections are usually self-limiting. Diagnosis can also be difficult when the lesions of a pre-existing bullous disorder delay recognition of the punched-out erosions of the varicelliform infection.

Disease course and prognosis
The fever subsides after 4 or 5 days and the pustules become crusted and slowly heal, leaving little permanent scarring. Rarely, there may be progression to potentially fatal systemic infection, such as encephalitis [520,521]. Secondary bacterial infection with staphylococci or streptococci is a risk and may lead to sepsis.

Recurrences of eczema herpeticum can occur. In a European study of 214 patients, recurrent infection occurred in 26.5% [522]. Recurrences are commonly milder than the initial episode, but sometimes are of comparable severity [**499**].

Investigations
If possible, blister fluid or a surface swab should be analysed for HSV (see earlier). Serum collected at onset and 10 days later will permit HSV serological testing. Skin biopsy shows the usual features of an acute HSV lesion in eczema herpeticum.

Management
Awareness of the possibility of widespread herpetic infection should be encouraged in atopic eczema patients or their parents.

Antiviral treatment is recommended in all ages and should be started as soon as possible after diagnosis, as delay in treatment can lead to prolongation of the illness [523].

Less ill patients respond well to oral aciclovir [524], valaciclovir or famciclovir. Severe cases should receive intravenous aciclovir [525] and this should also be considered early in patients who are immunosuppressed. If any immunosuppressive medication is non-essential, it should be reduced or stopped during the infection. Eczema herpeticum in pregnancy has been treated with aciclovir without an adverse effect on the baby [526]. Periocular lesions may lead to conjunctival infection and damage, so warrant urgent eye examination and treatment.

Bacterial infection and the underlying eczema or other dermatosis should be treated in the usual way. If antiviral therapy is given, the use of topical steroids does not appear to lead to a longer disease course [527].

Frequently recurrent disease may benefit from low-dose prophylactic aciclovir or valaciclovir [528].

> **Treatment ladder for eczema herpeticum**
>
> **First line**
> - Oral aciclovir, 400 mg 5 times a day, for 5 days, for adult
> - Oral valaciclovir, 500 mg BD for 5 days, for adult
> - Oral famciclovir, 250 mg TDS for 5 days, for adult
>
> **Second line**
> - Intravenous acyclovir, 5 mg/kg every 8 hours for 5 days or until lesions clearing
>
> **Third line**
> - Consider prophylactic oral antiviral therapy for recurrent eczema herpeticum
>
> Dose and duration are recommended to be minimal, because there are no trials to confirm optimum regime.

Resources

Patient resources
https://www.bad.org.uk/shared/get-file.ashx?id=197&itemtype=document
https://nationaleczema.org/eczema/related-conditions/eczema-herpeticum/
(Both last accessed August 2023.)

POLYOMAVIRUS INFECTIONS

Definition and general description of disease domain

Polyomaviridae (PyV) encompasses a family of small (45 nm) non-enveloped icosahedral viruses with 5 kb double-stranded, circular DNA genomes encoding early non-structural proteins, small tumour antigen (sTAg) and large tumour antigen (TAg), and the late virion proteins (VPs) VP1, VP2 and VP3. Unlike the 200 or more HPVs, there appears to be a smaller number of PyVs that infect humans (HPyV) (Table 25.7) [**1**]. Although HPyV infections occur in most individuals, HPyV-mediated diseases are rare and primarily occur in patients who are immunocompromised [**1**].

HPyVs were first described in 1971 when BK and JC polyomaviruses were identified in immunosuppressed individuals with ureteric obstruction and progressive multifocal leukoencephalopathy, respectively [**1,2**]. Merkel cell carcinoma polyomavirus (MCPyV), identified in 2008, was the first HPyV associated with a skin disease [**3**]. Subsequently, trichodysplasia spinulosa virus (TSV) was found to be associated with the rare dermatosis, trichodysplasia spinulosa; HPyV-6 and -7 were identified in pruritic and dyskeratotic dermatosis (PDD); HPyV-9 was found in widespread hyperkeratotic cutaneous lesions in organ transplant recipients; LIPyV is the most recently discovered HPyV and is also detected in skin but not yet associated with skin disease [**1**].

Merkel cell polyomavirus infection

Introduction and general description
A polyomavirus detected in Merkel cell carcinoma (MCC) of both immunosuppressed and immunocompetent individuals in 2008 was named Merkel cell polyomavirus (MCPyV) and emerging data suggest that there are several genotypes [3,4].

Epidemiology
Incidence and prevalence
Serological studies indicate that exposure to MCPyV is very common [**1,2**]. Primary exposure begins in childhood after transient

Table 25.7 Human polyomaviruses [1,2].

Polyomavirus	Abbreviation	Disease in humans	Site of detection
BK polyomavirus	BKV, HPyV-1	Renal allograft nephropathy	Mononuclear blood cells; urine
JC polyomavirus	JCV, HPyV-2	Progressive multifocal leukoencephalopathy	Mononuclear blood cells
Karolinska Institute polyomavirus	KIV, KIPyV	–	Respiratory secretions
Washington University polyomavirus	WUV, WUPyV	–	Respiratory secretions
Merkel cell carcinoma-associated polyomavirusvirus	MCV, MCPyV	Merkel cell carcinoma	Skin
Human polyomavirus 6	HPyV-6	Pruritic and dyskeratotic dermatosis; keratoacanthoma	Skin
Human polyomavirus 7	HPyV-7	Pruritic and dyskeratotic dermatosis	Skin
Trichodysplasia spinulosa-associated polyomavirus	TSV, HPyV-8	Trichodysplasia spinulosa	Skin; urine; renal tissue
Human polyomavirus 9	HPyV-9	Hyperkeratotic lesions in organ transplant recipients	Serum; urine; skin
Malawi polyomavirus; human polyomavirus 10	MWPyV HPyV-10	–	Stool; skin; respiratory
Mexico polyomavirus	MxPyV	Diarrhoeal illness	Stool
Saint Louis polyomavirus	STLPyV	–	Stool
Lyon IARC polyomavirus	LIPyV	–	Skin; oral

immunity from maternal antibodies [5]. Seroprevalence rises from early childhood until adulthood: 10% of preschool-age children are seropositive, rising to at least 40% of the normal population by age 18; further slow increase in seroprevalence occurs during adult life, so that 60–96.2% of the adult population are estimated to have been exposed to MCPyV [1,5–7]. MCPyV seropositivity is found more commonly in serum of immunocompromised patients [8,9]. Viral DNA is present in 2.6% of healthy blood donors [10] and MCPyV appears to be the cutaneous HPyV most frequently shed from the skin, with some studies indicating rates up to 61.5% in healthy individuals [11,12] and 90% of patients with MCC [13]. There is a correlation between the presence of viral DNA in skin and circulating antiviral antibodies [14,15].

Merkel cell carcinoma and MCPyV (Chapter 146)

MCPyV is strongly implicated as a cause of MCC [1,2,16,17,18]. MCC develops in only a minority of those infected with MCPyV and the virus is detected in approximately 80% of MCCs [3,16,17,18]. Virus-positive MCCs occur more frequently in the northern hemisphere [19], have a lower tumour mutational burden, harbour clonally integrated MCPyV and express polyomavirus oncoproteins that are highly immunogenic and required for ongoing tumour growth [16,17,18]. Virus-negative MCCs are more common in white patients living in areas of high UV exposure; these tumours are characterised by a high tumour mutational burden with a prominent UV-mutational signature and encode tumour-specific UV-neoantigens [16,17,18].

MCPyV status in MCC is associated with specific clinicopathological features, with virus-negative tumours demonstrating mostly pleomorphic nuclei and abundant cytoplasm [20]. There is emerging evidence that MCC in the context of immunosuppression may be more frequently virus negative [21,22] and that virus-negative MCC may be more aggressive [23].

Antibody and T-cell responses to MCPyV T-antigen oncoproteins are strongest in patients with MCC [24]. MCPyV T-antigen antibody titres have also been correlated with MCC tumour burden [25] and may be helpful in MCC prognostication and surveillance: it is proposed that the seronegative cohort is at higher risk and may require more intensive radiological imaging, whereas disease status can be tracked in part by T-oncoprotein antibody titres in lower-risk seropositive cohorts [15].

Pathophysiology

Predisposing factors

MCC is more common in older individuals and in immunosuppression, such as after organ transplantation or with HIV infection [16,22]. Merkel cell polyomavirus has been reported in cases of epidermodysplasia verruciformis (EV) [26].

Pathology

MCPyV replicates in human cells but may cause little observable disease [1,2]. In MCC, the virus is integrated into the host genome and is neither able to replicate nor produce viral capsid proteins, but the MCPyV-encoded early transforming viral T proteins – large and small T antigen (LT, ST) – are produced [1,2,16]. This is discussed in detail in Chapter 146 but, in brief, LT and ST abrogate function of the critical tumour suppressors RB and p53, respectively. Viral integration leads to expression of a truncated LT antigen which facilitates tumour maintenance and cell growth. LT contains the LXCXE motif which binds RB protein and inactivates its tumour-suppressor function. Virus-positive tumours also express MCPyV ST antigen which is the main transforming gene with a major role in metastasis: ST binds Fbxw7 (a ubiquitin-proteasome system protein and a critical tumour suppressor), leading to accumulation of oncogenic proteins such as cyclin-E, c-Jun, mTOR and truncated LT-Ag [1,16,17].

Clinical features

Infection with the virus is not known to produce any symptoms or signs. It may be many years between infection, seroconversion and the potential development of MCC. Clinicopathological features of MCC are discussed in detail in Chapter 146.

Management

No treatment is needed for the presence of virus on the skin.

Resources

Further information
https://www.skincancer.org/skin-cancer-information/merkel-cell-carcinoma/

Patient resources
https://www.cancerresearchuk.org/about-cancer/neuroendocrine-tumours-nets/merkel-cell-skin-cancer
(Both last accessed August 2023.)

Trichodysplasia spinulosa

Definition and nomenclature
Trichodysplasia spinulosa polyomavirus (TSV, HPyV-8) causes a rare folliculocentric skin disease with prominent hyperplastic epidermal inner root sheath structures and abundant TSV virion production. It was first described in immunocompromised transplant recipients and a viral aetiology was confirmed in 2010 [1,28,29].

> **Synonyms and inclusions**
> - Follicular digitate keratoses

Causative organisms
TSV was discovered in the skin lesions of an immunosuppressed patient with trichodysplasia spinulosa (TS) at high copy number of approximately 10^6 copies per cell [28,30]. TS is thought to result from a primary TSV infection of the inner root sheath keratinocytes rather than reactivation of latent infection [1,31,32]. The infection also appears to be systemic, with TSV found in blood, cerebrospinal fluid, respiratory tract, urinary tract, faeces, cardiac tissue and renal allografts [1,30]. Children are born with maternal antibodies to TSPyV and begin producing antibodies in the first year after primary exposure, which may occur via respiratory secretions [1]. Adult seroprevalence rates are 60–80%, but the average in preschool-age children is 5–10% [33,34]. Prevalence of viral DNA on skin swabs is low at 0–3.8% in adults. Viral DNA is also present in renal tissue and urine [35].

Epidemiology
Incidence and prevalence
Trichodysplasia spinulosa is extremely uncommon. Even among long-term immunosuppressed transplant recipients, it is reported very rarely [27]. Children and adults may be affected. Both immunosuppression following transplantation and immune compromise due to haematological malignancy can predispose to the condition.

Clinical features
Presentation
TS is characterised by numerous, mildly pruritic, filiform flesh-coloured to pink folliculocentric papules, with central keratotic spines that are most evident over the nose and cheeks. Alopecia, particularly involving the eyebrows, and skin thickening causing 'leonine' facies may also occur [1,27].

Pathology
The follicles are expanded with keratinocytes enlarged with cytoplasmic inclusion bodies and trichohyaline granules. The hyperkeratotic material projects in a spicule from the follicular ostium. Electron microscopy shows densely packed viral particle arrays in the keratinised cells within the follicle. Hair shafts are poorly formed [1,29].

Patients with TS mount a high antibody response against the virus. Seropositive individuals also mount a cellular immune response against the virus [36].

Management
First line
Clearance with reduction in immunosuppression has been reported [31]. Topical antiviral treatment with cidofovir (1% or 3% cream) has been reported to produce improvement in some cases [28,37–39]. Physical approaches (e.g. shaving or plucking) have also been successful [38,39].

Second line
Oral valganciclovir may improve the appearance of the lesions [40]. Improvement with acitretin and leflunomide has also been reported [38,39].

Human polyomavirus-6- and -7-associated pruritic and dyskeratotic dermatoses (PDD)

Definition and nomenclature
A pruritic skin eruption in immunocompromised patients with a distinctive histological pattern associated with human polyomaviruses 6 and 7 [1].

Causative organisms
Human polyomavirus-6 (HPyV-6) and human polyomavirus-7 (HPyV-7) were discovered in 2010 in swabs from healthy skin of immunocompetent and immunocompromised individuals [11]. Seroepidemiological studies show that these viruses are ubiquitous, with seroprevalence in healthy adults of 88% and 72% and detection in healthy skin samples of 14–28% and 11–13% for HPyV-6 and HPyV-7, respectively [11,41].

Epidemiology
Incidence and prevalence
The first cases of PDD associated with HPyV-7 were described in two lung transplant recipients in 2015 through genomic sequencing techniques [42]. Subsequently HPyV-6- and -7-associated cases were reported in 2017 in a kidney/pancreas transplant recipient, a patient living with HIV infection and an apparently immunocompetent individual [43].

Clinical features
Presentation
The rash is usually intensely pruritic, with brownish pink, velvety and fine scaly plaques on the lower back, buttocks, gluteal cleft, neck, chest, axillae and legs, but often sparing acral areas and the face [42,43]. Lichenified plaques with follicular-based papules and pits and alopecia are also described [44].

Pathology
Biopsy specimens from lesional skin showed a characteristic pattern of dyskeratosis and irregular columns of parakeratosis described as 'peacock plumage', with plump, eosinophilic keratinocytes containing viral inclusions at different levels of the epidermis [42–44].

Management
No specific antiviral treatment has been identified [1]. Acitretin may be helpful [44,45] as may topical cidofovir [46].

Human polyomavirus-9 and hyperkeratotic skin lesions in organ transplant recipients

Definition and nomenclature
An entity in which painful, progressive, hyperkeratotic skin lesions and pulmonary failure in organ transplant recipients are associated with HPyV-9 infection was first described in 2022 [47].

Causative organisms
HPyV-9 was first isolated in an organ transplant recipient [48] and seropositivity increases post-transplant [49,50]. It was found in lesional skin, serum and lung autopsy tissues in three organ transplant recipients with this condition [47].

Clinical features
All patients initially had acral lesions that spread to proximal extremities and trunk. Facial involvement was also seen. Lesions were pink-brown or violaceous, hyperkeratotic, progressive and painful. All patients died from pulmonary and multiorgan failure around 1 year from onset of the rash [47].

Pathology
Skin biopsy demonstrated hyperkeratosis, acanthosis, dyskeratosis, scattered necrotic and vacuolated keratinocytes, and a patchy lymphocytic infiltrate in the superficial dermis. A high HPyV-9 viral load was found in the skin with viraemia and HPyV-9 mRNA in lung tissue [47].

Management
Changes in immunosuppression were unhelpful. Skin lesions appeared to improve in one case with acitretin and intravenous cidofovir.

Malawi polyomavirus; human polyomavirus-10

Initially discovered in stool from a healthy child in Malawi (Malawi polyomavirus, MWPyV) [51], an almost identical species, human polyomavirus-10 (HPyV-10), was independently identified in warts on the buttock of a patient with WHIM (warts, hypogammaglobulinemia, infections and myelokathexis) syndrome [52]. The seroprevalence of MWPyV/HPyV-10 is very high (42–99%) in adults [53] and it is most often detected in stool, but is also present on the skin in 3.4% of healthy individuals and 9.3% of HIV-infected men [41]. However, it remains unclear whether it represents skin contamination or whether HPyV-10 is a true skin pathogen [1].

Human polyomaviruses and keratinocyte skin cancers

A role for HPyVs in the pathogenesis of keratinocyte cancers has been investigated, particularly in the context of immunosuppression-associated keratinocyte cancers, but their contribution remains uncertain. In general, the viral loads of HPyVs detected in most studies are low, with few significant differences in skin viral DNA prevalence or copy number detected in benign versus cutaneous SCC (cSCC), cSCC *in situ* or actinic keratoses [54–59]. These findings are possibly more consistent with HPyV latency in skin rather than an active carcinogenic role, but a possible contribution cannot currently be excluded.

HUMAN PAPILLOMAVIRUS INFECTIONS

Definition

Human papillomaviruses (HPVs) are small, 50–55 nm diameter DNA viruses that infect squamous epithelia, causing cell proliferation. The commonest effect of HPV infection is the development of warts (verrucae). These virus-induced tumours are pleomorphic and can affect a wide variety of sites, principally the skin of the extremities, genital skin and mucosa, and oropharyngeal mucosa.

The family *Papillomaviridae*, which includes HPVs and papillomaviruses that infect other species including fish and mammals, are all included within the recently renamed order of *Zurhausenvirales*.

The HPVs form a large group of closely related viruses, distinguished one from another on the basis of their DNA. Since 1995, a distinct genotype has been defined as a specific type if there is greater than 10% difference in nucleotide homology within the *L1* gene compared with other papillomavirus types [1,2]. To date, over 200 types have been recognised and characterised [3]. However, a large number of putative new types have been detected, which are yet to be completely evaluated. The human viruses are divided into five genera: α, β, γ, μ and ν papillomaviruses (alpha, beta, gamma, mu and nu). Most of the newly defined types in recent years have been in the beta and gamma genera [4]. This classification and main clinical associations of the different HPV types are shown in Table 25.8.

All papillomavirus types have a tropism for stratified squamous epithelial cells, but they vary in their specificity for different anatomical sites [5]. For example, HPV-1 replicates in heavily keratinised skin of palms and soles, whereas HPV-16 has a preference for mucosal areas and HPV-11 replicates in genital and laryngeal epithelium.

General description of disease domain

HPVs can infect and cause disease at any site in stratified squamous epithelium, either keratinising (skin) or non-keratinising (mucosa). They are frequently found on skin and in hair follicles of normal skin. The clinical problems encountered with such infections can be broadly divided into benign lesions such as cutaneous

Table 25.8 Human papillomaviruses (HPV). The main clinical lesions caused by different HPV types.

HPV type	Genus	Associated clinical conditions/where HPV detected
1	μ	Deep plantar and palmar warts
2	α	Common warts, filiform warts, plantar warts, mosaic plantar warts
3	α	Plane warts
4	γ	Common warts, plantar warts
5	β	Warts in EV and immunosuppressed, SCC in EV and immunosuppressed
6	α	Ano-genital warts, laryngeal papillomas
7	α	Butchers' warts
8	β	Warts in EV and immunosuppressed, SCC in EV and immunosuppressed
9	β	Warts in EV and immunosuppressed, rarely SCC in EV and immunosuppressed
10	α	Plane warts
11	α	Ano-genital warts, laryngeal papillomas, verrucous carcinoma
12	β	Warts in EV and immunosuppressed, SCC in EV and immunosuppressed
13	α	Focal epithelial hyperplasia
14	β	Warts in EV and immunosuppressed, SCC in EV and immunosuppressed
15	β	Warts in EV and immunosuppressed, rarely SCC in EV and immunosuppressed
16	α	Ano-genital warts, AGIN, cervical carcinoma
17	β	Warts in EV and immunosuppressed, rarely SCC in EV and immunosuppressed
18	α	Genital warts, AGIN, cervical carcinoma
19	β	Warts in EV and immunosuppressed, SCC in EV and immunosuppressed
20	β	Warts in EV and immunosuppressed, SCC in EV and immunosuppressed
21	β	Warts in EV and immunosuppressed, SCC in EV and immunosuppressed
22, 23	β	Warts in EV and immunosuppressed, rarely SCC in EV and immunosuppressed
24, 25	β	Warts in EV and immunosuppressed, SCC in EV and immunosuppressed
26	α	Cutaneous lesions in immunosuppressed, genital lesions including carcinoma
27	α	Common warts, ano-genital warts in children
28	α	Flat and common warts in normal and immunosuppressed
29	α	Cutaneous warts (rare)
30	α	Ano-genital lesions, laryngeal carcinoma
31	α	Ano-genital warts, CIN, cervical carcinoma
32	α	Focal epithelial hyperplasia, oral papillomas
33	α	CIN, VIN, cervical cancer
34	α	Oro-genital warts, AGIN
35	α	Ano-genital warts, CIN, cervical cancer
36	β	Warts in EV and immunosuppressed, SCC in EV and immunosuppressed
37, 38	β	Warts in EV and immunosuppressed, rarely SCC in EV and immunosuppressed
39	α	Ano-genital warts, AGIN, cervical cancer
40	α	Ano-genital warts, skin and mucosal lesions in immunosuppressed, AGIN
41	ν	Plane warts, SCC skin
42, 43	α	Ano-genital warts
44	α	Oro-genital warts
45	α	Ano-genital warts, AGIN, cervical cancer
46		Reclassified
47	β	Warts in EV and immunosuppressed, SCC in EV and immunosuppressed
48	γ	Cutaneous warts (rare)
49	β	Cutaneous warts, warts in EV
50	γ	Cutaneous warts, warts in EV
51	α	Ano-genital warts, ano-genital intraepithelial neoplasia
52	α	Ano-genital warts, AGIN, cervical cancer
53	α	Ano-genital warts, CIN, cervical cancer
54	α	Ano-genital warts, Buschke–Löwenstein tumour (rare)
55		Reclassified as subtype of HPV-44
56	α	Ano-genital warts, CIN, cervical cancer
57	α	Common warts, oro-genital warts in children, skin lesions in immunosuppressed, epidermoid cyst of sole
58	α	Ano-genital warts, AGIN, cervical cancer
59	α	Oro-genital warts, AGIN, cervical cancer
60	γ	Plantar epidermoid cysts, pigmented plantar warts
61, 62	α	Low-risk ano-genital lesions
63	μ	Cutaneous warts (rare), multiple punctate keratoses of foot
64		Reclassified
65	γ	Common warts, plantar warts, pigmented plantar warts
66	α	Ano-genital warts, CIN, cervical cancer
67	α	Ano-genital warts, AGIN, cervical carcinoma
68	α	Ano-genital warts, AGIN, cervical cancer
69	α	CIN, plantar wart in HIV
70	α	Ano-genital warts, AGIN, ano-genital cancers
71	α	Ano-genital warts
72	α	Ano-genital warts, cervical lesions
73	α	Ano-genital warts, AGIN, ano-genital cancers
74	α	Ano-genital warts
75, 76	β	Cutaneous warts, warts in EV
77	α	Cutaneous warts, dysplasia and SCC
78	α	Cutaneous warts
79		Reclassified
80	β	Warts in EV and immunosuppressed, rarely SCC in EV and immunosuppressed
81	α	Low-risk ano-genital lesions
82	α	CIN
83, 84	α	Low-risk ano-genital lesions
85	α	AGIN, ano-genital cancers
86, 87	α	Low-risk ano-genital lesions
88	γ	Cutaneous warts
89	α	Low-risk ano-genital lesions
90	α	Ano-genital warts
91	α	Cutaneous warts, ano-genital warts
92	β	Cutaneous dysplasia and SCC
93	β	Warts in EV and immunosuppressed, SCC in EV and immunosuppressed
94	α	Cutaneous warts
95	γ	Common warts, plantar warts, pigmented plane warts
96	β	Cutaneous dysplasia and SCC in EV
97	α	Cervix
98	β	Skin, HNSCC
99	β	Skin. HNSCC
100	β	Skin
101	γ	Cervix, male genitalia
102	α	Genital skin/mucous membranes
103	γ	Cervix, male genitalia
104	β	Skin, HNSCC
105	β	Skin
106	α	Genital skin/mucous membranes
107	β	Actinic keratosis
108	γ	Low-grade CIN
109	γ	Skin & mucosa
110	β	Actinic keratoses
111	β	Actinic keratoses
112	γ	Genital warts
113	β	Skin, HNSCC
114	α	Skin & mucosa
115	β	Skin & mucosa
116	γ	Rectal swab
117	α	Cutaneous wart
118	β	Cutaneous wart in immunosuppressed
119	γ	Genitalia, skin, keratoacanthoma, mouth

HPV type	Genus	Associated clinical conditions/where HPV detected
120	β	Mouth, skin, genital area
121	γ	Mouth, male genitalia
122	β	Skin
123	γ	
124	β	
125	α	Cutaneous wart
126	γ	Cutaneous wart
127	γ	Skin
128	γ	Cutaneous wart
129	γ	Cutaneous wart
130	γ	Cutaneous wart, actinic keratosis, genitalia, nose
131	γ	Cutaneous wart
132	γ	Cutaneous wart, skin
133	γ	Cutaneous wart, skin, genitalia
134	γ	Cutaneous wart
135	γ	Skin, mouth, nasal cavity, genitalia
136	γ	Mouth, skin
137	γ	Mouth
138	γ	Mouth
139	γ	Mouth
140	γ	Mouth
141	γ	Mouth
142	γ	Oral & nasal cavity, skin
143	β	Mouth
144	γ	Mouth, genitalia
145	β	Mouth
146	γ	Mouth
147	γ	Oral, nasal
148	γ	Cutaneous wart
149	γ	Cutaneous wart
150	β	Skin
151	β	Skin
152	β	
153	γ	Genital wart
154	γ	Cutaneous wart, skin
155	γ	Actinic keratosis
156	γ	Skin
157	γ	Skin
158	γ	Anal swab
159	β	
160	α	Plane wart
161	γ	Skin
162	γ	Skin
163	γ	Skin
164	γ	Skin
165	γ	Skin
166	γ	Skin
167	γ	Skin
168	γ	Skin
169	γ	Skin
170	γ	Skin
171	γ	Mouth
172	γ	Mouth
173	γ	Mouth
174	β	Skin SCC
175	γ	Genital wart
176	γ	
177	α	
178	γ	Skin
179	γ	Cutaneous wart
180	γ	Genital wart

AGIN, ano-genital intraepithelial neoplasia, includes AIN, CIN, PIN, VIN, and vaginal intraepithelial neoplasia; CIN, cervical intraepithelial neoplasia; EV, epidermodysplasia verruciformis; HNSCC, head and neck squamous cell carcinoma; PIN, penile intraepithelial neoplasia; SCC, squamous cell carcinoma; VIN, vulval intraepithelial neoplasia.

warts, ano-genital warts, oral warts and laryngeal warts, and pre-malignant or malignant lesions such as intraepithelial neoplasia and squamous cell cancers of the ano-genital area and upper respiratory tract.

Basic biology

The virus infects the basal layer of the epithelium, probably the stem cells, but viral replication takes place only in fully differentiated keratinocytes – cells of the upper stratum spinosum and stratum granulosum. The viral DNA is functionally divided into early (E) and late (L) regions; the early genes are responsible for DNA replication, transcriptional regulation and transformation, while the late genes code for the structural proteins of the viral capsid [6]. Expression of the late genes of the virus is dependent upon the differentiation of the host cell. Propagation of papillomaviruses in tissue culture *in vitro* is therefore extremely difficult as it is hard to mimic all the necessary requirements for the completion of the virus life cycle [7].

Papillomas caused by HPVs are initially benign. In these lesions, viral genomes replicate as extrachromosomal episomes. A small percentage can progress to dysplasia or neoplasia. This occurs only with certain so-called 'high-risk' or 'cancer-associated' types of HPV, and under certain circumstances, genetic and environmental, some of which are incompletely understood. The strongest association between papillomavirus infection and the development of malignancy is in the case of cervical carcinoma. In the majority of malignantly transformed cells (i.e. those affected by high-risk genital HPVs), the viral DNA is integrated into the cellular chromosomes, usually with the loss of large sections of the viral genome. Viral replication does not occur, but the viral regulatory genes, *E6* and *E7*, are always retained. The oncogenic potential of the high-risk HPV types depends upon the expression of these early genes whose products play a role in cell transformation and immortalisation. This is because the E6 protein inactivates the cell's tumour suppressor protein p53 and the E7 protein inhibits the cell's pRb protein from its normal function as a negative regulator of cell cycle proliferation. These viral proteins and others can also interact with several other cellular proteins, with additional effects on cell behaviour.

These clinically evident infections with HPVs are described later, but there is also evidence that after initial infection, HPVs may persist in a latent form and may be subsequently reactivated.

Subclinical and latent human papillomavirus infection

Evidence has accumulated, mainly from studies of genital skin and mucosa, for subclinical and latent HPV infection. It has been estimated that up to 70% of genital HPV infections may be subclinical (i.e. unnoticed by the patient) but detectable by full clinical examination, histology, cytology or molecular analysis. In a latent infection, there may be no morphological changes, but the viral DNA is present.

Genital HPV infection can often be subclinical but may be detected during routine cervical smear tests or on vulval or penile examination. Of 545 students attending an annual gynaecological examination in an American university, 1% were aware that they had signs of genital warts, but a further 16% had evidence of HPV infection from colposcopy, cytology or detection of HPV antigen or DNA assessed by hybridisation [8]. Of over 9000 women routinely screened by cervical cytology in Germany in 1987, 2.1% had simple HPV infection (koilocytosis), and 3.7% had signs of dysplasia or neoplasia; of the other (cytologically normal) cases, HPV DNA was detected by hybridisation in 9% [9].

The highly sensitive PCR has revealed apparently very high rates of HPV cervical infection in the general population [9,10]. Longitudinal studies have suggested that many infections are transient and individuals may lose or acquire different HPV types over time, but persistent, high-grade HPV infection in the cervix is a risk factor for the development of cervical intraepithelial neoplasia (CIN) [11,12].

HPVs are frequently detected on the skin, under the nails and in the hair follicles of immunosuppressed and also immune-competent individuals [13–15].

Immunity to human papillomavirus [16,17]

The relative sequestration of the virus in the upper reaches of the epidermis, the lack of an animal model for HPV, the difficulty of finding never-infected control subjects and the large number of HPV types have delayed research progress and our understanding of the immune mechanisms in relation to this virus. Over recent decades, however, the ability to clone the viral genes and to produce recombinant capsid proteins and early (E) gene peptides has led to many advances including work with animal models.

Primary infection can be prevented by circulating antibodies against the viral coat protein and this has led to the development of effective vaccines. Prophylactic vaccination against HPV types 6, 11, 16 and 18 is now in clinical use in many countries [18–20] and a vaccine covering nine HPV types is available in a more limited number of countries.

The principal mechanism for the rejection of warts is via the cell-mediated immune system. Warts can disappear when the immune response is stimulated, while in persistent disorders of cell-mediated immunity, the prevalence and severity of warts and the incidence of HPV-related malignancy are increased [21]. In addition, the histological changes in regressing warts are consistent with cell-mediated attack; a study of resolving plane warts showed lymphocytic and phagocytic infiltrates including helper and suppressor T cells, Langerhans cells and satellite-cell necrosis [22]. A more detailed dissection of the immunological events occurring in resolving genital warts has shown that the lymphocytic infiltrate is predominantly of CD8+ cells [23], with an activation profile in keeping with a T-helper type 1 (Th1)-biased immune response.

The apparent failure of the immune system in otherwise healthy individuals to clear warts for months or years remains incompletely understood. A subdued local immune response is suggested by the observations that Langerhans cell numbers are reduced within warts [24] and T lymphocytes are rare within the epidermal compartment. In these patients and also those who harbour high-risk genital HPVs with the development of cancer, it is possible that there may be inability by the immune system to target certain HPV proteins, possibly due to poor antigen presentation, poor effector response or virally induced local immunosuppression resulting in the development of tolerance [25]. The initial success of the virus in establishing infection may similarly depend in part on the avoidance of detection by the innate immune response and certain immunomodulatory effects of the viral proteins.

Cutaneous warts

Definition and nomenclature

Skin warts are benign tumours caused by infection of keratinocytes with HPV, visible as well-defined hyperkeratotic protrusions.

> **Synonyms and inclusions**
> - Common wart: verruca vulgaris
> - Plane wart: verruca plana

Epidemiology
Incidence and prevalence

Warts are common throughout the world. Cutaneous warts occur at any age, but are unusual in infancy and early childhood. In various studies, it has been estimated that 2–30% of school-age children and young adults have warts [26–28].

Age

The incidence increases during the school years to reach a peak in adolescence and early adulthood [29], then declines rapidly through the twenties and more gradually thereafter.

Associated diseases

Warts are more common and more persistent in conditions of immune compromise.

Pathophysiology
Predisposing factors

Warts are spread by direct or indirect contact. For infection to occur, the wart virus particle may need to come into contact with a stem cell in the basal epidermal layer. Thus, impairment of the epithelial barrier function, by trauma (including mild abrasions), maceration or both, greatly predisposes to inoculation of the virus, and is generally assumed to be required for infection at least in fully keratinised skin, as in the following examples:

1. Plantar warts are commonly acquired from swimming pool or shower room floors, whose rough surfaces abrade moistened keratin from infected feet and help to inoculate virus into others, skin softened by water immersion.
2. Common hand warts may spread widely round the nails in those who bite their nails or periungual skin, over habitually sucked fingers in young children, and to the lips and surrounding skin in both cases.
3. Shaving may spread wart infection over the beard area.
4. Occupational handlers of meat, fish and poultry have high incidences of hand warts, attributed to cutaneous injury and prolonged contact with wet flesh and water.
5. Immune compromise can reduce initial protection against infection.

The time of acquisition of the infection can seldom be ascertained for common and plantar warts, but the incubation period has been estimated to range between a few weeks and more than a year [30], and experimental infections have taken as long as 20 months to produce clinical warts [31].

Iatrogenic transmission. Because of the long incubation period, iatrogenic spread would be difficult to establish and seems not to have been reported, though the possibility exists. Human papillomavirus DNA has been detected on instruments used for the examination of women with clinical or subclinical HPV infection [32] and in the environment of a genito-urinary medicine clinic [33]. Human papillomavirus DNA is found in the smoke plume from warts treated with laser or electrocautery [34]. The practice of dipping cotton wool swabs for a series of patients into the same flask of liquid nitrogen could transfer herpes simplex virus (used as a model, and by implication HPV) between patients [35].

Infectivity. There is no reliable information on the infectivity of common and plantar warts, but it seems to be substantially less than genital warts.

Pathology [36] (Figure 25.19)

Viral warts show acanthosis and hyperkeratosis, usually with the characteristic feature of koilocytosis of upper keratinocytes. In most warts there is also papillomatosis. In koilocytes and other granular layer cells, there may be basophilic nuclear inclusion bodies, which are seen ultrastructurally to be composed of arrays of viral particles. These upper epidermal cells have eosinophilic inclusions representing irregular clumped keratohyaline granules. This cytopathic effect may show detailed features typical of the HPV type involved [37,38].

Common and plantar warts. These are characterised by hyperplasia of all layers of the epidermis. There is gross hyperkeratosis with areas of parakeratosis, especially above the papillomatous projections, and both spinous and granular layers are conspicuously thickened. Elongated and flattened rete ridges are bent inwards towards the centre of the wart. The granular layer may be disordered with foci of koilocytes. These vacuolated cells have a dark nucleus which often appears flattened or twisted. Residual features of vacuolated cells or abnormal keratohyaline granules may be seen within the parakeratotic stratum corneum. In deep palmoplantar warts caused by HPV-1, the cytopathic changes are more marked and may be visible in the lower stratum spinosum. Plantar warts have a more endophytic growth pattern and a very thick cornified layer. Common warts on the face, limbs or near mucous membranes often have a morphology similar to genital warts with exophytic growth and a variable amount of hyperkeratosis.

Plane warts. The hyperkeratosis is of a loose lamellar type and there is acanthosis without papillomatosis. Vacuolated epidermal cells are more conspicuous and contain numerous viral particles [39].

Causative organisms

See Table 25.8. Common warts (excluding plantar warts) are due mainly to HPV-2, but also to the closely related types 27, 57 and types 1 and 4.

Plantar warts are caused by HPV-1, -2, -4, -27 or -57. The deep 'myrmecia' form is due to HPV-1. Smaller lesions may contain HPV-2, -4, -27 or -57, while mosaic warts are commonly caused by HPV-2.

Plane warts are due mainly to HPV-3 and -10.

Clinical features

Presentation

Warts on the skin may present in a number of different morphological forms, dependent on virus type, body site, immunological status of the patient and environmental influences. Of 1000 children under 16 with warts referred to hospital clinics in Cambridge, UK,

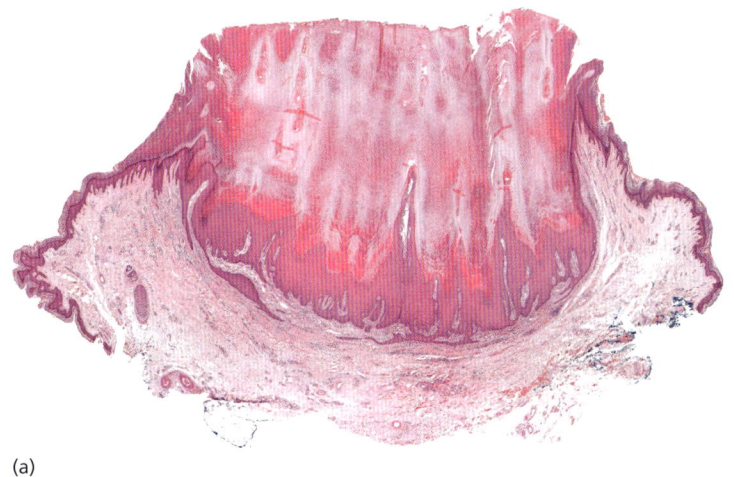

(a)

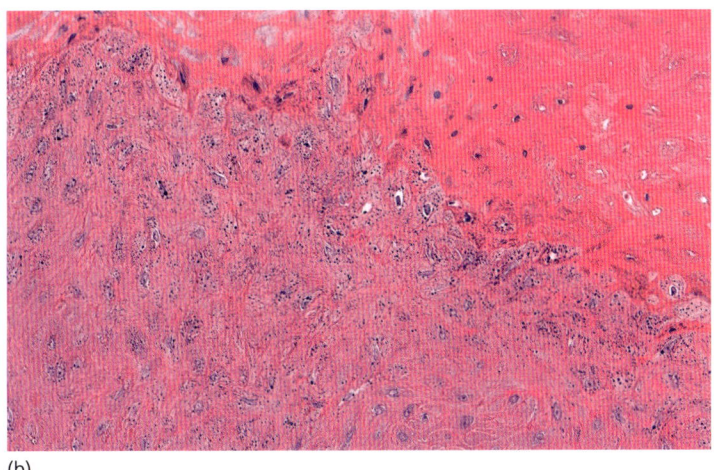

(b)

Figure 25.19 Histology of viral wart. (a) Low power, ×40, showing morphology of wart lesion with papillomatous acanthosis and hyperkeratosis. (b) Higher magnification highlights hypergranulosis and clumping of keratohyalin granules along with focal koilocytosis. Courtesy of Dr J Eduardo Calonje, St John's Institute of Dermatology, King's College London, UK.

in the 1950s, 70% had common warts, 24% plantar warts, 3.5% plane warts, 2.0% filiform warts and 0.5% ano-genital warts [40]. A more recent study from the Netherlands showed that plantar warts were the most common, present in 70% of the primary school-age children who had warts, while common warts were present in 42% of the affected children [28].

Common warts (Figure 25.20). These present as firm papules with a rough horny surface. They range in size from less than 1 mm to over 1 cm in diameter, and by confluence can form large masses. They are most commonly situated on the backs of the hands and fingers, in children on the knees, but may occur anywhere on the skin. A single wart may persist unchanged for months or years, or large numbers may develop rapidly or after an interval. New warts may form at sites of trauma, though this Koebner-like isomorphic phenomenon is usually less marked than in plane warts.

Common warts are usually symptomless, but may be tender on the palmar aspects of the fingers, when fissured or when growing beneath the nail plate; warts on the eyelids may be associated with conjunctivitis or keratitis. Common warts account for only 1 or 2% of warts on or around the genitalia in adults; in the male, they are almost always confined to the shaft of the penis. They often retain their usual morphological characteristics with dry hyperkeratosis and frequently do not resemble soft acuminate (genital) warts. In children, HPVs causing common warts may account for up to two-thirds of ano-genital warts [41].

Periungual warts (Figure 25.21). Common warts around the nails, especially at the nail folds or beneath the nail, can disturb nail growth. Nail biting may increase the risk of infection at this site.

Plantar warts. A plantar wart at first appears as a small shining 'sago-grain' papule, but soon assumes the typical appearance of a sharply defined rounded lesion, with a rough keratotic surface surrounded by a smooth collar of thickened horn. If the surface is gently pared with a scalpel, the abrupt separation between the wart tissue and the protective horny ring becomes more obvious, as the epithelial ridges of the plantar skin are not continued over the surface of the wart. If the paring is continued, small bleeding points, the tips of the elongated dermal papillae, are evident.

Most plantar warts are beneath pressure points, the heel or the metatarsal heads. Individuals may be affected by single or numerous lesions. Sometimes, a cluster of small satellite warts, the smallest of pinhead size, having at first an almost vesicular appearance, may develop around a large wart. Mosaic warts are so described from the appearance presented by a plaque of closely grouped small warts (Figure 25.22). The angular outlines of the tightly compressed individual warts are seen when the surface is pared.

Pain is a common but variable symptom. It may be severe and disabling but may be absent, and many warts are discovered only on routine inspection. Mosaic warts are often painless.

The duration of plantar warts is very variable. Spontaneous regression occurs sooner in children than in adults and is delayed if hyperhidrosis or orthopaedic defects are present. In children before puberty the average duration is probably less than a year, but in older children and adults a longer duration is not uncommon and persistence for several years is not exceptional. The number of warts

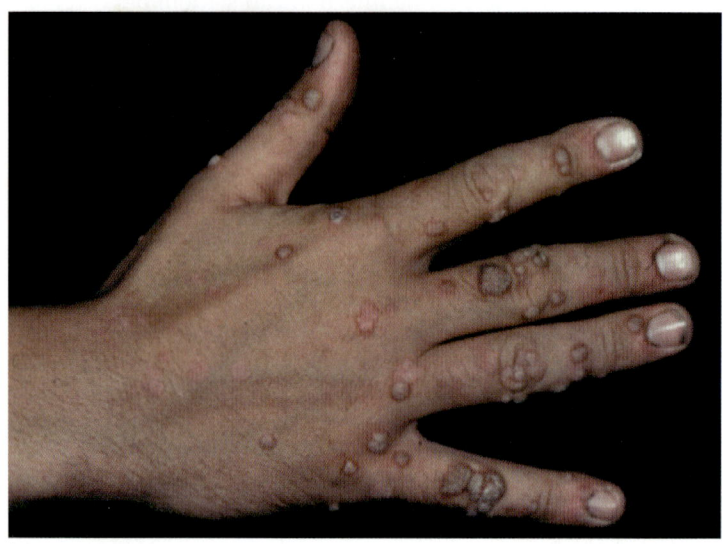
(a)

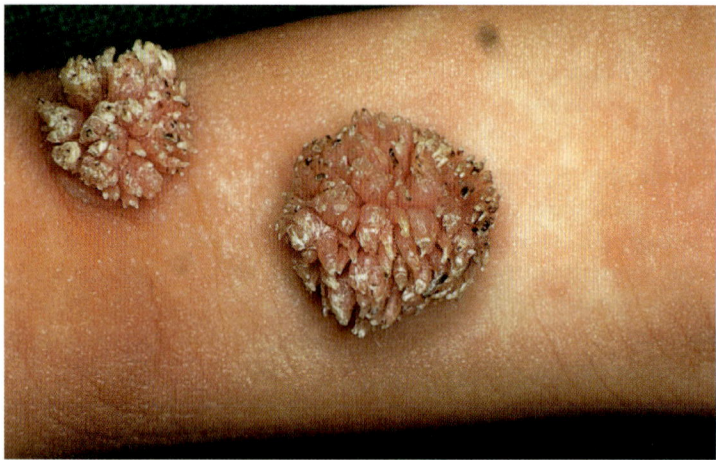
(b)

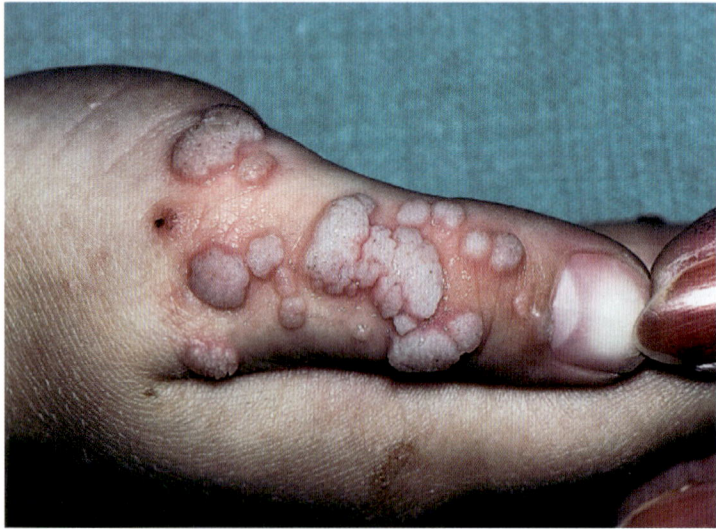
(c)

Figure 25.20 Common warts. (a) Hand. Courtesy of Addenbrooke's Hospital, Cambridge, UK. (b) Dorsum of the finger, filiform warts. Courtesy of Dr A. S. Highet, York District Hospital, UK. (c) Warts on the thumb spread by thumb-sucking. Courtesy of Dr A. S. Highet, York District Hospital, UK.

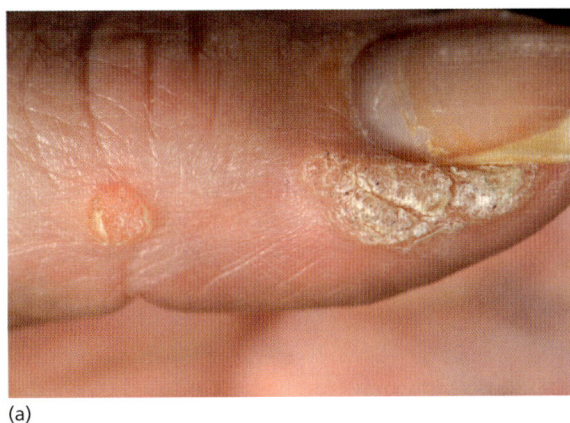
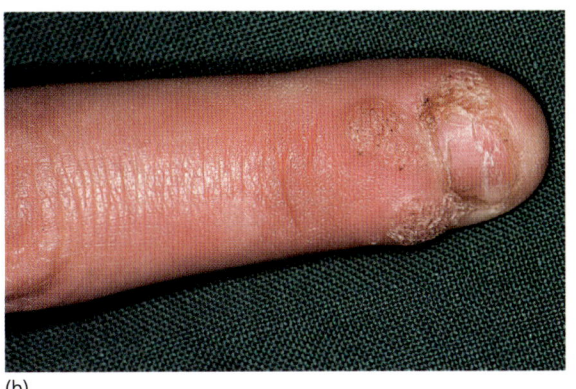

Figure 25.21 (a) Periungual warts. Courtesy of Addenbrooke's Hospital, Cambridge, UK. (b) Periungual warts in a nail-biter. Courtesy of York District Hospital, UK.

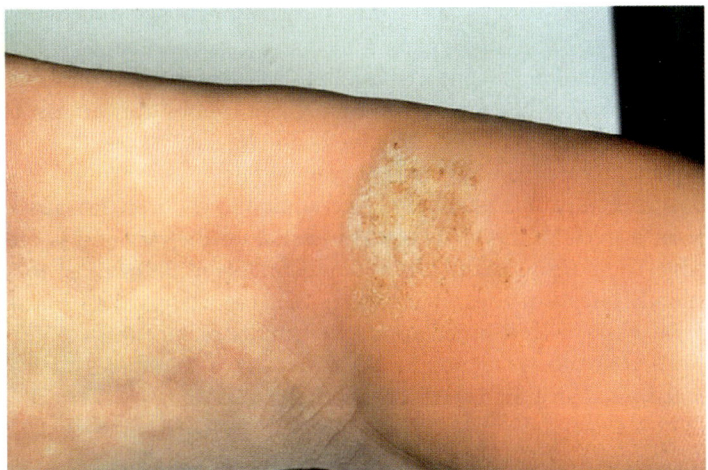

Figure 25.22 Mosaic plantar wart. Courtesy of Addenbrooke's Hospital, Cambridge, UK.

present does not influence the prognosis, but mosaic warts tend to be especially persistent.

Plane warts (flat warts) (Figure 25.23a). Plane warts are smooth, flat or slightly elevated and are usually skin coloured or greyish yellow, but may be pigmented. They are round or polygonal in shape and vary in size from 1 to 5 mm or more in diameter. The face and the backs of the hands and the shins are the sites of predilection and the number present ranges from two or three to many hundreds. Contiguous warts may coalesce and a linear arrangement in scratch marks is a characteristic feature (Figure 25.23b). Although all warts present are usually of the same type, a few common warts may be associated, especially on the backs of the hands.

Clinical variants

Filiform and digitate warts (ICD-10: B07) (Figure 25.24). Filiform and digitate warts occur commonly in the male, on the face and neck, irregularly distributed, and often clustered. Digitate warts, often in small groups, also occur on the scalp in both sexes, where they are occasionally confused with epidermal naevi. Isolated warts on the limbs often assume a filiform shape.

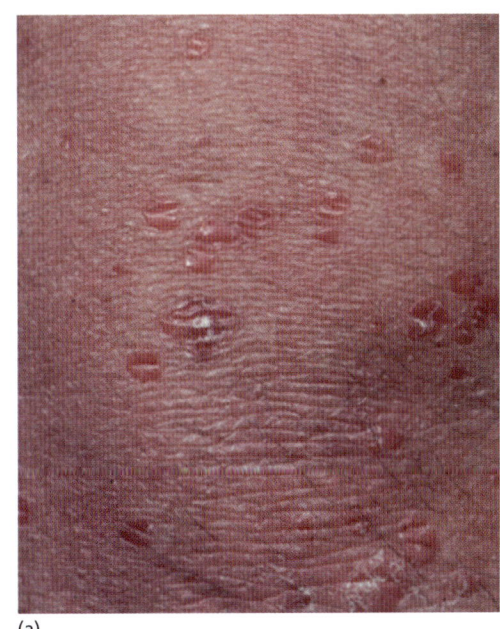
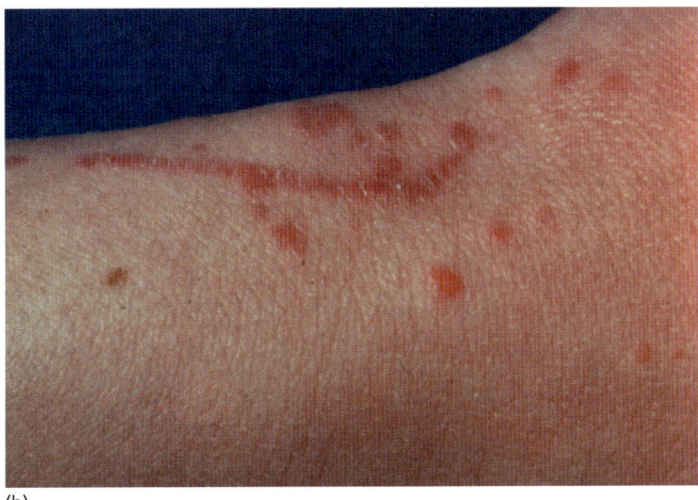

Figure 25.23 Plane warts. (a) Warts on the knee. (b) Warts on the arm with spread into a scratch. Courtesy of Addenbrooke's Hospital, Cambridge, UK.

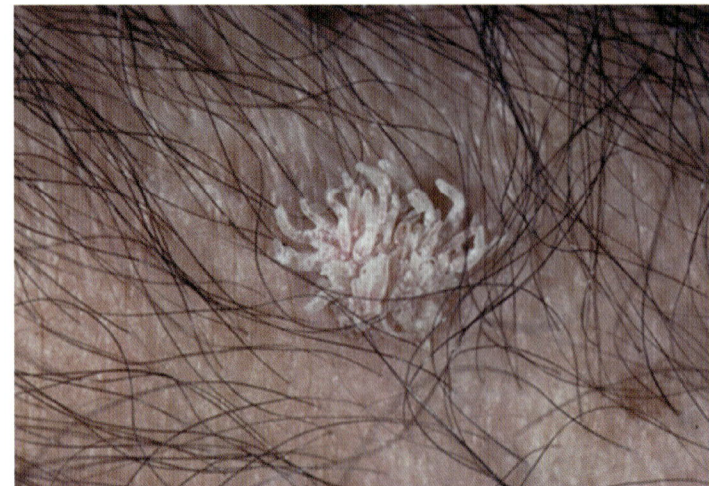

Figure 25.24 Filiform wart on the forearm. Courtesy of Addenbrooke's Hospital, Cambridge, UK.

Huge hyperkeratotic warts. Very rarely, warts can be both extensive and extremely hyperkeratotic, retaining long horny projections. There may be some degree of underlying immune compromise as well [42,43].

Butchers' warts (*ICD-10*: B07). Occupational handlers of meat, poultry or fish have a high incidence of hand warts where the skin is in prolonged contact with moist animal flesh. Among 1480 New York meat trade workers, 23% of those directly handling meat had warts, compared with 10% of those employed in other tasks [44]. In a Polish study, warts affected 49% of slaughterhouse workers who had direct contact with flesh, but only 9% of those working in an automated slaughterhouse where little handling of meat took place [45].

These lesions affect the hands, are often larger than common warts, and have a high risk of recurrence even after successful treatment. HPV-2 is frequently found in butchers' warts, but HPV-7 is present in a third to a half of lesions [45–48]. HPV-7 initially seemed specific to meat handlers. However, it has been reported occasionally in warts of non-meat handlers [47,49], in facial and oral warts of patients with HIV disease [50], in toe web warts and in ano-genital warts [51].

Epidermoid plantar cysts (*ICD-10*: B07). Epidermoid cysts of weight-bearing areas of the sole have been found to contain papillomavirus (HPV-60 and more rarely HPV-57) in several Japanese patients [52,53]. The cysts, which are thought to arise either by implantation or by infection of the eccrine duct [54], show histological features of HPV infection in the stratifying squamous wall. The upper epidermal cells produce large cytoplasmic granules and abundant viral particles.

Pigmented warts. Warts with pigmentation have been reported mainly on the palms and soles in Japanese patients [55]. Melanosomes are increased within the lesions, which are associated with HPV-65 (64%), -4 (23%) and -60 (13%).

Psoriasis. The use of sensitive PCR amplification has revealed HPV sequences in patients with psoriasis and it is speculated that the virus may have a role in the disease process [56,57]. Alternatively, the abnormal barrier function or local microbiota of psoriatic skin may permit subsequent higher carriage and detection rate of HPV DNA [58].

Differential diagnosis

Hand warts. Conditions that may be confused with hand warts include epidermal naevus, Bowen disease, actinic keratosis and callus.

Plantar warts. As well as the distinction from corns and calluses, plantar warts may rarely be confused with the discrete horny papules of punctate keratoderma of genetic origin (Chapter 63) which develop during childhood or early adult life, are irregularly scattered over the palms and soles, and are often largest in pressure areas. Dermoscopy can also help to distinguish a plantar wart from a corn or a callosity [59]. In warts, the plantar ridges of the epidermis are seen to be pushed apart and the mosaic and papillomatous features, sometimes with dark pinpoints of thrombosed capillaries, are visible. A callus or corn has a more amorphous appearance, but the central keratotic 'seed' may be seen in a corn.

In the differential diagnosis of plane warts, lichen planus causes most difficulty. It is relatively less common in children, favours the flexor aspects of the forearms, is unusual on the face and is often itchy. The mucous membranes may be involved. In contrast to the smooth, purplish, polygonal papules of lichen planus, the surface of plane warts has a stippled appearance under magnification.

In acrokeratosis verruciformis numerous warty papules are symmetrically distributed on the backs of the hands.

Disease course and prognosis

Spontaneous clearance of warts can occur at any time from a few months to years and it is impossible to offer a reliable prognosis in the individual patient. Clearance is usually quicker in children but warts may persist for many years in adults. In primary school-aged children, about half will clear within a year [28]. About 65% of warts disappear spontaneously within 2 years [60] and 95% within 4 years [61].

Regression of common warts is asymptomatic and occurs gradually over several weeks, usually without blackening [62]. Regression of plane warts is usually heralded by inflammation in the lesions [63], causing itch, redness and swelling, such that previously unnoticed warts may become evident. Depigmented haloes may appear around the lesions. Resolution is usually complete within a month, and appears to be HPV type specific as it generally occurs in all plane warts at all body sites, though not in any coexisting warts of other types.

Regression of plantar warts is occasionally clinically inflammatory, and often culminates in blackening from thrombosed blood before the lesion separates [64], but in many cases simply takes the form of apparent drying and gradual separation.

Malignant change in warts is extremely rare but has been reported in immunosuppression [65].

Malignant change in lesions with features of periungual warts is extremely rare but has been reported in immunosuppression, and in association with bowenoid hyperkeratotic plaques or with genital

HPV disease [66–68]. HPV-16 or other high-risk genital virus types are frequently found in such lesions [69].

Investigations
Clinical diagnosis of warts is often sufficient, but atypical, subclinical or dysplastic lesions may need laboratory confirmation of HPV infection. Methods available are as follows:
1 Histology.
2 Immunohistochemistry or immunocytochemistry using type-common or type-specific antibodies.
3 Non-routine laboratory techniques: PCR for HPV DNA or DNA *in situ* hybridisation.

Management [70–72]
Not all warts need treatment as many give little inconvenience and will resolve spontaneously. In addition, patients may need encouragement to persevere with long-term daily use of simpler preparations and more aggressive therapies, such as cryotherapy or surgery, have potential disadvantages. Gentle reduction of the layer of hyperkeratotic epidermis by regular filing or paring down will usually make the lesion more comfortable, especially for plantar warts.

Advice on simple measures to limit the spread of the infection will be appreciated. Plantar warts should be covered with adequate plaster strapping, or the foot with close-fitting rubber 'verruca socks', or pool-side sandals worn at swimming pools or communal baths or showers. The spread of periungual and perioral warts is often due to biting of nails or periungual skin, and this practice must be strongly discouraged if attempted treatment is to be worthwhile; the use of adhesive strapping after the application of a 'wart paint' helps to break the habit. In addition, simple domestic hygiene, such as cleaning of baths and showers after use and avoidance of shared towels, may reduce spread.

The most commonly used treatments for warts involve destruction of the area of epidermis infected with the virus. Such treatments usually initially involve application of a topical preparation. Other therapies aimed at modifying the growth of the epidermis or to stimulate an immune response require either a topical or a systemic approach. Combination therapies are often used.

Whatever method is used there will be failures and recurrences. Treatment usually needs to continue for up to 3 months and may be improved by a combination of therapies. There is some evidence that treatments are less successful in adults compared with children and in those with more warts or warts of longer duration [73]. The best clinical guide to cure is the restoration of normal epidermal texture, including the epidermal ridge pattern where appropriate. Where treatment trials have been placebo controlled, a 20–30% response rate generally is observed for placebo treatment.

Where skin healing is markedly impaired or in neuropathy, as in diabetes and peripheral vascular disease, treatments that cause erosion of the epidermis may lead to prolonged ulceration and are best used very cautiously if at all.

First line
Topical treatments that can be used by the patient at home can be regarded as first line.

Salicylic acid. The keratolytic effect of salicylic acid helps to reduce the thickness of warts and may stimulate an inflammatory response. A preparation containing 12–26% salicylic acid in a quick-drying collodion or gel base, applied daily, is the treatment of first choice for common and plantar warts. A review of 16 placebo-controlled trials confirmed an earlier impression of efficacy [74], with 49% cured (range 0–69%) compared with 23% of placebo-treated patients [75]. Removal of surface keratin and the remnants of the previous application by gentle use of a pumice stone, emery board or foot file is a helpful preliminary in all warts and essential in very hyperkeratotic plantar warts. However, overenthusiastic abrasion is a common, if understandable, mistake, which may enhance spread of the virus by inoculation into adjacent skin. It is conceivable that abrasion of warts may help to stimulate an immune response [76]. Accurate application of a salicylic acid preparation, avoiding normal skin, will minimise subsequent local discomfort. After drying, a whitish deposit remains.

Penetration into thick keratin, as on the sole, is enhanced by adhesive plaster occlusion, which promotes maceration of the keratin layer and a reduction in barrier function. Occlusion can improve the response rate for treatment with salicylic acid [77]. Adhesive plaster containing 40% salicylic acid is useful for plantar warts. It is applied daily, cut to the shape of the wart or group of warts and held in place by plain adhesive plaster.

Salicylic acid ointment 40%, in direct comparison with cryotherapy, has been shown to be equal [78] or less effective (15% or 49% cure rate respectively) [79], but more effective than placebo.

The regular use of salicylic acid preparations on warts may need to be continued for at least 3 months and often longer. They can be used in combination with many other treatments (see other treatments later) helping to reduce the thickness of the epidermal layer and improve penetration of other agents. Combinations in common use are salicylic acid with lactic acid [80], with 5-fluorouracil (5-FU), with 5-FU and cantharidin, with cryotherapy or laser and with imiquimod.

Salicylic acid in the usual concentrations is best avoided on facial warts, but less irritant concentrations in cream formulations can be helpful, especially for plane warts.

Glutaraldehyde. Proprietary preparations of this virucidal compound contain 10% glutaraldehyde in aqueous ethanol [74] or in a gel formulation, but there have been no controlled trials. Treated skin hardens and stains brown which limits acceptability on the hands, but as it dries into the skin without being rubbed off, it is a useful application for warts on the feet. The lack of an erosive effect can be of use in patients with slow healing. A preparation of 20% glutaraldehyde in aqueous solution produced a 72% cure rate for a variety of different cutaneous warts in 25 individuals [81]. Allergic contact dermatitis to the glutaraldehyde occurs occasionally and cutaneous necrosis is a rare complication of the strong solution.

Formalin. Formalin is virucidal, but also dries and hardens the skin, facilitating paring. Soaks or compresses of 2–3% formalin in water (formalin is about 37% formaldehyde in water) may be effective for plantar warts [82] with a reported cure rate of 80% in children, but is time consuming and difficult to limit to affected skin. The affected area must be soaked in the solution for 15–20 min daily, using soft paraffin as a barrier application to protect adjacent or more sensitive skin from irritant dermatitis. A comparative study of formalin soaks with either water soaks or oral saccharose showed no difference in clearance [83]. Formaldehyde in a 0.75% gel and 5 or 10% solution applied directly to the wart has been used with apparent effect [84,85].

Occlusion. Continuous duct tape occlusion of common warts for up to 2 months compared favourably with cryotherapy every 2–3 weeks in children [86], but placebo-controlled or comparator trials have not confirmed any significant effect in either adults or children [87,88]. Occlusion is often used in conjunction with topical therapy and the combination may enhance clearance.

5-fluorouracil. A 5% cream or ointment of 5-FU carefully applied daily under occlusion for a month is more effective than placebo [89,90]. Hyperpigmentation as well as redness and erosion can be limiting side effects and, if used periungually, may cause onycholysis. As a 5% solution needled into warts monthly for up to 3 months, a response rate of 87% was reported in randomised comparator studies [91,92]. Intralesional injection of 40 mg/mL 5-FU weekly for up to 4 weeks produced clearance in over 60% of warts [91,93], but this is a painful treatment.

A combination of 5% 5-FU and 10% salicylic acid tested in several studies cleared 63% of warts, compared with 23% when using salicylic acid alone [94], and an uncontrolled study of 0.5% 5FU with 10% salicylic acid also suggested a useful effect [95]. When used in combination with cryotherapy, the clearance rate was similar to that of cryotherapy alone [96].

Caustics and irritants. Monochloroacetic acid [97], trichloroacetic acid [98], silver nitrate [99,100], cantharidin [101], phenol [102], formic acid [103], potassium hydroxide [104], hydrogen peroxide [105] and other highly irritant chemicals can be used with effect but may cause painful reactions. If not applied carefully and accurately, these can cause chemical burns [106].

A study from the Netherlands showed a higher clearance rate of plantar warts treated fortnightly with saturated MCA solution alone (46%) compared with cryotherapy plus daily salicylic acid (39%) [107]. The peeling agents pyruvic acid [108,109] and glycolic acid [110] can be helpful, especially in the treatment of plane warts.

Retinoids. This treatment topically may be tried in plane warts, but the best results are claimed for higher than usual concentrations and irritation is common. The therapy can be effective in immunosuppressed patients [111]. In a study of children with plane warts treated with 0.05% tretinoin cream, 85% of 25 cleared their warts compared with 32% of controls [112]. Adapalene 0.1% gel applied under occlusion for up to 2 months cleared all plantar warts in 25 patients and was comparable to cryotherapy in an open comparative study [113].

Vitamin D analogues. Maxacalcitol alone or in combination with salicylic acid has been reported to be effective in the clearance of common warts [114,115]. The successful use of calcipotriol and calcitriol has been reported in a few anecdotal cases [116,117] and vitamin D3 has been used intralesionally with potential efficacy [118].

Second line

Treatments that are physician administered, more time consuming or expensive can be classed as second line.

Cryotherapy. Dimethyl ether spray, carbon dioxide snow and liquid nitrogen all produce cold thermal damage to the skin. Liquid nitrogen produces the coldest freeze and is commonly used in hospital practice, applied either by a cotton wool bud or from a cryospray. Both methods seem to be equally effective [119]. The rate of application of freeze is affected by the size of the hole in the spray nozzle or by the size, shape and density of the cotton wool at the tip of the bud. Dipping cotton buds for different patients into a common flask containing the liquid nitrogen may carry a risk of cross-infection.

Any thick keratin should be pared off, especially in plantar warts [120], and the surface dried before freezing begins. In standard treatment, the application is continued until a rim of iced tissue (easily seen as a white discoloration) about 1 mm in width develops in the normal skin surrounding the wart. The freeze is maintained for 5–30 s depending on the size and site of the wart. This may require a continuous or pulsed spray for between 5 and 20 s, depending on the size and thickness of the wart. Longer freezing (over 2 s of continual freeze) is more likely to leave scarring, possibly damage underlying structures and not improve clearance rates [121]. A gentler or 'traditional' freeze involves freezing until the 1 mm rim of frozen skin is visible and then stopping. This milder method seems to be less efficacious in clearance [122]. After thawing, a second freeze cycle will improve the cure rate in plantar warts, although the benefit is less marked in hand warts [123]. As well as damaging cells, cryotherapy may lead to clearance by stimulating the development of an immune response [124].

The response to treatment with cryotherapy is comparable or slightly better than that achieved with salicylic acid [78,79]. Treatment repeated every 3 weeks gives a 30–70% cure rate for hand warts after 3 months [74,125]. More frequent treatments are likely to improve responses although will induce more pain, and longer intervals are less effective [73].

If this fails, or when a wart is particularly painful or deep, or both, as may occur over a bony prominence on the foot, more prolonged application, typically up to 30 s, perhaps repeated after thawing, may be used to achieve a greater destructive effect at the cost of significantly greater blistering and pain. For such treatment, local or even general [126] anaesthesia may be considered. Topical anaesthetic post-procedure can improve tolerability in children [127] but the use pre-procedure is not of proven benefit.

The main disadvantage of freezing is pain. This is unpredictable and surprisingly variable between patients, but in some cases, especially with longer freezing times, it may be severe and persist for many hours or even a few days. Oral painkillers and strong topical steroids may help. Swelling of the treated area and the surrounding skin begins within minutes, and where tissues are lax, as in the periorbital area, it may be dramatic. A blister, sometimes haemorrhagic, may ensue within a day or two. After the usual short freezing times, the reaction will be likely to have resolved and healing occurs within 2–3 weeks. Scarring is unlikely with freezing times under 30 s. Occasionally, damage to underlying tissues may result, for example to a tendon [128] or the nail matrix, and excessive freezing times should be avoided over nerves, for example on the sides of the fingers. Depigmentation often occurs, and can be a significant cosmetic disadvantage in patients with darkly pigmented skin.

Laser. The pulsed dye laser has been used to treat warts with cure rates of approximately 32–100%, using a minimum of two treatments [129–131]. Facial plane warts can respond [132]. Other lasers such as the erbium:yttrium aluminium garnet (Er:YAG) and the neodymium:yttrium aluminium garnet (Nd:YAG) can also be used [133,134]. Overall, the efficacy of these laser therapies appears comparable to other treatments such as cryotherapy [135], but fewer laser treatments may be required to achieve clearance [136].

The carbon dioxide laser has a greater risk of producing more postoperative pain and scarring [137,138] but has been used to treat a variety of different forms of wart, both cutaneous and mucosal [137]. It can be effective in eradicating some difficult warts, such as periungual and subungual warts which have been unresponsive to other treatments. Clearance of cutaneous warts at 12 months is reported to be 55–70% [139,140]. Infectious virus can be detected in the plume during carbon dioxide laser use [141], so an operator mask and air extraction system are advised.

Laser treatment for other indications has been associated with the spread of facial warts [142,143].

Hyperthermia. Localised heat of up to 30 min at 44°C can also speed wart clearance, with 54% clearance compared with that of 12% with placebo [144]. Devices to produce such localised sustained heat without necrosis have not been readily available and vary between studies. Using a thermosurgery device held just above anaesthetised warts for 1 min produced clearance in 80% of the warts after one treatment in a randomised controlled trial [145]. Early attempts to use an adhesive heat patch applied for 2 hours show some promise [146].

Heat to a level of tissue destruction is produced by electrocautery, infrared coagulation and microwaves. The reported cure rate in two series totalling 71 warts treated with infrared coagulation was 69% [147,148] which compares favourably with cryotherapy. Heat damage due to localised microwave energy given to 34 patients in up to five treatments over a year has given a response rate of 76% even in warts of long duration [149].

Surgery. Excision is usually to be avoided since scarring is inevitable and recurrences of the wart in the scar are frequent. However, curettage can be effective as treatment for filiform warts. Curettage and cautery/electrocoagulation, usually in combination, may be used for painful or resistant warts, but carry a risk of scarring. Cautery or electrocoagulation can produce a plume containing active virus particles, so smoke extraction is advised and operator and assistant personal protection should be worn.

Photodynamic therapy (PDT). A number of open or placebo-controlled studies have shown clearance rates of 75–90% for hand and foot warts [150], plane warts [151] and even periungual warts [152] with PDT using aminolaevulinic acid. Methyl aminolevulinate PDT (MAL-PDT) with a pulsed dye laser light source is an alternative regime, with a reported clearance rate of 53% of warts [153]. The treatment may need to be repeated two or three times but can be limited by pain [154]. Paring of warts or treatment with topical salicylic acid pre-treatment can increase efficacy of PDT [155].

Third line

Third line treatments include those that might be considered in situations of severe and recalcitrant infection and also those treatments with less evidence base that might be considered when first and second line treatments have produced no effect.

Podophyllin and podophyllotoxin. Podophyllin and purified podophyllotoxin act as antimitotics, disrupting the formation of the spindle on which chromosomes align at mitosis. They are used mainly for the treatment of ano-genital warts but can also have an effect in cutaneous warts, although penetration into keratinised skin may be poor.

They have been used with caution under prolonged occlusion [156] or in a strength of 5% in combination with salicylic acid 30% and cantharidin 1% applied every 2 weeks for up to 10 weeks [157,158]. Although clearance rates may be high, acute pain can occur with intense local inflammation. Podophyllin and podophyllotoxin are contraindicated in pregnancy [159] and are not licensed for use in children.

Topical immunotherapy

Imiquimod. Topical immunomodulation with imiquimod 5% cream is licensed for treatment of genital warts, superficial basal cell carcinoma and actinic keratoses. Cutaneous warts have also responded to imiquimod treatment [160], although poor penetration through the keratinised surface may necessitate twice daily application for up to 24 weeks, or combination with salicylic acid to achieve useful results [161,162]. The addition of occlusion has been shown not to affect clearance rate [163]. Butchers' warts, facial filiform warts and plane warts [164–166] may all respond and immunosuppression does not appear to block the therapeutic effect [166,167]. The treatment can cause irritation, discomfort and occasionally erosion at the point of application with a small risk of causing vitiligo-like depigmentation [168].

Contact dermatitis immunotherapy. Diphenylcyclopropenone (diphencyprone, DPC) is used as a potent immunogen [169]. Cure rates of between 44% and 88% of patients were obtained at the end of treatment [170–172], often with apparent greater efficacy than cryotherapy [173]. The treatment can be used with a chance of success in the immunosuppressed [174]. The side effect of itching at treatment sites is generally tolerated, but some patients develop dermatitis in other areas or widespread urticaria [175]. The use of squaric acid dibutylester as a contact allergen in such regimens may be equally efficacious and better tolerated [176]. Allergens used for immunisation such as bacilli Calmette–Guerin (BCG) have also been used topically [177] and intralesionally (see later).

Intralesional immunotherapy. A number of studies over recent years have shown that intralesional injection of known antigens, usually used as vaccines, can stimulate the clearance of warts [177,**178**]. Trials using intralesional *Candida* antigen to produce a local hypersensitivity reaction suggest that this approach could speed wart resolution in recalcitrant cases [179] and can be used in immune compromise. The immunogens for mumps or tuberculosis (PPD) and the measles, mumps and rubella (MMR) vaccine have been applied as intralesional therapy [180]. Using the MMR vaccine, clearance can occur after one to four injections with reported clearance rates of 47–85% [181,182].

The possibility that the trauma of the injection alone stimulates the immune response is not supported by saline-controlled MMR injection studies, which report 60–85% clearance in the active group and 10–28% clearance in the placebo group [178].

Interferon. Different interferons have been administered by different routes to patients with refractory warts in various sites. These studies are seldom directly comparable, and the use of interferons in warts is still experimental. The majority of studies have involved patients with refractory genital warts and interferon use has mostly been disappointing. The most encouraging report is of complete clearance of injected warts in 11/12 patients with recalcitrant common and plantar warts treated with human IFN-α [183]. Cutaneous warts on the palms and soles have been treated with intralesional interferon, using a needleless injector [184].

Systemic immunotherapy.
H_2 receptor antagonists. Results from the use of oral cimetidine in wart treatment in adults have been conflicting. In open studies of high-dose cimetidine (30–40 mg/kg/day for 3–4 months), two-thirds demonstrated improvement or complete resolution without recurrence [185,186], but in placebo-controlled trials, no significant benefit of cimeditine therapy has been observed [187,188]. In children, cimetidine may produce slightly greater benefit [189,190] and combination treatment with levamisole may enhance the effect [191]. Ranitidine has been assessed in an open study in which 49% of patients with common or plane warts cleared while taking 300 mg twice daily [192].

Zinc. Oral zinc has a mild effect on the immune system. In one study comparing zinc sulphate with cryotherapy to cryotherapy alone, there was no added benefit to the oral treatment [193], but others have reported that oral zinc sulphate (10 mg/kg/day) produces a 50–80% cure rate of warts, although gastrointestinal side effects are common and often lead to discontinuation of therapy [194]. Topically, zinc sulphate as a 10% aqueous solution applied three times daily for 4 weeks in a double-blind trial produced a cure rate of 86% for plane warts [195]. Zinc oxide 15–20% ointment may also be used [196,197] and intralesional zinc sulphate 2% has also been reported to be of use [194].

HPV immunisation. A number of anecdotal reports have suggested clearance of cutaneous warts after the quadrivalent HPV vaccine [198,199] and a small retrospective observational study of 30 patients has shown clearance in 47% and improvement in a further 17% [200], but no placebo-controlled study has yet been conducted.

Oral retinoids. Oral retinoids, by reducing epidermal proliferation, can help to debulk warts, although the infection may persist making relapse likely. Acitretin and isotretinoin have been reported to be helpful in cases of extensive and hyperkeratotic warts in immunosuppressed patients [201,202]. Hyperkeratotic warts in otherwise healthy patients can respond to oral retinoid therapy either alone [203,204] or in combination with other standard treatment [205,206]. This effect may be temporarily useful, perhaps in relieving pain or disability due to exceptionally hyperkeratotic warts, or in facilitating the use of other treatments. Plane warts appear to respond better and may clear with isotretinoin 0.5 mg/kg/day for 2 months [207,208] or low-dose acitretin therapy.

Intralesional cytotoxics
Bleomycin [209]. Doses of intralesional bleomycin are given in units or in milligrams; 1 mg contains 1500–2000 U. Protocols vary, but typically bleomycin sulphate 0.25–1 mg/mL is injected up to three times to a maximum total dose of 4 mg [210]; or 1000 U/mL to two injections and a maximum total dose of 2000 U [211]. Lower concentrations of 100–500 U/mL seemed as effective [212,213]. Injections, in volumes ranging between 0.2 and 1.0 mL per wart, are very painful and preceding or concurrent local anaesthesia should be considered [214]. A haemorrhagic eschar develops; 2–3 weeks later, it is pared down if it has not detached spontaneously. Used in this way, there has been no evidence of systemic toxicity.

In open studies, cure rates for previously refractory warts are reported to be between 20 and 100% [212,213,215], with superiority over cryotherapy as well as placebo [216,217]. Local complications include nail loss [218] or dystrophy [219] following periungual injections, Raynaud phenomenon in treated fingers and local pigmentation [220] or urticaria [218]. Flagellate hyperpigmentation, more commonly a feature after systemic administration, has been reported after local injection [221] and this potential risk of systemic absorption is a contraindication for intralesional bleomycin in pregnancy [212].

Hayes and O'Keefe [212] give useful guidance on method and contraindications. Implantation of the bleomycin from a surface application using a sterile lancet [222] or the Dermojet® [223] may be better tolerated.

5-Fluorouracil. 5-FU has also been used as an intralesional injection or needled into warts in a few studies with clearance rates reported between 45% and 93% [224,225]. Side effects include pain, hyperpigmentation and numbness.

Cidofovir. By incorporating into replicating DNA, this nucleoside analogue damages dividing cells. It is licensed for treatment of CMV retinitis, but has been used with success intravenously (3–5 mg/kg as a single dose given every 1–2 weeks) for very severe warts [226] and can also be injected intralesionally, diluted from 375 mg/mL to 15 mg/mL and injected monthly [227,228] or, when applied as a 1–3% cream, with variable clearance [229,230]. Cidofovir can be used in immune compromise [231–233]. Side effects, mainly seen with systemic administration, include nephrotoxicity, metabolic acidosis and bone marrow suppression. Local application, especially on mucosal surfaces, can produce erosion and pain, but topical treatment of skin lesions is generally well tolerated [229].

Plant extracts. Sinecatechins extracted from green tea as Polyphenol E are licensed for use for ano-genital warts and have been used with anecdotal success in a cutaneous plantar wart [234].

Traditional Chinese herbal medicine has also been reported to clear warts using mixtures containing multiple plant extract ingredients applied topically [235].

Psychological methods. Many myths and some studies claiming that warts can be effectively treated by suggestion or 'magic' have been inadequately controlled for spontaneous regression [236]. Formal hypnosis, however, was reported to clear warts on the suggested (the more severely affected) side only, in 9 of 10 patients who achieved a satisfactory depth of hypnosis, the other side of the body acting as an internal control [237]. Children appear to have a higher rate of success than adults. Persistent refractory warts disappeared following hypnosis in an uncontrolled study of three immunodeficient children [238].

Resources

Further information
Kwok CS, Gibbs S, Bennett C *et al*. Topical treatments for cutaneous warts. *Cochrane Database Syst Rev* 2012:Issue 9:CD001781.

Treatment ladder for cutaneous warts

See details for treatment in text

First line
- Salicylic acid
- Glutaraldehyde
- Formalin
- Occlusion
- Topical 5-fluorouracil
- Caustics
- Retinoic acid
- Vitamin D analogues

Second line
- Cryotherapy
- Laser
- Hyperthermia
- Surgery
- Photodynamic therapy

Third line
- Podophyllin and podophyllotoxin
- Imiquimod
- Topical immunotherapy
- Intralesional immunotherapy
- Interferon
- H2 receptor antagonists
- Zinc
- Oral retinoids
- Intralesional bleomycin
- Intralesional 5-fluorouracil
- Cidofovir
- Psychological methods

Ano-genital warts

Synonyms and inclusions
- Condyloma acuminatum (singular)
- Condylomata acuminata (plural)

Epidemiology
Incidence and prevalence
In countries with highly developed medical services, referral rates of genital warts have greatly increased in the last 50 years. In the UK, there was a marked increase in the incidence of ano-genital warts (condylomata acuminata) from the 1970s to the 1990s [239], with a continuing rise over the next two decades [240]. There has been a slight decrease in the incidence of ano-genital warts in developed countries over the last 10 years, attributed to the introduction of the HPV vaccine, as rates of other sexually transmitted diseases such as chlamydia have continued to rise [241,242,**243**].

The overall population incidence worldwide is approximately 200/100 000 [244].

Age
The incidence is highest in the age group 20–34 years [245] and for young adults is estimated to be 700/100 000 [246].

Sex
The incidence and prevalence in males were higher than in females, but recent calculations suggest equality [**243**,244].

Pathophysiology
Predisposing factors
Genital warts have a high infectivity. The thinner mucosal surface is presumably more susceptible to inoculation of virus than thicker keratinised skin, but in addition lesions are commonest in sites subject to greatest coital friction in both sexes.

Human papillomavirus transmission has been most closely studied in the case of ano-genital warts. Acquisition most commonly follows sexual contact, but it is generally agreed that ano-genital warts are not always transmitted sexually. Perianal warts may accompany genital warts, either due to local spread of infection or to direct contact during anal coitus.

In prospective studies, approximately two-thirds of sexual contacts of patients with genital warts developed lesions themselves within 24 months; infectivity seemed highest early in the course of the disease [247,248]. Close inspection by penoscopy of male sexual contacts of women with genital HPV disease has shown that 69% [249] or 88% [250] have at least small lesions. Prospective studies of sexual contacts of patients with genital warts indicated that the incubation period between contact and diagnosis of genital warts is 3 weeks to 24 months, with a median of 3–10 months [247,248].

Occasional non-sexual acquisition of ano-genital warts in adults is assumed to be possible. The sensitivity of PCR analysis has shown that HPV DNA may be present on underwear and the fingers of patients with genital warts [251,252], suggesting that transmission could occur by a number of routes.

Transmission of ano-genital warts in children [253,254]. Ano-genital warts are uncommon in children, but their occurrence frequently stimulates discussion of the possibility of sexual transmission. This should always be considered, but there remains insufficient information to offer a reliable estimate of the relative frequency of sexual abuse in such cases.

Infection from the mother's genital tract at delivery [255,256] is regarded as a frequent source of childhood ano-genital warts, probably including those presenting up to 2 years of age. Genital papillomavirus transmitted from mother to baby at birth may persist in childhood [257,258], as shown by the retention of the DNA and/or a humoral response against the viral proteins. It is thought that perinatally acquired HPV infection may not manifest as genital warts for some years.

Postnatally, transmission from adults with genital warts may occur non-sexually [259]. Reviews of reports published between 1976 and 2018 [260,261] found that the route of infection was believed or confirmed to be sexual in a minority (5–20%).

Absence of other physical evidence of molestation, location of the warts on fully keratinised skin as opposed to genital or anal mucosa, a clinical resemblance to common warts and young age of the child, perhaps up to 1–2 years at the onset of the warts, would tend to support non-sexual transmission. Where sexual abuse is suspected, the case should be referred to a paediatrician or child abuse specialist. In addition, HPV typing is not routinely of use but might be forensically useful; the same type in child and in suspected abuser would be consistent with but not proof of sexual transmission, while different types would be strong evidence against the possibility.

Pathology [37]

Genital warts show extreme acanthosis and papillomatosis, but the horny layer is parakeratotic and not very thick. Koilocytes may be limited in distribution and not found in all sections. The epidermal processes are wide and rounded, with a well-defined lower border. The connective tissue is frequently very oedematous and the capillaries tortuous and increased.

Causative organisms

The low-risk HPVs are most often the cause of ano-genital warts, most commonly HPV-6 (in about 45–90%) [262–264] or HPV-11 and less frequently other types, as indicated in Table 25.8. Multiple types may be detected within a single wart, including both high- and low-risk types [265,266]. HPV-1 and HPV-2 may occur in genital warts [267,268]. The incubation period between infection and clinical disease is between 3 and 12 months.

In children, warts in the ano-genital area are often more hyperkeratotic than in adults and may be caused by HPV types associated with cutaneous disease as well as HPV-6 and -11. Studies involving HPV typing of childhood ano-genital warts have produced somewhat varying conclusions, but overall, approximately 50% have been found to harbour mucosogenital HPV with the cutaneous types 2, 27 and 57 also commonly detected [269,270].

Clinical features

Presentation (Figure 25.25)

They are often asymptomatic, but may cause discomfort, discharge or bleeding. The typical ano-genital wart is soft, pink, elongated and sometimes filiform or pedunculated. The lesions are usually multiple especially on moist surfaces, and their growth can be enhanced during pregnancy [271], or in the presence of other local infections [272]. Large malodorous masses may form on vulvar and perianal skin (Figure 25.26) and have been reported beneath the abdominal apron in obesity [273]. This classical 'acuminate' (sometimes called papillomatous or hyperplastic) form constitutes about two-thirds of ano-genital warts. The commonest sites, the area of the frenulum,

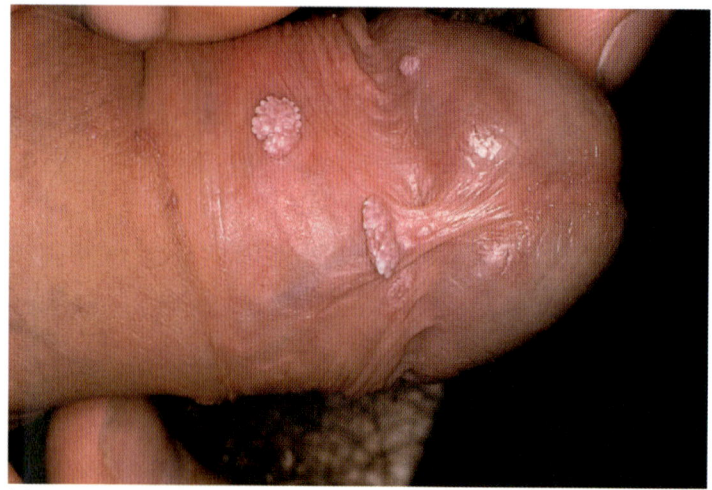

(a)

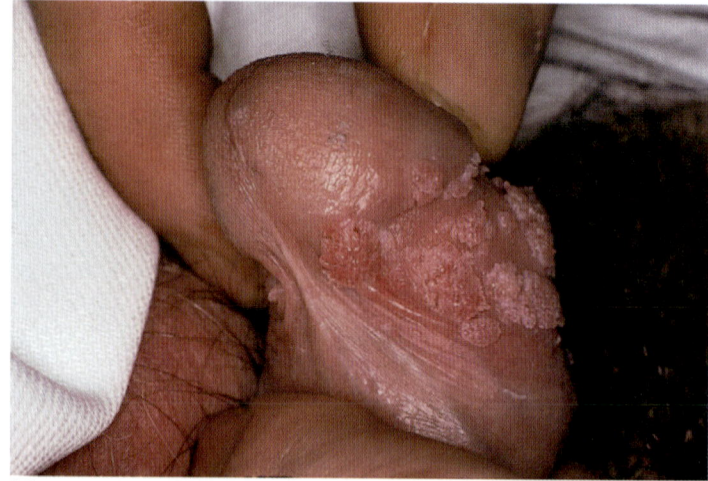

(b)

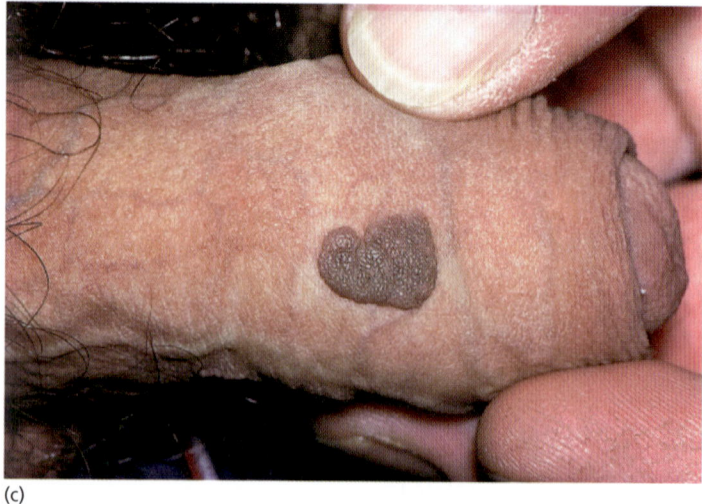

(c)

Figure 25.25 Penile warts. (a,b) Classical condylomata acuminata. (c) This pigmented lesion was confirmed histologically to be a viral wart. Courtesy of York District Hospital, UK.

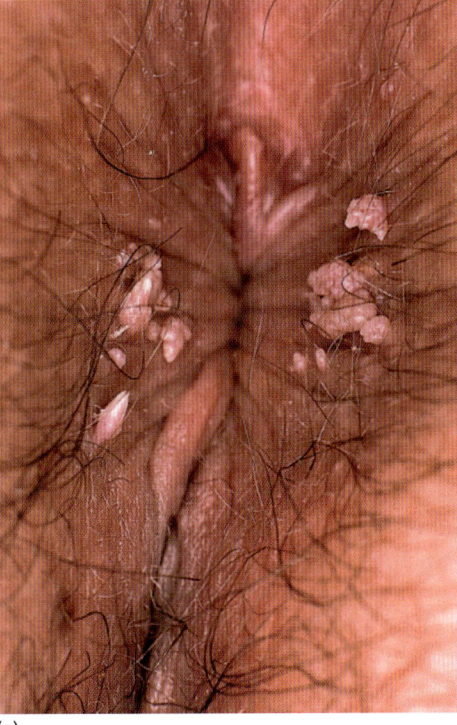
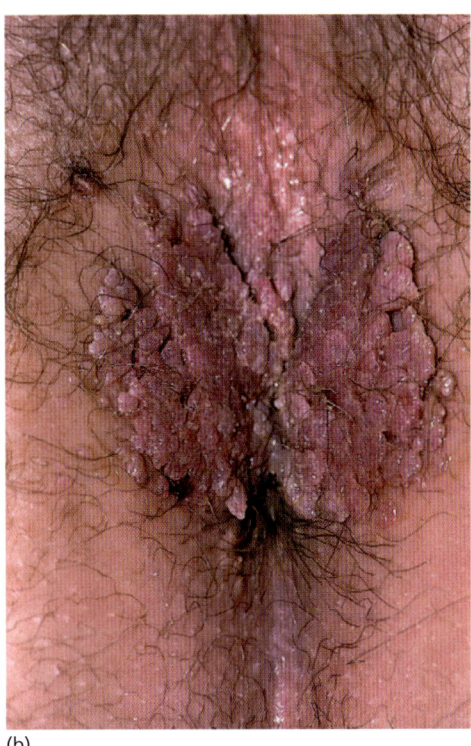

Figure 25.26 (a,b) Perianal warts. Courtesy of York District Hospital, UK.

corona and glans in men, and the posterior fourchette in women, correspond to the likely sites of greatest coital friction [271]. Most other lesions are flat, though more conspicuous than plane warts elsewhere, and some of these, generally on non-mucosal surfaces such as the penile shaft, pubic skin, perianal skin and groins, may be sufficiently pigmented to resemble seborrhoeic keratoses. Both acuminate and flat types may coexist.

Clinical variants

The mucosal HPV types responsible for ano-genital disease can cause disease at mucosal surfaces of the oropharynx, nose and eye.

Oropharyngeal warts and cancer. Oral warts, including some which appear to have been sexually transmitted [274], usually contain HPV-6 or -11 [275] and more rarely HPV-2, -57 or -16 [276]. They are common in association with HIV disease when a greater variety of HPV types may be found, including HPV-7, more usually associated with butchers' warts [50,51]. Antiretroviral treatment may lead to worsening of the warts rather than improvement [277]. HPV-13 and -32 seem to be almost specific for lesions of the rare benign familial disorder focal epithelial hyperplasia (Heck disease) [278]. High-risk genital HPVs have been detected in over 80% of cases of oral leukoplakia, and in at least 70% of cases of oropharyngeal carcinoma, with variation between countries [279].

Respiratory papillomatosis [280,281] is due most commonly to HPV-11, but also associated with other common genital types such as HPV-6 and rarely with high-risk HPV-16 [282]. Childhood cases are believed to result from maternal infection, probably at birth during vaginal delivery. Latent or subclinical infection in the laryngeal mucosa presumably explains recurrences after successful treatment, and might explain adult-onset cases, although some of these may be due to sexual transmission [283]. Treatment usually involves recurrent debulking of lesions. Malignant transformation occurs very rarely and is most commonly associated with HPV-11 [284].

Other sites. Low- and high-risk mucosal HPVs are detected in conjunctival papillomas [285] and nasal inverting papillomas [286].

Differential diagnosis

Seborrhoeic keratosis and ano-genital intraepithelial neoplasia can also produce pigmented warty lesions in the genital area [287]. Histological features and immunostaining for HPV and cell cycle-associated proteins can help to distinguish the lesions. The development of large protuberant masses, induration, pain or serosanguinous discharge should arouse suspicion of malignant change requiring prompt excision or biopsy and also assessment of immune status. Histologically, differentiation from malignant condylomas may be difficult after treatment with podophyllin or podophyllotoxin due to increased mitotic index.

Verrucous carcinoma (Buschke–Löwenstein tumour) (Chapter 111) is often initially misdiagnosed as genital warts.

Condylomata lata and lymphogranuloma venereum (Chapter 30) should be considered. Metastatic Crohn disease involving the vulval or perianal area often presents with skin tags on an oedematous or indurated background.

Vulval papillomatosis, with a diffuse velvety or granular appearance in the vaginal introitus, and pearly penile papules may cause confusion with the possibility of warts.

Complications and co-morbidities

Patients with genital warts frequently have other sexually transmitted genital infections [288]. The presence of any type of ano-genital wart should raise the possibility that the patient may also be infected with high-risk HPVs and prompt screening for ano-genital intraepithelial neoplasia.

Very florid warts should warrant consideration of an underlying immune deficiency.

Disease course and prognosis

The duration of ano-genital warts varies from a few weeks to many years. Recurrences can be expected in about 25% of cases, the interval varying from 2 months to 23 years [289]. Human papillomavirus DNA can be demonstrated in clinically and histologically normal skin adjacent to warts and intraepithelial neoplasia, and this latent infection correlates well with recurrence after clinical cure [290].

Management [291,292,**293**]
Prevention

The introduction of the anti-HPV vaccine has resulted in a reduction of incidence of ano-genital warts. In countries such as Australia, where there was early adoption of the tetravalent vaccine in 2007, which is prophylactic for HPV-6, -11, -16 and -18, a decrease in attendances for ano-genital warts was observed by 2014 [294]. This decrease has subsequently been observed elsewhere in men as well as women [295–297]. Extension of the vaccine to males over the last few years is expected to result in even greater effect.

First line

Podophyllotoxin is the most common treatment used, with expected clearance rates of over 50%. It is applied as a 0.15% cream or 0.5% solution by the patient twice daily for 3 consecutive days in a week for 4 consecutive weeks [298,299]. Podophyllin is contraindicated in pregnancy [300]. Podophyllotoxin appears to be safer but should still be avoided in pregnancy.

An alternative home-applied treatment is imiquimod, used as 5% or 3.75% cream [301]. The 5% cream is applied three times per week for up to 16 weeks [302], but the 3.75% cream applied twice daily for 2 weeks and repeated 2 weeks later seems to be equally effective. Skin irritation is common for both these treatments.

Second line

Other home treatments include sinecatechins (Polyphenol E from green tea), which can also be applied by the patient [303,304].

Other treatments used in the clinic include cryotherapy, electrocautery, surgery, photodynamic therapy, laser, trichloroacetic acid, 5-FU and cantharidin [**293**,305–308].

Third line

In severe cases of extensive or giant warts, often in immunosuppressed patients, more aggressive cytotoxic or antiproliferative treatments have been used [309,310].

Interferon may be considered, administered either systemically or intralesionally, but studies are few and results are variable. Overall, the effect is better than placebo [311]. Intralesional IFN-α or -β as monotherapy gives an overall response rate of 36–63% [312] for genital warts, but oral warts may respond slightly better [313].

Resources

Further information

https://www.cdc.gov/std/treatment-guidelines/anogenital-warts.htm
https://www.bashhguidelines.org/current-guidelines/skin-conditions/anogenital-warts-2015/

Patient resources

https://patient.info/sexual-health/sexually-transmitted-infections-leaflet/anogenital-warts
(All last accessed August 2023.)

Treatment ladder for ano-genital warts

See text for details

First line
- Podophyllotoxin
- Imiquimod

Second line
- Cryotherapy
- Surgery
- Laser
- Caustics
- Photodynamic therapy

Third line
- Interferon

Human papillomavirus-associated intraepithelial and invasive neoplasias of genitalia and mucosae

Definition

HPVs have been associated with several different dysplastic or malignant conditions [**314**]. An aetiological association between infection with high-risk HPVs and the development of cervical carcinoma is well established, and evidence for a causative effect in other ano-genital and head and neck cancers has emerged over the last two decades [315].

General description of disease domain

Squamous cell premalignancy and malignancy of the skin, ano-genital area, oro-pharynx [316], nasal cavities [317], larynx [318], oesophagus [319], lung [320] and conjunctiva [321] may harbour high-risk α or β HPVs.

Basic biology

In ano-genital lesions, type 16 is found most commonly and, together with HPV-18, accounts for 70–80% of HPV-positive cervical lesions, although approximately 30 different HPV types can infect this site. In cervical carcinoma cells, the HPV DNA is almost always integrated into the host cell genome, in contrast to its extrachromosomal location in benign and early premalignant lesions [322]. Premalignant and malignant disease at other mucosal sites usually involves these high-risk HPV types, while the types found most frequently in cSCC are the β types which are found in the episomal state.

Cervical intraepithelial neoplasia and invasive carcinoma [323]

Epidemiology

These conditions are epidemiologically associated with sexual activity, including age of first sexual intercourse, multiplicity of partners and a history of sexually transmitted diseases, in both the female patient and her male partner(s). Cervical intraepithelial neoplasia (CIN) is associated with a personal history of overt genital warts [324], and with penile warts [325] or penile intraepithelial neoplasia [326] in the partner.

Pathophysiology

HPV is commonly detected in dysplastic cervical lesions and is found in 90–100% of cervical cancers [**327**].

High-risk HPVs can also be detected by sensitive PCR in approximately 10% of cytologically normal cervices [**243**,328], with some variation between countries and continents. This association is highest in young sexually active women [329] in whom infection may be transient. The persistent finding of a high-risk HPV type in the cervix of a woman increases the likelihood of progression of the disease [330].

Management

The introduction of vaccination against HPVs from 2007 is already showing signs of reducing the incidence of CIN [331–333]. The premalignant ano-genital disorders are best managed by or in association with gynaecology, urology or colorectal surgery. For vulvar intraepithelial neoplasia, see Chapter 110; penile intraepithelial neoplasia, see Chapter 109; perianal intraepithelial neoplasia, see Chapter 111; and verrucous carcinoma, see Chapter 110.

Cutaneous squamous cell carcinoma without immunosuppression

With the advent of sensitive DNA detection methods by PCR, the HPV genome has been found in approximately 25–50% of keratoses and non-melanoma skin cancers of immunocompetent individuals [334]. It is DNA of the EV-associated types, the β HPVs, which is present in these lesions. The viral DNA is not exclusive to dysplasia – it can also be found in normal skin and hair follicles in 45% of healthy people tested [335]. The exact molecular role of the virus in the development of skin cancers remains a subject of intense debate [336,337,**338**], but evidence is mounting for their role early in this carcinogenic pathway [339,340].

The high- and low-risk HPV types that cause genital disease are also reported in certain extragenital warts and carcinomas. Although such cases are more common among the immunosuppressed, immunocompetent individuals may also be affected. Squamous cell carcinoma or Bowen disease of the fingertip and nail bed has been associated with high-risk genital HPVs [341–344], especially when in association with genital HPV disease. Cutaneous intraepithelial carcinoma of the skin (Bowen disease) has been found occasionally to harbour HPV-2 [345] and a number of ano-genital HPV types [346–348].

Malignant change may rarely develop in apparently normal warts, usually when very longstanding [349,350], but the accuracy of the original diagnosis must always be in question [351].

Ionising radiation may act as a c-factor for malignant change in warts [352]. Widespread actinic keratoses and cSCCs arising after PUVA photochemotherapy may also be associated with HPV infection [353].

IMMUNODEFICIENCY AND HPV INFECTION

Overview

Severe cutaneous and mucosal HPV infection may be a manifestation of underlying immunodeficiencies which may broadly result from either primary inborn errors of immunity (IEI) or acquired immunodeficiencies [1,2,**3**,**4**]. The major immunological defects underlying primary or acquired HPV susceptibility are either defects of keratinocyte-intrinsic immunity (particularly for β-HPVs) or errors of T-cell-mediated adaptive immunity (affecting both T cells, particularly CD4+ T cells, and antigen-presenting cells (APCs)), or a combination of both (Table 25.9). Defects of adaptive B-cell immunity do not appear to predispose significantly to severe HPV infection (despite the preventative effect of HPV vaccination), nor do defects of myeloid or lymphoid leukocyte-mediated innate immunity [1,2,**3**,**4**].

The spectrum of HPV clinical presentations described in immunodeficiency includes:
- Epidermodysplasia verruciformis (genetic and acquired)
- Persistent and/or recalcitrant viral warts (including 'tree-man' syndrome)
- Generalised verrucosis
- HPV-associated anogenital, head and neck and cutaneous squamous cell neoplasia

Inborn errors of immunity and HPV infection

Identification of the genetic basis of human IEIs predisposing to HPV infections has provided important clues to understanding the immune response to HPV. Presentation may be in early life, or not develop or become apparent until adult life. Cutaneous and mucosal HPV infections vary in severity, as does susceptibility to non-HPV mucocutaneous infections and HPV-associated malignancy (Table 25.10).

Epidermodysplasia verruciformis

Epidermodysplasia verruciformis (EV) is characterised by persistent and widespread cutaneous infection with beta HPVs (beta-HPV)

Table 25.9 Classification of immunodeficiencies predisposing to human papillomavirus (HPV) infection. Details of each condition are presented in Table 25.10

Immune mechanisms			Examples/gene involved	Dominant HPV type[a]
Inborn error of immunity	Keratinocyte intrinsic immunity		EVER1, EVER2 CIB1	Beta
	Adaptive immunity (T cell/APC)	T-cell differentiation/number	LCK, DCLRE1C, MST1, TPP GATA2, STK4, IL7/IL7R, IL2RG, JAK3, RHOH, CORO1A SASH3, NHEJ1, ATM, LIG4, ADA, ZAP70	Beta Alpha, gamma, beta Alpha, gamma
		T-cell migration	DOCK8, STK4 CXCR4, WAS	Alpha, gamma, beta Alpha, gamma
		T-cell activation	RHOH CD4, CD28, TAOK2, CARMIL2, CARD11, MAGT1	Alpha, gamma, beta Alpha, gamma
		APC differentiation/number	GATA2, CXCR4	Alpha, gamma
		APC migration	DOCK8	Alpha, gamma, beta
Acquired immunodeficiency	Adaptive immunity (T cell/APC)		HIV; haematological malignancy; organ transplantation; other iatrogenic immunosuppression.	Alpha, gamma, beta

[a] HPV types: alpha, cutaneous/mucosal; beta, cutaneous; gamma, cutaneous; APC, antigen-presenting cell.

[1,2,3–5] causing disseminated hypo- and hyperpigmented plane warts, pityriasis versicolor-like lesions, red plaques and seborrhoeic keratosis-like lesions with characteristic histological features. Progression to cSCC on UV-exposed sites may occur.

Three main forms of EV are recognised [6]:

1 *Classic genetic (typical) EV*: EV is considered classic/typical when cutaneous beta-HPV infection is an isolated clinical feature resulting from mutations in genes critical for keratinocyte intrinsic immunity (*EVER1/TMC6*, *EVER2/TMC8* and *CIB1*). Patients are otherwise healthy with no evidence of compromised T-cell-mediated immunity and an absence of other infectious manifestations.
2 *Non-classic genetic (atypical) EV*: this form of EV results from inborn errors of T-cell immunity in genes including *RHOH*, *MST-1* and *CORO1A*. These patients are also vulnerable to other infections.
3 *Acquired EV* describes an EV-like syndrome that develops in patients with acquired immunodeficiency such as HIV, haematological malignancy and iatrogenic immunosuppressive drugs.

Genetic EV (classic/typical and non-classic/atypical)

Definition and nomenclature
Classic/typical EV is a rare genodermatosis and was first described in 1922 [7]. Patients are otherwise healthy and resistant to mucosal HPV and other skin microorganisms. It is usually inherited in an autosomal recessive pattern of transmission. Approximately 30–40% will go on to develop cSCC on UV-exposed sites.

> **Synonyms and inclusions**
> - Lewandowski and Lutz dysplasia

Non-classic/atypical EV-like syndromes are observed in certain other IEIs affecting T-cell and APC function, with possible additional effects on keratinocyte intrinsic immunity [6].

Epidemiology
Incidence and prevalence
Classic/typical EV is rare with about 500 patients reported globally in 2017 [5], although seropositivity for beta-HPVs occurs in 20–65% of the population [8].

Pathophysiology
Causative organisms
At least 25 different beta-HPVs have been identified in EV lesions and patients are typically infected with multiple HPV types of which HPV-5 is the most prevalent [9]; types, 8, 9, 12, 14, 15, 17 and 19–25 are also frequent (Table 25.8). Cutaneous alpha-HPVs -3 and -10, which cause plane warts, are also found in EV [10] and genital alpha-HPVs may occasionally also be found [11,12]. HPV-5 and -8 are the main types associated with malignancy, with types 14, 17, 20 and 47 occasionally involved [5,9,13].

Histopathology
The histological picture is similar in the different clinical lesions. Characteristically, hyperkeratosis and acanthosis are associated with keratinocytes displaying hyperchromatic nuclei, coarse keratohyalin granules and vacuolation or ballooning with a blue-grey pallor in the perinuclear area of keratinocytes and may affect the upper half to three-quarters of the spinous layer. HPV DNA may be detected in these vacuolated or 'clear' cells by *in situ* hybridisation and PCR. Viral particles can be identified ultrastructurally not only in the Malpighian cells, but also in basal cells. The viral cytopathic changes persist in Bowenoid lesions and early cSCC [5,13,14].

Genetics and immunopathogenesis
Studies of the genetic aetiologies of classic/typical and non-classic/atypical EV have shown that beta-HPV infection control requires skin-intrinsic viral restriction and a functional T-cell adaptive immune response.

Classic (typical) EV. Classic EV is caused by mutations of genes encoding proteins of the CIB1–EVER1–EVER2 complex, selectively

Table 25.10 Primary inborn errors of immunity associated with human papillomavirus (HPV) disease. Adapted from Béziat 2020 [3].

Syndrome	Gene	Inheritance	EV classic/typical (T); non-classic/typical (A)	Cutaneous warts	Ano-genital or oral warts	HPV-associated malignancy	Other mucocutaneous phenotype	Immune phenotype
IEIs which include EV clinical features								
Epidermodysplasia verruciformis	EVER1	AR	+++ (T)			Cutaneous SCC	Isolated EV	Normal T cell count; small proportion naïve T cells
Epidermodysplasia verruciformis	EVER2	AR	+++ (T)			Cutaneous SCC	Isolated EV	Normal T cell count; small proportion naïve T cells
Epidermodysplasia verruciformis	CIB1	AR	+++ (T)			Cutaneous SCC	Isolated EV	No immunological abnormalities
CORO1A deficiency	CORO1A	AR	+ (A)	+			Severe susceptibility to infections – HSV-1, molluscum, staphylococcal tuberculoid leprosy, EBV	CD4+ T-cell lymphopenia Low naïve CD4+ and CD8+ T cells Impaired NK function
RHOH	RHOH	AR	+++ (A)	+			Molluscum, HSV1, gingivostomatitis, Burkitt lymphoma	Low naïve CD4+ and CD8+ T cells
STK4 deficiency	STK4	AR	++ (A)	+ (25%)			Superficial bacterial/viral infections	CD4+ T cell, CD8+ T cell, and B-cell lymphopenia
LCK	LCK	AR	+ (A)				Broad susceptibility to infections	Impaired TCR signalling; CD4+ T-cell lymphopenia
DCLRE1C	DCLRE1C	AR	+ (A)		+		Broad susceptibility to infections	Low B cells and CD3+ T cells Hypogammaglobulinemia
MST1 deficiency	MST1	AR	+ (A)				Dermatitis, oral candida, HSV1-2, VZV, molluscum, EBV	CD4 T-cell lymphopenia
TPP2	TPP2	AR	+ (A)				Susceptibility to viral infections	Low CD4 and CD8 T cells Low B cells
Severe combined immunodeficiency	IL2RG	XLR	+ (A)	+ (+++ post-HSCT)		Cutaneous SCC Ano-genital SCC	Patients with deficiencies of IL-2Rγ and JAK3 AND IL7R develop disseminated warts (common, EV) after HSCT	T–B+NK– phenotype CD4 lymphopenia post-HCST (but not correlated with warts)
	*LIG4	AR	–	+				
	*ADA	AR	–	+				
	JAK3	AR	+ (A)	+ (+++ post-HSCT)				
	*ZAP70	AR	–	+				
	IL7	AR	+ (A)	+				
	IL7R	AR	+ (A)	+++				
DOCK 8 (dedicator of cytokinesis 8) deficiency	DOCK-8	AR	+ (A)	+++ (40%)		Cutaneous SCC Ano-genital SCC	Eczema, abscesses, mucocutaneous candidiasis, chronic cutaneous viral infections	High serum IgE levels, eosinophilia, and T- and NK-cell lymphopenia
IEIs with no prominent EV clinical features								
GATA-2 haploinsufficiency	GATA-2	AD	–	+++ (50%)	+++	Ano-genital SCC	Severe infections (viral, bacterial, fungal)	Pancytopenia (neutrophils, monocytes, DCs, T cells, NK cells); modest impact only on LCs
WHIM syndrome (warts, hypogammaglobulinaemia, infections, myelokathexis)	CXCR4	AD GOF	–	+++ (80%)	+++	Ano-genital SCC (16%)		Pancytopenia; restricted TCR repertoire
SASH-3 deficiency	SASH-3	XL	–	+++ (75%)				Neutropenia, B-, T-, and NK-cell lymphopenia and defective TCR signalling

(continued)

Table 25.10 (continued)

Syndrome	Gene	Inheritance	EV classic/typical (T): non-classic/typical (A)	Cutaneous warts	Ano-genital or oral warts	HPV-associated malignancy	Other mucocutaneous phenotype	Immune phenotype
Complete magnesium transporter 1 deficiency (XMEN)	MAGT1	XLR	–	++ (30%)	+		EBV infection, molluscum	Low NKG2D expression on NK and CD8+ T cells, low IgG, and CD4 lymphopenia
CARMIL-2 deficiency	CARMIL2	AR	–	++ (30%)	+		Molluscum contagiosum, bacterial and fungal infections, dermatitis	Low Treg cells, central memory CD4 and CD8 T cells, and memory B cells
CARD-11	CARD11	AD	–	++ (30%)				lymphopenia in ¼ cases
CD28 deficiency – 'tree man syndrome' (TMS)	CD28	AR	–	+++ (HPV2 and 4)	+		Generalised severe hyperkeratotic cutaneous papillomatosis	
TAOK2 deficiency	TAOK2		–	+++				
Complete CD4 deficiency	CD4	AR	–	++				Absence of CD4 expression on CD8– TCRαβ+ T cells
ICOS deficiency (common variable immunodeficiency-like disease)	ICOS	AR	–	++ (14%)	+	Ano-genital SCC		Low B cell, hypogamma globulinemia Low T-follicular helper cells
ADA2 deficiency	ADA2	XLR	–	+			Autoinflammation, polyarteritis nodosa-type vasculitis	Variable leukopenia or lymphopenia
Netherton syndrome	SPINK5	AR	–		+	Cutaneous SCC (including Buschke–Lowenstein tumour)	Ichthyosis, bamboo hair, atopic diathesis, recurrent skin infections	Low B cells with immature phenotype; impaired NK cell cytotoxic activity
Wiskott–Aldrich syndrome	WAS	XLR	–	+ (4%)	+	Head and neck SCC	Eczema, cancer, autoimmune	Lymphopenia; impaired myeloid and lymphoid function
Ataxia-telangiectasia	ATM	AR	–	++ (20%)			Opportunistic infections	Broad lymphopenia – B cells, CD4 and CD8 T cells, restricted TCR and BCR repertoires
Fanconi anaemia	21 FA genes	AR (XLR)	–			Ano-genital SCC Head and neck SCC		
WILD syndrome: warts, immune depression, lymphoedema and ano-genital dysplasia	?	?	–	+++ (80%)	+++	+ (14%)	Lymphoedema (including genital), epidermal naevi	CD4 lymphopenia
Primary intestinal lymphangiectasia	?	?	–	+++				

AD, autosomal dominant; AGIN, ano-genital intraepithelial neoplasia, includes AIN, CIN, PIN, VIN and vaginal intraepithelial neoplasia; AR, autosomal recessive; BCR, B-cell receptor; DC, dendritic cells; EV, epidermodysplasia verruciformis; GOF, gain-of-function; HSCT, haematopoietic stem cell transplant; LC, Langerhans cells; NK, natural killer cells; SCC, squamous cell carcinoma; TCR, T-cell receptor; XLR, X-linked recessive. *Subtypes of SCID not usually associated with EV-like features.

disrupting keratinocyte-intrinsic immunity to these viruses [13,15]. In 2002, the first two IEIs underlying classic EV were identified as autosomal recessive deficiencies in EVER1 and EVER2 which are endoplasmic reticulum transmembrane proteins encoded by *TMC6* and *TMC8*, respectively, adjacent genes located on chromosome 17q25 [16]. EVER1/2 mutations account for approximately 75% of EV-affected individuals worldwide. In 2018, a third IEI was discovered – CIB1 (encoding calcium- and integrin-binding protein-1) deficiency [**15**,17]. Although abnormal zinc homeostasis due to EVER1/2 deficiency was initially thought to underlie the lack of control of beta-HPV infection, since the identification of CIB1 it is postulated that the pathogenesis of the beta-HPV-driven skin lesions involves disruption of a skin-restricted, keratinocyte-intrinsic restriction factor (the CIB1–EVER1–EVER2 complex) which confers immunity against beta-HPVs: it does this through interaction with two HPV proteins, E8 and E5, which are absent from beta-HPVs [**5**,12,16,17]. Beta-HPV infections are widespread and asymptomatic in the general population but cause disease only in EV patients lacking EVER/CIB1 complex-dependent keratinocyte-intrinsic immunity. The resulting inability to control beta-HPV-driven keratinocyte proliferation allows beta-HPV-driven lesions to develop, but EV patients are not more prone to developing common HPV warts, due to non-beta-HPVs [**15**]. The clinical and virological phenotypes of EVER1-, EVER2- and CIB1-deficient patients are indistinguishable.

Non-classic (atypical) EV. Patients with non-classic EV have primary T-cell immunodeficiencies resulting in CD4 T cell lymphopenia and impairment of circulating T-cell response to CD3 stimulation [**5**]. The T-cell deficit, common to all non-classic EV, highlights the importance of full T-cell development and function in protective immunity to beta-HPVs. Mutations in genes including *MST1*, *RHOH*, *CORO1A*, *TPP2*, *DCLRE1C*, *LCK*, *RAS GRP1*, *DOCK8*, *IKBKG*, *ITK*, *RASGRP1*, *SMARAL1*, *STK4* and *IL7* are all reported in association with atypical EV [**3**] (Table 25.10). In some cases, the genetic defect is unknown [18]. An EV phenotype is also described in patients with severe combined immunodeficiency due to mutations of *IL2RG* and *JAK3* who have had allogeneic haematopoietic stem cell transplantation but in whom this deficiency in keratinocytes is not corrected despite being otherwise healthy [19]. Persistent infection with beta-HPVs causes skin lesions identical to those of classic EV, but these patients are also susceptible to other viral, bacterial, fungal and parasitic infections, autoimmune disease and other malignancies, particularly haematological, depending on the mutated gene and the nature of the T-cell deficit [**5**].

Clinical features
Presentation of typical EV [**5**,6,**13**,20–22]
The onset of skin lesions in genetic EV is usually in infancy. Lesions on the face and neck are generally indistinguishable from plane warts, although flat, scaly, reddish hypopigmented macules, resembling pityriasis versicolor, may be located on the forehead, and seborrhoeic keratosis-like lesions are also seen. On the trunk and limbs, larger red, hypo- or hyperpigmented pityriasis versicolor-like areas tend to predominate. Thicker plaques are pink-red, violet or brown in colour and may resemble seborrhoeic keratoses or pigmented warts, and in darker skins hypopigmentation is often more obvious (Figure 25.27). Warts develop rapidly in childhood but may first appear at any age. They are most numerous on the face and neck and backs of the hands and feet, and may be restricted to these sites, but there are often scattered lesions elsewhere and the warts may be generalised over the entire body surface. Irregular confluence of lesions to form lines or large plaques is often seen. Typical common warts are often present, especially on the sides of the fingers and on the palms and soles, and small warts on the vermilion border of the lips or in the urethra have occasionally been noted, although mucous membranes are usually spared. Clinical penetrance of the classic EV phenotype is complete at the age of 10 years in patients with EVER and CIB1 deficiencies.

Differential diagnosis
Acrokeratosis verruciformis is superficially very similar to EV. Flat warty papules on the backs of hands and feet and on the knees and elbows are present from infancy. The palms are diffusely thickened and show small keratoses and punctiform breaks in the papillary ridges. Histologically there is no vacuolation. In lichen planus the papules, which are usually pruritic, are pink or lilac in colour and distinctive mucosal lesions are often present. The histology is diagnostic.

Complications and co-morbidities
Dysplastic and malignant changes occur most often on UV-exposed sites, commonly as actinic keratoses and Bowen disease, suggesting that UV radiation is an important factor. cSCC may develop on UV-exposed sites – particularly the forehead – in up to 60% of patients from the third decade onwards. They tend to develop slowly and may be locally destructive, but rarely metastasise [**5**,**13**,20–22].

Investigations
The characteristic histopathology findings for EV are usually diagnostic. Identification of beta-HPVs by PCR or *in situ* hybridisation within lesions can indicate the possibility of EV and this will be strengthened by detection of multiple types in both benign and, if present, malignant lesions. However, the presence of beta-HPV as part of the normal skin microbiome is common [23,24,**25**] and seropositivity for beta-HPVs occurs in 20–65% of the population [8,26]. The presence of beta-HPVs is therefore not diagnostic.

Management
Treatment of EV is challenging. If a diagnosis of EV is suspected or confirmed, avoidance of excessive sun exposure and UV-protective measures should be instigated. Monitoring for cutaneous malignancy is advisable [27].

First line
Treatment for the benign lesions of EV is often not very effective. Imiquimod has been of benefit in only some patients [28,29]. Photodynamic therapy can reduce lesions, but treatment may need to cover large areas and be repeated [30]. Cryotherapy can be used on non-pigmented skin but gives only a temporary response. Other

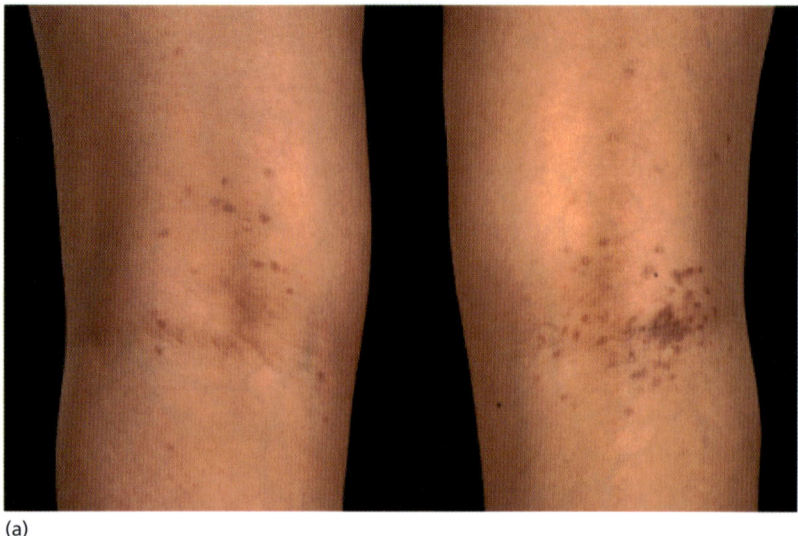

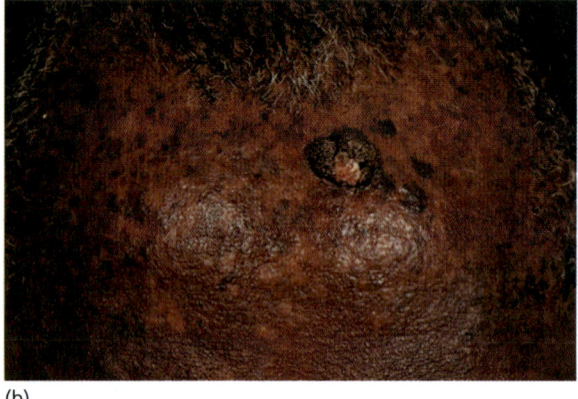

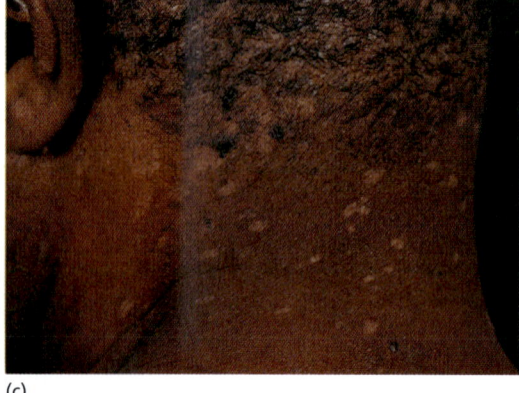

Figure 25.27 Epidermodysplasia verruciformis. (a) Pigmented flat warty lesions in popliteal fossae. Courtesy of Addenbrooke's Hospital, Cambridge, UK. (b) Multiple, confluent flat warts with a seborrhoeic keratosis-like lesion on the forehead and (c) neck. Courtesy of Barts Health NHS Trust, UK.

treatments that have shown occasional but inconsistent benefit include topical vitamin D analogue [31], topical immunotherapy with squaric acid dibutylester [32], oral cimetidine [33,34] and oral zinc [35]. The role of HPV vaccination is unclear, although it has been reported as partially helpful in a case of non-classic EV [36]. Management of suspected skin cancer is by histological diagnosis and surgical removal. Use of photodynamic therapy for EV-associated actinic keratosis and SCC *in situ* has also been reported [37].

Second line
More widespread and disfiguring lesions may warrant systemic therapy with oral retinoids. These can produce cosmetic improvement [38], but the effect is dose dependent and relapse occurs if the drug is stopped [39]. Oral isotretinoin can also reduce the benign lesions and may be effective as longer-term low-dose treatment [40]. Acitretin can improve skin manifestations [36,41,42] and may reduce the risk of development of SCC, as in transplant recipients, but this is not yet proven.

Third line
Combination therapy with acitretin and interferon or acitretin and photodynamic therapy has been suggested and may give better response than either therapy alone [41,43].

Treatment ladder for epidermodysplasia verruciformis

First line
- Imiquimod
- Photodynamic therapy
- Cryotherapy

Second line
- Acitretin
- Isotretinoin

Other inborn errors of immunity and recalcitrant viral warts

In addition to IEIs presenting with typical and atypical EV, other primary immunodeficiencies may predispose to persistent, extensive and recalcitrant cutaneous and anogenital warts and, in some cases, cutaneous, mucosal or anogenital malignancies [1,2,3]. Patients with IEIs have been a frequent source for identification of new HPV types [44]. The genetic basis, immunological and clinical features of these IEIs are summarised in Tables 25.9 and 25.10. They are broadly associated with mutations of genes affecting the number or function of cells in multiple leukocyte compartments and include GATA-2 haploinsufficiency [45], CXCR4 deficiency in WHIM syndrome [45–48], SASH-3 deficiency [49], complete magnesium transporter 1 (MAGT1) deficiency [50], CARMIL-2 deficiency [51], CARD-11 deficiency [52], TAOK2 deficiency [53], complete CD4 deficiency [54,55], ICOS deficiency (common variable immunodeficiency-like disease) [56,57], ADA2 deficiency [58], Netherton syndrome [59], Wiskott-Aldrich syndrome [60], ataxia–telangiectasia [61], Fanconi anaemia [62], WILD syndrome (warts, immune depression, lymphoedema and ano-genital dysplasia) [63,64] and primary intestinal lymphangiectasia [65]. Although patients with IL2RG and JAK3 SCID genotypes may develop severe warts including atypical EV, particularly post-haematopoietic stem cell transplant [66], other SCID genotypes including ILG-4, ADA and ZAP70 are associated with warts but not EV-like changes [2,3]. Similarly, severe warts may be more prominent than atypical EV changes in other conditions including DOCK8 deficiency [67–69].

In 2021 a key role for the CD28 T-cell co-stimulation pathway in control of cutaneous HPV infection emerged through investigation of patients with widespread recalcitrant warts not explained by known IEIs [70]. CD28 recognises CD80/CD86 on APCs and IEIs that impair this pathway result in a predisposition to alpha- and gamma-HPV infections. Three patients with complete CD28 deficiencies inherited in an autosomal recessive manner were reported to have severe, recalcitrant common warts [4]. One patient had benign but giant and disseminated cutaneous horns – described as 'tree man syndrome' – with warts specifically harbouring HPV-2 and -4, alpha- and gamma-HPV types respectively [70]. These patients are otherwise healthy and it appears that CD28 is largely redundant in protective immunity to infection and only slightly impairs T-cell development and function. Cutaneous warts have also been reported in 30% of patients with MAGT1, CARD11 and CARMIL2 deficiencies, which all impair CD28 expression or signalling in T cells and are associated with recalcitrant warts [2,3].

Human papillomavirus in acquired immunodeficiency

Severe mucocutaneous HPV infections are more frequent in patients with acquired immunodeficiencies, particularly those associated with adaptive T-cell immunity. The most common acquired immunodeficiencies are those resulting from HIV infection, haematological malignancy and iatrogenic immunosuppression. Clinical presentations include common warts, acquired EV, and premalignant and invasive mucocutaneous SCC.

HIV infection (Chapter 31)
The incidence of warts is reported to be between 5 and 27% in PLWH. Common and plantar warts are increased in frequency and severity but are not a major problem in most patients. There is also an increased incidence of facial and intraoral warts, some of which contain HPV-7 ('butchers' wart' virus) [71]. Beta-HPV types are also over represented in warts from PLWH and specific HLA immunogenotypes may be associated with susceptibility [72]. An acquired EV phenotype is well recognised in PLWH and cSCCs may arise in this context [73]. Cutaneous HPV disease may worsen with the immune reconstitution syndrome [74–76] and this may be triggered by HPV vaccination [77]. Perianal warts, especially in men who have sex with men (MSM), may be florid and refractory to treatment [78]. HPV-associated ano-genital intraepithelial neoplasia and progression to malignancy are increased in incidence but may be reduced by antiretroviral therapy in PLWH [79–81]. Benign HPV-related oral lesions include multifocal epithelial hyperplasia, warts and papillomatosis [82,83] and HPV-associated oropharyngeal cancers are increased in PLWH [84].

Haematological malignancies
Warts are more common in patients with Hodgkin disease and, to a lesser extent, in those living with other malignant lymphomas and chronic lymphatic leukaemia [85,86].

Immune-mediated inflammatory disorders (IMIDs)
Intrinsic dysregulated immunity independent of immunosuppressive drugs in IMIDs such as systemic lupus erythematosus may have an increased risk of cutaneous warts and HPV-associated ano-genital disease [87,88].

Iatrogenic immunosuppression
Long-term immunosuppressive drug treatment is an important factor predisposing to severe HPV infection (Figure 25.28). One of the largest patient groups receiving long-term immunosuppressive drugs is solid organ transplant recipients: at one-year post-transplant, 15% of 120 kidney transplant recipients had warts [89], but this can rise to 90% by the end of the fifth year [90]. Warts harbouring HPV-2 and HPV-4 infections are the most frequent and both children and adults are affected [91]. Warts are often refractory to standard methods of treatment; in addition to the standard treatments used in the general population, reduction of immunosuppression may be considered on a case-by-case basis in close dialogue with both transplant clinicians and patient. A contributory role for HPV in the pathogenesis of keratinocyte cancer in the context of iatrogenic immunodeficiency is discussed in detail in Chapter 147. The incidence of ano-genital HPV infection and intraepithelial neoplasia and malignancy is also significantly increased [92,93].

Acquired epidermodysplasia verruciformis (AEV)
Acquired EV is a condition in which similar lesions to those seen in typical/classic genetic and atypical/non-classic genetic EV are described in association with acquired immunodeficiency (Table 25.11; Figure 25.29) [6,73,94–113]. Both intrinsic immune dysregulation and immunosuppressive medications affecting T-cell function can contribute to AEV. Those at risk of AEV include patients with lymphoma, HIV/AIDS (including vertically acquired HIV), patients receiving long-term immunosuppressive drugs after organ and bone marrow transplantation and for inflammatory diseases [6,73]. However, AEV appears to be reported infrequently despite increasing numbers of immunodeficient individuals and it

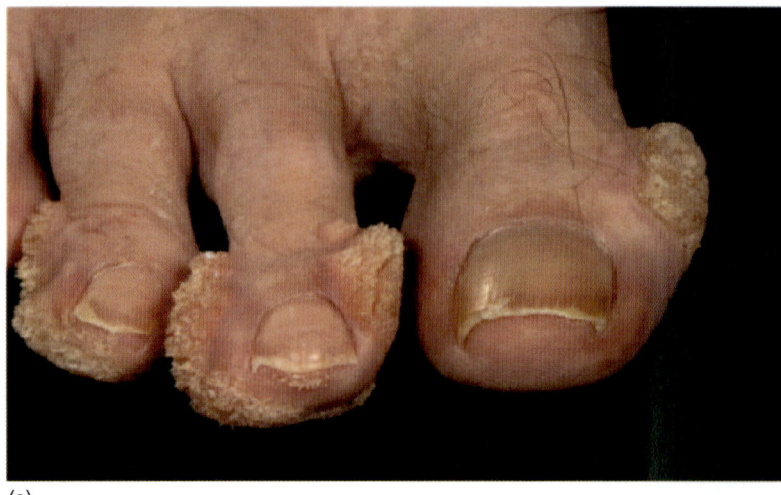
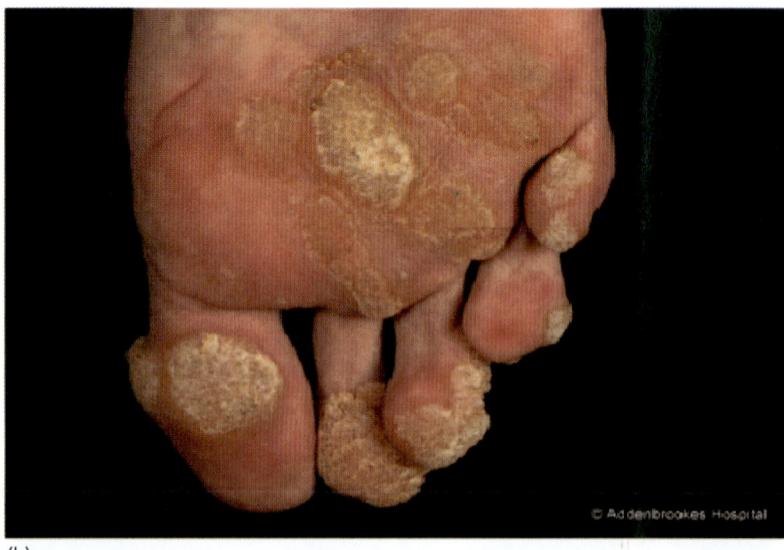
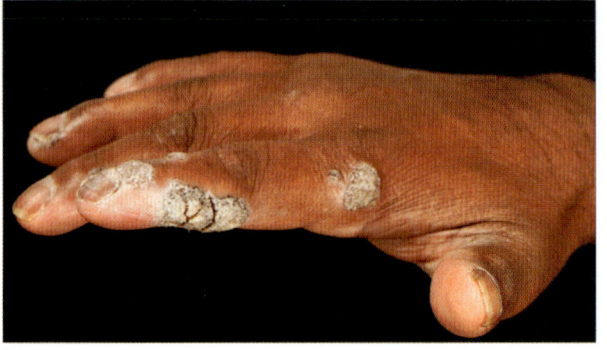
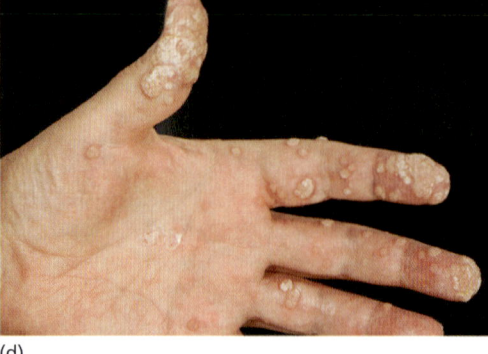

Figure 25.28 Extensive plantar warts in a kidney transplant recipient. (a) Toes. (b) Sole. Courtesy of Addenbrooke's Hospital, Cambridge, UK. (c,d) Warts on hands of kidney transplant recipients. Courtesy of Barts Health NHS Trust, UK.

is proposed that there are possible additional genetic susceptibilities that predispose some patients to developing EV following an acquired immunodeficiency [6,13].

Treatment

In AEV, the risk of malignant progression seems to be lower than in genetic EV, but surveillance for malignancy of skin, upper respiratory tract and genital tract is advised, as is consistent sunscreen use. For HIV-associated AEV, antiretroviral therapy may lead to remission [99], but responses are not consistent [113]. Treatments with cryotherapy, imiquimod cream, oral retinoids and interferon can be used, as in classic/genetic EV, but the responses are unpredictable [6,73,114–116] and the role of HPV vaccination is currently unclear [109].

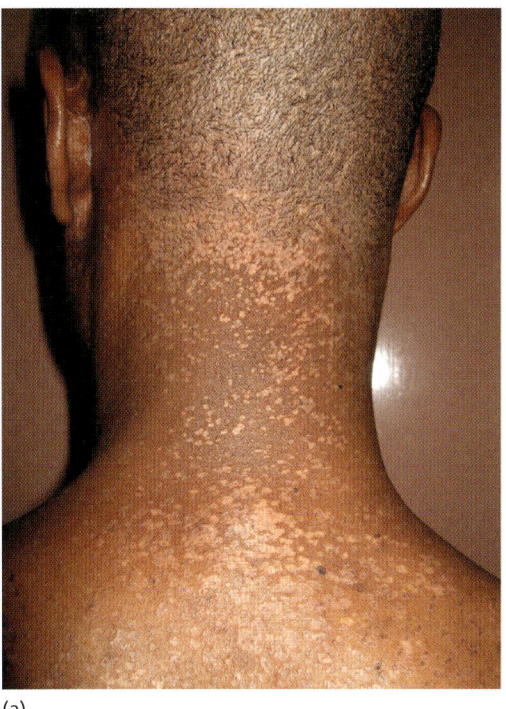
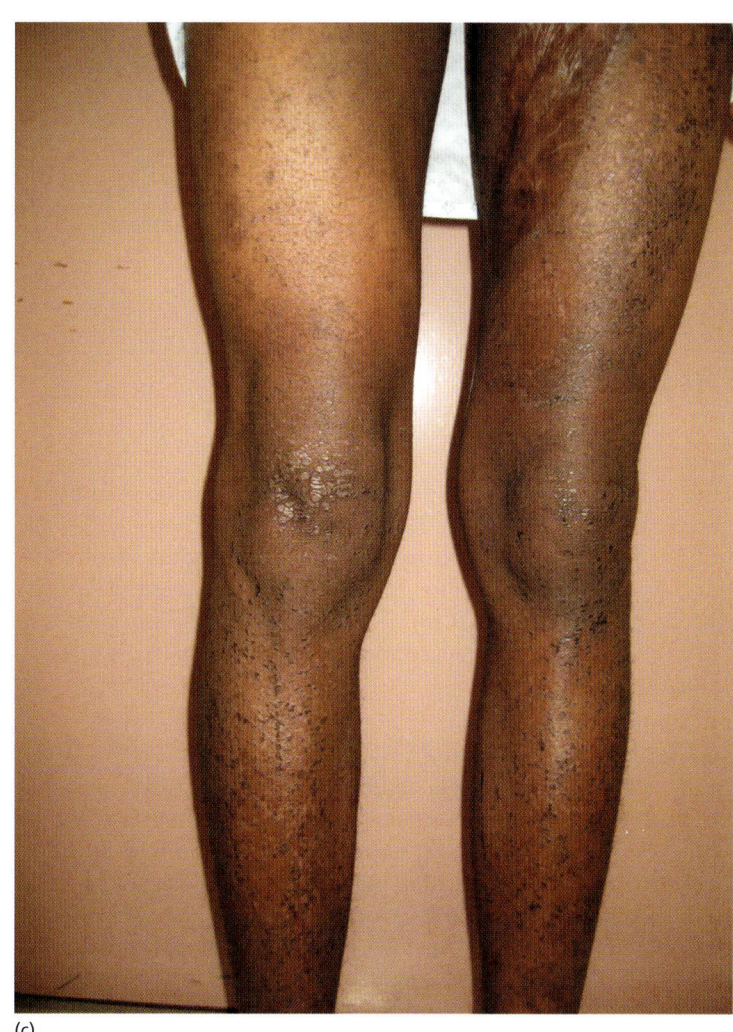
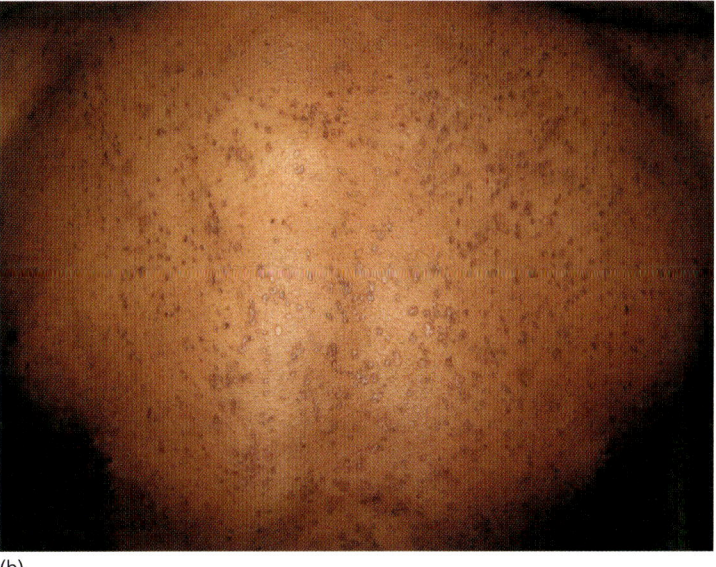

Figure 25.29 Acquired epidermodysplasia verruciformis. Widespread flat hyper- and hypopigmented lesions affecting the whole body: (a) neck, (b) back and (c) legs. Courtesy of Dr K. W. Shum, University Hospitals of Derby and Burton, UK.

Table 25.11 Conditions associated with acquired epidermodysplasia verruciformis.

Condition	Examples
HIV infection in children/adolescents	[94,95]
HIV infection in adults	[96–99]
Haematological malignancy (lymphoma, leukaemia, myelodysplastic syndrome)	[100–103]
Organ transplantation	[104–109]
Bone marrow transplantation and graft-versus-host disease	[110]
Atopic eczema (severe and immunosuppressed)	[111]
Systemic lupus erythematosus (with immunosuppression)	[112]
Leprosy (lepromatous)	[113]

HEPATITIS INFECTIONS

Many viruses infect the liver, but it is the primary target organ for only five: hepatitis A virus (HAV), hepatitis B virus (HBV), hepatitis C virus (HCV), hepatitis D virus (HDV) and hepatitis E virus (HEV). HDV is a defective virus and replicates only when coinfected with HBV.

Viral hepatitis infections may be associated with a wide spectrum of cutaneous manifestations which occur in three main contexts: during the acute disease phase; during chronic infection; as a consequence of adverse reactions to vaccines and antiviral therapies. HBV and HCV infection status is also relevant to skin disease in the context of screening prior to initiating immunosuppressive or biologic therapies, as chronic active infection can have a direct clinical impact on treatment selection (Chapter 19).

Cutaneous associations with hepatitis are best established for HBV and HBC [1,2–5,6,7]. Limited data are available for HAV and there are even fewer reports for skin disease associated with HEV infection [6,7].

Hepatitis B

Introduction and general description

HBV causes an acute hepatitis before potentially establishing chronic persistent infection. Together with HCV, chronic HBV infection leads to cirrhosis and hepatocellular carcinoma resulting in more than 1.3 million deaths in 2015, as high as those of TB, HIV infection and malaria [8,9,10]. Skin manifestations associated with HBV can appear in both acute and chronic infection [1,2–4,6,7].

Epidemiology
Incidence and prevalence

In 2019 approximately 296 million people worldwide were living with chronic HBV infection (with hepatitis B surface antigen (HBsAg) positivity), with an estimated 1.5 million new infections each year and 820 000 deaths, mostly from cirrhosis and hepatocellular carcinoma [8]. Only a proportion (7–40%) carry HBeAg (the soluble extracellular form of hepatitis B core antigen) and are infectious. The infection is endemic in many parts of the world and HBsAg is found in about 8% of individuals in hyperendemic areas such as sub-Saharan Africa and East Asia, with lower levels of carriage in other endemic areas as South America, Eastern and Central Europe. In these areas, the most usual route of transmission is from mother to child, but transmission via blood transfusion, needle-sharing and sexual contact is most common in non-endemic areas. Earlier age of acquisition of HBV is associated with an increased risk of chronic infection. About 10–15% of people with chronic HBV infection are coinfected with hepatitis C and 1% are also infected with HIV; the prevalence of HBV infection in PLWH is 7.4% [10].

Pathophysiology
Causative organisms and pathology

Human HBV is a member of the *Hepadnaviridae* family [9]. There are 10 HBV genotypes (A–J), classified according to difference in the full-length genome sequence. These genotypes have different geographic distributions but whether they are associated with different disease is debated [9]. HBV is a small, enveloped DNA virus. The icosahedral nucleocapsid – the virus core – contains the partially double-stranded relaxed circular DNA (rcDNA) of approximately 3200 bp, covalently linked to the HBV polymerase that has reverse transcriptase activity. Several surface proteins expressed externally on the envelope are important for binding and entry into host cells. After viral entry into the nucleus, it is converted into fully double-stranded DNA, which is then converted into covalently closed circular DNA (cccDNA), the stable HBV DNA responsible for its persistence. As the virus replicates it is detectable in serum by PCR: HBeAg is found in blood and antibodies develop against the nucleocapsid protein (core antigen, HBcAg). Electron microscopy of serum during this replicative phase reveals complete virus particles (Dane particles) and excess surface (envelope) protein formed into small spheroids and cylinders.

If a cytotoxic immune response develops against HBcAg, symptoms and signs of an acute hepatitis develop. HBV DNA disappears from the blood but HBeAg and HBsAg are still detectable and antibodies against both HBcAg and HBeAg are detectable. If the virus is cleared effectively, neither HBV DNA nor HBV antigens are detectable, but antibodies to the surface or envelope protein (HBsAg, Australia antigen) develop and persist, providing protection against reinfection. Persistence of viral replication for 6 months indicates chronic infection which involves a dynamic interaction between the virus and the host immune responses. The likelihood of becoming a chronic carrier is highest if infection occurs perinatally rather than as an adult. Different phases of chronic HBV infection have been described, with differing biochemical and virological profiles. A substantial proportion of patients with chronic infection develop cirrhosis and hepatocellular carcinoma, whereas others have lifelong quiescent disease activity and will not require antiviral therapy.

Hepatocyte damage in HBV infection can be caused directly by viral infection, but is more commonly due to the immunological response by cytotoxic lymphocytes to the virally infected cells [9].

Clinical features related to skin

In addition to generic cutaneous symptoms related to cholestatic liver disease (including pruritus, jaundice, hypermelanosis, spider naevi, nail changes), a range of skin manifestations are described in association with acute and chronic HBV infection [1,2–4,6,7].

Serum sickness-like reaction (SSLR). Acute HBV infection most commonly manifests in the skin as immune complex hypersensitivity (type III hypersensitivity). Such signs may be seen in 15–30% of cases, approximately 6 weeks before hepatitis becomes apparent. SSLR presents with general malaise, fever, proteinuria or haematuria, arthropathy, angioedema, and skin involvement including urticarial-type rashes (with corresponding leukocytoclastic vasculitis on histology), angio-oedema, morbilliform rashes, lichenoid dermatitis, palpable purpura and erythema multiforme-like lesions [1,7].

Gianotti–Crosti syndrome (papular acrodermatitis of childhood). In children, both acute and chronic HBV infections have been associated with Gianotti–Crosti-like skin changes with non-pruritic, non-coalescing papules (see later) [1,2,11].

Polyarteritis nodosa (PAN). Chronic HBV infection is associated with vasculitis and PAN is one of the more common presentations [1,7,12–14] (Chapter 100). Livedoid vasculopathy is also observed [15]. This association is greater in areas where hepatitis B is not endemic and may be related to a higher viral load. Up to two-thirds of cases of PAN may be HBsAg positive [7,13].

Lichen planus (LP). An association with LP is reported, including oral LP, but not confirmed in all studies [1,7,16,17].

Other cutaneous manifestations. Essential mixed cryoglobulinaemia has been described with HBV infection although it is most common with HCV [2,7]; an association with chronic spontaneous urticaria is controversial [18]. An increased risk of SCC of the skin has been reported in a north European population [19].

Vaccination and skin disease

Recombinant HBV vaccination was first introduced in 1981, and the WHO now recommends that all infants receive vaccination at birth and this dose, followed by two additional booster doses, induces protective anti-HBs antibodies in more than 95% of infants [8,9,10]. This global pre-exposure prophylaxis strategy aims to eliminate HBV and reduce liver cancer incidence; by 2015, the global HBsAg prevalence had decreased in children under 5 years from 4.7% to 1.3%. Post-exposure vaccination for non-immunised people or in those who have failed to respond to the vaccine after accidental exposure (e.g. needlestick injury) consists of a combination of HBV immunoglobulin and vaccination [8,9,10].

A wide range of skin conditions have been reported to follow HBV vaccination [2]. These include urticaria, maculopapular rash, pityriasis rosea-like rash [20], erythema nodosum [21], erythema multiforme, vasculitis and polyarteritis nodosa [22], systemic lupus erythematosus [23], dermatomyositis [24], Reiter syndrome [25], morphoea profunda [26], granuloma annulare [27], solitary mastocytoma [28], pseudolymphomatous hyperplasia [29], lichen planus [30], anetoderma [31], Gianotti–Crosti syndrome [32], erythema elevatum diutinum [33,34], scleromyxoedema and lichen myxoedematosus [35].

Antiviral treatment and skin disease

Oral nucleos(t)ide analogue therapy is the main form of anti-HBV treatment worldwide. Entecavir and two prodrugs of tenofovir are recommended as first line and have now replaced older-generation nucleos(t)ide analogues (lamivudine, adefovir and telbivudine) [9,10]. Subcutaneous pegylated IFN-α for 12 months remains possible as first line therapy in chronic HBV infection, but its unfavourable side-effect profile and the low likelihood of sustained viral suppression after discontinuation compared with long-term nucleos(t)ide analogue therapy have restricted its use [9]. HBV reactivation is a potentially fatal complication of immunosuppressive therapy such as rituximab (although not lower-risk drugs such as azathioprine and methotrexate) and a finite duration of prophylactic therapy with a nucleos(t)ide analogue, irrespective of serum HBV DNA concentration, may reduce risk. Tenofovir may also be used prophylactically to prevent perinatal transmission if there is a risk of maternal HBV vaccine failure [9,10].

Antiviral therapy (possibly in combination with immunosuppression) can lead to clearance of HBV-associated polyarteritis nodosa [1,36] and vasculitis [2,32]. Some severe skin reactions have been reported during antiviral treatment of HBV including toxic epidermal necrolysis with adefovir [37]. Entecavir has been associated with lichenoid and maculopapular rashes [38,39] and granulomatous reactions [40].

Resources

Further information

https://cks.nice.org.uk/topics/hepatitis-b/
https://www.cdc.gov/hepatitis/hbv/index.htm
https://www.who.int/news-room/fact-sheets/detail/hepatitis-b
(All last accessed August 2023.)

Hepatitis C

Introduction and general description

HCV, first described in 1989, causes acute and chronic liver disease associated with high morbidity and mortality and is a major global health problem [10,41]. As with HBV infection, skin manifestations are associated with both acute and chronic infection [1,3–5,6,7,42,43].

Epidemiology
Incidence and prevalence

Hepatitis C has a worldwide distribution. In 2019 approximately 58 million people had chronic infection, with 1.5 million new cases and 290 000 deaths globally [41]. It is endemic in many areas of the world: infection rates are up to 20% in Egypt, while in non-endemic areas, such as northern Europe, infection rates are of the order of 0.5%. Horizontal transmission is via blood and body fluids. Injection drug use is the major source of new HCV infections in most high-income regions of the world. Outbreaks among men living with HIV who have sex with men have been reported worldwide. Transmission through transfusion has essentially been eradicated where blood donations are screened for HCV [9]. Vertical transmission perinatally from an infected mother is associated with a 1–10% transmission rate. Acute HCV infection is asymptomatic in approximately 75% of patients, but 70–80% of adults develop chronic infection, of whom up to 20% develop cirrhosis and are at risk of hepatocellular carcinoma, both accounting for most associated deaths [41].

Pathophysiology
Causative organism and pathology

HCV is a small enveloped single-stranded positive-sense RNA virus and a member of the flavivirus family (*Flaviviridae*), genus *Hepacivirus*. There are seven known genotypes: type 1 causes about 70% of infections and genotype 2 approximately 20% and the genotype may influence response to available antiviral treatment. Extrahepatic manifestations are common and are proposed to result from both the host immune response to HCV infection and direct viral cytopathic effects [1].

Clinical features
Presentation

In acute HCV infection, reported skin manifestations include jaundice, vasculitis, urticaria, erythema multiforme and erythema nodosum. Skin manifestations of chronic HCV are more frequent, with the four most common being mixed cryoglobulinaemia, lichen planus, porphyria cutanea tarda and necrolytic acral erythema.

Mixed cryoglobulinaemia (MC). MC is a systemic vasculitis of small and medium vessels characterised by the presence of serum cryoglobulins generated by an expansion of B cells. These are detected in up 30–40% of chronic HCV infections, but only 5–30% are symptomatic with features of mixed cryobuliaemia syndrome (MCS) [43]. Conversely, more than 80–90% of patients with MC have chronic HCV infection [43]. Immune complexes precipitate mainly in the skin, joints, kidneys and peripheral nerve fibres, activating complement and causing tissue damage. There may be general features of fatigue, arthralgia and hepatosplenomegaly. Palpable purpura with or without livedo is the most common feature in the skin, most often on the lower legs. Raynaud phenomenon, pruritus, urticaria and leg ulcers are also seen [42,43]. Leukocytoclastic small vessel vasculitis is the main histological feature [42].

Lichen planus (LP). Although some studies have suggested a 2.5–4.5-fold increased risk of LP in HCV-positive patients and a 5-fold increased risk of HCV in patients with LP, this association varies widely with geographic region and study design. In patients with oral LP, HCV increases the risk of oral SCC [1,7,42,43,44,45].

Porphyria cutanea tarda (PCT). PCT is associated with liver disease, but detection of antibodies in a high proportion of non-familial cases suggests an aetiological link. There is geographic variation, with reports of 20–90% of cases of PCT being HCV seropositive [43,44,45]. Although the relative risk of HCV infection in patients with PCT is increased up to 275-fold in case–control studies [42], PCT is relatively rare with a reported prevalence of between <1% and 5% [42].

Necrolytic acral erythema (NAE) [1,3,7,42,43]. NAE is distinguishable from other forms of necrolytic erythemas by its acral location, most often on the dorsal feet. It has been reported in 0.2–1.7% of HCV-infected patients and was initially considered pathognomonic for infection [46]. In endemic areas, 10–30% of patients may also be HBV positive. NAE runs a relapsing and remitting course with lesions evolving from red and violaceous papules, vesicles, erosions and plaques into hyperkeratotic plaques which can become hyperpigmented and may be painful. Histology demonstrates psoriasiform epidermal hyperplasia [3]. Serum zinc levels are frequently low [47,48].

Pruritus and pruritic eruptions. In chronic HCV infection pruritus affects up to 15% of patients, either as generalised pruritus without skin lesions or associated with secondary changes such as lichenification, lichen simplex chronicus and nodular prurigo [42,49].

Other skin disorders. Associations between HCV infection and other skin manifestations are reported [43]. In addition to LP, the risk of immune-mediated chronic inflammatory skin disorders including psoriasis, vitiligo, alopecia areata and cutaneous lupus erythematosus is also increased [5]. Polyarteritis nodosa [50,51], erythema nodosum [52], Sjögren syndrome [53], erythema multiforme [54], erythema induratum [55], disseminated superficial actinic porokeratosis [56], granuloma annulare [57], morphoea [58], drug hypersensitivities [59] and bullous pemphigoid [60] are also reported.

Management

There is currently no vaccine against HCV [10,40]. Previous pegylated IFN-based treatment regimens were associated with substantial toxicity. In 2011, boceprevir and telaprevir – first-generation NS3/4A HCV protease inhibitor direct-acting antivirals (DAAs) – were licensed for use in combination with IFN and ribavirin ('triple therapy') for genotype I infections. Although this revolutionised HCV treatment in terms of improved virological cure rates, triple therapy is associated with significant side effects. In 2014 three HCV DAAs (sofosbuvir, simeprevir and daclatasvir) were introduced in IFN-free regimens, with sustained virological response and improved tolerability. Further NS3/4A protease inhibitors, NS5A inhibitors, NS5B nucleoside analogue inhibitors and NS5B non-nucleoside inhibitors have followed [10,43]. The WHO now recommends therapy with DAAs for all adults, adolescents and children from 3 years of age with chronic HCV infection and treatment for 12–24 weeks cures more than 95% of people [10,41,43].

HCV-associated skin diseases respond variably to antiviral treatments [42,43]. In HCV-associated mixed cryoglobulinaemia, elimination of HCV infection with DAA treatment together with suppression of associated B-cell clonal expansions using rituximab may be beneficial [61]. Although treatment is associated with rapid control of most vasculitis manifestations, cryoglobulins remain positive in about 50% of patients, a small proportion remain at risk of clinical relapse and severe vasculitis may not respond [62]. Although data remain limited, DAA treatment has also been reported to result in improvements in skin disease in a significant proportion of patients with pruritus [63,64], lichen planus [63,65], NAE [64], PCT [66], psoriasis [63,67], eczema [64] and LE [68] have all been reported.

Adverse cutaneous effects of HCV antiviral treatment

Interferon/ribavirin regimens have high rates of cutaneous side effects including exacerbation of immune-mediated inflammatory skin conditions: dermatitis is the most common pattern, but psoriasis, lichen planus, discoid lupus and alopecia areata are also reported [67,69,70].

The addition of HCV protease inhibitors telaprevir and boceprevir as part of triple therapy increases the risk of cutaneous adverse effects to approximately 50–70%; rashes are most frequently eczematous with a spongiotic dermatitis as the most common reaction pattern, and in many cases therapy can be continued with appropriate treatment [71,72]. However, severe cutaneous adverse reaction syndromes which necessitate modification or discontinuation of antiviral treatment have been described, including DRESS, Stevens–Johnson syndrome and toxic epidermal necrolysis, including some resulting in fatalities [71–78].

The risk of adverse cutaneous effects with second generation DAAs appears to be lower compared with first generation protease inhibitors, especially in patients not treated with IFN or ribavirin in whom rates of less than 5% are reported [79]. Symptomatic treatment with antihistamines and corticosteroids may provide adequate control and it is not usually necessary to suspend DAA treatment [79,80]. Together with eczematous reactions, also reported are leukocytoclastic vasculitis [81], photosensitivity [82], photodistributed lichenoid eruptions [83] and subacute cutaneous LE [84].

Resources

Further information

https://www.who.int/news-room/fact-sheets/detail/hepatitis-c
https://www.cdc.gov/hepatitis/hcv/index.htm
https://cks.nice.org.uk/topics/hepatitis-c/
(All last accessed August 2023.)

PARVOVIRUS INFECTIONS

Until 2005, parvovirus B19 was the only member of the *Parvovirus* family known to be a human pathogen. Molecular analysis of viruses isolated from humans has since revealed other parvoviruses that can infect humans, although their prevalence and role in disease are not yet clearly defined (Table 25.1).

General description of disease domain

Human parvoviruses are widespread, affecting all ages, worldwide.

Erythema infectiosum

Synonyms and inclusions
- Parvovirus B19 infection, acute B19V infection, fifth disease

Epidemiology

Incidence and prevalence

Parvovirus B19 infection is very common but often undiagnosed, with most individuals becoming infected in childhood. Transmission is mainly by droplets, but parenteral and intrauterine infection can occur. The majority of adults are seropositive [1,2]. Parvovirus B19 DNA has been found in the skin in a number of conditions including erythema infectiosum, although causality is unproven (see Clinical variants later).

Pathophysiology

Causative organisms

Parvovirus B19 (Figure 25.30) has been reclassified as primate erythroparvovirus 1 in the genus *Erythroparvovirus* within the *Parvoviridae* family [3,4]. The genome of the virus is single-stranded DNA of 5–6 kb. Three genotypes are recognised, but most acute infections are due to type 1 [5].

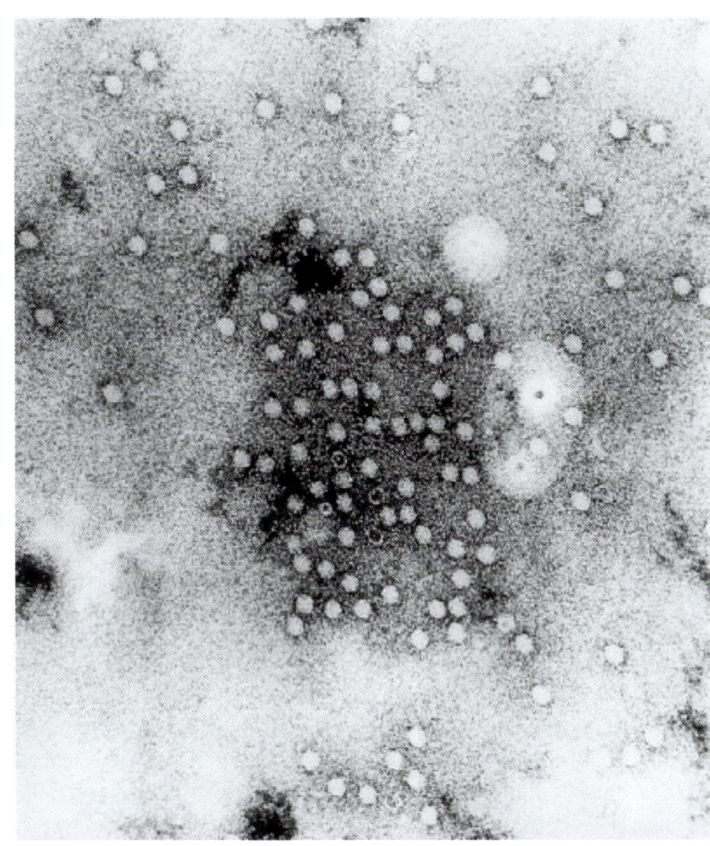

Figure 25.30 Human parvovirus (B19) in the serum of a patient with aplastic crisis. Negatively stained electron micrograph, ×200 000. Courtesy of Mr T. W. Lee, John Radcliffe Hospital, Oxford, UK.

Clinical features

Presentation

In children, the exanthem commonly develops suddenly without prodromal symptoms, although there may be mild malaise, myalgia, sore throat, headache or fever [6,7,8]. Rose-red papules on the cheeks rapidly coalesce to form a hot turgid redness, almost erysipeloid, giving a 'slapped cheek' appearance. There is often perioral pallor. During the next 2–4 days, maculopapules appear on the proximal extremities and extend distally to the hands and feet and proximally to the trunk, often forming a lace-like pattern. The palms and soles may be involved and acral lesions may be petechial. There may be dark red macules on the buccal and genital mucous membranes. Lymphadenopathy is not common.

In adults, acute infection is seen more commonly in women than men. Polyarthralgia is often the predominant symptom of infection [9] and systemic symptoms are more marked. When the exanthem does occur, the features of facial redness are usually less marked than in children [10] and the eruption is frequently purpuric [11].

Clinical variants

Rarely, lesions may be vesicular or pustular [12]. The eruption may be petechial or purpuric in children, often generalised [13], but sometimes acral or flexural. An acral pattern of purpuric lesions, amounting to papular-pruritic gloves and socks syndrome (see later), is the commonest skin association or variant of parvovirus B19 infection [14].

Table 25.12 Cutaneous conditions with possible association with parvovirus B19 (acute or reactivated).

Condition	References
Urticaria/angio-oedema	[15]
Vasculitis	[16,17]
Sweet syndrome	[18]
Pityriasis lichenoides (pityriasis lichenoides et varioliformis acuta)	[19,20]
Hydroa vacciniforme	[21]
Red baby syndrome	[22]
Systemic sclerosis	[23]
Behçet disease	[24]
Psoriasis	[25]
Wells syndrome	[26]
Acute generalised erythematous pustulosis (AGEP)	[27,28]

Other conditions associated with B19 are listed in Table 25.12.

Complications and co-morbidities

During the early stages, there is leukocytosis with relative lymphopenia; later an eosinophilia may be accompanied by a lymphocytosis. Mild anaemia is common but aplastic anaemia occurs rarely, most commonly in those with pre-existing haematological disorders or immunosuppression [29]. Rare complications such as haemophagocytic syndrome, myocarditis and severe liver damage have been reported [30].

Acute parvovirus infection in pregnancy, especially first trimester, can result in fetal death or hydrops fetalis [31].

Disease course and prognosis

The facial redness abates within a few days and the eruption usually fades in 6–10 days, but evanescent recurrences on previously affected sites may continue for 2 weeks or longer [32].

While the arthropathy common in adults usually resolves in a few weeks, joint symptoms can persist for more than 2 months in 10% of infected women. In some cases, the combination of parvovirus infection with rash and arthritis is accompanied by other features diagnostic of connective tissue disease such as systemic lupus erythematosus or rheumatoid arthritis [33], but a causative association has not been proved [34].

Investigations

Confirmation of infection is usually made by serology. IgM antibodies against the capsid proteins VP1 and VP2 are detectable during the second week of acute infection and for up to 2 months, while IgG antibodies develop as lasting evidence of past infection. False negative results can occur.

Parvovirus DNA can be detected by PCR in the early stages of disease in serum. This can be quicker and of use if clinical suspicion is high but the immune test negative [35]. In later stages of the infection, the viral DNA is found in tissues such as skin, bone marrow, heart and joints, and may persist throughout life [36]. Up to 25% of skin samples may harbour residual viral DNA [37,38].

Management

As the infection is usually mild and self-limiting, no specific treatment is needed. In pregnant women, rapid diagnosis is essential. In immunosuppression or haematological disease such as sickle cell disease, review for bone marrow failure is needed.

Resources

Further information

https://www.gov.uk/guidance/parvovirus-b19
https://cks.nice.org.uk/topics/parvovirus-b19-infection/
https://www.cdc.gov/parvovirusb19/index.html

Patient resources

https://www.nhs.uk/conditions/slapped-cheek-syndrome/
https://dermnetnz.org/topics/erythema-infectiosum/
(All last accessed August 2023.)

Other parvoviruses

Within the family of *Parvoviridae*, viruses in three other genera have been detected in humans [39]. The geographic prevalence varies, but more extensive studies are needed to determine potential importance in human disease.

Of the primate bocaparvoviruses, human bocavirus 1 (HBoV-1) has been found most commonly in respiratory tract infections while HBoV-2, -3 and -4 are more closely associated with gastrointestinal upset. Over 90% of adults are seropositive for HBoV-1 and antibodies to the other bocaviruses are also common [40]. An associated red maculopapular eruption on the chest or face has occasionally been observed during acute infection [41,42].

In the *Tetraparvovirus* genus, the human parvovirus 4 (PARV4) appears to be spread parenterally and may be detected in combination with other blood-borne viruses, especially in immunosuppressed individuals [43]. The acute infection usually presents with non-specific features, respiratory illness or gastrointestinal upset, and in some infection may become persistent [44]. An associated rash has rarely been reported with seroconversion [45].

Human infection with viruses in the genus *Protoparvovirus* has only been detected in the last decade. Bufavirus (BuV) and Tusavirus (TuV) may be detected in the faeces of children with diarrhoea. Cutavirus (CuV) has been discovered in the faeces and in a proportion of skin biopsies of cutaneous T-cell lymphoma patients, but appears to be absent from skin of healthy individuals [46].

HUMAN RETROVIRUS INFECTION

General description of disease domain

Human retroviruses are single-stranded RNA viruses that replicate in host cells following DNA production via reverse transcription using a viral reverse transcriptase and insertion of this DNA into the host genome using a viral integrase. This DNA, once incorporated within the host cell DNA, is known as a provirus. Retroviruses exclusively infect vertebrates and there are three main groups: oncogenic retroviruses, which cause cancer in some species; lentiviruses, which can cause severe immunodeficiency and death in humans and other animals; spumaviruses, which are benign and not linked to disease. Human retroviruses include HIV-1 and HIV-2, which cause acquired immunodeficiency syndrome and are discussed in detail elsewhere (Chapter 31). Human T-lymphotropic viruses are also important human pathogens causing haematological, neurological and skin disease [1].

HUMAN T-CELL LYMPHOTROPIC VIRUSES

General description of disease domain

Human T-cell lymphotropic viruses (HTLVs) are closely related to their simian counterparts and are believed to have arisen following cross-species transfer from monkeys to humans [1]. HTLV-1 was the first human oncogenic retrovirus to be discovered in 1977 followed by HTLV-2 in 1982 [2,3]. In 2005, two further retroviruses, HTLV-3 and HTLV-4, were identified [4]. HTLV-1 causes adult T-cell leukaemia/lymphoma (ATL), HTLV-1-associated myelopathy or tropical spastic paraparesis (HAM/TSP) and infective dermatitis. HTLV-2 was isolated from patients with a T-cell variant of hairy cell leukaemia and may be associated with myopathy. HTLV-3 and -4 have not yet been conclusively linked to human disease [1].

Epidemiology and transmission

Estimates for total numbers of people living with HTLV-1 infection range from 5 to 20 million [5,6], but this is likely an underestimation due to the scarcity of reliable data. The virus is endemic in the Caribbean, Central and South America (especially Brazil and adjacent countries), south-west Japan, sub-Saharan Africa and northern Iran [7]. There are smaller foci of incidence in South-East Asia, South Africa, Europe and central Australia. The seroprevalence is between 0.1 and 15% in endemic areas with rates of up to 30% in affected families. In non-endemic areas, seroprevalence is below 0.03% with most positive individuals being immigrants from endemic areas or intravenous drug users [8].

At least six different subtypes of HTLV-1, A–G, have been identified by molecular sequence analysis. Subtype A is more widely distributed in the world, while the subtypes B and D–G are found in Africa, with subtype C detected in Australia and Oceania [9]. Although it is found more commonly in areas of poverty and poor health, the incidence is increasing in urban areas and regions not previously associated with the infection [10].

HTLV-1 is transmitted primarily through cell-containing bodily fluids including blood, breast milk, semen and cervical secretions. The major route of transmission of HTLV-1 is via breast milk, with estimated mother to child transmission rates of 3.9–27%. Horizontal spread is by sexual transmission (mainly from male to female) and by blood (leukocyte transfer is necessary, with transmission rates of up to 63% from a positive donor).

HTLV-2 is endemic in intravenous drug users throughout the western hemisphere.

Basic biology

The human T-lymphotropic viruses belong to the *Deltaretrovirus* genus of the *Retroviridae* family, *Orthoretrovirinae* subfamily [1,11].

HTLV-1 infects CD4+ T lymphocytes. After entering the cell, the virus makes a DNA copy of its genome, using virally encoded reverse transcriptase. This integrates randomly into the cell genome. The integrated or proviral DNA produces proteins, most notably Tax, which regulate not only viral but also cellular promoters in adjacent genes and at a distance (a *trans*-activation mechanism). HTLV-1 also encodes a protein called Hbz from the antisense strand of the proviral genome that counters many Tax functions in the infected cell, but also promotes cellular proliferation, inhibits apoptosis and disrupts genomic integrity. Overall, these processes result in cellular transformation and virus-mediated oncogenesis [12].

Haematological and neurological disease associated with HTLV-1

Most HTLV-1 infections are apparently asymptomatic, although the virus probably exerts subtle effects on long-term health [12].

In 2–5% of those infected, HTLV-1 is associated with an aggressive form of ATL first described in Japan [5,13], also referred to as ATL-lymphoma (ATLL) because it usually begins as a lymphoma which progresses to a late leukaemia phase (Chapter 139). ATL is classified into smouldering, primary cutaneous tumoral, chronic, lymphoma and acute subtypes, and cutaneous lesions are common.

In 0.25–3% of infections, HTLV-1 is also associated with a chronic neurological disease – HTLV-1-associated myelopathy/tropical spastic paraparesis (HAM/TSP) [14]. It is not known what determines the form of disease HTLV-1 infection can take.

The risks of both complications are greater in those with a higher proviral load [15] and the development of HAM/TSP is linked with immunological response [16]. The interval between infection and disease is considerably shorter for TSP: 6 months to 3 years has been recorded following blood transfusion. HTLV-1 is also associated with uveitis.

Infective dermatitis associated with HTLV-1

Synonyms and inclusions
- HTLV-1-associated infective dermatitis
- Infective dermatitis

Introduction and general description

There is a high prevalence of skin disease in people living with HTLV-1 infection. This includes xerosis, ichthyosis and seborrhoeic dermatitis [17,**18**]. Infective dermatitis associated with HTLV-1 infection (IDH) is a specific inflammatory disease of childhood which develops in a minority of individuals with HTLV-1 infection [19,20]. Although the disease may clear spontaneously in adolescence, it is also seen in adulthood [21,**22**,23]. There is a high risk of development of TSP/HAM, with between 30 and 47% showing signs of the disease in later life, and also a risk of ATLL [24,25].

Epidemiology
Incidence and prevalence
Infectious dermatitis develops in HTLV1-positive children and seems to be more common in the Caribbean and in Brazil than in other areas of HLTV-1 endemicity [20]. The onset is most frequent between the age of 2 and 3 years, but may be as early as a few months or as late as age 11 years. The disease has been reported in adults [**22**,23,26] when the skin disease may present together with or after the development of ATLL [27]. The disease is more common in females [28].

Associated diseases
As well as an increased risk for TSP/HAM, there is also a much lower risk for the development of ATLL [29,30]. Patients with TSP/HAM may have other associated immunological manifestations such as uveitis and myositis, and these may rarely be seen in children with infective dermatitis.

Pathophysiology
Predisposing factors
Vertical acquisition of HTLV-1 via breastfeeding from an infected mother is the main predisposing factor.

Presentation
The dermatitis is often most marked on the scalp, around the ears and the nares, in the axillae and groin and on the neck. In these areas, but especially around the nostrils, there are often erosions and crusting [25]. There may be a watery nasal discharge. Blepharitis and conjunctivitis are very common.

The dermatitis is mildly to moderately pruritic and lichenification is not a major feature.

Differential diagnosis
Seborrhoeic dermatitis, atopic eczema, contact dermatitis [**22**].

Pathology
It is not known what leads to the development of the disease in only some HTLV-1 infected children. There is some evidence to support a high proviral load [27,31] and a marked Th1 response [32], but an undefined genetic predisposition is also suggested [33]. Histologically it has two patterns: a superficial perivascular dermatitis or a lichenoid dermatitis, and epidermal hyperplasia may mimic psoriasis. The infiltrate is composed of a predominance of CD8-positive lymphocytes [**22**].

Complications and co-morbidities
Lymphadenopathy, anaemia.

Disease course and prognosis
If the child remains well without development of TSP/HAM, the infective dermatitis often improves and disappears in the teenage years [25].

Investigations
If HTLV-1-associated infective dermatitis is suspected, serology or PCR for HTLV-1 should be performed. Skin swabs to confirm bacterial infection and guide antibiotic therapy are needed. Infection with *Staphylococcus aureus* or *Streptococcus* is very common, especially in the skin around the nostrils.

Management
Appropriate antibiotic treatment leads to disease improvement, but relapse occurs when antibiotics are discontinued [34]. Therefore, prolonged antibiotic therapy against *Staph. aureus* and/or *Strep. pyogenes* is usually needed.

Symptomatic treatment of the dermatitis with emollients and application of mild to moderate potency topical steroids is of use.

Resources

Further information
https://www.who.int/news-room/fact-sheets/detail/human-t-lymphotropic-virus-type-1 (last accessed August 2023).

VIRAL INSECT-BORNE AND HAEMORRHAGIC FEVERS

Viral haemorrhagic fevers (VHFs) are caused by RNA viruses from seven different families: *Arenaviridae, Peribunyaviridae, Hantaviridae, Nairoviridae, Phenuiviridae* (all of the order *Bunyavirales*), *Filoviridae* (order *Mononegavirales*) and *Flaviviridae* (order *Amarillovirales*) (Table 25.13).

The insect-borne viruses of the family *Togaviridae* cause a variety of infections that are less severe than VHFs.

General description of disease domain

Most VHFs are severe, multisystem diseases in which fever, vascular damage and haemorrhage are prominent features and mortality is frequently high. They are seen mainly in tropical areas where they are endemic, but with increasing global travel, cases are now not uncommonly seen outside these areas [**1**,2].

Suspected cases of VHF should be isolated. Definitive diagnosis is usually made at a reference laboratory with advanced biological containment capabilities and handling of specimens for testing must only be carried out after discussion with the microbiologist [**1**].

Basic biology

Most of these viruses cause zoonotic infections, the human being an accidental host, but human-to-human transmission also occurs.

Thrombocytopenia is present in all VHFs and reduced levels of coagulation factors in many [3]. Additional mechanisms which may apply in some cases are platelet dysfunction, disseminated intravascular coagulation, circulating anticoagulants and vascular injury. All can result in circulatory shock with high mortality [3].

Table 25.13 Viruses causing haemorrhagic fevers in humans and related viruses.

Family	Genus	Species	Disease	Virus abbreviation
Arenaviridae	Old World	Lassa virus	Lassa fever	LASV
		Lujo virus	Lujo haemorrhagic fever	LUJV
		Lymphocytic choriomeningitis virus	Lymphocytic choriomeningitis	LCMV
	New World (Tacaribe complex viruses)	Junin virus	Argentinian haemorrhagic fever	JUNV
		Mapucho virus	Bolivian haemorrhagic fever	MACV
		Guanarito virus	Venezuelan haemorrhagic fever	GTOV
		Sabia virus	Brazilian haemorrhagic fever	SABV
		Chapare virus	Bolivian haemorrhagic fever	CHPV
		Latino virus	Bolivian haemorrhagic fever	LATV
		Whitewater Arroyo virus	Haemorrhagic fever with liver failure	WWAV
Peribunyaviridae	Orthobunyavirus	Bunyamwera virus	Bunyamwera fever	BUNV
		Bwamba virus	Bwamba fever	BWAV
		Oropouche virus	Oropouche fever	OROV
Hantaviridae	Orthohantavirus	Hantaan virus	Haemorrhagic fever with renal syndrome	HTNV
		Sin Nombre virus	Hantavirus pulmonary syndrome	SNV
Nairoviridae	Orthonairovirus	Crimean–Congo haemorrhagic fever virus	Crimean–Congo haemorrhagic fever	CCHFV
Phenuiviridae	Phlebovirus	Rift valley fever virus	Rift valley fever	RVFV
Filoviridae	Orthomarburgvirus	Marburg marburgvirus	Marburg haemorrhagic fever	MARV
	Orthoebolavirus	Bundibugyo ebolavirus	Ebola virus disease	BDBV
		Sudan ebolavirus	Ebola virus disease	SUDV
		Taï Forest ebolavirus	Ebola virus disease	TAFV
		Zaire ebolavirus	Ebola virus disease	EBOV
Flaviviridae	Orthoflavivirus	Yellow fever virus	Yellow fever	YFV
		Dengue fever virus	Dengue fever	DENV 1–4
		Kyasanur forest disease virus	Kyasanur forest disease	KFDV
		Omsk haemorrhagic fever virus	Omsk haemorrhagic fever	OHFV
		Zika virus	Zika fever	ZIKV

ARENAVIRUS INFECTIONS

There are two groups of arenaviruses that cause severe VHF in humans – Old World and New World viruses – based on genetic differences as well as where the viruses are geographically distributed [2]. Lymphocytic choriomeningitis virus causes a meningoencephalitis, not VHF.

General description of disease domain

Rodents are the natural hosts for these viruses. Contact with urine, droppings or other secretions from infected animals can lead to human disease after an incubation period of 1–3 weeks. Person-to-person transmission occurs with certain arenaviruses (Chapare, Lassa, Machupo and Lujo viruses) when there is direct contact with the blood or other body fluids of infected individuals or contact with contaminated objects.

Lassa fever and Lujo haemorrhagic fever have a high mortality when severe. The New World viruses all produce very similar diseases [4].

Lassa fever

Introduction and general description

This disease was first recognised in humans in 1969 in Nigeria [5]. Although most cases occur in sub-Saharan Africa, especially in West Africa (including Sierra Leone, Liberia, Guinea and Nigeria), imported cases in travellers are diagnosed occasionally [6].

Epidemiology
Incidence and prevalence
In West Africa, there are at least 500 000 infections per year with 5–10 000 deaths annually [6]. Serological surveys in endemic areas have shown that up to 50% of the population of some villages have had past infection.

Pathophysiology
Causative organisms
The natural host is the multimammate rat, *Mastomys natalensis*, a common rodent in West African villages [7]. Transmission to humans occurs most commonly in the wet season, producing short-lived outbreaks or epidemics, with secondary infections by human-to-human spread in households and hospital staff [8].

Clinical features
Presentation
The incubation period of Lassa fever is 2–21 days. Fever, malaise, headache and non-productive cough herald the onset of disease [6].

A maculopapular or petechial rash over the face, arms and thorax may be seen. There is usually joint, retrosternal and lumbar pain with a developing painful sore throat. Conjunctivitis and periorbital oedema are common. High fever and severe prostration follow [9–11].

Classification of severity
In severe cases, features may include diarrhoea, leading to hypovolaemia, renal damage with proteinuria, central nervous system involvement with confusion, coma, convulsions and respiratory complications. These are most likely in the first week of illness.

Complications and co-morbidities
Bleeding is rare but indicates a poor prognosis. Symptoms can be difficult to distinguish from malaria and typhoid and these should be considered in an individual returning from an endemic area with an appropriate history [7]. Misdiagnosis at the onset of infection may be more common since the Covid-19 pandemic in early 2020 [10].

Disease course and prognosis
Recovery begins in the second week of illness but in severe cases, deterioration is evident at about day 7. The overall mortality rate is 2–4% but rises in severely affected hospitalised patients to 10–20%. Lassa fever in the third trimester of pregnancy is associated with a greater than 30% mortality rate. In survivors, about a quarter develop deafness in one or both ears, which may be permanent, or may slowly resolve [7].

Investigations
Diagnosis is dependent on an accurate history and an understanding of the geography of the disease, supported by laboratory investigations: IgM and IgG ELISA and RT-PCR in the early stages of disease. These may not be available in some endemic areas and the ReLASV Antigen Rapid Test has been developed for bedside use in resource-limited regions [11]. Lassa fever is a notifiable disease in many countries [7].

Management
Currently, there are no approved vaccines or treatments for Lassa fever. Off-label therapeutics for acute infection used include ribavirin (given IV within 6 days of symptom onset) and convalescent plasma, but efficacy is suboptimal. Ribavirin is occasionally used as post-exposure prophylaxis for high-risk exposure to Lassa virus. Newer agents such as favipiravir, taribavirin, arevirumab-3, pegylated interferon and LASV-specific monoclonal antibodies are under evaluation. Supportive measures are essential. Given the limited treatment options, prevention of infection should be prioritised, particularly in endemic regions [7,11,12].

Resources

Further information
https://www.gov.uk/guidance/lassa-fever-origins-reservoirs-transmission-and-guidelines
https://www.who.int/health-topics/lassa-fever#tab=tab_1

Patient resources
https://www.cdc.gov/vhf/lassa/index.html
(All last accessed August 2023.)

Lujo virus haemorrhagic fever

Definition and nomenclature
Lujo virus was first identified in West Africa in 2008 and was the second African haemorrhagic fever virus to be described [13].

Synonyms and inclusions
- Zambian haemorrhagic fever

Epidemiology
Incidence and prevalence
A series of five cases has been described, starting with a patient in Zambia whose source of infection was unknown: four health care workers were subsequently infected [13].

Causative organisms
As with other arenaviruses, Lujo virus has a rodent host as its reservoir and humans are infected by direct or inhalational contact with urine or faeces of infected rodents. Person-to-person infection is most likely the result of direct contact with the body fluids of an infected person. The Lujo virus is related to Lassa fever virus [14].

Clinical features
Presentation
After an incubation period of 1–2 weeks, the illness starts with fever, headache, pharyngitis, diarrhoea and myalgia. A morbilliform eruption, widespread but mainly affecting the face and trunk, can be accompanied by facial swelling [15,16].

Classification of severity
In severe and potentially fatal disease, respiratory failure and neurological decline develop. Haemorrhagic features with profound bleeding can occur [15,16].

Disease course and prognosis
In five reported cases, the mortality was 80%, usually occurring 10–13 days after onset [13].

Management
First line
General supportive measures with fluid balance and blood transfusions.

Second line
Ribavirin may be of use both in acute infection and as post-exposure prophylaxis.

Resources

Further information
https://www.cdc.gov/vhf/lujo/index.html (last accessed August 2023).

Argentinian, Bolivian, Brazilian and Venezuelan haemorrhagic fevers

Synonyms and inclusions
- Jujin haemorrhagic fever (Argentinian haemorrhagic fever)
- Machupo haemorrhagic fever (Bolivian haemorrhagic fever)
- Chapare haemorrhagic fever (Bolivian haemorrhagic fever)

Table 25.14 Haemorrhagic fevers and the natural hosts of the virus.

Disease	Virus	Host	Geographic distribution
Argentinian haemorrhagic fever	Junin virus	Drylands vesper mouse (*Calomys musculinus*)	Argentina
Bolivian haemorrhagic fever	Machupo virus	Large vesper mouse (*Calomys callosus*)	Bolivia
Bolivian haemorrhagic fever	Chapare virus	Unknown	Bolivia
Bolivian haemorrhagic fever	Latino virus	Large vesper mouse (*Calomys callosus*)	Bolivia
Brazilian haemorrhagic fever	Sabiá virus	Unknown	Brazil
Venezuelan haemorrhagic fever	Guanarito virus	Short-tailed cane mouse (*Zygodontomys brevicauda*)	Venezuela
Haemorrhagic fever	Whitewater Arroyo virus	White-throated woodrat (*Neotoma albigula*)	South-western USA

Introduction and general description

These arenaviruses are closely related and are grouped together as the New World or Tacaribe complex viruses as the diseases they cause are clinically alike [16,17–19,20,21].

The viruses and their natural hosts are listed in Table 25.14.

Epidemiology

Incidence and prevalence

The viruses and the diseases they cause are currently limited to the areas in which they were first described.

Clinical features

History

Spread from rodent to human can occur directly, as via a bite or handling animals, or indirectly by harvesting food crops in areas contaminated by rodent urine.

Presentation

The 3–21-day incubation is followed by a high fever, headache, malaise and myalgia, redness or a petechial eruption of the face, neck and upper chest, a pharyngeal enanthem and petechiae. Epistaxis and haematemesis may also occur in the first week of the illness. Shock ensues in over half the patients.

Disease course and prognosis

These infections are associated with about a 15–60% mortality rate if untreated [20].

Investigations

Diagnosis is usually by detection of viral antigens by ELISA. RT-PCR can be helpful but is not in routine diagnostic use [1].

Management

Preventative measures include rodent control and avoidance of rodent contact. The incidence of Argentinian haemorrhagic fever has reduced following the use of live attenuated JUNV vaccine and other vaccines are in development [20,22].

First line

Supportive measures are the mainstay of treatment [20].

Second line

Current treatment for Argentinian haemorrhagic fever includes transfusion of immune plasma and possibly ribavirin [20,23]. Ribavirin can be used for all infections, but no real measure of its efficacy has been made [24]. Other treatments in development include the antiviral favipravir, monoclonal antibodies and leflunamide [20,25].

Resources

Patient resources

https://www.cdc.gov/vhf/virus-families/arenaviridae.html (last accessed August 2023).

BUNYAVIRUS INFECTIONS

General description of disease domain

A number of arthropod members of the Bunyaviruses, Flaviviruses, Hantaviruses, Phleboviruses and Nairoviruses cause febrile illnesses (Table 25.13). These may be severe, as in tick-borne Crimean Congo haemorrhagic fever [16,26–31], the mosquito-borne zoonosis Rift Valley fever [32] and the febrile illness associated with Oropouche viruses [33] and Kayanur Forest disease (a filovirus) [34]. There may be hepatitis and haemorrhagic features. In severely affected individuals, skin and mucosal signs of petechial rashes, bruising, mucosal petechiae and bleeding are indicators of a higher mortality risk [16,35].

Some related viruses found predominantly in sub-Saharan Africa, such as Bwamba fever virus [36] and Bunyamwera virus [37], can cause very mild or subclinical infections. When symptomatic, there is mild fever, myalgia and occasionally a rash.

Hantaviruses have a rodent reservoir and are transmitted directly from animal to human [38,39]. Most infections are subclinical, but two types of illness are recognised:
1. Haemorrhagic fever with renal syndrome (HFRS) presents abruptly after a 2–4-week incubation period as a flu-like illness followed by a hypotensive phase on day 5, which can be followed by acute renal failure. Petechial bleeding and substantial haemorrhage are recorded in <10% of the cases. Mortality varies with the infecting strain from <1 to 10% and occurs typically in the oliguric phase.
2. Hantavirus pulmonary syndrome develops after inhalation of the virus and has a sudden onset with fever, cough, myalgia and headache. Pulmonary oedema and respiratory failure (adult respiratory distress syndrome) rapidly ensue and are associated with a high mortality rate.

Diagnosis
IgG and IgM ELISA and RT-PCR can be used to confirm infection [1].

Treatment
Treatment is primarily supportive. There are no approved treatments or vaccines. However, ribavirin has been used in Crimean Congo haemorrhagic fever with some benefit and in the early stages of HFRS [29]. Vaccines are in development.

Resources

Further information
https://www.cdc.gov/vhf/virus-families/bunyaviridae.html (last accessed August 2023).

FILOVIRUS INFECTIONS

General description of disease domain

The *Filoviridae* cause two serious human diseases, Marburg haemorrhagic fever and Ebola virus disease (formerly Ebola haemorrhagic fever) [40,41].

Marburg and Ebola haemorrhagic fevers

Definition and nomenclature
The Marburg and Ebola viruses produce very similar diseases and so are considered together here. Both cause severe haemorrhagic fever with a high mortality rate. They infect humans and non-human primates (monkeys, gorillas and chimpanzees).

Synonyms and inclusions
- Marburg virus disease
- Ebola virus disease

Introduction and general description
Marburg virus disease (MVD) was first observed in 1967 simultaneously in laboratories in Marburg and Frankfurt, Germany and Belgrade, Yugoslavia when 30 infections (seven of which were fatal) followed the importation of African green monkeys (*Ceropithecus aethiops*) from Uganda [42,43]. Further outbreaks of Marburg disease have occurred in Africa, Kenya, Zimbabwe, Uganda, Democratic Republic of Congo and Angola.

The closely related but antigenically distinct Ebola virus was first identified near the Ebola River in Democratic Republic of Congo (formerly Zaire) in 1976 [44]. Outbreaks of Ebola virus disease (EVD) have since occurred sporadically in Central Africa, Congo, Uganda, Gabon, South Sudan and the Ivory Coast. In 2014–16 a prolonged outbreak started in Guinea and became a global epidemic within months, mainly spread between family members, but also in travellers returning to the USA [40,45]. In the 2018 outbreak in eastern Democratic Republic of the Congo, more than 32 000 people were infected and 13 600 deaths were reported [40,41].

Epidemiology
Causative organisms
These filoviruses are found only in Africa. Four species of Ebola virus cause human disease: Bundibugyo, Sudan, Zaire and Taï Forest [46]. Reston ebolavirus causes disease in non-human primates and pigs and it is unknown whether Bombali ebolavirus, discovered in bats in Sierra Leone in 2018, causes human disease [40,41].

Incidence and prevalence
African fruit bats (*Rousettus aegyptiacus*) are the natural host for Marburg virus. Occasional cases are reported in visitors to caves or mines inhabited by bats via contact with bat faeces or aerosols, but infection usually occurs from handling infected animals or contact with non-human primates infected with the virus. Bats and non-human primates are also the likely source for Ebola virus. Once humans are infected there is a risk of person-to-person spread via blood and bodily fluids (including sexual contact) or contaminated objects including needles and syringes. Health care workers are at particularly high risk. The virus can persist in some bodily fluids for as long as 80 days [40,41].

Pathophysiology
Ebola virus enters through mucous membranes, skin and parenterally. It infects monocytes, macrophages, dendritic cells, endothelial cells, fibroblasts, hepatocytes, adrenal cortical cells and epithelial cells. Hepatocellular necrosis is associated with dysregulation of clotting factors and subsequent coagulopathy. Adrenocortical necrosis is associated with hypotension and impaired steroid synthesis. Release of pro-inflammatory cytokines causes vascular leak and clotting impairment, ultimately resulting in multiorgan failure and shock [41].

Clinical features [40,41,42,47–50]
Presentation [51]
The incubation period is usually 2–21 days (average 8–10 days) followed by the sudden onset of headache, high fever and myalgia. Towards the end of the first, early generalisation phase (days 1–5), a morbilliform rash commonly develops, more obvious on paler skins and most prominent on the buttocks, trunk and upper arms. Initially perifollicular red macules occur which progress to maculopapular lesions and become confluent. An enanthem may be present as a dark red palatal discoloration and vesicles may occur on the soft palate simultaneously or preceding the exanthem. In severe cases, the rash may become petechial or purpuric, with a diffuse livid redness over the face, trunk and limbs.

Disease course and prognosis
In the second or early organ phase (days 5–13), diarrhoea and dehydration, hepatitis and renal damage occur. Haemorrhage, commonly gastrointestinal and mucosal, begins on about the fifth day of illness.

After 2 weeks, the patient enters the third phase – either the convalescent phase or, if severe and progressive, the late organ stage. Death is usually preceded by severe haemorrhage and multiorgan dysfunction between days 8 and 17. In survivors, desquamation of the rash occurs about a week after its onset.

Fatality rates for MVD are 23–90% [16] and for EVD are 80–90% [41].

Diagnosis and investigations

Clinical diagnosis of MVD and EVD may be challenging, as many signs and symptoms are similar to other infectious diseases endemic in these areas (e.g. dengue, malaria and typhoid fever) as well as Covid-19 during the recent pandemic.

RT-PCR and antigen ELISA are used during MVD disease to diagnose cases within a few days of symptom onset. Antibody ELISA can show IgM during the disease and IgG for up to 5 months after disease. Virus isolation should only be done in high biocontainment laboratories. EVD is usually diagnosed by RT-PCR [1].

Management

Suspected cases must be isolated and extreme care taken to avoid spread to family, health care workers and other contacts. Virus excretion continues for days to weeks in survivors and all items contaminated with body fluids should ideally be incinerated or disinfected thoroughly.

Early supportive care improves survival. Ribavirin has no effect on filoviruses. Two monoclonal antibody therapies (Inmazeb® and Ebanga™) were approved for the treatment of Zaire EVD in 2020 [52]. A vaccine against Zaire ebolavirus (rVSV-ZEBOV) was approved in 2019 and is recommended as pre-exposure prophylaxis in adults at occupational risk of exposure [53].

Resources

Further information
https://www.cdc.gov/vhf/ebola/
https://www.who.int/en/news-room/fact-sheets/detail/ebola-virus-disease
https://www.gov.uk/government/collections/ebola-virus-disease-clinical-management-and-guidance
(All last accessed August 2023.)

FLAVIVIRUS INFECTIONS

This family contains the largest group of antigenically related arthropod-borne viruses (arboviruses), transmitted by both mosquitoes and ticks [54]. More than 50% of these viruses cause disease in humans, including yellow fever, dengue and Zika viruses [55,56,57,58,59]. The causes for the increasing incidence and geographic expansion of these diseases in recent years are likely to include migration of humans and animals, development of air transport and travel, global land use change, climate change, deforestation and urbanisation [60,61]. This has been a cause for international concern and there is an urgent need for development of vaccines, better diagnostic tests and vector control tools [56,58,59,62].

General description of disease domain

Although yellow fever, dengue and Zika virus infection are all associated with cutaneous manifestations, most flavivirus infections, including the tick-borne encephalitides complex, are not. Hepatitis C virus is also a flavivirus (see earlier in this chapter).

Yellow fever

Introduction and general description

Yellow fever is an acute viral haemorrhagic disease transmitted by infected mosquitoes. 'Yellow' refers to the jaundice that occurs in some patients. The clinical illness manifests in three stages: infection, remission and intoxication [59,63]. After an incubation period of 3–6 days, infection causes general malaise, fever, headache, musculoskeletal aches and nausea. This is followed by a period of remission when most patients fully recover. However, in 15–20% symptoms recur after 24–48 hours, with progression to the intoxication stage consisting of hepatitis causing jaundice, abdominal pain and vomiting. Severe leukopenia and thrombocytopenia may develop with haemorrhage from the mouth, nose, eyes or stomach [59,63,64].

Epidemiology

Incidence and prevalence

The virus is endemic in subtropical South America and Africa, with increasing incidence recently in West Africa. Imported cases are reported in travellers [59,63,64].

Pathophysiology

Causative organisms

The virus is transmitted by mosquitoes of the *Aedes* and *Haemogogus* species.

Diagnosis

Yellow fever may simulate malaria, leptospirosis, viral hepatitis and other haemorrhagic fevers. PCR testing of blood and urine can detect the virus in the early stages and ELISA is used to identify antibodies in the later stages.

Management

Supportive treatment improves survival. There is no specific antiviral drug for yellow fever. Prophylactic vaccination with the live attenuated vaccine provides lifelong protection, but should be used with caution in immunocompromised individuals and those over 60 years [65]. In epidemics it is used together with vector control measures to eradicate the mosquito vectors.

Resources

Further information
https://www.gov.uk/government/uploads/system/uploads/attachment_data/file/306941/Green_Book_Chapter_35_v3_3.pdf
http://www.who.int/mediacentre/factsheets/fs100/en/
https://www.cdc.gov/yellowfever/index.html

Patient resources
https://nathnacyfzone.org.uk/factsheet/66/yellow-fever-factsheet
(All last accessed August 2023.)

Dengue

Synonyms and inclusions
- Break-bone fever

Introduction and general description
Dengue is perhaps the most important mosquito-borne infection in humans, affecting 100 million people annually worldwide. The virus causes a range of infections from asymptomatic to dengue haemorrhagic fever which has a high mortality [56,57,66].

Epidemiology
Incidence and prevalence
Since the 1980s, the disease has spread widely in Africa, Central and South America, the Indian subcontinent, Queensland in Australia and Oceania, as well as South-East Asia, where annual epidemics are common and increasing in size. The infection is endemic in more than 100 countries, particularly the South-East Asia region, western Pacific region and the Americas, and almost half of the world population lives in areas with a risk of dengue [67].

Pathophysiology
Causative organisms
There are four antigenically distinct dengue viruses – serotypes DENV 1–4; infection is followed by lifelong immunity to the specific serotype and infection up to four times is possible. The second dengue virus infection is most likely to cause severe disease and hospitalisation.

The virus is spread via mosquitoes, mainly *Aedes aegypti* but also *A. albopictus*.

Clinical features
Infection can be asymptomatic or cause an acute self-limiting febrile illness or lead to a severe haemorrhagic fever which is associated with a 1–10% mortality. The usual form after primary infection in childhood is asymptomatic.

Presentation
Dengue fever starts after an incubation period of 3–14 (average 7) days as a fluctuating fever with nausea, vomiting, headache, myalgia, arthralgia, bone pain, eye pain and severe backache. A rash develops on the third to fourth day of the fever in about half the patients. There may be generalised redness, but usually the rash is maculopapular or scarlatiniform and can be itchy. It may start on the legs and spread caudally or on the chest and trunk and spread to the face, arms and legs [57,68,69]. The rash fades as the fever subsides (day 7) but can pass through a phase with petechiae on the arms and legs due to mild thrombocytopenia. In people with skin of colour, the rash may be more difficult to appreciate.

Mucosal involvement with oro-pharyngeal or conjunctival injection is seen in about 30%.

Clinical variants
Dengue haemorrhagic fever and dengue shock syndrome occur, most commonly in children, in areas where dengue is hyperepidemic and there is co-circulation of multiple serotypes of the virus.

People who have been infected with one serotype and subsequently have a second infection with a different serotype are at greater risk of developing dengue haemorrhagic fever/dengue shock syndrome. The acute high fever is followed by a prolonged vasculopathy, in which fluid is lost to tissue spaces causing hypovolaemic shock. The capillary leak also leads to thrombocytopenia and clotting disturbances, causing a haemorrhagic diathesis, which is manifest as petechiae and can be demonstrated by a positive tourniquet test. The permeability increases which leads to further plasma loss, some of which collects as effusions in the pleural and abdominal cavities. Dengue shock syndrome is usually fatal without meticulous fluid replacement and plasma expansion [57].

Differential diagnosis
Certain clinical diagnosis from other arbovirus infections may not be possible, but the combination of thrombocytopenia and haemoconcentration is highly suspicious. Measles and other exanthemata may require exclusion [57].

Classification of severity
Around 500 000 patients per year have severe dengue fever or dengue haemorrhagic fever/dengue shock syndrome necessitating hospital admission.

Severe dengue is classified as illness with features of systemic vascular leakage. Early warning signs of development of severe dengue include abdominal pain, persistent vomiting, oedema, lethargy, hepatomegaly and increasing haematocrit with decreasing platelet count and rising serum albumin, aspartate aminotransferase (AST) and alanine aminotransferase (ALT) concentrations [57,70]. Disease can be more severe in pregnant women with adverse fetal outcomes [57,71].

Investigations
Confirmation of dengue infection is obtained by culture or detection of the virus in blood by RT-PCR or ELISA for the NS1 antigen in the acute phase or by serological studies on acute and convalescent sera [57].

Management
Prevention
Vector control is important in endemic areas. A live-attenuated dengue vaccine (Dengvaxia) against all four serotypes (DENV1–4) is approved for use in children aged 9–16 years with laboratory evidence of previous dengue virus infection and living in areas where dengue is endemic [72,73].

First line
There is no specific antiviral treatment, so management is symptomatic and supportive [57,58]. Non-steroidal anti-inflammatory drugs are avoided due to the risk of bleeding. Paracetamol can be used as an antipyretic and analgesic.

Second line
In dengue haemorrhagic fever/dengue shock syndrome, oral and intravenous fluids must be managed carefully to balance fluid lost through vascular leakage [57,70].

Resources

Further information
https://www.cdc.gov/dengue/index.html

Patient resources
https://www.who.int/news-room/fact-sheets/detail/dengue-and-severe-dengue
https://www.gov.uk/government/collections/dengue-fever-guidance-data-and-analysis
(All last accessed August 2023.)

Zika virus

Introduction and general description
Zika virus was isolated in 1947 from the blood of a sentinel rhesus monkey in the Zika Forest, Uganda. Serological evidence of infection was subsequently found in Africa and Asia and the first large human outbreak occurred in 2007. Zika virus infection was considered a mild disease until 2015 when severe neurological complications were identified during an epidemic with its epicentre in Brazil [55,56,74].

Epidemiology
Incidence and prevalence
Outbreaks of Zika have been reported in tropical Africa, South-East Asia and the Pacific Islands. Because the symptoms of Zika are similar to many other diseases, cases may not have been recognised [56,74].

Pathophysiology
Causative organisms
Zika virus (ZIKV) is usually transmitted to humans by mosquitoes, *Aedes* species (*Ae. Aegypti* and *Ae. albopictus*), which breed in domestic water-holding containers. Non-human primates and humans are the main reservoirs, and during outbreaks human-to-vector-to-human (anthroponotic) transmission occurs. Non-vector vertical transmission is reported perinatally and *in utero* [75,76]; sexual and transfusion-related transmission have also been reported and ZIKV persists in bodily fluids [77]. ZIKV co-circulates with other flaviviruses such as dengue and high antibody titres to DENV were associated with reduced risk of ZIKV infection and symptoms in Brazil [78].

Clinical features
Presentation
The incubation period is 3–14 days. Infection may be asymptomatic. Fever with maculopapular rash, arthralgia, conjunctivitis myalgia and headache is characteristic of acute infection. This is usually mild and lasts for 3–7 days. The rash is similar in adults, children and pregnant women, and is itchy, may have a marked papular component and often starts on the chest and spreads to the rest of the body. Conjunctivitis and petechiae on the palate are rare [79].

Clinical variants
Severe disease is uncommon and mortality is low. However, severe neurological complications may occur and Guillain-Barré syndrome, acute myelitis and meningoencephalitis have all been reported. ZIKV infection during pregnancy confers an increased risk of miscarriage and stillbirth. It is teratogenic, causing microcephaly and other severe fetal brain defects (congenital Zika syndrome), and mortality is increased in childhood [75].

Differential diagnosis
The differential diagnosis is broad, based on clinical features, and includes dengue, chikungunya, malaria, rickettsia, leptospirosis, group A streptococcus, rubella, measles, parvovirus, enterovirus and adenovirus.

Investigations
RT-PCR in serum is the main test for ZIKV detection in the first 5 days of disease. PCR positivity of urine persists for longer. Because viraemia is short lived, a negative RT-PCR does not rule out Zika infection and serological tests for IgM antibodies should also be performed. Because of similar symptoms and geographic distribution, patients with suspected ZIKV infections also should be investigated for possible dengue or chikungunya virus infection. However, there is strong cross-reactivity between ZIKV, DENV and other flaviviruses.

Management
First line
Treatment is generally supportive. No specific antiviral treatment is available. NSAIDs should be avoided until dengue is excluded to avoid haemorrhage.

Prevention
ZIKV vaccines are not currently available but are in development [80–82]. As with dengue and chikungunya, people with ZIKV infection should be protected from further mosquito exposure during the initial illness to prevent infection of other mosquitoes and reduce the risk of local transmission.

Resources

Further information
https://www.cdc.gov/zika/index.html
https://www.who.int/news-room/fact-sheets/detail/zika-virus
https://www.gov.uk/government/collections/zika-virus-zikv-clinical-and-travel-guidance
(Last accessed August 2023.)

TOGAVIRUS INFECTIONS

General description of disease domain

Viruses of the *Alphavirus* genus of the *Togaviridae* family are mostly mosquito-borne arbovirus infections. The Old World alphaviruses, which include Sindbis virus, chikungunya virus and Ross River virus, cause a clinical syndrome characterised by an acute febrile illness, maculopapular rash and polyarthritis (Table 25.15). New World alphaviruses, including Venezuelan equine encephalitis virus, eastern equine encephalitis virus and western equine encephalitis virus, induce encephalomyelitis but no exanthem. Following recovery from the acute infection, debilitating arthralgia

Table 25.15 Togaviruses of *Alphavirus* genus causing human diseases with cutaneous involvement.

Alphavirus species	Abbreviation	Disease	Vertebrate reservoir	Distribution
Sindbis virus	SINV	Rash, arthritis	Birds	North Europe, Africa, Australia
Chikungunya virus	CHIKV	Rash, arthritis	Primates, humans	Africa, Latin America, India, South-East Asia
O'Nyong-Nyong virus	QNNV	Rash, arthritis	Primates, humans	Africa
Mayaro virus	MAYV	Rash, arthritis	Primates, humans	South America
Ross River virus	RRV	Rash, arthritis	Mammals, humans	Australia, South Pacific
Barmah Forest virus	BFV	Rash, arthritis	Mammals, humans	Australia

and neurological complications may persist [83]. As with other arbovirus infections, climate change may be changing the epidemiology of many alphavirus infections [60].

The *Rubivirus* genus of *Togaviridae* includes Rubella virus (RUBV, see later).

Basic biology

Togavirus infections may be differentiated by their virus-specific IgM response in an ELISA or by molecular detection of viral RNA in blood by RT-PCR.

Sindbis virus infection

Definition and nomenclature
The Sindbis virus (SINV) was first isolated in 1952 in Cairo, Egypt, and can be regarded as the prototype togavirus causing a mosquito-borne viral fever [84].

Synonyms and inclusions
- Ockelbo disease (Sweden)
- Pogosta disease (Finland)
- Karelian fever (Russia)

Epidemiology
SINV infection can occur in any individual in contact with mosquitoes. However, the incidence is highest in northern Europe where SINV is endemic [84,85].

Predisposing factors
In Sweden, the disease is more common in rural areas and in individuals with obesity, hypertension or with a history of cerebrovascular disease [84].

Causative organisms
SINV has a worldwide distribution. Epidemics have been reported in Europe (Finland, Sweden, Norway, Germany, Slovakia), Asia, North Africa and South Africa, the Middle East and Australia. The virus vectors are mosquitoes of several species (*Culex*, *Culiseta*, *Anopheles*, *Aedes*) [86]; birds are the vertebrate reservoir.

Genetics
There is some evidence that HLA type can influence susceptibility to infection, with HLA-DRB1*01 being more common in affected members of a population [87].

Environmental factors
European outbreaks have been most common in summer and early autumn, when mosquitoes are most abundant. In Finland, epidemics have occurred in a 7-year cycle. There is no evidence of human-to-human transmission [84].

Clinical features
History
The disease occurs in places and at times of mosquito breeding. The features of the infection appear between 1 and 2 weeks after inoculation by mosquito bite [86].

Presentation
Non-specific features of malaise, mild fever, headache and musculoskeletal aches can be followed rapidly by a more definite peripheral arthritis and a widespread rash which is often itchy [84]. The eruption consists of small papules and macules up to 1 cm in diameter, most abundant on the trunk, thighs and limbs. There is relative sparing of the hands, feet and face.

Disease course and prognosis
The rash clears within a week. Arthralgia often lasts for several months and persists for over a year in half those affected [88].

Investigations
Evidence of infection can be confirmed by rising titres of IgM (within 8 days) and IgG antibodies (within 11 days). RT-PCR to detect viral RNA in blood or skin is a more rapid test but may not be readily available in routine laboratories.

Management
There is no specific antiviral treatment or vaccine available for SINV infection. Treatment is symptomatic (antihistamines, non-salicylate analgesia). Personal protective measures should be taken to reduce the risk of mosquito bites [84].

Resources

Further information
https://www.ecdc.europa.eu/en/sindbis-fever/facts (last accessed August 2023).

Chikungunya fever

Definition
Chikungunya means 'bending up', which reflects the severe joint pains that are a major feature of this virus infection. Rash is seen in 20–80% of cases [89].

Introduction and general description
Chikungunya virus (CHIKV) infection is a mosquito-borne arbovirus infection which is endemic in Africa, southern Europe, South-East Asia and islands in the Indian and Pacific Oceans [58,**89**,90].

Epidemiology
Infection with CHIKV occurs after a mosquito bite usually in an endemic area. There have been epidemics in the last 15 years in Reunion Island [91], India and Sri Lanka [92], Italy [93], France [94], and China and Bhutan [95]. In 2013, CHIKV infection was found for the first time on islands in the Caribbean.

Pathophysiology
Causative organisms
CHIKV is spread by mosquitoes either directly between humans or via monkey intermediate hosts. The virus can transmit vertically from mother to child. The *Aedes aegypti* and *Aedes albopictus* mosquitoes are the most common vectors and over recent years the latter has adapted to life in southern Europe [96]. The virus has also developed a mutation which facilitates life in the *Aedes albopictus* mosquito [97].

Clinical features
Presentation
The incubation period is 3–7 days (range 1–12 days). The illness begins with an acute onset of fever, symmetrical polyarthralgia (often in the hands and feet), headache, anorexia and nausea. A rash develops in about half of those affected and is usually maculopapular and occasionally petechial or purpuric and may be itchy. It is most pronounced on the trunk and to a lesser extent on the limbs and may be accompanied by facial flushing. External ear redness may reflect chondritis and conjunctivitis also occurs. Ano-genital and oral ulceration is occasionally observed [98]. Acute symptoms generally resolve within 7–10 days.

Classification of severity
In more severe disease, complications may include encephalopathy and haemorrhagic features, and respiratory or liver failure [89]. Infection *in utero* or neonatally has a high chance of leading to severe infection. Risk is also increased in those over 65 years and with co-morbidities including hypertension, diabetes and cardiovascular disease. Rare complications include uveitis, retinitis, myocarditis, hepatitis, nephritis, bullous skin lesions, haemorrhage, meningoencephalitis, myelitis, Guillain-Barré syndrome and cranial nerve palsies.

Clinical variants
In children, especially infants, lesions may be vesicular or pigmented [99]. Presentation may be atypical in pregnancy [100].

Differential diagnosis
Dengue, malaria and other mosquito-transmitted arbovirus infections including other alphavirus infections should be considered.

Complications and co-morbidities
Some cases of psoriasis apparently triggered by chikungunya fever have been reported [101].

Disease course and prognosis
The fever and general malaise subside after about 3 days. The rash can be transient or last up to a week, sometimes leaving postinflammatory hyperpigmentation. The joint pains usually clear within a few days to weeks but are often persistent and more than 50% have arthralgias for more than 12 months. Most recover satisfactorily. In large epidemics, such as that in Reunion Island in 2005–7, the mortality is approximately 1/1000 but can be higher in severe or atypical cases [102].

Investigations
Viral culture to detect virus in the first 3 days of illness may be used. Detection of reverse-transcribed viral RNA from blood by PCR or hybridisation is the fastest diagnostic test in the first 8 days of illness [103]. Serological IgG and IgM antibody detection by ELISA tests after the first 4 days of illness is more readily available.

Management
The risk of CHIKV infection in endemic areas can be reduced by mosquito control. As with dengue, affected individuals should be protected from further mosquito exposure during the first week of illness to reduce the risk of further transmission. No prophylactic vaccine or specific antiviral therapies are currently approved [104,105]. General supportive measures for a virus-induced fever are used. NSAIDs can help persistent arthralgia, but should be avoided in the acute phase until dengue fever is excluded.

Resources

Further information
https://www.who.int/news-room/fact-sheets/detail/chikungunya
https://www.gov.uk/guidance/chikungunya
https://www.cdc.gov/chikungunya/index.html

Patient resources
https://www.cdc.gov/chikungunya/pdfs/chikv_fact%20sheet_cdc_general%20public_cleared.pdf
(All last accessed August 2023.)

O'Nyong-Nyong fever

Introduction and general description
O'Nyong-Nyong virus (QNNV) and the illness it causes are very similar to Sindbis virus [106,107]. The virus was first isolated in 1959 in Uganda and O'Nyong-Nyong means 'weakening of the joints'. It is spread via the *Anopheles funestus* and *Anopheles gambiae* mosquitoes.

Clinical features

Presentation

An acute onset of fever with headache, nausea and malaise is associated with musculoskeletal pains and arthralgia especially in the knees, ankles and feet. In about 80% there is an associated maculopapular eruption that is often itchy. In up to 50% of affected individuals, there is cervical lymphadenopathy and mild conjunctival injection, making clinical distinction from measles difficult.

Differential diagnosis

Other arbovirus infections, measles.

Investigations

Diagnosis is by serology or RT-PCR [108].

Ross River virus

Introduction and general description

Ross River virus (RRV) infection is spread to humans by a variety of mosquito species. The natural reservoir for RRV is suspected to be kangaroos, marsupials and other wild rodents [109].

Synonyms and inclusions
- Epidemic polyarthritis

Epidemiology

Incidence and prevalence

RRV was first identified in Townsville, Australia. It is the most common arbovirus infection in Australia where approximately 5000 cases are notified annually [109]. The virus is endemic in tropical Australia and also in Papua New Guinea and the Pacific islands. Isolated cases occur elsewhere in travellers returning from these parts of the world [110].

Age

The most common group affected is 30–40-year-olds and illness is rare under the age of 10 years.

Clinical features

Presentation

The infection is characterised by fever, polyarthritis, myalgia, rash, general malaise and lymphadenitis [111]. After an incubation period of 3–21 days (mean 9 days) a mild fever with headache and myalgia occurs. A polyarthritis of the ankles, knees, fingers and wrists is very common and rash occurs in over half. The rash is usually a non-itching, maculopapular eruption on the limbs and trunk, but can occasionally be vesicular or purpuric; it may begin several days before to 11 days after the arthritis and lasts 2–10 days [112].

Clinical variants

Chronic arthritis and tiredness can persist for up to 6 months with acute exacerbation and relapses. Recovery is universal and followed by lasting immunity.

Differential diagnosis

This infection must be distinguished from acute rubella and other arbovirus infections. In its chronic form, rheumatoid arthritis should be considered.

Investigations

In the acute phase, infection can be detected by molecular identification of the viral RNA or a rising antibody titre to RRV [112].

Management

Treatment is supportive. There are no antiviral medications or vaccines. Vector control and personal protection against mosquitoes are important in endemic areas.

Resources

Patient resources

https://wwwnc.cdc.gov/travel/diseases/ross-river-virus-disease
https://www.betterhealth.vic.gov.au/health/conditionsandtreatments/ross-river-virus-disease
https://www.health.nsw.gov.au/Infectious/factsheets/Pages/ross-river-fever.aspx (Last accessed August 2023.)

Barmah Forest virus

Definition

Barmah Forest virus (BFV) is a mosquito-borne arbovirus and was first identified near the Murray River in New South Wales, Australia. The illness it causes is similar to, but milder than, RRV [113].

Epidemiology

Incidence and prevalence

The infection is endemic in northern Queensland, Australia, where the incidence of the disease is increasing, possibly due to changes in land and irrigation practices which allow increased mosquito breeding [114].

Clinical features

Presentation

The illness presents with arthralgia and myalgia and occasionally fever, but these general symptoms may be absent. The rash, which occurs in about 90% and may be the presenting feature, is often florid and generalised. It is maculopapular but may be vesicular. Facial urticaria and oedema may be seen [115].

Differential diagnosis

In endemic areas, the main differential is with RRV infection which is more common than BFV infection. A rash is more common and arthritis less common in BFV compared with RRV.

Disease course and prognosis

Prolonged arthralgia occurs infrequently.

Investigations
Serology to detect IgM, usually by ELISA, is used to confirm the viral infection.

Resources

Patient resources

http://conditions.health.qld.gov.au/HealthCondition/condition/14/217/190/barmah-forest-virus

https://nt.gov.au/wellbeing/health-conditions-treatments/viral/barmah-forest-virus

(Last accessed August 2023.)

Mayaro virus infection

Synonyms and inclusions
- Mayaro fever
- Uruma fever

Introduction and general description
Mayaro virus (MAYV) infection causes a self-limiting illness with similarities to other mosquito-borne arbovirus infections.

Epidemiology
Incidence and prevalence
The virus is found in tropical South America [116], Central America and the Caribbean. Brazil has the highest number of reported cases. Occasional cases in returning travellers may be seen in other parts of the world.

Pathophysiology
Causative organisms
The reservoir host of the virus is believed to be monkeys with spread of the infection to humans via a number of mosquito species, especially *Haemagogus* and *Aedes*.

Clinical features
Presentation
After an incubation period of 1–14 days, the illness starts with fever, headache, myalgia and arthralgia, particularly wrists, ankles, fingers and toes. There may be lymphadenopathy and gastrointestinal upset [117]. A transient non-pruritic maculopapular rash appearing 5 or more days after the onset of illness is seen in 30–50% of cases, affecting variable areas of the body [118,119]. Desquamation may be seen as the rash clears.

Disease course and prognosis
The illness is self-limiting and lasts a few days to a few weeks, although arthralgia may persist for a year or more. However, severe manifestations have been reported including neurological complications, haemorrhage and myocarditis [120].

Differential diagnosis
Symptoms may be similar to other arboviral diseases endemic in the same areas as dengue, chikungunya and Zika virus infections. Coinfections with dengue or chikungunya viruses have been reported.

Investigations
Diagnosis is by serology or RT-PCR.

Management
Analgesia and antipyretics can be used. NSAIDs should be avoided until dengue is excluded.

Resources

Patient resources

https://www.cdc.gov/mayaro-virus/ (last accessed August 2023).

Rubella

Definition and nomenclature
Rubella infection causes a well-recognised exanthem, of particular importance and risk to the fetus if infection occurs during pregnancy.

Synonyms and inclusions
- German measles

Introduction and general description
Rubella infection causes one of the common exanthems of childhood or adolescence. The incidence has been greatly reduced in areas where immunisation is routine.

Epidemiology
Incidence and prevalence
The disease occurs throughout the world and is endemic in large cities. Epidemics occur at irregular intervals, usually during the spring. Transmission is by droplets from the nasopharynx and infectivity is greatest at the end of the incubation period and falls rapidly during the 4 days after the appearance of the rash.

There is a worldwide drive to increase immunisation programmes with the aim of eradicating rubella and the congenital rubella syndrome [1], but even in countries where immunisation has been routine for decades, epidemics can occur, either related to immigration or to individual or community choice to avoid immunisations [2].

Age
Infection is most common among older children and young adults.

Pathophysiology
Pathology
No distinctive pathological changes have been described in the skin.

Causative organisms

Rubella virus is the only member of the *Rubivirus* genus of the family *Matonaviridae* known to infect humans. It does not require an insect vector to spread. Thirteen genotypes have been identified so far [3] but of these, four types (1E, 1G, 1J and 2B) account for over 70% of infections.

Clinical features [4]
Presentation

The rash appears after an incubation period of about 14 days (range 12–21 days). Children rarely experience prodromal symptoms but adults have a brief prodromal illness lasting 1–5 days, consisting of fever up to 39°C, headache and malaise, sore throat without coryza and suffusion of the conjunctivae with a gritty sensation. The symptoms subside as the rash develops.

An enanthem of dull red macules or petechiae confined to the soft palate (Forschheimer sign) is present in up to 20% of patients during the prodromal period or on the first day of the rash. Enlargement of lymph glands begins 5–7 days before the rash appears whether or not there are prodromal symptoms, and reaches a maximum on the first or second day of the rash. The enlargement is generalised but characteristically involves the suboccipital, postauricular and cervical glands. However, these glands are not invariably affected and their involvement is not pathognomonic of rubella. The tenderness of the glands subsides after a day or two but palpable enlargement may continue for several weeks.

The rash appears first on the face and spreads rapidly downwards to the trunk and limbs. It consists of pink macules, at first discrete, but soon becoming confluent on the face as a diffuse redness. During the second day, the face begins to clear and the macules on the trunk show some coalescence, those on the limbs remaining discrete.

The blood count may be normal, or there may be a leukopenia with an inconstant increase in plasma cells.

Complications and co-morbidities

These are few in childhood. In older children and adults, arthritis is not uncommon and affects up to 70% of females and 5% of males. The clinical picture is variable and the arthritis usually resolves within a month.

Rarely, purpura – thrombocytopenic or non-thrombocytopenic – occurs as a complication of rubella. Very rarely encephalitis is reported. Haemophagocytic syndrome has rarely been diagnosed in association with rubella infection, with most cases being in women [5].

Rubella in pregnancy. The prenatal damage produced by rubella in early pregnancy was first noted by Gregg in Australia in 1941. The overall risk of fetal damage appears to be about 85% for primary maternal infection during the first 11 weeks [4]. Infection at this stage usually results in multiple defects. Between weeks 12 and 16, the risk of a rubella defect is about 35% and is principally that of deafness. Thereafter, although fetal infection occurs it does not result in damage.

The features of congenital rubella syndrome are mainly neurological [4,6]. Heart and eye damage is most frequent in embryos infected under 6 weeks; deafness and mental deficiency occur in embryos of all ages up to about 16 weeks. Intellectual disability and microcephaly may not be apparent until a year or more after prenatal infection [7]. During the neonatal period congenital rubella may give rise to a number of manifestations which are self-limiting in those infants which survive [8,9]. The most frequent is thrombocytopenic purpura, which may be manifest as a transient purpuric rash. Other features are jaundice and bone lesions which may simulate congenital syphilis.

Disease course and prognosis

By the third day the rash on the trunk has cleared and by the fourth the eruption on the limbs has also faded. The rash may be absent in some 40% of cases.

Investigations

Laboratory investigations must be carried out to confirm a diagnosis in pregnancy or immunosuppression. Serology remains the appropriate technique and the first clotted blood should be taken as soon as possible after the rash is noted. A second blood sample is required after 7–10 days. Antirubella antibodies can be detected from the time when the rash appears. IgM antibodies suggest acute or recent rubella infection while IgG antibodies appear 2–3 weeks later or may indicate prior exposure and immunity. In neonates, the presence of IgM and continued antibody production are indicative of congenital infection [10] and should be sought if congenital rubella syndrome is suspected, especially in countries where rubella is not eradicated.

Rapid diagnosis and distinction from other viral infections producing a rash can be achieved by RT-PCR amplification of viral RNA from saliva and throat swabs [11], but this is not routine practice in most diagnostic laboratories.

Management
Prophylaxis

Active immunisation by inoculation with live attenuated rubella virus is employed in many countries. It was introduced in the UK in 1970 and is now routinely offered to infants aged 1–2 years as a triple vaccine (MMR: measles, mumps, rubella). A preschool booster of MMR is also recommended. If they are found to be susceptible, rubella vaccine is also given to selected groups of women who require protection, such as medical and nursing staff and schoolteachers. A quadruple vaccine including varicella has recently become available but there has been concern, though not confirmation, that this combination leads to a slight increase in convulsions [12,13] (see Measles later).

Pregnancy is a contraindication to the vaccine and should be avoided for 4 weeks after its administration. There have, however, been no reports of damage to the fetus following inadvertent vaccination of pregnant women [14]. Arthralgia is common in adult women 2–4 weeks after vaccination and in children a rubelliform rash may occur [15]. A case of post-vaccination encephalitis has been reported [16]. Vaccinated females do not seem to be infectious.

No specific treatment is needed.

Table 25.16 Picornaviruses commonly causing human disease.

Genus	Species	Genotype	Abbreviation	Disease
Aphthovirus	Foot and mouth disease virus			Foot and mouth disease
Enterovirus	Enterovirus A	Coxsackievirus A5	CV-A5	Gastroenteritis
	25 serotypes	Coxsackievirus A6	CV-A6	Upper respiratory tract infection, pneumonia
		Coxsackievirus A16	CV-A16	Myocarditis
		Enterovirus A71	EV-A71	Meningitis, encephalitis
				Herpangina, hand, foot and mouth disease
	Enterovirus B	Coxsackievirus B1	CV-B1	
	63 serotypes	Echoviruses	E1 etc.	
	Enterovirus C 23 serotypes	Poliovirus	PV-1, -2, -3	Poliomyelitis
	Enterovirus D–J			
	Rhinovirus 80 serotypes	Rhinovirus A–C	RV A, B, C	Coryza
Hepatovirus		Hepatitis A virus		Hepatitis
Parechoviruses	Parechovirus A	Human parechovirus 1	PeV1 (formally echovirus 22)	Gastroenteritis
		Human parechovirus 2	PeV2 (formally echovirus 23)	Upper respiratory tract infection
		Human parechovirus 3	PeV3	Meningitis
		Human parechoviruses 4–16		Encephalitis

PICORNAVIRUS INFECTIONS (ENTEROVIRUSES)

General description of disease domain

There are over 30 genera in the *Picornaviridae* family, with human disease represented within four. In the *Aphthovirus* genus, foot and mouth disease is mainly a disease of animals but can occasionally cause disease in humans. The *Enterovirus* genus includes coxsackieviruses, enteroviruses, echoviruses, rhinoviruses and polioviruses and several cutaneous manifestations are reported. The *Hepatovirus* genus, which includes hepatitis A virus, and the *Parechovirus* genus are also within the *Picornaviridae* family (Table 25.16).

Skin manifestations are commonly seen with coxsackie and echovirus infections, which usually present with gastroenteritis or respiratory tract symptoms.

Basic biology

The enteroviruses are spread mainly via the faeco-oral but also the respiratory route. Cases occur sporadically or during epidemics, when many unaffected individuals may carry and shed the virus. Hand washing with a detergent can help to reduce spread between individuals.

Foot and mouth disease

Definition

Foot and mouth is a common and serious epidemic virus disease affecting farm animals in Europe, Asia and Africa. It rarely infects humans.

Introduction and general description

True foot and mouth disease has occurred in both adults and children in direct contact with infected stock [1,2].

Pathophysiology
Pathology

Histology of a lesion shows loculated vesicles in the deeper layers of the epithelium of the mucous membranes and intranuclear inclusions in neighbouring cells.

Clinical features
Presentation

The incubation period ranges from 2 to 18 days. Malaise, headache and fever, with burning of the oral mucous membranes, are followed after 2 or 3 days by vesicles of the buccal mucous membrane, tongue and lips, and occasionally on the palms, soles and interdigital skin. The vesicles are followed by ragged ulcers and may be accompanied by pain and oedema. Sometimes only the mouth or the hands are involved. The disease tends to be more severe in infants and children than in adults.

Disease course and prognosis

The temperature falls after a few days to a week and the lesions heal within 2 weeks.

Investigations

The viral nucleic acid may be detected in blood or vesicles by RT-PCR. Alternatively, the diagnosis can be confirmed by detection of antibody in the serum by ELISA tests.

Management

Symptomatic treatment is all that is needed.

Enterovirus infection

Introduction and general description

Infection with coxsackieviruses, enteroviruses or echoviruses can be accompanied by a maculopapular eruption with or without vesiculation or oral involvement.

Epidemiology

Incidence and prevalence
Incidence of sporadic cases and epidemics is more common in summer and autumn months and in warmer, humid areas of the world. Person-to-person spread can be rapid.

Pathophysiology

Causative organisms [3]
Human infections due to enterovirus (EV) infection are most commonly caused by EV A species. Six groups of genetic variations of EV A are identified and those in A, B or C genogroups are found most commonly. Coxsackieviruses (CV) A1–A24 and B1–B6 are now classified within the EV A, B and C species. The echoviruses are classified within the EV B species. In epidemics, several variants circulate.

Clinical features

Presentation
A febrile illness with gastroenteritis or respiratory tract infection is the usual presentation and an accompanying short-lived rash is a common feature. The rash usually appears after the onset of fever, but rarely may precede or appear simultaneously. Infection can be subclinical. At the more severe end of the spectrum, a prostrating and sometimes fatal illness with myocarditis, respiratory failure or meningoencephalitis may occur.

Clinical variants
The rash is usually maculopapular without diagnostic features but vesicles and oral ulcers may be present. If vesicular stomatitis is the predominant feature, the illness may be described as herpangina, and, if an acral eruption is also present, as hand, foot and mouth disease.

A large number of variations of eruption have been reported, sometimes attributed to a species of EV (Tables 25.17, 25.18 and 25.19), but no assumptions should be made about the causative agent or agents, based on clinical features alone.

In individuals, especially children, who have atopic eczema, a widespread eruption can vesiculate and be more pronounced on areas of dermatitis. This eruption, termed eczema coxsackium, is most commonly associated with CV-A6 and -A16.

Investigations
RT-PCR is used to detect and type the virus from stool, throat swab, nasal secretions or vesicle fluid.

Echovirus and rubella infections are often present simultaneously in a community, and the eruptions they produce may be indistinguishable. It is therefore essential for any woman developing a rash in the early stages of pregnancy to be investigated for both EV and rubella infection.

Hand, foot and mouth disease

Definition and nomenclature
An acute infection caused by enterovirus infection, usually coxsackievirus, leading most commonly to mild malaise, with oral ulcers and hand and foot vesicular eruption.

Table 25.17 Skin manifestations of coxsackievirus infections.

Coxsackie A4	Herpangina
	Papular or papulovesicular eruption over hands, feet, buttocks [4]
	A widespread vesicular eruption lasting for up to 2 weeks [4,5]
Coxsackie A6	Hand, foot and mouth disease
	Herpangina; papulovesicular eruption of anticubital fossae [6]
	Eczema coxsackium
	Generalised eruption with perineal involvement in pregnant woman [7]
	Generalised eruption with large blisters [8]
	A Gianotti-Crosti-like syndrome [8]
Coxsackie A9	A short-lived, central maculopapular eruption [9]
	Generalised maculopapular eruption [10]
	Morbilliform, urticarial or petechial eruption [10]
Coxsackie A14	A papular eruption [11]
Coxsackie A16	Hand, foot and mouth disease
	Papular or petechial eruption
	Eczema coxsackium
	A Gianotti–Crosti-like syndrome [12]
Coxsackie B3	A prolonged papular eruption [13]
	A papular or papulovesicular eruption of hands, feet, buttocks [4]
	Congenital infection with florid papulovesicles with nodules and ulceration, plus associated pneumonia, carditis and hepatitis [14]
Coxsackie B4	Herpangina
	A papular or papulovesicular eruption of hands, feet, buttocks [4]
Coxsackie B5	A vesicular stomatitis involving the anterior portions of the oral cavity and the lips, associated with erythema multiforme [15], which can also give a morbilliform exanthem [16]

Table 25.18 Skin manifestations of echovirus infections.

Echovirus 9	Rubelliform or morbilliform eruptions [17]
Echovirus 16	The 'Boston eruption', large pink macules on face and trunk, occasionally widespread including palms and soles, following a brief febrile illness in children or adults [18]
Echovirus 2	Rubelliform rash [19]
Echoviruses 11, 19	Petechial rash [20]
Echoviruses 6, 11, 18, 25	Maculopapular rashes [21,22]
Echoviruses 23, 32	Telangiectatic macular lesions [23]
Echovirus 19	Punctate macular rash in infants [24]
Echovirus 11	Vesicular eruptions [25–10]

Table 25.19 Skin manifestations of enterovirus infections.

E-A71	Hand, foot and mouth disease with smaller vesicles than CV-A16 [27]
	Herpangina
	A papular eruption sometimes with diffuse erythema or petechiae [28,29]
EV-D68	Painful exanthema in adolescents [**30**]

Synonyms and inclusions
- Enteroviral vesicular stomatitis with exanthem

Epidemiology

Incidence and prevalence
Sporadic cases and epidemics occur throughout the world, with peaks in the summer, spring and autumn months.

Age
Children aged below 10 years are those most commonly affected. Adults are not infrequently affected.

Pathophysiology
Pathology [6]
Histology is not usually performed, but shows spongiosis, intraepidermal splits progressing to vesicle formation, mononuclear cells entering the epidermis and necrosis of individual keratinocytes. There is a lymphocytic upper dermal and perivascular infiltrate. Viral particles are detectable with electron microscopy [31].

Causative organisms
Outbreaks had previously been caused most commonly by CV-A16, but in South-East Asia and also in other areas, more recent epidemics have been caused by CV-A6, CV-A10 and EV-A71 [6,32]. Other species found during epidemics and in sporadic cases include CV-A2, CV-A4, CV-A5, CV-A9, CV-B1, CV-B4 and CV-B5 [33].

Clinical features
Presentation
The illness is usually mild, starting 5–7 days after infection and lasting a week. In children, the onset is with a low-grade fever, sore throat and malaise, but in adults, a painful stomatitis is an early feature. Blisters in the mouth soon break down to superficial ulcers. Children are more likely than adults to develop flaccid greyish 2–5 mm oval vesicles on the palms and slightly less frequently on the soles (Figure 25.31). They occur on the sides or backs of the fingers and toes, especially around the nails, and around the margins of the heels, but may be seen in the finger flexures, on the palms and soles and sometimes the buttocks [34]. They are usually few in number but rarely up to 50. They fade after 2–3 days. It is not uncommon for there to be lesions elsewhere, especially on the buttocks and legs and less commonly on the arms and torso [35]. Infection can be subclinical.

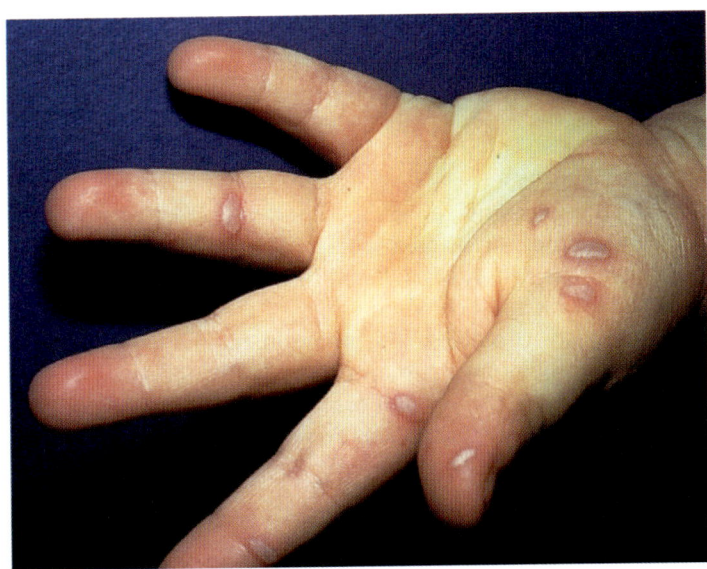

Figure 25.31 Hand, foot and mouth disease. Courtesy of Addenbrooke's Hospital, Cambridge, UK.

Clinical variants
Very rarely, a widespread vesicular eruption occurs over the buttocks, trunk and perioral area [36]. Severe disease with a generalised eruption is more common in CV-A6 infections [37]. In some, the eruption may be papular or maculopapular without vesicles [10]. In infants the disease can be more severe, but in adults, atypical presentations are more common and are more likely in association with CV-A6 and EV-A71. In atopic individuals with even mild eczema, eczema coxsackium can develop.

Differential diagnosis
Oral lesions may suggest herpes simplex or Stevens–Johnson syndrome. If skin lesions are widespread, chickenpox or, in atopics, eczema herpeticum should be considered. Bullous impetigo, vasculitis or immunobullous disease may also be suspected in some presentations.

Complications and co-morbidities
Severe disease may be apparent by a high fever and can include neurological symptoms and signs of lethargy, myocarditis, pneumonitis, meningitis, encephalitis, Guillain–Barré syndrome and flaccid paralysis. In recent epidemics in South-East Asia caused by EV71, mortality rates up to 5% have been reported [38]. In a number of epidemics, in Asia, the USA and Europe, nail changes of Beau lines, onycholysis [39] or nail shedding (onychomadesis) has followed 2–4 weeks after the acute infection [40,41].

Disease course and prognosis
Relapses are rare and a chronic intermittent course is exceptional. Viral shedding persists for an average of 3 weeks after infection but may be more prolonged after severe disease [42].

Investigations
Samples are best collected from multiple sites: swabs from vesicle fluid, the throat, rectum and skin, blood and cerebrospinal fluid when available. PCR analysis provides rapid diagnosis or culture a slower option. Enteroviral typing can be made with RNA sequence analysis of the VP1 region of the genome which is highly conserved [43,44]. Serology can assist in retrospective investigation in epidemics [45].

Management
Supportive. Severe cases with neurological symptoms may be treated with intravenous immunoglobulin [46]. Vaccines against EV71 are in development.

Herpangina [47]

Synonyms and inclusions
- Enteroviral vesicular stomatitis with exanthem

Epidemiology
Incidence and prevalence
Occurs throughout the world with epidemics and sporadic cases most common in summer and autumn [48].

Age
Mainly affects children aged 1–10 years but may occur in adults, especially during epidemics [49].

Associated diseases
Herpangina commonly occurs together with hand, foot and mouth disease epidemics.

Pathophysiology
Causative organisms
Many picornaviruses are associated, but the most commonly isolated viruses are enteroviruses A and B (especially species CV-A2, -A5, -A6, -A9, -A10, -A16, A-24; CV-B3, -B4; E-6, E-9 and EV-A71) [49–53].

Clinical features
Presentation [47]
The first manifestation is sudden onset of fever, which may last up to 5 days. Sore throat and dysphagia develop soon after onset and may be accompanied by cough, rhinitis, nausea, vomiting and diarrhoea. Up to 15 or 20 tiny vesicles, 1–2 mm in diameter, with a vivid red areola, develop on the pharynx, tonsils, uvula and soft palate.

Disease course and prognosis
The vesicles erode into shallow ulcers, 2–4 mm diameter, which enlarge for 2 or 3 days and heal in 4 or 5 days. Complete recovery is expected within 7 days.

Management [47]
Management is supportive with temperature control. Topical anaesthetic, such as lidocaine gel, can help when ulceration is making swallowing difficult [54]. Transmission should be avoided with isolation at home for most cases.

Parechovirus infection

Synonyms and inclusions
- Human parechovirus infection

Introduction and general description
Human parechoviruses (HPeV) have been identified within the *Picornaviridae* family on the basis of their genomic organisation [55]. They usually cause gastroenteritis but may also cause respiratory symptoms, meningoencephalitis and rash.

Epidemiology
Incidence and prevalence
Studies of seroprevalence suggest that exposure to these viruses is extremely common throughout the world. Of adults in Finland, 99% have antibodies to HPeV1 [56]. In Japan, where HPeV3 was first reported, 85% of children are seropositive [57]. HPeV1 is the genotype found most commonly, followed by HPeV2, although there is geographic variation for the prevalence of types 2, 3, 4 and 5.

Age
Young children, especially neonates, are most commonly affected.

Pathophysiology
Causative organisms
Within the genus *Parechovirus*, the species Parechovirus A causes disease in humans and to date, 19 genotypes have been identified [58].

Clinical features
Presentation
In HPeV1 or -2 infection, the usual manifestations are gastroenteritis or respiratory symptoms, but a transient, non-specific maculopapular rash occurs in about 20% of cases [59,60]. Neurological symptoms are less common. In HPeV3 and HPeV5, sepsis and meningococcal features are more frequent.

In severe infections with sepsis and meningoencephalitis, rash occurs in most cases at about day 3 of the febrile illness. It may frequently show a pattern of palmoplantar redness and usually lasts about 3 days [61].

In adults, infection is frequently asymptomatic, but can present with many of the features shown in children, although skin involvement is not reported [62].

Investigations
The quickest diagnostic test is by RT-PCR [63].

Management
Treatment is supportive, using rehydration and antipyretics.

Hepatitis A infection

Epidemiology
Incidence and prevalence
The virus is highly endemic in developing countries where almost all the population is likely to be infected and immune by the age of 10 years [64]. The infection is often subclinical in children. Developed countries with good water and sewage systems have very low rates of hepatitis A infection but occasional outbreaks are reported, usually due to contaminated foodstuffs. Travellers from low-risk countries to areas of high endemicity are at risk of infection.

Pathophysiology
Causative organisms
Hepatitis A virus is classified within the genus *Hepatovirus*. There are three human genotypes, I, II and III, each with subtype A and B. Subtype IA is the most common.

The virus is very stable in the environment and is spread by the faeco-oral route, by ingestion of contaminated food and water or through close person-to-person contact. During the prodrome and the early icteric phase, the patient excretes virus in the faeces and is infectious, although only a transient viraemia occurs.

Clinical features
Presentation
The average incubation period is 30 (15–40) days. Most people suffer a prodrome of a flu-like illness, anorexia and arthralgia in the week

preceding the jaundice. Occasionally, in about 10% of cases, there is a transient eruption [65], usually maculopapular, petechial or urticarial. Other reported skin manifestations are a morbilliform eruption with predominance in sun-exposed sites [66]; a Gianotti–Crosti-like eruption in a child [67]; haemophagocytic lymphohistiocytosis [68]; a vasculitic eruption attributed either to Henoch–Schönlein purpura [69] or cryoglobulinaemia [70]; a localised skin inflammation associated with parotitis [71]; and chronic urticaria [72]. Conditions developing soon after acute hepatitis A infection and possibly related to liver function include variegate porphyria and DRESS [73,74].

Differential diagnosis
Hepatitis A must be distinguished from other causes of jaundice.

Disease course and prognosis
Jaundice is uncommon in children, occurring in about 10%, but occurs in about 90% of adults. Fulminant hepatitis rarely occurs. Death can occur later due to chronic hepatitis.

Investigations
The diagnosis is confirmed by detecting hepatitis A IgM antibody. The presence of IgG antibody indicates past infection (or immunisation) and gives protection. Molecular detection of virus in stool or saliva is possible and permits analysis of variants [75].

Management
Active immunisation with inactivated or attenuated virus or short-lived passive protection using human immunoglobulin are both available for travellers or susceptible contacts.

Symptomatic measures are usually sufficient. The infection is of a few weeks' duration and no chronic carrier state exists. Alcohol should be avoided during the convalescent period.

Resources

Further information
http://www.who.int/mediacentre/factsheets/fs328/en/
https://www.health.nsw.gov.au/Infectious/factsheets/Pages/parechovirus.aspx
(Both last accessed August 2023.)

RHABDOVIRUS INFECTIONS

Vesicular stomatitis virus infection

Synonyms and inclusions
- Indiana vesiculovirus

Definition
Vesicular stomatitis virus or vesiculovirus is an arbovirus which infects horses and cattle in the Americas, Asia and Africa. It is generally mild but can mimic foot and mouth disease. It is occasionally transmitted to humans by direct or indirect contact with infected animals [1].

Pathophysiology
Pathology
The infection can cause vesicles which are intraepithelial. Intranuclear inclusions are present in infected cells. The virus has been used as recombinant vector for several vaccines, including Ebola virus. In such studies, the viral proteins are detected in perivascular infiltrates in the dermis and subcutis [2].

Clinical features
Presentation
The incubation period is 2 days after which there is a flu-like illness with fever, myalgia and malaise. This is occasionally followed by mild stomatitis with vesicles on the gums and buccal and pharyngeal mucosa and lymphadenitis. Some patients develop vesicles of the fingers.

Complications and co-morbidities
Encephalitis has been reported [3].

Disease course and prognosis
Recovery is usually complete within a week. Antibodies against the virus are detectable at about 10 days, with neutralising antibodies persisting for at least 1 year [4].

PARAMYXOVIRUS INFECTIONS

The *Paramyxoviridae* family comprises four genera:
1. *Morbillivirus* (includes measles morbillivirus).
2. *Metapneumovirus* (includes human metapneumovirus) and *Orthopneumovirus* (includes human orthopneumovirus and respiratory syncytial virus, RSV).
3. *Respirovirus* (includes human parainfluenza virus 1 and 3).
4. *Orthorubulavirus* (includes human orthorubulavirus or mumps virus).

MEASLES AND RESPIRATORY SYNCYTIAL VIRUS

General description of disease domain

Within the family of paramyxoviruses, cutaneous manifestations are usually only produced in measles and occasionally in RSV infections. Other genera of the myxoviruses are shown in Table 25.1.

Measles [1]

Definition and nomenclature
Measles is a highly infectious disease caused by the measles morbillivirus of the genus *Morbillivirus*.

Synonyms and inclusions
- Morbilli
- Rubeola
- First disease

Introduction and general description [1]

The development of a maculopapular eruption in a person with prodromal cough, coryza and conjunctivitis should prompt the consideration of measles. In areas of the world where measles vaccination has been established for many years, the diagnosis is often overlooked.

Measles is still a notifiable disease in the UK.

Epidemiology
Incidence and prevalence

Measles is distributed throughout the world and occurs throughout the year. In temperate regions, the incidence is highest in late winter and spring. In 1999, there were an estimated 873 000 deaths from measles, but two decades later, the estimate was 140 000 deaths worldwide [2,3]. The incidence has been greatly reduced in countries where measles vaccination is offered to all children and it is estimated that 84% of all children worldwide receive immunisation.

The introduction of vaccination against measles is extending worldwide, with impressive reduction in mortality, but the prospect of global eradication of the disease is some time away. Concerns relating to the safety of vaccination since the 1990s have led to a reduced proportion of vaccinated children in several countries, with subsequent increases in incidence and reports of isolated outbreaks of the disease [2,4].

Measles infection occurs from human to human via the upper respiratory tract where initial replication occurs before wide dissemination throughout the body. Infection can also be spread via semen, saliva and mucus. An infected individual is infectious from approximately 4 days before to 4 days after the onset of the rash.

Age

Where measles is endemic, children are most commonly affected. In areas where vaccination is routine, but without 100% uptake, infection in young adults may be seen more frequently.

Pathophysiology
Predisposing factors

The disease is highly contagious and contact of a non-immune person with a person with measles infection or with their secretions is likely to result in infection.

Pathology [5,6]

During the prodromal period, there is establishment of infection in the reticuloendothelial system; there is also lymphoid hyperplasia with formation of fused multinucleate giant cells. The prodromal rash appears to be the result of viraemia with antigen and virus deposits in the capillaries. Cells in the Koplik spots also contain viral nucleocapsids. The conspicuous macular eruption on the fourth day is the result of the cell-mediated immunity response against the viral proteins.

Shortly after the rash appears, measles virus causes a transient depression of the T-cell-mediated immune responses that is an important feature of the infection [7] and can persist for 1–2 months.

Causative organisms

The measles virus is a morbillivirus, of the *Paramyxoviridae* family. The cellular receptors for the virus in natural infection are the CD150 (signalling lymphocyte activation molecule, SLAM) and the nectin 4 (poliovirus receptor-like 4, PVRL4) molecules and also CD46 for cultured virus strains [6,8]. Initial replication in upper respiratory tract epithelial cells is followed by spread to regional lymph nodes and subsequent viraemia.

Clinical features
History

After contact, the incubation period is about 10 days.

Presentation [9,10]

The onset is acute with prodromal symptoms of fever, malaise and upper respiratory symptoms of pharyngitis and rhinitis. The conjunctivae are injected and there may be photophobia. From the second day, Koplik spots are usually present on the buccal mucous membrane opposite the premolar teeth – bluish white spots with bright red areolae (Figure 25.32). Fever, catarrh and cough increase for 3–5 days. The exanthem characteristically develops on the fourth day on the forehead and behind the ears, and spreads within 24 h to the rest of the face, the trunk and the limbs. The palms and soles are affected. The rash, which can be slightly itchy, is at first macular but soon forms dull red papules, which tend to coalesce in irregularly concentric patterns but may be more diffusely confluent.

Not all features of the illness may be present, but the presence of Koplik spots is an almost diagnostic feature of measles infection [11].

Clinical variants

In very severe forms, the rash may be haemorrhagic. An extensive bullous eruption may rarely develop during the acute stage of measles. In some cases, this eruption has the features of Stevens–Johnson syndrome, but in others it resembles epidermal necrolysis.

Differential diagnosis

The features of other infective exanthems, such as dengue or enterovirus, should be considered. Kawasaki disease and toxic shock syndrome may have similar features. Drug eruptions should not cause confusion as the upper respiratory catarrh and conjunctival suffusion are absent.

Classification of severity

Infection in an individual with profound defects of cell-mediated immunity is usually severe and carries a high risk of mortality.

Complications and co-morbidities

Complications occur in about 30% and are more common in young children, the very elderly, the malnourished and the chronically ill [10]. Secondary infections leading to bronchopneumonia, enteritis and otitis media are most commonly reported. The most serious complication is encephalitis which occurs in 1/1000 cases [12]. If the immune response is severely defective there may be no rash but

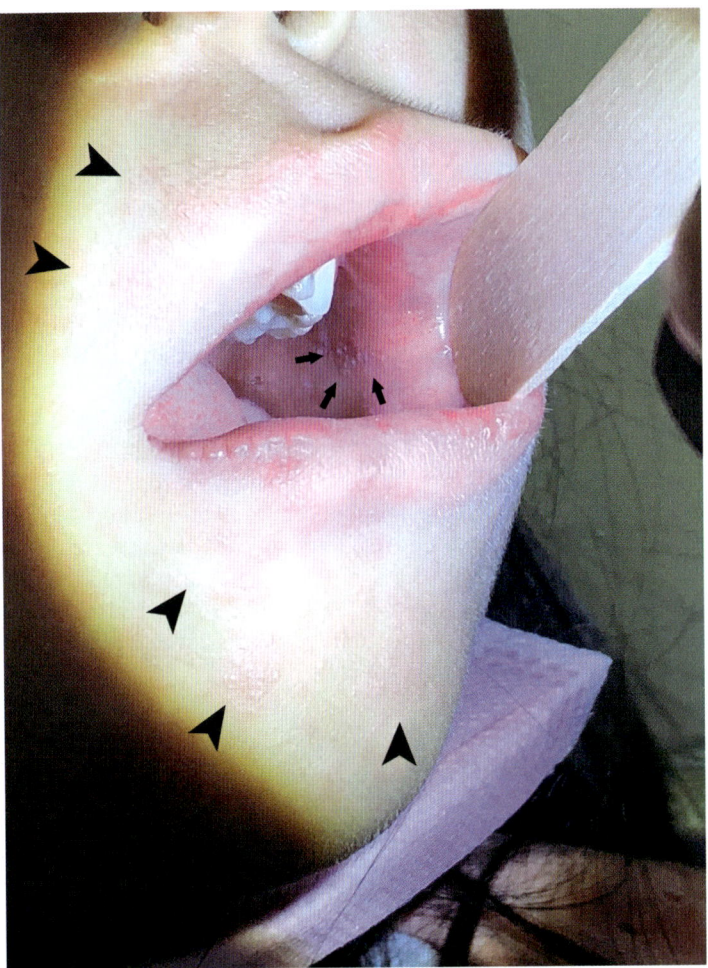

Figure 25.32 Koplik spots on the buccal mucosa in measles. Reproduced with permission of CDC/Heinz F. Eichenwald, MD.

viral replication progresses to produce a giant-cell pneumonia or a fatal encephalopathy.

Very rarely, the late complication of subacute sclerosing panencephalitis (SSPE) can develop 7–10 years after infection. SSPE is more common when infection has occurred in individuals under 1 year of age.

Infection during pregnancy can lead to spontaneous abortion, premature delivery and may carry a risk of more severe disease for the mother [13].

Disease course and prognosis
The rash starts on the head and neck, and spreads from the upper to lower body. From the fourth to the tenth day the rash fades, to leave some brownish staining and fine desquamation. The transient immunosuppression lasting for a few weeks can increase the risk of bacterial infections in the recovery period. Lifelong immunity follows recovery.

Investigations
Specific measles IgM antibodies are usually detectable in serum or saliva 3 or 4 days after the appearance of the rash, and maximum titres of IgG are reached 2–4 weeks later. Virus culture and isolation are possible but not easy. Molecular diagnosis and phylogenetic analysis of measles RNA are not routine but may be done in acute cases and localised outbreaks [1,14].

Management
Prevention
Passive protection is possible using normal human immunoglobulin given within 5 days of exposure, which prevents or attenuates the infection in contacts and is reserved for those children at special risk or for non-immune pregnant mothers after exposure to an infected contact.

Active immunisation with live attenuated viral vaccine has greatly reduced the incidence of measles infections, although infection can rarely occur in fully vaccinated individuals during outbreaks [15]. A mild illness with a rash is common during the 3 weeks following the vaccine and there are occasional reports of other eruptions post-vaccination such as Stevens–Johnson syndrome [16], pityriasis lichenoides [17] and Gianotti–Crosti syndrome [18].

The vaccine is available as a single vaccine, but is used more commonly as the triple vaccine (MMR) or as the newer quadruple vaccine which includes varicella (MMR-V) (see Rubella earlier).

First line
The patient should be confined to home and bed and given symptomatic treatment. Antibiotics may be required to control secondary bacterial complications.

Second line
Children with measles, especially in areas of high mortality, should be given vitamin A (two doses of 200 000 IU for older children with lower doses for those under 1 year of age) [19].

Third line
Measles pneumonia may be helped by ribavirin [20].

Resources

Further information
https://www.gov.uk/government/collections/measles-guidance-data-and-analysis
https://www.cdc.gov/measles/hcp/index.html
https://www.who.int/health-topics/measles#tab=tab_1

Patient resources
http://www.nhs.uk/conditions/Measles/Pages/Introduction.aspx
http://www.cdc.gov/measles/about/index.html
https://www.who.int/en/news-room/fact-sheets/detail/measles
(All last accessed August 2023.)

Respiratory syncytial virus

Definition
Human RSV infection is very common and may cause coryza, bronchiolitis, bronchitis or pneumonia. It has rarely been associated with cutaneous signs.

Epidemiology
Incidence and prevalence
Human RSV causes annual epidemics during the winter months in temperate regions or in the rainy season in the tropics [21]. Most people have been infected by the age of 1 or 2 years and may suffer repeated infections throughout life.

Pathophysiology
Causative organisms
Human RSV (human orthopneumovirus) has two antigenic subtypes, A and B, which differ most in their surface glycoprotein G. Group A viruses are more frequently detected.

Clinical features
Presentation
Infection occurs after an incubation period of 4–5 days. The virus is especially associated with bronchiolitis in babies and infants, with bronchitis and pneumonia occurring in a proportion of infections. In older children and adults, upper respiratory symptoms occur that are indistinguishable from a common cold. Again in old age, RSV pneumonia is not uncommon and in the immunosuppressed is associated with a high rate of mortality [22]. A transient fine pink macular rash on the face and trunk has been observed in a few instances in children, occurring in one study in up to 10% of children affected with RSV-B but in only 1% of those with RSV-A [23]. Occasionally, it is more extensive and involves the arms, shoulders, chest, back and buttocks [24].

Investigations
Diagnosis can be achieved by rapid antibody detection or by RT-PCR to detect viral nucleic acid. Viral culture is slow but can be confirmatory.

Management
There is no specific antiviral therapy, so treatment is supportive.

In severe cases, such as RSV pneumonia in immunosuppression or chronic lung disease, ribavirin or palivizumab may be considered.

HUMAN CORONAVIRUS INFECTION

General description of disease domain

Human coronaviruses (HCoVs) are important human pathogens and belong to the *Coronaviridae* family of the *Nidovirinae* order of viruses. These are enveloped, single-stranded, positive sense RNA viruses with a genome length of approximately 30 kb and are among the largest known RNA viruses [1,2]. Seven HCoVs are currently recognised: HCoV-229E, HCoV-NL-63, HCoV-HKU, HCoV-OC43, SARS-CoV, NL63, severe acute respiratory syndrome (SARS-CoV), Middle East respiratory syndrome (MERS-CoV) and severe acute respiratory syndrome-2 (SARS-CoV-2).

HCoVs cause human respiratory diseases which range from asymptomatic to mild respiratory tract infections to epidemics with significant morbidity and mortality, including the SARS-CoV epidemic in 2002–2003, the MERS-CoV epidemic in 2012 and the SARS-CoV-2 pandemic in 2019 [1,2,3]. However, only SARS-CoV-2 has been associated with significant mucocutaneous disease [4].

Severe acute respiratory syndrome coronavirus-2 (SARS-CoV-2)

Introduction
In December 2019, the first cases of unexplained, severe pneumonia were reported in Wuhan, Hubei Province, China [5,6]. The pathogen isolated from lower respiratory tract samples of infected patients proved to be a novel zoonotic HCoV – SARS-CoV-2 – and the disease was termed Coronavirus Disease 2019 (Covid-19) [5]. SARS-CoV-2 was first transmitted to humans as a zoonotic infection and human-to-human transmission occurs via respiratory droplets and aerosols [2]. By the end of January 2020, cases were already being reported outside China and subsequently spread rapidly across the globe [7]. In March 2020, Covid-19 was declared a pandemic by the WHO and subsequently became a major public health challenge affecting every aspect of life [8].

Epidemiology
Incidence and prevalence
As of September 2023, the WHO estimates over 770 million confirmed Covid-19 cases, including over 6.9 million deaths [9].

Age
Covid-19 infection affects all age groups with differing degrees of severity, ranging from asymptomatic carriers to fatal infections [10–12].

Pathophysiology
Causative organism
SARS-CoV-2 is an HCoV. HCoVs are of zoonotic origin and most have originated in bats or rodents [2]. Intermediate reservoir hosts for several HCoVs have been identified, for example dromedary camels and palm civets for MERS and SARS-CoV, respectively. SARS-CoV-2 is unique in that zoonotic transmission from infected humans back to a variety of mammalian species (including farmed minks, wild white-tailed deer, dogs, cats, lions and tigers in zoos) is also recognised [2].

Transmission. Human-to-human transmission is by airborne respiratory droplets/aerosols, contaminated fluids splashed in eyes, nose or mouth and, rarely, via contaminated surfaces. SARS-CoV-2 is highly transmissible: its basic reproductive number (the number of secondary infections when an index case is introduced into a fully susceptible population) early in the pandemic was 3.28 – higher than those of SARS-CoV and MERS-CoV (2.0–3.0 and 0.9, respectively). Infectivity begins 4–5 days before the onset of symptoms, with upper respiratory tract peak viral load around the time of symptom onset, declining 7 days after symptom onset, but with duration of viral shedding and infectiousness for up to 10 days in mild to moderate Covid-19 and up to 20 days with severe Covid-19, including immunocompromised people [2].

SARS-CoV-2 virology. SARS-CoV-2 has 16 non-structural proteins including the spike, membrane, envelope and nucleocapsid proteins. Virions enter host cells by binding of their viral spike protein to host cell angiotensin-converting enzyme 2 (ACE2) receptors which are most abundant in the lungs (alveolar type II cells), but also present in cardiovascular, renal and gastrointestinal systems, and skin [2,5]. The efficiency of this binding is a key determinant of transmissibility and SARS-CoV-2 appears to bind with greater affinity than other virulent HCoVs, which may explain its higher transmissibility [2,12,13]. SARS-CoV-2 is also unusual in the frequency with which it is associated with mucocutaneous manifestations compared with other HCoVs: despite phylogenetic analysis of SARS-CoV-2 showing that it is closely related to both MERS and SARS, significant mucocutaneous manifestations have not been reported in association with these infections nor with other common respiratory viruses such as influenza [4]. Expression of ACE2 in the skin is highest in keratinocytes, followed by sweat glands, and the widespread expression of ACE2 in the skin and binding affinity of SARS-CoV-2 may contribute to this increased prevalence [14,15].

SARS-CoV-2 variants. In spring 2020 the original virus transitioned to a variant with four genomic mutations, including a single D614G point mutation in the spike protein that conferred a fitness advantage. Since then, multiple waves of variants have emerged, often showing greater antibody escape and higher transmissibility [2,13]. In late 2020, alpha (B.1.1.7), beta (B.1.351) and gamma (P.1) variants were identified in the UK, South Africa and Brazil, respectively. These were replaced by the delta (B.1.617.2) variant first detected in India in the summer of 2021. The omicron (B.1.1.529) variant emerged in Africa in late 2021 and became the most prevalent virus globally. Omicron is highly transmissible and has more than 50 mutations, at least 30 of which are in the spike protein, which has allowed significant escape from vaccination or prior non-omicron infection-elicited neutralising antibody responses. Omicron subvariants BA.1, BA.1.1, BA.2, BA.2.12.1, BA.4 and BA.5 have subsequently emerged; BA.5 neutralising antibody titres are approximately threefold lower than those against BA.1 and BA.2, and by 2022 BA.5 was the most prevalent type in the USA [13], but new variants are constantly emerging and in August 2023 the most dominant variant was EG.5 (https://covid.cdc.gov/covid-data-tracker/#variant-proportions).

Predisposing factors

Co-morbidities increasing susceptibility to infection include older age, high body mass index (BMI), diabetes, hypertension, cardiovascular disease, chronic obstructive pulmonary disease and immunosuppression. Sex differences, lifestyle differences such as smoking, pregnancy, SARS-CoV-2 variants and levels of exposure to the virus may also confer increased susceptibility to infection and risk of severe infection [12,16,17]. Genetic risk factors have been identified in genome-wide association studies: genes associated with severe illness include those broadly involved with failure to control viral replication and an enhanced tendency towards pulmonary inflammation and intravascular coagulation genes, and include genes such as those with a role in interferon signalling, B and T lymphopoiesis, myeloid cell differentiation, coagulation factors and platelet activation [16,18,**19**,20].

Immune response

The immune response to SARS-CoV-2 infection plays a key role in influencing disease severity by mediating both protective and immunopathogenic processes [21,22], although current understanding is incomplete [23]. The innate immune response is triggered immediately following SARS-CoV-2 viral exposure, with activation of the complement cascade and production of type I interferons. Early and robust interferon production is associated with reduced viral titres and mild clinical disease. In contrast, patients with severe/critical Covid-19 may have suppressed interferon expression and a parallel increase in tissue and systemic inflammation. The adaptive immune response takes several days to weeks to manifest [24]. SARS-CoV-2 infection activates a T-helper lymphocyte-1 immune response with spike protein-specific CD4+ lymphocytes. The resulting neutralising antibodies primarily responsible for blocking acquisition of SARS-CoV-2 infection are those binding to the receptor-binding and N-terminal domains of spike proteins that prevent virus attachment to host cells. IgM, IgG and IgA antibodies are produced during infection: IgG in the bloodstream and extracellular spaces is the main isotype associated with protection against infection, but IgA in respiratory tract secretions, serum and saliva also plays an important role [24]. Although patients with severe Covid-19 disease tend to generate higher titres of antibodies, some patients develop antibody responses even with mild or asymptomatic disease [21]. Viral replication is suppressed by CD8+ T-cell responses which are also highly cross-reactive against SARS-CoV-2 variants and contribute to protection against severe disease [13]. SARS-CoV-2-specific and neutralising antibodies decrease over about 8 months, although T-cell immunity may persist in those with mild Covid-19 infection who are subsequently seronegative [13]. Dysregulation of these immune responses may contribute to Covid-19 pathology, including mucocutaneous manifestations [21,22,25].

Key mechanisms contributing to multiorgan injury secondary to infection with SARS-CoV-2 broadly include direct viral toxicity, endothelial cell damage and thrombo-inflammation, immune dysregulation and hyperinflammation caused by viral inhibition of interferon signalling, T-cell lymphodepletion, production of autoantibodies and proinflammatory cytokines (particularly IL-6 and TNF-α) and dysregulation of the renin–angiotensin–aldosterone system [12,**21**,25]. It has been proposed that three main pathophysiological pathways underpin mucocutaneous Covid-19 disease: (i) complement cascade-mediated thrombotic, cell-poor, vascular injury syndromes in which deployment of the alternative and mannan binding lectin complement pathways of the innate immune response results in production of cytokines such as IL-6 from endothelium and activation of the coagulation cascade; (ii) robust T-cell-driven and type I interferon-driven inflammatory cutaneous reactions; (iii) B-cell-driven immune complex and autoantibody-mediated processes [**21**,25]. The relative contribution of these pathogenetic processes to specific mucocutaneous disorders is considered in more detail in later sections.

Clinical features

It is characterised by respiratory symptoms, fever, myalgia, fatigue and anosmia, but it is a multisystem disease: cardiovascular, neurological, haematological, renal, gastrointestinal, hepatobiliary, endocrinological, ophthalmological and dermatological involvement may also occur and reflect either extrapulmonary dissemination and replication of SARS-CoV-2 or the immunopathological sequelae of infection [11,12,26] (Table 25.20). Overall, approximately 80% of those infected experience mild to moderate symptoms, 15% severe symptoms and 5% progress to critical disease. A complication of severe disease – the 'cytokine storm' – is an uncontrolled cytokine and chemokine response to SARS-CoV-2 infection with hyperactivation of effector T cells and production of pro-inflammatory cytokines (IL-1, IL-2, IL-6, TNF-α and IFN-γ). It can lead to acute respiratory distress syndrome (ARDS) associated with increasing plasma leakage, vascular permeability, disseminated intravascular coagulation, thromboembolic events and multiorgan failure [11,12].

Mucocutaneous involvement was recognised early in the Covid-19 pandemic, with initial reported prevalence ranging from 0.2% in China to 20% in Italy [6,27]. More recent systematic reviews and meta-analyses indicate approximately 6–8% overall of those with Covid-19 infection will experience mucocutaneous disorders with a spectrum of presentations spanning early viral exanthems to later vasculopathies [4,28,29,30,31,32,33,34]. SARS-CoV-2 in skin health and disease is covered in more detail later.

Investigations

There are three main methods for the detection of SARS-CoV-2 infection and host response [23,35]:

- Molecular test – PCR: these are highly sensitive and specific for detection of viral RNA in nasal or nasopharyngeal swabs. They are recommended by the WHO for confirming diagnosis in individuals.
- Antigen rapid detection tests (Ag-RDT): these detect viral proteins in nasal or nasopharyngeal swabs. They are less sensitive than PCR but are easier, faster, cheaper and able to detect infection in those at risk of transmitting virus to others, and are used as a public health tool for screening individuals at increased risk of infection.
- Antibody tests: serology tests detect response to infection or vaccination and are useful public health surveillance tools, but the correlation with protection is unclear and they are not used to provide proof of immunity.

High concentrations of virus are present in the nasal passages of infected individuals and SARS-CoV-2 infections may be asymptomatic, pre-symptomatic or symptomatic. Viral RNA in upper respiratory tract samples is detectable up to 6 days before symptoms, peaks around the time of symptom onset, and is usually undetectable about 2 weeks after symptom onset. RNA positivity may persist for weeks, but live virus cannot be cultured later. The mean period of infectiousness is approximately 2–3 days before and 8 days after symptom onset [23]. Development of both IgM and IgG antibodies peaks at day 11–14 after onset of symptoms. Optimal timing for testing is therefore usually within 2 weeks for PCR and Ag-RDT and 7 days or more after symptom onset for antibody tests [23].

Table 25.20 Pulmonary and extrapulmonary manifestations of Covid-19 [11,12]

Organ	Manifestation
Lung	Cough; sore throat; upper respiratory tract infection; anosmia; ageusia
	Pneumonia
	Silent hypoxia
	Acute respiratory distress syndrome
Renal	Acute kidney injury; acute tubular necrosis
	Electrolyte abnormalities (e.g. hyperkalemia, hyponatremia, hypernatremia)
	Metabolic acidosis
	Proteinuria; haematuria
Neurological	Anosmia; ageusia; headaches; dizziness; myalgia; fatigue; insomnia
	Stroke
	Encephalopathy; encephalitis; Guillain–Barré syndrome; acute haemorrhagic necrotising encephalopathy
	Ophthalmoplegia; polyneuritis
Gastrointestinal	Diarrhoea; nausea/vomiting; abdominal pain; anorexia
	Mesenteric ischaemia; gastrointestinal bleeding
	Hepatic dysfunction: elevated aminotransferases; elevated bilirubin
	Pancreatic injury
Haematological	Venous thrombotic complications (deep vein thrombosis, pulmonary embolism)
	Arterial thrombotic complications (myocardial infarction, ischaemic stroke, acute limb and mesenteric ischaemia)
	Catheter-related thrombosis (arterial/venous catheters, extracorporeal circuits)
	Cytokine-release syndrome ('cytokine storm'): high-grade fevers, hypotension, multiorgan failure
Cardiovascular	Myocardial ischemia; type II myocardial infarction
	Cardiac arrhythmias (including atrial fibrillation); sudden cardiac death
	Myocarditis
	Cardiomyopathy; Takotsubo cardiomyopathy
	Cardiogenic shock
Endocrine	Hyperglycemia
	Diabetic ketoacidosis (in previously undiagnosed diabetes)
	Euglycemic ketosis
	Abnormal thyroid function
	Adrenal insufficiency
Musculoskeletal	Myalgia
	Myositis; myopathy
	Rhabdomyolysis
Psychiatric	Psychosis
	Anxiety; depression; suicidal ideation
Mucocutaneous	See Tables 25.21–25.31

SARS-COV-2 IN SKIN HEALTH AND DISEASE: OVERVIEW

The Covid-19 pandemic has had far-reaching implications for many aspects of skin disease and dermatological practice.

Mucocutaneous manifestations of Covid-19 infection

Introduction and general description

A wide range of mucocutaneous manifestations has been reported in association with SARS-CoV-2 infection in adults and children.

Initial reports appeared as early as February 2020 and many thousands of publications have appeared subsequently. Although they have rapidly informed scientific knowledge and medical practice in many aspects of Covid-19 and skin disease, there are considerable variations in reporting and heterogeneity between studies [36,37]. While the role of SARS CoV-2 infection – direct, indirect (e.g. due to reactivation of other viruses) or coincidental (e.g. due to drug hypersensitivity) – remains uncertain for many mucocutaneous conditions, they may potentially assist in early Covid-19 diagnosis in some cases and provide predictive information regarding likely disease severity and outcomes [4,33,38,39]. Skin diseases not related to SARS-CoV-2 infection, other infections and drug reactions should all be considered in the differential diagnosis of mucocutaneous changes in Covid-19, especially for non-specific manifestations such as urticaria or maculopapular eruptions.

Epidemiology

Covid-19 dermatology registries were created in the early stages of the pandemic (Table 25.21) and have provided important information on many aspects of SARS-CoV-2 and skin health and disease. These include mucocutaneous presentations associated with acute and chronic ('long') SARS-CoV-2 natural infection and vaccination; outcomes of SARS-CoV-2-positive patients with pre-existing dermatological diseases; the safety of systemic treatments during Covid-19 infection. Limitations of registry data include lack of information on the total population, and under representation of populations of colour and those living in low-income countries, as most cases entered in registries to date have been white patients from North America and Europe [40].

Incidence and prevalence

The reported incidence of mucocutaneous involvement in patients with acute Covid-19 is highly variable, and few population-level data or large cohort studies with a known denominator exist [31,41]. Multiple factors make the true prevalence difficult to assess and include the severity (asymptomatic, non-hospitalised, hospitalised, admitted to ICU) of Covid-19 in the population reported; the expertise of the clinical assessor (dermatology specialist, non-specialist, patient-reported); how assessment was performed (e.g. face to face or virtual; full skin examination or limited examination in critically ill patients or while trying to maintain strict infection prevention techniques); the stage of Covid-19 infection (early, concurrent, late); whether SARS-CoV-2 infection was suspected or laboratory proven (particularly early in the pandemic when access to SARS-CoV-2 diagnostic resources was generally more limited [4]); differences between populations in terms of access to care and/or reporting; other factors related to geography and ethnicity/race [42,43]; the presence of pre-existing dermatoses [40]; and the presence of other possible non-Covid-19 causes (e.g. iatrogenic due to concurrent medication or other viral infections) [44,45].

For example, an incidence of 0.2% was reported in an early study from China of 1099 hospitalised patients examined by non-specialists [6]. In contrast, a study published the following month found changes in 20% of virus-positive in-patients in a single-centre study in Italy who were screened by dermatologists [27], whereas a prevalence of 7.25% was subsequently reported from India in hospitalised patients also screened by a dermatologist in a single centre [46]. An estimated incidence of almost 9% was reported in a UK community-based study of more than 300 000 of 4 million self-reporting contributors to the ZOE COVID Symptom Study smartphone application; a subset of approximately 11 500 of these contributors also responded to an independent online survey of skin-specific symptoms, with more than 2300 providing clinical photographs [32]. The largest systematic review and meta-analysis of 240 publications to December 2020 included 2056 patients and estimated an overall prevalence of approximately 6% [31], consistent with earlier systematic reviews [47–49]. Using this estimate and extrapolating to the 600 million people infected by SARS-CoV-2 globally to September 2022 [9], it is therefore possible that around 36 million will have been affected by mucocutaneous manifestations of Covid-19.

Table 25.21 Selected international Covid-19 dermatology registries. Adapted from Freeman et al. 2021 [40].

Registry		Provider/patient-facing	Website
AAD/ILDS	American Academy of Dermatology/International League of Dermatological Societies Covid-19 Dermatology Registry	Provider	https://www.aad.org/member/practice/coronavirus/registry
HS-COVID	Global Hidradenitis Suppurativa Covid-19	Both	https://hscovid.ucsf.edu/
PeDRA	Pediatric Dermatology Research Alliance (COVID-Acral ischaemia/perniosis)	Provider	https://pedraresearch.org/2020/04/20/covid-acral-ischemia-perniosis-in-children/
PsoProtect	Psoriasis Registry for Outcomes, Therapy and Epidemiology of Covid-19 Infection	Provider	www.psoprotect.org
PsoProtectMe	Psoriasis Registry for Outcomes, Therapy and Epidemiology of Covid-19 Infection – patient reported registry	Both	https://psoprotectme.org/
SECURE-AD	Surveillance Epidemiology of Coronavirus Under Research Exclusion-Atopic dermatitis	Both	www.covidderm.org
SECURE-Alopecia	Surveillance Epidemiology of Coronavirus Under Research Exclusion-Alopecia	Provider	https://secure-derm.com/secure-alopecia/
SECURE-Psoriasis	Surveillance Epidemiology of Coronavirus Under Research Exclusion-Psoriasis	Provider	https://school.wakehealth.edu/departments/dermatology/secure-psoriasis

Ethnicity

Covid-19 disproportionately affects populations with skin of colour (SOC) in terms of both infection rates and disease severity and significant disparities in health care have been brought into stark focus by the pandemic [42]. The lack of data on patients with SOC has been recognised in many studies [29,32,40,50], and the lack of clinical images of Covid-19 in SOC has also been highlighted as an important concern. In one review, only 4% of 130 published images were Fitzpatrick phototypes IV and none was V or VI [51] and such underrepresentation of different races, ethnicities and skin colour in the medical literature may have a significant impact on early diagnosis and outcomes [29,41,42,43,51,52].

Despite these challenges, there are emerging differences in both the prevalence and phenotypes of Covid-19-associated skin manifestations in terms of both geography and race/ethnicity [4,41,50]. The reported prevalence of skin disorders was only 0.6–2.59% of hospitalised SARS-CoV-2-positive patients in two separate studies in India [53,54], although in another the rate was 7.25% [46]. Similarly, prevalence was 0.2% in one early study of hospitalised patients in China [6] and 0.56% in a single-centre study in Japan [55], also possibly suggestive of a lower prevalence compared with US and European populations. The frequency of specific phenotypes may also vary [50]. For example, a chilblain-like lesion (CBLL) is the most common skin problem in white populations [31], but there are fewer reports in those of African or Hispanic descent in the USA [56–58] and in patients of South Asian descent in India [46]. The prevalence of other vaso-occlusive disorders also appears to be lower in Asian compared with white populations [41,43,46]. Pathophysiological explanations include genetic polymorphisms predisposing to inflammatory events (e.g. resulting from differences in interferon production) and thromboembolic events (e.g. increased levels of lipoprotein A and Factor V Leiden in some populations) [33,42]. However, other factors such as reporting bias, socioeconomic and cultural disparities may contribute to these discrepancies. For example, access to care, care-seeking behaviour and self-reporting biases may exist between different racial/ethnic groups. Health care provider biases may also exist, for example underrecognition of redness in people with darker skin tone may contribute to underreporting of some skin manifestations, as may reporting biases in different countries [41,42,50,52].

Pathophysiology

SARS-CoV-2 binds to ACE2 receptors expressed in the subcutaneous fat and epithelial cells and direct viral invasion is proposed to contribute to the development of mucocutaneous manifestations in Covid-19. Dysregulation of the humoral immune response and resulting inflammatory cascade and autoantibody formation (including to vasculature, connective tissue and skin) is a hallmark of SARS-CoV-2 infection and this also contributes to development of mucocutaneous disorders. Other potential contributory pathogenetic mechanisms include reactivation of other viruses (e.g. herpes virus) and hypersensitivity reactions to drugs used during treatment of Covid-19 infections [21,24,25,59].

Clinical features

No standardised classification of the clinical morphology of mucocutaneous presentations associated with Covid-19 has been consistently used in the literature. One of largest case series published early in the pandemic from a nationwide, prospective study in Spain included 375 patients and proposed a consensus classification of five main clinical patterns [28], subsequently modified to six in a study from Italy [34,60]. A broader classification into two mechanistic categories has also been proposed, specifically eruptions related to virally triggered inflammatory responses (as in other viral exanthems) and vasculopathy-related cutaneous changes secondary to Covid-19 systemic consequences (especially vasculitis and thrombotic vasculopathy) [29]. However, numerous additional presentations which cannot be easily included in these broader classifications have been reported (Tables 25.22 and 25.23) [4,28,29,30,31,32,33,34,38,39,41,60–65,66,67] and some patients display more than one phenotype [29,31,34,60].

The relative frequencies of specific presentations reported by different studies varies, but there is general agreement that pernio-like lesions or CBLLs, red/maculopapular/morbilliform exanthems and urticaria are the most common phenotypes (Table 25.22) [28,29,31,32,34,60]. However, reliably distinguishing entities which are directly associated with SARS-CoV-2 infection from those occurring during Covid-19 but associated with other causes is challenging. Iatrogenic drug reactions, exanthems due to viruses other than SARS-CoV-2 and pre-existing dermatoses are examples of possible confounders and there are also important variations between countries and skin types (see later).

Table 25.22 Clinical phenotypes of mucocutaneous manifestations described in association with Covid-19. Adapted from Agnihothri 2021 [4]; Galván Casas 2020 [28]; Freeman 2020 [29]; Marzano 2021 [30]; Holmes 2022 [31]; Visconti 2021 [32]; Do 2021 [33]; Genovese 2021 [34]; Bassetti 2022 [38]; Huynh 2022 [39]; Tan 2021 [41]; Marzano 2020 [60]; Mohseni 2021 [61]; Brandini 2021 [62]; Seebacher 2022 [63]; Rekhtman 2021 [64]; Nguyen 2022 [65]; Neale 2021 [66]; La Rosa 2021 [67].

Category	Morphology
Inflammatory/ exanthematous	Urticarial rash
	Confluent red/maculopapular/morbilliform exanthem
	Papulovesicular/vesiculobullous exanthem
Vasculopathic	Chilblain-like acral pattern
	Livedo reticularis
	Purpura/petechiae
	Vaso-occlusive (livedo racemosa; retiform purpura; acro-ischaemia; pressure-associated ulceration and necrosis)
Other cutaneous	Multisystem inflammatory syndrome (children, adults)
	Erythema multiforme-like rash
	Pityriasis rosea-like rash
	Herpes zoster reactivation
	Neutrophilic dermatoses (Sweet syndrome)
	Erythema nodosum/panniculitis
	Grover disease-like eruption
	Gianotti–Crosti-like eruption
	Erythema elevatum diutinum-like lesions
	Symmetrical drug-related intertriginous and flexural exanthema (SDRIFE)-like eruption
	Eruptive pyogenic granulomas
	Vitiligo
Hair and nails	Alopecia (telogen/anagen effluvium; androgenic; alopecia areata)
	Trichodynia
Mucosal	*Oral:* aphthous-like ulcers; tongue depapillation; angular cheilitis; blisters; white plaques; hyperpigmentation
	Genital: acute genital ulcers (Lipschütz ulcers)

Table 25.23 Clinicopathological features of mucocutaneous manifestations described in association with COVID-19. Adapted from Agnihothri and Fox 2021 [4]; Do, Stewart and Harp 2021 [33]; Holmes et al. 2022 [31]; Genovese et al. 2021 [34]; Galván Casas et al. 2020 [28]; Marzano et al. 2021 [30]; Marzano et al. 2020 [60]; Visconti et al. 2021 [32]; Desai, McMichael and Khanna 2021 [42]; Freeman et al. 2020 [29]; Mohseni Afshar et al. 2021 [61]; Bassetti et al. 2022 [38]; Brandini et al. 2021 [62]; Huynh et al. 2022 [39]; Seebacher, Kirkham and Smith 2022 [63]; Tan, Tam and Oh 2021 [41]; Rekhtman et al. 2021 [122]; Nguyen and Tosti 2022 [65]; Neale and Hawryluk 2021 [66]; La Rosa et al. 2021 [67].

Cutaneous manifestation	%*	Age range	Clinical features	Timeline with Covid-19 symptoms	Association with Covid-19 severity	Histopathology reported specifically in Covid-19-associated cases	Management reported in Covid-19 cases
Chilblain (perniosis)-like acral lesions (pseudo-pernio, 'COVID toes/fingers')	54.2 Significant variation with geography/race/ethnicity	Children, young adults	Asymmetrical dusky red-violaceous-purpuric patches, oedematous papules, plaques or less frequently bullae predominantly affecting the toes, lateral aspects of the feet, and/or less frequently fingers and elbows. Associated with itching and a painful/burning sensation	Late	Asymptomatic Mild	Necrotic epidermal keratinocytes; perivascular and periadnexal dermal lymphocytic infiltrate of CD3+/CD4+ T cells; dermal oedema; vascular changes (endotheliitis and microthrombi)	Resolve over 2–8 weeks; expectant management; topical corticosteroids
Maculopapular/morbilliform rash	13.6	50s–60s	Generalised, symmetrical, erythematous macules and papules initially truncal with centrifugal progression; purpuric lesions may coexist from the onset or develop during course of eruption; often pruritic	Concurrent	Moderate	Spongiotic dermatitis with eosinophils and superficial perivascular lymphocytic and/or neutrophilic infiltrate in early lesions with histiocytes in later lesions	*Mild*: topical corticosteroids *Severe*: systemic corticosteroids
Erythema†	3.9						
Urticarial rash	8.3	40s	Itchy urticarial rash predominantly affecting trunk and limbs; angioedema may also rarely occur	Concurrent	Moderate	Superficial perivascular lymphocytic infiltrate; scattered eosinophils; upper dermal oedema; epidermal dyskeratosis	Antihistamines; low-dose oral corticosteroids
Papulovesicular-vesiculobullous rash	6.3	40s–60s	*Widespread*: polymorphic pattern with small papules, vesicles and pustules (varicella-like). May be itchy *Localised*: papulovesicular lesions involving mid-chest/upper abdomen and back	Early/concurrent	Moderate	Prominent acantholysis and dyskeratosis; unilocular, suprabasal intraepidermal vesicles; vacuolar degeneration of basal layer; endotheliitis in dermal vessels	Expectant
Purpura/petechiae	3.4	30s–70s	Purpura may be generalised, acral or intertriginous. Lesions may evolve into haemorrhagic blisters and leading to necrotic-ulcerative lesions	Late	Moderate Severe	Leukocytoclastic vasculitis, severe perivascular neutrophilic and lymphocytic infiltrate, fibrin and endothelial swelling	*Mild*: topical corticosteroids *Severe*: systemic corticosteroids
Erythema multiforme-like rash	3.3	Children–young adults	Targetoid, confluent macules, papules and plaques of varying size with haemorrhage and central crusting. Oral involvement (palatal macules and petechiae; chelitis) may occur	Concurrent/late	Mild	Interface dermatitis; superficial and deep perivascular and peri-eccrine CD3+/CD4+/CD8+ lymphocytic infiltrate; vasculopathic changes; positive immunohistochemistry for spike protein in vessel endothelium	
Livedo reticularis	2.4	40s–60s	Mild, transient, symmetrical, lace-like, dusky patches forming complete rings with a pale centre; trunk and limbs	Concurrent/late	Moderate	Pauci-inflammatory microthrombotic vasculopathy	Expectant
Vaso-occlusive disorders (livedo racemose; retiform purpura; acro-ischaemia)	1.8	60s	*Livedo racemosa*: large, irregular, asymmetrical, violaceous, annular lesions in patients with severe coagulopathy *Retiform purpura*: extremities and buttocks; often asymptomatic	Late	Severe	Epidermal necrosis; superficial and deep dermal thrombosis; vasculopathy in small and medium-sized vessels; perivascular lymphocytic infiltrate; complement deposition in vessel walls	Expectant Widespread: systemic corticosteroids

(continued)

PART 3: INFECTIONS & INFESTATIONS

Table 25.23 (continued)

Cutaneous manifestation	%*	Age range	Clinical features	Timeline with Covid-19 symptoms	Association with Covid-19 severity	Histopathology reported specifically in Covid-19-associated cases	Management reported in Covid-19 cases
Multisystem inflammatory syndrome in children (MIS-C) and adults (MIS-A)	0.3	More common in children	Polymorphic maculopapular eruption; trunk and flexural; acral erythema; extremity swelling and desquamation; mucositis; fissured lips (see Table 25.25)	Concurrent	Severe	*Children*: varies from leucocytoclastic vasculitis to erythema multiforme-like histology. *Adults*: varies from superficial, perivascular, lymphocytic infiltrate with occasional neutrophils and extravasated red cells to superficial and deep perivascular and periadnexal lymphocytic infiltrate	See text
Hair and nails							
Telogen effluvium	1.1	40s	Most common form of alopecia occurring after Covid-19	Late	–	–	
Trichodynia	–		Commonly associated with telogen effluvium	Late	–	–	
Alopecia areata	–		Usually in pre-existing disease; less commonly new onset	Late	–	–	
Androgenic alopecia	–		Usually precedes Covid-19	Pre-Covid	Severe	–	
Nails	–		Beau lines; onychomadesis; red-white discoloration with distal onycholysis; other discolorations of lunula and nail plate	Late	–	–	
Oral/genital lesions							
Oral lesions	0.7	–	Aphthous-like ulcers; erythema multiforme-like lesions; other oral ulcers; enanthems; oral submucous fibrosis; tongue depapillation; angular cheilitis, necrotising gingivitis; white plaques; hyperpigmentation; erythema; petechiae; dysgeusia/ageusia	Early Concurrent	–	Lesion-type dependent	Lesion-type dependent
Acute genital (Lipschütz) ulcers	–	40s	Necrotic ulcers labia minora; sharply demarcated borders with no evidence of 'kissing lesions'; associated oral ulceration	Concurrent	Mild	–	Oral corticosteroids
Others							
Pityriasis rosea-like	4	Young adults	Both classic pityriasis rosea (papulosquamous eruption with ovoid patches and plaques with fine collarettes of scale and preceding herald patch) and atypical digitate papulosquamous variants described	Concurrent	–	Mild spongiosis; spongiotic vesicles containing lymphocytes and Langerhans cells; parakeratosis; mild papillary oedema and dermal lymphohistiocytic infiltrate; SARS-CoV-2 spike protein detected in endothelium of dermal blood vessels in affected skin	Expectant; topical corticosteroids if symptomatic

Condition		Age	Clinical presentation	Timing	Severity	Histology	Treatment
Reactivation of herpes zoster	–	–	Clinical presentation similar to non-Covid-19 disease	Concurrent	–	–	–
Sweet syndrome	–	60s	Red painful nodules on scalp, extremities, trunk; oral ulcers; fever; elevated neutrophil count	Late	Moderate	Neutrophilic infiltrate with vascular proliferation	Expectant; regression with recovery from Covid-19
Erythema nodosum/panniculitis	–	–	Clinical presentation similar to non-COVID-19 disease				
Gianotti–Crosti-like rash	–	Young adult	Pruritic papules and vesicles coalescing into plaques; elbows, thighs and bilateral popliteal fossa			Subacute spongiotic dermatitis; patchy parakeratosis; focal spongiotic vesiculation; acanthosis with elongation of the epidermal ridges; papillary dermal oedema; perivascular upper dermal lymphocytic	Expectant
Symmetrical drug-related intertriginous and flexural exanthema (SDRIFE)-like rash	–	70s	Red rash in axillae and antecubital fossae, extending to trunk and inner thighs	Concurrent	Moderate–severe	Subcorneal pustules and superficial infiltrates of lymphocytes and eosinophils	Expectant
Grover disease-like	–	50s	Truncal papules and papulovesicles; possible overlap with papulovesicular eruptions	Concurrent	Mild	Focal acantholysis; dyskeratotic epidermal keratinocytes; mild dermal perivascular lymphocytic infiltration with some eosinophils; SARS-Cov-2 spike protein positive in endothelium and eccrine sweat gland epithelium	
Erythema elevatum diutinum-like	–	30s	Firm, symmetrical, smooth, pink-red nodules on extensor surfaces including dorsum hands; itchy and burning	Concurrent–late	Mild	–	
New-onset vitiligo	–	40s	Typical vitiligo affecting limbs, trunk, face 2 weeks after Covid-19	Late	Mild	–	–
New-onset bullous pemphigoid (BP)	–	80s	Maculopapular and acral vesicular rash evolved into BP	Late	Mild	As for non-Covid-19-associated BP	Oral corticosteroids and doxycycline

*Based on systematic review by Holmes et al. 2022 [31]. †Erythema grouped separately by Holmes et al. 2022 [31].

Timeline relative to Covid-19 systemic symptoms

There are emerging differences in the timing of some mucocutaneous manifestations relative to onset of Covid-19 systemic symptoms. These differences were first reported in a large case series from Spain [28] (Table 25.23). In the UK community-based ZOE COVID Symptom Study, self-reported mucocutaneous symptoms were the first presentation of the disease in 17% and a more powerful predictor of infection than fever (odds ratio for rash 1.67 and for fever 1.48) [32]. Mucocutaneous changes similarly occurred before other Covid-19 signs in 12% of patients in a dermatologist-reported US registry study [29] and approximately 7% overall in a systematic review [31] and may therefore be an important predictor of infection. Onset tends to be during the earlier inflammatory phase for vesiculobullous rashes (5.6 days), urticarial rashes (7 days), maculopapular rashes (9 days) and red rashes (10.6 days); in the later inflammatory phase for livedo reticularis (14.1 days), CBLL (15.9) and acral ischaemia (23 days); and most delayed for hair and nail disorders (50 days) [31]. The duration of disorders is also variable, with a mean of 13 days, ranging from 6.7 days for urticaria to 32 days for acral ischaemia [4,30,31,49,63].

Relationship with Covid-19 disease severity

In up to 21% of cases, mucocutaneous manifestations may be the only clinical sign of Covid-19 infection [31,32]. Certain trends are emerging between specific mucocutaneous manifestations and Covid-19 disease severity (Table 25.23). This may partly relate to the varying immune response following SARS-CoV-2 infection, and it is proposed that specific disease patterns may potentially help in predicting Covid-19 prognosis [4,28,31,33,38,60,68]. Vaso-occlusive presentations (livedo racemosa, retiform purpura, acro-ischaemia) are seen in older age groups and are associated with severe and critical disease, including ICU admission and mortality. Conversely, maculopapular, urticarial and papulovesicular eruptions appear to be associated with less severe disease although are more common in hospitalised patients. At the other end of the spectrum, CBLL – which is more frequent in younger age groups – is often associated with asymptomatic or pauci-symptomatic Covid-19 [28,29,30,31,41].

Clinical variants

The clinicopathological characteristics and treatment of the most frequent mucocutaneous disorders reported in association with Covid-19 are summarised in Table 25.23. Selected conditions are discussed in brief next.

Chilblain-like lesions (CBLL, pseudo-pernio, 'Covid toes/fingers'). Perniosis (chilblains) is a cold-sensitive inflammatory disorder that presents at sites of cold exposure (usually toes or fingers and occasionally other acral sites such as the ear) as pink-red-violaceous macules, papules, plaques or nodules which may blister and ulcerate in severe cases and are associated with pain and/or a burning sensation (Figure 25.33). They may be idiopathic or associated with autoimmune conditions (e.g. chilblain lupus), haematological

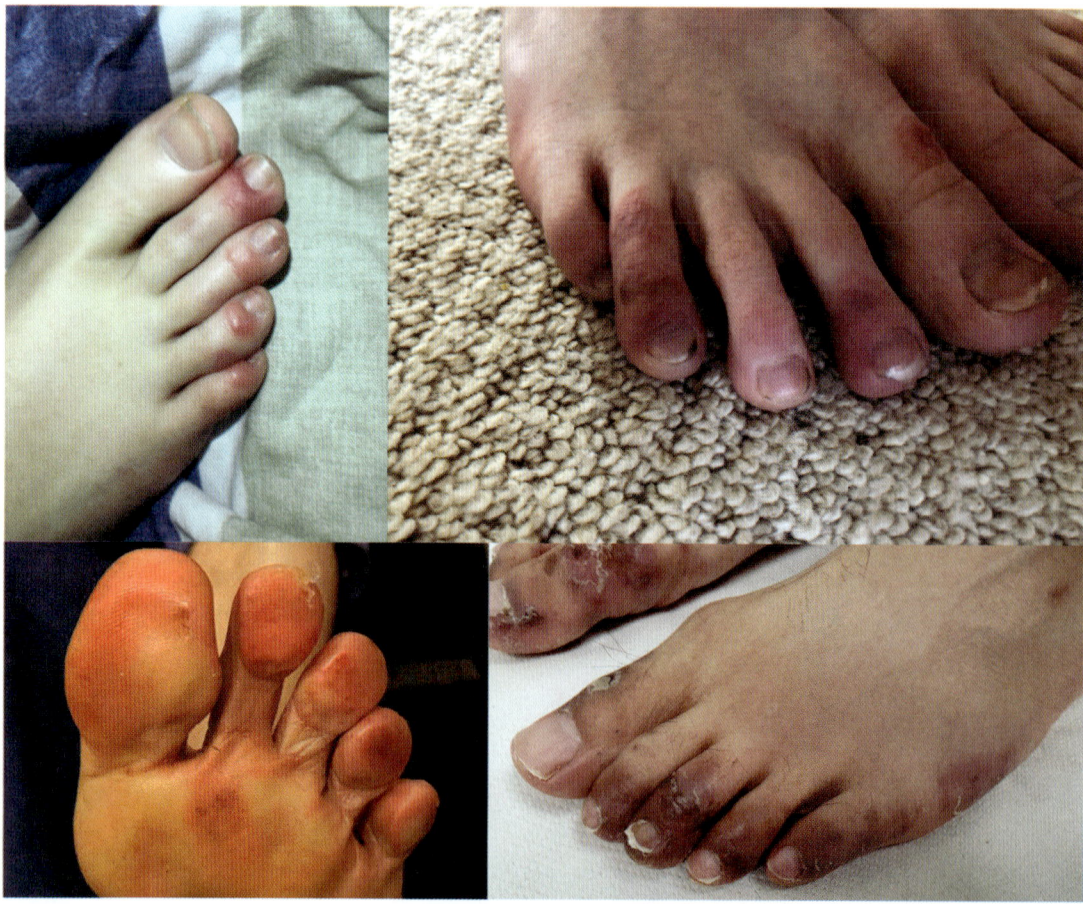

Figure 25.33 Examples of chilblain-like lesions associated with SARS-CoV-2 infections. (a,b) Examples in white subjects from the UK provided by subjects via the ZOE COVID application. Courtesy of Dr Veronique Bataille (British Association of Dermatologists COVID Atlas (www.covidskinsigns.com)). (c,d) Examples in South Asian subjects living in the UK. (c) Courtesy of Dr Abha Gulati. (d) Courtesy of Dr Anshoo Sahota.

malignancies, specific genodermatoses and other infections such as Epstein–Barr virus [4,29,33,50].

The first report of pernio-like lesions in association with Covid-19 was in an Italian adolescent [69] and subsequent reports from Spain suggested they occurred mainly in later stages of disease [28]. The marked rise in cases of a previously uncommon condition, at an atypical time of year (spring), in temperate areas and in patients apparently at low risk initially pointed to an association: clustering of cases in families and close contacts and subsequent larger cohort studies also support this association, as does identification of SARS-CoV-2 viral particles in endothelial cells of CBLL by electron microscopy [70,71]. However, the absence of Covid-19 symptoms, negative SARS-CoV-2 nasopharyngeal RNA on RT-PCR and lack of positive serology in many patients with CBLL led to theories that CBLL was an epiphenomenon and only indirectly related to infection with the virus [56,72].

It is now clear that a negative test does not rule out an association and may simply reflect the timing and type of laboratory testing undertaken. There is a window between cleared infection (median time to undetectable RNA on nasopharyngeal swab RT-PCR is 14 days, so that 50% are negative before this) and detectable antibodies (average time to mount an antibody response is 7–14 days) [4,21,33,73]. In addition, there is a relationship between disease severity and antibody levels: those who develop CBLL have relatively mild clinical courses and may not mount a marked antibody response, but are nonetheless able to elicit *in vitro* neutralising antibodies that prevent viral entry into epithelial cells. Furthermore, these antibodies may be IgA rather than IgG or IgM that are the usual antibodies assessed in commercial tests. A robust type I interferon response to viral nucleotide sensing may also enhance the early innate immune response to viral infection, resulting in mild disease and suppressed antibody formation and later development of CBLL. Consistent with this, pernio-like lesions are also observed in type 1 interferonopathies (e.g. Aicardi–Goutieres syndrome and STING-associated vasculopathy), and CBLL and severe Covid-19 are thought to lie at two ends of a type I interferon spectrum [74]. Genetic predisposition is also emerging as a possible contributor to susceptibility [19]. For example, in genome-wide association studies, the 3p21.31 region is associated with Covid-19 severity and also contains the *TREX1* gene, missense mutations in which are responsible for familial chilblain lupus [75].

Histopathology of CBLL is similar to non-Covid-19 perniosis, with vascular changes, dermal oedema and a superficial and deep perivascular lymphocytic infiltrate [4,33]. In some cases, immunohistochemistry has confirmed vasculitis in dermal vessels with deposition of immunoglobulins or complement and platelet aggregation, but lesions are primarily inflammatory and not suggestive of systemic coagulopathy, unlike vaso-occlusive disorders such as livedo racemosa or retiform purpura. Microthrombi seen in a small subset are likely to be secondary to the inflammation and correlate with a bullous or necrotic phenotype.

CBLLs are more common in children and young adults and there are possible differences in the prevalence of CBLL by geographic areas and population ethnicity/race. Lesions are typically self-limiting, lasting 1–3 weeks, with excellent prognosis, although may be recurrent [76]. First line management is expectant. Topical corticosteroids, topical antibiotics and NSAIDs have all been used for acute inflammation. If pain is more problematic, use of topical anaesthetics and analgesics is also described [66].

Maculopapular rashes. Maculopapular rashes (encompassing macular redness and morbilliform rashes), the second most common cutaneous manifestation after CBLL, are usually concurrent with Covid-19 symptoms, have a median duration of 7 days and are associated with moderate severity Covid-19 disease [31,77]. They are frequently itchy and often initially truncal with centrifugal progression to become generalised, consisting of symmetrical, red macules and papules (Figure 25.34). In some cases, purpuric changes may coexist from the outset or develop during the course of the eruption. Skin biopsy often shows spongiosis, basal cell vacuolation and perivascular lymphocytic infiltrate, which are features typical of other viral-induced skin lesions. Although likely to be secondary to the immune response to viral infection, maculopapular rashes are also a potential side effect of many medications used in Covid-19 treatment and this should be considered in their differential diagnosis. As they are usually self-limiting, treatment is not generally required, but topical corticosteroids or systemic steroids in severe cases have been used [4,33,38].

Urticarial eruptions. Urticarial rashes are common and occur early in the course of Covid-19 – in some cases as a prodromal sign – with a median duration of 4–7 days and in association with moderate severity disease [78,79]. They typically involve the trunk and limbs, with pruritus being the main symptom (Figure 25.35). Treatment includes antihistamines or low-dose oral corticosteroids. Proposed mechanisms include viral IgM/IgG cross-reacting with mast cell IgE and causing mast cell degranulation [80]. As with morbilliform rashes, urticarial eruptions are also a common side effect of drugs used in Covid-19 treatment.

Papulovesicular/vesiculobullous eruptions. These exanthems also usually occur early after the onset of Covid-19 symptoms [30] and are associated with moderate severity disease [31]. Generalised and localised forms are described and are usually more truncal and associated with minimal pruritus compared with true varicella [30,81]. The rash may also simulate Grover disease and some histological overlap including acantholysis has been reported [82]. In other cases, basal vacuolar degeneration with multinucleate, hyperchromatic keratinocytes and dyskeratotic cells is consistent with viral infection [30,81,83] and it has been proposed that the direct pathogenic effects of SARS-CoV-2 on basal layer keratinocytes lead to acantholysis and dyskeratosis [82].

Petechiae and purpura. These are the most common vascular lesions, usually occur late relative to Covid-19 symptoms and are associated with moderate to severe disease [31] (Figure 25.36). An early report described a patient with a petechial rash misdiagnosed as dengue [84] and acral, intertriginous or diffuse presentations occur. Aetiology includes thrombocytopenia/platelet dysfunction, clotting abnormalities and vasculitis (which may progress to blisters and ulcerated lesions). Henoch-Schönlein purpura and IgA vasculitis have also been reported [85,86].

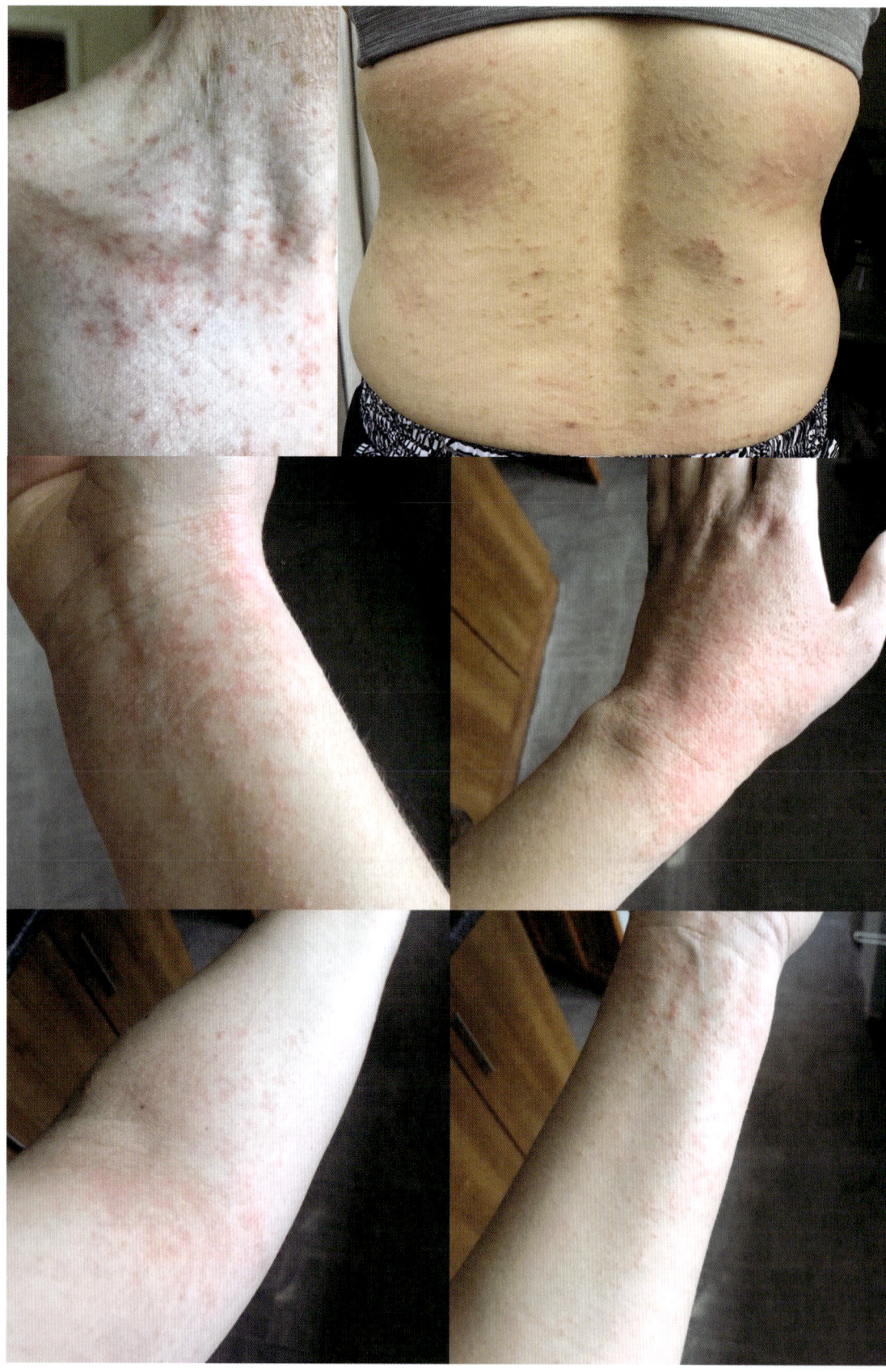

Figure 25.34 Examples of red and maculopapular rashes associated with SARS-CoV-2 infection. Examples provided by subjects in the UK via the ZOE COVID application. Courtesy of Dr Veronique Bataille (British Association of Dermatologists COVID Atlas (www.covidskinsigns.com)).

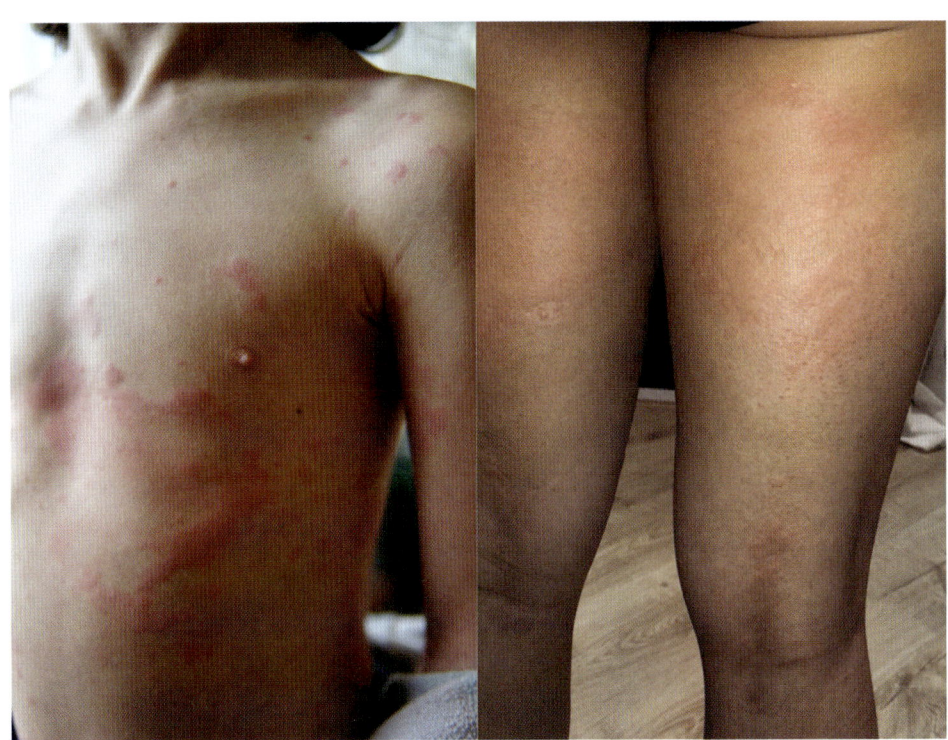

Figure 25.35 Examples of urticarial rashes associated with SARS-CoV-2 infection. Examples provided by subjects in the UK via the ZOE COVID application. Courtesy of Dr Veronique Bataille (British Association of Dermatologists COVID Atlas (www.covidskinsigns.com)).

Livedo reticularis. Livedo reticularis occurs concurrently or late relative to Covid-19 systemic symptoms and consists of symmetrical, annular, violaceous patches involving trunk and limbs caused by partial or intermittent blood flow reduction to the skin. Histology shows pauci-inflammatory microthrombotic vasculopathy [29] and thus microthromboses or low-grade vascular inflammation resulting from SARS-CoV-2-associated endothelial cell damage are possible pathomechanisms [33]. Livedo reticularis is usually associated with moderate rather than severe disease [33,39].

Vaso-occlusive disorders (fixed livedo racemosa; retiform purpura; acro-ischaemia; pressure-associated ulceration and necrosis. Covid-19 is associated with a hypercoagulable state resulting in venous and arterial thrombosis. Vaso-occlusive skin lesions are rare, occur late in the course of Covid-19, are most often seen in older patients with severe Covid-19, often with systemic thromboembolic complications, and have the highest mortality rate of all COVID-associated skin manifestations [28,29,33,49]. Pathomechanisms may involve hyperactivation of the complement system possibly through local immune stimulation by SARS-CoV-2 spike protein present in the cutaneous microvasculature; this may synergise with antiphospholipid autoantibodies found in patients with severe Covid-19, leading to increased coagulation with formation of occlusive thrombi in small dermal vessels resulting in microvascular injury and necrosis [33,87]. *Livedo racemosa* consists of persistent, large, irregular, violaceous, broken annular patches indicating significantly reduced cutaneous blood flow. *Retiform purpura* are on a spectrum with livedo racemosa, but are associated with more severe vascular occlusion leading to stellate, purpuric skin lesions with incipient or frank ulceration, seen most often as *acral ischaemia* on the extremities. *Pressure-associated ulceration and necrosis* has been described in critically ill patients and particularly occurs on the sacral/buttock areas, with areas of ulceration often surrounded by livedoid plaques and retiform purpura and evidence of thombotic vasculopathy and pressure necrosis [88–90]. *Acrofacial purpura and necrosis* is described in association with minor pressure injury, for example due to direct contact with medical devices and during the process of proning to improve oxygen status [91].

Erythema multiforme-like lesions. Erythema multiforme-like eruptions with acral and truncal distributions are reported in both children and young adults [31,77,92]. Lesions are pruritic or painful and appear as red macules and plaques consisting of two (atypical targets) or three (typical targets) rings, usually on the extremities with central crusting in some cases (Figure 25.37). Oral mucosal changes may be present (erosive cheilitis and palatal macules/petechiae). Positive immunohistochemistry for SARS-CoV-2 spike protein has been identified in vascular endothelium in erythema multiforme [93], but possible drug causes should also be considered (see later).

Pityriasis rosea (PR)-like eruption. PR-like rashes with both classic and atypical presentations appear to occur at greater frequency in Covid-19 [31,77]. Proposed mechanisms include direct effects of SARS-CoV-2 in the skin, as SARS-CoV-2 spike protein has been detected in the endothelium of dermal vessels in PR [94], or indirect effects including dysregulated immunity and reactivation of other viruses such as HHV-6 or -7 [68,95].

Reactivation of herpes zoster. An increased incidence of herpes zoster in patients with confirmed Covid-19 has been observed, but it is uncertain whether this is coincidental or a direct effect of SARS-CoV-2-associated immune dysregulation [28].

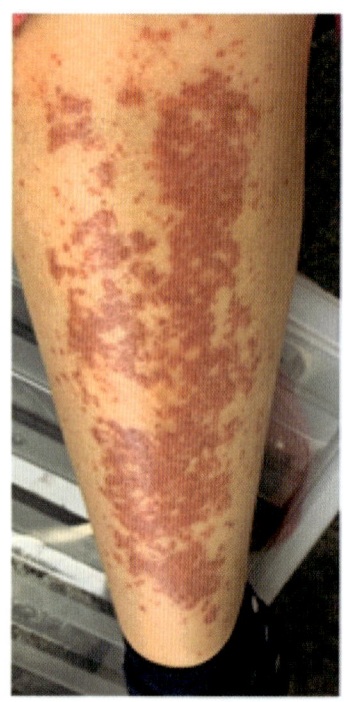
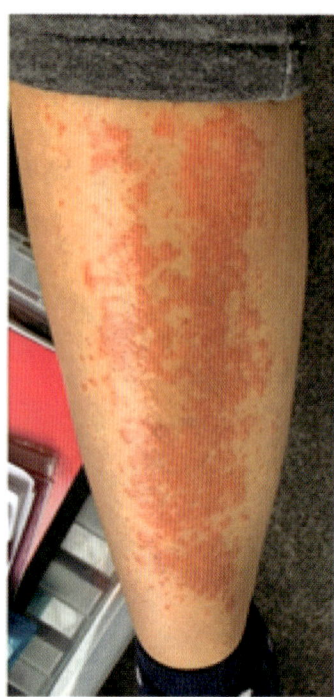
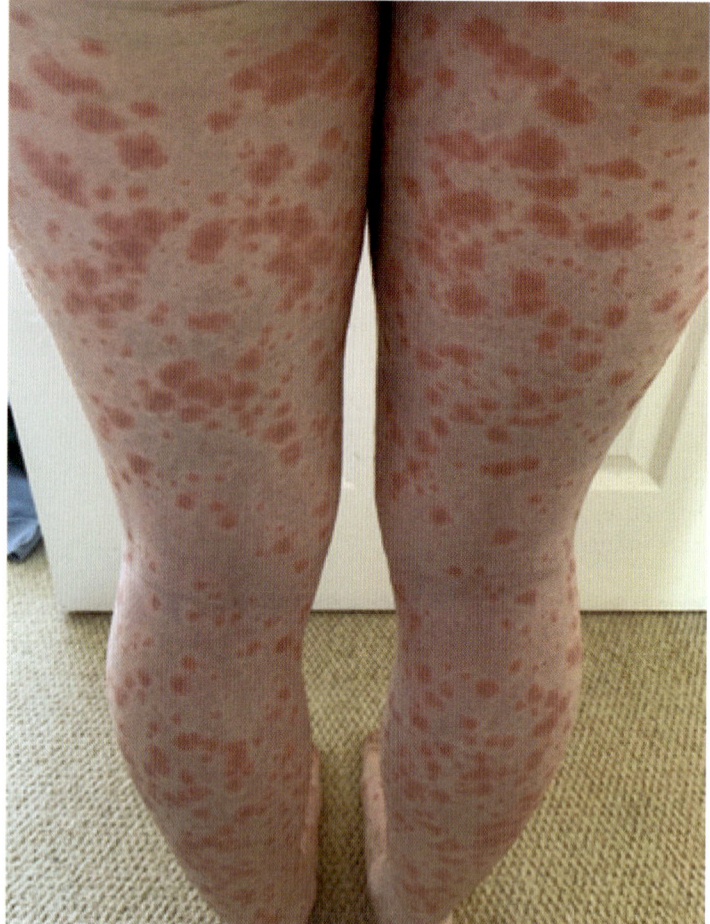

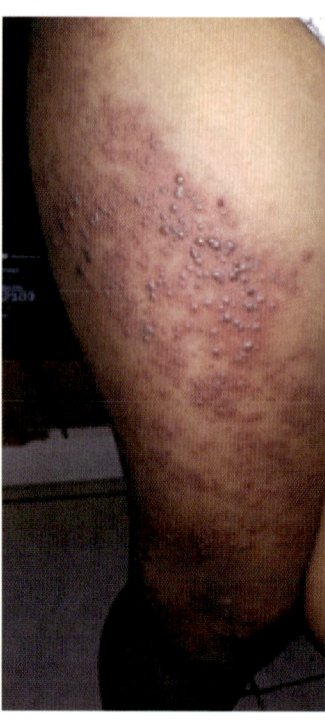

Figure 25.36 Examples of purpuric and vasculitis rashes associated with SARS-CoV-2 infection. Examples provided by subjects in the UK via the ZOE COVID application. Courtesy of Dr Veronique Bataille (British Association of Dermatologists COVID Atlas (www.covidskinsigns.com)).

Figure 25.37 Example of erythema multiforme-like rash associated with SARS-CoV-2 infection. Example provided by subject in the UK via the ZOE COVID application. Courtesy of Dr Veronique Bataille (British Association of Dermatologists COVID Atlas (www.covidskinsigns.com)).

Sweet syndrome. Elevated neutrophil count is a consistent finding in Covid-19 and may contribute to reported cases of Sweet syndrome that regress during recovery from Covid-19 without specific treatment [96].

Multisystem inflammatory syndrome in adults (MIS-A). MIS is a severe hyperinflammatory condition associated with SARS-CoV-2 and although most common in children, it is also recognised in adults (MIS-A) [97]. The five criteria for MIS-A include severe illness requiring hospitalisation for patients >21 years of age; positive laboratory tests for SARS-CoV-2 infection in the past 12 weeks; severe dysfunction of one or more extrapulmonary organ systems; laboratory evidence of severe inflammation (ESR, CRP, neutrophilia, D-dimer, fibrinogen, ferritin, LDH, procalcitonin, IL-6); absence of other causes for severe respiratory illness [98]. Hyperinflammation is proposed to result from hyperactivation of the innate immune system, probably due to aberrant interferon responses [99]. Mucositis is common and polymorphic rashes are also described and include urticarial macules and plaques, morbilliform eruptions, purpura, petechiae and retiform purpura [97,98,100]. Histology varies from superficial, perivascular, lymphocytic infiltrate with occasional neutrophils and extravasated red cells to superficial and deep perivascular and periadnexal lymphocytic infiltrate [100]. *In situ* hybridisation for SARS-CoV-2 is usually negative. At least half of all patients with MIS-A required ICU admission and treatments include intravenous immunoglobulin, corticosteroids and tocilizumab, an interleukin-6 inhibitor [97].

Mucosal lesions. Various mucosal manifestations have been described, many in association with cutaneous lesions.

Oral. Reported disorders include aphthous-like ulcers, tongue depapillation, angular cheilitis, blisters, white plaques, hyperpigmentation and enanthems (e.g. macular and petechial changes). The aetiology is likely to be multifactorial and proposed mechanisms include direct action of SARS-CoV-2 on oral mucosal cells, dysregulated immunity, coinfection with other organisms and adverse drug reactions [62,67,92].

Genital. Acute genital (Lipschütz) ulcers have been described in association with Covid-19 [101], as has a reactive infectious mucocutaneous eruption with shallow erosions of the periurethral glans penis, lips and hard palate [102].

Hair and nail disorders. Covid-19 is reported to be associated with telogen effluvium, alopecia areata and androgenetic alopecia [65]. As with other mucocutaneous manifestations of Covid-19, the causes are likely to be multifactorial and include direct virus-induced and delayed immunological responses to infection.

Telogen effluvium (TE). A systematic review of more than 1800 patients with Covid-19 and alopecia found TE to be the most common type presenting after Covid-19 infection [65]. In a series of 214 patients from Spain, 14% with TE were asymptomatic in terms of Covid-19 infection [103]. Early-onset TE (within 4 weeks) has been reported in more than 60% of patients, but onset is later ($\geq$12 weeks) in the remainder [104]. It is proposed that early-onset TE is possibly a consequence of upregulated pro-inflammatory cytokines (e.g. IL-1b, IL-6, TNF-α, IFN-γ) during more severe infection which triggers induction of an immediate anagen release [104]. However, the contributions of drugs used in Covid-19 treatments (e.g. heparinoids) and both physiological and psychological stress have also been highlighted [103,104].

Trichodynia. Scalp dysaesthesia is a common accompanying symptom and was reported in 42% of patients presenting with TE in one series [104].

Alopecia areata (AA). AA usually occurs in patients with pre-existing disease (as is also seen with other viruses such as Epstein–Barr virus and cytomegalovirus). However, Covid-19 may rarely trigger new-onset AA [65,105]. The mechanism underlying this association with SARS-CoV-2 infection may be autoimmune, with loss of immune privilege of hair follicles in anagen [65].

Androgenetic alopecia (AGA). In one systematic review, AGA was more common than TE and AA, but almost always preceded Covid-19 [65]. It is proposed to be a marker of susceptibility to more severe disease, possibly related to androgen-mediated upregulation of the transmembrane serine protease 2, facilitating entry of SARS-CoV-2 into cells via the ACE2 receptor [65,106].

Nail changes. CBLL, acral vascular changes and periungual desquamation in MIS may all affect the nail apparatus. Other late nail changes reported in association with Covid-19 include Beau lines, onychomadesis and variable pigmentation of the nail plate and lunula, for example in the 'Covid red half-moon' sign in which half-moon-shaped red bands surround the distal part of the lunula [107].

Other mucocutaneous presentations (Tables 25.22 and 25.23). Case reports of other conditions associated with Covid-19 include Grovers [108–110] and erythema elevatum diutinum-like eruptions [77]; eruptive pyogenic granulomas [111]; new-onset vitiligo [112]; and new-onset autoimmune bullous disorders including bullous pemphigoid [113] and pemphigus [114].

Chronic ('long') Covid-19. SARS-CoV-2 infection associated with prolonged symptoms has been termed 'long Covid' or 'long-haul Covid' [115]. Between 66% and 87% of patients continued to experience one or more Covid-19 symptoms 2 months after PCR positivity and approximately 30% at 6 months [116–118]. In one registry study, mucocutaneous symptoms persisting for at least 60 days included CBLLs in 6.8% and livedo reticularis [119]. Alopecia may also be persistent [21]. Some of these disorders may be mediated by autoimmune responses, but the full implications of long Covid for mucocutaneous disease remain to be established [21,119].

Covid-19 and skin disease in children

General description of disease domain

Children have less frequent infection, generally with a milder course, with higher frequencies of asymptomatic infection, fewer respiratory sequelae and fewer severe complications compared with adults [66,120]. The contrasting presentation in children is likely to be multifactorial and includes [66,121,122]:
- Reduced viral entry and infection due to fewer ACE receptors in nasal/lung epithelium.
- Stronger innate and adaptive antiviral immunity (increased cytokines, interferon production and CD4+/CD8+ T cells; more vigorous CD8+ T-cell responses).
- Healthy vascular endothelium.
- Fewer predisposing factors for severe disease.

Epidemiology

Cutaneous manifestations reported in children are diverse and include most phenotypes seen in adults. They may be the main or only clue to infection in mild or asymptomatic disease [66]. Mucocutaneous lesions have been described in more than 8% of hospitalised children and may be associated with better prognosis [66,122]. However, the more robust immune responses in children may also underlie some of the differences seen in the pattern of cutaneous responses compared with adults, such as the increased frequency of CBLLs and multisystem inflammatory syndrome in children (MIS-C) [66].

Clinical features
Chilblain-like lesions (CBLL, pseudo-pernio, 'Covid toes/fingers') in children. Prior to the Covid-19 pandemic, chilblains/pernio was relatively uncommon in children. Rates of new-onset chilblains/pernio increased dramatically coinciding with the pandemic, with 29% of all cases reported in children [56]. Hypotheses to explain this increased prevalence have focused on differences in levels of interferon production. Interferon provides innate immunity against

viruses and it is proposed that healthy children and young adults mount robust interferon responses to SARS-CoV-2 which clear the virus but lead to delayed pernio-like lesions, which are effectively a post-viral manifestation of Covid-19 infection [21,74,123,124]. As in adults, CBLLs affect toes, feet, ankles, fingers and hands and present as asymptomatic or painful and/or pruritic, red and purpuric papules, macules and plaques with vesicles and bullae in some cases [66,124].

Multisystem inflammatory syndrome in children (MIS-C)/ paediatric inflammatory multisystem syndrome temporally associated with SARS-CoV-2 infection (PIM-TS). MIS-C/PIMS-TS is one of the most severe consequences of Covid-19 in children and is a novel hyperinflammatory condition that shares features with toxic shock syndrome and Kawasaki disease, including fever, skin, mucous membrane and distal extremity changes [4,125].

Definition. MIS-C is defined by the Centers for Disease Control and Prevention (CDC) as a hyperinflammatory response to current or recent SARS-CoV-2 infection or exposure in an individual under 21 years with a fever lasting more than 24 hours, elevated laboratory inflammatory markers (ESR, CRP, neutrophilia, D-dimer, fibrinogen, ferritin, LDH, procalcitonin, IL-6), dysfunction of more than two organs (cardiac, respiratory, gastrointestinal, renal, haematological, neurological and skin), requiring hospital admission and not explained by other illness [126]. PIM-TS is similarly defined by the WHO as a child presenting with persistent fever, inflammation and evidence of single or multiorgan dysfunction, with additional features which include a rash or bilateral non-purulent conjunctivitis or mucocutaneous inflammation signs [127].

Pathophysiology. This is unclear but may be the result of a hyperinflammatory immune response driven by SARS-CoV-2. Immune-complex development from viral antigens (type III hypersensitivity) is postulated to initiate a cytokine storm with systemic inflammation and autoantibody development may also play a pathogenic role [21,128]. Genetic predisposition towards a pro-inflammatory immune response to infection has been identified in some studies [129–131].

Clinical features. Intensive care and circulatory support are frequently required, and mortality is approximately 2% [66]. The earliest cases were reported in the UK [131] and most are previously healthy children, with a median age of 5–11.5 years, with black or Asian race/ethnicities most frequently affected [66,120,121,132]. As with CBLL, MIS-C is thought to be a late or post-viral complication, with antibody titres higher than levels of RNA detection [121]. Skin and/or mucosal changes are present in 50–83% of children with MSI-C, which is higher than that generally reported in children with Covid-19 infection [66,121,133]. Generalised or localised skin involvement is described with a wide array of morphologies (Table 25.24). Mucosal involvement, particularly oral and conjunctival, is common and was the most frequent manifestation in one series [121]. The exact relationship between mucocutaneous involvement and disease severity remains uncertain [66,122,134].

Table 25.24 Mucocutaneous findings reported in multisystem inflammatory syndrome in children. Adapted from Neale and Hawryluk 2021 [66]; Dondi et al. 2022 [125].

Eyes	Oral	Hands and feet	Non-acral skin
Periorbital oedema	*Lips:* Fissuring	Oedema	Urticaria
Hyperaemia	Redness	Redness	Macular and maculopapular exanthems
Discharge		Desquamation	Morbilliform exanthem
	Mouth:	Purpura	Scarlatiniform exanthem
	Papillitis	Petechiae	Erythema infectiosum-like exanthem
	Strawberry tongue	Vesicles	
		Erythema multiforme-like	Erythema multiforme-like
		Beau lines	Purpura, petechiae, livedo, Henoch Schönlein purpura/vasculitis
		Perniosis-like	Gianotti–Crosti-like
			Erythema nodosum
			Severe cutaneous adverse reactions

Table 25.25 Kawasaki disease compared with multisystem inflammatory syndrome in children. Adapted from Neale and Hawryluk 2021 [66].

	Multisystem inflammatory syndrome in children (MIS-C)	Kawasaki disease (KD)
Demographics		
Age	Mean age 9 years	90% ≤5 years
Sex	Slightly more males	Male predominance
Race/ethnicity/geography	Black, hispanic/Latino	More common in Asia (Japan, South Korea and Taiwan)
Clinical signs		
Unexplained fever	>24 hours	≥5 days
Respiratory	41%	35%
Cardiovascular shock	66%	10%
Gastrointestinal	87%	61%
Oral mucosal change		
Distal extremity changes		
Rash		
Conjunctivitis	<50% meet criteria for KD	Diagnostic criteria for KD = 4/5
Cervical lymphadenopathy		

Differential diagnosis. These features may be diagnostically challenging, particularly in the context of a child with fever and a negative Covid-19 test. Many simulate those of Kawasaki disease, making this an important differential diagnosis (Table 25.25). In addition, toxic shock syndrome, bacterial sepsis, scarlet fever, drug hypersensitivity, other viral infections, vasculitis and systemic illnesses such as macrophage activation syndrome should also be considered [66,133].

Management. In addition to supportive care that requires ICU admission in up to 80% of cases, treatment of MIS-C includes systemic corticosteroids, intravenous immunoglobulins and antiviral agents; cytokine inhibitors and immunomodulators have also been used [66].

Table 25.26 Other potential cutaneous manifestations of Covid-19 infection in children. Adapted from Neale and Hawryluk 2021 [66].

Urticaria
Maculopapular rash
Vesicles/papulovesicular rash
Petechiae
Purpura
Retiform purpura
Livedo reticularis
Ecchymotic-like lesions
Erythema multiforme-like lesions
Herpetiform oral eruption
Plantar papules
Roseola-like rash
Lingual papillitis
Eccrine hidradenitis
Erythema nodosum

Co-morbidities and complications. Although most children with MIS-C recover, post-hospitalisation sequelae include coronary artery abnormalities in 16–21% [135]. Hair abnormalities including alopecia areata and telogen effluvium are also described [136].

Other mucocutaneous manifestations of Covid-19 infection in children. In addition to CBLL and MIS-C, a range of other inflammatory, vascular and non-specific cutaneous changes have also been reported in children (Table 25.26) [4,21,66,76,121,122,134].

Effects of SARS-CoV-2 infection on pre-existing mucocutaneous disease

Disease exacerbation by SARS-CoV-2 infection

Viral infections may be associated with exacerbations of autoimmune and other pre-existing skin conditions and are also reported for SARS-CoV-2 infection (Table 25.27). Multiple factors are likely to account for such disease flares and include those directly related to SARS-CoV-2 infections (e.g. due to dysregulation of cytokines and chemokines such as interferon, IL-36, CXCL8), as well as factors related to the pandemic including non-adherence to treatment and socioeconomic factors [137]. For example, a systematic review of publications to July 2021 reported exacerbation of pre-existing psoriasis, subacute lupus erythematosus, pemphigus vulgaris,

Table 25.27 Pre-existing dermatoses reported to be exacerbated by SARS-CoV-2 infection.

Psoriasis
Atopic dermatitis
Alopecia areata
Subacute lupus erythematosus
Pemphigus vulgaris
Bullous pemphigoid
Systemic sclerosis
Sézary syndrome
Acrodermatitis continua of Hallopeau

systemic sclerosis, Sézary syndrome and acrodermatitis continua of Hallopeau [137]. In a registry-based study of atopic dermatitis, 18% experienced a flare of atopic dermatitis during Covid-19 [29] and in a separate patient-reported study of adults with atopic dermatitis and psoriasis in the Netherlands, 26% experienced worsening during symptomatic infection with SARS-CoV-2 [138]. In Italy, 42.5% of patients with alopecia areata experienced a relapse approximately 2 months after Covid-19 compared with 12.5% in the absence of Covid-19 [139].

Covid-19 outcomes in patients with pre-existing mucocutaneous diseases

Outcomes of patients with Covid-19 who are receiving systemic immunosuppressive or biologic treatments for dermatological conditions have been of particular concern during the Covid-19 pandemic. Registries have been an important source of information on this question. For example, data from the SECURE-AD registry showed that Covid-19 duration and resolution were not significantly influenced by type of systemic medication for atopic dermatitis (dupilumab versus conventional immunosuppressives) and that complication rates were low [40]. Similarly, the PsoProtect and SECURE-Psoriasis registries have reported that patients with psoriasis receiving biologics had a lower risk of hospitalisation compared with those on non-biologic systemic therapy, with most patients recovering fully [140]. Patient reporting to the PsoProtectME registry has indicated differences in behaviour between treatment groups, with greater risk-mitigating behaviour by those on targeted therapies compared with standard systemic agents that may contribute to differences in outcomes [140]. Evidence from provider and patient-reported cases from the HS COVID Registry [111] has also shown that biologic therapy is not associated with worse Covid-19 outcomes in patients with hidradenitis suppurativa, nor is there a difference between patients who continue versus discontinue biologic treatment [40]. In a retrospective study of Covid-19 outcomes for patients with autoimmune blistering disorders, mortality was higher compared with the general population, although rituximab use was not associated with a higher rate of SARS-CoV-2 positivity [142].

However, it is important to point out that evidence is rapidly evolving in this area. In a large nationwide cohort study in the UK which included more than 1.1 million adults with immune-mediated inflammatory diseases affecting the joints, bowel and skin, 19 000 of whom were receiving targeted immune-modifying therapy and 182 000 standard systemic therapy, the overall risk of Covid-19-related critical care admission or death was increased compared with the general population after adjusting for confounders such as age, sex, deprivation, smoking, high BMI and cardiovascular disease, and this was higher in ethnic groups other than white [143]. There was no increased Covid-19-related mortality associated with use of TNF inhibitors, IL-12/IL-23 inhibitors, IL-17 inhibitors, IL-6 inhibitors, or Janus kinase inhibitors compared with those on standard systemic therapy, with the exception of rituximab which was associated with increased Covid-19-related death (HR 1.68, 95%CI 1.11–2.56) [143]. These and other conditions are discussed in more detail in relevant chapters.

Table 25.28 World Health Organization guidelines on drug treatment in Covid-19 and associated mucocutaneous reactions. Adapted from Agrawal 2020 [144].

Covid-19 severity	Drug	Class	Examples of mucocutaneous adverse effects
Critical/severe	Dexamethasone**	Corticosteroid	Pruritus, skin infection, acneiform eruptions, skin atrophy, telangiectasia, purpura, oedema, hirsutism, striae
	Tocilizumab or sarilumab**	IL-6 receptor blocker	Maculopapular rash, urticaria, skin infections, pruritus, psoriasiform dermatitis, pustular eruptions, necrotising fasciitis
	Baricitinib**	Janus kinase (JAK) inhibitor	Urticaria, angioedema, palmoplantar pustulosis-like eruption, herpes zoster, herpes simplex reactivations, skin cancers
	Remdesivir (severe only)*		Maculopapular rash, exfoliative erythroderma, Stevens–Johnson syndrome, toxic epidermal necrolysis, erythema multiforme, urticaria, lichenoid drug eruption, lipodystrophy, annular erythema, photosensitivity, hyperpigmention of nails, oral mucosa and skin, pruritus, alopecia, xerosis, paronychia, insect bite hypersensitivity
	Ruxolitinib and tofacitinib (only if IL-receptor blocker or baricitinib unavailable) X	JAK inhibitors	See above for baricitinib
	Convalescent plasma (research only) X		Urticaria, maculopapular rash, eczema, erythema multiforme, purpura
	Ivermectin (research only) X	Anti-parasitic	Urticaria, pruritus, papulopustular rash, oedema, toxic epidermal necrolysis, Stevens–Johnson syndrome, drug reaction with eosinophilia and systemic symptoms (DRESS) syndrome
Non-severe but highest risk of hospital admissions	Nirmatrelvir with ritonavir**	Antiviral	See above for remdesivir
	Molnupiravir*	Antiviral	See above for remdesivir
	Remdesivir*	Antiviral	See above for remdesivir
	Corticosteroids X		See above for dexamethasone
	Ivermectin (research only) X	Anti-parasitic	See above for ivermectin
	Fluvoxamine (research only) X	Selective serotonin reuptake inhibitor and σ-1 receptor agonist	Morbilliform rash, pruritus, ecchymoses, flushing
	Convalescent plasma XX		See above for convalescent plasma
Strong recommendations against use regardless of severity	Hydroxychloroquine XX	Antimalarial, anti-inflammatory	Maculopapular rash, acute generalised exanthematous pustulosis, exacerbation of psoriasis, urticaria, pruritus, Stevens–Johnson-like syndrome, DRESS syndrome, alopecia, hair bleaching, mucocutaneous dyspigmentation
	Lopinavir-ritonavir XX	HIV-1 antiviral	See above for remdesivir
	Colchicine XX	Anti-inflammatory	Morbilliform rash, lichenoid drug eruption, alopecia, toxic epidermal necrolysis-like reaction, bullous and erythema-nodosum-like lesions
	Casirivamab and imdevimab #	Monoclonal antibodies	Pruritus, urticaria, anaphylaxis
	Sotrovimab #	Monoclonal antibody	Erythema, morbilliform rash, pruritus, anaphylaxis

**Strong recommendations in favour; *weak or conditional recommendations in favour; X, weak or conditional recommendations against use; XX, strong recommendations against use (# with omicron variant).

Mucocutaneous manifestations of treatment for Covid-19 infection

Covid-19 disease severities are defined by the WHO as:
- *Critical:* acute respiratory distress syndrome, sepsis, septic shock or other conditions requiring life-sustaining therapies (e.g. invasive/non-invasive mechanical ventilation or vasopressor therapy).
- *Severe:* oxygen saturation <90% on room air, pneumonia, severe respiratory distress.
- *Non-severe:* absence of these criteria.

Most patients with Covid-19 have relatively mild illness and require only symptomatic measures. Specific treatments are available for those with severe or critical disease or with non-severe disease at high risk of hospitalisation with more severe disease (e.g. organ transplant recipients; PLWH; haematological malignancies; other immunocompromise; sickle cell disease; certain neurological, autoimmune or inflammatory conditions). The evidence base for these treatments is evolving rapidly with numerous RCTs completed or in progress [144]. The current WHO recommendations for drug treatment of Covid-19 with reported mucocutaneous reactions are summarised in Table 25.28.

Drug reactions should be considered in the differential diagnosis of mucocutaneous disorders arising in the context of Covid-19 and it is likely that at least some of the mucocutaneous manifestations reported in association with Covid-19 are drug related [44,45,145,146].

Table 25.29 Approved SARS-CoV-2 vaccines (September 2022).

Platform	Vaccine
Messenger RNA (mRNA)	Moderna Spikevax mRNA-1273
	Pfizer–BioNTech Comirnaty BNT162b2
Adenovirus vector–based	AstraZeneca Vaxzevria and Covishield ChAdOx1
	Johnson & Johnson–Janssen Ad26.COV2.S
Inactivated virus	Sinopharm Covilo BBIBP-CorV
	Sinovac CoronaVac; Bharat Biotech Covaxin
Adjuvanted protein	Novavax Nuvaxovid
	Covovax NVX-CoV2373

MUCOCUTANEOUS REACTIONS TO SARS-COV-2 VACCINES

General description of disease domain

As of October 2022, more than 300 Covid-19 vaccines for prevention of both Covid-19 and viral transmission were in preclinical or clinical development [22]. Ten Covid-19 vaccines have been approved by the WHO for global use and involve four separate vaccine platforms (Table 25.29). It is estimated that by September 2022, more than 12.5 billion vaccine doses had been given globally [9], although their use in developing countries has been limited, highlighting stark global health inequities [13]. Real-world effectiveness data have shown that mRNA vaccines (BNT162b2 and mRNA-1273) induce high initial antibody titres that wane after a few months, whereas adenovirus vector-based vaccines (Ad26.CoV2.S) induce lower initial antibody responses but have greater durability. Subsequent cellular immune responses induced by both vaccine types are more durable than serum antibody titres. As CD8+ T-cell responses control viral replication after infection, it is predicted that SARS-CoV-2 vaccines will continue to protect against severe infection even after such waning of humoral immunity and potential reduced effectiveness against blocking infection with emerging variants such omicron [13].

Epidemiology

As with many vaccines, constitutional symptoms are frequently observed with SARS-CoV-2 vaccines and include fever, headache, fatigue, chills, muscle pain, diarrhoea and local injection-site reactions. Myocarditis and pericarditis have also been reported together with the rare vaccine-induced immune thrombotic thrombocytopenia (VITT), but both thrombosis and myocarditis are significantly more frequent after natural Covid-19 infection [13].

Although reported prevalence in SARS-CoV-2 vaccine trials is low, a greater number of cutaneous adverse events have been reported in real-world data accruing from observational studies during Covid-19 mass vaccination, including registry data (e.g. AAD/ILDS, PsoProtect, SECURE-AD, SECURE-Alopecia and HS COVID) [40,147]. In a systematic review and meta-analysis of 300 studies published up to December 2021, global prevalence was estimated at 3.8% (95%CI, 2.7–5.3%) and highest for mRNA vaccines at 6.9% (95%CI, 3.8–12.3%) [148]. A broad spectrum of disorders has been described and many simulate skin conditions associated with natural Covid-19 infection, such as chilblains, erythromelalgia and pityriasis-rosea like reactions (Table 25.30) [147,**148**,149–164]. Registry data suggest reactions are reported less frequently with booster vaccinations [165]. As with mucocutaneous disorders arising with natural Covid-19 infection, there may be difficulty in distinguishing between causation and coincidental presentation and the temporal relation to Covid-19 vaccination.

Pathophysiology

A range of pathomechanisms are implicated and – as with natural Covid-19 infection – many are the result of vaccine immune/autoimmune responses rather than direct viral effects [**148**,150,155]. This may explain the variation in prevalence across vaccine platforms, with higher prevalence after mRNA vaccines explained by their stimulation of more robust immune responses [**148**,149, 150,155,158].

Clinical features

Local injection site reactions. The most frequent cutaneous manifestations of Covid-19 vaccination in clinical trials were local injection site reactions. These are similar to patterns of reaction commonly seen with other vaccines and are less often reported in non-trial observational studies, although they were the second most common skin reaction in one registry study [153]. These usually occur within 7 days of injection and present with pain, redness, swelling, tenderness, induration and pruritus, and are more common after the first dose and in those under the age of 60 years [149,159]. They occasionally present atypically with patches and plaques which may become vesicular [166].

Delayed local reactions. In real-world settings, the most frequent reaction is the delayed large local reaction ('Covid arm'), with redness, induration and tenderness which may mimic cellulitis and occurs 7 or more days after vaccination. This was initially reported in the phase III trial with Moderna mRNA-1273 in 0.8% of participants after the first dose and 0.2% after the second [167]. In a single-centre study of the Pfizer–BioNTech BNT162b2 vaccine it was observed in 2.1% of patients [168]. It appears to be restricted to mRNA vaccines [169], particularly females under 65 years of age. It is usually mild, resolves after 4–5 days and most cases are reported after the first dose, but it may recur after second vaccination [149,152]. Histology is consistent with a delayed-type, T-cell-mediated hypersensitivity reaction with superficial and deep perivascular lymphocytic infiltrates, scattered mast cells and occasional eosinophils [168,169]. The precise aetiology is uncertain, but hypotheses include a delayed hypersensitivity to the excipient PEG found in both BNT162b2 and mRNA-1273 vaccines [149] or related to the delayed appearance of the spike protein at the injection site, which corresponds with the timing of onset of delayed local reactions [152].

Urticaria and angioedema. In one large registry study, urticaria was the second most common vaccine-related skin reaction after local injection site reactions [154]. Although it is reported as an immediate hypersensitivity reaction (i.e. within 4 hours of vaccination), in most observational studies it has a more delayed onset. This is a significant distinction as an immediate severe reaction

Table 25.30 Mucocutaneous reactions reported in association with SARS-CoV-2 vaccines and their possible pathomechanisms. Adapted from Sun 2021 [149]; Tan 2022 [152]; Washrawirul 2022 [148]; Magro 2021 [150]; McMahon 2021 [153]; McMahon 2022 [154]; Avallone 2022 [156]; Avallone 2022 [157]; Freeman 2022 [147]; Gambichler 2022 [158].

Reaction pattern	Possible pathomechanisms	Examples
Type I immediate hypersensitivity	Allergic reaction to Covid-19 vaccine components (polyethylene glycol and polysorbate 80) leading to mast cell degranulation	Urticaria Angioedema Anaphylaxis
Type IV delayed hypersensitivity	Increased Covid-19 vaccine-mediated immune recruitment in the presence of secondary allergens	Delayed large local skin reaction ('Covid arm') Morbilliform rashes (including V-REPP) Erythema multiforme Inflammatory reactions in dermal filler sites, previous radiation sites and old BCG scars
Autoimmune reactions	Molecular mimicry (cross-reactivity to viral antigens): e.g. genetic similarities between the SARS-CoV-2 spike protein components and endogenous cross-reactive human antigens	Vaccine-induced immune thrombocytopenia Lupus erythematosus Vasculitis Bullous pemphigoid
	Bystander effect (viral-induced release of sequestered self-antigens)	Vitiligo Alopecia areata
Others	Functional angiopathies Reactivation of viral conditions	Chilblain-like lesions Pityriasis rosea Pityriasis rosea-like eruptions Herpes zoster, herpes simplex
	Vaccine immunogenicity	Flares of pre-existing dermatoses, e.g. psoriasis

with anaphylaxis may potentially represent a contraindication to a second vaccination [148,149,153]. Angioedema is less common, but both are almost always associated with mRNA vaccines, and it remains unclear whether the excipient PEG is responsible for these urticarial reactions [152].

Morbilliform/maculopapular and papulovesicular rashes. Morbilliform and maculopapular rashes are reported in multiple observational studies and appear to share similarities to those described with natural Covid-19 infection [149]. They usually occur within 2–3 days of vaccination, resolve within one week, but may recur after the second vaccine [152]. The exact mechanism is unclear, but histology suggests an immune process rather than direct viral effects, with spongiosis and mild dermal perivascular infiltrates. In one series, reported from the AAD/ILDS registry, 58 of 803 (7%) of all skin reactions had biopsies and the most common histopathological reaction pattern was spongiotic dermatitis. The term V-REPP (vaccine-related eruption of papules and plaques) was used to describe the corresponding clinical spectrum ranging from papules with subtle scaling through to pityriasis rosea-like and papulovesicular changes [154].

Delayed inflammatory reactions (DIRs). Viral illnesses and influenza vaccines are among the known triggers of DIRs to hyaluronic acid fillers and SARS-CoV-2 vaccines appear to have a similar potential [149]. Although uncommon, these DIRs have occurred to fillers injected at least 1–2 years before Covid-19 vaccination, often develop within 24–48 hours, present with pain, redness, swelling and induration in areas previously treated with fillers and may occur after first or second injections. Similar reactions at the sites of old BCG scars and previous radiotherapy have also been described [148,152]. Most fillers are injected in adipose tissue which contains a high concentration of ACE2 receptors. It has been proposed that, as in natural Covid-19 infection, interaction of the SARS-CoV-2 spike protein releases a pro-inflammatory cascade which may explain this inflammation. These reactions are usually resistant to antihistamines and hyaluronidase, but ACE inhibitors promote an anti-inflammatory response and oral lisinopril is described as an effective treatment, leading to resolution within 24–72 hours [170].

Chilblain-like reactions (pseudo-perniosis). Chilblain-like reactions are well recognised with natural Covid-19 and have also been described with SARS-CoV-2 vaccination, particularly after the first dose of mRNA vaccines, with a 3-day median duration of onset [152]. Although the mechanisms are unclear, this suggests that vaccines and SARS-CoV-2 activate similar immune pathways rather than direct viral effects involving strong IFN-I responses [149,154].

Petechial and purpuric rashes. A range of clinical patterns are reported including new-onset vasculitis, immune thrombocytopenic purpura, Henoch-Schönlein purpura, pigmented purpuric dermatosis, purpura fulminans, livedo racemosa and cutaneous thrombosis/skin necrosis [154].

Bullous eruptions. New onset of bullous pemphigoid, pemphigus vulgaris and bullous fixed drug eruption have all been described after mRNA vaccines and 60% after the first dose [114,152,171,172].

Viral reactivation. Herpes zoster reactivation has also been reported, particularly in patients with autoimmune disorders. The cause is uncertain, but it has been hypothesised that it may represent a dysregulation of cell-mediated immunity unmasked by vaccine immunomodulation, with paradoxical worsening of latent infection, similar to immune reconstitution syndrome [152,154].

Pityriasis rosea. The median duration of the onset of the eruptions of PR following vaccination is 5.5 days and most cases have been reported after mRNA vaccination [152]. The exact pathomechanisms are unclear: while PR may represent reactivation of latent herpes viral infection, similar to natural Covid-19 infection, it may alternatively result from a delayed hypersensitivity response to the vaccine [152,154].

Severe cutaneous adverse reactions (SCARs). SARS-CoV-2 vaccination has rarely been associated with anaphylaxis, with frequency rates of 2.5–11.1 per million. Other SCARs such as acute generalised exanthematous pustulosis and Stevens–Johnson syndrome have also been reported [**148**,169,173–176].

Flares in pre-existing dermatoses. Vaccine immunogenicity may also result in altered levels of chemokines and cytokines that may contribute to flares in pre-existing dermatoses (e.g. psoriasis, atopic dermatitis, lichen planus, autoimmune blistering disorders, Behçet disease, systemic lupus erythematosus, dermatomyositis) and may unmask these conditions for the first time in genetically predisposed individuals [159].

Other dermatoses. A wide spectrum of other cutaneous reactions has been reported more rarely, although distinguishing a coincidental onset with genuine vaccine-related disorders may be challenging (Table 25.31) [147–149,152–163,177].

Table 25.31 Other cutaneous manifestations reported in association with SARS-CoV-2 vaccination. Adapted from Freeman 2022 [147]; Washrawirul 2022 [**148**]; Sun 2021 [149]; Tan 2022 [152]; McMahon 2021 [153]; McMahon 2022 [154]; Niebel 2021 [155]; Avallone 2022 [156]; Avallone 2022 [157]; Gambichler 2022 [158]; Seirafianpour 2022 [159]; Shakoei 2022 [160]; Shafie'ei 2022 [161]; Bawane 2022 [162]; Shawky 2022 [163]; Darrigade 2022 [177].

Erythema multiforme-like lesions
Erythromelalgia
Lichen planus
Alopecia
Neutrophilic dermatoses/Sweet syndrome
Erythema nodosum
Livedo reticularis
Rowell syndrome
Urticarial vasculitis
Raynaud phenomenon
Eruptive angiomatosis
Eosinophilic cellulitis
Acantholytic dermatosis
Vitiligo
Acneiform eruption
Pityriasis lichenoides et varioliformis acuta
Rosacea/rosacea-like
Fixed drug eruptions
Symmetrical drug-related intertriginous and flexural exanthema
Granuloma annulare
Pityriasis rubra pilaris
Tattoo sarcoidal reaction
Prurigo nodularis
Regression of viral warts
Regression of lymphoproliferative disorder
Cutaneous mucormycosis

COVID-19 vaccination and skin disease

Previous skin reactions to vaccination. In general, most cutaneous reactions are mild and self-limiting. They are rarely a contraindication to subsequent vaccination but should be considered on a case-by-case basis. Most guidelines and recommendations point out the compelling safety profiles of Covid-19 vaccines and the importance of allaying fears about such reactions and encouraging vaccine completion [**148**,149,152,158]. Patients with SCARs after previous vaccination should be assessed on a case-by-case basis [164]. Immediate, severe allergic reactions/anaphylaxis to a previous Covid-19 vaccine or its components are regarded as the only major contraindication to vaccination [159].

Allergy testing. Criteria for allergy testing prior to vaccination in local and national guidelines include severe type I allergies (e.g. urticaria, angio-oedema and anaphylaxis) to the first vaccination dosage and/or to ingredients of the vaccine; a history for allergies to PEGs and polysorbates; patients with a history of anaphylaxis to other drugs or vaccinations; patients with systemic mastocytosis or idiopathic anaphylaxis [158,159].

Other pre-existing dermatological disorders and patients on biologic/immunomodulatory treatments. Vaccine immunogenicity may be directly affected by disorders such as autoimmune inflammatory diseases, or indirectly affected by immunosuppressive and immunomodulatory treatment. It is recommended that vaccination should be encouraged in almost all cases, but certain precautions may be necessary regarding the type of vaccine platform and modifications of vaccination and/or treatment schedules may be required to optimise immunisation, maintain control of underlying disease and avoid severe adverse reactions [159]. There is evidence from the PsoProtect registry that only a minority of people with psoriasis are hesitant about vaccination [178]. Consensus elements of recommendations will evolve as more evidence emerges [159].

Skin disorders resulting from use of personal protective equipment (PPE)

During the Covid-19 pandemic, the use of PPE (e.g. medical masks, goggles, face shields, gowns and gloves) and frequent handwashing have presented a significant burden of occupational dermatoses to health care workers in particular [179–184], but this has also been evident in the general population [184] (see Chapter 128).

Regular basic skin care education, early access to specialty clinics [182] and better-fit PPE have been proposed as feasible approaches to mitigating PPE-related occupational dermatoses [185–189] (see Chapter 128).

Altered health care delivery during the Covid-19 pandemic on diagnosis and prognosis of skin cancer

Disruptions to dermatology services during the Covid-19 pandemic and patient-related factors have affected rates of diagnosis and delivery of treatment with potential impacts on patient outcomes. This is particularly relevant for skin cancer care [190,191].

Many publications, particularly from Europe and the USA, report a reduction of approximately 30–70% in skin cancers diagnosed and treated during Covid-19 pandemic lockdowns compared with equivalent periods pre-lockdown both at skin cancer centres [192–202] and nationally in England [203] and the Netherlands [204]. For keratinocyte cancers (KC), cSCC were generally prioritised over BCC with the greatest decreases therefore in BCC [194,203,204]. Surgical activity was reduced with, for example, 49–77% of Mohs micrographic surgeons reporting discontinuing procedures in the UK during these periods [194,205]. Subsequent modest increases in diagnoses of KC and melanoma have been reported in post-lockdown recovery periods but these have not necessarily returned to pre-pandemic rates [192,199,203,204].

There has been concern that this decline in incidence represents patients who will present later, with poorer outcomes in terms of morbidity and mortality. Data are currently limited because of the relatively short follow-up. A study from Italy reported a significant increase during the pandemic in advanced skin cancers diagnosed, defined as melanomas stage T1b or higher and KC with high-risk clinicopathological features [206], and similar findings were reported from Spain [201] and Ireland [207]. In contrast, a study from the UK reported improved detection of earlier-stage melanomas during lockdown and highlighted the importance of maintaining urgent skin referral pathways during pandemics [208]. Encouragingly, a recent large population-based cohort study from the Netherlands evaluating cSCC and melanoma outcomes pre and post first and second Covid-19 lockdowns did not identify more unfavourable primary tumour characteristics [209]. However, as with many skin diseases, longer-term follow-up studies in coming years will be required to assess the potential impact of delayed diagnosis and treatment during the Covid-19 pandemic.

Resources

General information
World Health Organization: https://www.who.int/emergencies/diseases/novel-coronavirus-2019
World Health Organization Coronavirus (Covid-19) Dashboard: https://covid19.who.int/
Centers for Disease Control and Prevention: https://www.cdc.gov/coronavirus/2019-ncov/index.html
Johns Hopkins Coronavirus Resource Center: https://coronavirus.jhu.edu/map.html
NHS Covid-19 website: https://www.nhs.uk/conditions/coronavirus-Covid-19/

Covid-19 resources relevant to dermatology
British Association of Dermatologists: https://covidskinsigns.com
COVID acral ischemia/perniosis in children: https://redcap.chop.edu/surveys/?s=TR8FTHF9KW
American Academy of Dermatology: https://www.aad.org/member/practice/coronavirus/registry
Alopecia: https://securealopecia.covidderm.org/login/?next=/insight/
Atopic dermatitis: https://www.covidderm.org/login/
Psoriasis: https://psoprotect.org/
Hidradenitis suppurativa: https://hscovid.ucsf.edu/
Connective tissue or vasculitis (not psoriasis): https://rheum-covid.org/
Reynolds SD, Mathur AN, Chiu YE et al. Systemic immunosuppressive therapy for inflammatory skin diseases in children: expert consensus-based guidance for clinical decision-making during the Covid-19 pandemic. *Pediatr Dermatol* 2020;37:424–34.
Wiley compiled literature: https://novel-coronavirus.onlinelibrary.wiley.com/
University of Nottingham Centre for Evidence Based Dermatology compiled literature: https://www.nottingham.ac.uk/research/groups/cebd/resources/coronavirus-resource/coronavirushome.aspx
AAD: https://www.aad.org/member/practice/managing/coronavirus
MDS: https://www.meddermsociety.org/Covid-19-medical-inpatient-dermatology-responses-patients/
(All last accessed August 2023.)

OTHER CUTANEOUS PROBLEMS ASSOCIATED WITH VIRAL INFECTIONS

General description of disease domain

Several patterns of cutaneous reaction are associated with viral (and other) infections and may be grouped together as paraviral eruptions.

These include acute generalised exanthematous pustulosis (Chapter 117), asymmetrical periflexural exanthem of childhood, erythema nodosum (see Chapter 97), erythema multiforme (Chapter 47), vasculitis (Chapter 100), urticaria (Chapter 42), Gianotti–Crosti syndrome, Kikuchi–Fujimoto disease (Chapter 148), papular-pruritic gloves and socks syndrome, pityriasis lichenoides (Chapter 133), pityriasis rosea, polyarteritis nodosa (Chapter 102), Sweet syndrome (Chapter 49) and TORCH syndrome and, recently, the many features observed closely with SARS-Cov-2 infections (see earlier).

Papular-pruritic gloves and socks syndrome

Introduction and general description
Papular-pruritic gloves and socks syndrome was first described in 1990 [1]. It presents as an acute acral dermatosis, occurring predominantly in young adults. It is regarded as an idiosyncratic reaction, usually to a viral infection [2].

Epidemiology
Incidence and prevalence
Usually occurs as an isolated case but has been reported in families [3].

Age
Mainly young adults. Less commonly in children and rare in older adults [4].

Table 25.32 Infections associated with papular-purpuric gloves and socks syndrome.

	References
Viral infections	
Parvovirus B19	[9]
Epstein–Barr virus	[10]
Cytomegalovirus	[10,11]
Human herpesvirus type 6	[12]
Human herpesvirus type 7	[13]
Hepatitis B	[14]
Rubella	[15]
Measles	[16]
SARS-CoV-2	[17]
Bacterial	
Mycoplasma	[18]

Pathophysiology
Pathology
Epidermal acanthosis and patchy basal cell degeneration with subepidermal oedema and a patchy mixed inflammatory cell infiltrate and extravasated red blood cells are seen [5]. The viral structural protein may be detected in the walls of dermal blood vessels [6]. Molecular detection of parvovirus B19 DNA may be detectable in the serum and skin of associated cases [7,8].

Causative organisms
Parvovirus B19 infection is the most commonly associated infection [9]. In children, EBV or CMV may be more common than in adults [10]. Other infectious triggers for the syndrome are listed in Table 25.32, although in some cases no specific cause can be identified.

Clinical features
Presentation
The hands, wrists, feet and ankles are intensely pruritic and are affected with macular and papular redness and associated oedema. Lesions may be violaceous in darker skin types. The features are often most intense on the palmar and plantar surfaces. There may also be associated purpura and rarely petechiae. There is often a distinct cut-off at wrists and ankles. The cutaneous features are frequently accompanied by oral inflammation with petechiae, vesicopustules and ulceration [19]. Malaise and fever can follow a few days after the onset of the eruption and there may be lymphadenopathy.

Clinical variants
The eruption can occasionally involve the perioral and perianal or other flexural skin [20]. Unilateral or more generalised eruptions are occasionally seen [21].

Disease course and prognosis
The rash and associated features settle within 1–2 weeks but in children the eruption may last a month. Skin clearance usually involves desquamation. There are rare instances of prolonged or recurrent disease [22].

Investigations
Evidence of an infective trigger can be sought. In acute papular-pruritic gloves and socks syndrome associated with parvovirus, antiviral IgM is usually detectable at the time of the eruption and IgG is detectable later [23].

Management
Treatment is supportive.

TORCH syndrome

Introduction and general description
The term TORCH syndrome was originally used to encompass infection acquired congenitally or perinatally from the mother caused by several aetiological agents (*Toxoplasma gondii*, 'others' including syphilis, *r*ubella, *c*ytomegalovirus and *h*erpes simplex types 1 and 2) in which the clinical presentation was somewhat similar [24]. In practice, there are some distinctions between the manifestations of the various infections, although all may cause cutaneous and disseminated abnormalities. Skin abnormalities of jaundice, purpura and petechiae are most common. Vesicles and mucosal ulceration may occur with herpes infection. Since the acronym was first used, many more infections (coxsackie, enteroviruses, parvovirus B19, VZV, HIV, HTLV-1, hepatitis B, Zika virus, *Borrelia burgdorferi* and chlamydia) have been included in the 'others' and although the use of TORCH screening is still useful [25], the concept of TORCH syndrome is now of limited value.

Gianotti–Crosti syndrome

Synonyms and inclusions
- Papular acrodermatitis of childhood
- Papular infantile acrodermatitis

Introduction and general description
Gianotti–Crosti syndrome [26,27,**28**] is a characteristic, self-limiting cutaneous reaction usually to a viral infection, in which red papules appear on the limbs and face, occurring mainly in children.

Epidemiology
Age
The syndrome mainly affects children between the ages of 6 months and 12 years, though occasional adult, usually female, cases have occurred [29,30]. Small epidemics or clustering of cases is often observed.

Pathophysiology
Pathology
The epidermis shows spongiosis with some acanthosis and parakeratosis. There is a patchy, perivascular, mainly lymphocytic or lymphohistiocytic infiltrate in the dermis. These features are more marked in vesicular lesions.

Table 25.33 Infections associated with Gianotti–Crosti syndrome.

	References
Viral infections	
Herpes simplex virus	[32]
Epstein–Barr virus	[33–35]
Cytomegalovirus	[36]
Human herpesvirus type 6	[37]
Coxsackie A16	[38]
Coxsackie B4 and B5	[33]
Echovirus 7 & 9	[39,40]
Hepatitis A	[41]
Hepatitis B	[31]
Coronavirus, SARS-CoV-2	[42]
Rotavirus	[43]
Echovirus	[44]
Milker's nodule	[45]
Molluscum contagiosum	[46]
Parvovirus B19	[47]
Respiratory syncytial virus	[48]
Mumps	[49]
Influenza	[50]
Parainfluenza	[51]
HIV	[52]
Bacterial	
Mycoplasma	[53]
Streptococcus A	[48]
Bartonella	[54]
Borrelia burgdorferi	[55]

Table 25.34 Immunisations associated with Gianotti–Crosti syndrome.

Immunisation	References
Measles, mumps, rubella	[58]
Diphtheria, pertussis	[51,59]
Influenza	[60]
Influenza, H1N1	[61]
Hepatitis A	[62]
Hepatitis B	[63]
Polio	[48]
Yellow fever	[64]
Varicella-zoster	[65]

Causative organisms

The majority of the early cases reported had hepatitis B infection [31], but several other viral and non-viral infections have been implicated (Table 25.33) and EBV infection is now the most common association. Cases following immunisation are also reported [56,57] (Table 25.34). In a minority of cases, no evidence of viral infection can be found.

Clinical features
Presentation
Over the course of 3 or 4 days, a profuse eruption of pink to red, flat-topped papules develops first on the thighs and buttocks, then may extend down the legs (Figure 25.38), to the extensor aspects of the arms, and finally the face. There may be a few short-lived lesions on the trunk but the torso is usually spared, as are scalp, palms and

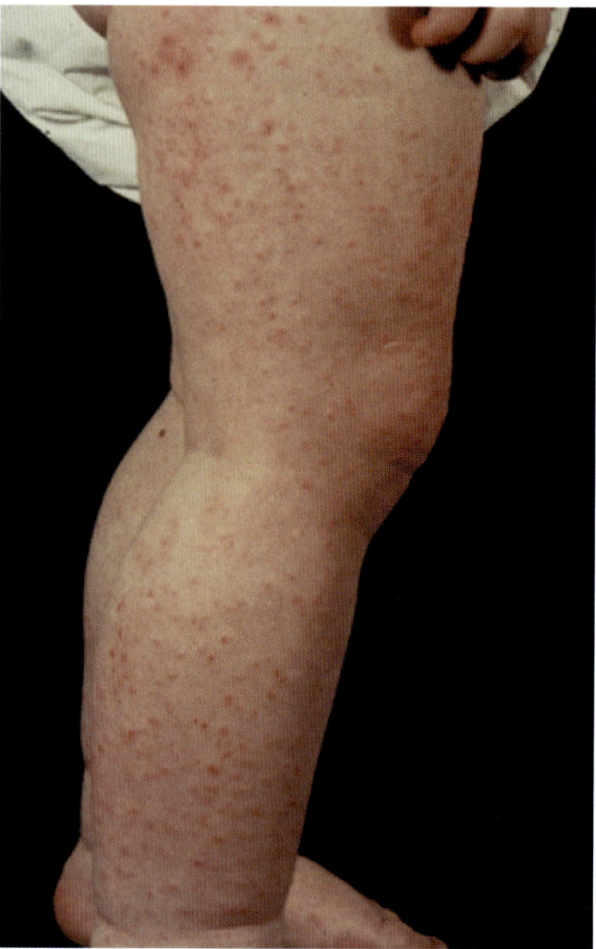

Figure 25.38 Gianotti–Crosti syndrome. Papular eruption on the leg. Courtesy of Dr N. P. Burrows, Addenbrooke's Hospital, Cambridge, UK.

soles. The distribution is often asymmetrical. The individual papules are 5–10 mm in diameter, and their characteristic deep red-brown colour on pale skin, which may be less distinct on darker skin, may later be modified by purpuric staining, especially on the legs. Itch is said not to be a feature of the hepatitis B cases, but may occur in those due to other viruses.

Generalised lymphadenopathy, mostly axillary and inguinal, is common and can persist for months after the rash. Constitutional complaints are not usually marked, although there may be mild fever, upper respiratory tract symptoms, diarrhoea and lassitude.

Clinical variants
Lesions may be vesicular.

Differential diagnosis
The skin lesions are sufficiently distinctive in morphology, distribution and duration. Differential diagnoses to consider include lichen planus, lichenoid drug eruptions, scabies and erythema multiforme.

Complications and co-morbidities
With hepatitis B, liver involvement is common and usually, but not invariably, mild and anicteric. Hepatomegaly and liver function abnormalities each occasionally occur in HBsAg-negative cases.

Disease course and prognosis
The eruption fades in 2–8 weeks with mild desquamation and rarely with a more prolonged course. Hypo- or hyperpigmentation may be transient, especially in darker skins. Recurrence has been reported rarely with infection or immunisation [57,66,67].

Investigations
Evidence of a triggering infection should be sought and liver function should be assessed. The changes in the peripheral blood are inconstant: there may be a leukopenia or a slight leukocytosis with 2–15% of monocytes; the erythrocyte sedimentation rate is not raised.

Management
There is no specific treatment. Emollients or topical steroids can give symptomatic relief.

In recurrent or severe cases, ribavirin can be considered [68].

Resources

Patient resources
https://dermnetnz.org/topics/papular-acrodermatitis-of-childhood (last accessed September 2021).

Asymmetrical periflexural exanthem of childhood

Synonyms and inclusions
- Unilateral laterothoracic exanthem
- Unilateral mediothoracic exanthem
- Superimposed lateralised exanthem

Epidemiology
Age
Most common in young children aged 1–5 years but also reported in adults [69,70].

Pathophysiology
Causative organisms
The association with an identified infective agent is not as strong as in Gianotti–Crosti or papular-purpuric gloves and socks syndrome, but evidence of concurrent influenza, parainfluenza, adenovirus, parvovirus B19, EBV, HHV-7 or SARS-CoV-19 infections has been reported [71–77].

Clinical features
Presentation
The eruption starts asymmetrically, affecting the axilla, groin or trunk, and then spreads centrifugally [78]. There are small papules or macules which can be slightly itchy. There is often associated lymphadenopathy. In adults the distribution can be limited to the medial anterior chest [79].

Disease course and prognosis
A low-grade fever can develop, usually after the onset of the eruption, although malaise and fever can precede the rash [80]. After 2–4 weeks, the rash fades with desquamation.

Eruptive pseudoangiomatosis and eruptive hypomelanosis

These two eruptions have been described in association with infections, but a causal link is unproven.

Eruptive pseudoangiomatosis may follow a number of possible triggers and presents with small, red, telangiectatic papules, often surrounded by a pale halo, on exposed areas or more widespread. Suggested viral associations are enteroviruses or an infection spread by insect bites [81,82].

Eruptive hypomelanosis appears as multiple small hypopigmented areas in a guttate pattern mainly on extensor surfaces of limbs. It is asymptomatic and fades within a month. It has been reported in children in association with coryzal symptoms and rarely in small outbreaks [83,84].

Pityriasis rosea

Definition and nomenclature
Pityriasis rosea is an acute self-limiting disease, probably infective in origin, affecting mainly children and young adults and characterised by a distinctive skin eruption and minimal constitutional symptoms.

Synonyms and inclusions
- Pityriasis circinata et maculata of Vidal

Introduction and general description
Pityriasis rosea is a relatively common eruption, occurring throughout the world [85,86,**87**].

Epidemiology
Incidence and prevalence
The estimated annual incidence is 170/100 000 [88]. In temperate climates, there may be a seasonal variation.

Although the cause of pityriasis rosea is uncertain, many epidemiological and clinical features suggest that an infective agent may be implicated. True epidemics have not been reported, but the reported epidemiological evidence for infectivity includes occasional family or household outbreaks, seasonal and year-to-year fluctuations [89–91], with some evidence for clustering in space and time [92]. The natural history of the disease, with a primary lesion that could correspond to the site of inoculation, a disseminated secondary eruption after an interval, mild constitutional symptoms, a self-limiting course and the infrequency of second attacks are all features paralleled by many diseases of proven infective origin.

Age
Most cases of pityriasis rosea occur between the ages of 10 and 35 years and it is uncommon, but not unreported, in infancy, early childhood or old age [93].

Sex
It is slightly more common in females [88].

Ethnicity
Susceptibility to the disease appears not to be influenced by race or atopy.

Pathophysiology
Predisposing factors
The eruption has been reported during immunosuppressive treatment [94,95], but it is not obviously more common in immune compromise.

A pityriasis rosea-like reaction has been reported for several drugs (Table 25.35).

Table 25.35 Drugs associated with a pityriasis rosea-like eruption (synonyms: pityriasiform drug reaction; pityriasis rosea-like drug eruption).

Drug	References
ACE inhibitors	
• Captopril	[96]
• Lisinopril	[97]
Aspirin/acetylsalicylic acid	[98]
Allopurinol	[98]
Barbiturates	[99]
β-blockers	
• Atenolol	[100]
Biologics	
Adalimumab, omalizumab, rituximab	[101–103]
Ibrutinib, imatinib	[104,105]
Clonidine	[96]
Ergotamine	[106]
Gold salts	[107]
Griseofulvin	[108]
Isotretinoin	[109]
Ketotifen	[110]
Lamotrigine	[111]
Levamisole	[112]
Meprobamate	[108]
Metronidazole	[113]
Nortriptylene	[114]
Omeprazole	[115]
Ondansetron	[116]
Penicillin	[108]
D-penicillamine	[117]
Terbinafine	[118]
Vaccines	
BCG	[119]
Diphtheria toxoid	[120]
Pneumococcal vaccine	[121]
Hepatitis B	[122]
Yellow fever	[123]
SARS-CoV-2	[124,125]

Pathology [126,127]
The herald patch and secondary lesions show similar histological features but these are not diagnostic. In the epidermis, spongiosis, vesicles and patchy parakeratosis are common. Some apoptotic keratinocytes may be seen in the upper epidermis. The upper dermis shows mild papillary oedema and a mononuclear cell perivascular infiltrate with focal invasion of inflammatory cells into the epidermis, where they may form pustules, mainly subcorneal. The infiltrate comprises mainly CD4+ helper T lymphocytes but also Langerhans cells. HLA-DR antigens are expressed on the keratinocyte surface. Occasional dyskeratotic keratinocytes are seen, sometimes adjacent to a Langerhans cell.

Causative organisms
Many infectious agents have been suspected as causative, but evidence is strongest for a viral aetiology with herpesvirus-like particles found in 71% of pityriasis rosea lesions [128].

Involvement of two herpesviruses, HHV-6 and HHV-7, has been suggested as a cause for the eruption, most likely in reactivation after an asymptomatic primary infection [87]. The viral DNA is present in peripheral blood mononuclear cells and lesional and unaffected skin of the majority of individuals with acute pityriasis rosea. HHV-7 is detected slightly more frequently than HHV-6, but often both viruses are found [129,130]. However, evidence of HHV-6 or HHV-7 presence and activity is also found in a proportion (10–44%) of unaffected individuals, suggesting that if there is a causal relationship, infection with the viruses does not always lead to disease.

Other viruses that may act as a trigger for pityriasis rosea are HHV-8 [131], herpes simplex virus type 2 [132], hepatitis C [133], H1N1 influenza [134] and SARS-CoV-2 [135,136].

Clinical features
History
Prodromal symptoms are usually absent but up to 5% have vague complaints of headache, slight malaise, athralgia or fatigue.

Presentation (Figure 25.39)
The first manifestation of the disease is usually the appearance of the herald patch, which is larger and more conspicuous than the lesions of the later eruption and is usually situated on the thigh or upper arm, trunk or neck. Rarely, the herald patch may appear on the face, scalp, penis, palm or sole [137].

It is a sharply defined, red, round or oval plaque, soon covered by fine scale. It rapidly reaches its maximum size, usually 2–5 cm in diameter but occasionally much larger. Rarely, there may be more than one herald patch. After an interval, which is usually between 5 and 15 days, but may be as short as a few hours or as long as 2 months, the general eruption begins to appear in crops at 2–3-day intervals over a week or 10 days. Less often, new lesions continue to develop for several weeks. In its classical form the eruption consists of discrete oval lesions, dull pink in colour and covered by fine dry silvery-grey scales. The centre tends to clear and assumes a wrinkled, atrophic appearance and a tawny colour, with a marginal collarette of scale attached peripherally, with the free edge of the scale internally. The long axes of the lesions characteristically follow

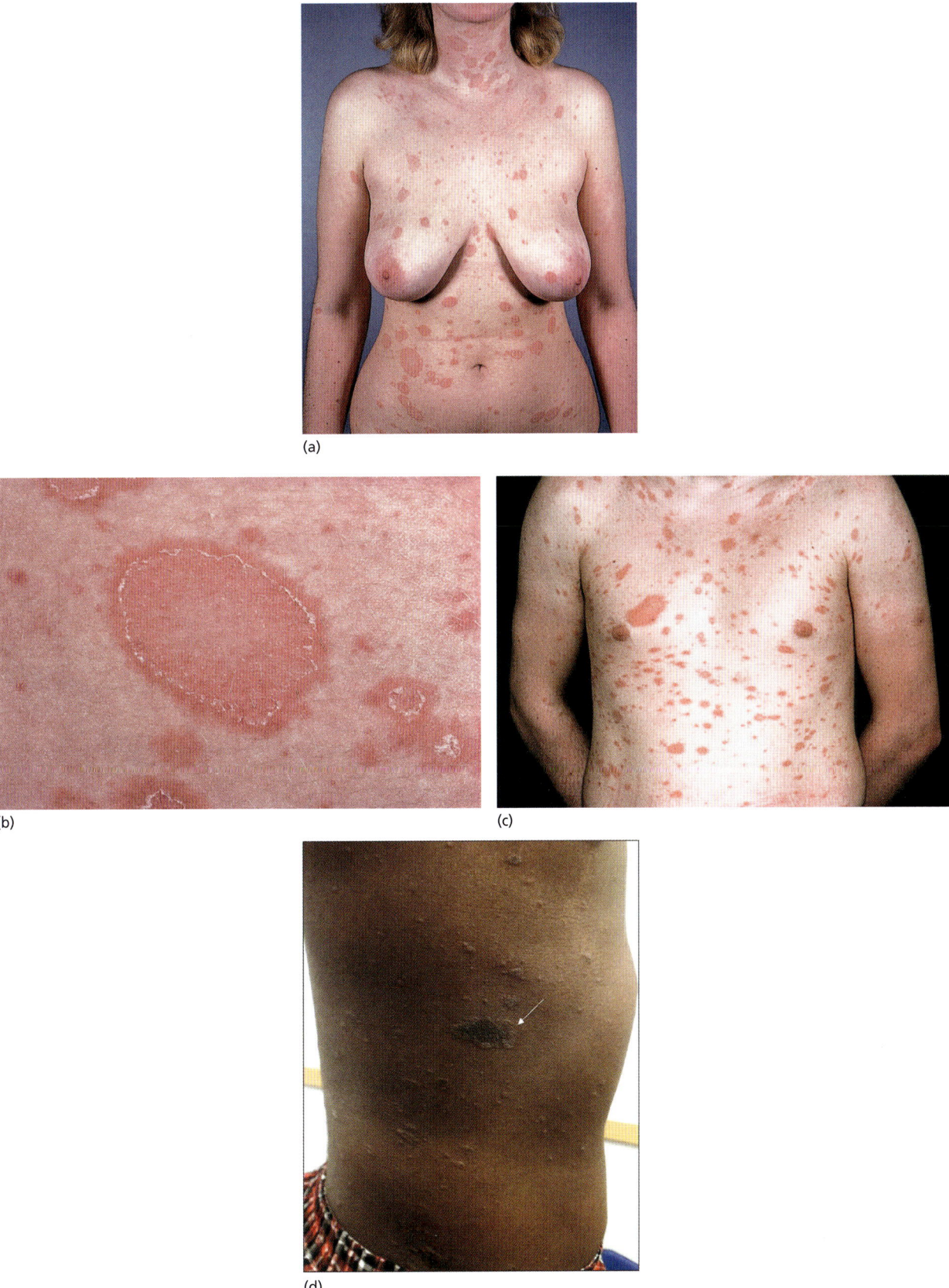

Figure 25.39 Pityriasis rosea: (a) with herald patch on the right of the abdomen, shown in close-up in (b). Courtesy of York District Hospital, UK. (c) With herald patch on the right of the chest. Courtesy of Dr A.S. Highet, York District Hospital, UK. (d) Second recurrence of pityriasis rosea – herald patch indicated by the white arrow. Reproduced from Senthilkumar et al. (2014), *Indian Journal of Dermatology, Venereology, and Leprology*.

the lines of cleavage parallel to the ribs in a Christmas tree pattern on the upper chest and back. The scaly lesions are commonly associated with pink macules of varying size and the eruption may be exclusively macular.

The lesions are usually most numerous on the trunk, base of the neck and upper third of the arms and legs. Involvement of the face and scalp is quite common, especially in children, and in one large series of cases lesions were found on the forearms and lower legs in about 12% and 6%, respectively. Lesions on the palms are exceptional, but can occur. There may be discrete scaly red patches, diffuse redness and scaling or scattered small vesicles. Oral lesions are present in a quarter of cases [138] and can consist of ill-defined red patches with some erosion or with punctate haemorrhages, or bullae. Oral lesions are more common in severe, persistent or relapsing disease. Rarely, there may be lesions on the vulva.

Subjective symptoms are usually absent but there may be slight or moderate pruritus. Occasionally, slight fever, malaise and enlargement of the lymph nodes, generalised or confined to the cervical glands, may be present and, exceptionally, more severe constitutional symptoms have been recorded.

Clinical variants

Pityriasis rosea may be atypical in the appearance or distribution of the lesions or in its course [139,140]. The herald patch is absent or undetected in about 20% of cases. The more widespread eruption may be almost generalised or may be limited to a few lesions, often around the herald patch. In some cases, the eruption is confined to a single region, or may be maximal on the extremities, almost sparing the trunk [141,142]. Unilateral pityriasis has been reported [143].

Especially in children, the lesions may be predominantly papular or urticarial in the early stages, but they are soon surmounted by an inconspicuous ring of fine scales. This papular variant may be more common in pregnant women.

Papulovesicular, vesicular, purpuric, erythema multiforme-like lesions, follicular and pustular forms may rarely occur [144–146]. In a variant of the papular form, more common in Africans than Europeans, small lichenoid papules are thickly set in the edges of the lesions [147].

In pityriasis (rosea) circinata et marginata of Vidal [148], sometimes regarded as a special form of pityriasis rosea and seen mainly in adults, the lesions are few and large, and are often localised to one region of the body, especially the axillae or groins [149]. They tend to become confluent and may persist for several months.

Differential diagnosis

An eruption almost identical to classical pityriasis rosea can occur as a drug reaction (Table 25.20). In addition to the timing of the eruption and drug intake, other features to support this diagnosis would be the absence of constitutional symptoms, an acute onset of the rash without a herald patch, pruritus and a tendency for the lesions to become very inflamed or lichenoid in appearance. The pattern may be variable in a patient taking a drug which is known to produce reactions of this nature, with a pityriasiform eruption being atypical, progressive and irritable. Other patterns of drug reaction may have to be excluded. Histologically, apoptotic keratinocytes in the epidermis and eosinophils in the dermis may be seen.

Seborrhoeic dermatitis may be pityriasiform, but small scaly follicular papules may be present and there is no herald patch. Dry discoid eczema may cause confusion, but lesions are usually more numerous on the limbs. The hypopigmented patches with dry, branny scales of pityriasis alba are most frequent on the face, and are seen mainly in young children. The pigmented form of pityriasis versicolor does not show marginal scaling and the chronicity would be very atypical.

Secondary syphilis is the classic trap but the resemblance is not very close. There is no herald patch and the lesions are roseolar or maculopapular.

Guttate psoriasis and pityriasis lichenoides may sometimes need exclusion. In both, the lesions are papular and persistent. In psoriasis they are surmounted by silvery scales. In pityriasis lichenoides they are polymorphic, some showing haemorrhagic crusting and some adherent scales.

The herald patch and the localised forms such as pityriasis circinata are easily, and in practice frequently, confused with ringworm. The lesions of ringworm are red and oedematous and may show marginal vesiculation. In case of doubt, scrapings from the edge of the lesions should be examined microscopically for mycelium.

Complications and co-morbidities

Pityriasis rosea occurring in the first trimester of pregnancy may be associated with a higher than normal risk of spontaneous abortion or premature delivery of an infant with hypotonia and hyporeactivity [150]. Effects on the fetus are more likely if the disease is severe in the mother, if oral lesions are present or if there is reactivation of HHV-6.

Disease course and prognosis

The skin lesions commonly fade after 3–6 weeks, but some clear in 1 or 2 weeks and a few persist for as long as 3 months. A longer duration, except in localised forms, is unusual. Such persistent pityriasis rosea may be associated with persistent HHV-6 or -7 infection [151]. There may be temporary hyper- or hypopigmentation, but usually the lesions vanish without trace.

Second attacks of pityriasis rosea occur in about 3–4% of cases after an interval of a few months or many years, and rarely a partial or complete relapse of a fading eruption may be seen. Multiple recurrences are rare [149].

Investigations

Diagnosis is usually made on clinical grounds, but where there is uncertainty, skin biopsy may help to distinguish from other possible diagnoses.

Management

The common asymptomatic and self-limiting cases require no treatment. Mild symptoms may benefit from an oral antihistamine and topical calamine lotion or emollient.

First line

If itch is troublesome, or the appearance distressing, a topical steroid, usually of moderate potency or UVB, can be helpful [152].

Second line

Based on the concept of HHV-6 or HHV-7 as a cause of the eruption, trials of antiviral drugs are reported. The standard dose regimen of aciclovir (400 mg five times a day for 1 week) or higher doses (800 mg five times daily for 1 week), used early after the onset of the eruption, may lead to a more rapid resolution of skin lesions and reduction in level of itch [153]. Antiviral treatment may also be useful in relapsing cases.

The use of oral erythromycin antibiotic (1 g four times a day for 2 weeks for adults) was reported to clear the disease within 2 weeks of treatment [154], but subsequent studies with erythromycin, clarithromycin and azithromycin have not confirmed any clear effect [153,155,156].

Resources

Patient resources

https://jamanetwork.com/journals/jamadermatology/fullarticle/2711244 (last accessed August 2023).

Key references

The full list of references can be found in the online version at https://www.wiley.com/rooksdermatology10e

Introduction

2 Howley PM, Knipe DM, eds. *Field's Virology*, 7th edn. Philadelphia: Wolters Kluwer, 2021.
4 Burrell CJ, Howard CR, Murphy FA. Laboratory diagnosis of virus diseases. In: Burrell CJ, Howard CR, Murphy FA, eds. *Fenner and White's Medical Virology*, 5th edn. Cambridge, MA: Academic Press, 2016:135–54.

Poxvirus infections

3 Breman JG. Smallpox. *J Infect Dis* 2021;224(12 Suppl. 2):S379–86.
5 Oliveira JS, Figueiredo PO, Costa GB et al. Vaccinia virus natural infections in Brazil: the good, the bad, and the ugly. *Viruses* 2017;9:340.
20 Bryer J, Freeman EE, Rosenbach M. Monkeypox emerges on a global scale: a historical review and dermatologic primer. *J Am Acad Dermatol* 2022;87:1069–74.
28 Poland GA, Kennedy RB, Tosh PK. Prevention of monkeypox with vaccines: a rapid review. *Lancet Infect Dis* 2022;22(12):e349–58.
31 Thornhill JP, Barkati S, Walmsley S et al. Monkeypox virus infection in humans across 16 countries – April–June 2022. *N Engl J Med* 2022;387:679–91.
44 Bellinato F, Gisondi P, Girolomoni G. Monkeypox virus infection: what dermatologist needs to know? *J Eur Acad Dermatol Venereol* 2022;36:e656–8.
77 Gronemeyer L-L, Baltzer A, Broekaert S et al. Generalised cowpox virus infection. *Lancet* 2017;390:1769.
90 Caravaglio JV, Khachemoune A. Orf virus infection in humans: a review with a focus on advances in diagnosis and treatment. *J Drugs Dermatol* 2017;1:684–9.
122 Chen X, Anstey AV, Bugert JJ. Molluscum contagiosum virus infection. *Lancet Infect Dis* 2013;13:877–88.
178 van der Wouden JC, van der Sande R, Kruithof EJ et al. Interventions for cutaneous molluscum contagiosum. *Cochrane Database Syst Rev* 2017;Issue 5:CD004767.

Herpesvirus infections

1 Corey L. First-episode, recurrent, and asymptomatic herpes simplex infections. *J Am Acad Dermatol* 1988;18:169–72.
52 Cernik C, Gallina K, Brodell RT. The treatment of herpes simplex infections: an evidence-based review. *Arch Intern Med* 2008;168:1137–44.
92 Raborn GW, McGaw WT, Grace M et al. Treatment of herpes labialis with acyclovir. Review of three clinical trials. *Am J Med* 1988;85:39–42.
97 Rooney JF, Straus SE, Mannix ML et al. Oral acyclovir to suppress frequently recurrent herpes labialis. A double-blind, placebo-controlled trial. *Ann Intern Med* 1993;118:268–72.
110 Brugha R, Keersmaekers K, Renton A et al. Genital herpes infection: a review. *Int J Epidemiol* 1997;26:698–709.
120 Tronstein E, Johnston C, Huang ML et al. Genital shedding of herpes simplex virus among symptomatic and asymptomatic persons with HSV-2 infection. *JAMA* 2011;305:1441–9.
126 Patel R, Kennedy OJ, Clarke E et al. 2017 European guidelines for the management of genital herpes. *Int J STD AIDS* 2017;28:1366–79.
130 Groves MJ. Genital herpes: a review. *Am Fam Physician* 2016;93:928–34.
150 Corey L, Wald A. Maternal and neonatal herpes simplex virus infections. *N Engl J Med* 2009;361:1376–85.
168 Hammad WAB, Konje JC. Herpes simplex virus infection in pregnancy – an update. *Eur J Obstet Gynecol Reprod Biol* 2021;259:38–45.
180 Nardone A, de Ory F, Carton M et al. The comparative sero-epidemiology of varicella zoster virus in 11 countries in the European region. *Vaccine* 2007;25:7866–72.
190 Sauerbrei A, Wutzler P. The congenital varicella syndrome. *J Perinatol* 2000;20:548–54.
194 Tunbridge AJ, Breuer J, Jeffery KJ et al. Chickenpox in adults – clinical management. *J Infect* 2008;57:95–102.
212 Leung J, Harpaz R, Baughman AL et al. Evaluation of laboratory methods for diagnosis of varicella. *Clin Infect Dis* 2010;51:23–32.
225 Breuer J, Fifer H. Chickenpox. *BMJ Clin Evid* 2011;2011:0912.
226 Shrim A, Koren G, Yudin MH et al. Management of varicella infection (chickenpox) in pregnancy. *J Obstet Gynaecol Can* 2012;34:287–92.
238 Sampathkumar P, Drage LA, Martin DP. Herpes zoster (shingles) and postherpetic neuralgia. *Mayo Clin Proc* 2009;84:274–80.
247 Weinberg JM. Herpes zoster: epidemiology, natural history, and common complications. *J Am Acad Dermatol* 2007;57(Suppl. 6):S130–5.
257 Kost RG, Straus SE. Postherpetic neuralgia – pathogenesis, treatment, and prevention. *N Engl J Med* 1996;335:32–42.
261 Forbes HJ, Bhaskaran K, Grint D et al. Incidence of acute complications of herpes zoster among immunocompetent adults in England: a matched cohort study using routine health data. *Br J Dermatol* 2021;184:1077–84.
282 Anon. Varicella and herpes zoster vaccines: WHO position paper, June 2014. *Wkly Epidemiol Rec* 2014;89:265–87.
297 Sangueza-Acosta M, Sandoval-Romereo E. Epstein-Barr virus and skin. *An Bras Dermatol* 2018;93:786–99.
314 Berry PA, Bernal W, Pagliuca A et al. Multiple organ failure and severe bone marrow dysfunction in two 18 year-old Caucasian patients: Epstein–Barr virus and the haemophagocytic syndrome. *Anaesthesia* 2008;63:1249–54.
332 Picard D, Janela B, Descamps V et al. Drug reaction with eosinophilia and systemic symptoms (DRESS): a multiorgan antiviral T cell response. *Sci Transl Med* 2010;2:46ra62.
341 Kimura H, Cohen JI. Chronic active Epstein-Barr virus disease. *Front Immunol* 2017;8:1867.
351 Tokura Y, Ishihara S, Tagawa S et al. Hypersensitivity to mosquito bites as the primary clinical manifestation of a juvenile type of Epstein–Barr virus-associated natural killer cell leukemia/lymphoma. *J Am Acad Dermatol* 2001;45:569–78.
364 Agut H, Bonnafous P, Gautheret-Dejean A. Laboratory and clinical aspects of human herpesvirus 6 infections. *Clin Microbiol Rev* 2015;28:313–35.
370 Wolz MM, Sciallis GF, Pittelkow MR. Human herpesviruses 6, 7, and 8 from a dermatologic perspective. *Mayo Clin Proc* 2012;87:1004–14.
385 Asano Y, Yoshikawa T, Suga S et al. Clinical features of infants with primary human herpesvirus 6 infection (exanthem subitum, roseola infantum). *Pediatrics* 1994;93:104–8.
399 Wang X, Patel SA, Haddadin M, Cerny J. Post-allogeneic hematopoietic stem cell transplantation viral reactivations and viremias: a focused review on human herpesvirus-6, BK virus and adenovirus. *Ther Adv Infect Dis* 2021;8:1–20.
412 Lesher JL, Jr. Cytomegalovirus infections and the skin. *J Am Acad Dermatol* 1988;18:1333–8.
413 Drago F, Aragone MG, Lugani C et al. Cytomegalovirus infection in normal and immunocompromised humans. A review. *Dermatology* 2000;200:189–95.
450 Prieto-Barrios M, Aragón-Miguel R, Tarragó-Asensio D et al. Human herpesvirus 8-associated inflammatory cytokine syndrome. *JAMA Dermatol* 2018;154:228–30.
462 Cattamanchi A, Saracino M, Selke S et al. Treatment with valacyclovir, famciclovir, or antiretrovirals reduces human herpesvirus-8 replication in HIV-1 seropositive men. *J Med Virol* 2011;83:1696–703.

472 Leung DY. Why is eczema herpeticum unexpectedly rare? *Antiviral Res* 2013;98:153–7.
473 Wollenberg A, Zoch C, Wetzel S et al. Predisposing factors and clinical features of eczema herpeticum: a retrospective analysis of 100 cases. *J Am Acad Dermatol* 2003;49:198–205.
499 David TJ, Longson M. Herpes simplex infections in atopic eczema. *Arch Dis Child* 1985;60:338–43.

Polyomavirus infections
1 Nguyen KD, Chamseddin BH, Cockerell CJ et al. The biology and clinical features of cutaneous polyomaviruses. *J Invest Dermatol* 2019;139:285–92.
2 DeCaprio JA, Garcea RL. A cornucopia of human polyomaviruses. *Nat Rev Microbiol* 2013;11:264–76.
16 Becker JC, Stang A, DeCaprio JA et al. Merkel cell carcinoma. *Nat Rev Dis Primer* 2017;3:17077.
28 van der Meijden E, Janssens RW, Lauber C et al. Discovery of a new human polyomavirus associated with trichodysplasia spinulosa in an immunocompromised patient. *PLOS Pathog* 2010;66:e1001024.
30 Kazem S, van der Meijden E, Feltkamp MC. The trichodysplasia spinulosa-associated polyomavirus: virological background and clinical implications. *APMIS* 2013;121:770–82.

Human papillomavirus infections
3 Mühr LSA, Eklund C, Dillner J. Towards quality and order in human papillomavirus research. *Virology* 2018;519:74–6.
16 Tyring SK. Human papillomavirus infections: epidemiology, pathogenesis, and host immune response. *J Am Acad Dermatol* 2000;43:S18–26.
17 Stanley MA, Sterling JC. Host responses to infection with human papillomavirus. *Curr Probl Dermatol* 2014;45:58–74.
70 Sterling JC, Gibbs S, Haque Hussain SS et al. British Association of Dermatologists' guidelines for the management of cutaneous warts 2014. *Br J Dermatol* 2014;171:696–712.
71 Soenjoyo KR, Chua BWB, Wee LWY et al. Treatment of cutaneous viral warts in children: a review. *Dermatol Ther* 2020;33:e14034.
72 García-Oreja S, Álvaro-Afonso FJ, García-Álvarez Y et al. Topical treatment for plantar warts: a systematic review. *Dermatol Ther* 2021;34:e14621.
178 Muse ME, Stiff KM, Glines KR et al. A review of intralesional wart therapy. *Dermatol Online J* 2020;26:2.
243 Kombe Kombe AJ, Li B, Zahid A et al. Epidemiology and burden of human papillomavirus and related diseases, molecular pathogenesis, and vaccine evaluation. *Front Public Health* 2021;8:552028.
293 Gilson R, Nugent D, Werner RN et al. 2019 IUSTI-Europe guideline for the management of anogenital warts. *J Eur Acad Dermatol Venereol* 2020;34:1644–53.
314 zur Hausen H. Papillomaviruses in the causation of human cancers – a brief historical account. *Virology* 2009;384:260–5.
327 Walboomers JM, Jacobs MV, Manos MM et al. Human papillomavirus is a necessary cause of invasive cervical cancer worldwide. *J Pathol* 1999;189:12–19.
338 Harwood CA, Toland AE, Proby CM et al. The pathogenesis of squamous cell carcinoma in organ transplant recipients. *Br J Dermatol* 2017;177:1217–24.

Immunodeficiency and HPV infection
3 Béziat V. Human genetic dissection of papillomavirus-driven diseases: new insight into their pathogenesis. *Hum Genet* 2020;139:919–39.
4 Uitto J, Saeidian AH, Youssefian L et al. Recalcitrant warts, epidermodysplasia verruciformis, and the tree-man syndrome: phenotypic spectrum of cutaneous human papillomavirus infections at the intersection of genetic variability of viral and human genomes. *J Invest Dermatol* 2022;142:1265–9.
5 de Jong SJ, Imahorn E, Itin P et al. Epidermodysplasia verruciformis: inborn errors of immunity to human beta-papillomaviruses. *Front Microbiol* 2018;9:1222.
13 Przybyszewska J, Zlotogorski A, Ramot Y. Re-evaluation of epidermodysplasia verruciformis: reconciling more than 90 years of debate. *J Am Acad Dermatol* 2017;76:1161–75.
15 de Jong SJ, Matos I, Crequer A et al. The human CIB1-EVER1-EVER2 complex governs keratinocyte-intrinsic immunity to β-papillomaviruses. *J Exp Med* 2018;215:2289–310.
25 McBride AA. Human papillomaviruses: diversity, infection and host interactions. *Nat Rev Microbiol* 2022;20:95–108.
73 Moore S, Rady P, Tyring S. Acquired epidermodysplasia verruciformis: clinical presentation and treatment update. *Int J Dermatol* 2022;61:1325–35.

Hepatitis infections
1 Akhter A, Said A. Cutaneous manifestations of viral hepatitis. *Curr Infect Dis Rep* 2015;17:452.
6 Maslennikov R, Ivashkin V, Efremova I et al. Immune disorders and rheumatologic manifestations of viral hepatitis. *World J Gastroenterol* 2021;27:2073–89.
7 Cozzani E, Herzum A, Burlando M et al. Cutaneous manifestations of HAV, HBV, HCV. *Ital J Dermatol Venerol* 2021;156:5–12.
9 Seto WK, Lo YR, Pawlotsky JM et al. Chronic hepatitis B virus infection. *Lancet* 2018;392:2313–24.
10 Thomas DL. Global elimination of chronic hepatitis. *N Engl J Med* 2019;380:2041–50.
42 Garcovich S, Garcovich M, Capizzi R et al. Cutaneous manifestations of hepatitis C in the era of new antiviral agents. *World J Hepatol* 2015;7:2740–8.
43 Wiznia LE, Laird ME, Franks AG, Jr. Hepatitis C virus and its cutaneous manifestations: treatment in the direct-acting antiviral era. *J Eur Acad Dermatol Venereol* 2017;31:1260–70.

Parvovirus infections
1 Mossong J, Hens N, Friederichs V et al. Parvovirus B19 infection in five European countries: seroepidemiology, force of infection and maternal risk of infection. *Epidemiol Infect* 2008;136:1059–68.
2 Röhrer C, Gärtner B, Sauerbrei A et al. Seroprevalence of parvovirus B19 in the German population. *Epidemiol Infect* 2008;136:1564–75.
7 Servey JT, Reamy BV, Hodge J. Clinical presentations of parvovirus B19 infection. *Am Fam Physician* 2007;75:373–6.
10 Hayakawa H, Tara M, Niina K et al. A clinical study of adult human parvovirus B19 infection. *Intern Med* 2002;41:295–9.
37 Bonvicini F, La Placa M, Manaresi E et al. Parvovirus B19 DNA is commonly harboured in human skin. *Dermatology* 2010;220:138–42.

Human retrovirus infection
1 Peeters M, D'Arc M, Delaporte E. Origin and diversity of human retroviruses. *AIDS Rev* 2014;16:23–34.
12 Hirons A, Khoury G, Purcell DFJ. Human T-cell lymphotropic virus type-1: a lifelong persistent infection, yet never truly silent. *Lancet Infect Dis* 2021;21:e2–10.
18 Dantas L, Netto E, Glesby MJ et al. Dermatological manifestations of individuals infected with human T cell lymphotropic virus type I (HTLV-I). *Int J Dermatol* 2014;53:1098–102.
22 Bravo FG. Infective dermatitis: a purely cutaneous manifestation of HTLV-1 infection. *Semin Diagn Pathol* 2020;37:92–7.

Viral insect-borne and haemorrhagic fevers
1 Racsa LD, Kraft CS, Olinger GG et al. Viral hemorrhagic fever diagnostics. *Clin Infect Dis* 2016;62:214–19.
6 Brisse ME, Ly H. Hemorrhagic fever-causing arenaviruses: lethal pathogens and potent immune suppressors. *Front Immunol* 2019;10:372.
7 Houlihan C, Behrens R. Lassa fever. *BMJ* 2017;358:j2986.
20 Frank MG, Beitscher A, Webb CM et al. South American hemorrhagic fevers: a summary for clinicians. *Int J Infect Dis* 2021;105:505–15.
41 Jacob ST, Crozier I, Fischer WA, 2nd et al. Ebola virus disease. *Nat Rev Dis Primers* 2020;6:13.
56 Paixão ES, Teixeira MG, Rodrigues LC. Zika, chikungunya and dengue: the causes and threats of new and re-emerging arboviral diseases. *BMJ Glob Health* 2018;3(Suppl. 1):e000530.
57 Kularatne SA. Dengue fever. *BMJ* 2015;351:h4661.
59 Paules CI, Fauci AS. Yellow fever – once again on the radar screen in the Americas. *N Engl J Med* 2017;376:1397–9.
74 Wikan N, Smith DR. Zika virus: history of a newly emerging arbovirus. *Lancet Infect Dis* 2016;16:e119–26.
89 Weaver SC, Lecuit M. Chikungunya virus infections. *N Engl J Med* 2015;373:94–5.

Rubella
4 Best JM. Rubella. *Semin Fetal Neonatal Med* 2007;12:182–92.
9 Cooper LZ, Ziring PR, Ockerse AB et al. Rubella. Clinical manifestations and management. *Am J Dis Child* 1969;118:18–29.

Picornavirus infections (enteroviruses)

3   Nikonov OS, Chernykh ES, Garber MB et al. Enteroviruses: classification, diseases they cause, and approaches to development of antiviral drugs. *Biochemistry (Mosc)* 2017;82:1615–31.

30 Chang Y-K, Chen K-H, Chen K-T. Hand, foot and mouth disease and herpangina caused by enterovirus A71 infections: a review of enterovirus A71 molecular epidemiology, pathogenesis, and current vaccine development. *Rev Inst Med Trop São Paulo* 2019;60:e70.

34 Wang SM, Liu CC, Tseng HW et al. Clinical spectrum of enterovirus 71 infection in children in southern Taiwan, with an emphasis on neurological complications. *Clin Infect Dis* 1999;29:184–90.

35 Hubiche T, Schuffenecker I, Boralevi F et al. Dermatological spectrum of hand, foot and mouth disease from classical to generalized exanthema. *Pediatr Infect Dis J* 2014;33:e92–8.

47 Yu H, Li X-W, Liu Q-B et al. Diagnosis and treatment of herpangina: Chinese expert consensus. *World J Pediatr* 2020;16:129–34.

61 Shoji K, Komuro H, Miyata I et al. Dermatologic manifestations of human parechovirus type 3 infection in neonates and infants. *Pediatr Infect Dis J* 2013; 32:233–6.

Paramyxovirus infections

1   Moss WJ. Measles. *Lancet* 2017;390:2490–502.

5   Sheikine Y, Hawryluk EB, Burgin S et al. Histopathology of measles exanthem: a case with characteristic features and eosinophils. *J Cutan Pathol* 2012;39:667–70.

9   Battegay R, Itin C, Itin P. Dermatological signs and symptoms of measles: a prospective case series and comparison with the literature. *Dermatology* 2012;224:1–4.

10 Strebel PM, Orenstein WA. Measles. *N Engl J Med* 2019;381:349–57.

14 Hübschen JM, Bork SM, Brown KE et al. Challenges of measles and rubella laboratory diagnostic in the era of elimination. *Clin Microbiol Infect* 2017;23:511–15.

19 D'Souza RM, D'Souza R. Vitamin A for preventing secondary infections in children with measles – a systematic review. *J Trop Pediatr* 2002;48:72–7.

Human coronavirus infection

2   Solomon M, Liang C. Human coronaviruses: the emergence of SARS-CoV-2 and management of COVID-19. *Virus Res* 2022;319:198882.

4   Agnihothri R, Fox LP. Clinical patterns and morphology of COVID-19 dermatology. *Dermatol Clin* 2021;39:487–503.

19 Gupta K, Kaur G, Pathak T et al. Systematic review and meta-analysis of human genetic variants contributing to COVID-19 susceptibility and severity. *Gene* 2022;844:146790.

21 Gallman AE, Fassett MS. Cutaneous pathology of COVID-19 as a window into immunologic mechanisms of disease. *Dermatol Clin* 2021;39:533–43.

28 Galván Casas C, Català A, Carretero Hernández G et al. Classification of the cutaneous manifestations of COVID-19: a rapid prospective nationwide consensus study in Spain with 375 cases. *Br J Dermatol* 2020;183:71–7.

29 Freeman EE, McMahon DE, Lipoff JB et al. The spectrum of COVID-19-associated dermatologic manifestations: an international registry of 716 patients from 31 countries. *J Am Acad Dermatol* 2020;83:1118–29.

31 Holmes Z, Courtney A, Lincoln M et al. Rash morphology as a predictor of COVID-19 severity: a systematic review of the cutaneous manifestations of COVID-19. *Skin Health Dis* 2022;2:e120.

32 Visconti A, Bataille V, Rossi N et al. Diagnostic value of cutaneous manifestation of SARS-CoV-2 infection. *Br J Dermatol* 2021;184:880–7.

42 Desai SR, McMichael AJ, Khanna R. Coronavirus disease 2019 and race in dermatology. *Dermatol Clin* 2021;39:569–74.

66 Neale H, Hawryluk EB. COVID-19 pediatric dermatology. *Dermatol Clin* 2021; 39:505–19.

143 MacKenna B, Kennedy NA, Mehrkar A et al. Risk of severe COVID-19 outcomes associated with immune-mediated inflammatory diseases and immune-modifying therapies: a nationwide cohort study in the OpenSAFELY platform. *Lancet Rheumatol* 2022;4:e490–506.

148 Washrawirul C, Triwatcharikorn J, Phannajit J et al. Global prevalence and clinical manifestations of cutaneous adverse reactions following COVID-19 vaccination: a systematic review and meta-analysis. *J Eur Acad Dermatol Venereol* 2022;36:1947–68.

Other cutaneous problems associated with viral infections

2   Gutermuth J, Nadas K, Zirbs M et al. Papular-purpuric gloves and socks syndrome. *Lancet* 2011;378(9786):198.

28 Leung AKC, Sergi CM, Lam JM et al. Gianotti–Crosti syndrome (papular acrodermatitis of childhood) in the era of a viral recrudescence and vaccine opposition. *World J Pediatr* 2019;15:521–7.

78 Coustou D, Léauté-Labrèze C, Bioulac-Sage P et al. Asymmetric periflexural exanthem of childhood: a clinical, pathologic, and epidemiologic prospective study. *Arch Dermatol* 1999;135:799–803.

79 Chuh A, Zawar V, Sciallis GF et al. Pityriasis rosea, Gianotti-Crosti syndrome, asymmetric periflexural exanthem, papular-purpuric gloves and socks syndrome, eruptive pseudoangiomatosis, and eruptive hypomelanosis: do their epidemiological data substantiate infectious etiologies? *Infect Dis Rep* 2016;8:6418.

87 Drago F, Broccolo F, Rebora A. Pityriasis rosea: an update with a critical appraisal of its possible herpesviral etiology. *J Am Acad Dermatol* 2009;61:303–18.

93 Leung KC, Lam JM, Leong KF et al. Pityriasis rosea: an updated review. *Curr Pediatr Rev* 2021;17:201–11.

150 Drago F, Ciccarese G, Herzum A et al. Pityriasis rosea during pregnancy: major and minor alarming signs. *Dermatology* 2018;234:31–6.

153 Contreras-Ruiz J, Peternel S, Gutiérrez CJ et al. Interventions for pityriasis rosea. *Cochrane Database Syst Rev* 2019;Issue 10:CD005068.

CHAPTER 26
Bacterial Infections

Catriona Wootton and Ivo Elliott

Dermatology Department, Churchill Hospital, Oxford, UK; Department of Infection, John Radcliffe Hospital, Oxford, UK

Introduction: normal skin bacteria and bacterial microbiome, 26.2
Normal microbial ecology, 26.2
Flora of specialised areas, 26.4
Adherence, 26.5
Skin and defence, 26.5

GRAM-POSITIVE BACTERIA, 26.5
STAPHYLOCOCCUS AUREUS, 26.5
COAGULASE-NEGATIVE STAPHYLOCOCCI, 26.9
STREPTOCOCCI, 26.9
STAPHYLOCOCCAL AND STREPTOCOCCAL INFECTIONS, 26.12
Impetigo, 26.13
Ecthyma, 26.16
Cellulitis and erysipelas, 26.17
Folliculitis, 26.21
Furuncle (boil, abscess), 26.23
Carbuncle, 26.25
Sycosis, 26.26
Staphylococcal scalded skin syndrome, 26.27
Toxic shock syndrome, 26.29
Recurrent toxin-mediated perineal erythema, 26.31
Streptococcal vulvovaginitis, 26.32
Perianal streptococcal cellulitis, 26.33
Blistering distal dactylitis, 26.33
Toxin-mediated streptococcal disease, 26.34
Scarlet fever, 26.34
Streptococcal toxic shock-like syndrome, 26.36
CORYNEFORM BACTERIA, 26.36
Diphtheria, 26.37
Erythrasma, 26.38
Trichomycosis axillaris, 26.41
Pitted keratolysis, 26.41
ARCANOBACTERIUM HAEMOLYTICUM INFECTION, 26.42
TRUEPERELLA PYOGENES INFECTION, 26.43
CUTIBACTERIUM (FORMERLY PROPIONIBACTERIUM), 26.43
BACILLUS, 26.43
Anthrax, 26.43
LISTERIA MONOCYTOGENES, 26.45
Listeriosis, 26.45
ERYSIPELOTHRIX RHUSIOPATHIAE, 26.46
Erysipeloid, 26.46
CLOSTRIDIUM, 26.47
Gas gangrene (clostridial myonecrosis), 26.47

GRAM-NEGATIVE BACTERIA, 26.48
NEISSERIA MENINGITIDIS, 26.48
Meningococcal infection, 26.49
Gonococcal infection, 26.50
ACINETOBACTER, 26.50
MORAXELLA, 26.50
PSEUDOMONAS AERUGINOSA, 26.50
Pseudomonas infection, 26.50
BURKHOLDERIA, 26.53
Melioidosis, 26.53
Glanders, 26.54
STENOTROPHOMONAS MALTOPHILIA, 26.55
KLEBSIELLA PNEUMONIAE RHINOSCLEROMATIS, 26.55
Rhinoscleroma, 26.55
FRANCISELLA TULARENSIS, 26.57
Tularaemia, 26.57
PASTEURELLA, 26.58
Pasteurella multocida and related infections, 26.58
YERSINIA, 26.58
Plague and Yersinia infections, 26.59
Yersinia enterocolitica, 26.60
BRUCELLA, 26.60
Brucellosis, 26.60
BARTONELLA, 26.61
Trench fever, 26.61
Cat scratch disease, 26.62
Bacillary angiomatosis, 26.63
Oroya fever and verruga peruana, 26.64
VIBRIO VULNIFICUS INFECTIONS, 26.65
EHRLICHIA AND ANAPLASMA, 26.66
Ehrlichiosis and anaplasmosis, 26.66
OTHER GRAM-NEGATIVE BACILLI, 26.66

ANAEROBIC BACTERIA, 26.67
Tropical ulcer, 26.67
Granuloma inguinale, 26.68

SPIROCHAETES AND SPIRAL BACTERIA, 26.68
TREPONEMES, 26.69
Endemic (non-venereal) treponematoses, 26.69
Endemic syphilis or bejel, 26.69
Yaws, 26.69
Pinta, 26.70
BORRELIA, 26.71

Relapsing fever, 26.71
Borrelia burgdorferi and Lyme disease, 26.71
LEPTOSPIRA, 26.74
Leptospirosis (including Weil disease), 26.74
RAT-BITE FEVERS, 26.74
Spirillum minus rat-bite fever or sodoku, 26.74
Streptobacillary rat-bite fever and Haverhill fever, 26.75

LEGIONELLOSIS, 26.75

MISCELLANEOUS, 26.75
Botryomycosis, 26.75
Necrotising subcutaneous infections, 26.76

MYCOPLASMA INFECTIONS, 26.77

CHLAMYDIAE, 26.78
Psittacosis, 26.78

RICKETTSIAL INFECTIONS, 26.79
TYPHUS GROUP, 26.79
Epidemic typhus, 26.79
Brill–Zinsser disease, 26.80
Murine typhus, 26.80
SPOTTED FEVER GROUP, 26.80
Rocky Mountain spotted fever, 26.81
Tick typhus, 26.81
TRANSITIONAL GROUP, 26.82
Rickettsialpox, 26.82
Flea-borne spotted fever, 26.83
SCRUB TYPHUS GROUP, 26.83
Scrub typhus, 26.83

ACTINOMYCETE INFECTIONS, 26.83
Actinomycosis, 26.83
Nocardiosis, 26.85

DERMATOSES POSSIBLY ATTRIBUTABLE TO BACTERIA, 26.86
Chancriform pyoderma, 26.86
Pyoderma vegetans, 26.87
Dermatitis gangrenosa infantum, 26.87
Kawasaki disease, 26.88

Key references, 26.89

Rook's Textbook of Dermatology, Tenth Edition. Edited by Christopher Griffiths, Jonathan Barker, Tanya Bleiker, Walayat Hussain and Rosalind Simpson.
© 2024 John Wiley & Sons Ltd. Published 2024 by John Wiley & Sons Ltd.

Introduction: normal skin bacteria and bacterial microbiome

The human skin is an interface between the body and the external environment. In this role it provides a unique and delicate ecosystem; this results from colonisation of the skin by a diverse array of microorganisms that includes viruses, fungi and mites alongside bacteria. This symbiotic collection is known as the skin microbiome. A delicate balance exists between the host and these microorganisms and disruption to the equilibrium may lead to skin disease or infection. Aside from the arrival of frankly pathogenic organisms, a wide range of bacteria arrive on the skin surface and stay briefly in small numbers before disappearing, unable to multiply and thrive in this relatively inhospitable environment. Bacteriological sampling will reveal the presence of these otherwise unsuspected 'transients' [1]. Organisms not normally considered as resident members of the skin flora may sometimes colonise and become established in modest numbers for relatively long periods. Bacteria of this intermediate category have been labelled temporary residents. Furthermore, certain sites such as the skin of the face may be recolonised from the nostrils or mouth by *Staphylococcus aureus* or β-haemolytic streptococci, giving the false impression that these organisms are members of the normal facial flora whereas they are transients. The ability to use whole sequencing techniques has begun to revolutionise the study of skin flora, although unravelling the role of different populations of bacteria in skin disease is at an early stage.

When the skin is inflamed or otherwise abnormal, it is often difficult to determine whether an organism found on its surface is causing or contributing to the observed pathology [2,3]. Bacteriology reports must be interpreted with caution in the light of the known capabilities of the organism isolated. If the skin is damaged or the immune status of the subject impaired, bacteria usually regarded as non-pathogenic on the body surface may become opportunist pathogens. Equally, it appears that under certain conditions some resident bacteria may trigger defence mechanisms thereby contributing to the pathogenesis of some skin diseases. The number of organisms in the inoculum is of considerable importance. Within a given species, there are also strain differences in virulence. Some strains have a particular tendency to cause disease, perhaps due to greater adherence to epithelial cells, perhaps because of differences in enzyme production. The underlying mechanisms are not fully understood, but the principle is well recognised.

From the point of view of host defence, there are three aspects to be considered: first, the integrity of the skin barrier plus epidermal growth; second, the interactions between commensal organisms of the resident microbiome and the potential invader; and third, the classical immune and innate resistance mechanisms.

Even on the skin, the most accessible of body sites, the complexities of host–parasite relationships remain incompletely understood. Detailed culture-independent studies and DNA sequencing techniques of pathogens and commensals, and investigations of epidermal replication and of the immune capabilities of the host, however, have advanced our understanding. For example, examination of the forearms of six healthy volunteers, using sequence analysis of the bacterial *16S* gene, has shown a significant diversity of microorganisms. The number of species identified was much greater than any identified by standard cultural procedures, and several unknown phyla were also reported [4].

There is now a considerable literature on the microbiology of human skin of which these references are some of the most important texts: [5–7]. For general microbiology and infectious disease, Mandell *et al.* [8] and Collier and Balors [9] are recommended.

Normal microbial ecology
Methods of sampling

Numerous conventional methods have been used to sample the normal or commensal flora of the skin, especially when large numbers of subjects must be sampled; these are usually performed by swabbing in a standardised manner. The number of organisms is increased by the duration of rubbing, pressure exerted and moistening the swab. Semiquantitative data and some information as to the spatial distribution of bacteria are provided by sticky tape sampling, roll tubes or replica plating. The best quantitative estimates of the total bacterial flora are determined by applying an open-ended cylinder of known cross-sectional area to the skin, introducing a small known volume of suitable liquid vehicle (phosphate buffer plus Triton X-100®) and scrubbing the surface of the skin to free the organisms. However, it is very time-consuming, and gives a poor yield of the intrafollicular anaerobes. Full-thickness skin biopsy material should in theory provide a better sample [5].

The disposal of organisms from the skin can be studied quantitatively by air sampling techniques using either settle plates or an impaction sampler while the subject performs a specified activity, for example undressing in a small room [10].

The media used for isolation clearly influence the results of sampling. Noble, although recognising the special value of selective media, recommends in general the use of ordinary blood or serum agar for aerobic organisms and solid Brewer's thioglycolate medium without indicator but with 1% Tween 80® for *Cutibacterium* (formerly *Propionibacterium*) *acnes* [5].

For culture-independent studies using molecular genetic methods, the DNA of the organisms has to be extracted, processed and amplified. Broad-range polymerase chain reaction (PCR) primers identify the conserved universal genes found in all organisms within the target taxonomy; bacteria are most commonly classified by the amplification of their small subunit 16S rRNA gene sequence. The methods have been described previously [4,6,11].

Whole-genome shotgun metagenomics side-steps the need for amplification and allows for assessment of the structure of the whole microbiome without the biases inherent in 16S sequencing. This technique stands to develop further our understanding of the skin and its flora [6,12].

Normal flora

The concept of a stable normal resident flora composed of large numbers of organisms belonging to relatively few species is well established [1]. However, anatomical and environmental differences across the body lead to topographical variation in the microbiota [13]. Genetic studies show that there are variations from subject to subject, within an individual, with time and with site [9,13].

The previously established flora have been largely confirmed by the newer genetic techniques, but many new organisms have also been observed. The skin's ecological characteristics have been expanded by these new findings and the role of these microorganisms in skin health and disease is becoming clearer [4,13].

Temporary resident bacteria may confuse the picture, being less easy to distinguish from stable commensal organisms than obvious transients. It is possible, however, to describe a basic pattern of colonisation of healthy human skin from which some variations may be observed. In simple terms, dry skin supports a low level of colonisation, while moist areas and those well supplied with sebaceous glands are heavily populated. Most organisms reside on the surface of the stratum corneum in the crevices between squames in the looser outermost layers. These surface dwellers are not evenly distributed but are aggregated into microcolonies of varying sizes comprising perhaps 50 or several hundred cells. Their composition also varies with epidermal depth. Sebaceous sites are inhabited by anaerobes (*Cutibacterium* species) in their deeper parts and aerobic cocci in addition to *Malassezia* species of yeasts nearer the surface.

The resident aerobic flora that have been identified consist of Gram-positive cocci of the *Firmicutes* such as *Staphylococcus* species, actinobacteria like *Micrococcus* species and a variety of Gram-positive rods, the coryneforms or diphtheroids. These coryneform organisms are mainly *Corynebacterium* species but some are *Brevibacterium* species. The only significant Gram-negative residents are *Acinetobacter* species. Actinobacteria dominate on sebaceous follicle-rich areas and *Firmicutes* in the axillae. However, there are substantial regional and interpersonal differences; as stated earlier, bacterial populations also vary with the depth of the epidermis and in the presence of diseased skin.

Cutibacteria are regularly found in the follicles and sebaceous glands of adult skin and are the main anaerobic residents. The species *Staphylococcus saccharolyticus* is an anaerobic *Staphylococcus* and is a member of the normal flora in about 20% of subjects. Streptococci are notable by their absence, although they may frequently be found as transients (from the mouth) on perioral skin, or other sites prior to the onset of impetigo [14].

The genus *Staphylococcus* comprises more than 40 different species [15], and about 10 of these are regularly found on normal skin. The coagulase-positive species *Staph. aureus*, however, should not be considered as a resident on healthy skin in most subjects, although it is frequently found in the anterior nares. It occurs there as a resident in about one-third of most populations and is carried on perineal skin in up to 20%. Healthy axillary skin, and toe clefts in shoe-wearing populations, may also harbour it in a smaller percentage of subjects. On damaged skin, for example in eczema or psoriasis, *Staph. aureus* may be found, sometimes widely over the skin surface, with evidence suggesting that more than 90% of people with atopic eczema are colonised with *Staph. aureus* [16].

Of the coagulase-negative resident *Staphylococcus* species, *Staph. hominis* and *Staph. epidermidis* (moist sites) are the most important numerically, but *Staph. capitis*, *Staph. cohnii*, *Staph. haemolyticus*, *Staph. saprophyticus* and *Staph. warneri* have also been isolated from many subjects. Interestingly, *Staph. xylosus* has also been found to be fairly common on North American skins but does not seem to be a cutaneous resident in the UK. *Staph. simulans* is another recognised but uncommon cutaneous *Staphylococcus* on both sides of the Atlantic [7].

Organisms of the genus *Micrococcus* are less numerous than *Staphylococcus* species on healthy skin but are relatively more important on sparsely populated, dry sites and in childhood. *M. luteus* and *M. varians* appear to be the dominant species but *M. kristinae* and *M. sedentarius* are accepted as residents and *M. lylae* may be significant in infancy [6].

Coryneforms

The coryneform (or diphtheroid) organisms are mostly aerobic, Gram-positive pleomorphic rods. Several different genera of organisms fall under the coryneform umbrella including *Cutibacterium* (formerly *Propionibacterium*) species, *Brevibacterium* and *Actinomyces* [17]. Classification of the *Corynebacterium* genus is challenging and involves consideration of cell wall components; the Centers for Disease Control (CDC) have also developed a classification system for the coryneform group to aid recognition.

Brevibacterium species are clearly separable from the genus *Corynebacterium* by molecular and cell wall composition studies, nutritional requirements and by the production of methane thiol. These relatively recently recognised organisms have now been established as normal inhabitants of the skin (at least in a sizeable minority of subjects) and are particularly associated with (but not confined to) moist sites. They are related to *Brevibacterium* species isolated from dairy products, and by the production of methane thiol are the probable cause of the cheesy odour of sweaty feet [18].

Three species of *Cutibacterium* (formerly *Propionibacterium*), which are anaerobic, Gram-positive, rod-shaped organisms, are now generally acknowledged as members of the resident flora in adults. *C. acnes* and *C. granulosum* are widespread, but particularly associated with follicles that have large sebaceous glands over the face and upper trunk. They have both been associated with acne lesions in which their role is a matter of considerable interest. Another species, *C. avidum*, is found in moist sites, particularly the axillae and groins, and it is an opportunistic pathogen [19].

Quantitative cultural studies

Using cultural methods, the population of Micrococcaceae per square centimetre of the skin has been estimated as 600 for the hand, 60 for the forearm, 300 for the scapular region and 500 000–1 000 000 in the axilla [7]. Total anaerobic organisms, that is including diphtheroids as well, were reported by Williamson as averaging 1.46×10^6 for the scalp, and 2.41×10^6 for the axilla [20]. The number of organisms on a particular subject's skin varies little with time. There is, however, considerable variation within the population [21,22]. Some individuals habitually carry high, and others very low, numbers of bacteria but this distribution does follow a 'log normal' curve.

Modifying factors

The influence of various factors on the microbial population has been investigated by using a quantitative sampling technique and molecular analysis. Abstinence from washing does not increase the count. Taking a shower probably produces a brief temporary reduction in the bacterial flora, but because it leads to the break-up of the microcolonies on the skin and a more even distribution of bacteria, it may actually cause increased dissemination of bacteria for an hour or two afterwards [7].

The effects of increased hydration have been studied [2]. The total flora increases greatly; in the early stages, coagulase-negative staphylococci and micrococci predominate but, later, lipophilic coryneforms become numerous and micrococci diminish in importance. Gram-negative rods increase steadily with time. In humid tropical conditions, *Pseudomonas aeruginosa* is commonly isolated from moist areas, and in neonates nursed in high-humidity atmospheres, colonisation and infection with *P. aeruginosa* occur with increased frequency [23].

Age, sex and ethnic differences

The human skin becomes colonised from birth. Neonates are covered with vernix caseosa which has been shown to contain the antimicrobial peptide cathelicidin and also lysozyme, both of which have antibacterial properties. This suggests that the infant has the capacity to secrete these substances, perhaps in preparation for bacterial colonisation after birth [24]. In infants, the bacterial flora is somewhat unstable and varied, being more likely to include, probably as temporary residents, streptococci and spore-forming bacilli [25].

The mode of delivery influences the skin microbiota in a neonate; vaginal delivery results in colonisation of bacteria similar to those in the mother's vagina (*Lactobacillus*, *Prevotella*, *Sneathia* spp.) whereas Caesarean section confers normal adult skin flora such as *Corynebacterium*, *Staphylococcus* and *Cutibacterium* spp. [6].

Micrococcus species appear to be more prominent than on the adult skin, but *Cutibacterium* species require the increased skin lipid levels of puberty before becoming established, and are present at very low levels, if at all, before the onset of puberty. In elderly subjects, streptococci make an appearance as residents, and in this age group enteric organisms are found more often, particularly in moist sites. There is evidence that males carry higher numbers of bacteria, at least of aerobic organisms, than females [7], a fact which probably accounts for the observation that men are more likely to be disseminators of *Staph. aureus*, if they are perineal carriers, than are women [26,27].

Ethnic differences have been demonstrated in the nasal carriage of *Staph. aureus* – non-Hispanic white and Hispanic individuals (33%) were found to be more likely than non-Hispanic black individuals (27%) to carry this organism in the USA [28]; but comparative data on the densities of the bacterial populations of the main groups of resident organisms are lacking.

Changes in normal flora, including an increase in the number of subjects carrying Gram-negative organisms, may occur in seriously ill patients, apparently to an extent that cannot be accounted for by the treatment they are receiving [29]. Antiseptics applied to the skin, as in the preparation of operation sites, generally remove the transient flora and reduce the resident organisms [5]. The application of agents that specifically inhibit Gram-positive cocci is generally followed by an increase in the population of Gram-negative rods [30]. Carriage of *Staph. aureus* may also be affected by cold weather, duration of hospital stay or multiple injections [31].

Role of normal flora

The normal flora of the skin appears to have several functions, of which the most important is probably defence against bacterial infection through bacterial interference. *Cutibacterium acnes* releases free fatty acids through hydrolysing triglycerides in sebum, thereby generating an acidic milieu, which inhibits the growth of common pathogens such as *Staph. aureus* and *Streptococcus pyogenes* [32–34], which then favours the growth of corynebacterial and Gram-negative staphylococci.

Apocrine sweat is sterile and odourless when secreted. The odour develops due to bacterial action, mainly attributable to corynebacteria. Deodorants are effective largely through their antibacterial activity [35].

The skin appears able to discriminate between commensal organisms and harmful pathogens; the process of discrimination, however, is not fully elucidated. The skin microbiome appears to play an important role in immunity and Toll-like receptors (TLRs) on the skin surface may become desensitised through prolonged exposure to commensals. It has been demonstrated that *Staphylococcus epidermidis* is able to produce compounds which can modulate the host innate immune response either by means of a direct effect on pathogenic organisms or via TLR signalling [**14**].

Flora of specialised areas

Certain areas of skin have specific floras when cultured, which differ quantitatively or qualitatively from the general picture just outlined and are therefore worthy of special consideration.

Nasal vestibule

The nasal microbiome of healthy individuals typically includes *Corynebacterium*, *Staphylococcus*, *Streptococcus*, *Bifidobacterium*, *Dolosigranulum* and *Moraxella*. The percentage incidence varies greatly with different populations but, as nasal carriers sometimes disseminate large numbers of organisms, their detection and treatment are most important in the control of staphylococcal and streptococcal infections. Twin studies have demonstrated that the nasal microbiota are environmentally derived. However, women appear to have significantly reduced nasal bacterial density compared with men [36].

External auditory meatus

In addition to coagulase-negative staphylococci and coryneforms, *Proteus* species, *Escherichia coli*, *Neisseria catarrhalis* and *N. flora* have been isolated in small but significant numbers from normal ears.

Axilla

This site supports a very high level of bacterial colonisation, mostly staphylococci, micrococci and coryneforms.

Toe clefts

When wearing shoes, the fourth toe cleft is often hyperhydrated and the skin macerated. Such conditions sustain an extraordinarily large number of bacteria, mainly the common organisms of the general resident flora, but Gram-negative organisms are also found in this site. The toe web is an important site for *Brevibacterium* species, and not surprisingly *Acinetobacter* species are often isolated, as are *Alkaligenes* species. In the elderly and in tropical climates, coliforms and other organisms of the intestinal flora may be present [37].

Vulva

Organisms regularly isolated from this area include the expected coagulase-negative staphylococci, micrococci and coryneforms, with coliforms and enterococci occurring frequently as residents and as transients from faecal sources. Group B streptococci may be cultured from this site, usually in small numbers.

Perineum and groin

Staphylococci and coryneforms predominate in the perineum and groin, as they do in all moist skin sites. Gram-negative organisms of the intestinal flora may also be found in this site, due to faecal contamination, but should rapidly disappear in most healthy individuals.

Umbilicus

The umbilicus of the newborn is frequently colonised by *Staph. aureus* shortly after birth. The incidence varies greatly, but for infants born in hospital it is probably not very different from the nasal colonisation rate. The umbilicus of the newborn may also be colonised by *Strep. pyogenes* and look normal. The organisms can readily spread from infant to infant in a hospital nursery. Searches for the source of staphylococcal and streptococcal infection in a maternity unit should always include umbilical swabs from the babies.

Adherence

The ability of bacteria to stick to the skin surface, the process of adherence, has been extensively investigated. On wet surfaces, the hydrophobic nature of many bacterial walls promotes close apposition between the bacterium and human cells. In addition, there are smaller elements of the outer surface, adhesins, which also promote adhesion [38]. These are usually specific and interact with the host cell via a receptor site. Examples of bacterial adhesins include lipoteichoic acid [39], found in both staphylococci and streptococci; in the latter this is located in fine cell wall projections or fibrillae. Similar filamentous structures, fimbriae or pili, occur in many Gram-negative bacteria. Adhesins not only allow the organisms to remain on the epithelial surface, they may also regulate the relationship between different bacteria, such as the composition of microcolonies, via the interaction of complex excreted material covering the bacterial surface. The secretion of extracellular material, such as slime, allows bacteria to adhere to foreign surfaces as well as the stratum corneum [40]. Where this involves suture materials or plastics such as percutaneous cannulae, heavy colonisation may then be followed by invasion, resulting in abscess formation or septicaemia. In addition, organisms such as *Staph. aureus* can secrete peptidoglycan and form protective biofilms.

Skin and defence

The epidermis provides a barrier from which contaminating organisms are constantly being removed by desquamation. Investigators have spread organisms on the skin surface, studied their disappearance and attempted to elucidate the factors concerned. The early theories that the acid pH of most of the skin surface was an important defence mechanism against bacteria have now been completely rejected [7]. Desiccation appears to account for the difference in the rate at which implanted bacteria disappeared from acid and alkaline areas, the alkaline areas being moister.

The survival of several species of bacteria on the forearm skin has been studied [41] using plastic films of differing permeability to water and it is likely that a chemical mechanism was largely responsible for the destruction of *Strep. pyogenes*, whereas drying was responsible for the destruction of *E. coli* and *P. aeruginosa*. Both factors appeared to contribute to the elimination of *Staph. aureus*. Extraction of the fatty acids from the skin diminishes resistance to colonisation by staphylococci, and fatty acids may be neutralised to some extent by binding with an antibiotic such as neomycin [42].

The skin participates very actively in defence by producing antimicrobial peptides such as cathelicidin, *cis*-6-hexadecenoic acid and the various defensins [43]. These are produced by keratinocytes, but neutrophils, mast cells and platelets which are recruited to the area may also be involved in the production of antimicrobial peptides [44]. Other molecules present on the skin and in sweat such as dermcidin and histone H4 also aid in the control of epidermal bacteria. Defective control of these peptides in response to the microbiome may contribute to a number of different skin diseases [45].

The phenomenon of bacterial interference is sufficiently closely related to skin defence to be mentioned here. Colonisation of some sites by one strain of staphylococci interferes with the subsequent colonisation by a different strain. Competition for available nutrients is thought to explain this phenomenon. The organisms also produce bacteriocins (antibiotic substances) which may inhibit the growth of others [46]. When pathogens invade, the host response is via the adaptive and innate immune systems, which are interrelated. There is an important role for variations in TLR signalling in determining levels of colonisation particularly for potential pathogens such as *Staph. aureus*.

GRAM-POSITIVE BACTERIA

Staphylococcus and *Streptococcus* are Gram-positive bacteria that can cause cutaneous infections through adherence to the skin surface, proliferation and invasion. Superficial epidermal infections include impetigo and ecthyma, whereas deeper infections include cellulitis and necrotising fasciitis. Invasion through the hair follicle leads to folliculitis and furunculosis, and toxin production leads to cytokine cascades resulting in diffuse skin injury seen in staphylococcal scalded skin syndrome (SSSS) and scarlet fever. The characteristics of the Gram-positive organisms are discussed in detail and the mechanisms by which they lead to cutaneous infections.

STAPHYLOCOCCUS AUREUS

Definition

Staphylococcus is a Gram-positive cocci bacterium that usually forms into clusters (from 'Staphylo', like a 'bunch of grapes'). *Staph. aureus* is one of the many pathogenic species of *Staphylococcus* that cause specifically skin infections such as impetigo, boils, wound infections and septicaemia.

Introduction and general description

Staph. aureus is a coloniser and pathogen of humans and mammals. A significant proportion of the general population are colonised with *Staph. aureus* on their skin/nasal mucosa and in the majority this is not associated with disease. However, the scope of *Staph. aureus*-mediated disease is broad and it can commonly cause skin disease by infecting breaks/wounds in the skin and may lead to folliculitis, impetigo, secondary infection of underlying inflammatory skin diseases (dermatitis), boils/abscesses, cellulitis, septic arthritis and osteomyelitis, infections of prosthetic devices as well as systemic infections such as endocarditis, pneumonia and life-threatening bacteraemia. Disease can also result from *Staph. aureus* toxin production such as occurs in SSSS, toxic shock syndrome (TSS), Panton–Valentine leukocidin (PVL) necrotic skin lesions and necrotising pneumonia as well as food poisoning from toxin ingestion. The widespread use of broad spectrum antibiotics is thought to have contributed to the increasing global incidence of antibiotic-resistant strains of *Staph. aureus* including meticillin-resistant *Staph. aureus* (MRSA). Box 26.1 shows how *Staph. aureus* is involved in cutaneous disease.

Box 26.1 Involvement of *Staphylococcus aureus* in cutaneous disease

Direct infection of skin and adjacent tissues
- Impetigo
- Ecthyma
- Folliculitis
- Furunculosis
- Carbuncle
- Sycosis
- Occasionally in cellulitis
- Others

Secondary infection
- Eczema, infestations, ulcers, etc.

Cutaneous disease due to effect of bacterial toxin
- Staphylococcal scalded skin syndrome
- Toxic shock syndrome
- Staphylococcal scarlatina
- Recurrent toxin-mediated perineal erythema

Epidemiology

Incidence and prevalence

Recent studies have shown that *Staph. aureus* is the most commonly isolated pathogenic bacteria from nosocomial infections in the USA and the second most common in the out-patient setting [1]. Between 40% and 50% of bacteraemia isolates in North America are MRSA, with rates in Europe in 2007 ranging from 0.8% in Germany to 35% in the UK and 48% in Portugal [2]. Awareness and efforts to tackle MRSA have resulted in a downward trend in the EU/EEA population-weighted mean of MRSA infections, from 19% of *Staph. aureus* infections in 2015 to 15.5% in 2019 [3]. Community-acquired MRSA (CA-MRSA) prevalence has also significantly increased over the past few decades and is responsible for severe skin infections, in often otherwise healthy individuals. CA-MRSA is spread by direct contact and is more commonly associated with toxin production than nosocomial MRSA. However, the artificial boundary between community and hospital is becoming increasingly blurred in many settings where CA-MRSA leads to nosocomial infections replacing traditional hospital-acquired MRSA (HA-MRSA). Additionally, the detection of livestock-associated MRSA (LA-MRSA) [3] highlights that this is an evolving picture and therefore distinctions previously based on clinical epidemiology are becoming less relevant, leading to more genotypic definitions.

Age

Neonates tend to be rapidly colonised by *Staph. aureus* in their nose and around the umbilical stump [4] with higher rates in infants born in hospital (72%) than at home and lower rates in those receiving regular disinfectant to the umbilicus [5]. Nasal carriage rates then fall to a minimum of 10–15% at 1 year of age before rising to adult levels by the age of 5 years [5]. Most of the data relating to *Staph. aureus* at different ages have been gleaned from studies determining rates of MRSA infections. For example, there is evidence that rates of meticillin-sensitive *Staph. aureus* (MSSA) and MRSA are equally prevalent in children from 4 to 59 months of age, that those aged 11–18 years are more likely to be affected by MSSA and that older age (>60 years) is more associated with MRSA than MSSA. However, these age-related differences more reflect underlying diseases and/or the state of the patient's immune system rather than age itself. Generally, patients with MRSA are significantly older and have more underlying disease than those with MSSA, and mortality is higher in the MRSA group except for infections leading to pneumonia.

Sex

Males and females are equally affected by *Staph. aureus* infections; however, outbreaks of CA-MRSA occur more commonly in males (sports team associated, men who have sex with men). However, being female is independently associated with a higher mortality from *Staph. aureus* bacteraemia than being male [6].

Ethnicity

Outbreaks of CA-MRSA are common in ethnic minority groups living in overcrowded conditions. Reports in the literature have shown increased prevalence of MRSA in African Americans (USA), Hispanics (USA), Aborigines (Australia) and those of Pacific ethnicity (New Zealand) and lower rates in Asians (USA) [7].

Associated diseases

Staph. aureus infections occur in association with reduced skin barrier function. This may result from minor skin trauma (cuts, scratches, abrasions, burns, etc.), chronic skin breaches (ulceration), inflammatory skin disease (dermatitis), associated with other primary skin infections such as viruses (chickenpox/shingles, herpes simplex virus), fungi (tinea capitis with a kerion, *Candida* paronychia) and mycobacterial infections (*M. abscessus*, *M. marinum*). Type 1 diabetes, renal haemodialysis, liver disease and prosthetic implants are all associated with higher rates of *Staph. aureus* infections, which may in some cases result in bacterial endocarditis.

Pathophysiology
Predisposing factors
Studies suggest that 10–20% of the general population are persistent carriers of *Staph. aureus* with up to 50% intermittent carriers and 20–30% non-carriers [8]. The overall prevalence of *Staph. aureus* nasal carriage in healthy adults is 27% [9]. Host and bacterial factors are thought to play a role in staphylococci carriage [10] in particular the production of cell wall lipoteichoic acid (LTA) by the *Staph. aureus* strain [11]. However, studies have demonstrated that after inoculation with a mixture of *Staph. aureus* strains up the nose, individuals reverted to type, i.e. to persistent carriers (often with their original strains and not the strains inoculated) or non-carriers (most reverted within 2 weeks of inoculation) and intermittent carriage continued [12]. Persistent carriers are a significant source of *Staph. aureus* that results in infections in both hospital and community settings. Children have higher persistent rates of nasal carriage than adults. Among hospital staff, 25% are colonised by *Staph. aureus* in their nasal mucosa [13]. Patients at greatest risk of *Staph. aureus* infections including life-threatening bacteraemia include those with ulcers/chronic wounds, previously documented *Staph. aureus* infections/colonisation, central venous/urinary catheters, surgical wounds, intravenous drug users, patients with liver disease, immunocompromised/suppressed individuals and those taking systemic corticosteroids. CA-MRSA is most commonly spread by direct contact and therefore is most prevalent in those living in overcrowded conditions, low socioeconomic groups, young children, in the context of poor hygiene and associated with individuals who have minor breaks in their skin. Outbreaks of CA-MRSA are reported among athletes, military recruits, in day care facilities, intravenous drug users and men who have sex with men.

Carriage. Genetic factors, perhaps involving bacterial adherence and immune responses, are suggested by higher nasal carriage rates in white than black-skinned individuals, by studies of families and twins, by higher than normal rates in patients with phenylketonuria, by increased adherence in atopic eczema and by an association of nasal carriage with human leukocyte antigen (HLA)-DR3 [14–17]. In those susceptible to nasal colonisation, the overall rate depends on the extent to which the many transient carriers acquire the organism by contact with persistent carriers. This at least partly underlies the increase in carriage rates following hospital admission [18], higher rates in urban than in rural areas [19] and variation in carriage rates with age. High rates of nasal carriage in atopic eczema (79%) [20] may partly derive from the heavy load of *Staph. aureus* on the skin, but increased adhesion of the organism to nasal mucosal cells may be relevant [17]. As a primary reservoir of *Staph. aureus*, nasal carriage has been identified as a major risk factor for the subsequent development of community-acquired and nosocomial infections. Those patients on ambulatory peritoneal dialysis or haemodialysis who carry *Staph. aureus* in the nose are much more likely to get infection of the exit sites, usually with the same bacterial strain [18]. Patients with HIV infection and AIDS-related diseases have higher carriage rates of *Staph. aureus* than those unaffected, even when intravenous drug users are excluded among the HIV-positive individuals, and this is a risk factor for subsequent severe infection with *Staph. aureus* [21]. The underlying mechanism for this is as yet unclear.

Various surface components of *Staph. aureus*, such as teichoic acid, LTA, fibronectin-binding proteins and type 5 and type 8 capsular polysaccharides, have all been implicated as substances responsible for, or contributing to, binding of the organism in the nose [18]. However, not all have been successfully confirmed. Intestinal carriage of *Staph. aureus* is particularly common among hospitalised patients, and this may be associated with transmission of the organism to the skin. The organism was identified not only in the nose (45%) but also in the stool (36%) of 71 hospitalised subjects [22]. The majority of these patients were persistent stool carriers. Furthermore, swabs taken from environmental surfaces, such as bedside tables, showed contamination of these surfaces too. Molecular typing of the organisms showed some of the isolates from the nose and stool were clonally identical to those from the environmental sources [22].

Suppression of carriage. Although there are no long-term studies to identify the best method of reducing carriage, regular long-term application of chlorhexidine cream to the appropriate sites (anterior nares, perineum or axillae) and use of an antiseptic, typically chlorhexidine or povidone–iodine, in a detergent base for daily bathing or showering including hair washing are effective in clinical practice, although recolonisation occurs soon after treatment is stopped. Oral or topical antibiotics may contribute to elimination of the organism, but in general recolonisation occurs soon after the treatment is stopped [23], with two main exceptions. Intranasal mupirocin eliminated nasal *Staph. aureus* after a 5-day course in all patients treated, and 50% remained free of the organism after 5 months [24]. In haemodialysis patients, oral rifampicin, 600 mg daily for 7–10 days, cleared the organism for 3 months in 80% of cases [25]. Good results also were obtained with long-term low-dose clindamycin, 150 mg daily for 3 months [26]. The staphylococci have become resistant to many antibiotics over the past few decades while therapeutic options have decreased.

Pathology
Staph. aureus has the ability to produce numerous surface factors and proteins that help it to survive and evade host immunity. The most highly characterised surface defence of *Staph. aureus* is protein A which is composed of five homologous immunoglobulin/antibody binding domains, each able to bind to the Fc region of antibodies and the Fab region of the human VH3 family. This binding inhibits the antibodies from fixing complement or directing macrophages which results in disruption of opsonisation and phagocytosis. Higher levels of protein A are more commonly associated with strains leading to persistent nasal colonisation. *Staph. aureus* synthesises another protein called coagulase which triggers the clotting cascade, leading to the production of a mesh of plasma proteins which effectively surrounds the bacteria giving it an immunological cloak of disguise. The ability of *Staph. aureus* to invade deep tissues is facilitated by the production of collagenases and hyaluronidase.

Causative organisms
There are 40 different species of *Staphylococcus* defined by their Gram-positive staining and their ability to form a 'cluster of

grapes'. Different species are subclassified by their ability to produce coagulase enzymes, which can cause blood to clot. Most species are harmless to humans and are part of the normal commensal flora of the skin, such as coagulase-negative *Staph. epidermidis*. In the immunocompromised patient, however, this species of *Staphylococcus* can cause life-threatening infections especially in association with central venous catheters. The genitourinary tract is colonised by the commensal *Staph. saprophyticus* and the stomach by *Staph. leei*. The main pathological species in humans is *Staph. aureus*, which is mainly but not exclusively coagulase positive.

Antibiotic resistance. Evidence suggests the application of topical antibiotics to the skin increases the likelihood of the development or the transfer of antibiotic resistance [27]. Of special importance is gentamicin resistance, which can be transferred between strains of *Staph. aureus*, and also between coagulase-negative staphylococci and *Staph. aureus* [28]. Topical fusidic acid and mupirocin were previously associated with a low incidence of resistance; however, this is no longer the case with resistant strains being widely reported [29,30].

Meticillin-resistant *Staph. aureus*. Resistance to the antibiotic meticillin was reported first in 1961 [28]. Over the past few decades, epidemics of MRSA infection have increased in frequency worldwide. Many hospitals have had to institute control measures to contain the spread of the infection [31]. Once established in hospitals, its survival seems to be promoted by the widespread use of antibiotics. New clones of MRSA may follow changes in antibiotic usage [32]. Resistance to antibiotics occurs when an organism acquires a gene that allows the microbe to inactivate the antibiotic. This may occur spontaneously as a genetic mutation, or involve the acquisition of a mobile genetic element such as a plasmid, transposon, integron or gene cassette [33]. Unfortunately, MRSA carriage on the skin may persist for years, and increases the risk of spread if patients who are carriers are readmitted to hospital [34]. The risk factors identified for patients developing MRSA infection include previous antibiotic use, contact with a health care worker or nursing home resident, residence in a long-term care facility, admission to an intensive care unit, intravenous drug use, indwelling devices, haemo- or peritoneal dialysis, nasogastric or other invasive tubes, immunosuppression and surgical procedures. Outcomes for patients infected with MRSA are worse than for those with MSSA. Identifying patients with MRSA as they are admitted to hospital would allow isolation, in an attempt to reduce exposure of other patients. However, this requires significant resources, and perhaps screening high-risk groups of patients, with some of the risk factors already mentioned, would target the investigations and be more cost-effective [35]. In the UK, most MRSA infections occur in older patients (82% over 60 years of age); the vast majority of strains are resistant to fluoroquinolones and macrolides, and are mupirocin resistant [32]. Vancomycin has traditionally been the drug of choice for treating these infections, but as treatment has to be given intravenously the duration of hospital stay is often prolonged. This increases the cost of the hospital stay, and also exposes the patient to further nosocomial infections [31]. Furthermore, the appearance of strains of staphylococci with clinical resistance to vancomycin and teicoplanin is increasing in frequency. Guidelines for the treatment of MRSA infections have been published [32] and are regularly updated.

CA-MRSA infections have become common recently, with infections reported worldwide including among military personnel, prison inmates, intravenous drug users, athletes and homeless people [36]. The majority of infections present as abscesses or folliculitis. The staphylococci are genetically distinct from those acquired in the hospital setting and often carry the *PVL* virulence gene, although there is now much crossover in the strains isolated from patients in hospital. These organisms are probably best described respectively as 'community-type' and 'health care/hospital-type' strains without specific regard for where the infection was actually acquired. Although most patients presenting with community-type staphylococcal infections will respond to drainage of the abscess, some develop bacteraemia, which may require systemic antibiotic therapy [28]. The choice of antibiotic should reflect the sensitivities, and many strains are still sensitive to trimethoprim-sulfamethoxazole and tetracycline. Resistance to fluoroquinolones and erythromycin, and thus clindamycin, limits their use. Linezolid is still currently beneficial although it is expensive. Unfortunately, multidrug-resistant CA-MRSA has been reported [37].

Genetics

Staph. aureus was one of the first bacteria to have its entire genome sequenced (2001). Since then, more extensive genomic data have been amassed and these have helped to define divergent species and strains of *Staphylococcus* through identification of their specific surface proteins and toxins produced. Molecular typing of *Staphylococcus* strains has led to a better understanding of how outbreaks of staphylococci occur and how the bacteria can be spread in the community and in hospitals. The pathogenic capacity (virulence) of each strain of *Staph. aureus* depends on several factors; however, the most important appears to be its armamentarium of exotoxins, which include PVL, exfoliative toxins, phenol-soluble modulins and superantigens. Most toxin-encoding genes are located on mobile genetic elements (MGE) which leads to vast heterogeneity [38]. For example, the cause of meticillin resistance, the *mecA* gene, is situated on MGE, the staphylococcal cassette chromosome mec (SCCmec), and within that there are seven major variants, I–VII [39]. CA-MRSA harbours SCCmec type IV, V or VII and has a genetically distinct background from HA-MRSA. Other genetic elements associated with MRSA expression include murE and femA but these mechanisms remain poorly understood [40].

Environmental factors

Staph. aureus has the ability to survive and colonise a number of different environments through sophisticated stress response mechanisms that result from the regulation and expression of their genes. *Staph. aureus* has the ability to withstand quite high temperatures (up to 50°C), acidity and salt. Consequently, *Staph. aureus* can colonise the axillae, inguinal regions, throat and anterior nares in a significant proportion of the population.

COAGULASE-NEGATIVE STAPHYLOCOCCI

Definition
Coagulase-negative staphylococci (CoNS) comprise a broad group of species that are found commensally on the skin and mucous membranes (*Staphylococcus hominis*, *Staphylococcus epidermidis*) and vaginal tract (*Staphylococcus saprophyticus*). In the past, they have been somewhat dismissed as low-virulence organisms that have been thought to represent 'contaminants' in microbiological cultures. However, there is a growing body of evidence that suggests these CoNS persist on hospital surfaces and devices and lead to clinically relevant infections in up to 30% of health care-related sepsis episodes [1].

Introduction and general description
Staph. epidermidis [2] is the main pathogen of the group. In the otherwise healthy patient, it is probably an occasional cause of minor skin infections, including superficial folliculitis, although its significance in an individual case may be difficult to judge.

Epidemiology
Associated diseases
Secondary infection of pre-existing dermatoses, such as atopic eczema, seems not to occur. *Staph. epidermidis* may cause infections in wounds and especially around implanted surgical devices. It has been increasingly recognised as a cause of major internal infections, including endocarditis [3] and septicaemia, especially in patients with immune deficiencies. A case of cellulitis in a woman with acute myelocytic leukaemia was reported [4], and the organism has been associated with vasculitis in a patient on cytotoxic therapy for ovarian carcinoma [5].

Pathophysiology
Predisposing factors
The ability to adhere to foreign bodies and produce extracellular slime during the course of colonisation is thought to be important for pathogenicity [6]. The organism is able to adhere initially to the device and then also produces clusters which are multilayered. The glucosamine polymer polysaccharide intercellular adhesin (PIA) is a major contributor. The mechanisms involved in the epidemiology and pathogenesis of infection caused by CoNS have been discussed in detail by Becker *et al.* [6].

Causative organisms
A single isolate of *Staph. epidermidis* from blood culture could be due to contamination, but if found repeatedly it may be regarded as probably significant. *Staph. saprophyticus* is a recognised cause of urinary tract infection, especially in young women [7]. More recently *Staphylococcus lugdunensis*, a CoNS, was found to cause 16 cases of abscesses and wound infections in Greece [8].

Genetics
The genes encoding for the biosynthesis of glucosamine polymer PIA are well recognised as enabling CoNS to adhere to tissues and cause disease.

Environmental factors
The biofilm produced is important for the pathogenesis as it seems to be tolerant of antibiotics and may contribute to its persistence. Multiple antibiotic resistance is common and may be transferred to *Staph. aureus*. Workplace surfaces and hands of health care workers swabbed in a hospital in Italy demonstrated higher levels of antibiotic resistance in the CoNS isolated than the MRSA isolates [9].

STREPTOCOCCI

Definition
The streptococci are Gram-positive catalase-negative cocci characteristically arranged in pairs or chains. They are nearly all facultative anaerobes, that is they can grow aerobically or anaerobically [1].

Introduction and general description
Strep. pyogenes or 'group A streptococci' are extracellular bacterial pathogens which cause disease in humans involving the mucous membranes, tonsils, skin and deeper tissues. Specifically, they cause pharyngitis, impetigo, cellulitis, erysipelas, necrotising fasciitis, TSS, scarlet fever, septicemia, pneumonia and meningitis.

Strep. pyogenes is one of the most common pathogens of humans. Between 5% and 15% of the population are colonised by the bacteria, usually in their respiratory tract. This commensal usually causes disease when the balance between host immunity (immunosuppression) and bacterial factors (virulence) is altered. The most common skin disease associated with *Strep. pyogenes* is cellulitis or erysipelas usually of the lower limb or face. More rarely, TSS and necrotising fasciitis are also mediated by *Strep. pyogenes* in the skin and can be life threatening.

Box 26.2 summarises the main cutaneous infections associated with streptococci.

Epidemiology
Incidence and prevalence
Strep. pyogenes is the most common cause of acute pharyngitis and is responsible for between 15% and 30% of cases in children and 5–10% of cases in adults [2]. Infection rates are dependent on geographic location, climate, season and age. Between 12% and 23% of school-aged children are estimated to be pharyngeal carriers. Public health agencies in 11 countries in northern Europe found that severe streptococcal infections reached 3/100 000 population per year [3]; similar rates are reported in Australia/USA (3–4/100 000) with higher rates in the low and middle income nations (12/100 000 in Kenya). The risk of infection was highest among the elderly and males. Skin wounds/lesions were the most common predisposing factor occurring in 25% of cases. Of patients, 32% had cellulitis and 8% necrotising fasciitis. Overall case fatality at 1 week was 19% and 44% among patients with streptococcal toxic shock syndrome (STSS) [3]. Resurgence of streptococcal infections over the past 30 years is thought to be partly due to changes in virulence as well as evolving antibiotic resistance.

> **Box 26.2 Involvement of streptococci (mostly group A) in cutaneous disease**
>
> **Direct infections of skin or subcutaneous tissue**
> - Impetigo
> - Ecthyma
> - Erysipelas
> - Cellulitis
> - Vulvovaginitis
> - Perianal infection
> - Streptococcal ulcers
> - Blistering distal dactylitis
> - Necrotising fasciitis
> - Others
>
> **Secondary infection**
> - Eczema, infestations, ulcers, etc.
>
> **Tissue damage from circulating toxin**
> - Scarlet fever
> - Toxic-shock-like syndrome
> - Recurrent toxin-mediated perineal erythema
>
> **Skin lesions attributed to allergic hypersensitivity to streptococcal antigens**
> - Erythema nodosum (Chapter 99)
> - Vasculitis (Chapter 102)
>
> **Skin disease provoked or influenced by streptococcal infection (mechanism uncertain)**
> - Psoriasis, especially guttate forms (Chapter 35)
> - Kawasaki disease (see later)

Age

Streptococcal pharyngitis is uncommon under the age of 3 years and is thought to be mainly a disease of school-aged children, which reflects patterns seen in acute rheumatic fever where the highest prevalence is in those aged 5–15 years. In low and middle income countries, poststreptococcal glomerulonephritis (PSGN) is most common in children <11 years and is thought to result from *Streptococcus* associated with scabies infestations. The average prevalence of scabies in tropical countries is 5–10% of children and studies have shown a significant proportion of these individuals have chronic haematuria [4] as a result of PSGN. In higher income countries, PSGN is most common in white males more than 50 years of age and is associated with diabetes, malignancy, alcoholism, HIV infection and intravenous drug use.

Sex

Males and females are equally affected across all types of streptococcal infections.

Ethnicity

Streptococcal infections do not show any predilection to any particular ethnic group.

Associated diseases

Scabies infestations (Chapter 34) frequently lead to excoriated skin, which is vulnerable to streptococcal as well as necrotising secondary infection. The streptococcal infections following scabies have been shown to be linked to symptomatic PSGN and asymptomatic chronic haematuria. Guttate psoriasis (Chapter 35) is thought to be associated with streptococcal pharyngitis and perianal streptococcal dermatitis 2–3 weeks prior to the onset of the psoriatic lesions. The exact pathophysiological mechanism is not fully understood but the guttate psoriasis phenotype is more common in HLA-Cw*0602-positive patients. *Streptococcus* dysregulates the interactions between HLA-C and natural killer cells resulting in inflammatory changes [5]. Sydenham chorea, Tourette syndrome, obsessive compulsive disorder and paediatric autoimmune neuropsychiatric disorders associated with streptococcal infection (PANDAS) have all been linked to neurological damage resulting from streptococcal infections [6]. There is evidence that antibodies induced by group A streptococcal infections react with basal ganglia neurons in Sydenham chorea and PANDAS. Antibasal ganglia antibodies (ABGA) are present in most cases of acute Sydenham chorea, and in Tourette syndrome 91% of patients with positive ABGA had a raised antistreptolysin O titre (ASOT) [7].

Erythema nodosum (Chapter 97) is most frequently idiopathic; however, among the necrotising triggers, streptococcal pharyngitis is the most common cause. Scleredema of Buschke (Chapter 57) has also been linked with streptococcal infection of the throat in children and adults and treatment with high-dose antibiotic seems to reduce the resultant fibrosis [8].

Pathophysiology
Predisposing factors

The major streptococcal skin pathogen in humans is group A *Streptococcus* or *Strep. pyogenes*. The surface of *Strep. pyogenes* is highly complex and chemically variable and accounts for many of the bacteria's virulence factors. These include capsular polysaccharides (C-substance), cell wall peptidoglycans, LTA, fimbrial proteins, fibronectin binding proteins (FBP) and surface proteins M, R and T. The capsule is composed of hyaluronic acid which is chemically similar to that found in human connective tissue, allowing the bacteria to evade recognition by the host's immune system. Adhesion to host tissue is facilitated through LTA, fibronectin binding and M protein. The M proteins also protect the organism against phagocytosis and aid necrotising, consequently markedly increasing pathogenicity. Currently, at least 80 different M protein sequence types have been identified using molecular approaches to identify the *emm* (M protein) genes. The *emm* gene superfamily includes antiphagocytic molecules and immunoglobulin binding proteins. M protein interacts with TLR2 on monocytes in the peripheral blood stimulating them to release cytokines interleukin (IL)-6, IL-1B and tumour necrosis factor (TNF)-α. This response is amplified in the presence of neutrophil-derived heparin binding protein (HBP) which co-stimulates monocytes by interacting with CD18/CD11 [9]. The presence of M protein expressing *Streptococcus* in necrotising fasciitis triggers recruitment of monocytes and neutrophils into the infected tissue in combination with HBP, and this synergistically results in a severe acute inflammatory response and extensive tissue destruction. The predominant M1 protein subtype has been implicated in the resurgence of acute rheumatic fever in children since the 1980s. T protein is present on the surface of group A but not group C/G streptococci. T typing identification has been useful in investigating outbreaks due to streptococcal infections where M protein has not been identified. Four of the 25 T antigens identified are pilus-like structures on the bacterial surface similar to those found in Gram-negative bacteria. R protein has yet to be properly characterised, but is thought not to be a virulence factor. C5a peptidase, a proteolytic enzyme on the surface of group A *Streptococcus*, inhibits the recruitment of phagocytic cells to the site of infection, and thus plays a role in the pathogenesis of streptococcal disease [4].

The majority of STSS cases have been associated with the presence of streptococcal pyrogenic exotoxins (SPE), particularly A and C. Through genome sequencing projects, SPEs A–J have been identified so far [10]. The SPEs are part of a larger group of pyrogenic toxin superantigens (PTSAgs) that can activate the immune system directly, bypassing antigen-mediated immune stimulation, by binding invariant regions and specific receptors. Up to 20% of T cells are directly stimulated [11], resulting in a massive detrimental surge in cytokine levels, which in turn leads to capillary leak, tissue damage, cardiovascular shock and ultimately multiorgan failure seen in STSS.

The Lancefield group antigens have been used historically to help classify streptococci in the laboratory alongside haemolysis by strains on blood agar. However, Lancefield group (A–R) does not correlate to streptococcal species and haemolysis is imprecise (β-haemolytic, α-haemolytic and non-haemolytic (γ-haemolytic) organisms). Nevertheless, more detailed identification is now possible with molecular genetics and some streptococci have consequently been reclassified [1].

Carriage. *Strep. pyogenes* carriage in the oropharynx affects about 10% of the general population and 20% of schoolchildren in the winter/spring. In carriers, there is no host immune response to the bacteria and persistence can last for many months [12]. Streptococci can invade human cells by multiple mechanisms including FBPs, which engage with α5β1 integrin receptors on epithelial cells [13]. Failure to eradicate *Strep. pyogenes* from the throat following pharyngotonsillitis occurs in 30% of cases, and the isolated strains more commonly expressed the FBP gene *prtF1*, which also resulted in higher rates of antibiotic treatment failure. On screening family members of an index case of streptococcal pharyngitis, 25% were found to be carriers of *Strep. pyogenes* in the throat. Carriers had a low antistreptolysin O (ASO) titre level compared with those with both invasive and non-invasive streptococcal disease [14]. The normal skin does not provide a favourable habitat for *Strep. pyogenes*, perhaps due partly to a bactericidal effect of skin lipids [15], and transient skin carriage is found in only 0.5–1.0% of individuals [16]. However, the duration of survival of streptococci on the normal skin of patients with infections, and on the hands and arms of those handling such patients, may be sufficient to allow their dispersal by this route. Asymptomatic anal carriage is an occasional source of significant infection in contacts [17]; this was highlighted by Semmelweis and his observations which led to significant reductions in deaths from puerperal fever and the dawn of infection control practices [18]. Streptococci colonise damaged skin, although less readily than staphylococci. They can frequently be isolated from eczematous and other moist lesions, although the borderline between colonisation and infection is often difficult to define.

Pathology

Strep. pyogenes causes disease through numerous pathological mechanisms. The primary factors include the ability of the organism to invade epithelial cells and remain in the intracellular state evading the host immune system. The bacteria can adhere to the surface of cells through a complex matrix of cell wall and surface structures that also inhibit phagocytosis. One surface structure, protein M, is ever changing and is responsible for most of the organism's antigenic shift and drift. Toxins and extracellular products lead to direct inflammatory responses which ultimately result in host cell damage.

Causative organisms

Streptococcal bacteria are classified into groups α, β and γ according to their ability to haemolyse red blood cells. α-Haemolytic streptococci species include *Strep. viridans* (mainly present in the mouth and leads to dental caries, gingival infections and endocarditis usually following dental extraction), *Strep. pneumoniae* (causes community-acquired pneumonia, sinusitis, otitis media, conjunctivitis, osteomyelitis, endocarditis, cellulitis, meningitis). β-Haemolytic species include groups A–H: *Strep. pyogenes* (group A, leads to pharyngitis, impetigo, scarlet fever, STSS, necrotising fasciitis, pneumonia, bacteraemia, as well as acute rheumatic fever and acute glomerulonephritis); *Strep. agalactiae* (group B, which is responsible for disease mainly in neonates and the elderly including pneumonia and meningitis, also colonisation of the vagina during pregnancy can lead to premature rupture of membranes leading to fetal morbidity/mortality. In the USA, Canada and Australia women are screened in the antenatal period for group B *Streptococcus*); group B *Streptococcus* can also cause cellulitis; *Strep. dysgalactiae* (group C, pharyngitis, cellulitis and septicaemia); *Strep. bovis* (group D, can cause endocarditis) and *Strep. anginosus* group (formerly *Strep. milleri*, groups A, C, G, F; are part of the normal gut flora but can cause liver and brain abscesses and lung empyema). *Enterococcus* species such as *E. faecalis* and *E. faecium* may be γ-non-haemolytic or haemolytic group D. These *Enterococcus* bacteria are part of the normal bowel commensals; however, they can cause disease in the form of root canal and urinary tract infections, endocarditis, bacteraemia and meningitis.

Genetics

Different isolates of *Strep. pyogenes* are now identified using *emm* typing [19] which has superseded the Lancefield group classification. More than 150 *emm* types have been characterised at the 5′ end locus (including the first 220 bases of the sequence) present on all *Strep. pyogenes* isolates; this region includes the M protein which is an important virulence factor. *Emm* amplicon restriction digest analysis has been shown to be a valuable tool for rapid analysis of streptococcal outbreaks.

Environmental factors

It is widely accepted that skin damage needs to precede cutaneous streptococcal pyoderma. On experimental application under occlusion to intact normal skin, several strains of *Strep. pyogenes* failed to cause disease and indeed rapidly died; localised superficial infection occurred only if the skin had been scarified [20]. For infection to occur, the streptococci need to adhere to the skin and at least 11 adhesins have been recognised including M protein, LTA and serum opacity factor, among others. Spread of streptococcal bacteria is facilitated by conditions of overcrowding, particularly in school dormitories and nursing homes. Contaminated foods have also led to outbreaks and there are reports of late-onset neonatal group B streptococcal sepsis resulting from streptococci in breast milk [21].

Investigations

The ASOT is an indicator of previous infection by streptococci of groups A, C or G. The upper limit of normal is 200 units/mL and highest titres range from 2000 to 3000 units/mL. In streptococcal skin infection, however, the ASO response is weak and an unreliable guide to diagnosis. Recent studies showed no correlation between the ASOT level and clinical severity of acute rheumatic fever including the extent of cardiac involvement [17]. Antibodies to deoxyribonuclease (DNase) B [22] and to hyaluronidase are more regularly raised in streptococcal skin disease. DNase B antibodies are probably specific for group A *Streptococcus*. One hyaluronidase antibody is specific for group A, and another for groups C and G jointly [23]. Susceptibility of neonates to group B streptococcal infection is related to the level of capsular type-specific antibodies in the maternal serum [24].

In some countries where streptococcal infection is common, the ASO titre may be persistently elevated so that raised titres may not be indicative of recent infection. More specific investigations may thus be required.

STAPHYLOCOCCAL AND STREPTOCOCCAL INFECTIONS

Staphylococci and streptococci produce infections by various routes, including direct invasion, by haematogenous spread of the organisms or by the toxins they produce (Boxes 26.1 and 26.2).

Clinical history

Skin infections with *Staph. aureus* are more common in patients with breaks in the skin such as scratches, wounds and ulcers, those who have other skin infections such as tinea pedis and herpesvirus or an underlying inflammatory skin disease such as atopic eczema. More than one family/group member may be affected either simultaneously or sequentially. Other risk factors to consider in the history include contact sports, travel abroad, contact with animals, previous history of MRSA, immunosuppression, men who have sex with men, health care workers, renal/liver disease, prosthetic implants and intravenous lines. In cutaneous infections with *Staph. aureus*, patients usually report the onset of a focal area of redness on the skin that may initially be asymptomatic; however, within days the affected skin usually becomes tender or even painful and may become associated with blistering, pustule/boil formation and eventually golden crusting and ulceration. Patients may variably feel otherwise well in themselves or may complain of fever, malaise, cough, diarrhoea, etc., depending on the strain of *Staph. aureus* implicated and the specific tissue sites infected.

Skin infections related to streptococcal species are prevalent globally with a higher incidence of pyoderma infections in the tropics. Group A *Streptococcus* is highly transmissible, passing from person to person through direct skin contact, respiratory droplets and nasal discharge. Streptococci residing in the perianal skin and under fingernails are more frequently spread in conditions of overcrowding and poor hygiene. There is usually a history of skin trauma, abrasion, wounds or underlying skin disease for *Strep. pyogenes* to cause a cutaneous infection. Impetigo secondary to streptococci passes between family members and children at school, leading to clustering of cases. Erysipelas and cellulitis usually start from a small break in the skin from an insect bite reaction, a minor scratch, wound, tinea pedis or xerotic cracked skin. Necrotising fasciitis can also result from minor skin trauma but may also follow any surgical intervention. The initial skin changes are usually manifested by acute redness with a papule which may develop into blistering, pustules and oedema. Depending on the type of cutaneous infection there may be some tenderness and pain.

Staphylococcus and *Streptococcus* in atopic eczema. *Staph. aureus* is frequently isolated from lesional and non-lesional skin of patients with atopic eczema (Chapter 41) and is widely accepted as having a pathogenic role [1]. Secondary colonisation and carriage rates are high for both *Staphylococcus* and *Streptococcus* in atopic eczema. Staphylococci have been shown to adhere more readily to the skin of atopic individuals, even on non-lesional skin, compared with non-atopic individuals. There is also evidence that high bacterial density (over $10^6/cm^2$) on lesions, which may be insufficient to produce overt signs of clinical infection, nonetheless significantly aggravates the eczema [2]. In a recent study of children with clinically infected atopic eczema, 72% had a significant growth of *Staph. aureus*, 16% streptococcal species and 14% had mixed cultures [3]. Atopic eczema patients infected with *Strep. pyogenes* were more likely to be pyrexial, have facial involvement, cellulitis, bacteraemia and be hospitalised [3]. Following systemic antibiotic treatment for infective episodes of atopic eczema, skin swabs show decreased levels of *Staph. aureus* and *Strep. pyogenes* but increased levels of *Strep. epidermidis*, *Cutibacterium* and *Corynebacterium* species [4]. In true infective eczema, bacteria, including *Staph. aureus*, are regarded as the primary stimulus for an eczematous response, although the mechanisms are uncertain. Cytotoxic antibody and immunoglobulin E (IgE) reactions against bacterial (including *Staph. aureus*) antigens may be important in atopic and discoid eczema [5]. *Staph. aureus* was isolated from 14 of 20 children with infantile seborrhoeic dermatitis, but its pathogenicity was uncertain [6].

The staphylococci produce exotoxins with superantigenic properties, which cause T-cell activation, cytokine release and mast cell degranulation [1,7]. Superantigens trigger Langerhans cell migration into regional lymph nodes, where they interact with T cells, which recirculate into the skin, causing augmentation of the skin immune response. These superantigens are thought to negate the effects of topical steroids. This may in part explain why treating the infection and the atopic eczema simultaneously is more effective than treating either in isolation [1].

In atopic eczema, there also seems to be a reduction in the level of antimicrobial peptides which lyse the outer membrane of microbes. This in turn leads to a reduction in innate immunity and diminishes the ability of atopic individuals to react to the staphylococcal load. Whether this is a genetic abnormality or secondary to other factors remains to be determined [1]. Atopic eczema is characterised by a complex of immunological abnormalities, involving interactions between IgE-bearing antigen-presenting cells, T-cell activation, mast cell degranulation and a combination of immediate and cellular immune responses [8]. Following exposure, T and dendritic cells are recruited to the area, and induce inflammation. One of the chemokines expressed is CC chemokine ligand 18. This was shown to be relevant in the recruitment of the pro-inflammatory cells [9].

Impetigo

Definition
Impetigo is a contagious, superficial pyogenic infection of the skin. Two main clinical forms are recognised: non-bullous and bullous impetigo.

Introduction and general description
Impetigo is a common superficial skin infection resulting mainly from staphylococcal and, less frequently, streptococcal infections that may occur in isolation or secondary to any kind of underlying skin disease or breach in the epidermis.

Epidemiology
Incidence and prevalence
Pure staphylococcal non-bullous impetigo [1,2] is relatively frequent worldwide and large outbreaks often occur. The peak seasonal incidence is in late summer [3]. The incidence in a Dutch survey was between 0.017 and 0.021 and in the UK 0.01 events per person-year [1,2]. Preschool and young school-age children are most often affected. In adults, males predominate and large outbreaks may be troublesome in barracks and similar communities [4]. Although overcrowding, poor hygiene and existing skin disease, especially scabies, predispose to infection [5], many cases occur in previously healthy subjects with good living standards.

Bullous impetigo is usually sporadic, but clusters of cases may occur in families and other groups, and larger outbreaks are occasionally seen in institutions [6]. It is most frequent in the summer months. Minor abrasions and other skin lesions may predispose to infection if the patient or a contact carries an appropriate strain of *Staphylococcus* [7]. An increased incidence in hospital workers has been noted [8].

Age
Impetigo is most common in children. Bullous impetigo occurs at all ages; although it is more commonly reported in children it is thought adult cases are probably underreported [9]. In the newborn, bullous impetigo may be especially widespread and was formerly called pemphigus neonatorum, as it resembles the clinical picture of pemphigus, with widespread blistering.

Sex
Males and females are equally affected by impetigo.

Associated diseases
Infective complications are uncommon in the absence of systemic disease or malnutrition, although deeper infections such as cellulitis occasionally occur with streptococcal infection [10]. Streptococcal impetigo accounts for the majority of cases of poststreptococcal acute glomerulonephritis [11]. The incidence of acute glomerulonephritis in different series of patients with streptococcal impetigo depends on the nephritogenic potential of the infecting strain. Some never induce nephritis [3], but 25% of patients with pyoderma due to *Strep. pyogenes*, type M-49, are affected. The overall incidence of poststreptococcal acute glomerulonephritis has declined in recent decades. The latent period for development of nephritis after streptococcal pyoderma is 18–21 days, compared with about 10 days for throat infection, raising the unproven possibility that early treatment of skin infection might offer a better chance of preventing renal disease. Poststreptococcal nephritis is a significant risk factor for chronic renal disease in later life [12]. Scarlet fever, urticaria and erythema multiforme may follow streptococcal impetigo [13]. Rheumatic fever is not a complication of streptococcal impetigo [14].

Pathophysiology
Predisposing factors
Non-bullous impetigo may be caused by both *Staph. aureus* and streptococcal bacteria [15], but recent evidence suggests in most parts of the world *Staph. aureus* is usually implicated, with *Strep. pyogenes* mainly predominating in warmer climates. However, there are occasional infections with group G and group C organisms [16]. Often there may be a mixed picture with reports of impetigo being primarily caused by *Strep. pyogenes* with *Staph. aureus* a secondary coloniser. The preponderance of group II phage types seen in bullous impetigo seems also to apply to the non-bullous staphylococcal disease [17].

Bullous impetigo is a superficial cutaneous infection with *Staph. aureus*. The organism can generally be cultured from blister fluid. Injections of bacterial isolates from affected patients into newborn mice result in a generalised SSSS [18]. Exfoliative (epidermolytic) toxin has been recovered from the blister fluid of some cases and is thought to act as a trypsin-like serine protease and cleave desmoglein 1 [19] to form the blister. The toxin is produced commonly, but not exclusively, by staphylococci of phage group II. In addition, both exfoliative toxins A and B act as superantigens, and stimulate B and T cells to proliferate [20]. The localisation of the epidermal splitting in bullous impetigo compared with the widespread involvement in the generalised form is probably related to local production of the toxin, whereas in SSSS the toxin is disseminated haematogenously [21].

Pathology
In bullous impetigo, the *Staphylococcus* strain responsible synthesises an exfoliative toxin (ET) that selectively digests one of the intracellular adhesion molecules, desmoglein 1, resulting in superficial blisters [13,22]. Staphylococcal strains most commonly produce either ETA (encoded on a phage genome) or ETB (encoded on a large plasmid). ETA strains are frequently associated with bullous impetigo and ETB with SSSS. More recently, ETC has been identified from a horse with a skin infection and ETD from patients with localised staphylococcal skin infections. ETD is thought to be an important virulence factor in epithelial disruption allowing local invasion of the skin. Histology from bullous impetigo classically

demonstrates an epidermal split just below the stratum granulosum, neutrophils migrating through a spongiotic epidermis into the blister cavity, which may also contain cocci (seen on special stains). Occasional acantholytic cells may be seen, perhaps due to the action of neutrophils. The upper dermis contains an inflammatory infiltrate of neutrophils and lymphocytes.

Causative organisms
- *Staph. aureus.*
- *Strep. pyogenes.*

Clinical features
Presentation
In non-bullous impetigo, the initial lesion is a very thin-walled vesicle on a red base [16]. The vesicle ruptures so rapidly that it is seldom seen as such [17]. The exuding serum dries to form yellowish brown crusts (Figure 26.1), which are usually thicker and 'dirtier' in the streptococcal form (Figure 26.2). Gradual irregular peripheral extension occurs without central healing, and multiple lesions, which are usually present, may coalesce. The crusts eventually dry and separate to leave redness in less pigmented skin and grey, brown or purple discoloration in skin with darker pigmentation, which fades without scarring [23]. In severe cases, there may be regional adenitis with fever and other constitutional symptoms. The face especially around the nose and mouth and the limbs are the sites most commonly affected, but involvement of the scalp is frequent in tinea capitis, and lesions may occur anywhere on the body, especially in children with atopic eczema or scabies. Involvement of the mucous membranes is rare. There is a tendency to spontaneous cure in 2–3 weeks but a prolonged course is common, particularly in the presence of underlying ectoparasitic infestations or eczema, or in hot and humid climates. In heavily pigmented skin, the lesions may be followed by temporary hypopigmentation or hyperpigmentation.

In bullous impetigo, the bullae are less rapidly ruptured and become much larger; a diameter of 1–2 cm is common but they

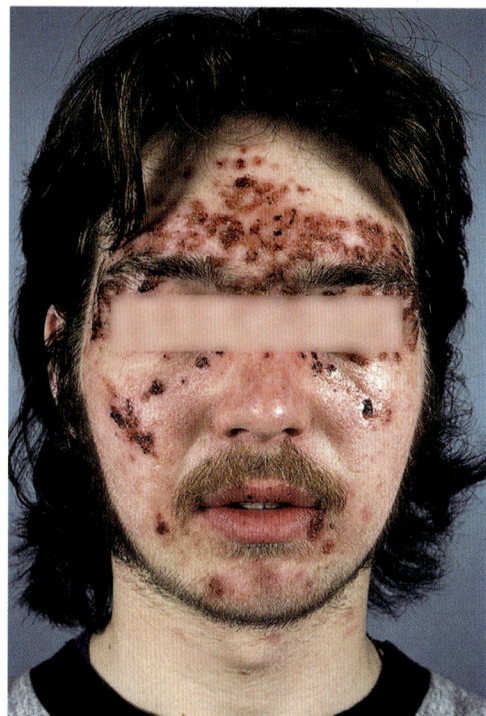

Figure 26.2 Streptococcal (group A) pyoderma.

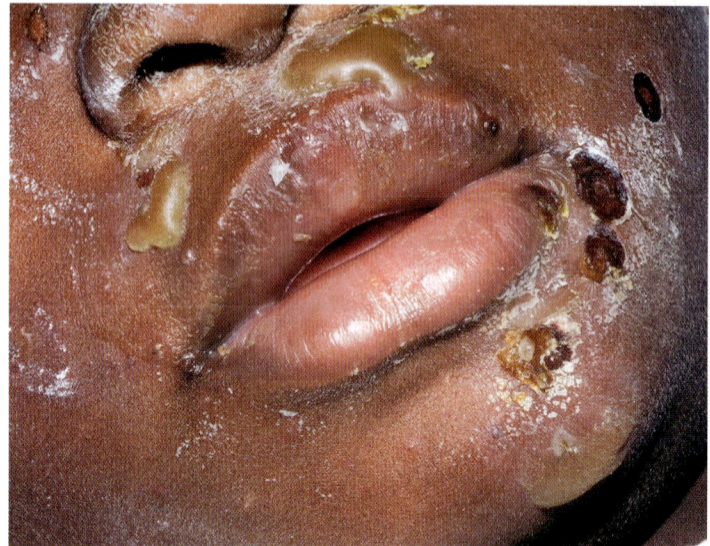

Figure 26.3 Bullous impetigo. Courtesy of King's College London.

may be of very considerable size, and persist for 2 or 3 days (Figure 26.3). The contents are at first clear, later cloudy. After rupture thin, flat, brownish crusts are formed. Central healing and peripheral extension may give rise to circinate lesions which are eroded (Figure 26.4). Although the face is often affected, the lesions may occur anywhere, and may be widely and irregularly distributed, often favouring the sites of existing skin disease, especially miliaria or trivial injuries such as insect bites. The buccal mucous membrane may be involved. Commonly, rather few lesions are present, but the picture is very variable. Regional adenitis is rare.

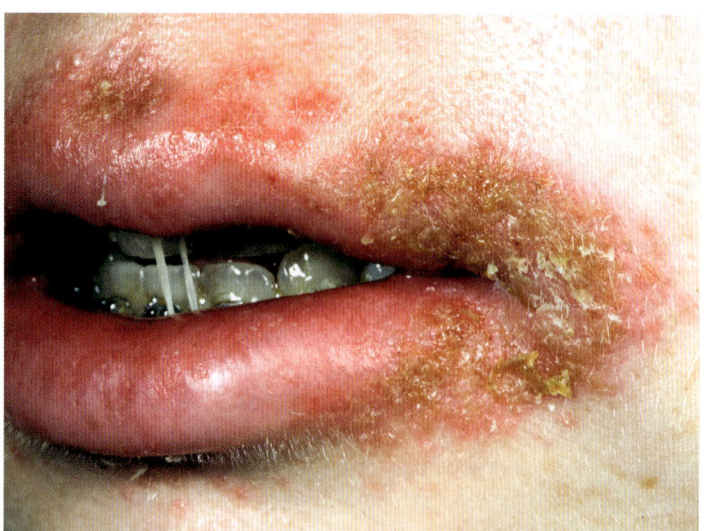

Figure 26.1 Staphylococcal impetigo. Courtesy of King's College London.

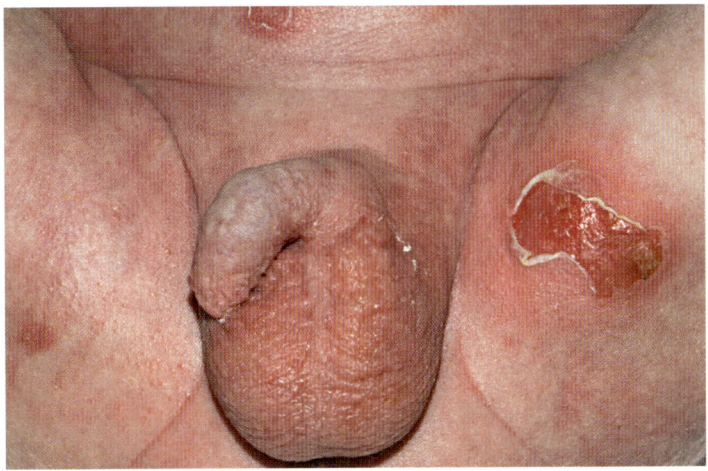

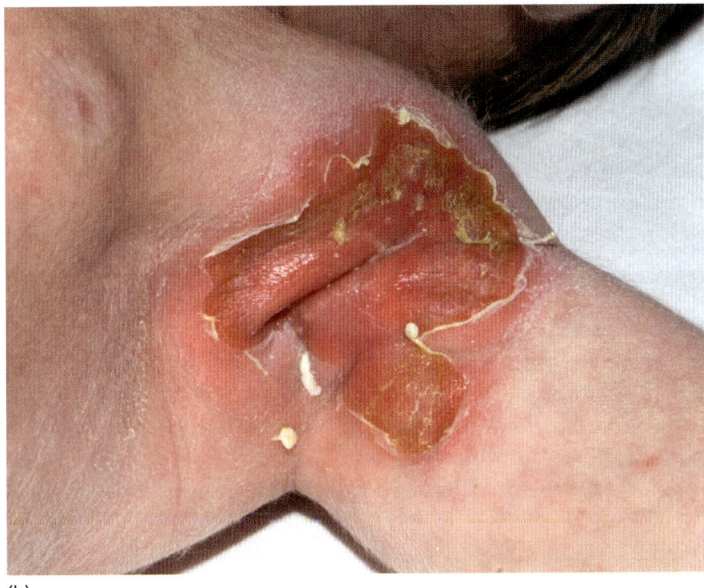

Figure 26.4 (a,b) Erosive bullous impetigo in a neonate. Courtesy of King's College London.

Clinical variants
Bullous and non-bullous impetigo.

Differential diagnosis
Immunobullous diseases, localised SSSS, contact dermatitis (irritant or allergic) and herpes simplex infections.

Disease course and prognosis
Impetigo is usually self-limiting and resolves within days to weeks with the appropriate use of topical cleansers and antibiotics. Spread to others in close contact with the index case is common and relapse is more frequently seen in individuals with underlying skin diseases and in staphylococcal carriers.

Investigations
Microbiological skin swabs taken from affected skin.

Management
A recent Cochrane review concludes that there is no generally accepted standard therapy for the treatment of impetigo [24]. Studies failed to demonstrate any significant difference in outcomes between topical fusidic acid and mupirocin, although some studies found topical mupirocin superior to oral erythromycin. Topical antibiotics were superior to disinfectants alone, although the latter can be a useful adjuvant. There was no superior outcome when comparing topical versus oral antibiotics; however, there was evidence that not all oral antibiotics are equally effective. Penicillin was inferior to erythromycin and cloxacillin. Newer topical antibiotics such as retapamulin and ozenoxacin have been shown to be effective in treating impetigo. However, they are expensive and the former is no longer licensed in Europe [25]. If the infection is widespread or severe, or is accompanied by lymphadenopathy, then an oral antibiotic such as flucloxacillin or erythromycin is indicated [26]. Local patterns of resistance need to be considered, as resistance of *Staph. aureus* to penicillin is now common worldwide. The addition of a topical antibiotic or antiseptic may hasten the response and help to limit the spread of infection, although this has not been confirmed [27]. Antiseptics would be a rational sole therapy for impetigo where antibiotics are unavailable. Chlorhexidine and povidone–iodine would each be suitable, but controlled trials on their efficacy are not available. Removal of infected crusts is bacteriologically and cosmetically helpful. Frequent application of an ointment, preferably containing an antibacterial agent, and washing with soap and water are beneficial.

Where impetigo is endemic among children, measures to reduce the transmission frequency of infections should be adopted. These include installing indoor water supplies, encouraging hand washing, distributing medical resources more efficiently, health education and instituting treatment early in the course of the disease. When hand washing was promoted, the prevalence of impetigo dropped significantly [28]. Emphasis should be placed on identification of predisposing factors such as insect bites, pediculosis, scabies and minor trauma.

A summary of the management of impetigo is given in Figure 26.5.

Wash the affected skin daily with disinfectants such as chlorhexidine, povidone–iodine or sodium hypochlorite. All close contacts and the patient should wash their hands with antibacterial soap to reduce onward transmission. Topical antibiotic should be applied twice daily to the affected skin for 5–7 days, the most effective of which include mupirocin, fusidic acid and 2% clindamycin cream. If the impetigo is extensive, or there is a marked bullous component to the clinical picture or there is palpable lymphadenopathy, then in addition give systemic antibiotics for 1 week. The choice of antibiotic will depend on local resistance patterns and any known antibiotic hypersensitivities of the patient. First line antibiotics include antistaphylococcal penicillins (e.g. flucloxacillin, dicloxacillin, cloxacillin), co-amoxiclav, clindamycin and doxycycline. Second line antibiotics include macrolides such as erythromycin and clarithromycin (macrolide resistance can be quite high in *Staph. aureus*) and co-trimoxazole (high resistance rates in *Strep. pyogenes*). Third line antibiotics include linezolid and fluoroquinolones.

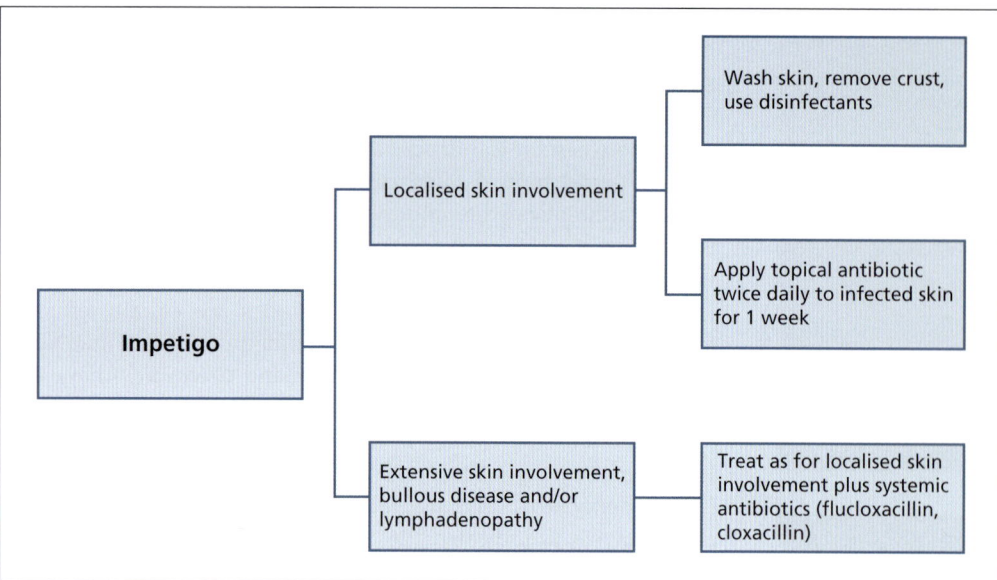

Figure 26.5 Management of impetigo.

Ecthyma

Definition
Ecthyma is a pyogenic infection of the skin characterised by the formation of adherent crusts, beneath which ulceration occurs. Ecthyma most commonly results from group A *Streptococcus* and causes a deeper infection than in impetigo.

Epidemiology
See earlier section on *Staph. aureus* and *Strep. pyogenes*.

Age
Extremes of age are most commonly affected.

Pathophysiology
Predisposing factors
Group A *Streptococcus* may lead to ecthyma on normal skin or may opportunistically penetrate through damaged skin (trauma or underlying dermatitis) and more commonly affects vulnerable patients with immunocompromise (HIV, neutropenia) or diabetes, and outbreaks in the military are reported [1]. It also more frequently occurs in high-humidity environments and in the context of poor hygiene. Pharyngeal carriers of *Strep. pyogenes* are also more susceptible to recurrent disease.

Pathology
The infection and resultant inflammation are much deeper in ecthyma than in impetigo and thus there is loss of the epidermis and dermis leading to ulceration and the lesions heal with scarring.

Causative organisms
- *Strep. pyogenes* (group A *Streptococcus*).
- *P. aeruginosa*.
- *Staph. aureus*.

Environmental factors
Warm moist environments and overcrowding are predisposing factors leading to higher rates of ecthyma infection.

Clinical features
Presentation
Small bullae or pustules on a red base are soon surmounted by a hard crust of dried exudate (Figure 26.6), which increases in size by peripheral accretion, with an indurated base. The crust is thicker than that formed in impetigo and is only removed with difficulty, to reveal a purulent, irregular ulcer [2]. The lesions are usually few but new lesions may develop by autoinoculation over a long period. The buttocks, thighs and legs are most commonly affected.

Differential diagnosis
- Pyoderma gangrenosum.
- Ecthyma gangrenosum.
- Tick bites.

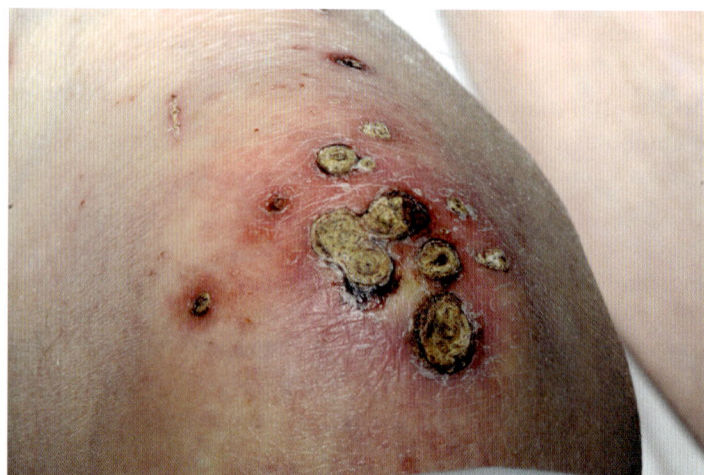

Figure 26.6 Ecthyma. Courtesy of King's College London.

Complications and co-morbidities
Autoinoculation may occur causing increased numbers of skin lesions.

Disease course and prognosis
Healing usually occurs after a few weeks with scarring.

Investigations
Microbiological swabs should be taken from affected skin.

Management
Improved hygiene and nutrition, and treatment of scabies and any other underlying diseases, are important. The antibiotic chosen should be active against *Strep. pyogenes* and *Staph. aureus*. If *P. aeruginosa* is suspected a second antibiotic agent should be added (oral fluoroquinolone) or an intravenous agent with a broad spectrum of activity. Necrotic infected adherent crust should be gently removed after soaking with a disinfectant and softening with an oily cream. Topical antibiotics such as fusidic acid and mupirocin can be applied twice daily to localised lesions. Topical therapy either with sulconazole or miconazole cleared lesions satisfactorily over 1 week [3]. Oral antibiotics for 1–2 weeks may be required in the context of multiple lesions or immunocompromised vulnerable patients. Penicillin-derived agents can be used. If staphylococcal bacteria are suspected to be implicated then erythromycin, clindamycin and doxycycline may also be used. If ecthyma gangrenosum is suspected then piperacillin, gentamicin, amikacin, ciprofloxacin and ofloxacin can be administered intravenously.

Treatment ladder for ecthyma

First line
- Topical fusidic acid
- Topical mupirocin
- Oral flucloxacillin

Second line
- Topical sulconazole
- Topical miconazole
- Oral clindamycin
- Oral doxycycline
- Oral erythromycin/clarithromycin
- Oral linezolid

Third line (with anti-pseudomonal activity)
- Piperacillin/tazobactam IV
- Ciprofloxacin/ofloxacin IV
- Gentamicin IV
- Amikacin IV

Cellulitis and erysipelas

Definition
Cellulitis is strictly an acute, subacute or chronic inflammation of loose connective tissue. Erysipelas is a bacterial infection of the dermis and upper subcutaneous tissue; its hallmark is a well-defined raised edge reflecting the more superficial (dermal) involvement. However, cellulitis may extend superficially and erysipelas deeply, so that in many cases the two processes coexist and it is impossible to make a meaningful distinction. Current usage tends to regard erysipelas as a form of cellulitis rather than a distinct entity, so that the definition of cellulitis would include inflammation of dermal as well as subcutaneous tissue. The closely similar bacteriology of the two conditions [1,2], and the demonstration of streptococcal antigens in both dermis and subcutis in both conditions [1], support this view. However, the two terms are still sometimes used in the traditional sense, especially when their typical distinctive features are being contrasted.

Introduction and general description
Painful diffuse inflammatory skin infection in the deep skin layers and the subcutaneous fat usually affecting a lower limb or the face.

Epidemiology
Incidence and prevalence
Cellulitis is common: lower-limb cellulitis accounted for over 55 000 hospital admissions in one year in England and is responsible for around 3% of emergency department attendances [3].

Age
Patients most affected are between the fourth and sixth decades.

Sex
Males and females are equally affected by cellulitis [3].

Ethnicity
In a UK-based study, white ethnicity patients were at higher risk of developing cellulitis than patients from other ethnic groups [4].

Associated diseases
Associated diseases and complications can occur if cellulitis/erysipelas is inadequately treated, leading to fasciitis, myositis, subcutaneous abscesses, septicaemia and, in some streptococcal cases, nephritis – and the more severe infections may be fatal, especially in infants and in the debilitated or immunosuppressed.

Childhood facial cellulitis due to *Haemophilus influenzae* type b is typically unilateral, and often associated with ipsilateral otitis media, the presumed source in those cases. The patient presents with systemic illness, and the affected cheek or periorbital tissue shows induration and discoloration which is characteristically purplish blue [5,6]. With the introduction of *H. influenzae* type b vaccination, this condition is becoming increasingly rare.

Otherwise, periorbital (preseptal) cellulitis follows trauma to the eyelids or local skin sepsis and is usually streptococcal, occasionally staphylococcal. If the infection is behind the orbital septum (postseptal), in the deeper orbital tissues, the term orbital cellulitis applies, and it is commonly a sequel to sinusitis. In addition to cutaneous signs, proptosis, ophthalmoplegia and loss of visual acuity may occur. Periorbital and orbital cellulitis may be complicated by cavernous sinus thrombosis, orbital, subperiosteal or cerebral abscess formation, or meningitis [7,8].

Severe myocardial depression has been reported in a previously healthy young woman with streptococcal cellulitis [9].

Cellulitis of the tongue in neutropenic patients may cause upper airways obstruction [10]. In the immunodeficient, the presentation may be atypical, as in two cases of erysipelas without redness [11], and previous antibiotic treatment may modify the clinical appearances in the otherwise healthy patient. Recurrent streptococcal cellulitis (or erysipelas) is attributed to lymphatic damage, which, although sometimes initially clinically inapparent, predisposes to further infection and further lymphatic impairment manifesting as lymphoedema (see Figure 26.9). Venous insufficiency often predisposes to recurrent erysipelas of the leg [12]; however, equally in the context of dermatosclerosis an acute inflammatory phase (hypodermitis) can be misdiagnosed as erysipelas [13].

Pathophysiology
Predisposing factors
Bacteria are present in affected tissue in small numbers, and attempts to culture them, from biopsy material, from swabs of biopsy sites, from needle aspiration of saline-injected tissue, and even from fluid from blisters or erosions when present, are often unsuccessful. Blood cultures and swabs from possible entry sites, for example wounds or inflammatory lesions, generally situated distally to the infection, occasionally yield presumably relevant organisms. Cultures of biopsy specimens, needle aspirates and probable sites of entry fail to provide positive results in the majority of cases. Streptococcal serology may be helpful retrospectively [2], and immunofluorescence may identify streptococcal group antigens in biopsy specimens [1].

Pathology
In cellulitis there is marked oedema, dilated superficial capillaries and extravasation of red blood cells in the dermis with scattered inflammatory cells, mainly neutrophils and lymphocytes.

Causative organisms
Cellulitis and erysipelas in the immunocompetent patient are predominantly streptococcal diseases, usually involving group A *Streptococcus*. Group B *Streptococcus* is seen especially under the age of 3 months [14]. In adults, group B streptococci may cause pelvic erysipelas especially after surgery [15]. In cellulitis, *Staph. aureus* is occasionally implicated alone or together with a *Streptococcus*. *Staph. aureus* should be regarded as an occasional cause of cellulitis, but rarely if at all of classical erysipelas.

H. influenzae type b is an important cause of facial cellulitis in young children especially up to the age of 2 years [5,6]; however, this is now increasingly rare due to vaccination in infancy against *H. influenzae* and *Pneumococcus*. *H. influenzae* cellulitis is rare in adults [16].

In cellulitis in a setting of venous or lymphatic compromise, including limbs on which saphenous venectomy has been performed, or following surgery to the breast, non-group-A streptococci, especially groups B and G, predominate. Periorbital cellulitis is similar to that in other sites; however, orbital cellulitis, usually secondary to sinusitis, involves the major sinus pathogens such as *Streptococcus pneumoniae*, other streptococci, *Staph. aureus*, *H. influenzae* and penicillin-sensitive anaerobes [2]. Cellulitis due to *Aeromonas hydrophila* can complicate injuries contaminated by water (usually fresh) or soil [17]. A case of cellulitis due to the marine organism *Vibrio alginolyticus* has been recorded [18]. Cellulitis is part of the spectrum of infection due to *Pasteurella multocida* inoculated by animal bites [19]. Erysipelas-like infections and cellulitis due to *Strep. pneumoniae* [20,21], *P. aeruginosa* [22] and *Campylobacter jejuni* [23] have been reported, mostly in the immunocompromised. In such patients, *P. aeruginosa* may cause gangrenous cellulitis and ecthyma gangrenosum [24]; and cellulitis may be caused by *Acinetobacter calcoaceticus* [25] and *Strep. epidermidis* [26]. A case of *Bacteroides fragilis* cellulitis responding to metronidazole has been reported [27]. *Yersinia enterocolitica*, an intestinal pathogen, may also cause cellulitis [28]. The fish pathogen, *Streptococcus iniae*, has also led to cases of cellulitis following minor injuries while handling fish [29].

Clinical features
Presentation (Figure 26.7)
Colour change (purple or darkening of the skin in more pigmented skin types or redness in less pigmented skin), heat, swelling and pain or tenderness are constant features. In erysipelas the edge of the lesion is well demarcated and raised, but in cellulitis it is diffuse, although cases showing both types of edge or an intermediate picture are not uncommon. In erysipelas blistering is common, and there may be superficial haemorrhage into the blisters or in intact skin especially in elderly people. Severe cellulitis may show bullae (Figure 26.7b) and can progress to dermal necrosis (Figure 26.8), and uncommonly to fasciitis or myositis. Lymphangitis and lymphadenopathy are frequent. Except in mild cases, there is constitutional upset with fever and malaise. Classical erysipelas starts abruptly and systemic symptoms may be acute and severe, but the response to treatment is more rapid.

The leg is the commonest site, and here there is usually a wound even if superficial, an ulcer, or an inflammatory lesion including tinea pedis or bacterial infection, which can be identified as a possible portal of entry. The next most frequent site for classical streptococcal erysipelas is the face (Figure 26.7c, d), where a traumatic entry site is less commonly seen, and where bilateral infection occasionally occurs.

Differential diagnosis
- Necrotising fasciitis.
- Venous insufficiency of the lower leg.
- Acute contact dermatitis.

Complications and co-morbidities
Recurrent episodes may lead to lymphatic damage leading to chronic lymphoedema (Figure 26.9) of the affected site. Rarely necrotising fasciitis may develop.

Disease course and prognosis
Usually the disease settles over 1–2 weeks with appropriate systemic antibiotics. However, recurrence can occur and some patients required secondary preventative prophylaxis with a daily dose of penicillin V (500 mg daily).

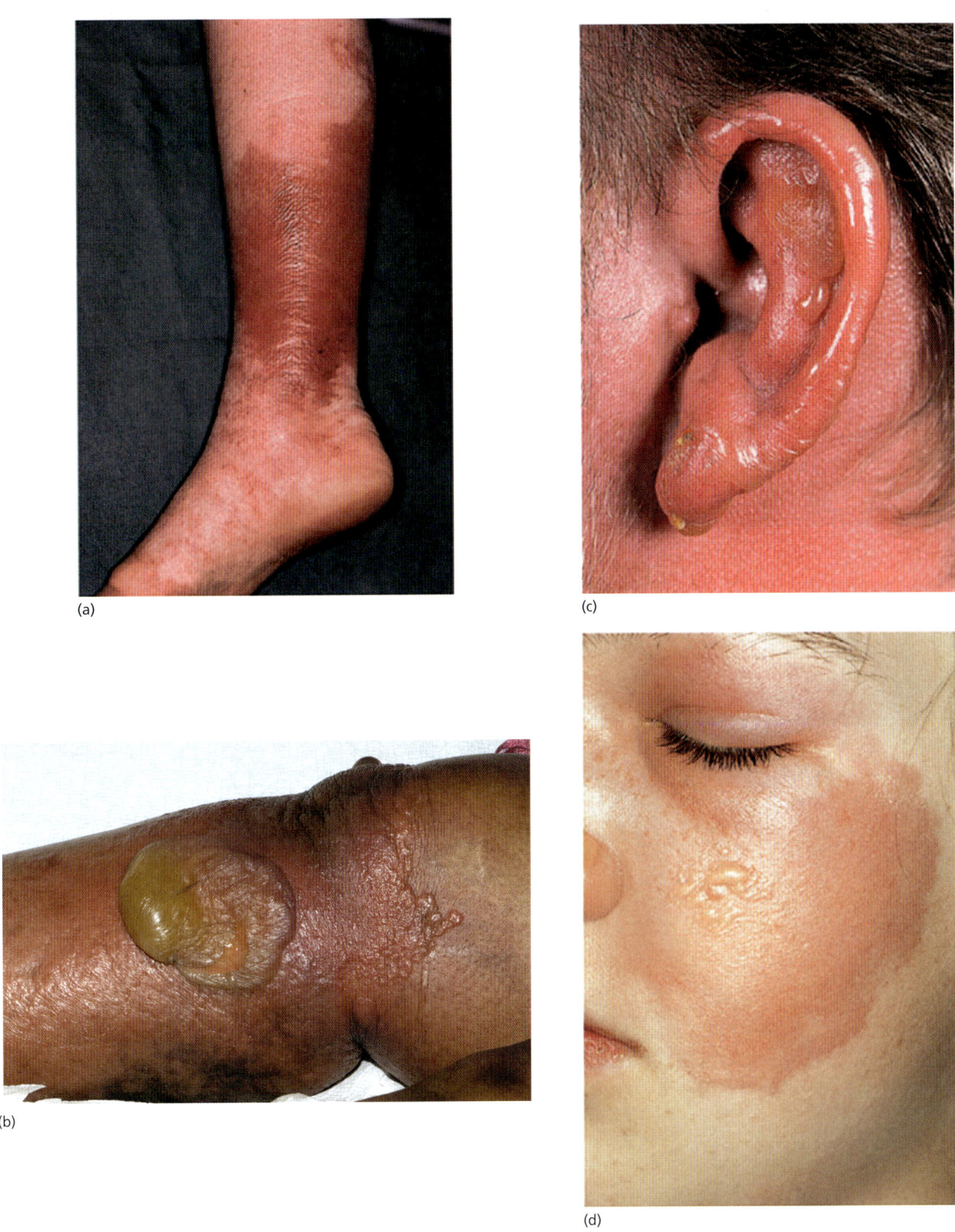

Figure 26.7 Cellulitis/erysipelas. (a) Lower leg. (b) Bullous cellulitis of the leg. Courtesy of King's College London. (c) Pinna. (d) Face.

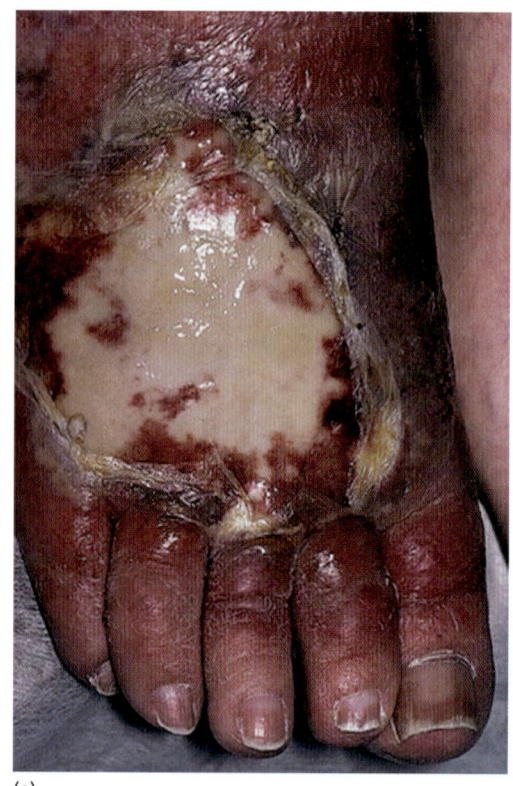
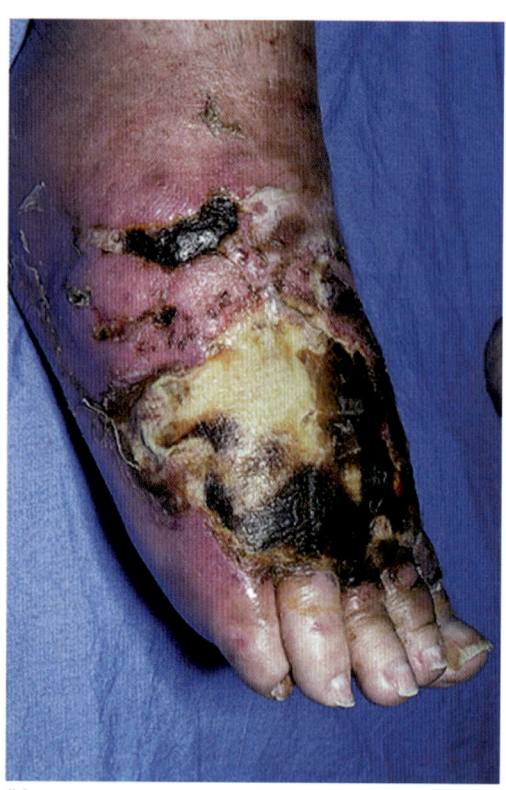

(a) (b)

Figure 26.8 (a) Cellulitis with early dermal necrosis. (b) The same foot after 11 days; the dermis is forming a black eschar, which eventually sloughed off; the resulting ulcer healed rapidly.

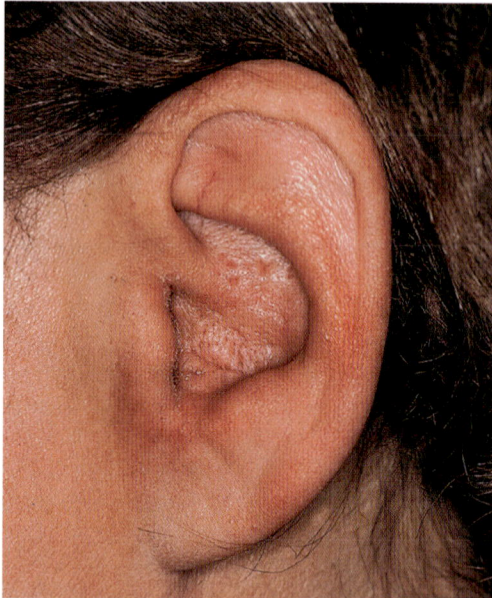

Figure 26.9 Poststreptococcal lymphoedema of the pinna; this patient had frequent recurrences of cellulitis requiring long-term penicillin.

Investigations

Specimens for bacteriological examination can be taken from vesicle fluid or eroded or ulcerated surfaces, in addition to blood cultures. Exudative, fissured or traumatised sites distal or adjacent to limb infections may yield relevant organisms. Surface swabs from intact skin are unlikely to be helpful, but in the case of facial infections the pathogen should be sought in nose, throat, conjunctiva and sinuses. Identification of soluble streptococcal antigens may be effective, but is rarely performed in the clinical setting [1]. However, even a combination of sampling techniques commonly fails to yield the pathogen [1,2].

Serological studies may provide evidence of streptococcal, and less commonly staphylococcal, infection. An initial high titre may be regarded as suggestive, especially in a patient presenting several days or more after the onset, but paired sera from days 1 and 14 would be more reliable in retrospective diagnosis. Early use of antibiotics may, however, limit the antibody response. The antibodies and their significance are discussed later.

Differentiating cellulitis of the leg from deep vein thrombosis is important and Doppler ultrasound examination, venous angiography and plethysmography may add diagnosis.

Management

A clinical assessment as to the likely pathogen(s), as discussed earlier, should guide the initial choice of treatment. Appropriate antibiotic(s) should be given in full dosage, by the intramuscular or intravenous route in the more severe cases that are associated with septicaemia, arthritis or suspected fasciitis, although oral treatment may suffice for milder, uncomplicated infections [30]. In all cases, initial treatment should cover streptococci, and for facial infections in young children, *H. influenzae*.

First line

Anti-staphylococcal penicillins exert a bactericidal effect on streptococci as well as staphylococci, and for this reason have been suggested as oral monotherapy in adults without systemic toxicity or co-morbidity. Flucloxacillin at a dose of 500 mg–1 g four times daily; clarithromycin 500 mg twice daily may be substituted in case of penicillin allergy. In patients admitted to hospital, flucloxacillin 1 g four times daily intravenously, increased to 2 g in severe disease or in patients weighing >90 kg or cefazolin 1–2 g 8-hourly intravenously; in the case of penicillin allergy, ceftriaxone 2 g daily intravenously (non-severe allergy) or clindamycin 450 mg 8-hourly intravenously (severe allergy) has been advocated. For presumed streptococcal infections, penicillin is the treatment of choice, given as benzylpenicillin 600–1200 mg 6-hourly intravenously in the more severe cases. In peri-orbital cellulitis co-amoxiclav 1.2 g 8-hourly intravenously is suggested; substituted by ceftriaxone 2 g daily intravenously in non-severe penicillin allergy or clarithromycin 500 mg twice daily in severe allergy. The duration of treatment remains undefined. A randomised double-blind placebo-controlled trial for uncomplicated cellulitis showed that 5 days of antibiotic therapy was as good as 10 days of treatment [31]. Treatment should be continued for longer if there are any clinical indications such as extension of the cellulitis, abscess formation which may need drainage or an adverse reaction to the drug administered. Peri-orbital cellulitis may also require longer courses. Co-trimoxazole, linezolid, vancomycin and other agents are likely to be effective alternatives [32].

Anticoagulant therapy should be considered if there is associated thrombophlebitis or reduced mobility. A wider range of organisms should be considered in patients with deficient immunity, in the special situations discussed earlier and in those not responding to initial treatment. Early consultation with colleagues in microbiology is advisable.

PATCH study II showed that patients given penicillin 250 mg twice daily for 6 months following a single episode of cellulitis had fewer episodes of recurrent cellulitis during the following 3 years [33].

Second line

In recurrent cases of cellulitis, long-term phenoxymethyl penicillin (penicillin V), 500 mg to 2 g daily, can prevent recurrent attacks and is cost-effective; however, if the secondary penicillin prophylaxis is then stopped within 1 year any protective effect from recurrent episodes is lost [33]. Vigorous treatment of any local skin damage is important to prevent recurrent disease, although 50% of cases relapsed in a study on prophylaxis where tinea pedis was specifically treated early. In patients allergic to penicillin, an alternative drug, commonly erythromycin, should be taken. Some patients may require lifelong prophylaxis. Recurrent episodes of cellulitis have also been associated with post-cellulitic oedema, and oedema is a risk factor for recurrent disease. Reduction of the oedema is likely to be beneficial [34]. Despite efforts to prevent recurrent disease with long-term prophylaxis, many patients still suffer recurrent disease [35,36].

Treatment ladder for cellulitis/erysipelas

First line
- Flucloxacillin
- Clarythromycin
- Clindamycin
- Benzylpenicillin (if streptococcal infection only)

Second line
- Co-trimoxazole
- Linezolid
- Vancomycin

Prophylactic treatment for recurrent infection
- Penicillin
- Erythromycin

Folliculitis

Definition

Folliculitis refers to inflammation of the hair follicles; this may be caused by infection, occlusion, irritation, drugs or alterations in immune function.

Introduction and general description

Staph. aureus, coagulase-negative staphylococci and physical or chemical irritation are common causes of superficial folliculitis.

Epidemiology

Incidence and prevalence

Folliculitis is very common, but the exact incidence is not known as most patients do not seek medical attention.

Age

Superficial *Staph. aureus* folliculitis can be seen in any age group. Adult males are most commonly affected by folliculitis in the beard area.

Pathophysiology

Predisposing factors

Staph. aureus superficial folliculitis (follicular impetigo of Bockhart) is an infection of the follicular ostium; however, superficial folliculitis is not always primarily or exclusively infective in origin. Physical or chemical injury to the skin may be associated with a folliculitis, the pustules of which may be sterile or may contain coagulase-negative staphylococci (as part of the skin flora). Occupational contact with mineral oils or therapeutic or occupational exposure to tar products often results in folliculitic lesions, which in the case of oil folliculitis are associated with conspicuous oil plugging of many follicles. Other chemical irritants can cause folliculitis, which may be the only visible change, or may accompany an eczematous reaction. Beneath adhesive plasters or adhesive dressings, a sterile folliculitis is common. Following epilation, a traumatic folliculitis may develop [1].

Causative organisms
- *Staph. aureus*, including community-acquired meticillin-resistant *Staph. aureus* (CA-MRSA).
- Coagulase-negative staphylococci.
- *P. aeruginosa*.
- *Pityrosporum* yeast and occasionally dermatophytes.

Clinical features
Presentation
Isolated intermittent follicular lesions are so frequent on the neck and beard, and heal so rapidly, that they are commonly ignored. Also frequent, but more persistent, are papules or pustules on the thighs and buttocks of adolescent and young adult males and occasionally females, especially those with acne. Clinically, the lesions present as small, follicular papules or pinhead pustules. They are rarely painful but can be pruritic. Sometimes, small crusts cover a red, pouting, follicular orifice. In *Staph. aureus* superficial folliculitis the individual lesions are domed yellow pustules, sometimes with a narrow red areola. The pustules develop in crops (Figure 26.10) and may heal within 7–10 days, but sometimes become chronic. In older children and adults, the infection may extend more deeply in some follicles as furuncles or as sycosis. In some cases, recurrent or chronic staphylococcal folliculitis may merge imperceptibly with folliculitis decalvans. However, acute staphylococcal folliculitis is common and the many clinical variants of cicatrising folliculitis are rare.

A chronic symmetrical superficial folliculitis has been described, which typically affects the legs of young males resulting in alopecia and atrophy of the involved skin [2]. The presence of *Staph. aureus* is a feature of the condition, which has been termed dermatitis cruris pustulosa et atrophicans, and resistance to therapy is also common. In many cases hypergammaglobulinaemia has been identified but no other systemic features have been recorded. No cases have been described in white skin and a humid environment appears to be associated. The condition has been reported on the arms and face as well and in females, but this is much less common.

CA-MRSA may present with folliculitis or an abscess and can progress to severe infections. Athletes participating in team sports may spread the infection to other members of the team, as may military personnel, prisoners and others who are often involved in close contact with individuals [3].

Differential diagnosis
Follicular pustules can be confused with the non-follicular lesions of pustular miliaria, which should be considered when a widespread papulopustular eruption develops in hot and humid conditions, on previously normal skin, or studding an existing inflammatory dermatitis. Follicular pustules are also a feature of subcorneal pustular dermatosis, in which the lesions appear recurrently on the trunk and resolve to leave fine scale. Follicular pustules may occur in tinea infections. The more or less simultaneous development of pustules on a circumscribed, red and oedematous or scaling plaque should arouse suspicion of acute pustular psoriasis or a pustular adverse reaction to medications. In the context of bone marrow transplantation, the possibility of follicular graft-versus-host disease should be considered. Folliculitic eruptions can develop due to certain medications: corticosteroids, hormones, lithium, protein kinase inhibitors, BRAF inhibitors, anticonvulsants, halogens and immunosuppressants (especially ciclosporin and sirolimus). Pseudofolliculitis is an irritant condition resulting from the sharp tips of shaven hairs or ingrowing hairs and secondary infection can occur.

Disease course and prognosis
Folliculitis is usually self-limiting, settling within a few days; however, it can be recurrent and persistent depending on the underlying cause.

Investigations
These are usually not required; however, where CA-MRSA is suspected, swabs should be taken to check the sensitivity of the organism.

Management
Superficial folliculitis of external chemical or physical origin will settle if the irritant is removed. Mild staphylococcal folliculitis is often self-limiting, or may respond to cleansing or topical antiseptics. In more severe cases, antibiotics, topical or systemic, may be required. If the infection is persistent or recurrent, the usual sites of staphylococcal carriage should be swabbed in the patient and his or her contacts and decolonisation treatment prescribed. Because CA-MRSA can be spread by skin-to-skin contact, prevention of further infections is advisable. Hand washing is the single most important behaviour modification in the prevention of spread. Sports participants should shower regularly and personal clothing should not be shared [3]. Daily application of 6.25% aluminium chloride hexahydrate in completely anhydrous ethyl alcohol was reported to be very effective treatment for chronic folliculitis of unspecified type, except for scalp lesions [4].

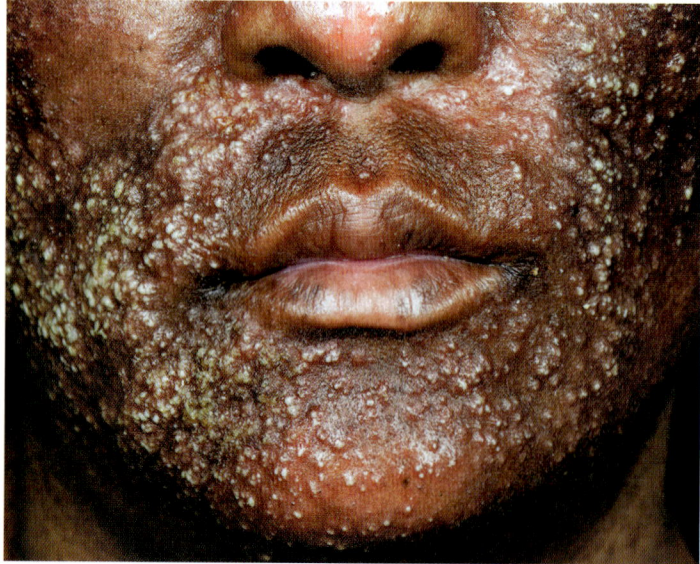

Figure 26.10 Acute folliculitis on the face. Courtesy of King's College London.

> **Treatment ladder for folliculitis**
>
> **First line**
> - Cleanse the affected skin once daily with an antiseptic wash. Avoid heavy occlusive ointments
> - Topical antibiotics twice daily to the affected areas, using fuscidic acid, mupirocin or clindamycin 2% cream
>
> **Second line**
> - Anti-staphylococcal penicillin (e.g. flucloxacillin)
> - Clindamycin
> - Cephalexin
>
> **Third line**
> - Tetracyclines
> - Erythromycin

Furuncle (boil, abscess)

Definition
A furuncle (or boil) is an acute, usually necrotic, infection of a hair follicle with *Staph. aureus*. Sterile furuncles can, however, occur secondary to injected, usually oil-based, drugs into the skin. Often the terms furuncle/boil/abscess are used interchangeably; however, abscesses are not necessarily centred on the hair follicle, but for convenience will be included here.

Introduction and general description
Skin abscesses are collections of pus in the dermis and adipose tissue that usually result from infection. However, injection of foreign material into the skin can result in sterile abscesses.

Epidemiology
Incidence and prevalence
Recent epidemics of furunculosis attributable to specific strains of staphylococci have occurred [1]. Many of these have been associated with community-acquired staphylococcal infections. A French study of patients with furunculosis showed staphylococci in the majority of swabs, and 42% of the isolates had PVL genes present [2]. These were associated with epidemic furunculosis. Clinically, the lesions were more inflamed and multiple. Nasal carriage of staphylococci was strongly associated with recurrent disease but not simple furunculosis (one attack) [2]. The cutaneous and nasal isolates were identical. A similar study from Japan showed 40–60% of isolates were PVL gene positive [3]. Although the PVL locus is thought to be a strong marker for community-acquired meticillin-resistant *Staph. aureus* (CA-MRSA), the study from Japan showed that many PVL-producing strains are meticillin-sensitive *Staph. aureus* (MSSA) [3]. From the very common, milder, persistent and recurrent cases, a wide variety of strains common to many types of staphylococcal infection may be grown, and predisposing factors must be assumed to be of relatively greater significance, although their nature is often difficult to establish. The observation of families over a period of years showed that the same phage type may be responsible for irregular episodes of infection between long intervals of clinical quiescence [4,5].

Age
Furuncles are relatively uncommon in early childhood in temperate climates except in atopic subjects, but increase rapidly in frequency with the approach of puberty, and in adolescence and early adult life are a common occurrence [4]. In adolescence, boys are affected more than girls and the peak incidence parallels that of acne vulgaris.

Pathophysiology
Predisposing factors
The infecting strain of *Staph. aureus* isolated from the furuncle is usually also present in the nares or the perineum [6], which may imply that the repeated and heavy inoculation that occurs in the chronic carrier may be a necessary condition for the development of furunculosis. The surface defence mechanism, and hence the normal balance of microflora, may be disturbed in favour of the staphylococci, which may be carried for some months in the vicinity of recently healed lesions. From the sites of carriage, the infection is disseminated by the fingers and by clothing. Simple mechanical friction of collars and belts may determine the distribution of the lesions. Malnutrition is an important predisposing factor in some countries. Diabetes is widely believed to predispose to furunculosis, although the published evidence does not uniformly confirm this [7,8]. Furunculosis is common in patients infected with HIV. However, in a high proportion of cases in healthy young adults, no convincing predisposing factor can be incriminated.

Pathology
A furuncle is an abscess of a hair follicle, usually of vellus type. The perifollicular abscess is followed by necrosis with destruction of the follicle. The exact pathogenic mechanism by which staphylococci produce the abscess is not clear, but injection of PVL into rabbit skin produced necrotising lesions. This suggests that the cytotoxin produced may have a role to play [9].

Causative organisms
Staph. aureus, which may be MSSA or MRSA and may be PVL positive.

Environmental factors
Furuncles in the UK are most common during the early winter months [10]. As with other superficial staphylococcal infections, the factors responsible for the outbreak and its persistence are unknown. There is seldom any evidence of impairment of the immune response. Reports on the possibility of impairment of neutrophil function are conflicting [11,12].

Clinical features
Presentation
A furuncle first presents as a small, follicular, inflammatory nodule, soon becoming pustular and then necrotic (Figure 26.11), healing after discharge of a necrotic core to leave a violaceous macule and,

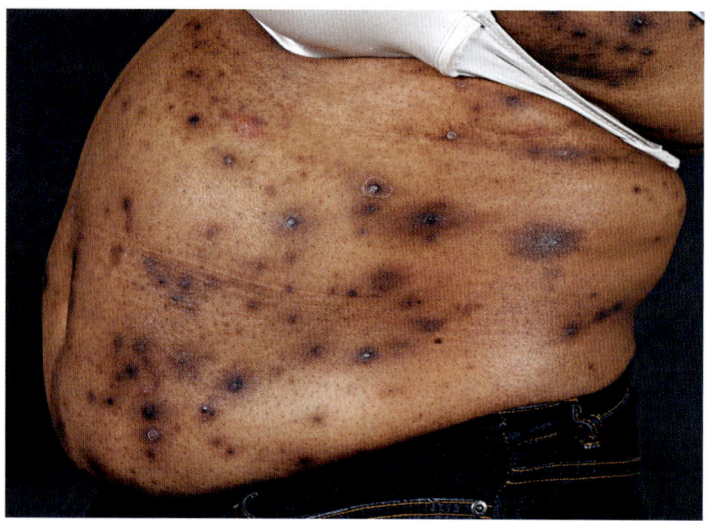

Figure 26.11 Staphylococcus aureus abscesses. Courtesy of King's College London.

ultimately, a permanent scar. The rate of development varies greatly and necrosis may occur within 2 days or only after 2–3 weeks. Tenderness is invariable, and in the more acute and larger lesions there may be throbbing pain. Lesions in the nose or external ear canal can cause very severe pain. The lesions may be single or multiple and tend to appear in crops. Occasionally, there may be fever and mild constitutional symptoms. Malnutrition increases the risk of septicaemia. On the upper lip and cheek, cavernous sinus thrombosis is a rare and dangerous complication. The sites commonly involved are the face and neck, the arms, wrists and fingers, the buttocks and the anogenital region. Attacks may consist of a single crop, or of multiple crops, at irregular intervals with or without periods of remission. The prognosis cannot be reliably determined during a first attack. In some individuals, crops continue to develop for many months or even years. In HIV disease, furuncles may coalesce into violaceous plaques [13]. Systemic infections such as bacterial endocarditis may complicate furunculosis, particularly with CA-MRSA strains [14].

Clinical variants

In patients with multiple and/or recurrent boils/abscesses, PVL-positive *Staph. aureus* infections (MSSA/MRSA) should be suspected (Figure 26.12), or when more than one member of a household is affected either consecutively or simultaneously. Risk factors for PVL infections include overcrowding/close contact, poor hygiene and skin breaks. High-risk groups include health care/care home/nursery workers, military personnel, those playing contact sports (rugby, judo, wrestling), athletes and food handlers. PVL lesions tend to be >5 cm in diameter, are more likely to be necrotic and are more painful than would normally be expected [15].

Differential diagnosis

Other pustular lesions must be differentiated. Furuncles are deep-seated nodules, in contrast to the lesions of superficial staphylococcal folliculitis. The vesicopustules of disseminated herpes simplex are umbilicated and appear simultaneously in large numbers on sites of active or healed eczema. The pustules of acne

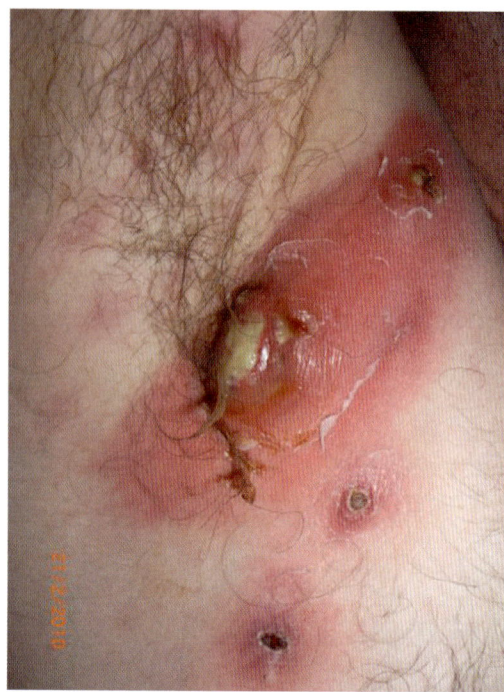

Figure 26.12 Panton–Valentine leukocidin multiple necrotic recurrent abscesses. Courtesy of King's College London.

are but one type of lesion in a polymorphic syndrome. They are associated with papules and comedones, and are usually confined to the face and trunk. Pustules can also occur in halogen eruptions, usually symmetrical and of rapid onset. Nodules and abscesses occur mainly in the axillae and perineum in hidradenitis. Single or few, large, suppurating nodules on exposed skin raise the possibility of myiasis.

Investigations

In settings such as the USA, where PVL-positive MRSA is common, PVL toxin testing is not routinely recommended. Conversely, in settings where a high proportion of PVL cases are associated with MSSA, toxin testing is only recommended for recurrent skin and soft-tissue infection caused by *Staph. aureus* [16]. The rationale for this is that because PVL strains are common and not usually pathogenic, testing and subsequent decolonisation are only required in the context of recurrent or invasive disease.

Management

Simple *Staph. aureus* furuncles. Each episode may need to be treated systemically with an anti-staphylococcal penicillin or another penicillinase-resistant antibiotic. A topical antibacterial agent reduces contamination of the surrounding skin. Recurrent cases where new boils develop at the end of each course of antibiotic should raise the suspicion of a PVL-producing strain. Nasal and perineal carriage of *Staph. aureus* in the patient and other household members should be sought.

PVL *Staph. aureus* furuncles. Purulent collections should undergo surgical drainage where appropriate. Anti-staphylococcal penicillins and other β-lactam antibiotics enhance PVL production *in vitro* at subinhibitory concentrations [17]. Clindamycin, linezolid and fusidic acid inhibit PVL production, while vancomycin has no effect. There are no data to support treating non-necrotic PVL-producing *Staph. aureus* with combinations of antibiotics typically used in invasive necrotising infections. Therefore, in the absence of high MRSA prevalence rates, standard therapy with adequate dosing of anti-staphylococcal penicillin is recommended. Alternative agents in penicillin allergy or PVL-MRSA include clindamycin, doxycycline, linezolid and co-trimoxazole. Decisions on antibiotics should be further guided by antibiotic susceptibility testing and local guidance. In severe infections with evidence of toxic shock, necrotising fasciitis or purpura fulminans, a combination of two or three agents (including those with toxin-inhibitory effects) is recommended, including intravenous agents such as vancomycin, daptomycin, tigecycline and teicoplanin. Intravenous immunoglobulin (IVIg) can be given in severe necrotising invasive infections [15]. Once the PVL infection has been treated then decolonisation of the index case plus any affected/high-risk close contacts should be undertaken simultaneously. Nasal mupirocin (matchstick head-sized amount) on the end of a cotton bud should be applied to the inner surface of each nostril TDS for 5 days plus chlorhexidine 4% or triclosan 1% wash (applied to wet skin, used as a soap and left on for 1 min) daily for 5 days [15].

Treatment ladder for furuncle

Simple furunculosis: first line
- Flucloxacillin
- Erythromycin

PVL *Staph. aureus* furunculosis: seek local guidance
- Anti-staphylococcal penicillin at adequate dosing
- Clindamycin
- Doxycycline
- Linezolid

Severe PVL *Staph. aureus*
- Vancomycin with clindamycin or rifampicin
- Rifampicin and clindamycin
- Rifampicin and linezolid

NB
Any large painful necrotic fluctuant abscess may require incision and drainage under local anaesthetic in addition to the above antibiotics.

Carbuncle

Definition
A carbuncle is a deep infection of a group of contiguous follicles with *Staph. aureus*, accompanied by intense inflammatory changes in the surrounding and underlying connective tissues, including the subcutaneous fat.

Introduction and general description
Carbuncles tend to be larger than abscesses/boils as they represent a cluster of coalescing boils connected under the skin surface.

Epidemiology
Incidence and prevalence
Carbuncles usually occur in otherwise healthy individuals but are more common in the presence of diabetes, malnutrition, cardiac failure, drug addiction or severe generalised dermatoses, obesity and during prolonged steroid therapy. Patients who are *Staph. aureus* carriers in the anterior nares are also at greater risk of developing a carbuncle than non-carriers. Generally, carbuncles are not common, as demonstrated in a military setting where carbuncles/furuncles accounted for only 6% of bacterial skin infections in the US armed forces compared with cellulitis accounting for about 50% [1].

Age
Carbuncles occur predominantly in middle or old age.

Sex
Males are more commonly affected than females.

Pathophysiology
Causative organisms
- *Staph. aureus*.

Clinical features
Presentation
The term carbuncle is derived from the Latin word for a small fiery coal and describes the painful hard red lump that is the initial stage of the infection. It is at first smooth, dome-shaped and acutely tender. It increases in size for a few days, to reach a diameter of 3–10 cm or occasionally more. Suppuration begins after some 5–7 days, and pus is discharged from the multiple follicular orifices. Necrosis of the intervening skin leaves a yellow slough surmounting a crateriform nodule. In some cases, the necrosis develops more acutely without a preliminary follicular discharge, and the entire central core of the lesion is shed, to leave a deep ulcer with a purulent floor. Most lesions are on the back of the neck, the shoulders or the hips and thighs, and although usually solitary, may be multiple or associated with one or more furuncles. Constitutional symptoms may accompany, or even precede by some hours, the development of the carbuncle. Fever may be high, and malaise and prostration may be extreme if the carbuncle is large or the patient's general condition poor. In favourable cases, healing slowly takes place to leave a scar. In the frail and ill, death may occur from septicaemia or from metastatic infection.

Differential diagnosis
The differential diagnoses are similar to those of furuncles. Orf and anthrax are also important differentials. However, the overlying eschar seen in classical cases of anthrax should aid diagnosis. A swab should be taken, but treatment should not be postponed until bacteriological confirmation is available.

Disease course and prognosis
Carbuncles usually settle with a combination of incision/drainage and oral antibiotics. Lesions usually heal with scarring.

Investigations
Skin swabs for microbiology.

Management
An anti-staphylococcal penicillin antibiotic should be given. Incision and drainage or saucerisation under local anaesthetic may be required to help remove pus and necrotic tissue and expedite healing [2].

Sycosis

Definition
Sycosis is a subacute or chronic pyogenic infection involving the whole depth of the follicle and usually refers to disease in the beard area, sycosis barbae.

If the follicles are destroyed with clinically evident scarring, the term lupoid sycosis, or ulerythema sycosiforme, is applied. Folliculitis decalvans is essentially the same process involving the scalp. Many sites may be involved in the same individual.

Epidemiology
Age
Post adolescence.

Sex
Males are most commonly affected.

Pathophysiology
Predisposing factors
Sycosis occurs mostly in males after puberty and commonly involves the follicles of the beard. Most cases begin in the third or fourth decade. The infecting organism is *Staph. aureus*, the same phage type of which can often be isolated from the nose [1], but unknown constitutional factors must be accorded the major role in determining susceptibility, for the staphylococci do not normally penetrate more deeply than the follicular ostia. Many patients have seborrhoea, with a greasy complexion and chronic blepharitis. Indoor workers are affected more often than those who work in the open air.

Pathology
The affected follicle is packed with polymorphonuclear leukocytes, which infiltrate its wall. Around the follicle there is a chronic granulomatous infiltrate in which lymphocytes, plasma cells, histiocytes and foreign-body giant cells are conspicuous. The sebaceous gland, or the whole follicle, may be destroyed and replaced by scar tissue.

Causative organisms
- *Staph. aureus*.

Clinical features
Presentation
The essential lesion is an oedematous red follicular papule or pustule centred on a hair [2]. The individual papules remain discrete, but if neighbouring follicles are involved the perifollicular oedema may coalesce, to produce the raised plaques studded with pustules which suggested the appearance of a ripe fig to the ancient author who coined the term sycosis. In the common subacute forms, the lesions may be scattered irregularly over the beard or grouped, especially on the upper lip and below the angles of the jaw. Attacks of varying duration occur at irregular intervals over months or years. In more chronic forms, the lesions are typically clustered into plaques, especially on the upper lip and chin, and may persist for very long periods – nearly 20 years in one case [3]. There is often some crusting and scaling, but the hairs are retained and there is no evident scarring.

In lupoid sycosis, the follicles are destroyed by scarring, and active papules and pustules fringe the advancing margin around a pink atrophic scar. Granulomatous inflammatory changes may give the papules a lupoid appearance. The process usually begins in front of one ear or under the chin and extends irregularly in any direction. The scalp may be extensively involved. Rarely, a similar process affects axillary and pubic hair, or the lower legs, thighs and arms. Lupoid sycosis tends to persist indefinitely, although the rate of extension may vary from time to time.

Differential diagnosis
The most frequent misdiagnosis is pseudofolliculitis (Figure 26.13) caused by ingrowing hairs. The papules and pustules are irregularly scattered over the sides of the neck and the angles of the jaw and are not grouped but may lie in skin folds. Tinea barbae, a dermatophyte infection in the beard, usually occurs on the chin, mandibular areas or upper lip. There is an oedematous plaque of grouped pustules of acute onset which is relatively asymptomatic. Typically, tinea barbae is caused by zoophilic dermatophytes encountered through contact with farm or domestic animals and mycological analysis is recommended. Lupus vulgaris is an important, if rare, differential; the presence of pustules, however, is highly suggestive of lupoid sycosis but a biopsy should be undertaken if doubt remains.

Disease course and prognosis
The condition may be relapsing and remitting.

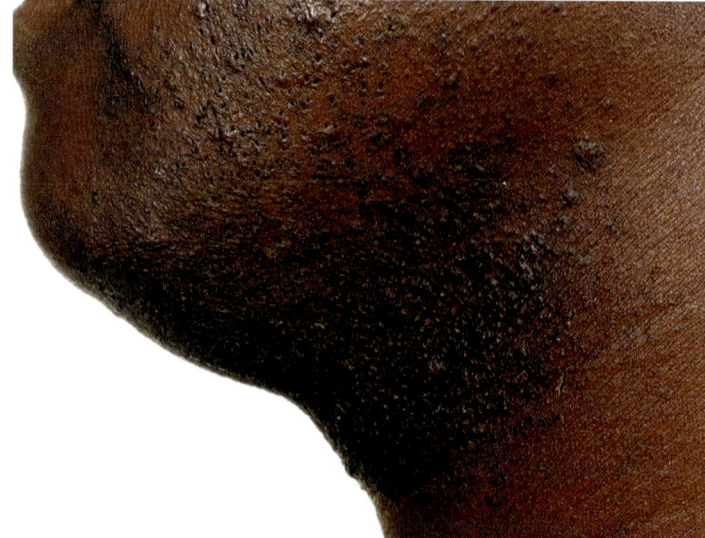

Figure 26.13 Pseudofolliculitis.

Investigations
Swabs from affected skin and from the anterior nares for microbiology.

Management
The subacute forms are relatively easily controlled by antibiotic ointments but tend to relapse when the application is stopped. If a nasal swab indicates a chronic carrier state, the antibiotic should also be applied to the nasal vestibules. In resistant cases, a course of systemic antibiotic may be effective. Alteration to the shaving regime (single blade disposable or electric razor, leaving the hair longer, shaving in the direction of the hair follicle and avoid daily shaving) may help prevent episodes in the longer term. Permanent hair removal is also worth considering in chronic cases. Case reports suggest photodynamic therapy may be effective in the treatment of recalcitrant folliculitis barbae [4].

Treatment ladder for sycosis

First line
- Topical antibiotic therapy
- Consider letting beard hair grow or changing shaving practice

Second line
- Systemic antibiotics such as flucloxacillin, cloxacillin or erythromycin
- Oral retinoids

Third line
- Laser hair removal
- Photodynamic therapy

Staphylococcal scalded skin syndrome

Definition and nomenclature
Staphylococcal scalded skin syndrome (SSSS) is an exfoliative dermatosis in which classically most of the body surface becomes tender and red and the superficial epidermis strips off. The syndrome was first described in children (Ritter disease), but adults may be affected. Outbreaks of SSSS in nurseries and neonatal units have been reported, spread from carers who are asymptomatic staphylococcal carriers [1,2].

Synonyms and inclusions
- Ritter disease

Epidemiology
Age
Children (under the age of 6 years) and neonates are most commonly affected by the generalised form of SSSS; rarely adults may be affected. The localised form of the disease may be more frequent in older children and adults than the current literature suggests.

Associated diseases
Renal failure (exfoliative toxins (ETs) are usually eliminated through the kidneys), malignancy, immunosuppression and alcohol abuse have all been reported to predispose adults to the disease [3], although otherwise healthy individuals may be affected [4].

Pathophysiology
Predisposing factors
Approximately 5% of *Staph. aureus* strains (from all phage groups) produce an exfoliative toxin (ETA, ETB) [5]. The initial infection may be very trivial such as an area of impetigo, bacterial conjunctivitis, iatrogenic wound or a streptococcal throat. More significant infections such as staphylococcal pneumonia, septic arthritis or endocarditis can also lead to SSSS. The more extensive and dramatic epidermal changes are then triggered by the ETs which target the cell adhesion protein desmoglein 1 (DG1) resulting in separation of keratinocytes just beneath the granular layer in the epidermis (intraepidermal). In bullous impetigo the ETs remain local in the infected skin, but in SSSS the ETs are spread haematogenously resulting in widespread skin involvement.

Pathology
Histologically, there is splitting of the epidermis between the granular and spinous layers, which does not usually contain inflammatory cells. A few lymphocytes surround the superficial blood vessels. The disease is caused by one or more ETs, usually A or B, which are serine proteases [6] that selectively cleave the cellular adhesion molecule DG1 [7] found on epidermal keratinocytes. Antibodies to desmoglein may develop in some patients with SSSS [8]. The same toxins are involved in bullous impetigo, which may be regarded as a localised form of SSSS although patients with bullous impetigo do not seem to develop the same level of antibody. This may be due to the shorter duration of the disease [8]. Toxin A is chromosomally encoded on a phage genome whereas toxin B is encoded on a large plasmid [9]. ETA-producing strains are more commonly isolated from patients with bullous impetigo and ETB from patients with SSSS [10]. Regulation and expression of ETA and ETB are complex and not fully elucidated [10] and the role of ETs as superantigens in SSSS is speculated [11].

Causative organisms
Staph. aureus strains producing ETs are the causative organisms. Initially, phage group II was implicated; however, there is evidence that all phage groups can cause SSSS. There are increasing numbers of reports of CA-MRSA causing SSSS in neonates.

Clinical features
Presentation
The initial event is usually a localised staphylococcal infection (Figure 26.14) [4]. This may be in the skin or at a distant or 'occult' site. A few days later, patients develop fever, irritability and skin tenderness. A widespread red eruption follows which is usually accentuated in the flexures (neck, axillae, inguinal creases and gluteal cleft) (Figure 26.15) and progresses rapidly to superficial blister formation (Nikolsky positive). The tender skin becomes gathered into folds and, as it shrinks, leaves raw areas which are

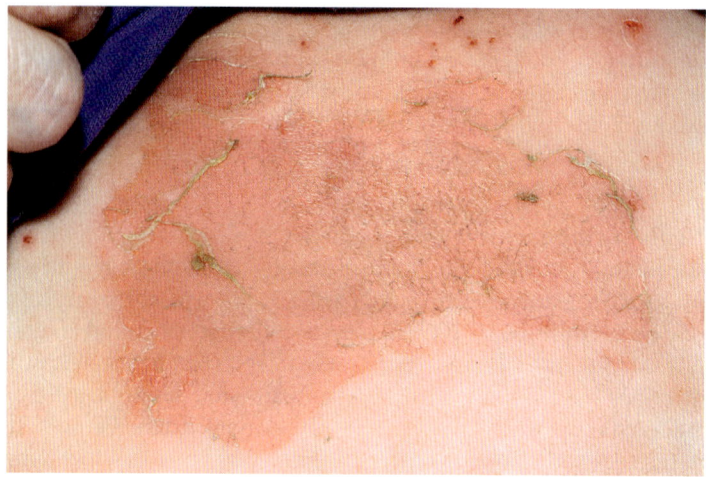

Figure 26.14 Staphylococcal scalded skin syndrome in a child. Courtesy of King's College London.

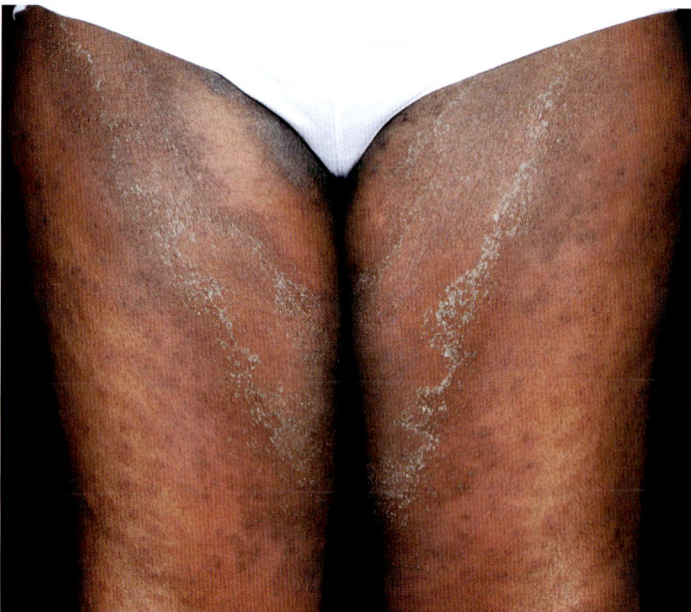

Figure 26.15 Staphylococcal scalded skin syndrome in an adult. Courtesy of King's College London.

extremely painful. Mucosal membrane involvement is absent. Thick crusting and fissuring are common around the eyes, nose and mouth. The condition usually heals within 7–14 days.

Clinical variants

SSSS can be generalised or localised. Localised SSSS seems to favour the flexures, in particular the axillae (Figure 26.16a), groin and limb flexures. Healing of the localised form of the disease classically leaves wrinkled desquamating skin with hyperpigmentation (Figure 26.16b).

Differential diagnosis

'Scalded skin syndrome' historically has been used as a synonym for toxic epidermal necrolysis (TEN) (Chapter 117). However,

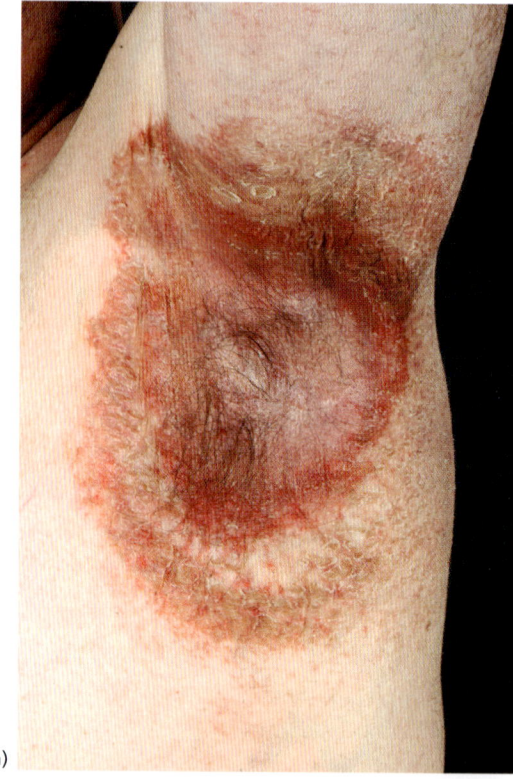

(a)

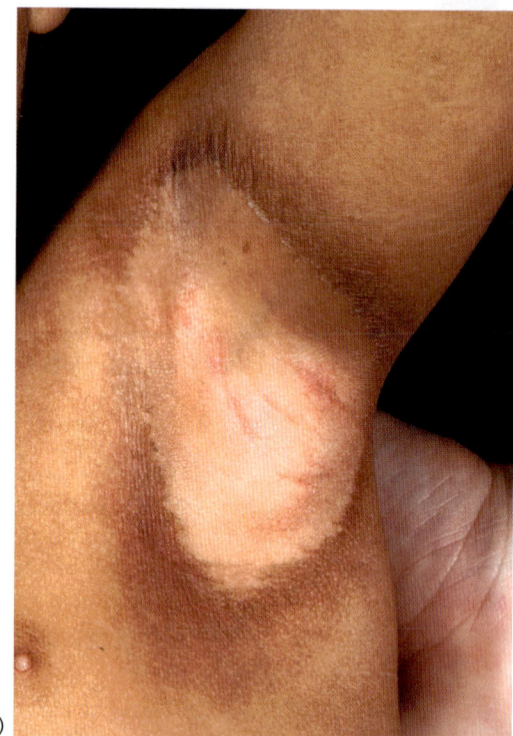

(b)

Figure 26.16 (a) Localised staphyloccocal scalded skin syndrome (SSSS). (b) Localised SSSS healing with wrinkling desquamation and hyperpigmentation. Courtesy of King's College London.

cell necrosis does not occur in the staphylococcal disease, and it is widely accepted that the term 'staphylococcal TEN' is inappropriate. Both TEN and Stevens–Johnson syndrome are the most important differential diagnoses to consider and they can be differentiated from SSSS on biopsy, where instead of the superficial blistering of SSSS there is subepidermal blistering and full-thickness epidermal necrosis. Other differential diagnoses include TSS, scarlet fever, Kawasaki disease, drug hypersensitivity, thermal or chemical burns, pemphigus and genetic blistering disorders.

Classification of severity
The generalised form of the disease is considered to be more severe than the localised form.

Disease course and prognosis
SSSS usually settles within a few weeks when treated with appropriate systemic antibiotics. However, the localised form of the disease may be prolonged with episodes of relapse over several months. Postinflammatory hyper- or hypopigmentation may occur following healing.

Investigations
Swabs and cultures of blister fluids do not usually grow *Staph. aureus*, as the blisters are mediated by the toxins which are disseminated haematogenously. The staphylococci may, however, be isolated from the original septic site if identified. Typing of *Staph. aureus* and PCR for toxin production may be possible in some laboratories. In adults with generalised SSSS, blood cultures are often positive for *Staph. aureus*, whereas this is rarely the case in children.

Management
Parenteral anti-staphylococcal antibiotics such as flucloxacillin, cefazolin, clindamycin, tigecycline or daptomycin should be used as first line therapy. First generation cephalosporins, penicillin G or erythromycin may be used if a susceptible strain of *Staph. aureus* has been identified. Clindamycin may be given orally or parenterally alone (or in combination with rifampicin or tetracyclines), or parenteral vancomycin or tobramycin if MRSA is suspected. If antibiotics are administered early, children usually recover within 7 days and the mortality rate is low at 4%. In adults, the overall mortality rate is higher, around 60%, which is likely to reflect that in adults, SSSS is more common in those with underlying health conditions [12]. Those patients without underlying disease recover more rapidly.

Treatment ladder for SSSS

First line
- Anti-staphylococcal penicillins
- Cefazolin
- Clindamycin
- Daptomycin

First line treatments if MRSA is suspected
- Vancomycin
- Linezolid
- Tigecycline

Toxic shock syndrome

Definition and nomenclature
This is a serious life-threatening illness characterised by fever, acute redness followed by desquamation, circulatory shock and multisystem disease which is mediated by one or more bacterial toxins elaborated by *Staph. aureus* or *Strep. pyogenes*.

Synonyms and inclusions
- Staphylococcal TSS
- Streptococcal TSS

Introduction and general description
Toxic shock syndrome (TSS) was first reported in significant numbers of patients shortly after the introduction of super-absorbent tampons in the 1970s. Thousands of menstruating women using these highly absorbent tampons presented acutely unwell with fever, low blood pressure and multiorgan failure leading to a death rate of 15%. This particular type of tampon is no longer manufactured and the number of cases has consequently declined dramatically.

Epidemiology
Incidence and prevalence
Toxic shock syndrome is thought to be rare and has been reported to affect approximately 1–17/100 000 tampon users per annum.

Age
Any age can be affected but in general the condition is more common at the extremes of age and in menstruating women (15–40 years)

Sex
Historically, it is more common in females.

Ethnicity
Black women between the ages of 13 and 40 years in the USA had lower antibody titres to TSS toxin 1 (TSS-1) than white or Hispanic women, suggesting the former are more at risk of menstrual TSS [1].

Associated diseases
Recent chickenpox infection, cellulitis and necrotising fasciitis, underlying HIV or internal malignancy, alcohol misuse and diabetes have all been associated with an increased risk of TSS.

Pathophysiology
Predisposing factors
Nearly all cases have been infected or colonised by *Staph. aureus*. Staphylococcal infection of any severity, at any site, at any age and in either sex may cause TSS [2]. However, in most of the early cases, the organism was isolated from the vagina of menstruating women using high-absorbency tampons in the USA; in these cases, symptomatic vaginitis was common but not invariable. It seemed likely that staphylococci, perhaps introduced by hand or from perineal skin, found appropriate conditions for growth in the medium of the

menstrual blood, facilitated in some way by the tampon. A strong association with absorbency, and especially with one brand, was noted. Avoidance of these materials in tampons was followed by a dramatic fall in the incidence, so that after 1985 the majority of USA cases were non-menstrual [3]. Women are also at risk post-partum and if using internal barrier-type contraception such as the diaphragm.

Toxic shock syndrome toxin 1, previously identified as staphylococcal enterotoxin F or as pyrogenic exotoxin C [4], is produced by 80–90% of *Staph. aureus* isolates from affected cases and is believed to be the main bacterial mediator of the disease. More recently, staphylococcal enterotoxin B was also identified from cases of TSS [5,6]. This toxin belongs to a family of bacterial pyrogenic toxin super antigens (PTSAgs), which are able to stimulate T-lymphocyte proliferation in a non-antigen-specific manner. This results in fever, inflammation and shock. Most of these PTSAgs are encoded by a series of distinct mobile elements referred to as staphylococcal pathogenicity islands, which are located at specific sites in the genome and can be mobilised and transferred by other phages to other strains [7]. A similar disease has been associated with severe infections with *Strep. pyogenes* [8] and may be mediated by re-emergent scarlet fever toxin A [9].

Pathology

There are no specific histological features. A perivascular mononuclear cell infiltrate and papillary oedema may occur in the dermis. In cases with blister formation the split is subepidermal [10].

Causative organisms
- *Staph. aureus*.
- *Strep. pyogenes*.

Clinical features
History
In menstrual TSS, women are usually about 5 days into their menstrual bleeding when they present with malaise and fever.

Presentation
The onset is acute with fever and rash. Vomiting and diarrhoea are common early features, and involvement of the muscle, liver, kidneys and central nervous system may follow. Circulatory shock (which does not respond to intravenous fluid replacement) is often rapid in onset and severity, and acute renal impairment frequently coexists. Multiorgan failure follows soon afterwards with at least three systems needed to be involved to fulfil the diagnostic criteria (gastrointestinal, renal, hepatic, central nervous system, muscular, haematological and mucous membranes). The rash may be the presenting feature or may develop within the first day. A widespread macular redness, sometimes faint, and clearing within 3 days is commonest, but scarlatiniform and papulopustular eruptions are also described. In more pigmented skin types, the rash may be more difficult to discern or may look more hyperpigmented or purpuric rather than red. Oedema of the hands and feet may be marked with indolent associated blistering (Figure 26.17). There is generalised mucous membrane redness, especially intense in the conjunctiva, under which there may be haemorrhage. Oral, oesophageal, vaginal and bladder mucosae may ulcerate. Occasionally, vesicles and

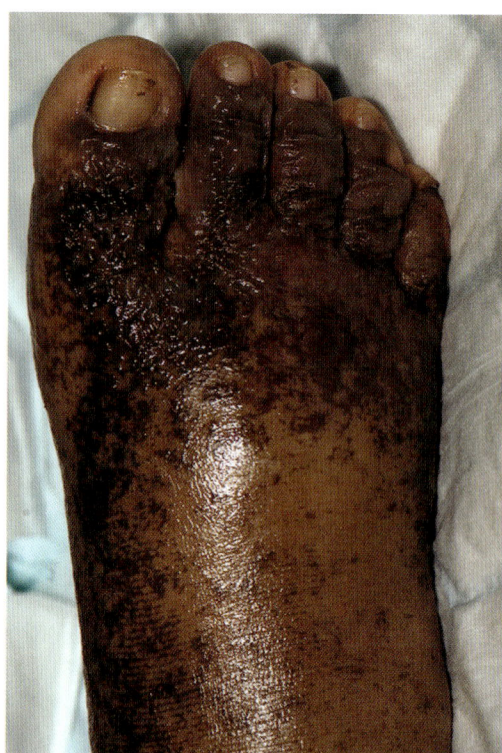

Figure 26.17 Indolent blistering associated with toxic shock syndrome.

bullae may form. Towards the end of the second week, the majority of patients develop a widespread, itchy, maculopapular sometimes urticarial rash, which is thought not to be drug induced in most cases. Thrombocytopenia may cause purpura in a retiform pattern at the peripheries (Figure 26.18). Desquamation is highly characteristic. It occurs 10–21 days after onset, and may be confined to the fingertips, may affect all the palmar and plantar skin or may be generalised. Reversible patchy alopecia or telogen effluvium and transverse ridging and partial loss of nails are later non-specific findings.

Differential diagnosis
Septic shock and other infections should be excluded by appropriate investigations. Some reported adult cases of Kawasaki disease may have had TSS. The diseases have features in common, but Kawasaki disease can usually be differentiated by prolonged fever, cardiac involvement, generalised lymphadenopathy and absence of peripheral shock. Reports of staphylococcal scarlatina may represent milder cases of TSS. Ehrlichosis may present with a life-threatening illness similar to TSS [11]. *Clostridium sordellii* infection may be associated with TSS and a high mortality rate. The disease resembles the staphylococcal syndrome and it may result from postpartum infections [12], gynaecological procedures or intravenous drug use.

Complications and co-morbidities
TSS results in multiorgan failure which may manifest as adult respiratory distress syndrome, acute and in some cases chronic renal failure and disseminated intravascular coagulation.

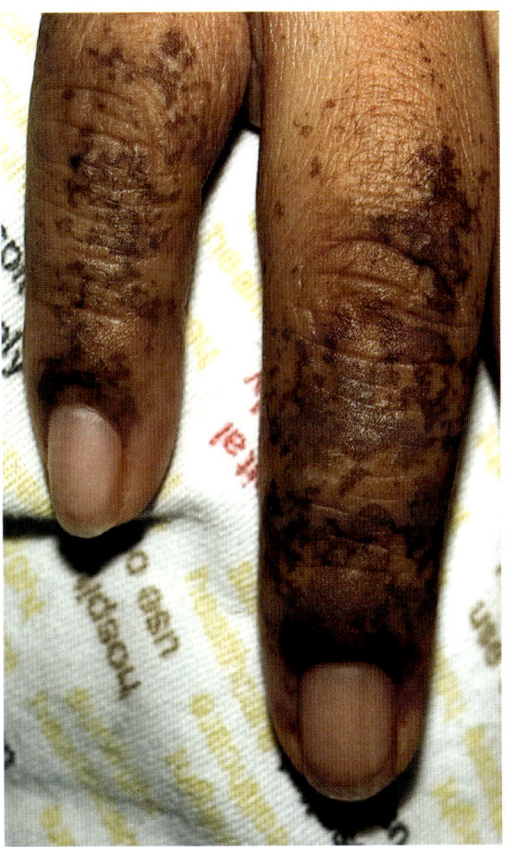

Figure 26.18 Retiform purpura in toxic shock syndrome.

Disease course and prognosis
If treated in a high-dependency unit with prompt use of appropriate intravenous antibiotics, most patients recover over about 3 weeks; however, the mortality rate remains at about 7% [10,13].

Investigations
The diagnosis is primarily clinical, supported by the confirmation, in the great majority of cases, of *Staph. aureus* infection through microbiological cultures. Several sets of blood cultures should be taken (more commonly positive in group A streptococcal disease than staphyloccocal infections). Microbiological swabs from wounds and from the vagina of menstruating or postpartum females should also be taken. Routine biochemistry may show raised creatinine which frequently precedes hypotension.

Management
Tampons should be sought by clinical examination and removed if present and infected wounds debrided. Appropriate systemic antibiotic therapy should be given. Intensive general supportive measures are essential such as fluid resuscitation and ventilatory support. In addition, patients may require noradrenaline circulatory support and dialysis. The use of systemic corticosteroids and IVIg still remains controversial in the management of septic shock including TSS. A Cochrane review concluded that there was evidence that polyclonal IVIg reduced mortality in adults; however, this benefit was not demonstrated in trials [14]. There was no proven benefit in neonates. There was insufficient robust benefit demonstrated with the use of IgM enriched IVIg [14]. Studies have shown that the use of low-dose systemic corticosteroids reduced the duration and dose of vasopressor agents in septic shock [15] and ameliorates septic shock but does not reduce mortality at day 28 [16]. There is some evidence from animal studies that the expression of glucocorticoid receptors is progressively decreased in experimental sepsis leading to reduced translocation of dexamethasone into cells, which may explain why steroid treatment only appears to be beneficial when administered early in septic shock [17]. Synthetic human monoclonal antibodies against staphylococcal enterotoxin B have been shown to be protective against TSS in mice [18] and enhanced survival [19].

Intravenous clindamycin should be given as first line treatment as this is highly effective against most strains of *Staph. aureus* and *Strep. pyogenes* and is known to reduce toxin production. In addition, benzylpenicillin sodium (penicillin G) to cover *Strep. pyogenes* is recommended. When *Staph. aureus* is known or suspected, an anti-staphylococcal penicillin or vancomycin (for MRSA) should be added to ensure adequate cover.

Treatment ladder for TSS

First line
- Haemodynamic resuscitation
- IV clindamycin (600–900 mg three times daily) +/− benzylpenicillin sodium (penicillin G) (2.4–4.8 g daily in four divided doses) or vancomycin (1–1.5 g every 12 h). Intravenous antibiotics are usually continued for up to 1–2 weeks depending on the clinical response

Second line
- For severe cases, consider additional intravenous immunoglobulin (initial dose 2 g/kg, then 4 days of 0.4 g/kg)

Recurrent toxin-mediated perineal erythema

Definition
Recurrent perineal erythema is mediated by superantigen toxins produced by strains of *Staph. aureus* and *Strep. pyogenes*.

Introduction and general description
Strep. pyogenes infection of the throat leads to perineal redness and subsequent rapid desquamation resulting from bacterial toxins. The condition is often recurrent.

Epidemiology
Incidence and prevalence
Not known.

Age
Young children usually under the age of 12 years but adults may occasionally be affected [1].

Sex
Males and females are equally affected.

Pathophysiology
Predisposing factors
Group A streptococcal throat infections and impetigo often precede the onset of the disease. Superantigens produced by *Staph. aureus* and *Strep. pyogenes* lead to non-specific T-cell activation and toxin-mediated redness at distant skin sites [2].

Causative organisms
- *Strep. pyogenes*.
- *Staph. aureus*.

Clinical features
History
Recurrent episodes of pharyngotonsillitis followed by redness in the perineum and occasionally the axillae.

Presentation
After a sore throat, patients develop an eruption in the perineal area. The rash resembles erysipelas (Figure 26.19) with macular redness or inflammation but settles more quickly with desquamation, and is associated with very little in the way of systemic features [3]. Other cutaneous areas may also be red including the hands, feet and axillae [4,5]. Some patients also have a strawberry tongue.

Disease course and prognosis
The disease is recurrent but settles rapidly with appropriate antibiotics.

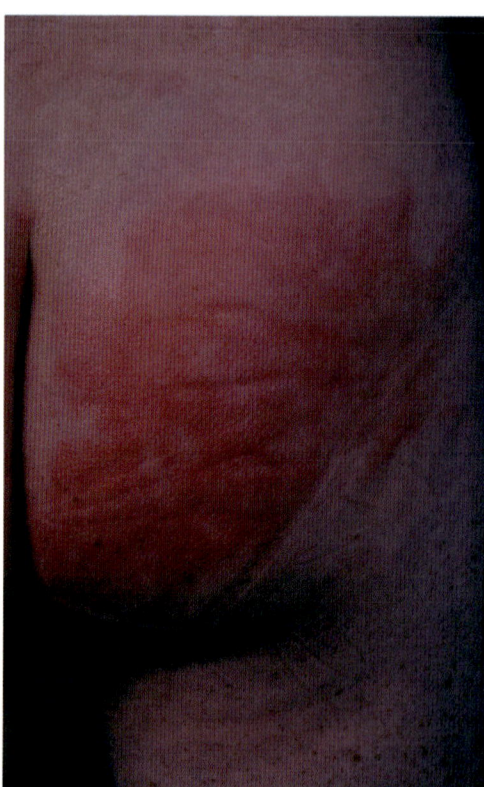

Figure 26.19 Recurrent toxin-mediated perineal erythema.

Investigations
The diagnosis is made on clinical grounds. Patients are usually well, with a history of a sore throat. Swabs from the perineal area do not grow any specific organisms, but throat swabs may yield *Staph. aureus* or *Strep. pyogenes*.

Management
Patients respond well to a short course of antibiotics, which covers *Strep. pyogenes* and *Staph. aureus*, with few sequelae.

Streptococcal vulvovaginitis (Chapter 112)

Definition
Vaginal infection with group A streptococci, mainly affecting prepubescent girls.

Introduction and general description
Patient complains of irritation or soreness in the genital area.

Epidemiology
Incidence and prevalence
Not known.

Age
Mainly affects prepubescent girls but women may also be affected.

Sex
Females.

Associated diseases
Perianal infection occasionally coexists.

Pathophysiology
Predisposing factors
Personal or family member with a cutaneous or respiratory infection with group A streptococcal disease. In older women, sexual contact with an infected person.

Causative organisms
- *Strep. pyogenes* accounts for 10% of cases of vulvovaginitis in prepubertal girls [1].
- Other bacterial causes of vulvovaginitis in prepubertal girls, including *E. coli, Enterococcus faecalis, H. influenzae, Proteus mirabilis* and *Staph. aureus,* cannot be distinguished clinically [2,3].

Clinical features
History
Young girl usually complains of irritation or soreness in the vaginal area with associated pain on passing urine.

Presentation
The child complains of genital soreness or irritation and the skin is acutely red. There may be purulent/watery or yellow vaginal discharge or dysuria.

Differential diagnosis
Candida infections and sexually transmitted diseases.

Disease course and prognosis
The symptoms usually settle with appropriate systemic antibiotics; however, recurrence may be problematic.

Investigations
Swabs from the vulvo-vaginal area for microbiology.

Management
The infection responds to oral penicillin or clarithromycin. Some authors report rapid cure with vaginal clindamycin 2% cream [4]. There is some evidence that there may be concomitant group A streptococci and *Candida* in women, therefore treatment with antibiotics plus fluconazole may be indicated [5].

Perianal streptococcal cellulitis

Definition and nomenclature
The term 'cellulitis' [1,2] seems inappropriate for this superficial infection that lacks fever and other systemic symptoms, although surface swabs yield group A streptococci in all cases.

Synonyms and inclusions
- Perianal streptococcal dermatitis

Introduction and general description
An uncommon superficial cutaneous infection in the perianal area almost exclusively in young children.

Epidemiology
Age
Most patients are children aged between 6 months and 10 years [3], but occasional adult cases are seen.

Associated diseases
Guttate psoriasis and, in girls, vulvovaginitis are occasionally associated.

Pathophysiology
Predisposing factors
Some, but not all, patients were found to harbour *Strep. pyogenes* in the throat, usually of the same strain, and sometimes there is a recent history of pharyngitis or impetigo in a family member [4]. In some reported cases, there had been symptoms for many weeks or months, suggesting that chronic infection may occur.

Causative organisms
- *Strep. pyogenes*.
- *Staph. aureus* has been reported to cause a similar clinical appearance with satellite pustules at the periphery [5].

Clinical features
Presentation
Perianal soreness or irritation, pain on defecation and sometimes secondary faecal retention are typical presenting symptoms. The affected skin is bright red and may be fissured. The genital skin may also be additionally affected [6].

Differential diagnosis
The diagnosis of perianal streptococcal cellulitis is often delayed due to consideration of other diagnoses in the affected children including diaper dermatitis, seborrhoeic dermatitis, scarlet fever, candidiasis and even sexual abuse [7].

Disease course and prognosis
Usually clears rapidly with appropriate antibiotic treatment.

Investigations
Perianal swab for microbiology.

Management
The condition responds to an oral antibiotic. Penicillin is often successful [3,4], but recurrences in some patients respond to a macrolide and topical mupirocin [3,8,9] for 10–14 days. A 2-week course of oral antibiotic treatment is usually recommended [2].

Blistering distal dactylitis

Definition
A distinct entity presenting with localised group A streptococcal infection of the distal phalanx usually in a child.

Introduction and general description
Blistering distal dactylitis manifests as multiple bullae on the volar aspects of the hands and fingers usually in young children. Lesions appear over a few days and may leave superficial erosions secondary to usually group A *Streptococcus* but also *Staph. aureus* infections.

Epidemiology
Age
Children between the ages of 2 and 16 years of age are most commonly affected but there are cases reported in adults [1]. Rarely cases have been reported in children a few months of age [1,2].

Pathophysiology
Causative organisms
Group A streptococci and other organisms have been identified, including group B streptococci [3] and *Staph. aureus* [4]. More recently *Staph. aureus* has been noted to be implicated in adults [5].

Clinical features
Presentation
A large blister or blisters containing thin seropurulent fluid forms on the distal phalanx, usually of a finger, and typically on the

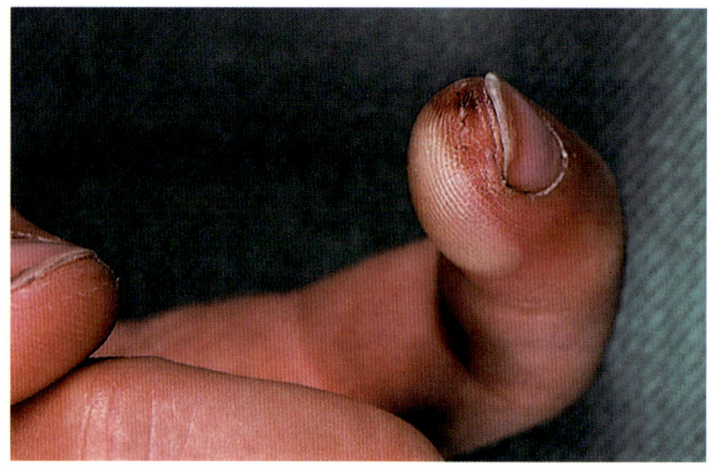

Figure 26.20 Blistering distal dactylitis.

palmar pad (Figure 26.20), although it may extend to the nail folds, and more proximal involvement of the palmar skin is sometimes seen [6]. An upper respiratory tract infection is sometimes present. One recurrent case occurred beside an ingrowing toenail [7].

Differential diagnosis
- Herpetic whitlow.
- Bullous impetigo.
- Pompholyx eczema.

Disease course and prognosis
Usually settles rapidly with the appropriate antibiotics.

Investigations
The organism is cultured from blister fluid.

Management
If bullae are tense, they may be disrupted gently with a sterile needle, leaving the blister roof intact [2]. A course of anti-staphylococcal penicillin antibiotics (flucloxacillin, dicloxacillin, cloxacillin) is usually effective [5]. Topical therapy with wet dressings may be helpful [5].

Toxin-mediated streptococcal disease

There has been a resurgence over the past decade of invasive streptococcal diseases many of which are mediated by toxin production. The following section includes toxin-mediated streptococcal diseases that affect the skin including scarlet fever and a toxic shock-like syndrome.

Scarlet fever

Definition and nomenclature
A disease manifested by pharyngitis caused by toxin-producing group A streptococci, fever and a distinctive scarlatiniform rash.

Synonyms and inclusions
- Scarlatina

Introduction and general description
Scarlet fever is mainly a disease of young children who do not have protective antibodies against streptococcal exotoxins. Scarlet fever is characterised by an acute streptococcal pharyngitis with fever, with a rash occuring in about 1 in 10 cases.

Epidemiology
Incidence and prevalence
The disease occurs worldwide but the full syndrome is uncommon in the tropics, where surveys suggest that subclinical infections must be frequent [1]. There has been a dramatic resurgence of cases over the past decade with epidemics reported in China, Hong Kong and Poland [2,3,4]. Scarlet fever is endemic in large towns but the incidence varies greatly from year to year. The incidence in the Oxford (UK) region at a time of greater frequency of the disease was 0.3 confirmed, and 1.25 suspected, cases per 1000 per year [5]. In the last few decades, scarlet fever has been less severe than in the late 19th and early 20th centuries, perhaps because of the virtual disappearance of type A toxin [6].

Age
Most cases occur between the ages of 5 and 15 years although infections are reported in infancy and adults [4].

Sex
Equal numbers of males and females are affected.

Ethnicity
Scarlet fever is not reported more commonly in any particular ethnic groups; however, it has been reported to be more common in conditions of overcrowding and high rates are reported in the least affluent populations [7].

Associated diseases
Rheumatic fever, poststreptococcal glomerulonephritis, osteomyelitis.

Pathophysiology
Predisposing factors
Scarlet fever is an acute infection caused by strains of *Strep. pyogenes* producing pyrogenic exotoxin (erythrogenic toxin, erythrotoxin), of which there are three antigenically unrelated types, A, B and C [8,9–11]. All three are capable of producing scarlet fever. Toxin production appears to depend on the presence of a temperate bacteriophage and is exclusive to group A streptococcal infection, a single strain of which may produce none, one, two or all three toxins [12]. In the 1970s and 1980s, type B was the most frequent toxin in the USA, Germany and England, and type C was also seen; type A is believed to have been responsible for the severe disease seen several decades ago. Whether an infected individual develops scarlet fever or a septic streptococcal illness, such as tonsillitis or cellulitis, depends on the level of antitoxic immunity, normally acquired by previous exposure.

Pathology

The upper respiratory tract is the usual portal of entry and, although infection of surgical and other wounds may sometimes be responsible, most reports of this association have not included bacteriological examination of the throat. Droplet infection is the most common but the disease may also be spread by fomites.

Group A streptococci are classified by M antigens, which are encoded by *emm* genes. At least 200 *emm* types have been identified so far and these are associated with different geographic locations, virulence and resistance patterns. One study from Taiwan confirmed a shift in *emm* genotype over a 20-year period, with a significant increase in prevalence of macrolide resistant disease [13]. The fluctuation in genotypes has been reported following various outbreaks in different countries and the increasing prevalence of antibiotic resistant strains is a recurrent theme [2,14].

The erythrogenic toxin is responsible for cutaneous vasodilatation, which may be associated with oedema and a perivascular cellular infiltrate. The toxin may also produce a degenerative myocarditis. The bacterial component of the syndrome consists of septic lesions in many organs, with abscess formation. Glomerulonephritis depends on an immunological mechanism. An attack with a rash confers permanent, specific antitoxic immunity. The toxin produced by other strains is not neutralised, hence second attacks, although rare, can occur. Bacterial immunity is temporary and there is therefore no permanent protection against the septic manifestation of infection by the same or related strains of *Strep. pyogenes*.

Causative organisms
- *Strep. pyogenes*.

Environmental factors
Overcrowding, poor sanitation.

Clinical features
Presentation
After an incubation period, which is usually 2–5 days, fever, anorexia and vomiting usher in the infection [15]. If the throat is the portal of entry, there is an acute follicular or membranous tonsillitis, with painful lymphadenopathy. If the infection has entered a wound, there may be increased tenderness and some serous discharge. The rash, which appears on the second day, first on the upper trunk, is made up of fine, red punctate lesions, and has been likened to 'sunburn with goose pimples' or 'sandpaper'. In more deeply pigmented skin, the rash will be less visible but the texture change should be discernible. It generalises within a few hours or over 3 or 4 days. Transverse red streaks in the skin folds due to capillary fragility are known as Pastia lines. The face is flushed and relative pallor around the mouth is characteristic. The lower legs are involved last and least. After 7–10 days, the rash is succeeded by desquamation, bran-like in most areas but in large lamellar scales on the palms and soles.

The oral mucous membranes are bright red and there may be deeper red puncta on the palate. The tongue is at first heavily coated, but by the second or third day scattered swollen red papillae give the 'white strawberry tongue' appearance. As the epithelium is shed, the tongue becomes smooth and dark red ('red strawberry tongue') before returning to normal. Fever usually settles in 7–10 days. The typical course of the mild or moderate case may be modified if either the toxic or septic manifestations are severe.

In the severe toxic form, the eruption is very intense and may be purpuric. Fever is high and the patient is delirious or comatose. Myocarditis may be present. In the septic forms, the local pharyngeal lesions are severe and there may be extensive oedema. Otitis media and peritonsillar abscesses are frequent.

Differential diagnosis
Rubella, the early stage of smallpox, and some drug reactions can simulate scarlet fever. The lack of pharyngeal lesions and the distribution of the exanthem will usually enable the diagnosis to be established. Rarely, staphylococcal infections are accompanied by a scarlatiniform erythema.

In the so-called recurrent scarlatiniform erythema, repeated attacks of a somewhat similar rash, followed by exfoliation, occur without discoverable cause. Far East scarlet-like fever occurred in epidemics in East and South East Asia during the 1950s. The aetiological agent has been identified as *Yersinia pseudotuberculosis* IP31758, and the complete genome has now been sequenced, showing its evolution from the typical strain of *Y. pseudotuberculosis* [16].

Complications and co-morbidities
Complications are caused either by the toxin, or by bacterial invasion of the tissues by local extension or by haematogenous dissemination, or by a probably allergic reaction. Of the toxic manifestations, myocarditis is the most important. The suppurative complications include hepatitis, arthritis, meningitis and osteomyelitis. Rheumatic fever and glomerulonephritis are presumed to be allergic in origin.

Disease course and prognosis
At present, the prognosis is good and the mortality of treated cases is under 1%. Second attacks are more frequent in patients in whom early antibiotic control of the initial attack has impaired an adequate immune response [17].

Investigations
The classical form of the disease associated with tonsillitis is unlikely to be misdiagnosed if it is considered. The diagnosis may be supported by culture of a group A *Streptococcus* and a rising ASOT.

Management
Penicillin remains the mainstay of antibiotic treatment of scarlet fever [18] and should be given in adequate dosage for 10 days as soon as the diagnosis is suspected, to reduce the communicability of the infection. Recent cases and outbreaks have included large numbers of strains resistant to erythromycin, tetracycline and clindamycin [2,19], and cases associated with CA-MRSA [20] and PVL [21] have been reported.

> **Treatment ladder for scarlet fever**
>
> **First line**
> - Penicillin
> - Amoxicillin
> - Cephalosporins (first generation)
>
> **Second line**
> - Clindamycin
> - Clarithromycin
>
> **Third line**
> - Vancomycin
> - Linezolid

Streptococcal toxic shock-like syndrome

Definition
Fever, myalgia and flu-like symptoms are followed by pain in an extremity, or the abdomen. A rash followed by desquamation, circulatory shock and multisystem disease characterise the streptococcal toxic shock-like syndrome (STSLS).

Epidemiology
Age
The disease may occur in children or adults.

Pathophysiology
Predisposing factors
This disorder has been associated with the recent re-emergence of invasive group A streptococcal infections. Group A streptococci are usually cultured from the blood. The streptococcal toxins are likely to be responsible for this condition, although the exact pathogenic mechanisms are currently still unknown. Slightly more atypical species of *Streptococcus* have recently been reported to cause STSLS [1–4].

Causative organisms
- *Strep. pyogenes.*
- *Strep. suis.*
- *Strep. dysgalactiae.*
- *Strep. agalactiae.*

Environmental factors
Some of the recent epidemic outbreaks have been associated with zoonotic species of streptococci such as via contact with pigs [1,5].

Clinical features
Presentation
The disease is similar to staphylococcal TSS, although there may be some differences. Cases of streptococcal TSLS are associated with severe invasive group A streptococcal disease, whereas staphylococcal TSS may be associated with either severe or trivial infection. Surgical wounds, throat infections, vaginal infections postpartum or soft-tissue infections due to group A *Streptococcus* may be followed by the STSLS [6,7]. The onset of the illness is usually rapid with high fever, a rash that desquamates, ensuing hypotension and ultimately multiorgan failure. Virulent strains of *Streptococcus* produce potent exotoxins that are highly destructive of particularly skin and muscle.

Differential diagnosis
Staphylococcal TSS.

Complications and co-morbidities
Complications include myositis, endophthalmitis, peritonitis and renal failure [8].

Disease course and prognosis
The disease is associated with a mortality rate of 25%.

Investigations
Blood cultures are frequently positive, and swabs from the site of clinical infection almost always yield group A *Streptococcus* M types 1, 3, 12 and 28. The streptococcal pyrogenic exotoxins (SPEs) A and B are produced in the majority of these cases.

Management
Penicillin, clarithromycin or clindamycin would be the treatment of choice for most soft-tissue infections caused by group A streptococcal disease. Where necrotising fasciitis or myositis has developed, rapid debridement, fasciotomy or amputation may be required. IVIg may be helpful to neutralise the toxin [9].

> **Treatment ladder for streptococcal toxic shock-like syndrome**
>
> **First line**
> - Penicillin
> - Clindamycin
>
> **Second line**
> - Cephalosporin (first generation)
> - Clarithromycin
>
> **Third line**
> - Vancomycin
> - Linezolid

CORYNEFORM BACTERIA

Definition
The term coryneform bacteria is currently used to describe Gram-positive, non-sporing, rod-shaped, pleomorphic organisms commonly referred to as diphtheroids [**1**,**2**].

This heterogeneous group has a wide distribution in nature and is of considerable importance to the dermatologist. It includes the aerobic cutaneous *Corynebacterium* species (among which *C. diphtheriae* is most well-known), *Brevibacterium*, *Arcanobacterium* and *Actinomyces* species, as well as the anaerobic but aerotolerant *Cutibacterium* species (formerly *Propionibacterium*) [3,4] (Box 26.3).

Box 26.3 Coryneform bacteria

Human commensals or pathogens

Aerobic
- *Corynebacterium diphtheriae* – primarily throat
- *C. ulcerans*
- *C. pseudotuberculosis*
- *C. striatum*
- *C. pseudodiphtheriticum*
- *C. minutissimum*
- *C. jeikeium*
- *C. propinquum*
- *C. amycolatum*
- *C. urealyticum*
- *Arcanobacterium* (formerly *Corynebacterium*) *haemolyticum*
- *Brevibacterium epidermidis*

Anaerobic (aerotolerant)
- *Cutibacterium* (formerly *Propionibacterium*) *acnes* – primarily follicular
- *Truperella* (formerly *Corynebacterium*) *pyogenes* – primarily skin
- *Cutibacterium granulosum*
- *Cutibacterium avidum*

Box 26.4 Diseases caused by *Corynebacterium*

- Diphtheria
- Erythrasma
- Trichomycosis axillaris
- Pitted keratolysis

Introduction and general description

Many different species of aerobic coryneform bacteria may be isolated from the normal human skin. Their classification remains unsatisfactory, but attempts to divide them into a six-species complex on the basis of obligate lipophilicity, glucose fermentation, tyrosine clearance and nitrate reduction provides some clarity [1]. Taxonomic advances have resulted in the renaming and reclassification of several species [4]. Apart from *Corynebacterium* species, it is now clear that *Brevibacterium* species, non-lipophilic coryneform organisms, can be isolated regularly from most human skin, especially the toe clefts [2]. It is generally accepted that trichomycosis axillaris and erythrasma are caused by an overgrowth of resident coryneforms, and there are grounds for suggesting that one of the organisms involved in pitted keratolysis is also a resident coryneform (Box 26.4). In trichomycosis, a variety of different strains of aerobic coryneforms have been implicated, not a single species (*Corynebacterium tenuis*) as originally thought. In erythrasma, the term *Corynebacterium minutissimum* is still used, but it is probably wise to recognise that this label implies a species complex of fluorescent aerobic coryneforms capable of initiating, alone or with others, the characteristic scaling and pigmentary changes of that condition. As with so many other skin microorganisms, corynebacteria have also become resistant to many antibiotics [5]. *Corynebacterium jeikeium*, *Corynebacterium amycolatum* and *Corynebacterium urealyticum* are highly resistant to most antimicrobial agents, and these organisms are regularly found on the skin and mucous membranes. They may be associated with systemic infections, particularly in patients with catheters or those who are immunosuppressed [6]. Carriage of these organisms occurs on many different skin sites, especially the perineal area, suggesting that the antibiotic resistance originates in the gastrointestinal tract and then passes to the skin [6].

Diphtheria

Definition

This is an acute disease caused by toxin-producing strains of *Corynebacterium diphtheriae*. Two other zoonotic species (*Corynebacterium ulcerans* and *Corynebacterium pseudotuberculosis*) may also produce toxin and lead to the condition. Currently many diphtheria cases recorded are caused by *C. ulcerans* [1]. A milder form of the condition can result from non-toxin-producing *C. diphtheriae*. While classically diphtheria is a throat and systemic infection, isolated skin infections, cutaneous diphtheria, are seen.

Epidemiology

Incidence and prevalence

C. diphtheriae is widespread, especially in the tropics, but outbreaks in more temperate climates are not uncommon. The infection is typically spread from affected cases or carriers via nasopharyngeal secretions. Generally, the rates of infection are considerably less in individuals receiving adequate courses of immunisation, and where infections occur they are usually less severe in these groups than in the non-immunised [2]. It is likely that widespread immunisation programmes have been in part responsible for the decreased incidence of diphtheria. When immunisation coverage is reduced, outbreaks of diphtheria re-emerge, as in the former Soviet Union countries in the late 1990s [3]. One interesting observation is that isolates of *C. diphtheriae* from immunised subjects are less likely to be toxigenic than those from the non-immunised.

Cutaneous diphtheria is rarely reported in temperate climates, but the diagnosis is easily overlooked [4]. An outbreak occurred in Vancouver, Canada, in all numbering 44 cases. Another report from northern Canada has stressed the persistence of diphtheria in spite of high immunisation rates, and the more frequent isolation of *C. diphtheriae* from Native Americans than from other ethnic groups [5]. In the tropics, especially where hygiene standards are low, the infection is more readily established in pre-existing skin lesions, and in the southern USA cutaneous infections have been shown to be significant in the epidemiology of diphtheria, particularly in poor communities [6]. In the UK, 17 cases of cutaneous diphtheria reported from 1995 to 2002 were all travel related [7]. It has also been seen in pig handlers [8].

Age
All ages.

Sex
Both sexes.

Pathophysiology

The diphtheria toxin consists of two fragments: the A polypeptide, which is the active segment, and the B fragment, which binds to cell surface receptors. The A segment inactivates transfer RNA translocase, preventing protein synthesis. Strains of *C. diphtheriae* differ in toxigenicity, and those isolated from chronic skin lesions often produce little toxin. All strains are lysogenic for temperate phages: strains which lose their phage lose their ability to produce toxin. As the toxin inhibits cellular protein synthesis, this results in local tissue destruction and the formation of the pseudomembrane. Haematological spread of the toxin is responsible for the potential complications, most commonly myocarditis and neuritis.

The association of *C. diphtheriae* with yaws in the Pacific area is statistically significant and suggests that the lesions produced by the spirochaete may provide particularly suitable conditions for colonisation by diphtheria. Colonisation of skin lesions by a strain of low virulence may not modify their morphology or produce any remote toxic effects. Such strains may provide a sufficiently strong antigenic stimulus for immunity to develop. A toxigenic strain induces local necrotic changes and systemic effects.

Causative organisms
- *C. diphtheriae*.
- *C. ulcerans*.
- *C. pseudotuberculosis*.

Clinical features [4,5]
Presentation
The typical early lesion is a superficial ulcer, rounded, oval or irregularly linear, with a clearly defined, overhanging edge.

Exudate from the ulcer floor tends to form a tough grey or brownish grey, adherent membrane. Later, the ulcer may deepen, and its edge become rolled, raised and avascular. There may be moderate enlargement of the regional lymph nodes. In temperate climates, the lesions occur most commonly at the umbilicus, behind the ears, in the genito-crural flexures, in a toe cleft or in a finger or toe, where a whitlow may be simulated. They may, however, develop in any pre-existing skin lesion and in the tropics commonly complicate such conditions as desert sores. The diagnosis may be suspected in persistent ulcers with an adherent membrane.

A rare clinical form has been described in children with eczema: varicelliform vesicles or pustules are succeeded by diphtheritic ulcers. For this reason the role of *C. diphtheriae* in the pathogenesis of skin lesions has been questioned, particularly as other potentially pathogenic bacteria, such as staphylococci and streptococci, may be present [4].

Clinical variants
Faucial diphtheria may be associated with adherent haemorrhagic crusts around the nose and mouth.

Differential diagnosis
In many cases, the lesions are less distinctive and may simulate impetigo or ecthyma.

Complications and co-morbidities
Systemic manifestations are characteristically absent or mild in cutaneous diphtheria, but are occasionally severe, especially in infants. In all forms, neurological complications, on which the retrospective diagnosis of diphtheria is sometimes based, occur in some 30% of cases and myocarditis in 5–10%.

Disease course and prognosis
Cutaneous diphtheria may persist for 6–12 weeks, healing with scar formation.

Investigations
Swabs should be sent for culture; if a pseudomembrane is present the swab should be taken from under the membrane. The toxigenicity can be determined using the Elek test or PCR testing for the *rpoB* gene and the A-subunit of the *tox* gene, and this should be performed by the national reference laboratory.

Management
Specific antitoxin should be administered to confirmed or probable cases of diphtheria in a hospital setting. A dose of 20 000–50 000 units should be given intramuscularly. Macrolides and benzylpenicillin are the antibiotics of choice and are required alongside the antitoxin. Antibiotic treatment should be given for 14 days and elimination of the organism confirmed microbiologically. The subsequent management will depend on whether there is neurological or cardiac involvement, and will be facilitated if the toxigenicity of the infecting strain can be established. With cutaneous disease the risk of significant toxin absorption is low, so the benefits of diphtheria antitoxin must be weighed against the risks. Antibiotic therapy, again with macrolides or benzylpenicillin, is required and thorough cleaning of the wound should be performed. Cases should be isolated in hospital for at least the first 24 h of antibiotic treatment or have restricted contact in the community. All cases should be immunised once stable as infection does not always induce adequate levels of anti-toxin. The disease is notifiable to public health authorities and management of close contacts is important to prevent onward transmission. Close contacts should self-monitor for disease and be excluded from work in high-risk occupations (e.g. health and social care workers), be swabbed for asymptomatic carriage, receive 7 days of a macrolide or a single intramuscular dose of benzylpenicillin and be immunised [9].

Erythrasma

Definition
Erythrasma is a mild chronic localised superficial infection of the skin caused by a group of closely related aerobic coryneform bacteria, usually known as *C. minutissimum*. It is a common disease affecting the axillae, groins and toe webs which may be symptom free or show mild discomfort and itching.

Epidemiology
The epidemiology of erythrasma has not been fully elucidated. There seems to be little doubt that the organisms responsible are

frequently members of the normal flora, at least in the toe clefts, and that some shift in the host–parasite relationship results in the development of classical erythrasma [1].

Age
Clinical infection may occur at any age but is more common among adults than children.

Sex
Both sexes.

Associated diseases
Erythrasma may be the presenting feature in patients with diabetes [1].

Pathophysiology
Predisposing factors
Excessive sweating, obesity, poor hygiene and advancing age may predispose individuals to the condition. Individuals living in institutions (college dormitories, army barracks, nursing homes) are more likely to develop erythrasma [2].

Pathology
It is now recognised that the Gram-positive rods and filaments found in the scales of erythrasma are coryneforms. Among normal populations, mild toe cleft scaling with pink fluorescence is common. Clinically important infections of the groins are much less frequent and those of the axilla are even more uncommon. A more generalised form of erythrasma (also described as disciform) can occur on the trunk.

Causative organisms
The name *C. minutissimum* has been given to the organisms, but possibly more than one species may be involved.

Environmental factors
A warm humid climate is a predisposing factor.

Clinical features
History
This is generally a chronic disease which presents in the groins or axillae (Figure 26.21). Erythrasma, as detected by Wood's light examination, involves the toe clefts more frequently than any other site (Figure 26.22).

Presentation
As clinically manifest lesions, erythrasma occurs most commonly in the groins, axillae and the intergluteal and submammary flexures. The patches are of irregular shape and sharply marginated, at first red, but later becoming brown. New lesions are smooth, but older lesions tend to be finely creased or obviously scaly. In the generalised form, the sharply marginated, reddish brown plaques may cover extensive areas of the trunk and limbs.

In temperate climates most lesions are symptomless, but in the tropics, particularly, irritation of the lesions in the groins may lead to scratching and lichenification. Involvement of the perianal skin may present as pruritus ani, of which erythrasma is an uncommon cause.

Clinical variants
Toe cleft infections are often asymptomatic; the scaling, fissuring and maceration that may be present are not necessarily caused by the corynebacteria. Rarely, *C. minutissimum* has been associated

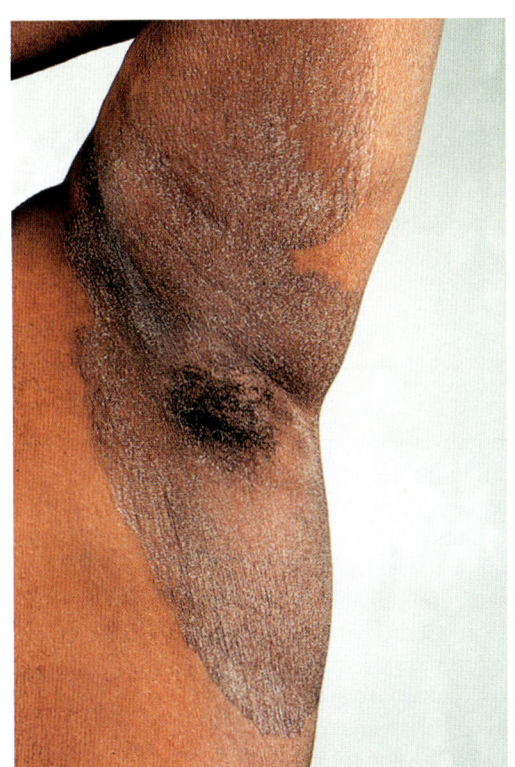
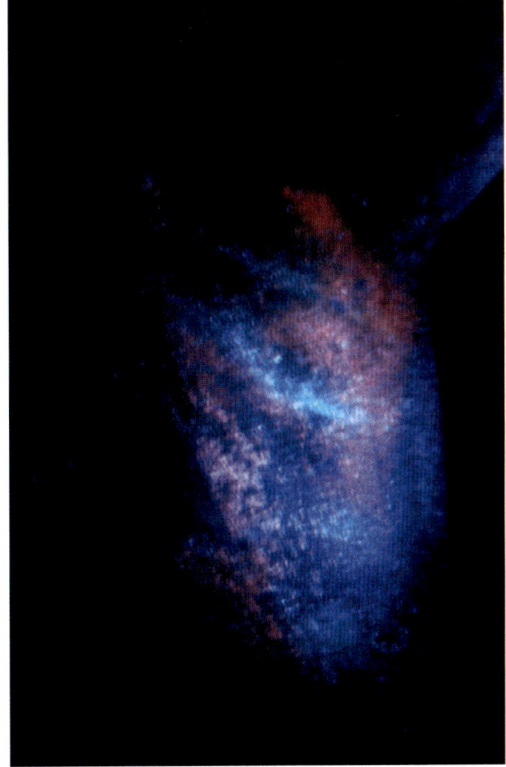

Figure 26.21 (a) Erythrasma in the axilla. Courtesy of St John's Institute of Dermatology. (b) Fluorescence with Wood's light. Courtesy of King's College London. (a) (b)

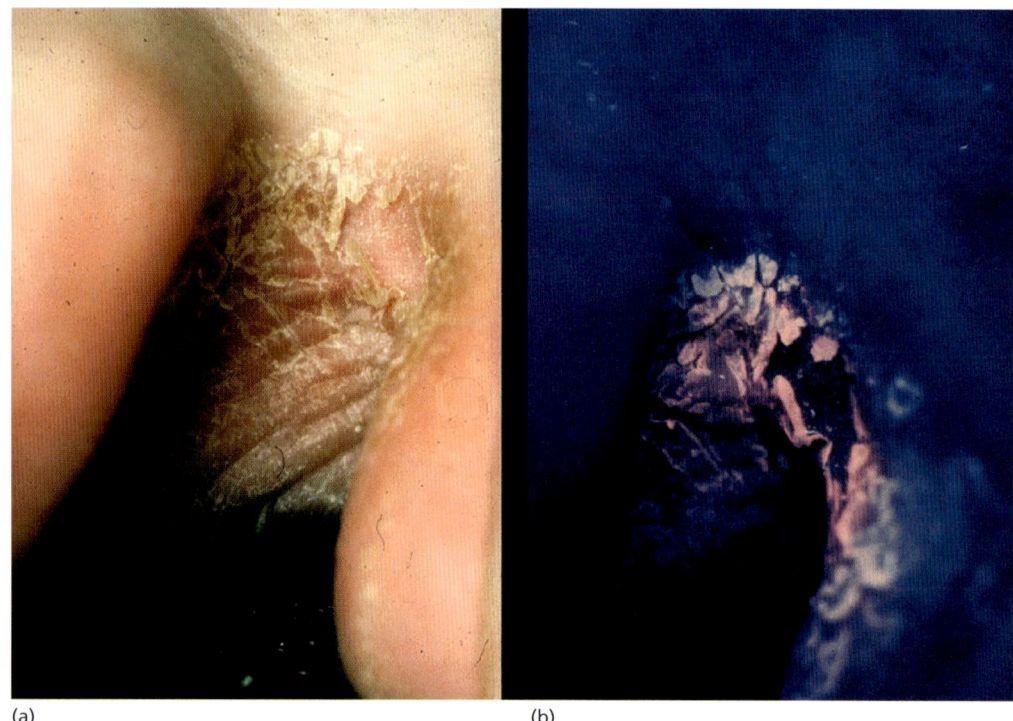

Figure 26.22 (a,b) Erythrasma of the toe cleft. (b) Fluorescence with Wood's light. Courtesy of King's College London.

with systemic disease, such as recurrent abscesses or endocarditis in immunocompromised individuals [3].

Differential diagnosis
Pityriasis versicolor is most commonly confused with erythrasma, but it occurs predominantly on the upper trunk, and the individual lesions are small and are not red. On the thighs, groins and pubic area, tinea cruris may be simulated, but the relative lack of inflammation, complete absence of vesiculation and absence of satellite lesions point against tinea. It is difficult to differentiate erythrasma of the toe clefts from tinea pedis or *Candida* infection, but, as in all varieties of erythrasma, the presence of coral-red fluorescence under Wood's light is diagnostic. Since many patients have both tinea pedis and erythrasma, mycological examination of scales is important. Flexural psoriasis is an important differential that may need to be excluded.

Disease course and prognosis
Chronic without treatment.

Investigations
Coral-red fluorescence with Wood's light is attributable to coproporphyrin III and strongly suggests erythrasma, although it does not necessarily indicate active infection. The persistence of fluorescence after eradication of the coryneforms may depend on the thickness of the horny layer, as it is common at the margins of the toe webs. Pink fluorescence is also demonstrable in some necrotic tumours and on the normal tongue, where it is not apparently caused by coryneforms. It is seen in the follicular openings of the normal skin of the face and the upper trunk, where corynebacteria or cutibacteria are the likely cause. In the groins and axillae, acanthosis nigricans may fluoresce a brilliant pink colour, presumably due to heavy colonisation with fluorescent coryneforms, although other bacteria may show pink fluorescence. Scrapings from the affected skin may show bacteria if stained with Gram or Giemsa or even with simple potassium hydroxide clearance. Cultural confirmation is not necessary as the clinical appearance is typical and Wood's light examination of the patient shows the characteristic changes.

Management
Without treatment the condition tends to persist indefinitely, although there may be spontaneous fluctuations in severity. Although several treatments have been recommended for erythrasma, there are no studies comparing their effectiveness [4].

Erythrasma responds well to most topically applied azole antifungal agents, such as clotrimazole and miconazole [5]. The duration of therapy varies, but 2 weeks is usually sufficient. For more extensive lesions, erythromycin is probably the most effective treatment. Alternatives include topical fucidin and oral tetracycline. Good results have also been reported with a single dose of 1 g clarithromycin [6]. Relapse is a problem in some patients. In these cases the usual approach adopted is to give long-term antiseptics, such as povidone–iodine, and to use drying agents, such as powders, in the affected areas.

Treatment ladder for erythrasma

First line
- Topical azole antifungal
- Erythromycin

Second line
- Tetracyclines
- Clarithromycin

Trichomycosis axillaris

Definition and nomenclature
This is a superficial infection of axillary hairs with the formation of adherent granular nodules or concretions, which can be yellow, black or red in colour, on the hair shaft. These are commonly malodourous. The term 'trichomycosis' is misleading as the causative agents are bacteria not fungi [1]. It is important to distinguish trichomycosis axillaris from trichomycosis nodosa or Piedra.

Synonyms and inclusions
- Trichobacteriosis

Epidemiology
Trichomycosis is a common but underrecognised condition.

Age
Uncommon before puberty as the infection generally affects axillary and pubic hair.

Sex
No specific sex predilection. However, probably less frequently seen in females due to removal of axillary hair.

Pathophysiology
Pathology
Studies using transmission and scanning electron microscopy [2] have shown that the concretions consist almost exclusively of tightly packed bacteria. They grow within and between the cuticular cells and may invade the cortex [2].

Causative organisms
Several species of *Corynebacterium* have been implicated including *C. flavescens* (most common), *C. propinquum* and *C. tenuis*. These biotypes probably reflect the range of resident coryneform types in the normal axilla. It has been shown that changes in the chemical environment of these organisms may induce pigment production, perhaps explaining the different colours of the nodules, which are not attributable to different bacterial strains [3].

Environmental factors
More common in hot and humid environments.

Clinical features
History
It is usually asymptomatic and the patient is often unaware of its presence. Some patients complain of malodour.

Presentation
Yellow, black or red concretions are present on the hair shaft and these may be hard, or soft and nodular, or more diffuse. In the nodular varieties, the hair may be brittle and easily broken [2]. The underlying skin is normal. The axillary sweat may be yellow, black or red according to the colour of the concretions, and the clothing may be stained. The yellow type is the most common. The few figures available on the prevalence of trichomycosis show it to be common. Axillary infection was present in 27% of adult male students in one UK survey, and in 42% of male patients but only 7% of women patients in a hospital setting [4]. Pubic infection is less common but can occur [5].

Differential diagnosis
Pediculosis pubis, which may affect axillary as well as pubic hair, and piedra should be considered. Examination under Wood's light is helpful. Microscopical confirmation of the diagnosis is desirable.

Complications
Trichomycosis axillaris is a benign condition with no associated complications.

Disease course and prognosis
Chronic but fluctuates in severity.

Investigations
Potassium hydroxide mounts show the bacteria as narrow bacillary organisms in the yellow or red concretions. They are Gram positive. For culture, the hairs must be surface sterilised, and this may be done by immersion in 70% alcohol. Incubation at 37°C in blood agar is recommended. Light and ultrastructural studies, together with various stains, have shown that a variety of coryneforms adhere to the hair shaft and some are encapsulated in an extracellular encasing. This was thought to be an analogue of glucan synthesised by streptococci and responsible for the adhesion [6].

Management
Removal of hair from affected areas is the most efficient treatment option. Topical antibiotics such as clindamycin are effective. The use of an antiperspirant such as aluminium chloride is an effective way to reduce sweating, creating a less favourable environment. Antiseptics such as benzyl peroxide are useful for treatment and prevention [7].

Pitted keratolysis

Definition and nomenclature
A superficial infection of the skin apparently caused by various species of *Corynebacterium* and producing circular erosions on the soles [1–3].

Synonyms and inclusions
- Keratolysis plantare sulcatum

Epidemiology
There are few studies of the prevalence of the condition. However, it is felt to be a common condition; it occurs in barefoot populations in the tropics as well as more familiarly in the context of occlusive footwear and hyperhidrosis. Military personnel, farmers and athletes appear to be more at risk of the condition [4].

Age
All ages.

Sex
More commonly seen in males [4].

Pathophysiology
Pathology
Pits and erosions in the keratin of the soles or palms with minimal inflammation.

Causative organisms
Various bacterial species have been identified in this condition; *Corynebacterium* ssp. are most commonly isolated but others include *Dermatophilus congolensis*, *Kytococcus sedentarius* and *Actinomyces keratolytica*. The bacteria are thought to invade the keratin when it is softened by sweat [1–3].

Clinical features (Figure 26.23)
History
There are numerous superficial erosions of the horny layer of the soles and the undersurfaces of the toes.

Presentation
All parts of both soles may be affected, but pressure-bearing or friction areas are most commonly affected. Conspicuous, discrete, shallow, circular lesions with a punched-out appearance coalesce in places to produce irregular erosions. There is occasionally green or brown discoloration of the horny layer. Hyperhidrosis is often associated, sometimes with maceration, stickiness and a foul odour [4,5]. Soaking the feet in water for 15 min causes swelling of the horny layer and accentuates the lesions. Pain, irritation and/or a burning sensation are commonly described [4].

Clinical variants
Similar changes affecting the palms have been described rarely [6].

Differential diagnosis
The lesions are easily recognisable, but tinea pedis should be considered.

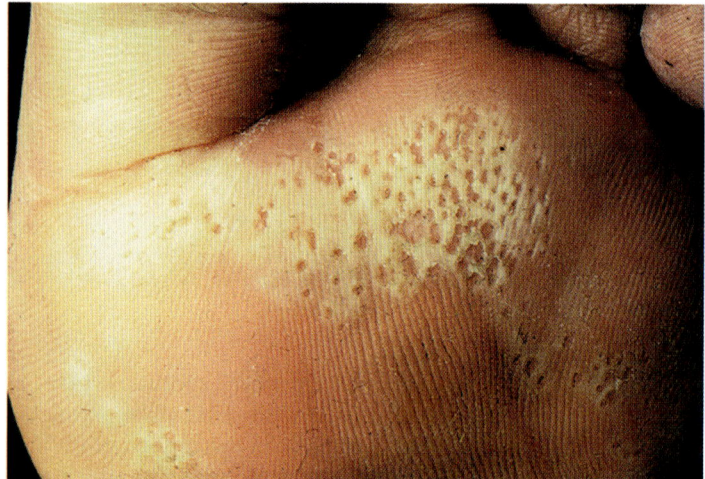

Figure 26.23 Pitted keratolysis. Courtesy of St John's Institute of Dermatology.

Investigations
Generally, this condition is diagnosed by its clinical appearance.

Histology
A mixture of bacillary bacteria and filamentous microorganisms may be seen in abundance in the most superficial parts of the stratum corneum and extending downwards between keratinocytes. There is associated lysis of the keratin.

Laboratory identification
The organisms are not always easy to find in potassium hydroxide mounts but are more easily detected in Gram-stained scrapings. Culture can be performed. However, given the existing confusion over the identity of the causative species, it is generally not a useful diagnostic process.

Management
Measures to promote foot hygiene, such as wearing cotton socks, which are changed frequently and appropriately laundered, and avoiding long periods in occlusive footwear help to manage the condition. Treatment of hyperhidrosis slowly brings the condition under control including potassium permanganate soaks, aluminium chloride and iontophoresis.

First line
A more rapid response may be obtained with fucidin ointment. Other topical antibiotics and imidazoles such as clotrimazole are reputed to be effective [1].

Second line
Botulinum toxin which reduces the hyperhidrosis has been helpful [7].

ARCANOBACTERIUM HAEMOLYTICUM INFECTION

Infection with this Gram-positive bacillus (formerly known as *Corynebacterium haemolyticum*) [1] usually affects the throat and may be associated with a maculopapular rash. Patients usually present with sore throats, mild to moderate in severity with little malaise or fever, and approximately half the patients developed a maculopapular rash [1,2]. The rash, consisting of red papules, typically starts distally and spreads to affect the trunk with sparing of the face, palms and soles. In immunocompromised patients, it may cause a diphtheria-like infection and septicaemia. Cutaneous infections can present as ulcers, abscesses or cellulitis and can result in osteomyelitis. Co-infection with other Gram-positive bacteria such as staphylococci and streptococci is common [3]. Lepromatous ulcers are frequently colonised with these organisms [4]. The organism produces soluble toxins including sphingomyelinase D and phospholipase D, which contribute to its virulence. The swab needs to be cultured on 5% human blood agar for isolation and identification [1]. The diagnosis may be missed if there is co-infection with streptococci because *Arcanobacterium* haemolyse more slowly [3]. *Arcanobacterium* are sensitive to many antibiotics and treatment with appropriate antibiotics is effective.

TRUEPERELLA PYOGENES INFECTION

Trueperella pyogenes (previously known as *Actinomyces* or *Corynebacterium pyogenes*) is an animal pathogen but there are reports of purulent lesions, abscesses and leg ulcers with this bacterium as well as endocarditis, pneumonia and sepsis [1]. Outbreaks of skin ulceration have been documented in Thailand [2]. The clinical appearances of lesions closely resemble those seen with other forms of pyoderma including tropical ulcers. The mode of transmission of the infection has not been established but may involve flies or ectoparasites.

CUTIBACTERIUM (FORMERLY PROPIONIBACTERIUM)

Cutibacterium (previously known as *Propionibacterium*) [1] are anaerobic, but aerotolerant, coryneforms of the resident normal flora. These Gram-positive pleomorphic bacilli are found in large numbers and are widely distributed over the whole skin.

Though historically all termed *Corynebacterium acnes*, it is now recognised that they are more properly classified as *Cutibacterium* and may be divided into three main species. *C. acnes* and *C. granulosum* are found predominantly in the pilosebaceous follicles of those sites where sebum is plentiful, and *C. avidum* is mainly isolated from moist intertriginous zones [2].

From its location, it is unlikely that *C. avidum* has any part in the causation of acne. The importance of *C. acnes* and *C. granulosum* in acne is considered in Chapter 90. Recently, the genomic sequence of a bacteriophage of *C. acnes* has been characterised [3].

In addition to its association with acne, *C. acnes* is capable of biofilm formation [4] and has been isolated from cases of prosthetic valve endocarditis, prosthetic joint infection, postoperative endophthalmitis and shunt infections [5]. It has also been proposed as a cause of indolent scalp folliculitis [6].

BACILLUS

Bacillus anthracis is a Gram-positive encapsulated organism which can survive as spores for over 20 years in soil and is the cause of anthrax. Rarely, other species of the genus *Bacillus*, predominantly *B. cereus*, may cause deep subcutaneous infections resembling necrotising fasciitis, a variety of different infections of the eye ranging from conjunctivitis to panophthalmitis, food poisoning and systemic diseases [1,2].

Anthrax [1,2]

Definition
Anthrax is a zoonotic infection with *B. anthracis*. It is primarily an infection of herbivorous animals, but occasional outbreaks occur in other species and infection in humans is seen.

Epidemiology
Animals are infected by ingesting the spores. *B. anthracis* spores are able to survive in soil for decades. In endemic areas (Africa, central Asia, Middle East and South America) animal infections, and hence human infections, are still a serious problem [3]. Only occasional cases are seen in other areas, and these sporadic cases are easily overlooked as the diagnosis is not considered [4]. In endemic areas, humans are infected directly from animals or animal products, and male adults are most at risk, but in some rural communities children minding cattle may be infected. There are no known cases of human-to-human spread.

Anthrax often follows occupational exposure during care of livestock or the handling of products. In western Europe, most cases of anthrax formerly occurred among workers in the wool, hair or bristle industries, or those handling animal materials imported from India, Pakistan or Africa. In many countries, stricter codes of practice for hygiene in the workplace resulted in a decline even in sporadic infections. Unsterilised imported bone meal, or sacks contaminated with it, remains a potential hazard, although warning labels on this product appear to be effective in reducing the danger still further. It has also been associated with the injection of heroin, thought to be contaminated with the organism [5].

Age
All ages.

Sex
Both sexes.

Associated diseases
Deliberate and accidental dissemination of anthrax spores has been recorded resulting in both respiratory and cutaneous forms of anthrax. For this reason, *B. anthracis* is classified as a weapon of bioterrorism and handling is subject to regulation in many countries [6].

Pathophysiology
Pathology
Human resistance to infection is normally high. Cutaneous inoculation is favoured by minor trauma or pre-existing skin lesions. However, hair follicles may also provide a portal of entry to the organism [7]. Pulmonary and intestinal forms result from the inhalation or ingestion of spores. Disseminated disease involves massive bacteraemia and is often fatal; it can occur irrespective of the portal of entry. The anthrax bacillus induces an inflammatory tissue response in which haemorrhage and necrosis are associated with a gelatinous oedema, which contains large amounts of bacterial capsular material.

Causative organisms
B. anthracis is present in large numbers in skin lesions and in the blood in systemic infections. The major virulence factors are the binary exotoxins, oedema and lethal toxins, which are encoded on two virulence plasmids pX01 and pX02. Oedema toxin, calmodulin-dependent adenylate cyclase A, is known to inhibit neutrophil function, and is responsible for the oedema which develops locally, and lethal toxin, a zinc metalloprotease, is an inhibitor

of mitogen-activated protein kinase kinases. It leads to stimulation of macrophages to release TNF-α and IL-1β, which are in part responsible for sudden death in systemic disease [2].

Environmental factors
Presence of infected animal vectors (e.g. sheep, goats, cattle).

Clinical features [1,2]
History
The lesion of cutaneous anthrax follows after introduction of endospores into the skin. The exposed skin, especially the face, neck, hands or arms, are affected most often. There may be a single lesion or multiple lesions. Although sometimes referred to as the 'malignant pustule', the lesion is not purulent and is often relatively painless.

Presentation
After an incubation period of typically 5–7 days, an irritable papule develops at the site of inoculation. A bulla on an inflamed, oedematous base soon follows. The bulla ruptures and forms a haemorrhagic crust around which is a zone of oedema (Figure 26.24) in which may be several small vesicles. The surrounding tissues are oedematous, and although the regional lymphatic glands may be tender, their involvement is slight in relation to the severity of the lesion and lymphangitis is unusual. In some cases, particularly when the face is involved, malignant oedema, characterised by severe swelling, induration and multiple bullae, may develop, and the localised pustule is inconspicuous or absent. The clinical picture is very variable and purely or predominantly bullous lesions have been reported.

Constitutional symptoms may begin 3 or 4 days after the onset of the pustule. Anthrax meningitis is a rare complication of cutaneous disease. Overall, the mortality of untreated cutaneous anthrax is between 5% and 20%, but most cases are mild and healing follows in 2–3 weeks. Severe oedema or toxaemia is of poor prognostic significance. With early and adequate antibiotic treatment, all cases are curable.

Clinical variants
Anthrax may also cause respiratory, oropharyngeal and gastrointestinal disease. In the respiratory type, mild prodromal symptoms (myalgia, malaise, fever) lasting around 4 days are followed by progressive respiratory symptoms including severe dyspnoea and shock. The gastrointestinal type may follow ingestion of endospore-contaminated meat from infected animals. Symptoms include haematemesis and diarrhoea with abdominal pain. Oesophageal involvement may give rise to dysphagia, local adenopathy and marked swelling of the neck [4].

Differential diagnosis
Staphylococcal infection, vaccinia, ecthyma gangrenosum, cat scratch disease (formerly named para-anthrax), blastomycosis and sporotrichosis may need exclusion. Both staphylococcal infections and pox infections (e.g. orf) can simulate anthrax very closely. Both may show the central black haemorrhagic crust and the zone of oedema. The history, rapid course, clinical appearance and lack of lymphangitis should suggest the diagnosis, which must be confirmed by bacteriological examination [5].

Disease course and prognosis
In severe untreated cases, malaise, high fever, toxaemia and prostration may be followed by delirium, collapse and death.

Investigations
Chains of Gram-positive bacilli can be seen in smears of lesions. Swabs should be taken from vesicle fluid or the base of lesions (under any eschar) and sent for culture and PCR testing. Biopsies should also be taken from any skin lesions for both histopathology and culture. Blood cultures are usually positive in systemic disease, although treatment should not be withheld while awaiting bacteriology results, as rapid deterioration may result in death. A lumbar puncture should be performed if there is any concern regarding systemic involvement. A serological test to the capsular antigens and exotoxin components is available, and a rising antibody titre to the protective and capsular antigens is indicative of recent infection or vaccination. However, these tests have little value in the acute illness. An anthraxin skin test may be suitable for the retrospective analysis of anthrax infections [1].

Management [1,2]
Treatment should not be withheld until bacteriological confirmation has been obtained.

In systemic anthrax or cutaneous lesions affecting the head or neck, treatment should include at least two agents, one with bactericidal activity against *B. anthracis* and a protein synthesis

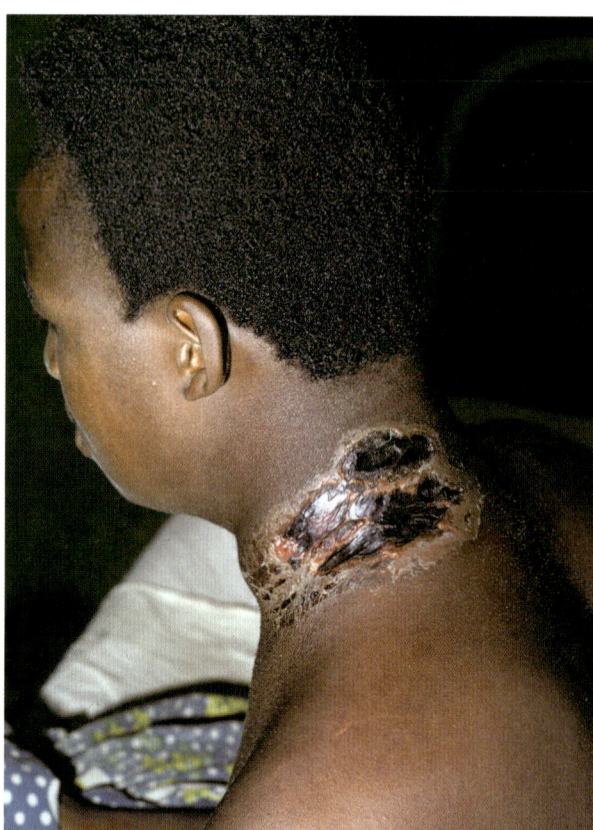

Figure 26.24 Anthrax. © D.A. Warrell.

inhibitor to suppress toxin production. Therapy should be given intravenously for at least 2 weeks and until clinically stable. Once the initial treatment phase is completed, the patient can be switched to a single oral agent for 60 days which is used to prevent relapse from surviving spores. Fluoroquinolones or doxycycline combined with macrolides, clindamycin, carbapenems, penicillins, chloramphenicol and rifampicin are all potential treatment options, but it is important to ensure susceptibility if relying on penicillins as *B. anthracis* possesses β-lactamase genes.

For cutaneous anthrax lesions without systemic involvement, monotherapy with either a fluoroquinolone or tetracycline for 14 days should be sufficient but the course should be extended to 60 days if exposure was due to aerosol.

Three anthrax anti-toxin antibody preparations have received approval from the Food and Drug Administration (FDA) but these are not yet routinely used in practice [8].

Vaccination gives some protection [9] and should be offered to those who are exposed in the course of their occupations, but prevention should be directed primarily at control of the disease in animals and disinfection of animal products. Prophylaxis for asymptomatic patients exposed to anthrax spores includes a 6-week course of doxycycline or ciprofloxacin.

Anthrax is a notifiable disease and therefore steps must be taken to inform the public health department when there is clinical or laboratory suspicion of anthrax.

Treatment ladder for cutaneous anthrax without systemic involvement

First line
- Ciprofloxacin
- Doxycycline

Second line
- Clindamycin
- Amoxicillin (if penicillin susceptible)

LISTERIA MONOCYTOGENES

Listeria monocytogenes is a Gram-positive microaerophilic motile bacillus easily confused with coryneform organisms. It can survive low temperatures and will grow at 4°C. It is a facultative intracellular pathogen, inducing its own uptake into non-phagocytic cells, and spreads from cell to cell by an actin-based motility process. In addition, most strains express internalin A, a protein required for invasion of host cells [1]. It is the cause of listeriosis.

Listeriosis

Epidemiology
Listeriosis is an uncommon cause of skin signs and symptoms. The organism is found in water and soil, and has been isolated from sewage sludge and inferior silage [2]. It infects wild, domestic and laboratory animals, and direct infection from cattle and sheep is a hazard to veterinary surgeons and farmers [3]. However, listeriosis is mainly a food-borne disease, and milk, cheese and poultry are the main sources of human disease [4].

Age
All ages but more common in neonates or older age groups.

Sex
Both sexes.

Pathophysiology
Predisposing factors
Most cases of listerial infections occur in individuals with predisposing conditions which include pregnancy, glucocorticoid therapy and other immunocompromising conditions.

Pathology
Transmission is by ingestion of or contact with contaminated products. Transplacental and birth canal infections are a well-recognised hazard to the fetus and neonate [5]. Infection of a baby from the mother's milk has been reported [6]. Otherwise, direct transfer from human to human does not seem to occur. However, *L. monocytogenes* may be carried asymptomatically in the human gut as well as the cervix and vagina, at least for short periods, so the potential for transfer of infection does exist.

Causative organisms
- *L. monocytogenes*.

Environmental factors
General and soil, but also milk, milk products and processed meats.

Clinical features [7]
History
Although most cases of listeriosis are sporadic, there have been several outbreaks reported over the past 10 years. Most adult infections are now thought to be subclinical, but a mild febrile illness with gastrointestinal symptoms and loin pain may occur in otherwise healthy individuals. More serious infections with a meningitis or glandular fever-like illness are well known and in immunocompromised patients, meningitis or pneumonia may dominate the picture.

Presentation
Cutaneous lesions are uncommon in these cases, but when present are purpuric. During pregnancy, an indeterminate febrile illness, not necessarily severe, may occur. This may not arouse any suspicions, but the fetus may be aborted or the infant may be stillborn or premature. Neonates may develop a combination of respiratory and gastrointestinal symptoms with granulomas of the posterior pharynx, generalised redness and dark red or bluish papules, especially on the trunk and leg. Meningitis and septicaemia may be seen later in the neonatal period [8].

Clinical variants
In veterinary surgeons, a mild predominantly cutaneous form of the disease may occur 1–3 days after contact with an infected animal [3]. Fever and malaise are followed after a day or so by an

eruption of discrete dull-red papules, some of which later show central pustulation.

Differential diagnosis
Acute febrile conditions such as meningococcal infections presenting with purpura.

Disease course and prognosis
In serious adult infections, in the immunocompromised patient and in the neonate, the prognosis is poor without treatment, at least 30% of cases being fatal [1].

Investigations
As there are no specific clinical features, the diagnosis will be missed unless it is borne in mind in unexplained fevers, glandular fever-like illness and meningitis. As the incubation period can be quite long (6–8 weeks) mild symptoms may be forgotten. In those at risk through occupation, or predisposing states, the diagnosis is established by blood culture and, if a high index of suspicion towards diphtheroids is maintained, through isolation from other sites. The organism grows easily on blood or nutrient agar but cold enrichment may help.

Management
First line
The drug of choice is ampicillin or amoxycillin, but the organism is also susceptible to penicillin, erythromycin and tetracycline. Gentamicin may be used with ampicillin or penicillin, particularly in immunocompromised individuals, as synergism occurs.

Infection control
Prevention of contamination of foods is vital to reduce the number of outbreaks of listeriosis. Individuals at high risk of infection should be informed about cross-contamination of foods, thorough cooking of foods and storage of perishable foods [9].

ERYSIPELOTHRIX RHUSIOPATHIAE

Erysipelothrix rhusiopathiae is a Gram-positive rod. It is widespread in nature as a commensal or pathogen in a wide variety of animal species and is the cause of erysipeloid.

Erysipeloid [1–3]

Definition
Erysipeloid is an acute, rarely chronic, infection with *E. rhusiopathiae*. This is now a very rare infection mainly confined to the skin.

Epidemiology
The causative organism can persist in soil for many months, causing infection long after the contamination. It colonises a wide variety of animals worldwide, including mammals, birds, fish and shellfish, and causes disease in many of these, especially in pigs.

Age
Any age.

Sex
Both sexes.

Pathophysiology
Pathology
Human infection is contracted by direct contact, occasionally from living animals, but more commonly from carcasses, so that erysipeloid usually affects those working in slaughterhouses and the fishing industry, butchers, farmers and veterinary surgeons.

Causative organisms
E. rhusiopathiae: the existence of L forms might explain the occasional chronic or recurrent infections [1]. The organism, *E. rhusiopathiae*, produces a neuraminidase and a hyaluronidase, both of which are believed to be virulence determinants. The presence of a capsule may also aid the organism's survival.

Clinical features [1–4]
History
Three clinical syndromes have been distinguished in humans: localised cutaneous, which is the most common (erysipeloid of Rosenbach), generalised cutaneous and systemic, in which skin lesions may occur. Most human infections are localised and self-limiting.

Presentation
Following an incubation period of 2–7 days, a tender violaceous red rash develops around the inoculation site and extends centrifugally, but irregularly, with a sharp and sometimes gyrate border, which may be vesicular. Most lesions are on the hand, fingers or forearms, but any exposed area may be involved. Erysipeloid can occur following a cat or dog bite. Fever and mild constitutional symptoms such as arthralgia are present in only 10% of cases but up to 30% may have some local lymphangitis. Extension continues for 3 or 4 days, rarely for as long as a week, but the area eventually involved is seldom more than 10 cm in diameter. Without treatment, healing normally occurs spontaneously in 2 weeks without desquamation or suppuration.

Clinical variants
Diffuse cutaneous infection is rare, with progression of violaceous lesions proximally from the site of inoculation. Additional sites may also be involved. There may be systemic symptoms with fever and arthralgia most common, but blood cultures are typically negative. This form is also usually self-limiting, but runs a more protracted course with the possibility of recurrences.

Systemic infection with *E. rhusiopathiae* is uncommon but risk factors include immunosuppression, diabetes and chronic liver or kidney disease [5]. Cutaneous erysipeloid lesions are seen in around 40% of patients with systemic infection [2]. Ingestion of contaminated meat can result in systemic infection but cutaneous inoculation can also result in systemic disease. Endocarditis (usually affecting the aortic valve), joint, bone, brain and pleural involvement have been described. Congestive cardiac failure, myocardial abscesses and aortic valve perforation may follow. Patients are ill, lose weight and may show localised cutaneous swellings with central necrosis, or scattered perifollicular papules. Blood cultures are usually positive with appropriate techniques.

Differential diagnosis
Causes of cellulitis such as group A *Streptococcus* infections, although the lesions are seldom highly symptomatic and fever is often mild, if present.

Disease course and prognosis
Uncomplicated lesions resolve spontaneously.

Investigations
Culture
Blood cultures in systemic disease should confirm the diagnosis; historically *E. rhusiopathiae* may have been misinterpreted as *Lactobacillis* spp. or *Actinomyces* spp. However, MALDI-TOF (matrix-assisted laser desorption/ionisation-time of flight mass spectrometry) or PCR should now reduce this risk [6]. The diagnosis of the cutaneous disease is mainly clinical and is based on exposure risk, the violaceous colour of the lesions, and a subacute course with limited constitutional symptoms.

Pathology [4]
Cultures of deep biopsy material from the advancing edge of recent lesions occasionally yield the organism, which is Gram positive, non-motile and non-sporulating. However, cultures are often negative. Histology shows epidermal spongiosis or vesiculation, dermal oedema, lymphangitis, capillary engorgement and infiltration with neutrophils and eosinophils. Organisms have only rarely been detected by light microscopy. However, electron microscopy has demonstrated cell wall deficient bacteria (L forms), which may explain the difficulty of demonstrating the bacteria by conventional methods.

Management [1–4]
Most isolated skin lesions heal spontaneously in about 4 weeks. Healing is facilitated by antibiotic therapy. The organism is typically sensitive to penicillins, cephalosporins, fluoroquinolones and clindamycin. Tetracyclines and macrolides are potential treatment options but the sensitivity of the organism is variable. For severe or systemic infections, intravenous penicillin is required. As the organism may persist on environmental surfaces, thorough cleaning with antiseptics helps with decontamination (e.g. fishing boats etc.) [7].

The organism is resistant to vancomycin, which is often used as empirical therapy in endocarditis due to Gram–positive organisms.

> **Treatment ladder for erysipeloid**
>
> **First line**
> - Penicillin
> - Cephalosporins
> - Ciprofloxacin
>
> **Second line**
> - Clindamycin

CLOSTRIDIUM

The clostridia are anaerobic, Gram-positive, spore-forming bacilli, widely distributed in the soil and in the gastrointestinal tracts of humans and other mammals. They are the main causes of gas gangrene.

Gas gangrene (clostridial myonecrosis)

Definition and nomenclature
Gas gangrene is a clinical syndrome caused by the infection of wounds with various species of *Clostridium* [1,2] but most commonly *C. perfringens*. However, other clostridia are occasionally identified: *C. septicum*, *C. novyi* and *C. histolyticum* [3].

> **Synonyms and inclusions**
> - Clostridial myonecrosis

Introduction and general description
Gas gangrene is a potentially fatal infection if unrecognised. It mainly occurs when wounds are contaminated with soil or water after trauma [1,2]. Although localised, toxaemia can be very severe.

Epidemiology
C. perfringens can be isolated from the skin of the thighs, groins and buttocks of many healthy persons [1]. The infection can occur in any part of the world.

Age
Mainly in adults.

Sex
Both sexes.

Associated diseases
Trauma, especially following natural disasters or gunshot/knife wounds, orthopaedic or bowel surgery and obstetric complications.

Pathophysiology
Pathology
The α-toxin produced by *C. perfringens* is a zinc-containing molecule with phospholipase C and sphingomyelinase activity, which is haemolytic and thought to be the main virulence factor in gas gangrene [4]. The toxin has been shown to affect neutrophil migration, platelet aggregation and may also modulate host cell metabolism [4].

A high proportion of war wounds are contaminated by clostridial spores, but clinical infection usually develops only in the presence of severely damaged anoxic muscle. Gas gangrene used to be an infection of the greatest importance in war time; better management of casualties has reduced its incidence enormously. It is an uncommon but well-documented complication of orthopaedic surgery, particularly above-knee amputations in ischaemic limbs. In these latter patients, the organism usually originates in the patient's own bowel [1].

Causative organisms
The most important species of *Clostridium* involved are *C. perfringens*, *C. septicum*, *C. novyi* and *C. histolyticum*, but other species may also play a role [1]. Heroin used by drug users may be contaminated with *C. sordellii*, which may cause life-threatening myonecrosis and fulminant shock syndrome [2].

Environmental factors
Clostridium species may be found in soil, decaying vegetation and the human or animal gastrointestinal tract.

Clinical features
History
Traumatic gas gangrene typically presents with severe pain at the site of traumatic injury or surgery. The incubation period is often fewer than 24 hours but may be up to several days.

Presentation
Deep and dirty wounds in the muscular regions of the body are most susceptible. However, abdominal and intrauterine infections also occur. Oedema develops around the wound, continues to spread and is associated with pallor and mottling of the skin. The skin is described as having a bronzed appearance before becoming purpuric. The skin is exquisitely tender, often with overlying bullae and later with the formation of black sloughs. It is important to note that occasionally there is anaesthesia of the skin when there is destruction of underlying nerves [5]. Toxaemia is severe; tachycardia and prostration develop rapidly and the patient is pale but often not febrile [1], followed by shock and multiorgan failure. Crepitation from gas in the tissues is classical but inconstant.

Differential diagnosis
Necrotising fasciitis due to other pathogens (Figure 26.25).

Disease course and prognosis
There is a high mortality where diagnosis is delayed. Complications include renal failure and liver necrosis.

Investigations
A clinical diagnosis can be made based on the degree of pain at a site of traumatic injury with associated signs of systemic toxicity and the presence of gas in the deep tissues (which can be confirmed on CT or MRI scanning). Blood and tissue culture should reveal the organisms; the organisms may also be seen on microscopy of affected tissue.

Management [3,5]
Prompt surgical debridement of all devitalised tissue is essential.

Broad spectrum empiric antibiotic therapy should be initiated while awaiting confirmation of the organisms involved. High-dose intravenous penicillin in combination with clindamycin is the definitive treatment once *Clostridium* spp. has been identified.

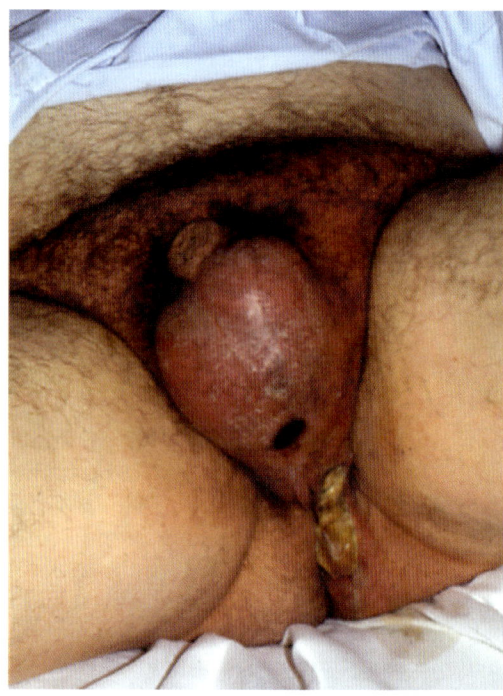

Figure 26.25 Fournier necrotising fasciitis of the groin. Courtesy of King's College London.

Alternatives include metronidazole and imipenem [2], but antimicrobial therapy is only an adjunct to surgery. The role of hyperbaric oxygen remains controversial: while some studies have found significant survival benefit, others have found no benefit [6].

Treatment ladder for gas gangrene

First line
- Surgical debridement
- Intravenous penicillin plus clindamycin

Second line
- Metronidazole
- Imipenem

GRAM-NEGATIVE BACTERIA

The skin may be infected by Gram-negative bacteria either as a result of systemic spread from another site via haematogenous dissemination or by direct local invasion.

NEISSERIA MENINGITIDIS

Neisseria meningitidis is a Gram-negative diplococcus. It can be divided into different serotypes on the basis of capsular polysaccharides, types A, B and C being the most important. All types are pathogenic.

Meningococcal infection

Synonyms and inclusions
- Meningococcal septicaemia
- Meningococcaemia

Introduction and general description
N. meningitidis colonises the human upper respiratory tract and is transmitted by droplet from patients or healthy carriers. It may cause localised infections, such as conjunctivitis and otitis media, or severe and potentially fatal disease with septicaemia and meningitis.

Epidemiology
Although at present there are 12 serogroups of *N. meningitidis*, over 90% of disease is caused by serogroups A, B, C, W-135, X and Y. The highest burden of disease is seen in the 'meningitis belt' of sub-Saharan Africa. Infection carries an overall mortality rate of up to 20% [1]. *N. meningitidis* carriage in the nasopharynx occurs in up to 10% of the population [2].

Age
Any age but two peaks recognised: children aged less than 1 year and adolescents/young adults aged 16–23 years.

Sex
Either sex.

Pathophysiology
Predisposing factors
Individuals living in group settings such as student accommodation are at increased risk of becoming infected. Complement deficiencies, either inherited or secondary to medication, and asplenia also increase the risk of developing meningococcal disease.

Pathology
In order to cause disease, the organism has to bind to the epithelium through surface-expressed proteins, such as pili, the polysaccharide capsule and lipo-oligosaccharide (LOS) [3]. Severe meningococcal disease affects mainly children under the age of 10 years, but epidemics or sporadic cases in adults may occur, for instance in institutions such as military barracks or university lodgings. Bacteraemia is believed to be the primary event in all forms of the infection and the route by which the organism reaches the meninges.

The early petechial skin lesions result from the presence of the organisms in capillary endothelium accompanied by disseminated intravascular coagulation, with necrosis of the vessel wall or thrombosis [4]. The skin lesions occurring late in the course of acute infections or in chronic infections show a vasculitis thought to be produced by soluble antigen–antibody complexes [5].

Causative organisms
- *N. meningitidis*.

Historically group B is commoner in Europe and group A in tropical regions. However, with the increasing introduction of effective vaccines targeting different subgroups, the epidemiological picture may change over time [1].

Clinical features
History
Although most patients have classical onset, in some children it may evolve very rapidly and with minimal warning signs.

Presentation
Acute meningococcal septicaemia with or without meningitis may present as a fulminating illness, and the rash may be a very useful clue to early diagnosis. The incidence of rash is estimated at between 40% and 90%, perhaps depending on the thoroughness with which lesions in the more sparsely affected cases are sought [4]. Early skin lesions are not always haemorrhagic and may take the form of discrete pink macules or papules a few millimetres in diameter on any part of the body, including the palms and soles [6]. Purpura follows in many cases. Transient red, morbilliform or urticarial eruptions are occasionally seen.

A purpuric eruption is characteristic, and occurs mainly on the trunk and limbs. The petechiae are usually small and scanty, but vary in size and number. In severe cases, larger purpuric lesions may occur, including extensive ecchymoses and necrotic ulceration, particularly in dependent areas and under pressure sites, and are associated with a high mortality [7,8].

Vasculitis may occur during the acute illness, beginning 5–9 days after the onset, even if adequate antibiotic treatment has been given. Nodules or bullae may be sparse and confined to the limbs, or may be more numerous and widespread; the lesions may ulcerate [8]. Arteritis and episcleritis may be associated. Similar vasculitic lesions occur in chronic septicaemic infection [9] in which milder maculopapular eruptions are also seen.

Clinical variants
There is a rare form of chronic meningococcaemia which can present with a rash, low-grade fever and arthritis identical to that described for chronic gonococcaemia (see later).

Differential diagnosis
Includes causes of acute vasculitis, viral haemorrhagic fevers such as Ebola and Marburg, dengue and Rocky Mountain spotted fever.

Complications and co-morbidities
Disseminated intravascular coagulation and purpura fulminans may occur which can lead to gangrene and autoamputation of distal extremities; this is more common in young children. Waterhouse–Friderichsen syndrome results from adrenal gland failure secondary to haemorrhagic destruction caused by the *N. meningitidis* infection. Skin infarction may also occur and can lead to contractures and severe scarring.

Disease course and prognosis
The infection can be rapidly fatal and death can occur before the development of the rash.

Investigations
The diagnosis is confirmed by isolation of *N. meningitidis* from blood or cerebrospinal fluid or by PCR.

Management
- Circulatory support and intravenous fluids.
- Intravenous ceftriaxone or benzylpenicillin in high doses is the first line treatment of choice.
- Cefotaxime, meropenem or chloramphenicol (in the context of severe allergy to cephalosporins and penicillin) are suitable alternatives.

Infection control
Meningococcal meningitis and septicaemia are notifiable diseases. In the UK, a single dose of ciprofloxacin is recommended as prophylaxis for close contacts; rifamipicin is a suitable alternative. Vaccines are available for meningococcal infections caused by groups A, B, C, Y and W-135. Meningococcal B and C vaccines form part of the childhood vaccination programme in the UK and the quadrivalent MenACWY vaccine is offered to young adults. Vaccines may also be deployed in at-risk groups [10].

Treatment ladder for meningococcal infection

First line
- Ceftriaxone
- Intravenous benzylpenicillin

Second line
- Cefotaxime
- Meropenem
- Chloramphenicol

Gonococcal infection

Gonococcal infection, including disseminated, is discussed in Chapter 30.

ACINETOBACTER

Acinetobacter species are a group of bacteria commonly found in the environment. Most of the infections are caused by *A. baumannii* but *A. calcoaceticus*, *A. lwoffii* and *A. haemolyticus* are also recognised human pathogens. These closely related *Acinetobacter* organisms are found as members of the resident skin flora in the axilla and groin in about 20% of normal subjects, and may occur in the toe webs and on drier sites [1–3]. They have been isolated from skin pustules and from cellulitis [4], but their main importance lies in their role as uncommon opportunistic pathogens. *Acinetobacter* spp. were primarily responsible for nosocomial pneumonia and bacteraemia. Meningitis, osteomyelitis, synovitis, burn sepsis and wound infections are also reported. *Acinetobacter* spp. was a major cause of wound, soft-tissue and invasive infection in soldiers in Afghanistan and Iraq, particularly after traumatic injury. In the very young and the very old particularly, the source of infection may be exogenous but endogenous infection clearly occurs, and indwelling intravenous catheters are likely routes in septicaemia. Community-acquired infection, particularly pneumonia, but more rarely meningitis, cellulitis or bacteraemia, is more prevalent in warm, humid environments including Asia, Australia and Oceania. Highly resistant strains have emerged in critical care settings [5].

MORAXELLA

The genus *Moraxella* includes an important respiratory pathogen *M. catarrhalis*. *M. osloensis* has been reported as a cause of gonococcaemia-like systemic infection with skin lesions [1] and bacteraemia with a petechial rash [2]. These cases apart, *Moraxella* are more closely associated with respiratory or middle ear infection or conjunctival inflammation than cutaneous colonisation or disease [3].

PSEUDOMONAS AERUGINOSA [1,2]

P. aeruginosa (*P. pyocyanea*; *Bacillus pyocyaneus*) is an aerobic, Gram-negative rod, which occurs only as a transient member of the skin flora, mainly in the ano-genital region, axillae and external ear, and is normally kept in check by the dominant Gram-positive cocci.

Pseudomonas infection

Synonyms and inclusions
- Gram-negative folliculitis
- Ecthyma gangrenosum

Epidemiology
Pseudomonas species produce a variety of different infections in the skin depending on the site and underlying condition of the patient. It is a saprophytic organism that occurs in soil and water and has a predilection for humid environments. It is present in the intestine of a small percentage of adults and a high proportion of infants. Widespread colonisation is not uncommon after hospital admission or antibiotic treatment. It readily colonises burns, ulcers or other moist skin lesions, and often contaminates fomites as well as showers, sinks and respiratory equipment in intensive care units. Jars of ointment may also be contaminated [3]. *P. aeruginosa* is typically an opportunistic pathogen, commonly seen as a nosocomial infection in patients with impaired defence mechanisms such as burn wounds, mechanical ventilation, urinary catheters, neutropenia and cystic fibrosis. Outbreaks of pseudomonal (also known as Gram-negative) folliculitis are not uncommon among users of overcrowded heated swimming pools or jacuzzis.

Sex
Both sexes.

Age
Any age, but predisposing conditions more important.

Associated diseases
Neutropenia, intubated patients, burns, cystic fibrosis, necrotising otitis externa.

Pathophysiology
Pathology
Pseudomonas spp. are able to produce a vast array of enzymes and other putative virulence factors. Antibiotic usage and prolonged maceration both favour the establishment of *Pseudomonas* even in previously healthy adults, and clinical infections eventually develop in a large proportion.

Experimental superhydration of the skin for 7 days with water-soaked cotton pads produced a vesiculopustular rash from which *Pseudomonas* was isolated [4].

Under experimental conditions, *Pseudomonas* is pathogenic only in massive dosage or in damaged tissue [5], a pattern of behaviour that parallels that observed in humans, although the relationship between dose and pathogenicity is not well understood [6]. *Pseudomonas* appears to play a part in modifying and perpetuating some paronychial infections. It is commonly isolated from chronic leg ulcers and from many other persistently moist lesions, including chronic external otitis, and, although its presence may be clinically apparent, it is uncertain to what extent it is pathogenic under these conditions. It is believed to be capable of maintaining the inflammatory changes after other organisms have been eliminated. Typical strains produce two pigments, the blue–green pyocyanin, a phenazine derivative, and a greenish yellow pyoverdin.

Causative organisms
Usually *P. aeruginosa*.

Environmental factors
Soil and water, including household or hospital bathroom appliances (e.g. sinks).

Clinical features [2,7,8]
Presentation
Pseudomonal infections can present in many different ways depending on the immunocompetency of the host and location of the infection. Mild skin infections tend to present in healthy individuals and may resolve without specific antibacterial therapy; these include nail infections, interdigital infections and folliculitis.

P. aeruginosa infection of the nail usually results in a green discoloration of the nail due to pyocyanin pigment production (Figure 26.26). This is typically seen in the context of chronic paronychia.

The damp, humid environment that can develop as a result of maceration or antibiotic use in the interdigital spaces facilitates colonisation by pseudomonal species. Inhibition of the Gram-positive flora or dermatophytes by this maceration or antibiotic use allows the development of a distinctive *Pseudomonas* infection of the toe webs [1,8] (Figure 26.27), also referred to as tropical immersion foot. It is characterised by sharply demarcated areas of maceration and tender erosions, sometimes tinged with green, and showing green fluorescence under Wood's light. The

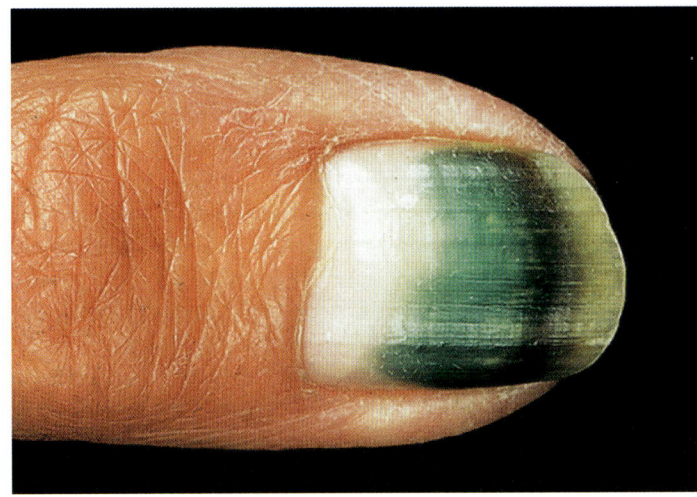

Figure 26.26 *Pseudomonas* infection of the nail. Courtesy of St John's Institute of Dermatology.

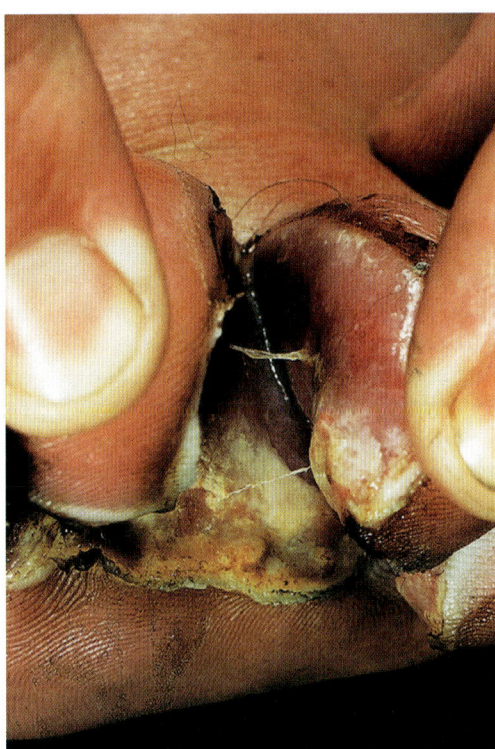

Figure 26.27 *Pseudomonas* infection of the foot. Courtesy of St John's Institute of Dermatology.

sodden plaque tends to break down, and secondary invasion by *Candida* may follow [5].

Gram-negative folliculitis seen in swimming pool or jacuzzi users is a well-documented entity [9,10]. It may include macular, papular or pustular lesions which are tender. Some are urticarial, suggesting insect bites. Any part of the body that has been immersed may be affected, but often the worst areas are those in contact with bathing costumes. In most cases, the rash occurs spontaneously roughly 24 hours after exposure and settles spontaneously within 7–10 days in the absence of re-exposure.

Clinical variants
Pseudomonas can cause localised infection in infancy in the periumbilical area, with a foul-smelling bluish green discharge and spreading redness. In some cases, usually under conditions of high humidity, widely scattered pustules may break down to form necrotic ulcers.

Pseudomonas can also invade superficial wounds, particularly burns [11]. This complication still carries a high mortality as large quantities of these organisms may thrive in burn eschar, and secondary septicaemia may result. Secondarily infected burns show discoloration of the slough with extensive surrounding oedema. Fever and shock may supervene. However, careful management and use of debridement in burns units have reduced the incidence. In a survey of patients with severe burns, only 1% had an episode of *Pseudomonas* bacteraemia [11]. Cutaneous features of pseudomonal septicaemia include subcutaneous nodules, ecthyma gangrenosum and gangrenous cellulitis [2].

P. aeruginosa can also cause infection of the ear, which ranges from mild superficial infection to life-threatening necrotising (malignant) otitis externa. Swimmer's ear is the term used for the mild, self-limiting external otitis typically seen as a result of maceration of the external auditory canal resulting from swimming and/or loss of the acidic cerumen, which usually protects from infection and maceration. This presents with pain, redness and swelling of the canal and occasionally involves the pinna as well. Necrotising otitis externa occurs when pseudomonal infection of the external auditory canal persists, penetrating the epithelium, invading the surrounding soft tissue and ultimately leading to osteomyelitis of the skull base. This condition is more common in the context of diabetes or immunocompromise and presents with severe ear pain, purulent discharge, oedema of the ear canal and potentially cranial nerve palsies.

Ecthyma gangrenosum is a cutaneous manifestation of pseudomonal septicaemia and it most commonly occurs in the severely compromised host [2,12,13]. Skin lesions may not be a feature of pseudomonal septicaemia or there may be non-specific inflammation, which can be tender or spontaneously painful [14], purpura or a cellulitis-like picture. Bullae may form, particularly in moist areas such as the axillae, perineum and the buttocks. The classical presentation of ecthyma gangrenosum is of a gunmetal grey, infarcted macule with surrounding erythema, which then evolves into a necrotic ulcer with black eschar and surrounding redness (Figure 26.28) [2].

P. aeruginosa is recognised as a rare cause of necrotising fasciitis. Typically affecting the elderly or immnocompromised, the condition starts insidiously with a localised area of pain and swelling which rapidly progresses to widespread inflammation and destruction of tissue. Pseudomonas has also been implicated in Fournier gangrene, which is a clinical variant of necrotising fasciitis, predominantly affecting the male genitalia, but also seen in females.

Pseudomonas spp. have also been implicated in severe exacerbations of acne vulgaris [15].

Pseudomonas is an important cause of ventilator- and hospital-acquired pneumonia, catheter-associated urinary tract infections and respiratory tract infection in patients with cystic fibrosis.

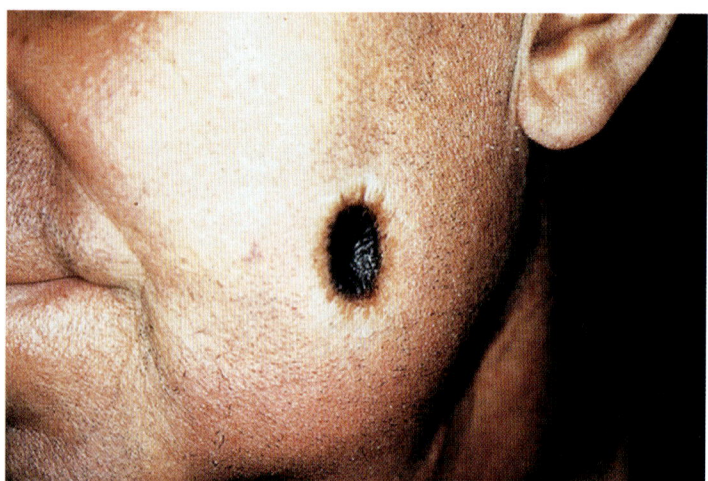

Figure 26.28 Ecthyma gangrenosum. Courtesy of Dr G. Scott.

Differential diagnosis
The differential diagnoses vary with the location and severity of the presentation but may include staphylococcal, streptococcal or Gram-negative skin infections, anthrax (eschars), rickettsial infection (eschar), fungal or dermatophyte infection (nail and interdigital infection).

Complications and co-morbidities
Pseudomonal septicaemia, especially in immunocompromised hosts, carries a significant risk of mortality.

Disease course and prognosis
The prognosis of systemic infections is poor, unless there is early treatment. Local infections in infants or patients with debilitating illnesses should be regarded as potentially dangerous, as systemic extension occurs readily. The invasion of damaged skin in the otherwise normal subject may be difficult to control permanently until the lesions are healed, but usually has no serious significance.

Investigations
Bacteriological confirmation of the diagnosis is readily obtained by cultures from the skin lesions or blood. The significance of the isolation of *Pseudomonas* from non-specific lesions must be carefully evaluated with the clinical findings.

Management
Pseudomonas has a propensity for antimicrobial resistance [2,16], requiring vigilance when determining therapeutic options.

For superficial lesions, drying of macerated skin is the first step of treatment. This can be achieved with acetic acid (1%) compresses, potassium permanganate soaks, povidone or silver sulfadiazine cream.

In the case of burns, extensive debridement followed by topical applications of silver sulfadiazine therapy is useful.

Nail involvement can be managed with acetic acid soaks (1%) or topical preparations of aminoglycosides or fluoroquinolones. If these are ineffective then an oral fluoroquinolone may be required. Nail avulsion may be used in the context of onychodystrophy.

In every case where antibiotics are required, it is vital to base ongoing therapy on the results of *in vitro* sensitivity tests.

In septicaemia or where a severely compromised patient has superficial infection, systemic therapy using intravenous antibiotics should be started promptly. Potential antibiotic options include antipseudomonal penicillins, aminoglycosides, certain cephalosporins (e.g. ceftazidime), carbapenems and fluoroquinolones, some of which may be used in combination.

BURKHOLDERIA

Burkholderia are aerobic Gram-negative bacteria. Those relevant to cutaneous infection are *B. mallei* and *B. pseudomallei*, the causes of glanders and melioidosis, respectively.

Melioidosis

Definition and nomenclature [1]
Melioidosis is the disease caused by a saprophytic environmental bacterium called *B. pseudomallei*, which is found in soil and fresh surface water.

Synonyms and inclusions
- Whitmore disease
- Nightcliff gardener's disease

Introduction and general description
Melioidosis is a clinically diverse disease which can result in the development of skin lesions particularly abscesses. *B. pseudomallei* is recognised as a biothreat.

Epidemiology
Melioidosis predominates in South-East Asia (especially northern Thailand), northern Australia, India and China. Sporadic cases have been reported in Africa, the Middle East, Caribbean and South and Central America, and imported cases in travellers also occur. In endemic areas such as northern Thailand and northern Australia, cases of melioidosis rise sharply in the monsoon season, highlighting the importance of water and wet soil for transmission. Person-to-person spread is rare but laboratory-acquired and iatrogenic infections have been reported [2].

Sex
Affects males more than females.

Age
Any age can be affected but systemic disease is more common in adults with a peak around 40–60 years; in northern Thailand 80% of children have antibodies by age 4 years [2].

Associated diseases
Diabetes, chronic renal disease, other causes of immunosuppression (e.g. steroid use, malignancy, etc.) and chronic lung disease, especially cystic fibrosis, are risk factors for melioidosis.

Pathophysiology
Pathology
Infection in humans can occur through environmental contamination of a minor skin injury, percutaneous inoculation, inhalation, aspiration or ingestion. There is a high seroprevalence of *B. pseudomallei* in individuals living in endemic areas, suggesting subclinical infection is common.

Causative organisms
- *B. pseudomallei*.

Environmental factors
Water and soil associated; peaks occur in the wet season in endemic areas and following severe weather or other events such as the 2004 tsunami in the Indian Ocean.

Clinical features [1]
History
The disease may run an acute, subacute or chronic course. The incubation period following exposure can range from 1 to 21 days but in cases of significant exposure (such as near-drowning) the onset of disease may be very rapid. Acute disease is most common but chronic disease (lasting beyond 2 months) can occur. Latent infection can also occur and has been reported up to three decades after exposure. Travel to endemic areas and exposure risk are important to ascertain.

Presentation
Melioidosis typically presents as either a localised skin infection or pneumonia. Pneumonia is the most common presentation and may be acute with pyrexia, cough and respiratory distress or more chronic with a similar presentation to tuberculosis. Skin infections present with ulceration or abscess formation; frequently this will progress to systemic involvement with abscess formation in other organs and septicaemia. In many cases the clinical picture is variable, with unexplained fever and disseminated pyogenic lesions.

Clinical variants
Melioidosis may present with parotitis (especially common in children), osteomyelitis or septic arthritis, encephalomyelitis or as a genitourinary infection. Subacute, chronic and latent melioidosis are well described.

Differential diagnosis
Other causes of abscesses such as staphylococcal infection, nocardiosis and tuberculosis.

Disease course and prognosis
Untreated systemic melioidosis is fatal; with early diagnosis and prompt treatment overall mortality is 10–35% depending on the clinical syndrome.

Investigations

Culture is the mainstay of diagnosis and appropriate samples should be sent for culture; for cutaneous lesions this would include a swab of any purulent material or the base of an ulcer or tissue from a non-ulcerated lesion. Blood cultures should also be sent. It is important to alert the laboratory if melioidosis is suspected as selective media may be required and there is also a risk of laboratory-associated infection. The Gram-negative bacilli may be seen on microscopy of aspirated pus but the sensitivity is poor with Gram staining. However, immunofluorescence may be helpful. Serology alone is not sufficient for diagnosis, partly because of high background seropositivity in endemic areas [3] but also false-negative serology in acute sepsis [4]. Imaging such as chest radiography and computed tomography (CT) or ultrasound scanning of the abdomen should be performed to look for evidence of disseminated disease.

Management [5]

Management involves appropriate parenteral antibiotics in the acute phase (minimum 10 days), followed by an eradication phase with oral antibiotics, with the total treatment time lasting at least 12 weeks [6]. Ceftazidime is the drug of choice for the acute phase but meropenem and imipenem are suitable alternatives; amoxicillin–clavulanic acid (co-amoxiclav) is considered second line therapy. Trimethoprim-sulfamethoxazole (co-trimoxazole) is the oral agent used for the eradication phase and co-amoxiclav would be second line; doxycycline could be used as an alternative to co-amoxiclav if required. Surgical drainage of abscesses should be performed where possible. Testing samples for antibiotic sensitivities is advised as there are reports of antibiotic resistance. In the context of localised disease, oral therapy alone may be sufficient but expert advice should be sought in this instance.

Treatment ladder for melioidosis

First line
- Ceftazidime (acute phase)
- Co-trimoxazole (eradication phase)

Second line
- Meropenem/imipenem or co-amoxiclav (acute phase)
- Co-amoxiclav (eradication phase)

Glanders

Definition and nomenclature [1,2]

Glanders is the result of infection with *B. mallei*; typically the infection affects horses and donkeys but it can be passed to humans.

Synonyms and inclusions
- Farcy
- Equina

Introduction and general description

A rare infection, mainly confined to parts of the tropics, which presents with ulcerating lesions on the skin and mucous membranes. *B. mallei* is a host-adapted clone of *B. pseudomallei* (which causes melioidosis); as a result the clinical manifestations are very similar in both diseases.

Epidemiology

It is now extremely rare worldwide; sporadic cases still occur in Africa, Asia, the Middle East and South and Central America. Humans are infected by direct contact with horses, the bacillus usually gaining entry through a skin abrasion or through mucosal surfaces of the eyes, nose or mouth; inhalation is also a potential mode of transmission. Human-to-human transmission is rare but has been reported [1]; infection in laboratory personnel is a risk and *B. mallei* is recognised as a biothreat.

Age
Any age.

Sex
Both sexes.

Pathophysiology
Pathology

B. mallei gives rise to a local adenitis, followed by necrosis and abscess formation. The infection spreads by the regional lymphatics and by metastasis.

Causative organisms
- *B. mallei*.

Environmental factors

Individuals in close contact with infected horses and other equines are at risk of glanders.

Clinical features [2]
History

Glanders may be an intensely acute, rapidly fatal disease or may run a chronic relapsing course over months or years.

Presentation

In the acute form of glanders the incubation period is between 1 and 14 days, following which a localised infection develops with cellulitis, which soon breaks down to form an irregular ulcer with an offensive haemorrhagic purulent discharge. Malaise, headache and fever are associated features. If the primary site is cutaneous, the regional lymphatics become swollen and tender, and dull-red nodules along their course break down to form abscesses and sinuses. If the nasal or oral mucous membrane is the site of inoculation, there is extensive necrosis and destruction of the septum and palate. After a variable interval – a few days or many weeks – metastatic lesions begin to appear: grouped, dull-red papules, pustules or bullae, especially over the joints and face, are followed by ulcers that enlarge and coalesce. Deep subcutaneous abscesses with multiple sinuses may also occur.

Clinical variants
Pneumonic disease may lead to acute abscess formation, pleural effusion and lobar infiltration. The onset is rapid and without prompt treatment leads to death within several weeks.

Differential diagnosis
Melioidosis, staphylococcal infection, sporotrichosis, pyoderma gangrenosum, tuberculosis.

Complications and co-morbidities
Pneumonia and septicaemia.

Disease course and prognosis
Although some cases survive for long periods with intermittent bacteraemia with severe constitutional symptoms and metastatic manifestations, others are rapidly fatal, and in general the mortality without treatment is very high. Interestingly there appears to be a window of improvement after the first wave of symptoms and this seems to last for a variable length of time [1]. This may be interpreted as eradication leading to premature treatment cessation.

Investigations
The clinical history of exposure to equines (which may have subclinical infection) is vital in order to suspect the diagnosis. Isolation of the organism is required for diagnosis; serology can be useful but does cross-react in melioidosis.

Management [1]
As glanders in humans is rare, no formal treatment regime exists, but a similar therapeutic regime to that used in melioidosis seems logical: acute parenteral treatment with ceftazidime, meropenem or imipenem followed by oral eradication treatment with trimethoprim–sulfamethoxazole (co-trimoxazole), amoxicillin–clavulanic acid (co-amoxiclav) or possibly doxycycline for around 12 weeks.

STENOTROPHOMONAS MALTOPHILIA [1]

Stenotrophomonas maltophilia, previously classified as a *Pseudomonas* species, is a rare cause of opportunistic infection typically seen in the context of prolonged hospital stays, mechanical ventilation, broad spectrum antibiotics, neutropenia or malignancy. It can cause pneumonia or septicaemia. However, *Stenotrophomonas maltophilia* can also cause cellulitis and ecthyma gangrenosum [1,2]. The cutaneous lesions are typically nodular and may accompany septicaemia. Trimethoprim–sulfamethoxazole, tigecycline, minocycline and levofloxacin have all been used for treatment, but multidrug resistance is a growing problem [3,4].

KLEBSIELLA PNEUMONIAE RHINOSCLEROMATIS

Klebsiella pneumoniae rhinoscleromatis is a subspecies of *K. pneumoniae* and the cause of a distinctive infection of the upper respiratory tract mainly seen in the tropics.

Rhinoscleroma

Definition and nomenclature
Rhinoscleroma is a chronic granulomatous, slowly progressive and potentially fatal infectious and mildly contagious disease caused by the bacterium *K. pneumoniae* subspecies *rhinoscleromatis* (*Klebsiella rhinoscleromatis*) that affects the upper and lower airways.

Synonyms and inclusions
- Scleroma

Introduction and general description
This infection is originally localised in the nasal fossae and invades the upper respiratory tract and lacrimal apparatus, where it produces an infiltrating granuloma with a marked tendency to sclerosis and subsequent obstruction. It is a condition difficult to cure.

Epidemiology [1,2]
The disease occurs sporadically almost all over the world, but is endemic (although still rare) in parts of Central and North Africa, Central and South America, South-East Asia, the Middle East and eastern Europe. The disease is acquired by direct or indirect contact with the nasal exudate of an infected person. It is more common in rural areas where social and hygiene standards are lower.

Age
The infection can occur at any age, but it is more frequent between the ages of 20 and 50 years.

Sex
Both sexes but slight female predisposition [2,3].

Pathophysiology
Pathology [3–5]
Rhinoscleroma is caused by *K. pneumoniae* subsp. *rhinoscleromatis*. This bacillus measures about 3 μm in length and appears isolated, in pairs or even in short chains, and is encapsulated, non-motile and Gram negative. *K. rhinoscleromatis* has a mucopolysaccharide capsule that helps to protect it from phagocytosis, facilitating intracellular survival. The mucopolysaccharide in the capsule of the bacterium is thought to be responsible for most of the damage caused by the infection. The cell-mediated immunity in individuals with rhinoscleroma is impaired and there is a decrease in the number of CD4 lymphocytes.

Causative organisms
- *K. pneumoniae* subsp. *rhinoscleromatis*.

Environmental factors
Lower socioeconomic status, poor hygiene and poor nutrition are risk factors for rhinoscleroma [5].

Clinical features
History
The first manifestations are usually nasopharyngeal, but the disease may also affect the larynx, trachea, bronchi and lacrimal duct [2].

Since the disease runs a very slow progressive course and the lesions are indolent, the patient tends to seek medical advice only when it has been present for several years, as general health is not impaired.

Presentation
The disease progresses through three overlapping stages [3,5]:
1. Exudative (catarrhal), rhinitic or atrophic stage. This begins with symptoms of a common cold. There is headache and difficulty in breathing, a fetid purulent rhinorrhoea of long duration (weeks or months), with scabs, dryness of the throat and occasional epistaxis. Hypertrophy of the mucous membrane can be observed, especially on the septum.
2. Proliferative or granulomatous stage. Initially, there is the infiltrative period which may involve the nose and mouth. As the symptoms of coryza begin to subside, infiltration and obstruction of the lower portion of the nasal fossae occur, with an exuberant, friable granulation tissue, crusting and induration, which later extends to the pharynx and larynx. Breathing may become difficult and painful, and tracheotomy is sometimes necessary.
3. Fibrotic (sclerotic) stage. Clinical improvement occurs. The previously inflamed tissue is replaced by dense collagen. The healing process (spontaneous or after therapy) leads to anatomical distortion (e.g. of the nose) and stenosis of the structures affected during the proliferative stage.

Differential diagnosis
Rhinoscleroma must be differentiated from other diseases involving the nasal fossae and upper respiratory tract. At the early stages, chronic bacterial rhinosinusitis and atrophic rhinitis should be considered. At the late stages, the following enter the differential diagnosis: mucocutaneous leishmaniasis, which is highly destructive but not as proliferative or obstructive as scleroma, and paracoccidioidomycosis, which affects especially the mucous membranes of the mouth and is accompanied by marked adenopathy and granulomatous lesions that bleed easily ('blackberry' stomatitis). Granulomatosis with polyangiitis and malignant epithelial tumours and sarcomas can be differentiated by their rapid evolution. Other diseases that must be considered are sarcoidosis, nasal tuberculosis, yaws, leprosy, lymphomas and nasal polyps.

Complications and co-morbidities
Progressive pharyngeal and nasal scarring.

Disease course and prognosis
Seldom fatal but disfiguring and recurrences are not uncommon.

Investigations [1]
The identification of the bacterium is not easy and is based on its biochemical activity, which distinguishes it from other *Klebsiella* species or on molecular diagnostic testing. Diagnosis is usually based on clinical and histopathological data [2]. While culture is diagnostic, it is only positive in up to 60% of cases.

Histopathology [1,4]
The histopathological picture is pathognomonic. A dense infiltrate is observed consisting mainly of plasma cells and two types of highly characteristic cells, the association of which allows this process to be distinguished from other granulomas. These cells are Mikulicz cells and Russell bodies. A Mikulicz cell is a large round vacuolated histiocyte measuring 100–200 μm in diameter containing Giemsa or Gram-positive bacilli (A granules) or amorphous clusters of mucopolysaccharide (B granules). The Russell body or colloid body, measuring 20–40 μm, is a structure in the cytoplasm of the plasma cells, elliptical in shape, homogeneous and extremely eosinophilic, and as such stains bright red. Inside the Mikulicz cells, the bacilli are protected from the cell-mediated immune system, and hence there is a need for long-term therapy to be active against the bacteria when they are released.

Radiographic findings
Computed tomography findings can help identify rhinoscleroma from other malignant and granulomatous disorders. Characteristic findings include homogeneous, non-enhancing nasal and nasopharyngeal soft-tissue masses which have distinct edges, nasal turbinate atrophy, transglottic narrowing, vocal cord thickening, crypt-like changes in the trachea and discrete subglottic narrowing, as well as calcification, wall thickening and nodules [6,7].

Endoscopic examination may be required to determine the extent of involvement [5].

Management [8,9]
This is essentially a chronic disease with a slowly progressive course. Relapses are frequent after apparent bacteriological cure. Involvement of the trachea or bronchi inevitably worsens the prognosis. The disease is rarely associated with AIDS [10]. Treatment is typically a combination of prolonged antimicrobial therapy and surgical debridement [5]. Various antibiotics have been used to treat rhinoscleroma and where possible treatment should be based on antimicrobial sensitivities. Agents used (either alone or in combination) include trimethoprim–sulfamethoxazole, streptomycin, tetracyclines, fluoroquinolones, rifampicin and second and third generation cephalosporins. Antimicrobial therapy is likely to be required for at least 3 months and this is an important consideration with respect to the therapeutic choice [11].

During the healing process, scarring affects the upper respiratory tract, nose, pharynx and larynx. In the inactive fibrotic stage, surgical treatment may be required to correct severe structural and functional abnormalities, such as the narrowing of the nasal vestibule, nasopharyngeal stenosis and laryngeal web formation. Nasal endoscopic techniques and the carbon dioxide laser have been used for the treatment of obstructive scars [5,10].

Treatment ladder for rhinoscleroma

First line
- Fluoroquinolones
- Tetracyclines

Second line
- Second/third generation cephalosporins
- Trimethoprim–sulfamethoxazole

FRANCISELLA TULARENSIS

Francisella tularensis is a Gram-negative bacteria responsible for tularaemia, a zoonotic infection. It is a pleomorphic non-motile Gram-negative coccobacillus which produces a powerful endotoxin. It is a facultative intracellular parasite.

Tularaemia

Definition and nomenclature [1,2]
Tularaemia results from systemic infection with *F. tularensis*.

Synonyms and inclusions
- Deer-fly fever

Introduction and general description
This is a systemic infection in which skin features include an inflammatory reaction at the site of entry with tissue necrosis and secondary exanthemata.

Epidemiology
Wild lagomorphs (rabbits and hares) and rodents are the main reservoir of infection. However, the organism can infect many species of wild and domestic vertebrates as well as invertebrates. The organism can survive in an animal carcass as well as soil and water for several weeks. Transmission to humans can occur either directly or indirectly from animal contact and via bites from ticks (usually *Dermacentor* species) or other arthropods [2]. The epidemiological pattern is extremely variable; infected food and water have been responsible for outbreaks. However, most cases are sporadic. Airborne transmission is also possible, leading to pneumonic disease. The combination of aerosol transmission and high virulence resulting in severe pneumonia means that *F. tularensis* is categorised as a biothreat. The disease is endemic in the northern hemisphere, including the USA and many parts of northern and eastern Europe apart from the UK. It is also seen in Asia and the Middle East. Outside of North America, *F. tularensis* subsp. *holarctica*, which is less virulent, is more common.

Age
Any age.

Sex
Both sexes, but more common in males due to risk of exposure.

Pathophysiology
Pathology
F. tularensis is a highly virulent organism; inhalation of only 10 live organisms can lead to potentially lethal disease. Following inoculation, the infection spreads to the regional lymph nodes before spreading systemically. *F. tularensis* replicates within the macrophages leading to macrophage death; it also infects neutrophils where it is able to suppress the oxidative burst and inhibit neutrophil apoptosis [3]. *F. tularensis* also exhibits several virulence factors such as lipopolysaccharides, type IV pili and siderophore. A cluster of genes known as the *Francisella* pathogenicity island (FPI) appear to determine the virulence of the organism [4].

Causative organisms
- *F. tularensis*.

Environmental factors
Individuals exposed to animals, for example farmers, veterinarians, hunters and meat handlers, are at increased risk.

Clinical features
History
The incubation period varies from 1 to 10 days. The clinical manifestations depend on the portal of entry: the skin, eye, or respiratory or gastrointestinal tract.

Presentation
Six clinical manifestations of tularaemia are recognised; most sporadic cases are of the ulceroglandular, glandular or oculoglandular type:

1. Ulceroglandular – this accounts for around 90% of cases [4]. Typically, a single, painful, red nodule develops at the site of inoculation. This lesion then ulcerates and a central eschar will form. Associated tender regional lymphadenopathy occurs and may become suppurative. Subcutaneous nodules spreading along the draining lymphatics in a sporotrichoid pattern can occur [5]. The symptoms are accompanied by fever. Transmission from animals usually results in lesions on the arms or hands whereas arthropod transmission more commonly results in lesions on the head, trunk or legs.
2. Glandular – this refers to tender regional lymphadenopathy without an identifiable skin lesion.
3. Oculoglandular – this occurs when infection with *F. tularensis* occurs through exposure to the conjunctiva and results in unilateral pain, infection of the conjunctiva and conjunctival oedema with associated regional lymphadenopathy.

Secondary skin manifestations are common to all presentations of tularaemia and can take many forms including maculopapular exanthema, vesicular lesions, Sweet syndrome, erythema multiforme, urticarial reactions and erythema nodosum [6].

Clinical variants
Oropharyngeal, pneumonic and typhoidal forms of tularaemia are also recognised. Oropharyngeal disease appears to be more common in Europe [6] and typically occurs from oral exposure. Pneumonic disease may be primary, from inhalation, or secondary due to haematogenous spread. Typhoidal disease describes a systemic illness without localising features.

Differential diagnosis
Differential diagnoses include acute staphylococcal or streptococcal infection, rickettsial infections, *Bartonella* infections, sporotrichosis, syphilis, plague, anthrax, Q-fever and melioidosis.

Complications
Complications from untreated disease include sepsis, renal failure, hepatitis, endocarditis, mastoiditis, meningitis and osteomyelitits.

Disease course and prognosis
Untreated, the course may be prolonged; the mortality of the typhoidal and pulmonary forms exceeds 30%, and that of the oculoglandular form is about 5%.

Investigations
The organism may be cultured from the primary lesion, the lymph nodes or gastric or pharyngeal washings. As *Francisella* is slow growing, it may take up to 2 weeks to observe growth. Specific agglutinins appear in the serum after about 10 days and increase in titre for around 4 weeks. Cross-agglutination with the *Brucella* antigen is a possible source of error. An enzyme-linked immunosorbent assay (ELISA) is available in some laboratories. As laboratory-associated infections can occur it is important that *Francisella* is identified as the possible organism on any samples sent for analysis.

Management
All cases are likely to require antimicrobial treatment. Aminoglycosides, tetracyclines and fluoroquinolones have established efficacy in treating tularaemia; ciprofloxacin and doxycycline are commonly used [7].

A live attenuated, unlicensed vaccine against tularaemia is available, restricted to laboratory workers at risk, but it does not appear to generate robust protection against pneumonic disease [8] so research is ongoing to develop further vaccines.

Treatment ladder for tularaemia

First line
- Ciprofloxacin
- Doxycycline
- Gentamicin (severe disease)

PASTEURELLA

Pasteurella multocida and related infections

Definition
P. multocida is a small Gram-negative bacillus widely distributed as a member of the normal flora of the respiratory tract or intestines of many domestic and wild animals, in which it may cause haemorrhagic septicaemia if the resistance of the host is low [1].

Introduction and general description
The organism does not normally occur in humans, but may be demonstrable in the sputum of patients with bronchiectasis. Most human infections follow bites by cats, dogs or other animals, and

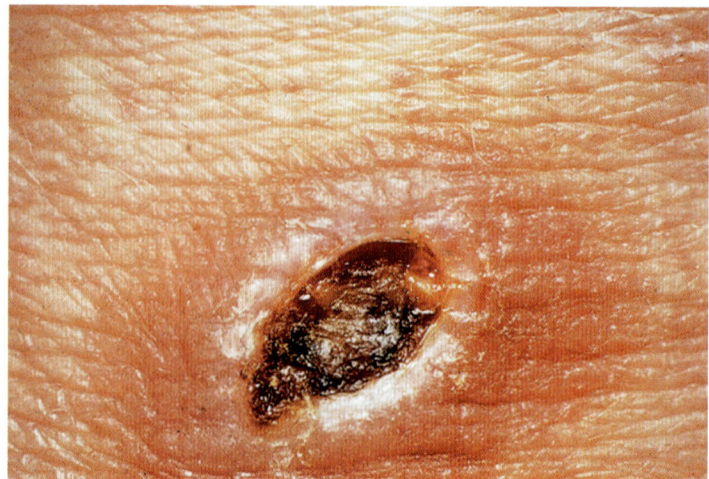

Figure 26.29 *Pasteurella multocida* infection. Courtesy of St John's Institute of Dermatology.

scratch injuries (usually from cats) may also become infected. There are two main subspecies, *P. multocida multocida* and *P. multocida septica*. Other species which can cause wound infections include *P. canis*, *P. stomatis* and *P. dagmatis*.

Clinical features
Most lesions are on the hands, arms or lower legs [1–3] (Figure 26.29). The clinical picture is influenced by the extent and depth of the bite. Redness and swelling around the wound may spread rapidly over a wide area and may break down to discharge greyish yellow, haemorrhagic pus through one or more sinuses. In other cases, the inflammatory changes, often associated with great tenderness, remain localised to the edges of the wound. If the bite is deep, there may be osteomyelitis or synovitis. Of patients 10–15% are febrile and localised lymphadenopathy often develops. About 15% of patients, particularly those patients with internal disease affecting the abdominal cavity or lung, have no history of exposure to animals.

Investigations
The diagnosis will be suggested by the history and is confirmed by the isolation of the slow-growing Gram-negative bacillus.

Management
The infection responds to penicillin, ampicillin and cephalosporins, for example cefuroxime. However, β lactamase-producing strains are not infrequent and as bite wounds are often polymicrobial, agents containing β lactamase inhibitors such as clavulanic acid are recommended [4,5]. Alternatives include fluoroquinolones and tetracyclines.

YERSINIA

The main skin pathogens are *Yersinia pestis*, causative organism of the plague, and *Y. enterocolitica*, which causes Yersiniosis, a gastrointestinal infection. *Y. pestis* [1] is a small Gram-negative non-sporing and non-motile bacillus; with Giemsa it shows characteristic bipolar staining.

Plague and *Yersinia* infections

Definition and nomenclature
This is a zoonotic infection caused by *Y. pestis*, spread by fleas found on rats, which is well recognised as the cause of large outbreaks of infection both historically and in the present day.

Synonyms and inclusions
- Black Death
- Bubonic/pneumonic plague

Introduction and general description
A disease of great historical significance, plague was responsible for several major epidemics in Europe, North Africa and the Middle East in the middle ages and later. The largest of these, known as the Black Death, is thought to have killed around one-third of the population of Europe [2].

Epidemiology
It is a zoonotic infection that predominantly affects a wide variety of rodents, especially urban and domestic rats, *Rattus rattus* and *R. norvegicus*, and is conveyed from them to humans by the bites of fleas or humans may be infected after contact with contaminated material. *Y. pestis* has been shown to contaminate soil, which may be a source of infection for animals [2]. In pneumonic disease, droplet transmission from person to person can occur. Plague is endemic in parts of India and East and South East Asia, and in Madagascar and Southern and Central Africa [3,4]. Sporadic outbreaks occur in North Africa and the Middle East and there are foci of infection in the USA [5]. Occasional cases are recognised elsewhere in travellers from endemic areas.

Age
Any age.

Sex
Both sexes.

Pathophysiology
Pathology
Following inoculation of the organism by a flea bite, the regional lymph node becomes swollen (the classic bubo of bubonic plague), and systemic spread, typically with a severe febrile illness, develops, frequently leading to death within days, without appropriate antimicrobial therapy. Lung involvement occurs in some cases, with sputum that is highly infectious. If *Y. pestis* is inhaled, it is likely to lead to primary pulmonary infection (pneumonic plague), which is almost invariably fatal within 3 or 4 days. In plague epidemics, mild bubonic infections with no systemic spread and truly subclinical infections both occur. Conversely, a patient may rapidly die of flea-transmitted plague without ever developing a bubo. In some instances, cerebral symptoms may be severe.

Causative organisms
- *Y. pestis*.

Clinical (cutaneous) features
History
The incubation period is 3 or 4 days, but it may occasionally be over 7 days.

Clinical presentation
Bubonic plague is the most recognised and common form of the disease. Although typically there is no distinct lesion at the site of the initial flea bite, an erythematous plaque may appear, become bullous and then crusted like an anthrax lesion. Such primary cutaneous lesions may occur in 10% of patients. The bubo arises in the regional lymph nodes several days later. The bubo is a swollen lymph node that becomes acutely painful (Figure 26.30). During the bacteraemic phase, a macular, erythematous or petechial rash may develop; this is sometimes frankly purpuric (the Black Death). Necrotic lesions that closely resemble ecthyma gangrenosum may develop [6]. These are the result of vasculitis and occlusion of vessels with fibrin thrombi. In a few cases, umbilicated vesicles or pustules are seen, particularly over the trunk [4]. This atypical eruption has been a notable feature of certain epidemics and is generally associated with a high mortality. If bubos are excluded, cutaneous lesions probably occur in about 10% of cases in most epidemics.

Clinical variants
Several clinical manifestations of plague are recognised in addition to bubonic: pneumonic, septicaemic, meningitic, pharyngeal and gastrointestinal.

Differential diagnosis
Differential diagnoses include anthrax, lymphoma, brucellosis, *Bartonella* infection, chancroid, lymphogranuloma venereum, rickettsial infections, syphilis and tularaemia.

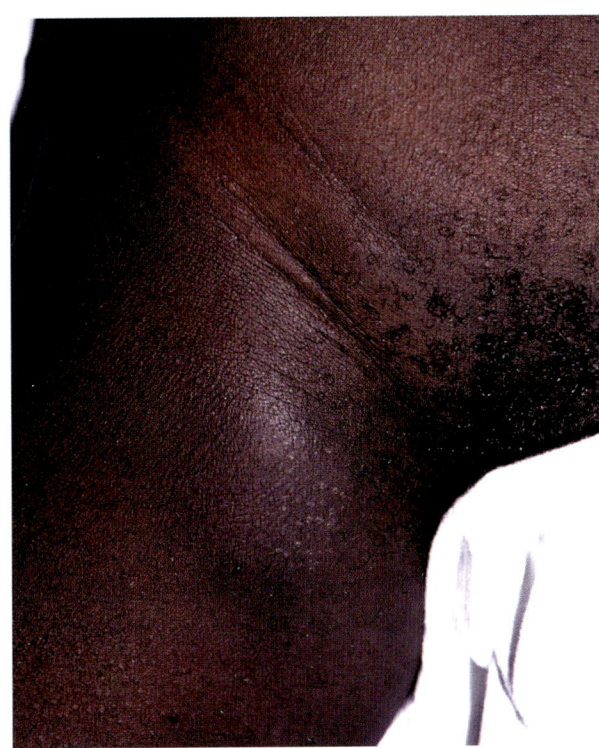

Figure 26.30 Bubo in *Yersinia pestis* infection. © D.A. Warrell.

Disease course and prognosis
Untreated plague is a fatal illness. With appropriate antibiotics the mortality from bubonic plaque drops to around 5% [2].

Investigations
Despite the short incubation period, air travel may carry infected individuals to any part of the world. Even in endemic areas, sporadic cases are often misdiagnosed. The adenitis is the most characteristic feature. Aspiration of a bubo and direct examination of smears and culture confirm the diagnosis. The culture of blood and sputum should also be undertaken.

Management
All cases require prompt antibiotic therapy. Streptomycin, gentamicin, fluoroquinolones, doxycycline and chloramphenicol are all appropriate therapeutic options [2] and treatment should last 10–14 days.

Yersinia enterocolitica

Yersinia enterocolitica is an important cause of a syndrome in which diarrhoea and pain similar to appendicitis occur. In some reported cases there is polyarthritis, and a high proportion of patients, 30% in some series, also have erythema nodosum. Lesions appear from 2 to 20 days after the onset of abdominal symptoms [1,2].

BRUCELLA

Brucella are Gram-negative bacteria responsible for the zoonotic infection brucellosis.

Brucellosis

Definition and nomenclature
Brucellosis is a zoonosis and a disease of domestic and farm animals which can be transmitted to humans.

Synonyms and inclusions
- Undulant fever
- Mediterranean fever
- Malta fever

Introduction and general description
Cases of brucellosis in humans are sporadic and often remain unrecognised due to its protean manifestations.

Epidemiology
Brucellosis is a widespread infection of cattle, sheep, goats, pigs and dogs with *Brucella abortus*, *B. melitensis*, *B. suis*, and *B. canis* respectively. Human cases are seen mainly in countries of the Mediterranean basin as well as the Middle East, sub-Saharan Africa, South and Central Asia and Latin America.

Age
Any age.

Sex
Both sexes.

Pathophysiology
Pathology
Humans are infected by the ingestion of contaminated unpasteurised milk or milk products, or by direct contact with infected animals. The incidence is therefore highest in veterinary surgeons and farmers. Human-to-human transmission is rare but has been reported. There are also species confined to causing disease in animals.

The organism, a Gram-negative aerobic coccobacillus, colonises the cells of the reticuloendothelial system and induces a granulomatous tissue response.

Causative organisms
- *B. abortus*.
- *B. melitensis*.
- *B. suis*.
- *B. canis*.

Environmental factors
Individuals working in occupations requiring close contact with animals such as veterinarians, abattoir and dairy workers and farmers are at increased risk of acquiring brucellosis. The consumption of unpasteurised dairy products is the most common mode of transmission.

Clinical features
History
After an incubation period, which is usually between 2 and 4 weeks, but may be longer, malaise, headache, myalgia and night sweats accompany the onset of an intermittent fever.

Presentation
Brucellosis tends to run a chronic, granulomatous course and can affect any organ system [1]. Various non-specific features may develop including anorexia, dizziness, organomegaly and lymphadenopathy. Skin lesions develop in up to 10% of cases but are not pathognomonic and include morbilliform, scarlatiniform and roseolar exanthems, vasculitis lesions and ulceration. Erythema nodosum-like lesions of the legs have also been reported [2,3].

Clinical variants
Contact brucellosis [2,3]. Veterinary surgeons, and others who are in frequent contact with infected animals, may develop a high degree of allergic sensitivity to *Brucella* antigens. Contact with the secretion of an infected animal, usually during delivery, gives rise to pruritus, erythema and urticarial wheals within a short time of contact, often followed within 48 h by a profuse eruption of follicular papules, many of which become vesicular or pustular, and heal in 10–14 days to leave small scars. Secondary eruptions of erythema multiforme type may develop remotely from the sites of contact. The contamination of abrasions by *B. suis* may cause indolent ulcers.

Differential diagnosis
Brucellosis should be considered in the differential diagnoses of fevers of unknown origin and these include typhoid fever,

tuberculosis, leptospirosis, dengue, toxoplasmosis, Epstein–Barr virus, cytomegalovirus, HIV and lymphoma. In contact brucellosis, transmissible diseases including herpes simplex and zoster as well as zoonoses such as orf and poxvirus infections should be considered.

Complications
Brucellosis can result in focal osteoarticular disease in up to 70% of cases with peripheral arthritis, sacroiliitis and spondylitis. Focal genitourinary, neurological, cardiovascular or pulmonary involvement may occur, leading to significant morbidity and potential mortality (especially with endocarditis) [1,4].

Disease course and prognosis
The course of brucellosis is variable [2]. The illness usually lasts for 3 or 4 months, but both acute fulminating and chronic forms occur. In the latter, there may be persistent infection of the bone, gallbladder or other organs. Relapse following treatment is not uncommon [1,2].

Investigations
Cultures can take up to 3 weeks to grow and may require special techniques. Therefore, it is important to notify the laboratory staff if brucellosis is suspected. Culture may be taken from blood and body fluids such as cerebrospinal fluid, synovial fluid or tissue.

Serological tests may be useful. However, in endemic countries high antibody titres (>1:640) may be required to confirm causality and a lack of correlation between serological findings, clinical outcomes and culture positivity has been demonstrated [5]. PCR-based methods are helpful for confirming the diagnosis.

Management
Patients should receive appropriate antibiotic therapy. The recommended course of treatment for brucellosis includes doxycycline and either rifampicin or an aminoglycoside, both of which should be given for at least 6 weeks [1,6,7]. Shorter periods of therapy increase the risk of relapse.

Fluoroquinolones or trimethoprim–sulfamethoxazole (co-trimoxazole) could be used in combination with first line antimicrobials if required.

> **Treatment ladder for brucellosis**
>
> **First line**
> - Doxycycline plus either rifampicin, gentamicin or streptomycin
>
> **Second line (in combination with first line agents)**
> - Trimethoprim–sulfamethoxazole
> - Ciprofloxacin

BARTONELLA

Definition
Originally classified as rickettsiae, *Bartonella* species are now regarded as bacteria more closely related to *Brucella* than to other genera [1]. *Bartonella* spp. have been reclassed from the genus *Rochalimaea* [2]. *Bartonella* species are Gram-negative bacilli, which are capable of infecting and surviving inside erythrocytes.

Introduction and general description
The human diseases associated with these organisms are trench fever due to *B. quintana*, bacillary angiomatosis (*B. henselae*, *B. quintana*), cat scratch disease (*B. henselae*) and Oroya fever (*B. bacilliformis*). Other described *Bartonella* spp., such as *B. elizabethae*, have rarely been associated with human disease, for example bacteraemia. Those organisms that cause vascular proliferation (e.g. *B. bacilliformis*) are known to stimulate the production of vascular endothelial growth factor (VEGF), its receptors VEGFR-1 and VEGFR-2, and angiopoietin 2 in host cells. *Bartonella* species may also remain in endothelial cells in a vacuole-like structure called an invasome.

Trench fever

Definition and nomenclature
Trench fever is caused by *B. quintana*, which is transmitted to humans by the human body louse (*Pediculus humanus corporis*) [3].

> **Synonyms and inclusions**
> - Quintana fever

Epidemiology
It has been diagnosed in many different countries, usually under conditions where there have been very poor levels of hygiene. The name trench fever stems from its identification among soldiers during the First World War.

Pathophysiology
Humans are the only known reservoir. Transmission is by inoculation with contaminated louse faeces via skin or conjunctiva.

Clinical features
The clinical manifestation of infection can range from a mild febrile illness to debilitating disease. The nature of the fever can be episodic or persistent, and the synonym quintana (or 5-day) fever refers to the paroxysmal exacerbations which can occur after asymptomatic periods [4]. Malaise, headache, gastrointestinal symptoms and bone pain are common. Most cases have a widespread maculopapular eruption, most prominent on the trunk, which fluctuates with the fever.

Disease course and prognosis
The illness is usually mild with spontaneous recovery. Chronic bacteraemia may occur, particularly in the immunocompromised, and the organism is a cause of culture-negative endocarditis.

Management
Uncomplicated bacteraemia should be treated with doxycycline or a macrolide for 4–6 weeks. For severe or chronic disease, doxycycline

in combination with gentamicin or a third generation cephalosporin is recommended [5].

Cat scratch disease

Definition and nomenclature
Infection due to *B. henselae*.

Synonyms and inclusions
- Inoculation lymphoreticulosis
- Subacute regional lymphadenitis
- Teeny disease

Introduction and general description
This is a syndrome characterised by the development of peripheral lymphadenopathy after a cat scratch or bite. Patients with the syndrome usually have antibodies to this organism, which has also been isolated from lymph nodes.

Epidemiology
Cats are the natural reservoir for the *B. henselae* and they may have a persistent bacteraemia for many months [6] without clinical signs of disease. *B. henselae* has been found in other domestic animals such as dogs, guinea pigs and rabbits [4]. The disease is worldwide in distribution and appears to be more common in autumn and winter. Cat scratch disease, as the name suggests, develops after a scratch or bite from an infected cat. Cat fleas (*Ctenocephalides felis*) are responsible for transmission between felines but it is not clear if this is a source of infection for humans. Contact with infected cat saliva via mucous membranes or broken skin may account for cases without the classical scratch or bite.

Age
It affects all ages, but mostly children and teenagers.

Sex
Both sexes.

Pathophysiology
Pathology
After inoculation, *B. henselae* invades endothelial cells causing a localised inflammatory reaction and regional lymphadenopathy [7]. There is a granulomatous response to the infection in the immunocompetent host; in the immunocompromised, vasculoproliferative changes may occur. In some cases the infection may become disseminated and in an unknown number the infection is asymptomatic.

Causative organisms
- *B. henselae*.

Clinical features [8,9]
History
As already stated not all infected cases become symptomatic. There is a history of cat contact, not necessarily prolonged or close, and usually a local wound. In many cases, it is believed that the cat is the source of the organism and the wound is the portal of entry. A scratch by a cat fulfils both requirements and is the commonest mode of infection. The cat is usually young but not ill. Occasionally, more than one member of a family may be affected.

Presentation
Up to 10 days after the inoculating event, a papule (occasionally a group of papules) may form, which progresses through vesicular and crusting stages in 2 or 3 days, and may ulcerate. This lesion may be inconspicuous or may take several weeks to regress and may leave a superficial scar [4]. Identification of the inoculation wound is of diagnostic importance, and examination should include the scalp, ears and fingers. About half are on the hands and arms and one-quarter on the head and neck. Constitutional symptoms are usually mild, but fever is present in 60% of cases, persisting from a few days up to 2 weeks. Illness lasting more than 2 weeks is uncommon [10].

Lymphadenopathy is present in all cases, and usually develops within 1 or 2 weeks of the initial papule, although it may not be noticed until later. The affected node is in the drainage path of the primary lesion but there is no lymphangitis. It is solitary in 85% of patients; two or three are seen occasionally [9]. Uncommonly, bilateral lymphadenopathy is seen, but this can be explained by separate inoculations or a single one close to the midline. The glands are painful and tender and occasionally progress to suppuration and discharge before regressing in a period of weeks or months; persistent enlargement is uncommon. Recurrent lymphadenopathy is exceptional [10].

Clinical variants
Primary inoculation of the eye may occur as a result of contact with cat saliva or self-inoculation from another site. This can result in granulation, usually painless, and usually on the palpebral conjunctiva, followed by enlargement of the preauricular gland, constituting one of the forms of Parinaud oculoglandular syndrome [11].

Unusual cutaneous manifestations include a maculopapular rash, urticaria, thrombocytopenic purpura, erythema nodosum, erythema multiforme and erythema marginatum; they appear to be more common among patients with severe or systemic disease [10].

Differential diagnosis
Sporotrichosis, atypical mycobacterial infection, pyogenic adenitis, viral infections such as Epstein–Barr virus, cytomegalovirus and HIV, toxoplasmosis, tularaemia, lymphoma and sarcoidosis must be considered.

Complications and co-morbidities
Rarely, hepatomegaly or splenomegaly with granuloma formation can occur, most commonly in children, which may be associated with persistent fever [12]. Arthralgia and myalgia can occur but are most common in older age groups.

Cat scratch disease is recognised as a cause of neuroretinitis, which can lead to oedema of the optic nerve and acute visual loss. Other neurological complications are also described in cat scratch disease including encephalopathy and transverse myelitis.

Disease course and prognosis
Cat scratch disease, even when accompanied by the more severe complications, is generally benign and self-limiting.

Investigations
Unilateral lymphadenitis is the usual presenting feature. A history of a cat scratch days or weeks previously resulting in a granulomatous nodule distal to the gland would immediately confirm the diagnosis, and the importance of actively seeking these two features has been emphasised [9]. If they are lacking, the clinical diagnosis is made by exclusion.

Serology can be performed but has poor sensitivity and specificity. *B. henselae* is slow growing and fastidious so when sending samples for culture it is essential that the laboratory is informed of the suspected diagnosis so the sample can be managed appropriately; however, even with optimal techniques, positive culture from blood and tissue samples may be elusive.

Both the primary lesions and the regional lymph nodes show characteristic, although non-specific, changes on histology. In the early stages, there is focal reticulum cell hyperplasia, which forms granulomas of the sarcoid type. Later, there are microabscesses surrounded by a palisade of epithelioid cells and occasionally Langhans giant cells. The earlier a lymph node is biopsied, the greater the numbers of bacilli visible with the Warthin–Starry silver stain; they are usually undetectable by the time suppuration has occurred [13].

Immunohistochemistry demonstrates the bacilli in the inoculation lesion or, more commonly by the time of presentation, in the lymph node, and would confirm the diagnosis. However, the organisms are increasingly difficult to detect as the disease progresses. Otherwise, histology is not specific, and biopsy is not routinely recommended.

Historically, skin testing with cat scratch disease antigen, made from pus from affected lymph nodes, was used but is no longer performed.

PCR testing for *Bartonella* is useful for distinguishing between species but it is not very sensitive; PCR is more likely to be positive in the first 6 weeks of the disease [14].

Management
In most cases, the disease is mild and self-limiting. However, for patients with lymphadenitis, a 5-day course of azithromycin is generally recommended, although there is a lack of randomised trials [15]. Alternatives include clarithromycin, rifampicin, ciprofloxacin and trimethoprim–sulfamethoxazole. In more severe disease, including neurological and ocular disease and endocarditis, combinations of these antibiotics for prolonged periods are required.

Fluctuant glands may be aspirated but should not be incised as chronic drainage may occur. Excision of lymph nodes is not justified therapeutically, although it may occasionally be indicated for histology.

Bacillary angiomatosis

Definition and nomenclature
Bacillary angiomatosis is an uncommon disease found in AIDS patients and occasionally other patients with severe immunosuppression [16]. Rarely, bacillary angiomatosis can occur in immunocompetent individuals [17]. It is characterised by the development of friable angiomatous papules and nodules. Two *Bartonella* spp. have been associated with this infection: *B. henselae* and *B. quintana* [18]. The appearance of these lesions follows a septicaemia, which is usually mild and often passes unnoticed.

Synonyms and inclusions
- Epithelioid angiomatosis

Introduction and general description
The disease presents with small proliferative blood vessel-containing lesions on the skin surface.

Epidemiology
The disease has been most commonly described in North America but has been reported in most parts of the world. The infection is sporadic and there is not necessarily a history of exposure to cats or of skin injury.

Age
Any, but usually seen in adults.

Sex
Both sexes.

Associated diseases
- HIV/AIDS
- Severe immunocompromise

Pathophysiology
Pathology
The skin lesions follow early and symptomatic blood dissemination of the microorganisms. The bacteria can invade erythrocytes as well as endothelial cells and are able to stimulate angiogenesis in the vascular endothelium.

Causative organisms
B. henselae and *B. quintana*. The reservoirs for *B. henselae* and *B. quintana*, respectively, are cats and humans; the latter bacterium is probably transmitted by the body louse. There are no known differences between skin infections caused by the two species of *Bartonella*.

Clinical features
History
Commonly, there is no history of exposure or obvious entry point.

Presentation
The lesions of bacillary angiomatosis are very variable [19]. They appear as either solitary or crops of red to purpuric vascular papules, which may then expand into nodules. Superficial lesions closely resemble pyogenic granulomas. Ulceration and bleeding can occur. They may involve any site including mucosal surfaces. Local lymphadenopathy occurs infrequently. Very extensive lesions may cover parts of the face or trunk.

There is lobular proliferation of small blood vessels that contain swollen endothelial cells. These contain granular material, which consists of clumps of bacteria seen with the Warthin–Starry stain.

Differential diagnosis
The lesions need to be distinguished from pyogenic granulomas, molluscum contagiosum, Kaposi sarcoma, cutaneous lymphoma and deep fungal infections disseminated to the skin. The lesions are very similar to those of verruga peruana.

Complications and co-morbidities
Complications include bacillary peliosis, where vascular lesions develop in internal organs especially the liver. Again, the endothelial cells lining these spaces contain large numbers of organisms. Bacillary peliosis is typically seen with *B. henselae* infection and can be fatal. Subcutaneous and osseous lesions can occur and these are more frequently seen in infection with *B. quintana*.

Disease course and prognosis
The skin lesions remain if the patient does not receive treatment and the disease may be fatal if left untreated, especially if there is visceral disease.

Investigations
The diagnosis is made by the appearance of the typical lesions and biopsy, which should reveal the presence of large clusters of bacteria on Warthin–Starry staining. *Bartonella* spp. can be difficult to culture. Serology is not very sensitive or specific and PCR may be useful, especially for distinguishing between different *Bartonella* species. If bacillary angiomatosis is suspected, imaging should be performed to exclude peliosis.

Management
There are no controlled studies of treatment of this condition. Doxycycline or erythromycin is usually given. It may be necessary to use long periods of treatment for 12 weeks or longer. Peliosis, as well as cutaneous lesions, typically responds to antimicrobial therapy, but may require a longer treatment course. Relapses are common after cessation of therapy.

Surgical removal of solitary lesions may be appropriate but should be done under antibiotic cover.

Oroya fever and verruga peruana

Definition and nomenclature
Oroya fever is an infectious disease transmitted by *Phlebotomus* spp. (sandfly) and caused by the small rod-shaped organism *B. bacilliformis*.

Synonyms and inclusions
- Carrión disease [20]

Introduction and general description
Infection with *Bartonella bacilliformis* can result in two distinct clinical manifestations which may occur in isolation or sequentially [21]. Oroya fever, as the name suggests, is a febrile illness which may be followed by the appearance of multiple angiogenic skin papules, verruga peruana. The link between Oroya fever and verruga peruana was only made in 1885 when Daniel Carrión, a medical student, injected himself with exudate from a verruga lesion. He subsequently developed Oroya fever, from which he died.

Epidemiology
The disease is endemic in the inter-Andean valleys between 500 m and 3200 m above sea level, especially Peru, but outbreaks have occurred in neighbouring Latin American countries.

Age
In the endemic areas, most individuals are infected in childhood and acquire a permanent immunity.

Sex
Both sexes.

Pathophysiology
Pathology
The disease is transmitted via bites from infected female sandflies of the genus *Lutzomyia*. The organism is flagellate and can adhere to and invade red blood cells. *B. bacilliformis* is able to colonise the entire circulatory system [21]. Persisting forms in circulating cells act as a reservoir for new infections spread by sandflies. The bacteria can also penetrate endothelial cells *in vitro* and produce an endothelial cell stimulating factor.

Causative organisms
B. bacilliformis; case reports exist of other *Bartonella* species resulting in similar clinical manifestations: *B. rochalimae* and *Candidatus Bartonella ancashensis* [20,22].

Clinical features
History
The incubation period is usually about 60 days following a bite from an infected sandfly.

Presentation
Two forms of infection are recognised: Oroya fever and verruga peruana; these are now known to represent two stages of infection.

Oroya fever is the first stage of disease: there is a sudden onset of pyrexia accompanied by a rapidly progressive, haemolytic anaemia, due to the destruction of infected red blood cells [23]. Hepatosplenomegaly and generalised lymphadenopathy occur and a petechial or ecchymotic rash may develop. The mortality is high, especially in pregnant women. Secondary infections are common and include salmonella, toxoplasmosis, malaria, shigellosis, histoplasmosis and pneumocystosis; these are also potentially life threatening [21].

Verruga peruana is the second disease state recognised with *B. bacilliformis* infection. It may develop without previous Oroya fever, or may follow it weeks or months later. The eruption is composed of red papules, which appear in crops and often become nodular or pedunculated. Some lesions become very large, others may be haemangiomatous or haemorrhagic. Lesions may be

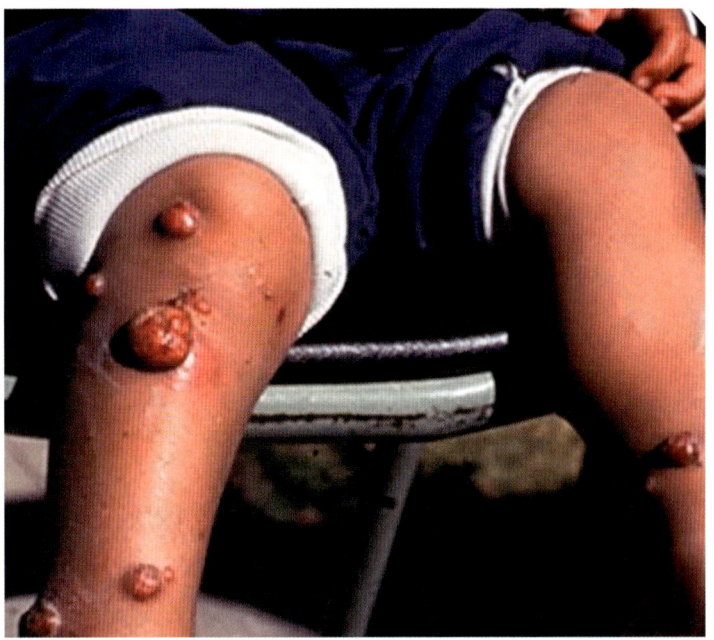

Figure 26.31 Nodular and mular lesions of verruga peruana. Image courtesy of Dr Ciro Maguiña.

classed as either miliary (multiple small, red papules), mular (blood-filled nodules) or diffuse (groups of larger subdermal nodules) (Figure 26.31) [24]. They are most numerous on the face, neck and limbs but may also involve the mucous membranes. Constitutional symptoms of fever, malaise, myalgia and lymphadenopathy may coexist in this form of infection, which may settle spontaneously. Lesions may persist for months or years and may heal with scarring. Verruga peruana is rarely fatal but lesions can bleed [21].

Differential diagnosis
Verruga peruana must be distinguished from yaws, acquired haemangiomas, disseminated deep mycoses and Kaposi sarcoma.

Complications and co-morbidities
Haemolytic anaemia in the acute phase of Oroya fever.

Disease course and prognosis
Oroya fever is potentially fatal with a high case fatality rate. Verruga lesions generally settle spontaneously over time.

Investigations
The diagnosis should be considered only if the patient has visited the endemic areas. In Oroya fever, the organism can be seen in blood films or isolated in blood cultures.

The biopsy appearances of verruga peruana show lesions containing numerous small blood vessels with endothelial proliferation and *B. bacilliformis* may be seen in the cytoplasm of endothelial cells with Warthin–Starry or Giemsa staining. There is a variable infiltrate of chronic inflammatory cells, and lesions heal with fibrosis [25].

Management
All febrile cases should receive antibiotic therapy. In Oroya fever, ciprofloxacin is the most commonly used agent [20]. Ciprofloxacin is also active against common secondary infections such as salmonella, making it a sensible therapeutic option. Other potential treatment options include chloramphenicol, penicillin, doxycycline and trimethoprim–sulfamethoxazole. Ceftriaxone should be added in severe cases [20].

In verruga peruana, response to antibiotics is unsatisfactory; most lesions evolve and eventually settle uninfluenced by treatment.

VIBRIO VULNIFICUS INFECTIONS

Definition
Certain non-cholera vibrios have been found to cause severe cellulitis. *Vibrio vulnificus* is the best known of these organisms. *V. vulnificus* is a flagellated Gram-negative curved rod-shaped organism.

Epidemiology
V. vulnificus is a marine pathogen, found in warm seawater areas such as around the Gulf of Mexico, South America, Asia and Australia. It can invade via the gastrointestinal tract following ingestion (typically raw oysters) or contaminate superficial wounds [1,2].

Clinical features
In immunocompromised patients, such as those with diabetes, HIV or chronic renal or liver disease, and occasionally in the otherwise healthy, *V. vulnificus* infection may cause a septicaemic illness of rapid onset. A characteristic is the appearance, in almost two-thirds of patients, of acute onset cellulitis and haemorrhagic bullae which ulcerate and may progress to necrotising fasciitis. These typically appear on the lower extremities. Systemic signs include hypotension and rigors leading to multiorgan failure. The infection is often rapidly progressive and fatal.

Primary wound infections due to *V. vulnificus* will present with cellulitis, necrotising fasciitis and ulceration at the site of injury, which may then progress to septicaemia [3]. *V. vulnificus* has also been found to survive for over 24h on skin and then infect an abrasion [4].

Disease course and prognosis
V. vulnificus infection can be fatal; mortality from a primary wound infection is around 25% but is significantly higher in those with underlying conditions or primarily septicaemic disease.

Investigation
Clinical suspicion of *V. vulnificus* is based on exposure to the marine environment or ingestion of raw shellfish. Although *V. vulnificus* grows readily on a variety of culture media it is important to liaise closely with the laboratory so the diagnosis is not overlooked. Culture and microscopy of skin lesions should reveal the organism and PCR from blood or wound exudate is helpful.

Management
Treatment should be initiated as early as possible as there is a case fatality rate of 50%.

Various antimicrobial therapy options exist but ceftazidime in combination with either ciprofloxacin or doxycycline is recommended. Combined antibiotic regimes are generally recommended as antibiotic resistance is not uncommon.

Surgical debridement of necrotic lesions is required and any abscesses should be drained.

EHRLICHIA AND ANAPLASMA

Ehrlichia spp. are small, round or ovoid Gram-negative bacteria [1]. They are the cause of ehrlichiosis, which is a tick-borne zoonosis, predominantly infecting domestic and wild animals. The bacteria form clusters of intracellular inclusion bodies known as morulae [1]. *Anaplasma phagocytophilum* is an obligate intracellular bacterium, which is also transmitted to humans via ticks, and causes human granulocytic anaplasmosis.

Ehrlichiosis and anaplasmosis

Definition and nomenclature
Tick-borne zoonotic infections caused by *Ehrlichia* spp. and *A. phagocytophilum*, respectively.

Synonyms and inclusions
- Human monocytic ehrlichiosis
- Human granulocytic ehrlichiosis

Epidemiology
Most cases have been described from the USA [2], although patients with this infection have been recognised in Europe and South America. In the USA, the distribution of the American dog tick, *Dermacentor variabilis*, and the lone star tick, *Amblyomma americanum*, coincide with the distribution of human cases. Natural hosts include wild vertebrates such as white-tailed deer but domestic animals including dogs may be infected.

Age
Any age.

Sex
Both sexes.

Pathophysiology
A number of different *Ehrlichia* species have been recognised in humans. *Anaplasma phagocytophilum* is a related member of the Anaplasmataceae family, to which *Ehrlichia* belongs, and it can result in a similar clinical disease known as human granulocytic anaplasmosis.

Pathology
Ehrlichia and *Anaplasma* are rickettsia-like, obligate intracellular bacteria which invade white blood cells. Ehrlichia are transported into cells via the host cell filopodium during the initial stages of infection but in later stages of the disease they are released when the host cell membrane ruptures [1].

Causative organisms [3]
- *E. chaffeensis*.
- *E. ewingii*.
- *E. muris eauclairensis*.
- *A. phagocytophilum*.

Environmental factors
Disease peaks are timed with tick activity so most cases are seen between late spring and early autumn.

Clinical features
The clinical features of ehrlichiosis are non-specific [4]. The median incubation period following the tick bite is 7 days and patients generally present with fever, malaise, headache and myalgia. Over 30% of patients have a diffuse maculopapular rash and in some this becomes petechial [5]. Rashes are much less common with *Anaplasma* infections [6]. Leukopenia and thrombocytopenia may develop.

Differential diagnosis
The differential diagnosis includes other tick-borne rickettsial diseases such as Rocky Mountain spotted fever and anaplasmosis.

Investigations
The diagnosis is difficult as cultural techniques are complicated and PCR-based diagnosis or serological assay using immunofluorescence is employed instead. The clinical history is also important.

Management
First line treatment is doxycycline, as it is for other tickborne rickettsial infections [3].

OTHER GRAM-NEGATIVE BACILLI

The aeromonads may occasionally cause cellulitis. These bacteria are inhabitants of water and cause infections in fish and reptiles. Cellulitis or necrotising fasciitis caused by *Aeromonas* spp. is rare, but may follow contamination of a wound in contact with fresh water [1]. It may also occur in immunocompromised patients. *Aeromonas* spp. have inducible β-lactamases and are frequently resistant to penicillins and some cephalosporins. Quinolones, ceftazidime and meropenem are usually active, and sensitivity to co-trimoxazole and chloramphenicol is variable [2]. Cellulitis can spread rapidly and may involve muscle tissue or periosteum unless treated promptly [3]. *A. hydrophila* has been reported to cause ecthyma gangrenosum [4].

Bacteria such as *Capnocytophaga canimorsus*, known originally as dysgonic fermenters (DF), may also cause severe cellulitic skin lesions. These organisms are Gram-negative rods that grow poorly on most culture media. They are zoonotic and have been isolated from the oral cavity of dogs. *C. canimorsus* causes infections in patients who have undergone splenectomy or have other predisposing conditions, where it causes an acute septicaemic illness. More indolent infections including cellulitis are seen in otherwise healthy patients [5]. However, septicaemia may also develop in this group.

Eikenella corrodens, an anaerobic Gram-negative bacillus, may cause abscesses of the skin in intravenous drug abusers. It has also been isolated from wounds caused by human bites [6].

ANAEROBIC BACTERIA

Definition
Anaerobic bacteria are organisms that cannot grow on a solid surface in the presence of oxygen. Anaerobic bacteria can be divided into those that are obligate (strict) anaerobes, such as *Treponema* spp., and the moderate anaerobes such as *B. fragilis*. They include both Gram-positive (e.g. *Cutibacterium* spp.) and Gram-negative (e.g. *Bacteroides* spp.) organisms and certain spiral bacteria. Most of the bacteria considered in this section are Gram negative.

The family Bacteroidaceae consists of Gram-negative rod-shaped bacilli with rounded or pointed ends. Some are fusiform. They are non-motile, do not form spores and are strict anaerobes [1]. Within the family are four genera: *Bacteroides*, *Prevotella*, *Porphyromonas* and *Fusobacterium*. These include the *B. fragilis* group, many of which are gastrointestinal tract commensals. The *Prevotella* spp. includes the organisms formerly known as *B. melaninogenicus* and *B. oralis*, now *P. melaninogenica* and *P. oralis*, respectively. The different genera can be classified according to nutritional requirements, pigmentation and morphology. Classification within the genus, *Fusobacterium* spindle-shaped bacilli, is unsatisfactory and, although a few species have been clearly defined, many isolates of commensal fusiform bacteria from animals and humans cannot be reliably identified as named species.

Fusobacterium organisms, although a well-known cause of infections in animals, are less often isolated today from human pathological material. In the past, *F. necrophorum* was regarded as an uncommon but important human pathogen among those in contact with animals. The term necrobacillosis or Lemierre syndrome was applied to such infections, characterised as they were by necrosis and abscess formation. *F. nucleatum* can be found in severe intraoral infections such as acute necrotising ulcerative gingivitis or Vincent's angina.

In common with many anaerobic bacteria, *Fusobacterium* spp. appear to synergise with other organisms, including spiral bacteria, to produce disease. They have been implicated in the pathogenesis of cancrum oris (noma) as well as tropical ulcer (*F. ulcerans*) [2], where the production of butyric acid by these organisms contributes to tissue necrosis.

Leptotrichia spp. are long, Gram-negative, rod-shaped organisms with pointed ends, not truly spindle shaped, sometimes forming lengths of separate filaments. They are part of the oral, intestinal and urogenital flora. *L. trevisanii* is particularly associated with septicaemia in the immunocompromised and other *Leptotrichia* species are reported to cause cellulitis after bites, oropharyngeal infections and chorioamnionitis [3].

Bacteroides spp. are now recognised as common causes of Gram-negative bacteraemia and abscesses. They are occasionally implicated in suppurative hidradenitis and in infected pilar cysts. Mixed infections are characteristic of this group of bacteria.

In diabetic ulcers, in particular, *Bacteroides* spp. may be isolated and appear to be contributing to the clinical condition [4].

Prevotella infections dominate in intraoral infections, including pyorrhoea. In many cases, they may act in concert with other bacteria.

Clinical features
This group of organisms are important causes of a variety of infections from sinusitis and oral abscesses to endocarditis. *Bacteroides*, *Prevotella*, *Porphyromonas* and *Fusobacterium* spp. in combinations may also cause abscesses below the waist area. They have also been associated with other severe cutaneous infections such as necrotising subcutaneous infection.

Management
Treatment of anaerobic Gram-negative infections is largely empirical and testing the organisms for sensitivity is difficult. The choice of drugs includes metronidazole, clindamycin, imipenem and amoxicillin–clavulanate. However, advice should be sought before selecting therapy.

Tropical ulcer

Definition and nomenclature
Tropical ulcer is a synergistic bacterial infection that follows invasion of the skin by at least two organisms: a *Fusobacterium* spp. (usually *F. ulcerans*) plus a spirochaete or other anaerobic bacterial species [1,2].

Synonyms and inclusions
- Tropical phagedenic ulcer
- Tropical phagedena

Introduction and general description
Tropical ulcers occur in the tropics and present as acute or chronic ulcers.

Epidemiology
Tropical ulcer occurs very commonly throughout the hot and humid tropical regions. In some areas, northern Papua New Guinea for example, it is the commonest skin disease [3]. The disease has been described in countries from sub-Saharan Africa, India, South-East Asia and the West Pacific region. Tropical ulcers may also be seen as imported cases [4].

It has acquired numerous local names, but there are few minor differences in its clinical features and course.

Age
Commonest in children.

Sex
Both sexes.

Pathophysiology
Predisposing factors
There is no clear evidence that host-predisposing factors play a part in the pathogenesis of this condition. Previously, malnutrition was thought to be critical to the development of tropical ulcers, but it is likely that social factors such as overcrowding are equally important. Studies have failed to demonstrate a correlation between nutritional indices and the development of tropical ulcer [5], although the possible role of micronutrient deficiencies is unknown. Zinc therapy, however, does not appear to hasten healing of lesions [6].

Causative organisms
F. ulcerans plus a variable combination of other bacteria including spiral bacteria.

Environmental factors
Humid tropics where night-time temperature does not fall to low levels. While the reservoir of *F. ulcerans* is not known, it has been isolated from mud and stagnant water in endemic areas [7].

Clinical features (Figure 26.32)
History
Most tropical ulcers develop at a site of potential trauma, a scratch, cut or insect bite, and are therefore commonest on the lower legs and on the unshod foot. They are not unusual on the arms and may occur anywhere.

Presentation
The ulcers develop as a small papule or bulla, which may be haemorrhagic, and which breaks down rapidly to form a sharply defined ulcer, with a slightly indurated edge that may be undermined. An important feature is the rapid breakdown of the pre-ulcerative papule to form a tropical ulcer [7].

The floor of the ulcer is covered by a foul-smelling, greyish, purulent slough. Tropical ulcers are painful in the acute phase and there may be fever and constitutional symptoms. There is usually no regional lymphadenitis. If the lesion is treated promptly, even with careful dressing, the spread is limited to a lesion 2–4 cm in diameter, which heals slowly.

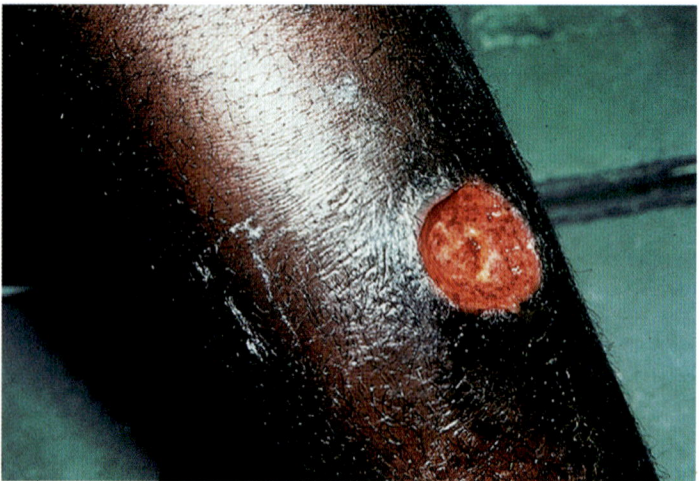

Figure 26.32 Tropical ulcer. Courtesy of St John's Institute of Dermatology.

Differential diagnosis
Differential diagnoses include yaws, venous ulcers, cutaneous leishmaniasis, ecthyma, pyoderma gangrenosum and Buruli ulcers.

Complications and co-morbidities
Squamous cell carcinomas may develop in chronic ulcers [8]. Squamous epithelioma may develop after 10 or more years.

Disease course and prognosis
Ulcers may involve deeper structures such as the tendons and periosteum [7]. Chronic ulceration can occur as can recurrent ulceration, which is more common in children [8].

Investigations
While pleomorphic fusiform and spiral bacteria are important pathogenic organisms, their presence or absence is not diagnostic and their isolation in culture not always possible.

Clinical features are the mainstay of diagnosis: rapid onset, clinical appearance and clustering of cases in the locality. Sores due to infected skin lesions are more indolent and smaller in size.

Management
Rest, elevation of the limb and adequate diet are of great importance. Any underlying chronic disease should be treated.

Antimicrobial therapy with metronidazole, tetracyclines or penicillin in the early stages is recommended.

Surgical debridement may be beneficial and early skin grafting has been successful in the rapid treatment of tropical ulcers, but it is dependent on the availability of the necessary expertise and patient compliance [3].

Granuloma inguinale

Granuloma inguinale or donovanosis is genital ulcer caused by *Klebsiella* (*Calymmatobacterium*) *granulomatis*. It is a sexually transmitted infection and is discussed in Chapter 30.

SPIROCHAETES AND SPIRAL BACTERIA

Definition
Spirochaetes are long flexible spiral organisms, motile but without external flagella. Many exist in nature in aquatic habitats [1,2]. Three genera exist and include important human pathogens and commensals: *Treponema*, *Borrelia* and *Leptospira*.

Treponema pallidum causes syphilis (Chapter 29); *T. pertenue* causes yaws; *T. carateum* causes pinta; and *T. endemicum* causes endemic syphilis (Bejel). *Borrelia recurrentis* causes louse-borne relapsing fever; *B. duttoni* and other species cause tick-borne relapsing fever; and *B. burgdorferi* and other species are the cause of Lyme borreliosis with associated erythema chronicum migrans (ECM), transmitted by *Ixodes* spp. ticks. *Leptospira interrogans* complex causes leptospirosis, including Weil disease. Commensal spirochaetes occur in the mouth (*T. microdentium* and *T. macrodentium*) and around the genitalia (*T. refringens*), as well as in the intestine. They appear to have no pathogenic potential but they are important as they may be confused with *T. pallidum*, from which they differ morphologically.

Spirillium minus, the cause of one form of rat-bite fever, is a spiral bacterium which is short, rigid and has bipolar flagella.

TREPONEMES

Endemic (non-venereal) treponematoses [1–3]

The endemic treponematoses comprise endemic syphilis or bejel, yaws and pinta, whose causative treponemes are morphologically and serologically indistinguishable.

Transmission is by skin-to-skin or mouth-to-mouth contact, and children are at greatest risk of infection. They are not sexually transmitted and congenital infection does not appear to occur. These diseases are similar to venereal syphilis in that they have an early stage, which includes primary and secondary lesions, and a late (tertiary) stage. The early stage is highly infectious and can persist for weeks to months. Cutaneous lesions are prominent, and mucous membranes and bones are involved in endemic syphilis and yaws.

Diagnosis is based on clinical features, identification of treponemes in mucocutaneous lesions, and serology; serological tests are identical to those for venereal syphilis. Specific molecular diagnostics are becoming increasingly available. Specific treponemal tests usually remain positive for life. Treponemes are easily identified in primary and secondary lesions by dark-ground microscopy and silver stains.

Following mass treatment campaigns in the 1950s and 1960s, the incidence of the endemic treponematoses was greatly reduced [3], but these diseases have not been totally eradicated.

Endemic syphilis or bejel

Definition and nomenclature
Endemic syphilis is a rare disease caused by *T. pallidum* subsp. *endemicum* [1].

Synonyms and inclusions
- Bejel
- Firjal
- Loath

Epidemiology
It occurs predominantly in the southern border of the Sahara desert and parts of the Middle East. It is still seen occasionally and usually in remote communities isolated from medical care.

Pathophysiology
Pathology
Transmission is thought to be via mucosal or skin contact [4].

Causative organism
- *T. pallidum* subsp. *endemicum*.

Clinical features
The *primary* lesion, which is frequently a papule or small ulcer [2], usually occurs in the mouth, where it often goes undetected, or on the nipples of breastfeeding women nursing infected children.

Secondary lesions, which are similar to those of venereal syphilis, include mucous patches on the buccal mucosa or lips, a generalised non-pruritic maculopapular rash, condylomata lata and generalised lymphadenopathy; painful periostitis and osteitis may affect the long bones and hands [4]. Untreated, secondary lesions last for 6–9 months.

The late (*tertiary*) stage is characterised by gummata, which can affect the nasopharynx (causing local destruction (gangosa)), skin, mucosa and bone.

Differential diagnosis
Differential diagnoses include herpetic infections, leprosy, aphthous ulcers, cutaneous leishmaniasis, rhinoscleroma, histoplasmosis, mycobacterium infections and syphilis.

Investigation
Serological reactions in endemic syphilis are identical to those seen in venereal syphilis. Both rapid plasma reagin (RPR) and the Venereal Disease Research Laboratory (VDRL) tests are widely available but can yield false positive results due to unrelated infections or disorders and false negative results in early disease. Both RPR and VDRL are referred to as non-treponemal tests and need to be combined with a treponemal test to confirm the result [4]. Treponemal tests can involve a variety of techniques such as immunofluorescence and agglutination assays, for example the *Treponema pallidum* haemagglutination (TPHA) test, but it is important to note that they remain positive even after successful treatment. The non-treponemal tests, however, can allow for monitoring treatment response with decreases in antibody titre [4]. Rapid, point-of-care tests are available and useful in low-resource settings. However, they cannot detect between treated and untreated disease, like the other treponemal tests.

Dark-field microscopy allows for direct identification of treponemes from lesion exudates but cannot differentiate between species. Treponemes cannot be easily cultured. The genomes of *T. pallidum* subspecies are highly conserved with <0.2% sequence variation between subspecies [5]. PCR-based assays are now available in high-income settings, with combined PCR and sequencing or whole genome sequencing proving to be most specific [6].

The histopathology of early endemic syphilis resembles venereal syphilis with a dermal infiltrate composed of lymphocytes and plasma cells and the presence of granulomas.

Management
Treatment is similar to that conducted for venereal syphilis (Chapter 29). In general, treponemes respond to parenteral penicillin and azithromycin.

Yaws

Definition and nomenclature
Yaws is caused by *T. pallidum* subsp. *pertenue*.

> **Synonyms and inclusions**
> - Framboesia (German and Dutch)
> - Pian (French)
> - Buba (Spanish)
> - Bouba (Portuguese)
> - Parangi (Sinhalese)

Introduction and general description
Yaws is an endemic disease that mainly presents with skin lesions. It is the subject of a number of international control programmes and is listed as a neglected tropical disease by the World Health Organization (WHO).

Epidemiology [1]
It is a disease of tropical rural populations, occurring in the Caribbean, Central and South America, throughout tropical Africa, South-East Asia and the Pacific islands. Transmission is favoured by overcrowded conditions. It used to be one of the commonest tropical diseases of the skin prior to the WHO's treatment campaigns in the 1950s and 1960s and in 2012, the WHO launched a new initiative aiming to eradicate yaws by 2020. In 2012, 84% of the 256 343 cases reported to the WHO came from just three countries: Papua New Guinea, Solomon Islands and Ghana [7]. One of the main challenges in eliminating the disease is probably related to the difficulty of managing those with latent phase disease in remote areas [3].

Age
Commonest in children but can affect adults.

Sex
Both sexes.

Pathophysiology
Pathology
Although many of the features of the overall pathogenesis of this disease resemble those of syphilitic disease (e.g. latency), the initial lesions are thought to follow direct entry of bacteria into non-genital skin.

Causative organisms
- *T. pallidum* subsp. *pertenue*.

Clinical features
History
There is seldom a history of injury preceding the appearance of the initial lesions.

Presentation
In the *primary* stage, the initial lesion ('mother yaw') is usually a solitary firm papule, although multiple lesions sometimes occur, at the point of entry of the treponemes [1,2]. This later ulcerates and is covered by a yellowish crust and granulating edge and centrally it is moist and red. The lesion is said to resemble a raspberry (hence the name framboesia) and is teeming with treponemes. Mother yaws are most common on the leg and may persist for several months before healing spontaneously to leave an atrophic, sometime hypopigmented scar [4]. Lymphadenopathy and arthralgia may also occur at this stage.

'Daughter yaws' are multiple lesions that develop in the *secondary* stage, often after the initial lesion has healed, sometimes up to 2 years later [4]. These smaller lesions occur in successive crops and often occur adjacent to body orifices. The lesions expand and then ulcerate and are also highly infectious. They are variable in appearance; papules, exuberant exophytic lesions, ulcers and hyperkeratotic plaques have all been described [1,4]. These secondary lesions also heal spontaneously within weeks to months although relapses can occur [4]. Fever, malaise and osteitis may accompany this stage [4].

A small proportion with untreated disease may enter late (*tertiary*) stage yaws, characterised by gummata, most commonly in the skin, bones and nose. As with other tertiary treponomal infections, this can lead to bowing of the tibia (sabre tibia), saddle nose deformities and destructive lesions of the nasopharynx and palate (gangosa).

Differential diagnosis
The differential diagnosis includes impetigo, ecthyma, pyoderma gangrenosum, cutaneous leishmaniasis, mycobacterium infections, leprosy, tropical ulcer and syphilis.

Disease course and prognosis
The disease can be disabling but is not fatal.

Investigations
As the organisms are closely related, serological tests used in syphilis are also employed in yaws. As with *T. pallidum*, *T. pertenue* is non-cultivable by conventional laboratory methods. Molecular diagnostic methods are likely to supersede serology, but remain limited to a few laboratories worldwide.

Biopsy is not a confirmatory diagnostic procedure. Early lesions show acanthosis, spongiosis and papillomatosis, with intraepidermal microabscesses. There is a moderate to dense dermal inflammatory infiltrate consisting of plasma cells, lymphocytes, macrophages, neutrophils and eosinophils. Numerous treponemes can be identified with silver stains. Late lesions are similar to those of tertiary cutaneous syphilis with the presence of granulomas and necrotic areas [4].

Management
All cases require antibiotic treatment. As with other forms of syphilis, typically parenteral penicillin or azithromycin is first line treatment.

Pinta

> **Synonyms and inclusions**
> - Carate
> - Mal de pinto
> - Morado Azul
> - Lota

Introduction and general description
Pinta is a disease exclusively of the skin caused by *T. pallidum* subsp. *carateum*.

Epidemiology
Although there has been a marked decline in its prevalence over the last century, it is still thought to be focally endemic in tropical Central and South America [4].

Pathophysiology
Pathology
Transmission is thought to be via skin contact [4].

Causative organism
- *T. pallidum* subsp. *carateum*.

Clinical features
In the *primary* stage of pinta, a few papules or erythematosquamous plaques develop. After an interval of months or years, the *secondary* stage features more extensive lesions, which are similar in appearance to the initial lesions. These are known as 'pintids'. Their initial red colour changes to brown, slate blue, black or grey, and eventually there is depigmentation intermixed with hyperpigmentation.

In the late (*tertiary*) stage, which takes several years to develop, there is irregular pigmentation, vitiligo-like hypochromia, areas of hyperkeratosis and cutaneous atrophy.

Pinta lesions are considered infectious with the exception of the late stage depigmented lesions [4].

Differential diagnosis
The differential diagnosis includes erythema dyschromicum perstans (ashy dermatosis), pityriasis alba, vitiligo, atrophic lichen planus and tuberculoid leprosy.

Investigations
The diagnosis is similar to that used in yaws with dependence on serology. *T. carateum* is also non-cultivable and there are now molecular tests able to distinguish *T. pallidum* and *T. pertenue*.

The histopathological findings are similar in primary and secondary lesions. There is migration of lymphocytes through an oedematous and acanthotic epidermis. Some areas show lichenoid changes. There are numerous melanophages in the upper dermis. In the hypopigmented lesions of the tertiary stage, there is epidermal atrophy and loss of melanin in the basal layer. Treponemes may be demonstrable in lesions of all stages.

Management
As with the other endemic treponematoses, treatment with penicillin is first line therapy.

BORRELIA

Relapsing fever

Definition
There are two forms of this disease: louse-borne or epidemic relapsing fever due to *B. recurrentis*, for which the human body louse (*Pediculus humanus corporis*) is the vector, and tick-borne endemic relapsing fever caused by various species of *Borrelia*, for example *B. duttoni* and *B. hermsi*. These spirochaetes are so genomically similar that they are now considered ecotypes of a single genomospecies [1].

Epidemiology
The louse-borne epidemic form is found in Ethiopia, the Sudan, other parts of sub-Saharan Africa and South America. It has also been diagnosed in Europe, in refugees from the Horn of Africa who had passed through Libya [1]. It is associated with overcrowding and poor hygiene, conditions which enable the human body louse to flourish. The milder, sporadic tick-borne cases occur worldwide [2]. The very variable symptom complex develops after an incubation period of about a week [1,2].

Clinical features
High fever, headache, myalgia, vomiting and respiratory symptoms usher in the acute attack. Jaundice and hepatosplenomegaly with liver tenderness are common, and a petechial or purpuric rash, predominantly on the trunk, is found in up to 60% of patients. In severe disease, hyperpyrexia, myocarditis, acute respiratory distress syndrome and splenic rupture can occur [1]. A remission occurs after a few days, to be followed by a relapse, and this pattern may continue for weeks. The cutaneous eruption does not, however, recur after the initial episode.

Differential diagnosis
Differential diagnoses include dengue fever, yellow fever, Lassa fever, brucellosis, leptospirosis, rat bite fever and *Bartonella* infection.

Investigations
Diagnosis is best confirmed by demonstration of the spirochaete in blood films using stained preparation or dark-ground illumination. PCR can be used for species diagnosis [1]. It is important to note that patients with tick-borne relapsing fever may have false positive serology for Lyme disease [2].

Management
The usual treatment is either tetracycline or erythromycin. Penicillin is an alternative. In louse-borne infections, a single dose may be adequate [3]. Because treatment failures are more frequent in the tick-borne group, the course of therapy is usually prolonged, typically up to 10 days.

A severe Jarisch–Herxheimer reaction may occur at the outset of treatment, particularly in louse-borne relapsing fever treated with penicillin [4].

Borrelia burgdorferi and Lyme disease

Definition and nomenclature
Lyme disease is a tick-borne zoonotic disease caused by spirochaetes of the *B. burgdorferi* sensu lato complex. Nine species of this *Borrelia* complex have been found to cause human disease, most commonly *B. afzelii* and *B. garinii* as well as *B. burgdorferi* sensu stricto, which was the original isolate and most common causative agent in North

America [1]. Henceforth, *B. burgdorferi* sensu stricto will be referred to as *B. burgdorferi*.

Synonyms and inclusions
- Lyme borreliosis

Introduction and general description
Lyme disease is named after the town of Lyme in Connecticut, USA, where the disease was first recognised in 1977. The characteristic eruption, ECM, which occurs at the site of inoculation, is a common early manifestation. Dissemination of the infection may cause disease of the nervous system, heart and joints, in addition to other dermatoses. Differences in the disease spectrum in different geographic areas have been noted and may be due to variation within the bacterial species [2] or to differences in diagnostic criteria and treatment practices [3].

Epidemiology [2]
The principal vector of *B. burgdorferi* infection is the *Ixodes* tick, different species of which predominate in different parts of the world, their distribution corresponding to that of Lyme disease. Patients usually live close to, or have visited, woodland areas, where small mammals are necessary hosts for immature stages in the life cycle of the tick. Adult ticks may infest larger mammals, especially deer. Humans are incidental, dead-end hosts for the spirochaetes [1].

Lyme disease has been reported in most temperate parts of the world but especially in the USA, where it is the commonest vector-borne infection, and in Europe, particularly in Scandinavia and central Europe. Positive *B. burgdorferi* serology without clinical disease is not uncommon in endemic areas and those with occupational risk factors [1,5].

Infection may occur at any time of year. Young nymphal ticks feed in early summer, when there is a marked peak in incidence of acquisition of human Lyme disease. The smaller autumn peak noted in some studies is associated with bites from adult ticks [4,5]. Deer, in particular, appear to harbour the infection in endemic areas.

Age
Any age.

Sex
Both sexes.

Pathophysiology
Pathology
The spirochaetes are transmitted into human skin when an infected tick takes a blood meal. The spirochaetes undergo significant transcriptomic and proteomic changes during feeding in preparation for inoculation [1]. Once in the human dermis, the spirochaetes replicate and migrate outwards along the plane of the dermis, explaining the characteristic feature of ECM with its gradually expanding annular formation.

The spirochaetes may spread via the bloodstream to other sites such as the central nervous system, joints and heart. There is evidence that surface *Borrelia* antigens may change during infection and thereby evade recognition and that the organism may bind host antigens such as plasmin.

After *B. burgdorferi* infection, specific antibodies are produced, but if the patient is treated early in the course of the disease, antibodies may disappear within a period of months and reinfection may occur.

Causative organisms
- *B. burgodorferi*.
- *B. afzelii*.
- *B. garinii*.

Environmental factors
The risk of acquiring Lyme disease is increased in individuals spending time outdoors, whether for work or recreation, especially if in areas with suitable tick habitat such as woods or dense vegetation [1], although increasingly cases are being reported from urban environments [6].

Clinical features
History
Of patients ultimately diagnosed as having Lyme disease, about 50% recall a tick bite; a bite by the autumn and winter feeding adult tick is more likely to be noticed than a bite by the summer feeding nymphs.

Presentation
Typically ECM will develop at the site of inoculation, usually within 7–14 days (Figure 26.33). ECM usually presents as a gradually expanding, red ring, enlarging at a rate of several centimetres per week. In some cases the redness is intense, in others barely detectable; it may be entirely flat or show elevation at the centre, the periphery or both [7]. The rash may be more difficult to detect in more pigmented skin types. Slight scaling is occasionally seen. Older areas of residual erythema may become dusky blue. There may be a zone of clearing behind the advancing ring producing a target-like morphology. Moderate burning or itching occurs in one-third of cases. If untreated, the lesion fades, usually within a few weeks, but the duration may vary between 1 day and 14 months. Regional lymphadenopathy and constitutional symptoms may occur. These are more common in North American disease than in Europe [1].

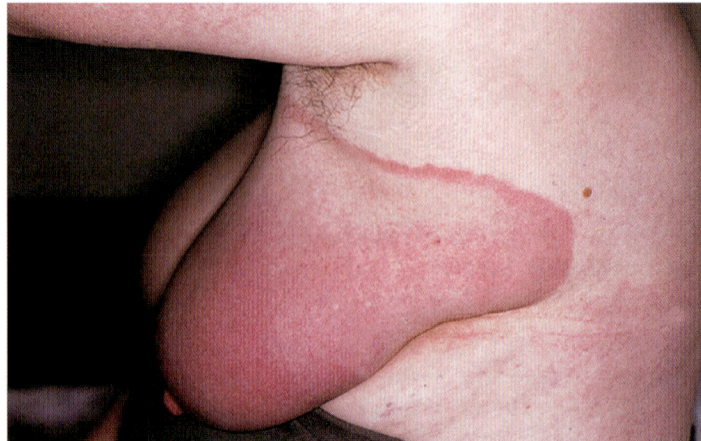

Figure 26.33 Erythema chronicum migrans. Courtesy of Dr A.S. Highet.

Dissemination of the infection may occur within days or weeks of inoculation. Spirochaetes have been detected in affected organs, although immunological processes may also contribute. Systemic features of Lyme disease include arthritis, neural involvement and heart disease including myocarditis, pericarditis and conduction defects. Migratory joint pains, myositis, conjunctivitis, hepatitis, generalised lymphadenopathy and splenomegaly may also occur. Neurological disease appears to be more prominent in European disease [1].

Clinical variants

With dissemination of the infection, secondary lesions of ECM are seen in about 20% of patients [1], and are typically smaller and less migratory than the original lesion. Malar erythema in febrile cases, and a diffuse maculopapular rash, may occur. Localised urticaria, generalised urticaria, urticarial vasculitis [8] and septal panniculitis have been reported.

Lymphocytoma cutis (also known as lymphadenosis benigna cutis) may present concurrently with ECM or develop later. It is typically a solitary nodule, seen mainly on the earlobe or on the breast areola. *B. burgdorferi* serology is usually positive, spirochaetes can be demonstrated in affected tissue, and the lesion subsides within 5 weeks of antibiotic therapy.

Acrodermatitis chronica atrophicans (ACA) is a late cutaneous manifestation of infection and has been associated primarily with *B. afzelii* infection. It is seen mainly in northern, central and eastern Europe [1,2]. Initially there is an erythematous plaque which slowly enlarges and gradually becomes violaceous and atrophic. Typical sites are the hands, feet, knees and elbows and there may be associated arthritis and polyneuropathy [1]. Spirochaetes have occasionally been cultured, but *B. burgdorferi* serology is strongly positive in all cases. Lesions respond to appropriate antibiotic therapy.

Lyme neuroborreliosis refers to the neurological manifestations of the infection and may occur early or late in the disease process. Presentations include cranial nerve palsies, peripheral neuropathy, meningitis and encephalopathy.

The possibility of *B. burgdorferi* having an aetiological role in morphoea and lichen sclerosus has been raised, based on the clinical association of these conditions with ACA and positive *B. burgdorferi* serology in some patients with morphoea [9,10]; however, the association has not been confirmed.

Asymptomatic or subclinical infection appears to be more common in Europe compared with North America, with substantial proportions of individuals living in endemic areas having *B. burgdorferi* antibodies without clinical disease [1]. An unknown number, however, may be at risk of late complications [11].

Differential diagnosis

The differential diagnosis of ECM includes arthropod-bite reactions, granuloma annulare, tinea infection, cellulitis, erythema multiforme and drug eruptions.

Disease course and prognosis

Chronic infections are recognised regularly both in the skin and associated with disease in the central nervous system and joints. Reinfection is possible, defined as ECM occurring at a distant site from the initial lesion with appropriate exposure. Those without detectable antibodies following prior infection are thought to be most at risk [1].

Investigations

Confirmation of *B. burgdorferi* infection is mainly by serology, although this is often negative in the first few weeks after inoculation. Serological testing conventionally uses a two-tiered testing protocol, where an enzyme immunoassay (ELISA) or indirect fluorescent antibody test (IFA) is followed by immunoblots. False negative tests may be due to the sequestration of antibody in immune complexes [12]. Serological testing is the preferred investigation for Lyme disease. Non-serological tests such as PCR and culture are generally not useful nor practical and should only be used as adjuncts to serological tests [13]. However, if clinical suspicion is high despite negative serology, there may be a place for performing PCR and culture on a biopsy from ECM [14].

Biopsy of acute lesions shows a superficial and deep perivascular and interstitial lymphohistiocytic infiltrate containing plasma cells, which is characteristic of ECM. The histology of lymphocytoma cutis is characterised by a dense polyclonal lymphocytic infiltrate. In ACA, plasma cells are prominent within the lymphohistiocytic infiltrate; the epidermis is atrophic and there may be liquefaction degeneration of the basal layer and telangiectasia of the papillary dermis. Spirochaetes may be identified by the Warthin–Starry stain.

Management

In the first instance, if attached ticks are discovered, they should be mechanically removed with tweezers or a similar device, ensuring the head section is included.

In the early stages of disease, serology is rarely positive and the focus should be on prophylactic antibiotics (ideally within 72 hours) for a high-risk tick bite. High-risk tick bites include those from highly endemic areas or where the tick was attached for over 36 hours [13]. Single-dose doxycycline (200 mg for adults; 4.4 mg/kg for children) is recommended as chemoprophylaxis in certain settings [13].

For patients presenting with ECM, oral antimicrobial therapy with doxycycline, amoxicillin or cefuroxime is recommended. The standard treatment course ranges from 14 days (Infectious Disease Society of America) [13] to 21 days (National Institute for Health and Care Excellence). Azithromycin would be a suitable second line option [13].

After dissemination has occurred, the results of even intensive therapy are less impressive; whether this is due to incomplete eradication of the organism or to an immunological pathogenesis is not known. Systemic disease should be treated as described, although the course length may be increased depending on the clinical manifestations. Neuroborreliosis and cardiac disease may require intravenous ceftriaxone or benzylpenicillin. However, depending on the severity, oral doxycycline may also be a suitable therapeutic option [13].

Preventing tick exposure with the use of protective clothing and repellents along with careful inspection of the skin after walking in endemic areas and prompt removal of attached ticks are the mainstays of Lyme disease avoidance.

> **Treatment ladder for Lyme disease**
>
> **First line**
> - Doxycycline
> - Intravenous ceftriaxone in neuroborreliosis or cardiac involvement
>
> **Second line**
> - Azithromycin

LEPTOSPIRA

Leptospirosis (including Weil disease)

Definition
Leptospirosis is an infection caused by organisms of the *Leptospira interrogans* complex and other genetically defined *Leptospira* species [1].

Epidemiology
Leptospira have a worldwide distribution. These spiral bacteria are commonly carried by rodents, particularly rats, but also pigs, dogs, cattle and wild animals, such as hedgehogs and moles. Rodents especially can excrete the organism in urine due to renal infection. Transmission to humans occurs via two routes: direct contact with an infected animal or indirect contact via contaminated substrate such as soil or water [2]. Therefore infections occur mainly in sewer workers and in those handling animals but occasionally result from exposure during watersports or fishing in a contaminated environment. Outbreaks can occur after heavy rainfall. Human-to-human transmission is extremely rare but has been reported [2].

Pathophysiology
Pathology
The portal of entry is usually the gastrointestinal tract, following consumption of infected water, but the infection can also penetrate through skin abrasions and mucous membranes. The spirochaetes cause extensive damage to endothelial cells.

Clinical features
After an incubation period of 1–2 weeks, an acute febrile illness begins abruptly. The most distinctive features are severe muscular pain and tenderness, and intense conjunctival infection. Headache, abdominal pain and respiratory symptoms are frequent. A transient truncal rash can occur, which can be maculopapular, urticarial or purpuric.

Weil disease occurs when following the initial phase a more severe illness develops with jaundice, renal failure, purpura and confusion [2].

A leptospiral form of pretibial fever is another clinical manifestation of leptospirosis, in which erythema may develop, most commonly on the legs.

Disease course and prognosis
In Weil disease the mortality rate is around 10% but can increase beyond 50% when there is lung involvement [3]. In milder forms spontaneous recovery typically occurs after about a week.

Investigations
The diagnosis is usually established by serology. PCR is useful but multiplex PCR, using two sets of primers, is recommended due to the risk of false positive results [2].

Management
Treatment for mild leptospirosis is usually doxycycline but azithromycin and amoxicillin would be suitable alternatives [3]. In more severe disease, benzylpenicillin or ceftriaxone would be recommended. Renal support with dialysis may be required. Treatment may induce a Jarisch–Herxheimer reaction.

RAT-BITE FEVERS

Spirillum minus rat-bite fever or sodoku

Definition
This form of rat-bite fever is caused by a spiral flagellate organism *Spirillum minus* (also called *Spirillum minor*), and it is usually transmitted, as the name suggests, by a bite from a rat.

Epidemiology
This is rare, with most cases being reported in Japan. It may cause disease in animal technicians bitten during the course of their work [1].

Clinical features
Up to around 10 days after the bite, the wound becomes indurated and may ulcerate, and an eschar may form. A fever develops accompanied by malaise and regional lymphadenopathy [2]. A violaceous, macular rash may become widespread, extending from the original lesion; rarely plaques are seen [3]. A recurrent course with remissions and relapses accompanied by increasingly severe local inflammation and a generalised cutaneous eruption is characteristic. Arthritis, however, is rare in this type of rat-bite fever.

Differential diagnosis
Sodoku may be differentiated from streptobacillary fever by finding the spiral organism in exudate or blood. Spirillum cannot be cultured on standard media in the laboratory.

Management
Untreated, most patients with *S. minus* infections recover without complication, although recovery may be prolonged. Penicillin is first line treatment; doxycycline would be a suitable alternative.

Streptobacillary rat-bite fever and Haverhill fever

Definition
Streptobacillus moniliformis is a natural inhabitant of the nasopharynx of rats and is the cause of the commoner and more severe form of rat-bite fever. When infection with this organism occurs in the absence of a rat bite, the term Haverhill fever is often used in recognition of an epidemic in Haverhill, Massachusetts, USA, when raw milk was thought to be the source of infection.

Streptobacillosis is also known by the descriptive term epidemic arthritic erythema.

Epidemiology
Streptobacillary rat-bite fever is more commonly seen in children, where lower socioeconomic status is likely to be relevant. While most reported cases occur in the USA, it has been reported in many other countries in Europe, Australia and Africa. Most cases in Asia are thought to be due to *Spirillum minus* [1]. In addition to rat bites, the disease may also be transmitted via contact with infected rat urine or other bodily fluids. The disease can be transmitted by pet rats, not just wild animals.

Pathophysiology
Causative organisms
The organism is a pleomorphic microaerophilic bacillus, sometimes showing beaded swellings.

Clinical features
When a rat bite is the origin of infection with this bacillus, the incubation period is short, usually less than a week. Typically, there is no sign of inflammation at the site of injury but a macular haemorrhagic, vesicular or petechial rash develops and involves the extremities, particularly the palms and soles [2]. The disease is manifested by an acute relapsing fever and migratory polyarthralgia, which affects the large joints as well as small joints of the extremities [1]. Other manifestations of this infection include endocarditis and, particularly in children, diarrhoea [2]. Lymphadenopathy is rare.

The clinical picture is similar in Haverhill fever, in which papules, vesicles, pustules and crusted lesions have been described along with late-onset pharyngitis.

Investigations
The diagnosis may be confirmed by blood culture, but clinical suspicion is required as culture can be challenging. Skin lesions demonstrate a leukocytoclastic vasculitis on histology [1].

Management
Without treatment, most cases eventually settle, but chronic arthritis and complications such as liver abscesses, pneumonia and endocarditis have been recorded. Untreated the mortality rate is around 10% [1].

Penicillin is the drug of choice, continued for at least a week with high-dose therapy in patients with complications [1]; doxycycline is a suitable alternative.

LEGIONELLOSIS

Definition
Legionellosis is an acute respiratory infection caused by a variety of different species of the genus *Legionella*, of which *L. pneumophila* accounts for over 90% of cases [1].

Epidemiology
One of the major features of the infection is the clustering of cases, often associated with exposure to organisms in the environment such as water-cooling systems, showers and humidifiers.

Clinical features
The disease may present with a flu-like illness without pneumonia (Pontiac fever) or with pneumonia. A variety of cutaneous features have been described in both pulmonary and non-pulmonary legionellosis, including abscesses, nodules, cellulitis, ulceration, bullae, pustules, panniculitis, pretibial erythema and a diffuse red rash [2]. These features are not diagnostic [3].

MISCELLANEOUS

Botryomycosis

Definition and nomenclature
Botryomycosis is a rare, chronic granulomatous reaction to bacterial infection, containing granules resembling the sulphur granules of actinomycosis [1,2].

Synonyms and inclusions
- Actinophytosis
- Bacterial pseudomycosis

Introduction and general description
Most cases of botryomycosis are caused by *Staph. aureus*; *P. aeruginosa* is implicated in around 20% of cases [3,4] and much less frequently other organisms may be isolated. Botryomycosis may develop in the skin or viscera and a variety of underlying predisposing factors have been described.

Epidemiology
This is a rare condition with a sporadic worldwide distribution.

Age
Any age.

Sex
Both sexes.

Associated diseases
Rarely seen in apparently healthy individuals, botryomycosis is associated with several predisposing disorders, especially diabetes, HIV/AIDS and liver disease [4,5].

Pathophysiology
Pathology
Skin injury may be the route of entry in some cases. The presence of a foreign body is thought to be predisposing to the condition [1]. Low-virulence strains of the causative microorganisms seem to be key and the size of bacterial inoculation may be crucial, resulting in a delicate balance between host and pathogen [5]. Impairment of the host's cellular immune response is thought to be relevant but the process of granule formation is not well understood [4]; through the Splendore–Hoeppli phenomenon [6] the bacteria are surrounded by eosinophilic material resulting from the host's immune response. This prevents phagocystosis and leads to chronic infection [7].

Causative organisms
- *Staph. aureus.*
- *P. aeruginosa.*
- More rarely *E. coli*, *Micrococcus*, *Streptococcus* and *Neisseria* species among others.

Clinical features
History
The infection may follow skin injury, but this is not typically the case.

Presentation
The resemblance to actinomycosis is clinically evident. Most lesions are on the extremities, especially feet and hands, but other sites including the perianal region and the face may be affected. In the primary cutaneous form, single or multiple abscesses of the skin and subcutaneous tissues break down to discharge serous fluid through multiple sinuses and heal after a course of many months to leave atrophic scars [1]. Vegetative verrucous lesions can occur as can nodular lesions [4]. Patients are generally well, afebrile and with minimal symptoms, although itch and tenderness may occur [4].

Clinical variants
Most cases are localised, but widespread involvement can occur [4].

Visceral botryomycosis is endogenous and typically seen in the immunosuppressed or in surgical patients. This most commonly affects the lungs, especially in the context of cystic fibrosis [4].

Differential diagnosis
- Mycetoma.
- Furunculosis.
- Actinomycosis.

Disease course and prognosis
The infection becomes chronic unless treated.

Investigations
Diagnosis should be based on microscopy, histopathology and culture. The key to the diagnosis is the presence of a small cluster of microorganisms on biopsy. This cluster resembles the grain of a mycetoma or sulphur granule of actinomycosis. The granules contain basophilic bacterial granules with a surrounding eosinophilic tissue reaction [2]. Gram staining may identify the bacteria but culture should also be performed.

Management
Treatment depends on the nature of the organism and, where appropriate, antibacterial sensitivities should be determined. For *Staph. aureus* infections, anti-staphylococcal penicillin and erythromycin would be first line agents. Antimicrobial therapy may have to be prolonged. Surgical excision and drainage may also be required.

Necrotising subcutaneous infections

Definition and nomenclature
This is a group of infections, caused by various aerobic and anaerobic bacteria, in which the principal focus of disease is the soft tissues of the deep dermis, adipose tissue and subcutaneous fascia, where the hallmark of infection is extensive necrosis accompanying cellulitis [1,2].

Synonyms and inclusions
- Necrotising fasciitis
- Fournier gangrene
- Progressive bacterial synergistic gangrene
- Meleney synergistic gangrene

Introduction and general description
In addition to an initially focal site of skin oedema, inflammation and subsequent clinically apparent necrosis, the affected patient is usually severely ill and toxic, and there is a high mortality rate with these infections [3]. The extent of infection is clearly variable; in some cases the pathology is restricted to a zone bound by fascia, while in others the infection extends to involve the muscle and deep vessels.

Epidemiology
Necrotising subcutaneous infections occur worldwide. Several different clinical entities are encompassed by this term but all of these conditions carry a significant mortality risk and require prompt recognition and treatment.

Age
Rare in children.

Sex
Both sexes.

Associated diseases
- May follow surgical procedures.
- Diabetes.

Pathophysiology
Pathology
The clinical classification of these infections is challenging and various pathogens may be associated but are not always isolated. It has been suggested [4] that there are at least two distinct groups of infections – those caused by β-haemolytic, usually group A, streptococci and others that depend on an infection with multiple

organisms, one of which is usually an anaerobe. The presence of a streptococcal aetiology is often difficult to establish with certainty, and infections without a proven cause may show striking increases in antistreptococcal antibody titres, suggesting that this may have been the original or a contributory cause [5]. The pathogenesis of the mixed bacterial infections is not well understood. Other variations include the presence or absence of muscle involvement.

While a complete and taxonomically valid list is difficult to compile, these infections include the following proposed types:
1. Clostridial cellulitis (gas gangrene).
2. Necrotising cellulitis or fasciitis due to:
   - β-haemolytic streptococci, or
   - other bacteria.
3. Progressive bacterial synergistic gangrene.
4. Gangrenous cellulitis due to other pathogens such as *Pseudomonas* spp. or zygomycete fungi (mucormycosis). These are mainly seen in the immunocompromised patient or after severe trauma.

To complicate the issue, eponymous titles have been used, and Meleney's name has been associated both with streptococcal necrotising cellulitis [6] and with progressive bacterial synergistic gangrene [7]. Similarly, Fournier gangrene, which describes a specific cellulitic necrotising process originally affecting the lower anterior abdominal wall and the scrotal fascia, probably includes at least two aetiologically different conditions, all affecting this specific site [8].

Clinical features
History
The clinical hallmark of all these infections is the appearance of necrosis in addition to cellulitis, which is often accompanied by a rapid course and considerable toxaemia. In practice, the main features of these infections are difficult to separate on clinical grounds, although there are some variations due to site of infection, and it is possible that they are part of a continuum of disease from cellulitis to myonecrosis. Death is a frequent outcome in such cases. Predisposing factors include trauma, infection, diabetes and previous surgery.

Clinical variants
Necrotising fasciitis, including streptococcal necrotising cellulitis, may follow entry of group A *Streptococcus*, *Staph. aureus*, *A. hydrophila*, *Vibrio vulnificus* or a mixture of other bacteria into the skin, most commonly on the head, neck or limbs [3]. The site of entry may not always be apparent. Patients usually present with a hot, tender, erythematous area of swelling; gradually the skin becomes dusky [3,9]. Bullae and necrosis of underlying tissue may supervene and the overlying skin may become anaesthetic. Unfortunately, the often indolent onset can give rise to a false sense of lack of urgency [10].

Progressive synergistic gangrene is usually seen in association with abdominal or other surgery where there is contamination of the wound by leakage of bowel contents. It may occur without apparent injury to the skin surface [11]. The organisms vary but microaerophilic streptococci, *Bacteroides* spp. or other anaerobes as well as Gram-negative bacteria are found. The wound becomes extended with surrounding necrosis and oedema, and the patient becomes toxic and unwell. The extending infection may affect muscle. Rapid deterioration of the patient's clinical state occurs with dehiscence of the surgical wound and toxaemia.

Fournier gangrene (see Figure 26.25) occurs where there is infection around the lower abdominal fascial plane in men, with tracking of the infection into the scrotum [8]. It may be caused by group A *Streptococcus* or multiple organisms, although it is commoner with the latter. The management is identical to that used for these infections in other sites.

Differential diagnosis
The differential diagnosis includes gas gangrene, mucormycosis, cellulitis, pyoderma gangrenosum and ecthyma gangrenosum.

Complications and co-morbidities
Deep invasion with progressive necrosis and infarction of subcutaneous tissue, toxaemia and septicaemia.

Disease course and prognosis
This is fatal unless treated.

Investigations
Although swabs from the skin surface are usually negative, culture from swabs and tissue should be requested. However, therapy should not be delayed by waiting for results. The presence of gas in the tissue may suggest the diagnosis, but its absence does not exclude this disease process. Computed tomography is a more precise method of demonstrating gas in tissues than X-ray [12]. It is important to consider other potential causes of acute necrosis and toxaemia, particularly in the neutropenic patient, where cellulitis associated with single, such as *Pseudomonas*, or multiple organisms can occur. The zygomycete fungal infection, mucormycosis, should also be considered and impression smears taken from the wound edges or biopsy material may be helpful in excluding this possibility.

Management
This is an acute emergency warranting management in an intensive care unit. The most important step in diagnosis and management is surgical exploration and debridement [13], in which subcutaneous tissues down to the fascia are found to be necrotic. The overlying skin is usually surgically removed, although in some cases this has been laid back as a flap once the necrotic tissue has been removed.

Empiric antimicrobial treatment should be initiated while awaiting culture and sensitivity results. Intravenous penicillin and clindamycin would be suitable if either *Strep. pyogenes* (group A streptococcal disease) or *Clostridium* spp. is strongly suspected; if the causative agent is not apparent, however, broader coverage with ceftriaxone and metronidazole or piperacillin-tazobactam or a carbapenem with clindamycin is recommended [11,**14**]. However, if antibiotics are given without surgical intervention, therapy is rarely successful.

MYCOPLASMA INFECTIONS

Mycoplasmas, formerly known as pleuropneumonia-like organisms, are members of the smallest free-living bacterial class, Mollicutes [1].

They lack a rigid cell wall but can grow, although slowly, on artificial media.

Several *Mycoplasma* species are associated with humans. Some are commensals in the mouth, such as *M. orale* and *M. salivarium*; others are found in the healthy genital tract, such as *M. hominis* and the closely related *Ureaplasma urealyticum*, but may also lead to pathological states, like urethritis, in the case of *U. urealyticum* and pelvic inflammatory disease with *M. genitalium* [2].

M. pneumoniae is endemic worldwide and is spread by respiratory droplets. Year-round infections occur but peaks are seen in late summer and early autumn traditionally [1].

Clinical features
M. pneumoniae is a well-recognised cause of minor upper respiratory tract infections and pneumonia, particularly in young people [3]. The organism has also been associated with various systemic manifestations including meningoencephalitis, aplastic and haemolytic anaemia, polyarthritis and acute glomerulonephritis [1].

About one-third of patients with *M. pneumoniae* upper respiratory tract infections will develop skin features [1,4]. The majority of these cutaneous manifestations are erythematous exanthems. However, erythema nodosum and urticaria are also fairly common [1]. Stevens–Johnson syndrome occurs in around 5% of patients [1,5,6]. Erythema multiforme has been attributed to *M. pneumoniae* infection even without clinical evidence of lower respiratory tract infection by a rising antibody titre and isolation of the organism from skin lesions.

Investigations [1]
PCR-based diagnostic methods provide the most rapid and reliable means of identifying the cause. Cold agglutinins are produced in the majority of patients in response to the infection and antibody tests are available but have low sensitivity and specificity. In addition, complement-fixing antibodies can be demonstrated but may take over a week to develop. Culture is slow and should be done from nasopharyngeal aspirates ideally.

Management
Macrolides such as azithromycin and clarithromycin, tetracyclines and fluoroquinolones are effective in *M. pneumoniae* infections [1]. There is no evidence that the use of antibiotics triggers the appearance of skin rashes.

CHLAMYDIAE [1,2]

Chlamydiae are obligate intracellular bacterial parasites; in their infectious form they have a cell wall, contain both DNA and RNA, replicate by fission, and are susceptible to broad spectrum antibiotics, notably tetracyclines; they are therefore classed with the bacteria. There is a single genus with three subgroups or species.

Chlamydia trachomatis is spread by direct contact and can cause trachoma, an endemic ocular infection in many developing countries, frequently leading to blindness; and when sexually transmitted it can cause urethritis, but also deeper infections such as cervicitis, endometritis and salpingitis [3]. Eye infection may result from contact with infected genital secretions. Other serotypes predominantly infect lymphatic tissue and cause the sexually transmitted disease lymphogranuloma venereum (Chapter 30).

C. pneumoniae infection leads to outbreaks of respiratory infections and has been detected in some chronic skin ulcers [4] but its role is not clear.

C. psittaci is endemic in many species of birds and occasionally causes an interstitial pneumonitis in humans known as psittacosis or ornithosis [5].

Psittacosis

Synonyms and inclusions
- Ornithosis

Introduction and general description
The name 'psittacosis' was introduced because human infections were acquired from parrots (psittacines). Subsequently, many non-psittacine birds, for example domestic and sea birds, were found to carry the infection and 'ornithosis' was introduced as a more general term. The terms are now used synonymously.

Epidemiology
The disease is endemic not only in the parrot family, but also in over 120 species of birds, including pigeons, domestic fowl, ducks and finches, all of which have caused human infection; transmission occurs from inhalation of infected dust from excreta of sick or latently infected birds. It is caused by *C. psittaci*.

However, in many cases no bird source can be identified. Human-to-human spread by infected respiratory tract droplets is known to occur and may be commoner than previously recognised [1,2].

Clinical features
The incubation period is typically between 5 and 14 days. The manifestations are very variable [3–5]. Severe pneumonia, with cyanosis and collapse, myocardial involvement, jaundice, encephalitic symptoms and even death can occur. Most cases, however, present with high fever, malaise, headache, myalgia and respiratory symptoms [3]. Even milder attacks are probably frequent.

Exanthems occur occasionally [3], and erythema nodosum and erythema multiforme have also been reported [4–6].

Investigations
Confirmation of the diagnosis can be made using PCR or serology [3]. Culture is not usually recommended due to the risk of laboratory transmission.

Management
Tetracyclines are the drugs of choice and early administration can be life saving; response is usually noted in about 48 h and treatment should be continued for 10 days. Erythromycin or azithromycin is recommended for children and in pregnancy.

RICKETTSIAL INFECTIONS

Rickettsiae are regarded as small bacteria and most are obligate intracellular parasites. They are spread by the bites of arthropods and cause widespread infection in endothelial cells, which may result in vascular infarcts, extravascular fluid loss and disseminated intravascular coagulation.

The genus *Rickettsia* is broadly subdivided into the typhus group, the spotted fever group (SFG), the scrub typhus group (STG), the transitional group and the non-pathogenic ancestral group [1]. The spotted fever group are transmitted by ticks, whereas the typhus and transitional groups are transmitted by fleas, lice and mites and the scrub typhus group by mites.

Rickettsial infections classically present with a triad of fever, headache and myalgia; many will also present with a widespread rash and some a painless eschar.

Advancing age and glucose-6-phosphate dehydrogenase (G6PD) deficiency are risk factors for more severe manifestations with rickettsial infections.

Various serological techniques and other methods are available for the diagnosis of rickettsial infections, but are generally of retrospective value, and treatment should be started on the basis of a clinical diagnosis. Direct or indirect immunofluorescence, ELISAs, western blot and PCR diagnostic tests are available depending on the disease. Culture is not routinely performed because successful culturing can be challenging but also requires a higher biosafety level laboratory.

While the features of the main rickettsial diseases will be considered individually, management will be described for all the infections (Box 26.5).

TYPHUS GROUP

Epidemic typhus

Definition and nomenclature
Epidemic typhus is caused by *R. prowazekii* and is transmitted by the human body louse, *Pediculus humanus corporis* [2].

Synonyms and inclusions
- Louse-borne typhus

Epidemiology
It occurs worldwide but epidemics are mainly associated with the displacement of populations by war or natural disasters. Epidemic typhus is more common in the colder months. Humans are the only known reservoir of infection.

Age
Any age.

Sex
Both sexes.

Box 26.5 Management of rickettsial infections

- All patients should be treated with antibiotics
- First line of treatment: doxycycline is the drug of choice and treatment should be started as soon as the clinical diagnosis is made. The drug is usually given in full dose as a course of 7 days, although there is some evidence suggesting shorter courses may be as effective [3]
- Alternative treatments: azithromycin and chloramphenicol are possible alternatives to doxycycline. Chloramphenicol was previously recommended for rickettsial infections in pregnant women and children aged 8 years and under due to concern over dental staining, enamel hypoplasia and fetal bone malformations; however, evidence suggests this is unlikely with short courses of doxycycline [4,5]
- General supportive measures are necessary in severe cases
- With louse-borne disease (e.g. epidemic typhus, trench fever), isolation and effective delousing are necessary to control the spread of infection

Pathophysiology
Pathology
R. prowazekii multiplies in the gut endothelium of the human body louse and is released in its faeces. The rickettsiae are then transmitted to the human when skin abrasions are contaminated with louse faeces. The rickettsiae multiply in small blood vessel endothelial cells, leading to increased vascular permeability and vasodilation. Vascular obstruction, thrombosis, haemorrhage and perivascular inflammatory infiltration may also occur. The lesions are widely distributed but are often numerous in the skin, brain and heart.

Causative organisms
- *R. prowazekii*.

Clinical features
History
After an incubation period of 7–14 days, the disease presents with the abrupt onset of fever, severe headache, myalgia and malaise.

Presentation
The symptoms increase in severity for several days. A rash develops in over 80% of cases, initially presenting on the trunk, within a few days of the fever starting. It consists of crops of red to brown macules about 5 mm in diameter; the rash spreads centrifugally, but spares the palms and soles (Figure 26.34). The face is also spared but is often flushed with intensely injected conjunctivae. During the second week, the rash becomes deeper red and often frankly purpuric, and in severe cases may be confluent.

Differential diagnosis
- Septicaemia (especially typhoid fever).
- Malaria.
- Leptospirosis.
- Murine typhus.
- Viral haemorrhagic fevers.
- Meningococcal septicaemia.

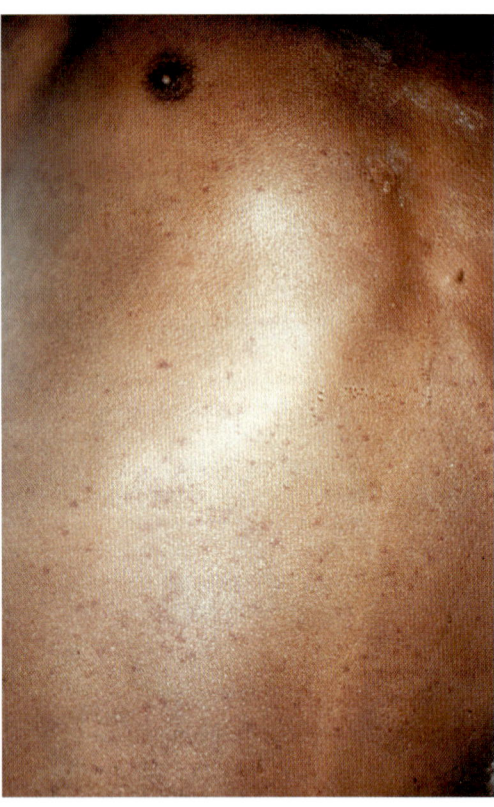

Figure 26.34 *Rickettsia prowazekii* louse-borne typhus in Ethiopia. © D.A. Warrell.

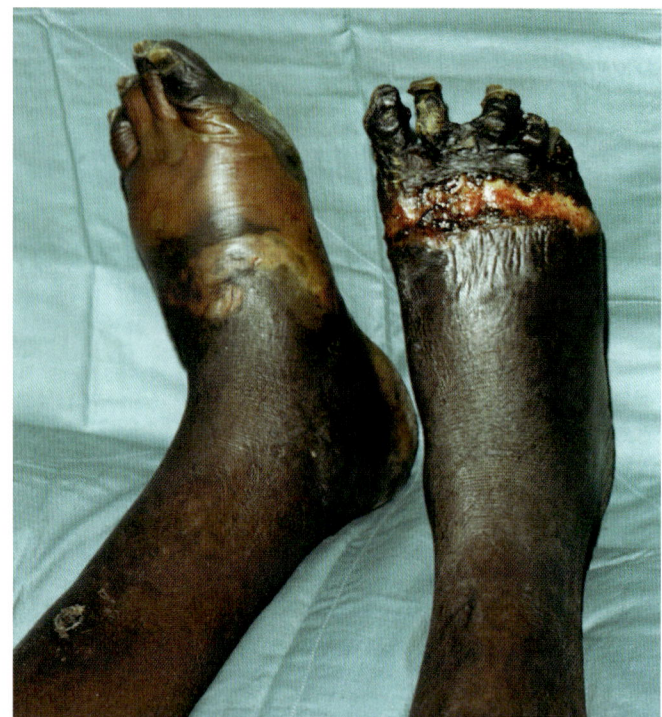

Figure 26.35 Gangrene resulting from *Rickettsia prowazekii* louse-borne typhus in Ethiopia. © D.A. Warrell.

Complications and co-morbidities

The other clinical manifestations and the outcome depend on the degree of involvement of the myocardium and the central nervous system. Gangrene of the fingers, toes, genitalia or nose may result from vascular obstruction (Figure 26.35).

Latent disease is well reported; see Brill–Zinsser disease [2,6].

Sylvatic typhus refers to typhus cases resulting from contact with flying squirrels rather than transmission via human body lice, although the exact mode of transmission in these cases is yet to be defined [2,7]. In these cases, the disease is less severe with a much lower mortality risk.

Disease course and prognosis

Untreated, up to 40% of cases are fatal, but serious sequelae are unusual in those who recover. Death, or recovery, occurs between the second and third weeks.

Management
See Box 26.5.

Brill–Zinsser disease [6]

Synonyms and inclusions
- Sporadic typhus

This is the recrudescence of epidemic typhus, sometimes after decades, in individuals who have previously recovered from an attack. The clinical features are those of the primary attack, but often milder, and the rash may be evanescent or absent.

Murine typhus

Synonyms and inclusions
- Endemic typhus

Murine typhus is caused by *R. typhi* (formerly *R. mooseri*) [8]. It is transmitted to humans from the rodent reservoir, most commonly by the Oriental rat flea, *Xenopsylla cheopis*. The infection occurs worldwide although murine typhus is more common in tropical and subtropical regions [8]. The pathological changes are similar to those described in epidemic typhus.

The clinical features parallel those of epidemic typhus, but milder. The rash is variable, often starting in the axillae. It is seldom haemorrhagic and may go undetected. The condition is typically self-limiting but complications may occur in up to 25% of patients and include myocarditis, respiratory failure, meningoencephalitis and renal failure [8].

SPOTTED FEVER GROUP

The infections in this group (Table 26.1) are generally transmitted by ticks and the group consists of over 30 species found worldwide [9]. Similar infections caused by distinct species occur in the tropical and subtropical regions of all continents. The incidence of spotted fever rickettsioses has increased over recent decades [10]; the reasons for this are likely to be multifactorial but include the expanding geographic distribution of ticks.

Table 26.1 Classification of the rickettsial spotted fever and transitional groups.

Organism	Main geographic area	Name
Rickettsia rickettsia	Americas (mainly USA)	Rocky Mountain spotted fever
R. conorii	Mediterranean region, SW Asia, India	Mediterranean spotted fever
R. sibirica	Russia, Central Asia, China	Siberian tick typhus
R. australis	Australia	Queensland tick typhus
R. japonica	Japan	Japanese spotted fever
R. africae	Sub-Saharan Africa	African tick typhus
R. felis	Americas, Europe, Australia	Flea-borne spotted fever
R. akari	USA, Russia, Central Asia	Rickettsialpox

Rocky Mountain spotted fever

Definition
Caused by *R. rickettsii*, Rocky Mountain spotted fever (RMSF) is the most common and severe of the rickettsial spotted fever infections. Transmitted via the bite of an infected tick, it results in an acute febrile illness accompanied by an exanthem.

Synonyms and inclusions
- Brazilian spotted fever

Epidemiology
Most cases are reported in the south-eastern and south-central USA, but the disease has also been reported from Central and South America. Various tick species transmit the infection; *Dermacentor* spp. are the most common vectors but *Rhipicephalus sanguineus* and *Amblyomma* spp. have been reported.

Age
Any age.

Sex
Both sexes.

Pathophysiology
Pathology
This is the most virulent of the rickettsial spotted fever infections. Widespread inflammatory and destructive changes are produced in the small blood vessels, especially in the skin and central nervous system.

Causative organisms
- *R. rickettsii*.

Clinical features
History
Within 14 days of a tick bite, there is an abrupt onset of severe headache, fever and myalgia. Prolonged tick contact is not required for transmission of infection and there may be no knowledge of a tick bite.

Presentation
After 3 or 4 days, a maculopapular eruption appears on the wrists and ankles and soon spreads centrally to the limbs, trunk and face. The palms and soles are usually involved. Except in the mildest cases, the rash becomes haemorrhagic, and in the most severe may be confluent. Eschars (tache noir) are not commonly seen in RMSF compared with other forms of tick typhus. Neurological symptoms may be a prominent feature and encephalitis may ensue [11].

Differential diagnosis
- Viral haemorrhagic fevers.
- Meningococcal septicaemia.
- Other rickettsial infections.

Complications and co-morbidities
Complications include the formation of thrombi and microinfarcts in the skin, brain and gastrointestinal tract. Gangrene of the fingers, toes, genitalia or nose may result from vascular obstruction. Other severe manifestations may include renal failure, pulmonary and cerebral oedema and disseminated intravascular coagulation.

Disease course and prognosis
Without prompt treatment with doxycycline, the mortality exceeds 20%.

Investigations
In RMSF diagnosis is confirmed serologically or by direct immunfluorescence detection of *R. rickettsii* antigen in the vascular endothelium of a skin biopsy. PCR testing can also be done on biopsy specimens.

Management
See Box 26.5.

Tick typhus

Definition and nomenclature
The term tick typhus refers to disease caused by several different rickettsial species, which vary with geographic location (Table 26.1) [12]. Most commonly it refers to the rickettsial infection caused by *R. conorii*, transmitted to humans via the bite of an infected dog tick (*Rhipicephalus sanguineus*). The synonym *boutonneuse* comes from the French word for spotty, referring to the classical rash.

Synonyms and inclusions
- Mediterranean spotted fever
- Boutonneuse fever
- Fièvre boutonneuse
- Kenya tick typhus
- African and Indian tick typhus
- Queensland tick typhus
- Astrakhan fever

Epidemiology
In many countries, tick typhus is caused by *R. conorii*, which is transmitted by the bites of a variety of ixodid ticks. Different genetic clades (strains) are endemic in the countries around the

Mediterranean and in many parts of Africa, Asia and India. Other rickettsial species, such as *R. africae*, *R. sibirica*, *R. australis* and *R. japonica*, among others, have been identified as causative agents of tick typhus-like disease. *R. felis* results in a similar disease process but is transmitted via fleas rather than ticks (flea-borne spotted fever).

The diagnosis is important to consider in returning travellers; the diagnosis is aided by identifying an eschar but this may need to be sought on thorough examination. African tick typhus caused by *R. africae* is the most frequently imported rickettsiosis and is characterised by the presence of multiple eschars and frequent absence of rash, contrary to other rickettsioses [13].

Age
Any age.

Sex
Both sexes.

Pathophysiology
As with other rickettsial infections, the rickettsiae multiply in the small blood vessel endothelial cells, leading to vascular obstruction, thrombosis and haemorrhage.

Clinical features
History
After an incubation period, which is usually between 5 and 7 days, the onset of fever is accompanied by headache, malaise, myalgia and occasionally mental confusion. Typically, the fever lasts for 7–14 days.

Presentation
In the majority of cases, an eschar (tache noire) may be found at the site of the tick bite. The ulcer, which is 2–5 mm in diameter, has a black necrotic centre and a red areola. The regional lymph nodes may be enlarged and tender. Three or four days later, a pink maculopapular eruption develops first on the forearms and then rapidly generalises, involving the face, palms and soles. It increases in density for a few days and in severe cases may be haemorrhagic; rarely more severe reactions such as digital necrosis and pneumonia have been described.

Differential diagnosis
- Viral haemorrhagic fevers.
- Meningococcal septicaemia.
- Other rickettsial infections.

Complications and co-morbidities
While typically more benign than RMSF, complications can occur and include myocarditis, meningoencephalitis, neuropathies, digital necrosis and renal failure.

Disease course and prognosis
Apart from weakness and lassitude, convalescence is uneventful and recovery with doxycycline is usual, except in the severe forms in frail or elderly people. The rash fades slowly after the fever subsides.

Investigations
The diagnosis is confirmed serologically and species-specific diagnosis may be achieved by PCR. If an eschar is present, a swab or biopsy from this lesion for PCR may be helpful.

Management
See Box 26.5.

TRANSITIONAL GROUP

Rickettsialpox

Definition
R. akari is transmitted to humans from rodents by the mouse mite, *Liponyssoides* (formerly *Allodermanyssus*) *sanguineus*. Rickettsialpox is classified as a member of the transitional group of rickettsia as it shares features from both the spotted fever group and typhus group.

Epidemiology
It was first identified, in 1946, in New York City but cases have since been widely reported. Mite bites in humans most commonly occur after attempts to reduce the rodent population, as there are fewer rodent hosts available.

Age
Any age.

Sex
Both sexes.

Pathophysiology
Pathology
Unlike other rickettsiae, *R. akari* targets macrophages rather than endothelial cells. Vacuolar degeneration in the basal layer results in blurring of the dermal–epidermal junction and vesiculation best regarded as subepidermal, although regenerating epidermis may give an impression of intraepidermal separation. The superficial and middle dermal layers contain a neutrophilic and mononuclear cell infiltrate, but light and electron microscopy fail to demonstrate the organisms.

Causative organisms
- *R. akari*.

Clinical features
History
After an incubation period of 7–14 days, a papule appears at the mite bite site. This enlarges, becomes vesicular and dries to form a crust. The regional lymph nodes are enlarged.

Presentation
A triad of fever, vesicular rash and eschar is classical. The patient often fails to notice the initial lesion. Constitutional symptoms including myalgia and headache may develop, accompanied, or soon followed, by a generalised eruption of papules surmounted

by small vesicles, which crust and heal within 2–3 weeks. The distribution and extent of the eruption are very variable, but palms and soles are spared. The lesions heal without scarring.

Differential diagnosis
- Varicella infection.
- Other rickettsial infections.

Disease course and prognosis
The illness is usually mild and spontaneous recovery is expected within 2–3 weeks. Doxycycline shortens the duration of symptoms.

Investigations
Laboratory confirmation is by serology and PCR.

Management
See Box 26.5.

Flea-borne spotted fever

R. felis results in a similar disease process but is transmitted via fleas rather than ticks (flea-borne spotted fever).

SCRUB TYPHUS GROUP

Scrub typhus

Definition
The infective agent of scrub typhus, *Orientia tsutsugamushi* (previously *R. tsutsugamushi*), is conveyed to humans by bites from *Leptotrombidium* spp. mites, which are usually hosted by small mammals. The mites do not feed on blood, but on digested epithelioid tissue. The term *tsutsugamushi* comes from the Japanese words *tsutsuga* (illness) and *mushi* (insect).

Synonyms and inclusions
- Tsutsugamushi fever

Epidemiology
The disease was historically distributed within the 'Tsutsugamushi Triangle', extending from Japan to northern Australia and across to Pakistan. Increasingly there are reports of scrub typhus from sites well outside this area including Africa and Chile [14].

Pathogenesis
Orientia differ from other rickettsiae as they lack lipopolysaccharide and peptidoglycan structures. The pathological changes are a focal vasculitis, involving the skin, lungs, heart, brain and kidneys.

Causative organisms
- *O. tsutsugamushi*.

Clinical features
The ricksettsial triad of fever, rash and headache develops after an incubation period of around 10 days (6–21 days). An eschar may be present, but the frequency appears to vary with geographic location and they are often in hidden sites so can be easily missed. The regional lymph nodes are enlarged and tender. After about a week, a generalised macular or maculopapular eruption develops and may fade rapidly or persist for 7–10 days [15].

Disease course and prognosis
The clinical picture varies with the virulence of the strain and previous exposure. The majority of disease is mild and frequently goes unrecognised. Pneumonitis and meningoencephalitis are not infrequent and without treatment the mortality risk may be up to 60%. In less severe cases, the fever subsides and recovery occurs during the second or third week. Treatment with doxycycline is effective.

Investigations
As with other rickettsial infections the diagnosis can be confirmed with serology and PCR.

Management
See Box 26.5.

ACTINOMYCETE INFECTIONS

The actinomycetes are higher bacteria whose members cause two uncommon but important human infections: actinomycosis and nocardiosis. They show a number of unusual characteristics. *Actinomyces* spp. usually form large granules *in vivo* and *Nocardia* spp. are partially acid fast. Both form branching filaments *in vitro* and *in vivo*.

Actinomycosis

Definition and nomenclature
A chronic spreading suppurative and granulomatous disease caused primarily by *A. israelii*: draining sinuses are formed through which the characteristic sulphur granules are discharged [1].

Synonyms and inclusions
- Lumpy jaw (cattle)

Introduction and general description
This is a rare infection, commonly presenting in the skin, although other clinical forms such as pelvic actinomycosis are important and should be included in the differential diagnosis of pelvic tumours and inflammatory disease.

Epidemiology
The disease is worldwide in its distribution but is uncommon with a higher incidence of the disease in rural tropical areas and in

agricultural workers. The increased risk in people living in remote areas is most likely due in part to poor dental hygiene and less access to antibiotics, to which the organisms are extremely sensitive. Full-blown actinomycosis is also rare now in most countries where dental care is readily available. It is possible that it may cause minor dental infections, which are treated with antibiotics before major pathology can develop or a definitive diagnosis be established.

Age
Any age, but rare under the age of 10 years.

Sex
Adult males are more commonly affected than females, but the sex incidence is equal in childhood.

Associated diseases
Actinomycosis is associated with immunosuppression, diabetes, HIV infection and recent trauma or surgery. Actinomycetes are thought to have a role in bisphosphonate-related osteonecrosis of the jaw [1].

Pathophysiology
Actinomycetes are bacteria producing filamentous branching rods. Most of the pathogenic actinomycetes occur in nature and belong to the soil saprophytic flora. Pathogenic anaerobic actinomycetes are normal inhabitants of the human mouth and actinomycosis is therefore acquired endogenously.

In some respects, actinomycosis and mycetoma are similar. Actinomycosis differs from mycetoma in being caused by endogenous and anaerobic agents, and in having no tendency to be confined to the extremities.

Actinomycetes gain access to humans through damage to the mucosal barrier: trauma, surgical procedures such as dental extractions, foreign bodies (such as intrauterine devices) and pyogenic abscess formation [2].

Pathology [3]
The usual appearance is that of a suppurating fibrotic inflammatory process. Small abscesses and pus-filled sinus tracts are formed. Haematogenous spread to distant organs is unusual. In the tissues, the organism forms granular colonies from which radiate delicate branching filaments, some of which bear club-shaped processes ('ray fungus'). Surrounding the colonies, a chronic neutrophil and lymphocytic infiltrate extends towards the skin, irrespective of where the primary lesion is, and this readily breaks down to form multiple fistulae from which pus containing the granules may be discharged. These so-called sulphur granules are lobulated masses of intertwining filaments. Lesions of actinomycosis almost always contain other bacteria besides *Actinomyces*, and it is thought that some of these associated organisms have a synergistic role in the development of the infection.

Causative organisms
- *A. israelii*.

Many other species of *Actinomyces* have been associated with human infection including *A. gerencseriae*, *A. naeslundii*, *A. odontolyticus*, *A. viscosus*, *A. meyeri* and *A. turicensis*.

Clinical features
History
Actinomycosis can affect any organ or body tissue [3]. Characteristic features are chronic changes with abscess formation, sinus tracts and purulent discharge containing sulphur granules [3]. Several clinical variants are recognised.

Clinical variants
Cervico-facial actinomycosis [4]. This is the most common form, accounting for around half of all cases, and is typically seen by dentists. Poor oral hygiene and smoking are thought to be associated [2]. It presents as a dull-red indurated nodule on the cheek or submaxillary region. Multiple sinuses, puckered scarring and the formation of new nodules produce an uneven lumpy surface. The sinuses may close temporarily and later reopen or they may be replaced by other sinuses. The characteristic sulphur granules may be found in the discharging pus. The primary lesion is usually in the mandible or maxilla, and probably arises as a direct extension from a periodontal abscess formed in turn as the result of carious teeth, dental extraction or trauma to the jaw. Board-like induration of the skin is described. Maxillary lesions may extend to the orbit, bones of the skull and brain. Involvement of bone occurs early, usually before sinuses are formed. Periostitis is followed by osteomyelitis with cystic spaces within the bone.

Thoracic actinomycosis. The thoracic form of actinomycosis is thought to result from aspiration of oropharyngeal secretions [2] and it may present in a similar way to active tuberculosis with cough, haemoptysis, night sweats and weight loss. It is doubtful whether the normal lung can be infected, and most cases are thought to result from secondary infection of a lung abscess, tuberculosis, lung cancer and bronchiectasis, among others. The organism may extend outwards from the lung to the skin through the thoracic wall, sometimes with osteomyelitis of the ribs and eventually with multiple draining sinuses [5].

Abdominal actinomycosis [3]. This form usually occurs as a consequence of surgery or abdominal infection [2]. It can present with intra-abdominal abscess formation or a slow-growing mass, with constitutional disturbance. It is thought that the organisms reach the gastrointestinal tract from the oropharynx. Extension to the liver with resulting jaundice is frequent. Likewise, extension to the ovaries, kidneys, bladder or spine may occur. The organism may extend into the abdominal wall with the resultant sinus tracts appearing on the skin surface. Haematogenous spread to distant organs occurs but is rare.

Cutaneous actinomycosis. This form is usually a secondary process, originating from an underlying, deeper infection or as a result of haematogenous spread from a more distant site [2]. Primary cutaneous actinomycosis does occur but is very uncommon and is thought to occur through implantation. Subcutaneous nodules extend slowly and break down to form sinuses [6] and the regional lymph nodes may be affected.

Pelvic actinomycosis [7]. Recognised as a distinct form of the disease, pelvic actinomycosis is associated with the use of intrauterine contraceptive devices [7]. The skin is not affected in pelvic actinomycosis but the infection may spread to abdominal sites [8].

Musculoskeletal, cerebral and disseminated actinomycosis are also distinct clinical forms [1,2].

Differential diagnosis
Actinomycosis has a fairly typical appearance, but as the disease is rare, the diagnosis may not be suspected. Differential diagnoses, depending on the clinical presentation, include other chronic infectious diseases, such as tuberculosis, syphilis, nocardia and botryomycosis; appendicitis, osteomyelitis and liver abscesses; and also lung, uterine and intestinal cancer.

Prognosis
The prognosis of any form of actinomycosis without treatment is generally poor but the cervico-facial and primary cutaneous varieties may remain localised for long periods.

Investigations
The diagnosis is established by identifying the sulphur granules in the pus and on histological examination but should be confirmed by culture or PCR. Actinomyces are slow growing, so culture may take up to 3 weeks [1]. The granules can generally be seen macroscopically, as yellow granules up to 1–2 mm in diameter, often adherent to gauze dressings. When crushed and examined microscopically, narrow bacillary forms and elongate filaments with occasional branching may be found.

Imaging may be required, depending on the presentation, but the features are usually non-specific [1].

Management
Actinomycosis is a chronic disease producing a marked fibrotic reaction and it is difficult to obtain effective drug levels where required. Therefore, a quick response to treatment should not be expected [8].

Actinomyces spp. are generally sensitive to β-lactam agents [2] and first line treatment is usually penicillin. Typically, long courses of antibiotics are prescribed, extending up to a year or more [3]. Wide surgical excision has been used in addition to antimicrobial therapy. There is now a move away from this to more limited procedures when required and a greater reliance on targeted antibiotic therapy [1].

Alternatives to penicillin include tetracyclines, macrolides, clindamycin and carbapenems, but it is important to note that sensitivities appear to vary considerably within *Actinomyces* species [1,2].

Nocardiosis

Definition
This is an acute-to-chronic suppurative disease caused by the Gram-positive, aerobic actinomycete *Nocardia*. The primary infection is usually pulmonary, but there may be haematogenous spread to other organs. The central nervous system is frequently attacked. Primary cutaneous nocardiosis as well as mycetoma due to *Nocardia* spp. are both well described.

Introduction and general description
Nocardiosis can affect many different areas of the body but is most commonly seen in the skin or pulmonary system [1]. It generally presents with single or multiple abscesses. The actinomycetomas caused by *Nocardia* species are considered in Chapter 32.

Epidemiology
This rare, sporadic infection has a worldwide distribution, although primary cutaneous infections have mainly been reported from the tropics or North America.

Nocardia is a ubiquitous saprophyte, found in soil as well as fresh and salt water. It is an opportunistic pathogen primarily in immunocompromised individuals. Pulmonary forms of the disease are most likely due to inhalation, whereas cutaneous infections are most commonly due to traumatic inoculation.

Age
Any, although very rare in childhood.

Sex
Both sexes, although more common in males.

Associated diseases
As an opportunistic pathogen, *Nocardia* is most often found in the context of chronic disease or impaired T-lymphocyte mediated immunity, including HIV/AIDS, in those receiving some biological agents such as anti-TNF antibodies [2], and in solid-organ transplant recipients. It has also been reported with Cushing syndrome, diabetes and following the use of corticosteroids.

Pathophysiology
Pathology
Mild subclinical nocardiosis may occur, but since the organism is known to cause fatal infections in humans, isolation of *Nocardia* in patient samples should not be disregarded [1].

Nocardia spp. can cause localised skin infections, typically after traumatic implantation. *N. asteroides* may cause a localised abscess without dissemination (primary cutaneous nocardiosis). *N. brasiliensis*, and occasionally other species, is a common cause of actinomycetoma, following entry via a wound.

Causative organisms
- *N. asteroides* complex.
- *N. brasiliensis*.
- *N. otitidiscaviarum*.
- Rarer species include *N. farcinica* and *N. transvalensis* [1].

Environmental factors
Soil-associated infections occur after cutaneous injury. Nosocomial outbreaks of nocardiosis associated with contamination of ventilation systems have been described [3].

Clinical features
History
Onset is usually rapid with a febrile illness in systemic infections. Cutaneous injury typically precedes cutaneous disease.

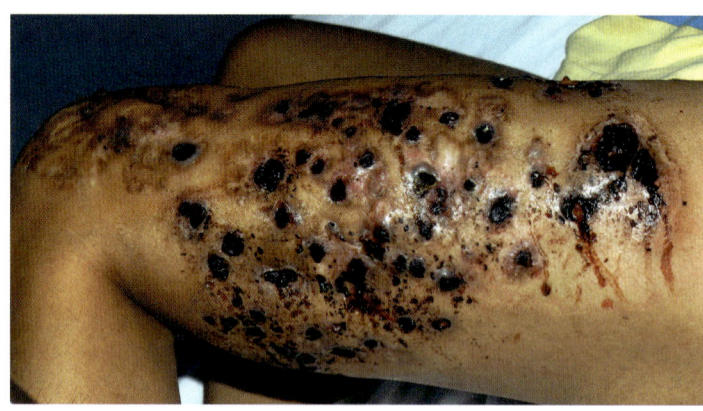

Figure 26.36 Nocardiosis. © D.A. Warrell.

Presentation
Pulmonary nocardiosis is the most common clinical manifestation and has a similar presentation to tuberculosis, with cough, dyspnoea, haemoptysis, fever and night sweats [4,5]. Involvement of the brain or meninges is present in 30% of cases, and the skin in 30%. Spread to the skin and subcutaneous tissue produces solitary or multiple abscesses, which may involve the muscles and bones [6] (Figure 26.36). Disseminated disease, with deep abscesses at any site, may develop.

Clinical variants
Cutaneous nocardiosis is usually seen in immunocompetent hosts and commonly presents with cellulitic changes at the site of traumatic injury [1]. Tender nodules or abscesses with purulent discharge may develop. Ascending regional lymphadenopathy may accompany cutaneous nocardiosis (termed lymphocutaneous nocardiosis) [7,8]; the lymph nodes can suppurate and may become necrotic.

Actinomycetoma due to *Nocardia* spp. is described elsewhere (Chapter 32).

Differential diagnosis
The differential diagnosis for pulmonary nocardiosis includes tuberculosis, histoplasmosis, aspergillosis, actinomycosis, other forms of pneumonia as well as lymphoma. The differential diagnosis for cutaneous nocardiosis includes cellulitis, actinomycosis, sporotrichosis and cutaneous tuberculosis.

Disease course and prognosis
The prognosis of disseminated nocardiosis without treatment is poor. In primary cutaneous infection, resolution is usual but disseminated nocardiosis is fatal if untreated and there is a mortality, even with treatment, of over 20%.

Investigations
Diagnosis requires confirmation of the organism, which may be achieved with microscopy and culture. Pus or sputum smears may reveal the narrow (less than 1 μm) branching filaments, which are only partially acid fast with a 'beaded' appearance [1]. As with *Actinomyces*, *Nocardia* spp. are slow growing, so the suspected diagnosis should be discussed with the laboratory.

Imaging will be required in pulmonary and cerebral infection. However, the findings are non-specific.

Management
All cases require antibiotic treatment. Primary cutaneous lesions typically require only one antimicrobial and trimethoprim–sulfamethoxazole (co-trimoxazole) is typically first line [1]. Up to 3 months of treatment may be required [9]. Severe pulmonary or disseminated infection may require a combination of agents and the treatment course may be 6–12 months. Suitable antibiotics include carbapenems (imipenem or meropenem), third generation cephalosporins, minocycline, co-amoxiclav, linezolid and amikacin [1]. Second line agents should be based on *in vitro* susceptibility testing.

Abscesses may require surgical incision and drainage.

DERMATOSES POSSIBLY ATTRIBUTABLE TO BACTERIA

There are many distinctive clinical syndromes in which bacteria appear to play a principal or secondary pathogenic role, but in which the lesions cannot be correlated with the known infections due to the species isolated. An abnormal response of the tissues or immunity of the host has therefore been postulated.

In some such syndromes, allergic hypersensitivity to the infecting organisms or their products has been demonstrated, and in others it is believed to be an important factor in determining the altered response to the bacteria.

The clinical features of many infections are modified by defects, inherited or acquired, in the host's capacity to produce a normal antibody and leukocytic response. Chronic granulomatous disease of childhood, for example, results from the failure of leukocytes to destroy certain species of ingested bacteria.

Chancriform pyoderma

Definition
This uncommon condition can mimic primary syphilis and occurs more often in children than in adults.

Epidemiology
Cases have been reported from Europe and from North and Latin America [1].

Pathophysiology
The aetiology is uncertain, but a necrotising reaction to a strain of *Staph. aureus*, inoculated by minor trauma, has been suspected.

Clinical features
The lesion, which is usually solitary, is often situated around the eyelids or near the mouth, or occasionally on the genitalia [1,2]. A sharply marginated ulcer, sometimes exceeding 1 cm in diameter, with an indurated base and a bright-red areola, enlarges slowly for a few days. The regional lymph nodes are enlarged and tender; the ulcer is relatively painless.

Differential diagnosis
It is important to exclude other conditions including syphilis, primary tuberculosis, atypical mycobacterium infection, leishmaniasis, Behçet syndrome and malignancy.

Disease course and prognosis
Without treatment the ulcer may persist for several weeks before healing to leave a superficial scar. Recurrent episodes may occur.

Management
Treatment with antibiotics shortens the duration but the response in our experience is not dramatic.

Pyoderma vegetans

Definition and nomenclature
Pyoderma vegetans is a rare mucocutaneous condition of uncertain aetiology characterised by the development of epithelial hyperplasia and pustular lesions. Crusting, sinus tract formation and ulceration may also occur [1].

Synonyms and inclusions
- Dermatitis vegetans
- Pyodermatitis-pyostomatitis vegetans
- Pyodermite vegetante of Hallopeau

Pathogenesis
Pyoderma vegetans is difficult to define and almost certainly the name has been used to describe a number of differing skin rashes, such as blastomycosis-like pyoderma [2] and possibly superficial granulomatous pyoderma [3]. As the aetiology of the disease is unknown, it is not known whether these share a common pathogenesis.

Commonly, either *Staph. aureus* or group A *Streptococcus* is isolated from lesions but, as the rash does not usually respond to antibiotics alone, the role of these bacteria in the pathogenesis of the condition is unclear. The disease has been most commonly described in the context of inflammatory bowel disease, especially ulcerative colitis [4,5], but has also been reported with a variety of underlying conditions including alcoholism, lymphoma [6] and HIV infection.

Pathology
The disease process is not fully understood and it has been suggested that it is a response to heavy bacterial colonisation or epidermal invasion in a patient with defective immunity [7].

Clinical features
Pyoderma vegetans may develop at any site, but the flexures are often involved. In some cases, encrusted and hyperplastic plaques appear on the skin surface [6,8]. These may break down and weep and there is often central clearing. Where a prominent edge with crust formation is seen, the lesions may mimic blastomycosis. Alternatively, there may be ulceration, the condition resembling a form of pyoderma gangrenosum. Lesions may heal spontaneously but generally this is a chronic disease.

Pyostomatitis vegetans refers to the disorder when it affects the mucosa, usually the oral cavity, and it typical presents with small pustules which may rupture leaving erosions in a characteristic 'snail track' appearance [4,9].

Differential diagnosis
The differential diagnosis includes pyoderma gangrenosum, pemphigus vegetans, verrucous carcinoma, halogenoderma, botryomycosis and deep fungal infections such as blastomycosis and coccidioidomycosis.

Investigations
Diagnosis is difficult and largely depends on the exclusion of other conditions, such as specific infections, iododerma, pyoderma gangrenosum and pemphigus vegetans. It is partly the absence of other diagnostic features that supports the diagnosis of pyoderma vegetans. Immunofluorescence may help to differentiate pyoderma vegetans from pemphigus vegetans. Cultures should be taken and may reveal *Staph. aureus*. Repeat biopsies from the skin lesion may be necessary and typical features include epithelial hyperplasia and abscess formation in the epidermis and dermis, comprising neutrophils or eosinophils [9]. It is important to exclude underlying diseases such as ulcerative colitis, lymphoma or leukaemia.

Management
There are no treatment guidelines for pyoderma vegetans. Topical and systemic corticosteroids can be helpful but recurrence can occur upon cessation. Oral antibiotics and immunosuppressants have been used with varying success, often with the addition of surgical management (excision, curettage or laser debridement) [10,11]. There has been a report of an excellent response to etanercept in a patient who also had psoriatic arthritis [12].

Dermatitis gangrenosa infantum

Definition
This is a rare condition in which the infant presents with multiple necrotic ulcers on the skin surface.

Epidemiology
It is mainly reported to occur within the first 2 years of life, in some cases developing after viral infection or vaccination.

Pathophysiology
The aetiology of this rare condition is unknown.

Pathology
The histology of the few reported cases shows an acute necrotic reaction involving the dermis and epidermis similar to that seen in pyoderma gangrenosum.

Clinical features
While these may arise *de novo*, they often appear on a pre-existing rash such as varicella or severe seborrhoeic dermatitis. The affected child is usually acutely ill with a high pyrexia and rapid deterioration follows [1], often ending in death. While it is possible that, in some cases, this may be a form of infantile pyoderma gangrenosum, secondary complications, such as septicaemia, dominate the clinical picture. *Staph. aureus* may be isolated from cutaneous ulcers, but it is not clear whether this is a secondary event.

Kawasaki disease

Definition and nomenclature
Kawasaki disease is an acute vasculitic syndrome of unknown aetiology seen in childhood.

Synonyms and inclusions
- Mucocutaneous lymph node syndrome

Introduction and general description
This condition is a disease usually seen in children, typically affecting those under 5 years of age. It presents with fever and a generalised exanthem with lymphadenitis. Complications include myocarditis and arthritis. The aetiology is unknown, although it has been suggested it could be an abnormal immune reaction to an infectious trigger in the context of a genetically susceptible individual [1].

Epidemiology
The disease was first described in Japan by Kawasaki in 1967 [2], and the highest incidence of the disease is still seen in Japan, Korea and Taiwan [3]. There appears to be a genetic predisposition because in the USA, Kawasaki disease is more common in those with Asian, Pacific Islander and African lineage [3].

Age
The disease occurs in childhood, often under the age of 5 years, and cases are rarely seen in adults [2].

Sex
Males are more commonly affected, and the condition is seen more often in siblings than in the general population, suggesting the possibility of transmission; however, epidemics of the disease have not been recorded [4].

Associated diseases
Kawasaki disease appears to be more common in children with allergic diseases: atopic dermatitis, asthma and allergic rhinitis [5].

Pathophysiology
Pathology
The disease leads to inflammation of medium-sized arteries throughout the body, especially the coronary arteries, leading to aneurysms and further complications including thrombosis, calcification and ultimately myocardial ischaemia [6].

Immune system dysfunction is thought to play an important part in the disease process. Imbalance in the T lymphocyte subsets has been demonstrated in Kawasaki disease and it has been suggested this may be in response to activation by superantigen production from *Staph. aureus* or *Strep. pyogenes* [7]. A variety of other pathogens have been implicated as potentially having a role in the development of Kawasaki disease including measles, human herpesvirus-6, parvovirus B19, Epstein–Barr virus and more recently SARS-CoV-2 [6]. Some studies have suggested the disease is IgA driven [8], with increased concentrations of IgA and absence of IgM and IgG at affected sites [6].

Clinical features
History
The onset is acute, with a high fever which lasts for at least 5–7 days.

Presentation
The child presents with injected conjunctivae, dry and fissured lips, a red tongue with prominent papillae (strawberry tongue) and a red throat. Redness and oedema of the hands and feet can occur, resolving with desquamation once the fever has abated. Kawasaki disease is associated with a polymorphous exanthem, which usually occurs within 5 days of the onset of fever [3]; the rash may be morbilliform or erythema multiforme-like. There is accompanying cervical lymphadenopathy in many patients, although it is not always present, and may only involve a single node.

Fever resolves after 1–2 weeks, but conjunctival injection and lassitude may persist. In about one-quarter of cases there is accompanying myocarditis, which may be followed by symptomatic coronary artery disease and in 1–2% by myocardial infarction. Myocarditis presents with arrhythmia or tachycardia; pericarditis and valve incompetence may also occur. Coronary disease occurs secondary to aneurysms of the coronary arteries, which may thrombose. However, these also regress over a couple of years in most patients.

Clinical variants
Multisystem inflammatory syndrome in children (MIS-C) is a clinically distinct disease from Kawasaki and has been described as a postinfectious syndrome of SARS-CoV-2 infection. A proportion of children with this condition meet the criteria for Kawasaki disease [3].

Differential diagnosis
While this condition may resemble a number of virus-associated exanthems, the presence of the typical rash and accompanying myocarditis are characteristic.

Complications and co-morbidities
In addition to coronary arterial aneurysms, other complications include arthralgia, arthritis, severe erythema multiforme, iritis, proteinuria, hepatitis and aseptic meningitis.

Disease course and prognosis
There is slow resolution although lassitude persists, but myocarditis may result in complications which can be life threatening.

Investigations

Kawasaki disease is diagnosed on clinical features and there are specified criteria for diagnosis [3]. Abnormalities on investigation may include leukocytosis, raised alanine aminotransferase (ALT) and anaemia. Thrombocytosis is most often seen in the post-acute phase. There is no specific diagnostic test for this syndrome, but if it is suspected an electrocardiogram (ECG) and echocardiogram should be performed.

Management

There are no definitive treatments for Kawasaki disease. IVIg in high dosage is first line, and reduces the overall mortality and complications of the disease, including the risk of coronary aneurysms [9]. The treatment appears to work rapidly with resolution of fever and should ideally be given within the first 10 days of illness. Aspirin is also helpful in reducing the risk of platelet aggregation, and is given alongside IVIg [3]; it may also be used long term if there is evidence of coronary aneurysms.

Corticosteroids may be beneficial, especially in patients at risk of IVIg resistance [10]. Infliximab, etanercept and ciclosporin have been used in refractory cases [3].

Additional resources

Centers for Disease Control and Prevention (CDC): https://www.cdc.gov. (Last accessed July 2023.)

Key references

The full list of references can be found in the online version at https://www.wiley.com/rooksdermatology10e

Introduction
5 Noble WC. *Microbiology of Human Skin*. London: Lloyd-Luke Medical Books, 1981.
6 Hannigan GD, Grice EA. Microbial ecology of the skin in the era of metagenomics and molecular microbiology. *Cold Spring Harb Perspect Med* 2013;3(12):a015362.
7 Chen YE, Tsao H. The skin microbiome: current perspectives and future challenges. *J Am Acad Dermatol* 2013;69:143–55.
14 Maddox JS, Ware JC, Dillon HC. The natural history of streptococcal skin infection. *J Am Acad Dermatol* 1985;13:207–11.
18 Sharpe ME, Law BA, Phillips BA et al. Methanethiol production by coryneform bacteria; strains from dairy and human skin sources and *Brevibacterium linens*. *J Gen Microbiol* 1977;101:345–9.
43 Kenshi Y, Gallo RL. Antimicrobial peptides in human skin disease. *Eur J Dermatol* 2008;18:11–21.
45 Zeeuwen PL, Kleerebezem M, Timmerman HM et al. Microbiome and skin diseases. *Curr Opin Allergy Clin Immunol* 2013;13:514–20.

Gram-positive bacteria
Staphylococcus aureus
1 Styers D, Sheehan DJ, Hogan P et al. Laboratory-based surveillance of current antimicrobial resistance patterns and trends among *Staphylococcus aureus*: 2005 status in the United States. *Ann Clin Microbiol Antimicrob* 2006;5:2.
3 European Centre for Disease Prevention and Control. Antimicrobial resistance in the EU/EEA (EARS-Net) – Annual Epidemiological Report 2019. Stockholm: ECDC, 2020.
11 Weidenmaier CJ, Kokai-Kun F, Kristian SA et al. Role of teichoic acids in *Staphylococcus aureus* nasal colonization, a major risk factor in nosocomial infections. *Nat Med* 2004;10:243–5.
28 Cohen PR. Community-acquired methicillin-resistant *Staphyloccocus aureus* skin infections: a review of epidemiology, clinical features, management and prevention. *Int J Dermatol* 2007;46:1–11.
32 Gould FK, Brindle R, Chadwick PR et al. MRSA Working Party of the British Society for Antimicrobial Chemotherapy. Guidelines (2008) for the prophylaxis and treatment of methicillin-resistant Staphylococcus aureus (MRSA) infections in the United Kingdom. *J Antimicrob Chemother* 2009;63:849–61.
38 Grumann D, Nubel U, Broker BM. *Staphylococcus Aureus Toxins – Their Functions and Genetics. Infection, Genetics and Evolution*. Oxford: Elsevier, 2013.

Streptococci
4 Hay RJ, Steer CA, Engelman D et al. Scabies in the developing world – its prevalence, complications and management. *Clin Microbiol Infect* 2012;18:313–23.
10 McCormick JK, Pragman AA, Stolpa JC et al. Functional characterization of streptococcal pyrogenic exotoxin J, a novel superantigen. *Infect Immun* 2001;69:1381–8.
11 Cunningham MW. Pathogenesis of group A streptococcal infection. *Clin Microbiol Rev* 2000;13:470–511.
17 Roodpeyma S, Kamali Z, Zare R. Rheumatic fever: the relationship between clinical manifestations and laboratory tests. *J Paediatr Child Health* 2005;41:97–100.
19 Steer AC, Law I, Matatolu L et al. Global *emm* type distribution of group A streptococci: systematic review and implications for vaccine development. *Lancet Infect Dis* 2009;9:611–16.

Staphylococcal and streptococcal infections
Impetigo
1 Rortveit S, Rortveit G. Impetigo in epidemic and nonepidemic phases: an incidence study over 41/2 years in a general population. *Br J Dermatol* 2007;157:100–5.
13 Ladhani S. Understanding the mechanism of action of the exfoliative toxins of *Staphylococcus aureus*. *FEMS Immunol Med Micro* 2003;39:181–9.
19 Amagai M, Matsuyoushi N, Wang ZH et al. Toxin in bullous impetigo and staphylococcal scalded-skin syndrome targets desmoglein 1. *Nature Med* 2000;6:1275–7.
20 Monday SR, Vath GM, Ferens WA et al. Unique superantigen activity of staphylococcal exfoliative toxins. *J Immunol* 1999;162:4550–9.
22 Kato F, Kadomoto N, Iwamoto Y et al. Regulatory mechanisms for exfoliative toxin production in *Staphylococcus aureus*. *Infect Immun* 2011;79:1660–70.
24 Koning S, Van der Sande R, Verhagen AP et al. Interventions for impetigo. *Cochrane Database Syst Rev* 2012;Issue 1:CD003261.
26 Stevens DL, Bisno AL, Chambers HF et al. Practice guidelines for the diagnosis and management of skin and soft-tissue infections. *Clin Infect Dis* 2005;41:1373–406.
28 Luby S, Agboatwalla M, Feikin D et al. Effect of hand washing on child health: a randomised controlled trial. *Lancet* 2005;366:225–33.

Cellulitis and erysipelas
1 Swartz MN. Clinical practice: cellulitis. *N Engl J Med* 2004;350:904–12.
4 Halpen J, Holder R, Langford NJ. Ethnicity and other risk factors for acute lower limb cellulitis: a UK-based prospective case-control study. *Br J Dermatol* 2008;158:1288–92.
30 Kilburn SA, Featherstone P, Higgins B et al. Interventions for cellulitis and erysipelas. *Cochrane Database Syst Rev* 2010;Issue 16:CD004299.
32 Raff AB, Kroshinsky D. Cellulitis: a review. *JAMA* 2016;316:325–37.
33 Mason JM, Thomas KS, Crook AM et al. Prophylactic antibiotics to prevent cellulitis of the leg: economic analysis of the PATCH I and II trials. *PLOS One* 2014;9:e82964.
34 Cox NH. Oedema as a risk factor for multiple episodes of cellulitis/erysipelas of the lower leg: a series with community follow-up. *Br J Dermatol* 2006;155:947–50.

Furuncle (boil, abscess)
1 Zetola N, Francis JS, Nuermberger EL et al. Community acquired methicillin-resistant *Staphylococcus aureus*: an emerging threat. *Lancet Infect Dis* 2005;5:275–86.
2 Durupt F, Major L, Bes M et al. Prevalence of *Staphylococcus aureus* toxins and nasal carriage in furuncles and impetigo. *Br J Dermatol* 2007;157:1161–7.
3 Yamasaki O, Kaneko J, Morizane S et al. The association between *Staphylococcus aureus* strains carrying Panton-Valentine leukocidin genes and the development of deep-seated follicular infection. *Clin Infect Dis* 2005;40:381–5.
15 Health Protection Agency. *Guidance on diagnosis and management of PVL associated Staphylococcus aureus infections (PVL-SA) in England*, 2008. https://www.gov.uk/government/collections/panton-valentine-leukocidin-pvl-guidance-data-and-analysis (last accessed February 2023).

16 Shallcross LJ, Fragaszy E, Johnson AM et al. The role of the Panton-Valentine leucocidin toxin in staphylococcal disease: a systematic review and meta-analysis. *Lancet Infect Dis* 2013;13:43–54.

17 Stevens DL, Ma Y, Mcindoo E et al. Impact of antibiotics on expression of virulence-associated exotoxin genes in methicillin-sensitive and methicillin-resistant *Staphylococcus aureus*. *J Infect Dis* 2007;195:202–11.

Staphylococcal scalded skin syndrome

4 Patel GK, Varma S, Finlay AY. Staphylococcal scalded skin syndrome in healthy adults. *Br J Dermatol* 2000;142:1253–5.

6 Bukowski M, Wladtka B, Dubin G. Exfoliative toxins of *Staphylococcus aureus*. *Toxins (Basel)* 2010;2:1148–65.

10 Kato F, Kadomoto N, Iwamoto Y et al. Regulatory mechanisms for exfoliative toxin production in *Staphylococcus aureus*. *Infect Immun* 2011;79:1660–70.

11 Courjon J, Hubiche T, Phan A et al. Skin findings of *Staphylococcus aureus* toxin-mediated infection in relation to toxin encoding genes. *Pediatr Infect Dis J* 2013;32:727–30.

12 Patel GK, Finlay AY. Staphylococcal scalded skin syndrome: diagnosis and management. *Am J Clin Dermatol* 2003;4:165–75.

Toxic shock syndrome

1 Parsonnet J, Hansmann MA, Delaney Ml et al. Prevalence of toxic shock syndrome toxin 1-producing *Staphylococcus aureus* and the presence of antibodies to this superantigen in menstruating women. *J Clin Microbiol* 2005;43:4626–34.

9 Parsonnet J. Mediators in the pathogenesis of toxic shock syndrome: overview. *Rev Infect Dis* 1989;11(Suppl. 1):S263–9.

10 Chesney PJ. Clinical aspects and spectrum of illness of toxic shock syndrome: overview. *Rev Infect Dis* 1989;11(Suppl. 1):S1–7.

14 Alejandria MM, Lansang MA, Dans LF et al. Intravenous immunoglobulin for treating sepsis, severe sepsis and septic shock. *Cochrane Database Syst Rev* 2013;Issue 16:CD001090.

Toxin-mediated streptococcal disease

2 You YH, Song YY, Yan XM et al. Molecular epidemiology characteristics of *Streptococcus pyogenes* strains involved in an outbreak of scarlet fever in China, 2011. *Biomed Environ Sci* 2013;26:877–85.

7 Ralph AP, Carapetis JR. Group A streptococcal diseases and their global burden. *Curr Top Microbiol Immunol* 2013;368:1–27.

8 Hallas G. The production of pyrogenic toxins by Group A streptococci. *J Hyg* 1985;95:47–57.

18 Van Driel ML, De Sutter AI, Keber N et al. Different antibiotic treatments for group A streptococcal pharyngitis. *Cochrane Database Syst Rev* 2013;Issue 30:CD004406.

Coryneform bacteria

1 Funke G, von Graevenitz A, Clarridge JE et al. Clinical microbiology of coryneform bacteria. *Clin Microbiol Rev* 1997;10:125–59.

2 Chen YE, Tsao H. The skin microbiome: current perspectives and future challenges. *J Am Acad Dermatol* 2013;69:143–55.

Trichomycosis axillaris

7 Blaise G, Nikkels AF, Hermanns-Le T et al. Corynebacterium-associated skin infections. *Int J Dermatol* 1986;14:993.

Gram-negative bacteria
Pseudomonas aeruginosa

1 Morrison AJ, Wenzel RP. Epidemiology of infections due to *Pseudomonas aeruginosa*. *Rev Infect Dis* 1984;6(Suppl.):627–44.

2 Wu DC, Chan WW, Metelitsa AI et al. *Pseudomonas* skin infection: clinical features, epidemiology, and management. *Am J Clin Dermatol* 2011;12:157–69.

Burkholderia

1 Wiersinga WJ, Virk HS, Torres AG et al. Melioidosis. *Nat Rev Primers* 2018;4:17107.

2 Dance DA. Ecology of *Burkholderia pseudomallei* and the interactions between environmental *Burkholderia spp.* and human-animal hosts. *Acta Trop* 2000;74:159–68.

5 Dance D. Treatment and prophylaxis of melioidosis. *Int J Antimicrob Agents* 2014;43:310–18.

Bartonella

4 Lins KA, Drummond MR, Velho PENF. Cutaneous manifestations of bartonellosis. *An Bras Dermatol* 2019;94:594–602.

15 Rolain JM, Brouqui P, Koehler JE et al. Recommendations for treatment of human infections caused by *Bartonella* species. *Antimcrob Agents Chemother* 2004;48:1921–33.

Spirochaetes and spiral bacteria
Treponemes

1 Antal GM, Lukehart SA, Meheus AZ. The endemic treponematoses. *Microbes Infect* 2002;4:83–94.

2 Engelkens HJ, Vuzevski VD, Stolz E. Non-venereal treponematoses in tropical countries. *Clin Dermatol* 1999;17:143–52.

3 Walker SL, Hay RJ. Yaws – a review of the last 50 years. *Int J Dermatol* 2000;39:258–60.

Borrelia

Borrelia burgdorferi and Lyme disease

1 Radolf JD, Strle K, Lemieux JE et al. Lyme disease in humans. *Curr Issues Mol Biol* 2020;42:333–84.

2 Steere AC. Lyme disease. *N Engl J Med* 2001;345:115–19.

3 Stanek G, Wormser GP, Gray J et al. Lyme borreliosis. *Lancet* 2012;379:461–73.

14 Eldin C, Raffetin A, Bouiller K et al. Review of European and American guidelines for the diagnosis of Lyme borreliosis. *Med Mal Infect* 2019;49:121–32.

Miscellaneous
Necrotising subcutaneous infections

1 Anaya DA, Dellinger EP. Necrotizing soft-tissue infection: diagnosis and management. *Clin Infect Dis* 2007;44:705–10.

3 Brook I. Microbiology and management of soft tissue and muscle infections. *Int J Surg* 2008;6:328–38.

14 Stevens DL, Bryant AE. Necrotizing soft-tissue infections. *N Engl J Med* 2017;377:2253–65.

Rickettsial infections

12 Parola P, Paddock CD, Socolovschi C et al. Update on tick-borne rickettsioses around the world: a geographic approach. *Clin Microbiol Rev* 2013;26:657–702.

CHAPTER 27

Mycobacterial Infections

Stephen L. Walker[1] and Richard O. Phillips[2]

[1] Faculty of Infectious and Tropical Diseases, London School of Hygiene and Tropical Medicine, London, UK
[2] Kumasi Centre for Collaborative Research in Tropical Medicine, Kwame Nkrumah University of Science and Technology, Kumasi, Ghana

---

Introduction, 27.1

MYCOBACTERIAL INFECTION, 27.2
Classification, 27.2
Epidemiology, 27.2
Mycobacterium tuberculosis infection, 27.2
HIV and *Mycobacterium tuberculosis* co-infection, 27.2
Non-tuberculous mycobacterial infections, 27.3
Basic biology, 27.3
Immunology of tuberculosis, 27.3
Protective immunity to *M. tuberculosis*, 27.3
Immunopathology, 27.4
Diagnostic tests for tuberculosis, 27.4
Tuberculin skin test, 27.4
Interferon γ release assays for the diagnosis of latent tuberculosis, 27.4
Diagnosis of mycobacterial infections, 27.5

TUBERCULOSIS OF THE SKIN, 27.5
Classification, 27.5
Clinical spectrum of cutaneous tuberculosis, 27.5
Classification difficulties, 27.6
General description, 27.6
Basic biology, 27.6
Pathogenesis, 27.6
Development of the granuloma, 27.6

Histopathology, 27.7
Disease-specific changes, 27.7
Differential diagnosis, 27.7
Diagnostic tests for cutaneous tuberculosis, 27.8
Nucleic acid amplification tests, 27.8
Treatment, 27.9
General measures, 27.9
Drug therapy, 27.9
Current treatment regimens, 27.9
Prognosis, 27.10
BCG vaccination, 27.10
Complications, 27.11
Therapeutic use, 27.11
Tuberculosis and anti-TNF-α treatment, 27.11
Primary inoculation tuberculosis, 27.12
Scrofuloderma, 27.13
Orificial tuberculosis, 27.16
Acute cutaneous miliary tuberculosis, 27.17
Metastatic tuberculous abscess, 27.17
Warty tuberculosis, 27.19
Lupus vulgaris, 27.20

TUBERCULIDS, 27.24
Classification, 27.24
General description, 27.24

Basic biology, 27.25
Lichen scrofulosorum, 27.25
Papulonecrotic tuberculid, 27.27
Erythema induratum of Bazin, 27.29
Other nodular tuberculids, 27.31
Erythema nodosum, 27.31
Nodular vasculitis, 27.31
Lupus miliaris disseminatus faciei, 27.31
Tuberculous mastitis, 27.31

NON-TUBERCULOUS (ATYPICAL) MYCOBACTERIA, 27.32
Classification, 27.32
General description, 27.32
Basic biology, 27.32
Mycobacterium marinum infection, 27.32
Mycobacterium kansasii infection, 27.35
Mycobacterium ulcerans infection, 27.36
Mycobacterium avium complex (*M. avium* and *M. intracellulare*) infection, 27.40
Mycobacterium haemophilum infection, 27.41
Mycobacterium scrofulaceum infection, 27.42
Mycobacterium szulgai infection, 27.43
Infection with fast-growing mycobacteria, 27.43

Key references, 27.45

Introduction

The genus *Mycobacterium* contains more than 190 species of which over 25 are pathogenic in humans and other vertebrates [1]. The most important obligate human pathogens are *M. tuberculosis* and *M. leprae*, but others such as *M. avium* complex (*M. avium* and *M. intracellulare*) and *M. ulcerans* are also significant. Disease-causing mycobacteria other than those of the *M. tuberculosis* complex (including *M. tuberculosis*, *M. bovis*, *M. bovis* bacillus Calmette–Guérin (BCG) and related species) and *M. leprae* are referred to as non-tuberculous mycobacteria (NTM), although the terms atypical, environmental or opportunistic mycobacteria are also used [1].

Mycobacterium tuberculosis DNA has been isolated from ancient Hungarian and pre-Colombian Peruvian human remains with signs compatible with antemortem tuberculosis [2,3]. Tuberculosis is the leading cause of death from an infectious and is an enormous global health problem [4]. Approximately one-third of the world's population is infected with *M. tuberculosis* bacteria. It is estimated that globally there were approximately 10 million new tuberculosis cases in 2020 and that 1.5 million deaths were attributable to the disease [4]. Tuberculosis is primarily a disease of poverty, with 93% of cases occurring in low- and middle-income countries. The World Health Organization (WHO) reports that mortality and incidence rates are falling in most parts of the world but co-infection with human immunodeficiency virus (HIV) and drug-resistant tuberculosis, both

---

Rook's Textbook of Dermatology, Tenth Edition. Edited by Christopher Griffiths, Jonathan Barker, Tanya Bleiker, Walayat Hussain and Rosalind Simpson.
© 2024 John Wiley & Sons Ltd. Published 2024 by John Wiley & Sons Ltd.

multidrug resistant (MDR) and extensively drug resistant (XDR), and the impact of Covid-19 on services represent considerable challenges [4]. Globally, rifampicin-resistant and MDR tuberculosis (defined as being resistant to rifampicin and isoniazid) are thought to account for 3–4% of newly diagnosed cases, although this rate rises to 20% in some countries in Asia and Europe. The prevalence is significantly higher in individuals who have previously received antituberculosis therapy (ATT). XDR tuberculosis (defined as being resistant to rifampicin, any fluoroquinolone and one of bedaquiline or linezolid) is estimated to account for 1.2% of bacteriologically confirmed pulmonary cases (those which were tested) [4].

This chapter will deal first with the general properties and characteristics of the mycobacteria, before discussing tuberculosis and infections by NTM. Leprosy is considered separately in Chapter 28.

Table 27.1 Mycobacteria of dermatological interest.

Rate of growth	Species
Slow growers	M. marinum
	M. kansasii
	M. avium
	M. intracellulare
	M. haemophilum
	M. ulcerans
	M. szulgai
	M. scrofulaceum
	M. tuberculosis
Rapid growers	M. abscessus (group)
	M. chelonae
	M. fortuitum (group)
	M. mageritense
	M. wolinskyi
	M. smegmatis
	M. mucogenicum
Non-culturable	M. leprae
	M. lepromatosis

Adapted from Atkins and Gottlieb 2014 [7].

MYCOBACTERIAL INFECTION

The term 'mycobacterium' was given in 1896 to a large group of bacteria producing mould-like pellicles when grown on liquid media. All are slender, non-motile, aerobic, non-sporing rods with a waxy coating that makes them resistant to most stains. Once stained, however, they are not easily decoloured (acid-fast).

Classification

The genomes of *M. tuberculosis* [1], *M. bovis*, *M. bovis* BCG, *M. leprae* [2] and some NTM including *M. ulcerans* [3], *M. marinum* [4] and *M. avium* have all been sequenced. Molecular techniques have also resulted in the delineation of the phylogeny of the mycobacteria. In general, the obligate mycobacterial pathogens (*M. tuberculosis* complex and *M. leprae*) and the most virulent NTM are more susceptible to antibiotics than other NTM [5]. It is hypothesised that these more virulent species, which are more closely related phylogenetically and are most adapted to humans, have lost resistance mechanisms through lower selection pressures [5]. The other NTM are consequently of less clinical significance but are often more difficult to treat.

The mycobacteria were classified previously according to their rate of growth and production of pigment [6]. This classification retains some utility for classifying mycobacteria that cause clinical disease (Table 27.1) [1,7].

The cell wall of the mycobacteria, which is responsible for their acid-fast staining properties, has a complex structure. The typical peptidoglycan backbone of a Gram-positive bacterial cell abuts onto a typical phospholipid plasma membrane. Outside the peptidoglycan layer, and covalently bonded to it, there is a branched polymer arabinogalactan. Onto this are attached the long chain fatty acids termed mycolic acids. Numerous other lipids and glycolipids are non-covalently inserted into this lipophilic outer layer. Lipoarabinomannan (LAM; a phosphatidylinositol mannoside) is inserted into the plasma membrane and reaches out through the layers of the wall to the exterior [8,9].

Epidemiology

Mycobacterium tuberculosis infection
The WHO describes the burden of tuberculosis as 'enormous' [1]. In 2020, India, China, Indonesia, the Philippines, Pakistan, Nigeria, Bangladesh and South Africa accounted for 86% of the estimated cases.

One component of Millennium Development Goal 6 to stop and reverse the increasing incidence of tuberculosis by 2015 was achieved but this trend has been reversed due to the impact of Covid-19 [1]. The mortality rates from tuberculosis are falling in all the WHO regions. WHO's 'End TB Strategy' has a target to reduce mortality to 90% of its 2015 level by 2030.

In England in 2019, 4725 cases of tuberculosis were reported. London accounted for more than one-third of cases and the majority of the burden remains in the conurbations and large urban areas [2]. The majority of cases (73.6%) occurred in individuals born outside the UK, with a rate of 40 per 100 000 population compared with 2.5 cases in UK-born individuals. Pulmonary disease was the most common and 28.4% of these patients also had extrapulmonary involvement. The most common co-morbidity was diabetes mellitus.

Cases of MDR and XDR tuberculosis continue to be a major challenge. Outcomes are suboptimal in this group of patients, with only 59% of patients being successfully treated in 2018 [1].

Molecular diagnostic tests using nucleic acid amplification techniques can detect the presence of *M. tuberculosis* DNA and also the marker of rifampicin resistance, and are now widely available [3].

HIV and *Mycobacterium tuberculosis* co-infection
It is estimated that one-third of the world's population have latent *M. tuberculosis* infection, which is defined as the presence of viable bacilli in an individual without the symptoms and signs of disease [4]. The immunosuppression caused by HIV infection (Chapter 31) greatly increases the risk of developing clinical disease,

and tuberculosis is the leading cause of mortality in HIV-infected individuals [5,6]. The WHO estimated that 17.3% of the 1.2 million people who died of tuberculosis in 2019 were infected with HIV [1].

HIV-associated tuberculosis mortality is reduced by effective ATT, concurrent antiretroviral therapy (ART) and the administration of co-trimoxazole [5]. Tuberculosis can be prevented in people living with HIV by the use of ART (although the risk of developing tuberculosis is still higher than in HIV-negative individuals) and, where appropriate, isoniazid preventative therapy (IPT) [6].

The UK guidelines recommend universal HIV testing in health care services for the diagnosis of tuberculosis [7]. Since 2007, the WHO has recommended provider-initiated testing and counselling for HIV infection and this has improved the rates of HIV testing in people diagnosed with tuberculosis [5]. The WHO recommends that HIV-infected infants should not receive BCG vaccination due to the high rates of BCG-associated disease [8].

Non-tuberculous mycobacterial infections

Non-tuberculous mycobacteria are widely distributed in the environment with high isolation rates worldwide. Organisms can be found in the soil and water, including treated water sources; in fact *M. kansasii*, *M. xenopi* and *M. simiae* are recovered almost exclusively from municipal water sources. There is no evidence of animal to human or human to human transmission of NTM and these organisms may cause both asymptomatic infection and symptomatic disease. HIV infection and iatrogenic immunosuppression has resulted in an increase in the incidence of NTM-associated disease. Cosmetic procedures, both surgical and non-surgical, and other types of body modification are increasingly being reported in association with NTM infection [9]. Antitumour necrosis factor (anti-TNF) therapies appear to increase the risk of NTM infection [10] although there was no increase in the risk of serious skin infections in patients with rheumatoid arthritis treated with these drugs.

The rate of NTM reporting in England, Wales and Northern Ireland increased from 0.9 per 100 000 population in 1995 to 2.9 per 100 000 in 2006 [11]. The most frequently reported were *M. avium* complex, *M. malmoense*, *M. kansasii* and *M. gordonae*. It has been suggested that this increase may reflect reporting practices and increased detection and identification of NTM due to improved laboratory techniques. It is important to determine the clinical relevance of any NTM isolate and there are accepted criteria for this [12].

In high-income settings, *M. avium* complex infection in those with profound immunosuppression secondary to HIV is associated with reduced survival [13]. In resource-limited settings, patients with HIV starting ART have a higher risk of mortality compared with patients in high-income settings [14]. A diagnosis of NTM infection is classified as WHO stage 4 of HIV infection. NTM infection is significantly associated with mortality in this group, with approximately a twofold increased risk of death [14].

Basic biology

Immunology of tuberculosis

Three factors in the immunology of tuberculosis remain poorly explained: the latent state, the balance between protection and immunopathology after previous exposure, and the failure to eliminate persistent mycobacteria.

Following infection, only 5–10% of individuals develop progressive disease, but some bacteria remain viable in the tissues of subclinically infected individuals. *M. tuberculosis* DNA can be identified not only in macrophages, but also in cells such as fibroblasts and type II pneumocytes, located in lung tissue devoid of lymphocyte infiltration in healthy individuals living in tuberculosis endemic countries [1]. Neutralisation of TNF for the treatment of inflammatory disorders such as rheumatoid arthritis or psoriasis can lead to reactivation and progressive disease [2,3] as can other immunosuppressive drugs, HIV, stress and starvation.

Immunocompetent individuals with tuberculosis usually develop a necrotising skin test response to *M. tuberculosis* antigens. The immunopathological response is thought to account for much of the tissue damage associated with tuberculosis. Robert Koch demonstrated in the late 19th century that guinea pigs with tuberculosis would develop a severe necrotic reaction at the site of injection of killed bacteria and also in existing tuberculous lesions – the 'Koch phenomenon' [4]. The differences between protection and immunopathology are highlighted by the fact that protection correlates with small skin reactions to tuberculin rather than with exaggerated necrotic responses [5].

The inefficiency of the immunopathological response as a microbicidal mechanism has a second important consequence. In patients with tuberculosis, most of the organisms are killed rapidly by antimicrobial chemotherapy. However, there are 'persisters' that may be biologically distinct from the bacteria that are associated with latency and these are not eliminated by the drugs or by the immune response. The failure of the immune response to eliminate persisters is attributable to the fact that the immunopathological response does not quickly switch to the non-necrotic protective mechanism characterised by the responses seen in successfully BCG vaccinated individuals. The result is that treatment must continue for at least 6 months or relapse will occur [6].

Protective immunity to *M. tuberculosis*

The cell wall of the mycobacterium is resistant to damage mediated by antibodies and complement and immunity depends on an intact T-lymphocyte response. Initial host resistance to *M. tuberculosis* is led by the innate immune systems pattern recognition receptors (PRRs) such as Toll-like receptor 2 (TLR-2), which recognises a wide variety of mycobacterial ligands, and TLR-9, which senses mycobacterial DNA and C-type lectins. The transmission of *M. tuberculosis* is via aerosol and once inhaled the organism is recognised and phagocytosed by a range of cells including macrophages, dendritic cells, monocytes and neutrophils [7]. The recruitment of these cells facilitates the establishment of the organism within the host by providing the intracellular niche it requires. The collection of phagocytes leads to granuloma formation, and the recruitment of uninfected macrophages into the granuloma has been shown in zebrafish to be a means of increasing the number of infected cells and disseminating the infection [8]. This has undermined the notion of the granuloma as solely a host-protective structure [9].

Pathogenic mycobacteria once established are able to manipulate the cells and their organelles and thus avoid deleterious intracellular mechanisms. *M. tuberculosis* in mice is able to leave the phagosome and enter the cytosol by inhibiting the expression of genes in the TLR-2 and MyD88 signalling pathway [10]. Gene deletions of the MyD88 or CARD9 adaptor proteins in mice leads to fulminant and lethal infection [11,12].

The activation of the PRRs leads to the expression of proinflammatory cytokines, chemokines and adhesion molecules, leading to the formation of antigen-specific CD4+ lymphocytes in the draining lymph nodes. These lymphocytes are essential for the development of the effector systems in the killing of mycobacteria; CD8+ lymphocytes are also involved in mice and non-human primates [13]. γδ T cells also play a role in the host defence against M. tuberculosis [14]. The development of effective, adaptive immunity halts bacterial progression and individuals do not shed bacteria. At this stage, an individual is considered to have latent tuberculosis and exhibits an immunological equilibrium [7]. However, the precise interplay of the various mechanisms that are responsible for this protective immunity remains unclear. TNF and interferon γ (IFN-γ) are essential in the immune control of tuberculosis and are well described in humans due to the effects of anti-TNF therapies and IFN-γ gene receptor deficiency. IFN-γ and interleukin 12 (IL-12) control TNF, which is produced by monocytes and macrophages.

The adaptive immune response to M. tuberculosis is delayed. Humans do not become tuberculin skin test (TST) positive for up to 6 weeks after exposure [15,16]. Understanding and overcoming this delay is a primary goal of vaccine research [17]. In mice infected with M. tuberculosis, antigen-specific T-regulatory cells delay the migration of effector T cells to the lung [17]. T-regulatory cells can also reduce the expression of co-stimulatory molecules such as CD80 on dendritic cells, which are required for the priming of naive T lymphocytes [18].

Immunopathology

There is accumulating evidence for the role of neutrophils in contributing to the pathology associated with infection with M. tuberculosis. This was demonstrated in genetically susceptible mice [19] and more recently this has been supported in a study in humans with active and latent tuberculosis [20]. There was a significant increase in the expression of genes related to IFN-γ and type I IFN-αβ. The former is protective in active tuberculosis but the latter are associated with more virulent strains of M. tuberculosis and reactivation of tuberculosis. The increase in type I IFNs was neutrophil driven. It was also demonstrated that approximately 10% of individuals with latent tuberculosis in the study had a similar profile to those with active tuberculosis. This is the same proportion of patients with latent tuberculosis whom one would anticipate might eventually develop active tuberculosis. There is also evidence that IFN-γ acts directly on neutrophils to decrease their lifespan [21], and a lack of IFN-γ leads to an increase in IL-17-producing cells and increased numbers of neutrophils that are IL-17 dependent [22].

Diagnostic tests for tuberculosis

Tuberculin skin test

The TST has been in use for over 100 years [1] and depends upon delayed-type hypersensitivity to mycobacterial antigens, following an intradermal injection of purified protein derivative (PPD). PPD is a culture filtrate of tubercle bacilli containing over 200 antigens shared with M. bovis BCG and many NTM [2]. This lack of specificity is a major drawback in populations vaccinated with BCG. A positive test can result from clinical or latent infection due to M. tuberculosis, from BCG vaccination or from contact with environmental mycobacteria. As the TST depends on a lymphocyte-induced delayed hypersensitivity reaction it is of low sensitivity in immunosuppressed patients. Individuals with severe illness, including those with some forms of active tuberculosis, with HIV infection and those on immunosuppressant drugs including corticosteroids, may have false negative reactions [3].

Tuberculin testing should be done by the Mantoux method as this is the only technique that has been standardised and extensively validated. PPD (0.1 mL = 5 tuberculin units) is injected into the volar aspect of the forearm using a 27-gauge needle to raise a small weal. The diameter of the induration is measured after 48–72 h. Normally a cut-off of 5 mm induration is used to determine those at high risk of infection, for example close contacts of an active case, patients with radiographic abnormalities consistent with tuberculosis, those with HIV infection and those immunosuppressed with corticosteroids or other agents. A cut-off of 10 mm is used in migrants from endemic areas, health care workers, the homeless and residents of some urban areas, and those patients with diabetes, renal disease, silicosis and other conditions associated with an increased risk of latent tuberculosis. Finally a cut-off of 15 mm is used in those with no risk factors.

Tuberculin sensitivity appears within a few weeks of the onset of an infection with M. tuberculosis and is usually lifelong, although rarely tuberculin reactions may decrease in size (reversion) [4]. In any community, the number of individuals who react strongly to tuberculin relates to the prevalence of active tuberculosis. The risk of developing clinical tuberculosis in tuberculin-positive children is roughly proportional to the strength of their tuberculin reaction [5] and protection consistently correlates with small non-necrotising responses, while large necrotic responses indicate susceptibility or actual disease [6].

Weaker reactions do not correlate with the amount of active tuberculosis in a community. Some are due to infection with other mycobacteria, and others are due to the waning of reactivity under various influences such as ageing.

Interferon γ release assays for the diagnosis of latent tuberculosis

Interferon γ release assays (IGRAs) are T-cell-based blood tests that measure the host response to M. tuberculosis by utilising antigens that are much more specific for M. tuberculosis than tuberculin. IGRAs are more specific than the TST in the diagnosis of latent M. tuberculosis infection in adults and children [7,8], however the sensitivity is no better than that of the TST. In the UK, IGRAs are not recommended for the routine diagnosis of active tuberculosis [9]. However, the US Food and Drug Administration (FDA) has approved IGRAs as indirect tests of M. tuberculosis infection, including that causing active disease, when used in conjunction with other clinical and diagnostic methods [10]. IGRAs were reported to be helpful in supporting the diagnosis of tuberculid in three patients [11].

The two commercially available IGRAs, QuantiFERON®-TB Gold In-Tube test (QFT-GIT) (Qiagen, Valencia, CA, USA) and T-SPOT®

TB test (T-Spot) (Oxford Immunotec, Abingdon, UK), both employ early secretory protein 6 and culture filtrate protein 10. In addition the QFT-GIT also uses TB7.7. These antigens are absent in most NTM and all strains of BCG, making these tests useful in individuals who have received BCG vaccination. The QFT-GIT assay uses an enzyme-linked immunosorbent assay (ELISA) to measure the concentration of IFN-γ in the plasma supernatant following incubation of blood with the antigens and both negative and positive controls. The T-Spot assay measures the number of IFN-γ-producing T cells after overnight incubation in tissue culture plates.

The UK National Institute for Health and Care Excellence (NICE) recommends that the use of IGRAs should be considered in people who are contacts of someone with tuberculosis whose TST is positive or those in whom a TST would be less reliable. IGRAs either alone or in combination with a TST are recommended in HIV-positive individuals with CD4 counts of 200–500 cells/mm^3 and other people who are immunosuppressed [9]. The British Association of Dermatologists' guidelines for the use of biological therapy for psoriasis advise that prescribers consider assessing patients using IGRAs alone or in conjunction with a Mantoux test [12].

In a study of individuals with psoriasis who were being considered for anti-TNF therapy there was only moderate agreement between the two different IGRAs (indeterminate results having been excluded) and the authors suggested that in some situations it may be useful to use a TST in conjunction with both IGRAs [13]. Other authors have expressed a preference for IGRAs rather than a TST in screening for latent tuberculosis in these individuals [14].

Diagnosis of mycobacterial infections

Some mycobacterial infections may be suspected from their clinical features, geographic location or the interests or occupation of the patient. For example, *M. marinum* infections are seen in tropical aquarium owners. Others such as *M. ulcerans* may not be recognised so easily. Any obscure granulomatous or ulcerative lesion of the skin should be biopsied and cultured for mycobacteria. This can take several weeks in the case of 'slow growers'.

Light and fluorescence microscopy using Ziehl–Neelsen stain and auramine, respectively, are used to visualise mycobacteria in specimens. It is not possible to distinguish between different species of mycobacteria using microscopy. Mycobacterial culture can be performed on solid or liquid media. The optimal culture temperature for NTM is at 30°C and so is lower than that of *M. tuberculosis*, which is 35°C and is often routinely used in laboratories for all mycobacterial cultures [15]. This may adversely affect the yield of NTM by culture unless culture at the lower temperature is requested.

Mycobacterium species identification utilises DNA amplification from isolates using whole genome sequencing (WGS), which can also be used to predict resistance to first and some second line agents. WGS may be used to determine isolate relatedness and transmission dynamics as well. Xpert® MTB/RIF (Cepheid, USA) is a cartridge-based molecular diagnostic test that can detect the presence of *M. tuberculosis* DNA and also the marker of rifampicin resistance [16]. It has been shown to be sensitive and specific in the diagnosis of pulmonary tuberculosis using sputum [17]. A WHO-funded systematic review and meta-analysis has also confirmed its utility in extrapulmonary tuberculosis, although none of the studies included in the analysis used skin specimens [18].

Mass spectrometry has been reported to be a rapid technique for mycobacterial identification [19], and the utility of detecting urinary LAM as a diagnostic test for tuberculosis is being studied [20].

TUBERCULOSIS OF THE SKIN

Cutaneous tuberculosis comprises only a small proportion of all cases of tuberculosis; nevertheless, considering the high prevalence of tuberculosis in many developing countries these numbers become significant. In western Europe, tuberculosis of the skin has become uncommon [1].

Classification

Clinical spectrum of cutaneous tuberculosis

The wide clinical spectrum of cutaneous tuberculosis is dependent on the route of infection (endogenous or exogenous), the immune status of the patient and whether or not there has been previous sensitisation with tuberculosis.

Primary inoculation of the skin, usually following trauma, produces a tuberculous chancre in the non-immune host, whereas the so-called 'prosector's wart' or tuberculosis verrucosa cutis, occurs in primary infection in the immune host. Lupus vulgaris occurs mainly through haematogenous, lymphatic or contiguous spread but can occur following inoculation. Scrofuloderma results from contiguous involvement of the skin overlying tuberculosis in a deeper structure, most commonly lymph nodes, bone or joint disease or epididymitis. Metastatic tuberculous abscesses (tuberculous gumma) can occur due to haematogenous spread from a primary focus. This usually occurs when host resistance is suppressed, it can be part of miliary tuberculosis, and results in single or multiple lesions. Orificial, perioral or perianal tuberculosis can occur following ingestion of mycobacteria from either swallowed respiratory secretions or from milk contaminated with *M. bovis*.

The tuberculids are thought to be the result of immunological reactions to haematogenously spread antigenic components of *M. tuberculosis*, usually occurring in individuals with high levels of immunity, with an extracutaneous source of *M. tuberculosis*. *M. tuberculosis* complex DNA has been identified in some instances by polymerase chain reaction (PCR) [1]. There are three main forms: lichen scrofulosorum, papulonecrotic tuberculid and erythema induratum of Bazin. A variant nodular tuberculid has recently been described [2,3].

The incidence of the different forms of cutaneous tuberculosis varies globally. Scrofuloderma was the commonest form in the most recent UK series [4], whereas lupus vulgaris occurred most commonly in a study from South Africa [5]. Serial reviews from Hong Kong have shown a change in the commonest form of skin tuberculosis in recent years from tuberculosis verrucosa cutis in 1968 [6] to tuberculid erythema induratum in 1995 [7] and 2006 [8]. In India, scrofuloderma and lichen scrofulosorum [9–11] were the most frequently found forms in childhood, whereas lupus vulgaris was the commonest form in adults [10,11], and also in a series from Pakistan [12]. In Japan, there appears to be a trend towards an increasing incidence of the tuberculids, particularly in older patients [13]. Scrofuloderma was found in 70% of 202 cases of skin tuberculosis in a 2008 study from Tigray, northern Ethiopia, of whom 29% had coexisting HIV [14]. Scrofuloderma was also the most common form (72%) identified in a series from Morocco [15]. In a recent study from Nepal, tuberculosis verrucous cutis had a higher incidence (44%) than other types of cutaneous tuberculosis [16].

Classification difficulties

No entirely satisfactory classification exists, reflecting the difficulty in classifying a disease whose diverse manifestations are dependent on so many factors, such as the host's cell-mediated immunity and the route of infection. In 1896, Darier separated proven tuberculosis lesions from the remainder. This led, inevitably, to a number of conditions being accepted as 'tuberculids' on circumstantial evidence. Confusion between true tuberculosis and a less specific 'tuberculoid' histology compounded the difficulty until the advent of effective antituberculosis drugs, when the lack of response of many of the so-called tuberculids, and their tendency to resolve spontaneously, led to a more critical evaluation of their aetiology. With the advent of new methods to detect *M. tuberculosis* complex DNA, the position of the tuberculids has become clearer.

In 1981, Beyt et al. [17] classified the disease into inoculation tuberculosis, secondary tuberculosis, haematogenous tuberculosis and eruptive tuberculosis. This did not take into account immunological considerations. More recently, it has been suggested that a useful concept is the mycobacterial load [18] and that tuberculosis can be classified into multibacillary forms where there are abundant mycobacteria (e.g. scrofuloderma, tuberculous chancre, acute miliary tuberculosis) and paucibacillary forms where mycobacteria are difficult to isolate (e.g. lupus vulgaris, tuberculosis verrucosa cutis) (Table 27.2). In this classification the tuberculids would sit at the extreme end of the paucibacillary spectrum [19].

General description

Cutaneous tuberculosis made up 4.4% of all cases of tuberculosis notified in one UK district between 1981 and 1995 [1], and 3.5% of 370 patients with tuberculosis reported from Turkey in 2003 [2].

In India in the 1950s and 1960s, cutaneous tuberculosis affected 2% of all skin out-patients. By the 1980s, this had fallen to 0.15% [3] and in two series published around the millennium this had fallen to 0.1% [4,5]. More recent reports from Morocco and India suggest that cutaneous tuberculosis is again becoming more prevalent with incidence rates of 2% and 0.7%, respectively [6,7].

A current problem is that atypical and even standard presentations may be overlooked through lack of familiarity with the various patterns that may occur.

Basic biology

Pathogenesis

Mycobacterium tuberculosis and *M. bovis* and occasionally *M. bovis* BCG, an attenuated form of *M. bovis*, are pathogenic to humans. The majority of human disease is due to *M. tuberculosis*, *M. bovis* being found in only 1–1.5% of isolates [1]. *M. bovis* has a broad host range and is the principal agent responsible for tuberculosis in domestic and wild mammals [2].

Transmission of infection within and between species is mainly by inhalation of air-borne droplet nuclei particles containing *M. tuberculosis* complex, resulting in pulmonary infection. *M. bovis* may also penetrate the gastrointestinal mucosa and lymphatic tissue of the oro-pharynx when ingested in milk. Direct inoculation of the skin by *M. tuberculosis* complex also occurs particularly if there is any defect in the skin barrier. Survival of *Mycobacterium* species in aerosols generated from human saliva is usually less than an hour, indicating that close and prolonged contact is required for transmission of infection [3]. Studies of contact tracing have shown that 1% of close contacts are affected [4]. *M. tuberculosis* is not a virulent organism and only 5–10% of infections will lead to clinical disease, although this risk increases substantially with immunosuppression (e.g. with HIV infection or treatment with TNF-α inhibitors). Other predisposing factors for cutaneous tuberculosis include poverty, malnutrition, poor living conditions and the emergence of drug-resistant *M. tuberculosis*.

Development of the granuloma

Dissemination of the bacteria takes place via the lymphatics and bloodstream. In persons with intact immunity this initiates

Table 27.2 Classification of cutaneous tuberculosis.

Host immunity	Method of inoculation	Disease
Multibacillary forms		
Naive host	Direct inoculation	Tuberculous chancre (primary inoculation)
Low	Contiguous spread	Scrofuloderma
Low	Autoinoculation	Orificial tuberculosis
Low	Haematogenous spread	Acute miliary cutaneous
Low	Haematogenous spread	Tuberculous gumma (abscess)
Paucibacillary forms		
High	Direct inoculation	Warty tuberculosis (verrucosa cutis)
High	Direct inoculation	Lupus vulgaris (some)
High	Haematogenous spread	Lupus vulgaris
High	?Haematogenous spread	Tuberculids: Lichen scrofulosorum, papulonecrotic tuberculid, erythema induratum (Bazin)

granuloma formation. For decades the tuberculous granuloma was considered to be a host-driven mechanism formed to control infection. The recent ability to visualise cellular events of granuloma formation at the whole animal level in zebrafish has provided new insights into the mechanisms and consequences of granuloma formation. These studies indicate that rather than having a protective function, granuloma formation contributes to bacterial multiplication and spread [5]. It has now been shown that the RD1 locus in virulent mycobacteria releases the early secreted target 6 (ESAT-6) protein, which stimulates epithelial cells to produce metalloproteinase 9 (MMP-9). MMP-9 secretion promotes the recruitment of new macrophages to the granuloma where they become infected and expand the granuloma. The host responds by producing CD4 and CD8 T cells that attempt to control bacterial growth. The mature granuloma therefore represents an equilibrium between mycobacterial growth and the host immune response [6], and in this way *M. tuberculosis* can persist for decades within the granuloma structures.

Overt tuberculous disease can result from either early progression of a primary granuloma during the infection process or reactivation of an established granuloma in a latently infected person. Such reactivation is usually due to a dysregulation in the immune response (e.g. HIV infection, diabetes, cancer, malnutrition, ageing, TNF-α inhibitors).

To the epidemiologist, 'primary' tuberculosis means any lesions developing within 5 years of the original infection [7], while later lesions are considered as 'secondary'. There is always a difficulty in determining whether post-primary lesions are due to the reactivation of existing disease, for example as in patients with HIV infection or during TNF-α inhibitor treatment, or due to reinfection, particularly since BCG protection diminishes with time. Exogenous reinfection is probably rare, but does occur [8], and the reactions seen in a host already sensitised by a previous infection differ from those of the non-sensitised. A primary infection in the skin, for example, will be manifest as a cutaneous chancre whereas inoculation into a previously sensitised host may lead to tuberculosis verrucosa cutis (see 'Warty tuberculosis' later in this chapter).

The tuberculin test becomes positive after 3–8 weeks. This may be accompanied by fever or erythema nodosum (see Chapter 97), which is therefore a sign of a recent primary infection.

Histopathology

Mycobacterium tuberculosis can cause skin infection by direct inoculation into the skin, by haematogenous spread from an internal lesion and by direct contact with tuberculosis in an underlying deeper structure [9]. Early, non-specific inflammatory changes give rise after 3–6 weeks to a characteristic tubercle or granuloma. At this stage tubercle bacilli are rarely found, although inoculation cultures may be positive.

The fully formed granuloma consists of a focus of epithelioid cells containing a variable, but usually sparse, number of Langhans giant cells and a surrounding infiltrate of mononuclear cells. The centre of the tubercle undergoes caseation necrosis and sometimes calcifies. Endovascular or perivascular changes in the vicinity of the tubercle become more marked as necrosis proceeds, and are accompanied by a cellular reaction leading to fibrosis. Granulomas vary in appearance and are influenced by the virulence of the organism and the immune status of the patient. Where cellular immunity is impaired, the resulting pathology is less granulomatous (due to fewer activated macrophages) and there are greater numbers of bacteria found. Typical or less well-developed tuberculoid granulomas occur in many conditions other than tuberculosis.

Disease-specific changes

Differences in the histopathological appearances depend on the balance between infection and immunological response. In the tuberculous chancre (see 'Primary inoculation tuberculosis' later in this chapter), an acute, necrotic, neutrophilic reaction changes to a mononuclear infiltrate and, after 3–6 weeks, into typical tubercles in which the bacilli may no longer easily be seen. In miliary and orificial forms, the typical tubercle does not form or is imperfect or necrotic [10]. Bacilli are normally numerous, except in the milder neonatal form of miliary tuberculosis [11].

In scrofuloderma, the skin is destroyed by non-specific abscess formation and ulceration. Tubercle formation and caseation necrosis occur at the periphery and bacilli can, with diligence, be found. In warty tuberculosis, the classic hallmarks are often missing, but there is marked hyperkeratosis, acanthosis and papillomatosis (which may be pseudoepitheliomatous) and an intense dermal infiltrate of neutrophils, lymphocytes and some giant cells (Figure 27.1). Bacilli are rarely demonstrable; typical tubercles are uncommon and caseation is rare.

The appearances in lupus vulgaris (Figure 27.2) are variable and may give rise to diagnostic difficulty. The typical changes are those of well-marked tubercle formation with epithelioid nodules embedded in sheets of lymphocytes. Occasionally, the epidermal changes resemble those of warty tuberculosis. Caseation is usually sparse or even absent, and the amount of lymphocytic infiltrate is variable. Bacilli are seldom demonstrated, although they can sometimes be cultured. As the lesions heal, increasing fibrosis strangles the remaining small foci of tubercle bacilli or epithelioid cells, which slowly become absorbed by the reparative process. Squamous and basal cell epithelioma may arise in longstanding lesions.

Differential diagnosis

The typical features are characteristic, but the variations may cause confusion with many other diseases, especially if caseation necrosis is absent or the subject's immune response is minimal.

It is impossible on histological grounds to differentiate the lesions of other mycobacterial infections. In sarcoidosis, all the features except caseation necrosis may be present, and differentiation from lupus vulgaris may be impossible, although the epithelioid cell foci tend to be more scattered and well defined and are surrounded by relatively fewer lymphocytes and by reticulin. In tuberculoid leprosy, a neural and perineural involvement is the only distinguishing feature. In leishmaniasis, one must rely on finding the causative organism; similarly with blastomycosis and chromoblastomycosis. Tertiary syphilis shows more pronounced vascular changes and a plasma cell infiltrate.

A non-specific tuberculoid infiltrate, with irregular groups of epithelioid cells in an inflammatory infiltrate but without the formation of typical tubercles – as seen, for example, in rosacea or panniculitis – may also cause confusion.

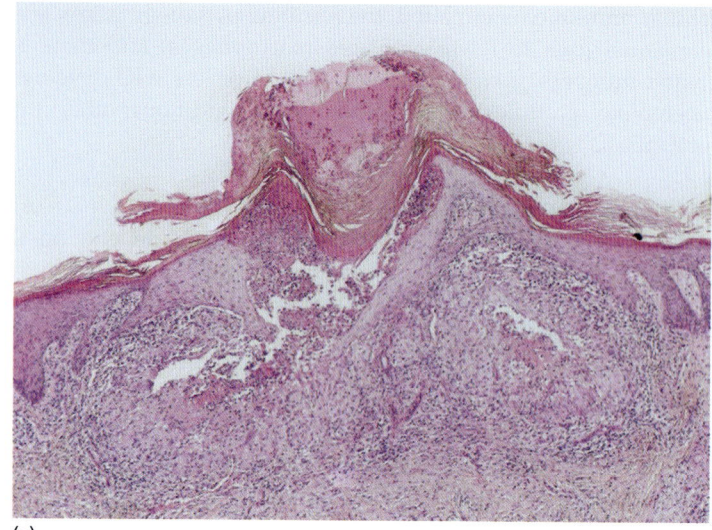

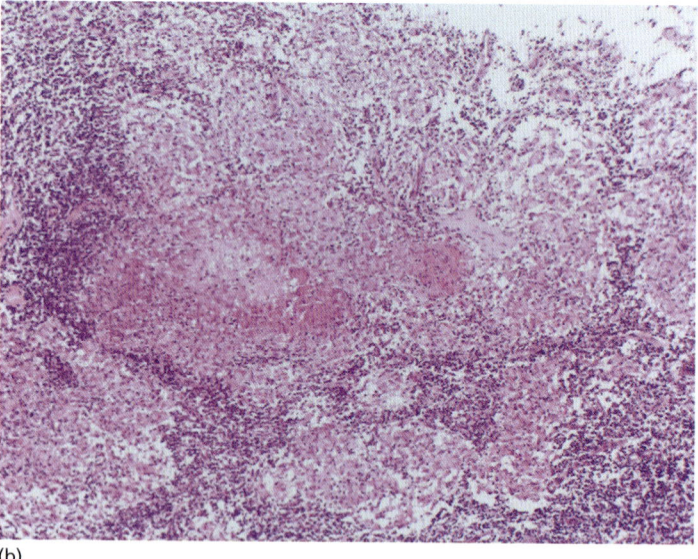

Figure 27.1 Warty tuberculosis. (a) Epidermis showing hyperkeratosis and acanthosis, with acute inflammation and abscess formation in the upper dermis. Ill-defined caseating granulomas with Langerhans giant cells are present in the mid-dermis. Magnification 120× (H&E). (b) Deep dermis showing a granulomatous inflammatory cell infiltrate. The granulomas contain epithelioid histiocytes with prominent Langhans giant cells and caseation. Magnification 140× (H&E). Courtesy of Dr M. Bamford and Dr A. Fletcher.

Diagnostic tests for cutaneous tuberculosis

The diagnosis of skin tuberculosis may be suggested by clinical features and typical histological findings but the only absolute criterion is the demonstration of *M. tuberculosis* in either tissue culture from skin biopsy or cytological smear, or the demonstration of mycobacterial DNA by PCR. This may be very difficult in paucibacillary lesions such as lupus vulgaris.

Other indications toward the diagnosis, which are by themselves unreliable, include the following:

1 The presence of active, proven tuberculosis elsewhere in the body.
2 The presence of acid-fast bacilli in the lesion itself – this will also be seen in infections with other mycobacteria.

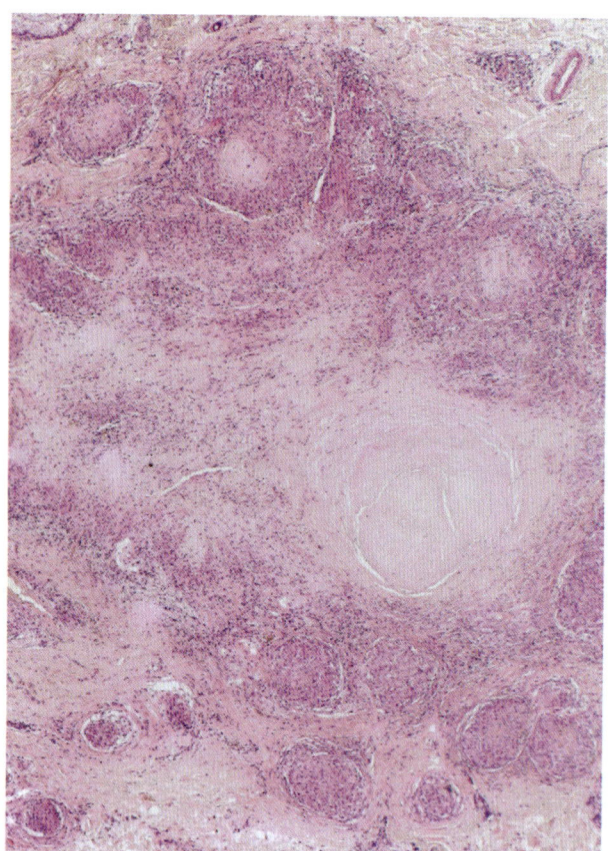

Figure 27.2 Lupus vulgaris. Extensive caseous granulomatous inflammation in the deep dermis in lupus vulgaris (H&E). Courtesy of Dr M. Bamford and Dr A. Fletcher.

3 A positive reaction to tuberculin – a strongly positive reaction of >15 mm in diameter may be considered of diagnostic value [1] although there is not total agreement on this [2].
4 Positive IFN-γ release assay [3].
5 The effect of specific therapy – in areas of high tuberculous prevalence a therapeutic trial of antituberculous therapy should be considered [4–6].

The difficulties in separating tuberculosis from a 'tuberculoid reaction' seen in leprosy (Chapter 28), leishmaniasis (Chapter 33), deep mycoses (Chapter 32), infections with NTM (see 'Non-tuberculous (atypical) mycobacteria' later in this chapter), syphilis (Chapter 29) and sarcoidosis (Chapter 96) are dealt with elsewhere.

Nucleic acid amplification tests [7,8]

The *in vitro* amplification of specific DNA sequences using the PCR has become a valuable tool in the rapid detection of slow-growing organisms such as *M. tuberculosis*. Several systems have been reported for the molecular detection of mycobacterial DNA using different parts of the mycobacterial genome to generate highly sensitive and specific probes [9–11]. Most studies use an assay system based on the insertion sequence IS6110 because of the repetitive nature of this element in the *M. tuberculosis* genome [12]. Other gene targets used include the 16s rRNA gene or genes encoding MPB-64, 38 kDa and 65 kDa proteins. IS6110 has zero or low copy numbers in some *M. tuberculosis* strains and the combination of two or more gene targets has been employed in multiplex PCR, for example

IS6110 + MPB-64 or IS6110 + 38 kDa + MPB-64 [7]. As few as two colony-forming units of *M. tuberculosis* cells, or as little as 15 fg of DNA, can be detected [13].

Using the PCR technique, mycobacterial DNA has been demonstrated in all the different histopathological variants of cutaneous tuberculosis including the tuberculids [13–19]. Tan *et al.* showed that the PCR technique was 100% sensitive and specific in multibacillary cutaneous tuberculosis, but in paucibacillary tuberculosis DNA PCR positivity rates were 55% for tuberculosis verrucosa cutis (38 cases) and 60% for lupus vulgaris (five cases). The overall sensitivity was 73% [20]. In other studies sensitivity was found to be less [21], and in this context it should be noted that sensitivities among different laboratories may vary [8].

The technique reduces the time required for diagnosis in those cutaneous lesions where bacteria can be cultured easily, and may be particularly useful in paucibacillary lesions such as lupus vulgaris. The technique can be used in a variety of pathological specimens, including archival formalin-fixed tissue sections. A generic criticism of this technique lies in its sensitivity; tissue samples containing bacterial DNA may be positive because of bacteraemia and not necessarily because the organism is involved in the pathogenesis of the tissue lesion [14]. Both false positive and false negative results can be obtained and the issue of contamination also represents a big potential pitfall.

Treatment

General measures

In the UK, all patients with tuberculosis must be notified as this is a statutory requirement [1] and contact tracing must be initiated if appropriate [2]. Attention to the patient as a whole is an essential part of the proper management of any cutaneous tuberculous lesion and involves a careful search for an underlying focus of disease and coexistent infections. Because of the rising incidence of drug-resistant tuberculosis, it is vital to confirm the diagnosis bacteriologically whenever possible and to obtain drug susceptibilities [3]. Tuberculosis, pulmonary or extrapulmonary, is an acquired immune deficiency syndrome (AIDS) defining illness. HIV testing should be offered to all individuals. If pulmonary, bone, lymph node or renal tuberculosis is found, a combined approach with other specialists is essential, as management will depend upon the organs involved, the extent of the lesions and the patient's immunity.

Drug therapy

Treatment of cutaneous tuberculosis should follow the same drug regimen as that for pulmonary tuberculosis [4]. The NICE 2016 guidelines [5] recommend that the treatment of all patients should be supervised by physicians with full training in the management of tuberculosis and with direct working access to tuberculosis nurse specialists or health visitors.

Patient non-adherence is currently one of the most important factors limiting successful treatment. Directly observed therapy (DOT), where the ingestion of every drug dose is witnessed, has shown improved cure rates in a number of countries [6,7]. Treatment completion rates of over 90%, however, have been reported from both the USA and UK using mainly self-administered therapy and only selective – not universal – DOT [8].

Patients should have a risk assessment for adherence and DOT considered for those patients who have adverse factors. These include patients who are homeless or who have a substance or alcohol use disorder, mental illness, multiple drug resistances and those with a previous history of non-adherence with antituberculous medication [9]. DOT can be daily, but an intermittent regimen is often more convenient. Fixed-dose combination tablets should be used to improve adherence and prevent monotherapy, which can lead to acquired drug resistance within weeks in active disease.

Current treatment regimens

The antituberculosis drugs currently used in first line treatments are around 60 years old. The regimen that is recommended by WHO and NICE for new cases of drug-susceptible tuberculosis is highly effective, with cure rates of around 90% in HIV-negative patients [8,10]. The standard recommended regimen is 6 months of treatment with four first line drugs: a combination of rifampicin, isoniazid, ethambutol and pyrazinamide for 2 months, followed by a 4-month continuation phase of rifampicin and isoniazid (the 6-month four-drug regimen) [11]. Attempts have been made to shorten the total duration of treatment by reducing the length of the continuation phase. The Centers for Disease Control and Prevention (CDC) recently recommended the use of a 4-month regimen of rifapentine, isoniazid, pyrazinamide and moxifloxacin in individuals older than 12 years with drug-susceptible tuberculosis [12].

There are 10 new or repurposed antituberculosis drugs currently in late phases of clinical development [8]. Bedaquiline was approved for use in the treatment of patients with MDR tuberculosis in 2012 and pretomanid was approved in 2019 for use with bedaquiline and linezolid [13].

Drug dosing schedule and common side effects

The standard recommended regimen consists of four drugs:

1. Isoniazid (300 mg daily) for the full 6 months.
2. Rifampicin (450 mg daily for those weighing less than 50 kg; 600 mg daily for those above this weight) for the full 6 months.
3. Pyrazinamide for the first 2 months (1.5 g daily for those weighing less than 50 kg; 2.0 g daily for those above this weight).
4. Ethambutol for the first 2 months (15 mg/kg body weight daily).

All the drugs are taken on an empty stomach once daily.

Isoniazid remains the standard drug, given in all regimens because of its efficacy, cheapness and low toxicity. Its commonest side effects are peripheral neuropathy (most common in elderly people), which can be countered by giving pyridoxine (10 mg daily) prophylactically from the start of treatment, and hepatitis in adults over 35 years of age.

Rifampicin can commonly cause elevated serum transaminases during the first 2 months of treatment, but therapy can usually be continued except in severe cases. Urine, sweat and tears may be coloured orange. The induction of liver enzymes by rifampicin may reduce the effectiveness of oral contraceptives.

Pyrazinamide causes hepatitis in 1%, and arthritis and the precipitation of gout and cutaneous hypersensitivity in 3.5%.

Ethambutol may cause visual disturbances and rarely a retrobulbar neuritis, which is reversible if detected early. Patients should be warned of this risk and advised to stop the drug if visual symptoms develop. Visual acuity using a Snellen chart should be carried out before treatment starts. The drug is best avoided in young children and in those with renal impairment.

In summary, all antituberculous drugs may cause adverse reactions. In one study, reactions occurred in 10% of patients treated. Reactions were significantly more common in those not receiving standard antituberculosis chemotherapy [14].

HIV disease

In HIV-infected patients, there have been no controlled trials of sufficient power to detect differences in efficacy between regimens and currently the same 6-month regimen is recommended [8,15]. Drugs used to treat tuberculosis may interact with some antiretroviral drugs. HIV-positive tuberculosis patients continue to have worse outcomes than HIV-negative tuberculosis patients. The treatment success rate for all new HIV-positive tuberculosis patients was 73% compared with 87% among HIV-negative tuberculosis patients. If it is assumed that HIV-positive tuberculosis patients who defaulted from treatment would have died from tuberculosis, the death rate was 19% among HIV-positive tuberculosis patients compared with 3% among HIV-negative tuberculosis patients. Such findings are consistent with two autopsy studies in South Africa, which showed that undiagnosed tuberculosis remains the main cause of death among HIV-positive people [8].

Multidrug-resistant tuberculosis

This is defined as resistance to rifampicin and isoniazid [16,17]. MDR tuberculosis is important because there is loss of both the main bactericidal drug (isoniazid) and the main sterilising drug (rifampicin). The consequences of this situation are considerable. Patients who are sputum smear positive remain infectious for much longer than those with susceptible organisms and have a higher death rate from, and a lower cure rate for, their tuberculosis [5].

In 2020, about 132 000 new cases of MDR tuberculosis were confirmed, but this is an underestimate as not all countries are testing for drug resistance [8].

In 2010, the WHO endorsed the first rapid molecular test that can be used to simultaneously test for pulmonary tuberculosis and rifampicin resistance: Xpert® MTB/RIF [18,19]. Though not a complete surrogate for MDR tuberculosis, particularly in settings where levels of drug resistance are low, rifampicin resistance is the most important indicator of MDR tuberculosis and can be used as an initial screening test and to identify those requiring further testing to be performed at national or supranational tuberculosis reference laboratories.

Extensively drug-resistant tuberculosis

Extremely drug-resistant tuberculosis was first reported from South Africa in patients with HIV infection [20,21]. By the end of 2012, XDR tuberculosis had been reported by 92 countries [8]. On average, an estimated 9.6% of MDR tuberculosis cases have XDR tuberculosis. The proportion of MDR tuberculosis cases with XDR tuberculosis is highest in Azerbaijan (12.8%), Belarus (11.9%), Latvia (16.0%), Lithuania (24.8%) and Tajikistan (21.0%). Treatment of such patients is complex, and is difficult in many countries that lack adequate primary care facilities and the necessary tools to detect drug resistance promptly. Ideally, treatment should only be carried out by experienced physicians in hospitals with appropriate isolation facilities and in consultation with appropriate mycobacterial reference laboratories [5,8].

Modification for dermatological practice

Yates and Ormerod have shown that the standard 6-month regimen is effective in treating cutaneous tuberculosis [4]. In their series of patients, over 50% had coexisting disease elsewhere, all had a good clinical response and there were no relapses following treatment. Historically, some forms of skin tuberculosis have been treated by isoniazid alone [22]. This is no longer appropriate as drug resistance is likely to develop with monotherapy – and if drug resistance to isoniazid is already present, it means, in effect, that no therapy is being given.

The excision of small lesions of lupus vulgaris or warty tuberculosis, if diagnosed early, may be effective. Surgery may be helpful in scrofuloderma, sometimes shortening the time needed for chemotherapy. Plastic surgery may help the disfigurement left by treated lupus vulgaris.

Prognosis

Now revolutionised by modern therapy, the prognosis depends largely on early and accurate diagnosis. When tuberculosis has become generalised or has affected the meninges, the prognosis must be doubtful. The mortality in patients with dual tuberculosis/HIV infection is higher than in HIV-negative patients and the same applies in all forms of drug-resistant tuberculosis. In infants and young children, tuberculosis is always a serious disease. Tuberculosis confined to the skin usually responds well to multiple therapy and a clinical response will usually occur within 4–6 weeks, with lupus vulgaris showing a faster response time than scrofuloderma.

BCG vaccination

The BCG vaccine for the prevention of tuberculosis is almost 100 years old [1]. Calmette and Guérin, at the Pasteur Institute in Lille developed the vaccine from 1908 onwards using *in vitro* attenuation by repeated passage of an isolate of *M. bovis*. It was finally tested in humans in 1921 [2]. There are several different commercial BCG vaccines in use today, which differ in virulence and immune response induced due to genomic differences in the vaccine [3,4], although there are currently insufficient data to favour or recommend one BCG vaccine strain. Strategies for the development of new vaccines are concentrating on both a new replacement vaccine and booster vaccines given in addition to BCG [5]. A recent trial of MVA85A, a new tuberculosis vaccine in infants, showed no additional protection was conferred compared with BCG alone [6].

While current BCG vaccines protect against severe forms of tuberculosis in children (tuberculosis meningitis and miliary tuberculosis), its efficacy in preventing pulmonary tuberculosis in adults is highly variable [7]. Several studies have shown that BCG does not appear to prevent skin tuberculosis [8]. The protective effect of BCG in children is likely to last at least 15 years [9]. In the UK, BCG is only offered to individuals at higher risk of exposure to tuberculosis. It is recommended for babies born in areas of the UK where the rates of tuberculosis are high, those who have a parent or grandparent who was born in a country with a high rate of tuberculosis and those who live with, or are close contacts of, someone with infectious tuberculosis. BCG is not recommended for use in infants known to be infected with HIV, due to the risk of disseminated BCG disease [7].

Complications

After BCG vaccination, a local reaction usually occurs 2–6 weeks later as a small papule that may slowly enlarge and discharge purulent material to leave a shallow ulcer. Tuberculin conversion normally takes place within 12 weeks.

Complications are rare in relation to the number of vaccinations carried out. Excluding abnormal BCG primary complexes, all reported localised or generalised reactions among nearly 1500 million persons vaccinated between 1948 and 1974 made up less than 2 per million [10]. Of these, keloids, rashes and ocular manifestations accounted for 1.35 per million, and 'tuberculosis-like' lesions for 0.16 per million.

Non-specific reactions to BCG include urticaria and erythema multiforme [11]. Unusual reactions have also occurred, such as generalised maculopapular or purpuric eruptions associated with arthralgia and abdominal pain or myalgia, usually after repeated vaccination [12,13]. Extensive or protracted ulceration sometimes occurs.

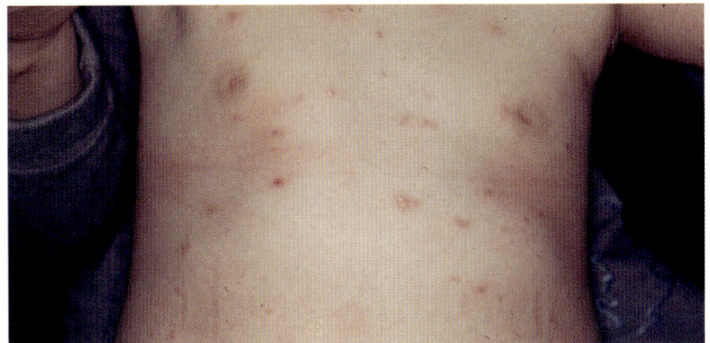

Figure 27.4 Atypical papular tuberculid following BCG vaccination. Courtesy of Dr J. Muto.

Specific complications include tuberculous processes caused by the BCG organism. Lupus vulgaris may develop at the vaccination site, usually a few months after vaccination, but cases have been reported as long as 3 years after vaccination (Figure 27.3) [14–16]. This can be a recurrent problem [17] and is more likely to occur after multiple vaccinations [18]. Scrofuloderma has also been reported [19]. Several of the tuberculids including lichen scrofulosorum [12], an atypical papular tuberculid thought to be a variant of papulonecrotic tuberculid (Figure 27.4) [20] and erythema induratum of Bazin [21] have followed vaccination. As these are hypersensitivity reactions to M. bovis, antituberculous therapy is not necessary other than in immunocompromised patients. The development of basal cell carcinoma in a BCG scar has been reported [22]; squamous cell carcinoma also developed in BCG-induced lupus vulgaris in a 7-year-old child [23]. Disseminated cutaneous granulomas have been noted in infants with immunodeficiency syndromes [24,25].

Therapeutic use

The BCG vaccine is used as immunotherapy in the management of superficial and in situ transitional cell carcinoma of the bladder. It is usually instilled into the bladder on a monthly basis. Primary infection of the glans penis by M. bovis BCG has been described after intravesical BCG treatment (Figure 27.5) [26]. Distant cutaneous granulomas have been described after BCG immunotherapy for melanoma [27].

Tuberculosis and anti-TNF-α treatment (see Chapter 35)

As TNF-α has an integral part in the pathway leading to granuloma formation and maintenance, blockade of this factor would logically lead to an increased risk of mycobacterial infections [1]. Reactivation of tuberculosis should be considered a risk with all anti-TNF agents, although most reports are related to infliximab [2,3]. Recent findings have shown that the physiological TNF-mediated signalling is somehow impaired by TNF antagonists, leading to the exacerbation of chronic infection associated with aberrant granuloma formation and maintenance. Although both receptor and antibody agents appear to pose an equally high risk in causing the development of new tuberculosis infections, monoclonal anti-TNF-α antibody seems more likely to reactivate latent tuberculosis infection [4].

Miliary tuberculosis has been reported [5,6] and reactivation has occurred during antibiotic prophylaxis [7]. Non-tuberculous

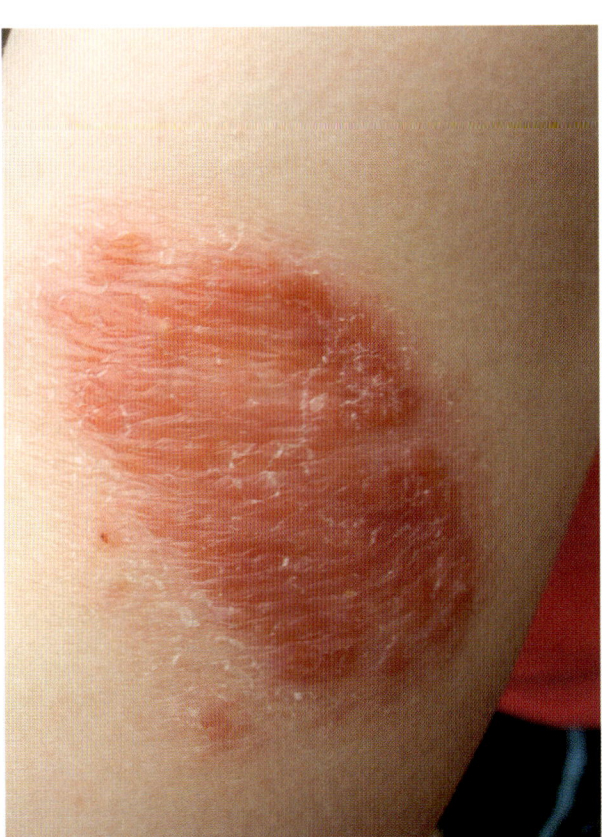

Figure 27.3 Plaque of lupus vulgaris measuring 50 × 30 mm at the site of a previous BCG vaccination. Courtesy of Dr Stephen L. Walker.

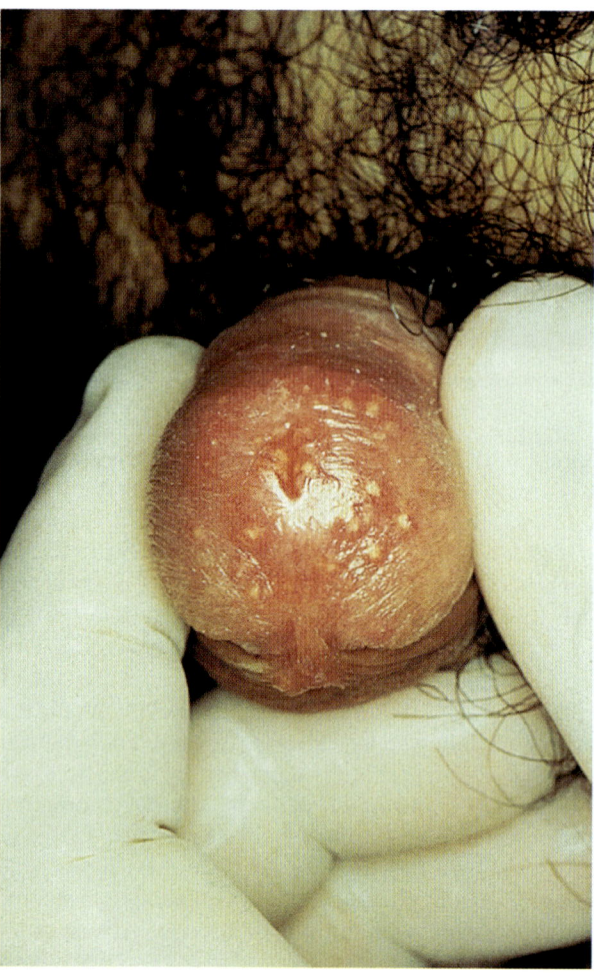

Figure 27.5 *Mycobacterium bovis* BCG infection of the glans penis, showing an infiltrated red plaque containing small, deep-seated, yellow papules. Courtesy of Dr M. Ribera.

mycobacterial disease has also been associated with anti-TNF-α treatment [8,9]. The increase in active tuberculosis in association with anti-TNF-α treatment has led to a requirement for patient screening for active and latent tuberculosis before anti-TNF treatment is given [10,11]. Guidelines for assessing risk and for managing *M. tuberculosis* infection and disease in patients due to start anti-TNF-α treatment have recently been updated by NICE [12]. Higher numbers of patients are at risk of developing tuberculosis with anti-TNF-α therapy in Asia compared with western Europe and North America. The relatively lower risk of tuberculosis with etanercept may be particularly relevant in regions with a high incidence of tuberculosis [13].

Primary inoculation tuberculosis

Definition and nomenclature
A tuberculous chancre is the result of the inoculation of *M. tuberculosis* into the skin of an individual without natural or artificially acquired immunity to this organism. The initial lesion contains many organisms (multibacillary).

Synonyms and inclusions
- Tuberculous chancre
- Tuberculosis primary complex

Introduction and general description
Primary inoculation tuberculosis develops as a result of inoculation of mycobacteria into the skin or mucosa of an individual not previously infected or having no natural or artificially acquired immunity to tuberculosis. Some form of injury is mandatory for the initiation of the infection, as the tubercle bacillus cannot penetrate the normal intact skin or mucosal barrier. The bacillus enters the skin through abrasions and minor injuries, usually on the face or limbs and commonly in children. The disease also occurs in at-risk occupations such as health care workers, particularly in areas of high prevalence for tuberculosis [1,2].

Tuberculous chancres have followed ritual circumcision [3], infections with inadequately sterilised syringes and needlestick injuries [4–6], wounds [7], operations (e.g after blepharoplasty and also following scalpel injury to a surgeon) [8–10], ear piercing, mouth to mouth artificial respiration [11] and tattooing [12]. More recently cases have occurred after acupuncture [13]. In regions where tuberculosis is prevalent in the community, lesions may occur anywhere on the body from contact with sputum or following insect bites [14] or pyococcal infections of the skin. Sexual transmission has been reported [15,16] and following a vehicular accident [17]. *M. bovis* has been reported as the causative organism of a tuberculous chancre in a patient with HIV infection [18].

Epidemiology
Incidence and prevalence
This is believed to be an uncommon form of skin tuberculosis [19], but the incidence may be underestimated, particularly in areas with a high prevalence of tuberculosis. There are approximately 35 cases reported in the English literature.

Age
It commonly affects children.

Associated diseases
Lupus vulgaris may develop at the site of inoculation. Warty tuberculosis and scrofuloderma have also been described and occasionally systemic tuberculosis can develop.

Pathophysiology
Predisposing factors
Children are most at risk, particularly those who have not received BCG vaccination, and who are exposed to pulmonary tuberculosis from another household member or caregiver. Laboratory and health care workers may also be at risk [2].

Pathology
The early changes are those of acute neutrophilic inflammation with necrosis occurring in both the skin and affected lymph nodes. Numerous bacilli are present. After 3–6 weeks, the infiltrate becomes more granulomatous and caseation appears, coinciding with the disappearance of the bacilli.

Causative organisms
- *Mycobacterium tuberculosis*.
- *Mycobacterium bovis*.
- Bacille Calmette–Guérin.

Environmental factors
Overcrowding, low socioeconomic status and poor living conditions are all predisposing factors.

Clinical features
History
Any painless, non-healing ulcer or lesion with localised lymphadenopathy, especially in a child, should arouse suspicion.

Presentation
The earliest lesions occur 2–4 weeks after inoculation and may appear as a brownish papule, nodule or ulcer with an undermined edge and a granular haemorrhagic base. In time, the edge becomes firmer and an adherent crust develops. When obvious trauma is absent, the initial lesion is often small with a central silvery scale, and may show 'apple jelly' nodules on diascopy. The lesions are commonest on the face, hands and lower extremities [20]. Apparent healing may conceal active infection below the surface and the development of a cold abscess. Regional lymphadenopathy often develops after 4–8 weeks. The complex of the tuberculous chancre and regional lymphadenopathy is the cutaneous equivalent of the Ghon focus in the lung. Occasionally, lupoid nodules occur around the healed ulcer or deeper infection simulates scrofuloderma. Lesions closely simulating paronychia have been described on the fingers [21].

Clinical variants
Several forms of mucosal lesions have been described. Conjunctival lesions may cause oedema and irritation [22]. Ulceration and oedema of the lids, with preauricular lymphadenitis, has been described [23]. Oral lesions are uncommon [11], but painless lesions, often misdiagnosed, may form in a tooth socket or on the gums simulating gingivitis. Oral lesions may be an expression of oral primary tuberculosis [2].

Differential diagnosis
The differential diagnosis includes other causes of ulceration, other mycobacteria (e.g. *M. marinum*), *M. ulcerans* disease, actinomycosis, cutaneous leishmaniasis and malignancies [24]. It also includes other disease with sporotrichoid patterns such as sporotrichosis, cat scratch disease and tularaemia.

Classification of severity
Severity is variable.

Complications and co-morbidities
In rare instances, it may lead to disseminated tuberculous disease.

Disease course and prognosis
If untreated the chancre will heal slowly over many months. Lupus vulgaris or tuberculosis verrucosa cutis may develop at the site of the original lesion. Occasionally, haematogenous spread of the organism can occur with development of tuberculosis elsewhere, including miliary tuberculosis [18]. Erythema nodosum (Chapter 97) developed in four out of 40 patients in one series [22]. The enlarged draining lymph nodes usually subside slowly, often calcifying; less often, cold abscesses and sinuses develop producing scrofuloderma.

Investigations
The diagnosis is usually established on the history, clinical picture, histology and microbiological findings. Acid-fast bacilli are seen in the primary skin lesion and in draining nodes in the early stages of the disease. The tuberculin test is usually negative at the beginning of the course but may become positive later.

Management
First line
Antituberculous therapy should be commenced promptly (see 'Current treatment regimens' earlier in this chapter). Treatment should follow the appropriate current guidelines for treatment of tuberculosis of other organs, taking into account the degree of systemic involvement, the immune status of the patient and the existence of MDR forms of tuberculosis.

Scrofuloderma

Definition and nomenclature
Scrofuloderma results from the direct invasion of the tubercle bacillus into the skin from an underlying contiguous tuberculous focus.

Synonyms and inclusions
- Tuberculosis colliquativa cutis

Introduction and pathogenesis
Scrofuloderma results from the involvement and breakdown of the skin overlying a contiguous tuberculosis focus. This is usually a lymph gland, infected bone or joint, lacrimal gland or duct, breast or testes (Figure 27.6) [1–5]. In one report, which included details of 23 patients with scrofuloderma [2], the condition occurred most commonly with cervical, epitrochlear and retroauricular gland infection. The face and neck were again the most frequently affected sites for lesions in another series of 27 patients [6]. It was consistently the commonest form of cutaneous tuberculosis in childhood and adolescents in three large series from India [3,4,7] and in another series of adults from the UK [8] and in a recent study from northern Ethiopia (71% of 202 cases) [9].

In the Ethiopian study, the lesions most frequently involved the cervical and axillary lymph nodes but also nodes in the groins and chest. Lesions were also associated with osteomyelitis of the scalp, ribs or limbs; sometimes giving rise to areas of extensive ulceration (Figure 27.7). Four patients had breast involvement and two had testicular disease. Coexisting HIV infection was present in 22% of the patients [9].

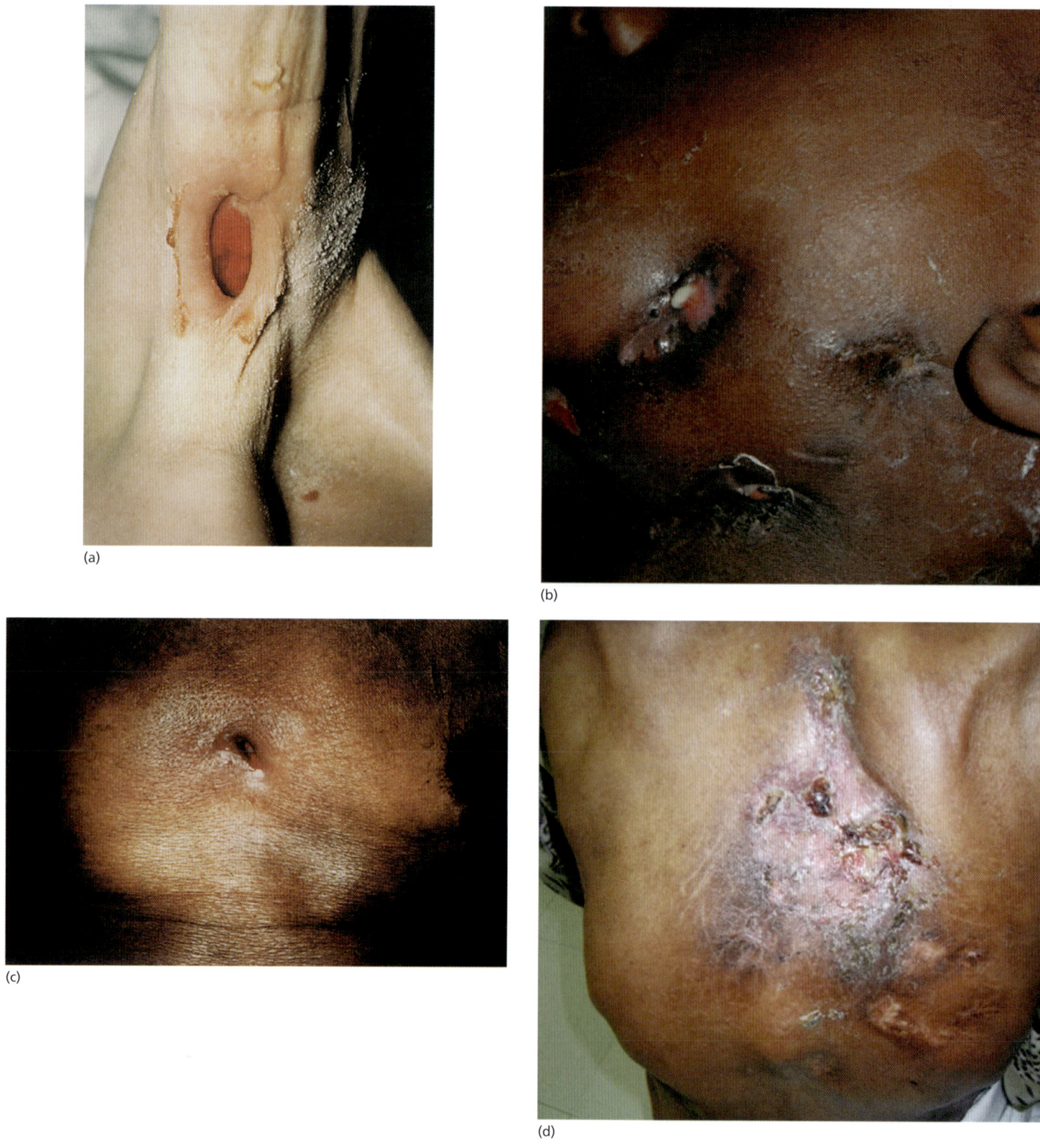

Figure 27.6 Scrofuloderma. (a) Associated with tuberculosis of the axillary glands occurring in a 74-year-old man prior to antituberculous therapy. (b) Associated with sternal tuberculosis occurring in a 62-year-old man. (c) Involving the cervical glands. (d) Associated with tuberculosis of the spine. (a, b) Courtesy of British Journal of Dermatology.

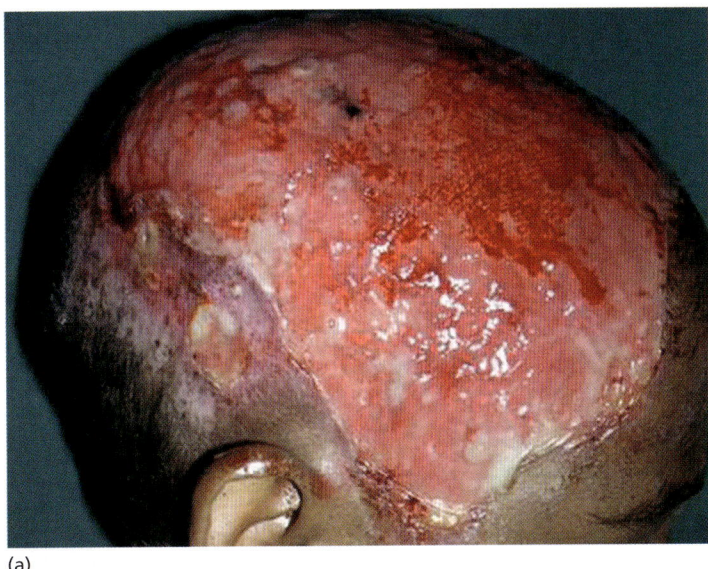
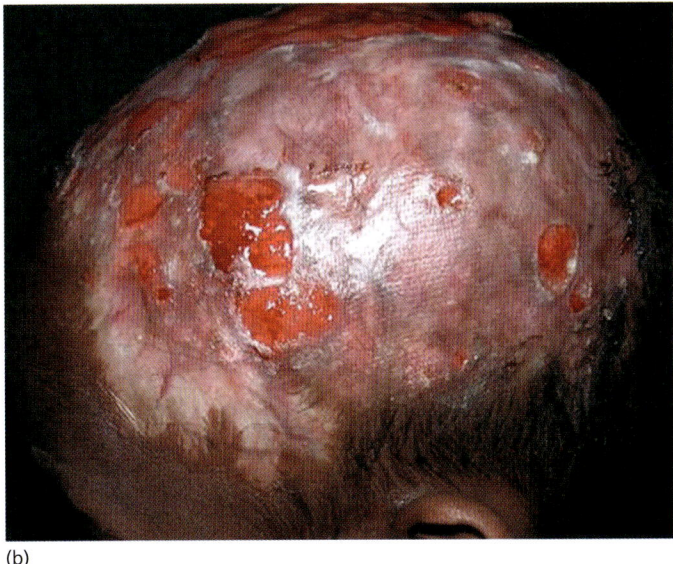

Figure 27.7 (a) Ulcerative form of scrofuloderma in an Ethiopian child secondary to tuberculous osteomyelitis of the skull. (b) The same child after several months of antituberculous treatment showing healing of the lesion. Courtesy of Dr Valeska Padovese.

Epidemiology
Incidence and prevalence
Worldwide, it is the commonest form of cutaneous tuberculosis.

Age
It is most common in children and within the first three decades of life.

Sex
Males were affected 1.5 times more than females in a recent series from India [10].

Associated diseases
Systemic tuberculosis and Sweet disease can coexist [11].

Pathophysiology
Predisposing factors
These include poor life conditions and coexisting HIV infection [9].

Pathology
There is usually an ulcerated dermal abscess with an ill-defined histiocytic component. Marked caseation necrosis, in which there are usually numerous bacteria, is seen in the deeper structures [2].

Causative organisms
- *Mycobacterium tuberculosis*.

Clinical features
History
There is usually asymptomatic swelling or ulcer or discharging sinus. The history may be protracted.

Presentation
Typically, scrofuloderma begins as asymptomatic, bluish red, subcutaneous swellings that persist for several months and overlie an infected gland or joint. They break down to form undermined ulceration with granulating tissue at the base. Numerous fistulae may intercommunicate beneath ridges of bluish skin. Progression and scarring produce irregular adherent masses, densely fibrous in places and fluctuant or discharging in others. Excessive granulation tissue may give rise to fungating tumours. Sporotrichoid spread has been reported [12]. After healing, characteristic puckered scarring marks the site of the infection.

Clinical variants
Extensive ulcerative lesions, particularly on the scalp, may give rise to diagnostic difficulties.

Differential diagnosis
Non-tuberculous mycobacterial infection especially *M. avium* complex lymphadenitis, and the more benign *M. scrofulaceum*, need to be excluded by culture [13]. Other differential diagnoses include sporotrichosis, actinomycosis, syphilitic gummata, hidradenitis suppurativa, melioidosis and bacterial abscess [14].

Disease course and prognosis
Spontaneous healing can occur, but the course is very protracted and leaves typical, cord-like scars.

Investigations
A skin biopsy should be taken from the edge of the sinus or ulcer. Tubercle bacilli can usually be easily identified on biopsy specimens or cytology smears from fine-needle aspirations, the latter being very useful in a low resource setting and can be used as a first line investigation [9]. Mycobacterial culture should be performed if available.

The Mantoux test is normally positive. HIV infection and other causes of immunosuppression need to be excluded.

Management
First line
Antituberculous therapy should be commenced promptly (see 'Current treatment regimens' earlier in this chapter). Treatment should follow the appropriate current guidelines for the treatment of tuberculosis of other organs, taking into account the degree of systemic involvement, the immune status of the patient and the existence of MDR forms of tuberculosis.

Orificial tuberculosis

Definition and nomenclature
Orificial tuberculosis is characterised by painful ulcerated lesions due to tuberculous infection of the mucosa or the skin adjoining orifices. The patient will usually have advanced internal tuberculosis. The most commonly affected area is the oral mucosa, especially the tongue.

Synonyms and inclusions
- Tuberculosis cutis orificialis

Introduction and general description
Orificial tuberculosis is a rare multibacillary form of cutaneous tuberculosis. The lesions occur where there is advanced pulmonary, intestinal or genito-urinary disease from which large numbers of mycobacteria are shed. Lesions can occur anywhere on the buccal mucosa and around the anus, vulva or penis [1,2]. Oral lesions are usually secondary to tuberculosis affecting the upper airway or lungs, whereas perineal lesions are normally secondary to intestinal or genito-urinary disease [3]. Most lesions are produced by autoinoculation of organisms into a break in the mucosal surface. In oral lesions they will commonly follow ingestion of bacilli in sputum. However, some lesions may be caused by haematogenous spread or direct spread from adjacent organs [4]. Perianal lesions have been reported without pulmonary or gastrointestinal involvement [5].

Epidemiology
Incidence and prevalence
This is rare form of cutaneous tuberculosis.

Age
It is rare in children and usually affects middle-aged and elderly males [2].

Sex
Most of those affected are males.

Associated diseases
Systemic tuberculosis can coexist.

Pathophysiology
Predisposing factors
Advanced systemic tuberculous disease, immunosuppression and malnutrition are all predisposing factors.

Pathology
The histopathological changes are variable and are often of a non-specific inflammatory type. In most cases a tuberculoid infiltrate with pronounced necrosis is found in the deep dermis. Tubercle bacilli are usually easy to demonstrate.

Causative organisms
- *Mycobacterium tuberculosis*.

Clinical features
History
Patients give a history of painful ulceration around orifices and may have constitutional symptoms such as fever, malaise, weight loss and night sweats.

Presentation
The affected individual is usually a severely ill adult with advanced visceral tuberculosis who may have impaired cell-mediated immunity. Lesions occur most commonly in the mouth (Figure 27.8a). Small, red, oedematous nodules rapidly break down to form painful, shallow ulcers with undermined bluish edges. The ulcers seldom exceed 2 cm in diameter and show no tendency to heal spontaneously; they may involve the tongue, particularly the tip and lateral margins [2] and may be associated with granulomatous swelling of the lips (Figure 27.8b). Gingival involvement has also been reported [6], as has the occurrence in a tooth socket after extraction [2]. In the perianal area, ulcers may be sharply demarcated with red borders and a purulent base [7,8]. Vulval lesions have a similar appearance and are often very painful [9].

Clinical variants
Plaques similar to lupus vulgaris or a hypertrophic lesion similar to tuberculosis verrucosa cutis can occur [3].

Differential diagnosis
Oral lesions need to be differentiated from Crohn disease, mucocutaneous leishmaniasis, oral paracoccidioidomycosis and rhinoscleroma. Ano-genital lesions must be differentiated from malignancy, nicorandil-induced ulceration, Crohn disease, cutaneous amoebiasis, anal paracoccidioidomycosis, chronic herpes simplex infection and syphilis.

Disease course and prognosis
The lesions themselves will not heal spontaneously and can be slow to respond to antituberculous treatment.

Investigations
Histology from a skin biopsy sample, and occasionally smear cytology from the base of a purulent ulcer, will usually show multiple acid-fast bacilli. Cultures of tissue are normally positive within 6 days. If available, PCR may give a result within 24 h. As patients often have severely impaired cell-mediated immunity, the tuberculin test is often negative. Patients should be screened to exclude associated systemic tuberculosis particularly of the lungs, intestinal tract and genito-urinary system; 79% of one series had associated pulmonary disease [1]. Causes of immunosuppression such as HIV infection should be excluded.

Tuberculosis of the skin

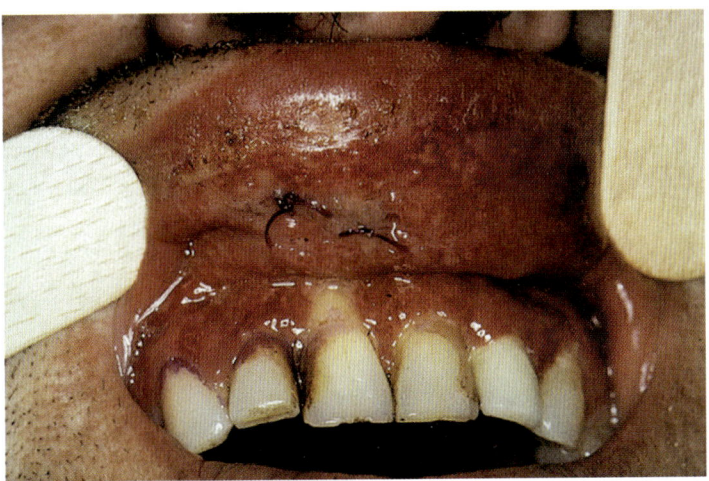

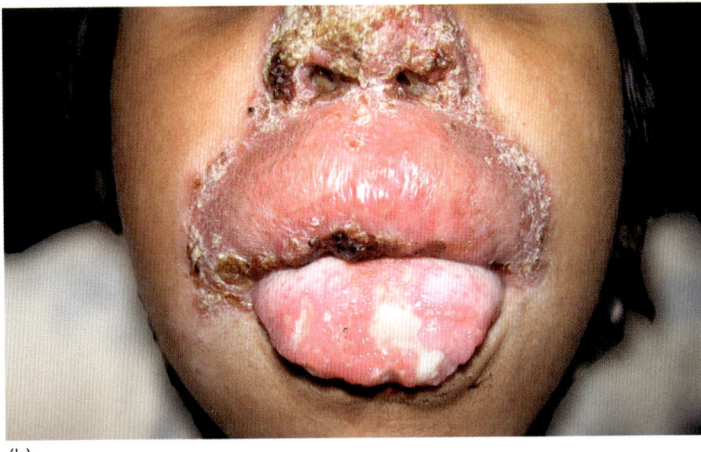

Figure 27.8 Periorificial tuberculosis. (a) Crusty erosions are evident on the gingival surface and mucosal surface of the lip. (b) Granulomatous enlargement of the upper lip and lesions extending to the nose. The tongue shows red erosions and ulceration. (a) Courtesy of Dr F. Nachbar. (b) Courtesy of Dr V. Ramesh.

Management
First line
Antituberculous therapy should be commenced promptly (see 'Current treatment regimens' earlier in this chapter). Treatment should follow the appropriate current guidelines for the treatment of tuberculosis of other organs, taking into account the degree of systemic involvement, the immune status of the patient and the existence of MDR forms of tuberculosis.

Acute cutaneous miliary tuberculosis

Definition and nomenclature
Acute miliary tuberculosis is due to the haematogenous spread of tubercle bacilli into the skin.

Synonyms and inclusions
- Tuberculosis cutis miliaris disseminata
- Tuberculosis cutis miliaris acuta generalisata

Introduction and general description
Acute miliary tuberculosis of the skin is rare and is usually seen in advanced pulmonary or meningeal and disseminated tuberculosis. It affects infants and young children or immunosuppressed patients such as those with concurrent HIV infection [1,2] or following viral infections such as measles [3] or malnutrition.

Epidemiology
Incidence and prevalence
Acute miliary tuberculosis of the skin is rare.

Age
It is usually found in infants and children.

Pathophysiology
Pathology
Histology shows necrotising tuberculous granulomas with multiple acid-fast bacilli.

Causative organisms
- *Mycobacterium tuberculosis*.

Clinical features
Presentation
The cutaneous lesions consist of crops of minute bluish papules, vesicles, pustules or haemorrhagic lesions in a patient who is obviously ill. The lesions can occur all over the body but are most frequently found on the trunk, thighs, buttocks and genitalia [4]. The vesicles may become necrotic to form small ulcers [5]. Red nodules have been described [6]. Neonates born to tuberculous mothers may develop a milder form of the disease with limited visceral involvement and a few scattered papules [7].

Disease course and prognosis
The prognosis is poor, but response to treatment is possible.

Investigations
The development of an unusual exanthematic rash in an ill person with known tuberculosis or tuberculous contacts suggests the diagnosis, which should be confirmed by skin biopsy. The tuberculin test is negative. Appropriate investigations should be made to determine the extent of internal tuberculous infection [8].

Management
First line
Antituberculosis therapy should be started immediately if there is a strong suspicion (see 'Current treatment regimens' earlier in this chapter). This type of tuberculosis may be complicated by MDR tuberculosis [9].

Metastatic tuberculous abscess

Definition and nomenclature
Metastatic tuberculous abscesses or tuberculous gummata result from the disseminated haematogenous spread of mycobacteria

and present as single or multiple dermal subcutaneous nodules which may become fluctuant or break down to form ulcers. Unlike scrofuloderma, there is no involvement of underlying tissue.

> **Synonyms and inclusions**
> - Tuberculous gumma

Introduction and general description
This form of tuberculosis is the result of haematogenous dissemination from a primary focus during periods of lowered resistance, resulting in single or multiple lesions. It is seen particularly in malnourished children [1] or in immunodeficient adults [2], and has been noted after venepuncture [3] and in association with underlying lymphoma [4] and systemic immunosuppressant treatment such as corticosteroids [2].

Epidemiology
Incidence and prevalence
It occurred in 9% of 202 patients in a study from northern Ethiopia [5], but generally the incidence is lower.

Age
This form of tuberculosis usually occurs in children but there is a wider age range in the immunocompromised.

Pathophysiology
Predisposing factors
Malnutrition and immunosuppression are predisposing factors.

Pathology
Histology shows massive necrosis with copious amounts of bacteria.

Causative organisms
- *Mycobacterium tuberculosis*.

Environmental factors
Poor living conditions are associated with its occurrence.

Clinical features
Presentation
A tuberculous gumma presents either as a firm, subcutaneous nodule or as a non-tender, fluctuant abscess (Figure 27.9). The extremities are more often affected than the trunk. The overlying skin may break down to form an undermined ulcer, often with sinuses or fistulous tracts (Figure 27.10) [4,6]. Lesions may be multiple. Unusual and transitional forms may occur [7]. Rarely, multiple abscesses have been noted during the treatment of miliary tuberculosis [8]. Lesions causing carpal tunnel syndrome have been well documented [9].

Differential diagnosis
These abscesses can be difficult to differentiate from pyogenic bacterial infections, syphilis, non-tuberculous mycobacterial infections, pyoderma gangrenosum and some fungal infections [10].

Complications and co-morbidities
Carpal tunnel syndrome may coexist.

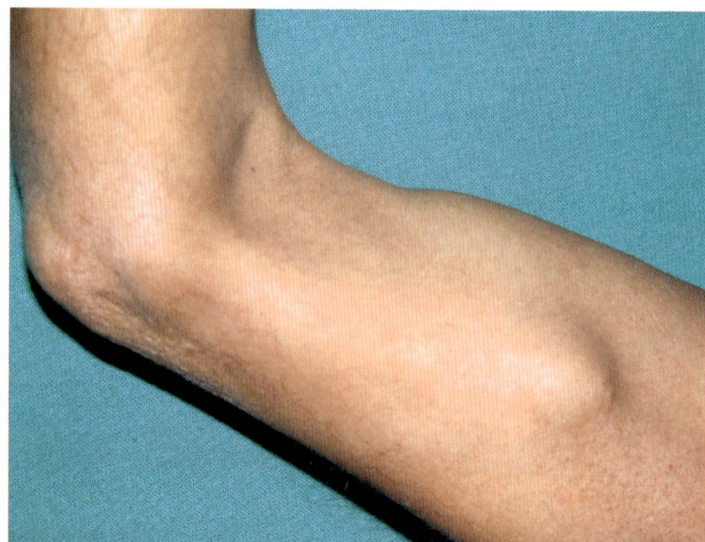

Figure 27.9 Tuberculous gumma (metastatic cold abscess) in a patient with a pleural effusion. Courtesy of Dr V. Ramesh.

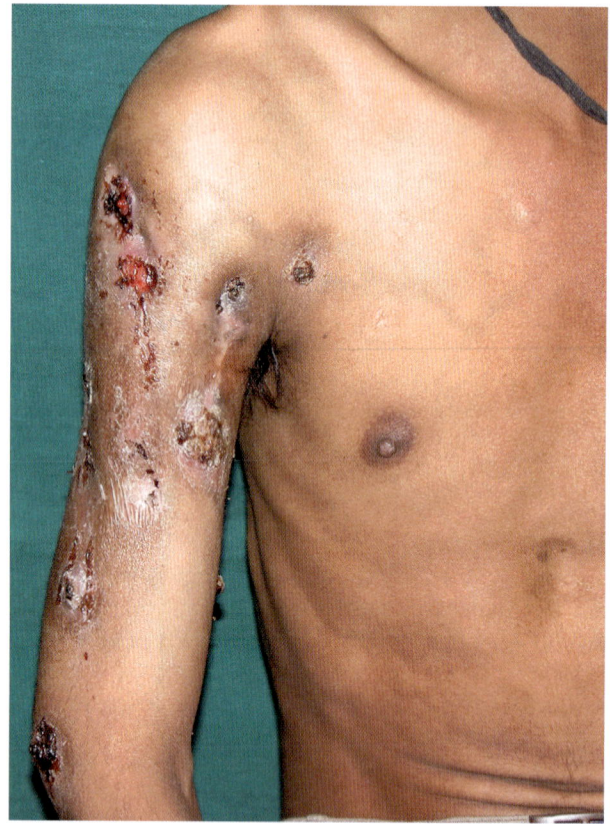

Figure 27.10 Multiple metastatic abscesses (gummas) on the right arm. Courtesy of Dr V. Ramesh.

Disease course and prognosis
Cutaneous lesions gradually improve on treatment.

Investigations
The diagnosis is confirmed by culture. The patient should be screened for an underlying focus of tuberculosis and causes of immunosuppression. The tuberculin test is usually positive but

can be negative if associated with a poor general condition of the patient.

Management
First line
Full antituberculous treatment should be given, which should be guided by culture (see 'Current treatment regimens' earlier in this chapter).

Warty tuberculosis

Definition and nomenclature
This is an indolent, warty, plaque-like form of tuberculosis caused by exogenous inoculation of *M. tuberculosis* into the skin through open wounds or abrasions in previously infected or sensitised individuals who will have a moderate or high degree of immunity [1]. There are usually few organisms in the lesion (paucibacillary).

Synonyms and inclusions
- Tuberculosis verrucosa cutis

Introduction and general description
Warty tuberculosis occurs by exogenous inoculation of bacteria in previously sensitised individuals. This commonly occurs by accidental inoculation from extraneous sources particularly in health care workers; it also known as 'anatomist's warts', 'prosector's warts' and 'verruca necrogenica' [2]. It can also occur by autoinoculation with sputum in a patient with active tuberculosis. It was the predominant form of tuberculosis in Hong Kong in the 1960s when children were nursed with open nappies and became infected from sputum from sitting on the ground [3]. Persons walking barefoot where the organism is present may similarly become infected [4,5].

Epidemiology
Worldwide the incidence of tuberculosis verrucosa cutis is extremely variable but appears to be commonest in Asia. It was the commonest form of tuberculosis in a 2010 study from Nepal, at 48% [6], and 18% in studies from Pakistan [7] and Bangladesh [8]. In most other studies it has accounted for between 3% and 7% of patients with cutaneous tuberculosis [9–12].

Pathophysiology
Pathology
There is a striking pseudoepitheliomatous hyperplasia with superficial abscess formation, and an intense, mixed infiltrate with granulomas in the deeper dermis and occasional necrosis. Bacilli are seen only occasionally.

Causative organisms
- *Mycobacterium tuberculosis*.

Clinical features
History
The history is usually that of a slowly enlarging lesion, which in some cases can remain undiagnosed for many years [13,14].

Presentation
Lesions occur on those areas exposed to trauma and to infected sputum or other tuberculous material. In Europe, the lesions are most likely to occur on the hands, but in Asia, the knees, ankles and buttocks are mainly involved [5,15].

The lesions are typically asymptomatic and start as a small, indurated, warty papule with a slight inflammatory areola. By gradual extension, a verrucose plaque is formed. Irregular extension at the edges leads to a serpiginous outline with finger-like projections. The centre may involute, leaving a white atrophic scar, or the whole lesion may form a massive, infiltrated, papillomatous excrescence (Figure 27.11). The colour is purplish, red or brown. The consistency is generally firm, but there may be areas of relative softening. Pus may sometimes be expressed from these soft areas or from fissures. The lesions may resemble lupus vulgaris [16], but the sites are different. The appearance may be psoriasiform

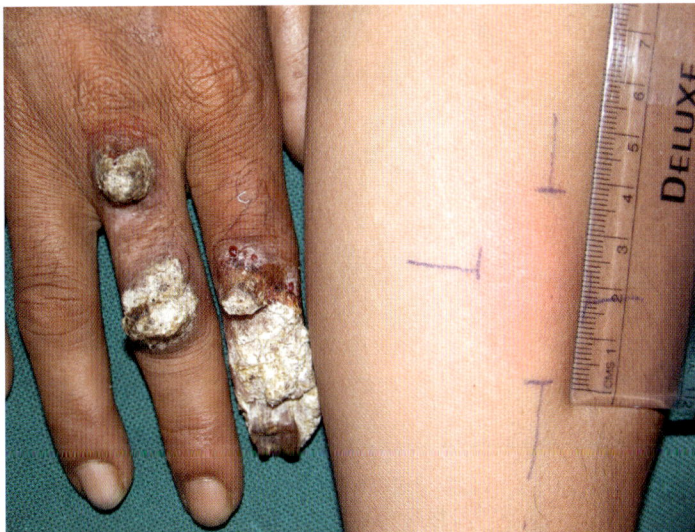

(a)

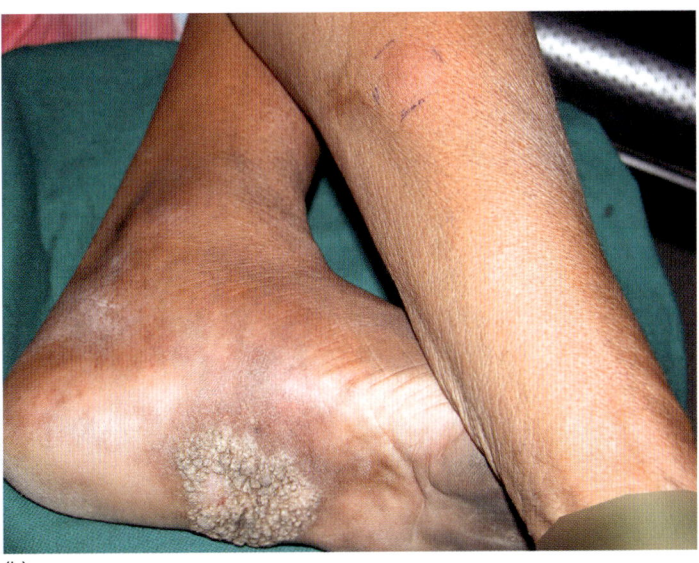

(b)

Figure 27.11 Warty tuberculosis with strong tuberculin reactions. (a) The right ring and middle fingers. (b) Sole of the left foot. Courtesy of Dr V. Ramesh.

(Figure 27.12) or keloidal. Occasionally, exudate and crusting are predominant. Very rarely, multiple lesions implying multiple inoculations [17], sporotrichoid spread (Figure 27.13) [18] and also tuberculous lymphadenitis can occur [19].

Clinical variants
Deeply destructive papillomatous and sclerotic forms may cause deformity of the limbs [13]. A generalised form, associated with papulonecrotic and lupoid lesions [20], occurs in patients with active disease, but is best regarded as a haematogenous form with a variable tissue response. An exuberant granulomatous form was described in Hong Kong [5] and has also be seen in other reports from Asia [15]. Tumour-like forms can occur [21,22].

Differential diagnosis
Subungual and digital lesions must be distinguished from warts, and those on the hands from keratoses. Blastomycosis, chromoblastomycosis and actinomycosis may simulate exuberant forms, and crusted lesions may resemble leishmaniasis. Tertiary syphilis may be confused when the central scarring is surrounded by a serpiginous edge. Hypertrophic lichen planus and lichenification occasionally cause difficulty, but lesions of these disorders are multiple or itchy. Lupus vulgaris is not usually hyperkeratotic and shows 'apple jelly' nodules on diascopy.

The lesions caused by NTM can usually only be distinguished by microbiological culture. *M. marinum* poses particular difficulties (see '*Mycobacterium marinum* infection' later in this chapter).

Complications and co-morbidities
Active disease of other organs should be sought, as bone tuberculosis, tuberculous lymphadenitis [19] or pulmonary tuberculosis may coexist [5]. Miliary tuberculosis has also been reported [23] as has coexistence with scrofuloderma [24].

Disease course and prognosis
The condition responds to antituberculosis treatment; without it, extension is usually extremely slow and lesions may remain virtually inactive for months or years [13,14,25]. Spontaneous remission may occur and usually results in atrophic scars.

Investigations
Histopathology of the lesion will usually differentiate it from inflammatory lesions but lesions due to NTM are more difficult and ideally require culture of the organism. Commercial IFN-γ assays may help to differentiate lesions due to NTM and *M. bovis* and are also not affected by BCG vaccination [26,27]. PCR may be helpful if positive but is often negative in paucibacillary forms of cutaneous tuberculosis.

Management
First line
Treatment should follow the appropriate current guidelines for the treatment of tuberculosis of other organs, taking into account the degree of systemic involvement, the immune status of the patient and the existence of MDR forms of tuberculosis (see 'Current treatment regimens' earlier in this chapter).

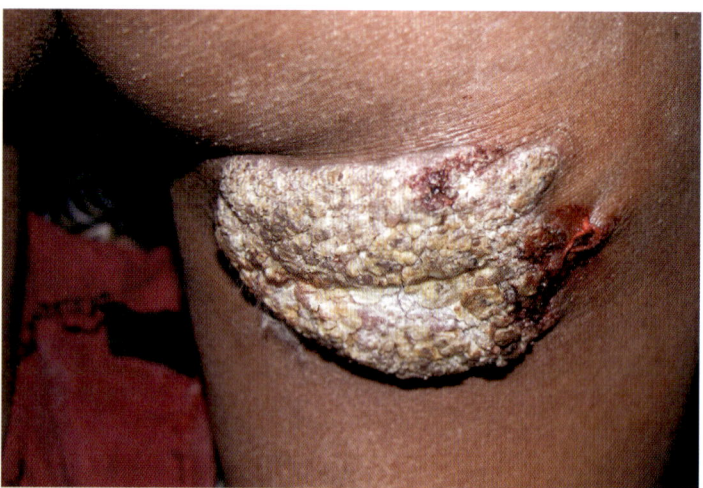

Figure 27.12 Warty tuberculosis of the right thigh. Courtesy of Dr V. Ramesh.

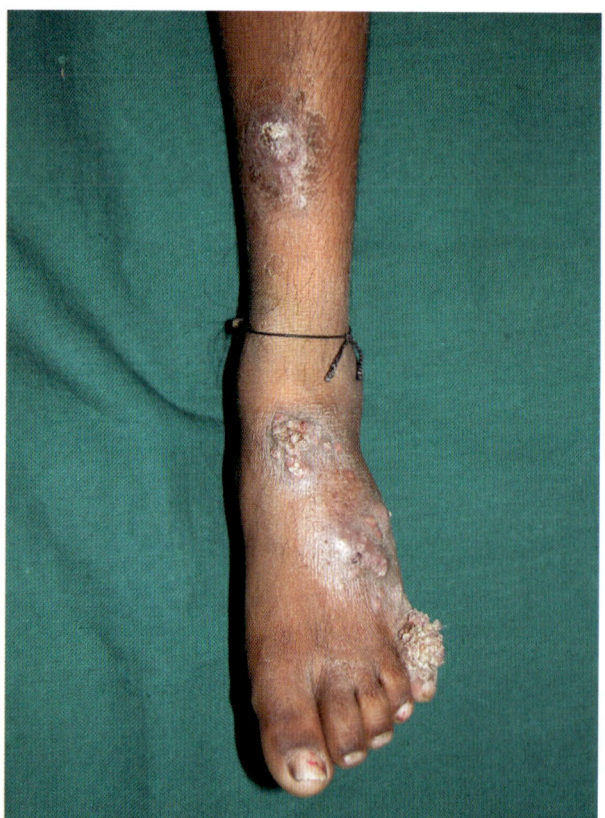

Figure 27.13 Sporotrichoid spread of warty tuberculosis. Courtesy of Dr V. Ramesh.

Lupus vulgaris

Definition
This is a chronic, progressive, paucibacillary form of cutaneous tuberculosis, occurring in a previously sensitised individual with a high degree of immunity to tuberculin. The characteristic lesion is a plaque, composed of soft, reddish brown papules, the appearance on diascopy being said to resemble apple jelly.

Introduction and general description

Lupus vulgaris is one of the most prevalent forms of cutaneous tuberculosis and occurs in previously sensitised individuals. A characteristic lesion is a slowly enlarging plaque with an elevated border and central atrophy. The edges of the lesion gradually extend in some areas and heal with scarring in others, sometimes causing considerable tissue destruction over many years. There are many clinical variants including tumour-like and ulcerated forms, which may pose diagnostic difficulties. The lesions are acquired either by haematogenous spread from an underlying tuberculous focus or by direct inoculation. Those on the face are usually thought to be due to haematogenous spread, while those located on the extremities are more likely to be due to reinoculation [1].

Epidemiology
Incidence and prevalence

Lupus vulgaris was the most common form of cutaneous tuberculosis in adults in published series from India, South Africa and Pakistan [2–4]. In Tunisia there has been an increase in the proportion of cases with lupus vulgaris, presumably reflecting greater immunity to tuberculosis in the community [5,6]. Lupus vulgaris was also the commonest presentation in a recent publication from Spain [7].

Sex
The condition appears to be more common in women than men.

Pathophysiology

Lupus vulgaris originates from an underlying focus of tuberculosis, typically in a bone, joint or lymph node, and arises by either contiguous extension of the disease from underlying affected tissue or haematogenous or lymphatic spread. Sometimes the underlying focus is not clinically apparent, and in such cases reactivation of a latent cutaneous focus secondary to a previous silent bacteraemia is postulated [8]. It can also arise after exogenous inoculation [9] or as a complication of BCG vaccination [10,11,**12**].

Pathology

The histological features are variable. Normally, tubercles with scanty or absent central caseation, surrounded by epithelioid histiocytes and multinucleate giant cells, are present in the superficial dermis. Peripheral lymphocytes are often prominent. Occasionally, tubercle bacilli may be numerous [13]; more often, they are hard to demonstrate or are absent. The epidermis may be ulcerated with an associated mixed inflammatory infiltrate, atrophic or acanthotic. If the acanthosis is severe, giving rise to pseudoepitheliomatous hyperplasia, differentiation from squamous cell carcinoma may be difficult [14].

Causative organisms
- *Mycobacterium tuberculosis*.
- *Mycobacterium bovis* [15].
- Bacille Calmette–Guérin [10,11,**12**].

Clinical features
Presentation

Lupus vulgaris commonly appears in normal skin as a solitary lesion, although it can arise at the site of a primary inoculation such as after a tattoo [9], in the scar of scrofuloderma or at the site of a BCG vaccination [10,11,**12**]. In Europe, over 80% of lesions are on the head and neck, particularly around the nose [16,17]. Next in frequency are the arms and legs, but involvement of the trunk is uncommon. In India, the face is affected less often and the buttocks and trunk more frequently [18]. In children the lesions are often on the lower limbs and buttocks; they usually occur by reinoculation and may relate to playing without clothing or shoes [19].

The initial lesion is a small, reddish brown, flat plaque of soft, almost gelatinous, consistency. On diascopy, the diagnostic 'apple jelly' nodules may be demonstrated. The lesion gradually becomes elevated, infiltrated and brown and grows by slow peripheral extension to become gyrate or discoid in shape with areas of atrophy. There is usually only a single lesion, except in disseminated forms, which usually occur in association with active pulmonary tuberculosis [20]. Sporotrichoid-like spread has also been reported [21].

There is great variability in clinical presentation but the many clinical forms fall into five general patterns, depending on the local tissue response to the infection.

1 *Plaque form* (Figure 27.14). Flat plaques are found with an irregular or serpiginous edge. The surface of the lesion may be smooth or covered with psoriasiform scale. Large plaques may show irregular areas of scarring with islands of active lupus tissue. The edge often becomes thickened and hyperkeratotic.
2 *Ulcerative and mutilating forms* (Figure 27.15). Scarring and ulceration predominate. Crusts form over areas of necrosis. The deep tissues and cartilage are invaded and contractures and deformities occur. In milder forms, keratotic plugs overlying pinpoint ulcers are associated with slow scar formation.
3 *Vegetating form* (Figure 27.16). This is characterised by marked infiltration, ulceration and necrosis with minimal scarring. Mucous membranes are invaded and cartilage is slowly destroyed. When the nasal or auricular cartilage is involved, extensive destruction and disfigurement ensue.
4 *Tumour-like forms* (Figure 27.17). The hypertrophic form presents either as soft tumour-like nodules or as epithelial hyperplasia with the production of hyperkeratotic masses. In the 'myxomatous' form, huge soft tumours occur predominantly on the ear lobes, which become grossly enlarged [22]. Lymphoedema and vascular dilatation are sometimes marked.
5 *Papular and nodular forms*. Multiple lesions occur simultaneously in disseminated lupus-true 'miliary lupus'. This usually occurs after temporary immunosuppression as described in postexanthematous forms, such as after measles [23].

Mucosal involvement. The nasal, buccal or conjunctival mucosa may become involved, either primarily by a papule, nodule or ulcer, or by spread from a contiguous skin lesion. Nasal lesions start as nodules, which bleed easily and then ulcerate, leading sometimes to cartilage destruction. A dry rhinitis may be an early symptom. Granulating, vegetating or ulcerating lesions of the buccal mucosa, palate, gingiva or oro-pharynx may occur by direct extension or by lymphatic spread from nasal lesions. These can produce stenosis of the larynx and scarring deformities of the soft palate.

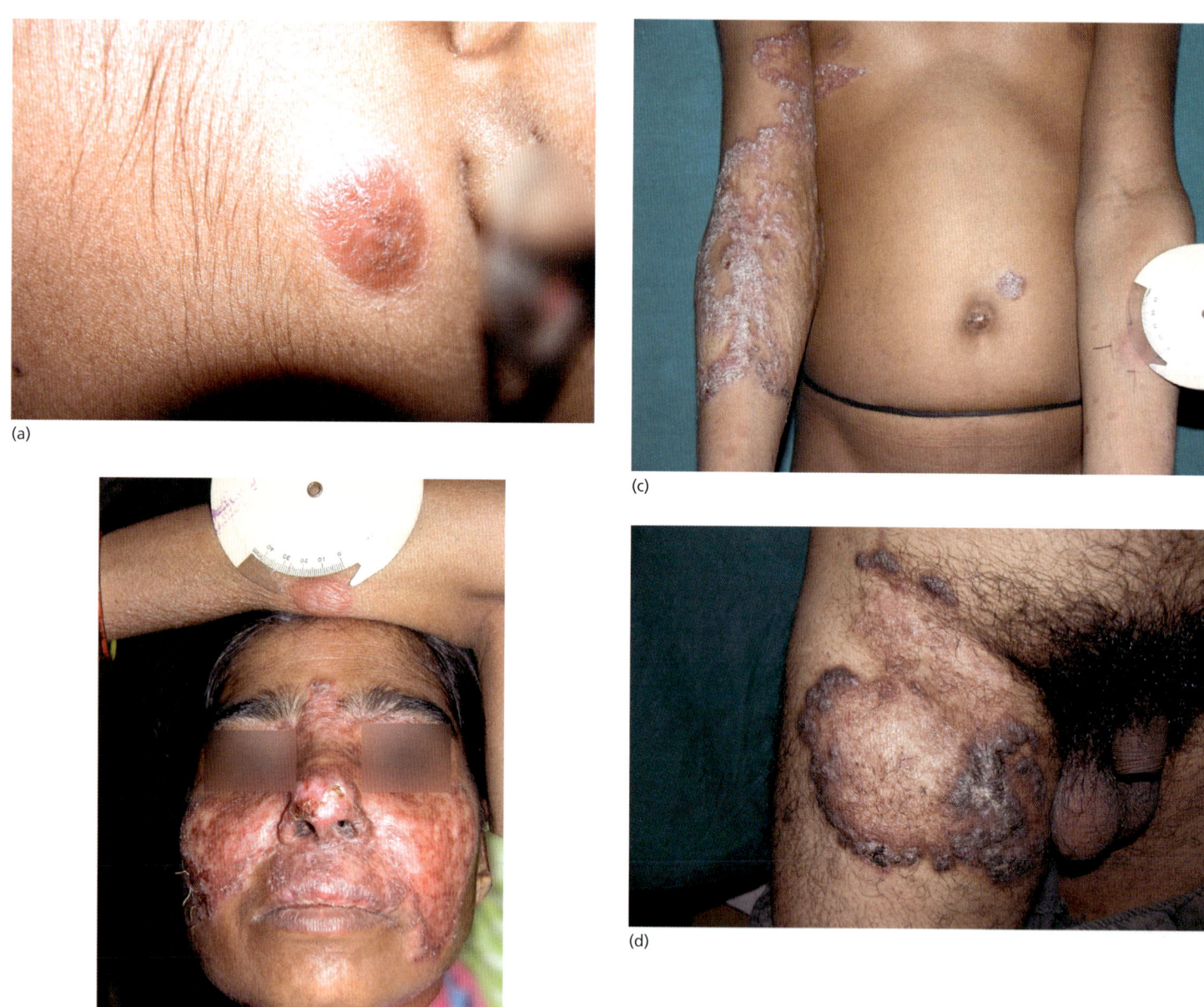

Figure 27.14 Lupus vulgaris. (a) A solitary plaque on the left cheek. (b) Lesions of the face resembling discoid lupus erythematosus. Note the strong tuberculin reaction. (c) Lupus vulgaris showing typical central atrophy and a serpiginous edge. (d) Lupus vulgaris showing a thickened and hypertrophic edge. Courtesy of Dr V. Ramesh.

Clinical variants

There is a great variability in clinical presentation and atypical forms including giant forms are becoming more common [24,25].

Differential diagnosis

Because of its rarity in countries such as the UK, the index of suspicion may be low [26]. The well-established plaque with central scarring presents few difficulties, but in the early stage, lupus vulgaris may easily be confused with lymphocytoma, Spitz naevus or lupus erythematosus. In appropriate patients, syphilis must be excluded. The histological features and culture results will differentiate lupus vulgaris from the deep mycoses, which may closely resemble the vegetating and crusted type. The lupoid form of leishmaniasis may be impossible to distinguish clinically. On the face, it may be mistaken for rosacea [26] or for a port-wine stain [27], and on an extremity for other mycobacterial infections.

Leprosy and sarcoidosis, however, are the chief causes of diagnostic difficulty. The nodules of leprosy are firmer, and other signs are present. The nodules of sarcoidosis resemble grains of sand rather than 'apple jelly'; this applies to the feel on probing rather than to the colour, which is often greyish.

Lupus vulgaris may resemble psoriasis, but is more infiltrated and usually solitary; Bowen disease can resemble both. Lupus vulgaris of the perianal area mistaken for lichen simplex chronicus and Crohn disease has also been reported (Figure 27.18) [28,29]. Warty tuberculosis usually affects the hand and is more scaly and verrucous than lupus and the histological features are different.

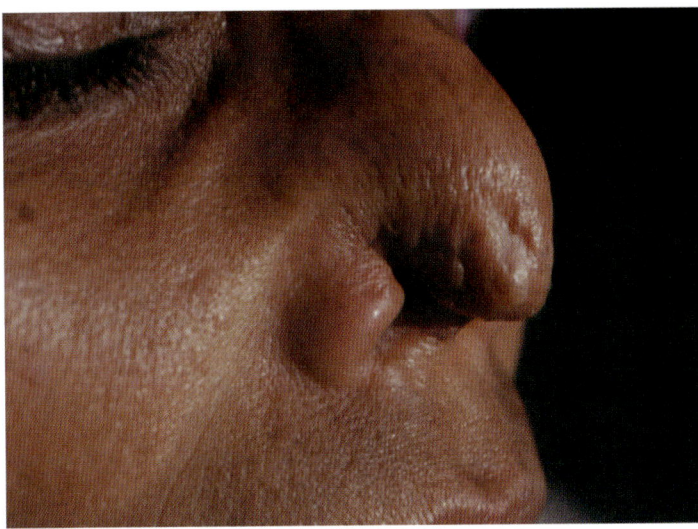

Figure 27.15 Nasal deformity as a late sequela of lupus vulgaris. Courtesy of Dr V. Ramesh.

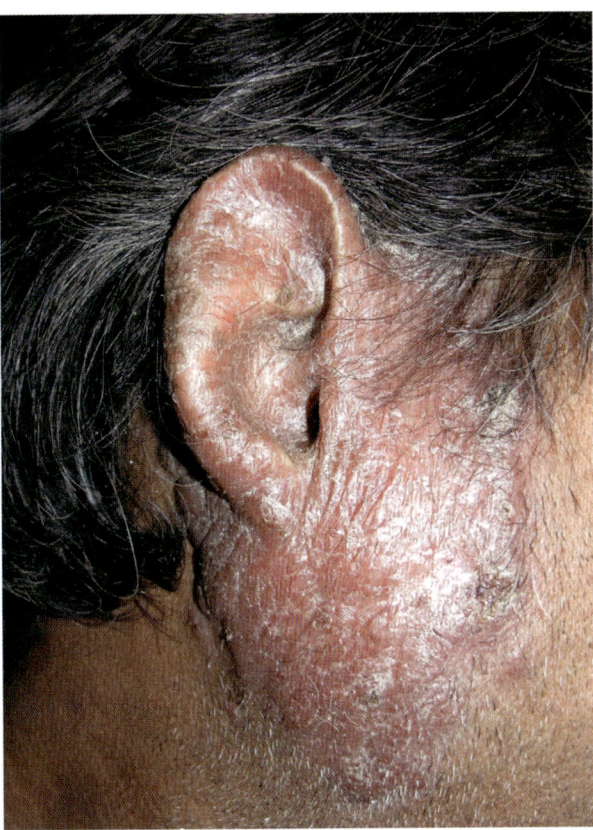

Figure 27.17 Tumour-like form of lupus vulgaris on the ear lobe and face. Courtesy of Dr V. Ramesh.

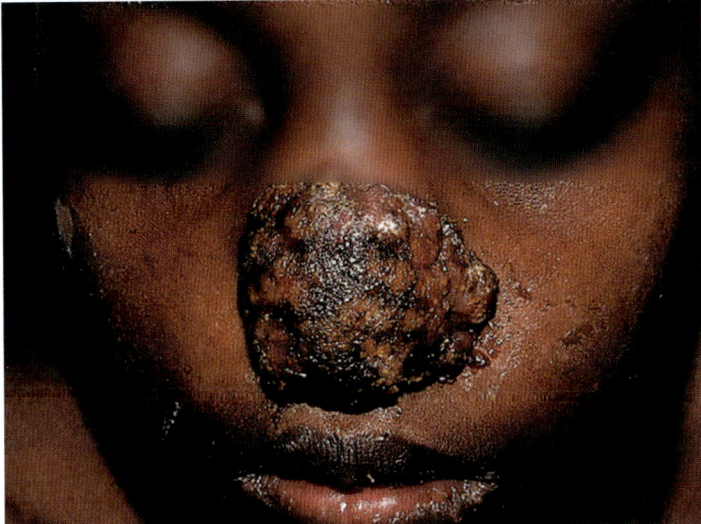

Figure 27.16 Vegetating lupus vulgaris on the nose. Courtesy of Dr J. E. Bothwell.

A therapeutic trial of antituberculous therapy may be considered in cases where the diagnosis is difficult. A clinical response should be expected within 4–6 weeks [30,31].

Complications and co-morbidities

Scarring, contractures and tissue destruction are prominent features. The scars are usually thin, white and smooth, but are unstable and may break down or become keloidal. Contraction may lead to ectropion or microstomia, which may require plastic surgery. Active lupus vulgaris frequently reappears in scar tissue.

Malignant changes are well known to arise in longstanding lupus vulgaris. *In situ* or invasive squamous cell carcinomas are the most common tumours and may occur insidiously in between 0.5% and 10% of patients [32–34] and may be confused with renewed activity of the lupus itself (Figures 27.19 and 27.20). Basal cell and syringoid eccrine carcinomas and also melanomas, lymphomas and sarcomas have been reported [35,36]. Squamous cell carcinoma as a complication of lupus vulgaris usually takes about 25–30 years to develop and normally occurs in patients in their fourth and fifth decades [37]. Some early cases may relate in part to ultraviolet light therapy, which was a treatment modality in use before chemotherapy [33], however a case was reported in a child following BCG-induced lupus vulgaris [38].

Disease course and prognosis

Despite long periods of indolence, the natural course of an untreated lesion is progressive. With appropriate treatment there is often a clinical response as early as 5 weeks into treatment and usually marked improvement by 10 weeks. Failure to respond within 4–6 weeks may suggest an alternative diagnosis [31].

Investigations

The paucibacillary nature of lupus vulgaris, along with its many clinical variants, presents a diagnostic challenge. Skin biopsy is usually helpful but as the quantity of bacilli encountered in cutaneous lesions is small, stains for acid-fast bacilli are usually negative [24,39]. Culture may be more helpful and was positive in 12.5% of samples from a study in India [19], and in 40% of a series from Spain [7]. PCR has been successfully used to confirm the diagnosis of lupus vulgaris [40,41]. The tuberculin test is usually positive and IFN-γ assays may also be helpful.

Management
First line

Standard multidrug antituberculosis therapy should be given (see 'Current treatment regimens' earlier in this chapter). Isoniazid has in the past been used as monotherapy, but this practice is strongly discouraged as up to 26% of patients have clinical evidence of tuberculosis at other sites [2] and if the patient is resistant to the drug, effectively no treatment is being given. A case report of lupus

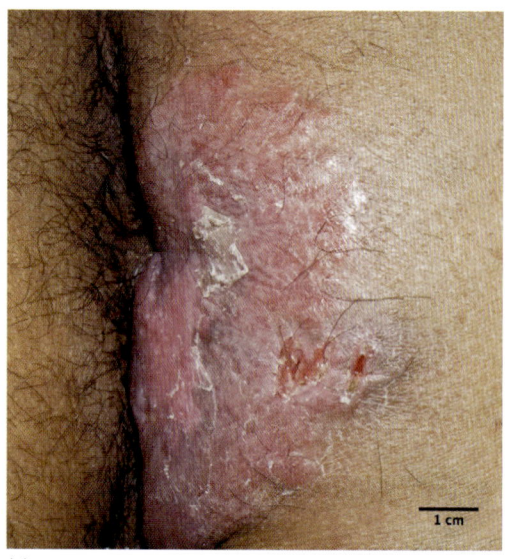
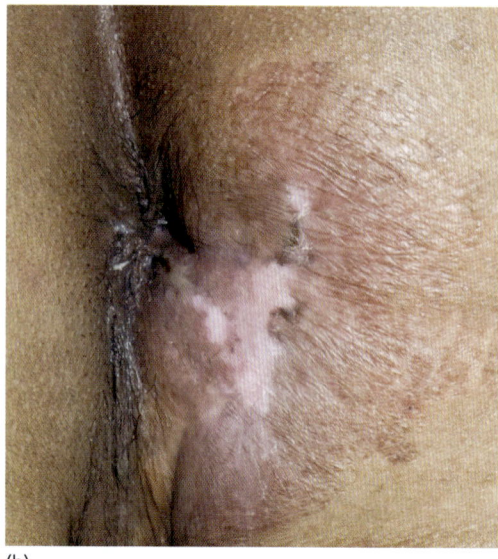

Figure 27.18 Perianal lupus vulgaris (a) before and (b) after treatment. Courtesy of Dr Julia Rhodes.

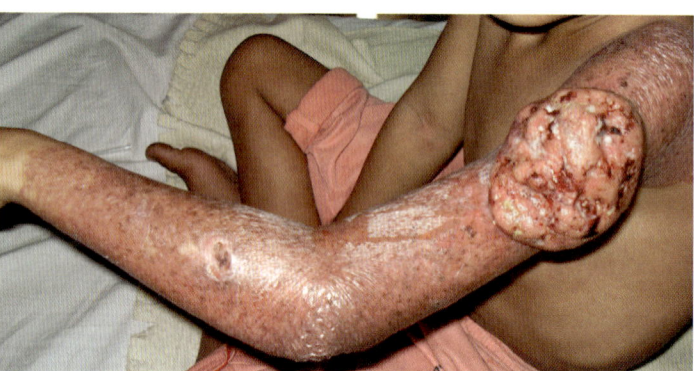

Figure 27.19 Extensive BCG-induced lupus vulgaris in a child complicated by squamous cell carcinoma. Courtesy of Dr Binod Kr Thakur and Dr Shikha Verma.

vulgaris caused by isoniazid-resistant *M. tuberculosis* emphasises this point [42].

TUBERCULIDS

Tuberculids can be considered to be cutaneous hypersensitivity reactions to haematogenous dissemination of *M. tuberculosis* or its antigens from a primary source in an individual with strong antituberculous cell-mediated immunity. The diagnostic criteria include tuberculoid histology on skin biopsy, a strongly positive Mantoux reaction, the absence of *M. tuberculosis* in the smear and negative culture and resolution of the skin lesions with antituberculous therapy.

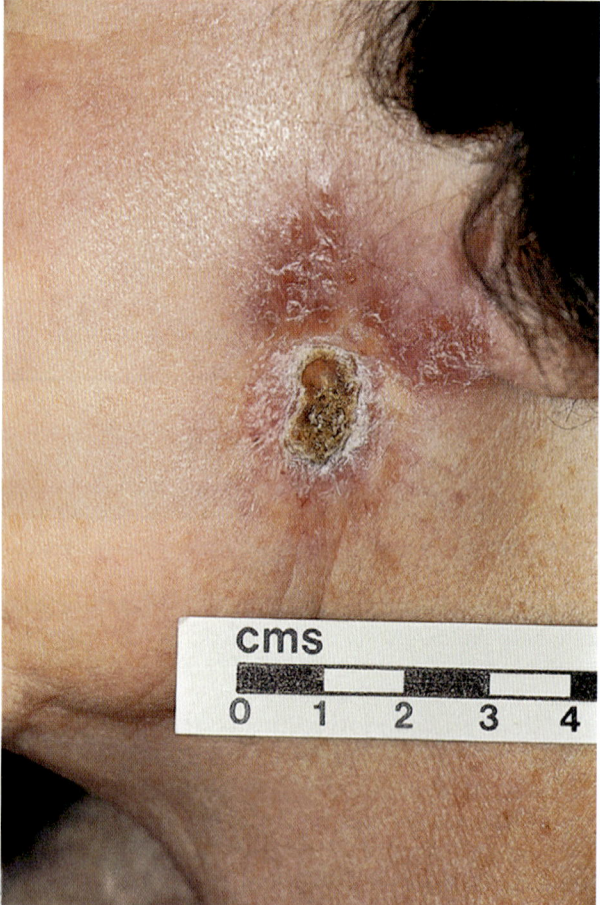

Figure 27.20 A basal cell carcinoma arising in an old area of lupus vulgaris.

Classification

True tuberculids can be grouped as follows:
1 *Micropapular*: lichen scrofulosorum.
2 *Papular*: papulonecrotic tuberculid.
3 *Nodular*: erythema induratum of Bazin or nodular tuberculid.

General description

In 1896, Darier introduced the concept of tuberculids to explain a group of dermatoses with tuberculoid histopathology occurring in individuals with manifest or past tuberculosis, a strongly positive tuberculin test but an absence of bacilli in skin biopsy specimens and negative culture. Included initially were lichen scrofulosorum, papulonecrotic tuberculid, erythema induratum of Bazin, rosaceiform tuberculid and lupus miliaris disseminatus faceii. Later, when effective treatment for tuberculosis became available it was also required that tuberculids should have a good response to antituberculous treatment and rosaceiform tuberculid and lupus miliaris disseminatus faceii were excluded from the group.

Basic biology

Currently, there is still controversy concerning the pathogenesis of the tuberculids and their association with *M. tuberculosis* as supporting evidence is often circumstantial. However, the demonstration of *M. tuberculosis* DNA by PCR in lichen scrofulosorum, papulonecrotic tuberculid and erythema induratum of Bazin would seem to be fairly hard evidence in favour of a definite association [1,2–4]. Evidence is perhaps greatest in papulonecrotic tuberculid as some cases have evolved into lupus vulgaris [5] and for lichen scrofulosorum where around 75% of cases have a proven underlying focus of tuberculosis [6]. Most authors currently feel that erythema induratum of Bazin – a nodular vasculitis – is a multifactorial disorder with many different causes, tuberculosis being one of them [7]. Similarly, erythema nodosum can be considered a facultative tuberculid with tuberculosis being just one of many causes [8].

Fluctuations in the immunological state of the patient may determine the development and features of the eruption. The onset of lichen scrofulosorum has been noted to occur after the initiation of antituberculous treatment and probably represents a shift in the cell-mediated immune status of the patients [9]. Papulonecrotic tuberculid developed in a patient with HIV infection after an increase in the CD4 T-lymphocyte count occurred following the addition of a second antiretroviral drug [10].

In the most recent study from Hong Kong, in which 131 patients with cutaneous tuberculid were identified, erythema induratum was by far the commonest tuberculid identified ($n = 127$, 96%), followed by papulonecrotic tuberculid ($n = 4$, 3%) [11]. In several recent studies from India the incidence of lichen scrofulosorum appears to be increasing and is particularly common in children [12].

Lichen scrofulosorum

Definition and nomenclature
Lichen scrofulosorum is a rare tuberculid first described by Hebra in 1868. It presents as a lichenoid eruption of minute papules occurring predominantly in children and adolescents with active tuberculosis. It is usually associated with a strongly positive tuberculin reaction.

Synonyms and inclusions
- Tuberculosis cutis lichenoides

Introduction and general description
Lichen scrofulosorum classically occurs in children and adolescents with a strong immune sensitivity to *M. tuberculosis* and is thought to result from an immune response to haematological spread from an underlying tuberculous focus. Patients typically show a strong positive reaction to PPD, eruptions often measuring 18 mm or larger, and the site may ulcerate. Prior vaccination with BCG does not prevent this condition developing [1].

The lesions typically consist of asymptomatic, tiny, follicular papules, which vary from skin coloured to red and often closely resemble lichen nitidus.

Lichen scrofulosorum is a cutaneous marker for underlying tuberculosis and up to 73% of patients have an associated focus of tuberculosis elsewhere, commonly in the cervical, hilar and mediastinal lymph nodes (up to 65%). Other foci include the lung, bone or intracranial sites [1–4]; in one series 15% had evidence of tubercular foci at multiple sites [1]. Up to 30% of patients may have no obvious underlying focus of tuberculosis. Lichen scrofulosorum has also been reported with *M. avium* infection [5,6], with *M. szulgai* [7] and also after BCG vaccination [8]. Other forms of cutaneous tuberculosis, such as lupus vulgaris, tuberculous gumma, papulonecrotic tuberculid [9] and tuberculosis verrucosa cutis, may coexist [1,10].

Epidemiology
Incidence and prevalence
Lichen scrofulosorum is now rarely seen in Europe although in 1976 a series of four cases were reported in the UK [11]. There is some evidence that the incidence is increasing in India [12]. In two series of cutaneous tuberculosis in Indian children, lichen scrofulosorum was the second most common disorder, seen in 23.5% and 33% of the cases, respectively [4,13]. This compares with a much earlier study that included 75 Indian children with cutaneous tuberculosis where only one case of lichen scrofulosorum was reported over a 25-year period [14]. In the largest published series of 39 Indian patients with lichen scrofulosorum this represented 7.6% of 513 patients with cutaneous tuberculosis [1], and in a study reported from Ethiopia [15] in 2008, 7.7% of 202 patients with cutaneous tuberculosis had lichen scrofulosorum.

Age
Lichen scrofulosorum appears to be commonest in children and adolescents. In one large series from India, 84% of patients were less than 15 years of age [1].

Sex
There is no sexual predisposition.

Ethnicity
The highest incidence is found in the Indian subcontinent and Africa south of the Sahara.

Associated diseases
Other forms of cutaneous tuberculosis, such as lupus vulgaris, tuberculous gumma and tuberculosis verrucosa cutis, may coexist [1,10].

Pathophysiology
The exact pathogenesis is unknown but may be the result of a type III hypersensitivity reaction to a haematogenous spread of

mycobacteria from an active internal site of infection. This seems to occur in persons with a high sensitivity to tuberculin and the continued formation of antigen–antibody complexes may lead to a type IV hypersensitivity reaction and granuloma formation. Its onset in some patients may be linked to an upregulation of their immune system and has been described in two patients with AIDS after starting ART and antibacterial treatment, respectively, probably due to the inflammatory response with an increase in cell-mediated immunity that may follow treatment of a multibacillary infection [16,17].

Predisposing factors
Overcrowding and close contact with others infected with *M. tuberculosis* are predisposing factors. In one series, 62.7% of children had a family member with tuberculosis [13].

Pathology
Superficial dermal granulomas surround hair follicles and sweat ducts, and may occupy several dermal papillae. Epithelioid cells, lymphocytes and occasional giant cells are seen. Usually there is no caseation. Mycobacteria are not seen in the sections and cannot be cultured from biopsy material. Mycobacterial DNA has been detected by PCR in two patients [7,18].

Causative organisms
- *Mycobacterium tuberculosis*.
- *Mycobacterium bovis*.
- *Mycobacterium avium*.
- *Mycobacterium szulgai*.

Environmental factors
These include low socioeconomic status and overcrowding [13].

Clinical features
History
The skin lesions are usually subtle and asymptomatic but the patient may have symptoms related to an underlying focus of tuberculosis elsewhere, such as lymphadenopathy.

Presentation
The eruption consists of symptomless, 0.5–3.0 mm diameter, closely grouped, lichenoid papules. The lesions are usually skin coloured (Figure 27.21), but may be yellowish or reddish brown. They are often perifollicular and can appear in groups or in an annular arrangement or coalesce into confluent plaques (Figure 27.22). The papules may have an adherent crust or small pustule. A few rare cases of bullous lesions and lesions at the site of a Mantoux test have also been described [1,11,19]. They are mainly found on the abdomen, chest, back and proximal limbs, but may occur on the face (Figure 27.23) [20], palms and soles [21] as well as the vulval area [22,23].

Clinical variants
Lichenoid (Figure 27.24) [19], psoriasisform [24] and granuloma annulare-like [25] variants have been described.

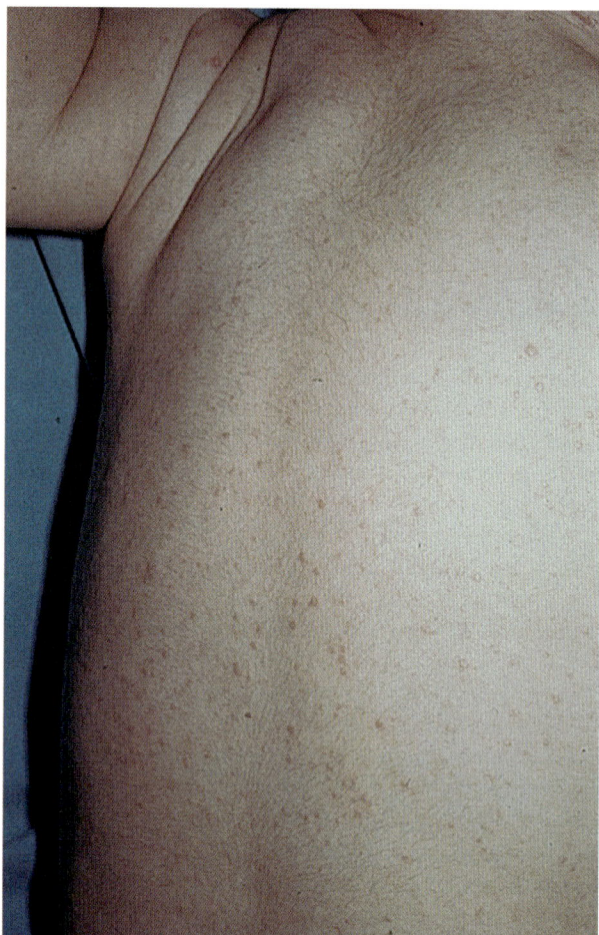

Figure 27.21 Lichen scrofulosorum of the trunk showing subtle skin-coloured papules. Courtesy of Dr Antonio Torrelo.

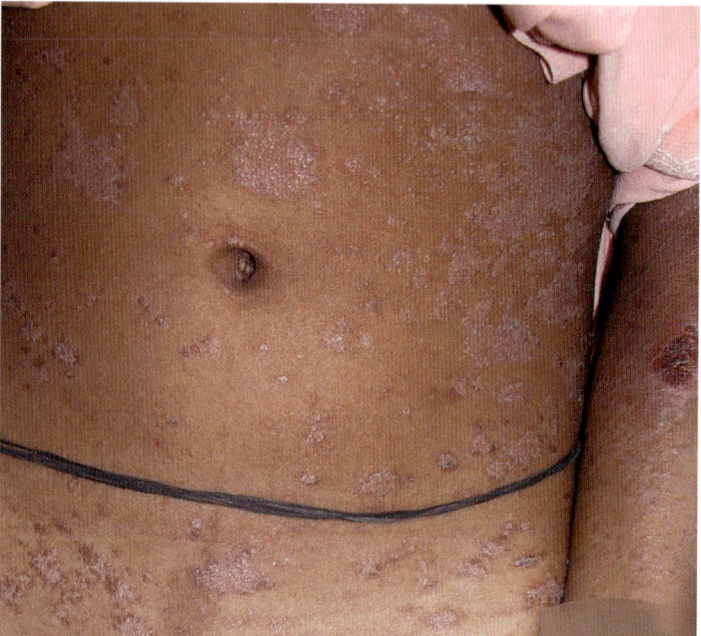

Figure 27.22 Lichen scrofulosorum showing annular and plaque-like lesions with strong tuberculin reaction. Courtesy of Dr V. Ramesh.

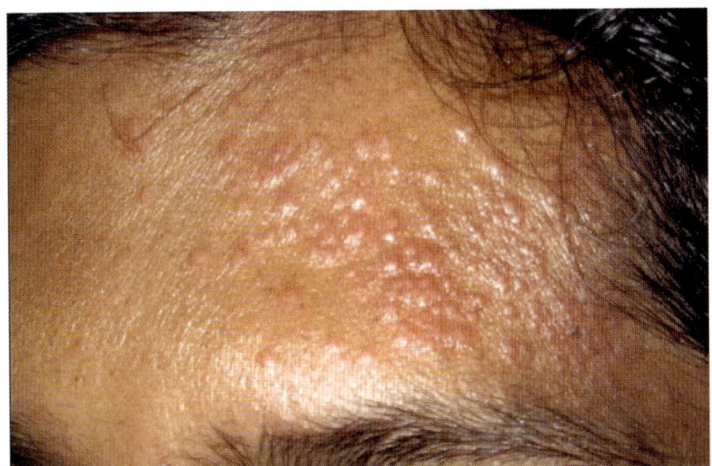

Figure 27.23 Lichen scrofulosorum on the forehead. Courtesy of Dr Yogesh S. Marfatia.

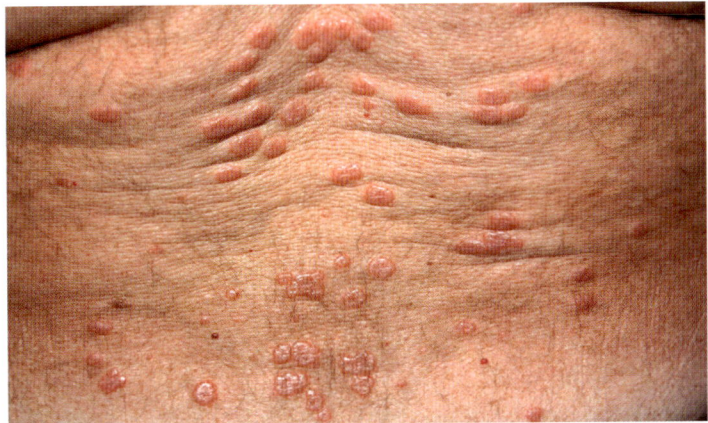

Figure 27.24 Lichenoid variety of lichen scrofulosorum. Courtesy of Dr Luis Requena.

Differential diagnosis
The differential diagnosis includes all asymptomatic follicular lesions where the lesions demonstrate a tendency to group together. These include: lichen nitidus, in which the lesions are more shiny and tend to be peripheral; keratosis spinulosa, in which the lesions have spiny projections over lichenoid papules; keratosis pilaris, where the lesions are non-inflammatory and usually on the upper thighs and arms; and papular or lichenoid sarcoidosis, secondary syphilis and drug eruptions. Annular lesions may closely resemble pityriasis rosea.

Classification of severity
The severity of the rash is variable.

Complications and co-morbidities
An underlying systemic tuberculosis infection may be found.

Disease course and prognosis
With specific antituberculous therapy, the lesions usually clear within 4 weeks and sometimes as early as 2 weeks [4,13]. They heal without scarring.

Investigations
A high index of suspicion is necessary for diagnosis as the lesions may be subtle and asymptomatic [26]. As the majority of patients will have a focus of tuberculosis elsewhere, they should be extensively screened [13]. The tuberculin reaction is normally strongly positive and may even be ulcerative, but can be negative in patients with immunosuppression such as in HIV infection [19]. Mycobacteria are not usually seen in a skin biopsy with acid-fast stains and they cannot be cultured from the lesions. Mycobacterial DNA has been detected by the PCR in rare cases [7,18].

Management
First line
Treatment of lichen scrolulosorum should follow the appropriate current guidelines for the treatment of tuberculosis of other organs, taking into account the degree of systemic involvement, the immune status of the patient and the existence of MDR forms of tuberculosis (see 'Current treatment regimens' earlier in this chapter) [27].

Papulonecrotic tuberculid

Definition and nomenclature
Papulonecrotic tuberculid is a chronic, recurrent and symmetrical eruption of necrotising skin papules arising in crops, involving primarily the buttocks and extensor surfaces of the arms and legs. Lesions usually heal with varioliform and pitting scarring.

Synonyms and inclusions
- Tuberculosis papulonecrotica

Introduction and general description
The papulonecrotic subtype of tuberculid mainly affects children and young adults. It classically presents with asymptomatic clusters of small, inflammatory, red papules that may go on to become pustular or necrotic and evolve into discrete crusted ulcers that heal over weeks with varioliform scarring. The lesions are usually symmetrically distributed, mainly on perniotic areas such as the ears, acral parts of the limbs and extensor surfaces of the joints, but may occur on the lower abdomen, trunk, buttocks [1] and scalp [2]. Localised forms are rare and mainly involve the genitalia [3–6].

An associated focus of tuberculosis can be demonstrated in many patients; this ranged from 38% to 75% of patients in three different studies [7–9]. The rapid response to antituberculous therapy usually leaves no doubt of the aetiology when a tuberculous focus cannot be found. In a series of 91 patients, papulonecrotic tuberculid evolved into lupus vulgaris in four patients [7]. Papulonecrotic tuberculid has also been described after BCG vaccination [10–13], indicating possible haematogenous mycobacterial spread as a cause of this tuberculid. Mycobacteria are rarely demonstrated in skin lesions, although they were found in two of the patients who had associated lupus vulgaris in the series discussed above [7] and in a recent case report of two patients [14] in whom M. tuberculosis DNA sequences were also confirmed by PCR. There are indeed several reports that show that *M. tuberculosis* DNA can be detected by PCR in lesions of papulonecrotic tuberculid [9,15,16]. Papulonecrotic tuberculid has occurred with *M. avium* complex in a patient with HIV infection [17] and also in conjunction with erythema induratum [18,19]. The tuberculin test is normally positive, often with a severe and even necrotic reaction appearing within 8–12 h.

Epidemiology
Incidence and prevalence
Papulonecrotic tuberculid is uncommon and accounts for approximately 4% of patients with cutaneous tuberculosis [20–22].

Age
It usually affects young adults and occasionally children. In a series of 91 patients, over 65% of patients developed the lesions before the age of 30 years [7].

Sex
There is no sexual predisposition.

Ethnicity
The highest incidence is in south Asia and countries south of the Sahara in Africa.

Associated diseases
In several documented cases lesions have both coexisted with [23] and developed into lupus vulgaris [7]. Coexistence with other forms of cutaneous tuberculosis such as erythema induratum has also been noted [15,18,19,24].

Pathophysiology
The pathophysiology is similar to the other tuberculids, that is, a cutaneous immunological reaction to the presence of occult tuberculosis in a patient with moderate to high immunity. However, papulonecrotic tuberculid has been described after BCG vaccination [10–13], indicating possible haematogenous mycobacterial spread as a cause of this tuberculid. Mycobacteria have also been found in a few patients with papulonecrotic tuberculid [7,14] and *M. tuberculosis* DNA can be detected fairly frequently by PCR [15,16,25].

Predisposing factors
These include systemic tuberculosis.

Pathology
The primary lesion is a subacute lymphohistiocytic vasculitis that causes thrombosis and destruction of small dermal vessels. These changes lead to a wedge-shaped infarct-like lesion with a large central zone of coagulation necrosis surrounded by inflammation extending from the superficial to the deep dermis, and sometimes into the subcutaneous tissues. A histiocytic palisade, similar to that of granuloma annulare, is seen around larger lesions. The involvement of adjacent small vessels is striking, ranging from a mild lymphocytic vasculitis to fibrinoid necrosis and thrombotic occlusion [8,9].

Causative organisms
The vast majority of cases occur in patients infected with *M. tuberculosis*, although there have been reports of papulonecrotic tuberculid associated with *M. kansasii* [26], *M. avium* complex [17] and *M. bovis* infections [27].

Environmental factors
These include poverty and overcrowding.

Clinical features
History
The lesions may be generally asymptomatic but there may also be symptoms of associated tuberculous disease elsewhere.

Presentation
The eruption consists of recurring crops of symmetrical, hard, dusky red papules. These crust or ulcerate, leaving pigmented, sometimes atrophic, varioliform scars over the course of a few weeks (Figure 27.25). New crops may continue over months or years. In some cases, showers of rapidly healing lesions occur, in others a chronic open ulcer may last for some months [8]. In children, phlyctenular conjunctivitis may be present [9]. The legs, knees, elbows, hands and feet are the sites of predilection, but the

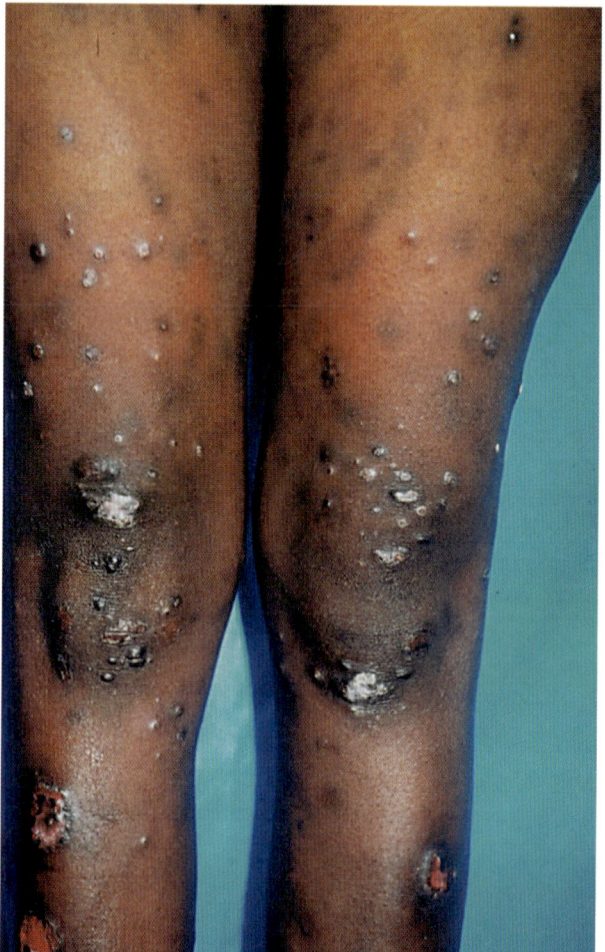

Figure 27.25 Papulonecrotic tuberculid of the legs. Courtesy of Professor J. Aboobaker.

ears, face, scalp [2], buttocks and penis and vulval areas – sometimes alone [3–6] – may be involved. Perniotic areas may be favoured.

Clinical variants
Isolated lesions on the genitalia, particularly the penis, may occur [3–6]. A verrucous variant mimicking Kyrle disease has been described [28].

Differential diagnosis
The differential diagnosis includes pityriasis lichenoides, where the lesions may be more widespread and affect the palms and soles; leukocytoclastic vasculitis, whose lesions are more pleomorphic; and nodular prurigo.

Classification of severity
The severity of skin lesions is variable.

Complications and co-morbidities
Lesions usually heal with scarring and hyperpigmentation.

Disease course and prognosis
With appropriate antituberculous therapy the lesions usually start to clear as early as 3–4 weeks.

Investigations
A lesional biopsy and tuberculin testing should be carried out. The tuberculin test is usually strongly positive. Mycobacteria have only rarely been demonstrated in skin lesions [7,14], but the PCR is frequently positive [15,16,25] and may be helpful. An IFN-γ release assay has been shown to be helpful in detecting latent tuberculous infection when the PCR was negative [29]. Patients should be screened for an underlying focus of tuberculosis. A therapeutic trial of specific antituberculous therapy is usually decisive in doubtful cases.

Management
First line
Treatment of papulonecrotic tuberculid should follow the appropriate current guidelines for treatment of tuberculosis of other organs, taking into account the degree of systemic involvement, the immune status of the patient and existence of MDR forms of tuberculosis (see 'Current treatment regimens' earlier in this chapter) [30].

Erythema induratum of Bazin

Definition and nomenclature
Erythema induratum of Bazin is the most commonly reported form of tuberculid and represents a tuberculosis-associated panniculitis. Around 80–90% of affected patients are young to middle-aged females, who classically present with crops of small, tender and painful red or dusky nodules or deep-seated plaques on the calves which may ulcerate. Most patients will have a positive tuberculin test or IGRA and respond well to antituberculous therapy.

> **Synonyms and inclusions**
> - Nodular vasculitis
> - Bazin disease
> - Tuberculosis cutis indurativa

Introduction and general description
Erythema induratum [1] was first described by Ernest Bazin in 1861 as a condition occurring 'on the legs of female laundresses and in young and plump well nourished women with the typical phenotype of those with the scrofula'. Recurrent nodular and ulcerative lesions that are usually localised to the lower legs, but can affect other areas, characterise the lesions. Typical patients are young to middle-aged women [2–5]. The histopathology demonstrates a lobular panniculitis with vasculitis [6]. It has been regarded as a tuberculid occurring secondary to tuberculosis elsewhere in the body. However, this pattern of nodular vasculitis does not occur exclusively in association with tuberculosis and some authors would now consider erythema induratum of Bazin to be a multifactorial disorder with several different causes, tuberculosis being just one of them [4]. Those patients without evidence of associated tuberculosis would be classified as having nodular vasculitis. Supporting this concept are reports of nodular vasculitis in association with chronic hepatitis C infection [7,8] and a recent report where *M. chelonae* was identified as the causative organism [9]. Erythema induratum has also been reported in an infant after BCG vaccination [10]. There is a growing opinion that the term erythema induratum of Bazin should be used solely where the association with tuberculosis is proven, which in some instances may require determining the clinical response to antituberculous treatment [4,5].

Epidemiology
Incidence and prevalence
Worldwide, the prevalence of erythema induratum is quite variable. It is rare in the UK, accounting for five out of 47 cases of cutaneous tuberculosis in a series of patients, all of whom were from the Indian subcontinent [11]. It is now the commonest form of cutaneous tuberculosis found in Hong Kong [12], where it accounted for 86% of patients in a published series, and also in Japan, where 40% of a large case series were affected [13]. In a South African series of 92 patients, 21% had erythema induratum [14]. In contrast only two out of 202 patients in a series from northern Ethiopia were found to have Bazin disease [15].

Age
The disease mainly affects the young and middle aged and is rare in children [16].

Sex
The disease occurs predominantly in females, and in three published series women accounted for between 78% and 90% of the cases [2,12,17].

Ethnicity
The disease is most commonly found in China, south Asia and Africa south of the Sahara.

Associated diseases

An association with clinically overt tuberculosis is uncommon but has been reported with naso-pharyngeal, renal and endometrial tuberculosis [18,19]; in one Japanese series 25.8% of patients had tuberculous lymph node involvement and 15% had lung invovement [20]. A search should be made for active and latent tuberculosis elsewhere. Coexistence with other forms of cutaneous tuberculosis such as papulonecrotic tuberculid and lichen scrofulosorum has been described [21].

Pathophysiology
Predisposing factors

Past or active foci of tuberculosis are usually present and the tuberculin test is usually positive. It has been suggested that PPD-specific T cells capable of producing IFN-γ may be involved in the formation of erythema induratum as a type of delayed hypersensitivity response to mycobacterial antigens at the site of skin lesions. Immune complex deposition may play a role in the vasculitic component [22].

Pathology

The histological features are those of either focal or diffuse, lobular or septolobular, granulomatous panniculitis in association with neutrophilic vasculitis of either large or small blood vessels. There are areas of coagulative and caseation necrosis and, usually poorly developed, granulomas – although mixed, pallisading and lipophilic granulomas can occur [23–25]. The exact histological pattern very much depends on the time at which the biopsy was taken during disease evolution [4]. *M. tuberculosis* is seldom recovered from the lesions, but mycobacterial DNA can be found in up to 77% of skin biopsy specimens [23,24,26–28].

Causative organisms
- *Mycobacterium tuberculosis*.
- *Mycobacterium bovis* [10].
- *Mycobacterium chelonae* [9].

Environmental factors
These include poverty and overcrowding.

Clinical features
History
The lesions are generally asymptomatic but acute nodules can be painful. There may be symptoms of associated tuberculosis elsewhere, for example lymphadenopathy.

Presentation
The disease presents as an indolent eruption of ill-defined nodules or subcutaneous plaques, usually affecting the posterior aspect of the lower legs of young or middle-aged women. However, lesions may affect other body areas, such as the upper limbs, thighs, buttocks and trunk. The plaques are usually indurated with a scaly surface (Figure 27.26). Follicular perniosis may be present. Lesions may ulcerate, usually centrally, and this may be precipitated by cold weather or venous stasis. The ulcers are ragged, irregular and shallow, with a bluish edge. The lesions heal with atrophic, hyperpigmented scarring [2–5].

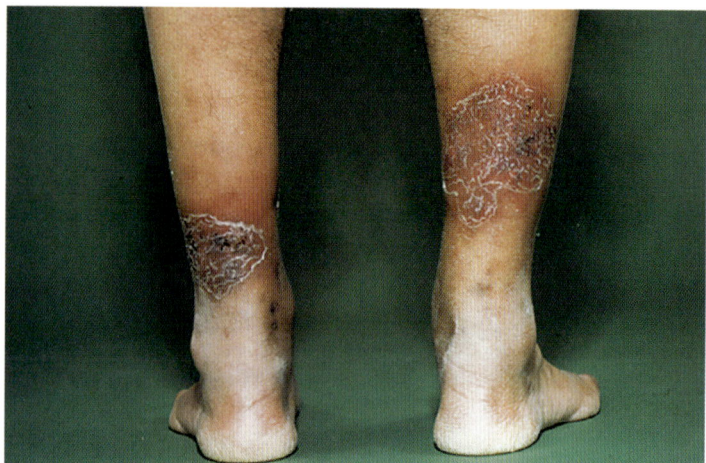

Figure 27.26 Erythema induratum of the legs.

Clinical variants
A variant, in which the pathology is at the junction of the dermis and subcutaneous fat, has been described and the term nodular tuberculid has been proposed for this pattern [29,30]. A second variant has been described where non-ulcerating subcutaneous nodules are distributed along the course of the great saphenous vein, and this has been termed nodular granulomatous phlebitis or superficial thrombophlebitic tuberculid [31,32].

Differential diagnosis
The differential diagnosis includes other conditions presenting as nodules on the lower extremities such as erythema nodosum, pancreatic panniculitis, polyarteritis nodosa, lupus profundus, subcutaneous sarcoid, cutaneous T-cell lymphoma and perniosis (chilblains).

Classification of severity
Severity is variable.

Complications and co-morbidities
Lesions may heal with hyperpigmented scarring.

Disease course and prognosis
Untreated, the disease course is chronic with recurrent crops of new lesions sometimes over many years. Response to antituberculous therapy may take between 1 and 6 months and resolution may be slow, even with adequate therapy [33], particularly if there are associated erythrocyanotic features.

Investigations
The diagnosis is made on characteristic clinical morphology, a positive tuberculin test and circumstantial evidence of tuberculosis elsewhere in the body, supplemented by histopathological findings. Detection of *M. tuberculosis* DNA by PCR on a skin biopsy specimen may be positive but a negative result does not exclude the diagnosis. IGRAs may be helpful in the diagnosis of latent tuberculosis [34,35]. Although cases of active tuberculosis are rare in erythema induratum, the patient should be fully investigated for subclinical active tuberculosis infection. The diagnosis can be confirmed by

a good response to antituberculous therapy. In cases where the diagnosis of tuberculosis seems unlikely, testing for hepatitis C and other infections is recommended.

Management
First line
Full specific antituberculous therapy should be given according to current recommended guidelines for systemic tuberculosis (see 'Current treatment regimens' earlier in this chapter). There is no place for monotherapy as has been recommended in the past [36] as drug resistance is likely to develop, which effectively means that no treatment is being given. In a series of 32 patients from Korea there was an 18% relapse rate in 22 patients who were treated with isoniazid alone [17]. Schneider and colleagues [23] treated 20 patients with a standard multiple drug regimen for 9 months and reported clearance of all patients within 1–6 months.

Second line
In some patients simple measures such as resting, non-steroidal anti-inflammatory drugs and compression bandaging may be helpful [4].

Other nodular tuberculids

Erythema nodosum
This is fully discussed in Chapter 97. Tuberculosis is now a rare cause in western Europe and the USA, but is a more frequent one in countries where the disease is still common. A tuberculous cause should always be considered in children. It occurred in nine out of 113 children with non-respiratory tuberculosis reported in the UK in 1978–79 [1].

Nodular vasculitis
This is clinically and histologically indistinguishable from erythema induratum although the lesions do not usually ulcerate. Most authors would now accept those of tuberculous origin to be categorised as erythema induratum and to be separated from those of non-tuberculous origin. An exhaustive search for underlying tuberculosis should be made before commencing oral steroids or other immunosuppressive agents.

Lupus miliaris disseminatus faciei
This is generally thought to be a variant of rosacea (see Chapter 89). However, in areas with an extremely high tuberculosis prevalence it is possible to find patients who have papulonecrotic lesions on the face and ears leading to varicelliform scarring (Figure 27.27). Mycobacteria can sometimes be seen in the lesions, the histology of which is granulomatous. There is a positive tuberculin test and the skin lesions improve on antituberculous therapy. Such cases would seem to be real lupus miliaris affecting the face [2]. One may have to keep an open mind about such cases.

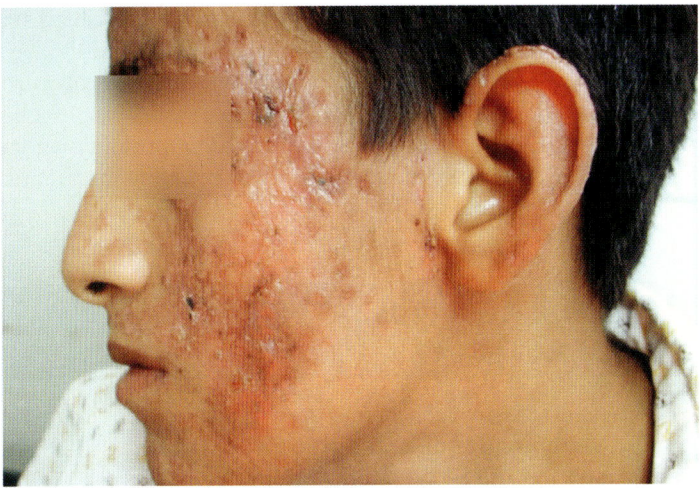

Figure 27.27 Acneform-like lesions with scarring on the face and ears. Tuberculoid histology with acid-fast bacilli is seen demonstrating a true lupus miliaris disseminatus faciei. Courtesy of Dr F. G. Bravo.

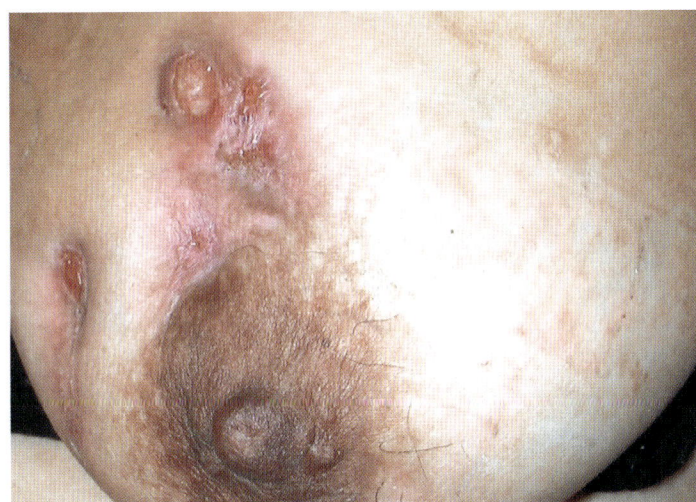

Figure 27.28 Granulomatous mastitis due to tuberculosis. Courtesy of Dr F. G. Bravo.

Tuberculous mastitis
Tuberculous mastitis is one of the causes of granulomatous mastitis (Figure 27.28) and is an important diagnosis to make as it is clinically and radiologically indistinguishable from breast cancer. The disease is most often unilateral and consists of ulcerative plaques, nodules, abscesses and occasionally sinuses on the breast of a female, usually in their twenties. A retrospective study from the UK in London of 44 women and three men (median age 33 years) with breast tuberculosis reported 'fistulation' in 26% [3].

The disease follows a chronic course [2,4–6]. Although rare, comprising approximately 0.025–0.1% of all surgically treated diseases of the breast, the ratio is higher in low and middle income countries [7] and in people who are immunocompromised [8,9].

On histology, often performed on specimens from fine-needle aspiration, granulomas are seen with fat necrosis but acid-fast bacilli are rarely found. The tuberculin test is normally positive and PCR is sometimes positive [4,10]. Tuberculosis-related granulomatous mastitis has been considered to be a form of nodular tuberculid affecting the breast tissue [2] but some cases are associated with involvement of the axillary lymph nodes and with scrofuloderma and may be culture positive [11,12]. One recent case report occurred with erythema nodosum [10]. The disease shows an excellent response to antituberculous therapy and is an important diagnosis to make in order to avoid an unnecessary mastectomy or treatment with oral corticosteroids [13].

NON-TUBERCULOUS (ATYPICAL) MYCOBACTERIA

Non-tuberculous mycobacteria are typically environmental organisms residing in soil and water. Of the more than 140 NTM species reported in the literature, 25 species have been strongly associated with NTM diseases in humans; the remainder are environmental organisms rarely encountered in clinical samples.

Classification

The NTM can be divided into slow-growing and rapidly growing types (see Table 27.1). Several slow-growing NTM produce disease in humans. The species of rapidly growing mycobacteria capable of producing disease in humans are the *M. fortuitum* group (including *M. margaritense*), the *M. abscessus* group, *M. chelonae* and *M. smegmatis*. Others include *M. wolinskyi*, *M. goodii* and *M. mucogenicum*. These mycobacteria can cause skin, soft tissue, bone, lymphadenitis and pulmonary infection as well as disseminated disease [1,2]. Other manifestations such as chronic otitis media, otomastoiditis and musculoskeletal infections have also been described [3].

General description

The NTM are *Mycobacterium* species other than *M. tuberculosis* and *M. leprae*. In the late 1950s and 1960s, these organisms were referred to as 'atypical', as they were thought to be unusual *M. tuberculosis* strains [1].

Non-tuberculous bacteria cause disease much more frequently in immunocompromised hosts, and with the advent of the AIDS epidemic and increasing use of anti-TNF therapy [2–4], their clinical importance and incidence has increased [5]. This has led to recent major advances in our understanding of their biology, epidemiology and clinical presentations, and the issue of diagnostic and treatment guidelines from both the American and British thoracic societies [6]. Pulmonary disease remains the commonest clinical presentation following infection with this group of organisms. The commonest NTM that cause cutaneous infection are members of the *M. fortuitum* complex (*M. fortuitum*, *M. peregrinum*, *M. chelonae*, *M. abscessus* and *M. mucogenicum*), *M. marinum* and *M. ulcerans*. The *M. avium* complex, *M. haemophilum*, *M. scrofulaceum* and *M. szulgai* are also of dermatological interest.

In immunocompetent patients, cutaneous infection is usually a consequence of trauma, and skin lesions tend to be localised. Immunocompromised hosts show a tendency to develop widespread or disseminated lesions [7].

Basic biology

Correct species identification is important because NTM species differ in their clinical relevance, growth rate, temperature tolerance, chromogenic characteristics and drug susceptibility. The diagnosis of NTM disease is complex and requires good communication between clinicians, radiologists and microbiologists [1]. PCR-based methods for identifying the *hsp65* gene differentiate closely related species [2,3].

Mycobacterium marinum infection

Definition and nomenclature

Mycobacterium marinum causes disease in many fish species and human infection follows contact with fishes or contaminated water. The commonest presentation is a nodule on the hand or upper limb that may demonstrate sporotrichoid spread. Spread of infection to deeper structures occurs in up to a third of patients. The sporotrichoid or rapidly disseminating form is commoner in the immunocompromised [1].

Synonyms and inclusions
- Swimming pool granuloma
- Fish tank granuloma

Introduction and general description

Mycobacterium marinum (formally *M. balnei* and *M. platypoecilus*) was first isolated in 1926 by Aronson from saltwater fish carcasses in the Philadelphia Aquarium [2]. In 1942, Baker and Hagan showed that the bacteria caused tuberculosis in freshwater platy fish and named the organism *M. platypoecilus*. The first report of human disease appeared in 1951 [3], when the organism was found to be the cause of granulomatous skin lesions in those using a contaminated swimming pool in Sweden and was named *M. balnei*. Subsequently, *M. balnei* and *M. platypoecilus* were shown to be the same organism, and they are now called *M. marinum*. In the late 1950s, *M. marinum* was found to be the cause of infections acquired from aquariums in humans [4].

The natural habitat of *M. marinum* is fresh or salt water, particularly enclosures of water that are not often replenished, such as swimming pools and aquariums [5]. Its distribution is worldwide, but the organism is especially prevalent in heated water in temperate climates and in the sea, natural pools and rivers and on beaches. Its vectors include fresh- or saltwater fish, snails, shellfish, dolphins and water fleas [6]. It can also be isolated from cracks in masonry and mud and from water even where chlorination appears to be sufficient [7].

On immunodiffusion analysis, the organism can be shown to possess antigens characteristic of the slow-growing mycobacteria [8], although its growth is more rapid than that of most members in that group. It will grow on ordinary laboratory media in 7–10 days if cultured at 30–33°C; significant inhibition of growth occurs at 37°C.

M. marinum is probably only pathogenic on abraded skin, although a history of trauma cannot always be elicited [9]. Strain characteristics may be important in the virulence of the organism [10].

Epidemiology

Occupational or recreational exposure to salt or fresh water has occurred in the majority of cases. Most of the early proven cases of *M. marinum* infections were described in individuals frequenting swimming pools [11]. The first two cases of 'swimming-pool granuloma' in the UK were reported from Yorkshire in 1964 [12]. In one outbreak, over 300 cases were traced [13]. Similar outbreaks have occurred in Wales [14] and France [15]. The infection has also been contracted in natural bathing pools by the Dead Sea [16] and in the sea in the USA [17].

In many recent cases, the source of infection has been tropical fish tanks [18], but outbreaks with multiple cases have also been described in fish farms [19]. In a national survey of 63 culture-confirmed cases occurring in France between 1996 and 1998, inoculation related to fish tank exposure was documented in 84% of cases [20]. Ornamental fish such as the Siamese fighting fish *Betta splendens* and the snakehead *Channa striata* are often hosts of the mycobacteria [21], but the organism has been shown to infect at least 150 species of fish [22].

Fish tuberculosis is a chronic infection that causes wasting of the fish, but may take up to 12 months to cause death (Figure 27.29). Most infections in humans are acquired while cleaning out the tanks. *M. marinum* survives readily in water and can be cultured from dead fish, the sides of tanks and sand and water samples [23]. One child developed the infection indirectly after bathing in the bath in which his father had recently cleaned a tropical fish tank [24]. Risk factors for individuals with HIV are similar. Disseminated infection can occur in immunocompromised patients [25,26].

Incidence and prevalence

Mycobacterium marinum infections are rare, and estimates of the annual incidence varies from 0.27 cases per 100 000 persons in the USA to 0.04 per 100 000 in France [27].

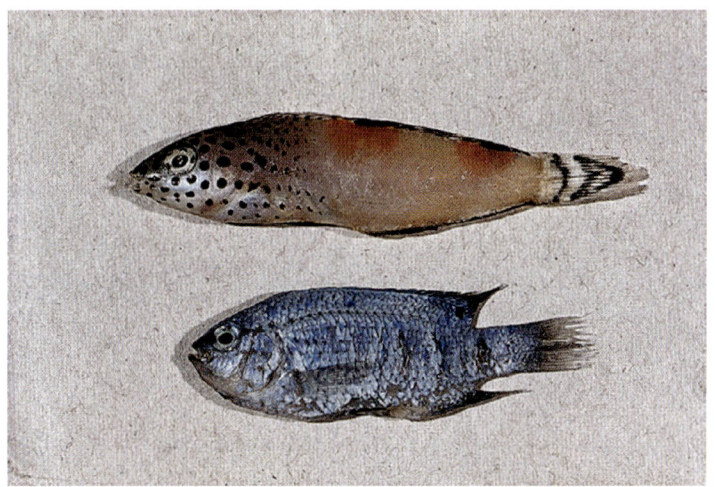

Figure 27.29 Fish infected with *Mycobacterium marinum*. Courtesy of Professor J. A. A. Hunter.

Pathophysiology
Predisposing factors

Keeping and rearing tropical fish predisposes to infection and exposed professions include fishworkers, fishmongers and cooks. Ang *et al.* [9] noted that 44.7% of infected patients were engaged in fish-related activities.

Pathology

Lesions may show non-specific inflammation in the first few months, while older lesions show well-formed tuberculoid granulomas [28] with fibrinoid masses rather than caseation. Langhans giant cells are not always present. Intracellular acid-fast bacilli – longer and broader than tubercle bacilli – are detectable in only approximately 10% of cases [29]. Epidermal changes including ulceration and pseudoepitheliomatous hyperplasia may occur in chronic lesions.

Causative organisms

- *Mycobacterium marinum.*

Clinical features
History

There may be a history of trauma and water-/fish-related hobbies or occupations.

Presentation

Skin lesions develop after an average incubation period of 2–3 weeks following inoculation of the organisms onto abraded skin. Occasionally, the incubation period can be as long as 9 months [30], leading to delays in diagnosis, as important clinical clues in the patient's history may be overlooked. The initial lesion is either a solitary nodule or pustule that may break down to form an ulcer or abscess, or that may remain as a verrucous plaque. Lesions are most common on the elbows, knees and feet of swimmers, and on the dominant hand and fingers of fish fanciers. The inhibition of *M. marinum* growth at 37°C accounts for its ability to infect the cooler body extremities while rarely spreading systemically [31].

Lesions are often multiple. In the sporotrichoid form, which occurs in approximately 20% of cases [20], nodules may extend along the line of lymphatic vessels (Figure 27.30) [9,32]. The regional lymph glands may be enlarged, but never break down. Deeper infections occurred in 29% of patients in one series [33] and resulted from direct extension of the cutaneous infection.

M. marinum infections in patients with HIV have been reported in the pre-ART era but are uncommon in the post-ART era. Disseminated infection can also occur in non-HIV immunocompromised hosts.

Differential diagnosis

Cutaneous nodular infections may mimic fungal and granulomatous infections such as blastomycosis, coccidioidomycosis, cryptococcosis and histoplasmosis. Other differential diagnoses includes leishmaniasis, nocardiosis and sporotrichosis in endemic areas, as well as other NTM infections such as from *M. kansasii*, *M. chelonae* and *M. gordonae*, all of which may spread in a sporotrichoid manner. Cultures are of particular value in the exclusion of other diagnoses. Skin tests using antigens specific to *M. marinum* are of little value.

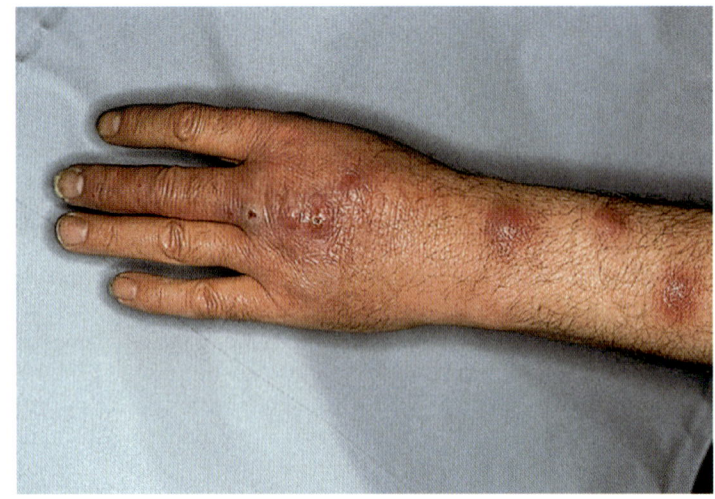

Figure 27.30 *Mycobacterium marinum* infection showing sporotrichoid spread from the hand to the forearm in an aquarist. Courtesy of Dr I. H. Coulson.

Classification of severity
Severity is variable.

Complications and co-morbidities
Chronic complications of the disease are minimal with early diagnosis and adequate treatment. Some patients may develop persistent ulceration at the site of initial exposure. With delayed treatment or improper selection/duration of antibiotic therapy, patients may develop deeper infections. Deeper infections may be complicated by tenosynovitis, osteomyelitis bursitis and septic arthritis [34]. Immunocompromised patients may develop disseminated lesions [35–37].

Prognosis
The prognosis is excellent in most cases, especially in patients with immunocompetent status. Treatment failure may result in ulcerative forms and when deeper structures are involved. Clinical outcomes of *M. marinum* infections in patients with HIV infection do not differ from those without HIV infections. A continued immunocompromised state and ongoing risk of exposure can increase the risk of disease. Some patients may need lifelong suppression therapy [38].

Investigations
As with all mycobacterial disease, the diagnosis requires a high index of suspicion. A history of contact with water, fish tanks, aquariums, etc., combined with granulomatous histology, is suggestive of the diagnosis. A positive culture can be obtained in some 70–80% of cases if the organism is grown between 30 and 33°C. It is important to alert the microbiologist to the suspicion of *M. marinum* infection so that specimens are cultured in the appropriate manner. Cultures should be observed for 6 weeks, but generally colonies will be seen in 10–28 days. The positivity rate of cultures ranges from 70% to 80%. Lesions have a very low concentration of microorganisms; hence cultures should be obtained even in the absence of microscopic evidence of bacilli.

PCR amplification techniques using *Mycobacterium* genus-specific primers can help diagnose *M. marinum* infection directly in the biopsy sample. A Ziehl–Neelsen stain of biopsy specimens or yellowish discharge is only rarely positive since the number of mycobacteria in clinical specimens is low.

TSTs using purified protein derivative are positive in 67–100% of cases. QuantiFERON®-TB Gold and ELISA may also be positive in *M. marinum* infections but are unhelpful for diagnosis [38].

Species-specific monoclonal antibody against 56 kDa *M. marinum* antigens may have potential use in rapid culture identification [39]. *M. marinum* infection has also been identified using PCR–reverse cross blot hybridisation assay with species-specific gene probes [40]. This may lead to more rapid diagnosis, but cultures will still be necessary to assess the antibiotic sensitivities of different strains.

Typical tuberculoid granulomas are seen in only two-thirds of cases, and the histopathology of nodules can be confused with rheumatoid nodules. *M. marinum* infections can mimic other histopathological patterns such as a sarcoid-like granuloma or granuloma annulare [41].

Positive blood culture findings have also been reported in disseminated infections.

Management
There have been no comparative trials of treatment regimens for infections with *M. marinum* of sufficient power to guide optimal management; thus therapeutic decisions must be made on the basis of susceptibility testing [42,43] and outcomes reported in case series and anecdotal reports [20]. *M. marinum* is susceptible to clarithromycin, sulphonamides, trimethoprim/sulfamethoxazole, rifampicin, rifabutin and ethambutol, and variably susceptible to doxycycline, minocycline, linezolid and streptomycin. It is resistant to isoniazid and pyrazinamide.

There is no consensus on the regimen or the duration of therapy in *M. marinum* infections. Whereas most experts recommend treatment with two active agents, minimal disease has been successfully treated with monotherapy [27] but one needs to bear in mind that *M. marinum* is a naturally drug-resistant species [44]. A retrospective study of 16 cases of culture-positive *M. marinum* showed that clarithromycin, both on *in vitro* testing and on clinical response, was the drug of choice [45]. The authors also pointed out that clarithromycin seems to be superior to other drugs in terms of lack of significant side effects.

Clarithromycin and ethambutol are a reliable combination that provides an optimal balance of efficacy and tolerability for most patients without the need to wait for susceptibility testing results. Rifampicin should be added in cases of osteomyelitis or other deep structure infection. Azithromycin is a reasonable alternative to clarithromycin [20,27]. Drugs need to be continued for 1–2 months after the resolution of symptoms, typically 3–4 months in total [46].

Susceptibility testing is not routinely recommended but should be requested in cases of treatment failure [18]. Treatment failure is more usually related to the involvement of deeper structures, delay in diagnosis and inappropriately administered intralesional steroids [47]. Amikacin has been used in a refractory disseminated case [48].

Deep *M. marinum* infection involving the hand can be aggressive and may result in permanent disability. Specialists in infectious diseases and hand surgery should be consulted [49]. Surgical debridement of lesions is somewhat controversial, but may be considered when deeper structures are involved [50]. Photodynamic therapy may have some role to play [51] although more data are needed.

Fish fanciers and fish salesmen are seldom aware of, or ignore, the risk of mycobacterial infection from their hobby/occupation [52]. Simple preventative measures, such as the use of gloves or covering cuts and grazes, should be recommended to fish handlers [23]. Public health authorities should be notified when a public source of infection is identified, and other cases should be looked for. Maximum chlorination of swimming pools is effective [15].

Patients who are immunocompromised will need to be treated with two agents for at least 6 months. In one report, a patient with AIDS was successfully treated with rifampin and ethambutol for 6 months. The lesion recurred after stopping therapy, so therapy was restarted with a clarithromycin regimen. Sometimes chronic lifelong suppressive therapy may be necessary [53,54].

Mycobacterium kansasii infection

Definition
Mycobacterium kansasii is primarily a pulmonary pathogen, usually causing a tuberculosis-like illness in patients with underlying pulmonary disease such as chronic obstructive pulmonary disease and cystic fibrosis [1]. Cutaneous infection is rare and more likely to occur in immunocompromised patients. The clinical pattern of skin lesions varies widely and includes papules, nodules and verrucous plaques – sometimes in a sporotricoid pattern and sometimes also cellulitis and abscesses.

Introduction and general description
Mycobacterium kansasii is a slow-growing, photochromogenic bacterium of Runyon group I that grows optimally at 37°C. It is one of the most pathogenic and most frequent NTM isolated from humans [2]. Buhler and Pollack first described this slow-growing mycobacterium in 1953 [3]. Under light microscopy, *M. kansasii* appears as thick rectangular, beaded, Gram-positive rods which are longer than those of *M. tuberculosis* [4].

It is found worldwide, but exhibits clustering in urban and industrial areas [5,6] such as southern and central USA, southeast England and Wales and northern France. Tap water is the major reservoir of infection for this organism and person to person contact has not been reported [7]. *M. kansasii* exhibits heterogeneity, and of the seven subtypes identified by PCR–restriction fragment length polymorphism (RFLP) of the *hsp65* gene, type 1 has been most strongly associated with clinical disease [8]. Subtype 1 has been shown to have an active ESX-1 virulence factor, whereas this system was inactive in subtype 5, which seems to be non-pathogenic [9,10].

In immunocompetent patients, *M. kansasii* infection commonly produces a granulomatous pulmonary infection with cavities resembling tuberculosis. This usually occurs in association with underlying lung disease [11]. Primary cutaneous infection is rare [12] and first reports of the organism as a cutaneous pathogen were not made until 1965 [13]. It most commonly affects persons exposed to contaminated water, particularly after local trauma [14]. The majority of patients with cutaneous lesions have some impairment of their immune status [15].

Epidemiology
Incidence and prevalence
Mycobacterium kansasii is one of the most commonly reported species of non-tuberculous bacteria isolated [**2**,16]. Cutaneous lesions are rare but are more common in patients with impaired immunity and in disseminated disease [17]. *M. kansasii* infections are more likely to occur in urban areas than rural areas and several studies have reported an association with mining practices [18]. *M. kansasii* infections are also prevalent in areas where HIV infection is common due to the susceptibility of the hosts.

Age and sex
This infection primarily affects middle-aged white men but it can affect adult patients of any sex, race or age [19].

Pathophysiology
Predisposing factors
Pulmonary disease is associated with chronic lung disease, including chronic obstructive pulmonary disease, bronchiectasis, pneumoconiosis and cystic fibrosis. Other underlying conditions predisposing to *M. kansasii* infection include malignancy particularly haematological, previous mycobacterial infection, alcohol abuse and immunocompromised situations including HIV infection, immunoglobulin A deficiency [20], solid organ transplantation and the use of corticosteroids.

Pathology
As with the clinical picture, the histology can be very variable, but a granulomatous histology and a mixed inflammatory infiltrate with acid-fast bacilli in the histiocytes is often noted. Histopathology is identical to tuberculosis in some cases and there may also be abscess formation and epidermal, subcutaneous or deep dermal necrosis [12,14].

Causative organisms
- *Mycobacterium kansasii*.

Environmental factors
Chronic occupational exposure to dust, which can occur in miners, welders, sandblasters and painters, is a common environmental factor [5,21].

Clinical features
Presentation
The second most frequent organ involved in *M. kansasii* infection after pulmonary disease is the skin [22]. As a primary cutaneous disease, *M. kansasii* produces a variety of lesions, usually confined to a distal extremity. Lesions are commonly composed of papules and pustules, often forming verrucous or granulomatous plaques or nodules, which may ulcerate. A sporotrichoid pattern [23], cellulitis [24], rhinophyma [25] and single and multiple abscesses have all been reported. Papulonecrotic tuberculid skin lesions have been reported in one patient [26].

Skin lesions associated with disseminated *M. kansasii* have increased since the onset of the AIDS epidemic [27]. In non-HIV-infected patients, disseminated disease is most commonly associated with haematological malignancy although 23% of published cases were in previously healthy patients with no underlying disease [17]. Disseminated visceral infection can be life-threatening. In HIV and immunocompromised patients, the presentation can be atypical and include bacteraemia, osteomyelitis, abscesses and cellulitis. Pericarditis with cardiac tamponade has been reported in HIV patients [28].

Clinical variants
Tenosynovitis [29,30], bursitis [31], arthritis, osteomyelitis [32] and carpal tunnel syndrome have all been reported [13].

Differential diagnosis
The main differential diagnoses are cutaneous tuberculosis, other NTM infections, bacterial infections, fungal infections, *Actinomyces* group infections, cancer, granulomatosis with polyangiitis and sporotricosis.

Complications and co-morbidities
The disease may become disseminated. Bone involvement, such as vertebral osteomyelitis and sacroiliitis, are common with disseminated diseases [33]. Pneumothorax, psoas abscess, bone marrow granuloma, liver granuloma and possible spleen abscesses have also been described in the literature [34]. Central nervous system complications like meningoencephalitis are very rare and are usually fatal.

Disease course and prognosis
The natural course of non-disseminated skin infection by *M. kansasii* is one of non-serious indolent progression and the outcome of treatment is usually good. However, skin infection associated with systemic dissemination carries a poor prognosis with around 60% mortality.

With appropriate treatment, the prognosis is usually good [35].

Investigations
Histology of biopsy specimens with staining for acid-fast bacilli should be carried out and representative clinical specimens from either biopsy specimens, exudates or fine-needle aspiration should be cultured. The laboratory should be advised to provide appropriate culture conditions to detect slow-growing mycobacteria. PCR analysis may be helpful in overcoming difficulties in culture [10,36,37].

Management
Mycobacterium kansasii is typically susceptible to conventional antituberculous drugs (rifampicin, ethambutol, streptomycin and isoniazid) with the exception of pyrazinamide. There are no separate guidelines for the treatment of cutaneous infections.

Rifampicin is the cornerstone of *M. kansasii* therapy. The first line therapy recommended by the Infectious Diseases Society of America/American Thoracic Society (IDSA-ATS) guidelines for *M. kansasii* is rifampicin, ethambutol and isoniazid plus pyridoxine [38–40]. The recommended duration of therapy is at least 12 months or more with the goal to have culture negative results for 12 months on therapy.

First line
The current recommended treatment for pulmonary disease includes isoniazid, rifampicin and a third agent, usually ethambutol, for 18 months [11]. In order to optimise therapy, *in vitro* susceptibility sensitivity testing should be performed [41].

Rifampicin-containing regimens have low failure rates (1.1%) and low long-term relapse rates (<1%).

Second line
In severe disease, with resistant isolates or adverse drug reactions, the addition of streptomycin or amikacin for the first 3 months followed by an intermittent therapy with one of these drugs for 6 months is recommended [19].

Third line
Rifampicin is the cornerstone of current therapy but acquired resistance to this and isoniazid can occur. In these cases, clarithromycin, levofloxacin, moxifoxacin and in particular linezoloid seem to be the best alternatives [42].

Mycobacterium ulcerans infection

Definition and nomenclature
Mycobacterium ulcerans is a slow-growing, environmental *Mycobacterium* that affects the skin and subcutaneous tissues. Skin lesions begin as a papule, nodule, plaque or oedema and then develop into large, indolent ulcers with undermined edges.

Synonyms and inclusions
- Buruli ulcer (Uganda)
- Bairnsdale ulcer or Searls ulcer (Australia)
- Kasongo (Democratic Republic of Congo)
- Many other local names

Introduction and general description
Mycobacterium ulcerans is an environmental *Mycobacterium* that grows slowly and infects the skin and subcutaneous tissues. This gives rise to a painless nodule, papule, plaque or oedema that evolves into a painless ulcer with undermined edges, often leading to disabling sequelae [1,2]. It grows optimally on routine mycobacteriological media at 32°C.

Over 150 years ago in 1897, Sir Albert Cook working in Kampala, Uganda, first described large ulcers, almost certainly caused by *M. ulcerans* [3,4]. However, the bacterium was not isolated until 1948, when MacCallum and colleagues were investigating a cluster of patients with unusual ulcers in Victoria, Australia [5]. In the 1960s, the disease was noted to be endemic in refugee camps in Buruli, Uganda, near the Nile [6]. A breakthrough came in 1999 when Small and his colleagues discovered mycolactone A/B, a diffusible, necrotising, immunosuppressive, polyketide-derived macrolide toxin, responsible for the dramatic necrosis of fat and subcutaneous tissue characteristic of the disease [7]. More recently, comparative genomic analysis has revealed that *M. ulcerans* arose from *M. marinum* by horizontal transfer of a virulence plasmid that carries a cluster of genes for mycolactone production, followed by reductive evolution [8].

M. ulcerans has now been reported in over 33 countries in Africa, the Americas, Asia and the western Pacific [9]. It prevails in rural tropical wetlands, especially areas with stagnant water, including ponds and swamps. However, *M. ulcerans* is also acquired without wetland exposure [2].

M. ulcerans is now the third most important pathogen of man after *M. tuberculosis* and *M. leprae*. Its emergence in several West African countries over the past two decades has been dramatic, notably in Benin, Cote d'Ivoire and Ghana [10], with other important foci in French Guiana, Papua New Guinea and Australia [1]. The rapid re-emergence of *M. ulcerans* may be attributable to man-made alterations to the environment, such as deforestation and other topographic alterations, which increase the amount of wetlands. Changes in global temperature and precipitation patterns may further promote the re-emergence of *M. ulcerans* [2]. In some African communities, *M. ulcerans* has replaced tuberculosis and leprosy as the most prevalent mycobacterial disease. The rising incidence of the disease, its predilection for poor rural communities, the cost of complex surgery, the lost production during illness and the reduced fitness after recovery combine to make *M. ulcerans* a major socioeconomic burden in areas of prevalence [11].

Epidemiology

There is evidence that *M. ulcerans* is not usually transmitted from person to person but that it is mainly acquired from its aquatic niches [12]. Portaels and colleagues were the first to use PCR-based detection methods to investigate a role for insect vectors in transmission [13]. *M. ulcerans* DNA has been recovered from aquatic insects, fish, molluscs, water filtrate and plant materials in endemic areas [14–17]. Marsollier and colleagues showed that *M. ulcerans* is carried and multiplies in the water bug *Naucoris cimicoides* [18–20]. Although these insects are predators of small molluscs and fish and have been shown under experimental conditions to transmit the pathogen to mice after biting [18], they do not normally bite humans. However, in a serological survey of healthy individuals in a *M. ulcerans* endemic region, high titres of antibodies were found to *N. cimicoides* salivary proteins, which could be accounted for by the exposure of humans to water bug bites [21].

In a landmark study from Benin, *M. ulcerans* was isolated from the water strider (*Gerris* species, from the aquatic order Hemiptera) in pure culture and shown to be genetically and phenotypically identical to that isolated from patients living in the same region [22]. However, the water strider generally avoids humans. Mammals, such as possums and koalas, as well as mosquitoes [23,24] have been proposed as hosts of *M. ulcerans* in Australia, although the fact that mosquitoes are active vectors of the infection has been challenged [25]. In Africa, terrestrial mammals are also being investigated as reservoirs of *M. ulcerans* [26]. In addition, *Acanthamoeba* species have been implicated as reservoirs and possible vectors for infection [27].

The most likely mode of transmission would appear to be local, minor, often unnoticed skin trauma that permits the inoculation of *M. ulcerans* [2]. Person to person transmission has only rarely been documented [28]. Risk factors for *M. ulcerans* within endemic areas include failure to wear protective clothing, exposure to unprotected natural water sources and inadequate care of minor skin wounds [29,30]. HIV seropositivity is thought to increase the risk for *M. ulcerans* and to be associated with aggressive disease [31]. An increase in risk has not been shown in other areas [31,32].

Incidence and prevalence

The disease has been reported from 33 countries, primarily in subtropical and tropical regions of Africa, Asia, Australia [33] and Latin America, but 15 regularly report cases to the WHO. The majority of affected places are in the tropical regions of West and Central Africa where access to health services remains a challenge. At national and subnational levels, the disease is highly focal.

Adequate surveillance data are missing for most of the endemic areas, therefore the incidence and prevalence of *M. ulcerans* are not precisely defined. In Ghana, an overall national prevalence rate of active lesions of 20.7 per 100 000 is reported, but the rate was as high as 150.8 per 100 000 in districts where the disease was more endemic. The figures are likely to be a gross underestimation as many cases are undiagnosed because of the geopolitical and socioeconomic factors in endemic countries and in areas where there is no surveillance.

Age

Children (5–15 years old) have the highest incidence of *M. ulcerans*, with most lesions on the lower extremities. In contrast, most of the patients in Australia and Japan are adults, and children under 15 years of age constitute less than 20%.

Sex

Males and females are equally affected by the disease.

Pathophysiology

Pathology

There is a latent period of around 4 months or more before an infection becomes overt [34]. After inoculation into the skin, *M. ulcerans* proliferates and produces the polyketone toxin mycolactone [4]. The physiopathology of *M. ulcerans* is closely associated with diffusion of the toxin from bacterial foci. The temperature requirement of *M. ulcerans* favours the development of lesions in cooler tissues, especially the skin and subcutaneous tissue. Mycolactone destroys tissues by apoptosis and necrosis and suppresses host immune responses [35]. The earliest change is an acute necrosis of dermal and subcutaneous tissue; characteristically, there is extensive involvement of the subcutaneous fat as a septal panniculitis. The fat becomes necrotic and may calcify. Mycobacteria can be found, in spherical clumps, outside cells, in the layer of exudate on the ulcer floor and in the fatty septae. Some organisms show signs of degeneration and lose their usual rod-like shape. Necrosis of the dermis extends laterally, leading to the characteristic undermining of the ulcer edge [36]. The organism selectively destroys those tissues within its own viable temperature range [37]; muscle is usually spared, perhaps because of its higher temperature. In the deeper dermis, a leukocytoclastic vasculitis is seen, affecting small and medium-sized vessels. After some months, healing starts and is accompanied by a lymphocytic or granulomatous reaction. Fibrosis and scarring complete the sequence.

Causative organisms
- *Mycobacterium ulcerans*.

Genetics
Gene sequences of the 3′ end of the 16S rRNA of *M. ulcerans* vary by geographic origin, dividing *M. ulcerans* broadly into African, American, Asian and Australian strains, with many substrains on each continent [38]. Each major strain generally differs in clinical presentation, mycolactone type and virulence, and host immune responses [39]. Mycolactone type coding by geographic origin includes A/B (Africa, the most pathogenic), C (Asia, Australia) and D (Asia) [35].

Environmental factors
The organism is prevalent in rural tropical wetlands.

Clinical features
History
There may be a history of a visit to an endemic area.

Presentation
The estimated mean incubation period of *M. ulcerans* in Victoria, Australia is 135 days or 4.5 months (range 34–264 days) [34,40]. Although uncommon, cases of *M. ulcerans* disease have been reported in neonates suggesting that the incubation period could be shorter in this age group [41,42]. *M. ulcerans* presents as a spectrum of localised or disseminated clinical forms, with variable natural history [43].

About 70% of patients are children below 15 years of age. Early lesions are papular, nodular or oedematous and are usually on an arm or leg, but can be on the trunk or head. Some cases do not progress further, but usually a nodule will break down to form a shallow necrotic ulcer, which extends rapidly and irregularly, with deeply undermined edges (Figure 27.31). Most ulcers are painless unless secondarily infected. Well-demarcated, painless plaques can also occur. An ulcer may reach a diameter of several centimetres over the course of a few weeks. The floor of the ulcer is formed of necrotic fat, and there may be a clear mucoid discharge. Ulcers are usually single, although satellites may develop. Large lesions may be surrounded by extensive induration (Figure 27.32). There is little

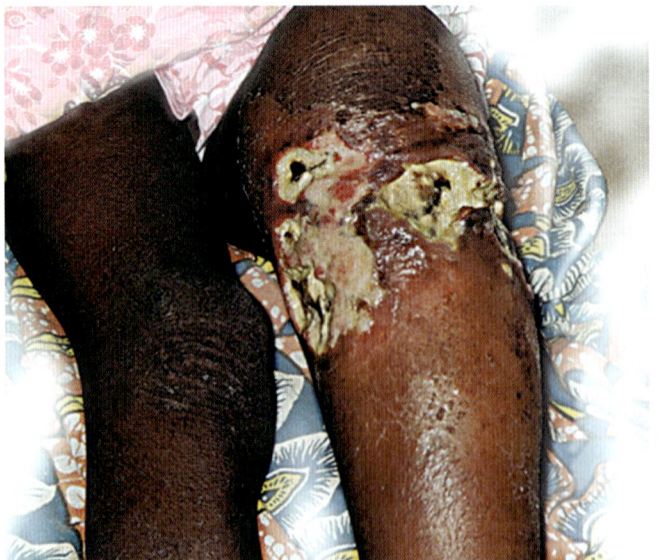

Figure 27.31 *Mycobacterium ulcerans* in an 8-year-old child. Courtesy of Professor F. Portaels.

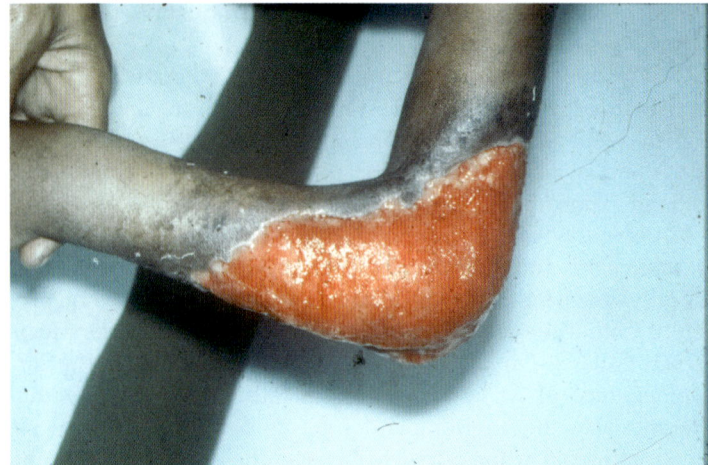

Figure 27.32 Extensive *Mycobacterium ulcerans* of the elbow in a child. Courtesy of Dr P. L. A. Niemel.

or no constitutional disturbance such as fever or lymphadenopathy, even with severe local disease. Disseminated disease has occurred in association with HIV infection [44]. Unfortunately, because the ulcers are painless and victims often live in remote areas, most patients do not receive medical attention until the damage is extensive.

Differential diagnosis
Differential diagnosis of an established lesion includes ulcerated tuberculosis lesions, blastomycosis or other deep fungal infections, cellulitis and pyoderma gangrenosum, necrotising faciitis and other causes of ulcers. In early lesions, foreign body granulomas, epidermoid cysts, appendage tumours and other causes of panniculitis will come into the differential diagnosis.

Complications and co-morbidities
Approximately 10% of patients develop involvement of bone adjacent to the skin lesions or metastatic osteomyelitis from lympho-haematogenous spread of *M. ulcerans* [2]. The involvement of other organs is rare. The fibrosis and calcification that accompany healing may lead to contractures and severe deformity.

Disease course and prognosis
The course is variable, but usually prolonged without antibiotic treatment. Healing may occur after 6–9 months but some lesions persist for longer. A review of 102 patients in Ghana in 1998 indicated that the average length of hospital stay was more than 100 days. The infection led to 10 amputations, 12 joint contractures and two deaths from tetanus and sepsis [11]. Developments in medical treatment since 2004 have improved treatment outcomes, especially in early lesions.

Investigations
In endemic areas, suspicion should allow an early diagnosis to be made. However, sporadic or anomalous cases with ulcerating lesions, presenting when the patient has left the area, may make diagnosis more difficult [45]. The four diagnostic laboratory tests for *M. ulcerans* are: (i) direct smear (with acid-fast stains auramine O or Ziehl–Neelsen); (ii) culture at 32°C; (iii) histopathology; and (iv) PCR [2]. Lesion sampling techniques include swabbing, punch biopsy and, as a less invasive alternative to biopsy, fine-needle

aspiration [46]. IS2404 PCR is the gold standard for confirmation and it has the highest sensitivity with results possibly available within 48 h [47,48]. The WHO has a programme to improve access to the test globally (70% access by the end of 2014) but direct smears are useful at the community level where PCR is not available.

The availability of point-of-care testing for *M. ulcerans* disease will potentially have a positive impact on case management. Recently, recombinase polymerase amplification (RPA) and loop-mediated isothermal amplification (LAMP) have been evaluated as point-of-care assays. RPA assay for *M. ulcerans* (Mu-RPA), available in a portable suitcase has been used as an alternative to PCR, especially in areas with limited infrastructure [49]. A BU-LAMP assay based on the LAMP technique is being investigated as it may be easier and faster to use in the field than conventional PCR [50].

Pharmacological assays to detect mycolactone in tissues infected with *M. ulcerans* may become a diagnostic adjunct to culture [51,52]. Regardless of the test or sampling method, at least two sites per lesion suspicious for *M. ulcerans* should be sampled; this process increases sensitivity over a single sample by up to 25% [2].

Management

Historically, skin lesions have been excised, although the recurrence rate approaches 16% at 1 year for small lesions [53] and reaches 28% among late severe cases, which often require extensive radical surgery and grafting and may result in significant morbidity [1,54]. Significant progress has been made since WHO introduced a regimen of rifampicin plus streptomycin in 2004 following encouraging preliminary data [55]. In 2010, a randomised controlled trial from Ghana showed no significant difference in the proportion of patients with moderate lesions achieving cure after receiving the WHO recommended 8-week course of rifampicin and streptomycin chemotherapy, compared with the proportion who achieved cure after receiving 4 weeks of streptomycin and rifampicin followed by 4 weeks of rifampicin plus clarithromycin [56].

Combination antibiotic therapy with intramuscular streptomycin (15 mg/kg) and oral rifampicin (10 mg/kg) daily for 8 weeks was used to treat *M. ulcerans* disease, dramatically improving healing and reducing relapses [57,58]. Streptomycin required prolonged intramuscular injections and was associated with a risk of ototoxicity [59]. This combination is no longer recommended.

Following successful clinical trials, daily oral treatment with rifampicin and clarithromycin is now recommended [60]. The current recommended treatment for *M. ulcerans* disease is a full oral antibiotics regimen comprising rifampicin 10 mg/kg body weight daily (maximum 600 mg) combined with clarithromycin 7.5 mg/kg body weight twice daily (maximum 1000 mg) daily for 8 weeks (56 doses).

First line
Oral rifampicin 10 mg/kg and oral clarithromycin 15 mg/kg should be given for 8 weeks. Surgery should be considered in addition after antibiotic therapy.

Second line
Rifampicin and moxifloxacin may be given daily for 8 weeks in adults.

Paradoxical reaction
The paradoxical reaction is an immune-mediated phenomenon observed in some patients with *M. ulcerans* disease that is characterised by worsening of the existing lesion(s) with attendant pain and occurrence of new lesions during or after antibiotic therapy following an initial period of clinical improvement (Figure 27.33). The paradoxical reaction is thought to be due to an immunological response to residual *M. ulcerans* antigens which are known to persist for many months after successful treatment [61]. The exact pathogenesis of the paradoxical reaction remains unknown but one hypothesis is that it is caused by an inflammatory reaction that, prior to antibiotic treatment, is suppressed by mycolactone. As the *M. ulcerans* organisms are killed by antibiotics, mycolactone production ceases and its suppressive effect is lost causing a rebound of inflammation. The paradoxical reaction is analogous to paradoxical reactions in tuberculosis and HIV coinfected patients when ART restores the immune response. The prevalence rates of paradoxical reaction varies from 8% to 22% in Africa and Australia, with time to development of paradoxical reaction following treatment initiation also varying widely from a few weeks in some patients to several

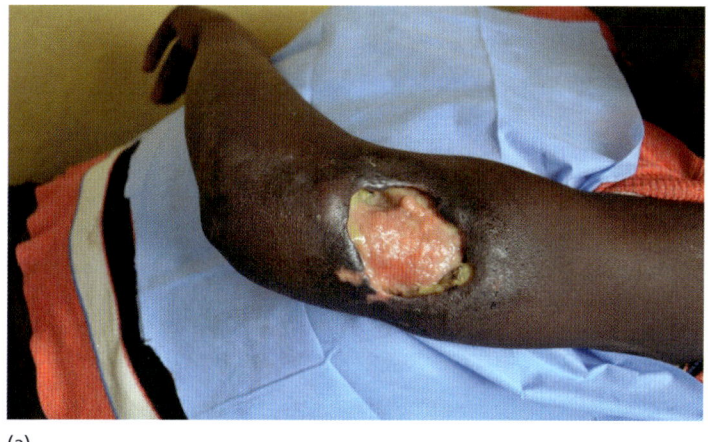 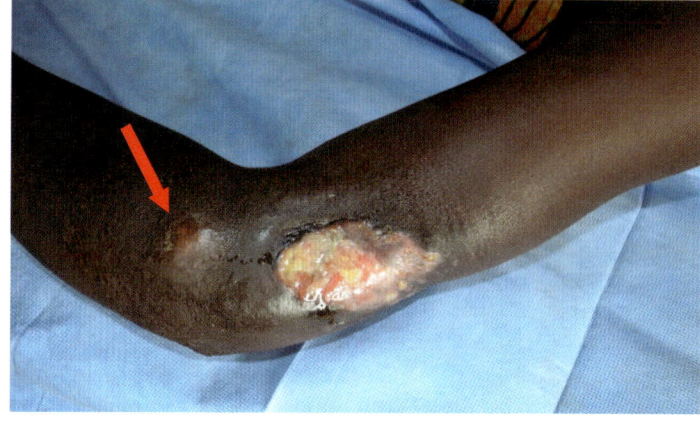

(a) (b)

Figure 27.33 *Mycobacterium ulcerans* infection. (a) Ulcerative form of *M. ulcerans* disease before antibiotic initiation. (b) The paradoxical reaction developed 3 weeks after completion of 8 weeks of combination rifampicin and streptomycin. A new lesion can be seen close to the original ulcer. Courtesy of Dr Richard Phillips.

months in others [62–65]. Paradoxical reactions are thought to be associated with high bacterial load [65].

Awareness of this may prevent unnecessary treatment change. Some cases have been treated with corticosteroids [66]. BCG vaccination appears to offer some short-term protection against *M. ulcerans* and may protect against osteomyelitis [67].

Stigma, mental health and social burden of *M. ulcerans* disease

The debilitating impact of *M. ulcerans* disease negatively affects not only patients but also their caregivers to a significant degree. The lesions may heal with severe disfiguring scars, leading to contractures and functional limitations. These can be common sequelae especially in the absence of appropriate early medical treatment and measures aimed at preventing disability. The disabling and disfiguring scarring as well as stigma associated with the disease reported results in mental distress in affected persons and can result in persisting social participation restrictions even among patients with past infection [68,69]. The debilitating nature of *M. ulcerans*, the young median age of disease occurrence, the significant financial burden and frequent hospital visits leads to a wide-ranging role for caregivers such as relatives and family [70]. Thus, *M. ulcerans* disease caregivers face substantial physical, psychological and financial distress and a reduced quality of life as a result of their caregiving role [70].

The social and mental health impact of *M. ulcerans* disease highlights the importance of national control programmes to work to integrate psychosocial and other support services in the management of *M. ulcerans* patients in their countries.

Mycobacterium avium complex (*M. avium* and *M. intracellulare*) infection

Introduction and general description

Chronic pulmonary infection is the most common form of human disease, with lesions similar to tuberculosis. In immunocompetent hosts, infection usually occurs in patients with predisposing lung conditions, which include pneumoconiosis, silicosis and cystic fibrosis. The prognosis is strongly influenced by the associated disease [1,2]. Osteomyelitis [3] and granulomatous tenosynovitis [4] have both been reported, and in countries with low rates of tuberculosis, *M. avium* complex (MAC) is the commonest cause of cervical lymphadenitis in children [5,6].

Epidemiology
Incidence and prevalence

Disseminated infections with MAC were rare before the emergence of HIV infection and peaked before the widespread use of ART [7]. Prior to the use of ART, MAC affected up to 50% of individuals with AIDS [8,9]. MAC remains an important cause of opportunistic infection in the immunosuppressed and may also cause an immune reconstitution inflammatory syndrome (IRIS) in those individuals with HIV being treated with ART [10].

Pathophysiology
Predisposing factors

Immunosuppression is most commonly due to HIV infection. A review of the published cases in patients without HIV infection emphasises the frequent association with haematological malignancies (particularly hairy cell leukaemia), connective tissue disease and corticosteroid or cytotoxic therapy [11,12].

Causative organisms

This complex comprises the closely related organisms *M. avium* and *M. intracellulare*, which can be differentiated using PCR-aided DNA–DNA hybridisation or LAMP [13]. They are slow-growing organisms with optimal growth at 37°C and are ubiquitous saprophytes, found in tap water, soil, dairy products, animals and house dust [1]. Both the respiratory and gastrointestinal tracts serve as portals for systemic infection, and as many as 30% of normal faecal samples yield isolates of MAC [14]. Skin involvement secondary to disseminated disease is uncommon and primary skin infection is rare [15].

Clinical feature
Presentation

Involvement of the skin is uncommon, but can occur either following traumatic skin inoculation in cervical lymphadenitis, in which case sinus formation is indistinguishable from tuberculous scrofuloderma, or in immunocompromised hosts, in whom MAC may disseminate from primary visceral lesions. Skin lesions are of variable appearance and include multiple ulcers [16], nodules (Figure 27.34a) [17], ulcerated nodules, abscesses [18], painless nodules and plaques resembling lepromatous leprosy [19] or lupus vulgaris (Figure 27.34b) [20] as well as lesions resembling prurigo nodularis [21]. Sporotrichoid spread [22] and lichen scrofulosorum have been reported with MAC infection [23].

In HIV-infected patients, the most common manifestation of MAC infection is mycobacteraemia, but skin lesions may provide a clue to the presence of disseminated MAC infection. Infection tends to occur late in HIV disease and most frequently in patients whose CD4+ cell counts have fallen below 50 cells/μL [9]. The incidence is decreasing due to ART and the use of prophylactic antibiotics where indicated [24]. On starting ART, some patients may experience MAC IRIS due to restoration of delayed hypersensitivity and cytokine production. Symptoms include fever, lymphadenitis and cutaneous lesions [10,25].

Investigations

The diagnosis may be made by blood culture or by the culture of MAC from the bone marrow or a liver biopsy. In patients with cutaneous lesions, the culture of skin biopsy specimens or aspirated seropurulent fluid may give positive results. Tissue staining for acid-fast bacilli is often negative. Histology shows non-caseating granulomas, and sometimes acid-fast bacilli within giant cells or extracellularly. Identification of MAC DNA in affected tissues using PCR may be useful in cases where the organism cannot be grown [26].

Management

The treatment of MAC has greatly improved with the use of the macrolide antibiotics clarithromycin and azithromycin and of

Non-tuberculous (atypical) mycobacteria

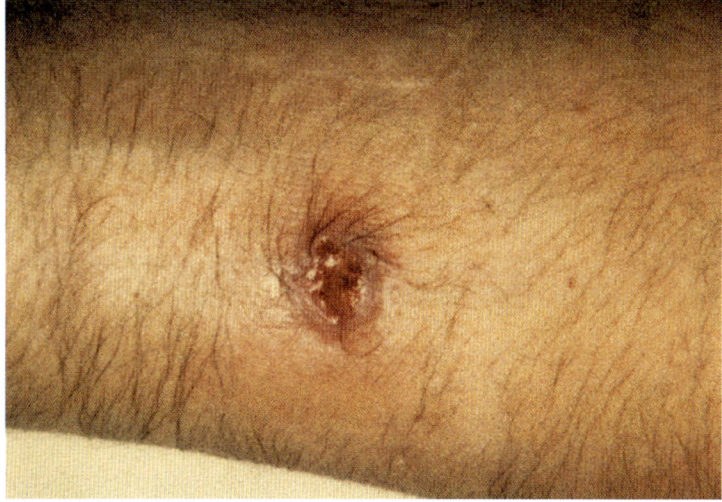

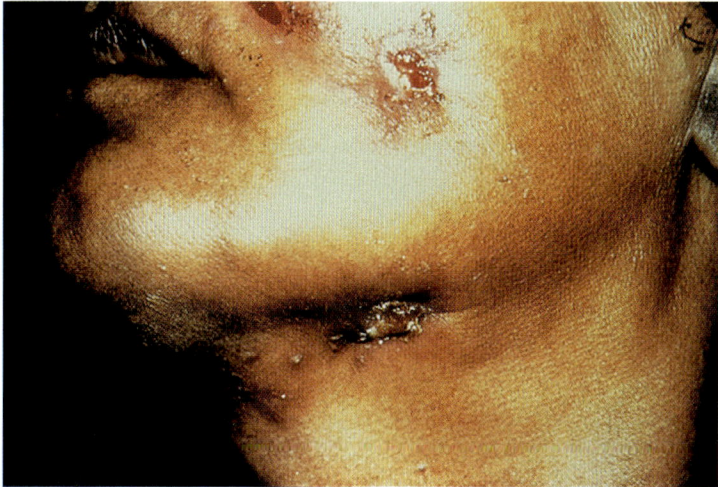

Figure 27.34 *Mycobacterium avium* complex infection. (a) Presenting as a red nodule with central ulceration on the extensor aspect of the forearm in an immunosuppressed patient with systemic lupus erythematosus. (b) Infection of the left cheek and submandibular area, showing sinuses and resembling lupus vulgaris. Courtesy of Dr P. Kullavanijaya.

rifabutin. HIV-positive individuals with a CD4+ count of less than 50 cells/µL should be considered for prophylaxis with azithromycin or clarithromycin if they are not able to accept ART or ART is failing [27].

First line
Patients with lymphadenitis are treated with surgical excision of the affected nodes [28]. Surgical excision has also been used in some patients with localised skin lesions [17]. In HIV-associated MAC disease, a macrolide in combination with ethambutol is the minimum recommended treatment. The addition of rifabutin is advised in cases where there is profound immunosuppression, marked symptoms or no viable ART options [27]. It is recommended that treatment be continued lifelong or until there is an adequate response to ART. In immunocompetent patients with extrapulmonary disease, chemotherapy should probably be continued for 18–24 months.

Mycobacterium haemophilum infection

Introduction and general description
Mycobacterium haemophilum was first described in 1978 in a patient with Hodgkin disease [1]. It is an increasingly recognised pathogen in immunocompromised patients, including those with HIV infection, following organ transplantation and in patients with haematological malignancies or those requiring prolonged immunosuppression including with biologic agents [2].

Pathophysiology
Pathology
Histologically, suppurative granulomas containing acid-fast bacilli are usually seen, but occasionally granulomas may be poorly formed and have varying amounts of necrosis [3].

Causative organisms
- *Mycobacterium haemophilum*.

Environmental factors
The natural habitat and means of acquisition of *M. haemophilum* are unknown although water sources are strongly suspected [4].

Clinical features
Presentation
Mycobacterium haemophilum typically causes red or violaceous papules and nodules that enlarge to become painful abscesses or ulcers (Figure 27.35) and occasionally may present as annular plaques [4,5] or panniculitis. Lesions typically occur on the extremities and are often situated over joints. This may reflect the low optimal growth requirements and a predilection to grow on cooler areas of the body. Systemic features such as weight loss, tenosynovitis, joint effusions, osteomyelitis or respiratory tract symptoms may coexist.

This pathogen causes cutaneous, synovial and less frequently pulmonary or disseminated infections [4]. It has also been isolated from otherwise healthy, immunocompetent children with lymphadenitis [6], and in one series was recovered from 18% of children with cervico-facial lymphadenitis [7]. There are case reports of cutaneous *M. haemophilum* infection associated with tattooing in immunocompetent adults [8,9].

Differential diagnosis
The differential diagnosis includes *M. marinum* and MAC infections, other bacterial infections and Kaposi sarcoma.

Investigations
Mycobacterium haemophilum may be cultured from the skin or other tissues or secretions, but has unique growth requirements and therefore may be underrecognised and underreported. It grows optimally at 30–32°C and the growth medium must contain iron. The organism can be identified by sequencing of the 16S rRNA *rpoB* and *hsp65* genes [4].

Management
There are currently no standardised guidelines for the treatment of *M. haemophilum* infection. The most recent comprehensive review of

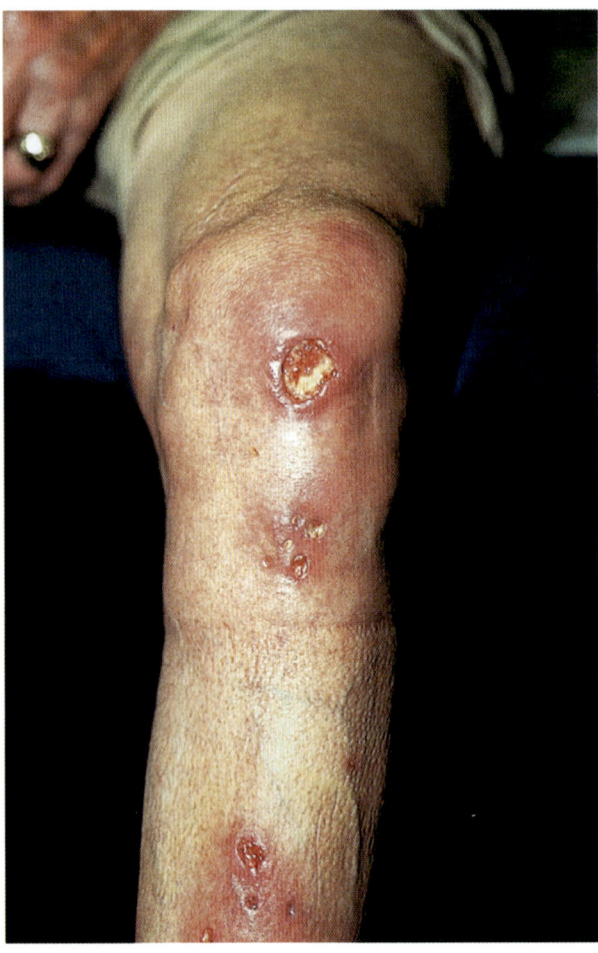

Figure 27.35 *Mycobacterium haemophilum* infection producing ulcerated nodules on the left knee and shin, with a non-ulcerated nodule on the medial aspect of the knee. Courtesy of Dr J. C. Murray.

the subject states that there is general agreement that patients should be treated with multiple antibiotics for 12–24 months.

First line
The regimen usually consists of at least three drugs. The antibiotic combination favoured is clarithromycin, ciprofloxacin and a rifamycin [4]. The organism is resistant to isoniazid and ethambutol. Treatment is difficult. Lesions may persist despite therapy or relapse after treatment is stopped. In immunocompetent children with lymphadenitis, surgical excision is the treatment of choice. People diagnosed with HIV are usually started on ART.

Mycobacterium scrofulaceum infection

Definition
Mycobacterium scrofulaceum has been primarily associated with cervical lymphadenitis in children. It can also cause disseminated infection, pulmonary disease and skin lesions. Its incidence has been declining and cases are now rarely documented [1].

Introduction and general description
Mycobacterium scrofulaceum is a slow-growing scotochromogen. Historically, *M. scrofulaceum* has been associated with cervical lymphadenitis in young children and was the most common cause of lymphadenitis in children until the 1970s. In recent years, the frequency of this infection has declined and there are now more cases caused by MAC [2]. Recent studies have shown that the newly described species *M. parascrofulaceum* may account for many of the clinical isolates [3]. Cutaneous infections are rare and are usually part of disseminated infection.

Epidemiology
Incidence and prevalence
The organism is most prevalent in southeastern USA. It has been isolated from water, raw milk, other dairy products, pooled oysters and soil [4]. The route of infection is primarily by ingestion or inhalation. The numbers of organism isolates from drinking water in the USA have been declining and *M. scrofulaceum* is now rarely recovered [5].

Skin lesions due to *M. scrofulaceum* are extremely rare.

Age
This infection most commonly affects young children.

Pathophysiology
Predisposing factors
Impaired immunity as occurs in HIV infection, haematological malignancies, amyloidosis and being on immunosuppressive drugs are all predisposing factors for infection [6].

Pathology
Abscess formation is seen in the lymph nodes and can be difficult to differentiate from tuberculosis. Acid-fast bacilli are usually noted. Skin lesions may show central necrosis with abscess formation surrounded by granulomatous inflammation with lymphocytes, epithelioid histiocytes and foamy macrophages and, occasionally, acid-fast bacilli [7]. Hyperkeratosis and acanthosis may be seen in the epidermis [6].

Causative organisms
- *Mycobacterium scrofulaceum*.

Clinical features
Presentation
Patients usually present with swelling and sometimes sinuses of the submandibular and submaxillary glands. These evolve slowly and are often unilateral with few constitutional symptoms apart from mild neck pain [8]. They may resolve spontaneously. Skin lesions can present as a nodule, abscess, plaque or ulcerative lesion [6,9]. A patient with sporotrichoid lesions has been reported [10] and chronic ulcerative and nodular skin lesions associated with pulmonary infection were seen in a patient with HIV infection [11]. Disseminated infection in a child with IFN-γ receptor 1 deficiency has recently been reported [12].

Differential diagnosis
Other causes of cervical lymphadenopathy including scrofuloderma due to *M. tuberculosis* and MAC infection should be excluded.

M. marinum infection should be included in the differential in cases demonstrating sporotrichoid spread.

Investigations
Biopsy specimens should be taken for culture and histology. Cultures may also be performed on fine-needle aspirates from infected lymph nodes and sputum in cases with pulmonary involvement. PCR examination may be necessary to differentiate *M. scrofulaceum* from *M. parascrofulaceum* [1].

Management
There are no clear guidelines for treatment, emphasising the need to perform susceptibility testing on confirmed disease-producing isolates of *M. scrofulaceum* [1,8].

First line
Surgical treatment of infected lymph nodes is probably the treatment of choice as *M. scrofulaceum* exhibits *in vitro* resistance to numerous antibiotics [13]. Treatment of more widespread disease is similar to that for MAC as isolates of *M. scrofulaceum* have a similar susceptibility pattern [14]. One patient had resolution of skin lesions after 9 months of therapy with isoniazid and rifampicin [9]. Clarithromycin has been shown to have *in vitro* activity against *M. scrofulaceum* [4], and localised cutaneous infection in a previously healthy child was successfully treated with monotherapy with clarithromycin for 6 months [6].

Mycobacterium szulgai infection

Introduction and general description
Mycobacterium szulgai was first described in 1972 and has a worldwide distribution. Infection is principally pulmonary, but infections have also involved bursae, tendon sheaths, bones, lymph nodes and skin. Skin lesions include diffuse cellulitis, nodules and sinuses [1], and multiple inflammatory skin lesions [2]. In one case report an individual who presented with an isolated skin ulcer subsequently developed acute respiratory distress syndrome secondary to pulmonary involvement [3]. In one series intralesional and systemic corticosteroids were shown to be a risk factor for the development of skin lesions [4].

Management
First line
Isoniazid, rifampicin, ethambutol and streptomycin have been used for the treatment of *M. szulgai* infection [5].

Infection with fast-growing mycobacteria

Definition
These mycobacteria are very common in the environment and are fast growing in humans. They include the *M. abscessus* group, *M. chelonae*, *M. fortuitum* group and *M. smegmatis*. They can infect healthy individuals, but most frequently cause disease in the immunosuppressed.

Epidemiology
Incidence and prevalence
A review of 63 patients with skin or soft-tissue infections due to rapidly growing mycobacteria showed that patients with *M. chelonae* and *M. abscessus* were more likely to be older than 45 years, to be taking immunosuppressive medication and to have multiple disseminated lesions. This was in contrast to patients with *M. fortuitum* infection who were more likely to have a single lesion following surgery or injury at the infected site [1]. Conditions associated with disseminated infection include organ transplantation, rheumatoid arthritis, renal failure and autoimmune disorders. Disease due to *M. chelonae* is strongly associated with concomitant corticosteroid therapy [2].

Pathophysiology
Pathology
Abscess formation in the dermis and subcutis is the rule, but tuberculoid granulomas with or without necrosis may occur (Figure 27.36).

Causative organisms
These organisms are widely distributed in the environment in soil and water and may also be commensal organisms of human skin. They are extremely hardy; members of the *M. fortuitum* group and *M. smegmatis* can grow at 45°C, and *M. chelonae* and members of the *M. abscessus* group and *M. mucogenicum* resist the activity of organomercurials, chlorine, 2% concentrations of formaldehyde and other commonly used disinfectants [3]. These organisms are commonly isolated from municipal tap water [3,4]. *M. chelonae* has been found as a contaminant in a solution of gentian violet [5] and tattoo ink [6]. *M. abscessus* has been isolated from contaminated lidocaine [7] and histamine solutions [8]. Clusters of cases (and pseudo-outbreaks) have most commonly related to contaminated bronchoscopes and endoscopic cleaning machines and to contaminated hospital water supplies [3].

Clinical features
Presentation
Clinical cutaneous disease with these pathogens seems to follow two patterns. In the immunocompetent host, a traumatic injury (including tattooing and surgical procedures) is followed by the development of localised abscess formation [9]. In the immunocompromised individual, there may be no history of trauma and patients may present with disseminated disease, with multiple subcutaneous nodular lesions, positive blood cultures, cervical lymphadenitis, keratitis and occasionally endocarditis and central nervous system involvement [10,11].

The *M. fortuitum* group accounts for 60% of community-acquired, localised cutaneous infection caused by rapidly growing mycobacteria, but is a rare cause of pulmonary disease. This group is also responsible for the majority of health care associated (nosocomial) cases of postsurgical wound infections and catheter infections [11]. *M. fortuitum* infection has been reported in the sternum after open heart surgery [12], as a cause of peritonitis in patients receiving continuous ambulatory peritoneal dialysis [13], after localised microinjections (mesotherapy) for pain control [14] and after some cosmetic procedures such as liposuction [15] and prosthetic

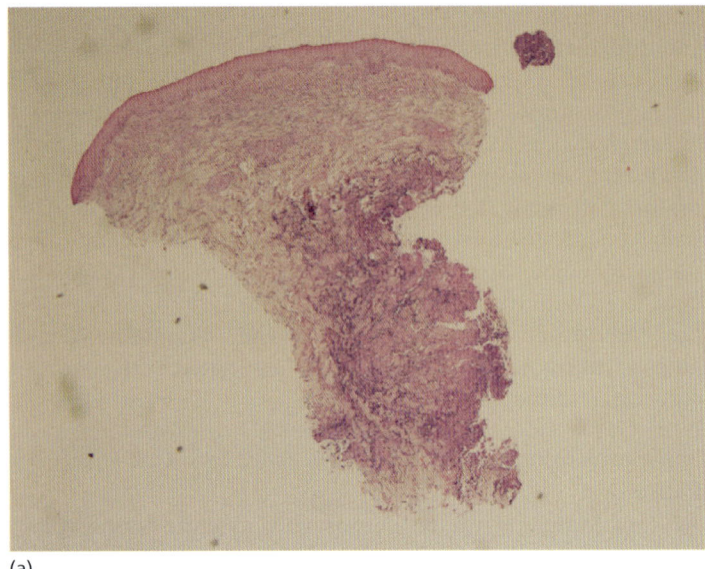 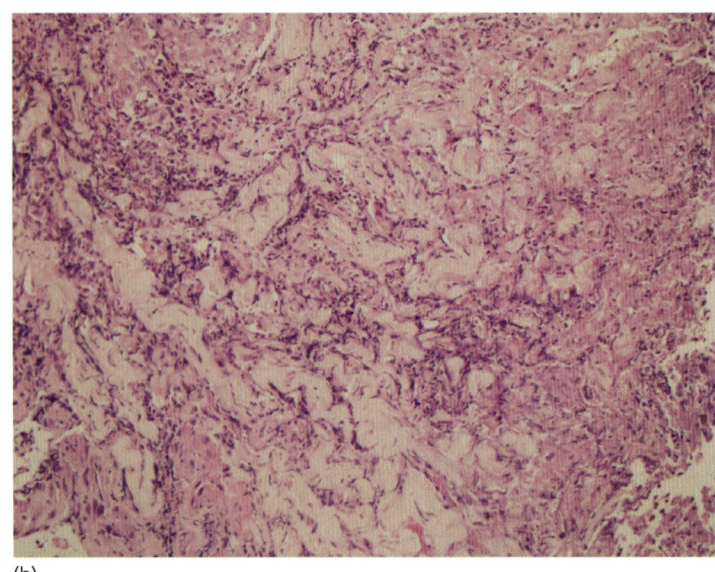

Figure 27.36 *Mycobacterium abscessus* infection. (a) Cellular infiltrate in the mid and deep dermis. (b) A heavy infiltrate of neutrophils and nuclear dust in the mid and deep dermis with abscess formation. Courtesy of Dr D. Rozenman.

breast implants [16]. An outbreak of over 60 cases of *M. fortuitum* furunculosis was caused by infected whirlpool footbaths in a nail salon [17]. A patient with lupus vulgaris-like lesions has also been described [18].

M. chelonae and the *M. abscessus* group are responsible for approximately 95% of disseminated cutaneous infections caused by rapidly growing mycobacteria [10]. These organisms also cause chronic lung disease and are one of the most common isolates from cystic fibrosis patients. Postinjection abscesses are probably the commonest skin lesions caused by *M. abscessus*, which is the most pathogenic and chemotherapy resistant of the rapidly growing mycobacteria [19,20] (Figure 27.37). An outbreak in 12 patients at an ear, nose and throat clinic in 1969 was due to contaminated histamine injections [8]. Two hundred and thirty-two individuals in Colombia were infected with *M. abscessus* following intradermal injections performed by an alternative medical practitioner [7]. Infections have been reported after liposuction and liposculpture [15] and in medical tourists returning to the USA after cosmetic procedures undertaken abroad [21]. Haemodialysis is also a risk factor [19]. A survey in the USA found that NTM were recovered from 83% of water supplies to dialysis units [4]. Two employees at a hot spring bath in Korea developed sporotrichoid lesions due to *M. abscessus* and were assumed to have been contaminated from the bath water [22].

M. chelonae causes community-acquired disease – for example, post-traumatic skin or soft-tissue infection, bone infection and disseminated cutaneous infection; after surgery and related catheter use [2]; and after injections (including acupuncture [23]). Implanted porcine heart valves themselves may be contaminated with *M. chelonae* [24]. Disseminated red subcutaneous nodules are the commonest manifestation, most commonly seen on the distal parts of the limbs (Figure 27.38), or in a sporotrichoid pattern [25]. Localised cellulitis, subcutaneous abscesses and osteomyelitis (usually following skin injury) are also seen. Sixty-two per cent of patients infected with *M. chelonae* in one series were receiving corticosteroids and 72% were immunosuppressed [1]. Widespread infection is rare, although recently there was a report of an immunocompetent individual who succumbed to complications of *M. chelonae* endocarditis [26]. It has also been reported in association with hidradenitis suppurativa and diabetes [27]. HIV infection does not appear to increase the risk of *M. chelonae* infection.

Infections involving *M. smegmatis* have included cellulitis, localised abscesses, osteomyelitis following trauma and rarely pneumonia [28]. There have been no reports of disseminated cutaneous infection. Sporadic cases of catheter sepsis and infection after plastic surgery have been noted [10].

Investigations

These infections are easily missed; lesions may be attributed to foreign bodies, deep mycoses or osteitis. The median time from onset of symptoms to diagnosis was 86 days in the largest series available [1]. They should be considered in the differential diagnosis of chronic relapsing nodules and abscesses in immunocompromised individuals. Diagnosis is usually made by the culture of biopsy

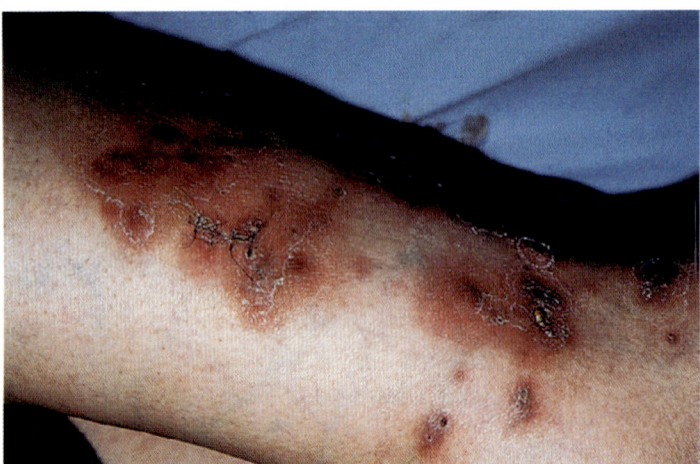

Figure 27.37 *Mycobacterium abscessus* infection causing abscesses. Courtesy of Dr A. G. Smith.

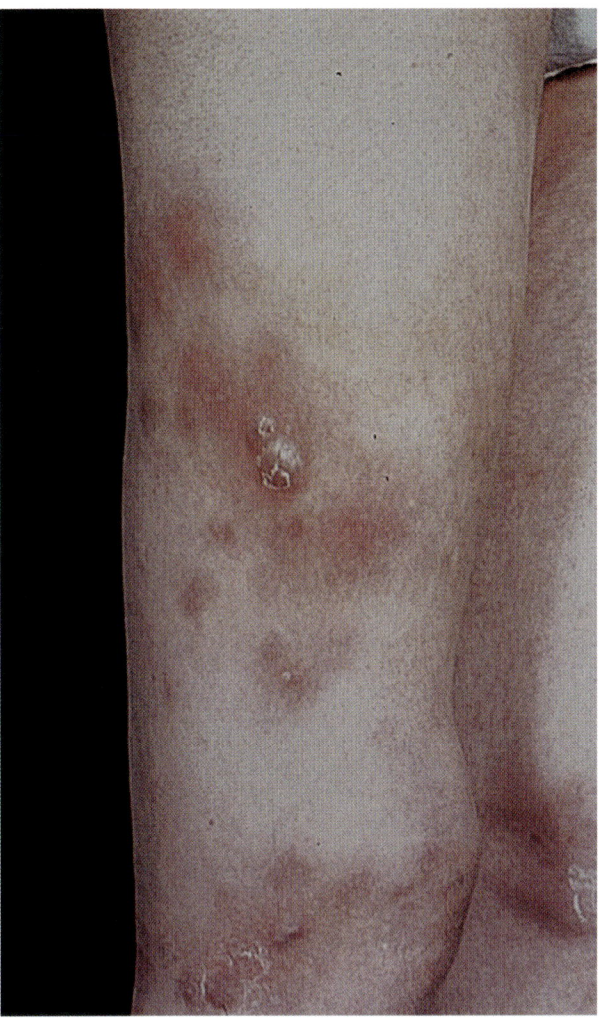

Figure 27.38 *Mycobacterium chelonae* infection of the lower limb. Courtesy of Dr R. D. Ead.

material; in the case of abscesses, a biopsy from the wall is more likely to yield the organism than is aspirated pus. They all have the distinctive ability to produce visible colonies between 5 and 7 days at temperatures ranging between 22 and 45°C, but some strains may fail to grow at 37°C. Their identification is possible by differences in culture requirements, biochemical tests and DNA homology. Clinically, the lesions are not specific to the species involved [9].

Management

There are no available studies that compare different antibacterial regimens. Susceptibility testing of isolates is recommended with the use of empirical therapy until susceptibilities are known. Single lesions may respond to monotherapy but disseminated cutaneous or pulmonary disease requires multidrug therapy. Localised and disseminated infection both usually require prolonged therapy [20].

First line

The *M. fortuitum* group is much less drug resistant than *M. chelonae* or the *M. abscessus* group. The recommended antibacterials with high activity against each species are shown in Table 27.3. The resistance of *M. abscessus* appears largely intrinsic rather than acquired [20]. Surgical debridement of cutaneous lesions may be a useful adjunct to treatment in some patients [29].

Key references

The full list of references can be found in the online version at https://www.wiley.com/rooksdermatology10e

Tuberculosis of the skin
General description

1 Yates VM, Ormerod LP. Cutaneous tuberculosis in Blackburn district (UK): a 15 year prospective series. *Br J Dermatol* 1997;136:483–9.
4 Kumar B, Rai R, Kaur I *et al*. Childhood cutaneous tuberculosis: a study over 25 years from northern India. *Int J Dermatol* 2001;40:26–32.

Table 27.3 Antimicrobials with high activity against different *Mycobacterium* species.

Rapidly growing mycobacteria	Resistance mechanisms	Antimicrobials (with 100% activity)
M. fortuitum group	Tetracycline resistance erm 39 ?Aminoglycoside phosphotransferases	Ciprofloxacin/levofloxacin/moxifloxacin Trimethoprim-sulfamethoxazole Linezolid Imipenem Amikacin Tigecycline
M. abscessus group	erm 41 ? arr	Clarithromycin/azithromycin Linezolid Amikacin Tigecycline
M. chelonae	?	Clarithromycin/azithromycin Linezolid Amikacin Tigecycline
M. smegmatis	erm 39	Sulphonamides Doxycycline Imipenem Amikacin

Adapted from Brown-Elliott *et al*. 2012 [20].

BCG vaccination

5 Evans TG, Brennan MJ, Barker L, Thole J. Preventive vaccines for tuberculosis. *Vaccine* 2013;31S:B223–6.

6 Tameris MD, Hatherill M, Landry BS *et al*. Safety and efficacy of MVA85A, a new tuberculosis vaccine, in infants previously vaccinated with BCG: a randomised, placebo-controlled phase 2b trial. *Lancet* 2013;381:1021–8.

Lupus vulgaris

12 Walker SL, Lozewicz S, Sood R *et al*. Lupus vulgaris due to *Mycobacterium bovis* bacillus Calmette-Guérin at the site of previous BCG vaccination. *Clin Exp Dermatol* 2008;34:e213–15.

Tuberculids
Basic biology

1 Victor T, Jordaans HF, van Niekerk DJ *et al*. Papulonecrotic tuberculid. Identification of *Mycobacterium tuberculosis* DNA by polymerase chain reaction. *Am J Dermatopathol* 1992;14:491–5.

6 Singal A, Bhattacharya SN. Lichen scrofulosorum: a prospective study of 39 patients. *Int J Dermatol* 2005;44:489–93.

Erythema induratum of Bazin

34 Angus J, Roberts C, Kulkarni K. Usefulness of the QuantiFERON test in the confirmation of latent tuberculosis in association with erythema induratum. *Br J Dermatol* 2007;157:1293–4.

Non-tuberculous (atypical) mycobacteria
Mycobacterium marinum infection

27 Harris DM, Keating RK. *Mycobacterium marinum*: current recommended pharmacological treatment. *J Hand Surg Am* 2009;34:1734–5.

Mycobacterium kansasii infection

2 Esteban J, Garća-Pedrazuela M, Muñoz-Egea M C *et al*. Current treatment of nontuberculous mycobacteriosis: an update. *Expert Opin Pharmacother* 2012;13:967–86.

8 Alcaide F, Richter I, Bernasconi C *et al*. Heterogeneity and clonality among isolates of *Mycobacterium kansasii*: implications for epidemiological and pathogenicity studies. *J Clin Microbiol* 1997;35:1959–64.

Mycobacterium ulcerans infection

8 Demangel C, Stinear TP, Cole ST. Buruli ulcer: reductive evolution enhances pathogenicity of *Mycobacterium ulcerans*. *Nat Rev Microbiol* 2009;7:50–60.

57 Phillips RO, Sarfo FS Abass MK *et al*. Clinical and bacteriological efficacy of rifampin-streptomycin combination for two weeks followed by rifampin and clarithromycin for six weeks for treatment of *Mycobacterium ulcerans* disease. *Antimicrob Agents Chemother* 2014;58:1161–6.

60 Phillips RO, Robert J, Abass KM *et al*. Rifampicin and clarithromycin (extended release) versus rifampicin and streptomycin for limited Buruli ulcer lesions: a randomised, open-label, non-inferiority phase 3 trial. *Lancet* 2020;395:1259–67.

65 Frimpong M, Agbavor B, Duah MS *et al*. Paradoxical reactions in Buruli ulcer after initiation of antibiotic therapy: relationship to bacterial load. *PLOS Negl Trop Dis* 2019;13:e0007689.

Mycobacterium scrofulaceum infection

4 Weitzul S, Eichhorn PJ, Pandya AG. Nontuberculous mycobacterial infections of the skin. *Dermatol Clin* 2000;18:359–77.

13 Bartralot R, Garcia-Patos V, Sitjas D *et al*. Clinical patterns of cutaneous nontuberculous mycobacterial infections. *Br J Dermatol* 2005;152:727–34.

CHAPTER 28

Leprosy

Diana N. J. Lockwood and Stephen L. Walker

London School of Hygiene and Tropical Medicine, London, UK

| Leprosy, 28.1 | Key references, 28.17 |

Leprosy

Definition and nomenclature
Leprosy is a chronic granulomatous disease caused by *Mycobacterium leprae*, principally affecting peripheral nerves and skin.

Synonyms and inclusions
- Hansen's disease
- Hanseniasis
- Names in local languages in endemic areas

Introduction and general description
Mycobacterium leprae, discovered by Armauer Hansen in Norway in 1873, was the first bacillus found to be associated with a human disease [1]. Previously, the slow spread of the disease and its familial association suggested that it was inherited. This belief, and the fear of the deformities that leprosy may cause, have contributed to the stigma associated with leprosy and remains a major obstacle to leprosy control. Advances in bacteriology, chemotherapy and epidemiology mean patients today can be reassured that their bacterial infection is readily treatable with antibiotics although associated nerve damage is more difficult to treat. In series of patients seen in London from 1995 to 2018, patients came from 34 different countries with 51% acquiring their infection in South Asia and 19% acquiring their infection in Africa [2].

Epidemiology
Incidence and prevalence
About 4 million people have, or are disabled by, leprosy. Prevalence has fallen due to a combination of effective antibiotic therapy. Incidence, however, remains stable and 202 185 new cases of leprosy were reported to the World Health Organization (WHO) in 2019, from more than 120 countries; the vast majority occurring in South and South-East Asia, South America and Africa. The countries that reported the most new cases were India, Brazil and Indonesia [3]. Leprosy has not always been a tropical disease; for example, it was endemic in Norway until the early 20th century. Nearly all the new cases now seen in Europe and North America acquired their infection abroad [4].

Although leprosy is rarely a primary cause of death, patients have a standardised death rate at least twice that of the general population due to the indirect secondary effects of the disease [5]. It is estimated that 1 million disability-adjusted life years (DALYs) are lost globally each year due to leprosy, with 6.3 years of healthy life being lost per patient.

Age
Leprosy can occur at all ages but there is a peak in the teens and early twenties.

Sex
Leprosy occurs equally in both sexes until puberty then an excess of male cases has regularly been found, although this may be due to women being reluctant to present to health workers with skin lesions [6].

Pathophysiology
Predisposing factors
Living in a leprosy endemic area, age, sex and household contact are risk factors for acquiring leprosy [7]. Bacille Calmette–Guérin (BCG) vaccination protects against leprosy, and clustering of cases is well recognised [8]. Although poor nutritional status was thought to predispose to leprosy, no good evidence substantiates this; improved socioeconomic conditions reduce the risk of leprosy.

Various genes and regions in the human genome have been linked to or associated with susceptibility to leprosy *per se* or with a particular type of leprosy but these are not all reproducible in different populations. Mira *et al.* have identified that certain alleles in the *PARK2* and *PACRG* region on chromosome 6 are associated with susceptibility to leprosy in Vietnamese and Brazilian cohorts [9]. *PARK2* is expressed by both Schwann cells and macrophages. It is a ubiquitin E3 ligase and is involved in the delivery of polyubiquinated proteins to the proteosome complex involved in protein degradation [10]. In an Indian cohort, homozygotes for the different alleles of the vitamin D receptor (*VDR*) gene were associated with tuberculoid or lepromatous disease [11]. Upregulation of the *VDR* gene on macrophages is associated with increased intracellular killing of *M. tuberculosis*.

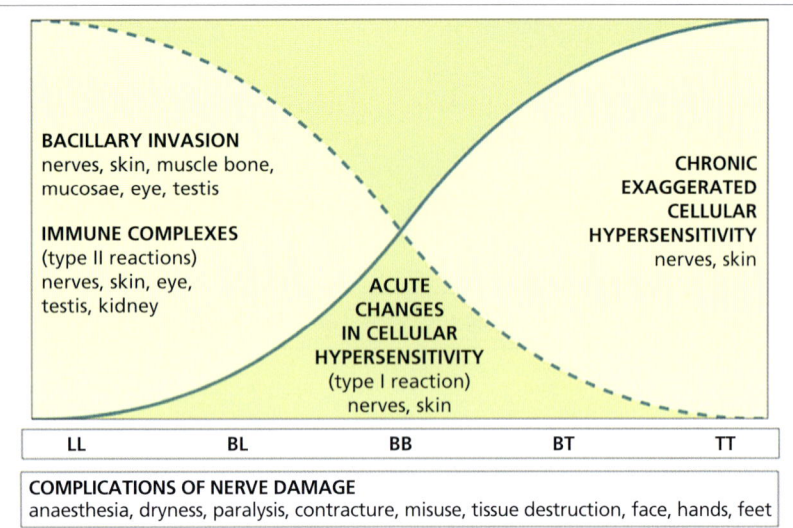

Figure 28.1 Mechanisms of damage in leprosy, and tissues affected. Mechanisms under the broken line are characteristic of disease near the lepromatous end of the spectrum, those under the solid line of the tuberculoid end. They overlap in the centre where, in addition, instability predisposes to type 1 reactions. Abbreviations are given in text.

Polymorphisms of the tumour necrosis factor α (TNF-α) promoter region were shown to be associated with increased susceptibility to lepromatous leprosy (LL) [12], while in a cohort from southern Brazil the same allele was protective against leprosy *per se* [13]. A study of Malawians did not find any association of this TNF promoter with leprosy [14]. Brazilian and Indian groups have demonstrated that polymorphisms of the interleukin 10 (IL-10) promoter are associated with resistance to leprosy [15,16]. The differing and sometimes conflicting results of genetic studies may be attributed to differences in study design and sample size. It is also possible that different populations have distinct genetic susceptibilities.

Early in the human immunodeficiency virus (HIV) epidemic it was predicted that HIV infection would worsen leprosy outcomes with more patients developing lepromatous disease, an impaired response to multidrug therapy (MDT) and fewer reactions. However, none of these has happened and instead HIV immune dysregulation rather than immune suppression dominates the clinical picture in patients with leprosy and HIV. HIV infection does not appear to confer increased susceptibility to leprosy.

Subclinical infection with *M. leprae* is probably common, but the development of established disease is rare. There is no reliable test for determining whether a person has encountered *M. leprae* and has mounted a protective immune response. In contacts of leprosy patients, there is frequently evidence of specific sensitisation to *M. leprae*, using markers of infection such as serum antibody levels, *in vitro* lymphocyte transformation tests (LTTs) and skin test responses to soluble *M. leprae* antigen [17]. Contacts of an untreated elderly man with borderline lepromatous (BL) leprosy in a British residential home showed that 23/30 and 25/30 had positive Mitsuda skin test and positive LTT responses, respectively, to *M. leprae* sonicate, but only two contacts had positive antibody (immunoglobulin M phenolglycolipid (PGL) antigen) responses. Self-healing often occurs in early tuberculoid cases. Leprosy is probably analogous to tuberculosis, in which only 10% of infections manifest as clinical disease [18]. In the 20th century, there were only two reported cases of secondary transmission within Britain, both cases acquired from a known case of leprosy [19].

Nasal discharges from untreated LL patients, who are often undiagnosed for several years, are the main source of infection in the community [20,21]. In Indonesia and Ethiopia, *M. leprae* DNA has been detected in nasal swabs in up to 5% of the population. Infection probably also occurs through the nose. *M. leprae* is inhaled, multiplies on the inferior turbinates and has a brief bacteraemic phase before binding to Schwann cells and macrophages. In patients with the tuberculoid types of leprosy, *M. leprae* remains within the skin and nerve compartments and these patients are probably never infectious.

The skin is unimportant in leprosy transmission. Bacilli are rarely found in the epidermis and are only excreted by untreated LL patients. The only evidence of bacilli entering via the skin comes from case reports of direct inoculation from procedures such as tattooing. There is no evidence that biting arthropods transmit leprosy.

Pathology

Pathogenesis of leprosy [22]. The pathogenesis, and thus the clinical features, reflect four principal causes of tissue damage (Figure 28.1):

1 The degree to which cell-mediated immunity (CMI) is expressed [23]. LL represents a failure of CMI specifically towards *M. leprae* with resultant bacillary multiplication and spread and the accumulation of antigen in infected tissues. The absence of activated lymphocytes and macrophages means that nerve damage is slow and gradual in onset. In tuberculoid leprosy, CMI is strongly expressed, so that the infection is restricted to one or a few skin sites and peripheral nerves. Lymphocytic infiltration rapidly causes nerve damage. Between those two polar forms lie the borderline forms of disease, with the extent of disease reflecting the balance between CMI and bacillary load.

2 The extent of bacillary spread and multiplication. In LL, haematogenous spread of bacilli occurs [24] to cool, superficial sites, including the eyes, upper respiratory mucosa, testes, small muscles and bones of the hands, feet and face, as well as the peripheral nerves and skin. In tuberculoid leprosy, bacillary multiplication is restricted to a few sites and bacilli are not readily found.

3 The appearance of tissue-damaging immunological complications: leprosy reactions [25]. Borderline patients (borderline

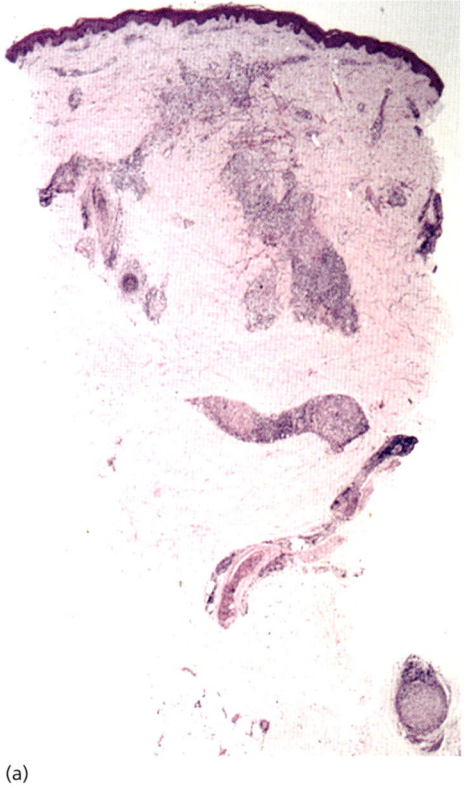
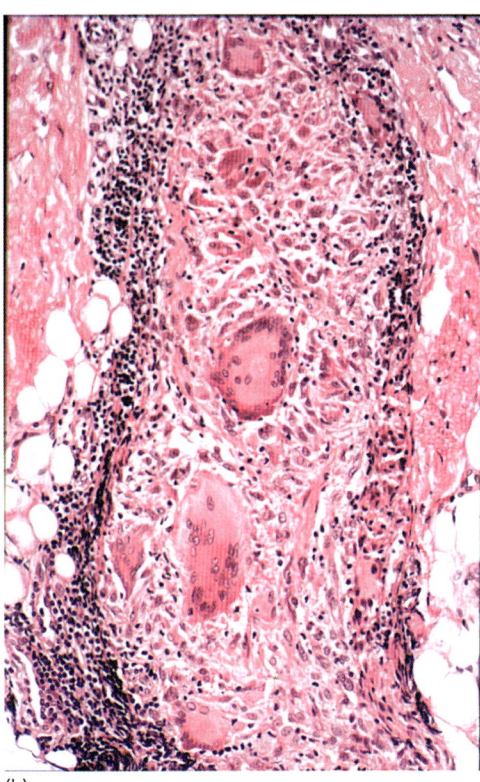

Figure 28.2 (a) Low-power view (H&E) showing tuberculoid granulomas around nerve and skin appendages in the mid-dermis and a swollen, deep dermal nerve. There is no epidermal erosion. Around the granulomas there is a dense lymphocytic infiltrate. (b) Medium-power view (H&E) of a different case showing a deep nerve in tuberculoid leprosy with granulomatous disruption of the nerve with surrounding lymphocytic infiltrate. Courtesy of Professor S. Lucas, Kings College, London, UK.

tuberculoid (BT), borderline borderline (BB) and BL) are immunologically unstable and at risk of developing immune-mediated reactions. Type 1 (reversal) reactions are delayed hypersensitivity reactions caused by an increased recognition of *M. leprae* antigens in skin and nerve sites. Type 2 reactions, erythema nodosum leprosum (ENL), are due in part to immune complex deposition and occur in BL and LL patients who produce antibodies and have a large antigen load.

4 The development of nerve damage and its complications. Nerve damage occurs in two settings, in skin lesions and in peripheral nerve trunks. In skin lesions, the small dermal sensory and autonomic nerve fibres supplying the dermal and subcutaneous structures are damaged, causing local sensory loss and loss of sweating within the area of the skin lesion [26]. Peripheral nerve trunks are vulnerable at sites where they are superficial or are in fibro-osseous tunnels. At these points, a small increase in nerve diameter leads to raised intraneural pressure, with consequent neural compression and ischaemia. Damage to peripheral nerve trunks produces characteristic signs, with dermatomal sensory loss and dysfunction of muscles supplied by that peripheral nerve. Physiological evidence of central and peripheral autonomic nerve involvement has also been reported [27,28].

Nerve damage leads to anaesthesia, muscular weakness and contracture, and autonomic dysfunction. These permit trauma, bruising, burns, cuts and, especially, tissue necrosis from prolonged, inappropriate or repetitive trauma, which in turn lead to ulceration, secondary cellulitis and osteomyelitis and loss of tissue, so that deformity is added to disability.

Histology [22]. *Mycobacterium leprae* has a predilection for neural tissue, and the first evidence of infection is often found in the peripheral nervous system. Patients with early leprosy of both tuberculoid [29,30] and lepromatous types have abnormalities in nerve conduction studies and a histological picture of small fibre loss, with segmental demyelination and remyelination [31]. Bacilli probably enter the nerves via endoneural blood vessels [32], the target cell being the Schwann cell. In the dermis, the type and degree of cellular infiltrate reflects the degree of CMI. The classification of Ridley and Jopling [33] describes five groups on the immunological spectrum designated tuberculoid tuberculoid (TT), BT, BB and BL leprosy and LL. In this classification, epithelioid cells and lymphocytes at the tuberculoid end of the spectrum give place to macrophages, which appear increasingly foamy as the lepromatous pole is reached.

Tuberculoid leprosy. Tuberculoid granulomas collect in foci surrounding neurovascular elements (Figure 28.2). The granuloma invades the papillary zone and may even erode the epidermis, but acid-fast bacilli (AFB) are not seen. Cutaneous nerves that are not destroyed appear greatly swollen by epithelioid cell granulomas and surrounded by a zone of lymphocytes; occasionally there may be caseation within the nerve.

Lepromatous leprosy. Histological examination of skin lesions shows thinning of the epidermis and flattening of rete ridges (Figure 28.3). The papillary layer of the dermis appears as a clear band, while deeper in the dermis lies the typical diffuse leproma consisting of foamy macrophages, with the addition of a few lymphocytes and plasma cells. The dermis contains enormous numbers of AFB, singly or in clumps (globi). With treatment, the leproma shows increased foamy change, vacuolates and breaks

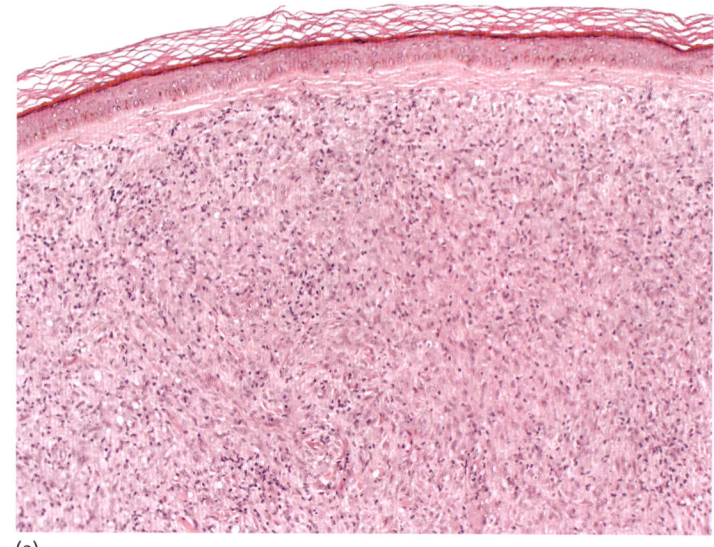

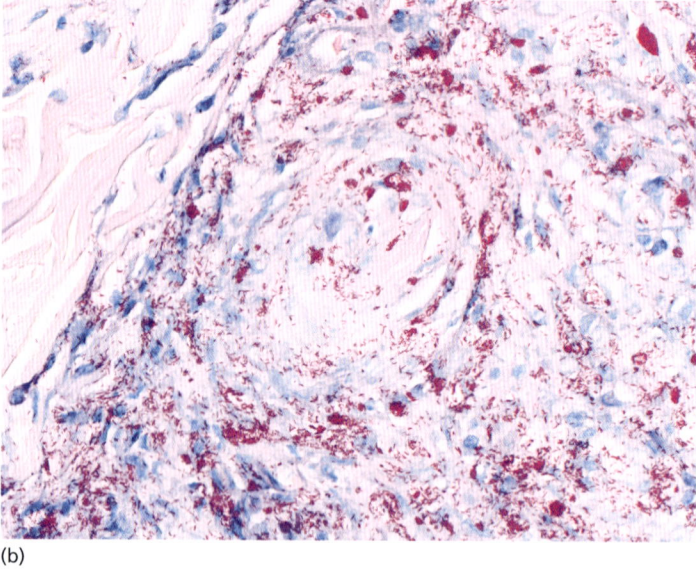

Figure 28.3 (a) Lepromatous leprosy. Medium-power view (H&E) showing a thin epidermis, a clear subepidermal zone and a dense, uniform macrophage infiltrate in the dermis. (b) High-power view (Wade–Fite stain) showing single and clustered acid-fast bacilli, part solid, part fragmented. Courtesy of Professor S. Lucas, Kings College, London, UK.

up into discrete foci with fibrocytes at the periphery. These foci shrink as treatment is continued and bacilli become fragmented and granular. In lepromatous neuropathy, there is quiet asymptomatic bacillation of Schwann cells leading to foamy degeneration of these cells. Demyelination, damage and destruction of the axis cylinder are prominent features and later Wallerian degeneration occurs [34]. Despite the large numbers of organisms in the nerve there is only a small inflammatory response; ultimately the nerve fibroses and is hyalinised [35].

Borderline leprosy. In BT leprosy, the epithelioid cell granuloma is more diffuse than in TT leprosy with a free, but narrow, papillary zone. Giant cells tend to be foreign body rather than Langhans in type, and dermal nerves are moderately swollen by cellular infiltration, or may show only Schwann cell proliferation. AFB are usually absent or scanty. In mid-BB leprosy, there is diffuse epithelioid cell granuloma with scanty lymphocytes and no giant cells; the papillary zone is clear, nerves are slightly swollen by cellular infiltrate and AFB are present in moderate numbers. In BL leprosy, macrophages may show slight foamy change. Lymphocytes are present in dense clumps or are widely distributed in parts of the granuloma; a few epithelioid cells may be seen occasionally. The formation of small granulomas is characteristic of borderline leprosy and granulomatous regions may abut strands of normal looking but heavily bacillated Schwann cells [36]. Nerve damage in borderline leprosy results from a combination of bacillary invasion and inflammation producing widespread nerve damage. Acute neuritis damage occurs particularly during reversal reactions: oedema of the epithelioid cell granuloma compresses the remaining Schwann cells causing rapid functional loss in an already compromised nerve.

Indeterminate leprosy. This early and transitory stage of leprosy occurs in those whose immunological state has not yet been determined, and histologically there is a scattered, non-specific histiocytic and lymphocytic infiltration with some concentration around skin appendages (Figure 28.4). Rarely, a single bacillus will be found within a dermal nerve. The indeterminate phase may last for months or years before resolving or progressing to one of the determinate types of leprosy described earlier.

Reactions: type 1 and erythema nodosum leprosum. Type 1 reactions are characterised by an increase in lymphocytes within lesions, severe oedema with disruption of the granuloma, giant cell formation and human leukocyte antigen (HLA) expression [37,38]. In type 2 (ENL) reactions, neutrophils infiltrate the granuloma and there is vasculitis and macrophage degeneration together with breakdown of foam cells (Figure 28.5).

Immunology [39]. The immune response to *M. leprae* determines not only whether disease will develop, but also which type of leprosy. The highly conserved Toll-like receptors on the surface of monocytes and macrophages recognise mycobacterial lipoproteins [40]. For *M. leprae* the TLR2/1 heterodimer is activated with monocyte differentiation into macrophages and dendritic cells [41]. The latter present antigen and activate naive T cells by IL-12 secretion [42]. The IL-12βR2 portion of the IL-12 receptor is expressed more on T helper 1 (Th1) lymphocytes, preferentially shifting the immune response further towards a Th1 response.

In addition, IL-2 stimulates the expansion of α/β CD8 T cells and antigen non-specific natural killer cells in the lesion. All three types of cell can produce interferon γ (IFN-γ), the major cytokine responsible for activating bactericidal mechanisms within the macrophage [43].

In tuberculoid leprosy, there is good evidence of a strong CMI response. Tests of T-cell function such as LTTs show that tuberculoid leprosy patients respond to *M. leprae* antigens as in whole *M. leprae*, separated *M. leprae* antigens and cloned antigens (18 and 65 kDa) [44]. Skin tests with lepromin, a heat-killed *M. leprae* sonicate preparation, are strongly positive in these patients. Staining of skin biopsies from tuberculoid lesions with T-cell markers shows highly organised granulomas composed predominantly of CD4 cells and

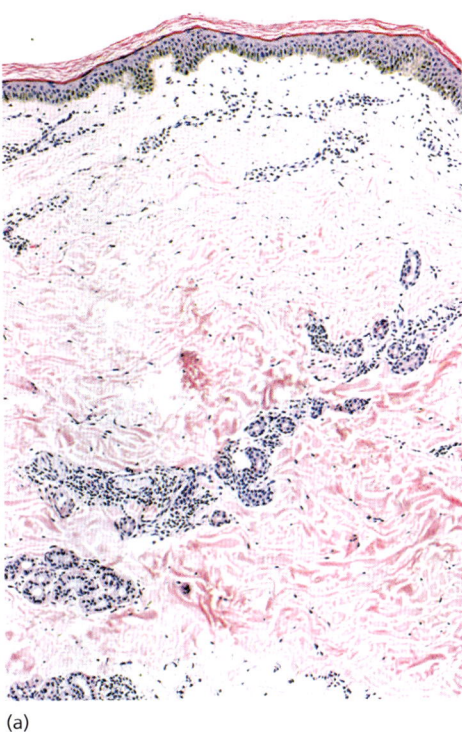
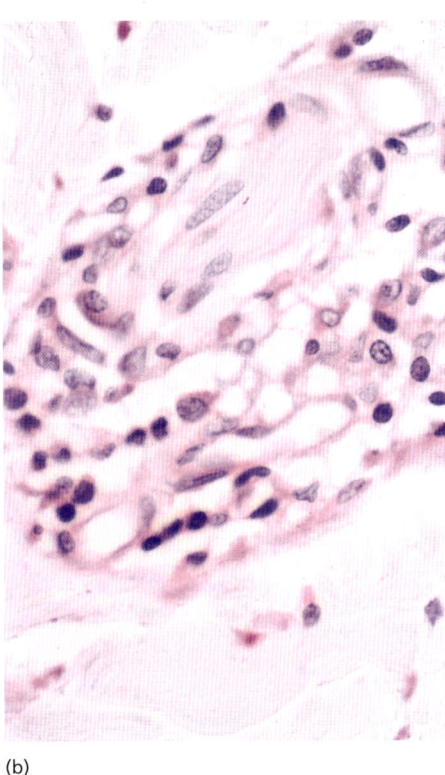

Figure 28.4 (a) Indeterminate leprosy. Low-power view (H&E) showing minimal perineurovascular inflammation in the mid-dermis. (b) High-power view (Wade–Fite stain) showing one acid-fast bacillus in a Schwann cell. Courtesy of Professor S. Lucas, Kings College, London, UK.

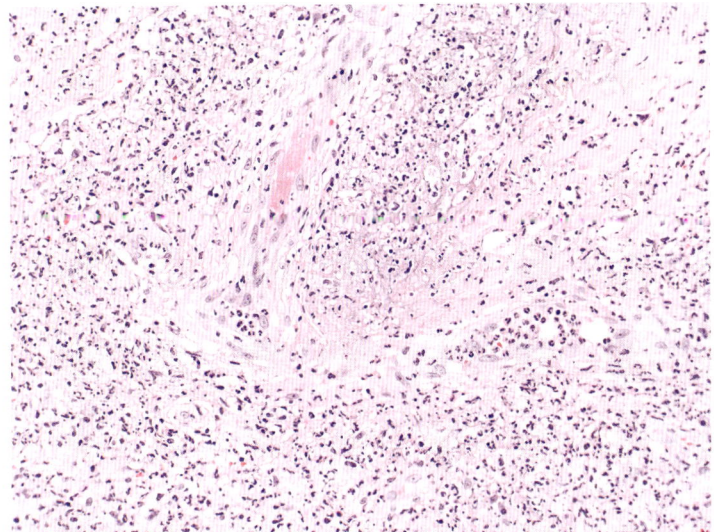

Figure 28.5 Erythema nodosum leprosum. Medium-power view (H&E) showing foamy macrophages with infiltrating polymorphs. There is also a swollen small artery in the centre of the photograph. Courtesy of Professor S. Lucas, Kings College, London, UK.

macrophages, with a peripheral mantle of suppressor/cytotoxic CD8 cells [45]. This strong CMI response has been misdirected at some stage and the result is a late, strong cell-mediated response that clears antigen at the expense of local tissue destruction.

LL patients are unable to mount a CMI response to *M. leprae*, with a failure of the T-cell response, and lymphocytes from LL patients respond poorly in LTTs to whole *M. leprae* and cloned antigens. Similarly, LL patients fail to mount a skin test response to intradermal challenge with lepromin. The anergy of the lepromatous patient is striking because it is specific for the leprosy mycobacterium. Lepromatous patients can respond to antigens of other mycobacteria such as *M. tuberculosis*, both in *in vitro* and in skin tests [46,47]. Identification of cell types in LL granulomas shows them to be a disorganised mixture of macrophages and T cells, mainly CD8 cells [48].

Both T-cell and macrophage dysfunction occur in lepromatous patients. The T-cell failure may be due to clonal anergy or active suppression. Regulatory T cells are increased in LL [49]. Defects in cytokine production have been demonstrated in lepromatous patients; the addition of IL-2 to T-cell culture media restored the proliferative response to *M. leprae* in lepromatous patients [50], and intralesional injections of recombinant IL-2 reconstituted the local immune response with elimination of *M. leprae* from macrophages [51]. Macrophage defects described in LL disease include defective antigen presentation and recognition, defective IL-1 production, a failure of macrophages to kill *M. leprae* and a macrophage suppression of the T-cell response [40].

Studies of circulating cytokines in leprosy patients, and cytokine production in skin lesions, show that tuberculoid patients have a Th1-type response to *M. leprae* with predominant IL-2 and IFN-γ production, while lepromatous patients have low cytokine production, mainly of a Th2 type.

The inflammation seen in type 1 reactions is due to T-cell activity, with enhanced T-cell proliferation towards *M. leprae* antigens, increased numbers of CD4 and IL-2-producing cells in granulomas and local production of cytokines such as IFN-γ and TNF-α [52]. Type 1 reactions are associated with an overproduction of Th1-type cytokines [53]. ENL has classically been regarded as an immune complex disorder. This is supported by the presence of immunoglobulin and complement in the lesions and circulating immune complexes, however evidence for the consistent deposition of immune complexes in affected tissues is lacking [54–56].

There is also evidence of enhanced T-cell activity during ENL episodes, with increased numbers of CD4 cells [57] in the lesions, and production of the cytokines TNF-α and IL-6, increased circulating IL-2 receptors and high levels of circulating TNF-α [58] in acute episodes.

Serology. Specific anti-*M. leprae* antibodies are produced against lipoarabinomannan, PGL and the protein antigens of *M. leprae*. No single antigen has been identified for use in detecting early subclinical infection. For all three types of antigen, multibacillary patients produce antibodies prolifically, while paucibacillary patients show a variable, often undetectable, response.

LL is a hypergammaglobulinaemic state and false positive serological tests of autoantibodies such as rheumatoid factors, anti-DNA, cryoglobulins and cardiolipin may be found.

Causative organisms

Mycobacterium leprae has never been grown *in vitro*. Limited growth has been achieved in the mouse footpad [59], and more widespread growth and disease in immunosuppressed and nude mice [60] and the nine-banded armadillo [61]. Leprosy is a zoonosis in the southern part of the USA for a small number of cases. The latter has provided mycobacteria for genetic and biochemical analysis and the production of trial vaccines. *M. leprae* grows at 30–33°C, with a doubling time of 12 days and remains viable in the environment for up to 10 days [62]. The *M. leprae* genome was sequenced in 2001 and has a 3.27 Mb genome that displays extreme reductive evolution [63]. *M. lepromatosis* has a similar sized genome and causes leprosy in a proportion of cases [64]; less than half the genome contains functional genes and many pseudogenes are present. One hundred and sixty-five genes are unique to *M. leprae*, and functions can be attributed to 29 of them. A comparison of biosynthetic pathways with *M. tuberculosis* shows that *M. leprae* has only two genes for lipolysis (*M. tuberculosis* has 22). *M. leprae* has lost many genes for carbon catabolism, and many carbon sources (e.g. acetate and galactose) are unavailable to it. *M. leprae* growth may be restricted to a few carbon sources on which it can maintain a balanced carbon metabolism. It has also lost anaerobic and microaerophilic electron transfer systems. *M. leprae* has many genes for haem and iron-based proteins, but it is severely limited in its iron uptake capacity since it cannot produce iron scavenging sideropores [65]. Recent genomic analysis of *M. leprae* shows that there are four main strains of the mycobacterium. Recent skeletal evidence shows that *M. leprae* has had a stable genome for at least 10 centuries [66–68].

M. leprae has a complex antigenic cell wall composed of lipids, carbohydrates and proteins. The organism also synthesises a species-specific lipid, PGL [69]. Several polymerase chain reaction (PCR) probes (18, 36 and 65 kDa and ribosomal RNA sequences) have been developed for the detection of *M. leprae* DNA in tissues from leprosy patients [70]. Although these are specific, they are not yet sensitive enough to be useful in diagnosing patients whose skin is bacteriologically negative on staining for AFB. The molecular basis for rifampicin resistance has been elucidated and it is now possible, using a PCR–single-strand polymorphism technique, to identify rifampicin-resistant isolates within hours [71].

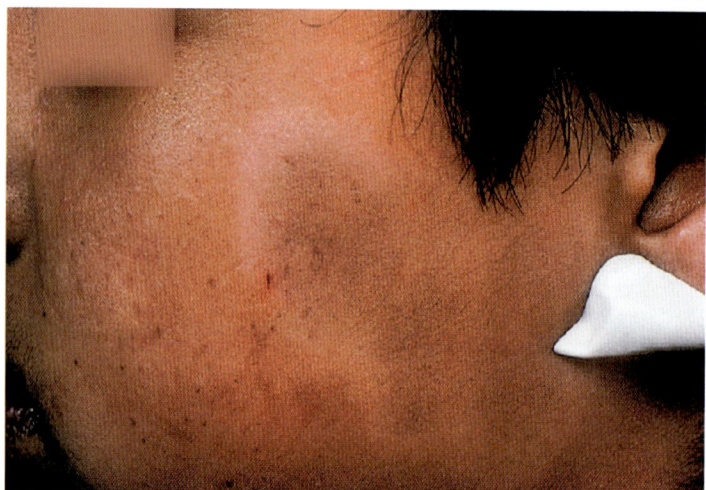

Figure 28.6 Indeterminate leprosy. The face of a Nepali child showing vague hypopigmented patch with some central healing. Note the mark of a recent slit-skin smear.

Clinical features

History

Leprosy is a chronic disease with a long incubation period. Tuberculoid cases have an average incubation time of 2–5 years, and one of 8–12 years for lepromatous cases. American servicemen who developed leprosy after serving in the tropics presented up to 20 years after their presumed exposure [72].

Presentation [73]

Early lesions and presenting symptoms. The classic early skin lesion is of indeterminate leprosy on the face, extensor surface of the limbs, buttocks or trunk (Figure 28.6) [74]. Scalp, axillae, groins and lumbar skin tend to be spared. Indeterminate lesions comprise one or more slightly hypopigmented or red macules, a few centimetres in diameter, with poorly defined margins. Hair growth and nerve function are unimpaired. A biopsy may show the periadenexal infiltrate and only a prolonged search will reveal scanty acid-fast organisms. Alternatively, the initial skin lesion has features of one of the established forms of the disease. The commonest early lesion is an area of numbness on the skin.

Patients frequently present with signs of nerve damage: weakness or anaesthesia due to a peripheral nerve lesion, or a blister, burn or ulcer in an anaesthetic hand or foot. Borderline patients may present with nerve pain, sudden palsy, multiple new skin lesions, pain in the eye or a systemic febrile illness [75,76].

Features of established leprosy. Table 28.1 lists the clinical features of tuberculoid and lepromatous leprosy.

Clinical variants

Tuberculoid leprosy. Only nerves and skin show clinical evidence of disease; lesions are few, often solitary. A skin lesion appears with or without evidence of nerve involvement. The typical lesion is a plaque that is conspicuous, red, copper coloured or purple, with raised and clear-cut edges sloping towards a flattened and

Table 28.1 Characteristics of lesions of polar leprosy.

	Tuberculoid	Lepromatous
Number of lesions	1–10	Hundreds, confluent
Distribution	Asymmetrical, anywhere	Symmetrical, avoiding 'spared' areas
Definition and clarity	Defined edge, markedly hypopigmented	Vague edge, slight hypopigmentation
Anaesthesia	Early, marked, defined, localised to skin lesions or major peripheral nerve	Late, initially slight, ill-defined but extensive, over 'cool' areas of body
Autonomic loss	Early in skin and nerve lesions	Late, extensive as for anaesthesia
Nerve enlargement	Marked, in a few nerves	Slight but widespread
Mucosal and systemic	Absent	Common, severe during type 2 reactions
Number of *Mycobacterium leprae*	Not detectable	Numerous in all affected tissues

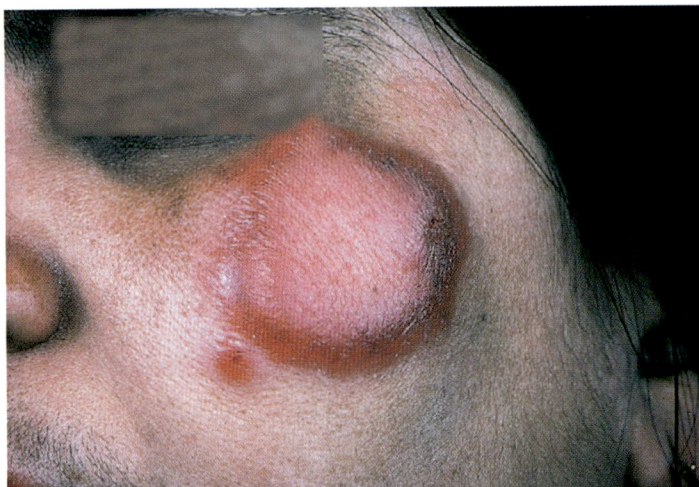

Figure 28.7 Tuberculoid leprosy. The face of a Pakistani woman showing a reddish plaque with a well-defined active edge, and a small satellite lesion. On the face, such lesions may not be anaesthetic.

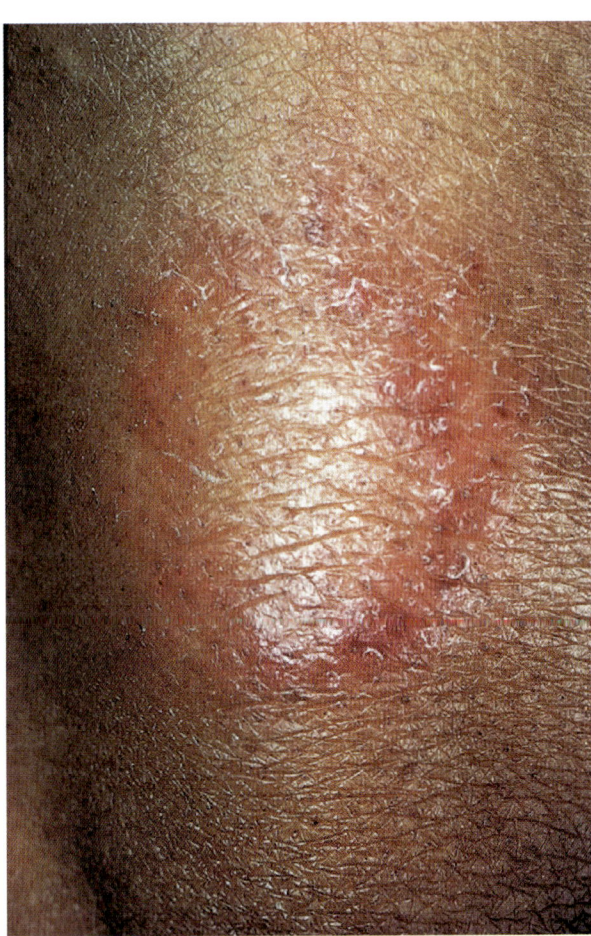

Figure 28.8 Tuberculoid or borderline tuberculoid leprosy. The upper arm of an Indian man, showing a typical dry, hairless, hypopigmented plaque with a scaly, red edge. Such lesions are usually anaesthetic.

hypopigmented centre (Figures 28.7 and 28.8). Redness may not be seen on pigmented skins. The surface is dry, hairless and insensitive, and sometimes scaly. Sensory impairment may be absent on the face because of the large supply of sensory nerve endings. A thickened sensory nerve may be palpated or a thickened nerve trunk felt locally, for example a thickened ulnar nerve with an arm lesion. Less commonly the lesion is a macule, red in light skins and hypopigmented (never depigmented) in dark skins (Figure 28.9). Such macules have a dry, hairless and insensitive surface.

Lepromatous leprosy. The first clinical manifestations are dermal with macules, diffuse papules, infiltration or nodules, or all four. Macules are small, multiple, red or faintly hypopigmented, with vague edges and shiny surface (Figure 28.10). Papules and nodules usually have a normal skin colour but sometimes are red (Figure 28.11), with a bilaterally symmetrical distribution on the face, arms, legs and buttocks, but may be anywhere apart from the hairy scalp, axillae, groins and perineum (i.e. regions of the skin with the highest temperature). Hair growth and sensation are not initially impaired over the lesions. In polar LL, diffuse infiltration and gradual thickening of the dermis may precede nodule formation by months or years (Figure 28.12). Lesions of the oral mucosa occur as papules on the lips and nodules on the palate (which may perforate), uvula, tongue and gums (Figure 28.13). The nasal mucosa may be hyperaemic, and epistaxis is now rare (Figure 28.14).

The longest peripheral sensory nerve fibres are first affected, causing numbness and anaesthesia on the dorsal surfaces of the hands and feet, and later on the extensor surfaces of the arms and legs, and finally over the trunk. Infiltration of corneal nerves causes anaesthesia, which predisposes to injury, infection and blindness if there is also lagophthalmos due to damage to the facial nerve.

In untreated LL, the lines of the forehead become deeper as the skin thickens (leonine facies), the eyebrows and eyelashes become

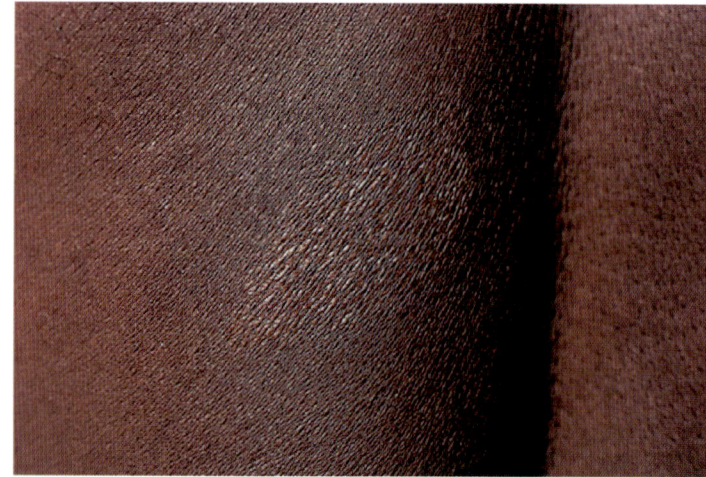

Figure 28.9 Tuberculoid or borderline tuberculoid leprosy. The back of a Nigerian child showing well-defined hypopigmented macule with altered skin texture. The lesion was anaesthetic.

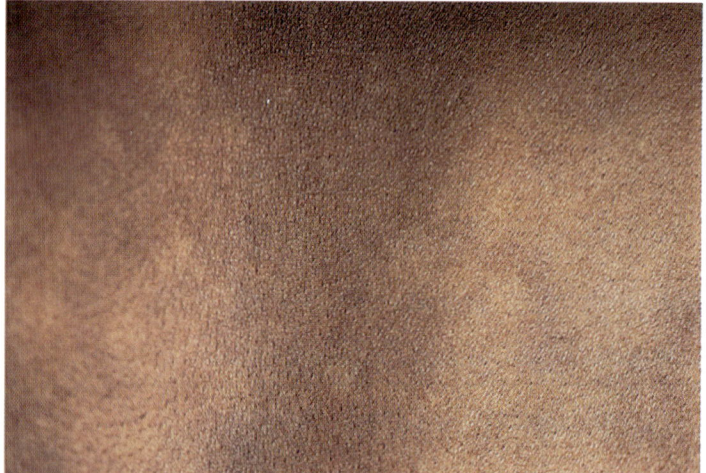

Figure 28.10 Lepromatous leprosy (borderline lepromatous/lepromatous). The back of a Bangladeshi boy showing numerous, often confluent hypopigmented macules, with relative sparing of the midline.

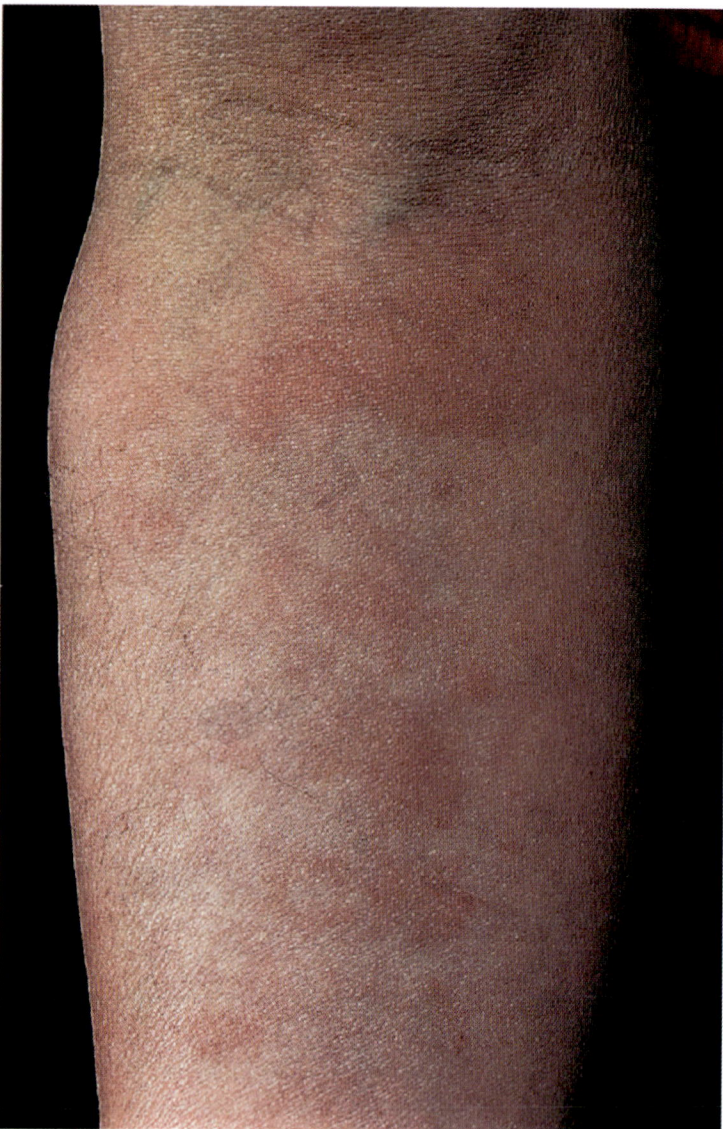

Figure 28.11 Lepromatous leprosy. The forearm of an English man showing red macules and infiltration, which characterise a relapse of dapsone-resistant lepromatous leprosy.

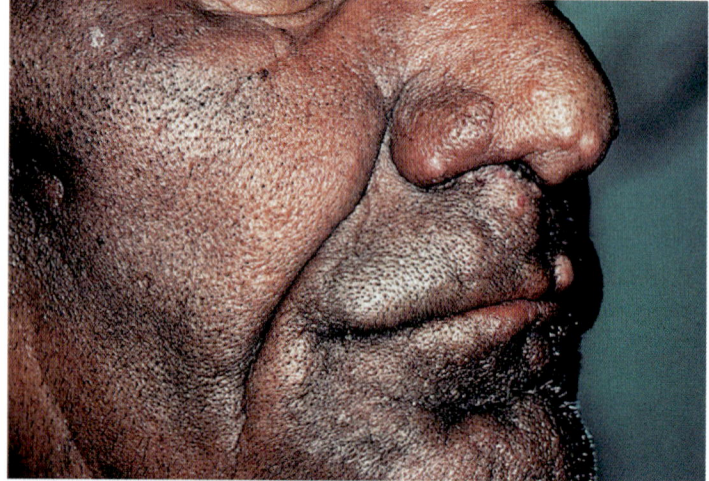

Figure 28.12 Lepromatous leprosy. The face of a man showing diffuse infiltration of the skin and appearance of nodules on the nose and lip.

thinned or lost (madarosis), the ear lobes are thickened, the nose becomes misshapen and may collapse due to septal perforation and loss of the anterior nasal spine, the voice becomes hoarse and the upper incisor teeth loosen or fall out [77]. A slow fibrosis of the peripheral nerves results in nerve thickening and bilateral 'glove and stocking' anaesthesia. Testicular atrophy causes sterility, impotence and gynaecomastia. Leprous deposits in the eyes cause keratitis, iridocyclitis and iris atrophy, also now rare.

Histoid lesions are distinctive round, regular, cutaneous nodules that stand out on normal skin [78].

The pure diffuse type was described by Lucio and Alvarado in Mexico in 1852. Patients have impaired sensation in the hands and feet, and gradual loss of the eyebrows, eyelashes and body hair. The skin of the whole body becomes diffusely thickened with alopecia, nasal and laryngeal involvement, and small telangiectases, but cutaneous nodules and plaques do not develop. The eyes have a shining appearance [79].

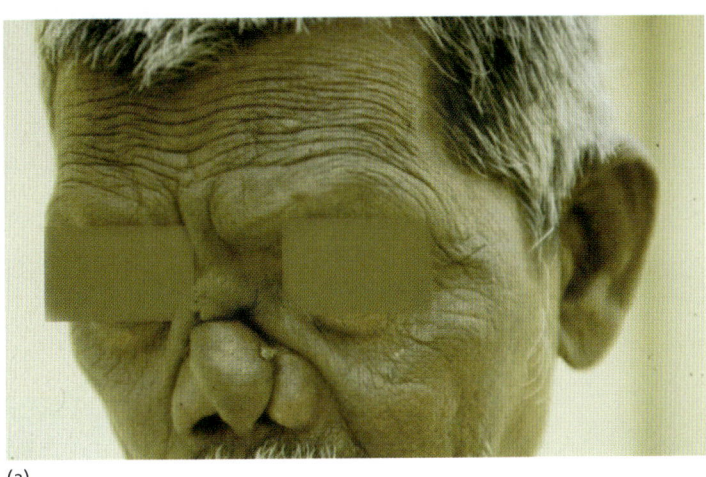
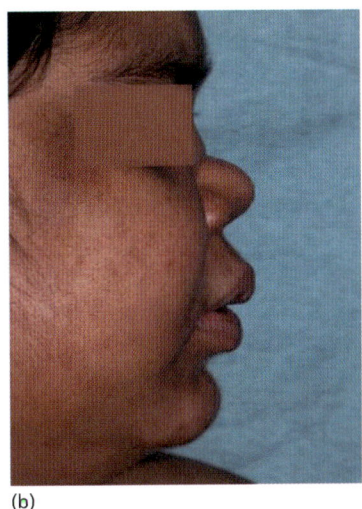

Figure 28.13 Lepromatous leprosy. (a) Man with nasal collapse and forehead wrinkling. (b) Woman with nasal collapse.

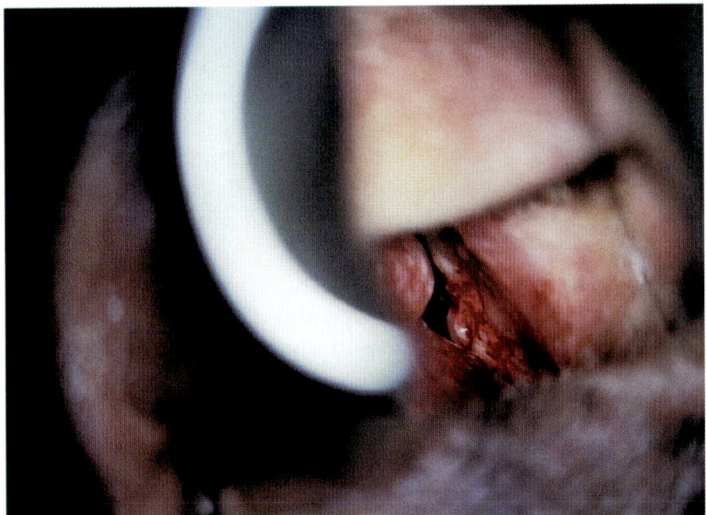

Figure 28.14 Lepromatous leprosy. Examination via a nasal speculum shows a pale septal nodule and bleeding. Such lesions in untreated lepromatous patients constitute a major source of infection.

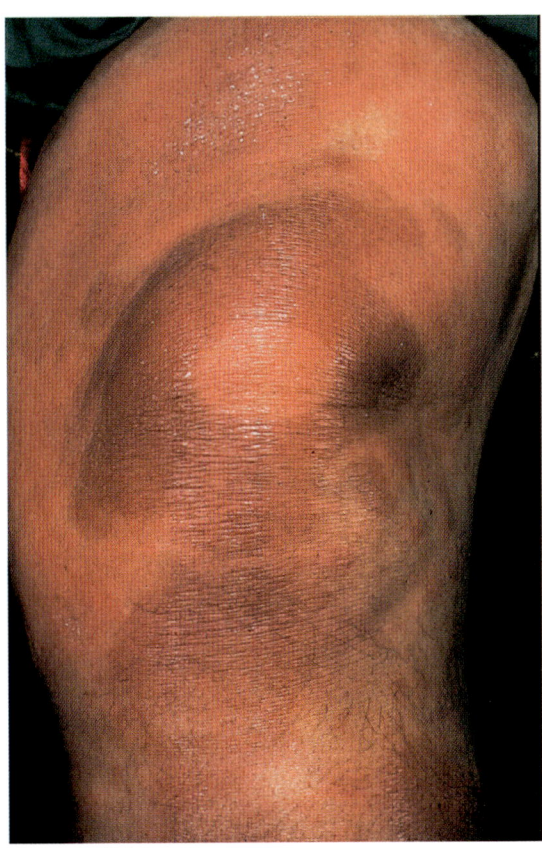

Figure 28.15 Borderline leprosy. The knee of a Saudi Arabian woman, showing classic annular lesions with well-defined centres with possible healing old borderline tuberculoid lesions, contrasting with spreading red infiltration. Slit-skin smears showed acid-fast bacilli.

Borderline leprosy. Skin lesions are intermediate in number between those of the two polar types already described, depending on the position of the patient on the borderline spectrum, and are distributed asymmetrically. They may take the form of macules, plaques, annular lesions or bizarre-shaped bands. Plaques with a 'punched-out' appearance are characteristic of the middle of the spectrum (Figure 28.15). Towards the tuberculoid end of the spectrum, lesions are fewer and drier (Figures 28.16 and 28.17), have more hair loss and anhidrosis and are more insensitive. One or more nerves are likely to be thickened and have nerve function impairment (Figure 28.18). Neural symptoms may precede the appearance of skin lesions by as much as 8 years [80]. When a patient's disease of borderline leprosy downgrades to lepromatous, the resulting subpolar LL (designated LLs) patients can be differentiated from polar lepromatous (LLp) patients because, in addition to typical lepromatous skin lesions, there are several asymmetrical, thickened nerves and one or more typical borderline skin lesions. Damage to structures other than the skin and nerves will not be manifest clinically in borderline leprosy, even though bacilli may be present in other tissue. Borderline leprosy is the commonest type of disease encountered and is unstable and 'downgrades' towards lepromatous, especially if untreated, or 'upgrades' towards tuberculoid. The clinical change lags the immunological and histological changes (Figure 28.19).

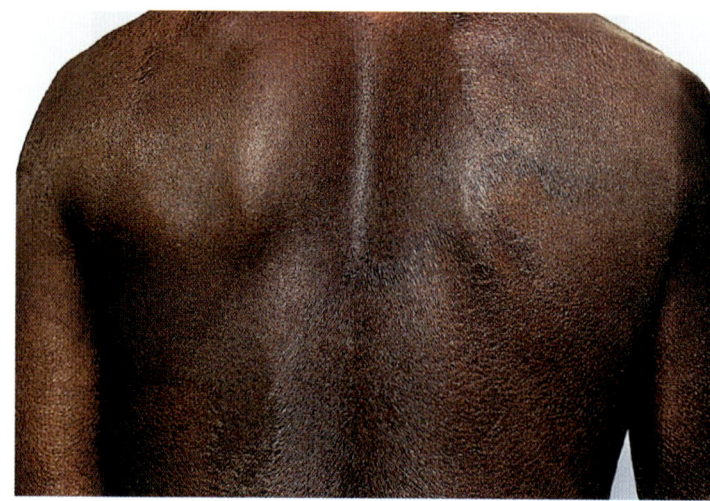

Figure 28.16 Borderline tuberculoid leprosy. The back of a Nigerian man showing large well-defined scaly macules with some marginal elevation. Extensive disease, such as this, may seriously impair sweating and heat control.

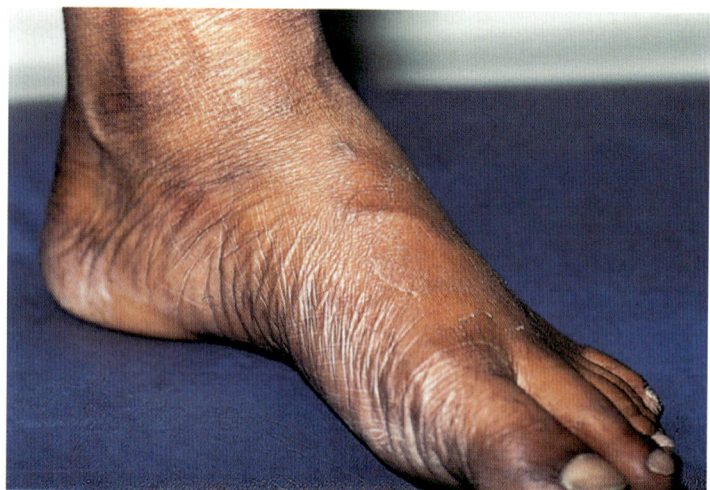

Figure 28.18 Borderline leprosy. The foot of a Bangladeshi child showing enlargement of posterior tibial and anterior tibial nerves.

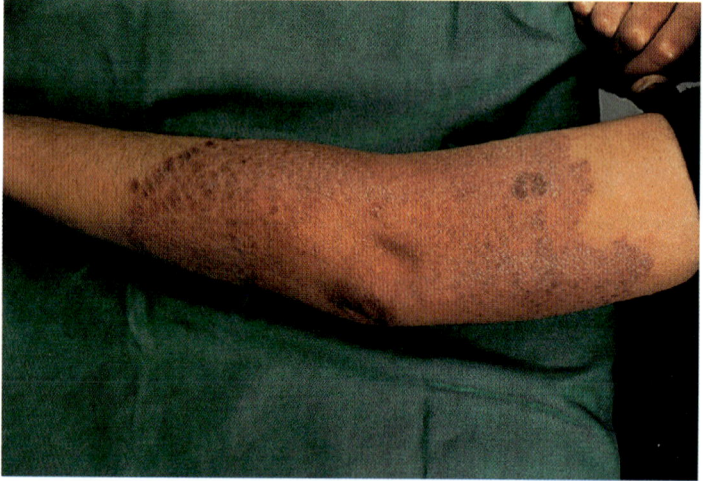

Figure 28.17 Borderline tuberculoid leprosy. The arm of an Indian woman. A large scaly macule is developing secondary ichthyotic change.

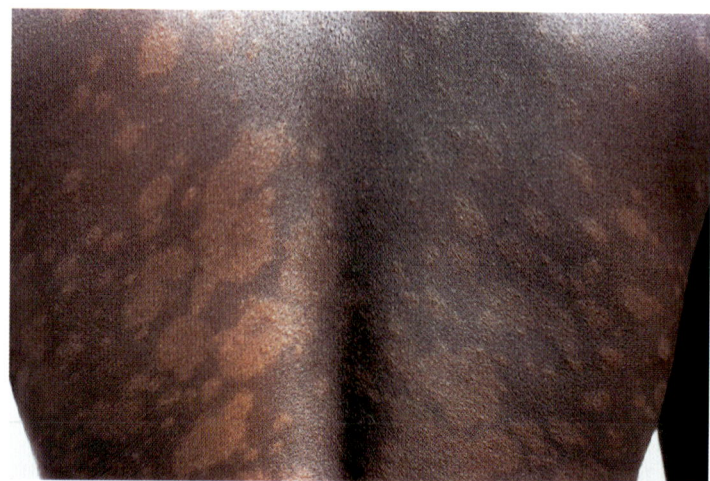

Figure 28.19 Borderline tuberculoid leprosy downgrading to borderline leprosy. The back of a Nigerian woman, showing typical well-defined hypopigmented macules of borderline tuberculoid leprosy and many small lesions, some of which are papular. Slit-skin smears showed acid-fast bacilli.

Pure neural leprosy. Pure neural leprosy occurs in 5–10% of patients with asymmetrical involvement of the peripheral nerve trunks and no visible skin lesions. On histology of a cutaneous nerve biopsy, all types of leprosy are seen [81].

Leprosy in pregnancy. Women may present with all types of leprosy during pregnancy. They are at high risk of type 1 reactions in the postpartum period and may present with leprosy then [82].

Leprosy in HIV infection. HIV infection is associated with the full spectrum of clinical and histopathological features of leprosy [17,83]. HIV-infected individuals have normal granuloma formation even with low numbers of circulating CD4 lymphocytes. Coinfected patients appear to be at increased risk of developing leprosy reactions and the borderline types of leprosy dominate the clinical picture. Leprosy may also present as an immune reconstitution inflammatory syndrome (IRIS) in HIV-infected patients after starting active antiretroviral therapy [84,85].

Leprosy in non-endemic settings. Leprosy may be underdiagnosed in non-endemic countries. Of new patients seen in the period 1995–99 at the Hospital for Tropical Diseases, London, diagnosis had been delayed in over 80% of cases [4]. Patients had been misdiagnosed by dermatologists, neurologists, orthopaedic surgeons and rheumatologists, because leprosy was not considered as a cause of peripheral neuropathy in patients from leprosy-endemic countries. These delays had serious consequences for patients, with over half of them having nerve damage and disability. A retrospective study spanning a 23-year period showed that some individuals developed symptoms and were diagnosed many years after leaving an endemic region and there were no cases of secondary transmission [2].

Differential diagnosis

Macular lesions. Hypopigmented congenital lesions do not exhibit reduced sensation. Vitiligo is depigmented; leprosy lesions are never completely depigmented. Hypopigmented lesions of pityriasis alba in children are difficult to distinguish from lepromatous macules, but their surface is often scaly and smears do not contain AFB. Pityriasis versicolor is not always scaly, but a central distribution on the trunk and the presence of numerous distinct macules are contrary to the characteristics of lepromatous macules. Lesions of tinea corporis are pruritic and scrapings often demonstrate the causative dermatophyte.

Plaques and annular lesions. In addition to ringworm, granuloma multiforme, sarcoidosis and cutaneous tuberculosis may resemble tuberculoid leprosy, having a similar immunological basis and often indistinguishable histological pattern. However, the lesions are not anaesthetic. Peripheral nerves may rarely be enlarged in sarcoidosis [86].

Nodules. Cutaneous leishmaniasis causes nodules, but they usually have some epidermal change and the majority ulcerate after some weeks or months. They are seldom as numerous as those of LL. Slit-skin smears, appropriately stained, reveal *Leishmania*. Lesions of the rare diffuse cutaneous leishmaniasis may be confusing until slit-skin smears have been examined [87]. Post-kala-azar dermal leishmaniasis in India and East Africa has a similar distribution and appearance to the skin lesions of LL [88].

Nerves. Peripheral nerve thickening is rarely seen except in leprosy. Hereditary sensory motor neuropathy type III is associated with palpable peripheral nerve hypertrophy. Amyloidosis, which can also complicate leprosy, causes thickening of the peripheral nerves. Peroneal muscular atrophy (Charcot–Marie–Tooth disease) is an inherited neuropathy that causes distal atrophy and weakness; the nerve biopsy is characteristic. The causes of other polyneuropathies such as HIV infection, diabetes mellitus, alcohol, vasculitides and heavy metal poisoning should all be considered where appropriate [89].

Eye disease. Likewise, there are many causes of eye disease in endemic countries which may cause signs that in isolation mimic leprosy, especially trachoma, in which trichiasis and entropion follow scarring of the lids, and onchocerciasis, which causes uveitis and its complications.

Classification of severity

All new leprosy patients need to be classified according to either the Ridley–Jopling classification or the WHO classification. Patients should be assessed to determine whether they have new nerve damage. Finally, they should be assessed for being in a reaction.

Complications and co-morbidities

Reactions: type 1, erythema nodosum leprosum and neuritis.

Type 1 reactions occur in borderline disease and are characterised by acute neuritis and/or acutely inflamed skin lesions [90]. Nerves often become tender with a loss of sensory and motor functions. Existing skin lesions become red or oedematous and may desquamate or rarely ulcerate. New lesions may appear (Figure 28.20). Occasionally, oedema of the face, hands or feet is the presenting symptom, but constitutional symptoms are unusual. Patients often

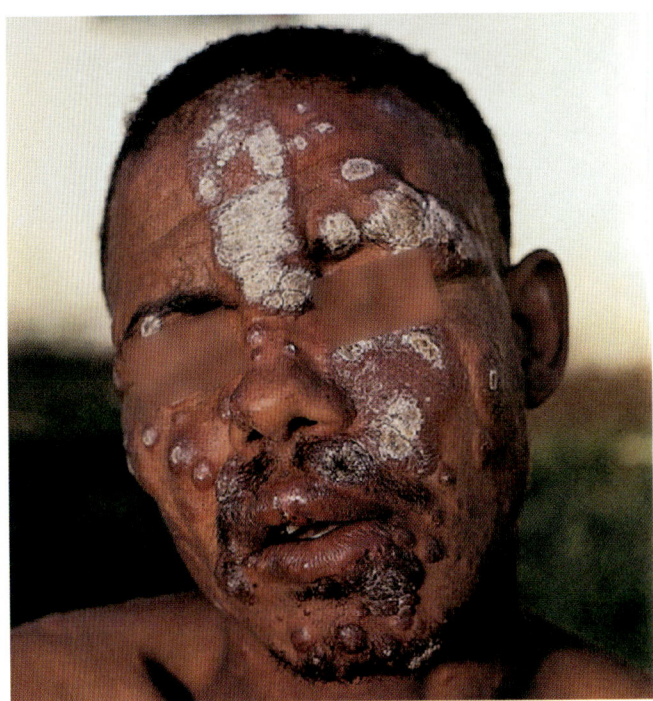

Figure 28.20 Type 1 reaction in borderline leprosy in an Ethiopian man. The existing lesions become acutely inflamed, and will scale and threaten ulceration. Many small new lesions have appeared. The histology shows a borderline tuberculoid pattern.

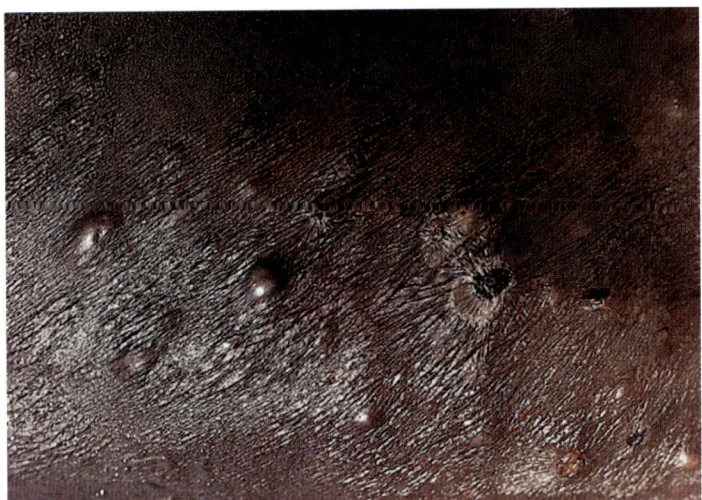

Figure 28.21 Type 2 reaction in lepromatous leprosy in a Nigerian man: erythema nodosum leprosum. Several of the reaction nodules have broken down, releasing pus.

first present for medical advice when a previously quiescent BT lesion develops a spontaneous type 1 reaction. A recent cohort study in India found that most type 1 reactions occurred in the first 12 months after starting treatment [91]. Women are also at risk during the puerperium.

Type 2 (ENL) reactions occur in patients with multibacillary disease (LL and BL). They may occur before, during or after treatment. Up to 50% of LL patients and 15% of BL patients may experience ENL reactions [92]. Attacks are often acute at first but may be prolonged or recurrent over several years. ENL manifests as painful red nodules on the face and extensor surfaces of the limbs. The lesions may be superficial or deep, with suppuration

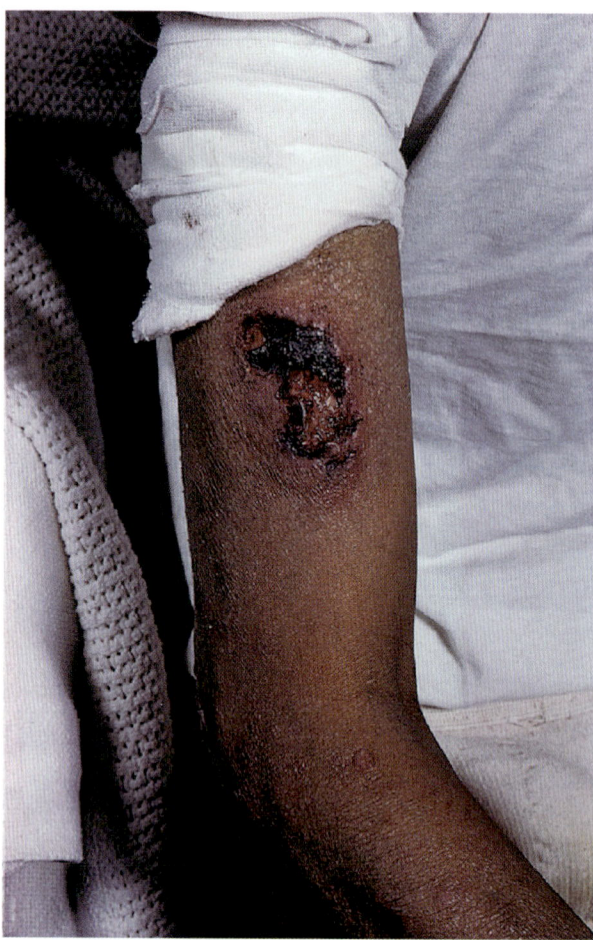

Figure 28.22 Type 2 reaction in lepromatous leprosy in a Bangladeshi man: severe necrosis and ulceration. Erythema nodosum leprosum tends to be more severe in people from Asia than from Africa.

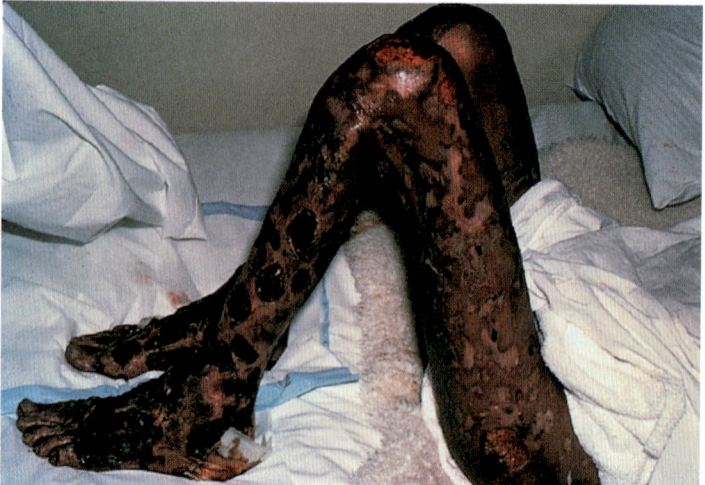

Figure 28.23 Lucio phenomenon in a Mexican man. The severe recurrent ulceration due to deep subcutaneous vasculitis may be fatal. Courtesy of Dr J. Keystone, the Toronto Hospital, Toronto, Canada.

(Figure 28.21), ulceration (Figure 28.22) or brawny induration when chronic. Acute lesions crop and desquamate, fading over several days (Figure 28.22). ENL is a systemic disorder producing fever and malaise and may be accompanied by uveitis, dactylitis, arthritis, neuritis, lymphadenitis, myositis and orchitis [93,94]. Peripheral nerve neuritis and uveitis with its complications of synechiae, cataract and glaucoma are the most serious complications of ENL.

The Lucio phenomenon only occurs in patients with Lucio leprosy [95]. It is due to infarction caused by obstructive vasculopathy and leading to the appearance of irregularly shaped red patches which become dark and heal, or form bullae and then necrose, leaving deep painful ulcers that are slow to heal (Figure 28.23). The systemic upset is severe and can be fatal. This form of leprosy has been associated with *Mycobacterium lepromatosis*.

Nerve damage [96]. Of the three physiological functions of nerves, the sensory component is commonly the first and most severely affected, but occasionally there is a pure motor lesion. Autonomic dysfunction is always present in severe nerve damage [97]. In skin lesions this is associated with loss of hair growth and of sebaceous and sweat secretion, and poor pigment formation. In a limb it causes capillary stasis, cyanosis and dryness, which predispose to fissuring. Two large cohort studies with systematic nerve examination at entry showed that the posterior tibial nerve is the most frequently affected nerve, followed by the ulnar, median, lateral popliteal and facial nerves [98,99]. Ulnar and median nerve lesions are usually low, causing small muscle but not deep flexor weakness, and anaesthesia of the two halves of the hand. Isolated median nerve lesions are unusual. Common peroneal nerve lesions cause difficulty in dorsiflexion and eversion of the foot and anaesthesia of the outer border of the foot, a combination which predisposes to traumatic damage and plantar ulceration (Figure 28.24). Posterior tibial nerve damage is serious because it causes paralysis and contracture of the small muscles of the foot and anaesthesia of the sole.

Eye involvement. Blindness due to leprosy is a serious complication, especially for a patient with anaesthetic hands and feet. Eye damage results from both nerve damage and bacillary invasion, and a recent cohort study found that 2.8% of multibacillary patients were blind at diagnosis, and a further 11% of patients had potentially blinding ocular pathology [100]. Lagophthalmos results from paresis of the orbicularis oculi due to involvement of the zygomatic and temporal branches of the facial (VIIth) nerve. Facial lesions cause a 10-fold increase in the risk of facial nerve damage [101]. In lepromatous disease, lagophthalmos occurs later and is usually bilateral. Damage to the ophthalmic branch of the trigeminal (Vth) nerve causes anaesthesia of the cornea and conjunctiva, which results in drying of the cornea, a reduction in blinking and leaves the cornea at risk of minor trauma and ulceration. Bacillary invasion of the iris and ciliary body makes them extremely susceptible to reactions.

Investigations [102]

The diagnosis is usually made clinically based on two out of three characteristic findings, or by the demonstration of AFB in slit-skin smears, or by histology typical of leprosy. The cardinal signs are:
- Hypopigmented, anaesthetic skin lesions.
- Thickened peripheral nerves.
- Acid-fast bacilli in the skin.

The AFB load of a patient is determined by modified Ziehl–Neelsen staining of slit-skin smears. Suspect lesions, and sites commonly affected in LL, should be sampled (e.g. the forehead,

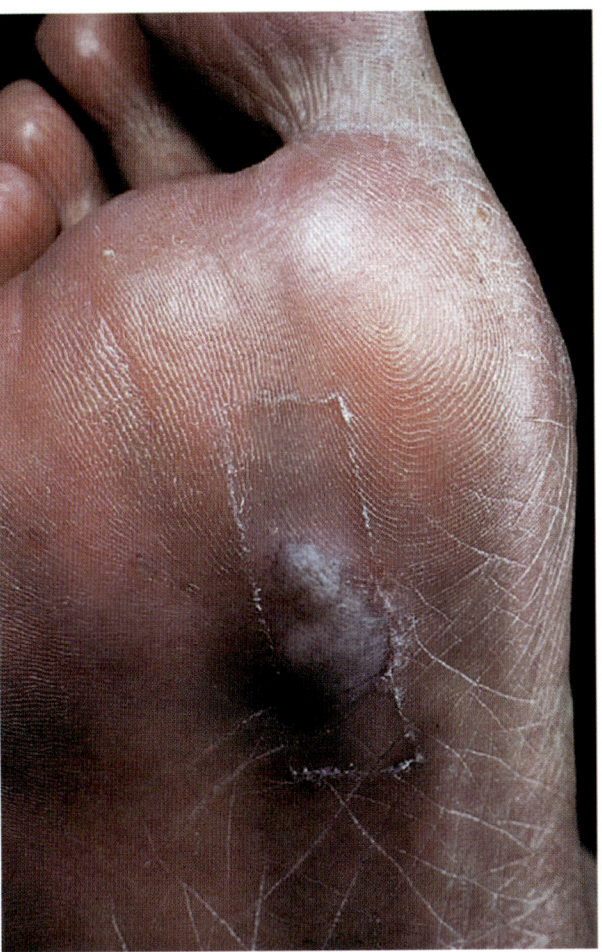

Figure 28.24 Necrosis blister in an anaesthetic foot. Necrotic material has tracked to soft skin from the site of trauma, beneath the metatarsal heads.

earlobes, chin, extensor surface of the forearm, buttocks and trunk). The density of bacilli is expressed using a logarithmic scale, which ranges from 1+ (1–10 bacilli per 100 high-power fields) to 6+ (>1000 bacilli per single high-power field). A mean score, the bacterial index (BI), is derived by adding the scores from each site and dividing by the number of sites sampled [103]. In untreated LL, the BI is 5 or 6. The BI is zero in TT disease. Slit-skin smears only detect bacilli present at a concentration greater than 10^4/g tissue, and so cannot be used as a test of microbiological cure. With treatment, bacilli disappear from BB lesions in a few months and from BL lesions in a year or two.

Slit-skin smears [104]
The lesion is cleaned with ether or alcohol, and a fold is gripped firmly between the thumb and forefinger to render it blood free. An incision 5 mm long and 3 mm deep is made with a small-bladed scalpel (size 15); the blade is turned at right angles to the cut, and without relaxing the finger pressure, the wound is scraped several times in one direction. Fluid and pulp from the dermis, collected on one side of the blade, are gently smeared onto a glass slide. The smear is then fixed over a flame and stained.

Skin biopsy [105]
The incision should be made down to and including the subcutaneous fat.

Nerve biopsy
In pure neural leprosy a nerve biopsy is necessary to establish the diagnosis. A purely sensory thickened peripheral nerve should be sampled, for example the radial cutaneous at the wrist, or the superficial peroneal or sural nerve at the ankle.

Serology
The evaluation of PGL serology in extensive field studies shows that more than 90% of untreated multibacillary patients have positive serology in comparison with 40–50% of paucibacillary patients and 5–10% of healthy controls [106]. PGL-1 antibodies can now be detected using a dipstick-type test (so-called lateral flow). This has been evaluated in field settings and seropositivity correlates with bacterial load measured by slit-skin smears [107].

Management
There are five main principles of treatment:
1. Stop the infection with chemotherapy.
2. Treat reactions and reduce the risk of nerve damage.
3. Educate the patient to cope with existing nerve damage, in particular anaesthesia.
4. Treat the complications of nerve damage.
5. Rehabilitate the patient socially and psychologically.

These objectives are best achieved with a multidisciplinary, patient-centred approach. Individuals will require accurate information, reassurance and time to come to terms with a life-changing diagnosis.

Antibacterial treatment for leprosy is highly effective, with low relapse rates, but needs to be taken over 6 or 12 months. New patients can be reassured that their infection is curable and that the aim of treatment is to minimise further nerve damage. Patients should not develop the mutilating sequelae seen previously.

Left untreated, borderline patients will downgrade towards the lepromatous end of the spectrum, and lepromatous patients will suffer the consequences of bacillary invasion. Borderline patients are at risk of developing type 1 reactions, which may result in devastating nerve damage. Many patients present with established nerve damage, which cannot be reversed. Treatment of the neuritis is challenging; some patients with active neuritis will develop permanent nerve damage despite treatment with corticosteroids. It is not possible to determine which patients will develop reactions or nerve damage. Nerve damage and its complications may be severely disabling, especially when all four limbs and both eyes are affected.

First line
Chemotherapy. The WHO proposed multidrug therapy (MDT) for the treatment of leprosy in 1982 [108] to avoid monotherapy. The first line antileprosy drugs are rifampicin, dapsone and clofazimine; paucibacillary patients are treated for 6 months and multibacillary patients for 12 months [109]. Previously, patients diagnosed with paucibacillary leprosy did not receive clofazimine. Table 28.2 gives the details of drug dosages and duration of treatment. The outcomes of treatment are very good with a relapse rate of approximately 1%. The BI falls by approximately one log unit per year. The skin lesions may take months to improve, and hypopigmentation, atrophy and nodules may persist. Blister packaging for better treatment

Table 28.2 World Health Organization (WHO) multidrug therapy regimen.

Age group	Drug	Dosage and frequency	Duration	
			MB	PB
Adult	Rifampicin	600 mg once a month	12 months	6 months
	Clofazimine	300 mg once a month, 50 mg daily		
	Dapsone	100 mg daily		
Children 10–14 years old	Rifampicin	450 mg once a month	12 months	6 months
	Clofazimine	150 mg once a month, 50 mg daily		
	Dapsone	50 mg daily		
Children <10 years old or <40 kg	Rifampicin	10 mg/kg once a month	12 months	6 months
	Clofazimine	6 mg/kg once a month, 1 mg/kg daily		
	Dapsone	2 mg/kg daily		

From WHO, 2018 [109].
MB, multibacillary; PB, paucibacillary.

adherence and worldwide donor funding of leprosy treatment have facilitated huge improvements in the availability of treatment and successful completion rates.

Rifampicin is a potent bactericidal for *Mycobacterium leprae*. Four days after a single 600 mg dose, bacilli are no longer viable [110]. It acts by inhibiting DNA-dependent RNA polymerase, thereby interfering with bacterial RNA synthesis. Rifampicin is well absorbed orally. Hepatotoxicity may occur with a mild transient elevation of hepatic transaminases, but this is rare at the dosage and intervals recommended for leprosy and is not an indication for stopping treatment. Because *M. leprae* resistance to rifampicin can develop as a one-step process, rifampicin should always be given in combination with other antileprotics [111].

Dapsone (4,4-diaminodiphenylsulphone) acts by blocking folic acid synthesis. It is only weakly bactericidal. Oral absorption is good, and it has a long half-life, averaging 28 h. Dapsone, in the doses recommended for leprosy, commonly causes mild haemolysis, and rarely anaemia or psychosis. Glucose-6-phosphate dehydrogenase deficiency seldom causes a problem and is not routinely looked for. The 'dapsone hypersensitivity syndrome' – a form of DRESS (drug reaction with eosinophilia and systemic symptoms) – occurs 6 weeks after commencing dapsone and manifests as exfoliative dermatitis associated with lymphadenopathy, hepatosplenomegaly, fever and hepatitis, and may be fatal [112]. HLA-B*13:01 is associated with the development of the dapsone hypersensitivity syndrome [113]. Agranulocytosis, hepatitis and cholestatic jaundice occur rarely with dapsone therapy [114].

Clofazimine is a brick-red, fat-soluble crystalline dye. The mechanism of its weakly bactericidal action against *M. leprae* is not known. High drug concentrations are found in the intestinal mucosa, mesenteric lymph nodes and body fat. The most noticeable side effect is skin discoloration, ranging from red to purple-black, the degree of discoloration depending on the dose and leprosy infiltration. The pigmentation usually fades within 12 months of stopping clofazimine, although traces of discoloration may remain for up to 4 years. Urine, sputum and sweat may become pink. Clofazimine also produces a characteristic ichthyosis on the shins and forearms. Gastrointestinal side effects, ranging from mild cramps to diarrhoea and weight loss, may occur because of clofazimine crystal deposition in the wall of the small bowel.

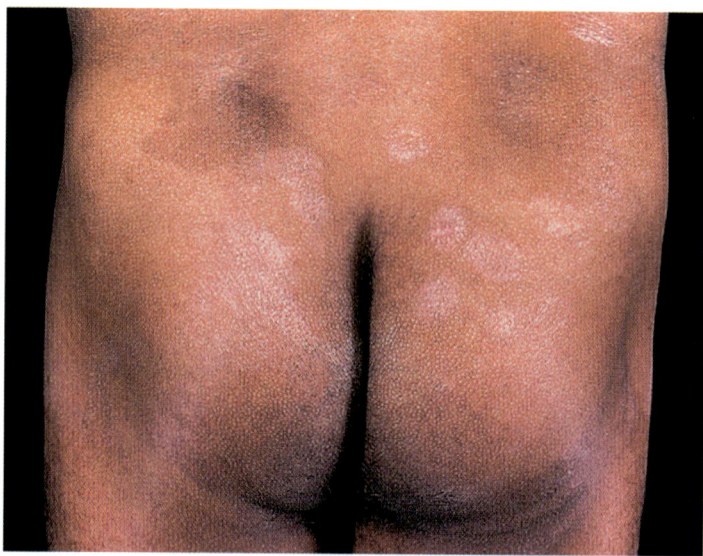

Figure 28.25 Borderline lepromatous (BL) leprosy upgrading to borderline tuberculoid (BT) leprosy. The buttocks of an Indian man who 'relapsed' 3 years after completing multidrug therapy for BL leprosy. The lesions here are typical hypopigmented, red, scaly plaques of BT leprosy in reaction. No acid-fast bacilli were seen on slit-skin smears. In this situation, the distinction between (bacterial) relapse and simple reversal reaction may be impossible.

Relapse treatment. Relapsed multibacillary patients are also retreated with MDT regardless of any change in classification [115]. The distinction between reinfection, relapse and reaction may be difficult (Figure 28.25). Therefore, paucibacillary patients require 2 years, and multibacillary patients at least 5 years, of monitoring after treatment. Patients can be discharged if there is no evidence of activity or reaction but should be advised to return if new symptoms develop, especially in the hands, feet or eyes. Patients with reactions or physical or psychological complications may need much longer care.

Published clinical outcomes for patients treated with the paucibacillary regimen show that 2–44% of patients had clinically active skin lesions at the end of treatment [116]. Nerve impairment occurred *de novo* in 2.5% of patients, and visible disabilities increased from 4% at enrolment to 7% at 8–10 years of follow-up. Relapse rates are low, ranging from 0% in Ethiopia [117] to 2.5% over 4 years in Malawi [118]. For patients treated with the multibacillary regimen for 24 months, one study in Thailand found that 29% of lesions were still active after 3 years and that visible disabilities increased from 5% at enrolment to 13% at 8–10 years of follow-up [119]. Relapse rates have been reported from six observational studies varying from zero in China and Ethiopia to 2.04/100 person-years in India. Observational studies done after 12 months of MDT show relapse rates of 1% in patients in Bangladesh and Brazil [120,121]. Susceptibility testing of *M. leprae* strains from relapsed multibacillary patients has shown them to remain drug sensitive.

Second line

Several other drugs are bactericidal for *M. leprae*: fluoroquinolones, minocycline and clarithromycin [109]. The fluoroquinolones pefloxacin and ofloxacin have high bactericidal activity, with 22 daily doses killing 99.99% of viable *M. leprae* present in multibacillary cases at the start of treatment [122]. Daily minocycline (100 mg) treatment of multibacillary patients for 3 months resulted in killing all viable *M. leprae* organisms [123]. Clarithromycin, given in 500 mg daily doses to multibacillary patients, has a similar bactericidal effect [124]. Antagonism between these new drugs has not been demonstrated [125]. Ofloxacin, minocycline and clarithromycin are established second line drugs, and may replace dapsone and clofazimine. Minocycline may also cause hyperpigmentation of skin lesions, and so may not be an appropriate substitute for clofazimine if pigmentation is to be avoided [126].

A triple-drug combination (rifampicin, ofloxacin and minocycline) which can be given as a single monthly dose for 6 or 12 months can be used to treat patients with adverse effects to one of the components of standard MDT [127].

Treatment of reactions and neuritis [128]

Nerve damage occurs before diagnosis and during and after MDT. It may occur during a reaction or without overt signs of nerve inflammation (silent neuropathy). In field cohort studies 16–56% of newly diagnosed patients had nerve damage [129]. In a Bangladeshi study, 25% of multibacillary patients developed nerve damage during treatment [130]. This study also showed that 65% of patients with multibacillary leprosy who had nerve damage at diagnosis developed new nerve damage over a 5-year follow-up; therefore, this group should be closely monitored. Analysis from a large cohort study in Ethiopia showed that standardised nerve function testing was needed monthly to detect new nerve damage early [131].

Patients frequently seek medical advice for their leprosy only when a type 1 reaction develops in a previously quiescent skin lesion, or when they develop pain, weakness or numbness. Awareness of the early symptoms of reactions by both patient and physician is important, because if left untreated severe nerve damage may occur. The peak time for type 1 reactions is in the first 6 months of treatment [132], so it is important to warn patients about reactions. The sudden development of reactional lesions soon after starting treatment is distressing and may affect adherence to MDT.

The treatment of reactions is aimed at controlling acute inflammation, easing pain, reversing nerve and eye damage and reassuring the patient. MDT should be continued. Neuritis (e.g. nerve tenderness, new anaesthesia and/or motor loss) or inflamed skin lesions should be treated with corticosteroids. Standardised courses of prednisolone have been used, starting at 40 mg daily, reducing by 5 mg every 2–4 weeks [133]. Patients with borderline reactions commonly need 20 weeks of steroids. An Indian study compared different starting doses (60 versus 30 mg) and durations (12 versus 20 weeks) and showed that the longer durations gave the best outcomes. A study looking at cytokine profiles in reactional patients showed that, even after 6 months of steroid treatment, some patients still had high levels of pro-inflammatory cytokines in their skin lesions [134]. In another approach, the prevention of reactions has been explored. In one study, multibacillary patients were randomised to either prednisolone 20 mg daily or placebo for the first 3 months of their MDT. Reactional episodes were significantly lower in the prednisolone-treated group at 4 months, but the protective effect was lost by 12 months. These studies all demonstrate that reactions are difficult to prevent and to switch off once established. Other immunosuppressants have also been studied to assess their effect in reactions: 3 days of 1 g methylprednisolone did not reduce the recurrence rate [135]. Adding azathioprine to prednisolone did not improve nerve function or reduce recurrence rate [136].

Erythema nodosum leprosum is a difficult condition to treat, and frequently requires therapy with high-dose steroids (80 mg daily, tapered down rapidly) or thalidomide. The severity and response to treatment is assessed clinically using the 10 item ENLIST ENL Severity Scale [137]. Since ENL frequently recurs, steroid dependency can easily develop. Thalidomide (400 mg daily) is superior to steroids in controlling ENL and is the drug of choice in severe ENL [138]. Women with severe ENL may benefit from thalidomide treatment. This is a potentially challenging decision for the woman and her physician and needs careful discussion of the benefits and risks (e.g. phocomelia when thalidomide is taken in the first trimester of pregnancy). Women should use double contraception and report immediately if menstruation is delayed. This requires access to contraception and a robust pregnancy prevention programme. Unfortunately, thalidomide is unavailable in several leprosy-endemic countries despite its undoubted value. High-dose clofazimine (300 mg/day) has been used in ENL. Anti-TNF blockers have been used with some success in a few reported cases [139].

Acute iridocyclitis is treated with 4-hourly instillation of 1% hydrocortisone eye drops and 1% atropine drops twice daily.

Additional aspects of management

Education of the patient. Educating a leprosy patient about their disease is the key to successful management. The patient can be reassured that within a few days of chemotherapy they will not be infectious and can lead a normal social life. A clear explanation of the disease and refutation of myths about leprosy will help the patient come to terms with their diagnosis and may improve compliance. Care and awareness of their limbs is as important as chemotherapy. Anxieties about transmission and reactions, as well as issues about compliance, should be addressed.

Complications of nerve damage [140,141]. The complications of nerve damage, which are the major causes of disability and deformity in leprosy, are preventable by early diagnosis, correct treatment and education of the patient. Monitoring sensation and muscle power in the patient's hands, feet and eyes should be part of the routine follow-up, so that new nerve damage is detected early.

Dry skin should be treated by soaking in water, followed by rubbing with emulsifying ointment or petrolatum. Calluses should be rubbed down with pumice or an abrasive nylon pad and fissures need to be covered to allow them to heal.

The morbidity and disability associated with leprosy is secondary to nerve damage. A major goal in the prevention of disability is to create patient self-awareness, so that damage is minimised. The patient with an anaesthetic hand or foot should understand the importance of daily self-care, especially protection when doing potentially dangerous tasks, and inspection for trauma. For each patient, potentially dangerous situations such as cooking, car repairs or smoking should be identified. Soaking dry hands and feet followed by rubbing with oil keeps the skin moist and supple.

Anaesthetic feet need protecting with appropriate shoes. For anaesthesia alone, a well-fitting 'trainer' with firm soles and shock-absorbing inners will provide adequate protection. When there is deformity, such as clawing, shoes must be tailored to ensure protection of pressure points and even weight distribution.

The patient should question the cause of any injury so that the risk can in the future be avoided. Plantar ulceration occurs secondary to increased pressure over bony prominences. Ulceration is treated by rest. Unlike ulcers in diabetic or ischaemic feet, ulcers in leprosy heal only if they are protected from weight-bearing. No weight-bearing is permitted until the ulcer has healed. Appropriate footwear should be provided to prevent recurrence.

Neuropathic pain. Neuropathic pain is an increasingly recognised complication of leprosy, reported in up to 20% of treated patients; having a reaction is a risk factor. The pain should be assessed using tools such as the DN4 questionnaire. Patients should be treated using an analgesic ladder starting with paracetamol, then a non-steroidal anti-inflammatory such as ibuprofen. Many patients need treatment with amitriptyline or gabapentin [142].

Weakness or paralysis. These patients require physiotherapy, with the objective of permitting the return of function while preventing the formation of contracture. Patients with contractures are taught exercises to prevent fixation. Contractures of hands and feet, foot drop, lagophthalmos, entropion and ectropion are amenable to reconstructive surgery.

Social, psychological and vocational rehabilitation. The social and cultural background of the patient determines the nature of many of the problems that may be encountered. The patient may have difficulty in coming to terms with leprosy. Their community may reject the patient. Education, gainful employment, confidence from family, friends and doctor, and plastic surgery to correct stigmatising deformity, all have a role to play.

Prevention and control

Dermatologists play a key role in diagnosing and treating leprosy patients. For much of the 20th century, leprosy patients were detected and treated within vertical programmes dedicated to leprosy. Although these were effective, they also became inefficient as the numbers of leprosy patients declined. The management of leprosy patients is now being integrated into a range of health services including combined leprosy and tuberculosis programmes, dermatology programmes and full integration with general health services. The current WHO strategy emphasises the importance of quality services that are accessible and patient-centred, provide free treatment with MDT, undertake appropriate prevention of disability and refer patients on for the management of complications. There are now huge needs to train people to recognise leprosy. The development of referral services is also a critical need if an integrated approach is to work well.

Chemoprophylaxis. Single-dose rifampicin is being used as chemoprophylaxis. The current evidence for efficacy is weak. In the COLEP trial in Bangladesh, household and social contacts of leprosy patients were given a single 600 mg dose of rifampicin or placebo. Rifampicin did not protect against the development of leprosy in household members. It only protected significantly in social contacts of leprosy patients, protection was only against the development of PB disease and lasted only for 2 years [143]. These findings suggest that rifampicin is effective only when the mycobacterial load is low at early disease stages. Despite this weak and short-lived protection, this prophylaxis is now being recommended by WHO [109]. There is a risk that by giving out this ineffective protection, *M. leprae* will develop resistance to rifampicin.

Vaccines against leprosy. BCG vaccine provides protection against leprosy because the antigens are closely related in all the locations where it has been studied, but this effect varies [144]. The protection is thought to be greatest for close contacts.

Stigma

Stigma continues to be strongly associated with leprosy and needs to be combated at many levels including the individual, community and national level. A new initiative called a New Face for Leprosy is working to improve the images of leprosy that are found on the web, with images of affected people who have jobs and successful social lives including families (https://newfaceleprosy.com/; last accessed May 2023). There are also new approaches that involve developing links with other people who experience stigma [145]. Community-based rehabilitation (CBR) is now recognised as a key part of leprosy work and new guidelines will help promote this work.

Leprosy patients continue to present in many countries and will need diagnosis and treatment. Leprosy is unlikely to be eradicated until there is considerable improvement in general health, wealth, living conditions and education.

Resources

Public Health England, *Memorandum on Leprosy 2012*: https://assets.publishing.service.gov.uk/government/uploads/system/uploads/attachment_data/file/334363/Memorandum_on_leprosy_2012.pdf.

World Health Organization, *Leprosy (Hansen's disease)*: https://www.who.int/health-topics/leprosy#tab=tab_1.

(Both last accessed May 2023.)

Key references

The full list of references can be found in the online version at https://www.wiley.com/rooksdermatology10e

2 Lockwood DN, McIntosh A, Armstrong M, Checkley AM, Walker SL, McBride A. Diagnosing and treating leprosy in a non-endemic setting in a national centre, London, United Kingdom 1995–2018. *PLOS Negl Trop Dis* 2020;16:e0010799.

4 Lockwood DN, Reid AJ. The diagnosis of leprosy is delayed in the United Kingdom. *Q J Med* 2001;94:207–12.

7 Fine PE. Leprosy: the epidemiology of a slow bacterium. *Epidemiol Rev* 1982;4:161–88.

8 Feldman RA, Sturdivant M. Leprosy in Louisiana, 1855–1970. An epidemiologic study of long-term trends. *Am J Epidemiol* 1975;102:303–10.

10 Ciechanover A. The ubiquitin proteolytic system. *Neurology* 2006;66(Suppl. 1):1–13.

12 Roy S, McGuire W, Mascie-Taylor CG et al. Tumor necrosis factor promoter polymorphism and susceptibility to lepromatous leprosy. *J Infect Dis* 1997;176:530–2.

16 Malhotra D, Darvishi K, Sood S et al. IL-10 promoter single nucleotide polymorphisms are significantly associated with resistance to leprosy. *Hum Genet* 2005;118:295–300.

34 Job CK, Desikan KV. Pathologic changes and their distribution in peripheral nerves in lepromatous leprosy. *Int J Lepr Other Mycobact Dis* 1968;36:257–70.

53 Yamamura M, Wang X-H, Ohmen JD et al. Cytokine patterns of immunologically mediated tissue damage. *J Immunol* 1992;149:1470–5.

62 Truman R, Singh P, Sharma S. Probable zoonotic for leprosy in the Southern United States. *N Engl J Med* 2011;364:1626–33.

63 Cole ST, Eiglmeier K, Parkhill J et al. Massive gene decay in the leprosy bacillus. *Nature* 2001;409:1007–11.

91 Van Brakel WH, Nicholls PG, Das L et al. The INFIR Cohort Study: assessment of sensory and motor neuropathy in leprosy at baseline. *Lepr Rev* 2005;76:277–95.

119 Dasananjali K, Schreuder PA, Pirayavaraporn C. A study on the effectiveness and safety of the WHO/MDT regimen in the northeast of Thailand: a prospective study, 1984–96. *Int J Lepr Other Mycobact Dis* 1997;65:28–36.

CHAPTER 29

Syphilis and Congenital Syphilis

George R. Kinghorn[1] *and Rasha Omer*[2]

[1] University of Sheffield, Sheffield, UK
[2] Rotherham NHS Foundation Trust, Rotherham, UK

| Global overview of sexually transmitted infections, 29.1 | Syphilis, 29.2
Congenital syphilis, 29.22 | Key references, 29.29 |

Global overview of sexually transmitted infections

The global health burden of sexually transmitted infections (STIs) and human immunodeficiency virus (HIV) remains large and is increasing in many regions. The World Health Organization (WHO) estimates that more than 1 million people acquire chlamydia, gonorrhoea, syphilis or trichomoniasis each day [1]. If the major viral STIs are included, then prevalence may be increased threefold. However, the true prevalence is still unknown, because surveillance is inadequate in many countries, especially in low- and middle-income countries (LMICs) in sub-Saharan Africa, South-East Asia and the Americas, where the sexual ill health burden is greatest.

The incidence of STIs depends as much upon social and economic factors as upon biology and behaviour. STIs thrive in situations where communities are disrupted by conflict and war, where there is a high dependence upon migrant labour that disrupts families, and where commercial sex work is prevalent. They are also promoted by stigmatisation, which delays presentation for treatment and reduces the resources employed for their control. High-income countries have also seen an increase in STIs since 2000, especially in marginalised communities including men who have sex with men (MSM), ethnic minorities and young people.

STIs are caused by a diverse group of microorganisms recently expanded by newly recognised sexually transmissible pathogens such as *Mycoplasma genitalium* and the Zika and Ebola viruses [2]. The traditional bacterial STIs continue to evolve and clinical presentations of some, such as lymphogranuloma venereum, have changed. While chancroid and granuloma inguinale have become rare, gonorrhoea and syphilis have re-emerged as major public health concerns due to increased transmission among MSM and the spread of antimicrobial-resistant gonorrhoea.

Many individuals have asymptomatic early infections, and this favours onward transmission. The later complications are a serious cause of morbidity and mortality. STIs adversely affect reproductive health, especially in women, and are a major cause of infertility because of damage to the fallopian tubes from ascending infections. Adverse pregnancy outcomes in terms of ectopics, miscarriage and stillbirth are common. Postabortal and postpartum infections related to STIs are thought to cause around one-third of maternal deaths worldwide. Fetal morbidity and mortality may also occur from preterm birth associated with many STIs and from vertical transmission causing congenital infections. Premature death in adults of both sexes may also result from genital cancers associated with human papillomavirus (HPV) infections and liver disease associated with sexually transmitted hepatitis B and hepatitis C.

Before the advent of highly active antiretroviral therapy, the greatest loss of life was associated with HIV infection. The biological and behavioural synergy between STIs and HIV, which favours both acquisition and transmission, emphasises the need for coordinated public health control measures [3]. STI rates remain high in those living with HIV and in those using pre-exposure prophylaxis (PrEP).

The WHO has set global targets for reducing the incidences of both syphilis and gonorrhoea by 90% from their 2016 baseline values by 2030 (Figure 29.1) [4]. In addition, it has set an ambitious aim to abolish congenital syphilis cases in over 80% of countries.

Success in these objectives will require a coordinated, multi-agency approach involving multiple government departments including public health, education and social services. Improved surveillance is the basis for the development of national and local strategic planning. Behaviour change and promotion of condom use can reduce individual risk. Diagnostic laboratory testing services should underpin clinical services. Antimicrobial resistance, especially in *Neisseria gonorrhoeae* and *Mycoplasma genitalium*, is an increasing cause for concern and requires ongoing monitoring. The wider use of new sensitive and specific point-of-care rapid testing can improve early diagnosis in relevant settings especially in LMICs where diagnostic services have limited availability.

Partner notification and contact tracing have long been key components of comprehensive patient management. During the past decade, the increasing use of dating apps on the internet has facilitated sex with anonymous partners thereby reducing the efficacy of partner notification. To counteract this, innovative ways to use the Internet to promote health education and partner notification will be needed.

Rook's Textbook of Dermatology, Tenth Edition. Edited by Christopher Griffiths, Jonathan Barker, Tanya Bleiker, Walayat Hussain and Rosalind Simpson.
© 2024 John Wiley & Sons Ltd. Published 2024 by John Wiley & Sons Ltd.

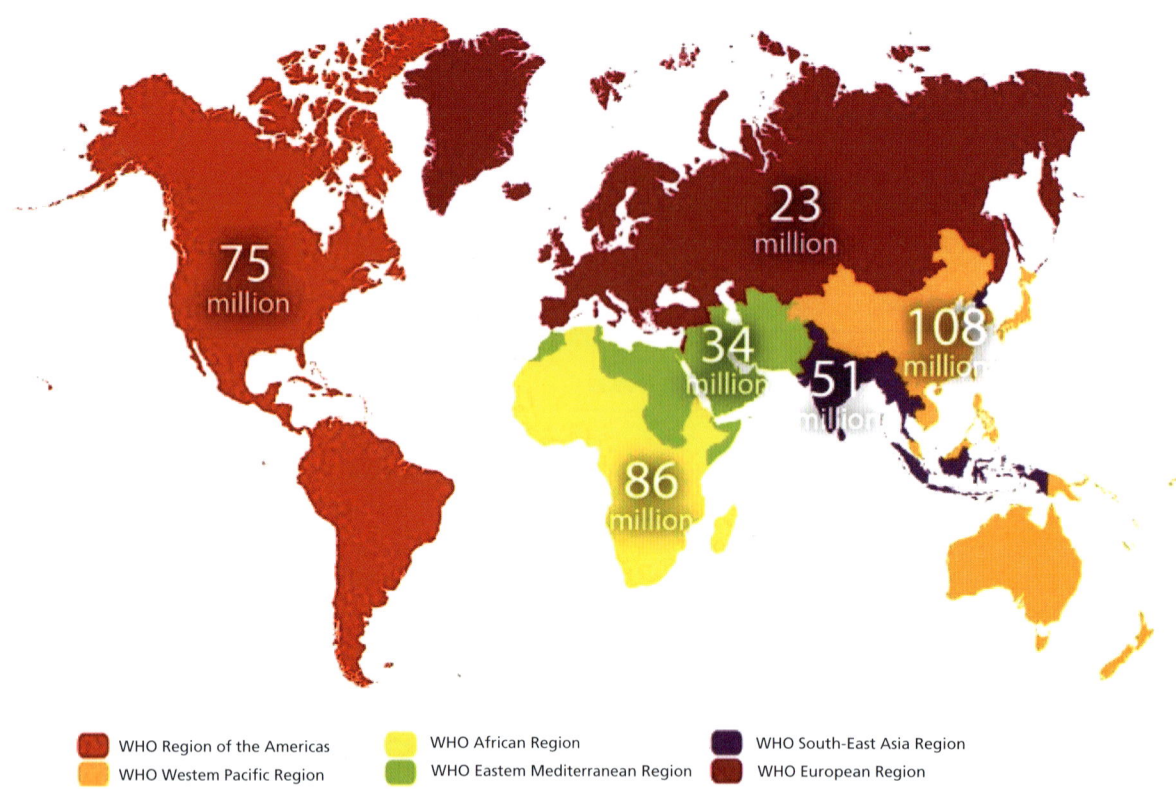

Figure 29.1 Estimated new cases of curable sexually transmitted infections (gonorrhoea, chlamydia, syphilis and trichomoniasis) by WHO region, 2016. Reproduced from WHO 2016 [4] with permission.

The effect of the Covid-19 pandemic has yet to be clearly defined. This has exposed the vulnerabilities resulting from inadequate resourcing of public health services in many countries. Such inadequacies have also favoured STI spread. Although lockdowns and restriction of social interactions temporarily reduce the opportunities for new sexual relationships, the move to virtual medical consultations has also deterred many individuals from presenting for STI screening and early diagnosis. History has shown that any temporary improvements in STI incidence are likely to be short-lived unless there is sustained commitment to control efforts when social constraints are lifted.

However, the remarkable success in the rapid development of effective vaccines against SARS-CoV-2 also gives renewed hope that recent technological advances could be extended to other infections, including the STIs, for which vaccine development has so far proved elusive. Innovation in interventions and service delivery will continue to be necessary to meet changing population needs, reduce health inequalities and keep pace with the continuing evolution of its causative microorganisms.

Syphilis

Definition and nomenclature

Syphilis is an infectious disease caused by the spirochaetal bacterium *Treponema pallidum* subsp. *pallidum*. The disease is usually acquired through sexual contact. Congenital syphilis (CS) occurs through transplacental transmission. Untreated syphilis infection can evolve through several stages, each separated for variable times by periods of latency in which there are no clinical manifestations.

> **Synonyms and inclusions**
> - The name syphilis was coined by Fracastoro, an Italian physician and poet, in 1530. His poem titled 'Syphilis *sive morbus gallicus*' tells of a shepherd named Syphilus who was smitten with the disease by the god Apollo as punishment for his defiance [1]
> - Among the many names that syphilis has acquired through the ages, it was dubbed the 'great imitator' due to its florid systemic manifestations that often caused confusion with other diseases. In the 16th century it was also called the 'great pox' to distinguish it from smallpox as syphilis produced a similar rash in its early stages

Epidemiology

Incidence and prevalence

Socioeconomic factors play an important role in the prevalence of syphilis. In developing countries, the disease has remained a prominent cause of genital ulcer disease in heterosexual men and women, and cause of stillbirth and neonatal morbidity and mortality [2,3].

In 2018, the WHO estimated that there were 6 million new syphilis cases and a global prevalence of 0.53 per 1000 individuals aged 15–49 years in both sexes; there was a marked geographic variability in prevalence rates ranging from 0.11 in the European region to 1.58 in the African region [4]. Prevalence rates were also higher than average in the Americas and eastern Mediterranean regions and lower than average in South-East Asia and the western Pacific regions.

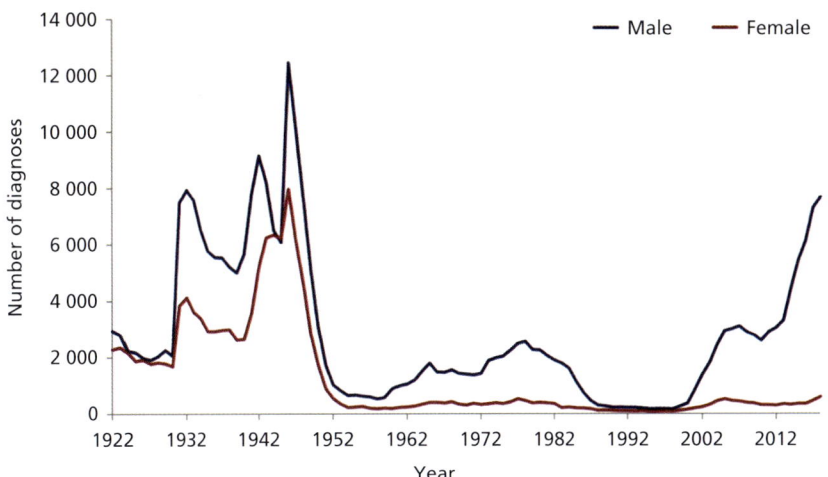

Figure 29.2 Number of syphilis diagnoses by sex: UK, 1922–2018. Reproduced from Public Health England 2019 STI slide set Version 1.0; published 2 September 2020.

Both the UK [5] and the USA [6] have maintained effective national STI monitoring systems since the pre-antibiotic era of the last century. The high incidence of syphilis in World War II peaked as thousands of demobilised men and women returned home to resettle. The period of relative socioeconomic stability of the early 1950s saw a decline in all STIs, including syphilis. Syphilis outbreaks were seen in association with crack cocaine during the 1990s. Since 2000, syphilis rates have again risen, especially in MSM where high-risk sexual behaviours have increased following the advent of effective antiretroviral treatment. Incarceration, sexual activity associated with illicit drug use and accessing multiple anonymous sexual partners by internet dating apps are recognised risk factors. There are high rates of associated HIV infection, and reinfections are becoming more common. Rates in heterosexuals had declined to low levels but have more than doubled in the past 10 years, especially in socially marginalised individuals with poor access to health care, raising renewed fears of the re-emergence of CS. Similar observations are seen in other high-income countries in Europe [7].

Age
Syphilis occurs in sexually active individuals of all ages and recent acquisition is commoner in young adults.

Sex
Although there is marked preponderance of cases in males, this sex difference relates to patterns of sexual behaviour (Figure 29.2). It is generally considered that male to female transmission is more efficient.

Ethnicity
The disease occurs in all racial groups. No racial or genetic predisposition has been shown.

Associated diseases
Acquired syphilis commonly coexists with other STIs, hence comprehensive screening is advised when syphilis is detected.

Pathophysiology
The causative spirochaete usually enters the body via microscopic dermal abrasions. Subsequently, it enters the lymphatics and blood to disseminate widely.

Pathology
A local inflammatory response to the causative organisms is the basis of all clinical manifestations. Precise details of the mechanisms causing tissue damage and of host defences remain ill defined.

The fundamental pathological changes in syphilis are the same in early and late disease. They occur in and around the blood vessels in the form of a perivascular infiltration of lymphocytes and plasma cells, accompanied by intimal proliferation in both the arteries and veins (endarteritis obliterans).

In early lesions, perivascular infiltration by lymphocytes and plasma cells is accompanied by intimal proliferation in the arteries and veins. This leads to ischaemia and ulceration. Organisms are most numerous in the walls of the capillaries and lymphatic vessels. They can be demonstrated by the Levaditi silver stain, by the fluorescent antibody technique and by immunohistochemistry [8]. The papular skin lesions of secondary syphilis also show endothelial swelling in dermal vessels. In addition, there is often psoriasiform hyperplasia of the epidermis with a multifocal interface change associated with lymphocytes and particularly plasma cells (Figure 29.3). Immunohistochemistry for treponema shows numerous microorganisms, which in secondary syphilis tend to be more prominent within the epidermis (Figure 29.4).

In late lesions, the characteristic lesion of mucocutaneous surfaces is the syphilitic gumma. Granulation tissue forms with histiocytes, fibroblasts and epithelioid cells. Endarteritis obliterans and necrotic areas are pronounced. Gummata most often originate in subcutaneous tissues and spread in all directions. Spirochaetes are not readily demonstrable in these lesions.

Heubner arteritis occurs in cardiovascular and meningovascular syphilis. It is characterised by lymphocytic and plasma cell infiltration of the vasa vasorum and the adventitia of large and medium-sized vessels. Occlusion of the vasa vasorum results in medial necrosis and fibroblast proliferation. There is associated subintimal proliferation, which leads to luminal occlusion and thrombosis.

Causative organisms
The causative spirochaete of syphilis, *Treponema pallidum* subsp. *pallidum*, was discovered by Schaudinn and Hoffmann in 1905 and originally was called *Spirochaeta pallidum*.

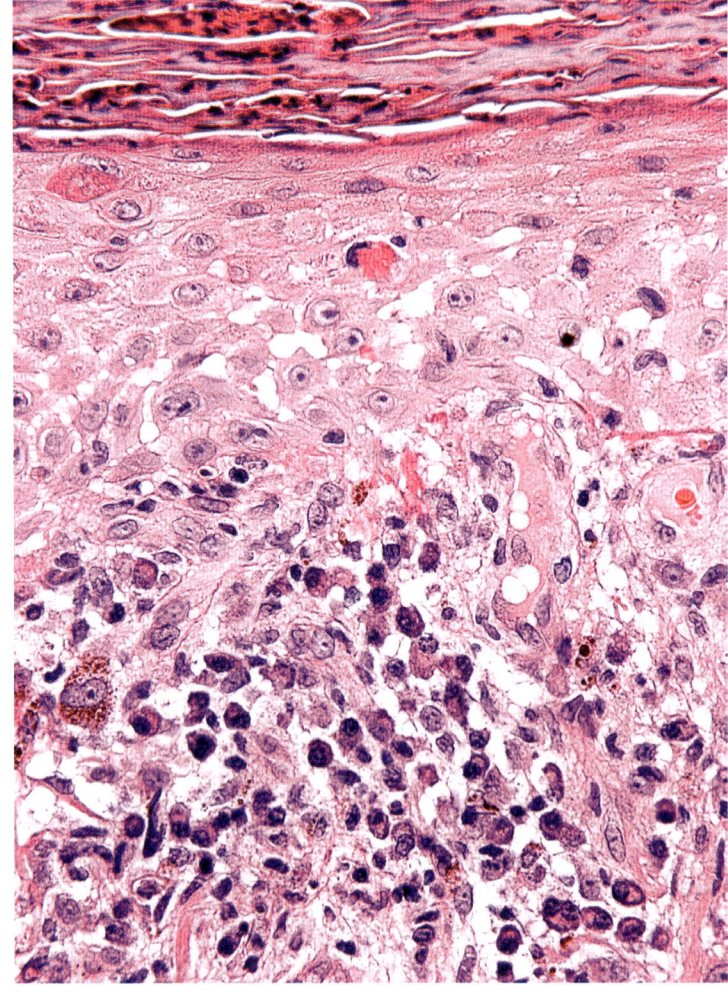

Figure 29.3 Secondary syphilis showing psoriasiform hyperplasia of the epidermis with spongiosis and interface change with abundant plasma cells.

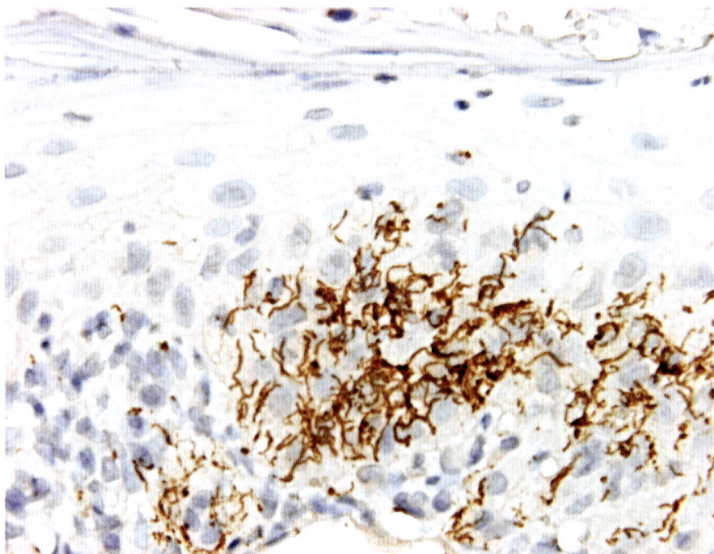

Figure 29.4 Secondary syphilis. Immunohistochemistry shows numerous spirochaetes within the epidermis.

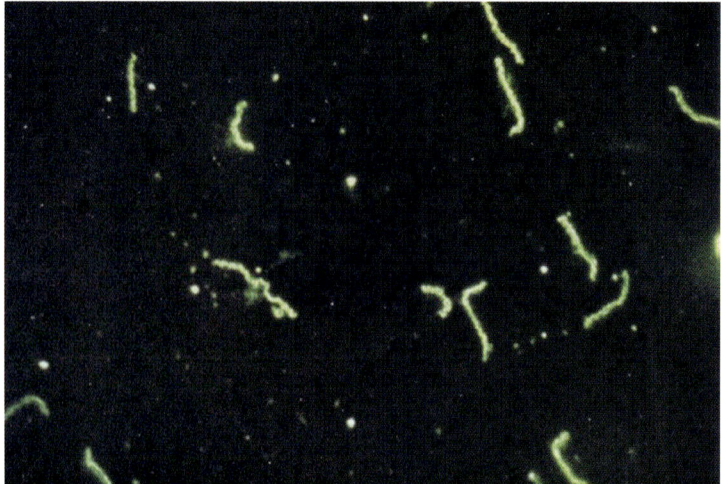

Figure 29.5 *Treponema pallidum* on dark ground microscopy.

T. pallidum cannot be grown in the laboratory on any biochemical medium. Not all animals are susceptible to it. The rabbit is commonly used in laboratory studies and as a source of the *T. pallidum* used in diagnostic tests. *T. pallidum* cannot be differentiated from those treponemes involved in other forms of treponematosis, nor from the Nichol strain, which was isolated in 1912 from the brain of a patient and kept alive by passage through many generations of rabbits. Another experimental treponeme, the Reiter strain, is said to have been isolated in 1922. In contrast with the Nichol strain, it is avirulent and can be cultivated on a relatively simple medium. Freeze-dried extracts were used for many years in the Reiter protein complement fixation test.

Morphology. In daily practice, *T. pallidum* is demonstrated by dark-field microscopy (Figure 29.5). It appears as a pale, white, fine, corkscrew organism with close and very regular coils (Figure 29.6). Its length varies from 6 to 15 µm and its coils from 0.09 to 0.18 µm. There are between eight and 20 coils. As a practical guide, to help differentiate the organism from others like it, there are about seven to eight coils per diameter of a red blood corpuscle. It contains a

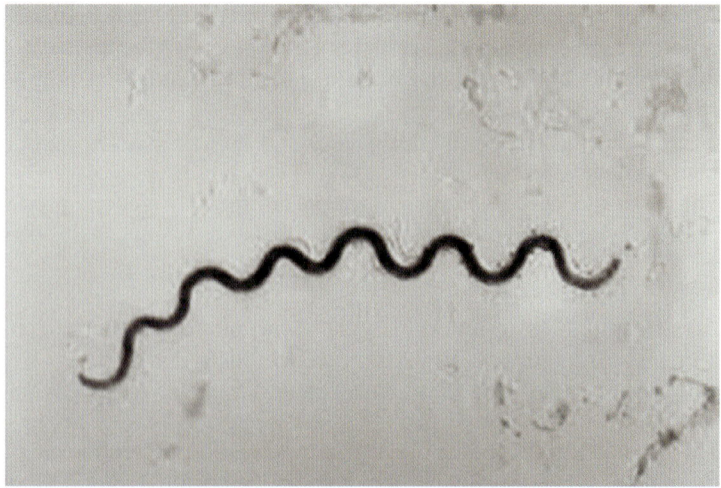

Figure 29.6 *Treponema pallidum* showing typical morphology.

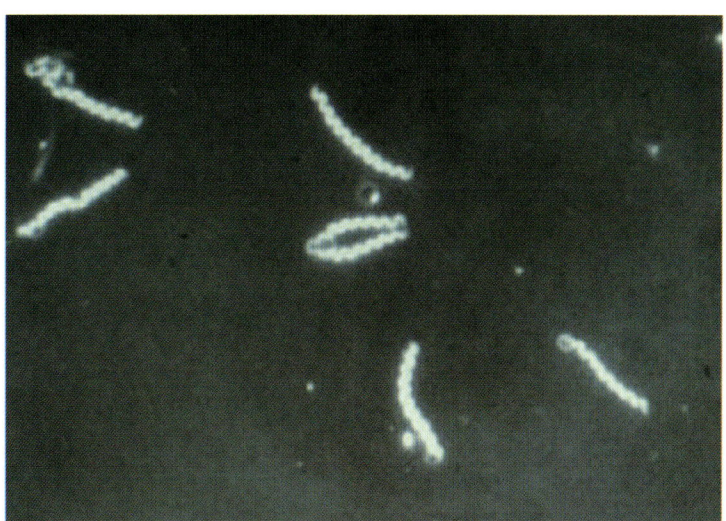

Figure 29.7 Immunofluorescent image of *Treponema pallidum*.

periplasmic flagellum and is actively motile [2]. The movements of *T. pallidum* are pathognomonic. It rotates around its long axis and thus appears to quiver and screw slowly backwards and forwards; it shows a highly typical angling movement, forming both acute and obtuse angles. It shows both grace and elegance and these help to distinguish it from other genital or oral spirochaetal organisms. Treponemes can also be demonstrated by the direct fluorescent antibody method [9–11] and by rapid immunofluorescent staining of smears [12] from lesions (Figure 29.7).

Of the several spirochaetes found in the genital area and requiring differentiation from *T. pallidum*, the most important are *Borrelia refringens* and *B. balanitidis*. Both are thicker than *T. pallidum* and have fewer coils, which are irregular. In addition, they move with more fidgety, snake- and eel-like movements. *B. gracilis* is finer than *T. pallidum*, with closer coils and a lack of typical movements. It can be found at the gum margins between teeth.

Microbiology. The organism is microaerophilic and has evolved to become a highly invasive and persistent pathogen with little toxigenic activity and an inability to survive outside the mammalian host [13]. It has extreme nutritional requirements due to deficiencies in its biosynthetic pathways and has a narrow equilibrium between oxygen dependence and toxicity. It cannot be cultured on artificial media, but it can be propagated in organ culture, such as rabbit testes. It has a slow growth rate, optimal at 33–35°C, with a doubling time of 30–36 h. The organism shares extensive DNA homology with three other pathogenic treponemes which cause yaws, bejel and pinta.

Analysis of the genome, which is contained on a single circular chromosome of 1138 kbp, shows that the organism lacks lipopolysaccharide and lipid biosynthesis mechanisms, as well as many metabolic pathways including, for the tricarboxylic acid cycle, components of oxidative phosphorylation and for most amino acids and vitamins. It requires D-glucose, maltose and mannose but cannot utilise other sugars. It can use exogenously supplied amino acids and is dependent upon serum components such as fatty acids.

T. pallidum initiates an inflammatory response at the site of inoculation and is disseminated during the primary infection. The organism has a surface-associated hyaluronidase enzyme, which may play a role in this process. Phagocytosis by cytokine-activated macrophages, as part of a predominant T-helper 1 (Th1) type early response, aids bacterial clearance and resolution of the primary lesion [14]. Virulent organisms promote the adhesion of lymphocytes and monocytes to human vascular cells, and this is important in immunopathogenesis [15]. As with other organisms that cause chronic disease, *T. pallidum* has evolved mechanisms for evading immune responses. A Th1–Th2 switch occurs with macrophage suppression caused by prostaglandin E2 down-regulation; however, the molecular mechanisms remain poorly understood [16]. Depressed cell-mediated responses occur during the later stages of syphilis, and a lowered CD4+ lymphocyte count has been reported [17].

Molecular features. Relatively few genes are involved in pathogenesis. It has been postulated that the immunoevasiveness of *Treponema pallidum* is the result of the organism's unusual molecular architecture. The outer membrane lacks lipopolysaccharide and contains few, poorly immunogenic transmembrane proteins. The highly immunogenic proteins are lipoproteins anchored predominantly to the periplasmic leaflet of the cytoplasmic membrane [2]. The *T. pallidum* repeat protein genes (TpR) occupy 2% of the genome and encode for a group of potential virulence factors, which are targets for strong cellular and humoral responses [18]. The TpR-K proteins demonstrate marked antigenic variation [19].

Clinical features
Natural history
Stages. The clinical presentation of syphilis is extremely diverse and may occur decades after the initial infection. Syphilis, if untreated, may pass through four stages: primary, secondary, latent and late. The first two stages are contagious. They seldom last more than 2 years and do not exceed 4 years. Latency may last from 5 to 50 years. Only 25–30% of patients present with late, chronic, crippling or fatal manifestations. The frequency of these late manifestations continues to decline, and in many countries they are now rare.

Incubation period. The incubation period of syphilis is generally given as 9–90 days and varies inversely with the size of the spirochaete inoculum. Typically, most genital primary sores appear 3 weeks after exposure. Inguinal lymphadenopathy, initially unilateral, occurs after a further week and usually becomes bilateral by 5 weeks after infection. Reactive reaginic serological tests are detectable at 5.5–6 weeks, the macular rash at 8 weeks, papular lesions at 3 months and condylomata lata at 6 months.

Course of untreated syphilis. Several investigations have helped to elucidate the natural history of untreated syphilis, for example the Oslo study of untreated syphilis [20] and the Tuskegee study [21]. Regarding the first of these, Caesar Boeck believed that *no* treatment was better than using mercury. He therefore kept some 2000 infectious patients with syphilis in hospital for 1–12 months (average 3–6 months), until all traces of their infection had gone.

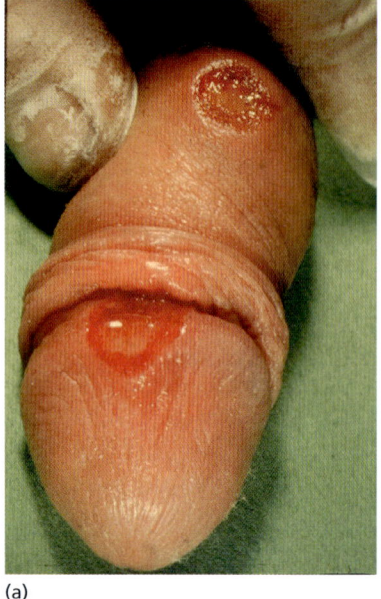 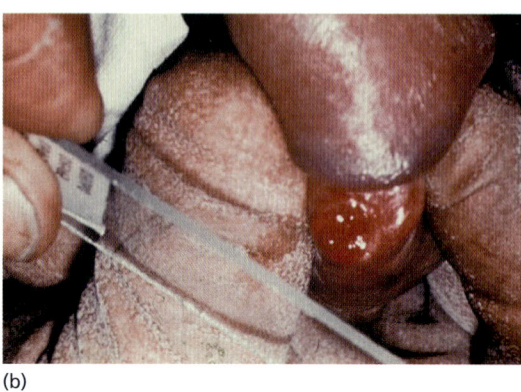 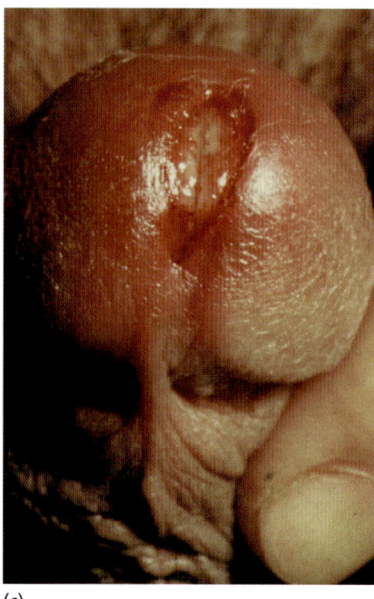

Figure 29.8 Penile chancres. (a) Primary syphilis showing chancres on the glans and shaft of the penis. (b) Taking specimens for dark ground microscopy from a penile chancre on the coronal sulcus. (c) A penile meatal chancre, which may be mistaken for meatitis associated with urethritis.

Gjestland [20] made a follow-up study of 1147 patients and summarised the findings as follows:
- 24% developed mucocutaneous relapses.
- 11% died of syphilis.
- 16% developed benign late manifestations, usually cutaneous nodules or gummata.
- 10% developed cardiovascular syphilitic lesions.
- 6% developed neurosyphilis.

It would appear therefore that long before the arsenicals and penicillin were introduced, at least 60% of people with syphilis lived and died without developing serious symptoms of their infections.

Presentation of primary syphilis

The primary chancre appears at the site of the initial treponemal invasion of the dermis. Initial lesions are papular but rapidly ulcerate. It may occur on any skin or mucous membrane surface and is usually situated on the external genitalia.

The typical primary sore appears as a regularly edged, regularly based, hard and button-like ulceration measuring up to 1 cm in diameter. Unless secondarily infected, primary sores are not painful. The ulcer is often surrounded by a narrow, red border, 1–2 mm wide (Figure 29.8). This marks the limits of the inflammatory reaction and is most productive of *T. pallidum*. The lesion may be crusted due to drying of serous exudate. Induration of the ulcer is characteristic, but it should be remembered that all lesions in the coronal sulcus of the penis are indurated. 'Kissing ulcers', sometimes hourglass in shape, are not uncommon. About 50% of lesions are atypical and lack one or more of the classic features. If the infection is inoculated into pre-existing lesions such as anal fissures, genital herpes or balanitis, the chancre may assume the shape of these conditions. In most cases, there is only a single chancre. Multiple chancres may appear simultaneously or within a few days of each other. Untreated, the chancre persists for a variable period but seldom, if ever, exceeds 3 months. As a rule, it heals spontaneously in 3–8 weeks. In about one-third of cases, it leaves a regularly edged, slightly depressed, thin, depigmented, atrophic scar.

The appearance of the genital and perianal chancre is followed by swelling of the inguinal lymph nodes, initially unilateral. Maxillary and submental lymph nodes enlarge when infection is in or around the oral cavity. Wherever they appear, the enlarged glands are discrete, rubbery and free from fixation to the skin or underlying tissues.

In men, the chancre most usually occurs on the glans penis, near the frenulum or on the underside of the prepuce. Less commonly, the primary lesion appears on the shaft of the penis. If near the hilt, it may be called a 'condom chancre'. Less common sites are the pubic region or the external urinary meatus where it may masquerade as non-specific urethritis with scanty serous discharge. Lesions are often surrounded by oedema. Subpreputial lesions may be accompanied by acquired phimosis and lymphangitis dorsalis penis may occur; it is felt as an indolent 'string', some 2 mm in diameter.

In MSM, the anus and rectum may be sites of primary infection (Figure 29.9) and may often be unnoticed by the affected person. Anal lesions may present as an indurated fissure. Pain may be a feature, as may itch and bleeding, especially after defaecation. Like genital primary lesions, extragenital sores are accompanied by regional lymphadenitis.

In women, most cases of early syphilis have reached the secondary stage when diagnosed [22]. A chancre is less frequently demonstrated, partly because the primary lesion may be on or in the cervix. The most common sites for a vulvar chancre are the labia minora or majora (Figure 29.10a), around the urethral orifice, on the clitoris or, quite commonly, on the posterior commissure where it may masquerade as an indurated irregular fissure. Surrounding vulval oedema is common (Figure 29.10b). A chancre very rarely occurs on the vaginal wall.

Extragenital chancres may be found on the lips (Figure 29.11a) as a result of kissing, cunnilingus or fellatio. The indurated ulcer

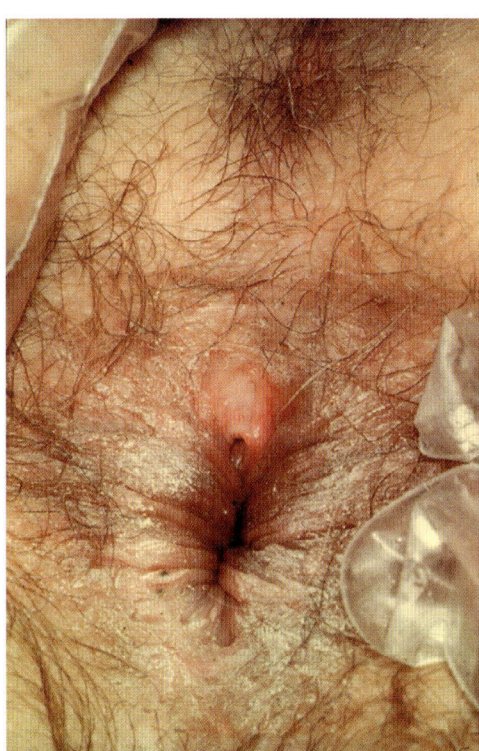

Figure 29.9 Anal lesion in syphilis.

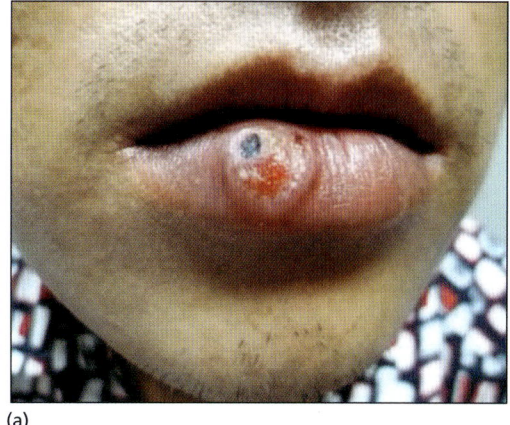

(a)

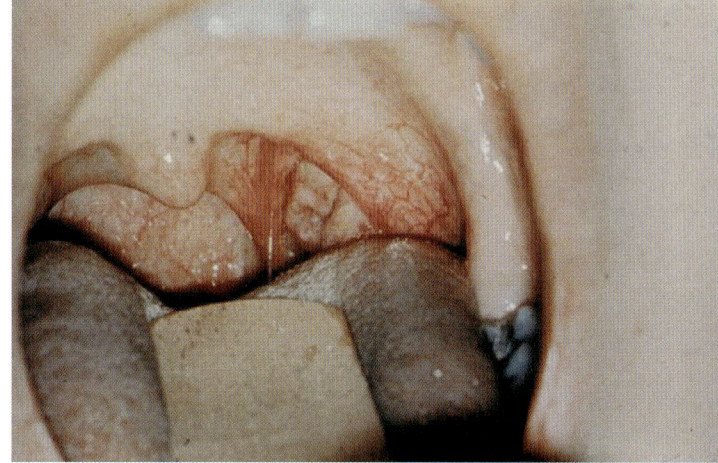

(b)

Figure 29.11 (a) A non-tender, non-purulent, oval ulcer with a clean base and raised rolled border on the lip of a 24-year-old man. (b) Primary chancre of the left tonsil. (a) Reproduced from Qiao and Fang [84].

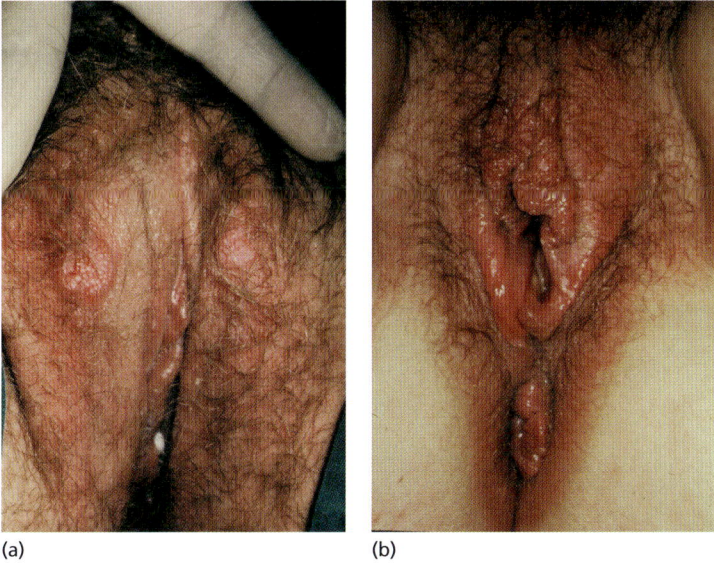

(a)   (b)

Figure 29.10 (a) Bilateral early chancres of the labia majora. (b) Chancre of the fourchette with surrounding oedema. This patient also had accompanying gonorrhoea, genital *Chlamydia* and trichomoniasis causing the accompanying vulvovaginitis. This illustrates how STIs frequently occur as multiple infections in the same patient.

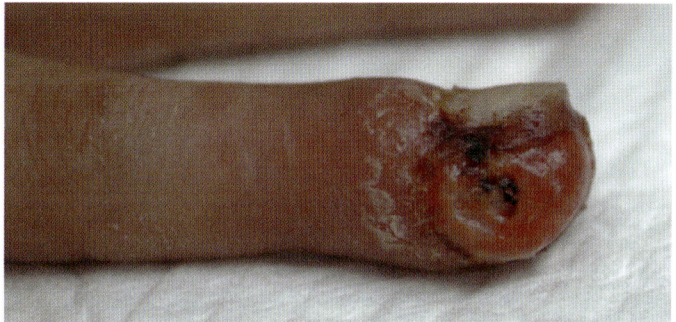

Figure 29.12 Primary syphilis of the fingers. Red to violaceous erosive nodule around the nail fold of the left index finger with secondary onychomadesis. Reproduced from Marcantonio *et al.* 2021 [85] with permission of BMJ Publishing.

may be surrounded by oedema. Chancres of the tongue and tonsil (Figure 29.11b) and primary lesions of the fingers (Figure 29.12), acquired in sexual foreplay, also occur. Other extragenital chancres may follow from nibbling or biting the nipple, ear, neck or arm.

Presentation of secondary syphilis

Secondary syphilis is the stage when generalised manifestations occur on the skin and mucous membranes. Serological tests are always positive in immunocompetent persons. Rashes in secondary syphilis have three common features:
- They are non-itchy.
- They are coppery red in colour.
- Symmetrical distribution.

The manifestations of generalised treponemal dissemination first appear at around 8 weeks. Constitutional symptoms consist of fever, headache and bone and joint pains that are more pronounced

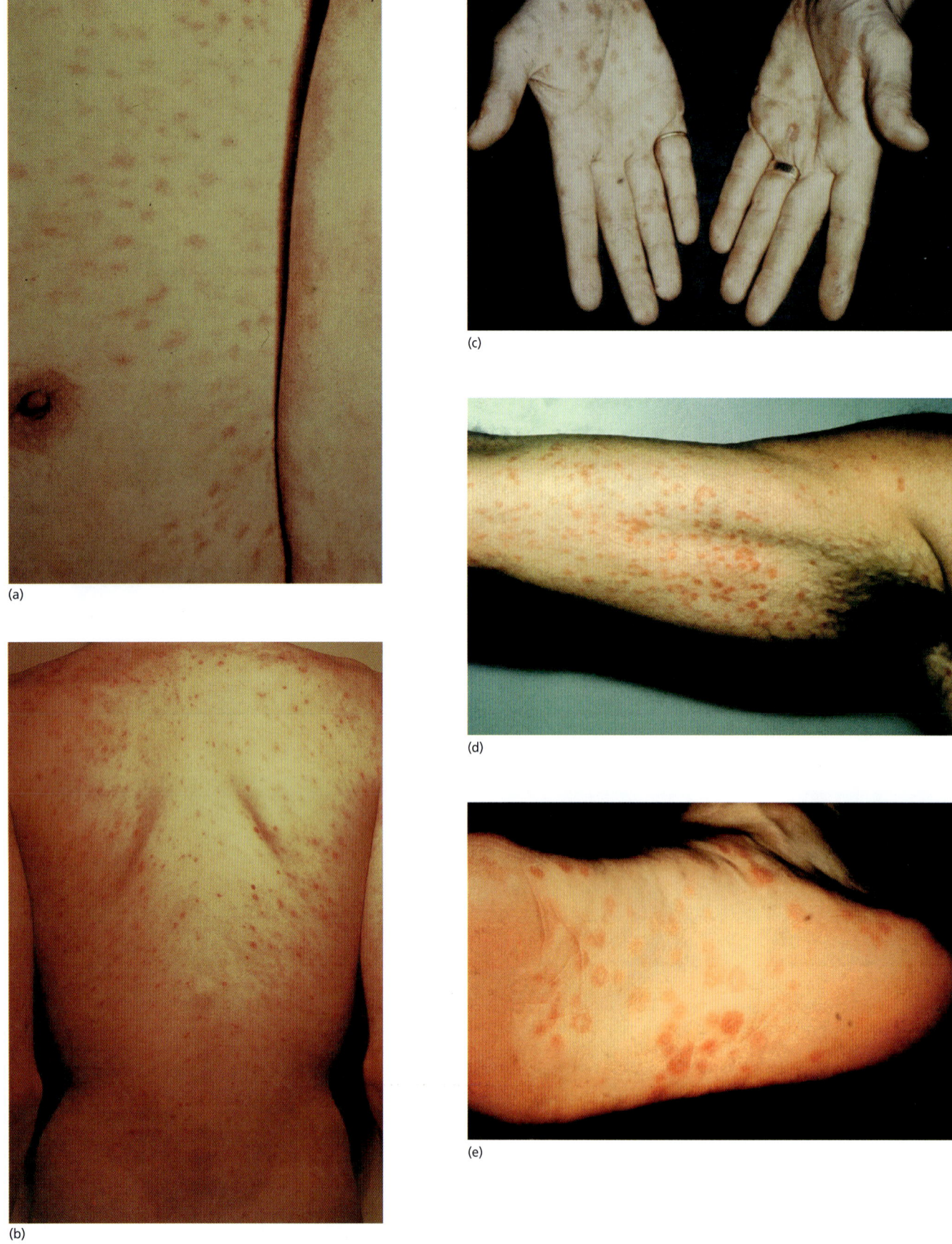

Figure 29.13 Secondary syphilis. (a) Extensive truncal maculopapular rash. (b) Macular rash with lesions following the skin lines of cleavage. (c) Papulosquamous palmar rash. (d) Axillary maculopapular lesions showing a classic coppery colour. (e) Papulosquamous lesions on the sole of the foot.

at night. There is wide diversity in physical features although rashes are the commonest feature. They are initially macular and become papular by 3 months. The features of secondary syphilis are diverse.

Macular syphilide (roseolar rash) (Figure 29.13). This is the earliest generalised syphilide; it is easily overlooked and seldom diagnosed in patients with deeply pigmented skin. The patient should be examined in daylight as it is easy to overlook an early or fading rash. It appears as symmetrical, coppery red, circular and oval spots. On the back, the lesions clearly follow the lines of cleavage of the skin. The roseolar spots do not scale or itch and, being in some patients sparse and evanescent, may pass unnoticed. When a roseola is fading, it sometimes leaves a pattern of depigmented spots on a hyperpigmented background. Such a leukoderma syphiliticum (Figure 29.14) is most commonly located on the back or sides of the neck and was formerly known as the 'necklace of Venus'.

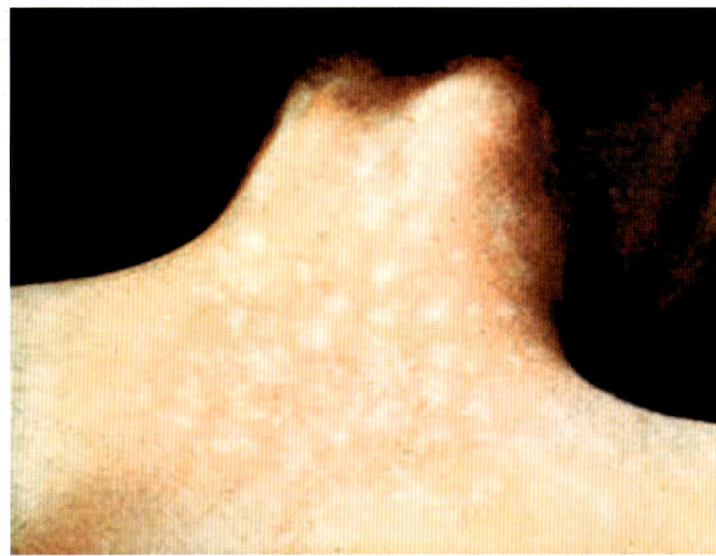

Figure 29.14 Syphilitic leukoderma showing depigmentation at sites of healed secondary lesions on the neck and upper back.

Papular syphilide (Figure 29.15). The papule is the basic lesion of secondary syphilis. Individual papules seldom exceed 0.5 cm in diameter. Its form of presentation can vary widely depending on the nature and colour of the patient's skin, the site affected and the climate, hygiene and clothing. Papular rashes may recur and be punctuated by spells of apparent latency. More usually, early papular rashes are in fact maculopapular and they have an even and generalised distribution all over the body. However, a purely coppery red papular rash, widely and symmetrically distributed, may also be seen. The typical papule is firm and round, although the largest may be oval. Early papules tend to be shiny, but gradually a thin layer of scale forms and is quickly shed. This is the typical papulosquamous syphilide. Older lesions tend to be more pigmented. In the late phases of a papular syphilide, nummular lesions, 1–3 cm in diameter and covered by massive layers of scales, may closely resemble psoriasis. Because the underlying lesions are exuding serum, the scales are easily removed. Psoriasiform papules of the palms and soles are especially common in more richly pigmented skin (Figure 29.16) as are annular and circinate papular rashes. Such rashes may resemble granuloma annulare, annular sarcoid or scaly varieties of tinea.

On macerated skin surfaces and mucous membranes, eroded weeping papules with a tendency to hypertrophy often appear. On the genitals, for example, at the peno-scrotal junction, there may be

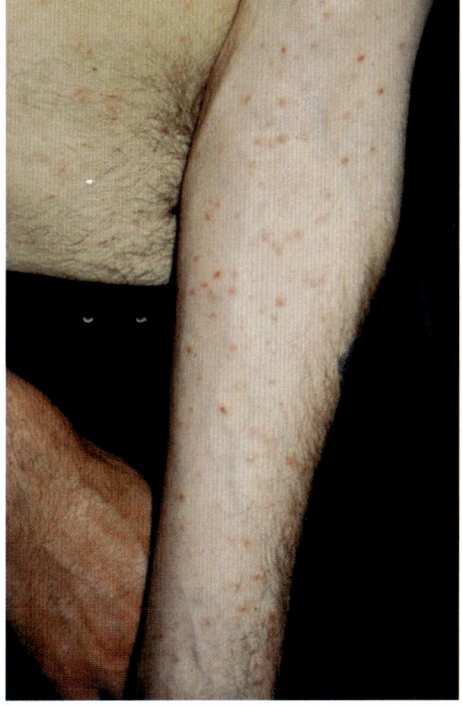 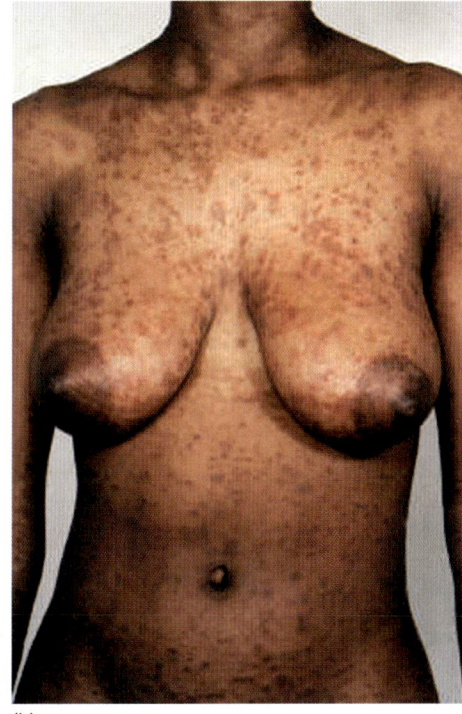

Figure 29.15 Secondary syphilis showing papular syphilides on (a) the forearms and (b) the trunk.

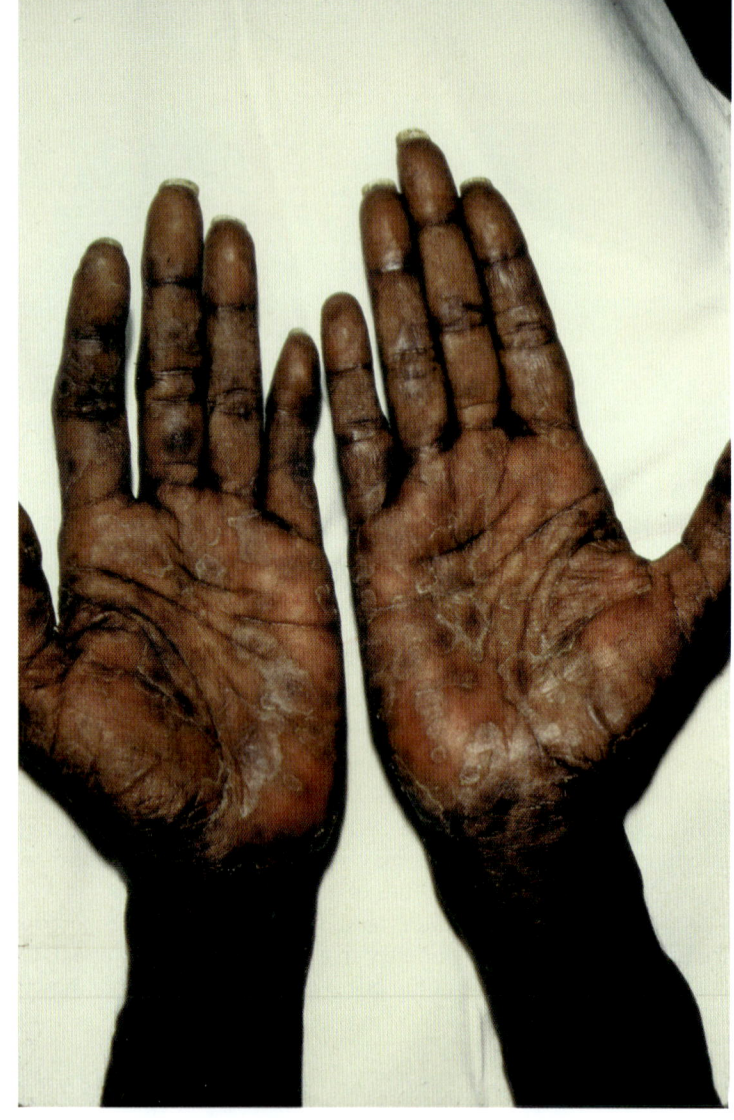

Figure 29.16 Secondary syphilis showing psoriasiform lesions of the palms.

same as those involved in acne vulgaris and seborrhoeic dermatitis. Sometimes, the papules form a line along the hair margin, the corona veneris.

Hyperkeratotic lesions of the palms and soles may flake, peel and fissure. Hypertrophic papules between the toes may resemble severe tinea pedis.

Micropapular and miliary eruptions are especially seen late in the second stage, about a year or more after infection. Characteristics of such a lichenoid syphilide include small conical or spinular elements, which tend to be arranged in groups of varying size over the body. A corymbose syphilide is one with a large central papule surrounded by small satellite papules.

Pustular ulcerative syphilide. This characterised the 16th century epidemic but is now all but unknown. Lesions that most nearly resemble this nowadays are the crusted papule of the scalp where brushing and combing tears papules, which ooze serum and may become secondarily infected. Such lesions, unlike other syphilides, may leave scars. Atypical facial plaques or ulcerated nodules (lues maligna) are more common with coexisting HIV infection [23].

Nails. Syphilitic paronychia with secondary onychia is sometimes seen in the secondary stage. It has no special characteristics.

Lesions of the mucous membranes. On the mucous membranes the basic papular eruptions are less distinctive, but they tend to be symmetrically distributed. As the surface epithelium dies, it turns grey and forms round or oval mucous patches on the palate or inner aspects of the lips and cheeks (Figure 29.18b). These mucous patches may coalesce to form 'snail-track' ulcers although ulceration is not common. Sharply defined, round or oval lesions devoid of dead epithelium may appear on the tongue and may be associated with flattened papillae. Bilateral syphilitic tonsillitis may coexist, as may syphilitic laryngitis associated with eroded papules and hoarseness.

Syphilitic alopecia. Patchy hair loss is characteristic of syphilis. The hair falls out leaving small, scattered, irregularly thinned, 'moth-eaten' patches of semibaldness (Figure 29.19). The eyebrows and beard may be affected [24,25]. Syphilitic alopecia may be accompanied by a more generalised, diffuse alopecia associated with generalised infection and anaemia.

Generalised lymphadenopathy. This occurs in 50% of secondary syphilis cases. As in the localised lymphadenopathy of primary infection, the nodes are painless, discrete, mobile and rubbery, and vary in size from about 0.5 to 2 cm.

Neurological involvement. During the secondary stage, the central nervous system may be invaded. Abnormalities in the cerebrospinal fluid (CSF), such as raised cell count and increased protein, can be found in at least 15% of cases. Less often, serological tests are positive in the CSF. The patient may complain of headache only. Occasionally, meningitis may present as paralysis of one

small, eroded papules flush with the skin or hypertrophic, coalesced papules (condylomata lata). Such lesions more commonly occur around the anus, groin and vulva (Figure 29.17a–d). In men, the papules frequently occupy the entire surface of the glans penis, the coronal sulcus and the inner aspect of the prepuce (Figure 29.17e). Partial or complete acquired phimosis is not infrequent in such cases. The free margin of the prepuce may be a circle of tender, fissured ('split') papules. In women, in the axillae and beneath the breasts, small, superficial, eroded, lentil-sized (about 0.3 cm) papules are sometimes seen, but more typical are hypertrophic papules, which may affect the adjacent mucous membrane. In the last stages of pregnancy, hypertrophic, coalesced, sodden-surfaced papules may be very pronounced. Later, the papules are more irregularly distributed but show a predilection for certain sites, such as the corners of the mouth (Figure 29.18a), angles of the nose, the palms and soles and body folds such as beneath the breasts or in the axillae. The face is often affected, particularly if the patient has greasy skin. The seborrhoeic areas involved are the

(a) (b) (c) (d) (e)

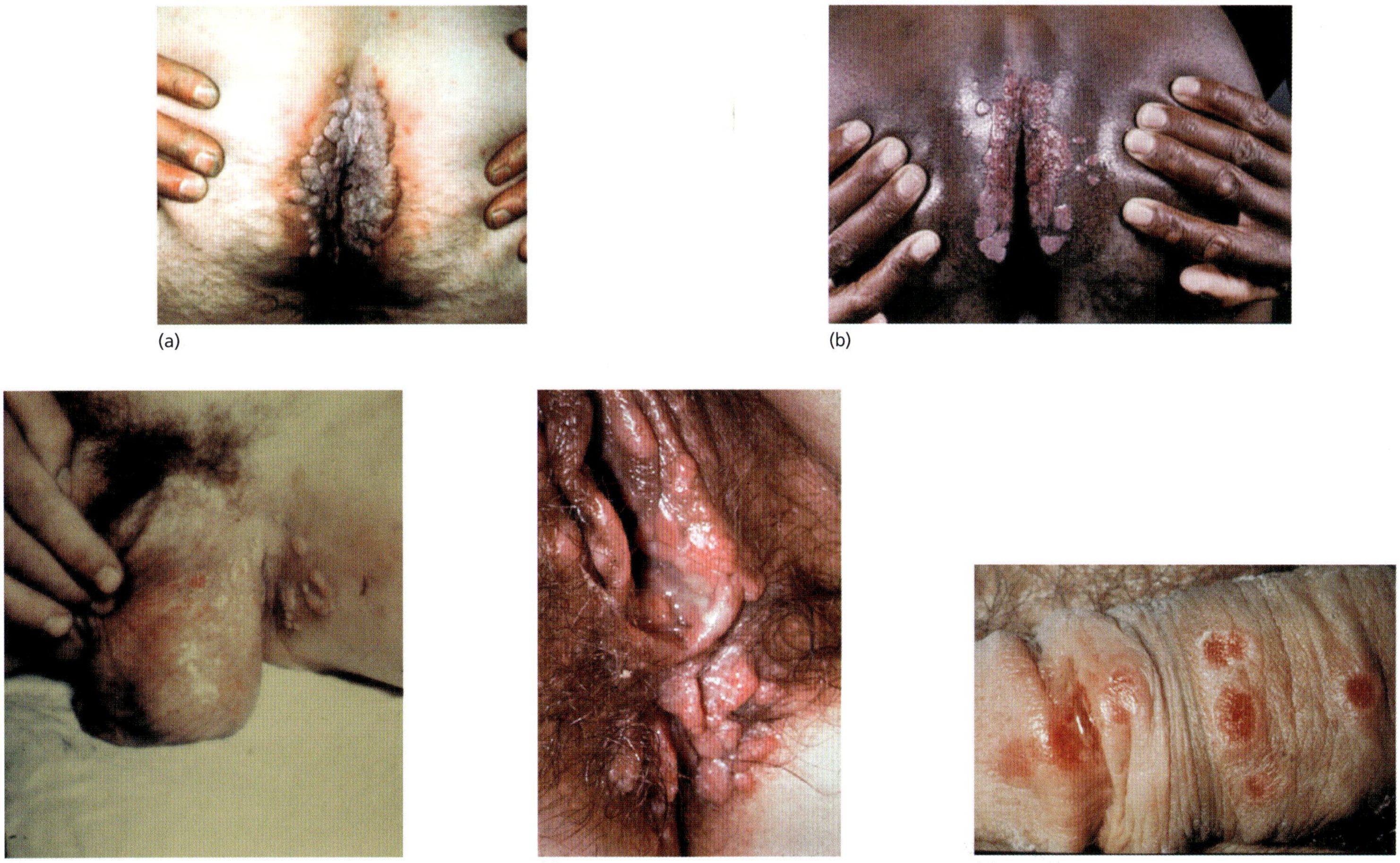

Figure 29.17 Condylomata lata of secondary syphilis: (a, b) perianal; (c) round the groin; (d) perivulval; (e) on the penile shaft with surrounding depigmentation (with a persistent primary in the coronal sulcus).

(a) (b)

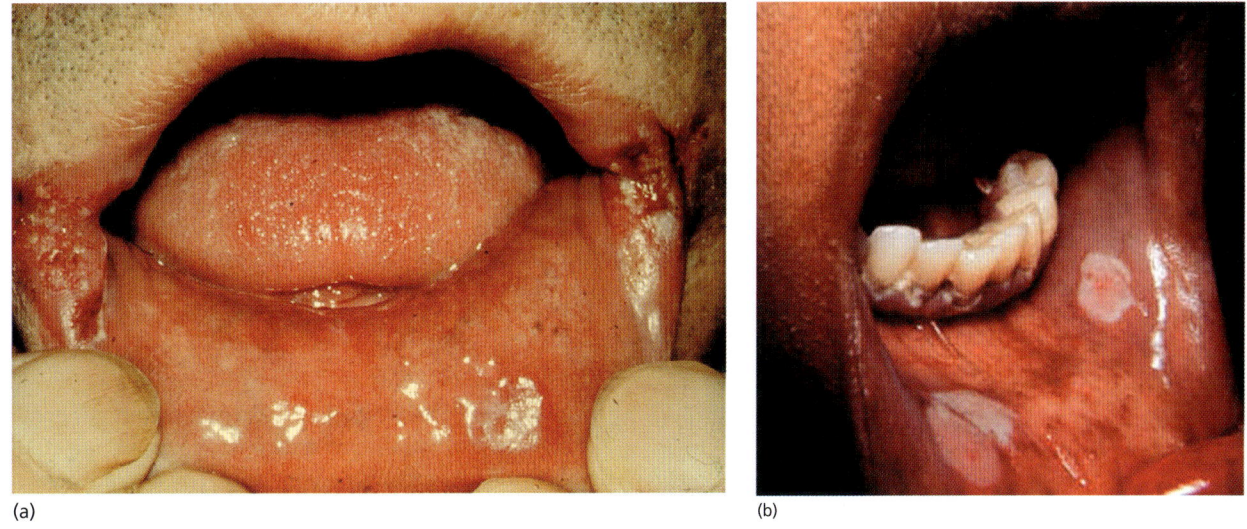

Figure 29.18 Oral lesions of secondary syphilis. (a) Split papules at the angle of the mouth. (b) Mucous patches on the buccal mucosa.

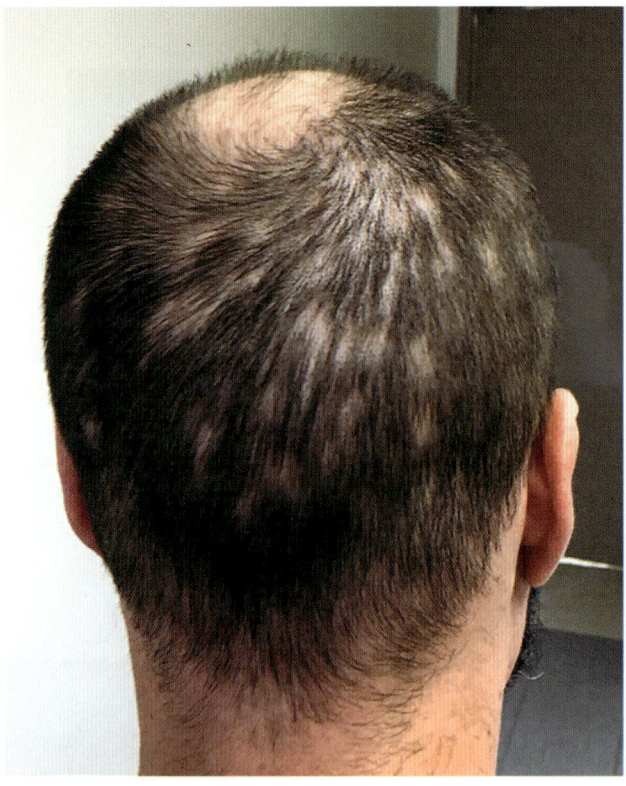

Figure 29.19 Thirty-four-year-old male with moth-eaten alopecia of secondary syphilis. Reproduced from Moshiri and Moxam 2018 [86].

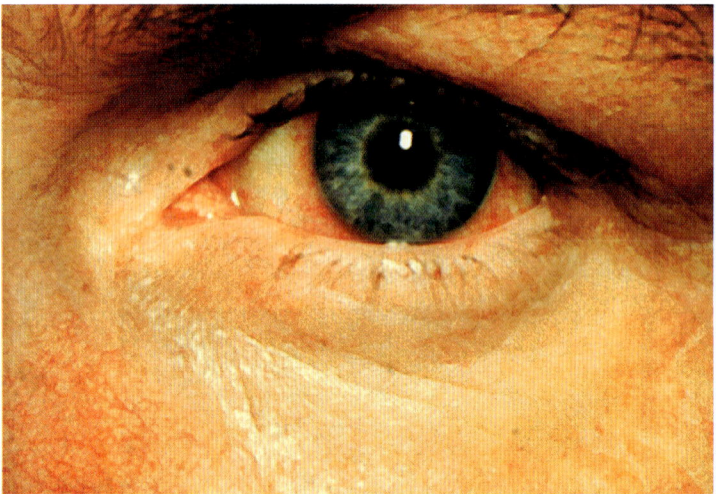

Figure 29.20 Syphilitic iritis causing circumcorneal injection of the blood vessels.

or more cranial nerves. Meningomyelitis with paraplegia and double incontinence is rare.

Other systemic features. Other systemic features of secondary syphilis include panuveitis (Figure 29.20) [26], periostitis and joint effusions, glomerulonephritis, hepatitis, gastritis and myocarditis.

The lesions of secondary syphilis resolve spontaneously in a variable time and most patients enter the latency stage within the first year of infection. In some, especially the immunocompromised, primary or secondary lesions may recur.

Presentation of latent syphilis

In latent syphilis there are no clinical stigmata of active disease, although disease remains detectable by positive serological tests. In early latency, within 2 years of infection, vertical transmission of infection may still occur, but sexual transmission is less likely in the absence of mucocutaneous lesions. The late manifestations of syphilis subsequently arise, often decades later, in about 25% of those who have latent syphilis.

To establish a diagnosis of latent syphilis, there are strict criteria. Clinical evidence of active, early, late or congenital syphilis must be absent; the CSF must be normal and a chest X-ray (preferably posteroanterior and left oblique, to view the aorta at a right angle) must also be normal. Positive (reactive) serological tests for syphilis (STS) must be confirmed by examination of a second specimen.

The differential diagnosis may be from biological false positive reactions or from other treponematoses, particularly yaws in immigrants to westernised countries. The presence of a scar of a primary chancre or leukoderma syphiliticum at the back of the neck may be helpful. Yaws is usually acquired by children living in poor rural conditions in the tropics. Presenting in adulthood with positive STS, they may give a history of yaws or chronic sores or bone pains, or they may know of the disease in their family, school or parish. Some have clinical or radiological evidence of old periostitis in their long bones [27]. Much the same may apply to bejel [28].

Yaws was targeted for eradication by the WHO in the 1950s but has re-emerged in warm, humid, forest areas in some countries in Africa, Asia, Latin America and the Pacific. It is associated with poverty and low socioeconomic conditions. The WHO has renewed global efforts to eradicate the disease since 2012.

Presentation of tertiary syphilis

After a period of latency of up to 20 years, manifestations of late syphilis can occur. However, screening for syphilis in blood donors and pregnant women has contributed greatly to the prevention of late syphilis. In addition, since the commencement of the antibiotic era, many people with latent and asymptomatic late syphilis have happened to receive penicillin or other treponemicidal antibiotics in circumstances unconnected with syphilis ('happenstance antibiotic therapy'). Such inadvertent therapy has also contributed to the decline of late syphilis, so that it is becoming rare in many parts of the western world including the UK and USA.

Late skin syphilis. Late skin syphilis appears in two types: the superficial or nodular syphilide and a deeper gummatous syphilide. Transitional forms also occur.
- *Nodular or tubercular syphilide.* The lesions are protruding, firm, coppery red nodules (larger than 0.5 cm diameter) (Figure 29.21a). On dependent limbs, they may be cyanotic. The nodules appear in groups with a tendency to a circinate arrangement – that is, forming interwoven circles and part of circles. As the disease heals centrally, it extends peripherally. The spread does not take place equally in all directions, so that the outline may be horseshoe shaped, tongued, kidney shaped or serpiginous. Some nodular eruptions resemble granuloma annulare or annular forms of sarcoid. Their histology resembles secondary syphilis. In other

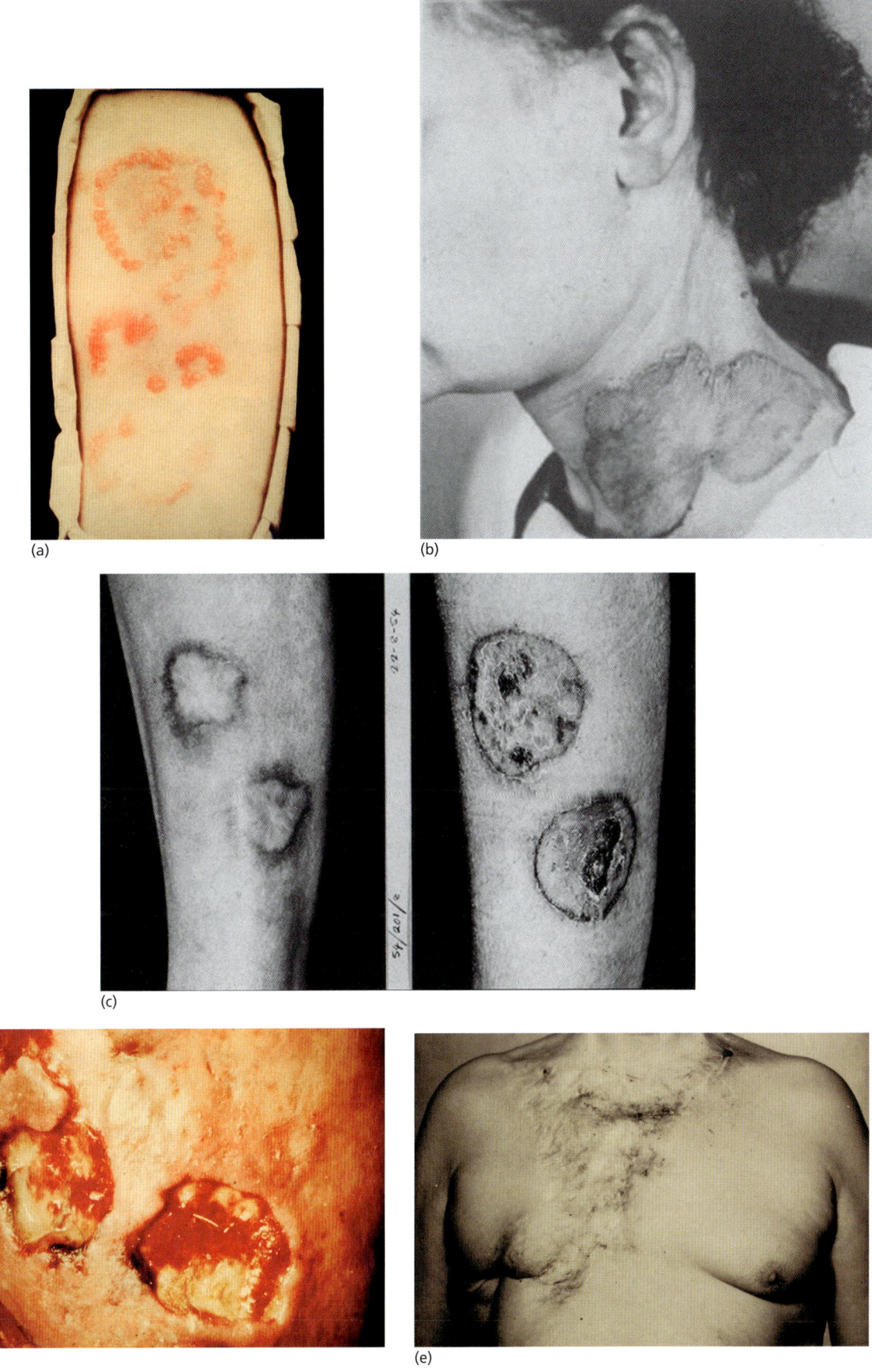

Figure 29.21 Skin lesions in tertiary syphilis. (a) Nodular gummata of the arm. (b) Psoriasiform gummata on the neck. (c) Psoriasiform gummata of the leg before (right) and after (left) treatment. (d) Ulcerated gummata on the leg showing wash-leather slough. (e) Extensive gummata of the chest wall showing peripheral healing and scarring.

cases, the abundance of waxy scales gives the eruption a psoriasiform appearance (Figure 29.21b, c). Most frequently, serpiginous nodulo-ulcerative eruptions are covered by massive crusts. Even the smallest ulcers have a punched-out appearance.

Lesions of nodular syphilis can appear anywhere on the body, but favour the extensor surfaces of the arms, back and face. They are symptomless. Where they have spread extensively, smooth, soft, finely wrinkled ('cigarette paper') central scarring is a feature. In their early stages, these scars may be pink, but after a year or two they are white. Nodular syphilis spreads slowly but more rapidly than lupus, producing a lesion of similar size in months rather than years.

- *Gummata*. The characteristic lesions of tertiary syphilis appear 3–10 years after infection and consist of granulomas or gummata. The granulomas appear as cutaneous plaques or nodules of irregular shape and outline and are often single lesions on the arms, back and face. They have a tendency for central necrosis and ulceration and for peripheral healing with tissue-paper scarring (Figure 29.21d). They most often originate in the subcutis, growing in all directions, into the dermis and epidermis as well as the deeper tissues. Gummata that start in bone or muscle also tend to ulcerate the skin, and their true origin may be difficult to determine. Gummatous changes sometimes take place more superficially with scattered, small ulcerations along the margins. This form is difficult to differentiate from a nodular syphilide.

Gummata are usually painless even when they ulcerate. Their central necrotic tissue may turn into a slimy, stringy mass, and it is this that gives rise to the name 'gumma'. Multiple gummata tend to coalesce, the bridges of skin between them gradually undergoing necrosis. Such ulcerations offer a wide variety of scalloped and geometrical patterns. A punched-out appearance is characteristic. Gummata vary in size from 2 to 10 cm. They favour the scalp, face, sternoclavicular areas of the chest and lateral calf. Gummata can be extensive and show healing with tissue paper scarring at their periphery (Figure 29.21e).

Late mucous membrane lesions. These lesions not infrequently attack the palate, both the hard and soft palate, with tissue destruction that may lead to loss of the uvula and scarring or perforation of the hard palate (Figure 29.22). In cases of congenital syphilis, destruction of the nasal septum may also occur, producing a saddle-nose deformity. They may also cause: (i) painless testicular swelling, mimicking a tumour [29]; (ii) portal hypertension and portosystemic anastomoses (Figure 29.23); and (iii) diffuse interstitial glossitis. Late syphilis of the tongue may present with localised or diffuse changes: a solitary gumma or diffuse gummatous infiltration. The latter often passes through a stage of chronic interstitial glossitis with fissuring and, later, obvious leukoplakia with patchy necrosis, sometimes associated with trauma from the teeth (Figure 29.24). In other cases, changes are more superficial, with red, smooth, glazed areas and the loss of papillae. Although sometimes painless, these changes may be accompanied by discomfort on eating hot or acid foods. All the forms of tongue involvement described are recognised as precancerous, so that even after adequate antisyphilitic treatment, regular observation of the patient is an essential element of sound management.

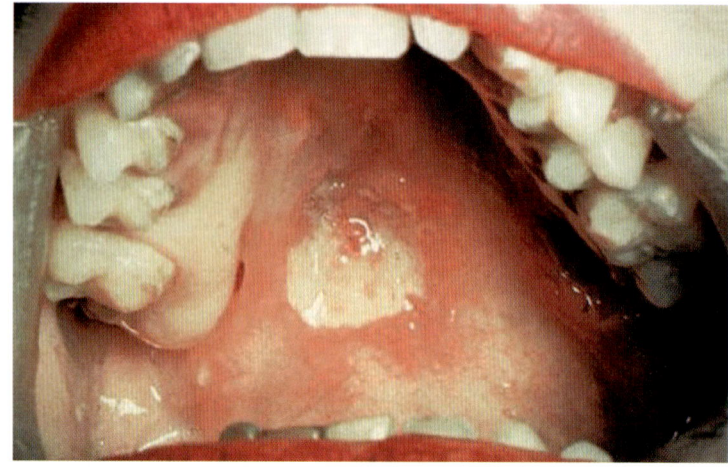

(a)

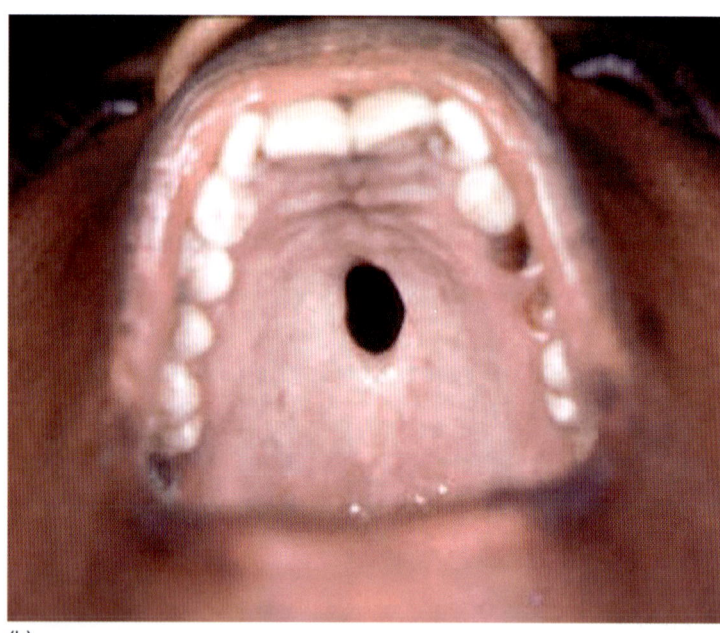

(b)

Figure 29.22 Mucosal lesions of tertiary syphilis. (a) Early gumma of the hard palate. (b) Perforated gumma of the hard palate.

Cardiovascular syphilis and neurosyphilis. These late manifestations, although detectable earlier, may take 20 or more years to become clinically evident.

The typical lesion of cardiovascular syphilis is aortitis affecting the ascending aorta and appearing 10–30 years after infection. The aortitis may be asymptomatic and detected as dilatation of the ascending aorta on a chest X-ray, often accompanied by linear calcification of the aortic wall (Figure 29.25a), or it may lead to stretching and incompetence of the aortic valve, left ventricular failure or aneurysm formation (Figure 29.25b). Aneurysms may be associated with a variety of syndromes caused by pressure on adjacent structures in the mediastinum, and they may cause sudden death from rupture. Other symptoms include angina pectoris from associated coronary ostial stenosis. Cardiovascular syphilis is more commonly associated with neurosyphilis than with gummatous disease.

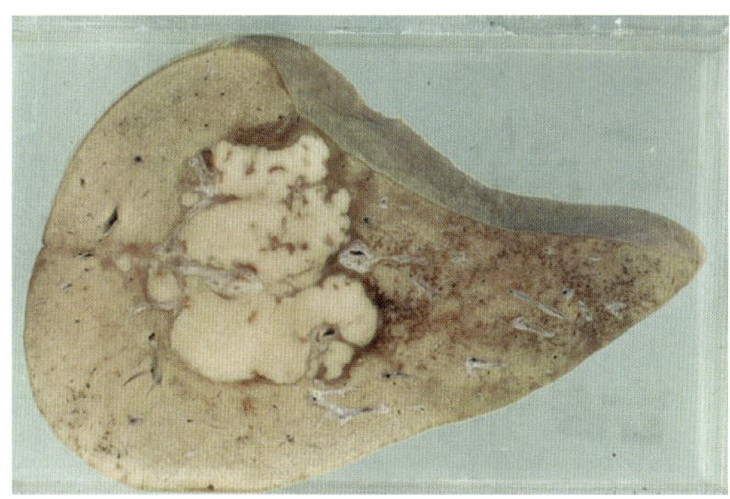

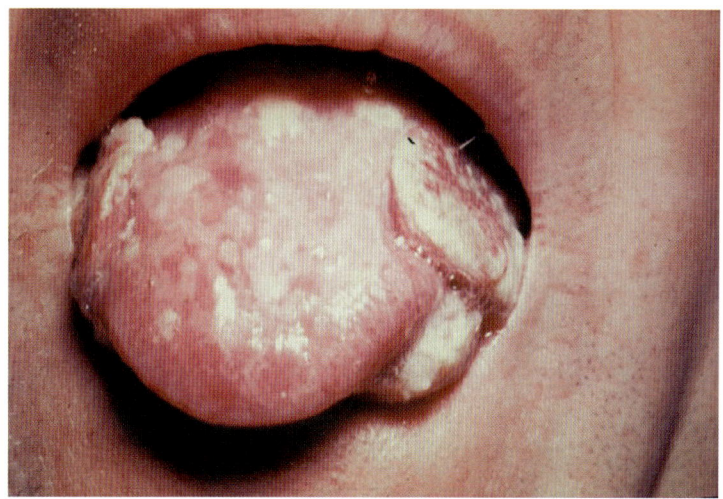

Figure 29.24 Chronic interstitial glossitis with bilateral squamous carcinoma.

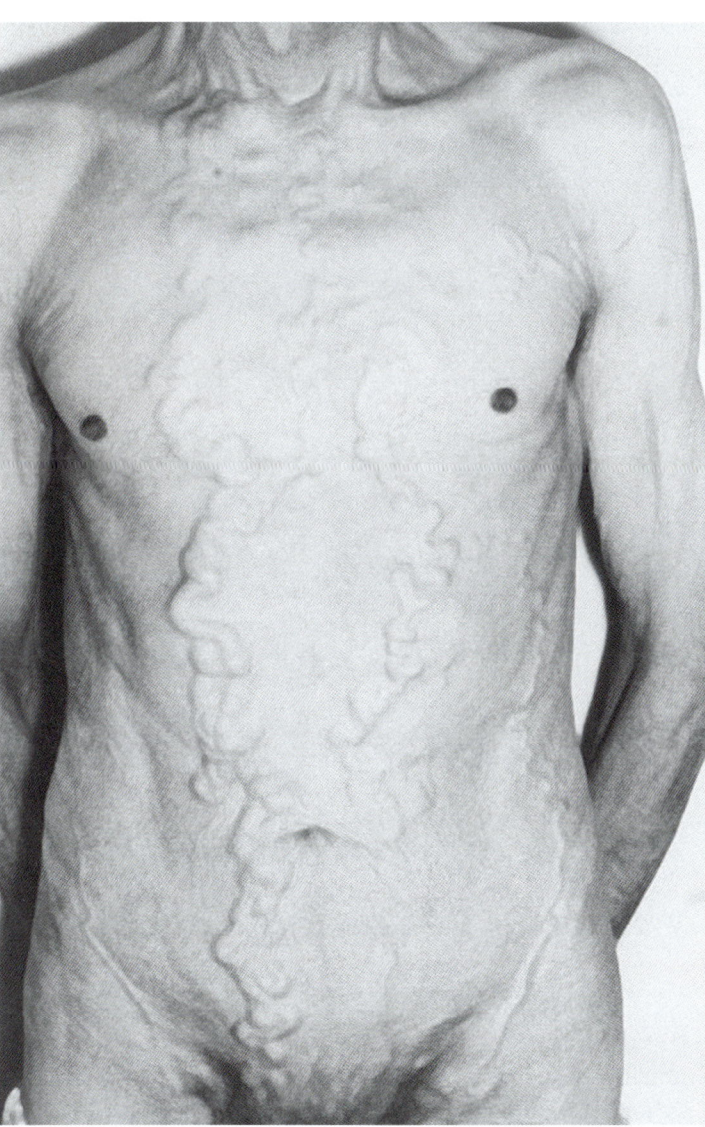

Figure 29.23 Visceral lesions of tertiary syphilis. (a) Gumma of the liver causing portal vein obstruction. (b) Portal hypertension with caput medusa caused by hepatic gummata.

Neurosyphilis is characterised by several heterogeneous syndromes [30,31]. The differential diagnosis of neurosyphilis covers the whole spectrum of neurological and psychiatric conditions. The onset can occur weeks or decades after treponemal dissemination.

- *Asymptomatic neurosyphilis* precedes the development of clinically apparent disease and accounts for one-third of all neurosyphilis. It occurs in 10% of those with latent disease and has a peak incidence at 12–18 months after infection. It reverts spontaneously in 70% of patients.
- *Meningeal neurosyphilis* usually has its onset during secondary disease and is characterised by symptoms of headache, confusion, nausea and vomiting, neck stiffness and photophobia. There may be focal seizures, aphasia, delirium and papilloedema. Cranial nerve palsies cause unilateral or bilateral facial weakness and sensorineural deafness [32].
- *Meningovascular syphilis* occurs most frequently between 4 and 7 years after infection. The clinical features of hemiparesis, seizures and aphasia reflect multiple areas of infarction from diffuse arteritis.
- *Gummatous neurosyphilis* results in features typical of a space-occupying lesion.
- *Parenchymatous syphilis* appears later and has become rare in its classic forms in the antibiotic era. The peak incidence of general paralysis from parenchymatous disease of the brain used to be 10–20 years after infection. The onset is insidious with subtle deterioration in cognitive function and psychiatric symptoms that mimic those of other mental disorders. As the disease progresses neurological signs develop, including pupillary abnormalities, hypotonia of the face and limbs, intention tremors and hyperreflexia.
- *Tabetic neurosyphilis* was the most common form of neurosyphilis in the pre-antibiotic era, with an onset 15–25 years after primary infection. The most characteristic symptom is of lightning pains – sudden paroxysms of lancinating pain affecting the lower limbs. Other early symptoms include paraesthesia, progressive ataxia and bowel and bladder dysfunction. Tabes also causes neuropathic (Charcot) joints in the spine, hips, knees

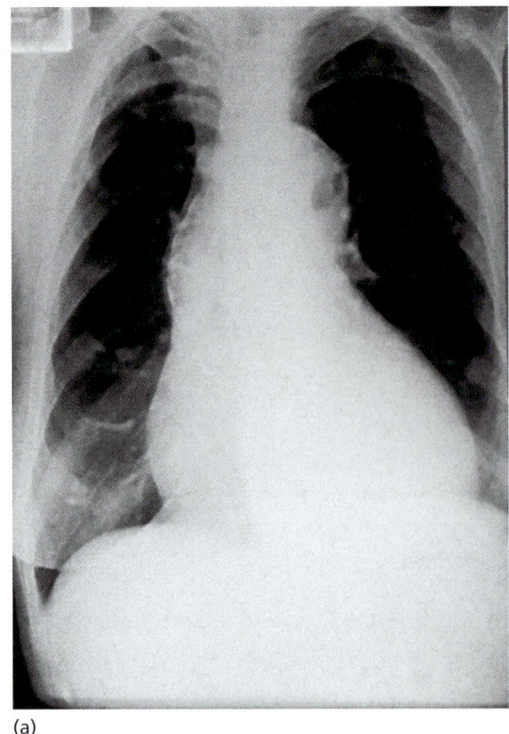
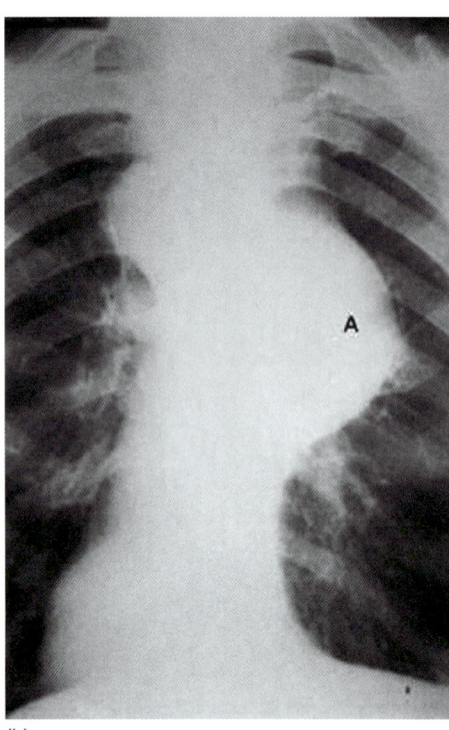

Figure 29.25 Cardiovascular syphilis. (a) Chest X-ray showing a dilated aorta with linear calcification in the wall of the ascending aorta. (b) Chest X-ray showing an aneurysmal swelling (A) of the ascending aorta.

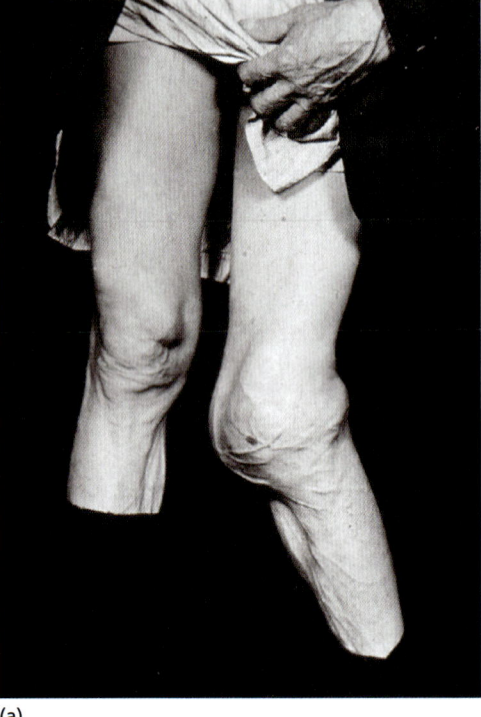
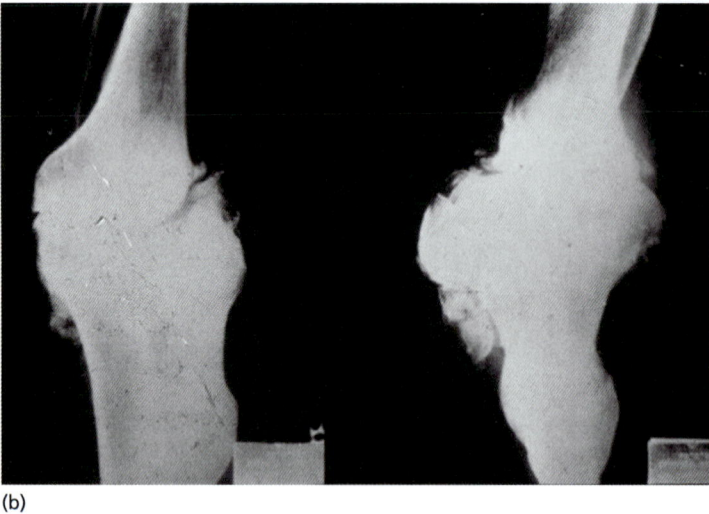

Figure 29.26 Tabes dorsalis. (a) Charcot (neuropathic) joints of the knee. (b) X-ray of Charcot joints of the knee showing a loss of normal alignment with multiple osteophytes formation.

(Figure 29.26) and feet. Perforating ulcers of the feet, now much more commonly seen in diabetics, also occur.
- *Ocular syphilis* may occur at any stage of the disease and has re-emerged as an important cause of uveitis during the past 20 years, especially in HIV-positive MSM. Any eye structure can be involved. Posterior uveitis and panuveitis in association with impaired visual acuity are most common. It is recommended that treatment should follow that for neurosyphilis.
- *Otic syphilis* presents with sensorineural hearing loss, tinnitus and vertigo from treponemal infection of the cochlea-vestibular system. Although it had become rare, more cases may occur as early syphilis cases increase.

Syphilis and HIV infection

There is epidemiological synergy between HIV and other sexually transmitted infections [33]. Syphilis increases the risk of HIV acquisition and onward transmission. HIV infection may alter the natural history of syphilis [34].

Early syphilis has increased since the advent of antiretroviral therapy and pre- and postexposure prophylaxis in association with unsafe sexual practices. In most patients with early HIV infection, the clinical features, serological test results and response to treatment are like those in non-HIV-infected persons [35]. With advancing immunosuppression, all of these may be significantly altered. Lues maligna and neurological and ocular involvement [36–39] have been reported more commonly.

Differential diagnosis

Primary syphilis. A wide variety of diseases can affect the genitals and must be considered (Table 29.1). Genital herpes and balanoposthitis have typical clinical features, although they may occur with a chancre. Secondarily infected traumatic sores may look like chancres. Classic chancroid has become rare but sporadic cases still occur, often within ulcers with mixed infections [40]. Likewise, classic lymphogranuloma venereum has become less common. The 'inflammatory bubo' may resemble the unilateral and bilateral adenitis of early syphilis. Unlike syphilis, the glands are usually matted, adherent to the inflamed skin and show a tendency to central fluctuation. Excoriated secondary syphilitic papules in women can be confused with multiple small chancres. Chancre redux is a recurrence of the primary sore at its original site [41]. Tertiary syphilis, tuberculous ulceration, cancer or pre-cancerous dermatoses such as erythroplasia of Queyrat and Bowen disease can occasionally cause difficulty. The papules of scabies on the glans or on the shaft of the penis may arouse strong suspicions. Any lesion at the site of a healed primary has been labelled pseudochancre redux [42]. On the cervix, a chancre may easily be taken for an 'erosion' or a cancer [43], especially when suspected syphilis is not the reason for examination.

Oral and rectal lesions should give rise to a suspicion of possible syphilis. Anal fissures and anal warts, 'haemorrhoids', anal discharge and irritation or a finding of some form of sexually transmitted proctitis, for example due to gonorrhoea, herpesvirus or *Chlamydia trachomatis*, should alert the physician to the possibility of concomitant syphilis [44]. In the rectum, a chancre may be mistaken for a cancer.

With a chancre on the lip, the most important differential diagnosis is facial herpes simplex. Apart from the appearance, the recurrent nature of herpes is helpful in its diagnosis. Secondarily infected traumatic lesions with oedema may closely resemble a chancre, as may cancer of the lip. Traumatic ulcers of the tongue can sometimes be infiltrated. Behçet syndrome with both oral and vulvar lesions may present a problem. Tonsillar chancres may be mistaken for tonsillitis, glandular fever or Vincent angina. When the accompanying angular or submental adenopathy is painless, syphilis should be seriously considered.

A longstanding whitlow or paronychia ought to lead to examination for both herpes virus and *Treponema pallidum*. Where epitrochlear or axillary adenitis is painless, STS are indicated.

Secondary syphilis. The skin manifestations of secondary syphilis are so variable that it must be considered in the diagnosis of all dermatoses that are in any way atypical (Table 29.2).

With a macular rash, drug eruptions must first be considered. The history, itching and lack of adenopathy aid differentiation. Measles and rubella may cause difficulty, but it is pityriasis rosea that is most often called into question. The presence of a herald patch and the collarette of scales distinguish this condition from macular syphilis.

With papular eruptions, many diseases can cause difficulty in diagnosis, and it must be remembered that people with seborrhoeic dermatitis or psoriasis can also have syphilis. Lichen planus with its shiny, angled, violaceous lesions should seldom cause difficulty. Acne vulgaris and seborrhoeic dermatitis may confuse the unwary, as may impetigo and occasionally leprosy or tuberculosis if the face is affected. In the ano-genital region, condylomata lata have been incorrectly diagnosed as haemorrhoids and as condylomata acuminata. Balanitis circinata, hyperkeratotic lesions of reactive arthritis and genital herpes may also lead to misdiagnosis.

The micropapular varieties of syphilis can be confused with keratosis pilaris, lichen scrofulosorum, trichophytide and lichen planopilaris. Eruptions of the palms and soles may bear a striking resemblance to psoriasis and scaling mycoses.

Table 29.1 Differential diagnoses of primary syphilis in different genital areas.

Genital area	Other STIs	Trauma	Dermatoses	Inflammatory conditions	Drugs	Neoplasia
Penile	Genital herpes Chancroid Lymphogranuloma venereum Granuloma inguinale Scabies HPV infection Other stages of syphilis	'Zip injury'	Lichen planus Lichen sclerosis Psoriasis Balanitis	Plasma cell balanitis Behçet disease	Fixed drug eruption	Squamous carcinoma Bowen disease
Cervical	Cervical ectopy or metaplasia					Cervical cancer or CIN
Anal	HPV infection	Anal fissure Haemorrhoids				Squamous carcinoma
Oral				Tonsillitis Behçet disease		

CIN, cervical intraepithelial neoplasia; HPV, human papillomavirus; STI, sexually transmitted infection.

Table 29.2 Differential diagnoses of secondary syphilis.

Other STIs	Dermatoses	Other inflammatory conditions	Drugs	Neoplasia
Genital herpes	Seborrhoeic dermatitis	Behçet disease	Systemic drug eruptions	Squamous carcinoma
Scabies	Pityriasis rosea	Infectious mononucleosis	Stevens–Johnson syndrome	Bowen disease
HPV infection	Psoriasis	Angular cheilitis		Kaposi sarcoma
Circinate balanitis (reactive arthritis)	Lichen planus Mycoses			

HPV, human papillomavirus; STI, sexually transmitted infection.

Table 29.3 Differential diagnosis of tertiary syphilis in different parts of the body.

Facial	Truncal	Legs
Lupus vulgaris	Psoriasis	Chronic venous ulcer
Rosacea	Mycosis fungoides	Bazin disease
Lupus erythematosis		
Leukaemic infiltrations		
Neoplasia		

With oral lesions, the question of aphthae has first to be considered. The painful nature of the lesions contrasts with syphilis and the aphthous lesions are markedly areolated [45,46]. Tonsillitis or tonsillar papules with lymphadenopathy may make differential diagnosis from infectious mononucleosis a difficult clinical problem. An accompanying morbilliform rash, perhaps precipitated by the administration of ampicillin, may add to the confusion, especially as the condition is sometimes accompanied by false positive STS.

Tertiary syphilis. Skin reactions to bromides and iodides commonly deceived the physician in the past. On the face, lupus vulgaris, epithelioma and Bowen disease can cause diagnostic difficulties (Table 29.3). Midline granuloma, sycosis barbae, infiltrated forms of rosacea and lupus erythematosus have all been confused with late syphilis. On the trunk and limbs, it can resemble circinate psoriasis, leukaemic infiltrations and mycosis fungoides. On the legs, gummatous ulceration can look very like a venous ulcer. Bazin disease may also be simulated.

Changes in the tongue should not be confused with the congenital deformity of scrotal tongue, when the tongue remains quite soft. Where leukoplakia is associated with interstitial glossitis, or fibrotic nodules, biopsy is necessary to exclude carcinoma.

Prognosis

The cure rates with initial treatment of early syphilis are better than 95%. The long-term outcome of adequately treated cases is excellent. In late syphilis, infection can usually be arrested although some treponemes may persist in less accessible sites (e.g. the eye and nervous system). If immune function is normal, this rarely has clinical sequelae.

Investigations

The tests used to diagnose syphilis continue to evolve and will vary in different parts of the world according to the laboratory resources available. Microscopic identification of the causative organism is possible in specimens obtained from lesions but requires the availability of dark-field microscopes and experienced operators. Serological testing remains the bedrock of screening, but the choice of tests will vary in different locations; enzyme immunoassay (EIA) tests are now the most used screening tests. In developed countries, polymerase chain reaction (PCR) based tests are becoming more widely available as are rapid point-of-care tests that can give rapid results on fingerprick specimens.

Dark-field microscopy

Treponema pallidum can be identified from lesions of primary, secondary or early congenital syphilis by dark-field microscopy. In primary syphilis, it makes the diagnosis possible before measurable antibodies appear. In secondary syphilis, it provides immediate confirmation of a clinical diagnosis. The organism has a characteristic morphology and motility, with a sinusoidal profile and a wavelength and amplitude of 1.1 and 0.4 μm, respectively [47].

Lesions are initially cleansed with a saline-soaked gauze swab then abraded with a dry gauze swab. The edge of the lesion is gently squeezed and the exudate collected with the edge of a coverslip and placed on a slide. Healing ulcers and papular lesions often require initial abrasion with the blunt edge of a scalpel blade. Patience is needed to identify *T. pallidum*. Repeat testing on consecutive days may be necessary. In all highly suspect genital and/or oral lesions where it proves impossible to demonstrate *T. pallidum*, lymph node puncture material, mixed with injected sterile saline (0.5 mL), should be examined. Any treponeme found will always be *T. pallidum*.

The organism can also be identified by direct immunofluorescent antibody testing where no facilities for dark-field microscopy exist.

In biopsy specimens from late syphilis, or in atypical early lesions, it may be possible to identify the organism using silver stains such as Warthin–Starry preparations or by direct immunofluorescent antibody testing.

Molecular amplification tests

Polymerase chain reaction diagnosis has been based on primers and probes prepared from the 47 kDa gene. After a 40-cycle series of denaturing, annealing and extension, the PCR products can be visualised by electrophoresis or Southern blot hybridisation with a ^{32}P-labelled probe and then autoradiography. This technique should be of greatest value in detecting the low numbers of treponemal products in neurosyphilis; it should also be useful in CS, in which the interpretation of serological test results may be difficult. Molecular amplification tests have also been successfully used in multiplex systems to investigate the aetiology of genital ulcers [48] and lymph node biopsy specimens [49].

There is no internationally approved commercially available test so PCR testing is usually confined to specialised reference laboratories [50].

Table 29.4 Sensitivities of serological tests at different stages of untreated syphilis.

Test	Stage of disease (% positive (range))			
	Primary	Secondary	Latent	Tertiary
VDRL	78 (74–87)	100	95 (88–100)	71 (37–94)
RPR	86 (77–99)	100	98 (95–100)	73
FTA-ABS[a]	84 (70–100)	100	100	96
TPPA[a]	76 (69–90)	100	97 (97–100)	94
EIA	93	100	100	

Courtesy of Centers for Disease Control and Prevention, Atlanta, GA.
[a] FTA-ABS and TPPA are generally considered to be equally sensitive in the primary stage of the disease.
EIA, enzyme immunoassay; FTA-ABS, fluorescent treponemal antibody absorption; RPR, rapid plasma reagin; TPHA, *Treponema pallidum* haemagglutination test; TPPA, *Treponema pallidum* particle agglutination; VDRL, Venereal Disease Research Laboratory.

Serological tests

Serological tests for syphilis and serological tests for other treponematoses can be divided into reaginic or non-treponemal tests, and specific or treponemal tests. The immune responses in all the treponematoses appear to be the same, and there is no test that will differentiate one treponematosis from another [51]. The sensitivity of the different tests varies according to the stage of the syphilis (Table 29.4).

Standard non-treponemal tests. The non-treponemal tests detect immunoglobulin M (IgM) and IgG antibodies to lipoidal material released from damaged host cells and to lipoidal-like antigens of *T. pallidum*. There are four tests available that use the Venereal Disease Research Laboratory (VDRL) antigen (consisting of cardiolipin, cholesterol and lecithin) as the principal component. These tests are quantitative and are useful in assessing the response to treatment. Reactivity to these tests does not develop until 1–4 weeks after the chancre appears in primary syphilis. Titres are highest in secondary syphilis. The prozone phenomenon occurs in 2% of sera; undiluted sera give negative results because of antibody excess, the presence of blocking antibodies, or both. The titre slowly declines after the secondary stage, and it may spontaneously become negative in some cases of late latent syphilis and neurosyphilis.

The VDRL slide test is widely used and requires the microscopic demonstration of antigen–antibody flocculation in heat-inactivated serum.

The unheated serum reagin (USR) test is like the VDRL test but does not require preheated serum, because the antigen has been stabilised.

The rapid plasma reagin (RPR) test and toluidine red USR (TRUST) use either charcoal or red paint pigment added to the USR reagent to enhance visualisation of the antigen–antibody flocculation. The flocculation is visible macroscopically. This test can be performed in consulting rooms, clinics and laboratories where facilities, experience and personnel are limited. An automated RPR test is available.

Treponemal tests. Specific treponemal antibody tests detect antibodies to antigenic determinants of treponemes. They are qualitative procedures and are not helpful in assessing treatment responses. Once positive, they tend to remain positive for life, irrespective of treatment.

The *T. pallidum* immobilisation (TPI) test was first developed in 1949 after Nelson and Mayer [52] showed that serum from syphilitic patients contains an antibody that, in the presence of complement, inhibits the normal movements of virulent *T. pallidum*. This test required virulent *T. pallidum* (Nichol strain) obtained from rabbits. Although sensitive and specific [53,54], it has been superseded by newer, less time-consuming tests.

The fluorescent treponemal antibody absorption (FTA-ABS) test [55–57] and the FTA-ABS double staining (FTA-ABS DS) test are both indirect immunofluorescent tests. The double stain test employs a fluorochrome-labelled counterstain for *T. pallidum* and an antihuman IgG conjugate labelled with tetramethylrhodamine isothiocyanate to detect antibody in the patient's serum. False positive results may occur in about 1% of sera. Possible causes include technical error, Lyme borreliosis, pregnancy, genital herpes, alcoholic cirrhosis and connective tissue diseases such as systemic lupus erythematosus and scleroderma.

The *T. pallidum* haemagglutination assay (TPHA) was first described by Rathlev in 1967 [58]; a variant microtechnique has since gained popularity. In all forms, the TPHA is simple to perform and results are readily reproducible [59]. The test is very sensitive and specific [60,61]. The microhaemagglutination assay for antibodies to *T. pallidum* (MHA-TP) detects passive haemagglutination of erythrocytes sensitised with ultrasonicated Nichol strain *T. pallidum*. In many laboratories, the TPHA has been replaced by the similar *T. pallidum* particle agglutination (TPPA) test that uses gelatine particles rather than erythrocytes as the carrier. It is more sensitive than the FTA-ABS test.

More recently, sensitive treponemal immunoassays have been developed using a variety of techniques including EIA, chemiluminescence immunoassay (CIA) and microbead immunoassay (MBIA) [62,63]. These tests can be easily automated and thereby improve turnaround times. Many laboratories are now employing a reverse testing algorithm whereby initial screening is by these tests with subsequent testing by quantitative non-treponemal tests.

It is essential to confirm the presumptive serological diagnosis of syphilis on a second specimen from the patient.

Rapid point-of-care tests for syphilis

The resurgence of syphilis worldwide and limited laboratory diagnostic facilities in high-prevalence countries has stimulated the development of rapid point-of-care tests [64]. These can be performed outside a laboratory setting with minimal training and no equipment, using a fingerprick blood sample. The tests are simple, are not affected by prozone effects and can be transported and stored at temperatures <30°C. Their sensitivity is 85–98% and their specificity 93–98%. They are used for targeted screening in resource-poor countries, especially for the screening of pregnant women and other high-risk groups. In developed countries, their use is also being studied in outreach settings with MSM and sex workers and their clients [65,66].

Biological false positive reactions

All the tests in use can produce biologically false positive (BFP) results (Table 29.5). Some apparently healthy persons produce reagins in excess. They are classified as BFP reactors. BFP reactions may be acute or chronic, that is they last less than or more than

Table 29.5 Biological false positive reagin tests for syphilis in acute and chronic diseases.

Acute	Chronic
Infections:	Autoimmune diseases
Malaria	Dysgammaglobulinaemias
Leprosy	
Typhus	
Viral pneumonia	
Infectious mononucleosis	
Filariasis	
Trypanosomiasis	
Lyme disease	
Pregnancy	

6 months. The same occurs in association with acute and chronic diseases. Persistently low-titre-positive reagin tests with repeatedly negative treponemal tests are the rule in acute BFP reactions. They rarely last more than 3 months. Strongly positive reactions are more common in chronic BFP reactors.

The following are among the commonest associations with acute BFP reactions: malaria, leprosy (especially the lepromatous form) [67–69], typhus, respiratory tract infection (especially viral pneumonia), infectious mononucleosis, active pulmonary tuberculosis, hepatitis, subacute bacterial endocarditis, measles, chickenpox, filariasis, trypanosomiasis, leptospirosis and relapsing fever. BFP reactions are also reported in connection with pregnancy [70] and narcotic addiction.

Chronic BFP reactions are associated with autoimmune diseases and dysgammaglobulinaemia. Chronic BFP reactions may exist for some time and herald the onset of connective tissue disease by some years, for example systemic lupus erythematosus (especially in Rhesus-negative women), polyarteritis nodosa and rheumatoid arthritis [71,72].

The FTA and FTA-ABS tests may also give BFP reactions in the elderly, in autoimmune disorders [73], and in Lyme disease [74].

Examination of the cerebrospinal fluid

Indications for the examination of CSF in syphilis include the following:
- Neurological, ophthalmic or auditory symptoms and signs.
- Other clinical evidence of active infection – aortitis, gumma or iritis.
- Treatment failure.
- HIV infection.
- A non-treponemal serum titre of more than 32 if the duration of syphilis is over 1 year.
  The typical CSF findings of neurosyphilis consist of:
- Moderate mononuclear pleocytosis (10–400 cells/mL).
- Elevated total protein (0.46–2.0 g/L).
- Positive CSF VDRL test.

The CSF VDRL test is highly specific and false positive results are rare in the absence of blood contamination. A negative CSF VDRL test does not exclude neurosyphilis, although non-treponemal serological tests usually remain positive in both serum and CSF in such cases.

CSF can also be subject to treponemal antibody and PCR testing. The TPPA test is often used for confirmatory testing.

Management

Parenteral penicillin G is the preferred drug at all stages of syphilis; the preparations used, the dosage and the duration of treatment depend on the clinical stage and disease manifestations. Penicillin remains not only the most effective treponemicide, but it is easy to administer, has few side effects and is relatively inexpensive. Results continue to be excellent for all forms and stages of treponemal disease, and there are no signs that *T. pallidum* has developed resistance to this antibiotic. Injectable penicillins are generally preferred to oral preparations because of problems of patient compliance and uncertain absorption from the gastrointestinal tract.

> **Treatment ladder for syphilis**
>
> **First line**
>
> **Early syphilis (primary, secondary and early latent)**
> - Benzathine penicillin G 2.4 mega units IM single dose or ×2 (days 1 and 8)
> - Procaine penicillin G 0.6–1.2 mega units IM OD for 10–14 days
>
> **Late latent and cardiovascular**
> - Benzathine penicillin G 2.4 mega units IM weekly ×3 (days 1, 8 and 15)
> - Procaine penicillin G 0.6–1.2 mega units IM OD for 14–20 days
>
> **Neurosyphilis (including neurological/ophthalmic involvement in early syphilis)**
> - Procaine penicillin 1.8–2.4 mega units IM OD plus probenecid 500 mg PO QDS for 14–20 days
> - Benzyl penicillin 10.8–24 g daily, given as 1.8–2.4 g IV every 4 h for 14–20 days
>
> **Second line**
>
> **Early syphilis (primary, secondary and early latent)**
> - Doxycycline 100 mg PO BD for 14 days
> - Ceftriaxone 500 mg IM OD for 10 days (if no anaphylaxis to penicillin)
> - Erythromycin 500 mg PO QDS for 14 days
> - Azithromycin 2 g stat or 500 mg PO OD for 10 days
>
> **Late latent and cardiovascular**
> - Doxycycline 100 mg PO BD for 28 days (if penicillin allergic)
> - Amoxicillin 2 g PO TDS plus probenecid 500 mg PO QDS for 28 days
>
> **Neurosyphilis**
> - Doxycycline 200 mg PO BD for 28 days
> - Amoxicillin 2 g PO TDS plus probenecid 500 mg PO QDS for 28 days
> - Ceftriaxone 2 g IV or IM for 10–14 days
>
> **Steroids**
>
> Steroids should be given with all antitreponemal antibiotics for cardiovascular syphilis and neurosyphilis:
> - Prednisolone 30–60 mg daily for 3 days, beginning 1 day before first antibiotic dose

Adequate treatment requires the maintenance of serum concentrations more than 0.03 penicillin units/mL for at least 10 days. UK [75,76] and European [77] guidelines generally recommend a daily dose of 0.6 mega units whereas the WHO [78] and USA [79] recommend double this amount. A single intramuscular dose of 0.6 mega units of aqueous procaine penicillin gives an effective serum concentration for at least 24 h; in comparison, a single intramuscular dose of 2.4 mega units of benzathine penicillin G maintains effective levels for about 2 weeks. As this preparation may cause pain on injection, 1.2 mega units are usually given in the upper and outer quadrant of each buttock.

Treatment of late syphilis theoretically may require a longer duration of therapy because organisms are dividing more slowly, but the validity of this concept has not been addressed. The penetration of aqueous procaine penicillin into the CSF (as into the aqueous humour) is poor; that of erythromycin is poorer and that of benzathine penicillin poorest of the three [80].

For treatment of neurosyphilis, high dosages of crystalline benzyl penicillin G, plus probenicid, should be considered. Desensitisation of penicillin-allergic patients is recommended.

In patients who are hypersensitive to penicillin, regimens based on ceftriaxone, doxycycline and erythromycin have all been successfully used to treat syphilis; however, success is less assured than with penicillin. Azithromycin, given in dosages of 500 mg daily for 10 days, or in a single 2 g dosage, has recently been successful, but there are concerns about the emergence of antimicrobial resistance [81,82].

All patients with syphilis should be offered screening for other sexually transmitted infections and HIV. Serological testing for HIV should be repeated after 3 months in those persons presenting with primary syphilis who initially test negative.

HIV-seropositive individuals
It is recommended that CSF examination be performed in all patients with syphilis who are HIV seropositive. Generally, recommended regimens are the same as those in HIV-negative individuals if CSF examination is normal [83].

Pregnant women
Only penicillin-based regimens have documented efficacy, and desensitisation should be considered in those who are allergic. Those women who have had documented treatment for syphilis in the past do not need retreatment in current or subsequent pregnancies as long as there is no clinical evidence of syphilis, and the VDRL or RPR titre is negative. First line treatment is with benzathine penicillin.

Macrolides are no longer a treatment option.

Penicillin reactions
Accidental deaths following treatment are very rare and mainly due to anaphylactic shock reactions to penicillin. If penicillin is used in patients with a history of allergy, it is advisable to keep the patient under observation for 15–20 min after the injection. An emergency kit should always be available.

Treatment ladder for syphilis in pregnancy

First line

Early syphilis (primary, secondary and early latent)

Trimesters 1 and 2 (up to and including 27 weeks' gestation)
- Benzathine penicillin G 2.4 mega units IM single dose

Trimester 3 (from 28 weeks' gestation)
- Benzathine penicillin G 2.4 mega units IM on days 1 and 8
- Procaine penicillin G 0.6–1.2 mega units IM OD for 10–14 days

Late latent, cardiovascular and gummatous syphilis (all three trimesters)
- Benzathine penicillin G 2.4 mega units IM on days 1, 8 and 15

Second line

Early syphilis (primary, secondary and early latent) (all three trimesters)
- Procaine penicillin G 0.6–1.2 mega units IM OD for 10–14 days
- Amoxicillin 500 mg PO QDS plus probenecid 500 mg PO QDS for 14 days
- Ceftriaxone 500 mg IM OD for 10 days (if no anaphylaxis to penicillin)

Late latent, cardiovascular and gummatous syphilis (all three trimesters)
- Procaine penicillin G 0.6 mega units IM OD for 14 days
- Amoxycillin 2 g TDS and probenecid 500mg QDS for 28 days

Steroids
Steroids should be given with all antitreponemal antibiotics for cardiovascular syphilis and neurosyphilis:
- Prednisolone 40–60 mg daily for 3 days, beginning 1 day before first antibiotic dose

---

Treatment ladder for neurosyphilis in pregnancy

First line
- Procaine penicillin G 1.8–2.4 mega units IM OD plus probenecid 500 mg PO QDS for 14 days
- Benzyl penicillin 10.8–14.4 g daily, given as 1.8–2.4 g IV every 4 h for 14 days

Second line
- Amoxicillin 2 g PO TDS plus probenecid 500 mg PO QDS for 28 days
- Ceftriaxone 2 g IM (with lidocaine as diluent) or IV (with water for injection as diluent) for 10–14 days (if no anaphylaxis to penicillin)

Steroids
Steroids should be given with all antitreponemal antibiotics for neurosyphilis:
- Prednisolone 40–60 mg daily for 3 days, beginning 1 day before first antibiotic dose

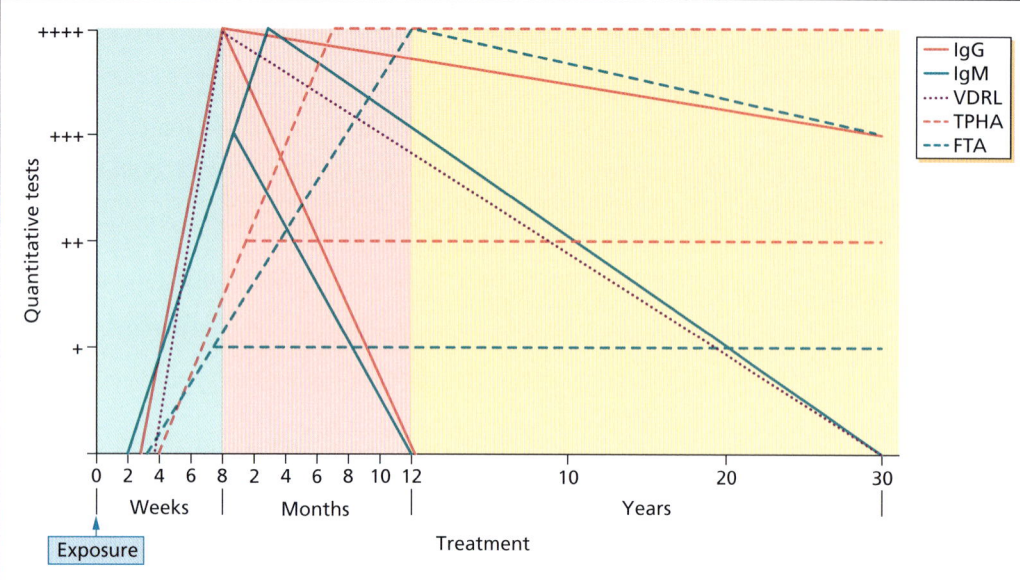

Figure 29.27 Typical serological responses at different stages and in response to treatment of syphilis. FTA, fluorescent treponemal antibody; Ig, immunoglobulin; TPHA, *Treponema pallidum* haemagglutination assay; VDRL, Venereal Disease Research Laboratory. Courtesy of Centers for Disease Control, Atlanta, GA, USA.

Hoigne reactions (acute psychotic symptoms due to inadvertent intravenous injection of procaine in procaine penicillin) are recognised.

The *Jarisch–Herxheimer reaction* is an acute febrile reaction that occurs in many patients within 24 h of commencing treatment. It is mediated by cytokines. Headache, myalgia, bone pains and an exacerbation of skin lesions may accompany the fever. It must be differentiated from penicillin allergy. Patients should be advised that it might occur. Symptoms may be controlled by antipyretics. The fever (38–40°C) rarely persists more than 8 h.

In pregnant women the reaction may induce early labour or cause fetal distress. In late neurosyphilis and cardiovascular syphilis, the Jarisch–Herxheimer reaction can be more serious and may be associated with life-threatening sequelae. Many clinicians advocate a short course of corticosteroids to lessen its effects in these patients. One such regimen is to prescribe oral prednisolone 30–60 mg daily for 3 days, beginning syphilis treatment 24 h after the first dose.

Follow-up

Follow-up for clinical and serological assessment should be carried out at 3, 6 and 12 months after the completion of treatment in early syphilis (Figure 29.27). Recurrence is due more often to reinfection than to relapse.

Reinfections are more likely during the first year after penicillin therapy. non-treponemal test titres correlate with disease activity and will usually become negative with time after successful treatment. In some patients, who are described as being 'reagin fast', low titre positivity in these tests may persist for life. Apart from up to 25% of patients treated for primary syphilis, the treponemal tests will continue to remain positive after successful treatment.

In late latent or tertiary benign syphilis, a 2-year follow-up is adequate. Quantitative non-treponemal tests are repeated at 3 and 6 months, and each 6 months thereafter. Follow-up of cardiovascular and clinical neurosyphilis should be for life.

Treatment failure is suggested by a fourfold increase in titres, less than a fourfold decrease in pre-treatment titres within 12–24 months, and the development of symptoms or signs attributable to syphilis. All treatment failures require CSF examination. In cases of serological or clinical relapse, retreatment with double doses is recommended.

In latent syphilis, a 2-year follow-up is adequate. The same applies to late benign syphilis. In neurosyphilis it is usual to repeat the CSF examination every 6 months until the cell count has become normal. There is a slower response of the CSF VDRL criteria and total protein. Retreatment should be considered if the cell count shows an inadequate response or if all these parameters have not returned to normal by 2 years. In cases of serological or clinical relapse, retreatment with double penicillin doses is recommended. Patients treated for neurological or cardiovascular syphilis should be followed up for many years.

Management of sexual contacts

Attempts should be made to identify, trace and offer further investigation to at-risk sexual contacts. In early syphilis, these are contacts occurring within 3 months plus the duration of symptoms for primary syphilis, within 6 months plus the duration of symptoms for secondary syphilis and within 1 year for early latent disease. All long-term partners of patients with late syphilis should be offered investigation.

Many clinicians also recommend presumptive treatment of all sexual contacts within the 90-day period preceding patient presentation of early syphilis if serological test results are not immediately available and if follow-up cannot be assured.

Congenital syphilis

Definition

Congenital syphilis results from transplacental passage of *Treponema pallidum* from an infected pregnant woman to her fetus but may also occur during delivery in the presence of maternal genital lesions. If untreated during pregnancy, syphilis can lead to fetal loss or stillbirth or, in a live born infant, neonatal death, prematurity, low birth weight and infant disorders such as deafness, neurological impairment and bone deformities. It is largely preventable by good prenatal care and timely penicillin treatment [1–3].

Introduction and general description

Transmission of *T. pallidum* from mother to fetus can occur during any stage of maternal syphilis but the risk is higher in women with primary or secondary stage syphilis [4]. Fetal infection can occur during any trimester of pregnancy. A wide spectrum of severity exists, and only severe cases are clinically apparent at birth.

Epidemiology
Incidence and prevalence

In recognition that CS is the second most common cause, after malaria, of preventable stillbirth worldwide, the WHO launched a global initiative in 2007 to eliminate transmission during pregnancy.

Precise data on the incidence of CS among live born infants are limited, especially for countries without surveillance or reporting systems. In 2008, the WHO estimated that 1.86 million cases of syphilis occurred globally among pregnant women each year. A large proportion of them were untreated or inadequately treated. Up to one-third of women attending antenatal care clinics were not tested for syphilis. It was estimated that annually there were approximately 215 000 stillbirths or early fetal loss, 90 000 cases of neonatal death, 65 000 cases of low birth weight and 150 000 infections in newborns resulting from syphilis infections among pregnant women.

By 2016, the global rate had declined to 473 cases per 100 000 live births and several countries reported elimination of CS because of enhanced surveillance and treatment in pregnancy [5].

In the USA, CS reported rates had declined to their lowest ever in 2014 but have since doubled, reflecting the increase in early syphilis cases in women, notably in socioeconomically deprived blacks or Hispanics, the homeless and substance abusers [6].

In Western Europe, CS rates have remained lower than the WHO global elimination target of <50 cases per 100 000 live births. In the UK, there were 21 cases in total during 2011–2017 [7]. While routine antenatal screening rates exceed 97%, seroconversion in late pregnancy is a persisting concern. Repeat serological screening for syphilis is recommended for at-risk women at 30 weeks' gestation. Where return for test results cannot be assured, point-of care tests at antenatal screening are recommended. Dual screening for both syphilis and HIV is more cost-effective than either alone at preventing adverse pregnancy outcomes [8].

Only severe cases present at or shortly after birth. Most cases will present during childhood although the diagnosis in some may not be made until adulthood. The disease is seen equally in both sexes. There is no racial predisposition. Cases reflect the socioeconomic status and adequacy of health care systems in their countries of origin.

Pathophysiology
Pathology

The histological lesion of CS, as with acquired syphilis, is that of obliterative endarteritis, consisting of mononuclear and plasma cell infiltration surrounding the blood vessels with intimal hyperplasia and swollen, hyperplastic endothelial cells. Fibrosis and gummata are frequently observed in the infected tissue. Fibrosis can be relatively fine in character, consisting of collagen disposition around the blood vessels, or it may distort and replace the parenchyma of the affected organ. Gummata consist of a thin peripheral rim of mononuclear cell infiltrate, central 'gummy' necrosis, and fibrosis – but any of these features may predominate [9]. Any fetal organ can be involved. Liver, kidneys, bone, pancreas, spleen, lungs, heart and brain are most frequently affected.

Causative organisms

Congenital syphilis is caused by *Treponema pallidum* subsp. *pallidum*.

Clinical features (Table 29.6)
Presentation

The clinical manifestations are a consequence of active infection with *T. pallidum* and the inflammatory response induced in various organs. The severity is variable, ranging from life-threatening involvement of multiple organs to isolated radiological or laboratory abnormalities [10].

Congenital syphilis can be divided into:
1 Early disease, presenting within the first 2 years of life.
2 Late disease, presenting from age 3 onwards.
3 Stigmata of CS, the scars and deformities associated with the infection that may be seen in adults.

Early congenital syphilis

Many infants are asymptomatic. The placenta may show proliferative vascular changes and there may be acute inflammation of the umbilical cord (funisitis) [11]. In about two-thirds of untreated cases, clinical signs may begin to appear in the third to eighth week of life. In nearly all cases the signs appear within 3 months. Early CS can manifest as rhinitis with serosanguinous nasal discharge, vesiculobullous eruptions of the skin, oral mucous patches, bony abnormalities, chorioretinitis and visceral lesions.

- *Mucous membranes*. Syphilis rhinitis, generally described as 'snuffles', is the most important and frequent sign (Figure 29.28a). It manifests as a profuse, serous, nasal discharge that contains a high concentration of *T. pallidum*. The inflammatory process can lead to severe nasal cartilage and bone destruction that can lead to the 'saddle-nose' deformity of late CS (Figure 29.28b). Mucous patches can also be found on the tongue and palate.
- *Skin*. The coppery red rash resembles the acquired papular rash of secondary syphilis. Individual lesions, which can be relatively large, can typically be seen on the extremities, especially the palms and soles (Figure 29.29). Lesions on the face may also present as deeply fissured ('split') papules at the angles of the mouth or lateral to the external nares. The eruptions often become papulosquamous and anal condylomata may be present. Paronychia is said to be typical. *T. pallidum* can be demonstrated in the serum from any of these lesions. Skin lesions on the lips, nostrils and anus heal with radiating scars (rhagades). 'Pemphigus syphiliticus' occurs in some babies presenting with bullae, desquamation or erosions (Figure 29.30). Bullae most commonly occur on red, infiltrated palms and soles; their serous contents

Table 29.6 Features of congenital syphilis.

	Early features	Late features
Birth weight	Low birth weight: may be <2500 g	
Mucocutaneous	Snuffles	Rhagades
	Maculopapular rash	Gummata
	Pustules	Palatal perforation
	Mucous patches	
	Condylomata lata	
	Vesiculobullous lesions	
	Rhagades	
	Desquamation	
	Alopecia	
Dental		Hutchinson teeth
		Mulberry molars
Laryngeal	Hoarse cry	
Ocular	Chorioretinitis	Interstitial keratitis
	Uveitis	Uveitis
	Glaucoma	Glaucoma
Gastrointestinal	Hepatosplenomegaly	
	Pancreatitis	
	Enteritis	
Renal	Nephritis	
	Oedema and ascites	
Lymphatics	Lymphadenopathy	
Haematological	Thrombocytopenia	
	Anaemia	
	Disseminated intravascular coagulation	
Central nervous system	Aseptic meningitis	Mental delay
	Chronic meningovascular syphilis	Eighth nerve deafness
	Cranial nerve palsies	Convulsive disorders
	Hydrocephalus	Paresis and paralysis
		Tabes dorsalis
Skeletal	Periostitis	Periostitis causing frontal and parietal bossing
	Osteochondritis causing pseudoparalysis	Sabre tibiae, scaphoid scapula
	Osteitis	Thickening of medial part of clavicle
		Short maxilla and protuberant mandible
		Saddle nose
		Clutton joints

Adapted from Parish 2000 [23].

contain abundant active treponemes. Napkin dermatitis is sometimes mistaken for syphilis. The syphilitic papules are generally less 'hypertrophic' and their appearance less eczematous than in napkin dermatitis.

- *Other features*. There are often bone abnormalities, characterised by diaphyseal periostitis, osteochondritis and a positive Wimberger sign (Figure 29.31), which may present with limb pseudoparesis. Osteochondritis, which is a common early sign, occurs at the end of the long bones, particularly the lower end of the tibia and fibula (Figure 29.32) [12]. The zone between the bone and the cartilage becomes broad and irregular. It shows as a very tender, painful swelling and may lead to Parrot pseudoparalysis. Even without treatment, it tends to disappear within the first year of life. It may be confused with rickets or trauma from physical abuse.

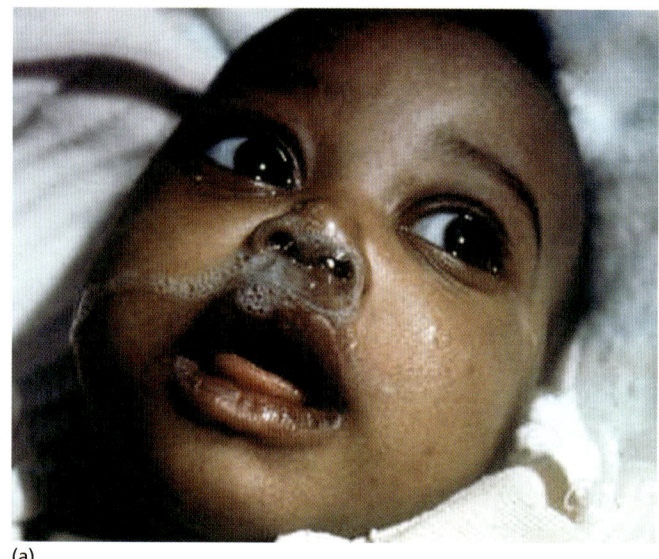

(a)

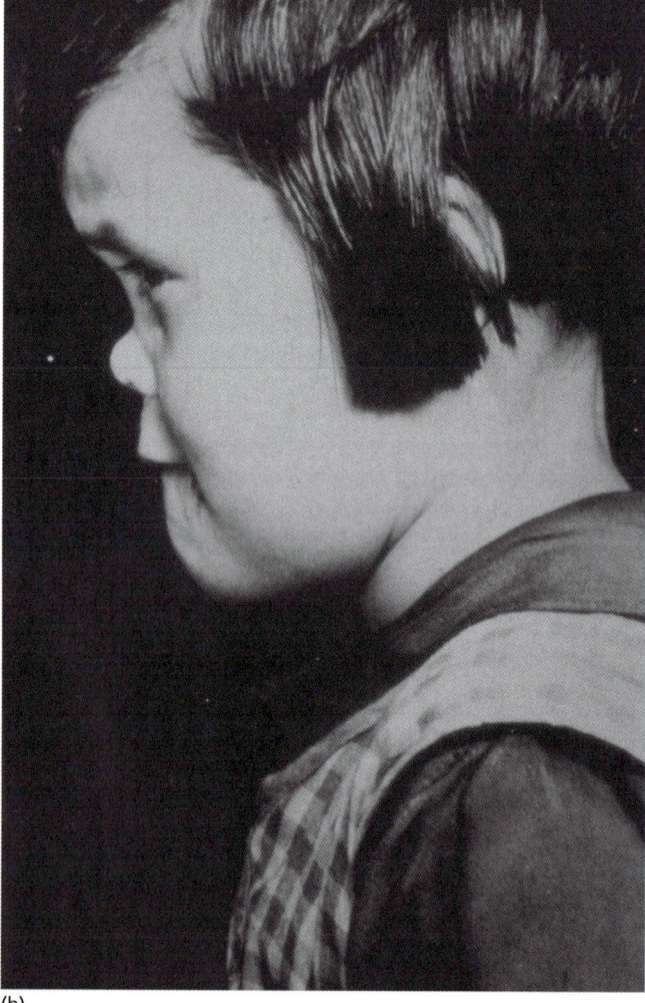

(b)

Figure 29.28 (a) Early congenital syphilis showing serous nasal discharge from nasopharyngitis – 'syphilitic snuffles'. (b) Congenital syphilitic facies with saddle nose deformity and frontal bossing of late congenital syphilis resulting from earlier nasopharyngitis and impaired development of the maxilla.

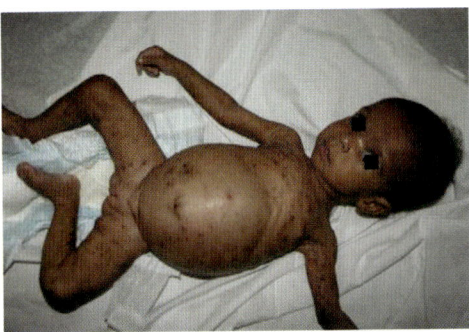

Figure 29.29 Infant with hepatosplenomegaly and a generalised maculopapular rash. From Rodríguez-Cerdeira and Silami-Lopes 2012 [87] with permission of Elsevier.

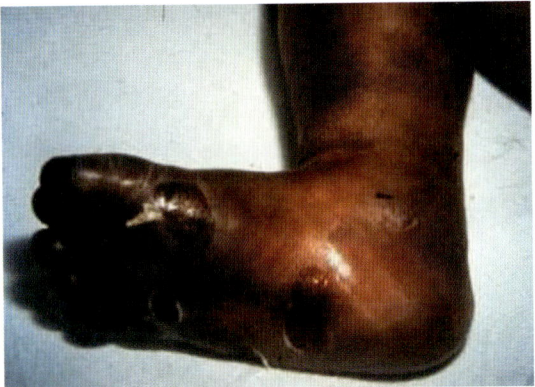

Figure 29.30 Early congenital syphilis ('pemphigus syphiliticus') with ruptured bullae on the soles, resembling bullous pemphigoid. From Rodríguez-Cerdeira and Silami-Lopes 2012 [87] with permission of Elsevier.

Later, there may be periosteal changes or, more rarely, a characteristic osteomyelitis syphilitica in one or more phalanges (syphilitic dactylitis) (Figure 29.33). Visceral lesions causing pneumonia alba, hepatomegaly and splenomegaly, sometimes with jaundice, are common, as is anaemia and thrombocytopenia [13]. Meningitis and meningoencephalitis with convulsions have been described, with bulging of the fontanelle, neck stiffness and, later, hydrocephalus and severe intellectual impairment. Choroiditis and chorioretinitis may occur, but anterior uveitis is rare.

Late congenital syphilis

The manifestations of late CS represent the consequences of the inflammatory response at the sites of treponemal infection during the early stages of the disease. Late CS can present as a variety of skeletal developmental defects and a characteristic facies. Dental abnormalities occur. Other features include hydrocephalus and mental retardation, as well as other typical lesions of gummatous syphilis (Figure 29.34) and neurosyphilis.

The common problem is to differentiate latent or late acquired syphilis from late CS. The possibility of non-venereal treponematoses can further complicate the situation in some patients; the results of STS are of marginal help. A thorough history, including antibiotic history and clinical examination is needed to establish a diagnosis of late CS.

Late CS eruptions of the skin and mucous membranes can closely resemble the nodular syphilides, gummata and periostitis

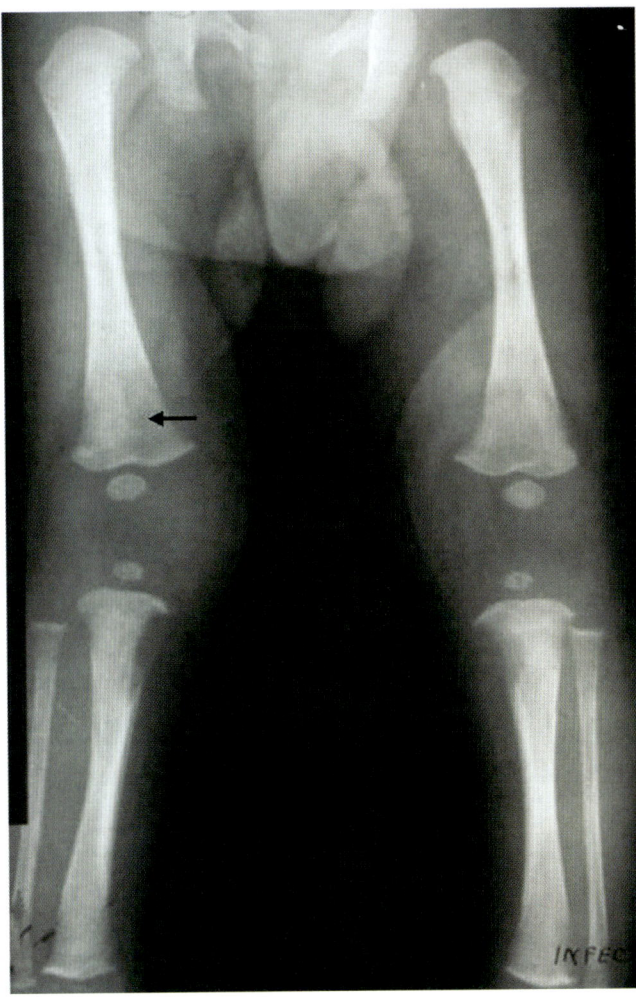

Figure 29.31 Wimberger sign (arrow) – destruction of the proximal metaphyses of the tibiae.

of late acquired syphilis. Signs characteristic of CS alone must therefore be sought. They are of great diagnostic importance as they generally appear in children from 5 to 16 years of age.

- *Interstitial keratitis.* This is the commonest and most serious late lesion [14]. It is rare in patients before 6 years of age and over 40 years [15]. Both eyes are usually affected, and recurrences are recognised. Attacks may have a 3-month course. There is spotty or diffuse clouding of the cornea, with pronounced ciliary and pericorneal injection. Brush-like vessels are seen penetrating from the sclera into the deeper layers of the cornea, which is best seen with a slit lamp [16]. Vision is soon affected. Photophobia and pain are marked features. Iridocyclitis and choroidoretinitis may coexist. The condition is not directly influenced by antisyphilitic treatment. Patients must be referred to an ophthalmologist. Corticosteroid therapy in the form of eye drops or subconjunctival injections is indicated and may have to continue for up to 3 months to prevent the relapse of this 'allergic' phenomenon [17]. If well supervised, it will almost certainly eliminate the danger of blindness.
- *Clutton joints.* This is a painless synovitis affecting the knees (Figure 29.35). The condition resolves spontaneously over several months. It is uninfluenced by antisyphilitic treatment [18].

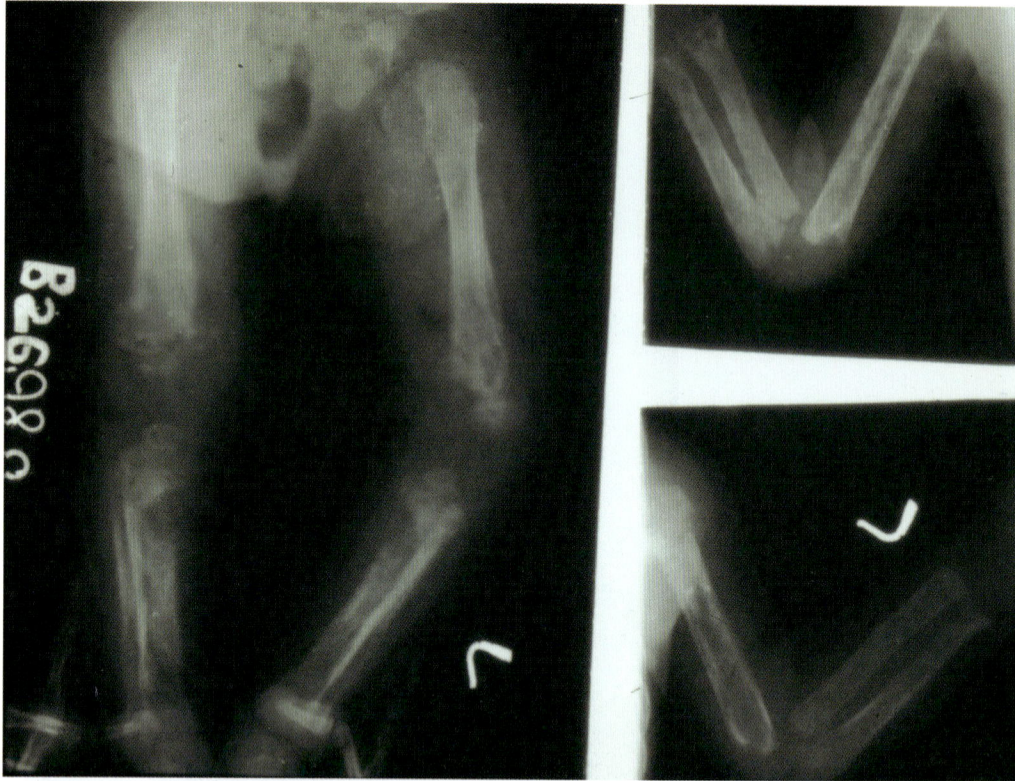

Figure 29.32 Widespread syphilitic osteitis, periostitis and destructive metaphysitis of the long bones.

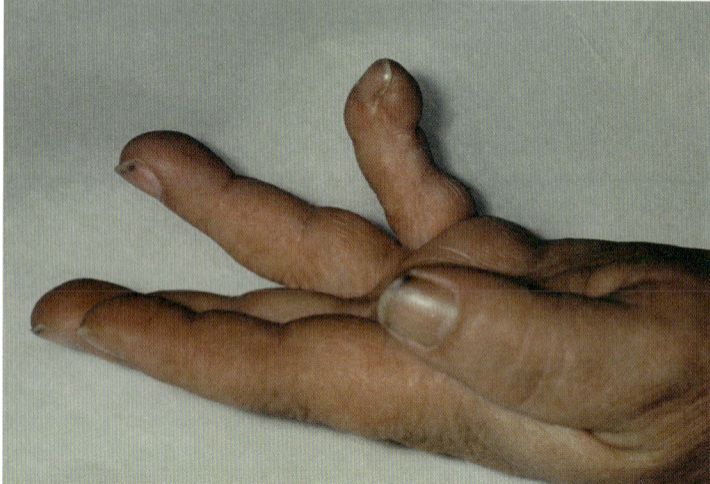

Figure 29.33 Dactylitis of the little finger in late congenital syphilis.

- *Bone involvement.* Periostitis of the long bones is common, particularly of the tibiae, which may become thickened and bent anteroposteriorly (sabre tibiae). Rarely, there may be changes in the inner ends of the clavicles or localised destruction of the outer table of the skull (Figure 29.36). Gummata of the palate are common, with residual perforation of the hard palate.
- *Eighth nerve deafness (neurolabyrinthitis).* This is a characteristic and moderately common complication. It is eventually bilateral in most cases. It may follow interstitial keratitis after some years. Tinnitus and vertigo are common prodromal symptoms and may continue and accompany the increasing perceptive deafness. The condition is uninfluenced by antisyphilitic treatment [19].

- *Cardiovascular syphilis.* If it occurs at all, it is extremely rare [20,21].
- *Neurosyphilis.* Cerebrospinal changes are not rare. Juvenile general paralysis may start between 6 and 21 years. Tabes is less frequent.

Stigmata

Scars and defects caused by CS have diagnostic importance in distinguishing it from acquired syphilis.
- *Teeth.* One of the characteristic stigmata of CS is deformity of the upper, central incisor teeth [22]. These so-called Hutchinson teeth are due to defective development of the permanent teeth buds and are often associated with abnormalities in the development of the upper jaw (Figure 29.37). The incisors are conical or barrel shaped, with a degree of notching at the free edge. Another deformity, not so characteristic, is the 'mulberry molar' (Figure 29.38), usually the first molar, which has a flat, occlusive surface with only poorly enamelled rudiments of the usual cusps
- *Hutchinson triad.* Interstitial keratitis, Hutchinson teeth and eighth nerve deafness form the Hutchinson triad.
- *Other stigmata.* Other stigmata are rhagades at the corner of the mouth, a broad-based saddleback nose, a 'dish face', Parrot nodes on the skull, the 'pepper and salt' fundus due to scarred choroiditis and optic atrophy (Figure 29.39).

Investigations

The diagnosis of CS can prove to be difficult for the following three reasons:
1. *Treponema pallidum* is non-cultivatable and often difficult to demonstrate in clinical specimens.
2. Serological analysis is complicated by the presence of transplacentally acquired maternal antibodies.
3. Most neonates have no evidence of infection at birth [23].

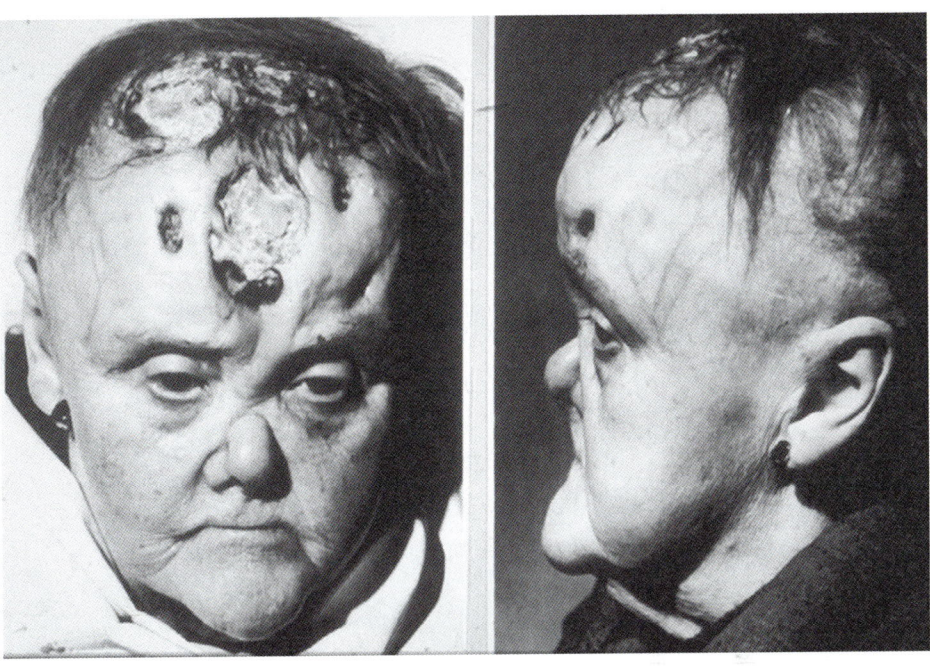

Figure 29.34 Late congenital syphilis with gummata on the forehead and scalp.

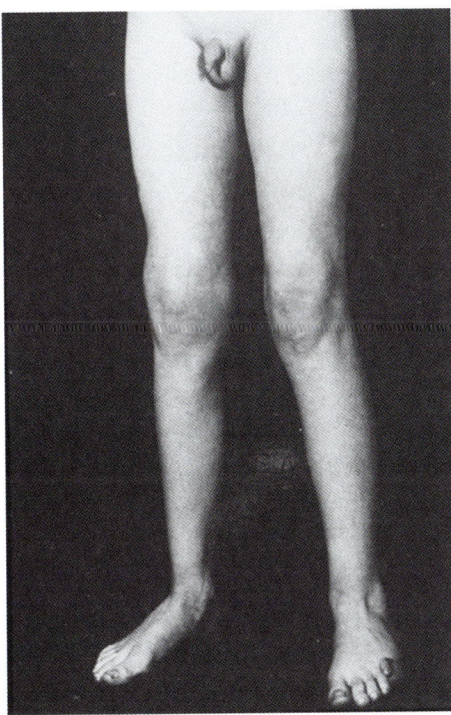

Figure 29.35 Clutton joints in late congenital syphilis.

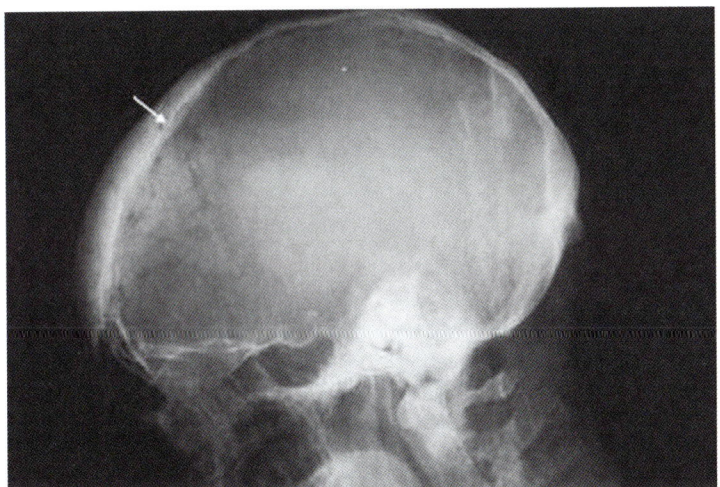

Figure 29.36 Early congenital syphilis showing osteitis of the skull bones (arrow) causing a worm-eaten appearance.

Evaluation of neonates for congenital syphilis

The following investigations should be carried out in children born to seropositive mothers with no documented treatment at least 4 weeks before delivery, if a non-penicillin regimen was administered, or if relapse or reinfection is suspected:

- Examination for stigmata of CS.
- X-ray of the long bones for evidence of periostitis.
- CSF examination.
- Dark-field microscopy and/or PCR from exudates of suspicious lesions or fluids.

Infection of the neonate is also suggested if the serum non-treponemal antibody titre is four or more times more than the mother's, or if specific IgM treponemal antibody tests are positive.

Passively transferred maternal IgG antibody can persist in the infant's serum for up to 12 months.

Management

Treatment decisions must be made on the basis of:
- Identification of syphilis in the mother.
- Adequacy of maternal treatment.
- Presence of clinical, laboratory or radiographic evidence of syphilis in the infant.
- Comparison of maternal (at delivery) and infant non-treponemal serological titres using the same test, preferably conducted by the same laboratory.

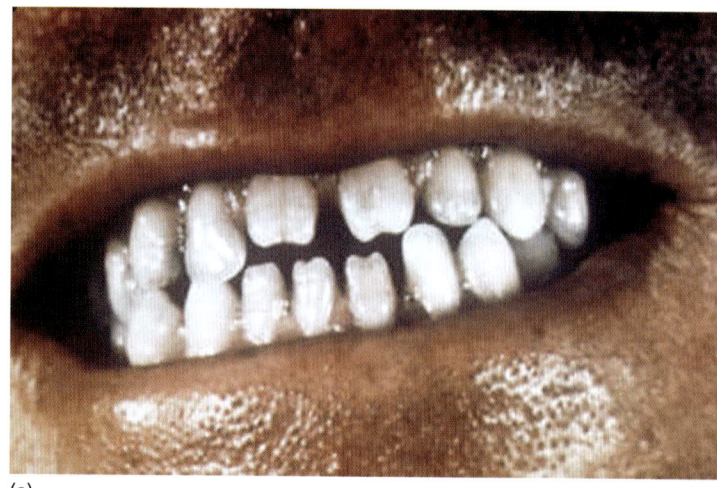

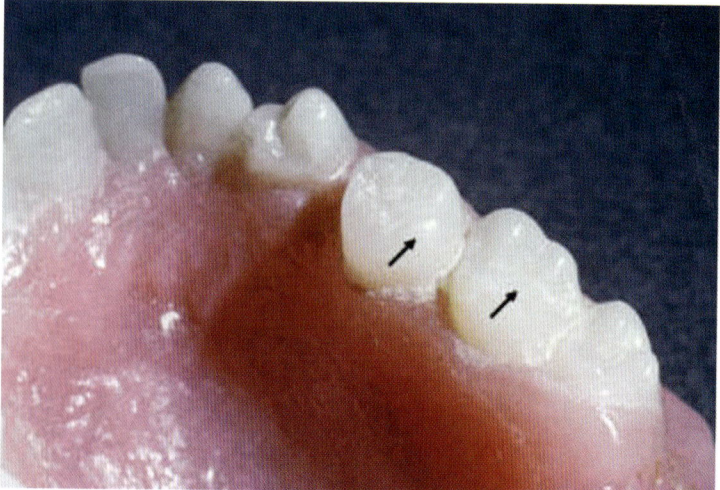

Figure 29.38 Moon molars showing a dome-shaped malformation and loss of cusps (arrows).

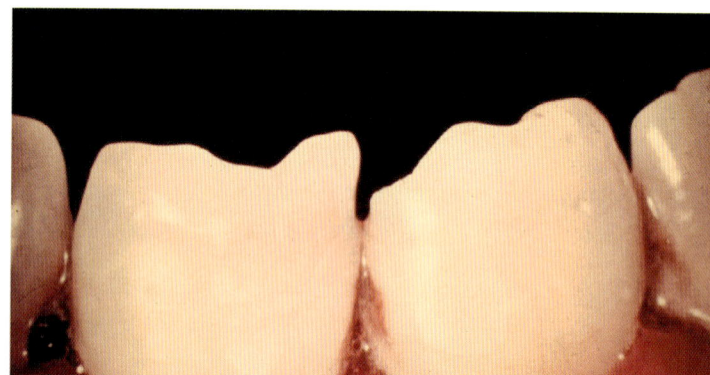

Figure 29.37 Malformations of the secondary dentition in late congenital syphilis. (a) Hutchinson teeth. (b) Close-up of Hutchinson incisors.

Lack of assured supply of benzathine penicillin [24] and other practical issues [25] continue to make progress towards the ambitious WHO strategy of eradicating CS extremely challenging in many low-income countries.

Treatment ladder for congenital syphilis

First line
For neonates
- *Aqueous crystalline penicillin G* 60 000–150 000 units/kg/day, administered as 30 000–50 000 units/kg/dose IV every 12 h during the first 7 days of life and every 8 h thereafter for a total of 10 days
  Or
- *Procaine penicillin G* 50 000 units/kg/dose IM in a single daily dose for 10 days

IV therapy is preferable due to the pain associated with IM injections

For older infants and children
- *Aqueous crystalline penicillin G* 0.2–0.3 mega units/kg/day IV, administered as 50 000 units/kg every 4–6 h for 10 days

In infants with a normal examination, a non-treponemal serological titre the same or less than fourfold the maternal titre, the mother was treated during pregnancy, treatment was appropriate for the stage of infection, and treatment was administered >4 weeks before delivery, plus if the mother has no evidence of reinfection or relapse, close monitoring is recommended, and treatment is optional

Where given, the recommended regimen is:
- *Benzathine penicillin G* 50 000 units/kg/day in a single IM injection

Second line
Data are insufficient regarding the use of other antimicrobial agents. In cases of shortage or penicillin allergy then ceftriaxone can be used. However, if a non-penicillin agent is used, close serological and CSF follow-up are indicated

For infants aged ≥30 days
- *Ceftriaxone* 75 mg/kg IV/IM OD in a single daily dose for 10–14 days

For older infants
- *Ceftriaxone* 100 mg/kg OD in a single dose

Infants and children who require treatment for syphilis but who have a history of penicillin allergy or develop an allergic reaction presumed secondary to penicillin should be desensitised, if necessary, and then treated with penicillin

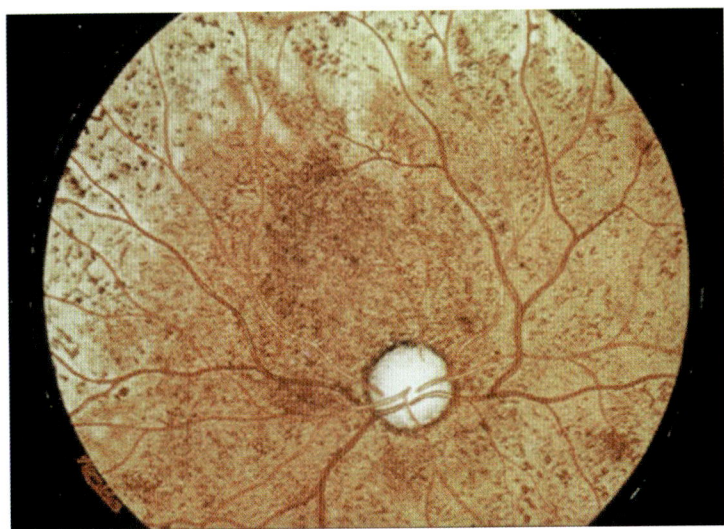

Figure 29.39 Congenital syphilis with chorioretinitis and optic atrophy.

Follow-up

All seroreactive infants (or infants whose mothers were seroreactive at delivery) should receive careful follow-up examinations and serological non-treponemal testing every 2–3 months until the test becomes non-reactive or the titre has decreased fourfold.

Non-treponemal antibody titres should decline by the age of 3 months and should be non-reactive by 6 months if the infant is not infected (i.e. if the reactive test result was caused by passive transfer of maternal IgG antibody) or was infected but adequately treated.

The serological response after therapy might be slower for infants treated after the neonatal period. If these titres are stable or increase after age 6–12 months, the child should be evaluated (e.g. given a CSF examination) and treated with a 10-day course of parenteral penicillin G.

Resources

Guidelines and data

British Association for Sexual Health and HIV (BASHH): https://www.bashh.org/guidelines.
Centers for Disease Control and Prevention (CDC), syphilis information: https://www.cdc.gov/std/syphilis.
International Union Against Sexually Transmitted Infections (IUSTI): https://iusti.org/wp-content/uploads/2020/07/Syphilis2020guideline.
Prochazka M, Evans J, Thorn L, Sinka K, and contributors. *Tracking the Syphilis Epidemic in England: 2010 to 2019*. London: Public Health England, 2021.
World Health Organization (WHO), guidelines for the treatment of *Treponema pallidum*: https://www.who.int/publications/i/item/9789241549714.

Patient resources

British Association for Sexual Health and HIV (BASHH): https://www.bashhguidelines.org/patient-information-leaflets.
Centers for Disease Control and Prevention (CDC), syphilis fact sheet: https://www.cdc.gov/std/syphilis/default.htm.
International Union Against Sexually Transmitted Infections (IUSTI): https://iusti.org/patient-information/.
National Health Service (NHS), syphilis: https://www.nhs.uk/conditions/syphilis (All last accessed February 2023.)

Key references

The full list of references can be found in the online version at https://www.wiley.com/rooksdermatology10e

Syphilis

2 Peeling RW, Mabey D, Kamb ML et al. Syphilis. *Nat Rev Dis Primers* 2017;3:17073.
5 Mohammed H, Blomquist P, Ogaz D et al. 100 years of STIs in the UK: a review of national surveillance data. *Sex Transm Infect* 2018;94:553–8.
7 Spiteri G, Unemo M, Mårdh O, Amato-Gauci AJ. The resurgence of syphilis in high-income countries in the 2000s: a focus on Europe. *Epidemiol Infect* 2019;147:e143.
13 Radolf JD, Deka RK, Anand A et al. *Treponema pallidum*, the syphilis spirochete: making a living as a stealth pathogen. *Nat Rev Microbiol* 2016;14:744–59.
64 Park IU, Fakile YF, Chow JM et al. Performance of treponemal tests for the diagnosis of syphilis. *Clin Infect Dis* 2019;68:913–18.
70 Catterall RD. Collagen disease and the chronic biological false positive phenomenon. *Q J Med* 1961;30:41–55.

Congenital syphilis

1 World Health Organization (WHO). *The Global Elimination of Congenital Syphilis: Rationale and Strategy for Action*. Geneva: WHO, 2007.
2 World Health Organization (WHO). *Report on Global Sexually Transmitted Infection Surveillance, 2018*. Geneva: WHO, 2018.
3 World Health Organization (WHO). *Global Guidance on Criteria and Processes for Validation: Elimination of Mother-to-Child of HIV and Syphilis*, 2nd edn. Geneva: WHO, 2017.
25 Taylor M, Gliddon H, Nurse-Findlay S et al. Revisiting strategies to eliminate mother-to-child transmission of syphilis. *Lancet Glob Health* 2018;6:e26–8.

CHAPTER 30

Non-syphilitic Bacterial Sexually Transmitted Diseases

George R. Kinghorn[1] *and Nadi K. Gupta*[2]

[1] Sheffield Teaching Hospitals NHS Foundation Trust, Sheffield, UK
[2] Rotherham Hospital NHS Foundation Trust, Rotherham, UK

Gonorrhoea, 30.1	Chancroid, 30.18	Key references, 30.26
Genital *Chlamydia* infection, 30.8	Granuloma inguinale, 30.21	
Lymphogranuloma venereum, 30.14	*Mycoplasma genitalium* infection, 30.23	

Gonorrhoea

Definition and nomenclature
Gonorrhoea is a bacterial infection caused by *Neisseria gonorrhoeae* that principally causes purulent inflammation of the genital mucous membranes. It is primarily sexually transmitted but vertical transmission during childbirth is important. It is, after genital *Chlamydia trachomatis* infection, the second most common bacterial sexually transmitted infection (STI) in the UK and other developed countries. Antimicrobial resistance is an increasing cause of global concern.

Synonyms and inclusions
- Sexually transmitted infection (STI)
- Oro-pharyngeal gonorrhoea
- Rectal gonorrhoea
- Gonococcal conjunctivitis
- Ophthalmia neonatorum

Introduction and general description
Gonorrhoea results in several clinical syndromes including urethritis, cervicitis, epididymo-orchitis, pelvic inflammatory syndrome, disseminated gonococcal infection and ophthalmia neonatorum.

Epidemiology
Incidence and prevalence
Disease rates are unknown for most countries because of inadequate surveillance and reporting systems. In 2016, the World Health Organization (WHO) estimated there were 87 million cases worldwide with global incidence rates of 20 per 1000 females and 26 per 1000 males [1]. Higher rates occur in the low- and middle-income countries (LMICs) of Africa, the Americas and western Pacific regions. In the high-income countries (HICs) of Europe and North America, where the highest rates occur in marginalised populations within large conurbations, infection rates are again increasing. International travel can facilitate spread including of antimicrobial resistant strains across international borders [2].

In the UK, the annual number of diagnosed cases has been increasing since 2005 and reached historic highs in males in 2018 (Figure 30.1) [3]. One-third or more of the infections in males are homosexually acquired.

Age
The highest rates of infection occur in young people, especially in teenage women and men in their early twenties. Currently in the UK, rates are highest in males aged 20–34 years and females aged 16–19 years (Figure 30.2). Infection rates have also been increasing in older age groups.

Ethnicity
Although black ethnic groups are disproportionately affected in the UK and USA, there is no known racial predisposition to gonorrhoea.

Associated diseases
Individuals diagnosed with gonorrhoea are at risk of other coexistent STIs including human immunodeficiency virus (HIV) infection, therefore a full sexual health assessment is warranted.

Pathophysiology
Predisposing factors
Gonorrhoea has a high infectivity and is easily transmitted before symptoms appear. Socioeconomic and behavioural factors and patterns of sexual mixing affect its spread.

Pathogenesis
The causative organism shares common ancestry with other commensal *Neisseria* and has developed multiple mechanisms to combat host innate and adaptive immunity [3]. These include:
1. Prevention of complement activation, opsonisation and bacterial killing.
2. Modulation of the activities of macrophages, dendritic cells and neutrophils.

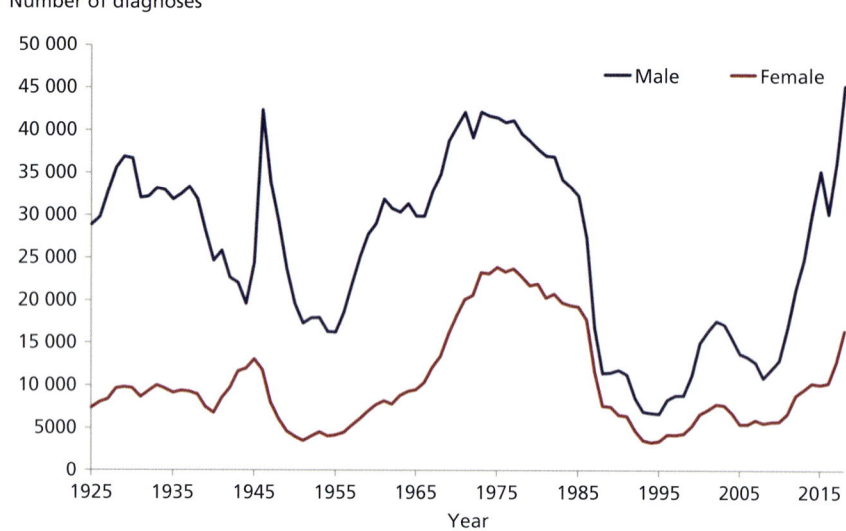

Figure 30.1 Number of gonorrhoea diagnoses by sex in the UK, 1925–2018. Public Health England 2019 slide set (version 1.0, published 2 September 2020).

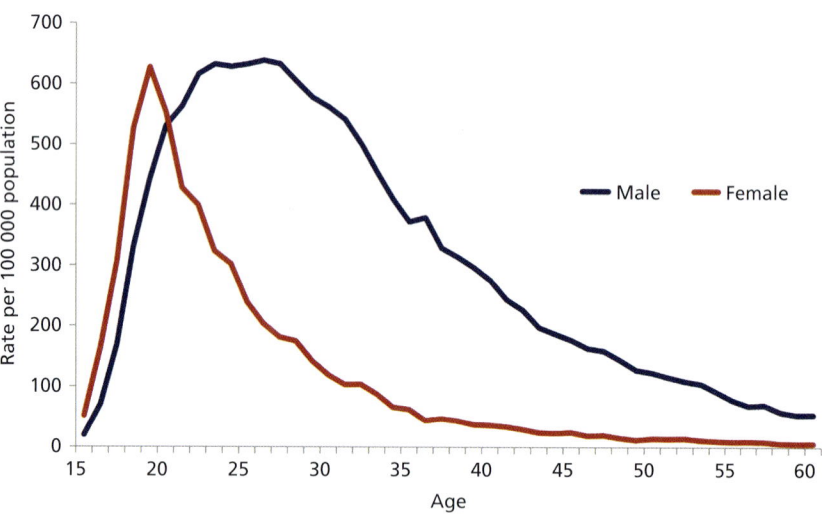

Figure 30.2 Rate of gonorrhoea diagnoses by sex and age in England, 2019. Adapted from Public Health England 2019 slide set (version 1.0, published 2 September 2020).

3 Modulation of T-cell function.
4 Variation in surface components of the organism to avoid the adaptive immune system.
  Reinfection after successful treatment is common.

It has been estimated that in 0.5–3% of cases, haematogenous spread from the mucous membranes can lead to disseminated gonococcal infection [4]. Strains that have the ability to resist the activity of antibodies and complement predispose to dissemination [5]. Host factors predisposing to disseminated gonococcal infection include:

- Female sex.
- Men who have sex with men (MSM).
- Pregnancy.
- Menstruation.
- Systemic lupus erythematosus.
- Complement deficiency.
- Intravenous drug use.
- HIV infection.

Pathology
Humans are the only natural host for gonococci. The gonococci attach to host mucosal cells with the aid of pili, which cover the entire outer cell surface, and outer membrane proteins. The pili undergo antigenic variation in which strains change their antigenic type. The gonococci then penetrate between cells into the subepithelial space. They may also be able to multiply intracellularly and exit from the basal surface of the cell. The host mounts an acute inflammatory response that leads to epithelial sloughing, submucosal microabscesses and purulent discharge.

Causative organisms
Gonorrhoea is caused by the Gram-negative, aerobic, intracellular diplococcus, *Neisseria gonorrhoeae*, that principally infects host columnar epithelium. Outside the human host the organism is delicate and susceptible to drying, but within the body it has a large capability to effect antigenic variation, which helps it evade the host immune response and to develop antimicrobial resistance. Repeated reinfections by the same strain can occur.

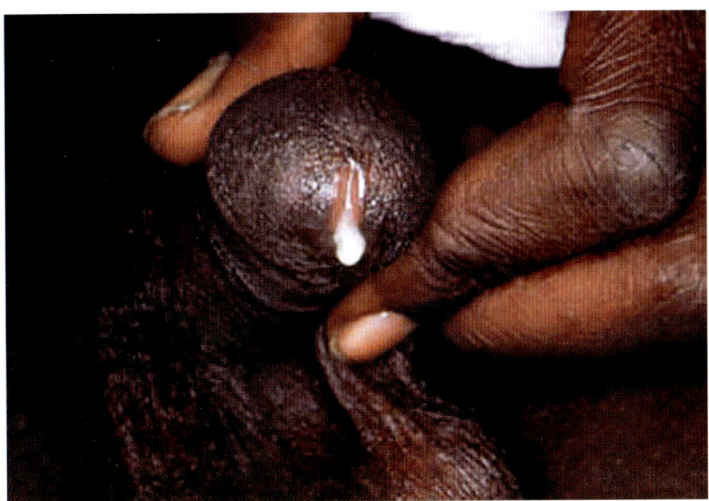

Figure 30.3 Acute urethritis with a purulent discharge.

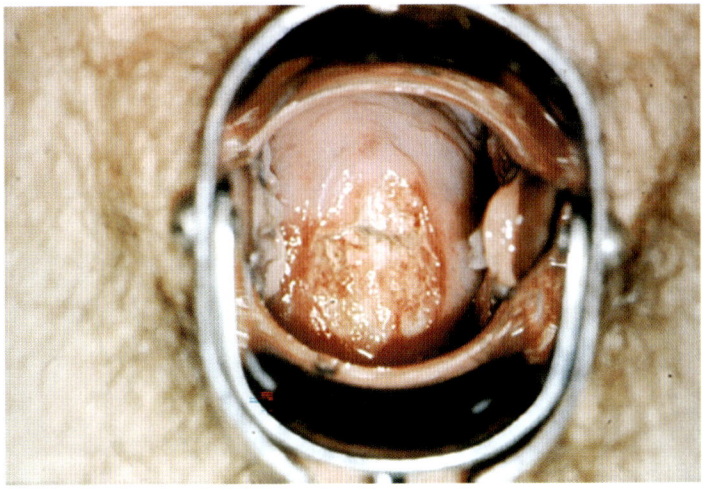

Figure 30.5 Gonococcal cervicitis showing a mucopurulent discharge with redness.

Clinical features

History
In symptomatic cases the incubation period is generally short, and symptoms typically have their onset 1–5 days after sexual contact with an infectious person.

Presentation
Infection may be asymptomatic in both sexes when it is diagnosed as a result of opportunistic testing or contact tracing.

The common presentation in men is with acute urethritis. There is rapid onset of dysuria accompanied by a purulent discharge, which is often profuse (Figure 30.3). Some may only develop a

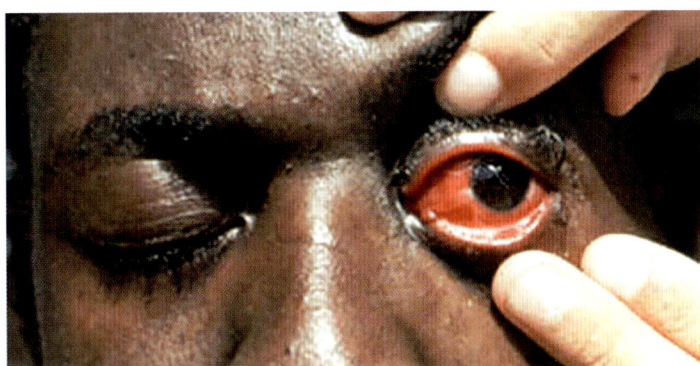

Figure 30.6 Gonococcal conjunctivitis showing an acute, severe, purulent discharge with irritation and a red eye.

scant or minimally purulent discharge. In MSM, there may also be rectal and pharyngeal infections. Gonococcal proctitis may be asymptomatic but may present with rectal pain, tenesmus and discharge (Figure 30.4). Infection of the oro-pharynx may present with exudative pharyngitis and cervical lymphadenopathy but is usually asymptomatic [6].

The primary site of infection in women is the cervix but the urethra, rectum and pharynx may be involved. Symptomatic infections manifest as excessive vaginal discharge, dysuria, deep dyspareunia, postcoital bleeding and intermenstrual bleeding. However, most women with early infections report no symptoms. On examination there may be evidence of cervicitis with cervical discharge, redness and contact mucosal bleeding (Figure 30.5).

A less common site of infection in adults is the eye, where autoinoculation of the organism from infected ano-genital sites leads to acute conjunctivitis. This presents as an acutely painful red eye (Figure 30.6) with purulent discharge that may progress to panophthalmitis and loss of vision. Gonococcal conjunctivitis is more often associated with newborn babies as ophthalmia neonatorum, which usually occurs in the first week after birth (Figure 30.7). Prompt recognition and treatment are essential to prevent permanent visual damage.

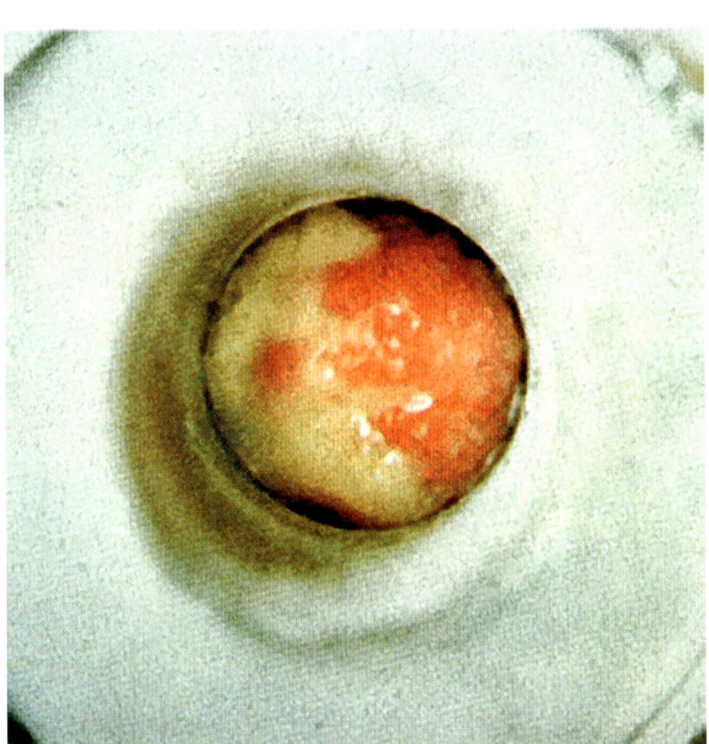

Figure 30.4 Gonococcal proctitis: proctoscopy reveals an inflamed mucosa and a purulent discharge.

30.4   Chapter 30: Non-syphilitic Bacterial Sexually Transmitted Diseases

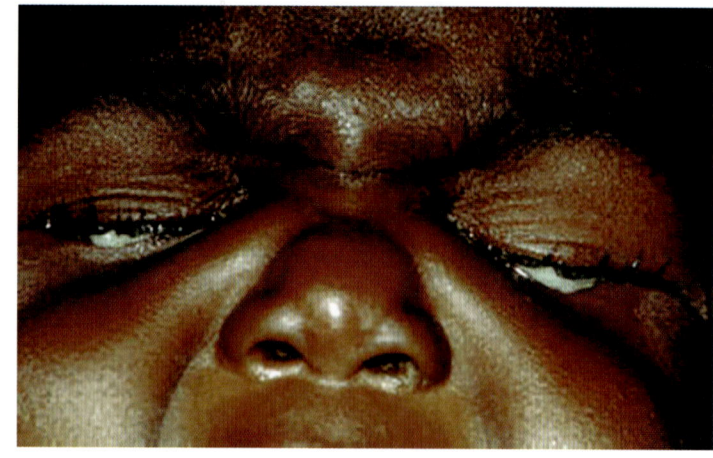

Figure 30.7 Gonococcal ophthalmia neonatorum: the purulent discharge may be profuse.

Differential diagnosis
Differential diagnoses include the following:
- Lower genital tract infections – *Chlamydia trachomatis, Mycoplasma genitalium, Trichomonas vaginalis,* non-specific urethritis and genital herpes.
- Urinary tract infection.
- Pelvic inflammatory disease (PID).
- Ectopic pregnancy.
- Cervical or endometrial neoplasia.
- Other causes of intermenstrual bleeding

Complications and co-morbidities
Complications may occur from local abscess formation, ascending infections or haematogenous spread. There are also those associated with pregnancy and the neonatal period. Figure 30.8 shows the main sites of gonococcal infection.

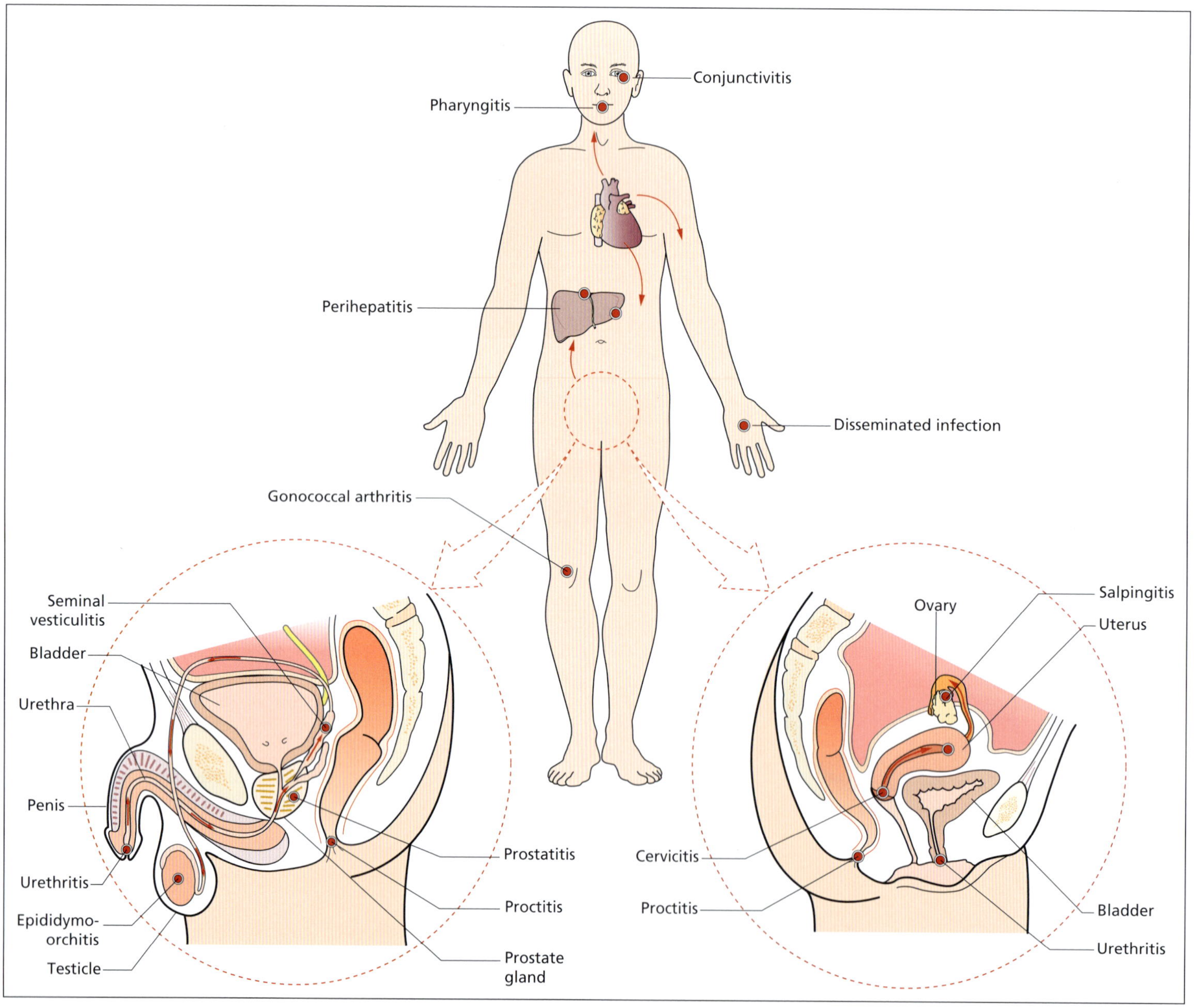

Figure 30.8 Points of entry and route of dissemination of gonococci.

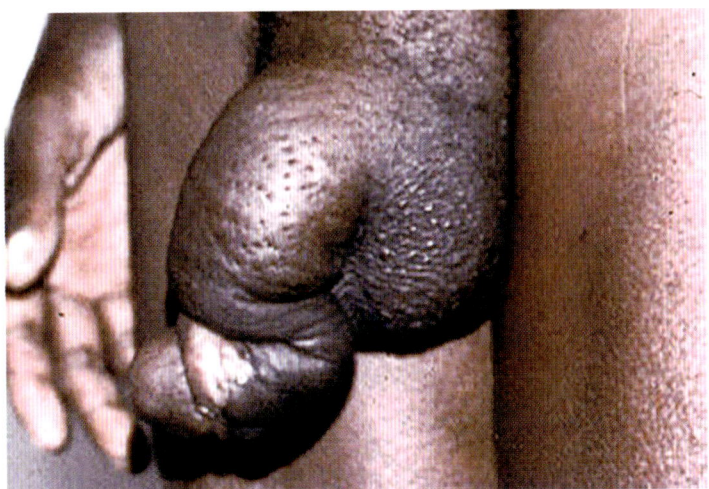

Figure 30.9 Saxophone penis caused by a periurethral abscess.

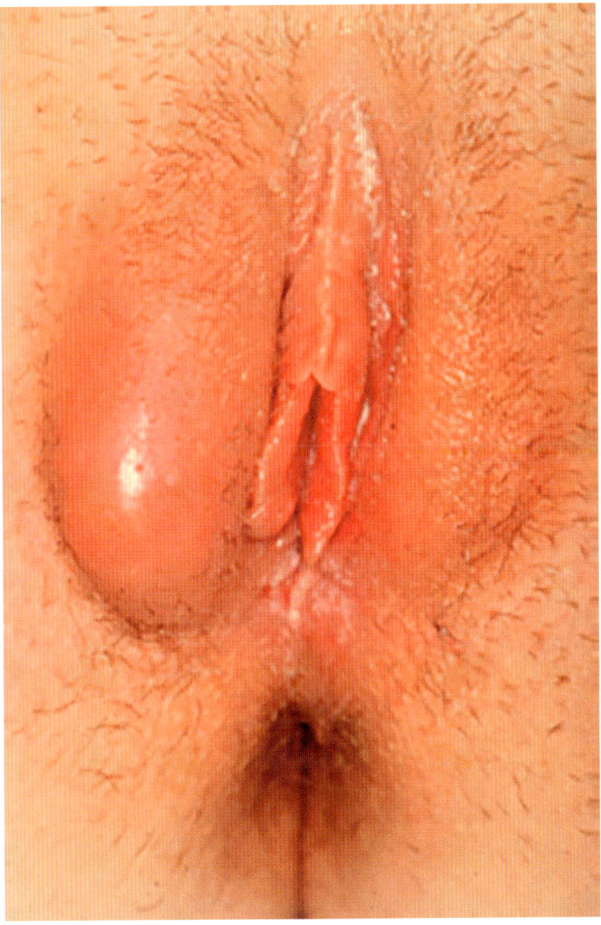

Figure 30.10 Bartholin abscess: the Bartholin glands are located on either side of the vaginal opening and can become obstructed and/or infected. Gonorrhoea should be considered as a cause.

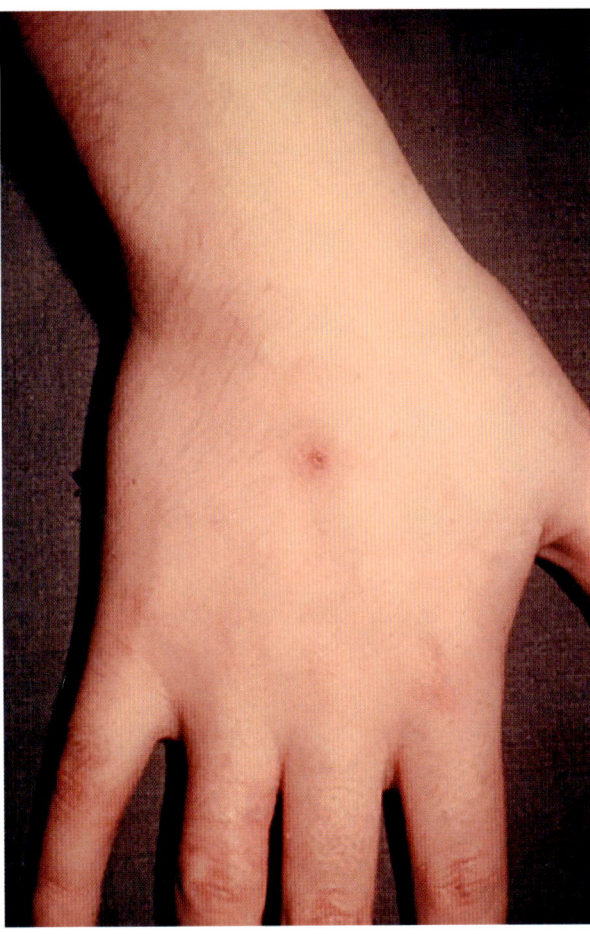

Figure 30.11 Disseminated gonococcal infection showing a macular lesion with central necrosis on the dorsum of the hand.

Periurethral abscess may occur in either sex and leads to fistula formation and subsequent urethral stricture. In males, it may cause a saxophone penis deformity (Figure 30.9). Gonorrhoea should also be considered as a possible cause for a Bartholin abscess (Figure 30.10).

Ascending infection in men causes acute prostatitis, with symptoms of urinary frequency, strangury and back or perineal pain. It may also present as unilateral or bilateral painful testicular swelling resulting from acute epididymo-orchitis.

In women, ascending infections cause PID. This is usually acute in onset, with lower abdominal and pelvic pain, fever and marked adnexal and cervical motion tenderness on bimanual pelvic examination. Acute salpingitis may develop into a tubo-ovarian abscess. Scarring after healing may result in scarring of the fallopian tubes and tubal factor infertility.

Acute perihepatitis (Fitz-Hugh–Curtis syndrome) [7] may also occur with gonorrhoea, chlamydia or mixed infections. It presents as fever and right upper quadrant pain and tenderness that mimics acute cholecystitis. Perihepatitis, resulting from inflammation of the liver capsule, generally occurs in much younger women than in those who typically suffer from cholecystitis. Periappendicitis, which may also be caused by either gonorrhoea or chlamydial infection, has a similar pathogenesis. Pregnancy and neonatal complications may include premature rupture of the membranes, premature delivery and acute chorioamnionitis and ophthalmia neonatorum. PID is less likely to occur than in the non-pregnant state.

Disseminated gonococcal infection. The classic presentation is with a dermatitis–arthritis syndrome in a patient with mild fever. The skin lesions are small, tender and initially maculopapular (Figure 30.11). A central vesicle or pustule (Figure 30.12) appears,

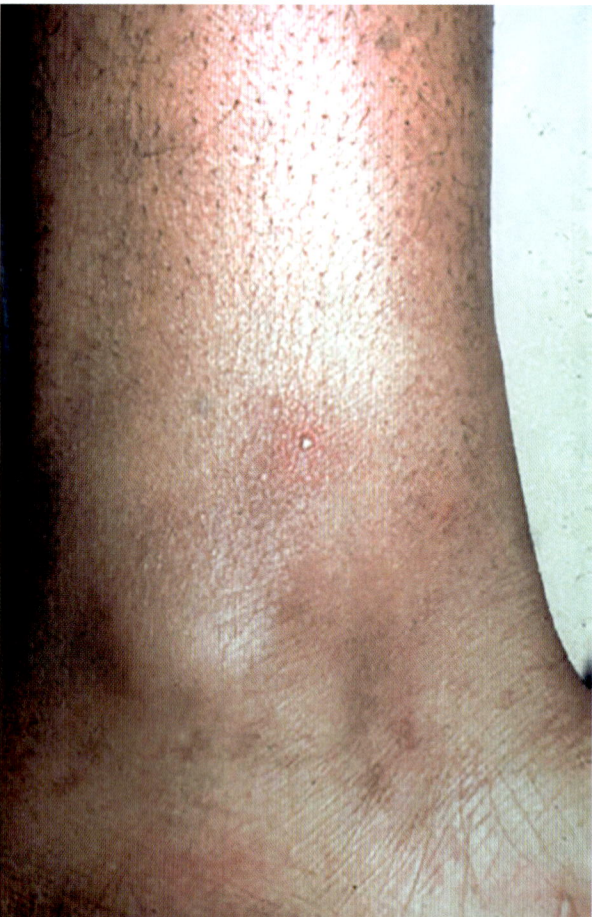

Figure 30.12 Disseminated gonococcal infection showing a pustule surrounded with redness above the lateral malleolus.

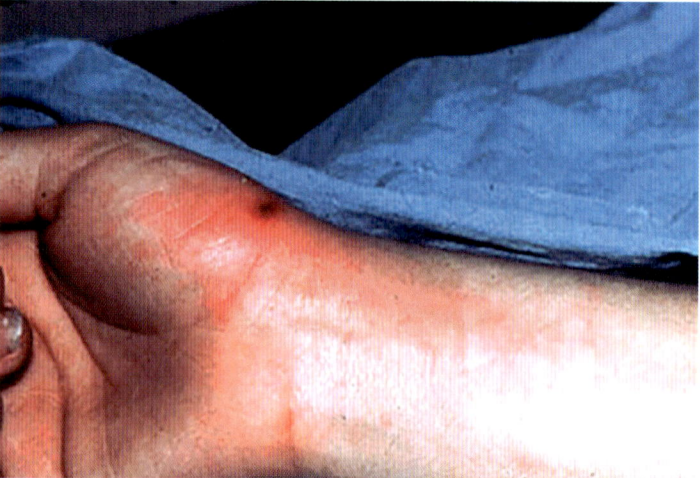

Figure 30.13 Disseminated gonococcal infection showing early macular lesions that progress to pustules and haemorrhagic lesions.

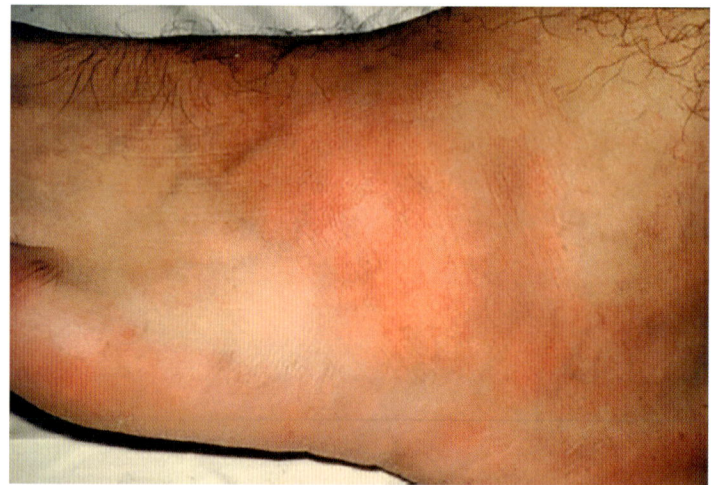

Figure 30.14 Gonococcal arthritis in the metatarsal joints.

and haemorrhage and necrosis commonly ensue. Lesions occur in crops, usually between 5 and 40, and are commonly seen peripherally near affected joints. They may also occur on the torso and the palms and soles.

Joint or tendon pain is the most common accompanying feature. Tenosynovitis often affects the hands and fingers (Figure 30.13). It may be accompanied by a migratory polyarthralgia, affecting the knees, elbows, wrists, metacarpo-phalangeal joints, ankle joints and metatarso-phalangeal joints (Figure 30.14). There is a high yield of positive blood cultures in such cases.

Later, one-third of cases will develop a suppurative arthritis, which most commonly affects the knee. By this stage, skin lesions have usually disappeared and blood cultures are often negative. Rarely, pericarditis and endocarditis may also occur at this later stage. The latter is more common in men, usually affects the aortic valve and presents with a subacute onset of chest pain, fever, chills and malaise. Meningitis, similar to that caused by meningococci but with a less rapid course, is rare but well recognised.

Disease course and prognosis

If untreated, 95% of people with uncomplicated urethritis are asymptomatic after 6 months. However, the rate of complications may be more than 20%. Similarly, pharyngeal infection has a spontaneous rate of clearance close to 100% at 12 weeks. Uncomplicated infections treated with appropriate antimicrobial therapy resolve completely. Urethral strictures, common in the pre-antibiotic era, are now rare.

Investigations

Microscopy

A rapid presumptive diagnosis can be made by the identification of Gram-negative intracellular diplococci within phagocytes in stained smears from ano-genital sites (Figure 30.15). This allows one-stop diagnosis and treatment and is most useful in men with a urethral discharge where sensitivity is 90–95% [8]. It is far less reliable for diagnosing infections of the rectum, pharynx and cervix.

Culture

Confirmation is by culture of the organism and differentiation from other *Neisseria* species by antigenic or biochemical testing. The gonococcus is a fastidious organism and requires appropriate methods of specimen collection and transportation to the laboratory. Specimens are plated onto nutritive, selective media and incubated in a humid atmosphere containing 5% CO_2. Culture

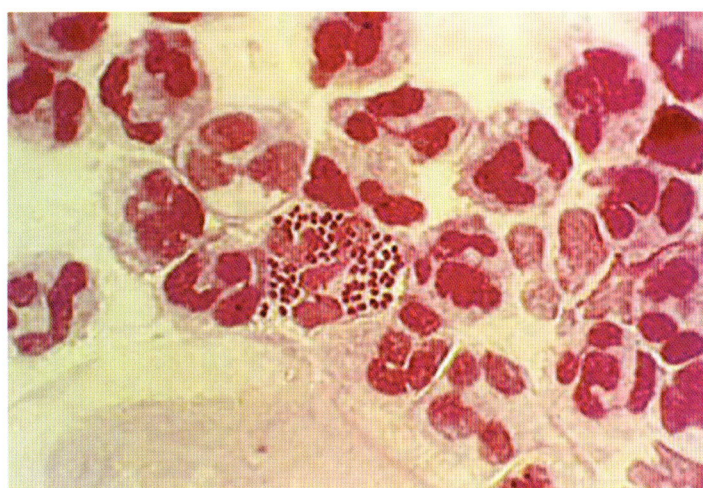

Figure 30.15 Gram staining of a urethral smear demonstrating intracellular and extracellular Gram-negative diplococci.

remains the gold standard for diagnosing gonorrhoea. Importantly, culture is close to 100% specific and allows the testing of isolates for antimicrobial sensitivities.

Nucleic acid amplification tests

Nucleic acid amplification tests (NAATs) for the diagnosis of gonorrhoea are commonly combined with those for *Chlamydia* in commercial assays. They are more sensitive than culture because of the problems associated with specimen collection, transportation and culture requirements. There are a variety of platforms and test methodologies, including polymerase chain reaction (PCR), strand displacement assay, transcription-mediated amplification assay and 16s RNA detection [9,10]. They do not produce isolates that allow antimicrobial sensitivity, have lower sensitivity when used on urine specimens in women and can produce false positive results from cross-reactions with other pathogenic and commensal *Neisseria* species. Thus, it is advisable that when such tests are used for screening, especially in low prevalence populations, results are viewed as being presumptive, and confirmation is sought by repeat sampling for culture. In high-risk persons and contacts, specimens for culture should be taken alongside those for NAATs testing.

NAATs can also be modified to allow molecular analysis of isolates that are useful in epidemiological studies and network analysis [11,12].

Management

The gonococcus has a marked propensity to develop antimicrobial resistance (Figure 30.16) which is a major worldwide threat to efforts to reduce the impact of STIs. Gonococcal isolates now show high rates of quinolone resistance, increasing azithromycin resistance and emerging resistance to extended-spectrum cephalosporins [13,14].

A recent major change in UK guidelines is the move away from routine combination antimicrobial therapy. Monotherapy with either ceftriaxone IM, where antimicrobial sensitivity is unknown, or with oral ciprofloxacin if the causative isolate is known to be sensitive, is now first line therapy. The Centers for Disease Control and Prevention (CDC) likewise recommends ceftriaxone as first line treatment.

Where concurrent *Chlamydia* infection is present, additional therapy with either doxycycline (or azithromycin in pregnancy) is given. Pharyngeal infection is more difficult to eradicate.

Complicated infections require longer courses of treatment.

Patients with gonorrhoea should always be fully assessed and screened for other STIs and HIV. Both verbal and written information should be given about the infection, its transmission and prevention. Patients should be asked to assist with partner notification efforts, and to avoid further sexual contact until at least 7 days after they and their partners have received treatment and all symptoms have resolved.

A test of cure (TOC) at 3 days after treatment by culture is no longer routine and is only undertaken if there are persistent symptoms. In asymptomatic patients, TOC by NAAT test is performed at 2 weeks after treatment completion.

Epidemiological treatment is often recommended for contacts presenting within 14 days of their most recent sexual exposure to the index case. Otherwise, it is recommended that the need for treatment is delayed until the results of diagnostic tests are known.

Gonococcal vaccine

The first potential vaccine-induced protection against gonorrhoea in humans has been reported, with decreased rates of gonorrhoea described among individuals vaccinated with the *Neisseria meningitidis* serogroup B vaccine, MeNZB. This has reinvigorated efforts to develop new vaccines to combat the ongoing threat to public health posed by antimicrobial-resistant gonorrhoea [15,16].

Treatment ladder for gonorrhoea

Uncomplicated infection

First line
- Ceftriaxone 1 g IM single dose
- Ciprofloxacin 500 mg PO single dose (only when antimicrobial sensitivity known prior to treatment)

Second line
- Cefixime 400 mg PO + azithromycin 2 g PO (significant treatment failure reported)
- Spectinomycin 2 g IM + azithromycin 2 g PO (spectinomycin does not clear pharyngeal gonorrhoea)
- Gentamycin 240 mg IM + azithromycin 2 g PO

Pregnancy and breastfeeding
- Ceftriaxone 1 g IM single dose
- Spectinomycin 2 g IM single dose
- Azithromycin 2 g PO single dose, if antimicrobial sensitivity is known before treatment

Complicated infection

Gonococcal epididymo-orchitis
- Ceftriaxone 1 g IM + regimen chosen to treat epididymo-orchitis

Gonococcal pelvic inflammatory disease (PID)
- Ceftriaxone 1 g IM + regimen chosen to treat PID

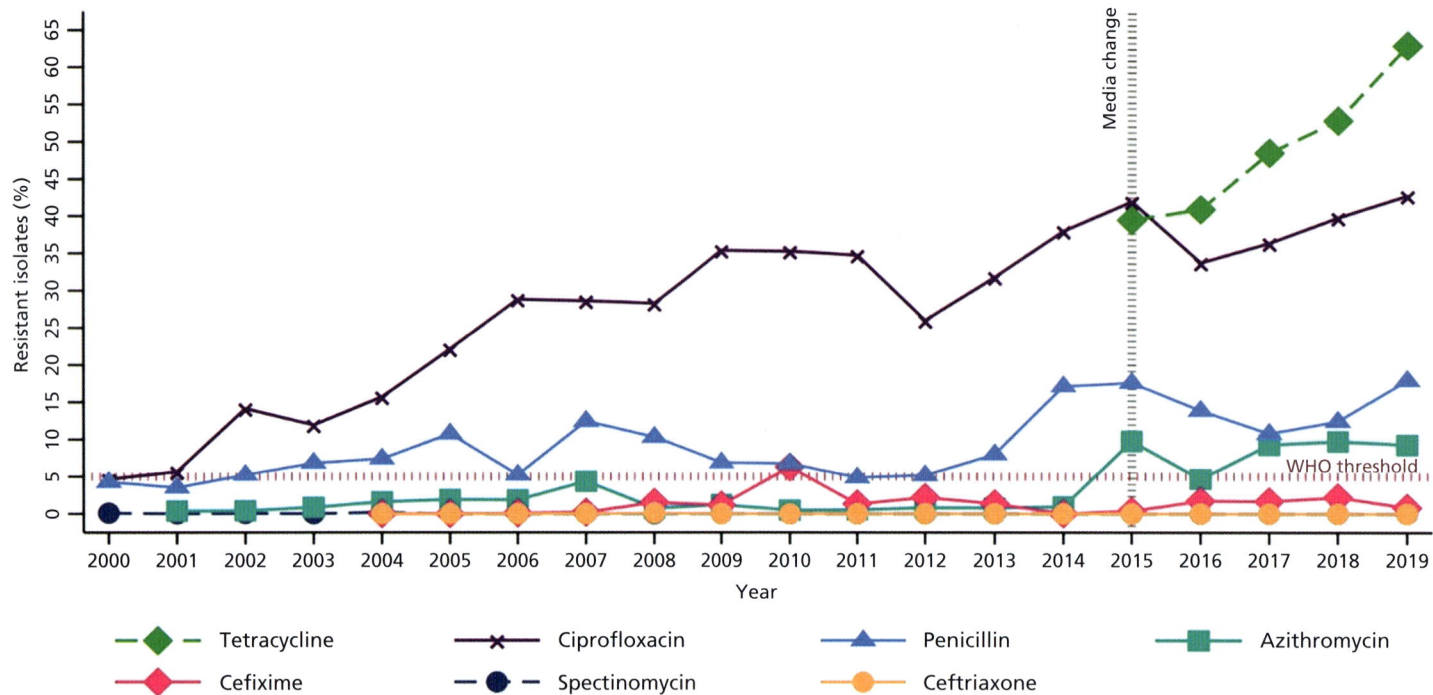

Figure 30.16 Percentage of *Neisseria gonorrhoeae* isolates in the GRASP sentinel surveillance system that were resistant to selected antimicrobials: England and Wales 2000–19. Due to changes in the diagnostic sensitivity test medium used to test antimicrobial susceptibility of sentinel surveillance isolates, minimum inhibitory concentrations for the 2015–19 collections are not directly comparable with those from previous years. Trends from 2000 to 2014 compared with 2015–19 must be interpreted with caution (point of change indicated by vertical dashed black line), particularly for azithromycin and tetracycline (data for tetracycline are only included from 2015 onwards due to this issue). The 5% threshold (≥5% of infections resistant to the first line therapy) at which the World Health Organization (WHO) recommends that first line treatment guidelines should be changed is indicated by the horizontal dashed red line. From Public Health England (PHE). Antimicrobial resistance in Neisseria gonorrhoeae in England and Wales. Key findings from the Gonococcal Resistance to Antimicrobials Surveillance Programme (GRASP 2019).

Gonococcal conjunctivitis
- Ceftriaxone 1 g IM single dose

Disseminated gonococcal infection
- Ceftriaxone 1 g IM or IV every 24 h
- Cefotaxime 1 g IV every 8 h
- Ciprofloxacin 500 mg IV every 12 h
- Spectinomycin 2 g IM every 12 h

Treatment to continue for 7 days. May switch to oral therapy, guided by antimicrobial sensitivities, 24–48 h after symptom improvement, with:
- Cefixime 400 mg PO
- Ciprofloxacin 500 mg PO twice daily
- Ofloxacin 400 mg PO twice daily

Resources

Further information
Fifer H, Saunders J, Soni S, Sadiq ST, FitzGerald M. 2018 UK national guideline for the management of infection with *Neisseria gonorrhoeae*. *Int J STD AIDS* 2020;31:4–15.

Public Health England (PHE). *Gonococcal Resistance to Antimicrobials Surveillance Programme Report*. https://www.gov.uk/government/publications/gonococcal-resistance-to-antimicrobials-surveillance-programme-grasp-report.

Public Health England (PHE). *Sexually Transmitted Infections (STIs): Annual Data Tables*. https://www.gov.uk/government/statistics/sexually-transmitted-infections-stis-annual-data-tables.

St Cyr S, Barbee L, Workowski KA *et al*. Update to CDC's treatment guidelines for gonococcal infection, 2020. *MMWR Morb Mortal Wkly Rep* 2020;69:1911–16.

Unemo M, Ross J, Serwin A, Gomberg M, Cusini M, Jensen J. 2020 European guideline for the diagnosis and treatment of gonorrhoea in adults. *Int J STD AIDS* 2020;956462420949126.

Patient resources
British Association for Sexual Health and HIV (BASHH), patient information leaflets: https://bashh.org/guidelines.

Centers for Disease Control and Prevention (CDC). *Gonorrhoea – CDC fact sheet*. http://www.cdc.gov/std/gonorrhea/stdfact-gonorrhea.htm.

International Union against Sexually Transmitted Infections (IUSTI), patient information leaflets (in different languages: https://iusti.org/patient-information/.

National Health Service (NHS). *Overview: Gonorrhoea*. https://www.nhs.uk/conditions/gonorrhoea.

(All websites last accessed May 2023.)

Genital *Chlamydia* infection

Definition
Genital chlamydia only became widely recognised during the 1970s but is now the most common bacterial STI worldwide. It causes inflammation of the genital and rectal mucous membranes as well as the conjunctiva. Asymptomatic infections are common in both sexes and promote ongoing sexual transmission. Vertical transmission during childbirth also occurs. The causative organism, *Chlamydia trachomatis*, is an exclusively human, obligate, intracellular bacterial pathogen with a complex life cycle.

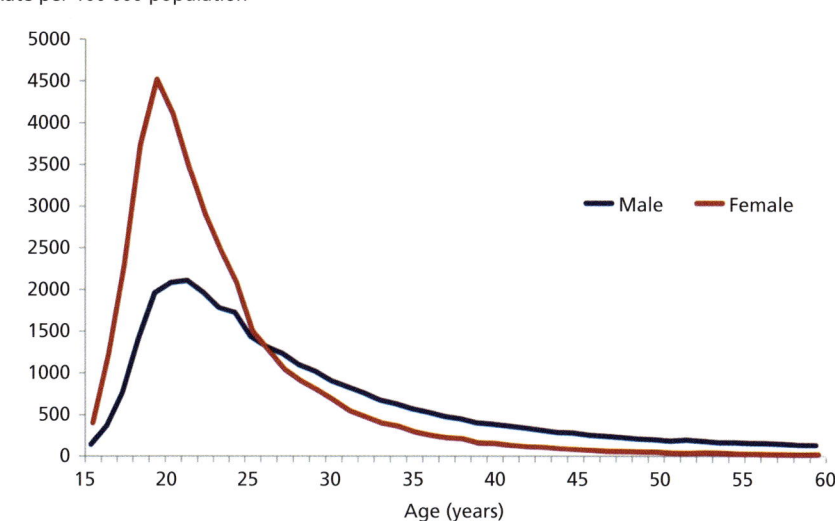

Figure 30.17 Rates of chlamydia diagnoses by sex and age. From Public Health England 2019 slide set (version 1.0, published 2 September 2020).

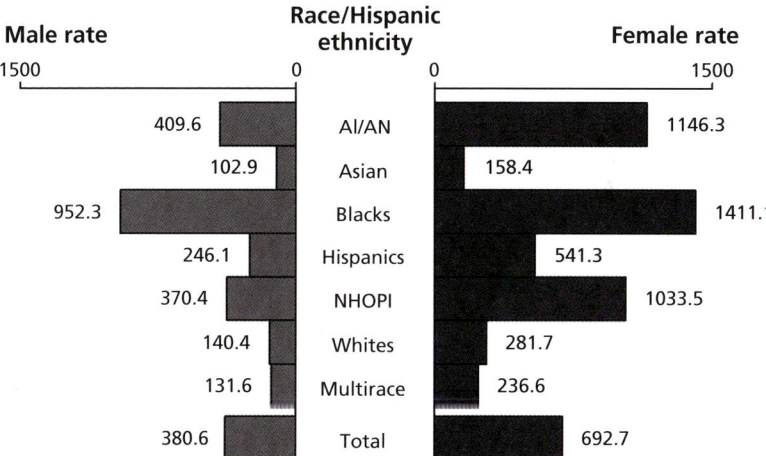

Figure 30.18 Chlamydia rates (per 100 000) of reported cases by ethnicity and sex: USA, 2018. AI/AN, American Indian/Alaskan native; NHOPI, native Hawaiian/other Pacific Islander. From Sexually Transmitted Diseases Surveillance 2018. Chlamydia. https://www.cdc.gov/std/stats18/STDSurveillance2018-full-report.pdf.

Introduction and general description

Chlamydia trachomatis serovars A–C are responsible for ocular trachoma, which is a major cause of blindness worldwide. Genital *C. trachomatis* D–K strain infections are considered the world's most common sexually transmitted bacterial pathogens. *C. trachomatis* serovars L1–L3 cause lymphogranuloma venereum (LGV).

This section describes *C. trachomatis* infections caused by strains D–K only; these cause clinical syndromes including urethritis, cervicitis, epididymo-orchitis, pelvic inflammatory syndrome, seronegative reactive arthritis and ophthalmia neonatorum.

Epidemiology

Incidence and prevalence

In 2016, WHO calculated that the global prevalence of genital chlamydia in people aged 15–49 years in 2016 was 3.8% in females and 2.7% in males. The highest prevalence rates were in the African, Americas and western Pacific regions [1,2]. In the European region the prevalence rates were 3.2% in females and 2.7% in males.

The UK and USA both have opportunistic screening programmes [3].

Age

Age is the most significant risk factor for genital chlamydia, with the highest rates being found in those under 25 years old and a decreasing prevalence with increasing age (Figure 30.17). Other risks include a new sexual partner or more than one sexual partner in the past year and lack of consistent condom use.

Sex

The number of cases in females exceeds that in males. In England, the number of cases in both sexes has increased as more screening has been undertaken, and the sex gap has reduced.

Ethnicity

There is no racial or ethnic predisposition to genital chlamydial infection. In both the UK and USA, disparities persist in chlamydia and other STI rates which are reflective of broader inequities in social and economic conditions for minority ethnic communities (Figure 30.18).

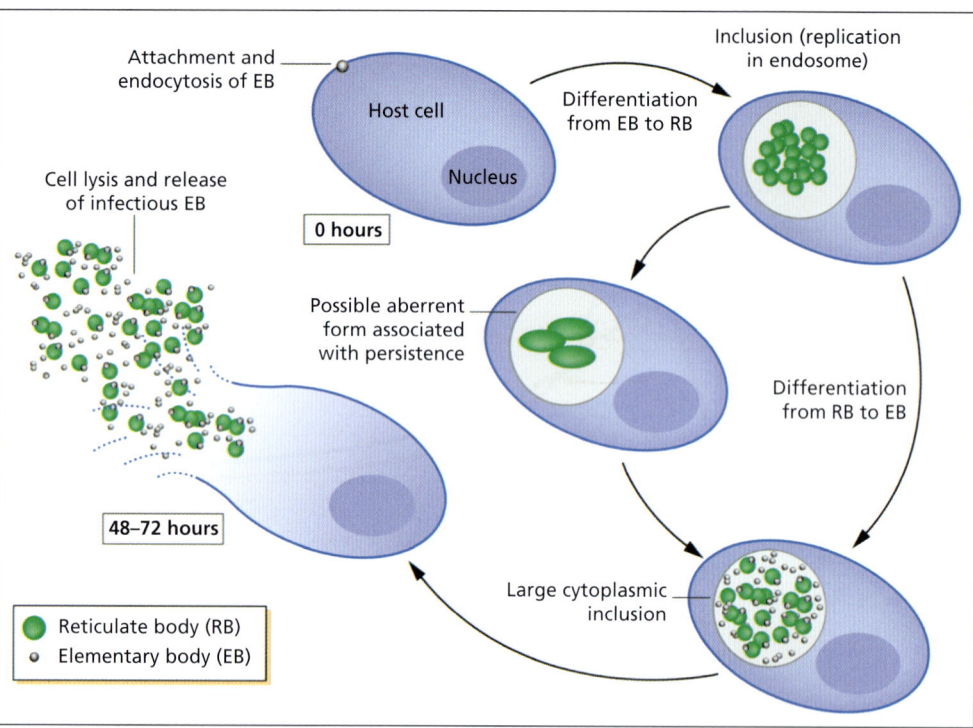

Figure 30.19 The life cycle of *Chlamydia trachomatis*.

Associated diseases

Individuals diagnosed with genital chlamydia are at risk of other coexistent STIs, therefore a sexual health assessment is warranted. Chlamydia may also be a causal factor in sexually acquired reactive arthritis.

Pathophysiology

Subacute or chronic asymptomatic infection is common, and the infection can persist for many months or years if untreated [4]. The clinical manifestations of *Chlamydia* infection are probably a direct result of tissue damage as well as host immune response, resulting in scarring of the affected mucous membranes. Repeated infections have higher rates of sequelae than those with single infections. This is true for trachoma as well as genital chlamydia.

The organism can manipulate an array of host processes to support its persistence. It also upregulates synthesis of a 60 kDa heat shock protein (hsp60) which is released from the infected cell. The immune response to this hsp60 is thought to contribute to upper genital tract pathology.

Specific type 1 T-cell responses appear important in both the control of infection and the development of pathology [5]. There is no evidence that natural immunity can provide the complete, long-term protection necessary to prevent chronic pathology.

Pathology

Histological examination of tissue samples from women with PID caused by *C. trachomatis* revealed neutrophils in the endometrial surface epithelium and gland lumens, dense subepithelial stromal lymphocytic infiltration, stromal plasma cells and germinal centres containing transformed lymphocytes.

Causative organisms

Chlamydiae are obligate intracellular parasites and cannot be cultured on artificial media. They exhibit a unique, two-stage developmental cycle with two forms:
- An extracellular, infectious elementary body (EB).
- An intracellular, replicative reticulate body (RB).

This cycle begins when infectious, metabolically inert EBs attach to and stimulate uptake by the host cell. The internalised EB remains within a host-derived vacuole, termed an inclusion, and differentiates into a larger, metabolically active RB. The RB multiplies by binary fission, and after 8–12 rounds of multiplication the RBs differentiate to EBs asynchronously. At 48–72 h postinfection, EB progeny are released from the host cell to initiate another cycle (Figure 30.19).

C. trachomatis strains A–K primarily infect squamocolumnar epithelial cells.

Clinical features

History

Asymptomatic infection occurs in up to 90% of women and more than 50% of men. Infection may be diagnosed as a result of opportunistic screening, contact tracing or self-referral for a test following partner change.

Presentation

Men commonly present with signs and symptoms of anterior urethritis, consisting of mucopurulent urethral discharge and dysuria, with an onset 1–3 weeks after intercourse with an infected partner (Figure 30.20). In men practising receptive anal intercourse, rectal infections may occur. These are often without symptoms, but some will have proctitis, which will manifest as anal discharge,

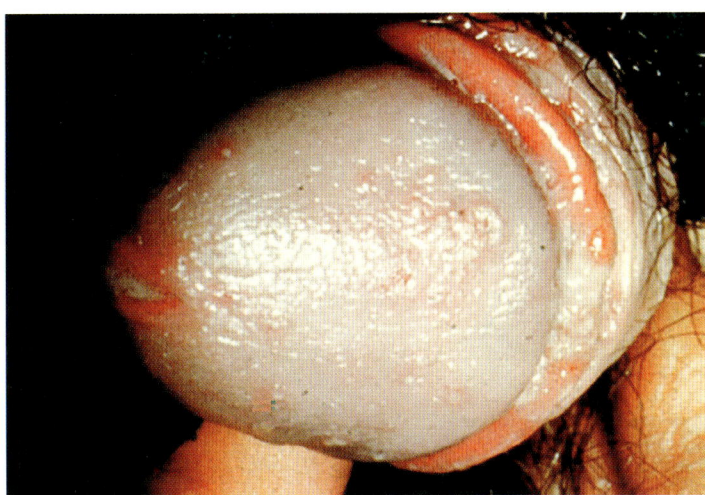

Figure 30.20 Chlamydial urethritis with meatal redness and a mucopurulent discharge.

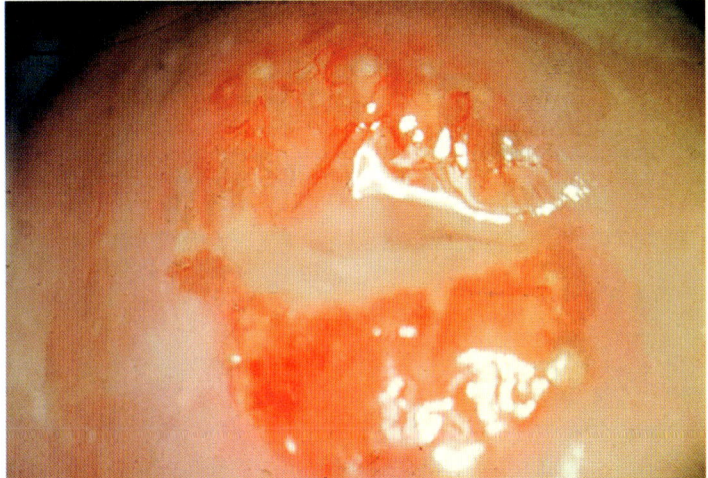

Figure 30.21 Follicular cervicitis with raised, white, rounded swellings – this may raise the index of suspicion for chlamydia.

bleeding and discomfort [6]. It is important to exclude LGV if rectal symptoms are present.

Women may present with a variety of symptoms including postcoital or intermenstrual bleeding, lower abdominal pain, vaginal discharge and dysuria. Typically, in such patients there are signs of mucopurulent cervicitis and/or contact bleeding (Figure 30.21). Rectal infection may occur even in the absence of history of receptive anal intercourse.

Extragenital infections also occur. Pharyngeal infections are usually asymptomatic. Infection of the eye causes acute follicular conjunctivitis, which is usually, but not always, associated with genital infection (Figure 30.22). Neonates born to an infected mother may develop conjunctivitis and/or pneumonia with failure to thrive. Chlamydia in pregnancy may be associated with premature labour and preterm birth.

Differential diagnosis

The common presenting symptoms are non-specific and can have a wide range of causes:

- Lower genital tract infections with non-specific urethritis, *Neisseria gonorrhoeae*, *Mycoplasma genitalium*, *Trichomonas vaginalis* or genital herpes.
- Urinary tract infection.
- Rectal lymphogranuloma venereum.
- Pelvic inflammatory disease.
- Ectopic pregnancy.
- Other causes of intermenstrual bleeding.
- Cervical or endometrial neoplasia.

Complications and co-morbidities

Complications mostly occur from ascending infections. They are also associated with pregnancy and the neonatal period. Ascending infection in men causes epididymo-orchitis. Epididymo-orchitis in those under 35 years old is most likely to be caused by a sexually transmitted organism. In those over 35 years, urological pathogens such as *Escherichia coli*, *Klebsiella* sp. or enterococci are more likely.

C. trachomatis should be considered as a possible cause for a Bartholin abscess, with or without concurrent gonococcal infection. In the absence of treatment, 10–40% of women infected with *Chlamydia* will develop PID, with a significant proportion of these cases being asymptomatic or having mild, atypical symptoms. PID can result in tubal factor infertility, ectopic pregnancy and chronic pelvic pain (Figure 30.23). The risk of developing PID increases with each recurrence of *C. trachomatis* infection, as does the risk of reproductive sequelae. Fitz-Hugh–Curtis syndrome presents as upper right-sided abdominal pain caused by perihepatitis [7]. Fibrinous 'violin-string' adhesions can be seen at laparoscopy (Figure 30.24). It is associated with extensive tubal scarring and adhesions.

Chlamydia is strongly associated with sexually acquired reactive arthritis (SARA). Reactive arthritis can be defined as a sterile inflammatory arthritis following bacterial infection elsewhere (Figure 30.25). Around 80% have a history of urethritis or genital chlamydia, and SARA occurs in 0.8–4% of those infected with *C. trachomatis*. Predisposing factors include male sex, human leukocyte antigen (HLA) B27 genotype and HIV infection [8]. It is a seronegative, asymmetrical, spondyloarthropathy with or without extra-articular features, and includes the following:

- Mucocutaneous manifestations including circinate balanitis (Figure 30.26), erosions affecting the buccal and rectal mucosa and keratoderma blenorrhagica (Figure 30.27).
- Iritis and conjunctivitis.

There is some evidence that *Chlamydia* may persist in a metabolically active state in the synovial tissue of patients and, although long-term antibiotic treatment is controversial, a small randomised controlled trial has demonstrated there may be some value in this approach [9].

Investigations

Iodine-stained inclusion bodies within epithelial cells infected with *C. trachomatis* can be seen (Figure 30.28) but microscopic diagnostic techniques have low sensitivity and have been superseded [10].

NAATs are now the only recommended diagnostic tests for *Chlamydia*. There are a variety of test types and platforms, which generally have a sensitivity of >90%. In 2006, in Sweden, a new genetic variant of *C. trachomatis* was reported that contained a 377 bp deletion in the cryptic plasmid contained by all genital

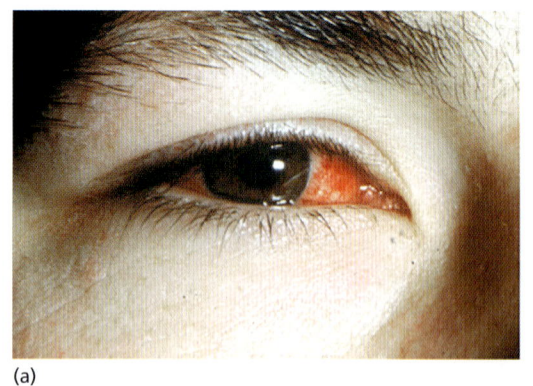
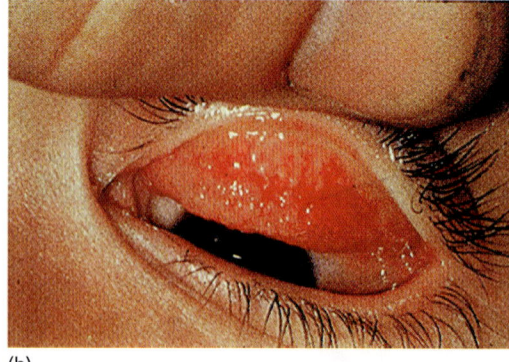

Figure 30.22 (a) Chlamydial conjunctivitis can present as a non-specific, red and irritated eye. (b) Acute follicular conjunctivitis is usually associated with viral infection or chlamydia. Chronic conjunctivitis may be seen in trachoma or lymphogranuloma venereum.

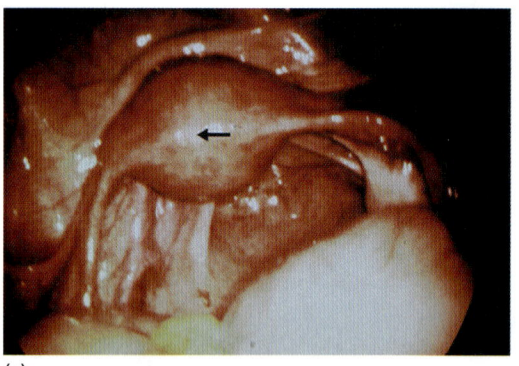
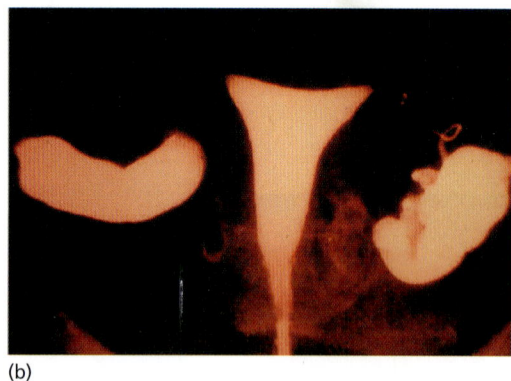

Figure 30.23 (a) A tubo-ovarian swelling (arrow) as a consequence of repeated chlamydial infection. (b) Hysterosalpingogram showing scarred fallopian tubes and bilateral hydrosalpinx.

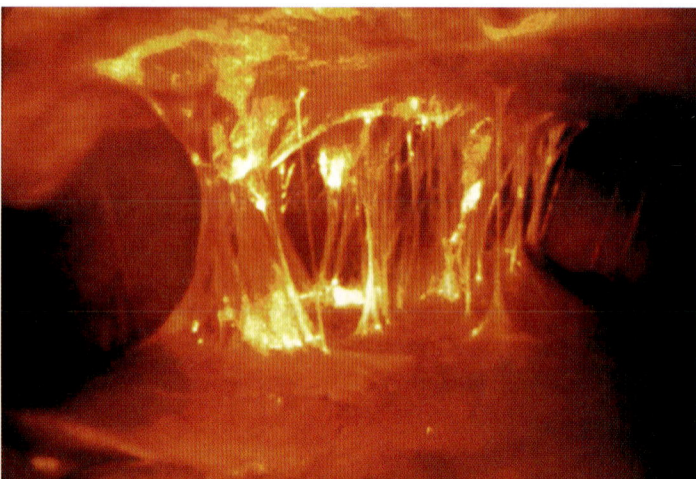

Figure 30.24 Fitz-Hugh–Curtis syndrome is a complication of pelvic inflammatory disease and results in violin-string adhesions of the liver capsule as a consequence of perihepatitis.

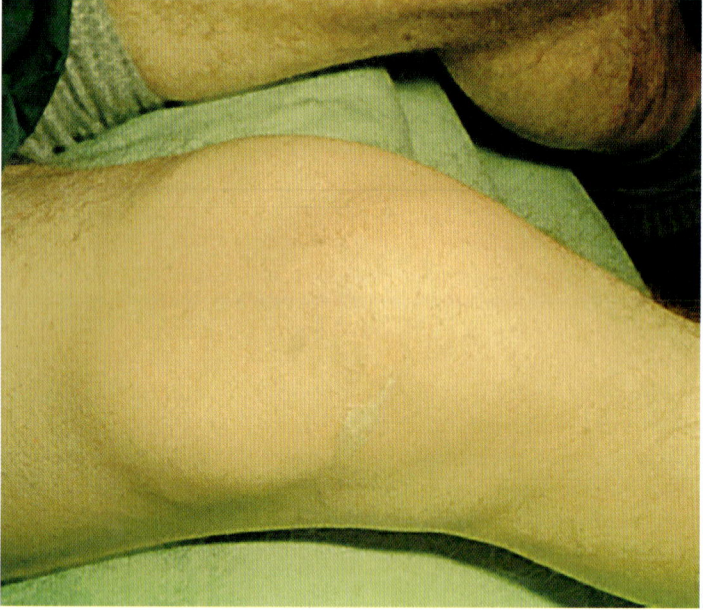

Figure 30.25 Sexually acquired reactive arthritis with knee involvement causing joint swelling.

Chlamydia strains and resulted in negative tests on some commercial assays [11].

All NAATs will detect LGV-positive samples as *Chlamydia* positive but will not differentiate between LGV and non-LGV types. Genotyping to identify LGV infection should be undertaken on *Chlamydia*-positive samples according to local guidelines.

A first-void urine sample is the sample of choice in men, and in females a self-taken vaginal swab or an endocervical swab is acceptable. In MSM and commercial sex workers, pharyngeal and rectal testing may also be indicated.

Cell culture is no longer recommended for routine screening or diagnosis.

Serological tests for *Chlamydia* include the older microimmunofluorescence test and the newer enzyme immunoassays. They do not have a clinical role in the routine management of non-LGV *C. trachomatis* infection.

NAAT-based point-of-care tests (POCTs) which enable patients to be tested and treated at the same clinical visit have the potential to reduce time to treatment, improve patient care and facilitate partner notification and control efforts. These can be fully automated and independent of central laboratories [12,13].

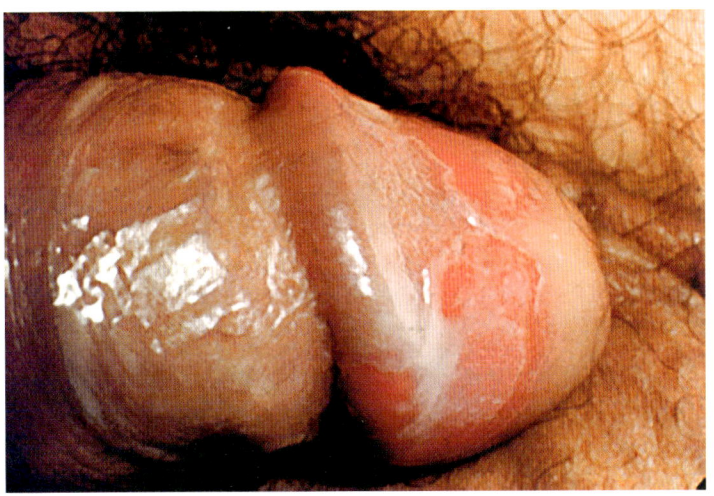

Figure 30.26 Serpiginous and annular lesions with slightly raised borders on the glans penis of a patient with sexually acquired reactive arthritis.

Management

Treatment is indicated whenever genital chlamydia is diagnosed or suspected on epidemiological grounds where there is a history of contact with a person known to be infected. Patients with genital chlamydia should always be fully assessed and screened for other STIs and HIV, asked to assist with partner notification efforts and be offered non-judgemental education, counselling and support. They should be asked to abstain from sexual contact until they and their partners have completed treatment and their symptoms have resolved.

Single-dose azithromycin is no longer recommended because it is less effective than doxycycline in treating rectal infections, which also occur in women, and because of concerns about increasing macrolide resistance in *Mycoplasma genitalium* and other STIs that are commonly concurrent with genital chlamydia infections.

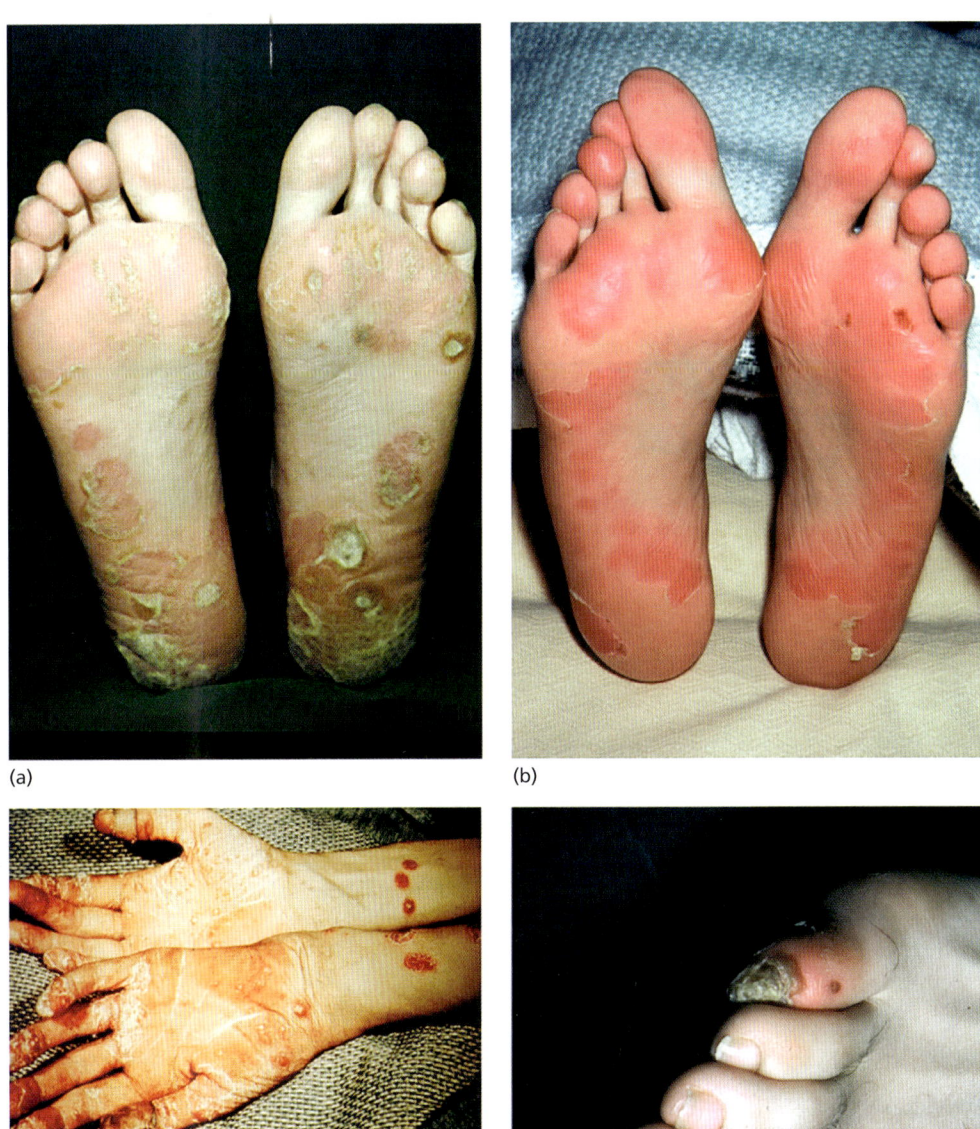

Figure 30.27 (a) Keratoderma blenorrhagica (KDB) is seen in reactive arthritis and can be a result of sexually transmitted or gastrointestinal pathogens. (b) Resolving lesions of KDB. (c) Severe KDB affecting the hands and arms. (d) Nail involvement in KDB.

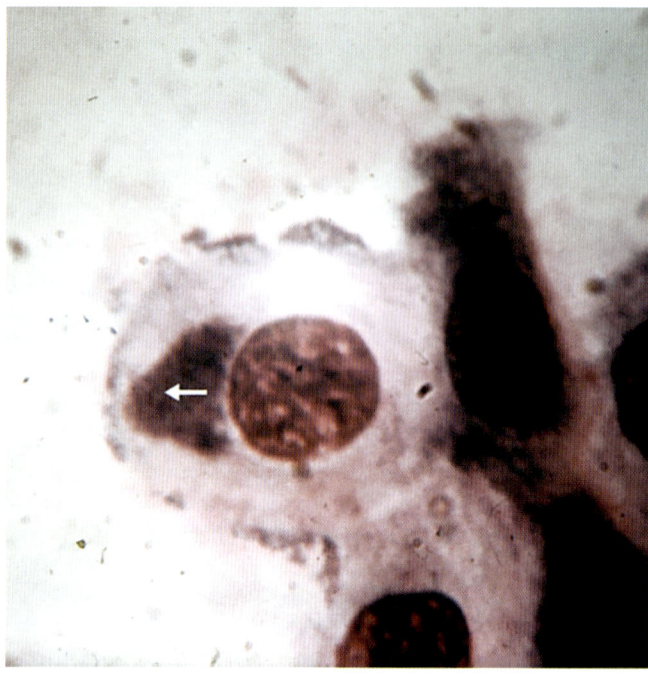

Figure 30.28 An inclusion body (arrow) in the cytoplasm of an epithelial cell stained with iodine.

In pregnant women, doxycycline is contraindicated [14]. Three-day azithromycin treatment has fewer reported side effects than with other alternative regimens.

In complicated infections, more prolonged courses of treatment are employed, and specialist advice may be required.

Vaccine

The limited success of national screening programmes to reduce *Chlamydia* prevalence has stimulated ongoing research to develop an effective human vaccine [15], one of which has progressed to phase I clinical studies [16].

Treatment ladder for genital *Chlamydia* infection

Uncomplicated uro-genital and pharyngeal infection

First line
- Doxycycline 100 mg twice daily for 7 days
- Azithromycin 1 g single dosage, then 500 mg daily for 2 days

Second line
- Erythromycin 500 mg twice daily for 10–14 days
- Ofloxacin 200 mg twice daily or 400 mg once daily for 7 days

Pregnancy and breastfeeding
- Azithromycin 1 g single dosage, then 500 mg daily for 2 days
- Erythromycin 500 mg twice daily for 14 days
- Erythromycin 500 mg four times daily for 7 days
- Amoxicillin 500 mg three times daily for 7 days

Complicated infection

Chlamydial PID
- Ceftriaxone 500 mg IM single dose + oral doxycycline 100 mg twice daily and metronidazole 400 mg twice daily for 14 days

Or
- Ofloxacin 400 mg PO twice daily + metronidazole 400 mg PO twice daily for 14 days (if gonorrhoea is unlikely)

Epididymo-orchitis
- Ceftriaxone 500 mg IM single dose + doxycycline 100 mg PO twice daily for 10–14 days

Or
- Ofloxacin 200 mg PO twice daily for 14 days (if gonorrhoea is unlikely)

Chlamydia-associated reactive arthritis
- Rest
- Non-steroidal anti-inflammatory drugs
- Seek specialist advice

Resources

Further information

British Association for Sexual Health and HIV (BASHH), guidelines: https://bashh.org/guidelines.

Centers for Disease Control and Prevention (CDC). *Chlamydia Statistics.* https://www.cdc.gov/std/chlamydia/stats.htm.

International Union against Sexually Transmitted Infections (IUSTI). *STI Treatment Pocket European Guidelines 2019.* https://www.iusti-europe.eu/web/images/guidelines/PocketGuideline2019.pdf.

National Institute for Health Care and Excellence (NICE). *Chlamydia – uncomplicated genital.* https://cks.nice.org.uk/topics/chlamydia-uncomplicated-genital/.

Patient resources

British Association of Sexual Health and HIV (BASHH), patient information leaflets: https://bashh.org/guidelines.

Centers for Disease Control and Prevention (CDC). *Chlamydia – CDC fact sheet.* http://www.cdc.gov/std/chlamydia/stdfact-chlamydia.htm.

International Union against Sexually Transmitted Infections (IUSTI), patient information leaflets (in different languages): https://iusti.org/patient-information/.

National Health Service (NHS). *Overview: Chlamydia.* http://www.nhs.uk/conditions/Chlamydia/Pages/Introduction.aspx.

(All websites last accessed May 2023.)

Lymphogranuloma venereum

Definition and nomenclature

Lymphogranuloma venereum is a sexually transmitted infection caused by one of three serovars (L1–L3) of the obligate intracellular bacterium *Chlamydia trachomatis*. L2 is the most common strain involved.

Synonyms and inclusions
- Tropical or climatic bubo
- Lymphopathia venereum
- Strumous bubo
- Poradenitis inguinalis
- Durand–Nicholas–Favre disease
- Lymphogranuloma inguinale
- Poradenitis inguinalis

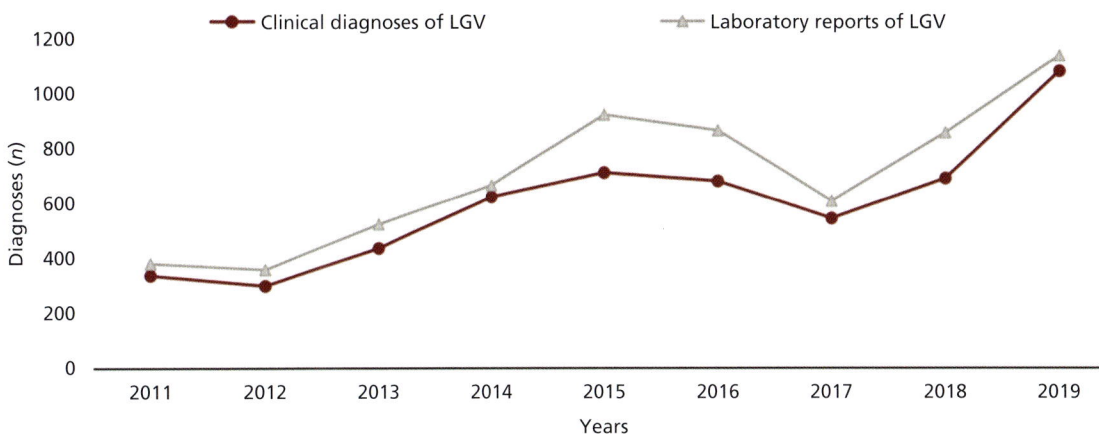

Figure 30.29 Number of lymphogranuloma venereum (LGV) reports among men by data source, England 2011–19. From Public Health England 2020 [1]. Clinical diagnoses of LGV as reported in GUMCAD STI Surveillance System. Laboratory reports of LGV refer to combined data from CTAD Chlamydia Surveillance System and Modular Open Laboratory Information System (MOLIS)

Introduction and general description
Lymphogranuloma venereum was rare in industrialised countries prior to 2003. Since then, it has re-emerged as a significant disease in MSM [1]. Many are HIV-positive and also have a high rate of hepatitis C coinfection. LGV is now hyperendemic among MSM in the UK. Most cases in the UK present with a proctitis/proctocolitis syndrome (mimicking inflammatory bowel disease), rather than the classic inguinal (bubonic) form.

Epidemiology
Incidence and prevalence
Lymphogranuloma venereum has long been prevalent in tropical countries of Africa, Asia, the Caribbean and Central and South America. Classic disease is usually acquired heterosexually and is manifest as genital ulceration with suppurative regional lymphadenopathy. It had been rare in developed countries, being seen mainly as an imported infection in travellers returning from endemic countries. However, since 2003, a series of LGV cases presenting with proctocolitis have been reported, mostly affecting HIV-positive MSM (Figures 30.29 and 30.30) [1]. This presentation has now become more common in Europe than the classic bubonic form seen in the tropics. Classic LGV is seen more commonly in tropical countries including southern Africa, West Africa, Madagascar, India, South-East Asia and the Caribbean.

Age
Lymphogranuloma venereum may occur in sexually active adults of all ages.

Sex
The classic form may occur in either sex. LGV proctitis has been described almost exclusively in MSM, the majority of whom were HIV positive [1]. A small number of cases have been described in heterosexuals, including women, in Europe [2,3].

Ethnicity
There is no known racial predisposition.

Associated diseases
Lymphogranuloma venereum proctitis in MSM is commonly associated with HIV and hepatitis C coinfection.

Pathophysiology
Predisposing factors
Many MSM report high-risk sexual behaviour, including unprotected anal intercourse, fisting and sharing sex toys; it is often connected to group sex parties [4].

Pathology
The organism spreads from the site of the initial lesion to the regional lymph nodes. The main pathological process is a thrombolymphangitis and perilymphangitis. Multiple necrotic foci appear within the lymph nodes (Figure 30.31). There is an infiltrate of polymorphonuclear lymphocytes and plasma cells. The necrotic areas enlarge and coalesce to form stellate abscesses. Subsequent periadenitis can lead to loculated abscesses, fistulae and sinus tract formation. The inflammatory process lasts weeks to months and is followed by fibrosis. Fibrosis causes disruption of the lymph node architecture leading to chronic oedema and induration.

The pathological process in the rectum consists of ulceration of the mucosa, the formation of granulomatous tissue, cryptitis and crypt abscesses without distortion of the crypt architecture. The granulomatous process may affect the bowel wall and the ensuing fibrosis may lead to stricture formation.

Causative organisms
Lymphogranuloma venereum is an STI caused by serovars L1–L3 of the obligate intracellular bacterium *Chlamydia trachomatis*. *C. trachomatis* is classified into 15 serovars based on immunogenic epitope analysis of the major outer membrane protein. Only serovars L1–L3 cause LGV, probably due to their tropism for the lymphatic system [5]. The L2 serovar has several subtypes distinguishable according to amino acid differences [6].

Clinical features
History
Patients present with complaints of genital ulceration and inguinal swelling or rectal discharge and bleeding. Late-stage disease presents with chronic oedematous genital swelling.

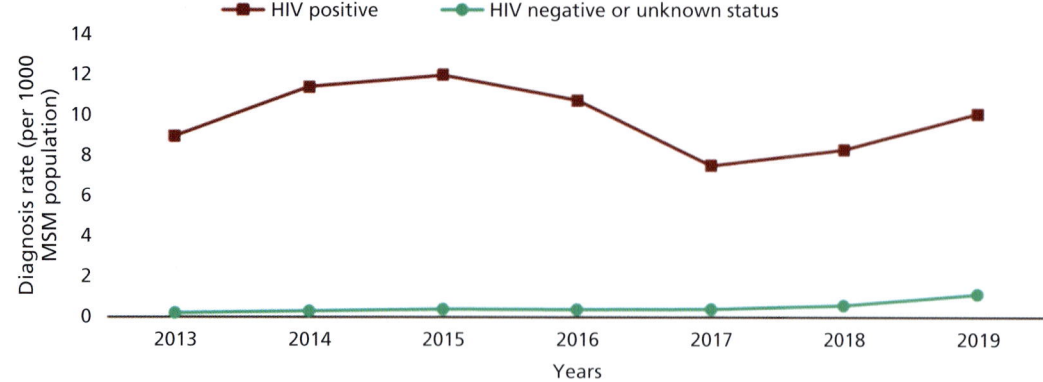

Analysis using GUMCAD STI Surveillance System data. Analysis restricted to men who have sex with men (MSM) which includes men who were reported as being gay or bisexual. Men include transgender men. ONS population estimates based upon the 2018 estimates by sexual orientation. 2018 data used for all years and available for aged 16+ only. Number of HIV positive MSM calculated as the number of MSM seen for HIV care that reside in England (from 'Key Population groups HIV data tables': https://www.gov.uk/government/statistics/hiv-annual-data-tables). The number of MSM who are HIV negative or of unknown status calculated as the difference between the total number of MSM in England and number of HIV positive MSM in England

Figure 30.30 Lymphogranuloma venereum diagnosis rates per 1000 population among men who have sex with men (MSM) by HIV status, England 2013–19. From Public Health England 2020 [1].

Presentation

Lymphogranuloma venereum occurs in three stages (Table 30.1): primary (transient ulceration, proctitis), secondary (inguinal) and tertiary (genito-ano-rectal syndrome). Many infections in the primary and secondary stages may go undetected.

Primary stage. The primary stage presents about 3–30 days after infection. It is characterised by transient papules or ulcers at the site of inoculation which may go unnoticed (Figure 30.32). The lesion is usually a single, non-indurated, shallow ulcer or pustule or papule. It may be painful or painless, heals rapidly and leaves no scar. It is often found on the coronal sulcus in men and on the posterior vaginal wall, fourchette or vulva, and occasionally on the cervix. The lesion may go unnoticed by the patient particularly if inoculation occurs during anal intercourse. Extragenital lesions have been described such as ulcers and fissures in the perianal area in MSM [7], the lip or oral cavity and in extragenital lymph nodes. Cases of pharyngeal infection have been reported in MSM. LGV can present with symptomatic pharyngeal ulceration as well as asymptomatic carriage [8].

Haemorrhagic proctitis is the primary manifestation of infection seen in those engaging in anal intercourse. This presents as proctitis/proctocolitis, which may be haemorrhagic. The patient may experience purulent, mucoid or bloody anal discharge, rectal pain, tenesmus and constipation. Examination with a proctoscope may show ulcerative proctitis. There may be accompanying constitutional symptoms such as fever and malaise. Asymptomatic rectal *C. trachomatis* infection in the UK is usually with non-LGV *Chlamydia*.

Secondary stage. The secondary stage occurs on average 2–6 weeks after the primary stage. The secondary stage may present with the classic form in heterosexuals with tender inguinal and/or femoral lymphadenopathy. The lymphadenopathy is usually unilateral, and buboes develop which are enlarged, tender, painful glands in the groin (Figure 30.33). About one-third of patients may

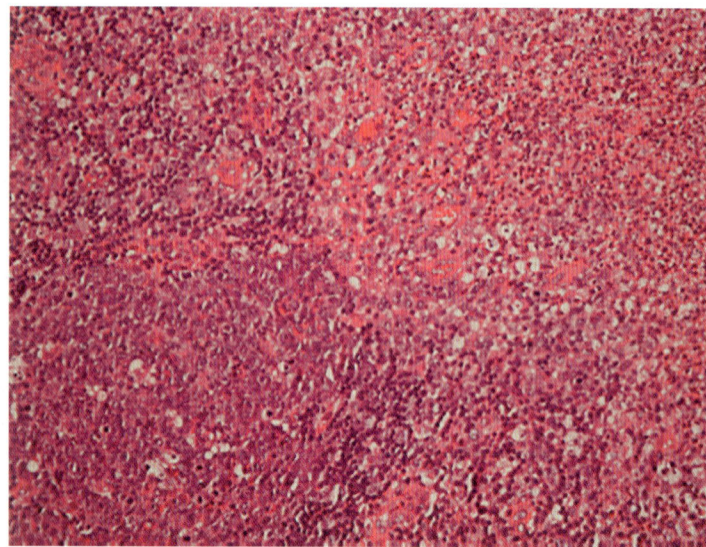

Figure 30.31 Part of a reactive lymph node with a follicle centre (lower left) seen alongside an inflammatory and necrotic focus of polymorph neutrophils (centre and upper right). Courtesy of Dr K. Suvarna.

have the characteristic 'groove sign' – a groove-like depression caused by femoral and inguinal lymph node enlargement above and below the inguinal ligament (Figure 30.34). The groove sign is considered pathognomonic of LGV but occurs in only 20% of cases. Inguinal buboes may suppurate and rupture, causing discharge from multiple points, creating chronic fistulae.

In women, inguinal/femoral lymphadenopathy is less common than in men. This is probably because primary involvement is usually in the vagina, cervix, posterior urethra or rectum, which drain into the perirectal or deep iliac lymph nodes. In females, the presence of lymphadenopathy may emulate the presenting features of pelvic inflammatory disease, appendicitis or tubo-ovarian abscess.

Table 30.1 Stages of lymphogranuloma venereum.

Stage	Incubation period	Clinical features
Primary	3–30 days	Small papule/pustule/ulcer at the site of inoculation which heals spontaneously with no scarring
		Haemorrhagic proctitis may occur in those engaging in anal intercourse
Secondary	Days to weeks	Lymphatic involvement of nodes that drain the primary lesion
		Classic form: tender unilateral or bilateral inguinal and/or femoral adenopathy ('groove' sign)
		If primary infection is in the rectum, the deep iliac lymph nodes are affected but remain unnoticed. This can also occur in women due to drainage of the cervical or upper vaginal area to the perirectal lymph nodes
		The lymph nodes may coalesce to form a 'bubo' or abscesses that may rupture spontaneously with the development of fistulae or sinus tracts
		There may be systemic features such as malaise and fever
Tertiary	Years after chronic untreated infection	Chronic granulomatous inflammatory process with lymphatic obstruction leading to fistula formation, strictures and disfiguring conditions such as genital elephantiasis and esthiomene, which refers to hypertrophic enlargement with ulceration of the external genitalia

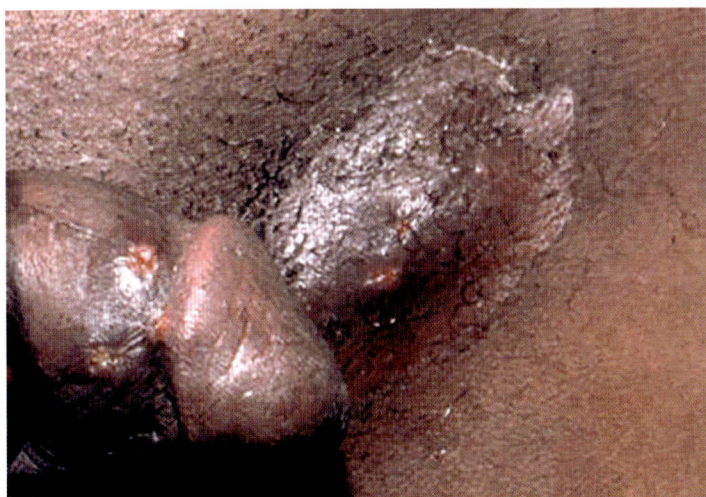

Figure 30.32 Primary stage of lymphogranuloma venereum, showing genital ulceration.

Systemic symptoms such as fever, chills, malaise, anorexia, weight loss, myalgia and arthralgia may feature. Reactive arthritis in MSM following LGV proctitis has been reported in several cases [9].

Most patients recover after the secondary stage without sequelae.

Tertiary stage. The tertiary stage follows chronic untreated infection in a few patients. *C. trachomatis* incites a chronic inflammatory response and destruction of tissue in the involved areas including proctitis and proctocolitis. This may occur any number of years after infection. The resultant fibrosis leads to lymphatic obstruction and genital lymphoedema. Women may develop oedema (elephantiasis) of the vulva with the formation of polypoid growths, fistulae, ulceration and chronic granulomatous disfiguring fibrosis and scarring of the vulva with esthiomene (Greek meaning 'eaten away'). These conditions occur most frequently in women, reflecting the involvement of the retroperitoneal lymphatics rather than inguinal lymphatics. Elephantiasis may affect the male genitalia, leading to oedema and deformity of the penis.

Differential diagnosis

Lymphogranuloma venereum must be considered in the differential diagnosis in patients presenting with genital ulceration, inguinal lymphadenopathy, proctocolitis or rectal stricture.

LGV may mimic and be misdiagnosed as inflammatory bowel disease as patients may present with proctocolitis without characteristic lymphadenopathy and have similar endoscopic and histological findings [10]. The diagnosis of LGV proctocolitis must be considered if there is a failure of response to inflammatory bowel disease therapy, particularly for MSM or if a rectal *Chlamydia* test result is positive.

Genital ulceration due to LGV is not dissimilar to that of genital herpes, primary syphilis or chancroid. These conditions must be carefully differentiated.

Inflammatory bowel disease is an important differential diagnosis of proctitis. Other differential diagnoses include anal fissure, enteric infections, other STIs such as gonorrhoea, syphilis, herpes simplex, *C. trachomatis* serovars D–K and human papillomavirus (warts) and, in patients who are HIV positive, cytomegalovirus infection.

Complications and co-morbidities

Late complications include rectal strictures with or without proctitis and colitis, perianal abscess and perineal, recto-vaginal or urethral fistulae. Intestinal obstruction may result from stricture formation. An association with rectal cancer has been reported.

Disease course and prognosis

Early treatment improves the prognosis and reduces onward transmission.

Investigations

The diagnosis is confirmed by the detection of L serovars of *C. trachomatis* from the site of infection. The diagnostic method of choice is detecting *C. trachomatis* nucleic acid using NAATs and confirmation by real-time PCR assays for LGV-specific DNA. These assays have high sensitivity and specificity and have therefore superseded traditional methods. PCR testing has performed well on specimens from a variety of sites including from the ulcer, rectum, bubo aspirates, pharynx, lymph node aspirates, biopsy specimens and first-void urine samples.

Elevated numbers of polymorphonuclear leucocytes detected upon microscopy of rectal swabs are predictive of LGV proctitis.

Serology using complement fixation tests or microimmunofluorescence assays has been superseded by *C. trachomatis* NAATs. Serology cannot necessarily distinguish past infection from current infection. The Frei test, which was based on a positive hypersensitivity reaction to purified chlamydial antigen, is now obsolete and of historical interest only.

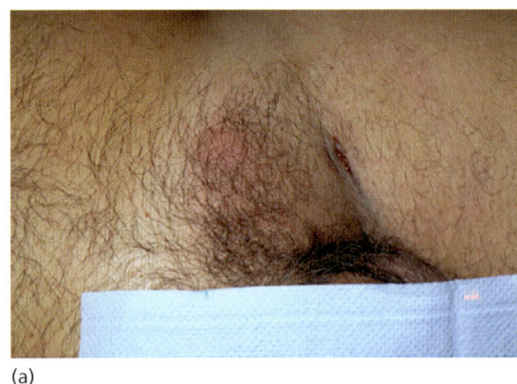
(a)

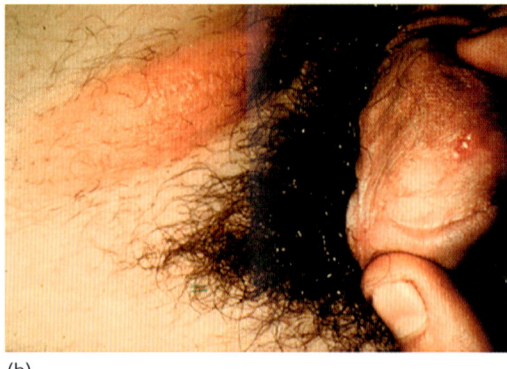
(b)

Figure 30.33 (a, b) Lymphogranuloma venereum buboes. (a) Courtesy of Dr E. Powles.

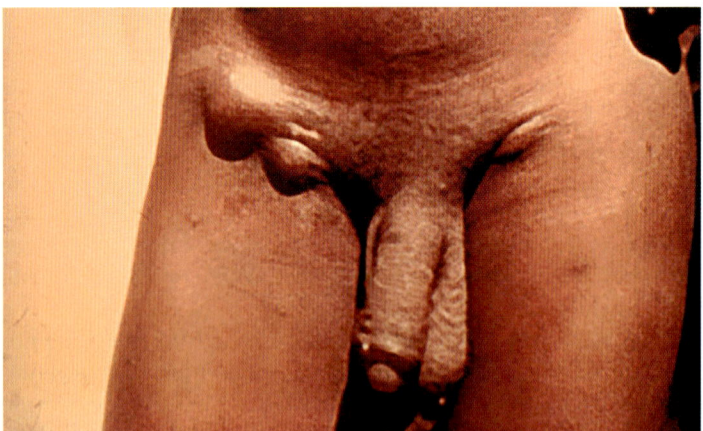

Figure 30.34 Lymphogranuloma venereum inguinal syndrome showing the 'groove sign'.

Management

There should be detailed investigation to exclude other STIs. Early treatment is important to prevent the chronic phase. Prolonged courses of antibiotics (at least 3 weeks) are required. Fluctuant buboes may require aspiration through healthy adjacent skin, although surgical incision is usually contraindicated due to the risk of complications such as sinus formation. Longer-term complications such as fistulae and strictures may require surgery to alleviate symptoms. Partner notification should be undertaken.

Treatment ladder for lymphogranuloma venereum

First line
- Doxycycline 100 mg PO twice daily for 21 days

Second line
- Erythromycin 500 mg PO four times daily for 21 days

Third line
- Azithromycin 1 g PO weekly for 3 weeks (although clinical data are lacking it is probably effective based on its chlamydial antimicrobial activity)

Resources

Further information

British Association for Sexual Health and HIV (BASHH), guidelines: https://bashh.org/guidelines.

Centers for Disease Control and Prevention (CDC). *Sexually Transmitted Disease Treatment Guidelines, 2021.* https://www.cdc.gov/std/treatment-guidelines/default.htm.

De Vries HJC, de Barbeyrac B, de Vrieze NHN *et al.* 2019 European guideline on the management of lymphogranuloma venereum. *J Eur Acad Dermatol Venereol* 2019;33:1821–8.

Patient resources

British Association for Sexual Health and HIV (BASHH), patient information leaflet: https://www.bashhguidelines.org/media/1033/lgv_pil_digital_2_2015.pdf.

International Union against Sexually Transmitted Infections (IUSTI), patient information leaflet: https://iusti.org/wp-content/uploads/2019/11/LGVleaflet2017.pdf.

Terence Higgins Trust. *LGV (Lymphogranuloma Venereum).* https://www.tht.org.uk/hiv-and-sexual-health/sexual-health/stis/lgv-lymphogranuloma.

(All websites last accessed May 2023.)

Chancroid

Definition and nomenclature

Chancroid, one of the three venereal diseases originally defined in the 1917 UK legislation, is a genital ulcer disease (GUD) caused by the bacterium *Haemophilus ducreyi*. Although previously endemic, it has become rare in most developed countries. In the UK, it is usually imported by travellers returning from resource-poor parts of the world.

Synonyms and inclusions
- Ulcus molle
- Soft chancre
- Ducreyi disease

Introduction and general description

Chancroid is an acute ulcerative condition affecting the ano-genital region and is often associated with visible lymphadenitis (buboes).

Epidemiology
Incidence and prevalence
Chancroid used to be one of the commonest causes of genital ulcers in many developing countries in Africa and Asia but is now becoming rarer, except for North India and Malawi [1,2,3]. This may be related to the introduction of syndromic management protocols for GUD in resource-poor countries where diagnostic laboratory facilities are not available and to diagnostic advances in genital herpes detection.

Chancroid is now rare in the industrialised world. Sporadic cases have been reported after being initially misdiagnosed as genital herpes [4–6]. Heightened awareness is required in those presenting with genital ulceration following travel to endemic areas.

Although cases of genital ulcer disease caused by *H. ducreyi* are in decline, it has become recognised as a common cause of non-genital cutaneous ulceration, especially in children, in the South Pacific [7,8,9].

Age
The condition may be seen in sexually active individuals of all ages.

Sex
The condition is diagnosed more often in males. Subclinical infections may be more common in females.

Ethnicity
It is usually seen in patients of African or Asian origin but there is no known racial predisposition.

Associated diseases
Coinfections of *H. ducreyi* with *Treponema pallidum* or herpes simplex virus are well recognised. Chancroid is also an important cofactor in the transmission of HIV.

Pathophysiology
Pathology
Trauma or microabrasion to the skin or mucosa allows for penetration of the organism into the epidermis. There is a subsequent local tissue reaction resulting in an initial intraepithelial lesion consisting of lymphocytes, macrophages and granulocytes. The cellular immune response is predominantly mononuclear with infiltrates containing CD4+ and CD8+ T lymphocytes and macrophages. Lymphadenitis associated with chancroid is predominantly a pyogenic inflammatory response. The intraepidermal lesion results in a red papule, which eventually pustulates. The pustule undergoes central necrosis and enlarges, forming a pathognomonic, tender, non-indurated ulcer with undermined margins and grey or yellow, necrotic, purulent exudates covering the base.

Causative organism
The causative organism is *H. ducreyi*, a Gram-negative facultative anaerobic coccobacillus.

Genetics
The organism has similar growth requirements and biochemical properties to other *Haemophilus* species but shows differences by rRNA analyses that suggest it is more closely linked to the *Actinobacillus* cluster of the Pasteurellaceae family. It has a single 1.7 Mb chromosome. The organism has considerable potential to develop antimicrobial resistance via both plasmid and chromosomally mediated mechanisms. It remains extracellular in clinical lesions, can avoid phagocytosis by granulocytes and macrophages, and mediates damage by the production of various toxins and by cytokine induction.

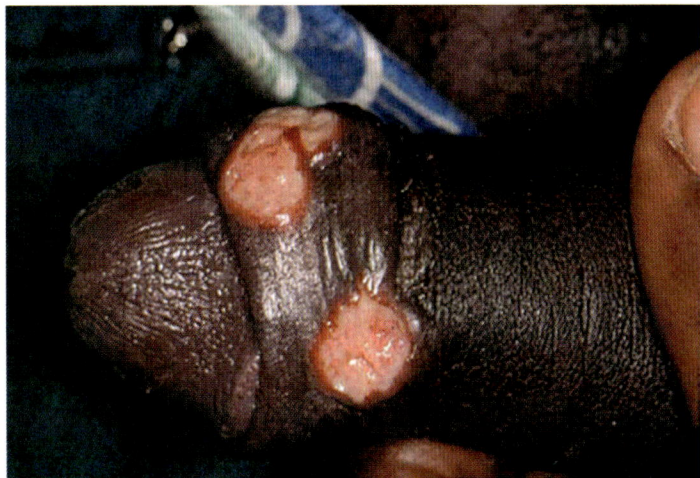

Figure 30.35 Chancroidal penile ulceration. Courtesy of Dr D. Lewis.

Clinical features
History
The incubation period is usually short, between 3 and 10 days. There may be a history of recent sexual exposure with someone from an endemic area, possibly a commercial sex worker. Chancroid is characterised by painful ano-genital ulceration and lymphadenitis with progression to bubo formation.

Presentation
The primary lesion starts as an inflammatory papule at the site of inoculation, in which micropustules develop and progress to form ulcers (Figure 30.35). Central necrosis of the pustule leads to characteristic painful, non-indurated ulceration with undermined edges. Autoinoculation from the primary ulcer may lead to the development of multiple or kissing ulcers on opposing skin surfaces. Lesions are more common in uncircumcised men and may be located on the prepuce, frenulum, coronal sulcus, glans penis and penile shaft. Perianal lesions may occur in MSM. In females, lesions may be recognised at the vaginal introitus or on the labia; vaginal and cervical lesions often go unnoticed (Figure 30.36). In over one-third of cases, there is accompanying inguinal lymphadenitis which may progress to suppurating bubo formation (Figure 30.37). These are usually unilateral and may become fluctuant and rupture spontaneously to form inguinal ulcers and sinuses (Figure 30.38). Extragenital lesions can occur via autoinoculation. Lesions of the lips and oral cavity have been described.

Clinical variants
In HIV-positive patients with more advanced immunosuppression, chancroidal lesions may be more persistent and slower to heal, more

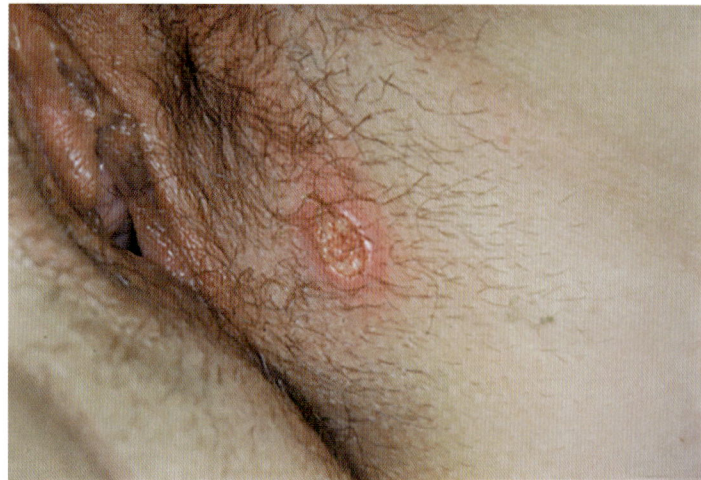

Figure 30.36 Chancroidal ulceration in a female.

numerous, and may fail to respond to single-dose treatment regimens. Prompt diagnosis and treatment of chancroid may abrogate increases in HIV replication [10].

Differential diagnosis
The differential diagnosis includes syphilis and herpes simplex, which also cause genital ulceration.

Complications and co-morbidities
Complications include phimosis and phagadenic ulceration following secondary infection, which may result in genital deformity. Chronic cutaneous ulceration, usually without genital lesions, has also been reported [7,8,9]. It can coexist with yaws [11].

Disease course and prognosis
Left untreated, patients may develop complications as well as chancroid enhancing HIV transmission.

Investigations
The diagnosis should be suspected if there is a history of painful ulceration following the requisite incubation period and subsequent formation of unilateral buboes with or without sinus formation. Testing for *H. ducreyi* is not routinely available in most UK diagnostic laboratories.

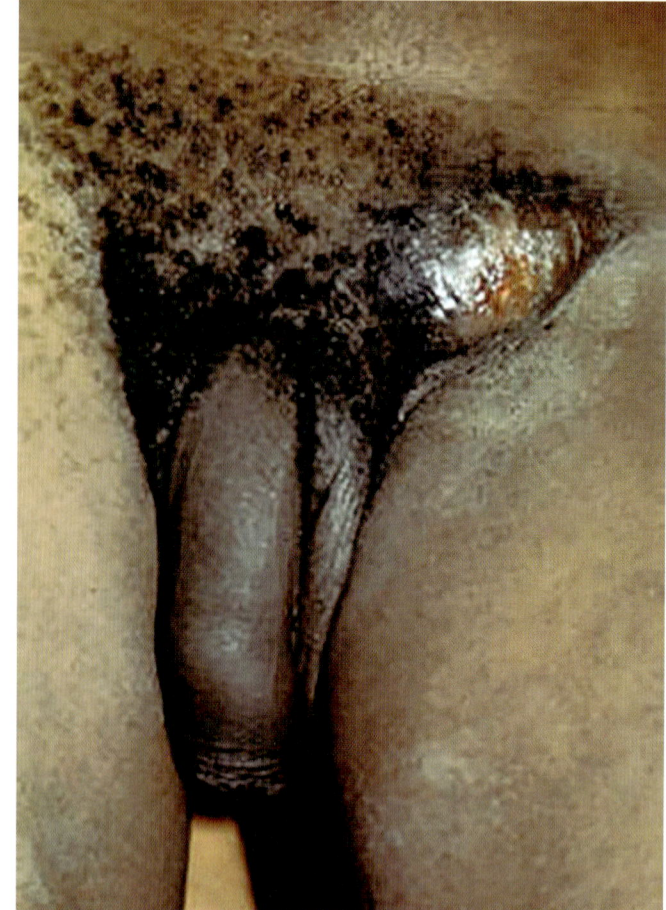

Figure 30.38 Discharging inguinal bubo.

Direct detection by microscopy of smears from chancroidal lesions typically shows sheets of the organism in a 'shoal of fish' pattern, but this has low sensitivity and specificity and is no longer recommended.

H. ducreyi is a fastidious bacterium and is very difficult to culture. Culture of material obtained from the ulcer base or bubo pus is poorly sensitive and specific transport media and culture facilities are not widely available in the UK.

The use of PCR has revolutionised the laboratory diagnosis of chancroid. Some of these tests have the advantage of

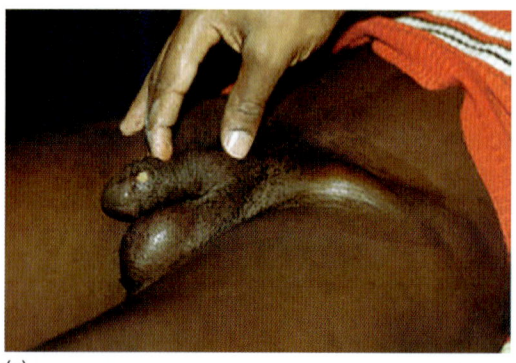

(a)

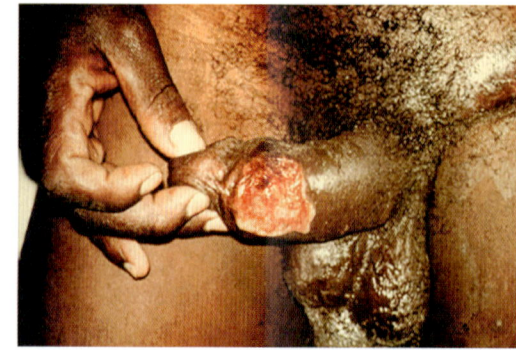

(b)

Figure 30.37 (a) Penile chancroid with inguinal bubo. (b) Giant penile chancroid with inguinal bubo.

simultaneously testing for other relevant pathogens, in particular *Treponema pallidum* and herpes simplex virus. PCR should be requested where appropriate facilities are available in patients with suspicious lesions returning from endemic countries and for their partners [12].

GUD often has a mixed aetiology so tests for other genital pathogens are essential and follow-up serological testing for syphilis and HIV should be performed. Serological tests have been described that may be useful in epidemiological studies, but these have no role in routine patient management.

Management

Prompt antibiotic treatment is essential to reduce the risk of complications as well as the risk of acquisition and onward transmission of HIV. Partner notification should be undertaken.

Single-dose treatment with either ciprofloxacin, azithromycin or ceftriaxone is associated with cure rates of over 90% [13,14]. Single-dose regimens have the advantage of ensuring compliance, however HIV seropositivity is associated with treatment failure and single-dose regimens should be avoided in coinfected patients. Thiamphenicol is another therapeutic drug option [15]. The WHO has proposed syndromic approaches for the treatment of genital ulcers to be used in settings where appropriate laboratory diagnosis is not available. Fluctuant buboes should be aspirated to avoid complications of spontaneous rupture, with care being taken to introduce the needle through adjacent areas of healthy skin.

Treatment ladder for chancroid

First line
- Azithromycin 1 g PO in a single dose
  Or
- Ceftriaxone 250 mg IM in a single dose

Second line
- Ciprofloxacin 500 mg PO twice a day for 3 days
  Or
- Erythromycin base 500 mg PO four times a day for 7 days

Resources

Further information

British Association for Sexual Health and HIV (BASHH), guidelines: https://bashh.org/guidelines.
Centers for Disease Control and Prevention (CDC). *Sexually Transmitted Disease Treatment Guidelines, 2021.* https://www.cdc.gov/std/treatment-guidelines/default.htm.
Lautenschlager S, Kemp M, Christensen JJ *et al*. 2017 European guideline for the management of chancroid. *Int J STD AIDS* 2017;28:324–9.

Patient resources

NSW Government. *Chancroid Fact Sheet*. https://www.health.nsw.gov.au/Infectious/factsheets/Pages/chancroid.aspx.
(All websites last accessed May 2023.)

Granuloma inguinale

Definition and nomenclature

Granuloma inguinale is a genital ulcerative condition found in endemic foci in certain tropical countries. It is rare in the UK. The causative bacterial organism is *Klebsiella granulomatis* (formerly known as *Calymmatobacterium granulomatis*).

Synonyms and inclusions
- Donovanosis (granuloma inguinale was first described by McLeod in 1882 but the synonym donovanosis was proposed to honour Donovan who first demonstrated the causative organism)

Introduction and general description

Granuloma inguinale is now a rare infection and there has been a continued decline in cases globally. It is seen in small endemic foci in certain tropical countries. It is a cause of GUD, it may be followed by genital disfigurement and it has the potential for malignant change [1]. Much about the condition is imperfectly understood. Granuloma inguinale is generally regarded as being an STI because of the usual genital location of the lesions, increased incidence in those individuals and age groups with the highest sexual activity and its association with other STIs. Non-venereal spread has been reported in children, as has transmission to the neonate during vaginal delivery.

Epidemiology

Incidence and prevalence

The prevalence of granuloma inguinale has decreased markedly in recent times and the condition can almost be classed as sporadic. Cases are still reported in Papua New Guinea, South Africa, India and Brazil. The condition has virtually been eradicated in Australia [2]. It occurs mostly in marginalised populations with poor access to health care. Small epidemics have occurred in Europe, particularly among migrants [3].

Age

The condition usually affects sexually active adults, mainly between the ages of 20 and 40 years.

Sex

There does not seem to be a predilection for a particular sex.

Ethnicity

The condition is most often reported in black ethnic races.

Associated diseases

Granuloma inguinale may occur with other STIs and has been identified as a risk factor for the acquisition of HIV. Studies have shown that the probability of HIV infection increases with longer duration of lesions [4].

Pathophysiology

Predisposing factors

Poor hygienic conditions have been associated with the condition.

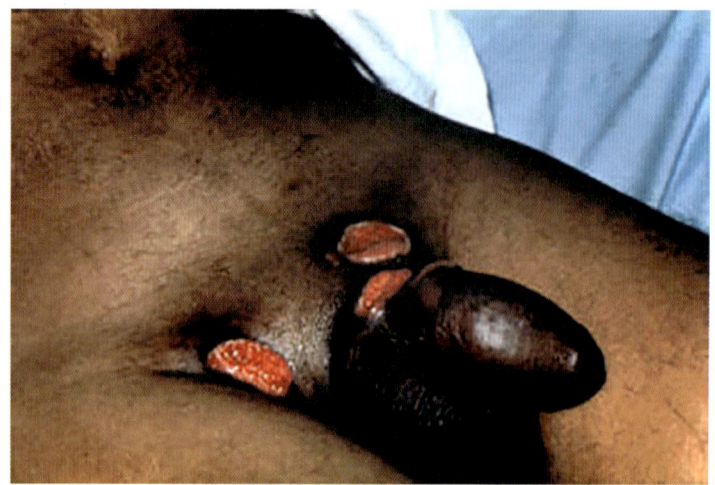

Figure 30.39 Granuloma inguinale with beefy red granulomas.

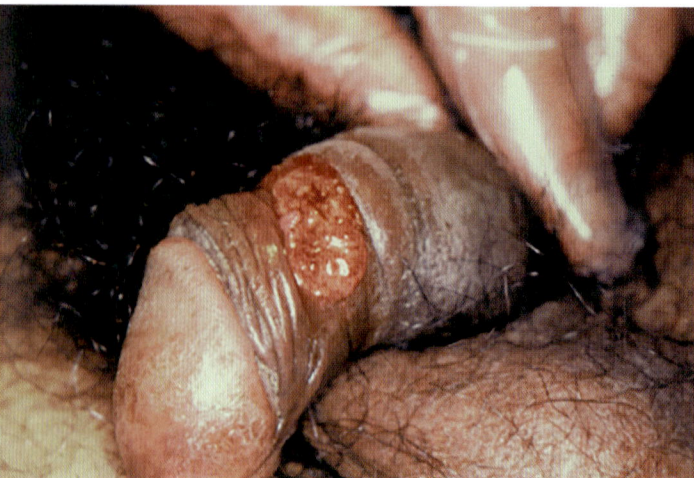

Figure 30.40 Granuloma inguinale with a hypertrophic lesion.

Pathology
Histological examination shows epithelial proliferation with heavy infiltration of plasma cells and neutrophils with few lymphocytes.

Causative organisms
The causative organism *K. granulomatis* is a Gram-negative intracellular coccobacillus.

Clinical features
History
The incubation period is not precisely known but is considered to be between 1 and 360 days. Lesions appear in an average period of 50 days.

Presentation
Four types of lesions have been described:
- Ulcerogranulomatous: the most common type with beefy red ulcers that bleed when touched.
- Hypertrophic: usually with a raised irregular edge.
- Necrotic: offensive-smelling ulcers causing tissue destruction.
- Sclerotic or cicatricial: with fibrous or scar tissue.

At the site of primary inoculation, one or more papules or subcutaneous nodules develop into friable ulcers or hypertrophic lesions. Granuloma inguinale causes ulcerative granulomatous lesions, which may be multiple, bleed readily and extend (Figure 30.39). Raised lesions with a hypertrophic, irregular edge may occur (Figure 30.40). The ulcers grow slowly and are highly vascular with a beefy red appearance. Lesions tend not to be painful. Lymphadenopathy is not usual unless there are other ulcer pathogens present, but subcutaneous extension of granulomas may mimic enlarged lymph nodes (pseudobuboes).

Secondary infection can result in necrotic, foul-smelling, deep ulceration. Untreated infections may either resolve spontaneously (leaving dry, fibrotic lesions and scarring) or may persist and slowly spread. Lesions commonly occur on the coronal sulcus or inner aspect of the penile prepuce in uncircumcised men, on the anus in MSM and the labia or introitus in females (Figure 30.41).

Primary lesions have also been reported in extragenital sites such as the upper arms, chest, legs, jaw, mouth, cervix and bones

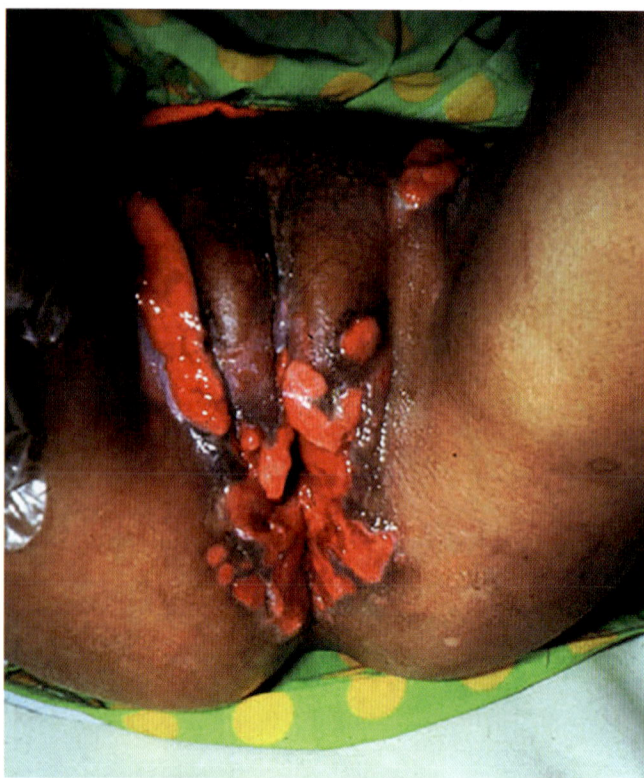

Figure 30.41 Granuloma inguinale in a female patient.

(particularly the tibia). Primary lesions of the cervix may mimic carcinoma. Dissemination into the abdominal cavity, intestines, spleen, liver, lungs, uterus and ovaries has been reported. It may present as a pelvic mass mimicking carcinoma [5].

Differential diagnosis
The differential diagnosis includes other causes of GUD such as primary syphilis and some secondary forms (such as condylomata lata), chancroid (particularly in its phagedenic form), chronic herpes simplex and lymphogranuloma venereum, which may coexist. Other infective conditions include genital amoebiasis and cutaneous tuberculosis, other granulomatous lesions such as Crohn disease, and genital cancers.

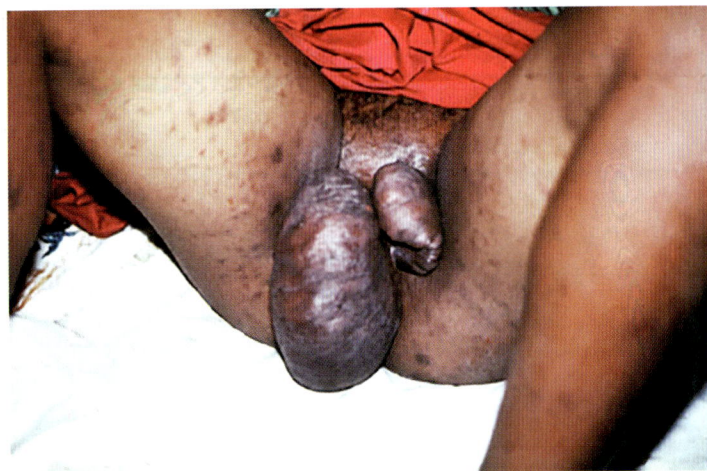

Figure 30.42 Pseudo-elephantiasis.

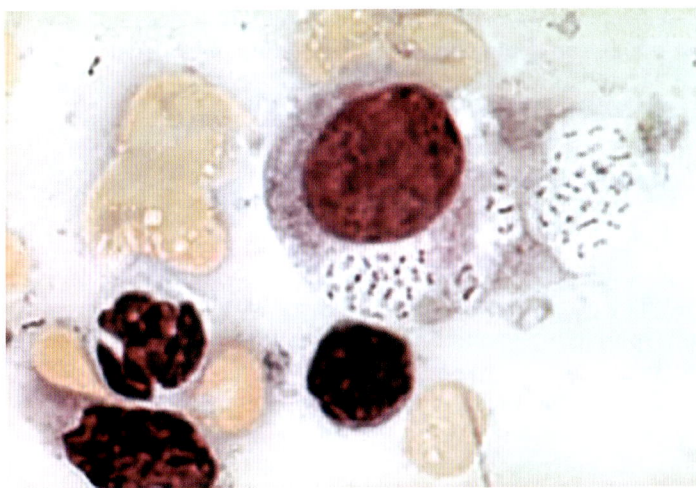

Figure 30.43 Biopsy smear showing mononuclear cells containing the causative organism with bipolar staining.

Complications and co-morbidities

Granuloma inguinale causes a wide range of lesser-known complications. It may be followed by pseudo-elephantiasis (Figure 30.42) [6] resulting from persistent granulomas that may constrict lymphatics. Genital scarring and disfigurement may ensue. Other complications include haemorrhage, genital mutilation, cicatrisation, development of squamous cell carcinoma, haematogenous dissemination to the bone and viscera (particularly during pregnancy), psoas and perinephric abscess, spinal cord compression and vertical transmission. Lesions affecting the ears of infants may occur [7,8].

Disease course and prognosis

Untreated lesions tend to be persistent, slowly extending and destructive. HIV augments continuation of the lesions with persistent ulcers for prolonged periods.

Investigations

The diagnosis is generally made by microscopic identification of Donovan bodies. These are found in large mononuclear cells of the monocyte/macrophage lineage, whose cytoplasm contains numerous organisms, 0.5–0.7 by 1–1.5 μm in size, that show bipolar staining ('safety-pin appearance') (Figure 30.43). Giemsa, Wright or Leishman stains are usually used. Specimens may be obtained from pinched-off tissue fragments taken directly from the lesion or from biopsy specimens.

Successful culture of the causative organism has been reported in human peripheral blood monocytes and in the Hep-2 cells [9,10]. PCR tests have been described but are not yet routinely available.

Management

Prolonged antibiotic treatment is often necessary. Patients should be thoroughly investigated for accompanying STIs and partner notification should be undertaken.

Long-term antibiotic treatment is recommended for at least 3 weeks or until the lesions have completely healed. Other alternative antibiotics include erythromycin, ciprofloxacin and gentamicin [11].

> **Treatment ladder for granuloma inguinale**
>
> All regimes are for at least 3 weeks or until lesions have completely healed.
>
> **First line**
> - Azithromycin 1 g PO weekly or 500 mg PO daily on the first day followed by 500 mg daily
>
> **Second line**
> - Doxycycline 100 mg PO twice daily
>   Or
> - Co-trimoxazole 960 mg PO twice daily

Resources

Further information

British Association for Sexual Health and HIV (BASHH) Clinical Effectiveness Group. *United Kingdom National Guideline for the Management of Donovanosis (Granuloma Inguinale) 2018*. https://www.bashhguidelines.org/media/1219/donovanosis-2018.pdf.

Centers for Disease Control and Prevention (CDC). *Sexually Transmitted Disease Treatment Guidelines, 2021. Granuloma Inguinale (Donovanosis)*. https://www.cdc.gov/std/treatment-guidelines/donovanosis.htm.

O'Farrell N, Moi H. 2016 European guideline on donovanosis. *Int J STD AIDS* 2016;27:605–7.

Patient resources

NSW Government. *Donovanosis Factsheet*. http://www.health.nsw.gov.au/Infectious/factsheets/Pages/Donovanosis.aspx.

(All websites last accessed May 2023.)

Mycoplasma genitalium infection

Definition and nomenclature

Mycoplasma genitalium is a sexually transmitted bacterium belonging to the mollicutes class. It is the smallest prokaryote capable of self-replication, with a genome of 580 kB. It does not have any peptidoglycan-containing cell wall and thus is inherently resistant to β-lactam antibiotics.

Introduction and general description

First discovered in 1981 [1], *M. genitalium* has emerged over the last few decades as an important sexually transmitted pathogen causing adverse health outcomes in both men and women. It is a cause of non-gonococcal urethritis in men, and cervicitis and PID in women. However, past efforts to identify this organism on a routine basis found difficulty due to the fastidious nature of the bacterium. Furthermore, limited molecular diagnostics and the use of widespread empirical antibiotic treatment have led to the emergence of multidrug resistant strains worldwide. Surveillance has only recently been possible following the availability of diagnostic PCR.

Epidemiology
Prevalence
In a systematic review and meta-analysis of 63 studies, the summary prevalence estimate was 1.3% in HICs and 3.9% in LMICs [2].

Age
A large prospective multicentre study in the USA found that the overall prevalence of *M. genitalium* was significantly higher in those aged 15–24 years than in those aged 35–39 years [3].

Sex
Both sexes may be affected. Prevalence is similar in women and men [2].

Ethnicity
The risk for *M. genitalium* infection is higher in those of black ethnicity [3,4].

Associated diseases
Coinfection with other STIs is common. A New Orleans study in women presenting to a sexual health clinic showed that coinfection was common with *Chlamydia trachomatis* (22/70, 31.4%), *Trichomonas vaginalis* (22/70, 31.4%), *Neisseria gonorrhoeae* (17/70, 24.3%) and any of the three pathogens (39/70, 55.7%) [5].

Increased numbers of sexual partners in the preceding 12 months and other high-risk sexual behaviour increase risk of acquisition of *M. genitalium* and other STIs [5,6].

Pathophysiology
Mycoplasma genitalium is a flask-shaped organism. It causes inflammation in the uro-genital tract by adhesion to host epithelial cells eliciting acute inflammatory signals via highly expressed innate immune sensors. Binding of these receptors to *M. genitalium* and its lipoproteins results in activation of pro-inflammatory signals including potent chemokines, ultimately resulting in leukocyte recruitment to the site of infection. Multiple factors to aid pathogenesis include the ability for adhesion, gliding motility and cell invasion [7]. Knowledge about the organism and host factors that contribute to pathogenicity continues to evolve.

Clinical features
Most patients are asymptomatic. In a UK population survey, no symptoms were reported by 94.4% of men and 56.2% of women [8]. Box 30.1 lists the main clinical features found.

Box 30.1 Clinical features of *Mycoplasma genitalium* infection

Males
- Asymptomatic
- Urethral discharge (Figure 30.44)
- Dysuria
- Penile irritation
- Urethral discomfort
- Urethritis (acute, persistent, recurrent)
- Balanitis and/or posthitis [9]
- Proctitis (in MSM)

Females
- Asymptomatic
- Dysuria
- Postcoital bleeding
- Painful intermenstrual bleeding
- Cervicitis
- Lower abdominal pain

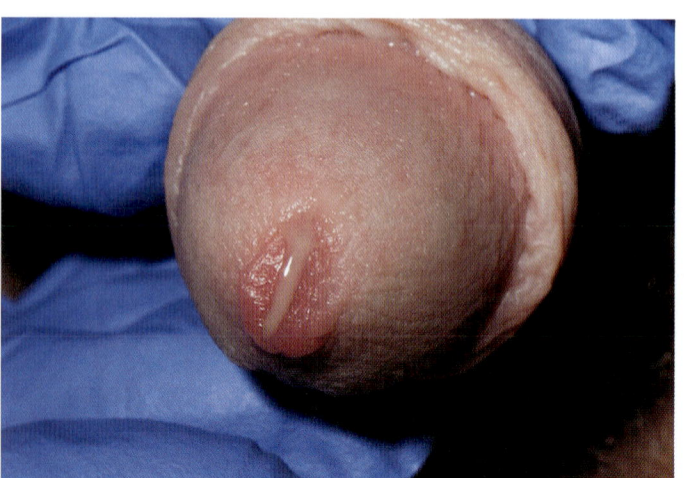

Figure 30.44 Urethral discharge in male with *Mycoplasma genitalium* infection.

Differential diagnosis
These include the following:
- *Chlamydia trachomatis*.
- *Neisseria gonorrhoeae*.
- *Trichomonas vaginalis*.
- Urinary tract infection.
- Pelvic inflammatory disease.
- Other causes of intermenstrual bleeding.
- Gynaecological pathology.

Complications and co-morbidities
Complications in males included epididymo-orchitis. There are conflicting data from studies of the association of *M. genitalium* with

male infertility [10], and a possible association of reactive arthritis with *M. genitalium* urethritis has been described [11].

Complications in females include PID, tubal factor infertility (uncertain association), sexually acquired reactive arthritis and preterm delivery. An Australian study from 2018 found 5.5% cases of PID were due to *M. genitalium* where no other pathogen was detected [12], with similar clinical characteristics to women with PID caused by *C. trachomatis* infection.

Disease course and prognosis

There is still much to learn about the natural history of *M. genitalium* infection. Persistence of infection has been documented. A US study of 147 infected women found persistent *M. genitalium* PCR positivity in 42% throughout the 12-month follow-up period [13]. There are no similar cohort studies in untreated men as yet. There are studies in men that confirm that it may persist after antibiotic therapy. Spontaneous clearance may also occur, as with other STIs [14,15].

Investigations

The introduction of diagnostic *M. genitalium* NAATs (PCR) including antimicrobial resistance testing has led to improved detection and antibiotic stewardship. There is current debate about the need for routine asymptomatic screening. Because there is no convincing evidence that asymptomatic infection warrants treatment, and many patients will spontaneously clear the organism [16], asymptomatic screening is not currently recommended.

The British Association of Sexual Health and HIV (BASHH) published the first UK national management guideline in 2018. BASHH recommends testing only symptomatic individuals such as men with non-gonococcal urethritis and women with PID, with consideration for testing in those with other clinical syndromes, such as cervicitis, epididymo-orchitis and proctitis. Current guidance recommends testing current sexual partners and only treating if they are confirmed positive, to prevent reinfection of the index case. In 10 studies measuring *M. genitalium* infection status in couples, 39–50% of male or female sexual partners of infected participants also had *M. genitalium* detected [17].

M. genitalium does not possess a cell wall and so cannot be seen upon Gram stain of genital secretions and requires weeks to months to culture. Therefore, conventional methods of culture and susceptibility testing are not feasible. Serology testing is affected by cross-reactivity to other mycoplasmas, including *Mycoplasma pneumoniae*.

NAATs for *M. genitalium* are now commercially available and are the investigation of choice. Simultaneous testing for genotypic resistance is recommended to inform treatment, given the high rate of antimicrobial resistance. However, not all UK sexual health services currently have the facilities for *M. genitalium* PCR, despite widespread concerns about increasing resistance.

First-void urine is the specimen of choice in males. Vaginal swabs (either clinician taken or self-taken) are the specimen of choice for females.

Management

General principles of management

Mycoplasma genitalium is an STI that shares some clinical and epidemiological characteristics with *C. trachomatis*, but its propensity to develop antimicrobial resistance poses a significant challenge. Different strategies are used worldwide in the treatment of *M. genitalium*, including pre-treatment with doxycycline with the aim of reducing bacterial load [18], followed by an extended course of azithromycin, such as in the BASHH guidelines, with the use of resistance testing where available. Moxifloxacin is recommended for those who fail first line treatment, those with known macrolide resistance and for women with PID. In a systematic review and meta-analysis of 59 studies, the summary prevalence of mutations associated with azithromycin resistance in *M. genitalium* increased from 10% before 2010 to 51% in 2016–17 [19]. Limited data from a London study suggest a prevalence of 30–40% [20]. There is no clear evidence for the optimum regimen, but first line treatment with single-dose macrolides is not recommended and has been removed as first line empirical therapy for *C trachomatis* from the BASHH national treatment guidelines for this reason. Test of cure is currently recommended in some guidelines (BASHH guidance recommends 5 weeks after treatment) as resistance can emerge during treatment.

Treatment ladder for *Mycoplasma genitalium* infection

Uncomplicated infection
- Doxycycline 100 mg two times daily for 7 days followed by azithromycin 1 g PO as a single dose, then 500 mg PO once daily for 2 days (where the organism is known to be macrolide sensitive or where resistance status is unknown)
- Moxifloxacin 400 mg PO once daily for 10 days (if organism is known to be macrolide resistant or where treatment with azithromycin has failed)

Complicated infection (PID/epididymo-orchitis)
- Moxifloxacin 400 mg PO once daily for 14 days
  Alternative treatment regimens:
- Doxycycline 100 mg PO twice daily for 7 days followed by pristinamycin 1 g PO four times daily for 10 days
- Pristinamycin 1 g PO four times daily for 10 days
- Doxycycline 100 mg PO twice daily for 14 days
- Minocycline 100 mg PO twice daily for 14 days

Resources

Further information

British Association for Sexual Health and HIV (BASHH). *British Association for Sexual Health and HIV National Guideline for the Management of Infection with Mycoplasma Genitalium (2018)*. https://www.bashhguidelines.org/media/1198/mg-2018.pdf.

Jensen JS, Cusini M, Gomberg M, Moi H. 2016 European guideline on Mycoplasma genitalium infections. *J Eur Acad Dermatol Venereol* 2016;30:1650–6.

Patient resources

British Association for Sexual Health and HIV (BASHH). *Mycoplasma Genitalium – the Basics*. https://www.bashhguidelines.org/media/1226/mgen_pil_digital_p2_2019.pdf.

(All websites last accessed May 2023.)

Key references

The full list of references can be found in the online version at https://www.wiley.com/rooksdermatology10e

Gonorrhoea
2 Kirkcaldy RD, Weston E, Segurado AC, Hughes G. Epidemiology of gonorrhoea: a global perspective. *Sex Health* 2019;16:401–11.
3 Public Health England. *Sexually transmitted infections (STIs): annual data tables*. https://www.gov.uk/government/statistics/sexually-transmitted-infections-stis-annual-data-tables (last accessed May 2023).

Genital *Chlamydia* infection
1 Mitchell H, Allen H, Sonubi T et al. *Sexually Transmitted Infections and Screening for Chlamydia in England, 2019*. London: Public Health England, 2020.

Lymphogranuloma venereum
1 Public Health England. *Trends of Lymphogranuloma Venereum (LGV) in England: 2019*. Health Protection Report Vol. 14, No. 23. London: Public Health England, 2020.
5 Martin-Iguacel R, Llibre JM, Nielsen H *et al*. Lymphogranuloma venereum proctocolitis: a silent endemic disease in men who have sex with men in industrialised countries. *Eur J Clin Microbiol Infect Dis* 2010;29:917–25.
8 Riera-Monroig J, Fuertes de Vega I. Lymphogranuloma venereum presenting as an ulcer on the tongue. *Sex Transm Infect* 2019;95:169–70.

Chancroid
3 Lewis DA, Müller E, Steele L *et al*. Prevalence and associations of genital ulcer and urethral pathogens in men presenting with genital ulcer syndrome to primary health care clinics in South Africa. *Sex Transm Dis* 2012;39:880–5.
7 Gonzalez-Beiras C, Marks M, Chen CY *et al*. Epidemiology of Haemophilus ducreyi infections. *Emerg Infect Dis* 2016;22:1–8.
11 Ndzomo Ngono J-P, Tchatchouang S, Noah Tsanga MV *et al*. Ulcerative skin lesions among children in Cameroon: it is not always yaws. *PLoS Negl Trop Dis* 2021;15:e0009180.

Granuloma inguinale
6 Narang T, Kanwar AJ. Genital elephantiasis due to donovanosis: forgotten but not gone yet… *Int J STD AIDS* 2012;23:835–6.

Mycoplasma *genitalium* infection
9 Horner PJ, Taylor-Robinson D. Association of *Mycoplasma genitalium* with balanoposthitis in men with non-gonococcal urethritis. *Sex Transm Infect* 2011;87:38–40.
16 Kirby T. *Mycoplasma genitalium*: a potential new superbug. *Lancet Infect Dis* 2018;18:951–2.
17 Cina M, Baumann L, Egli-Gany D *et al*. Mycoplasma genitalium incidence, persistence, concordance between partners and progression: systematic review and meta-analysis. *Sex Transm Infect* 2019;95:328–35.

CHAPTER 31

HIV and the Skin

Christopher B. Bunker[1] and Vincent Piguet[2]

[1] University College London Hospitals and Chelsea and Westminster Hospitals, London, UK
[2] Division of Dermatology, Department of Medicine, University of Toronto; Division of Dermatology, Women's College Hospital, Toronto, Ontario, Canada

---

HIV INFECTION AND AIDS, 31.1

DERMATOLOGICAL MANIFESTATIONS OF HIV INFECTION, 31.11
Introduction, 31.11
PRURITUS, XEROSIS, ICHTHYOSIS AND PRURIGO, 31.12
PIGMENTARY DISORDERS, 31.12
COAGULOPATHIES, 31.12
INFLAMMATORY DERMATOSES, 31.12
Erythroderma, 31.12
Seborrhoeic dermatitis, 31.12
Atopic eczema, 31.15
Psoriasis, 31.15
Eosinophilic folliculitis, 31.17
Pruritic papular eruption, 31.17
Granuloma annulare, 31.18
Porphyria cutanea tarda, 31.18
Drug reactions, 31.18
INFECTIONS, 31.20

BACTERIAL INFECTIONS, 31.20
Other bacterial infections, 31.22
VIRAL INFECTIONS, 31.23
Herpes simplex, 31.23
Varicella-zoster virus, 31.23
Cytomegalovirus, 31.24
Human papillomavirus, 31.25
Mollusca, 31.26
Other viral infections, 31.26
FUNGAL INFECTIONS, 31.26
Candidosis, 31.26
Dermatophytosis, 31.26
Histoplasmosis, 31.27
Cryptococcosis, 31.28
Talaromyces marneffei infection (penicilliosis), 31.28
Other fungal infections, 31.28
PROTOZOAL INFECTIONS, 31.29

SCABIES, 31.29
MISCELLANEOUS INFECTIONS, 31.29
NEOPLASMS, 31.30
Kaposi sarcoma, 31.30
Melanoma and non-melanoma skin cancer, 31.31
Lymphoma, 31.32
Other neoplasms, 31.33
SPECIAL SITUATIONS, 31.33
Hair and nails, 31.33
Oro-pharynx, 31.34
Ano-genital, 31.35
Women, 31.36
Children, 31.36
Haemophilia, 31.37
Intravenous drug use, 31.37
IRIS/IRD/IRAD, 31.37

Key references, 31.39

HIV INFECTION AND AIDS

Definition
Human immunodeficiency virus (HIV) infection is acquired sexually, from blood or blood products, or vertically from an infected mother during pregnancy, birth or breastfeeding. The virus infects immunocompetent cells including CD4+ T cells and macrophages. It creates variable patterns of disease in individuals, groups and races but all are characterised by evolving, sometimes fulminant immunodysfunction affecting many systems of the body.

Introduction and general description
It is now over 40 years since acquired immune deficiency syndrome (AIDS) was first recognised as a novel disease. Within 2 years of defining AIDS as a distinctive syndrome in 1981, HIV was identified as the causative agent.

Dermatological involvement in AIDS has been appreciated since the disease was first recognised as a cryptic acquired immune deficiency illness in homosexual men and before the causative virus was identified. Mucocutaneous involvement establishes criteria for diagnosis and staging; the prognostic significance of some complications, for example pruritic papular eruption/eosinophilic folliculitis, hairy leukoplakia and Kaposi sarcoma (KS), was well recognised before specific treatments were introduced. The proportion of patients with skin complications and the number of these manifestations in any one patient increase as HIV infection progresses and AIDS develops. The incidence and severity of several common cutaneous diseases (such as mollusca, herpes simplex and seborrhoeic dermatitis) are increased in patients with HIV and this correlates in many instances with the absolute numbers of CD4+ T cells. The effect HIV infection may have on some dermatological conditions such as psoriasis and leprosy is less clear-cut. Since the recognition of AIDS there have been many case reports of uncommon dermatoses in HIV-positive patients where an association is speculative. The skin and mucosae are important in HIV infection as they represent routes for infection and potential targets for prevention (e.g. by male circumcision, topical microbicides or vaccination). HIV has been demonstrated in the dermis of infected individuals and may be present in Langerhans cells and other subsets of dendritic cells in the skin. Different cytokine expression patterns distinguish different cutaneous manifestations. The advent of highly active combined antiretroviral therapy (ART; HAART was the original acronym, then cART, but ART is now preferred) has been incalculably beneficial to patients with HIV, but novel side effects of these drugs (such as lipodystrophy) have emerged, and the skin can be affected by manifestations of the immune reconstitution inflammatory syndrome/immune reconstitution associated disease.

The dermatological complications of HIV and AIDS may be distressing to patients and difficult for dermatologists to diagnose and manage. Also, many dermatoses presenting in the population at large need to be regarded as 'indicator conditions' to prompt advice about, and initiation of, HIV testing. A move to 'normalisation' of HIV testing through 'opt out protocols' is advocated in clinical practice to decrease the number of patients presenting with more advanced disease and to diminish the scale of unsuspecting forward transmission. Immediate therapy is now recommended on diagnosis of HIV. This is important because patients successfully treated with ART can achieve the same mortality rates as the general population. Increasingly, HIV dermatology in the developed world is concerned with the consequences of antiretroviral (ARV) treated stable HIV disease. For example, although AIDS-related cancers are decreasing, non-AIDS-defining cancer is on the increase, particularly non-melanoma skin and ano-oro-genital cancer.

However, the dermatological manifestations of HIV are of further interest in that the 'experiment of nature' sheds light on both the immunopathological natural history of HIV infection and the aetiology of common and rarer dermatoses that happen to be found with a higher incidence in HIV-infected than non-HIV-infected patients. Their occurrence emphasises the importance of the skin as a dynamic immunological organ.

Epidemiology
Incidence and prevalence

AIDS was first described as a distinct clinical entity in 1981 [1]. HIV-1 infection now represents a global pandemic. In 2006, there were an estimated 2.9 million deaths from AIDS worldwide. In 2012 an estimated 35.3 million people were believed to be living with HIV infection [2,3], while in 2020, 37.7 million people were living with HIV and 1.5 million people were newly infected [3].

Global trends in the HIV pandemic can be sourced from the Joint United Nations Programme on HIV/AIDS (UNAIDS) [3], who take estimates available from published studies and combine them with unpublished data, collected as part of AIDS control programmes in many countries, to provide national estimates of prevalence and deaths. About 95% of AIDS cases occur in non-industrialised countries and 75% in sub-Saharan Africa. One recent threat to the fight against HIV/AIDS has been the Covid-19 pandemic, through the diversion of attention and resources, both human and fiscal, and uncertain interactions [4].

In the UK, more than 2500 new HIV infections were reported each year between 1991 and 1997 – two-thirds of these from London – whereas in 2012, 6360 people were newly diagnosed with HIV in the UK, nearly half of whom were diagnosed at a late stage with a CD4 count below 350 cells/mm^3. By the end of 2014, there were an estimated 110 000 people living with HIV (PLWH) in the UK [5,6]. In 2017 there were 101 600 PLWH, 4363 new HIV infections and 428 deaths [7]. In 2018, the UK reached the United Nation's 90-90-90 target with more than 90% of PLWH diagnosed, more than 90% of those receiving treatment and more than 90% of those with an undetectable viral load [8].

Table 31.1 Clades of HIV.

Clade	Estimated incidence 2000 (%)	Primary geographic distribution
A	27	East, West and Central Africa, eastern Europe
B	12.3	USA, UK, Australia
C	47.2	South Africa, India, China
D	5.3	East Africa
A/E	3.2	South-East Asia
F, G, H, J, K	5.0	Central Africa, Caribbean, Latin America

Sex
Women and children represent the fastest growing subpopulations of HIV-infected patients in the developed world.

Ethnicity
Different subtypes of HIV-1 are predominantly found at different geographic locations (Table 31.1).

Pathophysiology
Virology

Two main types of HIV infect humans: HIV-1 and HIV-2. Worldwide, HIV-1 is by far the commonest cause of AIDS. HIV-2, which differs in a number of its regulatory genes and is found predominantly in West Africa, apparently causes immune deficiency and AIDS more slowly than HIV-1 and is less infectious with lower rates of both sexual and mother-to-child transmission.

Phylogenetic analyses of many samples of HIV-1, isolated from diverse geographic origins, have revealed that they can be divided into *groups*, *subtypes* (or *clades*), *sub-subtypes* and *circulating recombinant forms* (CRFs) [1–4]. Groups are the distinctive HIV-1 lineages: M (major), N (new) and O (outlier). The vast majority of HIV-1 strains found worldwide and responsible for the pandemic belong to the M lineage. Group O is endemic in Cameroon and neighbouring countries, and group N has been identified in west Central Africa.

Within group M there are further genetic subtypes or clades which are approximately equidistantly related to each other and represent a homogeneous group not resembling any other subtype across their entire genome. There are at present nine subtypes of HIV-1 identified: A–D, F–H, J and K. All known representatives of what was initially described as subtype E appear, in fact, to be recombinants of subtypes A and E, and are now designated CRF01-AE. Within some subtypes further phylogenetic structure can be identified, for example subtype or clade F is divided into two sub-subtypes or sub-clades F1 and F2. It is also clear that clades B and D might be better considered as subclades of a single subtype, but for historical reasons it is difficult to change these descriptions [5].

Different subtypes of HIV-1 are predominantly found at different geographic locations, although in no country of the world does a single subtype circulate alone. The contribution of the different clades to the worldwide pandemic has been calculated (Table 31.1) [6–8].

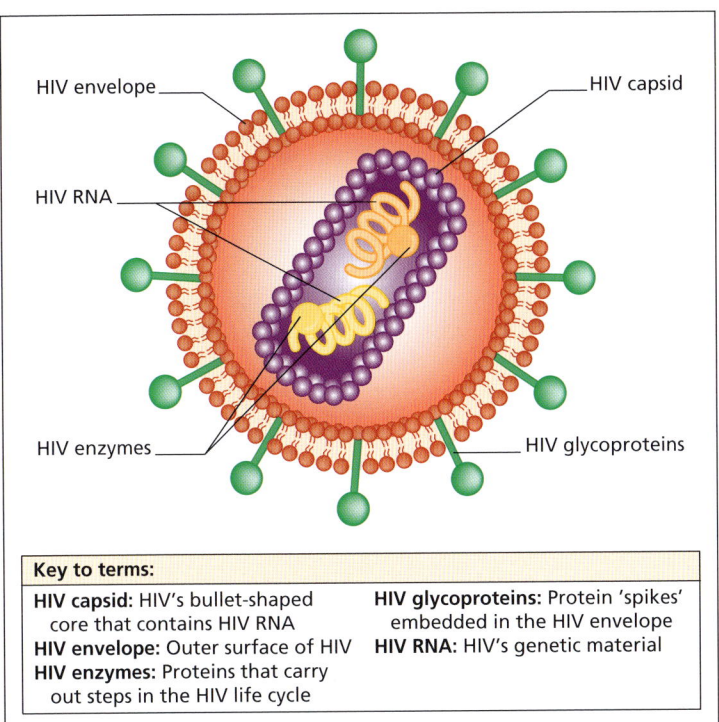

Figure 31.1 Structure of HIV. Adapted from AIDS Info 2014 [39].

HIV is a single-stranded RNA virus (Figure 31.1). The structure of the virus is complex (Figure 31.2), with three major structural genes: *gag* (coding for nuclear proteins), *pol* (coding for reverse transcriptase) and *env* (coding for the envelope). The rate of transcription of the genome is controlled by a number of regulatory genes including *rev*, *tat* and *nef*, and there are a number of other small accessory genes important for infection (*vif*, *vpu*, *vpr*).

The virus gains access to cells by docking the envelope protein on the CD4 receptor and on the co-receptors (primarily CCR5 on monocytes/macrophages, and CXCR4 on T cells) [9]. Tissue mononuclear phagocytes, including human ano-genital monocyte-derived dendritic cells and langerin-expressing conventional dendritic cells (DC2), are major HIV target cells [10]. The process of fusion and inward passage of the genetic material of the virus is accomplished by the transmembrane envelope protein gp41 coming into contact with the cell surface. Components of the Gag protein have an important chaperone function within the cell and allow reverse transcription to occur and the circular DNA product to be transported to the nucleus of the cell. There, a virally encoded enzyme, integrase, cleaves the circular DNA and inserts it into the host DNA, repairing the insertion sites. Proviral DNA may remain integrated for a substantial period of time before viral transcriptional events are triggered when the cell becomes activated. Initial transcriptional products are the regulatory proteins Rev, Tat and Nef. The Tat protein increases viral transcription, and Rev acts in *cis* to enhance replication by interacting with *rev* regulatory elements within the viral genome; *nef* has a number of putative functions, one of which may be to reduce the amount of major histocompatibility complex (MHC) class I antigen on the cell surface and thus impede recognition of the infected cell by cytotoxic T cells. The *vpr* gene is involved in nuclear transport and may downregulate cellular apoptosis.

The *vpu* gene may downregulate the amount of CD4 receptor protein being produced in the endoplasmic reticulum. Viral products of transcription are then transported to the cytoplasm, where the nuclear capsid proteins may again have an important chaperone function. Viral proteins are produced as a long polyprotein that is split into active proteins by the virally encoded protease enzyme. Viral RNA and viral proteins are then assembled around the nuclear capsid antigen and when the virus is fully assembled, it buds from the cell surface. Enormous amounts of viral RNA are continually released into the plasma ($>10^8$ viral particles per day) in untreated HIV-infected patients [11,12].

One of the major characteristics of HIVs is their extremely high genetic variability. This extensive heterogeneity is a result of the high error rate of reverse transcriptase [13] and the extremely fast turnover of virions in HIV-infected individuals [11,12]. In addition, the reverse transcriptase enzyme is highly recombinogenic [14], so that radically different genomic combinations may be generated in individuals infected by genetically diverse viruses. Recombination requires the simultaneous infection of a cell with two different proviruses, allowing the encapsidation of one RNA transcript from each provirus into the heterozygous virion. After the subsequent infection of a new cell, the reverse transcriptase, moving back and forth between the two RNA templates, generates a newly synthesised retroviral DNA sequence that is a recombinant between the two parental genomes [14–16]. It is now well established that recombination events between different subtypes or clades of HIV are relatively common and may result in CRFs of HIV. Members of one distinct CRF should resemble each other over the entire genome, with similar breakpoints reflecting similar ancestry from the same recombination event(s).

Immunology

The immune system is capable of mounting very strong attacks on invading pathogens and in many cases is able to eliminate them completely. Unfortunately, this does not seem to be the case with HIV infection, except perhaps in a very few individuals in whom exposure to the virus has resulted in specific cellular immune responses to the virus, but who have neither seroconverted nor become productively infected [17]. A few notable exceptions to this rule are a case of an infant who apparently cleared HIV infection at 18 months of age with ART and the long-term control of HIV being achieved in a patient after a CCR5 delta32/delta32 stem cell transplantation [18,19]. Although often strong and apparently useful anti-HIV responses are induced in HIV-infected individuals, these do not seem to have the capability of clearing viral infection. However, in some individuals, immune responses apparently play a role in allowing the host to coexist with the virus without progression to disease (long-term non-progressor patients) [20] (see 'Disease course and prognosis' later in this chapter).

Primary infection with HIV results in natural or innate immune responses that are mobilised within hours of infection and include inflammation, non-specific activation of macrophages, natural killer cells and complement, and the release of cytokines. After antigenic stimulation, acquired immune responses are primed. These responses emerge at the same time as clearance of viraemia, and rebound of CD4 T cells is seen. These HIV-specific responses include intrinsic immunity (restriction factors), specific humoral

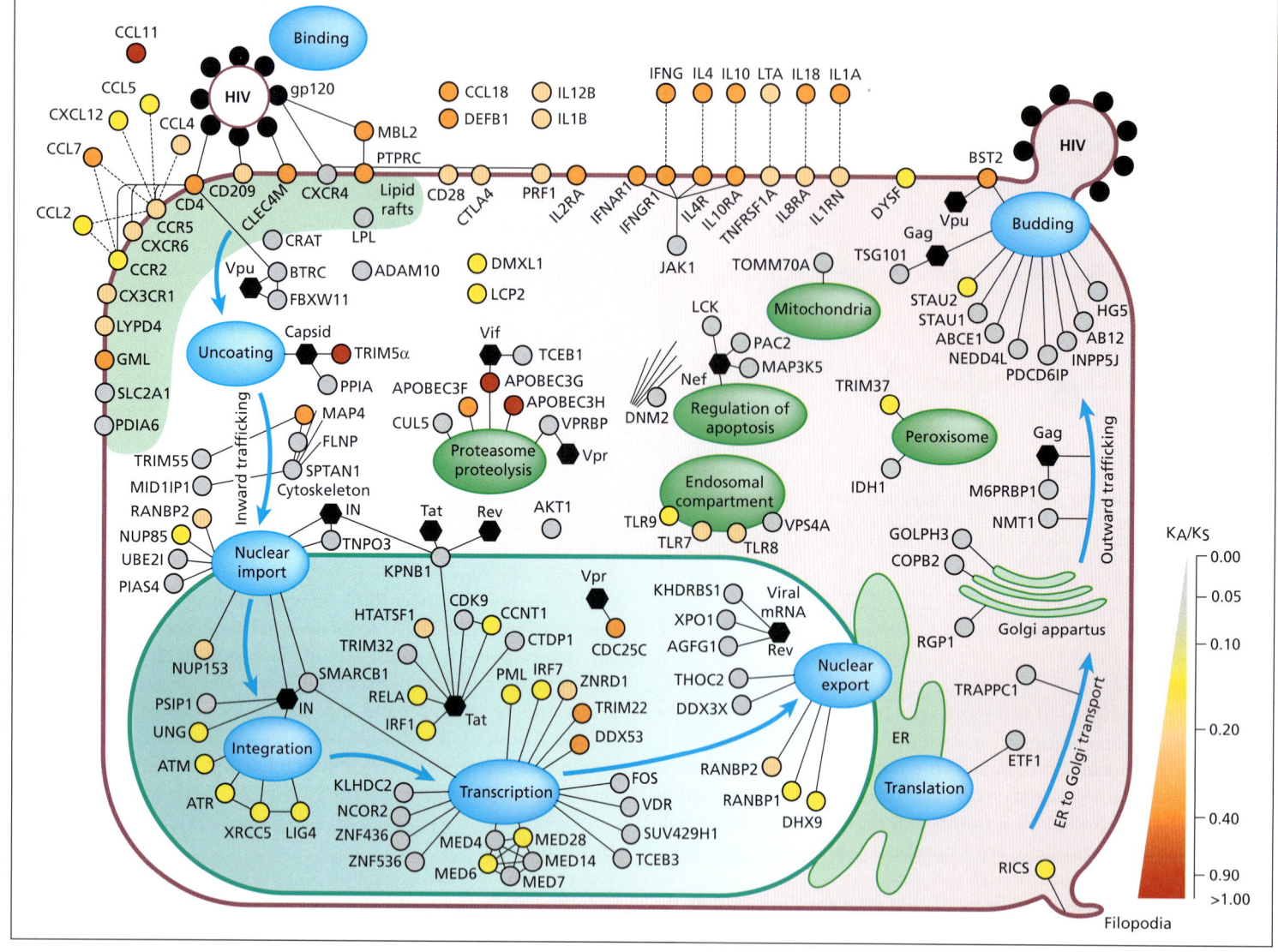

Figure 31.2 Stages in the HIV life cycle (blue ovals) showing location, interaction with and selective pressure of candidate cellular host factors/proteins that may be targeted for antiretroviral drug development. Host factors are localised in the cell using the different stages of the HIV-1 life cycle as a framework. The subcellular location, function and possible direct interaction with HIV-1 elements were determined using multiple databases and published studies. The degree of molecular evolution is classified in K_A/K_S quintiles: 0–0.11 (grey), 0.12–0.22 (yellow), 0.23–0.39 (bisque), 0.40–0.99 (orange) and ≥1 (red). Solid lines correspond to direct protein–protein binding. Dashed lines correspond to ligand–receptor interactions. Selected HIV-1 proteins (Gag, gp120, IN, Nef, Rev, Tat, Vif, Vpr, Vpu) are depicted in black. ER, endoplasmic reticulum. Reproduced from Ortiz et al. 2009 [9] with permission of Oxford University Press.

or antibody responses and specific cellular responses; these are outlined below.

Intrinsic immunity. In addition to innate and adaptive immune responses, cells express a number of factors that can confer some degree of resistance to HIV. These include APOBEC3G, TRIM5-alpha, tetherin, SAMHD-1 and the more recently identified interferon-induced *MX-2* gene [21–27]. These factors may provide opportunites for intervention as enhancing their function might confer greater resistance to the retroviral infection.

Specific humoral or antibody responses. These consist of neutralising antibodies to the envelope proteins of the virus and other non-neutralising antibodies to internal viral proteins such as *gag* [28]. Specific secretory immunoglobulin A (IgA) mucosal antibodies are also produced. Neutralising antibodies are usually measurable by 12 weeks after infection. One vaccine trial reported a modest success with 31.2% protection (the RV144 trial). A follow-up study of immune correlates suggested that IgG antibodies to variable regions 1 and 2 (V1V2) of HIV-1 envelope proteins may have contributed to protection against HIV-1 infection, while high levels of Env-specific IgA antibodies may have decreased the effects of protective antibodies. These studies suggest a critical role for antibodies in the success of a future HIV vaccine [29]. Recent animal studies underline the essential importance of antibody response in protection against HIV immunological and virological mechanisms of vaccine-mediated protection against simian immunodeficiency virus (SIV) and HIV [30].

Specific cellular (T-lymphocyte) responses. CD8 T lymphocytes or cytotoxic T lymphocytes (CTLs) form a primary component of the critical cellular immune response induced by HIV infection [31]. CTLs are differentiated from existing CTL precursors and express T-cell receptor molecules capable of recognising specific viral epitopes presented in the context of human leukocyte antigen (HLA) or MHC molecules at the surface of infected target cells. Mature CTLs are functional 5–10 days after antigenic stimulation, recognising, binding and then lysing the infected target cell. Virus-specific CTLs evolve faster than antibody responses and are often induced before seroconversion and before viral RNA has reached peak titres. Thus CD8 CTLs are temporally associated with a fall in viraemia during acute infection, and there is good evidence that CTLs play a major role in the control of HIV infection at this time and later in HIV disease. Evidence for strong CD8 antiviral pressure can be appreciated by the number and variety of strategies that viruses have evolved to avoid apoptosis and CTL recognition, thus prolonging the life of the virally infected cell and enabling viral replication and dissemination [32]. In addition to the lysis of infected cells, CD8 T cells can reduce viral replication by the production of soluble factors. These factors are not antigen specific but their production requires specific T-cell activation. Anti-HIV effects have been found for interferon γ (IFN-γ), interleukin 10 (IL-10), IL-13, IL-16 and the C-C chemokines macrophage inhibitory protein 1α (MIP-1α), MIP-1β and RANTES (regulated upon activation, normal T-cell expressed and secreted). Such soluble factors may also have profound effects on other opportunistic infections including those affecting the skin.

CD4 T-cell responses induced by HIV infection provide help to both HIV-specific CTLs and B cells. CD4 T-helper cells recognise antigen in the context of HLA class II molecules on the surface of antigen-presenting cells such as dendritic cells. CD4 responses to a variety of HIV proteins (including Env, Gag and Nef) have been demonstrated in early disease, but immunological abnormalities in T-helper function occur very early in HIV infection, even before CD4 T-cell numbers diminish in the peripheral blood. Furthermore, advances in our understanding of HIV-1 pathogenesis reveal that mucosal tissues, primarily in the gastrointestinal tract, are major sites for early viral replication and CD4 T-cell destruction, and may represent the major viral reservoir [33]. Reduced proliferative capacity and diminished IL-2 production in response to stimulation by exogenous antigens (including those from HIV and other pathogens) is one of the hallmarks of HIV disease.

On recognition of their specific antigen, naive CD4 T cells differentiate from a common (Th0) precursor into T-helper 1 (Th1) cells – which differentially secrete IL-2, IFN-γ, transforming growth factor β and IL-12 and can activate macrophages and 'help' CTLs – or into T helper 2 (Th2) cells – which secrete IL-4, IL-5, IL-6 and IL-10 that can activate B cells to proliferate and differentiate into antibody-producing plasma cells.

Central to the initiation of innate and adaptive immune responses is the dendritic cell, which is the most potent antigen-presenting cell. However, dendritic cells on mucosal surfaces (Langerhans cells and dermal dendritic cells) are likely to be some of the first targets in transmission. Dendritic cells, as well as transporting viral antigens across mucosal barriers and presenting them to CD4 cells, may themselves become infected with HIV and their function compromised [34]. Interestingly, while dendritic cell subsets tend to transfer HIV to CD4+ T cells without themselves being heavily infected, immature Langerhans cells might be able to degrade HIV via binding to a C-type lectin receptor called langerin [35–37]. In contrast, when Langerhans cells are activated, for instance by a co-infection with herpes simplex virus 2 (HSV-2), they become more infectable and transmit infection to CD4+ T cells more robustly [38].

It should be noted that the immunosuppressive nature of HIV infection, where CD4 T cells are infected and destroyed, may have a profound effect on immune responses to other pathogens, many of which result in dermatological disease and are described later in this chapter. It is interesting to observe that ART, which has a profound effect on HIV replication and enables some CD4 T-cell reconstitution, may also result in the re-emergence of useful opportunistic infection-specific cellular immune responses. Unfortunately, for reasons that are not well understood, HIV-specific responses are often not reconstituted. However, many AIDS-defining opportunistic infections, including diseases of the skin, may be resolved or avoided, and consequently ART has had a profound effect on morbidity and mortality in HIV disease.

Clinical features
Case definition of AIDS

As tests for HIV infection have become more accurate and our understanding of the infection's pathogenesis has become clearer, the need for an epidemiological definition of AIDS has diminished. However, it is of interest to consider the indicator conditions that have been used in the case definition of AIDS in adults, as shown in Box 31.1. The rank order of AIDS diagnoses reported to the US Centers for Disease Control in 1996 is shown in Table 31.2 [1,2].

Changes in the natural history of HIV that followed the introduction of ART in the mid 1990s include a sharp reduction in the frequency of KS and a decrease in *Pneumocystis jiroveci* (was *P. carinii*) pneumonia, reflecting the impact of prophylaxis and possible reconstitution of immune responses specific for opportunistic pathogens. The median CD4 T-cell count at the time of an AIDS-defining complication in those parts of the world where ART is available is now $67 \times 10^6/L$. However, it should be remembered that, at present, such efficacious therapy is not available to the vast majority of persons infected with HIV. It should also be noted that the AIDS case definition in children may be different from that in

Table 31.2 Rank order of AIDS diagnoses reported to the US Centers for Disease Control in 1996.

Diagnosis	Frequency (%)
Pneumocystis jiroveci pneumonia	20
Wasting	14
Cytomegalovirus disease	6
Kaposi sarcoma	6
Tuberculosis	5
Disseminated *Mycobacterium avium-intracellulare* infection	4
Chronic herpes simplex	4
Recurrent bacterial pneumonia	4
HIV-associated dementia	4
Toxoplasmosis	3

> **Box 31.1 Indicator conditions in the case definition of AIDS in adults**
>
> - Candidosis of the oesophagus, trachea, bronchi or lungs
> - Cervical cancer, invasive[a]
> - Coccidioidomycosis, extrapulmonary[a]
> - Cryptococcosis, extrapulmonary
> - Cryptosporidiosis with diarrhoea for >1 month
> - Cytomegalovirus of any organ other than the liver, spleen or lymph nodes
> - Herpes simplex with mucocutaneous ulcer for >1 month or bronchitis, pneumonitis or oesophagitis
> - Histoplasmosis, extrapulmonary[a]
> - HIV-associated dementia: disabling cognitive and/or motor dysfunction interfering with occupation or activities of daily living
> - HIV-associated wasting:[a] involuntary weight loss of >10% of baseline plus chronic diarrhoea (more than two loose stools per day for >30 days) or chronic weakness and documented enigmatic fever for >30 days
> - Isosporosis with diarrhoea for >1 month[a]
> - Kaposi sarcoma in patients younger than 60 years (or older than 60 years[a])
> - Lymphoma, non-Hodgkin of B-cell or unknown immunological phenotype and histology showing small, non-cleaved lymphoma or immunoblastic sarcoma
> - Lymphoma of the brain in patients younger than 60 years (or older than 60 years[a])
> - *Mycobacterium avium* or *M. kansasii*, disseminated
> - *Mycobacterium tuberculosis*, disseminated[a]
> - *Mycobacterium tuberculosis*, pulmonary[a]
> - Nocardiosis[a]
> - *Talaromyces marneffei* infection (penicilliosis)
> - *Pneumocystis jiroveci* pneumonia
> - Pneumonia, recurrent (bacterial)[a]
> - Progressive multifocal leukoencephalopathy
> - *Salmonella* septicaemia (non-typhoid), recurrent[a]
> - Strongyloidosis, extraintestinal
> - Toxoplasmosis of an internal organ
>
> [a] Requires positive HIV serology.

Table 31.3 Clinical manifestations of primary HIV infection.

Clinical manifestation	Frequency (%)	Mean duration (days)
Fever (>38°C)	77	17
Fatigue	66	24
Erythematous maculopapular rash	56	15
Myalgia	55	18
Headache	51	26
Pharyngitis	44	12
Cervical lymphadenopathy	39	15
Arthralgia	31	23
Oral ulcer	29	13
Odynophagia	28	16
Axillary lymphadenopathy	24	164
Weight loss	24	29
Nausea	24	18
Diarrhoea	23	13
Night sweats	22	15
Cough	22	18
Anorexia	21	15
Inguinal lymphadenopathy	20	9
Abdominal pain	19	15
Oral candidosis	17	10
Vomiting	12	10
Photophobia	12	11
Sore eyes	12	13
Genital ulcer	7	14
Tonsillitis	7	13
Depression	6	23
Dizziness	6	11

From Hawkins 2002 [5].

adults [3]. Furthermore, it is currently considered that in clinical care HIV disease should be viewed as a continuum, rather than just the presence or absence of AIDS. This continuum includes primary infection, symptomatic infection, early symptomatic state (previously known as AIDS-related complex), late symptomatic disease and advanced disease.

Presentation

Acute primary HIV infection may be clinically silent but up to 90% of patients develop a non-specific, symptomatic illness 1–6 weeks after exposure that lasts a few days to several months but usually less than a fortnight [4]. Symptoms and signs are often those of a non-specific viral infection, similar to infectious mononucleosis with lassitude, fever, arthralgia, myalgia and lymphadenopathy. Weight loss, nausea, vomiting and diarrhoea are common. Headache and photophobia may signify aseptic meningitis and cognitive dysfunction encephalitis, although other recognised neurological presentations include Bell palsy, brachial neuritis, radiculopathy, peripheral neuropathy and Guillain–Barré syndrome. Symptomatic primary HIV infection is a strong predictor of progression to AIDS [4]. Table 31.3 lists the frequency and duration of the principal clinical manifestations of primary HIV infection [5].

Dermatological manifestations of acute primary HIV infection

The principal dermatological manifestations of seroconversion are given in Box 31.2 [6]. A rash is found in up to 75% of people with symptomatic seroconversion. A symmetrical, maculopapular, red exanthem, notably of the face, palms and soles, occurs. Pale pink macules and erythematous, perifollicular papules have been described. Occasionally there may be urticarial or vesicular lesions and alopecia. The histology is characterised by an upper dermal, perimicrovascular and periappendageal CD8+ lymphocytic infiltrate with a mixed perivascular CD1a+ dendritic cell/CD8/CD4+ lymphocytic infiltrate. Epidermal changes may be absent or range from vacuolation and spongiosis to epidermal necrosis [7,8]. Painful oral ulceration, genital ulceration, erythema multiforme and Stevens–Johnson syndrome may occur [9–12]. Acute erosive genito-crural intertrigo has been described [13]. If the CD4 count falls precipitously, oral candidosis can develop. KS has been seen in primary HIV infection [14]. The exanthem may represent infection of cutaneous Langerhans cells, and the oro-genital lesions sites of viral inoculation [15].

> **Box 31.2 Dermatological manifestations of HIV seroconversion**
>
> - Exanthema
> - Enanthema
> - Urticaria
> - Erythema toxicum
> - Erythema multiforme
> - Oro-pharyngeal candidosis
> - Acute genito-crural intertrigo
> - Oral ulceration
> - Genital ulceration
>
> From Bunker and Staughton 2002 [6].

Table 31.4 Useful prognostic indicators around primary infection.

Clinical (soon after initial infection)	Laboratory (3–4 months after infection)
Presence of symptoms	CD4 T-cell count
Duration of symptoms (>14 days)	Quantitative viral load (HIV RNA measurement)
Number of symptoms (more than three)	Polymerase chain reaction
Candidosis	Branched chain DNA
Acquisition of HIV from an individual with advanced HIV disease	β_2-microglobulin
Neurological involvement	

From Hawkins 2002 [5].

Thus, primary infection, including non-specific dermatological reaction patterns, may go unnoticed, unreported or undiagnosed. Because the dermatological and other manifestations of seroconversion are non-specific, there are many differential diagnoses (Box 31.3). In the past, syphilis was the 'great imitator', perhaps now it is HIV [16]. It must also be appreciated that two (or more) illnesses may coexist.

> **Box 31.3 Differential diagnoses of primary HIV infection**
>
> - Erythema toxicum (and its differential diagnosis, drugs, infections, connective tissue disease)
> - Urticaria (and its differential diagnosis, drugs, infections, connective tissue disease, neoplasia)
> - Erythema multiforme (and its differential diagnosis)
> - Oro-genital ulceration (and its differential diagnosis, drugs, infections, connective tissue disease, immunobullous disease, Behçet syndrome, Stevens–Johnson syndrome)
> - Pityriasis rosea
> - Guttate psoriasis
> - Reactive arthritis
> - Still disease
> - Infections:
>   - Epstein–Barr virus
>   - Cytomegalovirus
>   - Parvovirus B19
>   - Herpes simplex virus
>   - Human T-lymphotropic virus type 1 and 2
>   - Hepatitis A, B and C
>   - Gonococcaemia
>   - Syphilis
>   - Rheumatic fever
>   - Toxoplasmosis
>   - Causes of meningoencephalitis and pneumonitis
> - Drug reactions
>
> From Bunker and Staughton 2002 [6].

The greater the number, severity and duration of the manifestations, the more likely a more rapid progression of HIV disease will occur in that individual (Table 31.4) [5,17,18].

Precise diagnosis and the exclusion of other causes can be complicated in the acute stage by the interpretation of bacteriological and virological results (e.g. serological diagnosis of syphilis). There may be lymphopenia (usually a modest fall in CD4 count, a mild rise in CD8 count and an inverted CD4/CD8 ratio) and thrombocytopenia and a biochemical hepatitis or cholestatic biochemical profile. A skin biopsy may not be helpful, showing non-specific histology: spongiosis, apoptosis, interface dermatitis and mild, perivascular, chronic, inflammatory infiltrate. Seroconversion illness is diagnosed by positive plasma HIV polymerase chain reaction (PCR) alongside negative or equivocal HIV antibody tests (see Box 31.4) [5].

> **Box 31.4 Diagnosis of HIV infection**
>
> **Essential assays**
> - Fourth generation HIV-1 and -2 immunoassay (includes HIV-1 p24 antigen testing)
> - HIV RNA polymerase chain reaction (PCR)
>
> **Supplementary tests after inconclusive ELISA results**
> - Quantitative RNA PCR if not previously performed
> - T-cell subset enumeration
> - Exclusion of other viral illnesses, e.g. cytomegalovirus (CMV), Epstein–Barr virus (EBV)
>
> **Point-of-care or rapid tests**
> - Finger pricking, saliva (antibody tests that require a subsequent confirmation by ELISA/western blot)
>
> From Bunker and Staughton 2002 [1], CDC 2013 [2] and Branson et al. 2014 [3]. ELISA: enzyme-linked immunosorbent assay.

Primary HIV infection should be promptly treated [19].

Clinical variants
Dermatological manifestations of HIV infection and variations in skin presentation according to age, sex and patient subtypes are covered in sections later in this chapter.

Complications and co-morbidities
Eosinophilia can be found in 65% of ART-naive HIV-infected patients. Patients with eosinophilia are more likely than patients

without eosinophilia to present with a rash. Extensive work-up for eosinophilia may not be necessary in most cases [20].

Antiretroviral therapy and subsequent immune restoration with ART can precipitate exacerbations of immune or inflammatory disease – the immune reconstitution inflammatory syndrome (IRIS) or immune restoration disease (IRD). The term immune reconstitution-associated disease (IRAD) is all embracing and preferred [21]. Immunorestoration may reactivate the host response to latent infections or unmask autoimmune diseases in genetically susceptible individuals. IRIS/IRD/IRAD results from immunopathology that is characterised by an increased production of multiple pro-inflammatory chemokines and cytokines associated with activation of myeloid cells (monocytes, macrophages and neutrophils). There are similarities with facets of Covid-19 and its complications due to SARS-CoV-2 [22]. Examples are progressive multifocal leukoencephalopathy, uveitis or vitritis in cytomegalovirus (CMV) retinitis, sarcoidosis, hepatitis C reactivation, post-streptococcal glomerulonephritis and lymphadenitis in tuberculosis and *Mycobacterium avium-intracellulare* infection [21,23]. Although IRIS/IRD/IRAD may transiently increase the risk of KS and non-Hodgkin lymphoma in HIV, this should not contraindicate the initiation of ART [24]. Distinct cytokine-mediated mechanisms contribute to IRIS/IRD/IRAD associated with herpesvirus and mycobacterial infections [25]. Paediatric IRIS/IRD/IRAD is common and has an appreciable mortality [26]. Approximately half of all IRIS/IRD/IRAD events are dermatological [27,28] (see later in this chapter).

Disease course and prognosis

Prospective epidemiological studies in HIV-infected but untreated individuals with known dates of seroconversion have allowed the quantification of many aspects of the natural history of HIV disease, and have shown that the course of HIV infection may vary considerably in different people. Thus, although some individuals develop AIDS within 2–3 years and are termed 'rapid progressors', others remain free from AIDS for more than 10–15 years and are termed 'long-term non-progressors' or 'long-term survivors'. In the absence of treatment, the average time from seroconversion to the development of AIDS is 8–11.6 years, with a median time of approximately 10 years. Interestingly, this median survival time was the same in the USA as it was in Uganda [29]. It should be noted that most existing data were obtained before the availability (in the west) of ARV drugs and prophylaxis for *Pneumocystiis jiroveci* pneumonia. Clearly, such drug treatment, when available, has a profound and beneficial effect on the natural history of HIV disease.

Certain clinical and laboratory factors are known to influence and help predict the rate of disease progression to AIDS in the HIV-infected individual. Rates of progression appear similar by gender, race and risk category after adjustment for access to health care. The predictors for progression to AIDS may be summarised as follows.

- *Transmission risk group*. Time from HIV seroconversion to AIDS is approximately 7 years in transfusion recipients, 10 years for haemophiliacs, 10 years for intravenous drug users and 10–12 years for homosexual men.
- *Age at onset of infection*. It has been reported that for patients aged 16–24 years at the time of HIV acquisition, the median time from seroconversion to AIDS is 15 years, whereas for those aged over 35 at seroconversion it is 6 years.
- *Clinical indicators*. Patients with symptomatic primary HIV infection (about 75% of all HIV patients) progress more rapidly than those with asymptomatic seroconversion. Other clinical markers of progression include the development of oral thrush, oral hairy leukoplakia, herpes zoster, constitutional symptoms and weight loss.
- *CD4 T-cell count*. CD4 T-cell counts and their decline over time are very important predictors of disease progression. On average, the CD4 T-cell count decreases by $40–80 \times 10^6$/L annually; an acceleration in CD4 T-cell decline heralds progression of disease. A CD4 T-cell count of $<200 \times 10^6$/L is diagnostic of AIDS, and the median survival time in an untreated patient with a CD4 T-cell count of $<200 \times 10^6$/L is 38–40 months. The average CD4 T-cell count for the most common AIDS-defining conditions is in the range of $20–100 \times 10^6$/L.
- *Viral load*. Plasma HIV RNA viral load correlates well with the extent of viral replication in an infected individual. Progressively increasing HIV RNA concentrations can signal the development of advancing immunodeficiency. A single measurement of plasma RNA viral load early in infection is a powerful predictor of the subsequent risk of progression to AIDS and death. The combined measurement of CD4 T-cell count and viral load is an extremely accurate method for assessing the prognosis of infected patients.

Other factors that may be predictive of HIV disease progression have not been well defined. Thus, coinfection with other pathogens such as CMV, Epstein–Barr virus, hepatitis B or malaria has not been shown conclusively to accelerate disease progression. Intriguingly, it has been suggested that coinfection with hepatitis G may reduce the rate of HIV progression. The genetic background of the patient has relevance. Genetic markers of progression that have been defined include polymorphisms in genes such as *CCR5*, which influences the ability of cells to become infected with HIV, and differences in HLA class I alleles, which may influence immune responses. The size and route of the initial inoculum of virus may have an important role to play, as may the pathogenicity, virulence, attenuation state or genotype of the infecting virus.

Investigations

The diagnosis of HIV can be established through a variety of tests detecting the presence of HIV in the serum, saliva or urine. These tests either detect antibodies, viral antigens or viral RNA. A key element is that these tests have to achieve a very high sensitivity and specificity. Typically, blood banks in western countries will use a combination of antibody, antigen and nucleic acid tests. Historically, in 2000, the World Health Organization (WHO) estimated that inadequate screening of blood products had led to over 1 million infections with HIV worldwide. Antibody tests include enzyme-linked immunosorbent assay (ELISA) or western blot. Rapid or point-of-care tests are also available, but as their results are less reliable than laboratory tests (ELISA/western blot), they typically require confirmation from more established methods. Currently, the chance of a false positive HIV test is approximately 1 in 250 000 when an ELISA with confirmation by western blot is performed. Antigen tests detect the presence of p24 (capsid or core antigen) but they tend to be replaced nowadays by nucleic acid-based tests in the USA and the European Union. Nucleic acid tests can detect one or several sequences from the virus such as HIV-1 *gag*, *env* and *pol* as well as HIV-2 genes. Various methods are used to detect viral loads in patients, including reverse transcription PCR and quantitative PCR. Finally, while not strictly part of HIV diagnosis, the measure of CD4+ T cell counts is often associated with viral load testing to measure the progression of HIV. It is also routinely performed at the time of diagnosis (Box 31.4).

Management
HIV prevention
Behavioural interventions are continually applied to HIV control and prevention, and risks are better quantified [1]. Biomedical prevention of HIV has entered a new era with evidence mounting from trials for the efficacy of circumcision, vaccines and topical and oral pre-exposure prophylaxis [2,3]. Most transmissions occur via sexual transmission but there is still a proportion of infections transmitted by people who inject drugs. Prevention efforts worldwide have been achieving results as the number of transmissions in LMICs has been reduced by 30% via a variety of strategies. ART can decrease the transmission of HIV by 96% [4]. Circumcision is also somewhat effective, with a 60% reduction [5]. Newer strategies include vaccines and microbicides; one vaccine trial showed a limited efficacy of 31.2% [6]. Microbicides are yet another avenue in the prevention of transmission. In one trial, the application of tenofovir topically conferred protection in approximately 40% of women who took part in the trial [7]. More recently, oral pre-exposure prophylaxis (PrEP) has been an excellent method of preventing HIV transmission. In 2020, over 120 countries had adopted the WHO PrEP recommendations into national guidelines [8]. In addition, the use of long-acting injectable regimens will probably simplify therapy for patients living with HIV-1 infection [9] as well as in the context of PrEP.

Antiretroviral treatment
Antiretroviral treatment of HIV began in the mid-1980s using monotherapy with the nucleoside analogue (nucleoside reverse transcriptase inhibitor, NRTI) zidovudine (or azidothymidine, also called AZT or ZDV) and the demonstration that this was better than placebo in the treatment of symptomatic disease. However, the treatment of HIV infection was revolutionised in developed countries as a result of the introduction of ART. This has reduced short-term mortality and markedly increased the quality of life by preventing opportunistic diseases [10]. ART has developed as a result of controlled trials showing that dual nucleoside analogue therapy improves survival compared with zidovudine (AZT, ZDV) monotherapy [11], and that three-drug therapy, consisting of two nucleoside analogues and a protease inhibitor, is superior to two drugs [12].

One of the causes of drug failure is the development of viral mutations displaying reduced sensitivity to drugs. Such mutations may arise either because of the selection of mutants already existing in the viral swarm or the *de novo* generation of new mutations as a result of selective pressure by the drugs. Avoiding the development of drug resistance requires drugs to be used in combination, making the selection or generation of new resistant mutations more difficult, and by the use of potent therapy, which suppresses viral replication as completely as possible.

The dramatic improvements in survival with the use of ART coincided with the development of two new potent classes of drugs. Following the incorporation of viral DNA into the host genome, viral progeny are produced as a result of the transcription of this DNA, which accompanies cell activation. This produces polyproteins, which to be effective have to be digested by a virally coded protease. A variety of inhibitors of this protease are now available to clinicians and all are extremely potent. The other potent class of compounds is that of the non-NRTIs. As described previously, the virus encodes for a unique enzyme, reverse transcriptase, that is responsible for converting viral RNA into a DNA copy, which is then incorporated in the host genome. The originally introduced therapies for HIV were all nucleoside analogues, which act as chain terminators of the growing DNA chain. Reverse transcriptase can also be inhibited very potently by a variety of chemicals that act in a pocket of the reverse transcriptase closely adjacent to the catalytic site. The potency of these drugs was only appreciated when they were given with nucleoside analogues to individuals who had not previously received treatment [13]. This combination inhibits viral replication sufficiently enough to prevent the selection of viral mutants with resistance to the non-NRTI class [14]. Novel ARV drugs include integrase inhibitors, fusion inhibitors and potential compounds that might target HIV proteins essential for efficient viral replication such as Vif, Vpr, Tat, Rev and Nef [15].

Current guidelines for when to start treatment can be obtained from the British HIV Association (BHIVA) **[16]**. The original hypothesis for the optimum treatment of HIV infection was 'hit hard and hit early' [17], that is to use potent regimens and to use them early in the disease course with the hope of completely eradicating evidence of infection within a finite period. Unfortunately, as our understanding of the pathogenesis of HIV infection has improved, this hypothesis has turned out to be unrealistic, perhaps most importantly because HIV is also incorporated into long-lived cells that generally divide very occasionally [18], and which may be relatively inaccessible to immune effector cells. It is only during the process of cellular replication that anti-HIV drugs are active, and therefore the early hopes of eradication within a 3–4-year period have not been realised. It is likely that present treatment will be required lifelong to continually suppress viral replication. Early treatment was also advocated because it was assumed that HIV caused irreversible deletions in the immune repertoire, so if treatment was started late patients would remain susceptible to opportunistic infections. Fortunately, this has been shown not to be the case. Even individuals treated in late disease show considerable reconstitution of the immune repertoire [19,20].

Perhaps the most important practical reason for renewed caution about the timing of initiating ART was the emergence of a variety of drug toxicities that were unsuspected at the time the drugs were originally licensed. For the nucleoside analogue class this includes mitochondrial toxicity and lactic acidosis [21], and for the protease inhibitors a variety of abnormalities of lipid metabolism. However, the greatest obstacle to a more complete understanding of these syndromes is that, of necessity, most of the present studies are observational and cross-sectional and represent the end results of processes that have been present in the patient for some years.

New drugs have been developed in the main classes – that is NRTIs, non-NRTIs and protease inhibitors. The main objective of such new drugs is to improve adherence to treatment by enhancing the convenience of the regimen or to diminish side effects. Thus the protease inhibitor atazanavir (ATV) appears to be free of blood lipid abnormalities in controlled trials [22], but whether this will translate into freedom from the lipid redistribution syndrome remains to be determined. Classes of drugs that attack new targets within the replication cycle of HIV are also being developed; the most advanced of these are those that inhibit the process of fusion. This is an important example of where an understanding of the detailed mechanisms involved in viral infection has led to the development of new drugs. The most advanced of these is enfuvirtide (ENF, T20). This drug inhibits the contraction of the helical coils associated with gp41, which normally contract and bring the surface of the envelope protein of the virus (gp120) into close contact with the cell surface. The disadvantage of this drug is that it has to be given by subcutaneous injection once or twice a day, and it therefore seems unlikely that this drug will be tolerated in the long term for naive patients. Its chief benefit is likely to be in patients who are failing other therapies. Additional drugs available are entry inhibitors such as CCR5 co-receptor antagonists (e.g. maraviroc (MVC)). In addition, HIV integrase strand transfer inhibitors are now in use, including raltegravir (RAL) and dolutegravir (DTG) [23,24].

New drugs, more tolerable regimens, the limited development of resistance in fully adherent patients and increasing recognition of non-AIDS-related morbidity (e.g. myocardial infarction, stroke, cirrhosis, renal failure) and non-AIDS-related cancers were some of the factors behind moves to the earlier introduction of treatment at CD4 counts of around $350 \times 10^6/L$ and then $500 \times 10^6/L$ [25]. Evidence suggested that early treatment of HIV reduces persistent inflammation, T-cell activation and dysfunction, with significant implications for disease progression, morbidity and mortality [26]. Newer molecules targeting the viral capsid are currently in development and might offer yet another way to control the virus [27]. Furthermore, the use of anti-HIV-1 antibodies is a promising area [28].

The overarching principles for the treatment of ART-naive patients derived from randomised clinical trials demonstrating virological, immunological and clinical efficacy, are to start with and maintain a triple regimen of two NRTIs and one from another class (i.e. non-NRTI, protease inhibitor or integrase inhibitor) [29–39]. Compliance and convenience is enhanced by combination formulations and less frequent dosing with single-tablet once-daily regimen the ideal.

The overall success of ART is such that HIV-infected adults with a CD4 cell count greater than $500 \times 10^6/L$ on long-term combination treatment now reach the same mortality rates as the general population [40]. However, there will always be challenging patients and clinical situations. Treatment may fail for many reasons – from poor compliance and adherence to drug resistance. The principles of second line, third line and salvage treatment are available from BHIVA [39].

Drugs are listed by class in Table 31.5. The principal non-dermatological side effects are beyond the scope of this chapter, however they remain important in HIV medicine not least because of their influence on compliance and adherence, these being important in individual treatment [41]. Mucocutaneous side effects are detailed in the sections on drug reactions and special situations, and in Box 31.8 and Tables 31.6, 31.7 and 31.8. Lipid abnormalities and lipodystrophy are discussed within the section on drug reactions. The cutaneous manifestations of IRIS/IRD/IRAD are covered at the end of the chapter.

The most serious dermatological side effects of ART used to be: (i) Stevens–Johnson syndrome/toxic epidermal necrolysis with nevirapine (less commonly, efavirenz) and drug reaction with eosinophilia and systemic symptoms (DRESS); and (ii) pharmacogenetic abacavir hypersensitivity [42]. However, the use of nevirapine has decreased and HLA-B*5701 testing has considerably reduced the abacavir hypersensitivity syndrome (previous incidence about 8%) [42].

Dermatologists should be aware of the risks of drug interactions in treating patients with HIV on ART, particularly because of the metabolism of protease inhibitors by the cytochrome P450 system in the liver.

Table 31.5 Antiretroviral drugs used in HIV by class of action.

NRTIs	Non-NRTIs	Protease inhibitors	Fusion inhibitors	Entry inhibitors	Integrase inhibitors	Pharmacokinetic enhancers
Abacavir (ABC)	Delavirdine (DLV)[a]	Amprenavir (APV)[a]	Enfuvirtide (ENF)	Maraviroc (MVC)	Bictegravir (BIC with TAF)	Cobicistat (COBI, /c)[c]
Didanosine (ddI, DDI)	Doravirine (DOR)	Atazanavir (ATV)			Cabotegravir	
Emtricitabine (FTC)	Efavirenz (EFV)	Darunavir (DRV)			Dolutegravir (DTG)	
Lamivudine (3TC)	Etravirine (ETR)	Fosamprenavir (FPV, prodrug of amprenavir)			Elvitegravir (EVG)	
Stavudine (d4T)	Nevirapine (NVP)	Indinavir (IDV, IND)			Raltegravir (RAL)	
Tenofovir (nucleotide) alefanamide/disoproxil (TAF/TDF)	Rilpivirine (RPV)	Lopinavir (LPV)				
Zalcitabine (ddC, DDC)[a]		Nelfinavir				
Zidovudine (AZT/ZDV)		Ritonavir (RTV, RIT, /r)[b]				
		Saquinavir (SQV, SAQ)				
		Tipranavir (TPV)				

[a] No longer available.
[b] Ritonavir (RTV, RIT, /r) in doses so low as to lack antiviral activity 'boosts' the activity of the other protease inhibitors.
[c] Cobicistat (COBI, /c) is used in combination with elvitegravir (EVG), emtricitabine (FTC) and tenofovir (TAF/TDF).

DERMATOLOGICAL MANIFESTATIONS OF HIV INFECTION

Introduction

Skin disease may provide the first suspicion of the diagnosis of HIV infection, cause significant morbidity as the disease progresses and point to a diagnosis with important systemic implications. The number of mucocutaneous diseases, like the CD4 T-cell count, is a prognostic indicator of the development of AIDS and overall survival [1]. Cutaneous manifestations of HIV can be considered as good clinical indicators to predict and assess the underlying immune status in resource-poor countries [2]. Some skin problems are less consequential than other manifestations of HIV infection, but many are very distressing to patients [3] and some potentially very serious or fatal [4–7]. Although some situations are clinically straightforward and readily amenable to satisfactory intervention, all of the dermatological complications of HIV infection can be a challenge to diagnose and manage. They may present with unusual symptoms and signs, coexist with other pathologies and be altered by treatment; drug reactions are common [3–7] and wound healing is impaired [8].

In general, HIV dermatology presents five broad challenges to the dermatologist. First is the opportunity to make the initial diagnosis of HIV in patients with a seroconversion illness or with subtle or florid manifestations of one or other dermatoses associated with underlying HIV infection. Next, there is differentiating whether a skin problem is caused by HIV infection or by HIV therapy [9,10]. Third, the dermatologist's therapeutic imagination and experience is occasionally tested. Then there is the imperative for clinicians to be aware of the risks and prevention measures of occupational exposure to HIV [11]. Lastly, there are the implications for what can be learnt from the study of HIV-associated skin disorders for the better understanding of the skin in HIV specifically, and in human health and disease generally. For example, the virus has been demonstrated in the cutis of infected individuals; cutaneous dendritic cells and Langerhans cells may be the main targets in acute HIV infection and contribute to the pathogenesis of skin disease in chronic infection [12–15]; immunogenotype and immunophenotype may distinguish different cutaneous manifestations [16–18]; involvement of cutaneous nerves [19–21] may contribute to the pathogenesis of HIV-related dermatoses [22]; and the skin and mucosae may be targets for prevention (e.g. by male circumcision) [23,24] or treatment of HIV (e.g. by Langerhans cell fusion inhibitors) [25].

In the early years of the epidemic, suspecting, or failing to suspect, that a patient presenting with a common dermatosis known to be associated with HIV infection might be HIV positive may not have been so important. Indeed, in the past, the patient's best psychological and fiscal interests might have been better served by relative ignorance. However, the benefits of earlier diagnosis that have ensued from ART place a greater onus on the clinician than hitherto to discuss HIV risk with patients presenting with skin diseases known to be associated with HIV and to recommend assessment, counselling and testing. A high index of suspicion is essential in all dermatological presentations (the concept of 'high' versus 'low' risk is outmoded), and this is facilitated by the move to 'normalisation' of HIV testing through 'opt out protocols' where classic and extended 'indicator conditions' (e.g. in the case of dermatology, seborrhoeic dermatitis, psoriasis, shingles, mollusca, warts and fungal infections) are diagnosed in the general populace. The aim of this approach is to decrease the number of patients presenting with more advanced disease and reduce the amount of unsuspecting forward transmission [26]. An alternative scenario is the evaluation of the patient already known to have HIV infection who presents with dermatological symptoms and whose physician is concerned that the skin condition is a complication of HIV or its treatment. ART has significantly reduced the cutaneous morbidity of HIV infection but adverse cutaneous reactions to treatment are common [9,27–29]. Up to 30% of patients with HIV are coinfected with hepatitis C, of which there may also be dermatological manifestations [30].

Conventional clinical dermatological history taking and examination are the beginning of the diagnostic endeavour. Some dermatoses can be diagnosed confidently on clinical grounds, but experience has shown that it is easy to be misled. Immunopathophysiological and neurovascular mechanisms in the skin determine the symptomatic and morphological presentation of all skin diseases, so it is not surprising that 'things look different' in HIV-infected patients. Several cutaneous conditions may coincide, sometimes within a single lesion. The commonest dermatological conditions associated with HIV infection are listed in Box 31.5. Some entities may be even commoner in certain ethnic groups, such as African Americans [31].

Box 31.5 Common dermatological conditions in HIV infection

- Pruritus/xerosis/ichthyosis
- Nodular prurigo
- Folliculitis
- Cellulitis
- Eosinophilic folliculitis
- Pruritic papular eruption
- Seborrhoeic dermatitis
- Psoriasis
- Granuloma annulare
- Drug eruptions
- Herpes simplex
- Herpes zoster
- Viral warts
- Mollusca
- Oral and vaginal candidosis
- Dermatophytosis (including onychomycosis)
- Scabies
- Basal cell carcinoma
- Squamous cell carcinoma
- Kaposi sarcoma

From Bunker and Staughton 2002 [7] and Bender *et al.* 2020 [31].

Investigations are frequently necessary. Swabs for bacteria and viruses and scrapings for fungi may be taken for laboratory microscopic examination and culture. Skin biopsy is often undertaken for histopathology and culture for fungi and acid-fast bacilli.

HIV dermatopathology is an expert area and clinicopathological correlation is important [32]. Two or more entities may coincide [33].

PRURITUS, XEROSIS, ICHTHYOSIS AND PRURIGO

The prevalence of pruritic conditions (xerosis, ichthyosis, prurigo) in PLWH may be as high as 40% and more common in African Americans than white populations [1–3,4,5]. HIV belongs in the differential diagnosis of generalised pruritus [4]. Itching patients must be evaluated and investigated carefully to exclude a specific pruritic dermatosis (e.g. scabies, tinea, atopic eczema, pruritic papular eruption of HIV, eosinophilic folliculitis) and the medical causes of generalised pruritus (e.g. hepatic and renal disease, lymphoma). Excoriations, eczematisation and impetiginisation can complicate scratching. Prurigo excoriée and prurigo nodularis may eventuate [1,6]. Pruritic symptomatology is not uncommon after ART and the commonest causes are xerosis, seborrhoeic dermatitis and tinea pedis [7] as well as the ARV drugs themselves (see Table 31.6).

The mechanism of HIV-related xerosis is uncertain but cutaneous peptidergic neuronal loss has been demonstrated [8]. Higher rates of atopy, a predominant Th2 immunophenotype, a disrupted skin barrier and lower CD4 nadirs may also contribute [4]. Severe intractable pruritus with eosinophilia may indicate a subset of HIV-infected patients with hyperactivation of humoral immunity and augmented viral load [9]. Pruritus and xerosis are also side effects of ARV drugs, especially the protease inhibitors [10].

Treatment follows conventional lines and includes phototherapy [1,2,11,12]. Thalidomide has been used for prurigo nodularis [13], and a specific significant therapeutic benefit has been propounded for raltegravir (RAL) [14].

PIGMENTARY DISORDERS

Hyperpigmentation of the skin and nails and mucosae is seen commonly in HIV-positive people. Explanations include the use of drugs such as zidovudine (AZT, ZDV), hydroxyurea and indinavir [1], opportunistic infections such as toxoplasmosis and hypoadrenalism. Generalised hyperpigmentation may be a sign of late infection in its own right [2]. Oral and anal hyperpigmentation are signs of low CD4 counts ($<200 \times 10^6/L$) and have been proposed as indicators for the initiation of ART in resource-poor settings, but may not be sensitive enough for this purpose [3]. Persistent serpentine supravenous hyperpigmentation has been described [4]. Acanthosis nigricans (Chapter 85) has been associated with untreated HIV and with the metabolic syndrome and insulin resistance due to ART and protease inhibitors [5–8].

Vitiligo (including its spontaneous and ART-related repigmentation) and extensive hypopigmentation (drug photosensitivity related) have been reported [1,9–16] down the years, and a case of disseminated vitiligo appearing around nodules of KS has also been described [17]; vitiligo has recently been established as a firm association with HIV/AIDS [18]. Congenital vitiligo has been reported in an HIV-negative child of HIV-infected, ART-treated parents [19].

COAGULOPATHIES

HIV-related thrombocytopenic purpura (Figure 31.3) may present to a dermatologist, and can be mistaken for KS [1,2]. Thrombotic thrombocytopenic purpura is also associated with HIV [3].

HIV-infected patients are at increased risk of venous and arterial thrombosis (smoking and hypertriglyceridaemia are associated risk factors [4]) and cutaneous ulceration or infarcts. Possible explanations include acquired protein S deficiency [5], antiphospholipid syndrome [6], calciphylaxis and HIV renal disease [7], Degos disease [8] and CMV viraemia [9,10]. Also described is warfarin-induced skin necrosis in six South African women with HIV, tuberculosis and venous thrombosis [11].

Acquired haemophilia is a severe bleeding disorder due to the development of autoantibodies to factor VIII that presents with haemorrhages in the skin, subcutis and muscles; HIV-associated cases have been reported [12].

INFLAMMATORY DERMATOSES

Some of the inflammatory dermatoses associated with HIV infection (Box 31.5) are specifically discussed here because they are common or of specific interest. Box 31.6 lists inflammatory dermatoses that have been less frequently observed in the context of HIV infection [1–166]. With many entities, associations remain speculative. In the US in-patient population, firm associations between AIDS and hidradenitis suppurativa, vitiligo and chronic urticaria have recently been established. AIDS was also associated with higher odds of lichen planus and leukocytoclastic vasculitis but these associations were not maintained after controlling for hepatitis B and C status [30].

Erythroderma

Erythroderma in HIV may have several causes, and the same differential diagnostic approach employed in general dermatology is recommended. Psoriasis, eczematous dermatoses (e.g. seborrhoeic dermatitis and exfoliative dermatitis), drug eruptions, mycosis fungoides, Sézary syndrome, atypical cutaneous lymphoproliferative disorder and paraneoplastic erythroderma are all possibilities [1–7]. In a young black patient, erythroderma may be a marker for HIV infection [8].

Seborrhoeic dermatitis

Only 1–3% of the general population has seborrhoeic dermatitis compared with 20–85% of patients with HIV (Chapter 40). Seborrhoeic dermatitis is commoner in seropositive than in seronegative

Table 31.6 Principal cutaneous side effects of antiretroviral drugs.

Drug	Side effect
Nucleoside reverse transcriptase inhibitors (NRTIs)	
All NRTIs	Pruritus, exanthem, urticaria
Abacavir	HLA-B*5701 hypersensitivity syndrome, SJS, TEN, Kawasaki syndrome, anaphylaxis, lipodystrophy
Didanosine (ddI, DDI)	Vasculitis, purpura, SJS, anaphylaxis, Ofuji papuloerythroderma, gynaecomastia, lipodystrophy, acral erythema, diaphoresis
Emtricitabine (FTC)	Hyperpigmentation, pustulosis, vesicobullous eruption
Lamivudine (3TC)	Vasculitis, anaphylaxis, angioedema, jaundice, allergic contact dermatitis, gynaecomastia, lipodystrophy, diaphoresis, SJS, TEN, pigmentation
Stavudine (d4T)	Lipodystrophy, gynaecomastia, neutrophilic eccrine hidradenitis, tendon xanthomas, diaphoresis, TEN
Tenofovir (nucleotide) alafenamide (TAF)/disoproxil (TDF)	Diaphoresis, lichenoid eruption, DRESS, SJS
Zalcitabine[a] (ddC, DDC)	Anaphylaxis, angioedema, acne, photosensitivity, erythroderma, granuloma annulare, bullous eruption, diaphoresis
Zidovudine (AZT, ZDV)	Erythema multiforme, SJS, TEN, polymyositis, erythroderma, porphyria cutanea tarda, purpura, vasculitis, insect bite reaction, discoloration of the skin (especially in skin of colour), neutrophilic eccrine hidradenitis, acne, bullous eruption, lipodystrophy, bromhidrosis, diaphoresis
Non-nucleoside reverse transcriptase inhibitors (non-NRTIs)	
All non-NRTIs	Pruritus, exanthem, SJS, TEN
Delavirdine (DLV)[a]	Xerosis, urticaria, angioedema, dermatitis, vesicobullous eruption, purpura, vasculitis, seborrhoea, gynaecomastia, diaphoresis
Doravirine (DOR)	Skin reactions [sic][b], pustulosis
Efavirenz (EFZ)	Pruritus, eczema, annular erythema, photosensitivity, gynaecomastia, leukocytoclastic vasculitis, urticaria, flushing, folliculitis, exfoliative dermatitis, DRESS, lipodystrophy, peripheral oedema
Etravirine (ETR)	Prurigo, xerosis, SJS, facial oedema, gynaecomastia, hyperhidrosis, lipohypertrophy
Nevirapine (NVP)	TEN, SJS, DRESS, angioedema, anaphylaxis, lipodystrophy, exfoliative dermatitis
Rilpivirine (RPV)	Rash [sic][b,c], Cushingoid features
Protease inhibitors (PIs)	
All PIs	SJS, TEN, exanthem, toxic pustoloderma, pruritus, xerosis, hypersensitivity syndrome, anaphylaxis, panniculitis, tendon xanthomas, lipomatosis, lipodystrophy, acanthosis nigricans
Amprenavir (APV)[a]	Toxic erythema (20–30%)
Atazanavir (ATZ)	Eczema, photosensitivity, seborrhoea, urticaria, vesicobullous eruption, purpura, gynaecomastia, diaphoresis, jaundice
Darunavir (DRV)	Rash c.10% [sic][c], urticaria, hyperhidrosis (with ritonavir (RTV, RIT, /r), toxic erythema, sulphonamide moiety
Fosamprenavir (FPV, prodrug of amprenavir)	Rash (c.20%) [sic][c]
Indinavir (IDV, IND)	Erythroderma, dermatitis, folliculitis, pigmentation, seborrhoea, urticaria, vasculitis, paronychia/pyogenic granuloma, striae, angiolipomatosis, porphyria, jaundice, gynaecomastia, paraesthesia, diaphoresis, bromhidrosis, flushing, HSV, HZV
Nelfinavir (NFV)	Rash (c.20%) [sic][c], urticaria, dermatitis, lichenoid reaction, palmar erythema, vasculitis, gynaecomastia
Ritonavir (RTV, RIT, /r)	Rash (27%) [sic][c], urticaria, IgA-mediated hypersensitivity, acne, seborrhoea, bullous eruption, eczema/dermatitis, psoriasis, peripheral oedema, facial oedema, folliculitis, granulomas, photosensitivity, ecchymosis, haematoma, paraesthesia, diaphoresis, flushing
Saquinavir (SQV, SAQ)	Photosensitivity, urticaria, acne, bullous eruption, dermatitis, seborrhoeic dermatitis, folliculitis, papulovesicular eruptions, furunculosis, HSV, HZV, verrucae, candidosis, hyperpigmentation, psoriasis, warts, fixed drug eruption, gynaecomastia, paraesthesia, diaphoresis
Tipranavir (TPV)	Photosensitivity, HSV, HZV
Fusion inhibitors	
Enfuvirtide (ENF)	Injection site reactions, xerosis, pruritus, exanthem, acne, folliculitis, HSV, papillomas, ecchymosis, paraesthesia
Entry inhibitors	
Maraviroc (MVC)	Rash (17%) [sic][c], pruritus, dermatitis, lipodystrophy, folliculitis
Integrase inhibitors	
Bictegavir (BIC with TAF)	Rash (<2%) [sic][c], angioedema, skin reactions (uncommon) [sic][b]
Dolutegravir (DTG)	Pruritus, rash [sic][c]
Elvitegravir (EVG)	Rash common [sic][b], pruritus, eczema, urticaria
Raltegravir (RAL)	SJS, DRESS, pruritus, rash [sic][c], diaphoresis, HZV
Pharmacokinetic enhancers	
Cobcistat (COBI, /c) with:	Skin reactions common or very common [sic][b]
EVG/FTC/TAF	Pustulosis and skin reactions common or very common [sic][b], rash 3% [sic][c]
EVG/FTC/TDF	

From Todd 2006 [4], Okwera *et al.* 1997 [6], Penneys 1990 [9], Ward *et al.* 2002 [33], Bhandarkar *et al.* 2011 [48], Shear 2021 [**105**], Anon 2021 [106], Terheggen *et al.* 2004 [107], Sevila *et al.* 1996 [108], Bessen *et al.* 1988 [109], Torres *et al.* 1992 [110], Introcaso *et al.* 2010a, 2010b [111,112], Zhang and Sun 2013 [113], Modak and Guha 2013 [114] and Isaacs *et al.* 2013 [115].
[a] No longer available.
[b] Anon 2021 [106].
[c] Shear 2021 [**105**].
DRESS, drug reaction with eosinophilia and systemic symptoms; HSV, herpes simplex virus; HZV, herpes zoster virus; SJS, Stevens–Johnson syndrome; TEN, toxic epidermal necrolysis.

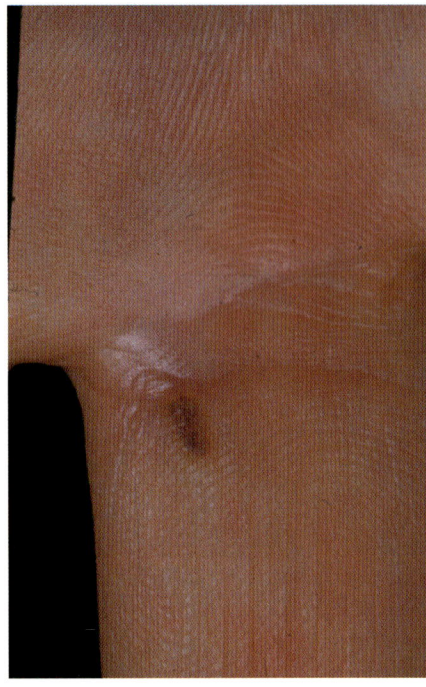

Figure 31.3 Thrombocytopenic purpura: purpuric macule on the finger. Courtesy of Medical Illustration UK Ltd.

Box 31.6 Inflammatory dermatoses less commonly associated with HIV

- Erythroderma [11]
- Photosensitivity/photodermatoses [12–17]:
  - With vitiligo-like hypopigmentation [18,19]
  - Chronic actinic dermatitis [20–22]
  - Porphyria cutanea tarda
  - Kwashiorkor [23]
- Allergic contact dermatitis [24–26]
- Prurigo nodularis [27–29]
- Chronic urticaria [30]
- Aquagenic urticaria [30,31]
- Erythema annulare centrifugum [32]
- Persistent insect bite reaction
- Hyperimmunoglobulin E syndrome [33]
- Hypereosinophilic syndrome [34–37]
- Papuloerythroderma [38]
- Pityriasis rosea (persistent) [39]
- Erythema dyschromicum perstans/ashy dermatosis of Ramirez [40]
- Pityriasis rubra pilaris [41–44]
- Lichen spinulosus [45]
- Acne vulgaris and variants/HIV follicular syndrome [41,46–48]
- Hidradenitis suppurativa [30,49–52]
- Lichen planus and lichen planopilaris [30,53,54]
- Perforating folliculitis [55]
- Kyrle disease [56]
- Neutrophilic eccrine hidradenitis [57,58]
- Lichen amyloid [59–61]
- Lichenoid granulomatous papular dermatosis
- Granuloma inguinale
- Granulomatous cheilitis [62]
- Erythema nodosum [63–65]
- Acroangiodermatitis/pseudo-Kaposi sarcoma [66]
- Varicose ulceration [67]
- Perniosis [68]
- Necrolytic acral erythema (and hepatitis C) [69]
- Pityriasis lichenoides acuta [70]
- Vasculitis [30,71–73]:
  - Associated with hepatitis C [74]
  - Henoch–Schönlein purpura and nephritis [75]; and hepatitis B [76]
  - Erythema elevatum diutinum [77–80]
  - Polyarteritis nodosa [81,82]
  - Parvovirus B19/papular purpuric gloves and socks syndrome [83,84]
  - Kawasaki-like syndrome [85]
  - Red finger syndrome [86–89]
  - Livedo reticularis/Raynaud phenomenon [90]
  - Cryoglobulinaemia; and with HCV [90,91]
  - Unilateral leukocytoclastic vasculitis [92]
  - Unilateral limb palpable purpura/occult abscess [93]
  - Degos disease [94]
  - Behçet disease [95–98]
  - Pyoderma gangrenosum [99–101]
  - Sweet syndrome (abacavir, arthritis, syphilis, opportunistic infections, influenza vaccine, IRIS/IRD/IRAD) [102–107]
  - Antiphospholipid syndrome [108]
  - Atypical neutrophilic dermatoses [109]
  - Cutaneous necrotising vasculitis [110]
  - Macular arteritis [111]; and hepatitis B [112]
- Systemic lupus erythematosus [113,114]
- Dermatomyositis [115–117]
- Systemic sclerosis [118–120]
- Relapsing polychondritis [89,94,121,122]
- Morphoea (Wolf isotopic response post VZV) [123]
- Anetoderma [124–128]
- Transient acantholytic dermatosis/Grover disease [129]
- Subcorneal pustular dermatosis [130]
- Darier disease [131]
- Autoimmune bullous diseases:
  - Commoner in African Americans than white populations [132]
  - Bullous pemphigoid [133,134]
  - Mucous membrane pemphigoid [135,136]
  - Pemphigus [137–140]
  - Paraneoplastic pemphigus [141]
  - Dermatitis herpetiformis [142,143]
- Acrodermatitis enteropathica [144,145]
- Eccrine squamous syringometaplasia (± cytomegalovirus) [146]
- Cutaneous mucinoses [147]:
  - Reticular erythematous mucinosis [148]
  - Lichen myxoedematosus/papular mucinosis [149–152]
  - Eccrine ductal mucinosis and follicular mucinosis (with scabies) [153]
  - Scleroedema [154]
- Lymphomatoid papulosis [155,156]
- Lymphomatoid granulomatosis [157]
- Atypical cutaneous lymphoproliferative disorders/CD8+ pseudolymphoma [158–163]:
  - Rosai–Dorfman disease (rosacea-like eruption) [164]
  - Palpable arciform migratory erythema [165]
- Dermatitis artefacta [166]

From Bunker 1996 [1], Bunker and Staughton 2002 [2], Penneys 1990 [3], Duvic 1991 [4], Cockerell 1991, 1993 [5,7], Cowley and Staughton 1991 [6], Rico *et al.* 1997 [8], Aftergut and Cockerell 1999 [9], Maurer 2005 [10].

homosexual men, and among infected patients it is more prevalent and has an earlier onset in homosexual and bisexual people compared with intravenous drug users [1]. Although found in seropositive individuals who are otherwise well, its severity is increased at CD4 T-cell counts below 100×10^6/L. This phenomenon is not adequately explained. The consensus is that classic seborrhoeic dermatitis represents an aberrant cutaneous reaction to commensal *Malassezia* yeast species. Possibly, the cutaneous immune dysfunction caused by HIV alters the host–organism relationship. The severity of seborrhoeic dermatitis may be related to yeast density or yeast strain [2–4]. There is a correlation between the numbers of yeast cells intimately associated with keratinocytes and the clinical severity of seborrhoeic dermatitis in patients with AIDS [5]. Patients taking ketoconazole have a lower prevalence of seborrhoeic dermatitis [6]. Also, imidazole treatment elicits clinical improvement, with a concomitant decrease in the numbers of *Malassezia* organisms per keratinocyte [7]. However, some studies have failed to demonstrate any fungal overgrowth in HIV-1 seropositive patients [5,8]. Abnormalities of skin surface lipids are not associated with the development of seborrhoeic dermatitis but are associated with HIV infection itself [9]. Seborrhoeic dermatitis has been related to low plasma zinc levels but this may not be significant [10]. Neuroendocrine and sebotropic factors are influenced by HIV infection, and seborrhoeic dermatitis and neurological disease may coexist in some patients. Seborrhoeic dermatitis is essentially a hyperproliferative dermatosis and keratinocyte stimulation may result from HIV infection because of either monocyte-derived lymphokines or a direct effect of the virus itself [11]. The nature of the relationship of seborrhoeic dermatitis with HIV suggests that *Malassezia*, although a factor, is not at the centre of the pathogenesis of the disorder [12].

Itchy, scaly patches are found at the classic sites for seborrhoeic dermatitis (Figure 31.4) and elsewhere. There may be folliculitis. Erythroderma has been reported [13,14]. An association of erythroderma, xerosis and seborrhoeic dermatitis with the development of dementia and spinal cord disease has been noted [11]. Extensive refractory seborrhoeic dermatitis appears to occur particularly in conjunction with pulmonary tuberculosis and AIDS in Zambia [15].

The differential diagnosis includes other causes of erythroderma and of folliculitis, eczema, psoriasis and dermatophytosis. Patients are often encountered with features of both seborrhoeic dermatitis and psoriasis–sebopsoriasis [16]. Scrapings can be examined for fungi to exclude tinea, and *Malassezia* species may be seen in large numbers. Skin biopsy may show hyperkeratosis, acanthosis, spongiosis, spotty keratinocyte necrosis, leukocytosis and subcorneal neutrophil infiltration. A deeper lymphocytic infiltration of the sebaceous glands and a more perivascular neutrophilic (with occasional leukocytoclasis) and plasma cell infiltrate is seen in HIV compared with classic seborrhoeic dermatitis [11,17,18]. The histology may be very similar to psoriasis.

Management follows conventional lines: emollients, topical steroids and antifungals and oral imidazoles. Topical pimecrolimus is effective [18]. Although clinical improvement of seborrhoeic dermatitis is often reported after immune reconstitution with ART, Schaub *et al*. [1] have opined that ART does not influence the prevalence, onset or disease-free survival times.

Atopic eczema

Atopic eczema or an atopic eczema-like condition has been thought to be common in children with HIV [1–3], but atopy is common anyway (see earlier and Chapter 41). One study has shown no increase in the prevalence of atopy in perinatally HIV-infected children compared with the general population [4]. In adults there have been reports of patients whose atopic eczema recurred or worsened during the course of HIV infection [5] and hyper-IgE syndrome has also been described [6]. HIV infection provokes a Th2-predominant immunophenotype, similar to that seen in patients with intrinsic atopic dermatitis and other allergic conditions [7]. Although some maintain that atopic eczema is not affected by HIV [8,9], it is much commoner in African American than white PLWH [10]. A decreased frequency of atopic diseases, fewer positive radioallergosorbent tests and lower average levels of IgE in HIV-positive compared with HIV-negative homosexual individuals has been found [11], as has dysregulation of IgE synthesis [12]. Fungal allergen-specific IgE responses may contribute to the pathogenesis of eczematous skin disease in HIV-infected individuals [13].

Psoriasis

Psoriasis (Chapter 35) is prevalent (2%) in the general population and can worsen or appear for the first time (often very severely) in HIV infection [1,2], but may regress preterminally [3]. It is more prevalent (*c*.5%) in PLWH [2,4,5] and even more so in AIDS [6]. HIV-associated psoriasis provides some insights into the pathogenesis of the disease, but the apparent paradox that a skin disease that involves activated T cells with a Th1 cytokine profile and responds to treatments that decrease T-cell counts should be associated with a systemic disease that manifests a Th2 cytokine profile and progressive T-cell depletion, is still not well explained [7–9]. It is now known that CD4 T cells producing IL-17 are central to the

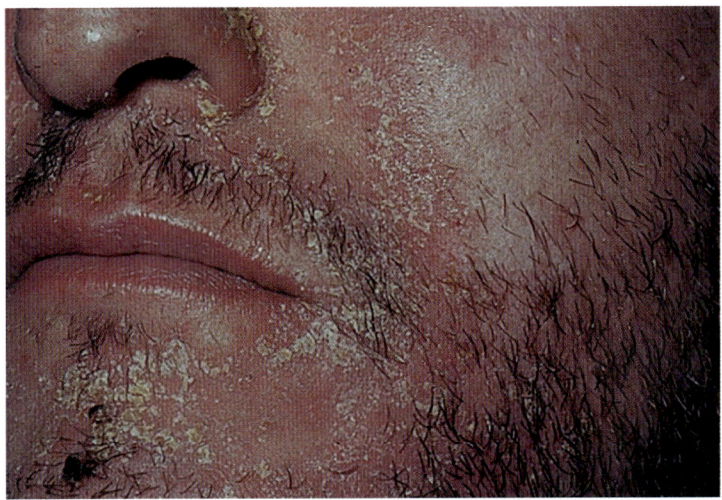

Figure 31.4 Seborrhoeic dermatitis on the face. Courtesy of Medical Illustration UK Ltd.

pathogenesis of classic psoriasis and this has to be accommodated by any explanation for the behaviour of psoriasis in HIV. Most patients with HIV-associated psoriasis are positive for HLA-Cw0602, as are HIV-negative patients with streptococcal-associated guttate psoriasis [8–11]. There are decreased numbers of epidermal Langerhans cells in the skin of HIV-infected individuals, as there may be, contentiously, in psoriasis [10–15]. Langerhans cells are infected by HIV and either the viral burden or HIV gene products may alter the antigen-presenting function of these cells. HIV gene products may have a role in the pathogenesis of proliferative epidermal disorders; transgenic mice that express some HIV genes in skin develop a diffuse psoriasiform epidermal hyperplasia [16]. There may be a selective defect in soluble antigen recognition by CD4 T lymphocytes, and numbers of CD8 memory T cells increase until just before death, creating an increased CD8/CD4 T-cell ratio in the skin. The depletion of suppressor CD4 T cells may result in unchecked pro-inflammatory pathways. Infections (e.g. streptococcal) that trigger psoriasis are common and the drive may be via superantigen-mediated autoimmunity; the HIV Nef protein has superantigenic properties. Autoreactive T cells bearing cutaneous lymphocyte-associated antigen may recognise autoantigens in the skin, initiating the molecular events that cause psoriasis, and once keratinocytes are activated, further antigenic epitopes can potentially be generated that maintain the T-cell response. Infections with viruses and bacteria, which are common in HIV, might contribute to epitope spreading. Polyclonal B-cell activation, increased numbers of γδ T lymphocytes, decreased natural killer cell function, increased macrophage nitric oxide production, hypercolonisation of the skin with *Staphylococcus aureus*, increased substance P production by infected immune cells, activation of human endogenous retroviruses, viral molecular mimicry perpetuating autoimmunity and immune dysregulation, defective reticuloendothelial cell function and enriched viral control alleles in the genome have all been mooted and discussed [7,9,17]. The last point has been interpreted to suggest the possibility that the excessive skin inflammation in psoriasis may be associated with an activation of antiviral immune pathways that were important to human ancestors who encountered viruses similar to HIV-1 [17].

Psoriasis in HIV-infected patients may be florid, severe and atypical (Figure 31.5). Psoriatic arthritis is held to be commoner in HIV psoriasis than in the general population of people with psoriasis [9]. Reactive arthritis (arthritis, urethritis, conjunctivitis), within the same clinical continuum as psoriasis in genetically predisposed individuals, occurs in HIV, sometimes very severely [18,19].

The differential diagnosis of psoriasis includes seborrhoeic dermatitis, atopic eczema, dermatophytosis, drug eruption and mycosis fungoides. Patients are often encountered with features of both psoriasis and seborrhoeic dermatitis – sebopsoriasis [20]. A psoriasiform eruption with the histological features of verruciform xanthoma has been described [21]. Investigations include mycology and skin biopsy.

Conventional treatment options for psoriasis serve most patients well [8,22]. Moderate to severe psoriasis (with or without arthritis) should be regarded as an indication for ART. Severe psoriasis can occur on cessation of ART [23].

There is no evidence that the theoretical risks and complications of phototherapy are clinically deleterious to individual patients

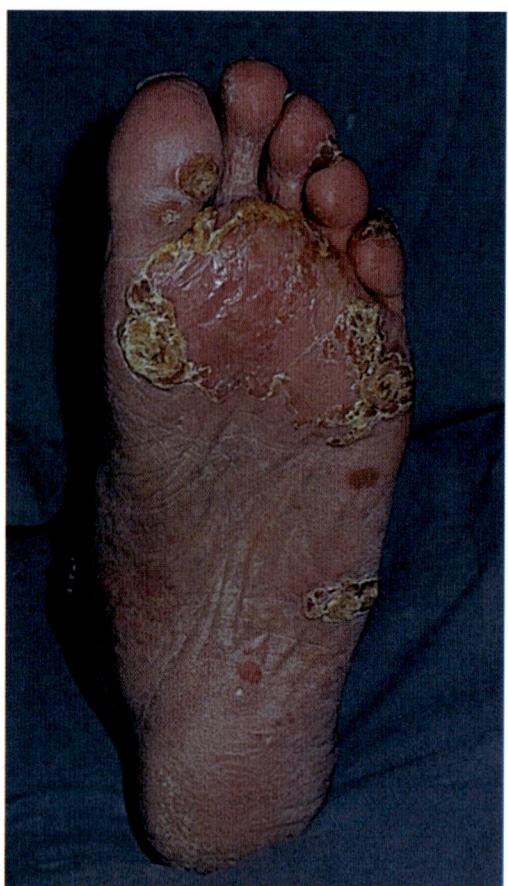

Figure 31.5 Severe plantar psoriasis in HIV infection. Courtesy of Medical Illustration UK Ltd.

[24–27]. T-cell numbers are unaffected and the Gag p24 antigen and HIV RNA levels may or may not increase [25,28]. Overriding the theoretical concerns about immunosuppression and photocarcinogenesis is the clinical need to relieve the morbidity of the severe, atypical, refractory psoriasis often seen in HIV [5]. Psoralen and ultraviolet A (PUVA) may be superior to UVB therapy [29].

The synthetic retinoid etretinate and its successor acitretin have been the most useful therapies for severe reactive arthritis and psoriasis in HIV infection, often alongside phototherapy; caution needs to be exercised alongside protease inhibitors with their retinoid-like side effects of xerosis, cheilitis and paronychia [1,8,18,19,22]. Ciclosporin and methotrexate have caused serious complications in HIV-infected patients, such as leukopenia and fulminant KS [30,31]. Methotrexate is probably best avoided; ciclosporin may have a place when urgent rapid control of potentially lethal generalised pustular or erythrodermic psoriasis is needed [8]. Claims have been made for the efficacy of cimetidine, carbamazepine, ranitidine, some antibiotics, ketoconazole and mycophenolate mofetil [8,32,33].

Treatment with zidovudine (AZT, ZDV) improves psoriasis [1]. Specific constituents of ART regimens, such as ritonavir (RTV, RIT, /r) and zalcitabine (dideoxycytidine (ddC, DDC), although this drug is no longer available), and ARV combinations appear to do likewise, with concomitant improvement of the clinical condition and virological status of the patient [8,34,35].

Theoretically, HIV infection might be thought to contraindicate the use of antitumour necrosis factor α (anti-TNF-α) directed therapy in psoriasis. However, etanercept and infliximab have been deployed [8,22,36,37], as have anti-IL-17 monoclonal antibodies and daclizumab (anti-CD25 IL-2 receptor antibody) in erythrodermic psoriasis [38,39]. Coates and Leslie [2] 'recommend that patients with newly diagnosed HIV/AIDS first be given an opportunity to respond to treatment with antiretroviral therapies given that restoration of the immune system is often associated with improvement in skin disease. In the interim, topical therapies, phototherapy, or systemic retinoids such as acitretin (or a combination of these) may be employed in an attempt to achieve disease control. ... [They] further suggest that, in patients whose skin disease is refractory to these interventions and in settings where regular follow-up is available to monitor for symptoms and signs of infection, severe and refractory psoriasis be treated with all available therapies, including biologic agents'.

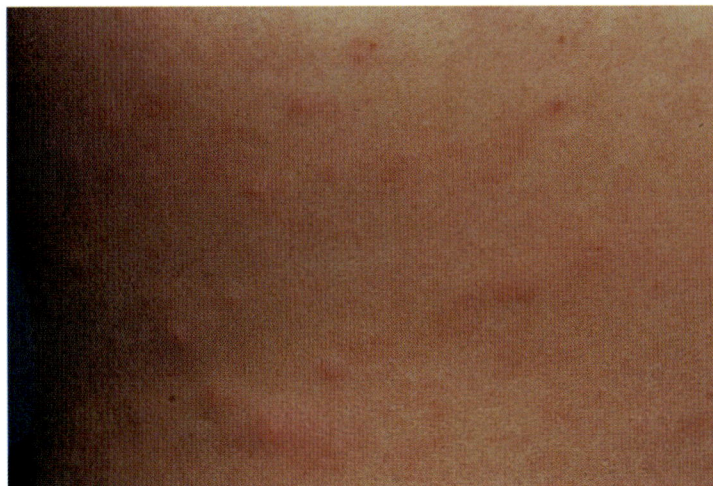

Figure 31.6 Eosinophilic folliculitis: excoriated papules on the trunk. Courtesy of Medical Illustration UK Ltd.

Eosinophilic folliculitis

Eosinophilic folliculitis is an HIV-specific disorder [1,2] related to Ofuji disease (Chapter 39). Originally thought to be an early sign of HIV infection, it is actually an uncommon presenting manifestation and especially rare in women [3]. It occurs at CD4 T-cell counts of $250–300 \times 10^6/L$, identifying patients at immediate risk of developing opportunistic infections, and can present during the immune reconstitution syndrome [4].

Clinical and histological overlap with the pruritic papular eruption (PPE) of HIV and bacterial, seborrhoeic or acneform folliculitis occurs [5,6], and this complicates interpretation of the earlier literature. The cause is unknown but Th2 cytokines (IL-4, IL-5), RANTES and eotaxin are increased in lesional skin [7] and there is a different cytokine and immunohistochemical profile compared with PPEs [6,8,9]. Foscarnet has been implicated in the development of eosinophilic folliculitis [10].

Eosinophilic folliculitis presents as a centripetal (face and trunk) eruption of pruritic, erythematous, perifollicular papules and pustules (Figure 31.6). Patients with eosinophilic folliculitis may be subclinically photosensitive [11]. It mimics staphylococcal or seborrhoeic folliculitis and acne vulgaris (especially acne excoriée), with which it can coexist. Histology can be characteristic, with degranulating eosinophils and mast cells in a perifollicular distribution [12].

The clinicopathological differential diagnosis is discussed in the section on bacterial infections, and in the following section on PPE. There may be a peripheral eosinophilia and elevated levels of IgE. Swabs are negative as the lesions are sterile.

Treatment can be problematic but the disease has virtually disappeared in the developed world in recent years with the introduction of ART, although immune reconstitution exacerbations have been reported [13,14]. Phototherapy is the most successful treatment modality but other treatments that have been tried include topical disodium cromoglycate, potent topical steroids, topical tacrolimus, oral antihistamines such as astemizole and cetirizine, oral antibiotics (erythromycin, tetracyclines, co-trimoxazole), oral itraconazole (for its antieosinophilic effect), oral dapsone, oral indometacin, oral isotretinoin and topical tacrolimus [4,15–22]. Eosinophilic folliculitis may be an indication for ART but may require treatment as above when exacerbated by ART as part of IRIS/IRD/IRAD.

Pruritic papular eruption

Pruritic papular eruption is globally a very common (if not the most common) cutaneous manifestation of HIV, the prevalence varying between 10% and 60% depending on geographic area [1–7]. It is most prevalent in Africa, India and South-East Asia. PPE is associated with eosinophilia and elevated IgE levels. It has some intriguing similarities with the papular eruption of pregnancy (Chapter 113). Insect bite hypersensitivity, as in papular urticaria (Chapter 34), is the likely pathomechanism [4,7–9]. The majority (e.g. 84% of Ugandan patients) have histology characteristic of arthropod bites and patients blame mosquitoes [4], 95% in one study [7]. Interestingly, in another paper, 75% had circulating bullous pemphigoid autoantibodies and up to 30% met the diagnostic criteria for bullous pemphigoid on histology, western blotting, immunofluorescence and immunoelectron microscopy [10]. Although increased CD8 lymphocytes, increased IL-5 and abundant eosinophils point to a Th2 response, the immunophenotypic profile of PPE differs from that of eosinophilic folliculitis [5,9,11–14]. PPE is a sign of an advanced degree of immunosuppression and may often be the first sign of HIV, occurring at CD4 T-cell counts below $100–200 \times 10^6/L$ (median $46 \times 10^6/L$) in one study [4], with the severity of the rash inversely proportional to the CD4 count [4,15].

PPE presents as excoriated, red, urticarial papules. Exposed parts of the body, especially the upper and lower limbs, are sites of predilection [6]. Scars from scratching and infection can be disfiguring and stigmatising [4,7]. The clinical differential diagnosis includes nodular prurigo, prebullous pemphigoid, scabies, papulonecrotic tuberculid, drug eruption, photodermatitis, secondary syphilis, onchodermatitis and eosinophilic, seborrhoeic, bacterial and acneform folliculitis. There is significant clinical overlap and this can cause difficulty in interpreting the literature.

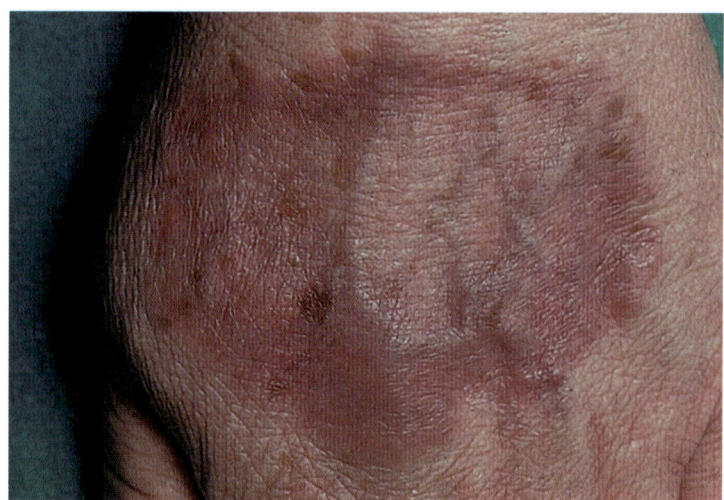

Figure 31.7 Granuloma annulare on the hand. Courtesy of Media Resources UCL.

Histology shows wedge-shaped, moderately dense, superficial and deep perivascular and interstitial lymphocytic and eosinophilic infiltrates. The epidermis is hyperplastic and there may be a spongiotic punctum [4]. It can be challenging to differentiate histologically from eosinophilic folliculitis but immunohistochemistry may be helpful [13].

The approach to the treatment of PPE is similar to that of eosinophilic folliculitis, with phototherapy the lynch pin; thalidomide and pentoxifylline (oxpentifylline) have been claimed to be efficacious [16–18]. Oral antihistamines are superior to topical steroids [19]. PPE is a strong clinical indication for initiating ART.

Granuloma annulare

Localised, generalised, diffuse and atypical (including oral and perforating) forms of granuloma annulare (Chapter 95) occur in HIV infection (Figure 31.7) [1–5]. Violaceous lesions may mimic KS. Lesions simulated mollusca in one case [6]. An association with zalcitabine (ddC, DDC; no longer available) treatment has been mooted [7]. Cultures are negative [2]. There is a variable response to ART.

Porphyria cutanea tarda

Porphyria cutanea tarda (Chapter 58) has been considered polyfactorial in HIV [1,2]. Familial influences, viral hepatitis B and C (e.g. in haemophiliacs), alcohol and sunlight have all been implicated but current thinking emphasises the importance of coinfection with hepatitis C [3,4]. N-acetylcysteine has been used for treatment [5].

Drug reactions

Drug reactions are a common challenge in HIV dermatology (Chapters 117 and 118) [1–4]. The types of drug eruption that have been encountered are summarised in Box 31.7. A morbilliform toxic erythema is the usual reaction seen (with fever, arthralgia, abnormal liver function tests and eosinophilia). Erythema multiforme, Stevens–Johnson syndrome, toxic epidermal necrolysis/Lyell syndrome hypersensitivity syndromes, DRESS syndrome (Box 31.8), erythroderma, vasculitis, fixed drug eruptions, cutaneous photosensitivity, photocutaneous drug eruptions and skin sensitivity to radiotherapy have all been encountered [1,2,5–14]. Co-trimoxazole (sulfamethoxazole–trimethoprim), dapsone, pentamidine and antituberculous chemotherapy, especially with rifampicin, thioacetazone (thiacetazone) and ethambutol, pose particular risks [6,7]; isoniazid has recently been cited as a risk [15]. Phenytoin hypersensitivity syndrome can masquerade as pyrexia of unknown origin [16]. Probenecid (given to reduce the nephrotoxicity of cidofovir) can cause a hypersensitivity reaction [17].

Box 31.7 Cutaneous side effects of non-antiretroviral drugs in patients with HIV/AIDS

- Morbilliform toxic erythema
- Erythema multiforme, SJS, TEN, DRESS hypersensitivity syndrome (see Box 31.8)
- Erythroderma
- Anaphylaxis, urticaria, angioedema
- Jarisch–Herxheimer reaction (with IRIS/IRD/IRAD): doxycycline
- Xerosis, cheilitis
- Lichenoid reactions
- Psoriasis
- Photodermatoses
- Purpura
- Oro-genital ulceration
- Nicolau syndrome: paracetamol
- Vasculitis
- Fixed drug eruptions:
  - Pentamidine: also causes ulcers at the site of injection
  - Foscarnet: penile ulceration
- Generalised fixed drug eruption: ibuprofen
- Palmar/plantar keratoderma: glucan
- Flagellate erythema: bleomycin
- Eosinophilic folliculitis: foscarnet
- Acrocyanosis: butyl nitrite

From Todd 2006 [4], Okwera et al. 1997 [6] and Cockerell 1991 [97]. DRESS, drug reaction with eosinophilia and systemic symptoms; SJS, Stevens–Johnson syndrome; TEN, toxic epidermal necrolysis.

Of patients with *Pneumocystis jiroveci* pneumonia treated with co-trimoxazole, 60% experience fever, nausea, vomiting and a rash [18]. Amoxicillin–clavulanate causes a skin eruption in about half of HIV-infected patients who receive the drug compared with more than 90% of patients with acute lymphoblastic leukaemia or infectious mononucleosis and 3–10% of the general population [19].

Glucan has been implicated in causing palmoplantar keratoderma [20]. The striking flagellate erythema due to bleomycin has been observed in HIV [21,22], but this is relatively common in general oncological practice. Pustular psoriasiform reactions to pegylated doxorubicin (used for KS) have been seen [23]. Fixed drug eruptions are associated with pentamidine, which can also cause ulcers

> **Box 31.8 Drugs implicated in erythema multiforme, Stevens–Johnson syndrome (SJS), toxic epidermal necrolysis (TEN), hypersensitivity syndrome and drug rash with eosinophilia and systemic symptoms (DRESS) in patients with HIV/AIDS**
>
> - Abacavir (ABC)
> - Allopurinol
> - Amprenavir (APV)[a]
> - Carbamazepine
> - Clarithromycin
> - Co-trimoxazole (sulfamethoxazole–trimethoprim)
> - Efavirenz (EFV)
> - Etravirine (ETR)
> - Fluconazole
> - Griseofulvin
> - Indinavir (IDV, IND)
> - Isoniazid
> - Lamivudine (3TC)
> - Nevirapine (NVP)
> - Nitrofurantoin (in pregnancy)
> - Phenytoin
> - Probenecid
> - Pyrimethamine
> - Raltegravir (RAL)
> - Saquinavir (SQV, SAQ)
> - Stavudine (d4T)
> - Streptomycin
> - Sulfadiazine
> - Sulfadoxine
> - Thalidomide
> - Thioacetazone (thiacetazone)
> - Vancomycin
> - Zidovudine (AZT, ZDV)
> - Traditional Chinese medicines
>
> From Todd 2006 [4], Okwera et al. 1997 [6], Rustin et al. 1989 [8], Penneys 1990 [9], Rotunda et al. 2003 [10], Kong and Myers 2005 [34], Calista 2005 [38], Bourezane et al. 1998 [45], Vidal et al. 1992 [98], Girao et al. 2002 [99], Tebruegge and Pantazidou 2008 [100], Zhang et al. 2011 [101], Loulergue and Mir 2012 [102], Viswanath et al. 2012 [103], Mittmann et al. 2012 [104], Shear 2021 [**105**] and Anon 2021 [106].
>
> [a] No longer available.

at the site of injection [8,24], and foscarnet, which causes penile ulceration [25]. A generalised fixed drug eruption due to ibuprofen mimicking CTCL has been described [26]. One patient treated for bacillary angiomatosis with ART and doxycycline developed a Jarisch–Herxheimer reaction (and IRIS/IRD/IRAD) [27].

Interferons may precipitate ulceration at injection sites [28]. Hydroxyurea can result in mucocutaneous hyperpigmentation (and melanonychia) [29]. Butyl nitrite may produce acrocyanosis [30]. Nicalou syndrome has resulted from intramuscular paracetamol [31]. Warfarin-induced skin necrosis complicating venous thrombosis in the treatment of tuberculosis has been reported [32].

The principal cutaneous side effects of the ARV drugs are listed in Table 31.6. The side effects of these drugs on the oro-pharynx, hair and nails are discussed in the section on special situations later in this chapter.

Exanthems, erythema multiforme, Stevens–Johnson syndrome and toxic epidermal necrolysis can be complications of the components of ART [6,9,33–42]. HLA-C*04:01 has been suggested as a risk factor for nevirapine-induced Stevens–Johnson syndrome/toxic epidermal necrolysis in a Malawian HIV cohort [43]. As in other causes of toxic epidermal necrolysis, intravenous gammaglobulin may be an effective treatment [6,44,45]. The syndrome of DRESS has been reported with nevirapine [45] and other drugs used in HIV. Abacavir is associated with a hypersensitivity syndrome of fever, gastrointestinal symptomatology, malaise and in about 70% of patients a rash, but this has virtually disappeared following screening for HLA-B*5701 [31,46,47]. Nevirapine has been reported to cause exfoliative dermatitis [48]. An exanthematous pustulosis has been reported including with lopinavir–ritonavir (Kaletra) [49,50]. Nelfinavir can cause urticaria [51]. Erythroderma, abdominal pain and renal failure have been described with indinavir (IDV, IND) [52]. An anaphylactoid reaction and allergic contact dermatitis to lamivudine have been reported [53]. Ritonavir (RTV, RIT, /r) can cause an IgA-mediated hypersensitivity syndrome, haematoma formation and subcutaneous granulomas [33,53,54]. Didanosine (ddI, DDI) has been associated with papuloerythroderma of Ofuji [33]. Neutrophilic eccrine hidradenitis has been reported but causation (drug or disease) was not clear [55].

Xerosis and cheilitis are common with protease inhibitors [56]. Some cases of granuloma annulare have been blamed on zalcitabine (ddC, DDC) but this drug is no longer available. Fixed drug eruption has been reported with saquinavir (SQV, SAQ) [57]; photosensitivity and photoallergic dermatitis have been documented with saquinavir (SQV, SAQ) and efavirenz [58–60]. Gynaecomastia has complicated stavudine (d4T) and didanosine (ddI, DDI) treatment [61]. Indinavir (IDV, IND) has precipitated acute porphyria [62]. Panniculitis has been blamed on ritonavir (RTV, RIT, /r) and nelfinavir [63] and vasculitis on dolutegravir [64]. Painful perioral and peripheral paraesthesiae and bullae have been associated with ritonavir (RTV, RIT, /r) and peripheral paraesthesia with indinavir (IDV, IND) [65]. Enfuvirtide (ENF) causes injection-site reactions including pruritus, pain, redness, induration, nodules and scleroderma [66–68].

The mechanisms of common drug reactions are not clearly known but correspond to classic immunopathological models. Hypothetical pathomechanisms in HIV include acute or reactivated Epstein–Barr virus, CMV or other viruses, polyclonal B-cell activation, hypereosinophilia, hypergammaglobulinaemia, immune complex formation and the generation of autoantibodies and autoreactive T-cell clones that interact with drug or tissue complexes. However, glutathione deficiency, slow acetylation and active viral infections have been shown not to be correlated with sulphonamide sensitivity in patients with AIDS [69]. It has been proposed that the pattern of immune dysregulation (decreased Th1 cytokines; increased Th2 cytokines; increased IgE, IgA and eosinophils) predisposes to drug hypersensitivity. For example, co-trimoxazole exacerbates this hypersensitivity by decreasing Th1 responses; macrolides increase Th1 responses [4,6]. HIV infection confers distinct clinical phenotypes and immune inflammatory mechanisms in severe drug reaction. Sustained EBV and CMV activation, unbalanced Th2/Th1 and overactive CD8+ T cells create a pro-inflammatory environment [70]. HIV infection may predispose to toxic epidermal necrolysis via depletion of skin-directed CD4+ cells [71].

It is common experience that adverse reactions to co-trimoxazole may disappear with continued therapy and that some patients will tolerate rechallenge with amoxicillin–clavulanate. N-acetylcysteine pre-treatment may prevent co-trimoxazole hypersensitivity [72]. Prednisolone does not prevent sulphonamide- or nevirapine-induced cutaneous hypersensitivity [69,73]. Tolerance has been induced for nevirapine and nelfinavir [74]. Drug hypersensitivity can also disappear at very low CD4 T-cell counts ($<20 \times 10^6$/L) and before death occurs. Therefore, a prior drug reaction does *not* constitute an *absolute* contraindication to continued or further treatment with a particular drug.

The ability of all protease inhibitors and some NRTIs, especially stavudine (d4T), to cause lipodystrophy is a matter of both intense clinical frustration (because the appearances are distressing and stigmatising to patients [75]) and mechanistic fascination. Fat loss (lipoatrophy) from the naso-labial folds, cheeks and extremities occurs, with fat accumulation (lipohypertrophy) in the abdominal and dorsocervical (buffalo hump) and mammary regions. Up to 80% of patients on ART may develop facial lipoatrophy within 10 months of starting treatment [76], depending on the regimen. With newer regimens not containing stavudine (d4T) or zidovudine (AZT, ZDV), this is much rarer. The syndrome is completed by hyperlipidaemia, insulin resistance (including acanthosis nigricans) and lactic acidaemia. Mitochondrial toxicity is one proposed mechanism [46]. Overall, the mechanisms of fat alterations in PLWH are complex, multifactorial and not fully understood, although they are known to result in part from the direct effects of HIV proteins and ARV agents on adipocyte health, genetic factors, increased microbial translocation, changes in the adaptive immune milieu after infection, increased tissue inflammation and accelerated fibrosis [77]. There is concern about accelerated atherosclerosis and cardiovascular disease [78–81].

Benign symmetrical lipomatosis [82], tender or painful multiple angiolipomas [83], striae [84] and tendon xanthomas [85,86] have been reported. There has been one case report of associated scleroedema [87].

Also of interest to dermatologists are the retinoid-like effects of the protease inhibitors, particularly indinavir-induced paronychia, periungual pyogenic granuloma-like lesions, xerosis and cheilitis, and curly hair. The mechanism is uncertain [88–91] but experience shows that isotretinoin (for acne) can be used safely and effectively alongside protease inhibitors. Concomitant administration has paradoxically resulted in *lower* plasma retinoid levels [92].

Overall fat alteration in HIV will have an important effect on lifespan, healthspan and quality of life as patients age worldwide. Management in PLWH includes classic lifestyle alterations with a role for pharmacological therapies and surgery in some patients. Treatment of lipodystrophy is challenging, but some successful approaches include direct excision, ultrasonic-assisted liposuction, suction-assisted lipectomy, fat injections, soft tissue fillers, human growth hormone and releasing factor, leptin, metformin and thiazolidinediones [47,76,93–96]. Lipomas and angiolipomas can be treated by excision and liposuction [83].

INFECTIONS

BACTERIAL INFECTIONS (Chapter 26)

Skin and soft tissue infections are underappreciated complications of HIV infection. They are continuing causes of morbidity in the ART era and the majority (over 80%) will be community acquired [1]. Cellulitis is slightly commoner in African Americans than white PLWH [2]. Cutaneous bacterial infection poses the risks of bacteraemia and septicaemia (up to 25% of episodes) or may *signify* systemic infection. Central lines, concomitant chemotherapy, injectable drug abuse and the presence of other skin diseases present additional risks [1,3–5]. Skin flora (e.g. *Proprionibacterium acnes*) can be systemically pathogenic in the immunoincompetent patient, necessitating great circumspection in skin antisepsis prior to surgery and instrumentation [6]. The clinician must be alert to the dermatological signs of systemic bacterial infection, such as splinter haemorrhages and acral papulonecrotic lesions. A high index of suspicion and a low threshold for performing microbiological investigations and skin biopsies (including Gram stain and special stains and cultures) should be inculcated to allow precise diagnosis and specific treatment. *Staphylococcus aureus* (including meticillin-resistant *S. aureus* (MRSA)), *Pseudomonas* species, *Escherichia coli* and *Streptococcus pyogenes* are the commonest isolates in that order; polymicrobial infection may be present in up to 40% of cases [1]. Hospital- and community-acquired *Stenotrophomonas maltophilia* infections are being reported; this organism is a serious and emerging opportunistic pathogen [7]. *Staphylococcus lugdunensis* is a highly virulent coagulase-negative staphylococcal species implicated in endocarditis and joint infections but can be a significant pathogen in causing skin and soft tissue infections, with a clinical incidence that is likely to be underreported, including in HIV [8]. Systemic antibiotics should be chosen on the basis of the clinical situation and sensitivities when they become known; possible meticillin resistance should be anticipated. Abscesses should be treated by surgical drainage but also biopsied and cultured, including for mycobacteria and fungi [9].

Staphylococcal infection must be considered when a patient presents with the common scenario of folliculitis. Clinical differentiation between staphylococcal folliculitis, *Malassezia* folliculitis, dermatophyte folliculitis, eosinophilic folliculitis, demodex folliculitis and acne vulgaris or rosacea can be very challenging, and these entities may coexist. Very rarely, *Micrococcus*, *Acinetobacter baumanii* and *Clostridium perfringens* folliculitis and herpes simplex and zoster viral folliculitis have been encountered [10–15]. Cryptococcosis has presented as a corporeal pseudofolliculitis [16]. Intertriginous staphylococcal folliculitis may mimic candidosis. Histologically, other patterns of folliculitis may be recognised, for example a lymphocytic folliculitis or perifolliculitis with mixed inflammation are commonly seen, and more rarely follicular rupture with granulomatous inflammation [17].

Secondary staphylococcal infection of the skin may be a complication of many of the inflammatory dermatoses discussed earlier in this chapter. It is becoming an increasing problem, perhaps because of decreased usage of trimethoprim–sulfamethoxazole prophylaxis in the ART era [18].

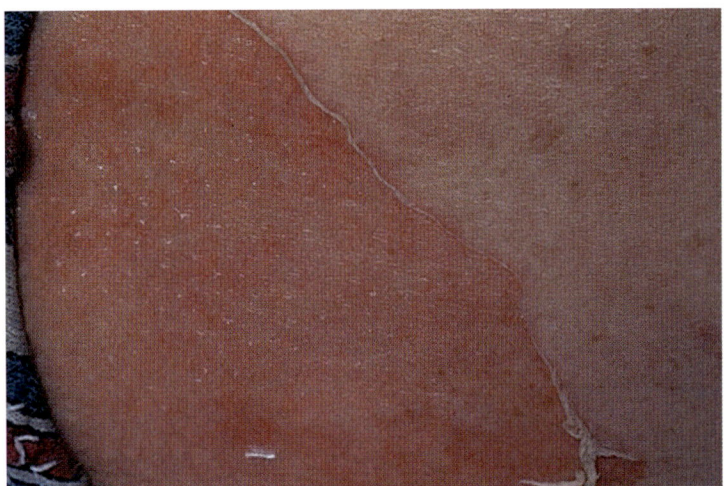

Figure 31.8 Staphylococcal scalded skin syndrome: staphylococcal pneumonia in an HIV-positive intravenous drug addict. Courtesy of Medical Illustration UK Ltd.

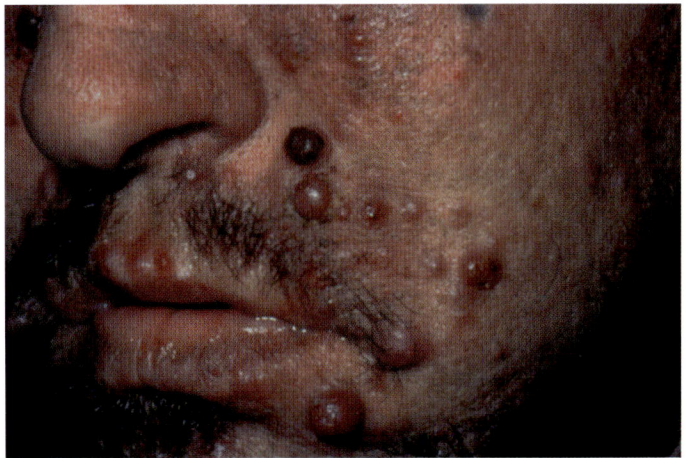

Figure 31.9 Bacillary angiomatosis: purple nodules on the face. Courtesy of Medical Illustration UK Ltd.

PLWH constitute a highly vulnerable population for MRSA colonisation [19–21]. Globally, 7% of such people are colonised with MRSA with substantial geographic variability, with the lowest prevalence in Europe and highest in the Americas and South-East Asia [21]. Nasal screening alone will underestimate the rate of colonisation by at least one-third [19]. MRSA skin infections have been increasing but may now be on the wane [22–34]. The most common type of MRSA infection among HIV-infected persons is skin or soft tissue infection caused by USA300, Panton–Valentine leukocidin (PVL) positive strains. HIV-infected people have an increased risk for both initial MRSA infections and recurrent infections compared with the general population [33]. Risk factors include prior exposure, hospitalisation, high-risk sex, injected drug use, poor HIV control, CD4 $<50 \times 10^6$/L, $\log_{10}$ HIV viral load copies/mL, absence of co-trimoxazole prophylaxis, partners with skin infections and recent receipt of a β-lactam or other antimicrobial [26,28,32,33,35–37].

Isolates are susceptible to co-trimoxazole, doxycycline, minocycline, ciprofloxacin, levofloxacin, vancomycin, linezolid, daptomycin and clindamycin but inducible resistance to clindamycin is increasing [28,32,33]. Recurrence rates can be as high as $c.25\%$ but minocycline treatment seems to be associated with a reduced risk of recurrence [34].

Besides folliculitis, manifestations of staphylococcal infections in HIV include bullous impetigo, ecthyma, cellulitis, abscesses, botryomycosis, staphylococcal scalded skin (Figure 31.8) and toxic shock syndromes [38–43]. Subcutaneous abscesses due to staphylococci may complicate injection or intravenous line sites. Surgical drainage is an important part of abscess management.

Group A *Streptococcus* erysipelas and lymphadenitis has been reported [44], as has pustulosis acuta generalisata [45].

A case of ecthyma gangrenosum (usually considered pathognomonic of *Pseudomonas* septicaemia) caused by coinfection by group A *Streptococcus* and *Staphylococcus aureus* has been described [46]; and another by meticillin-sensitive *S. aureus* (MSSA) [47].

Pseudomonas aeruginosa is an important potential cutaneous pathogen in HIV infection and AIDS. Ecthyma gangrenosum and panniculitis may be pointers to *Pseudomonas* septicaemia [48–51]; however even fatal cases of ecthyma gangrenosum may not show bacteraemia [52]. A rare case of ecthyma gangrenosum complicating psoriasis has been reported [53].

Bacillary angiomatosis, originally entitled 'epithelioid (haem) angiomatosisis', is caused by the Gram-negative cat-scratch disease organism *Bartonella* (previously *Rochalimaea*) *henselae* affecting the skin [1,54]. When it was first encountered, clinicians were intrigued by the similarity of bacillary angiomatosis to the cutaneous stigmata of chronic infection with *Bartonella bacilliformis*, the 'formular of verruga peruana'. These lesions may occur in the chronic phase of Oroya fever and are clinically and histologically very similar to those of bacillary angiomatosis. *Bartonella* seroprevalence is high in asymptomatic HIV patients in Brazil and is associated with breeding cats [55]. Bacillary angiomatosis presents with purple, papular and nodular vascular lesions resembling KS (Figure 31.9). Patients with bacillary angiomatosis do not appear to have an overt, acute, febrile haemolytic illness. Diagnosis is achieved by skin biopsy. Histologically, bacillary angiomatosis is distinguished from KS by being a lobular vascular proliferation where the abnormal, enlarged endothelial cells are epithelioid rather than spindled and by having a prominent neutrophilic infiltrate and neutrophil debris; there may be pseudoepitheliomatous hyperplasia [56]. The abnormal vascular spaces, lined with proliferating endothelium, contain *B. bacilliformis*. The clumps of organisms can be demonstrated by Warthin–Starry silver staining (Figure 31.10), immunoperoxidase staining of lesional tissue (where the bacilli are found within the abnormally proliferative cutaneous vasculature) or electron microscopy. Bacillary angiomatosis responds to oral erythromycin in most patients; isoniazid, rifampicin, ethambutol or clofazimine, either in addition to or instead of erythromycin, have also been used. IRIS/IRD/IRAD exacerbations have been seen, including a fatal case due to airway compression of the neck [57,58].

Syphilis (Chapter 29) may present atypically in HIV infection [3], confounding clinical recognition of the classic dermatological manifestations of primary chancre, papulosquamous eruption of secondary syphilis and gumma. The interpretation of serological tests can be complicated; they are not as sensitive in the immunoincompetent patient, so false negatives are a hazard

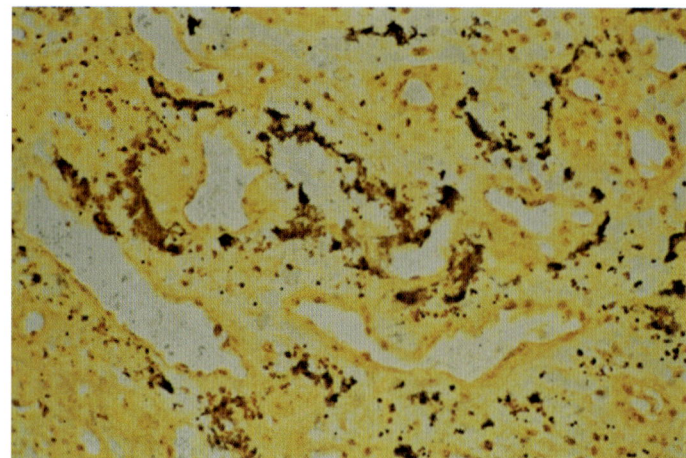

Figure 31.10 Bacillary angiomatosis: Warthin–Starry silver staining of *Bartonella bacilliformis* and proliferative vascular channels. Courtesy of Dr N. Francis.

[59–61]. Dermatologists should regard all genital, perianal and oral ulceration and any papulosquamous eruption with great suspicion and investigate them with circumspection [62]. Erythema multiforme and erythema multiforme-type eruptions can be the presentation of secondary syphilis [63,64]. Other rare manifestations of syphilis, not previously encountered by this generation of physicians, and other unusual presentations, such as keratoderma, finger nail involvement, leukoderma syphiliticum, necrotic red nodules and rupioid lesions (lues maligna), pityriasis lichenoides acuta, arthropod bite-like reaction, nodular syphilis (simulating lymphoma and KS), CD8+ pseudolymphoma in lues maligna, and gumma have all appeared in the literature [65–75]. A case masquerading as lupus vulgaris has been encountered [76]. Secondary syphilis IRIS/IRD/IRAD has been described [77]. Over the last few years rates of syphilis generally have been rising, and specifically in HIV-positive men who have sex with men (MSM) (rates have risen fivefold); this may be an unintended consequence of HIV PrEP [78,79]. Syphilis testing should be conducted at regular intervals in PLWH especially MSM, PrEP users and pregnant women [4].

Similar problems with yaws [80] have not been significant in clinical HIV practice. *Lyme borreliosis* pseudolymphoma [81] and a persistent erythema chronicum migrans (with meningoradiculitis) have occurred [82].

Reinfection with, or reactivation of, *Mycobacterium tuberculosis* (Chapter 27) seems to occur early in HIV infection, and extrapulmonary, including cutaneous [76], tuberculosis is common [83]. The clinical presentation is diverse, including lupus vulgaris [84], scrofula [85,86], scattered violaceous papules [87], acute miliary tuberculosis of the skin [88–91], keratotic papules, nodules and palmoplantar keratoderma [92], pilonidal sinus [93] and tuberculides [94,95]. Tuberculous lymphadenitis has been said to be a characteristic manifestation in HIV and in intravenous drug users coinfected with tuberculosis [96]. Management of tuberculous coinfection in about one-third of the estimated 30–40 million people infected with HIV poses particular challenges and is a specialist field [97,98].

Atypical mycobacterial skin disease in patients infected with HIV is usually due to *Mycobacterium avium-intracellulare*. This occurs as part of a disseminated infection in up to one-third of patients at CD4 T-cell counts below 50×10^6/L (rare below 200×10^6/L) [99]. Lesions described include violaceous papules, nodules, ulcers, cold abscess and simulating histoid leprosy [100–102]. Concomitant *M. tuberculosis*, *M. avium-intracellulare* and CMV has been seen [103]. *M. avium* complex has been isolated from an HIV-positive woman with erythema multiforme [104]. Skin involvement has also been reported with *M. kansasii* [87], *M. haemophilum* [105–107], *M. fortuitum* [108], *M. lentiflavum* [109] and *M. marinum* [110]. In these instances, the eruption probably occurred after primary infection of the skin by the organism, but a fatal case of disseminated *M. marinum* has occurred [111]. Sporotrichoid spread can involve an affected limb emanating from a distal primary site [112,113]. Aggressive multifocal Buruli ulcer due to *M. ulcerans* has been described [114].

The diagnosis of mycobacterial infection can be problematic because characteristic histopathological features such as caseating granuloma may be absent due to diminished cell-mediated immunity [115]. Spindle cell pseudotumours may be seen [116]. All biopsies where tuberculosis and/or atypical mycobacterial infection are suspected should be stained for acid-fast bacilli (which may be very numerous because of diminished cell-mediated immunity), and a separate portion sent for mycobacterial culture under appropriate laboratory conditions.

Prophylaxis and treatment of tuberculosis and atypical mycobacterial disease depends on the clinical scenario (including CD4 count) and the results of microbiological investigations (including sensitivity testing), and is an expert area. ARV and specific conventional antituberculous drugs are used. Atypical mycobacterial infection is treated with a macrolide and ethambutol.

Unlike other mycobacterial disease, the epidemiological and clinical features of leprosy have not been signally modified by the HIV pandemic [117–120] with the exception of reported manifestations of IRIS/IRD/IRAD [121–125].

Other bacterial infections

Donovanosis (*Calymmatobacterium granulomatis*) is known to coexist with HIV: extragenital donovanosis [126] and transformation to squamous cell carcinoma (SCC) have been reported [127]. Cutaneous granulomas due to *Corynebacterium minutissimun* [128], a subcutaneous abscess in one patient and rubbery skin nodules in another due to *Rhodococcus equi* [129,130], an unusual presentation of chancroid [131], a paranasal ulcer due to *Chryseomonas luteola* [132], rickettsial pox [133], an abscess due to *Peptostreptococcus ivorii* [134], a disseminated papular eruption caused by *Serratia marcescens* [135] and red plaques on the legs due to *Campylobacter* [136] have been described.

Botryomycosis is a rare, chronic, suppurative, bacterial infection that primarily affects the skin and subcutaneous tissues and has been associated with HIV since the early days of the epidemic [137].

HIV predisposes to necrotising fasciitis and Fournier gangrene [138,139]. Fournier gangrene is a hazard with a high mortality in AIDS and may complicate chemotherapy [140].

Dermatological manifestations of HIV infection

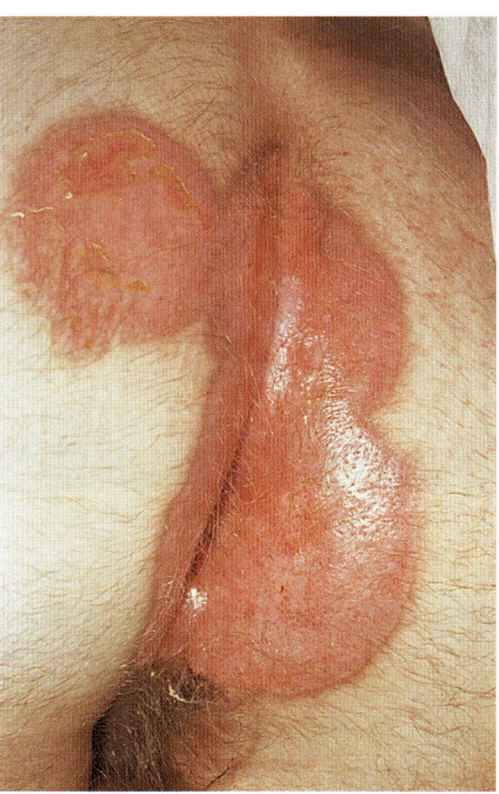

Figure 31.11 Chronic perianal ulceration in herpes simplex infection before the era of highly active antiretroviral therapy.

VIRAL INFECTIONS (Chapter 25)

Herpes simplex

Severe, chronic, ulcerative, perianal disease (Figure 31.11) caused by HSV-2 (human herpesvirus 2, HHV-2) was one of the first features of AIDS to be reported [1]. HSV-1 and HSV-2 infections are extremely common during the course of HIV illness [2,3]. PLWH with HSV-2 infection are also two to three times as likely to transmit HIV [3]. Although ano-genital involvement is frequent, any site can be affected with acute lesions that are vesicobullous but which become chronic, eroded and crusted, vegetative or ulcerating. HSV infection may not be self-limiting as it is in normal individuals. Persistent necrotic digits [4] and perioral ulceration may occur. A facial folliculitis (sycosis) has been reported [5], as has Kaposi varicelliform eruption after laser resurfacing [6]. A granulomatous exophytic lesion of the hand due to both HSV-1 and HSV-2 has been described [7]. Secondary bacterial infection is very common. Coinfection with *Candida* can contribute to atypical presentations [8]. Concomitant infection with CMV has also been seen [9]. Resolution can occur with specific treatment for HSV and general HIV treatment. However, herpetic lesions recur; the impact of ART has been to improve this situation, although HSV IRIS/IRD/IRAD is now a recognised phenomenon, and can be difficult to diagnose and treat being chronic, erosive, verrucous and pseudotumoral (see Figure 31.28) [10–13].

Diagnosis depends on clinical suspicion and laboratory virology (Chapter 25); additionally, acute and convalescent sera may be examined for HSV antibodies (immunoglobulin M and G). A skin biopsy may show typical cytopathic signs and positive immunostaining for HSV. In the USA, the Tzanck test is popular for rapid identification of multinucleate giant cells, which are not pathognomonic because they are seen also in varicella, herpes zoster and pemphigus [14,15].

The treatment of HSV infection in HIV requires systemic antiviral drugs (of which aciclovir is the prototype), including prophylactically [2]. The approach should be aggressive because HSV activates HIV replication [16]. Topical and systemic treatments for secondary bacterial infection are often necessary. HSV mutants (i.e. those with mutant or absent viral thymidine kinase) are responsible for HSV resistance, although progressive HSV-2 infection has been reported despite aciclovir therapy and demonstrable sensitivity of isolates to aciclovir. Concern is growing about the rise of aciclovir-resistance rates (as high as 10%) in HIV [3]. Intravenous vidarabine has been effective in aciclovir-resistant herpes simplex, but foscarnet (trisodium phosphoformate), which is a direct inhibitor of HSV DNA polymerase, is better for severe HSV-2. Famciclovir [17] and valaciclovir are alternatives to aciclovir. Cidofovir is a DNA polymerase inhibitor used in CMV infection, but is also effective against HSV. Vaccine developments for HSV have been disappointing to date [3].

Varicella-zoster virus

Reactivation of varicella-zoster virus (VZV, HHV-3) frequently accompanies HIV infection and can be severe [2,3,18]. Recurrences of VZV also occur in HIV-negative people and in up to 20% of HIV-negative immunocompromised patients. The frequency of recurrence in HIV-positive individuals is unknown. It is controversial whether all patients presenting with dermatomal VZV should be counselled about HIV testing, but it is regarded as a predictor of HIV infection in African patients [19]; one recommendation is that anyone under 50 presenting with VZV be tested for HIV [3]. Reactivation of VZV is the commonest cutaneous manifestation of immune restoration disease [20].

The distribution of the eruption is characteristically dermatomal but differentiation from herpes simplex may not always be clinically certain. Ophthalmic zoster may be complicated by conjunctivitis or optic neuritis, so ophthalmological input is advised. The involvement of the sacral nerves may cause acute retention of urine, haemorrhagic cystitis and constipation. Other manifestations include motor zoster, zoster encephalomyelitis and purpura fulminans. A non-bullous folliculitis has been described [5]. A chronic, verrucous dermatomal form can occur (Figure 31.12). An atypical, sometimes protracted, disseminated VZV eruption of sparse but ecthymatous necrotic lesions is occasionally seen, but there is usually a concomitant dermatomal recurrence. Linear Darier disease with chronic zoster superinfection has been reported [21]. The differential diagnosis includes *Pseudomonas* ecthyma gangrenosum and disseminated infection with atypical mycobacteria, fungi, vaccinia or HSV. Central nervous system and pulmonary or central neurological involvement should be suspected. The clinical diagnosis is supported by virological methods and occasionally by biopsy.

An important component of management is the treatment of pain. Potent analgesia may be supplemented by carbamazepine

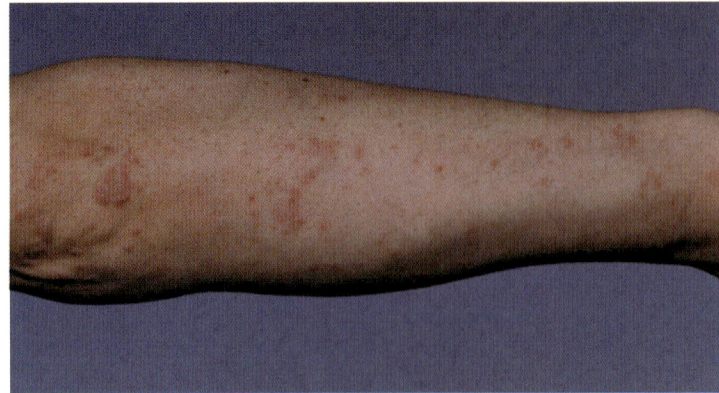

Figure 31.12 Chronic verrucous herpes zoster. Courtesy of Medical Illustration UK Ltd.

and dosulepin. Intractable postherpetic neuralgia may require specialised pain control. A topical or systemic antibiotic is often needed for secondary infection. Oral prednisolone is given by some. Systemic parenteral therapy with aciclovir is indicated in HIV-associated herpes zoster especially when sight, sphincteric function and facial expression are threatened and where pulmonary or neurological involvement is suspected. Disseminated VZV infection can be severe with a poor prognosis. Intravenous high-dose aciclovir is the treatment of choice. Intercurrent intramuscular VZV immunoglobulin has been used to prevent recurrences and may be used intravenously if aciclovir fails. Emerging aciclovir resistance may become a problem but vidarabine and recombinant IFN-α are possible alternatives [22]. Varicella immune globulin can prevent or modify the clinical illness and vaccination may boost immunity; the new recombinant vaccine is increasingly recommended for PLWH depending on age [3,18,23].

Cytomegalovirus

Reactivation of CMV in HIV infection occurs with a CD4 count below 50×10^6/L. Despite the frequency of ocular (blindness), gastrointestinal (dysphagia, diarrhoea), neurological (encephalopathy) and adrenal (postural hypotension) disease, skin involvement with CMV is relatively uncommon in HIV, but when CMV affects the skin, the mortality can be about 85% in 6 months [24]. It is possible that cutaneous involvement goes unnoticed and hence is underdiagnosed. Purpura, papules, nodules, verrucous plaques and painful ulcers (Figure 31.13), including of the perineum, coagulopathies (see the section on coagulopathies earlier in this chapter) and nodular prurigo (Figure 31.14) have been described [25,26]. The differential diagnosis of these clinical possibilities is broad. HSV and CMV skin involvement may be seen concurrently [15], and concomitant CMV, *Mycobacterium tuberculosis*, *M. avium-intracellulare* and mucormycosis have been documented [27,28]. It has been argued that CMV does not play a significant role in most of the cutaneous lesions where it is found [29].

CMV infection should be suspected histologically if dermal capillary neoangiogenesis, fibrinoid thrombi, necrotic endothelial cells, epidermal hyperplasia, acantholysis and keratinocyte degeneration are seen. Keratinocytes and endothelial cells contain characteristic

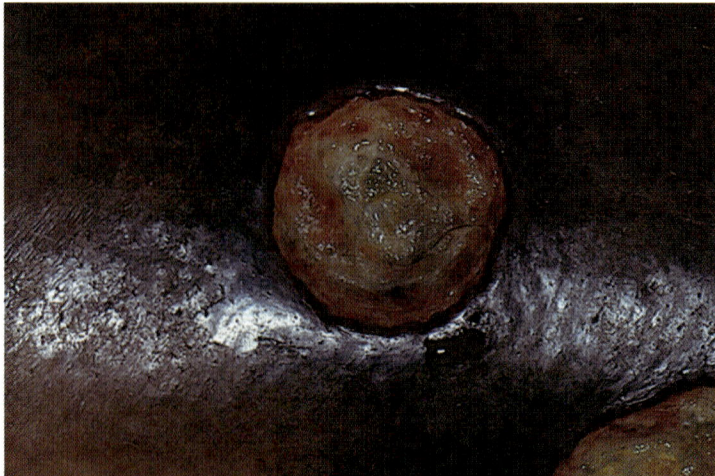

Figure 31.13 Cytomegalovirus vasculitis: leg ulcers. Courtesy of Medical Illustration UK Ltd.

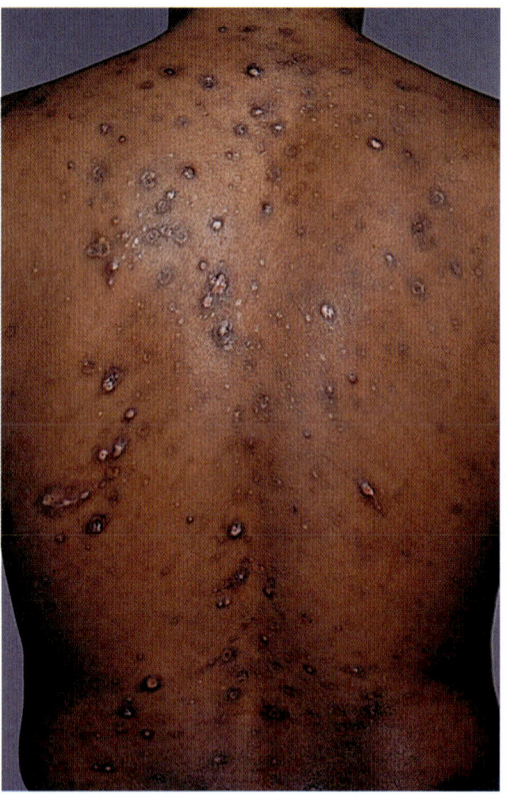

Figure 31.14 Cytomegalovirus infection: nodular prurigo-like eruption on the back. Courtesy of Medical Illustration UK Ltd.

CMV inclusions. Syringosquamous metaplasia has been observed [30,31]. PCR, immunohistochemistry, *in situ* hybridisation and electron microscopy may be employed. Skin biopsy material can be cultured with human fibroblasts to demonstrate the cytopathic effect; the demonstration of CMV viraemia can be similarly achieved by the co-culturing of a patient's leukocytes [32]. Serological testing may be difficult to interpret.

Treatment and prophylaxis centres on immunoreconstitution with ART, although a severe cutaneous ulcerative eruption has been reported after the initiation of ART and possibly represents

IRIS/IRD/IRAD [33]. Intravenous foscarnet, ganciclovir and cidofovir are specific treatments [34]. Mutations in the viral kinase allow the development of drug resistance.

Human papillomavirus

Warts are found in about 5–30% of patients with HIV [2,3,35,36]. Ano-genital warts (condylomata acuminata) may be a non-specific and insensitive marker for HIV infection. Around 40% of MSM diagnosed with HIV may have genital warts at presentation [37]. Human papillomavirus 6 (HPV-6) and HPV-11 (not associated with malignant potential) have been identified as the types most frequently found [38]. Ano-genital HPV infection is a risk factor for ano-genital cancer particularly of the anus (and cervix) yet it is rare for condylomata to contain HPV-16, which has a well-documented association with anal carcinoma. MSM have a higher incidence of both perianal warts and in situ and invasive anal carcinoma. Yet genital warts are more frequent in seropositive intravenous drug users. HIV infection may alter and worsen the expression and consequences of ano-genital HPV infection [39–41]. Anal HPV is a risk factor for asymptomatic bacterial sexually transmitted infections in HIV-positive MSM [42]. HPV-16 and other oncogenic types have been found in carcinoma in situ and high-grade dysplasia has been found in genital warts from HIV-positive individuals [43,44]. The risk of progression of anal intraepithelial neoplasia associated with anal HPV infection to invasive SCC was originally thought to be low [45] but the odds of developing anal cancer following ano-genital warts in HIV are approximately 13 [46]. Overall, anal cancer may be 50 times and penis cancer 5–6 times commoner in HIV (Chapter 109). Invasive cervical cancer is possibly more common but does behave more aggressively and is an AIDS-defining diagnosis. It has been suggested that all HPV-associated cancers should be included as AIDS-defining illnesses [47].

The clinical diagnosis of warts is straightforward when classic sites are involved with lesions of typical morphology. In patients with HIV, warts may be extensive, numerous, exuberant and admixed with other pathologies (e.g. mollusca) (Figure 31.15). HPV contributes to the causation of Bowen disease [48], erythroplasia of Queyrat and Bowenoid papulosis (clinically like viral warts, often pigmented, with the histology of Bowen disease/SCC in situ), and invasive penile, anal and cervical cancer. A presentation resembling the rare, inherited condition, epidermodysplasia verruciformis, can occur (Figure 31.16) [49–54], clinically resembling pityriasis versicolor in some cases. It may not improve with ART and is associated with mucosal HPV and lymphoproliferative disease. Epidermodysplasia verruciformis is also increasingly seen as an acquired HPV (types 1, 2, 5, 6, 16 and 52) related dermatosis in many vertically infected HIV children in sub-Saharan Africa. It is disfiguring and stigmatising and unresponsive to ART, as in adults [55,56]. CD4 T-cell estimation and HIV testing should be considered in any patient with atypical clinical presentations of viral warts. Occasionally, a skin biopsy may be necessary, particularly if in situ or invasive squamous cell malignancy is suspected but the risks of SCC in acquired epidermodysplasia verruciformis are not established [18].

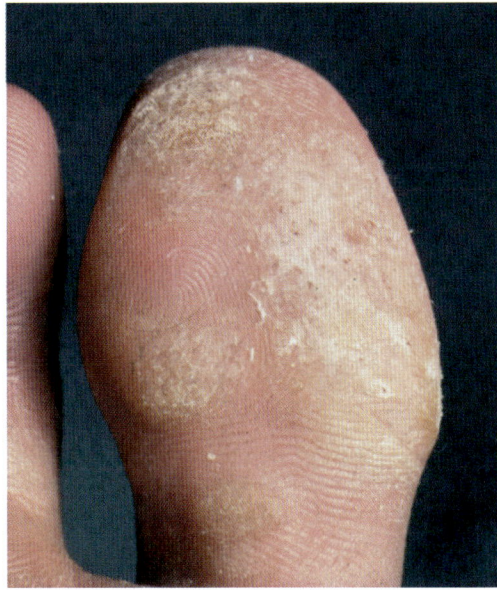

Figure 31.15 Human papillomavirus infection: myrmecia on the great toe. Courtesy of Media Resources UCL.

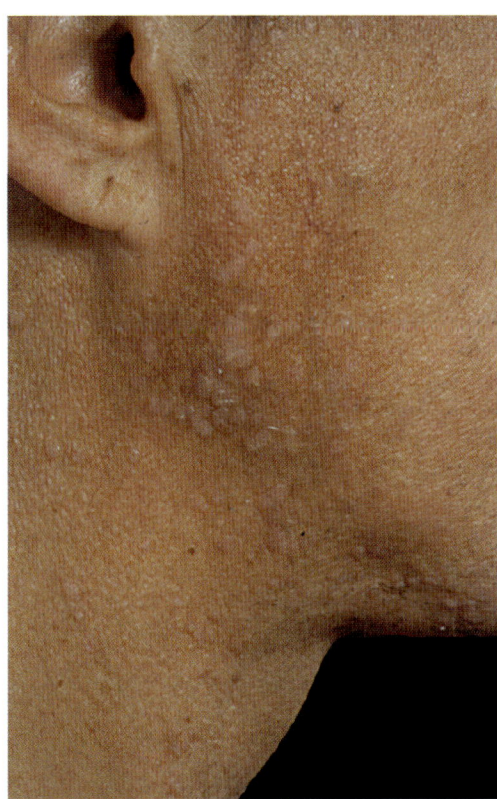

Figure 31.16 Epidermodysplasia verruciformis in human papillomavirus infection: discrete and confluent warty papules on the right cheek and neck. Courtesy of Imperial College School of Medicine.

Conventional treatments for warts may fail. Topical imiquimod and topical and intravenous cidofovir have been used [57–60]. ART can lead to the regression of warts, but some patients have been seen whose warts persist or return after many years of remission; this seems to be related to low nadir or mean CD4 count [61–65] and/or is a manifestation of IRIS/IRD/IRAD [10]. The future for

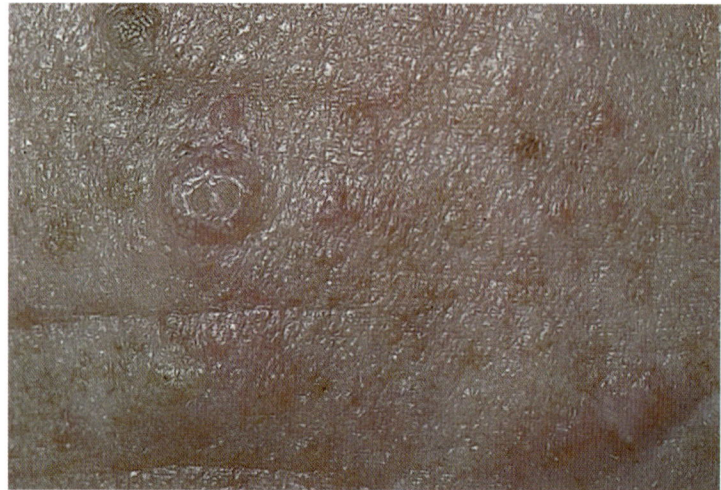

Figure 31.17 Atypical mollusca: flesh-coloured papules and nodules on the forehead. Courtesy of Media Resources UCL.

the containment of HPV-related disease including cancer generally, but especially in HIV, looks brighter with the development and introduction of effective vaccines [18,66,67]. HPV vaccination may be therapeutic [68–70].

Mollusca

Mollusca are caused by infection with four closely related molluscipoxviruses, MCV-1 to -4, and frequently affect the skin of patients with HIV [71], in homosexual seropositive patients more in than intravenous drug users [39]. Virtually all paediatric infections are caused by MCV-1, yet in HIV patients MCV-2 causes 60% of the infections [72,73] suggesting that HIV-associated mollusca does not represent the recurrence of childhood mollusca. There may be several or many papular or larger, 'giant', nodular lesions, particularly on the face and neck. Often, in the context of HIV infection, the lesions do not manifest pathognomonic classic morphology (Figure 31.17) and are not typically domed in shape and lack the characteristic central umbilication or delling [74,75]. A cheek abscess has been described [76]. Florid, extensive, genital lesions with cellulitis have been reported [77]. The differential diagnosis includes sebaceous hyperplasia, syringoma, warts, cryptococcosis, histoplasmosis and basal cell carcinoma. Mollusca can coincide with all of these entities. Mollusca are diagnosed with the greatest confidence by skin biopsy because the clinical morphology in the HIV-positive patient may not be pathognomonic. The classic histological features are usually present. A molluscum involving an epidermoid cyst and causing a xanthogranuloma-like reaction has been described [78]. Mollusca may represent an immunoreconstitution phenomenon.

Mollusca vary widely in response to conventional treatment [2]. The introduction of ART can elicit resolution, but an increased incidence and as a manifestation of IRIS/IRD/IRAD have also been reported [61,65,75]. Topical imiquimod, topical and systemic cidofovir [59,79,80], electron beam therapy [81] and diphencyprone [82] have been used.

Other viral infections

Parvovirus B19 can cause cutaneous vasculitis [83] and a persistent papular purpuric gloves and socks syndrome with anaemia [84]. Measles in children may behave atypically and with more complications [85]; it has been reported in vaccinated HIV-positive adults [86]. EBV-positive mucocutaneous ulcers and lymphoproliferative lesions have been described in HIV [87]. Human polyomavirus 6 and 7 have been incriminated in a pruritic and dyskeratotic dermatosis [88].

The data available to date indicate that PLWH infected with Covid-19 are largely affected by similar features of disease risk and progression as HIV-uninfected patients. Older age and co-morbidities appear to be the main factors for severe Covid-19 morbidity and mortality [89].

FUNGAL INFECTIONS (Chapter 32)

Candidosis

Oral candidosis has classically been associated with immunosuppressive states and was one of the first features to be recognised in the early days of the HIV epidemic before the syndrome was clearly defined and the causative agent identified [1]. Oesophageal candidosis is an AIDS-defining diagnosis. It is commoner in homosexual seropositive patients than intravenous drug users [2]. Pseudomembranous disease is the commonest oro-pharygeal manifestation but red patches are also seen. *Candida albicans* is the most frequent species isolated. Treatment is with single-dose oral fluconazole [3] or localised oral miconazole [4,5]. Resistance can occur. Long-term prophylaxis with azoles is avoided. Oral candidosis predicts AIDS in a median of 2 years and so is an indication for the institution of prophylaxis for *Pneumocystis jiroveci* and ART. In the past, practically everyone with HIV infection would have had *Candida* as a pathogen at some stage in their disease [6], but this may not be the case now in western countries with earlier diagnosis. Vaginal candidosis can occur early in HIV infection [7] and is the commonest presentation of HIV in women in the USA. In HIV, *Candida* can also be responsible for paronychia, onychodystrophy, angular cheilitis and intertriginous candidosis [8,9]. A generalised cutaneous eruption of papules and nodules has been described [10]. *C. krusei* fungaemia has been reported in HIV/AIDS patients previously exposed to azole antifungals and skin lesions may be common [11]. Cutaneous candidosis, systemic candidosis or invasive candidosis including candidaemia, *Candida* disease due to species other than *C. albicans* and resistance to azoles and other antifungals, are all becoming more common [12]. Finally, candidosis is recognised as an immunoreconstitution phenomenon.

Dermatophytosis

Generally, dermatophytes are only occasionally responsible for significant cutaneous infection in immunocompromised patients [13],

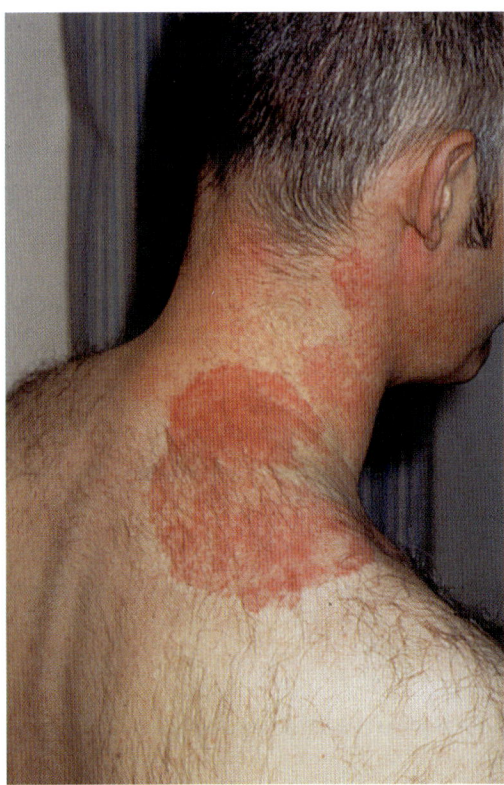

Figure 31.18 Tinea corporis and faciei. Courtesy of Medical Illustration UK Ltd.

Esoteric superficial fungal infections have also been reported. A patient presented with 'dirty' brown spots on the scrotum from which were co-cultured the dematiaceous fungi *Bipolaris* and *Curvularia* [28]. A new species, *T. eboreum*, has been isolated from an HIV patient with tinea pedis [29]. A case of fingernail proximal subungual onychomycosis with associated skin infection caused by an opportunistic mould, *Aspergillus sydowii*, has been published [23].

Dermatophyte infection is treated with conventional topical and systemic therapy (Chapter 32) depending on clinical assessment and the results of mycology. Oral terbinafine is safe and efficacious [30].

Histoplasmosis

Extrapulmonary infection with histoplasmosis is an indicator condition in the case definition of AIDS (see Box 31.1). Histoplasmosis is very rare in the UK and Europe so a travel history is important, but some autochthonous HIV-associated cases have occurred in Europe. In endemic areas, such as North, Central and Latin America, Africa, India or the Far East, 20–50% of patients with AIDS will develop histoplasmosis at CD4 counts below 200×10^6/L. The systemic presentation can mimic tuberculosis. There is fever, lymphadenopathy, hepatosplenomegaly, lung disease and pancytopenia. Patients may also be alcoholics and heavy smokers. It may be fatal (compared with the self-limiting bronchopneumonia seen in immunocompetent individuals). Disseminated histoplasmosis may produce skin involvement in up to 10% of patients in the USA but in between 38% and 85% of Latin American cases. The skin may be the most frequent site of localised infection (8.3%). A wide morphological spectrum of lesions is seen. Macules, papules, plaques, crusted/eroded/ulcerated papules and plaques mainly located on the face and chest, as well as oral involvement with erosions and ulcers, are the commonest presentations, with more variation in lesions associated with higher CD4 counts. An exanthem, lesions resembling molluscum contagiosum, acneform folliculitis, nodules and tumours, psoriasiform eruptions including keratotic plaques, varicelliform lesions, vasculitic lesions, erythema multiforme-like lesions, an exfoliative dermatitis, an atypical ecthyma and depressed pits on the palms and soles and lesions admixed with KS, have been described. Two-thirds of patients with skin disease may have pulmonary involvement and in one series of disseminated cutaneous histoplasmosis approximately 40% of the cases died [14,31–41]. Cutaneous histoplasmosis may be seen as an immunoreconstitution phenomenon.

Systemic diagnosis is by chest X-ray, Wright staining of a blood film (demonstrating intracellular fungi), blood cultures, lymph node, liver or skin biopsy or Tzank cytology [42,43] and culture. *Histoplasma capsulatum* can be demonstrated by Gomori methenamine silver stain of a skin biopsy section. A wide variety of unusual cutaneous histopathological findings have been described [41].

Treatment is by ART and itraconazole and/or amphotericin, with long-term itraconazole as secondary prophylaxis because relapse is so common [14,36,44].

but the situation is subtly different in HIV infection [14]. Homosexual men are very likely to have a superficial fungal infection regardless of their HIV status. For example, in Sweden, Torssander *et al.* [15] showed that 37% of seropositive homosexual men had mycologically proven toe cleft dermatophytosis, usually *Trichophyton rubrum*, compared with about 30% of seronegative homosexual men and about 9% of heterosexual men. Clinical findings, for example interdigital scaling, similar to those of tinea pedis are very common in men. Dermatophytes can be isolated from normal toe clefts in about 7% of homosexual men (regardless of HIV status) but not from clinically normal toe clefts in heterosexual men. Tinea incognito secondary to chronic potent topical steroid misuse for another dermatosis may develop. Widespread dermatophytosis is not common in HIV/AIDS; Torssander *et al.* found dermatophytes only in the groins, toe clefts and toenails. However, atypical tinea corporis (Figure 31.18), folliculitis, palmoplantar hyperkeratosis, erythroderma and extensive and deep, invasive dermatophytosis, including Majocchi granuloma, can occur [14,16–20]. Overall, dermatophytosis is significantly commoner in African American than white PLWH [21].

Onychomycosis in HIV-infected patients can occur in 15–40%, that is four times more often than in the general population [22–24]. It is also commoner in African American than white PLWH [21]. There is some evidence that these rates are falling [25]. *T. rubrum* is the commonest pathogen [26]. Psoriasis and the yellow nail syndrome should be considered in the differential diagnosis of nail discoloration and dystrophy. Mycological confirmation should be obtained. Improvement of onychomycosis with ART in the absence of specific antifungal treatment has been observed [27].

Cryptococcosis

Cryptococcus neoformans infection affects 5–10% of patients with AIDS in the UK and USA and 30–40% in Africa. The brain, lung and skin are sites of predilection. Up to 20% of patients with disseminated disease may have skin involvement. In HIV/AIDS, cryptococcal skin involvement should be suspected when papulonodular necrotising skin lesions with central umbilication, like molluscum contagiosum (Figure 31.19), are encountered in the context of neurological or pulmonary disease. Herpetiform lesions, violaceous lichenoid lesions, an acneform papulopustular and nodular eruption on the chin, rhinophyma, a warty tumour on the foot, a pseudofolliculitis, cellulitis and *Cryptococcus* admixed with, and mimicking, KS have also been described [45–49]. Cutaneous cryptococcosis may occur as an IRIS/IRD/IRAD.

Systemic diagnosis is by serology, blood culture, urine culture and lumbar puncture (including serology, culture and India ink staining). Cutaneous diagnosis is by skin biopsy with special stains for the cryptococcal capsule (e.g. mucicarmine) and culture, or Tzanck preparation [43].

Treatment aims to eradicate the disease in the immunocompetent patient and to control symptoms in the patient with advanced HIV disease. Intravenous liposomal amphotericin and oral fluconazole are the mainstays of treatment. Primary and secondary prophylaxis is with oral fluconazole. Cryptococcal meningitis has a poor prognosis even with treatment.

Non-*neoformans* cryptococcal opportunistic infections can involve the skin [50,51].

Talaromyces marneffei infection (penicilliosis)

Talaromyces marneffei infection (penicilliosis) is an AIDS-defining diagnosis and causes fever, lymphadenopathy, hepatosplenomegaly and anaemia with cutaneous involvement [52–56]; it can be an immunoreconstitution phenomenon. Skin lesions range from flesh-coloured follicular papules with or without central umbilication, nodules and acne-like lesions evoking a differential diagnosis of syringoma, steatocystoma multiplex and trichoepithelioma (Figure 31.20). Dermoscopy can be useful revealing a circular or quasi-circular, whitish, amorphous structure with a central brownish keratin plug [57].

Other fungal infections

The superficial and systemic mycoses encountered in HIV have been well reviewed [58,59]. Coccidioidomycosis is endemic in southwest USA; extrapulmonary disease is an AIDS-defining

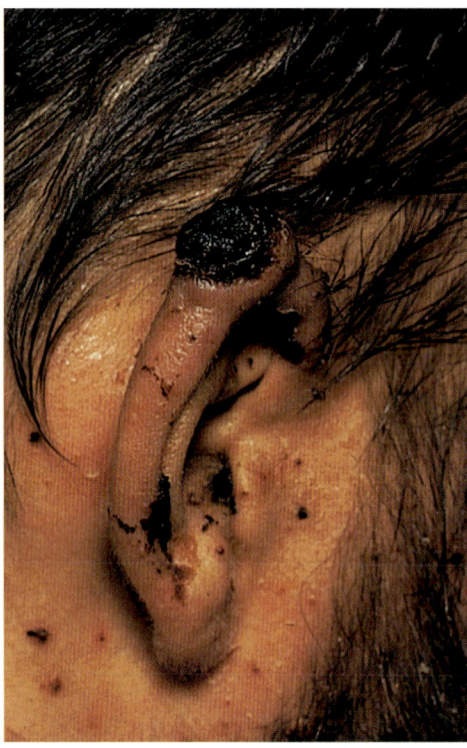
(a)

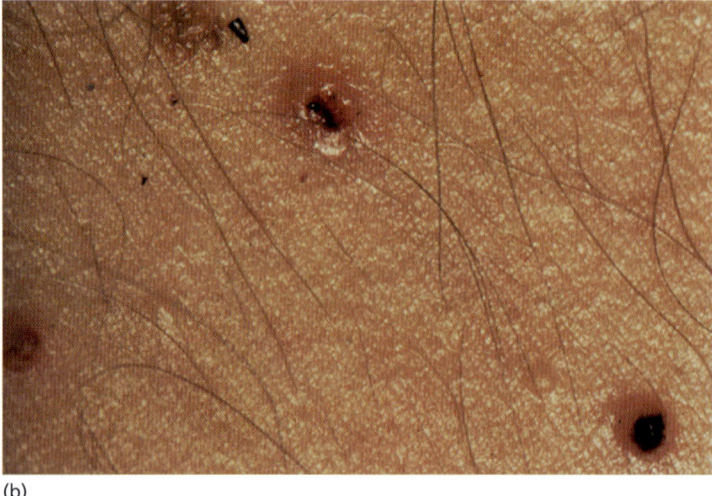
(b)

Figure 31.19 Cryptococcosis. (a) Necrotising papules and nodules on the right ear and neck. (b) Close up of necrotising papules. Courtesy of Medical Illustration UK Ltd.

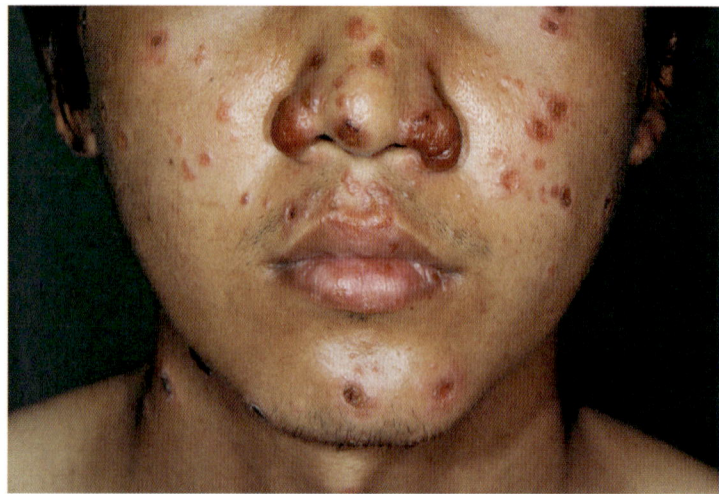

Figure 31.20 *Talaromyces marneffei* infection (penicilliosis). Courtesy of Professor Vesarat Wessagowit.

diagnosis but skin lesions seem rare [14]. Cutaneous sporotrichosis [6,60,61], paracoccidioidomycosis (50%) [62–66], blastomycosis [67], nocardiasis [68–71], rhinosporidiosis [72], primary cutaneous aspergillosis [73–75], mucormycosis [76,77], *Paecilomyces lilacinus* infection [78], cutaneous protothecosis [79–81], fusariosis, [82], *Emergomyces africanus* (emergomycosis) [83,84], basidiobolomycosis [85], emmonsiosis [86] and primary cutaneous actinomycosis [87] have all been reported in HIV/AIDS. *Malassaezia* species may cause a folliculitis (including during immunoreconstitution) and pityriasis versicolor may be more extensive in HIV and also possibly occur as an IRIS/IRD/IRAD [58,59,88].

PROTOZOAL INFECTIONS (Chapter 33)

Pneumocystis jiroveci pneumonia is common in HIV infection but disseminated disease and cutaneous involvement are rare [1,2]. Two patients have been described with mass lesions in the external auditory canal; spread from middle ear infection (itself due to retrograde spread from the pharynx via the Eustachian tube) was the probable mechanism. Lesions masquerading as KS have been described [3].

Cryptosporidiosis and microsporidiosis can cause skin lesions [4,5]. Disseminated amoebiasis may rarely cause skin manifestations but the dermatological involvement may lead to diagnosis of the systemic illness. A solitary papule of the thigh, a soleus muscle abscess, disseminated skin lesions and cutaneous ulceration have been described [6–9]. Ano-genital ulceration due to amoebiasis should lead to the suspicion of underlying HIV infection [10,11].

Endemic protozoal diseases such as leishmaniasis may behave differently in the HIV-infected patient and may also mimic or complicate KS and dermatofibroma. Cutaneous nodules and ulcers, digital necrosis, linear brown macules of the digits and palms, ulceration of the tongue, a tattoo reaction and cutaneous hyperpigmentation and atypical disseminated leishmaniasis resembling post-kala-azar dermal leishmaniasis have been described [12–26]. Four cases of a dermatomyositis-like presentation have been published with lesions limited to the dorsum of the hands, wrists and elbows and histology showing tuberculoid granulomas [27]. Patients have a higher rate of recurrence or reinfection and their disease is more difficult to treat compared with HIV-negative individuals [21]. However, cutaneous detection of *Leishmania* is frequent in individuals with visceral leishmaniasis (and very rarely skin involvement such as infiltrative leukocytoclastic purpura and maculopapular exanthem [28] has been reported) and sometimes *Leishmania* is associated with skin changes attributable to other pathogenic processes including rheumatoid nodulosis, so its presence does not imply a causative role [23,29]. IRIS/IRD/IRAD-associated leishmaniasis is recognised.

Reactivation of American trypanosomiasis (Chagas disease) in AIDS may manifest with skin lesions [30].

SCABIES (Chapter 34)

Scabies occurs frequently in HIV-infected patients [1,2] and may have unusual clinical features (Figure 31.21), for example the skin

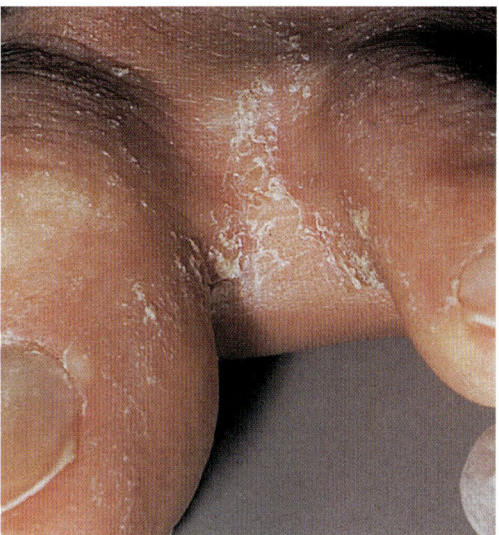

Figure 31.21 Norwegian scabies: interdigital scale.

of the head and neck is often involved, which is highly unusual in non-HIV-infected adults. It is important to have a high index of suspicion. Scabies has been endemic in the HIV population in London and there are occasional epidemic outbreaks on HIV wards, in hospices and in the community. Transmission is by sexual intercourse, nursing, comforting and massage. Norwegian/crusted scabies [3] is highly contagious and its diagnosis should arouse suspicion of underlying HIV infection [4]. Crusted scabies in HIV infection may be localised to the soles [5] or the genitals [6]. Eccrine ductal and follicular mucinosis have been found on histology [7]. Treatment follows conventional lines but eradication may be difficult. Topical sulphur and oral ivermectin can be useful [8,9].

MISCELLANEOUS INFECTIONS

Demodex (Chapter 34) can cause dermatological morbidity in HIV-infected patients. A pruritic, papulonodular folliculitic eruption of the face and neck, upper limbs and torso is recognised, responsive to acaricides including ivermectin [1–3]. Also described have been a rosaceal eruption [4] and an ivory white, poorly defined, indurated plaque on the temple [5]. Demodicosis can also occur during immunoreconstitution with ART [3,6].

Cutaneous larva migrans has presented with fever in an HIV-infected individual after the commencement of treatment with zidovudine (AZT, ZDV) and didanosine (ddI, DDI) [7], and as a red plaque on the cheek [8].

HIV-positive patients with oncocerciasis have higher onchocercal skin scores than those who are not HIV infected [9].

Malakoplakia is an uncommon granulomatous reaction to infection (bacteria, mycobacteria and fungi) usually of the genital tract and cases in HIV have been reported [10,11].

Extraintestinal strongyloidosis is an indicator condition for the case definition of AIDS. Fatal hyperinfection with *Strongyloides stercoralis* has been described, the skin signs being centripetal, reticulated petechiae and purpura with numerous larvae found on skin biopsy [12].

A 49-year-old HIV-positive Namibian man presented with multiple cutaneous nodules confirmed as cysticercomas which led to the diagnosis of asymptomatic neurocysticercosis due to *Taenia solium* [13].

Myiasis affecting the face and mouth has been reported [14,15].

NEOPLASMS

Kaposi sarcoma

Classic sporadic KS, African endemic KS, Greek (Peloponnesian) endemic KS, iatrogenic immunosuppression-associated KS and AIDS-related KS are recognised [1,2]. KS has been considered an AIDS-defining diagnosis in patients with low CD4 counts and high viral loads, but cases have been encountered at CD4 counts >300 × 10^6/L and low or undetectable viral loads, either on ART or ART naive patients (Chapter 137) [3]. KS has been seen in HIV-negative homosexual men [1,4,5]. It is commoner in African American than white PLWH [6].

The prevalence of KS in patients infected with HIV has declined throughout the epidemic [1]. KS is caused by infection with the oncovirus HHV-8 (KS herpesvirus (KSHV)). It is probably transmitted sexually, more by the faecal–oral route or ejaculate than by blood, in HIV-positive homosexual men [7–11]. However, KS is also seen in non-homosexuals and in children arising from other routes of transmission, for example saliva [12,13]. The pathogenesis of KS is thought to involve angiogenic and pro-inflammatory effects on endothelial cells that proliferate to form characteristic spindle-cell tumours [14]. KS appearing at the sites of application of topical tacrolimus prescribed for seborrhoeic dermatitis in a patient undergoing treatment with ART has been reported [15].

HIV/AIDS-related KS may be a disseminated disease with gastrointestinal and pulmonary involvement. Cutaneous KS is multicentric and often involves the face, oral mucosa, palate (Figure 31.22a) and genitalia. Lesions may be multiple, follow skin creases and may be grouped or linear and koebnerise (Figure 31.22b). Lymphoedema may eventuate [16,17]. The classic lesion in HIV is a purple patch, plaque or nodule, which may ulcerate; phimosis may occur [18]. There may be diagnostic difficulty with morphologically banal lesions in at-risk or worried individuals or with clinically atypical presentations (e.g. yellow-green penile plaques have been reported [19]), and the importance of having a high index of suspicion and taking a skin biopsy must be stressed.

The differential diagnosis (Box 31.9) [20] includes naevi, histiocytoma, lymphangioma [21] and granuloma annulare [22], although cryptococcosis [23,24], histoplasmosis [25], leishmaniasis [26,27], lesions due to *Pneumocystis* [28] and dermatophytosis [29] may also mimic and/or complicate KS. *Candida* has been found within KS lesions [30]. Pyogenic granuloma and bacillary angiomatosis masquerading as KS are important to consider and confirm or exclude. Pseudo-Kaposi sarcoma (acroangiodermatitis) has been reported in HIV [31]. The differential diagnosis of oral lesions is discussed in the section on the oro-pharynx in HIV later in this chapter and includes the other causes of mouth ulcers and tumours, candidosis, lichen planus, drug eruption and angina bullosa haemorrhagica. The differential diagnosis of genital lesions includes psoriasis, lichen planus, lichen sclerosus, fixed drug eruption, Zoon balanitis and erythroplasia of Queyrat.

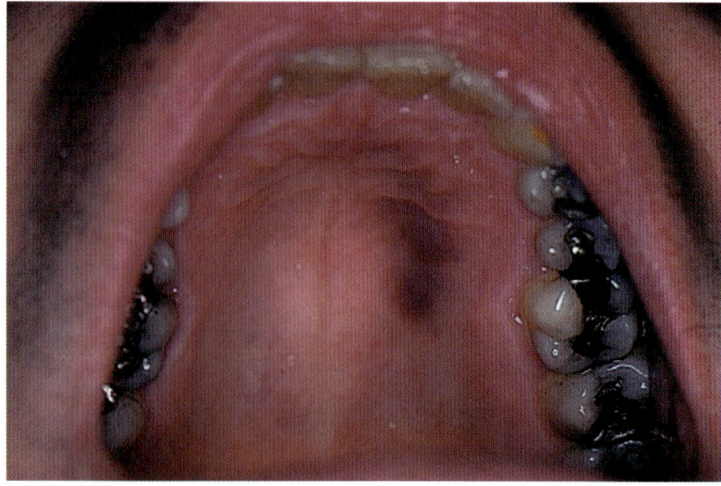

(a)

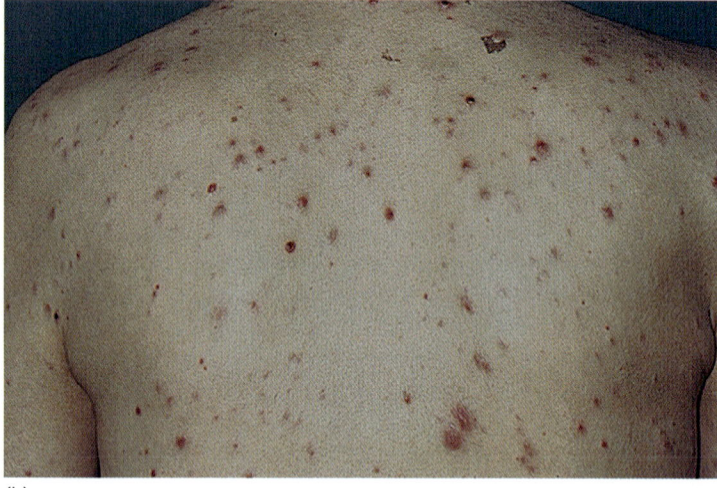

(b)

Figure 31.22 Kaposi sarcoma. (a) Purple nodules on the palate. (b) Multiple purple nodules and plaques on the back. Courtesy of Medical Illustration UK Ltd.

Box 31.9 Differential diagnosis of Kaposi sarcoma

- Naevus
- Angioma
- Histiocytoma
- Pyogenic granuloma
- Melanoma
- Bacillary angiomatosis
- Cryptococcosis
- Histoplasmosis
- Leishmaniasis
- *Pneumocystis* lesions
- Dermatophytosis

From Bunker and Staughton 2002 [20] and other sources.

Diagnosis is either clinical or clinicopathological. The histological features of KS are well described [30,32] and consist of dilated, irregularly shaped, vascular structures that are typically slit-like in a fully developed nodular lesion; epithelioid morphology has been described [33]. The differential diagnosis may be clarified by immunohistochemical techniques.

The staging of KS takes into account tumour bulk [34–37], systemic illness and immunosuppression (Chapter 137).

Systemic and local treatments that have been employed in KS are summarised in Box 31.10. ART itself is very effective for early-stage KS [3,35–39]. Indeed, ART has reduced the incidence of KS and prolongs relapse-free and overall survival in AIDS KS [3,35–37]. However, IRIS/IRD/IRAD-related KS occurs, and men with unremitting cutaneous KS have been reported despite ART, raising the question of immunosenescence [3,40–44]. Radiotherapy can cause significant adverse sequelae, for example radiodermatitis, in survivors. Systemic chemotherapy is needed for advanced-stage KS or those with progressive KS despite ART including IRIS/IRD/IRAD KS [35–37]. The future may be in vaccination against KHSV and targeted therapies with monoclonal antibodies or kinase inhibitors [37,45].

Melanoma and non-melanoma skin cancer

While the incidence of AIDS-defining cancers is decreasing, the incidence of non-AIDS-defining cancers (NADCs) (melanoma, Hodgkin lymphoma, leukaemia, and liver, respiratory, anal, oro-pharyngeal and prostate cancers) is increasing. It has been debated whether this reflects a true increase in incidence or is a consequence of increased surveillance, detection and reporting [1–6]: in the USA it seems to be driven by an increase in the size of the HIV-infected population and ageing [7]. Primary skin malignancies constitute the most frequent NADCs among HIV-positive people [8]. HIV/AIDS patients have a 2–5-fold risk of developing a non-melanoma skin cancer (NMSC); the relative risk of NMSC in PLWH is not as high as in solid organ transplant patients and the ratio of SCC to basal cell carcinoma (BCC) in HIV-infected individuals is 1 : 7, compared with 1.8 : 1 in renal transplant patients [1,9,10]. Intriguingly African Americans with HIV have an increased risk of SCC [11]. Melanoma is probably c.2.5 times more common, although one UK study has found a decreased incidence and others no association [1,2,5,8,12–15,**16**]. Anal cancer has been increasing since the introduction of ART [2] and is the fourth most common cancer in MSM [17]. Penile cancer is 5–6 times commoner, despite ART. Recreational ultraviolet exposure is possibly more important in the causation of NMSC than immunosuppression, although a low CD4 count nadir confers an increased risk of developing SCC [1,18,**19**,20]. The role of HPV in ano-genital and oral cancer, epidermoplasia verruciformis and nail unit SCC is established. It has been suggested that all HPV-associated cancers should be included as AIDS-defining illnesses [21] but HPV is unlikely (although controversial) to be pathogenic in most cutaneous HIV-associated SCC [1,3,9,22,23]. Genital ulceration due to donovanosis has been reported to progress to SCC [24]. Long-term voriconazole therapy has been associated with multiple SCCs [25].

Clinically, actinic keratoses are very common; atypicality should prompt more vigorous assessment and more aggressive treatment. Bowen disease and SCC may present atypically, at a younger age, at unusual sites (e.g. the digit and nail fold, where diverse high-risk oncogenic HPV types may be implicated [26,27]) and be multifocal, extravagant and aggressive with a high risk of recurrence and metastasis and a high mortality (Figure 31.23) [9,23,28–37]. BCC presents at a younger age, it may be multiple and eruptive and is commonly of the superficial type. Aggressive, infiltrative, infundibulocystic, micronodular, neurotropic and morpheiform histological variants and even metastatic BCC have been reported. Generally, BCC was *not* thought to behave more aggressively clinically in the HIV-infected population, but increasingly high rates of recurrence are being reported [9,34,35,38–42]. As with SCC this does not seem to be related so much to immunosuppression as

---

Box 31.10 Treatments for Kaposi sarcoma (KS)

Local treatment
- Cryotherapy
- Radiotherapy
- Topical retinoids: alitretinoin [46]
- Topical antivirals: cidofovir, docosanol [47]
- Topical β-blockers: propranolol, timolol [48]
- Intralesional, e.g. IFN-α, TNF-α, vinca alkaloids
- Electrochemotherapy: bleomycin [49]
- Surgery, e.g. curettage, cautery, infrared coagulation [50]
- Laser
- Photodynamic therapy [51]
- Cosmetic camouflage

Systemic treatment
- ART
- Isotretinoin
- Cidofovir
- Intravenous chemotherapy, e.g. anthracyclines such as liposomal daunorubicin, liposomal doxorubicin, bleomycin, paclitaxel, vincristine, etoposide [35,52]
- Human chorionic gonadotrophin [53]
- Interleukin 4 [54]
- Imatinib mesylate (platelet-derived growth factor/c-Kit receptor inhibitor) [55]
- Thalidomide, lenalidomide [56]

Summary of current recommendations
- Early-stage KS (T0 stage):
  - ART
  - Consider local radiotherapy or liposomal anthracycline for rapidly progressing or cosmetically disfiguring disease
- Advanced-stage KS (T1 stage):
  - ART and liposomal anthracycline
- Anthracycline-refractory KS:
  - ART and paclitaxel

From Bunker and Staughton 2002 [20], Bower and Portsmouth 2002 [34], Gbabe et al. 2014 [35], Anglemyer et al. 2014 [36], Cesarman et al. 2019 [37] and Bower 2014 [45]. ART, antiretroviral therapy; IFN, interferon; TNF, tumour necrosis factor.

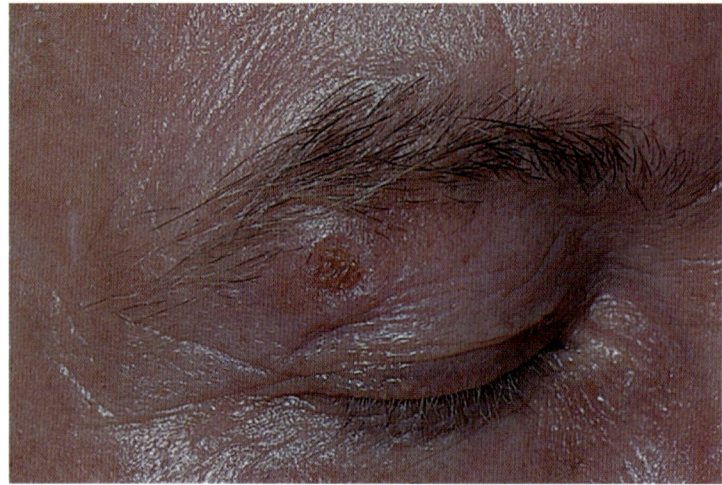

(a)

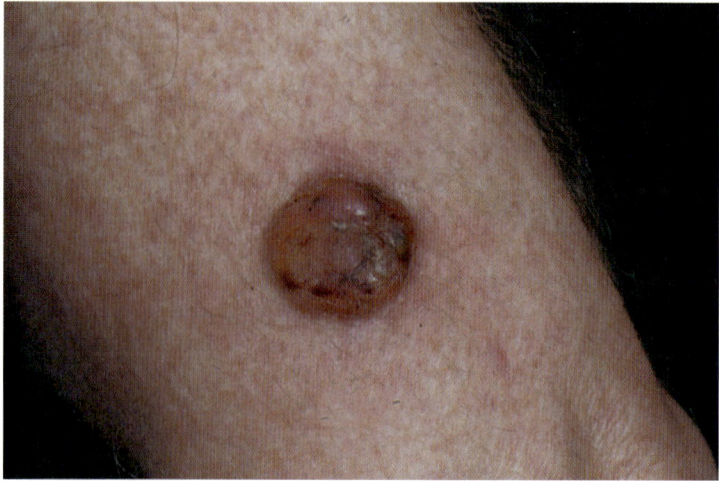

Figure 31.24 Melanoma: 2-month history of rapidly growing amelanotic nodule on the left arm; Breslow thickness >10 mm. Courtesy of Medical Illustration UK Ltd.

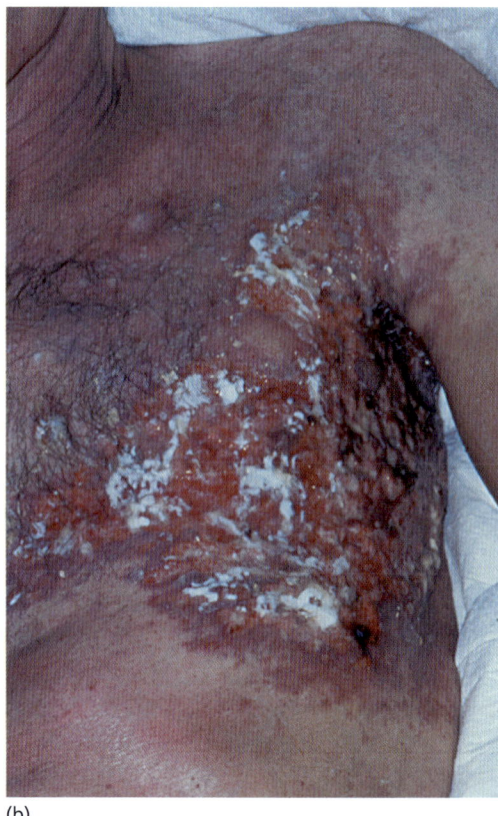

(b)

Figure 31.23 Squamous carcinoma. (a) Ulcerated nodule on the right upper eyelid. (b) Metastatic zosteriform ulceration of the left axilla and chest. Courtesy of Medical Illustration UK Ltd.

to ultraviolet exposure, but has implications for treatment and follow-up [33]. Porokeratosis is associated with immunosuppression, sun damage and HIV [43]. Ano-genital squamous cancer and precancer and their relationship to HPV and HIV are discussed here and in Chapters 109, 110 and 111 [8,44,45].

Melanoma may present atypically, appearing as 'normal naevi' or 'benign macules' or multiple 'naevoid lesions' (Figure 31.24) and may behave more aggressively with decreased disease-free and overall survival rates [16]. Low CD4 counts indicate a poorer prognosis although the Breslow thickness is unrelated to the CD4 count at presentation [9,46–49].

Conventional treatment protocols should be followed for the management of BCC, SCC and melanoma in HIV practice; conventional Mohs micrographic surgery should not be regarded as contraindicated [50]. However, mindful of the potential aggressivity of SCC and melanoma, assiduous attention to local excisional margin control, more extensive investigation for regional or disseminated disease, and closer follow-up in patients with SCC and melanoma are advocated [16,48,51]. The specific place for deployment of immune checkpoint-based immunotherapy of melanoma in PLWH is under evaluation [16]. BCC and SCC have been reported to remit with ART [52,53]. Topical imiquimod has been used for treatment of BCC in HIV [54] and is useful for the common scenario of multifocal superficial BCCs. Vismodegib has been used safely in HIV [55].

Patients receiving ART and therefore surviving HIV longer, even for a natural lifespan, need to be counselled about sun avoidance [1] and have careful dermatological evaluation and follow-up, including of the ano-genital skin and mucosa and of the oro-pharynx. Patients with a history of severe immunosuppression (CD4 count of $<200 \times 10^6/L$) or those with prior NMSCs (or both) should be seen annually [1]. All new or changing skin lesions should be evaluated assiduously, with a low threshold for biopsy. More widespread HPV vaccination offers a promising preventative tactic [56].

Lymphoma

A wide spectrum of involvement of the skin with lymphoma is seen in HIV/AIDS [1]. Non-Hodgkin B-cell lymphomas are common in HIV [2] and can cause skin lesions [3–5]. The majority of lymphomas are monomorphic, but some polymorphic types may be seen as in post-transplant patients [6]. Burkitt lymphoma is one of the most common non-Hodgkin lymphomas in HIV-infected patients, associated with EBV in about half of cases; skin involvement might be with disseminated or solitary lesions [7]. The very rare primary cutaneous B-cell lymphoma–leg type presenting as a painful leg ulcer in HIV has been reported in a young adult male with HIV [8]. Intravascular lymphomatosis may be associated with HIV and involve the skin, for instance with telangiectatic, indurated, slightly red plaques on the trunk [9]. Primary cutaneous presentation of extracavitary primary effusion lymphoma is exceedingly rare, but a panniculitis like-presentation has been reported in HIV [10].

Plasmablastic lymphoma is a rare, EBV-associated variant of diffuse large-cell lymphoma that often involves the oral cavity in HIV-positive patients but can affect the skin. It is usually refractory to treatment but may be self-healing [11–15]. EBV-positive mucocutaneous lymphoproliferative lesions have been described affecting the oro-pharynx, skin and rectal and/or genital mucosa, which broadens the concept of EBV-positive mucocutaneous ulcer [16]. HHV-8 can be associated with solid lymphomas [17].

The relationship of Hodgkin disease to HIV has been controversial [3,18,19]; several hundred cases have been reported. HIV-associated Hodgkin disease differs from non-HIV-associated disease by manifesting 'B' symptoms more commonly, a more advanced stage at presentation, extranodal disease, a higher incidence of EBV in affected tissue, predominant mixed cellularity and lymphocyte-depleted histologies, a less complete response rate, a higher relapse rate and a significantly shortened median survival [18]. It can manifest as a panniculitis [20]. Multiple myelomas have presented in the skin with primary cutaneous plasmacytomas [21]. Chloroma (granulocytic sarcoma) has also been reported [22].

Cutaneous T-cell lymphoma (mycosis fungoides and Sézary syndrome) may be associated with HIV/AIDS [23–25]. A case of cutaneous extranodal natural killer/T-cell lymphoma mimicking cellulitis has been described [26]. Subcutaneous panniculitis-like T-cell lymphoma has been reported [27]. A 61-year-old Haitian male with HIV on ART presented with waxing and waning, multiple, painful pink papules on his distal fingers and back for more than a year. Adult T-cell lymphoma/leukemia (ATLL) due to HTLV-1 was diagnosed on biopsy and further investigations [28]. HTLV-1 and HIV-1 are frequent co-pathogens; however, despite its potential for accelerated progression of HIV disease and the risk of developing ATLL, HTLV-1 is seldom considered and sought in the HIV-1 positive individual [29].

Multicentric Castleman disease is discussed in Chapter 25 [30–33]. It is frequently associated with HHV-8, especially in HIV. Optimal treatment has not been established. Rituximab may confer survival benefit for HHV-8-associated disease, but it is related to exacerbations of KS [34].

The rare HIV-associated atypical cutaneous lymphoproliferative disorder (ACLD) is an itchy, generalised eruption of patches, plaques or erythroderma, and is clinically suggestive of mycosis fungoides or Sézary syndrome. A polyclonal CD8+ T-cell infiltrate on biopsy is seen: the condition usually responds to ART [35]. HIV-associated cutaneous pseudolymphoma presents with intensely pruritic, extensive, infiltrative skin involvement, alopecia universalis, weight loss and eosinophilia; it also responds to ART [36].

Lymphomatoid papulosis has been described [37,38], as has lymphomatoid granulomatosis, which is a rare EBV-associated lymphoproliferative disease [39]. Cutaneous mucinoses, ACLD and CD8+ pseudolymphomas are listed in Chapter 35.

Other neoplasms

The benign and malignant skin neoplasms that have been reported in association with HIV are listed in Box 31.11 [1–45].

> **Box 31.11 Benign and malignant cutaneous neoplasms reported in association with HIV**
>
> **Common or classic associations**
> - Kaposi sarcoma
> - Actinic keratosis
> - Basal cell carcinoma
> - Squamous carcinoma
> - Melanoma
> - Lymphoma
>
> **Rare or speculative associations**
> - Eruptive seborrhoeic keratoses (Leser–Trélat) [1]
> - Eruptive dysplastic naevi [2,3]
> - Histiocytoma/dermatofibroma: solitary, multiple and eruptive; exclude leishmaniasis [4–8]
> - Xanthomas [9–12]
> - Porokeratosis of Mibelli [13,14]
> - Pilomatrixoma (in association with myotonic dystrophy) [15]
> - Trichodysplasia spinulosa (and variants; and associated with HIV follicular syndrome) [16–18]
> - Facial miliary osteoma [19]
> - Lipomas and angiolipomas (with protease inhibitors) [20]
> - Acquired progressive lymphangioma [21]
> - Neurofibromatosis [22]
> - Metastatic tufted angioma [23]
> - Leiomyoma, angioleiomyoma, leiomyosarcoma (including Epstein–Barr virus-associated) [24–28]
> - Multiple low-grade fibroblastic sarcomas with epidermodysplasia verruciformis [29]
> - Atypical fibroxanthoma [30]/pleomorphic dermal sarcoma [31]
> - Dermatofibrosarcoma protuberans [32]
> - Sebaceous carcinoma [33]
> - Pilomatrical carcinoma [34]
> - Porocarcinoma [35]
> - Extramammary Paget disease [36]
> - Merkel cell carcinoma [37–43]
> - Cutaneous metastases (lung cancer) [44,45]

SPECIAL SITUATIONS

Hair and nails

The abnormalities of hair and nails associated with HIV infection and their treatments are listed in Box 31.12, Figure 31.25 and Table 31.7 [1–6] (Chapters 87 and 93). Acquired trichomegaly of the eyelashes may be a marker of advanced HIV infection [5,7]. A striking case of kwashiorkor with hair and nail changes has been documented [8].

Up to 70% of HIV-infected individuals can have nail changes [2]. Up to 36% may have clubbing [9]. Grey nails and distal banded nails are associated with low CD4 counts of $<200 \times 10^6/L$ and these signs have been suggested as a low-cost way of identifying patients needing ART but their sensitivity is low [10]. Onychomycosis is usually due to *Trichophyton rubrum* or uncommon *Candida* species [2]. Some African patients with the yellow nail syndrome [11] have AIDS *and* tuberculous pleural effusion or pneumonia; the yellow nail syndrome is a recognised association of chronic pulmonary disease. Paronychia and ingrown toenails are particular complications of indinavir (IDV, IND), and probably not lamivudine, as had been suggested [12,13].

Box 31.12 Abnormalities of the hair and nails in HIV infection

Hair
- Patchy and diffuse alopecia/telogen effluvium [14]
- Fine hair
- Eyelash trichomegaly [7]
- Alopecia (non-specific)
- Alopecia areata (Figure 31.25) and universalis [15]
- Lichen planopilaris [16]

Nails
- Clubbing [9]
- Half and half nails
- Transverse (Beau) lines
- Longitudinal ridging
- Distal banding [10]
- Loss of the lunula
- Leukonychia
- Grey nails [10]
- Blue nails [17]
- Longitudinal melanonychia
- Yellow nail syndrome [11]
- Periungual erythema [18]
- Onycholysis and onychoschizia
- Onychomycosis

From Prose *et al.* 1992 [1], Cribier *et al.* 1998 [2], Bunker and Staughton 2002 [3], Ward *et al.* 2002 [4], Mirmirani *et al.* 2003 [5] and Shear 2021 [6].

Oro-pharynx

Many oral manifestations have been reported in acute HIV infection and seroconversion [1]. Transient intraoral redness, erosions and ulcers and candidosis are all described. Xerostomia is common. HIV infection must be excluded in the differential diagnosis of Sjögren syndrome [2]. Salivary gland swelling is frequently seen in children but less so in adults infected with HIV [3].

Oral symptoms and signs are common in established HIV infection; their presence may be an indicator of HIV disease severity [4]. Smoking and alcohol ingestion contribute to the morbidity [1,5]. Oral hyperpigmentation is a sign of low CD4 counts ($<200 \times 10^6/L$) and has been proposed as an indication of eligibility for ART but it may not be sensitive enough for this purpose [6]. Distressing mouth ulceration occurs frequently. The differential diagnosis includes

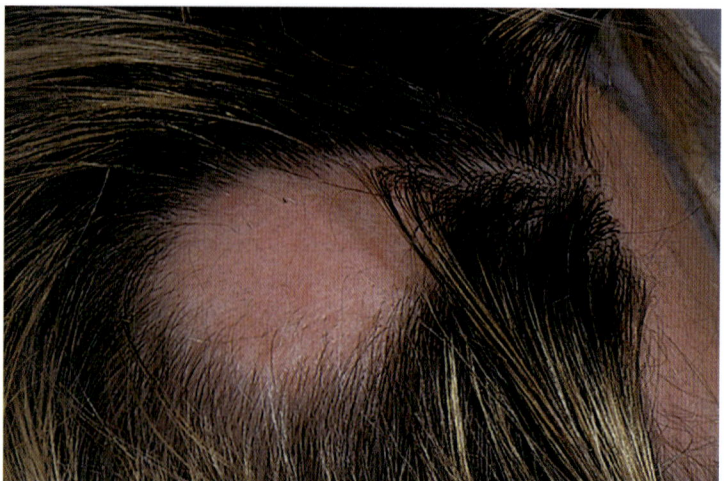

Figure 31.25 Alopecia areata. Courtesy of Medical Illustration UK Ltd.

malignancy (KS and lymphoma), HSV, CMV, fungal infections, Behçet disease, drug-induced ulceration (e.g. didanosine (ddI, DDI)) and idiopathic aphthous ulceration. Thalidomide has proved useful for the last of these [7] at a dose of 100 mg nightly for 2 weeks followed by maintenance therapy of 100 mg every 5 days, with monitoring to avoid peripheral neuropathy [8]; however, ART is also effective [9].

Oral candidosis is very common in HIV-positive individuals and almost universal in AIDS. The extent and persistence of the disease are responsible for much morbidity in patients with HIV and AIDS. Sometimes the entire oro-pharynx, larynx and oesophagus may be involved, but mild forms with just angular cheilitis and/or focal red or white patches on the oral mucosa, palate or tongue are also seen [1,4,5,10,11].

Severe periodontal disease is also not unusual [1,4,5]. Gangrenous stomatitis, due to opportunistic anaerobic organisms and *Candida*, *Pseudomonas* and *Staphylococcus*, causes severely symptomatic perioral ulceration complicated by pain, bleeding and inability to feed [12]. Necrotising ulcerative stomatitis with histology resembling extranodal Kikuchi disease [13] has also been described, as has cancrum oris (noma) [14,15]. Hairy leukoplakia is a new clinical entity that has emerged during the HIV epidemic and is probably associated with EBV infection [1,3,4,5]. It is particularly important because it is an early specific sign of HIV infection, with the sinister implication that if untreated 75% of patients developed AIDS within 2–3 years. It is much commoner in African American than white PLWH [16]. It is usually asymptomatic, although patients have often noticed the appearance of a roughened patch along the lateral margin of the tongue (Figure 31.26). To the patient it may feel rough and to the physician it may look craggy but it is not truly 'hairy'. Other intraoral sites have been reported. The differential diagnosis includes trauma, *Candida*, leukoplakia, lichen planus and white sponge naevus. Hairy leukoplakia has not yet been shown to involve other mucosal or extramucosal sites. White sponge naevus may be familial and may occur on the tongue. Intriguingly, oral hairy leukoplakia and oral warts rarely coexist [17]. Biopsy may be necessary. Hairy leukoplakia is now known to occur in other immunocompromised people and has even been reported in healthy individuals. Treatment options include topical

Table 31.7 Abnormalities of the hair and nails due to drugs in HIV infection.

Drug	Abnormality
Drugs affecting the hair	
Zidovudine (AZT, ZDV)	Eyelash hypertrichosis
Atazanavir (ATV), delaviridine (DLV)[a], didanosine (ddI, DDI), efavirenz (EFZ), indinavir (IDV, IND), lamivudine (3TC), lopinavir (LPV), ritonavir (RTV, RIT, /r), saquinavir (SQV, SAQ), stavudine (d4T), zalcitabine (ddC, DDC)[a], zidovudine (AZT, ZDV) [19–22]	Alopecia (non-specific)
ART	Curly hair
Indinavir (IDV, IND) [23]	Pigmentation
Drugs affecting the nails	
Zidovudine (AZT, ZDV), indinavir (IDV, IND) [23]	Pigmentation
Zidovudine (AZT, ZDV) [24], doxorubicin [25]	Longitudinal melanonychia
Hydroxyurea [26,27]	Melanonychia
Indinavir (IDV, IND), ritonavir (RTV, RIT, /r), zidovudine (AZT, ZDV); lamivudine (3TC) (disputed and rare) [12,13]	Paronychia/pyogenic granuloma
Indinavir (IDV, IND)	Onychocryptosis (ingrown nail)
Delaviridine (DLV)[a]	Not specified

From Prose *et al*. 1992 [1], Cribier *et al*. 1998 [2], Bunker and Staughton 2002 [3], Ward *et al*. 2002 [4] and Shear 2021 [6].
[a] No longer available.

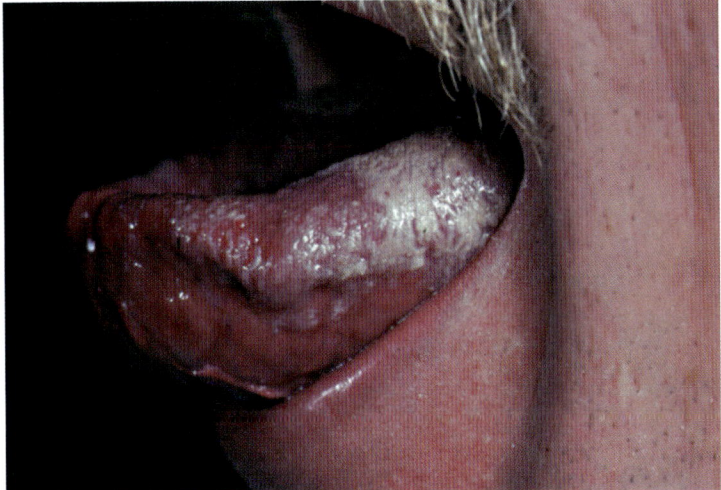

Figure 31.26 Hairy leukoplakia. Courtesy of Media Resources UCL Trust.

podophyllin, topical retinoids, topical gentian violet, cryotherapy, surgical excision, oral aciclovir, valciclovir and famciclovir [18,19], but it responds to ART.

HSV infection is common in and around the mouth. Painful, red, eroded lesions are characteristic and the extent and chronicity, or frequency of recurrences, cause much debility [20]. CMV may present similarly. A nodular form of intraoral HSV has been described in the context of IRIS/IRD/IRAD [21].

Just over 1% of HIV-infected individuals have oral HPV infection [3]. An increased number of benign HPV-related oral lesions are seen in HIV patients on ART and may be related to the longer life expectancy of individuals with an impaired immune system rather than a direct effect of ART [22]. However, there has been a dramatic increase in oncogenic HPV oro-pharyngeal carcinomas and they occur in a younger group of patients compared with the classic smoking- and alcohol-related cancers. HPV transmission is through high levels of oral sexual practice. Tumours arise deep within tonsillar crypts or at the base of the tongue and so can be difficult to detect clinically. Nodal involvement is early [23–25].

All HIV patients under follow-up should have their oral cavity examined regularly.

KS occurs frequently in the mouth, often in the palate. It appears as red patches, plaques or nodules (see Figure 31.22a). The early red lesions may be mistaken for HSV or *Candida*. The differential diagnosis also includes the other causes of mouth ulcers and tumours, lichen planus, drug eruptions and angina bullosa haemorrhagica.

Other problems that can affect the oral cavity include petechiae due to thrombocytopenia [3], tuberculosis [26], disseminated histoplasmosis [27,28], sporotrichosis [22,29], paracoccidioidomycosis (40%) [24,30,31], myiasis [32], hyperpigmentation and oral and labial melanotic macules [3,33], primary amyloidosis [34], lymphoma (for example plasmablastic lymphoma [36] and EBV-associated mucosal ulcer and lymphoproliferative lesions [37]) and other rare malignancies such as Merkel cell carcinoma, salivary lymphoepithelial carcinoma, naso-pharygeal carcinoma and EBV-related SCC [25], and the side effects of radiotherapy and drugs (Table 31.8) [3,37–40]. Cheilitis, mouth ulceration and xerostomia are the commonest side effects. Cheilitis (Figure 31.27) is thought to be a common consequence of protease inhibitors but is mainly associated with indinavir (IDV, IND), ritonavir (RTV, RIT, /r) and saquinavir (SQV, SAQ).

Ano-genital

Ano-genital disorders are discussed in detail in Chapter 111. Sexually acquired infections in PLWH are discussed earlier in this chapter and in Chapters 29 and 30.

Balanoposthitis, proctitis, piles, perianal ulceration, abscess, fissure and fistula are prevalent in homosexual men and in HIV infection [1–4]. In the US in-patient population, a firm association between AIDS and hidradenitis suppurativa has now been established [5]. HIV is a risk factor for Fournier gangrene [6].

HIV-positive MSM have a high risk for HPV-induced condylomata, premalignant ano-genital lesions and ano-genital cancers. Screening for HPV-induced dysplasia is held to be crucial to avoid progression to invasive carcinomas [7,8] although there is no

Table 31.8 Oral side effects of drugs and radiotherapy given for HIV infection.[a]

Drug	Oral side effect
Abacavir (ABC)	Oral ulceration, perioral paraesthesia
Amprenavir (APV)[b]	Dysgeusia, perioral paraesthesia
Atazanavir (ATV)	Oral ulceration, dysgeusia
Delaviridine (DLV)[b]	Oral ulceration, xerostomia, gingivitis, stomatitis, sialorrhoea, lingual oedema, dysgeusia
Didanosine (ddI, DDI)	Oral ulceration, dysgeusia, xerostomia
Doxorubicin	Lingual hyperpigmentation
Efavirenz (EFV)	Xerostomia
Enfuvirtide (ENF, T20)	Xerostomia, dysgeusia
Etravine (ETR)	Xerostomia, stomatitis
Fosamprenavir (FPV, prodrug of amprenavir)	Dysgeusia, perioral paraesthesia
Foscarnet	Oral ulceration
Hydroxyurea	Oral pigmentation
Indinavir (IDV, IND)	Cheilitis, xerostomia, oral ulceration, dysgeusia, gingivitis
Interferon (IFN)	Oral ulceration
Lopinavir (LPV)	Oral ulceration, xerostomia, gingivitis, sialadenitis
Maraviroc (MVC)	Stomatitis
Nelfinavir (NFV)	Oral ulceration, perioral paraesthesia
Nevirapine (NVP)	Oral ulceration, gingivitis
Ritonavir (RTV, RIT, /r)	Cheilitis, oral ulceration, xerostomia, gingivitis, ageusia and dysgeusia, perioral paraesthesia and pain, oral candidosis
Saquinavir (SQV, SAQ)	Oral ulceration, gingivitis, glossitis, stomatitis, perioral paraesthesia
Zalcitabine (ddC, DDC)[b]	Oral ulceration, xerostomia, ageusia and dysgeusia, gingivitis, stomatitis, glossitis, glossodynia
Zidovudine (AZT, ZDV)	Oral ulceration, oral pigmentation, dysgeusia, lichenoid eruption, gingivitis

From Schiodt 1997 [3], Moyle and Gazzard 2002a, 2002b [37,38], Abbasi and Wang 2008 [39] and Shear 2021 [40].
[a] Drugs without reported oral side effects are omitted from the table.
[b] No longer available.

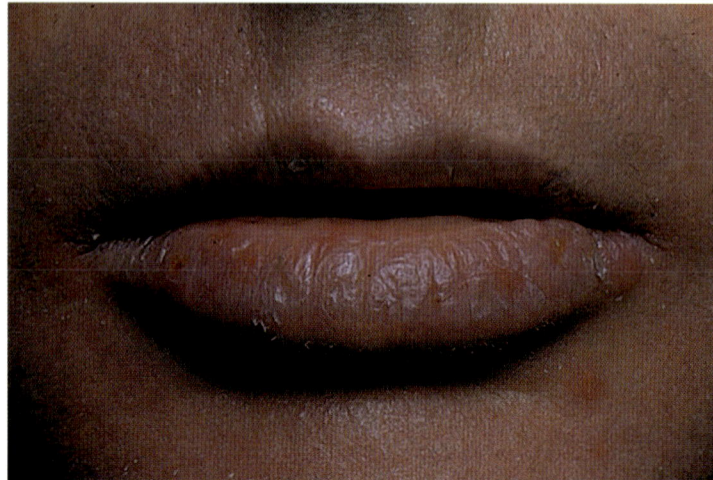

Figure 31.27 Cheilitis caused by indinavir (IDV, INR). Courtesy of Imperial College School of Medicine.

evidence that treating anal intraepithelial neoplasia prevents anal cancer [9]. Nevertheless, anal intraepithelial neoplasia and anal cancer remain common in MSM/PLWH despite awareness and screening and ART [10,11]. A high index of suspicion is necessary. A history of pain or bleeding should elicit careful examination; anoscopy, cytology and HPV typing have their places. HPV vaccination has increasingly been extended to high-risk populations and may be deployed as a treatment [12,13].

Miscellaneous conditions affecting the ano-genital area in PLWH include genito-gluteal porokeratosis [14] and EBV mucocutaneous ulcer [15].

Women

Women and children represent the fastest growing subpopulations of HIV-infected patients in the developed world. Women are more susceptible than men to the acquisition of HIV and often sustain more damage to their health from the disease [1]. There are few significant differences in dermatological morbidity between HIV-infected men and women save that women have less KS and oral manifestations including hairy leukoplakia and possibly onychomycosis, and that mollusca may appear earlier in women [2,3]. Eosinophilic folliculitis is held to be very rare in women [4]; it predominantly affects the face and mimics acne excoriée [5]. Antibiotics such as nitrofurantoin given during pregnancy may be more risky for Stevens–Johnson syndrome [6]. Thrombotic thrombocytopenic purpura may complicate pregnancy [7], but pregnancy does not generally seem to affect the occurrence of HIV-associated dermatoses [8]. For example, KS may regress or disseminate and be associated with IRIS/IRD/IRAD in pregnancy [9,10]. Cutaneous manifestations in HIV-infected women are improved by ART [11].

Children

Paediatric HIV infection is increasing in incidence but shows differences compared with adults. Vertical transmission from an infected mother is the usual mode of infection. There is a challenging and broad differential diagnosis of immunosuppression in children (Box 31.13) [1]; all of these conditions may have cutaneous manifestations.

> **Box 31.13 Differential diagnosis of childhood immunosuppression**
>
> - Di George syndrome
> - Ataxia–telangiectasia
> - Wiskott–Aldrich syndrome
> - Agammaglobulinaemias
> - T-cell and B-cell immunodeficiencies
> - Malnutrition
> - Malignancy
> - Congenital infections
> - Iatrogenic immunosuppression
> - Graft-versus-host disease

Dermatological disease is common in children with HIV/AIDS [2–6]. Concomitant infection and malnutrition are important confounders [6]. Oral candidosis may affect up to one-third [5]. Atopic eczema is controversial; previously thought to be commoner, one study showed no increase in the prevalence of atopy in perinatally HIV-infected children compared with the general population [7]. Unclassified eczematous eruptions are certainly seen. An eruption resembling seborrhoeic dermatitis has been described. Widespread napkin dermatitis can occur. The pruritic papular eruption is common and, as in adults, so are drug eruptions. HIV can present with very high IgE levels [8].

Approximately 9% of children with HIV globally are colonised with MRSA (compared with about 1–3% of the normal population [9]). About half of children with advanced HIV disease can be expected to suffer a serious bacterial infection and 20% of these involve the skin. The commonest organism is *Staphylococcus aureus* and the usual clinical patterns are of cellulitis, impetigo, folliculitis and abscess formation; a persistent staphylococcal folliculitis may also be seen. Scrofuloderma seems to be the exclusive manifestation of cutaneous tuberculosis in HIV coinfected children in Ethiopia [10]. The risk of disseminated bacillus Calmette–Guérin infection is much higher in HIV-infected children than in the immunocompetent child [11]. The most common fungal infection is candidosis (c.75%). Dermatophyte infection is frequently encountered (tinea capitis, tinea corporis, onychomycosis). HSV infection of the skin and mucosae is common and may be very serious and chronic; likewise disseminated zoster infection [5]. Paediatric exanthematous diseases such as measles may behave atypically and with more complications [12]. Persistent verrucous varicella in a 3-year-old girl has been described as the first manifestation of HIV infection [13]. In HIV infection, molluscum lesions have a predilection for the face rather than the trunk. In a study of adolescent, vertically infected HIV children from Zimbabwe, Lowe *et al*. have reported a high prevalence of skin conditions, especially PPE (42%) and extensive epidermodysplasia verruciformis-like plane warts (24%) [14]. Epidermodysplasia verruciformis is an acquired HPV (types 1, 2, 5, 6, 16 and 52) related dermatosis and is disfiguring and stigmatising and unresponsive to ART, as in adults [15].

Juvenile dermatomyositis and systemic sclerosis have been reported [16,17].

KS in children has been rare (about 5%) but may be increasing in Africa [18]. It often affects other organs, with sparing of the skin.

The clinical presentation in children is commonly with oro-palatal and inguino-scrotal disease [18]. EBV-associated smooth muscle tumours and non-Hodgkin and other lymphomas are other common tumours in children with HIV, and cutaneous involvement can occur [6,19,20].

There have been reports of skin changes compatible with pellagra, scurvy and acquired zinc deficiency (acrodermatitis enteropathica), attributed to malnutrition and malabsorption associated with chronic infectious diarrhoea caused by opportunistic organisms [6,21]. Cancrum oris (noma) is seen in malnourished HIV-infected children [22].

Drug eruptions are common, as in adults [6]. ART-associated lipohypertrophy is rare; lipoatrophy is associated with a raised serum C-reactive protein [23]. Non-specific findings in paediatric HIV practice include exanthematous rashes and cutis marmorata or livedo appearance [24], cold urticaria and idiopathic urticaria, long eyelashes requiring frequent trimming, patchy alopecia (common), erythema dyschromicum perstans (ashy dermatosis) and pyoderma gangrenosum [25]. Children infected with HIV are at risk of abuse [4]. Cutaneous manifestations in HIV-infected children improve with ART [26] but treatment is not without morbidity, as in adults (see Tables 31.5, 31.6 and 31.8). Paediatric IRIS/IRD/IRAD affects about 5–20% and can have appreciable mortality, with the incidence higher and severity worse in resource-poor settings [27,28].

Haemophilia

Atopic eczema (in children), seborrhoeic dermatitis, candidosis, dermatophyte infection and folliculitis occur with increased prevalence in HIV-positive compared with HIV-negative people with haemophilia. These conditions may develop earlier in infected haemophiliacs than in MSM [1,2].

Intravenous drug use

Drug abusers may have severe ecthyma and abscesses complicating injection sites but there is often concomitant malnutrition and liver disease [1]. Oral candidosis and seborrhoeic dermatitis are the most common presentations; KS and oral hairy leukoplakia are rare [2]. MRSA is an increasing problem. Reynaud-Mendel *et al*. [3] found that genital warts were commoner in HIV-infected intravenous drug users than in male homosexuals. Tuberculous lymphadenitis has been said to be a characteristic manifestation in intravenous drug users coinfected with tuberculosis [4].

IRIS/IRD/IRAD

The immunopathology is discussed earlier. Approximately half of all IRIS/IRD/IRAD events are dermatological [1,2,3]. Reported dermatological IRADs are listed in Box 31.14, Figures 31.28 and 31.29. Treatment is disease-specific but incorporates topical and systemic immunosuppression.

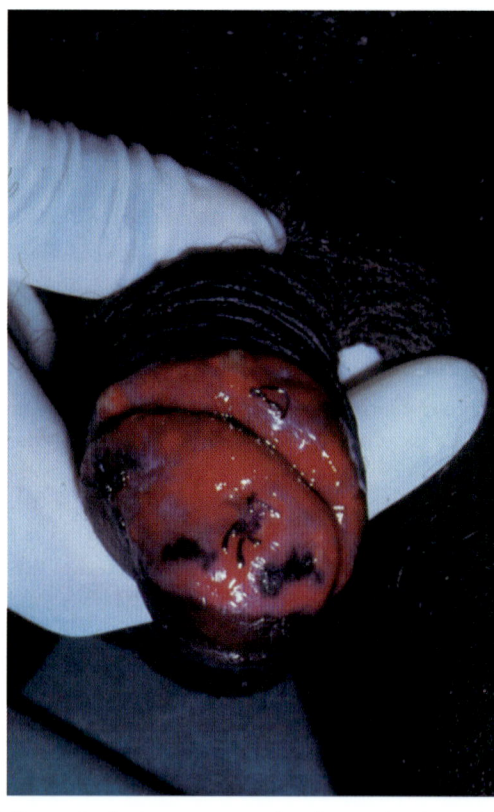

Figure 31.28 Herpes simplex immune restoration disease: chronic erosions on the penis. Courtesy of Medical Illustration UK Ltd.

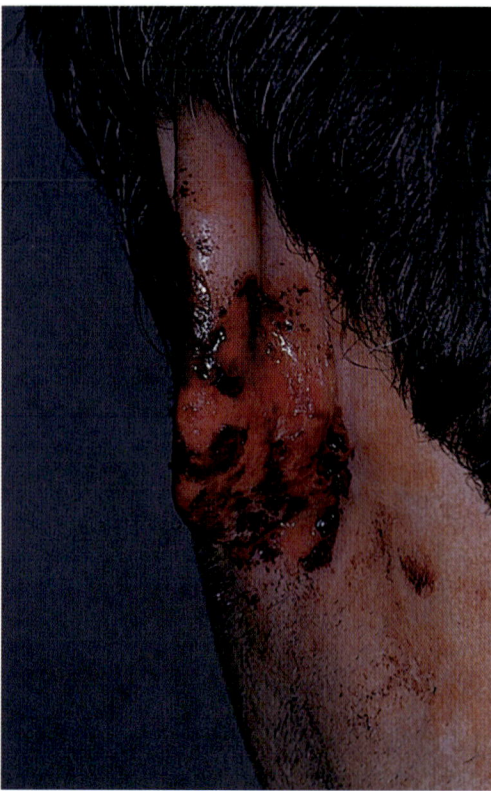

Figure 31.29 Cytomegalovirus immune restoration disease: necrotising impetiginised ulcer on the left ear. Courtesy of Imperial College School of Medicine.

Box 31.14 Dermatological manifestations of IRIS/IRD/IRAD

Human herpesviruses
- HSV-1 and -2: chronic oro-nasal and ano-genital disease (Figure 31.28) [4,5]
- Varicella-zoster virus (HHV-3)
- Epstein–Barr virus (HHV-4): hairy leukoplakia [6]
- Cytomegalovirus (HHV-6): acute multifocal cutaneous ulceration (Figure 31.29) [7], retinitis [8]
- Kaposi sarcoma herpesvirus (HHV-8) [9,10]

Other viruses
- HPV [11–13]: warts, oral warts, inflammation of existing warts, condyloma overgrowth
- Mollusca [14–16]

Bacteria
- Bacillary angiomatosis [17,18]
- Secondary syphilis [19]

Mycobacteria [20]
- Tuberculosis [21]
- Atypical mycobacterial infections [22,23]
- Leprosy [8,24–26]

Fungi
- Candidosis [6]
- Pityriasis versicolor [25,27]
- Tinea corporis [28]
- Cryptococcosis [29,30]
- Histoplasmosis
- Penicilliosis [31,32]
- Sporotrichosis [33,34]
- Leishmaniasis [27,35,36]
- Strongyloidiasis [37]
- Crusted scabies [38]

Inflammatory reactions related to infective agents
- 'Immune recovery folliculitis' – ?re-emergent hypersensitivity to *Demodex* and *Malassezia* [39–42]
- Severe seborrhoeic dermatitis – ?hypersensitivity to *Malassezia* [43]
- Alopecia
- Jarisch–Herxheimer reaction [18]

Idiopathic inflammatory reactions
- Photosensitivity [14]
- Papular pruritic eruption [25,44]
- Eosinophilic folliculitis [44–47]
- Sweet syndrome [47,48]
- Lupus erythematosus [49]
- Reactive arthritis
- Sarcoid [50,51]
- Granulomatous reactions to tattoos, foreign bodies and tribal medicines [52–54]
- Progressive supravenous granulomatous reaction [55]
- Alopecia universalis associated with Graves disease [37,56]
- Vitiligo and repigmentation of vitiligo [57,58]
- Acne vulgaris/rosacea [59,60]
- Relapsing polychondritis [61]
- Thrombophlebitis [62]

- Mid-dermal elastolysis [63]
- Oral ulceration [6]

Tumours
- Kaposi sarcoma (see HHV-8 above) [64]
- Non-Hodgkin lymphoma [64]
- Skin cancer (squamous cell carcinoma) progression [65]

Miscellaneous
- Eruptive dermatofibroma
- Eruptive naevi [66]
- Dyshidrosis
- Pseudoepitheliomatous hyperplasia [67]

From Meys et al. 2010 [1] and Lehloenya and Meintjes 2006 [3]. HHV, human herpesvirus; HPV, human papillomavirus; HSV, herpes simplex virus.

Key references

The full list of references can be found in the online version at https://www.wiley.com/rooksdermatology10e

HIV infection and AIDS
Epidemiology
7 Be in the Know. *Data*. https://www.beintheknow.org/understanding-hiv-epidemic/data (last accessed February 2023).
8 Public Health England (PHE). *Progress Towards Ending the HIV Epidemic in the United Kingdom. 2018 Report*. London: PHE, 2018. https://assets.publishing.service.gov.uk/government/uploads/system/uploads/attachment_data/file/821273/Progress_towards_ending_the_HIV_epidemic_in_the_UK.pdf (last accessed February 2023).

Pathophysiology
30 Roederer M, Keele BF, Schmidt SD et al. Immunological and virological mechanisms of vaccine-mediated protection against SIV and HIV. *Nature* 2014;505:502–8.

Management
16 British HIV Association (BHIVA). *Current Guidelines*. https://www.bhiva.org/guidelines (last accessed February 2023).

Dermatological manifestations of HIV infection
Pruritus, xerosis, ichthyosis and prurigo
4 Coates SJ, Leslie KS. What's new in HIV dermatology? *F1000Res* 2019;8:F1000 Faculty Rev-980.

Inflammatory dermatoses
Atopic eczema
7 Coates SJ, Leslie KS. What's new in HIV dermatology? *F1000Res* 2019;8:F1000 Faculty Rev-980.

Psoriasis
2 Coates SJ, Leslie KS. What's new in HIV dermatology? *F1000Res* 2019;8:F1000 Faculty Rev-980.

Drug reactions
105 Shear NH. *Litt's Drug Eruption and Reference Manual*, 27th edn. Oxford: CRC Press, 2021.

Neoplasms
Melanoma and non-melanoma skin cancer
16 Facciolà A, Venanzi Rullo E, Ceccarelli M et al. Malignant melanoma in HIV: epidemiology, pathogenesis, and management. *Dermatol Ther* 2020;33:e13180.
19 Asgari MM, Ray GT, Quesenberry CP Jr et al. Association of multiple primary skin cancers with human immunodeficiency virus infection, CD4 count, and viral load. *JAMA Dermatol* 2017;153:892–6.

Special situations
IRIS/IRD/IRAD
1 Meys R, Gotch FM, Bunker CB. Human papillomavirus in the HAART era of HIV: an immune reconstitution associated disease (IRAD)? *Br J Dermatol* 2010;162:6–11.
2 Seddiki N, French M. COVID-19 and HIV-associated immune reconstitution inflammatory syndrome: emergence of pathogen-specific immune responses adding fuel to the fire. *Front Immunol* 2021;12:649567.

CHAPTER 32
Fungal Infections

Roderick J. Hay
St John's Institute of Dermatology, King's College London, UK

Introduction, 32.2
Basic biology, 32.2
Reproduction, 32.3
Taxonomy and classification, 32.3
Nomenclature, 32.5
SUPERFICIAL MYCOSES, 32.6
Classification, 32.6
General description, 32.6
Identification, 32.6
Wood's light examination, 32.6
Collection of material, 32.7
Direct examination, 32.8
Culture, 32.8
Molecular diagnostics, 32.9
Identification of isolates, 32.9
SKIN DISEASE CAUSED BY *MALASSEZIA* SPECIES, 32.10
Pityriasis versicolor, 32.10
Malassezia folliculitis, 32.13
Other cutaneous disorders associated with *Malassezia* yeasts, 32.14
SUPERFICIAL MYCOSES CAUSED BY OTHER SPECIES, 32.14
Tinea nigra, 32.14
Black piedra, 32.15
White piedra, 32.16
Otomycosis, 32.17
Miscellaneous superficial mycoses caused by saprophytic moulds, 32.18
DERMATOPHYTOSIS, 32.18
Classification, 32.18
General description, 32.18
Basic biology, 32.20
Invasion of the epidermis, 32.20
Adherence, 32.20
Penetration, 32.20
Immunity, 32.21
Pathophysiology, 32.21
Other factors affecting infection, 32.22
Identification, 32.22
Genus *Microsporum*, 32.24
Genus *Trichophyton*, 32.26
Genus *Epidermophyton*, 32.30
Management, 32.30
General principles of management, 32.30

Therapeutic agents, 32.32
Treatment regimen, 32.34
Treatment failures, 32.34
SUPERFICIAL MYCOSES CAUSED BY DERMATOPHYTE INFECTION, 32.34
Tinea corporis, 32.35
Tinea capitis, 32.37
Tinea barbae, 32.40
Tinea faciei, 32.41
Tinea pedis, 32.42
Tinea manuum, 32.44
Tinea cruris, 32.45
Onychomycosis caused by dermatophytes, 32.46
Steroid-modified tinea, 32.49
Dermatophytide reactions, 32.50
SUPERFICIAL MYCOSES DUE TO OTHER HYPHAL FUNGI, 32.51
Superficial mycoses caused by *Neoscytalidium* species, 32.51
ONYCHOMYCOSIS CAUSED BY OTHER NON-DERMATOPHYTE MOULDS, 32.52
General description, 32.52
Identification, 32.53
Onychomycoses caused by *Scopulariopsis* infections, 32.53
Superficial onychomycosis caused by non-dermatophytes, 32.54
Onychomycosis caused by *Onychocola canadensis*, 32.55
Onychomycosis caused by miscellaneous moulds, 32.55
CANDIDOSIS, 32.55
Definition and nomenclature, 32.55
Classification, 32.55
General description, 32.56
Basic biology, 32.56
Candida ecology, 32.56
Pathophysiology, 32.57
Organisms, 32.57
Host factors, 32.57
Endocrine factors, 32.58
Immunological factors, 32.58
Candidosis and HIV/AIDS, 32.58
Identification, 32.58
Histology, 32.60

Management, 32.60
General principles of management, 32.60
Therapeutic agents, 32.60
First line, 32.60
CANDIDOSIS OF THE ORAL MUCOUS MEMBRANES, 32.61
Acute pseudomembranous candidosis, 32.61
Acute erythematous candidosis, 32.61
Chronic pseudomembranous candidosis, 32.61
Chronic erythematous candidosis, 32.62
Chronic plaque-like candidosis, 32.62
Chronic nodular candidosis, 32.62
Angular cheilitis, 32.62
Median rhomboid glossitis, 32.63
CANDIDOSIS OF THE SKIN AND GENITAL MUCOUS MEMBRANES, 32.63
Candida *intertrigo*, 32.63
Vulvo-vaginal candidosis, 32.63
Candidal balanitis, 32.64
Perianal and scrotal candidosis, 32.64
Perineal candidosis of infancy, 32.65
Nodular or granulomatous candidosis of the napkin area, 32.65
CANDIDOSIS OF THE NAIL AND PARONYCHIUM, 32.65
Candida *paronychia*, 32.65
Candida *onychomycosis*, 32.66
OTHER *CANDIDA* DISEASES, 32.66
Congenital candidosis, 32.66
Candida allergy, 32.67
Chronic mucocutaneous candidosis, 32.67
SUBCUTANEOUS MYCOSES, 32.69
Classification, 32.69
General description, 32.69
Identification, 32.69
Collection of samples, 32.69
Direct examination and histopathology, 32.69
Culture and identification of isolates, 32.70
Sporotrichosis, 32.70
Mycetoma, 32.72
Chromoblastomycosis, 32.75
Phaeohyphomycosis, 32.77
Lobomycosis, 32.78
Rhinosporidiosis, 32.79
Subcutaneous mycosis due to *Basidiobolus* and *Conidiobolus*, 32.79

SYSTEMIC MYCOSES, 32.80
Pathophysiology, 32.80
Identification, 32.80
Serological tests, 32.81
Direct examination and histopathology, 32.81
Culture and identification of isolates, 32.81
Histoplasmosis, 32.81
Blastomycosis, 32.84
Coccidioidomycosis, 32.86
Paracoccidioidomycosis, 32.88
Infections caused by *Talaromyces marneffei*, 32.89
Rare endemic mycoses, 32.90
Cryptococcosis, 32.90
Systemic candidosis, 32.92
Mucormycosis, 32.93
Unusual causes of skin lesions among opportunistic systemic mycoses, 32.93
Cutaneous infection caused by *Pneumocystis jiroveci*, 32.93
Infections caused by *Pythium insidiosum*, 32.94
Protothecosis, 32.94
Glossary of terms, 32.94
Acknowledgements, 32.95
Key references, 32.95

Introduction

Fungal infections or mycoses are common diseases. With the ease of worldwide travel, mycoses that were previously regarded as geographically limited can now be seen in any part of the world. Furthermore, in recent years the number of fungi recognised as human pathogens has risen, caused partly by an increasing population of immunocompromised patients as well as advances in molecular diagnosis. Fungi that were considered non-pathogenic are now being recovered as opportunistic pathogens. The routine identification of the majority of pathogenic fungi still relies on the direct observation of their morphology and this requires a knowledge of some of the fundamental features of fungal classification and structure, although increasing nunbers of laboratories are now using molecular identification methods. Over the last 20 years, a precise and complex terminology has been developed to describe the characteristic morphological features that may be observed [1,2–4] and an outline knowledge of this is useful in order to appreciate the often subtle differences that distinguish fungal pathogens (see the glossary at the end of the chapter).

Fungi are ubiquitous, capable of colonising almost any environment, and generally play an invaluable part in the decomposition and recycling of organic matter as well as playing a key role in plant nutrition. Fungi represent a distinct kingdom, and certain features of their metabolism, such as the pathway of lysine synthesis, are quite different from those found in bacteria and plants. With the use of molecular techniques, it is now recognised that the organisms originally included in this kingdom of Fungi contain at least three phylogenetically distinct groups, and some phyla have now been reclassified in the kingdoms Protozoa and Chromista. Almost all the fungi previously regarded as human pathogens, however, remain in the reclassified Fungi [5]. They have probably evolved from protozoan ancestors, and the kingdom Fungi is now believed to have originated before the separation of Animalia and Plantae. All fungi are heterotrophic and must exist as saprophytes or parasites. However, relatively few of the estimated quarter of a million species are pathogens of humans or other warm-blooded animals. The vast majority exist purely as saprophytes, commensals or plant parasites and, even among the few that do cause human disease, many have a well-established saprophytic or plant parasitic life cycle in which human infection has no role. At the beginning of this chapter, the principles and basic methods of medical mycology are described; subsequently, the sections describing the different groups of mycoses (superficial, subcutaneous and systemic) are each preceded by an introductory section.

Basic biology

Members of the kingdom Fungi show all the typical eukaryotic features, such as the organisation of genetic material into chromosomes enclosed within a membrane-bound nucleus, mitochondria and ribosomes. Unlike animal cells, however, their cells are enclosed by a rigid cell wall containing varying amounts of chitin, a polymer of *N*-acetyl glucosamine and β-glucans. The wall also contains mannans, glycoproteins and enzymes, some of which are secreted into the surrounding environment and break down complex organic compounds prior to their absorption. Fungi have an absorptive mode of nutrition. Within the cell wall, the cytoplasm is bounded by a plasma membrane in which the predominant sterol is not cholesterol, as in humans, but ergosterol.

The fungi may be broadly divided into two basic forms: moulds and yeasts (Table 32.1). Moulds are made up of long nucleate filaments called hyphae (singular: hypha), which are either largely aseptate (coenocytic) (see Figure 32.56) or divided into a series of cells by regular cross walls or septa (singular: septum) (see Figure 32.7a). Hyphae grow continuously at the apical tip, where the cell wall is constantly plasticised and new material added. This is the most metabolically active area of the cytoplasm. Further back, the cells may become vacuolated, and often the cytoplasm is reduced to a thin layer lining the cell membrane. Hyphae branch regularly, the branches diverging away from the parent hypha to utilise the environment to the maximum extent. Typically, the longest cell is at the apex of the hypha. The cytoplasm streams continuously, and the majority of septa contain pores that allow the movement of cytoplasm and even of organelles from one cell to another. An aggregation of hyphae is termed a mycelium, and the whole mass of the fungus is the thallus. The growth of a mould on solid media results in a circular colony, and in liquid media the mould forms a ball. Moulds produce cottony or velvety colonies in culture, and even large structures such as mushrooms are simply made up of a mass of hyphae.

In the yeasts, the main phase of the life cycle is unicellular, made up of ovoid to globose cells that usually reproduce by budding (see Figure 32.40) or, more rarely, by fission. After budding, when the daughter cell separates from the parent, a distinct bud scar is

Table 32.1 Morphology and diseases caused by the two main forms of fungi – yeasts and moulds.

Features	Yeasts	Moulds	Dimorphic fungi
Physical forms	Single-celled organisms that usually reproduce by budding	Multicellular fungi that often have complex life cycles and forms and produce different types of conidia (spores)	Fungi that can exist as either moulds or yeast or yeast-like forms. The transition between forms is associated with changes in temperature with the mould form seen at environmental temperature and the yeast or yeast-like form associated with human body temperature
Examples of diseases associated with these forms	*Candida* – candidiasis; including superficial oral or cutaneous disease and systemic candidiasis. *Malassezia* – pityriasis versicolor, seborrhoeic dermatitis, *Malassezia* folliculitis. *Cryptococcus* – cryptococcosis; including cryptococcal meningitis	*Aspergillus* – aspergillosis; including superficial aspergillosis (ear infections), allergic bronchopulmonary aspergillosis and disseminated invasive disease. Dermatophytes (including *Trichophyton*, *Microsporum*, *Epidermophyton*) – causing the various forms of dermatophytosis affecting skin, hair and nail. Mucoraceous moulds (including *Mucor*, *Rhizopus*, *Lichtheimia*) – causes of mucormycosis	*Histoplasma* – histoplasmosis. *Coccidioides* – coccidioidomycosis. *Blastomyces* – blastomycosis
Microscopic appearance	Round or oval cells, which may have prominent scars associated with separation from their progeny. Size 3–5 microns	Hyphae which may or may not have septa. Simple or specialised structures bearing spores of variable size and arrangement. Spores and hyphae may have inherent colour	Appearance varies with form. Yeast or yeast-like structures may be small and unicellular whereas moulds may have septate hyphae. Various spores are also formed by dimorphic fungi
Colony appearance	Usually white-cream colonies, rather like bacterial colonies. A few yeasts have inherent colonial colour. Cannot be identified by colonial appearance – require biochemical, molecular or other tests for identification	Colony morphology associated with colour, texture and growth rates characteristic of the species. Some moulds have diffusing pigment	Mould form is often a white or buff colony that may become darker with age. *Talaromyces marneffei* produces a diffusing red pigment. Yeast phases are often white-cream colonies as for other yeasts

left behind. In addition, however, some pathogens can also form filaments that may be true hyphae, similar to those of moulds, or pseudohyphae, which develop when two cells fail to separate after budding and simply elongate and lie end to end forming a chain. Pseudohyphae may be distinguished from true hyphae by the characteristic constrictions that may be seen at the points where two cells meet (see Figure 32.40) and the shortness of the apical cell. Yeasts produce soft, pasty or mucoid colonies.

Some fungi can completely switch their form of growth depending on the environmental conditions. These are termed thermally and nutritionally dimorphic fungi, and include several of the major respiratory pathogens, such as *Histoplasma capsulatum* and *Coccidioides immitis*. When cultured at room temperature or during growth in the environment, these fungi are typical moulds, yet in human tissues or on special media at 37°C they convert into yeasts or other non-filamentous forms.

Reproduction

Fungi reproduce both sexually and asexually, sometimes simultaneously. The sexual phase is termed the teleomorph and the asexual phase the anamorph; originally both types had separate taxonomic names, a potential source of confusion. In 2011 the naming rules were formally changed, fungi only have one name to cover both sexual and asexual phases. The process to determine which name has priority is on-going. Where names have changed recently, the older familiar names are retained in brackets throughout this chapter for ease of use. In the laboratory, sexual phases of pathogens are rarely seen, as the majority of fungi are heterothallic, which means that sexual reproduction requires the presence of two or sometimes four different mating types. Relatively few fungi can reproduce sexually by the mating of hyphae from a single mycelium, a condition termed homothallic.

Taxonomy and classification

In an attempt to reflect true phylogenetic relationships, the formal classification of fungi has previously been based upon the features of the sexual phase of growth. This involves the fusion of two nuclei followed by meiotic division. Unlike higher plants and animals, many of the fungi are haploid for the major part of the life cycle, the diploid phase being relatively short lived. Three groups or phyla of sexually reproducing fungi, *Glomeromycota* (previously *Zygomycota*), *Ascomycota* and *Basidiomycota*, contain human pathogens. A fourth, completely artificial group, the *Deuteromycota* or Fungi Imperfecti, was originally created to include those fungi with no known sexual phase, and the asexual phases of the *Ascomycota* and *Basidiomycota*. With the more sophisticated techniques available today, such as ultrastructural data on septa and genetic sequencing, these asexual 'mitosporic' species can now be placed within the recognised sexual groups, and the artificial form-phylum *Deuteromycota* will disappear from the literature. The asexual dermatophytes, for instance, will join the *Ascomycota* [6]. At present, fungal taxonomy is in a process of change and this is still reflected by the use of older terminology in many textbooks and publications.

The *Glomeromycota* are all moulds and reproduce sexually by the formation of thick-walled zygospores following the fusion of two outgrowths arising from the hyphae. The hyphae are very characteristic, being both extremely wide and often sparsely septate. The septa that are formed usually cut off sporing structures and old parts of the mycelium, and are complete, so that damage to any part of the hypha will result in the death of the whole aseptate length. Branching in this group is typically at right angles. Asexual reproduction is usually by means of sporangiospores formed by the cleavage of cytoplasm within a sporangium. This is a sac-like structure, which is supported by a specialised hypha, the sporangiophore.

The *Ascomycota* contains both moulds and yeasts. Sexual reproduction is by the production of ascospores, formed within a sac-like ascus. These asci may themselves be contained within a specialised fruiting body or ascoma, which may be large enough to be visible to the naked eye. The hyphae of the *Ascomycota* have a lamellate cell wall, with a thin electron-dense outer layer and a thicker electron-transparent inner layer. The hyphae are narrow and regularly septate, but the passage of cytoplasm and even nuclei from one cell to the next is made possible by the presence of a pore in the centre of each septum. When hyphae are damaged, however, this septal pore quickly becomes plugged by structures termed Woronin bodies, limiting the damage to those particular cells that were injured. A few of the *Ascomycota* have multiple pores in their septa.

In the *Basidiomycota*, sexual reproduction is by the production of basidiospores formed externally on sterigmata protruding from a club-shaped basidium. Many of this group produce the complex structures we know as mushrooms and toadstools, with gills, covered by basidia, raised above the ground to aid in airborne dispersal of the spores. Others, such as the rusts, smuts and basidiomycetous yeasts, are microscopic. The cell walls of the *Basidiomycota* are lamellate and electron dense. When present, the hyphae are narrow and septate. The septal pore structure in this group is more complex and characteristic, and usually comprises a lip-like extension termed a dolipore, which may be surrounded by perforated membranes called parenthosomes. These allow the passage of cytoplasm, but not nuclei, from one cell to the next. In the *Ascomycota* and the *Basidiomycota*, after the fusion of hyphal initials of opposite mating type, subsequent fusion of the two nuclei may be delayed, so that for part of the life cycle these cells contain two nuclei of opposite mating type, a state termed dikaryotic. For this reason, some workers combine these two groups into the *Dikaryomycota*. It is characteristic of the *Basidiomycota* that when a dikaryotic hyphal cell divides, a hook-like structure known as a clamp connection is formed between the two resulting cells as a way of allowing one daughter nucleus of each type to migrate into each cell.

The form-phylum *Deuteromycota* was artificially constructed as the phylogenetic relationships of many of the asexual fungi contained within it could not at that time be fully determined. Increasingly this phylum is no longer used by taxonomists. The asexual propagules of all the fungi classified in this group were called conidia. Three main divisions were recognised in the *Deuteromycota* and are still mentioned in the current literature: *Blastomycetes*, which are yeasts reproducing by budding; *Hyphomycetes*, which are moulds bearing the conidia exposed unprotected on the hyphae; and *Coelomycetes*, where the conidiogenous cells that produce the conidia are enclosed in a specialised protective fruiting structure, either a flask-shaped pycnidium or a saucer-shaped acervulus. The majority of fungi isolated in the laboratory are *Hyphomycetes*, and this group may be further subdivided according to colour into fungi that have dark hyphae – dematiaceous fungi – and those that are pale or brightly coloured – moniliaceous fungi. An amazing variety of conidia are formed by these fungi, and their laboratory identification still utilises the study of the method of conidial formation or ontogeny and conidial morphology, although this is increasingly replaced by molecular identification methods.

Spore (conidia) formation

Two main methods of conidial production are seen in the *Hyphomycetes*: thallic and blastic (Figure 32.1b–h). In thallic conidiation, a whole cell or section of a hypha is transformed into the conidium. The most common examples of this are arthroconidia (Figure 32.1b), when a hypha produces a series of septa, forming a chain of cells that separate at maturity, and chlamydoconidia (Figure 32.1c), which are formed when a single cell becomes thick walled and acts as a storage and survival cell but does not disarticulate at maturity.

In blastic conidiation, the conidium is formed by 'blowing out' or budding from only a small, weakened area of the cell wall of the conidiogenous cell. If both the outer and the inner cell wall are blown out to form the conidial wall, the budding is termed holoblastic. If the first conidium ruptures the outer cell wall, and only the inner cell wall is blown out as the conidial wall, the budding is termed enteroblastic. A large range of blastic conidia are produced, but certain basic patterns of conidial development may be recognised. Holoblastic conidia include solitary conidia, which may simply be produced by the blowing out of a small part of the hyphal wall, to form a lateral or terminal conidium. In other fungi, more specialised conidiogenous cells are found, and these may produce a succession of holoblastic conidia. Examples of this include those fungi with sympodial conidiogenous cells (Figure 32.1d), where after the first conidium has been formed, the conidiogenous cell continues to grow and produces a second conidium slightly ahead of and to one side of the base of the first conidium. It then repeats the process, forming a third conidium slightly ahead of and to the opposite side of the second conidium. This eventually results in a zig-zag appearance, with conidia coming off alternately on each side of the fertile cell. Such conidiogenous cells are very characteristic and are termed geniculate.

Many of the fungi with sympodial conidiation have multicellular conidia, either with transverse septa – phragmoconidia – or with both transverse and vertical septa – dictyoconidia.

Chains of holoblastic conidia may be formed by acropetal budding (Figure 32.1e), where, after the cell has budded, the cells remain attached and a further conidium is produced by the budding of the daughter cell. This continues building up a chain of cells with the youngest at the tip of the chain. The chains may branch.

Enteroblastic chains of conidia with the youngest cell at the bottom of the chain are termed basipetal and are formed by the repeated blowing out of the inner layer of the cell wall of specialised structures termed phialides and annellides. Phialides are often flask shaped and may have a pronounced collarette – a flaring ring of wall material surrounding the apex of the cell. The phialoconidia are formed by repeated budding at exactly the same point at the tip of phialide, which does not increase in length during this process (Figure 32.1f). In contrast, as a series of annelloconidia is formed, the cell apex proliferates slightly as each conidium is produced, leaving a series of ring-like scars at the tip of the cell, and the annellide becomes progressively narrower and longer (Figure 32.1g). Conidia produced by phialides and annellides may aggregate to form balls rather than chains.

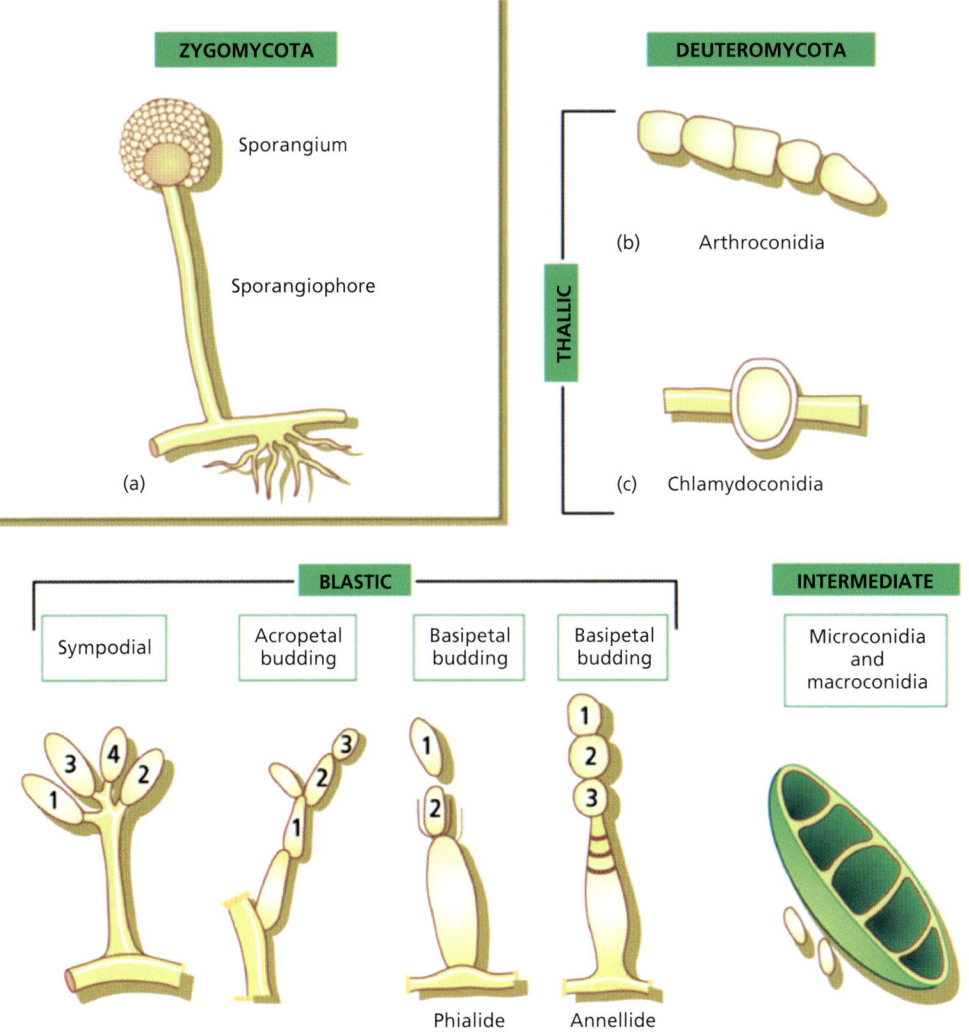

Figure 32.1 Asexual reproduction in fungi. (a) Zygomycota: the most characteristic form of asexual reproduction is the production of sporangia and sporangiospores. (b–h) Deuteromycota: asexual conidia may be formed by two main processes – thallic and blastic. Thallic conidiation results in the production of arthroconidia (b) and chlamydoconidia (c). Blastic conidiation may take several forms, including sympodial conidiogenous cells (d), acropetal budding (e) and basipetal budding from phialides (f) or annellides (g). The conidia of the dermatophytes do not fit in with this thallic–blastic division, but show features of both; they are also examples of fungi that produce two kinds of conidia simultaneously, which differ in size. These are termed microconidia and macroconidia (h).

A number of pathogens produce conidia that are not strictly thallic or blastic and which show a particular method of separation from the hypha. A specialised cell at the base of the conidium breaks, leaving a frill of wall material at the base of the conidium. These conidia are termed aleurioconidia.

Another feature that is seen in several fungal pathogens is polymorphism – the simultaneous production of more than one form of conidium. For instance, in the case of the dermatophytes, two types of conidia are formed that differ greatly in size; in such instances, the larger conidium is termed a macroconidium and the smaller a microconidium (Figure 32.1h).

Nomenclature

Nomenclature is the system whereby the correct names are applied to specific organisms and is a necessary adjunct to any system of classification. In mycology, as in other sciences, the lack of a uniform approach towards the recognition and description of new species of fungi led to the accumulation of a bewildering number and variety of names in the literature. As an example, *Candida albicans* has been described and redescribed many times since its original description in 1850. A classic taxonomical work [1] lists no fewer than 110 species in 22 genera for this fungus. The need to provide a single name for a single species becomes obvious, particularly when so many synonyms have been proposed for one and the same organism. In order to provide some conformity and stability to the naming of fungi (separate consideration is given to bacterial and zoological nomenclature), a series of principles, rules and recommendations have been incorporated into an internationally recognised code, whose authoritative guidance has done much to bring order to a state of confusion. Recent changes to this code should bring further streamlining to fungal naming rules [2].

As well as confusion in specific names, disease names have also given rise to controversy. As an increasing number of fungi have been shown to be capable of causing infection, particularly as opportunists in only a limited number of recorded cases, the habit of using the generic name of the fungus to produce a new disease name has become increasingly unwieldy, particularly when fungi are so frequently re-examined and often renamed. Well-established disease names have been retained, but where a new pathogen or pathology is involved the International Society for Human and Animal Mycology (ISHAM) [2] recommends that individual mycoses should be named as often as possible in the form 'pathology A caused by pathogen B'. Thus, the use of such terms as fusariosis and trichosporonosis is best discouraged and replaced by use of

Table 32.2 Organisms associated with superficial mycoses.

Type of mycosis	Fungi mainly associated
Diseases caused by *Malassezia*	*Malassezia globosa, M. sympodialis* and other *Malassezia* spp.
Tinea nigra	*Hortaea werneckii* and *Stenella araguata*
Black Piedra	*Piedraia hortaea*
White Piedra	*Trichosporon ovoides, T. inkin, T. asahii* and *T. mucoides*
Otomycosis	*Aspergillus niger* and other fungi
Miscellaneous superficial mycoses caused by saprophytic moulds	*Fusarium* spp., *Scopulariopsis brevicaulis* and other fungi
Dermatophytosis including dermatophyte onychomycosis	*Trichophyton* spp., *Microsporum* spp. and *Epidermophyton floccosum*
Onychomycosis caused by other non-dermatophyte moulds	*Neoscytalidium hyalinum, N. dimidiatum, Scopulariopsis (Microascus) brevicaulis, Fusarium* spp., *Aspergullus* spp., *Onychocola canadensis* and other fungi
Superficial candidosis	*Candida albicans, C. glabrata, C. tropicalis* and other *Candida* spp.

'eumycetoma caused by *Fusarium* species' or 'disseminated mycosis caused by *Trichosporon* species'.

Disease names used throughout this text are based on lists published independently by the Council for the International Organization of the Medical Sciences (CIOMS) [3], the ISHAM [4] and the World Health Organization (WHO) classification, ICD-10.

SUPERFICIAL MYCOSES

This section describes infections of the skin and mucosal surface – superficial mycoses. These are sometimes split into superficial and cutaneous mycoses.

Classification

The superficial fungal infections include *Malassezia* infections, dermatophytosis, candidosis and a range of non-dermatophyte infections of the skin and nails, such as dermatomycoses caused by *Neoscytalidium* species and onychomycosis caused by other non-dermatophyte moulds (Table 32.2).

General description

Some of the fungi causing these infections are present in the environment, but others, such as *Candida albicans* and *Malassezia* spp., have an intimate association with humans and are part of the normal microbiome of the gut and skin, respectively. A few, such as the anthropophilic dermatophytes, have evolved to the point where they have become almost completely reliant on the human host for survival.

Identification

The laboratory diagnosis of superficial fungal infections relies first on the direct microscopical observation of the pathogen in samples from the affected area. This is usually followed by culture and the specific identification of the fungus. For the laboratory to work optimally, the quantity and quality of the material examined is critical.

For most samples both culture and microscopic examination will be performed, so it is essential that as much clinical material as possible is submitted to the laboratory to allow both diagnostic methods to be carried out.

Wood's light examination

The recognition that hair infected by certain dermatophytes produces a characteristic fluorescence in UV light filtered by Wood's glass – which consists of barium silicate containing about 9% nickel oxide and transmits rays of wavelength above 365 nm – was an important advance in medical mycology. The nature and source of the fluorescent substances in infected hairs are not fully understood, but tryptophan metabolites produced by dermatophytes may be involved [1]. The hair remains fluorescent after the fungus has ceased to be viable. The fluorescent material can be extracted from the hair in hot water [2,3] or in a cold solution of sodium bromide [1]. The colour of the fluorescence is influenced by the pH of the solution [2]. Because fungi growing in culture or on hair *in vitro* do not fluoresce in this way, the phenomenon must be attributed to some substance produced by the interaction of the fungus and the growing hair. Its chemical nature has not been defined and the suggestion that it may be a pteridine has been challenged [3].

Only some of the dermatophytes capable of invading hair will induce fluorescence, but these include members of the genus *Microsporum* (e.g. *M. audouinii* and *M. canis*), which are common in a number of densely populated parts of the world. Hairs infected by these species produce a brilliant green fluorescence, easily recognised in a darkened room. Only the fully invaded portions of the shaft develop this property. In recent infections or at the spreading margin of early lesions, the fluorescent part of the hair may not yet have emerged from the follicle and can be detected only after the hair is plucked. Among other *Microsporum* species and variants, only *M. canis* var. *distortum* and *M. ferrugineum* regularly induce fluorescence, and *M. gypseum* and *M. nanum* occasionally do so. *Trichophyton schoenleinii* causes a paler green fluorescence of infected hair. In favus, the fluorescent hairs tend to be long, in contrast to the short, broken stumps characteristic of *Microsporum* infections.

In areas where *Microsporum* infections are prevalent, Wood's light is a useful tool in the diagnosis and treatment of an individual patient. The most common sources of error are the bluish or purplish fluorescence produced by ointments containing petrolatum, scales, serum, exudates, an insufficiently darkened room, light reflected from the examiner's clothing and the failure to remember that not all fungi cause fluorescence. Correctly performed and interpreted, the test is virtually specific, but absence of fluorescence in some infections with *M. audouinii* and *M. canis* has been reported [4]. The lamp can be used in the detection of subclinical infection and to assess response to treatment or spontaneous cure. The Wood's lamp is also of value in the diagnosis of pityriasis versicolor, where the scales fluoresce yellow in some cases. A similar yellow fluorescence, presumably because of the presence of yeasts of *Malassezia* species, may be seen in some cases of severe dandruff, in cradle cap in infants and in the follicular orifices of the face and upper trunk in normal subjects.

Collection of material

Material for examination must be collected from the most heavily infected area or active growing edge of the infection, wherever possible. Careful clinical examination may be helped by the use of Wood's light, especially in tinea capitis.

Skin

Disposable scalpel blades of the solid type, held vertically to the skin, are used to obtain scrapings. Alternatively, heat-sterilised, blunt, banana-shaped scalpels, which are available from chiropody firms, may be used. Cleaning of the skin with alcohol may be useful if the patient has applied ointment or powder but is not usually necessary. If the lesion has a definite edge, the material should be taken from the active margin, otherwise scraping from much of the area is adequate. In cases of partially treated pityriasis versicolor, when very little scaling is present, it is possible to take a sample by pressing a strip of sticky tape (Sellotape®) on to the lesion and then on to a drop of mounting fluid on a slide and use this for the direct examination. The method is less suitable for direct examination of samples from the cutaneous mycoses [1]. If it is difficult to obtain sufficient material for culture in cases of dermatophytosis, transport swabs are a good back-up, as is usual with candidiasis. When blisters are present, a pair of fine scissors may be used to cut off a blister roof for microscopical examination and culture; such samples are often packed with hyphae. The scrapings, hair or nail clippings should be collected and transported in specially designed flat transport packs, which keeps the specimen dry, thus preventing overgrowth of bacterial contaminants. Plastic containers are unsuitable as the skin adheres to the sides and is difficult to remove. The use of glass slides, which then have to be transported to the laboratory, is hazardous as they are frequently broken. Squares of brightly coloured or dark paper card are also useful; these may then be carefully folded and secured by a paper clip. The details of the patient, exact site of the lesion and time of sampling, animal contact or recent travel should then be clearly recorded. Dermatophytes in skin scrapings may remain viable for months and yeasts for several weeks.

Hairs

Hairs to be examined for the presence of black or white piedra may be simply cut off at skin level. If dermatophytosis is suspected, the hairs should be removed with the roots intact; cut hairs are unsuitable. In many instances, the affected hairs may be recognised because they are dull and broken but, if not, the fact that they slip out easily with fine forceps may also help in selecting the right material. This is particularly useful in examining scalp or beard kerions caused by *Trichophyton verrucosum*, where relatively little fungus may provoke a severe reaction, and it may be necessary to test many hairs before an infected hair is found. In those instances where the hairs break off very short, as in black-dot infections, a scalp scraping will yield the best material, with the infected roots appearing as tiny stumps among the skin scales. It should be noted that in cases of steroid-treated tinea corporis or tinea incognito, the examination of vellus hairs may be the easiest method of diagnosis as – although fungi such as *T. rubrum* rarely invade the hair shaft – they may colonise the hair follicle.

In addition to collecting scales and hairs, brush samples are excellent for the culture of scalp infections and may also be useful in testing suspected animal sources of infection [2–4]; however, microscopy cannot be performed on them. A sterile, plastic, scalp massager or disposable toothbrush is brushed firmly through the hair at least 10 times and is then pressed against the culture medium in a 90 mm Petri dish. This simple technique is an extremely sensitive culture method and is invaluable when screening large numbers of children. Several hundred children may be examined in a day by performing a Wood's light examination and taking a brush sample from each child, which can then be taken back to the laboratory for culture. Cultures from infected children produce a fungal colony from many of the inoculation points; contacts of infected children usually yield only a few colonies. In cases of kerion, when brush sampling may be unsuitable and painful, a transport swab wiped over the lesion will usually pick up enough conidia to give a positive culture.

Nails

The diagnosis of onychomycosis is complicated by the fact that the isolation of the pathogen in culture from nail material is more difficult to achieve than for skin and hair samples. In the majority of nail infections, the material for examination is taken from the distal end of the nail, despite the fact that the infection is advancing proximally. The hyphae at the distal end of the nail are less likely to be viable [5]. Unfortunately, it is usually not practicable to take deep samples from the proximal advancing edge without discomfort to the patient. The full thickness of the nail should be sampled, as most infections start in the hyponychium. Debris from under the nail is a fruitful source of material, which may be scraped out using the flat end of a dental probe. Superficial scrapings are inadequate, except in cases of superficial white onychomycosis or proximal subungual onychomycosis.

In cases of paronychia, the nail fold may be moistened with saline using a wet swab, and the flat end of a dental probe or blunt cautery tip may be gently pushed into the fold to withdraw material for direct examination and culture. After this, a swab should also be taken for culture.

As the isolation of fungi from nail material is difficult, samples should also be taken from any skin lesions that may be present, as these are very likely to be invaded by the same pathogen as the nail and cultures are more likely to be positive. It is essential when submitting nail material to the laboratory to specify whether the sample is a fingernail or toenail, as some pathogens are more prevalent in one than the other.

Mucous membranes

The mouth or vagina may be sampled using swabs. If the specimen is not to be examined immediately, swabs with transport medium are preferable as yeasts rapidly die in dry conditions. However, delays in the processing of transport medium swabs will allow multiplication of yeasts in the samples.

Ear

Scrapings from the external ear canal may be supplemented with swab samples.

Direct examination

For routine examination, specimens are usually mounted in 10–30% potassium hydroxide; the higher the percentage, the faster the specimen will clear. For skin scrapings and nails, warming gently over the pilot light of a Bunsen burner will speed up the process, but boiling should be avoided, if possible, as this tends to encourage the formation of artefacts, which may confuse the inexperienced observer. It is impossible to soften skin and nail samples too much, for the thinner the specimen, the easier it will be to observe the fungal elements. The cover slip should be pressed down firmly to obtain a monolayer of cells before microscopic observation. Excess potassium hydroxide will etch microscope lenses, so it must be removed by blotting with small squares of filter paper or tissue. A few minutes spent carefully preparing the specimen in this way are well spent. Nail specimens take longer to clear than skin, but if small pieces and debris are taken, they will usually soften within 10 min. In those instances where the nails do not soften satisfactorily, the slide may be put in a 37°C incubator for 1 h, and the material can then be flattened. In contrast to skin and nail samples, infected hairs are very delicate, and if heated or left in mounting fluid for more than a few minutes tend to disintegrate, obscuring the characteristic arrangement of the arthroconidia. They should therefore be examined as soon as possible after mounting. If examining specimens using bright-field illumination, the lighting is critical; overillumination, particularly when scanning the slide under low power (10×), will render the fungal elements invisible. The light should therefore be low initially and then raised when the presence of fungus is confirmed by examination with a higher power lens (20× or 40×). An alternative clearing agent, which does not require warming of the specimen, is 10% sodium sulphide solution [1,2].

With experience, bright-field examination of specimens cleared in this way is quick and relatively straightforward. However, several authors have recommended a variety of techniques to make observation of the fungal elements easier. Phase-contrast and dark-field microscopy can produce good results [3] but require that the specimen be really thin, and thus may need a longer period of softening of the material than bright-field microscopy. The addition of 35% dimethylsulphoxide to the potassium hydroxide may speed up softening, but overdigestion is then a problem, and the specimens should be examined within 1–2 h. Dimethylacetamide or dimethylformamide have been suggested as alternatives [4]. Several stains such as Congo red, methylene blue and cotton blue have been recommended to enhance the contrast between fungus and skin, but again these require a fully softened specimen.

Fluorescence microscopy using either acridine orange [5] or a fluorescent brightener such as Calcofluor white or Blankophor [1,2], which specifically stain polysaccharides in the fungal cell wall, is becoming increasingly popular. Comparative studies of different methods used in direct examination [2,6–8] concluded that most of the recommended staining procedures for direct microscopic examination were no better than the classic potassium hydroxide method, but that if a fluorescence microscope is available, the use of fluorescent brighteners does give superior results. One study [9] concluded that fluorescence microscopy using Blankophor P flussig in sodium sulphide solution was quicker and produced significantly fewer direct microscopy negative samples, which subsequently yielded fungus on culture, than bright-field microscopy using sodium sulphide solution alone.

Whatever method is used, the ability to find fungi on direct examination of samples is largely a matter of practice. The beginner may well be confused initially by the common artefacts that may be present, such as mosaic fungus – cholesterol-forming polygonal deposits around cells – air bubbles, fibres and crystals, but with practice it becomes progressively easier to find the fungi and distinguish the various infections.

Several workers advocate the histopathological processing of nail material and staining with a fungus-specific stain such as periodic acid–Schiff (PAS) as a routine measure [6]. It has been suggested that this not only confirms that the nail plate is actually invaded, but also reduces the number of false negative direct reports, where fungus is cultured from a microscopically negative nail. Although histological processing of samples has been shown to yield a higher rate of positivity than culture, the rates are similar to those obtained with potassium hydroxide microscopy in skilled hands [8,9]. As the facilities for histopathological processing may not be available in a small laboratory, routine microscopy supplemented by a fluorescent technique is still the method of choice.

Culture (Table 32.3)

For some of the superficial mycoses, the appearance of the fungal elements observed on direct examination is so characteristic that culture is not strictly necessary for diagnosis of the infection. Examples include pityriasis versicolor and, to a lesser degree, black piedra, white piedra and tinea nigra. For otomycosis, in contrast, culture is essential, as the range of organisms that can cause infection is large and the specific identification of the pathogen will have a profound effect on the therapy selected. Similarly, differences in the responses of the different pathogenic yeasts to some antifungals, such as fluconazole, necessitates identification down to species level, at least in patients on long-term treatment. The situation with dermatophyte infections is rather different because, although on direct examination of skin and nail samples the different species are indistinguishable, generally all the dermatophyte species apart from those causing tinea capitis respond similarly to the major systemic and topical antifungals available; treatment can be initiated on the basis of the direct examination. In addition, culture will provide valuable information on the possible source of infection and the likelihood of spread of the disease. Culture of specimens with negative direct microscopical results is also desirable, as it will allow the detection of the small percentage of cases where prolonged therapy, or a very inflammatory host reaction, may make the microscopical detection of the fungus in the skin difficult. The non-dermatophytic moulds capable of infecting the skin or nail,

Table 32.3 Cultural conditions for the isolation of superficial and cutaneous pathogens.

Disease	Causative organisms	Media		Antibiotics		Temperature		Maximum length of incubation (days)
		GP	MEA	Cyc	Chlor	26–28°C	37°C	
Black piedra	*Piedraia hortae*	+	+	+	+	+		28
White piedra	*Trichosporon* spp.	+	+	−	+	+		14
Tinea nigra	*Hortaea werneckii*	+	+	−	+	+		21
Dermatophytosis	*Trichophyton* spp. *Microsporum* spp. *Epidermophyton* spp.	+	+	+	+	+		21–28
Dermatomycoses caused by *Neoscytalidium* spp.	*Neoscytalidium dimidiatum Neoscytalidium hyalinum*	+		−	+	+		21
Onychomycosis caused by non-dermatophyte moulds	*Scopulariopsis* spp. *Sarocladium* (formerly *Acremonium*) spp. *Fusarium* spp., etc.	+	+	−	+	+		21
Candidosis	*Candida* spp.	+	+	−	+	+	+	7
Otomycosis	*Aspergillus* spp. *Candida* spp., etc.	+	+	−	+	+	+	21

Chlor, chloramphenicol 0.05 g/L; Cyc, cycloheximide 0.4 g/L; GP, glucose–peptone agar; MEA, malt extract agar; +, recommended; −, not recommended.

such as *Neoscytalidium* (*Scytalidium*) species and *Scopulariopsis brevicaulis*, can be diagnosed on the basis of direct microscopy, but this requires considerable expertise. In addition, mixed infections with dermatophytes do occur, so that it is advisable to always perform cultures in these cases.

Fungi grow readily on simple media containing glucose and preferably an organic nitrogen source; they are not particularly fastidious. The primary culture medium used therefore is largely a matter of personal choice. Many laboratories will select a simple glucose/peptone agar, either with 4% sugar, 1% peptone and an acid pH (Sabouraud's dextrose agar) or with 2% sugar, 1% peptone and a neutral pH (Emmon's modification). Antibacterial antibiotics such as gentamicin (0.0025%) and/or chloramphenicol (0.005%) may be added to reduce contamination and, if a dermatophyte infection has been diagnosed, the addition of cycloheximide at 0.04% will inhibit the growth of non-dermatophyte moulds. This antibiotic must be excluded, however, if infection by a non-dermatophyte mould such as *Neoscytalidium* or candidosis is suspected as, although *Candida albicans* is not affected, many of the less common species of *Candida* found particularly in nail and mucous membrane sites will be inhibited. For sites where non-dermatophyte moulds such as *Neoscytalidium dimidiatum* may be significant – palms, soles, toe webs and nails – it is simplest to perform duplicate cultures on media with and without cycloheximide. Sabouraud's dextrose agar is available from a number of different commercial sources. It should be noted, however, that variations in the different makes, particularly the type of peptone included, will affect the overall morphology of the isolates and cause differences in pigmentation and texture of the fungal colonies, particularly of dermatophytes. It is easiest therefore to become familiar with the morphology of these pathogens on one brand only. One should also note carefully which formulations have cycloheximide and/or chloramphenicol already incorporated (e.g. Mycosel® and Mycobiotic® agars) and which require their addition. Another medium that is frequently used for primary culture is 3–4% malt extract agar, which is also commercially available.

As incubation is much longer than for bacterial cultures, the medium should be poured relatively thickly to prevent drying out; a 30 mL/90 mm Petri dish is adequate. The majority of laboratories now perform their cultures in disposable plastic Petri dishes, but if screw-capped glass bottles or tubes are used, the tops must be left slightly loose to provide adequate aeration. For moulds, the temperature of incubation should be 26–28°C and cultures should be held for a maximum of 3–4 weeks, although routinely 2 weeks is used. For *Candida* species, the temperature of incubation should be 37°C, and plates may be discarded after 48 h. As some *Trichosporon* species will not grow at 37°C, incubation should be at 26–28°C for up to 2 weeks.

Molecular diagnostics

Increasingly, there has been an interest in diagnosing mycoses without the use of either classic microscopic examination or culture of samples, but by using molecular techniques. In the past 20 years, groups have reported the use of molecular techniques, including polymerase chain reaction (PCR) analysis, for the identification and classification of dermatophytes after culture [1–3]. More recently, methods have been developed for the primary diagnosis of dermatophytosis [4–7]. Molecular methods for primary diagnosis initially had limited success rates with only 30–40% of culture-positive samples being positive [5], but more recent studies have demonstrated sensitivity rates of 84% [5], with the added bonus that identification of the dermatophyte is performed concurrently. The time to diagnosis is substantially reduced in the absence of culture and is now achievable in 48 h [6,7]. For *Malassezia*-associated conditions, identification can also be performed directly from skin scales, without culture [8]. However, as speciation of *Malassezia* is not usually performed in routine laboratories, the relevance of this technique is likely to be limited. The introduction of commercially available kits for PCR diagnosis of dermatophytosis is allowing more laboratories to use this technique.

Identification of isolates
Yeasts

The identification of yeasts requires morphological data together with physiological and biochemical investigations. An examination of the yeast colony should include the recording of colour and texture. Microscopic features of note may include the size and shape of the budding cells (blastoconidia) and the presence of pseudohyphae, true hyphae, capsules, arthroconidia and ascospores. In the case of *Candida albicans*, the formation of terminal vesicles (chlamydospores) on cornmeal or rice agar supplemented with Tween 80, or the production of germ tubes after incubation in serum at 37°C for 2–3 h, allows specific identification. For speciation of other pathogenic yeasts, physiological tests must be performed. An increasing number of commercially produced yeast identification kits are available and widely used, including the API 32C® (bioMerieux) and the Auxacolor 2® (Sanofi Diagnostic Pasteur). Primary isolation media that allow the specific identification of certain species to be made by the production of a characteristic colour are also now available. On Albicans ID® medium (bioMerieux), *C. albicans* colonies develop a blue colour; on Chromagar® (Becton and Dickinson), *C. tropicalis*, *C. krusei* and *C. albicans* produce blue-, pink- and green-coloured colonies, respectively. These media facilitate the detection of mixed infections, which has become increasingly important because of the relative insensitivity of certain *Candida* species to some of the currently available antifungal drugs. However, it should not be used as the sole method of identification of yeast species.

Laboratories are increasingly using matrix-assisted laser desorption–time of flight spectrometry (MALDI-TOF) to carry out yeast identification. This technique allows the rapid identification of yeasts, within a matter of a few hours. As commercially available databases increase in breadth, the range of organisms that can be identified will also increase. The sequencing of isolates may be required for the definitive identification of some unusual yeasts but is only available in specialist centres.

Moulds

The identification of moulds relies almost entirely on the examination of the colonial and microscopic morphology. Examination of the fungal colonies should include noting the colour of the surface and reverse of the culture, and the presence of any pigment diffusing into the medium. The texture of the surface of the colony is also important, and terms such as downy, powdery, granular and glabrous are widely used (see the glossary at the end of the chapter). Hyphae that project above the surface of the agar – aerial hyphae – and growth completely submerged in the medium may also be characteristic. Folding may take very characteristic forms, either radial, circular or cerebriform (see the glossary at the end of the chapter). MALDI-TOF is also applicable to mould infections [1].

Microscopic features to note include the shape and size of the conidia, their colour, septation and the presence of wall thickenings or other ornamentation. The arrangement of the conidia on the conidiogenous cell and the type of conidiation is of critical importance. Such microscopic features may be observed using a needle mount, a sticky tape strip or a slide culture. The simplest method is a needle mount, when a portion of the growth is removed with a stiff wire needle and teased out in a drop of a suitable stain such as lactophenol cotton blue. A cover slip is applied and the sample examined microscopically. The disadvantage of this method is that, as it entails relatively rough handling of the material, it is inevitable that many of the conidia will become detached from the hyphae. A method that will retain more of the conidia in position is to apply a piece of sticky tape, sticky surface down, onto the surface of the colony, and then mount this in a drop of stain and examine the preparation directly through the back of the tape. Alternatively, the sticky tape can be placed sticky surface up so that the preparation is not observed through the tape itself, which will have poor optical characteristics. The sticky tape strip is extremely useful for the examination of colonies with many conidia. The most successful but time-consuming method for examining the details of conidial structure and formation, however, is the slide culture. In this method, the fungus is inoculated onto the four sides of a square of agar, sandwiched between a glass slide and cover slip, and maintained in a sterile Petri dish with a moist atmosphere. The fungus grows out from the agar block directly onto the glass of the cover slip and slide, which may be used to prepare two undisturbed mounts of the growing fungus. When sealed with nail polish, these form permanent preparations.

SKIN DISEASE CAUSED BY *MALASSEZIA* SPECIES

Pityriasis versicolor

Definition and nomenclature
This is a mild, chronic infection of the skin caused by *Malassezia* yeasts and characterised by discrete or confluent, scaly, discoloured or depigmented areas, mainly on the upper trunk.

Synonyms and inclusions
- Tinea versicolor
- Dermatomycosis furfuracea
- Tinea flavea
- Liver spots
- Chromophytosis

Introduction and general description
The normal microbiome of the skin includes a number of morphologically distinct lipophilic yeasts, *Malassezia* species, although in the older literature these are called *Pityrosporum*. However, genetic analysis has now demonstrated at least 22 separate species of lipophilic yeasts, of which eight occur relatively commonly on the human skin. The lipid-dependent species currently included within the genus are *M. sympodialis*, *M. globosa*, *M. restricta*, *M. slooffiae*, *M. furfur*, *M. obtusa* [1] and the more recently described *M. dermatis* [2], *M. japonica* [3], *M. yamotoensis* [4], *M. nana* [5], *M. caprae*, *M. equina* [6] and *M. cuniculi* [7]. One lipophilic but not totally lipid-dependent species, *M. pachydermatis*, is more often found on animal skin. The yeast previously known as *M. furfur* includes a complex of species, in particular *M. globosa*.

Colonisation by these species is especially dense in the scalp, the upper trunk and flexures – areas rich in sebaceous glands and their secretions. Various studies have examined the distribution of the different species in the skin microbiome from various sites and in lesional skin in various *Malassezia*-associated dermatoses. Some have included direct microscopical observation or counting of yeasts, some rely on cultures or molecular biome typing alone. However, as different workers have used different sampling techniques, few of them quantitative, and different culture media, the studies are not directly comparable. Some authors have found that *M. globosa* is most frequently associated with pityriasis versicolor [8], but others have found *M. sympodialis* [9] and *M. furfur* [10] as the predominant species. *M. sympodialis* is found most commonly on normal skin [11]. Microscopy of the scales of pityriasis versicolor nearly always reveals thick-walled, spherical yeast forms budding from a narrow base – compatible with *M. globosa* – and coarse, septate mycelium often broken up into short filaments. In some instances, however, more commonly in tropical zones [12–14], mycelium is observed together with oval yeasts budding from a broad base – a morphology more suggestive of *M. furfur* or *M. obtusa* [11]. Initially, it was found impossible to demonstrate the mycelial phase of *Malassezia* species *in vitro*, but three groups have succeeded in showing interconversion of the yeast and mycelial forms using a variety of substances [15–17].

Epidemiology
Age
In both tropical and temperate zones, the condition is rare in childhood but becomes more common in the late teens, with a peak in the early twenties.

Sex
The sexes are probably equally prone to this condition, but there are differences in susceptibility at different ages [18,19].

Ethnicity
No associations are known. Hypopigmented forms are more noticeable in skin type 3 and higher.

Associated diseases
Pityriasis versicolor has been claimed to be more common in various disease states; but only in Cushing syndrome, spontaneous and iatrogenic [20], and possibly in malnutrition are these suggestions reliably supported by evidence. Pityriasis versicolor does not appear to be more common in acquired immune deficiency syndrome (AIDS) patients [21].

Pathophysiology
Pityriasis versicolor in most cases represents a shift in the relationship between the host and the resident yeast flora. Factors contributing to the change are probably multiple.

Predisposing factors
There have been many attempts to explain susceptibility in terms of physical and biochemical abnormalities, such as application of oils to the skin or UV exposure, but a variety of differing and conflicting results leaves the problem unresolved. There is evidence of an antibody response to *Malassezia* species in subjects without pityriasis versicolor. There have been many studies on the humoral response to *Malassezia* species in patients with pityriasis versicolor and controls but, prior to the recognition of the new species, the antigens used were probably made from a number of different species, making the often conflicting results difficult to interpret. Similarly, studies of cell-mediated responses have also produced conflicting results with a wide range of antigens [22,23]. However, when mycelial phase antigens have been used there have been significantly greater lymphocyte transformation responses in pityriasis versicolor patients compared with controls [24]. The initial view that patients with pityriasis versicolor have a cell-mediated deficiency specific to *Malassezia* species or a depletion of specifically reactive T cells from the blood has been questioned [23]. Reviews of the immunology of diseases associated with *Malassezia* species are recommended to those interested in these aspects [25,26]. T-cell inhibition by a lipid component of the *Malassezia* cell wall has been reported [27].

Malassezia species do not attack the hair shaft, nails or mucous membranes, but pulmonary and systemic infections in infants on long-term intravenous lipid therapy caused by *Malassezia* are well documented [26].

Pathology
In those patients who produce a cellular response, the characteristic histological changes are of hyperkeratosis, parakeratosis and slight acanthosis, with a mild inflammatory infiltrate including mast cells in the upper dermis. Immunophenotyping of the infiltrates has revealed a dominance of memory T cells, an accumulation of macrophages and a lack of B cells [28]. A marked accumulation of Langerhans cells in the epidermis, a reduced expression of cellular activation markers and the presence of suppressor T cells were also demonstrated. The infecting organism is usually present in the upper layers of the stratum corneum and, on electron microscopy, may be seen to invade not only between but within the keratinised cells. Corneocyte counts have demonstrated an increased cell turnover in affected skin. There have been several mechanisms postulated for the alterations in pigmentation, including the production of dicarboxylic acids produced by *Malassezia* species (e.g. azaleic acid), which cause competitive inhibition of tyrosinase and perhaps a direct cytotoxic effect on hyperactive melanocytes [29]. However, such acids had no effect on normal melanocytes in tissue culture. The explanation for the hyperpigmentation seen in fair-skinned subjects remains obscure, although electron microscopy reveals abnormally large melanosomes in hyperpigmented lesions, and smaller than normal melanosomes in hypopigmented ones [30,31]. It has been noted that total epidermal pigmentation is reduced in hypopigmented lesions; a thicker keratin layer in hyperpigmented lesions may be significant [32].

Causative organisms
Pityriasis versicolor is usually caused by *M. globosa* and possibly *M. sympodialis* and *M. furfur*.

Environmental factors
It is known that some *Malassezia* species become mycelial more readily and have perhaps a slightly greater pathogenic potential. A positive family history among relations is found more often than chance would suggest in pityriasis versicolor but it is not known if this is due to genetic or environmental factors. Conjugal cases also occur and it is possible that in some instances, infection does not arise from the individual's own flora but by transmission from another individual [33].

The factors predisposing to the development of pityriasis versicolor are varied, but most attention has been devoted to environmental factors and individual host susceptibility. In a warm climate, more hyphae are associated with *Malassezia* yeasts in normal skin. In tropical climates, the condition is more common than in temperate zones, and as many as 40% of some populations may be affected [34]. Although no reliable figures are available for colder climates, the prevalence is fewer than 1%. In temperate zones, among patients who can give a reliable history, the onset is more often in the warmer months of the year or after travel to a warmer climate [18].

Clinical features [11,14,33]
Presentation
The patient usually has a patchy and varying change of skin colour, but mild irritation is sometimes noticed. The primary lesion is a sharply demarcated macule, sometimes slightly red, but characterised essentially by fine scaling (Figure 32.2a). Typically, the eruption shows large confluent areas, scattered oval patches and outlying macules. Where scaling is minimal, it may be emphasised by firm scraping or stretching of the skin, or with a sticky tape strip. The site most commonly affected is the upper trunk, but there is often spread to the upper arms, neck and abdomen. Lesions in the axillae and groins and on the thighs and genitalia occur, and extension down the forearms on to the backs of the hands and into the popliteal fossae is by no means rare; this is often associated with oval yeast forms in direct microscopy.

Clinical variants
Facial and scalp involvement are well recognised in the tropics, and occasional cases in which only these areas are affected are seen. Palmar lesions have been reported from the tropics, and rarely occur in temperate zones. A few unusual cases have been described where an anetoderma-like change follows infection [35].

The term versicolor is particularly apt. The colour of the scales may vary from pale ochre to medium brown. In untanned white skin, the affected areas are darker than normal, but they fail to respond to light exposure; in the suntanned subject, the abnormal skin is commonly paler; this is the pattern seen in type V or VI skin (Figure 32.2b). In ordinary cases that settle spontaneously or as a result of treatment, the residual depigmentation may remain for many months without any scaling. Under the Wood's lamp, the scaly lesions may show pale yellow fluorescence, and unsuspected, more widely scattered macular lesions are often revealed by this technique.

Differential diagnosis
Vitiligo and chloasma are normally distinguishable by their complete absence of scaling. Seborrhoeic dermatitis, pityriasis rosea, secondary syphilis, pinta and tinea corporis show more inflammatory change than pityriasis versicolor, and none of these ever has the even, fine scale of the latter condition. Erythrasma may closely mimic pityriasis versicolor with pigmentary change and scaling, but satellite lesions are less common and pink fluorescence under the Wood's lamp is often present. Erythrasma and pityriasis versicolor may occasionally coexist.

Complications and co-morbidities
Pityriasis versicolor is strikingly free from complications.

Disease course and prognosis
This is a chronic infection if untreated, although clinical expression such as extent may vary over time.

Investigations
The finding on direct examination of coarse mycelium, fragmented to short filaments 2–5 µm wide and up to 25 µm long, together with spherical, thick-walled yeasts 2–8 µm in diameter confirms the presence of the condition (Figure 32.3). Occasionally, oval yeasts may be seen. However, it is the mycelium that is the diagnostic feature and sometimes this predominates to the extent that there are few yeast forms. The characteristic appearance on microscopy has been likened to 'spaghetti and meatballs' or 'bananas and grapes'. As they are members of the normal flora, the isolation of *Malassezia* species from scrapings is of no diagnostic value and is not normally undertaken by diagnostic laboratories. Recently, molecular techniques and MALDI-TOF have opened the field to research at strain level [36].

Management
There are a number of different methods of treatment [11]. Relapse is very common, whatever the primary treatment. In all but the

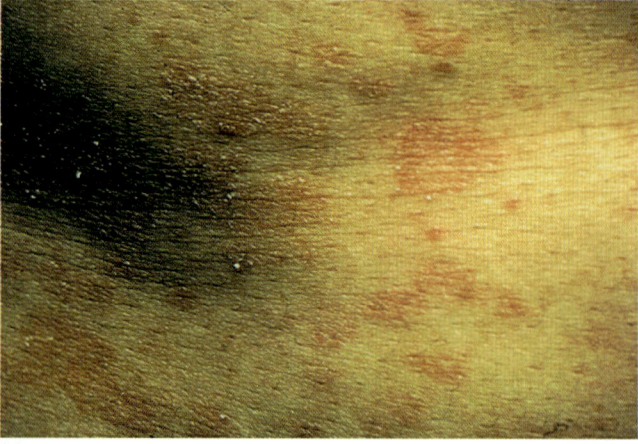
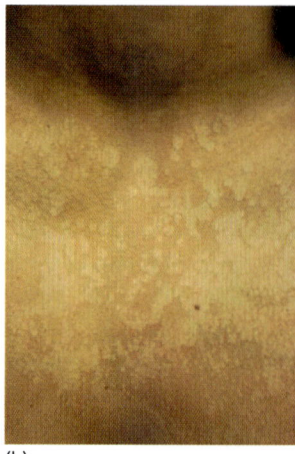

Figure 32.2 Pityriasis versicolor showing (a) typical fine scaling and (b) hypopigmentation in Type V skin.

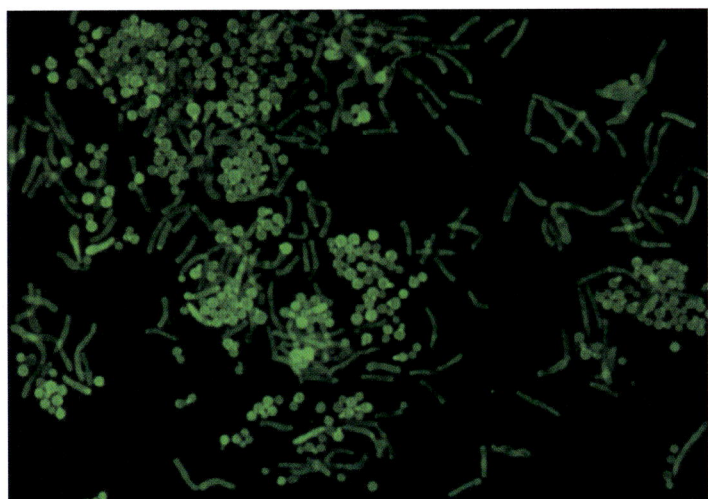

Figure 32.3 Pityriasis versicolor. Skin scales mounted in potassium hydroxide (KOH) and Calcofluor white UV illumination. The hyphae diagnostic of the condition have taken up the stain immediately. *Malassezia* yeasts are also present. Courtesy of the Department of Medical Mycology, St John's Institute of Dermatology, King's College London, London, UK.

most resistant cases it is probably simplest to re-treat each episode rather than resort to long-term suppressive therapy. Patients should be warned that repigmentation may take several months, as otherwise they will often report treatment failure, even when the organisms have been destroyed, simply because the hypopigmentation persists.

First line

The first line treatment is topical antifungal therapy. The topical azole antifungals work well in pityriasis versicolor and there is no significant difference in results achieved by different compounds [37]. The usual time to recovery is 2–3 weeks. However, there is increasing evidence that shorter application periods using appropriate formulations may work after only one or two applications. As has been shown with oral itraconazole, the organisms die rapidly after exposure to azoles, but in view of the thickened *Malassezia* cell wall they are not rapidly cleared from the epidermis, giving the false impression of a persistent infection [38,39]. Terbinafine 1% cream is also effective in pityriasis versicolor. The main problem with the use of topical antifungals is the difficulty of applying creams to such a wide body surface area. An alternative solution to this is provided by ketoconazole shampoo, and although it has not been fully evaluated in pityriasis versicolor, two or three applications of the shampoo appear to clear most infections.

A second, cheaper approach is the application of 2.5% selenium sulphide in a detergent base (Selsun® shampoo). It is applied to all the affected areas and left overnight. In many cases it is necessary to apply the material regularly (e.g. every other night over 2 weeks). In some patients, however, one or two applications may be sufficient. The shampoo is irritant if inadvertently applied to the face or genitalia, necessitating care in its application. It also stains clothes and bedding. Alternatives include 20% sodium hyposulphite solution and 50:50 propylene glycol in water. The latter has also been used intermittently as long-term suppressive therapy to prevent relapse [40].

Second line

The second line of treatment is oral antifungal therapy. While opinions differ as to the appropriate place for oral therapy, the authors usually reserve oral itraconazole for extensive or recalcitrant cases. Itraconazole is active against pityriasis versicolor in a total dosage of 800–1000 mg [39], usually given over 5 days. Fluconazole can also be used.

Treatment ladder for pityriasis versicolor

First line
- Topical azoles twice daily for 2–3 weeks
- Terbinafine 1% cream twice daily for 2–3 weeks
- Ketoconazole shampoo twice weekly for 2–3 weeks
- 2.5% selenium shampoo alternative days for 2–3 weeks

Second line
- Itraconazole 200 mg daily for 5 days

Malassezia folliculitis

Definition
This is a clinically distinct form of folliculitis on the back and upper trunk associated with *Malassezia* yeasts.

Epidemiology
Malassezia folliculitis is most often seen in teenagers or young adult males [1,2].

Pathophysiology
The exact pathogenesis of the condition is unknown.

Pathology
Biopsies taken from typical cases show clusters of yeasts within follicles surrounded by inflammatory cells; this is distinguishable from the colonisation of follicular openings that can be seen in normal individuals.

Environmental factors
Patients often report the development of lesions following a holiday in the sun or it may be found in patients who are acutely ill, for example in an intensive care unit.

Clinical features
Lesions are itchy papules and pustules, which are often diffusely scattered on the shoulders and back. The itching and distribution distinguish them from acne vulgaris.

Management
The condition responds well to oral itraconazole and less well to ketoconazole shampoo.

Other cutaneous disorders associated with *Malassezia* yeasts

Lipophilic yeasts of the genus *Malassezia* are part of the normal skin flora and therefore any evidence that they are either directly or indirectly implicated in the pathogenesis of skin disease is often difficult to assess.

For many years it has been known that *Malassezia* yeasts are found in large quantities in the scales of seborrhoeic dermatitis (SD), both on the scalp and elsewhere (Chapter 40). This was attributed to hyperproliferation of the epidermis, the assumption being that the organisms were merely colonising this particular site. The same was thought to be the case with skin-surface bacteria [1]. However, it has become apparent that most seborrhoeic dermatitis or scaling of the scalp (dandruff) clears on treatment with antifungal agents – coincidentally with the disappearance of the yeasts – and that if the patient relapses after therapy this occurs when the organisms reappear [2,3]. The circumstantial evidence, therefore, that the two events are causally related is very strong. In animals, it is possible to induce skin scaling that bears some resemblance to seborrhoeic dermatitis after the application of *Malassezia* yeasts [4]. Some but not all authors have reported that patients with seborrhoeic dermatitis have significantly raised levels of antibody to these organisms [5], but do not appear to develop contact sensitisation to antigenic extracts. One further finding is that seborrhoeic dermatitis is one of the earliest and most consistent abnormalities seen in patients with AIDS who are not on antiretrovirals (Chapter 31) [6,7]. Yet, as with seborrhoeic dermatitis in non-AIDS patients, there is no consistent correlation between colonisation and primary disease, although numbers of yeasts are higher in those with low CD4 counts.

Adult-type seborrhoeic dermatitis appears to be directly related to *Malassezia* yeasts but not to a single species [8]. The relationship between infant seborrhoeic dermatitis and these organisms is less well established. The mechanisms by which they induce skin changes are not fully known, although direct lipase activity [9] or inflammatory responses initiated by *Malassezia*-produced aryl hydrocarbon inhibitors such as malassezin and indolocar-bazole have been described [10,11]. It is also apparent that a small percentage of patients with typical seborrhoeic dermatitis do not respond to antifungals.

A further observation is that patients with an atopic background with eczema affecting the head and neck or head and neck dermatitis may also respond to topically applied azole antifungals, and they also show significantly raised IgE levels to antigens of *Malassezia* such as MGL 1304 or Mala s8/r8 [12]. Patients have usually had childhood eczema and the condition is most often seen in young adults.

Malassezia yeasts have also been associated with other skin conditions such as confluent and reticulated papillomatosis (Chapter 85) [13–15]. However, their presence in this condition is not invariable and their removal with antifungals not necessarily followed by significant changes in the skin lesions. In addition, some patients respond to minocycline. Finally, there is a variant of psoriasis that has been termed 'sebopsoriasis' where, it is speculated, lipophilic yeasts may have a pathogenic role [16]. Clinically, this condition shows features of both psoriasis and seborrhoeic dermatitis, and it is thought to represent an overlap syndrome between the two conditions.

SUPERFICIAL MYCOSES CAUSED BY OTHER SPECIES

Tinea nigra

Definition and nomenclature
Tinea nigra is an asymptomatic, superficial fungal infection caused by *Hortaea werneckii*. It generally affects the skin of the palms and is characterised by deeply pigmented, macular, non-scaly patches.

> **Synonyms and inclusions**
> - Tinea nigra palmaris
> - Keratomycosis nigricans palmaris
> - Pityriasis nigra

Epidemiology
Incidence and prevalence
This is a rare disease. It occurs sporadically in many parts of the world, including the Americas and the Caribbean, South Africa, Australia, Europe and the Far East. It is thought to be acquired by direct inoculation into the skin and can easily be reproduced experimentally by scarifying the skin and applying a pure culture of *H. werneckii* under a bandage.

Age
It can occur at any age but is rare in childhood.

Pathophysiology
Pathology
There is thickening of the stratum corneum in which hyphae are present. Inflammatory reaction in the dermis is minimal.

Causative organisms
Tinea nigra is generally caused by *H. werneckii* (synonyms *Exophiala werneckii* and *Phaeoannellomyces werneckii*) [1]. A different organism, *Stenella araguata*, has been isolated from some cases diagnosed in Venezuela [2,3]. The incubation period in separate studies was reported to be 10–15 days and 7 weeks, respectively.

Environmental factors
It is more commonly found in tropical climates.

Clinical features [4]
Presentation
This condition is asymptomatic. The lesions are macular, sharply defined and not scaly. The most distinctive feature is the brown or black colour, resembling a silver nitrate stain. The palms are most commonly affected [5,6] in cases reported in the western hemisphere, but other areas of the body such as the soles and, more rarely, neck and trunk have been recorded, particularly in Asia.

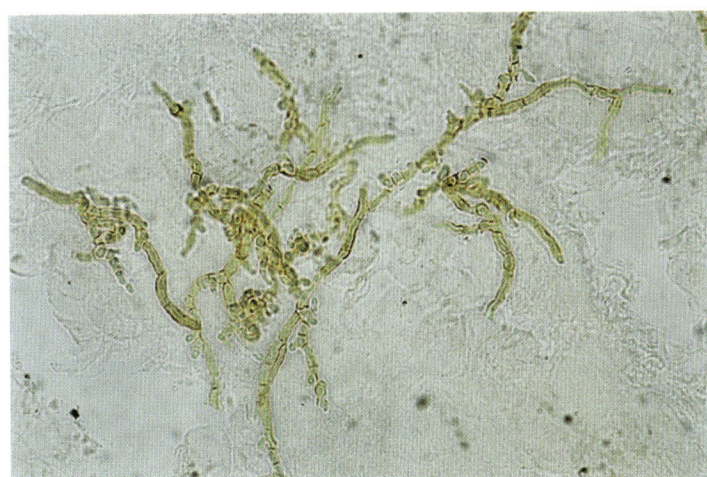

Figure 32.4 Tinea nigra. Skin scales mounted in 30% potassium hydroxide, bright field. The natural brown colour of the septate hyphae is apparent. Courtesy of the Department of Medical Mycology, St John's Institute of Dermatology, King's College London, London, UK.

Irregular outlines are produced by an uneven rate of spread or coalescence of lesions.

Differential diagnosis

The black colour and the absence of scaling differentiate the condition from pityriasis versicolor. The pigmented lesions of Addison disease, syphilis, pinta and junctional naevi of the palm may have to be differentiated and mycological examination of the scales is usually required.

Disease course and prognosis

Spontaneous clearance is very unusual.

Investigations

Dermoscopy of the skin lesions shows the presence of darkly pigmented and spiky strands, the hyphal clusters. Microscopy of infected epidermal scales in potassium hydroxide mounts reveals abundant brown, branched, closely septate hyphae up to 5 μm in diameter, and elongated budding cells (Figure 32.4). Inoculation of specimens onto Sabouraud's agar and incubation at 30°C yields slow-growing colonies.

Hortaea werneckii. Colony: cultures on glucose peptone agar may be relatively slow growing and initially yield a dirty white to grey, moist, yeast-like colony, which darkens to olive green to black, and over the course of several days becomes more filamentous and velvety. Microscopy: examination of young cultures reveals annellidic yeast-like budding cells, which are often uniseptate, the septum being dark in mature cells. The conidia are initially hyaline but become brown on maturity. Hyphae in older cultures produce intercalary and lateral conidiogenous cells, which are annellidic or sympodial.

Management

First line treatment is topical azole creams such as econazole and ketoconazole [7]. The condition also responds to the topical application of fungicidal preparations such as butenafine [8]. Benzoic acid compound ointment is also effective.

Black piedra

Definition and nomenclature

This is a fungal infection confined to the hair shafts and resulting in the formation of hard, dark, superficial nodules thereon. Black piedra is caused by the fungus *Piedraia hortae*.

> **Synonyms and inclusions**
> - Tinea nodosa
> - Trichomycosis nodularis

Epidemiology
Incidence and prevalence

This is a very rare infection. It occurs in humid wet tropical regions in the Americas and in South-East Asia [1], and affects monkeys as well as humans [2]. A study among the Zoro people of Brazil [3] showed a prevalence of infection of 57% in subjects over the age of 11 years.

Sex

The infection was thought to be more common in males than females, but one study showed no significant difference between the sexes [3].

Clinical features
Presentation

Lesions are asymptomatic. Black piedra is characterised by the presence of firmly adherent, black, gritty, hard nodules on the hairs of the scalp, or less frequently of the beard, moustache or pubic area. The nodules vary in size from microscopic to 1 mm or more in diameter, and their thickness often tapers, either from one end to the other or from the middle to the edge. They are usually multiple, and oval or elongate in shape. Subcuticular fungal growth may rupture the cuticle and the fungus may then grow on the outside of the cuticle, completely surrounding the hair shaft. Because the fungus grows into the hair shaft, the hair may fracture easily.

Disease course and prognosis

Untreated the infection is chronic.

Investigations

In histological sections or in potassium hydroxide mounts, the nodules are observed to be made up of closely packed brown hyphae held in a mass by a viscous or cement-like substance (Figure 32.5). At the edges of the nodule, regularly aligned hyphal strands and arthroconidia 4–8 μm in diameter can be seen, while in the thicker parts, club-shaped asci containing eight elongated ascospores may be formed. The ascospores have a polar filament at each end and can be observed by crushing or sectioning the nodule. *Piedraia hortae* is almost unique among the human pathogenic fungi in producing sexual spores in its parasitic phase.

Trichoscopy will show small brown black nodules around the hair shafts. The direct examination is so characteristic that culture is not absolutely necessary. If culture is performed, it should be noted that the fungus is not inhibited by cycloheximide.

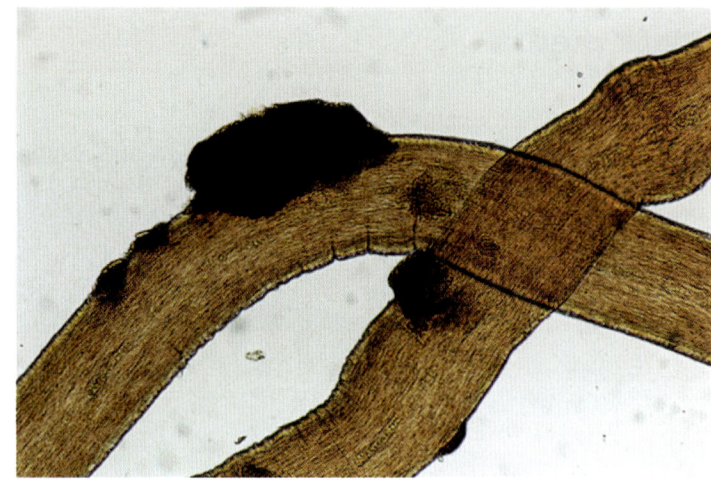

Figure 32.5 Black piedra. Hairs mounted in 30% KOH, bright field. The dark nodules are formed of dematiaceous hyphae cemented together to form a hard mass. Courtesy of the Department of Medical Mycology, St John's Institute of Dermatology, King's College London, London, UK.

Piedraia hortae. Colony: the culture is slow growing, compact, domed and black. Microscopy: this shows brown, thick-walled, septate hyphae and chlamydoconidia. Asci and ascospores may be present in the thicker portion of the colony [4] but are not formed by every isolate.

Management
Shaving or cutting the hair effects a cure. To prevent recurrence, antifungal preparations such as benzoic acid ointment compound BP can be applied. Treatment success with terbinafine has been reported [5].

White piedra

Definition and nomenclature
This is a fungal infection confined to the hair shafts and resulting in the formation of soft, white, grey or brown superficial nodules caused by *Trichosporon* species.

> **Synonyms and inclusions**
> - Trichosporosis nodosa

Epidemiology
Incidence and prevalence
The infection occurs in South America, Africa, central and eastern Europe and Japan [1,2]. The horse and certain species of monkey may also be affected. The cases occasionally observed in temperate countries have usually been visitors from the tropics, but cases have occurred in both Europe and the USA in individuals who have never left these regions [3–5]. A study in equatorial Africa demonstrated a prevalence of 18% in inguinal specimens from 449 female subjects [3].

Age
It occurs in adults.

Sex
There is no sex difference.

Pathophysiology
Predisposing factors
There is evidence that some cases may be sexually transmitted [6]. In addition, it has been postulated that the bacteria known to accompany the concretions of the fungi on hair, now identified as a new species of *Brevibacterium*, *B. mcbrellneri* [7], may have a synergistic role in the infection [8]. The strong proteolytic activity of the bacterium may facilitate hair shaft invasion by both yeasts and bacteria, while fungal by-products may stimulate bacterial growth. There is an increased carriage rate of perianal '*G. beigelii*' reported in HIV-positive individuals, suggesting that this region may provide a reservoir for carriage. Interestingly, there does not appear to be an increased incidence of hair shaft infection in these patients.

Pathology
There is hair shaft invasion.

Causative organisms
Until 1994, the aetiological agent of white piedra was considered to be the basidiomycetous yeast *Geotrichum* (*Trichosporon*) *beigelii*, but genetic analysis has now determined that this name covered a complex of different species [9]. The agent of white piedra in head hair is now considered to be *T. ovoides*, while organisms reported from crural white piedra include *T. inkin*, *T. asahii* and *T. mucoides*.

Clinical features
Presentation
This infection is asymptomatic. White piedra is characterised by the presence of soft, white or light brown nodules. The infection is more common on the hairs of the beard, moustache and genital areas than the scalp [4,5]. The fungus grows both within and outside the hair shaft, and the hair shaft may be weakened and break off. The nodules are transparent, easily detached from the hair and vary in size from microscopic to 1 mm in diameter. The underlying skin is not affected and there is no fluorescence under Wood's light.

Differential diagnosis
The presence of pruritus and the distinctive shape of egg cases of pediculi should serve to distinguish pediculosis from piedra, but microscopical examination is desirable.

Disease course and prognosis
If not treated this is a chronic infection.

Investigations
The nodules of white piedra are in the form of a sheath, which may extend around the hair shaft. These can be seen as white or semitransparent nodules with trichoscopy. With direct microscopy there may be extensive growth within the hair, giving rise to characteristic nodular swellings on the hair shaft. The hyphae segment into arthroconidia 2–4 μm in diameter and budding blastoconidia may also be seen (Figure 32.6). Most *Trichosporon* species are inhibited by cycloheximide, so this antibiotic should be excluded from the culture medium. As a few isolates fail to grow at 37°C, it is also advisable to incubate at 28–30°C.

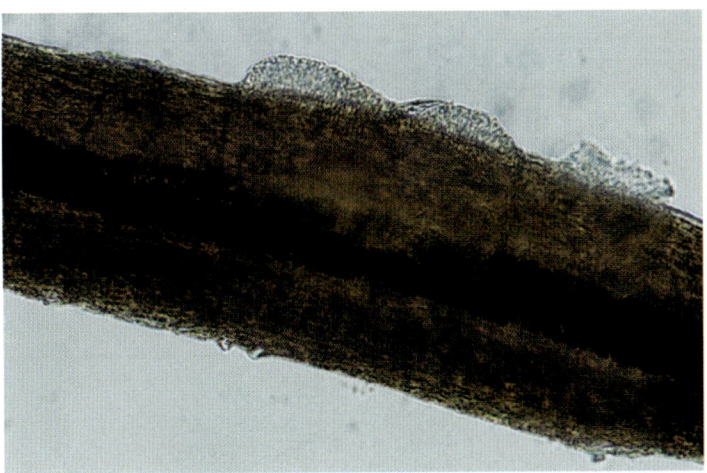

Figure 32.6 White piedra. Hair mounted in KOH, bright field. The gelatinous nodules formed by various *Trichosporon* species surround the hair. Courtesy of the Department of Medical Mycology, St John's Institute of Dermatology, King's College London, London, UK.

***Trichosporon* species.** Colony: the colonies of *Trichosporon* species develop rapidly and are soft, creamy and wrinkled, and sometimes mucoid [10]. Microscopy: the genus *Trichosporon* is characterised by the presence of hyphae, arthroconidia and budding cells. These are best observed with a deep cut streak on cornmeal or rice agar supplemented with Tween 80. Physiological tests: the species recently recognised using genetic analyses can be identified in the routine laboratory using their morphological characteristics, together with carbohydrate assimilation patterns determined by the commercial API 32C system, failure or ability to grow at 37°C and relative sensitivity to cycloheximide [9].

Management
As with black piedra, shaving or cutting the hair may effect a cure. Responses to concentrated topical antifungals, azoles and allyamines have been reported but are unpredictable.

Otomycosis

Definition and nomenclature
This is a chronic inflammatory condition of the external auditory canal caused by fungal infection. External otitis in general, including the differential diagnosis and management, is considered in Chapter 106.

Synonyms and inclusions
- Mycotic otitis externa

Pathophysiology
Causative organisms
In some patients with external otitis, fungi may be isolated from swabs or scrapings; indeed, material taken from the normal external ear may on occasion yield a variety of moulds [1]. Such isolates are more common in tropical regions. Very occasionally in external otitis, the fungus isolated appears to be playing a pathogenic part, perhaps even a primary one. The species most commonly accepted as pathogens in this situation include *Aspergillus niger*. Other species implicated as pathogens include *A. fumigatus* and other *Aspergillus* species [2,3], *Scedosporium apiospermum*, numerous other moulds and *Candida* species.

Clinical features
Presentation
The inflamed, itchy and sometimes painful external canal usually discharges a little serous fluid. In advanced cases of true mycotic otitis, an overgrowth of fungal hyphae may produce a mass of white material suggesting damp cotton wool, lodged in the external canal. Where *A. niger* is the causative organism, the mat of fungus is often covered by black fruiting heads [4].

Clinical variants
In severely immunocompromised patients, the external auditory meatus can be extensively eroded by fungal invasion to produce a necrotic form of otitis externa [5]. This form may spread to involve other sites including the middle ear and mastoids.

Differential diagnosis
The pinna may be the site of several mycotic diseases including chromomycosis [6], sporotrichosis [7] and tinea [4], but such infections usually spare the external auditory meatus.

Course and prognosis
It is chronic if not treated.

Investigations
Interpretation of the relevance of organisms recovered from swabs taken from the ear may be difficult and a light growth of a mould may be of little significance. *Rhizopus*, *Lichtheimia*, *Mucor* or *Penicillium*, or indeed *Aspergillus* species, in small amounts mean little, except in immunocompromised patients, where they may be more important. Similarly, a light growth of *Candida* may reflect colonisation or contamination, although this organism can cause external otitis. The criteria for accepting the fungus as having an aetiological role are the absence of any significant bacterial pathogens and the presence of large masses of fungi that may sometimes be seen on examination of the patient. If there is a considerable amount of fungal material in specimens taken for direct examination, this may be adequate evidence. Signs and symptoms present in otomycosis are largely similar to those of otitis due to other aetiological agents, although pruritus and discharge have been shown to be more common in fungal-associated disease in one study [2].

***Aspergillus niger*.** Colony: growing rapidly, the colony initially has a white or cream surface, which becomes black as the conidia are produced. The reverse remains pale cream to celadon green. Microscopy: the conidiophores arise at right angles to the supporting hyphae, and have a swollen globose vesicle at their tip, which is completely covered by a layer of supporting cells or metulae. These metulae support a layer of phialides, which produce chains of dark brown, rough-walled phialoconidia. The bottom end of the conidiophore ends in a foot cell inserted in the supporting hypha.

Management [4,8,9]

Careful cleaning, with removal of debris and fungal material from the ears, is of paramount importance. Various local applications have been suggested such as 2% thymol. Clotrimazole lotion has been employed with success in both *Aspergillus* and *Candida* infections. Bifonazole lotion and cream were effective in the majority of 35 patients included in a long-term study attempting to correlate the bacterial and fungal flora in patients with symptomatic otomycosis [9]. Oral itraconazole and voriconazole have both been used in the aggressive invasive form of otitis externa.

Miscellaneous superficial mycoses caused by saprophytic moulds

The normal skin, especially the scalp and toe clefts, is commonly contaminated with spores or even short lengths of mycelium of saprophytic species. If cycloheximide-free media are used, they may be readily cultured. Usually, such species are present in small amounts and may without difficulty be dismissed as contaminants that have impacted on the skin. From time to time, however, reports appear in the dermatological literature of cases in which species such as those of *Aspergillus* [1] appear to colonise damaged tissues, become firmly established and perhaps cause secondary tissue destruction. Most authors counsel caution before accepting any sort of pathogenic role for the moulds in these cases, but in immunocompromised patients or those with severe traumatic wounds the skin may become a portal of entry for invasive opportunistic fungal pathogens.

Investigations and management

In situations like these, it is important to use cycloheximide-free media in culture and then to weigh the facts carefully before assuming that the organism is anything more than a contaminant. In many cases, simple correction of local precipitating factors, such as maceration or occlusive dressings, may be all that is needed.

DERMATOPHYTOSIS

Synonyms and inclusions
- Tinea, ringworm

Classification

Dermatophytes are related fungi capable of causing skin changes of the type known as ringworm or dermatophytosis [1,2]. Thus defined, the ringworm species are all moulds belonging to three asexual genera: *Microsporum*, *Trichophyton* and *Epidermophyton*.

General description

Forty years ago, the sexual state of dermatophytes was unknown and this phase of the life cycle has still not been found for many of the common species. However, in those species where the sexual state has been identified, all the organisms are classified in the single genus *Arthroderma* in the phylum Ascomycota [3]. A list of synonyms of sexual and asexual names is included for reference (Table 32.4), although naming changes in the next few years mean that only one name will be maintained in the future. However, as sexual states are not routinely seen in the diagnostic laboratory, the name currently given to the asexual anamorph names will be used throughout this section.

In addition to the recognised pathogens, a number of fungi have been discovered that are keratinophilic and that are clearly close relatives of the ringworm fungi – indeed, some are even classified in the same three anamorph genera – but that are soil dwellers and non-pathogenic. Although some authors include these fungi within the dermatophytes, in the author's opinion they are better classified in the broader group of keratinophilic fungi, retaining the term dermatophyte for those species that can act as true superficial pathogens.

The taxonomy of dermatophytes is an ever-changing area and the use of molecular techniques to examine the relatedness of species has led to many controversies and conflicts in the literature. Gräser *et al.* suggested, on the basis of ribosomal internal transcribed spacers, that *Trichophyton equinum* var. *autotrophicum* should be considered synonymous with *T. tonsurans* [4]. However, this is a matter of conflict and debate among taxonomists in this area [5,6], and this synonymy was later formally rejected [7]. Detailed discussions on the molecular taxonomy of dermatophytes are beyond the scope of this volume and interested readers are referred to a review on this subject [8].

Three asexual dermatophyte genera are distinguished by the morphology of the large, multicellular macroconidia that are produced [9]. In the genus *Microsporum*, the macroconidia are rough, usually thick walled and range from fusiform to obovate in shape with 1–12 or more septa. Those of *Trichophyton* species are thin walled, smooth and may be cylindrical, fusiform or clavate in shape, with up to 12 transverse septa. In *Epidermophyton*, the macroconidium is clavate, broadened and rounded at its distal pole, thin walled and has up to five septa; the conidia are smooth when first formed, but as the colony ages, discrete wall thickenings may be observed.

Apart from the mycological classification of dermatophytes, it has been traditional for clinical and epidemiological reasons to group dermatophytes that infect humans according to their ecological niche: geophilic species originating in the soil (Table 32.5); zoophilic

Table 32.4 Asexual–sexual connections of dermatophytes.

Asexual state	Sexual state
Microsporum canis	*Arthroderma otae*
Microsporum fulvum	*Arthroderma fulvum*
Microsporum gypseum	*Arthroderma incurvatum*
Microsporum gypseum	*Arthroderma gypseum*
Microsporum nanum	*Arthroderma obtusum*
Microsporum persicolor	*Arthroderma persicolor*
Trichophyton mentagrophytes	*Arthroderma benhamiae*
Trichophyton mentagrophytes	*Arthroderma vanbreuseghemii*
Trichophyton simii	*Arthroderma simii*

Table 32.5 Geophilic and zoophilic dermatophytes.

Species	Geographical distribution	Major host
Geophilic species		
Microsporum (Nannizia) gypseum[a]	Worldwide	
Microsporum (Nannizia) praecox	USA, western Europe	
Zoophilic species		
Microsporum canis	Worldwide	Cat, dog
Microsporum canis var. *distortum* (now classed as part of *M. canis*)	New Zealand, USA	Cat, dog
Microsporum equinum (now classed as part of *M. canis*)	Worldwide	Horse
Microsporum gallinae	Worldwide	Fowl
Microsporum (Nannizia) nanum	Worldwide	Pigs
Microsporum (Nannizia) persicolor	Americas, Europe	Voles
Trichophyton equinum	Worldwide	Horse
Trichophyton mentagrophytes	Worldwide	Rodents
Trichophyton erinacei	Europe, New Zealand	Hedgehogs
Trichophyton quinckeanum	Worldwide	Mice
Trichophyton simii	India	Monkey
Trichophyton verrucosum	Worldwide	Cattle

[a] This asexual species is a complex of three sexual species.

Table 32.6 Anthropophilic dermatophytes.

Species	Geographical distribution
Epidermophyton floccosum	Worldwide
Microsporum audouinii	Worldwide
Isolates previously called *M. audouinii* var. *rivalieri* and var. *langeronii*	Africa
Microsporum ferrugineum	Far East, eastern Europe, Africa
Trichophyton concentricum	Pacific, South-East Asia, Latin America
Trichophyton gourvilii (now classed as part of *T. rubrum* of African origin complex)	Central Africa
Trichophyton interdigitale	Worldwide
Trichophyton megninii (now classed as part of *T. rubrum* of African origin complex)	Mediterranean
Trichophyton rubrum	Worldwide
Trichophyton schoenleinii	Worldwide
Trichophyton soudanense (now classed as part of *T. rubrum* of African origin complex)	Sub-Saharan Africa
Trichophyton tonsurans	Worldwide
Trichophyton violaceum	North Africa, India, Middle East
Trichophyton yaoundei (now classed as part of *T. rubrum* of African origin complex)	Central Africa

(), synonyms in recent classifications.

species with animal origins (Table 32.5); and anthropophilic species, which are largely restricted to human skin (Table 32.6). However, these three groups are not always sharply demarcated. Species that are clearly geophilic may contaminate or infect the coats of animals, especially small rodents, and may thus infect humans through an intermediate animal host. Similarly, animal species may shed infective material on to the soil and, although incapable of multiplying there, fungal elements may survive long enough to be isolated in a soil survey [10]. In the case of species affecting farm animals, their environment including cow sheds and fences may be contaminated by desquamated keratinocytes or hair containing fungal spores, just as the floors around swimming baths, school classrooms and the air of hospital clinics may be contaminated by anthropophilic species [10].

The distribution of the zoophilic species reflects that of the major animal hosts. Those geographically limited include *Microsporum canis* (including strains previously called *M. canis* var. *distortum*), *M. persicolor*, *Trichophyton erinacei* and *T. simii* (Table 32.5). Many of the anthropophilic species are also geographically limited and the classic endemic distributions are indicated in Table 32.6. However, to some degree these must reflect the distribution of diagnostic facilities and data for some areas are slight or outdated. Also, the anthropophilic dermatophytes are spread by movements of individuals and groups. For example, species classically thought of as African, such as *T. soudanense* (which is now classified as a *T. rubrum* of African origin), have been isolated in the USA and Europe with some regularity. The European infections have not been found among immigrants from the endemic areas alone, but also in children born in Europe of African immigrants and, more rarely, among the endemic European population. Some of the species that have been regarded as cosmopolitan, such as *T. schoenleinii*, are currently rarely isolated in the USA and western Europe, although in some areas, particularly parts of Africa, they remain endemic.

It must also be appreciated that these distributions are not static and the range of species in some areas may change dramatically and quickly. For instance, in one central London laboratory during the period between 1980 and 1990, the most common isolate from tinea capitis was the zoophilic organism *M. canis*. In contrast, during 2003 and 2004, *T. tonsurans*, a species that was rarely seen in the 1980s, was responsible for 87% of scalp infections and this has remained a dominant species (S. Howell, St John's Institute of Dermatology, King's College London, unpublished data). A review has highlighted the shifting epidemiology of dermatophytosis both in the UK and worldwide [11]. A more recent threat has been the spread from the Indian subcontinent of *T. indotineae* related to *T. mentagrophytes* that causes extensive tinea corporis/cruris and is resistant to some treatments including terbinafine. Spread has now been recorded outside India to other countries such as Bangladesh, Pakistan, the Middle East and countries in Europe.

From the evolutionary point of view, it is likely that the anthropophilic species represent the end of a line, starting with non-pathogenic, keratinophilic soil species, existing as saprophytes on keratinous debris, passing through the geophilic dermatophytes and the zoophilic species. The increased specialisation that this evolutionary trend implies seems to be accompanied by a progressive loss of the sexual state and a reduction in the production of conidia, particularly macroconidia, and a loss of certain mating types [12–14]. Virtually all the non-pathogenic, keratinophilic species and geophilic dermatophytes have demonstrable sexual states, as do a few of the zoophilic group, particularly those infecting animals living in burrows or dens and thus associated with soil. However, dermatophytes that infect larger animals, such as *T. verrucosum* from cattle, *T. equinum* from horses and the anthropophilic dermatophytes, have as yet no known sexual state. It has been suggested that this transition from sexual to asexual life cycles led to an unprecedented level of adaptive radiation among the anthropophilic dermatophytes, resulting in a large number of species and variants. Other factors that may have contributed to the adaptive radiation on humans include the separation of the human skin into distinct areas differing in the distribution of sebaceous glands and hairs, resulting in a marked affinity for particular body sites among the anthropophiles, which is not seen in zoophiles.

Basic biology

Characteristically, zoophilic species tend to produce highly inflammatory reactions in humans and this may lead to a spontaneous cure. Anthropophilic species produce mild but chronic lesions. There are many exceptions to this useful generalisation and the degree of inflammatory response depends in part on the site of infection – large follicles of scalp and beard are associated with an intense reaction – and the immune status of the host [1].

An important characteristic of the dermatophytes as parasites is their restriction to dead keratinised tissue. Although the inflammatory responses of ringworm infection involve the dermis and the Malpighian stratum of the epidermis, the fungus itself is found growing only within the stratum corneum of the epidermis, within and around the fully keratinised hair shaft, and in the nail plate and keratinised nail bed. Within these keratinised tissues, the fungus exists only as mycelium and arthroconidia. In this parasitic phase of fungal growth, there are no micro- or macroconidia and no specialised vegetative structures, such as spiral or pectinate hyphae. For these reasons, precise identification of the species of an infecting dermatophyte is generally impossible on direct microscopy of the skin or nail.

In dermatophyte infections involving hair, the fungus invades the follicle from the adjacent stratum corneum and follows one of several precise patterns of growth. In the case of *M. canis* and *M. audouinii*, for example, the fungus penetrates the keratinised hair at about mid-follicular level, having grown down on the hair surface [2]. It then grows downwards within the hair towards the bulb, until the zone of incomplete keratinisation is reached. Growth is then arrested, or rather slowed and resisted. An equilibrium is established, the fungal mycelium invading a new, fully keratinised hair shaft at the same rate as it is formed, but never growing down into the incompletely keratinised tissue. Further up the shaft, hyphae from the existing mycelium grow outwards from inside the hair and proliferate on its surface. These secondary, extrapilary hyphae are tortuous; they fragment into small arthroconidia, which rapidly round up to become spherical structures, and are seen as a packed mosaic of spores coating the surface of the hair. This is the small-spored ectothrix type of hair invasion.

Other species of dermatophytes show different patterns of hair invasion. *T. verrucosum* and *T. mentagrophytes*, like the *Microsporum* species, show arthroconidia on the surface of the hair and hyphae within it, but these conidia are larger and are arranged in straight chains. This is known as large-spored ectothrix hair invasion. *T. tonsurans* and *T. violaceum*, among others, produce an endothrix type of hair invasion, with the hyphae inside the hair fragmenting completely into a mass of relatively large arthroconidia, which are retained entirely within the hair shaft. *T. schoenleinii*, the cause of favus, is different again. The hyphae within the hair are fewer in number than in other endothrix infections and do not break up into a mass of arthroconidia but run intact through the hair, forming tunnels within its structure. When mounted in potassium hydroxide, these tunnels formed originally around the hyphae, which subsequently degenerate, create the characteristic air spaces seen. While in favus the infected hair commonly grows to normal lengths, in endothrix infections where arthroconidia are formed the hair shaft, being severely weakened, breaks at the skin surface. In small-spored ectothrix infections the shaft tends to fracture a few millimetres above the surface.

All these parasitic patterns are very different from the mode of growth of dermatophytes on hair *in vitro* [3]. If plucked hair is inoculated with any of the *T. mentagrophytes* varieties, for example, frond-like fungal hyphae develop on the surface and lift the cuticle cells. Conical pits are then formed perpendicular to the surface of the hair as penetration of the keratinised hair cortex occurs. Intrapilary growth follows along the hair shaft in both directions, and micro- and macroconidia may be produced. There are no linear chains of arthroconidia on the surface. Moreover, if a hair, parasitised *in vivo*, is plucked, and then cultured *in vitro*, the specialised growth pattern initially established will cease and the saprophytic phase, with the development of micro- and macroconidia, will rapidly follow.

Invasion of the epidermis
Invasion of the epidermis by dermatophytes follows a common pattern, starting with adherence between arthroconidia and keratinocytes, followed by penetration through and between cells and the development of a host response.

Adherence
On the stratum corneum, the first phase of dermatophyte invasion involves the adherence of infectious arthroconidia to keratinocytes. *In vitro*, this process is completed after about 2 h of contact, at which stage germination and penetration of the keratinocyte occurs [4]. Different dermatophytes show similar kinetics, which are also unaffected by the source of the keratinocytes. The germination of arthroconidia and hyphal prolongation that follows adherence proceeds radially, and *in vitro* there is evidence of the indentation of keratinocyte layers beneath the growing hyphae, possibly resulting from enzymic action [5]. The growing hyphae are thigmotropic and can sense surface changes in the underlying surface which may lead to penetration between corneocytes.

Penetration
Dermatophytes are keratinophilic. Evidence for this ranges from the ability of many dermatophytes to invade hair and nail *in vitro* to the demonstration of genetically regulated production of proteases with keratin specificity. *In vitro*, non-keratin substances extracted from keratinised tissues will support the growth of dermatophytes [6]. Dermatophytes produce a variety of proteolytic enzymes, which work in acid, alkali or neutral environments [7] and these protease genes are variably expressed with distinct enzyme patterns being found in infection versus cultured conditions [8]. Keratinase activity from certain dermatophytes is inducible by low-molecular-weight peptides released from the epidermis by the action of other fungal proteinases [9]. Other enzymes such as sulphur transporters are also involved [8]. Clinically, there appears to be a certain amount of heterogeneity in substrate preference as, while all dermatophyte species invade the stratum corneum of the skin, different species

vary widely in their capacity to invade hair and nail. *T. rubrum* rarely invades hair but frequently invades nail; *Epidermophyton floccosum* never invades hair and only occasionally invades nail. In addition, other factors, such as those concerned with host resistance (e.g. serum), have a role in limiting the ability of dermatophytes to penetrate further than the stratum corneum [10]. Genes encoding different proteinases such as fungalysins (MEP) or subtilisins (SUB) have been identified [11].

Immunity

Defence against the fungi causing ringworm depends on both innate and acquired immune mechanisms [12], the latter requiring the activation of immunological memory [13]. Serum factors appear to be able to inhibit the growth of dermatophytes *in vitro* and on cultured explants of skin. It is not entirely clear what is responsible for this, but unsaturated transferrin is one candidate, inhibiting the growth of dermatophytes by binding to the hyphae [14]. Its mode of action appears to be independent of iron-binding capacity. In experimental infections of skin grafted on to nu/nu mice, there is evidence of increased turnover of epidermis, which occurs in the absence of effective T-lymphocyte-mediated defence [15]. A further potentially important mode of defence is provided by the presence of fatty acids from sebaceous glands, which inhibit dermatophyte growth *in vitro*. This activity appears to reside in saturated fatty acids with chain lengths of 7, 9, 11 and 13 carbon residues. It has been postulated that their presence on the skin in postpubertal children may account for the spontaneous resolution of tinea capitis after this age and the rarity of new infections in adults. Undecenoic acid derivatives are a practical example where fatty acids have been used for the treatment of dermatophytosis. Whatever the influence of these factors, it is clear that in experimentally infected mice, the initial inflammatory changes occur as early in the process as 4 h after infection showing that endogenous mechanisms may attract leukocytes [16].

Skin also contains a range of antimicrobial peptides, including human β-defensins, cathelicidin LL-37 and dermicin [17]. These peptides are known to have activity against bacteria, viruses and fungi and to play a key role in protection against skin infections including dermatophytes as well as *Candida albicans* [18]. It has also been found that dermatophytes are chemotactic and that they can activate the alternative pathway of complement activation. This has been demonstrated for *T. rubrum*, *T. mentagrophytes* [16] and fungi causing endothrix scalp infections, such as *T. violaceum*. The production of cytokines, such as interleukin 1 (IL-1) by keratinocytes, is important in the mobilisation of neutrophil defences. It has been shown that neutrophils, and to a lesser extent monocytes, can kill dermatophyte conidia. This activity depends both on intra- and extracellular mechanisms, and the generation of the respiratory burst is an important stage in this process [19]. Dermatophytes produce catalase and superoxide dismutase, which may act as defence against the phagocyte-generated free radicals.

By contrast, there is little evidence that antibodies to dermatophytes are protective. Patients with widespread infections, such as tinea imbricata, may have high antibody titres [20]. The presence of elevated immunoglobulin E (IgE), in particular, is associated with chronicity [21]. The transfer of specific serum containing a high titre of antibody to irradiated mice does not confer immunity on recipients. It is still premature to rule out a role for antibody as dermatophytes show some cytological changes when grown in the presence of specific antibody *in vitro*. However, there is strong evidence that the development of cellular immunity via sensitised T lymphocytes (Th17) is a key factor in immunological defence. Lymphocytes bearing T-helper phenotypic markers are responsible for transferring immunity to infection to naive recipient mice [22]. In humans, the appearance of inflammation in ringworm correlates with the development of delayed-type skin reactivity to trichophytin [23–25] and cytokines such as interferon γ (INF-γ). Chronic infections are associated with poor T-lymphocyte-mediated response to specific fungal antigens, suggesting that depression of responses is responsible for the poor clinical response [23,26]. Langerhans cells can act as antigen-presenting cells for dermatophyte antigens.

The reason for the failure of immunity in persistent infections, and its relationship with chronicity, are still not well understood. There is an association between the presence of atopy and chronic dermatophytosis, with a high proportion of those with persistent disease having atopy (usually asthma or hay fever) as well as immediate-type hypersensitivity and raised IgE levels [23,26]. It has been suggested that modulation of T-lymphocyte activity either locally or systemically may be responsible. There is evidence of activation of a type 2 helper T (Th2) lymphocyte pathway, which might explain the spectrum of antibody responses; and although INF-γ is detected in infection, there is also evidence of the production of IL-4 associated with a Th2 pathway [27]. It has been found that dermatophyte antigens, including those that contain mannose residues, can reversibly suppress lymphocyte proliferation but not the expression of human leukocyte antigen (HLA) DR [28]. Patients with persistent infection have detectable levels of circulating antigen [29]. Both are possible factors in the regulation of immunity in dermatophytosis.

Pathophysiology

The clinical appearances of the various forms of ringworm infection are the result of the combination of direct damage to the keratinised tissues by the fungus (this applies mainly in hair and nail infections) and of the inflammatory host response. The latter varies widely. At one extreme there is the simple hyperkeratosis seen, for instance, in dry-type *T. rubrum* infections; at the other is the pustular, highly inflammatory kerion seen most frequently in zoophilic infections, such as those caused by *T. verrucosum*. *T. rubrum*, for instance, may provoke the epidermal changes seen in chronic dermatitis with hyperkeratosis, patchy parakeratosis, hyper- or hypogranulosis, spongiosis, mononuclear invasion and mild or moderate acanthosis. The accompanying dermal infiltrate of lymphocytes and histiocytes is largely perivascular. The picture may be more inflammatory with superficial crusting and the more acute inflammatory changes in the epidermis may at times become vesicular, to the extent of mimicking acute contact dermatitis. Other changes described include an erythema multiforme-like process with subepidermal bullae [1], and dermal blood vessel changes of vasculitis, accompanied by an infiltrate of lymphocytes, histiocytes, neutrophils and eosinophils. Another further histological pattern is a granuloma faciale type of reaction, in which the epidermis and the upper dermis are substantially normal, but the mid-dermis has an infiltrate of neutrophils, eosinophils, lymphocytes, histiocytes and plasma cells in close proximity to dilated blood vessels.

Pustular reactions may be subcorneal or follicular. The folliculitis and perifolliculitis are normally associated with fungal remnants in the follicles. Inflammatory changes range from spongiosis of the outer root sheath to deep perifollicular granulomatous inflammation showing areas of necrosis and foreign-body giant cells, perhaps induced by fragments of hair exuded from disrupted follicles. In cases of kerion, the histology is that of a combined subacute dermatitis and a marked folliculitis, with disrupted follicles and a diffuse granulomatous inflammatory response with many foreign-body giant cells, blood vessel changes and fibrosis.

In classic annular ringworm, the rim of the lesion is marked by clear inflammatory changes including a perivascular infiltrate of lymphocytes. By contrast, in the central zone, inflammation is usually less, possibly following elimination of the fungus in the stratum corneum. Through the persistence of immunological surveillance [2], previously infected skin remains free of fungal hyphae compared with uninfected skin, and fungal growth proceeds centrifugally. The epidermal turnover rate is normal within the ring, but more than four times as rapid in the zone where inflammation is maximal. Central clearance is often partial and, in tinea imbricata caused by *T. concentricum* and in some *T. indotineae* infections, successive waves of fungal growth occur in skin previously cleared of infection, but overall mycelial expansion is centrifugal.

Other factors affecting infection
Age, sex, genetic and racial factors
The known differences in the incidence of ringworm infection between the age groups and sexes seem, in general, to reflect differing rates of exposure and of sebum production, differing clothing and fluctuations of immunity with old age. There may be ethnic differences in susceptibility, for example in tinea capitis, but the pathogenetic mechanisms are not clearly established [3]. In tinea imbricata, a genetic susceptibility factor inherited as an autosomal recessive has been suggested [4]. Unusual or deep forms of dermatophytosis have been associated in families with mutations in the *STAT1* gene [5] – these families also have chronic candidosis and hypothyroidism – and *CARD9* gene where patients may have deep dissemination [6]. A survey of children with tinea capitis has uncovered nucleotide substitutions in genes involved in macrophage function, including epithelial barrier repair among other functions [7].

Patient co-morbidities
Patients with dermatophytosis are usually otherwise healthy. However, altered or chronic infections have been noted in a number of patient groups, such as those with chronic mucocutaneous candidosis or AIDS [8] and patients on corticosteroid therapy or with endogenous Cushing syndrome. There is also the raised incidence of atopy in patients with chronic infection, suggesting that host factors may well determine the clinical course. However, this is not the only factor, and it has been found that where there is ample facility for the spread of infection (e.g. among coalminers), the incidence of atopy is no different from that seen in uninfected co-workers [9].

There is no reliable evidence that diabetic patients are especially susceptible to dermatophyte infection, even though diabetes may affect the course of established infections; for example, diabetic patients with tinea pedis are more likely to develop onychomycosis.

Temperature and microenvironment
Dermatophytes grow poorly at 37°C. Although this factor may contribute to the lack of deeper penetration of the epidermis and dermis, intravenous injection will result in progressive infection in animal models of dermatophytosis. Raised carbon dioxide tension is known to facilitate arthroconidial formation and may also aid either adhesion or penetration [10]. Moisture is also important for the germination of arthroconidia on keratinocytes.

Competing organisms and co-pathogens
The ability of certain dermatophyte species to produce penicillin-like antibiotics may allow these fungi to regulate the bacterial flora [11]. Although there is some competitive interaction [1], *Staphylococcus aureus* may occasionally act as a co-pathogen, increasing the degree of inflammation in dermatophyte infections [1].

Identification

The isolation and identification of dermatophytes is a relatively simple process and needs only basic laboratory facilities. The features of the most common species will be outlined and illustrated when grown on 2% glucose, 1% mycological peptone (Oxoid) agar supplemented with 0.04% cycloheximide and 0.005% chloramphenicol at 26°C. Illustrations of the more unusual species are beyond the scope of this chapter and the reader is referred to more specialised texts [1,2].

All the dermatophyte species appear identical in skin and nail samples. Septate hyphae are observed, which may branch without constriction at the branching point and which display an even diameter along their length (Figure 32.7a). In some specimens the hyphae fragment into arthroconidia, which disarticulate when mature, and may then round up and increase notably in size (Figure 32.7b). These germinate to produce true hyphae. Hair invasion results in four distinct patterns: small-spored ectothrix, large-spored ectothrix, arthrosporic endothrix and favus endothrix (Figure 32.7c–f) and these are readily distinguishable by the arrangement and the size of the fungal elements. When trying to determine whether infection is endothrix or ectothrix, it is useful to note that the pigment in the hair clearly delineates the edge of the hair shaft and can be used as a marker to judge whether the fungus is entirely confined within the hair or has formed an ectothrix sheath of arthroconidia on the surface.

Most isolates can be identified directly from the primary culture, but if sporulation is poor a number of media may be used to encourage the production of conidia, including potato dextrose agar and lactritmel agar [3]. A few simple physiological tests, such as growth on polished rice grains, the production of urease, the ability to penetrate human hair *in vitro* and specific vitamin requirements, may be used to confirm the identification of certain species (Box 32.1).

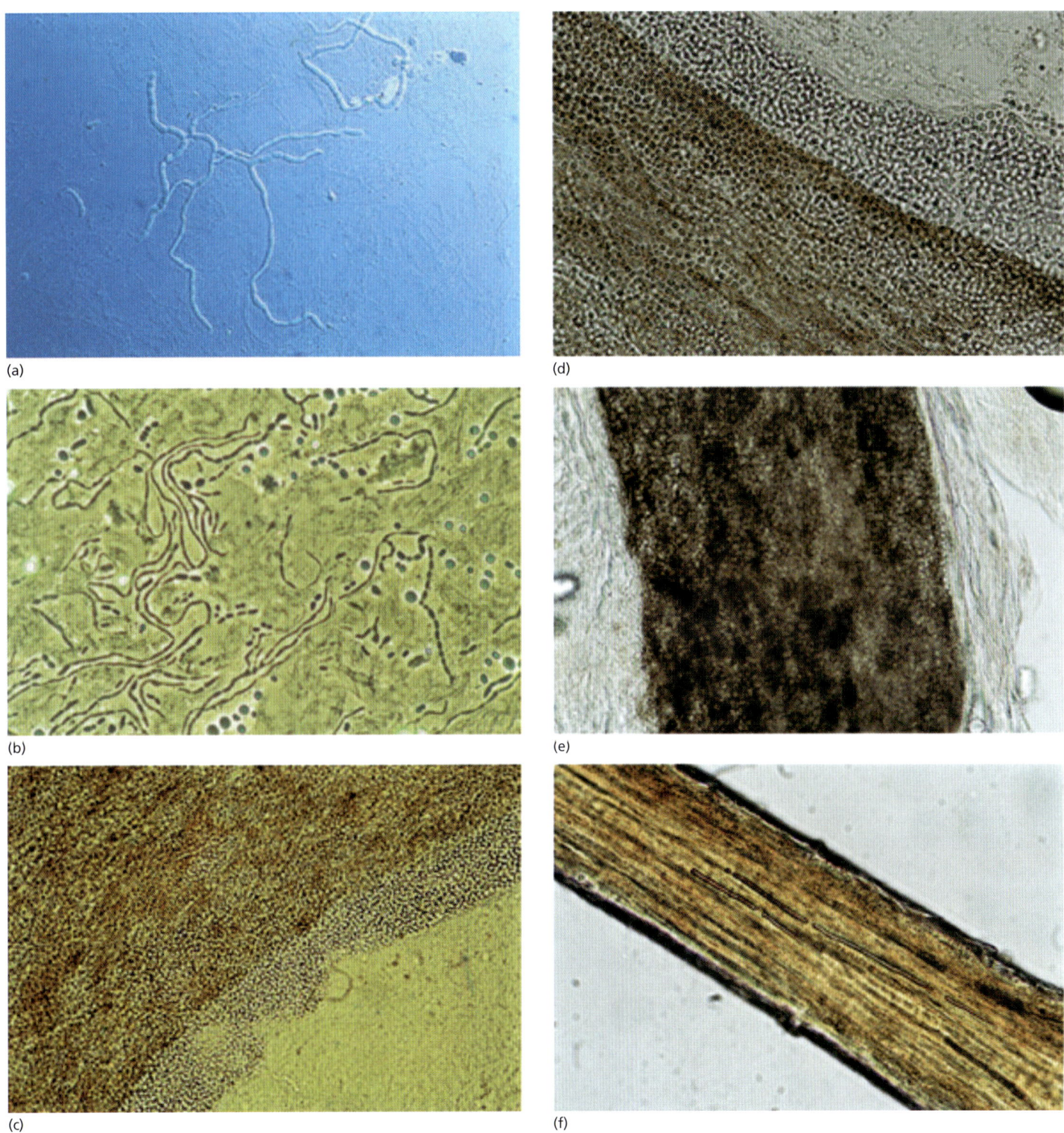

Figure 32.7 Dermatophytosis. (a) Skin scales mounted in 30% KOH, Nomarski illumination. The hyphae are very even in diameter and regularly septate. (b) Skin scales mounted in 30% KOH, phase contrast. The hyphae are fragmenting to form arthroconidia, which may increase notably in size and round up as they mature. (c) Small-spored ectothrix hair invasion, 30% KOH, bright field. The brown pigment delimits the edge of the hair, and the sheath of small arthroconidia that has formed on the surface of the hair is clearly visible. (d) Large-spored ectothrix hair invasion, 30% KOH, bright field. The sheath surrounding the hair is formed of arthroconidia, which are significantly larger than those seen in small-spored ectothrix infections. (e) Endothrix hair invasion, 30% KOH, bright field. The fungus inside the hair has broken up into a mass of large arthroconidia. These are retained entirely within the hair shaft. (f) Favus hair. The fungus is entirely confined within the hair shaft but does not fragment into arthroconidia. When first immersed in KOH, air is trapped around the hyphae forming the characteristic, long air spaces. These rapidly fill in with KOH, when the hyphae themselves become visible. Courtesy of the Department of Medical Mycology, St John's Institute of Dermatology, King's College London, London, UK.

Box 32.1 Physiological tests used in the identification of dermatophytes

Production of urease
Filter-sterilised urea agar base (Difco) is mixed with sterile molten agar and allowed to set. The medium is then inoculated with the test organism. After incubation at 26°C for 7 days, if urea is degraded, the colour turns from yellow to magenta red

Penetration of human hair *in vitro*
Sterile human hair is suspended in sterile distilled water supplemented with yeast extract. The test organism is inoculated onto the hairs. After 2 weeks' incubation at 26°C, hairs are mounted to look for wedge-shaped penetrations perpendicular to the hair axis

Vitamin tests
Trichophyton agars 1–7 (Difco) are used to determine vitamin requirements. Agar 1 is a casein-based, vitamin-free control; agar 2 is supplemented with inositol, agar 3 with thiamine and inositol, and agar 4 with thiamine alone. Agar 5 contains nicotinic acid. Agar 6 is an ammonium nitrate vitamin-free control for agar 7, which is supplemented with histidine. Small, agar-free inocula are transferred from Sabouraud's agar plates and incubated for 2–3 weeks at 26°C

Growth on rice grains
Ordinary white rice is covered with distilled water and autoclaved. The test organisms are then inoculated straight onto the surface and growth is assessed after 2–3 weeks' incubation at 26°C

Growth on 1% peptone agar
On this sugar-free medium, *Microsporum persicolor* will produce a pink surface colour, in contrast to *Trichophyton mentagrophytes*, which remains white

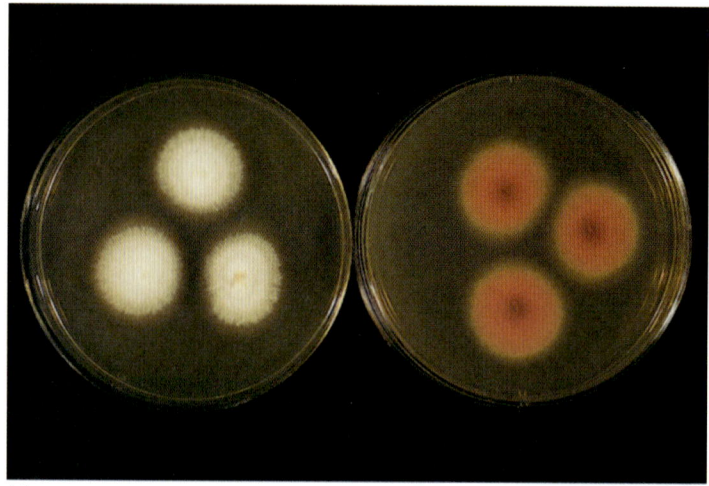

(a)

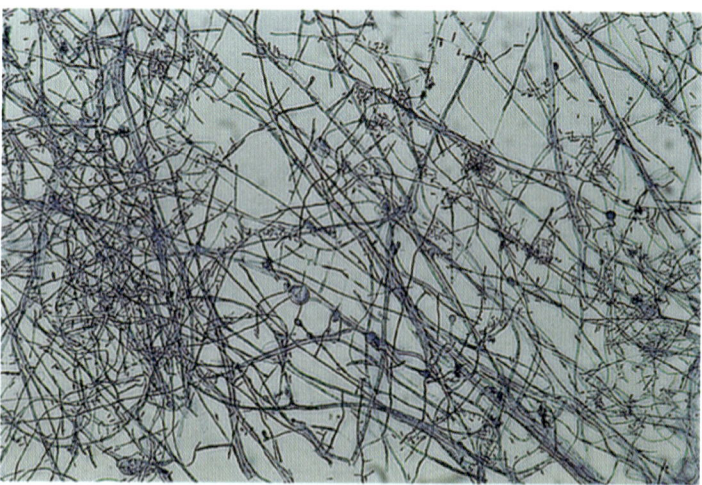

(b)

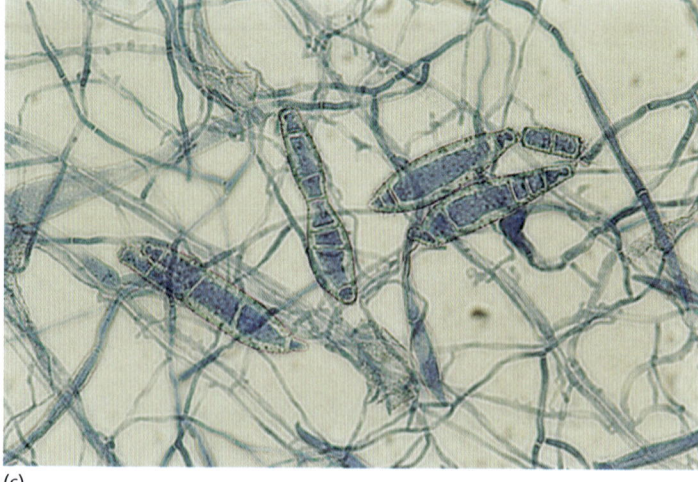

(c)

Figure 32.8 *Microsporum audouinii*. (a) Colony; the reverse of the colony is shown on the right. (b) Microscopy, bright field. In many isolates chlamydoconidia, racquet hyphae and microconidia may be the only features of note. (c) Microscopy, bright field. In some isolates, macroconidia are observed. These are large, unevenly septate and may have a waisted appearance. Courtesy of the Department of Medical Mycology, St John's Institute of Dermatology, King's College London, London, UK.

In recent years there have been numerous molecular studies of dermatophyte taxonomy. As a result, various changes have been recommended to the nomenclature and separation of the classically recognised species. Although not all the changes have been universally accepted, current studies suggest that there are many species complexes within the dermatophyte genera and have included many of the old 'varieties' of species within the complexes [4]. The area is still undergoing change and with the use of one name to designate both the sexual and asexual phases, more change is inevitable. Throughout this chapter, although newer names are used, the older names are included for ease of use.

In cases where cultures are completely atypical morphologically, however, molecular methods such as PCR and sequencing will allow species identification. As the cost of such analysis falls, more widespread use may become feasible.

Genus *Microsporum*
When present, macroconidia are species-specific; their production is enhanced by subculture on to lactritmel agar. Microconidia are similar in most species – clavate to elongate and borne along the sides of the hyphae – and thus not useful in species identification. The presence of specialised hyphae such as racquet hyphae where the cells are swollen at one end, and pectinate hyphae which bear unilateral, flattened, comb-like protrusions, may be helpful.

Microsporum audouinii (Figure 32.8). Colony: in many isolates the surface is white to tan with thin sometimes silky growth, which has been compared with mouse fur. Other strains may have a thicker, downy, white surface. The colour on the reverse of the colony is salmon pink to tan. Microscopy: in most isolates macroconidia are absent and the most characteristic features may be the presence of terminal and intercalary chlamydoconidia and racquet hyphae. However, in isolates where macroconidia are present, they are large, unevenly septate, variably rough and thick walled, and often have a constricted centre and irregular shape. Physiological tests: *M. audouinii* grows poorly or not at all on polished rice grains.

A variant found mainly in Africa (previously designated *M. audouinii* var. *rivalieri*) has also been reported from North America and Europe. The colony surface is white, with a distinctive ground-glass texture and radial or more complex cerebriform folding. Microscopically, macroconidia may be present, but the most characteristic feature is the presence of numerous pectinate hyphae. On primary culture, some isolates produce well-developed antler hyphae, which may cause confusion with *T. schoenleinii*. Subculture on to lactritmel agar may stimulate macroconidial production in these isolates and the characteristic small-spored ectothrix mode of *in vivo* hair infection will also aid in their correct identification.

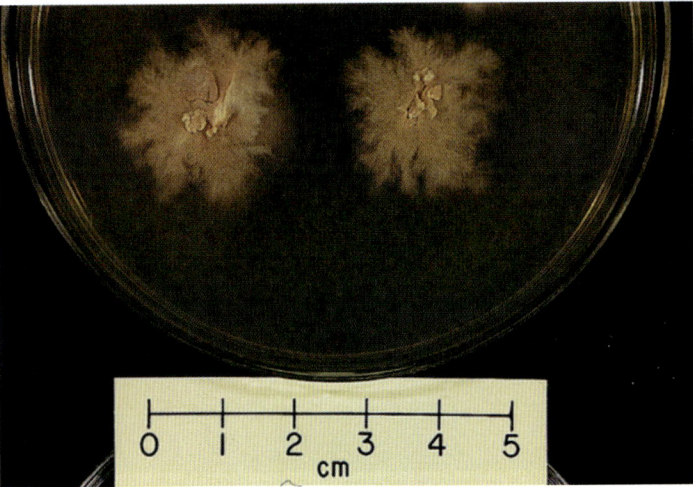

Figure 32.10 *Microsporum canis* glabrous form colony. Courtesy of the Department of Medical Mycology, St John's Institute of Dermatology, King's College London, London, UK.

Microsporum canis (Figure 32.9). Colony: the surface is white, thinning towards the edge to reveal the yellow or orange reverse pigment. The texture may be cottony, with a buff centre caused by the abundant production of macroconidia; alternatively, the surface may be thinner, silky or patchily cottony and entirely white. Radial folds may be present. Microscopy: macroconidia are rough, particularly at the tip, with thick outer walls and up to 16 cells. They are spindle shaped and may show a slightly bent apical beak. Physiological tests: *M. canis* grows well on polished rice grains. This medium also encourages macroconidial production.

A glabrous variant (Figure 32.10) has been described with heaped, leathery, yellow or orange-brown colonies with feathery edges [5]; this mutant quickly reverts to the normal colonial form and produces typical macroconidia if cultured on rice grains.

A variety found in Australia, New Zealand and the Americas was previously designated *M. audouinii* var. *rivalieri*. The rough, thick-walled macroconidia are grossly distorted and bent and abundant microconidia may be present.

Microsporum equinum (now included within *M. canis* sensu stricto). Colony: the short surface mycelium is white to pale buff with regular, deep, radial grooves. The reverse is pink or salmon. Microscopy: the macroconidia are characteristic. They are rough and thick walled but shorter and wider than those of *M. canis*, usually with one to four cells.

Microsporum ferrugineum. Colony: restricted, glabrous, heaped colonies, yellow to rust in colour or more spreading, downy colonies similar to *M. audouinii* may be seen. The pigment is often lost on subculture. Microscopy: thick 'bamboo' hyphae with prominent septa may be the only notable feature, although rare macroconidia resembling those of *M. canis* may be produced.

Microsporum (Arthroderma) gypseum (Figure 32.11). Mating studies have demonstrated that the fungus traditionally known as *M. gypseum* is actually a complex containing two separate species: *Arthroderma incurvatum* (anamorph *M. gypseum*) and *A. gypseum*

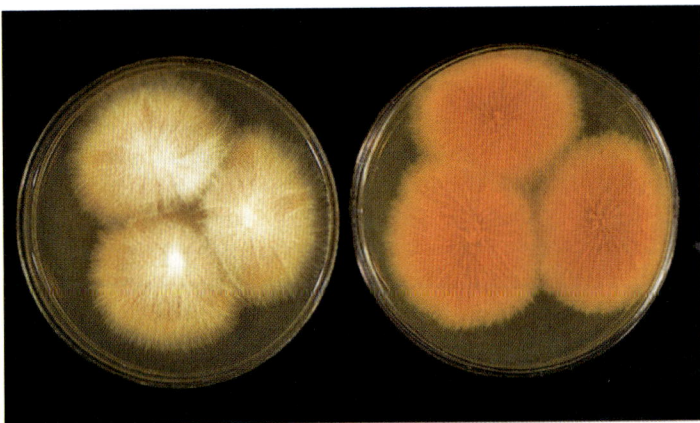

(a)

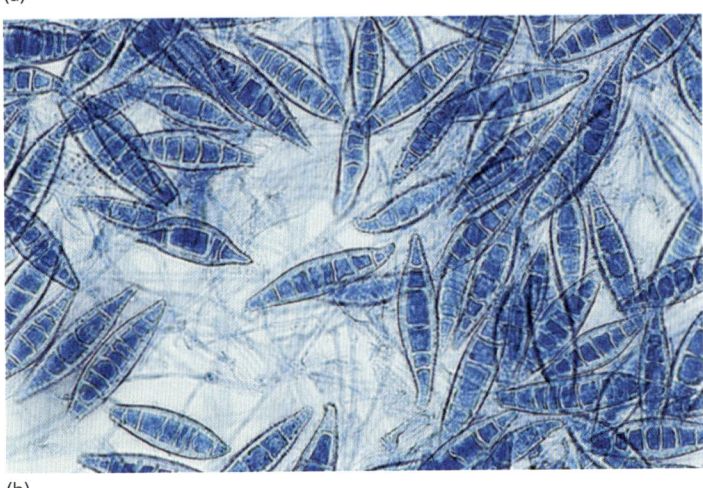

(b)

Figure 32.9 *Microsporum canis*. (a) Colony; the reverse of the colony is shown on the right. (b) Microscopy, bright field. The macroconidia are characteristic, thick-walled and fusiform, often with a tilted, apical beak. They are rough with the most pronounced thickenings at the apical tip. Courtesy of the Department of Medical Mycology, St John's Institute of Dermatology, King's College London, London, UK.

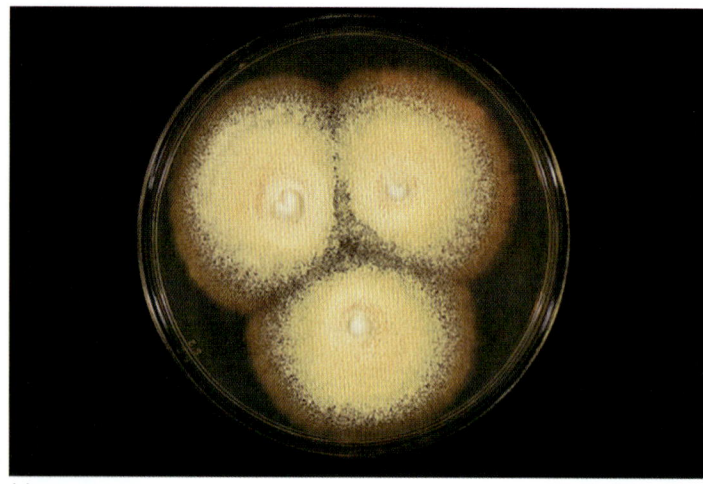

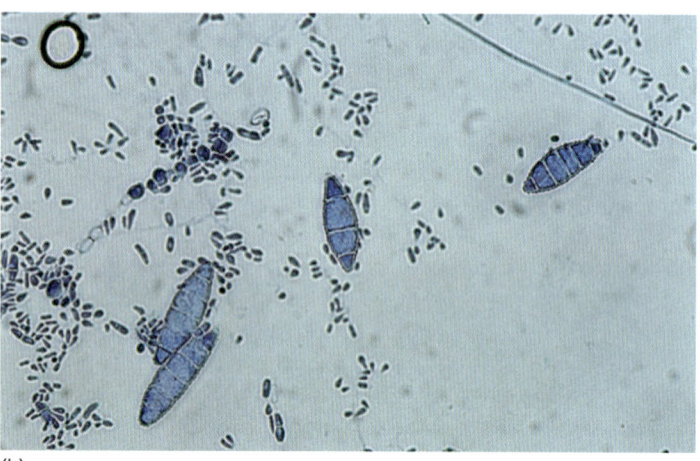

Figure 32.11 *Microsporum gypseum*. (a) Colony. (b) Microscopy, bright field. The macroconidia are abundant and characteristic, with a symmetrical cigar shape and thin, finely roughened cell walls. Courtesy of the Department of Medical Mycology, St John's Institute of Dermatology, King's College London, London, UK.

Microsporum (Nannizia) persicolor. Colony: the surface of the colony is creamy buff, sometimes with pale pink tones. The texture is noticeably thicker than that seen in *T. mentagrophytes*. The reverse is buff to brown and may also develop pink or reddish tones. Microscopy: this is very similar to *T. mentagrophytes*. Many clavate to spherical microconidia are present and are arranged in grape-like clusters and along the hyphae. Young microconidia are pyriform and matchstick hyphae with an elongated basal cell carrying a microconidium at its tip may be observed. Tightly coiled, spiral hyphae are usually present. Thin-walled, elongated macroconidia appear smooth on primary isolation media and usually contain six cells. Physiological tests: on medium free of sugar (1% peptone agar), *M. persicolor* colonies produce a rose-pink surface colour; *T. mentagrophytes* retains a white surface on this medium. On 3% salt agar, macroconidia are more obviously rough.

Genus *Trichophyton*

Macroconidia are rarely formed by most of the anthropophilic species and may not be particularly distinctive when they are. They are smooth and thin walled. The size, shape and arrangement of the microconidia is useful in species identification, together with the presence of features such as coiled spiral hyphae, abundant chlamydospore production and special physiological requirements.

Trichophyton concentricum. Colony: the compact, heaped, folded colonies have a grey, tan or brown surface; initially glabrous, a thin, short, surface mycelium may develop. The reverse may be tan, brown or have reddish tones. Microscopy: conidia are absent. The hyphae may be swollen and distorted with numerous chlamydospores and occasional antler hyphae or may be unremarkable. Physiological tests: 50% of isolates are stimulated by thiamine.

As the morphological features of this fungus are not very distinctive, it may be confused with other glabrous anthropophilic *Trichophyton* species, such as unpigmented isolates of *T. violaceum*. However, the clinical features of infection are so characteristic that they will aid in the identification.

Trichophyton equinum. Colony: in young cultures, the surface is very thin, revealing the reverse brown pigment. The reverse is initially brown in the centre with an outer yellow edge. As the culture matures, the surface texture thickens and becomes uniformly white and the reverse uniformly deep reddish brown. Microscopy: elongate to pyriform microconidia are arranged along the sides of the hyphae. Cylindrical, smooth, thin-walled macroconidia are rarely observed. Physiological tests: with the exception of some isolates from New Zealand and Australia, this fungus has a specific vitamin requirement for nicotinic acid.

Trichophyton gourvilii (now included within *T. rubrum* of African origin complex). Colony: the centre of the colony is garnet red to lavender, waxy, heaped, folded and surrounded by a flat, white, silky edge with an eyelash fringe. The reverse is cream to buff. Microscopy: clavate or pyriform microconidia are arranged along the sides of the hyphae.

Trichophyton megninii (now included within *T. rubrum* of African origin complex). Colony: the colony is very similar to downy

(anamorph *M. gypseum*). Colony: both species produce rapidly growing colonies with a cinnamon or brown, powdery surface. In *M. gypseum* the surface is almost completely flat. The reverse is yellow-buff to brown or may have red overtones. Microscopy: the numerous macroconidia are thin walled, finely roughened over their entire surface and have up to six septa. The shape is very symmetrical, broadly fusiform with rounded ends, and has variously been described as cigar or boat shaped.

Microsporum (Nannizia) fulvum. Colony: the appearance is similar to *M. gypseum* but there is typically a much thicker and more floccose surface texture. Microscopy: there are numerous macroconidia, thin walled, with 3–6 septa. They are longer and and more clavate than those of *M. gypseum*.

Microsporum (Nannizia) nanum. Colony: moderate to rapidly growing, flat, powdery colonies are seen with a buff surface and red-brown reverse. Microscopy: characteristic thin-walled, rough, obovate macroconidia with usually a single septum are abundantly produced.

T. rubrum isolates. The surface is white, developing pink or rose tones. The texture is velvety or downy, often with radial folds. The reverse is reddish brown to wine red. Microscopy: as in *T. rubrum*, pyriform microconidia are arranged along the sides of the hyphae. Physiological tests: when grown on a medium with an inorganic nitrogen source, this fungus has a specific requirement for l-histidine. It is urease positive.

Trichophyton mentagrophytes (Figure 32.12). Colony: the colonies are fast growing with an intensely granular surface, which may be entirely white or develop a cream centre. The edge of the colony is thinner and may be spiky or stellate. The reverse is yellow, tan or red to brown. Microscopy: the spherical microconidia are arranged in grape-like bunches and to a lesser extent along the hyphae. Coiled spiral hyphae are usually present and in many isolates thin-walled, cylindrical macroconidia with up to eight cells may be present. Physiological tests: the fungus is urease positive and penetrates human hair *in vitro*. *T. indotineae*, a new species associated with widespread treatment-resistant infection in India and other countries, is related to *T. mentagrophytes*, but it is identified using molecular tools.

Trichophyton erinacei. Colony: the rapidly growing colonies have a flat, white, intensely granular surface. The reverse is a bright canary yellow. Microscopy: elongate microconidia, even longer than those of *T. rubrum*, are arranged along the sides of the hyphae. Spiral hyphae and smooth, thin-walled macroconidia may be present in some isolates. Physiological tests: unlike other variants of *T. mentagrophytes*, the fungus is urease negative, but will penetrate human hair *in vitro*.

Trichophyton quinckeanum. Colony: the surface is white, velvety or downy and often folded in the centre. The reverse is buff to cream. The colony has been reported to have a distinctive sour smell. Microscopy: pyriform microconidia are arranged along the sides of the hyphae. Physiological tests: produces a Wood's light-positive hair infection in mice with characteristic scutula.

Trichophyton interdigitale (Figure 32.13). Colony: the most typical isolates are rapidly growing with a white, powdery surface, which develops a cream centre (Figure 32.13a). A few isolates may develop a pinkish surface. The reverse is tan or reddish brown, often with a

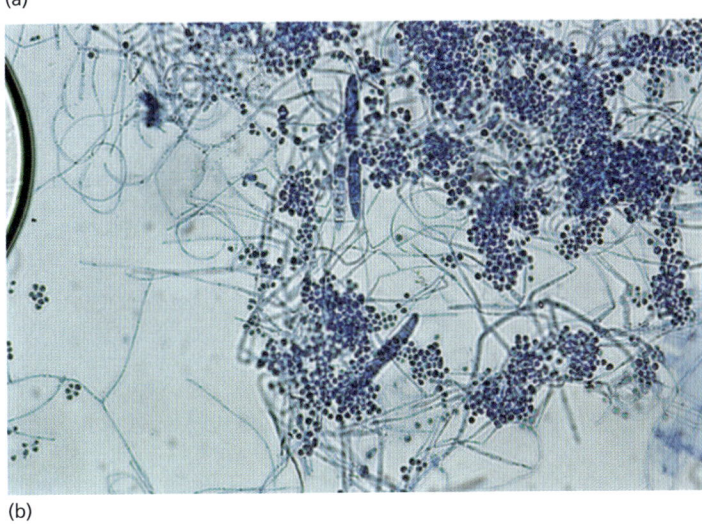

Figure 32.12 *Trichophyton mentagrophytes.* (a) Colony. (b) Microscopy, bright field. Round microconidia are arranged in clusters; spiral hyphae and thin-walled, smooth, cylindrical macroconidia may also be present. Courtesy of the Department of Medical Mycology, St John's Institute of Dermatology, King's College London, London, UK.

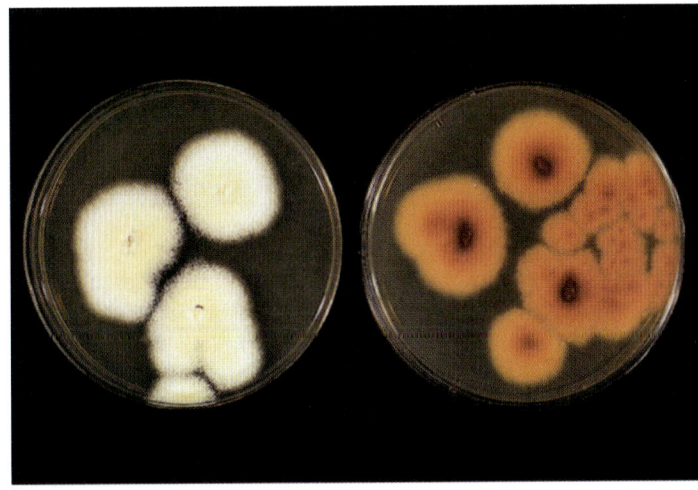

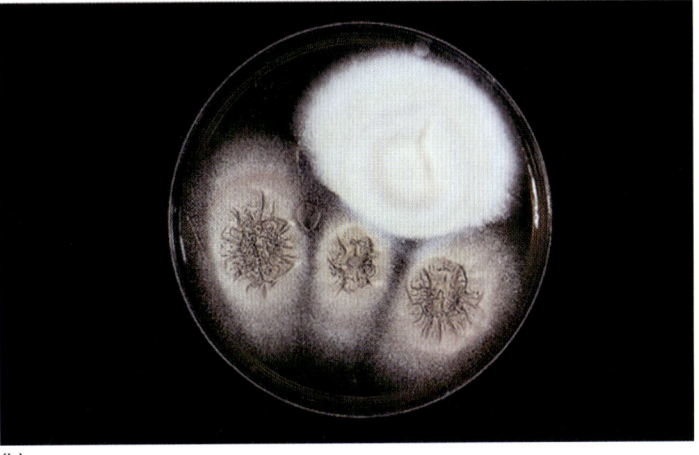

Figure 32.13 *Trichophyton interdigitale.* (a) Typical colony form; the reverse of the colony is shown on the right. (b) More unusual colony forms. The upper colony is of the downy white form and the lower colonies show an intricately folded, beige form. Courtesy of the Department of Medical Mycology, St John's Institute of Dermatology, King's College London, London, UK.

paler edge. Less typical downy forms have a fluffier white surface, sometimes slightly cream in the centre and folded (Figure 32.13b). The reverse is pale cream to buff. Microscopy: powdery isolates may be very similar to *T. mentagrophytes* with spherical microconidia arranged in bunches; spiral hyphae and macroconidia are present in some isolates. The fluffier downy isolates have pyriform microconidia arranged along the sides of the hyphae. Physiological tests: the fungus is urease positive and penetrates human hair *in vitro*.

The 'nodulare' form of *T. interdigitale* has a predominantly glabrous, waxy surface devoid of aerial hyphae and feathery sub-surface growth. Both the surface and reverse of the colony are orange-red in colour. Small areas of more typical white growth may be present. Nodular bodies are present on microscopical examination. This variety is relatively unstable and may quickly sector out into a powdery or downy colonial form.

Trichophyton rubrum. This is probably the most morphologically variable dermatophyte species and several distinct colonial forms are regularly isolated. Only the most common will be described here.

1 Downy form. This is the most commonly isolated form in temperate zones (Figure 32.14a, b). Colony: the surface of the colony is white, downy or cottony, and domed. The reverse of the colony is initially dark brown, usually with a paler cream border, but after incubation for 3–4 weeks produces the typical deep red pigment characteristic of this species. Microscopy: small, tear-shaped, clavate or elongate microconidia are arranged along the sides of the hyphae. In some isolates, microconidia may be scanty. Physiological tests: the fungus is urease negative and does not perforate human hair *in vitro*.
2 Melanoid form (Figure 32.14c). Colony: similar to the downy form, but characterised by producing a brown melanoid pigment that diffuses into the medium and masks any red pigment on the reverse of the colony. Microscopy: small, tear-shaped microconidia are arranged along the sides of the hyphae.
3 Dysgonic form (Figure 32.14d). Colony: slow-growing, tiny, deep red colonies with a brittle texture. This form is relatively unstable and will quickly revert to the more typical downy form.
4 Granular form (Figure 32.14e, f). Colony: the surface is powdery or granular, cream to pink and often raised and folded in the centre. The reverse is red-brown. Microscopy: numerous smooth, thin-walled, cylindrical or pencil-shaped macroconidia are produced; some macroconidia may have constricted septa. Typical tear-shaped microconidia are also present. Physiological tests: this form is urease positive and may penetrate human hair *in vitro*.
5 Yellow form. The surface may be similar to the more usual downy form or it may be smooth, leathery and yellow. The reverse is yellow; the red pigment characteristic of *T. rubrum* is completely absent. In instances where microconidia are not observed it may be difficult to show that this is indeed a dermatophyte. However, pigmentation and sporulation may be enhanced on lactritmel agar.

Trichophyton schoenleinii (Figure 32.15). Colony: on primary isolation, the colonies may be glabrous or velvety, usually heaped and folded, and often with a fringe of hyphae at the edge submerged in the culture medium. The surface is white to cream and the reverse is pale. On repeated subculture, most isolates become downy. Microscopy: conidia are usually absent. Characteristic dichotomously branching hyphae with flattened tips, termed chandelier or antler hyphae, are present in fresh cultures. These may be readily observed by focusing on the back of the primary culture plate with a ×10 objective. Swollen, distorted hyphae with many chlamydoconidia are also usually present.

Trichophyton simii. Colony: the surface is flat and granular, pale at the edges and buff or sometimes pink in the centre. The reverse is usually yellow to red-brown. Microscopy: many smooth-walled macroconidia are produced, often outnumbering the number of clavate to pyriform microconidia. The macroconidia are thin walled, cylindrical or torpedo shaped and are characterised by the development of constricted septa, and the fact that certain of the cells swell to produce endochlamydoconidia as they age.

Trichophyton soudanense (Figure 32.16). Colony: the colony is relatively slow growing, glabrous and leathery or brittle in texture, with a characteristic stellate or eyelash fringe around the edge. The colour is typically apricot to yellow, but isolates producing purple or red colonies are also common. Microscopy: when examined through the back of the primary culture plate using a ×10 objective, the hyphae appear stiff and 'brush-like'. They are very regularly septate and the formation of arthroconidia produces a zig-zag appearance. Reflexive branching back towards the centre of the colony is a characteristic feature. Pyriform microconidia may be present.

Trichophyton tonsurans (Figure 32.17). Colony: the colony surface is velvety or powdery and may be grey, cream or yellow in colour, more rarely brown in the centre. Some isolates produce very sparse surface mycelium, so that the reverse brown pigmentation shows through. Circular or radial folds are often present. The reverse is typically chocolate brown, mahogany or yellow. Microscopy: the most characteristic feature is that the microconidia are noticeably larger than those of *T. mentagrophytes* or *T. rubrum* and very variable in shape. They range from clavate to elongate, and swollen 'balloon' microconidia and stalked, matchstick microconidia are also observed. In the majority of isolates, chlamydoconidia are numerous and in some isolates spiral hyphae and macroconidia are present. Physiological tests: this fungus has a specific vitamin requirement for thiamine.

Trichophyton verrucosum (Figure 32.18). Colony: this is a very slow-growing fungus and after 2 weeks of incubation at 26°C the white or grey waxy colonies may still be barely visible. Growth is better at 37°C so, if cattle ringworm is suspected, incubation at both temperatures is recommended. Microscopy: examining the reverse of the primary plate under a ×10 objective, colonies incubated at 26°C show short hyphae with terminal chlamydoconidia. In contrast, colonies incubated at 37°C produce very characteristic long chains of chlamydoconidia. Clavate or elongate microconidia may be present along the sides of the hyphae. Rat-tailed macroconidia may be produced on depleted media. Physiological tests: most isolates have a requirement for thiamine and inositol. In a few, growth is enhanced by thiamine alone.

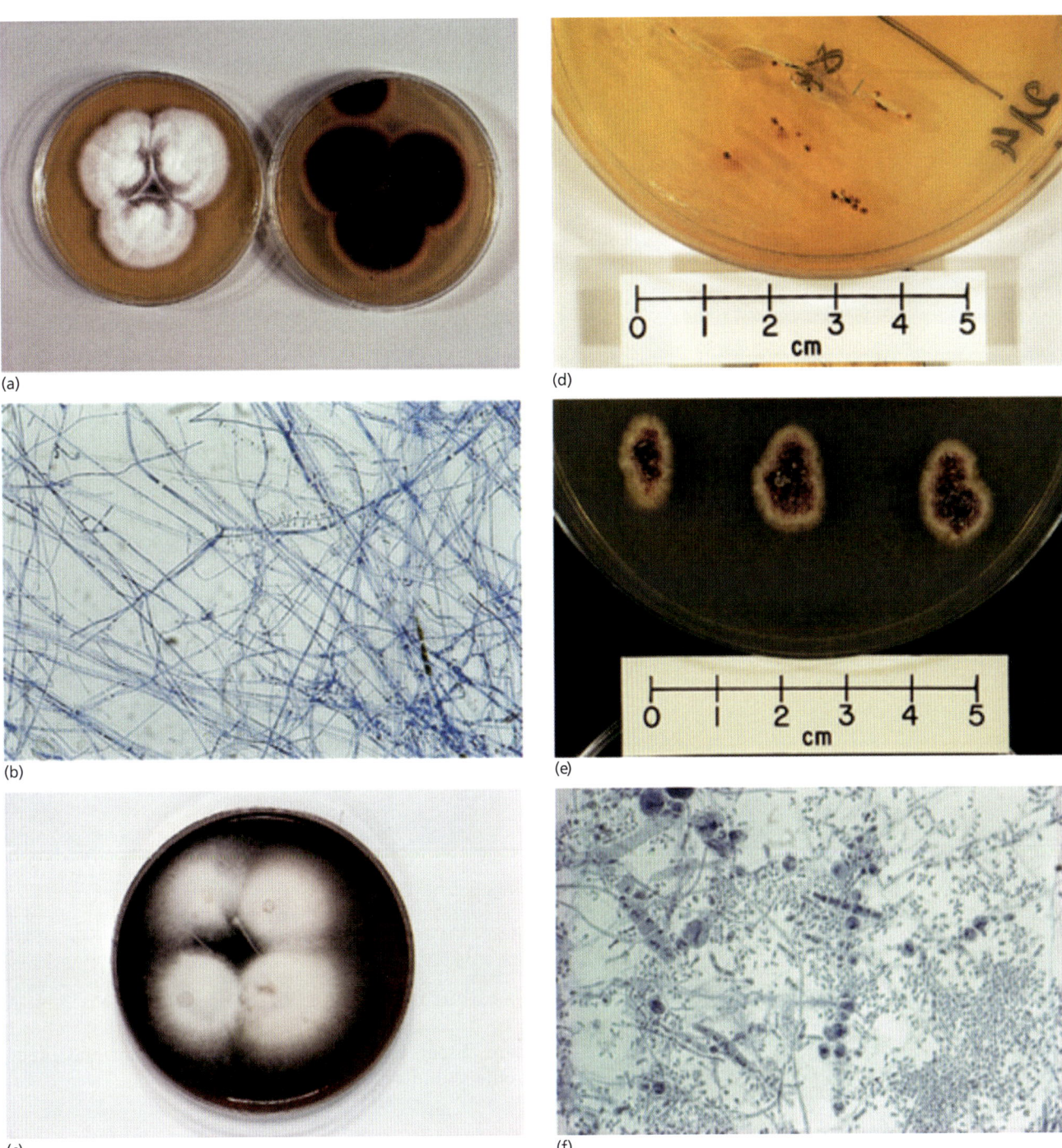

Figure 32.14 *Trichophyton rubrum*. (a) Downy colony; the reverse of the colony is shown on the right. (b) Downy form microscopy, bright field. Clavate to elongate microconidia are arranged along the sides of the hyphae. They may be scanty in some isolates. (c) Melanoid colony form. A brown pigment diffuses into the agar medium. (d) Dysgonic colony form. Growth is initially very restricted and the tiny colonies are a deep red. They usually revert to a more typical downy form within 2–3 weeks. (e) Granular form colony, with a powdery pink surface often raised and folded in the centre. (f) Granular form microscopy, bright field. Cylindrical, smooth-walled macroconidia are abundant and may become swollen as they mature with constricted septa. Microconidia and chlamydoconidia may also be abundant. Courtesy of the Department of Medical Mycology, St John's Institute of Dermatology, King's College London, London, UK.

Trichophyton violaceum (Figure 32.19). Colony: the slow-growing, glabrous colonies have a waxy or leathery texture. Characteristically they are deep purple-red in colour, but some isolates take several weeks to pigment, or retain unpigmented sectors. Occasionally, isolates fail to pigment at all. Microscopy: microconidia and macroconidia are usually absent. Chlamydoconidia and distorted hyphae may be present. Physiological tests: growth is stimulated by thiamine.

Trichophyton yaoundei (now included within *T. violaceum*). Colony: the colonies are initially glabrous and white to cream. As they age, the surface may develop a velvety texture and a tan

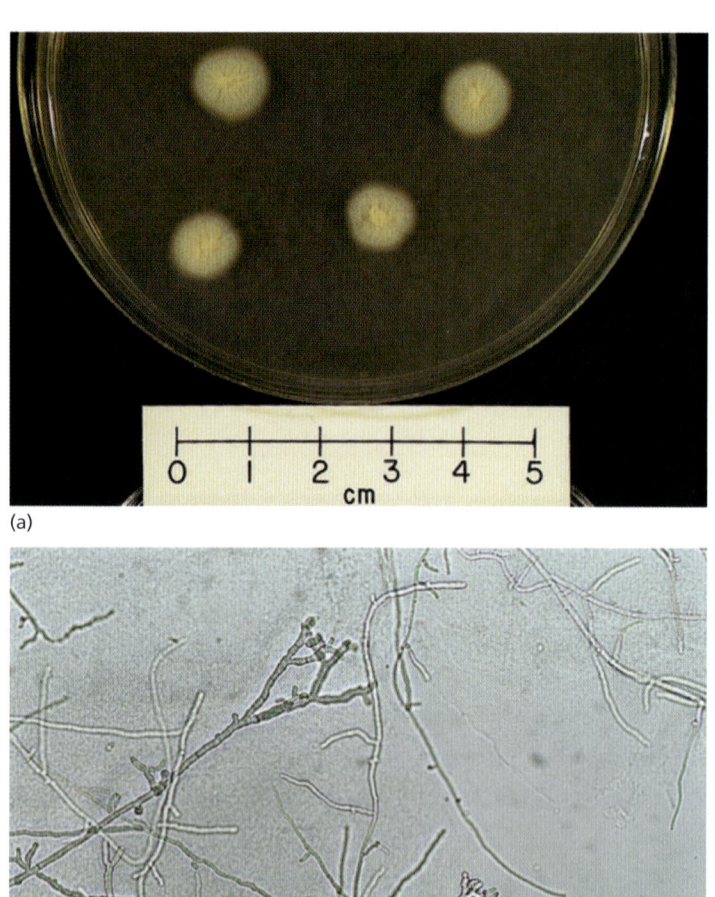
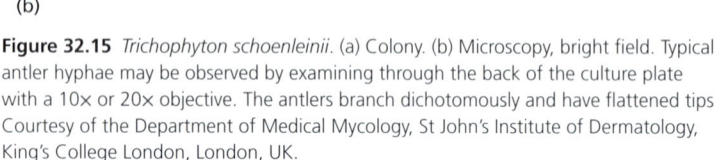

Figure 32.15 *Trichophyton schoenleinii*. (a) Colony. (b) Microscopy, bright field. Typical antler hyphae may be observed by examining through the back of the culture plate with a 10× or 20× objective. The antlers branch dichotomously and have flattened tips. Courtesy of the Department of Medical Mycology, St John's Institute of Dermatology, King's College London, London, UK.

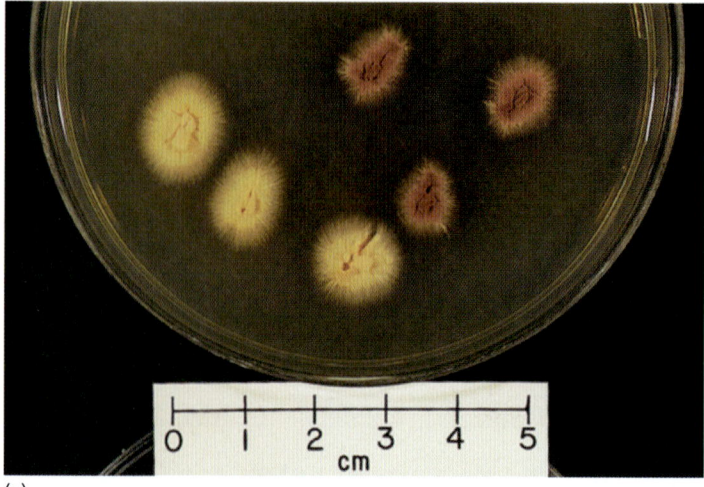
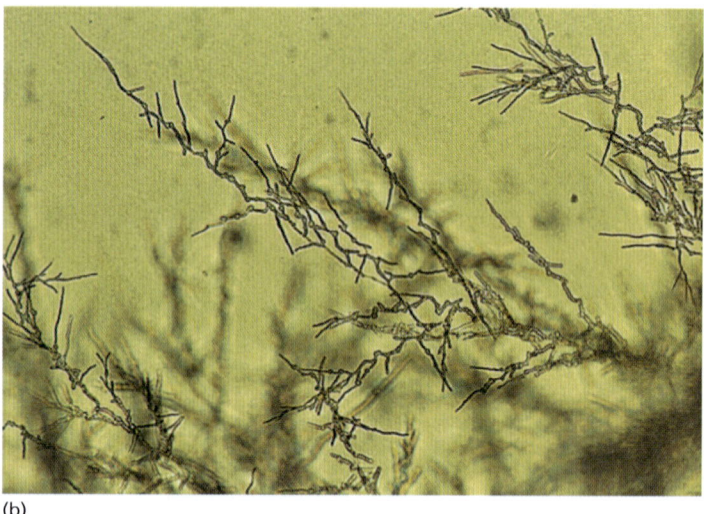

Figure 32.16 *Trichophyton rubrum* of African origin (formerly called *T. soudanense*). (a) Colony forms. A typical apricot yellow and a red isolate are illustrated. (b) Microscopy, bright field. The stiff hyphae with many arthroconidia and reflexive branching may be observed directly through the back of the culture plate. Courtesy of the Department of Medical Mycology, St John's Institute of Dermatology, King's College London, London, UK.

to brown colour; a diffusable brown pigment may be produced. Microscopy: irregular hyphae and chlamydoconidia may be present; clavate microconidia are rare. Physiological tests: the lack of vitamin requirements will distinguish this species from *T. verrucosum* and unpigmented isolates of *T. violaceum*.

Genus *Epidermophyton*
These are identified by their characteristic macroconidia and lack of microconidia.

Epidermophyton floccosum (Figure 32.20). Colony: this species grows rapidly to form velvety or suede-like colonies, which may remain flat or develop central or radial folds. The colour is typically khaki or olive green and some isolates produce tufts of floccose, sterile, white mycelium on the surface of the colony. Microscopy: large clavate macroconidia with a rounded apical end and up to six cells are rapidly formed. They are thin walled and initially smooth but may develop a few discrete thickenings as they age. Microconidia are absent. Chlamydoconidia are abundant and predominate in older cultures.

Management

General principles of management
The treatment of fungal infection is now comparatively straightforward and cure rates for many forms of dermatophytosis are over 90%. In addition to treatment, some other management measures are generally helpful.

The identification of the causative agent is useful, particularly in tinea corporis and tinea capitis where treatment of an infected animal source is important in order to prevent other infections. In the case of tinea capitis, it will also provide information on the risk of spread to other children at home or in school.

The prevention of dermatophytosis is not practicable except in situations where there is a high risk of spread to other individuals.

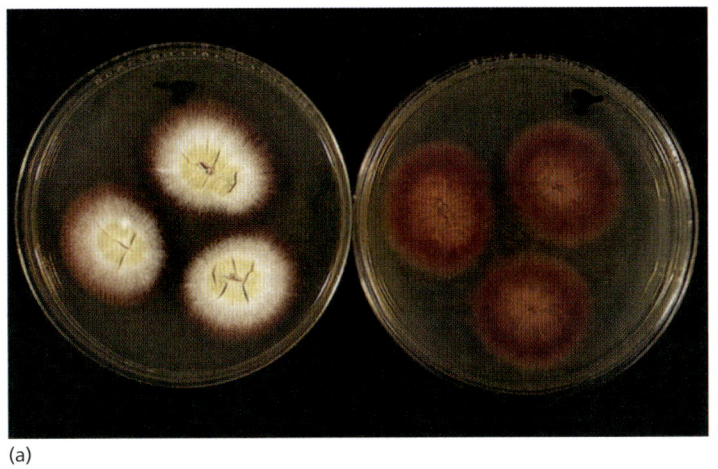

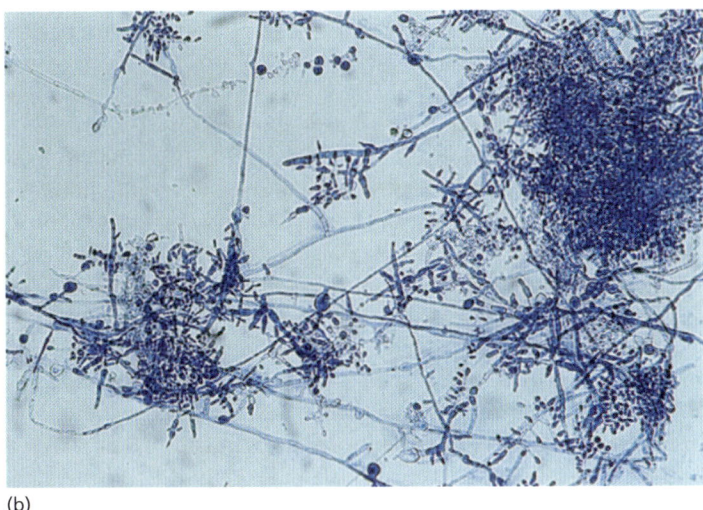

Figure 32.17 *Trichophyton tonsurans*. (a) Colony; the reverse of the colony is shown on the right. (b) Microscopy, bright field. The microconidia are large and vary considerably in their shape. Chlamydoconidia are often abundant; macroconidia and spiral hyphae are occasionally seen. Courtesy of the Department of Medical Mycology, St John's Institute of Dermatology, King's College London, London, UK.

These include shower rooms in industry or in the armed forces or schools. In the case of tinea pedis, improvement of hygiene in swimming baths may result in lower levels of infection. Frequent washing of changing room floors and walkways will remove infective material in skin scales. The provision of tolnaftate powder at swimming baths and encouragement to use it prophylactically has been shown to reduce levels of toe cleft tinea pedis caused by *T. interdigitale*, although it had little effect on *T. rubrum*. Clearly, infected individuals using these facilities should be encouraged to seek treatment. In industry or in schools, prompt treatment of infection combined with simple hygienic measures such as washing shower room floors with an antiseptic will be useful. It is less easy to prevent the spread of tinea pedis in households; treatment of infection and care in keeping to personal towels are both sensible measures. Even with less care, family members often remain free of infection in spite of the opportunities for exposure.

In the case of tinea capitis, it may be necessary to take preventative action [1]. This is particularly important if there is any evidence of an increasing number of cases of tinea capitis in schools. It is important to establish the nature of the infections and whether the organisms

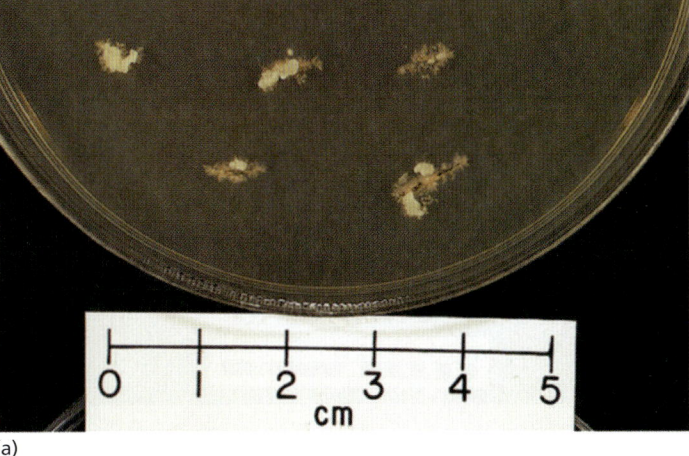

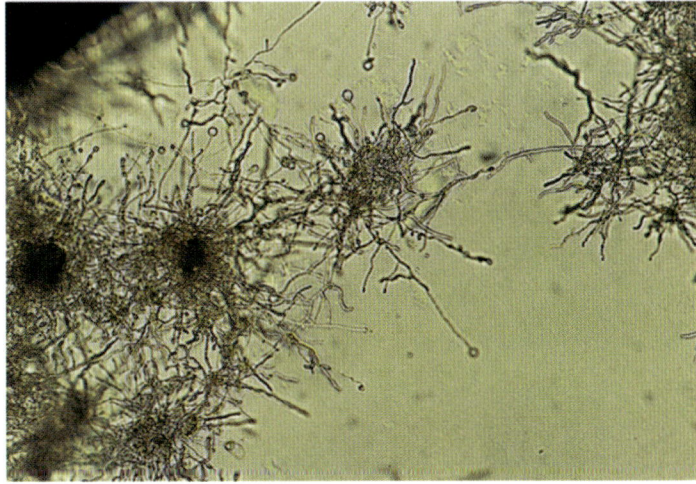

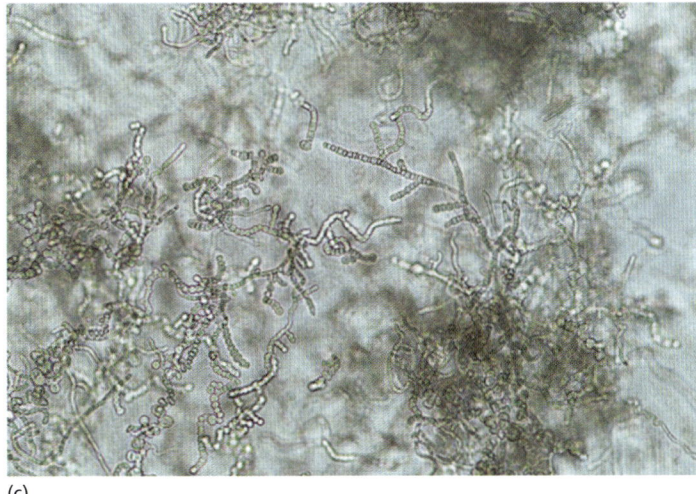

Figure 32.18 *Trichophyton verrucosum*. (a) Colony. (b) Microscopy at 26°C, bright field. Through the back of the culture dish, the small colonies are characterised by the development of hyphae with terminal swellings or chlamydoconidia. (c) Microscopy at 37°C, bright field. Grown at a higher temperature, characteristic long chains of chlamydoconidia are observed. Courtesy of the Department of Medical Mycology, St John's Institute of Dermatology, King's College London, London, UK.

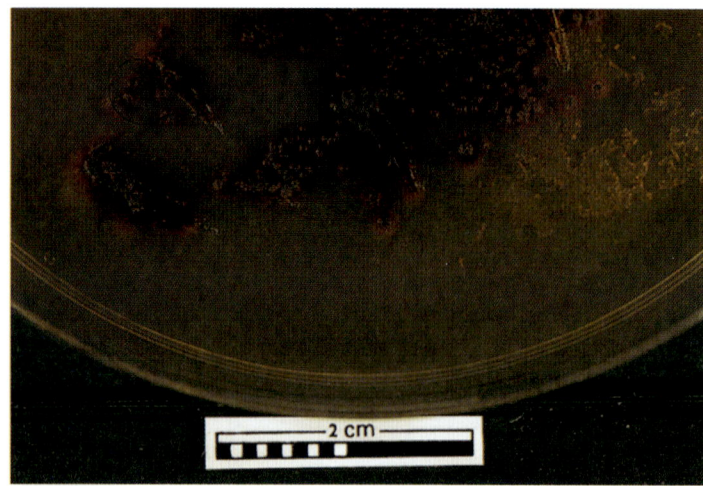

Figure 32.19 *Trichophyton violaceum* colony. Courtesy of the Department of Medical Mycology, St John's Institute of Dermatology, King's College London, London, UK.

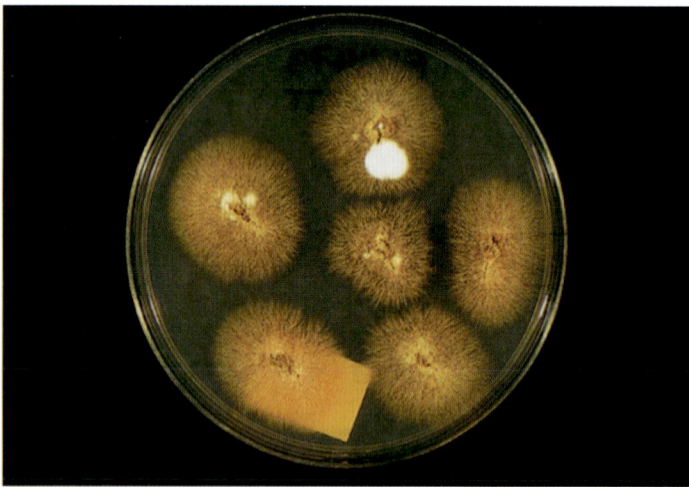

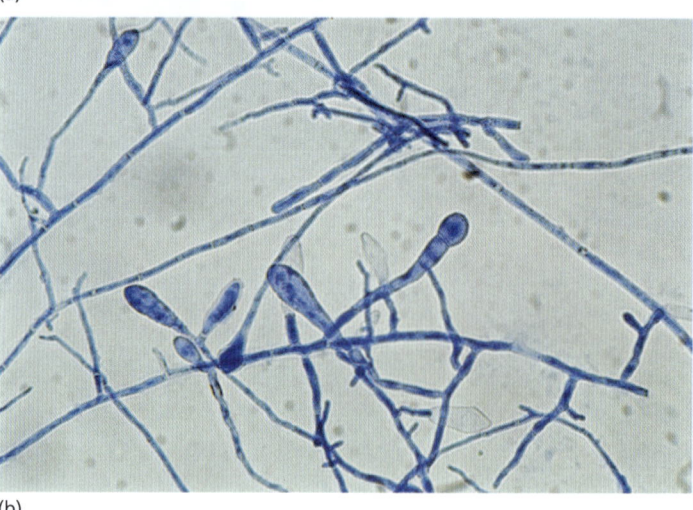

Figure 32.20 *Epidermophyton floccosum*. (a) Colony. (b) Microscopy, bright field. The clavate macroconidia are characteristic. Microconidia are absent but chlamydoconidia are very common. Courtesy of the Department of Medical Mycology, St John's Institute of Dermatology, King's College London, London, UK.

are anthropophilic. There are no proven methods of ensuring the eradication of infection in schools, but early identification of infected children and prompt treatment are probably the best approaches to adopt. An additional precaution is the use of a topical antifungal, which is likely to reduce spread while having little effect on the infection itself [1]. There is evidence that selenium sulphide or ketoconazole shampoo may reduce the incidence of positive cultures in children receiving griseofulvin. In most countries, infected children are not prevented from attending school but topical antifungal shampoos are often used in addition to treatment.

Therapeutic agents

The treatment of dermatophyte infections usually involves the use of oral terbinafine, fluconazole, itraconazole, griseofulvin or one of several well-tried topical preparations (Table 32.7). All those noted have been shown to be effective in a substantial majority of patients, provided they are used regularly.

Terbinafine [2,3]. Terbinafine is a member of the allylamine antifungals, a relatively newly developed group of drugs, that act by the inhibition of squalene epoxidase in the formation of the fungal cell membrane. This enzyme acts at an early stage in membrane biosynthesis and the accumulation of squalene is thought to destabilise the cell membrane. The two main antifungal compounds are naftifine and terbinafine. Both are active *in vitro* against dermatophytes in addition to other fungi; terbinafine is also active against *Sporothrix schenckii*, some *Aspergillus* species and *Histoplasma capsulatum*, in addition to other fungi. *In vitro* there is little difference between the dosage at which the drug inhibits cell growth and that at which the fungal cell is killed (the drug is fungicidal rather than fungistatic). Terbinafine can be given topically or orally. When given orally, it is rapidly taken up into the stratum corneum and it persists in nails at high concentrations for several months. These may exceed the minimum inhibitory concentration 80 days after the end of therapy [4]. Terbinafine is given orally in a dosage of 250 mg/day. It has produced rapid and long-lasting remissions in both nail disease [5,6] and persistent tinea pedis, as well as tinea corporis. A smaller tablet form of 125 mg is available in some countries for the treatment of children. The frequency of relapse is much lower than with griseofulvin. It also has activity against most of the agents of tinea capitis, particularly *Trichophyton* species, although it is not licensed for this indication in many countries [7]. There are few drug interactions reported for terbinafine and side effects are uncommon. Some patients describe abdominal fullness and nausea. Taste loss may occur occasionally but is reversible. Hepatic reactions, although reported, are exceptionally rare. Drug rashes including erythema multiforme or toxic epidermal necrolysis are also seen on occasion. A high level of terbinafine resistance due to a mutation in squalene epoxidase has been found in the *T. indotineae* strains.

Itraconazole [8,9]. This is an orally active azole of the triazole series. It has similar activity to ketoconazole, but without the risk of hepatotoxicity. Its mode of action is through the inhibition of the cytochrome P450-dependent demethylation stage in the formation of ergosterol on the fungal cell membrane. It is active *in vitro* against all the main superficial fungal pathogens including *Candida albicans*,

Table 32.7 Topical antifungal agents used in dermatophyte infections.

Compound	Available forms	Comments
Benzoic acid compound (Whitfield's ointment)	Ointment	Cheap, but may be difficult to source
Undecenoates: various brands available	Ointment, powder	Cheap
Tolnaftate	Cream, powder, lotion	Cheap
Imidazoles: miconazole, clotrimazole, econazole, sulconazole[a], ketoconazole, bifonazole[a]	Cream, powder, lotion, spray, shampoo (ketoconazole)	Broad spectrum including antibacterial (not ketoconazole)
Tioconazole nail solution[a]	Nail treatment	Expensive
Bifonazole urea[a]	Nail treatment	Expensive
Allylamines: terbinafine, naftifine[a]	Cream	Very rapid. Expensive
Amorolfine[a]	Cream, nail lacquer	Can be used on nails. Expensive
Cyclopyroxolamine[a]	Cream	Broad spectrum
Tavaborole	Nail treatment	Not available in many countries

[a] Availability varies in different countries.

as well as a wide range of fungi that cause deep infections from *Histoplasma capsulatum* to *Talaromyces* (previously *Penicillium*) *marneffei*. Itraconazole rapidly penetrates to the outer stratum corneum and is also found in sebum. It is avidly bound to keratin-containing tissues, and in nails, for instance, may persist long after cessation of therapy. It has been shown that after 3 months of 200 mg/day itraconazole, levels in the toenail persist for up to 6 months [10]. This feature allows a range of different dose regimens. These have evolved so that the initial treatments first described involving 100 mg/day itraconazole have been superseded by higher or intermittent (pulsed) therapy. It is active against a wide range of dermatophytes and is effective in regimens of 100 mg for 15 days in tinea cruris and tinea corporis, or 30 days in tinea pedis. The currently preferred regimen uses 400 mg/day, given as two daily doses of 200 mg. In tinea corporis, 1 week of therapy is sufficient, and in tinea pedis, 2 weeks. For onychomycosis, a regimen of 400 mg/day for 1 week every month for 3 months is usually given. Occasionally, longer periods of treatment are needed [11]. Although it is not licensed yet in many countries for the treatment of tinea capitis, it is effective in this indication [12]. There is some evidence that its absorption is impaired in the presence of phenobarbital. It also interacts with coumarin anticoagulants, ciclosporin, rifampicin, digoxin, statins and astemizole and terfenadine. It should not be given together with the latter antihistamines, as they may cause cardiac arrhythmias. Side effects are not common and mainly consist of nausea and abdominal discomfort. Hepatic reactions are exceptional.

Griseofulvin [13]. This is a metabolic product derived from several species of *Penicillium*, which was first isolated from *P. griseofulvum*. Its activity, which is fungistatic, is largely restricted to dermatophyte infections. The mode of action appears to be in part through inhibition of the formation of intracellular microtubules. Resistance to griseofulvin among dermatophytes is rare. The smaller particle size microcrystalline preparations of griseofulvin are better absorbed than those with larger particles, and the micronised form is now the standard preparation. Unlike itraconazole, griseofulvin is not firmly bound to keratin. The usual human regimen is 10 mg/kg/day given in tablet form or solution form for children. The solution form is not available in many countries. Treatment duration varies between 2 and 4 weeks for tinea corporis to over 1 year for onychomycosis of toenails. In tinea capitis, a single dose of 1–2 g griseofulvin has been reported to be effective in some patients with tinea capitis [14]. Drug interactions with phenobarbital and coumarin anticoagulants occur [13]. Headaches and nausea are common complaints in patients on griseofulvin; however, serious side effects have been extremely rare. There are a few reports of apparent precipitation or exacerbation of systemic lupus erythematosus and porphyrias by griseofulvin. Occasionally, urticarial rashes are seen and light sensitivity eruptions (distinct from lupus erythematosus and porphyria) have occasionally been reported. The use of griseofulvin has largely been superseded in many countries by terbinafine or itraconazole, except in tinea capitis.

Ketoconazole [15]. This orally active imidazole is a broad-spectrum antifungal agent. Hepatitis is a proven complication, occurring in one in 10 000 patients. Because of this, ketoconazole is now not recommended in most countries for superficial fungal infections.

Fluconazole [16]. Fluconazole is an orally active triazole antifungal used for the treatment of *Candida* infections and systemic mycoses. However, it also has activity against dermatophyte fungi. It is given in a regimen of 150 mg/week for 2–3 weeks for tinea corporis and tinea cruris, and somewhat longer for dry-type tinea pedis. It is also reported to be effective given in weekly doses in onychomycosis, although the exact length of treatment necessary is not clear as yet. There are fewer interactions than with itraconazole but, like the latter, side effects are rare and mainly confined to gastrointestinal discomfort. However, drug resistance in *Candida* species, particularly *C. krusei* and *C. glabrata*, has been described. There is also *C. albicans* resistance in some patients, particularly in those with HIV/AIDS [17].

There are few data at present on the use of posaconazole and voriconazole in dermatophytosis.

Topical applications. A great variety of topical applications have been used for the treatment of ringworm infections. The short list includes a few preferred preparations (Table 32.7) that have been soundly tested and are of comparable effectiveness [18–22]. In all cases, allergic contact dermatitis is rare. Irritant effects may occur with any of them, especially on raw skin and in fissures between the toes. Benzoic acid compound ointment (Whitfield's ointment) at full strength is not advised for tender skin, such as the scrotum or groins, and in such sites should only be used diluted to half strength with its vehicle (emulsifying ointment). Magenta paint (Castellani's paint) is still used in some cases of inflammatory tinea pedis, particularly when bacterial infection coexists, although potassium permanganate followed by a topical antifungal is preferred. Imidazoles for topical use, such as clotrimazole, econazole and ketoconazole, are now well established as effective remedies in ringworm infections with an extremely low incidence of adverse reactions. Other drugs in this group – miconazole, isoconazole, tioconazole and sulconazole – are equally effective [23,24]. Alternatives include topical terbinafine and amorolfine. Terbinafine applied topically has been shown to produce responses in some dermatophyte infections in very short periods. For instance, 1 week of topical terbinafine was found to be more effective than 4 weeks of clotrimazole in tinea pedis. Amorolfine, a morpholine, is mainly used as a treatment for onychomycosis in the form of a 5% nail paint [25] applied after abrading the nail once or twice weekly. It is more effective when used as combination therapy for onychomycosis with terbinafine or itraconazole. Other recent additions to the topical onychomycosis treatment range are luliconazole, efinaconazole and tavaborole.

Treatment regimen

The different syndromes of ringworm infections require different treatment regimens. The evidence base has only recently been reviewed in the case of some infections and among published clinical trials there are very few with long-term follow-up. Generally, topical therapies are used for localised or mild infections, and oral antifungals for hair, nail or more extensive infections. The newer oral azoles, such as fluconazole or itraconazole and terbinafine, are now the preferred oral treatments for extensive or severe dermatophytosis rather than griseofulvin. Although cheaper than the alternatives, griseofulvin is usually slower and, in many studies, less effective.

Treatment failures
Failure of topical therapy

Most failures of topical therapy are caused by inaccurate diagnosis or by inappropriate use of topical therapy (e.g. in hairy areas) or because the treatment is not used. Once or twice daily application for several weeks is usually required for success, and many patients, particularly if their symptoms are minor, will not achieve this unless they are carefully supervised and enthusiastically encouraged. Paradoxically, some non-fungal conditions may be improved considerably by one of the antidermatophyte preparations, although these remedies should not be used empirically to establish the diagnosis of ringworm infection. Many dermatoses respond, at least temporarily, to any bland application, and imidazole compounds in particular have considerable antibacterial properties.

Failure of oral therapy

When a patient fails to respond to terbinafine, fluconazole or itraconazole, the following points should be checked:

1. Is the diagnosis correct? If necessary, repeat scrapings.
2. Has the patient been taking the tablets regularly?
3. Is the patient taking any potentially competitive drugs?
4. In spite of taking them correctly, is the patient failing to absorb the antibiotic? An estimation of itraconazole levels, which is sometimes poorly absorbed, may be helpful.
5. In some patients with onychomycosis, poor penetration of drugs into defined linear streaks or nail edge areas of nail plate infection may account for treatment failure. Surgical removal of these abnormal nail areas, often after softening with urea ointment, may be useful.
6. Is there coexisting pathology such as HIV/AIDS or arterial disease?
7. Is a co-pathogen or secondary infection present? This should be considered in the feet and in the case of kerions, and perhaps in groin infections too. In nails, the coexistence of non-dermatophyte fungus should be considered. *Scopulariopsis brevicaulis*, apart from causing infections of the toenails in its own right, may coexist with *Trichophyton rubrum* or *T. interdigitale* and seems, at least on occasion, to cause failure of treatment. Nail removal may be indicated in this instance.
8. Antifungal resistance. This phenomenon is uncommon among dermatophytes [26], but where treatment failure occurs without any other explanation, it is possible to estimate the sensitivity of the causal organism. This should be performed by a specialist laboratory. Apart from true resistance, tolerance, in which the organism apparently becomes clinically resistant to the drug in the tissues but is sensitive *in vitro*, may also be important. Recently, strains of *T. indotineae* which show *in vitro* resistance to terbinafine, and some to azole antifungals have been reported, associated with widespread and treatment unresponsive tinea corpris/cruris [26]. Using higher and longer doses of itraconazole combined with a topical agent can lead to remission.
9. Reinfection. As ringworm fungi can frequently be isolated from the environment, when there are cases of ringworm of the scalp, and from clothing after laundering, it is highly likely that patients whose infection has been eradicated may be reinfected from these sources. Unfortunately, there is no proven way to avoid this.

Despite running through this checklist, dermatologists may not come up with an adequate explanation for treatment failure. In these situations, the use of one of the alternatives is a logical further step.

SUPERFICIAL MYCOSES CAUSED BY DERMATOPHYTE INFECTION

The wide variation in clinical presentation depends upon the species and probably the strain of the fungus concerned, upon the size of the inoculum, upon the site of the body infected and upon the immune status of the host. The traditional division of ringworm into different syndromes (Box 32.2) according to the site of the body infected is used because it is of considerable merit in terms of diagnosis and management.

> **Box 32.2 Ringworm syndromes**
>
> - Tinea corporis
> - Tinea capitis
> - Tinea barbae
> - Tinea faciei
> - Tinea pedis
> - Tinea manuum
> - Tinea cruris
> - Onychomycosis caused by dermatophytes
> - Steroid-related tinea
> - Dermatophytide reactions

Tinea corporis

Definition and nomenclature

Tinea corporis is ringworm of the glabrous skin. The clinical manifestations result from invasion and proliferation of the causal fungi in the stratum corneum. Terminal hair in the affected parts may be invaded. By definition, it includes lesions of the trunk and limbs, excluding ringworm of specialised sites such as the scalp, feet and groin, which are considered later.

> **Synonyms and inclusions**
>
> - Ringworm of the body
> - Tinea circinata

Pathophysiology

Natural infection is acquired by the deposition of viable arthrospores or hyphae on the surface of the susceptible individual. The source of infection is usually an active lesion on an animal or on another human, although fomite transmission is known to occur, and infection from soil is a well-established if unusual occurrence. In young children infected with *Trichophyton rubrum* and *Epidermophyton floccosum*, half of the infections may come from their parents. In geriatric wards, epidemics may occur [1]. Spread from existing localised infection (e.g. feet, groins, scalp and nails) is not uncommon. Invasion of the skin at the site of infection is followed by centrifugal spread through the stratum corneum. After this period of establishment (incubation), which lasts 1–3 weeks, the tissue responses to infection become evident. The characteristic annular appearance of many ringworm infections results from the elimination of the fungus from the centre of the lesion, and the subsequent resolution of the inflammatory host response at that site. This area usually becomes resistant to reinfection, although a second wave of centrifugal spread from the original site may occur with the formation of concentric red inflammatory rings. However, many lesions lack any tendency to central clearing. The natural history is variable. Some inflammatory cases of animal infection resolve spontaneously in a few months, while a typical case of *T. rubrum* tinea corporis may persist for years.

Causative organisms

For any part of the world, the causes of tinea corporis can be assessed by reference to the prevailing dermatophyte flora in the region [1–3]. All known dermatophytes can produce lesions of the glabrous skin. A comprehensive list of causal species thus corresponds to a complete list of dermatophytes. The most common are *T. rubrum*, *T indotineae* and zoophilic dermatophytes such as *Microsporum canis*. Some species have predilections for particular parts of the body; for example, *M. audouinii*, classically a cause of tinea capitis, and *T. rubrum*, which most commonly causes tinea pedis, can cause tinea corporis [4,5].

Environmental factors

Tinea corporis can occur in any climate although it is commoner in the tropics.

Clinical features

Presentation

The site of infection is typically on exposed skin, unless the infection represents an extension from a pre-existing infection. In such cases, infection may spread from the scalp, down the neck on to the upper trunk, or from the groins on to the buttocks and lower trunk.

Characteristic lesions are circular, usually sharply marginated with a raised edge (Figure 32.21). Single lesions occur, or there may be multiple plaques. The latter may remain discrete or become confluent involving wide areas. This clinical pattern is often modified in patients with defects in cellular immune responses [6]. The degree of inflammation is variable. This feature depends not only on the species of the fungus and the immune status of the host, but it is also roughly proportional to the extent of follicular invasion; thus, tinea corporis is generally less inflammatory than tinea capitis or tinea barbae. In inflammatory lesions, pustules or vesicles may dominate and even in mild infections close observation may reveal one or two small pustules. Rarely, frank bullae have been reported as an extreme expression of inflammatory change. In less inflammatory infections, scaling is a common but not constant finding. Central resolution, which is a common but not invariable feature of tinea

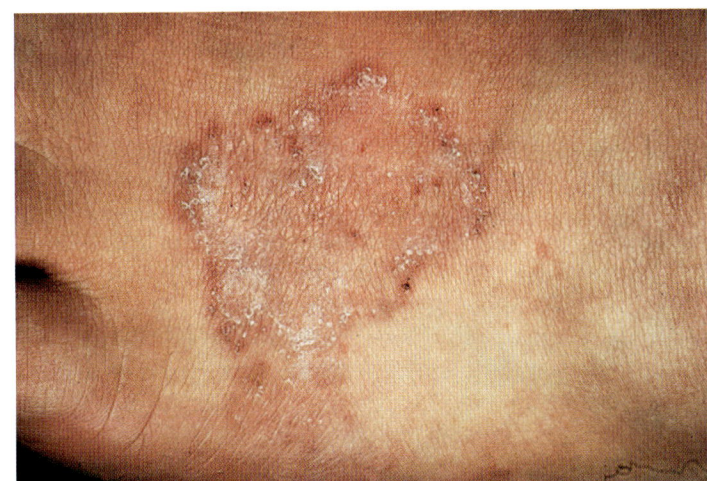

Figure 32.21 Tinea circinata: characteristic ringworm lesions.

corporis, is perhaps more frequent in inflammatory lesions, but it is by no means confined to them. The process is often incomplete, and the skin may show postinflammatory pigmentation, with a change of texture or residual red dermal nodules.

Clinical variants

Lesions of the glabrous skin caused by *M. canis* are not rare. They are as common in adults as in children and are characteristically annular. *M. audouinii* or *T. tonsurans* produce short-lived lesions of tinea corporis in some cases of scalp infection [7]. Zoophilic dermatophytes are all likely to cause inflammatory lesions of exposed skin. Although classically a cause of kerion, *T. verrucosum* can lead to extensive annular lesions of the upper trunk, especially in children [8]. These often start around the neck.

The anthropophilic species *T. rubrum* may invade the buttocks and lower back, as well as more distant sites of the trunk as an extension from tinea cruris. Very extensive and treatment unresponsive forms of tinea corporis and cruris are now common in India and neighbouring countries; these dominate the pattern of dermatophytosis seen [9]. Cases have also been seen in Europe and the Middle East. Lesions are widespread and, in some cases, there is concentric scaling. A newly characterised species *T. indotineae* (previously *T. mentagrophytes* (Type VIII)) accounts for many cases although some are caused by *T. rubrum* [9]. In infants, ringworm is rare, but the moist conditions of the perineal area may predispose to *E. floccosum* or *T. rubrum* infections [1].

T. rubrum may cause typical lesions with raised margins on the legs and usually extending from the feet, but rather psoriasiform lichenified plaques without central clearing may also occur, and a variety of vasculitis-like lesions are recognised. The perifollicular granulomatous nodules are classic, sometime referred to as Majocchi granuloma (Figure 32.22) [10,11], but erythema induratum-like plaques sometimes occur with an almost haemorrhagic appearance.

Tinea imbricata (Tokelau) resulting from *T. concentricum*, an anthropophilic dermatophyte found in southern Asia, the islands of the South Pacific and in Guatemala, southern Mexico and Brazil, causes a distinctive infection [12]. It seems to affect mainly the native peoples of these areas, and although susceptibility may be inherited as an autosomal recessive character [13], it occurs in both sexes and at all ages. Occasional cases may be seen elsewhere in travellers from these regions [14]. The infection begins as a scaling ring; centrifugal spread follows, but within the area of central clearing a second wave of scaling soon arises. The process is repeated to give numerous concentric rings (Figure 32.23) and, as the natural history is normally prolonged, the whole body may become affected. Pruritus is intense and may lead to lichenification. Hypopigmentation may accompany the lesions [15].

Atypical deep forms of tinea corporis occur. There are some reports of extensive and persistent cases of tinea corporis, in which dermal or subcutaneous involvement has been a feature [16,17]. Occasionally, a specific defect of immune function has been detected, such as a missing plasma factor. In other patients, depression of cellular immune responses is associated with the presence of a serum factor, possibly circulating antigen or immune complexes [6,18]. Such cases may present with dermal nodules, abscesses or draining sinuses [19]. A few particularly unusual dermatophyte

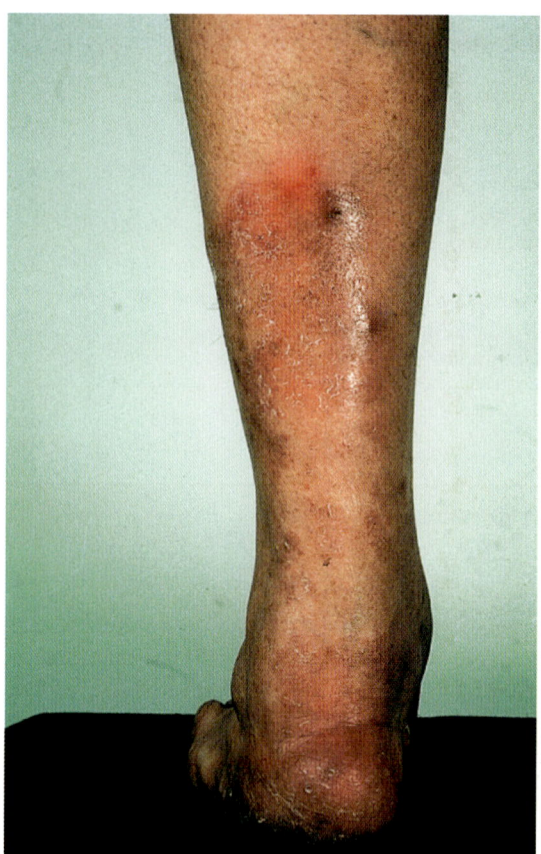

Figure 32.22 Nodular folliculitis caused by *Trichophyton rubrum*.

infections with invasion of bone, central nervous system and lymph nodes have been reported [16,20]; some are associated with *CARD9* mutations.

Differential diagnosis

Although tinea corporis can masquerade as any of a vast number of skin diseases, in practice the diagnosis is usually straightforward. The characteristic lesions seen with infection resulting from *M. canis* are easily diagnosed, but atypical infections caused by dermatophytes can, on occasion, cause great difficulty. Indeed, the possibility that any red, scaly rash on the body is a fungus infection should be considered, because lesions produced by fungi are so variable. Seborrhoeic dermatitis often causes difficulty, but the condition is symmetrical and there is often associated seborrhoeic dermatitis of the scalp and perhaps intertrigo in the body folds. Psoriasis can lead to confusion in those cases in which the distribution is not quite typical. Its presence on the knees, elbows and scalp, and associated psoriasis of the nails, particularly if pitting is present, is helpful. Patches of impetigo are often confused, particularly when dermatophytosis is of the circinate type. Growth of staphylococci from a skin swab does not, of course, exclude tinea. Lichenification of a patch of tinea (e.g. of the leg) can mimic lichen simplex. Discoid eczema is a common source of error. The plaques of papulovesicles tend to occur symmetrically on the limbs. Pityriasis rosea is also symmetrical and characteristically confined to the trunk and proximal parts of the limbs, but the herald patch, if seen, is almost impossible to differentiate from ringworm without microscopic may carry a squalene epoxidase gene mutation. Patients with these infections require treatment with higher doses of itraconazole, e.g. 200 mg daily and another topical antifungal for periods in excess of 2 months. With *T. concentricum*, treatment failures may occur with griseofulvin, but both terbinafine and itraconazole are effective although relapse is common.

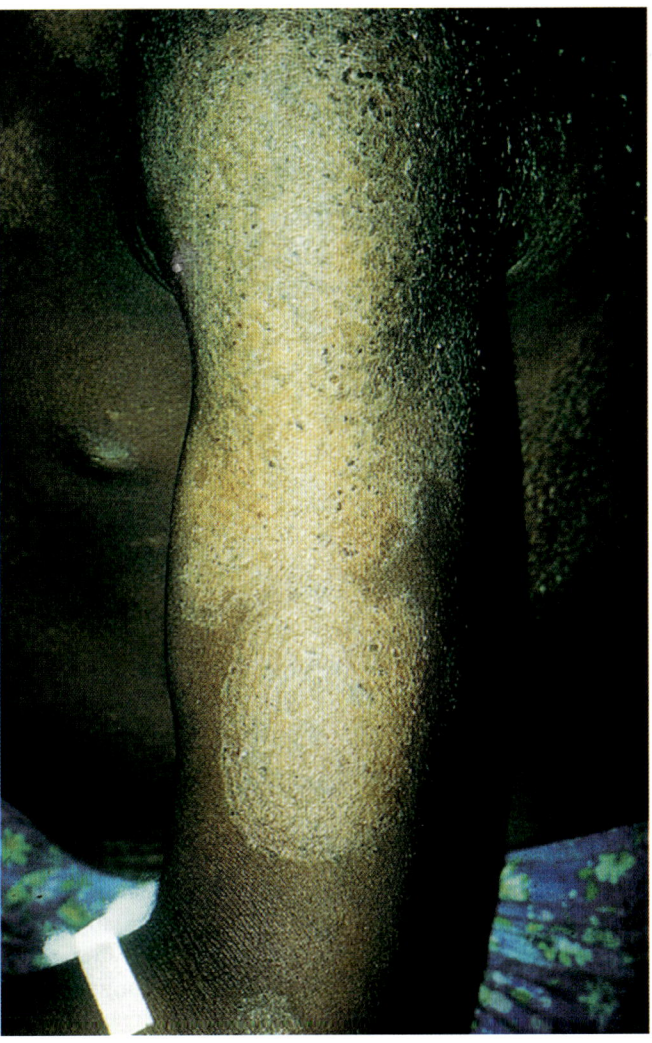

Figure 32.23 Tinea imbricata affecting the upper arm.

> **Treatment ladder for tinea corporis (see earlier for specific recommendations for the new strain of *T. mentagrophytes*)**
>
> **Localised disease, recent onset**
> - Topical terbinafine twice daily for 2 weeks
>   or
> - Topical azole once or twice daily for 2–4 weeks
>
> **Widespread disease**
> First line
> - Oral terbinafine 250 mg/day for 2–3 weeks
>   or
> - Itraconazole 100 mg/day for 2–4 weeks
>
> Second line
> - Griseofulvin 1 g/day for 4 weeks
> - For Indian variant infections, itraconazole 200-400 mg daily for up to 2 months

examination of scales. Candidosis, tertiary syphilis and pityriasis versicolor should be excluded.

Disease course and prognosis
Spontaneous resolution can occur but is uncommon.

Investigations
Direct microscopy and culture or PCR (see earlier) are the key elements of laboratory diagnosis

Management
Localised tinea corporis, especially of recent origin, commonly responds to topical therapy applied twice daily, usually for about a month. Topical terbinafine often works in a shorter time period (e.g. 2 weeks). In more widespread infections of recent onset, oral terbinafine or itraconazole will generally be preferred, and may be expected to clear the condition in about 2–3 weeks, depending on the dosage used. With griseofulvin, much longer term treatment is needed – up to several months with extensive infections. With infections associated with the Indian outbreak strains, many of the organisms are resistant to terbinafine and *T. indotineae* strains

Tinea capitis

Definition and nomenclature
This is ringworm of the scalp in which the essential feature is invasion of the hair shafts by a dermatophyte fungus. Ringworm of the beard area, although essentially similar, is discussed separately.

> **Synonyms and inclusions**
> - Ringworm of the scalp
> - Tinea tonsurans

Epidemiology
Those species of dermatophyte fungi most likely to cause tinea capitis vary from region to region [1,2,3,4,5]. Moreover, in any given location, the species may change with time, particularly as new organisms are introduced by immigration [6,7]. In tinea capitis, anthropophilic species predominate. The principal feature of tinea capitis in recent years has been the rise of *M. canis* as the dominant organism in infections in some parts of Europe [4], and the spread of *T. tonsurans* in urban communities in the USA [3], the UK [8] and in some other European countries [9].

Age
Tinea capitis is predominantly an infection of children, although adult cases are seen, particularly with *T. tonsurans* infections.

Ethnicity
Some species such as *T. tonsurans* show a predilection for African/Caribbean hair type.

Associated disease
Tinea capitis may also be seen in adults with AIDS.

Pathophysiology
Predisposing factors
The principles of hair invasion and the distinctions between *in vitro* and *in vivo* activity have been already outlined (see section on the basic biology of dermatophytosis). The spores of ringworm fungi causing tinea capitis can be demonstrated in the air in close proximity to patients with the condition. It is highly likely that scalp hair acts as a trapping device and it is known that contamination of hair without demonstrable clinical findings may occur among classmates of children with tinea capitis [10,11].

Pathology
From experimental work on *M. audouinii*, hair infection is preceded by invasion of the stratum corneum of the scalp skin [12,13]. This is followed, after approximately 3 weeks, by clinical evidence of hair shaft infection. Infection spreads to other follicles, then for a period of variable duration, although if it persists it does not spread further. Finally, there is a period of regression with or without an inflammatory phase.

There are several distinct types of hair invasion listed below.

Causative organisms
Most species of dermatophyte are capable of invading hair but some species (e.g. *T. tonsurans, T. schoenleinii* and *T. violaceum*) have a distinct predilection for the hair shaft. *E. floccosum, T. concentricum* and *T. interdigitale* seldom cause tinea capitis. All dermatophytes causing scalp ringworm can invade glabrous skin and many attack nails as well.

Ectothrix type. This may be a small-spored ectothrix caused by *M. audouinii* (including variants previously called *M. audouinii* var. *rivalieri*), *M. canis* (including variants previously called *M. canis* var. *distortum*), *M. equinum* or *M. ferrugineum*. In this type, the hair shaft is invaded mid-follicle. The intrapilary hyphae continue to grow inwards towards the bulb of the hair. Secondary, extrapilary hyphae develop and grow in a tortuous manner over the surface of the hair shaft, which is growing outwards continuously. These secondary, extrapilary hyphae segment to produce a mass of small arthroconidia (2–3 μm diameter), each one of which becomes rounded off and eventually spherical. The size of these conidia is such that they cannot easily be distinguished as separate structures under low-power microscopy. Fluorescence under the Wood's lamp is characteristically present in this type of hair invasion. A similar type of hair invasion occurs with other *Microsporum* species (e.g. *M. gypseum, M. fulvum, M. nanum* and *M. vanbreuseghemii*). The spores, although similarly arranged, are larger, in this case about 5–8 μm in diameter. Fluorescence has been reported in some cases.

Endothrix type. The endothrix type may be caused by *T. tonsurans, T. soudanense, T. violaceum, T. yaoundei, T. gourvilii* or *T. rubrum* (rare).

Intrapilary hyphae fragment into arthroconidia up to 8 μm in diameter, which are entirely contained within and completely fill the hair shaft. Hair thus affected is especially fragile and breaks off close to the scalp surface. This type is non-fluorescent.

Favus. Favic type is caused by *T. schoenleinii*. Broad, regularly septate hyphae and air spaces are seen in the hair shaft, but disarticulated arthroconidia are absent. The affected hair is less damaged than in other types and may continue to grow to considerable lengths. Greenish grey fluorescence is present [14]. Air spaces are characteristic and fungal hyphae form large clusters in the vicinity of hair follicles.

Clinical features
Presentation
The clinical appearance of ringworm of the scalp is variable, depending on the type of hair invasion, the level of host resistance and the degree of inflammatory host response [15,16]. The appearance varies from a few dull grey, broken-off hairs with a little scaling, detectable only on careful inspection, to a severe, painful, inflammatory mass covering most of the scalp. Itching is variable. In all types, the cardinal features are partial hair loss with inflammation to some degree (Figure 32.24). It is useful to recognise several basic clinical pictures, as described here.

Clinical variants
Small-spored ectothrix type. In *M. audouinii* [1] and *M. ferrugineum* infections, the basic lesions are patches of partial alopecia, often circular in shape, but showing numerous broken-off hairs, dull grey from their coating of arthrospores. Inflammation is minimal, but fine scaling is characteristic, usually with a defined margin. There may be several or many such patches arranged more or less randomly. In *M. canis* and the much rarer *M. canis* var. *distortum* infections, the picture is similar but there is typically more inflammatory change. In infections caused by all these species, green fluorescence under the Wood's light is usual, but occasional non-fluorescent cases have been reported, and may not be rare with *M. ferrugineum* (perhaps as many as 10%) [17]. Children are affected much more frequently than

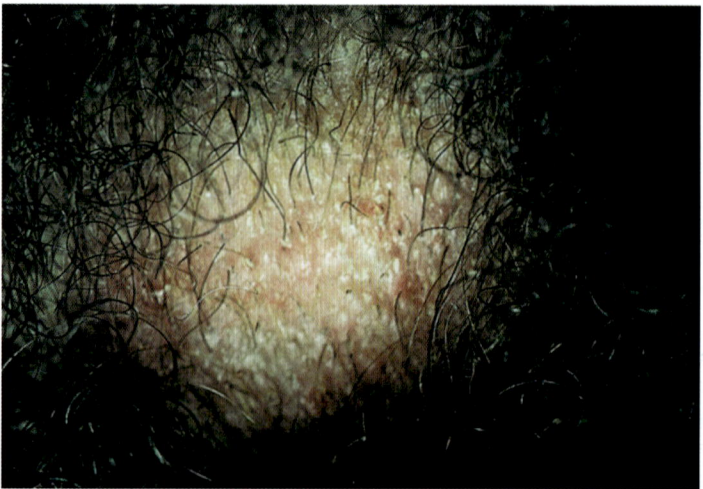

Figure 32.24 Tinea capitis caused by *Microsporum canis*.

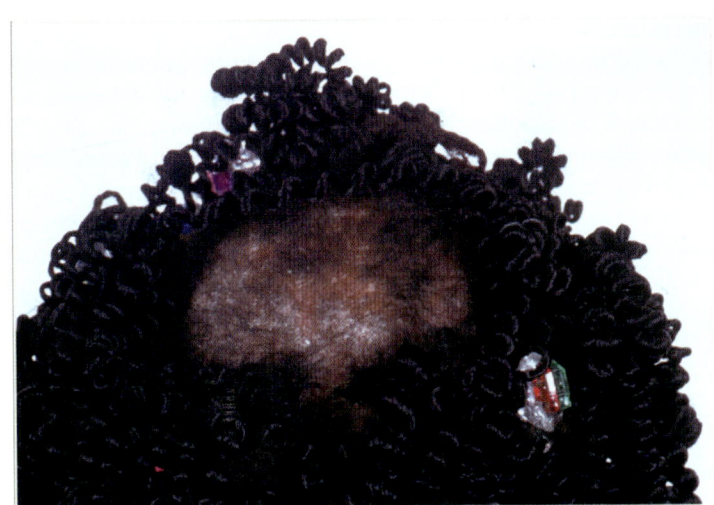

Figure 32.25 Kerion in a patient with *Trichophyton tonsurans* infection of the scalp.

adults, although the occasional case of tinea capitis in older patients must not be forgotten [18,19]. The attack rate for epidemic infections caused by anthropophilic species may be as high as 30%, within a school class for example, but it is commonly lower than that [20]. Infection rates of both *M. audouinii* and *M. canis* have been reported to be higher in boys than girls [1], often at least twice as high.

Kerion. The most severe pattern of reaction is known as a kerion (Figure 32.25). It is a painful, inflammatory mass in which such hairs as remain are loose. Follicles may be seen discharging pus, there may be sinus formation and on rare occasions mycetoma-like grains may be found [21]. Thick crusting with matting of adjacent hairs is common. The area affected may be limited, but multiple plaques are not rare, and occasionally a large confluent lesion may involve much of the scalp. Lymphadenopathy is frequent. Although this strong reaction is usually caused by one of the zoophilic species, typically *T. verrucosum* or *T. mentagrophytes*, occasionally a geophilic organism will be isolated, and anthropophilic infections that have been smouldering quietly for weeks may suddenly become inflammatory and develop into kerions if a high degree of hypersensitivity develops [22]. The possibility that a bacterial co-pathogen may be playing some part should not be ignored, and in this type of case a swab sent to the bacterial laboratory is a useful procedure in addition to the plucking of hairs for mycology. Generally, however, pustule formation represents an inflammatory response to the fungus itself [23].

Endothrix infections. In *T. tonsurans* [20,24,25] and *T. violaceum* [25,26] infections, a relatively non-inflammatory type of patchy baldness occurs. The formation of black dots (swollen hair shafts) as the affected hair breaks at the surface of the scalp is classic in this condition, but such findings may be inconspicuous [27]. The patches, which are usually multiple, may show minimal scaling, sometimes mimicking discoid lupus erythematosus, sometimes seborrhoeic dermatitis [28,29]. They are commonly angular in outline rather than round. Other forms include diffuse and patchy alopecia, some even with involvement of single isolated hair shafts and without scales. The common clinical types are grey patch (scaling with patchy hair loss), black dot and diffuse alopecia.

A low-grade folliculitis is also often seen, while sometimes a frank kerion may develop. The three African species, all now included within the African *T. rubrum* complex – *T. soudanense*, *T. yaoundei* and *T. gourvilii* – induce very similar lesions, in which the inflammatory reaction is usually mild but occasionally severe. Patients may have some nail involvement [30,31] or lesions on the face.

Favus. Infection with *T. schoenleinii* is now seen rarely and sporadically in a variety of countries, such as South Africa [32] and Ethiopia, where it is still endemic, as well as rare cases elsewhere. The classic picture of tinea capitis caused by this organism is characterised by the presence of yellowish, cup-shaped crusts known as scutula [33]. Each scutulum develops round a hair, which pierces it centrally. Adjacent crusts enlarge to become confluent and form a mass of yellow crusting. Many patients may show less distinctive changes, in early cases perhaps amounting to no more than perifollicular redness and some matting of the hair. Extensive, patchy hair loss with cicatricial alopecia and atrophy among patches of normal hair may be found in longstanding cases, where much of the hair loss is irreversible. In such patients, the glabrous skin is commonly affected by the development of similar yellowish crusts. Although childhood infection occurs in nearly all cases, it shows little if any tendency to clear spontaneously at puberty, particularly in women. Families with several generations affected are well recognised [14].

Differential diagnosis

The differential diagnosis of tinea capitis includes all conditions capable of causing patchy baldness with inflammatory changes of the scalp. Alopecia areata may show redness and, although of itself not a scaly condition, it may coexist with seborrhoeic dermatitis. Such cases can be confusing, although careful examination usually shows that the scaling and the hair loss are not co-extensive. Exclamation mark hairs must be distinguished from broken hairs of tinea capitis. Traumatic alopecia from hairdressing procedures and trichotillomania may also be confused [34]. Seborrhoeic dermatitis is usually more diffuse than tinea capitis, but in tinea amiantacea the changes are often localised. In this condition, the scaling is adherent to the hair, but breakage of the hair shaft does not normally occur. In psoriasis, hair loss is found only occasionally and again broken-off hairs are not usually present.

In impetigo, which may be secondary to pediculosis of the scalp, loosening of the hair is not normally present, but matting and crusting due to secondary staphylococcal infection may be present in inflammatory ringworm. A bacterial furuncle of the scalp is painful and usually situated on the neck area, and shedding of loosened hairs much less evident than in kerion. Discoid lupus erythematosus, lichen planus and other causes of cicatricial alopecia may sometimes have to be considered.

Disease course and prognosis

If untreated it may become chronic. Spontaneous recovery usually occurs at puberty.

Investigations

Using dermoscopy (trichoscopy), important clues to the diagnosis can be obtained. These include the presence of comma and corkscrew shaped hairs; other observable morphological changes are code-like hairs, zig-zag hairs and bent hairs. Direct microscopy and culture or PCR (see earlier) are the key elements of laboratory diagnosis.

Management
Topical therapy has little place in the management of this condition except as an adjunct to oral therapy.

Both itraconazole and terbinafine are licensed in some countries for use in children. Terbinafine is a good treatment choice for certain infections such as those caused by *Trichophyton* species, although it appears to be less effective in disease caused by *Microsporum* species. The best length of treatment for *T. tonsurans* and *T. violaceum* infections with terbinafine appears to be 1 month. There is some evidence that higher doses of terbinafine may be more effective for *Microsporum*. The appropriate length of treatment with either itraconazole or fluconazole is not established, although both appear to be effective against *T. tonsurans*.

Griseofulvin is also useful, particularly for *Microsporum* infections, but it is not available in all countries. Although massive single-dose therapy and intermittent dose regimens (25 mg/kg twice a week) have had some success, conventional continuous daily therapy (10 mg/kg) is advisable in general. In small-spored ectothrix infections, griseofulvin for at least 6 weeks is usually adequate. In some *T. tonsurans* and *T. schoenleinii* infections, much longer courses and sometimes higher dosage (20 mg/kg/day) of griseofulvin therapy may be needed.

With scalp kerions, the careful removal of crusts using wet compresses should not be neglected, and the possibility of coexisting bacterial infection should be considered. If confirmed by swabs, systemic antibacterial chemotherapy should be instituted. In general, the kerions are less painful than their inflammatory appearance suggests, but analgesics may be needed. Occasionally, in children with extensive kerions, frequent attendance at the out-patient clinic where skilled nursing is available may be of great value and is much appreciated by worried parents. Permanent hair loss from scarring is usually less than would be expected.

Ketoconazole shampoo or selenium sulphide can be used to prevent spread in the early phases of therapy when used in combination with an oral treatment. In severely inflammatory forms, there has been some argument in favour of using oral steroids to inhibit the inflammatory response. While this view has its supporters, we tend to review all cases early after the institution of antifungal therapy, and only use oral steroids in severe cases with widespread ide reactions.

Treatment ladder for tinea capitis

First line
- Terbinafine: 10–20 kg, 62.5 mg; >40 kg, 250 mg. All given daily for 4 weeks
- Itraconazole 2–4 mg/kg/day for 4–6 weeks
- Griseofulvin 10 mg/kg for 6 weeks (20 mg/kg considered in some *T. tonsurans* and *T. schoenleinii* infections)

Second line
- Itraconazole 5 mg/kg in weekly pulses for 2–3 rounds

Infection control [35,36]
It is of considerable importance with scalp ringworm to discover the species involved. Clearly, some information may be obtained from the clinical picture, the presence or absence of fluorescence, etc., but culture is required for this to be firmly established. Where animal species are concerned, the source should be proved mycologically; it is not always the expected one. Domestic pets can often be treated successfully and economically with griseofulvin. Cattle ringworm in calves will normally settle spontaneously. A group of highly infected laboratory mice should probably be destroyed.

With anthropophilic infections, careful investigation of the outbreak or epidemic is recommended, and exclusion of children from school is not recommended [36]. The latter may be resented by the parents and lead to non-compliance with treatment. With zoophilic infections such as *M. canis* ringworm, children can normally be allowed to remain at school as the risk of infection from human to human is low. The main treatments in all these conditions are terbinafine or griseofulvin. Topical therapy has little place, although it is sensible to remove matted crusts and to follow a routine of frequent shampooing.

Tinea barbae

Definition and nomenclature
This is ringworm of the beard and moustache areas of the face with the invasion of coarse hairs. It is thus a disease of the adult male. Tinea of the chin and upper lip in females and children are considered to be tinea faciei (ringworm of the glabrous skin of the face).

Synonyms and inclusions
- Ringworm of the beard

Epidemiology
Age
This condition predominantly affects male adults.

Pathophysiology
Predisposing factors
All the available clinical evidence points to a similar pathogenesis as that in tinea capitis.

Pathology
Infections with *T. verrucosum* and *T. mentagrophytes* lead to large-spored ectothrix invasion with the spores in chains. The other less commonly involved species produce their own characteristic types of hair invasion.

Causative organisms
The animal species *T. verrucosum* and *T. mentagrophytes* are responsible for the great majority of cases [1]. *M. canis* is an uncommon cause (eyelashes may be affected in some cases) as is *T. erinacei*. The anthropophilic species, *T. violaceum*, *T. schoenleinii* and *T. rubrum* [2], are recognised as occasional causes. *T. tonsurans* has been reported in wrestlers.

Clinical features

Presentation
The affected men are commonly farm workers in cases caused by the two main species: *T. mentagrophytes* and *T. verrucosum*. The clinical picture in these cases is that of a highly inflammatory, pustular folliculitis, often showing all the features of a kerion. Hairs of the beard or moustache regions are surrounded by red inflammatory papules or pustules, usually with exudation or crusting. Many hairs within the affected areas are loose and easily removed with forceps without causing pain. These inflammatory lesions, although tending eventually to settle spontaneously, often persist for some months. Some infections are less severe and consist of dry, circular, reddish, scaly lesions enclosing lustreless hair stumps, which are either broken off close to the surface of the skin or plug the follicles.

Differential diagnosis
The classic, highly inflammatory lesions are distinguished from boils by their relative lack of pain. The quieter cases of tinea must be distinguished from bacterial folliculitis, acne, rosacea and pseudofolliculitis. The presence of *Staphylococcus aureus* on a swab taken from lesions in this area does not exclude ringworm, as bacterial colonisation or frank co-infection may occur in tinea barbae. Unfortunately, mycological cultures are often negative.

Management
Beard infections usually respond satisfactorily to itraconazole or terbinafine, sometimes in combination with topical therapy over a period of 4–6 weeks. Fairly long-term follow-up is recommended and late recurrences undoubtedly occur.

Infection control
Early diagnosis and prompt treatment of the individual patient and the encouragement of high standards of hygiene in the livestock industry are as much as can be expected given the present state of knowledge. A vaccine against *T. verrucosum* in cattle has resulted in a reduced incidence of infection, not only in cows but also among their human contacts, in some countries in eastern Europe [3].

Tinea faciei

Definition and nomenclature
Tinea faciei is infection of the glabrous skin of the face with a dermatophyte fungus (the moustache and beard areas of the adult male are excluded).

Synonyms and inclusions
- Ringworm of the face
- Tinea faciale

Pathophysiology

Predisposing factors
Facial skin may be infected either by direct inoculation of a dermatophyte fungus from an external source (e.g. *T. mentagrophytes* from an infected pet mouse) or there may be secondary spread from pre-existing tinea of another body site. The latter pattern is likely to occur with *T. rubrum* as well as with *T. concentricum* infections.

Causative organisms
Trichophyton mentagrophytes and *T. rubrum* predominate, but *T. tonsurans*, *M. audouinii* and *M. canis* are also common causes worldwide. *T. concentricum* frequently spreads to the face in cases of tinea imbricata and, as with tinea corporis, all dermatophytes must be considered potentially capable of producing this condition. Wrestling-associated *T. tonsurans* infections are also recorded.

Clinical features

History
The prime reason for separating tinea faciei from tinea corporis in this account is to draw attention to the frequency of misdiagnosis in facial ringworm [1]. The clinical features vary considerably, but complaints of itching, burning and exacerbation after sun exposure are common. The last-mentioned symptom is a frequent source of diagnostic error [2]. There will often be a history of exposure to animals.

Presentation
The rash is usually red, but scaling is present in fewer than two-thirds of cases. Redness is more subtle in skin types IV–VI. A substantial proportion of patients do show annular or circinate lesions, and induration with a raised margin is present in about half (Figure 32.26). Simple papular lesions, and in some cases completely flat red patches, also occur. A few vesicles or pustules may be found, but these are rarely conspicuous. The application of topical steroids may be expected to modify the appearance still further. Facial infection may also be seen in Indian variant infections (see tinea corporis).

Differential diagnosis
Because of light sensitivity, the frequent absence of scaling and the somewhat nondescript appearance, this condition may be confused with discoid lupus erythematosus (DLE) [1] and polymorphic light eruption. Moreover, tinea faciei coexisting with DLE has

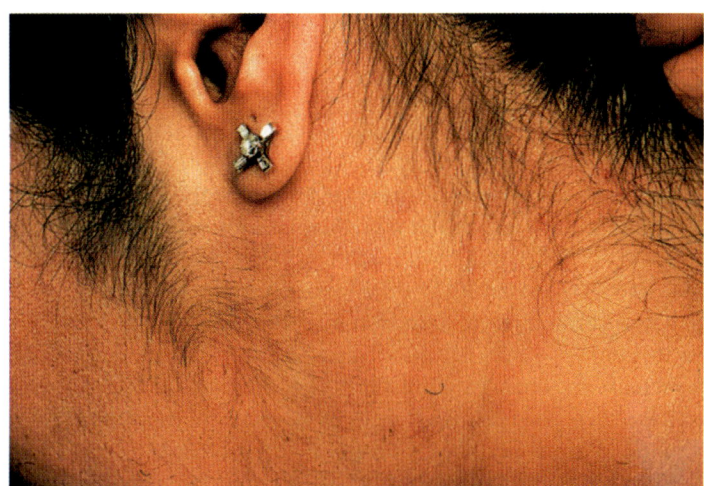

Figure 32.26 Tinea faciei caused by *Trichophyton rubrum*.

been described [3]. Bowenoid solar keratoses, psoriasis, impetigo, rosacea, seborrhoeic dermatitis [4] and benign lymphocytic infiltrates must also be considered. Reluctance to biopsy the face adds to the problem, but if the possibility of tinea faciei is remembered, careful examination and scrapings taken from the skin surface, even if this is not obviously scaly, should enable a diagnosis to be made. General examination of the skin, particularly the scalp, should not be forgotten. If topical steroids have been applied, a cessation of the therapy may be followed a few days later by a great increase in scaling and by appearances much more readily diagnosable.

Management
In localised cases, if promptly diagnosed, topical therapy seems to work well, especially with tolnaftate or one of the imidazoles. Where delay has occurred before the diagnosis is established, and especially when steroid therapy has modified the condition, terbinafine or itraconazole is generally preferred. Most cases will clear in 3 or 4 weeks, certainly in 6 weeks, but longstanding infections may occasionally need longer periods of treatment.

Infection control
Pets and laboratory animals may require treatment or elimination. It is customary to give short-term oral antifungal treatment, but the author has seen minimal lesions respond well to topical imidazoles.

Tinea pedis

Definition and nomenclature
This is infection of the feet or toes with a dermatophyte fungus. The term athlete's foot is used by some to imply any form of toe cleft intertrigo. In this account we therefore prefer the terms tinea pedis or foot ringworm, which clearly exclude infections caused by bacteria, *Candida* and non-dermatophyte moulds.

Synonyms and inclusions
- Foot ringworm
- Athlete's foot

Epidemiology
Incidence and prevalence
Tinea pedis is the most common form of dermatophyte infection in the UK and North America [1] and probably throughout the developed world. Overall prevalence within the community and including all age groups is not reliably known, but extrapolation from surveys [2,3] suggests that in industrialised countries at any one time as many as 10% of the total population may be expected to have dermatophyte infections of the toe clefts. Living in an institution, especially where washing facilities are shared, is likely to increase the chances of infection [3,4]. Prevalence figures as high as 80% have been reported among German miners, and in some wards of a long-stay hospital more than two-thirds of the patients were infected [4]. Nevertheless, tinea pedis may be transmitted within the family bathroom [5].

Age
The condition is more common in adults than children but may begin to occur in young children aged 6 or more. The mean age of onset was 15 years in one survey [3].

Sex
Adult males probably have about a 20% chance of developing tinea pedis, while among women only 5% are likely to become chronically infected.

Associated diseases
Among dermatological out-patients with *T. rubrum* infections there is a significant excess of atopic infections [6], but in a study of coal miners with recurrent *T. rubrum* tinea pedis this was not so [7], suggesting perhaps that reinfection from the environment, e.g changing rooms, is more important in industrial settings.

Pathophysiology
Predisposing factors
Occlusion of toe clefts through wearing shoes predisposes to this condition, which is in most cases initially a lateral web space infection.

Pathology
Experimental evidence [8] suggests the importance of maceration in dermatophyte infections of the toe clefts. These moist conditions probably favour growth of the fungus directly and damage the stratum corneum at the same time. A simultaneous increase in the bacterial flora is likely and may also play a part. There is growing evidence that during some symptomatic episodes in chronic tinea pedis, resident bacteria, such as large colony coryneforms, may act as co-pathogens, but whether or not they assist in initiating new infections remains, so far, unknown [9].

Causative organisms
Three anthropophilic species, *T. rubrum*, *T. interdigitale* and *Epidermophyton floccosum*, are together responsible for the vast majority of cases of foot ringworm throughout the world. Double infections with any two of these species occur and, for precision, especially in clinical surveys, it is useful to adopt a standard terminology to describe them. Combined infections are those in which different species are present in the same lesion. Concurrent infections are those in which different species are found in different lesions at the same time, and consecutive infections are those in which the same patient has a different organism at the single site on different occasions. Other species, including zoophilic ones, occur occasionally as a cause of tinea pedis. In countries where *T. violaceum* is common, foot involvement with this anthropophilic species is sometimes seen and may be very intractable [10]. The relative numerical importance of the three main species of dermatophyte can be discovered from the extensive published data on foot ringworm seen in dermatological clinics throughout the world. Although minor variations are frequent, an average clinic sample would be: *T. rubrum* infections, 70%; *T. interdigitale* infections, 15%; *E. floccosum* infections, <10%; mixed infections, 5%. The prevalence of *T. rubrum* infections has been growing over several decades [11]. Prior to 1970, in surveys of populations consisting of subjects in

institutions, coal mines [12] or swimming baths [2], the relative frequency of infections with T. interdigitale was higher than those caused by T. rubrum. T. interdigitale would outnumber T. rubrum by as much as eight to one [13]. Since 1980, surveys in industry have indicated that this pattern has changed, with over 80% of isolates being T. rubrum and children of a younger age being infected [14]. A proportion of patients also have Gram-negative bacterial infection of the web spaces [15,16].

Environmental factors
Although dermatophytes are occasionally isolated from clinically normal toe clefts, and a contrary situation exists in which mildly abnormal toe clefts yield no dermatophytes, it is now generally held that where dermatophytes are present (in perhaps 10% of the population) they do cause abnormalities and are not in the true sense members of the normal skin flora. The sex differences in the level of tinea pedis may be partly explained by different exposure to the causal fungi [17]. In this context, in one survey the level of infection among men who attended swimming baths was higher than in those who did not. In contrast, surveys at a swimming bath showed that the level of infection among girl swimmers was only one-quarter of that among boy swimmers [2]. However, further enquiry showed that the girls came to the baths less than the boys, so that there was, even in this instance, a true difference in exposure, although both groups went swimming.

Clinical features
Presentation
Itching is a common complaint in warm weather. The condition is highly persistent and the history is long. The most common form of tinea pedis is an intertriginous dermatitis characterised by peeling, maceration and fissuring affecting the lateral toe clefts, and sometimes spreading to involve the undersurface of the toes. This picture may be produced by any of the three species.

In T. rubrum infections, a scaling hyperkeratotic variety is often found that is particularly chronic and resistant to treatment and that affects the soles, heels and sides of the feet. The affected areas are pink and covered with fine, silvery white scales. If the foot is extensively involved, the term 'moccasin foot' or dry-type infection are sometimes applied (Figure 32.27). The dorsal surfaces of the toes and feet are not often affected (Figure 32.28), but associated nail infection is very common. As well as itching of the feet, the patient may also complain of their smell, and secondary bacterial infection, with fissuring in the toe clefts, may aggravate symptoms [9].

The changes produced by T. interdigitale vary from mild, insignificant scaling in the toe clefts to severe, acute, inflammatory reactions affecting all parts of the feet [18]. A vesiculobullous reaction is more likely to be caused by this species than by any other fungus (Figure 32.29). The reaction may occasionally extend over the whole sole. It may be preceded for months or years by maceration or fissuring in the toe clefts. Vesicles may become pustules and when they rupture they tend to leave collarettes of scaling with the intervening skin normal, or showing various degrees of scaling and inflammation. This variety of ringworm frequently goes on to apparent spontaneous cure, but tends to recur in warm weather; indeed, under hot humid conditions the inflammatory reaction may be extremely incapacitating. There may be associated hyperhidrosis.

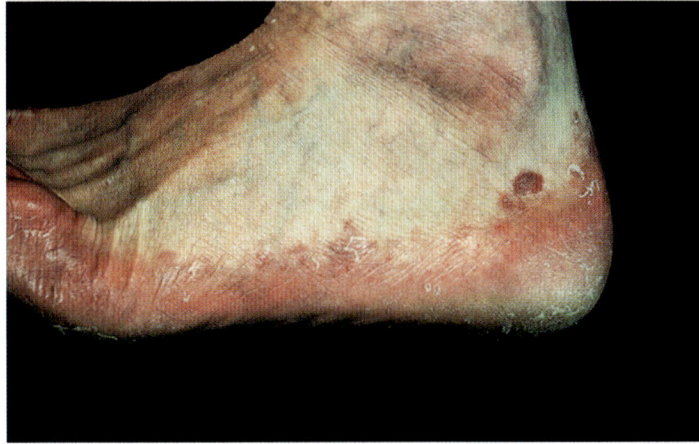

Figure 32.27 Dry-type *Trichophyton rubrum* infection.

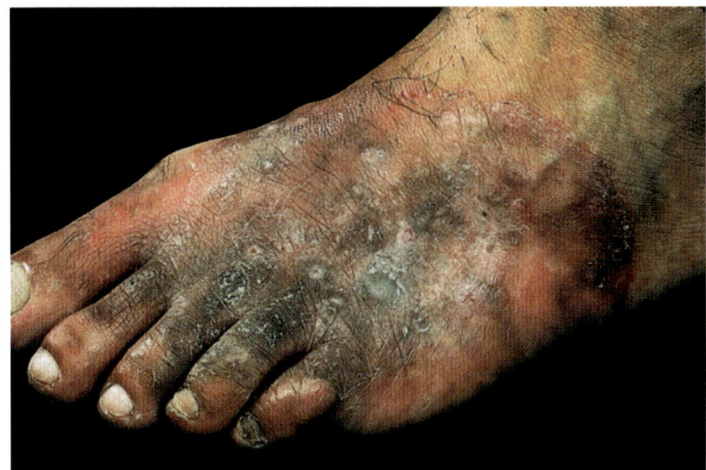

Figure 32.28 Tinea pedis spreading to the dorsum of the foot.

Apart from mild toe cleft intertrigo, E. floccosum may produce on occasion a vesicular infection of the sole similar to that typically produced by T. interdigitale, or a dry hyperkeratotic condition resembling infections caused by T. rubrum. With Epidermophyton infections, there is significantly less toenail involvement than with T. rubrum or T. interdigitale, but chronicity of the skin infection may be just as troublesome.

Clinical variants
When the lesions on the feet are acutely vesicular, irrespective of the fungus responsible, a vesicular allergic reaction (ide) may develop on the uninfected hands. This clinical picture, which closely simulates pompholyx, was vastly overdiagnosed in the past but is actually quite uncommon, and an ide reaction of this type should not be considered unless the primary foot condition is acutely inflammatory.

Differential diagnosis
Neoscytalidium and *Fusarium* infections may mimic interdigital tinea pedis; the former also produces dry-type infections. Where changes are largely restricted to the toe cleft, erythrasma (which is usually asymptomatic and rarely causes fissures) and candidosis (which is characterised by a build up of rather more white, macerated skin)

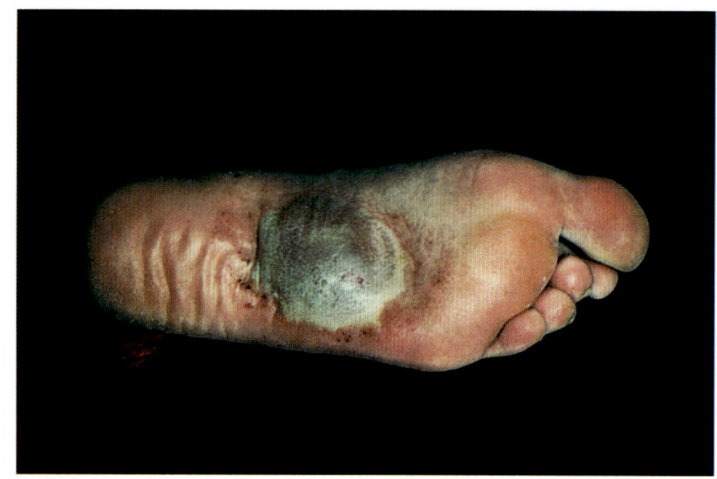

Figure 32.29 *Trichophyton interdigitale* infection: bullous lesion on the sole.

must both be considered. Other bacterial infections with staphylococci or streptococci or Gram-negative organisms, including *Acinetobacter* species, can produce inflammation and often odour. Any of these organisms may coexist with tinea pedis, contributing to a greater or lesser extent to the abnormalities seen. Apart from swabs and scrapings for bacteria and ringworm organisms, the Wood's lamp, which may show pink fluorescence for erythrasma and a greenish blue for *Pseudomonas* infections, may be useful.

Soft corns or callosities, sometimes with sinus formation, are common in the lateral toe clefts, especially in women. Younger children do not commonly suffer from foot ringworm but frequently have eczema of the foot such as juvenile plantar dermatosis. Where the sole of the foot is affected without obvious involvement of the toe cleft, a diagnosis of pustular psoriasis must be considered. The latter condition more commonly affects the heels than does tinea, but this is not a reliable criterion. Psoriasis, pityriasis rubra pilaris, reactive arthritis, contact dermatitis from nylon dyes or shoe materials, and tylosis may all need to be excluded. Scrapings by which a positive diagnosis of tinea pedis may be established should always be taken, and they may need to be repeated if an initial negative result is incompatible with the clinical features.

Complications and co-morbidities

The presence of interdigital tinea pedis is a risk factor for cellulitis in patients with lymphoedema.

Disease course and prognosis

The infection can be acute or chronic.

Investigations

Direct microscopy and culture or PCR (see earlier) are the key elements of laboratory diagnosis.

Management

For very mild toe cleft changes and for prophylaxis at swimming baths, one of the topical preparations is recommended. Tolnaftate powder, for instance, has proven value, and the imidazoles are likely to be equally effective. For toe cleft changes that are more than trivial, a cream is generally preferred and any of the listed preparations (see Table 32.7) can be confidently recommended for minor forms of tinea pedis. Azole preparations are cheap and are usually effective in a period of up to 30 days, but topical terbinafine can be effective in 7 days; there is also a formulation that can be applied as a single application across the soles of the feet. If the toe clefts are very inflamed and secondary bacterial infection is likely, a brief period with rest and bland applications may be necessary. Permanganate or aluminium chloride solution 20–30% twice daily can ease secondary infection. Clearly, if there is any evidence of serious bacterial infection, swabs should be taken; if there is clinical evidence of cellulitis, patients should receive a systemic antibacterial antibiotic.

In dry-type tinea pedis, usually caused by *T. rubrum*, terbinafine or itraconazole are of great value. Speed of recovery is faster and relapse rates less than with griseofulvin. Treatments using terbinafine 250 mg/day for 2 weeks or itraconazole 400 mg/day for 1–2 weeks are usually given.

> **Treatment ladder for tinea pedis**
>
> **Mild and moderate interdigital disease**
> - Topical imidazole twice daily for 4 weeks
> - Topical terbinafine twice daily for 7 days
>
> **Dry type tinea pedis**
> - Terbinafine 250 mg/day for 2 weeks
>   *or*
> - Itraconazole 400 mg/day for 1–2 weeks

Infection control

Clearly, if infected individuals avoided exposing others to their infection by not walking on the floors of communal changing rooms and by avoiding swimming baths, the level of infection in the community would fall. Because such large numbers of people are involved, many of whom are completely asymptomatic, this is usually not feasible. Moreover, eradication of these fungi from the toe clefts is often a long and tedious process and elimination of the organism may never be achieved. Among industrial workers using communal showers, it is virtually impossible to avoid continual exposure to infection. There are two simple measures that do seem fruitful. Frequent hosing of the floors of shower rooms and the sides of swimming baths does reduce the prevalence of dermatophytes on these surfaces, and probably would lead to a reduction of infection in time. This should certainly be encouraged. Effective antifungal powder is readily available, and encouragement of its use has been demonstrated to be effective in the long-term reduction of tinea pedis at swimming baths.

Tinea manuum

Definition and nomenclature

Any species of dermatophyte may affect the skin of the hand. Infections of the dorsal surface present no specific features and are considered as ringworm of the glabrous skin under tinea corporis.

This section is therefore concerned with ringworm of the palmar skin and with infections beginning under rings.

> **Synonyms and inclusions**
> - Ringworm of the hand

Pathophysiology
Predisposing factors
In most cases, apart from animal infections, there is pre-existing foot infection with or without toenail involvement. A special mention should be made of ringworm beginning under rings and wrist watches, and where anatomical deformities or occupational usage predispose to maceration between the fingers. Here, there may be a particular susceptibility to *T. interdigitale* infections, and in such cases infection may occur without obvious foot involvement [1]. Poor peripheral circulation and palmar keratoderma are other possible predisposing factors [2].

Causative organisms
For the most part, the organisms concerned are the three anthropophilic species involved in tinea pedis. Among cases coming to the skin clinics, *T. rubrum* is the most common cause by far. *E. floccosum* and *T. interdigitale* are involved in a minority of cases and mainly in the presence of pre-existing palmoplantar keratoderma such as tylosis. The anthropophilic species *T. violaceum* may also produce this clinical picture and animal species, e.g *T. erinacei*, may occasionally infect the palmar skin.

Clinical features
Presentation
Trichophyton rubrum infection may take several different clinical forms. Hyperkeratosis of the palms and fingers affecting the skin diffusely is the most common variety and is unilateral in about half of cases. The accentuation of the flexural creases is a characteristic feature. Other clinical variants include crescentic exfoliating scales, circumscribed vesicular patches, discrete red papular and follicular scaly patches, and red scaly sheets on the dorsal surface of the hand, which may be more subtle in type IV–VI skin. The latter forms are more likely to be zoophilic infections.

Differential diagnosis
Dermatophyte infections of the palm are often quiet and chronic, commonly passing unnoticed or misdiagnosed. Contact dermatitis, especially the primary irritant variety, psoriasis, pityriasis rubra pilaris, constitutional eczemas, keratoderma, syphilis and post-streptococcal peeling must all be considered. In ring infections and web space cases with anatomical deformity, candidosis and bacterial intertrigo should be excluded.

Unilateral scaling should always alert the clinician to the necessity of taking scrapings. Nail changes may help: pitting suggests psoriasis, but subungual hyperkeratosis if present should always be scraped. If the palmar infection spreads to the dorsal surface, more classic annular lesions may be seen, although this happens relatively infrequently. Tinea manuum, like tinea cruris and tinea faciei, is sometimes modified by inappropriate treatment with topical steroids leading to further diagnostic difficulties.

Disease course and prognosis
Chronic infection is usual.

Management
Chronic ringworm infections of the palm are not easily cleared and oral therapy is always needed. Itraconazole and terbinafine are both effective in this condition. Most cases clear with 2–4 weeks of treatment although it may be advisable to review the results a few months after the end of treatment. With griseofulvin, longer periods of treatment are necessary. Many patients will require 3 months of therapy and may even relapse after that.

Infection control
The prevalence of tinea manuum is directly related to the level of tinea pedis in the population. Prompt treatment of tinea pedis and the use of separate towels are sensible measures that can be recommended. However, it is likely that tinea manuum will continue to occur sporadically and a greater awareness of this condition, so that it may be recognised promptly, is of prime importance.

Tinea cruris

Definition and nomenclature
Tinea cruris is an infection of the groins by a species of dermatophyte.

> **Synonyms and inclusions**
> - Ringworm of the groin
> - Dhobie itch
> - Eczema marginatum

Epidemiology
Tinea cruris is commoner in adults and in males.

Pathophysiology
Predisposing factors
Apart from numerous cases of autoinfection from the foot to the groin [1], the sharing of towels and sports clothing is important [2]. In cases thus contracted, the toe clefts may be normal.

Causative organisms
The causal species are those implicated in foot ringworm but in different proportions. *T. rubrum* is the main cause [3]; *T, indotineae*, *T. interdigitale* and *E. floccosum* also account for some cases.

Environmental factors
It is more common in hot and humid climates.

Clinical features
Presentation
Whatever the causal species, itching is a predominant feature. The lesions in the early stages are red plaques, curved with sharp margins extending from the groin down the thighs. Scaling is variable

and occasionally may mask the inflammatory changes. Vesiculation is rare, but dermal nodules forming beading along the edge are commonly found in older lesions. Minute pustules are often detected if sought with care. Some central clearance is usually present but is often incomplete with nodules scattered throughout the affected area.

Satellite lesions, if present, are few in number and are relatively large. Spread to the scrotum is common, but scaling is minimal and inflammation is inconspicuous against a red background [4]. *E. floccosum* infections are clinically indistinguishable from *T. rubrum* infections but are often not associated with tinea pedis. *T. rubrum* cases are classically chronic and sometimes more nodular. The rarer *T. interdigitale* infections may be vesicular and inflammatory. A coinfection affecting the groins and other sites may also occur, particularly in *T. rubrum* and *T. indotineae* infections affecting the buttocks, the lower back and the abdomen (see tinea corporis). The penis is occasionally affected.

Differential diagnosis
Candidosis, which is more common in women, does not have a distinct raised margin. White pustules are often found, satellite lesions are numerous and small, and the frayed, peeling edge that occurs as the tiny pustules rupture is characteristic. Pityriasis versicolor may be localised to the groin but is usually non-inflammatory and asymptomatic, as is erythrasma. Central clearing is rarely found in either of these infections.

Intertrigo with heavy bacterial colonisation is common in the obese subject of either sex. It may show a sharp margin, but this edge is usually a simple curve where the opposed skin surfaces meet. In many cases, extension upwards from the groin is as prominent as that down the thigh, a feature usually absent in tinea cruris. The central skin is often macerated and the submammary, periumbilical and axillary skin may also be affected, resembling flexural seborrhoeic dermatitis. However, this feature is not a completely reliable distinguishing criterion, as *E. floccosum* in particular may involve the axillae and the submammary areas. Psoriasis and mycosis fungoides may occasionally mimic tinea cruris, but characteristic lesions in other sites can usually be found. In atopic eczema there may be lichenification, but these changes usually extend up towards the hip. Contact dermatitis from clothing or deodorants may confuse, and Hailey–Hailey disease and flexural Darier disease require consideration.

Topical steroids lead to suppression of the physical signs of tinea cruris.

Disease course and prognosis
The disease course is chronic.

Investigations
Direct microscopy and culture or PCR (see earlier) are the key elements of laboratory diagnosis.

Management
In cases of recent onset, topical therapy can be expected to be curative within 2–4 weeks. Any of the local applications listed in Table 32.7 are satisfactory, but benzoic acid compound ointment (Whitfield's ointment) should be prescribed at half strength.

Tolnaftate, terbinafine and the imidazoles are better tolerated in the flexural areas, and if the diagnosis is in doubt terbinafine and the imidazoles have the advantage of being effective against *Candida* as well. Where the condition has been present for many months, or has spread to the pubic area, the natal cleft or the buttocks, and where topical steroids have been used, systemic treatment is strongly recommended. Terbinafine and itraconazole usually produce a remission in 1–2 weeks [5]. Some patients relapse even after this therapy, although it appears less likely to occur than with griseofulvin. A longer course of therapy may work in these recalcitrant cases.

> **Treatment ladder for tinea cruris**
>
> **Recent-onset disease**
> - Topical terbinafine or imidazoles twice daily for 2 weeks
>
> **Chronic or extensive disease**
> - Oral terbinafine 250 mg/day for 1–2 weeks
>   *or*
> - Itraconazole 100 mg/day for 2–4 weeks

Infection control
Greater control of foot ringworm might lead to fewer cases of tinea cruris. A person suffering from tinea pedis or cruris should not lend towels to others, even if they have been laundered. In the tropics, light clothing and prompt treatment of tinea pedis are probably of importance. Topical therapy is often sufficient to control early cases, but long-established *T. rubrum* infection will require oral terbinafine or itraconazole.

Onychomycosis caused by dermatophytes

Definition and nomenclature
This is invasion of the nail plates by species of dermatophytes. A different category of onychomycosis is associated with certain other species of filamentous fungi that are frequently found in dystrophic nails; these are considered separately in the section Onychomycosis caused by other non-dermatophyte moulds [1,2].

> **Synonyms and inclusions**
> - Ringworm of the nails
> - Tinea unguium

Introduction and general description
Fungal nail disease or onychomycosis has been divided into seven main patterns depending on its location on the nail apparatus and how the fungal infection is initiated. Onychomycosis is divided into those caused by dermatophytes, *Neoscytalidium*, other non-dermatophyte moulds and *Candida* (see sections on onychomycosis later in this chapter). Table 32.8 provides a scheme for the

Table 32.8 The main patterns of onychomycosis.

Patterns of onychomycosis	Fungi
Distal and lateral subungual onychomycosis (DLSO)	Dermatophytes (*Trichophyton rubrum*, *T. mentagrophytes*), *Candida albicans*, *Fusarium* spp., *Neoscytalidium* spp., *Scopulariopsis brevicaulis*
Superficial onychomycosis (SO) (white or black): patchy	*T. mentagrophytes*, *T. rubrum*, *Fusarium* spp., *Acremonium* spp., *Neoscytalidium* spp.
Transverse	*T. rubrum*, *Fusarium* spp.
Proximal subungual onychomycosis (PSO) (patchy, striate (transverse) and longitudinal)	*T. rubrum*, *Fusarium* spp.
Endonyx onychomycosis	*T. soudanense*, *T. violaceum*
Totally dystrophic onychomycosis	Dermatophytes, *C. albicans*, *Neoscytalidium* spp.
Mixed onychomycosis; examples include the following on the same nail:	*T. rubrum*
DLSO plus SO	*T. rubrum*, *Fusarium* spp.
SO plus DLSO	*T. rubrum*, *Fusarium* spp.
SO plus PSO	*T. rubrum*
DLSO plus PSO	
Paronychia: with onychomycosis (usually DLSO or PSO)	*Candida* spp., *Fusarium* spp., *Neoscytalidium* spp.
Without onychomycosis	*Candida* spp., *Fusarium* spp., *Neoscytalidium* spp.

main infections and their methods of presentation, including the dermatophytes discussed in this section.

Epidemiology
Incidence and prevalence
The reported prevalence rates of dermatophyte onychomycosis are variable, with figures from 6% to 25% being found in northern Europe [1]. These depend on the methods of investigation, the higher figures being obtained by mycological sampling. However, in both Europe and Asia the highest prevalence rates are seen in the countries with the colder climates. Dermatophyte onychomycosis is less frequent in tropical climates.

Age
It is rare in children.

Sex
It is equally distributed.

Pathophysiology
Predisposing factors
It is likely that *T. rubrum* invades the nail plate with relative ease [2]. *T. rubrum* predominates in fingernail infections, owing no doubt to the prevalence of that species in tinea manuum. It is also the main cause of infection of the toenails. *T. interdigitale* is a less common cause and often only affects the great toenail. Invasion of the nail plate usually occurs either from the lateral nail fold or from the free edge and an elaborate network of channels and lacunae is formed [3], leading to opacity and eventually destruction and crumbling of the nail plate.

Pathology
Subungual hyperkeratosis frequently occurs but is sometimes difficult to distinguish from softening of the nail plate proper and the mechanism of its production is obscure. As might be expected from the age distribution of tinea pedis, onychomycosis is largely a disease of adults [4], but children, especially those in institutions and in households where the adults are infected with *T. rubrum*, may be infected from time to time. A poor peripheral circulation is frequently blamed for resistance to treatment [5]. It may also be a factor in susceptibility. Nails that have been traumatised and nails of elderly people, where linear growth is slow, are both unduly susceptible to infection.

Causative organisms
The principal dermatophytes concerned are: (i) associated with foot and hand infections (*T. rubrum*, *T. interdigitale* and *E. floccosum*); and (ii) associated with scalp infections (*T. tonsurans*, *T. violaceum* and *T. soudanense*). Ringworm of the nails occurs in all parts of the world, and almost all dermatophytes have been reported to infect nails at one time or another [2]. Although nail infections may be the only manifestation of fungus disease in a patient, in the great majority of cases they are associated with tinea pedis or tinea manuum, and the three dermatophytes most commonly implicated are therefore *T. rubrum*, *T. interdigitale* and, rarely, *E. floccosum* [6–8].

T. soudanense has been reported as a cause of onychomycosis, and other dermatophytes usually encountered as a cause of tinea capitis, such as *T. tonsurans* and *T. violaceum*, not infrequently infect fingernails. In regions or populations where tinea pedis is uncommon and tinea capitis caused by these fungi is frequent, they are likely to predominate as a cause of onychomycosis.

Clinical features [9]
Six distinct patterns of tinea unguium have been described (Table 32.8).

Distal and lateral subungual onychomycosis (DLSO). DLSO is the most common pattern of infection and usually presents as a streak or a patch of discoloration, white or yellow at the free edge of the nail plate, and often near the lateral nail fold. The initial invasion of the hyponychium shows through a relatively normal dorsal nail plate. It commonly spreads towards the base of the nail (Figure 32.30) and may occasionally become darker brown or black. The nail plate becomes obviously thickened and may crack as it is lifted up by the accumulation of soft subungual hyperkeratosis. A later phase of invasion may lead to massive destruction of the nail plate (total dystrophic onychomycosis). Although commonly starting with a single affected nail, other digits later become invaded. The variation in the severity of damage is sometimes marked, so that minor changes, a little discoloration or just fraying of the nails, may be all that is seen. Indeed, nail clippings may reveal fungus mycelium in nails that appear completely normal [10].

Superficial onychomycosis (SO). SO is a less common presentation and can produce a distinct form of nail invasion in which the dorsal surface of the nail plate is eroded in well-circumscribed, powdery white patches or as transverse linear streaks, often away from the free edge [11]. It is distinguishable from other causes of leukonychia

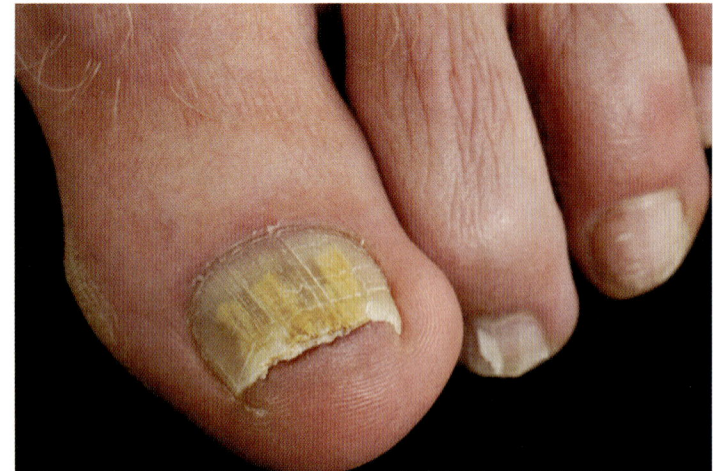

Figure 32.30 Onychomycosis caused by *Trichophyton rubrum*.

by the powdery nature of the white material, which can easily be scraped away; rarely, but not with dermatophytes, the colour of the infection is black (e.g. *Neoscytalidium*). The whole surface of the nail plate may be thus affected and occasionally this picture may also coexist with deep invasion of the nail plate of the ordinary type starting at the free edge. In some patients, superficial infection appears to originate from beneath the proximal nail fold and such cases respond poorly to topical therapy. Although more common with *T. interdigitale*, it can occasionally be seen in *T. rubrum* infections and also occurs with certain non-dermatophytes, for example *Fusarium* spp. Toenails are usually affected, but in AIDS patients superficial white onychomycosis of both toe- and fingernails has been reported [12]. In AIDS patients, superficial infection may coexist with proximal nail plate invasion.

Proximal subungual onychomycosis. This is a pattern that was very uncommon, but in the last 10 years has become particularly associated with immunosuppression including AIDS. Rapid invasion of the nail plate from the posterior nail fold may develop to produce a white nail with only a marginal increase in thickness [12]. The most common cause is currently *T. rubrum*, although in the past more unusual species such as *T. megninii* were associated with this picture. The origin of these infections is not clear. Clinically they appear as either linear bands or as patches of subungual infection emerging from under the proximal nail fold.

Endonyx onychomycosis. This is seen with infection caused by dermatophytes that cause endothrix scalp infections, notably *T. soudanense*. The nail plate is scarred with pits and lamellar splits. The invasion occurs from the top surface but penetrates deeply into the nail plate.

Totally dystrophic onychomycosis. This is the final common pathway for severe infection where the nail plate is completely destroyed.

Mixed onychomycosis. Patients often present with more than one pattern of nail plate invasion such as distal subungual and superficial nail invasion.

On occasion, patients with onycholysis alone may have positive cultures of dermatophytes, suggesting that carriage of dermatophytes without invasion is possible [13].

Differential diagnosis

The destructive changes of the nail plate and nail bed produced by dermatophytes can be mimicked closely by psoriasis. Fine pitting of the dorsal nail plate is never produced by fungal infections and strongly suggests psoriasis, as does the oil-drop sign away from the free edge. The irregularly buckled nail of eczema and the ridged or dysplastic nail of lichen planus must be distinguished. Paronychia, caused either by bacteria or *Candida*, usually affects the nail plate proximally and laterally, while the free edge is often spared, at least initially. Conversely, swelling of the nail fold is rare in dermatophyte infections, and purulent discharge is never a feature of uncomplicated tinea unguium. Onycholysis and other nail dystrophies must be considered. Dermatophyte of the nails is rarely symmetrical and it is common to find the nails of only one hand affected. The skin of the feet and of the palms should always be examined carefully.

Classification of severity

Generally, poorly responsive infections show involvement of the proximal nail bed and linear opaque streaks (dermatophytoma).

Disease course and prognosis

The disease course is chronic.

Investigations

Dermoscopy may show the appearance of a feathery margin at the borders of areas of onycholysis. Nail clippings or scrapings are essential, and direct microscopy should be carried out with great care as culture often fails with nail plate material [10,14]. For this reason, it is wise to sample any obvious skin lesions present, as these are usually infected with the same organism and will be more likely to yield a positive culture [15]. It must be remembered that double pathologies do occur and a nail, dystrophic from some other cause, may become invaded by a dermatophyte fungus. This is not uncommon with onychogryphosis. New molecular diagnostic methods may help to resolve some of these uncertainties [16].

Management

In general, fingernail infections with dermatophyte fungi respond satisfactorily to oral terbinafine 250 mg/day for 6 weeks or itraconazole 400 mg/day for 1 week, given monthly for 2–3 months. With griseofulvin, clearance may be expected in about 4 months, but longer treatment regimens up to 8 months or even 1 year are often needed [17]. In the case of toenails, longer periods of treatment may be necessary; for example, terbinafine 250 mg/day for 3 months or itraconazole 400 mg/day for 1 week given monthly for 3–4 months. One large clinical trial has shown better efficacy with terbinafine than itraconazole [18]. Some, possibly 15% of patients, fail to respond to these drugs, and there is a strong clinical impression that results are much better in younger patients in whom faster linear nail growth and relative absence of coexisting ischaemic or traumatic dystrophy are probably important factors. Poor peripheral circulation seems to have an adverse effect on treatment.

Avulsion of the nail or removal of the infected areas with a drill or burr as adjuncts to antifungals are occasionally valuable. Laser ablation is similarly useful but relapse rates are high and there have been few studies of the use of combined ablation techniques and antifungal therapy. The use of 40% urea cream under occlusive dressing is an alternative approach to treatment [19], particularly in oral treatment failures. The addition of the imidazole, 1% bifonazole, to the urea paste has produced good responses in some patients with involvement of the entire nail plate [20]. When a single great toenail is infected, these procedures are worthy of serious consideration. Unfortunately, there has been no reliable controlled evaluation of their worth and avulsion is certainly not without its drawbacks. Photodynamic therapy and iontophoresis have both been reported to produce remission in a small number of studies. Topical therapy for nail infections has been used in the past with poor results, except in superficial white onychomycosis caused by ringworm infection, where it may well be effective. Other topical agents reported to be effective – 28% tioconazole, ciclopyrox olamine and amorolfine nail paint, tavaborole, luliconazole and efinaconazole – have all produced remissions in some studies, although these are seldom frequent enough to encourage sole use of these preparations, except in early or superficial infections or as adjuncts to oral therapy. The use of combined treatment with either terbinafine or itraconazole with amorolfine may be more effective than oral therapy alone [21].

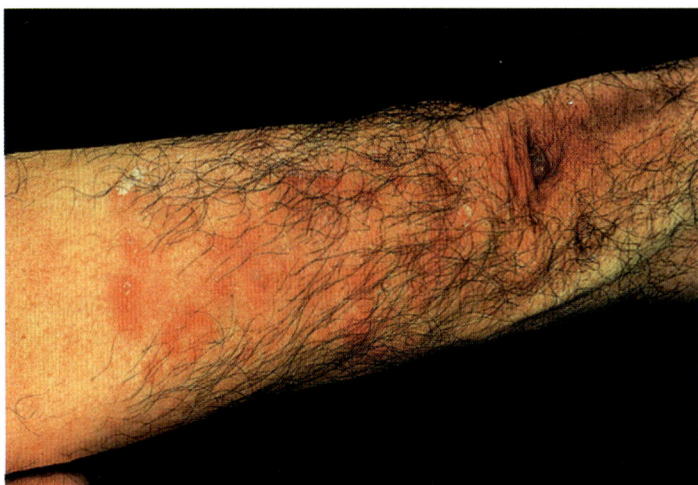

Figure 32.31 Tinea corporis in a patient on systemic corticosteroids.

> **Treatment ladder for onychomycosis caused by dermatophytes**
>
> **First line**[a]
> - Oral terbinafine 250 mg/day for 6 weeks for fingernails, for 3 months for toenails
>   *or*
> - Itraconazole 400 mg/day for 1 week, monthly for 2–3 months for fingernails, for 3–4 months for toenails
>
> **Second line**
> - Griseofulvin dose 1 g for 4–8 months (longer for toenails)
>
> [a]Topical treatment with amorolfine or ciclopirox olamine can be used in mild infections affecting the distal nail plate only or non-linear superficial onychomycosis.

Infection control
Proper early treatment of tinea pedis and tinea manuum would almost certainly reduce the prevalence of onychomycosis.

Steroid-modified tinea

Definition and nomenclature
These are ringworm infections modified by corticosteroids (systemic or topical) prescribed for some pre-existing pathology or given mistakenly for the treatment of misdiagnosed tinea.

Synonyms and inclusions
- Tinea incognito

Introduction and general description
Normally, the clinical diagnosis of tinea depends heavily on the inflammatory changes involved [1–3]. This inflammatory response may be almost totally suppressed by corticosteroids, systemic or topical. At the same time, it is probable that the resistance to infection mediated by the immune response, especially the cell-mediated response, is diminished by corticosteroids. In this situation, the infection is less likely to be diagnosed, and the patient is more susceptible to that infection.

With patients on systemic steroids (perhaps treated with additional immunosuppressive agents or irradiation [4]), the degree of modification is often minor, but even in these cases it may be sufficient to mislead (Figure 32.31), especially on the face. With topical steroids, the degree of modification can be profound. The usual sites where this problem occurs are the groins, lower legs, face and hands, but tinea circinata elsewhere may be steroid treated.

Clinical features
History
The history is characteristic. The patient is often satisfied initially with the treatment. Itching is controlled and the inflammatory signs settle, but there is a relapse on stopping treatment, with varying rapidity. Further applications bring renewed relief and the cycles are repeated. In the groins, the patient may develop few persistent nodules, which become unsuppressible by the steroid preparation.

Presentation
Typically, the raised margin is diminished. Scaling is lost and the inflammation is reduced to a few nondescript nodules. Often, a bruise-like brownish discoloration is seen, especially in the groins. On the face, the picture may be modified by a superimposed perioral dermatitis with papules and tiny pustules. Steroid-modified

eyelid infection may closely resemble a stye. With chronic use, atrophy, telangieciectasia and, in the groin and axillae, striae are likely to be observed. In some cases, concentric red rings are seen among the atrophy and telangiectasia; this may be seen with *T. indotineae* infections where topical corticosteroid misuse is common. Redness may be more subtle in skin types IV–VI. Presumably, these represent waves of fungal growth. The eruption remains localised but, especially in *E. floccosum* infections, it spreads more widely than one would expect in an unmodified case. Accumulation of fungal hyphae may lead to cross-infection, as has been reported with steroid-modified *T. violaceum* infection in a dermatology ward [1]. Strong fluorinated steroids seem most likely to produce this syndrome, but even 1% hydrocortisone cream can, on occasion, modify tinea to a confusing extent.

Differential diagnosis
The differential diagnosis of other steroid-modified infections in the groin, particularly candidosis, must be considered, and these may be indistinguishable without cessation of therapy and mycological investigations. A ready awareness that the face, groin and hands are sites of diagnostic error is important in alerting the physician, and the history is usually extremely suggestive.

Investigations
Scrapings may be difficult to obtain in a patient who is currently applying a steroid cream, but if he or she stops it for a few days an upsurge of inflammation with marked scaling often occurs, making clinical diagnosis easier and facilitating the taking of scrapings. In such samples, fungal mycelium is usually abundant but scrapings taken while steroids are still being applied may show very few fungal elements, unless a fluorescent whitener is used [5].

Management
Whatever site is affected, it is often best to treat steroid-modified ringworm with oral therapy, allowing a few applications of topical steroid to continue until the terbinafine or itraconazole has begun to take effect. It is wise to use 1% hydrocortisone cream or at least a weaker steroid than that originally prescribed, and also to warn the patient about a possible rebound in spite of these measures. Follow up to ensure steroid cream has been stopped and cure obtained is mandatory.

Dermatophytide reactions

Definition and nomenclature
This is a non-infective cutaneous eruption representing an allergic response to a distant focus of dermatophyte infection.

Synonyms and inclusions
- Microsporide
- Trichophytide or epidermophytide (according to genus)

Pathogenesis
Predisposing factors
A dermatophytide reaction was first observed in a patient with a kerion. Since then a great many cutaneous eruptions have been labelled unconvincingly as dermatophytides. The essential criteria required for the diagnosis of an ide reaction to a dermatophyte infection are the following [1]:
1. Proven dermatophyte infection, which usually becomes highly inflamed before the appearance of the secondary rash.
2. A distant eruption, which is demonstrably free of ringworm fungus.
3. Spontaneous disappearance of the rash when the ringworm infection settles, with or without treatment.

Even with these criteria, ide reactions may be overdiagnosed. An additional criterion has been recommended: the morphology of the ide eruption should match one of the well-recognised types.

Clinical features
History
The focus of infection is often a kerion, for instance caused by *T. verrucosum*, but the species is not important as long as it provokes inflammation. Highly inflammatory tinea pedis may be insufficient. The main ide reactions are well established:
1. A widespread eruption of small follicular papules grouped or diffusely scattered. The eruption is symmetrical, usually pronounced on the trunk, but in severe cases extending down limbs, even at times covering the face. Sometimes the follicular papules are topped by horny spines. The common cause of this type of ide reaction is a scalp ringworm kerion, typically caused by *T. verrucosum*. On occasion, *T. tonsurans* and *M. audouinii* may be responsible, when they produce inflamed ringworm. Treatment of the original ringworm lesion may play a part in initiating the process.
2. A pompholyx-like ide affecting the web spaces and palmar surfaces of the fingers, the palms and sometimes the dorsal surfaces of the hands. This eruption is characteristically associated with an acutely inflammatory tinea pedis, which may have arisen spontaneously or as a result of inappropriate treatment. The palmar and web space skin may be covered with itchy papules or vesicles. On occasion, bullae or pustules may occur. Clinically, this is indistinguishable from a constitutional eczema of the pompholyx variety, and the diagnosis of a dermatophytide in this clinical situation demands rigorous application of the criteria outlined above.
3. Of the many other suggested morphologies for ide reactions, erythema nodosum seems the most acceptable [2]. There are a few published accounts of this, and the authors are aware of other cases that fit the above criteria.

Clinical variants
It is possible that erythema multiforme, erythema annulare and urticaria may, on occasion, be manifestations of an allergic reaction to a ringworm infection, but such instances are rare.

SUPERFICIAL MYCOSES DUE TO OTHER HYPHAL FUNGI

Superficial mycoses caused by *Neoscytalidium* species

Definition
Neoscytalidium (previously *Scytalidium*) *dimidiatum* is a secondary pathogen of higher plants found mainly in tropical areas, but also in the USA and the Mediterranean region.

Introduction and general description
This grey to black mould is now recognised as the cause of ringworm-like infections of the palms, soles, toe webs and nails [1–4]. *Scytalidium hyalinum*, a variant non-pigmented form of *N. dimidiatum*, can also mimic tinea pedis and manuum and invade the nail plate [5]. Although logically this should be transferred to the genus *Neoscytalidium* as well, the formal proposal to do so has not been made as yet but it will be referred to here as *N. hyalinum*. These two moulds evoke the same clinical picture.

Epidemiology
Although these infections were first diagnosed in the UK in patients who were immigrants from the West Indies, East Africa and the Indian subcontinent, reports from areas where they may be truly endemic, such as the Caribbean [6], West Africa [7–9] and Thailand [10], have shown that infection by *Neoscytalidium* species is extremely common. Infection is mainly seen in those born in a tropical environment but has also been seen in Europeans who have merely visited an endemic area for a vacation.

Pathophyslology
Neoscytalidium species produce keratinases and therefore can penetrate the stratum corneum.

Clinical features
Presentation
Early infection is often asymptomatic.

These fungi can produce toe cleft changes and involvement of the palms and soles. In this, they closely resemble the dry-type infection caused by *T. rubrum* affecting the palms or soles [5]. Lesions are often asymptomatic and only discovered on routine inspection. In fingernails, the nail changes start at the lateral and distal edges, and there may be extensive undermining of the nail without corresponding thickening of the nail plate (Figure 32.32). The nails may fracture transversely in due course. Paronychia often accompanies these changes. Usually, yeasts are not present under the nail fold, suggesting that the changes are caused by *Neoscytalidium* alone. In the toenails, the changes are usually identical to those seen in dermatophyte infections. Occasionally, there may be increased pigmentation in the nail plate, but this should not be confused with idiopathic, longitudinal, pigmented streaking of the nail. This change is most prominent in white people with nail infections [11].

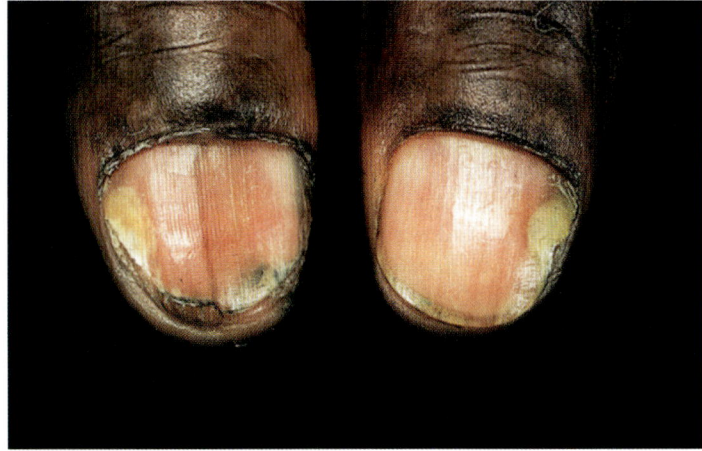

Figure 32.32 Onychomycosis caused by *Neoscytalidium dimidiatum*: early onycholysis.

The infection is confined to areas of thickly keratinised skin and involvement of less heavily keratinised areas, such as the groin, or dorsum of the hand or foot, is not found.

Differential diagnosis
This should include dry-type *T. rubrum* infections and, on the fingers, *Candida* paronychia.

Investigations
Although pigmented brown hyphae have occasionally been observed in skin and nail samples infected by *N. dimidiatum*, in the vast majority of cases the hyphae are hyaline and appear very similar to those of dermatophytes. Typically, however, they are more irregular, varying noticeably in width along the length of a single hypha (Figure 32.33) [12]. With experience, a preliminary

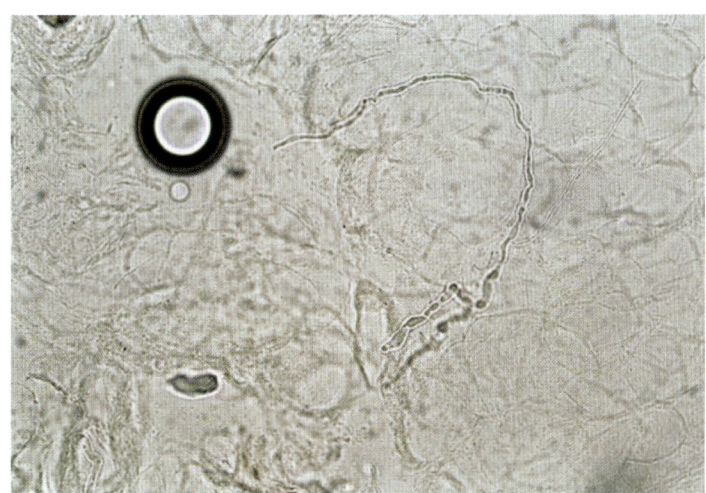

Figure 32.33 Infection by *Neoscytalidium species*. Skin scales are mounted in 30% KOH, bright field. The hyaline hyphae superficially resemble those of dermatophytes, but are very uneven in diameter. One- to two-celled arthroconidia may be observed. Courtesy of the Department of Medical Mycology, St John's Institute of Dermatology, King's College London, London, UK.

diagnosis of *Neoscytalidium* infection may be made on the basis of direct microscopy alone.

Both *N. dimidiatum* and *N. hyalinum* are sensitive to cycloheximide, and this antibiotic must be excluded from the culture medium. As mixed infections by *Neoscytalidium* species and dermatophytes have been recorded, duplicate cultures with and without cycloheximide are ideal, and will allow the isolation of both dermatophytes and non-dermatophytes. Mixed infections of dermatophytes and *N. dimidiatum* and *N. hyalinum* have also been reported.

Neoscytalidium dimidiatum. Colony: there is variable colonial morphology (Figure 32.34a) [13]. One form grows very rapidly and produces a high aerial mycelium, which completely fills a 90 mm Petri dish in a few days. The other common form grows more slowly, at about the same rate as a dermatophyte, and does not produce aerial hyphae, but has a velvety surface texture. Both are pale initially but darken to black and mouse grey, respectively, as they mature. Microscopy: branching chains of one- to two-celled brown arthroconidia are observed (Figure 32.34b). These are abundant in the fast-growing cultures but may be scanty in the slow-growing form. Coiled hyphae and rough-walled hyphae are usually present in the slow-growing cultures. *N. dimidiatum* produces melanin both in culture and *in vivo* [14].

Neoscytalidium hyalinum. Colony: the fungus grows rapidly, and in a few days produces a white to cream colony with a moderately high aerial mycelium and buff reverse (Figure 32.35). Microscopy: chains of hyaline one- to two-celled arthroconidia are produced.

Management

There is no reproducibly effective therapy, although individual patients may respond to treatment with topical azoles.

First line

Both organisms may be sensitive *in vitro* to itraconazole or terbinafine, but infections seldom respond to these drugs clinically.

ONYCHOMYCOSIS CAUSED BY OTHER NON-DERMATOPHYTE MOULDS

General description

Broadly, the term onychomycosis describes any fungal infection of the nail plate. Dermatophyte infections, *Candida* infections and *Neoscytalidium* infections are considered separately in this chapter and these organisms are considered to be primary pathogens (see Table 32.8). However, a wide variety of other non-dermatophyte moulds have been reported from abnormal nails, most often toenails, and in such cases their significance needs very careful assessment [1]. These are described below under the headings of onychomycoses caused by *Scopulariopsis* (assigned by some to the genus *Microascus*), superficial onychomycosis caused by non-dermatophytes, onychomycosis caused by *Onychocola canadensis* and onychomycosis caused by miscellaneous moulds.

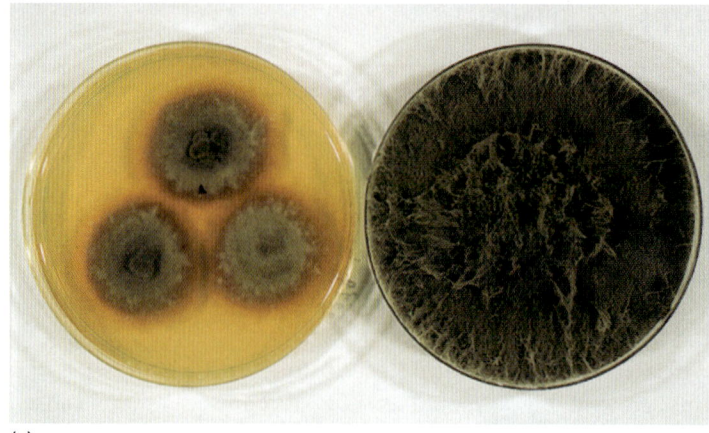

(a)

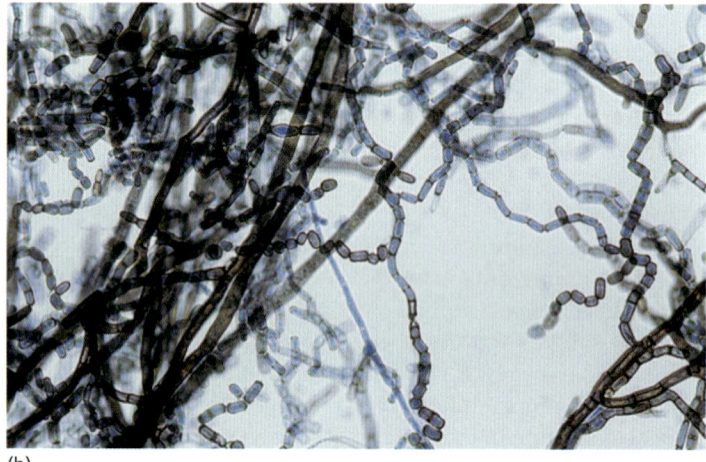

(b)

Figure 32.34 *Neoscytalidium dimidiatum.* (a) Colony forms. The fast-growing form (right) fills a 90 mm Petri dish in a few days and develops profuse aerial mycelium. The velvety, slow-growing form (left) grows at the same rate as a dermatophyte. (b) Microscopy, bright field. Chains of brown, one- to two-celled arthroconidia are characteristic. They may be scanty in the slow-growing form. Courtesy of the Department of Medical Mycology, St John's Institute of Dermatology, King's College London, London, UK.

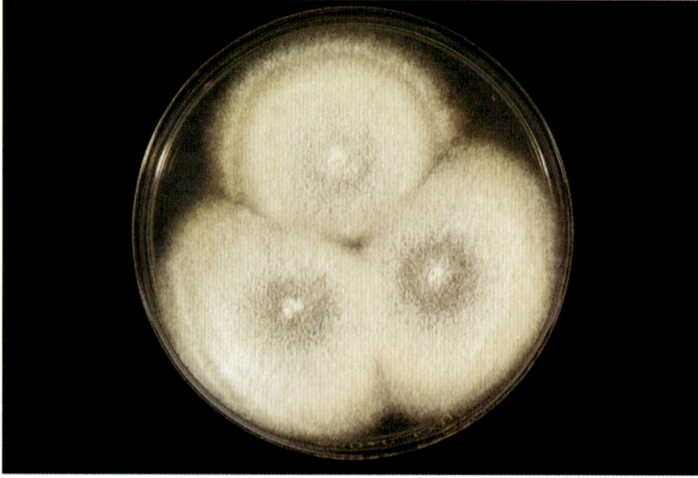

Figure 32.35 *Neoscytalidium hyalinum* colony. Courtesy of the Department of Medical Mycology, St John's Institute of Dermatology, King's College London, London, UK.

Identification

Many of these putative pathogens are common in the environment and may be isolated as contaminants, particularly on media free of cycloheximide. It is therefore essential in cases where such moulds are implicated in onychomycosis to correlate the morphological findings on direct microscopy with those of the isolate. A considerable proportion of dermatophyte-infected nails with typical hyphae present on direct microscopy will fail to yield a dermatophyte on culture. In these instances, the isolation of a few colonies of a contaminating mould may be misinterpreted. In other instances, a non-dermatophyte mould may be isolated in addition to a dermatophyte, and, once more, unless evidence suggestive of a mixed infection has been obtained on direct microscopy [2], in most instances this will represent simple contamination. Before the isolation of a non-dermatophyte can be considered significant, re-examination of the patient is essential in order to confirm the infection. A second direct examination will allow any unusual features of the fungus in the nail to be assessed. Atypical morphology, such as the presence of large numbers of fronding hyphae, or even the production of characteristic conidia within the nail, may be present. In such instances, a second culture on a medium free of cycloheximide may allow reisolation of the same mould and confirm the infection. Concurrent culture with cycloheximide is also recommended to confirm the absence of a dermatophyte – or it may in some instances prove the presence of a mixed infection – because nails rendered abnormal by a primary dermatophyte infection may occasionally be secondarily invaded by moulds. It is noteworthy that in unmixed infections these non-dermatophytes, unlike *Neoscytalidium* and *Fusarium* species, are incapable of producing concurrent skin infection.

Using reliable criteria, one survey in Canada of over 2500 isolates from infected nail samples found that *Scopulariopsis brevicaulis* made up 1.6% of the total and that species of *Aspergillus* and *Fusarium* comprised a further 0.3% of the total [3]. Similarly, a working group of the British Society for Medical Mycology [4] has estimated that approximately 5% of cases of onychomycosis are caused by non-dermatophyte moulds. Such data confirm the view that a few moulds are regularly reported from a small percentage of the total cases of onychomycosis and their isolation may suggest that they are playing some part in the pathology. However, whether their removal with antifungal therapy will result in clinical recovery remains to be established. By far the most common of these isolates is *S. brevicaulis*, which does appear capable of attacking undamaged nails or those with minor abnormalities. In cases of superficial white onychomycosis, species of *Acremonium*, *Fusarium* and *Aspergillus* may be isolated rather than *Trichophyton interdigitale*. *Onychocola canadensis* has been recognised as a cause of onychomycosis, after its original description in nine subjects from Canada and New Zealand [5,6].

Onychomycoses caused by *Scopulariopsis* infections

Clinical features

Scopulariopsis brevicaulis is a common saprophytic mould that does not attack the skin [2]. When it causes nail dystrophy, the clinical

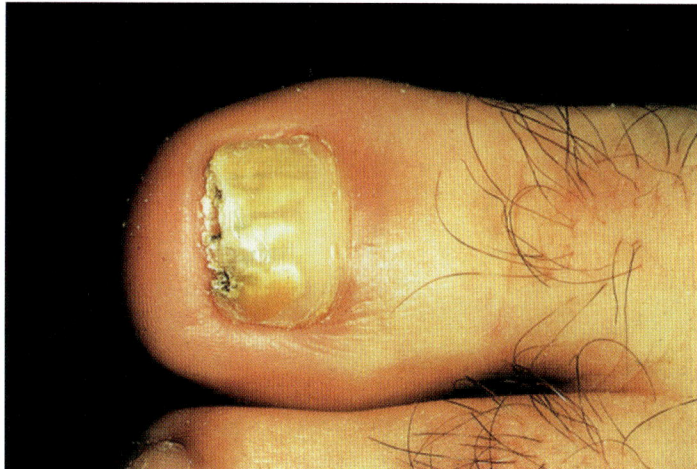

Figure 32.36 Onychomycosis caused by *Scopulariopsis brevicaulis*.

features may be indistinguishable from those of a dermatophyte infection, but where there is heavy invasion its brown spores may discolour the nail, producing a cinnamon colour (Figure 32.36). This is best seen end-on in the area of subungual hyperkeratosis. The great toenails are most often affected, but other toenails and very occasionally fingernails are also involved. Dermatophyte infections of the skin and of the *Scopulariopsis*-infected nail plate itself may coexist.

Investigations

The distribution of the fungus in the infected nail material is often patchy, but where conidia are found they are quite distinctive, being approximately spherical or lemon-shaped with one flat, basal facet. The thick cell walls and truncate bases of the conidia distinguish them from the arthroconidia of dermatophytes. The surfaces of the conidia appear smooth (Figure 32.37). The mould is partially sensitive to cycloheximide and, in most instances, if cycloheximide-containing medium is used for isolation, the

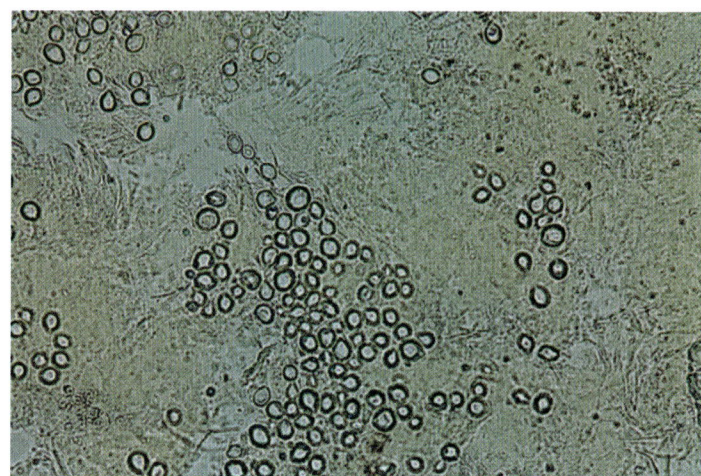

Figure 32.37 *Scopulariopsis brevicaulis*. Nail clipping mounted in KOH, bright field. The characteristic conidia are relatively thick-walled, oval or lemon-shaped with a truncate base. Courtesy of the Department of Medical Mycology, St John's Institute of Dermatology, King's College London, London, UK.

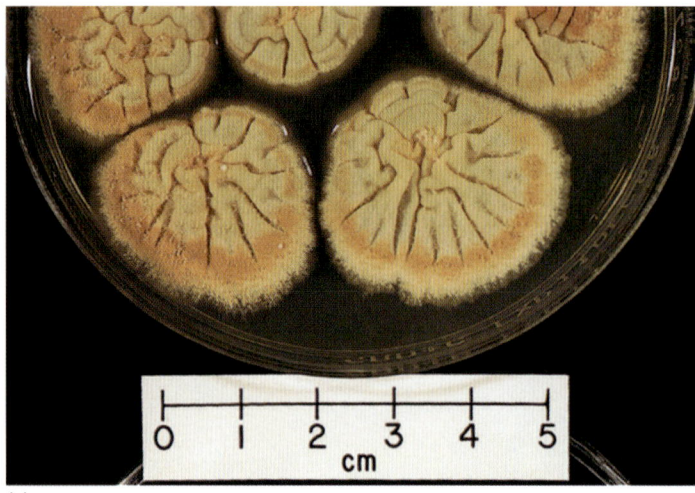

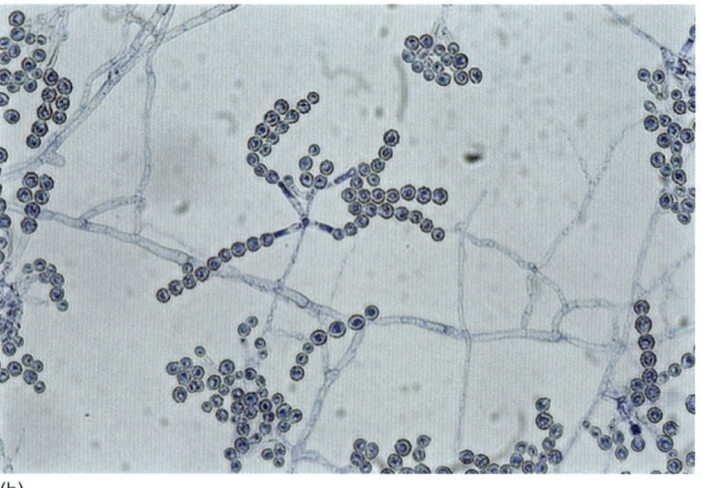

Figure 32.38 *Scopulariopsis brevicaulis*. (a) Colony. On media free of cycloheximide, the colonies are initially waxy and deeply folded, but the production of conidia rapidly produces a brown colour on the colony surface. (b) Microscopy, bright field. Chains of rough-walled conidia are formed from annellides. Courtesy of the Department of Medical Mycology, St John's Institute of Dermatology, King's College London, London, UK.

fungus will grow but remains compact, pale and intricately folded, producing few conidia.

Scopulariopsis brevicaulis (Figure 32.38). Colony: on cycloheximide-free medium the fungus grows rapidly to produce a powdery cinnamon brown surface, often with radial or cerebriform folds. The reverse is cream to brown. Microscopy: chains of basipetal conidia are formed from annellides. The conidia are rough, lemon-shaped or obovoidal with a truncate base.

Management

It is essential to search carefully for a coexisting dermatophyte infection, particularly if there are cutaneous changes. Treatment of pure *Scopulariopsis* infections is difficult. Occasionally, patients may respond to a topically applied lotion such as econazole. However, the most common approach is to use 40% urea paste as a method of chemical nail avulsion and, following removal of the infected plate, an azole antifungal cream or lotion is applied daily to the nail bed until the new nail has completely formed. Itraconazole 400 mg/day for 1 week per month for 3–4 months may be of help [7,8].

Superficial onychomycosis caused by non-dermatophytes

Clinical features

Non-dermatophyte moulds that cause superficial onychomycosis, which is generally white in colour, produce a clinical picture identical to that seen in superficial white onychomycosis caused by *T. interdigitale*. However, one distinguishing feature is the lack of accompanying skin lesions. Some forms of superficial onychomycosis present as cloudy superficial patches on the nail plate, others as transverse linear bands (striate leukonychia). The latter often emerge from beneath the proximal nail fold and seldom respond to topical antifungal therapy. A further form of superficial onychomycosis is followed by deep penetration of the nail plate. Rarely there is a superficial black onychomycosis.

Investigations

Direct examination of the nail material often reveals bizarre, atypical hyphal forms and extensive fronding hyphae (Figure 32.39). However, some degree of fronding may also be seen in dermatophyte infections. The most commonly isolated species, which include *Sarocladium* (*Acremonium*) *strictum*, *Aspergillus terreus* and *Fusarium* species, grow rapidly if cycloheximide is omitted from the culture medium.

Sarocladium (previously *Acremonium*) *strictum*. Colony: the rapidly growing colonies are slimy to waxy with a few central tufts of aerial mycelium and are pink, beige or orange in colour. Microscopy: elongate narrow phialides arise at right angles from

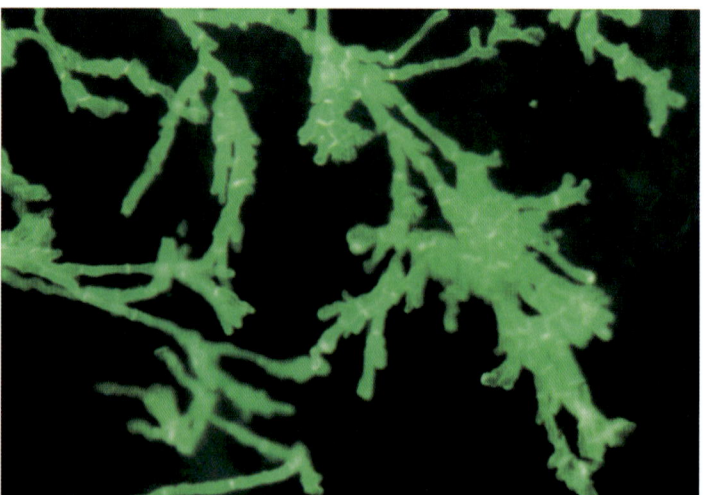

Figure 32.39 Superficial white onychomycosis caused by non-dermatophyte moulds. Nail clipping mounted in KOH and calcofluor white, UV illumination. Bizarre, fronding hyphae may be observed. Courtesy of the Department of Medical Mycology, St John's Institute of Dermatology, King's College London, London, UK.

the slender hyphae. The ellipsoidal conidia collect as a slimy ball at the apex of the phialide.

Aspergillus terreus. Colony: colonies are rapidly growing, powdery with a cinnamon brown surface and pale yellow reverse. Microscopy: the vesicle at the apex of the stout conidiophore bears metulae and phialides only on the upper two-thirds of its surface. Long chains of small, smooth, brown phialoconidia are produced, which form a columnar head.

Fusarium species. Colony: rapidly growing, woolly colonies may have a pink, purple or pale brown surface and reverse. Microscopy: the genus *Fusarium* is characterised by the production from phialides of curved multicellular macroconidia, with a distinct foot cell at the base. Microconidia are also formed and are unicellular or bicellular, ovoid to ellipsoidal. They collect as slimy balls or chains at the apices of the phialides. Chlamydoconidia may also be present.

Management
The results of treatment are unpredictable, but a trial of therapy with amorolfine 5%, tioconazole 28% or removal of the nail with surgery, 40% urea or laser is worth attempting.

Onychomycosis caused by *Onychocola canadensis*

Clinical features
This fungus was only recognised as a pathogen in 1990. Nails display yellow or grey discoloration and hyperkeratosis with a buildup of subungual debris.

Investigations
Direct microscopy reveals irregular hyaline, sometimes golden or brown hyphae, together with barrel-shaped or round arthroconidia. The fungus grows in the presence of cycloheximide as a very slowly developing, restricted, glabrous, pale grey mould, which after 5–6 weeks eventually produces delicate chains of hyaline, waisted arthroconidia.

Management
A single patient treated with griseofulvin showed some clinical improvement after 6 months, but the direct microscopy remained positive [6].

Onychomycosis caused by miscellaneous moulds

In contrast to the fungi described above, an enormous variety of other moulds have been implicated in one or only very few cases of onychomycosis. These include *Pseudeurotium ovalis*, *Pyrenochaeta unguius-hominis*, *Lasiodiplodia theobromae*, *Cochliobolus* (previously *Curvularia*) *lunata* and many others [9]. Investigations of abnormal toenails, especially in elderly people, have shown that an appreciable minority are colonised by non-dermatophyte fungi, usually moulds and often *Aspergillus* species. Fingernails are much less often invaded. These moulds are generally accepted as existing purely saprophytically. Although they may conceivably add to the primary damage caused by ischaemia, trauma or a dermatosis, they are, in general, of little practical importance to the patient. For the dermatologist, their significance lies in the fact that they must be distinguished from dermatophytes. Moreover, a dystrophic nail caused by ischaemia and secondarily colonised by *Aspergillus* species is likely to regrow abnormally even if the fungus is eliminated by avulsion. Unlike *Scopulariopsis* infections, secondary mould invasion often affects several nails and indeed all may be invaded.

Of all the other non-dermatophyte moulds that may cause nail disease, *Fusarium* is the most frequently associated. In addition to causing superficial onychomycosis, *Fusarium* species may also cause proximal subungual onychomycosis and other patterns of nail invasion; it can also cause interdigital infection.

CANDIDOSIS

Definition and nomenclature

Candidosis is an infection caused by the yeasts of the genus *Candida*. Superficial infections of the mucous membranes and skin are numerically most important, but deep invasive disease such as septicaemia, endocarditis and meningitis can also occur and these are considered in the section on systemic mycoses later in the chapter.

Synonyms and inclusions
- Candidiasis
- Moniliasis
- Thrush

Classification

Candida albicans is an oval yeast 2–6 × 3–9 µm in size that can produce budding cells, pseudohyphae and true hyphae [1]. This ability to simultaneously display several morphological forms is known as polymorphism. Although hyphae are likely to be produced during the process of tissue invasion, yeasts without hyphae may also occur in invasive disease, particularly in infections caused by non-*C. albicans* species. Apart from *C. albicans*, the genus *Candida* includes over 100 species, most of which are neither commensals nor parasites on humans. Other species of *Candida*, for example *C. tropicalis*, *C. dubliniensis*, *C. parapsilosis*, *C. guilliermondii*, *C. krusei*, *C. pseudotropicalis*, *C. lusitaniae*, *C. zeylanoides* and *C. glabrata*, are occasional causes of human candidosis, particularly in disseminated infections. The epidemiology of candidosis is changing and, where once *C. albicans* was the predominant species isolated from clinical samples, in some countries other species are now very common.

General description

Candida species cause a wide variety of different skin conditions, which are shown in Box 32.3.

> **Box 32.3 Clinical diseases (variants) caused by *Candida* species on the skin**
>
> **Candidosis of the oral mucous membranes**
> - Acute pseudomembranous candidosis
> - Acute erythematous candidosis
> - Chronic pseudomembranous candidosis
> - Chronic erythematous candidosis
> - Chronic plaque-like candidosis
> - Chronic nodular candidosis
> - Angular cheilitis
> - Median rhomboid glossitis
> - Candidosis, steroids and the mouth
>
> **Candidosis of the skin and genital mucous membranes**
> - *Candida* intertrigo (flexural candidosis)
> - Acute vulvo-vaginal candidosis
> - Chronic vulvo-vaginal candidosis
> - *Candida* balanitis
> - Perianal and scrotal candidosis
> - Perineal candidosis of infancy
> - Nodular or granulomatous candidosis of the napkin area
>
> **Candidosis of the nail and paronychium**
> - *Candida* paronychium
> - *Candida* onychomycosis
> - Congenital candidosis
>
> **Other *Candida* diseases**
> - *Candida* allergy
> - Chronic mucocutaneous candidosis

Basic biology

Candida ecology

Gastrointestinal tract carriage. *Candida albicans* is a frequent, but not invariable, normal member of the gastrointestinal microbiome [2]. Colonisation with *C. albicans* or another species may occur during birth directly from the birth canal, at some time during infancy or perhaps later in life. Colonisation of the mouth early in life is often followed by frank pathological changes, but if the organism is acquired later it is usually established asymptomatically.

The literature on oral carriage rates is extensive. Fewer than 26% of normal subjects [1] carry yeasts in the mouth, and *C. albicans* carriage rates are about 18%. Surveys of the oral flora of hospital patients show higher figures. Isolation rates of yeasts from faecal specimens and rectal swabs are also higher than those from oral samples. Figures of nearly 47% for yeast carriage and just under 41% for *C. albicans* have been suggested by published studies [1].

If molecular techniques or repeated sampling are used, the proportion of healthy adults carrying *Candida* in the gastrointestinal tract may be demonstrably higher, even rising to two-thirds. Moreover, if oral antibiotics that are effective against the resident gastrointestinal bacterial flora are given, *Candida* carrier rates rise [3]. The density and composition of the gastrointestinal yeast flora vary from individual to individual and influence the chances of isolation.

Studies of *Candida* serology and skin tests suggest that a substantial proportion of people not colonised by yeasts may have been exposed to *Candida* in the past. The practical implication of this is that normal individuals show a wide range in the density of carriage of *Candida* species in the oral microbiome. Extraneous factors such as oral antibiotic therapy are likely to increase not only the incidence of carriage, but also the number of organisms present and the chances of infection.

Vaginal carriage [4]. The healthy vagina may be colonised by yeasts – most commonly *C. albicans*, sometimes *C. glabrata* – in a proportion of women [5]. The percentage of vaginal carriers differs widely in different surveys, but a figure of 12.7% for *C. albicans* is probably accurate. Higher rates are found in hospital patients, even without vaginal disease [1]. Pregnancy, oral contraceptives and the use of intrauterine devices have all been associated with elevated carrier rates [6].

Cutaneous carriage. Generally, neither *C. albicans* nor any other species of *Candida* is a permanent member of the normal flora of the skin, although transient colonisation can occur in the neonatal period [7]. At the same time, skin adjacent to the body orifices and the skin of the fingers, which are in frequent contact with the mouth, often yield *C. albicans* and sometimes other species, particularly *C. auris*, *C. parapsilosis* and *C. guilliermondii*. *Candida* may be a persistent coloniser of moist intertriginous sites in individuals [8] as well as the subungual space in patients with pre-existing nail disease. Age and climate are important in this connection. Samples from the very young and the very old are more likely to yield *Candida*.

Carriage in other sites. The bronchial tree is not normally colonised by *Candida*, and where the organism is isolated from sputum specimens, at least in low amounts, it can be assumed that it has come from the mouth or oro-pharynx. It has been shown that swallowing a large quantity of *Candida* cells will result in the transfer of these yeasts rapidly through the gut wall into the circulation, presumably via the portal vein and the liver [9].

C. albicans can occasionally be cultured from the environment, usually in the vicinity of heavily infected subjects [1], human or animal; for example, it has been isolated from a nursery where there was an epidemic of oral thrush, from hospital bed linen and from the air of dermatology clinics. Normally, however, *Candida* is not part of the airborne microflora. Except for neonatal and conjugal infections, most cases of candidosis probably result from infection of the host by his or her own commensal yeasts. Studies using typing confirm the view that most infections are endogenous and generally infection follows a shift in the existing host–yeast relationship [10]. This shift from commensal to parasite results from a variety of influences. To date, an increase in yeast virulence has not been shown to be important. Isolates of *C. albicans* might be expected to differ in their capacity to cause damage in the human host [11]. In practice, such variations are hard to demonstrate, with the exception of a few specific mutations such as defective protease production.

Genetic methods of typing *Candida* strains have provided a means of investigating the spread of organisms within individual patients, groups or hospital wards [12]. They have indicated that the spread of predominant strains can occur either between individuals or in hospitals. In one well-documented outbreak, an isolate that resisted normal hand washing procedures was the cause of a number of infections in an intensive care unit [13]. This indicates that strains carried by patients may be replaced by others with different biological characteristics. These techniques can now be used to determine important issues, such as the acquisition of drug resistance [14]. *C. albicans* may also demonstrate an unusual phenomenon known as phenotypic switching, whereby a strain may change morphology or another phenotypic character such as drug sensitivity in response to a change in growth conditions; such changes are reversible and not associated with genetic variation [15].

Pathophysiology

Organisms

In animal experiments some *Candida* species have been shown to be less virulent than *C. albicans*, a finding that conforms with clinical experience. Generally, the most common pathogen in skin disease is *C. albicans*, although increasingly other species are isolated in vaginal infections and from immunocompromised patients. Factors such as the production of a secreted aspartyl protease by certain strains of *C. albicans* are also known to affect pathogenicity. Proteinase-negative strains are known to be less virulent [1]; laboratory-generated gene-defective strains have not been shown to be less virulent.

In oral and cutaneous candidosis, scrapings examined microscopically usually show *Candida* in both the budding and mycelial forms [2]. In histopathology of invasive candidosis, hyphae are usually present. This suggests that the production of hyphae may contribute to fungal virulence. *C. albicans* mutants that do not express hyphal-associated gene products, such as hypha-specific G1 cyclin-related protein, show attenuated virulence.

The ability of yeast forms to adhere to the underlying epithelial cells is also an important prequel of tissue invasion [3–5]. *C. albicans* is equipped to sense contact with an underlying human cell. Adherence of *Candida* to epithelial surfaces is mediated through a number of receptor interactions. *Candida* adhesins are either based on cell wall mannan or protein components [6]. The best studied adhesins are known as agglutinin-like sequence (ALS) proteins. It has also been shown that proteinase production is involved in adherence.

In vivo, a wide variety of factors have at various times been claimed to be important in stimulating mycelium formation [7]. Temperatures above 35°C, low oxygen tension, liquid media, non-sulphur-containing amino acids, a polysaccharide carbon source, serum and a pH of 7.5 are the most convincing factors in experimental studies [8]. However, it is difficult to relate these experimental results to the *in vivo* situation. *C. albicans* also produces melanin, a factor known to affect resistance to immunological responses. In order to penetrate human cells, it can both induce endocytosis as well as use hyphal-mediated penetration. *Candida*'s ability to form a biofilm on its own or with other micro-organisms on certain surfaces, including skin ulcers, may also lead to the expression of different genes affecting virulence or drug resistance such as drug efflux pumps.

The effects of ecological pressures from other organisms are of considerable importance [9]. Both in the gastro-intestinal tract and on the skin, the removal of competing bacteria leads to an increase in yeast numbers, an important prerequisite to invasion. Work on the competition between *Candida* and bacteria in saliva suggests that one factor is the amount of available monosaccharides such as glucose [9,10] and that if these are elevated, as in diabetes, bacterial flora will not inhibit the yeast [11]. Mechanisms other than nutrient depletion may also apply and *Candida* can shift to gluconeogenesis using different substrates in hostile environments such as the interior of a phagocyte. In other situations (e.g. the finger web), bacteria, especially Gram negatives, may act as co-pathogens rather than competitors, their presence enhancing the pathogenicity of the yeast. In addition, the presence of bacteria may impair the ability of *Candida* to adhere to the underlying substrate [12].

Host factors

Host factors involved in mucocutaneous candidosis are numerous. The elderly, the very young and ill patients are susceptible to oral thrush. However, a variety of other factors are also involved, and many patients have more than one predisposing factor. In the mouth, carbohydrate levels are important; food debris, likely to be present in the mouth of the severely ill patient with inadequate oral hygiene, should not be ignored and may be as significant as diabetic saliva. High glucose levels in urine, general tissue fluids and sweat may make people with diabetes more susceptible to candidosis [13]. Phagocytosis is also impaired in people with diabetes. In practice, infection in such groups is largely confined to *Candida* vulvovaginitis and balanitis.

Any form of local tissue damage may be important in the pathogenesis of candidosis [14]. Experimental removal of the stratum corneum facilitates the establishment of cutaneous candidosis and with a given inoculum increases the severity of the response [15], possibly by increasing the availability of adhesin receptors. In the mouth, dentures increase susceptibility; explanations include the formation of a dense biofilm. On the skin, maceration is of fundamental importance, and in experimental candidosis high moisture levels, usually provided by occlusion, are a prerequisite. Although several surveys have shown higher levels of *Candida* carriage on psoriatic and eczematous skin, and one other study [16] has claimed that *Candida* paronychia is more common in people with psoriasis, in general candidosis is not a common complication of either psoriasis or eczema.

In experimentally infected guinea pigs there is increased epidermal cell turnover, which develops after *Candida* infection, possibly through a T-cell-mediated mechanism. In this case, increased shedding of the stratum corneum correlates well with recovery from infection [17]. Higgs and Wells [18] showed that some patients with chronic mucocutaneous candidosis had iron deficiency. With iron replacement therapy, their resistance to *Candida* infection increased. On the other hand, *in vitro* experiments indicated that unsaturated transferrin acts as an inhibitor to *C. albicans*. Iron reverses this effect.

Apart from transferrin, the presence of persistent *Candida* infection has, on some occasions, led to the inhibition of T-cell function; an effect demonstrable with other leukocytes *in vitro*, and that was reversed by anti-*Candida* therapy [19]. *Candida* can interact directly with immune cells such as regulatory T cells (T_{reg} cells).

Endocrine factors [7,20]

Apart from diabetes, a variety of endocrinopathies have been mentioned as susceptibility factors in candidosis. In the syndrome of chronic mucocutaneous candidosis, mutations in the *AIRE* gene have been associated with endocrinopathies. There is also little doubt that Cushing syndrome, whether spontaneous or iatrogenic, increases susceptibility to a wide range of infections including candidosis. The mechanism seems to be a direct suppression of immune mechanisms, especially T-cell function.

Immunological factors

Intensive investigation of patients with the syndrome of chronic mucocutaneous candidosis, and studies of a wide range of patients with primary immune defects, indicate that in the defence against *Candida* infection, both superficial and deep seated, cell-mediated immunity is of paramount importance, coupled with normal phagocytosis and killing by polymorphs and macrophages [21,22]. Circulating antibodies or secretory IgA may have some role [23]. The induction of interleukins such as IL-12, -23, -27 and -35 are key steps in host defence. In children wearing orthodontic appliances, the risk of candidosis is higher in those with low salivary IgA levels.

While systemic corticosteroids act to increase susceptibility to candidosis by diminishing immune functions, the practical importance of topical steroids in this connection is not so well understood. However, there is evidence that an inflammatory response to *Candida* – which can be produced experimentally in humans but not in the rat [14] – by dead, disintegrated *Candida* cells, as well as by living organisms, can be suppressed by topical steroids. The description of large granulomatous lesions in the napkin or nappy (diaper) area of infants with candidosis treated with steroids suggests that it may also enhance the real susceptibility to the organisms, as might be expected if fewer lymphocytes and phagocytic cells are present.

The susceptibility of elderly and severely ill people, especially those with leukaemia, lymphomas or carcinomatosis, probably lies in large measure in the depression of cell-mediated immunity.

Patients with defective T-lymphocyte function, such as those with AIDS, appear to be particularly susceptible to mucosal or cutaneous candidosis, but not systemic infections [24,25]. Congenitally, T-cell-deficient mice (nu/nu) do not show reproducible increased susceptibility to systemic infection by *Candida*. In fact, some investigators have found heightened resistance, suggesting that T-lymphocyte activity alone does not account for resistance to systemic invasion [26]. By contrast, in patients with chronic mucocutaneous candidosis, the most consistent abnormalities have been those of T-lymphocyte function, particularly IL-17 expression [19]. Patients receiving treatment with IL-17 inhibitors are more susceptible to superficial *Candida* infection.

Patients with defective neutrophil or macrophage function are susceptible to both superficial and systemic candidosis. The activity of neutrophils and macrophages in phagocytosis and the killing of *Candida in vitro* has been demonstrated [27]. In addition, cytokines such as INF-γ appear to interact with these cells to enhance killing of the organism. It appears that there is therefore substantial interplay between different immune mechanisms in defence, including epidermally expressed peptides such as defensins against candidosis [28].

Candidosis and HIV/AIDS

In the untreated HIV-positive population, oral *Candida* carriage rates are generally high, and this has been confirmed by the finding that carriage rates are, for instance, higher in HIV-positive homosexual males than in a control group of HIV-negative homosexual men [29]. Another study of HIV-positive patients without clinical evidence of oral candidosis showed that 24% of 261 individuals were carrying *C. albicans* on the tongue or buccal mucosa. Colonisation rates were higher in intravenous drug abusers and in those with lymphopenia. In addition, patients with CD4 cell depletion and those with elevated $β_2$-microglobulin levels were more likely to be carriers [30]. Combination antiretroviral therapy usually reverses these findings.

The relationship between CD4 counts, as a guide to disease progression, and oral candidosis in AIDS patients has been studied by a number of authors. Oral thrush does appear to reflect viral load [31]. Both hairy leukoplakia and oral candidosis are markers for an increased rate of progression to AIDS [32]. The presence of oral candidosis may have implications for survival in some patients. For instance, HIV-positive patients with oral candidosis but who have no other features of AIDS have a poorer survival rate than those without it [33]. However, it is important to remember that immunologically related factors are not the only determinants of oral candidosis. The evidence that persistent vaginal candidosis is associated with AIDS is less convincing.

For further information see Chapter 31.

Identification

As *C. albicans* is a common commensal, the interpretation of cultural findings has to be related to the clinical appearances. A scanty growth of *C. albicans* from the skin or from a mucocutaneous site may be meaningless without evidence of infection from a positive direct microscopy.

On direct examination of skin or nail material, the oval, thin-walled yeasts bud on a narrow base and are usually accompanied by filaments, either true hyphae or pseudohyphae (Figure 32.40). When a non-*albicans* yeast is present, filaments may be absent. The size and shape of the yeasts observed may also suggest the presence of a non-*albicans* yeast; for example, the budding cells of *C. krusei* are noticeably larger and more elongate than those of *C. albicans*. Isolation and identification of *C. albicans* is simple. At 37°C, on media free of cycloheximide, colonies from swabs and skin samples usually appear within 1–3 days. However, growth from thicker skin and nail material can be slower, so plates should be held for a week before reporting as negative. Chromogenic agars have now been developed that sort species into differentially coloured colonies. On Albicans ID agar, the colonies of *C. albicans* are blue and all other yeasts are cream or white. On Chromagar, colonies

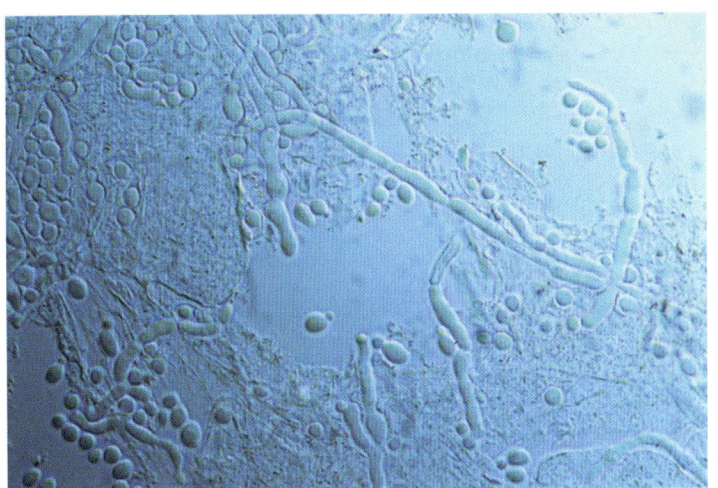

Figure 32.40 Candidosis. Skin scales mounted in 30% KOH, Nomarski illumination, oil. Budding yeasts and slender filaments are observed. Courtesy of the Department of Medical Mycology, St John's Institute of Dermatology, King's College London, London, UK.

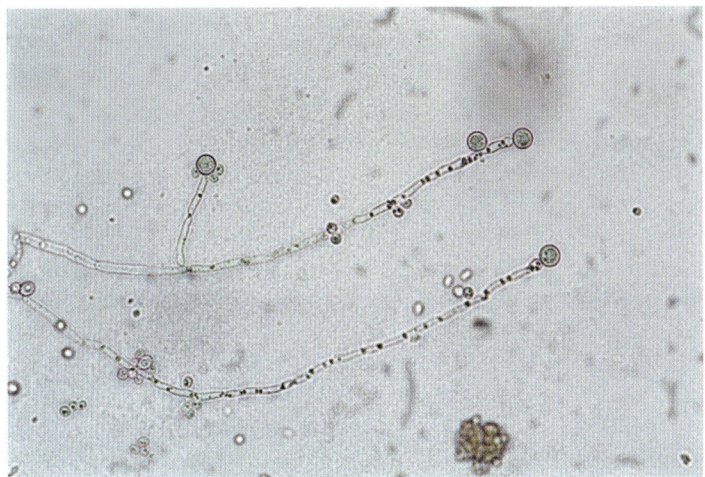

Figure 32.42 Specific identification of *Candida albicans* can be made by the observation of filaments with thick-walled terminal vesicles when cultured on a depleted medium such as rice–agar supplemented with Tween. Courtesy of the Department of Medical Mycology, St John's Institute of Dermatology, King's College London, London, UK.

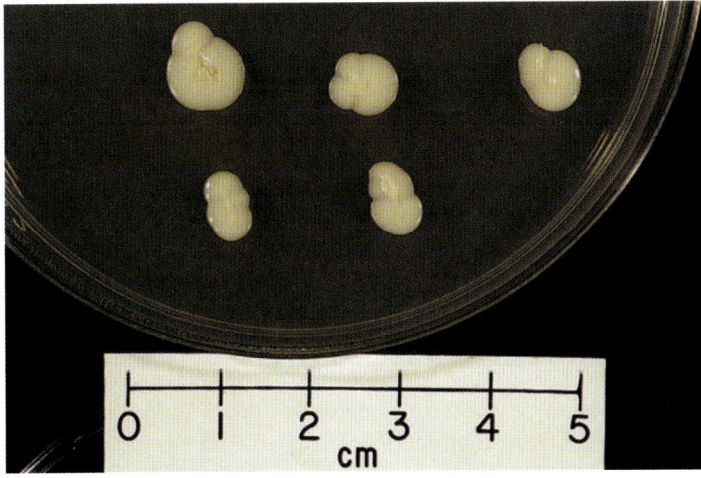

Figure 32.41 *Candida albicans* colonies showing a white to cream colour on glucose–peptone agar. Courtesy of the Department of Medical Mycology, St John's Institute of Dermatology, King's College London, London, UK.

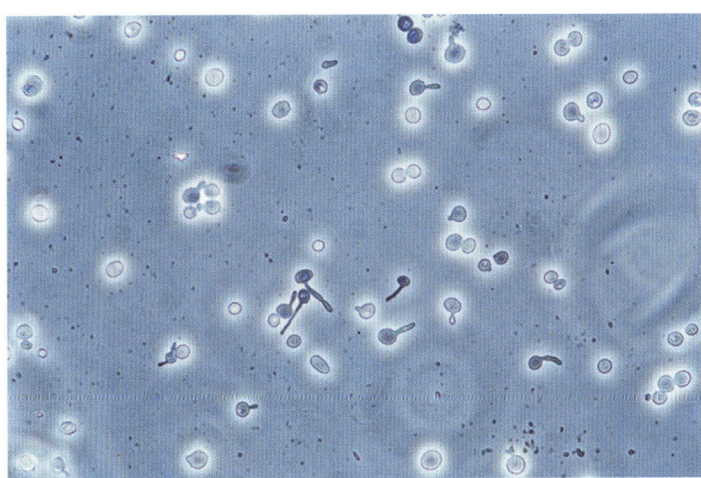

Figure 32.43 A second method for the specific identification of *Candida albicans* is the observation of germ tubes in serum after incubation at 37°C for 2–4 h. Courtesy of the Department of Medical Mycology, St John's Institute of Dermatology, King's College London, London, UK.

of *C. albicans*, *C. tropicalis* and *C. krusei* are green, blue and pink, respectively, although use of these media alone may not be reliable for differentiating species.

Candida albicans. Colony: the colonies on glucose–peptone agar are white to cream and soft in texture (Figure 32.41). Some isolates may produce wrinkled 'rough' colonies and some may produce an obvious fringe of pseudohyphae around the edge of the colony. Microscopy: mounts from primary culture plates will reveal predominantly budding yeast cells. The production of filaments is best examined on depleted media, such as cornmeal agar, or rice extract agar supplemented with Tween 80. The morphology of *C. albicans* on these media allows identification, for in addition to filaments and budding yeasts, *C. albicans* produces rounded refractile vesicles, usually erroneously termed chlamydospores (8–12 μm diameter), at the sides and ends of the filaments (Figure 32.42). These are produced within 24–96 h of incubation at 26°C. *C. albicans* also differs from most other species of *Candida* by the production of rudimentary true hyphae – germ tubes – when lightly inoculated into serum and incubated at 37°C for 2–4 h (Figure 32.43). The only other species that is germ tube positive and produces vesicles on depleted media is *C. dubliniensis*, a yeast originally described as being associated predominantly with oral infections in HIV-positive patients.

Other Candida species. Colony: the different species produce colonies that vary slightly in texture, colour and production of obvious pseudohyphae. With experience, these differences may be recognised on the primary culture plates, but specific identification always requires study both of the morphology and physiology of each isolate. Microscopy: the majority of pathogenic *Candida* species – *C. glabrata* is a notable exception – will produce filaments and budding yeasts, but not chlamydospores, on depleted media, and the appearance of these filaments and yeasts is subtly different and characteristic for each species. The presence or absence of filaments is a key characteristic that is necessary for the identification of all *Candida* yeasts. Physiological tests: a battery of physiological tests, such as sugar and nitrogen source assimilations, and determination of the presence or absence of urease, can be used.

The development of commercial yeast identification systems, such as the API 32C and Auxacolor, have greatly facilitated this task, and such kits are widely used. Recently, mass spectrometry (particularly MALDI-TOF) has increasingly been used for yeast identification. It has become particularly necessary to speciate non-*albicans* yeasts because of the realisation that some of these species may show innate resistance to some antifungals; for example, *C. glabrata* and *C. krusei* are often resistant to fluconazole.

Histology [1,2]

The range of clinical manifestations caused by *C. albicans* and other *Candida* species is paralleled by the variety of pathological changes seen in inflamed tissues. However, there are certain generalisations that can usefully be made about the histology of candidosis of epithelial surfaces. Fungal elements are almost always restricted to the outer layers of epithelium, including the stratum corneum. On the skin, particularly in acute infections, mycelium may be very sparse, and indeed yeast forms may be present in only small numbers. There is also less likelihood of finding mycelium in infectious species other than *C. albicans*.

Apart from the presence of the fungus, acute oral candidosis is characterised by inflammatory changes with the formation of a pseudomembrane of epithelial and inflammatory cells [1]. In the oral epithelium and cutaneous epidermis, the inflammatory infiltrate consists predominantly of polymorphs, which may form microabscesses or subcorneal pustules. Splitting of the epidermis often follows. In the dermis, the inflammatory infiltrate is a mixture of lymphocytes, plasma cells (especially in the mouth) and histiocytes. In chronic cases, hyperplasia with parakeratosis and acanthosis of the epithelium is associated with a mixed, chronic, inflammatory infiltrate. In chronic cutaneous lesions, hyperkeratosis with acanthosis may be seen, and in *Candida* granuloma of the skin, a dense mixed cell infiltrate may include giant cells [3]. Although the matter is still somewhat controversial, it seems probable that in chronic oral cases, neoplastic change secondary to candidosis may develop as a late feature [4].

Management

General principles of management [1]

In the treatment of candidosis it is important to be aware of the necessity of altering both localised and general susceptibility factors. In the mouth, for instance, this involves frequent toilet in the seriously ill and denture hygiene in other patients, whereas in *Candida* infections affecting the skin, careful drying of the affected sites is important. In many cases, topical antifungal therapy alone is sufficient to produce a response, but in immunocompromised patients with oro-pharyngeal candidosis, oral systemic therapy may be necessary to treat concomitant oesophageal infection, as well as being the most effective treatment for oral candidosis in immunosuppressed patients. In addition, oral antifungals are used to prevent systemic candidosis in neutropenic patients. Although the success of this approach is often contested, it is nonetheless a common practice. Apart from these indications, and chronic mucocutaneous candidosis (CMC) and onychomycosis, the main indications for systemic anti-*Candida* therapy are *Candida* septicaemia and deep-seated candidosis. Combination antiretroviral therapy in patients with AIDS improves the therapeutic outcome significantly.

Therapeutic agents

The polyene antibiotics amphotericin and nystatin are effective against *Candida* species and most other yeast pathogens. Even though the polyenes have been used over many years, resistance by *C. albicans* and other *Candida* species to these antibiotics is very rare, with the possible exception of *C. lusitaniae*. They are all safe to use topically, and contact dermatitis is rare. Of these drugs, only amphotericin is used systemically, and this must be given by intravenous infusion. Intravenous lipid-associated amphotericin B compounds, including a liposomal formulation (AmBi-some®, Gilead Sciences Inc., Foster City, CA, USA) and a lipid complex (Abelcet®, Zeneus, Eindhoven, The Netherlands), are also widely used in systemically ill patients. These compounds have the advantage of producing reduced renal toxicity. Gastrointestinal absorption of all the polyenes is limited; after oral administration, only 5–10% is taken up. The other important group of agents effective against *Candida* is the imidazoles. Clotrimazole, miconazole and econazole are the best known in topical use, and significant resistance to them has not developed in *Candida* species [2]. Contact allergy, although reported, seems to be almost as rare as reactions to the polyenes. The most useful oral treatments are the two triazoles, fluconazole [3] and itraconazole [4], that are also effective in these conditions and have the additional advantage that hepatotoxicity, seen with ketoconazole, is exceptionally rare with both drugs. The usual daily doses are itraconazole 100–200 mg and fluconazole 100–400 mg. In addition, fluconazole can be given for systemic candidosis as an intravenous compound. A formulation of itraconazole in cyclodextrin solution provides better absorption in severely immunocompromised patients. Resistance to fluconazole has been reported in HIV, AIDS or CMC patients receiving long-term therapy with the drug [5]. Similarly, primary resistance to fluconazole has been recorded with some *C. albicans* isolates, and particularly with *C. auris*, *C. krusei*, *C. dubliniensis* and *C. glabrata*. However, *Candida* infection and resistance is less common in patients receiving highly active antiretroviral (HAART) therapy [6]. Other azoles active against *Candida* species include voriconazole and posaconazole. Both have been used for severe oro-pharyngeal and oesophageal infection. In addition, caspofungin or anidulomycin, intravenous fungal cell wall inhibitors, are other anti-*Candida* agents used in systemic infections. Multidrug resistance has been seen particularly with *C. auris*.

Flucytosine is an agent that is absorbed from the gut, is relatively safe and very potent against those strains of *Candida* that retain their sensitivity. Unfortunately, resistance developing during treatment is not uncommon and this drug is now only occasionally used for candidosis.

First line

In infants, suspensions of nystatin, amphotericin or miconazole gel applied several times a day are usually adequate for treating oral thrush. In the adult patient, removal of dentures with careful hygiene at night is important. Amphotericin or nystatin lozenges, oral nystatin suspension or miconazole mucoadhesive tablets are effective in non-immunocompromised patients. The duration of the treatment varies with the condition: 10–14 days may be enough in acute cases. For treatment of unresponsive and chronic cases, such as those with hyperplastic candidosis, the responses to topical therapy are often poor, and either fluconazole (100–200 mg/day) [7,8] or itraconazole (100–200 mg/day) [9] are more effective. Voriconazole or posaconazole are alternatives. In patients with chronic oral candidosis, a biopsy may be justified to exclude leukoplakia. Angular stomatitis usually responds to treatment of the primary oral condition, although a topical antifungal applied to the area may speed recovery.

Oral candidosis in immunosuppressed patients frequently fails to respond to topical polyene therapy. In these conditions, the best approach is to use itraconazole [10] or fluconazole [11,12]. If possible, therapy should be given for short courses because of the risk of resistance developing with continuous therapy. Treatment is usually given until there is symptomatic recovery, which is usually quicker with fluconazole than the capsule formulation of itraconazole. A solution of itraconazole is an alternative to the capsule form and a new and better absorbed itraconazole formulation (Lozanoc) is available in some countries. Posaconazole or voriconazole are alternative treatments for these patients too.

CANDIDOSIS OF THE ORAL MUCOUS MEMBRANES

Candida is not uncommonly found in the normal mouth but candidosis is more likely to develop when there is local or general immunosuppression [1]. Apart from systemic steroid therapy, local applications of steroids in the form of steroid creams, mouthwashes and lozenges for the treatment of aphthosis or lichen planus of the mouth or steroid aerosols for asthma may predispose to candidosis, sometimes occurring as a secondary invasion of the primary pathology.

Candida can secondarily invade other oral conditions such as ulcerative lichen planus [2], leukokeratosis and white-sponge naevus. On the lips, invasion of traumatic cheilitis may complicate management. In all cases, the removal of *Candida* often speeds the recovery even though the yeast is only a contributory cause.

Acute pseudomembranous candidosis

Definition and nomenclature
The characteristic sign of this condition is a sharply defined patch of creamy, crumbly, curd-like, white pseudomembrane, which, when removed, leaves an underlying red base [3,4].

Synonyms and inclusions
- Oral thrush
- Acute pseudomembranous candidiasis
- Candidal stomatitis

Pathophysiology
Predisposing factors
It occurs most commonly in the first weeks of life and the preterm infant may be especially susceptible. Apart from in neonatal oral candidosis (as distinct from *Candida* carriage), acute pseudomembranous candidosis is usually secondary to local or general predisposing factors, notably in the neutropenic patient or those with HIV/AIDS [5–7] or IL-17 inhibitor therapy.

Pathology
The pseudomembrane consists of desquamated epithelial cells, fibrin, leukocytes and fungal mycelium that attaches it to the inflamed epithelium.

Clinical features
There may be one or many patches. The buccal epithelium on the cheeks, gums or palate may be affected. In immunocompromised patients with neutropenia or HIV/AIDS, the extension of lesions to the buccal mucosa, tongue and oesophagus is common. Erosion and ulceration are occasional complications and can lead to inadequate food intake due to pain. Coincidental oral infection with herpes simplex virus may occur in this group of patients [8]. Oral candidosis is the most common secondary infection in those with HIV/AIDS and recurrent or more prolonged episodes are to be expected in these patients [9].

Acute erythematous candidosis

Definition and nomenclature
In this condition, there is soreness and denuded, atrophic, red mucous membranes, particularly on the dorsum of the tongue [10]. It may follow pseudomembranous candidosis when traces of the residual membrane will often be found.

Synonyms and inclusions
- Acute atrophic oral candidiasis
- Antibiotic sore tongue

Pathophysiology
It is especially associated with antibacterial antibiotic therapy but may also develop in HIV-positive subjects and patients taking inhaled steroids. In these cases, the tongue is often markedly affected.

Chronic pseudomembranous candidosis

Definition
This does not differ clinically from the acute pseudomembranous variety but, as the name suggests, lesions are very persistent. It occurs principally in immunocompromised patients.

Chronic erythematous candidosis

Definition and nomenclature
Some soreness in the epithelium in the denture-bearing area is said to affect nearly one-quarter of all denture wearers and most, if not all cases appear to be caused by candidosis [11]. A similar problem may also occur in children wearing orthodontic appliances.

Synonyms and inclusions
- Chronic atrophic candidiasis
- Denture sore mouth
- Denture stomatitis

Epidemiology
The excess of female patients over males remains unexplained.

Pathophysiology
The elimination of *Candida* alone does not usually result in complete recovery, and it is likely that other factors such as chronic mechanical irritation and bacterial colonisation have a role in the pathogenesis of this condition.

Pathology
The epithelium is often shiny and atrophic, and there may be marked oedema, in some areas at least. In late cases, secondary papillomatosis may occur.

Clinical features
The condition is normally confined to the upper denture-bearing area, the palate and the gums. The affected mucous membranes show a variable bright or dusky red, fairly sharply defined at the margin of the denture. There is often an associated angular cheilitis and that is the feature that frequently brings the patient to seek dental or medical advice, for the symptoms from the palatal area are often minimal.

Co-morbidities
The vast majority of patients of either sex are otherwise fit. Underlying defects of immunity are not to be expected in this syndrome. However, HIV/AIDS patients with erythematous candidosis may enter a chronic phase.

Chronic plaque-like candidosis

Definition and nomenclature
Very persistent, firm, irregular, white plaques occur in the mouth, commonly on the cheek or the tongue [12].

Synonyms and inclusions
- Chronic hyperplastic candidiasis
- *Candida* leukoplakia

Epidemiology
Most patients are male and generally over the age of 30 years.

Pathophysiology
In most cases, serious predisposing factors are not present, although this appearance, particularly an extensive form, may occur in patients with chronic mucocutaneous candidosis. Smokers appear to be particularly prone to developing this form of oral candidosis [13].

Clinical features
The onset of the disorder is difficult to date, as symptoms are mild, with only slight soreness and roughness being noticed. Around the hyperplastic area, there may be a red margin. Unlike the pseudomembrane of oral thrush, this plaque cannot be easily removed.

Differential diagnosis
The significance of this condition lies in the fact that it must be differentiated from other types of leukoplakia as, although the affected areas may undergo malignant change [14,15], it may eventually clear with prolonged anti-*Candida* therapy.

Chronic nodular candidosis

Definition
This is a rare form of oral candidosis, where the clinical appearance that usually affects the tongue is cobbled. It is most often seen in certain patients with chronic mucocutaneous candidosis.

Angular cheilitis

Definition and nomenclature
Soreness at the angles of the mouth extending outwards in the folds of the facial skin is a well-known syndrome, not always associated with *Candida* infection [16].

Synonyms and inclusions
- Angular stomatitis
- Perlèche

Pathophysiology
It is perhaps best considered as an intertrigo in which different organisms may play a part, *Candida* being the most common. Nutritional status and mechanical factors (e.g. the depth of the fold), the presence of moisture from persistent salivation or licking the lips may also be important. The association with oral infection is important.

Clinical features
Although the condition may present acutely, it is common to find a long history of soreness and cracking at the angles of the mouth

and a fluctuating course is typical. Obviously, the oral cavity should be examined carefully in such cases and swabs taken from that site to establish the presence of *Candida* carriage, as well as from the affected skin at the angles.

Median rhomboid glossitis

This is an acquired condition, characterised by a more-or-less diamond-shaped area on the dorsum of the tongue with loss of papillae. It has been regarded in the past as a developmental abnormality but current opinion suggests that it is simply a variant of chronic plaque-like candidosis [17].

CANDIDOSIS OF THE SKIN AND GENITAL MUCOUS MEMBRANES

Most cases of cutaneous candidosis occur in the skin folds or where occlusion from clothing or medical dressings produces abnormally moist conditions. Areas close to the body orifices [1] and the fingers, which are frequently contaminated with saliva, are also at risk.

Candida *intertrigo*

Definition and nomenclature
Any skin fold may be affected, especially in the obese subject.

Synonyms and inclusions
- Flexural candidosis

Clinical features
Signs are typically redness with a little moist exudation starting deep in the fold (Figure 32.44). Redness is more subtle in skin types IV–VI. As the condition develops, it spreads beyond the area of contact, usually developing the typical features of candidosis with an irregular edge and subcorneal pustules rupturing to give tiny erosions, and then further peeling of the stratum corneum. Satellite lesions, pustular or papular, are classic. Soreness, and itching, which may on occasion be intense, is usual. Topical steroids, prescribed for relief of the latter symptoms, may modify the inflammatory signs and cause diagnostic confusion. Where the web spaces of the toes or fingers are affected, marked maceration with a thick, white, horny layer is usually prominent. In the case of the hands, some abnormality, including wide, fat fingers, appears to predispose to infection. In this particular syndrome (erosio interdigitalis blastomycetica or interdigital candidosis), *Candida* and Gram-negative bacteria are often co-pathogens [2]. Similar interdigital infections of the feet may occur in very hot climates, particularly in those with heavy footwear, for example army personnel. Apart from skin folds, macerated skin under rings and dressings may become infected with *Candida*.

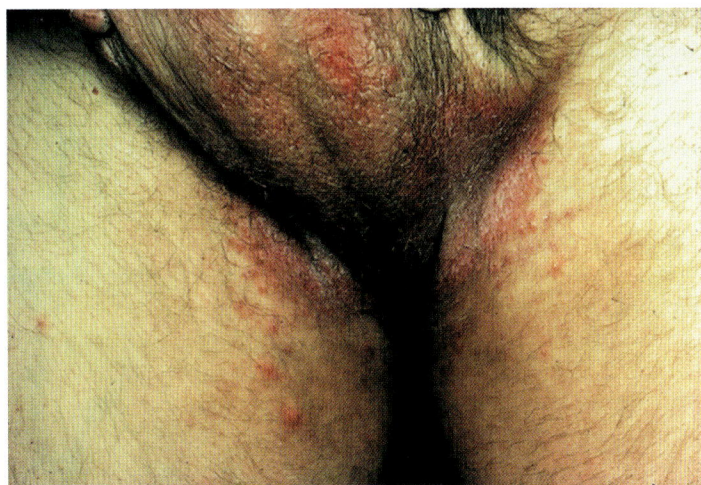

Figure 32.44 *Candida* infection of the groin.

Differential diagnosis
The differential diagnosis of intertriginous candidosis includes tinea, seborrhoeic dermatitis, bacterial intertrigo, flexural psoriasis, Hailey–Hailey disease and flexural Darier disease.

Investigations
It is important to establish that *Candida* species are present by taking a scraping or swab. Although it is useful to find mycelia, their absence does not exclude the diagnosis, and the culture of *Candida* from an inflamed lesion of a skin fold usually justifies instigation of anti-*Candida* treatment. Bacterial co-pathogens should be considered.

Management
First line
Candida intertrigo requires specific topical therapy (azole or polyene creams) usually continued for about 2 weeks, but treatment may be required for longer periods, and is likely to fail if attention is not given to drying the affected area. In some patients with moist *Candida* intertrigo, potassium permanganate soaks are more effective. Attention should be given to treating concomitant bacteria; once again, potassium permanganate is useful for this purpose. In finger or toe web infections, topical antifungal therapy, combined with the use of open footwear in the case of infections of the feet, is appropriate.

Vulvo-vaginal candidosis

Definition and nomenclature
This condition affects around 75% of women of child-bearing age and presents with itching and soreness, and with a thick, creamy white discharge [1,3]. Most women with vulvo-vaginal candidosis (VVC) have no evidence of underlying disease. See also Chapter 110.

Synonyms and inclusions
- Vulvo-vaginal thrush

Epidemiology
It is more common in pregnancy. In the non-pregnant, it is said to be more prevalent in the premenstruum, but a fluctuating course not clearly related to the menstrual cycle is frequent. Although commoner in sexually active subjects, it has been described in childhood and sexually inexperienced and elderly people.

Clinical features
Typically, there is reddening of the vaginal mucosa and the vulval skin, with curdy white flecks of discharge, but on occasion the only sign is reddening. The rash may extend onto the perineum and into the groin. The perianal area is often affected. In extensive cases, subcorneal pustules may be seen peripherally. In pregnancy, the picture is modified by marked physiological leukorrhoea.

Differential diagnosis
Trichomonas infection (although it usually produces watery brown discharge) and bacterial vulvovaginitis should both be considered in the differential diagnosis, and in pregnancy, physiological leukorrhoea. Dermatoses affecting the vulva may mimic this condition (e.g. psoriasis, contact dermatitis, lichen sclerosus).

Disease course and prognosis
Candidal vulvovaginitis may become recurrent and in around 5% of women it appears to be a chronic condition [3]. In chronic cases, the vaginal mucosa may become glazed and atrophic. There may be considerable vaginal soreness or irritation as well as dyspareunia.

Investigations
Management of the recurrent or chronic case is difficult; the condition causes considerable distress. It is important in such patients to evaluate the presence of *Candida* during repeated episodes where there are symptoms, to establish that recurrence of disease signs is associated with recurrence of *Candida* as other causes of vaginosis or *Chlamydia* infection are often confused. Molecular typing of isolates from women suffering from recurrent episodes has demonstrated that in most cases the same strain is responsible for the recurrences, suggesting that clearance of the organism was not achieved by standard courses of antifungal therapy [3,4]. Recently, deficiencies in IL-22 and *IDO1* gene products have been associated with susceptibility to recurrent VVC [5]. It is important to speciate isolates in recurrent VVC as non-*albicans* species that are treatment resistant such as *C. glabrata* may cause this infection. Although vaginal candidosis has been reported to occur with an increased frequency in women with HIV/AIDS, and in some cases the infection is resistant to therapy, this is not always the case; many patients present with an acute and treatable episode. In this it differs from oral candidosis.

Management
Acute vulvovaginitis can be treated with a single-dose topical preparation (pessary or ovule) such as clotrimazole, econazole or isoconazole. Longer courses of these compounds (e.g. 14 days), as well as polyenes such as nystatin, are also available in some countries. If there is coexistent involvement of the skin, a topically applied cream should also be used. However, single-day oral therapy with fluconazole 150 mg is widely available and both effective and convenient; itraconazole 600 mg is an alternative. Efficacy is similar to that seen with topical drugs.

Candidal balanitis

Definition
The skin of the glans penis, especially in the uncircumcised, may sometimes be colonised by *Candida* asymptomatically [6]. When candidal balanitis develops, it is usual to find either abundant vaginal *Candida* carriage or frank vulvovaginitis in the sexual partner, although this is variable.

Clinical features
In the mildest cases, transient tiny papules or pustules develop on the glans penis a few hours after intercourse and rupture, leaving a peeling edge. Some may settle spontaneously without going through the full evolution. This mild form is usually associated with a little soreness and irritation. In some men, the condition continues in this intermittent form. In more severe and chronic cases, the inflammatory changes become persistent over the glans and the prepuce (Chapter 109). Involvement of the groin sometimes coexists, especially in hot weather.

Differential diagnosis
In the case of balanitis, bacteria and herpes simplex require consideration, but few of the common sexually transmitted diseases are episodic in the way that candidosis is. Psoriasis and lichen planus, although sometimes fluctuating, should not be a cause of confusion, except with the chronic established lesion, in which case plasma cell balanitis and erythroplasia must be excluded, as must lichen sclerosus.

Investigations
The diagnosis in both sexes is confirmed by finding the organism, preferably in large numbers. However, even scanty amounts of *Candida* isolated from cases with typical clinical features demand active and sometimes prolonged therapy. In the male, failure to find the organism does not exclude the diagnosis if swabs or scrapings were not taken during the acute phase. It is wise to consider diabetes in cases of genital yeast infections, as florid persistent or recurrent lesions spreading beyond the genitalia seem most likely to be associated with that condition.

Management
Balanitis usually responds satisfactorily to topical antifungals applied several times a day, but if there is a source of infection in the sexual partner this should be treated appropriately and diabetes, if discovered, obviously requires management. Conjugal cases need simultaneous and often prolonged therapy.

Perianal and scrotal candidosis

Perianal and scrotal candidosis may occur with, or independently of, genital involvement (Chapter 109). Although usually starting around the anal margin with non-specific redness, soreness and irritation, subsequent spread along the natal cleft is common, with classic features developing as it extends. Involvement of the scrotum is usually in the form of a nondescript redness and subcorneal pustules are rarely seen. Candidosis must be included in the differential diagnosis of unexplained reddening of scrotal skin. Secondary infection of flexural psoriasis with *Candida* may have to be considered.

It has been suggested that a more objective assessment can be provided by taking quantitative cultures to determine the density of *Candida* more accurately [7]. For practical purposes this is not necessary, and dense growth of organisms on a swab culture or the presence of diagnostic clinical features such as satellite pustules are usually taken as indications for treatment.

Perineal candidosis of infancy

Definition and nomenclature
Candida albicans is commonly isolated from the moist skin of the buttocks and genitalia of the infant but is more prevalent where the skin is affected by napkin rash [7]. In some instances, the classic subcorneal pustules, a fringed irregular border and satellite lesions are found.

Synonyms and inclusions
- Diaper candidiasis
- Nappy candidiasis

Pathophysiology
In florid cases, there is little doubt that the organism is playing a pathogenic part, and it is likely to be found in the faeces [7,8]. In other nondescript cases of napkin area eruption from which the organism is isolated, the role of the yeast is in doubt. Steroid creams applied to this site not only modify the clinical features but they predispose to *Candida*. Moreover, if the bacterial flora has been suppressed by a topical antibiotic, this will also favour yeast growth. All these factors should be considered in any napkin rash.

Differential diagnosis
In acrodermatitis enteropathica, in which zinc deficiency plays a central role, there may be a secondary *Candida* infection, particularly of the napkin area.

Investigations
In all but the most trivial cases of napkin rash, a moistened swab or a scraping should be taken to discover whether or not *Candida* is present on the affected skin. If *Candida* is present, particularly in large numbers, even if the features are non-specific, a trial of anti-*Candida* therapy is generally indicated.

Management
First line
In infants, rashes in the napkin area should be investigated for *Candida* and, if present, this can be treated topically. The antifungal should be combined with a general regimen for napkin dermatitis, with frequent nappy changes. In seborrhoeic dermatitis, a weak topical steroid is appropriate for the disseminated dry lesions, but steroids should be avoided on the napkin area itself.

Nodular or granulomatous candidosis of the napkin area

Definition and nomenclature
This rare condition presents with an eruption over the buttocks, genitalia, upper thighs and pubis, within which develop nodules, sometimes as large as 2 cm across. These are bluish or brownish in colour and are reminiscent of Kaposi sarcoma [9,10].

Synonyms and inclusions
- Granuloma gluteale infantum

Pathophysiology
Histological changes are those of an intense dermal infiltrate with lymphocytes, eosinophils and histiocytes.

Clinical features
The primary napkin dermatitis may clear leaving only the nodules. Some examples have marked scaling and hyperkeratosis over the lesions, in others the epidermis appears to be normal. The natural history of this condition has not been elucidated.

Management
Successful management involves the removal of microorganisms, the avoidance of topical steroids and general measures to ensure adequate dryness in the region.

CANDIDOSIS OF THE NAIL AND PARONYCHIUM

Candida *paronychia*

Definition
Candida paronychium is a *Candida* infection of the nail fold.

Pathophysiology
Candida species, not always *C. albicans*, can be isolated from the majority of cases of chronic paronychia (Chapter 93) [1,2]. The yeast is thought to have an aetiological role in this condition, but bacteria and irritant or allergic contact dermatitis also play a part, although the contribution of each varies from patient to patient and with the chronicity of the disease.

Predisposing factors
This condition is chiefly found among those whose hands are frequently immersed in water. In chefs and pastry cooks, the presence of organic debris such as flour and other carbohydrates may be equally important. Toenail folds are not usually affected. Some experimental confirmation of the role of *Candida* has been

achieved by occluding the nail fold in the presence of the yeast, but fully developed, chronic paronychia has not been produced experimentally.

Clinical features

Typically, several fingers are chronically infected, but one or all may be involved. The nail fold is red and swollen, and there is loss of the cuticle and detachment of the nail fold from the dorsal surface of the nail plate, leading to pocketing. Occasionally, thick white pus may discharge; often force is needed to express it. The patient usually has marked tenderness and spontaneous pain is an occasional feature. Nail dystrophy with buckling of the nail plate and some discoloration and onycholysis around the lateral nail plate frequently occur, but massive destruction of the plate except in patients with chronic mucocutaneous candidosis is rare (see section on this disease later in the chapter). Many patients, particularly those who are resistant to treatment, appear to have a poor peripheral circulation. A link with psoriasis has been reported [3].

Treatment ladder for *Candida* paronychia

First line
- Azole solution twice daily for 2–4 months depending on clinical response
- Plus in chronic cases a medium strength topical steroid applied to the nail fold skin once daily
  or
- Itraconazole 100 mg daily for 1–2 months
- Fluconazole 100 mg daily for 1–2 months

Second line
- 4% thymol solution

Management
First line

Candida paronychia requires prolonged topical therapy with frequent applications of polyenes, imidazoles or non-specific remedies, such as 4% thymol in chloroform. Lotions are probably preferable to creams. There have been few studies of either itraconazole or fluconazole although they are effective in many cases of paronychia. Whatever anti-*Candida* regimen is chosen, it must be followed by general measures such as ensuring adequate drying of the hands. Even so, relapse is common in many patients, particularly in the chronic phases of paronychia. The continuing role of *Candida* is more contentious and other factors such as irritant or allergic contact dermatitis may play a part in the ongoing inflammatory response. For this reason, in chronic cases, the addition of a topical corticosteroid is a logical approach.

Candida *onychomycosis*

Definition

Candida onychomycosis is an infection of the nail plate caused by *Candida* species.

Pathophysiology
Predisposing factors

Two important predisposing conditions are Raynaud phenomenon or disease and Cushing syndrome.

Causative organism

The main clues that the yeast is a significant pathogen are erosion of the distal nail plate, the presence of yeasts and hyphae in the nail on direct microscopy and the isolation of *C. albicans*.

Clinical features

There are three main manifestations of *Candida* infection of the nail apparatus [4]. The most common is distal and lateral subungual onychomycosis (DLSO) associated with paronychia. Complete destruction of the nail plate is also seen in some patients with chronic mucocutaneous candidosis. In addition to these conditions, erosion of the distal and lateral nail plate of the fingernails, not usually progressing to total nail dystrophy, has been associated with *C. albicans* invasion of the nail [5]. This is not common, but when it occurs it is most often seen in women. Very rarely, *Candida* may invade the nail plate in the neonatal period, sometimes causing an isolated nail dystrophy with evidence of penetration of the superior aspect of the nail plate. In addition to these conditions, *Candida* is not infrequently isolated from the undersurface of the nail plate in patients with onycholysis resulting from other causes. Antifungal therapy in these circumstances does not produce any improvement.

See also the sections on onychomycosis caused by dermatophytes and onychymycosis caused by other non-dermatophyte moulds in this chapter.

Investigations

It is usual in chronic paronychia to establish which organisms are present, and a platinum loop introduced into the nail fold may be more valuable than a swab for this. It must be plated out promptly. When nail plate involvement is suspected, clippings should be taken.

Management

In proven *Candida* onychomycosis, fluconazole or itraconazole produce the best reponses [6].

OTHER *CANDIDA* DISEASES

Congenital candidosis

Definition and nomenclature

This, as the name implies, represents established candidosis, usually of the skin and birth membranes present at the time of birth, and following intrauterine infection [7].

Synonyms and inclusions
- Neonatal candidiasis

Pathophysiology

Factors associated with this condition have included prematurity and the presence of an intrauterine foreign body, usually a contraceptive device. It is believed to follow contamination of the skin surface during birth, and the high incidence of intrauterine infection or vaginal candidosis associated with this disease would support this contention. Such cases are distinct from the more common neonatal systemic candidosis, a septicaemic illness associated with extreme prematurity, where skin involvement is not common.

Clinical features

The amniotic fluid may be turbid at delivery [7,8]. The skin is the most common site for lesions, which are usually present at birth. The lesions are typically discrete vesicles or pustules on a red base. The face and chest are first affected by the rash, which generally spreads over the next few days after delivery. In over 10% there is evidence of spread to deep sites such as the lungs.

Disease course and prognosis

Although there has been a high level of mortality reported with such cases, the cause of death is usually related to other complications of prematurity rather than candidosis per se.

Management

In candidosis of the skin present at birth, topical therapy alone is required, but where there is systemic involvement, clearly amphotericin B or fluconazole should be considered.

Candida *allergy*

In normal subjects, skin testing for *Candida* antigens and serological studies may reveal evidence of antibodies to *C. albicans* and to other *Candida* species [1]. A variety of clinical features attributed to *Candida* allergy have been described and include urticaria, ordinary annular erythema, bullous annular erythema and generalised pruritus. Even palmoplantar pustulosis has been linked to delayed hypersensitivity to *Candida* antigen.

The term *Candida* allergy or *Candida* syndrome is also used to describe a constellation of symptoms ranging from headache to malaise and depression, allegedly secondary to colonisation of the gastro-intestinal tract with yeasts. However, there is no objective scientific evidence to connect these symptoms with the presence or absence of *Candida*.

Chronic mucocutaneous candidosis

Definition

Persistent *Candida* infection of the mouth, the skin and the nails, refractory to conventional topical therapy, is a distinct clinical pattern of infection. Sometimes it is associated with a variety of other infections, both cutaneous and systemic [1,2]. Many cases form part of the autoimmune polyendocrinopathy *Candida* ectodermal dystrophy syndrome (APECED) or CMC associated with hypothyroidism.

Pathophysiology

Patients with this syndrome comprise a heterogeneous group, which was originally classified [1,2] into several distinct categories using genetic and clinical criteria. It is probably best to exclude from the syndrome of chronic mucocutaneous candidosis those patients who present with a well-documented, underlying immune defect, such as severe combined immunodeficiency or agammaglobulinaemia, where severe candidosis may form a minor part of the secondary infectious complications. In these patients, mucosal candidosis is usually overshadowed by other serious infections, such as recurrent pneumonia or aspergillosis. In contrast, in patients with CMC, the skin and mucous membrane infections dominate the clinical pattern [3]. It is important to recognise that some patients with this syndrome may develop other infections, most commonly human papilloma virus infections (warts) and dermatophytosis, particularly those with associated hypothyroidism, in addition to other features, such as recurrent aphthous ulcers, seborrhoeic dermatitis and alopecia areata.

Most CMC patients develop signs in early childhood, and usually *Candida* infection is the presenting feature [4]. While a number of different forms of immune defect have been described in these patients [5], the abnormalities are neither constant nor diagnostic and may reverse with antifungal therapy. Within the childhood-onset group there are a number of different variants that show features in common. Such features should not be taken as inflexible markers of a particular type, as there is probably considerable overlap in clinical expression between the different groups. The different types are as follows but as genetic studies progress it is likely that more patients may be found to have underlying mutations:

1 *Autosomal recessive CMC* [6]. This usually starts in the first decade with persistent oral and nail plate infections. Generally, the health of these patients is good and they do not develop endocrine defects. They also tend to improve with increasing age.
2 *Autosomal dominant CMC* [7]. There are now a number of well-documented pedigrees of families with the dominant form of CMC. Generally, they are more severely affected than those with the recessive variety, and other infections, such as dermatophytosis, may be particularly troublesome.
3 *Idiopathic CMC* [2]. Some of the original group of patients labelled as 'idiopathic' have now produced affected offspring, and it is likely that some of these patients belong to the autosomal dominant group. Indeed, it is not possible to exclude the possibility that all may eventually be classified in this group. However, it remains a useful subgroup to describe patients, who may have other infections and often develop bronchiectasis and pulmonary bullae. Their candidosis is also very severe, with oesophageal involvement and the appearance of 'granulomas'. The term *Candida* granuloma was originally used to describe the condition suffered by these severely affected patients, who may produce sheets of hyperkeratosis caused by *Candida* infection on the skin and scalp. In practice, the main histological features are hyperkeratosis with only an occasional granuloma in the dermis. Rarely, patients have been reported from this group who develop other systemic diseases, such as cryptococcosis or miliary tuberculosis. Survival into adult life is still not universal in these children.

4 *CMC associated with endocrinopathy*:
   (a) Many of these patients appear to have the familial polyendocrinopathy syndrome [8,9]. Mutations of the autoimmune regulator gene appear to be correlated with this syndrome in many cases [9]. The condition is usually seen in early childhood, and occasionally the onset of *Candida* infection may predate the appearance of endocrine disease by as much as 10 years. The main cluster of endocrine abnormalities is hypoparathyroidism with hypoadrenocorticalism. In addition, other autoimmune abnormalities can occur, such as pernicious anaemia, vitiligo [10] and ovarian failure. This condition is also inherited as an autosomal recessive condition [11]. The severity of the patient's candidosis is variable, and it is not uncommon to find that one affected sibling has extensive infection while another has only mild but chronic oral candidiasis. This variety is associated with mutations in the autoimmune regulator gene pathway.
   (b) A further group of CMC patients has CMC with associated hypothyroidism [12] and type 1 diabetes. The inheritance of this abnormality is vertical, suggesting autosomal dominant transmission. The clinical features are similar to those of other patients with endocrinopathy but associated skin infections, including severe dermatophytosis, are more common. It is important to recognise this group in view of the different genetic risk. This form is associated with mutations in the *STAT1* gene [13].
5 *Late-onset CMC* [14,15]. Occasionally, adult patients are found to have the syndrome of CMC. The best documented cases have been associated with a thymoma [16], but the occasional sporadic infection in a patient with no detectable abnormality may be recognised. Patients with systemic lupus erythematosus occasionally develop the severe nail changes and oral manifestations of this condition. The sudden onset of chronic oral candidosis in an adult should be investigated as it may be the initial presentation of another condition such as HIV infection. Vaginal candidosis can occur but does not become chronic in these patients.

As genetic studies of patients with CMC continue it is possible that many patients with the first three types will be reclassified as belonging to the groups 4A and 4B with underlying endocrinopathy but with incomplete penetrance of clinical expression. One family group with CMC has been found to have no endocrinopathy but mutations in the *CARD9* gene [17].

Immunological abnormalities [3]

It is still not possible to correlate precisely defects of immune function with different clinical variants of the CMC syndrome. Indeed, with current investigative techniques, some cases have no demonstrable defect of immune function at all [4]. To date, a variety of defects of T-cell mediated immunity have been shown to be important. Defects of phagocytosis or killing in both macrophages and polymorphs, and defective Th17 cell responses have been found in patients with the chronic mucocutaneous syndrome. Raised levels of neutralising autoantibodies to INF-α subtypes have also been detected in a high proportion of patients with *Candida* endocrinopathy [5].

In addition, it is known that certain antigenic components of *C. albicans*, such as glycopeptides, are immunomodulatory [18].

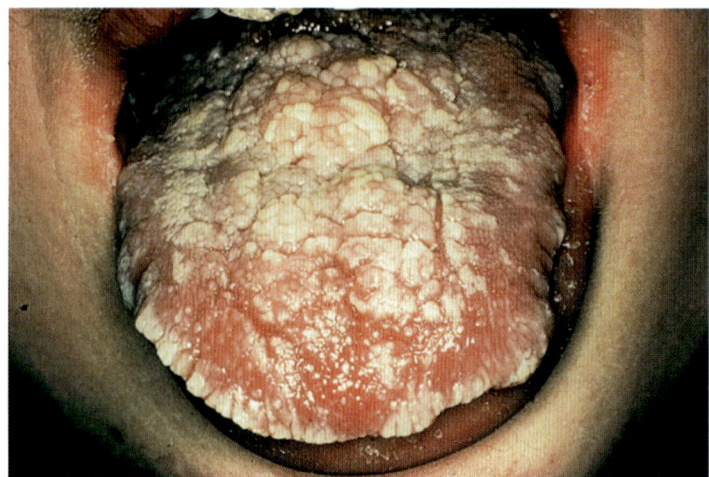

Figure 32.45 Chronic oral candidosis.

Reversal of some immune defects has been seen with successful clearance of candidosis in CMC patients.

Clinical features [1]

With minor variations, the syndrome consists of the following features, usually starting in infancy or early childhood:
1 Persistent oral thrush, responding only partially to conventional therapy, or relapsing promptly after apparently successful treatment. Chronic hypertrophic changes may follow (Figure 32.45). In other mucosal sites, although balanitis may occur, vulvovaginal candidiasis is less common.
2 Cutaneous candidosis. Often intertriginous skin is involved, but also the face and the hands, and sometimes the condition is widespread over the trunk and limbs. In longstanding lesions, the cutaneous changes are often atypical, suggesting ringworm. In some patients, markedly thickened areas with gross hyperkeratosis may form. However, lesions may also develop as deep dermal nodules or small macules. Scalp involvement is not rare in this syndrome. Dermatophytosis in such patients may present in a similar manner.
3 Paronychia is commonly a feature, often with extensive nail plate invasion and total dystrophic onychomycosis [16]. The important findings are nail invasion at an early age, often proceeding to complete nail involvement (Figure 32.46). Here, the nail plate is thickened and the whole terminal phalanx may become encased in hyperkeratotic infected skin.
4 Seborrhoeic dermatitis can be very persistent in some patients. Alopecia areata, vitiligo and other organ-specific inflammation such as keratitis are seen in patients with endocrinopathy.

Investigations

The diagnosis of this condition normally requires the elapse of time and a repeated failure to respond to conservative treatment. Confusion may occur with persistent ringworm infections, and indeed in some reported cases candidosis and dermatophytosis have coexisted. A family history is of obvious importance and special note should be taken of other infections, cutaneous or systemic. Full endocrine investigation is also indicated.

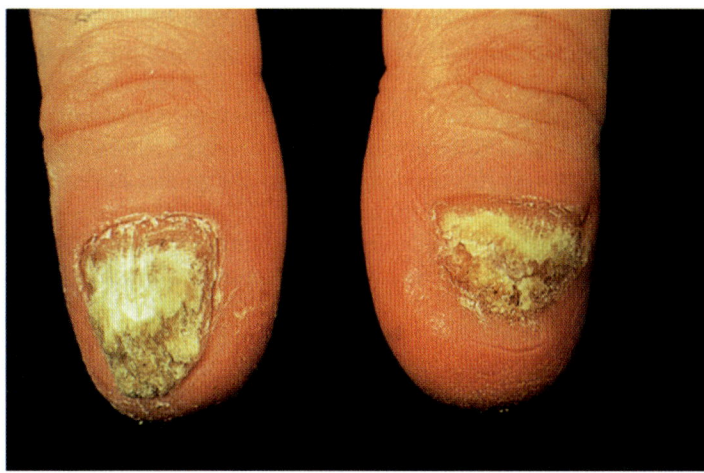

Figure 32.46 Candida onychomycosis in a patient with chronic mucocutaneous candidosis.

Management
First line
Treatment of this condition depends on antifungal chemotherapy [19]. Attempts have been made to restore T-cell function by the use of: (i) transfer factor [20]; (ii) thymosin; (iii) grafting compatible lymphocytes from blood or marrow; (iv) grafting fetal thymic tissue [21]; and (v) non-specific measures such as the restoration of normal iron stores when these are defective. Systemic anti-*Candida* therapy with fluconazole, itraconazole or voriconazole is usually necessary, and treatment may have to be prolonged and repeated.

Once a remission has been induced, maintenance therapy should be avoided where possible in view of the risk of antifungal resistance. Attention must be given to treating endocrine deficiencies, although such treatment does not lead to improvement in the candidosis. Endocrine screening tests should be repeated, even if initially negative, as patients with endocrinopathy may develop endocrine disease years after the first appearance of candidosis. Where appropriate, parents should be given genetic counselling. The possibility of coexisting dermatophytosis should not be forgotten, but it usually responds satisfactorily to oral treatment with itraconazole or terbinafine.

SUBCUTANEOUS MYCOSES

Subcutaneous mycoses, or mycoses of implantation, are sporadically occurring infections caused by fungi present in the natural environment that are directly inoculated into the dermis or subcutaneous tissue through a penetrating injury. They are seldom common even in endemic areas and are mainly seen in the tropics, although, as many have long incubation periods, they may be seen in countries outside these endemic areas in patients who were originally infected elsewhere. Mycetoma, chromoblastomycosis and sporotrichosis are now listed as neglected tropical diseases (NTDs) or skin NTDs by the World Health Organization (WHO).

Classification

The most common of these infections are sporotrichosis, mycetoma and chromoblastomycosis. Rarer infections are phaeohyphomycosis, lobomycosis, rhinosporidiosis and subcutaneous mycosis caused by *Conidiobolus* or *Basidobolus*.

General description

The diagnosis of subcutaneous mycoses is made initially by direct examination and examination of histopathological sections. Culture is not necessarily difficult, but identification of the more unusual pathogens may require the help of a reference mycological laboratory. Additionally, some isolates, particularly from cases of eumycotic mycetoma and phaeohyphomycosis, may fail to sporulate on primary isolation and special media or conditions of incubation may be required to encourage conidial production. The description of all the potential pathogens is outside the scope of this chapter, although brief descriptions of the most common isolates are included. Molecular identification methods are increasingly available, but usually only in specialist centres.

Identification

Collection of samples
Materials from patients thought to have subcutaneous mycoses are obtained from a variety of sources. Occasionally, superficial scrapings from a lesion may be useful, but generally pus or exudates discharging or obtained by aspiration, and biopsies, ideally both from the edge and from the centre of the lesion, are required for satisfactory diagnosis. All samples are placed in sterile containers for immediate despatch to the laboratory. To prevent drying out of the material tissue, biopsy specimens intended for culture must be placed in sterile saline or wrapped in moistened sterile gauze if they cannot be processed immediately. Delays in processing samples will increase the likelihood of bacteria or saprophytic fungi contaminating the samples.

Direct examination and histopathology
A simple potassium hydroxide mount may be enough to give a preliminary diagnosis in some cases. For example, typical organisms may be observed in superficial crusts from chromoblastomycosis lesions, and pus containing grains from mycetoma patients can be used to immediately differentiate fungi from actinomycetes. Generally, histopathology will be more informative. Of the specific fungal stains, the silver impregnation procedure (Grocott–Gomori stain) and PAS are most commonly used and give excellent results. However, in some instances, examination with haematoxylin and eosin (H&E) is valuable to determine whether the infecting fungus is naturally pigmented (dematiaceous). Details of the appearances of individual mycoses are dealt with more fully in the relevant sections of this chapter and are well reviewed in standard textbooks [1,2,3,4].

Culture and identification of isolates

Generally, tissue samples should be finely divided either by grinding or cutting into small pieces using sterile scalpel blades. The exception to this is material suspected of being infected with a mucoromycete, where the largely aseptate hyphae are particularly fragile and will not survive such fine division. Although glucose–peptone agar alone can be used for primary isolation of the subcutaneous pathogens, a number of other media are also commonly used, including inhibitory mould agar (BBL™) and brain–heart infusion agar (Difco™), with or without the addition of 5–10% sheep's blood. Antibacterial antibiotics such as chloramphenicol (0.005%) and gentamicin (0.0025%) are usually incorporated into the agar, and cycloheximide may be added for the culture of *Sporothrix schenckii* and the agents of chromoblastomycosis. If sufficient material is available, incubation at 26–30°C and 37°C on a variety of media is recommended. Although many organisms will grow quite quickly, cultures should be held for 6 weeks before being reported as negative. If isolates fail to sporulate on the primary culture plate, subculture onto potato dextrose agar (Oxoid™) or half-strength cornmeal agar (Oxoid) and incubation in the light may be necessary to encourage conidial production. Alternatively, molecular identification of isolates, often by sequencing, can be undertaken; this is becoming increasingly important for mycetoma and sporotrichosis.

Sporotrichosis

Definition

This is an acute or chronic fungal infection caused by a number of different species of *Sporothrix* [1]. There are both cutaneous and systemic forms of sporotrichosis.

Introduction and general description

Sporotrichosis is caused by the dimorphic fungus originally designated as *S. schenckii* [2]. It occurs in both temperate and tropical zones. Recently, under a major revision of nomenclature based on molecular sequencing, *Sporothrix* species pathogenic in man have been divided into a number of new species: *S. schenckii, S. braziliensis, S. mexicana, S. globosa* and *S. lurei*. These are based on both genetic and phenotypic markers. For instance, *S. braziliensis* is associated with infections spread from cats in a major focus of infection in Brazil and neighbouring countries. Because the application of molecular methods to *Sporothrix* is recent, it is likely that species identifications in older reports based on culture morphology will be inaccurate in some cases.

Epidemiology

Sporotrichosis is mainly seen in the tropics and subtropics. Fewer than 20 cases of sporotrichosis diagnosed in the UK have been published. The disease was common in France between 1905 and 1920, and occasional cases are reported from other European countries. It occurs sporadically in North, South and Central America [3], sub-Saharan Africa, India, Egypt, Japan and Australia [4] and has been particularly prominent in the mining areas of South Africa and, more recently, Rio de Janeiro state, Brazil. The incidence and possibly the geographical distribution are dependent on climate.

In Uruguay, it has been shown that the incidence is highest in the autumn and first half of the winter (high humidity and temperatures between 16°C and 22°C). These conditions favour saprophytic growth of *S. schenckii*. Sporotrichosis is rare in semi-arid areas. The fungus grows on decaying vegetable matter, for example the timber in mines. It has been shown that the timber harbours the fungus before being taken underground [5], and that the source is probably the soil in the vicinity of the mines. *Sporothrix* has also been recovered from the feet of mine workers who did not have sporotrichosis.

The disease may also occur in other groups occupationally exposed to the organism, such as workers using straw as packing material, forestry workers [6], florists or gardeners.

Unexplained areas of hyperendemicity have been described in certain countries, where unexpectedly high numbers of the local population develop cutaneous lesions of sporotrichosis and appear to be sensitised on skin testing with sporotrichin [7]. In one endemic zone originally in Brazil, spread of infection by infected cats has been seen [8]. This epidemic has now reached large numbers of patients and spread to adjacent states such as Argentina has been recorded. This outbreak is associated with *S. brasiliensis*.

Age

Sporotrichosis can occur at any age. On rare occasions it has been seen in young children. A family epidemic of cutaneous sporotrichosis was described among four children who became infected after playing in hay.

Sex

There is no sex predilection, although adult males are, by their occupation, most exposed to the risk of infection.

Ethnicity

This infection can occur in patients of any ethnic group.

Associated diseases

Sporotrichosis occurs in any individual. However, there are different clinical variants seen in immunocompromised patients and those with HIV/AIDS.

Pathophysiology

In most cases of cutaneous sporotrichosis the fungus is introduced into the skin or mucous membrane by trauma, as in a minor puncture wound caused by a thorn, a splinter or perhaps an insect bite. Sporotrichosis is not contagious, although transmission has been recorded from cats. Systemic sporotrichosis is rare, and the portal of entry is thought to be the lung in these cases. The incubation period is variable but is usually 8–30 days.

Pathology

Sporothrix may remain localised in the subcutaneous tissue, may spread locally in the subcutaneous lymphatics or, rarely, may be widely disseminated in the bloodstream after pulmonary infection. The underlying host immunity probably determines the form that the infection assumes. The fungus provokes a mixed granulomatous reaction with neutrophil foci. The fungus is present in the tissue,

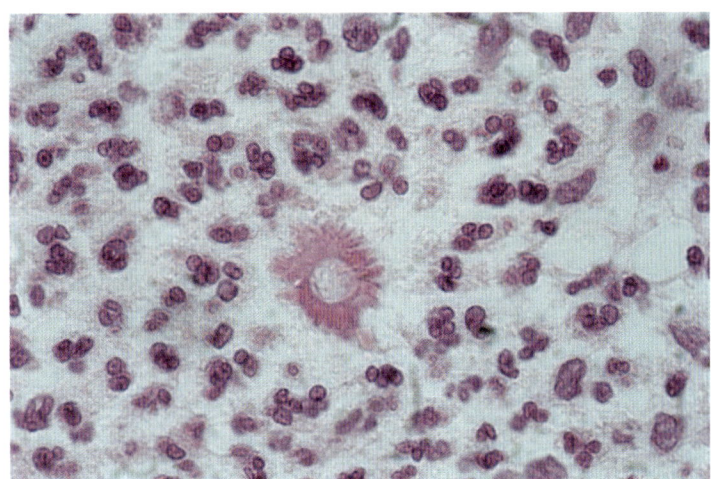

Figure 32.47 Sporotrichosis: tissue section stained with haematoxylin and eosin (H&E). Organisms are usually very scanty but asteroid bodies, representing a foreign body tissue reaction, may be observed. Courtesy of the Department of Medical Mycology, St John's Institute of Dermatology, King's College London, London, UK.

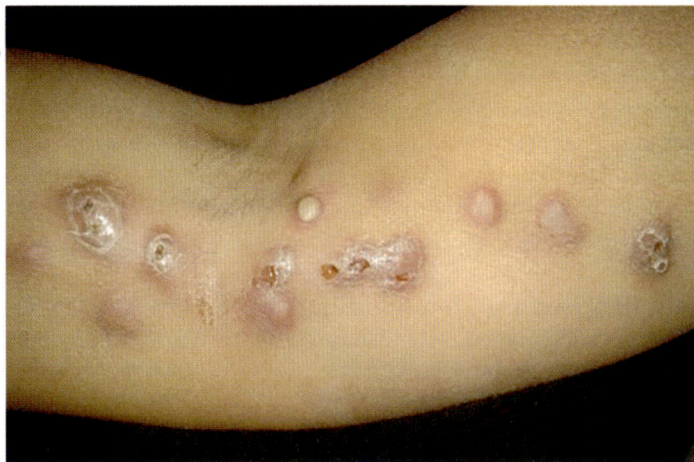

Figure 32.48 Cutaneous lymphatic sporotrichosis. Nodules draining seropurulent secretion, papules and pustules on the right upper limb along the ipsilateral lymphatic chain [12].

usually in the form of small (3–5 μm) cigar-shaped or oval yeasts, and these may, on occasion, be surrounded by a thick, radiate, eosinophilic substance that forms the distinctive asteroid bodies (Figure 32.47) [9]. A mycelial form of the fungus in tissue has occasionally been reported [10].

Causative organisms
These are *S. schenckii*, *S. braziliensis*, *S. mexicana*, *S. globosa* and *S. lurei*.

Environmental factors
None is known although they may be involved in hyperendemic disease. For instance, one well-documented hyperendemic focus of sporotrichosis occurred in mines in South Africa where pit props were contaminated with the fungus [5].

Clinical features
Presentation
Patients present with indurated and ulcerating nodules. The main clinical varieties of sporotrichosis are the cutaneous and systemic forms. In turn, cutaneous sporotrichosis is normally divided into two main types, the lymphangitic and fixed forms, but occasionally atypical varieties such as mycetoma-like or cellulitic forms may occur [2].

The most common type of sporotrichosis is the localised lymphatic variety, which follows the implantation of spores in a wound. This therefore usually occurs on exposed skin, often on the upper extremity [2,11] and is known as lymphangitic sporotrichosis. A nodule or pustule forms, which may break down into a small ulcer. Untreated, the disease usually follows a chronic course, which is characterised by involvement of the lymphatics from the draining area; a chain of lymphatic nodules develops (Figure 32.48). New nodules appear at intervals of a few days. These soften and ulcerate, and connecting lymphatic cords may be visible [13]. A thin purulent discharge may come from the primary lesion and the earliest lymphatic nodules. As the disease becomes chronic, the regional lymph nodes become swollen and may break down. The primary lesion may heal spontaneously leaving secondary nodules. The general health of the patient may not be affected.

The fixed variety, where the pathogen remains more or less localised at the point of inoculation, is less common [2,14]. The lesions may be acneform, nodular, ulcerated or verrucous; the latter form is occasionally very extensive. Less commonly, there may be infiltrated plaques or red scaly patches. An ulcer may be gummatous or may simulate an epithelioma. The plaques may suggest leishmaniasis or tuberculosis. It is thought that this variety may reflect a high degree of immunity on the part of the patient. The variable morphology of this type is notable.

The reason for the difference in clinical behaviour of the two principal forms of cutaneous sporotrichosis is unknown, although changes in temperature sensitivity of the organisms [15] or in the host's immune response [2] have both been suggested. It is possible that some sporotrichosis infections are self-healing. Others are chronic and may mimic mycetoma or stasis ulcers. In AIDS patients, multiple cutaneous lesions may develop, suggesting cutaneous spread. Infections associated with *S. brasiliensis* are often more extensive and require longer periods of treatment. They also may be accompanied by immunological reactions such as erythema nodosum or multiforme and arthralgia [8].

Clinical variants
The less common systemic form probably follows inhalation, and presents either with local pulmonary disease or focal or widely disseminated lesions in the joints, meninges and skin [16]. There is some evidence that systemic sporotrichosis occurs in patients with some type of defect in host defence, such as alcoholics. This is in contrast to the cutaneous variety, which occurs in perfectly healthy individuals. Where sporotrichosis has been reported in AIDS patients, the lesions have usually been widespread and have affected internal organs as well as the skin [17].

In the systemic type, which is rare, ulcerated nodules may develop anywhere on the body or mucous membranes, and visceral, joint and meningeal lesions may occur. Occasionally, vascular lesions resembling polyarteritis nodosa may be found. If untreated, this type is fatal.

Differential diagnosis

Sporotrichosis can simulate granulomatous lesions of almost any other origin and the diagnosis must be considered in cases when the initial lesions have followed an injury. The main conditions that may resemble sporotrichosis are mycobacterial infections and leishmaniasis. The mycobacterial infection caused by *Mycobacterium marinum* (fish-tank granuloma) may closely resemble lymphangitic sporotrichosis.

Complications and co-morbidities

Disseminated cutaneous disease can occur as described previously in patients with HIV/AIDS.

Disease course and prognosis

Cutaneous sporotrichosis is not life threatening. Although it may resolve spontaneously, chronic and persistent cases lasting for over 5 years are well known.

Investigations

In *Sporothrix* infections there are seldom large numbers of organisms visible in tissue samples or smears. Fluorescent antibody techniques have been successfully employed in locating the pathogenic phase *in vivo* [18] and serological tests are under development. The fungus grows readily on common agar media.

Sporothrix schenckii. Colony: the colonies are leathery, moist and initially white or cream with a wrinkled surface. As the colonies age, they may become progressively darker until they are brown or black. Microscopy: the slender (2 μm) hyphae bear small, oval to pyriform, hyaline conidia produced along the sides of the hyphae and sympodially at the ends of delicate conidiophores arising at right angles from the hyphae. The arrangement of the conidia at the apex of the conidiogenous cell is often described as palmate or flower-like, with each conidium attached by a denticle to the small vesicle. In many strains (particularly when freshly isolated), oval, round or triangular dark brown, thick-walled conidia are also produced, and it is partly the production of these conidia that results in the development of darkly pigmented colonies. However, pigmentation has also been reported to vary according to the culture medium and to increase with the addition of thiamine. Physiological tests: to confirm the identification, it is essential to convert this thermally dimorphic fungus to the yeast phase, as fungi that are non-pathogenic and morphologically very similar may be isolated as contaminants. This is best achieved on brain–heart infusion agar supplemented with sheep's blood and incubated at 37°C. The yeasts are typically oval or cigar-shaped.

Management

While cases have been described where spontaneous remission has been seen to occur [19], patients with sporotrichosis are treated with antifungals.

First line

Itraconazole 100–200 mg/day or terbinafine 250 mg/day are both effective and well tolerated. However, at these dosages the length of treatment is not significantly different from that used with potassium iodide [20]. In systemic cases, treatment with intravenous amphotericin B may also be helpful. Potassium iodide in large oral doses is effective in the localised types and should be continued for 3–4 weeks after clinical cure. It is cheap and effective, although side effects are common. A recommended schedule is five drops initially, increasing to 4–6 mL of saturated potassium iodide three times daily. Patient tolerance because of dry mouth, severe nausea and taste disturbance may require a lower maximum dose [21].

Treatment ladder for sporotrichosis

First line
- Itraconazole 100–200 mg/day until clinical recovery (at least 3 months)

  or
- Terbinafine 250 mg/day until clinical recovery (at least 3 months)

Second line
- Potassium iodide at an initial dose of five drops daily of saturated solution increasing slowly to 4–6 mL daily

---

Mycetoma

Definition and nomenclature

Mycetoma is a localised chronic infection caused by various species of fungi or actinomycetes and characterised by the formation of aggregates of the causative organisms (grains) within abscesses. This results in severe damage to the skin, subcutaneous tissues and bones of the feet, hands and other parts of the body. Grains are discharged to the surface through draining sinuses.

Synonyms and inclusions
- Maduromycosis
- Madura foot

Introduction and general description [1]

Mycetoma may be caused by various species of fungi (eumycetoma) and aerobic actinomycetes (actinomycetoma), which occur as saprophytes in soil or on plants [2]. From these sources, they are implanted subcutaneously, usually after a penetrating injury [3,4].

Epidemiology

The disease is largely confined to tropical and subtropical climates, usually among agricultural workers. A few cases have occurred in Europe and North America, but in many such cases the patients have originated from the tropics and the infection was imported. These cases also illustrate clearly that the disease may not become troublesome until many years (20–30 years) after the initial injury.

The relative frequency with which the different species are encountered varies from country to country [5,6]. Actinomycetomas caused by *Nocardia* species are most common in Central America and Mexico. In other parts of the world, the most common organism is a eumycetoma agent, *Madurella mycetomatis*. The actinomycete, *Streptomyces somaliensis*, is most often isolated from patients originating from Sudan and the Middle East [7].

Age
Mycetoma is rare in young children.

Sex
Adult males are most often infected.

Ethnicity
There is no ethnic predisposition.

Pathophysiology [4,8]
Critical to the survival of the fungus or actinomycete is its ability to form cell clusters or grains. The morphology of the grains aids survival either because in the case of actinomycetes there is a protective matrix, or with fungi there is cell wall thickening due in part to intrahyphal growth as well as linkage of adjacent cell walls. The deposition of melanin in the cell wall and as a surrounding matrix in the case of *M. mycetomatis* is a further protective mechanism. Melanin may also be protective against antifungal agents by binding these molecules.

Pathology
Histopathology is very important in diagnosis. The causal organisms produce a chronic inflammatory reaction leading to focal neutrophil abscess formation, with scattered giant cells and fibrosis. Grains in the form of white, yellow, red or black granules are found in the centre of the inflammatory response [9] and may be discharged in pus through multiple sinuses on to the skin surface. Secondary bacterial infection may occur, but this is not common [10]. The destructive process slowly extends deeply into the underlying tissues, and invades muscle and bones. An H&E preparation is sufficient to distinguish between eumycetoma and actinomycetoma.

Causative organisms
The condition, which is not contagious, is characterised by the presence of different coloured grains, which represent microcolonies of the organisms. The aetiological agents listed in Box 32.4 include only the most commonly isolated fungi.

Genetics
There is also evidence that populations with a high rate of susceptibility to mycetoma may have specific polymorphisms in cytokine genes [8].

Environmental factors
The causative organisms have been isolated from either soil or plant material, including thorns from *Acacia* bushes in endemic areas, or identified in soil using molecular probes.

Box 32.4 Main aetiological agents of mycetoma

Fungi: dark grain
- *Madurella mycetomatis*, *M. fahaliensis*, *M. pseudomycetomatis*
- *Trematosphaeria grisea*
- *Plenodomus senegalensis*
- *Medicopsis romeroi*

Fungi: pale grain
- *Scedosporium apiospermum*
- *Neotestudina rosatii*
- *Sarocladium* (formerly *Acremonium*) spp.
- *Fusarium* spp.

Actinomycetes
- *Actinomadura madurae*
- *Actinomadura pelletieri*
- *Streptomyces somaliensis*
- *Nocardia brasiliensis*
- *Nocardia otitidis-caviarum*
- *Nocardia asteroides*

Clinical features
Presentation
The clinical features are essentially the same no matter which fungus or actinomycete is concerned [11,12]. Because trauma favours infection, most lesions are on the foot and lower leg, but they may occur anywhere on the body [13]. The earliest stage is a firm, painless nodule but with time papules and pustules, which break down to form draining sinuses, appear on the skin surface (Figure 32.49). The whole area becomes hard and swollen, often without significant pain [14]. Extension to underlying bones and joints gives rise to periostitis, osteomyelitis and arthritis (Figure 32.50). In advanced cases, destruction of bone within an infected area may be almost complete, and gross deformity may result [15,16]. There are usually multiple sinus tracts draining pus. These may remain open for months or may close and reopen, or may be replaced by new sinuses. The discharge may be purulent or seropurulent. The

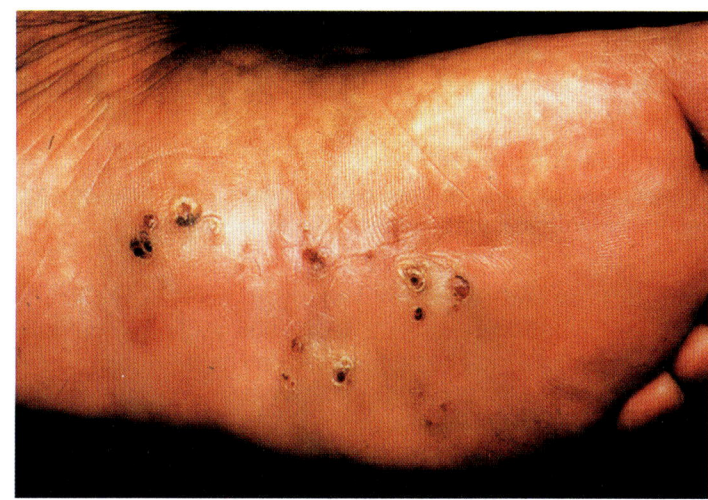

Figure 32.49 Mycetoma caused by *Madurella grisea*.

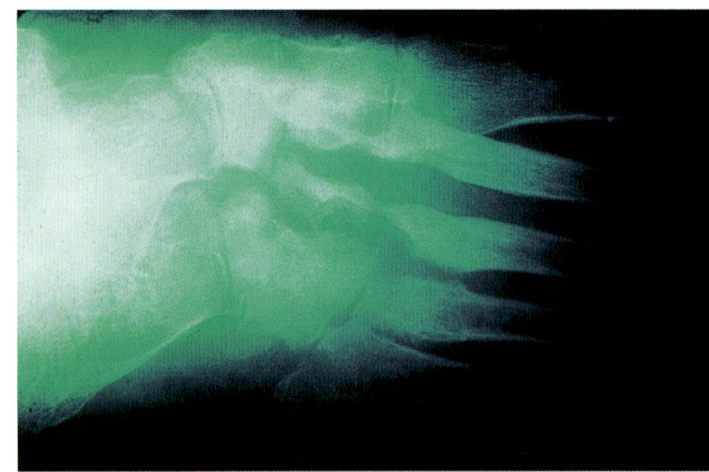

Figure 32.50 Erosive X-ray changes in a mycetoma.

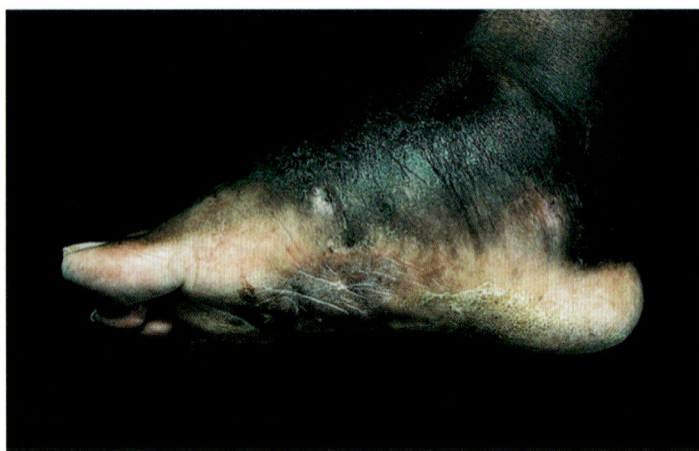

Figure 32.51 Eumycetoma affecting the foot.

condition is comparatively painless and usually develops slowly, but eventually results in gross swelling of the affected foot or other parts with serious deformity (Figure 32.51).

Clinical variants
Lymph node or disseminated infections are rare [17]. Rarely, bone disease without overlying subcutaneous or cutaneous signs can occur.

Differential diagnosis
Chronic osteomyelitis of bacterial or tuberculous aetiology may resemble mycetoma, particularly in the early stages.

Complication and co-morbidities
The main complication is bone destruction leading to deformity and osteomyelitis. Imaging techniques contribute greatly to assessment of the destruction. Magnetic resonance imaging (MRI) provides the most comprehensive method but X-ray and ultrasound can also be useful [16,18]. Where lesions are on the scalp or chest wall, deep extension can lead to skull penetration or lung invasion, respectively.

Disease course and prognosis
Mycetoma does not go into spontaneous remission and progression is slow but inevitable. However, the main outcome is deformity and reduced mobility, although in rare instances of very extensive disease the outcome may be fatal.

Investigations
In early mycetoma it may be necessary to incise pustules that represent foci of inflammation, necrosis and sinuses that have not yet ruptured through the skin; these pustules often contain grains. Pus from sinus discharge or needle aspiration should be examined under the microscope for the presence of grains, which may then be processed for histology or examined directly in potassium hydroxide. If the infection is eumycotic, when crushed under the cover slip the grains will be seen to consist of masses of fungal mycelium with hyphae 2–6 μm in diameter. Chlamydoconidia are frequently formed at the periphery or in the centre of the grains. Actinomycotic grains will be seen to consist of masses of much narrower bacterial filaments 0.5–1.0 μm in diameter. If there are no discharging sinuses, a biopsy may be required. In elephantiasis there are no sinus tracts.

A tentative diagnosis sufficient to initiate treatment may be made on the basis of grain colour, texture and direct microscopic appearance [4]. For instance, black grains are always caused by fungi and red grains by an actinomycete. Eumycetomas with black grains are termed dark-grain eumycetomas and many of the fungal species responsible produce hard or brittle grains with a brown, cement-like substance surrounding the hyphae. Eumycetomas with white or yellow grains are termed pale-grain eumycetomas and most contain no cement and have a soft texture (Figure 32.52).

In eumycotic disease, the final identification of the infecting fungus requires the isolation of the causal agent in culture or the application of molecular diagnostic techniques [19]. As the surfaces of the grains are frequently contaminated by bacteria, washing with saline containing antibacterials is recommended prior to inoculating the culture medium. Some grains may be non-viable. Primary

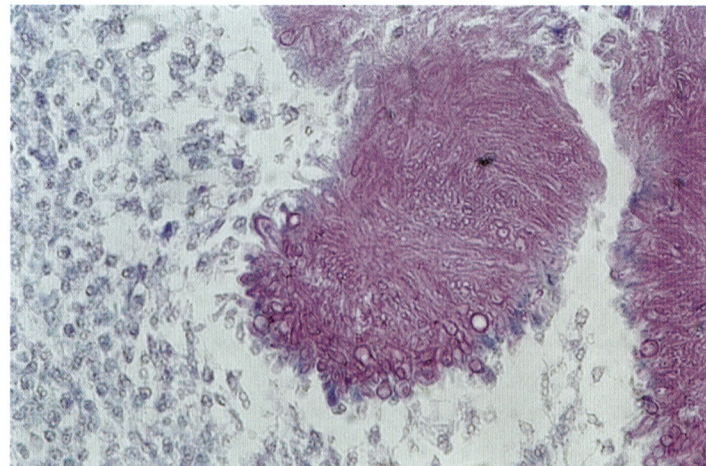

Figure 32.52 Mycetoma: tissue section. Distinct hyphal filaments, stained pink with periodic acid–Schiff (PAS), are clearly visible in a pale-grained eumycetoma. Courtesy of the Department of Medical Mycology, St John's Institute of Dermatology, King's College London, London, UK.

isolates may require subculture on nutritionally depleted media, such as half-strength cornmeal agar, to induce sporulation, and may fail to sporulate completely. Referral to a reference mycology laboratory for identification is recommended. Only the two most frequently isolated fungal species are described.

Madurella mycetomatis. Colony: the colonial form shows great variation. Colonies are initially pale and leathery, but after a few days become olive, ochre brown or grey in colour and may produce a diffusible brown pigment. Growth is faster at 37°C than at 28°C. Microscopy: on nutritionally poor media, spherical conidia may be formed from flask-shaped phialides. Primary cultures may produce large chlamydoconidia but are otherwise usually sterile. Increasingly diagnosis using molecular methods is advised particularly to distinguish this from other *Madurella* species

Scedosporium apiospermum (Pseudallescheria boydii). Colony: the colony grows rapidly with a floccose grey or brown-grey surface and white to dark grey reverse. Microscopy: oval, light brown, relatively thick-walled conidia with a truncate base are formed singly along the hyphae or in small groups from annellides. A second form of conidiation is seen in some isolates with the production of coremia – tufts of hyphae held together – which produce smaller hyaline annello-conidia at their tips. This is a homothallic species and the sexual phase with ascospores may be formed on primary culture.

Management
Localised lesions that can be excised without residual disability are best so treated. In other cases, medical treatment should first be attempted, although chemotherapy of mycetomas caused by fungi has, so far, been found to be quite unsatisfactory in most cases. This is despite the fact that certain fungi have been found to be relatively sensitive *in vitro* to therapeutic agents such as amphotericin B [1].

First line
Infection by species of actinomycetes may be susceptible to chemotherapeutic agents. The combination of dapsone with streptomycin or co-trimoxazole plus streptomycin has been reported to give good results [20]. An alternative second drug is rifampicin. Amikacin or imipenem may also be used in recalcitrant *Nocardia* infections.

Among the fungal causes of mycetoma, *M. mycetomatis* is the most sensitive to therapy as it responds to ketoconazole in some cases [1]. For the others, a trial of therapy with griseofulvin, terbinafine, voriconazole or itraconazole is worth attempting as, even though it may not be curative, the progress of the infection may be slowed [21]. This can be followed after 4–6 months by surgical excison of the remaining lesion.

Second line
Radical surgery, usually amputation, should be considered carefully. Removal of a limb may deprive the patient of livelihood in many countries and this will need to be taken into consideration. However, it remains the only effective means of removing very severe infections in some patients.

Treatment ladder for mycetoma

First line

Actinomycetomas
- Dapsone plus streptomycin or rifampicin
  or
- Co-trimoxazole plus streptomycin or rifampicin

Eumycetomas
- Azoles, e.g. itraconazole followed by surgery for remaining mycetoma

Second line
- Radical surgery

Chromoblastomycosis

Definition and nomenclature
This is a chronic fungal infection of the skin and subcutaneous tissues caused by pigmented fungi, which produce thick-walled single- or multicelled clusters (sclerotic or muriform bodies) in tissue. It is characterised by the production of slow-growing exophytic lesions, usually on the feet and legs [1,2].

Synonyms and inclusions
- Chromomycosis
- Verrucous dermatitis

Epidemiology
The condition is usually found in the tropics, particularly areas with medium to high rainfall, in rural communities [4]. It has been reported from Central, South and North America [3], Cuba, Jamaica and Martinique as well as from many other countries including India, South Africa, Madagascar, Australia and northern Europe. It is occasionally seen as an imported infection in Europe and the USA.

Age
Children are rarely affected.

Sex
Adult male agricultural workers are most often affected, but the condition has occasionally been reported in children.

Pathophysiology
The causal fungi have been isolated from wood and soil, and the infection usually results from trauma, such as a puncture from a splinter of wood [2,5].

Pathology
The histology is that of a foreign-body granuloma, with isolated areas of microabscess formation. In the organised granuloma, mainly within giant cells, groups of fungal cells may be seen. Because the

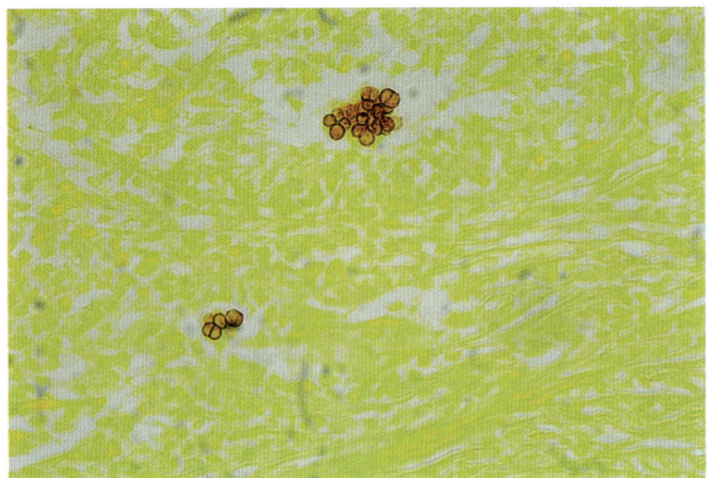

Figure 32.53 Chromoblastomycosis: tissue section. The natural brown pigment of the fungal muriform cells is clearly visible. The cells divide by fission and may form septa in more than one plane of division. Courtesy of the Department of Medical Mycology, St John's Institute of Dermatology, King's College London, London, UK.

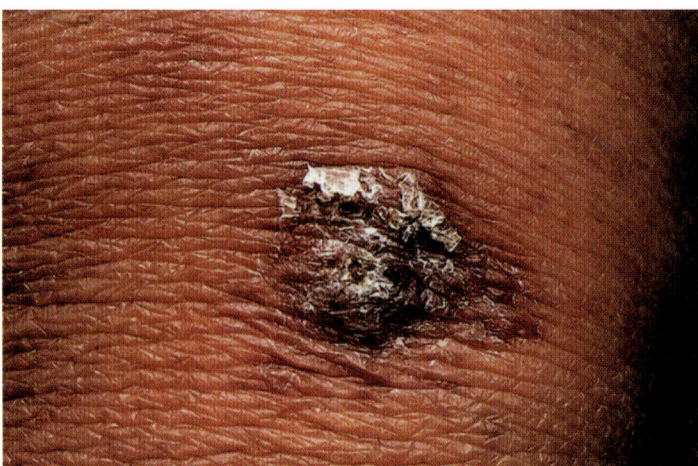

Figure 32.54 Early lesion of chromoblastomycosis.

cells are chestnut or golden brown in colour, they are easily distinguished in the infiltrate. The cells are characteristically divided in several planes of division by thick septa and are termed muriform or sclerotic cells (Figure 32.53). There is marked pseudoepitheliomatous hyperplasia in the epidermis and in some areas apparent transepidermal elimination of fungal cells, which can be found in the stratum corneum. The tissue between the granulomatous nodules shows chronic fibrosis.

Causative organisms
Chromoblastomycosis is caused by several fungi, the most common of which are *Phialophora verrucosa*, *Fonsecaea pedrosoi*, *F. compacta* and *Cladophialophora carrionii* (previously *Cladosporium carrionii*) [2]. Other rare causes include *Rhinocladiella aquaspersa*. The nomenclature of these fungi has been reviewed by McGinnis [6].

Clinical features [7,8]
History
The lesions are usually found on exposed sites, particularly the feet, legs, arms, face and neck (Figure 32.54). The disease develops over years rather than over a shorter period.

Presentation
A warty papule slowly enlarges to form a hypertrophic plaque [9,10]. In some lesions, the plaque is flat and expands slowly with central scarring. The early lesion may occasionally be an ulcer. Eventually, after months or many years, large hyperkeratotic masses are formed, and these may be as large as 3 cm thick (Figure 32.55). Secondary ulceration may occur. The lesion is usually painless unless the presence of secondary infection causes itching and pain. Satellite lesions are produced by scratching, and there may be lymphatic spread to adjacent areas.

Clinical variants
Some forms of the infection produce psoriasiform lesions. Haematogenous spread has occurred but is rare, and brain abscesses have been described.

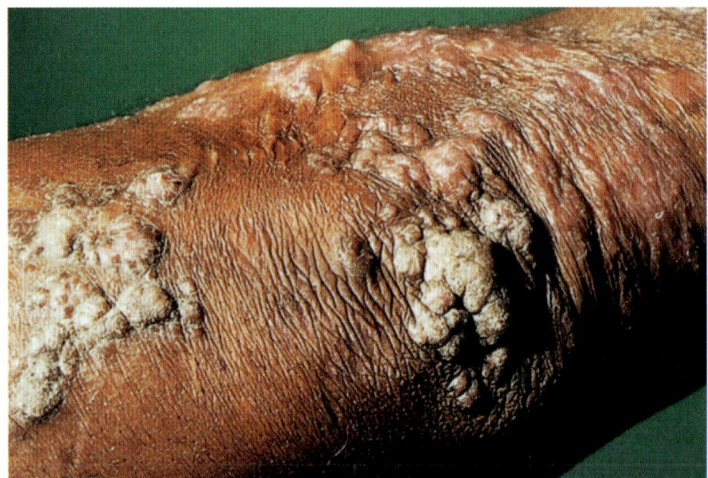

Figure 32.55 Plaque-type chromoblastomycosis.

Differential diagnosis
The disease must be differentiated from blastomycosis (by the absence of a sharp border containing minute abscesses) and also the absence of pulmonary lesions, cutaneous tuberculosis, leishmaniasis, syphilis and yaws.

Complications and co-morbidities
Secondary infection may eventually lead after several years to lymphatic stasis with the production of elephantiasis. Squamous carcinomas may develop in chronic lesions.

Disease course and prognosis
The course is chronic but non-fatal.

Investigations
Clusters of pigmented fungal cells can be seen with dermoscopy. Biopsy and culture of material for the associated fungi will establish the diagnosis. Irrespective of species, the pathogen can be seen in biopsy sections as deeply pigmented, thick-walled muriform or sclerotic cells in abscesses, giant cells or the epidermis. Occasionally, in superficial skin scrapings from the surface of the lesions,

pigmented hyphae rather than sclerotic cells are seen. Multiplication *in vivo* is by fission rather than budding, and this results in the production of single-, two- or multiple-celled clusters. In culture, the colonies of all species are dark grey-green to black and velvety or downy, with a black reverse.

Three forms of conidial production are observed in the most common agents of infection: acropetal budding, production of phialides and sympodial conidiation. Some agents are polymorphic, demonstrating more than one type of conidiation simultaneously, and this has caused some confusion in the nomenclature of these agents. They are named according to the dominant form of conidiation.

Phialophora verrucosa. Microscopy: the dominant form of conidiation is the production of flask-shaped phialides with a pronounced dark collarette at the apex. These are produced laterally or terminally. The hyaline, thin-walled, elliptical conidia are produced at the tip of the phialide in basipetal succession and collect as balls. On nutritionally weak media, a few sympodial or acropetal conidiogenous cells may also be observed.

Fonsecaea pedrosoi. Microscopy: the dominant form of conidiation is sympodial with the conidia confined to the upper part of the cell. The brown single-celled conidia are produced on short denticles and may in turn produce secondary conidia in a similar manner. Conidia produced by acropetal budding are also present in the majority of isolates, and some isolates will produce scanty phialides.

Cladophialophora carrionii. Microscopy: acropetal budding is dominant, producing long chains of pale, oval or lemon-shaped conidia. The chains branch at frequent intervals. On starvation media, such as half-strength cornmeal agar, bulbous phialides may be produced by the conversion of some of the cells within the branched chains.

Management
The main treatment of chromoblastomycosis involves the use of antifungal chemotherapy.

First line
Itraconazole (200 mg daily) or terbinafine (250 mg daily) is often successful, although responses to both are thought to be better if the causative organism is *C. carrionii* [11,12]. Flucytosine used on its own or combined with amphotericin B [13] may also be effective, but resistance to flucytosine may develop if it is used on its own.

Second line
Other approaches to treatment have included the use of cryotherapy or the local application of heat daily using a heat-retaining gel pack at a warm and comfortable temperature to induce shrinkage. This usually takes 2–3 months [14]. Surgery is only indicated for very small lesions, and even in these should be combined with chemotherapy. Photodynamic therapy has also been used.

Treatment ladder for chromoblastomycosis

First line
- Itraconazole 200 mg daily until clinical recovery

  or
- Terbinafine 250 mg daily until clinical recovery

Second line
- Heat application

Phaeohyphomycosis

Definition and nomenclature
Phaeohyphomycosis is a rare, and generally localised, subcutaneous or intramuscular infection, usually a cyst or abscess caused by hyphal brown-pigmented (dematiaceous) fungi [1]. Systemic forms of phaeohyphomycosis also exist.

Synonyms and inclusions
- Phaeomycotic subcutaneous cyst

Epidemiology
This infection is most often seen in patients from tropical areas. Some patients are immunocompromised, usually through steroid therapy. An ever-increasing number of fungi have been reported as agents of phaeohyphomycosis: a review lists 104 species [2]. The most common causative organisms are shown in Box 32.5.

Box 32.5 Major aetiological agents of phaeohyphomycosis

- *Exophiala jeanselmei*
- *Exophiala dermatitidis*
- *Cladophialophora bantiana*
- *Phialophora* spp.
- *Bipolaris* spp.
- *Exserohilum* spp.
- *Alternaria* spp.

Age, sex and ethnicity
This is an uncommon infection and relevant data on individual susceptibility are lacking.

Pathophysiology
The infection follows traumatic implantation of organisms from the environment.

Pathology
The fungi are found in a subcutaneous inflammatory cyst. There is usually a well-organised wall with surrounding fibrosis and a mixed

cellular infiltrate with multinucleate giant cells, lymphocytes and macrophages. Neutrophil infiltration also occurs. The fungi are usually found in the inner aspect of the cyst. They may be pigmented *in vivo* and visible in H&E stains but this is not always the case and specific fungal stains such as PAS are advised.

Causative organisms
These include *Exophiala jeanselmei*, *E. dermatitidis*, *Bipolaris* spp., *Alternaria alternata* and others that form pigmented hyphae in tissue (Box 32.5) [1].

Clinical features
Patients present with well-defined single cystic lesions on the trunk or limbs [3]. These are not painful but are unsightly and can grow large enough to warrant removal, at which stage the diagnosis is made.

Differential diagnosis
A Baker cyst or large pilar cyst should also be considered.

Course and prognosis
Although not fatal, this infection does not heal spontaneously.

Investigations
The organisms are not usually difficult to grow from the lesions, but the fact that so many different species may be involved, together with the failure of some primary isolates to sporulate, means that their identification may require the help of a specialist laboratory. The major dematiaceous pathogens are well illustrated and described in the review by Rinaldi [2].

Exophiala jeanselmei. Colony: this fungus belongs to the group sometimes termed 'black yeasts'. The colony is initially glabrous or moist, and black in colour. As the culture matures, it becomes more filamentous and eventually is covered with a grey velvety mycelium. Microscopy: initially, the culture is made up of single cells, which are annellides reproducing by budding. When the filamentous stage has developed, the septate brown hyphae bear slender annellides producing elliptical conidia, which collect in a mass at the tip of the conidiogenous cell or slide down to form a row along the side of the annellide. Physiological tests: will not grow at 40°C.

Bipolaris species. Colony: the colonies grow rapidly. Initially downy and pale grey, the colour darkens to olive grey or black on both the surface and reverse. Microscopy: the conidiogenous cells are geniculate, producing the brown multicellular phragmoconidia in a sympodial sequence. The hilum at the base of the conidium is only slightly protuberant.

Management
The usual treatment is excision, and although there are no published studies to establish efficacy, an appropriate antifungal such as itraconazole is often given after surgery.

Lobomycosis

Definition and nomenclature
This rare disease caused by *Lacazia loboi* is characterised by keloidal skin lesions that remain fairly well localised and do not affect the general health of the patient.

Synonyms and inclusions
- Keloidal blastomycosis
- Lobo disease

Epidemiology
The disease was first observed in 1931 in a patient from the Amazon valley. Other cases have also been seen there [1] and throughout central and northern South America.

Pathophysiology
It is thought that the agent might be associated with water and gain entry through a wound [2]. In most cases studied, the disease has been present for periods of many years. Infections have been reported in freshwater dolphins although here the infection shows distinct epidemiology extending to temperate waters and is likely to be due to a different clade (variety) [3].

Pathology
In H&E-stained sections there is a diffuse infiltrate of lymphocytes, macrophages and giant cells that contain the fungal cells, which are 5–10 µm in diameter. With fungal stains, these have a characteristic morphology, being aligned in short chains of 3–8 oval or round cells all joined by short tubular structures.

Causative organisms
The causal fungus, which has never been isolated in culture, is *Lacazia loboi* [4].

Clinical features
Lesions may be found anywhere on the body, but are usually on exposed parts – the legs, arms and face [1]. They can, in most instances, be associated with injuries to the skin, and spread from one site to another is thought to be by autoinoculation following injury. There is no marked lymphangitis and no visceral dissemination. Old chronic lesions present as elevated, crusted plaques.

Differential diagnosis
Clinically, the disease most closely resembles chromoblastomycosis.

Complications and co-morbidities
Squamous cell carcinoma may occasionally develop in chronic lesions [1].

Course and prognosis
This infection does not spread widely but remains localised or slowly expands over years.

Investigations
Microscopic examination of biopsy material will establish the diagnosis. The fungus has not been isolated in culture and mycological confirmation depends on recognition of the characteristic cells of *L. loboi* in tissue. This is easily performed with potassium hydroxide mounts of epidermal crusts or sections, which need not be specially stained.

Treatment
There is no effective medical therapy for lobomycosis and where possible lesions are excised surgically.

Rhinosporidiosis

Definition
This is a chronic granulomatous infection caused by *Rhinosporidium seeberi*, inducing polyps of the mucous membrane. The organism has never been isolated *in vitro*, but through genetic studies its taxonomic position is now clearer, and it is now considered an aquatic member of the Protista rather than a fungus.

Epidemiology
Rhinosporidiosis has occurred in many parts of the world rarely and sporadically, but it is endemic in India and Sri Lanka [1]. In one review, 51 cases were described from Uganda [2].

Age and sex
Adult male workers are the persons most likely to be infected.

Clinical features
Vascular polyps, which may be pedunculated, occur on any mucosal surface [3]. The mucous membrane of the nose, the naso-pharynx or the soft palate is involved in three-quarters of cases, and the conjunctiva or the lacrimal sac in a proportion of the others. Lesions are also found on other mucous membrane surfaces, such as the larynx, penis, vagina and rectum, and sometimes also on the skin, to which it is presumed to have spread from a primary site on the nearby mucous membrane [4]. The lesions become hyperplastic and may reach an enormous size, extending from the nostrils to the pharynx or outwards over the lip [5]. The pink or red surface is lobulated and cauliflower-like. Close examination of the surface reveals small white spots, which represent mature sporangia of the fungus. The disease may last for many years. Spontaneous resolution has been observed rarely. It is not contagious. Obstruction to breathing is usually the chief complaint. On the genitalia, the lesions look like condylomata. If the eye is involved there is conjunctivitis and photophobia, and the weight of the polyps may cause eversion of the lid.

Differential diagnosis
Typical lesions are easily recognised by their pink-purple colour, friable consistency and the presence of the white sporangia within the polyp itself. Atypical lesions should be differentiated from warts, condylomata and haemorrhoids.

Investigations
The causative organisms cannot be cultured and the diagnosis depends on histopathology – recognition of the sporangia seen on the surface of the polyp or in tissue sections. Depending on maturity, these may attain diameters of 0.5 mm, and can be readily seen by the naked eye as firm white cysts on or just below the surface. Microscopically, these are single, thick-walled and spherical, and when fully differentiated are packed with numerous rounded endospores, 6–7 μm in diameter. Immature and collapsed discharged sporangia are also present [6].

Management
Surgical removal resulting in complete eradication of the disease is the treatment of choice.

Subcutaneous mycosis due to *Basidiobolus* and *Conidiobolus*

Definition and nomenclature
This is a localised, subcutaneous and predominantly tropical mycosis characterised by chronic, woody swelling of subcutaneous tissue.

Synonyms and inclusions
- Subcutaneous zygomycosis
- Basidiobolomycosis
- Subcutaneous phycomycosis
- Conidiobolomycosis
- Rhinoentomophthoromycosis

Epidemiology
Subcutaneous infection caused by *Basidiobolus ranarum* was initially described in Indonesia [1,2], but cases have since been reported in Africa, Australia and South-East Asian countries. Subcutaneous infection caused by *Conidiobolus coronatus* (rhinoentomophthoromycosis) is another localised zygomycotic infection affecting animals and humans [3]. Reported from the West Indies, Africa, India and South America, infection may result in gross but non-painful facial swelling originating from the nasal mucosae or sinuses.

Pathophysiology
In their natural environment, both causative fungi *B. ranarum* and *C. coronatus* are associated with decaying vegetation and the gastrointestinal tracts of insects and frogs.

Clinical features
There is a slowly spreading, painless, subcutaneous swelling without other obvious clinical signs [4–6]. It may be single or there may be satellite lesions. The disc-shaped masses have a uniform non-pitting hard consistency [7]. The smooth rounded edge, which may be lobulated, can be raised by inserting the fingers underneath it. Pain and tenderness may be absent or, less often, pronounced. The overlying skin may be tense, oedematous, desquamating,

hyperpigmented or normal. Ulceration does not occur and the regional lymph glands are not often enlarged [8].

In *Basidiobolus* infections, the lesion usually involves the limbs or limb–girdle areas and the infection is most often seen in children. The clinical features of *Conidiobolus* infections are similar but affect the face, apparently spreading from the region of the inferior turbinates to involve the central facial tissues. It is mainly seen in young adults. Both subcutaneous infections are very disfiguring.

Differential diagnosis

Histological and mycological examinations are required for accurate diagnosis, but lymphatic oedema (which lacks the distinctive edge), subcutaneous malignant lymphoma (which grows more rapidly) and induration round an infection site (where there is pain and tenderness) have to be considered [9].

Complications and co-morbidities

Rarely, deep invasion with *Conidiobolus* has been described, and is usually not associated with skin lesions [10].

Investigations

The diagnosis is usually established histologically by biopsy, but culture is not difficult. The lesion is an eosinophilic granuloma lying deep in the subcutaneous tissue and largely replacing fat. Wide, sparsely septate hyphae, branching at right angles, are scattered throughout the granuloma (Figure 32.56) and there is often dense fibrosis [11,12].

Basidiobolus ranarum. Colony: on cycloheximide-free media at 30°C, *B. ranarum* grows very rapidly as waxy cream or yellow colonies with many radial folds. Microscopy: the hyphae are broad, 8–20 µm in diameter and have few septa. After 10–14 days, sexual zygospores with a prominent beak may be produced. In addition, unicellular sporangia – sporangiola – are formed, which are forcibly ejected into the air from the tip of the sporangiophore.

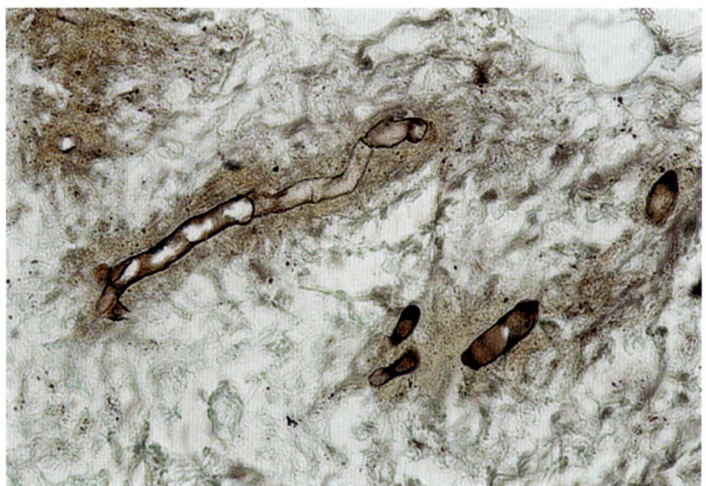

Figure 32.56 Subcutaneous *Basidiobolus* infection tissue section. Wide, aseptate hyphae stained black with Grocott methenamine silver (GMS) are characteristic of infection by a zygomycete. Courtesy of the Department of Medical Mycology, St John's Institute of Dermatology, King's College London, London, UK.

Conidiobolus coronatus. Colony: the colonies are waxy white to grey, becoming more powdery and beige as a short aerial mycelium develops. Microscopy: wide, sparsely septate hyphae are present. Sporangiola are forcibly discharged, and impact on the sides and lid of the Petri dish. Some sporangiola may form small protuberances or villi all over their surfaces.

Management

Itraconazole is useful in this condition. Lesions also usually respond to oral treatment with potassium iodide given in similar doses to those used in sporotrichosis. There is some evidence that co-trimoxazole can be used in addition in conidiobolomycosis.

SYSTEMIC MYCOSES

The systemic mycoses are fungal infections that involve deep structures and that have the propensity to disseminate, usually via the bloodstream, from the original focus of infection. They include two main groups of disease: the endemic mycoses and the opportunistic systemic mycoses.

Pathophysiology

Endemic mycoses are usually acquired via inhalation of the causative organisms. They therefore have a common mode of pathogenesis. In many cases, infections are asymptomatic and the primary infection can only be detected in retrospect by a positive skin test, as in tuberculosis. These mycoses have defined areas of endemicity, which may have a characteristic climate or flora and fauna. The main endemic mycoses are histoplasmosis (classic and African types), blastomycosis, coccidioidomycosis, paracoccidioidomycosis and infection caused by *Talaromyces* (previously *Penicillium*) *marneffei*. The clinical manifestations of these infections are affected by the underlying state of the patient, and many of them develop in the presence of particular immunodeficiency states, notably AIDS.

Cryptococcosis shares features of both endemic mycoses and the opportunistic infections. However, as it can affect the healthy and is a primary respiratory infection caused by a fungus that occupies a specific ecological niche, it will be considered here with the endemic infections.

The opportunistic systemic mycoses are those systemic infections that only occur in patients with some underlying predisposition. In contrast to the endemic mycoses, they may occur in any geographical area and their clinical manifestations are very variable, depending on the predisposition and mode of entry of the fungus.

Identification

The dimorphic fungi causing the endemic mycoses are extremely hazardous to the laboratory worker and must be handled in containment level 3 conditions. Laboratory infections and fatalities have been recorded. These organisms should never be cultured in Petri dishes, which pose too great a threat of aerosol dissemination.

Cultures should be performed in capped bottles or tubes. The laboratory must be alerted to the possibility of a dimorphic pathogen when the specimen is submitted for examination.

Serological tests

Serological tests are of considerable value in the diagnosis of the endemic mycoses. In the endemic infections, immunodiffusion tests may demonstrate the presence of specific precipitin bands, for example the H and M bands in histoplasmosis, and complement fixation tests are also routinely performed in suspected cases of histoplasmosis and coccidioidomycosis. The cross-reactivity of fungal antigens can be a problem, however, and this is true of antigens of *Blastomyces dermatitidis*, which cross-react with those of other dimorphic pathogens.

In the opportunistic systemic mycoses, serology is also useful but may be more difficult to interpret. Many normal individuals will have detectable antibodies to *Candida* species, resulting from exposure in the environment, so that changes in titre have more significance than a single positive test. Many patients with opportunistic infections caused by *Candida* or *Aspergillus* species will be unable to raise any antibody responses. For this reason, methods of detection of antigen or fungal metabolites are currently of most interest. However, antigenaemia is transient and detection may require serial samples.

The situation is reversed in cryptococcosis, however, where the detection of antigen rather than antibody has proved to be virtually diagnostic, and commercial latex particle agglutination, enzyme-linked immunosorbent assay (ELISA) or lateral flow tests for cryptococcal antigen are routinely used.

Direct examination and histopathology

As with the subcutaneous infections, in some instances a simple wet mount of samples such as sputum or broncho-alveolar lavage fluid can show characteristic fungal structures. For example, the observation of encapsulated yeasts in cerebrospinal fluid is diagnostic of cryptococcosis, and spherules of *Coccidioides immitis* may be detected in sputum. Histopathological investigations may allow the recognition of all the dimorphic fungi, zygomycetes and *Cryptococcus*, but cannot distinguish some of the rarer pathogens such as *Fusarium* species and *Scedosporium apiospermum* reliably from *Aspergillus*.

Culture and identification of isolates

Suitable media are similar to those described for the subcutaneous fungi. Incubation should be performed at around 30°C and also at 37°C if sufficient material is available. Many of the opportunistic pathogens will grow in a few days, but some of the dimorphic fungi grow relatively slowly, and cultures should be held for a minimum of 4–6 weeks.

The isolation of any of the dimorphic pathogens is always considered significant. The identification of the five major dimorphic agents may, however, be complicated by the fact that in some cases they can be morphologically atypical or sterile. Exoantigen tests and nucleic acid probes for specific identification of these pathogens have now been developed. These techniques involve less handling of these pathogens and are far quicker than the traditionally used methods for converting the organisms to their parasitic phase *in vitro*.

The situation is rather different with the opportunistic infections, where the pathogens are widespread in the environment. The isolation of a few colonies of *Aspergillus* from a non-sterile site such as sputum may be difficult to interpret. However, the isolation of an opportunistic pathogen from a normally sterile site should always be taken seriously.

The use of molecular diagnostic methods such as PCR-based methods for the diagnosis of systemic mycoses will increase, although such tests have seldom been standardised. At present they are used in a few laboratories for the commoner mycoses such as systemic *Candida* infections and candidaemia. They have good sensitivity and specificity and are likely to be used with increasing frequency in the future as they are more rapid than culture-based methods. At present they are more accurate for confirming the species rather than identifying the infection in pathological material.

Histoplasmosis

Definition and nomenclature

This is a highly infectious mycosis caused by *Histoplasma capsulatum* and affecting primarily the lungs, where it is generally asymptomatic [1]. The fungus is intracellular, parasitising the reticuloendothelial system and involving the spleen, liver, kidney, central nervous system and other organs. Rarely, the disease may become chronic, progressive and fatal.

Synonyms and inclusions
- Darling disease
- Histoplasmosis capsulati

Introduction and general description

Histoplasmosis results from infection with the dimorphic fungus, *H. capsulatum*. Previously two varieties of the fungus were differentiated: var. *capsulatum* or the closely related var. *duboisii*. The two varieties are differentiated on the basis of the yeast phase cell sizes, with var. *capsulatum* having smaller cells than those of var. *duboisii*. However, recent molecular studies demonstrated that there were multiple clades within *H. capsulatum* and that the assignment of three varieties (including var. *farciminosum* in horses and var. *duboisii*) were not phylogenetically relevant [2]. The African clade contained isolates previously classed as *H. capsulatum* var. *duboisii*, as well as *H. capsulatum* var. *capsulatum* and *H. capsulatum* var. *farciminosum*. However, despite this, there are important differences between the two morphological forms in their epidemiology and clinical manifestations. They show some subtle antigenic differences but their mycelial phases are identical. Therefore the old terminology, var. *capsulatum* and var. *duboisii*, will be used here until there is a clearer genetic explanation for these differences. Other species. *H. ohiense*, *H. mississipiense* and *H. suramericanum* cause pulmonary infections.

Epidemiology

The disease caused by *H. capsulatum* var. *capsulatum*, referred to here as histoplasmosis (small-form histoplasmosis), is widely distributed throughout the world, occurring in some 60 temperate and tropical countries in the Americas, Africa and Australasia [1]. It has been widely studied in the USA, where the number of human infections has been estimated at 30 million. It is highly endemic in the Mississippi and Ohio valleys. In certain areas, more than 80% of the population are known to have acquired the infection, as revealed by cutaneous reactivity to histoplasmin [3]. Infections with the *duboisii* form, known as African histoplasmosis or large-form histoplasmosis, have been reported only from Africa.

Age
Infants and children are frequently infected.

Sex
Among adults the rate is highest in male agricultural workers.

Ethnicity
There is no ethnic predisposition.

Associated diseases
Lymphoma appears to favour the development of the infection [4]. In addition, histoplasmosis is an important complicating infection in patients with AIDS [5,6].

Pathophysiology
Pathology
Histoplasmosis is normally a pulmonary infection which may spread through the bloodstream to affect other sites. Rarely the organism can be introduced by direct inoculation, usually as a result of a laboratory accident, to cause a local lesion with involvement of regional lymph glands (primary cutaneous disease).

Causative organsms
Histoplasma capsulatum exists as a saprophyte in nature and has often been isolated from soil, particularly when contaminated with chicken feathers or droppings. Other birds, such as starlings, and bats have also been implicated in the establishment of saprophytic reservoirs of infection.

Genetics
There is no known genetic predisposition.

Environmental factors
The fungus has been demonstrated in the soil of caves inhabited by bats and in endemic areas histoplasmosis is recognised as a hazard to cave explorers. *H. capsulatum* var. *capsulatum* has been isolated from the organs and faeces of house-dwelling bats in Panama. Its spores are infectious not only to humans, but also to small animals such as dogs, cats and rats. The disease is not transmitted from human to human or from animal to human, but by the inhalation of air-borne conidia. Epidemics have occurred from time to time among people exposed to spore-charged atmospheres when exploring caves or cleaning out sites rich in the excrement of birds. Infection may follow the introduction of spores through the skin and mucous membranes, as in laboratory workers.

Clinical features [1]
History
Benign forms of the disease, which heal by calcification, are indistinguishable on X-ray from tuberculosis. The spectrum of disease ranges from asymptomatic as well as symptomatic and benign infections to the progressive disseminated variety with blood spread to all organs. Primary coin lesions have been demonstrated as well as areas of cavitation. All varieties are reminiscent of tuberculosis.

Presentation
Skin lesions are more common with var. *duboisii* than with var. *capsulatum*. Indeed, whereas the skin is rarely affected in histoplasmosis except in AIDS patients, it is often involved in African histoplasmosis.

Although primary inoculation can rarely produce a local granuloma or ulcer, most skin lesions in histoplasmosis arise following dissemination from the primary pulmonary focus. Papules, ulcers, nodules, granulomas, abscesses, fistulae, scars and pigmentary changes may be seen, and there may be secondary involvement of the skin with osteomyelitis [7]. Involvement of the skin in some immunosuppressed patients may produce a condition resembling cellulitis [7].

Asymptomatic forms of histoplasmosis, indicated by the presence of positive skin test reactivity without evidence of infection, are common in endemic areas [3]. It is likely that this form of exposure is the dominant pattern, unless other factors such as a massive inoculum (exposure in a bat-infested cave) or defective host defence are present.

Clinical variants
Various clinical variants are discussed. The four main clinical varieties of histoplasmosis are acute pulmonary, acute disseminated, chronic pulmonary and chronic disseminated forms.

Acute pulmonary histoplasmosis. The patient has the usual symptoms of acute infection of the lungs and X-ray examination of the chest reveals diffuse mottling or localised infiltration. However, this acute pulmonary form must be considered uncommon, as a great majority of people in endemic areas who have shown reactions to histoplasmin testing and are assumed to have acquired their infection by the pulmonary route have done so without developing recognisable signs and symptoms. Even in such cases, the organism is not limited to the lungs but is disseminated throughout all parts of the reticuloendothelial system. Associated erythema multiforme or erythema nodosum have been observed. This skin reaction occurs very early in the disease, but the association with histoplasmosis may not be apparent for several weeks.

Acute disseminated forms. In this uncommon type, the lungs may be consolidated as a result of inhalation of many spores of *Histoplasma* and, although the pulmonary signs are prominent, there is also enlargement of the liver and spleen, fever, anaemia, loss of appetite and generalised enlargement of the lymph glands. In such circumstances, any of the manifestations listed may be prominent, and the clinical features can be infinitely variable. Pulmonary manifestations may simulate miliary tuberculosis.

Indurated granulomatous ulcers of the mouth, nose and larynx are often present and are distinctive [8]. Progressive emaciation, induced by gastrointestinal involvement, contributes to a fatal outcome after a course of weeks or months. Cutaneous or mucocutaneous granulomas are often seen in association with disseminated disease [9,10]. This is the form seen in patients with AIDS [11]. In AIDS patients, multiple small skin nodules may develop, the skin being more often involved than in other patient groups [4,5]. Often, papules have central softening.

Chronic pulmonary histoplasmosis. This usually occurs in adults and also closely resembles tuberculosis with pulmonary involvement.

Chronic disseminated forms. These may appear months or years after a patient has left an endemic area. The most common clinical presenting features are oral ulceration and Addison disease caused by adrenal infiltration. Mouth ulcers are large and may be chronic [8]; laryngeal involvement, ulceration or granuloma formation may also occur. Patients should be investigated for adrenal insufficiency, as this may appear for the first time during treatment. Ultrasound scans are useful for screening for adrenal enlargement [12].

Primary cutaneous histoplasmosis. This is very rare and appears after inoculation of the organism into the skin. The primary lesion is a nodule or indurated ulcer and there is often local lymphadenopathy [1].

Other forms of histoplasmosis. Other forms can be recognised. Dissemination may occur shortly after infection, or there may be a latent period of many years. Moreover, the severity of the condition may be influenced by various predisposing causes including leukaemia, corticosteroid treatment, lymphoma, diabetes, carcinoma, AIDS and systemic collagen disease [11,13].

African histoplasmosis. The clinical appearance of African forms of histoplasmosis are variable, and the disease is sporadic and uncommon [14]. It is confined to the areas south of the Sahara and north of the Zambezi river. The most common sites clinically involved in African histoplasmosis are the skin and bone, although lymph nodes and other areas including the lungs may be affected [15]. Skin lesions range from small papules resembling molluscum contagiosum, to abscesses or ulcers [16]. It is useful to screen patients with a bone scan or X-rays to exclude bone foci of infection [17]. The course of the disease is usually chronic, although some patients appear to develop a more rapidly progressive, disseminated type of infection. However, this form of histoplasmosis has only rarely been seen in AIDS patients. The diagnosis is confirmed by microscopy (direct or histopathology) and culture. Serology, using conventional tests, is often negative in African histoplasmosis.

Differential diagnosis
This includes other systemic mycoses such as *Talaromyces* infections and cryptococcosis. Skin lesions may resemble molluscum contagiosum.

Investigations
The diagnosis of histoplasmosis is established by identifying the small intracellular yeast cells (2–5 μm) of *Histoplasma* in sputum, peripheral blood, bone marrow or biopsy specimens. Lymph node aspiration may also be employed. Care should be taken in areas endemic for *Talaromyces marneffei* as the two organisms are of a similar size, although the latter shows characteristic septal formation rather than budding. *Histoplasma* is predominantly an intracellular parasite, growing within the cells of the reticuloendothelial system as an oval yeast (Figure 32.57). All phagocytic cells of the reticuloendothelial system are involved, including those in the liver, spleen, lymph nodes and bone marrow, so that the cytoplasm is swollen with masses of fungal cells. There is, at first, little tissue reaction; later, necrosis takes place to be followed by granulomatous changes and fibrosis. *H. duboisii* is usually distinctive in having a much larger tissue form. It often elicits an inflammatory response in which giant cells predominate. The intracellular yeasts are clearly seen with specific fungal stains such as methenamine silver and

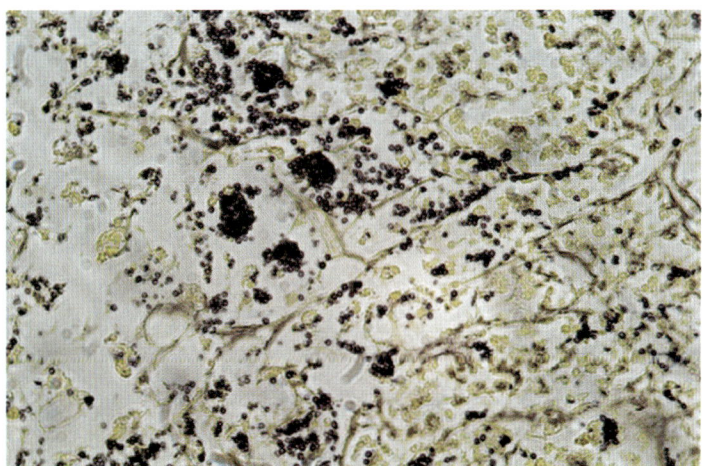

(a)

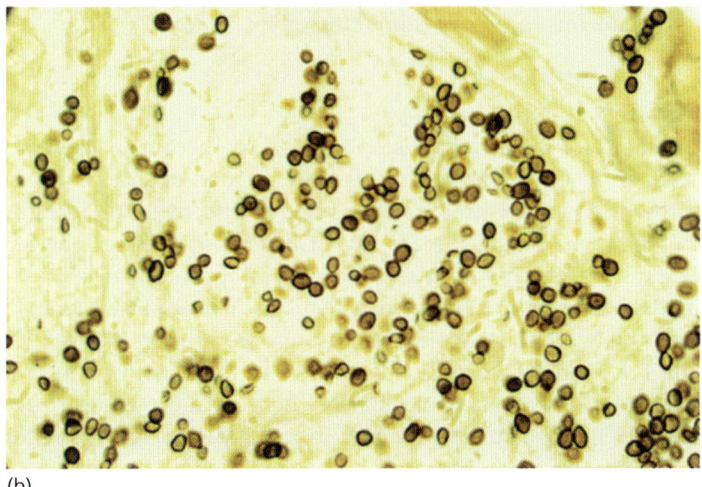

(b)

Figure 32.57 *Histoplasmosis capsulatum* var. *capsulatum*. (a) Tissue section. The tiny yeasts, stained black with GMS, are largely intracellular. (b) Oil immersion. The typical budding yeasts are clearly visible. Compare with *Talaromyces marneffei* infection (see Figure 32.62). Courtesy of the Department of Medical Mycology, St John's Institute of Dermatology, King's College London, London, UK.

PAS. The identity of the organism should be confirmed by culture. Some workers consider that cultures should be maintained for up to 12 weeks before reporting negative results, although more commonly they are kept for 4–6 weeks.

Histoplasma capsulatum. Colony: at 30°C the growth may initially be waxy, but surface mycelium usually develops to produce white or tan, cottony colonies. Microscopy: two types of conidia are formed: large (8–15 µm), rounded or occasionally pear-shaped, unicellular, tuberculate macroconidia; and small, oval, smooth or roughened microconidia. Physiological tests: ideally, cultural identification should be confirmed by demonstrating eluted *Histoplasma*-specific antigens by using an exoantigen test or a nucleic acid hybridisation test. However, if these techniques are not available, a suitable medium for conversion to the yeast phase is brain–heart infusion agar supplemented with 10% sheep's blood, 1% glucose and 0.1% cysteine.

Serological tests: the intradermal histoplasmin skin test is an epidemiological tool that is of no help in diagnosis because it is negative in many patients with disseminated histoplasmosis. A rising complement fixation titre indicates dissemination. Precipitins are also valuable because some antigens, designated H and M, correlate well with active or recent infection [18]. The histoplasmin skin test should not be performed before the serological test as it may produce a rise in the serological titre. Several serological kits are now sold commercially for both complement fixation and double diffusion tests. A significant development has been the use of a serological test for the detection of circulating *Histoplasma* antigens [19], which is particularly helpful in AIDS patients. The test can be used with serum or urine, although at the moment there is only one laboratory that offers commercial testing.

Management
All forms of histoplamosis require treatment with antifungal drugs, although in some acute forms of pulmonary histoplasmosis there is spontaneous recovery without treatment.

First line
The choice of therapy for histoplasmosis has become considerably wider in recent years. For many disseminated or localised forms of the disease, oral itraconazole is highly effective [20], including the treatment of the disease in AIDS patients, where long-term suppressive therapy is usually needed. It appears that the use of HAART may reduce the requirement for maintenance therapy in some cases. Posaconazole and fluconazole are alternatives [20]. Amphotericin B is useful and is used in those with widespread and severe infections, particularly where an intravenous drug is needed [3]. The acute pulmonary forms of histoplasmosis require no specific antifungal therapy.

In African histoplasmosis, there is evidence that itraconazole or ketoconazole are effective [21]. An alternative in severe cases is amphotericin B [16]. Some patients with solitary skin lesions may simply respond to excision without chemotherapy, although antifungals should be given where possible.

Treatment ladder for histoplasmosis

First line
- Itraconazole 100 mg daily until clinical remission
- For patients who are severely ill, amphotericin B 0.5–1 mg/kg daily (or liposomal amphotericin B 3 mg/kg daily) for 2 weeks. Itraconazole 200 mg once or twice daily may then be used for a further period depending on clinical response
- For mild disease, patients can be started straight on itraconazole 200 mg daily for a period determined by clinical response

Second line
- Fluconazole 800 mg daily for 3 months and then 400 mg daily until clinical remission is achieved
- There is insufficient evidence to recommend posaconazole at present

---

Blastomycosis

Definition and nomenclature
Blastomycosis is a chronic granulomatous and suppurative mycosis caused by *Blastomyces dermatitidis* and other species such as *B. percursus* and *B. emzantsi* (Africa). It affects primarily the lungs but disseminating forms also affect the skin, bones, central nervous system and other sites.

Synonyms and inclusions
- North American blastomycosis
- Gilchrist disease

Epidemiology
Incidence and prevalence
The condition was originally thought to be restricted to the North American continent where it extends from Canada, particularly Quebec, through the USA with occasional cases in Mexico and Central America. The largest number of cases is seen in the Mississippi valley [1]. Blastomycosis, however, is now known to be widely distributed in Africa, with the largest numbers of cases coming from Zimbabwe [2,3], and cases have also been reported from the Middle East [4], India [5] and Poland. The incidence of infections tends to be highest in rural areas [1] and in agricultural workers. Human–human transmission does not normally take place. The fungus has also been recovered from domestic animals (e.g. dogs).

Age
As with most of the systemic mycoses, adult males are most commonly affected, the majority being between the ages of 30 and 50 years. Indeed, some 86% of recorded cases are males.

Associated diseases
Blastomycosis is not common in patients with HIV/AIDS.

Pathophysiology

Blastomyces dermatitidis has only rarely been isolated from the environment. Studies suggest that its natural substrate may be wood debris or soil close to rivers or subject to flooding [6,7]. The fungus can grow in sterile soil in the laboratory, and it is believed that humans are infected by the inhalation of spores from a saprophytic source. However, primary skin infection also occurs, particularly in laboratory workers or pathologists.

Predisposing factors

Blastomycosis is an infection that can affect otherwise healthy individuals as well as the immunosuppressed.

Pathology

The tissue reaction, and ultimately the course and prognosis, are determined by the immunological response of the patient. Primary lesions, usually pulmonary, sometimes cutaneous, develop 1–3 weeks after infection and are associated with regional lymphadenopathy.

Clinical features [8]

History

As the source of exposure is not yet known there is no known incubation period.

Presentation

There are three forms of blastomycosis: primary cutaneous, pulmonary and disseminated.

Clinical variants

Primary cutaneous blastomycosis. This is very rare and follows trauma to the skin and introduction of the fungus. The condition has been seen mainly in laboratory workers (e.g. pathologists carrying out autopsy examinations) [9]. After inoculation, a red, indurated area with a chancre appears in 1–2 weeks with associated lymphangitis and lymphadenopathy. There may be some constitutional reaction. There is a strong tendency towards spontaneous recovery.

Pulmonary blastomycosis. This is very similar to pulmonary tuberculosis. There may be no symptoms, or there may be low-grade fever, chest pain, cough and haemoptysis. Occasionally, erythema nodosum develops [8]. The pulmonary lesion may resolve, or there may be cavity formation with lung abscess. In most cases, other organs are also affected [10]. The disease, if untreated, may frequently disseminate and often progresses to death. Mild, asymptomatic, self-limiting infections, common in histoplasmosis and coccidioidomycosis, may occur [11], but are probably uncommon.

Disseminated blastomycosis. When the infection spreads from the chest, lesions develop in many organs, commonly the skin, bones and central nervous system [12]. Mucous membranes are rarely involved. One or many skin lesions may be present [13]. These are often symmetrical and usually on the trunk rather than on the exposed parts. Each consists of a papule or nodule that may

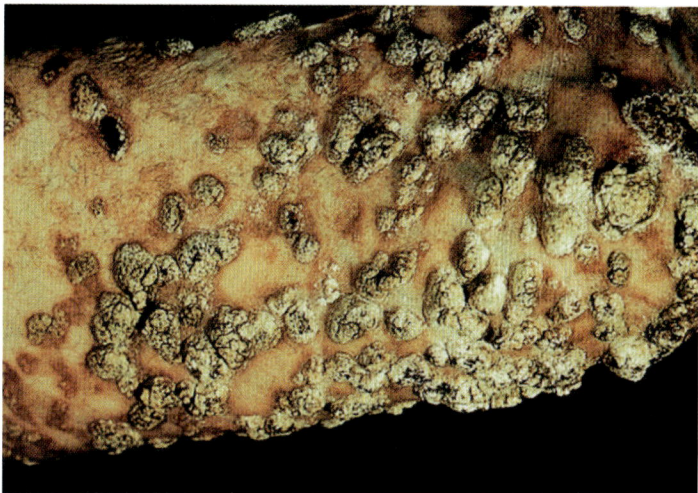

Figure 32.58 Cutaneous blastomycosis. Courtesy of Dr M. James, Royal Berkshire Hospital, Reading, UK.

ulcerate and discharge pus. The lesions enlarge at the periphery and tend to show central scarring, which may be dense. Eventually, after a relentless progress for months, the lesion is serpiginous in outline, the borders are raised and warty (Figure 32.58), and have a violaceous margin studded with miliary abscesses containing the organisms [8]. Other patients may present with nodules and abscesses. African patients with blastomycosis have a higher frequency of skin and bone involvement [2].

Differential diagnosis

The microabscesses are the distinctive clinical feature, but the chronic granulomas of the skin must be differentiated from tuberculosis, syphilis, leprosy, pyoderma gangrenosum and drug reactions resulting from bromides and iodides. Pulmonary lesions, which are invariably present, necessitate X-ray examinations of the chest and differentiation from tuberculosis and other infections, and from neoplasia. The diagnosis of the skin lesions is established by direct microscopy of pus in 10% potassium hydroxide and confirmed by culture or biopsy.

Investigations

The fungus can be observed in potassium hydroxide mounts of pus or scrapings as rather thick-walled, rounded, refractile, spherical yeasts with broad-based buds. Tissue sections must be scanned carefully to identify organisms (Figure 32.59). *B. dermatitidis* produces budding yeasts with a characteristic broad base to the bud in the tissues. The skin lesions that follow bloodstream dissemination show marked epidermal hyperplasia, which may be pseudoepitheliomatous in degree. Intra- and subepidermal polymorphonuclear abscesses and a granulomatous infiltrate are found in the dermis. These include giant cells of the Langerhans type, which contain the round or oval organisms with thick, refractile walls. Disseminated skin lesions may also take the form of abscesses with organisms in their walls or within giant cells, and a non-specific granulomatous infiltrate.

Blastomyces dermatitidis. Colony: mycelium develops in culture at 30°C, the colonies being initially waxy, then cottony and white to

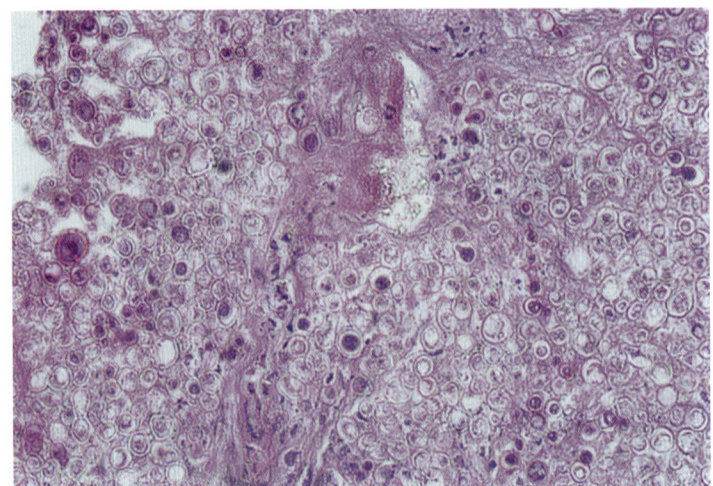

Figure 32.59 North American blastomycosis: tissue section. The large yeasts, stained pink with PAS, are characterised by the broad base of the buds. Courtesy of the Department of Medical Mycology, St John's Institute of Dermatology, King's College London, London, UK.

tan. Microscopy: small, rounded or pear-shaped conidia (2–5 μm) are produced on short stalks arising at right angles from the hyphae. Physiological tests: exoantigen tests or nucleic acid probes are available for safe and rapid identification of the organism. Alternatively, conversion to the yeast phase can be achieved on blood–glucose–cysteine agar. Other species are identified using molecular methods.

Serological tests: precipitating antibodies to *B. dermatitidis* are often present in the serum of infected subjects and a characteristic precipitin line, the E band, has been described in a high proportion of established cases [8].

Management
All variants of the disease require treatment.

First line
In most cases itraconazole appears to be effective and has the advantage that it can be given orally [14]. The best regimen is not clear, but at least 400 mg daily should be given initially.

Second line
Amphotericin B is still used for the treatment of widespread disseminated forms of blastomycosis [8]. Ketoconazole is an alternative therapy [15].

Treatment ladder for blastomycosis

First line
- Itraconazole 200–400 mg daily until clinical remission
- For patients who are severely ill, amphotericin B 0.5–1 mg/kg daily for 2 weeks followed by itraconazole for a further period depending on clinical response

---

Coccidioidomycosis

Definition and nomenclature
This is a (primary) respiratory fungal infection caused by *Coccidioides immitis* and *C. posadasii*, which may become progressive and disseminated, with severe or fatal forms.

Synonyms and inclusions
- Coccidioidal granuloma
- Valley fever
- San Joaquin valley fever
- Desert rheumatism

Epidemiology
Coccidioidomycosis is endemic in desert areas of the southwestern states of the USA and in parts of Central and South America [1]. Molecular studies have shown that there are two species of *Coccidioides*: *C. immitis* which occurs only in California and *C. posadasii* which occurs elsewhere [2]. However, on the basis of clinical and microbiological characteristics these two species cannot be differentiated routinely. Cases described outside this area are imported infections. The climate in endemic areas is characterised by high mean January and July temperatures and an annual rainfall of 12–50 cm. There is clear evidence that human infection may develop from a very short residence in, or even a journey through, an endemic area, so that with increasing travel, cases of coccidioidomycosis are found in many parts of the world. Skin tests have shown that the incidence in endemic areas may be as high as 95%. It is a widespread and important disease only within these regions.

Age
It affects any age.

Sex
There is a higher risk of dissemination in pregnant women.

Ethnicity
There is a higher risk of disseminated infection in patients with Latin, native American and African American backgrounds.

Pathophysiology
The fungus is a soil inhabitant; infection of humans and a wide variety of domestic and wild animals is acquired by inhalation of fungus-laden dust particles. The control of dust therefore becomes important in the prevention of the disease [3]. Primary infection of the skin is rare but is known to occur [4]. The inhaled spores (arthroconidia of the saprophytic mycelial phase) develop in the lung tissue to form spherules – large, round, endospore-containing structures, which when mature are usually 30–80 μm in diameter (Figure 32.60). Between 2 and 6 weeks after exposure, the patient becomes sensitive to an intradermal skin test using the fungal antigen, coccidioidin. The primary lesion is associated with regional lymphadenopathy, but usually there is no further spread. If secondary dissemination occurs, granulomatous lesions with giant cells and epithelioid cells are produced.

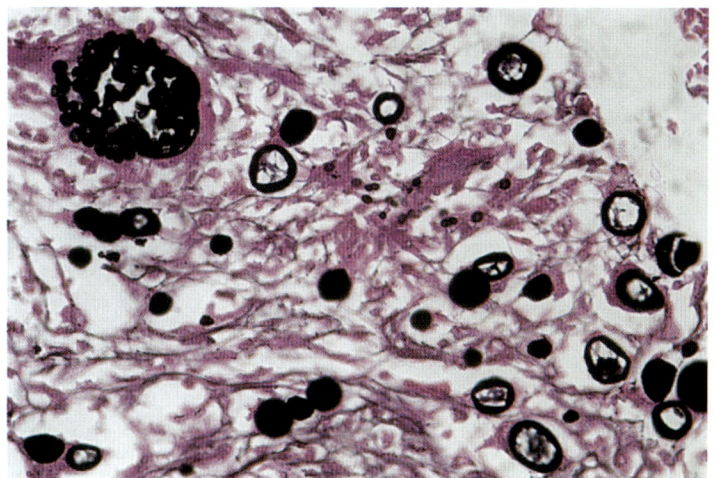

Figure 32.60 Coccidioidomycosis tissue section. Spherules of various sizes are stained black with GMS. In the top left-hand part of the slide, freshly released endospores are visible. Courtesy of the Department of Medical Mycology, St John's Institute of Dermatology, King's College London, London, UK.

Pathology

In histological sections of active lesions, spherules with endospores can usually be demonstrated with routine staining, but in lesions with immature, empty or degenerate fungal spherules this may be difficult or impossible. Spherules may be seen within the cytoplasm of histiocytes and in giant cells of the foreign-body type. The fungus can be easily demonstrated by the use of special fungus stains such as PAS or silver impregnation stains.

Causative organisms

The causative organisms are *C. immitis* and *C. posadasii*.

Clinical features [1]

History

The severity of coccidioidomycosis varies from a very mild, inapparent, upper respiratory tract infection to an acute, disseminated fatal disease.

Presentation

The primary pulmonary form, which is the most common form, is sometimes asymptomatic, but may simulate influenza (Chapter 47) or, occasionally, pulmonary tuberculosis. Erythema multiforme or erythema nodosum (Chapter 97) occurs from the third to the seventh week in some 3–25% of patients, particularly in females. In endemic areas, coccidioidomycosis is often the most common cause of erythema nodosum. There may be accompanying uveitis and arthralgia.

Pulmonary symptoms, when present, include pain resembling pleurisy, and often very sudden and acute shortness of breath, cough and associated pyrexia. Generalised aches, malaise and lassitude may occur, and there may be severe headache. An early, generalised, red, macular rash is seen in 10% of patients. The exceedingly rare primary skin lesions are painless, firm, indurated nodules often occurring 1–3 weeks after local trauma. Regional lymphadenopathy develops but spontaneous healing follows after a few weeks [5].

Clinical variants

Disseminated coccidioidomycosis is uncommon and develops in fewer than 0.5% of infected individuals, usually in black, Filipino or immunosuppressed patients [6]. It may develop rapidly by blood spread of endospores to all organs, or insidiously from a pulmonary lesion after a period of quiescence. The death rate in acute disseminated disease, or with meningitis, is very high [7]. Disseminated lesions may occur in the skin, subcutaneous tissues, bones, joints and all organs. The skin lesions may appear as abscesses, granulomas, ulcers or discharging sinuses, particularly if there is underlying bone or joint disease [4].

Persistent and progressive pulmonary involvement and dissemination of infection are seen, including the appearance of multiple skin lesions in patients with AIDS [8]. Prolonged and progressive pulmonary infection may also occur in AIDS patients.

Differential diagnosis

The clinical manifestations of the disease are so varied that the condition must be differentiated from most chronic infectious conditions. Residence in, or travel through, an endemic area might suggest the diagnosis.

Disease course and prognosis

The prognosis for the primary form is excellent; untreated, acute disseminated forms are fatal.

Investigations

The large (usually 30–80 μm, occasionally larger) globular spherules may be seen in potassium hydroxide mounts of sputum, cerebrospinal fluid or pus. Confirmation depends on the isolation of the fungus in culture.

Coccidioides immitis* and *C. posadasii*. Colony: cultures of *C. immitis* and *C. posadasii* are mycelial, fast growing, initially waxy then cottony, and white to tan [9]. Microscopy: characteristic thick-walled arthroconidia, separated from each other by alternate empty cells, are observed. Physiological tests: exoantigen testing and PCR probes are available for identification. If necessary, conversion can be achieved using the modified Converse medium [10].

Serological tests: these are of value in diagnosis and prognosis of the disease. Precipitins develop in up to 90% of infected individuals within 2–4 weeks but are short lived; complement fixing (CF) antibodies are characteristic of more severe infections and increase to a maximum after 6 months. A rise of CF antibodies indicates dissemination while a decrease parallels clinical improvement.

Skin tests with coccidioidin are of little value in diagnosing infections [1]. Patients with coccidioidomycosis may cross-react to histoplasmin, but responses are usually much milder, and seldom cause confusion with the specific reaction to coccidioidin. Spherulin, derived from the tissue form of *C. immitis*, is reported to be superior to coccidioidin in detecting cutaneous hypersensitivity in both epidemiological and clinical settings [11]. In severe infections, cutaneous anergy is common [12].

Management [1]

In the primary pulmonary infection, no specific therapy apart from rest is necessary. There is little evidence that the use of an oral azole, such as itraconazole, in patients with erythema nodosum is helpful in reducing symptoms, and it may aggravate the situation. For disseminated disease, the approach depends on the form of disease.

First line
Oral itraconazole (200–400 mg daily) and fluconazole (400–800 mg daily) are effective in some forms of localised infection such as solitary disseminated skin lesions [5] – the duration depending on the clinical response. Itraconazole may be effective in other disseminated forms of disease [13]. At present there is insufficient evidence on the most effective doses of the newer antifungal drugs voriconazole and posaconazole and these are second line treatments. Intravenous amphotericin B (0.5–1 mg/kg daily) or liposomal amphotericin (3 mg/kg daily) is used for many of the other clinical forms of coccidioidomycosis, including severe disease for periods of between 2 and 4 weeks [14]. The most difficult complications to treat at present are meningitis and joint infections. Neither of these responds well even to newer therapies, although temporary improvements may be achieved.

Paracoccidioidomycosis

Definition and nomenclature
This is a chronic granulomatous fungal infection caused by members of the species complex, *Paracoccidioides brasiliensis*, affecting the skin, mucous membranes, lymph nodes and internal organs [1].

> **Synonyms and inclusions**
> - South American blastomycosis
> - Paracoccidioidal granuloma

Epidemiology
Paracoccidioidomycosis has been reported from most Latin American countries, but the infection is most commonly found in Brazil, particularly in the state of Sao Paulo [2], Colombia and Argentina. The infection is not known in other continents. The disease is not transmitted directly from person to person. The condition is much more frequent in rural areas.

Age
It is rare in children.

Sex
Adult males between the ages of 20 and 50 years are most frequently infected, although exposure rates are equal across the two sexes [3]. The infection is very uncommon in women.

Pathophysiology
It is thought that the fungus occurs as a saprophyte on vegetation or in soil [4]. *P. brasiliensis* is likely to gain entry to the body after inhalation via the respiratory tract, as with the other dimorphic fungal infections. Susceptibility to *P. brasiliensis* may be related to HLA-A9. This antigen has been found more frequently in progressive pulmonary forms of the disease than in patients with extrapulmonary involvement. The inhibition of the yeast phase, the form seen in human infections, is at least partially dependent on the binding of oestrogen by the fungus, which may account for the marked sex difference in susceptibility [3].

Clinical features
History
The most common site of infection is the lung (pulmonary form), although skin and mucous membranes (mucocutaneous form) or lymph nodes (lymphatic form) are also often involved [4,5].

Presentation
Many patients have a mixed type of infection with involvement of different organ systems. In most patients, the disease is only slowly progressive.

Clinical variants
Patients with pulmonary lesions present with weight loss and chronic cough. The lesions may be bilateral and nodular on X-ray, and there is often extensive fibrosis [6]. Mucocutaneous lesions may be present in patients with lung disease or can occur on their own. Oral or circumoral lesions are common in the mucocutaneous forms of paracoccidioidomycosis, although they may also occur in the nose, conjunctivae or anus. Lesions may be localised or diffuse. If in the mouth, a severe, painful, ulcerating stomatitis occurs. The ulcers become granulomatous and spread over the mucous membranes (the so-called 'mulberry-like erosion'). Lesions of the gums are common: they loosen the teeth, which are usually lost. The tongue may be involved. The skin lesions may begin at the mucocutaneous junction by direct extension from the mouth, or there may be satellite lesions from autoinoculation [7]. Haematogenous or lymphatic spread results in subcutaneous abscesses. The cervical lymph nodes are sometimes enlarged early. They are palpable, painful, adherent to the overlying skin and may eventually suppurate with chronic sinus formation. If systemic spread occurs, the spleen, intestines, lungs and liver are involved; it is said that the intestines are often affected, with lesions eroding into the lumen. Bone lesions have been seen and the adrenals may be destroyed. The central nervous system may also be affected [1].

Untreated, the disease was fatal in a few months to a few years in 43% of proved cases [6,7]. The extensive, painful mouth lesions with loss of teeth interfere with feeding, and the patient becomes cachectic. Paracoccidioidomycosis is uncommon but does occur in AIDS patients, and widespread infections may develop in young adults or older children without recognisable predisposition.

Differential diagnosis
The frequency with which the mouth and gums are involved with a loss of teeth, the fact that there is no central scar formation, and the presence of marked lymphadenitis and lymphadenopathy differentiates paracoccidioidomycosis from blastomycosis. Other conditions to be considered are tuberculosis, syphilis, histoplasmosis, actinomycosis, sporotrichosis, rhinoscleroma and leishmaniasis. The organisms are readily found in biopsy specimens or in scrapings from the mucous membrane lesions. Aspiration of pus from lymph nodes will also provide material for microscopic examination and culture.

Complications and co-morbidities
See under clinical variants. Paracoccidioidomycosis is often associated with severe fibrosis, and in oro-pharyngeal lesions contractures or laryngeal strictures can occur during or after therapy.

Disease course and prognosis
The disease course is chronic and disseminated forms can be fatal.

Investigations
Pus, exudates and scrapings examined in potassium hydroxide mounts may show rounded refractile cells, which can be distinguished from *Blastomyces dermatitidis* when the characteristic multiple budding is seen. Yeasts range from 2 to 30 µm in diameter.

Paracoccidioides brasiliensis. Colony: growth is much slower and more restricted than that of *B. dermatitidis*. Initially flat or wrinkled and leathery, the colonies develop tufts of white to tan aerial mycelium. Microscopy: the hyaline, unicellular, pear-shaped conidia (3–4 µm) are borne directly on the hyphae or on short stalks. Very few conidia are produced. Physiological tests: an exoantigen test is available to identify the isolates; alternatively, conversion can be achieved on brain–heart infusion agar supplemented with 10% sheep's blood.

Serological tests: both complement fixation and immunodiffusion assays are useful in the diagnosis of this condition; antigen detection methods are in development [8]. In histological sections, the reaction resembles that seen in blastomycosis, namely granulomas with pyogenic inflammation. Giant cells are conspicuous and these frequently contain the rounded budding cells. Exceptionally, these may attain diameters of 60 µm. The tendency to produce many multilateral buds in tissue sections is diagnostic (Figure 32.61). In the skin and mucous membranes, there is pseudoepitheliomatous hyperplasia with severe granulomatous inflammation; intraepithelial abscesses occur and these frequently communicate with the surface.

Management
All forms require antifungal therapy.

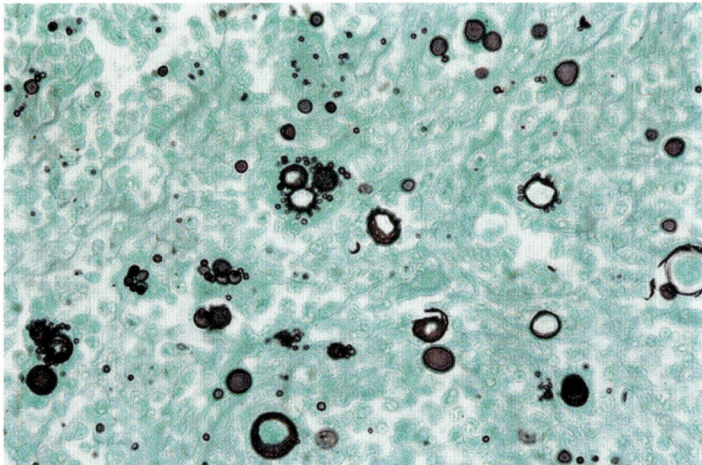

Figure 32.61 Paracoccidioidomycosis. The yeasts, stained black with GMS, are characterised by the numerous peripheral buds produced. Courtesy of the Department of Medical Mycology, St John's Institute of Dermatology, King's College London, London, UK.

First line
The treatment of choice in most cases is itraconazole 200–400 mg daily, which can produce remission in 3–6 months [9,10]. Ketoconazole 200 mg daily is an alternative. Relapse is common and long-term surveillance should be carried out. Some patients, particularly those with more rapidly progressive and extensive infections, may require amphotericin B 0.5–1 mg/kg for 2 weeks followed by oral itraconazole 200 mg daily [1].

Infections caused by *Talaromyces marneffei*

Definition and nomenclature
Talaromyces (previously *Penicillium*) *marneffei* is a recently recognised fungal pathogen that causes a disseminated mycosis in both healthy and immunocompromised patients [1]. There is a strong association with AIDS (Chapter 31).

Synonyms and inclusions
- Penicilliosis
- Talaromycosis

Epidemiology
Talaromyces marneffei infections in humans are confined to South-East Asia, particularly Thailand, southern China and Vietnam [2,3]. However, there are reports in other Asian countries, and imported cases have been seen in Europe and the USA [4]. Natural infections occur in bamboo rats, which are large, underground-dwelling rodents. Infections can occur in apparently healthy individuals, but it is a particular problem in severely immunocompromised patients in the endemic area.

It is rare in children and affects both sexes. HIV/AIDS or treatment with anti CD20 biologics may be associated.

Pathophysiology
Although the causative organism is thought to originate from soil, it has not been isolated from this source.

Clinical features
History
It is not known if there is a subclinical form of this infection (cf. histoplasmosis).

Presentation
Patients may present with respiratory symptoms, such as cough, chest pain and fever, or with signs of dissemination such as anaemia, multiple skin papules and hepatosplenomegaly. Skin lesions occur in over 50% of cases. They are small papules, ulcers or molluscum-like lesions. They are usually widely scattered on the face and trunk. *T. marneffei* infections are also seen in travellers to the endemic area.

Differential diagnosis
The main differential is with other disseminated mycoses, such as histoplasmosis and cryptococcosis, which can also be found in AIDS

patients in the endemic area. Biopsy and, where necessary, culture will distinguish between the different causes.

Complications and co-morbidities
These include fungaemia and dissemination to other sites.

Disease course and prognosis
Left untreated, this infection is fatal.

Investigations
Talaromyces marneffei forms characteristic cells that are divided by a septum in tissue (Figure 32.62). It does not produce buds. However, most cells in biopsy material are small, oval structures similar in size to *Histoplasma capsulatum*. Occasionally, larger banana-shaped cells are seen. The diagnosis can be made from appropriately stained biopsies, smears and blood films, although with experience the typical cells can be distinguished on simple stains such as leishmanin.

The organism can be isolated in culture and is usually identified by molecular probes. Serological tests such as Western blot are available in specialised centres.

Talaromyces marneffei. Colony: in culture, *T. marneffei* grows rapidly on glucose–peptone agar as a green or greyish mould. It produces a diffusible red pigment. Microscopy: typical *Penicillium* conidiophores and phialoconidia are produced. Physiological tests: on glucose–peptone agar after incubation for 14 days at 37°C, the organism produces dry, yeast-like colonies. The cells are oval to elliptical and reproduce by fission.

Management
All cases should be treated with antifungals.

First line
In severe cases, amphotericin B is necessary. There is usually a good response to itraconazole 200–400 mg/day, which is given until clinical remission, but this may have to be given for a long period to prevent relapse. With antiretrovirals it is possible to withdraw itraconazole once the lesions have healed.

Rare endemic mycoses

A new group of systemic infections caused by species of *Emergomyces* – *E. pasteurianus*, *E. africanus*, *E. orientalis*, *E canadiensis* and *E. europaeus* has been recognised. These are dimorphic fungi which invade following inhalation and can spread from the lung to other sites, particularly the skin, where they cause nodules, plaques or ulcers. These are often multiple. The source of *Emergomyces* is unknown although species DNA has been found in soil. The highest number of cases have been seen in South Africa but cases have also been recorded in China, Europe and North America. The infection usually occurs in severely immunosuppressed patients, including those with HIV. In tissue, the yeast fungi look identical to *Histoplasma capsulatum* but they can be grown in culture and identified by PCR. The infection responds to amphotericin B or an azole antifungal such as itraconazole or voriconazole [1].

Cryptococcosis

Definition
Cryptococcosis is an acute, subacute or chronic infection caused by the encapsulated yeast *Cryptococcus neoformans* or related species. There is a marked predilection for the brain and meninges, although the lungs and occasionally the skin and other parts of the body may be involved.

Epidemiology
Cryptococcosis, unlike many other systemic mycoses, occurs throughout the world [1]. The condition is not excessively rare, and the diagnosis is frequently unsuspected. It is particularly associated with AIDS and is now seen regularly in these patients if they are not receiving antiviral therapy.

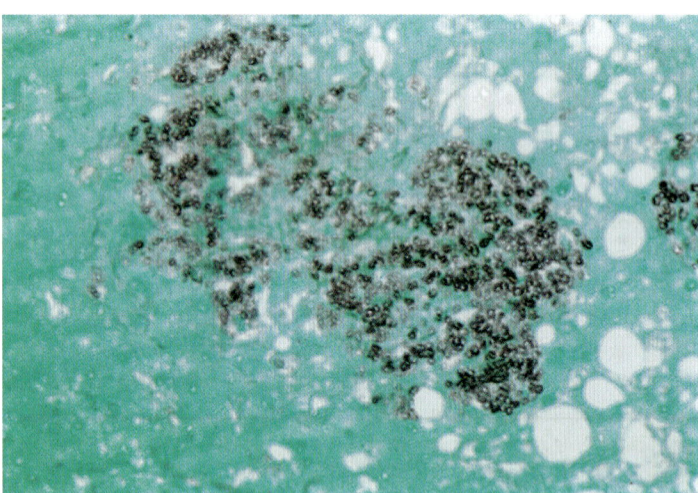

(a)

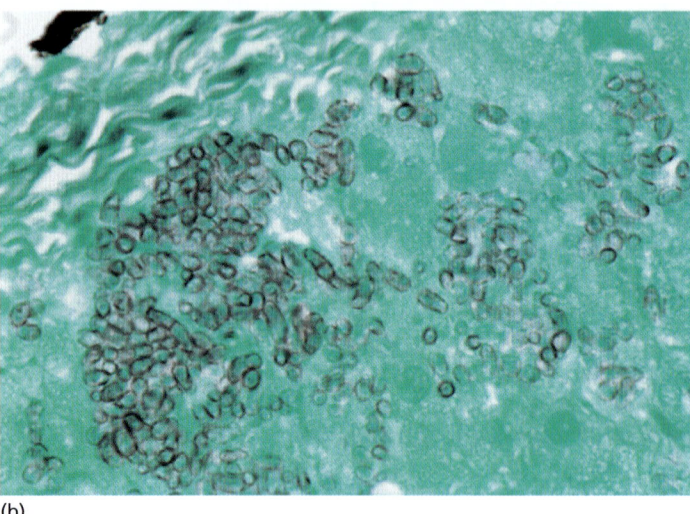

(b)

Figure 32.62 Infection by *Talaromyces* (previously *Penicillium*) *marneffei*. (a) Tissue section. The tiny organisms are largely intracellular and look very similar to histoplasmosis at this magnification. (b) Oil immersion. The organisms divide by a central septum, rather than by budding. Sausage-shaped cells are also clearly visible. Courtesy of the Department of Medical Mycology, St John's Institute of Dermatology, King's College London, London, UK.

Age
The disease usually occurs between the ages of 30 and 60 years, and is uncommon in childhood.

Associated diseases
Susceptibility is greatly increased by immunodeficiency states and neoplastic diseases, especially Hodgkin disease. Recognisable predispositions include AIDS, malignant lymphomas, sarcoidosis, collagen disease, carcinoma and systemic corticosteroid therapy [2]. Cryptococcosis has also been associated with immunosuppression in patients following renal transplantation. However, the main underlying disease is AIDS [3] (Chapter 31). The incidence of cryptococcosis in patients with established AIDS varies in different countries from 3–5% in the USA to 4% in the UK and over 12% in parts of Africa (e.g. Zaire) and Thailand. This resulted in an increase in the numbers of patients although this has now decreased with the wider availability of antiretrovirals.

Pathophysiology
The respiratory tract is the usual portal of entry, but primary cutaneous lesions may occur. *C. neoformans* is unusual among pathogenic fungi in its predilection for invasion of the central nervous system. Skin lesions occur in 10–15% of cases of disseminated cryptococcosis.

Causative organism
Cryptococcosis is caused by members of two species complexes, *C. neoformans* and *C. gattii*. These correspond to previous cryptococcal serotypes known as A, D, B and C [1]: *C. neoformans* var. *grubii* is serotype A [4], *C. neoformans gattii* is serotypes B and C, and *C. neoformans* var. *neoformans* is serotype D. Interest has been stimulated by the observation that in Europe and much of the USA the *neoformans* and *grubii* varieties were dominant, whereas in much of the tropics including Africa the *gattii* forms were more common [5]. With the spread of HIV infection, the *grubii*, in particular, and *neoformans* varieties are found in AIDS patients. The *neoformans* and *grubii* varieties exist as saprophytes in nature, being particularly abundant in soils enriched with pigeon droppings. By contrast, *C. gattii* has been isolated from leaf and bark debris from red gum trees. Unusual among pathogenic fungi, *Cryptococcus* is a basidiomycete. It is not known if spores produced by the sexual phase (basidiospores) constitute infectious propagules. Studies *in vitro* have shown that yeast cells of *C. neoformans* are susceptible to soil microorganisms, including bacteria and amoebae.

Animal–human or human–human transmission of the disease has not been reported. Bird droppings act as an excellent culture medium and probably play an important part in promoting multiplication of the fungus in contaminated soil and the provision of a significant reservoir of infection in the case of *C. neoformans*. The inhalation of small yeast forms that have been aerosolised is likely to be the main route of infection. It is assumed that *C. gattii* infections follow a similar route of infection, although the exact mode of pathogenesis is still not known.

Pathology
There may be minimal inflammatory reaction. The characteristic lesion consists of encapsulated budding cells mixed with a network

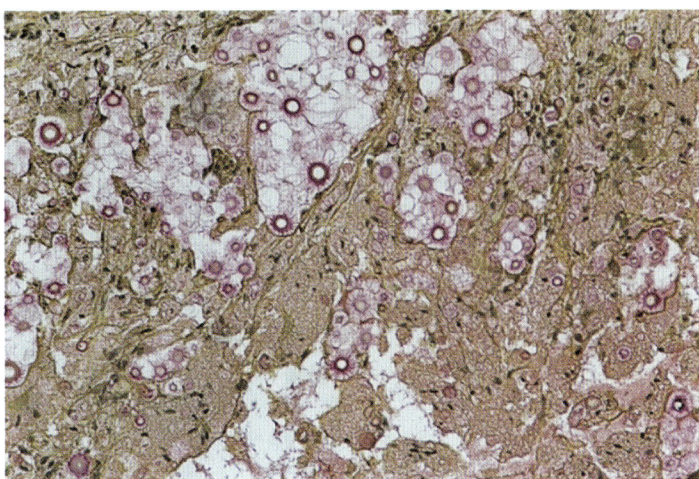

Figure 32.63 Cryptococcosis: tissue section. The mucicarmine stains the capsule specifically. The radiate spiny appearance is caused by shrinkage during processing. Courtesy of the Department of Medical Mycology, St John's Institute of Dermatology, King's College London, London, UK.

of connective tissue, which enlarges and compresses the surrounding tissues [6]. A specific stain for the capsule – mucicarmine – is available (Figure 32.63). Alternatively, a granulomatous reaction without caseation may be seen [7]. These clusters of cells are seen in most tissues of the body, but particularly in the central nervous system. In rare instances, cryptococci may proliferate in infected tissues in a non-encapsulated form.

Clinical features [2,3]
History
There is no known incubation period.

Presentation
Systemic involvement is usual. The central nervous system manifestations often predominate, presenting with meningitis or as focal brain lesions simulating a tumour. There is low-grade fever and general decline in health, ending in coma and death, usually within a few months or a year. Pulmonary or urinary tract cryptococcosis may occur without involvement of the central nervous system when the prognosis is believed to be favourable, as it is in the rare isolated cutaneous forms. In the disseminated disease, cutaneous lesions may precede or follow the signs of involvement of the central nervous system and lungs. These cutaneous and mucous membrane lesions, which occur in about 10% and 3% of cases, respectively, are seldom pathognomonic [6–10]. The most frequent types of lesions are firm or cystic, slow-growing, subcutaneous, erythema nodosum-like swellings. Acneform papules or pustules are characteristic of widespread systemic infection. They often occur around the nose and mouth. Any of these lesions may ulcerate or ulcers may develop in primarily unaffected skin, when they are often punched out with a rather distinctive rolled edge or are multiple and resemble molluscum contagiosum. Direct extension of infection to the skin from bony lesions may occur.

Clinical variants
Often, the term primary cutaneous cryptococcosis is used erroneously to describe a solitary lesion of *Cryptococcus* on the skin as

in many such cases there is evidence of systemic spread, implying that the skin lesion has developed after bloodstream spread from a primary lung focus [1]. Documented cases of primary cutaneous infection by inoculation occur but are rare.

In AIDS patients, the manifestations of cryptococcosis are not greatly different from those seen in other groups. However, often the symptoms of meningitis are minimal and there is evidence of dissemination, such as positive blood cultures or multiple skin lesions [1,11]. The skin lesions are often papules with central softening.

Differential diagnosis
Cryptococci may be recognised in smears of pus and of cerebrospinal fluid. When there is cutaneous involvement, cryptococci may be seen readily in and cultured from biopsy material. Their identity should be confirmed by culture. The diagnosis should particularly be considered when inflammatory nodules or ulcers develop in AIDS patients. However, similar lesions occur with other systemic mycoses, notably histoplasmosis and infections caused by *Talaromyces marneffei*.

Disease course and prognosis
It is chronic and fatal if untreated.

Investigations
The large (5–15 μm) budding cells with their characteristic capsules are best observed by direct microscopy of cerebrospinal fluid or pus in India ink or nigrosin mounts. Material suspected of containing *C. neoformans* should not be inoculated on to media containing cycloheximide, which inhibits growth. Incubation at 30°C for up to 4 weeks is sufficient.

Cryptococcus neoformans. Colony: the growth is soft, cream to pale brown and usually mucoid. Isolation of *C. neoformans* is facilitated by its tendency to form brown colonies on media made selective by the addition of various melanin precursors (e.g. *Guizotia* seed or caffeic acid media). Microscopy: yeasts alone are formed; no filaments are produced. Physiological tests: identification is based on such cultural characteristics as the ability to grow at 37°C, urease production, phenoloxidase production and the ability to assimilate creatinine and various carbohydrates. As with the identification of *Candida* species, commercial kits are widely used to identify *Cryptococcus neoformans*. *C. gattii* is identical using conventional culture techniques and can only be distinguished by molecular methods.

Serological tests: these are rapid, specific and useful, particularly in disseminated or central nervous system infections. Serodiagnosis is dependent on the detection of cryptococcal capsular antigen, using a latex agglutination test, an ELISA assay or a lateral flow device. High titres are found in AIDS patients in serum and cerebrospinal fluid. However, non-AIDS patients with single, localised skin lesions are often antigen negative.

Management
All patients should be treated with antifungal drugs.

First line
The mainstay of treatment in the non-AIDS patient is intravenous amphotericin B combined with flucytosine [12]. This should be used in most cases, except in the occasional patient without serious underlying disease, who has focal infections, such as a skin lesion, and in whom there is no evidence of systemic spread, where fluconazole 400–600 mg/day may be used. In AIDS patients, the situation is more complicated as although rapid control can be obtained, oral therapy is usually used after initial treatment, although most patients on HAART appear to achieve remission [13]. The current strategy adopted by most units is to use amphotericin B with or without flucytosine or fluconazole for 7–14 days to induce remission, followed by long-term oral fluconazole 200–400 mg/day given as out-patient therapy.

Second line
The use of higher doses of monotherapy with fluconazole 800–2000 mg daily is less effective.

Treatment ladder for cryptococcosis

First line
- Amphotericin B 0.5–1 mg/kg daily for 4–6 weeks or amphotericin B 0.2–1 mg daily (or liposmal amphotericin B 3 mg/kg daily) for 2 weeks
- Followed by fluconazole 400 mg daily for 4 weeks or until remission

Second line
- Fluconazole 800 mg daily for 6–8 weeks

Systemic candidosis

A general account of systemic candidosis is outside the scope of this text, but certain aspects impinge upon the dermatologist and are therefore considered [1,2]. There are also outbreaks of multi-drug resistant *Candida auris* in hospitals; this organism can be carried at skin sites but does not specifically cause skin lesions.

Definition
Systemic candidosis is an infection of deep organs, including the bloodstream, caused by *Candida* species.

Pathophysiology
In most cases of systemic candidosis, the causal organism originates in the patient's own gastrointestinal tract, and in patients with leukaemia or other serious illness prophylaxis with oral anti-*Candida* agents is indicated. Invasion by *Candida* along intravenous infusion lines is also important and maceration or signs suggestive of cutaneous candidiasis on adjacent skin should not be ignored.

Clinical features
Typical lesions start as macules, become papular or nodular, and may show a pale centre. Some are likely to be haemorrhagic and may break down to form ecthyma gangrenosum-like lesions. Subcorneal

pustules are not a feature, but follicular invasion by *Candida* leading to pustules and nodules in the scalp, beard, axilla and pubis may be characteristic of *Candida* septicaemia in heroin abusers [3]. Fever, diffuse muscle tenderness and a red macular rash are regarded as an indication for prompt skin biopsy in any compromised patient.

Investigations
The histology of a skin lesion showing *Candida* cells in the dermis provides a rapid diagnosis, often before a blood culture is positive. A minority of patients with *Candida* septicaemia manifest skin lesions, but, if suspected, lesions can be biopsied.

Management
The treatment of systemic candidosis with intravenous amphotericin B, caspofungin or azole drugs such as voriconazole or posaconazole is necessary. With fluconazole, isolates of the *Candida* strain should be tested for sensitivity if the patient fails to respond.

Mucormycosis

Definition and nomenclature
Mucormycosis is a systemic infection caused by mucoromycete fungi.

Synonyms and inclusions
- Zygomycosis
- Systemic mucormycosis
- Phycomycosis

Pathophysiology
Mucormycosis is caused predominantly by species of *Rhizomucor*, *Lichtheimia* (formerly *Absidia*) and *Rhizopus*. *Cunninghamella bertholletiae* and *Saksenaea vasiformis* are less common causes. Although these are frequent in the natural environment, they are rare causes of invasive disease in patients made susceptible by diabetes (sometimes in association with Covid-19 infection), neutropenia or renal disease [1,2]. Fatal infections have been reported in patients with burns. Apart from the invasion of necrotic burned areas or after severe trauma involving contact with soil, for example after a landslide, mucormycosis of the skin is uncommon. Necrotising infections of the skin associated with the application of dressings or wooden spatulas contaminated with *Rhizopus microsporus (rhizopodiformis)* [3,4] have been described. Cutaneous lesions have been described in patients with lymphoma and kidney transplants [2].

Clinical features
Lesions are progressive with necrotic ulcers similar to those described under necrotising fasciitis.

Investigations
Mucormycosis is usually diagnosed in autopsy or biopsy sections, based on the recognition of the broad and generally non-septate hyphae.

Management
As early treatment is essential, the use of frozen sections from skin lesions for rapid histopathological examination has been advocated. However, organisms can be grown from tissue. Infections may respond to intravenous amphotericin but mortality rates remain high.

Unusual causes of skin lesions among opportunistic systemic mycoses

Most of the organisms that can invade the immunocompromised patient may cause skin lesions. Some of these infections, such as candidosis, mucormycosis and cryptococcosis, have been described previously. However, other organisms that can cause skin disease include *Aspergillus* [1,2], *Trichosporon* [3] and *Fusarium* [4]; all of these may affect the neutropenic patient.

Aspergillus and *Trichosporon* usually produce large, scattered necrotic lesions, although with the latter, smaller papules and pustules have been seen. *Fusarium* and, more rarely, *Acremonium* infection, may produce target-like lesions, which may undergo central necrosis. In some cases of *Fusarium* infection, scattered skin lesions have been accompanied by digital cellulitis and superficial white onychomycosis caused by the same organism.

Skin involvement has also been described in a variety of invasive infections affecting the paranasal sinuses such as those caused by *Exophiala dermatidis*. Skin lesions in these infections develop in severely sick patients. However, skin biopsy will sometimes reveal the true diagnosis. Treatment for these infections is usually with amphotericin B. The response rates in both *Fusarium* and *Trichosporon* infections are low.

Cutaneous infection caused by *Pneumocystis jiroveci*

Definition
Pneumocystis jiroveci is an opportunistic fungal pathogen that is found in immunocompromised patients, including neonates, solid organ transplant recipients and AIDS patients.

Pathophysiology
Pneumocystis was previously regarded as a protozoan but molecular analysis has shown that it is best regarded as a fungus, although in certain structural features, such as its cell membrane, it differs from the fungal norm.

Clinical features
Usually a pulmonary infection, it has rarely been found to cause skin lesions in AIDS patients [1].

Investigations
The organisms stain with methenamine silver and appear as round, non-budding structures 5–10 μm in diameter.

Management
Treatment is with co-trimoxazole or pentamidine.

Infections caused by *Pythium insidiosum*

Definition and nomenclature
Infections caused by *Pythium* species were first recognised in animals in 1884, affecting mainly horses and mules. Since 1987, a number of cases of human infection have been reported, nearly all of them from Thailand and in farmers exposed to swampy areas.

Synonyms and inclusions
- Swamp cancer
- Florida horse leech

Pathophysiology
The organisms appear to invade blood vessels with large, sparsely septate hyphae, 3–20 μm in diameter, similar to those seen in zygomycosis. It is now recognised, however, that the organism is not a true fungus and is probably more closely related to the algae. It is possible to isolate *P. insidiosum* on glucose–peptone agar, but production of the characteristic motile biflagellate zoospores, necessary to speciate the isolate, requires special media and expertise [1].

Clinical features
Affected patients have usually had severe infections with ascending gangrene of the lower limbs. Most have had an underlying haemoglobinopathy such as thalassaemia [2].

Management
There is no known effective treatment, apart from high doses of amphotericin B and amputation.

Protothecosis

Definition
Prototheca is generally accepted as a genus of achloric algae embracing species of worldwide distribution. *P. wickerhamii*, *P. xanthoriae* (prev *P. zopfii*) and *P. stagnora* are rare opportunistic pathogens in humans [1]. Infections with green and blue-green algae, although recorded, are rarer still.

Clinical features
Lesions confined to the skin and subcutaneous tissues are generally located on exposed sites, and may be associated with trauma [2,3]. Papules, nodules, ulcers and multiple granulomatous lesions have all been described. In such cases, the organisms may be found in the dermis and epidermis. Protothecal bursitis, particularly of the olecranon bursa after injury, is also well documented, as are a few examples of widespread cutaneous, subcutaneous or deep infection in immunocompromised hosts including AIDS patients [4]. Colonisation of nails has been reported and *Prototheca* may occur as transients on the skin.

Management
Spontaneous recovery has occurred in one cutaneous infection. However, surgical excision is recommended for localised lesions and systemic amphotericin B, ketoconazole [5] or itraconazole have proved effective on occasions.

Glossary of terms

Anamorph	An asexual state.
Anthropophilic	Adapted to humans.
Arthroconidium	A spore resulting from the breaking up of a hypha into separate cells; characteristic of the parasitic form of ringworm fungi.
Asexual	Reproduction not involving prior union of two nuclei.
Blastospore	A spore formed by budding.
Cerebriform	Complex folding similar to the brain surface.
Chlamydospore	A thick-walled cell, intercalary or terminal containing stored food and able to function as a spore.
Clavate	Club shaped.
Cleistothecium	A reproductive structure associated with the sexual state of ringworm fungi.
Conidiophore	A specialised structure of varying complexity that bears conidiogenous cells.
Conidium	An asexual spore.
Dermatophyte	A ringworm fungus.
Dimorphic	Having two distinct forms, which often correspond to saprophytic and parasitic phases, respectively.
Downy	Fluffy.
Ectothrix	Dermatophyte hair infection with hyphae inside the hair and a sheath of spores outside the hair.
Endospore	A spore formed internally (e.g. sporangiospore).
Endothrix	Dermatophyte hair infection with fungus confined to the inside of a hair.
Faviform	Waxy, restricted, honeycomb-like growth of certain dermatophytes.
Floccose	Cottony.
Fusiform	Spindle shaped.
Geophilic	Soil inhabiting.
Glabrous	Smooth, leathery. Non hairy.
Grain	A compact agglomeration of fungal or actinomycete elements formed *in vivo*.
Granular	Texture similar to icing sugar.
Hypha	One of the branching filaments, septate or non-septate, that make up the vegetative mycelium of moulds.
Intercalary	Not terminal.
Kerion	An intensely inflammatory ringworm lesion.
Macroconidium	The larger of the two types of conidia in those fungi that bear large and small (microconidia) spores.

Microconidium	The smaller of the two types of conidia in those fungi that bear large (macroconidia) and small spores.
Mycelium	The collective name for a mass of hyphae.
Mycosis	A fungal disease.
Obovate	An inverted egg shape.
Pleomorphic	Strictly having two or more forms; used frequently to describe non-sporing (sterile) cultures of dermatophytes.
Powdery	With a texture like face powder.
Pseudohyphae	A hypha-like structure produced by elongation of budding yeasts lying end to end.
Pyriform	Pear shaped.
Sessile	Without a stalk.
Spiral	A vegetative hypha assuming spiral forms.
Sporangium	An asexual reproductive body in Zygomycetes.
Spore	A reproductive unit; formed sexually or asexually, and sometimes multicellular.
Sporophore	A spore-bearing structure.
Tuberculate	Covered with peg-like outgrowths.
Zoophilic	Adapted to an animal host.

Acknowledgements

The author acknowledges the valuable contributions made by Dr Ruth Ashbee to the previous edition of this chapter

Key references

The full list of references can be found in the online version at https://www.wiley.com/rooksdermatology10e

Introduction
2 De Hoog GS, Guarro J, Gene J, Figueras MJ. *Atlas of Clinical Fungi*. Baarn: Centraalbureau voor Schimmelcultures, Universitat Rovira I Virgili, 2000.
3 Sciortino CV. *Atlas of Clinically Important Fungi*. New York: John Wiley & Sons, Inc., 2017.
4 Kibbler CC, Barton R, Gow NAR, Howell S, MacCallum DM, Manuel RJ, eds. *Oxford Textbook of Medical Mycology* (Oxford Textbooks in Infectious Disease and Microbiology). Oxford: OUP, 2017.
5 Kirk PM, Cannon PF, Minter DW, Stalpers JA. *Ainsworth and Bisby's Dictionary of the Fungi*, 10th edn. Wallingford: CAB International, 2008.

Basic biology
Nomenclature
2 International Mycological Association. Taylor JW. One Fungus = One Name: DNA and fungal nomenclature twenty years after PCR. https://imafungus.biomedcentral.com/articles/10.5598/imafungus.2011.02.02.01 (last accessed August 2023).

Superficial mycoses
Skin disease caused by Malassezia species
Pityriasis versicolor
11 Crespo Erchiga V, Delgado Florencio V. *Malassezia* species in skin diseases. *Curr Opin Infect Dis* 2002;15:133–42.

Other cutaneous disorders associated with Malassezia yeasts
8 Saunte DML, Gaitanis G, Hay RJ. Malassezia-associated skin diseases, the use of diagnostics and treatment. *Front Cell Infect Microbiol* 2020;10:112.

Dermatophytosis
Basic biology
3 Mycology Online. *Dermatophytosis*. University of Adelaide. https://www.adelaide.edu.au/mycology/ (last accessed August 2023).

Identification
1 De Hoog GS, Guarro J, Gene J, Figueras MJ, eds. *Atlas of Clinical Fungi*. Baarn: Centraalbureau voor Schimmelcultures/Universitat Rovira i Virgili, 2000.

Superficial mycoses caused by dermatophyte infection
Tinea corporis
3 Elewski BE. Tinea capitis: a current perspective. *J Am Acad Dermatol* 2000;42:1–20.
Onychomycosis caused by other non-dermatophyte moulds
8 Gupta AK, Simpson FC. New therapeutic options for onychomycosis. *Expert Opin Pharmacother* 2012;13:1131–42.

Candidosis
Management
1 Lioakis MS Edwards JE. *Candida* species. In: Bennett JE, Dolin R, Blaser MD, eds. *Principles and Practice of Infectious Diseases*, 9th edn. Philadelphia: Churchill Livingstone, 2020:3087–102.

Subcutaneous mycoses
Identification
3 Carol A. Kauffman, Peter G. Pappas, Jack D. *Sobel Essentials of Clinical Mycology*. New York: Springer, 2011.
4 Anaissie EJ, McGinnis MR, Pfaller MA, eds. *Clinical Mycology*. Amsterdam: Churchill Livingstone, Elsevier 2009.

CHAPTER 33

Parasitic Diseases

Austinn C. Miller, Alfredo Siller Jr and Stephen K. Tyring
University of Texas Health Science Center, Houston, TX, USA

INFECTION WITH HUMAN NEMATODES, 33.1	Visceral larva migrans, 33.20	Sparganosis, 33.34
Onchocerciasis, 33.1	Gnathostomiasis, 33.21	**INFECTION WITH PROTOZOA, 33.35**
Mansonellosis, 33.6	Dirofilariasis, 33.23	Malaria, 33.36
Lymphatic filariasis, 33.7	Trichinosis, 33.24	Amoebiasis, 33.36
Loiasis, 33.10	**INFECTION WITH TREMATODES, 33.26**	Trichomoniasis, 33.38
Dracunculiasis, 33.12	Schistosomiasis, 33.26	Trypansomiasis, 33.39
Enterobiasis, 33.14	Cercarial dermatitis, 33.29	Leishmaniasis, 33.43
Ancylostomiasis, 33.15	Paragonimiasis, 33.30	Cutaneous leishmaniasis, 33.43
Strongyloidiasis, 33.17		Visceral leishmaniasis, 33.51
INFECTION WITH NEMATODES OF OTHER ANIMALS, 33.18	**INFECTION WITH CESTODES, 33.31**	Toxoplasmosis, 33.54
	Echinococcosis, 33.31	
Cutaneous larva migrans, 33.18	Cysticercosis, 33.32	Key references, 33.55

INFECTION WITH HUMAN NEMATODES

Nematoda is a diverse phylum that spans over 500 000 species of 'roundworms' and is considered to be the second largest phylum in the animal kingdom. Human nematode infections are often the result of a select group of species that includes angiostrongyliasis, ascariasis, dirofilariasis, enterobiasis, filariasis, strongyloides and trichinosis, among others.

In these infections, the human becomes an obligatory host at a stage in the parasite's life cycle. Helminths, including nematodes, may be long lived – up to 30 years for *Schistosoma* spp. and 17 years for *Onchocerca* spp. for example – and constant reinfection in endemic countries gives rise to heavy worm burdens. All nematodes must spend part of their life cycle outside the human body, either on soil or in water, or in an insect, crustacean or vertebrate intermediate host. *Strongyloides stercoralis* is the exception to this rule: autoinfection with this worm permits lifelong infections in humans. In some species of nematode, the worm is masked from immune recognition and large worm burdens may be tolerated with remarkably little clinical effect. For others, inflammation, often in response to naturally dying worms or their progeny, causes severe disease. By contrast, some helminths make excessive demands on the body's nutritional reserves.

A summary of the organisms and diseases caused by infection with human nematodes is provided in Table 33.1.

Table 33.1 Organisms and the diseases caused in nematode infection.

Disease	Organism
Onchocerciasis	*Onchocerca volvulus*
Streptocerciasis	*Mansonella streptocerca*
Lymphatic filariasis	*Wuchereria bancrofti*
	Brugia malayi
	Brugia timori
Loiasis	*Loa loa*
Dracunculiasis	*Dracunculus medinensis*
Enterobiasis	*Enterobius vermicularis*
Ancylostomiasis	*Ancylostoma duodenale*
	Necator americanus
	Strongyloides stercoralis (roundworm)
Strongyloidiasis	*Strongyloides stercoralis*

Onchocerciasis

Definition and nomenclature

Onchocerciasis, also known as 'river blindness', is caused by the filarial nematode, *Onchocerca volvulus*. The blackfly vector breeds near fast-flowing rivers and streams. The disease is second only to trachoma as an infectious aetiology of blindness worldwide. The disease typically affects rural communities and is a major cause of blindness and cutaneous disease, most notably in sub-Saharan Africa [1].

> **Synonyms and inclusions**
> - River blindness
> - *Onchocerca volvulus*
> - Blinding filariasis
> - Robles disease

Epidemiology

Incidence and prevalence

Worldwide, the number of infected people was estimated to be 20.9 million in the year 2017. More than 99% of cases originate in 31 countries in sub-Saharan Africa. Fewer cases have been identified in Yemen, Central America, Mexico, Columbia, Ecuador and Venezuela. Of the infected, approximately 14.6 million have skin disease and 1.5 million are affected with visual impairment or blindness due to the disease [2].

Pathophysiology

Pathology [3,4]

Mature worms and microfilariae are found in granulomatous dermal nodules (onchocercal nodules), often situated on the scalp of their hosts in Central America, but in Africa near bony prominences on the trunk and limbs or in the natal cleft. The nodules measure some 3–35 mm in diameter, and consist of an outer layer of fibroblasts, which contains the parasites in an organised fibrinous exudate. Inflammatory cells and sometimes giant cells tend to accumulate around the worms. Calcification may also occur.

Microfilariae migrate mainly in the dermis. Their death causes an inflammatory response. With chronic disease these changes are replaced by fibrosis and atrophy of dermis and epidermis [4,5].

The numbers of microfilariae can vary greatly. In some instances, there is a dense predominantly perivascular reaction with mononuclear cells and eosinophils, but few microfilariae [6]. At its severest, this is accompanied by marked acanthosis and hyperkeratosis. The reason for this extreme reaction is unknown, but specific antibody isotypic responses from patients with this form of onchocerciasis recognise a collagen antigen expressed by a specific nematode gene, which suggests that cross-reaction between antibodies to *Onchocerca* and human collagen might play a role in the pathogenesis of this condition [7]. Moreover, differences in severe and mild reactions related to the amount of *Wolbachia* symbiote found in different strains of *O. volvulus* [8]. Often in individuals with minimal clinical lesions and dermal inflammation, there is the highest density of dermal microfilariae (Figure 33.1). In these patients, there is evidence of defective T-lymphocyte stimulation by certain filarial antigens, which can be reversed by treatment [9]. Conversely, activation of T-cell mediated pathways is associated with the highly inflammatory forms such as lichenified onchodermatitis (LOD) [10].

Microfilariae also invade the eye, where they cause keratitis, posterior choroiditis, uveitis and optic neuritis, which can lead to blindness. Free microfilariae also penetrate superficial lymphatic vessels and may be found in the urine, tears, sputum, cerebrospinal fluid and, occasionally, in vaginal smears or irrigation sediment.

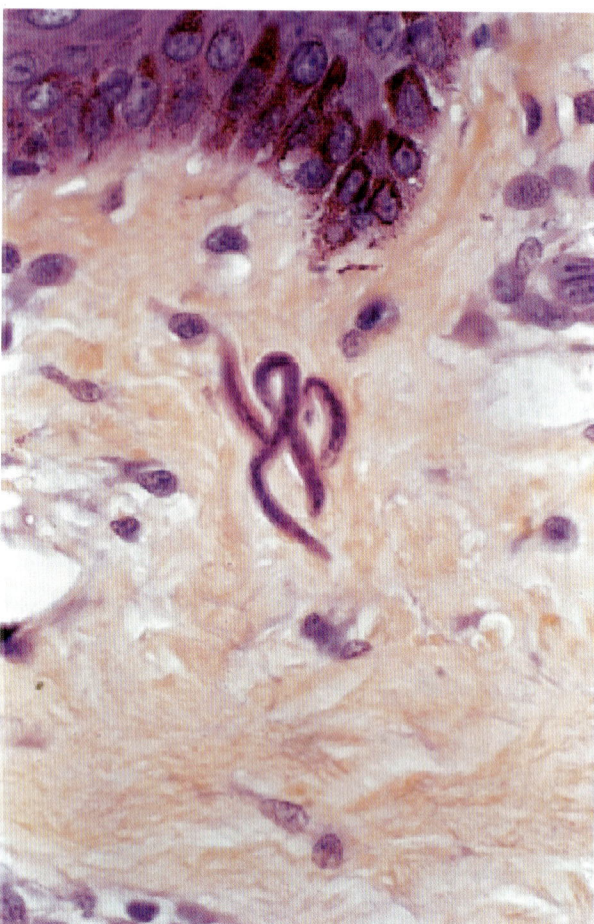

Figure 33.1 Microfilaria of *Onchocerca volvulus* in the upper dermis. Note the absence of inflammation around the live organism. Courtesy of Dr C. McDougall.

Causative organisms

- *Onchocerca volvulus*, a filarial nematode

Humans are infected with *O. volvulus* through the bite of a blackfly of the *Simulium* genus. Larvae develop in the thoracic muscles of the flies and 7 days after infection are fully developed in the labium of the proboscis. The blackfly deposit infective larvae into human skin, which mature over the next 6–12 months into mature adult parasites (macrofilariae). The females live in subcutaneous or intramuscular tissues and surround themselves with a fibrous capsule. The males do not stay dormant; instead, they migrate from one capsule to the next, fertilising the female larvae.

Some 10–12 months after initial infection, the adult female begins to reproduce. Offspring (microfilariae) migrate through subcutaneous tissue. Adults can live for up to 15 years and each female produces 1000–3000 microfilariae per day. Highly infected individuals can have over 100 million microfilariae in their skin [1,10] (Figure 33.2).

Clinical features

Presentation [4,11–14]

The most common signs and symptoms are pruritus, onchocercal dermatitis, nodules and, in areas of high endemicity, blindness. The disease may be detectable as early as 6 months of age, and presents with pruritus, often confined to a limb or other

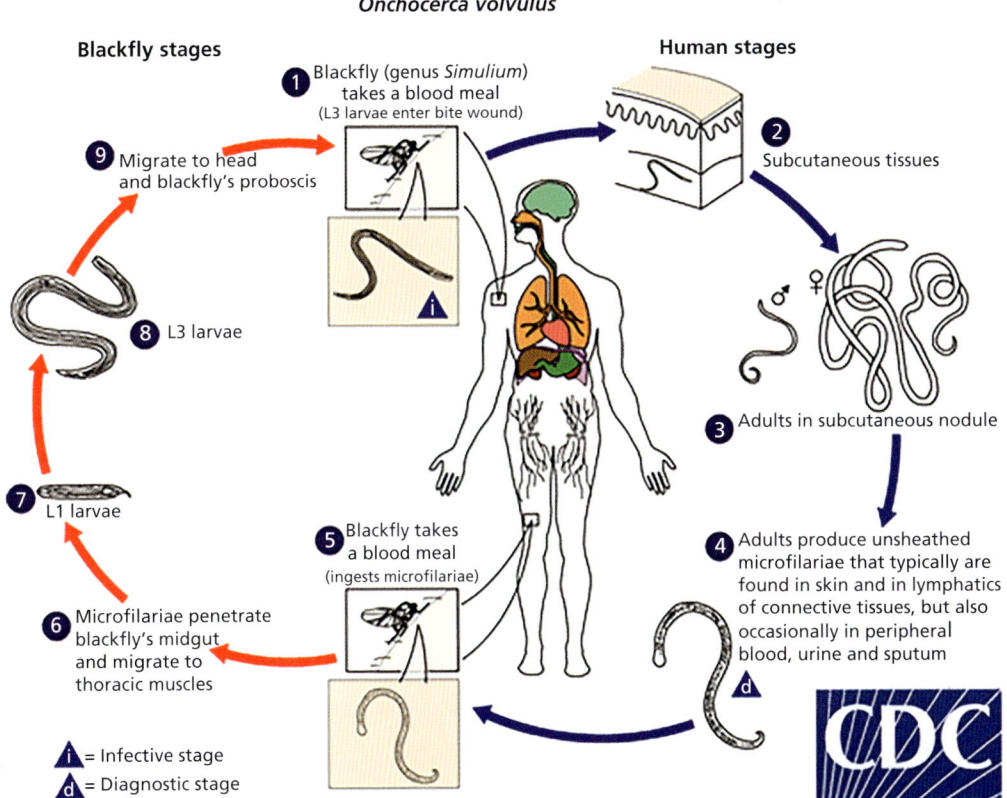

Figure 33.2 Life cycle of *Onchocerca volvulus*. Courtesy of the Centers for Disease Control and Prevention. https://www.cdc.gov/dpdx/onchocerciasis/index.html (last accessed February 2023).

circumscribed body site, and a non-specific papular rash worsened by scratching.

In some the skin may appear clinically normal, even when microfilarial counts in skin snips are found to be high. The skin changes seen in onchocerciasis vary with the age of the patient, the location of the infection on the skin surface and the geographical and climatic region where the infection occurs. Nonetheless, it is possible to define certain changes that are common features in onchodermatitis, although their prevalence varies from area to area. These changes have been classified as acute papular onchodermatitis (APOD) (Figure 33.3), chronic papular onchodermatitis (CPOD) (Figure 33.4), LOD, atrophy and hypopigmentation [13]. In children and in the earliest cases in endemic areas, the skin has an infiltrated appearance, with obliteration of surface markings. This is confined to one skin area and is often accompanied by the appearance of small itching papules or pustules (APOD). The oedematous features are often more pronounced in Europeans with the disease, when it may present with localised oedema [15]. In Europeans, red blotchy urticated papules are common early signs. The early rash is usually seen on exposed sites, such as the shoulders and around the pelvis. In Central America, acute swelling on the face and cheeks with redness and itching, known as 'erisipela de la costa,' is also a manifestation of this acute phase. Patients may continue to present with this pattern over months and years in the early phases of the disease.

As the infection evolves, localised areas of scarring and CPOD are seen. These may coexist with the acute papular eruption, but chronic lesions are excoriated papules and flat-topped scars with

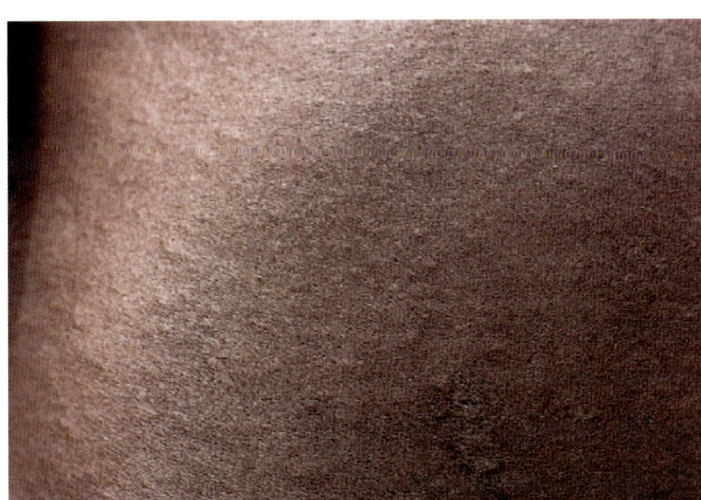

Figure 33.3 Acute papular onchodermatitis in a Nigerian. Early in the disease the papules are usually urticarial. These pruritic papules are usually 1–3 mm may progress into vesicles or pustules.

hyperpigmentation and some lichenification. The buttocks and shoulders are common sites for this rash.

Lichenified onchodermatitis may represent an extreme form of the last clinical pattern. When fully developed, it is a lichenified itchy rash confined to one limb or contiguous area (Figure 33.5), commonly the leg, although sometimes two or more areas are affected [6,9]. The rash is composed of itchy papules and nodules, which become confluent. The lesion is characteristically hyperpigmented, and it is known in Arabic-speaking areas as 'Sowda'.

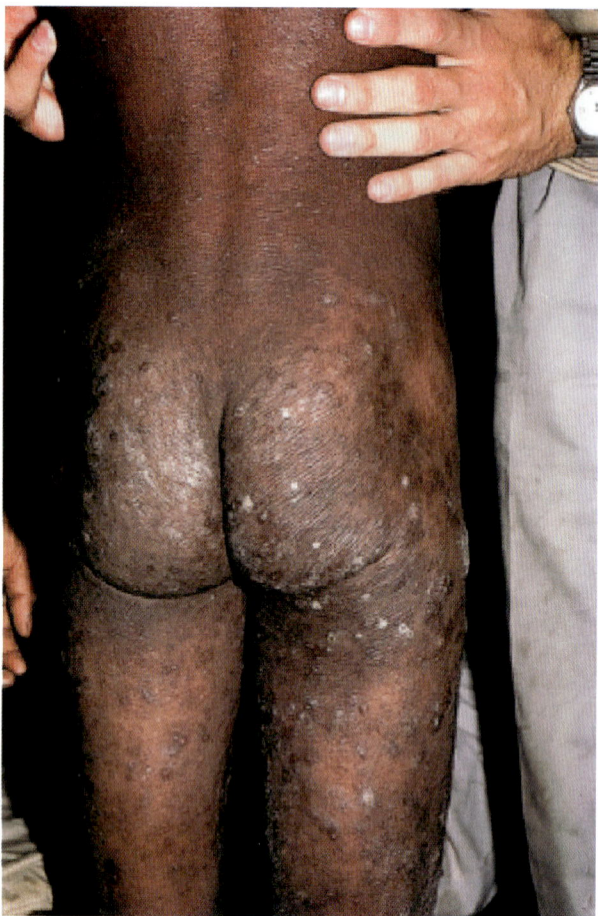

Figure 33.4 Chronic papular onchodermatitis. Lesions are starting to lichenify. These pruritic papules are typically flat-topped, hyperpigmented, and between 3 and 9 mm in size.

Gross enlargement of the regional lymph nodes is an important feature. Interestingly, it is found mainly in East Africa (Sudan [16], Ethiopia) and Yemen. It is less common in West Africa or South America. There is some evidence that this pattern of skin change is associated with very low microfilarial loads; it may also improve symptomatically over time with loss of itching and lichenification, but increasing microfilarial loads. LOD is mainly seen in teenagers and young adults.

Atrophy (Figure 33.6) is probably a consequence of long-standing onchocerciasis. It may develop after any of the patterns described previously or arise from apparently normal but infected skin sites. The most common sites to detect early atrophic changes are over the buttocks, shoulders or lower limbs. The skin becomes dry and shiny, with fine wrinkles resembling tissue paper. An extreme form of this secondary ichthyosis is known as 'lizard skin'. It is believed that degenerative changes leading to loss of dermal elastic fibres, combined with other factors, such as massive inguinal lymphadenopathy, may give rise to the 'hanging groin', which is an apron-like fold of skin in the inguinal region [17] containing lymph nodes. Depigmentation is a common feature of late-stage onchodermatitis [18]. It is most commonly seen bilaterally over the pretibial region, but may affect the inguinal regions, bony prominences and the shoulders (Figure 33.7). The patches of hypopigmentation are spotty, with islands of normal-appearing skin, but large coalescent

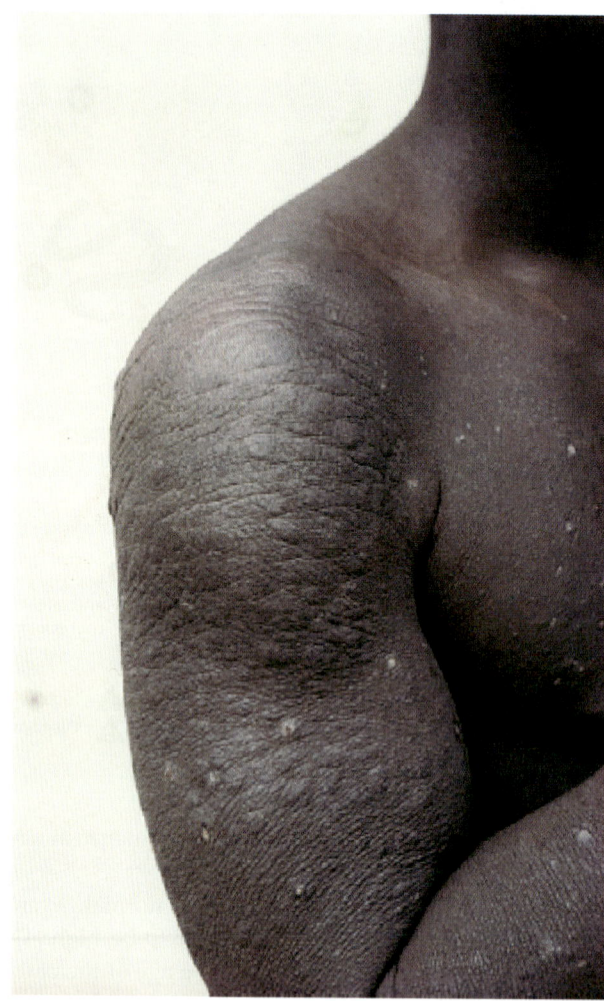

Figure 33.5 Late lichenified onchodermatitis (pachyderma).

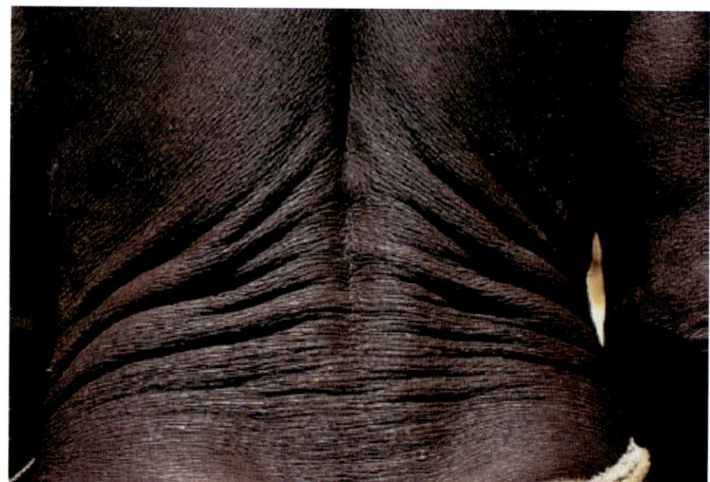

Figure 33.6 Late onchocerciasis. Atrophy of skin and damage to supporting tissue cause the skin to sag in folds (lizard skin).

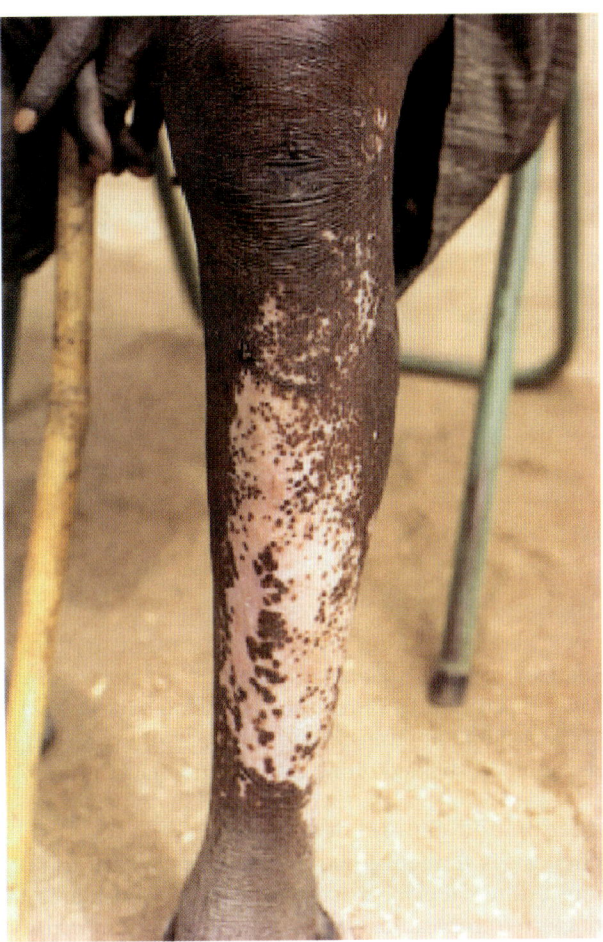

Figure 33.7 Depigmentation over the shin in late onchocerciasis (leopard skin). This is common in African endemic areas. Note the stick for the blind.

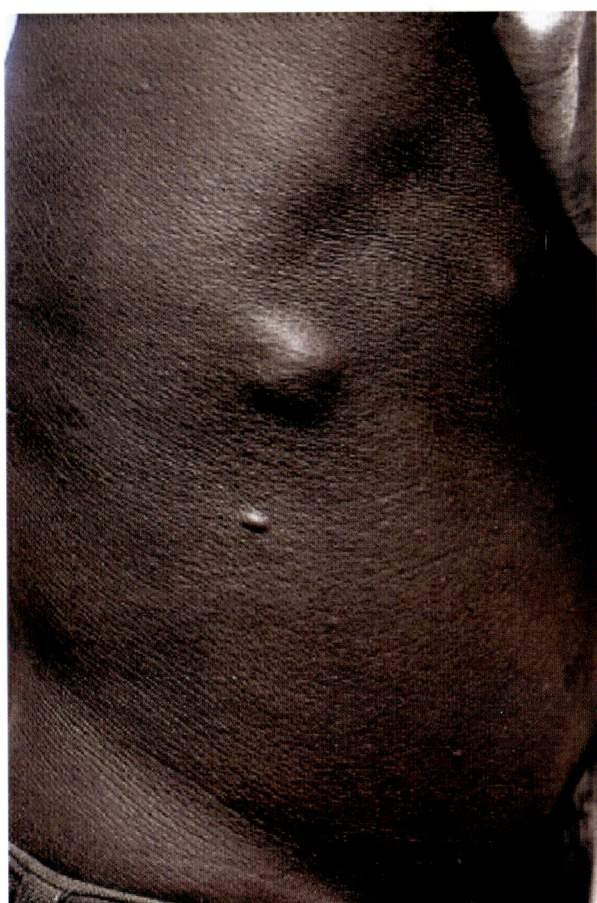

Figure 33.8 Cutaneous oedema and cutaneous and subcutaneous nodules in a Nigerian with onchocerciasis.

sheets of depigmentation are present in late-stage disease. The name 'leopard skin' is used to describe this change. While it is important to recognise that other causes of hypopigmentation, such as amyloid deposition, may also produce such changes in certain endemic areas, the presence of leopard skin in the community is used as an indicator of the prevalence of onchocerciasis in the population.

In many, if not most, patients with chronic onchocerciasis, it is possible to feel nodules containing the adult worms (Figure 33.8). They are usually found over the pelvic or pectoral regions, although the top of the natal cleft is often a good site to find them. In South and Central American cases, the nodules are often found on the head.

In endemic areas where onchocerciasis is found, the majority of the population may be affected; they will also have other skin diseases. There is little evidence that the presence of onchocerciasis affects the clinical appearances of these other conditions. However, it has been suggested that lepromatous leprosy [19] and widespread tinea corporis [12] are more common in certain patients with onchocerciasis.

Clinical variants
Other clinical variants of onchocerciasis may occur. These include an acute urticarial eruption seen in Zaire and, in Central America, an inflammatory rash accompanied by hyperpigmentation known as 'mal morado'.

Differential diagnosis
This includes leprosy, *Loa loa* infection, lymphatic filariasis, scabies, syphilis and yaws.

Complications and co-morbidities
The major complication of onchocerciasis is severe visual impairment and blindness. It is the most common cause of blindness in endemic areas. Ocular manifestations range from punctate and sclerosing keratitis, associated with the presence of microfilariae in the cornea and anterior chamber, to retinal pigmentation, optic atrophy, scarring and blindness. Onchocerciasis may result in blindness rates in endemic communities of 5–10% [20].

Disease prognosis
In endemic areas, the rate of infection increases up to the age of 50 years and no relative immunity is acquired. Symptoms increase in severity without treatment until atrophic changes are complete.

Investigations
Clinically, the diagnosis is usually evident, but other causes of prolonged pruritus and lichenification must be excluded, particularly scabies. Typical burrows may be hard to find in patients with scabies, and great tenacity is needed to demonstrate *Sarcoptes*. Skin snips for active microfilariae are taken with the corneoscleral

punch or by raising a little 'tent' of skin with a needle. This is then shaved off with a very sharp blade without bleeding, placed in normal saline in a microtitre well, covered with transparent adhesive tape, or placed under a cover slip and examined microscopically 30–60 min later. If microfilariae are not visualised, polymerase chain reaction (PCR) of the skin snip may allow for diagnosis, although PCR testing is not readily available nor commonly used. The buttocks and legs are often most heavily infected and are most likely to yield microfilariae. Nodules may be excised and examined histologically for adult worms and microfilariae. The white cell count shows a leukocytosis with relative eosinophilia. The filarial immunofluorescence test or enzyme-linked immunosorbent assay (ELISA) is positive in 60–90% of cases.

> **Treatment ladder for onchocerciasis**
>
> **First line**
> - Doxycycline, 100 mg every day PO × 6 weeks, followed by ivermectin 100–200 µg/kg, repeated every 6–12 months until asymptomatic
>
> **Second line**
> - Ivermectin 100–200 µg/kg, repeated every 6–12 months until asymptomatic
>
> **Third line**
> - Suramin, nodulectomy

Management

The treatment of onchocerciasis has been improved significantly by ivermectin, a microfilaricide. This drug is given orally in a single dose of 100–200 µg/kg [21]. This results in a prolonged suppression of microfilarial counts in skin snips, and improvement in skin symptoms and reversible eye changes [22]. Microfilarial counts remain very low for 6 months, then rise slowly but do not reach pretreatment levels within 1 year. Patients should be retreated every 6–12 months until they are asymptomatic. For patients in endemic areas, treatment may be required for 10 years or more. In patients with low parasite loads, such as travellers returning from an endemic country, about 30% will *not* relapse after each treatment [23]. The drug is well tolerated and side effects are seldom severe. Side effects that are seen include pruritus, skin oedema, arthralgia, malaise and fever. In particular, no acute eye changes accompany therapy [24]. Ivermectin has become the mainstay of population-based programmes for the control and elimination of onchocerciasis with striking effect [25].

Moxidectin, a drug closely related to ivermectin, has been recently approved to treat onchocerciasis. When comparing one 6 mg dose of moxidectin to one 150 µg/kg of ivermectin, it showed a greater reduction in microfilarial load over 18 months, with an 86% difference at month 12 [26]. Moxidectin is expected to reduce parasite transmission between treatment rounds more than ivermectin could, thus accelerating progress towards elimination.

Another new mainstay of therapy has been doxycycline, targeted against the endobacterium, *Wolbachia*, which results in sterilisation of female adult worms. A clinical trial using doxycycline has demonstrated that this approach in selected areas can result in an effective reduction in macrofilaria [27]. In a study of 93 patients with onchocerciasis, doxycycline (100 mg/day orally for 6 weeks) followed by a single oral dose of ivermectin resulted in clearance of microfilariae for up to 19 months, and complete elimination of the endobacterium [27].

Suramin is a drug that kills adult worms (macrofilaricide). However, it can cause severe adverse reactions and is now seldom used. Another approach now seldom used is nodulectomy, usually combined with a microfilaricide. In South America, some studies have shown that nodulectomy alone without drugs may reduce microfilarial levels by over 60% by 5 months after surgery [28]. It may reduce the burden of eye disease but it does not cure the disease, nor reduce transmission.

Mansonellosis

Definition

Mansonellosis describes a filarial disease caused by three species of parasitic nematodes (*Mansonella perstans*, *Mansonella streptocerca*, and *Mansonella ozzardi*). Humans are the primary definitive host for these parasites that are transmitted from person to person through the bites of blood sucking biting midges and blackflies.

Introduction and general description

Mansonellosis is thought to be the most prevalent form of filarial infections but remains the least studied and is considered to be the most neglected tropical disease. Originally, the term mansonellosis was used to refer exclusively to infection with *M. ozzardi*, and it was not until the mid-1980s that *M. perstans* and *M. streptocerca* were added to the genus.

Epidemiology

Incidence and prevalence

M. ozzardi is endemic to South and Central America, including several Caribbean islands. Humans are the only natural vertebrate host for *M. ozzardi*, while primates may serve as natural hosts for *M. perstans* and *M. streptocerca*.

M. perstans is estimated to infect 100 million people worldwide and is prevalent in places like sub-Saharan Africa, and in the Americas from Panama to Argentina. It is considered to be the most common of the mansonellosis infections [1].

Streptocerciasis is an infection caused by the filarial nematode, *Mansonella streptocerca*. The disease is seen mainly in parts of west and central Africa in rainforest areas, where it may be found in the majority of the population [2]. The exact prevalence of *M. streptocerca* is not known. The disease causes a subcutaneous filariasis, with *Loa loa* and *Onchocerca volvulus* being the other two causes in humans.

Pathophysiology

Pathology

M. ozzardi infections are often asymptomatic, but can include rash, fever, arthralgia, headache, lymphadenopathy and pulmonary symptoms. Microfilariae are present in both the blood and the skin. Adult worms often reside in lymphatics and within the thoracic and peritoneal cavities.

Similarly, *M. perstans* causes a mild infection with non-specific symptoms such as pruritus, urticaria, arthralgias and malaise. Unsheathed microfilariae can be found in the bloodstream and adult worms migrate to the subcutis, or pleura, pericardia, peritoneum and retroperitoneum.

Streptocerciasis causes a subcutaneous filariasis in humans. The disease is transmitted by biting midges (*Culicoides*). Adult worms reside in the dermis of the upper trunk and shoulder region and the microfilariae are found in the skin [2].

Causative organisms
- *Mansonella ozzardi*
- *Mansonella perstans*
- *Mansonella streptocerca*

Clinical features
Presentation [2,3]
Most individuals with mansonellosis are asymptomatic. The most common complaints include rash, pruritus, fever, arthralgia, headache, urticaria and malaise. In streptocerciasis, the rash is similar to that seen with onchocerciasis, with acute or lichenified pruritic papules (Figure 33.9). More widespread lichenification may also occur and hypopigmented macules are common. Secondary enlargement of the local lymph nodes is seen in many patients.

Investigations [2]
The diagnosis can be made by finding microfilariae in skin snips or in the blood. The microfilariae of *M. streptocerca* are less active than those of onchocerciasis and the microfilarial tip may curl in a typical 'shepherd's crook' appearance. Those of *M. perstans* have a blunt rounded tail with nuclei that extend to the tips of their tail; in contrast *M. ozzardi* have thin pointed tails and nuclei that do not extend to the tip.

Management [2]
Among the three types of human mansonellosis, the one caused by *M. perstans* is regarded as the most difficult to treat. Treatment studies have provided conflicting results, but diethylcarbamazine (DEC) plus mebendazole have proved effective in reducing microfilaraemia and is commonly used. Ivermectin and praziquantel did not prove to be useful in the treatment of *M. perstans* infections. Of the non-antihelminthic treatments, doxycycline has been shown to be curative of *M. perstans* in cases of concomitant *Wolbachia* bacteria endosymbiotic infection [4].

Ivermectin is effective against *M. ozzardi*. However, patients must be assessed for coinfection with *Loa loa* as ivermectin can cause severe reactions in these individuals. *M. ozzardi* is also known to harbour the endosymbiotic *Wolbachia*. Therefore, doxycycline may also be an effective treatment.

Ivermectin and DEC are effective for the treatment of *M. streptocera*, as it kills both the microfilariae and the adult worm. Both reduce microfilarial loads, but DEC is more commonly used. Currently, it is unclear whether *M. streptocera* harbours a *Wolbachia* endosymbiont.

> **Treatment ladder for mansonellosis**
>
> **First line**
> - Diethylcarbamazine 6 mg/kg/day for 12 days
> - Doxycycline 200 mg daily for 6 weeks (*M. perstans*/*M. ozzardi* strains with *Wolbachia* endosymbionts)
>
> **Second line**
> - Ivermectin (150 >µg/kg single dose)

Lymphatic filariasis

Definition and nomenclature
Lymphatic filiariasis is a globally neglected tropical disease caused by the worms *Wuchereria bancrofti*, *Brugia malayi* or *B. timori* [1]. *W. bancrofti* is the most common, accounting for approximately 90% infections, with person-to-person transmission spread by several different mosquito genera/species. These organisms occupy the lymphatic system in humans, and can lead to lymphoedema, hydrocoele, or in extreme cases elephantiasis.

> **Synonyms and inclusions**
> - Tropical elephantiasis

Epidemiology
Incidence and prevalence
Infection with filarial worms occurs between the latitudes of 40° north and 30° south. The areas with the highest incidence of infection are South-East Asia and sub-Saharan Africa. In the New World, there are fewer endemic foci: Guyana, Haiti and parts of Brazil. Control has been achieved in some other countries such as Taiwan and Japan. It is estimated that about 120 million people are infected

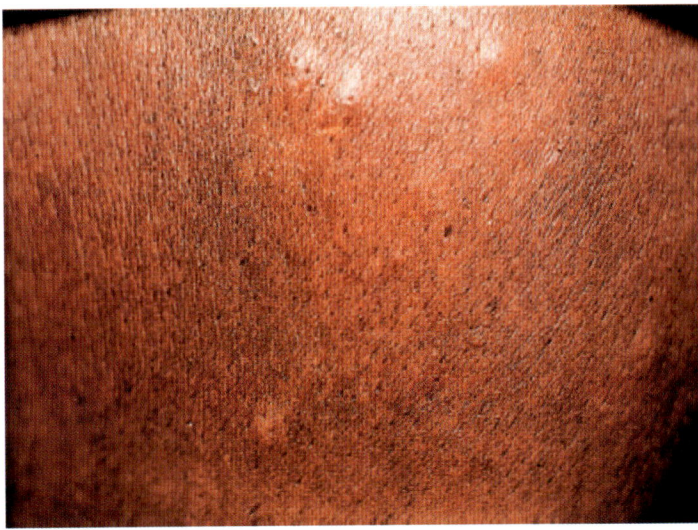

Figure 33.9 Streptocerciasis. Pigmentary changes and nodules in a patient from Zaire. Courtesy of the Armed Forces Institute of Pathology.

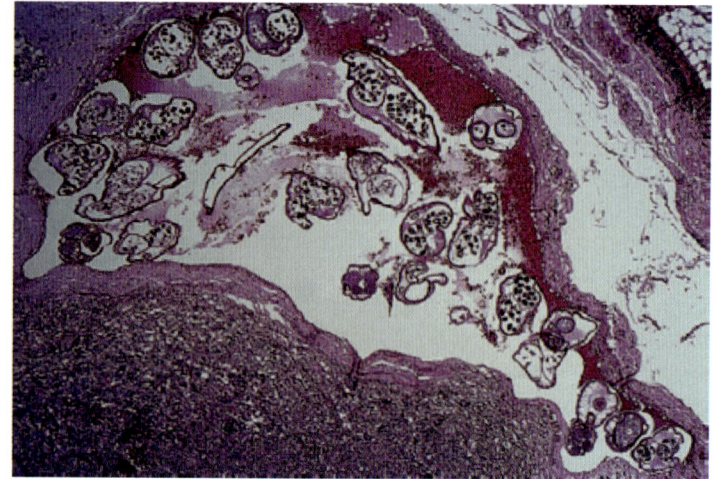

Figure 33.10 Lymphatic filariasis (low power, H&E). Female adult *Wuchereria bancrofti* within lymph node sinus. Multiple cross-sections of the worm are seen. Courtesy of Professor S.B. Lucas.

worldwide. *Brugia malayi* is mainly confined to South-East Asia and as far north as Korea, particularly in rural rainforest areas [1]. The most restricted of this group is *B. timori*, found only in certain Indonesian islands [1].

Pathophysiology

Pathology

The presence of adult worms in the lymphatics with an accompanying inflammatory response is the cause of the main pathological feature – lymphatic obstruction (Figure 33.10). Leakage of lymph may contribute to tissue damage. Circulation of microfilariae in the bloodstream has remarkably little effect, although their entrapment in the lungs may cause tropical pulmonary eosinophilia.

Causative organisms (Figure 33.11)
- *Wuchereria bancrofti*
- *Brugia malayi*
- *Brugia timori*

The disease is transmitted by many species of anthropophilic mosquitoes of the genera *Culex*, *Aedes*, *Mansonia*, *Anopheles* and *Coquillettida* [2]. In ingested human blood, where microfilariae are present, the organisms lose their sheaths in the mosquito's stomach and in less than 24 hours make their way into the thoracic muscles. Metamorphosis proceeds and mature larvae migrate to the labella 10 days after infection of the insect. Here they are ready to be transmitted to the next human by biting.

In humans, larvae pass through peripheral lymphatics, develop and migrate centrally and eventually grow into adults, which mate in the lymphatics proximal to the lymph nodes. Fertilised females

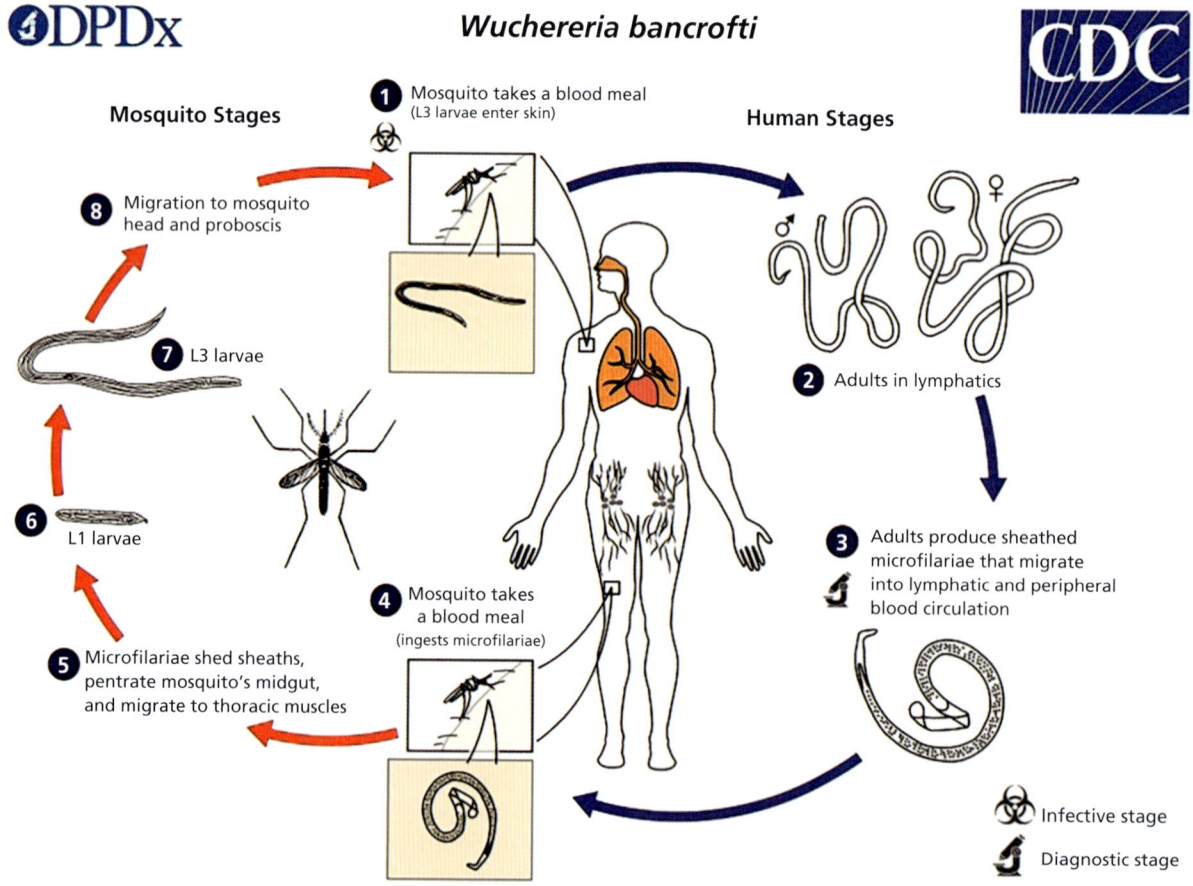

Figure 33.11 Life cycle of *Wuchereria bancrofti*. Courtesy of the Centers for Disease Control and Prevention. https://www.cdc.gov/dpdx/lymphaticfilariasis/index.html (last accessed February 2023).

discharge their microfilariae, which may be found in peripheral blood 12 months after the initial infection. Some microfilariae display periodicity and are only present in peripheral blood at certain times. The discharge is cyclical and occurs principally at night. These microfilariae can pass the placental barrier. The adults are found coiled up in dilated lymphatics. Adult worms are long-lived and can be reproductively active for 5–8 years, producing millions of larval or microfilarial stages that migrate from the lymphatic system to the blood [1].

Immunity to filarial infections is complex. Otherwise, healthy individuals from within the endemic area have both antibody and T-lymphocyte mediated immune responses. By contrast, those with active infections and episodic microfilaraemia may show reduced cellular immunity, suggesting that antigens from the organisms may modulate the immune response. In chronic disease, worms are encapsulated within inflammatory granuloma in the lymphatic system [3]. Another driver of inflammation is the bacterial endosymbiont *Wolbachia* which are potent inducers of innate and adaptive immune responses.

Clinical features
Presentation
Many of those infected do not appear to develop clinical signs of infection, therefore symptoms can vary considerably from patient to patient [4–6]. The first signs are often acute dermato-lymphangio-adenitis (ADLA) and acute filarial lymphangitis (AFL). In addition to systemic signs of fever, chills and headache, ADLA presents with swelling, tenderness and redness on the arms, legs or scrotum [7]. Swellings may be firm, and fixed nodules and urticaria have also been described at this stage. AFL involves acute inflammation of a lymphatic vessel with red streaks that progress distally and is caused by the death of the adult worm either spontaneously or following treatment. Patients present with small, tender nodules or cords at the site of the dying worms [8]. Cellulitis, which is common, may be mild or severe and is recurrent. In the severest form, it presents with fever and sweats and the painful enlargement of lymph nodes, particularly the inguinal group. Lymphangitis can accompany some attacks. Milder forms of cellulitis with more localised redness and tender swellings also occur repeatedly. Other complications include orchitis, which is commonly followed by hydrocoele and scrotal oedema, and recurrent epididymitis. Abscesses deep in the limb muscles, or more superficially located in lymphatics, occur.

Complications and co-morbidities
Repeated attacks of oedema and cellulitis, often associated with interdigital cracking, may be followed over a number of years by evidence of lymphatic obstruction (Figure 33.12). In males, complications commonly present as hydrocoeles, but lower leg oedema and elephantiasis may also develop. Hydrocoele or thickening of the scrotal skin is common in many endemic areas and may affect up to 25% of the adult male population [9]. Limb oedema of a varying extent and nature is also common and passes through several grades of severity before becoming gross elephantiasis. This may be followed by recurrent episodes of secondary infection and the appearance of warty thickening of the skin. The legs are usually affected, but the arms, breast and genitalia may also be involved. A further complication is rupture of dilated abdominal lymphatics.

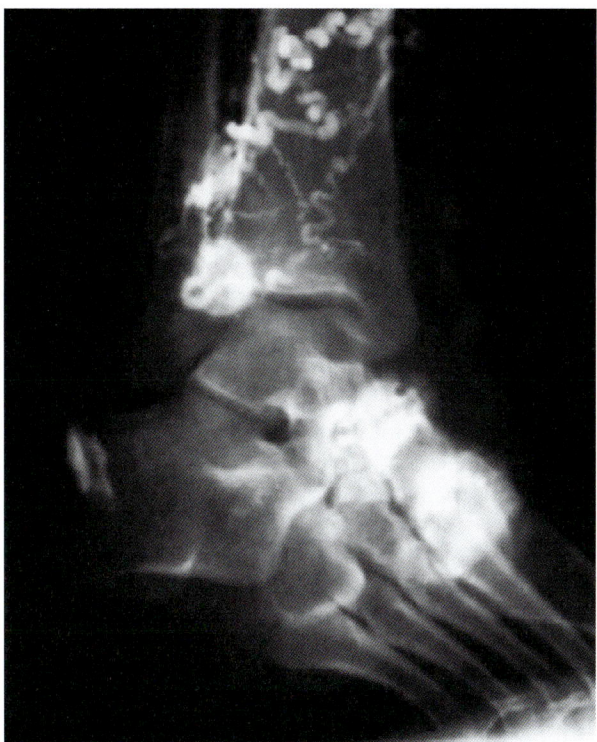

Figure 33.12 Lymphangiogram showing tortuous dilated lymphatic vessels in the leg of a patient with lymphatic filariasis from Mauritius.

Investigations
In an endemic area, it may be possible to make the diagnosis on clinical grounds, before the stage at which microfilariae appear in the blood, as well as in the chronic condition. Biopsy of an enlarged lymph node may be diagnostic.

Microfilariae are demonstrated in the blood especially in acute cases, either in a thick blood film or by passing heparinised blood through a millipore filter, which retains the microfilariae that can then be seen easily under the microscope and distinguished morphologically. When sampling blood, periodicity should be taken into account. Therefore, blood should be drawn between midnight and 02:00 hours, as microfilariae circulate in highest concentration at night.

An alternative procedure is to repeat blood films 1 hour after a single dose of DEC 100 mg. This releases more microfilariae into the circulation. However, some cases of filariasis do not appear to develop detectable filaraemia.

Another approach to diagnosis is the use of serology, where an indirect immunofluorescence or ELISA is positive in a high percentage of those affected, although it is not specific for each organism. An antigen detection system is also used, mainly with immunochromatographic card tests and is now the preferred method given rapid action and ability to detect latent infections [1,10]. A PCR based test has been applied to the detection of *W. bancrofti* genomic DNA in blood [11]. It is important to recognise the current deficiencies in the laboratory confirmation of this disease, as no single test is even 90% accurate.

Imaging studies can also aid in detection. Ultrasound with Doppler of the superficial lymphatics can demonstrate adult worms within dilated lymphatics [12]. Filaria motility *in vivo* has been termed the 'filaria dance sign'. In addition, radionuclide lymphoscintigraphic imaging of the extremities can demonstrate lymphatic dilatation and dysfunction in both asymptomatic persons and in those with lymphoedema (Figure 33.12).

Filarial lymphangitis must be distinguished from bacterial lymphadenitis, with its signs of a portal of entry. Genital lesions may resemble lymphogranuloma venereum with adenopathy and oedema.

Management

The management and elimination of lymphatic filariasis has become the focus of a group of research units, governmental organisations, non-governmental organisations (NGOs) and charities collectively known as the Global Alliance for the Elimination of Lymphatic Filariasis [13]. Two phases of their programme have been developed: parasite elimination and morbidity control. Parasite elimination depends on the use of chemotherapy through mass drug administration (MDA), which is also used for the treatment of individual patients. DEC has long been the main treatment [14,15], but is usually given with albendazole or as fortified salt in MDA programmes.

The dosage for individual patients is the same as for the treatment of onchocerciasis, although higher doses at monthly intervals have also been given. The predominant effect of the drug is on the viability of microfilariae, but it has relatively little impact on adult worms. It may be necessary to repeat the course after a few months if microfilariae reappear in the blood.

Side effects of DEC occur and include anorexia, nausea, vomiting, giddiness, headache, drowsiness and acute allergic reactions due to destruction of microfilariae and adult filariae.

Special care should be taken in areas where both lymphatic filariasis and onchocerciasis coexist, in view of the potentially serious nature of DEC reactions in the latter [9].

There is also experience with ivermectin, and it is effective in lymphatic filariasis. The drug works more rapidly than DEC, and microfilaraemia is reduced to 14–30% of pretreatment levels 6 months after therapy. There are also similar adverse reactions to ivermectin in patients with this condition. The dose is usually 200 μg/kg when given with albendazole. Because ivermectin does not kill adult worms, albendazole with DEC is thought to have better macrofilaricidal activity than albendazole with ivermectin. However, albendazole/ivermectin regimen is preferred for the treatment of lymphatic filariasis in areas that are co-endemic for onchocerciasis as DEC is contraindicated in patients with onchocerciasis.

Morbidity control is approached through a combination of lower limb exercise and regular cleansing, combined with treatment of potential portals of entry of bacteria, such as infected web spaces, which may be caused by fungal or bacterial infection [16]. There is evidence that this can reduce limb swelling considerably, even in late stages. These approaches are being developed across a range of endemic areas. Surgical approaches may improve the appearance of affected limbs either in the early stages by creating a lymph node to venous shunt, or by removing subcutaneous tissue and grafting of split-skin onto a muscle bed (Charles operation) [17] in established elephantiasis. Repeated drainage and surgery may be required for severe hydrocoeles.

Treatment ladder for lymphatic filariasis

First line
- Albendazole 400 mg PO × 1 dose annually plus diethylcarbamazine 6 mg/kg PO × 1 dose annually. Note: contraindicated in regions with co-endemic onchocerciasis. DEC is contraindicated in patients with onchocerciasis due to potential for severe inflammatory response

Second line
- Albendazole 400 mg PO × 1 dose annually plus invermectin 200–400 μg/kg PO × 1 dose (treatment of choice for regions with co-endemic onchocerciasis)

Loiasis

Definition and nomenclature

Loiasis is a filarial disease caused by the parasitic nematode *Loa loa*. The disease is transmitted by the bite of a *Chrysops* fly and is characterised by subcutaneous swellings and migration of the adult worm through the subconjunctival tissue of the eye.

Synonyms and inclusions
- Calabar swellings
- Fugitive swellings
- *Loa loa* filariasis
- African eye worm

Epidemiology

Human loiasis is restricted to the damp forest areas of west and central Africa from 8° north to 5° south of the Equator, and from the Gulf of Guinea to the African Great Lakes where it affects more than 10 million people [1,2]. It is particularly prevalent in the Cameroons and on the Ogowe River. Its distribution includes the coastal plain and follows the Zaire River approximately 800 km (500 miles) inland. It is also found in southern Sudan.

Pathophysiology
Causative organisms
- *Loa Loa*

Loa loa, the African eye worm, is transmitted to humans by blood-sucking tabanid flies of the genus *Chrysops* (deer fly, horse fly and mangrove fly), principally *C. silacea* and *C. dimidiate,* which bite by day. Infection is transmitted by the fly from person to person. Hill houses built at the level of the forest canopy or in cleared plantations are especially susceptible sites for the acquisition of the disease.

Larvae are liberated from *Chrysops* spp. when it presses the labella against the skin to take a blood meal [1,2]. They then enter the tissues through the puncture made by the proboscis. About 1 year after infection of the host, adult worms may appear under the skin or in the conjunctiva, but microfilariae in the blood are not discoverable until 5 months later [3]. The parasite migrates in fascial planes, from which microfilariae are released and travel up lymphatics to the bloodstream to be lodged in the lungs.

Each female adult worm can produce between 12 000 and 39 000 microfilariae per day in the absence of reproductive constraints [4]. Adult worms can live up to 15–21 years, although average lifespan is estimated to be 9 years [5,6].

Clinical features
Presentation
The adult makes frequent journeys through the skin connective tissues, and has often been seen on the fingers, trunk, scalp, lingual frenulum, loose penile skin, eyelids, beneath the conjunctiva and in the anterior chamber of the eye [7]. These migrations may cause a pricking, itching, a creeping sensation or may be symptomless; most individuals with *Loa loa* infection are asymptomatic or have few symptoms. However, when the parasite appears in the conjunctiva, considerable irritation is usual. When the eye is involved, unilateral palpebral oedema may develop and the worm may be seen actually crossing the eye (Figure 33.13).

In certain patients, including expatriates who come to live in an endemic area, these worm movements cause transient, migratory, oedematous swellings – Calabar or 'fugitive' swellings. These affect mainly the arm and hand (Figure 33.14), although they may appear on any part of the body. They develop rapidly and may be painful or itchy, lasting for several days.

Allergic manifestations, such as eosinophilia and angio-oedema, are often more severe in visitors who originate from a non-endemic area. They have been correlated with high immunoglobulin G (IgG) and IgE levels, and increased lymphocyte blastogenesis to filarial antigens [8].

In loiasis, when adult worms die and calcify, additional complications may occur including encephalitis, meningitis, glomerulonephritis, orchitis and scrotal swellings [9].

Investigations
Giemsa-stained blood smears can be used to make the diagnosis with a conventional light microscope when specific morphological features are present [10]. Periodicity should be taken into consideration when obtaining samples. Loiasis microfilariae circulate in highest concentration during the day so blood should be drawn between 12:00 and 14:00. Worms can also be identified if removed from subcutaneous of conjunctival tissue. ELISA and PCR testing are other viable methods [11].

Given ivermectin-associated serious adverse events in patients infected with *Loa loa*, MDA efforts to eliminate onchocerciasis and lymphatic filariasis in co-endemic regions have been suspended. To safely administer ivermectin in these regions, the 'LoaScope,' a mobile phone-based video microscope that automatically quantifies loiasis microfilariae has been developed [11]. This tool has demonstrated efficacy in screening out *Loa loa* in co-endemic regions, enabling ivermectin treatment for onchocerciasis and lymphatic filariasis without serious adverse events [12].

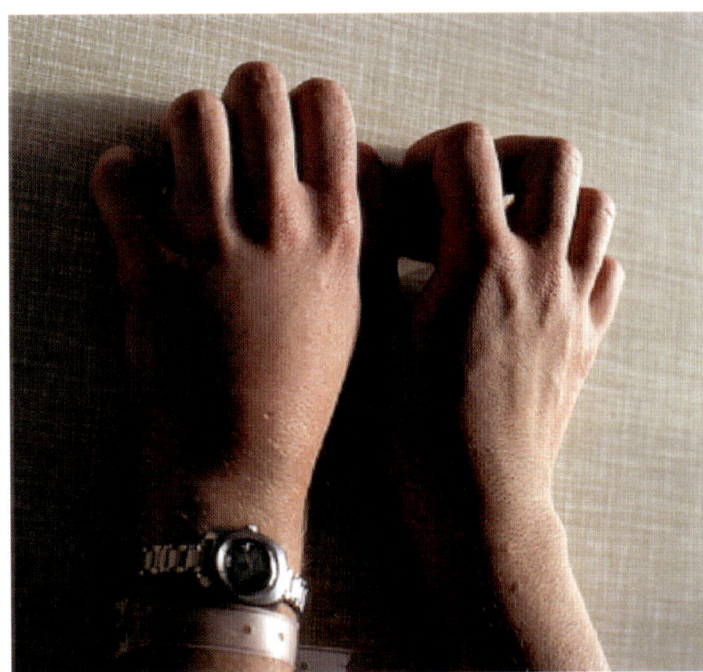

Figure 33.14 Calabar swelling of the dorsum of the left hand in a European patient with loaiasis. In this case no microfilariae were seen in the blood.

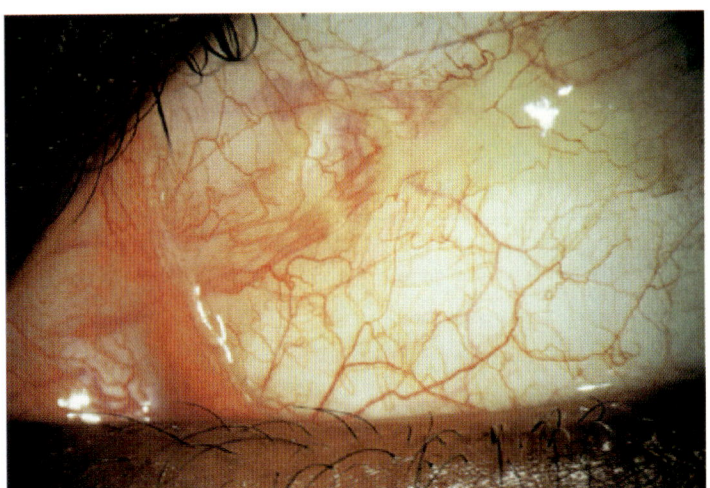

Figure 33.13 *Loa loa*. Creamy white adult worm crossing the conjunctiva of a Nigerian patient.

Management
One course of treatment with DEC is usually curative. Side effects are few and mild, although there may be an allergic reaction with one or more large Calabar swellings, fever, malaise, swelling of joints, joint pains and pruritus. There is a risk of encephalitis in heavy infections with headache, giddiness, vomiting, purpura and eosinophilia. After DEC therapy, elongated subcutaneous nodules, indicating the presence of adult worms, may appear [13].

Albendazole is a good second choice for therapy of loiasis [14]. There are fewer side effects with this medication. It has less microfilaricidal activity, so there is no massive antigen release associated with this therapy.

Ivermectin also produces good responses in loiasis and reduces microfilaraemia [15]. However, it does not kill adult worms. While it is generally well tolerated, adverse events, such as impaired conscious state and arthralgia, can be seen in those with high levels of microfilaraemia [16]. Moreover, those co-infected with onchocerciasis can have a life-threatening encephalitic reaction to ivermectin. Consequently, ivermectin should be used with caution and microfilarial load should be checked before administration. Apheresis can be used to reduce high microfilarial loads.

Adult worms can sometimes be removed from the conjunctiva surgically.

> **Treatment ladder for loiasis**
>
> **First line**
> - Diethylcarbamazine 8–10 mg/kg/day PO in three doses for 21 days
>
> **Second line**
> - Albendazole 200 mg PO BD × 21 days
>
> **Third line**
> - Ivermectin 200 µg/kg PO × 2 days

Dracunculiasis

Definition and nomenclature

Dracunculiasis, commonly referred to as Guinea worm disease, is a chronic parasitic infection due to the nematode, *Dracunculus medinensis*, which is among the longest nematodes to infect humans, growing up to 1 metre in length [1]. Mature female worms migrate along subcutaneous tissue, forming a painful ulcerating blister.

> **Synonyms and inclusions**
> - Dracontiasis
> - Guinea worm
> - Medina worm
> - Dragon worm

Epidemiology

While dracunculiasis was once very prevalent, its occurrence has been significantly reduced by eradication efforts since the start of the Guinea Worm Eradication Program in the 1980s. In the 1940s, estimates project 48 million people were affected through Africa, the Middle East and India. In 1986, the number of cases were approximately 3.5 million [2]. The World Health Organization (WHO) reports only 54 total cases in 2019 from Chad (48), South Sudan (4), Angola (1) and Cameroon (1) [3].

Pathophysiology

Causative organisms [4]
- *Dracunculus medinensis* (Figure 33.15)

The adult female worm matures over a 1-year period in humans and discharges larvae through an ulcerated skin lesion. Millions of these larvae are produced, particularly on contact with water;

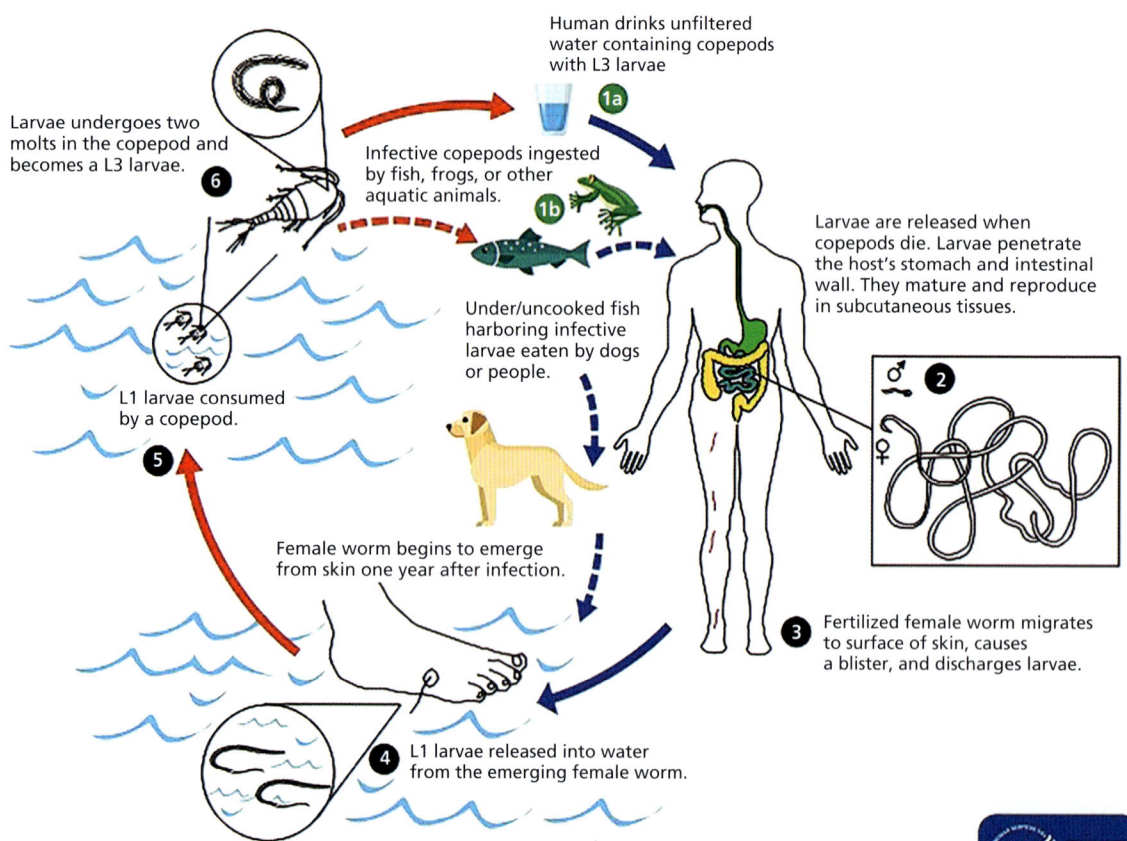

Figure 33.15 Life cycle of *Dracunculus medinensis*. Courtesy of the Centers for Disease Control and Prevention. https://www.cdc.gov/dpdx/dracunculiasis/index.html (last accessed February 2023).

these survive for 3–4 days and can develop further in copepods or water fleas (*Cyclops* spp. such as *C. leukarti*). After ingestion by the *Cyclops*, they pass through two developmental stages before reaching the infective third stage (L3) after 2 weeks. Humans are infected via drinking water containing infected *Cyclops* spp.; the larvae are released and penetrate the intestine. Further maturation occurs in the retroperitoneal space or other sites; mating occurs after about 3 months, and the males subsequently die. The females grow and migrate downwards, usually to the lower limbs. Aberrant migration can, however, occur [5]. The female penetrates the skin of the leg and can then discharge larvae after exposure to water. Each female contains 2–3 million larvae. Migration of the worm and larval forms is largely subclinical. Disease is associated with the presence of the adult female in subcutaneous tissue in the lower limbs.

Environmental factors
Dracunculiasis is a disease found in poor rural populations, most notably in Sudan and Chad. It can be spread in and around communal drinking, washing areas or wells.

Clinical features
Presentation [6]
Immediately before the appearance of part of the adult female through the skin, there may be generalised symptoms such as fever, pruritus, urticaria and oedema [7]. Dyspnoea and diarrhoea may also occur. Usually, however, the first sign of the infection is the appearance of a small papule or vesicle, which expands and bursts over 4–5 days. When this occurs, commonly on the lower limb, there is intense localised itching. This is often followed by the emergence of part of the female worm through the skin (Figure 33.16). The surrounding ulcer is covered with slough, which usually becomes secondarily infected. The worm itself is often palpable. Infections with two or more worms may also occur. Eventually, the worms may be resorbed or calcify.

Secondary infection is very common and may incapacitate the patient. It is a major cause of morbidity [7]. The common infecting organism is *Staphylococcus aureus*, but the open wound may also serve as a portal of entry for tetanus. Sometimes, *Dracunculus* may find its way into other sites, such as the knee joint, lung, pericardium and spinal cord, and cause localised infection.

Investigations
The appearance of the worm under the skin is typical. However, the adult can be induced to shed larvae onto a glass slide, which can be examined microscopically, by applying water to the extruded segment. Complete blood count with differential will demonstrate peripheral eosinophilia and immunoglobulin E, G1, and G4 levels are usually be elevated [8]. Worms may also calcify in tissue and can be visualised on radiography [9].

Management
There is no specific drug or vaccine to treat or prevent infection with *Dracunculus medinensis*. The object of treatment is the removal of the worm. This can be facilitated with an oral benzimidazole, such as metronidazole. After a few days, the inflammation lessens and it may be possible to extract the worm gently. It may be

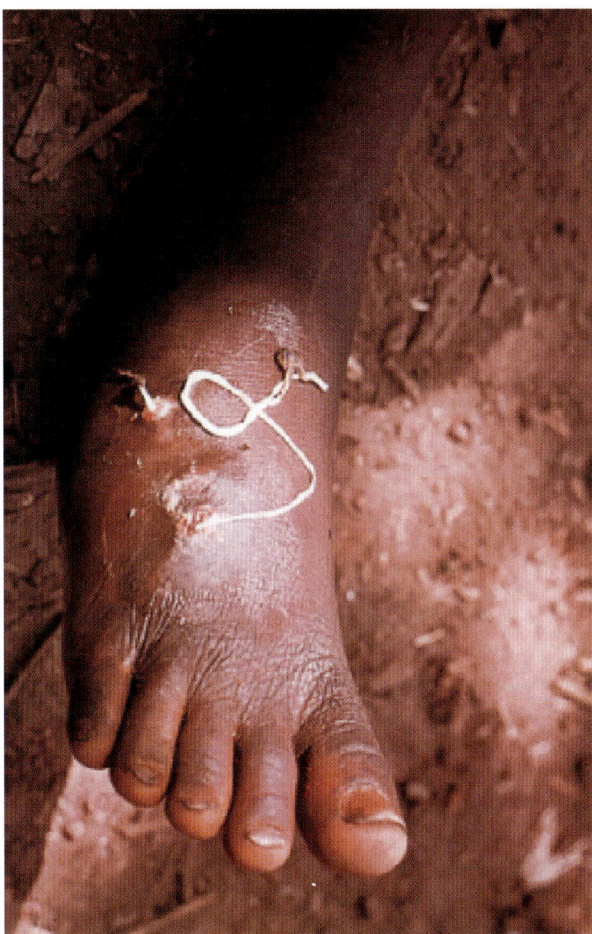

Figure 33.16 Guinea worm. Adult female *Dracunculus medinensis* emerging from the skin of a Nigerian patient. Courtesy of Dr R. Muller.

difficult to extract the worm if mebendazole is used [10]. The more traditional approach is to induce the worm to discharge larvae by applying water or ethyl chloride and to wind the free end around a matchstick or other small stick. By gradually winding more and more of the worm onto the spool, the whole nematode can be recovered. It is important not to exert tension or the worm will break and cause severe allergic cellulitis. The procedure is therefore carried out slowly over a few days. It has been suggested that the Rod of Asclepius represents *Dracunculus medinensis* extraction.

In addition, all cases should be treated with local antiseptics, tetanus toxoid and, if necessary, broad spectrum antibiotics [7]. The drug treatment described above does not affect the larvae or prevent transmission. The latter is best accomplished by public health programmes designed to provide clean drinking water, by sieving or filtration to remove *Cyclops*. Chemical control of *Cyclops* using larvicides such as temefos is also possible.

Considerable progress has been made in the past two decades in instituting effective public health measures for the control of dracunculiasis. Since 1986 the estimated prevalence has been reduced by 100% from an initial figure of 3.5 million. Goals were set for the complete eradication by 2020 [11] with an actual recorded figure of 27 cases worldwide in that year.

Enterobiasis

Definition and nomenclature
Enterobiasis, or pinworm, is one of the most common parasitic worm infections in the world. Its cause is infection by the roundworm *Enterobius vermicularis*. Usually a childhood disease, it can range from asymptomatic to causing severe anal and perianal itching. It is considered more a nuisance rather than a serious infection.

Synonyms and inclusions
- Pinworm
- Threadworm
- Seatworm
- Oxyuriasis

Introduction and general description
Enterobius vermicularis is the commonest human intestinal worm, with a worldwide distribution. It is prevalent in both temperate and tropical climates and is associated with crowding and poverty. Children are most commonly affected. Overall, males are affected twice as often as females, except in those aged 5–14, where females are predominantly affected. Whole families and communities, notably schools, may be infected as transmission can occur through contaminated clothing, bedding, furniture, or personal care products [1].

Epidemiology
Incidence and prevalence
It remains the most common helminthic infection in Western Europe and the USA, with a worldwide rate of infection over 1 billion [1]. An estimated 4–28% of children are infected globally [2]. The disease occurs in all socioeconomic groups; however, it more commonly occurs in overcrowded living conditions.

Age
The disease occurs most frequently in children between the age of 5 and 10.

Pathophysiology
Causative organisms (Figure 33.17)
- *Enterobius vermicularis*

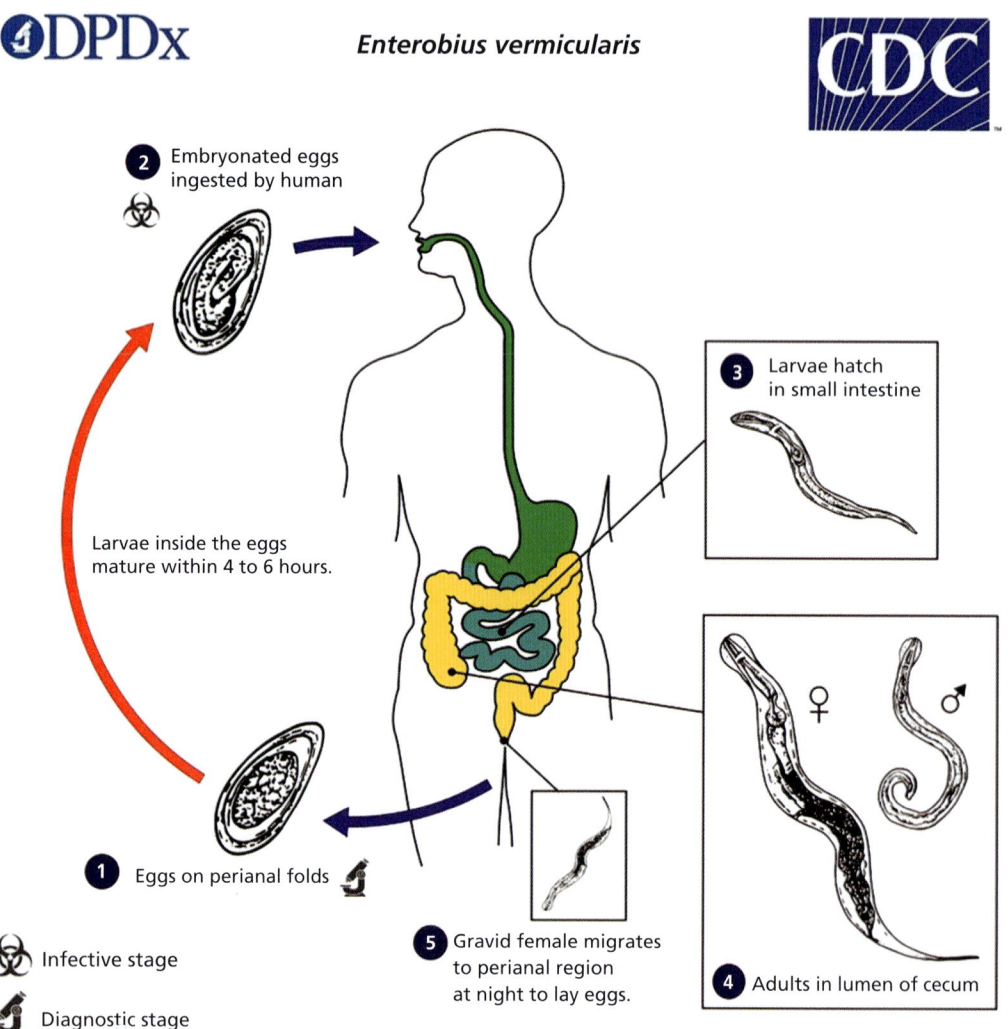

Figure 33.17 Life cycle of *Enterobius vermicularis*. Courtesy of the Centers for Disease Control and Prevention. https://www.cdc.gov/dpdx/enterobiasis/index.html (last accessed February 2023).

Male and female worms develop in the caecum, becoming mature 2–8 weeks after ingestion of fertile eggs. Gravid female worms migrate to the anus, and at night crawl on the perianal skin where they lay up to 16 000 eggs and expire. The eggs mature within a few hours. Transmission is by ingestion of eggs, most commonly carried by fingernails, following a scratch itch cycle often during sleep. Hands may also become contaminated through sharing a bed or bedroom. Occasionally, transmission may become airborne from infected dust, in which eggs may survive for up to 13 days. Adult worms live for 6–12 weeks.

Gravid female worms migrating on the skin cause intense itching, although not in all infected people. It is not known whether an allergic reaction is involved. Adult worms may burrow into the submucosa of the appendix or bowel and be associated with inflammation, although causation has not been clearly established. Female worms may migrate from the anus to the vagina, causing irritation and inflammation, and from there to the fallopian tubes or even peritoneal cavity, causing salpingitis and occasionally peritoneal nodules.

Clinical features
Presentation
Anal and perineal pruritus at night, with sleeplessness and irritability, are the leading symptoms. Perineal intertrigo, nocturia, secondarily infected excoriations, localised urticaria [3], vulval irritation and mucoid discharge may occur. Extraintestinal infection patterns in the vagina, urinary bladder, peritoneum, kidneys, liver and eye have been described in isolated cases [1,4,5]. It is important to realise, however, that a large number of infected children are asymptomatic.

Diagnosis
Diagnosis may sometimes be made by visualising the 10-mm long female worms on the perineum at night, on toilet paper or in the stools. When possible, worms should be positively identified in a laboratory, to avoid confusion with proglottids of *Dipylidium caninum*. However, the best procedure is to wind a 6-cm strip of adhesive cellulose tape over the butt end of a test tube or a wooden spatula, with the adherent side outward. This is then rubbed over the perianal skin (preferably on waking) and the diagnostic eggs and adults stick to it. A drop of toluene is placed on a microscope slide and the tape is spread on it and examined microscopically.

Management
Of the several antihelminthic drugs available, mebendazole or albendazole are probably the most effective with a 90–100% success rate, acting against all stages of the worm [1]. Treatment with both agents is a single dose, repeated after 2 weeks. A once-only dose has a high cure rate, although a second repeated dose achieves a cure rate of nearly 100%. The whole family or infected classmates should be treated to prevent reinfection. Scrupulous attention should be paid to cleanliness of hands and nails on rising, after defaecation and before eating. After each dosing, the bed linen should be changed and the bedroom vacuum cleaned. Even so, relapses may occur and periodic retreatment may be necessary. Pyrantel pamoate is also an acceptable alternative, with an efficacy around 90%. Its side effects are rare but include neurotoxicity and transient transaminitis. Ivermectin is generally not used for pinworm, although in one study it did have a 100% efficacy [6].

> **Treatment ladder for enterobiasis**
>
> **First line**
> - Albendazole, 200–400 mg PO for 1 day, then repeat dose in 2 weeks (some sources suggest repeating dose after 14 and 28 days)
> - Mebendazole 100–200 mg PO for 1 day, then repeat dose in 2 weeks (some sources suggest repeating dose after 14 and 28 days)
>
> **Second line**
> - Pyrantel pamoate: dose varies per weight (11 mg/kg; maximum 1 g); one time, then repeat dose in 2 weeks (some sources suggest repeating dose after 14 and 28 days)
>
> **Third line**
> - Ivermectin 0.2 mg/kg BD for 10 days

Ancylostomiasis

Definition and nomenclature
'Ground itch', 'dew itch' and 'uncinarial dermatitis' all describe a variable and transient eruption due to skin penetration by larvae of the hookworms *Ancylostoma duodenale* and *Necator americanus*, and the roundworm *Strongyloides stercoralis*. When the hookworms are present in large numbers, they produce an iron deficiency in the host, by feeding off blood in the intestinal wall.

> **Synonyms and inclusions**
> - Hookworm disease
> - Tunnel disease
> - Miner's anaemia
> - Ground itch
> - Dew itch
> - Uncinarial dermatitis
> - Cutaneous larva migrans

Epidemiology
Necator americanus and *A. duodenale* are human hookworms very widely distributed in the tropics and subtropics. *Necator americanus* predominates in Central and South Africa, southern Asia and Melanesia, and is almost the sole hookworm in the New World and Polynesia. In some communities, the impact of disease parallels that of malaria [1]. *Ancylostoma duodenale* is the only human hookworm in Europe, the Mediterranean coast, and central and northern Asia, and is more prevalent than *Necator* spp. in China, Japan and some parts of Indonesia. The global infection prevalence for any hookworm in 2016 was approximately 450 million [2].

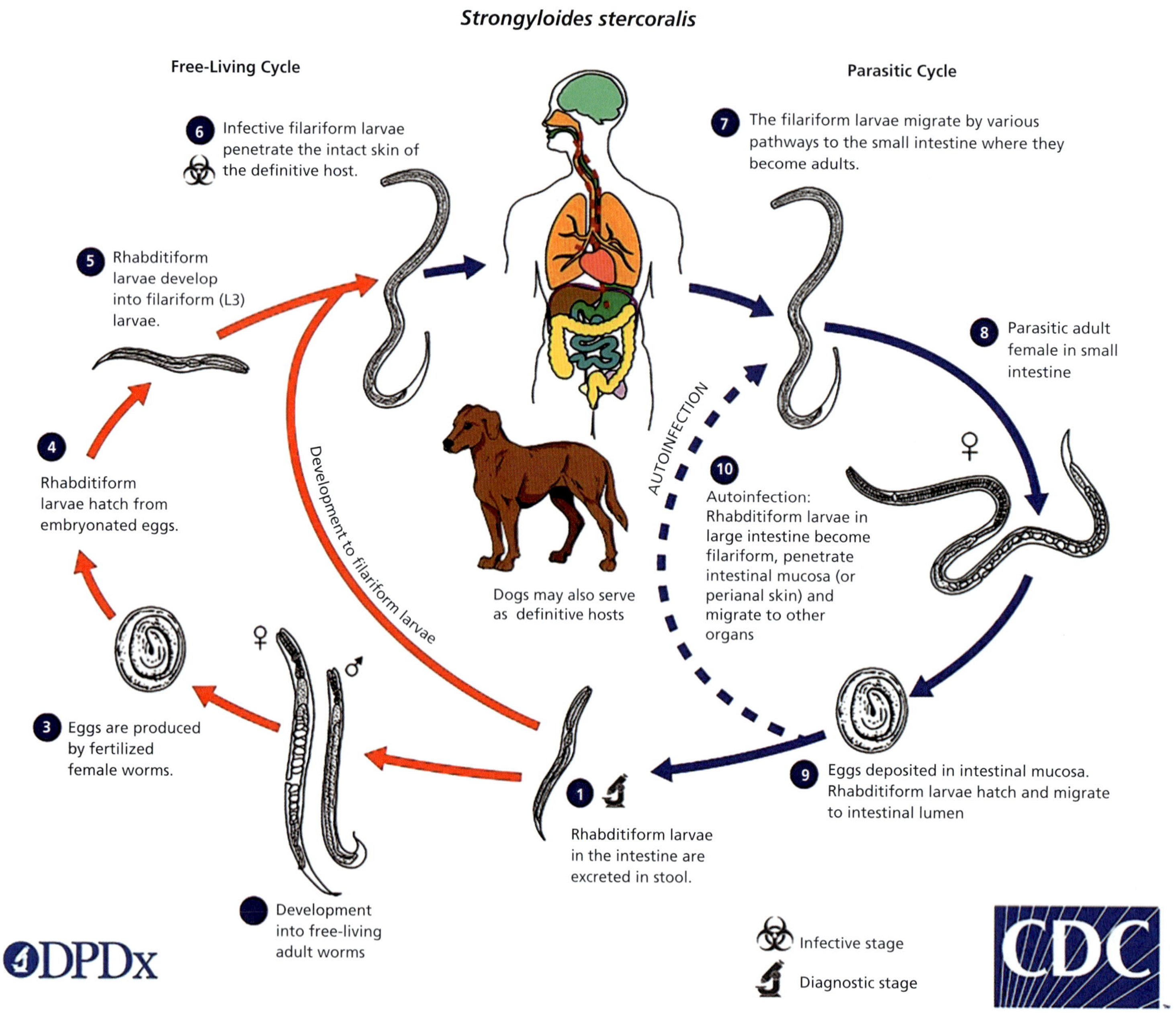

Figure 33.18 The life cycle of *Strongyloides stercoralis*. Courtesy of the Centers for Disease Control and Prevention. https://www.cdc.gov/dpdx/strongyloidiasis/index.html (last accessed February 2023).

Pathophysiology [3]
Causative organisms (Figure 33.18)
- *Ancylostoma duodenale*
- *Necator americanus*
- *Strongyloides stercoralis* (roundworm)

The adult worms live in the jejunum with the head firmly attached to the mucosa and cause bleeding: *N. americanus* 0.03 mL of blood per worm per day and *A. duodenale* 0.2 mL of blood per worm per day [4]. However, some reports estimate that *A. duodenale* is responsible for a 10-fold greater blood loss than *N. americanus* secondary to wasteful feeding (not all the blood *A. duodenale* ingests is digested) [3]. Bleeding leads to anaemia, hypoproteinaemia, digestive disturbances and stunted development. As many as 10 000 eggs are produced per day and are passed in the faeces. Eggs can survive varying periods of cold or drought, but under favourable conditions of warmth and humidity, hatch into motile rhabditiform larvae. After 5 days and further moults, the infective filariform larvae form. They migrate upwards through soil and grass and, after a period of contact of 5–10 min, can penetrate intact human skin. Walking barefoot is the commonest way of getting infected.

After penetrating the skin, larvae migrate within a day or two via the bloodstream to the lungs, pass up the bronchial tree, are swallowed and pass down the oesophagus, reaching the duodenum and jejunum, where they mature in 4–6 weeks. In passing through the lungs they cause acute alveolitis or pneumonitis. Life expectancy of adult *A. duodenale* worms is approximately 1 year and 3–5 years for *N. americanus*.

Environmental factors [5]
Favourable places for transmission include soil around houses, places of work such as plantations, cultivated fields and mines. Risk is further increased by warm and moist climate, walking barefoot, poor sanitation and personal hygiene. Children and pregnant women are at the highest risk.

Clinical features
Presentation
Larvae penetrating the skin cause ground itch: severe pruritus accompanied by redness and often a papular or papulovesicular rash [6]. The rash is most commonly on the feet and may be accompanied by a generalised urticaria. The rash is more common with *Necator* infections and may become secondarily infected as a result of scratching. Larvae passing through the lungs cause a syndrome of cough, wheeze and dyspnoea, which lasts for several days. Adult worms in the gut cause abdominal pain, diarrhoea and, occasionally, melaena. Later, features of iron deficiency anaemia, with haemoglobin levels as low as 5 g/dL, and hypoproteinaemia develop with pallor, oedema, puffy face and listlessness. Changes in the texture of skin and hair resemble those seen in kwashiorkor [7].

Clinical variants
Löffler syndrome. When passing through the lungs, the disease may cause Löffler syndrome, a disease in which eosinophils accumulate in the lung in response to a parasite load. Patients complain of a dry unproductive cough that usually resolves after 2–3 days, but may last up to 3 weeks.

Wakana syndrome [7]. With peroral infection, nausea, vomiting, pharyngeal irritation, cough and dyspnoea might occur.

Investigations
Clinical and circumstantial evidence point to a diagnosis of ground itch. Löffler syndrome is characterised by eosinophilia and patchy pneumonitis seen radiologically. Established infections are diagnosed by demonstrating characteristic eggs in the faeces.

Management
Ground itch is treated symptomatically with an antipruritic cream, such as crotamiton with 1% hydrocortisone, or oral antihistamines. Pulmonary symptoms, if severe, respond to a few days' corticosteroids. Established infections respond to albendazole or mebendazole or pyrantel pamoate [8]. Ivermectin has poor efficacy against hookworm. Oral iron is given for iron deficiency.

> **Treatment ladder for ancylostomiasis** [3]
> - Albendazole 400 mg PO × 1 dose
> - Mebendazole 100 mg PO BD × 3 days
> - Pyrantel pamoate 11 mg/kg/day for 3 days

Strongyloidiasis

Definition and nomenclature
Strongyloidiasis is an infection of the gastrointestinal tract with the parasitic roundworm *Strongyloides stercoralis*. Aside from abdominal symptoms, allergic reactions occur, commonly affecting the skin.

> **Synonyms and inclusions**
> - Strongyloidal ground itch
> - Larva currens

Introduction and general description
Strongyloides infection can be asymptomatic in about two-thirds of infected individuals and may therefore become chronic and potentially lifelong. Those who do develop symptoms or signs of infection present with features suggestive of atopy [1].

Epidemiology
Incidence and prevalence
Strongyloidiaisis occurs in warm, especially damp, climates such as West Africa, the Caribbean, the Amazon basin and is especially prevalent in South-East Asia. In endemic areas, especially in rural communities, up to 20% of the population can be infected. Globally, an estimated 30–100 million are affected across 70 countries [2].

Pathophysiology
Pathology [3,4]
Penetration of the skin by filariform larvae may cause dermatitis. Adult worms give rise to duodenitis and jejunitis, which may cause diarrhoea and malabsorption. Migrating larvae in the skin give rise to a weal-and-flare response, which follows the path of the larva. Hyperinfection causes severe enteritis with fluid loss, and paralytic ileus, pneumonia, meningoencephalitis and secondary Gram-negative bacterial septicaemia with shock and disseminated intravascular coagulation.

Causative organisms (Figure 33.18)
- *Strongyloides stercoralis*

  Strongyloides stercoralis is a widespread, parasitic roundworm with a life cycle and distribution similar to that of the hookworm, but with important differences [1]. Adult male and female worms, 3 mm long, live in the mucosal crypts of the duodenum and jejunum; eggs hatch quickly and rhabditiform larvae are passed in the faeces. In soil, they may either moult into infective filariform larvae, or set up a free-living cycle, with the production of more infective larvae. Infective larvae penetrate human skin, to establish new infections or augment existing ones. Alternatively, larvae mature in the gut and reinfect the patient by penetrating the mucosa or the perianal skin. This autoinfection is capable of maintaining the infection indefinitely and predisposes to hyperinfection syndrome [3].

Clinical features
Presentation
The ground itch caused by initial infection with *Strongyloides stercoralis* is similar to that seen in hookworm disease. Intestinal infection

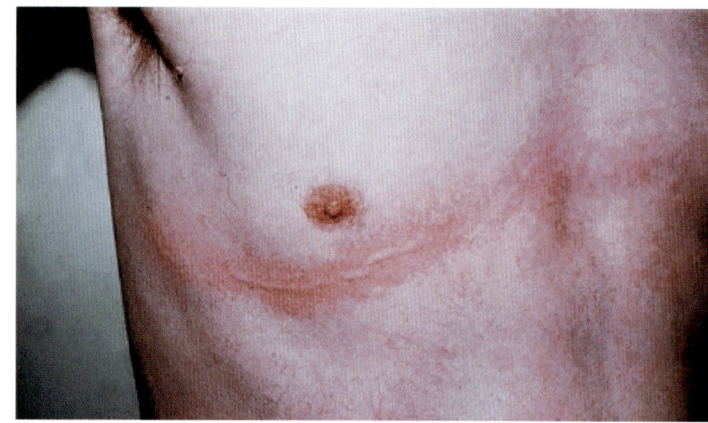

Figure 33.19 Larva currens rash of *Strongyloides stercoralis*. The weal and flare will have disappeared in a few hours.

causes abdominal pain, diarrhoea and, if severe, weight loss or stunting of growth in children [5]. Associated allergic phenomena are common. Urticaria and raised IgE levels occur in 66% of cases of strongyloidiasis among patients who have had the infection for over 45 years [6]. Thirty percent of these individuals also suffer from larva currens, the urticarial wheal and flare of migrating subcutaneous larvae. Tracks can be seen anywhere on the skin between the knees and nipples (Figure 33.19), but especially around the anus and buttocks. They move at a rate of 2–10 cm per hour and can traverse the abdomen in a single day and be gone the next day: features that distinguish the rash from that of larva migrans. Tracks may be several centimetres long or consist simply of one or more urticarial papules. Tracks may be linear or serpiginous but the rash may be less distinctive, mimicking a drug eruption [7].

Complications and co-morbidities

In hyperinfection or disseminated strongyloidiasis, extremely heavy worm loads build up and leave the confines of the gut, spreading through other organs. This severe syndrome may occur in patients who are immunosuppressed by corticosteroid drugs, lymphoma, leukaemia, infection with HIV or human T-cell leukaemia virus type 1 (HTLV-1), or debilitated by advanced age, tuberculosis or other severe infection, carcinomatosis, malnutrition or burns [4]. Heavy infection causes severe diarrhoea, with fluid and electrolyte loss; signs of ileus may develop. Fever, abdominal distension, cough, dyspnoea, mental changes and unconsciousness may develop, and the patient's body may go into shock. Shock commonly indicates a complicating Gram-negative septicaemia. Cough, dyspnoea and chest signs suggest pneumonia. A widespread petechial or purpuric rash may be seen [8]. In *Strongyloides* infections in HIV-positive patients, the immune reconstitution syndrome triggered by antiretroviral therapy has also been associated with increased generalised symptoms and pruritus [9].

Investigations [10,11]

Larvae and the ova of *Strongyloides* spp. are demonstrated in the faeces but the concentration may be low and the sensitivity of direct examination is often below 50%. This can be increased by one of several concentration or culture techniques. Serum *Strongyloides* antibody tests are available (ELISA and indirect immunofluorescent antibody test (IFAT)), but often confined to reference laboratories.

In severe or emergency situations, a good diagnostic yield can be obtained by more invasive methods such as examining samples of jejunal juice (most conveniently obtained by a 'string test' or entero-test capsule), jejunal biopsy or videocapsule endoscopy. Except in the hyperinfection syndrome, eosinophilia is common and tests for malabsorption may be positive.

Management

Ivermectin in an oral dose of 200 μg/kg body weight for two consecutive days, is the treatment of choice [11]. Albendazole is also effective in a dose of 400 mg/day twice a day for 3–7 days, and is free of toxicity. Thiabendazole is an alternative treatment, but its use is limited by gastrointestinal side effects. Ivermectin has been shown to be more efficacious than albendazole and better tolerated than thiabendazole [12].

For cases of hyperinfection, ivermectin is given daily until symptoms resolve. If there is a good response to treatment, eosinophil count and antibody levels should reduce. Faecal and possibly jejunal samples can be examined for larvae after 3 and 6 months.

Treatment ladder for strongyloidiasis

First line
- Ivermectin 200 μg/kg PO × 2 days

Second line
- Albendazole 400 mg PO BD × 3–7 days

INFECTION WITH NEMATODES OF OTHER ANIMALS

Nematodes that do not normally parasitise humans are often unable to mature or develop fully, or to home to within their normal site in the body. Biologically, the human is a dead-end host. The infective larvae tend to wander, causing one of several forms of larva migrans, or the adult worm migrates, causing migratory allergic phenomena. Worms reach unusual sites and give rise to eosinophilic granulomas, occasionally in important sites, such as the eye, causing blindness, or the lungs, causing radiological confusion. In other infections, full development may take place and humans act as accidental intermediate hosts.

A summary of the organisms and diseases caused by infection with nematodes of other animals is provided in Table 33.2.

Cutaneous larva migrans

Definition and nomenclature

Cutaneous larva migrans is often the clinical term used to describe a distinctive cutaneous eruption that may have numerous causes.

Table 33.2 The organisms and diseases in infection with nematodes of other animals.

Disease	Organism
Cutaneous larva migrans	Ancylostoma brasiliense
	Ancylostoma caninum
	Ancylostoma ceylonicum
	Unicararia stenocephala
	Bunostumum phlebotomum
Visceral larva migrans:	Toxocara canis
Toxocariasis	Toxocara cati
	Toxocara malayensis
Gnathostomiasis	Gnathostoma hispidium
	Gnathostoma nipponicum
Dirofilariasis	Subcutaneous disease: Dirofilaria tenuis, D. urii, D. subdermata and D. repens
	Pulmonary disease: D. immitis
Trichinosis	Trichinella spiralis

The prime features, as the name suggests, are that the lesions migrate or creep and that they are due to the presence of moving parasites in the skin. Visceral larva migrans also occurs.

Synonyms and inclusions
- Creeping eruption
- Sand worm eruption
- Plumber's itch
- Duckhunter's itch

Epidemiology
Incidence and prevalence
Infection is found most commonly in tropical and subtropical climates of Africa, South America, South-East Asia, the Caribbean and the southeastern USA, with larvae commonly found in sandboxes and beaches. Prevalence is often highest during wet seasons.

Pathophysiology
Causative organisms [1]
- *Ancylostoma brasiliense*
- *Ancylostoma caninum*
- *Ancylostoma ceylonicum*
- *Uncinaria stenocephala*
- *Bunostumum phlebotomum*

Causes of creeping eruption include *Ancylostoma brasiliense*, *A. caninum*, *A. ceylonicum*, *Uncinaria stenocephala* and *Bunostomum phlebotomum*. The aforementioned are all animal hookworms, of which the dog hookworm is the most common cause of creeping eruption in humans. *Anatrichosoma cutaneum*, a parasite of monkeys in East and South East Asia, is a rare cause. *Strongyloides stercoralis* causes a distinctive form of cutaneous larva migrans. *Dirofilaria repens* and *Spirometra* spp. cause a subcutaneous granuloma that may migrate very slowly. *Gnathostoma* spp. and *Loa loa* cause migratory evanescent subcutaneous swellings. Additionally, cutaneous myiasis due to larvae of flies of the genera *Gasterophilus* and *Hypoderma* may cause a creeping eruption similar to that caused by the animal hookworms. However, only the helminths that cause creeping eruption are considered further here.

Adult hookworms live in the intestines of dogs and cats, and their ova are deposited in the animals' faeces. Under favourable conditions of humidity and temperature, the ova hatch into infective larvae, which will penetrate human stratum corneum by secreting hyaluronidase. However, the larvae are unable to burrow through the basement membrane and are therefore unable to complete their lifecycle [2]. Thus, the worms die without reproducing and therefore it is a self-limited disease.

Environmental factors
Sandy, warm, moist and shaded areas are particularly favourable. Many infections are acquired by children in sandpits, plumbers under houses, farm workers under outbuildings, hunters in hides, gardeners from the soil and seabathers from the sandy shore. The condition is common in all warm climates and may occur in northern Europe during a hot summer. Outbreaks occur commonly in groups of holidaymakers who mostly acquired the condition by direct skin contact with infested sand while on tropical beach holidays [3].

Clinical features
Presentation [4]
The larvae may cause a pruritic red papule at the site of penetration where the skin has been in contact with infected soil, commonly the feet, hands and buttocks. The larvae can lie quiet for weeks or months, or immediately begin creeping activity with the production of a wandering thread-like line about 3 mm wide. This phenomenon is exceedingly itchy, slightly raised, flesh-coloured or pink, and forms bizarre, serpentine patterns. Large numbers of larvae may be active at the same time, with the formation of a disorganised series of loops and tortuous tracks (Figure 33.20).

The larvae advance at a rate of a few millimetres to a few centimetres daily, and are commonly found ahead of the track they leave behind. The wanderings of an individual larva are usually confined to a relatively small area, but it can travel exceptionally far. Itching leads to scratching and secondary changes of dermatitis and bacterial infection. In later stages, these tracks are difficult to see, the path being marked by small itchy and discontinuous nodules.

Cutaneous larvae migrans is self-limiting with estimates for the natural duration of the disease varying considerably. This variation almost certainly depends on the species of larva observed, and this is usually unknown. In one study, 25–33% of larvae died every 4 weeks, whereas in another (presumed due to *Ancylostoma brasiliense*) 81% of lesions disappeared in 4 weeks [5]. Others may persist for many months to years [6].

Clinical variants
In severe infestations, larva migrans may be accompanied by Löffler syndrome of pulmonary eosinophilia [7].

Differential diagnosis
The main differential diagnosis is the larva currens ('running larva') of strongyloidiasis. The main distinguishing factor between the two diseases is the speed at which the larvae travel. Larva currens is known for its distinct rapidity, with the larval track progressing at approximately 0.2 cm/min, with cutaneous lesions progressing up to 5–15 cm/h. In cutaneous larva migrans, the larval track

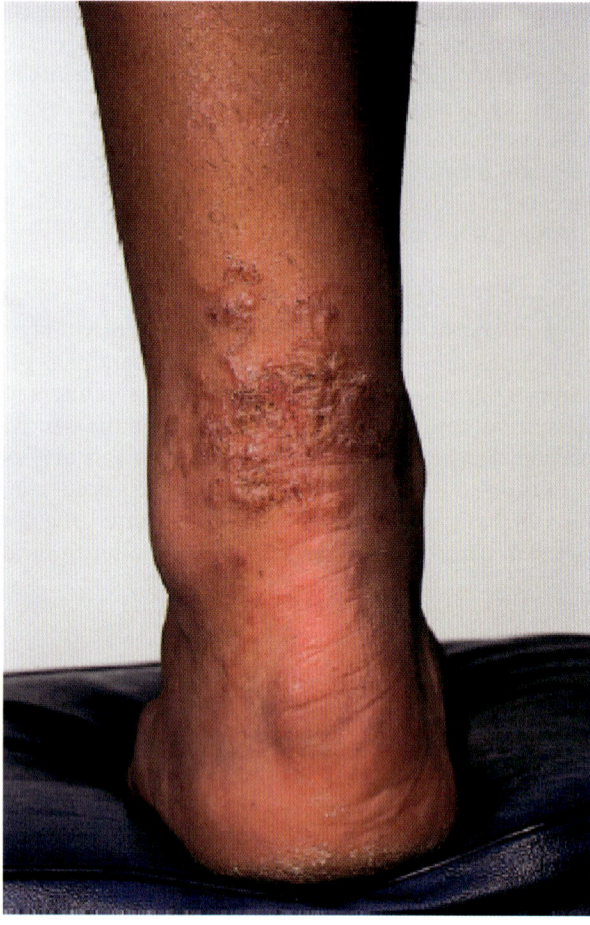

Figure 33.20 Cutaneous larva migrans (creeping eruption). There are several tortuous indurated inflamed worm tracks, in some of which may be seen a blister that marks the head of the track.

> **Treatment ladder for cutaneous larva migrans**
>
> **First line**
> - Ivermectin 200 µg/kg PO OD for 1 or 2 days
>
> **Second line**
> - Albendazole 400 mg PO for 3 days

progresses at approximately 1 cm/h with cutaneous lesions only progressing a few millimetres to a few centimetres daily.

Noninfectious causes of linear or serpiginous dermatoses includes phytophotodermatosis, jellyfish stings, zoster or lichenoid eruptions, but these can easily be ruled out by their non-creeping nature [8].

Diagnosis
The classic clinical picture of wandering, advancing, serpentine and itchy lesions is easily recognised, but may be atypical, hidden by vesicles and scaling, or spoiled by scratching and secondary infection.

Larva currens and migratory myiasis must be distinguished and, in the Orient, from gnathostomiasis. Biopsy in larva migrans is of little value, as the larvae have advanced beyond the clinical lesions.

Management
Antihelminthic treatment is warranted to relieve symptoms and reduce the likelihood of secondary bacterial infection. Ivermectin is the preferred treatment, and is given at 0.15–0.2 mg/kg every day PO × 1 or 2 days. Alternatively, albendazole 400 mg/day PO for 3 days is also effective, although in some cases the responses are poor. If localised, topical thiabendazole or ivermectin have proven effective [9,10].

Visceral larva migrans

Definition and nomenclature
Many non-human and human helminths may be found migrating in human organs at various stages in their life cycle, but the syndrome of visceral larva migrans is synonymous with the severe form of toxocariasis.

> **Synonyms and inclusions**
> - Toxocariasis

Epidemiology
Incidence and prevalence
Toxocariasis is prevalent worldwide, with concentrations greatest in areas with domestic dogs and cats. The disease is more common in developing countries with tropical and subtropical regions, and socioeconomically disadvantaged groups. Seroprevalences of *Toxocara canis* have been estimated at 1.6% in Japan, 2.4% in Denmark, 6.3% in Austria, 7% in Sweden, 14% in the USA and 19.6% in Malaysia, and greater than 80% of the population in Nepal and regions of Indonesia [1]. Children are at a higher risk of infection.

Pathophysiology
Pathology
In humans, the second-stage larvae migrate from the intestine to most parts of the body, but notably to the liver, lungs, muscles and brain where they eventually die in eosinophilic granulomas.

Causative organisms
- *Toxocara canis*
- *Toxocara cati*
- *Toxocara malayensis*

This infection is caused by *Toxocara canis*, *T. cati* and *T. malayensis*, the common roundworms of dogs, cats and wild carnivores. The domestic dog is thought to be the most important source of human infection. The prevalence of infection in dogs and cats may be high, reaching 51–100% in puppies of some countries (Nigeria, Portugal, India, and China) [1]. Eggs are passed in dog, cat, and wild carnivore faeces and remain infectious in soil for years outside these hosts.

Environmental factors
Humans are most commonly infected by ingesting eggs in soil, or in contaminated food or water. Children are especially at risk

when playing in parks or other areas frequented by dogs, or from domestic puppies that have not been regularly wormed.

Clinical features
Presentation
Most human infections are asymptomatic, or at least unrecognised. Persistent eosinophilia is, however, often present [2]; counts of over 25×10^9/L are common. In a proportion of infected children, the full syndrome of visceral larva migrans may develop. The essential features, apart from eosinophilia, are cough, dyspnoea and wheezing, failure to gain weight, muscle pains and sometimes fever. The liver is enlarged. Hyperglobulinaemia is frequent. The syndrome is self-limiting after a few months if reinfection is prevented.

Because so many cases are undiagnosed, the true incidence of cutaneous manifestations is unknown, but estimates suggest around 20% of patients with visceral larva migrans have cutaneous signs [3]. Generalised pruritus and urticarial or papular eruptions of the trunk and legs are most frequently reported. Hypodermatitis, Wells syndrome, Reiter syndrome and eosinophilic folliculitis have been documented [3]. Migratory panniculitis, although rarely reported, is distinctive and perhaps pathognomonic: substantial, tender, subcutaneous nodules vanish after 1 or 2 weeks [4,5].

Complications and co-morbidities
In a minority of infected individuals, who have never experienced visceral larva migrans, ocular larva migrans may also occur with larval migration through the posterior segment of the eye and is a predominant infectious cause of blindness in children in developed countries. A wandering larva causes an ocular granuloma simulating a neoplasm or may simulate a more vigorous inflammatory reaction such as that seen in uveitis [6]. In addition, patients may experience central nervous system disease with meningitis, encephalopathy with seizures and neuropsychiatric symptoms.

Investigations
Diagnosis is confirmed by morphometric assessment of larvae (if present) or detection of larval DNA from tissue or body fluid samples. Fluorescent antibody and ELISA techniques are helpful [7]. As serological or immunological methods alone do not allow for an unequivocal diagnosis of infection, PCR-based tools can assist in identification [1].

Management [1]
Treatment responses are often unsatisfactory given the requirement for drugs to reach larvae across a range of tissues. To date, there is limited data on the treatment of the disease. Individuals with mild symptoms may not require treatment, since they typically resolve in a few weeks. For patients requiring treatment, albendazole may prove to be the best agent; in the case of ocular infection, vitrectomy is often combined with medical treatment. In cases with central nervous system involvement, concomitant prednisolone is warranted. Mebendazole is an alternative agent to albendazole but it is not absorbed outside of the gastrointestinal tract. Cure rates are low with DEC.

Treatment ladder for visceral larva migrans

First line
- Albendazole 400 mg PO BD × 5 days
- With prednisolone if clinically warranted

Second line
- Mebendazole 100–200 mg PO BD × 5 days (not recommended in patients with ocular and neurological disease as it does not cross the blood–brain barrier)

Third line
- Diethylcarbamazine 4 mg/kg/day × 21 days

Gnathostomiasis

Definition
Gnathostomiasis is an infection caused by *Gnathostoma spinigerum*, *G. hispidium* and *G. nipponicum*, the definitive host of which are cats, wild felines, dogs and certain other animals that eat fish, snakes and frogs [1].

Epidemiology
Incidence and prevalence
Human gnathostomiasis occurs throughout South-East Asia, east of and including Bangladesh, China, Japan, Indonesia and the Philippines. The greatest number of cases are in Thailand, likely secondary to the custom of eating raw fish [2]. There are also reports from Mexico, Guatemala and Ecuador and in travellers returning from any endemic area [1,3]. About 5000 human cases have been reported worldwide since first described in 1889 [4].

Pathophysiology
Pathology
Larvae ingested by humans wander, mainly in subcutaneous tissues and muscles, causing deep tunnels, which form the sites of inflammation episodes or abscess formation. Histology shows intense infiltration with neutrophils, plasma cells, chronic inflammatory cells and especially eosinophils. Less common sites of infection include the brain and eye.

Causative organisms (Figure 33.21)
- *Gnathostoma hispidium*
- *Gnathostoma nipponicum*

Adult worms live in the stomach of the carnivore. Eggs are passed in the faeces, hatch in water and are ingested by *Cyclops*, a genera of tiny crustaceans or copepods, in which they transform further. When *Cyclops* is ingested by frogs, snakes or fish, the larvae develop to the third stage in the flesh of the animals, which in turn are eaten by the definitive host, thus completing the cycle. Humans are infected either by ingesting *Cyclops* in water or by eating inadequately cooked flesh of an intermediate host. Worms removed from a person are most commonly third-stage larvae or immature adults,

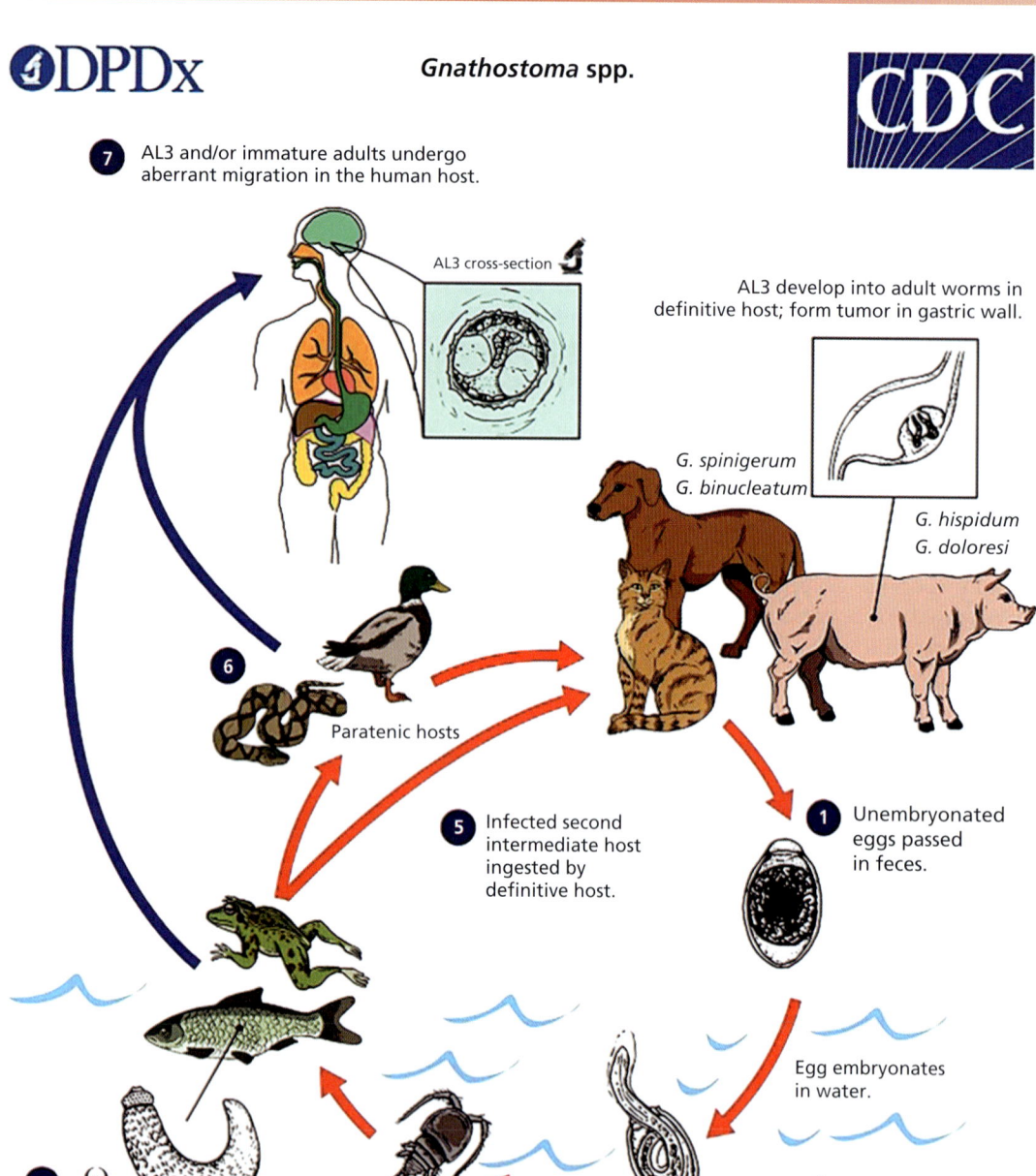

Figure 33.21 Life cycle of *Gnathostoma spinigerum* and *G. hispidum*. Courtesy of the Centers for Disease Control and Prevention. https://www.cdc.gov/dpdx/gnathostomiasis/index.html (last accessed February 2023).

which measure 2–4 mm long and are rust brown in colour due to ingested blood. The head of the worm is crowned by 4–8 rows of hooklets (Figure 33.22) and the anterior half of the body is covered in leaf-like spines. Rarely, a mature male worm, up to 12 mm long, has been found [5].

Clinical features
Presentation
Cutaneous gnathostomiasis presents as intermittent nodular migratory panniculitis, several centimetres in diameter [6]. Lesions are firm, warm, red and painful, lasting up to 4 weeks, before disappearing and returning nearby. They occur most commonly on the upper parts of the body, including the orbit. Abscesses may develop subcutaneously or in the muscle [7]. As the larvae migrate, they can also cause creeping eruptions or cutaneous larva migrans that are intensely pruritic.

Visceral gnathostomiasis occurs when larvae migrate throughout various internal organs and can affect almost any part of the body. Ocular, auricular, pulmonary, gastrointestinal, genitourinary and CNS manifestations have been reported [4].

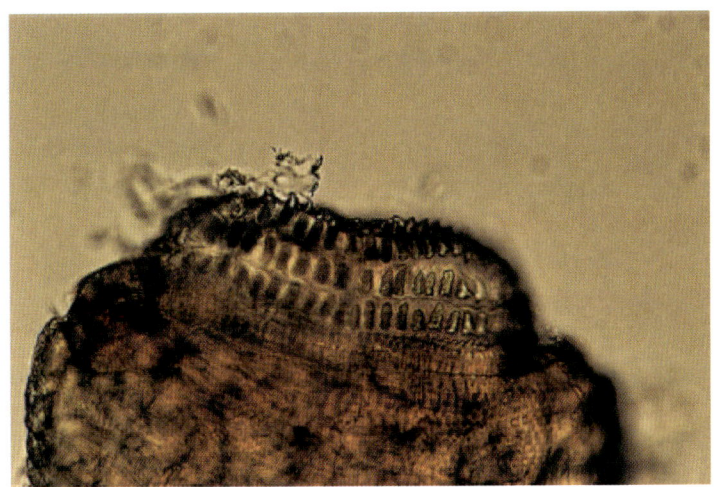

Figure 33.22 *Gnathostoma spinigerum*. Head of an adult worm that was extruded from a subcutaneous swelling in a patient from Bangladesh. The crown of hooklets is characteristic. Courtesy of Dr P.L. Chiodini.

Albendazole in a dose of 400 mg daily or twice daily for 21 days or ivermectin 200 μg/kg for either 1 or 2 days are effective. At present, data is insufficient to determine which regimen is superior, but albendazole is usually tried first. Other agents have not proven useful. Treatment of worms affecting the face is important, to prevent ocular involvement.

> **Treatment ladder for gnathostomiasis**
>
> **First line**
> - Surgical removal when feasible
> - Albendazole 400 mg PO OD or BD for 21 days (when surgical removal is not feasible)
>
> **Second line**
> - Ivermectin 200 μg/kg for 1–2 days

Larvae can survive in the human body for a very long period of time; episodes of swelling may become brief and less intense, and symptoms may recur intermittently for more than 10 years in untreated patients [4].

Differential diagnosis
Other nematodes that may cause similar clinical pictures include *Lagochilascaris minor*, a cause of subcutaneous abscesses in Surinam and Central America; *Thelazia callipaeda*, which parasitises the conjunctival sac in East and South East Asia; and *Gongylonema pulchrum*, a cosmopolitan parasite of pigs, bears, hedgehogs and monkeys that causes migratory lesions in the oropharyngeal submucosa of humans [8]. Isolated swellings may simulate inflammatory or neoplastic disease of other internal organs.

Complications and co-morbidities [4]
When larvae invade the eyes, permanent vision loss can occur. Invasion of the inner ear can result in hearing loss. Pleural effusions have been reported with pulmonary infections. Inflammation secondary to invasion of the gastric mucosa has caused gastric ulcers and perforation. Urinary tract disease is rare, but can result in haematuria. Neurognathostomiasis is the severest form of visceral disease. Fatal encephalomyelitis has also been described [9].

Diagnosis
The diagnosis is suggested by geographical history, clinical features and a peripheral eosinophilia, and is confirmed by surgical extraction of the worm. Occasionally, a worm is expelled through the skin. Reliable serological tests (PCR and ELISA) are available through some specialist centres [3]. Imaging studies can facilitate diagnosis in visceral disease.

Management [4]
There is no effective non-invasive treatment for gnathostomiasis. Surgical removal of worms is considered the most effective treatment, but this is often not feasible unless infections are cutaneous or superficial.

Dirofilariasis

Definition
Dirofilariasis is an infection by filarial nematodes of the genus *Dirofilaria*. There are two forms of the disease as follows.
1. Subcutaneous dirofilariasis caused by *D. tenuis* (*D. conjunctivae*), *D. urii*, *D. subdermata* and *D. repens*.
2. Pulmonary dirofilariasis caused by *D. immitis*, the dog heartworm.

Dirofilaria ursi and the related *D. subdermata* are natural parasites of bears and porcupines, respectively.

Epidemiology
Incidence and prevalence
Most cases of dirofilariasis are prevalent in warmer regions of the world where transmission can be sustained year round. *Dirofilaria repens* is a subcutaneous parasite of dogs and cats that is exclusive to the Old World, notably Europe, Asia and Africa. Greater than 3500 cases of human infection with *D. repens* have been reported in Europe from 1977 to 2016 [1]. *D. immitis*, *D. ursi* and *D. tenuis* are cosmopolitan in the New World and can be found in dogs, bears and raccoons, respectively, in the USA. Transmission to humans is thought to be by mosquitoes.

Pathophysiology
Causative organisms
- Subcutaneous disease: *D. tenuis*, *D. urii*, *D. subdermata* and *D. repens*
- Pulmonary disease: *D. immitis*

The dirofilarial life cycle, like other helminthic nematodes, consists of five developmental stages. Adult female worms produce thousands of microfilariae which are ingested by *Aedes*, *Anopheles*, *Culex* and *Mansonia* mosquitoes. Larvae mature within the mosquitoes in a temperature dependent process [2] and are passed to other hosts through bites. Definitive hosts include dogs, cats and other wild carnivores, where larvae further mature into adults

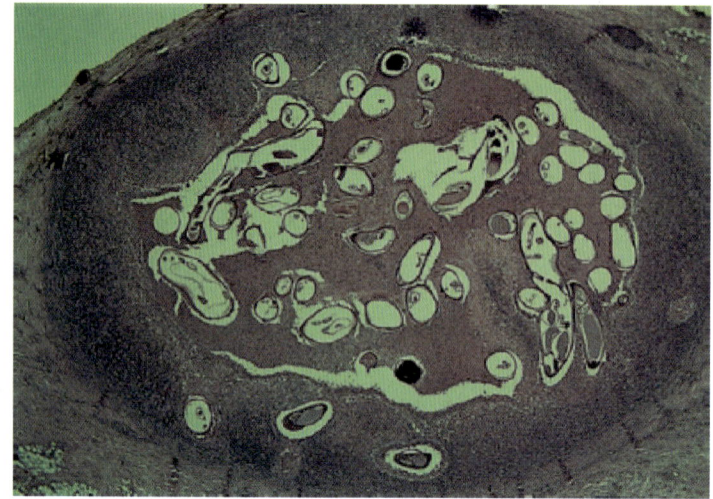

Figure 33.23 Dirofilariasis. Low-power view of cold abscess from the cheek. It shows degenerate coiled *Dirofilaria* worm within an abscess and surrounding lymphocytic infiltrate and fibrosis. Courtesy of Professor S.B. Lucas.

within the pulmonary arteries or heart (hence the name heartworm). Humans act as dead-end hosts as the worms do reach maturity and the disease is usually self-limiting.

Clinical features
Presentation
In subcutaneous disease, the lesion is usually a tender, occasionally migratory, nodule which develops over a few weeks. These clinical symptoms may be consistent with Wells cellulitis [3]. Common sites are the eyelid, scrotum, breast, arm and leg. The worm may also be seen in the conjunctiva and is present within a foreign-body granulomatous reaction in the nodule (Figure 33.23). Microfilariae are not found in the blood.

Patients with pulmonary disease are often asymptomatic. However, fever, chills, fatigue, cough with or without haemoptysis, wheezing and chest pain may occur.

Investigations
Diagnosis is made by extracting the worm from the lesion or by identifying it in an excised specimen. PCR and ELISA have also been useful in diagnosis.

Management
Definitive treatment is by surgical removal of the nodules. If surgical removal is not feasible, ivermectin can be used. Recently treatment with doxycycline has proven effective as it kills the bacterial endosymbiont *Wolbachia* that filariae depend on for growth, development, fertility and survival [4].

Trichinosis

Definition and nomenclature
Trichinosis, also known as trichinellosis, is an infection of the intestine and muscle, with *Trichinella spiralis*, a worldwide parasite of a wide range of carnivores. The human is normally an end host. A variety of allergic phenomena characterise human infection.

> **Synonyms and inclusions**
> - Trichiniasis
> - Trichinelliasis
> - Trichinellosis

Epidemiology
Incidence and prevalence
Trichinosis is distributed worldwide. It is an important disease both in Europe and in the USA, and has been found in Africa, south of the Sahara. It is estimated that 10 000 cases occur annually throughout the globe [1].

Pathophysiology
Predisposing factors
Humans acquire the disease by eating raw or undercooked meat infected by *Trichinella spiralis* – such as bush pig in Africa, bear and walrus meat in Alaska and the Arctic. Entire polar expeditions have died after eating an infected polar bear.

Pathology
Intestinal infection causes partial villous atrophy and mucosal and submucosal inflammation. The deposition of larvae in muscles is associated with oedema, loss of cross striations and basophilic degeneration (Figure 33.24). The coiled larvae are surrounded by an inflammatory infiltrate of lymphocytes and macrophages until they become encapsulated.

Causative organisms (Figure 33.25)
- *Trichinella spiralis*

The lifecycle of human trichinella follows three sequential phases: enteral phase, parenteral phase and encysting phase [2]. Encysted larvae of *Trichinella spiralis* are ingested in meat and hatch in the duodenum (enteral phase), penetrate the submucosa and within

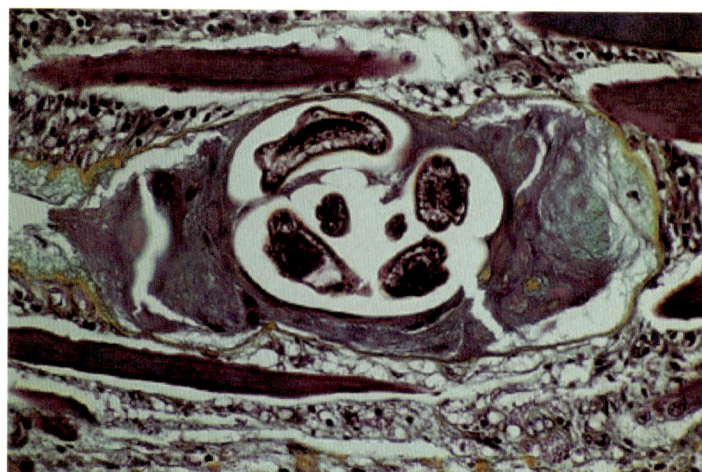

Figure 33.24 Trichinosis. Medium-power view, Movat stain, showing *Trichinella* worm within a 'nurse cell' in skeletal muscle. There is surrounding oedema, muscle disruption and lymphocytic infiltrate. Courtesy of Professor S.B. Lucas.

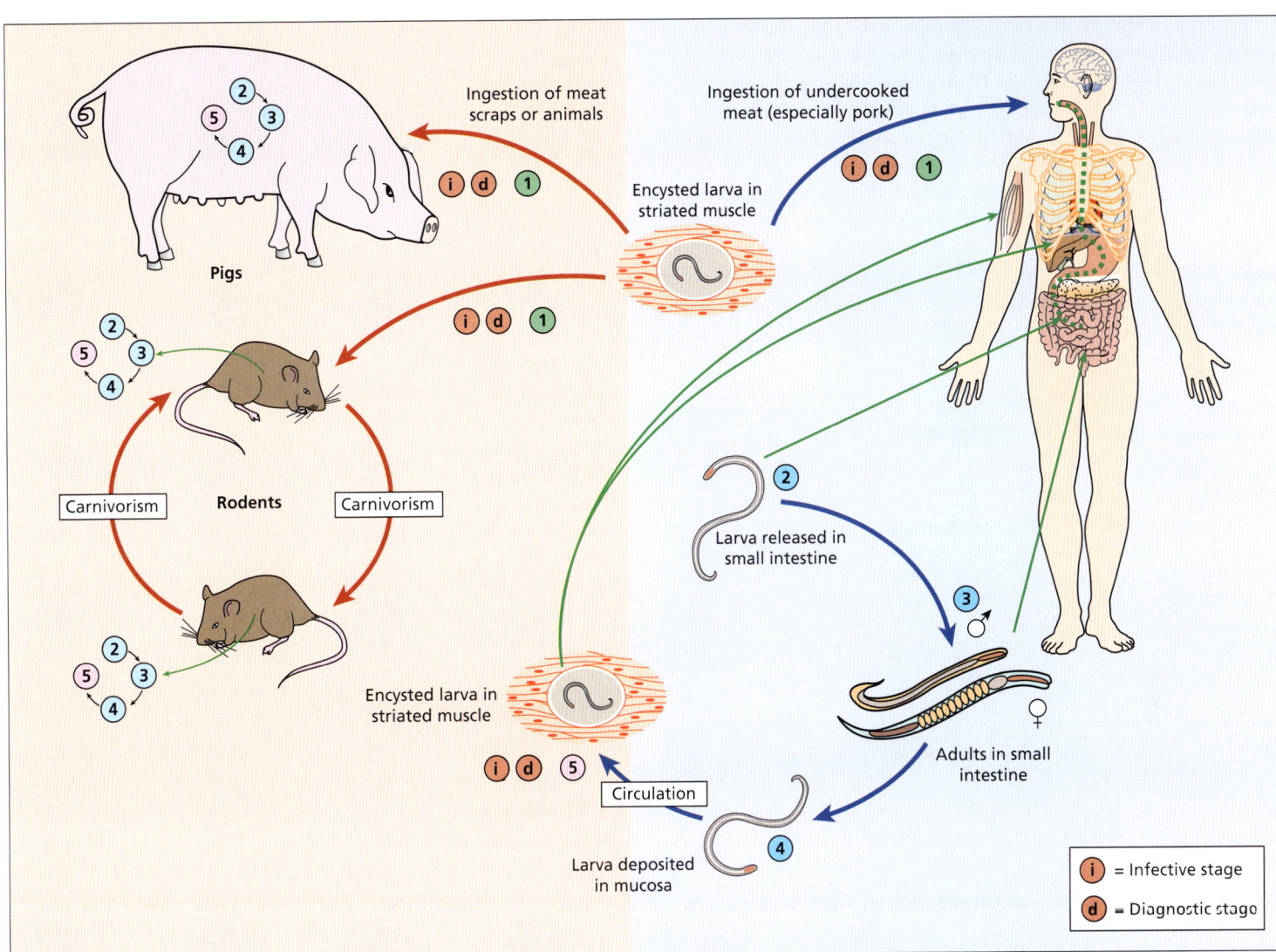

Figure 33.25 Life cycle of *Trichinella*. Courtesy of the Centers for Disease Control and Prevention. https://www.cdc.gov/dpdx/trichinellosis/index.html (last accessed February 2023).

5 days have matured, mated and started producing 200–2000 invasive larvae, which reach muscles (parenteral stage) where they become encysted and infective to a fresh host within 21 days. The adult worms live less than 2 months. Encystment and repair may occur for months to years after infection (encysting phase). Cysts may calcify, but the larvae remain viable for up to 40 years and can outlive their dead host by 10 days [3].

Clinical features
Presentation
The disease may be symptomless or mild, but generally, after a moderate infection with the 'muscle worms', severe symptoms resembling acute food poisoning ensue rapidly (intestinal phase). These are followed within a week by an acute illness with: fever; generalised muscle pain and tenderness; sweating; periorbital oedema; conjunctivitis; some paralysis of the muscles of the tongue, jaw and respiration; a transient maculopapular rash of the extremities; and splinter haemorrhages beneath the nails (invasive stage). Chronic symptoms include cachexia, oedema, and extreme dehydration (convalescent phase).

Clinical variants
In severe infections, there is involvement of the heart and central nervous system. A necrotising vasculopathy equivalent to classic polyarteritis nodosa is described [4].

Investigations
Clinical features can suggest the diagnosis within a week of eating inadequately cooked meat, especially pork. Worms may be found in faeces in the second to fourth week of the infection, and after 4 weeks in biopsied muscle. The eosinophil count, erythrocyte sedimentation rate and serum creatine phosphokinase are all raised. After 3 weeks, antibodies become detectable. ELISA and indirect fluorescent antibody tests are the most commonly used methods [5].

Management
The goal of management is to prevent systemic invasion. Therefore, treatment should begin as soon as the diagnosis is confirmed, ideally within the first 3 days of infection. Albendazole 400 mg twice daily for 8–14 days is the drug of choice [1]. Mebendazole is another option but requires more frequent monitoring and dosing. When

treated early, these medications are effective. Unfortunately, most infected people are diagnosed several weeks after the infection, when larvae have established themselves in the muscles. These larvae can survive for years despite treatment. As a consequence, advanced stages of infection should be treated for longer periods of time [5].

Management of the disease with systemic symptoms including central nervous system involvement, cardiac inflammation or pulmonary infiltration consists of combined use of a corticosteroid and an antiparasitic agent. Corticosteroids are lifesaving in suppressing allergic reaction at the height of larval spread and Jarisch–Herxheimer-type reaction with antiparasitics.

Treatment ladder for trichinosis

First line
- Albendazole 400 mg PO BD for 8–14 days

Second line
- Mebendazole 200–400 mg PO TDS for 3 days, then 400–500 mg PO TDS for 10 days

INFECTION WITH TREMATODES

Synonyms and inclusions
- Flukes
- Flatworms

Trematodes are non-segmented single-sex worms, flattened like a leaf and without a formal organ of attachment. Pairs of adult worms live in a hollow viscus (such as the vein, gut, bile duct or lung), from whence eggs make their way into faeces, urine or sputum. The eggs must enter water, hatch and infect a species of snail, in which a cycle of development and multiplication occurs, resulting in the release of motile cercariae. These either penetrate human skin or enter a resting stage in aquatic plants, fish or crustacea, and are later eaten. Trematodes are important and common parasites of humans, especially in Africa, and East and South East Asia. They cause skin disease either as a result of cercarial penetration, by the ectopic deposition of adult worms or their eggs, or by causing allergic phenomena.

A summary of the organisms and diseases caused by infection with trematodes is provided in Table 33.3.

Schistosomiasis

Definition and nomenclature
Schistosomiasis or bilharziasis is a serious systemic disease due to different species of human schistosomes or blood flukes. Rashes

Table 33.3 Organisms and diseases of infection with trematodes.

Disease	Organism
Schistosomiasis	Schistosoma mansoni
	Schistosoma japonicum
	Schistosoma haematobium
	Schistosoma mekongi (rare)
Cercarial dermatitis	Schistosoma japonicum (avian and mammalian species)
Paragonimiasis	Paragonimus westermani
	Paragonimus africanus
	Paragonimus peruviana
	Paragonimus szechuanensis

may occur during the invasive stage of this disease, when the skin is being penetrated by cercariae, and later there may be skin involvement at or near mucocutaneous surfaces, and less commonly at more distant sites on the trunk, following dissemination of ova.

A second group of non-human schistosomes cause cutaneous symptoms only. This situation follows penetration of cercariae into the skin, but further development of the flukes in humans is arrested and there are no sequelae. The condition 'swimmer's itch' or cercarial dermatitis is a prime example of this process.

Synonyms and inclusions
- Bilharziasis

Epidemiology
Incidence and prevalence [1]
Disease due to the commonest agent, *Schistosoma mansoni*, is endemic in Africa and South America (especially the Nile delta and north-east Brazil). *S. japonicum* occurs in China and South-East Asia, and *S. haematobium* extensively in Africa (especially in the Nile and Rift Valleys), Arabia, Madagascar and south-west India. Schistosomiasis affects almost 240 million people worldwide.

Pathophysiology
Causative organisms (Figure 33.26)
- *Schistosoma mansoni*
- *Schistosoma japonicum*
- *Schistosoma haematobium*
- *Schistosoma mekongi* (rare)
- *Schistosoma intercalatum* (rare)

Humans infected with *S. mansoni* and *S. japonicum* excrete eggs in the faeces, and with *S. haematobium* excrete eggs in the urine. On contact with water, these eggs develop into miracidia, which undergo further development in certain aquatic snails. From these, free-swimming cercariae are released, which are capable of penetrating human skin to produce the infection [2]. The organisms can pass rapidly through the epidermis and enter the venous blood within 24 h of contact with human skin. The larvae are then carried through the heart and lungs, and mature into flukes in the intrahepatic portion of the portal system.

Finally, the mature flukes pass from the portal system into the pelvic veins, where eggs are laid. *S. mansoni* and *S. japonicum* localise primarily in the mesenteric veins, while *S. haematobium* invades the

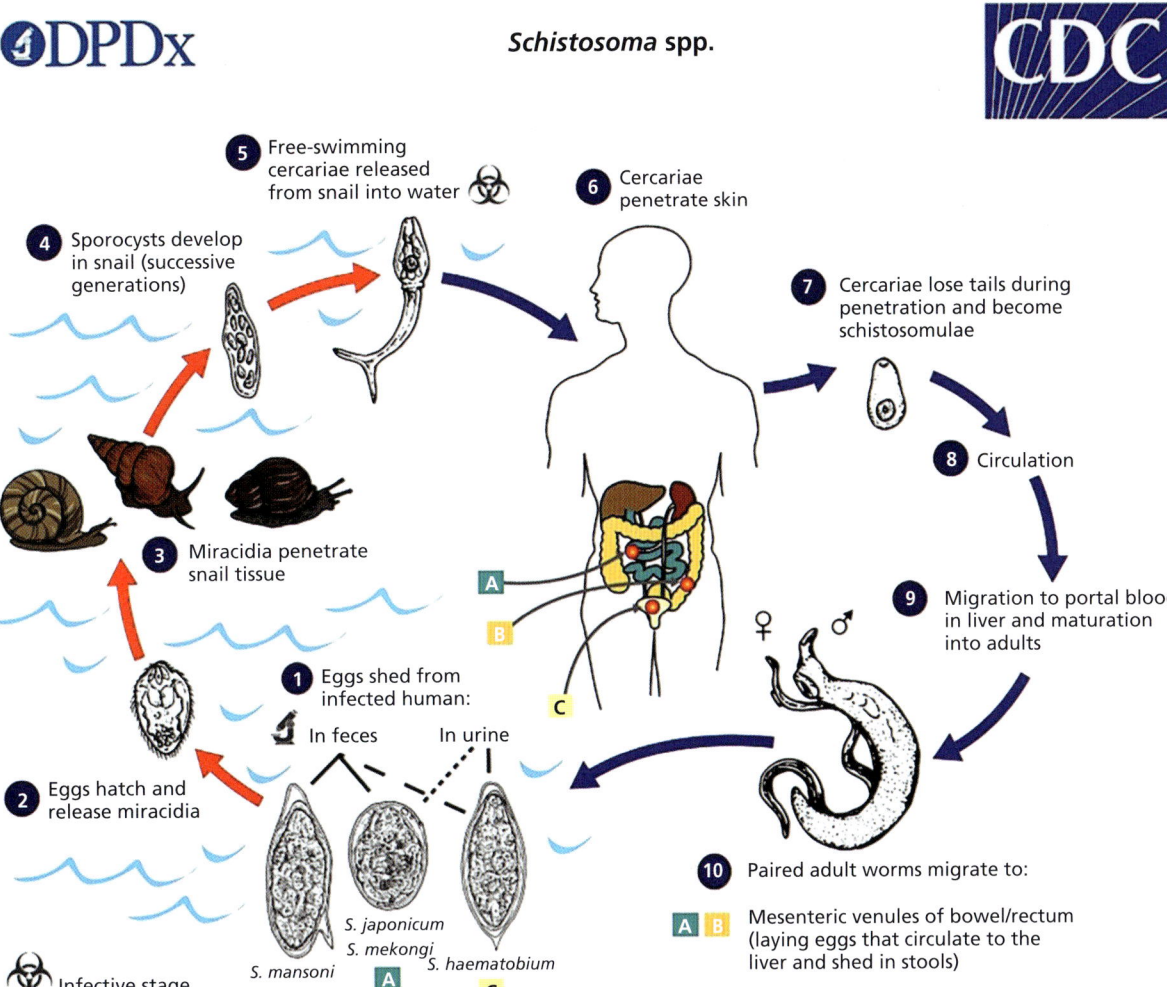

Figure 33.26 Life cycle of the *Schistosoma*. Courtesy of the Centers for Disease Control and Prevention. https://www.cdc.gov/dpdx/schistosomiasis/index.html (last accessed February 2023).

vesical and, sometimes, the rectal veins with the production of haematuria and other urinary symptoms. Ova work their way out of the veins into the tissues, where they cause the formation of granulomas in which there is a pseudotubercle arrangement of inflammatory cells rich in eosinophils and histiocytes, and occasional giant cells, surrounding the diagnostic ova [3].

Clinical features
Presentation
Skin manifestations of this common disease of tropical and subtropical distribution are incidental features of the underlying disease. They may be grouped as follows [4]:
1 Schistosomal dermatitis.
2 Urticarial reactions in the early weeks of the disease.
3 Paragenital granulomas and fistulous tracts.
4 Ectopic cutaneous schistosomiasis (lesions occurring away from the characteristic sites of egg deposition are termed 'ectopic'; Figure 33.27).

Ectopic sites of egg deposition probably arise through migration of adults via the paravertebral venous plexus.

Skin involvement may occur either as a result of the initial penetration of the skin by waterborne, free-living cercariae (an intermediate stage in the life cycle), during an immune-complex mediated phase of the infection, Katayama fever [5], or in the later stages of infection following ectopic localisation of worms or ova [6].

1 *Schistosomal dermatitis*. Penetration by cercariae of parts of the epidermis in contact with water may pass unnoticed or cause an itchy papular eruption indistinguishable from swimmer's itch (cercarial dermatitis due to non-human flukes). The symptom of itching usually lasts only for a few hours after leaving the water, although mild redness may persist for longer. In sensitised individuals, however, papules and itching persist for about a week [4].

2 *Urticarial reactions*. Four to eight weeks after penetration of the skin by cercariae, urticaria may occur. This is particularly severe in *S. japonicum* infection, together with fever, purpura, malaise, arthralgia, abdominal cramps, diarrhoea and enlargement of the liver and spleen. In some areas, for example China and Japan, this feature is so prominent that the disease is called 'urticarial

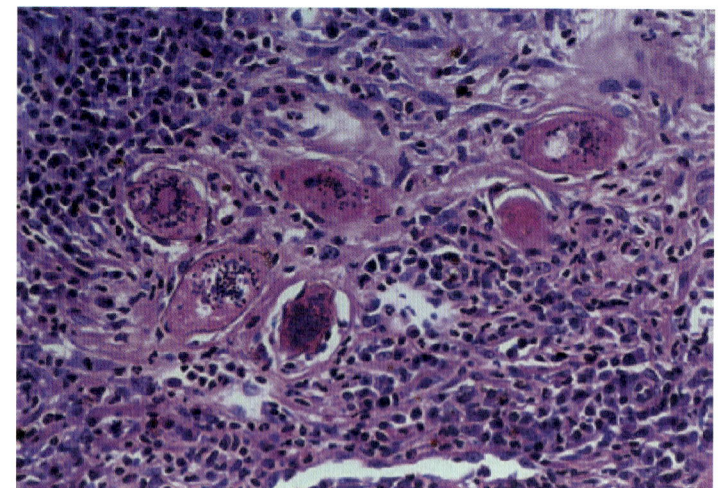

Figure 33.27 Schistosomiasis of the vulva (medium power, H&E) showing six schistosome eggs with surrounding lymphoplasmocytic infiltration. Courtesy of Professor S.B. Lucas.

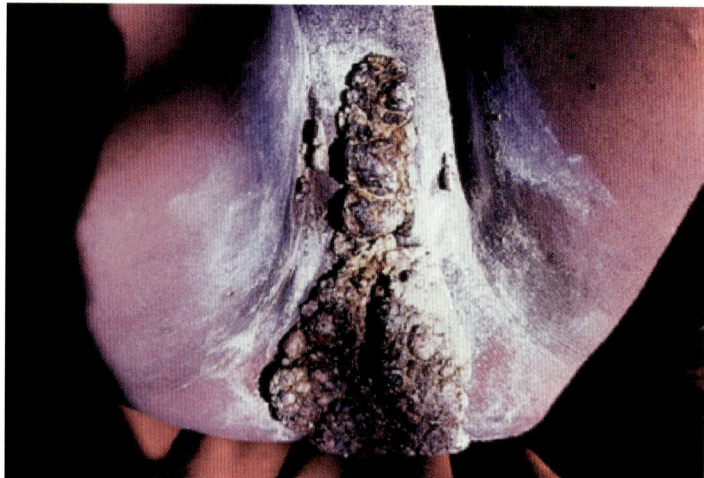

Figure 33.28 Schistosomiasis of the vulva and anus. Condylomatous lesions containing granulomas around schistosome ova. Courtesy of Professor G. Nelson.

fever' or Katayama disease. Eosinophilia is also typical. The symptoms resolve in about 4–6 weeks.

3 *Paragenital granulomas and fistulous tracts.* In areas of high endemicity, cutaneous bilharziasis of the perineum and external genital regions is not uncommon [7–9]. This follows direct spread of adult flukes to adjacent vasculature. Granulomatous genital condylomas occur and fistulous tracts with extensive firm masses, honeycombed by sinuses, are characteristically found on the perineum, groins or buttocks (Figure 33.28).

4 *Ectopic cutaneous schistomiasis* [10–14]. Ova may become deposited in the skin as well as in other ectopic sites, such as the conjunctiva, lungs and central nervous system. They arise following embolism of ova from adults, which are localised in abnormal sites, such as the paravertebral plexus [4]. The trunk is almost invariably the site of ectopic cutaneous involvement. The primary lesion is a flesh-coloured firm papule reaching a size of 2–3 mm and ovoid in shape. These papules agglomerate to form slightly raised plaques with irregular contours. Later still, some plaques develop a surface protuberance and deepen in colour but retain their irregular ovoid contours. The skin over old nodules may be deeply pigmented and scaly, and may later ulcerate. The para-umbilical area is a common site [10] but other areas may be involved (Figure 33.28), and, in some cases, the lesions have a segmental or zosteriform distribution [12–14]. With treatment, these lesions slowly disappear in about 5 months. A facial hypopigmented plaque is described.

Complications and co-morbidities

The major complications of schistosomiasis are due to infections affecting the liver (fibrosis), intestinal involvement and bladder infection, which may lead to carcinoma of the bladder. Other sites of involvement include the kidneys, heart, central nervous system and retina [2].

Investigations

The characteristic ova may be found in stools or urine (Figure 33.29). On occasions, rectal biopsy is an alternative method of finding ova. The latter have a characteristic morphology. Serology testing is

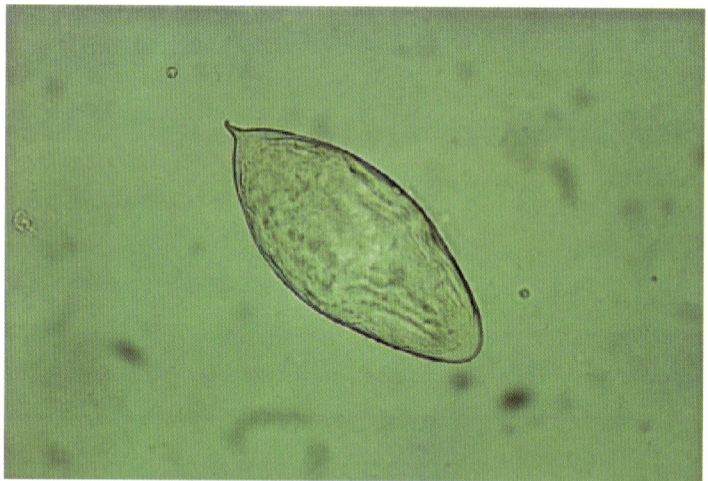

Figure 33.29 *Schistosoma haematobium* ovum in urine. Courtesy of Mr A.H. Moody.

useful for screening. Immunofluorescence, ELISA and PCR are commonly used. Ectopic cutaneous schistosomiasis is diagnosed by biopsy. Histology shows epithelioid cell granulomas containing degenerate ova (Figure 33.27).

Urinalysis can be used to identify those at risk with urogenital schistosomiasis. Imaging can also facilitate diagnosis.

Management

The treatment of choice for all schistosome species is praziquantel. The drug is given at a dose of 40 mg/kg divided into two doses for 1 day, except in infections due to *S. japonicum* and *S. mekongi*, where 60 mg/kg divided into three doses for 1 day is administered [15]. Cure rates are high with this regimen and there are few side effects such as abdominal discomfort and headache. However, there are increasing reports of treatment failures and resistance has been recorded in laboratory testing [16]. In early infections, the results of therapy are excellent, although reinfection is a continual risk. Many of the complications of the infection such as hepatic fibrosis, portal hypertension and ureteric stenosis are irreversible due to scar formation.

> **Treatment ladder for schistosomiasis**
>
> - Praziquantel 40 mg/kg PO divided into two doses for 1 day
> - Use 60 mg/kg PO divided into three doses for 1 day for *S. japonicum* and *S. mekongi*

Cercarial dermatitis

Definition and nomenclature
Cercarial dermatitis is a widely used term to describe a group of skin disorders having a common aetiology – an eruption resulting from waterborne penetration of the skin by free-living cercarial stages of non-human schistosomes. There are a number of local names for these conditions, such as swimmer's itch, clam digger's itch, sedge pool itch, koganbyo and sawah itch. Symptoms from this disease are mild and do not typically last more than 1 week.

> **Synonyms and inclusions**
> - Lake itch
> - Duck itch
> - Swimmer's itch
> - Sawah itch
> - Koganbyo
> - Clam digger's itch
> - Sedge pool itch

Epidemiology
The association between schistosomes and cercarial dermatitis has been known for many decades and cercarial dermatitis is reported in many countries. Geographic region, season, occupation and activity influence the frequency of cercarial dermatitis. However, there are no data on the number of afflicted persons per year [1].

Pathophysiology [2]
The pathogenesis of cercarial dermatitis is not completely understood but is believed to result from an allergic reaction secondary to skin penetration of schistosomes. The kinetics of the clinical response suggest that sensitisation is involved, with a more intense inflammatory reaction occurring in those sensitised. The first phase of epidermal penetration is accompanied by dermal oedema, which is followed by a brisk neutrophil reaction. Subsequent exposure results in a strong reaction characterised by lymphocytic vasculitis with lymphocytic dermatitis.

Causative organisms [3]
In general, species of schistosomes whose normal hosts are birds and non-human mammals shed eggs in bodies of water such as ponds, lakes and oceans. The eggs hatch and liberate miracida which then further develop in mollusca. Cercariae are then released and through chemotrophic reactions are drawn to human skin.
  See clinical variants for more details.

Environmental factors
Attempts to find common features connecting the likely locations for cercarial infections have not been entirely successful. It is apparent, however, that areas endemic for cercarial dermatitis usually have abundant submerged vegetation harbouring the intermediate hosts. Hot spells of weather have also been associated with a higher risk of the development of symptoms [4].

Clinical features
Presentation
Most forms of cercarial dermatitis have common features, although their intensity varies between individuals [5]. The first sign of an infection is the development of a tingling sensation after contact with water. This lasts for about 1 h and there may be a fine macular redness. After 10–15 h, there is usually a second phase with the appearance of multiple itchy papules with surrounding redness. These may evolve into vesicles or oedematous lesions. Bacterial superinfection may lead to pustules. In strongly sensitised hosts, papules may occur within 1 h. Massive infections may also cause fever, limb swelling, nausea and diarrhoea [1]. The whole reaction takes about a week to resolve. The papules closely resemble small insect bites. There are no long-term sequelae.

Clinical variants
Fresh-water avian cercarial dermatitis [5,6]. This follows penetration of the skin by cercariae of avian blood flukes. The intermediate hosts are freshwater molluscs. The flukes belong to the genera *Trichobilharzia*, *Gigantobilharzia* and *Ornithobilharzia*. The condition has been described from many different parts of the world including North America, particularly the lakes region of the USA, Canada, Europe, Africa, East and South East Asia [5,7]. In some countries, it affects patients with particular occupations such as rice farmers working in the paddy fields.

Sea-water avian cercarial dermatitis [8]. This follows invasion of the skin by blood flukes whose definitive hosts are sea birds. While it is recorded less frequently than infections caused by freshwater species, it accounts for the condition, seen in the Atlantic seaboard of the USA, known as clam-digger's itch. The intermediate hosts are marine molluscs. The term 'sea-bather's eruption' is used to describe a variety of different rashes that may develop after sea bathing. It is likely that it includes a number of different conditions from jellyfish dermatitis to eruptions due to toxic algae. A sea water form of cercarial dermatitis is therefore one cause of sea-bather's eruption [9].

Freshwater mammalian cercarial dermatitis [7]. This has been reported mainly from East and South East Asia, and the definitive hosts for the schistosomes in this condition are mammals such as water buffaloes.

Diagnosis [1]
History is most important in diagnosis. Affected patients usually meet three criteria: recent contact with a natural body of water, appearance of a papular skin eruption with severe itching 12–24 h after exposure, and lesions distributed only on parts of the body

immersed in water. Biopsy of papules within the first 24–72 h can assist in diagnosis with detection of schistosomulum.

Management
Treatment is entirely symptomatic. Although brisk rubbing with a dry towel seems sensible advice, there is no evidence that it prevents the second phase of responses [9]. Patients can be treated with antihistamines or topical applications of hydrocortisone. Preventative measures are seldom called for as infections tend to be sporadic. Control of vegetation in endemic areas or of the snail population are possibilities, but seldom practised unless the more serious problem of schistosomiasis is also present.

> **Treatment ladder for cercarial dermatitis**
> - Antipruritic cream (1% hydrocortisone) applied to the affected area twice daily × 1 week
> - Hydroxyzine 25 mg PO every 6 h as required for pruritus × 1 week

Paragonimiasis

Definition
Paragonimiasis is a trematode (fluke) infection caused by consumption of raw or undercooked crayfish or crab. It is a lung fluke that infects the lungs of the infected host. The disease is usually asymptomatic or presents with few and mild symptoms, but more serious cases can occur when the parasite travels to the central nervous system.

Epidemiology [1]
Infections caused by the lung fluke, *Paragonimus westermani*, are found in East and South East Asia, the West Pacific and in parts of India and central Africa. Similar species, *P. africanus*, *P. mexicanus* and *P. peruviana*, cause disease in the Cameroons and Central and South America, respectively. In China, two rare species, *P. szechuanensis* and *P. hueitungensis*, have been recorded as causes of migratory subcutaneous nodules in humans. *P. kellicotti* has been acquired in the USA. Given its broad distribution, over 292 million people are at risk of infection, with 23 million actually infected.

Pathophysiology
Causative organisms
- *Paragonimus westermani*
- *Paragonimus heterotremus*
- *Paragonimus philippinensis*
- *Paragonimus africanus*
- *Paragonimus uterobilateralis*
- *Paragonimus peruviana*
- *Paragonimus kellicotti*
- *Paragonimus szechuanensis*
- *Paragonimus hueitungensis*

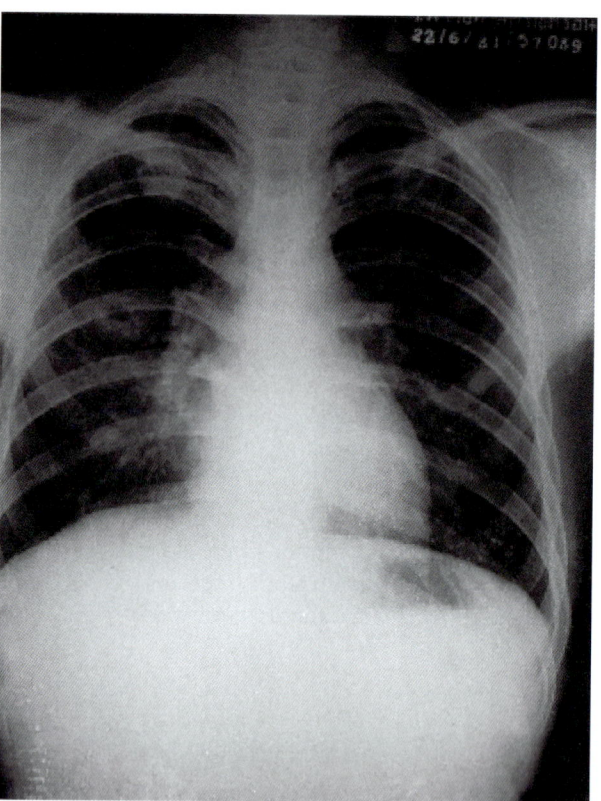

Figure 33.30 Paragonimiasis. Chest X-ray showing three discrete opacities, in two of which cavitation is present, characteristic of the disease in Thailand. Courtesy of Professor D.A. Warrell.

The adult worms are found in the respiratory tract, from which eggs are coughed up and swallowed, thus entering the faeces. Miracidia are released upon contact with water, and seek and penetrate snails. These in turn are the first intermediate hosts and liberate cercaria, which then enter the muscles of freshwater crustaceans such as crayfish. Human infection results from ingestion of inadequately cooked crabs and crayfish. Ingested metacercaria penetrate the intestinal wall and make their way through the diaphragm to the lungs.

Clinical features
Presentation
Adult worms encyst in the lungs (Figure 33.30) and cause a chronic cough with fever and sweats. Brown-stained sputum is characteristic. Flukes may also reach ectopic sites such as the peritoneum, brain or skin.

Skin lesions of paragonimiasis are large mobile subcutaneous nodules, often migratory, which develop into cold abscesses [2]. They can occur at any site including the conjunctiva and may enlarge rapidly to reach a diameter of 10 cm or more. The larger lesions are often painful and may rupture spontaneously.

Diagnosis [1]
Demonstration of fluke eggs in sputum, faeces, bronchial washing or surgical specimens provides a definitive diagnosis. However, immunologically based tests, such as ELISA, are regarded as more sensitive, given that eggs may be hard to find. Imaging

can facilitate diagnosis, although structural abnormalities are not always apparent even in active cases.

Management
Praziquantel given at 25 mg/kg/day in three doses for 2 days or one dose of triclabendazole, 10 mg/kg are the treatments of choice for this disease [3]. Mebendazole is not effective. Thiabendazole is an acceptable second line therapy for patients who cannot tolerate praziquantel. This drug is only available through the American Centers for Disease Control and Prevention. Anticonvulsant therapy and corticosteroids may be warranted in patients with cerebral paragonimiasis.

Treatment ladder for paragonimiasis

First line
- Praziquantel 25 mg/kg/day PO divided every 8 h × 2 days
- Triclabendazole 20 mg/kg, in two divided doses of 10 mg/kg

Second line
- Thiabendazole 10 mg/kg PO × 1 or 2 doses

INFECTION WITH CESTODES

Synonyms and inclusions
- Tapeworms

Tapeworms are flat ribbon-like helminths composed of a variable number of segments called proglottids. The anterior segment or scolex comprises the head, which carries hooks or suckers for attachment to the intestinal mucosa, and a narrow neck from which the proglottids develop. As the hermaphroditic proglottids mature, they become motile sacs full of eggs, which separate from the worm and pass in the faeces or wriggle through the anus. Adult tapeworms inhabit the intestinal lumen of a wide range of natural hosts. Eggs are taken up by an intermediate host and undergo often complex larval development; in some species, there may be two or more intermediate hosts, each supporting a different phase of larval development. The human is a natural host to certain tapeworms and may be an accidental host to others. Generally, infection with adult worms causes little or no disease, but infection with the larval stages may be serious [1].

Tapeworms that infect humans may be divided into two orders, Cyclophyllidea and Pseudophyllidea, within each of which certain species may cause skin disease (Box 33.1).

Echinococcosis

Definition and nomenclature
Two major species in the genus *Echinococcus* parasitise humans with the formation of hydatids, namely *E. granulosus* and

---

Box 33.1 Tapeworms infectious to humans

Cyclophyllidea
- *Echinococcus granulosus* and *E. multilocularis*. Tapeworms, respectively, of dogs and foxes. Larval stages cause echinococcosis, or hydatid disease in humans
- *Taenia saginata*. The beef tapeworm of humans. Causes taeniasis. No skin parasitisation
- *Taenia solium*. The pork tapeworm of humans. Causes taeniasis and cysticercosis
- *Multiceps multiceps*. A tapeworm of dogs and wolves. Its larval stage (coenurus) may parasitise the human brain and other organs [2]
- *Multiceps serialis*. A tapeworm of dogs, wolves and foxes, whose larval stages may parasitise human muscle or subcutaneous tissue [3]
- *Multiceps brauni*. A tapeworm of dogs whose coenurus may parasitise subcutaneous tissue and the eye in humans [2,4,5]

Pseudophyllidea
- *Spirometra* spp. Tapeworms of carnivores. The larval forms (spargana) cause sparganosis in humans
- *Diphyllobothrium latum*. The fish tapeworm of humans. Causes diphyllobothriasis

---

E. multilocularis. Adult *E. granulosus* lives in the intestine of the dog and, if ova are accidentally swallowed by humans or other animals, hydatid cysts develop. Sheep are the commonest intermediate hosts. Similarly, adult *E. multilocularis* lives in the bowel of red fox and arctic fox. Mice, voles and lemmings are the intermediate hosts.

Synonyms and inclusions
- Hydatid disease

Epidemiology [1]
Prevalence of echinococcal disease varies by species. *E. granulosus* occurs worldwide, with the highest incidence rates in Africa, Europe, Asia, the Middle East, Central and South America. It affects over 1 million people [2]. *E. multilocularis* is most prevalent in northern latitudes of Europe, Asia and North America.

Pathophysiology
Causative organisms
- *Echinococcus granulosus*
- *Echinococcus multilocularis*

Humans become infected by ingesting eggs in food or water that has been contaminated by, usually, dog faeces. In endemic countries, especially those where sheep rearing is not accompanied by strict regulations, children's hands readily pick up the eggs from the coats of dogs and are ingested. Eggs hatch in gastric acid and penetrate the wall of the duodenum, and are distributed via the bloodstream, mainly to the liver and lungs, but the bones and any other organ may also be infected. The larvae develop into fluid-filled cysts whose germinal layer produces numerous protoscolices, capable of becoming the scolices of adult worms after ingestion by the definitive host.

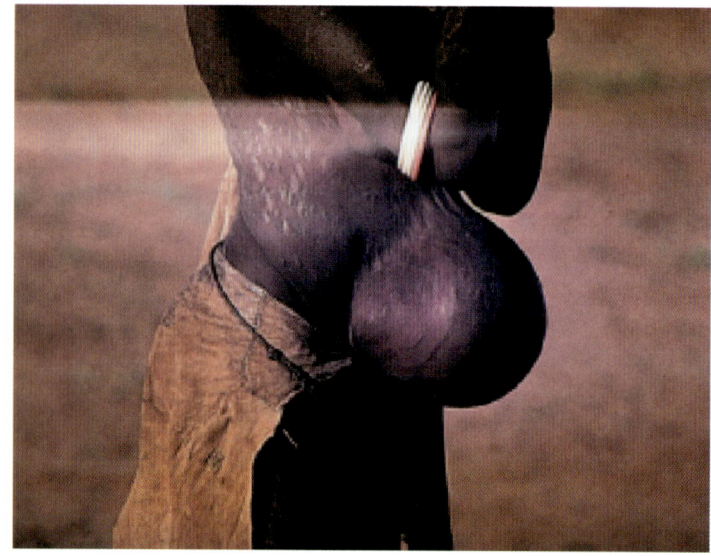

Figure 33.31 Hydatid disease. Subcutaneous hydatid cyst presenting as a hernia, in a woman from Turkana, Kenya. Courtesy of Dr C.N.L. MacPherson.

Cysts of *E. granulosus* tend to grow slowly and bud inwards, producing daughter cysts. Those of *E. multilocularis* may bud outwards, and thus spread through the tissues like a cancer.

Clinical features
Presentation
The commonest manifestation is an enlarged liver. Leakage of antigenic fluid from the cyst may cause cough, urticaria, abdominal pain and eosinophilia. The symptoms are dependent upon the location of cysts within the body. Rupture of the cyst may cause local signs and anaphylaxis. Hydatid cysts (Figure 33.31) may be palpable in muscle or subcutaneous tissues as firm painless swellings, often up to the size of an orange. They may be fluctuant. The overlying skin is normal.

Investigations
Clinical diagnosis is aided by radiography or computed tomography (CT) examination of the lungs and sonographic ultrasound of the liver [3]. On ultrasound, the evolution of cysts can be defined into stages according to a classification system developed by the WHO [4]. Hydatid lesions can appear as smooth round cysts that are anechoic, collapsed cysts or with the presence of multiple daughter cysts [5]. The pathognomonic 'water-lily' sign occurs with separation of the hydatid membrane from the cyst wall mimicking the appearance of a water lily. CT is the preferred method of detection for extrahepatic cysts. CT can accurately describe the number, size and location of cysts. CT is also frequently used during monitoring of patients during treatment. Excision of a subcutaneous cyst is conclusive. Great care must be taken not to spill any cyst fluid, which may give rise to further cysts. Complement fixation and ELISA are useful serological tests.

Management
Options for management include surgery, percutaneous drainage of cysts, drug therapy and observation. Management of disease is dependent on the size and classification of the cysts. The goal of surgery is to evacuate the cyst and obliterate the residual cavity. Relapse of disease does occur, so patients should be monitored for 3–5 years.

Cysticercosis

Definition and nomenclature
Taenia solium, the pork tapeworm, is responsible for producing human intestinal infection with the tapeworm (taeniasis), and the lodging of the larval stage (*Cysticercus cellulosae*) in numerous organs, especially the subcutaneous tissue, muscle and brain, with the production of the disease cysticercosis.

> **Synonyms and inclusions**
> - Larval taeniasis

Epidemiology
Incidence and prevalence
Taenia solium is an important human parasite with a wide, although shrinking, distribution. It is most frequent in Eastern Europe, China, Pakistan, India, Africa, Mexico and Central and South America. Its prevalence depends upon insanitary human faeces disposal and the eating of undercooked pork.

Pathophysiology
Pathology
The cysticerci are found most frequently in subcutaneous tissue and muscle, but may occur in any organ of the body, especially the brain. The growing cyst provokes a non-specific inflammatory reaction, which may be followed by fibrosis and eventual calcification.

Causative organisms
- *Taenia solium*

In taeniasis, the adult *T. solium* lives attached to the wall of the small intestine and may reach a length of 7 m. Inadequately heated or frozen pork is the sole source of human infection with the adult worm, but humans and other primates may harbour the cysticercus stage.

Human infections with *Cysticercus cellulosae* are due to: ingestion of eggs in contaminated food or drink; eggs from an individual's own intestinal infection being introduced into the mouth on dirty hands; or internal autoinfection as a result of vomiting – eggs must be digested in gastric acid.

Clinical features
Presentation
Adult worms in the intestine cause little or no reaction, although the passing of writhing fragments is distressing. The cysticerci form nodules in the subcutaneous tissue of the muscles (rarely with widespread muscular enlargement), eye [1], eyelid [2], lungs and brain and other organs, which may seriously interfere with function depending on their position. Major exacerbation

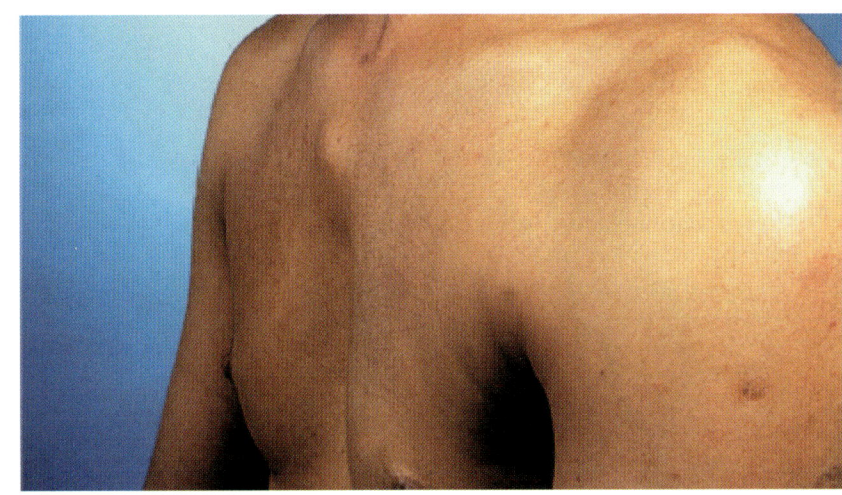

Figure 33.32 Cysticercosis in a man from North India. A subcutaneous cyst is seen over the sternum. Courtesy of Dr A.P. Hall.

of symptoms, such as epilepsy or intracranial obstruction, coincides with the death of the larvae. The disease in the skin is known as cysticercosis cellulosae cutis, and the subcutaneous nodules formed are 1–2 cm in diameter (Figure 33.32). They are rubbery and firm, rounded and painless and may remain unchanged for many years. Their numbers vary from one to hundreds, and when a lesion is identified, a search must be made for other accompanying lesions.

Prognosis is good in taeniasis, but in cysticercosis it is serious when vital organs are involved.

Differential diagnosis
Cysticercosis cellulosae cutis can be misdiagnosed as lipoma, epidermoid cyst, abscess, pyomyositis, tuberculous lymphadenitis, neuroma, neurofibroma, sarcoma, myxoma, ganglion or fat necrosis [3].

Investigations
Eggs in the stool cannot be differentiated morphologically from those of *T. saginata*, but examination of gravid proglottids allows for more precise identification. In cysticercosis, the histology of an excised cyst is diagnostic. Serology is helpful, but cross-reactions occur with hydatid disease.

X-ray examination frequently shows calcification in the muscle (Figure 33.33), although rarely in the brain. CT shows typical appearances in the brain and muscle. In the brain, cysticerci are typically found in the cerebral cortex or within the brainstem. CT imaging shows round non-enhancing hypodense lesions usually within 3–15 mm in diameter. As cysts degenerate, they may become hyperdense with increased density and oedema. In the muscle, calcified lesions typically described as cigar-shaped lesions are consistent with extraneural cysticercosis.

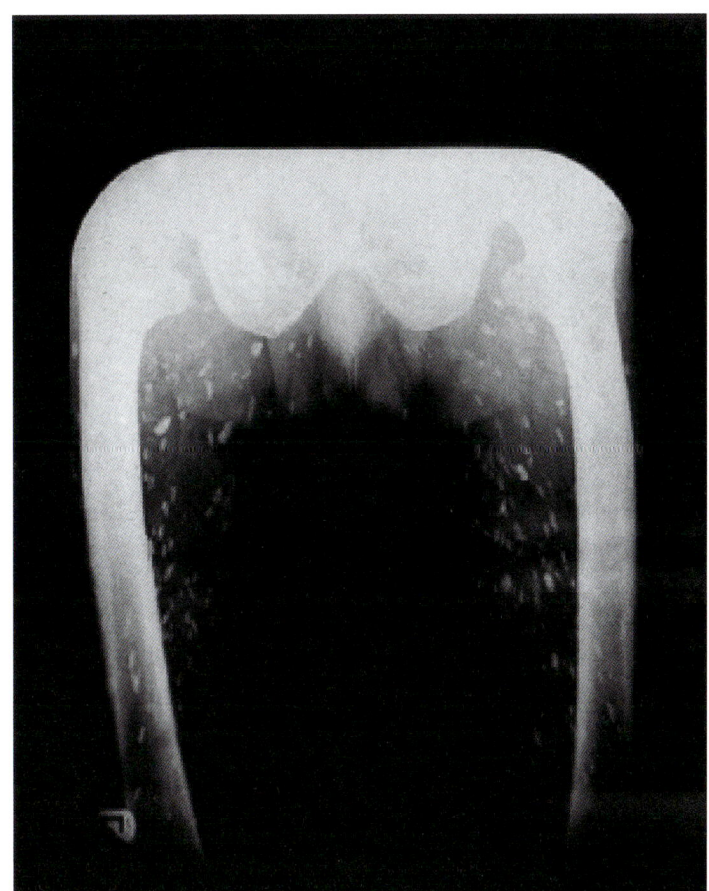

Figure 33.33 Calcified cysticercal cysts in the muscles of the thighs and pelvis.

Management
Subcutaneous cysticerci are important only in that they may point to a more serious cerebral infection, which should not be overlooked. Individual subcutaneous cysts may be removed surgically depending on location, or medically. Cerebral disease is treated with praziquantel 50 mg/kg daily for 10 days, under steroid cover. Steroids should be used to decrease the inflammation associated with the dying organisms. Patients may also require antiepileptic therapy if they present with seizures [4]. Adult tapeworms are treated with praziquantel in a dose of 10 mg/kg once. Obstructive lesions of the brain require surgical intervention.

Treatment ladder for cysticercosis [4]

- Albendazole 15 mg/kg/day (divided in two doses) for 7–14 days
- Praziquantel (50–100 mg/kg/day divided every 8 h) for 15 days
- Corticosteroids should be administered with antiparasitic therapy to decrease muscular or cerebral inflammation associated with the degenerating organism

Sparganosis

Definition

Sparganosis is a tissue infection with plerocercoid larvae or spargana of a number of species of pseudophyllidean tapeworms of the genus *Spirometra*. Patrick Manson described the first case, in Amoy, China in 1882. The Greek word sparganon means swaddling clothes and describes the slender ribbon-like character of the larval worm. Once a human becomes infected, the larvae migrate into the subcutaneous tissue and develop into painful nodules.

Epidemiology

The genus *Spirometra* has a worldwide distribution, although most human cases of sparganosis occur in South-East Asia and east Africa, where exposure to or consumption of infected intermediate hosts occurs most commonly [1].

Pathophysiology

Causative organisms (Figure 33.34)

- *Spirometra*

Adult *Spirometra* parasitise the gut of canines and felines. Eggs passed into water develop into procercoid larvae in copepod hosts of the genera *Diaptomus* and *Cyclops*. These are eaten by frogs, lizards, snakes, birds and some mammals, including mice and monkeys, in which the plerocercoid larvae develop, in muscle sheaths. Humans are infected either by the application of raw flesh to the skin or eye, usually as a medicinal poultice, or through

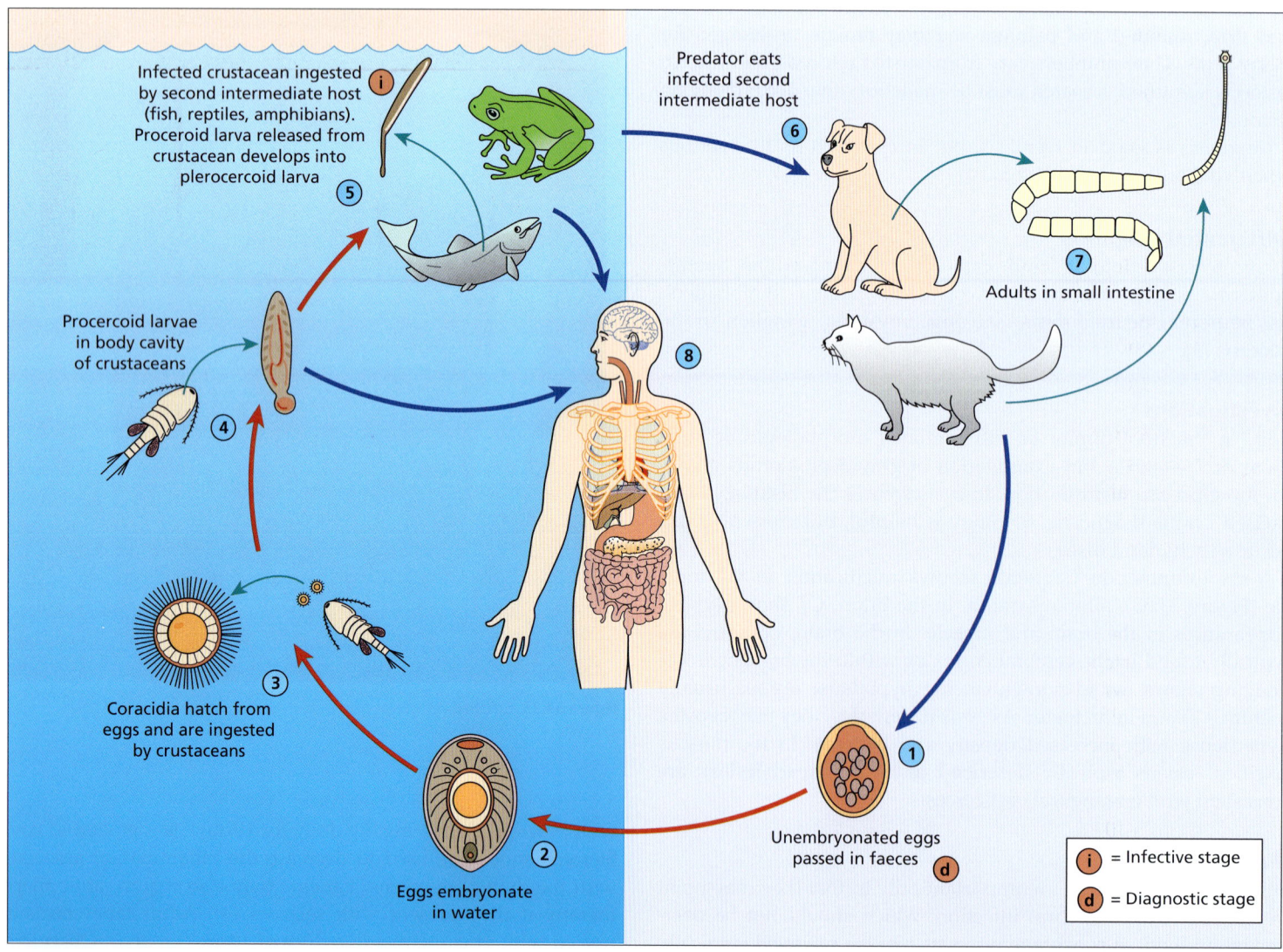

Figure 33.34 Life cycle of spargana. Courtesy of the Centers for Disease Control and Prevention. https://www.cdc.gov/dpdx/sparganosis/index.html (last accessed February 2023).

eating uncooked flesh or drinking water containing infected copepods.

Ingestion sparganosis occurs a variable amount of time after eating infected flesh or drinking infected copepods. The larvae penetrate the intestine and develop into sparagna, particularly in the subcutaneous tissues and muscle. The invaded areas become oedematous and form painful lumps, in the centres of which the white ribbon-like sparagna move [1]. Their death results in very intense inflammation with destruction of tissue and massive eosinophilia [2].

Clinical features
Presentation
Subcutaneous tissue involvement typically consists of a solitary, slow-growing often slowly migrating subcutaneous mass of the anterior abdominal wall [3]. Lesions may appear as clear, rubbery, irregular lumps or nodules between 0.5 and 5 cm in size [1]. The nodules may be asymptomatic or associated with pruritus, inflammation and pain. The epidermis appears normal. Ocular disease is the most common presentation, presenting as an extraocular (eyelid) mass, in perhaps one third to one half of cases.

Clinically, the lesions can assume a more nodular consistency with an insidious onset; they may last for several years and can also migrate. Lesions are typically painful. Localised elephantiasis also results due to lymphatic invasion.

Clinical variants
Application sparganosis. The sparagna migrate into the inflamed part causing an immediate severe local pruritus. Subsequently, signs of sparganosis may be very hard to differentiate from those of the primary inflammation for which the flesh poultice was applied. Redness, pain and swelling increase in severity over a few days or very few weeks, and the worms become localised in small nodules surrounded by pus (Figure 33.35). Ocular sparganosis frequently results in panophthalmitis and loss of the globe.

Sparganum proliferum. This is a rare form in which the sparganum branches and divides, producing thousands of mainly subcutaneous sparagna, which form subcutaneous nodules and itchy papules [4]. There may be a severe systemic illness with fever and eosinophilia.

Investigations
Diagnosis is made from the history and by recovery of sparagna after incision. Histologically, there is a granulomatous panniculitis and dermatitis, with a section of a sparganum [3]. Spirometra species are virtually indistinguishable, and therefore recognition of species by morphological appearance alone may prove difficult. Diagnosis is aided by the availability of ELISA serological studies using sparganum-specific monoclonal antibodies. The worm is usually less than 10 cm in length but can be up to 70 cm in size. The worm is typically white, wrinkled and ribbon shaped.

Management
Treatment is by surgical removal and drainage. Praziquantel has limited success in the treatment of the disease.

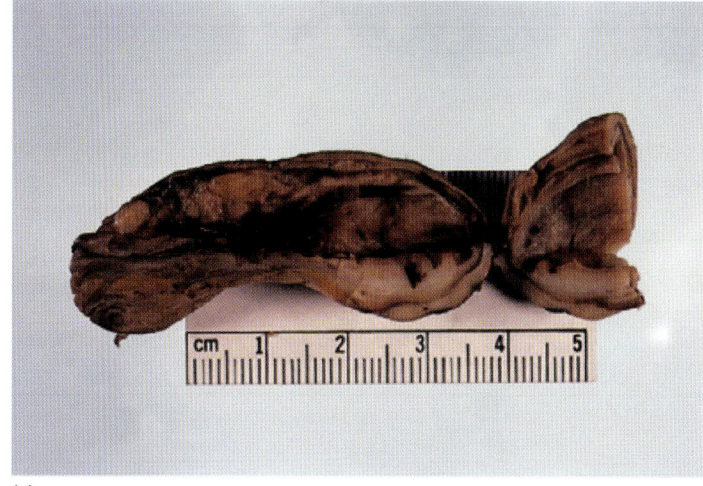

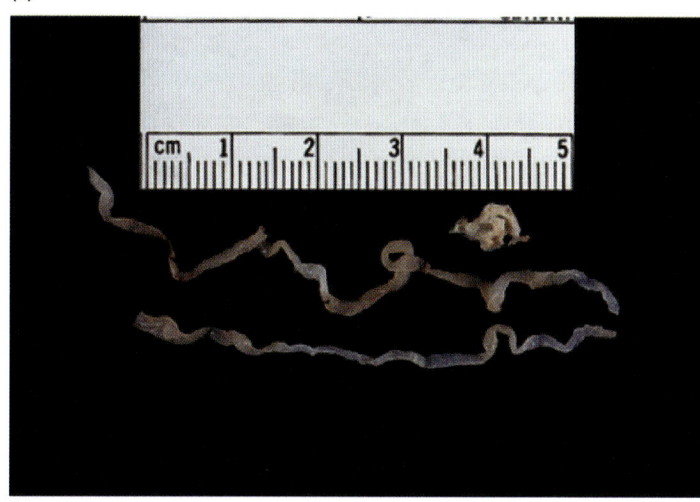

Figure 33.35 (a) Fibrous encapsulated cold abscess from the groin, which contained (b) a 22-cm long sparganum. Courtesy of Professor S.B. Lucas.

INFECTION WITH PROTOZOA

Of the protozoa that give rise to skin disease or may cause changes in the skin indirectly, only *Leishmania* are natural parasites of the skin, in the sense that part of their life cycle must be spent in it. Even so, humans are often simply an accidental host in a zoonotic infection. *Entamoeba histolytica* may occasionally invade the skin, usually as an extension of an existing visceral lesion. Free-living amoebae, of the genus *Acanthamoeba*, may cause a primary lesion in the skin, eye or ear, before invading the brain [1]. *Trypanosoma*, of the species that infect humans in Africa and America, may cause florid chancres soon after inoculation, but thereafter cause rashes indirectly. *Toxoplasma* causes an exanthem as part of the secondary stage of the infection and *Trichomonas*, a mucosal parasite, causes inflammation of the skin adjacent to the infected mucosa. Cutaneous manifestations of malaria, due to several species of *Plasmodium*, are simply a reflection of systemic infection severity, or of drug toxicity.

A summary of the organisms and diseases caused by infection with protozoa is provided in Table 33.4.

Table 33.4 Organisms and diseases in protozoa infection.

Disease	Organism
Malaria	*Plasmodium*
Amoebiasis	*Entamoeba histolytica*
Trichomoniasis	*Trichomonas vaginalis*
Trypansomiasis	African: *Trypanosoma gambiens, T. rhodesiense*
	American: *Trypanosoma cruzi*
Leishmaniasis	Old World: *Leishmaniasis major, L. tropica, L. aethiopica, L. infantum*
	New World: *Leishmaniasis braziliensis, L. vianna panamensis, L. mexicana Mexicana*
	Visceral: *Leishmania donovani donovani, L. donovani infantum*
Toxoplasmosis	*Toxoplasma gondii*

Malaria

Definition
Malaria is caused by parasites of the genus *Plasmodium* and is transmitted to humans by the bites of numerous species of mosquito belonging to the genus *Anopheles*. It causes a febrile systemic illness, which may be fatal in expatriates and children in endemic areas in the tropics and is a major cause of chronic illness.

Epidemiology [1]
Malaria is a disease of tropical and subtropical regions. *P. falciparum* and *P. vivax* are the predominant species worldwide with an estimated incidence of 229 million and 6.4 million cases respectively in 2019 [2]. The majority of falciparum occurs in sub-Saharan Africa. *P. malariae* and *P. ovale* have a global distribution. *P. ovale* is less common, found mainly in Africa and South-East Asia. The incidence of malarial infections depends on environmental suitability for local vectors in terms of altitude, climate, vegetation and implementation of control measures, and hence is inextricably linked to poverty, natural disasters and war.

Clinical features
Presentation
The mosquito bite can give rise to considerable skin reaction and the disease itself to numerous cutaneous manifestations. In the early cold stage of benign tertian malaria (*P. vivax*) there is vasoconstriction and gooseflesh; in the hot stage, flushing of the face and to a lesser extent other parts of the skin; and in the sweating stage, very profuse sweating. These manifestations are common to all diseases characterised by rigors caused by the release of endotoxin or 'endotoxin-like' substances. Malaria commonly causes jaundice and in the skin of Europeans and Asians may have a curious grey or greenish hue. In severe malaria, there may be bleeding from the gums or gastrointestinal tract and conjunctival petechiae may be seen, but cutaneous petechiae are rare. Herpes simplex and, occasionally, herpes zoster may develop.

Investigations [3]
Malaria is suspected primarily based on clinical features such as fever. However, there is no combination of signs or symptoms that reliably distinguishes malaria from other causes of fever. Therefore, diagnosis should be confirmed in all patients with suspected malaria through microscopy examination or rapid antigen based diagnostic tests of a blood sample.

Management
Several of the drugs used in the treatment of disease or for chemoprophylaxis cause skin problems. Chloroquine causes pruritus, especially in black skin, often severe enough to arrest treatment [4]. It responds to antihistamines, although the cause is unknown and there is never a rash. Various skin eruptions may occur, and it should be used with caution in patients with psoriasis, as it may exacerbate disease. Fansidar contains pyrimethamine and sulphadoxine. Epidermal necrolysis and Stevens–Johnson syndrome occur, sometimes fatally [5]. Quinine may also cause rashes, notably toxic erythema and urticaria.

Treatment is dependent upon where onset of disease occurred [3]. Chloroquine-sensitive areas include the Dominican Republic, Haiti and Central America north of the Panama Canal. There are several first line therapies for the treatment of chloroquine-resistant malaria. Artemisinin combination therapies (ACTs) result in the most rapid clearance time of all options. There are several oral artemisinin derivatives, including artesunate and artemether. These therapies should be given in combination to obviate resistance. The World Health Organization recommends the following combinations [3]:
- Artemether + lumefantrine.
- Artesunate + amodiaquine.
- Artesunate + mefloquine.
- Dihydroartemisinin + piperaquine.
- Artesunate + sulphadoxine-pyrimethamine.

Amoebiasis

Definition
Amoebiasis is an infection of the large intestine caused by the parasite *Entamoeba histolytica*. The disease causes bloody diarrhoea, and has been noted to spread to other organs such as the liver, lungs, brain and skin. The disease causes ulcers that may become necrotic with verrucous borders. Subcutaneous swellings may also occur.

Introduction and general description
Amoebiasis due to *Entamoeba histolytica* is arguably the third most important human parasitic infection, after malaria and schistosomiasis. It occurs worldwide, but is especially prevalent in South-East Asia and Central America, but the organism is found in all warm and temperate parts of the world where hygiene is inadequate [1].

Epidemiology
Globally, approximately 50 million people contract the infection each year [2]. All ages are affected. The vulva is particularly likely to be invaded in the infant with amoebic dysentery. Penile amoebiasis may occur in men who have sex with men [3], but invasive amoebiasis is not especially common in men who have sex with men or in patients with HIV infection [4].

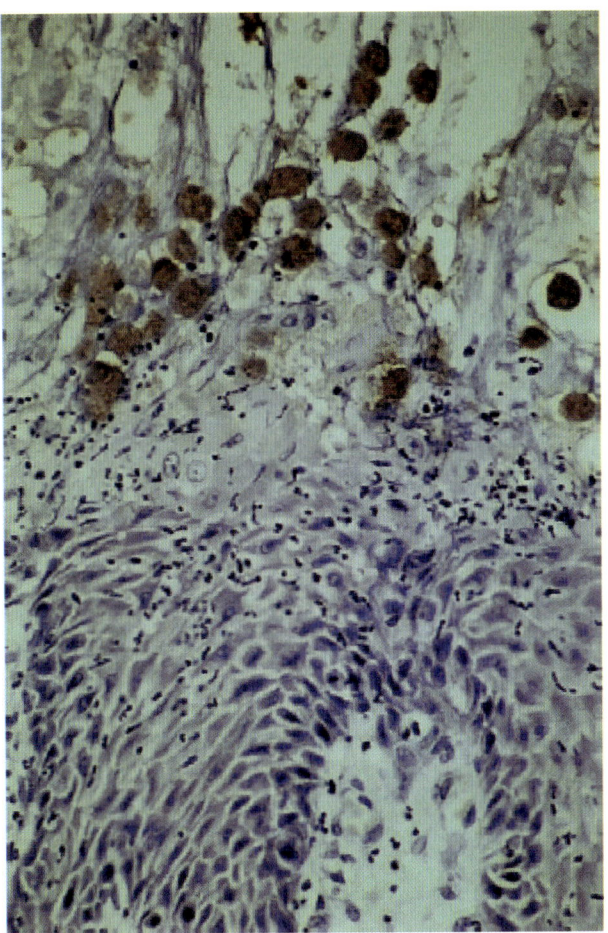

Figure 33.36 Cutaneous amoebiasis. High-power view of skin biopsy, showing *Entamoeba histolytica* trophozoites on the epidermis, causing necrosis. The amoebae are stained with immunoperoxidase and are brown. Courtesy of Professor S.B. Lucas.

Pathophysiology
Pathology
Trophozoites of a pathogenic zymodeme may, under conditions that have not been determined, invade the mucosa of the large bowel, causing amoebic dysentery [5]. Amoebae that escape the bowel into the bloodstream may spread and develop into abscesses, most commonly in the liver. Cutaneous amoebiasis (Figure 33.36) [6] develops when invasive amoebiasis escapes from the bowel to contiguous skin, usually around the anus or a colostomy, or after appendicectomy, or when amoebae are implanted in another mucosa, most commonly the vagina, cervix uteri or glans penis and rarely in the mouth. Rupture or surgical intervention of an amoebic abscess is a less common source of cutaneous infection. Amoebae lyse the skin and subcutaneous tissues and mucosae, producing necrosis and gangrenous sloughing. *Entamoeba histolytica* is one of the most powerful organisms in terms of its lytic capacity, and this is mediated through amoebapores following the binding to the host's tissue in a lectin-like manner [7].

Causative organisms
- *Entamoeba histolytica*

Entamoeba histolytica inhabits the lumen of the human caecum, colon and rectum. Free-living trophozoites 10–60 μm in diameter, encyst and divide. Cysts passed in the faeces may survive up to 30 days, depending upon conditions of humidity and temperature, and survive chlorination. They are transmitted in contaminated water or food, especially salads, or by hands or flies, or by anal intercourse. Ingested cysts that survive gastric acid complete the cycle. Isoenzyme electrophoretic analysis of cultured isolates suggests that pathogenic and non-pathogenic strains (zymodemes) of *E. histolytica* exist, but these cannot be distinguished morphologically [8].

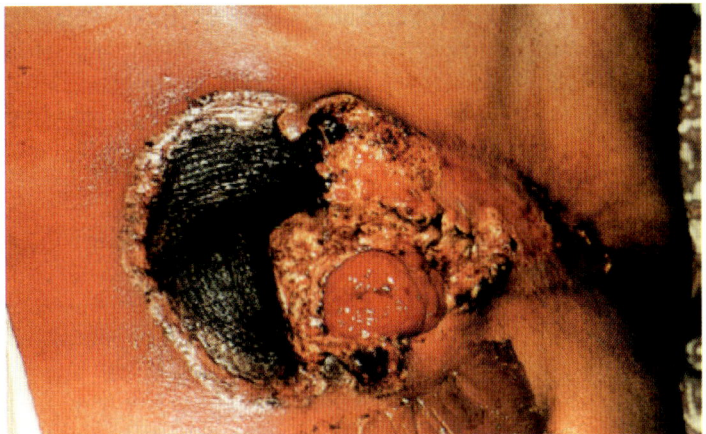

Figure 33.37 Cutaneous amoebiasis. Rapidly spreading ulcer around a colostomy in a patient with intestinal amoebiasis. Courtesy of Meddia (Medical and Diagnostic Services).

Clinical features
Presentation [6,9,10]
Cutaneous amoebiasis commonly presents with well-defined, indurated, painful, progressively enlarging plaques with overlying ulcers and sinuses draining pus [9]. Often, one or more lesions appear at the anus or on the buttocks and spread as sloughing coalescing ulcers [10] (Figure 33.37). The course of the disease varies from fewer than 2 weeks to as long as 2 years, the more rapid and destructive lesions tending to occur in the young. The skin lesion itself is not diagnostic and is either a deeply invading ulcer or an ulcerated granuloma (amoeboma). It is usually seen as a serpiginous ulcer with distinct raised thickened often undermined edges and with a red rim about 2 cm wide, haemopurulent exudate and necrotic slough. It is intensely painful. Regional adenitis is usual.

Differential diagnosis
A solitary lesion may be mistaken for an epithelioma or for tuberculosis verrucosa cutis. On the penis when regional lymphadenopathy is present, syphilis or lymphogranuloma venereum are considered in the differential diagnosis.

Disease course and prognosis
The prognosis is serious in the neglected case, particularly in infants, but with early diagnosis and treatment it is good. It is important to appreciate that a history of dysentery is not essential to the diagnosis of amoebiasis of the skin.

Investigations
Cutaneous amoebiasis can spread very rapidly and terminate fatally, so early diagnosis is important. Examination of fresh

material from the cutaneous lesion regularly discloses amoebae. Material should be taken from the edge of the ulcer avoiding necrotic tissue and examined at once under the microscope. The demonstration of motile trophozoites containing red blood cells is diagnostic. Histology of the ulcer edge will reveal amoebae, but the identification of the parasite in sections stained by H&E may be difficult (Figure 33.36). Amoebic trophozoites in faeces, biopsy, necropsy or abscess aspirate are revealed with much greater accuracy by immunofluorescence or immunoperoxidase staining. Serological tests are helpful, and the indirect immunofluorescent antibody test is positive in the serum of nearly 100% of patients with amoebic liver abscess, and in about 70% of patients with intestinal amoebiasis. Serial stool examinations should be performed.

Management
All infections should be treated, even if asymptomatic. The goal of therapy is to eliminate the invading trophozoites and to suspend carriage of the organism. Treatment of invasive amoebiasis is with metronidazole [11]. The recommended adult dose is 750 mg orally three times a day for 10 days. This should be followed by, or combined with, a luminal agent, e.g. paromomycin 750 mg orally three times a day for 10 days, or diloxanide furoate 500 mg three times a day, to eliminate intestinal cysts.

Local cleaning of cutaneous ulcers with antiseptic solutions may be necessary.

Where a hepatic abscess needs to be drained, this is most safely done by needle aspiration.

Effective treatment is usually followed by complete healing of the skin without the need for plastic surgery.

Treatment ladder for amoebiasis

First line
- Metronidazole, followed by a luminal agent such as paromycin, diiodohydroxyquin or diloxanide furoate

Second line
- Tinidazole 2000 mg PO OD for 3–5 days
- Nitazoxanide 500 mg PO BD for 3 days

Trichomoniasis

Definition
Trichomoniasis is the most common parasitic infection in humans in the industrialised world. Clinicians will recognise the disease as one of the most common vaginal complaints among female patients. Infection rates between men and women are identical; however, presentation in men is typically an asymptomatic urethritis.

Epidemiology
Age
Although most commonly seen in the second and third decades, the infection may occur at any age and has been reported in nearly 17% of babies aged from 1 day to 11 months. Many adults are asymptomatic carriers, particularly males. It can be isolated from up to 15% of men with non-specific urethritis. Discharge in males is scant.

Associated diseases
The condition is frequently associated with gonorrhoea [1] (Chapter 30). Transmission is usually by sexual intercourse, with an incubation period of 4–21 days. Occasional non-sexual transmission has been reported. In males, the condition occurs with non-specific urethritis in up to 5% of cases and balanitis may also occur [2]. The organism may be harboured in the prostate without symptoms.

Pathophysiology
Causative organisms
- *Trichomonas vaginalis*

Clinical features
Presentation
Trichomoniasis characteristically causes a copious discharge with vaginal soreness or irritation and urinary frequency. The odour of the discharge is often unpleasant, although this feature is not specific. In many cases, bubbles can be seen in the discharge and the vaginal mucosal and cervical surfaces are infected and sometimes covered with punctate haemorrhages; however, the 'strawberry cervix' is only seen in 2% of cases. The pH of the discharge is usually higher than the normal 4.5.

Investigations
In women, diagnosis is usually easily confirmed by examination of a wet film by phase contrast or dark-field microscopy [3], but culture, usually in Feinberg–Whittington medium, gives the most reliable results. Conversely, in males, examination of centrifuged urine or prostatic fluid following massage is only occasionally positive, and in many men it is not possible to confirm a clinical diagnosis. Examination of a stained dry film is neither easy nor reliable.

Sexual partners should always be examined and in both sexes, specimens taken to exclude other causes of sexually transmitted disease.

Management [4]
Standard treatment is with a single metronidazole 2 g oral dose. An alternate dose is metronidazole 500 mg orally twice a day for 7 days. Most clinicians prefer the single oral dose, as compliance is much higher. Regardless of treatment given, patients should avoid sexual contact for 7 days from last antibiotic dose. Gastrointestinal disturbances are common. Disulfiram-like reaction with alcohol may be counselled, although the evidence behind this is not well substantiated. Benzimidazole drugs should be avoided in the first 3 months of pregnancy.

Clotrimazole has been shown to provide symptomatic relief of disease, but does not eradicate the organism [2]. Tinidazole can be used for cases unresponsive to metronidazole, but is a more expensive alternative [5].

All sexual partners should be treated, because occurrence rates in partners are high. Identification of the organism in partners is not necessary. Patients should also be evaluated for concurrent gonorrhoea and *Chlamydia* infection.

> **Treatment ladder for trichomoniasis**
>
> **First line**
> - Metronidazole 2 g PO single dose
> - Tinidazole 2 g PO single dose (clotrimazole does not eradicate the organism)
>
> **Second line**
> - Metronidazole 500 mg PO BD for 7 days

Trypansomiasis

Definition and nomenclature

Trypanosomiasis is caused by protozoa of the genus *Trypanosoma*. There are African and American forms.

> **Synonyms and inclusions**
> - Sleeping sickness (African form)
> - Chagas disease (American form)

Epidemiology

Incidence and prevalence

African trypanosomiasis. The disease is endemic in a belt running across Africa, limited approximately by latitude 15°N and latitude 15°S. *Trypanosoma gambiense* is the culprit agent in West Africa, and the more virulent *T. rhodesiense* in East Africa to the east and south of Lake Victoria [1]. Occasional cases are imported into countries where the parasite is not endemic [2].

Age, sex, race and occupation have no influence on susceptibility to trypanosomiasis, except in how they may affect exposure to tsetse flies. *Trypanosoma gambiense* sleeping sickness tends to be an endemic disease, affecting rural communities, with localised outbreaks, while *T. rhodesiense* sleeping sickness causes sporadic infections in herdsmen, hunters and tourists. In some parts of the 'tsetse fly belt' the incidence is high, and, as the same flies transmit bovine trypanosomiasis to livestock, farmers cannot keep cattle, and poverty and malnutrition are rife. The number of cases has dropped dramatically over the past two decades. In 2018, only 977 cases were recorded [3].

American trypanosomiasis. The insect vectors are widely distributed in the American continent from latitude 42°N in the USA to latitude 43°S in Argentina [4]. *Trypanosoma cruzi* attacks humans and other mammals, and the disease it produces can be regarded as a zoonosis. The area of distribution of the disease is more limited than the range of the reduviid bugs that transmit it, since those found at the two extremes of the continent are wild species, while the domestic types, concerned in the transmission of the infection to humans, occur between latitude 25°N in Mexico and latitude 28°S in Argentina [4]. Approximately 7 million people are infected with *T. cruzi* worldwide [5].

Pathophysiology

Pathology

The tissues react almost immediately to the penetration of the metacyclic trypanosomes, producing oedema and cellular infiltration, which cause subcutaneous swelling. The infection spreads rapidly to the lymphatics, and the regional glands become oedematous and infiltrated with plasma cells and lymphocytes. The spleen and liver also enlarge. The trypanosomes penetrate immediately into the cells of the reticuloendothelial system at the site of the inoculation and transform into the leishmania form, later returning to the interstitial spaces and blood in the form of trypanosomes, penetrating again into the cells to repeat the cycle in different organs and systems. The most striking invasion is that of the spleen macrophages, the Kupffer cells of the liver and the cells of the striated muscles [6]. The inflammation and scarring that follows invasion of the myocardium may have serious consequences.

Causative organisms

African trypanosomiasis (Figure 33.38).
- *Trypanosoma gambiense* (West Africa)
- *Trypanosoma rhodesiense* (East Africa)

Trypanosomes develop, at the site of inoculation by the tsetse fly, from metacyclic forms to mature forms in about 10 days, and then enter the bloodstream. Within this time, the patient starts to develop an antibody response to the infection. The immunological reaction to the trypanosomes in the skin causes the chancre. The systemic clinical illness coincides with invasion of the bloodstream. The early pathology is, thereafter, mainly in the lymph nodes, at first those draining the sore and then generally, with an increase in lymphocytes and plasma cells, but the appearances are not specific, and trypanosomes are not easily seen histologically. In *T. rhodesiense* infections, the lymphoplasmocytic infiltrate is also found in the myocardium and this myocarditis may be fatal. In late trypanosomiasis, the meninges become invaded with the same infiltrate and then the brain, especially around the basal ganglia. Gliosis and cerebral atrophy follow. The cause of these pathological changes is poorly understood, although it is known that there is a polyclonal B-lymphocyte activation with the production of very high levels of IgM and circulating immune complexes [7].

American trypanosoma (Figure 33.39).
- *Trypanosoma cruzi*.

The disease is transmitted by blood-sucking insects of large size: hemipteran, reduviid bugs (assassin or kissing bugs), belonging to the family Triatomidae, particularly *Panstrongylus megistus* (Brazil), *Triatoma infestans* (southern Brazil, Uruguay, Paraguay, Bolivia, Southern Peru, Chile and Argentina) [4] and *Rhodnius prolixus* (Venezuela, Colombia, Guianas and Central America). The larva, nymph and the adult insect can transmit the infection. They are active during the night. After ingestion, the trypanosomes multiply in the vector's intestine by longitudinal division, and within 3 or 4 weeks transform into the metacyclic form, which is infective to humans. Once the insect has been infected, it remains so for the

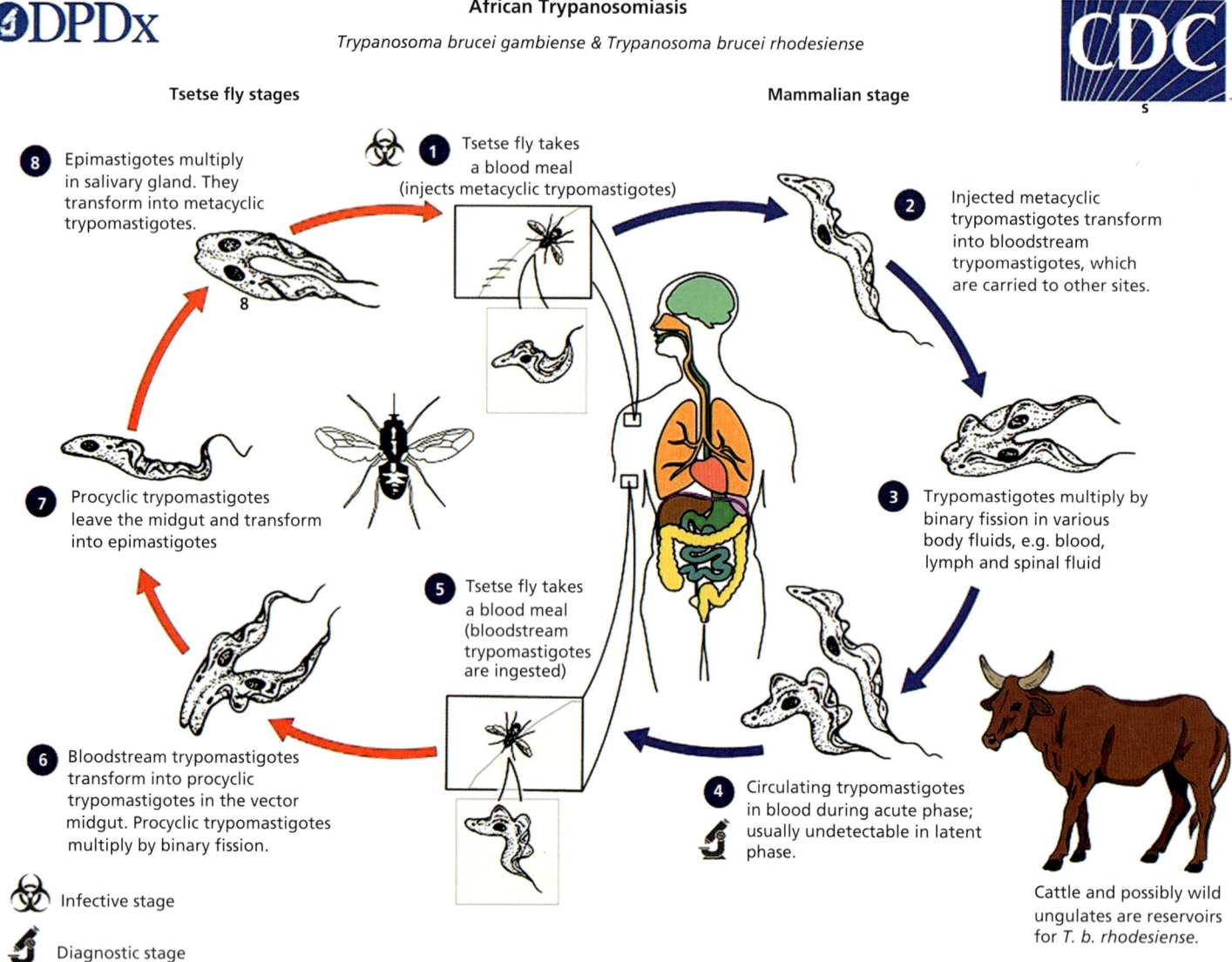

Figure 33.38 African trypanosomiasis parasite life cycle. (Courtesy of the Centers for Disease Control and Prevention. https://www.cdc.gov/dpdx/trypanosomiasisafrican/index.html (last accessed February 2023).

rest of its life. The disease has many non-human reservoirs, including cats, dogs, monkeys, pigs, squirrels, rats, skunks, raccoons, opossums, porcupines and armadillos. Transmission occurs by contamination through small cuts and abrasions on the skin, or through the normal mucous membranes of the eyes and lips when the vector, at the moment of biting, deposits its stools containing the infective metacyclic trypanosome. The bite wound itself may provide the portal of entry [4]. Less common modes of transmission include the ingestion of contaminated food, congenital transmission or transmission through contaminated blood or tissue [8].

Clinical features
Presentation [9,10,11]
African. The disease occurs in two stages: a haemolymphatic stage followed by a meningoencephalitic stage. Within a few days of the infected bite, a trypanosomal inoculation chancre starts to develop (Figure 33.40). It is a round, raised, red, hot and tender lesion, 2–5 cm or more in diameter, spreading to cover, for example, the entire surface of the forearm over the ensuing few days. There may be a tiny central punctum and a blister with fluid rich in trypanosomes may appear on its surface. The chancre is present in 70–90% of people infected with *T. rhodesiense*, less regularly with *T. gambiense*, but fades within a few weeks. It is usually accompanied by local lymphadenopathy.

The chancre heralds the onset of fever and systemic illness and generalised lymphadenopathy, which characterise the haemolymphatic stage. This is rapid and severe in *T. rhodesiense* infections, but gradual, mild, intermittent or even absent clinically in *T. gambiense* infections [12].

Early in the disease, lymphadenopathy may be particularly prominent in the posterior cervical chain, termed 'Winterbottom sign' [13]. During this phase of the illness, there may be oedema of the hands, feet and face and transient red or urticarial rashes, which are often circinate or annular, poorly defined, pale centrally

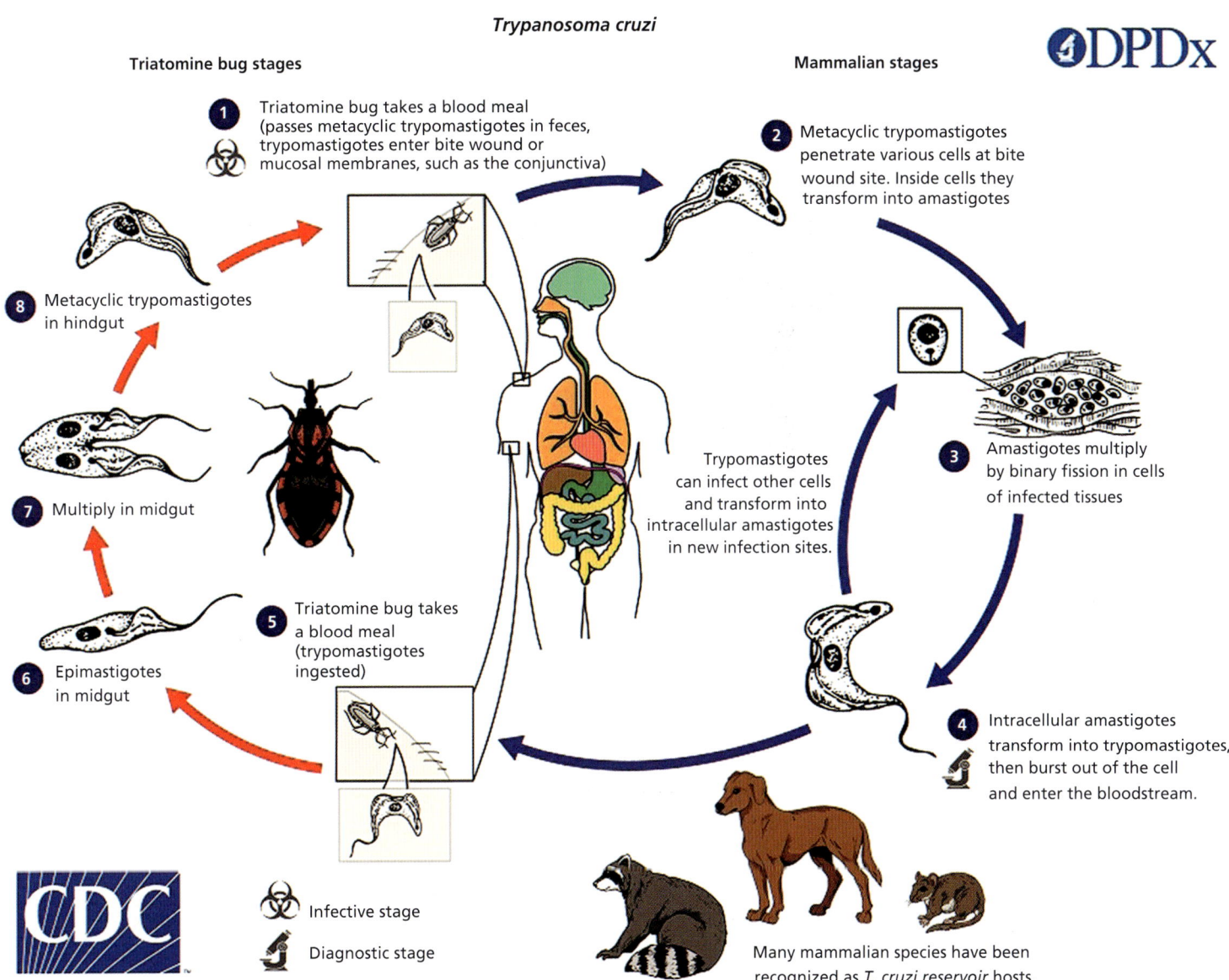

Figure 33.39 American trypanosomiasis parasite life cycle. Courtesy of the Centers for Disease Control and Prevention. https://www.cdc.gov/dpdx/trypanosomiasisamerican/index.html (last accessed February 2023).

and commonest on the trunk. The rash may be haemorrhagic (Figure 33.41). They are difficult to see in African skins.

When the central nervous system is invaded, the patient experiences behavioural changes, alterations in sleep patterns, extrapyramidal signs and ultimately coma. Neuropsychiatric involvement marks the onset of the meningoencephalitic stage. These occur months after the onset of *T. rhodesiense* infections, if the patient has not died earlier, and 1–3 years after the onset of *T. gambiense* infections. At this stage, pruritus and excoriations from scratching are common, and the patient is emaciated. Death is often due to intercurrent infection due to immune suppression.

American. The disease occurs in two stages: acute/early Chagas and chronic/late Chagas [14]. The great majority of infections do not present any clinical manifestations in the early phase. Signs of early disease appear on the fifth day after inoculation: these are both local and general. Eighty percent of the acute cases show the portal of entry in the conjunctiva, as evidenced by the 'eye sign' or 'Romaña's sign', also known as the 'ophthalmoganglionar complex' (oculoglandular complex), characterised by unilateral oedema of the eyelids and inflammation of the lacrimal gland (Figure 33.42). Cutaneous inoculation results in the 'cutaneous adenopathy complex' or 'inoculation chagoma' and is less common. The general manifestations consist of moderate to high fever accompanied by headache, myalgia and weakness, particularly pronounced in children, in whom the disease may end fatally from acute meningoencephalitis or myocarditis. Hepatosplenomegaly, oedema and various forms of exanthem ('schizotripanides') are frequent [4]. Forms called oedematous, neuropsychiatric, meningoencephalitic, respiratory, gastrointestinal and pseudotyphoid have been described [9].

The subacute and chronic forms almost always present with heart manifestations (chagasic myocarditis) and digestive manifestations (such as mega-colon and mega-oesophagus). 'Mega-syndromes' are

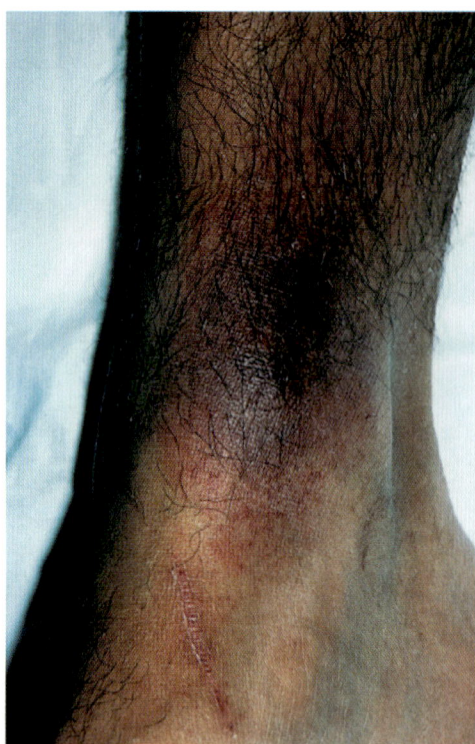

Figure 33.40 Trypanosomal chancre due to *Trypanosoma rhodesiense* infection, appearing 6 days after the bite of the tsetse fly. The lesion is swollen, inflamed and haemorrhagic.

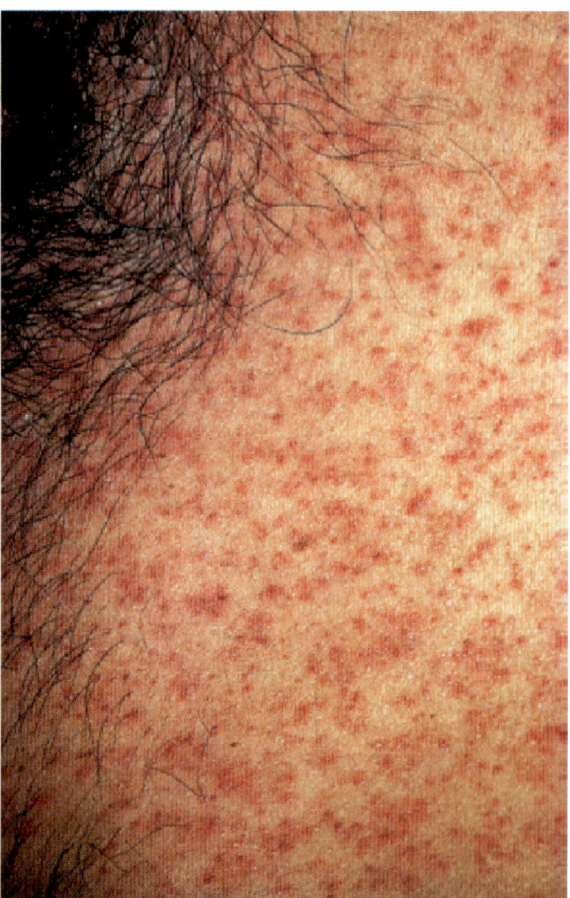

Figure 33.41 Trypanosomal rash. The maculopapular rash is becoming haemorrhagic.

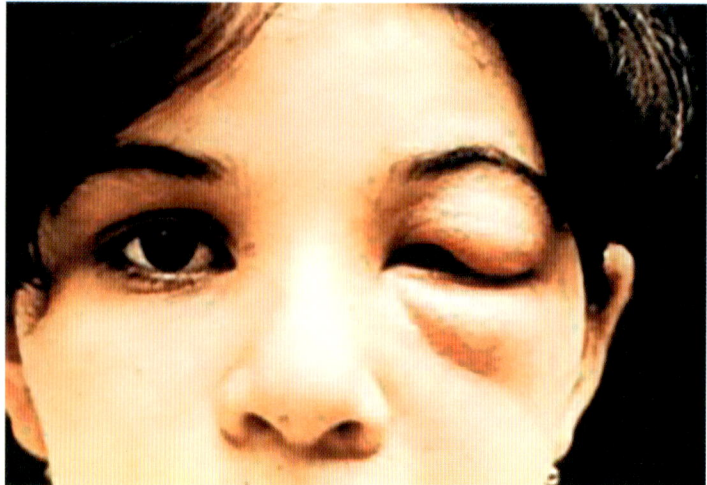

Figure 33.42 Chagas disease. Unilateral oedema of the eyelids and orbit (Chagas–Mazza–Romaña's sign).

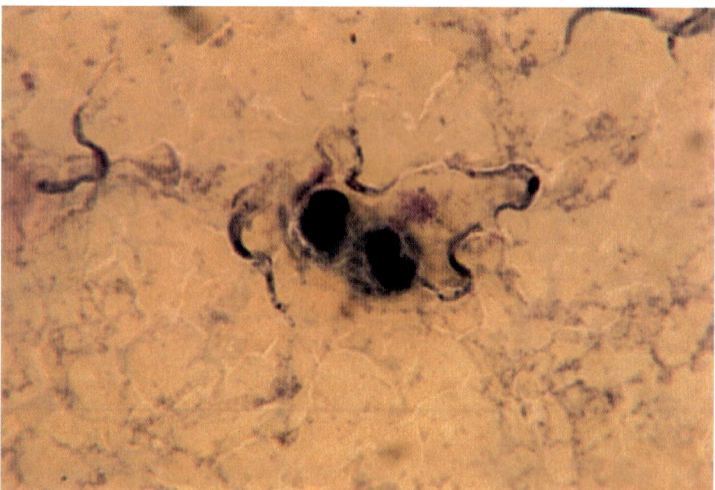

Figure 33.43 Trypanosomes in a thick blood film, stained with Giemsa. Courtesy of Dr P.L. Chiodini.

common in Brazil but absent in Venezuela. Congenital forms transmitted transplacentally or through lactation are rare.

Investigations

African. Within a few days of the onset of fever, trypanosomes may be demonstrated in simple thin blood films in *T. rhodesiense* infections. However, in *T. gambiense* infections, thick films (Figure 33.43) or concentration techniques [11] may be necessary. A more profitable approach is puncture and aspiration of the enlarged posterior cervical lymph nodes. Trypanosomes are seen undulating between the lymphocytes in the wet preparation, or well defined in a Giemsa-stained preparation. Cerebral involvement is characterised by raised protein in the cerebrospinal fluid, containing IgM, and a raised cell count comprising lymphocytes and morula cells (plasma cells distorted by vesicles of IgM). Serological tests, including ELISA and immunofluorescence, may be helpful. Serum IgM levels are often grossly elevated, and there may be anaemia. On diagnosis, a lumbar puncture is mandatory to establish whether the central nervous system has been invaded.

American. In the acute phase, the diagnosis is made by finding the parasite in the blood by direct examination, or by means of stained thick and thin smears, lymph gland biopsy, blood culture, animal inoculation and by the so-called xenodiagnosis of Brumpt: the reduviid bugs grown in the laboratory and free from infection are allowed to bite the forearm of the subject under suspicion and feed on the blood, after which the faeces of these insects are examined for metacyclic forms between 30 and 60 days later [9]. In the subacute and chronic forms, laboratory tests are of great help, particularly those based on the complement-fixation test using antigen from culture forms of *T. cruzi* (Machado–Guerreiro's test).

Management
African. A single course of suramin, preferably, or pentamidine isethionate is usually sufficient, if given before central nervous system invasion. Both drugs are seriously toxic [15].

American [16]. The acute stage (including congenital Chagas disease and transfusion acute disease) should be treated with a trypanocidal drug, either nifurtimox (Lampit®) or benznidazole (Rochagan®), oral dose. A rare side effect is an exfoliative dermatitis. Both drugs produce anorexia, weight loss, headache and dizziness, gastric irritation and, occasionally, peripheral neuritis (12–30%).

Treatment ladder for trypanosomiasis

African

First line
- Suramin sodium 200 mg IV (test dose), followed by 1 g/week for five doses

Second line
- Pentamidine isethionate 4 mg/kg IM on alternate days for five doses
- After central nervous system invasion, melarsoprol is used, often with corticosteroids [15]

American

First line
- Nifurtimox (Lampit) PO (8 mg/kg) for 60 or 90 days
- Or benznidazole (Rochagan), PO (6 mg/kg) for 30 or 60 days

Leishmaniasis

Cutaneous leishmaniasis

Definition
Leishmaniasis is a group of vector-borne diseases caused by a protozoan parasite from the genus *Leishmania*. The disease reservoirs include small mammals and parasite transmission occurs through the bite of an infected female sandfly vector.

The disease is endemic in approximately 90 countries, most commonly in tropical and subtropical regions. Clinical manifestations of disease range from aggressive cutaneous ulcers to systemic multiorgan disease.

Introduction and general description
Human leishmaniasis is usually classified as cutaneous or visceral, but the species that cause visceral disease may also cause skin lesions. In South and Central America, skin disease due to parasites of the *L. brasiliensis* complex may be complicated by the development of metastatic mucosal or mucocutaneous lesions. Mucosal disease is relatively rare with the other species [1].

Clinical patterns are poor indicators of species, although certain disease characteristics may be commonly associated with a particular species [2]. *Leishmania* spp. undergo a cycle of development in the gut of female sandflies, of the genera *Phlebotomus* in the Old World, and *Lutzomyia* and *Psychodopygus* in the New World. The species are morphologically identical, and are distinguished by isoenzyme pattern and DNA analysis. Monoclonal antibodies have also proved useful for rapid identification of isolates, especially in the field [3].

In its vertebrate host, the amastigote form of the parasite is found in cells of the reticuloendothelial system or in the dermis following severe parasite load and mononuclear cell necrosis. It is round or oval, 2–3 μm in diameter, with no protruding flagellum. The nucleus and kinetoplast stain deeply with the Romanovsky stains, giving the organism its characteristic appearance. In the sandfly and in artificial culture media, *Leishmania* spp. appear in the elongated promastigote stage, motile with an anterior flagellum.

Sandflies find their precise requirements for temperature and humidity in a wide variety of niches, commonly in rodent burrows and crevices and holes in banks, trees and houses in the Old World, and in tree canopies and forest litter in the New World [4]. Infection is transmitted by the bite of the fly, usually at night and outdoors; however, infected vectors can take a blood meal during the day if disturbed and also are responsible for inoculating parasites indoors within the household environment. Commonly, the infection is zoonotic; one species of *Leishmania* may be associated with one or many natural vertebrate hosts, which provide the reservoir of infection. Humans are commonly accidental hosts, although there are situations in which they may be the reservoir in an anthroponotic cycle. For these reasons, human leishmaniasis has a very wide geographical distribution and range of climate and altitude (Figure 33.44) and different epidemiological patterns (Table 33.5) [5].

Epidemiology
Incidence and prevalence
It has been estimated that 1.5 million new cases of cutaneous leishmaniasis occur annually and more than 80% of the total of cases affect individuals in developing countries [6]. Brazil, Iran, Afghanistan and Sudan suffer the highest prevalence and the disease is a priority for public health in all hyperendemic regions of the world. The disease is commonly imported into non-endemic countries by immigrants and returning travellers.

Old World. Cutaneous leishmaniasis of the Old World is due to *L. major*, *L. tropica*, *L. aethiopica* and *L. donovani infantum*, which

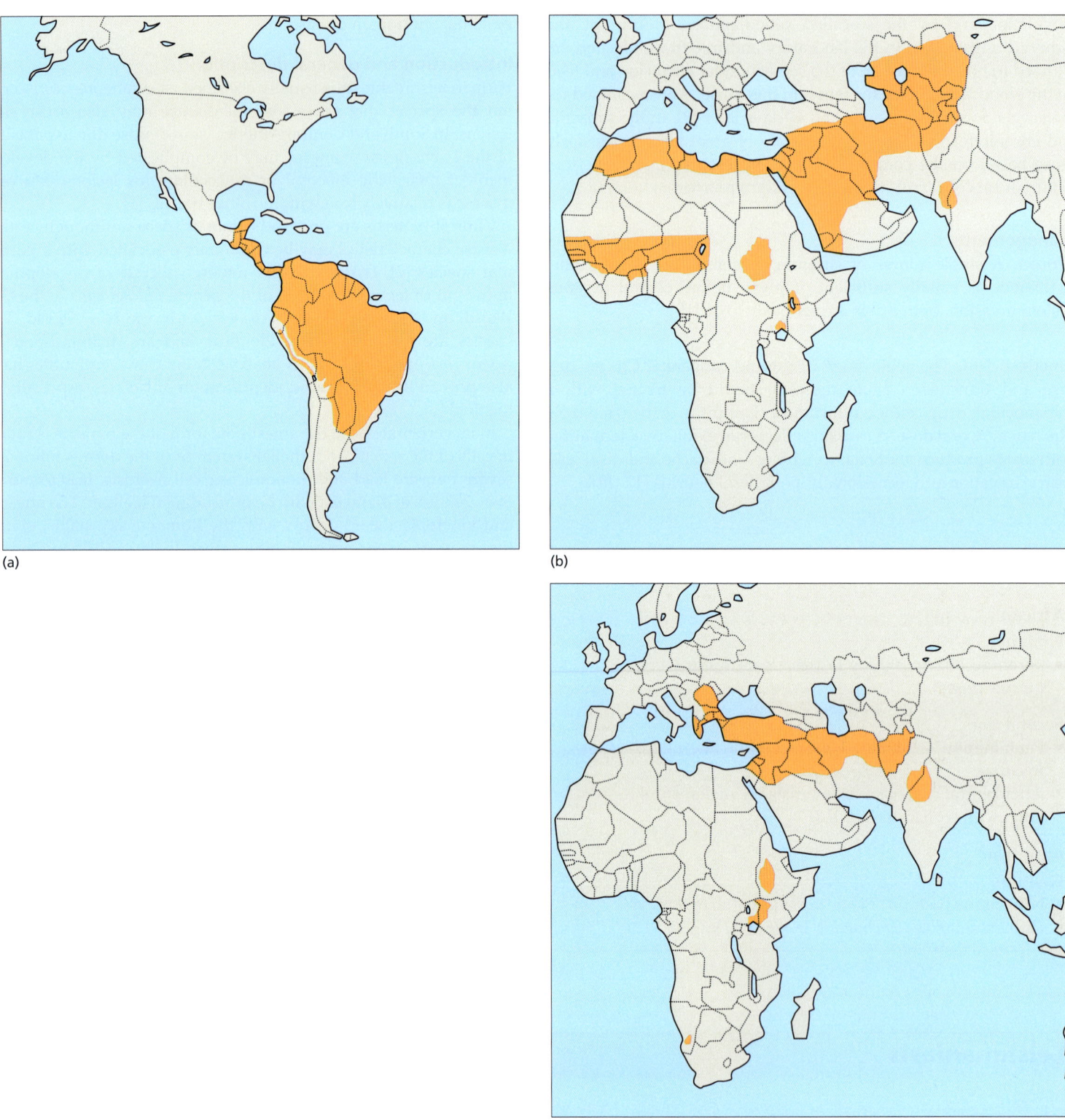

Figure 33.44 (a) Geographical distribution of cutaneous and mucocutaneous leishmaniasis in the New World. (b) Geographical distribution of Old World cutaneous leishmaniasis due to *Leishmania major*. (c) Geographical distribution of Old World cutaneous leishmaniasis due to *Leishmania tropica* and related species and *L. aethiopica*. Courtesy of the World Health Organization. http://www.who.int/leishmaniasis/leishmaniasis_maps/en/index.html (last accessed February 2023).

Table 33.5 Epidemiology of leishmaniasis. Courtesy of Weatherall et al. [5].

Organism	Clinical disease	Geography	Reservoir	Vector
Old World				
Leishmania donovani	VL, PKDL	North-East India, Bangladesh, Burma	Humans	Phlebotomus argentipes
L. infantum	VL, CL	Mediterranean basin, Middle East, China, Central Asia	Dogs, foxes, jackals	P. ariasi, P. perniciosus
L. donovani (Africa)	VL, PKDL	Sudan, Kenya, Horn of Africa, ?Senegambia	?Rodents in Sudan, ?canines, ?humans	P. orientalis, P. martini
L. major	CL	Semi-deserts in Middle East, North India, Pakistan, North Africa, Sudan, Central Asia	Gerbils (especially *Rhombomys, Meriones*)	P. papatasii
L. major	CL	Sub-Saharan savanna, Sudan	Rodents (especially *Arvicanthus, Tatera*)	P. duboscqi
L. tropica	LCL, VL	Towns in Middle East, Mediterranean basin, Central Asia	Humans, ?dogs	P. sergenti
L. aethiopica	LCL, DCL	Highlands of Kenya, Ethiopia	Hyraxes (*Procavia, Heterohyrax*)	P. longipes, P. pedifer
New World				
L. chagasi	VL, CL	Central America, northern South America, esp. Brazil, Venezuela	Foxes	Lutzomyia longipalpis
L. mexicana mexicana	LCL, DCL	Yucatan, Belize, Guatemala	Forest rodents (especially *Ototylomys* and *Peromyscus yucatanicus*)	Lu. olmeca, Lu. cruciata
L. m. amazonensis	LCL, DCL, MCL	Tropical forests of South America	Forest rodents (especially *Proechimys, Oryzomys*)	Lu. flaviscutellata
L. brasiliensis brasiliensis	LCL, MCL	Tropical forests of South and Central America	?Forest rodents	Psychodopygus wellcomei, Lutzomyia spp.
L. b. guyanensis	LCL, MCL	Guyanas, Surinam, Brazil, Venezuela	Sloths (*Choleopus*), arboreal anteaters (*Tamandna*)	Lu. umbratilis
L. b. panamensis	LCL, MCL	Panama, Costa Rica, Colombia	Sloths (*Choleopus*)	Lu. trapidoi
L. b. peruviana	LCL, MCL	West Andes of Peru, Argentine highlands	Dogs	Lu. verrucarum, Lu. peruensis

DCL, diffuse cutaneous leishmaniasis; LCL, localised cutaneous leishmaniasis; MCL, mucocutaneous leishmaniasis; NW, New World; OW, Old World; PKDL, post-kala-azar dermal leishmaniasis; VL, visceral leishmaniasis [10].

is responsible for all the cutaneous disease on the northern Mediterranean littoral west of Greece and for some of the disease in north Africa [7,8] (Table 33.5).

American cutaneous leishmaniasis and mucocutaneous leishmaniasis. The site of development of *Leishmania* in the gut of New World sandflies differs from that in Old World sandflies, and the parasites have been redesignated by the addition of the subgenus *viannia*, for example *Leishmania viannia brasiliensis* [9], but in this chapter the older, simpler terminology is retained, by which the parasites that cause disease in humans fall into the L. brasiliensis and L. mexicana complexes. American leishmaniasis is an endemic and mainly rural disease of damp forested terrain in South and Central America [9]; however, a growing number of autochthonous cases of L. mexicana have been reported in the USA in recent years, especially south-central USA.

It is typically epidemic among young people who work in the forests, 25% of young soldiers fighting in the jungle in certain areas and in villagers settled on land recently torn from the tropical forest. The optimum time for transmission is immediately after the rainy season.

Additionally, L. b. brasiliensis is becoming increasingly peri-urban [6], with a number of opportunistic hosts, including dogs and donkeys (whose true reservoir status is questionable). *Leishmania brasiliensis peruviana* is, by contrast, part of a mountainous zoonosis among peridomestic dogs, causing an endemic human infection that affects children especially. Vectors and reservoirs are given in Table 33.5. As increasing numbers of new species are identified, it is becoming clear that each is associated with its own complex of reservoir hosts and vector sandflies.

Age
In endemic areas where transmission is stable, children are especially affected, and the cumulative rate of infection as determined by the presence of scars and positive may approach 100%. In less stable situations, for example around oases, epidemics occur affecting all ages and sexes [11].

Pathophysiology
Pathology
Old World. Sandflies inoculate the infective metacyclic promastigotes when taking a blood meal from the superficial vascular network in the human dermis. Inoculated promastigotes are taken up by histiocytes and newly immigrated monocytes, in which they multiply. Most inoculations do not seem to result in clinical disease as phagocytosis and complement-mediated killing of *Leishmania* parasites results in clearing of the infection. A minority of successful parasite inoculations result in localised or disseminated clinical cutaneous leishmaniasis. After a period of time, which depends on parasite species, size of inoculum and the host's cellular immune response, a clinical lesion appears. This lesion comprises parasitised macrophages, lymphocytes and plasma cells, with little structure (Figure 33.45) [12,13]. With time, piecemeal and focal necrosis of parasitised cells is found, probably the result of antibody-dependent cell-mediated immunity. The overlying epidermis becomes hyperkeratotic and breaks down, causing an ulcer whose surface is covered in a crust composed of hyperkeratotic

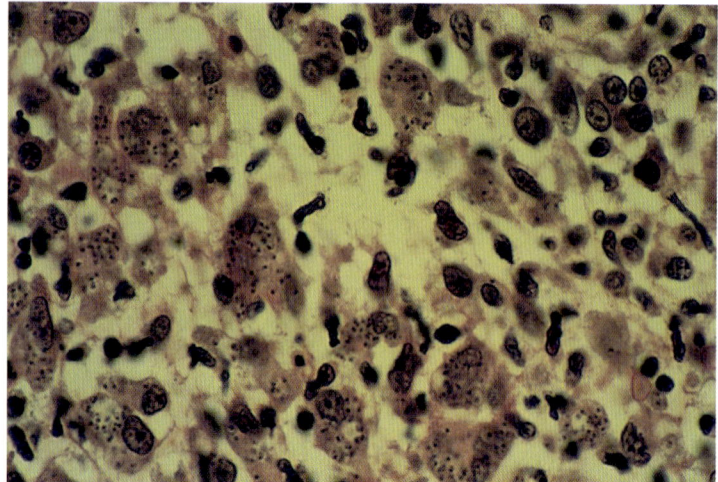

Figure 33.45 Cutaneous leishmaniasis (high power, H&E); biopsy of early lesion, showing abundant amastigotes in macrophages, and a few plasma cells. Courtesy of Professor S.B. Lucas.

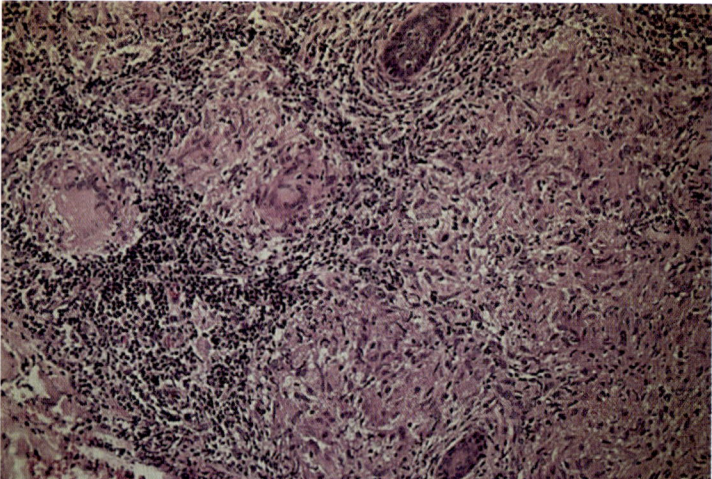

Figure 33.46 Chronic cutaneous leishmaniasis. Granulomatous dermatitis without necrosis. There are no amastigotes to be found in this case, and the differential diagnosis may be difficult between the other granulomatous dermatitides. Courtesy of Professor S.B. Lucas.

debris, dried exudate, dead cells, and live and dead parasites. This activity continues for several months, while the lesion appears clinically static. In other, especially chronic, cases the more classical epithelioid cell, and sometimes giant cell granuloma, develops with relatively little necrosis, but with similar epidermal changes (Figure 33.46). In these cases, parasites are difficult to find [14]. Rarely, when cell-mediated immunity fails to develop, as in diffuse cutaneous leishmaniasis, histology shows masses of parasitised, often vacuolated, macrophages, with little or no lymphocytic infiltrate and a normal or attenuated epidermis [15].

American cutaneous leishmaniasis and mucocutaneous leishmaniasis. The pathology of the skin lesions does not differ significantly from that of Old World disease. The necrotic pattern, with ulceration of the overlying epidermis, is common [12]. Although recovery from an infection confers lifelong immunity against reinfection with the same species of parasite, that immunity does not develop early enough or adequately to prevent the blood-borne metastatic spread of parasites of the *L. brasiliensis* complex, especially *L. b. brasiliensis* itself, to the mucosa of the nose, mouth, palate or larynx. Here, they may later start to multiply and cause severe destructive lesions, known as espundia (Portuguese: a sponge) [16]. Histology of the mucosal lesion [17] shows a collection of lymphocytes and plasma cells around small arterioles in the nasal submucosa. Occasional *Leishmania* are present in the vascular endothelial cells. Oedema, congestion and proliferation of vascular endothelium progress, leading to desquamation and necrosis of the overlying mucosa and underlying cartilage. Endarteritis and thrombosis add to the tissue destruction. Vascular supply is so reduced that only fibrous tissue remains.

Clinical features
Presentation
Old World [18]. Most previously uninfected individuals are susceptible. The incubation period is usually measured in months but ranges from a few days to over a year. One or more lesions occur on unclothed parts of the body, particularly on acral skin over bony prominences easily bitten by *Phlebotomus*, usually in a child. The face, neck and arms are the commonest targets. Lesions do not necessarily occur all at exactly the same time, but in endemic areas a family of children may all present with lesions and a history strongly suggesting infected sandfly bites all acquired in the same room on the same night.

The natural history of the lesions due to the four species tends to differ but there is much overlap, reflecting the variety in host response [2], so that lesions and their outcome are not always characteristic of the species (Table 33.6) [5]. The sequence of nodule, crusting, ulceration and healing with scar formation is common to all the self-healing sores.

Clinical variants
Old World.
Cutaneous leishmaniasis due to *L. major*: wet, rural or zoonotic cutaneous leishmaniasis [19,20]. After a short incubation period of less than 2 months, a red furuncle-like nodule appears at the site of inoculation (Figure 33.47). After 2 weeks a central crust forms. The crust may persist (Figure 33.48) or fall away revealing the underlying ulcer (Figure 33.49). The ulcer and the raised red margin enlarge over the next 2–3 months, and the lesion reaches a diameter of 3–6 cm. Multiple small secondary nodules (2–4 mm) sometimes occur around the lesion in lymphatics. Healing takes place in 2–6 months and leaves a scar. This type of cutaneous leishmaniasis is acquired in a rural area, where the infecting organisms are also rodent parasites and are poorly adapted to humans. It is an example of a zoonosis.

Cutaneous leishmaniasis due to *L. tropica*: dry, urban or anthroponotic leishmaniasis [21]. After an incubation period of more than 2 months, a small brownish nodule appears and transforms into a slowly extending plaque 1–2 cm in diameter in about 6 months. At this stage, shallow ulceration appears in the centre, which develops a closely adherent crust. Multiple secondary nodules occur much less frequently than in the 'wet' form. After 8–12 months, the lesion starts to regress and the ulcer heals, leaving a scar. The average time

Table 33.6 Clinical features of cutaneous leishmaniasis. Courtesy of Weatherall et al. [5].

Parasite and lesion	Natural outcome	Treatment
Leishmania major		
Self-healing rural sores	3–5 months Disabling scars	Physical/topical/IL/nil Sb 20 mg/kg/day × 2–3 weeks (?Some unresponsive)
L. tropica		
Self-healing urban sores	10–14 months	Physical/topical/IL/nil Sb 20 mg/kg/day × 2–3 weeks
Leishmaniasis recidivans	>10 years destructive	Sb 20 mg/kg/day × 3–6 weeks
L. aethiopica		
Self-healing, nodular	2–5 years	Physical/topical/nil
Mucocutaneous	>10 years destructive	Pentamidine 4 mg/kg/week × 8
DCL	Persists, disfiguring	Pentamidine 4 mg/kg/week × months
L. m. Mexicana		
Self-healing	6–8 months	Physical/topical/IL/nil
Chiclero ear	>10 years, destructive	Sb 20 mg/kg/day × 2–3 weeks Sb 20 mg/kg/day × weeks to months
L. m. amazonensis		
Self-healing	?Duration	?Sb 20 mg/kg/day × 3 weeks
DCL	Persists, relapses, disfiguring	Sb 20 mg/kg/day × months
L. b. brasiliensis		
Self-healing	?Duration, later mucocutaneous	Sb 20 mg/kg/day × 3–4 weeks
Mucocutaneous	Persists, destructive	Sb 20 mg/kg/day × 4 weeks, or amphotericin B
L. b. guyanensis		
Self-healing	?6–8 months	Sb 20 mg/kg/day × 3 weeks
Lymphatic nodules 'pian bois'	?Late espundia	If poorly responsive to Sb, use pentamidine
L. b. panamensis		
Self-healing	?Duration ?Late espundia	Sb 20 mg/kg/day × 3 weeks
L. b. peruviana		
Self-healing	?Duration	Physical/topical/nil Sb 20 mg/kg/day × 2–3 weeks

DCL, diffuse cutaneous leishmaniasis; IL, intralesional injection; Sb, antimony as pentavalent antimonial.

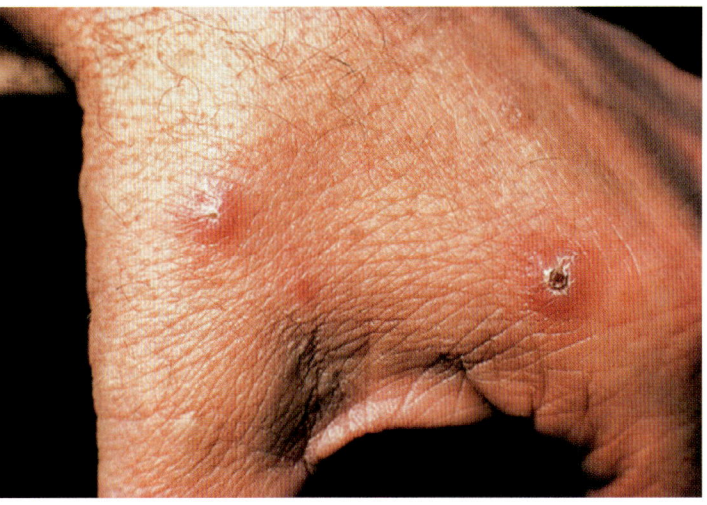

Figure 33.47 Cutaneous leishmaniasis due to *Leishmania major*: early papules, one of which is starting to show central crusting.

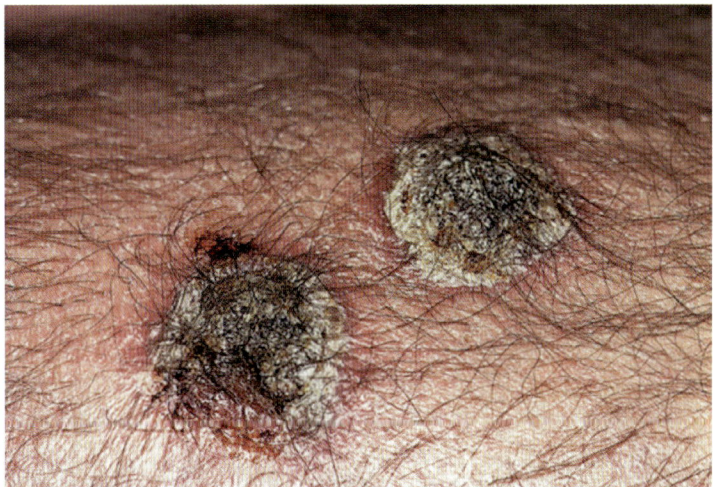

Figure 33.48 Cutaneous leishmaniasis due to *Leishmania major* from Saudi Arabia, showing marked and persistent crusting.

from nodule to scar is about 1 year, approximately twice as long as in the 'wet' form. Rare forms of viscerotropic infections by *L. tropica* have been described in war veterans who acquired the parasite in the Middle East and in cases of Indian kala-azar [22].

Cutaneous leishmaniasis due to *L. aethiopica* [15]. Lesions are most commonly central on the face and single. Satellite papules accuminate into a large spreading nodule that may not crust or ulcerate (Figure 33.50). Lesions are seldom much inflamed and heal over 2–5 years. If the sandfly bite has been on the mucosal border of the nose or mouth, primary mucocutaneous leishmaniasis may develop, producing swelling of the lips or nose and persist for many years (Figure 33.51), although without the gross destruction seen in Latin America caused by *L. brasiliensis*.

Cutaneous leishmaniasis due to *L. donovani infantum* [7]. Whereas infants infected with this parasite tend to get visceral leishmaniasis, adults are more likely to develop simple self-healing cutaneous disease, without concurrent or subsequent visceral involvement. The appearance and evolution of the lesions is typically slow and mild, when compared with that of *L. major*, with whom it coexists in North Africa [8] (Figure 33.52). Solitary mucosal lesions have occasionally been reported [1].

In addition to the classical self-healing sores, there are two types of cutaneous leishmaniasis that are chronic and may not heal spontaneously.

Leishmaniasis recidivans: chronic leishmaniasis, lupoid leishmaniasis [14]. It has been estimated that approximately 4% of *L. tropica* infections from Iran and Afghanistan will develop this chronic form of the disease. Brown-red or brown-yellow papules appear,

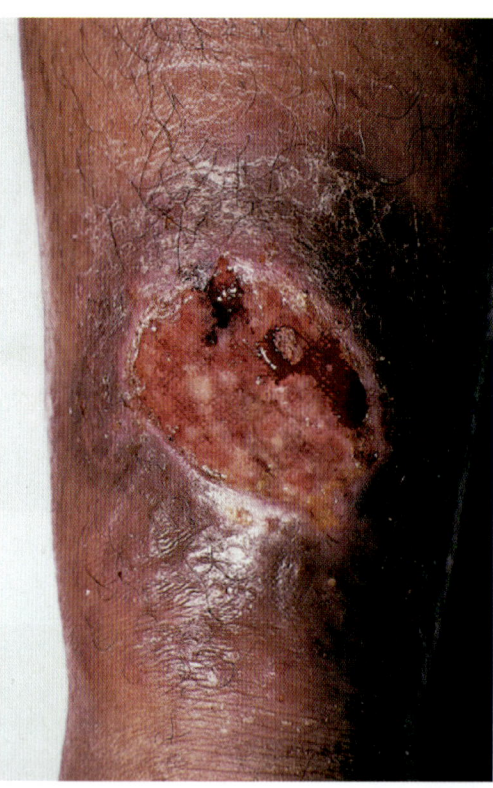

Figure 33.49 Cutaneous leishmaniasis due to *Leishmania major* from Sudan. An ulcer with a raised edge.

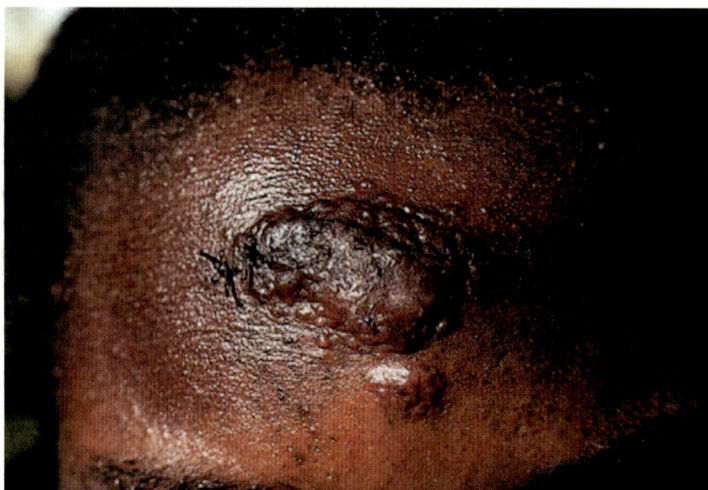

Figure 33.50 Cutaneous leishmaniasis due to *Leishmania aethiopica* from Kenya. A large nodule with many satellite papules and abundant parasites.

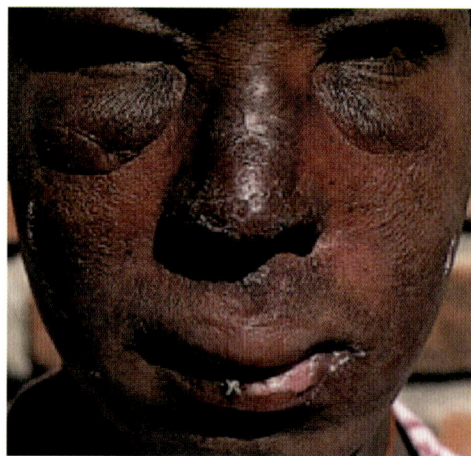

Figure 33.51 Nasal involvement, and marked inflammatory oedema in leishmaniasis due to *Leishmania aethiopica* in Ethiopia.

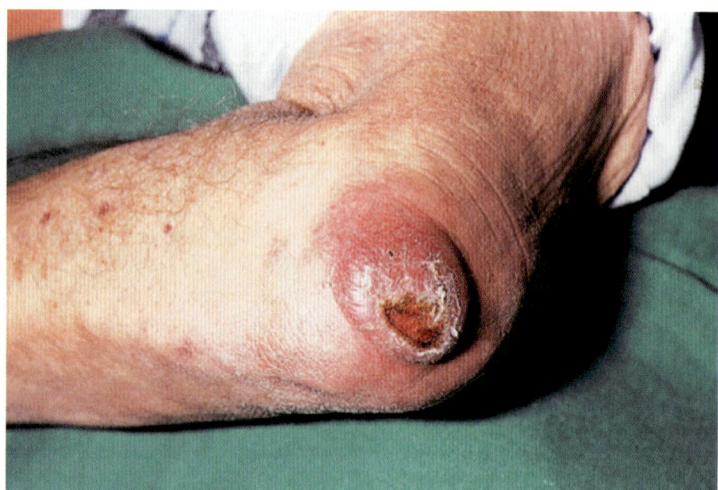

Figure 33.52 Cutaneous leishmaniasis due to *Leishmania infantum* in Spain. The fleshy nodule, with relatively little inflammation, is characteristic.

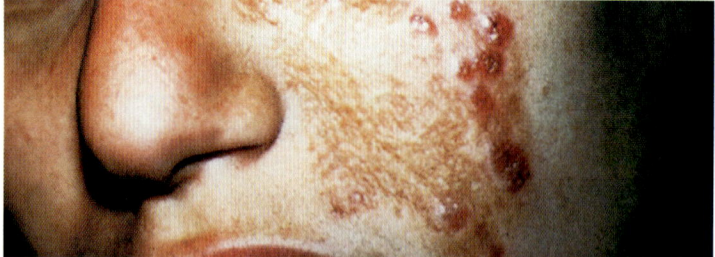

Figure 33.53 Leishmaniasis recidivans (lupoid leishmaniasis) in Baghdad, showing active papules cropping in the edge of the scar of the healed sore. Courtesy of Professor G. Rahim.

usually close to a scar of an old lesion of cutaneous leishmaniasis or actually in the scar. They coalesce and form a plaque closely resembling lupus vulgaris, even to the formation of apple-jelly nodules (Figure 33.53). The lesions frequently worsen in the summer and may ulcerate or form concentric rings. Rare keloidal and verrucous forms on the lower limbs are described. A psoriasiform type also occurs and may cover large areas of the body.

The recidivans lesion is the result of a peculiar host reaction in which cellular immunity fails to sterilise the lesion, despite the presence of exaggerated hypersensitivity. Although not as destructive as lupus vulgaris, lupoid leishmaniasis may persist and spread slowly for many years [23]. Investigations to demonstrate the parasite or leishmanial DNA in the affected skin are commonly negative.

Diffuse cutaneous leishmaniasis: disseminated cutaneous leishmaniasis, leishmaniasis cutis diffusa. In the Old World this form

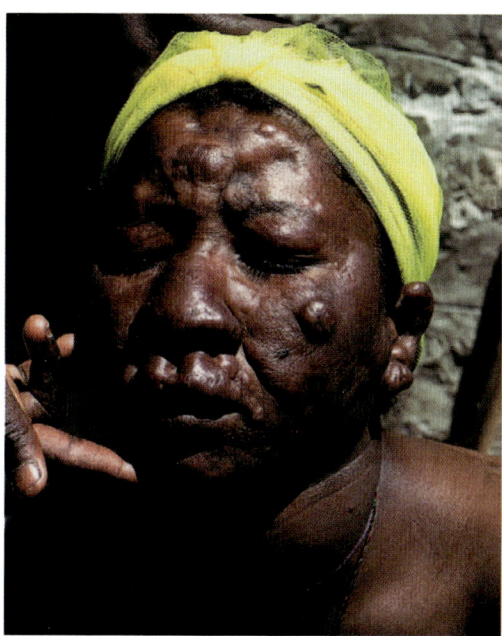

Figure 33.54 Diffuse cutaneous leishmaniasis due to *Leishmania aethiopica* in Ethiopia. The face is covered with infiltration and nodulation but there is no ulceration.

of the disease is due to *L. aethiopica* and has certain characteristic features [15]:
1 There is an initial lesion, which spreads locally, and from which the disease disseminates to other parts of the skin, often involving large areas (Figure 33.54).
2 The lesions are nodules that do not ulcerate.
3 There is a superabundance of parasites in the lesions.
4 The histology is characteristic in that macrophages full of amastigotes predominate.
5 Internal organs are not invaded and there is no history of kala-azar.
6 The leishmanin test and other tests of specific cellular immunity are negative.
7 The disease progresses slowly and becomes chronic.
8 Treatment produces only gradual improvement and relapse is the rule.

Under the influence of treatment, the histology changes towards the tuberculoid in a proportion of patients, and they may recover completely. Cases of coincident leishmaniasis and leprosy have been described, and show that the immune deficiency of each condition is specific [24].

American cutaneous leishmaniasis and mucocutaneous leishmaniasis.

Cutaneous leishmaniasis due to *L. mexicana* complex. The vector of *L. m. mexicana* bites humans reluctantly, so only those who spend long periods of time in the forest, such as chicle collectors, are at risk. The lesions behave like those of *L. major* or *L. tropica*. Most are on the side of the face or behind the ears (Table 33.6). Lesions on the pinna of the ear may invade cartilage, take many years to heal and destroy the pinna [25]. *Leishmania mexicana amazonensis* is extremely common in forest rodents, but the vector is not anthropophilic, so human infections are rare. A large proportion of them give rise to diffuse cutaneous leishmaniasis, which does not differ significantly from its counterpart in the Old World, due to *L. aethiopica* [26].

Cutaneous leishmaniasis due to *L. brasiliensis* complex [27]. Sores are often large deep ulcers, usually with a raised edge. Sores due to *L. b. guyanensis* are often fleshy and protuberant, usually on the limbs, often multiple, and resemble those of yaws, 'pian bois' [28]. This parasite and *L. b. panamensis* are especially associated with lesions along the draining lymphatics, but these may occur with any species. The lymphatic lesions may remain as discrete small nodules or may become inflamed and break through the skin to resemble the primary lesion. Lymphadenopathy is seldom marked.

Cutaneous leishmaniasis due to *L. b. peruviana*: 'uta' [29]. Lesions are less severe than those of *L. b. brasiliensis*. They heal spontaneously and are not known to cause mucocutaneous leishmaniasis.

Investigations

In endemic areas, or in travellers returned from endemic areas, the clinical diagnosis is not difficult in the case of typical sores. A positive diagnosis of cutaneous leishmaniasis (Old World and New World types) can be suggested, and in most cases confirmed, by the presence of one or more of the following criteria:
1 History of exposure to an endemic area in the previous weeks or months.
2 History of sandfly bites in the previous weeks or months.
3 History of high-risk activities such as sleeping outdoors, jungle or desert trekking.
4 Non-healing chronic nodular violaceous ulcer for 4–6 weeks or longer.
5 Demonstration of amastigotes in Giemsa-stained smears from infected skin by direct microscopy.
6 Demonstration of intracellular amastigotes in the dermis of H&E sections of skin.
7 Presence of leishmanial granulomas in the dermis in H&E specimens.
8 Growth of promastigotes in Nicolle–Novy–MacNeal (NNN) culture medium from lesional specimens.
9 Demonstration of leishmanial DNA by PCR.

Deeper subcutaneous sores (the so-called volcano lesion), sores arising from lymphatic spread or chronic sores in which scarring predominates may present difficulties. Confirmation is through the demonstration of the parasite. Usually, this is best achieved by making a smear of material from the sore and staining it with a Wright, a Giemsa or a Leishman stain on a microscope slide. The smear may be made from the exudate from the sore and is often positive even if purulent because secondary bacterial infection is unusual. Alternatively, a slit-skin smear is made, as for leprosy, being careful to avoid taking blood from the nodular part of the lesion. Parasites are usually readily seen in sores that have not yet started to heal but are difficult to see thereafter. Alternatively, material may be obtained through a needle or with a dental broach [30].

Ideally, material should also be cultured on NNN or similar medium. At the time of taking the lesional skin biopsy for histological examination, a portion of it should be cultured and dab smears made from the cut surface of the other portion before it is fixed.

Leishmania are harder to see and identify in sections than in smears. In chronic leishmaniasis especially, histology may not be able to distinguish leishmaniasis from sarcoidosis, tuberculosis or other tuberculoid pathologies. However, in acute forms with or without the presence of amastigotes, the presence of a granuloma has a high diagnostic sensitivity.

In all forms of cutaneous leishmaniasis, the leishmanin test will be positive once the stage of crusting has been reached [30]. The test is negative in the diffuse anergic forms. The leishmanin test, also called the Montenegro test, particularly in Central and South America, is a suspension of 5×10^6 cultured promastigotes of *Leishmania* spp. (*L. major* is commonly used for cutaneous diagnosis in Old World leishmaniasis) per millilitre of 0.5% phenol saline: 0.1 mL is injected into the volar surface of the forearm and the result read at 48–72 h. The antigen is normally standardised so that an induration of 5 mm or more, measured by the ballpoint technique, is positive [31]. While interpreting the result in an individual patient, it is important to take into consideration the prevalence rate in the control population. This intradermal skin test is not useful for the diagnosis of current cutaneous leishmaniasis as a positive result may indicate previous sensitisation. Moreover, there are also problems of cross-reactivity among different *Leishmania* spp., and therefore the Montenegro test is not useful for particular epidemiological settings where infections by different *Leishmania* spp. overlap.

Molecular diagnostic tests to detect leishmanial DNA by PCR have been available for several years. Assays can be carried out by using nuclear DNA and more recently the diagnostic sensitivity was significantly enhanced by using kinetoplast minicircle DNA [32]. The sensitivity of this test has been reported to be between 92% and 98% with 100% specificity by several authors [32]. A variety of clinical specimens, including cotton swabs and archival smears or paraffin-embedded skin sections, can be used as the DNA source for the PCR diagnosis. Ideally, the diagnosis of cutaneous leishmaniasis should achieve a species and subspecies specific level, as this has therapeutic and prognostic implications.

Management

Old World cutaneous leishmaniasis

Most sores will heal spontaneously, but their duration cannot be predicted in an individual case. It is reasonable to try topical methods of treatment for simple sores and to reserve the systemic use of pentavalent antimonials for problematic sores: these include sores where scarring would be disabling or severely disfiguring; sores that will not heal easily, for example on the lower leg or over a joint; sores involving mucosa or cartilage; or sores that might be due to parasites of the *L. brasiliensis* group. Thermotherapy is an effective, localised treatment: heating a sore to 50°C for 30 seconds over 1–3 sessions promotes healing but is technically difficult [33,34]. Small single sores may be frozen with cryotherapy [35], curetted under local anaesthetic [36] or infiltrated with 1–2 mL sodium stibogluconate or meglumine antimoniate, on one or two occasions a few days apart. Careful attention to technique is essential [37]. Local therapy using the aminoglycoside paromomycin in an ointment is another option [34].

Systemic treatment is with sodium stibogluconate or meglumine antimoniate by intravenous or intramuscular injection in a single daily dose of 20 mg antimony/kg, for as long as it takes to produce clinical and parasitological healing and a few days longer: usually 20 days for cutaneous leishmaniasis and 28 days for mucosal and visceral leishmaniasis [38]. Sores due to *L. brasiliensis* should be treated for the full 21 days [39]. *Leishmania aethiopica* is not sensitive to antimony at this dosage alone [26] and, when systemic treatment is justified, patients should also be treated with paromomycin in a dose of 15 mg/kg for 60 days or as long as necessary [34]. *L. major* can be treated with fluconazole 200 mg orally once daily for 6 weeks [34]. Patients with diffuse cutaneous leishmaniasis require treatment for many months beyond clinical and demonstrable parasitic cure [15]. Leishmaniasis recidivans (lupoid) may respond to local infiltration after nodulectomy or systemic antimonials. The additional use of steroids has helped some cases [20]. Severe scarring may require plastic repair. After healing, patients are normally immune to reinfection with the same species, although second sores in old age, or due to a parasite of a different zymodeme, have been reported. Cutaneous leishmaniasis in the immunocompromised host may manifest many years after exposure to the infective bite.

It is clear that the available treatments for cutaneous leishmaniasis are far from satisfactory. In addition, reported therapeutic failures with pentavalent antimonials have been described as an increasing problem in endemic regions for visceral leishmaniasis in India and also as an emerging problem in New World cutaneous leishmaniasis among returned travellers to the UK [40]. Novel approaches include combination therapeutic regimens using antimonials and immunostimulating agents. Intravenous treatment with pentavalent antimonials results in a number of common adverse reactions and side effects including hepatic, pancreatic, musculoskeletal and cardiac toxicity. Elderly patients seem to be more frequently and severely affected by these symptoms.

New World cutaneous leishmaniasis and mucocutaneous leishmaniasis [18]

This is summarised in Table 33.6. As with Old World leishmaniasis, intralesional antimonials, paromomycin ointment and thermotherapy are effective local therapies. *L. mexicana* is susceptible to ketoconazole 600 mg orally once daily for 4 weeks [34]. Lesions due to *L. b. guyanensis* are particularly liable to relapse. Lesions due to *L. b. brasiliensis* should be treated systemically for a week beyond parasitological cure, in order to prevent mucocutaneous leishmaniasis from developing [39]. Previously untreated patients with mucocutaneous leishmaniasis respond to pentavalent antimonials in a dose of 20 mg/kg/day, if given daily for 3–4 weeks [41]. Only 20% of relapsed patients will respond to the drug. Liposomal amphotericin B is the drug of second choice, given in a dose of 2–3 mg/kg for at least 20 days. Treatment that is inadequate in dose or duration leads to relapse and drug resistance. Secondary infection should be treated. Corticosteroids are useful to prevent laryngeal oedema that can otherwise complicate the start of treatment of laryngeal disease.

Miltefosine is an oral alkylphosphocholine drug that has activity against cutaneous, mucocutaneous and visceral leishmaniasis. A phosphocholine analogue, it is thought to interfere with cell-signalling pathways and it may interfere with parasite lipid biosynthetic enzyme synthesis. Miltefosine appears to have efficacy against *L. v. mexicana*, *L. v. panamensis*, *L. v. guyanensis* and *L. v. braziliensis* infection [34,42–45]. There is limited data available on miltefosine's efficacy against Old World leishmaniasis. Side effects of miltefosine include anorexia, nausea, vomiting and diarrhoea. The drug is contraindicated in pregnant women. The drug is given at 2.5 mg/kg (maximum 150 mg) orally once daily for 28 days. Additionally, the affordability of miltefosine continues to remain a critical issue making it an inaccessible treatment option for the majority of patients.

> **Treatment ladder for cutaneous leishmaniasis**
>
> Regimens for MCL from all species [34]:
> - Antimonials 20 mg/kg per day IV or IM OD for 30 days
> - Antimonials 20 mg/kg per day IV or IM OD for 30 days plus pentoxifylline 400 mg PO every 8 h for 30 days
> - Amphotericin B deoxycholate 0.7–1 mg/kg IV every other day up to 25–45 doses
> - Liposomal amphotericin B 2–3 mg/kg IV OD for up to a total dose of 40–60 mg/kg
> - Miltefosine 2.5–3.3 mg/kg PO OD for 28 days (in Bolivia)

Cutaneous leishmaniasis in the returned traveller. Common and rare forms of cutaneous leishmaniasis are increasingly being described in non-endemic regions of the world. A recent retrospective survey at the Hospital for Tropical Diseases in London disclosed more than 50 new cases, including Old and New World cutaneous infections by *L. tropica*, *L. v. braziliensis*, *L. major* and *L. donovani* complex. Patients with infections acquired in the New World manifested a more severe clinical picture and therefore sought medical referral at an earlier stage. The diagnosis was established by all four standard investigations including Giemsa smears for direct microscopy, H&E histology, parasitological culture and molecular diagnosis by PCR. Intravenous or intralesional treatment with sodium stibogluconate and other less frequently used agents resulted in cure for most of these patients. Daily oral itraconazole or allopurinol in combination with weekly intralesional sodium stibogluconate has been successful for most cases of simple cutaneous leishmaniasis. Educational strategies to increase the awareness of cutaneous leishmaniasis as an emerging problem in the UK are being directed at general practitioners, dermatologists and the public.

Visceral leishmaniasis

Definition and nomenclature
Leishmania donovani donovani and its close relative *L. donovani infantum* are, in contrast with the other species of *Leishmania* that infect humans, normally viscerotropic, and cause a severe systemic infection, which may be accompanied by cutaneous manifestations.

> **Synonyms and inclusions**
> - Kala-azar
> - Death fever
> - Dum-dum fever

Epidemiology
Incidence and prevalence
There are four main zoogeographical zones in which visceral leishmaniasis is found (Table 33.5). Transmission is peridomestic and tends to be stable in the Mediterranean. Dogs are the reservoir. Young children are most commonly affected.

Age
Infected adults tend to develop self-healing skin sores. In Brazil, peridomestic transmission from raiding foxes affects older children. A similar age group is affected in East Africa, where transmission of disease takes place outside the houses in the evenings. In India, where the human is the reservoir, epidemics occur every 15 years or so and all age groups, previously uninfected, are susceptible. Travellers and tourists of any age group are susceptible in any of the four zones.

Pathophysiology
Causative organisms (Figure 33.55)
- *Leishmania donovani donovani*
- *Leishmania donovani infantum*

In over 90% of cases, the infection is subclinical and cutaneous hypersensitivity and immunity develop [1]. In the others, especially in the malnourished, the parasite invades and multiplies in reticuloendothelial cells of the spleen, liver, lymphoid tissue, bone marrow and gut submucosa. This reticuloendothelial bombardment is associated with the overproduction of polyclonal IgG, specific antibody production and the formation of high titres of immune complexes and various autoantibodies.

Clinical features
Presentation [2,3]
After an incubation period of weeks to months, sometimes exceeding a year, fever develops, either insidiously or abruptly. The commonest additional symptoms are fatigue, discomfort from the presence of the enlarged spleen and cough, diarrhoea and epistaxis. Gross splenomegaly is the dominant physical sign; hepatomegaly, lymphadenopathy in some endemic zones and signs of malnutrition, including pedal oedema, red straight hair in Africans and wasting also occur. Hypersplenism causes anaemia, leukopenia and thrombocytopenia. Organ function is usually well preserved until late in the disease, but specific and non-specific indices of cell-mediated immunity are depressed, and secondary infections are common and often fatal [4]. In a few cases in Africa, a primary skin sore has been described, like those of cutaneous leishmaniasis. Rarely, there may be an accompanying mucosal lesion. In Indian people especially, the skin of the face, hands, feet and abdomen becomes hyperpigmented, even black: 'kala-azar' means black sickness. Despite epistaxis and sometimes jaundice, there is no evidence of cutaneous bleeding. In Iran, patients have been seen with numerous skin lesions [5].

Clinical variants
Post-kala-azar dermal leishmaniasis (PKDL) (dermal leishmanoid).
In 5% of east African patients and 20% of Indian patients, a rash develops after the visceral disease has healed, either spontaneously

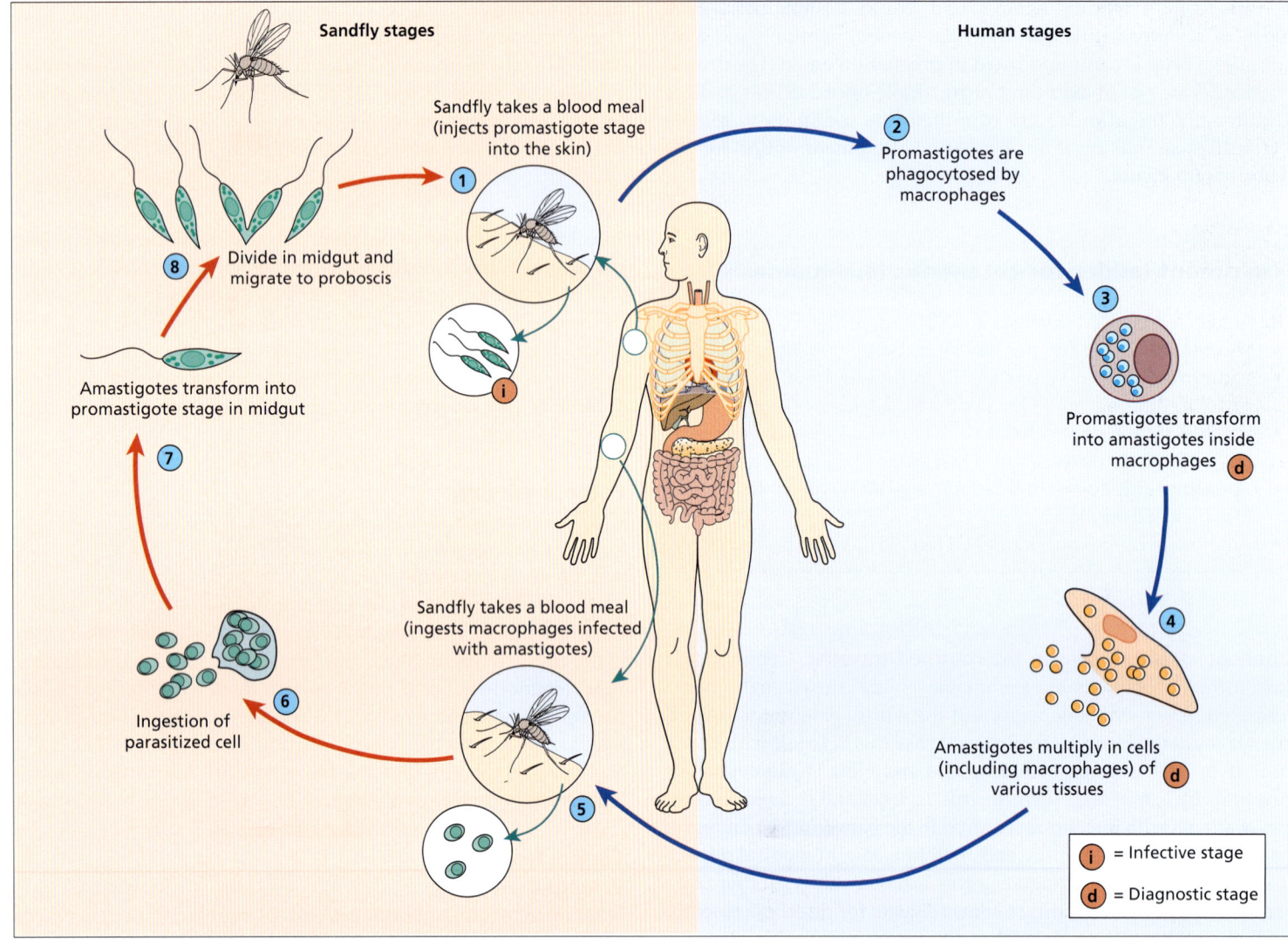

Figure 33.55 Life cycle of leishmaniasis parasite. Courtesy of the Centers for Disease Control and Prevention. https://www.cdc.gov/dpdx/leishmaniasis/index.html (last accessed February 2023).

or following treatment. A small proportion of patients with PKDL give no previous history of visceral disease. In Africa [6], the rash begins during convalescence, appearing on the cheeks, chin, ears and extensor aspects of the forearms, buttocks and lower legs (Figure 33.56). Usually, the rash comprises discrete papules, which on histological examination show a tuberculoid histology with scanty parasites. The leishmanin test is positive. The rash heals spontaneously over a few months. Presumably, it represents the acquisition of specific cellular immunity that is clearing up scattered parasites that remained in the skin. Both cellular immunity and pentavalent antimonials are less efficient in the skin than in the viscera.

In India, by contrast, the rash appears 1–2 years after recovery, as hypopigmented macules, similar in appearance and distribution to those of lepromatous leprosy (Figure 33.57). After a variable period of years or months, diffuse nodulation begins to develop in these macules (Figure 33.58). The rash is progressive over many years and seldom heals spontaneously. The tongue, palate and genitalia may be involved. There may be lymphadenopathy, but the viscera are spared and there are no features of relapse of the previous systemic infection. Presumably, this condition represents cellular immunity against a dermotrophic mutant of *L. donovani*. PKDL is thought to represent the intraepidemic reservoir of infection of visceral leishmaniasis in India.

The various lesions seen in PKDL are reflected in the histology of the type of lesion biopsied. Typically, histology shows a poorly differentiated infiltrate of chronic inflammatory cells, with a variable number of *Leishmania* in dermal macrophages [7]. A characteristic histomorphology in nodules is prominent follicular plugging with a dense plasma cell-rich lymphohistiocytic dermal infiltrate that shows an abrupt cut-off in the lower dermis [8]. The leishmanin test is usually negative but becomes positive after successful treatment [9].

Complications and co-morbidities

Visceral leishmaniasis in patients with HIV [10] (Chapter 31). The main area of overlap of these two infections is in southern Europe, especially Spain. Leishmaniasis may be acquired prior to or after

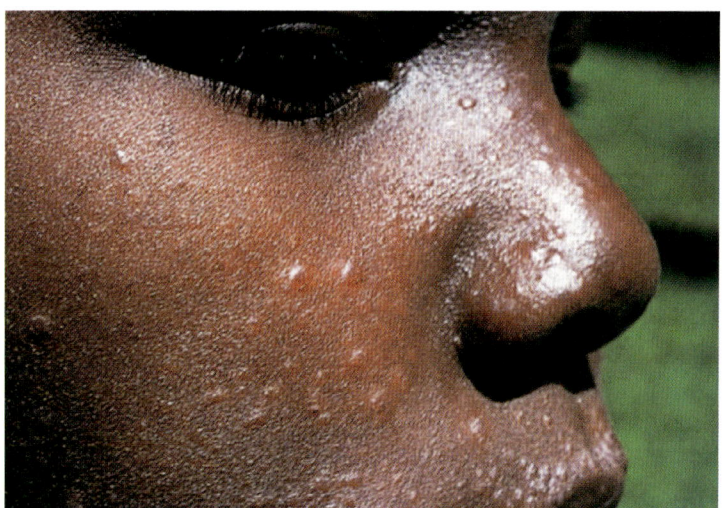

Figure 33.56 Post-kala-azar dermal leishmaniasis. Typical facial papules in a Kenyan arising 6 weeks after treatment and healing spontaneously. Courtesy of Dr J.D. Chulay.

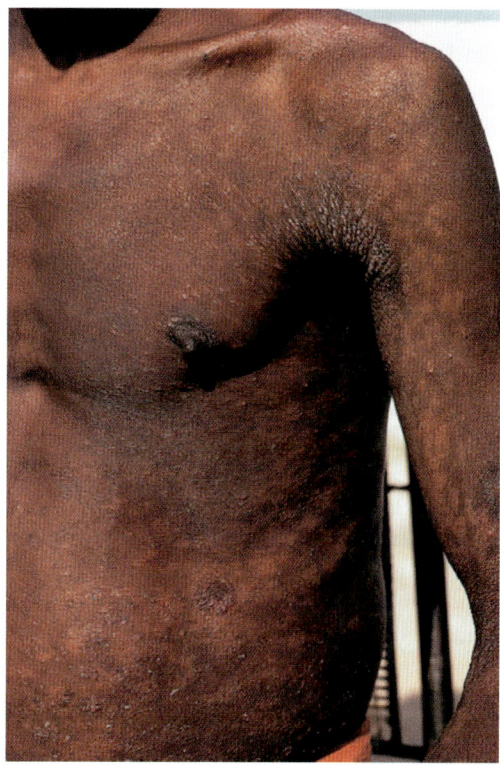

Figure 33.58 Post-kala-azar dermal leishmaniasis. A later stage than that shown in Figure 33.57. Papules are beginning to develop.

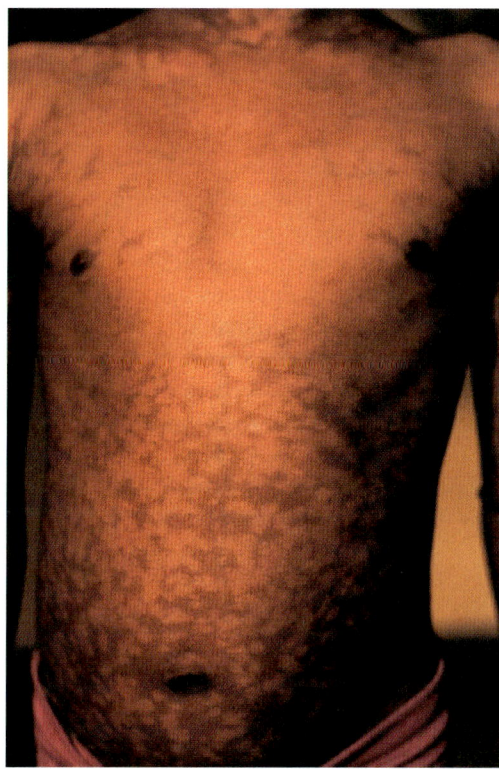

Figure 33.57 Post-kala-azar dermal leishmaniasis showing the extensive hypopigmented macular rash.

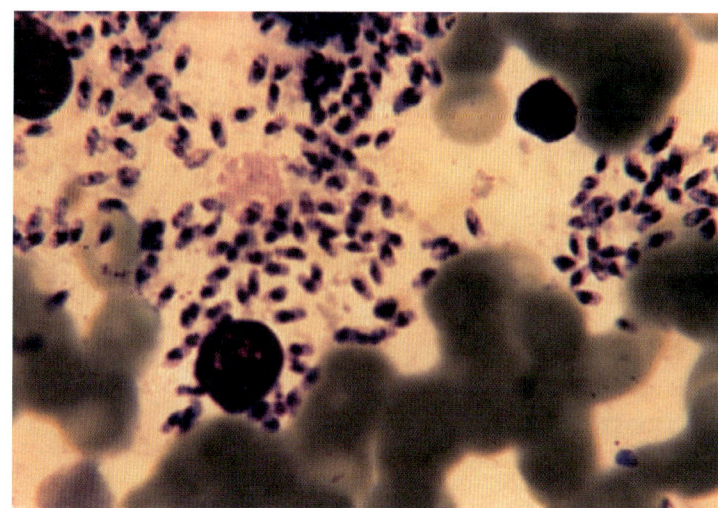

Figure 33.59 Amastigotes of *Leishmania infantum* in a bone marrow smear from a patient with visceral leishmaniasis and AIDS. Courtesy of Mr A.H. Moody.

the HIV infection and may thus be primary or secondary to the HIV infection. In some patients, typical characteristics of fever and splenomegaly have not been present and serological tests have been negative. On occasion, the parasite has been discovered by chance, for example in the biopsy of Kaposi sarcoma, and disseminated dermatofibroma-like lesions containing amastigotes have been described in a patient with AIDS co-infected with visceral *L. donovani* [11]. Aspirates of bone marrow and spleen show extremely heavy parasitisation. Relapse and mortality rates are high. Treatment should be prolonged and monitored by splenic aspirates.

Investigations

In visceral leishmaniasis, parasites may be demonstrated in aspirates of the spleen, bone marrow, liver or lymph node, in that order of likelihood (Figure 33.59). In PKDL, slit-skin smears are usually positive. Antibodies to *Leishmania* spp. may be demonstrated by a variety of techniques: indirect immunofluorescence, ELISA and direct agglutination tests are commonly performed [12]. The leishmanin test is negative, except in African PKDL.

Management

For visceral leishmaniasis, liposomal amphotericin B is the drug with the highest therapeutic value and best safety profile [13]. The antimonial drugs, such as sodium stibogluconate and meglumine antimoniate, remain the most widely used agents. Case fatality without treatment is over 90%. Supportive therapy to address concomitant anaemia, haemorrhage and secondary infection is all part of an optimal treatment regimen.

Miltefosine is an additional approved oral agent for the treatment of visceral leishmaniasis in adult patients infected with *L. donovani* who weigh at least 30 kg. The US Food and Drug Administration approved dose for patients 30–44 kg is 50 mg twice a day for 28 days and, for patients over 45 kg, the recommended dose is 50 mg three times a day for 28 days [14]. The mechanism of action of this therapy is not well understood. As a phosphocholine analogue, it is thought to interfere with cell-signalling pathways and it may interfere with parasite lipid biosynthetic enzyme synthesis [15]. In one clinical trial in India, the drug had a cure rate of 94% at 6 months in a cohort of 299 patients [16].

Treatment ladder for visceral leishmaniasis

First line
- Liposomal amphotericin B 3 mg/kg/day × 7–10 days
- Miltefosine for adult patients infected with *L. donovani* who weigh at least 30 kg: 30–44 kg, 50 mg twice daily × 28 days; 45 kg or more, 50 mg three times daily × 28 days

Second line
- Amphotericin B desoxycholate 0.75–1.0 mg/kg IV every other day for 30 days
- Sodium stibogluconate 20 mg/kg IV or IM OD for 28 days

Toxoplasmosis

Definition

Toxoplasmosis is caused by the intracellular protozoan *Toxoplasma gondii* that can cause acquired or congenital infections. Most persons infected are asymptomatic; cutaneous involvement is rare but described below.

Epidemiology

The prevalence of *Toxoplasma* infection in humans varies widely. Seroprevalence is low (10–30%) in North America, Northern Europe and Southeast Asia, moderate (30–50%) in Central and Southern Europe, and high in Latin America and tropical African countries [1]. Cutaneous toxoplasmosis is uncommon, occurring in less than 10% of acquired infections [2].

Pathophysiology
Pathology

The organism tends to invade the reticuloendothelial system and the endothelium of the blood vessels, forming granulomas with necrosis of affected tissues.

Causative organisms
- *Toxoplasma gondii*

The disease is caused by *Toxoplasma gondii*, a tiny sporozoon often assuming a crescentic shape, first identified in 1908 in a North African rodent, *Ctenodactylus gondii*. Cats are definitive hosts and a form of *Toxoplasma* cyst can be found in their faeces. Rodents and birds are the intermediate hosts. Larger mammals including humans are infected incidentally, by eating raw infected meat or by ingesting oocysts in contaminated food or water.

Clinical features
Presentation

Toxoplasmosis causes four types of disease in humans [3]:
1. An acute febrile lymphadenopathy.
2. Fetal infection, causing brain damage.
3. Ocular disease, usually due to reactivation of fetal infection.
4. Disseminated disease in immunocompromised patients, including those with HIV infection, causing fulminating encephalitis.

Skin changes are uncommon and non-specific. In the congenital disease [3], macular and haemorrhagic eruptions predominate. Occasionally, abnormal hair growth and exfoliative dermatitis have been seen. In the acquired disease, macular, maculopapular, papular and haemorrhagic eruptions also occur and may be followed by scarlatiniform desquamation. A dermatomyositis-like syndrome is described [4,5] and one case with clinical similarities to graft-versus-host disease has been reported [6]. A wide variety of other lesions have been described including vesicles and bullae [7], nodules [8,9], ulcers [10], livedo annularis, urticaria and an eruption-like pityriasis lichenoides; conclusive evidence of a causal relationship is not always clear.

Investigations

Diagnosis is made on clinical evidence and may be confirmed by demonstration of the organism in a biopsy of lymph node, liver or spleen, bone marrow, or in cerebrospinal and ventricular fluid. Routinely, the diagnosis is made serologically. Several methods are available including the following:
1. The Sabin–Feldman dye test, positive early and declining over 1–2 years, which measures mainly IgG antibodies.
2. Direct agglutination of formalinised parasites, useful for screening, detects IgM and IgG antibodies.
3. Indirect fluorescence, simple and safe, can be used to distinguish IgM from IgG antibodies, as can an IgM ELISA.

Management

The sulphonamides and pyrimethamine (Daraprim®) act synergistically and are effective [6]. Severe side effects may occur due to interference with folic acid metabolism. Folinic acid should be given to patients receiving pyrimethamine. Therapy is typically provided for

4–6 weeks with re-evaluation at the end of the treatment course. Infections in immunologically normal individuals are not usually treated.

Trimethoprim plus sulfamethoxazole is the treatment of choice for central nervous system toxoplasmosis in immunocompromised patients.

Treatment ladder for toxoplasmosis

First line
- Pyrimethamine (adult dose) 100 mg × 1 day as a loading dose, followed by 25–50 mg per day, plus sulfadiazine 2–4 g daily for 2 days, followed by 500 mg to 1 g dose four times per day, plus folinic acid (leucovorin) 5–25 mg with each dose of pyrimethamine
- Pyrimethamine (pediatric dose) 2 mg/kg × 1 day, followed by 1 mg/kg each day after, plus sulfadiazine 50 mg/kg two times per day, plus folinic acid (leucovorin) 7.5 mg per day

Congenital infection of newborns
- Pyrimethamine 2 mg/kg per day orally, divided twice per day for the first 2 days; then from day 3 to 2 months (or 6 months if symptomatic) 1 mg/kg PO OD every day; then 1 mg/kg PO OD, three times per week
- Sulfadiazine 100 mg/kg PO OD divided twice per day
- Folinic acid (leucovorin): 10 mg, three times per week
- Treatment described above typically followed for 12 months

Central nervous system involvement
- Parenteral trimethoprim-sulfamethoxazole (5 mg/kg and 25 mg/kg)

Key references

The full list of references can be found in the online version at https://www.wiley.com/rooksdermatology10e

Infection with human nematodes
Onchoceriasis
1 Brattig NW. Pathogenesis and host responses in human onchocerciasis: impact of *Onchocerca* filariae and *Wolbachia* endobacteria. *Microbes Infect* 2004;6:113–28.

10 Brattig NW, Cheke RA, Garms R. Onchocerciasis (river blindness) – more than a century of research and control. *Acta Trop* 2020;218:105677.

Lymphatic filariasis
1 Taylor MJ, Hoerauf A, Bockarie M. Lymphatic filariasis and onchocerciasis. *Lancet* 2010;376(9747):1175–85.
7 Shenoy RK. Clinical and pathological aspects of filarial lymphedema and its management. *Korean J Parasitol* 2008;46:119–25.

Infection with trematodes
Schistosomiasis
6 Torres VM. Dermatologic manifestations of *Schistosomiasis mansoni*. *Arch Dermatol* 1976;112:1539–42.

Infection with cestodes
Sparganosis
1 Liu Q, Li MW, Wang ZD, Zhao GH, Zhu XQ. Human sparganosis, a neglected food borne zoonosis. *Lancet Infect Dis* 2015;15:1226–35.

Infection with protozoa
Trypansomiasis
4 Romaña C. *Enfermedad de Chagas*. Buenos Aires: Lopez Libreros Editores, 1963.
9 Pifano F. *Aspectos de Medicina Tropical de Venezuela*. Caracas: OBE, 1964.

Leishmaniasis
Cutaneous leishmaniasis
5 Weatherall DJ, Ledingham JGG, Warrell DA, eds. *Oxford Textbook of Medicine*, 2nd edn. Oxford: Oxford University Press, 1987.

Visceral leishmaniasis
2 Rees PH, Kager PA. Visceral leishmaniasis and postkala-azar dermal leishmaniasis. In: Peters W, Killick-Kendrick R, eds. *The Leishmaniases in Biology and Medicine*, Vol. 2. London: Academic Press, 1987:114–22.

CHAPTER 34

Arthropods

Charlotte Bernigaud[1,2,3], Gentiane Monsel[3,4], Pascal Delaunay[5] and Olivier Chosidow[2,3,6]

[1] UPEC-Université Paris-Est Créteil Val de Marne, Department of Dermatology, AP-HP, Hôpital Henri-Mondor, Créteil, France
[2] Research group Dynamyc, EA7380, Faculté de Médecine de Créteil, Ecole nationale vétérinaire d'Alfort, USC ANSES, Université Paris-Est Créteil, Créteil, France
[3] GrIDIST, Groupe Infectiologie Dermatologique – Infections Sexuellement Transmissibles, Société Française de Dermatologie
[4] Sorbonne Université, Department of Infectious and Tropical Diseases, AP-HP, Hôpital Pitié-Salpêtrière, Paris, France
[5] Department of Parasitology-Mycology, Centre Hospitalier Universitaire de Nice, Hôpital de l'Ardet, Nice, France
[6] AP-HP, University Hospital La Pitié-Salpêtrière, Paris, France

SKIN DISEASE DUE TO ARTHROPODS, 34.1
Definition, 34.1
Pathophysiology, 34.2
Mechanical trauma, 34.2
Injection of irritant, cytotoxic or pharmacologically active substances, 34.2
Injection of potential allergens, 34.2
Secondary infection, 34.2
Invasion of the host's tissues, 34.2
Contact reactions, 34.2
Reactions to retained mouthparts, 34.2
Transmission of disease, 34.2
Environmental factors, 34.2
Pathology, 34.3
Clinical features, 34.3
Investigations, 34.4
Management, 34.5
Prevention, 34.5
General management, 34.5

CLASS INSECTA, 34.6
Mosquitoes, gnats, midges and flies (Diptera), 34.6
Myiasis, 34.9
Fleas (Siphonaptera), 34.13
Tungiasis, 34.15

Bees, wasps and ants (Hymenoptera), 34.15
Lice (Phthiraptera), 34.18
Head lice (*Pediculus capitis*), 34.18
Clothing/body lice (*Pediculus corporis*), 34.23
Crab lice (*Phthiriasis pubis*), 34.24
Bugs (Hemiptera), 34.25
Family Cimicidae, 34.25
Family Reduviidae, 34.29
Family Anthocoridae, 34.29
Family Pentatomidae, 34.30
Family Belostomatidae, 34.30
Thrips (Thysanoptera), 34.30
Beetles (Coleoptera), 34.30
Cockroaches (Dictyoptera), 34.32
Locusts (Orthoptera), 34.32
Butterflies and moths (Lepidoptera), 34.32

CLASS ARACHNIDA, 34.34
Spiders (Araneae), 34.34
Family Theridiidae, 34.34
Family Hexathelidae, 34.35
Family Sicariidae (formerly Loxoscelidae), 34.35
Family Lycosidae (wolf spiders), 34.36
Other venomous species, 34.36

Scorpions (Scorpiones), 34.36
Ticks (Acari), 34.37
Mites (Acari), 34.41
Family Sarcoptidae: human classical scabies, 34.41
Family Sarcoptidae: human crusted scabies, 34.48
Family Sarcoptidae: animal scabies, 34.50
Family Knemidokoptidae, 34.50
Family Psoroptidae, 34.50
Family Listrophoridae, 34.50
Mites of stored products, 34.50
House-dust mites, 34.51
Pyemotes mites, 34.51
Family Tydeidae, 34.52
Plant mites, 34.52
Cheyletiella mites, 34.53
Harvest mites (Trombiculidae), 34.54
Bird, rodent and reptile mites (Gamasida), 34.54
Follicle mites (Demodicidae), 34.55

CLASS CHILOPODA (CENTIPEDES) AND DIPLOPODA (MILLIPEDES), 34.57
Centipedes, 34.57
Millipedes, 34.57

Key references, 34.58

SKIN DISEASE DUE TO ARTHROPODS

Definition

Arthropods are among the oldest animals. They are characterised by segmented bodies; paired, jointed appendages (legs and antennae); an exoskeleton; and a bilateral symmetry. They can grow only by moulting. Usually, arthropods go through the following life stages: egg, larva or nymph and finally mature adult (male or female).

The arthropod phylum is the most diverse of all the animal phyla, most of the species being in the class Insecta.

Arthropods can be divided into two groups: mandibulates with antennae and chelicerates without antennae. The mandibulates include insects, Chilopoda and Diplopoda. The chelicerates include scorpions, spiders and mites.

Pathophysiology

Arthropods produce their effects on the skin by a variety of mechanisms [1–4], more than one of which may be implicated simultaneously.

Mechanical trauma
The puncture wound or laceration produced by the penetration of the skin seldom causes serious disturbance to the host. The nature of the trauma inflicted depends upon the structure of the mouthparts, which show wide variation between different species. There are two methods of feeding on blood: (i) 'vessel feeders' insert the tip of their mouthparts into a capillary, and (ii) 'pool feeders' lacerate the skin, damage blood vessels and feed on the extravasated blood. Vessel feeders include sucking lice (Anoplura) and most mosquitoes, and pool feeders include stable flies and tsetse flies.

Injection of irritant, cytotoxic or pharmacologically active substances
An injected substance may contain pharmacologically active agents that produce local or, if in sufficient quantity, systemic effects. Salivary secretions and sting venoms may contain various enzymes such as hyaluronidase, proteases, peptidases and phospholipases; kinins; histamine-liberating agents; histamine; 5-hydroxytryptamine; or acetylcholine.

Injection of potential allergens
The vast majority of reactions to arthropod bites or stings depend upon the presence in the host of specific antibodies to antigenic substances in the arthropod saliva or venom. Investigation of extracts of venom sacs and salivary glands from many species, using modern immunological techniques, has demonstrated the presence of numerous antigens, some specific for a single species and others common to several related species or even to related genera [5].

The type of reaction provoked by an arthropod bite or sting in an individual patient largely depends on previous exposure to the same or related species. When an individual is bitten for the first time by a species whose salivary secretions contain no directly injurious substance, there is commonly no reaction. After repeated bites, sensitivity starts to develop, manifest by an itchy papule developing about 24 h after each bite, and persisting for several days. With prolonged exposure, an immediate weal reaction occurs, to be followed by the delayed papular reaction. After a further period of exposure, the delayed reaction no longer occurs, and eventually there is no reaction at all. The patient is then said to be immune. Mellanby [6] demonstrated this sequence of events with mosquito bites and a similar response is seen with the bites of many other arthropods.

Some patients show a severe systemic hypersensitivity to arthropod allergens, manifested by anaphylaxis. The antigenic substances in the venoms of Hymenoptera (bees, wasps, hornets) are more likely to induce severe systemic hypersensitivity reactions than are the antigens of most other insects.

The capacity of a patient to respond to an antigenic stimulus is also an important factor in determining the reaction to an arthropod. The reactions of patients who are immunosuppressed, as a result of either disease or therapy, are modified. 'Exaggerated reaction of insect bite', also called 'insect-bite-like reaction' or 'eosinophilic eruption of haematoproliferative disease', is a relatively common and disturbing skin reaction in chronic lymphocytic leukaemia patients [7]. It may be related to the immune dysregulation accompanying chronic lymphocytic leukaemia and further exacerbated by external factors, including actual insect bites, chemoimmunotherapy and pyogenic infection. The diagnosis is based on the clinical characteristics and findings of dermatitis with an eosinophil-rich infiltrate on biopsy [8]. Other examples include the response to bites or common scabies in patients with HIV infection and Epstein–Barr virus-associated natural killer cell leukaemia/lymphoma or the occurrence of crusted scabies in immunosuppressed individuals. In HIV-infected individuals, pruritic papular eruption may be a reaction to arthropod bites. The most accepted hypothesis is that this condition reflects an altered and exaggerated immune response to arthropod antigens in a subset of susceptible HIV-infected patients [9].

Secondary infection
Bacterial infection may be introduced at the time of the bite, but commonly gains entry as a result of scratching, and may confuse the clinical picture. Compartment syndrome caused by streptococcal cellulitis complicating an insect bite has been described [10].

Invasion of the host's tissues
Certain flies cause myiasis, in which the host's tissues are invaded by larvae.

Contact reactions
Simple contact with the secretions of certain arthropods, or with their living or dead bodies, may provoke irritant or allergic contact reactions. For example, the secretions of blister beetles produce a severe irritant reaction and repeated handling of cockroaches may induce contact urticaria and dermatitis.

Reactions to retained mouthparts
Persistent granulomatous papules or nodules may be provoked by retained mouthparts, for example those of ticks.

Transmission of disease
Many diseases have arthropod vectors, for example malaria (mosquitoes), leishmaniasis (sandflies) and trench fever and typhus (lice) (Table 34.1).

Environmental factors
There are a number of environmental and social factors that determine the range of arthropod species to which an individual is exposed.

Persons living and working in tropical climates tend to wear fewer clothes and therefore expose larger parts of their body to bites and stings. Clothing itself is essential to the existence of the body louse and areas of constriction of clothing affect the distribution of the skin lesions caused by certain mites (e.g. harvest mites).

Certain occupations carry an increased risk of reactions to arthropods [11]. Forestry workers, for example, may be exposed to the urticating hairs of the caterpillars of certain species of Lepidoptera

Table 34.1 Main arthropod-transmitted diseases.

Arthropods	Transmitted diseases
Insecta	
Mosquitoes and flies	Malaria, yellow fever, dengue fever, West Nile fever, chikungunya, Zika fever, viral encephalitis, sleeping sickness, onchocerciasis, leishmaniasis
Fleas	Typhus, bubonic plague
Lice	Typhus, trench fever, relapsing fever, bacteria?
Reduviid bugs	Chagas disease
Cockroaches	Bacteria?
Arachnida	
Ticks	Lyme borreliosis, Rocky Mountain spotted fever, tick paralysis, Colorado tick fever, babesiosis, ehrlichiosis, Q fever, tularaemia
Mites	Scrub typhus

and dockworkers handling foodstuffs may be attacked by mites infesting the cargo.

In some societies, humans are exposed to attack by parasites of the domestic animals with which they cohabit.

Housing can influence exposure to arthropod attack in a number of ways. Overcrowded homes favour transmission of ectoparasites, such as lice and the scabies mite. Spiders and scorpions will take up residence in garages, outhouses and woodpiles.

The methods by which an arthropod is attracted to its host species include body heat, carbon dioxide in exhaled air (e.g. mosquitoes, ticks, fleas, bedbugs), the view (e.g. tsetse fly) and displacement of air or vibrations caused by the host (e.g. fleas) [12]. Human sweat contains mosquito attractants and anhidrotic subjects are unattractive to mosquitoes [13,14]. The human skin microflora may be responsible for producing compounds that attract mosquitoes and, as there is variation in the microflora between individuals, body odour probably contributes to susceptibility to biting [15,16]. Recently, it was shown that malaria-infected mosquitoes express enhanced attraction to human odour [17]. Human odour also appears to play a part in attracting sandflies [18]. Pregnant women appear to be more attractive to mosquitoes than the non-pregnant [19,20].

There is also a suggestion of increased susceptibility to mosquito bites in patients with HIV infection receiving antiretroviral therapy and suffering from lipoatrophy [21].

Alcohol ingestion also seems to promote mosquito attraction [22].

Certain species of flies are attracted to skin ulcers and purulent material, in which they lay their eggs.

Insect pheromones play a part in attacks by large numbers of Hymenoptera. Honeybees, when stinging, emit an alarm pheromone from glands in their sting chambers and this guides other bees to attack an intruder.

Pathology [23–25]

The histopathological changes associated with arthropod bites depend upon a number of factors, including the arthropod involved, the type of immunological reaction provoked and the duration of the lesion.

In the acute phase, there is a superficial and deep, perivascular and interstitial inflammatory infiltrate, which is characteristically wedge shaped. The infiltrate is usually mixed in composition with an abundance of lymphocytes and eosinophils, although neutrophils and histiocytes can also be seen. Neutrophils may predominate in reactions to fleas, mosquitoes, fire ants and brown recluse spiders. Sweet-like reaction to arthropod bites has also been reported [26]. Over the most prominent superficial infiltrates spongiosis can be seen, sometimes with progression to vesicle formation or epidermal necrosis.

In papular urticaria there is prominent papillary dermal oedema and a perivascular chronic inflammatory infiltrate with a significant admixture of eosinophils.

Bullous reactions develop beneath a more or less intact epidermis and may be multilocular.

In older lesions, excoriated areas may be altered by the scratching, resulting in parakeratosis and a dermal infiltrate with neutrophils and lymphocytes.

Chronic reactions often have a pseudolymphomatous appearance. The dermis contains a dense inflammatory infiltrate of lymphoid cells and histiocytes, with an admixture of eosinophils and plasma cells, and the presence of atypical mononuclear cells with hyperchromatic nuclei. Secondary lymphoid follicles with germinal centres are sometimes formed. Multinucleated cells may also occur. If retained mouthparts are present, there may also be giant cells of foreign-body type.

Additional histopathological features associated with particular arthropods are noted in the relevant sections of this chapter.

Clinical features

The very large number of species of biting and stinging arthropods, their different feeding habits and the variation in individual patients' responses to the various irritants and allergens injected determine the diversity of clinical features. Any arthropod bite can be totally asymptomatic. The type and distribution of lesions produced by individual arthropods are discussed in the relevant sections throughout this chapter. Table 34.2 shows the clinical and epidemiological features of the main arthropod bites. Clinical features of arthropod bites are not specific, so diagnosis relies on an array of arguments, none of which is specific by itself; it is the association of elements that is suggestive.

The most frequently encountered response is papular urticaria. Initially, an extremely itchy urticarial weal develops at the site of the bite and this is succeeded by a firm pruritic papule, which usually persists for several days. The weal and papule may show a central haemorrhagic punctum and the papule may be surmounted by a tiny vesicle. Lesions are often grouped in clusters and develop in crops at irregular intervals.

Table 34.2 Arthropod bites: main clinical and epidemiological features.

Arthropod	Clinical feature on examination	Location over the body	Timing of pruritus	Context
Bedbugs	3–4 bites in a line or curve	Uncovered areas	Morning	Travelling
Fleas	3–4 bites in a line or curve	Potentially anywhere, lower limbs	Daytime	Pet owners or rural living
Mosquitoes	Non-specific papules	Potentially anywhere	*Anopheles* spp. night; *Culex* spp. night; *Aedes* spp. day	Worldwide distribution
Head lice [28]	Eggs attached to hairs; live lice on the head associated with itchy, excoriated lesions	Scalp, ears and neck	Any	Children, parents or contact with children
Body lice [28]	Excoriated papules and hyperpigmentation; live lice inside clothes	Back	Any	Homeless people, low and middle incomes
Pubic lice	Pruritus on pubis, excoriated papules and non-specific secondary lesions, inguinal lymphadenopathy; live lice attached to pubic hairs ± eggs	Pubic hair, more rarely on armpits or eyebrows, eyelashes or beard	Any	Young adults, sexually transmitted
Scabies [28]	Vesicles, burrows, nodules and non-specific secondary lesions	Interdigital spaces, forearms, breasts, genitalia	Night	Sexually transmitted, households or institutions
Ticks	Erythema migrans or ulcer	Potentially anywhere	Asymptomatic	Pet owners or hikers
Harvest mites	Multiple urticarial papules, in a line or in a bouquet	Covered areas, under elastic bands in underwear or the pants belt	Daytime	Outdoor, gardening; summer or autumn
Pyemotes ventricosus [29]	Comet sign, a linear red macular tract	Under clothes	Any time when inside habitat	People exposed to woodworm contaminated furniture (*P. ventricosus* is a woodworm parasite)
Spiders	Two closely adjacent bite points ± necrosis (uncommon)	Face and arms	Immediate pain, no itching	Rural living

Adapted from Bernardeschi et al. [27]. Source and copyright holder: BMJ Publishing Group Ltd.

The number and distribution of skin lesions produced by the bites depend upon the type of exposure and the feeding habits of the arthropod involved. New bites by the same species will often cause a recrudescence of activity in existing lesions.

Bullous reactions are common on the lower legs (Figure 34.1), but may occur in other sites, especially in children. In the presence of lower limb venous hypertension, haemorrhagic or ulcerated lesions may develop. More severe local changes are sometimes found, with cellulitis and lymphangitis in the apparent absence of secondary infection. Eruptive pseudoangiomatosis-like lesions have also been reported as a response to arthropod bites [30,31].

Irritation is an almost constant symptom, and rubbing and scratching may increase the inflammatory changes and induce eczematisation. When the bites are very numerous, or if the local reaction is severe, there may be fever and malaise.

Secondary infection is a common complication and may manifest as impetigo, folliculitis, cellulitis and lymphangitis.

Anaphylactic shock is unusual except after Hymenoptera stings, but is occasionally seen with some other arthropods.

Bite reactions may persist for months. Tick attachment sites, in which the mouthparts may be retained, are the most likely to persist, but so may bites of mosquitoes and other arthropods.

Investigations

The diagnosis of arthropod bites is often self-evident, for example when the patient has spent the afternoon in the garden on a hot day in summer and subsequently develops typical lesions on exposed areas of skin. However, difficulty arises when the source of the bites is not immediately obvious. Only good clinical observation and specific questions will suggest a particular insect and collection of it is necessary for subsequent examination.

The distribution of the bites may provide a clue to their origin (see Table 34.2), for example localisation to the abdomen and thighs in cheyletiellosis or contact with sarcoptic mange in dogs, and involvement of the legs below the knees when the lesions are produced by cat or dog fleas. Patients should be asked about domestic pets; not only their own, but also those in the homes of close relatives who are visited regularly, as ectoparasites associated with pet animals are often the source of persistent arthropod bites. If the bites are not localised, but scattered all over the body, consider reactions to arthropods biting in the patient's bedroom, such as bird fleas, bird mites or bedbugs. Enquire if the patient has recently moved house. It may be that the previous owners of the new home kept pet animals and have left a legacy of domestic flea infestation. Even if the house remained empty for a considerable time before the new owners took up residence, the flea population will be waiting in cocoons to emerge when the new occupants arrive. Adult fleas can survive starvation for variable lengths of time depending upon species and environmental conditions [12,32] – a newly emerged and unfed dog flea, *Ctenocephalides canis*, will survive for approximately 60 days. In the absence of their natural hosts, such animal flea populations will not usually survive for more than a few months.

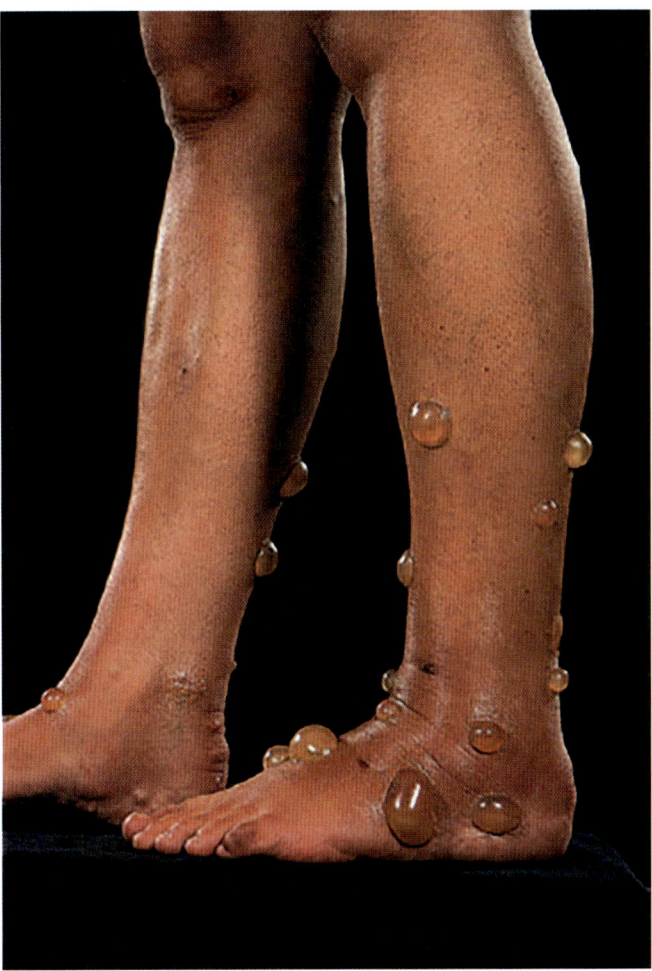

Figure 34.1 Bullous lesions in response to arthropod bites. Courtesy of Dr F. A. Ive, Durham, UK.

If the history and examination do not suggest a possible source for the problem, or if the dermatologist wishes to confirm a suspected source, the following procedures may be useful [33,34]:

1 The patient's pet animals should be examined, if possible, for signs of skin disease. Cheyletiellosis and canine scabies produce characteristic changes on an affected animal [35]. Vigorous combing of scale from the coat of a dog suffering from cheyletiellosis (Figure 34.2) will provide material in which *Cheyletiella* mites may be identified and skin scrapings will confirm sarcoptic mange. If the animal cannot be examined, the patient should be provided with a sheet of black paper and asked to collect brushings or combings from the animal's coat for subsequent examination.

2 If domestic infestation with cat or dog fleas is suspected, this can often be confirmed by examination of debris from the pet's bedding. The patient is supplied with a large polythene bag and instructed to place the pet's bedding in the bag and shake it vigorously for a few minutes. The bedding is then removed, the bag sealed and delivered to the dermatologist or parasitologist for microscopy of the debris. Macroscopically, flea eggs and faeces have a 'pepper and salt' appearance (Figure 34.3) and the larvae are grub-like. For identification, adult fleas should be 'cleared' in 10% potassium hydroxide for 24 h so that the majority of the pigment is removed and the anatomical details revealed. Cat and dog fleas are readily identified, but if unfamiliar species are encountered, the help of an entomologist with an interest in Siphonaptera should be sought. Correct identification of fleas is important so that proper control measures may be carried out [36].

3 If problems from bird fleas or bird mites are suspected, it is often of value to examine dust obtained with a vacuum cleaner from bedrooms. This is, however, time consuming and could require some entomological expertise.

4 It may be necessary to visit the patient's home to establish whether there are birds' nests under the eaves, which might be a source of fleas or mites, or to take specimens from household pets.

5 Mites that might have relevance to human dermatoses may be isolated from clothing, furnishings or bedding by the techniques described by Hewitt *et al.* [37].

An entomologist is often valuable in these situations, not only for identification of arthropods, but also to advise about their relevance to the situation. An arthropod discovered at the scene of the crime may only be an innocent bystander.

In some cases, in spite of extensive efforts, the source of the bites remains unknown, and the dermatologist can then only treat the problem symptomatically with oral antihistamines, topical antipruritics and insect repellents.

Management

Prevention [38,39,40,41]

There are several strategies that can be employed in attempts to avoid arthropod bites/stings and arthropod-related disease transmission, including protective clothing, insecticide-impregnated netting and repellents. With regard to the latter, there are two principal categories of commercially available insect repellents – plant-derived essential oils and synthetic chemicals. The former group includes citronella, oil of eucalyptus, peppermint, tea-tree oil, lavender, soybean oil and neem oil. DEET (N,N-diethyl-m-toluamide [or N,N-diethyl-3-methylbenzamide]), the most widely used repellent, is an example of the latter.

Recently introduced repellents include DEPA (N,N-diethyl phenylacetamide), PMD (*para*-menthane-3,8-diol) and picaridin, a synthetic derivative of pepper.

Unfortunately, with many of these agents, their volatility means that the repellent effect is transient (between 4 and 8 h) for the more efficient and benefit can only be sustained by repeated application. In addition, effectiveness is often limited to a narrow spectrum of susceptible arthropods detecting carbon dioxide (e.g. mosquitoes, ticks, sandflies).

General management

Species-specific treatment will be discussed in the relevant sections throughout this chapter.

General treatment principles include [42]:

- Local wound care by cleansing, removing of remaining arthropod parts.

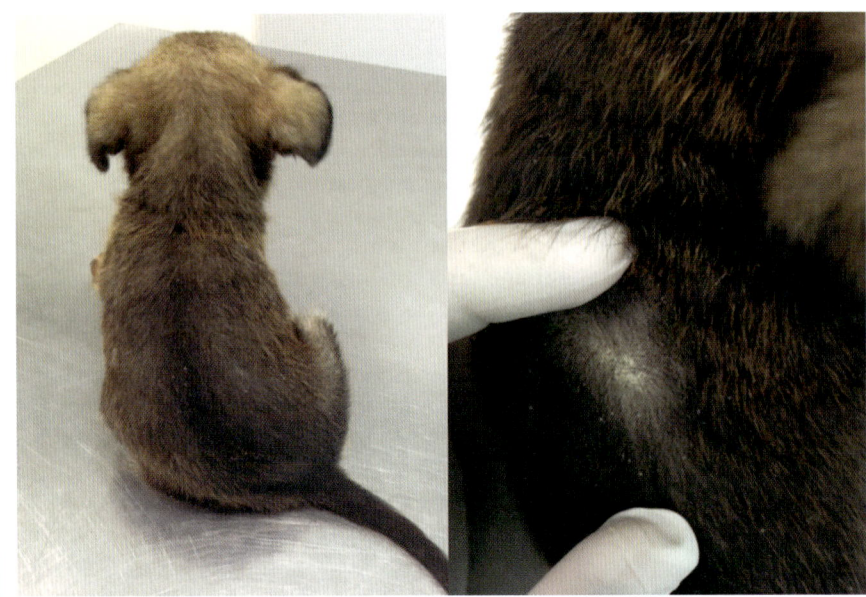

Figure 34.2 Itchy typical heavy white scale named 'walking dandruff' in the coat of a puppy suffering from *Cheyletiella* infestation. Courtesy of Ecole nationale vétérinaire d'Alfort, France.

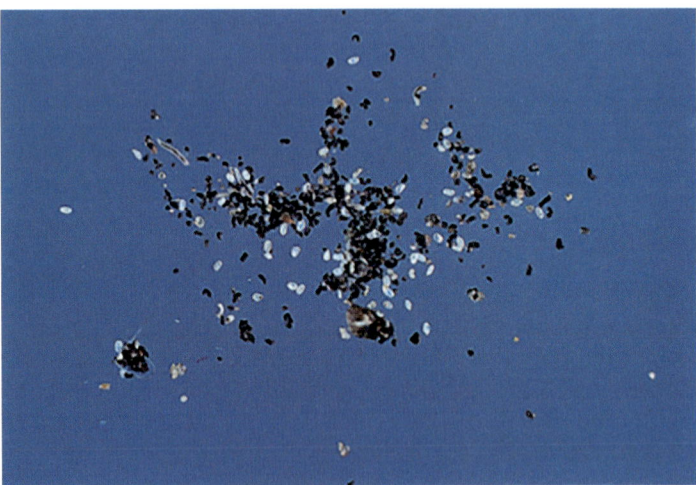

Figure 34.3 Typical 'pepper and salt' appearance of flea eggs and faeces in the debris from a cat's bedding.

- Management of pain and patient discomfort, by using ice packs, application of topical corticosteroids, systemic antihistamines, injection of local anaesthetics or sometimes the use of systemic analgesic.
- Institution of supportive measures such as adrenaline in case of severe allergic (anaphylaxis) or toxic reaction.
- Antibiotic therapy in case of secondary infection.
- Antivenom administration in case of envenomation from particular species.
- Tetanus prophylaxis if necessary.
- Desensitisation with venom immunotherapy using extracted insect venom. It may be an effective therapy for preventing further allergic reactions to insect stings, which can improve quality of life [43].

CLASS INSECTA

Mosquitoes, gnats, midges and flies (Diptera)

Definition
The order Diptera is one of the largest of the insect orders. Diptera are two-winged flies with a single pair of membranous forewings and with hindwings modified as balancing organs (halteres). Most feed on nectar, plant exudates or decaying animal and vegetable matter, but some are blood-sucking, and some have larvae parasitic on humans. To the dermatologist, the Diptera are important as biting insects and as the cause of myiasis, in addition to their capacity to transmit disease (Table 34.3).

The Diptera are currently usually classified in two suborders based on characteristics shown by larvae, pupae and adults – the Nematocera and the Brachycera. Detailed information on the morphology, biology and medical importance of Diptera is provided in comprehensive texts by Kettle [1] and Lane and Crosskey [2].

Classification
Suborder Nematocera (long-horned flies)
The Nematocera are small flies with long many-segmented filamentous antennae. With a few exceptions the medically important species are blood-suckers.

Family Culicidae (mosquitoes). Mosquitoes have a worldwide distribution. Three mosquito genera – *Anopheles*, *Aedes* (*Ochlerotatus*) and *Culex* – are responsible for the transmission of a number of human diseases, including malaria (Chapter 33), filariasis, yellow fever, West Nile virus, chikungunya, dengue fever and Zika virus.

Table 34.3 Main transmitted diseases by the insects of the order Diptera.

Suborder	Family	Species	Transmitted diseases
Nematocera	Culicidae (mosquitoes)	*Anopheles, Culex, Aedes*	Chikungunya, dengue fever, filariasis, Japanese encephalitis, malaria, Rift valley fever, West Nile virus, yellow fever, Zika virus
	Psychodidae (sandflies)	*Phlebotomus*	Cutaneous and visceral leishmaniaisis, Toscana fever
		Lutzomyia	Cutaneous and visceral leishmaniaisis, bartonellosis in New World (Carrion disease)
	Simuliidae (blackflies)	*Simulium*	Onchocerciasis, tularaemia
Brachycera	Glossinidae	*Glossina*	Sleeping sickness
	Tabanidae	*Tabanus* (horse flies)	Tularaemia
		Chrysops (deer flies)	Loiasis, tularaemia
	Muscidae	*Fannia*	Myiasis
		Musca	
	Calliphoridae	*Cochliomyia*	Myiasis
	Sarcophagidae	*Sarcophaga*	Myiasis
	Oestridae	*Dermatobia*	Myiasis
		Gasterophilus	
		Oestrus	
		Hypoderma	

Human malaria is transmitted exclusively by *Anopheles* species. Both male and female mosquitoes will imbibe sweet juices from flowers or ripe fruit, but only the females pierce the skin and suck the blood of vertebrate animals for production of eggs. Most mosquitoes are nocturnal feeders, but species from the genus *Aedes* (*Ochlerotatus*) are diurnal. The eggs of mosquitoes are deposited on or near water and adults develop via aquatic larval and pupal stages.

Family Psychodidae (sandflies). These are tiny (2–3 mm long) hairy flies with lanceolate wings and long legs. They are widely distributed, especially in the tropics and subtropics.

Genus *Phlebotomus*. Species of *Phlebotomus* are vectors of cutaneous and visceral leishmaniasis (Chapter 33) in the Old World. *Phlebotomus* species are also vectors of Toscana fever (TOSV), identified in 1971 [3]. *Phlebotomus* bites cause a condition known as harara (urticaria multiformis endemica) in Israel and the surrounding countries.

Genus *Lutzomyia*. *Lutzomyia* species are vectors of cutaneous and visceral leishmaniasis (Chapter 33) and bartonellosis in the New World.

Family Simuliidae [4]. Popularly known as blackflies, and with a worldwide distribution, these are small (2–6 mm) flies with a characteristic humped thorax and short broad wings. They breed only in areas of fast-flowing water and bite during the day.

Over large parts of the tropics, several species of blackfly are responsible for transmission of onchocerciasis (Chapter 33) – principally the *Simulium damnosum* complex (several closely related species) in West Africa, *S. neavei* in East Africa, *S. metallicum* in Venezuela and *S. ochraceum* in Guatemala. In temperate regions, the greatest problem caused by simuliids is their painful bites, and some species are such a persistent nuisance at certain times of the year that they may make large areas unpleasant to live or work in. In Serbia, the notorious Golubatz fly, *S. columbaschense* (*S. columbaczense*), which bred in the Danube at Golubatz, caused both mortality among livestock and human misery until environmental changes eliminated it. In North America, the most troublesome biting species are *S. venustum*, which is in the Holarctic and occurs from Alaska to Greenland and south to Texas and South Carolina, and *Prosimulium mixtum*, which occurs in the northeastern USA and eastern Canada. *Simulium posticatum* (the Blandford fly), formerly named *S. austeni* Edwards, is widely distributed throughout Europe and European Russia. In England, it is found in an arc running from East Anglia through Oxfordshire into Dorset. In the Stour valley area of Dorset, particularly in the region of Blandford Forum, the fly is notorious for the severity of the reaction to its bites [5,6]. It had not been known as a pest in the UK prior to the 1960s. The eggs are laid in cracks in vertical river banks, a short distance above the water [7]. The larvae are concentrated in stretches of fast-flowing water immediately downstream of barrages and weirs, where they attach themselves to weeds or stones and feed on phytoplankton. Adults hatch in May and are on the wing in May, June and early July. Females require a blood meal before oviposition, and although they will bite various wild and domestic animals, they appear to prefer humans and dogs. In the 1990s, biological control, using a bacterium (*Bacillus thuringiensis* var. *israelensis*) that selectively targeted the fly larvae, significantly reduced the severity of the problem.

Family Ceratopogonidae (biting midges; 'punkies'; 'no-see-ums'). These small flies (1–3 mm in length) have a worldwide distribution and are notorious as biting pests. The biting midges of the West Highlands of Scotland (the commonest species of which is *Culicoides impunctatus*), for example, are an intolerable nuisance and pose a problem to the Scottish tourist industry [8]. Males and females feed on nectar, but most females require a blood meal for maturation of the ovaries and egg production. There are four genera that suck blood: *Culicoides*, *Leptoconops*, *Austroconops* and *Forcipomyia* (subgenus *Lasiohelea*). They breed in rivers, swamps and marshes; they often occur in swarms and will readily attack any mammal in their vicinity. A few species enter homes and bite at night.

The genus *Culicoides* is widely distributed. *Leptoconops* species are largely restricted to the warmer parts of the Old and New World. *Austroconops* contains only one species, which is restricted to western Australia. *Lasiohelea* species are principally associated with tropical and subtropical rainforests.

Suborder Brachycera (circular-seamed flies, muscoid flies and short-horned flies)
The Brachycera are stout-bodied flies with short antennae, often composed of three segments, and never more than six.

Family Tabanidae. Many species of three genera of this family will attack humans – *Tabanus* (horse flies), *Chrysops* (deer flies) and *Haematopota* (clegs). They are large flies and have a worldwide distribution. Only females suck blood. Tabanid flies act as vectors for loiasis (Chapter 33) and tularaemia (Chapter 26), and some species may transmit anthrax mechanically [9].

Family Rhagionidae (snipe flies). Species of *Symphoromyia* occurring in the Palaearctic and Nearctic regions are vicious biters. *Atherix* is another blood-sucking genus in the Nearctic and neotropical regions, and *Spaniopsis* is troublesome in Australia.

Family Chloropidae (eye flies; frit flies). These flies are about 2 mm in length. The adults of some species are attracted to open sores, body secretions and the eyes, particularly eyes with a copious discharge. *Hippelates* and *Siphunculina* species are associated with humans and can act as mechanical vectors of yaws, conjunctivitis and streptococcal skin infection.

Family Muscidae (house flies; stable flies; tsetse flies). This family includes the familiar house fly *Musca domestica* and the lesser house fly *Fannia canicularis*. These do not bite but may act as mechanical vectors of disease. The muscids *Stomoxys calcitrans* (stable fly) and *Haematobia* species (horn flies) have mouthparts modified for sucking blood. They usually feed on large quadrupeds but can inflict painful bites on humans. Tsetse flies are vectors of trypanosomiasis (Chapter 33). They are confined to Africa south of the Sahara.

Family Hippoboscidae (flat flies; louse flies; keds). Members of this family are blood-sucking ectoparasites of birds and animals. Several species of ked have been recorded as biting humans [10,11].

Members of several other families of Diptera are important in that their larvae may cause myiasis.

Pathology
Diagnosis of mosquito bites is rarely performed in the acute phase. Histopathology will show an upper dermal perivascular infiltrate consisting of lymphocytes with histiocytes, eosinophils and mast cells. There may be mild oedema and a slight general increase in mast cells and eosinophils in the dermis. The overlying epidermis may show spongiosis sometimes amounting to vesiculation. In older lesions, excoriation often results in epidermal necrosis and crusting with a dermal infiltrate of lymphocytes and neutrophils. In addition, it is shown that saliva has a major role in the transmission of pathogens to the host agent [12].

Clinical features [13,14]
The clinical features of the bites of insects of this large and diverse order are variable. The nature of the pharmacologically active substances injected, and the degree of acquired allergic sensitivity to the antigenic substances in the saliva, are the main factors that determine the reaction. For most of the Diptera, the allergic component is by far the more important. The nature of any injected toxins is usually unknown and the effects attributable to them are usually slight. The clinical picture will also be influenced by the biting habits of the species concerned.

The reaction to mosquito bites is determined by previous exposure, and the sequence of events following multiple bites was elucidated by Mellanby [14]. In an individual not previously exposed, the bites produce no response. With subsequent bites, a delayed reaction occurs, consisting of pruritic papules, which develop approximately 24 h after the bites and persist for several days. After repeated bites for several weeks, the response changes, with the appearance of an immediate weal at the bite site. This resolves after about 2 h, to be replaced by the delayed reaction. Further exposure provokes the immediate reaction, but not the delayed response. Eventually, tolerance is acquired and no reaction occurs. Studies of the bite reaction in relation to age have shown an increase in immediate reactions from early childhood to adolescence and a decrease thereafter. The appearance and intensity of delayed reactions decrease with age [15]. It has been proved conclusively that the mosquito salivary glands are the source of the antigens responsible for the bite reactions [16].

Anaphylactic reactions to mosquito bites are rare [17]. Gaig *et al.* reported a patient with a serum sickness-like illness associated with mosquito bites [18]. Severe local reactions are not uncommon, and in highly sensitive subjects bullae, cellulitis and eczematisation are often seen, especially on the legs. Gravitational factors probably play a role in the development of bullae on the legs [19]. Exaggerated hypersensitivity responses to mosquito bites have been reported in patients suffering from chronic lymphatic leukaemia [20–23]. Although the lesions frequently appear months after the diagnosis of leukaemia and are unrelated to its course and therapy, they can also herald development or recurrence of leukaemia or lymphoma [24]. However, although the clinical picture and histological features are typical of arthropod bites, in many cases patients do not recall being bitten [22,25]. Exaggerated responses to mosquito bites have also been described in patients with HIV infection [26–28], and a chronic pruritic eruption in patients with AIDS in South Florida has been attributed to mosquito bites [29].

Over the past 20 years, there have been a number of reports from Japan of severe hypersensitivity to mosquito bites preceding the development of malignant histiocytosis [30,31]. This has now been characterised as a disease in which there is a triad of hypersensitivity to mosquito bites, chronic Epstein–Barr virus infection and natural killer cell leukaemia/lymphoma [32–35]. It affects predominantly Japanese people in the first two decades of life.

The skin lesions are bullae, which develop at mosquito bite sites, undergo necrosis, and heal with residual scarring [36]. Accompanying the skin lesions are systemic features, principally high fever and general malaise. Affected individuals die of haemophagocytic syndrome (malignant histiocytosis). Screening for haematological malignancies, latent Epstein–Barr virus infection and natural killer cell lymphocytosis should be considered in patients with unusual arthropod bite reactions [34,36].

The bites of Simuliidae, which may be numerous, are on exposed skin. The sites of the bites are often marked by a small blood crust with surrounding ecchymosis. Within a few hours, small pruritic papules develop, and these resolve after several days [37]. However, severe reactions with marked oedema of the limbs and constitutional upset occasionally occur, and in some cases nodules and discoid eczematous areas persist at the sites of the bites for several months [38]. The bites of the Blandford fly occur most frequently on the legs and women are principally affected [5,6]. The bites often produce a severe local reaction, with oedema and blistering, and may be accompanied by systemic manifestations, including pyrexia, arthralgia and meningism.

The biting midges of the family Ceratopogonidae generally cause small, papular lesions on exposed parts of the skin, but wealing and bulla formation may occur in sensitised individuals. Weal-like lesions, papules and persistent nodules have been described following bites from *Leptoconops torrens* in California [39].

Midges of the family Chironomidae are closely related to ceratopogonids. These midges do not bite, but hypersensitivity to their larvae, used as aquarium fish food and as bait, is well recognised [40,41], and includes contact urticaria [42] and protein contact dermatitis [43]. One study suggested that occupational exposure to chironomids may cause sensitisation with circulating IgE antibodies in sewage workers [44].

The bites of keds may be followed by the development of persistent pruritic papules [11].

The bites of horse flies and stable flies are often very painful and frequently become secondarily infected. Anaphylactic reaction to horse flies has also been reported in two patients already known to be allergic to stinging Hymenoptera venom, suggesting a cross allergen, between the Hymenoptera venom and the mosquito saliva [45].

Eruptive pseudoangiomatosis-like lesions have also been reported as a response to mosquito bites [46,47] and a relationship to *Culex pipiens* bites has been demonstrated [48].

Management [49–51]

Diptera bites should be cleansed thoroughly with water and soap to avoid secondary bacterial infection. A short course of topical steroids and systemic antihistamines may be used to control pruritus. Rare allergic reactions should be treated aggressively. Antihistamines taken prophylactically have been demonstrated in studies to decrease weal formations and subsequent pruritus following mosquito bites [52,53].

Prevention of mosquito and sandfly bites requires the use of protective clothing and chemical repellents, and methods to reduce the numbers of flies and mosquitoes in a given area. As the *Anopheles* species that carry malaria bite mostly at night, retiring to the indoors in the evening plays a major role in disease prevention. Transmission is also prevented by repellents and pyrethroid-impregnated mosquito netting. All travellers to malaria-endemic areas should take the recommended chemoprophylaxis. In contrast to *Anopheles* mosquitoes, *Aedes* mosquitoes that carry dengue, chikungunya or Zika virus tend to bite during the day. Repellents and protective clothing must be used to prevent transmission in endemic areas.

The hierarchy of measures against bites depends on the travel or the stay (e.g. place, season, length, modalities) and the persons (e.g. age, pregnancy, other pathology). The use of skin insect repellents is recommended, using an active ingredient which has been evaluated as innocuous (low toxicity, genotoxicity, ecotoxicity). Active ingredients currently being evaluated are DEET, picaridin (icaridin or KBR3023), 3-(*N*-acetyl-*N*-butyl) aminopropionic acid ethyl ester (IR35/35) and PMDRBO (mixture of *cis*- and *trans-para*menthan-3,8-diol) [54].

Myiasis

Definition

Myiasis is the infestation of body tissues of animals by the larvae (maggots) of Diptera [1–4]. Humans are sometimes infested depending on their behaviour, environment or clinical status. Parasitologically, flies may be classified into two main myiasis-producing groups: obligatory and facultative. Obligatory myiasis producers always pass their larval stage parasitically in the body of an animal. Larvae of facultative myiasis producers usually develop on decaying flesh or vegetable matter but may infest wounds.

Clinically, myiasis can be classified according to the part of the body that they affect. Cutaneous myiasis includes wound myiasis, furuncular myiasis and migratory myiasis, in which larvae penetrate and develop within the skin. The second form is cavitary myiasis. In nasopharyngeal myiasis, the nose, sinuses and pharynx are affected, and ophthalmomyiasis involves the eye, orbit and periorbital tissues. Intestinal and uro-genital myiasis involve invasion of the alimentary tract or uro-genital system.

Classification

All species of specific myiasis and most of facultative myiasis are classified within Calyptratae. Taxonomic division of the Calyptratae is presented in Table 34.4.

Family Muscidae. Eggs of *Fannia canicularis* (lesser house fly) and *Musca domestica* (house fly) may be deposited on ulcers and give rise to wound myiasis [6,7].

Family Calliphoridae (blowflies).
Genus *Cochliomyia* (*Callitroga*). These New World screwworms are distributed in the Americas, but are no longer established in North America, following intensive eradication efforts involving the release of a huge number of sterile male flies. Cases of myiasis involve the larvae of only two species of *Cochliomyia*: *C. macellaria* and *C. hominivorax* (*americana*). The larva of *C. macellaria* is a facultative parasite, which may be responsible for secondary infestation of wounds. Larvae of *C. hominivorax* are obligatory parasites, which feed on living tissue and can penetrate unbroken skin [8–10], but they may also infest wounds.

Table 34.4 Taxonomic division of the Calypratae.

Superfamily	Family	Subfamily or tribes	Species
Muscoidae	Muscidae		*Muscina* spp.
			Musca domestica (house fly)
	Fanniidae		*Fannia scalaris*
			Fannia canicularis
Oestroidea	Oestridae	Cuterebrinae	*Dermatobia hominis* (human botfly)
			Cuterebra spp.
			Alouattalyia baeri
		Gasterophilinae	*Gasterophilus* spp. (horse botflies)
		Hypodermatinaedae	*Hypoderma bovis* (cattle botfly)
			Hypoderma lineatum
			Hypoderma tarandi
		Oestrinae	*Oestrus* spp. (sheep nasal botfly)
	Sarcophagidae		*Wohlfahrtia magnifica* (spotted flesh fly)
			Wohlfahrtia vigil
			Wohlfahrtia opaca
			Sarcodexia lambens
	Calliphoridae		*Phormia regina*
			Protophormia terranovae
			Chrysomya bezziana
			Chrysomya megacephala
			Chrysomya albiceps
			Chrysomya rufifacies
			Cochliomyia hominivorax (New World screwworm)
		Auchmeromyiinae	*Auchmeromyia senegalensis* (Congo floor maggot)
		Luciliinae	*Lucilia* spp.
		Calliphorinae	*Calliphora* spp.
		Calliphorini	*Cordylobia anthropophaga* (tumbu fly)
			Cordylobia rodhaini (Lund's fly)

Adapted from Francesconi and Lupi [**5**]. Copyright holder of original artwork from which this table was adapted: American Society for Microbiology.

Genus *Chrysomya*. The Old World equivalent of *Cochliomyia*, *Chrysomya bezziana*, the Old World screwworm, is important medically as the larvae are obligate parasites in wounds.

Genus *Cordylobia*. *Cordylobia anthropophaga*, the 'tumbu' fly, is widespread in tropical Africa south of the Sahara [11], and most reported cases of tumbu fly myiasis are acquired in Africa [12,13,**14**]. There are, however, reports of myiasis acquired elsewhere, including Spain [15], Portugal [16] and Saudi Arabia [17]. Tumbu fly myiasis occurring in two boys who had never been to Africa might have been acquired as a result of their father, who made frequent visits to Africa, bringing tumbu fly eggs back among his possessions [18]. *Cordylobia* (*Stasisia*) *rodhaini*, the only other species of *Cordylobia*

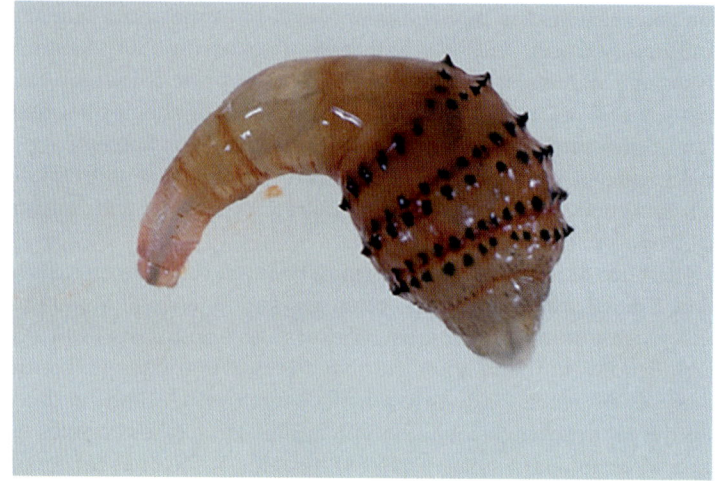

Figure 34.4 Third instar larva of *Dermatobia hominis* (the human botfly). Note the rows of backward-pointing spines.

known to infest humans, has a more limited distribution in tropical Africa, principally the rainforest areas. Extensive furuncular myiasis due to *C. rodhaini* has been reported in an Italian man who acquired the problem while working in Ethiopia [19], and in three Israeli travellers returning from Ghana [**14**]. Eggs are not laid on the host, but on sand or soil, especially if contaminated by urine or faeces. People are most commonly parasitised during the rainy season. Tourists can be infested by dressing with damp clothes that were lying on the ground, because adult flies tend to oviposit on soiled or damp clothing. After hatching, the larva raises its cephalic end searching for a suitable host. In the wild, rats are the usual host, but around human habitation, dogs and humans are common hosts. The larva attaches itself by means of its oral hooks (Figure 34.4) and rapidly penetrates the skin. When development is complete, usually in 14–16 days, it drops to the ground to pupate. Some of the factors that affect the distribution include unhygienic situations, high humidity, poverty and the use of soiled clothes [20].

Genus *Auchmeromyia*. Although strictly not a cause of myiasis, the larva of the fly *Auchmeromyia senegalensis*, the Congo floor maggot, is a blood-sucking parasite of humans. This fly occurs throughout tropical Africa, where it lives in huts and lays its eggs in the soil of the floor. The larvae lie buried in the soil during the day but emerge at night to feed on the sleeping occupants of the huts. Once engorged, they drop off the host and burrow back into the soil.

Other genera. Larvae of members of the genera *Phormia* (black blowflies) [21–23], *Lucilia* (greenbottle) and *Calliphora* (bluebottle) may also be secondary invaders of wounds in humans. In a study of wound myiasis in urban and suburban USA (in which homelessness, alcoholism and peripheral vascular disease were frequent cofactors) the majority of species identified were blowflies, the most common being *Lucilia sericata* [24]. Malignant wounds due to conditions such as non-melanoma skin cancer (squamous cell carcinoma or basal cell carcinoma) can be infested by *Lucilia sericata* maggots, mainly on the face or the legs [25].

There has been a recent resurgence of interest in the use of maggots (usually those of the greenbottle, *Lucilia sericata*) for wound debridement, especially diabetic ulcers or hard-to-heal wounds, an added bonus of which is their ingestion of antibiotic resistant bacteria such as meticillin-resistant *Staphylococcus aureus* [26]. The larvae must be prepared and maintained in sterile conditions before clinical use [27]. Maggot therapy has the following three core beneficial effects on a wound: facilitating faster and more effective debridement compared with standard dressings, disinfection and enhanced healing [28].

Family Sarcophagidae (flesh flies).
Genus *Sarcophaga*. There are occasional reports of members of this genus infesting wounds [29].

Genus *Wohlfahrtia*. These flies are similar to *Sarcophaga* and are important myiasis-causing flies in camels and sheep. The larvae of *Wohlfahrtia magnifica* may be deposited in the ear, eye or nose and cause extensive destruction of healthy tissue. Delir *et al.* reported an Iranian woman with a cavity in the left labium majus occupied by a number of *W. magnifica* larvae [30]. *W. magnifica* occurs in southeastern Europe, southern and Asiatic Russia, the Middle East and North Africa. *Wohlfahrtia vigil* and *W. opaca* are North American species whose females deposit larvae on the skin of young animals, resulting in furuncular myiasis. Lesions are identical to those of *Dermatobia* (see below). Human furuncular myiasis occurs only in young babies, as the larvae are unable to penetrate adult skin [31].

Family Oestridae.
Genus *Cuterebra* (rodent or rabbit botfly). Rabbits and rodents are the natural hosts for the larvae of these flies, which are sometimes responsible for human furuncular myiasis [32–34]. Baird *et al.* [35] reviewed 54 cases of North American cuterebrid myiasis.

Genus *Dermatobia* (human botfly). *Dermatobia hominis* is the only species in the genus. It is a bluebottle-like fly found in the neotropical areas of the New World, extending from southern Mexico to northern Argentina. It occurs in areas where temperature and humidity are relatively high, principally lowland forests. For example, the 'Madidi National Park' in Bolivia was mentioned as an important destination where travellers reported acquiring myiasis [14]. Rare cases have been reported on the east coast of the USA, in patients that did not report travelling to endemic regions [36,37]. These North American autochthonous cases might be explained by possible inoculation in travellers or by a change in the habitat of the fly, migrating northwards [38]. *Dermatobia hominis* causes cutaneous myiasis in a wide range of mammalian hosts, including humans, and is particularly important as a parasite of cattle.

The female fly does not deposit her eggs directly, but uses other insects, such as day-flying mosquitoes and blood-sucking flies, as vectors to carry her eggs to the host. This phenomenon is called 'phoresia' and explains the preferential localisation of lesions in non-covered areas of the body, unlike African myiasis caused by *Cordylobia anthropophaga* which contaminates covered areas. The female fly grasps the insect vector in midair and deposits a number of eggs on its abdomen. When the vector subsequently feeds on a potential host, the eggs hatch and the larvae rapidly burrow into the skin. Larval development lasts approximately 50–60 days, following which the larva emerges, drops to the ground and pupates. Human botfly myiasis should always be considered as a cause of boil-like lesions in patients who have recently returned from endemic areas [39–45].

Genus *Gasterophilus* (horse botfly). A form of migratory cutaneous myiasis known as 'creeping eruption' is caused by *Gasterophilus* larvae. The Gasterophilinae are mainly parasites of the alimentary tract of horses, but occasionally larvae of certain species of *Gasterophilus*, including *G. haemorrhoidalis* and *G. pecorum*, penetrate human skin.

Genus *Oestrus* (sheep nostril fly). *Oestrus ovis*, which develops in the nasopharyngeal passages of sheep and goats, and *Rhinoestrus purpureus*, which parasitises horses, are occasionally responsible for human myiasis, especially ophthalmomyiasis. The fly leaves its larvae (not eggs) directly in the eye and patients complain of mild or severe foreign-body sensation, redness, watery eyes or lid swelling. Larvae on the external surface of the eye can be detected and removed under dim light. Larvae can hide in the ocular fornices [46,47].

Genus *Hypoderma* (warble flies). The larvae of *Hypoderma* species are obligate parasites of cattle. The human is an abnormal host for *Hypoderma* and the larvae do not mature fully. After penetrating the skin, the larvae produce migratory subcutaneous swellings [48,49]. They may also invade the eye (ophthalmomyiasis), producing severe damage [49,50]. Marked eosinophilia may accompany infestation and Starr *et al.* [51] reported a cattle rancher in whom an illness due to infestation with *H. lineatum* and marked by pleuritis, pericarditis and myositis mimicked the hypereosinophilic syndrome. A recent epidemic of ophthalmomyiasis with ocular injury has been reported in five children who had visited reindeer (also called caribou) herding areas in Norway or Sweden, due to *Hypoderma tarandi*, a bumblebee-like fly that is common in subarctic regions [48]. Imported cases of human disease have also been reported [52].

Clinical features [1–4,40]
The habits of the flies and their larvae determine the variations in the clinical manifestations for which they are responsible.

Cutaneous myiasis
Traumatic or wound myiasis has been a serious complication of war wounds in tropical areas and is sometimes seen in neglected ulcers or wounds in most parts of the world [53]. *Cochliomyia hominivorax*, *Chrysomya bezziana* and *Wohlfahrtia magnifica* are the most common flies, worldwide, that cause obligatory human wound myiasis. Wound myiasis is most often initiated when flies oviposit in necrotic, haemorrhaging or pus-filled lesions [54]. In the presence of an open wound, the most important predisposing factors for wound myiasis are a lack of hygiene and poor socioeconomic status [54].

Obligatory cutaneous myiasis occurs in two main clinical forms (furuncular and migratory myiasis); in both there may be mild constitutional symptoms and eosinophilia. Both occur mainly on exposed skin – often the face, scalp, arms or legs [55]. In the furuncular form, boil-like lesions develop gradually over a few days. Each lesion has a central punctum, which discharges sero-sanguinous

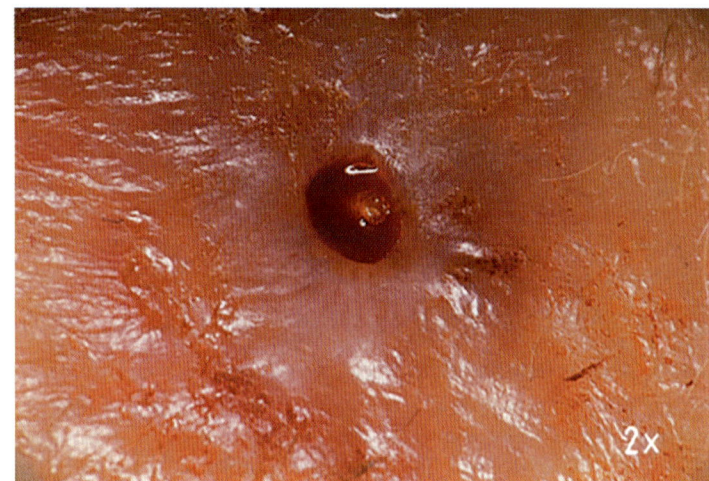

Figure 34.5 Furuncle-like lesion produced by *Dermatobia hominis*. The tail of the larva is visible in the centre of the lesion.

fluid. The posterior end of the larva, equipped with a group of spiracles, is usually visible in the punctum, and its movements may be noticed by the patient (Figure 34.5). The lesions are often extremely painful but sometimes not. Lesions due to *Dermatobia hominis* are most frequently unique on exposed body sites, whereas lesions due to *Cordylobia anthropophaga* can be multiple, on covered body areas [14]. The inflammatory reaction around the lesions may be accompanied by lymphangitis and regional lymphadenopathy and/or systemic symptoms [56]. Secondary bacterial infection is a possible complication. Once the larva has emerged, or has been removed, the lesions rapidly resolve. The flies causing furuncular myiasis in humans are *Dermatobia hominis*, *Cuterebra*, *Cordylobia anthropophaga*, *Cordylobia* (*Stasisia*) *rodhaini*, *Wohlfahrtia* species and *Hypoderma* species.

The second principal clinical form (migratory myiasis) is a creeping eruption, resembling cutaneous larva migrans (Chapter 33), in which a tortuous thread-like red line with a terminal vesicle marks the passage of the larva through the skin. The larva lies ahead of the vesicle in apparently normal skin [57]. The larva may live for months in human skin and may migrate 1–30 cm/day. Infestation may present with pustules, nodules or recurrent swelling [58]. This form of myiasis is produced by *Gasterophilus* larvae. The inflammatory nodular lesions produced by *Hypoderma* species are migratory.

Cavitary myiasis

The infestation of natural body cavities is called cavitary myiasis. Cavitary myiasis receive specific names, depending on the anatomical region affected. Internal organs may also be affected. *Eristalis tenax*, a fly called 'drone fly', can cause intestinal, gastric or urinary myiasis. It is an accidental myiasis related to ingestion of contaminated uncooked food or water containing fly larvae. Rare cases are mainly reported from India, Africa or Europe [59–61].

Investigations [5]
Furuncular myiasis
Clinical features are often sufficient to diagnose furuncular myiasis, especially in endemic regions. Dermoscopy may be helpful in difficult cases, showing a yellowish structure with black barb-like spines [5,62–64]. Ultrasound has also been used to confirm furuncular myiasis and may be useful to remove the larvae [65,66]. When ultrasound failed to detect larvae, colour Doppler sonography was able to visualise the continuous movement of internal fluids of the larva and confirm the diagnosis [67].

Migratory myiasis
The diagnosis relies on the identification of a dipteran larva. Magnification is used to visualise the parasite. In *Hypoderma* furuncular lesion, ultrasound may be helpful to detect the larva [52].

Wound myiasis
Diagnosis is easily made by the clinical inspection of the wound.

Management
Furuncular myiasis
The larva of *Cordylobia* can often be expressed by firm pressure around the edges of the lesion, but sometimes the punctum may require enlarging surgically.

The larva of *Dermatobia hominis* has a bulbous anterior end equipped with rows of spines (Figure 34.4) that help to anchor it in the skin and make its removal by manual pressure difficult [56]. Traditional methods of treatment include occluding the punctum with pork fat [68,69], blocking the spiracles of the larva and stimulating premature extrusion. A similar result may be obtained with mineral oil, petrolatum (Vaseline) or butter. Surgical management is most frequently recommended: the punctum is enlarged by cruciate incisions and this enables removal of an intact larva [70] (Figure 34.6). The injection of lidocaine (lignocaine) underneath the nodule may be sufficient to push the larva out [71], and Loong *et al.* [72] also found that injection of 2 mL of 2% lidocaine into the blind end of the cavity facilitated non-surgical removal of the larva.

Migratory myiasis [5]
After identification of its position, the larvae may be removed with a needle. The extraction of *Hypoderma* larvae may require a cruciform incision or only expression in case of furuncular lesions. However, in most cases, a surgical excision is necessary. Oral ivermectin or albendazole may be helpful if extraction is not possible because the larva is too deep into the tissue [52].

Wound myiasis
Wound myiasis requires debridement and irrigation to remove larvae, and treatment of secondary bacterial infection.

Ophthalmomyiasis
The treatment is simply based on the removal of all larvae. Antihistamine drops and/or topical antibiotics may also be used, as needed.

Ivermectin
Ivermectin has been used both topically and orally in the management of myiasis [38,46,47,73–78]. Oral treatment of human myiasis is based on anecdotal reports and most of the experience comes from veterinary medicine. Different therapeutic schemes have been adopted for ivermectin use in the treatment of myiasis. Ivermectin

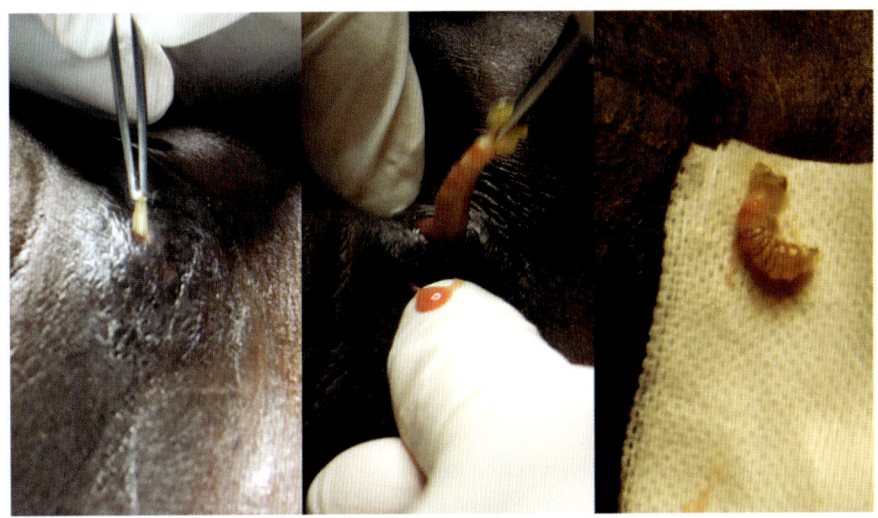

Figure 34.6 Extraction of *Dermatobia hominis* larva from a patient living in French Guyana. Courtesy of Dr C. Hotz, Henri Mondor Hospital, Créteil, France.

is not recommended for furuncular myiasis because it may kill the larva inside the lesion with a consequent inflammatory reaction.

Fleas (Siphonaptera)

Definition

Fleas are small (1–8 mm long) wingless insects, laterally compressed to facilitate moving between the animal hairs. Male and female adults are blood-sucking ectoparasites of mammals and birds. Approximately 2000 species and subspecies are known. Egg, larvae and cocoon stages occur on the ground. The larvae of fleas are not parasitic, but feed on organic material that they find in the nest or dwelling place of the host [1,2].

Classification

The order Siphonaptera contains three families of medical importance.

Family Tungidae

This family contains tropical species that burrow into human skin (see Tungiasis).

Family Pulicidae

Members of this family occur throughout the world, and some species transmit plague (*Yersinia pestis*) (Chapter 26) and murine typhus (*Rickettsia typhi*) (Chapter 26) [3–5]. Fleas also play a role in the transmission of rural epidemic typhus (*Rickettsia prowazekii*) in the USA [6]. In recent years, the flea-borne spotted fever agent *Rickettsia felis* has emerged and can be found throughout the world [7–9]. Cat fleas have been shown to be vectors of *Bartonella henselae*, the pathogen responsible for cat scratch disease and bacillary angiomatosis [10–12]. *Bartonella quintana* has been detected in cat fleas [13] and in *Pulex irritans* [14], although its main vector is the body louse. Infections from *Bartonella quintana* have re-emerged, predominantly among the alcoholic homeless populations in cities in both Europe and the USA [15]. The rabbit flea (*Spilopsyllus cuniculi*) may be a potential vector of *Bartonella alsatica*, which has been responsible for endocarditis and lymphadenitis in humans [16,17]. Many species are important only for the irritability of their bites. The species most frequently parasitising humans are the human flea, *Pulex irritans* (mainly in tropical areas), and the cat and dog fleas, *Ctenocephalides felis* and *Ctenocephalides canis* (mainly in occidental areas), but other species will bite humans in the absence of their normal host. The tropical rat flea, *Xenopsylla cheopis*, is the vector of bubonic plague.

The adult female flea lays her eggs during feeding on the host and the eggs fall to the ground, where an important food source for the larvae is the faeces of the adult flea. The larvae subsequently form cocoons and under suitable conditions of temperature and humidity the life cycle may be completed in a few weeks. However, the cocoon stage can sometimes last as long as a year and the flea may emerge only in response to vibrations produced by the movement of possible hosts.

In a household occupied by infested pet dogs or cats, fleas in various stages of development are found in the animals' bedding, and on carpets and soft furnishings. In a survey carried out in the UK in 2005, the prevalence of flea infestation in domestic cats was 21.1% (98.9% of fleas were *C. felis*) and in dogs 6.8% (93.1% of fleas were *C. felis*) [18]. The prevalences were stable in 2018, in another study from veterinarians in the UK, with 28.1% of cats and 14.4% of dogs that were flea-infested (>90% were *C. felis*) [12]. To date, no clinical case of murine typhus has been described in Spain, while the presence of *R. typhi* in cats and fleas has been demonstrated [19].

Family Ceratophyllidae

Species in this family are mainly parasitic on rodents and birds. Bird fleas overwinter in cocoons in birds' nests and emerge in spring. At this time, they can become household pests, as they may gain access to bedrooms from nests under the eaves.

Epidemiology

Infestation with the human flea, *Pulex irritans*, occurs mainly in congested and overcrowded communities with low standards of hygiene. It is now rare in developed countries. Cat and dog flea infestation in the home is, however, common.

Animal fleas are common throughout the world and persons in contact with domestic animals are frequently bitten. Severe attacks are sometimes experienced by individuals moving into premises long empty but previously occupied by pet cats or dogs. The vibration caused by footsteps triggers the emergence of fleas from their cocoons. Attacks are more likely to occur when the fleas do not have access to their usual host. Household infestations with bird fleas may occur from nests or nest boxes on or near the house [20], and similar problems may occur in the workplace [21]. An outbreak of papular urticaria in a nursery school was traced to an infestation with dog fleas from a fox's burrow beneath the building [22]. Similar problems were caused by *Ctenocephalides felis* entering houses from raccoons which had bred in the cavity between two houses [23].

Clinical features [6,24]

Flea bites usually provoke typical papular urticaria in a sensitised individual. Occasionally, the reaction is more severe and bullae may occur (Figure 34.1). The lesions may be grouped in lines or irregular clusters. Cat and dog flea bites occur predominantly on the legs or buttocks, and are most profuse around the ankles (Figure 34.7), most often at the posterior part, but they can also occur on the forearms. Adult women seem to be more often bitten than men, as trousers and socks might protect the legs [25,26]. Bites from bird fleas tend to be more extensive, as the sleeping occupants of bedrooms usually provide larger areas of exposed flesh.

Investigations [27]

If flea infestation from pet animals is suspected, this can be confirmed by microscopical examination of debris from the animals' bedding material (Figure 34.3).

The principal sign of flea infestation in an affected animal is the presence of dried concretions of flea faeces on the animal's coat. Some animals will also have signs of flea allergy dermatitis, with areas of crusting and alopecia, most frequently on the lower back and the base of the tail.

If fleas from another source are suspected of causing bites, it may be necessary to examine samples taken with a vacuum cleaner from rooms or to visit the suspect premises. It is important to identify the flea species responsible for an infestation so that efforts at eradication may be accurately directed at the source [28]. Cat fleas (Figure 34.8), dog fleas and common bird fleas may be readily identified after 'clearing' in 10% potassium hydroxide for 48 h [4], but the help of an entomologist should be sought.

Management [29]

The development of topical and oral agents such as fipronil, imidacloprid, lufenuron and selamectin has revolutionised domestic cat and dog flea control [30]. More recently, newer flea products have been marketed containing dinotefuran, metaflumizone, spinetoram or spinosad [31,32]. In addition, a new insecticide family has been discovered, the isoxazolines, with four products currently on the market containing afoxalaner, fluralaner, sarolaner or lotilaner [33]. However, flea control may remain difficult. Flea control programmes must also take into account the age, lifestyle and allergy status of the animal, the presence of other companions in the household and owner ability and resources.

Pest-control companies will deal with flea infestation from other sources. In private homes, personal action can be taken to investigate by meticulous cleaning with a vacuum and a floorcloth on resting

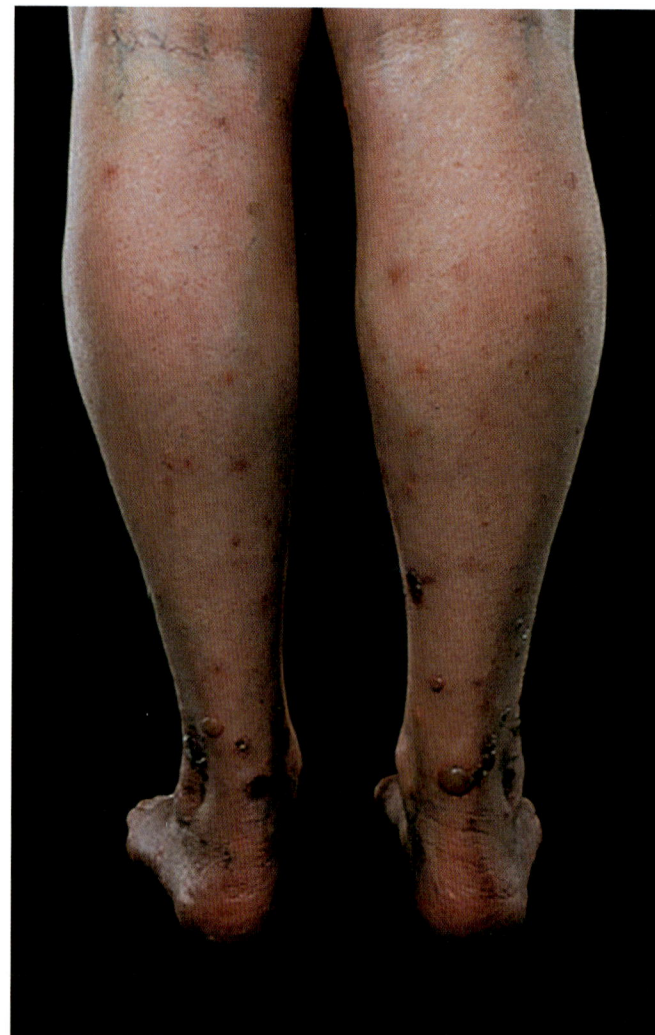

Figure 34.7 Typical distribution of cat or dog flea bites on the legs.

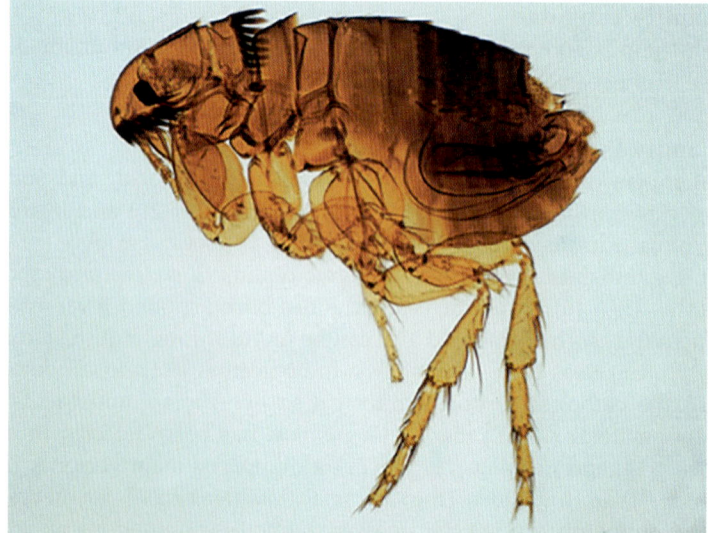

Figure 34.8 *Ctenocephalides felis*, the cat flea.

places of the cat or dog (bed, sofa, carpet) to remove eggs, larvae and cocoons.

Tungiasis

Introduction and general description
Tungiasis is caused by the sand flea *Tunga penetrans*, also known as the jigger or chigoe.

Epidemiology
Originally a native of South America, it subsequently spread to Africa [34,35], the Caribbean and India. Tungiasis has reappeared in Mexico [35] where it was previously last recorded in 1948. The ease of world travel has contributed to tungiasis being encountered in non-endemic areas [34–44]. Less frequently, another species, *Tunga trimamillata*, can infest humans, reported in Ecuador, Peru or Brazil [45]. Over 20 million individuals are estimated to be at risk in endemic regions, therefore tungiasis was recognised as a neglected tropical skin disease by the World Health Organization in May 2013.

Pathophysiology
Tunga penetrans is the smallest known flea (1 mm long). Its larvae develop in dry sandy soil and development from egg to adult takes about 3 weeks in favourable conditions. The impregnated female flea burrows into the feet of mammals, preferring humans and pigs. In humans, the fleas establish themselves between the toes, under the nails, on the lateral rim of the foot and on the soles, but other parts of the body may be affected. Once embedded in the skin, the flea's abdomen enlarges to the size of a pea, and large numbers of eggs are produced. The eggs are subsequently gradually extruded over a period of 2 weeks, and the female flea dies and is sloughed from the skin [46].

Pathology
Anatomical components of the flea are sufficiently distinctive to enable a diagnosis of tungiasis to be made histologically [47]. The distinguishing features are an eosinophilic cuticle with tracheal rings and adjacent eggs. The adjacent tissue exhibits basal epidermal hyperplasia [48].

Clinical features [34,49]
The presence of the fleas causes intense irritation. The typical appearance of an individual lesion is initially a black dot surrounded by a halo of redness, followed by enlargement to form a mother of pearl-coloured papule with a central dark punctum, produced by the enlarging flea abdomen. Secondary infections are common. Tungiasis lesions act as a portal of entry of bacterial superinfection that may be life-threatening, such as necrotising fasciitis [50], and tetanus has often complicated tungiasis in the past [51]. In severe cases, the feet may be honeycombed by multiple lesions, causing serious discomfort and disability (Figure 34.9) [52–54]. Repeated infections disfigure and mutilate the feet, potentially leading to impaired mobility. Indeed, tungiasis can be a serious health problem in resource-poor communities where children can be teased and stigmatised [50], and have a considerable impact on their quality of life, including absenteeisms from school. The differential diagnosis of tungiasis includes myiasis, verruca vulgaris, ingrowing toenail, acute paronychia, mycotic granuloma, malignant melanoma and arthropod bites [55]. Use of the dermoscope aids diagnosis by demonstrating the surface features [56–59].

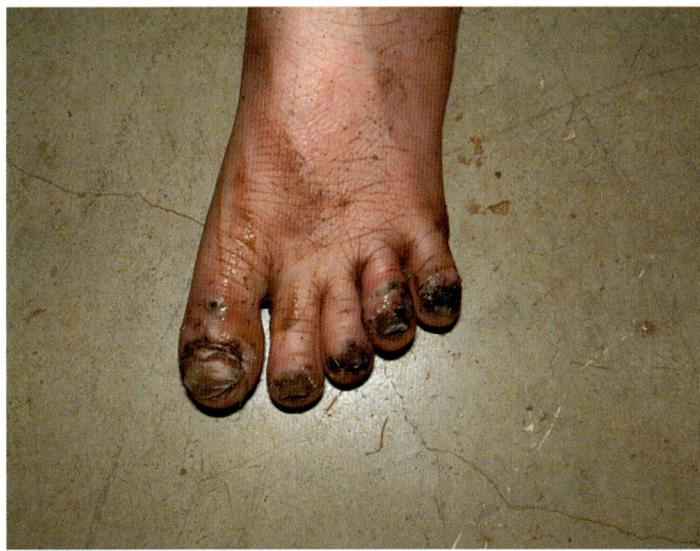

Figure 34.9 Tungiasis, showing a moderate to severe infestation of the foot. Courtesy of Dr C. Fuller, International Foundation for Dermatology.

Management [60,61,62]
The best procedure for dealing with tungiasis is blunt dissection of the intact parasite. Local people where the infection is endemic are very skilled at doing this, usually with a pin or splinter of wood. This can also be accomplished by enlarging the surface punctum and extracting the flea with tweezers, curettage and cautery, or excision. These procedures are often painful and poorly tolerated by young children. Ivermectin 0.8%, metrifonate 0.2% and thiabendazole 5% lotions have been tested topically but proven to be active but insufficiently effective [63]. Dimeticone, used for head lice infestation, might be promising [64], as well as a mixture of neem seed oil and coconut oil [65]. Prevention is essential, mainly based on regular application of a repellent. A plant-based repellent, assessed in Brazil, proved to be extremely effective in preventing infestation with *T. penetrans* [66], but has to be applied twice daily on the skin of the feet. Closed footwear use might be the most helpful and simplest way to prevent the disease in endemic areas [67].

The unwary traveller may well acquire tungiasis. Those visiting endemic areas should be warned to wear stout shoes and not to sit on the ground.

Bees, wasps and ants (Hymenoptera)

Definition
The adults of many species in this large order of insects have evolved a sting apparatus. The sting may or may not be barbed. Some use the sting in defence and others use it offensively in hunting for food. Males have no sting apparatus. Humans are frequently affected by these insects, as more than 94% of people will be stung at least once during their lifetime [1], with reactions varying from local discomfort, local to large reactions, to systemic anaphylactic reactions that can be fatal.

The Hymenoptera are readily recognised by the narrow waist (isthmus) connecting the abdomen to the thorax. Some of the more important families are described next.

Classification
Superfamily Apoidea (bees)
Honeybees (Apis mellifera). Honeybees possess a barbed sting. When humans are stung, the bee is frequently unable to remove the sting. The sting and venom apparatus are avulsed from the bee's abdomen in its struggles, but the venom apparatus continues to function and pump in more venom.

'Africanised' honeybees, the product of interbreeding between bees from southern Africa and European species, have caused significant problems [2]. These aggressive ('killer') bees, which have characteristics of their African antecedents including strong colony defensive behaviour, have migrated northwards from Brazil to the southern USA and more recently several North American states [3]. These Africanised bees may have negative impacts such as swarming, aggressive behaviour and the ability to mass attack, resulting in serious and fatal envenomation in humans and animals [3].

Humblebees; bumblebees (Bombus spp.). The sting is not barbed, and the bumblebee is therefore able to sting repeatedly. Most species are inoffensive and only sting defensively when severely provoked.

Superfamily Vespoidea
Family Vespidae (social wasps). This family includes wasps, yellow-jackets and hornets. Species of *Vespa*, *Vespula* and *Polistes* inflict painful stings. Wasps can also sting repeatedly, as they either have small barbs or none at all on their stings.

In Europe, *Vespa velutina*, also known as the 'Asian hornet', is a predator for honeybees, first detected in France in 2004. Since 2006 it has spread rapidly from the southwest of France into Europe, with conflicting data: some showing an associated increase in the number of stings in humans [4], and some showing that the increase of this Asian hornet population has not been correlated with an increase in the number of hymenoptera stings [5].

Superfamily Bethyloidea
These are small solitary wasps. They sometimes become abundant in houses infested by woodworm; indeed they are parasitic on the xylophagous beetle larvae of *Lepidoptera* and *Coleoptera*. They inject venom with their sting to paralyse the larvae and feed on their hemolymph before laying their own eggs on them. *Scleroderma domesticum* (Figure 34.10), *Epyris californicus* and *Cephalonomia gallicola* may inflict troublesome stings. Bites of *Scleroderma dosmesticum* can be aligned and have no typical localisation on the body. This house pest occurs usually in summertime, and is active in the evening and at night. Only the female is responsible for human lesions. They can be found near old wooden furniture in antique dealer stores. Management must be to treat furniture that has woodworm [6].

Superfamily Scolioidea
Family Formicidae (ants). Many ant species are equipped with powerful stings, including the Australian jumper and bull ants [7,8], and

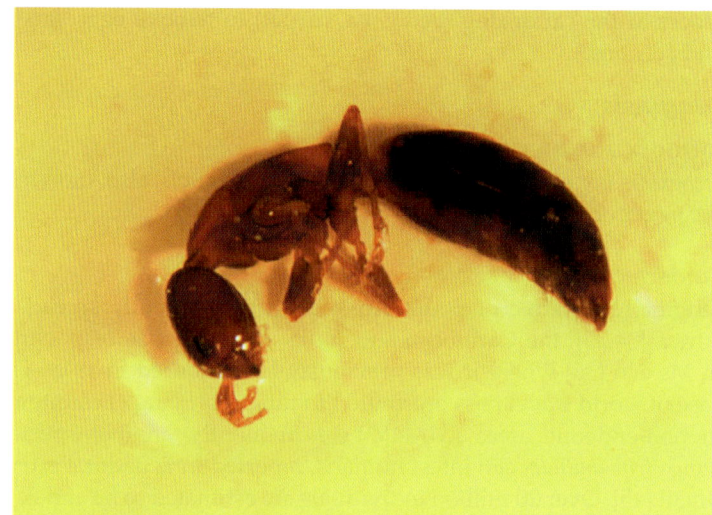

Figure 34.10 *Scleroderma domesticum*.

Solenopsis, the fire ant. Fire ants, so called because of the burning pain of their stings, have been particularly problematic in recent years in the USA. There are several native species of fire ant in the USA, but it is the red and black imported fire ants *S. invicta* and *S. richteri*, inadvertently brought to the USA from South America, that have become troublesome pests [5,9–12]. *Solenopsis invicta* is also well established in two locations in the Brisbane area, in Queensland, Australia [13]. Wood imported from South America was the source of fire ants responsible for anaphylaxis in a woman in Málaga, Spain [14], and more recently one case of imported fire ants caused anaphylaxis in Canada [15]. A child who had multiple fire ant stings presented with anaphylaxis and evolving signs of systemic envenomation, including rhabdomyolysis and renal failure, thus illustrating the potential for a significant Hymenoptera toxidrome [16].

The fire ant first uses its powerful mandibles to grip its victim and drives its non-barbed sting into the skin. It then rotates about the point of attachment of the mandibles and inflicts further stings in a circular pattern [10–12,17]. Although largely outdoor insects, fire ants may move into dwellings, causing problems for the inhabitants [18].

Species of *Pogonomyrmex* (harvester ants) may inflict multiple painful stings [6].

Pathophysiology
Venoms [19–30,31,32,33]
The composition of venoms is complex. Pharmacologically active and antigenic substances are both present, and an individual's reaction to the sting is determined partly by the quantity of the former, and partly by the degree of acquired hypersensitivity to the latter. Hymenoptera venom contains vasoactive amines, small polypeptides and larger protein molecules. The components of vespid (wasps, yellow-jackets and hornets) venoms include histamine, serotonin, mast cell degranulating peptide, wasp kinin, phospholipases, hyaluronidase and antigen 5. The three major allergens in vespid venoms are phospholipases, hyaluronidase and antigen 5. The venom of the honeybee contains histamine, mast cell degranulating peptide, melittin, phospholipase A_2, hyaluronidase and acid phosphatase. The three proteins in honeybee venom that

are important allergens are phospholipase A_2, hyaluronidase and acid phosphatase. In addition, the polypeptide melittin is also antigenic. Bumblebee venom appears to be chemically and antigenically related to honeybee venom [28].

Study of fire ant venom was impeded for many years by the extreme difficulty in obtaining sufficient amounts. The venom is composed of 90–95% water-insoluble piperidine alkaloids [29] that are not allergenic but are responsible for the immediate hive formation and the development of the sterile pustule at the sting site [34]. In recent studies, the alkaloid compositions have been reinvestigated and found to be much more complex than previously thought [35,36]. Alkaloid compositions vary among species of fire ants. When commercial-grade venom became available, several potent allergenic proteins were identified [11,26]. Antigenic similarity between fire ant venom, bee and wasp venoms and scorpion venom has been demonstrated [27,30].

Allergy to Hymenoptera venom is mediated by IgE antibodies. The antigenic substances in the venom of many Hymenoptera are more liable to induce high degrees of hypersensitivity of the immediate type than are the antigens of most other insects. Several risk factors are associated with the occurrence of severe systemic anaphylactic sting reactions [37]: vespid stings, older age [38], elevated tryptase concentration [38], male patient [38], specific medication (angiotensin-converting inhibitors) [38] and mastocytosis [39,40]. A preceding less severe systemic reaction may also predispose the patient to more severe reactions [38]. The prevalence of systemic anaphylactic reactions in epidemiological studies in Europe to hymenoptera stings ranged between 0.3% and 7.5% in adults and 0.15% and 3.4% in children [41]. Fortunately, case fatalities are rare, ranging from 0.03 to 0.48 fatalities per million inhabitants per year [1,42].

Clinical features [19,20,31,32]
Reactions to bee and wasp stings may be classified as local and systemic. Both may have a toxic or a hypersensitive mechanism. The typical local toxic reaction produced by pharmacologically active components of the venom is burning pain, which may be very severe, followed by redness and oedema. This local reaction subsides in a few hours. The systemic effects of multiple stings include hypotension, generalised vasodilatation, severe headache, vomiting, diarrhoea and shock, and the cumulative effect of a large number of stings may be fatal, particularly in children.

In some cases, hypersensitivity produces only a more intense local reaction manifest as increased oedema, usually developing within the first half hour, but occasionally delayed for several hours. If a generalised anaphylactic reaction occurs, this is usually within a few minutes of the sting. The manifestations of a generalised reaction may be classified as dermatological (pruritus, redness, urticaria and angio-oedema), respiratory (laryngeal oedema, bronchospasm) or vascular (tachycardia, hypotension, shock). These features may occur separately or in combination, and in varying degrees of severity.

Occasionally, late-onset reactions to stings occur [21]. In some patients, an urticarial reaction develops several hours after the sting, and in others a serum sickness-like reaction occurs, with urticaria, joint swelling and arthralgia.

A patient with a foreign-body granuloma and IgE pseudolymphoma following multiple bee stings has been reported [43], and another with an eosinophilic foreign-body granuloma after multiple self-administered bee stings as treatment in traditional Korean medicine [44].

Ocular lesions other than sting lesions (i.e. conjunctivitis, keratitis) have been reported due to liquid projections emitted by the yellow-legged hornet Vespa velutina. French poison control centres reported 29 cases over the period from 2004 to 2019, mainly in males working with hornet nests (e.g. firefighters, wasp exterminators) [45].

Skin lesions produced by fire ants typically occur in clusters [10–12]. The site of attachment of the mandibles may be marked by two minute haemorrhagic puncta. The initial reaction to the sting is the development of a weal, followed within a few hours by a vesicle. The fluid in the vesicle gradually becomes cloudy and after 8–10h the typical lesion is an umbilicated pustule on a red oedematous base. The pustule subsequently ruptures, forming a crust, and after several days the lesions heal, frequently leaving small scars. Specific histopathological features have been described [46]. Hand–foot syndrome associated with multiple fire ant stings has been described [47].

Systemic hypersensitivity reactions may also occur, and feature generalised urticaria and angio-oedema, wheezing, nausea and vomiting, and hypotension [10,48,49]. These manifestations may increase in severity with successive attacks and fatal anaphylaxis can occur [12,15,16].

Management [32,37,50,51]
Management of large local reactions
Conventional advice with regard to honeybee stings is that the sting should be immediately scraped off, never pinched because the remaining venom is inoculated; but a study by Visscher et al. [52] suggests that the method of removal does not affect the quantity of venom received and is therefore unimportant; the sting should simply be removed as rapidly as possible. The application of a potent topical corticosteroid to the sting site before the area is cooled with wet dressings or cool packs is usually recommended [37]. Oral antihistamine and/or systemic corticosteroids may be recommended even if there are no controlled studies; it is considered that this therapy should be initiated as soon as possible after the sting [37].

Management of systemic anaphylactic reactions
The treatment of choice for anaphylaxis in adults is intramuscular injection of adrenaline in the mid-outer thigh (1 mg/mL) at a dose of 0.01 mL/kg of body weight, repeated after at least a 5 min interval in the absence of clinical improvement or if deterioration occurs after the initial treatment, to a maximum dose of 0.5 mL. Patients who require repeated intramuscular doses of adrenaline may benefit from an adrenaline infusion. High-flow oxygen should be administered by face mask to all patients, as well as intravenous fluids; crystalloids given in boluses of 20 mL/kg in case of cardiovascular instability. Patients should be kept still and positioned lying on their back, with the lower extremities elevated to conserve circulation, or if unconscious placed in the recovery position. Patients should avoid sudden abrupt change to a more upright posture. Systemic antihistamines are commonly used in anaphylaxis but have only

been demonstrated to relieve cutaneous symptoms. Oral H1 (and H2) antihistamines are therefore only recommended for the relief of cutaneous symptoms of anaphylaxis. Oral or intravenous glucocorticosteroids are commonly used in anaphylaxis and are thought to possibly prevent protracted anaphylaxis symptoms; however, this has not been proven and they have a slow onset of action. Oral or parenteral glucocorticosteroids may be given once first and second line therapies have been administered [51]. Patients at risk of an anaphylactic response to Hymenoptera stings should wear a device such as a MedicAlert warning bracelet, in case they are discovered unconscious following a sting. All patients with a history of systemic anaphylactic reactions should also carry a sting emergency kit containing an autoinjector with adrenaline. Administration of a dose of 0.15 mg for patients weighing between 7.5 kg and 25 kg, and 0.3 mg for >25 kg, is recommended. They should therefore receive instruction in self-administration of adrenaline [51].

Venom immunotherapy

The introduction of venom immunotherapy has reduced the risk of anaphylaxis in Hymenoptera-sensitive patients. It is thought to exert its beneficial effect by stimulating the development of IgG (blocking) antibodies against the venom allergens. This prophylactic measure is indicated in patients with a history of life-threatening reactions to stings, positive skin tests and the presence of venom-specific serum IgE. However, such therapy should only be carried out in specialised units.

According to current European guidelines, venom immunotherapy is recommended only for patients with a history of moderate to severe reactions [53,54]. In cases of mild reactions, which are limited to the skin, venom immunotherapy is not considered mandatory. Golden *et al.* [55] suggested expanding the clinical indications for venom immunotherapy to include large local reactors where insect stings cause significant morbidity and impair the quality of life.

Lice (Phthiraptera)

Definition and nomenclature

Lice are members of the order Phthiraptera. They are wingless, dorsoventrally flattened insects, which are obligate ectoparasites of birds and mammals. The Phthiraptera are highly host specific and spend their entire lives on the host. Members of the suborder Anoplura are blood-sucking ectoparasites of mammals.

Synonyms and inclusions
- Pediculosis

Classification

Humans are parasitised by two species of Anoplura: *Pediculus humanus*, divided into *Pediculus humanus capitis* (head louse) and *Pediculus humanus humanus* (clothing or body louse); and *Pthirus pubis* (pubic or crab louse). Head lice and clothing lice are morphologically and biologically similar but have distinct ecologies. They have almost the same basic genetic content, i.e. being ecotypes of the same species (*Pediculus humanus*) [1], even if they differentially express certain genes. They are capable of interbreeding, but on the host they maintain their territorial preferences. *Pthirus pubis* is morphologically quite distinct from *Pediculus*. It is a louse that has only one close relative in the insect world, a species living on gorillas (*Pthirus gorillae*) and the ancestor of human pubic lice. It is thought that our human ancestors acquired pubic lice from gorillas, perhaps by sharing their bedding material or by humans feeding on gorillas. Interestingly, chimpanzees, our closest primate relative, are parasitised by *Pediculus* species (*P. schaeffi*) but not by *Pthirus*, and orangutans do not have lice.

Pthirus is the correct zoological name for the crab louse – the name should have been *Phthirus*, but a misprint was inadvertently accepted by the International Committee on Zoological Nomenclature [2].

The Anoplura are vessel feeders (solenophages), introducing their mouthparts directly into a blood vessel to withdraw blood [3,4]. The components responsible for probing the skin and piercing a blood vessel are a group of stylets, which are kept withdrawn within the head unless the insect is feeding. In the front of the head is a small snout-like tube, the haustellum, which is soft, eversible and armed with teeth. When the louse is about to feed, the haustellum is everted and the buccal teeth rotated outwards (Figure 34.11a). The teeth cut into the epidermis and the haustellum is driven into the skin. It eventually comes to rest with the buccal teeth fully everted, anchoring the mouthparts (Figure 34.11b). Once fixed in the skin, a bundle of stylets is pushed forward through the opening in the haustellum by protractor muscles within the head of the louse (Figure 34.11c). The stylets are advanced into the dermis as a single bundle or fascicle and probe for a small blood vessel.

Head lice (Pediculus capitis)

Epidemiology

Incidence and prevalence [5,6,7]
The head louse has a worldwide distribution, and head louse infestation (pediculosis capitis) is common both in high-, and in low- and middle-income countries. However, precise data on current prevalence are relatively sparse. The traditional perception of head lice as a parasitosis exclusively associated with schoolchildren of low socioeconomic status has now changed [8]. High rates of head louse infection have been reported from the USA, Canada and several other countries; a review by Gratz [5] provides a comprehensive survey of published information relating to prevalence. In the UK, prevalence has been reported to be 2%, with an annual incidence of 37% [9]. In Australia, the reported prevalence in schoolchildren is 13%. In Brazil, a prevalence of 43% in a slum and 28% in a fishing village was shown in 2005 [10]. In China, the prevalence is 14% (range of 0–52%) [11]. The numbers are stable, with a general estimation at 19%, the highest being in Central and South America (33%) and the lowest in Europe (5%) [12]. More recently, a decrease in the numbers of infestations has been described with the Covid-19 pandemic and associated mandatory lockdowns [13].

Age/sex
Head lice are more common in children, particularly in the age range 3–11 years, than in adults, and most surveys have shown that girls

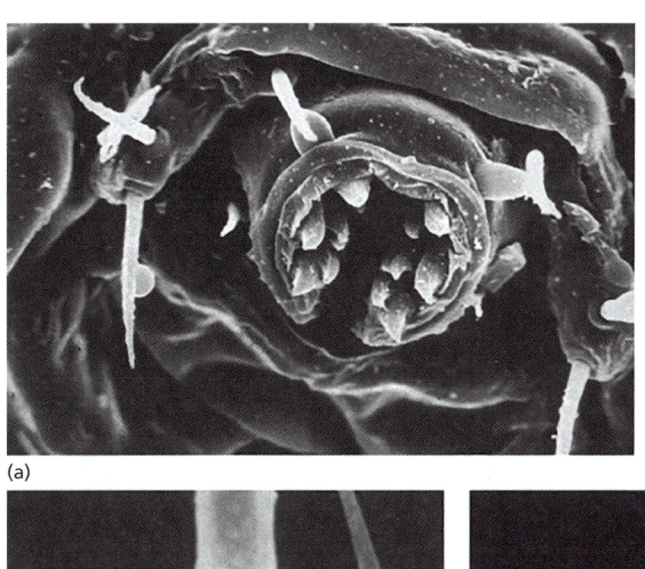
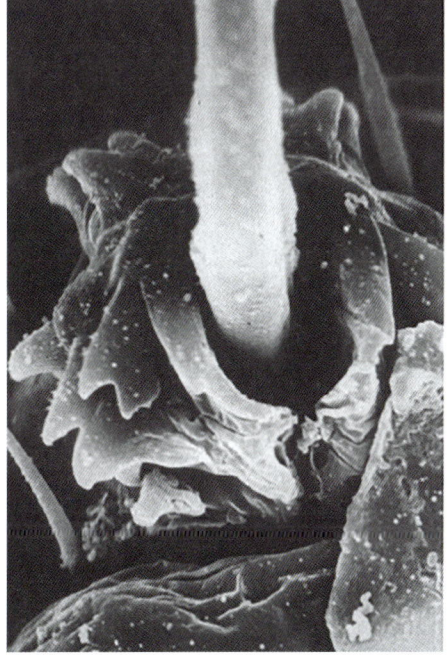
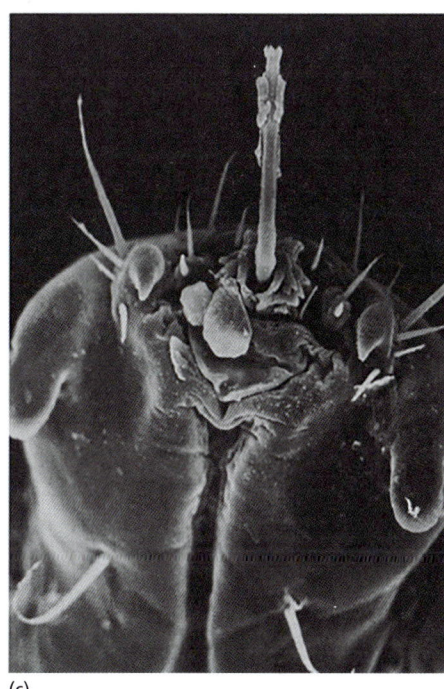

Figure 34.11 Scanning electron micrograph of a crab louse showing (a) haustellum with buccal teeth; (b) everted buccal teeth; and (c) the protruded stylet bundle.

are more frequently infected than boys [12]. Behaviour patterns in girls and boys at different ages probably influence rates of infection [14]. For example, in primary schools, children are organised into small groups around desks and head-to-head contact is frequent. In addition, hair contact is probably more likely between girls than boys. Older children tend to be more independent and more separated from their peers. The contribution of hair length to infection is contentious. Some studies have not shown any correlation between hair length and louse infection rates, but in others children with longer hair have had higher infection rates. A survey from Israel, in which detection of infection was by means of a louse comb rather than direct visual inspection, found a significantly higher infection rate in children with long and medium-length hair than in those with short hair [15].

Ethnicity

Several authors have noted a low incidence of head louse infection in black Americans [16,17], although infection rates in black Africans are high [5]. It has been suggested that the use of pomades by black Americans provides an environment unsuited to establishment of infestation [16], but head lice are quite common in the Indian subcontinent, where hair oils and creams are frequently used [18]. A survey in Brazil found the same prevalence in black as in white people [19].

Associated diseases

Head lice are not known to transmit any human pathogens. However, *Bartonella quintana* has been detected in the head lice of homeless individuals in San Francisco or more recently in Tokyo [20,21], in Nepalese slum children [22], but also in children in rural areas in Africa [23,24]. In a study in Paris in 2008–9, *Acinetobacter baumanii*, but not *B. quintana*, was detected in 95 samples (33%) from a total of 288 DNA samples from head lice collected from the heads of schoolchildren [25]. These results were consistent with a more recent study, perfomed in 2018 in the same area [26]. The significance of the finding of *A. baumanii* in head lice is uncertain [25], but since then the bacterium has been frequently associated with the head louse in different parts of the world [27–29].

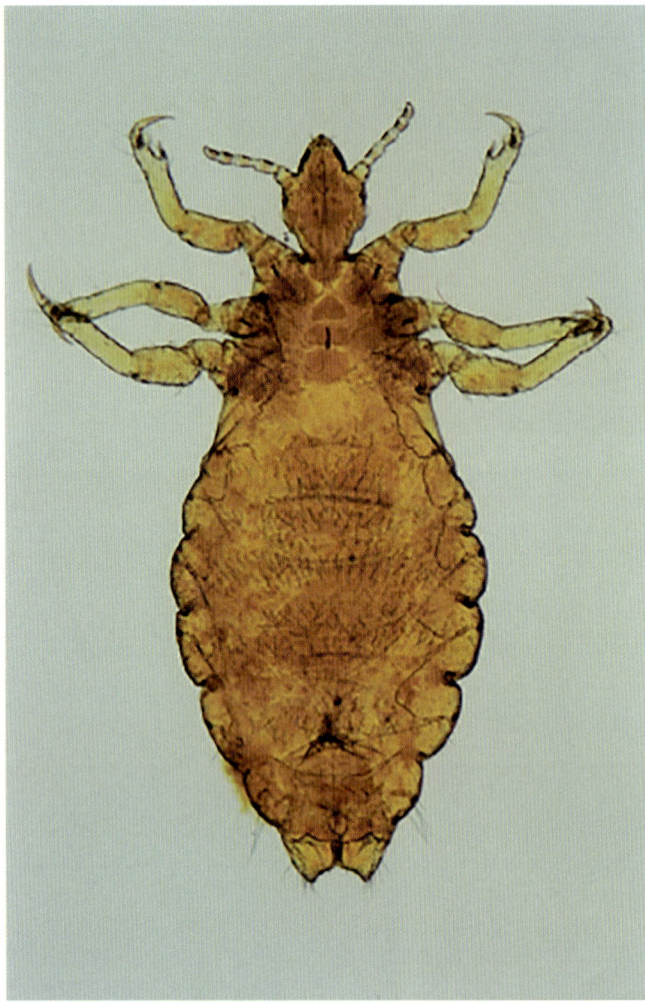

Figure 34.12 *Pediculus capitis*, the head louse.

Pathophysiology [2,7,30–32]

The adult female is a greyish white insect 3–4 mm long (Figure 34.12). The male is slightly smaller. The claws on the legs are adapted for clinging to hair. During her lifespan of approximately 40 days, the female lays an average of about seven eggs daily. The eggs are cemented to hair shafts with a chitinous cement material secreted by the female's accessory glands [32] (Figure 34.13a). In temperate climates, in order to provide a suitable temperature for incubation, the eggs are attached to hair close to the surface of the scalp. They are oval, flesh coloured and have a lid (operculum) capping the free end of the egg (Figure 34.13b). The operculum is pushed off by the emerging louse nymph. Once the louse has emerged, the empty egg case or 'nit' appears white and is easier to see than the intact eggs close to the scalp surface. Eggs hatch in about 8 days and, following three moults, the louse nymph reaches maturity in approximately 10 days.

It is thought that the majority of head louse infections are acquired by direct head-to-head contact, optimal conditions for transfer being when hairs are parallel and slow moving [33]. Burgess *et al.* estimated that it takes at least 30 seconds for lice to move from one head to another [34]. In low- and middle-income countries, spread of lice is encouraged by poverty, poor hygiene and overcrowding. Lack of hygiene alone does not encourage head louse infection.

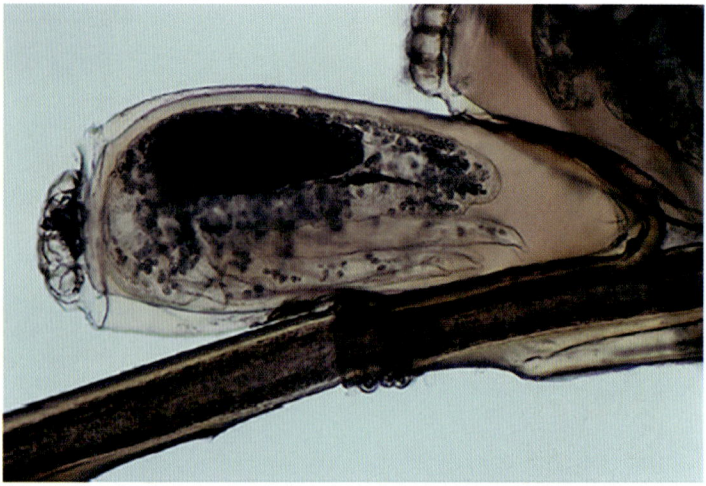

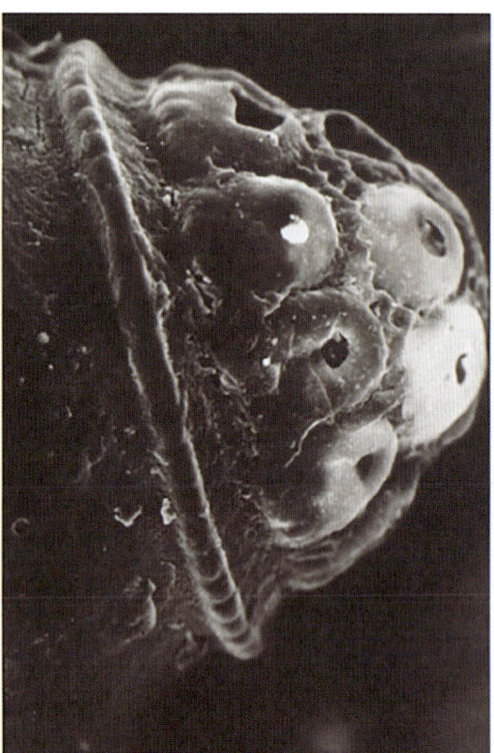

Figure 34.13 (a) Head louse eggs cemented to a hair shaft. (b) Scanning electron micrograph of the operculum on a head louse egg.

There are conflicting opinions about the importance of fomites in transmission of head lice [35–37], and in practice the putative role of caps, scarves, towels, pillowcases, combs and brushes is difficult to confirm or refute.

In Australia, an examination of classroom floors in schools in which there was an overall prevalence of head lice of 20.9%, employing a vacuum cleaner fitted with a filter, did not reveal any lice on the floors [38], suggesting that there is no requirement for anti-louse measures on carpets and floors.

Clinical features

Although many individuals are asymptomatic [39], scalp pruritus is the characteristic manifestation of head louse infection. Secondary

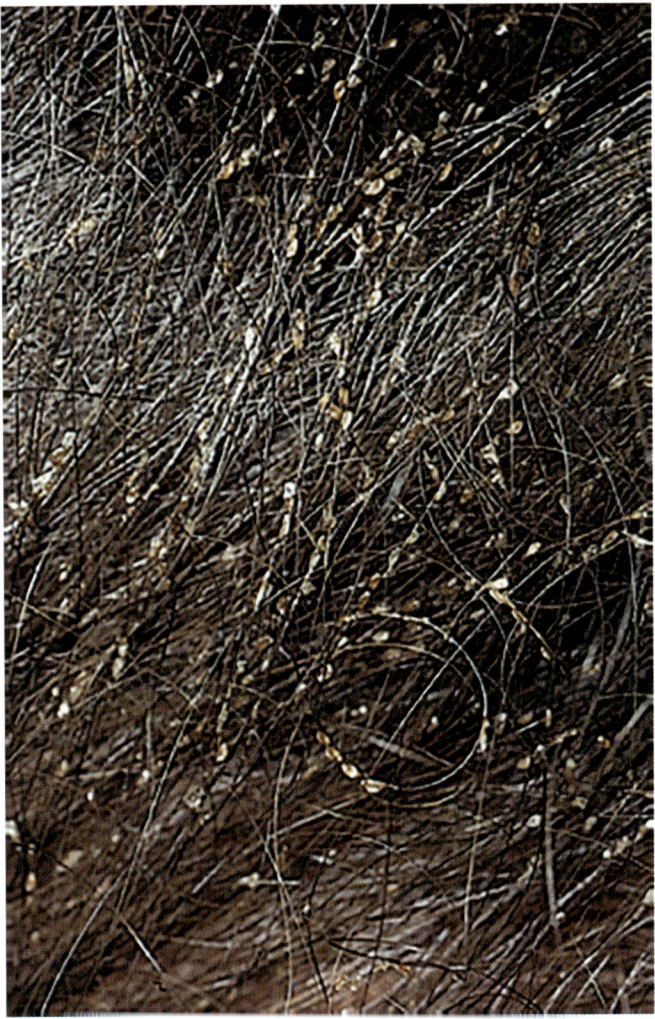

Figure 34.14 Numerous head louse eggs and empty egg cases.

bacterial infection may occur as a result of scratching and concomitant head louse infection must always be considered in cases of scalp impetigo. Pruritic papular lesions may occur on the nape of the neck and occasionally a generalised non-specific pruritic eruption develops [40]. In severe neglected cases, pus and exudate may produce matting of the hair – a state that has been termed 'plica polonica', from its prevalence in Poland in the early part of the 20th century. However, matting of the hair can occur in the absence of louse infection and it has been suggested that this term should be discarded [41].

The empty egg cases (nits) occur in greatest density on the parietal and occipital regions (Figure 34.14). However, on naked-eye inspection, they may be confused with peripilar keratin casts ('pseudonits'; hair muffs) [42,43] or dried globules of cheap hair lacquer.

Investigations
Detection of adult lice and nymphs provides evidence of an 'active' infestation, whereas the presence of eggs and egg cases alone merely indicates that infection has occurred at some time. The most reliable method of diagnosing current active infestation is by detection combing, which has been shown to be superior to direct visual examination of the hair and scalp [15,44–46], and also faster (57 s with the comb, versus 116 s with direct visual examination) [15]. Vacuuming the hair and scalp (with a voile inserted between the hose and the flat nozzle of the vaccum) could also be helpful. In a study performed in Southern Brazil, the vacuum method was less effective than visual inspection to diagnose overall infestation, but perfomed well at differentiating active infestation [47]. This is an important criterion for several reasons:

1 Individuals who do not have evidence of active infestation should not receive chemical treatment [46].
2 Participants in clinical trials of pediculicides should have live lice present on the head before enrolment, not just eggs alone.
3 Children who do not have evidence of active infestation may be inappropriately excluded from school [46,48,49].

Management
Principles of management [6,7,31,46,50,51–54]
Management of head louse infestation is difficult because good comparative effectiveness research is still lacking and louse resistance to pyrethroid has emerged. An initial Cochrane systematic review concerning pediculicides was withdrawn in 2007 [55], and again in 2018 [56].

The ideal treatment should be completely safe, free of harmful chemicals, readily available, easy to use and inexpensive. It should also be effective where there are local variations in resistance.

General guidelines for the use of chemical pediculicides have included advice to repeat treatment after 7–10 days [57] because of limited ovicidal activity, and that lotion and liquid formulations are preferable to shampoos as the latter expose the insects to relatively low concentrations of insecticide with subsequent poor efficacy, which, in the long term, might favour the development of resistance. Preparations with an aqueous base are less likely to irritate an excoriated scalp than alcoholic solutions, do not irritate the bronchi of asthmatics and are not flammable. Sprays are not suitable for people with asthma.

Family members should be examined and treated only if they show evidence of active infestation by the presence of live lice. Nits may be removed with a fine-toothed comb. Treatment has most chance of success if it is applied or undertaken correctly and if all affected individuals in the household are treated simultaneously. People should be advised to check whether treatment was successful by detection combing on day 2 after completing a course of treatment, and again after an interval of 7 days.

All materials that touched the heads of infested persons, such as hats, scarves, bedding and cushions, must be thoroughly washed in hot water (50°C at least) [58]. Any infested materials kept in plastic bags for 3 days may be safely used. Hair grooming aids, such as brushes, combs and curlers, should be discarded or decontaminated with an insecticidal powder.

Acquired resistance to insecticides
Classic insecticides like dichlorodiphenyltrichloroethane (DDT), lindane, carbaryl and malathion have been progressively replaced since the 1980s by pyrethrin and pyrethroid insecticides. These insectides are efficient, safe, convenient and cost-effective. Available formulations include 1% permethrin and pyrethrins plus piperonyl butoxide. However, lice with pyrethroid-resistant phenotype

emerged in the early 1990s [59]. There is now evidence of widespread pyrethroid resistance and less frequently malathion [59–66].

Pyrethroids are neurotoxins that modify the louse voltage-gated sodium channel (VGSC), causing spastic paralysis and death. Permethrin resistance in head lice is mostly conferred by the knockdown resistance (kdr) trait, conferred by three point mutations (M815I–T917I–L920F) in the VGSC α-subunit gene [67]. The prevalence of kdr-like louse alleles is not exactly known, but seems to be extremely variable, depending on the geographical area [68,69].

Alternative treatments

Resistance of head lice to insecticides led researchers to look for alternatives.

Physical treatment is an alternative to the use of chemical agents and, in the UK, the 'Bug Busting' (Community Hygiene Concern, London, UK) wet-combing method has been promoted as a treatment for head lice. The technique involves ordinary shampooing of the hair, followed by the application of generous amounts of conditioner, and combing using a fine-toothed comb to remove lice. This procedure is repeated every 4 days for 2 weeks [61–74]. Shaving the head is usually not acceptable because of psychosocial impact.

Dimethicone lotion (4% long-chain linear silicone in a volatile silicone base) [75–77] blocks the outer respiratory tract of lice and therefore water excretion, which causes physiological stress and death [78]. Coconut-derived emulsion shampoo, benzyl alcohol lotion 5% and spinosad cream rinse may be used too [79–81], as well as isopropyl myristate and cyclomethicone together [82].

Other readily available occlusive substances such as oils and margarine have been suggested but information on effectiveness is anecdotal. In one study that examined vinegar, isopropyl alcohol, olive oil, mayonnaise, melted butter and petroleum jelly, the use of petroleum jelly caused the greatest egg mortality, allowing only 6% to hatch [83].

Essential oils have been widely used in traditional medicine for the eradication of head lice, but because of the variability of their constitution, the effects may not be reproducible [84–86]. They can also cause toxic side effects such as irritation of the skin [87] or even neurological adverse events [88]. Several products including lavender, eucalyptus and tea-tree oils are marketed for the treatment of head lice and are in wide use. Although many plants naturally produce insecticides for their own protection that may be synthesised for use by humans, such as pyrethroids, some of these insecticidal chemicals produce toxic effects as well.

Ivermectin is a broad antiparasitic drug used for onchocerciasis, lymphatic filariasis (Chapter 33) or scabies. It induces arthropod and nematode paralysis and death by interrupting neurotransmission, acting on glutamate-gated or γ-aminobutyric acid–gated chloride channels. In a cluster-randomised controlled trial of patients with head lice refractory to insecticides, a single oral dose of ivermectin 400 µg/kg repeated within 7 days achieved higher louse-free rates on day 15 than 0.5% malathion (95.2% versus 85.0%) and their household members (92.4% versus 79.1%) [89]. This is an 'off-label' use of such dosage of ivermectin and its safety in patients with head louse infestation remains unknown. Topical ivermectin has shown greater efficacy than placebo in a randomised controlled trial and is now sold over the counter in the USA [90]. The lotion sounds convenient (i.e. applied to dry hair, left for 10 min, then rinsed with water, one single application), which should increase compliance. Surveillance is mandatory as recent treatment failures and possible resistance have been reported with ivermectin in geographical areas where the drug is widely administered for other parasites (onchocerciasis mass drug administration compaigns) [91]. Widespread use, including recent over-the-counter access, could be a concern [92].

Other interesting treatments are under development, especially drugs that could target all stages of the insect life cycle, including the egg stage. Abametapir, a metalloproteinase inhibitor, is a good candidate that could be given to patients as a single-dose topical treatment [93,94]. Isoxazolines (see paragraph on fleas earlier) are also considered [95]. Reliable trials are mandatory to generate high levels of evidence from randomised controlled trials and subsequently robust guidelines [96].

First line

The choice of a particular treatment strategy will depend on age, individual or parent preference, cost and success or failure with previous treatments. There is limited evidence to support the effectiveness of each treatment option recommended. No option is clearly superior or inferior to the others in terms of effectiveness and there are advantages and disadvantages for each method, and no method can guarantee success. There are different options: topical chemicals, topical oils, mechanical, topical physical, or systemic drugs. Topical chemical pediculicides that are still in use in Europe, the UK and the USA are permethrin, d-phenothrin, bioallethrin and synergised pyrethrins. Lindane and carbaryl were withdrawn in Europe in 2007. For malathion, following safety concerns, and a restriction to prescription-only from the French drug agency, the drug was withdrawn from the French market in 2018. It is also important to consider that most treatments that are used to treat head lice are medical devices and are not registered as 'drugs', and as such fewer regulatory requirements are mandatory for their commercialisation. In a French study performed in 2015, 21 over-the-counter head louse products bought from randomly selected pharmacies were tested *ex vivo* on 3919 lice and 4321 living eggs collected from the scalps of 400 children. Most products were poorly efficient [97]. The American Academy of Pediatrics recommends the use of 1% permethrin or pyrethrin insecticide as first line therapy [98], as do the Centers for Disease Control and Prevention (CDC) for over-the-counter medications, and either 5% benzyl alcohol, 0.5% ivermectin, 0.5% malathion or 0.9% spinosad lotions for prescription medications (https://www.cdc.gov/parasites/lice/head/treatment.html, last accessed July 2023). In case of therapeutic failure, before considering acquired resistance to insecticides, other options should be considered, e.g. low compliance, wrong formulation, insufficient regimen, reinfestation (Box 34.1). If resistance in the community has been proven or live lice are present 1 day after the completion of treatment, a switch to another class of drug may be necessary.

Second line

Second line treatment depends on the first line used. In the USA, second line options include wet combing or treatment with dimethicone or other topical agents, depending on the availability of the agents in the country.

Third or fourth line
Ivermectin if available (depending on the country) should be the last choice, whether topical (for still-infested persons) or oral (especially for mass treatment, off label).

> **Box 34.1 Causes of therapeutic failure for head lice**
>
> - Misunderstanding of instructions
> - Non-compliance
> - Resistance
> - Inappropriate instructions on head lice products or from health professionals
> - High cost of products
> - Misdiagnosis
> - Psychogenic itch
> - Incomplete ovicidal activity
> - Inappropriate preparation (e.g. shampoo)
> - Insufficient dose–time, frequency and/or quantity of product applied
> - Failure to retreat
> - Reinfestation
> - Live eggs not removed
>
> Adapted from Chosidow 2000 [6]. Copyright of original artwork: Elsevier.

Resources

Further information
www.cdc.gov/parasites/lice/head/
http://cks.nice.org.uk/head-lice
(both last accessed June 2023)

Clothing/body lice (Pediculus corporis)

Epidemiology [31]
Incidence and prevalence
Because body lice are associated with poor socioeconomic conditions, with infestation occurring only when clothes are not changed or washed regularly (pediculosis vestimenti), indigent, homeless and refugee-camp populations are predominantly affected. Body louse prevalence is underestimated in more developed countries and, as the number of homeless people increases, louse-borne infectious diseases are also on the rise. Molecular approaches are now convenient tools for epidemiological studies of louse-borne bacteria [99].

Associated diseases
Body lice may transmit several important diseases. The first is the epidemic typhus, caused by *Rickettsia prowazekii* (Chapter 26). Symptoms include headache, fever, confusion and rash. The disease usually becomes epidemic in populations living in poor crowded conditions. A huge outbreak of epidemic typhus (and trench fever but not relapsing fever) occurred in 1995–97 in Burundi, first affecting prison inmates, then more than 45 000 camp refugees [100]. Relapsing fever is caused by a spirochete, *Borrelia recurrentis*. Outbreaks occurred in Ethiopia and Southern Sudan in the 1990s [101]. Trench fever is related to *Bartonella quintana*. The disease was first

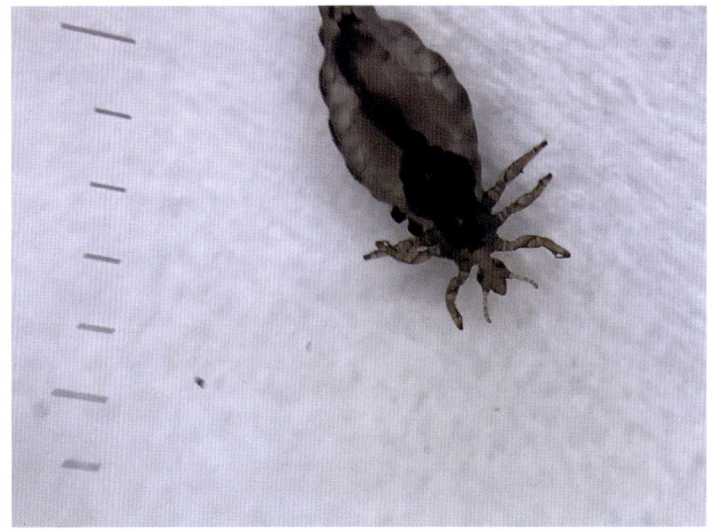

Figure 34.15 *Pediculus corporis*, the body louse, observed by dermoscopy (on the scale on the left the space between two lines corresponds to 1 mm).

recognised during World War I. Symptoms include fever, myalgias, headache, meningoencephalitis, chronic adenopathies and transient maculopapular exanthema, but it may be asymptomatic. Endocarditis may sometimes occur [102]. Homeless people with chronic alcoholism are at risk.

Pathophysiology
This louse is almost identical in appearance to the head louse, except that it is usually slightly larger, and its development is similar (Figure 34.15). Its natural habitat is the clothing of its host and it only visits the skin to feed. Its eggs are cemented to clothing fibres, with a preference for clothing close to the skin. Seams are a favoured site for oviposition. It thrives in situations where normal hygiene is lacking. The clothing louse and its eggs will not survive high-temperature washing and ironing and it is intolerant of temperature changes in its environment. It is therefore a parasite of individuals whose clothing is rarely changed or washed. The number of lice and eggs on the clothing varies greatly. In most infected individuals, the population is small, but in some there may be thousands of lice.

Clinical features [31,103]
In most infected persons, itching is the principal complaint. Pruritus is the result of sensitisation to louse salivary antigens. Others, who have not become sensitised or have acquired tolerance to the bites, are asymptomatic. The body is often covered in excoriations and there may be secondary bacterial infection. In those who have harboured clothing lice for long periods of time the skin is often hyperpigmented (so-called 'vagabonds' disease'; morbus errorum), and this is probably a postinflammatory phenomenon. Lice and eggs should be sought in the clothing.

Management [6,104]
Bed linens, towels and clothes used by the infested person should be decontaminated, and this action suffices for some physicians. Others recommend thorough washing of the body with soap followed by application of a pediculicide (the same as for head lice).

Ivermectin (3 doses of 12 mg each, given at 7-day intervals) was shown to reduce the number of body lice infesting a population of homeless men in 2006. Such treatment may be effective in limiting the viability of body lice in patients living in an institution or routinely returning to a treatment centre or shelter [105]. To prevent reinfestation, improving personal hygiene is important, including a regular change of clean clothes (at least weekly). Depending on the geographical location of the infested individual and his or her contact with other similarly infested individuals, the physician should consider the possibility of louse-borne disease, and antibiotics should be given if so. Infested furniture, mattresses and box springs should be discarded or fumigated to destroy lice and nits. Infested materials sealed in plastic bags may be used safely after 3 days.

Resources

Further information
www.cdc.gov/parasites/lice/body/ (last accessed June 2023)

Crab lice (Phthiriasis pubis)

Epidemiology [31]

Crab lice are transmitted by close physical contact, usually sexual, and infection with these lice occurs most frequently among sexually active young adults. It is standard practice in genito-urinary medicine (GUM) clinics to monitor prevalence rates of sexually transmitted infections, including crab lice. A marked decline in the number of female cases in one department in the UK led to the suggestion that waxing of pubic hair, particularly the fashion known as the 'Brazilian', was an important factor responsible for the decline [106].

Because many patients with crab louse infection who attend GUM clinics are found to be suffering from other sexually transmitted infections [107,108], screening for these is indicated.

Pathophysiology

The crab louse is quite distinctive in appearance (Figure 34.16) and habits from *Pediculus*. Its body is squat, and the second and third pairs of legs carry heavy, pincer-like claws. When static, the crab louse uses these huge claws to grip adjacent hairs close to the skin surface (Figure 34.17, see video published in [109]). Its eggs are squat and bulging compared with *Pediculus*. They are light brown in colour and, like those of the head louse, are cemented to the hair of the host. It is adapted to living in hair of a particular density. Scalp hair, except at the scalp margins, is too dense, but the crab louse will colonise axillary hair, eyebrows, eyelashes, beard hair, and hair on the trunk and limbs, in addition to pubic hair. It is mainly sedentary but becomes active at night when the host is sleeping [110]. It moves by transferring its grip from one hair to another. The crab louse has difficulty moving when taken from its host, whereas head and clothing lice are quite mobile off the host.

Crab lice are not known to transmit any human pathogens. However, DNA of *Bartonella quintana* was recently detected in pubic louse of homeless individuals in Marseille, a city located in the south of France, and in one individual seen at a parasitology consultation in Bobigny, a city close to Paris, between June 2017 and August 2018. Four species of *Acinetobacter* were also found (*A. baumannii, A. guillouiae, A. junii* and *A. schindleri*) [111].

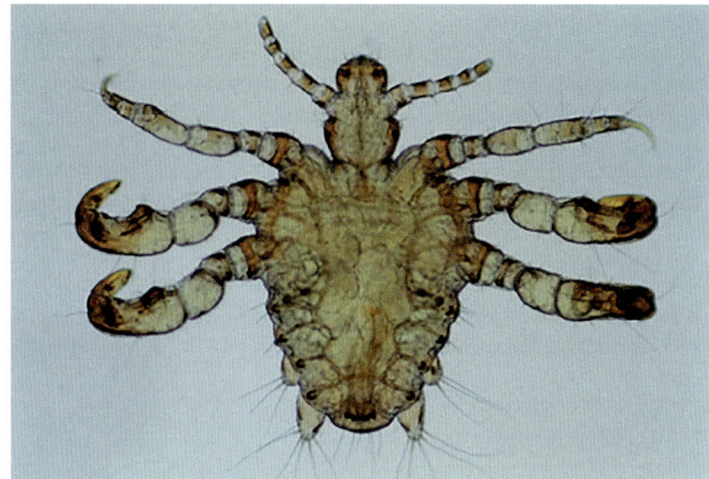

Figure 34.16 *Pthirus pubis*, the crab louse.

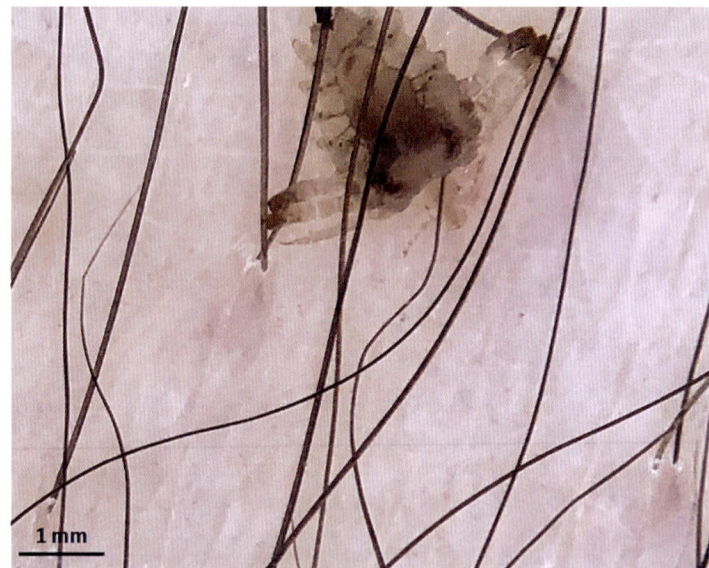

Figure 34.17 Crab louse clinging to pubic hairs.

Clinical features

Itching, mainly in the evening and at night, is the principal symptom. Close inspection of affected areas will reveal lice grasping hairs close to the skin surface and louse eggs attached to the hair shafts. Louse faeces are often visible as rust-coloured speckles on the skin and hair and the underclothes may be spotted with altered blood.

When crab lice are discovered on the pubic area, other hairy areas of the body should be examined, as these lice may colonise eyebrows, eyelashes (Figure 34.18), beard, axillae, areolar hair and the scalp margins [112,113]. In heavy infections in men, the hair on the trunk and limbs may be extensively colonised. A case has been reported in which the presence of an enormous population of lice was attributed to inappropriate use of topical steroids [110].

Blue-grey macules (maculae caeruleae) are occasionally seen on the skin [114], but their precise pathogenesis is unknown. Bullous lesions attributed to crab lice have been reported [115].

In children, crab lice may colonise the eyelashes and scalp [116]. Infection in children is usually acquired by close physical contact

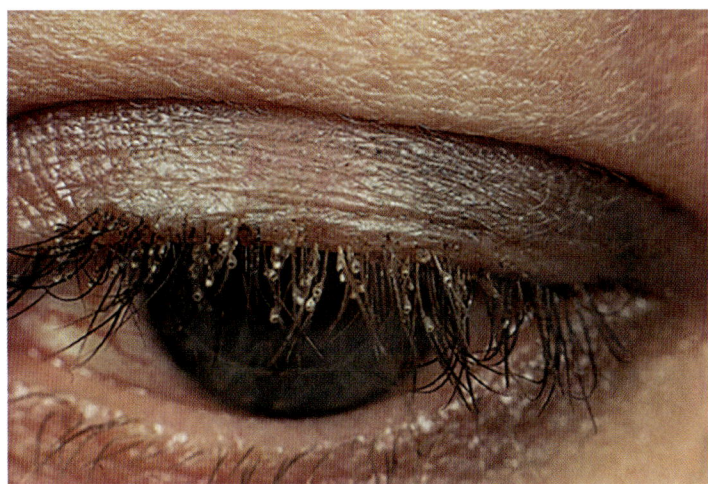

Figure 34.18 Crab louse eggs on the eyelashes.

with infected parents. As an isolated finding, it is not indicative of sexual abuse, although this may occasionally occur [117].

Management [104,118,119]

Pubic lice are treated with the same insecticidal creams or lotions as pediculosis capitis, with a second application after 7–10 days as the products have poor ovicidal activity. Resistance to pyrethrins has been shown [120]. All hairy areas of the body should be treated at the same time. Shaving is sometimes necessary when nits are plentiful. Infestations of the eyelashes should be treated with permethrin 5% cream (washed off after 10 min, to avoid corneal damage [121]) or only with petrolatum (applied twice a day for 8–10 days), followed by mechanical removal of the nits [122–124].

Oral ivermectin has been used by some authors at the regular dosage of 200 µg/kg repeated after 7 days [125–127], but some others have suggested a better and faster efficacy with the double dose of 400 µg/kg [128].

As in other louse infestations, all sexual contacts should be examined and treated when necessary. Bedding and clothes should be washed in hot water (>50°C). Prepubertal children presenting with pubic louse infestations should be evaluated with regard to possible child abuse [117]. Treatment failure is usually a result of an untreated hairy area or reinfestation from an untreated sexual contact. In addition, patients should also be screened for associated sexually transmitted disease.

Resources

Further information
www.cdc.gov/parasites/lice/pubic/
http://www.cdc.gov/mmwr/pdf/rr/rr5912.pdf
Department of Health, UK: http://cks.nice.org.uk/pubic-lice
(All last accessed June 2023)

Bugs (Hemiptera)

Definition

Hemiptera comes from the Greek hemi (half) and pteron (wing) because their wings are hardened near the base and membranous near the ends.

Classification

The suborder Heteroptera, the true bugs, has two families which are haematophagous and ectoparasitic for humans and three families with health impact in case of contact or bite:
- Cimicidae family (including bedbugs) with four major genera: *Cimex*, *Oeciacus*, *Leptocimex* and *Haematosiphon*.
- Reduviidae family (including kissing and assassin bugs) with three major genera: *Triatoma*, *Rhodnius* and *Panstrongylus*.
- Anthocoridae family commonly called minute pirate bugs or flower bugs.
- Pentatomidae family commonly called stink bugs.
- Belostomatidae family commonly called giant water bugs.

Haematophagous bugs (bedbugs and kissing bugs) are a minority compared with the high number of Hemiptera but they have a considerable impact on human health. A global resurgence of bedbugs has been observed since the 1990s, with clinical and pest control implications. The kissing bugs are vectors of *Trypanosoma cruzi*, the parasite of Chagas disease.

Family Cimicidae, including bedbugs

Classification [1–3]

This family includes 24 genera and 110 known species [4]. Cimicidae is a cosmopolitan family. Species are all ectoparasites of homeothermic vertebrates. All the stages of the life cycle are haematophagous. The host is often very specific and includes mainly birds and bats. It has been suggested that Cimicidae became adapted to feeding on humans when cave dwellers took up residence alongside bats. Bedbugs (*Cimex* spp.) are a small part of the family of Cimicidae.

Genus *Cimex*. *Cimex lectularius* (the common bedbug) is the species of bedbug that is cosmopolitan and will be discussed here.

Cimex hemipterus (the tropical bedbug) is less tolerant of low temperatures than *C. lectularius*. This bug is confined to tropical and subtropical regions, including India, Myanmar, Malaysia, South China and Central Africa, but infestation is possible in occidental countries because of world trade.

Cimex pipistrelli (the batbug), originating in a bat roost in a house, was responsible for itchy skin lesions in one of the house occupants [5].

Genus *Leptocimex*. *Leptocimex boueti* has a limited distribution in West Africa, where it parasitises humans and bats.

Genus *Oeciacus*. Several species are usually found on birds and in their nests, for example *Oeciacus hirundinis*, the martin bug [6], and *O. vicarius*, the swallow bug. They may invade houses from nests under the eaves and will bite humans readily, but it is unlikely that they can complete their life cycles on human blood or take up residence in houses as bedbugs do.

Genus *Haematosiphon*. *Haematosiphon inodorus*, the only species in this genus, is also known as the Mexican chicken bug. As the name suggests, its major host is the chicken, but it can be a serious pest in human domiciles if these are close to chicken roosts.

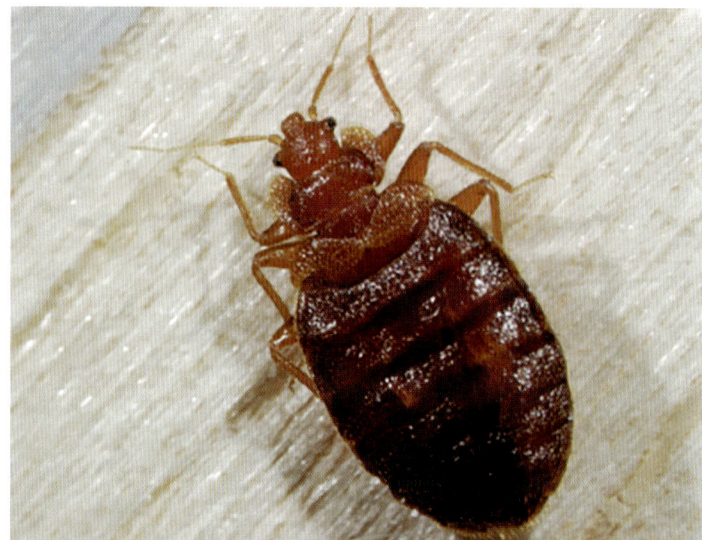

Figure 34.19 Bedbug adult (5–7 mm): *Cimex lectularius*.

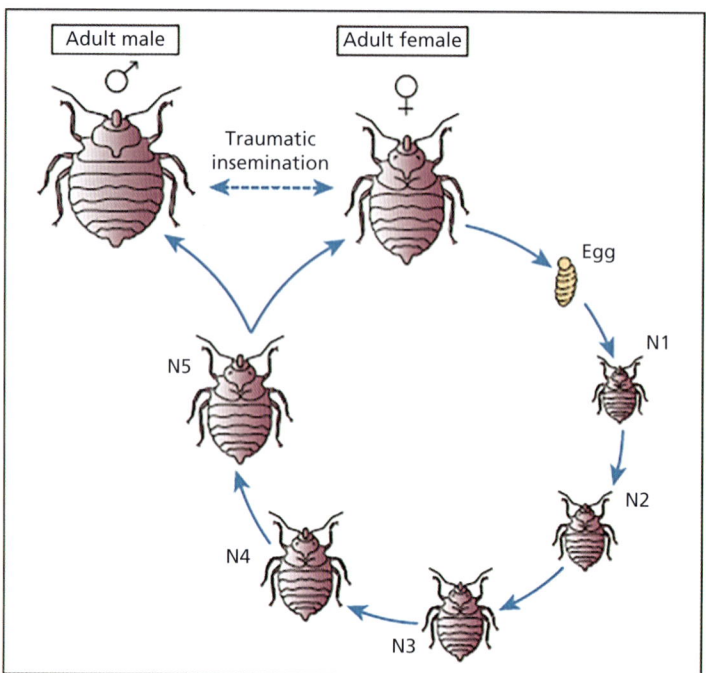

Figure 34.20 The life cycle of the bedbug. From Bernardeschi *et al.* 2013 [19]. Source and copyright holder: BMJ Publishing Group Ltd.

Introduction and general description

Bedbugs are resurging in developed countries [7], possibly due to international travel and changes in pest control practices [8]. Diagnosis of bedbug infestation relies on clinical manifestations of bites and direct observation of the arthropod, which is rarely recognised by those who are bitten [9] (Figure 34.19). Evidence is lacking on the bedbug's capacity to transmit disease, management of eradication and the economic impact of infestations.

Epidemiology [10,11]

Australian and European observational studies have shown increases in pest manager interventions in the past 30 years. There was a growing number of bedbugs identified in Australian laboratories between 2001 and 2004 [12–14]. In Europe, the British Pest Control Association's Executive Summary of 2014 showed that bedbug treatments by local authorities increased by 21% between 2010 and 2011 and 2013 and 2014 [11]. The reasons for this resurgence are not clearly understood and might be multifactorial. Different contributing factors may have played a role:
- The increase in domestic and international travel [15].
- The emergence of pyrethroid insecticide resistance [8,16], due to multiple mutations, which may also have contributed to dissemination [17].
- Using new techniques like bait to control other insects such as cockroaches, which may have permitted the growth of bedbug populations [18].

Sites of infestations are wide and include hotels, private homes, public transport vehicles and crafts (trains, cruise ships and aeroplanes), theatres, hospitals, long-term care facilities and armed-forces buildings [10,19,20]. In New York City, data (published in 2014) showed a prevalence as high as 12% in some neighbourhoods [10], and that at least 80% of hotels had dealt with bedbugs in 2015 (data from USA pest-control firms) [10,11]. Websites have been developed for travellers to check if their future hotel has had any reports of bedbug infestation (https://www.bedbugreports.com).

Because many disease pathogens have previously been reported in bedbugs [7,21,22], their role as potential vectors of infectious diseases is of interest. However, their full vectorial role has not yet been demonstrated [7], despite vectorial competence being demonstrated for *Borrelia recurrentis* [23], *Bartonella quintana* [24] and *Trypanosoma cruzi* [25]. Studies suggest that bedbugs may contain 'neutralising factors' that attenuate pathogen virulence and thereby decrease the ability of bedbugs to transmit infectious disease [26].

Pathophysiology [3,10]

Bedbugs are 4–5 mm in length, with dorsoventrally flattened, oval bodies, the forewings reduced to scale-like pads, and the hindwings absent. The mouthparts are modified into a proboscis adapted for piercing and sucking.

Female bedbugs deposit their pearly white, flask-shaped eggs in the crevices of floors and walls, in furniture, bedframes and mattresses. Each female lays about 300 eggs in her lifetime. The eggs hatch after about 10 days; the nymphal stage lasts approximately 6 weeks, during which time the bug moults five times (Figure 34.20) [19].

Bedbugs normally feed at night, usually about an hour before dawn, but they may feed during the day if circumstances are favourable [27]. They usually fear light and avoid glossy surfaces. During the day, they hide in dark places such as crevices in furniture and mattresses or peeling wallpaper. Searching for a food source is erratic and is probably at random at distances greater than a few centimetres, but in the final approach to the host, both temperature and odour play a part in guiding the bug. Feeding time is relatively short (3–12 min). During feeding, the bedbug injects saliva containing an anticoagulant and anaesthetic. A study performed in 2013 demonstrated that allergens causing itching and skin lesions are most likely contained in the saliva of bedbugs. Interestingly, bedbugs without salivary glands attempted to feed but were unable to do so, indicating that saliva is necessary for the feeding process. Furthermore, bedbug saliva was potent enough to cause pruritus and lesion development in a human volunteer by topical application alone, without breaking the skin [28].

Adult bedbugs that have a food source can live up to 4–5 months. In the absence of a suitable food supply, adult bedbugs can survive starvation, in ideal circumstances, an average of 70 days [29]. In the absence of its usual host, C. lectularius will attack other animals, and Cimicidae normally parasitic on other hosts are similarly prepared to attack humans, invading houses from birds' nests or chicken runs. The transmission of bedbugs may be passive, usually in clothing, luggage and furniture. Active dissemination also occurs using electric wiring or ventilation ducts.

Clinical features
Presentation
The initial bite is usually not felt because of the anaesthetic contained in the saliva of bedbugs. Allergic reactions to saliva may sometimes occur late. Although most patients do not have any symptoms after the first bites, reactions may occur 10 days later [30]. The most common reactions to bedbugs are pruritic maculopapular lesions centred by the bite, visible as a haemorrhagic punctum [8]. The distribution of the lesions may be evocative if the lesions are grouped on a line or a curve ('breakfast-lunch-dinner alignment', Figure 34.21a). However, this pattern of distribution is not specific for bedbugs and can be found in other arthropod infestations. Most of the lesions are distributed on uncovered areas of the body. Nodules (Figure 34.21b), bullous lesions (Figure 34.21c) or urticaria (Figure 34.21d) are less commonly found [8,31]. Few cases of systemic symptoms or anaphylaxis have been reported [8]. Bedbug infestation may also present as isolated pruritus. Patient questioning usually highlights similar symptoms in people who share the same bed or travel. Furthermore, lesions classically disappear when changing sleeping place. Bedbug infestation is confirmed by the identification of the insect, not requiring the assistance of an entomologist in most cases.

The bites of other Cimicidae are essentially similar, but their distribution depends on the method of exposure. Haematosiphoniasis is the name given to the cutaneous lesions caused by the bites of *Haematosiphon inodorus* (the Mexican chicken bug). Polymorphic lesions, consisting of weals, papules, vesicles, pustules and scabs, occur predominantly on exposed parts (uncovered) of the body [32].

Differential diagnosis
Various differential diagnoses can be made. The first is other arthropod bites [33], mainly scabies. However, the distribution of the lesions is not the same, as covered areas are commonly involved in scabies [**19,34**] (see Table 34.2). Furthermore, a central punctum corresponding to the bite site is not visible as in bedbug infestation. Flea infestation can be confounding, because of the same pattern of distribution of lesions, located on a line or curve.

Other dermatological differential diagnoses may require skin biopsy. They include Sweet syndrome, erythema multiforme or bullous dermatitis.

Complications and co-morbidities
Secondary bacterial infections (*Staphylococcus* or *Streptococcus*) of the cutaneous lesions are the main complications [35]. The psychological consequences may be important, leading sometimes to parasitophobia, but they are still underevaluated and underrecognised.

Management [10]
Management of bedbug bites
Management of bedbug bites is based on expert opinion. Topical steroids are used to relieve symptoms [36]. Systemic antihistamines may be helpful in cases of severe pruritus [36]. Secondary bacterial infections may require topical or systemic antibiotics, depending on the severity [37].

Management of bedbug infestation
Patient education. Patient and physician education by expert entomologists, parasitologists, dermatologists or expert pest managers is fundamental. Detection and identification of the arthropod (Figure 34.22a) or its faecal traces (Figure 34.22b) in suspected areas should be explained to physicians and patients [38].

Inspection and detection. The house of the patient has to be inspected meticulously including rest areas, beds, sofas and their surroundings, but also walls, wall cracks, tapestries, draperies and conduits for electric cables, to detect the insect or its dark faecal traces. As bedbugs emit a characteristic musty, sweet odour, trained sniffer dogs can be very efficient in detecting them [39]. This can be very helpful in large-scale facilities. Bedbug traps can also be used in cases of low-level infestation, although few of the commercialised kits have been seriously evaluated [40,41].

Non-chemical intervention. Bedbugs may be able to survive without feeding for 70 days; therefore, keeping infested places vacant cannot be recommended [7]. Early detection and control are recommended when possible. Entomologists and pest managers recommend the physical removal of bedbugs by using a vacuum cleaner with a disposal bag, which is immediately removed and sealed in plastic after use [10,42]. All life stages of bedbugs may be killed by washing at 60°C, dry cleaning or tumble drying at 40°C [43]. Placing items in a freezer for at least 2 h can be an option, but most domestic freezers are generally insufficient because insects should be frozen at -20°C to be killed [44]. Mattresses and furniture can be steamed at 60°C using affordable consumer-grade commercial steamers (conditions of use developed in [10]). Silicates and diatomaceous earth may be helpful in the management of bedbugs but need further investigation [45].

Chemical treatment. Bedbug infestations can be treated by insecticides, but this is not mandatory, especially when infestation of the dwelling is low. Pyrethroids are mainly used [46], as well as carbamates and insect growth regulators. Organophosphates are no longer used in Europe [47]. Bedbug resistance to all insecticides has been demonstrated [16,48]. In this situation, a combination of available products may be preferred. A second treatment is often necessary because of the low efficiency of insecticides against eggs. The delay between the two treatments is not clearly known, ranging from 4 to 20 days, depending on the temperature of the infested site.

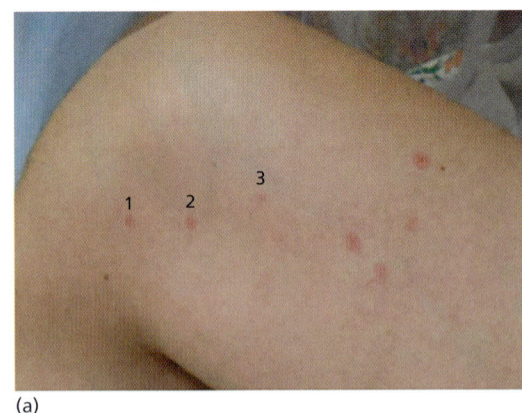
(a)

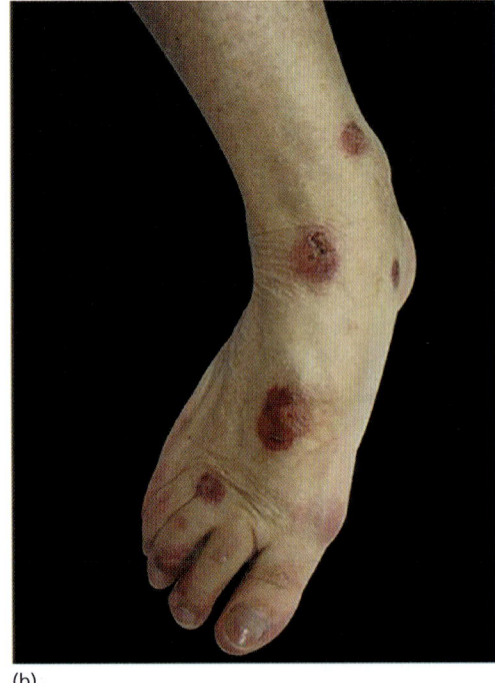
(b)

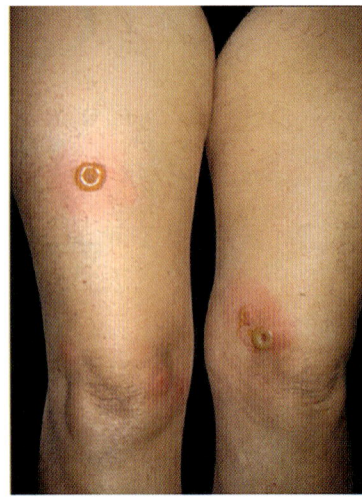
(c)

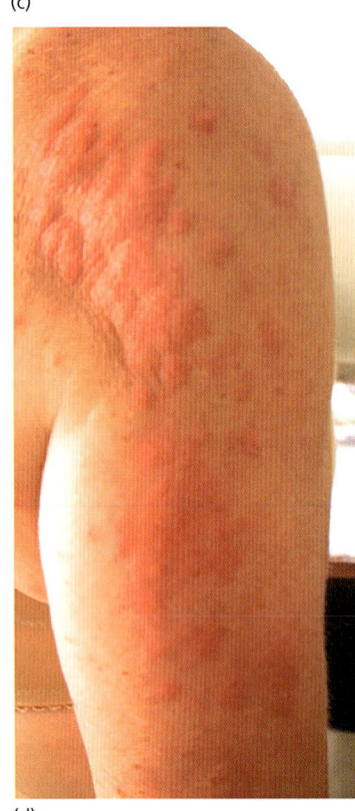
(d)

Figure 34.21 Clinical manifestations of bedbug bites: (a) three or four skin lesions are often seen in a 'breakfast (1), lunch (2), dinner (3)' distribution or (b) 'wheel' distribution. (c) Atypical bullous lesions and (d) urticarial. Bernardeschi et al. [19], BMJ Publishing Group Ltd.

Prevention of infestation [36]

The best way to prevent the spread of bedbugs is by early detection. It is recommended to wash mattress covers and bed linen at 60°C, seal cracks and crevices at home and regularly inspect furniture. Buying secondhand mattresses and furniture is a risk. Travellers should inspect their hotel room before sleeping and should not place their belongings such as suitcases on the floor, but consider placing them in a plasic trash bag or protective cover. Travellers who are exposed to bedbugs need to decontaminate luggage, clothes and belongings on returning home, using mechanical methods (brushing, vacuuming, heating, washing or freezing), rather than chemical methods, to eliminate eggs or bugs [15].

Resources

Further information

Doggett, S.L., Miller, D.M., and Lee, C.Y. (ed.) (2018). *Advances in the Biology and Management of Modern Bed Bugs*. Oxford: Wiley Blackwell.

University of Kentucky: https://www.ca.uky.edu/entomology/entfacts/entfactpdf/ef636.pdf – comprehensive lesson on bedbugs.

Centers for Disease Control and Prevention: https://www.cdc.gov/parasites/bedbugs/ – link to various articles on bedbugs.

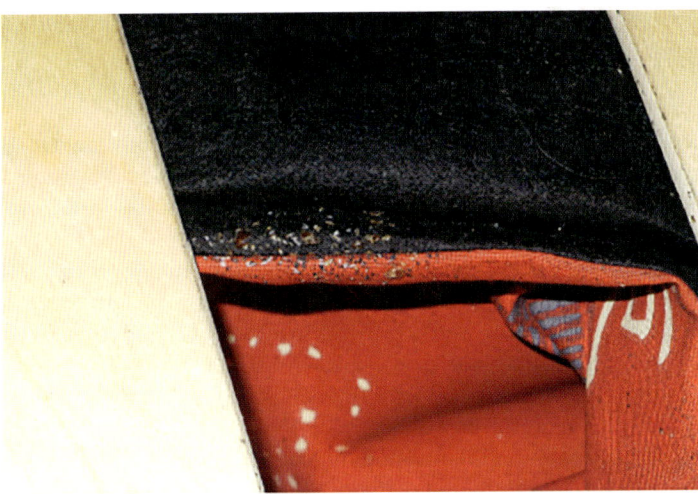

(a)

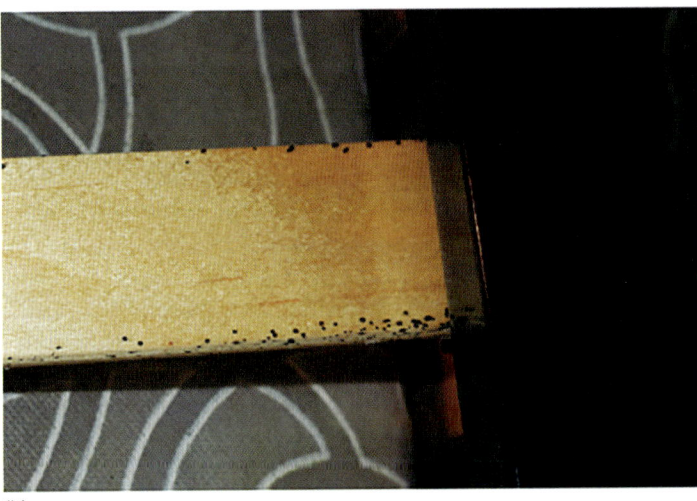

(b)

Figure 34.22 To educate patients to the 'search and destroy' strategy, general practitioners should show them pictures of (a) bedbugs and their typical hideouts (e.g. a fabric couch) and (b) bedbug faecal traces on the bedframe.

NHS Choices: http://nhs.uk/conditions/bites-insect/pages/introduction.aspx – clinical knowledge summary about insect bites.
(All last accessed June 2023.)

Patient resources
Up to Date:
www.uptodate.com/contents/bedbugs?source=search_result&search=bedbugs&selectedTitle=1~10 – provides accurate general knowledge about bedbugs.
Bed-Bugs.co.uk: http://bed-bugs.co.uk/ – provides an interesting picture gallery of bedbugs and their bites, together with practical tips for eradication.
Pest Control UK: http://pestcontrol-uk.org/ – DIY control of bedbugs.
Pest Control Australia, Victoria state: https://www.health.vic.gov.au/environmental-health/bedbugs-pest-control.
(All last accessed June 2023.)

Family Reduviidae (kissing bugs, assassin bugs and cone-nosed bugs)

Epidemiology
The majority of species of Reduviidae are predators on other insects and are commonly called 'assassin bugs' for this reason, but some attack humans and other animals. Most species are encountered in North, Central and South America, but some occur in Africa, the Middle East and South-East Asia, and in Australia. The subfamily Triatominae is the most important medically and includes the three major genuses *Triatoma*, *Rhodnius* and *Panstrongylus*. These genuses feed exclusively by sucking the blood of vertebrate animals. Adult Triatominae are large insects, commonly measuring 20–28 mm in length. They have an elongated head with a prominent proboscis and long four-jointed antennae.

The Triatominae are largely confined to the western hemisphere, with the majority of species being distributed in North, Central and South America. In the USA, *Triatoma sanguisuga* has the widest distribution, extending from the southeastern and mid-Atlantic states westwards, including Texas. Triatomines feed on a wide range of hosts, and domestic species feed on humans and domestic animals. They are of medical importance as vectors of *Trypanosoma cruzi* in Chagas disease [1,2]. This disease has been traditionally restricted to Latin America, but cases have been reported in the USA. Studies performed in 2010 and 2014 in Arizona and Louisiana showed that around 40% of collected kissing bugs ($n = 164$, 41.5% and $n = 49$, 40%, respectively) were infected with *T. cruzi*, indicating that the risk for infection in those regions may be higher than previously thought [3,4]. Changes in the geographical distribution of *Triatoma sanguisuga* are expected in the face of climate change, presumably through northward expansion of high-risk areas in North America [5].

Pathophysiology
In nature, triatomine bugs form colonies in the habitat of their host, for example a small mammal's nest or animal lair. In the southwestern USA, infestations are often found in the nests of wood rats. Some species, however, have become totally domesticated, and live and breed in human dwellings, laying their eggs in cracks and crevices in the floors and walls. The young hatch as nymphs, which are miniature versions of the adults. Nymphs and adults hide in crevices during the day and emerge at night to feed. Traditionally, it was believed that triatomine bugs only occurred in rural habitats, but recent studies have demonstrated evidence that they can also exist in highly developed urban environments [6].

Clinical features [7,8]
The bites of the predatory species of reduviid bugs (assassin bugs) are purely defensive and are usually extremely painful [9,10]. Triatome reduviids are known as kissing bugs because of their tendency to bite the face, especially around the lips. The bites of the blood-sucking Triatominae, however, are painless – this is essential to the parasite if it is to feed undisturbed. In an individual not previously exposed to the bites, there may be little reaction, but anaphylactic reactions are also a major concern [11]. With repeated exposure hypersensitivity develops, and reactions ranging from pruritic papules to haemorrhagic nodules and bullae may occur. A door-to-door survey showed that living in triatomine-exposed areas may be associated with a high prevalence of self-reported allergies [12].

Family Anthocoridae, commonly called minute pirate bugs or flower bugs

The Anthocoridae are related to the Cimicidae. Bugs of this family are mostly predacious on other insects but are known to bite humans occasionally. *Lyctocoris campestris* is a cosmopolitan species closely associated with humans, found for example in haystacks and granaries [1]. *Anthocoris kingi* and *Anthocoris nemorum* will also bite humans [2]. Another anthocorid bug, *Dufouriellus ater*, attacked many workers in a clothing factory in northeast England [3]. Human-biting potential of the predatory flower bug *Orius majusculus* has also been reported [4].

Family Pentatomidae, commonly called stink bugs

These bugs have glands in the thorax that emit a foul-smelling compound. This defence helps them to repel potential predators. Some insects of the family Pentatomidae, commonly known as marias-fedidas ('stink Mary'), can cause serious irritation to human skin, very similar to that produced by vesicant beetles. Areas of redness and vesiculation are accompanied by burning and pruritus [1]. There is no information on the pharmacological properties of substances secreted by the Pentatomidae but treatment is similar to that used after contact with *Paederus* or cantharidin.

Palomena prasina (the green shield bug), a member of this family, has been reported as the cause of perioral blistering in a small child [2].

Family Belostomatidae (giant water bugs)

Giant water bugs are rare cosmopolitan insects. They are typically encountered in freshwater streams and ponds. Alternate names include 'toe biters' because they can deliver an unpleasant sting and 'electric light bug' because they are attracted to lights. Giant water bugs may produce very painful lesions on humans and may carry infections [1,2]. Belostomatidae and another family (the Naucoridae) are carnivorous insects and are suspected to play a role in the transmission of Buruli ulcer and in the ecological expansion of the *Mycobacterium ulcerans* niche. The majority of cases of bites and suspected transmission of infection are localised in Africa occurring mainly in poor local communities. Other cases have been reported in Asia, Australia and South America [3–6].

Thrips (Thysanoptera)

Definition
Thrips (known as 'thunder flies') are tiny winged insects, 1–2 mm in length and usually yellowish brown or black in colour. The name thrips is derived from the Greek word meaning 'wood louse'. The order Thysanoptera ('fringe wing') comprises about 5000 species with a worldwide distribution. The majority feed on plant juices and some are important agricultural pests [1].

Pathophysiology
Some species are predatory on other arthropods. A few species appear able to suck blood and there are a number of reports that thrips can be responsible for skin lesions [2–6]. Cluster outbreaks can also occur, as reported in a series of 15 US Marines who presented with papular dermatitis secondary to bites from thrips [7]. Most thrips, however, are unable to penetrate the human epidermis and probably cause itching and prickling sensations only by their movement on the skin surface and their efforts to obtain water from perspiration.

Clinical features
Thrip bites, which occur on exposed skin, produce tiny puncta and small pink macules or papules [3]. Large numbers of American soldiers in Hawaii developed hypoanaesthetic papular lesions surrounded by blanched halos, which, it was suggested, were caused by Cuban laurel thrips [8]. Thrips infestation may sometimes be confused with delusional disorders because houseplants or ornamental plants can be infested by thrips. Patients may present with somewhat unusual stories and bizarre presentations. It is always important to make sure that there is not a genuine infestation of the skin (careful examination of the patient, home and even environment) before diagnosing delusional infestation (a persistent delusional disorder where patients believe they are infested despite all evidence to the contrary, Chapter 84) [9,10]. Thrips have also been mistaken for head lice [11].

Beetles (Coleoptera)

Definition
Beetles are insects whose forewings are modified to form hard wing cases for the membranous or reduced hindwings. There are over 370 000 known species, but it is likely that many more await discovery. They are mainly terrestrial and the majority feed on decaying animal or vegetable matter, but some are predaceous on other insects.

Classification
Vesicating and allergenic species are the main species of interest to dermatologists.

Vesicating species [1–3]
Family Meloidae (oil beetles; blister beetles). Most of the beetles in this group only cause problems when crushed on the skin, but some may emit their vesicating fluid without being crushed. The family is large and widely distributed. The beetles of this family feed on leaves of crops, such as tomatoes and potatoes, making interaction with humans likely. Many species contain the irritant cantharidin, which commonly is called 'Spanish fly'. Cantharidin is a vesicant that comes from more than 1500 species of 'blister' beetles. It is absorbed into the lipid component of keratinocyte membranes where it activates neutral serine proteases leading to the degeneration of desmosomes and resulting in vesicles and bullae [4]. Cantharidin has an undeserved reputation as an aphrodisiac, which is unfortunate for a chemical capable of producing severe toxicity. It has been used in blistering plasters and hair restorers, and in the treatment of warts and molluscum contagiosum.

Lytta vesicatoria (Figure 34.23) is perhaps the best known of the blister beetles. It is a large bright metallic green beetle that lives mainly in the Mediterranean region, mainly on ash trees, but is sporadically found further north, occasionally as far as England.

Other vesicating species include *Epicauta* spp. (USA, Mexico, India, Sudan and Senegal) [5] and *Mylabris* spp. (Nigeria, India) [6,7].

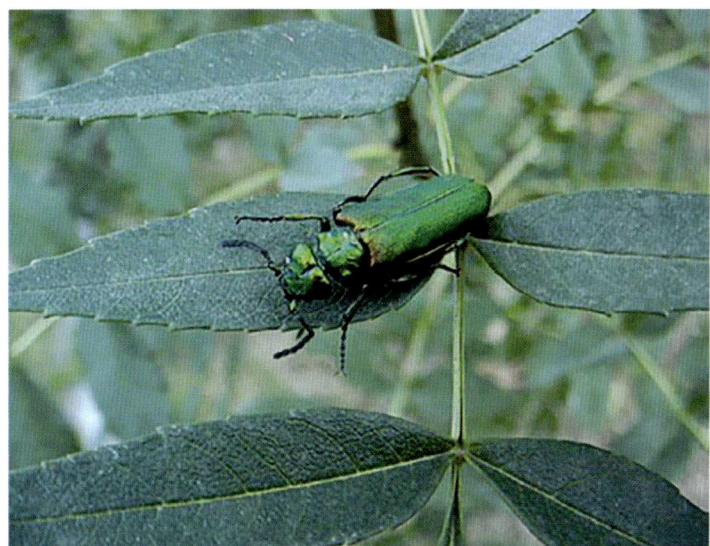

Figure 34.23 *Lytta vesicatoria* on an ash tree, the best known of the blister beetles. Courtesy of Dr M. Cornet, Nice, France.

Family Staphylinidae (rove beetles) [8–10]. The genus *Paederus*, found worldwide, includes many species containing a vesicant, pederin, which is chemically distinct from cantharidin. Pederin is released when the beetles are crushed, provoking an acute irritant contact dermatitis. Lesions may be plaque-like, linear (when a beetle has been brushed off the skin, leaving a streak of pederin on the skin surface) or 'kissing' (when a beetle has been crushed between two flexural surfaces). A major outbreak of vesicular dermatitis on Okinawa in 1966 was traced to contact with the beetle *Paederus fuscipes* [11] and a number of other reports have documented *Paederus* dermatitis from several parts of the world [12–19], including outbreaks that occurred in a military unit training in the Arizona desert during heavy rain and flooding [20], and in a military base in Iraq [21]. A plague of whiplash rove beetles (*Paederus australis*) forced evacuation of an Aboriginal community in the Northern Territory of Australia [22]. *Paederus sabaeus* has been responsible for several outbreaks of dermatitis in Africa at the end of the rainy season [23–26]. Indeed, beetle dermatitis is frequent in travellers [27–30].

You *et al.* [31] reported a case of bullous contact dermatitis following the use of crushed *Paederus* beetles for the treatment of vitiligo.

Histopathological changes of *Paederus* dermatitis include intraepidermal and subepidermal blistering, epidermal necrosis and acantholysis [32]. Mitotic figures and apoptotic changes such as chromatin condensation and DNA fragmentation have also been identified in the basal and suprabasal layers of the epidermis [19].

It has been proposed that the biblical third, fourth and sixth plagues of Egypt might have been related to rove beetles and the bullous lesions they cause [33].

Family Oedemeridae [2]. *Oxycopis vittata* has been reported as causing a blistering dermatitis in Puerto Rico [34]. *Sessinia* species (coconut beetles) have caused blistering in the Gilbert Islands [7].

Thelyphassa lineata produced a bullous dermatosis in a large number of New Zealand army personnel [35] and there is a report of blister beetle dermatosis in Hawaii caused by *Thelyphassa apicata* [36].

Family Tenebrionidae (darkling beetles). Many species inhabit wood, flour and grain stores. *Tribolium castaneum*, the 'rust-red flour beetle', has caused a pruritic eruption in workers handling infested jute packing bags [37]. The secretion of *Tribolium* species is mainly composed of quinones.

Species of *Blaps* can eject defensive secretions that are irritant and cause blistering.

Clinical features [1–3]. Usually, lesions are produced only when the beetle is crushed on the skin. A weal forms rapidly and is followed by a blister after 12–24 h. The blisters are sometimes linear 'whiplash dermatitis'. A characteristic feature is the development of kissing lesions, where a blister comes into contact with another area. Blisters induced in a small child by *Mylabris bifasciata* were associated with severe systemic manifestations of cantharidin poisoning [6]. In *Paederus* dermatitis, vesicles generally appear toward the centre of the plaque and frequently become pustular [18]. This is in contrast to cantharidin dermatitis, which is characterised by non-inflammatory vesicles and bullae [17]. *Paederus*-induced keratitis has also been reported [38]. The clinical differential diagnosis includes acute allergic or irritant contact dermatitis, thermal burns, chemical burns, herpes zoster, herpes simplex and bullous impetigo [17,21]. An important differential diagnosis to consider is phytophotodermatitis as there are many similarities between the two conditions including linear asymmetrical redness, blister formation and depigmentation [39].

Management. Experts agree that affected patients should be managed as irritant contact dermatitis, with removal of the toxin by immediate washing with soap and water. Primary prevention by increasing public awareness during outbreaks, decreasing the use of artificial lights at night and using mosquito nets is advocated by several authors [18,21].

Allergenic species

Family Dermestidae [40]. The beetles in this cosmopolitan family feed on hides, woollen materials and stored food. The females lay eggs during autumn, in dark places and cracks, often in furniture. The larvae, measuring 4 mm long, hatch at the end of winter or in spring. They usually live in dark places such as drawers or cupboards, but can also be found under carpets. The adult beetles are not known to be directly injurious to humans, but their larvae are covered with hairs, which may cause skin lesions.

Clinical features. The skin lesions are not distinctive. Dermatitis, urticaria and papular urticaria may occur. Papular urticaria in a child, caused by the larvae of *Dermestes maculatus* DeGeer, has been reported, but it was uncertain whether the reaction to the hairs was irritant or allergic [41]. *Dermestes peruvianus* was responsible for dermatitis, vasculitis, cervical lymphadenopathy and pulmonary nodular interstitial infiltrates in a man whose bed was colonised by the beetles [42].

The irritating hairs from the larvae of carpet beetles (*Anthrenus* spp.) may also cause skin lesions [43–45] (Figure 34.24). In a recent series of seven families (living in the area of Nice, in the south of France) affected by *Anthrenus* larvae, each individual had a median of 17 lesions on their skin. The lesions were mostly located under clothing [46]. There is also a report of the damaging effect of

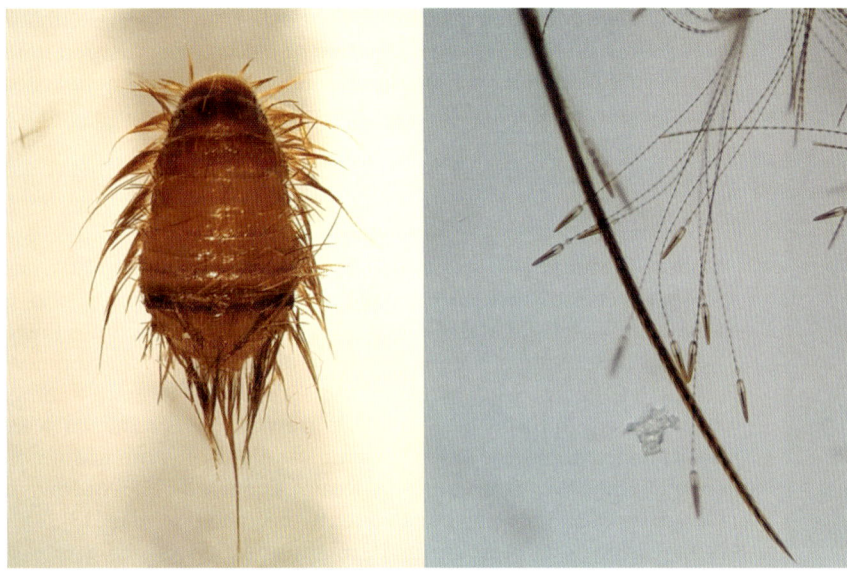

Figure 34.24 Larvae of *Anthrenus spp.* (binocular magnifier, ×40) and larvae hairs with spear-headed shape (magnification ×200). Simon *et al.* [46], US Department of Health and Human Services/Public Domain.

Anthrenus larvae on paraffin-embedded tissue specimens, especially the sectioned surface of hyperkeratotic lesions [47].

Cockroaches (Dictyoptera)

Definition
Cockroaches are members of the order Dictyoptera, suborder Blattaria. They belong to one of the primitive orders of insects, being allied to crickets, grasshoppers, praying mantids and stick insects. Cockroaches were originally adapted to hot climates, but a number of species have established themselves in cool climates by living inside warm human habitations. They are active nocturnally and are attracted to any organic material that may serve as food. This theoretically makes them potential mechanical vectors (by transportation, also called phoresy) of pathogenic organisms [1–3]. The main pest species are *Periplaneta americana*, *P. australasiae*, *Blatta orientalis* and *Blatella germanica*.

Clinical features [4,5]
Contact urticaria and dermatitis have been described in laboratory workers and others handling cockroaches constantly [6–8], and urticated papules developed in a medical records clerk exposed to copious insect debris containing fragments of *B. germanica* when clearing old case notes from a derelict hut [9]. Chronic urticaria in a child has been attributed to cockroach hypersensitivity [10].

Locusts (Orthoptera)

Definition
Sensitivity reactions, manifest as asthma and allergic rhinitis, are a recognised occupational hazard in those working with laboratory colonies of locusts [1–3]. The principal allergen appears to derive from the peritrophic membrane, which is present in the gut and surrounds faeces [2].

Clinical features
Contact urticaria to locusts has been reported by Monk [4] in a laboratory research worker who handled a large number of locusts. The patient produced a positive reaction to locust antigen on prick testing and a wealing reaction at the site of contact with a live locust. Similarly, worsening of asthma and urticaria in an atopic research laboratory worker on exposure to grasshoppers has been described [5].

Butterflies and moths (Lepidoptera)

Definition and nomenclature
Many members of this large order are of importance to the dermatologist because of the irritant properties of the hairs or spines of the caterpillars and sometimes of the adults. Skin lesions in the majority of cases are produced by a combination of mechanical and pharmacological effects [1,2]. The offending caterpillars are distributed through many different families [1,3].

Synonyms and inclusions
- Lepidopterism

Classification
The Lepidoptera order is one of the largest orders of insects. Caterpillars are the worm-like larval forms of Lepidoptera. The Lepidoptera contain probably between 125 000 and 150 000 different species of caterpillars, moths and butterflies [4].

Epidemiology
The true number of cases of caterpillar and moth reactions remains unknown, because few cases are reported in the literature and probably only the ones with severe reactions.

Epidemics of caterpillar dermatitis are frequent, depending on the seasonal abundance of the different species. For example, there

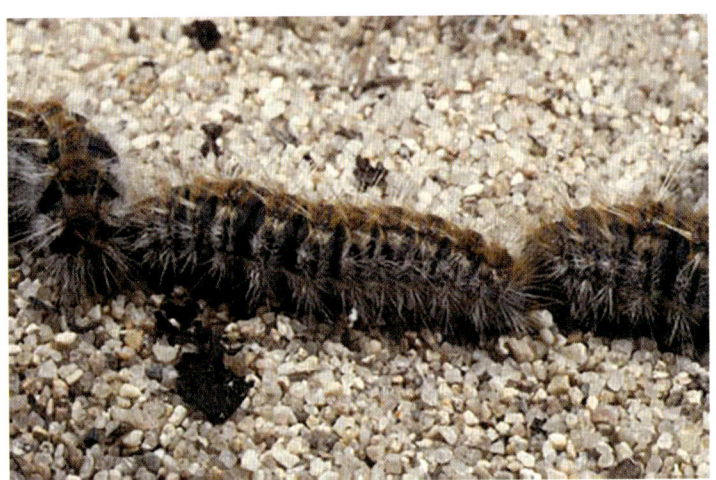

Figure 34.25 *Thaumetopoea pityocampa*. Courtesy of Dr M. Dutheil, Nice, France.

are periodic outbreaks of gypsy moth caterpillars (*Lymantria dispar*) [5,6], Douglas fir tussock moth caterpillar (*Orgyia pseudotsugata*) [7], puss caterpillars (*Megalopyge opercularis*), buck moth caterpillars (*Hemileuca maia*) [8], several *Euproctis* species [9] and several species of processionary caterpillars (*Thaumetopoea*) (Figure 34.25). Due to climate changes in recent years and a tendency towards warmer summers, an ongoing broadening from the southwest to the northeast of the UK is probable [10,11].

Some species have the capacity to be disseminated widely by wind dispersal. This phenomenon is also called 'ballooning' [12]. Winds can also disperse caterpillar 'hairs' (setae), which may cause dermatitis or ophthalmia nodosa [13,14]. A large outbreak of dermatitis caused by setae of the Asian mulberry tussock moth (*Euproctis flava*) has been described in China, using airborne dissemination [9].

Dermatitis caused by adult moths is less frequent. Caripito itch was described by Dinehart *et al.* in crew who docked their ship in Caripito, Venezuela. The dermatitis was secondary to the setae from female moths (*Hylesia*) [15]. Outbreaks of *Hylesia metabus* are sometimes notified in French Guyana [16].

Caterpillar dermatitis is quite frequent in children, but the reasons for this elevated frequency remain unknown, and may be due to parental concern and increased reporting [12,17].

Pathophysiology

Lepidoptera undergo four life stages: egg, caterpillar, pupa or chrysalis, and adult. The term 'lepidopterism' is applied to the ill effects on humans of a structure or product of some part of a moth or butterfly at any stage of its life history. Some authors apply the term 'erucism' to injurious effects from caterpillars and 'lepidopterism' to ill effects from adults. In the majority of cases, damage to human skin and mucosae occurs as a result of epithelial penetration by the setae of caterpillars. In addition to a foreign-body reaction, there is often an effect from venom. Setae develop from trichogen cells of the epidermis. They are hollow and may function as sensory receptors or communicate with a poison gland cell and contain venom. They commonly have barbs that hold them in place when they have penetrated the skin. In some families of moths, the caterpillars have clumps of much smaller setae known as 'dart hairs' or 'spicules' that are pointed at both ends and carry fine barbs. The point of attachment to the caterpillar is very narrow and easily fractured; hence, contact with the caterpillar may release huge numbers of these tiny darts. Such dart hairs are present in a number of species, including the brown tail moth (*Euproctis crysorrhoea*) and the pine processionary caterpillar (*Thaumetopoea pityocampa*) (Figure 34.25). Setae are also woven into cocoons and into the webs of the silk-spinning caterpillars.

Spines are an extension of the cuticle of the caterpillar and contain venom. The spines either have a terminal plug of inspissated material at their open ends that is released by pressure or a weak point at which the spine fractures to allow the venom to escape. Poisonous spines occur particularly on the caterpillars of the moth families Cochlididae (Eucleidae; Limacodidae), Saturniidae and Megalopygidae.

The venoms present in the setae and spines of caterpillars of a number of families of Lepidoptera have been studied but not fully elucidated. Some contain histamine, histamine liberators, serotonin and proteases. A protein, the thaumetopoein, has been isolated from pine processionary caterpillar hairs [18,19]. This has a direct effect on mast cells, leading to degranulation, and explains the urticating properties of these caterpillars. However, IgE-mediated hypersensitivity also appears to be responsible for some reactions to *Thaumetopoea* [20–22]. Moneo *et al.* [23] have demonstrated a 15 kDa IgE-binding protein in a larval extract. Immediate and delayed-type reactions to *Euproctis pseudoconspersa* caterpillar venom extracts have also been demonstrated [24].

In some species – for example, moths of the genus *Hylesia* (family Saturniidae) – irritating setae are carried by the adults. This genus is notorious for causing outbreaks of 'butterfly itch', 'moth dermatitis' or 'Caripito itch' [15] in tropical South America.

Pathology

The pathology of caterpillar dermatitis is usually non-specific [25,26]. Histology may be more specific when embedded spines are found [15]. Granulomas have been demonstrated in cases of ophthalmia nodosa [14], dendrolimiasis and pararamose.

Clinical features [1,2,27]

Presentation

Clinical features induced by caterpillars and moths are wide, ranging from localised stinging reactions, papular urticaria, urticarial weals, haemorrhagic diathesis, ophthalmia nodosa, dendrolimiasis, pararamose and oral exposure [27].

Localised stinging reactions consist of immediate mild to severe pain that lasts hours to days. Systemic symptoms are sometimes associated. Contact with *Megalopyge* caterpillars [28] produces immediate intense burning local pain accompanied by a spreading redness around the puncture sites. The affected area becomes oedematous, and there is often lymphangitis and regional lymphadenopathy. The local changes may be accompanied by pyrexia, headache, nausea and vomiting, particularly in children [29].

In papular urticaria, there are mild to moderate localised pruritic papules or eczematous lesions, predominantly in exposed areas. Lesions are caused by the setae from hairy or bristly caterpillars or from adult moths.

Urticarial weals and angio-oedema are seen with three species of processionary caterpillars (all belong to the genus *Thaumetopoea*). These lesions are secondary to type I hypersensitivity reactions [22,30–32]. Systemic symptoms have sometimes been reported [33–35].

The term 'lonomism' refers to a severe bleeding diathesis with intracranial haemorrhage, secondary to caterpillars found in Brazil and Venezuela (*L. obliqua* and *L. achelous*) [32].

Dendrolimiasis combines dermatitis and rheumatological involvement (arthralgia and arthritis) and is caused by contact with the Masson pine caterpillar (genus *Dendrolimus*) found in China [36]. Pararamose is quite similar, with skin eruption and arthritis, caused by contact with the Brazilian moth *Premolis semirufa* [10,37].

In the eye, caterpillar setae may cause a variety of changes ranging from conjunctivitis to ophthalmia nodosa [13,14,38] and even panophthalmitis.

Oral exposure is rare and the most common sites of exposure are the tongue and lips. Most cases occur in children [27].

Differential diagnosis
Differential diagnosis may be broad because cutaneous lesions and histology are not specific. Questioning of the patient should elicit a history of caterpillar exposure. This is key to the diagnosis.

Management [27]
Management of lepidopterism is mainly based on expert opinion and is largely symptomatic. Immediate washing with soap and water is classically recommended. Topical steroids and oral antihistamines should be used for mild reactions to control pruritus. Embedded setae should be removed, sometimes with the help of adhesive tape. Systemic steroids may be necessary in severe reactions. Opioid analgesia may be required in puss caterpillar stings.

Surgical removal of granuloma formation may be necessary in ophthalmia nodosa.

Specific antivenom against potentially fatal *Lonomia* genus envenomation is available [39].

CLASS ARACHNIDA

Arachnida are readily distinguished from insects, as the adults have no wings or antennae and possess four pairs of legs. Unlike insects, where the body is divided into three segments (head, thorax and abdomen), arachnids have only two, the cephalothorax, from which the legs arise, and the abdomen.

The Arachnida are classified into seven orders, only three of which are of medical importance:
1. Araneae (spiders).
2. Scorpiones (scorpions).
3. Acari (ticks and mites).

Spiders (Araneae)

Introduction and general description
The appearance of many of the larger spiders inspires terror or disgust, but very few of the many thousands of species are dangerous to humans [1,2]. This is why, when observing a large skin bite, many people suspect a spider bite with no scientific, clinical or entomological evidence. The myth that bites from various species cause necrotic ulceration may not be completely true [2]. In fact, bites by spiders from the genus *Loxosceles* can result in necrotic arachnidism and sometimes systemic illness, but many cases of necrotic arachnidism are only suspected and not proven [3]. Spiders are mostly shy and avoid contact with humans. Almost all are venomous and bite, but only a few have chelicerae strong enough to penetrate human skin and in most cases the bites are trivial. A recent Australian study describing 750 cases of spider bite, involving 26 spider families, showed that most of the time there were only a few symptoms [4]. The European tarantula, *Lycosa tarantula*, which inspired the tarantella in Italy in the Middle Ages, inflicts a temporarily painful but harmless bite. Some lycosid spiders in South America, for example *Lycosa antibucana*, cause severe swelling and lymphangitis. In the USA, the term 'tarantula' is erroneously applied to the large 'bird' or 'crab' spiders of the family Theraphosidae that attack only when vigorously provoked and whose bite may be painful but not dangerous. Some colourful species kept as pets, for example *Brachypelma smithi*, are among several that have urticating hairs capable of causing prolonged pruritus. Many spiders whose bites are dangerous and sometimes fatal are small, inconspicuous and unimpressive.

Clinical features
The clinical syndrome following the bite of a spider is known as arachnidism [5–8]. The form of arachnidism caused by species of the family Loxoscelidae is known as loxoscelism and that by widow spiders (*Latrodectus* species) latrodectism [9].

Air transport of crates of fruit and other materials may introduce exotic species to countries in which they are unable to multiply but can survive long enough to attack humans.

Diagnosis [2]
The diagnosis of spider bite is based on a clear history of a spider biting, ideally with collection and correct identification of the spider responsible, sometimes requiring the assistance of an entomologist. In areas where the spiders are recognised, the general population may identify a few spiders, such as widow spiders. The identification of spider venom in human tissue is not possible.

Differential diagnosis
Differential diagnosis may be broad including pyoderma gangrenosum, herpes simplex and zoster, staphylococcal (including Panton-Valentine toxin-related [10]) or streptococcal infection, lymphomatoid papulosis, chemical burn and squamous cell carcinoma.

Family Theridiidae

Genus *Latrodectus* (widow spiders).
Epidemiology
Spiders of this genus are widely distributed throughout the world. *Latrodectus mactans*, the black widow spider, occurs throughout subtropical and tropical regions. Other species have a similar but more limited range, although some extend to the temperate regions of Russia and Canada. It is the adult female spiders that produce the

most damaging bites in humans, but bites by male spiders have been reported in Australia [11].

Pathophysiology

The female of *L. mactans* is glossy black, with a body length of 1.5 cm and a leg span of up to 5 cm. She normally spins her web in empty burrows or under stones, but may be found in dark corners of barns, garages, store rooms or outdoor lavatories. She bites humans only in self-defence. *Latrodectus* venom is considered to be one of the most potent toxins, exceeding that of snake venoms, but the dose injected is minute in relation to the body weight of a human victim. The toxins of all species of *Latrodectus* that have been studied appear to be closely related and the symptoms from envenomation are similar.

Latrodectus hasselti, the red-back spider, is common in Australia [12,13]. *Latrodectus geometricus*, the brown widow spider, bites reluctantly, but is occasionally troublesome to vineyard workers in South Africa.

Clinical features (latrodectism) [5–7,14–16]

In the days of the outdoor lavatory, *Latrodectus* webs were often spun across the toilet seat, and this led to the frequent occurrence of bites on the buttocks and genitalia. The bite of *Latrodectus* species is fairly painless, but within a few minutes increasingly severe pain develops, usually at the site of the bite but also spreading to the adjacent region or even to the back, chest or abdomen. Cramp-like or colicky abdominal pain is particularly common. Puncta may be visible at the site of the bite, and there is local redness and oedema. There is frequently profuse sweating, and neuromuscular involvement causes paraesthesiae, incoordination and paralysis. The pain begins to subside within 24 h, and other symptoms resolve within 2–3 days, although weakness and lethargy may persist for longer. Myocardial damage, occasionally fatal, has been reported, but only from some species of widow spiders such as *Latrodectus tredecimguttatus* (Figure 34.26) [17,18].

Management [2]

There is no consensus concerning the management of latrodectism as evidence to support therapies is scarce and there are no controlled trials. Treatments that have been used include general measures such as analgesics and benzodiazepines, and more specific measures such as antivenom [19,20], calcium and magnesium. The effectiveness of widow spider antivenoms remains to be assessed [19,20]. Furthermore, there are some concerns regarding the tolerance of these antivenoms with reported cases of anaphylaxis following administration [21–23].

Family Hexathelidae

Genera *Atrax/Hadronyche* (Australia and South Pacific) and *Macrothele* (Taiwan and parts of eastern Asia) – funnel web spiders. Perhaps the best known of these is the Sydney funnel web spider, *Atrax robustus* [12], a large aggressive spider that is nocturnal and predominantly insectivorous. It normally lives under rocks and logs, but the spread of the Sydney suburbs into its habitat provided similar hiding places under houses. Funnel web spiders are the most deadly spiders worldwide.

Clinical features [8,24]

The bite of funnel web spiders is invariably painful. From the majority of bites, especially those of female spiders, no general symptoms follow, and recovery is uneventful. However, the large amount of venom from male spiders may cause severe systemic symptoms. Nausea and vomiting are early features, accompanied by abdominal pain, profuse sweating, piloerection, muscle fasciculation, lacrimation, excess salivation, dyspnoea and pulmonary oedema. Several fatalities were recorded prior to the development of an antivenom.

Management

The compression bandage-splinting method of first aid is effective in delaying onset of envenomation and may enhance local inactivation of venom. Severe reactions will require hospital admission and full supportive measures. Funnel web spider antivenom should be given urgently to any patient with severe envenomation, because it probably reduces the risk of death and the length of hospital stay [25].

Family Sicariidae (formerly Loxoscelidae)

Genus *Loxosceles* ('fiddleback' spider; 'violin' spider; 'brown recluse' spider). Over 100 species of *Loxosceles* are found in a worldwide distribution, but the majority are in North and South America, where loxoscelism is a major health problem.

Identification of a *Loxosceles* spider is based on six eyes in a curved row on the upper part of the body (the prosoma). It has been suggested that under future climate change scenarios, the spider's distribution may expand northwards, invading previously unaffected regions of the USA [26]. Several species are known to induce human skin necrosis: *L. reclusa*, *L. laeta*, *L. deserta*, *L. arizonica* and *L. rufescens* [3,8]. The most notorious is *L. reclusa*, the brown recluse spider, which is tan to brown in colour, with a dark brown, violin-shaped marking on the dorsum of the cephalothorax – hence the names 'fiddleback' and 'violin' spider. *L. reclusa* is active mainly at night and most bites occur when the spider is trapped against the person [3]. Its natural habitat is in dark areas beneath rocks and in holes and caves. It is also found in homes, in areas that are dark, dirty and undisturbed, such as attics, cupboards and garages.

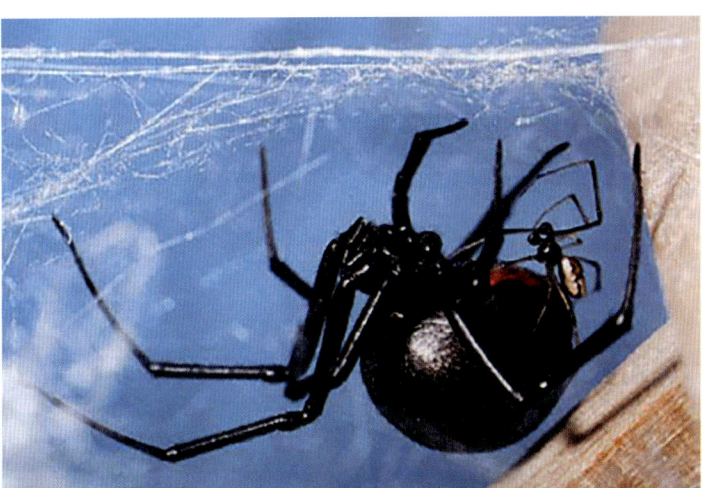

Figure 34.26 *Latrodectus tredecimguttatus* female, with the small male on her abdomen. Courtesy of Dr J. J. Peres, Peillon, France.

Loxosceles laeta also occurs widely in South America. *Loxosceles rufescens* is widespread in southern Australia and in Mediterranean regions [27].

Clinical features (loxoscelism) [5–8,15,28]

There are two distinct clinical forms of loxoscelism: necrotic cutaneous loxoscelism and the much less frequent viscerocutaneous loxoscelism. The clinical manifestations depend upon the age and health of the victim, the amount of venom injected and the site of the bite – fatty areas such as the proximal thigh and the buttocks show more cutaneous reaction and extensive involvement of the entire subcutaneous layer.

In necrotic cutaneous loxoscelism, there is local damage to the skin and subcutaneous tissues, but systemic symptoms are mild. The bite of the spider is usually relatively painless. However, after an interval of minutes or hours, severe pain develops at the site, accompanied by redness, oedema and a central bulla. In severe envenomation, a 'target' lesion is seen – central blue/purple discoloration surrounded by an ischaemic halo and an outer ring of redness (the 'red, white and blue' sign). After 3 or 4 days the central area becomes necrotic and an eschar develops. The eschar is eventually shed, leaving an ulcer, which may take a considerable time to heal. The size of maximum necrosis appears to be predictive of time to complete healing [28]. Robb *et al.* [29] described a patient with a generalised vasculitic exanthem following a brown recluse spider bite. Acute generalised exanthematous pustulosis following *L. reclusa* envenomation has also been reported [30].

In viscerocutaneous or systemic loxoscelism, which is more common in children than adults, general symptoms of pyrexia, severe malaise, restlessness and headache are marked. Within 24 h of the onset of general symptoms, ecchymoses, jaundice, haematuria and haemoglobinuria indicate massive intravascular haemolysis that may result in acute renal failure and death [31–36].

Management [3,8,15]

*R*est, application of *I*ce Compresses and *E*levation (RICE therapy) help to reduce inflammation and pain. Other treatments have been tried for loxoscelism, including antivenom, corticosteroids, dapsone, antihistamines, antibiotics, analgesics, hyperbaric oxygen therapy, electric shock, curettage and surgical excision [37–39]. However, there is no consensus concerning the efficacy of any of these treatments because they are not supported by controlled randomised trials. In this setting, the efficacy of antivenom and the timing of its use have not been clearly demonstrated [40,41]. In severe cutaneous loxoscelism with ulceration, negative pressure wound therapy may be helpful [42].

Family Lycosidae (wolf spiders)

There are a few reports of bites by members of the genus *Lycosa* [8,43,44]. They usually cause only local pain, swelling and redness, without cutaneous necrosis or significant systemic symptoms.

Other venomous species [7,8,12,45–48]

Spiders of several other families may cause unpleasant bites. Long-legged sac spiders of the genus *Chiracanthium* (family Miturgidae) that are found in many parts of the world may cause local pain, oedema and small areas of necrosis [8,47]. *Tegenaria agrestis* (family Agelenidae), the hobo spider (previously known as the aggressive house spider), is a cause of necrotic arachnidism in northwest USA [8,46,47]. Cases of bites from *Hololena* spiders, associated with headache and vomiting, have been recently reported [49]. Members of the families Gnaphosidae, Salticidae (jumping spiders), Sparassidae (huntsmen spiders) and Oxyopidae (lynx spiders) all occasionally bite humans, but the effects are usually mild, unless there is secondary bacterial infection.

Public concern with regard to the toxic effects of white-tailed spiders (*Lampona cylindrata* and *L. murina*) is not supported by studies, which have shown that these spiders are unlikely to cause necrotic arachnidism [50,51].

Scorpions (Scorpiones)

Definition

Scorpions are arachnids of the order Scorpiones. They are widely distributed in the tropics and subtropics. Approximately 1500 species of scorpions are described worldwide [1]. Only a few species are potentially dangerous for humans. The dangerous scorpions all belong, except one Scorpionidae, to the family of Buthidae, distributed in both the Old and New Worlds [1–5]. The venom is carried in the curved sting at the tip of the tail, which is swung over the scorpion's head to strike its prey. The principal components are neurotoxins [5,6], but some venoms also contain 5-hydroxytryptamine, histamine and kinins.

Epidemiology

Many scorpions are quite harmless and their stings of little consequence. There are areas of the world, however, where the risks from a scorpion bite are high and these include Africa (north Saharan, sub-Saharan, South Africa), the Near and Middle East, southern India and the Americas (in Mexico, and southern and eastern South America). Worldwide, the estimate of serious scorpion bites is over 1.2 million with 3250 deaths [1]. Species of *Androctonus* and *Buthus* (Figure 34.27) are important in the Middle East and North Africa, and *Centruroides* species cause problems in the southern USA and Mexico [7].

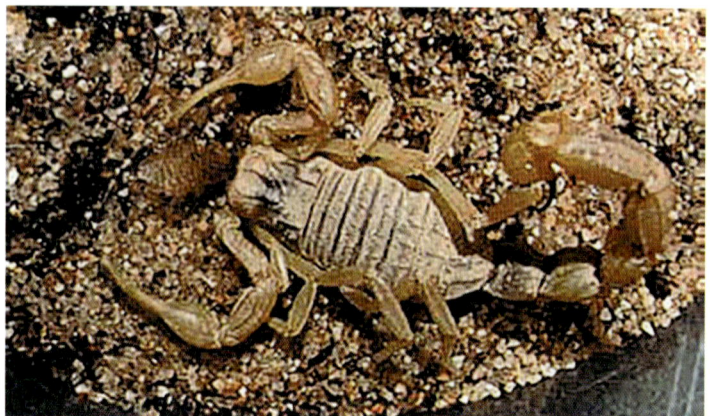

Figure 34.27 *Buthus occitanus*. Courtesy of Dr J. J. Peres, Peillon, France.

Pathophysiology

Tityus species are responsible for numerous episodes of envenomation in Brazil and Venezuela [8]. The venom of *Tityus serrulatus* is the most potent and results from tityustoxin. This toxin acts by binding to voltage-dependent sodium and potassium ion channels, leading to sialorrhoea, lacrimation and rhinorrhoea [9]. American troops stationed in Iraq and Afghanistan have suffered scorpion stings [10]. In this region, the sting of *Hemiscorpius lepturus* produces most cutaneous injury including purpura, necrosis and formation of bullae or ulcers [11]. *Hemiscorpius lepturus* also produces hemicalcin, which is a neurotoxin acting on ryanodine-sensitive calcium channels [12].

The incidence of scorpionism is low in Australia [13], where there are no dangerous species of scorpion [14].

Although adults are more often bitten, children experience more severe envenomations and their mortality is higher [1].

Clinical features [1,15–19]

The effects of scorpion stings may be local or systemic and they vary according to the species responsible. The local effects are usually immediate severe burning pain and hyperaesthesia, and there may be marked swelling. Pain remains often the only symptom. Appearance of digestive symptoms within the first few hours (in 5% of the cases) marks the entry of the patient into a serious stage of envenomation. Systemic effects include restlessness, profuse sweating, muscle spasms, difficulty with speech, marked increase in salivary and lacrimal secretion, nausea, vomiting, convulsions, hypertension, cardiac arrhythmias, myocarditis and pulmonary oedema. Death is usually due to respiratory or cardiac failure.

Management [1,14,16,18,20–23]

Prevention is important and is based first on individual precautions. People must check clothes and shoes while getting dressed. Collective measures are also important: house walls should be constructed with smooth coating to inhibit access of scorpions and doorways of houses should be checked and cleaned regularly. The benefit of insecticide has not been proven.

Once a bite has occurred, early treatment includes neutralising the circulating toxin as quickly as possible, combating the symptoms of envenomation and general supportive measures. Ice packs should be applied and the injection of local anaesthetic without vasoconstrictors around the sting site will help to reduce the pain. Specific antivenoms are available and indicated in all severe cases. Specific and symptomatic treatments may not be sufficient to prevent fatal outcome. However, in countries where scorpionism is a serious public health problem, antivenom and supportive treatments have significantly decreased mortality.

Ticks (Acari)

Definition [1]

Ticks are large acarines, which are blood-sucking ectoparasites of vertebrates. They are important vectors of diseases, such as tick-borne relapsing fever, and a number of viral, rickettsial (Chapter 26) and *Borrelia* (Chapter 26) infections (Lyme disease).

Classification

Ticks are typical arachnids, possessing mouthparts referred to as the capitulum, an unsegmented body and four pairs of legs in the adult. Larval ticks have three pairs of legs.

There are two major families: the Ixodidae (hard ticks) and the Argasidae (soft ticks). The term 'hard' refers to the dorsal chitinous shield or scutum, which is present in the Ixodidae but not in the Argasidae (Figures 34.28 and 34.29). In Ixodidae, the scutum covers the whole dorsum in the male but only a small anterior part in the female. In argasids there is little difference between the sexes. The mouthparts of ixodid ticks (capitulum) project forwards and are easily visible from above, whereas those of the argasid ticks can only be seen from below. A conspicuous component of the mouthparts is the toothed hypostome (Figure 34.30).

Introduction and general description

Ixodid ticks have four stages in their life cycle: egg, larva, nymph and adult. The larva and nymph require blood meals before further development can occur, and the adult female (Figure 34.31) also requires a blood meal before egg laying. The female lays one large batch of eggs and then dies. Some ixodids use one host for larval,

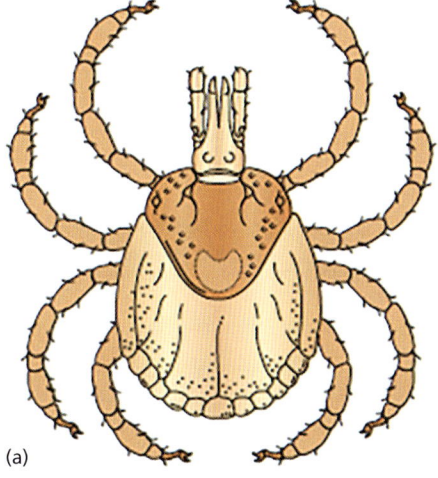 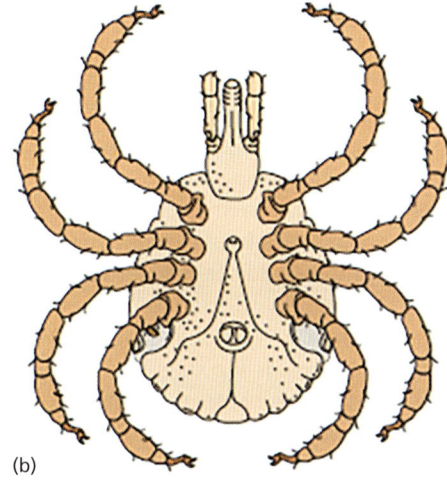

Figure 34.28 (a, b) Ixodidae: hard tick. The term 'hard' refers to the dorsal chitinous shield or scutum. The mouthparts (capitulum) of ixodid ticks project forwards and are easily visible from above. Adapted from Rodhain and Perez 1985 [36]. Copyright holder of original artwork: Maloine.

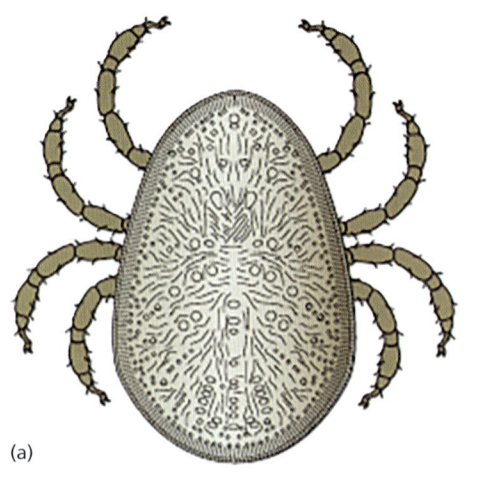
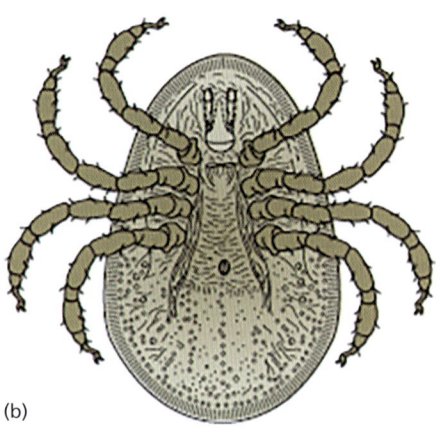

Figure 34.29 (a, b) Argasid: soft tick. The term soft refers to the absence of scutum. The mouthparts (capitulum) can only be seen from below. Adapted from Rodhain and Perez 1985 [36]. Copyright holder of original artwork: Maloine.

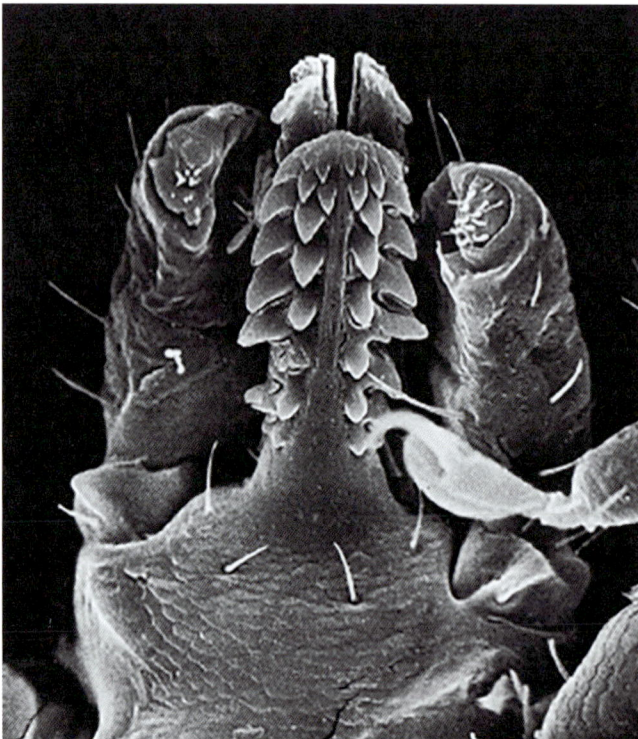

Figure 34.30 Scanning electron micrograph of tick mouthparts.

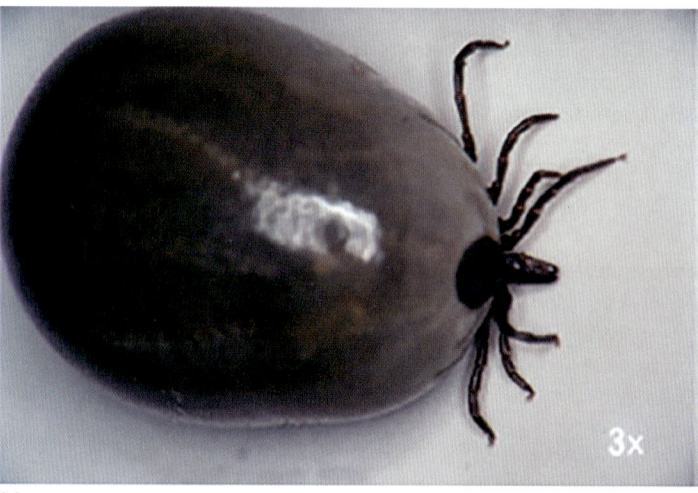

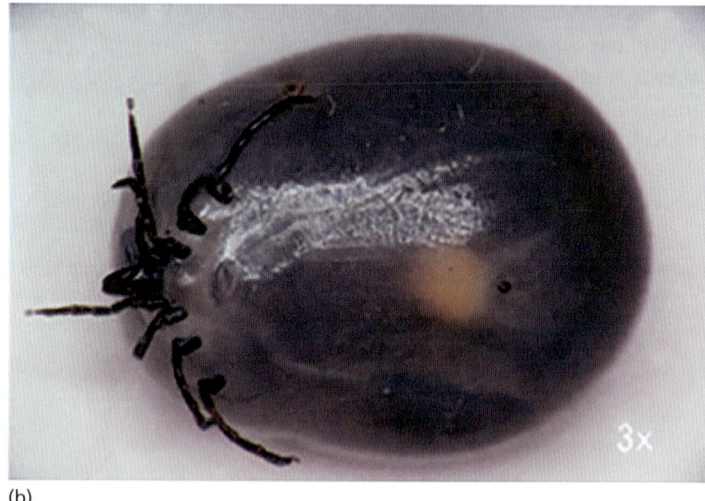

Figure 34.31 *Ixodes ricinus*, the sheep tick (engorged female). (a) Dorsal view. (b) Ventral view.

nymphal and adult stages (one-host ticks), whereas others require two or, more usually, three separate hosts.

To find suitable hosts, the larvae, nymphs and adults climb low vegetation and raise the first pair of legs ('questing'), which carry sense organs (Haller's organ). These organs are sensitive to a number of stimuli, including carbon dioxide in the exhalations of a potential host. If the host brushes past the vegetation, the tick will immediately grasp the animal's coat. Argasidae undergo several nymphal stages, and the adult female feeds a number of times during her lifetime, laying several batches of eggs. Ixodid ticks feed on the host, varying from several days (usually 2–4 days) to weeks, depending on such factors as life stage, host type and species of tick, whereas argasids visit their hosts nocturnally to feed for short periods of time, varying from several minutes (usually 1–2 h) to days, depending on the same factors (stage, host, tick). Argasids are mainly parasites of birds, bats and humans. Most ticks are essentially parasites of wild animals and humans are incidental hosts.

When attaching itself to the host, the tick uses its toothed chelicerae to cut into the epidermis, before thrusting the hypostome into the opening and gradually penetrating the dermis. The

Table 34.5 Important tick-borne diseases.

Disease	Agent	Vectors	Distribution
African tick bite fever	*Rickettsia africae*	*Amblyomma hebraeum* and *A. variegatum*	Sub-Saharan Africa, West Indies
Australian spotted fever	*Rickettsia marmionii* spp.	*Haemaphysalis novaeguineae*	Australia
Babesiosis	*Babesia microti*, *Babesia* strain WA-1	*Ixodes scapularis*	Eastern, midwestern, western USA, Europe
Crimean–Congo haemorrhagic fever	Nairovirus	*Hyalomma marginatum*	Asia, Africa and Europe
Human monocytic ehrlichiosis	*Ehrlichia chaffeensis*	*Amblyomma americanum*	Eastern, southern, midwestern USA, Europe and Africa
Human granulocytic ehrlichiosis	*E. ewingii* related to *E. equi*, *E. phagocytophila*	*Ixodes* spp.	Eastern, midwestern, western USA, Europe
Japanese spotted fever	*Rickettsia japonica*	*Ixodes ovatus*, *Dermacentor taiwanensis*, *Haemaphysalis longicornis* and *H. flava*	Japan
Lyme disease	*Borrelia burgdorferi*, *B. garinii*, *B. afzelii*	*Ixodes scapularis*	Northeastern, Pacific coast, midwestern, upper north central USA, northern Eurasia
Mediterranean fever	*Rickettsia conorii*	*Rhipicephalus sanguineus*	Mediterranean region and Africa to Indian subcontinent
Queensland tick typhus	*Rickettsia australis*	*Ixodes holocyclus* and *I. tasmani*	Australia, Tasmania
Rocky Mountain spotted fever	*Rickettsia rickettsii*	*Dermacentor variabilis*, *D. andersoni*, *Amblyomma* spp. and *Rhipicephalus* sp.	North, Central and South America
Siberian tick typhus	*Rickettsia sibirica*	*Dermacentor* spp., *Hyalomma* spp., *Haemaphysalis concinna*	Broadly distributed through north Asia (Siberia, Mongolia, Pakistan)
Southern tick associated rash illness	*Borrelia lonestari*	*Amblyomma americanum*	Southeastern, south central USA
Tick-borne relapsing fever	*Borrelia hermsii*, *B. Turicatae*, *B. parkeri*	*Ornithodoros* spp.	Western USA
Tick-borne lymphadenopathy (TIBOLA)	*Rickettsia slovaca*, *R. raoultii* and *R. rioja*	*Dermacentor marginatus*, *D. reticulatus*, *R. pumilio*	Southern and eastern Europe, Asia
Tularaemia	*Francisella tularensis*	*Amblyomma americanum* *Dermacentor andersoni* *Dermacentor variabilis*	Throughout USA, Europe and Asia

hypostome becomes anchored by a protein cement, produced by the salivary glands, which forms a cone around the hypostome and interlocks with its teeth [1,2]. Argasids, being rapid feeders, do not attach themselves as securely as ixodid ticks.

Ticks as vectors of disease [1,3,4] (Table 34.5)

Tick-borne diseases are highly regional and new diseases and geographical areas of prevalence continue to emerge [5]. Migratory birds have been implicated in the spread of diseases to new regions [6]. Within the large family of ixodid ticks, there are several genera of medical importance, including *Dermacentor*, *Haemaphysalis*, *Rhipicephalus*, *Amblyomma*, *Hyalomma* and *Ixodes*. Removal and identification of the tick can be a major step in the management of infectious diseases (Figure 34.32).

Dermacentor species act as vectors for a number of diseases, including Rocky Mountain spotted fever (Chapter 26), tick-borne lymphadenopathy (TIBOLA), also called *Dermacentor*-borne necrosis erythema lymphadenopathy (DEBONEL) [7], Siberian tick typhus, Colorado tick fever and several types of viral encephalitis.

Haemaphysalis species may also carry Rocky Mountain spotted fever, Siberian tick typhus and Colorado tick fever.

Rhipicephalus sanguineus (the brown dog tick) transmits *Rickettsia conorii*, the causative organism of boutonneuse fever (Mediterranean

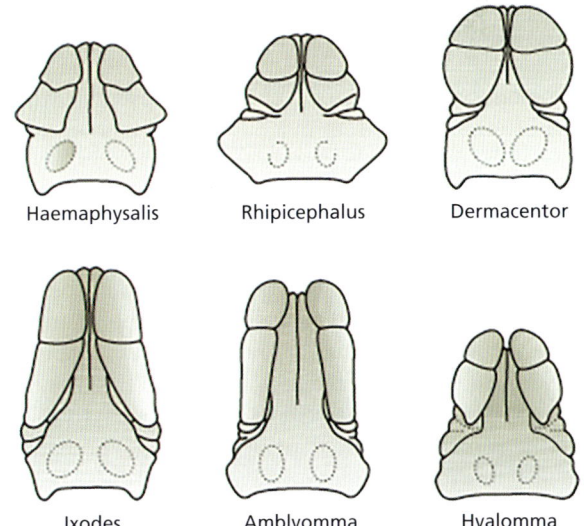

Figure 34.32 Morphology of capitulum and genera of Ixodidae hard tick. Within the large family of ixodid ticks, there are several genera of medical importance, including *Haemaphysalis*, *Rhipicephalus*, *Dermacentor*, *Ixodes*, *Amblyomma* and *Hyalomma*. Adapted from Rodhain and Perez 1985 [36]. Copyright holder of original artwork: Maloine.

spotted fever). *R. sanguineus* is normally confined to the tropics, but it may be encountered in temperate climates in centrally heated houses [8]. Ticks of the genus *Amblyomma* transmit *Rickettsia africae*, the organism responsible for African tick bite fever, tularaemia and human granulocytic anaplasmosis (ehrlichiosis) [9–11]. *Amblyomma americanum* (the lone star tick) has been recognised as a vector for *Borrelia lonestari*, the organism thought to be responsible for southern tick-associated rash illness (STARI), a Lyme disease-like infection [12], which is still an enigma despite years of research [13].

Ixodes species are important vectors of certain haemorrhagic fevers and viral encephalitis, and also of Lyme disease (Chapters 25 and 26). They may also transmit babesiosis to humans [14]. The principal vectors of Lyme disease are the sheep tick *Ixodes ricinus* in Europe, and *Ixodes dammini* (east coast) and *Ixodes pacificus* (west coast) in the USA.

Various species of Argasidae may also act as vectors of disease, the most important being *Ornithodoros* species, which transmit tick-borne relapsing fever. In Israel, *O. tholozani* (the cave tick), which is endemic in the Middle East, is the vector of *Borrelia persica*, a causative agent of relapsing fever [15].

Pathophysiology
The pathophysiology of acute tick bite lesions remains unclear. Tick biting parts can reach into the deep dermis, exposing these tissue layers to mouthpart and salivary antigens. Reactions may vary, depending on the interaction between the host and a particular tick species.

Pathology [3]
At the point of penetration of the tick mouthparts there is coagulation necrosis of the epidermis and papillary dermis [16]. Surrounding the hypostome is the homogeneous cement [17]. The punctured epidermis shows parakeratosis, spongiosis and frequently pseudoepitheliomatous hyperplasia. There is marked dilatation of upper dermal blood vessels, and a dense perivascular infiltrate of neutrophils and lymphocytes. Histology of the bite site several weeks after removal of the tick shows a perivascular and periadnexal infiltrate of lymphocytes, plasma cells and histiocytes [18,19]. Foreign-body giant cells may also be present in the infiltrate. If the hypostome has been damaged during removal of the tick, fragments of the mouthparts may be seen.

Clinical features [3,5,20]
In the case of ixodid ticks, it is usually the parasite itself that attracts the patient's attention. Larvae, nymphs or adults may be discovered attached to the skin and humans usually become accidental hosts when walking through, or sitting in, an area that contains ticks [21]. Larval ticks, sometimes referred to as 'seed ticks', are very small and may go unnoticed unless present in large numbers [22–24]. Bites from soft ticks may be particularly painful [25], perhaps because of their fast feeding or unique salivary contents. The colour of engorged ticks has led patients to suspect they had melanoma [26].

Several factors may be responsible for the type and intensity of tick bite reactions. They include feeding duration, mouthpart size, tick species, previous exposure and individual sensitivity. Dermatoses may be acute or chronic and may occur away from the site of the initial tick bite.

Acute lesions include red macules, papules or nodules, tissue necrosis and ulcers. Red plaques may be difficult to differentiate from erythema migrans, as they can expand to several centimetres. However, these red plaques do not have a tendency to clear in the centre like erythema migrans [16]. There may be focal necrosis leading to necrotic ulcers [25], but more commonly the reaction at the site of the bite is mild oedema, vesiculation or bullae formation [27,28]. Pruritic papules were a prominent feature of larval *Amblyomma* tick bites in a case reported by Fisher *et al*. [29]. A papular urticarial response to ticks has been reported in berry pickers [30] and papular urticaria has been observed developing within a few days of contact with numerous larval ticks of *I. ricinus*. The bites of the cave tick, *Ornithodoros tholozani*, produce characteristic deep red crusted papules or nodules, with a central punctum [15]. Postinflammatory hyperpigmentation may persist several months after acute lesions.

Acute lesions may sometimes persist and become chronic. Chronic lesions include plaques, papules and nodules [25]. The formation of tick bite granuloma is probably responsible for these lesions, which may persist for months or years [21]. The pathophysiology of the granuloma formation remains unclear but may be due to the persistence of tick mouthparts or cuticular fragments in the deep dermis [17].

Auto-eczematisation has been reported in association with a tick bite granuloma [31]. Temporary alopecia may develop around the sites of tick attachment to the scalp [19,32]. The aetiology of the alopecia remains unclear.

The main complication of tick bites is secondary infection (*Staphylococcus aureus* and group A *Streptococcus*), such as impetigo, ecthyma, erysipelas, cellulitis and superinfected necrotic ulcers [21,25]. These secondary infections may result from the persistence of tick material in the dermis or from host scratching.

Finally, tick bites can cause non-dermatological disease such as anaphylaxis, paralysis and other systemic symptoms [33]. Tick paralysis is an ascending flaccid paralysis probably caused by a neurotoxin injected by the feeding tick [34,35]. Occasionally, bulbar paralysis, respiratory failure and death occur. The site of action of the toxin appears to be in the region of the neuromuscular synapse. If the tick is removed, all the signs usually resolve rapidly, but sometimes recovery is slow. Children are more frequently affected than adults.

Tick paralysis occurs in particular localities in association with specific ticks [3]. Offending species include *Dermacentor andersoni* and *D. variabilis* (USA); *Ixodes holocyclus* (Australia); *I. pilosus* (South Africa); *I. ricinus*, *I. hexagonus* and *Rhipicephalus sanguineus* (Europe).

Management [5]
Tick removal
Removal of multiple ticks may be difficult. Ticks should not be removed by a sudden forcible movement, as this will often leave the mouthparts embedded in the skin. The tick should be removed intact with the help of tweezers or a special device designed for tick removal. The tick must be gripped as close to the skin as possible, with gentle traction usually succeeding. The risk of vector-borne disease transmission is minor if the tick is removed within 24 h. Application of fingernails, hot matches or isopropyl alcohol has been demonstrated to be efficient.

Treatment
Except for viral fevers and babesiosis, tetracycline is the antibiotic of choice for most tick-borne diseases. Delayed antibiotic therapy can be fatal, especially in Rocky Mountain spotted fever, and therefore therapy should be initiated quickly in cases of fever and headache in an endemic area, without waiting for laboratory confirmation.

Prevention
Avoidance of tick-infested areas, use of repellents and rapid tick removal are the key points of primary prevention. Secondary prevention is based on prophylactic antibiotics or rapid institution of antibiotics if symptoms appear.

Mites (Acari)

Family Sarcoptidae: human classical scabies

Definition
Scabies in humans and other animals is caused by mites of the family Sarcoptidae, which includes *Sarcoptes scabiei*, the scabies mite, *Notoedres cati*, a mange mite of cats and *Trixacarus caviae*, a mange mite of rodents.

The *Sarcoptes* causing scabies in humans and sarcoptic mange in many other animals are physiological variants of a single species, *S. scabiei*. Their host specificity is not complete, but they usually survive for only a short period on another host.

Introduction and general description [1–8,9,10–14]
Scabies is an ectoparasitic infection caused in humans by *Sarcoptes scabiei* var. *hominis*. The adult female measures approximately 0.4 mm long by 0.3 mm wide, and the smaller male 0.2 mm long by 0.15 mm wide. The body is creamy white and is marked by transverse corrugations, and on its dorsal surface by bristles and spines. There are four pairs of short legs; the anterior two pairs end in elongated peduncles tipped with small suckers. In the female, the rear two pairs of legs end in long bristles (setae) (Figure 34.33), whereas in the male, bristles are present on the third pair and peduncles with suckers on the fourth.

Copulation occurs in a small burrow excavated by the female or at the surface of the skin. The burrow is not confined to the stratum corneum, but is inclined downwards into the epidermis. Approximately 40–50 eggs are laid by each female during a lifespan of 4–6 weeks. Eggs hatch after 3–4 days into larvae, which dig new burrows closer to the skin surface. There, the larvae mature into adult mites in about 4 days. The adults may then either stay in that host or be scratched off and transmitted to a new host. Adult females can live in the host for up to a month. The life cycle lasts around 14–21 days (Figure 34.34) [9]. The mites show a preference for certain sites in which to burrow and appear to avoid areas with a high density of pilosebaceous follicles. The average number of adult female mites on an individual suffering from the common form of scabies is about 5 to 10. In crusted scabies large numbers of mites are present. Individually, pruritus represents a nuisance. The risk of contagiousness, impetiginisation, psychosocial impact and potential associated sexually transmitted diseases constitutes a concern.

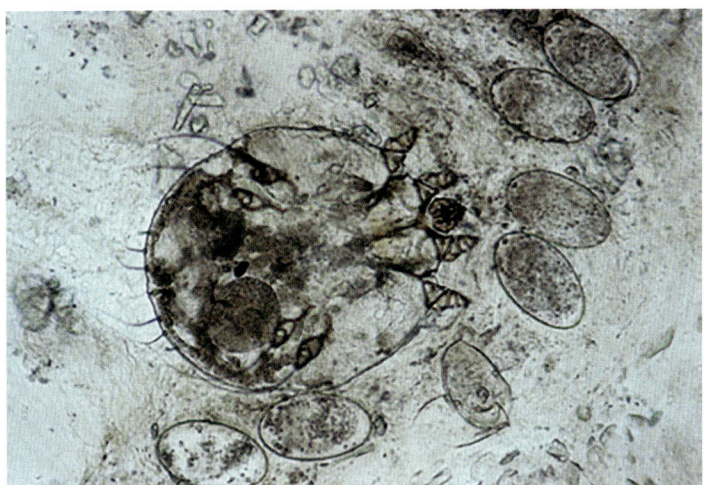

Figure 34.33 *Sarcoptes scabiei* var. *hominis*. Adult female with eggs present in a skin scraping.

Human scabies has played a modest but not insignificant role in history; the story of scabies has been related in detail by Hebra [1], Beeson [2], Heilesen [3], Friedman [4] and Parish [5].

Epidemiology [15,16–18,19]
Prevalence of the disease
There are substantial gaps in our knowledge of the epidemiology of scabies and its complications [20,21]. Nevertheless, recent initiatives driven by academic groups or consortiums such as the International Alliance for the Control of Scabies (IACS) or the Global Burden of Diseases (GBD) have regrouped international experts and have largely extended our awareness of this disease [16,22,23]. These recent efforts have led to the designation of scabies as a Neglected Tropical Disease by the World Health Organization in 2018 (www.who.int). Scabies is one of the commonest and most frequent skin infections worldwide and is estimated to affect between 177 and 237 million people globally at any single time. Measurement of the global burden of scabies has been recently performed in a cross-sectional analysis of the GBD 2015 big data [17]. They included 196 countries and territories and mapped scabies prevalence globally. They found that extreme scabies prevalence was seen in poor communities in tropical settings (Asia, Oceania and tropical Latin America), with crowded conditions and poor access to health care being major risk factors for outbreaks [17]. In a systematic review of prevalence studies of scabies published from 1985 to 2015, scabies prevalence ranged from 0.2% to 71.4% in different populations. Children, mostly under the age of 2, were at greater risk [18]. In high-income nations, high endemicity of scabies is often reported in closed communities and institutional settings, such as hospitals, child care and elderly care residential facilities, prisons, schools, homeless populations and refugee camps [19,24,25,26–28]. In low–middle-income countries, scabies occurs in overcrowded, often underprivileged, communities [29,30].

Pathophysiology [6,10,13,29,31,32]
Transmission of scabies occurs mainly via skin-to-skin contact and, less frequently, via fomites within a patient mite-contaminated environment (generally in the context of severe forms of scabies) [33].

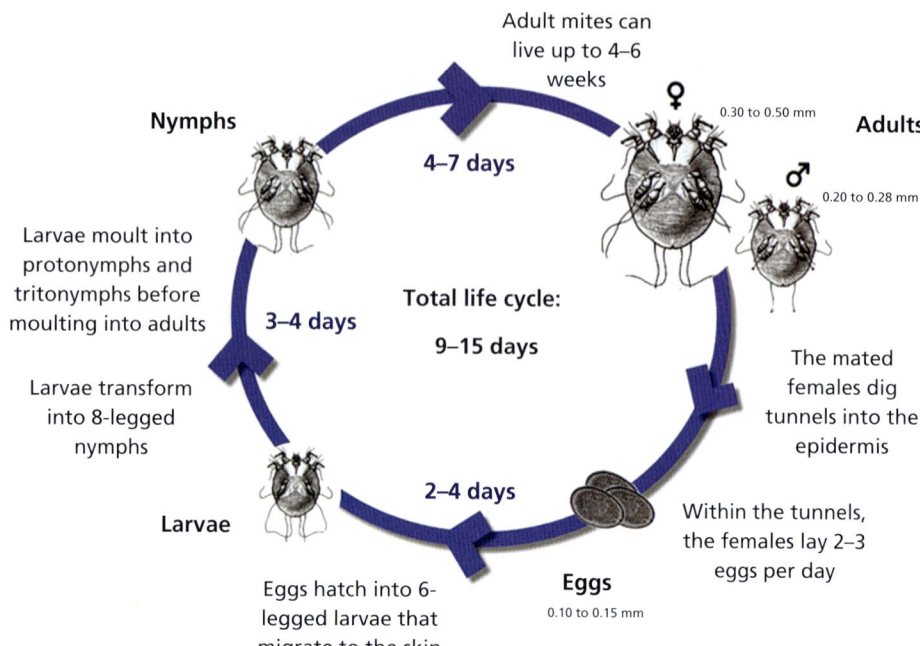

Figure 34.34 The life cycle of *Sarcoptes scabiei* var. *hominis*. From Thomas *et al*. [9]. Source and copyright holder: Elsevier. Adapted with permission of Elsevier from Bernigaud C., Chosidow O. Scabies [in French]. *Rev Prat* 2018;1:63–8.

As scabies is contagious, persons sharing the same household with patients may frequently be affected. This is especially the case in severe scabies, i.e. profuse or crusted scabies, in which the mite burden per person is dramatically increased, small epidemics around a single case can easily develop, and are fuelled by overcrowded households and transient lifestyles [15]. The risk of transmission is known to depend on the patient's mite load, household size and population concentration, and how individuals interact with each other. Indeed, people living in clustered communities or in crowded housing conditions are at higher risk of scabies and outbreaks. Away from the host, scabies mites can survive for 24–36 h at room conditions (21°C and 40–80% relative humidity), and have the capability of skin penetration and infectivity [34]. Females and nymphs survive longer than larvae and males in comparable conditions. Lower temperatures (10–15°C) and high relative humidity favoured survival [35]. Live mites have been demonstrated in dust samples collected in the homes of infected patients [36].

Allergic sensitivity to the mite or its products appears to play an important role in determining the development of lesions other than burrows and in producing pruritus. However, the sequence of immunological events is unclear and requires further elucidation. Evidence suggests that both immediate and delayed-type hypersensitivity are involved [31,32]. Skin tests with mite extracts have given equivocal results, although positive immediate-type reactions to intradermal tests have frequently been obtained in patients within a few months of scabies infection. Normal IgE levels were reported in one series of scabies patients [37], but later studies have shown significantly elevated levels in many individuals [38–40].

Susceptibility or resistance to *S. scabiei* infection shows some genetic predisposition. This is hypothesised to correlate susceptibility to severe disease with the dominance of an IgE-driven Th2 response or resistance to the infestation by an interferon-γ dominated Th1 response. This may be modulated by cytokine regulation in the skin and other immunological control mechanisms [41]. Recent developments in scabies mite biology have shown that scabies can now be considered to be a complex interaction between host, parasite and their associated microbiota [42]. Animal and *in vivo* models of infestation should facilitate a better understanding of these host–parasite interactions, which is critical to improving the treatment of scabies [43,44].

Clinical features [9,15,19]
Presentation
Itching is the most obvious manifestation of scabies, usually sparing the face in adult classical scabies. It is generally worst at night and when the patient is warm [45]. The onset occurs 3–4 weeks after the infection is acquired. Reinfection of a previously cured individual, however, may provoke immediate symptoms [19]. Typical locations of lesions are the finger webs (Figure 34.35a), the flexor surfaces of the wrists, the elbows, the axillae, the buttocks and genitalia (Figure 34.35b) and the breasts of women (Figure 34.42c). The typical lesions of scabies are burrows (Figure 34.35d,e), which appear as slightly raised brownish tortuous lesions. Inflammatory pruritic papules or nodules, sometimes surmounted by burrows, on the male genitalia are characteristic. The genitalia of males should be therefore systematically examined once scabies is suspected as these lesions may provide an important diagnostic clue if burrows are absent or difficult to find. Nodules are intensely itchy and may persist for weeks or months after the scabies has been effectively treated [19]. Secondary lesions are not specific. They include excoriations, eczematisation (Figure 34.35f) and impetiginisation, and may occur anywhere.

In sub-Saharan Africa, where prevalence of scabies is high, a report found that association of diffuse itching with cutaneous lesions and two typical locations or a household member with itching was highly sensitive (100%) and specific (97%) for a diagnosis

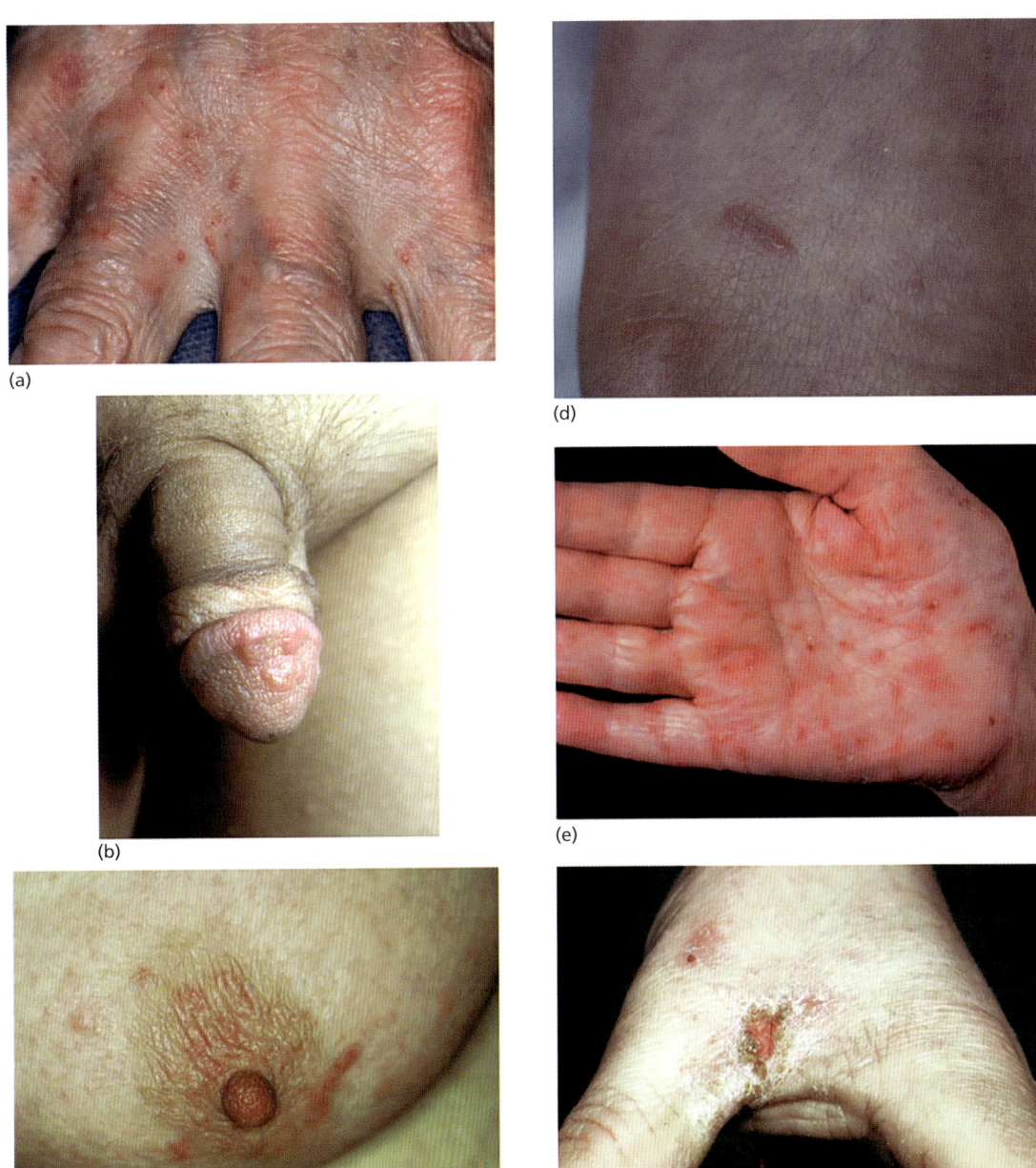

Figure 34.35 (a) Typical scabies in the finger webs. (b) Pruritic papules and nodules on the penis in scabies infestation. The genitalia should be examined in all instances of suspected scabies infestation, especially when the patient reports itching. (c) Papular lesions on the nipples and areolae are a common location for scabies in women. Given this woman's history of pruritus, scabies was easily identified by the finding of scabies in this location. (d) A typical linear burrow with a tiny vesicle at the distal end. (e) Numerous scabies burrows on the palm. Such obvious lesions are rarely seen, as they are usually obscured by eczema, impetigo or both. The more common presentation of scabies with eczematisation of the scratched lesion is shown in (f). The chronic pruritus of scabies rapidly leads to scratching and explains why eczema is frequently observed. Reproduced with permission from Chosidow et al. [15]. Copyright © Massachusetts Medical Society.

of scabies [46]. Consensus criteria for the diagnosis of scabies were published in 2020 following a Delphi process involving a panel of 34 international experts [47,48].

Clinical variants (Figure 34.36a–c)

Atypical forms of scabies (Table 34.6) may occur and be very difficult to diagnose. The clinical features of scabies in infants and young children differ in certain respects from those in older children and adults. In addition to the more extensive distribution of burrows already mentioned, vesicular and vesiculopustular lesions on the hands and feet are frequent, extensive eczematisation is often present, and there may be multiple crusted nodules on the trunk and limbs [49]. In the elderly, burrows commonly occur on the palms and soles, and may be very numerous. Truncal papulosquamous lesions, often surmounted by burrows, are common [25]. Secondary eczematisation is often troublesome. Crusted scabies is discussed separately (see later).

Complications

In addition to these primary manifestations, secondary features may occur and can confuse the clinical picture. Eczematous changes are common, and may be widespread and severe. The inappropriate use of topical corticosteroids may further modify the clinical picture to mimic other dermatoses (see section on crusted scabies later) – so-called 'scabies incognito' [29].

Recent epidemiological studies indicate increasingly substantial morbidity and even mortality [52] due to scabies infection, mostly caused by bacterial infections appearing after scratching of lesions. The discomfort caused by the intense itch can have direct consequences, i.e. depriving patients of sleep [53], interfering with concentration at work or school, leading to a negative impact on

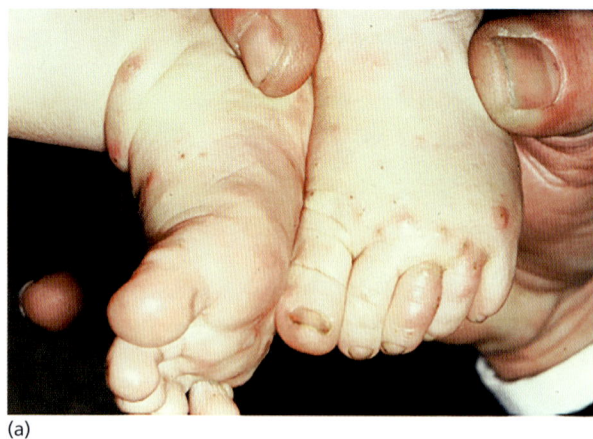
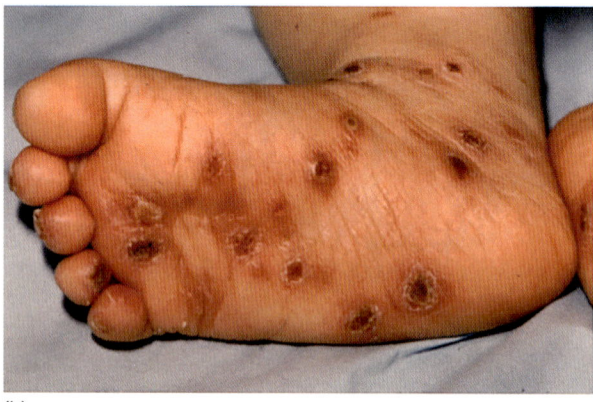
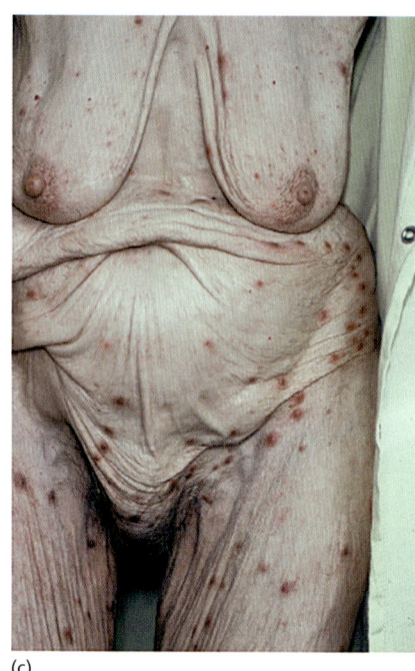

Figure 34.36 Scabies: clinical variants. (a) Scabies in an infant. Localisation on the sole is not atypical in this form of scabies, nor is involvement of the face, scalp and palms. (b) The foot of an infant with scabies superinfection presenting as impetigo. In such patients, the risk of glomerulonephritis associated with nephritogenic strains of *Streptococcus* is of concern in low- and middle-income countries. (c) Atypical papular scabies in an elderly woman who also had similar lesions on her back. Frequently, scabies goes unrecognised in such patients because itching is attributed to senile pruritus. Reproduced with permission from Chosidow et al. [15]. Copyright © Massachusetts Medical Society.

attendance, performance and quality of life [54]. Scratching scabies lesions themselves leads to breaches in the skin barrier that create an entry point for opportunistic commensal or pathogenic bacteria that can become invasive, such as group A streptococcus (GAS) and *S. aureus* [55]. These bacteria lead to secondary infection of the epidermis, also known as pyoderma or impetigo, which can become more severe and cause skin and soft-tissue infections (including necrotising fasciitis), septicaemia or more invasive bacterial infections. In some cases, immune-mediated diseases can occur following infection, such as glomerulonephritis [56] or acute rheumatic fever [57], both of which can become chronic. This association between scabies parasites and bacterial pathogens is observed mainly in tropical or subtropical areas of the globe and in remote locations [18], with some data suggesting that up to 40% of impetigo lesions can be linked with scabies, especially among young children [58,59]. This particular link was established early in the 1970s, with an epidemiological study showing epidemics of acute glomerulonephritis in Trinidad [60] contemporaneously with scabies outbreaks, or in interventional studies in the field showing reduction in childhood haematuria following scabies treatment [56], or reduction in impetigo or skin sores prevalence paralleling a reduction in scabies numbers during mass drug administration campaigns [61–63].

Investigations [15,48,64–67]

The typical history of pruritus with nocturnal exacerbations, the presence of contact cases within the family and the distribution of the eruption of inflammatory papules should suggest the diagnosis. The presence of genital lesions in men or breast nodules in women is strongly suggestive. Absolute confirmation can only be made by the evidence of burrows and/or mites, eggs, fragments of egg shells or scybala using light microscopy examination of skin samples [48]. A burrow is gently scraped off the skin with a blunt scalpel and the material placed in mineral oil on a microscope slide. Failure to find mites does not rule out scabies, as this technique is very specific but highly operator-dependent [15,64,65,68]. Parasitological confirmation of the diagnosis should be made in all cases if possible. It is essential in cases of crusted scabies or scabies in health care settings.

Dermoscopy is useful for detecting burrows and visualising their contents, the mite in its burrow resembling a 'jet-with-contrail' (40× magnification) [66]. With lower magnification (10×) with standard handheld dermoscopy, the circumflex accent-like image (as the French letter 'ô') represents the head and the two pairs of front legs of the mite scabies and is called the 'deltawing jet' sign [69,70] (Figure 34.37a). Dermoscopy is less time consuming than the skin scraping procedure and can be used in daily clinical practice by dermatologists. However, its use is limited by the cost of the device and the sensitivity may decrease in inexperienced hands, and on pigmented, eczematous or impetiginised skin [64,71]. Videodermoscopy utilises a dermoscope with a videocamera connected to a computer that allows very high magnification (80×) and can be used to assess the viability of living mites (Figure 34.37b). Confocal microscopy was recently employed for the confirmation of the

Table 34.6 Special forms of scabies.

Variable	Major clinical features
Involved subpopulation	
Infants and young children [49]	Lesions are vesicles, pustules and nodules, but their distribution may be atypical. Eczematisation and impetigo are common; scabies may be confused with atopic eczema or acropustulosis. Pruritus may be so severe that infants can be irritable and eat poorly
Homeless people	Eczematisation and impetigo are common. Extensive excoriated lesions are not necessarily indicative of scabies in homeless people but pruritus in a homeless shelter should suggest a diagnosis of scabies
The elderly	Atypical presentation is common. Scabies epidemics are reported frequently in nursing homes, where a single patient with crusted scabies may be the index patient leading to infection of other residents, as well as health care workers and their families
Immunocompromised patients	Severe scabies (i.e. atypical papular scabies or crusted scabies) develops predominantly in patients receiving topical or systemic corticosteroids, those with HIV infection, organ transplant recipients and patients of advanced age. Pruritus may be mild or absent (i.e. scabies incognito)
Indigenous communities	Scabies, whether crusted or not, may be endemic (e.g. risk factors include poor nutritional status, inadequate medical facilities and overcrowding). The burden of the disease may be very high among Aboriginal people in northern Australia, children in Africa or the Solomon Islands, and resettlement colonies in New Delhi, India, for example. Because of the high rate of scabies superinfection, Australian Aboriginal communities have the highest rate of poststreptococcal glomerulonephritis in the world
Atypical presentation	
Scabies of the scalp	Scabies may accompany or simulate seborrhoeic dermatitis or dermatomyositis on the scalp; infants, children, the elderly, patients with AIDS and patients with crusted scabies may be affected
Nodular scabies	A few violaceous, pruritic nodules are often localised on the groin, axillae and male genitalia; they represent a hypersensitivity reaction to mite antigens and persist weeks or months after treatment
Scabies mimicking immunologically mediated diseases	Bullous pemphigoid, urticaria, chronic lymphocytic leukaemia, B-cell lymphoma with monoclonal infiltrate, CD30+ lymphoid proliferations, necrotising vasculitis [50,51] and lupus erythematosus can all mimic scabies

Adapted from Chosidow 2006 [15] with permission. Copyright holder of original: Massachusetts Medical Society.

clinical diagnosis of scabies [72,73] (Figure 34.37c). The latter two of these techniques are expensive.

A skin biopsy may confirm the diagnosis of scabies if a mite or parts can be identified. However, in most cases the histology shows non-specific features, with epidermal spongiosis, papillary oedema, and superficial and deep perivascular inflammatory cell infiltrates with numerous eosinophils [74].

Some authors have tried to develop diagnostic techniques using molecular tools, such as matrix-assisted laser desorption ionisation–time of flight (MALDI-TOF), an antigen detection system or polymerase chain reaction (PCR) specifically targeting scabies DNA. With PCR, while most studies have found a very high specificity often close to 100%, sensitivity was continually low, ranging from 30% to 60% [75–77], much lower compared with parasite observation by either microscopic or dermoscopic examination [78]. Optimisation of the sampling procedure is necessary and might increase sensitivity [67]. To date, no biomarker-based diagnostic kits have been developed for use as a simple and rapid method to identify mite infection without dermatological skills. Recent metagenomics data using RNA-seq transcriptomics or proteomics might be useful to find candidate antigens and to develop rapid immunodiagnostic tests [79].

In the absence of confirmed mites, diagnosis is currently based entirely on clinical and epidemiological findings. Given the extensive differential diagnoses, the specificity of clinical diagnosis is poor, especially for those inexperienced regarding scabies. Furthermore, there are difficulties in distinguishing between active infestation, residual skin reaction and reinfestation. Despite the relatively low sensitivity of diagnostic testing, empirical treatment is not recommended for patients presenting with generalised itching [15].

Management [22,29,80–85]

Indication for therapy
Treatment should be prescribed to the patient and all close physical contacts, even without pruritus or cutaneous lesions.

Patient education
Patients should be advised to avoid close physical contact until they and their household members and sexual partners have been treated. Detailed verbal and written information about scabies infestation should be given to the patient [86].

Treatment options
Topical and oral products are available although rigorous studies to guide their use are lacking. Topical treatment includes 5% permethrin, 1% ivermectin, 1% lindane, 10–25% benzyl benzoate, 0.6% esdepallethrine (bioallethrin), 10% crotamiton and 6–33% precipitated sulphur. Topical scabicides have neurotoxic effects on mites. Table 34.7 summarises the doses and side effects of common agents used in scabies management. Topical agents should be applied to the entire skin surface, from 'head to toe', avoiding the eyes, nose and mouth [15]. The application period depends on the specific instructions from the manufacturer. Topical medicines were considered first line treatment until the arrival of oral ivermectin in 1981, which was, at first, reserved for recurrent, difficult-to-treat cases, those with superinfected or eczematous skin or for patients with crusted scabies [85].

Oral ivermectin is neurotoxic for many parasites, including mites, binding specifically to their chloride–glutamate and GABA receptors. It can be given at a dosage of 200 µg/kg in patients >2 years of age and >15 kg of body weight [85]. A second dose is necessary a week later due to the limited ovicidal activity of the drug [87] and the short half-life of ivermectin in the skin, which was shown in two experimental trials in a porcine scabies model [85,87–89]. Because ingestion of food increases the bioavailability of ivermectin by a factor of two [75], taking it with food might enhance the quantity of drug that penetrates into the epidermis. Ivermectin is apparently a safe drug with a low incidence of adverse effects and

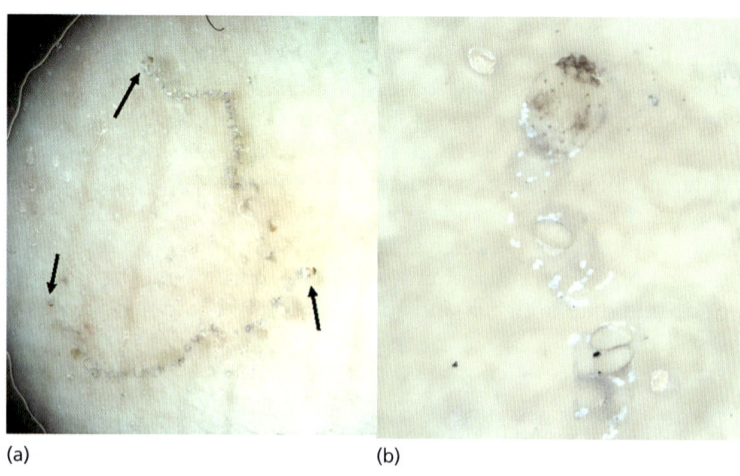
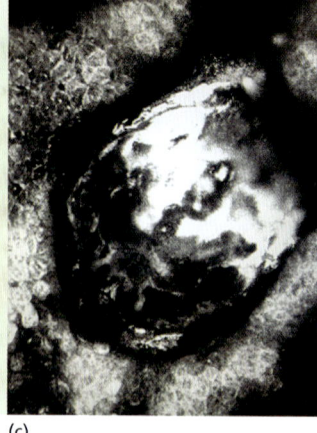

Figure 34.37 Two burrow lesions examined using dermoscopy (magnification ×10) showing three 'deltawing jet' signs (black arrows) (a). A burrow examined using videodermoscopy (magnification × 40) showing an adult female mite and eggs (b); and using reflectance confocal microscopy showing an adult female mite (c).

Table 34.7 Drugs commonly used to treat scabies.

Treatment	Dosage	Treatment regimen	Contraindication	Advantages	Disadvantages	Comments
Ivermectin*	Pills	200 μg/kg repeated after 7 days	Children <15 kg; pregnant or breastfeeding women (only approved in France)	Effective, easy, good patient compliance	Expensive in some countries	Not approved in many countries
Permethrin*	5% cream	Rinsed off after 8–12 h (overnight)	Safe in children >2 months of age	Effective, well tolerated, safe	Itching and stinging on application. Expensive in some countries	Second application often routinely prescribed 1 week after the first
Benzyl benzoate*	10–25% lotion or emulsion	Rinsed off after 24 h (one or several times)	Pregnant women and infants (only 12 h application) Safe in children >1 month of age	Effective, inexpensive	Can cause severe skin irritation	Not currently available in Canada, approved in Europe
Crotamiton*	10% ointment	Rinsed off after 24 h and then reapplied for an additional 24 h	–	Well tolerated, safe for infants	Questionable efficacy	Often used on scabies nodules in children
Esdepalletrin (bioallethrin)*	0.6% aerosol	Rinsed off after 12 h	People with asthma	–	–	**Withdrawn in the European Union**
Lindane*	1% lotion or cream	Rinsed off after 6 h	Pregnant women, infants, seizure disorders	Effective, inexpensive	Cramps, dizziness, seizures in children	**Withdrawn in the European Union because of neurotoxicity concerns**
Malathion*	0.5% aqueous lotion	Repeat after 7 days	Not approved in children <2 years of age	Easy to use	Skin irritation, dizziness, central nervous system toxicity	**Withdrawn in France**
Precipitated sulphur*	2–10% precipitate in petroleum base	Rinsed off after 24 h and then reapplied every 24 h for the next 2 days (with a bath taken between each application)	–	Safe for infants, pregnant and breastfeeding women	Questionable efficacy, skin irritation	–

*Available as generics.
Adapted from Chosidow 2006 [15] with permission. Copyright holder of original: Massachusetts Medical Society.

has been widely used for >30 years to combat neglected tropical parasitic diseases such as onchocerciasis, lymphatic filariasis and helminthiasis. Many of the reported adverse effects have occurred in individuals given ivermectin for the treatment of filariasis, in whom serious reactions were thought to be related to death of the parasites [50,90]. A report suggesting a pattern of excess deaths in elderly people in a residential unit, who were given ivermectin to control a scabies outbreak, raised concerns about its safety [51]. However, the conclusions of this report were challenged [91,92] and other authors' findings regarding its safety are reassuring,

Table 34.8 Treatment of scabies by clinical features or situation.

Purpose of therapy	Recommended therapy	Alternative therapy	Specific associated measures	Comments
Classical scabies	Two applications of permethrin 5% cream, or two doses of oral ivermectin, 200 µg/kg (a week apart)	Two applications of 10–25% benzyl benzoate	–	People in close physical contact, even without symptoms, should receive treatment at the same time (two applications/doses)
Children <2 years old	Permethrin or benzyl benzoate (only 12 h application)	Ivermectin is contraindicated in children <15 kg	Treat the face, except mouth and eyes	Treat scabies nodules with crotamiton
Pregnancy	Permethrin, benzyl benzoate (only 12 h application) and sulphur	Ivermectin is contraindicated in the USA, but authorised in France	–	–
Superinfected scabies	Prefer oral ivermectin if skin is affected	Topical or systemic antibiotherapy before topical treatment	–	Risk of poststreptococcal glomerulonephritis and systemic sepsis
Institutional outbreak of scabies	Treat clinical cases as for classical and crusted scabies	–	Simultaneously treat all cases and all exposed people	Formation of an outbreak management team

Adapted from Monsel and Chosidow 2012 [114].

even in the elderly population [93,94]. It has been suggested that conditions disturbing the blood–brain barrier integrity such as in young mammals may allow the drug to enter the central nervous system [95–97]. Therefore, some authors consider the drug must be contraindicated in children younger than 5 years of age or <15 kg, and during lactation. However, many recent publications and a systematic review reported ivermectin to be safe in children [98–101]. Its use in pregnant women is discouraged in the USA, but is possible in France [102,103]. The human central nervous system is protected against ivermectin accumulation by the membrane drug transporter ABCB1. Nevertheless, serious ivermectin toxicity was strongly suspected in a child carrying exceptional ABCB1-nonsense mutations; hence, pharmacovigilance remains necessary even if these events might be exeptional [104].

Finally, 5% permethrin cream or oral ivermectin (at a dosage of 200 µg/kg) may be used for the treatment of classical scabies. If permethrin is not available, 10–25% benzyl benzoate may be used. Oral ivermectin is more expensive and not licensed in most countries; however, this agent may be preferred for patients who cannot tolerate topical therapy or are unlikely to adhere to a therapeutic regimen. In classical scabies, the combination of topical therapy and oral ivermectin has never been compared with either treatment alone. Table 34.8 presents strategies of treatment according to the clinical picture.

Other interesting treatments are under development, especially drugs that could target all stages of the mite life cycle, including the egg stage [105]. Moxidectin is a good candidate that could be given to patients as a single-dose oral treatment [106,107]. A phase II trial has recently been completed (www.clinicaltrials.gov; NCT03905265).

Additional measures

Examination and laboratory investigation to search for sexually transmitted infection should be performed as scabies is considered to be a sexually transmitted disease [80].

Topical treatment must be applied to the entire skin surface, including the scalp, face, all folds, groin, navel and external genitalia, as well as the skin under the nails. Treating the face of babies is essential because transmission may occur by breastfeeding. Hands should not be washed during therapy, otherwise the topical treatment should be reapplied. If topical treatment is applied by another person, it is recommended that this person wears protective gloves.

All clothes and bedding must be washed at high temperature (>60°C) or must be kept in a plastic bag for several days. Simplified and generalised algorithms, based on high-throughput experimental data that can be used in a large range of settings, including resource-poor populations, were suggested recently [108]. Appropriate treatment should also be given for severe secondary bacterial infection (see later). There is no specific treatment for the itch. Antihistamines can assist, but it is their sedative properties that are effective, rather than an antipruritic mechanism [109]. Novel targets to manage the scabies itch are presented in [45].

Special treatment considerations

Table 34.8 presents the treatment of scabies according to the clinical feature or situation.

Children. Benzyl benzoate, esdepallethrin and permethrin may be used in infants. Benzyl benzoate and esdepallethrin are safe in children <2 years of age, but duration of use should be limited to 12 h. Ivermectin is contraindicated in children <15 kg.

Impetigo. Oral ivermectin should be preferred in this situation. If topical treatment is chosen, antibiotic therapy should be performed first. Topical antibiotic creams (e.g. mupirocin or fusidic acid) are not recommended in cases with profuse lesions. Systemic antibiotics have to target GAS and *S. aureus* (including MRSA in specific areas). Oral trimethoprim-sulphamethoxazole (cotrimoxazole) or intramuscular benzathine benzylpenicillin (penicillin G) are used in tropical endemic regions [110], whereas pristinamycin, amoxicillin/clavulanic acid or cephalexin may be used in non-tropical regions.

Table 34.9 Causes of persistent itching after scabicide therapy and management.

	Causes	Management
Cutaneous irritation	Overtreatment	Intensive use of emollient
	Eczematisation	Intensive use of emollient
	Contact dermatitis	Topical steroid
Treatment failure	Poor compliance; inappropriate or insufficient treatment	Further scabicide application
	Resistance to scabicide	Change scabicide
	Reinfestation or relapse	Further scabicide application
Psychogenic pruritus	Delusions of parasitosis	Antipsychotic drugs (prescribed by dermatologists and/or psychiatrists)
	Non-parasitic dermatosis	Treat the underlying cause

Adapted from Chosidow 2000 [19].

Pregnancy or breastfeeding. Permethrin, benzyl benzoate and sulphur appear to be safe in pregnancy, although the evidence is limited [111]. Oral ivermectin is not approved in the USA (ranked C in the United States Food and Drug Administration pregnancy category) but is permitted in France [102,103]. A recent systematic review and meta-analysis found that birth outcomes were not excessively abnormal in ivermectin-treated women compared with unexposed women [112], and some authors advocate for a widening of the access to ivermectin to scabies-infested pregnant women, especially in eczematous forms [113].

Institutional outbreaks. The management of institutional outbreaks is mainly based on consensus expert opinion. It requires coordination and adequate education of all involved personnel and a sustained effort to rapidly control the outbreak. Prompt recognition of the index case, formation of an outbreak management team, determining the extent of the outbreak and risk factors for transmission, immediate implementation of infection control practices, simultaneous treatment of cases and all exposed people, and concomitant environmental disinfection are key factors for controlling a scabies epidemic in health care settings [24,25].

Follow-up. Itching may persist several weeks after scabies and this should be clearly explained to the patient. Emollients may be helpful in cases of cutaneous irritation. The persistence of itching after 4 weeks should be reinvestigated (Table 34.9). Parasite resistance has been reported for both permethrin [115,116] and ivermectin [117,118], but its clinical importance remains a matter of debate. Studies are lacking and surveillance for better documentation is warranted.

Family Sarcoptidae: human crusted scabies

Synonyms and inclusions
- Norwegian scabies

Introduction and general description
The appellation 'Norwegian' derives from the description in Norway by Danielssen and Boeck [1] of a type of scabies in which huge numbers of mites were present in lepers. Von Hebra referred to this as 'scabies Norvegica Boecki' [2]. We strongly recommend that 'Norwegian' should be discarded and replaced by 'crusted' or hyperkeratotic, as others have [3,4].

Crusted scabies is a rare and severely debilitating form of the disease, characterised by the infestation of up to millions of mites and the development of a hyperkeratotic skin crust. An undiagnosed case of crusted scabies may be the source of an outbreak of common scabies.

Pathophysiology [5,6]
In common scabies, there are few mites, probably because scratching destroys the burrows. Crusted scabies occurs in people with an inadequate immune response to the mite, allowing them to multiply. It is a severe disease with a significantly higher morbidity than ordinary scabies.

Patients with intellectual disability or dementia may develop crusted scabies [7], and Down syndrome is a frequent association [3,8]. The reason for this association with intellectual disability is not completely understood, but lack of appreciation of pruritus may be important.

Crusted scabies may develop in patients who are immunosuppressed, either as a result of disease [9–11] or therapy [11–14], including with infliximab and tocilizumab [15,16]. In recent years, there have been numerous reports of its occurrence in patients with HIV infection; it has been reported in immune reconstitution inflammatory syndrome [17] and it is also an indicator of human T-cell lymphotrophic virus (HTLV-1) infection [18–20]. Crusted scabies has also resulted from the use of topical steroids [21] and pimecrolimus [22].

Crusted scabies sometimes occurs in otherwise healthy individuals [23,24], and in northern Australia, where crusted scabies is a problem in the Aboriginal population, 42% of a series of 78 patients had no identifiable risk factors [25]. In a more recent study of over 80 infested patients, half of them were diabetic and 23% were on dialysis for end-stage kidney failure. Sixteen per cent of patients had no co-morbidities and these were more likely to have a severe Grade 3 disease [26].

Clinical features [25–29]
Large warty crusts form on the hands (Figure 34.38a) and feet (Figure 34.38b,c), and the palms and soles may be irregularly thickened and fissured. The nail apparatus is frequently affected, with masses of horny debris accumulating beneath thickened and discoloured nails (Figure 34.38d). Redness and scaling occur on the face, neck, scalp (Figure 34.38e) and trunk, and may generalise. The extent of the erythroderma and the warty plaques varies greatly, and either may predominate. Crusted scabies may be localised, affecting only the scalp, face, fingers, toenails or soles [29]. Itching is

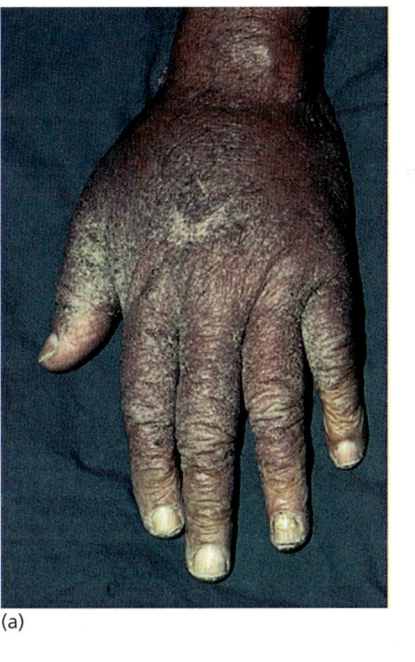
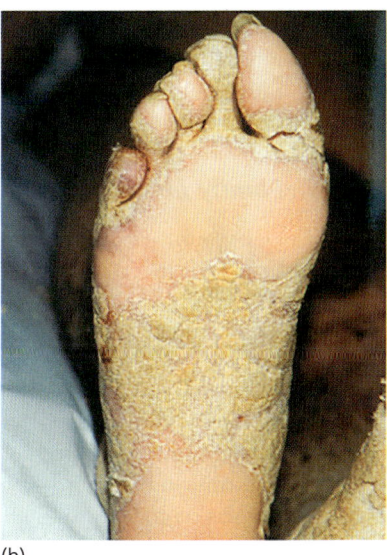
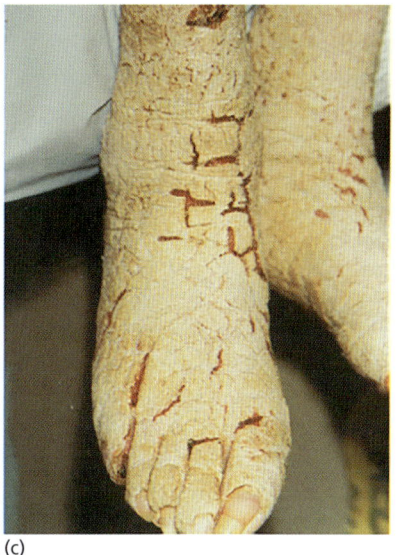
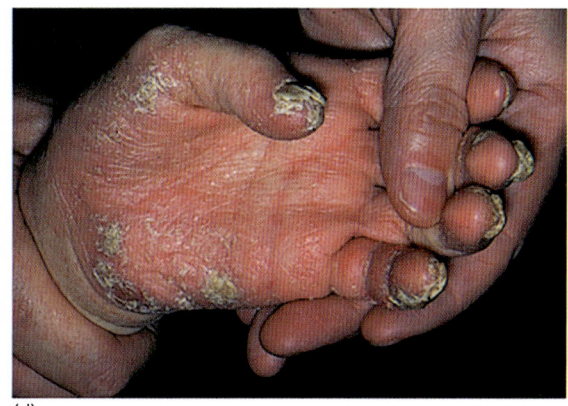
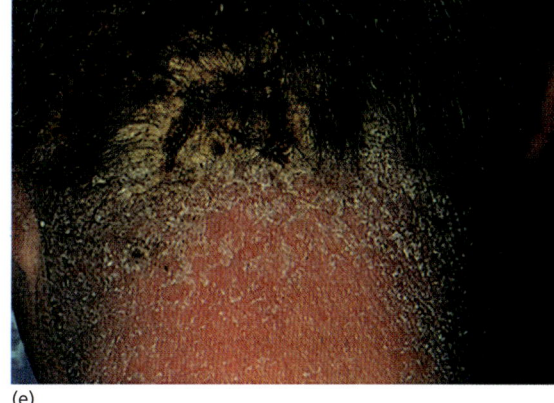

Figure 34.38 Crusted (Norwegian) scabies of the hand (a) and foot (b, c). (d) Grossly dystrophic nails in crusted scabies. (e) Severe scalp involvement in crusted scabies.

often absent or slight, but may occasionally be severe. Generalised lymphadenopathy is present in some cases, and blood eosinophilia and elevated IgE levels are common.

The diagnosis of this disease can be challenging and studies have shown a long delay in the diagnosis of severe scabies, lasting up to several months. For example, in a series of crusted scabies patients published in 2016, the delay was long, with a median of 7 months and an extreme of up to 16 months [30]. The delayed diagnosis may be explained by a lack of specific diagnostic criteria for severe scabies and insufficient knowledge of the clinical presentation by physicians. Crusted scabies may masquerade as hyperkeratotic eczema, psoriasis, Darier disease [31], contact dermatitis [32] and Langerhans cell histiocytosis [33]. Misdiagnosis can lead to incorrect prescriptions of treatments (mainly topical corticosteroids), initially improving pruritus but finally aggravating the infestation, which might cause life-threatening complications.

No diagnostic criteria for severe scabies have been established. Therefore, the diagnosis has to be confirmed by examination of scrapings, which will be teeming with mites and eggs.

Management [34–47]
General principles
Hospitalisation and isolation of the patient are required to manage crusted scabies because of the risk of transmission to people in physical contact. All individuals in contact should be treated. A keratolytic agent such as a salicylic acid preparation should be used to treat hyperkeratosis. Nails should be cut short and brushed with a scabicidal agent [36]. Expert consensus recommends combining topical and oral therapy [36], although this has never been evaluated. Only a few therapeutic studies for treatment of crusted scabies including more than five patients exist in the literature [25,42–44].

Some authors suggest that topical scabicide application should be repeated until two parasitological tests 3 days apart become negative. The administration schedule of ivermectin should be based on the severity of infection [45]; between three and seven doses have been proposed [28]. However, Currie et al. [46] reported evidence of resistance to ivermectin in two patients who had received multiple doses for recurrences of crusted scabies. Recently, a simple clinical grading scale to aid in the management of patients with crusted scabies has been proposed and may be useful [47].

Family Sarcoptidae: animal scabies
Introduction and general description [1]
Transmission of animal scabies to humans is probably rare because of the relative host specificity of the mites [2]. However, recurrent exposure to animal scabies mites can produce troublesome and diagnostically puzzling lesions.

Many varieties of *Sarcoptes scabiei* have been incriminated, including the following:
1. The mites causing sarcoptic mange in horses, cattle, buffalo, pigs, camels, monkeys, sheep and goats [3–8].
2. *Sarcoptes scabiei* var. *canis* commonly causes transient skin lesions in those in contact with infested dogs [9–15]. Exceptionally, scrapings from human skin have shown mites and eggs, and symptoms have persisted after contact with the animal has ceased [16]. Canine scabies has been experimentally transferred to humans [17]. Affected animals have areas of scaling and hair loss on the ears, face and limbs [18].
3. *Notoedres cati*, the cause of sarcoptic mange in cats, is almost unknown in the UK, but where it is endemic in the cat population, as in India [19] and Japan [20], human skin lesions may occur.

Clinical features
Skin lesions resulting from contact with animal scabies vary in extent and distribution, according to the mode of exposure. The eruption is usually composed of small pruritic weals or papules, which are frequently excoriated and resemble human scabies, but without burrows. Lesions from exposure to sarcoptic mange in dogs and notoedric mange in cats usually occur at sites of contact with the animal, principally the chest, abdomen, thighs and forearms.

Management
If contact with animal scabies is suspected, the diagnosis can only be confirmed by examining and taking scrapings from the suspect animal. Affected animals should be treated by a veterinary practitioner.

Human skin lesions are self-limiting and will resolve once exposure to the affected animal has ceased or it has been treated. Despite being self-limited, the skin eruption may be uncomfortable and topical treatment such as 5% permethrin cream will hasten recovery [21]. Oral ivermectin (200 µg/kg single dose) has been used [21,22], as well as topical corticosteroids, menthol preparations and oral antihistamines for symptomatic relief [23].

Family Knemidokoptidae
Knemidokoptes mutans causes scaly leg in domestic poultry and *Mesoknemidokoptes laevis* is a closely related mite that causes depluming itch in poultry; both have caused skin lesions in humans [1].

Family Psoroptidae
Mites of the family Psoroptidae cause mange in domestic animals. Species of *Chorioptes* and *Psoroptes* from cattle, horses and sheep have occasionally affected humans [1,2]. *Otodectes cynotis* is a common parasite in the ears of cats and dogs and has been discovered in the ears of a patient suffering from otitis externa [3,4]. It was also considered to be responsible for a pruritic dermatosis in a patient whose dog was infested. Psoroptic skin disease resembles scabies infestation. The distribution of the dermatitis is dependent upon the areas that come in close contact with the animals [5].

Family Listrophoridae
Listrophorus gibbus, a common parasite of the domestic rabbit [6], has been reported as causing papular urticaria in a child [7].

Mites of stored products [1,2]
Introduction and general description
Storage mite allergy is a well-recognised problem in certain occupations, including farmers, grain elevator workers and bakers. In addition to respiratory allergy, skin lesions can occur, secondary to bites or contact with allergens. These mites proliferate in a warm humid environment with relative humidity of 80% and a temperature between 25 and 30°C. Herbivorous and fungivorous, they subsist on fungi and are pests of stored food products with high moisture content.

Classification
Family Acaridae
These mites attack flour, grain, dried meat, cheese and dried fruit.

Acarus siro is the most important pest of storage premises and is found on flour, grain and, occasionally, cheese. It may cause skin lesions on those who handle these products.

Tyrophagus putrescentiae [3–6] is mostly found in stored food with a high fat and protein content such as dried eggs, ham, herring meal, cheese, nuts and copra. *Tyrophagus longior* is found on cheese, grain, hay and copra [7].

Suidasia nesbitti is particularly associated with wheat pollards and bran, and has been recorded as causing dermatitis in humans [8].

Rhizoglyphus species occur on flower bulbs and have caused dermatitis in persons handling stored bulbs.

Family Carpoglyphidae

Carpoglyphus passularum (*lactis*) is found on all kinds of dried fruit and may cause dermatitis [9,10].

Family Glycyphagidae

Glycyphagus domesticus is a widely distributed species, often found in large numbers on plant and animal remains in houses and stables. It has also been found in flour, wheat, hay, tobacco, cheese and ham. *Glycyphagus destructor* is often abundant in hay, straw and grain.

Pathophysiology

It has been suggested that the dermatitis caused by these mites, which are not haematophagous, results from irritation by mite products, either faecal or secretory [5]. Extracts from storage mites include endotoxins, which may modulate cell adhesion and secretion of cytokines by microvascular endothelial cells. These modulating properties vary among mite species [11].

Dockers and warehouse workers handling stored products are most at risk, but shopkeepers and domestic workers are occasionally affected.

Clinical features [12]

The eruption provoked by these mites is sometimes called 'copra itch' or 'grocer's itch', and is often composed of minute intensely pruritic papules or papulovesicles on exposed parts of the body, principally on the head and neck and forearms, but occasionally more widespread. The appearance of the eruption on the face may suggest an acute contact dermatitis.

House-dust mites

Introduction and general description

Dermatophagoides pteronyssinus, the house-dust mite, was first discovered by Trouessart in dust shaken from tanned mammal skins [1]. It was subsequently established that it is widely distributed in the human environment in house dust and beds [2,3].

Epidemiology

It occurs worldwide and has been reported from all inhabited continents [4]. It is commonly associated with *Euroglyphus maynei* and *Dermatophagoides farinae*, which are related species in the same family, the Pyroglyphidae. In the USA, *D. farinae* appears to be more plentiful in house dust than *D. pteronyssinus* [5].

Pathophysiology

The largest numbers of mites are found in houses that are damp and inadequately heated [4]. Numbers vary seasonally, increasing in early summer to reach a maximum by early autumn. In the UK, numbers are low in winter and increase in spring, when temperature and relative humidity rise [6].

The main food of *D. pteronyssinus* is human skin scales [7]. Xero-phylic moulds, especially *Aspergillus penicilloides*, are essential for the growth and survival of *D. pteronyssinus*. The moulds digest lipid in the scales which is toxic to the mites.

The major house-dust mite allergens (Der p1 and Der f1) are present in the faecal pellets.

Clinical features

The role of the house-dust mite in the pathogenesis of atopic eczema remains controversial [8–13] (Chapter 41). The allergens of *Euroglyphus maynei* are thought to play a role in the sensitisation and induction of clinical symptoms of atopic eczema [14,15]. The mites that most frequently induce atopic eczema are *D. pteronyssinus* and *D. farinae* [16].

Several studies have indicated that, in many individuals, the condition can be improved by techniques designed to reduce exposure to house-dust mite allergen [17–22], although the benefits on clinical status appear to be greater in children than in adults [14], and it is not possible to predict which patients will benefit. One study demonstrated that the houses of patients with moderate to severe atopic eczema had more house-dust mites than controls [23]. A critically appraised article published in 2013 concluded that there is unsufficient evidence to support house-dust mite reduction in the management of atopic eczema [24]. A systematic Cochrane review was published in 2015 [25].

Management

Measures employed to reduce the house-dust mite allergen load include regular vacuum cleaning of carpets, or their removal, using bedding covers made of material such as microporous Goretex® and the use of acaricides, including benzyl benzoate and permethrin [26].

Pyemotes mites

Introduction and general description

Pyemotes mites are all primarily parasites of insects or their larvae. They only affect humans when the latter come into contact with the food of their natural hosts.

The mite *P. tritici* preys on the larvae of many species of insect, infesting grain, straw or hay, and stored foodstuffs. Another species, *P. ventricosus*, preys on the larvae of wood-boring beetles, including the common furniture beetle *Anobium punctatum*.

Epidemiology

Pyemotes mites have been responsible for attacks of dermatitis in those shovelling grain or coming into contact with infested straw [1] and husk rice [2]. The dermatitis has been referred to by a number of terms, including 'barley itch', 'grain-shovellers' itch', 'grain itch', 'straw itch', 'cotton-seed dermatitis' and 'acarodermatitis urticarioides'. *Pyemotes* dermatitis has been reported in shop workers coming into contact with wheat used for decorative purposes [3–5]. Dermatitis in workers in a food mixing shed at a piggery was attributed to *P. herfsi* [6] and *P. zwoelferi* was incriminated in dermatitis acquired by contact with a package of everlasting flowers [7]. Dermatitis in a fisherman handling crab pots made of cherry wood was probably caused by *P. beckeri* [8].

An outbreak of dermatitis in a small hospital in Queensland, Australia, was attributed to *Pyemotes* mites originating in an adjacent grain storage facility [9]. Rodriguez-Casado et al. described a *Pyemotes* dermatitis outbreak associated with *A. punctatum*-infested wood desks in a school [10]. An outbreak of *P. ventricosus* (Figure 34.39) associated with *A. punctatum* was reported in southeastern France [11].

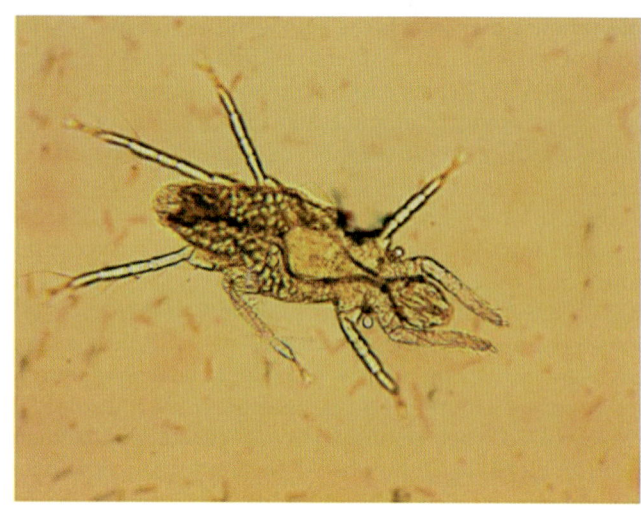
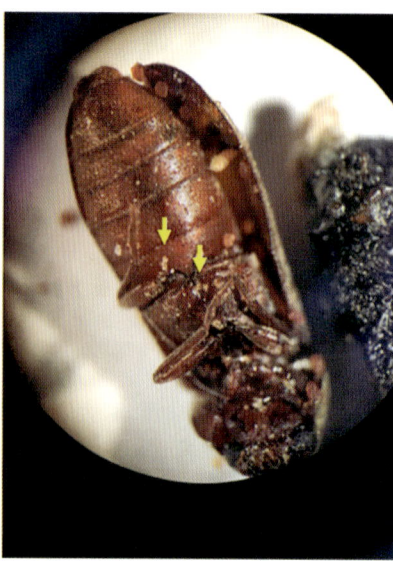

Figure 34.39 *Pyemotes ventricosus* (a) and *P. ventricosus* mites (yellow arrows) visible on *Anobium punctatum* (b).

Since the beginning of the 20th century, *Pyemotes* spp. have been recognised to cause dermatitis. In previously recorded outbreaks, ectoparasites of insect larvae feeding on plants were responsible for dermatitis in workers exposed to agricultural products [1,8,9]. Dermatitis caused by *Pyemotes* spp. is very rarely reported and has been associated with home interior infestations of *P. ventricosus* associated with *A. punctatum* [11].

Clinical features [12,13]

The lesions are red pruritic macules or urticated papules surmounted by vesicles; occasionally they may be bullous. These lesions are sometimes associated with a specific linear red macular tract, called the 'comet sign' [11,14,15] (Figure 34.40). This sign might represent the onset of specific lymphangitis but usually it is not. Whether this sign is specific to *Pyemotes* spp. or *P. ventricosus* remains unknown [11]. The lesions are often very numerous; their distribution is on covered places of the body and depends upon the mode of exposure. In grain handlers, they are usually on the forearms and neck, but they may be profuse around the waist and in the groin area. If the source of the mites is removed, the eruption is self-limiting and should resolve in 1–3 weeks. Systemic signs are rare but may include fever, chills, malaise and diarrhoea [4].

Management

Treatment is symptomatic with topical corticosteroids and antihistamines and resolution depends on the elimination of the source of the infesting mites [2]. To eliminate *Pyemotes* mites, infested areas may be treated with acaricides and/or the removal of infested furniture.

Family Tydeidae

Dermatitis in eight woodworkers in Perugia, Italy, was attributed to contact with *Pronematus davisi* mites on wood imported from North America [1]. This mite has a worldwide distribution and is widespread in North America where it usually lives under bark.

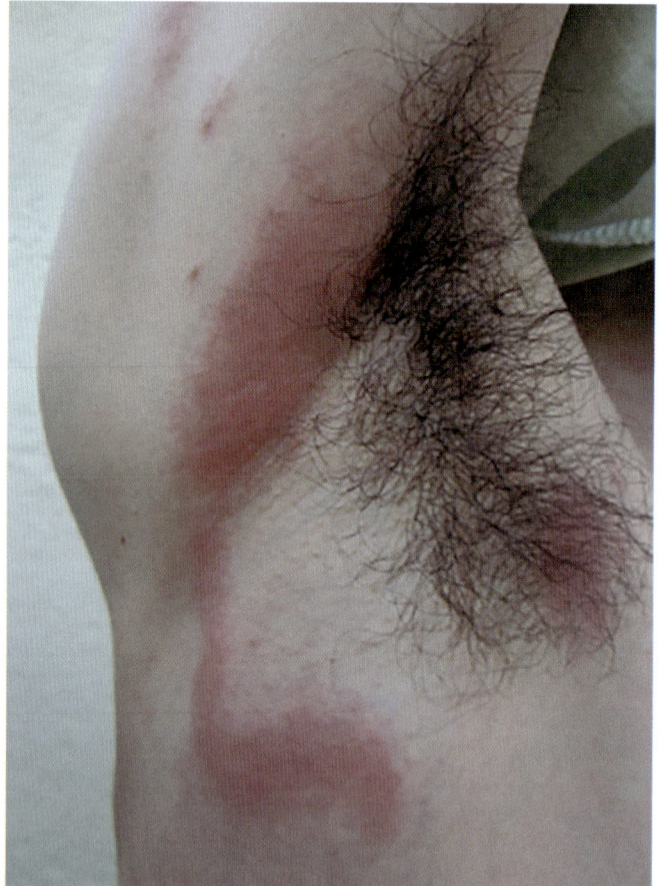

Figure 34.40 The 'comet sign'.

Plant mites

Some mites of the family Tetranychidae ('spider mites') cause cutaneous irritation or urtication in humans [1–4]. These mites are phytophagous and occur on every type of crop and ornamental plant [5]. The name 'spider mites' is derived from the silk webbing they produce from palpal glands.

Cheyletiella mites

Introduction and general description
Species of *Cheyletiella* mites are non-burrowing, obligatory parasites of certain mammals, predominantly dogs, cats and rabbits. The entire life cycle is completed on the host. Each egg is attached to a hair shaft by means of a fine thread, which is woven around it into a cocoon-like structure by the female mite. The adult mite develops via a larval and two nymphal stages. Adult mites move rapidly over the skin surface in pseudotunnels in keratinous debris. They use their hook-like palpi to attach themselves to the host while feeding on tissue fluids [1,2].

Epidemiology
Cheyletiella mites were first reported as attacking humans by Lomholt [3] of Copenhagen and in 1938 a case was reported from England [4]. It gradually became apparent that *Cheyletiella* infestation of dogs, cats and rabbits was common in most European countries, in the USA [5], in Canada [6] and in Australasia [7,8]. The distribution of these mites is worldwide. Many earlier reports incorrectly identified the species as *C. parasitivorax* when it was probably *C. yasguri*. It is now clear that *C. parasitivorax* is predominantly a parasite of rabbits, *C. yasguri* of dogs and *C. blakei* of cats [9,10]. The three species are morphologically very similar, but distinguishable by the shape of a special sensory organ on the dorsal surface of genu I [10–12].

It is not clear from the limited information available whether the incidence of these mites is increasing or whether infestation is becoming more frequently recognised. An investigation in the Netherlands [13] of 41 households in which two or more cats were kept showed *Cheyletiella* infestation of the animals in 27, with 20% of the human contacts having skin lesions. Any age, breed or sex of animal may be affected. In dogs, cheyletiellosis is particularly common in boxers.

Most affected animals are asymptomatic, but some may suffer from pruritus. The most obvious sign of infestation is excessive dandruff, especially on the back, which is often known as 'walking dandruff' [14] or 'mobile dandruff' by veterinary dermatologists (Figure 34.2).

Clinical features in humans [15–17]
The typical clinical picture is of large numbers of intensely itchy papules (Figure 34.41). Surmounting the papules there may be tiny vesicles and older lesions may show small areas of necrosis. Bullous lesions may occur [18,19]. The distribution of lesions corresponds to areas of contact with an infested animal, the abdomen and thighs being frequently involved as a result of an animal sitting on its owner's lap. The chest and arms may also be affected from carrying the animal. Dobrosavljevic *et al.* [20] reported a woman whose skin lesions were accompanied by eosinophilia, 'increased immune complexes' and rheumatological symptoms.

In a case with an extensive eruption, intradermal skin testing with an extract of *Cheyletiella* mites produced both immediate and delayed hypersensitivity responses [21].

Investigations [22]
The diagnosis may be confirmed by examination of combings from the animal's coat for the presence of mites. The suspect animal

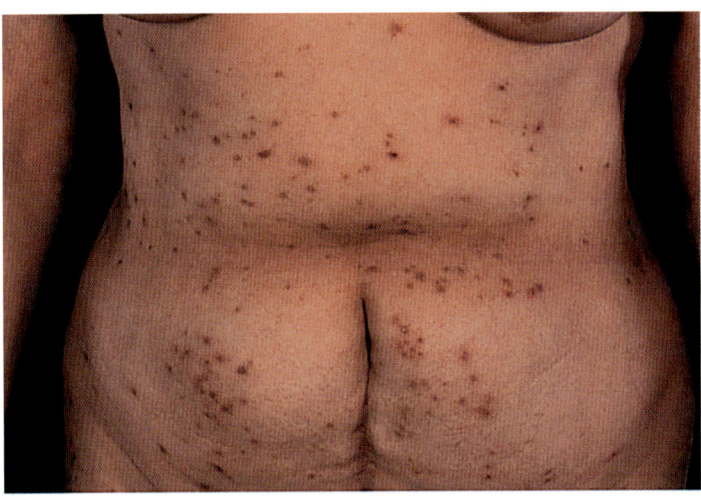

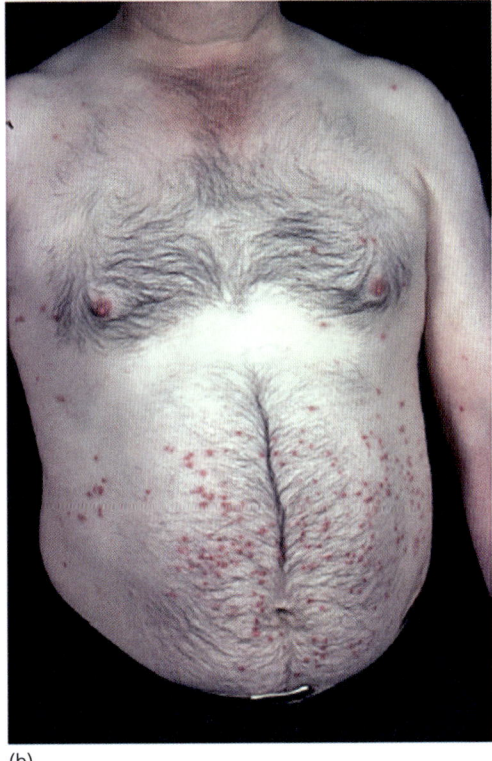

Figure 34.41 (a,b) Abdominal lesions in cheyletiellosis.

should be placed on a sheet of black paper and the coat, particularly along the back, vigorously combed, preferably with a fine-toothed comb. The debris collected can then be examined microscopically (Figure 34.42).

Management
The affected animal should be treated by a veterinary practitioner, using antiectoparasitic shampoos and dips. With reports of mites occasionally being found off the host animal, a thorough cleaning of the pet's sleeping area would be wise to prevent possible reinfection. Human skin lesions may be treated with a topical antipruritic. Once an animal has been treated effectively, there will be no further lesions on its owner within 3 weeks [23].

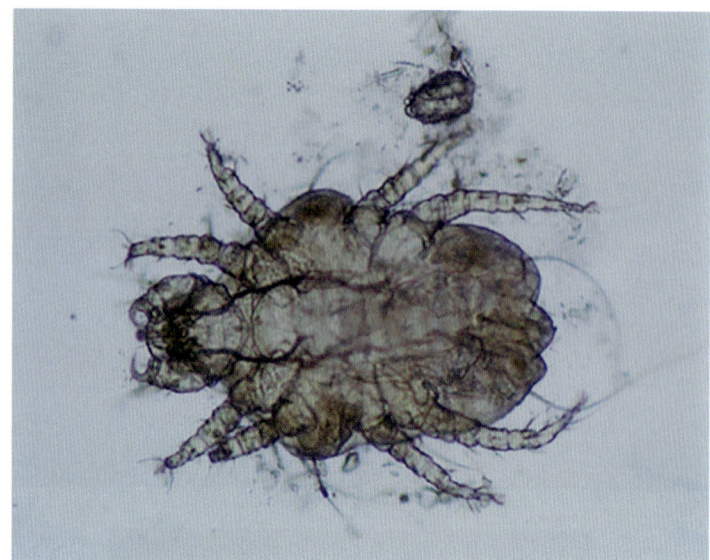

Figure 34.42 *Cheyletiella yasguri.*

Harvest mites (Trombiculidae)

Synonyms and inclusions
- Chiggers
- Harvest bugs
- Harvest lice
- Jiggers
- Red bugs

Introduction and general description
Harvest mites belong to the family Trombiculidae. More than 1200 species of trombiculids have been described and many may attack human beings or livestock [1].

Harvest mites are parasitic as larvae, but free living as nymphs and adults. The larvae may cause troublesome dermatitis (trombidiosis; scrub itch), and some are important vectors of rickettsial disease. They have many common names throughout the world, for example orange tawny (Ireland), chigger or red bug (USA).

The eggs are laid in soil. The six-legged larvae which emerge climb onto low vegetation to wait for suitable vertebrate hosts. On the host, the larvae move to areas where the skin is thin, such as the ears, axillae, groins and genitalia. There they pierce the skin with their cheliceral claws and inject saliva, which has cytolytic properties, into the epidermis [2]. This action forms a tube-like canal (stylosome) through which the mites feed on tissue fluids and cell debris. Once engorged, they fall to the ground and develop into eight-legged adults via a nymphal stage. Nymphs and adults feed on vegetable debris and the eggs of insects and other arthropods.

Epidemiology
Neotrombicula autumnalis, the European harvest mite, is widely distributed throughout Europe. In the UK [3], the larval mites are most numerous from May to October, with a peak in September. The most favoured natural host is the rabbit. *N. autumnalis* is not known to transmit disease.

Eutrombicula alfreddugesi and *E. splendens* are the most common chiggers attacking humans in the USA, and *E. batatas* is an important dermatitis-producing species in South America.

In South-East Asia, Australia and the Pacific Islands, trombidiosis is commonly caused by *E. wichmanni*, and species of *Odontacarus* and *Schoengastia* [4,5].

Species of *Leptotrombidium* including *L. akamushi*, *L. pallidum* and *L. deliense* are important vectors of scrub typhus (tsutsugamushi disease) caused by *Orientia tsutsugamushi* [6]. *L. akamushi* has a wide distribution, ranging from Japan and China southwards through South-East Asia to Indonesia and eastwards throughout the Philippines to New Guinea. *Leptotrombidium deliense* occurs in China, the Indian subcontinent, Malaysia, Indonesia, the Philippines, New Guinea and Australia. The natural hosts of *L. akamushi* and *L. deliense* are rodents and insectivores. *Leptotrombidium subquadratum* has been reported as a cause of pruritus and dermatitis in dogs and humans in South Africa [7].

Clinical features [4,8,9]
Humans are infested while working in or walking through grass or low vegetation. The response to the bites of harvest mites appears to be determined by the irritant effect of the mites' saliva and an acquired hypersensitivity to salivary antigens. Within a few hours, red macules appear at the sites of the bites, and these gradually develop into extremely itchy papules or papulovesicles.

The distribution of lesions is determined by the preference of mites for thin skin and the clothing of the host. Lesions commonly occur around the feet and ankles, the groins and genitalia, the axillae, the wrists and antecubital fossae, and areas constricted by clothing, such as the waistline. In heavy infestations, the whole body may be covered in lesions.

Chigger bites on the penis in children are responsible for a seasonal acute hypersensitivity reaction in the USA known as the 'summer penile syndrome' [10].

Trombiculid mite bites have provided evidence to implicate a suspect in a murder investigation [11].

Management [12,13]
Treatment of trombiculid mite bites is aimed at relief of the symptoms. Topical anaesthetics, topical antipruritics, topical or intralesional corticosteroids, oral antihistamines or counterirritants may be used.

Preventative methods include avoidance of high-risk areas and the use of insect repellent on both clothing and skin.

Bird, rodent and reptile mites (Gamasida)

Introduction and general description
Family Dermanyssidae [1,2]
Dermanyssid mites are haematophagous parasites of birds and mammals. *Dermanyssus gallinae* (chicken mite) (Figure 34.43), the red poultry mite, is a common parasite of domestic and wild birds. Poultry keepers, veterinary practitioners and others in direct contact with birds are sometimes attacked. Other dermanyssid mites responsible for dermatitis include *D. hirundinis* and *D. americanus*. Avian mites greatly increase during the hot season. They leave

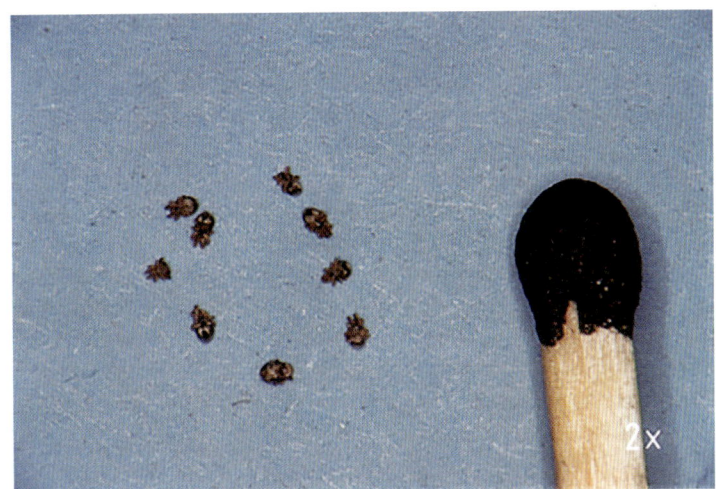

Figure 34.43 *Dermanyssus gallinae*: comparison in size with the head of a match.

feathers or nests to walk away. In this case, they may enter buildings via windows, ventilation grills or air conditioners, causing skin lesions on the occupants who observe hundreds of mites on the edges of windows or on furniture [3–8]. Lucky *et al.* [9] reported itchy papular lesions related to contact with pet gerbils infested with *D. gallinae* and *Ornythonyssus sylviarum*, and reviewed other reported cases of avian mite bites. *D. gallinae* may be a public health problem because of its potential role as a vector of disease (zoonosis): *Chlamydia psittaci*, *Erysipelotrix rhusiopathiae*, *Escherichia coli* and *Salmonella*, *Shigella* and *Staphylococcus* species have been isolated from the blood of mites, and it has been linked to cases of spirochaetosis, chicken pox, Newcastle disease, typhoid fever, fowl cholera and equine encephalitis, with transmission occurring between birds. No cases of transmission to humans have yet been reported [10,11].

Liponyssoides sanguineus, the house-mouse mite, is an ectoparasite of small rodents. It is of medical importance because it is the vector of *Rickettsia akari*, the agent causing rickettsial pox.

Family Macronyssidae [1]
Members of the Macronyssidae family are haematophagous ectoparasites of birds, mammals and reptiles.

Ornythonyssus sylviarum (the northern fowl mite) and *O. bursa* (the tropical fowl mite) are pests of domestic and wild birds, and occasionally attack humans [12–14]. *O. bacoti*, although known as the tropical rat mite, is cosmopolitan, occurring in both tropical and temperate areas of the world. There are a number of reports of its effects on humans in close proximity to infested rats, mice, hamsters and gerbils [15–21].

O. natricis, a snake mite, caused skin lesions in a family owning a pet python [22].

Clinical features [2,17,23,24]
The clinical effects vary according to the route and severity of infestation and the degree of the host's response. Most commonly, there is a profuse eruption of small intensely itchy weals or papules, sometimes grouped, and often asymmetrical. The lesions may have a central punctum and vesicles occasionally occur in the centre of the papules, especially in children. Because of the intense pruritus, excoriations are common and secondary infection may occur. Upon close inspection, the mite may be identified as a small red dot in the centre of the lesion.

There is no characteristic distribution because this is determined by the situation in which the bites are acquired. Those handling infested poultry tend to have lesions on the hands and forearms, whereas persons attacked by mites in bedding have more extensive bites. Occasionally, lesions are grouped adjacent to areas of tight clothing around the waistline. Rossiter [25] reported otitis externa associated with *D. gallinae* in two poultry catchers.

Investigations
In heavy infestations, the causative mites are often noticed by those affected. Any specimens obtained should be sent for identification to an entomologist familiar with Acari. When mite infestation is suspected, but no specimens are available, it may be necessary to visit the patient's home or workplace to determine the source of the problem.

Management
Avian mite dermatitis may be treated topically with corticosteroids. The itching may subside with oral antihistamines [3,8,9,14,24]. The use of topical acaricides is controversial because the mite does not live or reproduce on humans, but despite this some authors recommend applying 1–5% topical permethrin [26].

Follicle mites (Demodicidae)

Demodex folliculorum (Simon), the follicle mite, is an obligate parasite of the human pilosebaceous follicle. It was first discovered in cerumen by the anatomist Jakob Henle in 1841, but it was the dermatologist Gustav Simon who provided the first complete description of the parasite, under the name *Acarus folliculorum*, in 1842 [1,2]. The generic name *Demodex* was created for it in 1843 by the zoologist Richard Owen.

Introduction and general description [1,3]
D. folliculorum measures 0.3–0.4 mm in length, and has an elongated striated abdomen, giving it a worm-like appearance (Figure 34.44). A morphologically distinct species, *D. brevis* Akbulatova, has been recognised [4]. *D. folliculorum* occupies the hair follicle, and the smaller *D. brevis* the sebaceous and meibomian glands.

The lifespan of *D. folliculorum* is thought to be approximately 2 weeks. The heart-shaped eggs hatch to produce hexapod larvae and the eight-legged adults develop via two nymphal stages.

Follicle mites show a predilection for areas of high sebum production [5] and they have been shown to contain lipase [6]. They are most numerous on the forehead, cheeks, nose and nasolabial folds, but they are also found on the scalp, in the external ear, in eyelash follicles and meibomian glands, and on the upper chest and nipples. They have also been discovered on the penis, mons veneris, buttocks and in ectopic sebaceous glands in the buccal mucosa [7]. *D. folliculorum* assumes a head-down position in the

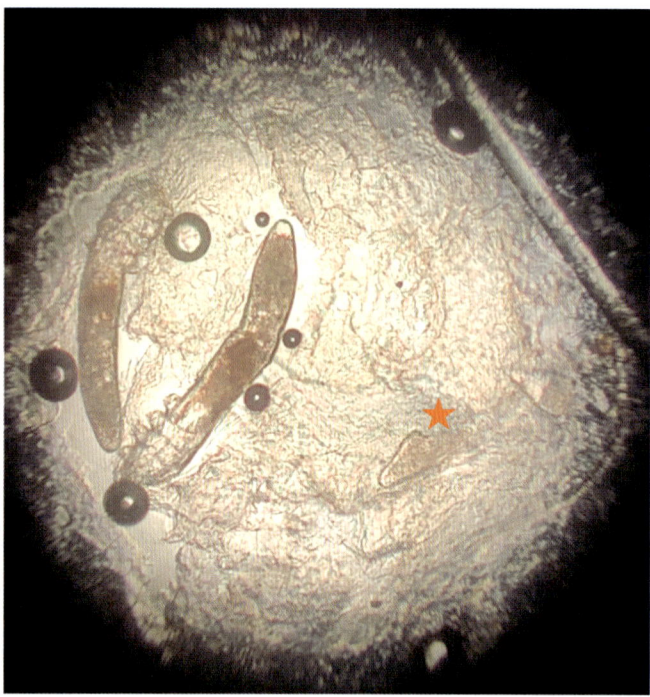

Figure 34.44 *Demodex folliculorum*, the follicle mite. Two adults and an egg (orange star) are visible.

follicle, often with the tip of the abdomen protruding from the follicular orifice. Follicle mites are quite motile and migrate from follicle to follicle. Most infested follicles contain two to six mites, but occasionally they are much more numerous. The prevalence of both *D. folliculorum* and *D. brevis* increases with age [8,9] and it is likely that with adequate sampling techniques mites could be discovered in some follicles in the entire adult population. The skin surface biopsy technique is a useful method of assessing the population density and distribution of *Demodex* mites [10,11]. New imaging techniques such as high-definition optical coherence tomography or confocal laser scanning microscopy may be helpful for the *in vivo* detection of *Demodex* mites. They enable fast and non-invasive recognition of *Demodex* mites and might become a useful tool in the diagnosis and treatment monitoring of *Demodex*-related skin diseases [12–14].

Pathophysiology

D. folliculorum has been implicated in the pathogenesis of a condition named pityriasis folliculorum [15,16]. This was originally described as occurring predominantly in middle-aged or older women who rarely washed their faces, but used large quantities of make-up and cleansing creams. The lack of washing and use of facial cosmetics were considered to be aetiological factors, but a similar appearance has subsequently been described in women who washed their faces regularly [16,17]. This dermatosis is characterised by diffuse facial redness, follicular plugs and vesiculopustules, which impart a 'nutmeg grater' appearance to the skin. These mites populate facial areas such as the forehead, eyebrows, eyelids, chin and nose. Occasionally, they may be found on the perioral mucosa, ear canal, chest and other body regions. In reported cases, skin scrapings have contained unusually large numbers of *Demodex* and the condition has responded to treatment with topical acaricides.

The question of the pathogenic role of *Demodex* in rosacea (Chapter 89) has always been debated [18–20]. Although studies employing skin surface biopsy have shown statistically significant increases in the density of *Demodex* mites in the facial skin of patients with rosacea compared with controls [10,11,21,22], it is still not clear whether rosacea merely provides a suitable environment for multiplication of the mites or whether the mites play a role in initiating the disease. Skin biopsies taken from patients with rosacea, following topical therapy with sulphur, failed to show any correlation between clinical improvement and reduction in mite population [23]. In large studies of the histopathology of rosacea [24,25], *Demodex* was conspicuously absent from areas of inflammation in sections in which it was present elsewhere. A recent report using meta-analysis of previous studies seemed to show a statistically significant association between *Demodex* species infestation and the development of rosacea [26].

It has been suggested that a local delayed hypersensitivity response to *Demodex* antigens might be partly responsible for the inflammatory component of rosacea [24] and the observation that most T cells in the granulomatous infiltrate surrounding extrafollicular *Demodex* are helper inducer T cells [27] lends support to the hypothesis that the pathogenesis of rosacea involves a cell-mediated immune response. A report has also noted that bacterial antigens associated with *Bacillus oleronius*, isolated from *D. folliculorum*, have the potential to stimulate an inflammatory response in patients with papulopustular rosacea [28].

Although extrafollicular *Demodex* or fragments of *Demodex* may be found in the granulomatous lesions of rosacea [29], its role in their induction has not been established. The mite may simply be displaced because the hair follicles have been destroyed by the inflammatory process.

A view that the beneficial effects of metronidazole in rosacea might be mediated through an action against *Demodex* [30] was not supported by the finding that mites can survive high concentrations of this drug *in vitro* [31].

Clinical features

Rosacea-like eruptions in which large numbers of mites could be demonstrated and which responded to therapy with acaricides [15,32–35] or metronidazole [36] have been described. The effectiveness of acaricidal treatment can be evaluated by skin surface biopsy [37].

Demodex has been implicated in the causation of papular and papulopustular lesions in immunosuppressed individuals, including children with leukaemia [38–41], a patient with tumour stage mycosis fungoides [42] and patients with HIV infection [43–46].

Facial lesions attributed to *Demodex* have been described in immunocompetent children, in the form of a localised scaly patch [47], rosacea-like and pityriasis folliculorum-like lesions [48] and scalp lesions mimicking favus in another child [49].

A study of *D. folliculorum* density in perioral dermatitis suggested that increased mite density was a secondary phenomenon related to topical steroids and also showed that mite density increased significantly in relation to the length of treatment [50].

Demodex is present in eyelash follicles and has been implicated in the pathogenesis of blepharitis in some patients, although its importance as a cause is disputed [51]. Oral ivermectin may be useful as a complement in the treatment of *D. folliculorum* infestation with ocular manifestation [52,53]. The value of topical ivermectin should be confirmed in a large real-life population.

CLASS CHILOPODA (CENTIPEDES) AND DIPLOPODA (MILLIPEDES)

Species within the classes Chilopoda and Diplopoda are classified in the mandibulate subphylum of the phylum Arthropoda.

Centipedes

Introduction and general description
Chilopoda is a class with approximately 2500 known species of chilopods. The common chilopod is the centipede, which is terrestrial, nocturnally active and carnivorous against other arthropods or worms. Some of the giant species also feed on small mice and birds. Centipedes are elongated arthropods, with bodies composed of many segments, each bearing one pair of legs. The first pair of legs is modified and provided with powerful hollow claws, which are used to grip prey and inject venom from poison glands in the basal segments of the legs (Figure 34.45).

Clinical features
The claws of smaller species of centipedes are unable to penetrate human skin, but some tropical and subtropical species, principally members of the orders Scutigeromorpha and the giant Scolopendromorpha, can inflict painful 'bites' [1–5]. The bites cause local pain, redness and oedema, which may persist for several hours. The bites may sometimes lead to necrosis or a delayed hypersensitive reaction [6]. Systemic symptoms include nausea, dizziness and pyrexia. There are rare reports of acute myocardial infarction following a centipede bite [7,8] and even human deaths [8–10]. Secondary infection is a major complicating factor of the envenomation.

Management
The site should be washed with soap and water to reduce the risk of wound contamination. Cold compresses and analgesia will help with pain control [11].

Millipedes

Introduction and general description
Diplopoda is a class with approximately 10 000 known species of diplopods. The common diplopod is the millipede, which is terrestrial on the forest floor. Millipedes also have multisegmented bodies and most segments bear two pairs of legs. They feed mainly on decaying vegetable matter and are generally regarded as harmless, but some large tropical species can cause injury to humans when acting defensively. The injurious effects of the defensive secretions of the giant Spirobolida millipedes of tropical and subtropical zones are well known to the indigenous populations of these areas.

Millipedes have numerous 'repugnatorial' glands distributed along the body segments, which provide a chemical defence system, and it is the corrosive secretions of these glands which may cause burns or allergy on the skin. In the majority of species, these secretions ooze out and form droplets around the foramina of the glands, but a few species are capable of squirting the fluid for some distance [12]. Millipede secretions contain benzoquinones and hydroquinones.

Clinical features [1,12–15]
Children often try to pick up millipedes and are therefore at most risk of burns from the corrosive defensive secretions. If millipede secretions enter the eye, they produce a severe irritant conjunctivitis. Contact with the skin produces a local burning sensation and a yellowish brown stain, which gradually darkens to deep mahogany or purple-brown [16]. This colour is produced by oxidation of the quinones in the secretions. The lesions blister within a day or two, but in the absence of secondary infection will heal and desquamate in 10–14 days. The discoloration may persist for months [17]. In dark-skinned individuals, persistent hypopigmentation is a common sequel.

Management [12]
Skin lesions should be washed with copious amounts of water to remove any remaining secretions and the area cleaned with alcohol (a solvent of benzoquinones) if available. Blisters should be treated with a topical antiseptic. Ocular injuries should be dealt with by an ophthalmologist, because severe envenomation can result in blindness [18].

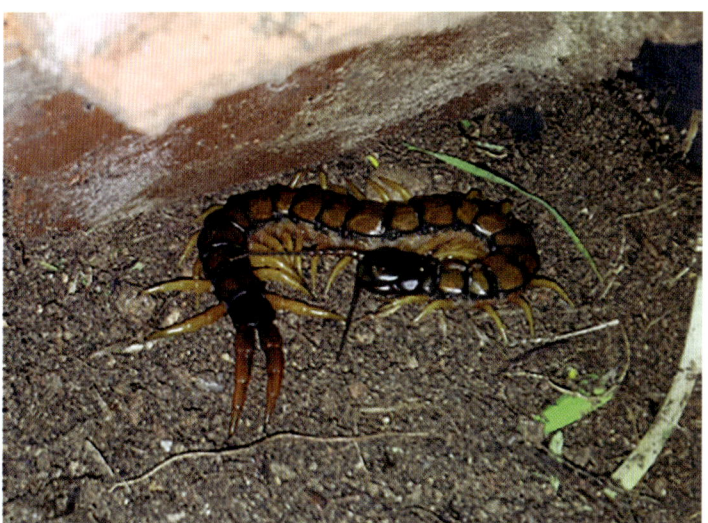

Figure 34.45 *Scolopendra cingulata* Latreille 1829, the most common scolopendromorph species in the Mediterranean area. Courtesy of Dr Botterman and Dr Melhem, Nice, France.

Key references

The full list of references can be found in the online version at https://www.wiley.com/rooksdermatology10e

Skin disease due to arthropods

15 Keystone JS. Of bites and body odour. *Lancet* 1996;347:1423.
27 Bernardeschi C, Le Cleach L, Delaunay P et al. Bed bug infestation. *BMJ* 2013;346:f138.
40 Elston DM. Prevention of arthropod-related disease. *J Am Acad Dermatol* 2004;51:947–54.
41 Debboun M, Frances SP, Strickman DA. *Insect Repellents: Principles, Methods and Uses*. Boca Raton: CRC Press, 2006.

Class Insecta
Mosquitoes, gnats, midges and flies (Diptera)

25 Barzilai A, Shpiro D, Goldberg I et al. Insect bite-like reaction in patients with hematologic malignant neoplasms. *Arch Dermatol* 1999;135:1503–7.

Myiasis

5 Francesconi F, Lupi O. Myiasis. *Clin Microbiol Rev* 2012;25:79–105.
14 Lachish T, Marhoom E, Mumcuoglu KY et al. Myiasis in travelers. *J Travel Med* 2015;22:232–6.

Fleas (Siphonaptera)

6 Bitam I, Dittmar K, Parola P et al. Fleas and flea-borne diseases. *Int J Infect Dis* 2010;14:e667–76.
60 Heukelbach J. Revision on tungiasis: treatment options and prevention. *Exp Rev Anti Infect Ther* 2006;4:151–7.
62 Coates SJ, Thomas C, Chosidow O et al. Ectoparasites: pediculosis and tungiasis. *J Am Acad Dermatol* 2020;82:551–69.

Bees, wasps and ants (Hymenoptera)

31 Reisman RE. Insect stings. *N Engl J Med* 1994;331:523–7.

Lice (Phthiraptera)

6 Chosidow O. Scabies and pediculosis. *Lancet* 2000;355:819–26.
50 Roberts RJ. Clinical practice. Head lice. *N Engl J Med* 2002;346:1645–50.
104 Coates SJ, Thomas C, Chosidow O et al. Ectoparasites: pediculosis and tungiasis. *J Am Acad Dermatol* 2020;82:551–69.
118 Salavastru CM, Chosidow O, Janier M et al. European guideline for the management of pediculosis pubis. *J Eur Acad Dermatol Venereol* 2017;31:1425–8.

Bugs (Hemiptera)

19 Bernardeschi C, Le Cleach L, Delaunay P et al. Bed bug infestation. *BMJ* 2013;346:f138.
34 Akhoundi M, Sereno D, Marteau A et al. Who bites me? A tentative discriminative key to diagnose hematophagous ectoparasites biting using clinical manifestations. *Diagnostics (Basel)* 2020;10:308.

Butterflies and moths (Lepidoptera)

4 Gullan PJ, Cranston P. *The Insects: An Outline of Entomology*, 3rd edn. London: Wiley-Blackwell, 2004.

Class Arachnida
Spiders (Araneae)

2 Isbister GK, Fan HW. Spider bite. *Lancet* 2011;378:2039–47.

Ticks (Acari)

5 Elston DM. Tick bites and skin rashes. *Curr Opin Infect Dis* 2010;23:132–8.

Mites
Family Sarcoptidae: human classical scabies

9 Thomas C, Coates SJ, Engelman D et al. Ectoparasites: scabies. *J Am Acad Dermatol* 2020;82:533–48.
15 Chosidow O. Clinical practices Scabies. *N Engl J Med* 2006;354:1718–27.
19 Chosidow O. Scabies and pediculosis. *Lancet* 2000;355:819–26.
25 Cassell JA, Middleton J, Nalabanda A et al. Scabies outbreaks in ten care homes for elderly people: a prospective study of clinical features, epidemiology, and treatment outcomes. *Lancet Infect Dis* 2018;18:894–902.

Pyemotes mites

11 Del Giudice P, Blanc-Amrane V, Bahadoran P et al. *Pyemotes ventricosus* dermatitis, southeastern France. *Emerging Infect Dis* 2008;14:1759–61.

Index

Note: Page numbers in *italics* refer to figures and those in **bold** refer to tables and boxes, where they fall outside the main text range. References are to pages within chapters, thus 58.10 is page 10 of Chapter 58.

22q11 deletion syndrome *see* velocardiofacial syndrome
25-hydroxy vitamin D₃   88.19

A

AA *see* Amyloid A
AAE *see* acquired angio-oedema
AAS *see* angioedema activity score
abacavir, hypersensitivity reactions to   **14.6**, 14.7
ABA criteria *see* American Burn Association criteria
abatacept, psoriatic arthritis treatment   35.46
ABC *see* atopic blepharoconjunctivitis; avidin–biotin–peroxidase complex method
ABCA12 gene
 harlequin ichthyosis   63.8
 ichthyosis   63.7
ABCD algorithm, melanoma diagnosis   142.9
ABCD mnemonic, melanoma diagnosis limitations   145.1
A-B-C model of habit disorders   84.12
ABD *see* Adamantiades–Behçet disease
abdomen
 atrophoderma of Pasini–Pierini   *55.19*
 connective tissue naevus   *73.18*
 Crohn disease, metastatic   *95.15, 95.16*
 heparin necrosis   *99.10*
 IgM pemphigoid   *50.54*
abdominal fistula   **112.3**
abdominal wall lymphoedema   103.51–103.52
ABHDS gene, neutral lipid storage disease with ichthyosis   63.36
ablative fractional resurfacing   161.1–161.3
 for acne scarring   *161.4*
 avoidance of bulk heating   161.4
 device names   **161.5**
 laser types   **161.5**
 for photodamaged skin   *161.3*
 for rhytids   161.5
 wound care   161.4
ablative lasers, hidradenitis suppurativa treatment   90.11
ABPI *see* ankle brachial Doppler pressure index
ABQOL *see* Autoimmune Bullous Disease Quality of Life
abrasions, sports injuries   122.16
ABS *see* acrylonitrile butadiene styrene
abscesses   3.43
 acne conglobata   *88.66*

dental abscess   108.9
dermal fillers, adverse reactions   *158.9*
see also furuncles
abscopal effects, radiotherapy on melanoma metastases   24.14
absorption, distribution, metabolism and elimination (ADME)   13.1–13.4
absorption of a drug
 clinical pharmacology   13.2
 topical medication   18.3, 18.5
AC *see* acne conglobata
acantholysis   3.38–3.39, 50.3
acanthomas
 benign proliferations of keratinocytes   132.1–132.8
 clear cell acanthoma   132.6–132.7
acanthome cellules claires of Degos and Civatte *see* clear cell acanthoma
acanthosis   3.39
 chronic actinic dermatitis   *126.14, 126.15*
 sensitisation   127.8
acanthosis nigricans (AN)   85.3–85.6, *140.14, 140.15*
 dermatoendocrinology   **150.10**, *150.11, 150.13*
 diabetic patients   62.3
 female genitalia   110.22
 oral lesions   108.67
acanthosis palmaris   148.15–148.16
acanthotic and ichthyotic epidermal disorders   148.14–148.17
acanthotic lesions, elastosis perforans serpiginosa   *94.55, 94.56*
Acari   34.37–34.57
ACC *see* American College of Chemosurgery
accelerated rheumatoid nodulosis (ARN)   97.16
accessory tragus   *106.8*
access to health care, initiatives for   7.8–7.11
ACD *see* allergic contact dermatitis
ACD by-proxy dermatitis ('conubial' dermatitis)   109.12
ACE *see* angiotensin-converting enzyme
acetylacetone test, formaldehyde   127.34
acetylcholine   2.9
 botulinum toxins, aesthetic use of   *159.2*
 pruritus   **81.3**, 81.4
acetylsalicylic acid, urticaria   117.5
ACH *see* acrodermatitis continua of Hallopeau
Achenbach syndrome (paroxysmal finger haematoma)   *94.19*, 99.5–99.6, 122.13–122.14
aciclovir
 pharmacological properties   19.49

 topical therapies   18.13
acid phosphatase   2.42
acids, burns   128.11
Acinetobacter   26.51
acitretin
 ichthyoses management   63.44–63.45
 psoriasis treatment   35.25–35.26
ACL *see* acquired cutaneous lymphangiectasia
aclovir-resistant herpes simplex virus   149.20, *149.21*
ACMS *see* American College of Mohs Surgery
acne   88.1–88.74
 acneform naevi   88.31
 agminata   88.34
 antiandrogens in management of   *88.50*
 assessment tools   16.4
 causative organisms   88.15–88.18
 chemical peel side effect   160.12
 comedonal   *4.19*, 88.1–88.2, *88.3, 88.14, 88.26, 88.27, 88.28*, 88.45–88.47, *88.45, 88.65*
  familial comedones   88.32
  prepubertal comedones   *88.69*
  senile comedones   88.31–88.32
 comprehensive acne severity system   88.38, **88.39**
 cosmetics use   88.25
 Cutibacterium   26.43
 depression   88.39
 detergent   88.25
 and diet   **88.20–88.24**, 88.26
 drug-induced   88.11–88.14
  drug classes   **88.12**
 ear dermatoses   **106.22**
 ectopic   88.31
 endocrinopathy   **88.42**
 environmental and lifestyle factors   88.18–88.26
 granulomatous   88.30
 heritable traits   **88.18**
 hormonal investigations   **88.42**
 infantile   88.68–88.74, 115.4–115.5
 inflammation   88.14–88.15, *88.17*
 inflammatory   *88.3, 88.27*
 isotretinoin treatment   5.3
 joint symptoms and arthritis association   155.10–155.11
 keloid-like   *88.30, 94.50*
 mechanical   88.30
 neonatal   88.68–88.74
 nodular   *88.29*
 and nutrition   **88.20–88.24**, 88.26
 occupational   88.66–88.68, **88.66**

 chloracne-inducing chemicals   **88.66**
 contaminated oil ingestion   88.68
 differential diagnosis   88.67, **88.68**
 dioxin accidents   **88.68**
papulopustular   *88.3*
penile   109.24
photodynamic therapy   22.7
pomade acne   88.25, *88.26*
predisposing medical conditions   **88.6**
prepubertal   88.68–88.74
 associated diseases   88.70
 clinical features   88.70–88.71
 complications and co-morbidities   88.72
 differential diagnosis   88.71
 disease course and prognosis   88.72
 epidemiology   88.69–88.70
 investigations   **88.72**
 isotretinoin treatment   **88.73**
 management   88.72–88.74
 pathophysiology   88.70
 psychological factors   15.3–15.4
 psychosocial effects   88.39
 pyogenic granulomas   88.41
 pyogenic sterile arthritis, pyoderma gangrenosum and acne syndrome   **45.6**, 45.13
 quality of life measurement   16.8, 88.38–88.39
 scarring
  ablative fractional resurfacing   *161.4*
  chemical peels   160.5, *160.6*
 severity measures   5.4
 suicide risk   88.39
 synovitis, acne, pustulosis, hyperostosis and osteitis syndrome   45.22, 88.7
 treatment options   **88.44**
 vulval   110.45
 see also chloracne
acne of chemical origin   129.7, 129.12–129.13
acne conglobata (AC)   87.50, *88.29*, 88.62–88.66
 abscesses and cysts   *88.66*
 associated diseases   88.63
 differential diagnosis   88.64
 features of   **88.65**
 genetics   88.64
 management   88.65–88.66, **88.67**
 predisposing factors   88.63
 sacroiliitis   155.10–155.11
 treatment options   **88.67**
Acne Core Outcomes Research Network (ACORN)   16.3
acné excoriée   84.20–84.22, 88.28–88.29, *88.30*

acne fulminans 88.59–88.62
  associated diseases 88.59
  causative organisms 88.60
  differential diagnosis 88.61
  features of **88.61**
  genetics 88.60
  investigations 88.61–88.62
  management 88.62, **88.63**
  musculoskeletal features 155.11
  presentation 88.60
  systemic treatments **88.63**
acneiform eruptions *91.3*
Acne Inversa Severity Index (AISI) 16.4–16.5
acne keloidalis 93.3–93.4
acne keloidalis nuchae (AKN) 87.50–87.51, 122.16–122.17
Acne Lesion Score Scale system (Echelle de Cotation des Lésions d'Acné/ECLA) 16.4
acne mechanica 122.15, 122.16
acne necrotica varioliformis 93.4–93.5
Acne-QoL *see* Acne-specific Quality of Life Questionnaire
Acne Quality of Life Scale (AQOL) 16.8
Acne-specific Quality of Life Questionnaire (Acne-QoL) 16.8
Acne Symptom and Impact Scale (ASIS) 16.8
acne tarda 88.4
acne treatment, use during pregnancy **113.20**
acne vulgaris 88.1–88.59
  acne agminata 88.34
  acneform naevi 88.31
  acromegaly association 88.7
  in adolescence 88.5
  age and sex 88.1–88.2, *88.4*
  alcohol use 88.25
  androgen receptor blockers 88.51
  anorexia nervosa association 88.30
  antiandrogen treatment *88.50*
  antibiotic therapy 88.46, 88.47, 88.48–88.49, 88.52
    adverse effects **88.49**
    gram-negative folliculitis *88.36*
    interactions with oral contraceptives 88.49
    prescribing policies **88.50**
    resistance to antibiotics **88.50**
  Apert syndrome association 88.10–88.11
  associated diseases 88.4–88.11
  azelaic acid treatment 88.47
  benzoyl peroxide treatment 88.46, 88.47
  and birth weight 88.26
  blue light therapy 88.58
  body dysmorphic disorder 88.30
  body mass index association 88.19
  causative organisms 88.15–88.18
  chemical peels 88.58–88.59, 160.5, *160.6*
  chloracne *88.14*
  clinical features 88.26–88.28
  clinical variants 88.28–88.30
  comedo extractor *88.58*
  complementary therapies 88.57–88.58
  congenital adrenal hyperplasia association 88.5–88.7, **88.10**
  corticosteroid treatment 88.57
  cosmetics use 88.25
  Cushing disease association 88.7
  dapsone treatment 88.46–88.47
  detergent acne 88.25
  devices and physical treatment 88.58
  diagnosis **88.42**
  and diet **88.20–88.24**, 88.26
  differential diagnosis 88.30–88.39
  disability-adjusted life years *88.5*
  disease course and prognosis 88.41
  drug-induced 88.11–88.14
    diagnosis **88.16**
    drug classes **88.12**
  eating disorders 88.30
  endocrinopathy **88.42**
  environmental and lifestyle factors 88.18–88.26
  epidemiology 88.1–88.14
  ethnicity 88.2–88.3
  female patients
    acne tarda 88.4
    hirsutism and hyperandrogenism 88.45
    polycystic ovary syndrome 88.4–88.5, **88.7**, 88.8, *88.9*
    premenstrual flare of acne **88.25**
  genetics 88.18
  granulomatous acne 88.30
  HAIR-AN syndrome association 88.7–88.8, *88.11*
  hirsutism 88.45
  hormonal investigations **88.42**
  hormonal therapy 88.49–88.52
  25-hydroxy vitamin D_3 88.19
  hyfrecation of macrocomedones *88.57*
  hyperandrogenism 88.45
  hypercortisolism association 88.7
  inflammation 88.14–88.15, *88.27, 88.28*
    inflammatory cascades *88.17*
  inflammatory papules *88.12*
  investigations 88.41–88.42
  isotretinoin treatment 88.51, 88.52–88.57
    adverse effects 88.54–88.57
    prescribing guidelines **88.53**
    relative success of **88.53**
  keloidalis *88.30*
  light therapy 88.58
  management 88.42–88.59
    aims of **88.43**
    comedonal acne 88.45–88.47
    complementary therapies 88.57–88.58
    devices and physical treatment 88.58
    first line therapy 88.44–88.45
    fixed combination therapy 88.46, 88.47
    general principles 88.42–88.43
    papulopustular acne 88.46, 88.47–88.52
    poor response to treatment **88.50**
    side effects of topical treatments 88.48
    systemic therapy 88.48
    treatment options **88.44**
  mechanical acne 88.30
  and menstrual cycle 88.25
  metformin treatment 88.57
  neurophysiology 88.15–88.18
  nicotinamide treatment 88.57
  nodular *88.29*
  and nutrition **88.20–88.24**, 88.26
  obesity association **88.23–88.24**
  occupational hazards 129.12
  oestrogen treatment 88.50–88.51
  PAPA (pyogenic sterile arthritis, pyoderma gangrenosum and acne) association 88.8–88.10
  papulopustular acne, treatment *88.46*, 88.47–88.52
  pathogenesis *88.17*
  pathophysiology 88.14–88.15
  photodynamic therapy 88.58
  pigment changes *88.3*
  polycystic ovary syndrome association 88.4–88.5, **88.7**, 88.8, *88.9*
  pomade acne 88.25, *88.26*
  postinflammatory macules *88.3*
  predisposing heritable traits **88.18**
  predisposing medical conditions **88.6**
  in pregnancy 88.26, 113.11–113.12
  premenstrual flares **88.25**
  presentation 88.26–88.28
  progestin treatment 88.50–88.51
  Propionibacterium acnes effect on human sebocytes *88.17*
  psychological problems 88.28–88.29
  psychosocial effects 88.39
  pustules *88.12*
  pyogenic granulomas 88.41
  quality of life measurement 88.38–88.39, **88.40**
  retinoid treatment 88.45–88.46, 88.47
  salicylic acid treatment 88.57
  SAPHO synovitis syndrome association 88.7
  scarring *88.3, 88.4, 88.29, 88.39–88.41*
  duration correlation *88.4*
  immune responses *88.40*
  mimics 88.38
  sebaceous glands, neuropeptide–cytokines/chemokine signalling *88.17*
  Sebutape analysis *88.28, 88.43*
  severe acne *88.3*, **88.42**
    management 88.52–88.57
    treatment algorithm *88.52*
  severity classification/definition 88.38–88.39, **88.43**
  in skin of colour 88.43–88.44, *88.45*
  sleep deprivation impact 88.25
  and smoking 88.19
  spironolactone treatment 88.51
  and stress 88.25
  sulphur treatment 88.57
  systemic therapy 88.52
  treatment options **88.44**
  UV radiation impact 88.25–88.26
  visible light treatment 88.58
  vitamin C treatment 88.57
  zinc treatment 88.51–88.52, 88.57
ACORN *see* Acne Core Outcomes Research Network
acquired angio-oedema (AAE) 43.1, 43.3, **43.6**
acquired autoinflammatory disorders 155.10
acquired cutaneous lymphangiectasia (ACL) 103.6
acquired cutis laxa 94.21–94.23
acquired digital fibrokeratoma 136.4
acquired disorders
  dermal connective tissue 94.1–94.58
  elastic tissue deposition 94.32–94.33
  epidermal keratinisation 85.1–85.31
  of hair 87.1–87.102
  pilosebaceous unit 93.1–93.13
acquired disorders with skin and renal involvement 154.6
acquired elastotic haemangioma 136.29
acquired epidermodysplasia verruciformis (AEV) 25.66, 25.71–25.72, *25.73*, **25.73**
acquired generalised lipodystrophy (AGL) 98.1–98.4
acquired hypermelanosis 86.9–86.33
acquired hypertrichosis 87.86–87.87
acquired hypomelanosis 86.34–86.47
acquired ichthyosis 63.47–63.50, 63.73, 85.1–85.3, 148.17
acquired idiopathic generalised anhidrosis 92.12
acquired idiopathic livedo reticularis 124.9–124.10
acquired immune deficiency syndrome *see* AIDS
acquired immunodeficiency diseases 149.18–149.20, **149.21**
  cytokine and signalling protein mutations **149.20**
  human papillomavirus infection 25.65–25.73, **25.66**, 25.71–25.73
  primary 149.18–149.20, **149.21**
  skin cancer 147.2–147.5
  skin manifestations 149.20–149.22
  see also AIDS; inherited immunodeficiency
acquired keratodermas 63.71–63.79
acquired lipodystrophy 98.1–98.13
acquired melanocytic naevi 131.17–131.21
  clinical presentation **131.16**
  compound naevus *131.19, 131.21*
  dermoscopic presentation **131.16**
  junctional naevus *131.18, 131.20*
  naevomelanocytic nests *131.18, 131.20*
  naevus cell types *131.19, 131.20*
  pathology **131.16**
acquired non-infective disorders, pilosebaceous unit 91.1–91.20
acquired pachydermatoglyphia (acanthosis palmaris) 148.15–148.16
acquired partial lipodystrophy (APL) 98.4–98.6, *98.5*
renal failure 154.2
acquired perforating dermatoses 63.76–63.77, 94.53–94.57
renal failure and dialysis complications 154.3–154.4
acquired pigmentary disorders 86.1–86.56
acquired poikiloderma 94.13
acquired progressive kinking of the hair 87.81
acquired progressive lymphangioma 136.38
acquired pseudo-ainhum 94.48
acquired pseudoxanthoma elasticum 94.30–94.31
acquired resistance, glucocorticoids 19.19
acquired resistance to insecticides, head lice 34.21–34.22
acquired syndromic hypomelanosis 86.42–86.47
acral acanthosis nigricans 85.5
acral arteriovenous tumour *see* cirsoid aneurysm
acral blistering
  epidermolysis bullosa simplex *69.10, 69.11*
  self-improving dystrophic epidermolysis bullosa *69.17*
acral fibromyxoma 136.59
acral lentiginous melanoma (ALM)
  melanoma classification 142.7, 142.8
  presentation 142.10, *142.14, 142.15, 142.17*, 142.19
acral lesions, PJT syndrome 68.13
acral melanoma (volar skin of palms and soles), dermoscopy *145.9*, 145.11–145.13
acral naevi 131.23–131.24
  compound acral naevus *131.23*
  on sole of foot *131.24*
acral peeling skin syndrome (APSS) 63.29, 69.19, *69.20*
  genes/proteins linkage 69.5–69.6
acral persistent papular mucinosis 57.6–57.7
Acremonium, skin lesions 32.93
acroangiodermatitis, purpura 99.4
acrocyanosis 79.9, 124.6–124.7
acrodermatitis 69.24
  Lyme disease/*Borrelia burgdorferi* role in B-cell lymphoma 139.37–139.38
acrodermatitis chronica atrophicans 94.15–94.16
acrodermatitis continua of Hallopeau (ACH) 35.39–35.41
  clinical features 35.40
  differential diagnosis 35.40–35.41
  genetics 35.40
  management 35.41
acrodermatitis enteropathica 79.15–79.16
  oral involvement 108.20
  zinc deficiency 61.25, 61.26
acrodermatitis pustulosa *see* infantile acropustulosis
acrodynia 121.5, 121.6
acrofacial purpura and necrosis, Covid-19 association 25.111
acrogeria (Grotton syndrome) 70.28
  clinical features of **70.26**
acro-ischaemia, Covid-19 association 25.111
acrokeratoelastoidosis 63.59, 63.60, 94.31–94.32
acrokeratosis paraneoplastica 148.19
acrokeratotic poikiloderma of Weary 75.2, 75.7
acromegaly 86.16
  acne vulgaris association 88.7
  dermatoendocrinology **150.11**, *150.12, 150.15,* 150.16
  ear dermatoses 106.22
acromelia, congenital pseudo-ainhum 94.48
acro-osteolysis with keratoderma (Bureau–Barrière syndrome) 63.71
acrospiroma
  use of term/hidradenoma relationship 137.23, 137.28

see also hidradenocarcinoma; hidradenoma
acrosyringeal naevus see eccrine syringofibroadenoma
acrosyringium, keratinisation of   63.71
acrylate resins   127.69–127.70
acrylates, contact allergy   127.47
acrylic nail systems   127.61
acrylonitrile butadiene styrene (ABS)   122.21
ACTG see AIDS Clinical Trial Group
ACTH see adrenocorticotrophic hormone
actin   3.25
actinic cheilitis (solar cheilosis)
  lip lesions   108.58
  photothermal ablation   23.21
actinic comedonal plaque   94.3
actinic elastosis   94.2–94.4
actinic folliculitis   91.6–91.8, 93.6
actinic granuloma see annular elastolytic giant cell granuloma   94.27–94.29
actinic keratoses (AK)   63.74, 141.1–141.12
  with Bowen disease, immunocompromised people   147.11–147.12
  chemical peels   160.5
  photodynamic therapy   22.4–22.6
  squamous cell carcinoma relationship   141.1
actinic lentigo (solar lentigo)   131.5–131.7, 160.7
actinic lichen planus   37.7, 37.17
actinic prurigo (AP)   126.2, 126.4, 126.10–126.21
  lip lesions   108.58–108.59
  photopatch testing   126.36
  polymorphic light eruption differentiation   126.7
actinic purpura   99.5
  ageing of skin   156.5, 156.6
actinic reticuloid   126.13
Actinomyces israelii, actinomycosis   26.84–26.86
Actinomyces keratolytica, pitted keratolysis   26.42–26.43
Actinomyces pyogenes see Trueperella pyogenes
actinomycetes   26.84–26.87
  mycetoma   32.73–32.75
  nocardiosis   26.86–26.87
actinomycosis   26.84–26.86
  botryomycosis similarity   26.77
actinophytosis see botryomycosis
action spectroscopy   10.4–10.5
active psoriasis see unstable psoriasis
active sensitisation, patch testing   127.32, 127.61
active sweating   2.9
acute adverse effects, photodynamic therapy   22.12–22.14
acute alcohol sensitivity   **104.9**
acute arsenical dermatitis   121.2
acute atrophic oral candidiasis see acute erythematous candidiasis
acute candidiasis
  oral involvement   32.61, 108.20, 108.31, 108.32
  see also oral candidiasis
acute contact dermatitis   127.12
  arsenic   121.2
acute cutaneous lupus erythematosus   89.8
acute cutaneous miliary tuberculosis   27.17
acute dermatolymphangioadenitis (ADLA)   103.16, 103.34–103.35
acute dermatomyositis   52.3, 52.5
acute diffuse otitis externa   106.16–106.17, 106.18
acute disseminated histoplasmosis   32.82–32.83
acute epidermal distension   85.28–85.30
acute erythema, solar urticaria   126.22
acute erythematous candidiasis   32.61
acute febrile neutrophilic dermatosis see Sweet syndrome
acute generalised exanthematous pustulosis (AGEP)   14.4, 118.1–118.4, 118.10
acute generalised pustular psoriasis of von Zumbusch   35.33–35.34, 118.4

acute genital ulcers see Lipschutz ulcers
acute graft versus host disease (aGvHD)   38.1, 38.2, 38.3–38.7
  clinical features   38.3–38.5
  epidemiology   38.1–38.2
  management   38.5–38.7
  pathology   38.2–38.3
  severity classification   38.4, **38.5**
acute guttate psoriasis   35.12–35.13
  lesions   35.13
acute haemorrhagic oedema, infants   115.9, 115.10
acute herpetic neuralgia (AHN)   82.4
acute inflammation, sports injuries   122.16
acute intermittent porphyria (AIP)   58.5
acute limb ischaemia, treatment options   **101.5**
acute liver disease, cutaneous features   153.4–153.5
acute localised exanthematous pustulosis (ALEP)   118.4
acute necrotising eosinophilic myocarditis (ANEM)   118.9
acute necrotising (ulcerative) gingivitis and noma (ANUG)   108.54–108.55
acute oedema
  allergic contact dermatitis   127.15
  blisters   85.28–85.30
acute otitis externa   106.15
acute perihepatitis (Fitz-Hugh–Curtis syndrome)   30.5
acute phototoxicity, PUVA phototherapy adverse effects   21.13
acute physiological reactions, heat/IR radiation   124.14
acute pseudomembranous candidiasis   32.61, 108.31, 108.32
acute pulmonary histoplasmosis   32.82
acute pulmonary insufficiency   125.4
acute radiation dermatitis   119.14
acute radiodermatitis   24.18, 24.19
acute scrotum   109.23, 109.25–109.26
acute selenium exposure   121.7
acute SJS/TEN   118.17
acute spongiotic dermatitis   126.15
acute spontaneous urticaria   42.5, 42.15–42.16
acute telogen effluvium   87.51, 87.56
AD see atopic eczema (dermatitis); autosomal dominant
ADA see adenosine deaminase
adalimumab
  hidradenitis suppurativa treatment   90.10
  psoriasis treatment   35.28
  psoriatic arthritis treatment   35.45
  scalp folliculitis   91.14
ADAM17 deficiency   45.16
Adamantiades–Behçet disease (ABD)   48.1–48.11, 97.9, 97.25, 97.51–97.52
  aphthous ulcers   48.5, **48.8**
  articular involvement   48.4, **48.8–48.11**
  autoimmune mechanisms   48.3
  bacterial agents   48.2
  causative organisms   48.2
  central nervous system involvement   **48.11**
  clinical features   48.4–48.6
  cytokine mediators   48.3
  differential diagnoses   **48.7**
  disease course and prognosis   48.6–48.7
  drug treatment   **48.9–48.10**
  endothelial cells   48.3–48.4
  epidemiology   48.1–48.2
  gastrointestinal involvement   **48.11**
  genetics   48.2–48.3
  genital ulcers   48.5, 109.23
  heat shock proteins   48.3
  immunogenetic factors   48.3–48.4
  international criteria for   **48.4, 108.40**
  International Study Group for Behçet syndrome   **108.40**
  investigations   48.7
  MAGIC syndrome   155.13
  management   48.7–48.8
  mechanical stimuli   122.3

  mucocutaneous involvement   48.4, **48.8**
  ocular disease   48.4, 48.6, **48.8**
  oral ulceration   48.2, 48.5, 108.40–108.41
    treatment   **48.8**
  pathology   48.2
  positive pathergy test   4.25
  prevention   48.11
  severity classification   48.6
  sex ratio   48.1
  skin and pulmonary involvement   152.4, 152.5
  systemic lesions   48.4–48.6
  treatment ladder   **48.8–48.11**
  uveitis   48.4, 48.6
  vascular involvement   **48.11**
  viral agents   48.2
  vulval ulceration   110.20
  see also Behçet-like disease entries
adamantinoid trichoblastoma   137.12
Adams–Oliver syndrome   **79.10**
ADAMTS metalloproteinases   2.32, 2.33
adapalene   18.25
AD (atopic dermatitis) see atopic eczema (dermatitis)
ADCs see AIDS defining cancers
ADCT see Atopic Dermatitis Control Test
addiction, illicit drugs   120.1
Addison disease   86.7, 86.17, 86.18
  adrenal function   86.17
  cytotoxic drugs   86.26
  ear dermatoses   **106.22**
  skin pigmentation changes   **150.7, 150.10,** 150.11, 150.13, 150.15, 150.18
adenoid cystic carcinoma   137.39–137.40
adenoma sebaceum   88.32
adenopathy and extensive skin patch overlying a plasmacytoma (AESOP) syndrome   149.11, 149.12
adenosine deaminase (ADA) deficiency   80.8
adenosine triphosphate (ATP) synthesis   121.2
adermatoglyphia   70.36
ADHD see attention-deficit hyperactivity disorder
adherens junctions   2.19–2.20
  keratinocytes   2.19
adipocytes   2.42, 97.1–97.2, 97.4
  cytotoxic T lymphocytes interaction   97.6–97.7
  erythema nodosum   97.22
  insulin sensitivity   97.5
  necrosis of   97.7–97.8, 97.44, 97.55
adipocytic necrosis, cold panniculitis   97.36
adipocytokines, obesity link   98.27
adipogenesis   97.5
adipokines   97.5–97.6
adiponecrosis e frigore   97.35
adiponectin   97.5
adipophilin   97.7
adipose tissue
  acquired generalized lipodystrophy   98.2
  CLOVES syndrome   72.9
  congenital (familial) lipodystrophies   72.1–72.3
  familial lipoedema   72.12
  familial partial lipodystrophies   72.3, **72.4**
  fibroadipose hyperplasia   72.9
  functions   98.27
  genetic disorders   72.1–72.13
  hemihyperplasia–multiple lipomatosis syndrome   72.9, 72.11
  hereditary obesity   72.3–72.9
  hereditary panniculitis   **72.11**
  lipodystrophies   72.1–72.3
  lipomatoses, hereditary   **72.10**
  pain   98.17
  physiology   97.3–97.4
  PIK3CA-related overgrowth spectrum   72.9–72.11
  types of   72.1
  see also obesity
adipose triglyceride lipase   63.36
adiposis dolorosa (Dercum disease)   **72.10,** 98.17–98.20

  benign symmetric lipomatosis contrast   98.16
  obesity association   98.17–98.18, 98.28
adjuvant and salvage radiotherapy, skin cancer   24.9–24.10
adjuvant systemic treatment, melanoma   144.6
ADLA see acute dermatolymphangioadenitis
ADLI see autosomal dominant lamellar ichthyoses
ADME see absorption, distribution, metabolism and elimination
adnexal carcinoma NOS   137.37–137.38
adnexal polyps, neonatal   114.19
adnexal structures   2.5–2.7
adolescents
  acne vulgaris   **88.5**
  measuring impact of skin disease   16.10
  psychological and social factors   15.3
  Skindex-Teen Dermatology Life Quality Index   16.10
  skin picking disorder   84.19
  trichotillosis   84.22–84.23, 87.32, 87.33
adrenal hyperfunction
  dermatoendocrinology   150.17–150.18
  see also congenital adrenal hyperplasia; Cushing disease/syndrome; hyperaldosteronism; hypercortisolism
adrenal insufficiency see Addison disease
adrenal steroid genesis pathway   **88.9**
adrenal suppression, systemic glucocorticoid therapy   19.19
adrenergic nerve supply, eccrine sweating   92.3
adrenocortical carcinoma   87.91
adrenocorticotrophic hormone (ACTH)
  ACTH administration, hypermelanosis   86.18–86.19
  hair follicle   87.11
adult colloid milium   94.5–94.6
adult eosinophilic pustular folliculitis   91.4
adult haemangiopericytoma   136.40
  see also myopericytoma
adult myofibroma   136.39–136.40
  see also myopericytoma
adult-onset Still disease (AOSD)   45.21, 53.8, 53.9, 100.29
adult progeria see Werner syndrome
adult T-cell leukaemia–lymphoma (HTLV-1 associated)   139.34–139.36
advanced glycation end-products (AGEs)   62.1
advancement flaps, surgical reconstruction   20.23, **20.24,** 20.25
adverse effects
  critical appraisal for evidence based medicine   17.17–17.18
  drug-induced pruritus   81.10–81.11
  drug-related   13.6, 13.9–13.11
  extracorporeal photochemotherapy   21.15
  isotretinoin acne treatment   84.42, 155.11
  patient education   21.16
  patient selection and assessment   21.15–21.16
  photodynamic therapy   22.12–22.14
  phototherapy   21.11–21.17
  pseudolymphoma   134.1, 134.2–134.3
  PUVA phototherapy   21.13–21.15, 21.16
  topical calcipotriol plus steroids   18.28, 18.29
  topical corticosteroids   18.15, 18.17–18.20
  topical therapy   18.4–18.5
  UVA-1 phototherapy   21.15
  UVB phototherapy   21.11–21.13
  see also cutaneous adverse drug effects; drug reactions
adverse immune reactions to drugs see immunological reactions to drugs
AE see atopic eczema (dermatitis)
aEDS see arthrochalasia Ehlers–Danlos syndrome
AEGCG see annular elastolytic giant cell granuloma
AEI see annular epidermolytic ichthyosis; annular erythema of infancy

AEIOU acronym, clinical characteristics of Merkel cell carcinoma 146.5, **146.7**
AEP *see* atopic eruption of pregnancy
AE-QoL *see* Angioedema Quality of Life Questionnaire
aerosolised cleaning fluid, inhalation of 120.4
AESOP syndrome *see* adenopathy and extensive skin patch overlying a plasmacytoma syndrome
aesthetic therapies
  laser resurfacing 161.1–161.6
  photodynamic therapy 22.8
  skin tightening 161.6–161.8
  see also cosmeceuticals; cosmetic treatments
AEV *see* acquired epidermodysplasia verruciformis
Africa, access to dermatologists 7.4
African eye worm (*Loa loa*) *see* loiasis
African histoplasmosis (*duboisii* form) 32.82, 32.83
African skin phenotypes, photoageing 156.2–156.3, 156.7
African trypanosomiasis (sleeping sickness) 33.39–33.43
  clinical features 33.40–33.41, *33.42*
  investigations 33.42
  management 33.43
  pathophysiology 33.39, *33.40*
Africa Teledermatology Project (ATP) 7.9
AFX *see* atypical fibroxanthoma
AGA *see* androgenetic alopecia
age
  drug pharmacokinetics and pharmacodynamics 13.7–13.8
  pruritus 81.2, 81.11
age effects
  basal cell carcinoma 140.2
  Merkel cell carcinoma risk 146.1–146.2
  seborrhoeic keratosis 132.1
ageing of skin 2.45–2.46, 156.1–156.12
  air pollution 156.8
  Barrier dysfunction 156.10–156.11
  Bateman purpura 156.5, *156.6*
  cellular changes 2.45
  chronic inflammation 2.45
  clinical features 156.1–156.6
  collagen fibril fragmentation 156.8–156.9
  cosmetic implications 156.11
  cutaneous nodular elastosis with cysts and comedones 156.4
  cutis rhomboidalis nuchae 156.5
  dermal connective tissue changes 94.1–94.6
  dermatoporosis 156.11
  dermatosis papulose nigra, skin of colour *156.3*
  DNA damage/repair 2.46
  dyspigmentation *156.2, 156.5*
  extrinsic ageing 156.1–156.4
    variants 156.3, *156.4*
  genetic diseases 2.46
  genetics of 156.6
  grading and measurement 156.6–156.7
  idiopathic guttate hypomelanosis 156.5, *156.6*
  implications of 156.10–156.11
  intrinsic ageing 2.46, 156.1, *156.2*
  medical implications 156.10
  menopausal skin ageing 156.6
  molecular mechanisms 156.10
  neck 156.4–156.5
  nodular elastosis with comedones and cysts *156.5*
  pathophysiology 156.7–156.10
  photoageing 2.45, 2.46, 156.1–156.4
    and natural ageing 156.10
  reactive oxygen species 156.4, 156.6
  sensory perception 2.45
  skin of colour 156.1–156.3
  skin structure and function 2.45–2.46
  smoking 156.4
  social implications 156.11

telomere shortening 2.45–2.46
transcriptomic analysis 2.46
UV exposure 2.46, 156.7–156.8, *156.10*
white skin 156.1
see also cosmeceuticals; premature ageing syndromes
AGEP *see* acute generalised exanthematous pustulosis
AGEs *see* advanced glycation end-products
aggrecan *2.38*
aggressive angiomyxoma *see* deep ('aggressive') angiomyxoma
aggressive digital papillary adenocarcinoma 137.34–137.35
aggressive systemic mastocytosis (ASM) 46.1, *46.9*, 46.10
AGL *see* acquired generalised lipodystrophy
agminated or segmental lentiginosis 131.3
agranulocytosis
  acute generalised exanthematous pustulosis 118.3
  dapsone 19.14
  oral involvement 108.71
AGS *see* Aicardi–Goutières syndrome
aGvHD *see* acute graft versus host disease
AHN *see* acute herpetic neuralgia
AI *see* artificial intelligence
Aicardi syndrome **72.10**
Aicardi–Goutières syndrome (AGS) **45.5, 45.6**, 45.13
AIDS
  case definition 31.5–31.6
  dermatological involvement 31.1
  eye disease **107.35**
  Kaposi sarcoma-associated herpesvirus 25.42, 25.43
  see also HIV infection
AIDS-associated eosinophilic pustular folliculitis 93.8
AIDS-associated Kaposi sarcoma 25.42, 25.43, 31.30–31.31, 31.35, 138.1, **138.2**, 138.4, 138.5, 138.6
AIDS Clinical Trial Group (ACTG), Kaposi sarcoma staging 138.4, **138.5**
AIDS defining cancers (ADCs) 147.2
AIDS patients
  biopsies 3.38
  hypermelanosis 86.25
AIDS wasting syndrome 98.7
AIN *see* anal intraepithelial neoplasia
ainhum 94.47–94.48
AIP *see* acute intermittent porphyria
airborne allergens 127.17–127.18
airborne contact dermatitis 126.18, 128.4
Aircast Walker's boot *83.16*
air pollution
  ageing of skin 156.8
  atopic eczema 41.7
airway oedema, burn injuries 125.2, 125.5
AISI *see* Acne Inversa Severity Index
AK *see* actinic keratoses
AKC *see* atopic keratoconjunctivitis
AKN *see* acne keloidalis nuchae
ALA *see* alpha-lipoic acid; 5-aminolaevulinic acid
Alagille syndrome (arteriohepatic dysplasia) 153.5
albinism 7.2, 68.5–68.8
  Griscelli–Pruniéras syndrome 68.9
  partial albinism in Chediak–Higashi syndrome 80.14
  skin cancer prevention and management 7.10–7.11, 7.12, *7.13*
albinism–deafness syndrome 68.9
Albright hereditary osteodystrophy **72.7**
  in infancy *72.9*
ALCL *see* anaplastic large-cell lymphoma
alcohols, topical therapies 18.9
alcohol sensitivity flushing **104.9**
alcohol services, psychosocial diseases 120.8
alcohol use
  and acne 88.25

BSL association 98.15, 98.16
cutaneous disease 84.39–84.40
oral squamous cell carcinoma 108.46
psoriasis association 35.4, 120.3
rosacea risk 89.3
Alcyonidium diaphanum stings 130.4
aldehydes, topical therapies 18.10
ALEP *see* acute localised exanthematous pustulosis
Alexandrite lasers, vascular lesions 23.7
alexithymia, identification and treatment importance 15.3
Alezzandrini syndrome 86.42
alginate dermal filler 158.5
ALHE (angiolymphoid hyperplasia with eosinophilia) *see* epithelioid haemangioma
Alibert, Jhaemmean-Louis 1.4, *1.5*
alitretinoin (9-cis retinoic acid) 41.29
  topical 18.25
ALK *see* anaplastic lymphoma kinase
alkalis, burns 128.11
alkali tests, irritant contact dermatitis 129.5
alkaptonuria 79.12, 86.50, *106.24*
alkyl glucosides 127.59
Allegemeines Krankenhaus, Vienna 1.6
alleles 8.3, 8.4–8.5, 8.9
Allen test 122.13
allergens 127.36–127.78
  arthropods 34.2
  bedbug bites 34.26–34.27
  beetle larval hairs 34.31–34.32
  binding to skin components 127.6–127.7
  contact cheilitis association **108.60**
  horse fly bites 34.9
  house dust mites 34.51
  hymenoptera venom 34.9, 34.16–34.18
  locusts 34.32
  mites 34.50, 34.51
  patch testing 129.7
  prevention strategies 127.2
  Reduviidae bug bites 34.29
  standard series lists **127.30**
  venom immunotherapy 34.18
allergic components, chemicals 128.6
allergic contact dermatitis (ACD) 9.10, 39.3, 39.21, 127.1–127.88, 128.2, 128.3, 128.5, 128.12, 129.5–129.7
  atopic eczema relationship 41.12, 41.22
  chemical peels, side effect of 160.13
  drug-induced eczema 117.3–117.5
  epidemiology 127.2–127.4
  erythroderma 39.35
  eyelids *39.22*
  male genitalia 109.12, **109.13**
  occupational 16.12, 129.5–129.7
  pathophysiology 127.6–127.7
  perianal skin 111.9
  peristomal skin 112.7–112.8
  population studies 127.3–127.4
  prevalence 127.3
  sensitising chemicals 127.6
  stings 130.4
  vulval 110.15
  see also contact dermatitis
allergic contact urticaria 127.82–127.86
  vulval 110.16
allergic disorders, involving respiratory system 152.1–152.2
allergic occupational hazards 129.8–129.11
allergic reactions 9.9–9.10
  clinical pharmacology 13.6
  dermatophyte infections 32.50
  IgE-related type 1 skin hypersensitivity 9.9–9.10
  patch testing technique 1.8
  sensitising agents used in topical therapies 18.33–18.34
  to insulin and glucose monitors 62.4
  topical therapy adverse effects 18.4, 18.5
  urticaria 42.5
allergic rhino-conjunctivitis, and atopic eczema 41.20
allergic transfusion reactions 149.15

allogeneic haematopoietic stem cell transplantation, graft versus host disease 38.1–38.12
allopurinol
  cutaneous adverse effects 155.9–155.10, 155.15
  hypersensitivity reactions **14.6**
allylamines, topical therapies 18.12
ALM *see* acral lentiginous melanoma
aloe, cosmeceutical use of 157.10–157.11
alopecia
  alopecia totalis 105.12
  biopsy 3.7
  cancer treatment 87.71–87.74
  chemotherapy-induced 119.5–119.6
  cicatricial *68.11*, 87.37, 87.38–87.53, *88.37*
  secondary 105.6–105.9
  cosmetic approaches 87.69, 87.97–87.101
  Covid-19 association 25.113
  cutaneous lesions 96.13
  cutaneous manifestations of Hodgkin disease 139.49
  diagnosis 87.13
  incontinentia pigmenti *68.11*
  lichen planopilaris 37.11
  linear morphoea en coup de sabre *55.24*
  lipoedematous 98.24–98.25, 105.10–105.11
  medical traumatic hair loss 87.30
  metastases to the scalp 148.5, 148.6
  monitoring/assessment 87.16–87.18
  neonatal 114.4
  non-scarring 87.28–87.35
  psoriatic 87.34, *105.3*
  radiotherapy-associated 119.14
  scarring 87.13–87.14, *87.19–87.20*, 87.36–87.38, 91.11, 107.4
  syphilis 29.10, *29.12*
  systemic lupus erythematosus *51.26*
  thallium poisoning 121.9
  topical use of sensitising agents 18.33–18.34
  vitamin D deficiency 61.10
  X-linked syndromes 63.69
  see also hair loss
alopecia areata (AA) 87.13–87.14, 87.16, 87.18–87.28
  Covid-19 association 25.113
  dupilumab 87.35
  eyebrows 107.4
  pigmentary disorders *87.92, 87.93*
  psychodermatology 84.3
alopecia areata incognita 87.23–87.24, 87.58–87.59
alopecia mucinosa (AM) 57.15–57.18, 87.47, 105.8, 139.14–139.15
alopecia neoplastica 148.5
alopecia totalis 87.24–87.27
alopecia universalis 87.24–87.27
ALOXE3 mutations 63.12, *63.13*
alpha-1 antitrypsin deficiency **72.11**
alpha-1 antitrypsin deficiency panniculitis 97.43–97.45
α_1-antitrypsin deficiency 152.5
alpha-hydroxyl acids, chemical peels 160.1–160.2
α-keratin intermediate filaments (α-KIF) 87.6
alpha-lipoic acid (ALA), cosmeceutical use of 157.1–157.2
alpha-mannosidosis, glycoproteinoses 79.3
alpha-N-acetyl-galactosaminidase deficiency 79.4
α_5-reductase inhibitors 87.96
alphaviruses
  mosquito borne togavirus infections 25.87–25.91
  viral arthropathies 155.3
Alstroemeriaceae dermatitis 127.73
Alström syndrome **72.7**
alternative treatments *see* complementary/alternative/traditional therapies; herbals
aluminium, allergic contact dermatitis 127.41

aluminium acetate 18.9
aluminium chloride, hyperhidrosis treatment 92.9
aluminium chloride hexahydrate
   caustic agent for skin surgery 20.47
   topical 18.9
ALUs *see* arterial leg ulcers
AM *see* alopecia mucinosa
amalgam fillings 127.41
amalgam tattoos 108.15
Ambras-type congenital hypertrichosis 87.85
ambulatory photodynamic therapy 22.11
AMD3100, wound healing *11.12*
amelanosis 86.8
amelanotic melanomas 142.14, *142.16, 142.17*
Amerchol L101 127.58
American Academy of Dermatology Resident International Grant Scheme 7.14
American Burn Association (ABA) criteria, burn injuries 125.2
American College of Chemosurgery (ACC) 20.32, 20.37
American College of Mohs Surgery (ACMS) 20.37
American cutaneous leishmaniasis *33.44, 33.45, 33.46, 33.49, 33.50–33.51*
American Joint Committee on Cancer (AJCC), Merkel cell carcinoma staging 146.5, 146.7, **146.8**
American Society of Tropical Medicine and Hygiene (ASTMH) 7.6
American trypanosomiasis (Chagas disease) 33.39–33.43
   clinical features 33.41–33.42
   investigations 33.43
   management 33.43
   pathophysiology 33.39–33.40, *33.41*
amicrobial, *see also* sterile
amicrobial pustulosis of the skin folds 49.20–49.21
   erosions and crusts involving the retro-auricular region *49.20*
amino acid metabolism and transport disorders **79.2**, 79.10–79.15
   alkaptonuria 79.12
   argininosuccinic aciduria 79.13–79.14
   dermatological features **79.11**
   Hartnup disease 79.14
   phenylketonuria 79.10–79.11
   prolidase deficiency 79.12–79.13
   serine, proline and glutamine synthesis defects 79.14–79.15
   tyrosinaemia type 2 79.11–79.12
amino acids, alpha-1 antitrypsin 97.43
amino acid supplements 88.12
amino formaldehyde resins 127.71
5-aminolaevulinic acid (ALA)
   contact allergy 22.13, *22.14*
   in photodynamic therapy 22.2–22.3, 22.4–22.6
amiodarone 86.25, 86.27–86.28
amnion, burn treatment 125.6
amniotic bands, and lymphoedema 103.29–103.30
amniotic membrane transplantation (AMT) 118.20
amobiasis 33.36–33.38
   clinical features 33.37
   epidemiology 33.36
   investigations 33.37–33.38
   management 33.38
   pathophysiology 33.37
amoebiasis, perianal skin 111.16
amorphous basophilic material, actinic elastosis 94.2
amphetamines, dermatoses induced by 120.2, *120.5*
ampicillin, exanthem caused by *117.2*
amputation stump neuromas 136.43
AMT *see* amniotic membrane transplantation
amylase, pancreatic panniculitis 97.41
Amyloid A (AA) amyloidosis, renal and skin involvement 154.2

amyloidoses 56.1–56.14, 86.22–86.23
   amyloid deposition in papillary dermis *56.5*
   amyloid, electron microscopy of *56.6*
   amyloidogenesis 56.1–56.2
   cardiac involvement 151.4
   classification 56.2
   clinical presentation 56.2
   cutaneous amyloidoses due to systemic disease 56.10–56.13
   ear dermatoses **106.22**
   electron microscopy 56.5, *56.6*
   eye disease **107.35**
   functional and disease-causing amyloids 56.2
   hereditary localised cutaneous amyloidosis **56.3**
   hereditary systemic amyloidoses with cutaneous involvement **56.4**
   hereditary systemic diseases with secondary cutaneous amyloidosis **56.4**
   histology 56.3–56.4
   immunohistochemistry 56.4, *56.5, 56.6*
   investigations 56.2–56.6
   localised cutaneous amyloidoses **56.3**, 56.6–56.10
      associated diseases 56.8–56.9
      clinical features 56.9–56.10
      clinical variants 56.10
      complications and disease course 56.10
      differential diagnosis 56.10
      epidemiology 56.7
      ethnicity 56.7–56.8
      pathophysiology 56.9
   management 56.13–56.14
   non-hereditary localised cutaneous amyloidosis **56.3**
   non-hereditary systemic amyloidoses with cutaneous involvement **56.4**
   oral involvement 108.69–108.70
   penile 109.25
   respiratory involvement 152.6
   systemic amyloidoses with cutaneous involvement 56.10–56.13
   ultrastructure 56.1
amyloidosis 86.22–86.23
amyopathic dermatomyositis 52.1
   see also clinically amyopathic dermatomyositis
amyotrophic lateral sclerosis 122.2
AN *see* acanthosis nigricans; atypical naevi
ANA *see* antinuclear antibody test
anabolic steroids, urticaria treatment 42.19
anaemia
   ancylostomiasis 33.15
   epidermolysis bullosa 69.26
   fanconi anaemia 76.11, **80.5**, 80.12–80.13
   skin signs 149.15–149.16
anaerobic bacteria 26.67–26.69
   aerotolerant coryneforms 26.37, 26.43
   Bacteroidaceae 26.67–26.68
   classification 26.67–26.68
   clostridia 26.48
   Eikenella corrodens 26.67
   normal skin flora 26.3, 26.4
   Peudomonas aeruginosa 26.51–26.53
   tropical ulcers 26.68–26.69
anaesthesia
   biopsy 3.2–3.3
   peripheral nerve damage in leprosy 28.3, 28.7
   photothermal ablation 23.21
   in pregnancy 113.24
anagen hair bulb 87.5, 87.8
anagen hair follicles 87.3, 87.7–87.8, *87.57*
   appearance *87.57*
   dermal papilla 87.5
   pathology 87.21
   pigmentation disorders *87.12*
   suprabulbar region 87.4
anagen release, telogen effluvium 87.53
anal abscess 111.27–111.28
   classification of *111.28*

anal canal 111.2
   internal haemorrhoids *111.32*
anal cancer 111.21–111.24
   clinical features 111.22–111.23
   epidemiology 111.22
   management 111.24
   pathophysiology 111.22
   perianal carcinoma *111.23*
anal fissure 111.30–111.31
anal fistula 111.28–111.30
   conditions associated with **111.29**
   development of an intersphincteric fistula *111.29*
   Parks classification *111.30*
analgesia
   hidradenitis suppurativa treatment 90.9
   SJS/TEN treatment 118.20
anal intraepithelial neoplasia (AIN) 111.19–111.21, 141.26
   histopathology *111.20*
anal orifice 111.2–111.3
anal/perianal/genital intraepithelial carcinomas 141.24, 141.26
anal sphincter 111.2–111.3
anal tags 111.32, *111.33*
anaphylaxis
   drug-induced 14.1–14.2, 117.5–117.7
   flushing **104.8**
   rubber latex allergy 127.84–127.85
   urticaria 42.1
anaplasia 3.39
Anaplasma phagocytophilum, tick-borne zoonotic infection 26.66–26.67
anaplasmosis 26.66–26.67
anaplastic large-cell lymphoma (ALCL) 139.28–139.29
anaplastic lymphoma kinase (ALK) 3.28
   positive/negative cutaneous lymphomas 139.1, 139.26, 139.28, 139.34
ANA screening *see* antinuclear antibody test
anatomical considerations, skin surgery 20.1–20.4
anatomy of skin 9.1
ANCA *see* antineutrophil cytoplasmic antibody
anchoring fibrils 2.26–2.27
ancient medical texts 1.1–1.3
Ancylostoma braziliense see cutaneous larva migrans
Ancylostoma caninum see cutaneous larva migrans
Ancylostoma ceylonicum see cutaneous larva migrans
Ancylostoma duodenale, ancylostomiasis 33.15–33.17
ancylostomiasis 33.15–33.17
   clinical features 33.17
   epidemiology 33.15
   management 33.17
   pathophysiology 33.16–33.17
androgenetic alopecia (AGA) 87.10, 87.60–87.71
   children/adolescents 87.66–87.67
   COVID-19 association 25.113
   FPHL with **87.67**
   treatment 87.68–87.70
androgen excess 87.88
androgen insensitivity syndrome 87.10
androgen receptor 87.10
androgen receptor blockers, acne vulgaris treatment 88.51
androgens
   for dyskeratosis congenita 67.15
   hair growth 87.9–87.10
   nail–patella syndrome 67.15
androgen-secreting tumours, hirsutism association 87.91
androgen-stimulated hair growth 87.10
androgen synthesis 87.10
ANEM *see* acute necrotising eosinophilic myocarditis
anetoderma 94.23–94.25
   of prematurity 114.9–114.10
aneurysmal fibrous histiocytoma 136.20, 136.21

anger, emotional effects of skin conditions 15.2
angina bullosa haemorrhagica, oral involvement 108.20
angioedema 152.2, *152.3*
   assessment tools 16.5, 16.9
   drug-induced 117.5–117.7
   oral involvement 108.10
   reactions to COVID-19 (mRNA) vaccines 25.117
angioedema activity score (AAS) 16.5
Angioedema Quality of Life Questionnaire (AE-QoL) 16.9
angioedema swellings, urticaria 42.1, *42.3*
angioedema without weals 43.1–43.7
   clinical features 43.4
   clinical variants 43.4–43.5
   definition and nomenclature 43.1
   disease course and prognosis 43.5
   epidemiology 43.2–43.3
   genetics 43.4
   investigations 43.5
   laboratory profiles *43.5*
   management 43.5–43.6
   pathophysiology 43.3–43.4
   treatment 43.5–43.6
angiofibromas
   non-ablative laser therapies 23.11
   photothermal ablation 23.21, *23.22*
   tuberous sclerosis complex 78.8, *78.10*
angiogenesis 101.1
   wound healing 11.5–11.6
angioimmunoblastic T-cell lymphoma 139.45
angiokeratoma circumscriptum 101.13–101.14
angiokeratoma corporis diffusum *see* Fabry disease
angiokeratomas 101.13–101.14, **101.17**
   dermoscopic view of *101.14*
   labia majora 110.3, *110.4*
   laser therapies 23.11, *23.12*
   lysosomal diseases associated with **79.7**
   male genitalia 109.6–109.7
   subtypes of **101.15**
angiolipoma 136.56
angiolupoid sarcoidosis 96.12
angiolymphoid hyperplasia with eosinophilia *106.24*
   ear dermatoses **106.22**
angiolymphoid hyperplasia with eosinophilia (ALHE) *see* epithelioid haemangioma
angiomas, laser therapies 23.11
angioma serpiginosum 71.4–71.5, 101.16, **101.17**, *101.18*, **101.18**
angiomatoid fibrous histiocytoma 136.62–136.63
angiomatosis, diffuse dermal *4.11*
angiomyofibroblastoma 136.9
angiomyolipomas, tuberous sclerosis complex 78.9
angiosarcoma 119.15, 136.34–136.36
   epithelioid angiosarcoma 136.37
   lymphangiosarcoma 103.7
angiotensin-converting enzyme (ACE) 127.10
angiotensin-converting enzyme (ACE) inhibitor-induced angio-oedema 43.2, 43.3, 43.4
angora hair naevus 73.21–73.22
angular cheilitis/angular stomatitis 32.62–32.63, 108.20, 108.59–108.60
angulated lines dermoscopy patterns, melanoma 145.7, *145.8*
anhidrosis
   eccrine gland disorders **92.11**
   hyperhidrosis and 92.11–92.12
animal bites *see* bites
animal parasites
   Cimicidae bugs 34.25–34.26
   mites 34.50, 34.54–34.55
animals, exposure to, and atopic eczema 41.8

animal-type melanoma *see* pigmented
      epithelioid melanocytoma/pigment
      synthesising melanoma
ankle
   familial Mediterranean fever   45.10
   hypertrophic lichen planus   37.7
   lichen planus pemphigoides   37.9
   lichen simplex   39.29
   lipoatrophic panniculitis in childhood
      97.56–97.57
   primary localised cutaneous amyloidosis
      56.7
   venous eczema   39.20
ankle brachial Doppler pressure index
      (ABPI)   101.4, **101.4**
   lower leg eczema   39.21
ankle flare (corona phlebectatica
      paraplantaris)   **101.43**, *101.44*
ankyloglossia
   epidermolysis bullosa   69.25
   oral involvement   108.87
annular elastolytic giant cell granuloma
      (AEGCG)   62.5, 94.27–94.30
annular epidermolytic ichthyosis (AEI)
      63.16
annular erythema of infancy (AEI)   47.9
   histopathology of lesional skin   *47.10*
annular lesions   4.7, *4.10*, 4.15, *63.75*
annular lichen planus   37.8
annular purpura   122.16
annular sarcoidosis   *96.10*
ano-genital cellulitis   111.14
ano-genital infections   32.63–32.65
ano-genital mammary-like gland tumours
   137.20
ano-genital pilonidal sinus   122.23
ano-genital region
   allergic contact dermatitis   127.16–127.17,
      127.22
   anatomy   109.3–109.4
   child abuse, signs of   109.9
   ecthyma gangrenosum   109.26
   embryogenesis of   111.3, *111.4*
   HIV   31.35–31.36
   hypo- and hyperpigmentation   **109.42**
   irritants   109.11
   staphylococcal cellulitis   109.26
   structure and function of   111.1–111.3
   see also perineal and perianal skin
ano-genital tumours
   anal/vulval/penile and perianal
      intraepithelial carcinoma   141.24,
      141.26
   hidradenoma papilliferum   110.31–110.33,
      137.20–137.21
ano-genital warts   25.61–25.64, 109.9
   cervical intraepithelial neoplasia
      association   25.65
   clinical features   25.62–25.64
   cutaneous squamous cell carcinoma
      association   25.65
   epidemiology   25.61
   male genitalia   109.29
   management   25.64
   pathophysiology   25.61–25.62
   vulva   *110.30*
   see also condylomata acuminata
ano-rectal abscess   111.27–111.28
   classification of   *111.28*
anorexia nervosa   84.26–84.27, 88.30
ANS *see* autonomic nervous system
antenatal procedures, neonatal
      complications arising from   **114.10**
anterolateral lower leg alopecia   87.29–87.30
Anthocidae (minute pirate/flower bugs)
      34.29–34.30
Anthozoa, stings from   130.1–130.2
anthrax   26.44–26.45
   clinical features   26.44–26.45
   epidemiology   26.44
   management   26.45
   pathophysiology   26.44
anthropophilic dermatophytes   32.19–32.20
anthroquinone dyes   127.65–127.66
anti-ageing cosmeceuticals   157.3–157.7

rhytid reduction   157.4–157.7
skin lightening   157.3–157.4
antiandrogens   87.70
   acne vulgaris treatment   *88.50*
   hair disorder treatment   87.95–87.97
   in pregnancy   **113.23**
antibiotics
   acne vulgaris treatment   88.46, 88.47,
      88.48–88.49, 88.52
      adverse effects of   **88.49**
      interactions with oral contraceptives
         88.49
   allergic contact dermatitis   127.45
   anti-inflammatory effects   19.48
   atopic eczema association   41.9
   atopic eczema treatment   41.27
   eye, side effects on   107.43
   'happenstance therapy'   29.12
   in pregnancy   **113.21**
   syphilis   29.12, 29.20–29.21
   systemic   19.46–19.48
   topical therapies   18.10–18.12
antibiotic sore tongue *see* acute erythematous
      candidiasis
antibody deficiencies   80.13
   inherited immunodeficiency   **80.5**
antibody probes, epidermolysis bullosa
      diagnosis   69.21
anticholinergic agents   18.38
anticonvulsant hypersensitivity syndrome
      118.5
antidepressants   84.43–84.44
   prescribing   84.43
   selective serotonin reuptake inhibitors
      84.43, **84.44**, 117.3
   switching   84.44
   tricyclic antidepressants   84.44, **84.45**
   types   84.43–84.44
antiepileptic drugs, acneform reaction
      88.13
antifungal agents
   dermatophyte infections   32.32–32.34
   in pregnancy   **113.20**
   seborrhoeic dermatitis management   40.8,
      40.9
   skin cancer risks in immunocompromised
      people   147.8
   systemic drugs   19.48, 40.9
   topical therapies   18.12–18.13,
      32.33–32.34, 40.8
anti-GBM *see* antiglomerular basement
      membrane vasculitis
antigenic tests   4.24–4.25
antigen mapping   69.21
antigen-presenting cells (APCs)   127.7, 135.2
   histiocytoses   135.1
   immune system   9.4–9.5
   T-cell receptors   118.5
antigens, epidermolysis bullosa   69.4
antiglomerular basement membrane
      vasculitis (anti-GBM)
      100.19–100.20
antihistamines
   adverse effects   42.17–42.18
   atopic eczema treatment   41.27
   in childhood   42.18
   mastocytosis treatment   46.9
   pharmacokinetic and clinical properties
      42.18
   in pregnancy   42.18, 113.19, **113.22**
   solar urticaria   126.24
   systemic   19.3–19.4
      cautions   19.4
      dose and regimens   19.4
      drug–drug interactions   19.4
      pharmacological properties   19.3–19.4
      potential adverse effects   19.4
   topical therapies   18.37
   urticaria treatment   42.17–42.18, 42.19
anti-inflammatory agents
   antibiotics   19.48
   cosmeceuticals   157.10–157.11
   mastocytosis treatment   46.9
   in pregnancy   **113.20**
   systemic therapy   19.2–19.46

antimalarial agents   19.4–19.7
   adverse effects   155.15
   cautions   19.6
   contraindication   19.6
   dermatological uses   19.4–19.5
   discoid lupus erythematosus treatment
      51.11
   dose and regimens   19.7
   drug–drug interactions   19.6
   hypermelanosis   86.26, 86.27–86.28
   monitoring   19.7
   ocular side effects   19.6, 107.43
   pharmacological properties   19.5
   potential adverse effects   19.5–19.6
   pre-treatment screening   19.7
   side effects   **51.11**, *51.25*
   systemic lupus erythematosus treatment
      51.37
antimicrobial agents
   allergic contact dermatitis   127.49–127.58
   burn injuries   125.10
   fast growing *Mycobacterium* species   **27.45**
   genital contact dermatitis   **109.13**
   in pregnancy   113.23–**113.24**
   systemic therapies   19.46–19.49
antimicrobial peptides, possible seborrhoeic
      dermatitis therapies   40.9
antimicrobial resistance
   corynebacteria   26.38
   gonococcus/*Neisseria gonorrhoeae*   30.1,
      30.2, 30.7, **30.8**
   impetigo management   26.16
   multidrug-resist tuberculosis   27.10
   Mycoplasma genitalium   30.24, 30.25
   STI coinfections   30.13
   topical fusidic acid use   18.11
   see also methicillin-resistant *Staphylococcus
      aureus*
antineoplastic and cytotoxic agents
      18.29–18.31
antineutrophil cytoplasmic antibody
      (ANCA) associated small vessel
      vasculitis   100.9, 100.13,
      100.20–100.28, 152.3–152.4
antinomy, dermatological reactions
      121.1–121.2
antinuclear antibody (ANA) test   126.6
   systemic lupus erythematosus
      51.34–51.36
antioxidants
   allergies   127.59
   cosmeceuticals   157.1–157.3
   resuscitation use   125.4
   topical medication   18.8
anti-p200 pemphigoid   50.38–50.42
   clinical features   50.40
   epidemiology   50.39
   histopathology   *50.40*
   investigations and diagnosis   50.40
   management   50.40–50.42
   pathophysiology   50.39–50.40
   serum autoantibodies against p200 antigen
      50.42
   treatment ladder   50.42
antiparasitic agents, topical therapies
      18.13–18.14
antiparasitic treatment
   lice   34.22, 34.25
   scabies   34.45–34.48, 34.50
   tungiasis   34.15
antiperspirants   18.37–18.38
antiphospholipid antibody syndrome
      (APLS)   51.42–51.45, 99.17–99.19
   associated diseases   51.42–51.43
   cardiac involvement   151.4
   clinical features   51.43
   complications and co-morbidities
      51.43–51.44
   criteria for   **99.17**
   cutaneous findings   **99.18**
   disease course and prognosis   51.44
   investigations   51.44
   management   51.44–51.45
   pathophysiology   51.43
   treatment ladder   51.45

antipsychotics   84.44–84.46
   body dysmorphic disorder   84.14
   delusional infestation management   84.7,
      84.8–84.9, 84.44
   types   84.45–84.46
antiretroviral-induced alopecia   87.35
antiretroviral therapy (ART)
   cutaneous side effects   31.13
   drug reactions   31.2, 31.8, 31.10, **31.13**,
      31.19, 31.20
   HIV/AIDS   31.2, 31.8, 31.9–31.10
   HIV-associated lipodystrophy   98.6–98.8
   reduction in AIDS defining cancers   147.2
antiseptics
   allergic contact dermatitis   127.45
   pressure ulcer treatment   123.11
   topical therapies   18.9–18.10
antistreptolysin O titre (ASOT)   26.11, 26.12,
      26.36
antisynthetase syndrome   52.8
anti-TNF-α treatment, mycobacterial
      infections   27.11–27.12
anti-TNF biologic therapy, pyoderma
      gangrenosum   49.7
α_1-antitrypsin deficiency   152.5
anti-type IV collagen pemphigoid   50.53
antivenom, cnidarian stings   130.3
antiviral agents   19.49
   adverse cutaneous effects, hepatitis
      treatments   25.75, 25.76–25.77
   hepatitis B treatment   25.75
   hepatitis C treatment   25.76–25.77
   herpes simplex infections   25.22,
      25.23–25.24, 25.25, 25.26, 25.27
   human herpesvirus 6 and 7   25.40
   pox viruses   25.7, 25.11, 25.18
   in pregnancy   **113.24**
   prophylaxis for immune suppressed
      patients   25.31, 25.42, 25.75
   prophylaxis for perinatal transmission
      25.31, 25.75
   prophylaxis to prevent HSV reactivation
      25.23, 25.24, 25.26, 25.27, 25.28
   topical therapies   18.13
   varicella-zoster virus   25.31, 25.32, 25.35
ants   34.16
ANUG *see* acute necrotising (ulcerative)
      gingivitis and noma
anus
   mucosal melanomas   142.11, *142.16*
   see also anal entries
anxiety
   acne vulgaris   88.39
   morphoea   55.29
   psoriasis   35.19
   skin-related health anxieties   15.2,
      84.25–84.26
anxiolytics   84.46
AOSD *see* adult-onset Still disease
AP *see* actinic prurigo
APCs *see* antigen-presenting cells
APECED *see* autoimmune
      polyendocrinopathy Candida
      ectodermal dystrophy syndrome
Apert syndrome   **106.7**
   acne vulgaris association   88.10–88.11
aphonia, vitamin B1 deficiency   61.14
aphthous-like ulcers
   oral ulceration   108.38–108.39
   systemic factors associated with   **108.39**
aphthous ulcers
   Adamantiades–Behçet disease   *48.5*, **48.8**
   female genitalia   110.19
   treatment   **48.8**
Aphthovirus infections   25.93
APL *see* acquired partial lipodystrophy
APLAID *see* autoinflammation and
      PLCG2-associated antibody
      deficiency and immune
      dysregulation
aplasia
   congenital pseudo-ainhum   94.48
   ocular features   **107.41**
aplasia cutis   87.30
APLS *see* antiphospholipid antibody
      syndrome

apocrine carcinoma 137.22–137.23
apocrine cystadenoma *see* apocrine hidrocystoma
apocrine glands 2.9, 2.43, 92.15–92.17
 changes in during pregnancy 113.2–113.3
 disorders 92.16–92.19
 function 92.1
 tumours 137.1, 137.2, 137.18–137.23
apocrine hidrocystoma 137.18–137.19
apocrine miliaria 92.18–92.19
apocrine tubular adenoma 137.22
apoeccrine glands 2.9, 92.1
apoptosis 3.39
appearance, social impacts 15.1
appendageal tumours *see* tumours of skin appendages
application sparganosis 33.35
applicators, brachytherapy 24.3
apps
 diagnosis 4.26, 5.13
 NLR SkinApp 7.12
apremilast
 discoid lupus erythematosus treatment 51.12
 immunomodulatory therapy 19.7–19.8
 psoriasis treatment 35.26
apron eczema 39.14, 39.15, 128.4
APS-1 *see* autoimmune polyendocrinopathy syndrome type 1
APSEA *see* Assessments of the Psychological and Social Effects of Acne
APSS *see* acral peeling skin syndrome
apthous lesions, autoinflammatory diseases **80.19**
AQOL *see* Acne Quality of Life Scale
AQP5 mutations, non-epidermolytic palmoplantar keratoderma 63.54
AQPs *see* aquaporins
aquagenic keratoderma 63.61–63.62
aquagenic urticaria **42.9**, 42.12, *42.13*
aquaporins (AQPs) 63.54
 eccrine glands 92.2
AR *see* autosomal recessive
Arachnida 34.34–34.57
 mites 34.41–34.57
 scorpions 34.36–34.37
 spiders 34.34–34.36
 ticks 34.37–34.41
Araneae (spiders) 34.34–34.36
Arao–Perkins bodies 87.64
arboviruses *see* arthropod-borne viruses
arbutin
 cosmeceutical use 157.3
 topical depigmenting agents 18.32
Arcanobacterium haemolyticum 26.43
ARCI *see* autosomal recessive congenital ichthyosis
ARC syndrome *see* arthrogryposis–renal dysfunction–cholestasis syndrome
arcuate lesions *4.11*
arenavirus infections 25.81–25.83
areola, microscopic examination of 3.33
Argentina, community dermatology 7.8
Argentinian haemorrhagic fever 25.82–25.83
argininosuccinic aciduria 79.13–79.14, 87.76
argyria 86.51–86.52, 121.8
ARIH *see* autosomal recessive ichthyosis with hypotrichosis
arm
 acne scarring 88.40
 acute generalised pustular psoriasis 35.33
 ageing of skin 156.2
 allergic contact dermatitis 127.14, 127.22
 Apert syndrome 88.11
 atopic eczema 41.19
 Bateman purpura 156.6
 bullous pemphigoid *50.16*
 capillary malformations 71.5
 carcinoma telangiectatica 103.15
 cicatricial pemphigoid *50.53*
 dermatitis herpetiformis *50.57*
 eczema 39.2
 elephantine psoriasis *35.14*

eosinophilic fasciitis *55.22*
erythema multiforme *47.2*
IgA vasculitis 100.15
interstitial granulomatous dermatitis *53.6*
keratosis pilaris *88.35*
lichenification of in patient with atopic eczema *39.28*
linear morphoea *55.26*
linear psoriasis with guttate psoriasis *35.15*
lymphatic malformations *71.22*
miliaria *114.7*
mucous membrane pemphigoid *50.29*
necrolytic migratory erythema *47.15*
pansclerotic morphoea *55.21*
pemphigus vulgaris *50.5*
psoriasis vulgaris *35.7, 35.11*
Rothmund–Thomson syndrome *75.5*
subcutaneous fat necrosis of the newborn *114.16*
swelling due to oedema 103.44–103.46
systemic lupus erythematosus *51.23, 51.24*
systemic sclerosis *54.4, 54.5*
urticaria *42.2, 42.11*
see also digital entries; finger; hand
armpit *see* axillary entries
ARN *see* accelerated rheumatoid nodulosis
arochordons *see* skin tags
arrector pili muscle
 degeneration in pattern hair loss 87.64
 hamartoma 136.52–136.53
 leiomyoma 136.53–136.54
arsenic
 acute toxicity 121.2–121.3
 agricultural chemicals 141.18
 dermatological reactions 121.1, 121.2–121.3
 groundwater contamination 141.13, 141.18
 historic medications 141.18
 hypermelanosis 86.25
 pigmentation effects 86.52
 predisposition to Bowden disease 141.18
 routes of exposure 141.13, 141.18
arsenical keratosis 141.13–141.14
arsenite 121.2
ART *see* antiretroviral therapy
artefacts 3.31–3.32
 due to blocking and sectioning 3.32
 due to poor biopsy technique 3.31–3.32
 due to staining techniques 3.32
 and fixation media 3.32
arterial/arteriolar disorders 101.1–101.31
 angiogenesis 101.1
 arterial leg ulcers 102.7–102.10
 arteriogenesis 101.1
 arteriovenous malformations 101.22–101.24
 cutaneous vascular malformations 101.26–101.31
 hypertensive ischaemic leg ulcers 102.10–102.13
 Klippel–Trenaunay syndrome 101.27–101.30
 livedo reticularis 124.9
 mixed leg ulcers 102.4–102.7
 neurovascular disorders 101.6–101.9
 Parkes Weber syndrome **101.28**, 101.30–101.31
 peripheral vascular disease 101.2–101.3
 telangiectases 101.10–101.22
 thromboangiitis obliterans 101.3–101.6
 ulceration 102.1–102.13
 vasculogenesis 101.1
 verrucous haemangioma 101.26, *101.27*
arterial leg ulcers (ALUs) 102.7–102.10
 clinical features 102.8–102.9
 epidemiology 102.8
 management 102.9–102.10
 pathophysiology 102.8
arterial occlusion, dermal filler, adverse reaction 158.10, **158.11**
arterial tortuosity syndrome **70.16**

arteries
 anatomy of head and neck 20.1–20.2
 subcutaneous fat 97.7
arteriogenesis 101.1
arteriohepatic dysplasia (Alagille syndrome) 153.5
arterioles 2.40, *2.41*
arteriolosclerosis, subcutaneous, hypertensive ischaemic leg ulcer *102.11*
arteriovenous disorders 71.11–71.14
 arteriovenous malformation 71.11–71.12
 hereditary haemorrhagic telangiectasia 71.12–71.13
 PTEN hamartoma tumour syndrome 71.13–71.14
arteriovenous malformations (AVM) 71.11–71.12, 101.22–101.24
 clinical features **101.23**
 conditions associated with **101.22**
 in infants *101.23*
 investigations 101.23
 management 101.24
 pathophysiology 101.23
arthritis
 acne association 88.63
 NLRP1-associated autoinflammation with arthritis and dyskeratosis 45.18
 osteoarthritis 155.8
 pachydermoperiostosis 155.14
 systemic lupus erythematosus 51.30
 systemic-onset juvenile idiopathic arthritis 45.21–45.22
 see also mixed connective tissue disease; psoriatic arthritis; reactive arthritis; rheumatoid arthritis; sexually acquired reactive arthritis
arthritis mutilans 35.42
arthrochalasia Ehlers–Danlos syndrome (aEDS) **70.4**, 70.9
Arthroderma species 32.18, 32.25–32.26
see also Microsporum gypseum
arthrogryposis–renal dysfunction–cholestasis (ARC) syndrome 63.30
arthropathies
 infective 155.2–155.5
 inflammatory 155.5–155.7, *155.8, 155.9*
arthropod bites, pseudolymphoma 134.2
arthropod-borne viruses (arboviruses)
 Bunyavirus infections 25.83–25.84
 flavivirus infections 25.85–25.87
 togavirus infections 25.87–25.91
arthropods 34.1–34.58
 arachnids 34.34–34.57
 attraction to humans 34.3
 centipedes and millipedes 34.57
 classification 34.1
 clinical and epidemiological features 34.3–34.4
 disease transmission 34.2
 environmental factors in exposure 34.2–34.3
 insects 34.6–34.34
 investigations of skin disease 34.4–34.5
 larval invasion of tissues/myiasis 34.2, **34.7**, 34.9–34.13
 management of skin disease 34.6
 pathology of skin effects 34.3
 pathophysiology of skin disease 34.2–34.3
 protective clothing and repellents 34.5
 see also louse-borne diseases
artificial hair implantation 122.23
artificial intelligence (AI) 4.26–4.27
 melanoma detection 142.16
 objective measures of skin properties 16.5
Ascher syndrome 94.27
Asclepius 1.2
ascorbic acid (vitamin C), topical depigmenting agents 18.33
aseptic abscess syndrome 49.21
Ashkenazi Jews, hyperhidrosis 92.5
ash-leaf-shaped macules, tuberous sclerosis complex 78.8

ashy dermatosis 86.32–86.33
Asian skin phenotypes, photoageing 156.2–156.3, 156.7
ASIS *see* Acne Symptom and Impact Scale
ASM *see* aggressive systemic mastocytosis
ASOT *see* antistreptolysin O titre
aspartylglucosaminuria 79.3–79.4
aspergillosis
 oral ulceration 108.56–108.57
 panniculitis due to 97.60–97.61
Aspergillus
 A. niger, otomycosis 32.17
 A. terreus, superficial onychomycosis 32.54–32.55
Aspergillus species, skin lesions 32.93
aspirin, urticaria 117.6
ASPRV1 encoding, autosomal dominant lamellar ichthyoses 63.20–63.21
assassin bugs 34.29
assessment *see* measurement
Assessments of the Psychological and Social Effects of Acne (APSEA) questionnaire 16.8
asteatosis 85.26–85.28
asteatotic eczema *see* eczema, asteatotic
asteroid bodies, sarcoidosis 96.3
asthma, and atopic eczema 41.11, 41.20
ASTMH *see* American Society of Tropical Medicine and Hygiene
Astrakhan fever *see* tick typhus
astringents 18.9
Astruc, Jean 1.3–1.4
asymmetrical cell division 2.44
asymmetrical hyperhidrosis 92.6–92.7
asymmetric periflexural exanthem of childhood 25.123
asymptomatic neurosyphilis 29.15
AT *see* ataxia telangiectasia
ataxia-pancytopenia syndrome 149.14
ataxia telangiectasia (AT) 76.10–76.11, **78.13**, **80.4**, 148.13–148.14
 bulbar telangiectasia *80.11*
 pulmonary involvement 152.5
ataxia with vitamin E deficiency (AVED) 61.11–61.12
atherosclerosis 101.2–101.3
athletes foot, *see also* tinea peddis
athlete's nodules 122.16
atlases, dermatology 1.4
atopic blepharoconjunctivitis (ABC) 107.16, 107.18, *107.22*
atopic cataract 41.21, *107.19*
atopic dermatitis (AD) *see* atopic eczema (dermatitis)
Atopic Dermatitis Control Test (ADCT) 16.3
atopic disease, hair loss presentation 87.20
atopic eczema/dermatitis (AE) 41.1–41.33
 acute 41.13
 adult phase 41.15
 age and sex 41.3
 air pollution 41.7
 allergens 127.12–127.13
 allergic contact dermatitis 41.12, 41.22, 127.10, 127.72, 127.83
 allergic rhino-conjunctivitis association 41.20
 allergy association 41.11
 animal exposure 41.8
 antibiotics association 41.9
 assessment tools 16.3–16.4, **16.4**
 asthma 41.11, 41.20
 'atopic march' 41.11
 atopic and non-atopic eczema 41.2–41.3
 autoimmune disease association 41.22
 autoimmunity 41.12
 bacterial infections 41.20
 bathing and showering 41.26
 biologic therapies 9.8–9.9
 breastfeeding and delayed weaning 41.7, 41.23
 calcineurin inhibitors 41.27
 cancer risk association 41.21–41.22
 cardiovascular disease association 41.21
 cheilitis 128.4–128.5

atopic eczema/dermatitis (AE) (*continued*)
  childhood infections and vaccinations 41.8–41.9
  childhood phase 41.15
  classification 41.1
  climatic conditions 41.6
  clinical features **41.1**, **41.2**, 41.12–41.16
  clinical variants 41.16
  community survey 5.2
  complications and associated diseases 41.20–41.22
  corticosteroids, topical 41.26–41.27
  cost studies 5.6
  developmental delay association 41.21
  diagnosis 5.4, **41.2**, 41.3
  diet 41.7, 41.23
  differential diagnosis 41.22
  discoid eczema lesions *41.17*
  disease endotypes 41.15
  disease prevention 41.23
  disease severity 41.3, 41.16, **41.18**
  drug endotypes 41.15
  dry skin 41.15
  ear dermatoses **106.22**
  economic burden of 6.10, 41.3–41.4
    psoriasis comparison 6.10
  emollients 41.26, 41.27
  endocrine factors 41.19
  endotoxin exposure 41.8
  endotypes 41.15
  environmental risk and protective factors 41.6–41.9
  epidemiology 5.4, 41.3–41.4
  and epidermal barrier 41.5–41.6
  erythema, papules, excoriations, crusting and secondary infection *41.15*
  ethnicity 5.10
  Filaggrin genetics and epidermal barrier 41.5–41.6
  financial cost of 5.6
  first line treatment 41.24, **41.25**
  flexural dermatitis *41.13*, *41.14*
  food allergy 41.11–41.12, 41.20
  general advice and education 41.24
  genetic factors 41.4–41.5
  global distribution **7.3**
  global prevalence *41.4*
  glucocorticoid sensitivity 41.19
  growth delay association 41.21
  gut microbiome 41.9
  habit reversal therapy 84.47–84.48
  hand involvement 41.16–41.17, *41.19*, 41.23
  helminth parasites 41.8
  history 41.12–41.13, **41.12**
  HIV 31.15
  house dust mite avoidance 41.23
  hygiene hypotheis 5.14, 41.7–41.8
  hyperpigmentation *41.14*, *41.17*
  ichthyosis vulgaris association 41.15
  immune dysregulation 41.9–41.10
  immunoglobulin E role 41.11
  incidence of 7.2
  infant feeding 41.23
  infantile phase 41.15, 115.2–115.3
  infantile seborrhoeic dermatitis 41.22
  infection and antibiotics 41.27
  inflammation in 2.17, 9.8
  initial assessment **41.12**, 41.24
  innate immune cells 41.11
  investigations 41.23–41.24
  itch and antihistamines 41.27
  JAK inhibitors 41.27, 41.30–41.33
  KP association 85.9
  lichenification *41.14*, *41.16*, *41.17*, *41.19*
  lipids 41.6
  lip-lick cheilitis 41.22
  maintenance therapy 41.27
  male genitalia 109.12
  malignancy risk association 41.21–41.22
  management 41.24–41.33
  mast cell role 2.16, 2.17
  maternal smoking during pregnancy 41.7
  microbial colonisation 2.13
  microbial exposure 41.7–41.8
  microbial responses 41.10
  mimics of atopic eczema **41.22**
  morbidity and cost 41.3–41.4
  novel therapies 41.30–41.33
  obesity 41.7
  occupational aspects 41.23
  ocular surface disorders 41.20–41.21
  papulovesicules *41.13*
  pathophysiology *41.3*, 41.4–41.12, *41.32*
  pets, exposure to 41.8
  phototherapy 21.4, *21.5*, 41.28
  physical inactivity 41.7
  pityriasis alba 41.17
  prevalence of 5.10, 5.11, 6.1, 41.4
  pruritus 41.12, 81.7–81.8
  psychodermatology 84.3
  psychological factors 15.4, 41.19
  psychosocial aspects 41.19–41.20
  quality of life impact 16.8, **41.18**
  as risk factor for allergic contact dermatitis 9.10
  sex steroids 41.19
  skin barrier dysfunction 41.23
  skin of colour 41.16
  skin microbiome 9.8, 41.9
  staphylococci/streptococci role 26.13
  subtypes 5.4
  subtypes of 5.4
  sweating 41.18–41.19
  synonyms and inclusions **41.2**
  targeting of pathophysiological pathways *41.32*
  third line therapy 41.28–41.33
    biologic therapy 41.29–41.30, **41.31**, **41.32**
    conventional systemic agents **41.31**
  tobacco smoke, exposure to 41.7
  topical therapy 41.26–41.27, **41.32**
    intensive topical treatment 41.28
  treatment algorithm *41.25*
  trigger factors *41.12*, 41.24–41.26
  unresponsive disease 41.28
  urban versus rural living 41.6–41.7, 41.8
  urticaria association 41.22
  UVA-1 phototherapy 21.4, 21.6
  viral infections 41.20
  and water hardness 41.23
  wet-wrap technique for control of 41.28
  white dermographism 41.17–41.18
atopic eruption of pregnancy (AEP) 113.15–113.16
  pruritus 81.11
atopic eye disease 107.16–107.23
  associated diseases 107.16
  clinical characteristics **107.21**
  clinical variants 107.17–107.18
  diagnosis **107.21**
  future therapeutic agents 107.23
  investigations 107.22
  management 107.22–107.23
  pathology 107.16–107.17
  severity classification 107.21
atopic hand eczema 128.2
atopic keratoconjunctivitis (AKC) 107.16, 107.17, 107.18, *107.19*–*107.20*, 107.21, 107.22
  with atopic eczema localised to eyelids *107.19*
  bacterial keratitis *107.19*
  inferior fornix and plical scarring *107.19*
  'polar bear rug' cataract *107.19*
  pseudogerontoxon *107.19*
  tarsal conjunctiva *107.19*
atopy 41.2, 41.23
  allergic contact dermatitis 127.10
  atopic eye disease 107.16–107.23
  Netherton syndrome 63.26
  obesity link 98.28
ATP *see* adenosine triphosphate; Africa Teledermatology Project
atrichia with papular lesions (APL) 87.28–87.29
atrophic morphoea, 'coup de sabre' paramedian form 94.21
atrophic parapsoriasis *see* large plaque parapsoriasis
atrophic photoageing 156.3, *156.4*
atrophic scars 94.13–94.15
atrophic skin
  Huriez syndrome 63.67
  rheumatoid arthritis 155.5
atrophic stria *94.8*
atrophie blanche
  chronic venous insufficiency **101.43**, *101.44*
  discoid lupus erythematosus *51.8*
  purpura 99.20–99.21
atrophies, ocular features **107.41**
atrophodermas 94.16–94.19
  follicular 94.16–94.17
  linear atrophoderma of Moulin 55.25–55.27, 73.22, 94.17
  of Pasini–Pierini 55.17, *55.19*, 94.18–94.19
  vermiculatum 85.11
atrophy of skin
  causes 94.6–94.21
  due to corticosteroids 94.6–94.9
  onchocerciasis 33.4
atropine-like drugs, hyperhidrosis treatment 92.9
attention-deficit hyperactivity disorder (ADHD) 63.6–63.7
ATTS *see* atypical trigeminal trophic syndrome
atypical adult-onset pityriasis rubra pilaris (type II) 36.2–36.4
atypical blotches, melanoma 145.7, *145.8*, 145.9
atypical decubitus fibroplasia 136.6
atypical dermal melanocytosis 73.21
atypical dots and globules, melanoma 145.7, *145.8*
atypical/dysplastic naevus syndrome 142.3–142.4
  see also dysplastic naevus syndrome
atypical fibrous histiocytoma 136.20, 136.21
atypical fibroxanthoma (AFX) 24.21, 136.22–136.23
atypical genital naevi, vulva 110.33
atypical intradermal smooth muscle neoplasm *see* leiomyosarcoma
atypical juvenile pityriasis rubra pilaris (type V) 36.4
atypical lipomatous tumour 136.58–136.59
atypical lymphocytes, chronic actinic dermatitis 126.14, *126.15*
atypical mycobacteria *see* non-tuberculous mycobacteria
atypical naevi (AN) **131.17**, 131.40–131.46
  clinical features 131.42–131.43
  dermoscopic images *131.44*–*131.45*
  disease course and prognosis 131.43
  epidemiology 131.41
  investigations 131.43
  management 131.43–131.46
  as melanoma precursors 142.2–142.3
  pathophysiology 131.41–131.42
  Spitz naevi **131.36**
atypical network patterns
  melanomas 145.7, *145.8*, *145.10*
  Spitz neavi 145.7
atypical (non-classical) epidermodysplasia verruciformis 25.66, 25.69
atypical post-radiation vascular lesion *see* atypical vascular proliferation after radiotherapy
atypical progeroid syndrome **72.5**
atypical smooth muscle tumour (dermal and subcutaneous type leiomyosarcoma) 136.54–136.55
atypical streaks, melanoma 145.7, *145.8*, 145.10
atypical trigeminal trophic syndrome (ATTS) *82.8*, *82.9*
atypical vascular lesions 103.32, 119.15
atypical vascular proliferation after radiotherapy (AVPRs) 136.38–136.39
atypical vascular structures/vessels, melanoma *145.8*, 145.9, 145.14
auricle (pinna) *see* ear, auricle

auricular haematoma 122.16
Auspitz sign, in psoriasis vulgaris *35.9*
Australia, skin cancer 6.1, 6.6, **6.7**
Austria, dermatology history 1.6
autoantibody screens, cutaneous photosensitivity diseases 126.6
autocrine factors, pigmentation regulation 86.5–86.7
autografts, burn wounds 125.5, 125.6
Autoimmune Bullous Disease Quality of Life (ABQOL) 108.8
autoimmune disorders
  acquired ichthyosis association 85.2
  APL association 98.4
  atopic eczema association 41.22
  bullous disease 85.30, 108.8
  dermatomyositis 52.1–52.13
  diabetic patients 62.4
  drug reaction with eosinophilia and systemic symptoms 118.11
  hair loss presentation 87.19–87.20, 87.22
  interstitial granulomatous dermatosis with musculoskeletal involvement 155.14
  involving respiratory system 152.2–152.3
  morphoea 55.7
  pregnancy 113.7–113.9
  skin and digestive system 153.3
  sweat glands 92.12
  urticaria association 42.3
  vitiligo association 86.35
autoimmune lymphoproliferative syndrome **72.11**, 80.14–80.15
autoimmune polyendocrinopathy Candida ectodermal dystrophy syndrome (APECED) 32.67
autoimmune polyendocrinopathy syndrome type 1 (APS-1) 87.20
autoimmune reactions, hair loss 87.74
autoimmunity
  in atopic eczema 41.12
  morphoea 55.8–55.9
autoimmunity defects, complement diseases 80.18–80.19
autoinflammation
  hidradenitis suppurativa 90.2–90.3
  panniculitis and dermatosis syndrome **72.11**
autoinflammation and PLCG2-associated antibody deficiency and immune dysregulation (APLAID) **45.5**, **45.7**, 45.12
autoinflammatory diseases with granuloma 45.11–45.12
  autoinflammation and PLCG2-associated antibody deficiency and immune dysregulation 45.12
autoinflammatory disorders 45.1–45.23, 80.17–80.18
  clinical features 45.1
  cutaneous manifestations **80.19**
  hereditary monogenic autoinflammatory syndromes 45.2–45.19
  urticarial or maculopapular rash 45.20–45.22
autoinflammatory granulomatosis of childhood (Blau syndrome) **45.5**, **45.7**, 45.11–45.12
autologous stem cell therapies 87.95
autonomic nervous system (ANS) 83.4–83.5
  adipose tissue 97.4
autosomal chromosome defects 74.1–74.3
  Behçet-like disease associated with trisomy 8 myelodysplasia 149.8
  chromosome 4, short-arm deletion syndrome 74.3
  chromosome 5, short-arm deletion syndrome 74.3
  chromosome 18, long-arm deletion syndrome 74.3
  Edwards syndrome (trisomy 18) 74.2
  Patau syndrome (trisomy 13) 74.2–74.3
  see also Down syndrome
autosomal dominant (AD) inheritance 8.3
autosomal dominant cutis laxa 77.5–77.6

autosomal dominant disorders
    disseminated superficial actinic
        porokeratosis   141.15–141.18
    Loeys-Dietz syndrome   141.42
    Muir–Torre syndrome   141.44–141.45
    multiple self-healing squamous
        epithelioma   141.41–141.42
autosomal dominant dystrophic
    epidermolysis bullosa   69.16
autosomal dominant epidermolysis bullosa
    simplex
    with migratory circinate redness
        69.9–69.10
    with mottled pigmentation   69.9
autosomal dominant familial partial
    lipodystrophy, AGL differentiation
    98.3
autosomal dominant IFAP2 syndrome
    63.25–63.26
autosomal dominant intermediate
    epidermolysis bullosa   69.15–69.16
autosomal dominant intermediate
    epidermolysis bullosa simplex
    69.8–69.9
    with cardiomyopathy   69.10
autosomal dominant lamellar ichthyoses
    (ADLI)   63.20–63.21
autosomal dominant localised epidermolysis
    bullosa simplex   69.8
autosomal dominant punctate porokeratosis
    63.59
autosomal dominant striate palmoplantar
    keratoderma   63.57
autosomal recessive agammaglobulinaemia
    80.5
autosomal recessive (AR) inheritance   8.3
autosomal recessive congenital ichthyosis
    (ARCI)   63.7–63.10
    management of   63.41, 63.44
autosomal recessive cutis laxa   77.6–77.7
autosomal recessive deafness, palmoplantar
    keratodermas   63.63
autosomal recessive dystrophic
    epidermolysis bullosa   69.16
autosomal recessive epidermolysis bullosa
    69.15–69.16
autosomal recessive epidermolysis bullosa
    simplex   69.10
    with BP230 deficiency   69.10
autosomal recessive ichthyosis with
    hypotrichosis (ARIH)   63.40
autosomal recessive intermediate
    epidermolysis bullosa simplex, with
    exophilin-5 deficiency   69.10–69.11
autosomal recessive localised epidermolysis
    bullosa simplex
    with exophilin-5 deficiency   69.10–69.11
    with muscular dystrophy   69.11
    with nephropathy   69.11
autosomal recessive mutations,
    erythrokeratoderma variabilis
    63.18
autosomal recessive PPK, gene mutations
    63.54
autosomal recessive severe epidermolysis
    bullosa simplex, with pyloric
    atresia   69.11
AVED see ataxia with vitamin E deficiency
avidin–biotin conjugate, immunoenzyme
    methods   3.15–3.16
avidin–biotin–peroxidase complex (ABC)
    method   3.16
AVM see arteriovenous malformations
AVPRs see atypical vascular proliferation
    after radiotherapy
axes of endocrine signalling   150.2
axilla
    abscess   90.4
    allergic contact dermatitis   127.16
    anti-p200 pemphigoid   50.41
    ectopic plaque   90.7
    hidradenitis suppurativa   88.38, 90.4
    microbiome   26.3, 26.4, 26.5
    staphylococcal scalded skin syndrome
        26.29

surgical treatment   90.11
axillary apocrine miliaria   92.19
axillary dermatitis, textile allergy   127.66
axillary fold, amicrobial pustulosis of the
    skin folds   49.20
axillary hair
    androgen-stimulated growth   87.10
    trichomycosis axillaris   26.41–26.42
axillary hyperhidrosis   92.3, 92.5–92.6
    management   92.9
    surgical treatment   92.10
axillary malodour   92.16–92.17
axillary skin
    childhood linear IgA disease   80.15
    microscopic examination of   3.33
    neurofibromatosis type 1   78.2
    pseudoxanthoma elasticum   70.32
azathioprine (AZA)   19.8–19.10
    atopic eczema treatment   41.29
    cautions   19.9
    contraindication   19.9
    dermatological uses   19.8
    dose and regimens   19.10
    drug–drug interactions   19.9
    monitoring   19.10
    pemphigus treatment   50.8
    pharmacological properties   19.8–19.9
    potential adverse effects   19.9
    pre-treatment screening   19.10
    systemic sclerosis treatment   54.24
azelaic acid
    acne vulgaris treatment   88.47
    chemical peels   160.2
    topical depigmenting agents   18.32
azo dyes   127.60, 127.61, 127.65–127.66

B
BA see benzyl alcohol; bioavailability
babies see infants; neonates
Baboon syndrome (BS)   **117.4**, 117.5, 121.6
BAC see benzalkonium chloride
bacillary angiomatosis   26.62, 26.64–26.65,
    109.28
bacille Calmette–Guérin (BCG)
    infection   27.1–27.4, 27.6, 27.11, *27.12*,
        80.8–80.9
    leprosy protection   28.16
    lupus vulgaris   27.23, *27.24*
    tuberculosis vaccination   5.3, 27.3–27.5,
        27.10–27.11, 27.20, 27.21, 27.25,
        27.27–27.29, 27.40, 80.8
    see also BCG vaccination
Bacillus anthracis   26.44–26.45
Bacillus cereus   26.44–26.45
Bacillus pyocyaneus see Pseudomonas
    infections, *P. aeruginosa / P. pyocyanea*
bacitracin   18.10
back
    acne conglobata   88.64
    acne fulminans   88.61
    acne-induced hyperpigmentation   88.41
    acne scarring   88.40
    acne vulgaris   88.27, 88.28
    annular erythema of infancy   47.10
    atopic eczema   41.17
    bullous pemphigoid   *50.17*, *50.18*, *50.20*
    diffuse cutaneous mastocytosis   46.6
    dysplastic naevus syndrome   131.41
    epidermolysis bullosa acquisita   50.45
    erythrodermic psoriasis   35.14
    linear morphoea   55.23
    naevus comedonicus   88.32
    pansclerotic morphoea   55.21
    pemphigus vulgaris   50.4
    pigmentary mosaicism   115.13
    pityrosporum folliculitis   88.37
    psoriasis vulgaris   35.8, 35.14
    roseola infantum   115.6
    spina bifida, tuft hair association   83.18
    steatocystoma multiplex   88.34
    subacute cutaneous lupus erythematosus
        51.15
    systemic lupus erythematosus   *51.23*,
        51.28
    systemic sclerosis   54.4

urticaria   *42.10*, *42.12*, *42.13*
bacteria
    adherence to the skin   26.5
    antibiotic resistance   18.11, 26.8
    dermatoses possibly attributable to
        infection   26.87–26.90
    molecular genetic identification methods
        26.2, 26.3
    normal skin microbiome   26.3–26.5
    possible role in chancriform pyoderma
        26.87–26.88
    sampling methods for skin microbes
        26.3
    temporary residents on skin   26.2
    see also microbial ecology of the skin; skin
        microbiome
bacterial antigen tests   4.24–4.25
bacterial arthropathies   155.4–155.5
bacterial colonisation, burn injuries
    125.9–125.10
bacterial decomposition, apocrine glands
    92.16
bacterial dysbiosis, lichen planus   37.3
bacterial infections   26.1–26.91
    actinomycetes   26.84–26.87
    anaerobic bacteria   26.67–26.69
    botryomycosis   26.76–26.77
    burn injuries   125.9
    chlamydiae   26.79
    ear piercing   106.11
    eyelids   107.38–107.39
    female genitalia   110.25–110.27
    gram-negative bacteria   26.49–26.67
    gram-positive bacteria   26.6–26.49
    HIV coinfection   31.20–31.22
    immunosuppressed renal allograft
        recipients   154.5
    legionellosis   26.79
    mycobacteria   27.1–27.46
    Mycoplasma   26.78–26.79
    necrotising subcutaneous infections
        26.77–26.78
    non-syphilitic sexually transmitted
        diseases   30.1–30.26
    opportunistic pathogens from skin   26.2,
        26.4, 26.17, 26.51, 26.55, 26.86
    perineal and perianal skin   111.13–111.15
    possible role in dermatoses   26.87–26.90
    protective role of normal skin flora
        26.4–26.5
    rickettsiae   26.80–26.84
    secondary to varicella   25.30
    skin defence mechanisms   26.5–26.6
    skin manifestations of primary
        immunodeficiencies   149.19
    spirochaetes   26.69–26.76, 109.27
    staphylococci and streptococci
        26.12–26.37
bacterial interference   26.6
bacterial isolates   90.3
bacterial panniculitis   97.47
bacterial pseudomycosis see botryomycosis
bacterial toxins
    diphtheria   26.38
    recurrent toxin-mediated perineal
        erythema   26.32
    scarlet fever   26.35
    streptococcal toxin-mediated disease
        26.35–26.37
Bacteroidaceae   26.67–26.68
Bacteroides   26.19, 26.67, 26.68, 26.78
    B. bacilliformis, Oroya fever and verruga
        peruana   26.65–26.66
    B. henselae, bacillary angiomatosis
        26.64–26.65
    cat scratch disease   26.62–26.64
BAD see British Association of
    Dermatologists
BADAS see bowel-associated
    dermatitis–arthritis syndrome
Bailey nylon monofilament   83.15
balanitis   109.4, 109.5
    Zoon balanitis   *109.14*
balanoposthitis   109.4–109.5
    non-specific balanoposthitis
        109.21–109.22

non-syphilitic spirochaetal ulcerative
    109.27
baldness cure, ancient Egypt   1.2
ballooning degeneration   3.40
balsam allergies   127.41–127.45
bandaging, lymphoedema therapy   103.58,
    103.59
band patterns, melanoma involving nail unit
    145.13
Bannayan–Riley–Ruvalcaba syndrome
    101.28
BAP-1 see BRCA1-associated protein
BAP1-inactivated melanocytic neoplasms
    (BIM), as melanoma precursor
    142.2
BAP1-inactivated naevus, scalp   *131.34*
BAP1 tumour suppressor gene, melanoma
    risk   142.4–142.5, 142.7
Barainelli–Seip syndrome see congenital
    generalised lipodystrophies
barber's hair sinus   122.22
Bardet–Biedel syndrome   **72.6**
baricitinib, atopic eczema treatment   41.30,
    41.31
Barmah Forest virus (BFV)   25.90–25.91
Barr body   8.7
barrier creams, allergic contact dermatitis
    127.35
Barrier dysfunction, ageing of skin
    156.10–156.11
Bartholin abscess
    chlamydia   30.11
    gonorrhoea   30.5
Bartholin cyst, vulval   110.31
Bartonella
    B. quintana, bacillary angiomatosis
        26.64–26.65
    infections   26.62–26.66
    trench fever   26.62
Bart–Pumphrey syndrome   63.64, 94.37
basal cell carcinoma (BCC)   140.1–140.21
    advanced/high risk disease   140.9,
        140.14, **140.15**, 140.16–140.17, 140.19
    ano-genital region   111.24
    auricle   106.21–106.27
        epidemiology   106.21–106.24
        management   106.26–106.27
        pathophysiology   106.25–106.26
    Bazex–Dupré–Christol syndrome
        140.20–140.21
    biopsy   3.4
    diagnosis   3.30, 3.31
    differential diagnosis   140.9–140.10
    drug/chemical photosensitivity   126.30
    epidemiology   140.1–140.2
    eyelid   107.47–107.48
    female genitalia   110.39
    histopathology   140.3, *140.4*
    immunocompromised people
        147.12–147.13, 147.16
    incidence of, in UK   6.1
    investigations   140.10, *140.11*, *140.12*,
        140.14
    lip   108.43–108.44
    male genitalia   109.42
    management   140.11–140.18
    margin assessment   140.14, **140.15**, 140.16
    Merkel cell carcinoma misdiagnosis
        146.5
    naevoid basal cell carcinoma syndrome
        140.3–140.4, 140.18–140.20
    pathophysiology   140.2–140.10
    photodynamic therapy   140.11,
        140.12–140.13
        contraindications   22.8
        Gorlin naevoid syndrome   22.2, 22.7
        superficial and thin nodular BCC
            22.6–22.7
    radiotherapy   24.12–24.13, *24.14*
        for ankylosing spondylitis as cause
            155.16
        indications   24.8–24.10
    risk factors   **140.2**
    risk stratification   140.11, **140.14**
    spectacle-frame acanthoma distinction
        122.14

basal cell carcinoma (BCC) (continued)
   superficial treatments 140.11, 140.12–140.14
   surgical treatments 140.14–140.16
   types 140.3
   see also keratinocyte cancer; naevoid basal cell carcinoma syndrome
basal cell papilloma see seborrhoeic keratosis
basal cells
   division of 2.44
   terminal differentiation 2.44
basal lamina 3.39
basaloid follicular hamartoma 137.12–137.13
Basan syndrome 63.66
base excision repair (BER) 10.6
baseline patch test series 127.29–127.30
basement-membrane region 122.4–122.5
basidiobolomycosis 32.79–32.80
Basidiobolus ranarum 32.79–32.80
basophilic, round tumour cell proliferations, Merkel cell carcinoma 146.3
basophilic amorphous deposits *97.61*
basophilic fat necrosis *97.8*
basosquamous (metatypical) basal cell carcinoma 140.3, 140.9
BAT see brown adipose tissue
Bateman purpura see actinic purpura
Bateman, Thomas 1.4
bathing, atopic eczema 41.26
'bathing cap' distribution, multivoltage X-ray techniques 24.3, *24.5*
bathing suit ichthyosis (BSI) 63.7, 63.8, 63.11
Bazex syndrome, ear dermatoses **106.22**
Bazex–Dupré–Christol syndrome **78.12**, 140.20–140.21
Bazin disease see erythema induratum of Bazin
BB-UVB see broad-band UVB
BCC see basal cell carcinoma
B-cell differentiation, lymphoid markers 3.29
B-cell directed biologic therapies 19.37–19.39
B-cell lymphoma
   external ear *106.34*
   radiotherapy 24.18
B-cell pseudolymphoma (lymphocytoma cutis) 134.1, 134.2, 134.8–134.10
B cells, immune system 9.6, 103.3
BCH see benign cephalic histiocytosis
BCS see brittle cornea syndrome
BD see Bowen disease
BDD see body dysmorphic disorder
BDI see Beck Depression Inventory
BDP see Bowen disease of the penis
BE see bioequivalence
beards
   pseudofolliculitis barbae 91.8, *91.9*, 122.23
   ringworm of the beard/tinea barbae 32.40–32.41
   sycosis 26.26–26.27
Beare–Stevenson syndrome 85.4
Beau lines 119.7, 119.8
becaplermin 18.39
Beck, Aaron T. 15.1–15.2
Beck Depression Inventory (BDI) 16.11
Becker melanosis, laser therapies 23.15–23.16
Becker naevus (or Becker melanosis) 73.18, 87.85, 87.86
Beckwith–Wiedemann syndrome *106.6*
bed bugs 34.25–34.29
   clinical features 34.27
   epidemiology 34.26
   management 34.27–28, *34.29*
   pathophysiology 34.26–27
'bed sores' 123.1
Beer's law, light absorption by skin 23.3
bees 34.16
Beetles (Coleoptera) 34.30–34.32
   allergenic species of 34.31–34.32

behaviour
   links to emotions and beliefs 15.1–15.3
   psychological factors in patients 15.2
Behçet disease see Adamantiades–Behçet disease
Behçet-like disease associated with trisomy 8 myelodysplasia 149.8
Behçet-like disease or inflammatory bowel disease-like autoinflammatory syndromes 45.15–45.16
Beighton score **70.8**
bejel (endemic syphilis) 26.70
beliefs
   links to emotions and behaviours 15.1–15.3
   psychological factors in patients 15.2–15.3
belimumab 51.12
Bell palsy 25.23
Belostomatidae (giant water bugs) 34.30
benign adnexal lesions, eyelid 107.45
benign calcifying epithelioma of Malherbe see pilomatricoma
benign cephalic histiocytosis (BCH) 135.17–135.18
benign cutaneous adverse reactions to drugs 117.1–117.9
benign cutaneous tumours and proliferations
   photothermal ablation 23.21
   see also capillary haemangiomas
benign cysts, eyelid 107.45–107.47
benign essential telangiectasia see hereditary benign telangiectasia
benign fibrous cutaneous nodules 94.43
benign keratinocytic acanthomas 132.1–132.8
   clear cell acanthoma 132.6–132.7
   dermatosis papulosa nigra 132.4–132.5
   lichenoid keratosis 132.7–132.8
   seborrhoeic keratosis 132.1–132.4
   stucco keratosis 132.4
   warty dyskeratoma 132.5–132.6
   see also inverted follicular keratosis
benign lesions
   dermoscopic patterns of naevi 145.1–145.7
   ear 106.33
   eyelid 107.44–107.47
benign lymphangioendothelioma 103.29
benign lymphoid proliferations see pseudolymphoma
benign melanocytic naevi, in pregnancy 113.9
benign nodular calcification 154.2
   see also metastatic cutaneous calcification
benign papillomatosis of the nipple see nipple, adenoma
benign proliferations 132.1–132.10
   benign keratinocytic acanthomas 132.1–132.8
   pseudoepitheliomatous hyperplasia 132.9–132.10
   skin tags 132.8–132.9
benign symmetrical lipomatosis (BSL) 98.15–98.17, *103.46*
benign tumours, male genitalia 109.29–109.31
benign vascular tumours 136.25–136.32
   classification **116.1**
benzalkonium chloride (BAC) 127.57
   topical therapies 18.10
1,2-Benzisothiazolin-3-one (BIT) 127.53, 127.54
benzo(a)pyrene *129.15*
benzocaine, patch testing 127.47
benzothiazole contact allergy 127.64
benzoyl peroxide (BPO) 88.46, 88.47
benzyl alcohol (BA) 127.58
BER see base excision repair
beriberi, vitamin B1 deficiency 61.14
Berloque dermatitis 86.28–86.30
beryllium, dermatological reactions 121.9
best evidence, evidence based medicine 17.4–17.8
β-adrenergic blockers, burn treatment 125.14

β-Carotene therapy 126.8
β rays 24.1
   see also electron beam therapy
beta-lactam allergy 117.7
beta-mannosidosis, glycoproteinoses 79.3
betamethasone, dose-vasoconstriction response profiles for *12.5*
betel nut chewing
   oral hyperpigmentation 108.17
   oral lichen planus 37.3
   oral squamous cell carcinoma 108.46
   teeth staining *108.15*
bexarotene 18.25
BFLS see Börjeson–Forssman–Lehmann syndrome
BFS see burning feet syndrome
BFV see Barmah Forest virus
BHA see butylated hydroxyanisole
BHD see Birt–Hogg–Dubé
bias
   Cochrane Collaborations risk of bias tool 17.9
   epidemiological studies 5.14
   types of bias in research studies 17.9–17.10
Bible, leprosy 1.3
'bib-sign', redness on chest in dermatomyositis 52.4, *52.6*
bicalutamide 87.96
Biett, Laurent 1.4–1.5
bilateral lymphoedema, lower legs *98.27*
bilharziasis see schistosomiasis
biliary tract disease 153.5
bilirubin 86.49
BIM see BAP1-inactivated melanocytic neoplasms
bimatoprost 18.39
bimekizumab
   psoriasis treatment 35.30
   psoriatic arthritis treatment 35.46
bioavailability (BA)
   clinical pharmacology 13.2–13.3, **13.2**
   of topical drugs 12.7–12.8
biobanking 8.1
biochemical functions, mechanical forces 122.1
biocides, formaldehyde-releasing 127.51–127.52
biodegradable dermal fillers 158.3–158.7
bioequivalence (BE), of topical drugs 12.7–12.8
biological dosimetry 10.2
biological elasticity 122.5
biologic registries, psoriasis treatment 35.29
biologic therapies 19.31–19.34
   atopic eczema 41.29–41.30, **41.31**, **41.32**
   C1-esterase inhibitor replacement therapy 19.39
   clinical pharmacology 13.1, 13.2
   definition 13.1
   directed against B-cells 19.37–19.39
   directed against cytokines 19.32–19.37
   eye, side effects on 107.44
   hidradenitis suppurativa 90.10, 90.11
   intravenous immunoglobulins 19.31, 19.40–19.41
   monoclonal antibodies (mAbs) 19.31–19.32
   morphoea 55.38–55.42
   omalizumab 19.39
   in pregnancy 113.21, **113.22**
   psoriasis treatment 35.27–35.31
   pyoderma gangrenosum 49.7
biomarkers 8.8–8.9
   prenatal testing and diagnosis *8.11*
biomechanical properties of skin 122.5–122.6
biomedical literature, evidence based medicine 17.2
biopsy of skin 3.2–3.10
   AIDs patients 3.38
   alopecia 3.7
   artefacts due to poor technique 3.31–3.32
   basal cell carcinoma 3.4
   blocking of specimens 3.6, 3.32

curettage 3.3–3.4
cysts 3.31
Darier disease *3.39*
direct immunofluorescence studies 3.12, 3.17
division of specimen 3.2, 3.4
electron microscopy 3.4
elliptical surgical biopsy 3.3, 3.6
epidermolysis bullosa diagnosis 69.20–69.21, 69.23
excisional biopsy 3.2
fetal skin 8.10
fixatives 3.4, **3.5**, 3.32
frozen sections 3.5
histochemistry 3.7–3.10
histological sections with little or no abnormality 3.44–3.45
identification labels 3.5
inadequate biopsy 3.1
inclusional/exclusional elliptical biopsies 20.8–20.9
indications for **3.2**
information provided with specimen 3.4
instruments for 3.3
interpretation problems 3.1
labelling of specimen 3.6
laboratory methods 3.5–3.10
little or no abnormality in histological sections 3.44–3.45
local anaesthetic 3.2
melanoma 143.1, 143.4–143.5
Michel medium 3.4–3.5, 3.12
microscopic examination of tissue sections 3.32–3.38
multiple biopsies 3.2
needle biopsy 3.4
painting margins of specimen 3.5–3.6
palm skin 3.33
photocopy procedure, blocking of specimens 3.6
planning 20.8–20.9
punch biopsy 3.3, 20.9–20.10
request form 3.4
retention of tissue specimens 3.6
section types 3.38
shave biopsy 3.4, 20.10–20.11
site selection 3.2, *3.12*
skin surface 4.22
sole skin 3.33
specimen preparation 3.4–3.7
squamous cell carcinoma 3.4
staining techniques 3.7–3.10
techniques 3.2, 3.3–3.4, 20.8–20.11
tissue processing 3.7
topical anaesthetic 3.2–3.3
transport media 3.4–3.5, **3.5**
urticaria 3.45
urticaria pigmentosa 3.2
see also histopathology of skin
biosimilars, psoriasis treatment 35.29
biotin
   deficiency 61.22–61.24
   metabolism disorders 79.15
   see also avidin–biotin conjugate
bipolar disorder 84.40
Bipolaris species 32.78
Birbeck granules 135.2
birthmarks
   naevus flammeus *101.10*
   see also naevi
birth weight, acne association 88.26
Birt–Hogg–Dubé (BHD) syndrome **78.14**, *78.15*
   differential diagnosis 88.30–88.31
   lesions of hair follicle mesenchyme 137.15–137.16
   pulmonary involvement 152.5
   renal/skin involvement 154.2
   skin tags 132.8
BIT see 1,2-Benzisothiazolin-3-one
bites 130.5–130.8
   animal bite injuries on infants/children 130–136, 115.14
   arthropods 14.2, 34.2–34.3, **34.4**, 34.14–34.15

by humans 130.6–130.7
clinical features 34.8–34.9
dogs/cats 130.6
infants 115.14
rodents 130.5
snakes 130.5–130.6
black death 26.59–26.60
blackflies 34.7
onchocerciasis vector 33.1, 33.2, *33.3*
Blackfoot disease 121.3
black hairy tongue 108.16, *108.17*
black heel/palm 99.6, 122.10–122.11, 122.16
black piedra 32.15–32.16
black rubber mix (sensitisers) **127.63**
black skin *see* skin of colour
blanchable redness 123.4
Blaschko lines 8.7, *8.8*
congenital epidermal naevi 73.5
Conradi–Hünermann–Happle syndrome 63.22
hypomelanosis of Ito 68.10
incontinentia pigmenti 68.11
keratinopathic ichthyoses 63.14
keratosis follicularis spinosa decalvans 63.24
linear and whorled hypermelanosis 68.12
Blashkoid lesions 4.16, *4.19*
blastic plasmacytoid dendritic cell neoplasm (CD4+/CD56+haematodermic neoplasm) 139.45–139.47
Blastomyces dermatitidis 32.85–32.86
blastomycosis 32.84–32.86, 109.28
oral lesions 108.57
Blau syndrome (autoinflammatory granulomatosis of childhood) **45.5**, *45.7*, 45.11–45.12
bleeding, complications after skin surgery 20.40–20.42
bleeding in skin and mucosa (purpura/petechiae/ecchymoses/epistaxis/gingival bleeding), liver disease association 153.9
Blegvad–Haxthausen syndrome 94.24
bleomycin, topical therapies 18.29–18.30
bleomycin-induced flagellate hyperpigmentation 119.8–119.9
blepharitis 107.7–107.15
associated skin disease **107.8**
causes *107.12*, 107.13
classification of chronic blepharitis **107.8**
complications and co-morbidities 107.13
conjunctival and corneal signs **107.8**
cutaneous *Leishmania* infection of eyelid *107.12*
demodex folliculorum infestation 107.10
diagnosis **107.13**
disease course and prognosis 107.13–107.14
eyelid signs **107.8**
incidence and prevalence 107.7–107.10
investigations 107.14
management 107.14–107.15
meibomian seborrhoea **107.8**
meibomitis **107.8**
ocular rosacea **107.8**, **107.10**, 107.11–107.12
pathology 107.10–107.12
Phthirus pubis causation *107.12*
predisposing factors 107.10
sebaceous carcinoma of eyelid *107.12*
seborrhoeic blepharitis **107.8**
staphylococcal blepharitis **107.8**, *107.9*, 107.10
symptoms **107.8**
treatment of chronic blepharitis **107.14**
ulcerative blepharitis *107.9*
blepharochalasis 94.26–94.27, 107.5
blepharoconjunctivitis *107.6*
blinding filariasis *see* onchocerciasis
blistering disorders 69.1–69.28
drug/chemical photosensitivity *126.29*
heat-associated diseases 124.15, *124.16*
internal malignancy association 148.22
juvenile springtime eruption 126.9
mechanical injuries 122.6, 122.8, 122.9–122.10, 122.16
PUVA phototherapy adverse effects 21.13
Stevens–Johnson syndrome/toxic epidermal necrolysis *118.14–118.15*
Tzanck smear 3.29
UVB phototherapy adverse effects 21.12
see also bullous diseases; paraneoplastic pemphigus; pemphigus
blistering distal dactylitis 26.34, 115.8
blisters
friction 122.6, 122.9–122.10
on the lips 108.60
oral ulceration **108.36**
'string of pearls' ring pattern *4.8*
vesicating beetles 34.30–34.31
Bloch, Bruno 127.1
blocking techniques, biopsy 3.6
blood eosinophilia 93.7, 93.9
blood-letting 1.3
blood supply, cones 124.8
blood tryptase, raised level of
mastocytosis 46.8
in patient without skin lesions **46.6**, *46.7*
blood vessels 2.40–2.42
anatomy of head and neck 20.1–20.2
Bloom syndrome **75.2**, **77.2**, 77.3–77.4, **78.13**, **80.5**, 148.12, 148.13
hyperpigmentation 80.11
blueberry muffin baby (dermal erythropoiesis) 114.21
blue-black lesions, melanoma 145.14
blue light therapy, acne vulgaris 88.58
blue naevus 3.44, **131.17**, 131.38–131.40
cellular **131.39**, *131.40*
common blue naevus *131.38*
congenital 73.15, *73.16*
dermoscopic image *131.40*
see also malignant blue naevus
blue rubber bleb naevus syndrome (BRBN) 71.2, 71.17–71.18, 136.42
blue toe syndrome *see* cholesterol embolus
blue-white veil, melanoma 145.7, *145.8*, 145.10
blushing 104.1–104.13
clinical presentation *104.10*
epidemiology 104.1
investigations 104.11
management 104.12
physiology 104.1
psychosocial aspects 104.2–104.3
typical distribution *104.2*
BMI *see* body mass index
BMPs *see* bone morphogenic proteins
BMS *see* burning mouth syndrome
BMZ *see* dermal–epidermal basement membrane zone
BNPD *see* 2-Bromo-2-nitropropane-1, 3-diol
body art 108.15–108.16
body/clothing lice 34.23–34.24
body contouring 161.8–161.9
body dysmorphic disorder (BDD) 84.12–84.15
and acne 88.30
by proxy 84.14
complaints and litigation 84.15
dislike of mole and freckles 84.26
male genitalia 109.6, 109.44
olfactory delusions 84.10
scales and screening questions **84.13**
body image 15.1
body mass index (BMI), and acne 88.19
body odour, olfactory delusions 84.10–84.11
Bohan and Peter classification, dermatomyositis 52.1
boils *see* carbuncles; furuncles
Bolivian haemorrhagic fever 25.82–25.83
bone disorders
diffuse lymphangiomatosis involving bone 136.39
Langerhans cell histiocytosis 135.8
systemic lupus erythematosus 51.30
bone dysplasia, nail–patella syndrome 67.15
bone marrow, mastocytosis 46.3, *46.4*, 46.8, *46.9*
bone marrow failure, dyskeratosis congenita 67.14–67.15
bone marrow transplantation
mastocytosis treatment 46.10
oral complications of 108.48
bone metastases, metastatic calcinosis cutis 59.5
bone morphogenic proteins (BMPs) 2.3, 2.4
bone scintigraphy, frostbite investigation 124.2
bony abnormalities, epidermolysis bullosa 69.26
borderline leprosy (BL/BB/BT) 28.2–28.3, 28.4, 28.6, 28.8, *28.9*, 28.10, 28.11, 28.13, *28.14*
Börjeson–Forssman–Lehmann syndrome (BFLS) **72.6**
Borrelia 26.72–26.74
B. afzelii 26.72, 26.73, 94.15–94.16
B. garinii 26.72, 26.73
B. recurrentis, louse-borne epidemic relapsing fever 26.72
Lyme disease 26.72–26.73
necrobiotic xanthogranuloma 97.17
Borrelia burgdorferi
complex of species 26.72
infective panniculitis 97.46
possible cutaneous B-cell lymphoma link 139.37–139.38
borreliosis 94.15–94.16
bosentan 124.12
botryomycosis 26.76–26.77
Botswana–UPENN partnership 7.7
botulinum toxin
aesthetic uses of 159.1–159.9
acetylcholine release blocking *159.2*
acquired resistance to botulinum toxins 159.8
adverse events 159.6–159.8
combination treatment 159.8
ethnic diversity and botulinum toxins 159.6
future botulinum toxins in development 159.8–159.9
history of clinical applications 159.2
history and early research 159.1–159.2
lower face 159.5–159.6
mid face 159.5
neck 159.6
side effects summary **159.7**
upper face 159.4–159.5
characteristics of **159.3**
clinical applications of for aesthetic conditions 159.3–159.6
eye, side effects on 107.44
pharmaceutical terminology **159.1**
pharmacology and action of neurotoxins 159.2–159.3
variation and equivalence 159.3
botulinum toxin A injection, hyperhidrosis treatment 92.9
botulism 159.1
Bouchard nodes 155.8
Bourneville disease *see* tuberous sclerosis complex
boutonneuse fever 26.82–26.83
bovine collagen dermal filler 158.5, 158.7–158.8
bowel-associated dermatitis–arthritis syndrome (BADAS) 49.15–49.17, 97.52, 153.3–153.4
acute inflammatory distal arthritis 49.16
clinical features 49.15–49.16
episcleritis 49.17
investigations 49.16
lesion appearance *49.16*
management 49.16–49.17
pathology 49.15
predisposing factors 49.15
pustules on trunk *49.16*
urticarial plaques *49.16*
bowel carcinoma, colostomy for *112.5*
bowel disease, dermatoses associated with 112.12–112.15
Bowen disease (BD) 141.18–141.24, *141.25*
and actinic keratoses, immunocompromised people 147.11–147.12
discoid skin lesions **39.10**
epidemiology 141.18
first line treatments 141.22–141.24
male genitalia 109.31–109.34
management 141.22–141.24, *141.25*
pathophysiology 141.18–141.22, *141.25*
perianal skin 111.20–111.21
photodynamic therapy 22.6
photothermal ablation 23.21
radiotherapy 24.14
second/third line treatments 141.24
see also anal/perianal/genital intraepithelial carcinomas; *in situ* carcinoma of the skin
Bowen disease of the penis (BDP) 109.31–109.34
bowenoid papulosis
Bowen disease comparison 141.19, 141.20–141.21, *141.22*
human papilloma virus 141.21
male genitalia 109.31–109.34
see also anal/perianal/genital intraepithelial carcinomas
box jellyfish stings 130.1–130.2
BP230 *see* bullous pemphigoid antigen
BP230 deficiency, autosomal recessive epidermolysis bullosa simplex with 69.10
BP *see* bullous pemphigoid
BPO *see* benzoyl peroxide
BRAC1-associated protein (BAP-1), germline mutations in 3.24
brachioradial pruritus (BRP) 81.12, 83.6–83.7
Brachycera (biting flies) 34.8
brachytherapy 24.3
bradykinin-induced angio-oedema 43.1, **43.2**, *43.3*, **43.6**
BRAF inhibitors
causing keratoacanthoma 141.38, 141.41
melanoma systemic therapy 144.4–144.5, *144.11*, **144.11**, 144.12
BRAF mutations, lobular capillary haemangioma/pyogenic granuloma within port-wine stains 136.26
BRAF-positive tumours 85.9
BRAF therapy *see* B-rapidly accelerated fibrosarcoma protein inhibitor therapy
BRAF V600E mutation
Erdheim–Chester disease 135.21
histiocytoses 135.3, 135.7, 135.9
juvenile xanthogranuloma 135.16
brain metastases 144.7
brain–skin axis
neuroendocrine stress response in skin 150.8–150.9
psychological factors in patients 15.2
branchial cyst 106.4
branchio-oto-renal syndrome 106.4, **106.7**
B-rapidly accelerated fibrosarcoma protein (BRAF) inhibitor therapy 85.23
Brazilian haemorrhagic fever 25.82–25.83
BRBN *see* blue rubber bleb naevus syndrome
breast
abscess, neonatal 114.25
diffuse dermal angiomatosis *4.11*
lymphangiomatous papules, benign *103.32*
lymphoedema 103.43–103.44
melanocytic naevi 131.22
morphoea 55.18
pansclerotic morphoea 55.21
swollen 103.43–103.44
breast cancer
breast lymphoedema 103.44
carcinoma telangiectatica on arm *103.15*

breast cancer (*continued*)
  radiotherapy side effects 119.15
  recurrent cellulitis in lymphoedema 103.14
  skin involvement 148.2–148.3
breastfeeding, and atopic eczema 41.7, 41.23
breast surgery, Mondor disease after 101.37
breathing exercises, lymphoedema 103.59
BRESEK/BRESHEK syndrome 63.24–63.25
Breslow thickness, melanomas 142.2, 142.8, 142.15–142.16, 142.21, 142.22, 142.24
Brevibacterium mcbrellneri, synergistic role with *Trichosporon* yeast in white piedra 32.16
Brief Symptom Inventory (BSI) 16.11
Brill–Zinsser disease 26.81
brimonidine 18.39
Britain, dermatology history 1.6–1.7
British Association of Dermatologists (BAD) 7.14
brittle cornea syndrome (BCS) **70.6–70.7**, 70.10
broad-band UVB (BB-UVB) phototherapy
  carcinogenesis risk 21.13
  efficacy 21.3–21.4, 21.7
  principles 21.1, 21.2
Brocq's acné excoriée 84.20–84.22
brodalumab
  psoriasis treatment 35.30
  psoriatic arthritis treatment 35.46
bromhidrosis 92.16–92.17
bromides, acneform reaction 88.13
bromidrosiphobia *see* olfactory delusions
2-bromo-2-nitropropane-1, 3-diol (BNPD) 127.52
bronchial epithelium, SJS/TEN involvement 118.20
bronchiolitis obliterans 118.17
bronchopneumonia, inhalation injury 125.4–125.5
bronchopulmonary injuries 125.5
bronze baby syndrome 86.49–86.50
Brooke's tumour *see* trichoepithelioma
Brooke–Spiegler syndrome
  cylindroma 137.30
  spiradenoma 137.31
  trichoepithelioma 137.10
brown adipose tissue (BAT) 72.1
brown fat 97.1–97.2
brown fat hypertrophy 98.15
brown pseudoscars, diabetic dermopathy 94.14
brown recluse spiders (Sicariidae) 34.35–34.36
brown tongue 108.16
brows
  botulinum toxin use 159.5
  see also eyebrows
BRP *see* brachioradial pruritus
Brucella 26.60–26.62
brucellosis 26.60–26.62
bruises/bruising *see* ecchymosis
Brunsting–Perry pemphigoid 50.51–50.52, 50.53
Bruton disease (X-linked agammaglobulinaemia) **80.5**, 80.13
Bryozoa, stings from 130.4
BS *see* Baboon syndrome
BSI *see* bathing suit ichthyosis; Brief Symptom Inventory; Burma Skincare Initiative
BSL *see* benign symmetrical lipomatosis
BSLE *see* bullous systemic lupus erythematous
bubble hair 87.77–87.78
buboes *see* inguinal buboes; lymphadenitis
bubonic plague 26.59–26.60
Bubostumum phlebotomum see cutaneous larva migrans
buccal fat-pad herniation 108.10
buccal mucosa
  cheek biting 108.32

epidermolysis bullosa acquista *50.45*
erythroplakia *108.24*
examination of 108.7
Fordyce spots *108.29*
homogeneous leukoplakia *108.34*
leiomyoma 108.13
leukoedema *108.29, 108.30*
lichen planus *37.5, 37.6, 108.76*
sarcoidosis 108.67
see also cheek
Buddhist texts 1.2–1.3
Buerger test, peripheral vascular disease 101.3
buffalo hump, HIV-associated lipodystrophy 98.7
bugs (Hemiptera) 34.25–34.30
bulbar telangiectasia 80.11
bulge region, hair follicle 87.4
bulimia nervosa 84.26–84.27
Bulkley, Henry D. 1.7
bullae 3.39
bullous dermatoses 4.8
  IP differential diagnosis 68.11
bullous diseases
  autoimmune, assessment 108.8
  diagnosis 3.11, 3.29, 3.30
  digestive system 153.6
  direct immunofluorescence *3.18*
  ear dermatoses **106.22**
  electron microscopy studies 3.30, 69.21–69.22
  female genitalia 110.20, **110.21**
  flexural sites **4.18**
  internal malignancy association 148.21–148.22
  microscopic appearance 3.29
  renal failure and dialysis complications 154.4
bullous eruptions, reactions to COVID-19 vaccines 25.118
bullous impetigo 2.19, 26.13–26.15
  neonates 114.24
bullous lesions, autoinflammatory diseases **80.19**
bullous lichen planus 37.8–37.9, 37.17
bullous lupus erythematosus 51.28–51.29
bullous pemphigoid (BP) 50.10–50.22, 148.22
  acute oedema blisters 85.30
  age of onset 50.11
  antigens 69.4, 69.5, **69.8**, 69.10
  associated diseases 50.11
  autoantibodies 50.11–50.12
  blisters, erosions, and haemorrhagic crusts *50.11, 50.16*
  cellular immune response 50.12
  in childhood *50.20*
  clinical features 50.15–50.16
  clinical variants 50.16–50.17
  cytokines and chemokines 50.12
  diagnosis 50.20, *50.21*, **50.22**, *50.24*
  differential diagnosis 50.17–50.18
  direct immunofluorescence microscopy *50.14*
  disease course and prognosis 50.18–50.19
  epidemiology 50.10–50.11
  genetics 50.15
  histopathology 50.13
  investigations 50.20, *50.21*, **50.22**
  localised bullous pemphigoid 50.17, *50.19*
  management 50.20–50.22
  oral involvement 108.81–108.82
  papule appearance *50.17*
  pathogenic mechanisms 50.12–50.13
  pathophysiology 50.11–50.13
  predisposing factors 50.13
  randomised controlled trials 50.20–50.21, **50.23**
  renal effects 154.6
  serum autoantibodies 50.14–50.15
    serological screening *50.14, 50.15*
  severity classification 50.18
  tissue-bound autoantibodies 50.13–50.14

treatment guidelines 50.21–50.22
urticarial and erythematous plaques *50.18*
vulval **110.21**
bullous porphyrias
  histopathology 58.4–58.5
  samples for laboratory testing 58.7
  typical subepidermal bulla in *58.6*
bullous pyoderma gangrenosum 49.4–49.5
bullous systemic lupus erythematous (BSLE) 50.48–50.51
  blisters on erythematosus *50.49*
  differential diagnosis 50.50
  epidemiology 50.48–50.49
  investigations and diagnosis 50.50
  management 50.50–50.51
  pathophysiology 50.49
  presentation 50.49–50.50
  serum autoantibodies *50.50*
  treatment ladder 50.51
  violaceous maculae *50.50*
Bunyaviruses, haemorrhagic fevers 25.83–25.84
buprenorphine, addiction prevalence 120.2
burden of skin disease 5.5, 5.6–5.7, 5.8, 5.9
Bureau–Barrière syndrome 63.71
Burkholderia 26.53–26.55
  B. mallei, glanders 26.55
  B. pseudomallei, melioidosis 26.53–26.54
Burkitt lymphoma 25.38
Burma Skincare Initiative (BSI) 7.11
burn depth
  assessment of 125.2
  clinical appearances **125.3**
  evaluation of 125.5–125.8
burning feet syndrome (BFS) 83.10–83.11
burning mouth syndrome (BMS) 82.1–82.3, 108.64–108.65, 127.18
  causes **108.64**
  epidemiology 82.2
  management 82.3
  pathophysiology 82.2–82.3
burning sensation, irritation 128.10–128.12
burns 125.1–125.15
  first-degree burns 125.5
  grafts 11.12
  hospital care 125.1
  oral lesions 108.31
  shock 125.2–125.4
Burton's lead line 121.5
Buruli ulcer 97.47
  genital 109.28
Buschke disease *see* scleroedema
Buschke–Löwenstein tumour
  male genitalia 109.39–109.40
  perianal skin 111.23
Buschke–Ollendorff syndrome 94.43
butterflies (Lepidoptera) 34.32–34.34
butterfly erythema pattern on face, dermatomyositis 52.3, *52.5*
butterfly sign (mid-back sparing), nodular prurigo 84.15
buttock
  bullous pemphigoid *50.16*
  capillary malformations 71.5
  cryoglobulinaemic vasculitis 100.16
  dermatitis herpetiformis *50.57*
  eruptive xanthomas *60.4*
  hemihyperplasia–multiple lipomatosis syndrome 72.11
  herpes simplex *4.8*
  linear IgA disease *50.37*
  morphoea *55.16*
  mucous membrane pemphigoid *50.29*
  necrolytic migratory erythema *47.15*
butylated hydroxyanisole (BHA) 127.59

C

C&C (curettage and cautery) *see* curettage and electrodessication
C1-esterase inhibitor (C1-INH) deficiency, angio-oedema due to 43.1, 43.4, 43.5–43.6
C1-esterase inhibitor (C1INH) replacement therapy 19.39

C3 nephritic factor, APL pathology 98.4
cacosmia *see* olfactory delusions
CACP (camptodactyly, arthropathy, coxa vara, pericarditis) syndrome 94.40–94.41
CAD *see* chronic actinic dermatitis; computer-aided diagnostic systems
CADIS *see* Childhood Atopic Dermatitis Impact Scale
CADM *see* clinically amyopathic dermatomyositis
café-au-lait macules (CALMs) 78.3, **131.1**
café-au-lait patches, laser therapies 23.15, *23.16*
caffeine
  cosmeceutical use of 157.11
  rosacea risk 89.3
  topical therapies 18.39
CAG repeats, hirsutism 87.88
CAH *see* congenital adrenal hyperplasia
CaHa *see* calcium hydroxylapatite
CAIN *see* CCAAT enhancer binding protein ε-associated autoinflammation and immune impairment of neutrophils
Calabar swellings *see* loiasis
calcaneal petechiae 122.16
calcification, lupus panniculitis 97.38
calcification of blood vessels *see* calciphylaxis
calcification of skin and subcutaneous tissues 59.1–59.10
  calciphylaxis 59.6–59.9
  dystrophic calcification 59.1–59.4
  idiotrophic calcification 59.4–59.5
  metastatic calcification 59.5–59.6
  secondary to trauma or injection/infusion of calcium-containing materials 59.3
  secondary to tumours and genetic disease 59.3–59.4
calcific panniculitis 154.2
  see also metastatic cutaneous calcification
calcific uraemic arteriolopathy *see* calciphylaxis
calcified cutaneous nodules of the heels, infants 115.15
calcifying aponeurotic fibroma 136.7–136.8
calcifying epithelioma of Malherbe (benign) *see* pilomatricoma
calcifying fibrous tumours/pseudotumours 136.7
calcifying nodules, ear dermatoses **106.22**, *106.24*
calcifying panniculitis *see* calciphylaxis
calcineurin inhibitors
  atopic eczema treatment 41.27
  mastocytosis treatment 46.10
  psoriasis treatment 35.22
  topical therapies 18.22–18.26, 41.27
calcinosis
  dermatomyositis 52.6
  systemic sclerosis 54.3, 54.17, **54.26**
  see also calcification of skin and subcutaneous tissues
calcinosis, scrotal 59.4, *59.5*, 109.30
calciphylaxis 59.6–59.9, 97.32–97.35, 99.23, 154.2, *154.3*
  penile 109.24
calcipotriol 18.28–18.29
calcitriol 18.28
calcium-containing injections/infusions 59.3
calcium enhancement indirect technique 3.14
calcium homeostasis, systemic abnormalities 59.5–59.6
calcium hydroxylapatite (CaHa) dermal filler 158.5, 158.6–158.7
calcium pump disorders 69.23–69.24
calibre-persistent artery, lip lesions 108.63
callosities 122.7–122.9
calluses 122.7–122.9, 122.16
CALMs *see* café-au-lait macules
calpains 94.38
calpastatin (*CAST*), skin fragility disorders 69.6

calponin 3.25
Calymmatobacterium granulomatis see Klebsiella granulomatis
Cambodia, clinical officer training 7.7–7.8
camouflage options
  alopecia 87.18, 87.69, 87.97–87.101
  hair disorders 87.101
camphor 18.38
camptodactyly 94.40–94.41
camptodactyly, arthropathy, coxa vara, pericarditis (CACP) syndrome 94.40–94.41
camptodactyly, tall stature and hearing loss (CATSHL) 94.40
CA-MRSA *see* community-acquired MRSA
CAMs *see* cellular adhesion molecules
Canada, psoriasis, economic burden of 6.8
Canale–Smith syndrome *see* autoimmune lymphoproliferative syndrome
cancer
  ectodermal dysplasias 69.18, 69.26–69.27
  hypermelanosis association 86.19, 86.20
  morphoea 55.7
  oral cancer 108.43–108.50
  palmoplantar keratodermas and 63.65–63.68
  photodynamic therapy 22.2
  radiotherapy principles 24.1–24.24
  systemic sclerosis 54.9–54.10
  urticaria association 42.3
cancer phobia 84.26
cancer-related lymphoedema 103.37–103.38
cancer risk, atopic eczema association 41.21–41.22
cancer treatment
  cutaneous side effects 119.1–119.15
  hair loss 87.71–87.74
Candida
  allergy 32.67
  antigen test 4.24
  classification 32.55
  colonisation sites in body 32.56–32.57
  cutaneous carriage 32.56
  identification 32.58–32.60
  intertrigo 32.63
  onychomycosis 32.66
  paronychia 32.65–32.66
  see also candidiasis
Candida albicans
  biology 32.55, 32.56
  identification 32.58–32.59
  versus other *Candida* species 32.55, 32.56
Candida infection
  hyper-IgE syndrome due to STAT3 loss of function mutations 80.17
  infants 115.8
  male genitalia 109.5, 109.11, 109.27
  peristomal skin 112.8, 112.9
  pustular psoriasis 118.4
candidal balanitis 32.64
candidal stomatitis *see* acute pseudomembranous candidiasis
candidal vulvo-vaginitis 110.27–110.28
candidiasis/candidosis 32.55–32.69
  biology 32.56–32.57
  chronic mucocutaneous candidiasis 80.17
  chronic oro-perineal candidiasis 80.7
  congenital candidiasis 114.28
  endocrine factors 32.58
  histology 32.60
  HIV/AIDS 31.6, 31.26, 31.34, 31.37, 32.58
  host factors 32.57–32.58
  identification 32.58–32.59
  immunological factors 32.58
  infants 32.65
  management 32.60–32.61
  nails and paronychium 32.65–32.66
  neonatal 114.28
  oral lesions 108.20–108.22, 108.31–108.32, 108.34, 108.57, 108.71
  oral mucous membranes 32.61–32.63
  organisms 32.55, 32.57
  pathophysiology 32.57–32.58
  penile 109.27
  perineal and perianal skin 111.15

in pregnancy 113.7
skin and genital mucous membranes 32.63–32.65
systemic 32.92–32.93
types of 108.57
CANDLE *see* chronic atypical neutrophilic dermatosis with lipodystrophy and elevated temperature
canities (hair greying) 87.91–87.93
cannabis
  dermatoses induced by 120.4–120.6
  drug interactions 120.3
  prevalence of use 120.2
  psychodermatology 120.2
cannabis arteritis 120.4
canthal lines, reduction of by botulinum toxin application 159.5
cantharidin (Spanish fly), vesicating beetles 34.30
Cantu syndrome 87.85
canula injection, dermal fillers 158.1–158.2, 158.3, 158.4
capecitabine, palmoplantar erythrodysaesthesia 119.2
capillaries 2.40, 2.41
capillaritis 86.47, 86.48, 86.49
capillary disorders 71.3–71.11
  angioma serpiginosum 71.4–71.5
  capillary marmorata telangiectatica congenita 71.6
  CLOVES syndrome 71.9, 71.10
  disseminated capillary malformation with overgrowth 71.7–71.8
  Klippel–Trenaunay–Weber syndrome 71.8–71.9
  macrocephaly–capillary malformation syndrome 71.8
  microcephaly–capillary malformation syndrome 71.7
  PI3K-related overgrowth syndromes 71.7–71.11
  Proteus syndrome 71.10-11child
  Sturge–Weber syndrome 71.3–71.4
capillary filtration, chronic oedema 103.4
capillary haemangiomas
  laser therapies, infants 23.8
  strawberry naevus on eyelid 107.16 107.17
  see also infantile haemangiomas; pyogenic granuloma
capillary loops 2.41
capillary malformation with dilated veins (CMDV) 71.4
capillary malformation with overgrowth (CMO) 71.7
capillary malformations (CMs) 71.3
capillary malformation–arteriovenous malformation (CM–AVM) 71.5–71.6
capillary marmorata telangiectatica congenita (CMTC) 71.6
capilleroscopy, acrocyanosis investigation 124.7
Capnocytophaga canimorsus 130.6
CAPS *see* cryopyrin-associated periodic syndrome
capsaicin 18.39
caput medusae 112.9
carbamazepine, hypersensitivity reactions 14.6, 14.7
carba mix (sensitisers) 127.63, 127.64
carbapenems 19.46
carbohydrate disorders 79.2
carbon dioxide lasers
  photothermal ablation 23.20–23.21
  skin resurfacing 161.1–161.3, 161.5
carbon monoxide (CO) inhalation 125.4
carbuncles 26.25–26.26
carcinogenesis
  heat/IR radiation 124.14
  PUVA phototherapy risks 21.14
  skin cancer surveillance after phototherapy 21.16–21.17
  UVA-1 phototherapy risks 21.15
  UVB phototherapy risks 21.13

carcinogenicity, azathioprine 19.9
carcinogens
  arsenic 141.13
  occupational skin cancer 129.14
  palmoplantar keratodermas 63.73
carcinoid syndrome (CS) 86.19–86.20
  flushing 104.1, 104.6, 148.25–148.26
carcinoid tumours
  dermatoendocrinology 150.10, 150.12, 150.19
  flushing 104.6
carcinoma
  apocrine carcinoma 137.23
  basal cell 4.22, 110.39
  causative viral agents, MCPyV human polyomavirus 146.2, 146.3
  extramammary Paget disease, female genitalia 110.37–110.39
  heat-associated 124.15
  keratinocytes *see* basal cell carcinoma; squamous cell carcinoma
  Merkel cell carcinoma 2.12, 146.1–146.10
  metastatic to the skin from other primaries, radiotherapy 24.15
  penile 109.35–109.39
  pilomatrical carcinoma 137.14–137.15
  sebaceous 88.33
  sweat glands 137.33–137.40
  trichilemmal 137.7
  verrucous carcinoma, female genitalia 110.37
carcinoma cells, carcinoma erysipeloides 148.3, 148.4
carcinoma en cuirasse 148.2, 148.3
carcinoma erysipeloides 148.2, 148.4
  genito-crural region 111.24
cardiac complications, drug reaction with eosinophilia and systemic symptoms 118.9
cardiac disorders 151.1–151.6
cardiac dysfunction, systemic sclerosis 54.23
cardiac embolus, purpura 99.15
cardiac function, striate keratoderma 63.63
cardiac pacemakers, cutaneous reactions 151.5–151.6
cardiac rhabdomyomas, tuberous sclerosis complex 78.9
cardiac-valvular Ehlers–Danlos syndrome (cvEDS) 70.3, 70.9
cardio-facio-cutaneous syndrome 78.9
cardiomyopathy
  autosomal dominant intermediate epidermolysis bullosa simplex with 69.10
  palmoplantar keratodermas and 63.62–63.63
cardiopulmonary disorders, systemic sclerosis 54.17–54.18
cardiorespiratory pulmonary fibrosis, systemic sclerosis 54.23
cardiotoxicity, antimalarials 19.6
cardiovascular disease
  atopic eczema association 41.21
  hidradenitis suppurativa association 90.2, 90.8
  psoriasis 35.19
  systemic lupus erythematosus 51.30
  systemic sclerosis 54.17–54.18
  UV radiation exposure 10.9
cardiovascular syphilis 29.14, 29.16
Carney complex 72.7, 78.13, 108.16, 131.3, 131.4, 148.11, 151.3–151.4
carnosine 157.7
carotenaemia 61.9
carotene 86.50
carotenoderma 61.9, 86.50
carotenoids 86.2
CARP *see* confluent and reticulated papillomatosis
Carpenter syndrome 72.6
carriage
  Staphylococcus aureus 26.7–26.8
  Streptococcus pyogenes 26.11–26.12

carrier peptides, cosmeceutical use of 157.6
cartilage, inflammatory chondopathies 155.11–155.13
cartilage excision, auricle melanoma 106.32
cartilage hair hypoplasia 78.14, 80.4, 80.11–80.12
Carvajal-Huerta syndrome 63.28, 63.63
Casal's necklace, pellagra 61.17
case–control studies about adverse events 17.17, 17.18
caseous necrosis 97.27
CASPAR *see* Classification of Psoriatic Arthritis
CASS *see* comprehensive acne severity system
catabolic states, adiponectin system 97.5
catagen phase of hair root 87.7, 87.8, 87.9, 87.57
cataract, atopic 41.21, 107.19
cat bites 130.6
catecholamines 97.4
caterpillar dermatitis 34.32–34.34
cathepsin B (*CTSB*), skin fragility disorders 69.6
cathepsin C 63.68
catheter-related bloodstream infections (CRBSI) 125.10
catheter-related infection (CRI) 125.10
cathinone derivatives 120.3
cationic detergents 87.98
cat scratch disease, *Bartonella henselae* 26.62–26.64
CATSHL *see* camptodactyly, tall stature and hearing loss
causative agents of disease 5.8–5.10
caustic agents, skin surgery 20.47, 20.50
CBAs *see* computer-based assessments
CBCL *see* cutaneous B-cell lymphoma
CBLL *see* chilblain-like lesions
CBT *see* cognitive behavioural therapy
CCA *see* clear cell acanthoma
CCAAT enhancer binding protein ε-associated autoinflammation and immune impairment of neutrophils (CAIN) 45.16–45.17
CCCA *see* central centrifugal cicatricial alopecia
CCLA *see* central conducting lymphatic anomaly
CCMs *see* cerebral cavernous malformation-associated cutaneous lesions
CCPDMA *see* complete circumferential peripheral and deep margin assessment
CCPWA *see* Comprehensive Care Programme with Persons with Albinism
CCTR *see* Cochrane Controlled Trials Registry
CD4+/CD56+haematodermic neoplasm (blastic plasmacytoid dendritic cell neoplasm) 139.45–139.47
CD8+ mycosis fungoides variant, epidermotropic/cytotoxic CD8+ T-cell lymphoma distinction 139.5
CD10 (endothelial cell marker) 3.26
CD30+ anaplastic large-cell lymphomas
  anaplastic lymphoma kinase expression 139.1
  primary cutaneous 139.28–139.29
CD30+ lymphoproliferative disorders
  Hodgkin disease relationship 139.26, 139.49
  primary cutaneous 139.25–139.29
  see also primary cutaneous CD30+ lymphoproliferative disorders
CD30-positive lymphoproliferative disorders 3.28
CD31 (glycoprotein) 3.26
CD34 (glycosylated transmembrane protein) 3.25, 3.26
CD34-positive fibrous tumours 136.7, 136.8, 136.9, 136.14, 136.15, 136.16, 136.17, 136.18

CD34-positive superficial fibroblastic tumour 136.16–136.17
CD40 deficiencies 80.9
CD56 (neural cell adhesion molecule) 3.28
CD151 antigen/tetraspanin (*CD151*) 69.4
CDAGS syndrome 85.22
CDC *see* Centers for Disease Control and Prevention
CDK4 *see* cyclin-dependent kinase 4 gene
CDKN2A *see* cyclin-dependent kinase inhibitor 2A gene
CDLE *see* chronic discoid lupus erythematosus
CDLQI *see* Children's Dermatology Life Quality Index
CDSN protein, peeling skin syndromes 63.28–63.29
CEA *see* cultured epithelial autografts
CEDNIK syndrome *see* cerebral dysgenesis–neuropathy–ichthyosis–palmoplantar keratoderma syndrome
cEDS *see* classical Ehlers–Danlos syndrome
CeHV-1 (cercopithecine herpesvirus 1) *see* herpes B virus infection
cell damage, pressure ulcers 123.2
Cellfina, cellulite laser treatment 161.9
'cellist's chest' 122.12
cell markers, immunocytochemistry panels of **3.10**
cell-mediated immunity (CMI), leprosy 28.2, 28.3, 28.4–28.5
cell therapy, epidermolysis bullosa 69.27–69.28
cellular adhesion molecules (CAMs) 127.7
cellular angiofibroma 136.9
cellular digital fibromyxoma *see* acral fibromyxoma
cellular fibrous histiocytoma 136.20, 136.21
cellular identification, electron microscopy studies 3.30
cellular neurothekeoma 136.48
Cellulaze, cellulite laser treatment 161.9
cellulite 98.25–98.27, **98.26**
  treatments 161.9, *161.10*
cellulitis 103.13–103.17
  ano-genital cellulitis 111.14
  definition and relationship to erysipelas 26.18
  gangrenous 26.78
  lymphadenitis 103.15
  lymphangitis 103.14–103.15
  perianal cellulitis 109.26, 111.14
  perianal streptococcal 26.33–26.34
  recurrent cellulitis (erysipelas) 103.13–103.14
  X-linked agammaglobulinaemia 80.13
cellulitis/erysipelas 26.18–26.22
  clinical features 26.19, *26.20–26.21*
  clinical investigations 26.19
  epidemiology 26.18
  investigations 26.19
  management 26.19, 26.21–26.22
  pathophysiology 26.18–26.19
  Staphylococcus aureus role 26.19
  Streptococcus role 26.18–26.19
cement-induced chromate sensitivity 127.40
CEN *see* congenital epidermal naevi
Centers for Disease Control and Prevention (CDC) 7.6
centipedes (Chilopoda) 34.57
CENTRAL *see* Cochrane Central Register of Controlled Trials
central centrifugal cicatricial alopecia (CCCA) 87.46–87.47, 87.68
central conducting lymphatic anomaly (CCLA) 103.32
central line associated infections, burn injuries 125.10
central nervous system (CNS)
  control of endocrine signalling axes 150.2
  drug reaction with eosinophilia and systemic symptoms 118.9

Erdheim–Chester disease 135.22
  incontinentia pigmenti 68.11
centrifugal lipodystrophy (CLD) 98.12–98.13
CEP *see* congenital erythropoietic porphyria
cephalic pustulosis, neonatal 88.69
Cephalopoda class, molluscs 130.4
cephalosporins 19.46
Ceratopogonidae (midges) 34.7–34.8, 34.9
cercarial dermatitis 33.29–33.30
cercarial organisms, jellyfish stings 130.2
cercopithecine herpesvirus 1 (CeHV-1) *see* herpes B virus infection
cerebral cavernous malformation-associated cutaneous lesions (CCMs) 71.2, 71.19
cerebral dysgenesis–neuropathy–ichthyosis–palmoplantar keratoderma (CEDNIK) syndrome 63.30
cerebro-oculo-facio skeletal syndrome (COFS) 76.8
cerebrospinal fluid examination, syphilis 29.20, 29.21
cerebrotendinous xanthomatosis 60.10
CERS3 deficiency 63.15
CERS3 gene, congenital ichthyosiform erythroderma 63.11
certolizumab pegol, psoriasis treatment 35.28–35.29
cerumen (wax), external ear 106.2–106.3
ceruminous glands, tumours of 106.34–106.35
cervical cancer 25.51, 25.64–25.65
  vulval lymphangiectasia 103.31
cervical intraepithelial neoplasia (CIN) 25.52, 25.65
cervical lymph nodes, drainage areas of **108.6**
cervical trophic syndrome (CTS) 82.8–82.9
cestodes, infections 33.31–33.35
cetearyl alcohol 127.59
cetrimide 18.10
cetuximb, papulopustular eruptions 119.3
CEVD *see* congenital erosive and vesicular dermatosis
CGH *see* comparative genomic hybridisation; congenital generalised hypertrichosis
CGL *see* congenital generalised lipodystrophies
CGPD *see* childhood granulomatous periorificial dermatoses
cGvHD *see* chronic graft versus host disease
CH *see* chlorhexidine
Chagas disease *see* American trypanosomiasis
chalazion (meibomian gland cyst) 107.11
  eyelid 107.45–107.46
chamomile 157.11
chancriform pyoderma 26.87–26.88
chancroid 30.18–30.21
  clinical features 30.19–30.20
  epidemiology 30.19
  investigations 30.20–30.21
  management 30.21
  pathophysiology 30.19
Chapare (Bolivian) haemorrhagic fever 25.82–25.83
chapping of the lips 108.60
Charcot arthropathy, diabetic patients 62.2
Charcot (neuropathic) joints, syphilis 29.15–29.16
CHARGE (coloboma, heart defects, atresia of the nasal choanae, retardation of growth/development, genital/urinary abnormalities and ear abnormalities and deafness) syndrome 80.4, 80.8, 106.4, **106.7**
CHB *see* congenital heart block
checkpoint inhibitors *see* immune checkpoint inhibitors
Chédiak–Higashi syndrome 68.8–68.9, **80.5**, 148.13
  partial albinism in 80.14

cheek
  biting 108.32
  dermal fillers 158.2, 158.4
  discoid lupus erythematosus 51.8
  erythropoietic protoporphyria 58.15
  impetigo 115.7
  pseudofolliculitis 93.2
  solar lentigo 131.6
  spontaneous atrophic scarring 94.14–94.15
  venous malformation 71.15
  volumisation of 158.4
  see also buccal mucosa
cheilitis 108.60–108.63, 127.15, 127.80, 128.4–128.5
  actinic cheilitis 108.58
  actinic prurigo 126.10, *126.11*
  angular cheilitis 108.20, 108.59–108.60
  contact cheilitis 108.60–108.61
  drug-induced cheilitis 108.61
  eczematous cheilitis 108.61
  exfoliative cheilitis 108.61–108.62
  foreign body cheilitis 108.62
  glandular cheilitis 108.62–108.63
  granulomatous cheilitis *108.73*
  infective cheilitis 108.63
  plasma cell cheilitis 108.63
  retinoid-induced 88.56
  Stevens–Johnson syndrome/toxic epidermal necrolysis 118.16
cheiroarthropathy, diabetic patients 62.5, *62.7*
chemical burns 128.11–128.12
  oral lesions 108.31
chemical depigmentation 86.45
chemical exposure, scleroderma-like syndromes 94.45
chemical peels 160.1–160.15
  acne treatment 88.58–88.59, 160.5, 160.6
  actinic keratoses 160.5
  alpha-hydroxyl acids 160.1–160.2
  azelaic acid 160.2
  caustic action peels 160.2–160.3
  chemistry of 160.1–160.4
  consent 160.8
  contraindications 160.6
  counselling 160.6–160.7
  deep peels 160.5
  depth of 160.4–160.5
  equipment for 160.8
  facial skin rejuvenation 160.5
  glycolic acid 160.2, *160.8*, 160.9–160.10
  histological level of controlled necrosis **160.4**
  indications 160.5–160.6
  Jessner solution 160.3, *160.7, 160.8*, 160.10, *160.11*
  lactic acid 160.2
  medium depth peels 160.4
  metabolic action peels 160.1–160.2
  peeling agents 160.9–160.11
  peeling technique 160.8–160.11
  phenol 160.3
  phenol-croton oil peel 160.10–160.11
  photodamaged skin 160.5
  photo documentation 160.8
  pigmentation 160.5–160.6
  post-peel care 160.11
  pre-peel procedure 160.6–160.8
  pyruvic acid 160.2
  retinoic acid 160.2
  salicylic acid 160.3–160.4, 160.10
  side effects and complications 160.11–160.14
    allergic contact dermatitis 160.13
    chemical burns 160.12, *160.13*
    infection 160.13
    milia and acneform eruption 160.12
    postinflammatory hyperpigmentation 160.12–160.13, *160.14*
    postinflammatory hypopigmentation 160.14
    premature peeling 160.12, *160.13*
    redness, persistent 160.11–160.12
    scarring 160.14

  systemic toxicity 160.13–160.14
  skin of colour 160.15
  skin pigmentation 160.5–160.6
  skin priming 160.7–160.8
  superficial peels 160.4
  toxic action peels 160.3–160.4
  trichloroacetic acid 160.2–160.3, 160.10, *160.11*
chemical photosensitivity 126.1, 126.27–126.32
chemical protection, glove materials **128.8**
chemicals
  acne-inducing 129.7, 129.12–129.13
  allergic components 128.6
  irritant properties 128.2–128.3, 128.6, 129.5
  occupational leukoderma 129.13–129.14
  phototoxic properties 128.9
  sensitisation 127.6
chemokines, bullous pemphigoid 50.12
chemoprophylaxis, leprosy 28.16
chemotactic factors, eosinophilic pustular folliculitis 93.7
chemotherapy
  cutaneous side effects 119.1–119.15
  cutaneous T-cell lymphoma 139.24
  hair changes 119.5–119.6
  hyperpigmentation 119.8–119.9
  hypertrichosis 119.6
  hypopigmentation 119.10–119.11
  leprosy 28.13–28.14
  Mee's lines *121.3*
  nail changes 119.6–119.8
  systemic sclerosis 54.25–54.26
  toxic erythema 119.1–119.2
chemotherapy-induced alopecia (CIA) 87.71–87.74, 119.5–119.6
chemotherapy-related eccrine syringosquamous metaplasia 92.15
ChemSex, drugs with sex 120.2–120.3
cherry angiomas 101.12–101.13, **101.17**
chest
  acne fulminans 88.61, *88.62*
  acne vulgaris 88.12, *88.13*
  Brunsting–Perry pemphigoid 50.53
  IgM pemphigoid 50.54
  linear morphoea 55.23
  lithium-induced acne 88.13
  macular cutaneous amyloidosis 56.7
  morphoea 55.5, 55.20, 55.21, 55.23
  pansclerotic morphoea 55.21
  plaque morphoea 55.20
  segmental psoriasis 35.15
  subacute cutaneous lupus erythematosus 51.15
  systemic sclerosis 54.4
chest wall, Mondor disease on 101.37
cheveux incoiffables *see* uncombable hair syndrome
Cheyletiella mites 34.53, *34.54*
CHHS *see* Conradi–Hünermann–Happle syndrome
chickenpox *see* varicella infection
chicken-wire reticulate erythema/urticaria 43.4
Chikungunya fever
  mosquito-borne togavirus infection 25.89
  oral involvement 108.50
chilblain-like lesions (pseudo-perniosis)
  COVID-19 association 25.108–25.109, 25.113–25.114
  COVID-19 vaccines 25.118
  internal malignancy association 148.25
chilblain lupus 51.6–51.7, *51.9*, 51.25
chilblains (perniosis) 97.37, 124.6
CHILD *see* congenital hemidysplasia–ichthyosiform naevus–limb defect syndrome
child abuse
  ano-genital signs of sexual abuse 109.9
  non-accidental injury 115.14
childhood, psychological and social factors 15.3, 15.4
Childhood Atopic Dermatitis Impact Scale (CADIS) 16.8

childhood granulomatous periorificial
    dermatoses (CGPD) 89.18–89.19
childhood HIV-associated lipodystrophy
    98.6
childhood linear IgA disease *50.36*, 80.14,
    80.15, 108.81
childhood lipoatrophic panniculitis
    97.56–97.57
childhood NEH *92.14, 92.15*
childhood rosacea 89.3
    idiopathic facial aseptic granuloma 89.16
    management 89.14–89.15
    ocular 89.6
children
    acne, prepubertal 88.68–88.74
    acrodermatitis enteropathica *61.26*
    actinic lichen planus 37.7
    acute scrotum 109.23, 109.25–109.26
    agminated or segmental lentiginosis
        131.3
    antihistamine treatment 42.18
    argininosuccinic aciduria *79.13*
    arteriovenous malformation *71.11*
    atopic eczema *41.13, 41.14, 41.15, 41.16,
        41.17, 41.18, 41.26*
        psychodermatology 84.3
    autoinflammatory granulomatosis of
        childhood **45.5, 45.7**, 45.11–45.12
    blistering distal dactylitis 26.34
    Bloom syndrome *77.3*
    bullous pemphigoid *50.20*
    calcifying aponeurotic fibroma
        136.7–136.8
    calcifying fibrous tumour/pseudotumour
        136.7
    capillary malformations *71.3, 71.5*
    cellular fibrous histiocytoma 136.21
    choanal atresia and lymphoedema *71.27*
    chronic bullous dermatosis *50.36*, 80.14,
        80.15, 108.81
    congenital blue naevi *73.16*
    congenital melanocytic naevi *73.12*
    cranial (nodular) fasciitis 136.5
    cutis laxa *70.17*
    DOCK8 deficiency *80.10*
    dog and cat bites 130.6
    epidermolysis bullosa acquisita *50.45,
        50.46*
    erythema infectiosum/fifth disease
        25.77–25.78, 115.6, *155.2, 155.3*
    erythropoietic protoporphyria *58.14*
    factitious nail disease 84.33
    flushing **104.10**
    fucosidosis *79.4*
    giant cell fibroblastoma 136.15–136.16
    granuloma annulare *95.5, 95.7*
    Griscelli syndrome *80.14*
    hair follicle naevus 137.7–137.8
    Hartnup disease *61.16*
    impact of skin disease assessment 16.8,
        16.9–16.10
    inherited immunodeficiency 80.2
    juvenile dermatomyositis *52.8*–*52.9*
    juvenile plantar dermatosis *39.23–39.24*
    juvenile springtime eruption, external ear
        106.25
    Langerhans cell histiocytosis
        115.15–115.16, 135.4, 135.5–135.7,
        135.9
    late-onset primary lymphoedema
        103.24–103.25
    lichen nitidus *37.10*
    lichen striatus *37.18*
    lip-lick cheilitis *41.22*
    lipofibromatosis 136.13–136.14
    lymphangioma 108.13
    Maffucci syndrome *71.20*
    malnutrition 61.2, 61.3, *61.4*
        severity classification 61.5–61.6
    mastocytosis *46.9*
    microbial ecology of the skin 26.4
    midface toddler excoriation syndrome due
        to pain insensitivity 83.12–83.13
    morphoea, diagnosis, assessment and
        treatment 55.39

mucopolysaccharidoses *79.3*
Münchausen syndrome by proxy
    84.37–84.38
neurocutaneous disorders, subgroups
    83.2
neurofibromatosis type 1, Manchester
    checklist *78.5*
normophosphataemic familial tumoral
    calcinosis *79.18*
paediatric HIV/AIDS 31.36–31.37
paediatric inflammatory multisystem
    syndrome temporally associated
    with SARS-CoV-2 infection 25.114
paediatric IRIS/IRD/IRAD 31.8
pansclerotic morphoea 55.19–55.21
papular acrodermatitis/Gianotti-Crosti
    syndrome 25.74
perianal streptococcal cellulitis
    26.33–26.34
perianal viral warts 111.18, *111.19*
phosphomannomutase 2 deficiency *79.10*
pilomatricoma 137.13
pityriasis rubra pilaris *36.4, 36.5*
plexiform fibrohistiocytic tumour 136.22
primary herpetic gingivostomatitis 25.21
pro-opiomelanocortin deficiency *72.8*
pruritus, idiopathic *111.6*
psoriasis vulgaris 35.15
PTEN hamartoma tumour syndrome
    71.13
purpura artefact 84.33
roseola infantum 25.39–25.40, 115.5–115.6
Rothmund–Thomson syndrome *75.5*
scarlet fever 26.35–26.36
severe combined immunodeficiency *80.8*
spindle cell haemangioma 136.31
staphylococcal scalded skin syndrome
    26.27, 26.28, *26.28*, 114.24–114.25,
    115.7–115.8
streptococcal vulvovaginitis in
    prepubescent girls 26.33
sun exposure as melanoma risk 142.6
syphilis, congenital 114.27–114.28
systemic juvenile idiopathic arthritis
    53.8, 53.9
systemic juvenile xanthogranuloma
    135.17
systemic lupus erythematosus *51.32*
systemic-onset juvenile idiopathic arthritis
    45.21–45.22
telangiectasia *75.5*
tinea capitis 32.31–32.32, 32.37–32.38,
    115.8–115.9
topical therapy application quantities
    18.3, 18.4
trichotillosis 84.22–84.23, 87.24, 87.32,
    87.33
urticaria pigmentosa *46.4, 46.5*
Williams–Beuren syndrome *70.18*
Wiskott–Aldrich syndrome *80.9*
wound healing 11.2
xeroderma pigmentosum *76.4*
X-linked lymphoproliferative diseases
    80.11
see also infants; juvenile...; neonates
Children's Dermatology Life Quality Index
    (CDLQI)
atopic eczema 16.8
questions **16.10**
usage 16.9–16.10
chillblains (perniosis) *97.36*, 124.5–124.6
type I cryoglobulinaemia 149.13, 149.14
Chilopoda (centipedes) 34.57
CHIME (coloboma–heart
    defect–ichthyosiform
    dermatosis–mental retardation–ear
    anomalies) syndrome 63.38–63.39
chin
    impetigo *115.7*
    numb chin syndrome/mental neuropathy
        148.23
    sinus related to dental abscess *108.9*
China, ancient medical texts 1.2
Chi-square test, statistical analysis of clinical
    studies 17.22

Chlamydia
    C. pneumoniae 26.79
    C. psittaci 26.79
Chlamydia pneumoniae, skin features 26.79
Chlamydia trachomatis 26.79
    life cycle 30.10
    serovars L1-L3, lymphogranuloma
        venereum 30.14–30.18
    strains D-K, genital infection 30.8–30.14
    see also genital chlamydia
chloracne (MADISH) *88.14, 88.15*,
    88.66–88.68, 129.7, 129.12–129.13,
    133.1, 133.7
    chemicals causing **88.66**, 129.12
chlorhexidine (CH) 127.57–127.58
chlorine-releasing agents 18.10
chloroacetate esterase stain *3.9*
chlorocresol 127.56
chlorophenols 129.12
chloroquine
    drug-induced pruritus 81.11
    eye, side effects on 107.43
    pruritus *117.3*
    sarcoidosis management 96.16
chloroquine pigmentation 86.26
chloroxylenol 18.10, 127.55–127.56
chlorpromazine
    hypermelanosis 86.26–86.27
    photosensitivity 126.30
choanal atresia and lymphoedema *71.27*
cholera, epidemiology 5.9–5.10
cholestasis 60.11–60.12, 153.5
cholestatic pruritus 81.9–81.10
cholesteatoma 106.21
cholesterol embolus, purpura 99.14–99.15
cholesterol sulphate
    acquired ichthyosis 63.47
    recessive X-linked ichthyosis 63.5
cholinergic urticaria **42.9**, 42.11–42.12
chondrodermatitis nodularis (CN)
    106.9–106.11
    clinical features 106.10
    epidemiology 106.9
    management 106.10–106.11
chondroid cells, juvenile hyaline
    fibromatosis 94.42
chondroid syringoma see mixed tumour of
    the skin
chondroitin sulphate (CS) *2.38*, **2.39**
chorionic villi, DNA-based prenatal
    diagnosis 8.10
chromate allergy 127.23
chromatograms, patch testing 127.33
chromhidrosis 92.18
chromium allergy 127.36, 127.39–127.41
chromium VI (CrVI) exposure 127.2
chromoblastomycosis 32.75–32.77
chromomycosis see chromoblastomycosis
chromophores
    light absorption by skin 23.3–23.4
    selective photothermolysis 23.5–23.6
chromophytosis see pityriasis versicolor
chromosomal disorders 8.6, 74.1–74.5
    autosomal chromosome defects
        74.1–74.3
    chromosomal mosaicism 74.5
    sex chromosome defects 74.3–74.5
chromosomal mosaicism 74.5
chromosome 4, short-arm deletion syndrome
    74.3
chromosome 5, short-arm deletion syndrome
    74.3
chromosome 18, long-arm deletion
    syndrome 74.3
chromosomes 8.3, 8.4
chronica atrophicans, cutaneous B-cell
    lymphoma 139.37–139.38
chronic acral dermatitis 39.14–39.15
chronic actinic dermatitis (CAD) 126.4,
    126.13–126.21, 126.31,
    126.32–126.35, *126.37*, 127.81
chronic active Epstein–Barr virus infection
    25.38
chronically sun-damaged skin 145.9,
    145.11, **145.11**

chronically swollen limb 103.9–103.10
chronic arsenic poisoning 121.2
chronic atrophic candidiasis see chronic
    erythematous candidiasis
chronic atypical neutrophilic dermatosis
    with lipodystrophy and elevated
    temperature (CANDLE) **45.5, 45.6**,
    45.14–45.15, **72.11,** *72.12*
chronic bulbous disease of childhood see
    childhood linear IgA disease
chronic bullous dermatosis (linear IgA
    disease of children) 108.81
chronic candidiasis 108.31–108.32
chronic cholestasis 60.11–60.12
chronic contact dermatitis *127.13*
chronic cutaneous leishmaniasis
    33.47–33.48
chronic diffuse telogen effluvium 87.54
chronic discoid lupus erythematosus (CDLE)
    87.43–87.44
chronic disseminated histoplasmosis 32.83
chronic erythema nodosum 97.25
chronic erythematous candidiasis 32.62
chronic graft versus host disease (cGvHD)
    38.1, 38.2, 38.3, 38.7–38.11
    clinical features 38.7–38.9
    epidemiology 38.2
    management 38.9–38.11
    pathology 38.3
    predisposing factors 38.2
    severity classification 38.9, *38.10*
    skin cancer risks 147.4–147.5
chronic granulomatous disease **80.5**
    eyelid, papular lesions around *80.15*
    malar erythematous photosensitive
        macular skin lesions *80.16*
chronic hyperplastic candidiasis see chronic
    plaque-like candidiasis
chronic infantile neurological cutaneous and
    articular syndrome (CINCA) **45.5,
    45.6**
chronic inflammation, and skin ageing 2.45
chronicity of disease 5.10
chronic kidney disease (CKD), pruritus
    association 81.8–81.9
chronic liver disease
    skin lesions 153.4
    vascular changes 153.8–153.9
chronic (long) COVID-19 25.113
chronic lymphocytic leukaemia (CLL)
    immunocompromised patients 147.1,
        147.3
    insect bite-like reactions 149.8–149.9
    skin infiltration as first sign 149.2
    see also non-Hodgkin lymphoma
chronic metabolic disease, acquired
    ichthyosis association 85.1
chronic mucocutaneous candidiasis (CMC)
    32.67–32.69, 80.17
    clinical features 32.68, *32.69*
    management 32.69
    oral lesions 108.32
    pathophysiology 32.67–32.68
chronic nodular candidiasis 32.62
chronic non-scarring folliculitis 91.13–91.14
chronic oedema 103.2, 103.3–103.5
    causes **103.4**
    clinical features 103.4
    epidemiology 103.3
    investigations 103.4–103.5
    lymphoedema comparison 103.3
    management 103.5
    pathophysiology 103.3–103.4
    penis 109.19–109.21
chronic oro-perineal candidiasis 80.7
chronic otitis externa 106.16, 106.17,
    106.18–106.19
chronic pain syndromes, male genitalia
    109.43–109.44
chronic panniculitis 97.30–97.32
chronic papillomatous dermatitis (CPD)
    112.8
chronic physiological reactions 124.14
chronic plaque-like candidiasis 32.62
chronic plaque psoriasis see psoriasis
    vulgaris

chronic pruritus (CP) 81.1–81.14
  atopic eczema 81.7–81.8
  clinical variants 81.7–81.12
  drug-induced pruritus 81.10–81.11
  epidemiology 81.1–81.2
  history taking 81.6
  inflamed skin/dermatoses 81.7
  investigations 81.13
  management 81.13–81.14
  presentation 81.6–81.7
  psoriasis vulgaris 81.8
  severity rating 81.12–81.13
  uncontrollable scratching 81.15
chronic pseudomembranous candidiasis 32.61
chronic pulmonary histoplasmosis 32.83
chronic radiation dermatitis 119.14
chronic radiodermatitis 24.18–24.20
chronic/recurrent self-healing eruptions, lymphomatoid papulosis 139.26–139.28
chronic red leg 103.16–103.17
chronic sarcoidosis 96.6
chronic scalp pain and dysaesthesia 82.12
chronic selenium toxicity 121.7
chronic spontaneous urticaria (CSU) 16.5
chronic superficial dermatitis, discoid skin lesions **39.10**
chronic superficial scaly dermatitis *see* small plaque parapsoriasis
chronic telogen effluvium 87.59–87.60
chronic ulcerative stomatitis 108.79
chronic ulcers, radiotherapy-associated 119.15
chronic urticaria 84.3
Chronic Urticaria Quality of Life Questionnaire (CU-Q$_2$oL) 16.9
chronic venous disease (CVD), venous leg ulcers 102.1–102.4
chronic venous insufficiency 101.40–101.46
  categories 101.40–101.41
  causes **101.41**
  clinical features **101.43**
  investigations **101.45**
  management 101.45–101.46
  pathogenesis **101.42**
  risk factors **101.41**
  treatment **101.45**
chronic wounds, elderly people 6.1
chrysiasis 86.52, 121.4
chrysoderma 86.52
Chrysops (tabanid flies) 33.12
  see also loiasis
Churg–Strauss syndrome *see* eosinophilic granulomatosis with polyangiitis
chylous disease 103.32
chymase 2.17
CIA *see* chemotherapy-induced alopecia
cicatricial alopecia 87.37, 87.38–87.53, 88.37
  central centrifugal 87.46–87.47, 87.68
  incontinentia pigmenti 68.11
  marginal 87.32
  non-specific 87.51
  secondary 87.52–87.53, 105.6–105.9
cicatricial pemphigoid 50.51–50.52, 50.53, 105.6
  diagnosis 50.24
  penile 109.25
cicatrising conjunctivitis 107.24–107.34
  management 107.29–107.32
ciclopirox olamine 18.12
ciclosporin 19.10–19.12
  dermatological uses 19.10
  dose and regimens 19.12
  drug–drug interactions 19.11–19.12
  monitoring 19.12
  morphoea treatment 55.38
  pharmacological properties 19.10–19.11
  potential adverse effects 19.11
  pre-treatment screening 19.12
  psoriasis treatment 35.25
  Stevens–Johnson syndrome/toxic epidermal necrolysis 118.11–118.12, 118.21

topical therapies 18.23
urticaria treatment 42.18
CIC-rearranged sarcoma (CIC-DUX4 sarcoma) 136.52
CIE *see* congenital ichthyosiform erythroderma; International Commission on Illumination
'cigarette face' 94.2
cigarette-induced keratoses 108.33
cigarette paper-like wrinkling 94.26
cigarette smoking *see* smoking
Cimicidae (including bed bugs) 34.25–34.29
CIN *see* cervical intraepithelial neoplasia
CINCA *see* chronic infantile neurological cutaneous and articular syndrome
circumcision, male 109.7
circumferential hyperkeratosis 63.64
circumscribed alopecias 87.30
circumscribed hyperhidrosis 92.6–92.7, 92.9
circumscribed juvenile pityriasis rubra pilaris (type IV) 36.4, *36.5*
circumscribed palmoplantar hypokeratosis 63.78
circumscribed plaque morphoea 55.17
  differential diagnosis **55.27**
cirrhosis 153.5, 153.8, 153.9
  hypermelanosis 86.22
cirsoid aneurysm 136.27
Civatte bodies 118.13
CKD *see* chronic kidney disease
CK syndrome 63.23
CLA *see* cutaneous lymphocyte antigen
Cladophialophora carrionii 32.77
clam digger's itch *see* cercarial dermatitis
CLAPO syndrome **101.28**
'clarinettist's cheilitis' 122.12
Clarkson syndrome 43.4
CLAs *see* complicated lymphatic anomalies
clascoterone, acne vulgaris treatment 88.49–88.50
Class A drugs 120.3
Class B drugs 120.3
Class C drugs 120.3
classic adult-onset pityriasis rubra pilaris (type I) 36.2, 36.4, *36.6*
classical adult eosinophilic pustular folliculitis 91.4
classical Ehlers–Danlos syndrome (cEDS) 70.2, **70.3**, *70.8*
classical eosinophilic pustular folliculitis 93.7, 93.8
classical epidermodysplasia verruciformis 25.66, 25.69
classical-like Ehlers–Danlos syndrome (clEDS) **70.3**, 70.9–70.10
classical-like type 2 Ehlers–Danlos syndrome (clEDS2) **70.3**
classic epidermolysis bullosa
  clinical subtypes 69.8–69.11
  genes/proteins implicated in 69.2–69.8
  molecular pathology 69.11–69.15
classic juvenile-onset pityriasis rubra pilaris (type III) 36.4, *36.5*
classic Sweet syndrome (CSS) 49.8, *49.11*
Classification of Psoriatic Arthritis (CASPAR) criteria **35.41**
classification of skin diseases 1.4, *1.6*
claudication, peripheral vascular disease **101.5**
claudin-1 junction, neonatal ichthyosis–sclerosing cholangitis 63.41
claudins 2.20
  gene mutations 2.21
CLCI *see* cumulative life course impairment
CLD *see* centrifugal lipodystrophy
cleansing of skin, neonates 114.2
clearance, clinical pharmacology **13.2**
clear cell acanthoma (CCA) 132.6–132.7
clear-cell hidradenoma *see* hidradenoma
clear cell sarcoma 136.64
cleavage resistant RIPK1-induced autoinflammatory syndrome 45.17
clEDS2 *see* classical-like type 2 Ehlers–Danlos syndrome

clEDS *see* classical-like Ehlers–Danlos syndrome
cleft lip/palate 108.83–108.85
  clinical features 108.84
  management 108.84–108.85
  pathophysiology 108.83–108.84
  predisposing factors 108.83–108.84
  syndromes associated with **108.84**
clenched fist injuries 130.6–130.7
Clericuzio-type poikiloderma with neutropenia 149.14
climate, and atopic eczema 41.6
climate change, and skin health 7.3–7.4
climatic bubo *see* lymphogranuloma venereum
clindamycin 18.10
clinical decision-making 16.6
clinical end point studies, topical bioavailability/bioequivalence assessment 12.7
clinically amyopathic dermatomyositis (CADM) 52.1, 52.7, 52.9, 52.11
clinical margins, melanoma excision 143.2–143.3
clinical officer training, Cambodia 7.7–7.8
clinical pharmacology 13.1–13.13
  absorption, distribution, metabolism and elimination of a drug 13.1–13.4
  adherence to treatment 13.9
  bioavailability 13.2–13.3, **13.2**
  clearance **13.2**
  drug actions, mechanisms underlying **13.4**, 13.5–13.6
  drug choice and medical decision making 13.7
  drug development and licensing 13.11–13.13
  drug interactions 13.9
  drug toxicity and adverse effects 13.6, 13.9–13.11
  drug types 13.1
  ethics and drug trial reporting 13.13
  medication errors 13.9–13.11
  molecular mechanisms underlying drug actions 13.5–13.6
  novel methods of drug delivery 13.3
  oral drug administration 13.2, 13.3
  'orphan' status of drugs 13.13
  parenteral drug administration 13.2–13.3
  personalised medicine 8.1, 13.11
  pharmacists' role 13.11
  pharmacodynamics **13.2**, 13.4–13.6
    factors affecting 13.7–13.9
  pharmacogenomics 13.11
  pharmacokinetics 13.1–13.4
  polypharmacy 13.8
  prescription-writing, medication errors 13.10, 13.11
  regulatory approval of drug applications 13.13
  'Swiss cheese model', drug-related patient harm 13.10
  terminology 13.1, **13.2**
  therapeutic outcome, factors affecting 13.7–13.11
  therapeutic window **13.2**
clinical questions, well-built questions in evidence based medicine 17.3–17.4
clinical research, evidence based medicine 17.1–17.2
clinical research papers
  adequate reporting 17.18–17.20
  data evaluation 17.18–17.25
  shortcut method for reading 17.24–17.25
  statistical methods 17.20–17.24
clinical trials
  critical appraisal for evidence based medicine 17.12–17.15
  see also randomised controlled clinical trials
clioquinol, patch testing 127.47
clitoris, structure and function of 110.2, 110.3
CLL *see* chronic lymphocytic leukaemia

CLND *see* completion lymph node dissection
clofazimine 86.26
clostridia 26.48–26.49
clostridial myonecrosis (gas gangrene) 26.48–26.49
Clostridium botulinum 120.7
Clostridium histolyticum, myonecrosis 26.48–26.49
Clostridium novyi, myonecrosis 26.48–26.49
Clostridium perfringens, myonecrosis 26.48–26.49
Clostridium septicum, myonecrosis 26.48–26.49
Clostridium sodellii, myonecrosis 26.48–26.49
clothing
  allergens 127.64, 127.65–127.67
  callosities 122.8
  dermatitis 127.16–127.17
  photoprotection 10.12
Clouston syndrome 63.68, 67.12, **78.13**
  oral lesions 108.28
  pachyonychia congenita 67.12
CLOVES (congenital lipomatous overgrowth, vascular malformations, epidermal naevi and skeletal/spinal anomalies) syndrome 71.2, 71.9, 71.10, 72.9, 72.11, 73.6–73.7, **101.28**, 103.23
clubbing of nails, internal malignancy links 148.18
clutton joints, congenital syphilis 29.25
CM *see* cutaneous mastocytosis
CMC *see* chronic mucocutaneous candidiasis
CMDV *see* capillary malformation with dilated veins
CMI *see* cell-mediated immunity
CMN *see* congenital melanocytic naevi
CMO *see* capillary malformation with overgrowth
CMs *see* capillary malformations
CMTC *see* capillary marmorata telangiectatica congenita
CMV *see* cytomegalovirus
CM–AVM *see* capillary malformation–arteriovenous malformation
CN *see* chondrodermatitis nodularis; cyanide
cnidarian stings 130.1–130.5
CNS *see* central nervous system; Comèl–Netherton syndrome
coagulase negative *Staphylococcus* 26.3, 26.9–26.10
coagulase positive *Staphylococcus* 26.3, 26.8, 93.2
coagulation defects, liver disease association 153.9
coagulopathies, HIV 31.12
coal tar 18.36–18.37, 35.21–35.22
cobalamin (vitamin B12) deficiency 61.19–61.21
cobalt allergy 127.38–127.39
cobalt spot test 127.33–127.34
cocaine
  death rates 120.1
  dermatoses induced by 120.2, 120.5
  pharmaceutical drug interactions 120.3
  prevalence of use 120.2
  soft-tissue infections 120.7
cocamide diethanolamide 127.59
coccidioidal granuloma *see* coccidioidomycosis
Coccidioides
  C. immitis 32.86, 32.87
  C. posadasii 32.86, 32.87
coccidioidin test 4.25
coccidioidomycosis 32.86–32.88
Cochrane, Archie 17.1, 17.6
Cochrane Central Register of Controlled Trials (CENTRAL) 17.6, 17.7
Cochrane Collaboration 17.2, 17.6–17.7
  risk of bias tool 17.9
Cochrane Controlled Trials Registry (CCTR) 17.9

Cochrane Library 17.6–17.7
Cochrane Skin Core Outcomes Initiative (CS-COUSIN) 17.14
cockade naevus 131.30, *131.31*
Cockayne syndrome (CS) 75.6, 76.5, 76.6–76.8, **77.2**
   bird-like facial appearance 76.7
   clinical features 76.7–76.8
   clinical variants 76.8
   genes and protein products **76.7**
   investigations 76.8
   management 76.8
   pathophysiology 76.7
cockroaches (Dictyoptera) 34.32
COCs *see* combined oral contraceptives
coding systems, diagnostic 4.2
coefficient of friction 122.6
coeliac disease
   oral involvement 108.72
   psoriasis association 35.18
   skin manifestations 153.3
coenzyme Q10 (CoQ10), cosmeceutical use of 157.2
Coffin–Lowry syndrome **72.7**
COFS *see* cerebro-oculo-facio skeletal syndrome
cognitive behavioural therapy (CBT) 84.47
cognitive models, beliefs/emotions/behaviours 15.1–15.3
Cohen syndrome **72.6**
cohort studies, adverse events 17.17–17.18
CO inhalation *see* carbon monoxide inhalation
COL1A1-USP6 gene rearrangement 136.6
colchicine 19.12–19.13
   dermatological uses 19.12
   pharmacological properties 19.12–19.13
   potential adverse effects 19.13
   safety precautions 19.13
cold
   cutaneous reactions to 124.1–124.16
   diseases caused/aggravated by 124.1–124.14
cold abscesses 33.24, 33.33, *33.35*
cold agglutinins 124.13–124.14
   cryogelling/cryoagglutination disorders 99.11–99.14
cold contact urticaria **42.9**, 42.10–42.11
cold-induced sweating syndrome 92.7
cold-induced vasoconstriction 124.1
cold-induced vasodilation 83.5
cold injury, neonatal 114.15, **114.18**
cold panniculitis 97.35–97.37, 114.14
cold sores *see* herpes labialis
Cole disease 63.61
Coleoptera (beetles) 34.30–34.32
collagen 2.2, 2.27–2.29
   basement membrane collagen 2.22–2.23
   biosynthesis 2.29–2.31, *2.30*
   cross-linking 2.31
   degradation 2.31–2.32, 10.10–10.11
   elastin interdependence 122.5
   epidermolysis bullosa 69.5, 69.16, 69.18–69.19, 69.21, *69.22*, 69.27
   fibril fragmentation in ageing 156.8–156.9
   gene expression 2.29–2.31
   genetic disorders 70.1–70.14
      Ehlers–Danlos syndromes 70.1–70.11
      osteogenesis imperfecta 70.12–70.14
      prolidase deficiency 70.11–70.12
   genetic heterogeneity **2.27**
   hydroxylation reactions 2.29, *2.30*
   light absorption/scattering by skin 23.4
   periodicity in collagen fibres 2.23
   scarring 11.8
   type I 2.22, 2.23, 2.28, 2.32
   type III 2.28, 2.32
   type IV 2.22–2.23, 2.28
   type V 2.28
   type VI 2.28
   type VII 2.26–2.27, 2.28, 2.32
   type XVII 2.28–2.29
   wound healing 11.7, 11.8

collagen bundles
   deep morphoea 97.13
   granuloma annulare 97.14
collagen dermal filler 158.5–158.6, 158.7–158.8
collagenoma 94.43
   Cowden syndrome 78.11
collagenosis nuchae *see* nuchal-type fibroma
collagenous colitis 153.3
collagenous fibroma *see* desmoplastic fibroblastoma
collagenous marginal plaques of the hands 94.4–94.5
collagen peptide supplements 122.6
collagen-stimulating dermal fillers 158.6–158.7
collarette scale *4.13*
collective teloptosis 87.53
Colliers' stripes 86.53
collodion baby 63.8, 63.12–63.13, 63.43–63.44, 114.19–114.21
collodions, vehicle choice for topical therapies 18.2
colloid body 3.40
colloid degeneration 94.5–94.6
   penile 109.31
colloid milium 94.5–94.6
coloboma–heart defect–ichthyosiform dermatosis–mental retardation–ear anomalies (CHIME) syndrome 63.38–63.39
colon, gastrointestinal polyposis 78.11
colophony 127.17–127.18, 127.45, 127.74–127.78
colostomy **112.3**
   Crohn ulceration 112.13, 112.14
   inflammatory polyps 112.6
   irritant skin reaction 112.2
   leakage and faecal dermatitis 112.4, 112.5
   localised bullous pemphigoid 112.12
colour dyes, specimen preparation 3.5–3.6
colour of skin *see* skin of colour
CoLQ *see* Course of Life Questionnaire
combined dyslipidaemia **60.2**
   type III hyperlipoproteinaemia 60.8–60.9
combined immunodeficiencies **80.4**, 80.7–80.13
   associated/syndromic features 80.11–80.13
combined melanocytic naevi 131.24–131.26
combined oral contraceptives (COCs)
   androgenic effect **88.13**
   antibiotic interactions 88.49
   hair disorder treatment 87.89, 87.95, **87.96**
comedo extractor 88.58
comedo naevus 73.7, 88.31, *88.32*, 137.5
comedonal acne *4.19*, 88.1–88.2, *88.3*, 88.14, 88.26, 88.27, 88.28, 88.45
   in acne conglobata 88.65
   comedo extractor 88.58
   cutaneous nodular elastosis with 156.4
   management 88.45–88.47
   nodular elastosis *156.5*
   prepubertal *88.69*
   submarine comedones *88.28*
   treatment algorithm 88.45
   see also chloracne
Comèl–Netherton syndrome (CNS) 63.26–63.28, **80.4**, 80.11
commensal skin flora 26.2–26.5
common acquired naevi **131.16**, 131.17–131.21
common naevi, low melanoma risk 142.2
common variable immunodeficiency (CVID) 80.1, **80.5**, 80.13, 147.2
common warts (verruca vulgaris) 25.52, 25.53, 25.54
   see also cutaneous warts
communication, holistic management of skin disease 15.6, 15.7
community-acquired MRSA (CA-MRSA) 26.6–26.7
community dermatology 7.7, 7.8, 7.11
community diagnosis 5.2
company-sponsored clinical trials 17.3

comparative genomic hybridisation (CGH), melanoma diagnosis 142.21
compensatory hyperhidrosis 92.7
   surgical treatment 92.10
complaints and litigation
   body dysmorphic disorder 84.15
   delusional infestation 84.9–84.10
   factitious skin diseases by proxy 84.38
complementary/alternative/traditional therapies
   acne vulgaris 88.57–88.58
   cosmeceuticals 157.7–157.10
   metal poisoning 121.1
   psychiatric problems 84.48
   topical 18.38
   wart treatments 25.60
   see also herbals
complement diseases, inherited immunodeficiency 80.18–80.20
complete circumferential peripheral and deep margin assessment (CCPDMA), basal cell carcinoma 140.16
completion lymph node dissection (CLND), melanoma 143.4, 143.5
complex aphthosis, oral ulceration 108.39–108.40
complex regional pain syndrome (CRPS) 83.20–83.23
   dermatological manifestations **83.22**
   diagnostic criteria **83.21**
   management 83.22–83.23
   treatment ladder 83.23
   triggers of **83.21**
complicated lymphatic anomalies (CLAs) 71.1, 71.22–71.23
Compositae (Asteraceae) allergy 127.11, 127.16–127.17, 127.19–127.20, 127.71–127.74
composite haemangioendothelioma 136.33–136.34
compound allergy 127.29
compound follicles 87.84
compound naevi
   acquired melanocytic naevi 131.19, *131.21*
   acral naevi *131.23*
   conjunctival naevus *131.25*
   definition **131.1**
   dysplastic melanocytic naevi *131.42*
   Spitz naevus *131.33*
comprehensive acne severity system (CASS) 88.38, **88.39**
Comprehensive Care Programme with Persons with Albinism (CCPWA) 7.10–7.11
compression syndromes, BSL association 98.15, 98.17
compression therapy, venous leg ulcer 102.5
computed tomography (CT) scans
   foreign body reactions 122.18
   morphoea 55.31
computer-aided diagnostic systems (CAD), melanoma diagnosis 142.10
computer-aided image analysis, skin properties 16.5
computer-based assessments (CBAs) 16.2
computerised dermoscopy devices, melanoma diagnosis 142.9
conception, drug pharmacokinetics and pharmacodynamics 13.8
conditioners (hair), alopecia management 87.98–87.99
condoms, genital contact dermatitis **109.13**
condyloma acuminata, human papillomavirus infection 113.4
condylomas, penis 109.39–109.40
condylomata acuminata 25.61–25.64
   see also ano-genital warts
condylomata lata, syphilis 29.5, 29.10, 29.11, 29.17
cones, blood supply 124.8
confetti ichthyoses 63.16, *63.18*
confetti-like macular atrophy 94.25

confidence intervals
   epidemiological studies 5.14
   statistical analysis of clinical studies 17.22–17.23
confluent hyperkeratosis *63.59*
confluent and reticulated papillomatosis (CARP) 85.6–85.8
confocal microscopy, basal cell carcinoma 140.10, *140.13*
congenital adrenal hyperplasia (CAH) 87.90–87.91
   acne vulgaris association 88.5–88.7
   adrenal steroid genesis pathway *88.9*
   clinical features **88.10**
   dermatoendocrinology 150.17–150.18
congenital alopecias 87.30
congenital anomalies, oral involvement 108.87–108.88
congenital biliary tract hypoplasia with consecutive cholestasis, jaundice 153.5
congenital candidiasis 32.66–32.67, 114.28
congenital cyanotic heart disease, associated finger clubbing 151.1, *151.3*
congenital cytomegalovirus infection 25.41
congenital dermatosis with reticulate scarring 94.14
congenital disorders
   and genetic syndromes, involving respiratory system and skin 152.5
   prenatal diagnosis 8.9–8.10
congenital epidermal naevi (CEN) 73.3–73.8
   Blaschko linear distribution *73.5*
   classification 73.2
   clinical features 73.4–73.5
   clinical variants 73.5–73.7
   complications and co-morbidities 73.7–73.8
   eccrine naevus 73.6
   epidermal thickening with hyperkeratosis and inflammatory reaction 73.4
   genetic basis of **73.3**
   investigations 73.8
   management 73.8
   pathophysiology 73.3–73.4
   sebaceous naevus 73.5, 73.6, 73.7, 73.8
   verrucous epidermal naevus 73.4, 73.5
congenital erosive and vesicular dermatosis, healing with reticulated supple scarring 114.9
congenital erosive and vesicular dermatosis (CEVD), neonates 114.9
congenital erythropoietic porphyria (CEP) 58.9–58.11
   clinical features 58.9–58.10
   genetic counselling 58.11
   investigations 58.10
   scarring of skin with resorption of terminal phalanges *58.10*
   treatment 58.10–58.11
congenital generalised fibromatosis *see* infantile myofibromatosis
congenital generalised hypertrichosis (CGH) 87.85
congenital generalised lipodystrophies (CGL) 72.2–72.3, 98.3
congenital haemangiomas, infants 116.7–116.9
congenital haemolytic anaemias 86.48–86.49
congenital heart block (CHB) 51.39–51.42
congenital hemidysplasia–ichthyosiform naevus–limb defect (CHILD) syndrome 63.23–63.24
congenital hypertrichosis 87.85
   lanuginosa 87.85
congenital ichthyoses
   management 63.41–63.46
   non-syndromic 63.7–63.13
   psychosocial aspects 63.46
   trichothiodystrophy 63.37
congenital ichthyosiform erythroderma (CIE) 63.10–63.13, *63.12*, *63.27*
congenital lax skin 94.21

congenital leptin deficiency 97.5
congenital lesions, oral involvement 108.28–108.31
congenital lipodystrophy 72.1–72.3, 98.2
congenital livedo reticularis 124.9
congenital localised hypertrichosis 87.85–87.86
congenital melanocytic naevi (CMN) 73.8–73.15, 131.15–131.17
    associated diseases 73.9
    benign proliferative nodule *73.11*
    bland naevus cells *73.9, 73.10*
    clinical features 73.11
    clinical presentation **131.16**
    clinical variants 73.11–73.12
    complications and co-morbidities 73.12–73.13
    dermoscopic presentation **131.16**
    differential diagnosis 73.12
    environmental factors 73.11
    facial features characteristic of 73.13
    genetics 73.10–73.11
    laser therapies 23.16
    management 73.14–73.15
    melanoma development *73.10*
    as melanoma precursors 142.2
    melanoma risk 73.13
    neurological abnormalities 73.12–73.13
    neurological investigation and patient follow-up *73.14*
    pathology **131.16**
    pathophysiology 73.9–73.10
    severity classification 73.12
    speckled lentiginous naevus 131.15–131.17
congenital midline hamartoma *see* rhabdomyomatous congenital hamartoma
congenital muscle hamartoma 73.19
congenital naevi 73.1–73.18
    blue naevus 73.15, *73.16*
    classification 73.1–73.2
    congenital epidermal naevi 73.2, 73.3–73.8
    congenital melanocytic naevi 73.8–73.15
    congenital naevus spilus 73.15–73.16
    connective tissue naevi **73.2**, 73.16–73.18
    fat naevus **73.2**, 73.16–73.18
    genetic classification 73.2
    histological classification 73.2
    inheritance of naevus mutations 73.3
    muscle 'naevi' **73.2**
    naevus phenotypes 73.1
    pigment cell naevi **73.2**
    Spitz naevi 73.15
    terminology **73.2**
congenital naevus spilus 73.15–73.16
congenital-onset primary lymphoedema 103.24
congenital palmoplantar and periorificial keratoderma with corneal epithelial dysplasia (Olmsted syndrome) 63.69–63.70, 108.30
congenital pilar/smooth muscle naevus *see* smooth muscle hamartoma
congenital poikiloderma 94.13
congenital pseudo-ainhum 94.48
congenital reticular ichthyosiform erythroderma (CRIE) 63.16, *63.18*
congenital rubella syndrome 25.92, 114.21
congenital self-healing reticulohistiocytosis (CSHRH) 135.5, *135.6–135.7*
congenital Spitz naevi 73.15
congenital superficial capillary malformations (port-wine stains) 73.20
    eyelids 107.47
    laser therapies 23.8–23.9, *23.10*, 23.11
    lobular capillary haemangioma/pyogenic granuloma within 136.26
    phakomatosis pigmentovascularis 73.22
congenital syphilis (CS) 29.2, 29.22–29.29
    clinical features 29.23–29.26
    definition 29.22–29.23
    early manifestations 29.23–29.25, *29.27*
    epidemiology 29.23
    investigations 29.26–29.27
    late manifestations 29.25–29.26, *29.27*
    management 29.27–29.29
    neonatal 114.27–114.28
    pathophysiology 29.23
congenital tuberculosis, neonates 114.28
congenital vellus hamartoma, hair follicle naevus 137.7
congestive heart failure, oedema 85.29
conglobate acne *see* acne conglobata
conidiobolomycosis 32.79–32.80
Conidiobolus coronatus 32.79–32.80
conjunctiva
    bulbar telangiectasia *80.11*
    UV radiation-exposure damage 76.5
conjunctival hyperaemia, mucous membrane pemphigoid 50.30
conjunctival naevi 131.24, *131.25*
conjunctivitis, actinic prurigo 126.10
connective tissue diseases (CTD) 3.44, 53.1–53.3
    acquired ichthyosis 63.47
    autoimmune disorders affecting skin and respiratory system 152.2
    direct immunofluorescence findings 3.19
    dystrophic calcification 59.1
    investigations 53.3
    management 53.3
    mechanical injuries 122.2
    ocular features **107.41**
    papular and nodular mucinosis 57.13–57.14
    skin fragility 69.20
    systemic sclerosis 54.8–54.9
connective tissue naevi **73.2**, 73.16–73.18
    haematoxylin and eosin stain *3.8*
    tuberous sclerosis complex 78.8
connective tissues, malignancy and rheumatological disorders 148.20–148.21
connective tissue septa *97.3*, 97.6
connexin 26, Vohwinkel syndrome 63.64
connexins, KID syndrome 63.33
connexons, gap junction 2.20
Conradi syndrome, follicular atrophoderma 94.17
Conradi–Hünermann–Happle syndrome (CHHS) 63.22–63.23
COnsensus-based Standards for the selection of health Measurement INstruments (COSMIN) checklist 16.3
Consolidated Standards of Reporting Trials (CONSORT) 17.14
constitutive pigmentation 68.1, 86.8–86.9
constitutive skin colour 86.1–86.2
constricting bands of the extremities 94.46–94.48
constriction artefact, oedema induction 84.33
consultants, referral rates 5.13
contact allergies
    musical instruments 122.12
    purpura **99.9**
    topical therapy 18.5
contact brucellosis 26.61
contact cheilitis 108.60–108.61
contact dermatitis 105.5, 127.1
    arsenic 121.2, 121.4
    cannabis-induced 120.4
    drug-induced eczema 117.3–117.5
    ear dermatoses **106.22**
    ear piercing 106.11–106.12
    erythromelalgia *101.9*
    eyelid 107.6
    irritants 128.1–128.13, 129.1–129.5
    lichen planus-like contact dermatitis 37.3
    patch testing technique 1.8
    perianal skin 111.12
    pseudolymphoma 134.1, 134.2
    vulval 110.14–110.15
    see also allergic contact dermatitis
contact hypersensitivity, Langerhans cells 2.14
contact immunotherapy, alopecia treatment 87.27
contact urticaria (CU) 42.13–42.14, 127.82–127.86
    non-immune 128.8–128.9
    occupational hazards 129.8–129.11
contagious pustular dermatitis *see* orf virus
contingency tables, statistical analysis of clinical studies 17.22
contour, principles of surgical design 20.19–20.20
contraception
    systemic lupus erythematosus 51.32
    see also combined oral contraceptives
contrite reaction, olfactory reference syndrome 84.10
contusion, external ear 106.8
conubial dermatitis (ACD by-proxy dermatitis) 109.12
Conus genus, stings from 130.4
conventional photodynamic therapy, actinic keratosis 141.10
cooling management, chemotherapy-induced alopecia 87.72
Copenhagen Psoriasis Severity Index 16.3
copper allergy 127.41
copper deficiency 2.34, 61.27–61.29
CoQ10 *see* coenzyme Q10
coral stings 130.1–130.3
core outcome measures 16.3
Core Outcome Set (COS), eczema outcome measures **16.3**
corkscrew hairs, vitamin C deficiency 61.21, *61.22*
cornea
    brittle cornea syndrome **70.6–70.7**, 70.10
    UV radiation-exposure damage 76.5
    vascularisation and scarring, herpes simplex virus 107.37
corneal argyria, silver exposure 121.8
corneal transplant, ocular rosacea 107.11
corneocytes 2.1, 2.6
corneodesmosin 69.6
cornification
    exfoliative disorders 63.26–63.30
    inherited disorders 63.1–63.80
cornoid lamella 85.20–85.21
    porokeratoses 63.75–63.76
corns 122.7–122.9, 122.16
corona phlebectatica paraplantaris (ankle flare), chronic venous insufficiency *101.43, 101.44*
coronary artery disease 51.30, 151.5
coronavirus *see* COVID-19
cortex, hair fibres 87.6, *87.7*
cortical cells 2.9
corticosteroid-induced rosacea-like facial dermatosis 89.17
corticosteroid injection, localised lipoatrophy due to 98.11–98.12
corticosteroid purpura 99.5
corticosteroids 1.8, 12.3, 12.8
    acneform reaction 88.11–88.12
    acne treatment 88.57, 129.12
    allergic contact dermatitis 127.45, 127.47
    allergic reactions 127.4
    atopic eczema treatment 41.26–41.27
    atrophy due to 94.6–94.10
    bronchopneumonia treatment 125.5
    chemical structure **18.14**
    cutaneous adverse effects 155.15
    drug reaction with eosinophilia and systemic symptoms 118.11–118.12
    eye, side effects on 107.40–107.43
    genital contact dermatitis **109.13**
    indications 18.15, **18.17**
    inflammatory peristomal skin diseases **112.4**
    intralesional injection 18.21–18.22
    local adverse effects 18.15, 18.17–18.19
    mastocytosis treatment 46.10
    mechanism of action 18.15
    morphoea treatment 55.36–55.37
    occlusion 18.21
    patch testing 127.47
    pemphigus treatment 50.8
    poststeroid panniculitis 97.58–97.59
    potency classification 18.14–18.15, **18.16**
    in pregnancy 113.19, **113.22**
    primary localised cutaneous amyloidosis treatment 56.13, 56.14
    psoriasis treatment 35.20, **35.21**
    side effects 18.15, 18.17–18.20
    Stevens–Johnson syndrome/toxic epidermal necrolysis 118.21
    systemic adverse effects 18.19–18.20
    tinea (ringworm) infections 32.49–32.50
    topical therapies 18.14–18.22
    urticaria treatment 42.18
corticosteroid-sparing agents, sarcoidosis management 96.15–96.16
corticotrophin-releasing hormone (CRH), hair follicle 87.11
Corynebacterium
    C. diphtheriae, diphtheria 26.38–26.39
    C. flavescens, trichomycosis axillaris 26.41–26.42
    C. minutissimum, erythrasma 26.39
    C. propinquum, trichomycosis axillaris 26.41–26.42
    C. pseudotuberculosis, diphtheria 26.38
    C. tenuis, trichomycosis axillaris 26.41–26.42
    C. ulcerans, diphtheria 26.38
    pitted keratolysis 26.42–26.43
Corynebacterium acnes see Cutibacterium
Corynebacterium haemolyticum see Arcanobacterium haemolyticum
Corynebacterium kroppenstedtii, rosacea 89.4
Corynebacterium pyogenes see Trueperella pyogenes
coryneform bacteria 26.37–26.43
    found on skin 26.4
    general description 26.37–26.38
    types 26.37
COS *see* Core Outcome Set
cosmeceuticals 157.1–157.13
    aloe 157.10–157.11
    alpha-lipoic acid 157.1–157.2
    anti-ageing
        rhytid reduction 157.4–157.7
        skin lightening 157.3–157.4
    anti-inflammatories 157.10–157.11
    antioxidants 157.1–157.3
    arbutin 157.3
    caffeine 157.11
    carnosine 157.7
    carrier peptides 157.6
    chamomile 157.11
    coenzyme Q10 157.2
    'cosmeceutical' term 157.1
    cysteamine 157.3
    efficacy of 157.1, 157.13
    glycine-glutamate-lysine-glycine 157.5
    glycosaminoglycans 157.4
    grape seed extract 157.7–157.9
    green tea (*Camellia sinensis*) 157.9
    herbals and phytochemicals 157.7–157.10
    hydroquinone 157.3–157.4
    hydroxy acids 157.4–157.5
    ingredients and potential uses, summary of **157.12–157.13**
    kojic acid 157.4
    lycopene 157.9–157.10
    neurotransmitter-affecting peptides 157.6
    origin of 157.1
    peptides 157.5–157.6
        mechanism of action **157.6**
    polyunsaturated fatty acids 157.5
    pomegranate 157.10
    regulation of 157.1, 157.13
    retinaldehyde 157.7
    retinoids 157.6–157.7
    retinol 157.7
    retinyl esters 157.7
    risks of using 157.13
    safety of 157.13
    signal peptides 157.5–157.6

soya 157.10
tranexamic acid 157.4
vitamin A (retinoids) 157.6–157.7
vitamin B 157.2
vitamin C 157.2–157.3
vitamin E 157.3
see also cosmetic treatments
cosmesis, alopecia treatment 87.18
cosmetic allergens 127.4–127.5, 127.12, 127.47–127.58, 127.59–127.60
    EU directives/regulations 127.35
cosmetic dermatitis 128.4
cosmetic exhaustion 128.4
cosmetic fillers, factitious panniculitis 97.48–97.49
cosmetic products, seborrhoeic dermatitis effects 40.4
cosmetics
    and acne 88.25, 129.12
    lead poisoning 121.5
    metal poisoning 121.1, 121.5
    photocontact facial melanosis 86.12
cosmetic subunit junction lines, principles of surgical design 20.20
cosmetic treatments 1.8, 1.9
    alopecia 87.69, 87.97–87.101
    APL management 98.6
    fat hypertrophy 98.15
    laser resurfacing 161.1–161.6
    in pregnancy 113.21, 113.24
    skin photoageing 156.11
    skin tightening 161.6–161.8
    see also cosmeceuticals
cosmetic vehicles/excipients 127.58–127.60
COSMIN *see* COnsensus-based Standards for the selection of health Measurement INstruments checklist
cost-benefit analysis, health economics 6.4
cost of disease *see* economic burden of disease
Costello syndrome 70.16, 78.9
cost-minimisation studies, health economics 6.4
counselling, chemical peels 160.6–160.7
Course of Life Questionnaire (CoLQ) 16.11
covert injections, dermatitis artefacta 84.33
COVID-19-induced perniosis, type I cryoglobulinaemia 149.14
COVID-19/SARS-CoV-2 (severe acute respiratory syndrome coronavirus 2) 1.8, 1.9, 25.100–25.120
    altered dermatological healthcare during pandemic 25.120
    clinical features 25.102
    cutaneous manifestations 152.4
    epidemiology 25.100
    exacerbation of pre-existing mucocutaneous diseases 25.115
    infants 115.5
    investigations 25.102
    irritant contact dermatitis 129.2
    mucocutaneous manifestations of infection 25.103–25.115
        children 25.113–25.115
        clinical features 25.104–25.115
        clinical variants 25.105–25.107, 25.108–25.113
        epidemiology 25.103–25.104, 25.113
        hair and nail disorders 25.113
        management 25.105–25.107
        pathophysiology 25.104
        relationship to disease severity 25.108
        timeline relative to systemic features 25.108
    mucocutaneous manifestations of treatment 25.116
    mucocutaneous reactions to vaccines 25.117
    occupational dermatoses 127.4
    outcomes in patients with pre-existing mucocutaneous diseases 25.115
    pathophysiology 25.100–25.101
    perniosis 124.5
    PPE-occupational dermatoses 25.119
    sexually transmitted infections, effect on 29.2

treatment, mucocutaneous manifestations 25.116
    vaccination considerations 25.117–25.119
    virology 25.101
    vitamin D deficiency 61.10
'Covid toes/fingers', chilblain-like lesions/pseudo-pernio associated with COVID-19 25.108–25.109
Cowden syndrome (PTEN hamartoma tumour syndrome) 71.2, 71.13–71.14, 72.10, 78.11, 78.14, 148.11–148.12
    oral involvement 108.85
    storiform collagenoma 136.3
    trichilemmoma 137.6
cowpox virus 25.12–25.13
    vaccinia virus relationship 25.7
coxsackieviruses 25.93–25.95
    vesicular exanthem 25.5
    see also eczema coxsackium
CP *see* chronic pruritus
CPD *see* chronic papillomatous dermatitis; cyclobutane pyrimidine dimer
crab lice 34.24–34.25
crack cocaine 120.1, 120.5
cradle cap 40.5, 115.1, 115.2
cranial dysraphism 87.86
cranial nerves, anatomical positions 20.2–20.4
cranial neuropathies 82.6
cranial (nodular) fasciitis 136.5
cranio-facial hyperhidrosis 92.6
craniosynostosis syndromes 70.17
CRBSI *see* catheter-related bloodstream infections
creams, topical drugs 12.3–12.4, 18.2
creep 122.3
creeping hair 122.22
CRH *see* corticotrophin-releasing hormone
CRI *see* catheter-related infection
cri du chat syndrome 74.3
CRIE *see* congenital reticular ichthyosiform erythroderma
crinkles 94.2, 94.26
crisaborole, atopic eczema treatment 41.27
Crisponi syndrome 94.40
Crohn disease (CD)
    cutaneous Crohn disease 95.13–95.16
    hidradenitis suppurativa association 90.2, 90.6, 90.7
    ileostomy for 112.5, 112.9
    leukonychia 121.7
    mucocutaneous features of 111.27
    oral involvement 108.72
    perianal 95.14, 111.26–111.27
    peristomal 112.13–112.15
    psoriasis in 35.18
    pyoderma gangrenosum 112.15
    skin involvement 153.2–153.3
    ulcerative colitis distinction 153.1–153.2
    vulval 110.23–110.24
cromoglicate 18.39
Cronkhite–Canada syndrome 87.58
Cross syndrome 68.9
croton oil, chemical peels 160.10–160.11
Crouzon syndrome 85.4, 106.7
Crown vessels, sebaceous gland hyperplasia 91.17
crow's feet (lateral periorbital lines), botulinum toxin injection 159.5, 159.6, 159.7
CRPS *see* complex regional pain syndrome
crude petroleum, acne 129.12
crust 3.40
crustacean vectors of parasitic disease, *Cyclops* species and dracunculiasis 33.13
CrVI *see* chromium VI
cryofibrinogenaemia, purpura 99.11–99.14
cryoglobulinaemia 124.13
    purpura 99.11–99.14
cryoglobulinaemic vasculitis 100.15–100.17, 124.13
    serum protein electrophoresis 100.17

cryoglobulins, cryogelling/cryoagglutination disorders 99.11–99.14
cryolipolysis, fat contouring 161.8–161.9
CryoModulation technology 161.6
cryopyrin-associated periodic syndrome (CAPS) 45.8–45.9
cryosurgery 20.46–20.47
    basal cell carcinoma treatment 140.11, 140.14–140.16
cryotherapy
    actinic keratosis 141.9
    Bowen disease 141.22–141.23
    cutaneous squamous cell carcinoma 141.35
    cutaneous warts 25.58–25.59
cryptococcosis 32.90–32.92
    oral involvement 108.57
cryptococcus infection, HIV 31.28
Cryptococcus neoformans 32.91, 32.92
crystal globulin vasculopathy 99.15
crystalloids, resuscitation use 125.3
crystal meth 120.4–120.5
crystal violet, tattoos 86.53
CS *see* carcinoid syndrome; chondroitin sulphate; Cockayne syndrome; congenital syphilis
cSCC *see* cutaneous squamous cell carcinoma
CS-COUSIN *see* Cochrane Skin Core Outcomes Initiative
CSHRH *see* congenital self-healing reticulohistiocytosis
CSS *see* classic Sweet syndrome; cultured skin substitute
CSU *see* chronic spontaneous urticaria
CSVV *see* cutaneous small-vessel vasculitis
CT *see* computed tomography
CTCL *see* cutaneous T-cell lymphoma
CTD *see* connective tissue diseases
CTLs *see* cytotoxic T lymphocytes
CTS *see* cervical trophic syndrome
CU *see* contact urticaria
Cubozoa (box jellyfish), stings 130.1
'cuff sign', lipoedema 98.22
cultured epithelial autografts (CEA) 125.6
cultured skin substitute (CSS) 125.6
culture-independent microbial studies, molecular genetic methods 26.2, 26.3
culturing samples
    quantitative bacterial studies 26.4
    skin flora 26.3
cumulative life course impairment (CLCI) 16.11
    impact of a long-term health condition over time 15.3
cupping, discoid hyperpigmentation 4.12
CU-Q₂oL *see* Chronic Urticaria Quality of Life Questionnaire
curettage 3.3–3.4
    Bowen disease treatment 141.23
    treating skin lesions 20.48
    unsuitable for basel cell carcinomas 20.35, 20.37
curettage and cautery (C&C) *see* curettage and electrodessication
curettage and electrodessication
    actinic keratosis 141.9
    basal cell carcinoma 140.14
    cutaneous squamous cell carcinoma 141.34–141.35
Curie, Marie 1.9
curlicue (storiform) pattern 3.40
Curry–Jones syndrome 73.7, 78.12
Cushing disease/syndrome 86.7, 86.18
    acne vulgaris association 88.7
    dermatoendocrinology 150.11, 150.13, 150.17
    striae 94.10, 94.11
cutaneo-mucosal venous malformation *see* venous mucocutaneous malformation
cutaneous adnexal tumours *see* tumours of skin appendages

cutaneous adverse drug effects
    allopurinol 155.9–155.10, 155.15
    antimalarials 19.5–19.6, 155.15
    antirheumatic therapies 155.15–155.16
    NSAIDs 155.15
cutaneous adverse events, reactions to COVID-19 vaccines 25.117
cutaneous amyloidoses *see* amyloidoses
cutaneous arteriovenous haemangioma *see* cirsoid aneurysm
cutaneous arteritis 97.9–97.11, 100.28–100.30
cutaneous atrophy
    causes 94.6–94.21
    perineal and perianal 111.12
    vascular Ehlers–Danlos syndrome 70.8
cutaneous B-cell lymphoma (CBCL)
    diffuse large B-cell lymphoma 139.37, 139.41–139.43
    follicle centre cell 139.37, 139.40–139.41
    marginal zone lymphoma 139.37–139.39
    primary 139.37–139.43
    secondary 139.43–139.45
    treatment algorithm 139.38
cutaneous bleeding
    causes 99.5
    see also ecchymosis (bruises); purpura
cutaneous burns, treatment 125.7–125.8
cutaneous Crohn disease 95.13–95.16
    clinical features 95.16
    lip swelling due to oro-facial granulomatosis 95.14
    management 95.16
    metastatic Crohn disease, 'knife-cut' fissures 95.15, 95.16
    pathology 95.14–95.16
    peno-scrotal lymphoedema 95.15
    peri-anal skin tags 95.14
    perivascular dermal infiltrates 95.15
    vulval swelling 95.15
cutaneous cylindroma, CYLD cutaneous syndrome 78.11
cutaneous cysts *see* chloracne; comedonal acne; cysts; dermoid cysts; metabolising acquired dioxin-induced skin hamartoma; vellus hair cyst
cutaneous effects of systemic therapies
    antimalarials 19.5–19.6, 155.15
    glucocorticoids 19.19
    hydroxycarbamide 19.21–19.22
cutaneous endometriosis, vulva 110.33
cutaneous epithelioid angiomatous nodule 136.28–136.29
cutaneous erythema *see* redness (erythema)
cutaneous Ewing sarcoma 136.51–136.52
cutaneous haemosiderosis 86.47–86.49
cutaneous histiocytoses 135.1–135.32
cutaneous histoplasmosis 32.82, 32.83
cutaneous horn 141.12–141.13
cutaneous hyperextensibility, classical Ehlers–Danlos syndrome 70.8
cutaneous infections
    panniculitis 97.46
    SJS/TEN complications 118.20
cutaneous juvenile xanthogranuloma 135.17
cutaneous keratocysts 133.6–133.7
cutaneous larva migrans 4.16
    clinical features 33.19–33.20
    definition/nomenclature 33.18–33.19
    management 33.20
    nematodes of other animals 33.18–33.20
    pathophysiology 33.19
    perineal skin 111.16
    see also ancylostomiasis
cutaneous laser therapy 23.1–23.24
cutaneous leishmaniasis 33.43–33.51
    chronic 33.47–33.48
    clinical features 33.46–33.49
    clinical variants 33.45, 33.46–33.49
    diffuse 33.48–33.49
    epidemiology 33.43–33.45
    investigations 33.49–33.50

cutaneous leishmaniasis (continued)
  management 33.50–33.51
  pathophysiology 33.45–33.46
cutaneous lesions 96.13, 96.15
  juvenile xanthogranuloma 135.16
  liver disease association 153.9
  panniculitis 97.6
  progressive nodular histiocytosis 135.19
cutaneous lupus 126.32, 126.33
cutaneous lymphadenoma see adamantinoid trichoblastoma
cutaneous lymphangiectasia 103.31–103.32
cutaneous lymphocyte antigen (CLA), primary cutaneous T-cell lymphomas 139.2
cutaneous lymphoid hyperplasia see pseudolymphoma
cutaneous lymphomas 139.1–139.50
  blastic plasmacytoid dendritic cell neoplasm 139.45–139.47
  classification 139.1, **139.2**, 139.37
  leukaemia cutis 139.47–139.48
  post-transplant lymphoproliferative disorder 139.47
  primary B-cell lymphoma 139.37–139.43
  primary T-cell lymphomas 139.1–139.37
  radiotherapy 24.15–24.18
  secondary B-cell lymphoma 139.43–139.45
  secondary T-cell lymphoma 139.45
  see also haematological malignancies
cutaneous macroglobulinosis 149.13
cutaneous markers of internal malignancy 148.1–148.28
cutaneous mastocytosis (CM) **46.2**, 46.3–46.5
  musculoskeletal involvement 155.13
cutaneous melanomas see malignant melanoma
cutaneous meningioma see meningothelial heterotopias
cutaneous metastases 148.4–148.6
cutaneous miliary tuberculosis, acute 27.17
cutaneous mucinosis 57.1–57.19
  classification 57.1, **57.2**
  connective tissue diseases 57.13–57.14
  dermal mucinoses 57.2–57.15, 57.16
  detection for research 57.1
  digital myxoid cyst 57.15, 57.16
  facial 57.14–57.15
  focal 57.14–57.15
  follicular mucinoses 57.15–57.18
  of infancy 57.6, 57.7
  lichen myxoedematosus 57.1–57.8
  myxoedema in thyroid diseases 57.11–57.14
  pinkus follicular mucinosis 57.16, 57.17
  primary mucinoses 57.2–57.18
  reticular erythematous mucinosis 57.8–57.9
  scleroedema 57.9–57.11
  secondary mucinoses 57.1, **57.2**, 57.18
  self-healing cutaneous mucinoses 57.14
  urticaria-like follicular mucinosis 57.16–57.17
cutaneous myoepithelioma 137.32–137.33
cutaneous necrosis, intravenous drug administration 120.7
cutaneous neoplasia, photodynamic therapy 22.6–22.7, 22.8
cutaneous neoplasms 3.21–3.29
  cytokeratin markers 3.21–3.22
  epithelial markers 3.21–3.23
  histiocytic markers 3.27
  keratin markers 3.21–3.23
  Langerhans cell markers 3.27, 3.28
  lymphoid markers 3.27–3.29
  melanocytic markers 3.23–3.25
  mesenchymal markers 3.25–3.26
  metastatic cutaneous tumours 3.26–3.27
  neuroendocrine markers 3.23
cutaneous (neuro-) endocrine signalling mechanism, key components **150.4**
cutaneous neurofibromas 78.3

cutaneous nodular elastosis with cysts and comedones, ageing of skin 156.4
cutaneous photosensitivity diseases 126.1–126.29
cutaneous polyarteritis nodosa 97.9–97.11
cutaneous porphyrias see porphyria
cutaneous radiation recall reactions, chemotherapy 119.12
cutaneous reactions
  cold and heat 124.1–124.16
  implanted metals 127.19
  surgical implants 151.5–151.6
cutaneous rhabdomyosarcoma 136.55–136.56
cutaneous rosacea 89.3, 89.13
cutaneous sarcoid-like reactions, tattoos 122.22
cutaneous sarcoidosis 96.3, 96.4, 96.6–96.7, 96.16
  rare forms 97.53–97.54
  treatment ladder **96.17**
cutaneous sarcoid reaction 96.17–96.18
cutaneous schwannoma 106.35
cutaneous small-vessel vasculitis (CSVV) 100.5–100.8
  blisters 100.7
  causes **100.5**
  leukocytoclastic vasculitis 100.6
cutaneous squamous cell carcinoma (cSCC) 106.27–106.28, 141.26–141.37
  associated diseases 141.1, 141.27
  causative organisms 141.30
  clinical features 141.30–141.34
  clinical variants 141.31
  definitions/nomenclature 141.26
  disease course and prognosis 141.32–141.34
  epidemiology 141.26–141.27
  first line treatment
    high/very high-risk disease 141.35, 141.37
    low-risk disease 141.34–141.35
  human papillomavirus association 25.65
  immunocompromised people
    clinicopathological features 147.10–147.11
    management 147.16–147.18
  investigations 141.34
  as a keratinocyte cancer 141.1
  management 141.34–141.37
  multiple self-healing **78.13**, 141.41–141.42
  pathology 141.29–141.30
  pathophysiology 141.27–141.30
  predisposing factors 141.29
  second line treatment 141.37
  severity classification/staging systems 141.31–141.32
  signalling pathways/networks 141.27–141.28, 141.29
  verrucous carcinoma of the foot/epithelioma cuniculatum 141.31
  see also keratinocyte cancer
cutaneous T-cell lymphoma (CTCL) 86.44
  acquired ichthyosis 63.48
  combination therapy 139.23–139.24
  extracorporeal photochemotherapy 21.7
  management 139.20–139.25
  origin of term 139.1
  phototherapy 21.4, 21.7
  primary 139.1–139.25
  rare primary cutaneous variants (non-MF) 139.29–139.37
  secondary 139.45
  systemic therapies 139.22–139.25
  topical therapies 139.21–139.22
  see also mycosis fungoides
cutaneous tuberculosis see tuberculosis of the skin
cutaneous tumours, WHO classification 142.8
cutaneous vascular malformations 101.26–101.31
  disorders associated with **101.28**

see also vascular disorders
cutaneous vasculitis see vasculitis, cutaneous
cutaneous warts
  clinical features 25.53–25.57
  cryotherapy 25.58–25.59
  epidemiology 25.52
  human papillomavirus 25.52–25.61
  hyperthermic therapy 25.59
  investigations 25.57
  laser therapy 25.59
  management 25.57–25.61
  pathophysiology 25.52–25.53
  photodynamic therapy 25.59
  surgery 25.59
  topical pharmacology 25.57–25.58, 25.59
cutibacteria
  in follicles and sebaceous glands 26.3
  infections 26.43
Cutibacterium (previously Propionibacterium)
  C. acnes 26.43
    effect on human sebocytes 88.17
    necrotising lymphocytic folliculitis 93.4
    sarcoidosis causation 96.4
    scalp folliculitis 93.5
  C. avidum 26.43
  C. granulosum 26.43
cuticle, hair fibres 87.6
cuticle defects, trichorrhexis nodosa 87.76
cuticular cells 2.9
cutis laxa 70.14–70.17, 77.5–77.7, 94.21–94.23
  autosomal dominant cutis laxa 70.17, 77.5–77.6
  autosomal recessive cutis laxa 77.6–77.7
  autosomal recessive type 1A cutis laxa 70.17
  causative genes **77.6**
  clinical features 70.15, **70.16**
  craniosynostosis syndromes **70.17**
  differential diagnosis 70.15
  elastin gene mutations 2.33–2.34
  glycosylation disorders **79.10**
  investigations 70.15
  management 70.17, 77.7
  molecular defect **70.16**
  pathophysiology 70.14–70.15, 77.5
  phenotypes **77.6**
  related syndromes **70.16**
  subtypes **77.6**
  types of **70.16**
cutis marmorata 114.3, 124.9
cutis marmorata telangiectatica congenita 124.9
cutis rhomboidalis nuchae, ageing of skin 156.5
cutis verticis gyrata (CVG) 98.25, 105.10
  dermatoendocrinology **150.10**, 150.12
CVD see chronic venous disease
cvEDS see cardiac-valvular Ehlers–Danlos syndrome
CVG see cutis verticis gyrata
CVID see common variable immunodeficiency
cyanide (CN), inhalation injury 125.4
cyanoacrylates 127.70
cyclin-dependent kinase 4 gene (CDK4), melanoma risk 142.4
cyclin-dependent kinase inhibitor 2A gene (CDKN2A) 3.24
  melanoma risk 142.4, 142.7
cyclobutane pyrimidine dimer (CPD), UV radiation exposure 10.6
cyclodopa 86.5
cyclophosphamide
  mucous membrane pemphigoid, management of 107.31
  pemphigus treatment 50.8
  systemic lupus erythematosus treatment 51.38
cyclo-phosphamide-induced alopecia 119.25
cyclophyllidea, infections 33.31–33.34
CYLD cutaneous syndrome 78.11, **78.12**

cylindroadenocarcinoma 137.35
cylindroma 137.29–137.30
  familial 137.30, 137.35
  malignant 137.35
  spiradenoma relationship 137.31
CYP1B1 variant 87.41
cyproterone acetate 87.96
cystatin A (CSTA), skin fragility disorders 69.6
cysteamine, cosmeceutical use of 157.3
cysticercosis 33.32–33.34
  clinical features 33.32–33.33
  management 33.33–33.34
  pathophysiology 33.32
cystic fibrosis
  sweat glands 92.3
  transient aquagenic keratoderma 63.62
cysts
  acne conglobata 88.66
  biopsy 3.31
  classification of cutaneous cysts 133.1, **133.2**
  cutaneous 133.1–133.7
  cutaneous keratocysts 133.6–133.7
  cutaneous nodular elastosis with 156.4
  dermoid cysts, infants 115.12, 115.13
  epidermoid 78.11, 88.33–88.34, 133.1–133.3
  with infundibular epithelial walls 133.1–133.4
  with isthmic epithelial walls 133.4–133.6
  milia 133.4
  mucocele 57.15, 57.16, 108.12, 109.30, 110.31
  nodular elastosis with 156.5
  pachyonychia congenita 63.52
  preauricular cysts, infants 115.12
  with sebaceous duct epithelial walls 133.6–133.7
  trichilemmal cysts 105.11, 133.4–133.5, 133.6, 137.5–137.6
  see also chloracne; comedonal acne; cysts; dermoid cysts; metabolising acquired dioxin-induced skin hamartoma; vellus hair cyst
cytodiagnosis 3.29–3.30
cytokeratin markers, cutaneous neoplasms 3.21–3.22
cytokine directed biologic therapies 19.32–19.37
cytokine mediators, Adamantiades–Behçet disease 48.3
cytokine mutations, immunodeficiencies **149.20**
cytokines
  antigen-presenting cells 127.7
  bullous pemphigoid 50.12
  hormone relationship 150.3
  macrophage secretion 97.5–97.6
  morphoea 55.10
  pruritus **81.3**, 81.4–81.5
  radiation dermatitis 119.14
  wound healing **11.4**, **11.5**
cytomegalovirus (CMV) 25.41–25.42
  HIV 31.24–31.25, 31.38
  infiltrating lipomatosis of the face association 98.19
  oral ulceration 108.51
  perianal skin 111.15
cytophagic histiocytic panniculitis 97.61–97.63
cytoreductive treatment, for mastocytosis 46.10
cytotoxic agents 18.29–18.31
  cutaneous T-cell lymphoma therapy 139.25
  factitious panniculitis 97.48
  hypermelanosis 86.26, 86.28
  intralesional treatment of cutaneous warts 25.60
cytotoxicity, UVA-1 phototherapy 21.2
cytotoxic protein expression, primary cutaneous aggressive epidermotropic CD8+ T-cell lymphoma 139.31–139.32

cytotoxic T lymphocytes (CTLs)
　adipocytes interaction   97.6–97.7
　drug-induced   118.12
　macrophages interaction   97.6–97.7

D
dabrafenib   141.38
Dabska tumour *see* papillary intralymphatic angioendothelioma
dactylitis, psoriatic arthritis   35.41
DADA2 *see* deficiency of adenosine deaminase 2
DALY *see* disability adjusted life year
DALYs *see* disability adjusted life years
danazol   97.32
dandruff   40.1, 40.4
　Malassezia yeast   32.14
dapsone   19.12–19.15
　acne vulgaris treatment   88.46–88.47
　adverse effects   19.14–19.15
　dermatological uses   19.13
　dose and regimens   19.15
　hypersensitivity syndrome   **14.6**, 19.15
　pharmacological properties   19.13–19.14
　safety precautions   19.15
　topical therapies   18.11
daptomycin   19.47
DARE (database of abstracts of systematic reviews)   17.7
Darier disease   3.41, 69.23–69.24, 110.6
　biopsy   *3.39*
　male genitalia   109.25
　oral lesions   108.28
Darier's sign, mastocytosis   *46.5*
dark-field microscopy, syphilis   29.18
Darling disease *see* histoplasmosis
database of abstracts of systematic reviews (DARE)   17.7
databases of controlled clinical trials   17.6–17.7
data protection, computer-based assessments   16.2
daylight photodynamic therapy   22.11–22.12, 141.10–141.11
DC *see* dissecting cellulitis; dyskeratosis congenita
DCMO *see* diffuse capillary malformation with overgrowth
DCOIT *see* dichloro-octylisothiazolinone
DCPs *see* deep chemical peels
DCs *see* dendritic cells
deafness
　albinism with   68.9
　congenital syphilis   29.26
　mitochondrial keratoderma with   63.65
　otic syphilis   29.16
　palmoplantar keratodermas with   63.63–63.65
　systemic lupus erythematosus   51.32
　Waardenburg syndrome   68.5
debridement, pressure ulcers   123.10
deceptive behaviour, factitious skin disease   84.29–84.38
decision making, holistic management of skin disease   15.6, 15.7
decongestion therapy, lipoedema management   98.23
decorin   2.38
'decubitus ulcers'   123.1
dEDS *see* dermatosparaxis Ehlers–Danlos syndrome
deep ('aggressive') angiomyxoma   136.62
deep burn wounds   125.6, 125.8
deep chemical peels (DCPs)   160.5
deep fibromatoses   139.33–139.34, *94.35*
deep folliculitis   91.8–91.15
deep morphoea   97.12–97.14, 97.30
　lupus panniculitis contrast   97.39, 97.64
deep partial-thickness burns   128.12
deep penetrating naevus (DPN)   142.2
deep perniosis   124.5
deep subcutaneous fat   97.3
deep-vein thrombosis (DVT)   101.31–101.34
　clinical features   101.32, **101.33**
　investigations   101.32–101.33

management   101.33–101.34
neoplasia association   148.26
risk factors   **101.32**
treatment   **101.34**
deer fly *see* Chrysops
deerfly fever *see* tularaemia
deficiency of adenosine deaminase 2 (DADA2)   **45.5**, **45.7**, 45.17
deficiency of interleukin 1 receptor antagonist (DIRA) syndrome   **45.5**, **45.6**, 45.12
deficiency of interleukin 36 receptor antagonist (DITRA)   45.12
deficiency states, oral features   108.70
degenerations
　dermal   3.40
　epidermal   3.40–3.41
degos acanthoma *see* clear cell acanthoma
Degos disease   99.21–99.22
dehydroepiandrosterone A (DHEA) supplements, acneform reaction   88.12
De Lange syndrome, oral involvement   108.85
delayed inflammatory reactions (DIRs), to COVID-19 vaccines   25.118
delayed pressure urticaria   42.9, 42.10
delayed reaction time, use of term   127.7
delayed tanning (DT), UV radiation exposure   10.8
delayed-type bacterial antigen tests   4.25
delayed-type stinging   128.10–128.11
deliberate self-harm   84.38–84.39
　with suicidal ideation   84.38
　without suicidal intent   84.38–84.39
deltanoids *see* vitamin D analogues
delusional beliefs
　Morgellons syndrome   84.11–84.12
　olfactory delusions   84.10–84.11
　psychodermatology   84.5–84.12
delusional disease by proxy, delusional infestation   84.5
delusional infestation (DI)   84.5–84.10
　associated diseases   **84.6**, 84.7
　clinical features   84.6–84.7
　complaints and litigation   84.9–84.10
　epidemiology   84.5–84.6
　investigations   84.7–84.8
　management   84.8–84.9
　pathophysiology   84.6
　thrip infestation confusion   34.30
demeclocycline, phototoxicity to   *126.29*
Demodex
　eosinophilic pustular folliculitis   93.7
　folliculorum infestation   107.10
　rosacea   89.3, 89.4–89.5, 89.10
dendrite surveillance extension and retraction cycling habitude (dSEARCH)   2.13
dendritic cells (DCs)
　allergic contact dermatitis   9.10
　dermal   2.15
　histiocytoses   135.1, 135.3
　immune system   9.3, *9.4*
　subtypes   9.4–9.5
dendritic epidermal T cells (DETCs)   9.7
dendritic keratitis, eyelid   *107.37*
dendritic melanocytes, naevus of Ota   *131.14*
dendrocytes, immune system   9.5
dengue, oral involvement   108.50
dengue haemorrhagic fever   25.86–25.87
denileukin diftitox (DAB389–IL-2 fusion toxin - Onzar/Ontak), cutaneous T-cell lymphoma   139.25
Denmark, non-melanoma skin cancer, incidence of   6.1
de novo post-transplant melanoma   147.13
dental abscesses   108.9
dental amalgam, oral lichen planus   37.3
dental care, epidermolysis bullosa   69.25
dental malformations, ectodermal dysplasias   69.18
dental plaque   108.5
dental sinus, acne nodule distinction   88.38

dental treatments, amalgam fillings   121.6, 121.8
dentition loss, Papillon–Lefèvre syndrome   63.69
dentogingival junction, anatomy of   108.4
denture-induced hyperplasia   108.10
denture sore mouth/denture stomatitis   32.62, 108.20–108.21
depigmentation   86.8
　acquired hypomelanosis differentiation   **86.42**
　allergic contact dermatitis   127.20–127.21
　melasma   *86.45*
　see also hypopigmentation
depigmenting agents, topical therapies   18.31–18.33
depilatories   18.33
deposition disorders, internal malignancy association   148.22–148.23
depot technique, dermal filler injection   158.2–158.3
depressed plaques
　centrifugal lipodystrophy   98.13
　insulin injection   98.11
depression
　acne vulgaris   88.39
　antidepressants   84.43–84.44, **84.44**, **84.45**, 117.3
　assessment   84.41
　dermatological patients   84.40–84.42
　emotional effects of skin conditions   15.2
　isotretinoin acne treatment   84.42
　morphoea   55.29
　psoriasis   35.19
　types   84.40
depth dose curves
　electron beam therapy   24.1–24.2
　proton beam therapy   24.2
　superficial X-ray therapy   24.1
Dercum disease (adiposis dolorosa)   **72.10**, 98.16, 98.17–98.18
　benign symmetric lipomatosis contrast   98.16
　obesity association   98.17–98.18, 98.28
dermal artefact   84.33
dermal atypical smooth muscle tumour (leiomyosarcoma)   136.54–136.55
dermal burns   125.6
dermal connective tissue, acquired disorders of   94.1–94.58
dermal degenerations   3.40
dermal deposition disorders, internal malignancy association   148.22–148.23
dermal deposits   3.30–3.31, 3.44
dermal–epidermal basement membrane zone (BMZ)   2.21–2.22
　basement membrane collagen   2.22–2.23
　hemidesmosomes   2.25–2.26
　immunofluorescence staining   *2.23*
　laminins   2.23–2.25
　molecular components   2.21
　structural components   2.22
　transmission electron microscopy image   *2.22*
dermal erythropoiesis (blueberry muffin baby)   114.21
dermal fillers   158.1–158.12
　adverse reactions and treatment for   108.62, 158.8–158.12
　management plan for   158.9
　alginate filler   158.5
　antidotes   158.8
　arterial occlusion   158.10
　treatment for   **158.11**
　biodegradable fillers   158.3–158.7
　bovine collagen filler   158.5, 158.7–158.8
　calcium hydroxylapatite filler   158.5, 158.6–158.7
　canula injection   158.1–158.2, **158.3**, *158.4*
　collagen-stimulating fillers   158.6–158.7
　combination fillers   158.7–158.8
　depot technique   158.2–158.3
　and different skin types   158.11–158.12

fanning technique   158.2–158.3
filler products   158.3–158.8
human collagen filler   158.6
hyaluronic acid filler   *158.9*
　immune response after   **158.11**
hydroxyethlmethacrylate and ethylmethacrylate microspheres suspended in hyaluronic acid   158.8
indications   158.1, **158.3**
inert fillers   158.3–158.6
injection errors   158.8
medical emergency following adverse reaction   158.10, **158.11**
multiple substance products   158.7–158.8
needle injection   158.1–158.2, **158.3**, *158.4*
non-biodegradable fillers   158.7–158.8
non-hyaluronic acid-based fillers   158.5–158.6
　immune response after   **158.11**
polyacrylamides   158.7
polyalkylamide   158.7
polycaprolacton filler   158.6
poly-L-lactic acid filler   158.6
polymethylmethacrylate and collagen   158.7–158.8
porcine collagen filler   158.5–158.6
risk assessment/reduction   158.9
silicones   158.7
single substance products   158.7
techniques   158.1–158.3
　injection errors   158.8
types of   **108.62**
dermal hyperneury   136.42–136.43
dermal infiltrate   3.44–3.45
dermal inflammatory infiltrate   126.3
　photothermal ablation   23.22
dermal leishmanoid *see* post-kala-azar dermal leishmaniasis
dermal mucin   94.44
dermal mucinoses   57.2–57.15, *57.16*
dermal nerve sheath myxoma   136.47–136.48
dermal non-neural granular cell tumour   136.60
dermal papilla   87.5, 87.8, 87.11
dermal pigmentation, laser therapies   23.16–23.17
dermal plaque, sarcoidosis   *96.8*
dermal plaque-like fibromatosis *see* dermatomyofibroma
dermal sheath, hair follicle   87.5
dermal-subcutaneous interface   98.24, 98.25–98.26
dermal substitutes, burn treatment   125.6
dermatan sulphate (DS)   **2.39**
dermatitis
　chronic actinic   4.6
　financial cost of   7.2
　'flaky paint' dermatitis in kwashiorkor   *61.4*
　herpetiformis   *4.8*
　Wilkinson's triangle (chronic actinic dermatitis)   4.6
　see also allergic contact dermatitis; atopic eczema (dermatitis); contact dermatitis; eczema; hand eczema; irritant contact dermatitis; photoallergic contact dermatitis
dermatitis artefacta   84.29–84.36
　by proxy (witchcraft syndrome)   84.33
　clinical features   84.31–84.35
　epidemiology   84.30
　male genitalia   109.9
　management   84.35–84.36
　pathophysiology   84.30–84.31
　skin picking disorder relationship   84.19
Dermatitis Family Impact questionnaire (DFI)   16.8, 16.10
dermatitis gangrenosa infantum   26.88–26.89
dermatitis herpetiformis (DH)   50.54–50.59
　associated diseases   50.56
　coeliac disease   153.3

dermatitis herpetiformis (DH) (continued)
  direct immunofluorescence microscopy
    3.18, *3.19*, *50.58*
  disease course and prognosis 50.57
  epidemiology 50.55–50.56
  genetics 50.56
  histopathology *50.58*
  internal malignancy association 148.22
  investigations 50.58
  management 50.58–50.59
  oral involvement 108.81
  pathophysiology 50.56
  presentation 50.56
  treatment ladder 50.59
dermatitis neglecta *see* dermatitis passivata
dermatitis passivata 84.36
dermatitis simulata 84.36
dermatitis veineuse *see* venous eczema
dermatochalasis 107.5
dermatoendocrinology 150.1–150.22
  biological basis 150.2–150.10
  clinical practice 150.10–150.21
  complexity of intraepithelial endocrine
    and neuroendocrine signalling
    milieu 150.8
  endocrinological considerations in skin
    therapy 150.12–150.14
  future perspectives 150.21
  key components in cutaneous (neuro-)
    endocrine signalling mechanism
    150.4
  (neuro-)endocrine contributions to
    cutaneous pathogenesis
    150.5–150.8
  patient evaluation for (neuro-) endocrine
    disorders 150.10–150.15
  signs and symptoms
    general endocrine disease seen in skin
      150.7
    hormone-based skin disease **150.7**
    indicative of endocrine disease 150.10,
      150.11
  skin and appendages as (neuro-) endocrine
    organs 150.3, **150.4**, 150.5
  skin and appendages as research models
    for general neuroendocrinology
    150.9
  specific endocrine conditions
    150.15–150.21
  stress responses 150.8–150.9
  see also endocrine disorders; hormones
dermatoepidemiology 5.1–5.2, 5.15–5.16
  see also epidemiology
dermatofibroma *4.19*, 136.19–136.21
dermatofibrosarcoma protuberans (DFSP)
  3.25, *3.26*, 24.15, 136.2, 136.14–136.15
dermatological pathomimicry 84.36
dermatology atlases 1.4
dermatology history 1.1–1.10
  ancient medical texts 1.1–1.3
  dermatology as global speciality in 20th
    century 1.7–1.10
  rational medicine, growth of 1.2–1.4
  scientific dermatology 1.4–1.7
Dermatology Index of Disease Severity 16.3
Dermatology Life Quality Index
  (DLQI/Skindex) 6.4, 15.3,
  16.6–16.7, 35.17
  adolescents 16.10
  descriptive score bandings **16.7**
  questions **16.7**
  usage 16.3, 16.7, 16.8, 16.12
Dermatology Quality of Life Scales 16.7
dermatomycosis furfuracea *see* pityriasis
  versicolor
dermatomyofibroma 136.8
dermatomyositis-associated panniculitis
  97.39, 97.40
dermatomyositis (DM) 52.1–52.13, 86.21,
  89.8
  cardiac involvement 151.4
  clinical features 52.3–52.8
  clinical variants 52.8–52.10
  definitions 52.1
  differential diagnosis 52.10

dystrophic calcification 59.1–59.2
epidemiology 52.1–52.2
eye disease **107.35**
internal malignancy association
  148.20–148.21
investigations 52.10–52.12
management 52.12, **52.13**
myositis-specific antibodies 52.2, 52.5,
  52.6, 52.11
oral involvement 108.67–108.68
pathophysiology 52.2–52.3
respiratory disease 152.2–152.3
severity classification 52.10
dermatopathia pigmentosa reticularis 68.12
dermatopathology
  examinations/national societies for 3.1
  terminology 3.38–3.43
dermato-pharmacokinetic (DPK) method
  12.8
Dermatophilus congolensis, pitted keratolysis
  26.42–26.43
dermatophyte infection
  perineal and perianal skin 111.15
  in pregnancy 113.7
dermatophytes 32.6–32.69
  anthropophilic 32.19
  asexual–sexual states **32.18**
  classification 32.18, **32.19**, 32.22–32.30
  collecting material 32.7–32.8
  geophilic 32.19
  identification 32.6–32.10
  non-dermatophyte hyphal fungi
    32.51–32.52
  Wood's light examination 32.6–32.7
  zoophilic 32.19
dermatophytide reaction (allergic response)
  32.50
dermatophytosis (ringworm) 32.18–32.34
dermatoporosis 94.1, 156.11
dermatoscopy *see* dermoscopy
dermatoses
  bullous dermatosis *4.8*
  chronic superficial scaly dermatosis *4.17*
  flexural sites **4.18**
  malignancy association 148.19–148.20
  in occupational groups **4.4**
  pruritus in inflamed skin 81.7
  sun-related 7.8
dermatosis papulosa nigra (DPN)
  132.4–132.5, *156.3*
dermatosparaxis Ehlers–Danlos syndrome
  (dEDS) **70.5**, 70.9
dermis 2.2
  anatomy 9.1
  chronological ageing/photoageing **10.10**
  collagen fibres 2.27
  embryonic development 2.3, 2.5
  immune cells 9.4–9.6
  immune surveillance 2.15, *2.16*
  mechanical properties 122.5
  microvessels in *2.41*
dermographism, urticaria 42.9–42.10
dermoid cysts
  infantile 115.12, *115.13*
  mouth 108.12
  penis 109.31
dermopathy, diabetic 62.2
dermoscopy 4.20–4.21
  acquired and small congenital naevi
    145.2, *145.3*, 145.4–145.6
  basal cell carcinoma 140.10, *140.11*
  benign patterns of naevi 145.1–145.7
  facial skin/chronically sun-damaged skin
    melanoma 145.9, *145.11*, **145.11**

intradermal naevi 145.6
melanoma diagnosis 142.9, 145.1–145.16
organised patterns in melanoma
  145.13–145.14, *145.15*
Spitz naevi 145.6
volar skin of palms and soles (acral)
  melanoma 145.9, 145.11–145.13
deroofing, lesions 90.10
desert rheumatism *see* coccidioidomycosis
designated patient irradiance (DPI) 21.3
desmin 3.25
desmocollin 3 (*DSC3*) 69.7
desmoglein-1 (*DSG1*) 69.6
desmoglein 3 (*DSG3*) 69.7
desmoglein (DSG) autoantibodies 3.14, *3.21*
Desmons syndrome 63.35
desmoplakin 69.7
  mutations, Carvajal-Huerta syndrome
    63.63
desmoplasia 3.41
desmoplastic basal cell carcinoma *see*
  morphoeic basal cell carcinoma
desmoplastic fibroblastoma 136.11–136.12
desmoplastic trichoepithelioma 73.7,
  137.10–137.11
desmosines 2.33, 2.34, *2.35*
desmosomal disorders 69.20
desmosomes 2.18–2.19, *2.19*, 63.57–63.58
desquamation, neonates 114.3–114.4
desquamative gingivitis 108.23, *108.82*
destructive/pro-inflammatory topical
  treatments, molluscum
  contagiosum infection 25.18
detached epidermis 118.14, 118.19
  Stevens–Johnson syndrome/toxic
    epidermal necrolysis *118.15*
DETCs *see* dendritic epidermal T cells
detergent acne 88.25
detergents
  alopecia management 87.98
  exposure regulations 127.2
  irritant properties 128.3
developing countries *see* low and middle
  income countries
developmental delay, atopic eczema
  association 41.21
dew itch *see* ancylostomiasis
dexpanthenol 127.59–127.60
DFI *see* Dermatitis Family Impact
  questionnaire
DFSP *see* dermatofibrosarcoma protuberans
DGEBF novolac resins *see* diglycidyl ether of
  bisphenol F resins
DH *see* dermatitis herpetiformis
DHA *see* dihydroxyacetone
DHEA *see* dehydroepiandrosterone A
dhobie itch *see* tinea cruris
DHT *see* dihydrotestosterone
DI *see* diabetes insipidus
diabetes 62.1–62.8
  acanthosis nigricans association 85.5
  acquired ichthyosis association 85.1–85.2
  acquired perforating dermatosis 94.53,
    94.54
  AGL association 98.2
  autoimmune disease 62.4
  bullae 62.7
  calluses 122.7
  cutaneous complications **150.11**
  dermopathy 62.2
  disease associations 62.4, *62.5*
  drug reaction with eosinophilia and
    systemic symptoms 118.9, 118.11
  eruptive xanthomas 62.3, *62.4*
  erysipelas-like reaction 62.2
  foot ulcer 62.2–62.3
  genetic syndromes 62.4–62.5
  granulomatous disorders 62.5
  hyperlipidaemia 62.3, *62.4*
  infections 62.3
  leg ulceration 62.1
  metabolic syndrome 62.4
  necrobiosis lipoidica *62.6*, *95.12*
  neurological damage 62.2–62.3
  obesity association 62.3, 98.28

perforating collagenosis (folliculitis)4
  62.5
pressure ulcers 123.4
pruritus 81.10
psoriasis association 35.18
retinopathy *62.5*
rubeosis 62.2
secondary dyslipidaemia 60.11
skin tags *62.3*
stiff skin and joints 62.5–62.6
systemic allergic contact dermatitis 117.4
treatment-related skin manifestations
  62.4
types of 62.1
vascular damage 62.1–62.2
wet gangrene of the foot 62.2
wound healing 11.9
see also insulin resistance
diabetes insipidus (DI), Langerhans cell
  histiocytosis 135.5, 135.8
diabetes mellitus *see* diabetes
diabetic bullae 62.7, 85.30
diabetic dermopathy 62.2
  brown pseudoscars *94.14*
diabetic foot ulcer 62.2–62.3
diabetic retinopathy *62.5*
diabetic scleroedema 57.9, 57.10, 62.5–62.6,
  62.7
diabetic thick skin 94.45
diacetylmorphine *see* heroin
diagnosis 4.1–4.27
  apps 4.26, 5.13
  artificial intelligence 4.26–4.27
  atopic eczema 5.4
  clinical investigations 4.19–4.20
  coding systems 4.2
  community diagnosis 5.2
  diascopy 4.19
  disease definition 4.1–4.2
  examination of skin 4.5
  fine-needle aspiration of lymph nodes
    4.22
  fundamentals 4.1
  history taking 4.2–4.5
  imaging examination 4.22–4.23
  imaging systems 4.20–4.22
  lesions, description of 4.5–4.20
  microscopy 4.20–4.22
  mobile smartphone applications 4.26,
    5.13
  palpation 4.17–4.18, *4.19*
  photography 4.19
  preimplantation genetic diagnosis
    8.10–8.11
  prenatal diagnosis 8.9–8.11
  presenting complaint 4.2–4.5
  in primary and secondary care 5.13
  quality of life assessment 4.5
  radiological examination 4.22–4.23
  simple clinical examination 4.18
  skin testing 4.23–4.25
  smartphone apps 4.26, 5.13
  store-and-forward consultations
    4.25–4.26
  teledermatology 4.25–4.26
  Wood's light 4.19–4.20
'Diagnostic Handbook', Mesopotamian 1.2
diagnostic test studies, critical appraisal for
  evidence based medicine
  17.15–17.17
diaper area *see* nappy/diaper/napkin area
diascopy 4.19
diazolidinyl urea 127.51
DIC *see* disseminated intravascular
  coagulation
dichloro-octylisothiazolinone (DCOIT)
  127.54
diclofenac 18.30
Dictyoptera (cockroaches) 34.32
diet
  and acne **88.20–88.24**, 88.26
  and atopic eczema 41.7
  diagnosis 4.4
  epidemiology 5.11
  and flushing **104.3**

low pseudoallergen diet **42.6**
seborrhoeic dermatitis 40.4
and urticaria **42.6**, 42.8
see also nutrition
dietary management
allergic contact dermatitis 127.35, 127.38
epidermolysis bullosa 69.25
lipoedema 98.23
Refsum disease 63.32
Sjögren–Larsson syndrome 63.33
subcutaneous fat disorders 98.26
trimethylaminuria 92.18
DIF *see* direct immunofluorescence
differentiated vulval intraepithelial neoplasia (VIN) 110.34, 110.35
diffuse alopecia areata 87.23–87.24
diffuse alopecias 87.28–87.35, 87.64
diffuse arterial disease 124.9
diffuse capillary malformation with overgrowth (DCMO) 101.28
diffuse cutaneous mastocytosis 46.6
diffuse/disseminated cutaneous leishmaniasis 33.48–33.49
diffuse fibrosis, causes 94.33–94.48
diffuse keratodermas 63.50–63.51
ectodermal dysplasias 63.68, *63.69*
woolly hair 63.63
diffuse large B-cell lymphoma (DLBCL) 25.39
diffuse lymphangiomatosis 136.39
diffuse melanosis 86.20, 86.22
diffuse neurofibroma 136.46–136.47
diffuse pigmentation, arsenic exposure 121.3
diffuse reticular pattern naevi *145.2, 145.3,* 145.4
diffuse telogen effluvium 87.54, *87.55*
diffusion enhancers, topical drug delivery 12.6
DiGeorge syndrome **80.4**, 80.8
digestive system disorders 153.1–153.9
digital clubbing, pachydermoperiostosis 155.14
digital fibromyxoma *see* acral fibromyxoma
digital ischaemia, internal malignancy association 148.24–148.25
digital mucous cyst 136.60
digital myxoid (mucous) cysts 57.15, *57.16*
digital necrosis, cannabis-induced 120.4
digital papillary adenocarcinoma 137.34–137.35
digital papular calcific elastosis 63.60
digital pathology 3.32
digital technology 1.9, 5.13
digital vasculitis, rheumatoid arthritis 155.6, *155.8*
digitate dermatitis *see* small plaque parapsoriasis
digitate hyperkeratoses 63.77
digitate lesions *4.17*
digits
blistering distal dactylitis 26.34
see also finger; toe
diglycidyl ether of bisphenol F (DGEBF novolac) resins 127.68
DIHS *see* drug-induced hypersensitivity syndrome
5α-dihydrotestosterone (DHT) 87.10
dihydroxyacetone (DHA) 18.39
dilated pore lesions, expanded follicular infundibulum 137.3
dimethylglyoxime test, nickel allergy 127.33, *127.34*
dimethylol dimethyl (DMDM) hydantoin 127.52
dimethyl sulfoxide (DMSO), irritant responses 128.3
dimeticone 18.14
dimorphic fungi, morphology and diseases **32.3**
dimples, commissural pit distinction 108.86
dinitrochlorobenzene (DNCB), allergic reactions 127.5–127.6
dioxin intoxication/poisoning

acne 88.68
acne vulgaris *88.15*
1,3-Diphenylguanidine (DPG) 127.63, 127.64
diphtheria 26.38–26.39
diploid/triploid mosaicism **72.7**
Diplopoda (millipedes) 34.57
Diptera 34.6–34.13
classification 34.6–34.8
clinical features of bites 34.8–34.9
myiasis 34.9–34.13
DIRA *see* deficiency of interleukin 1 receptor antagonist
direct immunofluorescence (DIF) 3.11–3.12, 3.17–3.19
bullous pemphigoid *50.14*
connective tissue diseases 3.19
dermatitis herpetiformis 3.18, *3.19*, 50.58
disease findings **3.17**
epidermolysis bullosa acquisita 3.18, *3.19*, 50.35
lichen planus 3.18, *3.19*, 37.15
linear IgA bullous dermatosis 3.18
linear IgA disease *50.35*
mucous membrane pemphigoid 107.28
pemphigoid 3.17–3.18
pemphigus 3.17, *3.18*, 50.3, 50.7
serration pattern analysis 3.17
direct tissue deformation damage, pressure ulcers 123.2
dirofilariasis 33.23–33.24
DIRs *see* delayed inflammatory reactions
disability, caused by skin disease 5.5–5.6
disability adjusted life years (DALYs) 5.6, *5.9, 6.3,* 6.4, 7.2, 16.9
acne vulgaris 88.5
disappearing/vanishing/phantom bone disease 136.39
see also Gorham syndrome; Gorham–Stout disease
discoid lesions *4.12*
discoid lupus erythematosus (DLE) 51.1–51.12, 87.43–87.44, *87.45*, 89.10, 97.38
antimalarial treatment **51.11**
associated diseases 51.2
atrophy of the epidermis 51.2
basal layer degeneration *51.2, 51.3*
chilblain lupus 51.6–51.7, *51.9*
clinical features 51.3–51.6
clinical variants 51.6–51.9
differential diagnosis 51.9–51.10
disease course and prognosis 51.10
disseminated DLE 51.4–51.6
emerging therapies 51.12
epidemiology 51.1–51.2
genetics 51.3
gyrate erythema *51.8*
histology *51.2, 51.3,* **51.3**
inflammatory infiltrate 51.2
investigations 51.10
lesion appearance *51.4, 51.5, 51.6, 51.24*
lichen planus 37.8, 37.16
lip lesions 108.64
localised disease 51.3–51.4
lupus erythematosus profundus (panniculitis) 51.7–51.8, *51.9*
lymphocytic infiltration *51.3*
management 51.10–51.12
oral agents in treatment of chronic DLE **51.11**
oral involvement 108.78, *108.79*
pathology 51.2–51.3
pathophysiology 51.2
predisposing factors **51.2**
rosaceous pattern *51.5*
scarring 51.4, *51.5, 51.7, 51.8*
severity classification 51.10
stem cells *51.3*
systemic lupus erythematosus relationship/comparison 51.6, **51.9**
discoid skin lesions
diagnosis of **39.10**
retinoid-induced *88.56*

discrete papular lichen myxoedematosus 57.6, 57.7
discrimination, institutionalised 1.9
disease, definition 5.4–5.5
disease associations 5.14
epidemiology 5.11–5.12
disease burden, global 7.2
disease frequency 5.7–5.11, 5.14
disease-modifying antirheumatic drugs (DMARDs), morphoea treatment 55.38
disease transmission, arthropods 34.2, **34.3**
disfigurement 4.3, 5.5
disorders of sexual development (DSDs) 110.5
disperse dyes 127.65–127.66
displaced persons camps (DPCs) 7.13
skin diseases diagnosed in **7.14**
dissecting cellulitis (DC) 87.50
localised swellings over the crown *105.7*
scalp 88.37, 105.7–105.8
disseminated blastomycosis 32.85
disseminated capillary malformation with overgrowth (DCMO) 71.7–71.8
disseminated disease
Mycobacterium tuberculosis complex 27.11, 27.13, 27.17–27.18, 27.21, 27.32, 27.33, 27.34, 27.35–27.36, 27.38, 27.40, 27.44
non-tuberculous mycobacteria 27.32–27.36, 27.38, 27.40–27.45
skin involvement 135.6
disseminated gonococcal infection 30.2, 30.4, 30.5–30.6
disseminated infundibulofolliculitis 91.14–91.15, 93.6–93.7
disseminated intravascular coagulation (DIC) 32.47
haemorrhage in patients with 99.17
neonatal purpura fulminans 114.21
disseminated palmoplantar porokeratosis 85.20, 85.22
disseminated superficial actinic porokeratosis (DSAP) 63.74–63.75, 85.20–85.22, 141.15–141.18
distal arthritis, in bowel-associated dermatosis–arthritis syndrome 40.16
distal and lateral subungual onychomycosis (DLSO) 32.47, **106.7**
distal nose, actinic prurigo *126.11*
distal symmetrical polyneuropathy **83.9**
distichiasis, lymphoedema–distichiasis syndrome 151.2
dithiocarbamates 127.63, 127.64
dithranol 18.39–18.41
psoriasis treatment 35.21
DITRA *see* deficiency of interleukin 36 receptor antagonist
DLBCL *see* diffuse large B-cell lymphoma
DLE *see* discoid lupus erythematosus
D-limonene 127.42–127.43
DLQI *see* Dermatology Life Quality Index
DLSO *see* distal and lateral subungual onychomycosis
DM *see* dermatomyositis
DMARDs *see* disease-modifying antirheumatic drugs
DMDM hydantoin *see* dimethylol dimethyl hydantoin
DM skin severity index (DSSI) 52.10
DMSO *see* dimethyl sulfoxide
DN *see* dysplastic naevi
DNA
human genome sequencing 8.8–8.9
methylation machinery 8.6
mutations and disease 8.5–8.7
prenatal diagnosis 8.9–8.11
DNA damage
skin ageing 2.46
tanning association 86.9
DNA photodamage, repair of 10.5–10.6
DNA repair disorders 76.1–76.12, **76.2**
ataxia telangiectasia 76.10–76.11
Cockayne syndrome 76.6–76.8

fanconia anaemia 76.11
inherited immunodeficiency **80.4–80.5**, 80.11
Muir–Torre syndrome 76.11
trichothiodystrophy syndrome 76.9–76.10
xeroderma pigmentosum 76.1–76.6
DNA sequencing, epidermolysis bullosa diagnosis 69.22–69.23
DNA viruses 25.6–25.78
hepatitis 25.73–25.77
herpesviruses 25.19–25.46
human papillomaviruses 25.49–25.73, **25.50–25.51**
parvoviruses 25.77–25.78
pathogenesis 25.2, 25.5
polyomaviruses 25.46–25.49
poxviruses 25.6–25.19
DNCB *see* dinitrochlorobenzene
DNS *see* dysplastic naevus syndrome
docetaxol treatment, palmoplantar erythrodysaesthesia *119.2*
DOCK8 deficiency 80.9, *80.10*
documentation/record keeping
biopsy information request form 3.4
ethics and drug trial reporting 13.13
histopathology skin report 3.38
phototherapy 21.17
dog bites 130.6
'dog ear' repair 20.22, *20.23*
Doll, Sir Richard 5.1
dominant dystrophic epidermolysis bullosa 94.43
donation of medicines 7.13
donor transmitted melanoma 147.13–147.14
donovanosis (granuloma inguinale), perineal skin 111.17
dopaquinone 86.5
Doppler ultrasound 4.22, *101.4,* **101.4**
dorsal hands, neutrophilic dermatosis of 49.12, *49.13*
dorsal nose, actinic prurigo 126.10, 126.12
dosimetry, UV radiation measurement 10.2
dots and globules dermoscopy patterns, melanoma 145.7
double lip 108.85
Dowling–Degos disease 68.13, 85.24
vulval lesions 110.23
Down syndrome (trisomy 21) 74.1–74.2, **106.7**
elastosis perforans serpiginosa 94.55, *94.56*
hair loss presentation 87.20
hidradenitis suppurativa association 90.2
oral involvement 108.85
doxepin, urticaria treatment 42.19
DPCs *see* displaced persons camps
D-penicillamine, cutaneous adverse effects 155.15
DPG *see* 1,3-Diphenylguanidine
DPI *see* designated patient irradiance
DPK *see* dermato-pharmacokinetic method
DPN *see* deep penetrating naevus; dermatosis papulosa nigra
dracontiasis *see* dracunculiasis
dracunculiasis 33.12–33.13
clinical features 33.13
management 33.13
Dracunculus medinensis (dracunculiasis) 33.12–33.13
dragon worm *see* dracunculiasis
draining lesions, Hurley stage III disease *90.9*
draining tunnels, hidradenitis suppurativa *90.5*
DRESS *see* drug reaction with eosinophilia and systemic symptoms
dressings
SJS/TEN treatment 118.19
skin surgery 20.37–20.38, 20.41
'drip sign', intentional damage by corrosive liquids 84.32, *84.34*
drug actions, mechanisms underlying **13.4**, 13.5–13.6
extracellular mechanisms 13.5

drug actions, mechanisms underlying (*continued*)
   intracellular mechanisms   13.5–13.6
   transmembrane mechanisms   13.5
drug allergens   127.4, 127.45–127.47, 127.54–127.58
   ano-genital region   127.16–127.17
   applied medicaments   127.45–127.47
drug-associated NEH   92.14–92.15
drug choice, and medical decision making   13.7
drug concentrations, topical therapies   18.1–18.2
drug delivery
   clinical pharmacology   13.2–13.3
   see also topical drug delivery
drug dependence, illicit drugs   120.1
drug development   13.11–13.13
   ethics and trial reporting   13.13
   preclinical drug identification   13.11–13.12
drug–drug interactions
   antibiotics with combined oral contraceptives   88.49
   antihistamines   19.4
   antimalarial agents   19.6
   azathioprine   19.9
   ciclosporin   19.11–19.12
   glucocorticoids   19.20
   hydroxycarbamide   19.22
   methotrexate   19.27
   mycophenolate mofetil   19.29
   pharmaceutical drugs with recreational drug   120.3
   polypharmacy   13.8
   retinoids systemic therapy   19.44
   tumour necrosis factor antagonist systemic therapy   19.34
drug hypersensitivity *see* immunological reactions to drugs
drug-induced hypersensitivity syndrome (DIHS)   118.5
drug injections, panniculitis   97.50
drug metabolism   13.3
drug reaction with eosinophilia and systemic symptoms (DRESS)   14.3–14.4, 14.7, 117.2, 118.1, 118.4–118.12
   musculoskeletal therapy effects   155.10, 155.15
drug reactions
   acanthosis nigricans   85.5
   acne vulgaris   88.11–88.14, **88.16**
   acrocyanosis   124.7
   anaphylaxis   117.5–117.7
   angioedema   117.5–117.7
   antiretroviral therapy   31.2, 31.8, 31.10, **31.13**, 31.19, 31.20
   benign cutaneous adverse reactions   117.1–117.9
   cheilitis   108.61
   chronic oedema   103.12–103.13
   clinical pharmacology   13.9
   dermatomyositis   52.9–52.10
   dermatoses, illicit drugs   120.4–120.6
   ear dermatoses   **106.22**
   eczema   117.3–117.5
   erythema multiforme   47.3–47.4
   exanthems   117.1–117.2
   HIV
      antiretroviral therapy   31.2, 31.8, 31.10, **31.13**, 31.19, 31.20, **31.36**
      non-antiretroviral therapy   31.18–31.20, **31.36**
   hypermelanosis   86.25–86.31, 86.53–86.54
   hyperpigmentation
      laser therapies   23.17
      oral involvement   108.17
   hypertrichosis   87.86–87.87
   lichen planus   37.3
   lupus erythematosus   117.7–117.9
   male genitalia   109.24–109.25
   morphoea   55.14–55.15
   neutrophilic eccrine hidradenitislsquo   149.7

neutrophilic panniculitis   97.52, **97.53**
oedema   103.12–103.13
oral ulcers   108.41
pemphigus   50.4
perineal and perianal skin   111.12–111.13
pruritus   81.10–81.11, 117.2–117.3
psoriasis vulgaris   35.3–35.4
purpura   **99.4**
scleroderma   94.45–94.46
seborrhoeic dermatitis   40.6–40.7
severe cutaneous adverse reactions   118.1–118.22
subacute cutaneous lupus erythematosus   **51.13–51.14**
Sweet syndrome   49.8, 49.10–49.11, 149.6
systemic lupus erythematosus   51.21, **51.22**
systemic therapy   19.2
telogen effluvium   87.56
urticaria   42.5, 42.8, 117.5–117.7
see also adverse effects; cutaneous adverse drug effects; drug–drug interactions; immunological reactions to drugs
drug-related links between skin and liver   **153.9**
drugs
   eccrine glands and   92.15
   and flushing   **104.3**
   licensing procedures   13.11–13.13
   ocular complications of drug therapy   107.40–107.44
   photosensitivity   126.1, 126.27–126.32
   secondary dyslipidaemia due to   60.12
   toxicity and adverse effects   13.6, 13.9–13.11
   types of   13.1
   see also clinical pharmacology; narcotic drugs
drug services, psychosocial diseases   120.8
dry beriberi, vitamin B1 deficiency   61.14
dry skin *see* xerosis cutis
DS *see* dermatan sulphate
DSAP *see* disseminated superficial actinic porokeratosis
DSDs *see* disorders of sexual development
dSEARCH *see* dendrite surveillance extension and retraction cycling habitude
DSG *see* desmoglein autoantibodies
DSH *see* dyschromatosis symmetrica hereditaria
DSSI *see* DM skin severity index
DT *see* delayed tanning
Duane reaction syndrome   **106.7**
Duckett Jones criteria, rheumatic fever diagnosis   **47.11**
duckhunter's itch, *see also* cutaneous larva migrans
duck itch *see* cercarial dermatitis
Ducreyi disease *see* chancroid
DUH *see* dyschromatosis universalis hereditaria
Duhring, Louis   1.7
dumping syndrome flush   **104.9**
Duncan disease *see* X-linked lymphoproliferative diseases
Dunnigan-type familial partial lipodystrophy (FPLD2)   98.9
dupilumab
   alopecia areata   87.35
   chronic actinic dermatitis   126.21
   systemic therapy   19.36
Dupuytren contracture (Dupuytren disease) *see* palmar fibromatosis
Durand–Nicholas–Favre disease *see* lymphogranuloma venereum
dutasteride   87.69, 87.96
DVT *see* deep-vein thrombosis
dye allergens   127.60–127.61, 127.65–127.67
   see also hair dyes
dyes
   antiseptic applications   18.38
   specimen preparation   3.5–3.6
dynein   86.4

dysaesthesia   83.7
   male genitalia   109.43–109.44
   neuropathic   83.5–83.6
dysaesthetic syndromes   82.1
   with/without neurological deficit   **82.1**
   see also mucocutaneous pain syndromes
dyschromatoses   68.1, 68.14–68.15
dyschromatosis symmetrica hereditaria (DSH)   68.14–68.15
dyschromatosis universalis hereditaria (DUH)   68.15
'dyshidrotic' eczema   129.1
dyskeratosis   3.41
dyskeratosis congenita (DC)   67.12–67.15, 68.12, 75.1–75.4, **78.12**, **80.5**, 80.12, 148.14, 149.14
   causative genes and modes of inheritance   **75.2**
   clinical features   **75.2**, 75.3–75.4
   co-morbidities   75.4
   cutaneous changes   67.13
   genetics   75.1–75.3
   investigations and diagnosis   75.4
   leukoplakia development   *75.3*
   management   75.4
   oral lesions   108.29
   skin cancer   147.2
   see also puritic and dyskeratotic dermatoses
dyskeratotic follicular epithelium, necrotising lymphocytic folliculitis   93.4
dyslipidaemias
   cerebrotendinous xanthomatosis   60.10
   classification   60.1, **60.2**
   combined dyslipidaemia   **60.2**, 60.8–60.9
   cutaneous features   **60.2**
   hypercholesterolaemia   **60.2**, 60.6–60.8
   hypertriglyceridaemias   **60.2**, 60.9–60.10
   primary dyslipidaemias   **60.2**, 60.6–60.10
   secondary dyslipidaemias   **60.2**, 60.11–60.12
   sitosterolaemia   60.11
dyslipidaemic plane (planar) xanthomas   60.4–60.6
dysmorphic disorders *see* body dysmorphic disorder
dyspigmentation
   ageing of skin   156.2, 156.5
   chemotherapy-induced   119.8–119.11
   occupational   129.13–129.14
dysplasia   3.41
   ocular features   **107.41**
   penis   *109.38*
dysplastic melanocytic naevi   *131.41*, *131.42*
   histological criteria   **131.43**
   microscopic images   *131.45*
dysplastic naevi (DN), as melanoma precursors   142.2–142.3
dysplastic naevus syndrome (DNS)   142.3–142.4, 142.7
   see also atypical/dysplastic naevus syndrome
dysproteinaemic purpura   99.6–99.7
dysthymia   84.40
dystonin epidermal isoform (BP230) (*DST*)   69.4
dystrophic anagen hairs   119.5
dystrophic calcification
   secondary to inflammatory disease/infections   59.1–59.3
   secondary to trauma or injection/infusion of calcium-containing materials   59.3
   secondary to tumours and genetic disease   59.3–59.4
dystrophic calcinosis, in systemic lupus erythematosus   51.28
dystrophic epidermolysis bullosa   69.2, 69.15–69.18
   cancer and   69.26–69.27
   connective tissue disorders   69.20
   diagnosis   69.21, *69.22*
   management   69.25–69.26

   molecular-based approaches   69.18–69.19
   systemic treatment   69.26
   type VII collagen   69.5
dystrophy *see* fingernail dystrophy; nail dystrophy; toenail dystrophy

E

EAC *see* erythema annulare centrifugum; external auditory canal
ear   106.1–106.35
   ageing changes   106.7–106.8
   allergic contact dermatitis   127.15–127.16
   anatomy   106.1–106.2, *106.3*
   antiphospholipid antibody syndrome   *99.18*
   arterial blood supply   *106.2*
   arteriovenous malformation   *71.11*
   auricle
      ageing changes   106.7–106.8
      anatomy   *106.1*, *106.3*
      basal cell carcinoma   106.21–106.27
      developmental anatomy   *106.3*
      infections   106.19–106.21
      lumpy scalp syndrome   106.6
      melanoma of   106.31–106.33
      pre-auricular anomalies   106.6–106.7, *106.8*
      squamous cell carcinoma   106.27–106.29
      terminal hair   *106.3*
      tumours of   106.21–106.35
      variations in shape of   106.5–106.6
   basal cell carcinoma of the auricle   106.21–106.27
   benign lesions   106.33
   cerumen (wax)   106.2–106.3
   cholesteatoma   106.21
   cicatricial pemphigoid   *50.52*
   cryofibrinogenaemia   *99.13*
   developmental disorders   106.3–106.7
      low-set ears   106.5
      macrotia (large ears)   106.5
      microtia (small ears)   106.4, *106.5*
   discoid lupus erythematosus   *51.5*, *51.7*
   earlobe creases   106.8
   elastotic nodules   94.3
   external auditory canal   106.1–106.3
      microbiome   26.5
      tumour management   106.29–106.31
   granuloma annulare   *95.7*
   ichthyoses   63.45
   infections   106.15–106.21
      otitis externa   106.15–106.19
      of the pinna   106.19–106.21
   inflammatory chondopathy effects   155.12
   involvement in skin disease and systemic disease   106.21, **106.22–106.23**
   keratosis obturans   106.21
   low-set ears   106.5
   macrotia (large ears)   106.5
   microbiology   106.2
   microtia (small ears)   106.4, *106.5*
   nerve supply   *106.2*
   otomycosis   32.17–32.18
   perforating disorders   **106.23**
   petrified ear   106.21
   physiology   106.1–106.2
   piercing
      keloids   106.14
      traumatic conditions   106.11–106.12
   premalignant lesions   106.33–106.34
   radiotherapy for skin cancer   24.11, *24.12*, *24.20*
   rheumatoid nodules   *53.6*
   squamous cell carcinoma of the auricle   106.27–106.29
   systemic lupus erythematosus   51.32
   traumatic conditions   106.8–106.15
      chondrodermatitis nodularis   106.9–106.11
      contusion   106.8
      ear piercing   106.11–106.12
      haematoma   106.8
      keloids   106.14–106.15

pseudocyst 106.8–106.9
split earlobe 106.12–106.14
tympanic membrane 106.2
see also perioral area
ear canal samples, superficial mycoses identification 32.8
earlobe
creases 106.8
keloid 94.50
piercing 106.11–106.12
split earlobe 106.12–106.14
repair techniques 106.13
early adulthood, psychological and social factors 15.3
early detection strategies, melanoma 142.15–142.18
EASI see Eczema Area and Severity Index
eating disorders 84.26–84.27
and acne 88.30
cutaneous co-morbidities 84.27
oral lesions 108.83
EB see epidermolysis bullosa
EBA see epidermolysis bullosa acquisita
Ebers Papyrus 1.2
EBM see evidence based medicine
Ebola haemorrhagic fever 25.84–25.85
EBP gene
Conradi–Hünermann–Happle syndrome 63.22–63.23
MEND syndrome 63.23
EBS see epidermolysis bullosa simplex
EBV see Epstein–Barr virus
ECCA see Echelle d'évaluation Clinique des Cicatrice d'Acné
ecchymosis (bruises)
causes **99.2**, **99.5**
diagnosis by lesion size **99.3**
primary ecchymotic haemorrhage syndromes 99.4–99.7
scurvy *61.22*
trauma injury 99.6
see also purpura
ecchymotic lesions, Hermansky–Pudlak syndrome 68.8
ECCL see encephalocraniocutaneous lipomatosis
eccrine angiomatous hamartoma 137.23
eccrine or apocrine/follicular carcinomas 137.35–137.40
eccrine or apocrine gland/follicular tumours 137.28–137.33
eccrine carcinoma, eyelid 107.49
eccrine dermal duct tumour 137.25
eccrine duct-blocking agents, hyperhidrosis 92.8–92.9
eccrine duct epithelium tumours, hidroacanthoma simplex 137.24–137.25
eccrine gland ablation, hyperhidrosis treatment 92.10
eccrine gland carcinomas 137.33–137.35
eccrine gland hamartomas and tumours 137.23–137.28
eccrine glands 2.2, 2.8–2.9, 92.1–92.4
disorders 92.4–92.15, **92.11**
drugs and 92.15
duct 92.2, 92.16
embryonic development 2.5
peptide histidine methionine immunoreactive fibres *83.4*
in pregnancy 113.2–113.3
tumours 137.2
vasoactive intestinal peptide immunoreactive fibres *83.4*
eccrine hidrocystoma 137.24
eccrine naevus 73.6
eccrine poroma *4.13*, 137.25–137.26
see also hidroacanthoma simplex
eccrine spiradenoma see spiradenoma
eccrine sweating
control of 92.3–92.4
neonates 114.3
eccrine syringofibroadenoma 137.26
eccrine syringosquamous metaplasia 92.15
ECD see Erdheim–Chester disease

ECDS see en coup de sabre
Echelle de Cotation des Lésions d'Acné (ECLA) 16.4
Echelle d'évaluation Clinique des Cicatrice d'Acné (ECCA) 16.4
echinocandin antifungals 19.48
echinococcosis 33.31–33.32
clinical features 33.32
management 33.32
pathophysiology 33.31–33.32
Echinoidea, stings from 130.3
echoviruses 25.93–25.94
ECLA see Echelle de Cotation des Lésions d'Acné
ECM see extracellular matrix
economic burden of disease 5.6, 6.5–6.10
definition 6.1
skin cancer 6.5–6.8
ECP see extracorporeal photopheresis
ecstasy (MDMA) 120.2, 120.4
'ecstasy pimples' 120.4
ecthyma
management 26.17–26.18
pathophysiology 26.17
role of *Staphylococcus aureus* and *Streptococcus pyogenes* 26.17–26.18
ecthyma contagiosum see orf virus
ecthyma gangrenosum
ano-genital region 109.26, 111.15
neonates 114.27
Pseudomonas aeruginosa 26.51, 26.52–26.53
ectodermal dysplasias (ED), palmoplantar keratodermas in 63.65, 63.68–63.70
ectodermal dysplasia–electrodactyly–macular dystrophy (EEM) syndrome 2.20
ectomesenchymal chondromyxoid tumour see cutaneous myoepithelioma
ectopic ACTH syndrome 148.17
ectopic calcification and abnormal mineralisation 70.31–70.36
fibrodysplasia ossificans progressiva 70.35
primary hypertrophic osteoarthropathy 70.35–70.36
pseudoxanthoma elasticum 70.31–70.35
ectopic disease, hidradenitis suppurativa association 90.6
ectopic glands 92.15
ectopic lesions, penis 109.6
ectopic plaque, axillae *90.7*
ectopic sebaceous glands 88.31
ectothrix type tinea capitis 32.38–32.39
eczema 39.1–39.7
acrodermatitis enteropathica 79.16
acute phase *39.2*, *39.3*, 39.4, 39.6
age and sex 39.2
allergic contact testing 1.8
asteatotic 39.9–39.12, 85.27, *85.28*, *85.29*, 85.30
associated diseases 39.10
clinical features and variants 39.11
craquelé appearance *39.11*
ear dermatoses **106.22**
environmental factors 39.11
management 39.11
pathology 39.10–39.11
predisposing factors 39.10
treatment 39.11
causative organisms 39.4
chronic *39.2*, *39.3*, 39.6–39.7
classification 39.1, **39.2**
clinical features 39.4–39.5
complications and co-morbidities 39.5, 127.22–127.23
conditioned hyperirritability 39.5
definition and nomenclature 39.1
discoid *4.12*
drug-induced 117.3–117.5
endogenous **39.2**
environmental factors 39.4, 39.11
epidemiology 39.1–39.2
exogenous **39.2**
genetics 39.4
house dust mites 34.51

investigations 39.5
male genitalia 109.11–109.13
management 39.6–39.7
patch testing 39.5–39.6
pathology 39.3–39.4
pathophysiology 39.3
psychological and social factors 15.4
secondary dissemination 39.4–39.5
severity classification 39.5
subacute *39.3*, 39.6
therapeutic agents **39.6**
treatment 39.7
unclassified 39.1
Wiskott–Aldrich syndrome *80.9*
see also atopic eczema; hand eczema; pompholyx eczema
Eczema Area and Severity Index (EASI) 16.3–16.4
eczema coxsackium 25.44, 25.94
eczéma craquelé see eczema, asteatotic
eczema herpeticum 25.43–25.46, 108.53
and atopic eczema 41.10, *41.20*
clinical features 25.44–25.46
management 25.46
pathophysiology 25.44
eczema marginatum see tinea cruris
eczematous cheilitis 108.61
eczematous dermatoses
contact dermatitis distinction 129.6
scrotum 109.11
eczematous disorders 39.1–39.36
apron eczema 39.14, *39.15*
assessment, investigation and management 39.1–39.24
chronic acral dermatitis 39.14–39.15
chronic superficial scaly dermatitis 39.27
discoid skin lesions, diagnosis of **39.10**
erythroderma 39.31–39.35
eyelid eczema 39.22–39.23
fingertip eczema 39.15
'gut'/slaughterhouse eczema 39.15–39.16
halo dermatitis 39.28
hyperkeratotic palmar eczema 39.14
infective eczemas 39.24–39.26
juvenile plantar dermatosis 39.23–39.24
lichenification 39.28–39.31
lichenoid chronic dermatitis 39.8–39.9
lichen simplex 39.28–39.31
lower leg eczema 39.19–39.22
Murray Williams warts 39.28
nummular dermatitis 39.7–39.9, **39.10**
patchy vesiculosquamous eczema 39.16
pityriasis alba 39.26–39.27
pompholyx eczema 39.14
recurrent focal palmar peeling 39.16
ring eczema 39.16
see also atopic eczema; eczema; hand eczema
eczematous skin diseases
primary immunodeficiencies 149.19–149.20
xerosis cutis in 85.26
eczema vaccinatum 25.44
ED see ectodermal dysplasias
EDC see epidermal differentiation complex
EDS see Ehlers–Danlos syndromes
education, see also patient education
educational partnerships 7.1–7.2, 7.14
see also training programmes/resources
education of general public, early melanoma detection 142.18
Edwards syndrome 74.2
Edwards syndrome (trisomy 18) 74.2
EECDRG see European Environmental and Contact Dermatitis Research Group
EEC syndrome **106.7**
EED see erythema elevatum diutinum
EEM see ectodermal dysplasia–electrodactyly–macular dystrophy syndrome
EFAD see essential fatty acid deficiency
EFFC see erythromelanosis follicularis faciei et colli
efficacy, influences on topical therapies 18.2

EGFR see epidermal growth factor receptor
EGPA see eosinophilic granulomatosis with polyangiitis
Egypt, ancient medical texts 1.2
eHFSCs see epithelial HF stem cells
Ehlers–Danlos syndromes (EDS) 70.1–70.11
arthrochalasia type **70.4**, 70.9
atrophic scars *94.13*
Beighton score **70.8**
brittle cornea syndrome **70.6–70.7**, 70.10
cardiac-valvular type **70.3**, 70.9
classical 70.2, **70.3**, *70.8*, 70.9–70.10
clinical variants 70.2–70.10
cutis laxa 94.22
dermatosparaxis type **70.5**, 70.9
diagnostic clinical criteria **70.3–70.7**
differential diagnosis 70.10
elastosis perforans serpiginosa 94.55, *94.56*
epidemiology 70.1
hypermobility type 70.2–70.8, **70.3**
inheritance mode **70.3–70.7**
investigations 70.10–70.11
kyphoscoliotic type **70.4**, 70.9
lax skin 94.27
management 70.11
molecular defect **70.3–70.7**
molecular subtypes **70.3–70.7**
musculocontractural type **70.6**, 70.9
myopathic Ehlers–Danlos syndrome **70.7**, 70.10
pathophysiology 70.2
periodontal Ehlers–Danlos syndrome **70.5**, *70.10*
piezogenic pedal papules 122.26
in pregnancy 70.11, 113.9
spondylodysplastic type **70.5–70.6**, 70.9
ultrastructural findings **70.3–70.7**
vascular type **70.4**, 70.8–70.9, 70.11
Ehrlichia, tick-borne zoonotic infection 26.66–26.67
ehrlichiosis 26.66–26.67
Ehrlich, Paul 1.7
eighth nerve deafness (neurolabyrinthitis), congenital syphilis 29.26
Ekbom disease see delusional infestation
EKV see erythrokeratoderma variabilis
elastic fibres 2.2, 2.32–2.33
assembly and cross-linking *2.35*
degradation disorders 2.34–2.35, 94.21–94.32
genetic disorders 70.14–70.21
cutis laxa 70.14–70.17
Marfan syndrome 70.20–70.21
Michelin tyre baby syndrome 70.19, 73.17
Williams–Beuren syndrome 70.18–70.19
transmission electron microscopy image *2.34*
elastic tissue deposition, acquired disorders 94.32–94.33
elastin 2.33–2.35
collagen interdependence 122.5
gene mutations 2.33–2.34
elastin-associated microfibrils 2.35–2.36
elastin degradation, UV radiation exposure 10.10–10.11
elastinopathies 70.14–70.19
cutis laxa 70.14–70.17
Michelin tyre baby syndrome 70.19
Williams–Beuren syndrome 70.18–70.19
elastoderma 94.33
elastofibroma dorsi 94.33, 136.10
elastogenesis 94.32
elastolytic conditions 94.27–94.30
elastolytic giant cell granuloma 94.27–94.29
elastorrhexis 94.31
annular elastolytic giant cell granuloma 94.29
elastosis perforans serpiginosa *4.11*, 63.76, 94.30, 94.55–94.57
renal failure and dialysis complications 154.3–154.4
elastotic degeneration 3.40

elastotic marginal plaques of the hands 94.4–94.5
elastotic nodules of the ear 94.3
elbow
  atrophic scarring, classical Ehlers–Danlos syndrome 70.8
  dermatitis herpetiformis 4.8
  lichenification of 39.30
  mixed connective tissue disease 53.4
  rheumatoid nodules 53.5
  Rothmund–Thomson syndrome 75.5
  tufted angioma 116.11
  xanthoma excised from 60.3
elderly people
  chronic wounds, incidence of 6.1
  microbial ecology of the skin 26.4
  pityriasis rubra pilaris 36.4
  psoriasis vulgaris 35.15
  psychological and social factors at older age 15.3
  systemic lupus erythematosus 51.32
  wound healing 11.10
electrocautery 20.42–20.43
electrochemotherapy (ECT) 20.48
  basal cell carcinoma 140.17
  melanoma 144.2
electrocoagulation 20.44
electrodesiccation 20.44
electrofulguration 20.44, 20.45
electromagnetic muscle stimulation (EMMS) 161.8
electromagnetic spectrum 10.1
electron beam therapy 24.1–24.2
  see also total skin electron beam therapy
electronic health records 5.11–5.12
electronic records
  disease outcome measurements 16.2
  see also computer-based assessments
electron microscopy 3.30–3.31
  amyloidoses 56.5, 56.6
  biopsy 3.4
  epidermis image 2.6
  epidermolysis bullosa diagnosis 69.21–69.22
  see also transmission electron microscopy
electrosection 20.44–20.45
electrosurgery 20.42–20.46
  characteristics 20.43
  effects 20.44–20.45
  equipment 20.43–20.44
  hazards and risks 20.45–20.46
  hidradenitis suppurativa treatment 90.11
  terminology 20.43
Elejalde syndrome 68.9
elephantiasis, ear dermatoses **106.22**
elephantiasis nostra verrucosa (ENV) 103.6
elephantine psoriasis 35.14
elicitation 127.6–127.7
elimination of a drug, clinical pharmacology 13.3–13.4
ELISA see enzyme-linked immunosorbent assay
elliptical surgical biopsy 3.3, 3.6
  principles 20.8–20.9
  technique 20.11–20.12
ELOVL4 deficiency 63.35
EM see erythema multiforme
EMA see epithelial membrane antigen
emapalumab 135.13–135.14
EMBASE (Elsevier's biomedical database) 17.7
embedding procedure, tissue processing 3.7
Emberger syndrome 103.25
emboli, purpura 99.14–99.19
embolic metastasis to digits 148.5, 148.6
embryonic development of skin 2.3–2.5
embryos, wound healing 11.2, 11.10
emergency treatment, burn injuries 125.1–125.2
Emergomyces infections, rare endemic mycoses 32.90
EMM see erythema multiforme major
EMMS see electromagnetic muscle stimulation

emollients 12.3, 18.3–18.4, 18.8–18.9
  atopic eczema treatment 41.26, 41.27
  ichthyoses management 63.42, **63.43**, 63.44
emotional disturbances, necrotising lymphocytic folliculitis 93.4
emotional sweating 2.9
emotions
  links to beliefs and behaviours 15.1–15.3
  psychological factors in patients 15.2
EMPD see extramammary Paget disease
emperipolesis, sinus histiocytosis with massive lymphadenopathy 135.27
emulsifiers, topical medication vehicles 18.5, 18.7
emulsions, topical drugs 12.3–12.4
EN see erythema nodosum
encephalitis, herpes simplex virus 25.23
encephalocraniocutaneous lipomatosis (ECCL) **72.10**, 98.20–98.21, 98.25
enchondromas, Maffucci syndrome 71.20
ENCODE see Encyclopedia of DNA Elements
en coup de sabre (ECDS) 87.52
  morphoea 55.23–55.24
Encyclopedia of DNA Elements (ENCODE) Project 8.1–8.2
endemic mycoses
  rare, systemic *Emergomyces* infections 32.90
  rare systemic *Emergomyces* infections 32.90
endemic (non-venereal) treponematoses 26.69–26.72
endemic relapsing fever, *Borrelia* spp. 26.72
endemic syphilis (bejel) 26.70
endocrine disorders 150.1–150.22
  causes 150.2
  hirsutism 87.91
  hypermelanosis 86.17–86.19
  lipodystrophy 98.8
  oral involvement 108.83
  signs and symptoms of general endocrine disease seen in skin **150.7**
  specific endocrine conditions 150.15–150.21
  tuberous sclerosis complex 78.9
  see also dermatoendocrinology; hormones
endocrine dysregulation, obesity 98.27–98.28
endocrine factors
  melanocyte regulation 86.7
  pigmentation regulation 86.5–86.7
endocrine mucin-producing sweat gland carcinoma 137.39
endocrine system
  drug reaction with eosinophilia and systemic symptoms 118.9
  nervous system relationship 150.2
endocrine therapies, hair loss 87.73
endocrinology
  principles 150.2–150.3
  role of skin and hair follicles 150.3
  signalling axes 150.2
  see also dermatoendocrinology
endocrinopathy
  acquired ichthyosis association 85.1
  chronic mucocutaneous candidiasis 32.68
endogenous eczema, contact dermatitis distinction 129.6
endogenous non-melanin pigmentation 86.47–86.51
endogenous ochronosis 86.50–86.51
endo-MT see endothelial-to-mesenchymal transition
endonyx onychomycosis 32.48
endophytic seborrhoeic keratosis see inverted follicular keratosis
endoplasmic reticulum (ER) 63.21
endothelial cells 2.40, 2.41, 2.42
  Adamantiades–Behçet disease 48.3–48.4
  microscopic examination of 3.37
  wound healing 11.6
endothelial-to-mesenchymal transition (endo-MT), systemic sclerosis 54.10

endothelin-1 86.10
  pruritus **81.3**, 81.5
endothelins 86.7
endothrix infection, periodic acid–Schiff stain 3.8
endotoxin exposure, and atopic eczema 41.8
endovascular lymphatic angioendothelioma see papillary intralymphatic angioendothelioma
energy fluence of lasers, selective photothermolysis 23.5
energy homeostasis, adipose tissue 97.4
England, skin cancer, economic burden of 6.5–6.6, **6.7**
enhancers, topical drug delivery 12.5–12.6
ENKTCL-NT see extranodal NK/T-cell lymphoma, nasal type
ENL see erythema nodosum leprosum
The Enlightenment 1.3–1.4
Entamoeba histolytica, amoebiasis 33.36–33.38
enterobiasis 33.14–33.15
  clinical presentation 33.15
  definition/nomenclature 33.14
  epidemiology 33.14
  management 33.15
  pathophysiology 33.14–33.15
Enterobius vermicularis 33.14–33.15
enteroviral vesicular stomatitis with exanthem see hand, foot and mouth disease; herpangina
enterovirus infections 25.93–25.96
  oral involvement 108.50
ENV see elephantiasis nostra verrucosa
envenomation see venoms
environmental acne see occupational acne
environmental allergens 127.4
environmental and drug-induced scleroderma 94.45–94.46
environmental factors
  acne 88.18–88.26
  arthropod exposure 34.2–34.3
  atopic eczema 41.6–41.9
  congenital melanocytic naevi 73.11
  eczema 39.4, 39.11
  epidemiology of skin disease 5.10–5.11
  generalised pustular psoriasis 35.32–35.33
  lichen planus 37.2–37.3
  melanoma 142.5–142.6
  neonatal lupus erythematosus 51.40
  nummular dermatitis 39.8
  palmoplantar pustulosis 35.37
  pemphigus 50.3–50.4
  psoriasis vulgaris 35.3–35.4
  pyoderma gangrenosum 49.4
  rural and urban environments 41.6–41.7, 41.8
  scleroderma 94.45–94.46
  seborrhoeic dermatitis 40.4, 40.7
  Sweet syndrome 49.10–49.11
  systemic lupus erythematosus 51.21
  systemic sclerosis 54.14–54.15
  urticaria 42.7
environmental mycobacteria see non-tuberculous mycobacteria
enzymatic fat necrosis 97.8, 97.42
enzyme-linked immunosorbent assay (ELISA) 3.16, 3.20–3.21
EORTC see European Organization of Research and Treatment of Cancer
EORTC QLQ-C30 see European Organisation for Research and Treatment of Cancer Core Questionnaire
eosinophilia
  drug reaction 118.1, 118.4–118.12
  gold toxicity 121.4
  HIV primary infection 31.7–31.8
eosinophiliamyalgia syndrome 94.30
eosinophilic cellulitis (Wells syndrome) 47.16
eosinophilic fasciitis (Shulman syndrome) **54.20**, 55.2, **55.3**, **55.4**, 55.21–55.23, 55.22, **55.27**, 97.13
eosinophilic folliculitis, HIV 31.17

eosinophilic globules 3.42
eosinophilic granulomatosis with polyangiitis (EGPA) 100.25–100.28, 152.3–152.4
eosinophilic pustular folliculitis 91.3–91.5, 93.7–93.10, 115.12
eosinophils
  lupus panniculitis 97.37–97.38
  microscopic examination of 3.35–3.36
EPDS see erosive pustular dermatosis of the scalp
ephelides 78.3, 86.2, 86.15–86.16, 131.1–131.3
  epidermis of 131.2
  hyperpigmentation 131.2
  melanoma risk 142.3
  oculocutaneous albinism 68.8
epidemic arthritic erythema see *Streptobacillus moniliformis*
epidemic polyarthritis see Ross River virus
epidemic typhus
  human body louse transmitted rickettsial infection 26.80–26.81
  rodent flea transmitted rickettsial infection (murine typhus) 26.81
epidemiology of skin disease 5.1–5.17
  association and causation 5.7–5.10
  burden of skin disease 5.5, 5.6–5.7, 5.8, 5.9
  causative agents of disease 5.8–5.10
  chronicity of disease 5.10
  clinical epidemiology 5.1
  community diagnosis and control 5.2
  comparisons and inferences 5.3
  continuum of disease 5.2–5.3
  definition 5.1
  dermatoepidemiology 5.1–5.2, 5.15–5.16
  diagnostic criteria 5.4
  dietary factors 5.11
  digital technologies 5.13
  disease associations 5.11–5.12, 5.14
  disease definition 5.4–5.5
  disease frequency 5.7–5.11, 5.14
  disease severity assessment 5.5
  early and later environment 5.10–5.11
  electronic health records 5.11–5.12
  epidemiological studies 5.15
  ethnicity 5.10
  genetic epidemiology 5.10
  Global Burden of Disease study 5.6–5.7, 5.8, 5.9
  health services research 5.12–5.14
  impairment, disability and handicap caused by disease 5.5–5.6
  incidence of disease 5.10, 5.14
  interpretation of results 5.14–5.15
  leisure factors 5.11
  medical need/supply and demand relationship 5.13–5.14
  and migration 5.10
  natural history of skin diseases 5.11–5.12
  needs assessments 5.12
  occupational groups 5.11
  population approach 5.2–5.4, 5.5
  prevalence of disease 5.10, 5.14
  prevention paradox 5.3–5.4
  public health approach 5.2, 5.4–5.7
  regional distribution of burden of disease 5.9
  relevance to dermatology 5.1–5.2
  risk factors 5.7–5.10, 5.14
  skin diseases as 'entities' in population 5.2–5.3
  Snow's epidemiological research 5.9–5.10
  socioeconomic factors 5.10–5.11
  terminology 5.14–5.15
  validity and repeatability 5.15
epidermal cysts
  formation, foreign body reactions 122.17
  vulva **110.32**
epidermal degenerations 3.40–3.41
epidermal detachment, in SJS/TEN 118.17, 118.20
epidermal differentiation complex (EDC) 2.7

epidermal dysplasia, photothermal ablation 23.21
epidermal growth factor receptor (EGFR) 87.73
epidermal growth factor receptor (EGFR) inhibitors 119.3–119.5, 119.7–119.8
  acneform reaction 88.14, *88.16*
epidermal growth factor receptor (EGFR) signalling 2.4
epidermal hyperplasia, calluses 122.7
epidermal inclusion cysts *see* epidermoid cysts
epidermal keratinisation, acquired disorders 85.1–85.31
epidermal keratins 63.13–63.18
epidermal lesions 3.44
epidermal melanin pigments **86.5**
epidermal melanin unit 86.2–86.3
epidermal naevi **73.2**, **73.3**, *73.4*
  see also congenital epidermal naevi
epidermal necrosis 118.13–118.14
epidermal neoplasia, photothermal ablation 23.21
epidermal pigmentation, Q-switched laser treatments 23.12–23.17, *23.18*
epidermal spongiosis, chronic actinic dermatitis 126.14, *126.15*
epidermal thickening, palmoplantar keratodermas 63.49
epidermis 2.1, *2.2*
  anatomy 9.1, *9.2*
  chronological ageing/photoageing **10.10**
  cornified cell envelope *2.7*
  dendritic epidermal T cells 9.7
  desmosomes 2.18–2.19
  differentiation *2.6*, 2.7, 2.8
  electron micrograph *2.6*
  embryonic development 2.3
  granular layer 2.5–2.6
  hyperproliferation 2.8
  immune cells 9.3–9.4
  lipids *2.8*
  Merkel cells 2.2, 2.11–2.12
  mesenchymal cells 2.4
  nail bed 2.11, 119.7
  stem cell proliferation *2.43*, 2.44
  stratum basale **2.5**
  stratum corneum 2.1, 2.6
  stratum lucidum 2.7
  structures of 2.5–2.7
  substance P immunoreactive nerve endings in 83.3
epidermodysplasia verruciformis (EV) 2.13, 25.65–25.66, **25.67**, 25.69–25.71
  classical/non-classical types 25.66, 25.69
  clinical features 25.69, *25.70*
  management 25.69–25.70
  pathophysiology 25.66, 25.69
  skin cancer 147.1–147.2
  see also acquired epidermodysplasia verruciformis
epidermoid cysts 78.11, 88.33–88.34, 133.1–133.3
  epidemiology 133.1
  management 133.2–133.3
  pachyonychia congenita 67.11
  pathophysiology/clinical features 133.2
  sebaceous duct epithelial walled cutaneous cysts 133.6–133.7
  surgical treatment 20.49
epidermolysis
  with glycolic acid peel *160.9*
  use of term 69.2
epidermolysis bullosa (EB) *8.8*, 8.10, 69.1–69.28, 94.43, 110.5
  clinical subtypes 69.8–69.11
  diagnosis 69.20–69.23
  digestive system 153.6
  friction blisters 122.10
  genes implicated in 69.2–69.8
  genito-urinary involvement 154.6
  innovative therapies 69.27–69.28
  oral involvement 108.23
  proteins implicated in 69.2–69.8

sweat glands 92.8
  treatment 69.24–69.28
epidermolysis bullosa acquisita (EBA) 50.42–50.48
  associated diseases 50.43
  in childhood *50.45*, *50.46*
  clinical features 50.44–50.46
  clinical variants 50.46
  diagnosis *50.24*
  differential diagnosis 50.46
  direct immunofluorescence findings 3.18, *3.19*, *50.35*
  epidemiology 50.43
  IgA EBA 50.36
  inflammatory variant *50.45*, *50.46*
  internal malignancy association 148.22
  investigations and diagnosis 50.46–50.47
  management 50.47–50.48
  mechanobullous variant *50.44*, *50.45*
  oral involvement 108.81
  pathophysiology 50.43–50.44
  perioral crusts and erosions *50.46*
  treatment ladder 50.48
  vulval **110.21**
epidermolysis bullosa simplex (EBS) 2.8, 69.2, 69.8–69.11
  management 69.25
  molecular pathology 69.11–69.15
epidermolytic hyperkeratosis 3.41, *63.16*–*63.17*
epidermolytic ichthyosis 63.14–63.16
epidermolytic palmoplantar keratoderma (EPPK) 63.50–63.51
epidermophytide, dermatophytide reaction 32.50
Epidermophyton, dermatophytosis 32.18, **32.19**, 32.21, 32.30, *32.32*
Epidermophyton floccosum **32.19**, 32.21, 32.30, *32.32*
epigenomics 8.6
epiluminescence microscopy *see* dermoscopy
epinephrine, urticaria treatment 42.18
episcleritis, BADAS-associated *49.17*
episodic angio-oedema with eosinophilia syndrome (Gleich syndrome) 43.4–43.5
Epistemonikos, finding systematic reviews 17.7
epithelial cysts *see* epidermoid cysts
epithelial HF stem cells (eHFSCs) 87.4
epithelial keratinocyte necrosis, drug-induced 118.12
epithelial markers, cutaneous neoplasms 3.21–3.23
epithelial membrane antigen (EMA) 3.22
epithelial necrolysis, acute SJS/TEN 118.17
epithelial sheath neuroma 136.50
epithelial stem cells *2.43*
  inflammatory memory 9.9
epithelioid angiosarcoma 136.37
epithelioid (bacillary) angiomatosis, oral infection 108.55
epithelioid haemangioendothelioma 136.36–136.37
epithelioid haemangioma 136.27–136.28
epithelioid sarcoma 97.15, 136.63–136.64
Epithelioid sarcoma-like haemangioendothelioma *see* composite haemangioendothelioma
epithelioma adenoides cysticum *see* trichoepithelioma
epithelioma cuniculatum (verrucous carcinoma of the foot) 141.31, **141.32**
epithiloid fibrous histiocytoma 136.20–136.21
epoxy resin, allergic contact dermatitis *127.14*, 127.68–127.69
EPP *see* erythropoietic protoporphyria
EPPK *see* epidermolytic palmoplantar keratoderma
Epstein–Barr virus (EBV) 14.4, 25.36–25.39, 126.25, 135.11
  angioimmunoblastic T-cell lymphoma 139.45

CD30+ lymphoproliferative disorders 139.26
diffuse large B-cell lymphoma 25.39
extranodal NK/T-cell lymphoma (nasal type) 139.36–139.37
lymphomatoid granulomatosis 139.44
lymphoproliferative disorders and malignancy 25.38–25.39
oral involvement 108.32, 108.51
post-transplant lymphoproliferative disorder 139.47
Epstein pearls, neonates 114.4
equestrian cold panniculitis *97.35*, 97.36, 97.37
equestrian panniculitis 124.6
equine disease, glanders 26.55
Er:YAG, photothermal ablation 23.21
Er:YAG lasers, skin resurfacing 161.1–161.3, **161.5**
ER *see* endoplasmic reticulum
erbium:yttrium-aluminium-garnet (Nd:YAG) lasers
  absorption spectra *23.4*
  tattoo removal 23.15
  vascular lesions 23.7, 23.10
Erdheim–Chester disease (ECD) 135.21–135.22
  BRAF V600E mutation 135.9
erectile dysfunction, systemic sclerosis 54.28
erethism 121.6
erisipeloid 26.46–26.48
erlotinib, papulopustular eruptions 119.3, *119.4*
erosions, oral ulceration 108.36
erosive adenomatosis of the nipple *see* nipple, adenoma
erosive pustular dermatosis of the scalp (EPDS) 105.13–105.14
erosive skin fragility disorders 69.20
erucism *see* caterpillar dermatitis
eruption cyst, over a primary tooth 108.10
eruptions
  diagnosis 4.3
  quinine-induced photo-lichenoid eruption *4.7*
  see also lesions
eruptive inflammatory psoriasis *see* unstable psoriasis
eruptive lentiginoses 86.17
eruptive melanocytic naevi 147.14
eruptive pseudoangiomatosis and eruptive hypomelanosis 25.123
eruptive vellus hair cyst 137.8
eruptive xanthomas 60.4
  diabetic patients 62.3, *62.4*
erysipelas 103.13–103.14, 106.19
  definition and relationship to cellulitis 26.18
  eyelid 107.38
  sclerosing panniculitis differentiation 97.32
erysipelas-like changes in skin, carcinoma erysipeloides 148.2–148.3, *148.4*
erysipelas-like reaction, diabetes mellitus 62.2
Erysipelothrix rhusiopathiae 26.46–26.48
erythema (redness)
  acne vulgaris *88.27*, *88.29*
  atopic eczema *41.15*
  chemical peels, side effect of 160.11–160.12
  chronic venous insufficiency **101.43**
  dermatomyositis 52.3, *52.4*, *52.5*, *52.6*
  differential diagnosis 89.7
  disease course 89.11
  drug/chemical photosensitivity *126.29*
  epidermolysis bullosa acquista *50.45*
  grading of in psoriasis vulgaris **35.17**
  hereditary angio-oedema *43.4*
  indicator of pressure ulcers 123.4
  irritant contact dermatitis 128.6
  laser therapies 23.9–23.11, 23.12, 23.13
  lichen planus *110.12*
  linear IgA disease *50.37*

morphoea *55.18*
non-blanchable 123.4, **123.5**, 123.8
transient *see* flushing
ultraviolet radiation *10.3*, *10.4*
UVB phototherapy adverse effects 21.11–21.12
UVR exposure 10.7
venous leg ulcer *102.5*
see also flushing; rosacea
erythema ab igne *4.16*, 124.14–124.16
erythema annulare centrifugum (EAC) *4.11*, 47.6–47.8
  associated diseases 47.7
  causes and associations **47.7**
  differential diagnosis 47.8
  histology *47.8*
  investigations 47.8
  lesion appearance *47.7*
  pathology 47.8
  predisposing factors 47.7
  treatment 47.8
erythema chronicum migrans (ECM) 47.9
  Lyme disease 26.69, 26.72, 26.73, *26.73*, 26.74
erythema dyschromicum perstans 86.32–86.33
erythema elevatum diutinum (EED) 100.8–100.10
  fibrosis *100.8*
  inflammatory cell infiltrate *100.8*
erythema gyratum repens 47.11–47.12
erythema induratum of Bazin 27.29–27.31, 97.26–97.30
  clinical features 27.30
  epidemiology 27.29–27.30
  investigations 27.30–27.31
  management 27.31
  pathophysiology 27.30
erythema infectiosum (fifth disease) 25.77–25.78, 115.6, 155.2, *155.3*
erythema marginatum 47.9–47.11
  associated diseases 47.10
  clinical features 47.11
  complications and co-morbidities 47.11
  Duckett Jones criteria for diagnosis of rheumatic fever **47.11**
  investigations 47.11
  pathology 47.10
  treatment 47.11
erythema multiforme (EM) 47.1–47.6, 127.19–127.20, 127.72
  classic target lesion *47.2*
  clinical features 47.5–47.6
  differential diagnosis 47.6
  drug reactions 47.3–47.4
    with eosinophilia and systemic symptoms 118.6
  epidermal necrosis 47.5
  erythema multiforme minor 47.5
  eye involvement *47.3*
  herpes simplex virus 25.23
  histopathology of a subepidermal blister *47.5*
  immunology 47.2–47.3
  management 47.6
  mucosal lesions *47.2*
  oral involvement 108.75
  pathology 47.5
  target lesions in *4.15*
  topical agents triggering erythema multiforme-like reactions 47.4–47.5
  triggering factors 47.3
erythema multiforme-like lesions, COVID-19 association 25.111
erythema multiforme-like PLE *126.4*, *126.5*
erythema multiforme major (EMM) 118.15
erythema neonatorum 114.3
erythema nodosum (EN) 27.31, 96.14, 97.18–97.25
  aetiological factors **97.19**–**97.20**, 97.21
  in pregnancy 113.12
erythema nodosum leprosum (ENL) 28.3, 28.4, **28.5**, 28.11, *28.12*, 28.15, 97.25–97.26

erythema nodosum-like lesions 97.51–97.52
erythematotelangiectatic rosacea 89.1
   microbiome 89.4
erythematous candidiasis
   acute 32.61
   chronic 32.62
   oral lesions 32.62, 108.20–108.22
erythematous rosacea, pathology 89.3
erythem (redness) 4.13, 126.1
erythrasma 26.39–26.41
   clinical features 26.39–26.41
   of groin 4.20
   investigations 26.41
   management 26.41
   pathophysiology 26.39
erythrocyanosis 124.7–124.8
erythrocytosis *see* polycythaemia vera; TEMPI syndrome
erythroderma
   allergic contact dermatitis 39.35
   causes of and prevalence in adults **39.31**
   chronic actinic dermatitis 126.18
   clinical features 39.32
   clinical variants 39.32–39.35
   complications and co-morbidities 39.35
   dermatophytosis 39.34
   disease course and prognosis 39.35
   drug reactions 39.33
      with eosinophilia and systemic symptoms 118.7, *118.8*
   eczematous dermatoses 39.32
   epidemiology 39.31
   HIV 31.12
   ichthyosiform erythroderma 39.33
   internal malignancy association 148.23
   leukaemia 39.32–39.33
   lichen planus 39.34
   lymphoma 39.32–39.33
   management 39.35
   Norwegian scabies 39.34
   papuloerythroderma of Ofuji 39.34–39.35
   pathology 39.31–39.32
   pemphigus foliaceus 39.34
   pityriasis rubra pilaris 39.33–39.34
   predisposing factors 39.31
   psoriasis 39.32
   severe combined immunodeficiency 80.7
   Sézary syndrome 39.33
   treatment 39.35
   unknown origin 39.33
erythrodermatous exfoliative 127.72
erythrodermic psoriasis 35.14, **35.16**
erythrodermic sarcoidosis 96.13
erythrogenic toxin, scarlet fever 26.35
erythrokeratodermas 63.18–63.20
erythrokeratoderma variabilis (EKV) 63.18–63.19
erythromelalgia 82.12–82.13, 101.6–101.9
   age of onset 101.7
   clinical features **101.8**
   ear dermatoses **106.22**
   epidemiology 101.7
   internal malignancy association 148.25
   investigations 101.9
   irritant contact dermatitis *101.9*
   management 101.9
   pathophysiology 101.7–101.8
   primary erythromelalgia 101.7–101.8
   secondary erythromelalgia 101.8
   associated diseases in 101.7
erythromelanosis follicularis of the face and neck 85.10, 86.14–86.15
erythromelanosis follicularis faciei et colli (EFFC) 85.10, 86.14–86.15
erythromycin 18.11, 19.47, 19.48
erythroplakia, oral involvement 108.23, *108.24*
erythroplasia of Queyrat
   penis 109.31–109.34
   see also anal/perianal/genital intraepithelial carcinomas
erythropoietic protoporphyria (EPP) 58.4, 58.14–58.17, *94.3*, 99.24, 126.7, 126.32–126.33
   acute reactions 58.15

bone health 58.16
clinical features 58.14–58.15
genetic counselling 58.16
investigations 58.15
liver disease in 58.16–58.17
oral involvement 108.85
osteoporosis 58.16
pathophysiology 58.14
photoprotection 58.15
escharotomy, burn management 125.8
essential fatty acid deficiency (EFAD) 61.31–61.34
   clinical features 61.32–61.33
   epidemiology 61.32
   genetics 61.32
   investigations 61.33
   management 61.33–61.34
   pathophysiology 61.32–61.33
essential thrombocythaemia (ET)
   thrombocytosis 99.10–99.11
etanercept
   psoriasis treatment 35.28
   psoriatic arthritis treatment 35.45
ethical issues
   drug trials, reporting of 13.13
   medical volunteer trips **7.15**
Ethiopia, medical schools 7.8
ethnicity
   botulinum toxins, aesthetic uses of 159.6
   chemical peels 160.15
   cutaneous squamous cell carcinoma in white and non-white populations 141.27
   dermatosis papulosa nigra 132.5
   diagnosis 4.4
   epidemiology 5.10
   mucocutaneous manifestations of COVID-19 infection 25.104
   neurobiological differences in pruritus 81.2
   rosacea 89.2
   seborrhoeic keratosis 132.1
ethylenediamine 127.19
ethylhexylglycerin 127.56–127.57
ethylmalonic encephalopathy 124.7
EU directives/regulations
   allergens 127.35
   MCI/MI preservatives 127.54
eumelanin 2.17, *2.18*, 86.5
Europe, skin cancer, economic burden of 6.6–6.8
European Environmental and Contact Dermatitis Research Group (EECDRG) 127.1–127.2
European Hidradenitis Suppurativa Foundation (EHSF) 16.5
European Organisation for Research and Treatment of Cancer Core Questionnaire (EORTC QLQ-C30) 16.9
European Organization of Research and Treatment of Cancer (EORTC), cutaneous lymphoma classifications 139.1, **139.2**, 139.6
EV *see* epidermodysplasia verruciformis
evidence based medicine (EBM) 17.1–17.25
   adverse events study evaluation 17.17–17.18
   applying evidence to specific patients 17.12, 17.16, 17.17
   clinical trial evaluation 17.12–17.15
   critically appraising evidence and applying it to individual patients 17.8–17.18
   definition 17.1
   diagnostic test study evaluation 17.15–17.17
   evaluating the data in clinical research papers 17.18–17.25
   experience-based decisions by physicians 17.5–17.6
   finding best evidence 17.2, 17.6–17.8
   five steps of practising 17.2
   formulating questions and finding evidence 17.3–17.8

hierarchy of evidence 17.4
levels of evidence **17.5**
limitations 17.2–17.3
meta analysis 17.4–17.5
presentation of data and basic statistics in clinical research papers 17.18–17.20
shortcut method for appraising clinical research papers 17.24–17.25
statistical methods in clinical research papers 17.20–17.24
systematic review evaluation 17.8–17.12
threats 17.3
validity of research 17.8–17.10, 17.12–17.16, 17.17
see also randomised controlled clinical trials
Ewing sarcoma, cutaneous 136.51–136.52
EWSR1-SMAD3-rearranged fibroblastic tumour 136.4
examination of skin 4.5
exanthema subitum *see* roseola infantum
exanthematous pustulosis 118.1–118.4
exanthems (rashes)
   COVID-19 association 25.109
   diagnosis 4.2
   drug-induced 117.1–117.2
   drug reaction with eosinophilia and systemic symptoms 118.7
   HIV acute primary infection 31.6, 31.7
   Langerhans cell histiocytosis 135.4, 135.6
   secondary syphilis 29.7–29.10
   viral infections 25.4–25.5, **25.4**
excessive hair growth 87.84–87.91
excessive washing
   obsessive–compulsive behaviour 84.26
   olfactory delusions 84.10
excisional biopsy 3.2
exclamation mark hairs 87.14–87.15, 87.23, *87.24*
excoriated nodular prurigo *see* prurigo nodularis
excoriée acné 84.20–84.22, 88.28–88.29, *88.30*
exercise, lymphoedema therapy 103.58
exercise-induced purpura 99.5, **99.9**
exercise-induced urticaria 42.12
exfoliative cheilitis 108.61–108.62
exfoliative dermatitis
   cutaneous manifestations of Hodgkin disease 139.49
   drug reaction with eosinophilia and systemic symptoms 118.7, *118.8*
   internal malignancy association 148.23
exfoliative disorders, cornification 63.26–63.30
exfoliative erythroderma, drug reaction with 118.10
exfoliative ichthyosis (EXI) 63.21–63.22
exocytosis 3.41
exogen 87.8
exogenous agents, perforating disease due to 94.55
exogenous androgens 87.91
exogenous drug- and chemical-induced photosensitivity 126.27–126.32
exogenous ochronosis 86.50–86.51
exogenous pigmentation 86.51–86.54
Exophiala jeanselmei 32.78
exophilin-5 deficiency, autosomal recessive EB simplex with 69.10–69.11
exophilin-5 epidermolysis bullosa 69.4
extensive dermal melanocytosis 73.21
external auditory canal (EAC) 106.1–106.3
   microbiome 26.5
   tumour management 106.29–106.31
external auditory meatus *see* external auditory canal
external carotid artery, anatomy of head and neck 20.1–20.2
external otitis, otomycosis 32.17–32.18
external root sheath tumours 137.5–137.7
   see also trichilemmal cyst
extracellular matrix (ECM) 2.27–2.28, 2.40
   wound healing 11.5

extracorporeal photochemotherapy *see* extracorporeal photopheresis
extracorporeal photopheresis (ECP)
   administration 21.11
   adverse effects 21.15
   conditions treated 21.7
   cutaneous T-cell lymphoma 21.7, 139.24–139.25
   graft-versus-host disease 21.7
   history 21.2
   principles 21.1
extracts
   allergic contact dermatitis 127.49
   patch testing 127.33
extracutaneous pyoderma gangrenosum 49.5
extracutaneous tumours, familial adenomatous polyposis 78.11
extragenital lichen sclerosus 94.25
extramammary Paget disease (EMPD) 110.37–110.39, 137.42–137.43, 148.7
   classification **110.38**
   immunocytochemical markers **110.38**
   male genitalia 109.40–109.41
   perianal skin 111.24
extramedullary haematopoiesis 149.5
extranodal NK/T-cell lymphoma, nasal type (ENKTCL-NT) 108.70, 139.36–139.37
extrapulmonary sarcoidosis 96.5
extravascular paraprotein deposition 149.13
extremities, constricting bands of 94.46–94.48
extremity escharotomies 125.8
eye 107.1–107.50
   acquired immune deficiency syndrome **107.35**
   amyloidosis **107.35**
   anatomy and physiology 107.1–107.2
   antibiotics, side effects 107.43
   antimalarials, side effects 19.6, 107.43
   atopic eye diseases 107.16–107.23
   biologic agents, side effects 107.44
   botulinum toxin, side effects 107.44
   cicatrising conjunctivitis 107.24–107.34
   conjunctival hyperaemia *50.30*
   contact dermatitis 107.6
   corticosteroids, side effects 107.40–107.43
   dermatomyositis **107.35**
   drug side effects 107.40–107.44
   epidermolysis bullosa 69.25–69.26
   episcleritis, BADAS-associated *49.17*
   erythema multiforme *47.3*
   extrapulmonary sarcoidosis 96.5
   filariasis (onchocerciasis) 107.40
   graft-versus-host disease 107.34
   granulomatosis with polyangiitis **107.35**
   herpes infection *1.10*
   histiocytoses **107.35**
   hypopyon, Adamantiades–Behçet disease *48.6*
   ichthyoses 63.45
   inflammatory bowel disease **107.35**
   inherited disorders **107.41–107.42**
   juvenile xanthogranuloma *135.16*, 135.17
   Kaposi sarcoma 107.49–107.50
   lacrimal apparatus *107.4*
   lacrimal glands 107.3
   leprosy 28.13, 107.39
   lupus erythematosus **107.35**
   Lyme disease 107.40
   malignant melanoma 107.49
   mucous membrane pemphigoid *50.30*, 107.24–107.32
   mycobacterial infections 107.39–107.40
   ocular complications of drug therapy 19.6, 19.15–19.16, *19.19*, 107.40–107.44
   ocular syphilis 29.16, 107.39–107.40
   onchocerciasis 33.2, 33.5
   ophthalmological terms **107.5**
   polyarteritis nodosa **107.35**
   porphyria **107.35**
   precorneal tear film 107.3

protozoal infections   107.40
pseudoxanthoma elasticum   70.33
psoralens, side effects   107.43–107.44
psoriasis   107.6
reactive arthritis   **107.35**
retinoids, side effects   107.43
river blindness (onchocerciasis)   107.40
sarcoidosis   **107.35**
Sjögren syndrome   **107.35**
Stevens–Johnson syndrome   107.32–107.34
syphilis   107.39–107.40
systemic diseases   **107.35**
systemic lupus erythematosus   51.32
toxic epidermal necrolysis   107.32–107.34
treponemal infections   107.39–107.40
tuberculosis   107.39
uveitis, Adamantiades–Behçet disease   48.4, 48.6
see also conjunctival entries; cornea; corneal entries; macular; ocular entries
eye area, use of lead shielding in radiotherapy for skin cancer   24.3, 24.4, 24.10–24.11
eyebrows
 anatomy and role   107.2
 disorders of   107.3–107.4
 hair density reduction   107.4
 hypertrichosis   107.4
 hypoplasia   107.4
 linear morphoea en coup de sabre   55.24
 synophrys   107.4
 syphilis of   105.12
 thinning of   107.4
 see also brows
eye colour, melanoma risk   142.3
eyelashes
 anatomy and physiology   107.2
 disorders of   107.4–107.5
 hordeolum   107.38, 107.39
 hypotrichosis   107.4
 madarosis   107.4–107.5
 Phthiriasis (lice) infestation   107.40
 trichomegaly   107.4
eyelids   107.1–107.50
 abnormalities of   107.5–107.6
 anatomy and physiology   107.2–107.3
 angioedema   42.3
 atopic eczema   41.20–41.21
 bacterial infections   107.38–107.39
 basal cell carcinoma   107.47–107.48
 benign adnexal lesions   107.45
 benign cysts   107.45–107.47
 benign lesions   107.44–107.47
 blepharitis   107.7–107.15
 blepharoconjunctivitis   107.6
 chalazion   107.45–107.46
 chronic granulomatous disease   80.15
 dendritic keratitis   107.37
 dermatitis   107.6, 127.15, 127.37
 eccrine carcinoma   107.49
 eczema of   39.22–39.23
 erysipelas   107.38
 haemangioma   107.46–107.47, 116.6
 herpes simplex virus infection   107.34–107.36, 107.37
 herpes zoster   107.36–107.38
 hordeolum   107.38, 107.39
 impetigo   107.38
 infantile haemangioma   116.6
 infections   107.34–107.40
 juvenile xanthogranuloma   107.45
 Kaposi sarcoma   107.49–107.50
 keratoacanthoma   107.47
 lipoid proteinosis   70.37
 malignant lesions   107.47–107.50
 malignant melanoma   107.49
 melanocytic naevi   107.46
 Merkel cell carcinoma   107.49
 microcystic adnexal carcinoma   107.49
 molluscum contagiosum   107.34, 107.36
 naevus of Ota   107.46
 necrotising fasciitis   107.39
 neonatal lupus erythematosus   51.40
 oedema   103.46, 103.47

ophthalmological terms   **107.5**
papular lesions around   80.15
parasitic infections   107.40
periorbital oedema   107.6–107.7
pigmentation changes   107.7
port-wine stain   107.47
psoriasis   107.6
scarring, long-term SJS/TEN   118.17
sebaceous carcinoma   107.49
seborrhoeic keratosis   107.44
skin cancer treatment   24.10, 24.11
squamous cell carcinoma   107.47, 107.48
swelling
 allergic contact dermatitis   129.6
 Stevens–Johnson syndrome/toxic epidermal necrolysis   118.14, 118.16
syringomas   4.8
urticaria   42.3
UV radiation-exposure damage   76.5
viral infections   107.34–107.38
warts   107.34, 107.36
xanthelasma   107.44
xanthelasma palpebrarum   60.4
eye protection, phototherapy   21.3, 21.10, 21.12, 21.15, 21.16
eye therapy, SJS/TEN   118.19–118.20

F
fabricated and induced illness, see also Münchausen syndrome by proxy
Fabry disease   79.6–79.8, 79.7, 79.8, 151.2–151.3, 154.1
 fucosidosis   79.4
face
 acne tarda   88.4
 acne vulgaris   88.3, 88.27, 88.28
 anti-p200 pemphigoid   50.41
 atopic eczema   41.15, 41.17
 blood vessels, position of   20.1–20.2
 bullous lupus erythematosus   51.28
 congenital adrenal hyperplasia   88.10
 discoid lupus erythematosus   51.5, 51.6
 eosinophilic pustular folliculitis   93.8
 granuloma faciale   100.12
 infantile acne   88.70
 infiltrating lipomatosis of the face   98.19–98.20
 Kikuchi–Fujimoto disease   51.33
 lichen planus actinicus   37.7
 linear morphoea, Blaschkoid nature of   55.23
 lupus erythematosus profundus   51.9
 motor nerves, position of   20.3–20.4
 neonatal acne   88.71
 neonatal lupus erythematosus   114.13
 oedema   103.46–103.49
 papular rashes, differential diagnosis   88.37–88.38
 pityriasis alba   39.27
 pityriasis rubra pilaris   36.4
 prepubertal acne   88.69, 88.70, 88.71
 progressive hemifacial atrophy   55.23, 55.24–55.25
 pyoderma faciale   88.36
 radiotherapy for skin cancer   24.10–24.12, 24.13, 24.14, 24.19
 rosacea   88.35
 sensory nerves, position of   20.2–20.3
 solid facial lymphoedema   88.41, 89.10, 89.16, 89.17, 103.47, 103.48
 Sweet syndrome   49.12
 swelling   98.19, 103.46–103.49
 systemic lupus erythematosus   51.23, 51.24
 systemic sclerosis   54.4
facial acne scar quality of life (FASQoL)   16.4
facial allergic contact dermatitis   127.14–127.15, 127.48
facial contact dermatitis   89.8
facial deformity, congenital syphilis   29.24, 29.26, 29.27
facial dermatoses, with uncertain nosological relationship to rosacea   89.15–89.17

facial dysmorphic features, Waardenburg syndrome   68.5
facial erythema, clinical features   89.5
facial hair, androgen-stimulated   87.10
facial hemiatrophy   94.20–94.21
facial hirsutism   87.90
facial hypertrichosis, porphyria cutanea tarda   87.87
facial infiltrating lipomatosis   72.11
facial lipoatrophy   98.7
facial lipomatosis, infiltrating   98.19–98.20
facial melanoses   86.9–86.15, 86.51
facial muscles, botulinum toxin injection sites   159.3
facial necrobiosis, atypical   95.12
facial nerve (CN VII), anatomy of head and neck   20.3–20.4
facial oedema
 drug reaction with eosinophilia and systemic symptoms   118.8
 minor features   89.6–89.7
facial pain syndromes   108.64–108.67
 burning mouth syndrome   108.64–108.65
 persistent idiopathic facial pain   108.65–108.66
 post-herpetic neuralgia   108.66
 trigeminal neuralgia   108.66–108.67
 trigeminal trophic syndrome   108.67
facial palsy, zoster   25.34
facial rejuvenation, laser resurfacing   161.1–161.6
facial sarcoidosis, photothermal ablation   23.22
facial skin
 ageing of skin   156.2, 156.3
 botulinum toxins, aesthetic uses of   159.3–159.6
 infantile haemangioma   116.3, 116.4
 melanoma, dermoscopy   145.9, 145.11, **145.11**
 microscopic examination of   3.33
 pyogenic granuloma   116.11
 see also chemical peels
facial surgery   20.1–20.52
facial telangiectasia, Rothmund–Thomson syndrome   75.5
facility-acquired pressure ulcers   123.1
FACS see fluorescence activated cell sorting
factitious disorders   84.29–84.38
 cheilitis   84.33, 108.61
 dermatitis artefacta   84.29–84.36
 dermatitis passivata   84.36
 dermatitis simulata   84.36
 dermatological pathomimicry   84.36
 malingering   84.36–84.37
 Münchausen syndrome by proxy   84.37–84.38
 Münchausen syndrome and pseudologia fantastica   84.37
 nails   84.33
 panniculitis   97.48–97.50
FACT-M see Functional Assessment of Cancer Therapy-Melanoma
facultative anaerobic bacteria   26.10
facultative (inducible) pigmentation   68.1, 86.2
FAE see fumaric acid esters
faecal dermatitis, colostomy leakage   112.4, 112.5
FALDH deficiency see fatty aldehyde dehydrogenase deficiency
false negative reactions, patch testing   127.28–127.29, 129.7
false positive reactions, patch testing   127.28, 129.7
famciclovir   19.49
familial acanthosis nigricans   85.4–85.5
familial adenomatous polyposis (FAP)   78.10–78.11
familial atypical/dysplastic naevus syndrome   142.4
familial body dysmorphic disorder   84.14
familial cerebelloretinal angiomatosis (von Hippel–Lindau syndrome)   148.9, 154.2

familial cold autoinflammatory syndrome (FCAS)   **45.5, 45.6**, 45.9
familial comedones   88.32
familial dysautonomia, respiratory system involvement   152.5
familial haemophagocytic lymphohistiocytosis (FHL)   135.11, 135.13
familial hypercholanaemia   2.21
familial hypercholesterolaemia (FH)   60.2, 60.6–60.8
 diagnosis of   60.7
 lipid concentrations in   60.7
familial infantile myofibromatosis   136.40
familial lipoedema   72.12
familial mandibuloacral dysplasia   70.28–70.29
 'tree-frog' appearance   70.29
familial Mediterranean fever (FMF)   **45.5, 45.6**, 45.9–45.10
 renal involvement   154.2
 Tel Hashomer criteria for diagnosis of   **45.10**
familial melanoma syndrome   142.3, 148.8–148.9
familial multiple KAs see multiple self-healing squamous epithelioma
familial partial lipodystrophy (FPL)   72.3, **72.4**
 Dunnigan-type   98.9
familial primary localised cutaneous amyloidosis   **56.3**, 56.9, 56.9
familial progressive hyper-hypopigmentation   68.10
familial progressive hyperpigmentation (FPH)   68.10
familial reactive perforating collagenosis   94.54–94.55
familial sea-blue histiocytosis   135.22–135.23
familial trichoepitheliomas, photothermal ablation   23.21
familial tumoral calcinosis   79.17–79.18
family
 measuring impacts of skin disease   16.10–16.11
 see also 'the Greater Patient' concept
Family Dermatology Life Quality Index (FDLQI)   16.10
family history, diagnosis   4.4
FamilyPso questionnaire   16.10
Family Reported Outcome Measure (FROM-16)   16.10
Fanconi anaemia   68.12, 76.11, **80.5**, 80.12–80.13, 148.14
FAP see familial adenomatous polyposis
FAPD see fibrosing alopecia in a pattern distribution
Farber disease   79.5–79.6
farcy see glanders
farm environments, and atopic eczema   41.8
fascial fibromatoses   94.34–94.36
Fas-Fas ligand, TEN interaction   118.21
FASQoL see facial acne scar quality of life
fat cell tumours   136.56–136.59
fat contouring   161.8–161.9
 bulk cooling/cryolipolysis   161.8–161.9
 bulk heating/thermolipolysis   161.9
fat homeostasis, lymphatic system   103.2
fat hypertrophy   98.13–98.15
fatigue, cold agglutinins   124.13
fat naevus   **73.2**, 73.16–73.18
fat necrosis, necrotic adipocytes   97.55
fat organ, adipokines   97.5
fat pads, glycosylation disorders   **79.10**
FATP gene, ichthyosis–prematurity syndrome   63.39
fat, subcutaneous see subcutaneous fat
fat tissue, composition   97.1–97.3
fatty acids
 acne   129.12
 and alcohols, topical medication vehicles   18.7
 energy homeostasis   97.4
fatty aldehyde dehydrogenase (FALDH) deficiency   63.32

fauces, examination of 108.7
Favre–Racouchot syndrome 88.31–88.32, 94.3–94.4
favus (favic type tinea capitis) 32.38, 32.39
FCAS see familial cold autoinflammatory syndrome
FCL see follicle centre cell lymphoma
FD see Flegel disease
FDEs see fixed drug eruptions
FDLQI see Family Dermatology Life Quality Index
febrile ulceronecrotic Mucha–Habermann disease (FUMHD) 134.3, 134.4
feet see foot
female androgenetic alopecia 87.68–87.70
female androgen physiology 87.88
female genital mutilation (FGM) 110.43
female pattern hair loss (FPHL) 87.13, 87.61, 87.62–87.66, 87.67
Female Sexual Function Index (FSFI) 16.12
Ferguson-Smith disease see multiple self-healing squamous epithelioma
Ferriman–Gallwey scoring system, hirsutism 87.88–87.89
ferritin 87.59, 87.70–87.71
fetal skin biopsy 8.10
fetal varicella syndrome 114.23
fetus
  hydrops fetalis 103.23
  lymphatic-related hydrops fetalis 103.23
feverfew (parthenolide) 157.8
FFA see frontal fibrosing alopecia
FGFR3 epidermal naevus syndrome 73.7
FGFRs see fibroblast growth factor receptors
FGFs see fibroblast growth factors
FGM see female genital mutilation
FH see familial hypercholesterolaemia; fibrous histiocytoma
FHL see familial haemophagocytic lymphohistiocytosis
fibreglass dermatitis 122.21, 129.1
fibrillinopathy 70.20–70.21
fibrillins 2.35–2.36
fibrinoid degeneration 3.40
fibroadipose hyperplasia 72.9
fibroblast growth factor receptors (FGFRs), acanthosis nigricans 85.4
fibroblast growth factors (FGFs) 2.3, 2.4
  wound healing 11.6
fibroblastic rheumatism (FR) 53.7–53.8, 155.7
  multicentric reticulohistiocytosis differentiation 135.25
fibroblastic tumours, EWSR1-SMAD3-rearrangement 136.4
fibroblasts 2.3, 2.39–2.40, 2.45
  collagen fibril fragmentation 156.8–156.9
  gene expression 2.40
  hair follicles 2.40
  microscopic examination of 3.37
  morphoea 55.10–55.11
  palmar fascial fibromatosis 94.34
  reactive oxygen species 156.4
  transmission electron microscopy 2.40, 156.9
  wound healing 11.6, 11.7–11.8
fibrodysplasia ossificans progressiva 70.35
fibroepithelial polyp see skin tags
fibrofolliculoma 137.16
  Birt–Hogg–Dubé syndrome 78.15
  differential diagnosis 88.30–88.31
fibrohistiocytic tumours 136.19–136.23
  diagnosis 3.25–3.26
  reclassification of angiomatoid malignant fibrous histiocytoma 136.17
fibroma
  tendon sheath 136.11
  vulval 110.32
fibroma-like epithelioid sarcoma see pseudomyogenic haemangioendothelioma
fibromatoses 94.33–94.48
  keloids association 94.49
fibromatous nodule, tuberous sclerosis complex 78.10

fibromyalgia, acne relationship 155.11
fibromyxoid sarcoma, low grade 136.18–136.19
fibro-osseous pseudotumour of the digits 136.6
fibrosing alopecia in a pattern distribution (FAPD) 87.43
fibrosis
  erythema elevatum diutinum 100.8
  mucous membrane pemphigoid 107.25, 107.32
  oral tissues 108.68
  in phyma 89.3
  subcutaneous sarcoidosis 96.3, 97.54
  systemic sclerosis 54.11–54.13
fibrous digital nodules 94.43
fibrous hamartoma of infancy 136.6–136.7
fibrous histiocytoma (FH) 4.19, 136.19–136.21
fibrous long-spacing collagen, CLD association 98.13
fibrous and myofiblastic tumours 136.1–136.19
fibrous papules of the face 136.2–136.3
fibrous papulosis of the neck 94.39–94.40
fibroxanthoma, atypical 106.34
fibulins 2.36
fiddleback/violin spiders (Sicariidae) 34.35–34.36
'fiddler's neck' 122.12
fifth disease see erythema infectiosum
'fight bites' 130.6–130.7
filaggrin 2
  peeling skin syndromes 63.30
  skin fragility disorders 69.6
filaggrin 2.6
  deficiency 85.2
filaggrin mutations
  allergic contact dermatitis 127.10
  ichthyosis vulgaris 63.3–63.4
  occupational contact dermatitis 129.3, 129.6
filarial elephantiasis see lymphatic filariasis
filarial worms 33.7–33.10
  see also lymphatic filariasis
filariasis (onchocerciasis) 107.40
filiform keratosis 63.77
filivirus infections, haemorrhagic fevers 25.85–25.87
fillers see dermal fillers
filovirus infections, haemorrhagic fevers 25.84–25.85
financial costs of disease see economic burden of disease
finasteride 87.69, 87.96–87.97
fine-needle aspiration of lymph nodes 4.22
finger
  acquired digital fibrokeratoma 136.4
  acral fibromyxoma 136.59
  allergic contact dermatitis 127.13, 127.14
  Apert syndrome 88.11
  arthritis mutilans 35.42
  atopic eczema 41.18
  blistering distal dactylitis 26.34
  bluish discoloration of fingertip 54.3
  callosities 122.12
  digital mucous cyst 136.60
  digital ulceration 54.3, 54.17, 54.25
  discoid lupus erythematosus 51.4, 51.9
  fibroblastic rheumatism 53.8
  fibro-osseous pseudotumour of the digits 136.6
  'finger pebbles', diabetes 62.5
  flexion contractures and calcinosis 54.3
  florid lichen planus 4.16
  fungal infection 80.12
  granulomatosis with polyangiitis 100.25
  hand, foot and mouth disease 115.6
  Kawasaki disease 115.10
  Orf-induced pemphigoid 50.55
  paroxysmal haematoma 94.19, 99.5–99.6, 122.13–122.14
  pompholyx eczema 39.15
  spindling, in discoid lupus erythematosus 51.9

  systemic sclerosis 54.3, 54.4, 54.5, 54.17, **54.25**
  ulceration and necrosis 54.3, 54.17, **54.25**
  vesicular eczema 129.6
  see also digits; phalanges
fingernail dystrophy
  nail–patella syndrome 67.15–67.16
  pachyonychia congenita 67.1, 67.11
  see also nails
fingertip
  eczema 39.15
  topical therapy application measure 18.3, 18.4
Finn patch test chamber 127.24–127.25
fire, hazards and risks of electrosurgery 20.45–20.46
FISH see fluorescence in situ hybridisation
fish odour syndrome (trimethylaminuria) 84.11, 92.17–92.18
fish stings 130.4–130.5
fish tank granuloma (*Mycobacteria marinum*) 27.32–27.35
fissured dermatitis 129.3
fissures
  hand eczema 128.4
  lip fissure 108.63–108.64
fistulae, complications of 112.1–112.16
Fitz-Hugh–Curtis syndrome 30.5
Fitzpatrick classification, acute and carcinogenic effects of UV radiation exposure 10.7
Fitzpatrick skin types I/II, cutaneous squamous cell carcinoma 141.30
fixatives
  biopsy 3.4, **3.5**, 3.32
  fragrances 127.42
fixed drug eruptions (FDEs) 14.4, 86.28, 86.29, 86.30–86.31
fixed-effects models 17.10
flagellate dermatitis 119.10
flagellate hyperpigmentation 119.8–119.9, 119.10
'flaky paint' dermatitis, kwashiorkor 61.4
flaps, surgical 20.22–20.29, **20.24–20.25**
flashlamps
  epidermal pigmentation 23.15
  selective photothermolysis 23.5
  therapeutic devices 23.3
  vascular lesion treatment 23.7, 23.10
flatworms see trematodes
flavouring agents, allergic contact dermatitis 127.41–127.45
flea-borne bacterial infections
  cat scratch disease 26.62–26.63
  murine typhus 26.81
  plague 26.59–26.60
  spotted fever 26.83, 26.84
fleas
  classification 34.13
  clinical features/investigations of bites 34.14
  epidemiology 34.13–34.14
  management of bites 34.14–34.15
  tungiasis 34.15
  see also *Tunga penetrans* (sand fleas)
Flegel disease (FD) 63.77–63.78, 85.17–85.18
flexibility (hypermobility), Beighton score **70.8**
flexural Dowling–Degos disease 68.13
flexural psoriasis (inverse psoriasis) 35.8, 35.9, **35.16**
flexures, allergic contact dermatitis 127.22
Florida horse leech see *Pythium insidiosum* infection
florid cutaneous papillomatosis 148.16, 148.17
  AN association 85.3–85.4
florid oral papillomatosis 108.45
florid papillomatosis of the nipple ducts see nipple, adenoma
flow cytometry, peripheral blood cell analysis 9.2
flucytosine antifungals 19.48
'fluid creep', resuscitation 125.3
fluid homeostasis, lymphatic system 103.2

fluid replacement, SJS/TEN treatment 118.20
flukes see trematodes
fluocinolone acetonide gel 12.3
fluorescence activated cell sorting (FACS) 9.2
fluorescence microlymphangiography 103.56
fluorescence in situ hybridisation (FISH), melanoma diagnosis 142.21
fluorescent lamps, cutaneous photosensitivity diseases 126.34
fluoroquinolones 19.47
5-fluorouracil (5-FU)
  basal cell carcinoma topical treatment 140.56
  Bowen disease topical treatment 141.23
  intralesional for keloids 94.52
  topical therapies 18.29, 140.12, 141.23
flushing (transient erythema) 89.6, 89.8–89.9, 89.12, 104.1–104.13
  associated disorders **104.4–104.9**
  causes of **104.3**
  characteristics of **104.4–104.9**
  in children **104.10**
  clinical presentation 104.10–104.11
  drug-induced **104.3**
  epidemiology 104.1
  food-induced **104.3**
  'geographical' pattern due to carcinoid tumour 150.12
  harlequin colour change **104.10**
  in infants **104.10**, 104.10
  internal malignancy association 148.25–148.26
  investigations **104.4–104.9**, 104.11
  management 104.11–104.12
  pathogenesis **104.4–104.9**
  pathophysiology 104.1–104.2
  physiology 104.1
  rosacea 89.1, **89.2**, 89.6, 89.8–89.9, 89.12, **89.14**
  symptoms and signs **104.4–104.9**
  treatment **89.14**, **104.4–104.9**
flutamide 87.70, 87.96
flux measurement, topical drug delivery 12.3, 12.4, 12.5
FMF see familial Mediterranean fever
focal acantholytic dyskeratoma see warty dyskeratoma
focal adhesions (focal contacts) 2.26
focal dermal elastosis, late-onset 94.32
focal epithelial hyperplasia, oral involvement 108.11
focal hyperhidrosis see gustatory hyperhidrosis
focal keratoderma, pachyonychia congenita 63.52
focal mucinosis, oral involvement 108.85–108.86
focal palmoplantar keratoderma 63.56–63.58
focal palmoplantar and oral hyperkeratosis syndrome 108.29
focal plantar keratoderma 63.52
foetal programming, maternal stress impacts 150.8
folate deficiency 61.18–61.19, 86.23–86.24
folate supplementation 19.27
folate synthesis inhibitors 19.47
folds, dermal fillers, indication for 158.1, **158.3**
foliaceus, in pregnancy 113.8–113.9
foliate papillae, anatomy of 108.4
foliate papillitis, oral involvement 108.11
folic acid depletion, UVB phototherapy adverse effects 21.12
follicle centre cell lymphoma (FCL) 139.37
follicle mites 34.55–34.57
follicular atrophoderma 94.16–94.17
follicular canal, eosinophilic pustular folliculitis 93.8
follicular eruptions, systemic medications 91.2–91.3

follicular hyperkeratoses
  keratosis circumscripta 85.13
  KP association 85.10
  pachyonychia congenita 67.12
follicular hyperkeratosis 3.41–3.42
follicular inflammation 93.7
follicular infundibulum
  dilated pore lesions 137.3
  tumours 137.3–137.4
follicular lichen planus 87.38–87.50
follicular miniaturisation 87.64, 87.65
follicular mucinosis 57.15–57.18, 87.47, 105.8, 139.14–139.15
follicular naevus 73.7
follicular occlusion tetrad 90.2
follicular papules 93.7
follicular pattern, hidradenitis suppurativa 90.6
follicular psoriasis 35.7, 35.9
follicular pustules 93.6
follicular units 87.64
folliculitis 26.22–26.23
  clinical features 26.22–26.23
  decalvans 87.48–87.50, 88.36–88.37
  deep 91.8–91.15
  diabetic patients 62.4, 62.5
  differential diagnosis 88.34–88.35
  HIV infection 87.35
  keloidalis 88.35–88.36, 88.37, 91.10–91.12, 93.3–93.4
  lymphocytic 91.12–91.13
  Malassezia yeast 32.13
  management 26.23
  pathophysiology 26.22
  perineal and perianal skin 111.13–111.14
  scalp 91.13–91.14
  superficial 91.1–91.8
folliculosebaceous cystic hamartoma 106.35
Fonsecaea pedrosoi 32.77
food allergies
  atopic eczema 41.11–41.12, 41.20, 41.23
  contact urticaria 127.84
  Netherton syndrome 63.26, 63.28
  oral allergy syndrome 42.13, 108.12, 127.84
  see also diet; nutrition
foot
  acral naevi 131.24
  allergic contact dermatitis 127.17, 127.22
  annular erythema of infancy 47.10
  anti-p200 pemphigoid 50.41
  arteriovenous malformation 71.11
  atrophie blanche 99.21
  blue naevus 131.40
  callosities 122.8
  calluses 122.7–122.8
  carotenoderma 61.9
  chronic acral dermatitis 39.14–39.15
  congenital blue naevi 73.16
  cryofibrinogenaemia 99.13
  cutaneous small-vessel vasculitis 100.7
  deformities 122.7
  diabetic 62.2–62.3
  discoid eczema 4.12
  discoid lupus erythematosus 51.4
  erysipelas-like reaction, diabetic patients 62.2
  erythromelalgia 82.12–82.13
  forefoot dermatitis 127.67
  freeze-induced damage 124.4
  glomuvenous malformation 71.18
  granuloma annulare 95.5
  granulomatosis with polyangiitis 100.25
  hair sinuses 122.22
  juvenile plantar dermatosis 39.23–39.24
  lichen planus pemphigoides 50.51
  lymphoedema 71.28
  mixed connective tissue disease 53.4
  neurofibroma, extensive plexiform 78.2
  neuropathic ulcer 83.13, 83.14, 83.15
  palisaded and neutrophilic granulomatous dermatitis 53.7
  pansclerotic morphoea 55.21
  podoconiosis 7.3, 103.36

  pretibial myxoedema 103.42
  serpiginous lesions 4.16
  STING-associated vasculopathy with onset in infancy 45.14
  wet gangrene in diabetes 62.2
  see also heel; sole; toe
foot calluses 122.7
foot and mouth disease 25.94
foot ringworm see tinea peddis
footwear
  allergies 127.67–127.68
  calluses caused by 122.7
Footwork: the International Podoconiosis Initiative 7.9–7.10
Fordyce, scrotal angiokeratoma of 109.6
Fordyce spots 91.15–91.17, 93.10–93.12
  labia minora/majora 110.3, 110.4
  oral lesions 108.29
forehead
  botulinum toxins, aesthetic uses of 159.4–159.5
  comedonal acne 88.2, 88.27, 88.28
  haemangioma, infantile 116.3, 116.6
  scarring, classical Ehlers–Danlos syndrome 70.8
  sebaceous gland hyperplasia 88.32
foreign bodies, hair as 91.10–91.11
foreign bodies/deposits
  detection of 3.38
  male genitalia 109.8
foreign body reactions 122.17–122.24
  cheilitis 108.62
  inflammatory 93.1–93.3
foreskin see prepuce
forest plots, meta-analysis of clinical trials 17.11
formaldehyde
  acetylacetone test method 127.34
  allergic contact dermatitis 127.49–127.51, 127.66
  cosmetic allergies 127.49–127.50
  resins 127.70–127.71
formaldehyde-releasing biocides 127.51–127.52
formaldehyde-releasing preservatives 127.50, 127.51–127.52
formalin, specimen preparation 3.5
formication, drug-induced 120.5
formulations, topical medication vehicles 18.2–18.3, 18.5–18.8, 18.21
fornix meter, ocular disease assessment 50.30
four humours theory, Galen 1.3
Fournier gangrene 26.77, 26.78
  male genitalia 109.26–109.27
Fox-Fordyce disease see axillary apocrine miliaria
FPH see familial progressive hyperpigmentation
FPHL see female pattern hair loss
FPL see familial partial lipodystrophy
FPLD2 see Dunnigan-type familial partial lipodystrophy
fractional ablative lasers
  for acne scarring 161.4
  device names 161.5
  laser types 161.5
  for photodamaged skin 161.3
  resurfacing 23.24
  for rhytids 161.5
  wound care 161.4
fractional non-ablative resurfacing 23.23–23.24
fractionated ablative lasers, skin resurfacing 161.2–161.3, 161.5
fragile X syndrome 72.7, 74.5, 106.7
fragrances see perfumes
framycetin 18.11
France
  dermatology history 1.4–1.5
  skin cancer, economic burden of 6.6, 6.7
Francisella tularensis, tularaemia 26.57–26.58
Franklin disease 108.70
freckles see ephelides

Fredrickson classification, dyslipidaemias 60.1
free margins, principles of surgical design 20.19
freeze-induced damage 124.2–124.4
Frey syndrome see gustatory hyperhidrosis
friction
  acne mechanica 122.15
  effects 122.6–122.7
  pressure ulcers 123.2, 123.3
  psoriasis 129.2
  sports injuries 122.16–122.17
  stratum corneum 122.4
frictional hypermelanosis 86.11
frictional trauma, mechanical stimuli 122.3
friction blisters 122.6, 122.9–122.10
FROM-16 see Family Reported Outcome Measure
frontal fibrosing alopecia (FFA) 87.41–87.43
frostbite 97.37, 124.2–124.4
frostnip 124.2
FSFI see Female Sexual Function Index
5-FU see 5-fluorouracil
fucosidosis
  angiokeratoma corporis diffusum 79.4
  glycoproteinoses 79.3
fugitive swellings see loiasis
fulminant liver failure 118.11
fumarates 19.15–19.17
  dermatological uses 19.16
  pharmacological properties 19.17
  potential adverse effects 19.17
  safety precautions 19.17–19.18
fumaric acid esters (FAE)
  discoid lupus erythematosus treatment 51.12
  psoriasis treatment 35.26
FUMHD see febrile ulceronecrotic Mucha–Habermann disease
Functional Assessment of Cancer Therapy-Melanoma (FACT-M) 16.9
fungal arthropathies 155.5
fungal biology 32.2–32.3
fungal cultures, superficial mycoses identification 32.8–32.9
fungal dysbiosis, lichen planus 37.3
fungal infections 3.44, 32.1–32.95
  burn injuries 125.10
  female genitalia 110.27–110.28
  hand dermatitis differentiation 128.5
  HIV coinfections 31.26–31.29, 31.35
  immunosuppressed renal allograft recipients 154.5–154.6
  inherited immunodeficiency 80.12
  male genitalia 109.28
  oral infections 108.56–108.57
  perineal and perianal skin 111.8, 111.15
  in pregnancy 113.7
fungal nail disease see onychomycosis
fungal panniculitis 97.47–97.48, 97.60–97.61
fungi
  asexual reproduction 32.4, 32.5
  classification/taxonomy 32.3–32.4
  morphology and diseases 32.3
  reproduction 32.3
  sexual reproduction 32.4–32.5
  spore formation 32.4–32.5
furocoumarins 86.29–86.30
furuncles (boils/abscesses) 26.23–26.25
  clinical features 26.24–26.25
  definitions 26.23
  epidemiology 26.23–26.24
  investigations 26.25
  management 26.25
  pathophysiology 26.24
furunculosis, perineal and perianal skin 111.13–111.14
Fusarium species
  skin lesions 32.93
  superficial onychomycosis 32.54–32.55
fusidic acid 18.11
Fusobacterium 26.67–26.68
  tropical ulcers 26.68

G

GA see glycolic acid; granuloma annulare
gadolinium chelates 94.44
GAGs see glycosaminoglycans
gain-of-function STAT1 mutation, oro-pharyngeal mucocutaneous *Candida* infection 80.17
Gaiter-like sclerosis 94.16
galactosialidosis 79.5
GALEF see Global Alliance to Eradicate Lymphatic Filariasis
Galen 1.3, 1.5
gallates 127.59
gall bladder, cutaneous features of biliary tract disease 153.5
Galli–Galli disease 68.13, 85.24
Gamasida mites 34.54–34.55
gamma heavy chain disease (Franklin disease) 108.70
gamma-hydroxybuyrate (GHB) 120.3
gangrene
  peripheral vascular disease **101.5**
  peristomal skin 149.7
  see also gas gangrene; necrotising subcutaneous infections; pyoderma gangrenosum
gap junctions 2.20
Gardner syndrome 108.86
GARFIELD acronym 80.2
garlic allergy 127.71, 127.73
gas gangrene 26.48–26.49
gastrointestinal bleeding 153.6–153.7
gastrointestinal cancer, syndromes linked with **78.14**
gastrointestinal diseases
  cutaneous features 153.1–153.4, **153.7**
  oral involvement 108.72–108.74
  systemic lupus erythematosus 51.31
  systemic sclerosis 54.17, **54.23**
gastrointestinal hamartomas 68.13–68.14
gastrointestinal involvement
  drug reaction with eosinophilia and systemic symptoms 118.9
  long-term SJS/TEN 118.17
gastrointestinal malabsorption
  associated skin conditions 153.6–153.7, **153.8**
  causes **153.8**
gastrointestinal polyposis, familial adenomatous polyposis 78.11
gastrointestinal symptoms, syndromic ichthyoses **63.39**
gastrointestinal toxicity
  antimalarials 19.6
  glucocorticoids 19.19
  methotrexate 19.26
gastrointestinal tract, epidermolysis bullosa 69.25
gastrointestinal ulcers 149.8
gastrointestinal venous malformations 71.17
gastro-oesophageal reflux disease 108.74
gastrostomy (G-Tube), bullous pemphigoid 50.19
GATA2 deficiency 149.14
Gaucher disease 79.5
  type II 63.30
GBD see global burden of disease
GBFDE see generalised bullous fixed drug eruption
GC see glucocorticoids
GCA see giant cell arteritis
GCs see glucocorticoids
GEH see generalised eruptive histiocytosis
GEKG see glycine-glutamate-lysine-glycine
gel nails 127.61
gels 12.3, 18.2
gender
  melanoma, trends in incidence and mortality 142.1
  women with HIV/AIDS 31.36
gender effects, Merkel cell carcinoma risk 146.1–146.2
gene mutations
  arsenic toxicity 121.2

gene mutations (continued)
  autosomal dominant lamellar ichthyoses 63.20–63.21
  autosomal recessive PPK 63.54
  CHILD syndrome 63.23–63.24
  Cole disease 63.61
  congenital ichthyoses 63.7–63.13
  Conradi–Hünermann–Happle syndrome 63.22–63.23
  Desmons syndrome 63.35
  disease 8.5–8.7
  dyskeratosis congenita **67.13**
  epidermolytic ichthyosis 63.15, *63.17*
  epidermolytic palmoplantar keratoderma 63.50
  exfoliative ichthyosis 63.21
  ichthyosis vulgaris 63.4
  ichthyosis–prematurity syndrome 63.39
  keratinopathic ichthyoses 63.13
  KID syndrome 63.33
  loricrin keratoderma 63.56
  Neu–Laxova syndrome 63.38
  pachyonychia congenita 63.51–63.52
  palmoplantar keratodermas 63.68
  recessive X-linked ichthyosis 63.5, 63.6
  Refsum disease 63.31
  see also genes; genetic disorders; genetics/genetic factors
General Health Questionnaire (GHQ-12), psychological impacts assessment 16.11
generalised anhidrosis, acquired 92.12
generalised bullous fixed drug eruption (GBFDE) 14.4
generalised cutaneous atrophy *94.10*
generalised diffuse Dercum disease 98.18
generalised Dowling–Degos disease 68.13
generalised elastolysis 94.21
generalised eruptive histiocytosis (GEH) 135.18
generalised eruptive keratoacanthoma 141.43–141.44
generalised essential telangiectasia **101.17**, 101.18–101.19
  branching with pressure *101.19*
  in pigmented skin *101.19*
generalised hyperhidrosis 92.4–92.5
generalised hypertrichosis 87.86–87.87
generalised lentiginosis without associated systemic symptoms 68.10
generalised lymphadenopathy, syphilis 29.10
generalised lymphatic anomaly (GLA) 103.28–103.29
generalised lymphatic dysplasia (GLD) 103.22
generalised nodular Dercum disease 98.18
generalised pigmentation, systemic sclerosis *86.21*
generalised plaque morphoea **55.3**, **55.4**, 55.17–55.19
generalised pruritus, neoplasia association 148.27
generalised pustular psoriasis (GPP) 35.31–35.36
  acute generalised pustular psoriasis of von Zumbusch 35.33–35.34
  age of onset 35.32
  clinical features 35.33–35.34
  co-morbidities 35.35
  differential diagnosis 35.34
  disease course and prognosis 35.35
  environmental factors 35.32–35.33
  epidemiology 35.32
  genetic factors 35.32
  histology 35.34
  investigations 35.35
  management 35.35–35.36
  pathogenic mechanisms 35.33
  in pregnancy 113.10–113.11
  severity classification 35.34–35.35
  subacute annular generalised pustular psoriasis 35.34
  systemic therapy 35.36
  topical treatment 35.36

generalised skin disease, linear manifestations of 73.22–73.23
general practitioners (GPs) 5.12–5.13
genes 8.3–8.4, *8.6*
  autosomal 8.4
  features of typical human gene *8.6*
gene therapy, epidermolysis bullosa 69.27
genetic counselling 8.9, 8.11
genetic disorders/syndromes
  adermatoglyphia 70.36
  of adipose tissue 72.1–72.13
    familial lipoedema 72.12
    fibroadipose hyperplasia 72.9
    hereditary panniculitis **72.11**
    lipomatoses **72.10**
    PIK3CA-related overgrowth spectrum 72.9–72.11
  basal cell carcinoma as an ancillary feature **140.7**
  Bazex–Dupré–Christol syndrome 140.20–140.21
  blistering diseases 69.1–69.28
  BSL differential diagnosis 98.16
  chromosomal disorders 74.1–74.5
    autosomal chromosome defects 74.1–74.3
    chromosomal mosaicism 74.5
  of collagen 70.1–70.14
    dystrophic calcification 59.3–59.4
    Ehlers–Danlos syndromes 70.1–70.11
    osteogenesis imperfecta 70.12–70.14
    prolidase deficiency 70.11–70.12
  congenital muscle hamartomas 73.19
  congenital naevi 73.1–73.18
  cornification 63.2
  DNA repair disorders with cutaneous features 76.1–76.12
  dystrophic calcification of skin and subcutaneous tissues 59.3–59.4
  of ectopic calcification and abnormal mineralisation 70.31–70.36
    fibrodysplasia ossificans progressiva 70.35
    primary hypertrophic osteoarthropathy 70.35–70.36
    pseudoxanthoma elasticum 70.31–70.35
  of elastic fibres 70.14–70.21
    cutis laxa 70.14–70.17
    Marfan syndrome 70.20–70.21
    Michelin tyre baby syndrome 70.19, 73.17
    Williams–Beuren syndrome 70.18–70.19
genetic disorders/syndromes, sex chromosome defects 74.3–74.5
  heterotrimeric G-protein mosaic disorders 73.19–73.21
  immunodeficiency, inherited 80.1–80.20
  infantile stiff skin syndromes 70.21–70.24
    hyaline fibromatosis syndrome 70.21–70.22
    restrictive dermopathy 70.24
    stiff skin syndrome 70.22–70.23
    Winchester syndrome 70.23–70.24
  inherited immunodeficiency 80.1–80.20
  inherited metabolic diseases 79.1–79.18
  inherited skin tumour syndromes 78.1–78.15
    familial adenomatous polyposis 78.10–78.11
    mosaic neurofibromatosis type 1 78.4–78.7
    neurofibromatoses 78.1–78.7
    RASopathies 78.7, **78.8**, **78.9**
    tuberous sclerosis complex 78.7–78.10
  keratins 2.8
  lipoid proteinosis 70.36–70.37
  metabolic diseases, inherited 79.1–79.18
  midface toddler excoriation syndrome 82.9
  miscellaneous dermal disorders 70.36–70.38
  naevi, congenital 73.1–73.18
  Naevoid basal cell carcinoma syndrome 140.3–140.4, 140.18

nails/nail growth 67.1–67.17
neutral lipid storage disease with ichthyosis 63.36
pigmentation 68.1–68.15
poikiloderma syndromes 75.1–75.8
premature ageing syndromes 70.25–70.31, 77.1–77.7
  acrogeria **70.26**, 70.28
  familial mandibuloacral dysplasia 70.28–70.29
  Mulvihill–Smith syndrome 70.29–70.30
  neonatal progeroid syndrome 70.30–70.31
  progeria 70.25–70.26, **70.26**
  Werner syndrome 70.26–70.27, **70.26**
pterygium syndromes 70.37–70.38
skin ageing 2.46
vascular disorders 71.1–71.28
  arteriovenous disorders 71.11–71.14
  capillary disorders 71.3–71.11
  lymphatic disorders 71.21–71.28
  venous disorders 71.14–71.21
genetic epidemiology 5.10
genetic mosaicism, lymphoedema 103.23
genetic risk score *see* polygenic risk score
genetics/genetic factors 1.9, 8.1–8.11
  adenoid cystic carcinoma 137.39
  angioma serpiginosum 101.16
  angiomatoid fibrous histiocytoma 136.63
  angiosarcoma 136.35
  apocrine carcinoma 137.23
  apocrine tubular adenoma 137.22
  arteriovenous malformations 101.23
  atypical lipomatous tumour 136.58–136.59
  autosomal dominant inheritance *8.3*
  autosomal recessive inheritance *8.3*
  basal cell carcinoma 140.3–140.5, 140.18
  basaloid follicular hamartoma 137.13
  biomarkers, prenatal testing and diagnosis *8.11*
  Blaschko lines *8.7*, *8.8*
  BRAF mutations, lobular capillary haemangioma/pyogenic granuloma within port-wine stains 136.26
  calcifying aponeurotic fibroma 136.7
  cellular angiofibroma 136.9
  chromosomal disorders 8.6
  chronic mucocutaneous candidiasis 32.67
  CIC-rearranged sarcoma 136.52
  classical epidermodysplasia verruciformis 25.66, 25.69
  clear cell sarcoma 136.64
  comedo naevus 137.5
  composite haemangioendothelioma 136.34
  congenital disorders 8.2
  cutaneous Ewing sarcoma 136.52
  cutaneous myoepithelioma 137.33
  cutaneous squamous cell carcinoma 141.27–141.28
  cylindroma 137.29, 137.30
  deep ('aggressive') angiomyxoma 136.62
  dermatofibrosarcoma protuberans 136.15
  desmoplastic fibroblastoma 136.12
  disseminated superficial actinic porokeratosis 141.15–141.17
  eccrine gland carcinomas 137.34
  eccrine poroma 137.25
  elastofibroma 136.10
  epithelioid angiosarcoma 136.37
  epithelioid haemangioendothelioma 136.37
  epithelioid haemangioma 136.28
  epithelioid sarcoma 136.63
  erythromelalgia 101.8
  EWSR1-SMAD3-rearranged fibroblastic tumour 136.4
  extramammary Paget disease 137.43
  fibroma of tendon sheath 136.11
  fibro-osseous pseudotumour of the digits 136.6
  fibrous hamartoma of infancy 136.7

gain-of-function mutations 8.6
genetic heterogenity 8.5
genetic linkage 8.9
genetic markers 8.8–8.9, *8.11*
gene tracking 8.9
genome sequencing 8.8–8.9
genomic imprinting 8.5
giant cell fibroblastoma 136.16
glomus tumours 136.42
granular cell tumours 136.49
haemosiderotic fibrolipomatous tumour 136.61
hidradenocarcinoma 137.36
hidradenoma 137.29
hidradenoma papilliferum 137.21
human genome *8.5*
Human Genome Project 8.1
human leukocyte antigens 8.7
inborn errors of immunity disposing to HPV 25.65, **25.66**, **25.67**–**25.68**, 25.70–25.71
infantile myofibromatosis/adult myofibroma 136.40
inherited disorders 8.8–8.9
Kaposi sarcoma 138.3
keratoacanthoma 141.39–141.40
Klippel–Trenaunay syndrome 101.27–101.28
leiomyoma 136.54
lichen planus 110.11
lipofibromatosis 136.14
Lyonisation 8.7–8.8
malignant peripheral nerve sheath tumour 136.51
melanoma risk 142.3–142.5
  familial atypical/dysplastic naevus syndrome 142.4
  identification of at risk population 142.7
  intermediate penetrance susceptibility genes 142.5
  major/high penetrance susceptibility genes 142.4–142.5
  phenotypic traits 142.3–142.4
microcystic adnexal carcinoma 137.37
mitochondrial disorders 8.5
mixed tumour of the skin 137.32
mosaicism 8.7–8.8
Muir–Torre syndrome 141.44
multifactorial disorders 8.2
multiple self-healing squamous epithelioma 141.41–141.42
mutations and disease 8.5–8.7
myoepithelial tumours 137.33
myopericytoma 136.41
nipple adenoma 137.22
nodular fasciitis 136.5
nosology 8.2–8.5
Paget disease of the nipple 137.41
Parkes Weber syndrome 101.30
perivascular epithelioid cell tumour 136.61
preimplantation genetic diagnosis 8.10–8.11
preimplantation genetic haplotyping 8.11
prenatal diagnosis 8.9–8.11
principles of medical genetics 8.2–8.5
pseudomyogenic haemangioendothelioma 136.34
reactive angioendotheliomatosis 136.24–136.25
rosacea risk 89.4–89.5
schwannoma 136.45
sebaceous adenomas and sebaceomas 137.17
secretory carcinoma 137.40
single-cell genomics 8.2
single-gene disorders 8.2, *8.3*, *8.4*
spindle cell haemangioma 136.31
spindle cell lipoma 136.58
spiradenoma 137.31
tenosynovial giant cell tumour 136.19
trichodiscoma 137.15
urticarial vasculitis 44.3
varicose veins 101.38–101.39, 101.42

venous malformations   101.25
X-linked dominant inheritance   *8.4*
X-linked recessive inheritance   *8.4*
genital area
  amicrobial pustulosis of the inguinal folds   *49.20*
  lymphoedema   103.49–103.51, *103.52*
  melanocytic naevi   131.22
  Stevens–Johnson syndrome/toxic epidermal necrolysis   *118.17*, 118.18
  swollen genitalia and mons pubis   103.49–103.51, *103.52*
genital chlamydia   30.8–30.14
  clinical features   30.10–30.11
  epidemiology   30.9–30.10
  gonorrhoea coinfection   30.7
  investigations   30.11–30.13
  management   30.13–30.14
  pathophysiology   30.10
genital dermatology   1.8
genital herpes   25.24–25.26, 109.28
genitalia, female   110.1–110.48
  acne, vulval   110.45
  angiokeratomas   110.3, *110.4*
  bacterial infections   110.25–110.27
    malakoplakia   110.26
    Mycobacterial infections   110.26
    Staphylococcal infections   110.25
    Streptococcal infections   110.25–110.26
  benign tumours   110.31–110.33
    atypical genital naevi   110.33
    Bartholin cysts   110.31
    cutaneous endometriosis   110.33
    mucinous cysts   110.31
    papillary hidradenoma   110.31–110.33, 137.20–137.21
  bullous disease   110.20, **110.21**
  clitoral variations   110.3
  congenital abnormalities   110.5
  Darier disease   110.6
  differentiated vulval intraepithelial neoplasia   110.34, 110.35
  disorders of sexual development   110.5
  epidermolysis bullosa   110.5
  female genital mutilation   110.43
  Fordyce spots   110.3, *110.4*
  fungal infections   110.27–110.28
    Candidal vulvo-vaginitis   110.27–110.28
    Tinea cruris   110.28
    Tinea incognito   *110.28*
  genital papular acantholytic dyskeratosis   110.45
  genodermatoses   110.5–110.6
  graft-versus-host disease   110.43–110.44
  Hailey–Hailey disease   110.5–110.6
  high-grade squamous intraepithelial lesions   110.34–110.36
  history and examination   110.2
  immunobullous disease   110.20, **110.21**
  inflammatory dermatoses of the vulva   110.6–110.18
    allergic contact dermatitis   110.15
    allergic contact urticaria   110.16
    irritant eczema   110.14–110.15
    lichen planus   110.10–110.13
    lichen sclerosus   110.6–110.10
    lichen simplex   110.16–110.17
    psoriasis   110.17–110.18
    reactive arthritis   110.18
    seborrhoeic eczema   110.14
    zoon vulvitis   110.13–110.14
  investigations   110.2
  labial variations   110.3
  malignant neoplasms   110.36–110.40
    basal cell carcinoma   110.39
    extramammary Paget disease   110.37–110.39
    Langerhans cell histiocytosis   110.40
    squamous cell carcinoma   110.36–110.37
    verrucous carcinoma   110.37
    vulval melanoma   110.39–110.40
  necrolytic migratory erythema   110.44–110.45

  non-sexually transmitted infections   110.24–110.31
  normal flora   110.3
  normal variants   110.3–110.4
  pain disorders   110.40–110.42
    classification of vulval pain   **110.41**
  papular acantholytic dyskeratosis   110.45
  pigmentary disorders   110.20–110.23
    acanthosis nigricans   110.22
    Dowling–Degos disease   110.23
    vitiligo   110.20–110.21
    vulval melanosis   110.21–110.22
  premalignant conditions   110.34–110.36
  structure and function   110.2–110.3
  traumatic lesions   110.42–110.43
    female genital mutilation   110.43
    mechanical hymenal fissures   110.42–110.43
  ulcerative disorders   110.18–110.20
    aphthous ulcers   110.19
    Behçet disease   110.20
    causes of vulval ulcers   **110.19**
    non-sexually acquired genital ulcers   110.19–110.20
  vaginal discharge, diagnosis of   110.24–110.25
  varicosities   110.4
  vestibular papillomatosis   110.4
  viral infections   110.28–110.31
    herpes simplex virus infections   110.29–110.30
    human papillomavirus infections   110.30–110.31
    poxvirus infections   110.28–110.29
    vulval warts   *110.30*
  vulval acne   110.45
  vulval oedema   110.23–110.24
  vulvo-vaginal adenosis   110.44
  see also vagina; vulvo-vaginal
genitalia, male   109.1–109.51
  acne   109.24
  acute scrotum   109.23
  allergic contact dermatitis   109.12, **109.13**
  amyloidosis   109.25
  anatomy   109.2–109.4
  angiokeratomas   109.6–109.7
  ano-genital warts   109.9
  artefactual conditions   109.8, 109.9
  atopic eczema   109.12
  bacillary angiomatosis   109.28
  balanitis   109.4
  balanoposthitis   109.4–109.5
  basal cell carcinoma   109.42
  benign tumours   109.29–109.31
  body dysmorphic disorder   109.6, 109.44
  Bowen disease of the penis   109.31–109.34
  bowenoid papulosis   109.31–109.34
  Buschke–Löwenstein tumour/giant condyloma   109.39–109.40
  Candida infection   109.5, 109.11, 109.27
  carcinoma of the penis   109.35–109.39
  child abuse, signs of   109.9
  chronic pain syndromes   109.43–109.44
  cicatricial (mucous membrane) pemphigoid   109.25
  condylomas of penis   109.39–109.40
  congenital and developmental abnormalities   109.7–109.8
  cutaneous genital conditions   109.42–109.44
  Darier disease   109.25
  dermatitis artefacta   109.9
  dermoid cysts   109.31
  drug reactions   109.24–109.25
  dysaesthesia   109.43–109.44
  ecthyma gangrenosum   109.26
  ectopic lesions on penile shaft   109.6
  eczema   109.11–109.13
  eczematous dermatoses   109.11
  erythroplasia of Queyrat   109.31–109.34
  extramammary Paget disease   109.40–109.41
  foreign body   109.8
  Fournier gangrene   109.26–109.27
  fungal infection   109.28

  genital herpes simplex   109.28
  genital pruritus, causes of   **109.2**
  genito-crural intertrigo   **109.3**
  haematoma and rupture, penile   109.8
  history and examination   109.4–109.5
  HIV infection   109.29
  human papillomavirus infection   109.29
  hyperpigmentation   **109.42**
  hypopigmentation   109.28, **109.42**, 109.43
  idiopathic lipogranuloma   109.43
  inflammatory dermatoses   109.9–109.26
  intraepithelial neoplasia, penile   109.31–109.34
  investigations   109.5
  irritant contact dermatitis   109.11
  Kaposi sarcoma   109.42
  keloid   109.31
  koro syndrome   109.44
  leishmaniasis   109.28
  lichen planus   109.18–109.19
  lichen sclerosus   109.15–109.18
  lichen simplex   109.11
  lipogranuloma   109.8–109.9, 109.43
  malignant melanoma   109.41
  median raphe cysts   109.30
  melanocytic naevi   109.6
  melanosis, penile   109.42–109.43
  Melkersson–Rosenthal syndrome   109.25
  metastases to the penis   109.42
  molluscum contagiosum   109.29
  MRSA   109.28
  mucoid cysts   109.30
  mutilation   109.9
  mycosis fungoides   109.42
  naevi on the penis   109.6
  non-sexually transmitted infections   109.26–109.28
  non-specific balanoposthitis   109.21–109.22
  non-syphilitic spirochaetal ulcerative balanoposthitis   109.27
  normal variants   109.5–109.7
  oedema, chronic penile   109.19–109.21
  pearly penile papules   109.6
  pemphigus   109.25
  penile horn   109.35
  penile lymphoma   109.42
  penile necrosis   109.22–109.24
  penoscrotal swelling   **109.20**
  perianal cellulitis   109.26
  perineal streptococcal dermatitis   109.26
  Peyronie disease   109.8
  phimosis   109.4, 109.16–109.17
  phthiriasis   109.29
  pilonidal sinus   109.24
  pityriasis rosea   109.28
  porokeratosis of Mibelli   109.35
  porokeratosis ptychotropica   109.35
  pre-cancerous dermatoses and carcinoma *in situ*   109.31–109.35
  pseudoepitheliomatous micaceous and keratotic balanitis   109.35
  psoriasis   109.9–109.10
  psychiatric disorders   109.44
  pubic hair   109.4, 109.27
  pyoderma gangrenosum   109.9, 109.23
  radiodermatitis   109.12
  sacral herpes zoster   109.28
  scabies   109.29, *109.30*
  sclerosing lymphangitis   109.8
  scrotal calcinosis   109.30
  scrotal panniculitis   109.23
  sebaceous gland prominence   109.6
  seborrhoeic dermatitis   109.12, 109.13
  self-instrumentation of   109.8
  self-mutilation of   109.9
  sexually transmitted diseases   109.28–109.29
  skin tags   109.5–109.6
  squamous carcinoma and malignant neoplasms   109.35–109.42
  squamous cell carcinoma, penile   109.31–109.34
  squamous hyperplasia   109.34–109.35
  squamous intraepithelial lesions   109.34–109.35

  staphylococcal cellulitis   109.26
  strangulation of the penis   109.8
  striae of Wickham   *109.19*
  structure and function   109.2–109.4
  syphilis   109.28
  tinea   109.27–109.28
  trauma   109.8–109.9
  trichomycosis pubis   109.27
  tuberculosis   109.27
  ulceration   109.5, 109.22–109.24, 109.28
    causes   **109.22**
  verruciform xanthoma   109.30–109.31
  viral warts   109.29
  warts   109.9, 109.29
  white patches and plaques, causes of   **109.34**
  yaws   109.27
  zoon balanoposthitis   109.14–109.15
  see also penis; scrotum
genital lentiginosis, laser therapies   23.15, *23.16*
genital melanosis   *131.10*
genital mucosa, lichen planus   37.6
genital mucosal lesions, COVID-19 association   25.113
genital pain
  penoscrotodynia   82.11–82.12
  vulvodynia   82.9–82.11
genital porokeratosis   85.21, *85.22*
genital psoriasis   35.10
genital sarcoidosis   96.14–96.15
genital skin, bowenoid papulosis   141.20–141.21
genital ulceration   30.18–30.19
  Adamantiades–Behçet disease   *48.5*
  Behçet-like syndrome associated with trisomy 8 myelodysplasia   149.8
  granuloma inguinale   30.21–30.23
  Lipschütz ulcers   25.37, 25.41, 25.113
  see also chancroid
genital warts *see* ano-genital warts
genito-femoral area
  Hurley stage I disease   *90.7*
  Hurley stage II disease   *90.8*
genitofemoral neuropathic pain/neuralgia   83.7
genito-urinary tract abnormalities   69.26
genodermatoses   8.2, 8.3, 8.4, 149.11
  associated with internal malignancies   148.7–148.13, 148.14
  blistering   69.1–69.28
  female genitalia   110.5–110.6
  with nail anomalies   67.2–67.3, 67.9
genome-wide score *see* polygenic risk score
genomic analysis of neoplasms, naevae as melanoma precursors   142.2
genomic analysis of squames, melanoma diagnosis   142.10
genomic imprinting   8.5
genomic medicine   8.1
genomics
  epigenomics   8.6
  immune system   9.2
  pharmacogenomics   13.11
  single-cell genomics   8.2
  skin ageing   2.46
  see also comparative genomic hybridisation
genophotodermatoses   126.1
genotype–phenotype correlations, congenital ichthyosiform erythroderma   63.7, 63.12
gentamicin   18.11
geographical factors, diagnosis   4.4
geographic tongue   108.24
geotrichosis, oral involvement   108.57
Germany
  health economic evaluations   6.2
  psoriasis, economic burden of   6.8–6.9
  skin cancer, economic burden of   6.6, **6.7**
germ line mosaicism, keratinopathic ichthyoses   63.14
gerodermia osteodysplastica   **70.16**
GG-NER *see* global genome nucleotide excision repair
GHB *see* gamma-hydroxybuyrate

ghost adipocytes
  infective panniculitis 97.46
  pancreatic panniculitis 97.41, 97.43
GHQ-12 *see* General Health Questionnaire
Gianotti–Crosti syndrome 25.121–25.123, 25.221–25.223
  Epstien-Barr virus association 25.37
  hepatitis B association 25.74
  infants 115.11
giant cell arteritis (GCA) 100.32–100.34
  oral involvement 108.69
  ultrasonographic image of superficial temporal artery *100.33*
  vessel wall involvement by granulomatous reaction *100.32*
giant cell fibroblastoma 136.15–136.16
giant cell granuloma 94.27–94.29
giant cells
  microscopic examination of 3.36, *3.37*
  multicentric reticulohistiocytosis 135.25
giant juvenile xanthogramuloma 135.16
giant porokeratoses 63.75
Giemsa stain 3.8
Gieson stain *3.8*
Gilchrist disease *see* blastomycosis
gingiva
  anatomy 108.4
  homogeneous keratosis *108.33*
  hypoplasminogenaemia 108.70
  melanotic macule 108.18
  oral lichen planus *108.7*
  proliferative verrucous leukoplakia 108.35
gingival erythema *110.12*
gingival lichen planus 108.77
gingival recession, lip/tongue piercing 108.16
gingival ulceration *108.55*
gingivitis
  acute necrotising (ulcerative) gingivitis and noma 108.54–108.55
  desquamative gingivitis 108.23, *108.82*
  plasma cell gingivitis 108.25
  vitamin C deficiency 61.21–61.22
gingivostomatitis, primary herpetic 25.20–25.22
Girimananda Sutra 1.2–1.3
GJB2 gene
  associated disorders 63.34
  KID syndrome 63.33, **63.34**
GLA *see* generalised lymphatic anomaly
glabella, botulinum toxins, aesthetic uses of 159.4
glabrous skin 2.43
glanders, *Burkholderia mallei* 26.55
glands of Tyson, Fordyce spots 93.11
glandular cheilitis 108.62–108.63
glandular fever *see* infectious mononucleosis
GLD *see* generalised lymphatic dysplasia
Gleich syndrome 43.4–43.5
glial heterotopic nodules 136.50
Global Alliance to Eradicate Lymphatic Filariasis (GALEF) 7.10
global burden of disease (GBD) 5.6–5.7, *5.8*, *5.9*, 7.2
global genome nucleotide excision repair (GG-NER) 76.2
global health dermatology 7.1–7.15
  academic capacity building 7.12
  access to health care initiatives 7.8–7.11
  burden of disease 7.2
  capacity development 7.7–7.8
  climate change and skin health 7.3–7.4
  community dermatology 7.7
  concept of global health 7.1
  educational capacity building 7.11–7.12
  educational partnerships 7.1–7.2, 7.14
  history of global health 7.1
  impact of common skin diseases **7.3**
  key stakeholders 7.4–7.6
  medical volunteerism 7.13, **7.15**
  migrant health dermatology 7.13, **7.14**
  needs assessments 7.12–7.13
  Sustainable Development Goals 7.1, 7.6–7.7

sustainable educational and health care partnerships 7.14
  teledermatology 7.8–7.9
  terminology 7.6–7.7
  volunteering opportunities 7.13, **7.15**
Global Programme to Eliminate Lymphatic Filariasis (GPELF) 103.35
globular patterns
  dermoscopy
    melanomas 145.7, *145.8*, *145.10*
    naevi *145.2*, *145.3*, 145.4–145.5, 145.6
GLODERM (International Alliance for Global Health Dermatology) 7.6
glomangioma/glomangiomyoma *see* glomus tumour
glomeruloid haemangioma 136.25
glomovenous malformations, oral involvement 108.25
glomus tumour 136.41–136.42
  diagnosis 3.25
glomuvenous malformation (GVM) 71.2, 71.18–71.19
glossitis 108.24–108.25
  atrophic glossitis *108.25*
  median rhomboid glossitis 108.22
glossodynia/glossopyrosis/glossalgia *see* burning mouth syndrome
glove materials, chemical protection **128.8**
GLP-1 *see* glucagon-like peptide-1
GLPLS *see* Graham-Little–Piccardi–Lassueur syndrome
glucagon and glucagonoma, dermatoendocrinology 150.10, 150.12, 150.19
glucagon-like peptide-1 (GLP-1) 125.14
glucagonoma syndrome, necrolytic migratory erythema 153.6
glucocorticoids (GCs) 19.17–19.21
  cautions 19.19–19.20
  contraindications 19.18
  dermatological uses 19.17
  dose and regimens 19.20–19.21
  drug–drug interactions 19.20
  monitoring 19.21
  pharmacological properties 19.17–19.18
  potential adverse effects 19.18, *19.19*
  pre-treatment screening 19.20
  sensitivity to, atopic eczema 41.19
glucocorticosteroids 2.31
glucose levels, burn injuries 125.14
glucose monitors, allergic reactions to 62.4
glue sniffer's rash 120.4
glutamine supplementation, hypermetabolism treatment 125.11–125.12
glutamine synthesis defects 79.14–79.15
glutathione-S-transferases (GSTs) 127.10
gluteal region *see* buttock
glyceryl trinitrate 18.41
  Raynaud phenomenon treatment 124.12
glycine-glutamate-lysine-glycine (GEKG) 157.5
glycine substitutions, dystrophic epidermolysis bullosa 69.19
glycolic acid (GA), chemical peels 160.2, *160.8*, 160.9–160.10
glycopeptides 19.47
glycoproteinoses 79.3–79.4, **79.4**
glycosaminoglycans (GAGs) 2.36–2.39
  cosmeceutical use 157.4
  gene location **2.39**
  molecular structure 2.36, *2.37*
  tissue distribution **2.39**
glycosaminoglycan synthesis 94.42
glycosylation
  CHIME syndrome 63.38
  congenital disorders of 79.9–79.10
glycyrrhetinic acid, topical therapies 18.41
glyphic wrinkles 94.2
glypicans 2.38
G_{M1} gangliosidosis 79.5
gnathostomiasis 33.21–33.23
  clinical features 33.22–33.23
  epidemiology 33.21

management 33.23
  pathophysiology 33.21–33.22
gold
  allergic contact dermatitis 127.40–127.41
  dermatological manifestations 121.3–121.4
Goldenhar syndrome **106.7**
golimumab, psoriatic arthritis treatment 35.45
gonadal mosaicism 8.7
gonococcal conjunctivitis 30.3, *30.4*, 30.8
gonococcal ophthalmia neonatorum 30.3, *30.4*
gonococcal vaccine 30.7
gonorrhoea 30.1–30.8
  antimicrobial resistance 30.7
  clinical features 30.3–30.6
  disseminated disease 30.5–30.6
  epidemiology 30.1
  gonococcal vaccine 30.7
  investigations 30.6–30.7
  management 30.7–30.8
  oral involvement 108.55
  pathophysiology 30.1–30.2
  perianal skin 111.16
gonosomal mosaicism 8.7
Gordon syndrome 103.24
Gorham syndrome
  diffuse lymphangiomatosis involving bone 136.39
  see also disappearing/vanishing/phantom bone disease
Gorham–Stout disease (GSD) 71.2, 103.28
  diffuse lymphangiomatosis involving bone 136.39
  see also disappearing/vanishing/phantom bone disease
Gorlin syndrome *see* naevoid basal cell carcinoma syndrome
gout **106.22**, 155.9–155.10
gouty panniculitis 97.60, *97.61*
gouty tophi 106.24
Gower panatrophy 94.19–94.20
GPA *see* granulomatosis with polyangiitis
GPCRs *see* G-protein-coupled receptors
GPELF *see* Global Programme to Eliminate Lymphatic Filariasis
GPP *see* generalised pustular psoriasis
G-protein-coupled receptors (GPCRs), transmembrane drug mechanisms 13.5
GPs *see* general practitioners
GR *see* granulomatous rosacea
Grading of Recommendations, Assessment, Development and Evaluations (GRADE) working group 17.11
grafts
  burn injuries *125.13*
  skin surgery 20.29–20.30, *20.34*, *20.35*
  wound healing 11.11–11.12
graft-versus-host disease (GvHD) 38.1–38.12, 98.9, 107.34
  acute 38.2, 38.3–38.7
  versus chronic distinction 38.1
  chronic 38.2, 38.3, 38.7–38.11
  clinical features 38.3–38.5, 38.7–38.9
  epidemiology 38.1–38.2
  extracorporeal photochemotherapy 21.7
  female genitalia 110.43–110.44
  management 38.5–38.7, 38.9–38.11
  oral involvement 108.48–108.49, 108.70
  pathology 38.2–38.3
  predisposing factors 38.2
  severity classification 38.4, **38.5**, 38.9, **38.10**
  skin cancer
    pathogenesis 147.9–147.10
    risks of chronic disease 147.4–147.5
    transfusion-associated 149.15
Graham-Little–Piccardi–Lassueur syndrome (GLPLS) 87.43
Gram-negative bacteria 26.49–26.67
Gram-negative folliculitis **88.36**
  Pseudomonas aeruginosa 26.51–26.53
  sports association 122.16

Gram-negative organisms
  burn wound infections 125.10
  Papillon–Léfèvre syndrome 63.68
Gram-positive bacteria 26.6–26.49
Gram-positive organisms, burn wound infections 125.10
Gram stain 3.9
granular cell myoblastoma, vulva **110.32**
granular cell tumours 108.45
  neural cells 136.48–136.49
granular fat 97.1–97.2
granulating wounds, postoperative care 20.37, 20.38–20.39
granulation tissue, peristomal skin *112.6*
granulocytic (myeloid) sarcoma
  infiltration of skin with malignant granulocyte precursor cells 149.2
  oral involvement 108.70
  see also leukaemia cutis
granuloma 3.41
  denture-induced granuloma 108.10
  erythema nodosum 97.22
  foreign body reactions 122.17, 122.21
  mercury 121.6
  peristomal skin *112.6*
  sarcoidosis 96.2–96.3
  subcutaneous tissue 97.12, 97.54
granuloma annulare (GA) 3.44, *4.10*, 95.1–95.8, 97.14–97.15
  associated diseases 95.1–95.2
  complications and co-morbidities 95.7
  diabetes association 62.5, *62.7*
  differential diagnosis 95.7
  disease course and prognosis 95.7–95.8
  drug-induced 95.2
  ear dermatoses **106.22**
  epidemiology 95.1
  generalised or disseminated 95.5, *95.6*
  HIV 31.18
  incidence and prevalence 95.1
  internal malignancy association 148.23
  interstitial or diffuse pattern *95.3*
  investigations 95.8
  localised 95.4–95.5
  management 95.8
  necrobiotic xanthogranuloma 97.18
  pathology 95.2–95.4
  pathophysiology 95.2
  perforating 95.3, *95.4*, 95.6, *95.7*
  presentation and clinical variants 95.4–95.7
  sarcoidal pattern 95.3, *95.4*
  subcutaneous 95.6–95.7
  sunlight exposure 95.2
  treatment ladder 95.8
granuloma faciale 89.10, 100.11–100.12
  ear dermatoses **106.22**
  inflammatory cell infiltrate *100.12*
  photothermal ablation 23.22
granuloma inguinale 30.21–30.23
  clinical features 30.22–30.23
  epidemiology 30.21
  investigations 30.23
  management 30.23
  pathophysiology 30.21–30.22
  perineal skin 111.17
granuloma multiforme 94.29–94.30
granuloma telangiectaticum *see* pyogenic granuloma
granulomatosis, orofacial 103.48, 108.72–108.74, 127.21
granulomatosis with polyangiitis (GPA) 100.22–100.25
  bilateral nodules *100.26*
  collagen degeneration *100.24*
  ear dermatoses **106.22**
  eye disease **107.35**
  inflammatory infiltrate *100.24*
  involving respiratory system 152.3–152.4
  oral involvement 108.69
  ulcerated lesions of cutaneous small-vessel vasculitis *100.26*
granulomatous acne 88.30
granulomatous disorders 95.1–95.16
  cutaneous Crohn disease 95.13–95.16

diabetic patients 62.5
granuloma annulare 95.1–95.8
necrobiosis lipoidica 95.8–95.13
orofacial granulomatosis 103.48, 108.72–108.74, 127.21
sarcoidosis 105.9
scalp 105.9
see also sarcoidosis
granulomatous (or nodular) candidiasis of the napkin area 32.65
granulomatous periorificial dermatoses, childhood 89.18–89.19
granulomatous reactions
 allergens 127.21
 annular elastolytic giant cell granuloma 94.29
 bacterial infection 26.76–26.77
granulomatous rosacea (GR) 88.34, 89.7, *89.8*, 89.9
granulomatous skin lesions
 necrotising skin *80.10*
 severe combined immunodeficiency 80.8
granulomatous slack skin disease 94.30, 139.16
granulomatous superficial pyoderma gangrenosum *49.5*, *49.6*
granulosis rubra nasi 92.10–92.11
grape seed extract (GSE) 157.7–157.9
Graves disease **150.7**, **150.10**, **150.11**, *150.14*, 150.20
gravitational purpura 99.4
'the Greater Patient' concept 16.10
Greece
 ancient medical texts 1.2
 Hippocrates 1.3
green tea (*Camellia sinensis*) 157.9
green zone 3.41
Grenz rays, kilovolt X-ray therapy 24.4, 24.7
grey lesions, melanoma 145.14
Griscelli syndrome 80.14
Griscelli–Prunièras syndrome types I and II 68.9
griseofulvin antifungals 19.48
 see also aciclovir; famciclovir; penciclovir; valaciclovir
groin
 chancroid 30.18–30.21
 erythrasma *4.20*
 hidradenitis suppurativa 88.38
 Langerhans cell histiocytosis 115.16
 linear IgA disease 115.11
 lymph drainage, obstruction of *103.8*
 microbiome 26.4, 26.5
 necrolytic migratory erythema *47.14*
 subcorneal pustular dermatosis *49.18*
groin rash, Langerhans cell histiocytosis 135.4
Grotton papules 52.5, *52.7*
Grotton syndrome **70.26**, 70.28
ground itch *see* ancylostomiasis; strongyloidiasis
groundwater contamination, by arsenic 141.13, 141.18
Group A streptococcus *see Streptococcus pyogenes*
Group B streptococci 26.12, 26.36–26.37
Group C streptococci 26.12, 26.36–26.37
Grover disease *see* transient acantholytic dermatosis
growth delay, atopic eczema association 41.21
growth factors
 hair disorder treatment 87.95
 wound healing **11.4**, *11.5*, **11.5**, *11.6*, 11.11
growth failure, ichthyoses 63.45
growth hormone, central nervous system controlled endocrine signalling axis 150.2
growth hormone deficiency, Netherton syndrome 63.26
growth hormone treatment, burn injuries 125.13
Grzybowski syndrome 141.43–141.44
GSD *see* Gorham–Stout disease

GSE *see* grape seed extract
GSTs *see* glutathione-S-transferases
G-Tube (gastrostomy), bullous pemphigoid *50.19*
GUD (genital ulcer disease) *see* genital ulceration
guinea pig maximisation test 127.8–127.9
Guinea worm *see* dracunculiasis
'guitar nipple' 122.12
gummas, syphilis 108.56
gummatous neurosyphilis 29.15
gummatous syphilide *29.13*, *29.14*, *29.15*
gums *see* gingiva
gustatory hyperhidrosis 83.24, 92.5–92.6, 92.8
 flushing in children **104.10**
 management 92.9
gut microbiome, and atopic eczema 41.9
'gut'/slaughterhouse eczema 39.15–39.16
guttate lichen planus 37.8, *37.9*
guttate morphoea 55.17
guttate psoriasis 35.15, **35.16**, 35.19
GvHD *see* graft-versus-host disease
GVM *see* glomuvenous malformation
gynaecomastia **150.10**, *150.12*, *150.13*, 150.14, 150.16, 150.17, 150.18

H
H&E *see* haematoxylin and eosin stain
HA20 *see* haploinsufficiency of A20
HA *see* hyaluronic acid
HAART *see* highly active antiretroviral therapy
habit disorders
 A-B-C model 84.12
 onychotillomania and onychophagia 84.25
 trichotillomania/trichotillosis 84.22–84.25, 87.14, 87.24, 87.32–87.34
 see also obsessive–compulsive behaviour/disorder
habit reversal therapies, psychodermatology 84.12, 84.15, 84.17, 84.18, 84.20, 84.21, 84.25, 84.47
HADS *see* Hospital Anxiety and Depression Scale
HAE *see* hereditary angio-oedema
haem
 biosynthesis of 58.2, 58.3, 58.4
 chemistry of 58.1–58.2
 molecular structure 58.2
haemangiomas 136.25–136.32
 capillary, laser therapies 23.8
 eyelid 107.46–107.47
 infants 23.8, 116.1–116.9
 oral involvement 108.25–108.26
haemangiosarcoma *see* angiosarcoma
haematological abnormalities, dyskeratosis congenita 75.4
haematological diseases
 necrobiotic xanthogranuloma association 135.24
 oral involvement 108.69–108.72
 skin manifestations 149.1–149.16
haematological malignancies
 eosinophilic pustular folliculitis 91.4
 graft-versus-host disease following allogenic haematopoietic stem cell transplantation 38.1–38.12
 human papillomavirus 25.71
 rare syndromes 149.14–149.15
 see also cutaneous lymphomas
haematological neoplasms
 infiltration of skin with neoplastic cells 149.2–149.5
 skin manifestations 149.1–149.15
haematological syndromes, ocular features **107.42**
haematoma
 external ear 106.8
 penile 109.8
 skin surgery 20.41–20.42
haematopoiesis 149.5
haematopoietic malignancies 148.2
haematopoietic stem cell transplantation (HSCT) 98.8–98.9

complications of 108.48
graft-versus-host disease 38.1–38.12
skin cancer risks 147.4–147.5
haematoporphyrin, photodynamic therapy history 22.2
haematoxylin and eosin (H&E) stain 3.7, *3.8*, *3.9*
haem disorders **79.2**
haemochromatosis 86.22, *86.23*, 86.48–86.49, 153.5
haemodialysis
 arteriovenous shunt site complications 154.5
 calciphylaxis 154.2
 cutaneous complications 154.4–154.5
 cutaneous signs 154.3–154.4
haemoglobin
 light absorption by skin 23.3–23.4
 vascular lasers 23.6
haemoglobinopathies 149.15–149.16
haemolytic anaemia/methaemoglobinaemia, dapsone side effect 19.14
haemophagocytic lymphohistiocytosis (HLH) 135.11–135.14
 infectious mononucleosis complication 25.37
haemophilia, HIV/AIDS 31.37
Haemophilus ducreyi, chancroid 30.18–30.21
haemorrhagic bulla, primary systemic amyloidosis 56.13
haemorrhagic crusting, hydroa vacciniforme 126.25, *126.26*
haemorrhagic fevers
 Bunyavirus infections 25.83–25.84
 filivirus infections 25.85–25.87
 filovirus infections 25.84–25.85
haemorrhagic lesions *4.12*
haemorrhagic onychomadesis, selenium exposure 121.7
haemorrhagic polymorphic light eruption 126.4, *126.5*
haemorrhagic proctitis, lymphogranuloma venereum 30.16
haemorrhagic rashes, measles 25.99
haemorrhoids 111.31–111.33
 origin of internal and external haemorrhoids *111.32*
 perianal skin tags *111.32*, *111.33*
 positions of internal haemorrhoids *111.32*
 prolapsed internal haemorrhoids *111.32*
 severity classification **111.33**
haemosiderin 86.47, *86.48*
haemosiderosis 94.10
haemosiderotic fibrolipomatous tumour 136.60–136.61
haemostasis
 open wounds 20.48
 wound healing 9.6
Hailey–Hailey disease (HHD) 69.24, 110.5–110.6
 ano-genital region 111.10
 perineal and perianal skin 111.10
Haim–Munk syndrome 63.68
hair 91.10–91.11, 122.22–122.24
 acquired disorders of 87.1–87.102
 anagen phase 87.8
 colour 86.5, 87.12–87.13, 87.73–87.74, 87.88, 87.99–87.101, 127.60–127.61, 142.3
 corkscrew hairs, vitamin C deficiency 61.21, *61.22*
 crab lice 34.24–34.25
 cyclical behaviour 87.9
 density on scalp 87.3
 external ear *106.3*
 follicular psoriasis 35.7, *35.9*
 foreign-body reactions 91.10–91.11, 93.1–93.2, 122.22–122.24
 fragility of 87.75–87.90
 greying 87.91–87.93
 head lice 34.18–34.23
 inherited immunodeficiency **80.4–80.6**
 internal malignancy effects 148.17–148.18
 iron deficiency 61.3, 61.4, 61.24, 87.59, 87.63, 87.70–87.71

keratins 2.10
lichen planopilaris *37.5*, 37.6, 37.11
metal poisoning signs 121.1
in pregnancy 113.1, **113.2**
psoriasis vulgaris 35.7, *35.9*
reddening of in protein-energy malnutrition *61.4*
regrowth, topical use of sensitising agents 18.33–18.34
sample collection in fungal infection 32.7
systemic lupus erythematosus 51.25–51.26
transplantation 87.97
types 87.2
variants, explanation for 2.10
see also arrector pili muscle; hirsutism; trichi...
HAIR-AN syndrome 85.4–85.5
 acne vulgaris association 88.7–88.8, 88.11
hair artefact, cutting/shaving to simulate disease 84.33
hair balls *see* trichobezoar
hair-bearing skin 2.43
hair bulb 87.4–87.5, 87.8
 scarring alopecia 87.37
hair changes
 associated with liver disease 153.9
 chemotherapy-induced 119.5–119.6
hair colour 87.99–87.101, 127.60–127.61
 melanoma risk 142.3
 pigmentation 87.12–87.13, 87.88
 trichochromes 86.5
 tyrosine kinase inhibitors 87.73–87.74
hair curl, classification 87.7
hair cycle 87.7–87.9
 dynamics 87.63
hair discs 2.12
hair disorders 87.1–87.102
 assessment/management 87.13–87.18
 common treatments 87.94–87.101
 cosmetic approaches 87.69, 87.97–87.101
 COVID-19 association 25.113
 excessive hair growth 87.84–87.91
 HIV 31.33–31.34
 ichthyoses 63.45
 ocular features **107.41**
 pigmentation disorders 68.6–68.7, 68.9, 87.91, 87.94
 structural defects 87.75–87.84
 syndromic ichthyoses **63.39**, 63.40–63.46
hair dyes, allergic reactions 127.5, 127.16, 127.33, 127.60–127.61
hair fall, increase in 87.53–87.71
hair fibres 87.6–87.7
hair-filled sinuses 122.23
hair follicle pigmentary unit (HFPU) 87.12–87.13
hair follicles (HF) 2.43, 87.2
 androgen action mechanism 87.10–87.11
 cysts and tumours, dystrophic calcification 59.3–59.4
 degeneration and regeneration 2.45
 density **87.3**
 development/distribution 87.2–87.3
 embryonic development 2.3–2.5, *2.5*
 fibroplasts 2.40
 growth phase 2.45
 as hormone-sensitive mini-organs 150.1, 150.3
 innervation 87.7
 light absorption 23.5–23.6
 melanocytes 2.17
 Merkel cells 2.12
 mesenchyme lesions 137.15–137.16
 miniaturisation 87.64, *87.65*
 naevi 137.7–137.8
 neuroendocrinology 87.11–87.13
 resting phase 2.45
 staphylococcal infections 26.22–26.27
 stem cells in 2.44–2.45
 suprabulbar region 87.4, 87.6
 tumours 137.2–137.5
 see also carbuncles; folliculitis; furuncles; sycosis
hair germ tumours and cysts 137.7–137.13

hair growth 87.9–87.11
  excessive 87.84–87.91
  phases of 2.10
hair immune system 87.11
hair loss
  assessment/management 87.13–87.18
  increased hair fall-associated 87.53–87.71
  infants 115.15
  infections 87.35–87.36
  presentations 87.18–87.74
  psychological and social factors 15.4
  scalp psoriasis 105.3
  see also alopecia
hair matrix tumours 137.13–137.15
hair presentation, Netherton syndrome 63.26–63.27
hair products
  allergic contact dermatitis 127.48
  effects on dandruff 40.4
hair pulling disorders (trichotillomania/trichotillosis) 84.22–84.25, 87.14, 87.24, 87.32–87.34
hair pull test 87.54–87.55, 87.65
hair reduction, laser treatment 23.5–23.6, 23.17–23.20
hair removal
  folliculitis keloidalis 93.4
  hidradenitis suppurativa treatment 90.11
  laser assisted 23.17–23.20, 93.4
  principles of light-assisted removal 23.5–23.6
  pseudofolliculitis 91.10, 93.1–93.2
hair shaft abnormalities, trichoscopy 87.74
hair shaft (HS)
  disorders of 87.14–87.15, 87.74–87.84
  fungal infections 32.15–32.16
  suprabulbar region 87.4
  white piedra 32.16–32.17
hair shedding, in infancy 114.4
hair sinus 122.22
hair styling, alopecia 87.99
hair systems 87.101
hair-thread tourniquet syndrome 122.23
  foot involvement 122.22
hairy leukoplakia, oral lesions 108.32–108.33, 108.34
half-and-half nails 154.3
halitosis, olfactory delusions 84.10–84.11
Hallermann–Streiff syndrome 77.2
hallucinations, delusional infestation 84.6
halo dermatitis 39.28
halo eczema naevus see Myerson naevus
halogen acne 129.12
halogenated aromatic hydrocarbons 129.12
halogenated salicylanilides 127.79–127.80
halo naevi 86.40–86.42, 131.27–131.28, 131.28, 131.29
  vitiligo association 86.34–86.35, 86.41
hamartoma of cutaneous adnexa and mesenchyme see rhabdomyomatous congenital hamartoma
hamartoma of the pilosebaceous follicle 137.8–137.9
hamartomas
  basaloid follicular 137.12–137.13
  dermoid cyst, mouth 108.12
  sclerosing epithelial see desmoplastic trichoepithelioma
hamartomatous polyps, PJT syndrome 68.13
Hamilton–Norwood scale, hair loss 87.65, 87.66
hand
  atopic eczema 41.16–41.17, 41.19, 41.23
  bullous eczema 39.14
  bullous pemphigoid 50.16
  callosities 122.8
  cheiroarthropathy 62.7
  cicatricial pemphigoid 50.52
  collagenous and elastotic marginal plaques 94.4–94.5
  deformity, epidermolysis bullosa 69.17–69.18, 69.26
  dermatomyositis 52.5, 52.7, 52.8
  discoid lesions, systemic lupus erythematosus 51.23

discoid lupus erythematosus 51.8
epidermolysis bullosa acquista 50.44
erythema elevatum diutinum 100.9
erythema multiforme 4.15, 47.2
erytropoietic protoporphyria 99.24
glomuvenous malformation 71.18
granuloma annulare 95.2, 95.5
Grotton papules in dermatomyositis 52.5, 52.7
IgA vasculitis 100.15
infrared thermograms 54.22
lichen planus 39.17
lichen striatus 37.18
Maffucci syndrome 71.20
mixed connective tissue disease 53.4
mucocutaneous venous malformation 71.16
mucous membrane pemphigoid 50.29
Nékam disease 37.11
neutrophilic dermatosis of dorsal hands 49.12, 49.13
oedema 103.21
palisaded and neutrophilic granulomatous dermatitis 53.7
pellagra, niacin deficiency 61.17
psoriasis vulgaris 35.11
Rothmund–Thomson syndrome 75.6
spindle cell haemangiomas 71.20
STING-associated vasculopathy with onset in infancy 45.14
systemic lupus erythematosus 51.23, 51.24
tinea nigra palmaris 32.14–32.15
tyrosinaemia type 2 79.12
xanthomatosis 60.6
see also palm
hand eczema 39.12–39.19, 127.13–127.14, 128.1–128.2, 128.3–128.4
  acute 39.19
  advice to patients 128.7
  aetiology 39.12
  apron eczema 39.14, 39.15
  associated diseases 39.13
  chronic 39.14–39.15, 39.18–39.19
  clinical features 39.14
  clinical variants 39.14–39.16
  complications and co-morbidities 39.17
  differential diagnosis 39.16–39.17, 127.22, 128.5
  disease course and prognosis 39.17–39.18
  environmental factors 39.13–39.14
  epidemiology 39.12–39.13
  fingertip 39.15
  genetics 39.13
  'gut'/slaughterhouse eczema 39.15–39.16
  hyperkeratotic 39.14
  inflammatory pathways 39.13
  investigations 39.18
  management 39.18–39.19
  morphological patterns 39.12
  nickel allergy 127.37–127.38
  occupational contact dermatitis 129.2, 129.6
  patchy vesiculosquamous eczema 39.16
  plant allergies 127.72
  pompholyx eczema 39.14
  population studies 127.3
  predisposing factors 39.13, 127.7
  preservatives 127.53–127.54
  prognosis 127.23
  recurrent focal palmar peeling 39.16
  ring eczema 39.16
  severity classification 39.17
  treatment 39.19
  Trichophyton infection 39.17
hand, foot and mouth disease 25.94–25.95, 108.50
  infants 115.6
handicap, caused by skin disease 5.5–5.6
hand–arm vibration syndrome (HAVS) 122.24–122.26
Hand–Schüller–Christian syndrome 135.6
Hansen, Gerhard 1.8
Hansen's disease/Hanseniasis see leprosy
Hapalochlaena maculosa, stings from 130.4

haploinsufficiency of A20 (HA20) **45.5, 45.7**, 45.15
haplotypes, mal de Meleda 63.55
Happle–Tinschert syndrome 73.7, **78.12**
haptenisation 118.5
hapten/pro-hapten model, T-cell recognition of drugs 14.5–14.6
haptens 127.8
harlequin colour change
  flushing in children 104.10, **104.10**
  neonates 114.3
harlequin ichthyosis (HI) 63.7–63.8, 63.9–63.10
  management of 63.43
Harmonising Outcome Measures for Eczema (HOME) **16.3**
Hartnup disease 61.16, 79.14
harvest mites 34.54
Hashimoto–Pritzker disease 135.5, 135.7
HAVS see hand–arm vibration syndrome
Haxthausen disease 63.71–63.72
HBV see hepatitis B virus
HC see hereditary coproporphyria
HCCVM see hyperkeratotic cutaneous capillary–venous malformations
HCoVs see human coronaviruses
HCV see hepatitis C virus
HDM see house dust mite
HD-OCT see high-definition optical coherence tomography
head, allergic contact dermatitis of 127.14, 127.21
Headington's anagen release 87.53
head lice 34.18–34.23
  clinical features 34.20–34.21
  epidemiology 34.18–34.19
  investigations 34.21
  management 34.21–34.23
  on mummified body 1.2
  pathophysiology 34.20
head and neck, anatomical considerations for skin surgery 20.1–20.4
head oedema 103.46–103.49, **103.47**
Heaf test 4.24
healing see wound healing
health anxieties, irrational/obsessional fears of skin problems 84.25–84.26
health care partnerships 7.14
health care settings 5.12–5.13
health economics 6.1–6.11
  decision-making in dermatology practice 6.10–6.11
  economic burden of disease 6.5–6.10
    atopic eczema 6.10
    definition 6.1
    psoriasis 6.8–6.10
    skin cancer 6.5–6.8
    studies on 6.10
  holistic perspective 6.2
  methods and approaches 6.1–6.5
    bottom-up/top-down approaches 6.3
    comparative/non-comparative studies 6.3, 6.4–6.5
    cost-benefit analysis 6.4
    cost-effectiveness analysis 6.4
    cost-minimisation studies 6.4
    cost-utility analysis 6.4
    evaluation perspectives 6.2
    friction cost approach 6.3
    human capital approach 6.3
    implementation of health economic findings in decision-making 6.5
    indirect costs 6.3
    intangible costs 6.3
    physician perspective 6.2
    prioritisation 6.5
    productivity costs 6.3
    rationalisation 6.5
    scaling 6.5
    secondary research 6.2–6.3
    types of health economic evaluation 6.2–6.5
    willingness to pay 6.4
  patient perspective 6.2
  psoriasis, economic burden of 6.8–6.10

  skin cancer, economic burden of 6.5–6.8
  societal perspective 6.2
  third-party payer perspective 6.2
health related quality of life (HRQoL) 6.2, 16.5–16.6
health services research 5.12–5.14
Health Systems Evidence (HSE) database 17.6, 17.7
hearing impairment
  palmoplantar keratodermas and 63.63–63.65
  see also deafness
heart
  congenital heart block 51.39–51.42
  Libman–Sacks endocarditis 51.18
  sarcoidosis 96.6
  systemic lupus erythematosus 51.30
  see also cardio … entries
heat
  cutaneous reactions to 124.1–124.16
  diseases caused by 124.14–124.16
  physiological reactions to 124.14
heat-associated carcinomas 124.15
heat contact urticaria **42.9**, 42.10
heat injuries 125.1–125.15
heat rash see miliaria
heat shock proteins (HSP),
  Adamantiades–Behçet disease 48.3
heavy coal-tar distillates 129.12
heavy metals, oral hyperpigmentation 108.17
Heberden nodes 155.8
Hebra, Ferdinand Ritter von 1.6
Heck's disease 108.11
hedgehog pathway inhibitors, hair loss 87.74
hEDS see hypermobile Ehlers–Danlos syndromes
heel
  black heel 99.6
  calcified cutaneous nodules of the heels 115.15
  mechanical injuries 122.10–122.11
  pedal papules of infancy 115.15
  piezogenic pedal papules 122.26
heel prick calcinosis 59.3
HEH see neutrophilic eccrine hidradenitis
Helicobacter pylori infection 153.1
heliodermatitis 89.7–89.8
heliotrope rash 52.3
helminth infestations
  and atopic eczema 41.8
  perineal and perianal skin 111.16
  see also cestodes; nematodes; trematodes
HEMA see hydroxyethlmethacrylate
2-HEMA see 2-hydroxyethylmethacrylate
hematidrosis 92.18, 92.19
hemidesmosomal inner plaques, keratins 69.4
hemidesmosomes 2.25–2.26
hemihyperplasia–multiple lipomatosis syndrome 72.9, 72.11
Hemiptera (bugs) 34.25–34.30
henna 87.100
Hennekam lymphangiectasia–lymphoedema syndrome 71.26
heparan 2.37
heparan sulphate (HS) **2.39**
heparan sulphate proteoglycans (HSPGs) 2.25
heparin 2.37
heparin-induced thrombocytopenia (HIT) 99.9–99.10
heparin necrosis, purpura 99.9–99.10
hepatic, see also liver disease
hepatic gummata, syphilis 29.15
hepatic haemangioma (HH), infants 116.5
hepatic sarcoidosis 96.5
hepatitis 25.73–25.77
  and lichen planus 37.2
  oral involvement 108.74
hepatitis A virus 25.96–25.97
  cutaneous features 153.4

hepatitis B virus (HBV) 25.74–25.75
  arthropathies 155.3
  cryoglobulinaemia 124.13
  cutaneous features 153.4–153.5
  human bite transmission 130.7
hepatitis C virus (HCV) 25.75–25.77
  cryoglobulinaemia 124.13
  cutaneous features 153.5
  human bite transmission 130.7
  polymorphic light eruption 126.2
  viral arthropathies 155.3
hepatobiliary disease 153.4–153.5
  cholestatic pruritus 81.9–81.10
  and psoriasis 35.19
hepatocellular carcinoma, PR association 85.8
hepatotoxicity, methotrexate 19.26
herbals
  acne vulgaris 88.57–88.58
  cosmeceutical use of 157.7–157.10
  psychodermatological uses 84.48
  traditional topical therapies 18.38
  wart treatments 25.60
  see also complementary/alternative/traditional therapies; plant extracts
hereditary angio-oedema (HAE) 43.1–43.2, 43.3–43.4
  clinical features 43.4
  reticulate prodromal erythema *43.4*
  treatment 43.6
hereditary anonychia 67.16–67.17
hereditary autoinflammatory disorders/syndromes
  arthralgia/arthritis 155.10
  renal involvement 154.2
hereditary benign intraepithelial dyskeratosis 108.29
hereditary benign telangiectasia **101.17**, 101.20, *101.21*
  aborising pattern *101.20*
hereditary coproporphyria (HC) 58.5, 58.7, 58.9, 58.12, 58.17
hereditary disorders/syndromes 8.2–8.5, 8.8–8.9
  acne plus musculoskeletal features 155.11
  cardiac involvement 151.1, 151.2–151.4
  pachydermoperiostosis 155.14
  prenatal diagnosis 8.9–8.11
  skin and renal involvement 154.1–154.2
hereditary fibrosing poikiloderma with tendon contractures, myopathy and pulmonary fibrosis **75.2**, *75.7*
hereditary haemorrhagic telangiectasia (HHT) *71.2*, 71.12–71.13, **78.14**, 153.7
  oral involvement 108.26
hereditary leiomyomatosis and renal cell cancer (HLRCC/Reed syndrome) **78.14**, *78.15*, 148.12, 154.2
hereditary lymphoedema type 1A (LMPH1A) 71.24–71.25
hereditary monogenic autoinflammatory syndromes 45.2–45.19, **155.10**
  autoinflammatory diseases with granuloma 45.11–45.12
  Behçet disease-like or inflammatory bowel disease-like autoinflammatory syndromes 45.15–45.16
  clinical features **45.6–45.7**
  dermatological signs and entities **45.3–45.4**
  epidemiology 45.2, **45.6–45.7**
  hereditary periodic fevers 45.8–45.11
  miscellaneous monogenic autoinflammatory syndromes 45.16–45.19
  pathophysiology 45.2–45.8
  related acquired sporadic or complex disorders **45.3–45.4**
  skin and/or mucosal manifestation **45.3–45.4**
  terminology **45.5**
  treatment **45.6–45.7**
  type 1 interferonopathies 45.13–45.15

hereditary mucoepithelial dysplasia (HMD) 63.25–63.26
hereditary neuropathies 83.11–83.24
hereditary non-polyposis colorectal cancer *see* Muir–Torre syndrome
hereditary obesity 72.3–72.9
  monogenic obesity with cutaneous features 72.4, **72.7**
  monogenic obesity without cutaneous features 72.3, **72.6**
  Prader–Willi syndrome 72.6–72.9
  pro-opiomelanocortin and prohormone convertase deficiency 72.4–72.6
  secondary skin complications of primary obesity **72.4**
hereditary panniculitis **72.11**, *72.12*
hereditary papulotranslucent acrokeratoderma 63.62
hereditary periodic fevers 45.8–45.11
  cryopyrin-associated periodic syndrome 45.8–45.9
  familial Mediterranean fever **45.5**, **45.6**, 45.9–45.10
  mevalonate kinase deficiency with recurrent fever and hyper-IgD syndrome 45.11
  pyrin-associated autoinflammation with neutrophilic dermatosis 45.10–45.11
  tumour necrosis factor associated periodic syndrome **45.5**, **45.6**, 45.9
hereditary progressive mucinous histiocytosis 135.23
hereditary sensory and autonomic neuropathies (HSANs) 83.12
hereditary syndromes *see* hereditary disorders/syndromes
Hermansky–Pudlak syndrome 68.8, **78.13**, **80.5**, 80.14
hermaphroditism 63.67
heroin
  addiction prevalence 120.2
  death rates 120.1
  dermatoses induced by 120.5–120.7
herpangina 25.95–25.96, 108.50
herpes-associated erythema multiforme 25.23
herpes B virus infection 25.43
herpes genitalis
  primary 25.24–25.25
  recurrent 25.26
herpes infection
  of eye *1.10*
  hair loss 87.35–87.36
herpes labialis
  primary herpetic gingivostomatitis 25.20–25.22
  recurrent oro-facial and cutaneous herpes 25.22–25.24
herpes simplex virus (HSV) *4.8*, 25.19–25.28, **25.44**
  antigenic types 25.19–25.20
  and atopic eczema 41.10
  cytology 3.29, *3.30*
  eyelid 107.34–107.36, *107.37*
  female genitalia 110.29–110.30
  genetically engineered for oncolytic virus therapy 144.1
  gingivostomatitis 25.20–25.22, 108.51–108.53
  guanosine analogue antivirals 19.49
  HIV 31.5, 31.23, *31.38*
  lingual recurrence *108.71*
  neonatal 114.22
  perineal and perianal skin 111.15, 111.16
  in pregnancy 113.4–113.5
  primary herpes genitalis 25.24–25.25
  primary herpetic gingivostomatitis 25.20–25.22
  primary/recurrent infections 25.19–25.20
  reactivation, PUVA phototherapy adverse effects 21.12, 21.13
  recurrent genital herpes 25.26
  recurrent oro-facial and cutaneous herpes 25.22–25.24

  subclinical viral shedding 25.20
herpes stromal keratitis (HSK), eyelid *107.37*
herpesviruses 1 and 2, human bite transmission 130.7
herpesviruses 6, 7 and 8, oral infection 108.53
herpesvirus infections 25.19–25.46, **25.20**
  Kaposi sarcoma 25.42, 25.43, 31.30
  oral infection 108.50–108.54
  reactivation of 14.4
  see also cytomegalovirus; eczema herpeticum; Epstein-Barr virus; human herpesvirus 6 and 7; human herpesvirus 8; inoculation herpes simplex; varicella-zoster virus; zoster
herpesvirus reactivation, drug reaction with eosinophilia and systemic symptoms 118.5–118.6
herpes zoster 25.32–25.36
  acute herpetic neuralgia 82.4
  clinical features 25.33–25.34
  cutaneous manifestations of Hodgkin disease 139.49
  epidemiology 25.32
  eyelid 107.36–107.38
  hair loss 87.35–87.36
  investigations 25.34–25.35
  management 25.35
  neuralgia 108.66
  neurogenic bladder dysfunction 154.6
  neurological complications 25.32, 25.33–25.34
  oral infection 108.53–108.54
  oticus 25.33–25.34
  pathophysiology 25.32
  postherpetic neuralgia 82.4–82.5
  reactivation after COVID-19 vaccination 25.118
  reactivation in COVID-19 patients 25.111
herpetic gingivostomatitis 25.21
herpetic whitlow 25.28
herpetiform ulceration 108.38, *108.39*
HES *see* hydroxyethyl starch
heterotopic sebaceous glands 91.15–91.17, 93.10–93.12
heterotrimeric G-protein mosaic disorders 73.19–73.21
  McCune–Albright syndrome 73.19–73.20
  phakomatosis pigmentovascularis 73.20–73.21
  Sturge–Weber syndrome 73.20
hexachlorophene 18.10
Hexathelidae (funnel web spider) 34.35
HF *see* hair follicles; hydrops fetalis
HFPU *see* hair follicle pigmentary unit
HFTC *see* hyperphosphataemic familial tumoral calcinosis
HGPS *see* Hutchinson–Gilford progeria syndrome
HH *see* hepatic haemangioma
HHD *see* Hailey–Hailey disease
HHT *see* hereditary haemorrhagic telangiectasia
HHV *see* human herpesvirus
HI *see* harlequin ichthyosis
hibernoma 136.57
hidradenitis suppurativa (HS) 87.50, 88.37, *88.38*, 90.1–90.11, 111.10–111.12
  acne conglobata association 88.63
  assessment tools 16.4–16.5
  clinical features 111.11–111.12
  epidemiology 111.10–111.11
  facial 23.23
  Hurley staging system 111.11, **111.12**
  inflamed nodules *90.5*
  management *90.10*, 111.12
  pathophysiology 111.11
  psychological factors 15.4
  quality of life assessment 16.8
  scarring *111.11*, *111.12*
  sexual function measures 16.12
Hidradenitis Suppurativa, Patient-Reported Outcome Measures 16.8

Hidradenitis Suppurativa Burden of Disease (HSBOD) 16.8
Hidradenitis Suppurativa Clinical Response (HiSCR) 16.4–16.5
HIdradenitis SuppuraTiva cORe outcomes set International Collaboration (HISTORIC) 16.3, 16.8
Hidradenitis Suppurativa Impact Assessment (HSIA) 16.8
hidradenitis suppurativa lesion, area and severity index (HS-LASI) 16.4
Hidradenitis Suppurativa Physician's Global Assessment (HS-PGA) 16.4
Hidradenitis Suppurativa Quality of Life (HiSQOL) questionnaire 16.8
Hidradenitis Suppurativa Quality of Life instrument (HS-QoL) 16.8
Hidradenitis Suppurativa Symptom Assessment (HSSA) 16.8
hidradenocarcinoma 137.35–137.40
hidradenoma 137.28–137.29
hidradenoma papilliferum (papillary hidradenoma) 110.31–110.33, 137.20–137.21
hidradénomes eruptifs *see* syringoma
hidroacanthoma simplex 137.24–137.25
hidrotic ectodermal dysplasia *see* Clouston syndrome
HIDS (hyperimmunoglobulinaemia-D syndrome) *see* mevalonate kinase deficiency
HID syndrome *see* hystrix-like ichthyosis and deafness
HIFU *see* high intensity microfocused ultrasound
high-definition optical coherence tomography (HD-OCT), basal cell carcinoma 140.10, *140.12*
high-grade squamous intraepithelial lesions (HSIL), female genitalia 110.34–110.36
high intensity microfocused ultrasound (HIFU) 161.7–161.8
highly active antiretroviral therapy (HAART) 91.5
  fibrous histiocytoma 136.21
  HIV-associated lipodystrophy 98.6–98.8
  lobular capillary haemangioma 136.26
high-molecular-weight kininogen (HMWK), bradykinin-induced angio-oedema 43.3
high-performance liquid chromatography (HPLC), porphyrias *58.8*
hindfoot anomaly 122.7
Hippocrates 1.3
Hirschsprung disease 68.5
hirsutism 87.84, 87.87–87.90
  acne vulgaris *88.45*
  depilatories 18.33
  disorders associated with 87.90–87.91
  laser-assisted hair removal 23.17, 23.19
HiSCR *see* Hidradenitis Suppurativa Clinical Response
HiSQOL *see* Hidradenitis Suppurativa Quality of Life
histamine 4 (H4) receptor, atopic eczema treatment 41.30–41.32
histamine
  release of in skin 14.1
  solar urticaria 126.21–126.23
histamine-evoked 'geographical' pattern of flushing, carcinoid tumours *150.12*
histamine receptors, pruritus **81.3**, 81.4
histiocytes
  function 135.1–135.2
  microscopic examination of 3.36
histiocytic disorders 149.16–149.17
histiocytic lymphoma 135.30–135.31
histiocytic markers, cutaneous neoplasms 3.27
histiocytic sarcoma (HS) 135.31–135.32
histiocytoid haemangioma *see* epithelioid haemangioma
histiocytoid Sweet syndrome 49.12, *49.14*, 97.22–97.23, 149.6

histiocytoma cutis *see* fibrous histiocytoma
histiocytoses 135.1–135.32
  eye disease 107.35
histochemistry, biopsy 3.7–3.10
histone deacetylase inhibitor therapy 139.25
histopathology of skin 3.1–3.46
  artefacts 3.31–3.32
  biopsy 3.2–3.10
  cytodiagnosis 3.29–3.30
  descriptive terms 3.38–3.43
  digital pathology 3.32
  electron microscopy 3.30–3.31
  foreign body reactions 122.18–122.19
  graft versus host disease 38.2, 38.3
  histological sections with little or no abnormality 3.44–3.45
  immunogenotyping 3.31
  immunopathology 3.10–3.29
  microscopic examination of tissue sections 3.32–3.45
  pseudoepitheliomatous hyperplasia mimicking squamous cell carcinoma 132.9–132.10
  reporting of 3.38
  Tzanck smears 3.29–3.30
  viral disease diagnosis 3.31
  see also biopsy of skin
Histoplasma capsulatum 32.81, 32.82, 32.84
histoplasmin test 4.25
histoplasmosis 32.81–32.84
  clinical features 32.82–32.84
  epidemiology 32.81–32.82
  HIV 31.27
  management 32.84
  oral lesions 108.57
  pathophysiology 32.82
HISTORIC *see* HIdradenitis SuppuraTiva cORe outcomes set International Collaboration
history of dermatology *see* dermatology history
history taking 4.2–4.5, 81.6
HIT *see* heparin-induced thrombocytopenia
hives *see* urticaria
HIV infection 31.1–31.39
  acute primary infection 31.6–31.7
  ano-genital disorders 31.35–31.36
  aphthous-like ulceration 108.71
  arthropathies 155.3, 155.4
  associated infections 31.20–31.30
  atopic eczema 31.15
  bacterial infections 31.20–31.23
  candidiasis 31.6, 31.26, 31.34, 31.37, 32.58, 108.21–108.22
  children 31.36–31.37
  clinical features 31.5–31.8
  coagulopathies 31.12
  coinfections 31.20–31.31
  complications and co-morbidities 31.7–31.8, 31.20–31.31
  as a continuum 31.6
  cryoglobulinaemia 124.13
  cryptococcus infection 31.28
  cytomegalovirus infection 31.24–31.25
  definition 31.1
  dermatological manifestations 31.11–31.39
    acute primary infection 31.6–31.7
    coinfections 31.20–31.31
    common conditions 31.11
    neoplasms 31.30–31.33
  dermatophytosis 31.26–31.27
  diagnosis 31.7
  drug reaction with eosinophilia and systemic symptoms 118.5–118.6
  eosinophilic folliculitis 31.17, 93.7, 93.8, 93.9
  eosinophilic pustular folliculitis 91.4–91.5
  epidemiology 31.2
  erythroderma 31.12
  fungal infections 31.26–31.29
  granuloma annulare 31.18
  hair abnormalities 31.33–31.34

hair loss 87.35
hairy leukoplakia, oral lesions 108.32, *108.33*
herpes simplex infection 31.23
histoplasmosis 31.27
history 31.1
HIV-associated lipodystrophy 98.2, 98.6–98.8
HIV-induced or exacerbated psoriasis 35.15–35.16
HIV-related pityriasis rubra pilaris (type VI) 36.4
human bite transmission 130.7
human papillomavirus infection 25.71, 31.25–31.26
immunology 31.3–31.5
immunosuppression causing lymphoproliferative disorders 139.47
infection and course 31.1–31.10
infection prevention 31.9
inflammatory dermatoses 31.12–31.20
initial diagnosis 31.7, 31.11
investigations 31.8–31.9, 31.11–31.12
Kaposi sarcoma 31.30–31.31, 31.35
leprosy 28.10
lip, warts on *108.14*
male genitalia 109.29
management 31.9–31.10
mollusca/molluscipoxvirus infection 31.26
mycobacterial infections 27.2–27.3, 27.9, 27.10, 31.22
nail abnormalities 31.33–31.34
neonates 114.24
neoplasms 31.30–31.33
  photodynamic therapy 22.7–22.8
  non-AIDS defining cancers 31.31
normalisation of testing 31.2, 31.11
oral hyperpigmentation 108.17
oral lesions 108.54
oro-pharyneal abnormalities 31.34–31.35, **31.36**
pathophysiology 31.2–31.5
penicilliosis 31.28
perineal and perianal skin 111.17
pigmentary disorders 31.12
porphyria cutanea tarda 31.18
posinophilic folliculitis 31.17–31.18
protozoal infections 31.29
pruritic conditions 31.12
psoriasis 31.15–31.17
recurrent genital herpes risk 25.26
scabies 31.29
scalp infection 105.12
seborrhoeic dermatitis 31.12, 31.15
seroconversion symptoms 31.5, 31.6–31.7, 31.11
skin cancer risks 147.2–147.3
skin manifestations of infection 149.20
staphylococcal infections 31.20–31.21
STI relationship 29.1, 29.3
striae 94.10
syphilis relationship 29.17, 29.21
trichodysplasia spinulosa 85.15
varicella-zoster infection 31.23–31.24
viral coinfections 31.23–31.26
viral warts, photodynamic therapy 22.7–22.8
virology 31.2–31.3, *31.4*
visceral leishmaniasis 33.52–33.53
women 31.36
see also people living with HIV
HIV-negative MSM (men who have sex with men), Kaposi sarcoma 138.1, **138.2**, 138.4
HLA *see* human leukocyte antigens
HLA-B* genes, drug reactions 118.6, 118.7
HLA-B27 haplotype 155.2, *155.3*, 155.5
HLA class II typing, cutaneous photosensitivity diseases 126.7
HLA-DR4 tissue type, actinic prurigo 126.10
HLH *see* haemophagocytic lymphohistiocytosis

HLRCC *see* hereditary leiomyomatosis and renal cell cancer
HLTS *see* hypotrichosis–lymphoedema–telangiectasia syndrome
HMD *see* hereditary mucoepithelial dysplasia
HMWK *see* high-molecular-weight kininogen
hoarseness
  disorders with skin and systemic manifestations 152.7
  pachyonychia congenita 67.12
hobnail endothelial cells 136.33
hobnail haemangioendothelioma *see* retiform haemangioendothelioma
hobnail haemangioma 136.29–136.30
Hodgkin disease
  cutaneous lymphoproliferative disorder relationship 139.26, 139.27, 139.34, 139.49
  cutaneous manifestations 139.48–139.49
  Epstein–Barr virus association 25.49
  infiltration of skin with malignant cells 149.4
  sarcoidosis association 96.1
Hoigne reactions, procaine penicillin 29.22
HOIL-1 deficiency 45.17–45.18
holistic management of skin disease 15.4–15.7
  effective communication 15.6
  key practical skills 15.6, **15.6**, *15.7*
  physical considerations 15.4–15.5
  psychological considerations 15.5
  social considerations 15.5
  spiritual considerations 15.5–15.6
holoprosencephaly **106.7**
holster sign, erythema on hips/lateral thighs in dermatomyositis 52.5, *52.9*
Holy Bible, leprosy 1.3
HOME *see* Harmonising Outcome Measures for Eczema
homeostasis 2.43–2.45, *9.4*, 9.6–9.7
home phototherapy 21.3, 21.8, 21.15, 21.18
homogeneous naevi *145.4*, 145.5–145.6
homogentisic acid 86.51
honey, topical application 18.38
honeycomb keratoderma 63.56
  Vohwinkel syndrome 63.63
hooking thumb 122.17
hookworm larvae
  ancylostomiasis 33.15–33.17
  see also cutaneous larva migrans
L'Hôpital St Louis, Paris 1.4–1.5
hordeolum 107.38, *107.39*
hormones
  effects on allergic contact dermatitis 127.6
  hidradenitis suppurativa 90.2
  lipoedema 98.21
  neuropeptide/neurotransmitter/cytokine distinctions 150.2–150.3
  secondary mediator generation in skin 150.7
  skin/appendage production *150.3*, **150.4**, 150.5
  skin as target *150.3*, 150.5–150.8
  treatment for acne vulgaris 88.49–88.52
  types of signalling 150.2
  see also dermatoendocrinology; endocrine disorders; endocrinology
hormone therapy-induced alopecia (HTIA) 87.73
Horner syndrome 83.23–83.24, 94.20
Hornstein–Knickenberg syndrome *see* Birt–Hogg–Dubé syndrome
horse fly *see* Chrysops
horseradish peroxidase 3.14, 3.15
Hortaea werneckii, tinea nigra 32.14–32.15
Hospital Anxiety and Depression Scale (HADS) 16.11
host defence, skin as barrier to pathogens 26.3
host–parasite relationship shift, erythrasma 26.38

house dust mite (HDM) 34.51
  atopic eczema association 41.23
housework dermatitis 129.3
housework-typeeczema 128.3
Howel–Evans syndrome 63.66, 148.7
Hoyeraal–Hreidarsson syndrome 67.15
HPA axis *see* hypothalamic–pituitary–adrenal axis
HPeV *see* human parechoviruses
HPLC *see* high-performance liquid chromatography
HPT axis *see* hypothalamic–pituitary–thyroid axis
HPV *see* human papillomavirus
HPyV *see* human polyomavirus
HRAS/KRAS mosaicism 73.5–73.6
  see also Schimmelpenning–Feuerstein–Mims syndrome
HR gene, atrichia with papular lesions 87.29
HRQoL *see* health related quality of life
HS *see* hair shaft; heparan sulphate; hidradenitis suppurativa; histiocytic sarcoma
HSANs *see* hereditary sensory and autonomic neuropathies
HSBOD *see* Hidradenitis Suppurativa Burden of Disease
HSCT *see* haematopoietic stem cell transplantation
HSE *see* Health Systems Evidence database
HSIA *see* Hidradenitis Suppurativa Impact Assessment
HSIL *see* high-grade squamous intraepithelial lesions
HSK *see* herpes stromal keratitis
HS-LASI *see* hidradenitis suppurativa lesion, area and severity index
HSP *see* heat shock proteins
HS-PGA *see* Hidradenitis Suppurativa Physician's Global Assessment
HSPGs *see* heparan sulphate proteoglycans
HS-QoL *see* Hidradenitis Suppurativa Quality of Life instrument
HSSA *see* Hidradenitis Suppurativa Symptom Assessment
HSV *see* herpes simplex virus
HTIA *see* hormone therapy-induced alopecia
HTLV *see* human T-cell lymphotropic virus
Hughes syndrome *see* antiphospholipid antibody syndrome
human bites 130.6–130.7
human body louse (*Pediculus humanus corporis*) 26.62, 26.64, 26.72, 26.80
  see also louse-borne diseases
Human Cell Atlas project 8.2
human coronaviruses (HCoVs) 25.100–25.120
  see also COVID-19/SARS-CoV-2
human genome 8.5
  sequencing of 8.8–8.9
Human Genome Project 8.1
human herpesvirus 6 and 7 (HHV-6/HHV-7) 25.39–25.40
  reactivation 25.40
  roseola infantum 25.39–25.40, 115.5–115.6
human herpesvirus 8 (HHV-8) 25.42–25.43
  Kaposi sarcoma 138.1–138.3, *138.4*, 138.5
  post-transplant lymphoproliferative disorder 139.47
human immunodeficiency virus *see* HIV infection
human leukocyte antigens (HLA) 8.7
  drug hypersensitivity reactions 14.6–14.7, **14.6**
  gold reactions 121.4
  rheumatoid nodules 97.15
human monocytic/granulocytic ehrlichiosis *see* ehrlichiosis
human papillomavirus (HPV) 2.13, 25.49–25.73, **25.50–25.51**
  acquired immunodeficiencies 25.65, **25.66**, 25.71–25.73
  Bowen disease 141.19

bowenoid papulosis 141.21
  cutaneous squamous cell carcinoma 141.30, 141.31
  epidermodysplasia verruciformis 25.65–25.66, 25.69–25.71
  female genitalia 110.30–110.31
  HIV 31.25–31.26, 31.31–31.32, 31.35–31.36
  inborn errors of immunity 25.65–25.71
  male genitalia 109.29
  neoplasia associations 25.64–25.65
  oral squamous cell carcinoma 108.46
  perineal and perianal skin 111.16, 111.17–111.19
  in pregnancy 113.4
  see also ano-genital warts; cutaneous warts
human parechoviruses (HPeV) 25.96
human polyomavirus (HPyV), Merkel cell carcinoma 146.2, 146.3, *146.4*
human polyomavirus-6 and -7 (HPyV-6 and HPyV-7) 25.48–25.49
human polyomavirus-8 (HPyV-8) *see* trichodysplasia spinulosa polyomavirus
human polyomavirus-9 (HPyV-9) 25.49
human polyomavirus-10 (HPyV-10) 25.49
human retrovirus infections 25.78–25.80
human T-cell lymphotropic virus 1 (HTLV-1)
  adult T-cell leukaemia–lymphoma association 139.3, 139.34–139.36
  haematological and neurological disease association 25.79
  infective dermatitis 25.79–25.80
human T-cell lymphotropic viruses 2/3/4 (HTLV-2-4) 25.79
humectants
  allergies 127.59
  topical medication vehicles 18.5, 18.7
hunter gatherer groups 1.1
hunting reaction of Lewis 124.1
Huriez syndrome 63.66, *63.67*, **78.13**
Hurley stage I disease
  chronicity 90.8
  genito-femoral area *90.7*
Hurley stage II disease
  genito-femoral area *90.8*
  inflamed nodules *90.5*
  non-inflamed nodules *90.4*
Hurley stage III disease, lesions *90.9*
Hurley staging system 90.1, 90.6
  definition of stages **90.7**
  hidradenitis suppurativa 16.4, 111.11, **111.12**
Hutchinson lupus 124.6
Hutchinson sign 145.13
Hutchinson, Sir Jonathan 1.6–1.7
Hutchinson triad, congenital syphilis 29.26
Hutchinson–Gilford progeria syndrome (HGPS) 70.25–70.26, **72.5**, 77.4–77.5
HUV *see* hypocomplementaemic urticarial; hypocomplementaemic urticarial vasculitis
HV *see* hydroa vacciniforme
HVLL *see* hydroa vacciniforme-like lymphoma
hyaline degeneration 3.40
hyaline fibromatosis syndrome 70.21–70.22, 94.42–94.43
hyalinising fat necrosis 97.8
hyaluronic acid (HA) 2.37, 2.39
  dermal filler *158.2*, *158.3*, 158.4–158.6, 158.8
    adverse reaction *158.9*, **158.11**
    haematoxylin and eosin staining of *158.10*
  skin elasticity 122.5
hydantoin, hypermelanosis 86.26–86.27
hydatid disease *see* echinococcosis
hydration
  irritant contact dermatitis 128.6
  mechanical injuries 122.6–122.7
hydroarsenicism 121.2
hydroa vacciniforme (HV) 126.24–126.27, 126.33
hydroa vacciniforme-like lymphoma (HVLL) 139.36

hydrocarbon-based formulations, topical drugs 12.3
hydrocortisone
  allergy 127.19
  topical therapies 18.14
hydrogels 12.3
hydrogen cyanide inhalation 125.4
hydrogen peroxide, topical therapies 18.10
hydropic degeneration 3.40
hydrops fetalis (HF) 103.23
hydroquinone
  cosmeceutical use of 157.3–157.4
  topical depigmenting agents 18.31–18.32
hydrotherapy, ichthyoses management 63.43
hydroxy acids 157.4–157.5
hydroxybenzoates 127.54–127.58
hydroxycarbamide 19.21–19.22
  dermatological uses 19.21
  drug–drug interactions 19.22
  potential adverse effects 19.21–19.22
  psoriasis treatment 35.26
  safety precautions 19.22
hydroxychloroquine
  eye, side effects on 107.43
  morphoea treatment 55.38
  sarcoidosis management 96.16, *96.17*
hydroxyethlmethacrylate (HEMA) and ethylmethacrylate microspheres suspended in hyaluronic acid, dermal fillers 158.8
hydroxyethyl acrylate 127.70
2-hydroxyethylmethacrylate (2-HEMA) 127.70
hydroxyethyl starch (HES), pruritus induction 81.11, 117.3
hydroxylation reactions, collagens 2.29, *2.30*
Hydrozoa, stings from 130.1
hyfrecation treatment, acne vulgaris *88.57*
hygiene
  atopic eczema 5.14, 41.7–41.8
  COVID-19 considerations 20.6–20.7
  pressure ulcer prevention 123.9
  skin surgery 20.5–20.7
hymenal fissures, mechanical 110.42–110.43
hymenoptera 34.15–34.18
  classification 34.16
  clinical features 34.17
  management 34.17–34.18
  pathophysiology of venom reactions 34.16–34.17
  systemic anaphylactic reactions 34.17–34.18
  venom immunotherapy 34.18
hyperacute dermatomyositis 52.5
hyperaldosteronism 150.17
hyperandrogenism 87.68, 87.88–87.89
  acne vulgaris *88.45*
  dermatoendocrinology 150.18
  pseudofolliculitis 91.9
hyperbaric oxygen (HBO), lymphoedema therapy 103.59–103.60
hypercalcaemia
  cutaneous metastatic calcification 59.5–59.6
  subcutaneous fat necrosis 97.57–97.58
hypercholanaemia, familial 2.21
hypercholesterolaemia **60.2**, 60.6–60.8
hypercoagulable states
  resulting in venous and arterial thrombosis 25.111
  superficial thrombophlebitis 97.9
hypercortisolism *see* Cushing disease/syndrome
hypereosinophilic syndrome, oral involvement 108.70
hypergammaglobulinaemic purpura 99.6–99.7
hyperglycaemia, burn injuries 125.14
hypergranulosis 3.41
hyperhidrosis 92.4–92.10
  anhidrosis 92.11–92.12
  eccrine gland disorders **92.11**
  epidermolysis bullosa simplex 69.8

gustatory 83.24, 92.5–92.6, 92.8, 92.9, **104.10**
  internal malignancy links 148.18–148.19
  management 92.8–92.10
  pachyonychia congenita 67.12
  shoe allergy 127.68
  skin disorders 92.8
  surgical treatment 92.9–92.10
  therapeutic use of antiperspirants 18.37–18.38
hyper/hypothyroidism **150.7**, **150.10**, **150.11**, 150.19–150.20
hyper-IgE syndrome due to STAT3 loss of function mutations 80.17
hyperimmunoglobulinaemia-D syndrome (HIDS) *see* mevalonate kinase deficiency
hyperinsulinaemia, obesity association 98.28
hyperkeratosis 3.41
  congenital epidermal naevi 73.4
  dermatomyositis 52.3, *52.8*
  'hystrix' like 63.17–63.18, *63.19*
  in ichthyoses 63.2, 63.10, 63.20
  inverted follicular keratosis 137.2–137.3
  of the nipple 63.79
hyperkeratosis lenticularis perstans *see* Flegel disease
hyperkeratotic cutaneous capillary–venous malformations (HCCVM) 71.2
hyperkeratotic disorders with skin fragility 69.20
hyperkeratotic lesions
  autoinflammatory diseases **80.19**
  elastosis perforans serpiginosa 94.55
  human polyomavirus-9 infection in organ transplant recipients 25.49
  tyrosinaemia type 2 *79.12*
hyperkeratotic palmar eczema 39.14
hyperkeratotic papules
  keratosis circumscripta *85.14*
  peristomal skin *112.7*
hyperkeratotic spicules, multiple minute digitate hyperkeratoses 63.77, *85.19*
hyperlipidaemia
  diabetes association 62.3, *62.4*
  granuloma annulare 95.1
  psoriasis association 35.18
hyperlipoproteinaemias
  classification **60.1**
  type I 60.9
  type III 60.8–60.9
  type IV 60.10
  type V 60.9–60.10
hypermelanosis 86.8
  acquired disorders 86.9–86.33
  drug origin 86.25–86.31, 86.53–86.54
  endocrine disorders 86.17–86.19
  solid malignant tumours 86.19, 86.20
  systemic disorders 86.19–86.25
  vitamin A deficiency 86.23–86.24
  see also hyperpigmentation
hypermetabolism, burn injuries 125.11–125.14
hypermobile Ehlers–Danlos syndromes (hEDS) 70.2–70.8, **70.3**
hypermobility (flexibility), Beighton score **70.8**
hyperoestrogenism 150.18
hyperparathyroidism
  dermatoendocrinology 150.20
  metastatic calcinosis cutis 59.5
hyperphosphataemia, cutaneous metastatic calcification 59.6
hyperphosphataemic familial tumoral calcinosis (HFTC) **79.10**, 79.17–79.18
hyperpigmentation
  acanthosis nigricans 62.3
  acne 88.41
  atopic eczema *41.14*, *41.17*
  autoinflammatory diseases **80.19**
  Bloom syndrome *80.11*
  chemical peels, side effect of 160.12–160.13, *160.14*

chemotherapy-induced 119.8–119.9
chronic venous insufficiency **101.43**, *101.44*
compound naevus *131.21*
dermal fillers, adverse reaction to 158.11–158.12
disorders of 68.1, 68.10–68.14
  due to cupping *4.12*
  dyskeratosis congenita 67.13, *80.12*
  freckle *131.2*
  from sun exposure in Whipple disease 153.4
  HIV 31.12
  ink-spot lentigo *131.8*
  lentigo simplex *131.4*
  linear morphoea en coup de sabre *55.24*
  male genitalia **109.42**
  melasma 86.10
    laser therapy 161.5–161.6
  morphoea *55.18*, 86.20–86.21
  mucosal melanosis *131.10*
  Nelson syndrome *86.7*
  neonates 114.4
  oral hyperpigmentation 108.14–108.19
  penile lentiginosis *131.10*
  peristomal skin *112.5*
  pigmentary mosaicism *115.13*
  pityriasis versicolor 32.11
  rheumatic diseases 86.20
  simple lentigo *131.4*
  systemic sclerosis 54.17
  vitamin B12 deficiency *61.20*
  see also hypermelanosis
hyperpituitarism 150.16–150.17
hyperplasia 97.5
  denture-induced hyperplasia 108.10
  Merkel cells 2.12
  ocular features *107.41*
  papillary hyperplasia 108.12, 136.23–136.24
  pseudoepitheliomatous 132.9–132.10
  Raynaud phenomenon 124.11
  sebaceous glands 91.17–91.18
  squamous 109.34–109.35
  see also PIK3CA-related overgrowth spectrum
hypersensitivity syndromes
  azathioprine 19.9
  dapsone 19.15
hypersensitivity to drugs *see* immunological reactions to drugs
hypertension
  nail–patella syndrome 67.16
  psoriasis association 35.18
hypertensive ischaemic leg ulcers (HYTILUs) 102.10–102.13
  clinical features 102.11–102.12
  epidemiology 102.10
  investigations 102.12–102.13
  management 102.13
  pathophysiology 102.10–102.11
hyperthermia, drug-induced 120.4
hyperthermic therapy, cutaneous warts 25.59
hyperthyroidism 86.19
  flushing **104.5**
hypertrichosis 87.84–87.87
  alopecia areata 87.35
  chemotherapy-induced 119.6
  congenital melanocytic naevi 73.12
  eyebrows 107.4
  medical disorders 87.87
  paradoxical hypertrichosis following laser-assisted hair removal 23.20
hypertriglyceridaemia **60.2**, 60.9–60.10
  haemophagocytic lymphohistiocytosis 135.12
  management 98.3
  type I hyperlipoproteinaemia 60.9
  type IV hyperlipoproteinaemia 60.10
  type V hyperlipoproteinaemia 60.9–60.10
hypertrophic photoageing 156.3
hypertrophic scars 11.9, 94.48–94.53
  laser therapies 23.12, 161.5
hypertrophy 97.5

hypoandrogenism 150.18
hypocalcaemia, vitamin D deficiency 61.10
hypocomplementaemic urticarial vasculitis (HUV) syndrome 44.1, 44.2, 44.3–44.4, 44.5, 100.18–100.19
hypoglycaemia, burn injuries 125.14
hypoglycaemic drugs, allergic reactions 62.4
hypohydrosis, ichthyoses 63.46
hypomelanosis 86.8
　acquired 86.34–86.47
　idiopathic guttate hypomelanosis-like hypopigmented macules and lentigines 21.12
hypomelanosis of Ito 68.9–68.10
hyponychial pigmentation, melanoma involving nail unit 145.13
hyponychium 2.11
hypo-oestrogenism 150.18–150.19
hypoparathyroidism 150.20–150.21
hypopigmentation
　actinic prurigo 126.12
　chemical peels, side effect of 160.14
　chemotherapy-induced 119.10–119.11
　Cole disease 63.61
　disorders of 68.1, 68.3–68.10
　HIV 31.12
　infantile seborrhoeic dermatitis 115.2
　male genitalia 109.28, **109.42**, 109.43
　onchocerciasis 33.4–33.5
　patch testing 127.31
　pityriasis versicolor 32.11, *32.12*
　systemic lupus erythematosus 51.28
hypopigmented sarcoidosis 96.12–96.13
hypopituitarism 150.7, **150.10**, **150.11**, *150.13*, 150.15–150.16
hypoplasia
　congenital pseudo-ainhum 94.48
　eyebrows 107.4
hypoplasminogenaemia, oral involvement 108.70
hypopyon, iritis 48.6
hyposensitisation, allergic contact dermatitis 127.35
hypostatic eczema *see* venous eczema
hypostatic haemosiderosis 86.47–86.49
hypothalamic–pituitary–adrenal (HPA) axis 87.11, 150.2
hypothalamic–pituitary–thyroid (HPT) axis, hair follicle 87.11
hypothalamopituitary–thyroid (HPT) axis 150.2
hypothenar hammer syndrome 122.13, 122.24
hypothyroidism
　acquired ichthyosis 85.2
　diffuse telogen effluvium *87.55*
　granuloma annulare 95.1
　heat-associated carcinomas 124.15–124.16
hypotrichosis
　eyelashes 107.4
　ichthyosis with 63.40
hypotrichosis–lymphoedema–telangiectasia syndrome (HLTS) 71.26, 103.23
hypoxia, neonates 114.3
hysteresis, stress-strain relationship 122.3
hystrix-like hyperkeratosis 63.17–63.18, *63.19*
hystrix-like ichthyosis and deafness (HID) syndrome 63.34–63.35
HYTILUs *see* hypertensive ischaemic leg ulcers

I

iatrogenic calcinosis 59.3
iatrogenic hypercarotenaemia 86.50
iatrogenic immunosuppression
　human papillomavirus 25.71
　viral infections 149.20, *149.21*
IBD *see* inflammatory bowel disease
ibuprofen, flux measurement 12.6
ICAS *see* International Alliance for the Control of Scabies
ICD *see* irritant contact dermatitis

ice pack dermatosis 97.37
ICH-GCP *see* International Conference on Harmonisation Good Clinical Practice
ichthyoses 63.2–63.3
　acquired forms 63.47–63.49
　common forms 63.3–63.7
　congenital forms 63.41–63.79
　glycosylation disorders **79.10**
　hypotrichosis 63.40
　keratinopathic forms **63.4**, 63.13–63.18
　management 63.41–63.46
　neuro-ichthyotic syndromes 63.30–63.39
　non-syndromic **63.3**, 63.20–63.22
　syndromic **63.3**, 63.39–63.47, *63.39*
　trichothiodystrophy 76.10
ichthyosiform atrophy 139.49
ichthyosiform erythroderma 39.33, *63.36*
ichthyosiform sarcoidosis 96.13
ichthyosis
　acquired 63.47–63.50, 63.73, 85.1–85.3, 148.17
　syndromic **63.3**, 63.22–63.62
ichthyosis Curth–Macklin (ICM) 63.16–63.17
ichthyosis follicularis–atrichia–photophobia (IFAP) syndrome 63.24–63.25
ichthyosis linearis circumflexa *63.27*
ichthyosis vulgaris 2.6, 63.3–63.5
　atopic eczema association 41.15
　KP association 85.9
ichthyosis–follicular atrophoderma– hypotrichosis–hypohidrosis (IFAH) 63.40
ichthyosis–prematurity syndrome (IPS) 63.39–63.40
ichthyotic disorders 3.44
ichthyotic epidermal disorders 148.17
ICI *see* immune checkpoint inhibitors
ICM *see* ichthyosis Curth–Macklin
ICU *see* immune contact urticaria
IDEOM *see* International Dermatology Outcome Measures
idiopathic acrocyanosis 124.7
idiopathic AGL 98.3
idiopathic circumscribed hyperhidrosis 92.7, 92.9
idiopathic cutaneous mucinoses 57.1, 57.2–57.18
idiopathic dermatitis 112.5
idiopathic facial aseptic granuloma (IFAG) 89.16
idiopathic generalised anhidrosis 92.12
idiopathic guttate hypomelanosis (IGH) 86.45–86.47
　ageing of skin 156.5, *156.6*
idiopathic guttate hypomelanosis-like hypopigmented macules and lentigines 21.12
idiopathic hirsutism 87.88, 87.90
idiopathic inflammatory myopathies (IIMs) 52.1–52.13
idiopathic livedo reticularis 124.8, 124.9–124.10
idiopathic lymphadenopathies 149.16–149.18
idiopathic mid-dermal elastolysis *94.25*, 94.26
idiopathic photodermatoses 126.1, 126.2–126.27
idiopathic thrombocytopenic purpura, oral involvement 108.70
idiotrophic calcification 59.4–59.5
IDN *see* intradermal naevi
idoxuridine 18.13
IDQoL *see* Infants' Dermatitis Quality of Life Index
IEI (inborn errors of immunity) *see* inherited immunodeficiency
IFAG *see* idiopathic facial aseptic granuloma
IFAH *see* ichthyosis-follicular atrophoderma–hypotrichosis– hypohidrosis
IFAP syndrome *see* ichthyosis follicularis– atrichia–photophobia syndrome

IFD *see* International Foundation for Dermatology
IFN-α2a *see* interferon α2a
IFN-α2b *see* intralesional interferon α2b
IFN α *see* interferon α
IgA pemphigus 50.6–50.7
IgA vasculitis 100.13–100.15
　fibrin deposition *100.14*
　leukocytoclasis *100.14*
　see also antineutrophil cytoplasmic antibody associated small vessel vasculitis
IgE *see* immunoglobulin E
IgE-related type 1 skin hypersensitivity 9.9–9.10
IgE test *see* immunoglobulin E test
IGF-1 *see* insulin-like growth factor
IgG4 disease, oral involvement 108.67
IgG4-related skin disease, ear dermatoses **106.22**
Iggo discs 2.12
IGH *see* idiopathic guttate hypomelanosis
IgM pemphigoid 50.53–50.54
IGRAs *see* interferon γ release assays
IHS4 *see* International Hidradenitis Suppurativa Severity Score System
IIEF *see* International Index of Erectile Function
IIF *see* indirect immunofluorescence
IIMs *see* idiopathic inflammatory myopathies
IL-1 antagonists, systemic therapy 19.37
IL-4/IL-13 antagonists, systemic therapy 19.36–19.37
IL-4/IL-13 inhibitors, atopic eczema treatment 41.29–41.30
IL-10 signalling disorders 45.16
IL-12/IL-23 p40 inhibitor, psoriasis treatment 35.29
IL-17 antagonists, systemic therapy 19.34, 19.35–19.36
IL-17 inhibitors, psoriasis treatment 35.30
IL-23 antagonists, systemic therapy 19.34, 19.35
IL-23/IL-17 antagonists, systemic therapy 19.34–19.35
IL-23p 19 inhibitors, psoriasis treatment 35.30–35.31
IL36RN gene, pustular psoriasis 118.2, 118.3
ILCs *see* innate lymphoid cells
ILD *see* interstitial lung disease
ILDS *see* International League of Dermatological Societies
ILE *see* lipid injectable emulsion
ileal metaplasia, urostomy 112.7
ileostomy **112.3**
　Candida infection *112.8*, *112.9*
　Crohn ulceration *112.13*, *112.14*
　granulation tissue with bowel metaplasia *112.6*
　'granulomas' beneath the stoma *112.6*
　leakage and eroded dermatitis due to corrosive faecal contents *112.4*
　leakage and hyperkeratotic papules *112.7*
　length of 112.5
　nicorandil ulceration *112.12*
　portal hypertension affecting peristomal skin *112.9*
　postinflammatory hyperpigmentation 112.5
　pyoderma gangrenosum *112.14*, *112.15*
　synergic gangrene *112.10*
　see also stomas
ILEP *see* International Federation of Anti-Leprosy Associations
IL-F *see* infiltrating lipomatosis of the face
ILFAD *see* intestinal failure-associated liver disease
iliac horns, nail–patella syndrome 67.16
iliohypogastric neuropathic pain/neuralgia 83.7
ilioinguinal neuropathic pain/neuralgia 83.7
illicit drugs
　ChemSex 120.2–120.3

dermatoses induced by 120.1–120.9
legal aspects 120.3–120.4
iloprost 124.12
ILP *see* isolated limb perfusion
IMACS *see* International Myositis Assessment and Clinical Studies
images, digital 1.9
imaging, melanoma diagnosis 142.9–142.10
imaging examination 4.22–4.23
imaging systems, diagnosis 4.20–4.22
imatinib, Erdheim–Chester disease treatment 135.22
imidazoles 18.12, 19.48
imidazolidinyl urea 127.51–127.52
IMIDs *see* immune-mediated inflammatory diseases
imiquimod 18.30
　basal cell carcinoma topical treatment 140.12, *140.16*
5% imiquimod cream, Bowen disease 141.23
immediate pigment darkening (IPD) 86.9
　UV radiation exposure 10.7
immediate-type reactions, contact urticaria 128.8
immediate-type stinging 128.10
immediate-weal tests 4.24
immobility, lymphoedema due to 103.40
immune cells 9.2–9.6
　chemical staining of 9.2
　dermal immune cells 9.4–9.6
　embryonic development of skin 2.3, *2.4*
　epidermal immune cells 9.3–9.4
　lymphoid lineage cells 9.5
　mucosal associated invariant T (MAIT) cells 9.5
　myeloid lineage cells 9.4–9.5
　peripheral blood 9.6
　plasma cells 9.6
　skin draining lymph node 9.6
　T cells 9.4, 9.5–9.7, 14.4, *14.5*, 50.2, 127.9
immune checkpoint inhibitors (ICI) 87.74
　cutaneous side effects of cancer immunotherapy 144.9–144.12
　cutaneous squamous cell carcinoma 141.33–141.34
　melanoma systemic therapy 144.2, *144.3*, 144.4, **144.6**, **144.8**, 144.9
immune complex small-vessel vasculitis 152.4
immune contact urticaria (ICU) 127.83–127.84, 127.86
immune dysregulation 80.13–80.15
　inherited immunodeficiency 80.2, **80.5**
immune ecosystem 2.12–2.13
immune function
　hidradenitis suppurativa predisposition 90.2–90.3
　and skin ageing 2.45
immune mechanisms, allergic contact dermatitis 127.6
immune-mediated inflammatory diseases (IMIDs)
　skin cancer risks 147.5
　systemic sclerosis 54.10–54.11
immune-modulating treatments, molluscum contagiosum infection 25.18
immune privilege, hair follicle 87.11, 87.22
immune reconstitution-associated disease (IRAD), antiretroviral HIV therapy effects 31.8, **31.38**
immune response, wound healing 11.2–11.3
immune surveillance 2.15, *2.16*
immune suppression, UV radiation in Merkel cell carcinoma 146.3
immune system
　dermatophytosis 32.21
　human papillomavirus 25.52
　in pregnancy 113.3–113.4
　skin disorders 149.16–149.22
　skin microbiome 26.5, 26.6
　see also immunology
immunoadsorption, pemphigus treatment 50.9

immunobullous disease 50.1–50.60
  anti-p200 pemphigoid 50.38–50.42
  bullous systemic lupus erythematous 50.48–50.51
  cicatrising conjunctivitis association 107.24–107.34
  dermatitis herpetiformis 50.54–50.59
  epidermolysis bullosa acquista 50.42–50.48
  female genitalia 110.20, **110.21**
  immunopathology **50.2**
  linear IgA disease 50.33–50.38
  mucous membrane pemphigoid 50.22–50.33
  oral involvement 108.80–108.82
  pemphigus 50.1–50.9
  rare pemphigoid disorders 50.51–50.54
  serological diagnosis *3.20*
  subepidermal diseases 50.9–50.59
immunocompromised patients
  antiviral agent prophylaxis 25.31, 25.42, 25.75
  cutaneous squamous cell carcinomas 147.10–147.11, 147.16–147.18
  cytomegalovirus infection 25.41
  haemophagocytic lymphohistiocytosis with infectious mononucleosis 25.37
  HPyV9 infection and hyperkeratotic skin lesions in organ transplant recipients 25.49
  Kaposi sarcoma 138.1, 147.2, 147.3, 147.14, 147.20–147.21, 147.23
  Kaposi sarcoma-associated herpesvirus 25.42, 25.43
  keratinocyte cancers 147.10–147.11, 147.16–147.21
  melanoma 147.13–147.14, 147.21, 147.23
  mpox infection 25.10
  non-tuberculous mycobacteria disseminated disease 27.32–27.36, 27.38, 27.40–27.45
  reactivation of human herpesvirus 6 and 7 25.39, 25.40
  reduced tumour immune surveillance, UV radiation related skin cancers 147.5–147.6
  skin cancer 147.1–147.26
    clinicopathological features 147.10–147.16
    management 147.16–147.24
    organisations 147.25
    pathogenesis 147.5–147.10
    primary and acquired immunodeficiencies 147.1–147.5
    risk of, drug effects on 147.5–147.8
    screening and surveillance 147.24–147.25
    ultraviolet radiation effects 147.5–147.6
  vaccinia infection 25.7–25.8
  varicella infection 25.30–25.31
immunodeficiency
  acquired *see* acquired immunodeficiency diseases
  neoplasia syndromes 148.13–148.14
immunodeficiency-associated eosinophilic pustular folliculitis 91.5
immunodeficiency, inherited *see* inherited immunodeficiency
immunodysregulation polyendocrinopathy enteropathy X-linked syndrome (IPEX) 80.14
immunoenzyme methods 3.14–3.16
  avidin–biotin coupling of antibody and enzyme 3.15–3.16
  chemical conjugation of peroxidase to antibody 3.14–3.16
  conjugates, use of 3.14–3.15
  controls 3.15
  enzyme-linked immunosorbent assay 3.16
  fixed frozen sections, examination of 3.15
  immunofluorescence comparison **3.14**
  paraffin sections 3.15
  technical limitations 3.14

immunofluorescence methods 3.10–3.14
  calcium enhancement indirect technique 3.14
  dermal–epidermal basement membrane zone 2.23
  direct immunofluorescence 3.11–3.12
  epidermolysis bullosa diagnosis 69.21, *69.22*
  and histopathology 3.11
  immunoenzyme methods comparison **3.14**
  indirect immunofluorescence 3.12–3.13
  photobleaching (fading) limitation 3.11
  specimen preparation
    DIF analysis 3.11–3.12
    IIF analysis 3.13
  specimen processing
    DIF analysis 3.12
    split-skin indirect technique 3.13–3.14
  specimen selection, DIF analysis **3.11**
  split-skin indirect technique 3.13–3.14
  types of 3.11
immunogenotyping 3.31
immunoglobulin E (IgE)
  atopic eczema 41.11
  IgE-mediated drug hypersensitivity 14.1–14.2
immunoglobulin E (IgE) test, contact dermatitis 129.7
immunoglobulin E test, contact dermatitis 129.7
immunoglobulin G4-related disease 149.17–149.18
immunoglobulin variable domains, naming conventions 19.31, **19.32**
immunohistochemistry, Merkel cell carcinoma 146.3, *146.4*, **146.5**
immunological abnormalities, chronic mucocutaneous candidiasis 32.68
immunological dysregulation, obesity 98.27–98.28
immunological photodermatoses 126.1, 126.2–126.27
immunological reactions to drugs 14.1–14.7
  clinical phenotype 14.6–14.7
  erythroderma 39.33
  hypersensitivity reaction, mechanisms and clinical correlations **14.2**
  IgE-mediated drug hypersensitivity 14.1–14.2
  pseudoallergic reactions 14.2–14.3
  T-cell-mediated drug hypersensitivity 14.3–14.4
  T-cell recognition of drugs 14.4–14.6
  type 4 hypersensitivity reaction, mechanisms and clinical correlations 14.2
immunological tolerance, allergic contact dermatitis 127.9
immunology 9.2–9.8
  atopic eczema 41.9–41.10
  erythema multiforme 47.2–47.3
  HIV 31.3–31.5
  immune cells in human skin 9.2–9.6, *103.14*
  and lymphatic system 103.2
  skin immune network in humans and mice 9.7
  and skin microbiota 9.7–9.8, *103.2*, 103.3
  systemic lupus erythematosus 51.20–51.21
  tissue homeostasis 9.6–9.7
  see also immune system
immunomodulation, UV radiation exposure 10.8–10.9
immunomodulators, in pregnancy **113.22–113.23**
immunomodulatory therapy 1.8
  risk reduction 19.3
  systemic therapy 19.2–19.46
  terminology 19.2
immunomodulatory therapy 3.10–3.29
immunopathogenesis, sarcoidosis 96.3–96.4
immunopathology 3.10–3.29
  applications of 3.16–3.29
    cutaneous neoplasms 3.21–3.29

direct immunofluorescence 3.17–3.19
enzyme-linked immunosorbent assay 3.20–3.21
indirect immunofluorescence 3.19–3.20
cell markers, immunocytochemistry panels **3.10**
immunocytochemistry panels of cell markers **3.10**
immunoenzyme methods 3.14–3.16
immunofluorescence methods 3.10–3.14
immunophenotyping, ichthyoses 63.45
immunostaining, oral mucosal vesiculobullous disorders **108.81**
immunosuppression
  actinic keratoses 141.1, 141.3
  Bowen disease 141.18
  ciclosporin 19.10–19.12
  cutaneous squamous cell carcinoma 141.3, 141.27, 141.29
  eosinophilic pustular folliculitis 91.3, 91.4–91.5, 93.7, 93.8–93.9
  infective panniculitis 97.46–97.47
  joint infections 155.4
  Merkel cell carcinoma 146.2, 146.9
  mucous membrane pemphigoid *107.31*
  oral candidiasis 32.58, 32.61
  renal transplantation, dermatological consequences of 154.5–154.6
  squamous cell carcinoma 141.6, 141.27, 141.29
  systemic amyloidoses treatment 56.14
  systemic lupus erythematosus treatment 51.37–51.38
  trichodysplasia spinulosa 85.15–85.16
  versus immunomodulatory drugs 19.2–19.3
  see also organ transplant recipients
immunosuppressive therapy
  acneform reaction 88.12–88.13
  post-transplant lymphoproliferative disorder 139.47
  skin cancer risks 147.5–147.8, 147.19–147.20
immunotherapy
  checkpoint inhibitors for melanoma therapy 144.2, *144.3*, 144.4, **144.6**, **144.8**
  combination therapies for melanoma 144.2–144.3
  cutaneous T-cell lymphoma 139.22–139.23
  melanoma 144.2–144.4
  Merkel cell carcinoma 146.9
  systemic, cutaneous warts 25.60
  topical, cutaneous warts 25.59–25.60
Impact of Chronic Skin Disease on Daily Life (ISDL) 16.7
Impact of Psoriasis Questionnaire (IPSO) 16.8
impacts of skin disease, measurement 16.5–16.13
impairment, caused by skin disease 5.5–5.6
impetigo
  clinical features 26.14–26.16
  epidemiology 26.13–26.14
  eyelid 107.38
  infants 115.7
  management 26.16
  oral infection 108.53
  pathophysiology 26.14
  Staphylococcus aureus and *Streptococcus pyogenes* 26.13–26.16
  see also bullous impetigo
implantable defibrillators, cutaneous reactions 151.5–151.6
implanted metals, cutaneous reactions 127.19
implants
  brachytherapy 24.3
  types of **108.62**
IMPSG *see* International Melanoma Pathology Study Group
IMRT *see* intensity modulated radiotherapy
inborn errors of immunity (IEI) *see* inherited immunodeficiency

inborn errors of metabolism *see* inherited metabolic diseases
incidence of disease 5.10, 5.14
inclusional/exclusional elliptical biopsies 20.8–20.9
inclusion body (digital) fibromatosis 136.10–136.11
incontinentia pigmenti (IP) *4.19*, 68.10–68.11, 69.24
indeterminate leprosy 28.4
indeterminate lymphocytic lobular panniculitis 97.39
index lesions, hidradenitis suppurativa 90.3–90.5
India, ancient medical texts 1.2–1.3
Indiana vesiculovirus *see* vesicular stomatitis virus
Indian skin phenotypes, photoageing *156.2*
indirect immunofluorescence (IIF) 3.12–3.13, 3.19–3.20
  mucous membrane pemphigoid 107.28
  negative and positive controls 3.14
  serological diagnosis of immunobullous disorders *3.20*
  substrates for 3.13
indolent systemic mastocytosis (ISM) 46.2–46.3, 46.10
infantile acropustulosis 114.8, 115.4
infantile digital fibromatosis 136.10–136.11
  see also inclusion body (digital) fibromatosis
infantile eosinophilic pustular folliculitis 91.3, 91.5–91.6, 93.7, 93.9–93.10
  differential diagnosis 93.**10**
infantile gluteal granuloma 115.3
infantile haemangiomas 116.1–116.7
  classification 116.2
  clinical variants 116.3–116.5
  complications and co-morbidities 116.5–116.6
  deep infantile haemangioma involving lateral neck *116.3*
  facial and neck plaque-type haemangiomas, evolution of *116.3*
  haemangioma precursor 116.2
  hepatic haemangioma 116.5
  laser therapies 23.8
  management 116.6–116.7
  multifocal cutaneous infantile haemangioma 116.5
  pathophysiology 116.2
  presentation 116.2–116.3
  propranolol treatment, protocol for *116.8*
  segmental infantile haemangioma **116.2**, 116.3–116.4
  treatment ladder for **116.7**
  ulceration 116.5, *116.6*
  vascular malformation comparison **116.1**
infantile haemangiopericytoma *see* infantile myofibromatosis
infantile/juvenile fibromatosis variant (non-desmoid type) *see* lipofibromatosis
infantile myofibromatosis 94.41–94.42, 136.39–136.40
infantile papular acrodermatitis *see* Gianotti–Crosti syndrome
infantile perianal pyramidal protusion 111.3
infantile Refsum disease 63.31
infantile sclerema neonatorum 97.60
infantile seborrhoeic dermatitis (ISD) 40.5, 41.22, 115.1–115.2
infantile stiff skin syndromes 70.21–70.24
  hyaline fibromatosis syndrome 70.21–70.22
  restrictive dermopathy 70.24
  stiff skin syndrome 70.22–70.23
  Winchester syndrome 70.23–70.24
infants 115.1–115.17
  acne 88.68–88.74, 115.4–115.5
  acropustulosis 114.8, 115.4
  acute haemorrhagic oedema 115.9, *115.10*
  acute scrotum 109.25–109.26
  Albright hereditary osteodystrophy *72.9*
  animal bite injuries 115.14

infants (*continued*)
annular erythema of infancy   47.9, *47.10*
arteriovenous malformations   *101.23*
atopic eczema   41.13, 41.14, 41.15, 41.26, 115.2–115.3
benign vascular tumours, vascular malformation distinction   **116.1**
bite injuries   115.14
blistering distal dactylitis   115.8
bronze baby syndrome   86.49–86.50
bullous pemphigoid   *50.20*
calcified cutaneous nodules of the heels   115.15
Candida infection   115.8
candidiasis of the napkin area   32.65
capillary malformations   *71.4*
chickenpox (varicella)   115.6–115.7
chronic infantile neurological cutaneous and articular syndrome   45.5, 45.6
circumcision, male   109.7
CLOVES syndrome   71.9, 72.11
cold panniculitis   97.36–97.37, 114.14
collodion baby phenotype   79.5
congenital candidiasis   32.66–32.67
congenital haemangiomas   116.7–116.9
congenital melanocytic naevi   73.12
COVID-19/SARS-CoV-2   115.5
cradle cap   115.1, *115.2*
cutis laxa   *70.17*
definition of infancy   115.1
dermoid cysts   115.12, *115.13*
developmental/genetic conditions   115.12–115.13
discrete papular lichen myxoedematosus   57.6
Ehlers–Danlos syndromes   70.11
eosinophilic pustular folliculitis   115.12
epidermolysis bullosa   69.24–69.25
eruption cyst, over a primary tooth   108.10
fibrous hamartoma of infancy   136.6–136.7
fifth disease/erythema infectiosum   115.6
flushing in   *104.10*, **104.10**
Gaucher disease   79.5
genetic conditions   115.12–115.13
Gianotti–Crosti syndrome   115.11
gluteal granuloma   115.3
haemangiomas   116.1–116.9
hair loss   114.4, 115.15
hand, foot and mouth disease   115.6
hepatic haemangioma   116.5
hereditary lymphoedema type 1A   *71.24*
human bite injuries   115.14
hyaline fibromatosis syndrome   70.21–70.22
impetigo   115.7
inclusion body (digital) fibromatosis   136.10–136.11
infective conditions   115.5–115.9
inflammatory conditions   115.1–115.5
iron deficiency   61.24, 61.25
JAK3-deficient severe combined immunodeficiency   *80.7*
juvenile xanthogranuloma   115.15
Kaposiform haemangioendothelioma   116.9–116.10
Kasbach–Merritt phenomenon   116.9–116.10
Kawasaki disease   115.9–115.11
koilonychia   115.14
Langerhans cell histiocytosis   115.15–115.16, 135.4, 135.5–135.7
linear IgA disease   115.11
linear morphoea   115.13
lipofibromatosis   136.13–136.14
lymphangioma   108.13
lymphangioma circumscriptum   103.25–103.28
lymphatic malformations   *71.22*
mastocytoma   *46.5*
mastocytosis   115.16–115.17
measles   115.7
Menkes disease   *79.17*
Michelin tyre baby syndrome   70.19, 73.17

midface toddler excoriation syndrome   82.9, 83.12–83.13
milia   115.13–115.14
molluscum contagiosum   115.9
multifocal cutaneous infantile haemangioma   116.5
napkin (diaper) dermatitis   115.3
neonatal lupus erythematosus   114.12–114.14
noma neonatorum (oro-facial gangrene)   114.27
non-accidental injury   115.14
non-malignant tumours   116.1–116.11
Omenn syndrome   80.7–80.8
papular urticaria   115.11–115.12
pedal papules of infancy   115.14, *115.15*
perianal pyramidal protusion   111.3
perianal streptococcal dermatitis   115.8
perianal ulcers, leukocyte adhesion deficiency type I   *80.16*
perianal viral warts   111.18, *111.19*
pigmentary mosaicism   115.13
pigmented neuroectodermal tumour   136.50–136.51
pityriasis alba   115.4
preauricular cysts and sinuses   115.12
psoriasis   115.3–115.4
pyogenic granuloma   116.10–116.11
raised linear bands of infancy   114.18–114.19
reactive conditions   115.9–115.12
restrictive dermopathy   70.24
roseola infantum   25.39–25.40, 115.5–115.6
scabies   115.9
seborrhoeic dermatitis   115.1–115.2
segmental infantile haemangioma   116.2, 116.3–116.4
severe combined immunodeficiency   *80.7*
staphylococcal scalded skin syndrome   114.24–114.25, 115.7–115.8
stiff skin syndrome   70.22–70.23
STING-associated vasculopathy   45.5, 45.6, 45.13–45.14, *80.18*
Sturge–Weber syndrome   *71.4*
tinea capitis   115.8–115.9
tinea corporis   115.8
tinea faciei   *115.8*
trichothiodystrophy syndrome   *76.10*
tufted angioma   116.10, *116.11*
Turner syndrome   *71.28*
urticaria   115.5
varicella   115.6–115.7
viral exanthems   115.5–115.7
Winchester syndrome   70.23–70.24
see also children; neonates
Infants' Dermatitis Quality of Life Index (IDQoL)   16.8, 16.10
Infants and Toddlers Quality of Life instrument (InToDermQoL)   16.10
infections
acquired ichthyosis   63.47, 85.1
burns   125.8–125.11, **125.10**
complications after skin surgery   **20.41**, 20.42
cutaneous lesions related to heart disease   151.5
dermatitis   39.25
dystrophic calcification   59.1
flexural sites   **4.18**
hair loss and   87.35–87.36
Helicobacter pylori associated with skin disorders   153.1
hidradenitis suppurativa differential diagnosis   90.5
HIV coinfections   **31.7**, 31.20–31.31
immune reconstitution-associated disease   31.8, 31.37–31.39
immunosuppressed renal allograft recipients   154.5–154.6
scalp   105.12
human immunodeficiency virus   105.12
syphilis   105.12
sexually transmitted infection overview   29.1–29.2
skin associated effects of respiratory tract infections   152.4

skin-related health anxieties   84.26
syphilis   29.1–29.29
Tropheryma whippelii/Whipple disease   97.47, 153.4, 155.5
infections of soft tissues, intravenous drug administration   120.7
infectious mononucleosis   25.36–25.37
infectious NEH   92.14
infective arthropathies   155.2–155.5
infective cheilitis   108.63
infective dermatitis   39.24–39.26
clinical features and variants   39.26
human T-cell lymphotropic virus 1   25.79–25.80
pathophysiology   39.25
treatment   39.26
infective eczematoid dermatitis   106.19
infective endocarditis, cutaneous lesions   151.5
infective panniculitis   97.46–97.48
infestations *see* myiasis; tungiasis
infiltrating lipomatosis of the face (IL-F)   98.19–98.20
infiltrative basal cell carcinoma   140.3, *140.4*
inflamed nodules, hidradenitis suppurativa   90.5
inflamed phyma, treatment   **89.13–89.14**
inflammation   9.8–9.9
acne vulgaris   **88.3**, 88.14–88.15, **88.27**, *88.28*
allergic inflammation   9.9–9.10
focal regression of melanoma   142.14
hand eczema   39.13
infants   115.1–115.5
inflammatory memory   9.9
pathological skin inflammation   9.8–9.9
pyoderma gangrenosum   49.3
viral exanthems   25.4–25.5
wound healing   9.6
see also delayed inflammatory reactions; multisystem inflammatory syndrome; pro-inflammatory topical treatments
inflammatory arthritides, oral involvement   108.68–108.69
inflammatory arthropathies   155.5–155.7, *155.8*, *155.9*
inflammatory bowel disease (IBD)
arthropathies   155.5
BADAS-associated   *49.16*
erythema nodosum in   97.21
eye disease   **107.35**
neonatal onset   45.16
psoriasis   112.10
skin complications of stomas   153.7
skin manifestations   153.1–153.3, **153.7**
see also Crohn disease; ulcerative colitis
inflammatory chondopathies   155.11–155.13
musculoskeletal features   155.11
inflammatory cutaneous lesions, laser therapies   23.12
inflammatory dermatoses
flexural sites   **4.18**
graft-versus-host disease   38.1–38.12
HIV   31.12–31.20
male genitalia   109.9–109.26
perineal and perianal skin   111.8–111.12
seborrhoeic dermatitis   40.1–40.10
transient acantholytic dermatosis   85.23–85.25
urticarial vasculitis   44.1–44.6
inflammatory diseases   1.8
Dermatology Index of Disease Severity   16.3
dystrophic calcification of skin and subcutaneous tissues   59.1–59.3
hidradenitis suppurativa association   90.2, 90.5–90.6
hypopigmentation   68.4
subcutaneous fat   97.6
inflammatory fibrosing conditions, internal malignancy association   148.21
inflammatory lesions, mouth   108.20–108.25
inflammatory myxohyaline tumour of the distal extremities with virocyte or Reed–Sternberg-like cells *see* myxoinflammatory fibroblastic sarcoma
inflammatory peeling skin syndromes   63.28, *63.29*
inflammatory plaques   **80.19**
inflammatory response
allergen exposure   127.7
melanoma   142.18
wound healing   11.2–11.3
inflammatory skin blistering, epidermolysis bullosa   *69.16*
infliximab
psoriasis treatment   35.27–35.28
psoriatic arthritis treatment   35.45
infraorbital lines, reduction of by botulinum toxin application   *159.7*
infrared (IR) radiation
disease causation   124.14–124.16
physiological reactions to   124.14
infudibulo-isthmicoma *see* pilar sheath acanthoma
infundibular cyst *see* epidermoid cysts
infundibular epithelial walled cutaneous cysts   133.1–133.4
infundibulofolliculitis   91.14–91.15, 93.6–93.7
infundibuloma, lesions/tumours of follicular infundibulum   137.3–137.4
infundibulomatosis, tumour of follicular infundibulum   137.3–137.4
infundibulum   87.3–87.4
ingenol mebutate   18.30–18.31
inguinal buboes, lymphogranuloma venereum   30.14, 30.15, 30.16, **30.17**, *30.18*
inguinal hyperhidrosis   92.6
inhalation injuries   125.4–125.5
inhalent-induced dermatoses   120.2, 120.4
inherited disorders   8.2–8.5, 8.8–8.9
cornification   63.1–63.80
of pigmentation   **68.2–68.3**
prenatal diagnosis   8.9–8.11
skin fragility   69.1–69.28
see also congenital entries; genetic disorders/syndromes; *hereditary entries*; inherited immunodeficiency; inherited metabolic diseases
inherited immunodeficiency   80.1–80.20
10 warning signs   80.2
antibody deficiencies   **80.5**, 80.13
autoinflammatory diseases   **80.19**
classification   80.3–80.4
clinical features   80.1–80.2
combined immunodeficiencies   **80.4**, 80.7–80.13
complement diseases   **80.6**, 80.18–80.20
autoimmunity defects   80.18–80.19
complement activation regulation defects   80.20
recurrent pyogenic infection   80.18
diagnostic laboratory tests   80.3
DNA repair defects   **80.4–80.5**
epidermodysplasia verruciformis   25.65–25.66, 25.69–25.71
GARFIELD acronym   80.2
human papillomavirus infection   25.65–25.71
immune dysregulation   80.2, **80.5**, 80.13–80.15
infectious disease-related manifestations   80.2
innate immunity defects   **80.6**, 80.16–80.18
management   80.3
neutrophil differentiation and adhesion defects   80.15–80.16
non-infectious non-specific manifestations   80.2–80.3
phagocytic defects   **80.5–80.6**, 80.15
severe combined immunodeficiency   **80.4**, 80.7–80.9
skin cancer   147.1–147.2

skin manifestations **80.4–80.6**, 149.18–149.20
warning signs 80.2
inherited metabolic diseases 79.1–79.18
 amino acid metabolism and transport disorders 79.10–79.15
 dermatological features **79.2**
 glycosylation disorders 79.9–79.10
 lipid metabolism disorders 79.15
 lysosomal storage disorders 79.1–79.8
 mitochondrial respiratory chain disorders 79.8–79.9
 vitamin and mineral disorders 79.15–79.18
inherited patterned lentiginosis 86.16
 oral hyperpigmentation 108.17
inherited skin tumour syndromes 78.1–78.15
 familial adenomatous polyposis 78.10–78.11
 neurofibromatoses 78.1–78.7
 skin syndromes linked with cancers 78.12–78.14
 tuberous sclerosis complex 78.7–78.10
inherited syndromes, Alagille syndrome 153.5
injecting drug use
 HIV 31.37
 localised lipoatrophy due to 98.10
 in pregnancy **113.21**
injections
 calcium-containing materials, dystrophic calcification of skin and subcutaneous tissues 59.3
 corticosteroid, localised lipoatrophy due to 98.11–98.12
 dermatitis artefacta 84.33
 insulin, fat hypertrophy due to 98.13–98.15
 intralesional corticosteroids 18.21–18.22
 sterile furuncles (abscesses) 26.23
injection techniques, local anaesthetics 20.8
injury healing *see* wound healing
ink-spot lentigo 131.8–131.9
 dermoscopic image *131.9*
 epidermis with lentiginous hyperplasia *131.8*
 hyperpigmentation *131.8*
innate immune cells, atopic eczema 41.11
innate immunity defects **80.6**, 80.16–80.18
innate lymphoid cells (ILCs) 2.12–2.13
 immune system 9.5
inner canthus, radiotherapy for skin cancer 24.10–24.11
inner root sheath (IRS) 2.9–2.10
 hair follicle 87.3–87.5
inoculation herpes simplex 25.28
insect bite-like reactions
 haematological malignancy association 148.23
 paraneoplastic manifestations of lymphoproliferative neoplasms 149.8–149.9
insecticides
 flea management 34.15
 head lice 34.21–34.22
insects 34.6–34.34
 bugs (Hemiptera) 34.25–34.30
 Diptera 34.6–34.13
 fleas/Siphonaptera 34.13–34.15
 hymenoptera 34.15–34.18
 larval invasion of tissues/myiasis **34.7**, 34.9–34.13
 lice (Phthiraptera) 34.18–34.25
 myiasis **34.7**, 34.9–34.13
 tungiasis 34.15
 see also mosquitoes
insensible sweating 2.9
in situ carcinoma of the skin 141.18–141.26
 anal/vulval/penile and perianal intraepithelial carcinoma 141.24, 141.26
 Bowen disease 141.18–141.24, *141.25*
 male genitalia 109.31–109.35
 see also Bowen disease

in situ melanomas, surgery 143.3
insulin
 allergic reactions to in diabetes 62.4
 lipodystrophy 62.4
insulin-induced fat hypertrophy 98.13
insulin-induced localised fat hypertrophy 98.14–98.15
insulin-induced localised lipoatrophy 98.10
insulin-like growth factor (IGF-1), burn treatment 125.13
insulin resistance (IR) 97.5
 acanthosis nigricans 85.3–85.6, **150.10**, *150.11*, *150.13*
 hirsutism association 87.90
 hypermetabolism 125.11
 secondary dyslipidaemia 60.11
insulin secretion 97.5
insulin sensitivity, adipocytes 97.5
integrins 2.24, *2.25*
 epidermolysis bullosa 69.4–69.5
intense pulsed light (IPL), hidradenitis suppurativa treatment 90.11
intensity modulated radiotherapy (IMRT) 24.3
intensive care treatment, and vitamin K deficiency 61.13
intention-to-treat (ITT) analysis, randomised controlled trials 17.12, 17.14
interdigital irritant contact dermatitis 128.4
interface dermatitis
 lichenoid exanthema *37.19*
 lichen planus *37.14*
interferon α2a (IFN-α2a), polymorphic light eruption 126.2
interferon α (IFN-α) therapy, cutaneous T-cell lymphoma 139.15, 139.16, 139.22–139.23, 139.25
interferon γ release assays (IGRAs), tuberculosis 27.4–27.5
interferons, melanoma immunotherapy 144.2
interleukin-16 polymorphisms 127.10
interleukins (2/4/13/31), pruritus **81.3**, 81.4–81.5
intermediate dystrophic epidermolysis bullosa 69.15
intermediate epidermolysis bullosa simplex 69.8–69.11
intermediate junctional epidermolysis bullosa, molecular pathology 69.12–69.13, 69.14
internal malignancy
 cutaneous markers 148.1–148.28
 PUVA phototherapy adverse effects 21.14
International Alliance for the Control of Scabies (ICAS) 7.9
International Conference on Harmonisation Good Clinical Practice (ICH-GCP) guidelines 13.13
International Criteria for Behçet Disease (ICBD) **108.40**
International Dermatology Outcome Measures (IDEOM) 16.3
International dermatomyositis classification of severity 52.10
International Federation of Anti-Leprosy Associations (ILEP) 7.10
International Foundation for Dermatology (IFD) 7.6
international health *see* global health dermatology
International Hidradenitis Suppurativa Severity Score System (IHS4) 16.5
International Index of Erectile Function (IIEF) 16.12
International League of Dermatological Societies (ILDS) 7.5–7.6
International Melanoma Pathology Study Group (IMPSG) 142.3
International Myositis Assessment and Clinical Studies (IMACS) group 52.7, 52.10, 52.12
International Society for Pharmacoeconomics and Outcomes Research (ISPOR) 16.2

International Study of Asthma and Allergies in Childhood (ISAAC) 41.3
internet phenomena, Morgellons syndrome 84.11–84.12
interpolation flaps 20.27
interstitial collagenase 2.31
interstitial granulomatous dermatitis
 musculoskeletal involvement 155.14
 rheumatoid arthritis involvement *53.6*
interstitial keratitis, congenital syphilis 29.25
interstitial lung disease (ILD)
 dermatomyositis 52.1, 52.2, 52.7, 52.11–52.12
 junctional epidermolysis bullosa with 69.15
intertriginous eruption associated with chemotherapy 119.2
intertrigo **109.3**
intestinal failure-associated liver disease (ILFAD) 61.32
intestinal lymphangiectasia 103.32
intestinal polyposis disorders 153.4
intestinal worms, enterobiasis 33.14–33.15
InToDermQoL *see* Infants and Toddlers Quality of Life instrument
intracutaneous neurohormone metabolism 150.7
intradermal injection 4.23
intradermal naevi (IDN), dermoscopic patterns 145.6
intradermal tests, for detection of delayed sensitivity to antigens 4.24–4.25
intraepidermal cleavage, epidermolysis bullosa diagnosis 69.22
intraepidermal sweat unit 92.2
intraepithelial carcinomas, anal/perianal/genital areas 141.24, 141.26
intraepithelial neoplasia
 human papillomavirus association 25.64
 see also cervical intraepithelial neoplasia
intrahepatic cholestasis of pregnancy 113.13–113.14
intra-individual comparative analysis of naevi
 dermoscopy 145.2
 melanoma diagnosis *142.9*
intralesional corticosteroids 20.47
 reactions to 122.19–122.21
 surgical indications 20.47
intralesional cytotoxics, cutaneous warts 25.60
intralesional injection, corticosteroids 18.21–18.22
intralesional interferon α2b (IFN-α2b) 140.13–140.14
intralesional therapies
 hidradenitis suppurativa 90.9
 skin malignancies 20.47–20.48
intralymphatic histiocytosis 155.14–155.15
intranodal MR lymphography 103.56
intravascular large B-cell lymphoma 139.43–139.44
intravascular papillary endothelial hyperplasia 136.23–136.24
intravascular paraprotein deposition 149.13–149.14
intravascular thrombi, Raynaud phenomenon 124.11
intravenous immunoglobulin (IVIG) 19.31, 19.40–19.41, 118.12, 118.21
 dose and regimen 19.41
 pemphigus 50.8
 pharmacological properties 19.40
 potential adverse effects 19.40–19.41
 pyoderma gangrenosum 49.7
 safety considerations 19.41
 systemic lupus erythematosus treatment 51.38
intravenous (IV) drug administration
 dermatoses induced by 120.6–120.8
 see also injecting drug use
invasive carcinoma, human papillomavirus association 25.65

invasive wound infection, burn injuries 125.9–125.10
inversa junctional epidermolysis bullosa 69.14
inversa recessive dystrophic epidermolysis bullosa 69.18
invertebrate vectors of disease
 blackfly (*Simulium* species) and onchocerciasis 33.1, 33.2, *33.3*
 Cyclops species and dracunculiasis 33.13
 leishmaniasis 33.43, **33.45**
 mosquitoes 25.87–25.91, 33.36, *103.34*
 sandflies and cutaneous leishmaniasis 33.43, 33.45, *33.52*
 tabanid flies and loiasis 33.12
 triatomidae bugs and American trypanosomiasis 33.39–33.40
 tsetse flies and African trypanosomiasis 33.39, *33.41*, *33.42*
inverted follicular keratosis 137.2–137.3
inverted nipple, glycosylation disorders **79.10**
in vitro tests 127.33
involucrin 2.7
involuting lichenoid plaque *see* lichenoid keratosis
iodides, acneform reaction 88.13
iodine, topical therapies 18.10
iodism, potassium iodide (systemic therapy) 19.30
iodopropynyl butylcarbamate (IPBC) 127.57
ion channels, transmembrane drug mechanisms 13.5
ionising radiation
 post-ionising radiation keratosis 141.14–141.15
 see also radiotherapy
iontophoresis, hyperhidrosis treatment 92.9
IP *see* incontinentia pigmenti
IPBC *see* iodopropynyl butylcarbamate
IPD *see* immediate pigment darkening
IPEX *see* immunodysregulation polyendocrinopathy enteropathy X-linked syndrome
IPL *see* intense pulsed light
IPPD *see* N-isopropyl-N-phenyl-p-phenylenediamine
IPS *see* ichthyosis–prematurity syndrome
IPSO *see* Impact of Psoriasis Questionnaire
IR *see* insulin resistance
IRAD *see* immune reconstitution-associated disease
iris
 juvenile xanthogranuloma of *135.16*
 Lisch nodules *78.2*
iritis, hypopyon *48.6*
iron, hair loss 87.59, 87.63, 87.70–87.71
iron deficiency 61.3, 61.4, 61.24–61.25, 87.59, 87.63, 87.70–87.71, 153.1
iron salts, tattoos 86.53
IR radiation *see* infrared radiation
irritable bowel disease (IBD) *see* inflammatory bowel disease
irritant contact dermatitis (ICD) 39.3, 128.1–128.13
 cannabis-induced 120.4
 male genitalia 109.11
 occupational 129.1–129.5
 occupational skin disease 16.12
 perineal skin 111.9
 peristomal skin 112.2–112.7
 prevalence 127.3
 vulval 110.14–110.15
irritant folliculitis 91.1
irritant occupational hazards 129.8–129.11
irritant reactions, topical therapy 18.4
irritants
 arthropod effects 34.2
 common types 128.2
 mechanism of action 128.3
IRS *see* inner root sheath
ISAAC *see* International Study of Asthma and Allergies in Childhood
ischaemic disorders, peripheral *see* peripheral vascular disease

ischaemic fasciitis 136.6
ischaemic fat necrosis 97.8
ischaemic heart disease 151.5
ischaemic toes, thromboangiitis obliterans 101.6
ischaemic ulcers 101.44, 123.1
    hypertensive ischaemic leg ulcers 102.10–102.13
ISD see infantile seborrhoeic dermatitis
ISDL see Impact of Chronic Skin Disease on Daily Life
Islamic medicine 1.3
island pedicle flaps, surgical reconstruction **20.24**, 20.25–20.26
ISM see indolent systemic mastocytosis
isobornyl acrylate 127.70
isocyanates, in polyurethanes 127.71
isolated dyskeratosis follicularis see warty dyskeratoma
isolated limb perfusion (ILP), melanoma 144.2
isolated striate palmoplantar keratoderma 63.56–63.57
isomorphic phenomenon see Koebner (isomorphic) phenomenon
isomorphic response, mechanical injuries 122.2
isoniazid, acneform reaction 88.13
isopropyl myristate 12.3
N-isopropyl-N-phenyl-p-phenylenediamine (IPPD) 127.63–127.64
isothiazolinones 127.53, 127.54
isotretinoin
    acne treatment 5.3, 88.51, 88.52–88.57
        adverse effects 88.54–88.57
        musculoskeletal adverse effects 155.11
        neuropsychological adverse effects 84.42
        prescribing guidelines **88.53**
        relative success of **88.53**
    childhood acne treatment **88.73**
    ichthyoses management 63.44–63.45
    prepubertal acne treatment **88.73**
    topical therapies 18.25
ISPOR see International Society for Pharmacoeconomics and Outcomes Research
isthmic epithelial walled cutaneous cysts 133.4–133.6
isthmus region of hair root 87.4
Italy
    psoriasis, economic burden of **6.8**, 6.9
    Renaissance medicine 1.3
itching
    antihistamines 41.27
    assessment tools 4.2, 16.5
    see also pruritus
itching purpura 99.7, 99.8, **99.9**
ITGA6, epidermolysis bullosa 69.4–69.5
ITGB4, epidermolysis bullosa 69.4–69.5
Ito, naevus of 68.9–68.10, 131.14–131.15
itraconazole 32.32
ITT see intention-to-treat
IV see intravenous
ivermectin 18.14
IVIG see intravenous immunoglobulin
ixekizumab
    psoriasis treatment 35.30
    psoriatic arthritis treatment 35.46

J

Jackson–Lawler type, pachyonychia congenita 67.1
Jacob disease, oral involvement 108.86
Jadassohn–Lewandowsky type, pachyonychia congenita 67.1
Jadassohn–Pellizzari-type anetoderma 94.23
JAK see janus kinases
JAKi see Janus kinase inhibitors
Janus kinase inhibitors (JAKi) 19.22–19.24, 87.27
    atopic eczema treatment 41.27, 41.30–41.33
    cautions 19.24

cutaneous adverse effects 155.15
dermatological uses 19.22
dose and regimens 19.24
monitoring 19.24
pharmacological properties 19.22–19.23
potential adverse effects 19.23–19.24
pre-treatment screening 19.24
pyoderma gangrenosum treatment 49.7
Janus kinases (JAK) 19.22–19.23
    transmembrane drug mechanisms 13.5
Japanese-form eosinophilic pustular folliculitis 93.8
Jarisch–Herxheimer reaction, penicillin 29.22
jaundice 86.49–86.50
    hepatitis A infection 25.97
    liver disorders 153.4, 153.5
    malaria 33.36
    yellow fever 25.85
jaws
    examination 108.6
    Gardner syndrome 108.86
    Gorlin syndrome 108.86
    pseudofolliculitis 93.2
JDM see juvenile dermatomyositis
Jeffrey Modell Foundation, warning signs of inherited immunodeficiency 80.2
jellyfish stings 130.1–130.3
Jessner's lymphocytic infiltrate 89.10, 134.10–134.11
    ear dermatoses 106.22
Jessner solution (JS), chemical peels 160.3, 160.7, 160.8, 160.10
Job syndrome see hyper-IgE syndrome due to STAT3 loss of function mutations
Jod–Basedow phenomenon, potassium iodide systemic therapy 19.30
jogger's nipples 122.16
jogger's toe 122.16
joint hypermobility (flexibility), Beighton score **70.8**
joint stiffness, in diabetes 62.5–62.6
JPHT see juvenile polyposis/HHT syndrome
JS see Jessner solution
JSE see juvenile springtime eruption
Jujin haemorrhagic fever (Argentinian haemorrhagic fever) 25.82–25.83
junctional epidermolysis bullosa 69.2
    laminin-332 69.5
    management of 69.25
    molecular pathology 69.12–69.15
    with pyloric atresia 69.13–69.14
junctional naevus
    acquired melanocytic naevi 131.18, 131.20
    definition **131.1**
JUP mutations, skin fragility disorders 69.7
juvenile chronic myeloid leukaemia 149.14
juvenile dermatomyositis (JDM) 52.6, 52.8–52.9, 52.11, 52.12
juvenile fibromatosis 94.41–94.43
juvenile hyaline fibromatosis 94.42–94.43
juvenile plantar dermatosis 39.23–39.24
juvenile polyposis/HHT syndrome (JPHT) 71.2
juvenile springtime eruption (JSE) 126.8–126.9
    external ear 106.25
juvenile xanthogranuloma (JXG) 115.15, 135.14–135.17, **135.20**, 149.14
    eyelid 107.45
juxta-articular Dercum disease 98.18
JXG see juvenile xanthogranuloma

K

KA see keratoacanthoma
Kabuki syndrome **106.7**
Kamino bodies 3.42
    compound naevus of Spitz 131.33
kaposiform haemangioendothelioma (KHE), infants 116.9–116.10
kaposiform lymphangiomatosis (KLA) 71.2, 103.29

Kaposi sarcoma-associated herpesvirus (KSHV/HHV-8) 25.42, 25.43, 31.30
Kaposi sarcoma (KS) 25.42, 138.1–138.6
    clinical features 138.3–138.5
    epidemiology **138.2**
    eyelid 107.49–107.50
    HIV/AIDS 25.42, 25.43, 31.30–31.31, 31.35, 138.1, **138.2**, 138.4, 138.5, 138.6
    immunocompromised patients
        clinicopathological features 147.14
        management 147.23
        non-Hodgkin lymphoma/chronic lymphocytic leukaemia patients 147.3
        people living with HIV 147.2
        systemic chemoprevention 147.20–147.21
        Wiskott–Aldrich syndrome 147.2
    male genitalia 109.42
    management 138.6
    oral involvement 108.26
    pathophysiology 138.1–138.3
    radiotherapy 24.15
    subtypes 138.1, **138.2**, 138.4
Kaposi varicelliform eruption see eczema herpeticum
Kaposi–Stemmer sign 103.6
kappa light chains, dermal deposition 56.6
Karelian disease see Sindbis virus
karyorrhexis 3.42
Kasbach–Merritt phenomenon (KMP) 116.9–116.10
Kashin–Beck disease 61.29–61.30
Kawasaki disease 100.30–100.32, 155.3–155.4
    cardiac involvement 151.4–151.5
    clinical features 26.89–26.90
    epidemiology 26.89
    infants 115.9–115.11
    management 26.90
    oral ulceration 108.41–108.42
    pathophysiology 26.89
    perineal and perianal skin 111.16
    possible bacterial role 26.89
Kaya and Saurat's classification of cutaneous adnexal cysts **133.2**
Kazal-type-related inhibitor, skin fragility disorders 69.6
KC see keratosis circumscripta
KCMC see Kilimanjaro Christian Medical Centre
KCs see keratinocyte carcinomas
kEDS see kyphoscoliotic Ehlers–Danlos syndrome
Kelch-like genes, epidermolysis bullosa 69.3–69.4
keloid 94.48–94.53
    penis 109.31
    radiotherapy 24.7–24.8
keloidal blastomycosis see lobomycosis
keloidalis, folliculitis 91.10–91.12
keloidal/nodular morphoea 55.15–55.16
keloidal papules 93.3
keloid-like scars, folliculitis 91.11
keloid reaction, tattoos 86.54
keloid scarring 11.9
    external ear 106.14–106.15
    hidradenitis suppurativa 111.12
Kenya, teledermatology 7.9
Keppen–Lubinsky syndrome **72.5**
keratan sulphate (KS) 2.37, 2.38, **2.39**
keratin aggregates, ichthyoses 63.13
keratin-associated proteins, hair follicle 87.6
keratin gene expression 2.7–2.8
α-keratin intermediate filaments (α-KIF) 87.6
keratinisation disorders 63.73–63.76, 85.18
    ocular features **107.41**
keratinised tissues, dermatophytes 32.20
keratin markers, cutaneous neoplasms 3.21–3.23
keratinocyte carcinomas (KCs)
    definition 141.1

immunocompromised patients
    clinicopathological features 147.10–147.11
    management 147.16–147.18
    prevention 147.18–147.21
    see also basal cell carcinoma; squamous cell carcinoma
keratinocytes 2.1, 2.5, 2.7–2.8
    adherens junction 2.19
    Cole disease 63.61
    differentiation process 9.1
    elatin gene expression 2.33
    grafts 11.12
    keratin filament network 2.8
    mechanical stretching 122.1
    melanocyte interface 86.3
    melanosome transfer to 86.4
    porokeratosis 85.19–85.20
    wound healing 11.4–11.5, 11.12
keratinocyte terminal differentiation, melanosomes 68.1
keratinocytic acanthomas, benign proliferations 132.1–132.8
keratinocytic disadhesion
    Carvajal-Huerta syndrome 63.63
    striate palmoplantar keratoderma **63.57**, 63.58
keratinopathic ichthyoses (KPIs) **63.4**, 63.13–63.18
    skin fragility 69.20
keratins
    epidermolysis bullosa 69.2–69.3, 69.7
    hair 2.10, 87.99
    hemidesmosomal inner plaques 69.4
    pachyonychia congenita 67.1
keratitis–ichthyosis–deafness (KID) syndrome 63.33–63.35, 108.29
keratoacanthoma (KA) 141.38–141.41
    associated conditions 141.38–141.45
    eyelid 107.47
    generalised eruptive keratoacanthoma 141.43–141.44
    lip 108.44
    multiple self-healing squamous epithelioma 141.41–141.42
    visceral malignancy 148.12
keratoderma blennorrhagicum, reactive arthritis 155.1
keratoderma climactericum (Haxthausen disease) 63.71–63.72
keratodermas
    acquired forms 63.71–63.79
    NIPAL4 mutations 63.14
    pachyonychia congenita 67.12
    palmoplantar keratodermas 63.49–63.71
    syndromic forms 63.62–63.71
keratoelastoidosis marginalis 63.60
keratolysis exfoliativa 85.25–85.26
keratolytics, ichthyoses management 63.42–63.43, **63.43**
keratolytics (topical), seborrhoeic dermatitis 40.8
keratolytic winter erythema 63.73–63.74
    genes/proteins linked to 69.6
keratomycosis nigricans palmaris see tinea nigra
keratoses
    NLRP1-associated autoinflammation with arthritis and dyskeratosis 45.18
    oral lesions 108.33
    PUVA phototherapy adverse effects 21.14
    seborrhoeic 132.1–132.4
    see also hyperkeratosis; seborrhoeic keratosis
keratosis alba see stucco keratosis
keratosis circumscripta (KC) 85.13–85.14, 85.14
keratosis follicularis spinulosa decalvans (KFSD) 63.24–63.25, 85.11, 87.48
keratosis linearis–ichthyosis congenita–sclerosing keratoderma 63.21
keratosis obturans 106.21
keratosis pilaris atrophicans 85.10–85.11

keratosis pilaris atrophicans faciei 85.10, *85.11*
keratosis pilaris (KP) 85.9–85.12, 88.34, *88.35*
keratosis pilaris rubra faciei 85.10
keratotic lichenification, KID syndrome 63.33
keratotic papules
 Flegel disease 85.17, *85.18*
 lichen spinulosus 85.12
 palmoplantar keratoderma punctata 63.58, *63.59*
keratotic plug, phrynoderma 85.14–85.15
kerion
 allergic reactions 32.50
 tinea capitis type 32.39
kerotic spicules, trichodysplasia spinulosa *85.16*
Keshan disease, selenium deficiency 61.29
ketoprofen allergy 127.79
KFD *see* Kikuchi–Fujimoto disease
KFSD *see* keratosis follicularis spinulosa decalvans
KHE *see* kaposiform haemangioendothelioma
KID *see* keratitis–icthyosis–deafness syndrome
kidneys *see* nephropathy; *renal entries*
α-KIF *see* α-keratin intermediate filaments
Kikuchi–Fujimoto disease (KFD) 51.33, 149.16–149.17
Kilimanjaro Christian Medical Centre (KCMC) 7.7
kilovoltage X-ray therapy 24.1, 24.3, 24.4, 24.7
Kimura disease 136.27, 149.17
Kindler epidermolysis bullosa (Kindler syndrome) 69.5, 69.19, **75.2**, 75.6, 108.86
Kindlin-1 (*KIND1/FERMT1*) 69.5
kinesin 86.4
kissing bugs 34.29
KIT gene 2.15
KIT receptor mutations, mastocytosis 46.1, 46.2
KLA *see* kaposiform lymphangiomatosis
Klebsiella (Calymmatobacterium) granulomatis 30.21–30.23
Klebsiella pneumoniae subsp. *rhinoscleromatis* 26.56–26.57
Klein–Waardenburg syndrome 68.5
KLHL24, epidermolysis bullosa 69.3–69.4
Kligman cream, topical depigmenting agents 18.32
Klinefelter syndrome 74.4
Klippel–Trenaunay syndrome (KTS) 101.27–101.30, 103.23
 spindle cell haemangioma 136.31
Klippel–Trenaunay–Weber syndrome *71.2*, 71.8–71.9
 oral involvement 108.26
KMP *see* Kasbach–Merritt phenomenon
knee
 atopic eczema *41.16*
 calcinosis *79.18*
 epidermolysis bullosa acquista *50.44*
 erythema elevatum diutinum *100.9*
 Gianotti–Crosti syndrome *115.11*
 nail–patella syndrome 67.16
 necrotising granulomatous lesions 80.10
 sarcoidosis 96.7
 tuberous xanthomas *60.3*
knuckle pads (subcutaneous fibroma) 94.37–94.38
 Bart–Pumphrey syndrome 63.64
 sports injuries 122.16
knuckles, granuloma annulare *95.5*
Koebner (isomorphic) phenomenon/Koebnerisation 86.36, 86.38, 119.14, 121.9, 128.5
 lichen planus induced by mechanical irritation 37.3
 linear lesions 4.7
 necrobiosis lipoidica 95.11, *95.12*
 psoriasis vulgaris *35.8*

Koebner (isomorphic) response, mechanical injuries 122.2–122.3, 122.22
Koenen tumours (periungual fibromas), tuberous sclerosis complex 78.8
koganbyo *see* cercarial dermatitis
Kogoj spongiform pustule 3.43
koilonychia, infants 115.14
kojic acid
 cosmeceutical use of 157.4
 topical depigmenting agents 18.32
Koplik spots
 measles 25.98, *25.99*
 oral lesions 108.33
koro syndrome, male genitalia 109.44
Kosaki overgrowth syndrome **72.5**
KP *see* keratosis pilaris
KPIs *see* keratinopathic ichthyoses
Kramer syndrome 68.9
KRT genes, epidermolysis bullosa 69.2–69.3, 69.7
KS *see* Kaposi sarcoma; keratan sulphate
KSHV *see* Kaposi sarcoma-associated herpesvirus
KTP *see* potassium titanyl phosphate lasers
KTS *see* Klippel–Trenaunay syndrome
Küster, Wolfgang 63.43
kwashiorkor 61.2, 61.3
 erythrodermic findings in *61.4*
 peripheral oedema and 'flaky paint' dermatitis *61.4*
 presentation 61.4
kyphoscoliotic Ehlers–Danlos syndrome (kEDS) **70.4**, 70.9
Kyrle disease 63.76, 63.77, 94.53, 154.3–154.4
Kytococcus sedentarius, pitted keratolysis 26.42–26.43

L

L *see* lichenoid keratosis
LA *see* lactic acid
labelling of tissue specimens 3.6
labial melanotic macules (labial lentigo) 131.11–131.12
labial mucosa 108.3, 108.6–108.7
labia majora
 angiokeratomas 110.3, *110.4*
 Fordyce spots 110.3
 structure and function of 110.2
labia minora
 Fordyce spots 110.3, *110.4*
 structure and function of 110.2
 vestibular papillomatosis 110.4
Lacazia loboi 32.78–32.79
lacrimal glands 107.3
lactate, eccrine sweating 92.3–92.4
lactation
 drug pharmacokinetics and pharmacodynamics 13.8–13.9
 rosacea and 89.15
 safe treatments in pregnancy 113.19–113.24
 transfer of toxic substances in 114.14
lactic acid (LA), chemical peels 160.2
lactiferous ducts of the nipple, nipple adenoma 137.21–137.22
LAD *see* linear IgA disease
LADD *see* laser-assisted drug delivery
lake itch *see* cercarial dermatitis
LAM *see* linear atrophoderma of Moulin; lymphangioleiomyomatosis
lambda light chains, dermal deposition of 56.6
LAMB (lentigines, atrial myxoma, blue nevi) syndrome *see* Carney complex
lamellar bodies, harlequin ichthyosis 63.8, *63.10*
lamellar granules/bodies 2.6
lamellar ichthyosis (LI) 63.10–63.13, *63.12*
lamellar scaling, trichothiodystrophy *63.37*
laminin-332 (*LAMA3*), (*LAMB3*), (*LAMC2*) 69.5, 69.14
laminin 411, wound healing 11.6

laminins 2.23–2.25
 chain composition **2.24**
 isoforms and domain organisations *2.24*
 laminin 332 2.25, 2.44
lamotrigine, hypersensitivity reactions to **14.6**
Langerhans cell histiocytoses (LCH) 2.15, 135.1, 135.2–135.11
 female genitalia 110.40
 infants/children 115.15–115.16, 135.4, 135.5–135.7, **135.9**
 oral involvement 108.70–108.71
Langerhans cell markers, cutaneous neoplasms 3.27, *3.28*
Langerhans cells (LCs) 2.1–2.2, 2.13–2.15
 antigen exchange 2.13, *2.15*
 epidermal immune cells *9.4*
 imaging of 2.13
 immune system 9.3
 skin ageing 2.45
 structure of 2.14, *2.16*
langerin 135.2
lanolin, topical medication vehicles 18.6–18.7
lanolin alcohols 127.58
lanolin allergy 127.58
large B-cell lymphoma (LBCL) 139.37, 139.41–139.44
large-cell lymphomas
 primary cutaneous anaplastic large-cell lymphoma 139.28–139.29
 primary cutaneous diffuse large B-cell lymphoma 139.37, 139.41–139.43
 secondary intravascular large B-cell lymphoma 139.43–139.44
large congenital melanocytic naevi, as melanoma precursors 142.2, *142.3*
large congenital naevi, melanoma detection 142.11
large plaque parapsoriasis (LPP) 134.6, 134.7–134.8
large-vessel vasculitis 100.32–100.35
larimal duct scarring, in erosive lichen planus 110.12
larva currens *see* strongyloidiasis
larval taeniasis *see* cysticercosis
larva migrans *see* ancylostomiasis; cutaneous larva migrans; visceral larva migrans
laryngo-onycho-cutaneous syndrome 69.14–69.15
laser-assisted drug delivery (LADD) 161.5
laser-assisted hair removal 23.17–23.20
 complications 23.19–23.20
 folliculitis keloidalis 93.4
 indications 23.19
laser-assisted lipolysis 23.24
Laser Doppler flowmetry (LDF) 128.6
laser resurfacing 161.1–161.6
 ablative and non-ablative fractional devices **161.5**
 for acne scarring *161.4*
 adverse effects 161.6
 avoidance of bulk heating 161.4
 carbon dioxide lasers 161.1–161.3, **161.5**
 device names **161.5**
 Er:YAG lasers 161.1–161.3, **161.5**
 fractionated ablative lasers 161.2–161.3, **161.5**
 management of patients 161.3–161.5
 non-ablative fractional resurfacing 161.2, **161.5**
 patient selection 161.3
 for photodamaged skin *161.3*
 postoperative course 161.4–161.5
 preoperative management and anaesthesia 161.3–161.4
 skin tightening 161.6
 wound care 161.4
lasers
 history 23.1
 principles 23.1–23.3
laser therapies 23.1–23.24
 basal cell carcinoma 140.16
 clinical applications 23.6–23.24

 cutaneous warts 25.59
 hair disorders 87.71, 87.95
 keloids/hypertrophic scars 94.52
 light-tissue interactions 23.4–23.5
 mechanical injuries 122.6
 selective photothermolysis 23.5–23.6
 theory 23.1–23.6
 tissue cooling to avoid epidermal heat damage 23.6
 tissue optics 23.3–23.4
 unrealistic expectations 23.6
 vascular lesions 23.6–23.12
 see also photothermal ablation
Lassa fever 25.81–25.82
latent syphilis 29.12
latent transforming growth factor beta binding proteins (LTBPs) 2.36
latent viral infections *see* reactivation of viruses; subclinical and latent viral infections
late-onset chronic mucocutaneous candidiasis 32.68
late-onset focal dermal elastosis 94.32
late-onset ichthyosis 63.47–63.50
late-onset junctional epidermolysis bullosa 69.14
late-onset primary lymphoedema 103.24–103.25
lateral canthal lines, reduction of by botulinum toxin application 159.5
latex *see* natural rubber latex; rubber allergy
latex–fruit syndrome 127.84
Latino skin phenotypes, photoageing 156.2–156.3
Lattice System Global Assessment, psoriasis 16.3
Laugier–Hunziker syndrome, oral involvement 108.18
lavender, cosmeceutical use of **157.8**
lax skin 94.21–94.23
 Ehlers–Danlos syndrome 94.27
lazy leukocyte syndrome *see* periodic fever, immunodeficiency and thrombocytopenia
LBCL *see* large B-cell lymphoma
LCH *see* Langerhans cell histiocytoses
LCs *see* Langerhans cells
LDF *see* Laser Doppler flowmetry
LDS *see* lipodermatosclerosis; Loeys-Dietz syndrome
LE *see* lupus erythematosus
lead, dermatological reactions 121.2, 121.4–121.5
lead shielding mask, radiotherapy for skin cancer near eyes 24.3, *24.4*, 24.10–24.11
leather
 chromium allergy 127.39–127.40
 shoe allergy 127.67–127.68
ledderhose disease *see* plantar fibromatosis
Leeds Acne Grading System 16.4
leg
 acquired cutaneous lymphangiectasia *103.6*
 acute haemorrhagic oedema in infancy *115.10*
 allergic contact dermatitis of 127.17, 127.22
 amniotic bands and lymphoedema *103.30*
 annular erythema of infancy *47.10*
 atopic eczema *41.14, 41.17,* 115.3
 bandaging, lymphoedema therapy *103.59*
 chronic red leg 103.16–103.17
 chronic venous oedema *103.10*
 congenital generalised lipodystrophies *72.2*
 congenital haemangioma 116.9
 cutaneous polyarteritis nodosa *100.29*
 cutaneous small-vessel vasculitis *100.7*
 dermatitis herpetiformis *50.57*
 eczema of the lower legs 39.19–39.22
  clinical features 39.20
  clinical variants 39.21

leg (continued)
    complications and co-morbidities 39.21
    disease course and prognosis 39.21
    management 39.21–39.22
    pathology 39.20
    treatment for 39.22
elephantiasis nostra verrucosa 103.6
eosinophilic fasciitis 55.22
eosinophilic granulomatosis with polyangiitis 100.27
eruptive xanthomas 60.4
granuloma annulare 95.6
hyperglobulinaemic purpura in patient with Sjögren syndrome 53.11
hypertrophic lichen planus 37.7
keloidal morphoea 55.16
laser therapies on veins 23.11
lichen simplex 39.29
linear IgA disease 50.37
linear morphoea 55.26
lipodermatosclerosis 103.17
lipoedema 72.12, 98.21–98.23, 103.54
livedo reticularis 4.11, 51.27, 53.3
lymphangioma malformation 103.27
lymphoedema–distichiasis syndrome 71.25
mixed connective tissue disease 53.3
morphoea 55.18, 55.20
necrolytic migratory erythema 47.15
Nékam disease 37.11
nummular dermatitis 39.8
palisaded and neutrophilic granulomatous dermatitis 53.7
pemphigus foliaceus 50.6
plaque morphoea 55.18, 55.20
podoconiosis (non-filarial lymphoedema) 103.36
psoriasis vulgaris 35.8, 35.13
pyoderma gangrenosum 49.2
rheumatoid arthritis-associated medium vessel vasculitis 53.8
small-vessel vasculitis 100.2, 100.3
STING-associated vasculopathy with onset in infancy 45.14
Sweet syndrome 49.12
swelling 103.9–103.10
ulcerated necrotic lesions 100.3
varicose veins 101.39
vasculitis 100.2, 100.3
veins, laser therapies 23.11
venous malformation 71.15
    see also ankle; knee; shin; thigh
legal issues
    drug use 120.3–120.4
    litigation by psychologically disturbed patients 84.9–84.10, 84.15, 84.36–84.38
Legionella pneumophila (legionellosis) 26.76
Legius syndrome 72.10, 78.9
leg ulcers 1.3
    aetiologies 102.1, **102.2**
    arterial leg ulcers 102.7–102.10
    diabetic patients 62.1
    hypertensive ischaemic leg ulcers 102.10–102.13
    mixed leg ulcers 102.4–102.7
    rheumatoid arthritis-associated 53.7, 155.6
    systemic lupus erythematosus 51.26
    venous leg ulcers 102.1–102.4
leiomyoma 136.53–136.54
    oral involvement 108.13
    vulva **110.32**
leiomyomatosis see hereditary leiomyomatosis and renal cell cancer; lymphangioleiomyomatosis
leiomyosarcoma/atypical smooth muscle tumour 136.54–136.55
leishmaniasis 33.43–33.54
    blepharitis 107.12
    cutaneous 33.43–33.51
    ear dermatoses **106.23**
    HIV 33.52–33.53
    male genitalia 109.28

    oral involvement 108.57
    parasitic organisms **33.45**, 33.46–33.49, 33.52
    vectors 33.43, **33.45**, 33.52
    visceral 33.51–33.54
    see also cutaneous leishmaniasis; visceral leishmaniasis
leishmaniasis cutis diffusa (diffuse/disseminated cutaneous leishmaniasis) 33.48–33.49
leishmaniasis recidivans (chronic/lupoid cutaneous leishmaniasis) 33.47–33.48
leisure factors
    diagnosis 4.4
    epidemiology 5.11
LEKTI see lymphoepithelial Kazal-type-related inhibitor
lentigines 131.3–131.9
    agminated or segmental lentiginosis 131.3
    familial lentiginosis syndromes **131.3**
    ink-spot lentigo 131.8–131.9
    lentiginosis profusa 131.3
    photochemotherapy (PUVA) lentigo 131.7–131.8
    PUVA phototherapy adverse effects 21.14
    RASopathies 151.3
    simple lentigo 131.3–131.5
    solar (or actinic) lentigo 131.5–131.7
    xeroderma pigmentosum 76.4
    see also mucosal melanotic lesions
lentiginoses 86.16–86.17, **131.3**
    oral involvement 108.17–108.18
lentiginosis profusa 131.3
lentigo, definition **131.1**
lentigo maligna (LM)
    facial and chronically sun-damaged skin 145.9, 145.11
    presentation 142.19
    radiotherapy 24.14–24.15
lentigo maligna melanoma (LMM) 106.33
    melanoma classification 142.7, 142.8
    presentation 142.10, 142.13, 142.19
    radiotherapy 24.14–24.15
    surgery 143.3–143.4
lentigo senilis (solar/actinic lentigo) 131.5–131.7
lentigo simplex 131.3–131.5
    dermoscopic image 131.5
    hyperpigmentation 131.4
Lenz–Majewski syndrome 70.16
LEOPARD syndrome (Noonan with multiple lentigines) **131.3**, 151.3
Lepidoptera (butterflies and moths) 34.32–34.34
lepidopterism
    use of term 34.33
    see also caterpillar dermatitis
lepromatous leprosy (LL) 28.2, 28.3–28.4, 28.5, 28.7–28.8, 28.9, 97.26
leprosy 28.1–28.17
    clinical features 28.6–28.13
    delayed diagnosis in non-endemic settings 28.10
    differential diagnosis of lesions 28.10–28.11
    drug treatments 1.8
    ear dermatoses **106.23**
    epidemiology 28.1
    erythema nodosum leprosum 28.3, 28.4, 28.5, 28.11, 28.12, 28.15
    eye infection 107.39
    genetic factors 28.1–28.2
    granuloma multiforme resemblance 94.30
    hair loss 87.36
    history 28.1
    HIV 28.10
    International Federation of Anti-Leprosy Associations 7.10
    investigations 28.13
    management 28.13–28.16
    oral involvement 108.55

    pathophysiology 28.1–28.6
    predisposing factors 28.1–28.2
    pregnancy 28.10
    in pregnancy 113.6
    prevention and control 28.16
    stigma 28.1, 28.16
    variants 28.2–28.3, 28.6–28.10
leprosy reactions, erythema nodosum leprosum 97.25–97.26
leptin, role of 97.4–97.5
leptin deficiency **72.7**
leptin receptor syndrome **72.6**
leptospirosis/Leptospira spp. 26.74–26.75
Leser–Trélat, sign of 148.16
lesional blistering, UVB phototherapy adverse effects 21.12
lesional erythema, versus persistent/diffuse erythema of rosacea 89.7
lesions
    annular lesions 4.7, 4.15
        granuloma annulare 4.10
        keratotic lesions 63.75
        porokeratosis 4.10
        tinea corporis 4.10
    arcuate lesions 4.11
    autoinflammatory diseases 80.19
    Blashkoid lesions 4.16, 4.19
    cocaine-induced 120.5
    colour of skin 4.13–4.15
    dermatomal distribution 4.16
    deroofing 90.10
    description of 4.5–4.20
        anatomical factors 4.5–4.6
        border of lesion 4.15
        colour of lesion **4.15**
        distribution pattern and arrangement 4.6–4.12
        external factors 4.6
        nomenclature 4.10–4.15, 4.16, 4.17
        shape of lesion 4.6–4.7, 4.8–4.10, **4.12**, 4.15, 4.16, 4.17
        size of lesion 4.10
    digitate lesions 4.17
    discoid lesions 4.12
    distribution of 4.16, **4.17**, **4.18**, 4.19
        anatomical factors 4.16
        Blashkoid distribution 4.16, 4.19
        dermatomal distribution 4.16
        external factors 4.16
    duration 4.3
    erythema 4.13
    erythrokeratoderma variabilis 63.18, 63.19
    flexural sites **4.18**
    haemorrhagic lesions 4.12
    hidradenitis suppurativa 90.3, 90.5
    history taking 4.2
    Hurley stage III disease 90.9
    linear lesions 4.15
        anatomical and causative factors **4.13**
        Koebner/isomorphic phenomenon 4.7
    livedoid lesions 4.11
    malar erythematous photosensitive macular skin lesions 80.16
    periodicity 4.3
    pityriasis rotunda 63.48
    polycyclic lesions 4.11
    reticulate lesions 4.16
    sarcoidosis 96.1, 96.6–96.7
    surface features 4.13
    target lesions 4.15
    tuberous sclerosis complex 78.8
le tic des lèvres (factitious cheilitis) 84.33, 108.61
Letterer–Siwe disease 135.6
leucocytoclastic vasculitis, urticarial vasculitis 44.1, 44.3
leucomelanoderma, drug/chemical photosensitivity 126.30
leukaemia cutis 139.47–139.48
    infiltration of skin with neoplastic cells 149.2–149.4
    purpura 148.2
    see also myeloid sarcoma

leukaemias
    erythroderma 39.32–39.33
    oral involvement 108.71
leukocyte antigen markers 3.27–3.28
leukocytoclasis, IgA vasculitis 100.14
leukocytoclastic vasculitis 100.6, 100.8
leukoderma 86.8
    hypomelanosis 86.45–86.47
    occupational 129.13–129.14
leukoderma acquisitum centrifugum 86.40
leukoedema, oral lesions 108.29, 108.30
leukonychia 119.7, 121.7
leukopenias, oral involvement 108.71
leukoplakia, dyskeratosis congenita 67.14, 75.3
leukoplakia, oral lesions 108.33–108.35
    chronic hyperplastic candidiasis (candidal leukoplakia) 108.34
    hairy leukoplakia 108.34
    malignancy risk **108.35**
    speckled leukoplakia 108.34
    sublingual keratosis 108.34
    syphilitic leukoplakia 108.34
leukotriene C4 (LTC4), release of in skin 14.1, 14.2
leukotriene receptor antagonists, urticaria treatment 42.19
leukotrienes, melanocyte regulation 86.7
levamisole-induced vasculitis 120.5, 120.6
Levulan®
    Kerastick®, Ameluz®, Alacare® 22.1
    see also 5-aminolaevulinic acid
Lewandowski and Lutz dysplasia see epidermodysplasia verruciformis
LF see lymphatic filariasis
LGV see lymphogranuloma venereum
LH3 see lysyl hydroxylase
LI see lamellar ichthyosis
Libman–Sacks endocarditis 51.18
lice (Phthiraptera) 34.18–34.25
    body/clothing lice 34.23–34.24
    classification 34.18
    crab lice 34.24–34.25, 34.25, 107.12, 107.40
    head lice 1.2, 34.18–34.23
    on mummified body 1.2
    see also louse-borne diseases
lichen amyloidosus 56.3
lichen aureus 3.9, 99.7, 99.8, **99.9**
lichen exanthematicus 37.4
lichenification/lichenoid reactions 3.42, 39.28–39.31
    allergens 127.20
    atopic eczema 41.14, 41.16, 41.17, 41.19
    familial primary localised cutaneous amyloidosis 56.9
    in ichthyoses 63.11
    irritant contact dermatitis 128.5
    nail changes 119.7
    pathogenesis 37.2
    tattoos 86.54
lichenified onchodermatitis (LOD) 33.3–33.4
lichen myxoedematosus (LM) 57.1–57.8
lichen nitidus 37.9–37.10
lichenoid chronic dermatitis 39.8, 39.9
lichenoid exanthema 37.19
lichenoid infiltrate, drug reaction with eosinophilia and systemic symptoms 118.6
lichenoid keratosis (LK) 132.7–132.8
lichenoid primary localised cutaneous amyloidosis 56.7
lichenoid sarcoidosis 96.13
lichen planopilaris (LPP) 37.5, 37.6, 37.11, 87.38–87.42
lichen planus-like drug eruptions 117.7–117.9
lichen planus-like keratosis see lichenoid keratosis
lichen planus (LP) 37.1–37.17, 127.20, 127.22
    actinic lichen planus 37.7, 37.17
    acute and subacute lichen planus with confluence of lesions 37.8
    amalgam fillings 127.41

annular lichen planus 37.8
associated conditions 37.13
associated with liver disease 153.4, 153.5, 153.9
bacterial or fungal dysbiosis 37.3
betel chewing 37.3
buccal mucosa 37.5, 37.6
bullous lichen planus 37.8–37.9, 37.17
classic eruption on wrist 37.3
clinical features 37.3–37.5
clinical variants 37.5–37.11, 37.16–37.17
complications and co-morbidities 37.11–37.12
dental amalgam 37.3
dermoscopy image of 37.13
direct immunofluorescence 37.15
direct immunofluorescence findings 3.18, 3.19
disease course and prognosis 37.13
drug causation 37.3
ear dermatoses **106.23**
environmental factors 37.2–37.3
epidemiology 37.1
erythrodermic lichen planus 39.34
florid 4.16
genetics 37.2
genital mucosa 37.6
guttate lichen planus 37.8, 37.9
hair 37.5, 37.6, 37.11
hand 39.17
hepatitis B association 25.75
hepatitis C association 25.76
hepatitis and other viruses 37.2
histology 37.13
hypertrophic lichen planus 37.6–37.7
interface dermatitis 37.14
internal malignancy association 148.23
investigations 37.13–37.15
keratoderma climactericum 63.72
lichen exanthematicus 37.4
lichen nitidus 37.9–37.10
lichen planopilaris 37.5, 37.6
lichen planus-like contact dermatitis 37.3
lichen planus pemphigoides 37.8–37.9, 37.17
lichen planus pigmentosus 37.7
male genitalia 109.18–109.19
management 37.15–37.17
mechanical irritation (Koebner phenomenon) 37.3
'mixed' lichen planus/discoid lupus erythematosus disease patterns 37.8, 37.16
mucous membranes 37.12
nails 37.11–37.12
Nékam disease 37.10–37.11, 37.16
palm 37.5, 37.7
pathology 37.1–37.2
penis 37.4
perianal skin 111.10
photomicrograph of 37.15
reticulate 4.16
scalp 37.5, 37.6
sole 37.7
treatment 37.15–37.16
vulva 110.10–110.13
 clinical features 110.11
 complications and co-morbidities 110.12
 epidemiology 110.10
 glazed erythema 110.12
 histology 110.10
 pathophysiology 110.10–110.11
 plaques 110.11
 vulvo-vaginal-gingival syndrome 110.12
 Wickham striae 110.11
Wickham striae 37.3, 37.13
wrist 39.17
see also oral lichen planus
lichen planus pemphigoides 37.8–37.9, 37.17, 50.51
oral involvement 108.78
lichen planus pigmentosus 37.7

lichens, allergic contact dermatitis 127.73, 127.74
lichen sclerosus (LS) 55.7
 ano-genital region 111.9–111.10
 liquefaction degeneration 3.40
 male genitalia 109.15–109.18
 perineal and perianal skin 111.9–111.10
 peristomal skin 112.10, 112.11, 112.12
 vulva 110.6–110.10
  clinical features 110.7–110.9
  complications and co-morbidities 110.8–110.9
  histology 110.7
  management of 110.9–110.10
  plaques 110.7
  scarring 110.9
  squamous cell carcinoma 110.9
lichen sclerosus morphoea 55.4, 55.5, 55.6, 55.7
lichen scrofulosorum (tuberculosis cutis lichenoides) 27.25–27.27
 clinical features 27.26–27.27
 epidemiology 27.25
 investigations 27.27
 management 27.27
 pathophysiology 27.25–27.26
lichen simplex 39.28–39.31
 male genitalia 109.11
 perineal and perianal skin 111.8
 vulva 110.16–110.17
lichen simplex chronicus (LSC) 81.18–81.20, 84.15, 105.5
 clinical features 81.20
 epidemiology 81.18
 management 81.19, 81.20
 pathophysiology 81.18–81.20
lichen simplex-like eczema 127.16
lichen spinulosus (LS) 85.12–85.13
lichen striatus 4.9, 37.17–37.19, 86.44
 management 37.18–37.19
 presentation 37.17–37.18
life course impairment assessment 16.11
Life Quality Index Occupational Dermatoses (LIOD) 16.12
lifestyle factors
 acne 88.18–88.26
 seborrhoeic dermatitis 40.4, 40.7
lifting flaps 20.26–20.27
LIG4 syndrome **80.4**
light
 absorption by skin 23.3–23.4
 amplification 23.2
 energy 23.4
 spontaneous and stimulated emission 23.1–23.2
 transmission through skin 23.4
 see also lasers; ultraviolet
light-assisted hair removal 23.5–23.6
 see also laser-assisted hair removal
light exposure
 Bowen disease 141.18, 141.19
 mechanical injuries 122.5
light therapy see laser therapies; phototherapy
light-tissue interactions 23.4–23.5
lilac, see also violaceous
lilac erythema, upper eyelids in dermatomyositis 52.3, 52.5
Liliaceae dermatitis 127.73
limbs
 anatomical considerations for skin surgery 20.4
 calciphylaxis 59.7
 dermatomyositis 52.5, 52.6, 52.9
 swelling 103.9–103.10, 103.16–103.17, 103.44–103.46
limonene 127.42–127.43, 127.44
linalool 127.44
lincosamides 19.47–19.48
Lind, James 5.1
linear atrophoderma of Moulin (LAM) 55.25–55.27, 73.22, 94.17
linear closure, skin surgery 20.21–20.22
linear epidermal naevus, oral lesions 108.30
linear furrows 94.2

linear IgA disease (LAD) 50.33–50.38, 149.13
 associated diseases 50.34
 bullous dermatosis 3.18, 50.36
 in childhood 50.36, 108.81
 clinical features 50.36
 clinical variants 50.36
 'cluster of jewels'/'string of pearls' sign 50.37
 diagnosis 50.24
 differential diagnosis 50.36
 direct immunofluorescence microscopy 50.35
 epidemiology 50.33–50.34
 histopathology 50.35
 infants 115.11
 internal malignancy association 148.22
 investigations and diagnosis 50.36–50.38
 management 50.38
 mixed immunobullous disease 50.36
 oral involvement in adults 108.81–108.82
 pathophysiology 50.34
 predisposing factors 50.34–50.35
 sub-lamina densa variant 50.36
 treatment ladder 50.38
 vesicle pattern along edge of lesion 50.37
 vulva **110.21**
linear IgA/IgG bullous dermatosis 50.36
linear keloids 94.50
linear lesions 4.7, **4.13**, 4.15
linear morphoea ('en coup de sabre') 55.3, 55.4, 55.23–55.27, 105.8–105.9
linear naevus syndrome (naevus sebaceous of Jadassohn) 108.29–108.30
linear porokeratosis 63.75, 85.20–85.21, 85.22
linear psoriasis 35.15
linear and whorled naevoid hypermelanosis (LWNH) 68.12
lines of Blaschko 8.7, 8.8
lingual erythema migrans 108.24
lingual thyroid 108.11
lingual tonsil 108.11
Linuche unguiculata stings 130.2
LIOD see Life Quality Index Occupational Dermatoses
lip
 actinic cheilitis (solar cheilosis) 108.58
 actinic prurigo 108.58–108.59
 acute/chronic enlargement of, differential diagnoses **108.74**
 allergic contact dermatitis of 127.15
 anatomy of 108.3
 angioedema 108.10
 angular cheilitis 108.59–108.60
 basal cell carcinoma 108.43–108.44
 blisters 108.60
 calibre-persistent artery 108.63
 'chapping' of 108.60
 cheilitis 108.60–108.63
 cleft lip/palate 108.83–108.85
 commissural pits 108.86
 contact cheilitis 108.60–108.61
 dermal fillers 158.3, 158.4
  adverse reaction to 158.9, 158.10
 dermal fillers and implants **108.62**
 discoid lupus erythematosus 108.64
 double lip 108.85
 drug-induced cheilitis 108.61
 enlargement of, acute/chronic **108.74**
 examination of 108.6–108.7
 factitious cheilitis 84.33, 108.61
 fissures 108.63–108.64
 granulomatous cheilitis 108.73
 haemorrhagic crusting of 108.61
 herpes labialis 108.53
 herpetic stomatitis 108.52
 HIV infection 108.14
 impetigo 115.7
 Kawasaki disease 115.10
 keratoacanthoma 108.44
 lesions 108.57–108.64
 lupus erythematosus 108.64
 mast cell mediator-induced angio-oedema 43.2

melanotic macule 108.18
melanotic macules 131.11–131.12
mucocutaneous venous malformation 71.16
multiple endocrine neoplasia 108.13–108.14, 108.13, 148.10
oedema 103.46, 103.48
Orf-induced pemphigoid 50.55
pits and sinuses 108.86
radiotherapy for skin cancer 24.12, 24.13
reactive perforating collagenosis 108.64
reticulate lichen planus 4.16
sarcoidosis 108.64
Sturge–Weber syndrome 108.27
swelling due to oro-facial granulomatosis 95.14
systemic amyloidosis with mucotaneous involvement 56.12
tattooing of 108.15–108.16
ulcerative lichen planus 108.77
venous lake 4.14, 108.28
vermilion 108.3
vermilionectomy repair 20.22
lipase, pancreatic panniculitis 97.41
lipid injectable emulsion (ILE), parenteral nutrition 61.32, 61.33–61.34
lipid metabolism disorders 60.1–60.12, 79.15
 dyslipidaemias, classification 60.1, **60.2**
 histiocytosis 135.22–135.23
 hypercholesterolaemia 60.6–60.8
 hyperlipoproteinaemias **60.1**, 60.8–60.10
 primary dyslipidaemias 60.6–60.10
 xanthomas 60.2–60.6
lipids
 atopic eczema 41.6
 barrier to prevent irritant contact dermatitis 128.3
 epidermal 2.8
 topical medication vehicles 18.5, 18.6–18.7
lipid vascules, neutral lipid storage disease with ichthyosis 63.36
lip-lick cheilitis 41.22
lipoatrophic panniculitis of the ankles in childhood 97.56–97.57
lipoatrophy 62.4
 HAART regimes **98.7**
 localised 98.9–98.13
lipoblastoma and lipoblastomatosis 136.57–136.58
lipodermatosclerosis (LDS) 39.21, 103.16–103.17
 champagne bottle leg appearance 103.17
 chronic venous insufficiency **101.43**
 mixed leg ulcer 102.7
lipodystrophies 72.1–72.3
 acquired 98.1–98.13
 localised 98.9–98.13
 total body irradiation association 98.8–98.9
lipoedema 98.21–98.25, 103.53–103.55
 clinical features 103.53–103.54
 differential diagnosis **98.22**, 103.54–103.55
 familial 72.12
 imaging characteristics **98.23**
 investigations 103.55
 of the lower limbs 98.21–98.23
 lymphoedema in 98.23
 management 103.55
 pathophysiology 103.53
 of the scalp 98.24–98.25
 stages of **103.55**
lipoedematous alopecia 98.24–98.25, 105.10–105.11
lipofibromatosis 136.13–136.14
lipofuscins secretion, chromhidrosis 92.18
lipogenesis 97.4
lipogranuloma, male genitalia 109.8–109.9, 109.43
lipohypertrophy 62.4
lipoid proteinosis 70.36–70.37
lipo-lymphoedema 98.23
lipolysis, regulation 97.4

lipoma 136.56–136.57
　oral involvement 108.13
　pain 98.18
　surgical treatment 20.49
　vulva **110.32**
lipomatoses
　benign symmetrical 98.15–98.17
　of the face 98.19–98.20
　fat hypertrophy distinction 98.13
　hereditary **72.10**
lipomembranous fat necrosis **97.32**
lipomyelomeningocele **72.10**
lipophagic granulomas, sclerosing postirradiation panniculitis 97.63
lipophagic granulomatous inflammation 97.8
lipophagic necrosis 97.7
liposarcoma 136.59
　see also atypical lipomatous tumour; well-differentiated liposarcoma
liposcution (suction lipectomy), lymphoedema 103.60–103.61
liposomes, vehicle choice for topical therapies 18.3
liposuction
　cellulite management 98.26
　fat hypertrophy 98.15, 98.16
　subcutaneous tissue 97.3
Lipschütz ulcers
　COVID-19 association 25.113
　cytomegalovirus infections 25.41
　infectious mononucleosis complication 25.37
liquefaction degeneration *3.40*
liquefactive fat necrosis 97.8
liquid nitrogen, cryosurgery 20.46
liquiritin, topical depigmenting agents 18.32
Lisch nodules (pigmented iris hamartomas) *78.2*, 78.3
Listeria monocytogenes 26.46
listeriosis 26.46
listeriosis, neonatal 114.26–114.27
lithium-induced acne 88.13
litigation *see* complaints and litigation; legal issues
livedo, sarcoidosis 96.13
livedoid lesions *4.11*
livedoid vasculopathy 124.10
　purpura 99.20–99.21
livedo racemosa *45.17*, 124.9
　COVID-19 association 25.111
livedo reticularis *4.11*, 124.8–124.10
　COVID-19 association 25.111
　in patient with mixed connective tissue disease *53.3*
　in systemic lupus erythematosus 51.26–51.27
liver, *see also* hepatic entries
liver disease
　arsenic 121.2
　cirrhosis 153.5, 153.8, 153.9
　cutaneous features 153.4–153.5, 153.7–153.9
　drug-related issues **153.9**
　in erythropoietic protoporphyria 58.16–58.17
　in porphyria cutanea tarda 58.13
　systemic lupus erythematosus 51.31
　see also hepatic entries; hepatitis; intestinal failure-associated liver disease
liver dysfunction
　drug reaction with eosinophilia and systemic symptoms 118.8–118.9
　juvenile xanthogranuloma 135.17
　sarcoidosis 96.5
liver failure, drug reaction with eosinophilia and systemic symptoms 118.9, 118.11
liver spots *see* lentigines; pityriasis versicolor
liver transplantation, alpha-1 antitrypsin 97.45
LL *see* lepromatous leprosy
LLLT *see* low-level laser light therapy
LM *see* lentigo maligna; lichen myxoedematosus

LMDF *see* lupus miliaris disseminatus faciei
LMIC *see* low and middle income countries
LMM *see* lentigo maligna melanoma
LMPH1A *see* hereditary lymphoedema type 1A
LMs *see* lymphatic malformations
LMWH *see* low-molecular-weight heparin
LMWK *see* low-molecular-weight kininogen
LMX1B mutations, nail–patella syndrome 67.15
LN *see* lupus nephritis
Loa loa filariasis *see* loiasis
loath *see* endemic syphilis
lobomycosis (lobo disease) 32.78–32.79
lobular capillary haemangioma *see* pyogenic granuloma
lobular panniculitis 97.8, 97.22, 97.50–97.53
local anaesthetics
　allergic contact dermatitis 127.45
　biopsy 3.2
　injection techniques 20.8
　skin surgery 20.7–20.8
　toxic reactions 20.7–20.8
local flaps, surgical reconstruction 20.22–20.23
localised anetoderma 94.23
localised atrophy, steroid injections *94.9*
localised blistering, epidermolysis bullosa simplex *69.11*
localised bullous pemphigoid 50.17, *50.19*
　peristomal skin 112.10, *112.12*
localised circumscribed hyperhidrosis 92.6–92.7
localised cutaneous amyloidoses 56.6–56.10
　associated diseases 56.8–56.9
　clinical features 56.9–56.10
　clinical variants 56.10
　complications and disease course 56.10
　differential diagnosis 56.10
　epidemiology 56.7
　ethnicity 56.7–56.8
　insulin injections 98.14
　pathophysiology 56.9
　types of amyloidosis **56.3**
localised dermatitis, plant allergies 127.72
localised dystrophic epidermolysis bullosa, molecular pathology 69.15–69.16
localised elastolysis 94.21
localised epidermolysis bullosa 69.8
localised epidermolysis bullosa simplex 69.11
localised hypertrichosis 87.85–87.87
localised junctional epidermolysis bullosa, molecular pathology 69.14
localised lichen myxoedematosus 57.6–57.8
localised lipoatrophy 98.9–98.13
　due to injected corticosteroid 98.11–98.12
　due to injected drugs 98.10
localised lipodystrophy 98.9–98.13
localised nodular Dercum disease 98.18
localised (pretibial) myxoedema, hyperthyroidism 57.11
localised pruritus, neoplasia association 148.27
localised scleroderma cutaneous assessment tool (LoSCAT) 55.33–55.34
locally injected agents, use during pregnancy **113.21**
local wound care, pressure ulcers 123.10
locusts (Orthoptera) 34.32
LOD *see* Lichenified onchodermatitis
Loeys-Dietz syndrome (LDS) 141.42
Löfgren syndrome 97.21, 155.7
　sarcoidosis 96.1, 96.4, 96.5–96.6, 96.15
loiasis 33.7–33.12
　clinical features 33.11
　definition/nomenclature 33.10
　epidemiology 33.10
　investigations 33.11
　management 33.11–33.12
　pathophysiology 33.10–33.11
long-arm deletion syndrome, chromosome 18 74.3
long Covid (chronic COVID-19), mucocutaneous manifestations 25.113

long-delayed (6-week) intradermal reactions 4.25
loose anagen syndrome 87.82–87.83, *87.83*
loricrin keratoderma 63.56
LoSCAT *see* localised scleroderma cutaneous assessment tool
loss-of-function mutations, results of 69.27
lotions, vehicle choice for topical therapies 18.2
Louis–Bar syndrome *see* ataxia telangiectasia
louse-borne diseases
　bacillary angiomatosis 26.64
　epidemic relapsing fever 26.72
　rickettsial epidemic typhus 26.80–26.81
　trench fever 26.62
lower limbs *see* leg
low-grade fibromyxoid sarcoma 136.18–136.19
low-level laser light therapy (LLLT) 87.71, 87.95, 103.59–103.60
low and middle income countries (LMIC)
　access to dermatological health services 5.13–5.14, 7.3, *7.4*
　scabies, incidence of 7.2
low-molecular-weight heparin (LMWH), management of Klippel–Trenaunay–Weber syndrome 71.9
low-molecular-weight kininogen (LMWK), bradykinin-induced angio-oedema 43.3
low power laser therapy 23.24
LP *see* lichen planus
LPP *see* large plaque parapsoriasis; lichen planopilaris
LS *see* lichen sclerosus; lichen spinulosus
LSC *see* lichen simplex chronicus
LTBPs *see* latent transforming growth factor beta binding proteins
LTC4 *see* leukotriene C4
lubricants, genital contact dermatitis **109.13**
Lucio phenomenon 97.26
Ludwig scale, hair loss 87.65, *87.67*
Lujo virus haemorrhagic fever 25.82
lumbosacral area, Mongolian spot *131.12*
lumbo-sacral hypertrichosis 87.86
lumpy scalp syndrome 106.6
Lund and Browder chart, burn injuries *125.2*, *125.3*
lungs *see* interstitial lung disease; *pulmonary entries*
lupus, dystrophic calcification 59.1, 59.2
lupus anticoagulant syndrome 99.17–99.19
lupus erythematosus (LE) 51.1–51.46, 86.21, *87.55*, 106.24, *106.25*, 126.2
　antiphospholipid antibody syndrome 51.42–51.45
　cardiac involvement 151.4
　discoid lupus erythematosus 51.1–51.12, *51.24*
　drug-induced 117.7–117.9
　ear dermatoses **106.23**
　eye disease **107.57**
　internal malignancy association 148.21
　keratoderma association 63.72
　lip lesions 108.64
　neonatal 114.12–114.14
　neonatal lupus erythematosus 51.39–51.42
　papular and nodular cutaneous mucinosis 57.13
　periodic acid–Schiff stain *3.8*
　perniosis 124.5–124.6
　subacute cutaneous lupus erythematosus 51.12–51.16
　systemic lupus erythematosus 51.1, 51.16–51.38
　UVA-1 phototherapy 21.6
lupus erythematosus profundus (lupus panniculitis) 51.7–51.8, *51.9*, 94.21, 97.37–97.40
lupus miliaris disseminatus faciei (LMDF) 27.31, 89.7, 89.10, 89.19
lupus nephritis (LN), classification **51.20**
lupus panniculitis *see* lupus erythematosus profundus

lupus pernio *89.10*, 96.8–96.11, 96.15, *96.17*
lupus vulgaris 27.20–27.24
　clinical features 27.21–27.23
　epidemiology 27.21
　management 27.23–27.24
　pathophysiology 27.21
　sarcoidosis differential diagnosis 96.3
LVA *see* lymphatico-venous anastomosis surgery
LWNH *see* linear and whorled naevoid hypermelanosis
lycopene, cosmeceutical use 157.9–157.10
Lyell syndrome *see* toxic epidermal necrolysis
Lyme disease (Lyme borreliosis) 26.73–26.74
　acrodermatitis chronica atrophicans 94.15–94.16
　Borrelia burgdorferi complex 26.72–26.73
　clinical features/variants 26.73–26.74
　cutaneous B-cell lymphoma 139.37
　definition/description 26.72–26.73
　epidemiology 26.73
　erythema chronicum migrans 26.69, 26.72, 26.73, *26.73*, 26.74
　eye involvement 107.40
　investigations 26.74
　management 26.74
　pathophysiology 26.73
lymphadenitis (buboes) 103.15
　chancroid 30.18, 30.19, 30.20, 30.21
　lymphogranuloma venereum 30.14, 30.15, 30.16, **30.17**, 30.18
lymphadenoma, *see also* adamantinoid trichoblastoma
lymphadenopathy, syphilis 29.10
lymphadenosis benigna cutis of Bafverstedt *see* lymphocytoma cutis/B-cell pseudolymphoma
lymphangiectasia 103.30–103.33
lymphangiogenesis 103.3
lymphangioleiomyomatosis (LAM) 103.28–103.29
　tuberous sclerosis complex 78.9
lymphangioma
　acquired progressive 136.38
　oral involvement 108.13
lymphangioma circumscriptum
　atruncular lymphatic malformation without lymphoedema 103.27
　clinical features 103.26–103.27
　differential diagnosis 103.27
　fluid-filled vesicles (frogspawn resemblance) 103.26
　genetics 103.26
　investigations 103.27
　management 103.27–103.28
　pathophysiology 103.26
　truncular lymphatic malformation with lymphangiectasia and lymphoedema 103.27
lymphangiomatosis 71.2, 103.28–103.29, 136.39
lymphangiomatous papules, benign 103.32
lymphangiosarcoma 119.15
lymphangitis 103.14–103.15
lymphatic filariasis (LF) 7.10, 33.7–33.10, 103.33–103.36
　causative organisms 103.34
　clinical features 33.9, 103.34–103.35
　definition/nomenclature 33.7
　differential diagnosis 103.35
　epidemiology 33.7–33.8, 103.33
　investigations 33.9–33.10, 103.35
　lifecycle of filarial nematodes in human and mosquito hosts 103.34
　management 33.10, 103.35–103.36
　pathophysiology 33.8–33.9, 103.33
lymphatic-like vascular channels, atypical vascular proliferation after radiotherapy 136.38–136.39
lymphatic malformations (LMs) 71.2, 71.21–71.22, 103.25–103.30
　amniotic band constriction-induced lymphoedema 103.29–103.30

Index

lymphangioleiomyomatosis 103.28–103.29
non-malignant lymphatic tumours 103.28–103.29
lymphatic obstruction, neoplasia association 148.27
lymphatico-lymphatic anastomosis surgery 103.61
lymphatico-venous anastomosis (LVA) surgery 103.61
lymphatic-related hydrops fetalis 103.23
lymphatic system
   anatomy of head and neck 20.2
   fat homeostasis 103.2
   fluid homeostasis 103.2
   function and structure 103.1–103.2
   and immunity 103.2
   lymphatic involvement in skin disease 103.2–103.3
   lymphatic vessel *103.14*
   lymph drainage routes *103.8*
   nutrition 103.2
   oedema and 103.2
   peripheral fat 103.2
lymphatic system disorders 71.21–71.28, 103.1–103.62
   abdominal wall lymphoedema 103.51–103.52
   acute dermatolymphangioadenitis 103.16
   arm swelling due to oedema 103.44–103.46
   atypical vascular lesions 103.32
   breast lymphoedema 103.43–103.44
   cancer-related lymphoedema 103.37–103.38
   cellulitis 103.13–103.17
   chronically swollen limb 103.9–103.10
   chronic oedema 103.2, 103.3–103.5
   chronic red leg 103.16–103.17
   chylous disease 103.32
   complicated lymphatic anomalies 71.1, 71.22–71.23
   congenital-onset primary lymphoedema 103.24
   cutaneous lymphangiectasia 103.31–103.32
   drug induced oedema 103.12–103.13
   facial oedema 103.46–103.49
   fluorescence microlymphangiography 103.56
   generalised lymphatic dysplasia 103.22
   genital lymphoedema 103.49–103.51, *103.52*
   hand oedema *103.21*
   head oedema 103.46–103.49
   histopathology 103.57
   hypotrichosis–lymphoedema–telangiectasia syndrome 103.23
   imaging techniques 103.7, *103.8*, 103.55–103.57
   immobility-induced lymphoedema 103.40
   intestinal lymphangiectasia 103.32
   intranodal MR lymphography **103.56**
   late-onset primary lymphoedema 103.24–103.25
   limb swelling 103.6, 103.9–103.10, 103.16–103.17, 103.44–103.46
   lipodermatosclerosis 103.16–103.17
   lipoedema 103.53–103.55
   lymphadenitis 103.15
   lymphangiectasia 103.30–103.33
   lymphangioma circumscriptum 103.25–103.28
   lymphangitis 103.14–103.15
   lymphatic filariasis 7.10, 33.7–33.10, 103.33–103.36
   lymphatic involvement in skin disease 103.2–103.3
   lymphatic malformations 71.2, 71.21–71.22, 103.25–103.30
   lymph fistula 103.32, 103.33
   lymphoceles 103.32, 103.33
   lymphography 103.55, **103.56**

lymphoscintigraphy (isotope lymphography) 103.7, *103.8*, 103.55, *103.56*, **103.56**
lymphovenous oedema 103.10–103.12
magnetic resonance lymphangiography **103.56**, 103.57
massive localised lymphoedema 103.52–103.53
mosaic lymphoedema associated with disturbed growth and/or cutaneous/vascular anomalies 103.23–103.24
multisegmental lymphatic dysplasia with systemic involvement 103.22
near infrared lymphangiography (ICG lymphography) 103.56–103.57
neck oedema 103.46–103.49
obesity-related lymphoedema 103.38–103.39
phlebolymphoedema 103.10–103.12
podoconiosis (non-filarial lymphoedema) 103.36–103.37
pretibial myxoedema 103.41–103.43
recurrent cellulitis (erysipelas) 103.13–103.14
regional swelling 103.43–103.53
Schimmelpenning–Feuerstein–Mims syndrome 71.23–71.24
secondary lymphoedema 103.33–103.43
seromas 103.32, 103.33
swollen breast 103.43–103.44
swollen limb 103.6, 103.9–103.10, 103.16–103.17, 103.44–103.46
syndromic lymphoedema 103.20–103.22
trauma-induced lymphoedema 103.40
venouos oedema 103.10–103.12
WILD syndrome 103.22
yellow-nail syndrome 103.21–103.22
see also lymphoedema
lymphatic tumours 136.37–136.39
see also lymphangioma circumscriptum
lymph drainage
   chronic oedema **103.4**
   management 103.57–103.61
lymph fistula 103.32, 103.33
lymph node metastasis, squamous cell carcinoma of the auricle 106.27–106.28
lymph nodes
   antigen-presenting cell migration 127.7
   drainage areas of cervical lymph nodes **108.6**
   examination of 108.6
   fine-needle aspiration of 4.22
   immune system 9.6
   Kikuchi–Fujimoto disease *51.33*
   lymphadenitis 103.15
lymph nodes and lymphatic drainage basins, in neck 106.28
lymph node transfer surgery 103.61
lymphoceles 103.32, 103.33
lymphocytes
   adipocytes interaction 97.6–97.7
   drug reaction with eosinophilia and systemic symptoms 118.5, 118.8
   microscopic examination of 3.34, *3.35*
   wound healing 11.3
lymphocytic alopecia 87.37, 87.38–87.50
lymphocytic folliculitis, scalp margin 91.12–91.13
lymphocytic infiltrates 134.1–134.11
   Jessner lymphocytic infiltrate 134.10–134.11
   lymphocytoma cutis 134.1, 134.2, 134.8–134.10
   parapsoriasis 134.6–134.8
   pityriasis lichenoides 134.3–134.5, *134.6*
   pseudolymphoma 134.1–134.3
lymphocytic lobular panniculitis 97.39
lymphocytic panniculitis, in childhood 97.56, *97.57*
lymphocytic perifollicular, necrotising lymphocytic folliculitis 93.4
lymphocytic vasculitis 97.38

lymphocytoma cutis (B-cell pseudolymphoma) 89.10, 134.1, 134.2, 134.8–134.10
lymphoedema 103.5–103.9
   abdominal wall 103.51–103.52
   acquired cutaneous lymphangiectasia *103.6*
   and amniotic bands 103.29–103.30
   bacterial/fungal infection 103.6, *103.7*
   bandaging 103.58, *103.59*
   breast lymphoedema 103.43–103.44
   breathing exercises 103.59
   cancer-related lymphoedema 103.37–103.38
   chronic oedema comparison 103.3
   chronic venous insufficiency **101.43**
   chronic venous oedema association *103.10*
   clinical features 103.6
   complications and co-morbidities 103.6
   diagnosis of 103.3
   elephantiasis nostra verrucosa *103.6*
   elevation and rest 103.59
   epidemiology 103.5
   excisional surgery 103.60
   exercise and movement 103.58
   external compression 103.58–103.59
   facial lymphoedema 103.46–103.49
   genital 109.19–109.21
   genitalia and mons pubis 103.49–103.51, *103.52*
   hyperbaric oxygen therapy 103.59–103.60
   imaging characteristics **98.23**
   immobility-induced lymphoedema 103.40
   infection 103.6, *103.7*
   prevention of 103.58
   intensive and maintenance treatment 103.60
   investigations 103.7
   Kaposi–Stemmer sign *103.6*
   limb swelling 103.6, 103.9–103.10, 103.16–103.17, 103.44–103.46
   in lipoedema 98.23
   lipoedema differential diagnosis 98.22
   liposuction (suction lipectomy) 103.60–103.61
   low-level laser therapy 103.59–103.60
   lymphangiosarcoma *103.7*
   lymphatico-lymphatic anastomosis surgery 103.61
   lymph node transfer surgery 103.61
   lymphovenous bypass (lymphatico-venous anastomosis) surgery 103.61
   macerated web-space skin *103.7*
   malignancy 103.7
   management 103.7–103.9, 103.57–103.61
   massage (manual lymphatic drainage therapy) 103.59
   massive localised lymphoedema 103.52–103.53
   medical assessment 103.58
   obesity 98.27
   obesity-related lymphoedema 103.38–103.39
   palmoplantar keratodermas with 63.72–63.73
   pathophysiology 103.5–103.6
   penoscrotal swelling **109.20**
   pharmacological therapies 103.60
   physical therapies 103.58–103.60
   postural exercises 103.59
   psychosocial issues 103.7
   skin care and infection prevention 103.58
   skin changes 103.6
   surgery 103.60–103.61
   syndromes associates with **103.20**
   systemic/visceral involvement 103.22–103.23
   trauma-induced lymphoedema 103.40
   weight loss 103.59
   see also primary lymphoedema
lymphoedema–distichiasis syndrome 71.25–71.26, 103.25, 151.2

lymphoepithelial Kazal-type-related inhibitor (LEKTI) 63.26–63.27, 69.6
lymphoepithelioma-like carcinoma 137.43–137.44
lymphogranuloma inguinale *see* lymphogranuloma venereum
lymphogranuloma venereum (LGV) 30.14–30.18
   clinical features/stages 30.15–30.17
   epidemiology 30.15
   investigations 30.17
   management 30.18
   pathophysiology 30.15
   perineal and perianal skin 111.16
lymphography, lymphatic system 103.55, **103.56**
lymphoid aggregates
   lupus panniculitis 97.37, *97.38*
   necrobiotic xanthogranuloma 97.18
lymphoid lineage cells, immune system 9.5
lymphoid malignancies, skin manifestations of paraneoplastic syndromes 149.8–149.9
lymphoid markers, cutaneous neoplasms 3.27–3.29
lymphoma
   acquired ichthyosis 85.2
   B-cell lymphoma, external ear *106.34*
   ear dermatoses **106.23**
   erythroderma 39.32–39.33
   external ear 106.34
   follicular mucinosis, association with *105.8*
   HIV 31.32–31.33
   hypermelanosis in 86.19–86.20
   oral involvement 108.71
   panniculitis-like 97.61–97.63
   pseudolymphoma relationship 134.1, 134.2
   see also cutaneous lymphomas
lymphomatoid eruptions 127.20
lymphomatoid granulomatosis
   respiratory involvement 152.6
   secondary cutaneous B-cell lymphoma 139.44–139.45
lymphomatoid papulosis 139.26–139.28, 149.9
   clinical features 139.27–139.28
   management 139.27
   pathophysiology 139.26–139.27
lymphomatous skin infiltrates 149.4
lymphoproliferative disorders
   Epstein–Barr virus association 25.38–25.39
   necrobiotic xanthogranuloma association 135.24
   post-transplant/immunodeficiency 139.47
   sarcoidosis association 96.1
lymphorrhoea *103.6*
lymphoscintigraphy (isotope lymphography), lymphatic system 103.7, *103.8*, 103.55, *103.56*, **103.56**
lymphovenous bypass (lymphatico-venous anastomosis) surgery 103.61
lymphovenous oedema 103.10–103.12
lymph vessels, subcutaneous tissue 97.2
lympthatic network 2.42
Lynch syndrome **78.14**, 148.12
   see also Muir–Torre syndrome
Lyonisation 8.7–8.8
Lyral allergy 127.44
lysosomal storage disorders 79.1–79.8
   Fabry disease 79.6–79.8
   glycoproteinoses 79.3–79.4
   mucolipidoses types II and III 79.4–79.5
   mucopolysaccharidoses 79.1–79.3
   sphingolipidoses 79.5–79.6
lysyl hydroxylase 3 (LH3) 69.7
lysyl oxidases 2.34, *2.35*

M

mAbs *see* monoclonal antibodies
macacine herpesvirus 1 *see* herpes B virus infection

McCune–Albright syndrome **72.7**, 73.19–73.20
machine learning, melanoma diagnosis 142.21
Machupo (Bolivian) haemorrhagic fever 25.82–25.83
macrocephaly–capillary malformation syndrome (M–CM) 71.8
macrocyclic chelating agents 94.44
macroglossia 108.11–108.12
　in amyloidosis 56.12, 108.69
macrolides 19.47
macrophages 135.1–135.3
　cytotoxic T lymphocytes interaction 97.6–97.7
　immune system 9.4, 9.5
　sarcoidosis 96.4
　secretion of cytokines 97.5–97.6
　tissue homeostasis 9.4, 9.7
　wound healing 11.3
macrophage–monocyte lineage, histiocytoses 135.1
macrotia (large ears) 106.5
macular effects, pseudoxanthoma elasticum 70.33
macular lymphocytic arteritis 97.9
macular primary localised cutaneous amyloidosis **56.6**, 56.7, 56.9
macular syphilide (roseolar rash) 29.8, 29.9
　see also roseola infantum
macules
　ash-leaf-shaped macules, tuberous sclerosis complex 78.8
　café-au-lait macules 78.3
　hypopigmented macules 76.4
maculopapular rash
　autoinflammatory diseases **80.19**
　complex and polygenic autoinflammatory diseases presenting with urticarial or maculopapular rash 45.20–45.22
　COVID-19 association 25.109, *25.110*
　drug-induced exanthems 117.2
maculopapular sarcoidosis 96.7
MADA *see* mandibulo-acral dysplasia with type A lipodystrophy
madarosis 107.4–107.5
MADB *see* mandibulo-acral dysplasia with type B lipodystrophy
Madelung disease (multiple symmetrical lipomatosis) **72.10**, 79.8, 98.15, *103.46*
MADISH *see* metabolising acquired dioxin-induced skin hamartoma
madura foot *see* mycetoma
Madurella mycetomatis 32.75
maduromycosis *see* mycetoma
Maffucci syndrome 71.20–71.21, 101.24, **101.25, 101.28**, 103.29, 136.31
MAGIC (mouth and genital ulcers with inflamed cartilage) syndrome 108.41, 155.11, 155.13
magnetic resonance imaging (MRI) 4.22, 4.23
　foreign body reactions 122.18
　morphoea 55.31, *55.32*
magnetic resonance lymphangiography (MRL), lymphatic system **103.56**, 103.57
MAGPs *see* microfibril-associated glycoproteins
Majeed syndrome 45.18
Majocchi disease *see* purpura annularis telangiectodes
major depressive disorder 84.40
major histocompatibility complex (MHC)
　class I deficiency 80.10
　class I-restricted drug presentation 118.12
　drug-binding 118.5
　histiocytoses 135.2
　molecule 14.4, 14.5, 14.6
Major Life Changing Decision Profile (MLCDP) 16.11

MAL *see* methyl aminolevulinate
malabsorption, acquired ichthyosis 63.47
malabsorption syndromes, hypermelanosis 86.23
malakoplakia 135.23–135.24
　female genitalia 110.26
　perianal skin 111.15
malaria 33.36
　clinical features 33.36
　epidemiology 33.36
　management 33.36
　see also antimalarial agents
Malassezia yeast species 86.43
　confluent and reticulated papillomatosis 85.6–85.7
　eosinophilic pustular folliculitis 93.7
　folliculitis 32.13, 88.35
　pustulosis in neonates 114.28–114.29
　scalp itch 105.15–105.16
　superficial mycoses 32.10–32.14
malathion, topical therapies 18.14
Malawi polyomavirus (human polyomavirus-10) 25.49
mal de Meleda 63.54–63.56
male angiomyofibroblastoma-like tumour 136.9
male *EBP* disorder with neurological defects (MEND syndrome) 63.23
male fertility, safe treatments in pregnancy 113.19–113.24
male pattern hair loss (MPHL/male androgenetic alopecia) 87.61–87.62, 87.64, *87.66*, 87.68–87.70
malignancies
　associated with dermatomyositis 2
　associated with seborrhoeic keratosis 132.1–132.2
　basal cell carcinoma 140.1–140.21
　Epstein–Barr virus association 25.38–25.39
　eyelid lesions 107.47–107.50
　human papillomaviruses 25.71
　immunosuppressants/immunomodulatory drug risks 19.2, 19.3, 19.8, 19.9, 19.11, 19.18, 19.21–19.22, 19.24, 19.26, 19.29
　Kaposi sarcoma-associated herpesvirus 25.42, 25.43
　paraneoplastic pruritus 81.10
　radiotherapy indications for skin disorders 24.8
　skin lesions with uncertain/unpredictable malignant potential 141.1–141.18
　zoster risks 25.34
malignancy, acquired ichthyosis 63.73
malignancy-associated generalised hypertrichosis 87.86
malignant acrospiroma *see* hidradenocarcinoma
malignant atrophic papulosis 99.21–99.22
malignant blue naevus, melanomas 142.14, 142.20, *142.21*
malignant cylindroma 137.35
malignant eccrine poroma 137.33–137.34
malignant fibrous histiocytoma *see* undifferentiated soft tissue sarcoma
malignant haemangioendothelioma *see* angiosarcoma
malignant hidradenoma *see* hidradenocarcinoma
malignant histiocytosis (MH) 135.29–135.32
malignant melanoma (MM)
　adjuvant systemic treatment 144.6
　ambiguous lesions 142.18–142.19
　ano-genital region 111.24
　atypical melanocytes in epidermis 3.24
　of the auricle 106.31–106.33
　basis for diagnosis 142.18–142.22
　biopsy 143.1
　blocking of transverse sections of 3.6
　BRAF inhibitors (vemurafenib and dabrafenib) treatment leading to keratoacanthoma 141.38
　classification 142.7–142.9
　clinical features 142.8–142.9

clinicopathology 142.1–142.25
colour of *4.14*
combination therapies with immunotherapy 144.2–144.3
combination therapies with targeted therapy 144.5
complete response after systemic therapy 144.8–144.9
completion lymph node dissection 143.4, 143.5
congenital melanocytic naevi 73.10, 73.13, 142.2
cost-of-illness meta-analysis **6.7**
cutaneous side effects of systemic therapies 144.9–144.12
cyclin-dependent kinase 4 gene 142.4
definition 142.1
dermoscopy 145.1–145.16
　benign naevus pattern comparison 145.1–145.7
　facial and chronically sun-damaged skin 145.9, *145.11*, **145.12**
　non-glabrous/non-facial skin 145.7–145.9
　organised patterns 145.13–145.14, *145.15*
　special locations 145.9–145.13
　volar skin of palms and soles 145.9, 145.11–145.13
detection 143.1
diagnostic tools 142.9–142.10, 142.18–142.21, 145.1–145.16
disease process 5.3
drug/chemical photosensitivity 126.30
early detection strategies 142.8–142.9, 142.15–142.18
electrochemotherapy 144.2
environmental factors 142.5–142.6
epidemiological classification 142.8
epidemiology 142.1–142.2
eyelid 107.49
follow-up 142.24–142.25
genetics 142.3–142.5
genomic link to naevi 142.2
histological subtypes 142.7
histopathological diagnosis 142.18–142.21
HIV 31.31–31.32
identification of at risk individuals 142.6–142.7
immunocompromised people
　clinicopathological features 147.13–147.14
　management 147.21, 147.23
immunotherapy 144.2–144.4
in situ, surgery 143.3
isolated limb perfusion 144.2
local therapies 144.1–144.2
macroscopic specimen of 3.6
management after surgery 142.22–142.25
metastatic disease systemic treatment 144.6–144.7
mole and cancer phobias 84.26
molecular classification 142.9
mortality rate 5.7
mucosal system treatment 144.7
neoadjuvant systemic treatment 144.6
oculocutaneous albinism 68.7
oncolytic virus therapy 144.1–144.2
oral melanoma 108.18
palmoplantar keratodermas 63.65
pathological criteria of malignancy 142.18–142.19
penis 109.41
phenotypic traits 142.3–142.4, 142.7
PRAME (PReferentially expressed Antigen in Melanoma) 3.25
precursors 142.2–142.3
predisposing factors 142.2–142.3
in pregnancy 113.9–113.10
presentation 142.10–142.15
prevention 142.6–142.7
prognostic markers 142.21–142.22
PUVA phototherapy adverse effects 21.14

radiotherapy 24.14, *24.15*, 144.2
sentinel lymph node biopsy 143.4–143.6
skin cancer, prevalence of 5.10
special circumstances for systemic treatment 144.7–144.9
staging 142.21–142.24
surgery 143.1–143.6
systemic treatment 144.1–144.12
targeted therapies 144.4–144.5, *144.11*, **144.11**, 144.12
therapeutic approach for systemic management 144.5–144.12
tissue sampling during surgery 144.1
trends in incidence and mortality 142.1
tumour kinetics and aggressiveness classification 142.8
uveal, system treatment 144.7–144.8
UVR exposure 10.9–10.10
vulval melanoma 110.39–110.40
wide local excision surgery 143.1–143.4
malignant otitis externa 106.19
malignant peripheral nerve sheath tumours (MPNSTs) 78.3, 136.51
malignant schwannoma *see* malignant peripheral nerve sheath tumour
malignant soft-tissue tumours 136.2, 136.14–136.15, 136.17–136.18
　see also sarcomas
malignant spiradenoma *see* spiradenocarcinoma
malignant Spitz tumour/malignant spitzoiid neoplasm *see* Spitzoid melanoma
malignant syringoma *see* microcystic adnexal carcinoma
malignant tumours
　misdiagnosed benign tumours 136.2, 136.5
　neurofibromatosis type 1 78.3–78.4
　sebaceous carcinoma 137.18
　uncertain malignancy of keratoacanthoma 141.38
　vascular 136.35–136.37
malingering
　definition 84.36
　factitial disease distinction 84.29, 84.36
　falsifying dermatological symptoms 84.36–84.37
malnutrition 61.1–61.7
　adiponectin system 97.5
　assessment 61.2
　in children 61.2, 61.3, *61.4*, 61.5–61.6
　classification 61.2, 61.5–61.6
　clinical features 61.3–61.4
　complications and co-morbidities 61.6
　diagnosis 61.5
　disease course and prognosis 61.6
　epidemiology 61.2
　ethnicity role 61.2–61.3
　incidence and prevalence 61.2
　investigations 61.6
　management 61.6–61.7
　predisposing factors 61.3
　protein-energy malnutrition 61.2, 61.3
　severity classification 61.5–61.6
　skin signs of nutritional disease **61.5**
MALT *see* mucosa associated lymphoid tissue
Malta fever *see* brucellosis
mammary glands 92.15
mammary-like gland adenoma of the vulva *see* hidradenoma papilliferum
mammary-like glands, tumours of ano-genital glands 137.40
mammary-type secretory carcinoma of the skin *see* secretory carcinoma
Manchester checklist, neurofibromatosis type 1 78.4, *78.5–78.6*
mandibuloacral dysplasia 98.3
mandibuloacral dysplasia with type A lipodystrophy (MADA) **72.5**, 77.5
mandibuloacral dysplasia with type B lipodystrophy (MADB) **72.5**, 77.5
manganese deficiency and excess 61.31
mangrove fly *see* Chrysops
MANIAC *see* melanocytic acral naevus with intraepidermal ascent of cells

mansonelosis 33.6–33.7
 definition 33.6
 epidemiology 33.6
 management 33.7
 pathophysiology 33.6–33.7
MAP kinase (MAPK) *see* mitogen-activated protein kinase
marantic endocarditis 99.15
marasmic kwashiorkor syndrome 61.2
marasmus 61.2, 61.3, *61.4*
Marburg haemorrhagic fever, filovirus infection 25.84–25.85
Marfan syndrome (MFS) 70.20–70.21, 94.11
marginal papular keratoderma (MPK) 63.60–63.61
marginal zone lymphoma (MZL)
 primary cutaneous B-cell lymphoma type 139.37
 see also primary cutaneous marginal zone lymphoma
marijuana *see* cannabis
marionette lines, dermal fillers *158.3*
Marshall syndrome 94.22
MART-1 *see* Melan-A
mascular amyloidosis 86.22, *86.23*
masking in clinical trials, evidence based medicine 17.12, 17.13
Mas-related G-protein-coupled receptor agonists (Mrgpr family), pruritus **81.3**, 81.5
Mas-related G protein–coupled receptor member X2 (MRGPRX2) 117.6
massage, manual lymphatic drainage therapy 103.59
massive localised lymphoedema 103.52–103.53
Masson ammoniacal silver nitrate technique 3.8
Masson pseudoangiosarcoma *see* intravascular papillary endothelial hyperplasia
Masson vegetant intravascular haemangioendothelioma *see* intravascular papillary endothelial hyperplasia
mast cell activation syndrome 46.7
mast cell degranulating stimuli, mastocytosis 46.9
mast cell disorders 3.45
mast cell leukaemia (MCL) 46.1
mast cell mediator-induced angio-oedema without weals 43.1, **43.2**
 clinical features 43.4
 incidence and prevalence 43.2
 pathophysiology 43.3
mast cells 2.15–2.17
 allergic-type response 9.9
 fibrosis 89.3
 granules 2.15, *2.17*
 immune cells in homeostasis *9.4*
 immune system 9.5
 immunity role 2.16–2.17
 microscopic examination of 3.37
 stabilising drugs 46.9
 staining technique 3.8–3.9
 urticaria 42.3–42.4
mast cell sarcoma **46.2**
mastitis
 neonates 114.25
 tuberculous 27.31–27.32
mastocytoma *46.3*, 46.5–46.6
mastocytosis 46.1–46.10
 aeitiopathogenesis 46.2
 associated diseases 46.2–46.3
 children *46.4, 46.5, 46.9*
 classification 46.1, **46.2**
 clinical features 46.3–46.7
 co-morbidities 46.7
 diagnostic work-up **46.8**
 disease course and prognosis 46.7
 epidemiology 46.2–46.3
 flushing **104.5**, 148.26
 genetics 46.3
 histopatholgy of skin lesions *46.3*
 infants 115.16–115.17
 investigations 46.7–46.8
 management 46.8–46.10
 mast cell degranulating stimuli **46.9**
 musculoskeletal involvement 155.13
 pathophysiology 46.3
maternal autoantibodies, transplacental transfer 114.11–114.12
maternal malignant disease, transplacental transfer 114.14
maternal milk *see* lactation
maternal transfer, *see also* teratogenicity
matrix metalloproteinases (MMPs) 2.31, 2.32
 collagen and elastin degradation, UVR exposure 10.10–10.11
 skin ageing 2.46
 wound healing 11.4, *11.5*, 11.8, **11.9**
mattress skin sutures 20.17–20.18
Mayaro virus (MAYV), Mayaro/Uruma fever 25.91
May–Gruenwald stain 135.22–135.23
MBT *see* 2-mercaptobenzothiazole
MC *see* mixed cryoglobulinaemia; molluscum contagiosum
MCAP *see* megalencephaly–capillary malformation syndrome
MCC *see* Merkel cell carcinoma
mcEDS *see* musculocontractural Ehlers–Danlos syndrome
MCI *see* methylchloroisothiazolinone
MCI/MI *see* methylchloroisothiazolinone and methylisothiazolinone
MCL *see* mast cell leukaemia
MCLID *see* microcephaly with or without chorioretinopathy, lymphoedema or intellectual disability
MCLMR *see* microcephaly with or without chorioretinopathy, lymphoedema and mental retardation
M–CM *see* macrocephaly–capillary malformation syndrome
MCPs *see* mucocutaneous pain syndromes
MCPyV *see* Merkel cell polyomavirus
MCTD *see* mixed connective tissue disease
MCV *see* molluscipoxvirus
MDA *see* Misuse of Drugs Act 1971
MDBGN *see* methyldibromoglutaronitrile
MDCPs *see* medium depth chemical peels
MDMA (N-methyl-3,4-methylenedioxymethamphetamine) *see* ecstasy
MDR *see* multidrug-resistant
MDTs *see* multidisciplinary teams
Meado Syndrome *see* Münchausen syndrome by proxy
measles 1.3, 25.97–25.98
 clinical features 25.98–25.99
 epidemiology 25.98
 infants 115.7
 management 25.99
 pathophysiology 25.98
measles/mumps/rubella vaccine *see* MMR
measurement 16.1–16.13
 aspects of most concern to patients 16.1–16.2
 challenges 16.1
 core outcome measures 16.3
 disease assessment tools 16.3–16.5
 disease impacts 16.5–16.13
 electronic delivery 16.2
 method validation 16.2–16.3
 objective measures of skin properties 16.5
 objective tools 16.2
 psychological impacts 16.11–16.12
 quality of life measures 16.5–16.11
 role in decision making 16.1
 self-assessment 16.2
 sexual functioning 16.12
 skin disease severity 16.1–16.3
 work impacts 16.12–16.13
mechanical acne 88.30
mechanical boundary-related risk factors, pressure ulcers 123.3–123.4
mechanical hymenal fissures 110.42–110.43
mechanical injuries 122.1–122.29
 biomechanical considerations 122.3–122.7
 foreign material effects 122.17
 reactions to 122.7–122.17
 vibration injuries 122.13, 122.24–122.26
mechanical irritation
 contact dermatitis 129.1
 lichen planus 37.3
 psoriasiform contact dermatitis *128.4*
 see also Koebner (isomorphic) phenomenon
mechanical load, pressure ulcers 123.2
mechanical properties of skin 122.4
mechanical stimuli, use of 122.3
mechanobullous diseases 69.2
mechlorethamine, topical therapies 18.31
MED *see* minimal erythema dose
medallion-like dermal dendrocyte hamartoma, neonates 114.11
median raphe cysts 109.30
median rhomboid glossitis 32.63, 108.22
medical devices, pressure ulcers 123.2
medical texts, ancient cultures 1.1–1.3
medical volunteerism 7.13, **7.15**
medicament contact dermatitis *127.11*, 127.12, 127.18–127.19
medication, *see also* clinical pharmacology; *drug entries*
medication adherence, behavioural effects of skin conditions 15.2
medication errors, clinical pharmacology 13.9–13.11
medication history, diagnosis of drug eruptions 4.3–4.4
medicines, donation of 7.13
Medicines Act 1968 120.4
Medina worm *see* dracunculiasis
Mediterranean fever *see* brucellosis
Mediterranean spotted fever *see* tick typhus
medium depth chemical peels (MDCPs) 160.4
medium-vessel vasculitis *100.3*, 100.28–100.32
MEDLINE (National Library of Medicine's bibliographic database) 17.7
MEDNIK syndrome *see* mental retardation–enteropathy–deafness–neuropathy–ichthyosis–keratodermia syndrome
MeDOCs *see* Mendelian disorders of cornification
mEDS *see* myopathic Ehlers–Danlos syndrome
medulla, hair fibres 87.7
medullary thyroid cancer (MTC), flushing **104.7**, 148.26
medusa stings 130.1
Mee's lines 121.2, *121.3*, 121.9
megalencephaly–capillary malformation syndrome (MCAP) **71.2**
megavoltage X-ray therapy 24.1, 24.3
meibomian gland cyst (chalazion) *107.11*
meibomian gland dysfunction (MGD) 107.7–107.15
meibomian seborrhoea **107.8**
meibomitis **107.8**, *107.11*
Meige disease 103.25
Meirowsky phenomenon 86.9
Meissner corpuscles, substance P fibres ending in *83.3*
MEK inhibitors *see* mitogen-activated protein kinase inhibitors
Melan-A (MART-1) (melanocyte marker) 3.23–3.24
melanin 2.42, 86.1
 biological significance 86.7–86.8
 disorder classification 86.8
 light absorption 23.3–23.4, 23.12
 photoprotection 10.11
 pigmentation disorders 68.1, 68.6, 87.93
 synthesis of 2.17
 trichochromes synthesis *86.6*
melanoblasts, migration/differentiation 86.3–86.4
melanocanthoma, oral melanocanthoma 108.18
melanocortin-4 receptor deficiency **72.6**
melanocortins, Addison disease 86.7
melanocytes 2.1, 2.5, 2.11, 2.17–2.18, 68.1, 86.1–86.9
 Cole disease 63.61
 culture 86.4–86.5
 differentiation *2.18*
 distribution 86.3
 endocrine regulation 86.7
 hair pigmentation 87.12
 skin pigmentation 86.1–86.9
 UV radiation response 86.5–86.7
melanocyte-stimulating hormone (MSH) 86.4, 86.10
melanocytic acral naevus with intraepidermal ascent of cells (MANIAC), use of term 142.19
melanocytic lesions 131.12–131.15
 histological sectioning of 3.7
 see also Mongolian spot
melanocytic markers, cutaneous neoplasms 3.23–3.25
melanocytic naevi 131.15–131.46
 acquired melanocytic naevi 131.17–131.21
 acral naevi 131.23–131.24
  compound acral naevus *131.23*
  on sole of foot *131.24*
 atypical naevi **131.17**, 131.40–131.46
 BAP1-inactivated naevus of the scalp *131.34*
 blue naevus **131.17**, 131.38–131.40
 breast 131.22
 cancer phobias 84.26
 clinical presentation **131.16–131.17**
 cockade naevus 131.30, *131.31*
 combined melanocytic naevi 131.24–131.26
 combined naevus *131.26*
 common acquired naevi **131.16**, 131.17–131.21
 compound naevus **131.1**, *131.19, 131.21, 131.25, 131.42*
 congenital melanocytic naevi 73.8–73.15, 131.15–131.17
 conjunctival naevi 131.24, *131.25*
 dermoscopic presentation **131.16–131.17**
 dysplastic melanocytic naevi *131.41, 131.42, 131.45*
 histological criteria of definition of **131.43**
 eyelid 107.46
 genital area 131.22
 halo naevus 131.27–131.28
  dermoscopic image *131.29*
  lymphocytic infiltrate with disruption of naevomelanocytic aggregates *131.28*
 intradermal/dermal naevus **131.1**, *131.21*
 junctional naevus **131.1**, *131.18, 131.20*
 laser therapies 23.16–23.17
 male genitalia 109.6
 Myerson naevus 131.28–131.29, *131.30*
 naevomelanocytic nests **131.1**, *131.18, 131.20*
 naevus cell types *131.19, 131.20*
 naevus of Ito 68.9–68.10, 131.14–131.15
 naevus of Ota 23.16, *23.17*, 107.46, 131.12–131.14
 oral melanocytic naevi, hyperpigmentation 108.19
 pathology **131.16–131.17**
 recurrent melanocytic naevi 131.26–131.27
 Reed naevus *131.34, 131.37*
 scalp 131.22–131.23, *131.34*
 Spitz naevus **131.16**, 131.32–131.37
 subtypes **131.16–131.17**
 targetoid haemosiderotic naevus 131.30–131.32
 with unusual morphology **131.16**, 131.24–131.32
 in unusual sites **131.16**, 131.21–131.24

melanocytic neoplasms
  diagnosis and classification 3.23–3.25
  terminology **131.1**
melanocytic tumours of uncertain malignant potential (MELTUMP), use of term 142.19
melanocytoma, melanoma precursor 142.2
melanocytosis, dermal 73.21, *73.22*
melanogenesis
  biochemistry 86.5
  UVR exposure 10.8
melanoma *see* malignant melanoma
melanoma of soft parts *see* clear cell sarcoma
melanoma–astrocytoma syndrome 148.9
melanoses, facial 86.9–86.15, 86.51
melanosomes
  keratinocyte terminal differentiation 68.1
  racial groups 86.8
  transport 86.4
melanotic macule, oral involvement 108.18
melanotic neuroectodermal tumour *see* pigmented neuroectodermal tumour of infancy
melanotic progonoma *see* pigmented neuroectodermal tumour of infancy
melasma 86.9–86.12
  depigmentation *86.45*
  on the face, dermatoendocrinology **150.6, 150.10**, *150.14*, 150.18
  Jessner solution peel *160.7, 160.8*
  laser therapies 23.17, *23.18*, 161.5–161.6
  treatment 86.33
melatonin, hair growth 87.9
Meleney synergistic gangrene 26.77, 26.78
melioidosis, *Burkholderia pseudomallei* 26.53–26.54
Melkersson–Rosenthal syndrome 109.25
MELTUMP *see* melanocytic tumours of uncertain malignant potential
membrane-bound transporters, drug pharmacokinetics 13.5
membranes, burn treatment 125.6
membranous fat necrosis 97.8, 97.12, 121.6
MEN *see* multiple endocrine neoplasia
Mendelian disorders of cornification (MeDOCs) 63.20–63.21, 63.45
Mendelian randomisation 5.8
MEND syndrome *see* male *EBP* disorder with neurological defects
meningeal involvement, xanthoma disseminatum 135.20
meningeal neurosyphilis 29.15
meningism, primary genital herpes infection 25.25
meningitis
  Acinetobacter 26.51
  anthrax 26.44
  listeriosis 26.46
  Neisseria meningitidis 26.49, 26.50
  streptococci 26.12
meningococcal infection 26.49–26.50
meningothelial heterotopias 136.49–136.50
meningovascular syphilis 29.15
Menkes syndrome/disease 2.34, 61.28, 61.29, 79.16, *79.17*, 87.93
menopause
  ageing of skin 156.6
  flushing **104.4**
menstrual cycle
  acne flares 88.25
  urticaria 42.8
mental/emotional sweating 2.9
mental health 1.9
  hair loss 87.21
  hidradenitis suppurativa association 90.2, 90.11
  psychiatric side-effects of systemic therapies 19.7, 19.18, *19.19*, 19.20, 19.43, 19.45
mentalis muscle 'creases', reduction of by botulinum toxin application *159.8*
mental neuropathy (numb chin syndrome), internal malignancy association 148.23
mental retardation–enteropathy–deafness–neuropathy–ichthyosis–keratodermia (MEDNIK) syndrome 63.30, 63.35, 79.17
menthol, traditional topical therapy 18.38
men who have sex with men (MSM)
  ChemSex 120.2–120.3
  Kaposi sarcoma in HIV-negative men 138.1, **138.2**, 138.4
  lymphogranuloma venereum 30.15
ME-PPD *see* 2-methoxymethyl-p-phenylenediamine
meralgia paraesthetica 83.7
2-mercaptobenzothiazole (MBT) 127.63–127.64
mercapto mix (sensitisers) 127.63
Mercurialis (Geronimo Mercuriale) 1.3
mercury
  allergic contact dermatitis 127.18, 127.41
  dermatological reactions 121.5–121.6
  pigmentation effects 86.52–86.53
Merkel cell carcinoma (MCC) 2.12, 146.1–146.10
  AEIOU diagnostic acronym 146.5, **146.7**
  clinical features 146.5–146.8
  course and prognosis 146.5
  diagnosis of *3.22*, 3.23
  epidemiology 146.1–146.2
  eyelid 107.49
  human polyomavirus-MCPyV 146.2, *146.3*
  immunocompromised people
    clinicopathological features 147.14–147.15
    management 147.23–147.24
    non-Hodgkin lymphoma/chronic lymphocytic leukaemia patients 147.3
    people living with HIV 147.2
  investigations 146.7–146.8
  management 146.8–146.10
  pathogenesis 146.2
  pathology 146.3–146.5
  polyomavirus infection 25.46–25.47
  predisposing factors 146.2
  radiotherapy 24.15
  staging 146.5, 146.7
Merkel cell polyomavirus (MCPyV) 25.46–25.47
  MCPyV-negative Merkel cell carcinoma 146.2, 146.3, *146.4*, 146.5, 146.9
  MCPyV-positive Merkel cell carcinoma 25.46–25.47, 146.2, 146.3, *146.4*
Merkel cells 2.2, 2.11–2.12
  disputed origins of Merkel cell carcinoma 146.2
  embryonic development 2.5
  hyperplasia 2.12
Merkel cell–neurite complexes 2.12
mesenchymal cells 2.4, 2.5
mesenchymal markers 3.25–3.26
mesenchyme, pre-adipocytes 97.1
mesoderm 2.3
Mesopotamia, ancient medical texts 1.2
meta analysis
  evidence based medicine 17.4–17.5
  see also systematic reviews
metabolic disorders
  acquired ichthyosis 63.47, 85.1
  AGL association 98.2
  blistering 69.24
  hair disorders 87.93
  ocular features 107.42
  primary dyslipidaemias 60.6–60.10
  xanthomas 60.2–60.6
  see also amino acid metabolism and transport disorders; inherited metabolic diseases; lipid metabolism disorders
metabolic syndrome
  diabetic patients 62.4
  hidradenitis suppurativa association 90.2
metabolising acquired dioxin-induced skin hamartoma (MADISH/chloracne) *88.14*, *88.15*, 88.66–88.68, 129.7, 129.12–129.13, 133.1, **133.2**, 133.7
metabolism
  androgen synthesis 87.10
  burn-induced changes 125.11
  hypermetabolic response to burn injuries 125.11–125.14
metabolism of drugs, clinical pharmacology 13.3
metabolism of prohormones to active metabolites 150.7
metabolism of steroid hormones *150.3*
metabolism of vitamins 59.5, 79.15
metaherpetic keratitis, eyelid *107.37*
metalloprotiens *see* ADAMTS metalloproteinase; matrix metalloproteinases; tissue inhibitors of metalloproteinases
metals
  allergies 127.19, 127.36–127.41
  oral hyperpigmentation 108.17
  pigmentation effects 86.51–86.53
  toxicity 121.1–121.10
metaplasia 3.42
  ileostomy 112.6
metastases
  from primary epidermal tumours 148.3
  penis 109.42
  scalp metastases 105.11–105.12
  to the skin from internal cancer 24.15, 148.4–148.6
metastatic calcinosis cutis 59.5–59.6, 154.2
  see also metastatic cutaneous calcification
metastatic carcinomas of skin 148.4
metastatic cutaneous calcification 97.33–97.34
  uraemic patients with combined hyperphosphataemia and hypercalcaemia 154.2
metastatic cutaneous tumour diagnosis 3.26–3.27
metastatic melanoma, systemic therapy 144.6–144.7
metastatic Merkel cell carcinoma 146.7, 146.9
metastatic oral neoplasms 108.45
metastatic pregnancy-associated melanoma (MPAM) 113.10
metastatic regressive melanoma 142.14
metastatic tuberculous abscess 27.17–27.19
metatypical (basosquamous) basal cell carcinoma 140.3
metformin
  acne vulgaris treatment 88.57
  hidradenitis suppurativa treatment 90.10
methacrylate allergic contact dermatitis 127.13, *127.14*
methacrylate nail systems 127.61–127.62
(meth)acrylate-related contact allergy 127.47
methaemoglobinaemia, dapsone side effect 19.14
methamphetamine, dermatoses 120.4–120.5
methicillin-resistant *Staphylococcus aureus* (MRSA) 26.8–26.9
  age effects 26.7
  community-acquired 26.6–26.7
  genetics 26.9
  HIV 31.21, 31.37
  male genitalia 109.28
methicillin-sensitive *Staphylococcus aureus* (MSSA), age effects 26.7
methotrexate (MTX) 19.24–19.28
  alopecia treatment 87.27
  atopic eczema treatment 41.29
  cautions 19.27
  contraindications 19.26
  dermatological uses 19.24–19.25
  dose and regimens 19.27
  drug–drug interactions 19.27
  folate supplementation 19.27
  monitoring 19.27–19.28
  morphoea treatment 55.37
  pemphigus treatment 50.9
  pharmacological properties 19.25–19.26
  potential adverse effects 19.26
  pre-treatment screening 19.27
  psoriasis treatment 35.23–35.25
  sarcoidosis treatment 96.16
  systemic lupus erythematosus treatment 51.38
2-methoxymethyl-p-phenylenediamine (ME-PPD) 127.61
N-methyl-3,4-methylenedioxymethamphetamine (MDMA) *see* ecstasy
methyl acrylate 127.70
methyl aminolevulinate (MAL), use in photodynamic therapy 22.2–22.3, 22.4, 22.5–22.7
methylchloroisothiazolinone (MCI) 127.53–127.54
methylchloroisothiazolinone and methylisothiazolinone (MCI/MI) 127.53–127.54
methyldibromoglutaronitrile (MDBGN) 127.55
methylisothiazolinone (MI) 127.53–127.54
methyl methacrylate (MMA) 127.70
metronidazole, topical therapies 18.11
Metvixia® *see* methyl aminolevulinate
Metvix® *see* methyl aminolevulinate
mevalonate kinase deficiency (MKD) **45.5, 45.6**, 45.11
mevalonate kinase (*MVK*) genes 85.20
mevalonic aciduria 63.74
Mexico
  community dermatology 7.8
  teledermatology training 7.9
MF *see* mycosis fungoides
MFAPs *see* microfibril-associated proteins
mFGS *see* modified Ferriman–Gallwey score
MFS *see* Marfan syndrome
MGD *see* meibomian gland dysfunction
MGUS *see* monoclonal gammopathy of uncertain significance
MH *see* malignant histiocytosis
MHC *see* major histocompatibility complex
MI *see* methylisothiazolinone
Mibelli porokeratosis 63.74, 63.75, 85.20, 85.21, 109.35
Michelin tyre baby syndrome 70.19, 73.17
Michel medium, biopsy 3.4–3.5, 3.12
microabscesses 3.43
microbial ecology of the skin 26.3–26.5
  age/sex/ethnic difference 26.4
  bacterial adherence 26.5
  modifying factors 26.4
  normal flora 26.3–26.5
  quantitative cultural studies 26.4
  role of normal flora 26.4–26.5
  sampling methods 26.3
  specialised areas 26.5
  temporary residents on skin 26.2, 26.3
microbial exposure, atopic eczema 41.7–41.8
microbiome
  gut 26.4, 26.5
  oral 108.5
  see also skin microbiome
microcephalic osteodysplastic primordial dwarfism type II **72.7**
microcephaly with or without chorioretinopathy, lymphoedema or intellectual disability (MCLID) 103.24
microcephaly with or without chorioretinopathy, lymphoedema and mental retardation (MCLMR) 71.27
microcephaly–capillary malformation syndrome (MIC–CAP) 71.7
microchimerism, rheumatoid nodules 97.15
microclimate 123.3
Micrococcus spp., normal skin flora 26.3
microcystic adnexal carcinoma 107.49, 137.36–137.37
microdialysis, topical bioavailability/bioequivalence assessment 12.8
microfibril-associated glycoproteins (MAGPs) 2.36

microfibril-associated proteins (MFAPs) 2.36
microneedling
  hair disorder treatment 87.95
  skin tightening 161.8
micronodular basal cell carcinoma 140.3, *140.4*
micronutrients, hypermetabolism treatment 125.12
microorganisms
  rosacea 89.4
  staining techniques 3.9–3.10
micropapular polymorphic light eruption 126.4, *126.5*
microscopic examination
  diagnosis 4.20–4.22
  superficial mycoses identification 32.8
microscopic examination of tissue sections 3.32–3.45
  areola 3.33
  axillary skin 3.33
  biopsy site and normal histological variation 3.33
  endothelial cells 3.37
  eosinophils 3.35–3.36
  examination of sections 3.33
  facial skin 3.33
  fibroblasts 3.37
  foreign bodies/deposits 3.38
  giant cells 3.36, *3.37*
  high-magnification examination 3.34
  histiocytes 3.36
  histopathology skin reports 3.38
  low-magnification histological pattern diagnosis 3.34
  lymphocytes 3.34, *3.35*
  mast cells 3.37
  monocytes 3.36
  mucous membranes 3.33
  myofibroblasts 3.37
  neutrophils 3.35
  palm and sole skin 3.33
  pericytes 3.37
  plasma cells 3.35
  preparing for microscopy 3.32–3.33
  rhabdomyocyte (striated muscle cell) 3.37
  scalp skin 3.33
  Schwann cells *3.37*
  scrotum skin 3.33
  smooth muscle cells 3.37
  tissue macrophages 3.36
  truncal skin 3.33–3.34
microscopic polyangiitis (MPA) 100.20–100.22, 152.4
microsponges, vehicle choice for topical therapies 18.2–18.3
microsporide *see* dermatophytide reaction
Microsporum infections, Wood's light examination 32.6
Microsporum species
  dermatophytosis 32.18–32.20, **32.19**, 32.24–32.26
  M. audouinii 32.24–32.25
  M. canis 32.25
  M. gypseum 32.25–32.26
microtia (small ears) 106.4, *106.5*
microvascular occlusion disorders, purpura 99.9–99.24
microvenular haemangioma 136.30
MIC–CAP *see* microcephaly–capillary malformation syndrome
mid-dermal elastolysis 94.25–94.26
middle age, psychological and social factors 15.3
midface toddler excoriation syndrome (MiTES) 82.9, 83.12–83.13
midges 34.7–34.8
Miescher radial granulomas 97.22–97.23
migrant health dermatology 7.13, **7.14**
migration, epidemiology 5.10
migratory circinate redness, autosomal dominant epidermolysis bullosa simplex with 69.9–69.10
migratory erythemas, internal malignancy association 148.19–148.20

migratory thrombophlebitis
  adenocarcinoma of the pancreas 153.6
  neoplasia association 148.26
milia
  chemical peel side effects 160.12
  cysts 133.4
  differential diagnosis 88.30, *88.31*
  infants 115.13–115.14
  neonates 114.4
miliaria 92.12–92.14
  management 92.13–92.14
  neonates 114.6–114.7
miliaria crystallina (sudamina) 92.12–92.13
miliaria profunda 92.12–92.13, 92.14
miliaria rubra (prickly heat) 92.12–92.13, 92.14
miliary calcinosis cutis 59.4, 59.5, 59.6
miliary tuberculosis, acute cutaneous 27.17
milk alkali syndrome, metastatic calcinosis cutis 59.5
milker's nodule 25.15
milker's sinuses 122.22–122.23
milk thistle (silymarin), cosmeceutical use of **157.8**, *157.9*
millipedes (Diplopoda) 34.57
Milroy disease 103.24
Milroy-like lymphoedema 103.24
mineral disorders 61.24–61.31, **79.2**, 79.15–79.18
  acrodermatitis enteropathica 79.15–79.16
  copper deficiency 2.34, 61.27–61.29
  familial tumoral calcinosis 79.17–79.18
  hair loss 59
  iron deficiency 61.3, 61.4, 61.24–61.25, 87.59, 87.63, 87.70–87.71, 153.1
  manganese deficiency and excess 61.31
  MEDNIK syndrome 79.17
  Menkes disease 79.16, *79.17*
  occipital horn syndrome 79.16
  selenium deficiency and excess 61.29–61.31
  skin manifestations of impaired absorption 153.1
  Wilson disease 79.17
  zinc deficiency 61.25–61.27, 69.24, 108.20, 153.9
mineralisation, abnormal 70.31–70.36
mineral oils/greases, topical medication vehicles 18.6
miner's anaemia *see* ancylostomiasis
'miniature puberty', neonates 114.4
miniaturised follicles 87.64, *87.65*
minimal erythema dose (MED), phototherapy 21.7–21.8
minimal phototoxic dose, PUVA 21.9
minocycline, sarcoidosis management 96.16
minocycline-induced hyperpigmentation 86.27–86.28
minoxidil 87.69–87.70, 87.73, 87.94
minoxidil acid, topical therapies 18.41
MIS-A *see* multisystem inflammatory syndrome in adults
MIS-C *see* multisystem inflammatory syndrome in children
Misuse of Drugs Act 1971 (MDA) 120.3–120.4
MiTES *see* midface toddler excoriation syndrome
mites (Acari) 34.41–34.57
  animal diseases 34.50
  bird/rodent/reptile mites 34.54–34.55
  Cheyletiella mites 34.53, *34.54*
  follicle mites 34.55–34.57
  harvest mites 34.54
  house dust mites 34.51
  plant mites 34.52
  Pyemotes mites 34.51–34.52
  rickettsial infection transmission 26.84
  scabies 34.41–34.50
  stored products 34.50–34.51
mitochondrial disorders 8.5
mitochondrial palmoplantar keratoderma 63.64–63.65
mitochondrial respiratory chain disorders **79.2**, 79.8–79.9

mitochrondria, damage from UVR exposure 10.11
mitogen-activated protein kinase (MAPK) pathway, targeted therapy for melanoma 144.4
mitogen-activated protein kinase (MEK) inhibitors
  chemotherapy cutaneous side-effects 119.3, 119.7–119.8
  melanoma systemic therapy 144.4–144.5, *144.11*, **144.11**, 144.12
mitogen-activated protein (MAP) kinase 87.73
mitten hand deformity, epidermolysis bullosa 69.17, 69.26
mixed connective tissue disease (MCTD) 53.1–53.3
  acral lesions 53.4
  cardiac involvement 151.4
  clinical features 53.2
  diagnostic criteria **53.2**
  investigations 53.3
  management 53.3
  pathophysiology 53.1–53.2
  and retiform purpura 53.4
mixed cryoglobulinaemia (MC) 25.76, 124.13
mixed immunobullous disease 50.36
mixed inflammatory infiltrate 87.50–87.52
mixed leg ulcers (MLUs) 102.4–102.7
  clinical features 102.7
  disorders associated with **102.6**
  epidemiology 102.5–102.6
  lipodermatosclerosis 102.7
  management of 102.8
  predisposing factors 102.6
mixed tumour of the skin 137.32
Mkar disease 94.30
MKD *see* mevalonate kinase deficiency
MLCDP *see* Major Life Changing Decision Profile
MLDSI *see* multisegmental lymphatic dysplasia with systemic involvement
MLUs *see* mixed leg ulcers
MM *see* malignant melanoma
MMA *see* methyl methacrylate
MMDK *see* multiple minute digitate keratoses
MMF *see* mycophenolate mofetil
MMP *see* mucous membrane pemphigoid
MMPs *see* matrix metalloproteinases
MMR (measles/mumps/rubella) vaccine
  intralesional immunotherapy for human papillomavirus infections 25.59–25.60
  prophylaxis 25.92, 25.99
  uptake of 115.7
MMR-V (measle/mumps/rubella/varicella) vaccine 25.92, 25.99
MMS *see* Mohs micrographic surgery
modified Ferriman–Gallwey score (mFGS), hirsutism 87.88–87.89
modified hidradenitis suppurativa score 16.4
modified Parkland resuscitation formula 125.2–125.3
modified Rodnan skin score (MRSS), systemic sclerosis **54.17**
modified Sartorius Score (MSS) 16.4
'Mogul skier's palm' 122.17
Mohs micrographic surgery (MMS) 20.30–20.37, 90.11
  basal cell carcinoma 140.16
  Boden disease 141.21
  cutaneous squamous cell carcinoma 141.33, 141.35, 141.37
  defect closure procedures 20.20–20.22, 20.26–20.29
  defect reconstruction 20.20–20.22, 20.26–20.29, 20.30–20.37
  definition 20.30–20.31
  history 20.31–20.32
  practical aspects and indications 20.35–20.37

procedure 20.33–20.34, *20.36*
results 20.34–20.35
skin cancer treatment comparisons 20.32–20.33
types of tumours **20.37**
moisture-associated skin damage 123.4
moisturisers, ichthyoses management 63.42
molecular amplification tests, syphilis 29.18
molecular-based approaches
  classic epidermolysis bullosa simplex 69.11–69.15
  classic junctional epidermolysis bullosa 69.15
  dystrophic epidermolysis bullosa 69.18–69.19
  pigmentation disorders *68.14*
molecular diagnosis, superficial mycoses identification 32.9
molecular genetic methods, culture-independent microbial studies 26.2, 26.3
moles *see* melanocytic naevi
Moll, cyst of 107.45
mollicutes, *Mycoplasma genitalium* infection 30.23–30.25
mollusca, stings 130.4
molluscipoxviruses (MCV-1 to MCV-4), HIV 31.26
molluscum contagiosum (MC) 25.15–25.19
  clinical features 25.16–25.17
  eczematisation around lesions 39.25
  epidemiology 25.15–25.16
  eyelid 107.34, *107.36*
  infants 115.9
  investigations 25.18
  management 25.18
  pathophysiology 25.16
  penis 109.29
  perianal skin *111.13*, 111.15
molluscum sebaceum *see* keratoacanthoma
moluscipoxviruses **25.6**, 25.15–25.18
molybdenum, dermatological reactions 121.9
MOMES syndrome **72.7**
MOMO syndrome **72.6**
'Mona Lisa smile', dermatitis artefacta 84.31, *84.32*
Mondor disease 101.36–101.37
  neoplasia association 148.26–148.27
  subtypes **101.38**
monetary costs of disease *see* economic burden of disease
Mongolian spot *73.22*, 79.3, 86.2, 131.12
monilethrix 87.78
monkey oesophagus substrate, indirect immunofluorescence *3.12*, 3.13–3.14, 3.19
monkeypox virus (MPXV) *see* mpox
monobenzyl ether of hydroquinone, topical depigmenting agents 18.32
monochromator phototesting 126.5–126.6, 126.12, 126.19, *126.20*, 126.23, *126.27, 126.31, 126.35*
monoclonal antibodies (mAbs) 19.31–19.32
  cutaneous T-cell lymphoma therapy 139.25
  WHO naming conventions 19.31, **19.32**
monoclonal gammopathy of clinical or cutaneous significance 149.10
monoclonal gammopathy of uncertain significance (MGUS)
  disorders of paraprotein activity 149.9–149.13
  disorders of paraprotein deposition 149.13, 149.14
  necrobiotic xanthogranuloma 135.24
  pyoderma gangrenosum 149.7
  skin disorders from cell infiltration 149.2, 149.4–149.5
monoclonal mast cell activation syndrome 46.6
monocytes
  immune system 9.5
  microscopic examination of 3.36

monogenic autoinflammatory syndromes *see* hereditary monogenic autoinflammatory syndromes
monogenic inherited pigmentation disorders **68.2–68.3**
monogenic obesity with cutaneous features 72.4, **72.7**
monogenic obesity without cutaneous features 72.3, **72.6**
monomorphic follicular papules, infundibulofolliculitis 93.7
monomorphic follicular papules/pustules, actinic folliculitis 93.6
monomorphic polymorphic light eruption 126.4
monosymptomatic delusional hypochondriasis
  delusional infestation 84.5–84.10
  olfactory reference syndrome 84.10–84.11
mons pubis
  cutaneous Crohn disease 95.15
  lymphoedema 103.49–103.51, *103.52*
mood disorders
  dermatological patients 84.40–84.42
  types 84.40
mood stabilisers 84.46–84.47
Moraxella spp. 26.51
Morbihan disease (solid facial lymphoedema) 88.41, 89.10, 89.16, *89.17*, 103.47, *103.48*
morbilliform eruption, drug reaction 118.7
morbillivirus 25.97–25.99
  see also measles
Morgellons syndrome 84.11–84.12
MORM syndrome **72.6**
morphine
  death rates 120.1
  drug-induced pruritus 81.11
  topical therapies 18.41
morphoea 55.1–55.42, 105.8
  age of onset 55.6–55.7
  associated diseases 55.7
  atrophoderma of Pasini–Pierini 55.17, *55.19*
  atrophodermas 94.18
  autoantibodies in relation to clinical features 55.9
  autoimmune diseases 55.7
  autoimmunity 55.8–55.9
  biologic therapies 55.38–55.42
  blood tests 55.30–55.31
  Borrelia antibodies 94.16
  cancer association 55.7
  causative organisms 55.12
  in childhood **55.39**
  circumscribed plaque morphoea 55.17, **55.27**
  classification 55.2–55.3
  clinical assessment **55.31**
  clinical features *55.9*, 55.15–55.27
  complications and co-morbidities 55.28–55.29
  CT scans 55.31
  cytokines and cellular signatures 55.10
  deep morphoea **55.3**, 55.16–55.17
  differential diagnosis 55.27
  disease course and prognosis 55.29–55.30
  disease modifiers **55.4**, 55.15–55.17
  drug reactions 55.14–55.15
  en coup de sabre 55.23–55.24
  environmental factors 55.13–55.15
  eosinophilic fasciitis **55.4**, 55.21–55.23, **55.27**
  epidemiology 55.6–55.7
  epidermal–dermal interaction 55.9
  erythematous plaque with telangiectases *55.6*
  extracutaneous manifestations 55.28–55.29
  fibroblast activation and sclerosis 55.10–55.11
  generalised plaque morphoea **55.3**, **55.4**, 55.17–55.19
  genetics 55.12–55.13
  guttate morphoea 55.17
  histology 55.5
  histopathology 55.11–55.12
  hyperpigmentation *55.18*, 86.20–86.21
  imaging modalities 55.31–55.32
  immunopathology 55.9–55.11
  incidence and prevalence 55.6
  investigations 55.30–55.35, *55.31*
  keloidal/nodular morphoea 55.15–55.16
  lichen sclerosus morphoea **55.4**, *55.5*, *55.6*, 55.7
  limited morphoea **55.3**, **55.4**, 55.17
  linear morphoea **55.3**, **55.4**, 55.23–55.27
    differential diagnosis 55.27
    head/neck variant 55.23–55.24
    linear atrophoderma of Moulin 55.25–55.27
    linear deep atrophic morphoea 55.27
    morphoea en coup de sabre 55.24
    progressive hemifacial atrophy 55.24–55.25
    trunk/limb variant 55.25
  localised scleroderma cutaneous assessment tool 55.33–55.34
  management 55.35–55.42
    biologic therapies 55.38–55.42
    corticosteroids 55.36–55.37
    phototherapy 55.36
    therapeutic algorithm *55.41*
    topical therapies 55.35–55.36
    treatments and levels of evidence **55.40**
  mixed type morphoea **55.4**, 55.27
  MRI imaging *55.31*, *55.32*
  outcome measures 55.32–55.35
  paediatric morphoea **55.39**
  pansclerotic morphoea 54.20, **55.4**, 55.19–55.21, **55.27**
  pathophysiology 55.8–55.15
  patient reported outcomes **55.35**
  plaque morphoea **55.3**
  predisposing factors 55.8
  presentation 55.15
  pressure sites from clothing *55.5*
  psychological manifestations 55.29
  radiation 55.14
  radiotherapy-associated 119.15
  redness (erythema) *55.18*
  sclerosis, causes of **55.14**
  severity assessment and classification 55.27–55.28
  skin biopsy 55.31
  synonyms and inclusions 55.1
  terminology 55.1–55.2
  therapeutic algorithm *55.41*
  topical therapies 55.35–55.36
  and trauma to skin 55.13–55.14
  and vaccination 55.13
  vascular activation and damage 55.9
  waxy plaques *55.5*
morphoeaform sarcoidosis 96.13
morphoea profunda 97.12–97.13
morphoeic basal cell carcinoma 140.3, 140.6, *140.8*, 140.9
morphogenesis 87.2
morpholines, topical therapies 18.12
Morton neuroma/metatarsalgia 136.43
mosaic acral keratosis 63.61
mosaicism 8.7–8.8, 74.5
mosaic lymphoedema associated with disturbed growth and/or cutaneous/vascular anomalies 103.23–103.24
mosaic neurofibromatosis type 1 78.4–78.7, **78.7**
mosaic pattern, piebaldism 68.4
mosaic RASopathies, lymphatic abnormalities 103.24
mosquitoes 34.6–34.7, 34.8–34.9
  lymphatic filariasis *103.34*
  malaria 33.36
  togavirus infections 25.87–25.91
mossy foot *see* podoconiosis (non-filarial lymphoedema)
moths (Lepidoptera) 34.32–34.34
motor nerves, anatomy of head and neck 20.3–20.4

mottled pigmentation, autosomal dominant epidermolysis bullosa simplex 69.9
mottling effect, livedo reticularis 124.9, *124.10*
moulds
  brachytherapy 24.3
  identification of isolates 32.10
  morphology and diseases 32.3
Moulin, linear atrophoderma of 55.25–55.27, 73.22, 94.17
moult cycle, hair 87.2
Moulting ('Mauserung') phenomenon, superficial epidermolytic ichthyosis 63.18
moult waves 87.9, 87.53
mouse studies, immune system 9.3, 9.7
mouth *see* oral cavity
Mozart ear 106.5
MPA *see* microscopic polyangiitis
MPAM *see* metastatic pregnancy-associated melanoma; *Mycoplasma pneumoniae*-associated mucositis
MPHL *see* male pattern hair loss
MPK *see* marginal papular keratoderma
M-plasty, skin surgery 20.21, *20.22*
MPNSTs *see* malignant peripheral nerve sheath tumours
mpox (formerly monkeypox) 25.8–25.12
  2022 outbreak 25.9–25.10
  clinical features 25.9, *25.10*
  complications and co-morbidities 25.10
  epidemiology 25.8–25.9
  investigations 25.10
  management 25.10–25.12
  pathology 25.10
  pathophysiology 25.9
  risk increased with waning smallpox immunity 25.6
MPSs *see* mucopolysaccharidoses
MPXV (monkeypox virus) *see* mpox
Mrgpr family *see* Mas-related G-protein-coupled receptor agonists
MRGPRX2 *see* Mas-related G protein–coupled receptor member X2
MRH *see* multicentric reticulohistiocytosis
MRI *see* magnetic resonance imaging
MRL *see* magnetic resonance lymphangiography
MRSS *see* modified Rodnan skin score
MSAs *see* myositis-specific antibodies
MSH *see* melanocyte-stimulating hormone
MS-LCH *see* multisystem Langerhans cell histiocytoses
MSM *see* men who have sex with men
MSS *see* modified Sartorius Score
MSSE *see* multiple self-healing squamous epithelioma
MTC *see* medullary thyroid cancer
MTS *see* Muir–Torre syndrome
MTX *see* methotrexate
muccous membrane changes, dyskeratosis congenita 67.14
Mucha–Haberman disease, oral ulceration 108.41
mucin
  skin deposition 57.1–57.19
  structure 57.1
  see also cutaneous mucinoses
mucinosis
  systemic lupus erythematosus 51.28
  see also cutaneous mucinoses
mucinous carcinoma 137.38
mucin-producing sweat gland carcinoma *see* endocrine mucin-producing sweat gland carcinoma
Muckle–Wells syndrome (MWS) **45.5**, **45.6**, 154.2
mucocele (mucous cysts)
  digital myxoid cysts 57.15, *57.16*
  male genitalia 109.30
  mouth 108.12
  vulva 110.31
mucocutaneous candidiasis, primary immunodeficiencies 149.18–149.19

mucocutaneous leishmaniasis
  New-World 33.43, *33.44*, 33.45, 33.46, 33.49
  Old-World 33.47, *33.48*
mucocutaneous lymph node syndrome *see* Kawasaki disease
mucocutaneous pain syndromes (MCPs) 82.1–82.14
  atypical trigeminal trophic syndrome 82.8, *82.9*
  burning mouth syndrome 82.1–82.3
  cervical trophic syndrome 82.8–82.9
  chronic scalp pain and dysaesthesia 82.12
  erythromelalgia 82.12–82.13
  midface toddler excoriation syndrome 82.9
  penoscrotodynia 82.11–82.12
  postherpetic neuralgia 82.4–82.5
  trigeminal neuropathic pain syndrome 82.5–82.7
  trigeminal trophic syndrome 82.7–82.8
  trophic syndromes 82.7–82.9
  vulvodynia 82.9–82.11
mucocutaneous venous malformation 71.16–71.17
mucoepithelial dysplasia 108.26–108.27
mucolipidoses types II and III 79.4–79.5
mucopolysaccharidoses (MPSs) 79.1–79.3
mucormycosis (zygomycosis) 32.93, 109.28
  oral involvement 108.57
  panniculitis due to 97.60–97.61
mucosa associated lymphoid tissue (MALT) lymphomas 139.37, 139.38
mucosal advancement flap, vermilionectomy repair 20.22
mucosal associated invariant T (MAIT) cells 9.5
mucosal lesions
  COVID-19 association 25.112–25.113
  psoriasis vulgaris 35.11–35.12
  systemic lupus erythematosus 51.29
mucosal melanoma
  presentation 142.11, *142.16*
  systemic treatment 144.7
  vaginal *145.12*, 145.13
mucosal melanotic lesions 131.9–131.12
  pigmented melanotic macules 131.9–131.11
  see also lentigines
mucositis (mucosal barrier injury), oral involvement 108.49–108.50
mucous cysts *see* mucocele
mucous membrane pemphigoid (MMP) 3.17, 50.22–50.33, 105.6, 107.24–107.32
  associated diseases 50.24
  biochip mosaic for detection of serum anti-laminin 332 IgG *50.31*
  classification of severity 107.26
  clinical features 50.26
  clinical features of ocular MMP 107.26
  clinical variants 50.26
  complications and co-morbidities 107.26
  conjunctival hyperaemia *50.30*
  diagnosis *50.24*, *50.32*, 107.26
  diagnostic problems in ocular MMP 107.26–107.28
  differential diagnosis 50.26
  direct immunofluorescence for 107.28
  epidemiology 50.24, 107.24–107.25
  European Consensus criteria for diagnosis of 107.28–107.29
  fibrosis prevention 107.32
  genital involvement *50.28*
  histopathology 50.25
  immunosuppression in *107.31*
  indirect immunofluorescence in 107.28
  investigations 107.26–107.28
  investigations and diagnosis 50.28–50.30, *50.31*
  lesions *50.29*
  management 50.30–50.31, 107.29–107.32
  ocular disease in *50.30*
  ocular pemphigoid 50.26
    classification **50.28**

ocular signs of 107.27–107.28
oral involvement 108.82
oral lesions 50.27
pathology 107.25–107.26
pathophysiology 50.24–50.25
predisposing factors 107.25
randomised controlled trials 50.30–50.31
serum autoantibodies 50.25–50.26
severity classification 50.26–50.28
tissue-bound autoantibodies 50.25
treatment guidelines 50.31
treatment ladder 50.31–50.33
vulva **110.21**
vulvar pemphigoid 50.26
mucous membranes
   allergic contact dermatitis 127.18
   congenital syphilis 29.23
   lichen planus 37.12
   microscopic examination of 3.33
   samples for superficial mycoses identification 32.8
   syphilis 29.10, 29.14, *29.15*
mudi-chood, ear dermatoses **106.23**
Muir–Torre syndrome (MTS/Lynch II syndrome) 76.11, **78.14**, 141.44–141.45
   sebaceous adenomas and sebaceomas 137.17
   sebaceous carcinoma 137.18
multicentric reticulohistiocytosis (MRH) 135.25–135.27, 155.14
   internal malignancy association 148.24
   oral involvement 108.71–108.72
   pleural effusion 152.6
multidisciplinary teams (MDTs)
   psychodermatology 84.2, 84.7, 84.8, 84.9, 84.12, 84.18, 84.35
   SJS/TEN treatment 118.19
multidrug-resistant (MDR) tuberculosis 27.10
multifocal cutaneous infantile haemangioma 116.5
multifocal epithelial hyperplasia (focal epithelial hyperplasia), oral involvement 108.11
multifocal venous malformation (MVM) *71.2*
multiple cutaneous neuromas *see* dermal hyperneury
multiple cutaneous and uterine leiomyomas syndrome *see* hereditary leiomyomatosis and renal cell cancer
multiple endocrine neoplasia (MEN) 108.13–108.14, 148.10–148.11
multiple endocrine neoplasia type 1 (MEN1) 148.10
multiple endocrine neoplasia type 2A (MEN2A) 148.10
multiple endocrine neoplasia type 2B (MEN2B) 108.13–108.14, 148.10–148.11
multiple glomangioma 136.42
multiple haemorrhagic sarcoma *see* Kaposi sarcoma
multiple hamartoma and neoplasia syndrome
   renal/urinary tract involvement 154.2
   trichilemmoma 137.6
multiple minute digitate hyperkeratoses 63.77
multiple minute digitate keratoses (MMDK) 85.18–85.19
multiple mucosal neuroma syndrome 108.13–108.14
multiple organ failure, hypermelanosis 86.21–86.22
multiple pigment sarcoma *see* Kaposi sarcoma
multiple primary hypersensitivities, patch testing 127.32
multiple self-healing squamous epithelioma (MSSE) **78.13**, 141.41–141.42
multiple symmetrical lipomatosis *see* Madelung disease

multipotent stem cell transplantation, *see also* haematopoietic stem cell transplantation
multisegmental lymphatic dysplasia with systemic involvement (MLDSI) 103.22
multisystem inflammatory syndrome in adults (MIS-A), COVID-19 association 25.112
multisystem inflammatory syndrome in children (MIS-C), COVID-19 association 25.114–25.115
multisystem Langerhans cell histiocytoses (MS-LCH) 135.2–135.9
multisystem sarcoidosis, acquired ichthyosis *63.48*
multisystem tumours, associated skin conditions 148.2
multivoltage X-ray techniques
   'bathing cap' distribution 24.3, *24.5*
   'stocking' distribution 24.3–24.4, *24.6–24.7*
Mulvihill–Smith syndrome 70.29–70.30
Münchausen syndrome 84.37
Münchausen syndrome by proxy 84.37–84.38
Munro microabscess 3.43, *35.6*
mupirocin, topical therapies 18.11
murine typhus 26.81
Murray Williams warts 39.28
muscle, *see also* dermatomyositis
muscle cells, smooth 2.40–2.41
muscle cell tumours 136.52–136.56
   skeletal muscle 136.55–136.56
   smooth muscle 136.52–136.55
muscle definition, electromagnetic muscle stimulation 161.8
muscle 'naevi' **73.2**
muscle signs, dermatomyositis 52.7
muscular dystrophy, autosomal recessive epidermolysis bullosa simplex with 69.11
musculocontractural Ehlers–Danlos syndrome (mcEDS) **70.6**, 70.9
musculoskeletal system 155.1–155.16
   epidermolysis bullosa 69.26
   history and examination 155.1–155.2
   ichthyoses 63.46
   sarcoidosis 96.5–96.6
   systemic sclerosis 54.18
musical instruments, skin reactions 122.11–122.13
mutations *see* gene mutations; genetic disorders/syndromes
mutilation, male genitalia 109.9
MVK genes *see* MeValonate Kinase genes
MVM *see* multifocal venous malformation
MWS *see* Muckle–Wells syndrome
Myanmar, skincare initiative 7.11
mycetoma 32.72–32.75
   clinical features 32.73–32.74
   epidemiology 32.72–32.73
   investigations 32.74–32.75
   management 32.75
   pathophysiology 32.73
mycobacterial infections 27.1–27.46
   eyelid 107.39–107.40
   female genitalia 110.26
   HIV coinfection 27.2–27.3, 27.10, 31.22
   non-tuberculous mycobacteria 27.3, 27.32–27.45
   panniculitides 97.46
   sarcoidosis causation 96.4
   types/classification 27.1, 27.2
   see also tuberculosis
Mycobacterium
   histology 28.3–28.4, *28.5*
   M. abscessus group 27.2, 27.43–27.45
   M. avium complex 27.2, 27.3, 27.32, 27.40–27.41
   M. balnei see *M. marinum*
   M. bovis 27.1, 27.2, 27.5, 27.6, 27.12
     see also bacillus Calmette–Guérin
   M. chelonae 27.2, 27.43–27.45, 97.47
   M. fortuitum group 27.2, 27.43–27.45

   M. goodii 27.2, 27.32
   M. gordonae 27.3
   M. haemophilum 27.41–27.42
   M. intracellulare 27.1, 27.2, 27.40
   M. kansasii 27.2, 27.3, 27.35–27.36
   M. leprae 27.1, 27.2, 28.1–28.6, *97.27*
     histology 28.3–28.4, *28.5*
     immunology 28.4–28.5
     serology 28.6
     see also leprosy
   M. malmoense 27.3
   M. marinum 27.2, 27.5, 27.20, 27.32–27.35
     sporotrichoid distribution *4.10*
   M. mucogenicum 27.2, 27.42, 27.43
   M. platypoecilus see M. marinum
   M. scrofulaceum 27.42–27.43
   M. simiae 27.3
   M. smegmatis 27.2, 27.32, 27.43–27.45
   M. szulgai 27.43
   M. tuberculosis 27.1, 27.2
     complex 27.5–27.24
     complex tuberculids 27.24–27.32
     erythema induratum 97.26, 97.29
     HIV combination 31.22
     nucleic acid amplification tests 27.8–27.9
     protective immunity 27.3–27.4
   M. ulcerans 27.36–27.40
     clinical features 27.38
     epidemiology 27.37
     investigations 27.38–27.39
     management 27.39–27.40
     pathophysiology 27.37–27.38
   M. wolinskyi 27.2, 27.32
   M. xenopi 27.3
   rapid growing species 27.2, 27.43–27.45
   slow growing species 27.2, 27.5–27.43
   see also tuberculosis of the skin
mycophenolate, morphoea treatment 55.37–55.38
mycophenolate mofetil (MMF) 19.28–19.30
   atopic eczema treatment 41.29
   dermatological uses 19.28
   dose and regimen 19.30
   drug–drug interactions 19.29
   monitoring 19.30
   pemphigus treatment 50.8
   pharmacological properties 19.28–19.29
   potential adverse effects 19.29
   safety precautions 19.29
   systemic lupus erythematosus treatment 51.38
Mycoplasma pneumoniae associated mucositis (MPAM) 118.16
Mycoplasma spp. 26.78–26.79
   M. genitalium 30.23–30.25
     clinical features 30.24–30.25
     epidemiology 30.24
     investigations 30.25
     management 30.25
     pathophysiology 30.24
   M. pneumoniae, in SJS/TEN 118.20
     Stevens–Johnson syndrome 118.15–118.16
mycoses (fungal infections) 32.1–32.95
   fungal biology and reproduction 32.2–32.5
   morphology of fungi *32.3*
   nomenclature 32.5–32.6
   pinna infection 106.21
   subcutaneous 32.69–32.80
   superficial 32.6–32.69
   systemic 32.80–32.94
mycosis fungoides
   discoid skin lesions **39.10**
   extracorporeal photochemotherapy 21.7
   male genitalia 109.42
   oral involvement 108.72
   phototherapy indications 21.4
   radiotherapy 24.15–24.16
   UVA-1 phototherapy 21.7
mycosis fungoides (MF) 139.2–139.25
   clinical features 139.8–139.12
   clinical variants/related conditions 139.9, 139.14–139.19

   epidemiology 139.3
   investigations 139.12–139.14
   management 139.20–139.25
   molecular features 139.19–139.20
   parapsoriasis relationship 134.6
   pathophysiology 139.3–139.8
   predisposing factors 139.3–139.4
   prognosis 139.10–139.12, *139.13–139.14*, **139.13**
   relationship to other lymphomas 139.1
   relationship to Sézary syndrome 139.2, 139.19–139.20
   staging/classification 139.6, **139.7**, **139.8**, 139.9–139.10
   T-cell receptor gene analysis 139.6–139.8
   typical 139.2–139.14
mycotic otitis externa *see* otomycosis
myelodysplasia
   oral involvement 108.72, 149.8
   VEXAS syndrome 45.19, 149.6, 149.7
myeloid disorders, leukaemia cutis 149.2–149.5
myeloid lineage cells 9.4–9.5
myeloid malignancies, skin manifestations of paraneoplastic syndromes 149.5–149.8
myeloid sarcoma (granulocytic sarcoma)
   infiltration of skin with malignant granulocyte precursor cells 149.2
   oral involvement 108.70
   see also leukaemia cutis
myeloma, oral involvement 108.72
myeloproliferative disorders, associated skin conditions 148.2
myelosuppression/myelotoxicity
   antimalarials 19.5
   azathioprine 19.9, 19.10
   hydroxycarbamide 19.21, 19.22
   methotrexate 19.26
Myerson naevus 131.28–131.29, *131.30*
MYH9-USP6 fusion gene, nodular fasciitis 136.5
myiasis, insect larvae **34.7**, 34.9–34.13
myoepithelial cells, eccrine glands 92.2
myoepithelial tumours 137.32–137.33
myofibroblasts 2.40
   microscopic examination of 3.37
   palmar fascial fibromatosis 94.34
   wound healing 11.7
myofibroma (adult) 136.39–136.40
myofibromatosis (infantile) 94.41–94.42, 136.39–136.40
myopathic Ehlers–Danlos syndrome (mEDS) **70.7**, 70.10
myopericytoma 136.40–136.41
myositis-specific antibodies (MSAs), dermatomyositis 52.2, 52.5, 52.6, 52.11
MYT1L deficiency **72.6**
myxoedema
   palmoplantar keratodermas with 63.72–63.73
   in thyroid diseases 57.11–57.14
myxofibrosarcoma 136.18
myxoid degeneration 3.40
myxoid liposarcoma, pleomorphic liposarcoma 136.59
myxoid malignant fibrous histiocytoma *see* myxofibrosarcoma
myxoid tumours, dermal nerve sheath myxoma 136.47–136.48
myxoinflammatory fibroblastic sarcoma 136.17
myxoma, mouth 108.14
Myxoma syndrome (Carney complex) **72.7**, **78.13**, 108.16, **131.3**, *131.4*, 148.11, 151.3–151.4
MZL *see* marginal zone lymphoma

N

NAC *see* N-acetylcysteine
N-acetylcysteine (NAC) 63.42–63.43
N-acetyltransferases (NATs) 127.10
NADCs *see* non-AIDS-defining cancers
NAE *see* necrolytic acral erythema

Naegeli–Franceschetti–Jadassohn syndrome 68.12
naevi
  acneform naevi 88.31
  Becker naevus 73.18
  blue naevus 3.44, 73.15, *73.16*, **131.17**, 131.38–131.40
  cancer phobias 84.26
  classification 73.1–73.2
  common dermoscopic patterns *145.2, 145.3*, 145.4–145.6
  congenital epidermal naevi 73.2, 73.3–73.8
  congenital naevi 73.8–73.16
  dermoscopy, benign patterns 145.1–145.7
  dynamic analysis for melanoma diagnosis 142.9
  epidermal 4.9
  fat naevus **73.2**, 73.16–73.18
  genetic classification 73.2
  hair follicles 137.7–137.8
  histological classification 73.2
  inheritance of naevus mutations 73.3
  intradermal, dermoscopic patterns 145.6
  intra-individual comparative analysis, melanoma diagnosis 142.9
  linear epidermal naevus, oral lesions 108.30
  linear naevus syndrome (naevus sebaceous of Jadassohn), oral lesions 108.29–108.30
  melanoma precursors 142.2–142.3
  melanoma presentation 142.10
  muscle 'naevi' **73.2**
  naevus phenotypes 73.1
  pigment cell naevi **73.2**
  prophylactic surgical excision to prevent melanoma not recommended 142.3
  reticular pattern naevi *145.2, 145.3*, 145.4, 145.6
  Spitz naevi 73.15, *145.5*, 145.6–145.7
  terminology **73.2**
  white sponge naevus, oral lesions 108.31
  see also melanocytic naevi; naevus-like entities
naevoid basal cell carcinoma syndrome (NBCCS/Gorlin syndrome) 22.2, 22.7, **78.12**, 140.3–140.4, 140.18–140.20, 148.7
  clinical features 140.18–140.20
  diagnostic criteria 140.19, **140.20**
  epidemiology 140.18
  genetics 140.3–140.4, 140.18
  management 140.20
  oral involvement 108.86
naevoid congenital hypertrichosis 87.85–87.86
naevoid hyperkeratosis 63.79
'naevoid melanoma', use of term 142.19
naevus acneiformis unilateralis *see* comedo naevus
naevus comedonicus 73.7, 88.31, *88.32*, 137.5
naevus depigmentosus *86.38*
naevus flammeus *101.10*
naevus folliculoris keratosus *see* comedo naevus
naevus of Ito 68.9–68.10, 131.14–131.15
naevus-like entities **73.2**, 73.21–73.23
naevus lipomatosus 98.25
naevus of Ota 131.12–131.14
  eyelid 107.46
  laser therapies 23.16, *23.17*
naevus phenotype (number and features of naevi), melanoma risk 142.3–142.4
naevus sebaceous (organoid naevus) 73.5, *73.6, 73.7, 73.8*, 87.30, 88.32, 105.11, *106.33*, 137.19–137.20
naevus spilus (speckled lentiginous naevus) *4.8*, 23.16, 73.15–73.16, 131.15–131.17
naevus zoniforme *see* comedo naevus
NAFR *see* non-ablative fractional resurfacing
Nagashima PPK 63.54
Nager syndrome **106.7**

NAI *see* non-accidental injury
NAIAD *see* NLRP1-associated autoinflammation with arthritis and dyskeratosis
Nail Assessment in Psoriasis and Psoriatic Arthritis (NAPPA) 16.3
nail bed epithelium 2.11, 119.7
nail biting (onychophagia) 84.25
nail changes
  chemotherapy-induced 119.6–119.8
  COVID-19 25.113
  during pregnancy 113.1, **113.2**
  HIV 31.33–31.34
  liver disease 153.9
  selenosis 121.7
nail disease, alopecia areata 87.23, *87.25*, 87.28
nail dysplasia 67.15
  nail–patella syndrome 67.15
  with triangular lunula 67.15, *67.16*
nail dystrophy
  dyskeratosis congenita 67.13, *67.14*
  epidermolysis bullosa *69.11, 69.13*, 69.15, 69.16
  gold toxicity 121.4
  melanoma 145.13
  pachyonychia congenita 63.51, 67.11
  peeling skin syndromes 69.20
  pigmentation disorders 68.12
  primary systemic amyloidosis 56.13
nail fold, mixed connective tissue disease 53.2
nail fold capillaroscopy 54.16
nail fold infection, candidiasis 32.65–32.66
nail fold necrosis, systemic lupus erythematosus 51.25
nail growth, genetic defects of 67.1–67.17
nail matrix epithelium 119.7
nail-patella-like renal disease 67.15, 154.1–154.2
nail–patella syndrome (NPS) 67.15–67.16, 154.1–154.2
nail picking (onychotillomania) 84.25
nail plate fungal infections *see* onychomycosis
Nail Psoriasis Severity Index (NAPSI) 16.3
nails 2.10–2.11
  acrodermatitis continua of Hallopeau 35.40
  allergic reactions 127.13, 127.15, 127.21, 127.47, 127.48, 127.49, 127.61–127.62
  anatomy and structure 2.11
  atopic eczema 41.18
  basal keratinocyte layers 2.11
  blue nail discolouration due to antimalarial therapy 51.25
  chloroquine pigmentation, systemic lupus erythematosus 51.23
  clubbing, internal malignancy links 148.18
  dermatomyositis 52.5, *52.9*
  embryonic development 2.5
  factitious nail disease 84.33
  genetic defects of 67.1–67.17
  hyperpigmentation, vitamin B12 deficiency 61.20
  inherited immunodeficiency **80.4–80.6**
  iron deficiency 61.24
  lichen planus 37.11–37.12
  lichen striatus 37.18
  melanoma 142.10–142.11, *142.15*, 145.12, 145.13
  metal poisoning signs 121.1
  mixed connective tissue disease 53.2
  nail bed 2.11, 119.7
  nail matrix 2.11, 119.7
  pigmentation effects of renal failure and dialysis 154.3
  pitting, psoriatic 35.12
  pityriasis rubra pilaris 36.3
  psoriasis vulgaris 35.10–35.11, *35.12*
  psoriatic subungual hyperkeratosis with distal onycholysis 35.12
  rheumatoid arthritis 53.7
  role of 2.43

salmon patches ('oil drops'), psoriasis vulgaris 35.12
sarcoidosis 96.13
selenium excess 61.30
subungual hyperkeratosis and splinter haemorrhages 36.3
syphilis 29.10
systemic lupus erythematosus *51.23*, 51.25
systemic sclerosis 54.16
yellow-nail syndrome 103.21–103.22, 152.6
see also onychomycosis
nail samples, superficial mycoses identification 32.7
'naked granuloma' 96.2
NAME (nevi, atrial myxoma, ephelides) *see* Carney complex
Nannizia species (*Microsporum*) **32.19**, 32.26
nano-pulse stimulation (NPS) technology 161.10
NAPPA *see* Nail Assessment in Psoriasis and Psoriatic Arthritis
nappy/diaper/napkin area
  dermatitis 40.5, 115.3, 128.5
  perianal candidiasis of infancy 32.65
NAPSI *see* Nail Psoriasis Severity Index
narcotic drugs, recreational use 120.1
narrow-band UVB (NB-UVB/TL-01) phototherapy
  adverse effects/risks 21.11–21.13, 21.15, 21.17
  combination therapy 21.10
  indications/efficacy 21.3–21.4, 21.5, 21.7
  polymorphic light eruption 126.7–126.8, *126.36*
  principles 21.1, 21.2–21.3
  psoriasis treatment 35.22–35.23
  regimen 21.8
nasal alar ulceration, trigeminal trophic syndrome 82.7, *82.8*
nasal glioma *see* glial heterotopic nodules
nasal type extranodal NK/T-cell lymphoma 139.36–139.37
nasal vestibule
  carriage of *Staphylococcus aureus* 26.4, 26.7–26.8
  microbiome 26.5
naso-labial fold, dermal fillers 158.2
nasopalpebral lipoma–coloboma syndrome 72.10
nasopharyngeal carcinoma, Epstein–Barr virus association 25.49
natal teeth, pachyonychia congenita 67.12
National Cancer Registration and Analysis Service (NCRAS), basal cell carcinoma incidence 140.1
national and international organisations, psychodermatology 84.2
National Library of Medicine's bibliographic database (MEDLINE) 17.7
NATs *see* N-acetyltransferases
natural gene therapy 8.8
natural history of skin diseases 5.11–5.12
natural killer (NK)/T cell extranodal lymphoma 139.36–139.37
natural rubber latex (NRL)
  allergy testing *4.24*, 129.7
  allergy to rubber gloves 39.14, 127.63
  contact urticaria 127.84–127.85
  genital contact dermatitis 109.13
nausea, PUVA phototherapy adverse effects 21.13
Naxos syndrome 63.62–63.63, 69.7
NBCCS *see* naevoid basal cell carcinoma syndrome
NB-UVB *see* narrow-band UVB
NCRAS *see* National Cancer Registration and Analysis Service
Nd:YAG *see* erbium:yttrium-aluminium-garnet lasers
near infrared lymphangiography (ICG lymphography), lymphatic system 103.56–103.57

neat (insoluble) cutting oils 129.12
Necator americanus, ancylostomiasis 33.15–33.17
neck
  ageing of skin 156.4–156.5
  allergic contact dermatitis of 127.14, 127.16
  atopic eczema 41.18
  botulinum toxins, aesthetic uses of 159.6
  bullous lupus erythematosus 51.28
  'dirty neck', atopic 41.18
  dyskeratosis congenita 75.3
  folliculitis keloidalis 88.37, 93.3
  granuloma annulare 95.2
  infantile haemangioma 116.3
  Kaposiform haemangioendothelioma 116.9
  lymph nodes and lymphatic drainage basins 106.28
  morphoea 55.23–55.24
  oedema 103.46–103.49
  perforating granuloma annulare 95.7
  plane xanthomatosis 60.5
  progressive hemifacial atrophy 55.25
  reticulate pigmentation, atopic eczema 41.18
  systemic lupus erythematosus 51.23
  white fibrous papulosis of 94.39–94.40
necrobiosis 3.42
necrobiosis-lipoidica-like lesions 96.13
necrobiosis lipoidica (NLD) 95.8–95.13, 97.11–97.12, 97.15
  associated diseases 95.9
  atrophy *95.11*, 95.13
  atypical facial necrobiosis *95.12*
  clinical features 95.11
  diabetic patients 62.5, *62.6*, 95.12
  differential diagnosis 95.11–95.12
  epidemiology 95.9
  incidence and prevalence 95.9
  management 95.12–95.13
  necrobiotic inflammation 95.10
  pathology 95.10, *95.11*
  pathophysiology 95.9–95.10
  rheumatoid nodule differentiation 97.16–97.17
  telangiectasia 95.11
  treatment ladder 95.13
necrobiotic palisading granulomas 95.2–95.3
necrobiotic xanthogranuloma (NXG) 97.17–97.18, 135.24–135.25, 149.11
necrolysis 3.42
necrolytic acral erythema (NAE), hepatitis C 25.76, 153.5
necrolytic migratory erythema (NME) 47.12–47.16, 110.44–110.45, 153.6
  clinical features 47.13–47.14
  clinical variants 47.15
  dermatoendocrinology **150.10**, 150.12, *150.14*, 150.19
  disease course and prognosis 47.16
  epidemiology 47.13
  histology *47.13*
  investigations 47.14, 47.16
  pathology 47.13
  presentation 47.14
  treatment for 47.16
necrosis 3.42
  chemical peels **160.4**
  diabetic foot with neurotrophic ulceration and necrosis ('mal perforans') 62.2
  drug-induced 120.7
  penis 109.22–109.24
necrotic adipocytes 97.7–97.8
  alpha-1 antitrypsin 97.44
  cold panniculitis 97.36
  fat necrosis 97.55
necrotic keratinocytes, acute generalised exanthematous pustulosis 118.2
necrotising fasciitis 26.77, 26.78, 111.15, 130.7
  eyelid 107.39
  neonates 114.26
necrotising granulomatous lesions *80.10*

necrotising infundibular crystalline folliculitis 63.76
necrotising lymphocytic folliculitis, scalp margin 91.12–91.13, 93.4–93.5
necrotising otitis externa 106.19
necrotising sarcoid granulomatosis, respiratory involvement 152.6
necrotising sialometaplasia, oral ulceration 108.42
necrotising soft-tissue infections, perineal and perianal skin 111.15
necrotising subcutaneous infections 26.77–26.78
needle biopsy 3.4
needle injection, dermal fillers 158.1–158.2, **158.3**, *158.4*
needs assessments
　access to dermatological health services 5.12
　global health dermatology 7.12–7.13
NEFAs *see* non-esterified fatty acids
negative network dermoscopy patterns
　melanomas 145.7, *145.8*
　naevi 145.6
Neglected Tropical Disease Non-Governmental Organisation Network (NNN) 7.6
neglected tropical diseases (NTDs) 7.2, 7.6, 7.7
　training guide for frontline health workers 7.11–7.12
NEH *see* neutrophilic eccrine hidradenitis
Neisser, Albert 1.6, 1.8
Neisseria gonorrhoeae 30.1–30.2, 30.8
Neisseria meningitidis 26.49–26.50
Nékam disease 37.10–37.11, 37.16
Nelson syndrome 86.7, 86.18, 86.19
Nematocera 34.6–34.7
nematocysts, stings 130.1–130.2
nematodes
　infection with human nematodes 33.1–33.18
　infection with other animal nematodes 33.18–33.26
NEMO, pigmentation disorders 68.10
neoadjuvant systemic treatment, melanoma 144.6
neoangiogenesis 101.1
neomycin
　patch testing 127.47
　topical therapies 18.11
neonatal acne 88.68–88.74
neonatal candidiasis 114.28
neonatal candidiasis *see* congenital candidiasis
neonatal cold panniculitis 97.36–97.37
neonatal erythroderma 63.40
neonatal herpes, primary HSV infection in mother 25.27
neonatal ichthyosis–sclerosing cholangitis (NISCH) 63.41
neonatal lupus erythematosus (NLE) 51.39–51.42
　associated diseases 51.39
　cardiac involvement 151.4
　cardiac problems 51.41
　clinical features 51.40–51.41
　disease course and prognosis 51.41
　environmental factors 51.40
　genetics 51.39–51.40
　haematological and hepatic problems 51.41
　pathophysiology 51.39
　pregnancy 51.41–51.42
　in pregnancy 113.7–113.8
　'racoon' eyelid lesions *51.40*
neonatal onset of pancytopenia, autoinflammation, rash and episodes of hemophagocytic lymphohistiosis syndrome 45.18–45.19
neonatal progeria syndrome **77.2**
neonatal progeroid syndrome 70.30–70.31
neonates 114.1–114.30
　acute pseudomembranous candidiasis 108.31

ADAM17 deficiency 45.16
adnexal polyp 114.19
alopecia 114.4
anetoderma of prematurity 114.9–114.10
antenatal procedures, complications arising from **114.10**
atrophic lesions of 114.11
bacterial infections 114.24–114.28
'blueberry muffin' baby 114.21
breast abscesses 114.25
bullous impetigo 114.24
cervico-facial oedema *71.28*
cleansing and moisturising of skin 114.2
cold injury 114.15, **114.18**
cold panniculitis 114.14
collodion baby 63.8, 63.12–63.13, 63.43–63.44, 114.19–114.21
congenital cytomegalovirus infection 25.41
congenital erosive and vesicular dermatosis 114.9
congenital heart block 51.39–51.42
congenital rubella 114.23
congenital syphilis 114.27–114.28
congenital tuberculosis 114.28
cutis marmorata 114.3
desquamation 114.3–114.4
eccrine sweating 114.3
ecthyma gangrenosum 114.27
epidermolysis bullosa 69.23–69.25
Epstein pearls 114.4
erosions in, differential diagnosis **114.24**
erythema neonatorum 114.3
fetal varicella syndrome 114.23
fungal infections 114.28–114.29
gonococcal ophthalmia neonatorum 30.3, *30.4*
gonorrhoea 30.3, 30.4, 30.5
harlequin colour change 114.3
herpes simplex virus infection 25.21, 25.27, 114.22
human immunodeficiency virus infection 114.24
hyperpigmentary disorders 114.4
hypoxia 114.3
infantile acropustulosis 114.8
infections 114.22–114.29
lentiginosis profusa 131.3
listeriosis 26.46, 114.26–114.27
lupus erythematosus 51.39–51.42, 114.12–114.14
Malassezia pustulosis 114.28–114.29
mastitis 114.25
maternal autoantibodies, transplacental transfer of 114.11–114.12
maternal malignant disease, transplacental transfer of 114.14
maternal milk, transfer of toxic substances in 114.14
medallion-like dermal dendrocyte hamartoma 114.11
medical procedures, complications arising from **114.10**
Michelin tyre baby syndrome 70.19, 73.17
microbial ecology of the skin 26.4, 26.5, 26.7
milia 114.4
miliaria 114.6–114.7
'miniature puberty' 114.4
necrotising fasciitis 114.26
noma neonatorum (cancrum oris/oro-facial gangrene) 114.27
nomenclature 114.1
Noonan syndrome *71.28*
occipital alopecia 114.4
omphalitis 114.26
oral findings 114.4
orbital cellulitis 114.26
pemphigoid gestationis, transplacental 114.12
pemphigus vulgaris 114.12
percutaneous absorption, toxicity risk 114.2
peripheral cyanosis (acrocyanosis) 114.3

periporitis staphylogenes 114.25
phytotherapy-induced rashes **114.11**
pityriasis rubra pilaris 36.4
postmature neonates 114.4
prematurity, complications of 114.9–114.10
preorbital cellulitis 114.26
purpura fulminans 114.21–114.22, 114.27
pustular eruptions **114.8**
raised linear bands of infancy 114.18–114.19
sclerema neonatorum 97.59–97.60, 114.17–114.18
sebaceous gland hypertrophy 114.4
sebaceous gland secretion 114.3
sepsis risk 114.2
skin appearance 114.3–114.4
skin barrier function 114.1–114.3
skin blistering *69.24*
skin disorders 114.5–114.9, 114.18–114.22
small-for-dates 114.4
staphylococcal cold abscesses of the large folds 114.25
staphylococcal scalded skin syndrome 114.24–114.25
subcutaneous fat disorders 114.14–114.18
subcutaneous fat necrosis 114.15–114.17, **114.18**
subcutaneous fat necrosis of 97.57–97.58
succulent gums 114.4
suction blisters 114.4
sweat gland abscesses 114.25
sweating 114.3
terminology 114.1
toxic erythema of the newborn 114.5–114.6
transepidermal water loss 114.2
transient myeloproliferative disorder 114.8
transient pustular melanosis 114.7–114.8
transplacental transfer/maternal milk-induced disorders 114.11–114.14
umbilical cord care 114.2–114.3
vernix caseosa 114.3, 114.4
viral infections 114.22–114.24
vitamin K deficiency 61.13
see also infants
neoplasia 86.19–86.20
　acquired ichthyosis association 85.1
　cutaneous metastases from gastrointestinal tract 153.1
　gastrointestinal and skin manifestations **153.7**
　infiltration of skin with neoplastic cells from haematological malignancies 149.2–149.5
　Merkel cell carcinoma 146.1–146.10
　musculoskeletal therapy relationship to skin cancer 155.15–155.16
　renal tumours related to hereditary syndromes 154.2
　rosacea 89.10
　skin manifestations of haematological neoplasms 149.1–149.15
　skin tumours in immunosuppressed renal allograft recipients 154.6
　umbilical metastases 153.1
neoplastic process, epithelioid sarcoma 97.15
neoprene allergy 127.64
Neoscytalidium species, superficial mycoses 32.51–32.52
nephritic factors, APL pathology 98.4
nephrocalcinosis 97.58
nephrogenic pruritus 81.8–81.9
nephrogenic systemic fibrosis **54.20**, 94.43–94.45
　differences from scleromyxoedema **57.5**
　renal dysfunction 154.5
nephropathic cystinosis, flushing in children **104.10**
nephropathy, autosomal recessive epidermolysis bullosa simplex with 69.11

nephrotic syndrome
　junctional epidermolysis bullosa with 69.15
　secondary dyslipidaemia and 60.12
　zinc deficiency associated with *61.26*
nephrotoxicity
　ciclosporin 19.11
　methotrexate 19.26
NEPPK *see* non-epidermolytic palmoplantar keratoderma
NER *see* nucleotide excision repair
nerve damage, skin surgery 20.42
nerve endings
　hair follicle 87.7
　hyperplasia 2.12
nerve entrapment syndromes 83.6–83.8
nerve sheath myxoma 136.47–136.48
nervous system
　anatomical considerations for skin surgery 20.2–20.4
　anatomy of head and neck 20.2–20.4
　anatomy of limbs 20.4
　autonomic 2.2–2.3, 83.4–83.5
　cutaneous innervation 83.2–83.4
　endocrine system relationship 150.2
　sensory innervation 83.2–83.4
　see also neurological disorders
NESS *see* Nottingham Eczema Severity Score
Netherton syndrome 63.26–63.28, **78.14**, 87.79, **87.80**
　pruritus in 63.46
　skin cancer 147.2
　SPINK5 69.6
　target therapy 63.45
network naevi *see* reticular pattern naevi
neuralgia
　genitofemoral neuropathic pain/neuralgia 83.7
　iliohypogastric neuropathic pain/neuralgia 83.7
　ilioinguinal neuropathic pain/neuralgia 83.7
　post-herpetic neuralgia 108.66
　pudendal neuropathic pain/neuralgia 83.7, 83.8
　trigeminal neuralgia 108.66–108.67
neural tissue tumours/neuromas *see* peripheral neuroectodermal tumours
neurocutaneous syndromes, ocular features **107.42**
neurodermatitis 127.15
neurodermatitis circumscripta *see* lichen simplex chronicus
neuroendocrine markers, cutaneous neoplasms 3.23
neuroendocrine stress response in skin, brain–skin axis 150.8–150.9
neuroendocrinology
　hair follicle 87.11–87.13
　(neuro-)endocrine contributions to cutaneous pathogenesis 150.9–150.10
　skin and hair as research models 150.9
neurofibromas 136.45–136.47
　cutaneous neurofibromas 78.3
　plexiform neurofibromas 78.3
　vulva **110.32**
neurofibromatoses 78.1–78.7
　mosaic neurofibromatosis type 1 78.4–78.7
　RASopathies 78.7, *78.8*, **78.9**
neurofibromatosis type 1 (NF1/von Recklinghausen disease) 78.1–78.4, **78.9**, 108.87, 148.9, 149.14
　clinical features 78.3
　diagnostic criteria **78.2**
　investigations 78.4
　lung disease 152.5
　malignant tumours in 78.3–78.4
　management 78.4, *78.5–78.6*
　Manchester checklist 78.4, *78.5–78.6*
　neurological disease 78.3
　oral involvement 108.87
　pathophysiology 78.1–78.3

neurofibromatosis type 1 (NF1/von Recklinghausen disease) (continued)
  renal involvement   154.1
  skeletal abnormalities   78.3
neurofibromatosis type 2   148.9
neurofibromin, juvenile xanthogranuloma   135.15
neurofibrosarcoma see malignant peripheral nerve sheath tumour
neurofilament, Merkel cell carcinoma   3.23
neurogenic pathways, rosacea   89.3
neuro-ichthyotic syndromes   63.30–63.39, **63.31**
neurokinin 1 receptor (NK1R), pruritus   81.4
neurolabyrinthitis (eighth nerve deafness), congenital syphilis   29.26
neurological abnormalities
  congenital melanocytic naevi   73.12–73.13
  secondary syphilis   29.10, 29.12
  xeroderma pigmentosum   76.5
neurological causes
  anhidrosis   **92.11**
  hyperhidrosis   **92.11**
neurological complications
  varicella infection   25.30
  zoster infection   25.32, 25.33–25.34
neurological disorders   83.1–83.25
  antibodies and targeted structures in skin biopsies   **83.6**
  autonomic nervous system   83.4–83.5
  brachioradial pruritus   83.6–83.7
  burning feet syndrome   83.10–83.11
  of childhood   **83.2**
  cold-induced vasodilation   83.5
  complex regional pain syndrome   83.20–83.23
  cutaneous innervation   83.2–83.4
  diagnosis   83.5
  distal symmetrical polyneuropathy, causes   **83.9**
  dysaesthesia   83.5–83.6, 83.7
  genetic neurocutaneous disorders   83.1–83.6
  genitofemoral neuropathic pain/neuralgia   83.7
  gustatory hyperhidrosis   83.24
  hereditary neuropathies   83.11–83.24
  hereditary sensory and autonomic neuropathies   83.12
  Horner syndrome   83.23–83.24
  iliohypogastric neuropathic pain/neuralgia   83.7
  ilioinguinal neuropathic pain/neuralgia   83.7
  mechanical injuries   122.1
  meralgia paraesthetica   83.7
  midface toddler excoriation syndrome due to pain insensitivity   83.12–83.13
  motor polyneuropathy   **83.8**
  nerve entrapment syndromes   83.6–83.8
  nervous system and the skin   83.1–83.6
  neuropathic pruritus   81.11–81.12
  neuropathic ulcer   83.13–83.19
  neurophysiological testing for skin innervation   83.5
  NF1-related tumours, secondary to   78.3
  notalgia paraesthetica   83.7
  oral involvement   108.83
  peripheral neuropathy   83.8–83.10
  pruritus   83.5–83.6
  pudendal neuropathic pain/neuralgia   83.7, 83.8
  restless leg syndrome   83.10–83.11
  scalp pruritus   **105.15**
  sensory innervation   83.2–83.4
  sensory polyneuropathy   **83.8**
  skin biopsy   83.5, **83.6**
  small fibre neuropathy   **83.9**
  spinal cord injury   83.19–83.20
  spinal dysraphism   83.17–83.19
  substance P immunoreactive nerve endings in the epidermis   83.3
  sympathetic nerve injury   83.20
  sympathetic skin response   83.5
  syringomyelia   83.16–83.17
  systemic lupus erythematosus   51.31–51.32
  triple response of Lewis   83.5
  tuberous sclerosis complex   78.8–78.9
neurological manifestations
  BSL association   98.15
  palmoplantar keratodermas   63.71
neuromuscular blocking agents (NMBA)   117.7
neuromuscular hamartoma   136.42
neuromuscular toxicity
  antimalarials   19.6
  glucocorticoids   *19.19*
neuropathic changes, burning mouth syndrome   82.2
neuropathic pain   123.10
  acute herpetic neuralgia   82.4
  IASP definition   82.5
  leprosy   28.16
  somatosensory system lesions/disease   82.5–82.6
  trigeminal neuropathic pain syndrome   82.5–82.7
neuropathic ulcer   83.13–83.19
  Aircast Walker's boot   *83.16*
  clinical features   83.13–83.14
  investigations   83.14
  management   83.14–83.16
  probing a neuropathic wound   *83.15*
  sensory loss assessment   *83.15*
  severity classification   83.14
  treatment ladder   83.16
  Wagner foot ulcer classification   **83.14**
neuropathy, see also peripheral neuropathy
neuropeptides
  pruritus   81.3, 81.4, 81.5, 81.8, 81.15, 81.20
  see also endothelin 1; substance P
neuropeptides/neurotransmitters, hormone relationship   150.2–150.3
neurosarcoidosis   96.5
neurosyphilis   29.15–29.16, 29.21
  congenital   29.26
neurothekeoma see cellular neurothekeoma; dermal nerve sheath myxoma
neurotransmitter-affecting peptides, cosmeceutical use of   157.6
neurotrophins, pruritus   81.3, 81.4
neurovascular disorders   101.6–101.9
neutral lipid storage disease with ichthyosis (NLSDI)   63.35–63.36
neutral lipid storage disease with myopathy (NLSDM)   63.36
neutropenia, haemophagocytic lymphohistiocytosis   135.12
neutrophil adhesion defects, inherited immunodeficiency   80.15–80.16
neutrophil differentiation defects, inherited immunodeficiency   80.15
neutrophilic cicatricial alopecias   87.48–87.50
neutrophilic dermatoses   49.1–49.22
  amicrobial pustulosis of the skin folds   49.20–49.21
  aseptic abscess syndrome   49.21
  bowel-associated dermatitis–arthritis syndrome   49.15–49.17
  internal malignancy association   148.23–148.24
  involving respiratory system   152.5
  pyoderma gangrenosum   49.1–49.8
  pyodermatitis-pyostomatitis vegetans   49.19–49.20
  subcorneal pustular dermatosis   49.17–49.19
  see also Sweet syndrome
neutrophilic dermatosis, rheumatoid arthritis   155.6, *155.8*
neutrophilic eccrine hidradenitis (NEH)   92.14–92.15, 119.2, 149.7–149.8
neutrophilic folliculitis   91.13
neutrophilic genital ulceration, Behçet-like syndrome associated with trisomy 8 myelodysplasia   149.8
neutrophilic granulomatous dermatitis, in patient with rheumatoid arthritis   *53.7*
neutrophilic lobular panniculitis   97.50–97.53
neutrophils   2.32
  immune cells in homeostasis   *9.4*
  microscopic examination of   3.35
  wound healing   11.2–11.3
neutrophil–macrophage colony-forming unit (NM-CFU)   135.1
Neu–Laxova syndrome (NLS)   63.38
nevoid basal cell carcinoma syndrome, basaloid follicular hamartoma   137.13
newborns see neonates
Newton law, viscoelastic materials   122.3
New-World cutaneous leishmaniasis   *33.44, 33.45, 33.46, 33.49, 33.50–33.51*
next generation sequencing (NGS)   69.23
NF1 see neurofibromatosis type 1
NF-kB pathway-related primary immunodeficiencies   80.16
NFTC see normophosphataemic familial tumoral calcinosis
NGS see next generation sequencing
niacinamide, topical depigmenting agents   18.33
niacin (vitamin B3) deficiency   61.15–61.17
NICH see non-involuting congenital haemangioma
nickel allergy   127.36–127.39
  dimethylglyoxime test   127.33, *127.34*
  prevention strategies   127.2
  prognosis   127.23
  sites of   127.16
  social factors   127.4–127.5
nicorandil ulceration, peristomal skin   112.10, *112.12*
nicotinamide   88.57, 121.3
nicotinamide-adenine dinucleotide (NAD), niacin deficiency   61.15, 61.16
nicotinamide and nicotinic acid, topical therapies   18.41
NICU see non-immune contact urticaria
nidogens   2.25
Niemann–Pick disease   79.5
Nightcliff gardener's disease see melioidosis
Nijmegen breakage syndrome   **80.4**
Nikolsky sign   118.14, 122.2–122.3
nintedanib, systemic sclerosis treatment   54.24
NIPAL4 mutations
  congenital ichthyosiform erythroderma   63.11, 63.12
  keratinopathic ichthyoses   *63.14*
nipple
  adenoma   137.21–137.22
  'guitar nipple'   122.12
  hyperkeratosis of   63.79
  inverted, glycosylation disorders   **79.10**
  jogger's nipples   122.16
  Paget disease   137.41
NISCH see neonatal ichthyosis–sclerosing cholangitis
nitrite and nitric oxide, topical therapies   18.41
'nitritoid' reaction, gold toxicity   121.4
nivirapine, hypersensitivity reactions   **14.6**
nivolumab, panniculitis induced by   97.53
NK1R see neurokinin 1 receptor
NK see natural killer
NLD see necrobiosis lipoidica
NLE see neonatal lupus erythematosus
NLRC4-associated autoinflammatory disease (NLRC 4-AID)   **45.5, 45.7**, 45.16
NLRP1-associated autoinflammation with arthritis and dyskeratosis (NAIAD)   45.8, 45.18
NLR SkinApp   7.12
NLS see Neu–Laxova syndrome
NLSDI see neutral lipid storage disease with ichthyosis
NLSDM see neutral lipid storage disease with myopathy
NM see nodular melanoma
NMBA see neuromuscular blocking agents
NM-CFU see neutrophil–macrophage colony-forming unit
NME see necrolytic migratory erythema
N-methyl-3,4-methylenedioxymethamphetamine (MDMA) see ecstasy
NMSC see non-melanoma skin cancer
NNN see Neglected Tropical Disease Non-Governmental Organisation Network
NNN Skin NTD CCG see Skin Related NTDs Cross Cutting Group
NNTs see numbers needed to treat
Nocardia spp., nocardiosis   26.86–26.87
NOCARH see neonatal onset of pancytopenia, autoinflammation, rash and episodes of hemophagocytic lymphohistiosis syndrome
nociceptive pain   123.10
nodular actinic elastosis   94.3–94.4
nodular basal cell carcinoma   140.3, *140.4, 140.8, 140.11*
nodular fasciitis   94.43, 108.12, 136.5
nodular or granulomatous candidiasis of the napkin area   32.65
nodular histiocytosis   135.19
nodular lesions, Langerhans cell histiocytosis   135.6
nodular lichen myxoedematosus   57.6, 57.7
nodular melanoma (NM)
  dermoscopic patterns   145.13, *145.14*
  melanoma classification   142.7
  presentation   142.10, *142.12*, 142.19
nodular morphoea   55.15–55.16
nodular prurigo see prurigo nodularis
nodular sarcoidosis   96.7–96.8
nodular (tubercular) syphilide   29.12–29.14
nodular (tumefactive) primary localised cutaneous amyloidosis   **56.3, 56.5, 56.8**
nodular vasculitis
  as a tuberculid   27.29, 27.31
  see also erythema induratum of Bazin
nodular–cystic fat necrosis   97.55
nodules
  hidradenitis suppurativa   *90.6*
  Merkel cell carcinoma   146.5, *146.6*
  onchocerciasis   33.5
  sarcoidosis   *96.8–96.9*
nodulocystic hidradenoma see hidradenoma
noma neonatorum (cancrum oris/oro-facial gangrene)   114.27
non-ablative fractional resurfacing (NAFR)   161.2, **161.5**
non-ablative lasers, hidradenitis suppurativa treatment   90.11
non-ablative resurfacing, laser therapy   23.23–23.24
non-accidental injury (NAI), infants   115.14
non-adherence to medical regimes   15.2
non-AIDS-defining cancers (NADC), people living with HIV   147.2–147.3
non-blanchable erythema   123.4, **123.5**, 123.8
non-bullous impetigo   26.13, 26.14
non-classical (atypical) epidermodysplasia verruciformis   25.66, 25.69
non-draining lesions, Hurley stage III disease   *90.9*
non-draining tunnel, hidradenitis suppurativa   *90.4*
non-eczematous responses, allergens   127.19–127.21
non-epidermolytic palmoplantar keratoderma (NEPPK)   63.53–63.56
non-esterified fatty acids (NEFAs)   97.4
non-follicular pustules, acute generalised exanthematous pustulosis   118.3
non-formaldehyde-releasing preservatives   127.52–127.53

non-Hodgkin lymphoma (NHL)
  AIDS defining cancer 147.2
  immunocompromised patients 147.1, 147.3
  infiltration of skin with neoplastic cells 149.4
  oral involvement 108.71
  see also chronic lymphocytic leukaemia
non-hyaluronic acid (non-HA) dermal fillers 158.5–158.6, **158.11**
non-immune contact urticaria (NICU) 127.83, 127.86, 128.8–128.9
non-inflamed nodules, Hurley stage II disease 90.4
non-inflamed phyma, treatment **89.14**
non-inflammatory disorders of subcutaneous fat 98.1–98.30
non-involuting congenital haemangioma (NICH) 71.2
non-Langerhans cell histiocytoses (non-LCHs) 135.14–135.21
non-LSH lesions 135.6
non-malignancy, generalised hypertrichosis association 87.86–87.87
non-malignant tumours, infants 116.1–116.11
non-melanin pigmentation 86.47–86.54
non-melanoma skin cancer (NMSC)
  arsenic exposure 121.3
  incidence of in Denmark/Slovakia 6.1
  PUVA phototherapy adverse effects 21.14
  recurrence in 6.5
  rheumatoid patients 155.15
non-scarring alopecia 87.28–87.35, 98.24
non-segmental vitiligo 86.34, 86.38
non-sexually acquired genital ulcers 110.19–110.20
non-sexually transmitted infections, male genitalia 109.26–109.28
non-specific balanoposthitis 109.21–109.22
non-specific cicatricial alopecia 87.51
non-specific hyperreactivity, patch testing 127.32
non-steroidal anti-inflammatory drugs (NSAIDs)
  allergic contact dermatitis 127.45, 127.79
  cutaneous adverse effects 155.15
  frostbite 124.3
  photosensitivity 126.27, 126.29, 126.31
  urticaria 117.6
non-syndromic autosomal recessive deafness 63.63
non-syndromic congenital ichthyoses 63.7–63.13
non-syndromic genodermatoses with nail anomalies **67.9**
non-syndromic ichthyoses **63.3**, 63.20–63.22
non-syndromic palmoplantar keratodermas 63.50–63.62
non-syphilitic bacterial sexually transmitted diseases 30.1–30.26
non-syphilitic spirochaetal ulcerative balanoposthitis 109.27
non-tuberculous mycobacteria (NTM) 27.1, 27.2, 27.3, 27.32–27.45
  classification 27.32
  disseminated disease 27.32–27.36, 27.38, 27.40–27.45
  disseminated tuberculous disease 27.32, 27.33, 27.34, 27.35–27.36, 27.38, 27.40, 27.42, 27.43, 27.44, 27.45
  infection diagnosis 27.5
Noonan with multiple lentigines syndrome (LEOPARD syndrome) **131.3**, 151.3
Noonan syndrome 78.9, 103.21, **106.7**
  granular cell tumours 136.49
  neonates 71.28
  oral involvement 108.86
noradrenergic and specific serotonergic antidepressants (NaSSAs) 84.43, **84.45**
norepinephrine reuptake inhibitors (SNRIs) 84.43

normocomplementaemic urticarial vasculitis (NUV) 44.1, 44.3, 44.4, 44.5
normolipaemic plane xanthoma 97.18
normolipaemic xanthoma, paraprotein activity 149.11
normophosphataemic familial tumoral calcinosis (NFTC) 79.17
North American blastomycosis 32.84, *32.86*
Norwegian scabies 39.34, *63.72*
nose
  fibrous papules 136.2–136.3
  granuloma faciale *100.12*
  inflammatory chondopathy effects 155.12
  primary localised cutaneous amyloidosis 56.8
  radiotherapy for skin cancer 24.11–24.12, *24.20*
  see also nasal entries; olfactory entries
nosological relationship, to rosacea 89.15–89.17
nosology 8.2–8.5
notalgia paraesthetica 83.7
  pruritus 81.12
notch signalling, hidradenitis suppurativa genetics 90.3
Nottingham Eczema Severity Score (NESS) 16.4
NPS see nail–patella syndrome; nano-pulse stimulation technology
NRL see natural rubber latex
NRS-11 see Numeric Rating Scale
NRTI see nucleoside reverse transcriptase inhibitor
NSAIDs see non-steroidal anti-inflammatory drugs
NSDHL mutations, CHILD syndrome 63.23–63.24
NTDs see neglected tropical diseases
NTM see non-tuberculous mycobacteria
nuchal-type fibroma 136.12
nuclear factor kappa-light-chain enhancer of activated B cells-autoinflammatory disease 45.16
nuclear hormone receptors
  hair growth 87.10
  intracellular drug mechanisms 13.5
nucleic acid amplification tests, *Mycobacterium tuberculosis* 27.8–27.9
nucleoside reverse transcriptase inhibitor (NRTI), HAART regimes 98.6–98.7
nucleotide excision repair (NER) 10.5–10.6, 76.2
numb chin syndrome (mental neuropathy), internal malignancy association 148.23
numbers needed to treat (NNTs), evidence based medicine 17.11, **17.12**
Numeric Rating Scale (NRS-11), peak itch over past 24 hours 16.3
nummular dermatitis 39.7–39.9
  associated diseases 39.7
  causative organisms 39.8
  clinical features 39.8, *39.9*
  differential diagnosis 39.8–39.9
  discoid skin lesions 39.10
  environmental factors 39.8
  epidemiology 39.7
  infected dermatitis *39.25*
  investigations 39.9
  management 39.9
  treatment for 39.9
nutrition
  acne **88.20–88.24**, 88.26
  epidermolysis bullosa 69.25
  hair disorders 87.93
  hypermetabolism treatment 125.11–125.12
  ichthyoses 63.46
  lymphatic system 103.2
  pressure ulcer prevention 123.9–123.10
  SJS/TEN management 118.20
  see also diet; dietary management; mineral disorders; vitamins

nutritional anaemias, skin signs 149.15
nutritional disorders 61.1–61.35
  essential fatty acid deficiency 61.31–61.34
  malnutrition 61.1–61.7
    assessment 61.2
    in children 61.2, 61.3, *61.4*
    classification 61.2, 61.5–61.6
    clinical features 61.3–61.4
    complications and co-morbidities 61.6
    diagnosis 61.5
    disease course and prognosis 61.6
    epidemiology 61.2
    ethnicity role 61.2–61.3
    incidence and prevalence 61.2
    investigations 61.6
    predisposing factors 61.3
    protein-energy malnutrition 61.2, 61.3
    severity classification 61.5–61.6
    skin signs of nutritional disease 61.5
  ocular features **107.41**
  see also mineral disorders; vitamins
NUV see normocomplementaemic urticarial vasculitis
NXG see necrobiotic xanthogranuloma

O

OA see ocular albinism
OAS see oral allergy syndrome
obesity
  acne association **88.23–88.24**
  adiposis dolorosa/Dercum disease 98.17–98.18, 98.28
  and atopic eczema 41.7
  BSL differential diagnosis 98.16
  cutaneous consequences 98.27–98.28
  diabetes patients 62.3
  hereditary obesity 72.3–72.9
  hidradenitis suppurativa association 90.2, 90.10
  lipoedema differential diagnosis 98.22, 98.23
  monogenic obesity with cutaneous features 72.4, **72.7**
  monogenic obesity without cutaneous features 72.3, **72.6**
  Prader–Willi syndrome 72.6–72.9
  pro-opiomelanocortin and prohormone convertase deficiency 72.4–72.6
  psoriasis association 35.18
  secondary skin complications of primary obesity **72.4**
  skin effects 98.27–98.28
  subcutaneous tissue 97.3
  visceral adipose tissue 97.5
obesity-related lymphoedema 103.38–103.39
obesity-related striae 94.11
objective measures, skin properties 16.5
Objective Severity Assessment Atopic Dermatitis (OSAAD) 16.4
obsessive–compulsive behaviour/disorder (OCD)
  acné excoriée 84.20–84.22
  body dysmorphic disorder 84.12–84.15
  hair loss 87.32
  lichen simplex chronicus 84.15
  nodular prurigo 84.15–84.18
  olfactory delusions 84.10
  psychodermatology 84.12
  skin picking disorder 84.19–84.20
  skin-related health anxieties 84.25–84.26
  trichotillomania/trichotillosis 84.22–84.25, 87.14, 87.24, 87.32–87.34
obstetric risk, pseudoxanthoma elasticum 70.33–70.34
obstetric trauma, perineal skin *111.7*, **111.8**
OCA see oculocutaneous albinism
occipital alopecia, neonates 114.4
occipital horn syndrome 2.34, 79.16
occipital scalp, hair transplantation 87.97
occludins 2.20
occlusive patch testing 127.32
occupational acne 88.66–88.68
  chloracne-inducing chemicals **88.66**, 129.12

contaminated oil ingestion **88.68**
differential diagnosis **88.67**, **88.68**
dioxin accidents **88.68**
occupational allergic contact dermatitis 129.5–129.7
  methylisothiazolinone 127.53
occupational argyria 86.52
occupational dermatology 129.1–129.17
  workplace visits 129.3–129.4
occupational dermatoses 127.12
  cement-induced 127.40
  classification 1.4
  data collection 127.3
  population studies 127.4
occupational dyspigmentation 129.13–129.14
occupational factors, epidemiology 5.11
occupational groups
  dermatoses occurring in **4.4**
  history taking 4.4
occupational irritant contact dermatitis 128.2, 128.6, 129.1–129.5
occupational leukoderma 86.45, 129.13–129.14
occupationally-induced skin tumours 129.14–129.15
occupational skin disease, work impact measures 16.12
occupational skin protection programme 128.7
occupational vitiligo 86.46
ochronosis 86.50–86.51
Ockelbo disease see Sindbis virus
OCP see oral contraceptive pill
OCT see optical confocal tomography; optimum cutting temperature
octopus stings 130.4
2-*n*-Octyl-4-isothiazolin-3-one (OIT) 127.53, 127.54
ocular albinism (OA) 68.6
ocular anomalies, infiltrating lipomatosis of the face association 98.21
ocular complications of drug therapy 19.6, 19.15–19.16, *19.19*, 107.40–107.44
ocular dermatoses see eye
ocular disorders
  Adamantiades–Behçet disease 48.4, *48.6*, **48.8**
  ophthalmic zoster 25.33, 25.34
  ophthalmological terms **107.5**
  tuberous sclerosis complex 78.9
ocular effects
  congenital syphilis 29.25, *29.28*
  extrapulmonary sarcoidosis 96.5
  long-term SJS/TEN 118.17
  palmoplantar keratodermas 63.70–63.71
  PUVA phototherapy adverse effects 21.14–21.15
  UVB phototherapy adverse effects 21.12–21.13
ocular juvenile xanthogranuloma 135.17
ocular larva migrans 33.21
ocular melanoma 142.11–142.12
ocular pemphigoid 50.26, **50.28**
ocular rosacea 89.1, *89.8*, **107.8**, 107.11–107.12
  clinical signs of **107.10**
  co-morbidities 89.10–89.11
  complications 89.10–89.11
  major features 89.6
  pathology 89.4
  treatment 89.13, **89.14**, **89.15**
ocular rosacea-like cutaneous rosacea 89.11
ocular signs, phrynoderma 85.15
ocular surface disorders
  atopic eczema 41.20–41.21
  cancers, xeroderma pigmentosum 76.5
  systemic lupus erythematosus 51.32
ocular syphilis 29.16, 107.39–107.40
oculocerebral syndrome with hypopigmentation 68.9
oculocutaneous albinism (OCA) 68.5–68.8, **78.13**
oculocutaneous tyrosinaemia (tyrosinaemia type II) 63.70–63.71

oculomucocutaneous syndromes 108.41
oculotoxicity
    antimalarials 19.6, 107.43
    dapsone 19.15–19.16
    glucocorticoids *19.19*
odds ratios (ORs), number needed to treat derivation 17.11, **17.12**
Odland bodies 85.17, 85.19
odonto-onycho-dermal dysplasia 63.68
ODSS *see* oral disease severity score
OE *see* otitis externa
oedema
    arm swelling 103.44–103.46
    chronic oedema 103.2, 103.3–103.5, 109.19–109.21
    chronic venous insufficiency *101.43*
    congestive heart failure 85.29
    constriction artefact 84.33
    drug induced oedema 103.12–103.13
    drug reaction with eosinophilia and systemic symptoms 118.8
    erythropoietic protoporphyria *58.14*
    eyelids 103.46
    facial oedema 103.46–103.49
    hand oedema *103.21*
    head oedema 103.46–103.49
    intravenous drug administration *120.7*
    kwashiorkor *61.4*
    lips 103.46, *103.48*
    lymphatic-related hydrops fetalis 103.23
    lymphovenous oedema 103.10–103.12
    neck oedema 103.46–103.49
    penis 109.19–109.21
    venouos oedema 103.10–103.12
    venous leg ulcer *102.5*
    vulval 110.23–110.24
    see also angioedema without weals; lymphoedema
oedema blisters 85.28–85.30
oedematous appearing striae *94.12*
oesophageal atresia, flushing in children **104.10**
oesophageal cancer, tylosis with 63.66, *63.67*, **78.13**
oesophageal involvement, epidermolysis bullosa 69.17–69.18, 69.25
oesophagus, gastro-oesophageal reflux disease 108.74
oesophagus tissue, monkey oesophagus substrate used in indirect immunofluorescence *3.12*, *3.13–3.14*, *3.19*
oestrogens
    acne vulgaris treatment 88.50–88.51
    pigmentation effects 86.7, 86.25
OFD1 *see* oro-facial–digital syndrome type 1
OFG *see* orofacial granulomatosis
Ofuji disease 91.3, 93.7
OHIP *see* Oral Health Impact Profile
oil hyperkeratoses 129.15
oils, contaminated, occupational acne **88.68**
ointments, vehicle choice for topical therapies 18.2
OIT *see* 2-*n*-Octyl-4-isothiazolin-3-one
old age spot *see* solar lentigo
older people *see* elderly people
Old-World cutaneous leishmaniasis 33.43–33.51
olfactory delusions 84.10–84.11
olfactory reference syndrome (ORS) 84.10–84.11
Olmsted syndrome (congenital palmoplantar and periorificial keratoderma with corneal epithelial dysplasia) 63.69–63.70, 108.30
OLP *see* oral lichen planus
omalizumab
    mastocytosis treatment 46.10
    systemic therapy 19.39
Omenn syndrome **80.4**, 80.7–80.8
omphalitis, neonates 114.26
Onchocerca volvulus 33.1–33.6
onchocerciasis (river blindness) 33.1–33.6, 94.13, 107.40
    ano-genital consequences 109.28

clinical features 33.2–33.5
    epidemiology 33.2
    investigations 33.5–33.6
    management 33.6
    pathophysiology 33.2
oncogenic viruses, skin cancer risks in immunocompromised people 147.8–147.9
oncolytic virus therapy, melanoma 144.1–144.2
Ontak *see* denileukin diftitox
onycholysis 127.21
onychomadesis 119.7
onychomycosis
    caused by *Candida* species 32.66
    caused by dermatophytes 32.47–32.49
    caused by miscellaneous moulds 32.55
    caused by *Neoscytalidium* species 32.51
    caused by non-dermatophyte moulds 32.52–32.55
    caused by *Onychocola canadensis* 32.55
    caused by *Scopulariopsis* species 32.53–32.55
    chronic mucocutaneous candidiasis *32.69*
    identification of causative organism 32.53
    patterns 32.47–32.48
    superficial 32.47–32.48, 32.54–32.55
onychophagia (nail biting) 84.25
onychotillomania (nail picking) 84.25
O'Nyong–Nyong fever, togavirus infections 25.89–25.90
Onzar *see* denileukin diftitox
open tests, allergic contact dermatitis 127.33, 127.86
ophthalmic zoster 25.33, 25.34
ophthalmological effects *see* eye; ocular effects
ophthalmological terms **107.5**
opiates
    pruritus 81.3, 81.4–81.5, 117.3
    psychodermatology 120.2
opportunistic bacteria on skin 26.2, 26.4, 26.17, 26.51, 26.55, 26.86
opportunistic mycobacteria *see* non-tuberculous mycobacteria
opportunistic systemic mycoses 32.93
optical coherence tomography
    basal cell carcinoma 140.10, *140.12*
    epidermal thickness measurement 16.5
optical confocal tomography (OCT)
    high-definition for basal cell carcinoma *140.10*, *140.12*
    melanoma diagnosis 142.9
optimism, adjusting to long-term health conditions 15.3
optimum cutting temperature (OCT) compound, biopsy for DIF examination 3.12
oral allergy syndrome (OAS) 42.13, 108.12, 127.84
oral cancer 108.43–108.50
    basal cell carcinoma of the lip 108.43–108.44
    complications of cancer treatment 108.48–108.50
    florid oral papillomatosis 108.45
    granular cell tumours 108.45
    keratoacanthoma of the lip 108.44
    metastatic oral neoplasms 108.45
    squamous cell carcinoma of the lip 108.44–108.45
    verrucous carcinoma 108.48
oral candidiasis 108.20–108.22, 108.31–108.32, 108.57, *108.71*
    acute pseudomembranous candidiasis 32.61, 108.31, *108.32*
    chronic candidiasis 108.31–108.32
    chronic hyperplastic candidiasis (candidal leukoplakia) 108.34
    chronic mucocutaneous candidiasis 32.68, 108.32
    HIV 31.6, 31.26, 31.34, 31.37
    oral lesions 108.20–108.22, 108.31–108.32, 108.34, 108.57, *108.71*

types of **108.57**
oral cavity 108.1–108.88
    abscesses 108.9
    acanthosis nigricans 108.67
    acquired lesions 108.31–108.35
    acrodermatitis enteropathica 108.20
    actinic cheilitis (solar cheilosis) 108.58
    actinic prurigo 108.58–108.59
    acute candidiasis 108.20
    acute necrotising (ulcerative) gingivitis and noma 108.54–108.55
    acute pseudomembranous candidiasis 108.31, *108.32*
    agranulocytosis 108.71
    allergic reactions in 127.18
    amalgam tattoos 108.15
    amyloidosis 108.69–108.70
    anatomical variants 108.7
    anatomy of 108.3–108.5
    angina bullosa haemorrhagica 108.20
    angioedema 108.10
    angular cheilitis 108.20, 108.59–108.60
    ankyloglossia 108.87
    aphthous-like ulcers 108.38–108.39
    aspergillosis 108.56–108.57
    bacterial infections 108.54–108.56
    basal cell carcinoma of the lip 108.43–108.44
    Behçet syndrome 108.40–108.41
    betel staining *108.15*, 108.17
    biology of 108.3–108.5
    black hairy tongue 108.16, *108.17*
    blastomycoses 108.57
    blisters, causes of **108.36**
    body art 108.15–108.16
    bone marrow transplantation, oral complications of 108.48
    brown tongue 108.16
    buccal fat-pad herniation 108.10
    buccal mucosa, examination of 108.7
    bullous pemphigoid 108.81
    burning mouth syndrome 108.64–108.65
    burns, oral lesions 108.31
    calibre-persistent artery, lip lesions 108.63
    cancer treatment, complications of 108.48–108.50
    Carney complex 108.16
    cervical lymph nodes, drainage areas of **108.6**
    'chapping' of the lips 108.60
    cheek biting 108.32
    cheilitis 108.60–108.63, *108.73*
    chemical burns, oral lesions 108.31
    chickenpox (varicella) 108.51
    chikungunya 108.50
    chronic bullous dermatosis of childhood 108.81
    cleft lip/palate 108.83–108.85
    Clouston syndrome 108.28
    coated tongue 108.16
    coeliac disease 108.72
    complex aphthosis 108.39–108.40
    congenital anomalies 108.87–108.88
    congenital lesions 108.28–108.31
    contact urticaria 42.13
    Cowden syndrome 108.85
    Crohn disease 108.72
    cryptococcosis 108.57
    cytomegalovirus infection 108.51
    Darier disease 108.28
    deficiency states 108.70
    De Lange syndrome 108.85
    dengue 108.50
    dental abscesses 108.9
    dentogingival junction, anatomy of 108.4
    denture-induced hyperplasia 108.10
    denture-induced stomatitis 32.62, 108.20–108.21
    dermatitis herpetiformis 108.81
    dermatological diseases 108.74–108.80
    dermatomyositis 108.67–108.68
    dermoid cyst 108.12
    desquamative gingivitis 108.23
    diagram of *108.4*

double lip 108.85
Down syndrome 108.85
drug-induced hyperpigmentation 108.17
dyskeratosis congenita 108.29
endocrine disorders 108.83
enteroviruses 108.50
epidermolysis bullosa 69.25, 108.23
epidermolysis bullosa acquisita *50.45*, 108.81
epithelioid (bacillary) angiomatosis 108.55
Epstein–Barr virus infections 108.51
erosions 108.36
eruption cyst 108.10
erythema multiforme *47.2*, *47.5*, 108.75
erythematous candidiasis 108.20–108.22
erythroplakia 108.23, *108.24*
erythropoietic protoporphyria 108.85
examination of 108.5–108.8
examinations 118.20
extranodal NK/T-cell lymphoma, nasal type 108.70
facial pain syndromes 108.64–108.67
fauces, examination of 108.7
fibrosis of oral tissues 108.68
fissured tongue 108.87–108.88
floor of mouth, examination of 108.7
florid oral papillomatosis 108.45
focal epithelial hyperplasia 108.11
focal mucinosis 108.85–108.86
focal palmoplantar and oral hyperkeratosis syndrome 108.29
foliate papillae, anatomy of 108.4
foliate papillitis 108.11
Fordyce spots 108.29
fungal infections 108.56–108.57, **108.56**
gamma heavy chain disease (Franklin disease) 108.70
Gardner syndrome 108.86
gastrointestinal diseases 108.72–108.74
gastro-oesophageal reflux disease 108.74
geographic tongue (benign migratory glossitis/erythema migrans) 108.24
geotrichosis 108.57
giant cell arteritis 108.69
gingiva (gums), anatomy of 108.4
gingival lichen planus 108.77
gingival recession, lip/tongue piercing 108.16
gingivitis
    acute necrotising (ulcerative) gingivitis and noma 108.54–108.55
    desquamative gingivitis 108.23, *108.82*
glomovenous malformations 108.25
glossitis 108.22, 108.24–108.25
gonorrhoea 108.55
Gorlin syndrome 108.86
graft-versus-host disease 108.48–108.49, 108.70
granular cell tumours 108.45
granulocytic sarcoma (myeloid sarcoma) 108.70
granulomatosis with polyangiitis 108.69
granulomatous cheilitis *108.73*
haemangioma 108.25–108.26
haematological diseases 108.69–108.72
haematopoietic stem cell transplantation, complications of 108.48
hairy leukoplakia 108.32–108.33, 108.34
hand, foot and mouth disease 108.50
hard tissue benign tumours 108.14
heavy metal induced hyperpigmentation 108.17
hepatitis 108.74
hereditary benign intraepithelial dyskeratosis 108.29
hereditary haemorrhagic telangiectasia (Osler–Rendu–Weber syndrome) 108.26
herpangina 108.50
herpes simplex gingivostomatitis 108.51–108.53
herpes simplex infections 25.20–25.24
herpesviruses 6, 7 and 8 108.53

herpesviruses 108.50–108.54
herpes zoster 108.53–108.54
herpetiform ulceration 108.38, *108.39*
histoplasmosis 108.57
HIV-associated candidiasis 108.21–108.22
HIV infection 108.17, 108.54
hypereosinophilic syndrome 108.70
hyperpigmentation 108.14–108.19
    causes of **108.15**
        drug, food, habits and heavy metal induced 108.16–108.17
hypoplasminogenaemia 108.70
idiopathic thrombocytopenic purpura 108.70
IgG4 disease 108.67
immune defects 108.25
immunity in 108.5
immunobullous disorders 108.80–108.82, **108.81**
impetigo 108.53
infections of 25.20–25.24, 108.50–108.57
inflammatory arthritides 108.68–108.69
inflammatory lesions 108.20–108.25
inherited patterned lentiginosis 108.17
intraoral examination 108.6–108.7
Jacob disease 108.86
jaws, examination of 108.6
Kaposi sarcoma 108.26
keratitis, icthyosis and deafness syndrome 108.29
keratoacanthoma of the lip 108.44
keratoses 108.33
Kindler syndrome 108.86
Klippel–Trenaunay–Weber syndrome 108.26
Koplik spots 108.33
Langerhans cell histiocytosis 108.70–108.71
Laugier–Hunziker syndrome 108.18
leiomyoma 108.13
leishmaniasis 108.57
lentiginoses 108.17–108.18
leprosy 108.55
lesions 78.3
lesions presentation 108.5
lesions that may cause lumps or swellings in the mouth **108.9**
leukaemias 108.71
leukoedema 108.29, *108.30*
leukopenias 108.71
leukoplakia 75.3, 108.33–108.35
linear epidermal naevus 108.30
linear IgA disease of adults 108.82
linear IgA disease of children 108.81
linear naevus syndrome (naevus sebaceous of Jadassohn) 108.29–108.30
lingual thyroid 108.11
lingual tonsil 108.11
lipoma 108.13
lumps and swellings 108.8–108.14
    lesion types **108.9**
        plant allergies 127.72
lupus erythematosus, lip lesions 108.64
lymphangioma 108.13
lymph nodes, examination of 108.6
lymphomas 108.71
macroglossia 108.11–108.12
MAGIC syndrome 108.41, 155.11, 155.13
malignant neoplasms 108.43–108.50
median rhomboid glossitis 108.22
melanocanthoma 108.18
melanoma 108.18
melanotic macule 108.18
metastatic oral neoplasms 108.45
microbiome 108.5
mixed connective tissue disease *53.3*
mucocele 108.12
mucoepithelial dysplasia 108.26–108.27
mucormycosis 108.57
mucosal immune system 108.5
mucosal melanomas 142.11, *142.16*
mucosal melanosis *131.10*
mucositis (mucosal barrier injury) 108.49–108.50

mucous membrane pemphigoid *50.27*, 108.82
multicentric reticulohistiocytosis 108.71–108.72
multiple endocrine neoplasia type 2B *108.13*, 148.10
multiple mucosal neuroma syndrome 108.13–108.14
mycosis fungoides 108.72
myelodysplastic syndromes 108.72, 149.8
myeloma 108.72
myxoma 108.14
neurological diseases 108.83
nodular fasciitis 108.12
non-Hodgkin lymphoma 108.71
Noonan syndrome 108.86
Olmsted syndrome 108.30
orocutaneous syndromes 108.83–108.87
orofacial granulomatosis 103.48, 108.72–108.74, 127.21
osteoma mucosae 108.14
pachyonychia congenita 108.30
papillary hyperplasia 108.12
papilloma 108.14
paraproteinaemias 108.72
pemphigoid (subepithelial immune bullous diseases) 108.81–108.82
pemphigus 108.80–108.81
perioral region, examination of 108.5–108.8
persistent idiopathic facial pain 108.65–108.66
Peutz–Jeghers syndrome 108.19
pigmentary incontinence 108.19
pigmented lesions 108.14–108.19
    causes of **108.15**
        drug, food, habits and heavy metal induced 108.16–108.17
plasma cell gingivitis 108.25
polyarteritis nodosa 108.69
post-herpetic neuralgia 108.66
premalignant lesions 108.42–108.43
presentation of oral lesions 108.5
protozoal infestations 108.57
pseudolymphoma 108.72
psoriasis 108.35
psychiatric disorders 108.83
purpura 108.27
pyodermatitis-pyostomatitis vegetans *49.19*
pyostomatitis vegetans 108.74
reactive arthritis (Reiter's syndrome) 108.68
reactive perforating collagenosis 108.64
recurrent labial HSV infection 108.52–108.54
red lesions 108.19–108.28
renal diseases 108.83
rhabdomyoma 108.14
rheumatoid arthritis 108.68
rheumatological diseases 108.67–108.69
salivary glands
    anatomy of 108.4
    examination of 108.6
sarcoidosis 108.64, 108.67
scarring of oral tissues 108.68
scleroderma 108.68–108.69
scrotal tongue *108.87*
sebaceous adenoma 108.30
soft tissue benign tumours 108.12–108.14
soft tissue swelling 108.9–108.12
squamous cell carcinoma of the lip 108.44–108.45
Stevens–Johnson syndrome *108.61*, 108.79, 118.20
stomatitis 25.97, 32.62–32.63, 108.20–108.21, *108.52*, 108.59–108.60
strawberry tongue 108.25
Sturge–Weber syndrome 108.27
Sweet syndrome 108.41
swelling 108.8–108.14, **108.9**, 127.72
syphilis 108.56
systemic diseases, oral manifestations 108.67–108.83
systemic lupus erythematosus 51.29

systemic sclerosis *54.4*
tattoos
    amalgam tattoos 108.15
    body art 108.15–108.16
teeth, anatomy of 108.4
telangiectasia 108.27
    hereditary haemorrhagic telangiectasia (Osler–Rendu–Weber syndrome) 108.26
tongue
    anatomy of 108.4
    examination of 108.7
trigeminal neuralgia 108.66–108.67
trigeminal trophic syndrome 108.67
tuberculosis 108.56
tuberous sclerosis 108.87
tylosis 108.30
Van der Woude syndrome 108.87
varicosities 108.27
vascular lesions 108.25–108.28
vascular proliferative lesions 108.27
vasculitides 108.69
velocardiofacial syndrome (22q11 deletion syndrome) 108.87
venous lake 108.28
venous mucocutaneous malformation 108.28
verruciform xanthoma 108.14
verrucous carcinoma 108.48
viral infections 25.20–25.24, 108.50–108.54
von Recklinghausen neurofibromatosis 108.87
Waldenström macroglobulinaemia 108.72
warty dyskeratoma (focal acantholytic dyskeratosis) 108.30–108.31
white lesions 108.28–108.35
white sponge naevus 108.31
Wiskott–Aldrich syndrome 108.28
xeroderma pigmentosum 108.87
see also lip; palate; perioral area; teeth; tongue
oral commissures, lips 108.3
oral contraceptive pill (OCP), hair disorder treatment 87.89, 87.95, **87.96**
oral disease severity score (ODSS) 108.8
oral drug administration 13.2, 13.3
oral dysaesthesia *see* burning mouth syndrome
oral epithelium, anatomy 108.3
oral hairy leukoplakia, reactivated Epstein–Barr virus 25.37–25.38
Oral Health Impact Profile (OHIP) 108.8
oral isotretinoin management, sebaceous gland hyperplasia 93.13
oral leukokeratoses, pachyonychia congenita 67.12
oral leukoplakia, dyskeratosis congenita 67.14
oral lichen planus (OLP) 37.3, 37.5–37.6, 108.76–108.79
    atrophic and ulcerative OLP 108.77
    betel chewing 37.3
    bullous OLP 108.78
    clinical features 108.76–108.78
    dental amalgam 37.3
    desquamative gingivitis 108.77
    differential diagnoses 108.78–108.79
    management of 108.78
    papular or plaque OLP 108.77
    pathophysiology 108.76
    postinflammatory hyperpigmentation *108.19*
    reticular OLP 108.76
    topical therapies **108.79**
oral melanocytic naevi 108.19
oral microbiome 108.5
oral minoxidil 87.70, 87.73, 87.94
oral mucosa
    acquired pigmentary disorders 86.24
    anatomy of 108.4
oral mucosal lesions 96.13
    COVID-19 association 25.113
    tylosis with oesophageal cancer *63.67*

oral pain, trigeminal neuropathic pain syndrome 82.5–82.7
oral pyogenic granuloma *113.3*
oral scarring, long-term SJS/TEN 118.17
oral squamous cell carcinoma (OSCC) 108.45–108.48
    classification of severity 108.47
    disease course and prognosis 108.47
    epidemiology 108.45–108.46
    features suggestive of **108.47**
    grades of carcinoma **108.47**
    history 108.46
    investigations 108.47–108.48
    management 108.48
    potentially malignant disorders **108.47**
    predisposing factors 108.46
    presentation 108.47
    TNM (tumour, node, metastases) classification 108.47, **108.48**
oral submucous fibrosis 108.42–108.43
oral therapy *see* systemic therapy
oral thrush *see* acute candidiasis
oral ulcers 108.36–108.42
    Adamantiades–Behçet disease *48.2, 48.5*, **48.8**
    agranulocytosis 108.71
    aphthous-like ulceration *108.71*
    aphthous-like ulcers 108.38–108.39, *108.71*
    aspergillosis 108.56–108.57
    Behçet-like syndrome associated with trisomy 8 myelodysplasia 149.8
    Behçet syndrome 108.40–108.41
    causes of **108.36**
    chronic ulcerative stomatitis 108.79
    complex aphthosis 108.39–108.40
    cryptococcosis 108.57
    drug-induced ulcers 108.41
    gingival ulceration *108.55*
    immune defects 108.25
    leukaemias 108.71
    leukopenias 108.71
    MAGIC syndrome 108.41, 155.11, 155.13
    mucormycosis 108.57
    necrotising sialometaplasia 108.42
    oral lichen planus 108.77
    recurrent aphthous stomatitis 108.37–108.38
    recurrent (episodic) ulceration 108.37–108.42
    single episode of ulceration 108.36–108.37
    superficial mucocoeles 108.42
    Sweet syndrome 108.41
    systemic disease association 108.41–108.42
    tongue *108.52*
    traumatic ulcerative granuloma with stromal eosinophilia 108.37
    treatment **48.8**
    ulcerative colitis 108.74
    ulcers of local aetiology 108.36–108.37
orange peel appearance (*peau d'orange*), infiltrative carcinoma skin 148.2, *148.3*
ORAS *see* otulin-related autoinflammatory syndrome
orbital cellulitis, neonates 114.26
orcein–Giemsa stain 3.8
Orf-induced pemphigoid 50.54, *50.55*
orf virus (ORFV) 25.13–25.14
organoid naevus (naevus sebaceous) *73.5, 73.6, 73.7, 73.8*, 87.30, 88.32, 105.11, *106.33*, 137.19–137.20
organ transplant recipients (OTRs)
    keratinocyte cancer risk factors 147.10
    melanoma 147.13–147.14
    pigmentation gene effects on skin cancer risks 147.4
    predisposition to cutaneous squamous cell carcinoma 141.3, 141.27, 141.29
    skin cancer
        management protocols **147.22, 147.23**
        radiotherapy 24.15
        risks 147.3–147.5

orificial tuberculosis 27.16–27.17
orocutaneous syndromes 108.83–108.87
oro-facial and cutaneous herpes, recurrent 25.22–25.24
orofacial granulomatosis (OFG) 103.48, 108.72–108.74, 127.21
oro-facial–digital syndrome type 1 (OFD1), abnormalities and renal involvement 154.2
orofaciodigital syndrome **106.7**
oro-genital ulceration, MAGIC syndrome 108.41, 155.11, 155.13
oro-pharyngeal abnormalities, HIV 31.26, 31.34–35, **31.36**
oro-pharyngeal mucocutaneous *Candida* infection, gain-of-function STAT1 mutation 80.17
oropyrosis *see* burning mouth syndrome
Oroya fever, *Bartonella bacilliformis* 26.65–26.66
'orphan' status of drugs, clinical pharmacology 13.13
ORs *see* odds ratios
ORS *see* outer root sheath
orthopoxviruses 25.6–25.13, **25.6**
  see also mpox; smallpox
Orthoptera (locusts) 34.32
OSAAD *see* Objective Severity Assessment Atopic Dermatitis
OSCC *see* oral squamous cell carcinoma
Osler–Rendu–Weber syndrome *see* hereditary haemorrhagic telangiectasia
osteoarthritis 155.8
osteogenesis imperfecta 70.12–70.14
  clinical variants 70.13
  differential diagnosis 70.13–70.14
  management 70.14
osteoma cutis 88.41
osteoma mucosae, oral mucosa 108.14
osteoporosis
  erythropoietic protoporphyria 58.16
  systemic lupus erythematosus 51.30
ostraceous psoriasis 35.14
Ota, naevus of 23.16, *23.17*, 107.46, 131.12–131.14
otic syphilis 29.16
otitis externa (OE) 106.15–106.19
  acute diffuse OE 106.16–106.17, 106.18
  acute localised OE 106.19
  acute OE *106.15*
  causative organisms 106.16
  chronic OE 106.16, 106.17, 106.18–106.19
  clinical features 106.16–106.17
  complications and co-morbidities 106.17–106.18
  investigations for 106.18
  necrotising OE 106.19
  pathophysiology 106.16
otomycosis 32.17–32.18, 106.20–106.21
otophyma, ear dermatoses **106.23**
OTRs *see* organ transplant recipients
otulin-related autoinflammatory syndrome (ORAS) 45.19
Oudtshoorn disease 63.73, *63.74*
outcomes
  core outcome measures 16.3
  digital recording 16.2
  see also measurement
outer root sheath (ORS), hair follicle 2.10, 2.44, 87.3–87.6
outlier lesions, atypical naevi for that individual 145.2
ovarian hyperthecosis 87.90
ovarian tumours, hirsutism association 87.91
overgrowth syndromes, infiltrating lipomatosis of the face differential diagnosis 98.19
overlap/coincident alopecias 87.51
overlap syndromes, dermatomyositis 52.8
OX40 deficiency 80.9–80.10
oxalate ebmolus, purpura 99.15
oxandrolone 97.32
  burn treatment 125.13–125.14
oxazolidinones 19.48
oxygenation factors, pressure ulcers 123.4
oxyhaemoglobin, erythema 128.6
oxyuriasis *see* enterobiasis
ozenoxacin, topical therapies 18.11

P

P4 (predictive, personalised, preventative, participatory) medicine 8.1
P13K/AKT/mTOR pathway, gene abnormalities within, lymphoedema association 103.23–103.24
PA *see* pyruvic acid
PAAND *see* pyrin-associated autoinflammation with neutrophilic dermatosis
PAC *see* perennial allergic conjunctivitis
PACD *see* photoallergic contact dermatitis
pachydermatoglyphy (acanthosis palmaris) 148.15–148.16
pachydermodactyly 94.38–94.39
pachydermoperiostosis 155.14
pachyonychia congenita (PC) 63.51–63.52, 67.1, 67.11–67.12
  friction blisters 122.10
  oral lesions 108.30
  skin fragility 69.20
  sweat glands 92.8
PAD13 gene 87.46
PAD (peripheral arterial disease) *see* peripheral vascular disease
paediatric autoimmune neuropsychiatric disorders associated with streptococcal infections (PANDAS) 26.11
paediatric dermatology 1.9
  see also adolescents; childhood; children; infants; neonates
paediatric inflammatory multisystem syndrome temporally associated with SARS-CoV-2 infection (PIM-TS) 25.114
PAF *see* platelet-activating factor
Paget disease 3.22, 137.40–137.42, 148.6–148.7
  see also extramammary Paget disease
pagetoid reticulosis 139.15–139.16
pagetoid spread of melanoma 142.18
pailloma 3.42
pain
  adipose tissue 98.17
  chemical burns 128.11
  diagnosis 4.3
  ectodermal dysplasias 69.27
  lipomas 98.18
  pressure ulcers 123.10
  PUVA phototherapy adverse effects 21.13
  stomas 112.6
pain disorders, female genitalia 110.40–110.42
painful hereditary callosities 63.52–63.53
painful plantar keratoderma, pachyonychia congenita 67.11
painful post-traumatic trigeminal neuropathy *see* trigeminal neuralgia
paints, vehicle choice for topical therapies 18.2
palaeodermatology 1.1
palate (roof of mouth)
  cleft lip/palate 108.83–108.85
  examination of 108.7
  leiomyoma 108.13
  melanotic macule 108.18
  mixed connective tissue disease 53.3
  papillary hyperplasia 108.12
  systemic lupus erythematosus 51.29
  torus palatinus 108.7, *108.8*
pale acanthoma *see* clear cell acanthoma
palisaded granulomatous dermatitis in patient with rheumatoid arthritis 53.7
palisading granulomas
classification 97.16–97.17
  necrobiotic xanthogranuloma 97.18
palisading necrobiotic granulomas 96.3
palladium allergy 127.40
palm
  acanthosis palmaris 148.15–148.16
  annular lesions of discoid lupus erythematosus *51.24*
  anti-p200 pemphigoid 50.41
  black palm 99.6
  congenital generalised lipodystrophies 72.2
  discoid lupus erythematosus *51.24*
  eccrine poroma 137.25–137.26
  hyperkeratotic palmar eczema 39.14
  keratolytic winter erythema 63.73, *63.74*
  lichen planus of *37.5*, 37.7
  microscopic examination of 3.33
  non-pustular palmoplantar psoriasis 35.10, *35.11*
  palmoplantar pustulosis 35.36–35.39
  pityriasis rubra pilaris *36.3*, 36.5
  pompholyx eczema 39.14, *39.15*
  recurrent focal palmar peeling 39.16
  xerosis cutis *85.26*
palmar creases
  ichthyosis vulgaris 63.4, *63.5*
  punctate keratosis of 63.60
palmar erythema
  internal malignancy association 148.25
  liver disease association 153.9
palmar fascial fibromatosis 94.34–94.35
palmar fibromatosis 93.34, 94.41–94.42, 136.12–136.13
palmar hyperhidrosis, surgical treatment 92.10
palmar keratoderma, pachyonychia congenita 67.12
palmar and plantar fibromatosis, superficial fibromatoses 136.12–136.13
palmar xanthomas 60.5–60.6
palmoplantar erythrodysaesthesia 119.2
palmoplantar hyperhidrosis 92.5, 92.6
palmoplantar hyperkeratosis 63.49
palmoplantar hyperlinearity, *ALOXE3* mutations 63.13
palmoplantar keratoderma punctata (PPKP) 63.58–63.59
palmoplantar keratodermas (PPKs) 36.3, *36.5*, 63.49–63.62, 79.8–79.9
  cancer and 63.65–63.68
  cardiomyopathy and 63.62–63.63
  in ectodermal dysplasias 63.68–63.70
  hearing impairment and 63.63–63.65
  neurological manifestations 63.71
  opthalmic manifestations 63.70–63.71
  sex reversal and 63.67–63.68
palmoplantar lesions, Stevens–Johnson syndrome/toxic epidermal necrolysis *118.14*
palmoplantar phenotype, non-syndromic ichthyoses 63.20
palmoplantar porokeratosis (of Mantoux) 63.75
palmoplantar pustulosis (PPP) 35.36–35.39, 93.8
  acute palmoplantar pustulosis *35.38*
  biologic therapy 35.39
  clinical features 35.37
  co-morbidities 35.38–35.39
  differential diagnosis 35.37
  environmental factors 35.37
  genetics 35.36–35.37
  histopathology 35.37
  management 35.39
  pathogenic mechanisms 35.37
  phototherapy 35.39
  pustulation in *35.38*
  severity classification 35.37–35.38
  systemic therapy 35.39
  topical treatment 35.39
palpation 4.1, 4.17–4.18, *4.19*
PAMS *see* paraneoplastic autoimmune multiorgan syndrome
PAN *see* polyarteritis nodosa
Panama, scabies, prevalence of **5.2**, 5.3
panatrophy 94.19–94.20
panatrophy of Gower 94.19–94.20
pancreatic carcinoma 97.41–97.42
pancreatic disease, cutaneous features 153.5–153.6
pancreatic enzymes, panniculitis 97.41
pancreatic neuroendocrine tumours (PNET) **104.8**
pancreatic panniculitis 97.41–97.43
pancreatitis 97.41–97.42
pancreatitis, panniculitis and polyarthritis (PPP) syndrome 97.42
pangeria (Werner syndrome) 70.26–70.27, **72.5**, 75.6, 77.1–77.3, **78.12**, 148.12, 148.13
panniculitis 97.1–97.64
  autoinflammatory diseases **80.19**
  biopsy 3.2
  classification **97.7**
  dermatomyositis 52.6
  hereditary **72.11**, *72.12*
  localised lipodystrophy secondary to 98.12
  pancreatic disease 153.6
  radiotherapy-associated 119.15
  of scleroderma 97.30
  scrotal panniculitis 109.23
  see also lupus erythematosus profundus
pansclerotic morphoea **54.20**, **55.4**, 55.19–55.21, **55.27**, 97.13
panthenol *see* dexpanthenol
Panton–Valentine leukocidin (PVL) virulence factor, Staphylococcal infections 111.13–111.14
PAP *see* peroxidase–antiperoxidase complexes
PAPA *see* pyogenic sterile arthritis, pyoderma gangrenosum and acne syndrome
papillary adenocarcinoma, aggressive digital 137.34–137.35
papillary dermis, anatomy 9.1
papillary eccrine adenoma *see* tubular adenoma
papillary endothelial hyperplasia, intravascular 136.23–136.24
papillary haemangioma 136.25
papillary hidradenoma (hidradenoma papilliferum) 110.31–110.33, 137.20–137.21
papillary hyperplasia, mouth 108.12
papillary intralymphatic angioendothelioma (PILA) 136.33
papillary tip microabscesses 3.43
papillomas
  milker's nodule/paravaccinia 25.15
  oral involvement 108.14
  see also human papillomavirus
papillomatosis 3.42
Papillon–Léfèvre syndrome 63.68, *63.69*
papular acrodermatitis *see* Gianotti–Crosti syndrome
papular elastorrhexis 94.33
papular facial rashes, differential diagnosis 88.37–88.38
papular keratoderma 63.60–63.61
papular lesions
  atrichia with 87.28–87.29
  drug-induced exanthems 117.2
papular (lichenoid) primary localised cutaneous amyloidosis **56.3**
papular mucinosis 57.6–57.7, 57.13–57.14
papular polymorphic light eruption 126.4, *126.5*
papular-pruritic gloves and socks syndrome, viral infections 25.120–25.121
papular syphilide 29.9–29.10
papular urticaria, infants 115.11–115.12
papular xanthoma 135.18–135.19
papules
  actinic prurigo 126.11
  conjunctival naevus 131.25
  eyelid 70.37

rosacea 89.6, *89.7*, *89.8*, 89.12, **89.14–89.15**
sarcoidosis 96.7–96.8
papuloerythroderma of Ofuji 39.34–39.35
papulonecrotic tuberculid (tuberculosis papulonecrotica) 27.27–27.29
papulopustular eruptions 119.3–119.5
   drug triggers **119.3**
   severity grading **119.4**
papulopustular rosacea 89.1
papulovesicular eruptions, COVID-19 association 25.109
papulovesicular polymorphic light eruption 126.4, *126.5*
parabens
   cosmetic allergies 127.52–127.53
   medicament allergies 127.54–127.58
parabens paradox 127.52–127.53, 127.55
parachlorometaxylenol (PCMX) 127.55–127.56
parachordoma *see* cutaneous myoepithelioma
paracoccidioidal granuloma *see* paracoccidioidomycosis
Paracoccidioides brasiliensis 32.89
paracoccidioidomycosis 32.88–32.89, 109.28
paracrine factors, pigmentation regulation 86.5–86.7
paradoxical hypertrichosis, following laser-assisted hair removal 23.20
paraesthetica, hypermelanosis *86.31*
paraffinoma 97.48, 97.49, 122.19
paraffin sections, immunoenzyme methods 3.15
paraffin wax, tissue processing 3.7
paragonimiasis 33.30–33.31
parakeratosis 3.42
parakeratosis ('shoulder parakeratosis'), pityriasis rubra pilaris *36.3*
parakeratosis variegata *see* large plaque parapsoriasis
parakeratotic hyperkeratosis 63.75
paramyxovirus infections 25.97–25.100
paraneoplastic acanthosis nigricans 85.5
paraneoplastic autoimmune multiorgan syndrome (PAMs) 50.6
paraneoplastic dermatoses 148.14–148.15, 148.19–148.20
paraneoplastic hypertrichosis lanuginosa 148.17–148.18
paraneoplastic pemphigus 50.3, 50.6, 148.21–148.22, 149.9
   oral involvement 108.76
paraneoplastic pemphigus (PNP), respiratory involvement 152.6–152.7
paraneoplastic phenomena involving the skin 148.14–148.20
paraneoplastic pigmentation 148.17, **148.18**
paraneoplastic pruritus 81.10, 148.27, 149.9
paraneoplastic syndromes
   lymphoid malignancies 149.8–149.9
   myeloid malignancies 149.5–149.8
   Sweet syndrome 149.6–149.7
paranichia (nail fold infection), candidiasis 32.65–32.66
paraphimosis 109.4, 109.16–109.17
parapoxviruses **25.6**, 25.13–25.15
paraproteinaemia
   granuloma annulare 97.18
   oral involvement 108.72
paraprotein-associated vasculitis 149.14
paraproteins
   plasma cell disorders 149.9–149.10
   skin manifestations/syndromes due to biological activity 149.10–149.13
   skin manifestations/syndromes due to paraprotein deposition 149.13–149.14
parapsoriasis 39.27, 134.6–134.8
'parasarcoidosis' syndromes 96.6
parasitic diseases 33.1–33.55
   cestodes 33.31–33.35
   nematodes - animal 33.18–33.26
   nematodes - human 33.1–33.18
   protozoa 33.35–33.55

trematodes 33.26–33.31
parasitic infections, eyelid 107.40
parasitophobia *see* delusional infestation
parastomal pyoderma gangrenosum 49.4, *49.5*
para-tert-butylphenolformaldehyde resin (PTBPFR) 127.67–127.68, 127.70–127.71
paravaccinia *see* milker's nodule
paraviral cutaneous eruptions 25.120–25.127
parechovirus infection 25.96
parenchymal injury 125.5
parenchymatous syphilis 29.15
parenteral drug administration 13.2–13.3
parenteral nutrition (PN), essential fatty acid deficiency 61.32, 61.33–61.34
Parents' Index of Quality of Life in Atopic Dermatitis (PIQoL-AD) 16.8
Parkes Weber syndrome 71.5, 71.7, 71.11, **101.28**, 101.30–101.31, 103.24
Parkland resuscitation formula 125.2–125.3
Parks classification of anal fistulae *111.30*
paronychia 119.7–119.8, **119.9**
paronychial herpes simplex *see* inoculation herpes simplex
paroxysmal finger haematoma 94.19, 99.5–99.6, 122.13–122.14
Parry–Romberg syndrome *see* progressive hemifacial atrophy
partial lipodystrophy, TBI/HSCT association 98.8
partial-thickness burns 125.6, 125.8
particulate matter (air pollution)
   ageing of skin 156.8
   atopic eczema 41.7
partitioning enhancers, topical drug delivery 12.5
parvovirus infections 25.77–25.78, 155.2–155.3
PAS *see* periodic acid–Schiff stain; pre-auricular sinus
PASH syndrome, acne conglobata association 88.63
PASI *see* Psoriasis Area and Severity Index
Pasini–Pierini, atrophoderma of 55.17, 55.19, 94.18–94.19
PASS syndrome, acne conglobata association 88.63
pastes, vehicle choice for topical therapies 18.2
Pasteurella multocida 26.59, 130.6
Patau syndrome (trisomy 13) 74.2–74.3
patch test artefacts, dermatitis artefacta 84.33
patch testing 127.1, 127.23–127.33
   age-related factors 127.5
   allergic contact eczema 1.8
   chronic actinic dermatitis 126.19, *126.21*, 126.34–126.35
   contact urticaria 127.86
   cosmetic allergens 127.49, 127.61
   drug impacts 127.6
   eczema 1.8, 39.5–39.6
   fragrance allergies 127.44–127.45
   medicament allergens 127.46–127.47
   metal allergies 127.41
   occupational contact dermatitis 129.7
   population studies 127.4
   sensitivity threshold 127.9
   stomas **112.9**
patchy alopecia 87.24, 87.26–87.27, 87.28–87.35
patchy reticular pattern naevi, dermoscopy *145.2*, *145.3*, 145.4
patchy vesiculosquamous eczema 39.16
patellar involvement, nail–patella syndrome 67.16
pathergy/pathergy testing 4.25, 122.2
Patient Benefit Index (PBI) 16.5
patient-centred care, key practical skills 15.6, **15.6**, *15.7*
patient education
   leprosy 28.15
   phototherapy 21.16

systemic therapy 19.2
patient follow-up, skin cancer surveillance after phototherapy 21.16
Patient Generated Index 16.9
patient involvement, measurement of disease state 16.1–16.2
patient organisations, ichthyoses 63.46, **63.47**
Patient-Oriented Eczema Measure (POEM) 16.3, 16.4
patient preparation for skin surgery 20.11
Patient-Reported Outcome Measures (PROMs) 16.2, 16.8
patient safety, phototherapy 21.16
patient selection
   sentinel lymph node biopsy for melanoma 143.5–143.6
   systemic therapy 19.1–19.2
patient specific measures, quality of life assessment 16.9
pattern hair loss 87.13–87.14, 87.60–87.71
   see also female pattern hair loss; male pattern hair loss
pattern recognition, melanoma diagnosis 142.9
paucibacillary cutaneous tuberculosis, lupus vulgaris 27.20–27.24
Paul of Aegina 1.3
Pautrier microabscesses 3.43
PB *see* pseudopelade of Brocq
PBI *see* Patient Benefit Index
PC1 deficiency **72.7**
PC *see* pachyonychia congenita
PCAs *see* primary cicatricial alopecias
PCBs *see* polychlorinated biphenyls
PCD *see* protein contact dermatitis
PCFCL *see* primary cutaneous follicle centre cell lymphoma
pCIA *see* persistent chemotherapy-induced alopecia
PCMX *see* parachlorometaxylenol
PCMZL *see* primary cutaneous marginal zone lymphoma
PCOS *see* polycystic ovary syndrome
PCPV (pseudocowpox) *see* milker's nodule
PCR *see* polymerase chain reaction
PCT *see* porphyria cutanea tarda
PD *see* periorificial facial dermatitis
PDCD *see* programmed cell death
PDD *see* puritic and dyskeratotic dermatoses
PDGF *see* platelet-derived growth factor
PDI *see* Psoriasis Disability Index
PDLs *see* pulsed dye lasers
PD-PSV *see* pyodermatitis-pyostomatitis vegetans
PDS *see* pleomorphic dermal sarcoma
PDT *see* photodynamic therapy
PEAG *see* pustulose exanthemique aiguë generalisés
peak itch over past 24 hours, NRS-11 16.3
pearly penile papules 109.6
peau d'orange (orange peel appearance), infiltrative carcinoma skin 148.2, *148.3*
'pebbling' of skin, mucopolysaccharidoses *79.3*
PECL *see* postinflammatory elastolysis and cutis laxa
PEComa *see* perivascular epithelioid cell tumour
pedal papules of infancy 115.14, *115.15*
Pediatric Symptom Checklist 16.10
Pediculus capitis (head lice) 34.18–34.23
Pediculus corporis (body/clothing lice) 34.23–34.24
pEDS *see* periodontal Ehlers–Danlos syndrome
peeling skin, leukonychia, acral punctate keratoses, cheiliti and knuckle pads syndrome (PLACK) 94.37–94.38
peeling skin syndromes (PSSs) 63.28–63.30, 69.5–69.6, 69.19–69.20
PeIN *see* penile intraepithelial dysplasia; penile intraepithelial neoplasia
pellagra 5.1–5.2, 86.23–86.24

Casal's necklace *61.17*
niacin deficiency 61.16, *61.17*
pelvic floor, muscles of (female) *111.3*
pelvic inflammatory disease (PID)
   chlamydia 30.10, 30.11, 30.14
   gonorrhoea 30.5, 30.7
PEM *see* pigmented epithelioid melanocytoma/pigment synthesising melanoma
PEMKB *see* pseudoepitheliomatous micaceous and keratotic balanitis
pemphigoid diseases
   autoantibodies **50.10**
   direct immunofluorescence findings 3.17–3.18
   oral involvement 108.81–108.82
   see also bullous pemphigoid
pemphigoid gestationis (PG) 113.17–113.19
   blister formation 113.18
   transplacental 114.12
   urticated red plaques *113.18*
pemphigus 50.1–50.9
   acantholysis 50.3
   age of onset 50.2
   antibodies 50.2–50.3
   associated diseases 50.2
   bullous pemphigoid 50.10–50.22
   clinical features 50.4–50.5
   clinical variants 50.5–50.7
   diagnosis **50.10**
   differential diagnosis 50.7
   direct immunofluorescence findings 3.17, *3.18*
   direct immunofluorescence microscopy *50.3*, 50.7
   disease course and prognosis 50.7
   division of 5.4
   drug-induced 50.4
   ELISA analysis 3.20, *3.21*
   environmental factors 50.3–50.4
   epidemiology 50.1–50.2
   genetics 50.3
   histopathology 50.7
   IgA pemphigus 50.6–50.7
   internal malignancy association 148.22
   investigations 50.7–50.8
   lesions in skin folds *50.5*
   management 50.8–50.9
      azathioprine 50.8
      corticosteroids 50.8
      cyclophosphamide 50.8
      immunoadsorption 50.9
      intravenous immunoglobulin therapy 50.8
      methotrexate 50.9
      mycophenolate mofetil 50.8
      plasmapherisis 50.9
      rituximab 50.9
      topical therapy 50.8
   oral involvement 108.80–108.81
   paraneoplastic 50.3
   pathophysiology 50.2–50.3
   penis 109.25
   serological assays 50.7–50.8
   severity classification 50.7
   T cells in 50.2
   see also paraneoplastic pemphigus
pemphigus foliaceus (PF) 39.34, 50.5, 50.6, *50.7*
pemphigus herpetiformis 50.6
pemphigus vegetans 50.5–50.6, 108.81
pemphigus vulgaris (PV) 50.4–50.5
   differential diagnosis 50.7
   neonatal 114.12
   oral involvement 108.80–108.81
   in pregnancy 113.8–113.9
   vulva **110.21**
PEN *see* porokeratotic eccrine ostial duct naevus
penciclovir, topical therapies 18.13
penetration enhancers, topical medication vehicles 18.5, 18.7–18.8
penetration injury, foreign bodies 122.17–122.18
D-penicillamine, cutaneous adverse effects 155.15

penicillamine, pseudoxanthoma elasticum 94.30
penicillin 1.8, 19.46
   cellulitis/erysipelas management 26.19, 26.21–26.22
   congenital syphilis 29.23, 29.28, 29.29
   cutaneous adverse effects of D-penicillamine 155.15
   reactions and allergies 29.21–29.22, 29.29, 117.7
   syphilis 29.20–29.22
penicilliosis (*Talaromyces marneffei* infections) 31.28, 32.89–32.90
penile fibromatosis 94.36–94.37, 136.13
penile horn 109.35
penile intraepithelial dysplasia (PeIN) 141.26
penile intraepithelial neoplasia (PeIN) 109.31–109.34
penile lentiginosis *131.10*
penile psoriasis *35.10*
penile squamous cell carcinoma (PSCC) 109.31–109.34
penis
   acne 109.24
   amyloidosis 109.25
   anatomy 109.2–109.3
   balanitis 109.4, 109.5
   Bowen disease of the penis 109.31–109.34
   bowenoid papulosis 109.31–109.34
   Buruli ulcer 109.28
   candidiasis 109.27
   carcinoma of 109.35–109.39
      classification **109.37**
         dysplasia and squamous carcinoma *109.38*
      risk factors **109.36**
   cellulitis 109.26
   chronic oedema 109.19–109.21
   cicatricial (mucous membrane) pemphigoid 109.25
   colloid degeneration 109.31
   condylomas 109.39–109.40
   dermoid cysts 109.31
   drug reactions 109.24–109.25
   ecthyma gangrenosum 109.26
   ectopic lesions 109.6
   erythroplasia of Queyrat 109.31–109.34
   fixed drug eruption 109.24
   Fordyce spots 93.11, 93.12
   foreign body 109.8
   haematoma and rupture 109.8
   keloid 109.31
   lentiginosis *131.10*
   lichen planus *37.4*
   lichen sclerosus *109.16*
   linear IgA disease *50.37*
   lipogranuloma 109.8–109.9
   lymphoedema 103.49–103.51, 109.19–109.21
   lymphoma 109.42
   malignant melanoma 109.41
   median raphe cysts 109.30
   melanosis 109.42–109.43
   Melkersson–Rosenthal syndrome 109.25
   metastases 109.42
   molluscum contagiosum 109.29
   mucous membrane pemphigoid *50.28*
   naevi on 109.6
   necrosis 109.22–109.24
   pearly papules 109.6
   pemphigus 109.25
   Peyronie disease 109.24
   pilonidal sinus 109.24
   porokeratosis of Mibelli 109.35
   psoriasis vulgaris *35.10*
   sclerosing lymphangitis 109.8
   squamous hyperplasia 109.34–109.35
   squamous intraepithelial lesions 109.34–109.35
   strangulation of 109.8
   striae of Wickham *109.19*
   tinea 109.27–109.28
   tuberculosis 109.27
   ulceration 109.22–109.24, 109.28

peno-scrotal lymphoedema, cutaneous Crohn disease *95.15*
penoscrotodynia (PSD) 82.11–82.12
PENS syndrome 73.7
Pentatomidae (stink bugs) 34.30
pentazocine panniculitis 97.48, 97.50
pentazocine ulcers 122.19, 122.21
Pentinnen syndrome **72.5**
people with albinism (PWA) 7.2, 7.10–7.11, 7.12, *7.13*
people living with HIV (PLWH)
   global trends 31.2
   infections 31.20–31.30
   inflammatory dermatoses 31.12–31.20
   Kaposi sarcoma 147.2
   Merkel cell carcinoma 147.2
   neoplasms 31.30–31.33
   non-AIDS-defining cancers 147.2–147.3
   pruritic skin conditions 31.12
   skin cancer risks 147.2–147.3, 147.12–147.16
PEP *see* polymorphic eruption of pregnancy
peptide repertoir model, T-cell recognition of drugs 14.6
peptides, cosmeceutical use 157.5–157.6
percentage concentrations of drugs, weight in weight or weight in volume 18.1
percutaneous absorption
   mechanisms of 12.1–12.2
   neonates 114.2
perennial allergic conjunctivitis (PAC) 107.16, 107.17, 107.18
perforating collagenosis *see* perforating folliculitis
perforating dermatoses 94.53–94.55
perforating disease due to exogenous agents 94.55
perforating disorders, renal failure and dialysis complications 154.3–154.4
perforating folliculitis (perforating collagenosis)
   diabetic patients 62.4, *62.5*
   renal failure and dialysis complications 154.3–154.4
perforating keratotic disorders 63.76–63.77
perforating pseudoxanthoma elasticum 94.30
perforin 135.11–135.12
perfumes
   allergies 127.41–127.45, 127.48, 127.79
   genital contact dermatitis 109.13
perfusion factors, pressure ulcers 123.4
perianal abscess 111.27–111.28
perianal candidiasis 32.64–32.65
perianal candidiasis of infancy 32.65
perianal carcinoma *111.23*
perianal cellulitis 109.26
perianal conditions, *see also* perineal and perianal skin
perianal dermatitis 128.5
perianal skin tags 111.32, *111.33*
perianal streptococcal cellulitis (dermatitis) 26.33–26.34
perianal streptococcal dermatitis, infants 115.8
perianal ulcers, leukocyte adhesion deficiency type I 80.16
peribuccal pigmentation of Brocq 86.15
pericytes *see* perivascular myoid cells
periderm 2.3
perieccrine calcium deposition, calcific arteriolopathy 97.33
perifollicular fibroma 137.15–137.16
perifollicular inflammation, rosacea 89.3
perifollicular papules, mid-dermal elastolysis 94.26
perifollicular purpura, scurvy *61.22*
perineal and perianal skin 111.1–111.34
   amoebiasis 111.16
   anal abscess 111.27–111.28
   anal fissure 111.30–111.31
   anal fistula 111.28–111.30
   anal intraepithelial neoplasia 111.19–111.21

   anal and perianal malignancy 111.21–111.24
   bacterial infections 111.13–111.15
      ano-genital cellulitis 111.14
      ecthyma gangrenosum 111.15
      folliculitis 111.13–111.14
      furunculosis 111.13–111.14
      necrotising soft-tissue infections 111.15
      perianal cellulitis 111.14
      perianal malakoplakia 111.15
      perianal tuberculosis 111.15
      Streptococcal dermatitis 111.14
   basal cell carcinoma 111.24
   Bowen disease 111.20–111.21
   carcinoma erysipeloides 111.24
   congenital and developmental abnormalities 111.3
   Crohn disease *95.14*, 111.26–111.27
   drug reactions 111.12–111.13
   embryogenesis of ano-genital region 111.3, *111.4*
   extramammary Paget disease 111.24
   fungal infection 111.8
   fungal infections 111.15
   haemorrhoids 111.31–111.33
   helminth infestations 111.16
   hidradenitis suppurativa 111.10–111.12
   history and examination 111.1
   human papillomavirus infection 111.16, 111.17–111.19
   infantile perianal pyrimidal protusion 111.3
   inflammatory dermatoses 111.8–111.12
      deep inflammatory dermatoses 111.10–111.12
      superficial inflammatory dermatoses 111.8–111.10
   investigations for 111.1
   melanoma 111.24
   obstetric trauma *111.7*, **111.8**
   perianal carcinoma *111.23*
   perianal sensory disturbances 111.3–111.8
   perianal skin tags 111.32, *111.33*
   perianal trauma 111.7–111.8
   perianal viral warts 111.18, *111.19*
   perineal and perianal pain 111.6–111.7
   pilonidal sinus 111.25–111.26
   pressure sores 111.7–111.8
   pruritus ani 111.3–111.6
   scabies infection 111.16
   sexually transmitted diseases 111.16–111.17
   squamous cell carcinoma 111.21–111.24
   structure and function of ano-genital region 111.1–111.3
   surgical management of conditions 111.25–111.33
   ulceration 111.12–111.13, 111.30–111.31
      HIV infection **111.17**
   viral infections 111.15–111.16
      cytomegalovirus infection 111.15
      herpes simplex virus infections 111.15
      Kawasaki disease 111.16
      molluscum contagiosum infection *111.13*, 111.15
perineal streptococcal dermatitis 109.26
perineum 111.1, *111.2*
   formation of *111.4*
   microbiome 26.3, 26.4, 26.5
   see also perineal and perianal skin
perineural invasion (PNI), advanced basal cell carcinoma 140.9
perineurioma 136.47
periodic acid–Schiff (PAS) stain 3.7, 3.8
periodic fever, immunodeficiency and thrombocytopenia (PFIT) 45.19
periodicity of lesion/eruption, diagnosis 4.3
periodontal Ehlers–Danlos syndrome (pEDS) **70.5**, *70.10*
perioral area, allergic contact dermatitis 127.15
perioral dermatitis 88.34, *88.36*, 89.10, *89.18*
perioral wrinkling, reduction of by botulinum toxin application *159.7*

periorbital bleeding, primary systemic amyloidosis with cutaneous involvement *56.11*
periorbital dermatitis *41.20*
periorbital lines, reduction of by botulinum toxin application *159.5*, *159.6*, *159.7*
periorbital oedema, eyelids 107.6–107.7
periorbital syringomas, photothermal ablation 23.21, *23.22*
periorificial facial dermatitis (PD) 89.10, 89.17–89.18
periostin, keloids 94.50
peripheral blood, immune system 9.6
peripheral cyanosis (acrocyanosis), neonates 114.3
peripheral fat, lymphatic system 103.2
peripheral globules, naevi 145.2, *145.3*, *145.4*–145.5
peripheral light brown structureless areas, melanoma *145.7*
peripheral network naevi with central hypo- or hyperpigmentation *145.2*, *145.3*, *145.4*
peripheral neuroectodermal tumours 136.42–136.52
peripheral neuropathy 83.8–83.10
   dapsone 19.14
   leprosy 28.1, *28.2*, 28.3–28.4, 28.6, 28.7, 28.9–28.10, 28.11, 28.12, 28.13, 28.15–28.16
   thallium poisoning 121.9
peripheral primitive neuroectodermal tumour *see* cutaneous Ewing sarcoma
peripheral streak patterns
   melanoma *145.7*, *145.8*
   Spitz naevi *145.6*, *145.7*
peripheral tan structureless areas, melanoma *145.9*, *145.10*
peripheral vascular disease (PVD) 101.2–101.3
   arterial leg ulcer *102.9*
   clinical features **101.2**
   investigations for **101.4**
   ischaemic foot *101.3*
   mixed leg ulcers 102.4–102.7
   platelet emboli *101.3*
   radiological investigations **101.4**
   treatment options **101.5**
   trophic changes *101.3*
   ulceration *101.3*
periporitis staphylogenes, neonates 114.25
peristomal dermatitis 128.5
peristomal pyoderma gangrenosum 49.4, *49.5*
peritonitis, acute scrotum 109.25
periungual allergic contact dermatitis 127.62
periungual fibromas (Koenen tumours), tuberous sclerosis complex 78.8
perivascular adipocytes 97.6
perivascular cell tumours 136.39–136.42
perivascular epithelioid cell tumour (PEComa) 136.61
perivascular myoid cells (pericytes) 2.40
   microscopic examination of 3.37
   myopericytoma 136.40–136.41
perlèche *see* angular cheilitis
perniosis *see* chilblain-like lesions; chilblains
peroxidase–antiperoxidase (PAP) complexes 3.14–3.16
per protocol analysis, randomised controlled trials 17.14
persistent chemotherapy-induced alopecia (pCIA) 87.72–87.74
persistent dento-alveolar pain disorder *see* trigeminal neuralgia
persistent erythema
   diagnostic features 89.5, *89.12*
   diffuse *89.7*
   treatment **89.13**
persistent human papillomavirus infections, primary immunodeficiencies 149.19

persistent idiopathic facial pain (PIFP) 108.65–108.66
persistent light reaction 126.29, 127.80–127.81
persistent light reactors 126.13–126.14
persistent pigment darkening (PPD) 86.9, 87.100
  UVR exposure 10.8
persistent superficial scaly dermatitis *see* small plaque parapsoriasis
persistent viral infections 25.4
  Epstein–Barr virus 25.36, 25.38
  herpesviruses 25.19
  human herpesvirus 6 and 7 25.39, 25.40
  see also recurrent entries
personal care products, genital contact dermatitis 109.13
personalised medicine, clinical pharmacology 8.1, 13.11
personality traits, beliefs/emotions/behaviours 15.3
personal protective equipment (PPE)
  allergic reactions 127.4
  irritant contact dermatitis 129.4
  occupational dermatoses in COVID-19 pandemic 25.119
persons with albinism (PWA) 7.2, 7.10–7.11, 7.12, *7.13*
perspiration, types of 2.9
PEST *see* Psoriasis Epidemiology Screening tool
petechiae
  COVID-19 association 25.109
  diagnosis by lesion size 99.3
  reactions to COVID-19 vaccines 25.118
  sports injuries 122.16
petrified ear 106.21
petrolatum, patch testing 127.25, *127.26*
pets
  arthropod infestation 34.4, 34.5, *34.6*, 34.13, 34.14
  atopic eczema 41.8
Peutz–Jeghers syndrome 78.14, **131.3**
  oral hyperpigmentation 108.19
Peutz–Jeghers–Touraine (PJT) syndrome 68.13–68.14
Peyronie disease 94.37, 109.24
PF *see* pemphigus foliaceus
PFIT *see* periodic fever, immunodeficiency and thrombocytopenia
PFR *see* phenol formaldehyde resin
PFS *see* post-finasteride syndrome
PG *see* pemphigoid gestationis; propylene glycol; pyoderma gangrenosum; pyogenic granuloma
PGA *see* Physician's Global Assessment
PGD2 *see* prostaglandin D2
PGD *see* preimplantation genetic diagnosis
PGH *see* preimplantation genetic haplotyping
PGs *see* proteoglycans
PHA *see* progressive hemifacial atrophy
PHACES syndrome (posterior fossa malformations, haemangiomas, arterial anomalies, cardiac anomalies, eye abnormalities, sternal pit and supraumbilical raphe) 116.3
phaeochromocytoma 86.19–86.20
  dermatoendocrinology 150.19
  flushing **104.7**
  pallor and rebound flushing 148.26
phaeohyphomycosis 32.77–32.78
phaeomelanin 2.17, *2.18*, 86.5
phaeomycotic subcutaneous cyst *see* phaeohyphomycosis
phagedena/phagedenic ulcer, *see also* tropical ulcer
phagocytes 135.1
phagocytic defects, inherited immunodeficiency **80.5–80.6**, 80.15
phagocytosis 135.2
phakomatosis pigmentokeratotica 73.5–73.6

see also HRAS/KRAS mosaicism; Schimmelpenning–Feuerstein–Mims syndrome
phakomatosis pigmentovascularis (PPV) 73.20–73.21
  phenotypic subclassifications **73.21**
  port-wine stain *73.22*
phalanges
  congenital erythropoietic porphyria 58.10
  familial mandibuloacral dysplasia *70.29*
  see also finger; toe
phantom tooth pain (trigeminal neuropathic pain) 82.5–82.7
phantosmia *see* olfactory delusions
pharmacists, clinical pharmacology 13.11
pharmacodynamics **13.2**, 13.4–13.6
  age 13.7–13.8
  conception, pregnancy and lactation 13.8–13.9
pharmacogenomics, clinical pharmacology 13.11
pharmacokinetics (PK) 13.1–13.4
  age 13.7–13.8
  conception, pregnancy and lactation 13.8–13.9
  topical bioavailability/bioequivalence assessment 12.8
pharmacological interaction (p-i) model, T-cell recognition of drugs **14.5**, 14.6
pharmacological modalities, burn injuries 125.13–125.14
pharmacotherapy (topical and systemic agents), phototherapy combination 21.10
pharmionics, clinical pharmacology 13.9
pharyngitis, *Streptococcus pyogenes* 26.10
phenol
  burns 128.11
  chemical peels 160.3
phenol-croton oil peel 160.10–160.11
phenol derivatives of hydroquinone, topical depigmenting agents 18.32
phenol formaldehyde resin (PFR), allergy 127.70–127.71
'phenoplastics' 127.70
phenothiazines, eczema 117.4
phenotype
  rosacea 89.1
  sweat glands 92.8
p-phenylenediamine (PPD) 127.60–127.61, 127.63–127.64, 127.66
p-phenylenediamine and toluene-2,5-diamine (PTD) 127.60–127.61
phenylketonuria (PKU) 79.10–79.11
phenytoin, palmar fascial fibromatosis 94.34
Phialophora verrucosa 32.77
philtrum 108.3
phimosis 109.4, 109.16–109.17
phleboliths, Maffucci syndrome *71.20*
phlebolymphoedema 103.10–103.12
PHN *see* postherpetic neuralgia
PHO *see* primary hypertrophic osteoarthropathy
phobias
  moles/skin cancer 84.26
  topical corticosteroids 84.26
  see also delusional infestation
pholcodeine hypothesis 117.7
phosphatase and tensin homologue (PTEN) hamartomatous syndromes **131.3**
  see also PTEN hamartoma tumour syndrome
phosphomannomutase 2 deficiency *79.10*
photoablation, UV radiation 23.5
photoactivation 127.79
photoageing 2.45, 2.46
  atrophic photoageing 156.3, *156.4*
  chemical peels 160.5
  collagen fibril fragmentation 156.8–156.9
  grading and measurement of 156.6–156.7
  hypertrophic photoageing 156.3

implications of 156.10–156.11
molecular mechanisms in *156.10*
and natural ageing 156.10
PUVA phototherapy adverse effects 21.13
in skin of colour 156.1–156.3
UVB phototherapy adverse effects 21.13
UV irradiation damage/episodic exposure 156.7–156.8, *156.10*
UVR exposure 10.10–10.11
in white skin 156.1
photoaggravated diseases 126.1, 126.32, *126.33*
photoallergic contact dermatitis (PACD) 127.78–127.82
photoallergic reactions
  chemotherapy 119.11–119.12
  polymorphic light eruption 126.2
  systemic drug-induced photosensitivity 126.28
  UV filters 127.62
photobiology 10.1–10.14
  normal effects of UVR on skin 10.5–10.11
  personal and population exposure to UVR 10.12–10.14
  photoprotection 10.11–10.12
  principles of 10.1–10.5
photobleaching, immunofluorescence 3.11
photochemical changes in skin
  laser therapies 23.4
  see also photodynamic therapy
photochemotherapy (PUVA)
  adverse effects 21.13–21.15
  history 21.2
  lentigo 131.7–131.8
  light source units 21.3
  mastocytosis treatment 46.10
  minimal phototoxic dose 21.9
  photosensitivity management 126.37
  PLE management 126.7–126.8
  principles 21.1
  psoralen choice and regimen 21.9
  UVA delivery 21.10
  UVB phototherapy comparison 21.5–21.6
  see also extracorporeal photopheresis
photocontact allergy 126.35, 127.11
photocontact facial melanosis 86.12–86.15
photodamage
  ablative fractional resurfacing therapy *161.3*
  dermal connective tissue 94.1–94.6
photodermatoses **106.23**
  acquired non-infective disorders 91.6–91.8
  pilosebaceous unit disorders 93.6
  PUVA phototherapy adverse effects 21.13
photodistributed erythema 89.9
photo documentation, chemical peels 160.8
photodynamic reactions, pigmentation 86.28–86.30
photodynamic therapy (PDT) 22.1–22.15
  acne vulgaris 88.58
  actinic keratosis 141.10–141.11
  acute adverse effects 22.12–22.14
  adverse effects **22.12**
  ambulatory 22.11
  basal cell carcinoma 140.11, 140.12–140.13
  Bowen disease 141.24
  chronic adverse effects 22.14
  clinical governance 22.15
  contraindications 22.8
  conventional methodology 22.9–22.11
  cutaneous squamous cell carcinoma 141.35
  cutaneous warts 25.59
  daylight 22.11–22.12
  history 22.1–22.2
  indications 22.4–22.8
  light sources 22.3–22.4
  methodology 22.8–22.12
  patient selection 22.8–22.9
  photosensitisers 22.2–22.3
  principles 23.4

process 22.1
see also phototherapy
photoepilation 23.17
  see also laser-assisted hair removal
photo-exposed skin, Jessner lymphocytic infiltrate 134.10
photographic assessment methods
  acne 16.4
  challenges 16.5
  diagnosis 4.19
  psoriasis 16.3
photography, development of dermatology 1.9
photomechanical interactions, laser therapies 23.5
photo-onycholysis 119.12
photopatch testing 126.34–126.35, 127.31, 127.78–127.79, 127.81–127.82
  chronic actinic dermatitis 126.19
  sunscreen chemicals *126.31*
photopheresis
  principles 21.1–21.2
  see also extracorporeal photopheresis
photophoresis *see* extracorporeal photopheresis
photoprotection 10.11–10.12
  cutaneous photosensitivity diseases 126.36
  erythropoietic protoporphyria 58.15
  keratinocyte cancer prevention in immunocompromised people 147.18
photosensitisation
  mechanisms 127.79
  photodynamic therapy 22.2–22.3
  see also 5-aminolaevulinic acid; methyl aminolevulinate
photosensitive eczema 126.13
  plant allergies 127.72
photosensitive psoriasis 126.2
photosensitivity 126.1
  allergic contact dermatitis 127.21
  chemotherapy-induced 119.11–119.12
photosensitivity diseases 126.1–126.39
  clinical assessment/management 126.32–126.37
  ocular features 107.42
photostimulation/photobiomodulation, laser therapies 23.4
phototesting, extracorporeal photochemotherapy 21.11
phototherapy 1.8, 21.1–21.18
  acne vulgaris 88.58
  adverse effects 21.11–21.15
    PUVA 21.13–21.15
    UVA-1 21.15
    UVB 21.11–21.13
  alopecia treatment 87.27
  at home 21.3, 21.8, 21.15, 21.18
  atopic eczema 21.4
  atopic eczema treatment 41.28
  audits 21.17
  carcinogenesis risks 21.13, 21.14, 21.15
  clinical governance 21.17
  combination therapy 21.10
  conditions treated 21.3–21.5
  contraindications 21.6
  cutaneous photosensitivity diseases 126.37
  cutaneous T-cell lymphoma 21.4
  delivery methods 21.8
  documentation/record keeping 21.17
  dosimetry 21.3, *21.4*, 21.17
  equipment maintenance 21.17
  equipment types 21.2–21.3
  history 21.2
  indications 21.3–21.5
  mastocytosis treatment 46.10
  minimal erythema dose 21.7–21.8
  modality choices 21.5–21.7
  morphoea 55.36
  new developments 21.18
  palmoplantar pustulosis 35.39
  patient education 21.16
  patient follow-up/skin cancer surveillance 21.16

phototherapy (continued)
  patient selection/assessment 21.15–21.16
  polymorphic light eruption 21.5
  principles 21.1–21.18
  psoriasis 21.3–21.4
  regimen variables 21.8
  risk management 21.16, 21.17
  safety of patients and staff 21.16
  setting up a phototherapy unit 21.17–21.18
  starting dose/increments/frequency and number of exposures 21.8
  topical and systemic agents combination 21.10
  types 21.1–21.2
  UVB versus PUVA 21.5–21.6
  UV calibration/dosimetry 21.3, 21.4
  vitiligo 21.4
  see also laser therapies; photodynamic therapy
phototherapy and photochemotherapy, cutaneous T-cell lymphoma 139.22
photothermal ablation
  complications 23.23
  devices 23.20–23.21
  indications 23.21–23.23
  skin disorder treatments 23.20–23.23
photothermal reactions, laser therapies 23.4–23.5
photothermolysis, selective 23.5–23.6
phototoxic contact dermatitis 127.78, 128.9–128.10
phototoxic drugs, photosensitivity diseases 126.28
phototoxic reactions
  chemotherapy 119.11–119.12
  pigmentation 86.28–86.30
  porphyrias 58.1
phototrichogram 87.14, 87.56
phrynoderma 61.8, 85.14–85.15
Phthiraptera (lice) 34.18–34.25
Phthiriasis pubis (crab lice) 34.24–34.25
  blepharitis due to 107.12
  eyelashes 34.25, 107.40
  male genitalia 109.29
PHTS *see* PTEN hamartoma tumour syndrome
phycomycosis *see* mucormycosis
phyma, fibrosis in 89.3
phymatous rosacea 89.1
  diagnostic features 89.5–89.6, 89.12
  differential diagnosis 89.10
  treatment **89.13–89.14**
Physalia, stings 130.1–130.3
physical dosimetry 10.2
physicians, experience based decisions versus evidence based 17.5–17.6
Physician's Global Assessment (PGA), psoriasis 16.3
physiological functions of skin 2.42–2.43
physiological hypermelanosis 86.9
physiological livedo reticularis 124.8, 124.9
physiological reactions, heat/IR radiation 124.14
phytanic acid 63.31
phytochemicals, cosmeceutical use of 157.7–157.10
phytophotodermatitis 86.28–86.30, 126.29–126.30
phytophotodermatosis 4.9
phytotherapy, psoriasis treatment 35.22–35.23
phytotherapy-induced rashes, neonates **114.11**
PI3Kδ deficiency 80.13
PI3K-related overgrowth syndromes 71.7
PI *see* protease inhibitor
piano paronychia 122.12
picker's acne *see* acné excoriée
picker's nodules *see* lichen simplex chronicus
PICO/PICOT acronyms of components for formulating well-built clinical questions 17.3, 17.4
Picornavirus infections 25.93–25.97

PID *see* pelvic inflammatory disease
piebaldism 68.3–68.4
Piedraia hortae, black piedra 32.15–32.16
piezogenic pedal papules 122.26–122.27
PIFP *see* persistent idiopathic facial pain
pigmentary disorders 3.44, 86.1–86.56
  electron microscopy studies 3.30
  female genitalia 110.20–110.23
  genetic disorders 68.1–68.15
  glycosylation disorders **79.10**
  haemochromatosis 153.5
  hair 87.12, 87.91–87.94
  HIV 31.12
  laser therapies 23.12–23.17, *23.18*
  ocular features **107.42**
  xeroderma pigmentosum 76.4–76.5
  see also hyperpigmentation; hypopigmentation
pigmentary incontinence 3.43
  incontinentia pigmenti 4.16, *4.19*, 4.22
  oral hyperpigmentation 108.19
pigmentary mosaicism, infants 115.13
pigmentation
  basal cell carcinoma 140.3, *140.4*, 140.6, *140.8*, 140.9, 140.10, 140.18, 140.21
  changes in during pregnancy 113.1, *113.2*, **113.2**
  chemical peels 160.5–160.6
  cutaneous manifestations of Hodgkin disease 139.49
  internal malignancy links 148.17, **148.18**
  liver disease association 153.8
  Merkel cell carcinoma risk 146.2
  pancreatic disease 153.5–153.6
  renal failure and dialysis effects 154.3
  seborrhoeic dermatitis effects 40.4–40.5
  UV light exposure 10.7–10.8
  UV light regulation 86.5–86.7
  variation in 2.18
  see also melanocytes; skin colour
pigmentation genes, skin cancer risks in immunocompromised people 147.6
pigmentation of hair 87.12–87.13, 87.88
pigmentation of hair nodules, trichomycosis axillaris 26.41–26.42
pigmentation of nails, renal failure and dialysis effects 154.3
pigment cell naevi **73.2**
pigmented dermatitis 127.20
pigmented epithelioid melanocytoma/pigment synthesising melanoma (PEM/animal-type melanoma) 142.2, 142.20
pigmented lesions
  surgical treatment 20.50
  see also malignant melanoma
pigmented melanotic macules 131.9–131.11
  genital melanosis *131.10*
  labial melanotic macules 131.11–131.12
  dermoscopic image *131.11*
  penile lentiginosis *131.10*
  squamous epithelium of oral cavity *131.10*
pigmented neuroectodermal tumour of infancy 136.50–136.51
pigmented purpura *see* capillaritis
pigmented purpuric dermatoses 99.7–99.9
pigmented purpuric lichenoid dermatosis of Gougerot and Blum 99.7, 99.8, **99.9**
pigment lasers
  complications 23.17
  tattoo and pigmented lesion treatments 23.12–23.17, *23.18*
PIK3CA-related overgrowth spectrum (PROS) 72.9–72.11, 98.19
  CLOVES syndrome 72.9
  facial infiltrating lipomatosis 72.11
  fibroadipose hyperplasia 72.9
  hemihyperplasia–multiple lipomatosis syndrome 72.9, *72.11*
PILA *see* papillary intralymphatic angioendothelioma
pilar cysts *see* trichilemmal cysts

pilar leiomyoma tumour *see* leiomyosarcoma/atypical smooth muscle tumour
pilar sheath acanthoma 137.4
pilar tumour of the scalp *see* proliferating trichilemmal tumour
pili annulati 87.80, *87.81*
pili multigemini 87.84
pili torti 87.78–87.79
pili trianguli et canaliculi 87.46
pilomatrical carcinoma 137.14–137.15
pilomatricoma 137.13–137.14
  dystrophic calcification 59.4
  familial pilomatrixoma **78.13**
pilomatrix carcinoma *see* pilomatrical carcinoma
pilomatrixoma *see* pilomatricoma
pilonidal sinus 87.50, 122.23
  penis 109.24
  perineal and perianal skin 111.25–111.26
pilosebaceous apparatus, tumours of skin appendages 137.1
pilosebaceous cysts, pachyonychia congenita 67.12
pilosebaceous naevoid disorders 88.31
pilosebaceous unit 2.9–2.10
  acquired disorders 93.1–93.13
  acquired non-infective disorders 91.1–91.20
  tumours of 105.11
pimecrolimus, topical therapies 18.23
p-i model *see* pharmacological interaction model
pinkus follicular mucinosis 57.16, *57.17*
pinna (auricle) *see* ear, auricle
pinta 26.71–26.72
  clinical features 26.71–26.72
  investigations 26.72
pin worm *see* enterobiasis
PIQoL-AD *see* Parents' Index of Quality of Life in Atopic Dermatitis
PiS allele 97.43–97.44
pited lips 108.86
pitted keratolysis 26.42–26.43
pitted skin, prolidase deficiency 70.12, *79.13*
pityriasis alba 39.26–39.27, 86.43–86.44
  atopic eczema 41.17
  discoid skin lesions *39.10*
  infants 115.4
  treatment for 39.27
pityriasis amiantacea 105.4
pityriasis capitis (dandruff) 40.1, 40.4
  Malassezia yeast 32.14
pityriasis circinata et maculata of Vidal *see* pityriasis rosea
pityriasis folliculorum 89.10
pityriasis lichenoides 134.3–134.5, *134.6*
pityriasis lichenoides chronica (PLC) 134.3–134.5, *134.6*
pityriasis lichenoides et varioliformis acuta (PLEVA) 134.3–134.4, 134.5
pityriasis nigra *see* tinea nigra
pityriasis rosea 25.123–25.127
  clinical features 25.124–25.126
  discoid skin lesions *39.10*
  epidemiology 25.123–25.124
  male genitalia 109.28
  management 25.126–25.127
  pathophysiology 25.124
  in pregnancy 113.6–113.7
  reactions to COVID-19 vaccines 25.119
pityriasis rosea-like eruption, COVID-19 association 25.111
pityriasis rotunda 63.47–63.49, 85.8–85.9, 148.17
pityriasis rubra pilaris (PRP) 36.1–36.6, 39.33–39.34
  associated diseases 36.1
  atypical adult-onset PRP (type II) 36.2–36.4
  atypical juvenile PRP (type V) 36.4
  circumscribed juvenile PRP (type IV) 36.4, *36.5*
  classic adult-onset PRP (type 1) 36.2, *36.4*, 36.6

classic juvenile-onset PRP (type III) 36.4, *36.5*
  clinical features 36.2
  clinical variants 36.2–36.4
  differential diagnosis 36.4
  disease course and prognosis 36.5
  epidemiology 36.1
  erythroderma 39.33–39.34
  genetics 36.2
  HIV-related PRP (type VI) 36.4
  hyperkeratosis with follicular plugging and parakeratosis *36.3*
  hyperkertotic follicular papules *36.3*
  irregular psoriasiform acanthosis showing alternating ortho- and parakeratosis ('checkerboard' pattern) *36.3*
  islands of sparing (areas of normal skin) *36.3*, *36.4*, *36.6*
  management 36.5–36.6
  palmoplantar keratoderma *36.3*
  pathophysiology 36.1–36.2
  psoriasis comparison **36.2**
  treatment ladder 36.6
pityriasis versicolor (tinea versicolour) 32.10–32.13, 86.43–86.44
  clinical features 32.12
  clinical investigations 32.12
  epidemiology 32.11
  management 32.12–32.13
  pathophysiology 32.11–32.12
pityrosporal dermatitis *see* seborrhoeic dermatitis
Pityrosporum see Malassezia
pityrosporum folliculitis 88.37
PiZ allele 97.43–97.44
PJT syndrome *see* Peutz–Jeghers–Touraine syndrome
PK *see* pharmacokinetics
PKDL *see* post-kala-azar dermal leishmaniasis
PKU *see* phenylketonuria
PL *see* primary lymphoedema
PLACK *see* peeling skin, leukonychia, acral punctate keratoses, cheiliti and knuckle pads syndrome
placode 87.3
plague, *Yersinia pestis* 26.59–26.60
PLAID *see* PLCG2-associated antibody deficiency and immune dysregulation syndrome
plain radiography, foreign body reactions 122.18
plakoglobin (*JUP*) 69.7
plakoglobin loss, palmoplantar keratodermas 63.63
plakophilin-1 (*PKP1*), skin fragility disorders 69.7
planar xanthomas 60.4–60.6
plane warts (verruca plana) 25.52, 25.53–25.54
  see also cutaneous warts
plant allergies 127.13, 127.16–127.17, 127.19–127.22, 127.43, 127.71–127.74
plantar callosities 63.52
plantar fascial fibromatosis 94.35–94.36
plantar fibromatosis 136.12–136.13
plantar hyperhidrosis 92.7
plantar keratoderma 63.51
  pachyonychia congenita 67.11–67.12
plantar pain, pachyonychia congenita 63.51–63.52
plantar phenotype, mal de Meleda 63.55
plant contact
  allergic contact dermatitis 129.6
  irritants 128.2
  photosensitivity 126.29
  poison ivy dermatitis 127.5–127.6, 127.20, 127.22, 127.71
plant extracts
  allergic contact dermatitis 127.49
  cutaneous wart therapy 25.60
  see also herbals
plant mites 34.52
plaque, dental 108.5
plaque-like CD34-positive dermal fibroma 136.8

plaque polymorphic light eruption   126.4, *126.5*
plaque psoriasis *see* psoriasis vulgaris
plaques
 actinic prurigo   *126.11*
 in periodontal Ehlers–Danlos syndrome   70.10
plaque sarcoidosis   96.7–96.8, *96.8–96.9*
plasma cell cheilitis   108.63
plasma cell disorders, skin manifestations   149.9–149.14
plasma cell gingivitis   108.25
plasma cell malignancies, infiltration of skin with neoplastic cells   149.4–149.5
plasma cells
 immune system   9.6
 microscopic examination of   3.35
plasmacytoid dendritic cells, blastic neoplasm   139.45–139.47
plasmacytoma-associated systemic amyloidosis with cutaneous involvement   56.11
plasmapheresis, pemphigus treatment   50.9
plastics, allergy to   127.68–127.71
plat dermatitis   127.11
platelet-activating factor (PAF), disease pathogenesis role   14.1, 14.2
platelet-derived growth factor (PDGF), wound healing   *11.6*
platelet disorders, purpura due to   99.2–99.4
platelet emboli, peripheral vascular disease   101.3
platelet plugging
 heparin necrosis   99.9–99.10
 thrombocytosis   99.10–99.11
platelet-rich plasma (PRP), hair treatment   87.27, 87.71, 87.95
platelets, wound healing   11.2–11.3
platinum, dermatological reactions   121.9
PLC *see* pityriasis lichenoides chronica
PLCA *see* primary localised cutaneous amyloidosis
PLCG2-associated antibody deficiency and immune dysregulation (PLAID) syndrome   **45.5, 45.7**
PLE *see* polymorphic light eruption
plectin (*PLEC*), epidermolysis bullosa   69.4
Plenck, Joseph Jacob   1.4
pleomorphic dermal sarcoma (PDS)   136.22–136.23
pleomorphic fibroma   136.4
pleomorphic lipoma   136.58
pleomorphic liposarcoma   136.59
pleomorphism   3.43
pleuropneumonia-like organisms *see Mycoplasma* spp.
PLEVA *see* pityriasis lichenoides et varioliformis acuta
plexiform fibrohistiocytic tumour (plexiform fibrous histiocytoma)   136.22
plexiform neurofibroma   78.3, 136.46
PLLA *see* poly-L-lactic acid [replace capital L with small cap L**]
plumber's itch *see* cutaneous larva migrans
Plumbe, Samuel   7.3
Plummer–Vinson syndrome, iron deficiency   61.24
PLWH *see* people living with HIV
plymers, isocyanates in polyurethanes   127.71
PMH *see* progressive macular hypomelanosis
PMMA *see* polymethylmethacrylate
PN *see* parenteral nutrition; prurigo nodularis
PNET *see* pancreatic neuroendocrine tumours
Pneumocystis jiroveci infections   32.93–32.94
pneumonia
 inhalation injury   125.4–125.5
 skin features   26.79
pneumonic plague *see* plague
PNH *see* progressive nodular histiocytosis
PNI *see* perineural invasion
PNP *see* paraneoplastic pemphigus
PNPLA2 gene, neutral lipid storage disease with ichthyosis   63.36

podoconiosis   *7.3*
 Footwork initiative   7.9–7.10
podoconiosis (non-filarial lymphoedema)   103.36–103.37
podophyllin/podophyllotoxin, topical therapies   18.13, 25.59, 25.64
POEM *see* Patient-Oriented Eczema Measure
POEMS syndrome (polyneuropathy, organomegaly, endocrinopathy, monoclonal protein and skin changes)   86.24–86.25, 149.11–149.12
Pogosta disease *see* Sindbis virus
poikiloderma of Civatte   86.13–86.14, 94.13
poikiloderma syndromes   75.1–75.8, 94.13
 acrokeratotic poikiloderma of Weary   **75.2**, 75.7
 dyskeratosis congenita   67.14, 67.15, 75.1–75.4
 hereditary fibrosing poikiloderma with tendon contractures, myopathy and pulmonary fibrosis   **75.2**, 75.7
 Kindler epidermolysis bullosa   69.5, 69.19, **75.2**, 75.6, 108.86
 poikiloderma with neutropenia, Clericuzio type   **75.2**, 75.7
 Rothmund–Thomson syndrome   75.4–75.6
poikilodermatous mycosis fungoides   94.13
poikilodermatous parapsoriasis *see* large plaque parapsoriasis
poikilodermatous plaque-like haemangioma   136.32
point mutations   8.6
poison ivy dermatitis   127.5–127.6, 127.20, 127.22, 127.71
poison/poisonous *see* toxic...; toxins
'polar bear rug' cataract, atopic keratoconjunctivitis   *107.19*
polar gel formulations, topical drugs   12.3
polarisable foreign bodies   122.17
poliosis   87.93
pollen allergy   127.84
pollen-fruit allergy syndrome *see* oral allergy syndrome
polyalkylamide, dermal fillers   158.7
polyangiitis, involving respiratory system   152.3–152.4
polyarteritis nodosa (PAN)   100.28–100.30
 eye disease   **107.35**
 hepatitis B   25.74
 hepatitis B virus infection   153.5
 oral involvement   108.69
 scrotal pain   109.26
polyarthritis, viral infections   155.2–155.3
polybrominated biphenyls   129.12
polycaprolacton dermal filler   158.6
polychlorinated biphenyls (PCBs), chloracne   129.12
polychondritis, relapsing/atrophic   155.11–155.13
polycyclic hydrocarbons, occupational skin cancer   129.15
polycyclic lesions   *4.11*
polycystic ovary syndrome (PCOS)   87.62, 87.88
 acne vulgaris association   88.4–88.5, **88.7**, **88.8**, *88.9*
 diagnosis criteria   **88.7**
 hidradenitis suppurativa association   90.2
 hirsutism association   87.90
 subtypes   **88.7**
polycythaemia vera (PV)
 pruritus   81.10
 thrombocytosis   99.10–99.11
polyendocrine disease   150.19
 see also autoimmune polyendocrinopathy
polyene antifungals   19.48
polyenes, topical therapies   18.12
polygenic risk score (PRS)   8.1
polyhydramion, Neu–Laxova syndrome   63.38
poly-L-lactic acid (PLLA), collagen-stimulating filler [replace capital L with small cap L**]   158.2, 158.6

polymerase chain reaction (PCR) test   3.9
polymers, allergic contact dermatitis   127.68–127.71
polymethylmethacrylate (PMMA) and bovine collagen, dermal fillers   158.7–158.8
polymicrobial flora, human bite wounds   130.7
polymorphic eruption of pregnancy (PEP)   113.16–113.17
polymorphic light eruption (PLE)   126.2–126.8, 126.32–126.33, *126.36*
 phototherapy   21.5, 21.12
 and psoriasis vulgaris   35.4
polymorphisms   3.43, 8.6
 HIV-associated lipodystrophy   98.7
 interleukin-16   127.10
 skin cancer risks   147.6
 thiopurine methyl transferase   19.8–19.9, 19.10
polymyositis
 dermatomyositis relationship   52.1
 internal malignancy association   148.20–148.21
polymyxin B, topical therapies   18.11
polyneuropathy, organomegaly, endocrinopathy, monoclonal protein and skin changes (POEMS) syndrome   86.24–86.25, 149.11–149.12
polyomaviruses (PyVs)   25.46–25.49, **25.47**, 85.15
 Merkel cell polyomavirus-positive carcinoma   25.46–25.47, 146.2, 146.3, *146.4*
 trichodysplasia spinulosa polyomavirus   25.48, 85.15–85.17, 87.36
polypharmacy   13.8
 see also drug–drug interactions
Polypodium leucotomos treatment   126.8
polypoid lesions *see* skin tags
polyposis disorders   153.4, **153.7**
 familial adenomatous polyposis   78.10–78.11
 gastrointestinal polyposis   78.11, 153.4
polyps
 hamartomatous polyps in PJT syndrome   68.13
 inflammatory intestinal polyps   *112.6*
 neonatal adnexal polyps   114.19
 see also skin tags
polytrichia   87.49
polyunsaturated fatty acids (PUFAs), cosmeceutical use of   157.5
polyurethanes (PUs), isocyanates in   127.71
pomade acne   88.25, *88.26*
POMC *see* pro-opiomelanocortin deficiency
pomegranate, cosmeceutical use of   157.10
pompholyx eczema   39.14
POP *see* progesterone-only pill
popsicle panniculitis   97.35
population approach, epidemiology   5.2–5.4, 5.5
poradenitis inguinalis *see* lymphogranuloma venereum
porcine collagen dermal filler   158.5–158.6
porcine dermal matrices   125.6
pore of Winer *see* dilated pore lesions
pork tapeworm, cysticercosis   33.32–33.34
porocarcinoma *see* malignant eccrine poroma
porokeratosis   3.44, *4.10*, 63.74–63.76, 85.19–85.23
 autosomal dominant punctate porokeratosis   63.59
 discoid skin lesions   **39.10**
 disseminated palmoplantar porokeratosis   85.20, 85.22
 disseminated superficial actinic porokeratosis   63.74–63.75, 85.20–85.22, 141.15–141.18
 genital   85.21, *85.22*, 109.35
 keratinocytes   85.19–85.20
 linear   63.75, 85.20–85.21, 85.22
 ptychotropic   63.75, 85.21, *85.22*, 109.35
 punctate palmoplantar   85.20–85.21

porokeratosis of Mantoux (palmoplantar porokeratosis)   63.75, 85.20–85.21
porokeratosis of Mibelli   63.74, 63.75, 85.20, 85.21, 109.35
porokeratotic eccrine ostial duct naevus (PEN)   63.33–63.34
poromas
 eccrine   *4.13*
 eccrine versus apocrine   137.25
porphyria   58.1–58.20
 acute attacks of   58.5–58.7
  precipitants of   58.6
  treatment   58.7
 bullous porphyrias, typical subepidermal bulla in   *58.6*
 causing cutaneous disease and acute attacks   58.17–58.18
 causing cutaneous disease but not acute attacks   58.9–58.17
 chemistry of porphyrins   58.1–58.2
 classification   58.2–58.4
 ear dermatoses   **106.23**, *106.25*
 enzyme deficiencies and   58.2
 eye disease   **107.35**
 haem
  biosynthesis of   58.2, *58.3*, *58.4*
  chemistry of   58.1–58.2
  molecular structure   58.2
 high-performance liquid chromatography analysis   *58.8*
 histopathology   58.4–58.5, *58.6*
 individual porphyrias   58.9–58.19
  acute intermittent porphyria   58.5
  congenital erythropoietic porphyria   58.9–58.11
  erythropoietic protoporphyria   58.4, 58.14–58.17
  hereditary coproporphyria   58.5, 58.7, 58.9, 58.12, 58.17
  porphyria cutanea tarda   58.11–58.14
  pseudoporphyria   58.18–58.19
  variegate porphyria   58.5, 58.7, 58.9, 58.12, 58.17–58.18
 laboratory testing   58.7–58.9
  biochemical findings in cutaneous porphyrias   **58.8**
  interpretation of results   58.8–58.9
  porphyrin analysis   58.8
  sample analysis   58.7
  screening of relatives   58.9
 management of skin disease   58.5
 pathogenesis   58.5
 pathophysiology   58.4
 photochemistry of porphyrins   58.2
 phototoxicity of porphyrins   58.1
 and the skin   58.4
 theoretical basis for understanding   58.1–58.2
porphyria cutanea tarda (PCT)   58.11–58.14, 126.7, 127.22
 associated with liver disease   153.7, 153.9
 clinical features   58.11
 clinical variants   58.11–58.12
 epidemiology and pathophysiology   58.11, *58.12*
 erosions, blisters, pigmentary changes and scarring   *58.12*
 facial hypertrichosis   *87.87*
 genetic counselling   58.14
 hepatitis C   25.76
 HIV   31.18
 investigations   58.12
 liver disease in   58.13
 mortality in   58.14
 renal failure and dialysis complications   154.4
 risk factors for   58.12–58.13
 scleroderma-like syndromes   *94.46*
 treatment   58.13–58.14
 see also pseudoporphyria
porphyrin/protoporphyrin, photodynamic therapy   22.2, 22.3, 22.4
porphyrins
 chemistry of   58.1–58.2
 photochemistry of   58.2
 phototoxicity of   58.1

port-wine stains (PWS) 73.20
  eyelid 107.47
  laser therapies 23.8–23.9, 23.10, 23.11
  lobular capillary haemangioma 136.26
  phakomatosis pigmentovascularis 73.22
posinophilic folliculitis, HIV 31.17–31.18
posterior fossa malformations *see* PHACES syndrome
post-finasteride syndrome (PFS) 87.96–87.97
post-herpetic neuralgia (PHN) 82.4–82.5, 108.66
  zoster 25.32, 25.34, 25.35
posthitis 109.4, 109.16–109.17
postinflammatory elastolysis and cutis laxa (PECL) 94.22, 94.23
postinflammatory hypermelanosis 86.30–86.31
postinflammatory hyperpigmentation, laser therapies 23.17, 23.18
postinflammatory hypomelanosis 86.43–86.44
post-ionising radiation keratosis 141.14–141.15
post-irradiation morphoea 119.15
post-kala-azar dermal leishmaniasis (PKDL) 33.51–33.52, 33.53–33.54, 155.5
post-operative care, skin surgery 20.37–20.40
postpartum telogen effluvium 87.56
post-radiotherapy alopecia 87.74
poststeroid panniculitis 97.37, 97.58–97.59
poststreptococcal glomerulonephritis (PSGN), scabies association 26.10
postsurgical artefact, induced non-healing for psychological reasons 84.33, 84.34
postsurgical wounds, induced non-healing for practical gain 84.37
post-thrombotic syndrome, venous leg ulcer 102.6
post-transfusion purpura 149.15
post-transplant lymphoproliferative disorder (PTLD) 25.39, 139.47
post-traumatic trigeminal neuropathy *see* trigeminal neuralgia
postural exercises, lymphoedema 103.59
potassium, thallium substitution 121.9
potassium iodide (systemic therapy) 19.30–19.31
  dermatological uses 19.30
  potential adverse effects 19.30
  safety issues 19.30–19.31
potassium permanganate, topical therapies 18.9
potassium sorbate (PS) 127.58
potassium titanyl phosphate (KTP) lasers
  absorption spectra 23.4
  tattoo removal 23.15
  vascular lesions 23.6, 23.7, 23.9, 23.12
povidone panniculitis 97.48, 97.50
powders, topical medication vehicles 18.2, 18.8
power of clinical trials, statistical analysis 17.22–17.23
poxvirus infections 25.6–25.19
  vulva 110.28–110.29
PPD *see* persistent pigment darkening; (*p*-)phenylenediamine
PPE *see* personal protective equipment
PPKP *see* palmoplantar keratoderma punctata
PPKs *see* palmoplantar keratodermas
PPP *see* palmoplantar pustulosis
PPP syndrome *see* pancreatitis, panniculitis and polyarthritis syndrome
PPV *see* phakomatosis pigmentovascularis
Prader–Willi syndrome (PWS) 72.6–72.9, **72.7**
  obesity association 98.28
  piezogenic pedal papules 122.26
PRAME (PReferentially expressed Antigen in Melanoma) 3.25
pravastatin-induced lichenoid drug eruption 117.8

pre-adipocytes 2.40, 97.1
pre-auricular cysts and sinuses, infants 115.12
pre-auricular sinus (PAS) 106.6–106.7
Preferred Reporting Items for Systematic Reviews and Meta-analyses (PRISMA), systemic review assessment 17.8
pregnancy 113.1–113.25
  acne 88.26
  acne vulgaris 113.11–113.12
  antihistamines in 42.18
  apocrine gland activity 113.2–113.3
  atopic eruption of pregnancy 113.15–113.16
  autoimmune skin diseases 113.7–113.9
  benign melanocytic naevi 113.9
  candidiasis 113.7
  cytomegalovirus infection 25.41
  dermatophyte infections 113.7
  drug pharmacokinetics and pharmacodynamics 13.8
  eccrine gland activity 113.2–113.3
  Ehlers–Danlos syndrome 70.11, 113.9
  eosinophilic pustular folliculitis 93.7
  erythema nodosum 113.12
  foliaceus 113.8–113.9
  fungal infections 113.7
  generalised pustular psoriasis 113.10–113.11
  glandular function **113.2**
  hair and nail changes in 113.1, **113.2**
  herpes simplex virus infection 113.4–113.5
  HIV 31.36
  human papillomavirus infection 113.4
  immune system changes in 113.3–113.4
  inflammatory skin diseases 113.10–113.12
  intrahepatic cholestasis of pregnancy 113.13–113.14
  itching 113.13–113.24
  leprosy 28.10, 113.6
  malignant melanoma 113.9–113.10
  maternal smoking during, and atopic eczema 41.7
  melasma 86.10, 86.12
  metastatic pregnancy-associated melanoma 113.10
  neonatal lupus erythematosus 51.41–51.42, 113.7–113.8
  obstetric trauma to perineal skin 111.7, **111.8**
  pemphigoid gestationis 113.17–113.19
  pemphigus vulgaris 113.8–113.9
  physiological skin changes in 113.1–113.4
  pigmentation changes in 113.1, 113.2, **113.2**
  pityriasis rosea 113.6–113.7
  polymorphic eruption of pregnancy 113.16–113.17
  postpartum telogen effluvium 87.56
  pregnancy-specific dermatoses and itching 113.13–113.24
  prenatal diagnoses 8.9–8.11
  pruritus 81.11, 113.13–113.14
  pseudoxanthoma elasticum 70.33–70.34
  psoriasis 35.19, 113.10–113.11
  rosacea 89.15, 89.16, 113.11–113.12
  rubella infection 25.92
  safe treatments in 113.19–113.24
  scabies 113.5–113.6
  sebaceous gland activity 113.2–113.3
  skin infections and infestations 113.4–113.7
  skin tumours 113.9–113.10
  STIs 30.6, 30.11, 30.14
  striae 94.11
  striae distensae 113.2, 113.3
  syphilis 113.6
  syphilis management 29.21, 29.22
  systemic lupus erythematosus 51.32, 113.7–113.8
  systemic therapies in 113.19–113.21, **113.22–113.24**
  topical therapies in 113.19, **113.20–113.21**

transplacental transfer of maternal autoantibodies 114.11–114.12
transplacental transfer of maternal malignant disease 114.14
urticaria 42.8, 42.18, 113.12
varicella zoster virus infection 113.5
vascular changes in **113.2**, 113.3
yeast infections 113.7
see also congenital…; teratogenicity
pre-haptens 127.8
preimplantation genetic diagnosis (PGD) 8.10–8.11
preimplantation genetic haplotyping (PGH) 8.11
prejudice regarding skin diseases 1.9
prelymphomatous eruption, discoid skin lesions 39.10
premalignant lesions
  external ear 106.33–106.34
  oral cavity 108.42–108.43
  vulva 110.34–110.36
premature ageing syndromes 70.25–70.31, 77.1–77.7
  acrogeria (Grotton syndrome) **70.26**, 70.28
  Bloom syndrome **77.2**, 77.3–77.4
  clinical features of **70.26**
  cutis laxa 77.5–77.7
  familial mandibuloacral dysplasia 70.28–70.29
  Hutchinson–Gilford progeria syndrome 70.25–70.26, **72.5**, 77.4–77.5
  mandibulo-acral dysplasia with type A lipodystrophy 77.5
  mandibulo-acral dysplasia with type B lipodystrophy 77.5
  Mulvihill–Smith syndrome 70.29–70.30
  neonatal progeroid syndrome 70.30–70.31
  pangeria (Werner syndrome) 70.26–70.27, **70.26**, **72.5**, 75.6, 77.1–77.3, **78.12**, 148.12, 148.13
  progeroid laminopathies and related conditions 77.4
premature greying of hair 87.92
premature teleptosis 87.53
prenatal diagnoses 8.9–8.11
preoperative preparation, skin surgery 20.11
preorbital cellulitis, neonates 114.26
prepubertal acne 88.68–88.74
  associated diseases 88.70
  clinical features 88.70–88.71
  complications and co-morbidities 88.72
  differential diagnosis **88.71**
  disease course and prognosis 88.72
  epidemiology 88.69–88.70
  investigations **88.72**
  isotretinoin treatment **88.73**
  management 88.72–88.74
  pathophysiology 88.70
prepubescent girls, streptococcal vulvovaginitis 26.33
prepuce
  anatomy 109.3
  balanoposthitis 109.4–109.5
  circumcision 109.7
  dorsal perforation **109.5**
  dorsal perforation of **109.5**
  paraphimosis 109.4, 109.16–109.17
  posthitis 109.4, 109.16–109.17
  structure and function 109.7
prescribing, topical therapies 18.1–18.4
prescription-writing, medication errors 13.10, 13.11
preservatives
  allergic contact dermatitis 127.48, 127.49–127.58
  genital contact dermatitis **109.13**
  topical medication 18.8
pressure-associated ulceration and necrosis, COVID-19 association 25.111
pressure dressings, skin surgery 20.38, 20.41
pressure erythema, chronic venous insufficiency **101.43**

pressure-induced alopecia 87.30–87.31
pressure injuries 123.1–123.12
pressure perception 2.12
pressure sores
  ischaemic fasciitis 136.6
  perineal and perianal skin 111.7–111.8
pressure ulcers 123.1–123.12
  classification systems 123.4–123.6
  COVID-19 association 25.111
  prevalence/incidence 123.1–123.2, **123.3**
  preventative measures 123.6–123.10
  risk factors 123.3–123.4, 123.6
pretibial myxoedema (PTM) 103.41–103.43
  clinical features 103.42–103.43
  hyperthyroidism 57.11
  investigations 103.43
  management 103.43
  pathophysiology 103.42
pre-transplant skin cancers 147.13, 147.18
prevalence of disease 5.10, 5.14
prevention paradox 5.3–5.4
prickly heat *see* miliaria rubra
prick tests 4.23–4.24
primary anetoderma 94.23–94.25
primary biliary cirrhosis (PBC) 86.21–86.22, 153.5
primary care 5.12–5.13
primary CD30+ lymphoproliferative disorders 139.25–139.29
primary chronic telogen effluvium 87.59–87.60
primary cicatricial alopecias (PCAs) 87.37, 87.38–87.50
primary congenital hypertrichosis 87.85–87.86
primary cutaneous acral CD8+ T-cell lymphoma (provisional) 139.33–139.34
primary cutaneous adenocystic carcinoma *see* adenoid cystic carcinoma
primary cutaneous aggressive epidermotropic CD8+ T-cell lymphoma 139.31–139.32
  CD8+ mycosis fungoides variant distinction 139.5
primary cutaneous anaplastic (CD30+) large-cell lymphoma 139.28–139.29
primary cutaneous B-cell lymphomas 139.37–139.43
primary cutaneous blastomycosis 32.85
primary cutaneous CD4+ small/medium pleomorphic T-cell lymphoproliferative disorder (provisional) 139.33
primary cutaneous CD30+ lymphoproliferative disorders 139.25–139.29
primary cutaneous diffuse large B-cell lymphoma 139.37, 139.41–139.43
primary cutaneous follicle centre cell lymphoma (PCFCL) 139.37, 139.40–139.41
primary cutaneous γδT-cell lymphoma 139.32–139.33
primary cutaneous histoplasmosis 32.82, 32.83
primary cutaneous lymphomas (PCLs), immunocompromised people 147.15–147.16
primary cutaneous mammary analogue secretory carcinoma *see* secretory carcinoma
primary cutaneous marginal zone lymphoma (PCMZL) 139.37–139.39
  clinical features/investigations 139.39
  definition 139.38
  management 139.39
  pathogenesis 139.37
  pathophysiology 139.37–139.38
primary cutaneous mucinoses 57.1, 57.2–57.18
primary cutaneous T-cell lymphomas 97.61, 97.62–97.63, 139.2–139.37

see also cutaneous T-cell lymphoma; mycosis fungoides
primary erythromelalgia 101.7–101.8
primary haemophagocytic lymphohistiocytosis 135.11, 135.13
primary herpetic gingivostomatitis 25.20–25.24
primary hypertrophic osteoarthropathy (PHO) 70.35–70.36
primary (idiopathic) cutaneous mucinoses 57.1, 57.2–57.18
primary immunodeficiency diseases *see* inherited immunodeficiency
primary localised cutaneous amyloidosis (PLCA) 56.2, **56.3**
  on ankle *56.7*
  on chest *56.7*
  management 56.13–56.14
  on nose *56.8*
  staining of amyloid *56.5*
  on toes *56.8*
  treatment 56.13–56.14
primary lymphoedema (PL) 71.24–71.28, 103.17–103.20
  causative genes and phenotypes **103.19**
  choanal atresia and lymphoedema 71.27
  clinical features 103.20
  congenital-onset primary lymphoedema 103.24
  epidemiology 103.19
  Hennekam lymphangiectasia–lymphoedema syndrome 71.26
  hereditary lymphoedema type 1A 71.24–71.25
  hypotrichosis–lymphoedema–telangiectasia syndrome 71.26
  late-onset primary lymphoedema 103.24–103.25
  lymphoedema–distichiasis syndrome 71.25–71.26
  microcephaly with or without chorioretinopathy, lymphoedema and mental retardation 71.27
  with myelodysplasia 71.27–71.28
  pathophysiology 103.19–103.20
  St George's classification algorithm *103.18*
  terminology **103.18**
primary (naevoid) congenital hypertrichosis 87.85–87.86
primary neutrophilic cicatricial alopecias 87.48–87.50
primary Raynaud phenomenon 124.10–124.12
primary syphilis 29.6–29.7, 29.17
primary systemic or amyloid light-chain amyloidosis (extravascular) 149.13
primary systemic amyloidosis
  haemorrhagic bulla *56.13*
  macroglossia *56.12*
  nail dystrophy *56.13*
  periorbital bleeding *56.11*
primary telangiectasias 101.16, **101.17**, **101.18**
primary tumours, Merkel cell carcinoma 146.6, 146.8
primin allergy 127.71, 127.73
primitive polypoid/non-neural granular cell tumour *see* dermal non-neural granular cell tumour
Primula dermatitis 127.5, *127.14–127.15*, 127.20–127.22, 127.71, 127.72–127.73
prioritisation, health economics 6.5
PRISMA *see* Preferred Reporting Items for Systematic Reviews and Meta-analyses
procollagen-lysine, 2-oxoglutarate 5-dioxygenase 3 (*PLOD3*) 69.7–69.8
proctitis/proctocolitis syndrome, lymphogranuloma venereum 30.15, 30.16, 30.17
productivity costs, health economic evaluation 6.3

proflavine, topical therapies 18.10
progeroid laminopathies 77.4
progeroid syndromes *see* premature ageing syndromes
progesterone-only pill (POP) 87.95
progestins
  acneform reaction 88.13
  acne vulgaris treatment 88.50–88.51
programmed cell death (PDCD) 71.2
progressive bacterial synergistic gangrene 26.77, 26.78
progressive hemifacial atrophy (PHA) 55.23, 55.24–55.25
progressive hyperpigmentation 68.10
progressive macular hypomelanosis (PMH) 86.44–86.45
progressive mucinous histiocytosis 135.23
progressive nodular histiocytosis (PNH) 135.19
progressive symmetrical erythrokeratoderma (PSEK) 63.19–63.20
pro-haptens 127.8
prohormones, transformation into active metabolite 150.7
pro-inflammatory cytokines, antigen-presenting cells 127.7
pro-inflammatory topical treatments, molluscum contagiosum infection 25.18
prolactin
  central nervous system controlled endocrine signalling axis 150.2
  hair follicle 87.11–87.12
prolidase deficiency 70.11–70.12, **72.7**, 79.12–79.13
proliferating trichilemmal tumour 137.5–137.6
proline synthesis defects 79.14–79.15
PROMs *see* Patient-Reported Outcome Measures
pro-opiomelanocortin deficiency (POMC) **72.7**
  C202T mutation *72.8*
  gene structure and post-translational processing *72.8*
pro-opiomelanocortin and prohormone convertase deficiency 72.4–72.6
prophylactic dressings, pressure ulcer prevention 123.9
prophylactic phototherapy, PLE management 126.7–126.8
prophylactic skin treatments, papulopustular eruptions 119.4
prophylactic surgical excision of naevi, not recommended to prevent melanoma 142.3
Propionibacterium see Cutibacterium
propolis 127.59, 127.74–127.78
propranolol
  burn treatment 125.14
  infantile haemangioma treatment 116.8
propylene glycol (PG) 12.3, 12.5, 127.59
PROS *see* PIK3CA-related overgrowth spectrum
Prospective Register of Systematic Reviews (PROSPERO) 17.8, 17.9
prostaglandin D2 (PGD2), release in skin 14.1
prostaglandins
  hair disorders 87.94–87.95
  male hair loss 87.62
prosthetic implants, cutaneous reactions 127.19
prosthetics, hair loss cover 87.69, 87.101
protease inhibitor (PI), HAART regimes 98.6–98.7
proteases
  Mas-related G-protein-coupled receptor agonists, endothelin 81.1
  pruritus **81.3**, 81.5
protein contact dermatitis (PCD) 127.10, 127.83, 127.85
protein C/protein S-related disease, purpura 99.15–99.17

protein-energy malnutrition 61.2, 61.3
  hair reddening *61.4*
  skin signs of nutritional disease **61.5**
protein fibre, types of 2.2
proteins
  in epidermolysis bullosa 69.2–69.8
  skin fragility link 69.5–69.8
proteinuria, nail–patella syndrome 67.16
protein–hyaluronic acid complex
  normal component of the dermal extracellular matrix 57.1
  see also cutaneous mucinoses; mucin
proteoglycans (PGs) 2.36–2.39
  functions of 2.38–2.39
  gene location **2.39**
  molecular characteristics and tissue distribution 2.38, **2.39**
Proteus syndrome 71.10–71.11, **72.10**, 73.6, **101.28**, 103.23–103.24
proton beam therapy 24.2–24.3
prototheocosis 32.94
protozoal infestations/infections 33.35–33.55
  eye 107.40
  HIV coinfections 31.29
  oral involvement 108.57
provocation testing, cutaneous photosensitivity diseases 126.4–126.6, 126.12, 126.19, 126.34
proximal subungual onychomycosis 32.48
PRP *see* pityriasis rubra pilaris; platelet-rich plasma
PRS *see* polygenic risk score
pruriginosa dystrophic epidermolysis bullosa 69.16
prurigo
  cutaneous manifestations of Hodgkin disease 139.49
  terminology 81.14
prurigo-like morphology, chronic actinic dermatitis 126.17
prurigo nodularis (PN) 81.14–81.18, 84.15–84.18
  clinical features 81.16–81.17, 84.16–84.17
  epidemiology 81.14, 84.16
  investigations 81.17–81.18
  lichen simplex chronicus relationship 84.15
  management 81.18, 84.17–84.18
  pathophysiology 81.15–81.16
  underlying diseases **81.17**
pruritic conditions (pruritus/xerosis/ichthyosis/prurigo)
  hepatitis C 25.76
  HIV 31.12
pruritus 81.1–81.21
  acetylcholine **81.3**, 81.4
  antihistamines 41.27
  atopic eczema 41.12, 81.7–81.8
  brachioradial 81.12, 83.6–83.7
  central transmission of itch 81.3
  chronic 81.1–81.14
  chronic kidney disease related 81.8–81.9
  clinical features 81.6–81.13
  cutaneous induction of itch 81.2–81.3
  cutaneous manifestations of Hodgkin disease 139.49
  definitions/nomenclature 81.1
  diabetes 81.10
  diabetic patients 62.6–62.7
  drug-induced 81.10–81.11, 117.2–117.3
  fibreglass dermatitis 122.21
  friction blisters *122.9*
  genital pruritus **109.2**
  gold toxicity 121.4
  hepatobiliary disease/cholestasis 81.9–81.10
  histamine/histamine receptors **81.3**, 81.4
  in ichthyoses 63.46, 63.47
  inflamed skin/dermatoses 81.7
  itching purpura 99.7, 99.8, **99.9**
  lichen simplex 81.18–81.20
  lichen simplex chronicus 84.15
  liver disease association 153.8
  localised 81.12

  malignancy manifestation 81.10
  mediators of itching in skin diseases **81.3**, 81.4–81.8
  methamphetamine-induced 120.5
  neoplasia association 148.27
  neurological aspects 81.2–81.4, 81.11–81.12
  neuropathic 83.5–83.6
  neuropathic pruritus 81.11–81.12
  non-atopic causes 84.16
  notalgia paraesthetica 81.12
  opioid peptides **81.3**, 81.4–81.5
  peripheral and central neuronal sensation 81.4
  phototherapy adverse effects 21.12
  polycythaemia vera 81.10
  in pregnancy 81.11, 113.13–113.24, **113.20**
  prurigo nodularis 81.14–81.18
  psoriasis vulgaris 81.8
  psychiatric and psychosomatic diseases/psychogenic pruritus 81.12
  psychogenic 84.27–84.29
  PUVA phototherapy adverse effects 21.13
  renal failure and dialysis complications 154.3, *154.4*
  scalp 105.14–105.17
  scratching 81.3–81.4
  senescence 81.11
  systemic diseases 81.8–81.10
  systemic sclerosis 54.16, **54.26**
  tachykinins **81.3**, 81.4
  thyrotoxicosis 81.10
  trophic syndromes 82.7–82.9
  see also itching
pruritus ani 111.3–111.6
  clinical features 111.5–111.6
  epidemiology 111.5
  excoriations and lichenification, idiopathic pruritus *111.6*
  management of 111.6
  medicament allergens 127.46
  pathophysiology 111.5
  secondary causes of **111.4–111.5**
PS *see* potassium sorbate
PSCC *see* penile squamous cell carcinoma
PSD *see* penoscrotodynia
PSEK *see* progressive symmetrical erythrokeratoderma
Pseudallescheria boydii see Scedosporium apiospermum
pseudo-ainhum 63.55, 63.56, *63.61*, *94.18*
pseudoallergic reactions
  drug hypersensitivity 14.2–14.3
  urticaria 42.5, 42.6, 42.8
pseudochromhidrosis 92.18
pseudocowpox (PCPV) *see* milker's nodule
pseudocyst, external ear 106.8–106.9
pseudoedematous-appearing striae *94.12*
pseudoepitheliomatous hyperplasia 132.9–132.10
pseudoepitheliomatous micaceous and keratotic balanitis (PEMKB) 109.35
pseudofolliculitis 26.27, 91.8–91.10, 93.1–93.2
pseudofolliculitis barbae 91.8, *91.9*, 122.23
pseudohypoaldosteronism, miliaria association 92.13
pseudo-Kaposi syndrome *see* acroangiodermatitis
pseudologia fantastica 84.37
pseudolymphoma 134.1–134.3
  B-cell/lymphocytoma cutis 134.1, 134.2, 134.8–134.10
  external ear 106.34
  oral involvement 108.72
  pathophysiology 134.1–134.2
  T-cell origin 134.1–134.2
pseudomembranous candidiasis 32.61
Pseudomonas infections 26.51–26.53
  botryomycosis 26.76–26.77
  clinical features and variants 26.52–26.53
  colonisation of wounds, colour *4.14*

Pseudomonas infections *(continued)*
  epidemiology 26.51
  management 26.53
  P. aeruginosa/P. pyocyanea 26.51–26.53
  pathophysiology 26.51
  see also ecthyma gangrenosum; *Stenotrophomonas maltophilia*
pseudomyogenic haemangioendothelioma 136.34
pseudopelade of Brocq (PB) 87.44–87.46
pseudo-pernia *see* chilblain-like lesions
pseudophotodermatitis 127.72
Pseudophyllidea, infections 33.31, 33.34–33.35
pseudopods, melanomas 145.7, *145.8*
pseudoporphyria 58.18–58.19
  bullous eruption due to renal failure/dialysis 154.4, *154.5*
  drug-induced 126.29
pseudopyogenic granuloma *see* epithelioid haemangioma
pseudosarcomatous fasciitis/pseudosarcomatous fibromatosis *see* nodular fasciitis
pseudosarcomatous fibroblastic/myofibroblastic proliferations, ischaemic fasciitis 136.6
pseudoxanthoma elasticum (PXE) 70.31–70.35, 94.30–94.31, 97.30
  associated diseases 70.31
  of axillary skin *70.32*
  cardiovascular changes 70.33
  'chicken skin' appearance *70.32*
  clinical variants 70.34
  diagnostic criteria **70.32**
  differential diagnosis 70.34
  gastrointestinal changes 70.33
  investigations 70.34
  management of 70.34–70.35
  obstetric risk 70.33–70.34
  ocular changes 70.33
  pathophysiology 70.31–70.32
  skin changes 70.32–70.33
PSI *see* Psoriasis Symptom Inventory
psittacosis 26.79
psoralen photosensitisers
  adverse effects 21.9, 107.43–107.44
  development of PUVA 21.2
  natural sunlight therapies 21.2
  oral and topical regimens 21.9
  photochemotherapy principles 21.1
  used in PUVA 21.9
psoralen and ultraviolet A (PUVA) 86.17, 126.6
  cutaneous T-cell lymphoma 139.21, 139.22, 139.23
  development 21.2
  lentigines 86.17, 131.7–131.8
  mastocytosis treatment 46.10
  palmoplantar pustulosis 35.39
  psoriasis treatment 35.23
  UVB phototherapy comparison 21.5–21.6
  see also phototherapy
psoriasiform dermatitis 85.14
psoriasiform irritant contact dermatitis 128.4
psoriasiform palmar phenotype, Papillon–Léfèvre syndrome 63.69
psoriasiform plaques, zinc deficiency *61.26*
psoriasiform sarcoidosis 96.13
psoriasis 35.1–35.48
  acute generalised exanthematous pustulosis distinction **118.4**
  alcohol misuse relationship 84.40
  alopecia 87.34, *105.3*
  ano-genital psoriasis 109.9–109.10
  assessment tools 16.3, **16.3**
  atopic eczema cost comparison *6.10*
  biologic therapies 9.8–9.9
  classification **35.2**
  diagnosis 4.1
  disease associations 5.11
  ear dermatoses **106.23**, *106.25*
  economic burden of 6.8–6.10

erythrodermic psoriasis 39.32
eyelid 107.6
genetic factors 8.1
global distribution **7.3**
gold reactions 121.4
hand dermatitis differentiation 127.22, 128.5
HIV 31.15–31.17
hypopigmentation *86.44*
infantile psoriasis 115.3–115.4
inflammation mechanism 9.8
irritant contact dermatitis 129.1, *129.2*
keratoderma climactericum 63.72
male genitalia 109.9–109.10
mechanical injuries 122.2
oral lesions 108.35
perineal and perianal skin 111.8
peristomal skin *112.9*, 112.10, 112.11
phototherapy 21.3–21.4
pityriasis rubra pilaris comparison **36.2**
polymorphic light eruption 126.2
in pregnancy 113.10–113.11
psychodermatology 84.3
psychological and social factors 15.4
PUVA-induced lentigines in patient with *131.7*
quality of life assessment 16.7–16.8
radiation dermatitis differentiation 119.14
recreational drug-related 120.3
scalp 105.2–105.4
susceptibility genes and pathways **35.3**
vitamin D analogue topical treatment 18.27–18.28
vulva 110.17–110.18
see also psoriasis vulgaris (chronic plaque psoriasis); psoriatic arthritis; pustular psoriasis
Psoriasis Area and Severity Index (PASI) 16.3, 35.16–35.17, **35.27**
Psoriasis Disability Index (PDI) 16.8
Psoriasis Epidemiology Screening tool (PEST) 16.3
Psoriasis Family Impact 16.10
psoriasis gyrata *1.5*
Psoriasis Symptom Inventory (PSI) 16.5
psoriasis vulgaris (chronic plaque psoriasis) 35.1–35.31
  acute guttate psoriasis 35.12–35.13
  age at onset 35.2
  alcohol misuse 35.4
  atypical forms of 35.14
  Auspitz sign *35.9*
  biologic therapies 35.27–35.31
    adalimumab 35.28
    bimekizumab 35.30
    biosimilars 35.29
    brodalumab 35.30
    certolizumab pegol 35.28–35.29
    etanercept 35.28
    IL-12/IL-23 p40 inhibitor 35.29
    IL-17 inhibitors 35.30
    IL-23p 19 inhibitors 35.30–35.31
    infliximab 35.27–35.28
    ixekizumab 35.30
    registries 35.29
    secukinumab 35.30
    short-term efficacy in randomised trials **35.27**
    TNF-alpha inhibitors 35.27
  cancer association 35.18
  cardiovascular disease 35.19
  in childhood 35.15
  cigarette smoking 35.4
  clinical features 35.6–35.12
  clinical variants 35.12–35.14
  complications and co-morbidities 35.17–35.19
  differential diagnosis 35.16
  disease course and prognosis 35.19
  drug reactions 35.3–35.4
  elephantine psoriasis 35.14
  environmental factors 35.3–35.4
  epidemiology 35.1–35.2
  epidermal hyperplasia with suprapapillary thinning *35.6*

erythema, scaling and induration, grading of **35.17**
erythrodermic psoriasis 35.14, **35.16**
flexural psoriasis (inverse psoriasis) 35.8, *35.9*, **35.16**
follicular psoriasis 35.7, *35.9*
genetics 35.2–35.3
genital psoriasis 35.10
guttate psoriasis 35.15, **35.16**, 35.19
hepatobiliary disease 35.19
histopathology 35.5, *35.6*
history 35.6
HIV-induced or exacerbated psoriasis 35.15–35.16
immune-mediated inflammatory disease association 35.18
incidence and prevalence 35.1–35.2
infection 35.3, 35.18
intraepidermal spongiform pustule *35.5*
investigations 35.19–35.20
linear psoriasis 35.15
management 35.20–35.31
metabolic syndrome association 35.18
molecular genetics 35.2–35.3
mucosal lesions 35.11–35.12
Munro microabscess formation in lesional stratum corneum *35.6*
nail psoriasis 35.10–35.11, *35.12*
non-pustular palmoplantar psoriasis 35.10, *35.11*
in older age groups 35.15
ostraceous psoriasis 35.14
pathogenic mechanisms 35.4–35.5
physical trauma 35.4
phytotherapy 35.22–35.23
pityriasis rubra pilaris comparison **36.2**
plaques
  changes in fully developed plaques *35.5*
  encircled by clear peripheral zone (halo or ring of Woronoff) *35.7*
  fiery red plaques of unstable psoriasis *35.13*
  with gross hyperkeratosis *35.14*
  red scaly plaques *35.7*
  silvery white scaling *35.8*
pregnancy outcomes 35.19
presentation 35.6
pruritus 81.8
psychological distress 35.4
psychological/psychiatric morbidity 35.19
PUVA photochemotherapy 35.23
remissions from 35.19
scalp psoriasis 35.7, *35.9*
seborrhoeic psoriasis (sebopsoriasis) 35.7–35.8
segmental psoriasis 35.15
severity classification 35.16–35.17
sunlight exposure 35.4
systemic therapy 35.23–35.27
  acitretin 35.25–35.26
  apremilast 35.26
  ciclosporin 35.25
  fumaric acid esters 35.26
  hydroxycarbamide (hydroxyurea) 35.26
  methotrexate 35.23–35.25
  properties of **35.24**
  tofacitinib 35.27
  tyrosine kinase 2 inhibitor 35.27
topical treatment 35.20–35.22
  calcineurin inhibitors 35.22
  coal tar 35.21–35.22
  corticosteroids 35.20, *35.21*
  dithranol 35.21
  novel agents 35.22
  vitamin D analogues 35.20–35.21
unstable psoriasis 35.13, *35.14*, 35.35
vascular bleeding points *35.9*
psoriatic alopecia 87.34, *105.3*
psoriatic arthritis 35.41–35.46
  age at onset 35.42
  assessment tools 16.3
  associated diseases 35.42

biologic treatment 35.45–35.46
Classification of Psoriatic Arthritis (CASPAR) criteria **35.41**
clinical features 35.43
distal interphalangeal involvement *35.42*
epidemiology 35.42
genetics 35.42
investigations 35.43
management *35.44*
pathophysiology 35.42–35.43
severity classification 35.43
systemic therapy 35.44–35.45
treatment 35.43–35.46
PSS-AD *see* Psychosomatic Scale for Atopic Dermatitis
PSSs *see* peeling skin syndromes
psychiatric disorders
  male genitalia 109.44
  oral effects 108.83
  see also anxiety; body dysmorphic disorder; depression; stress
psychiatric side-effects of systemic therapies 19.7, 19.18, *19.19*, 19.20, 19.43, 19.45
psychiatric therapies
  alternative therapies 84.48
  combined somatic/psychological disorders 84.47–84.48
  drug therapies 84.43–84.47
  psychological therapies 84.47–84.48
  use in dermatology 84.42–84.43
  see also talk therapies
psychoactive drugs *see* psychotropic drugs
Psychoactive Substances Act 2016 120.4
psychodermatolgy
  atopic eczema 41.19
  urticaria 42.8
psychodermatology 1.8–1.9, 84.1–84.49
  "by proxy" disorders 84.5, 84.14, 84.26, 84.29, 84.33, 84.37–84.38
  classification 84.2
  deliberate self-harm 84.38–84.39
  delusional beliefs 84.5–84.12
  eating disorders 84.26–84.27, 108.83
  factitious skin disease 84.29–84.38, 97.48–97.50, *108.61*
  'golden rules' 84.2–84.3
  illicit drug use 120.2
  models of service provision 84.2
  multidisciplinary teams 84.2
  national and international organisations 84.2
  obsessive–compulsive behaviour 84.12–84.26
  psoriasis 35.19
  psychoemotional stress role in skin disease 150.8
  psychogenic itch 84.27–84.29
  psychogenic pruritus 81.12
  quality of life assessment 84.4–84.5
  skin-related health anxieties 84.25–84.26
  stigmatisation 1.9, 5.5, 16.8, 28.1, 28.16, 84.3–84.4
  therapies for psychological disorders 84.42–84.48
  treating skin condition concomitantly with psychological disease 84.2, 84.14
  see also suicidality
psychoemotional stress, role in skin disease 150.8
psychogenic itch 84.27–84.29
psychogenic pruritus 81.12, **105.15**
psychological care, stepped approach **15.5**
psychological distress
  acne 88.28–88.29
  morphoea 55.29
  psoriasis vulgaris 35.4
psychological and emotional factors, exacerbating cutaneous disorders 84.1, 84.2
psychological factors, diagnosis 4.5
psychological impacts, measurement 16.11–16.12
psychological methods, cutaneous wart therapy 25.60–25.61
psychological and social factors

see also cutaneous T-cell lymphoma; mycosis fungoides
primary erythromelalgia 101.7–101.8
primary haemophagocytic lymphohistiocytosis 135.11, 135.13
primary herpetic gingivostomatitis 25.20–25.24
primary hypertrophic osteoarthropathy (PHO) 70.35–70.36
primary (idiopathic) cutaneous mucinoses 57.1, 57.2–57.18
primary immunodeficiency diseases see inherited immunodeficiency
primary localised cutaneous amyloidosis (PLCA) 56.2, **56.3**
   on ankle 56.7
   on chest 56.7
   management 56.13–56.14
   on nose 56.8
   staining of amyloid 56.5
   on toes 56.8
   treatment 56.13–56.14
primary lymphoedema (PL) 71.24–71.28, 103.17–103.20
   causative genes and phenotypes **103.19**
   choanal atresia and lymphoedema 71.27
   clinical features 103.20
   congenital-onset primary lymphoedema 103.24
   epidemiology 103.19
   Hennekam lymphangiectasia–lymphoedema syndrome 71.26
   hereditary lymphoedema type 1A 71.24–71.25
   hypotrichosis–lymphoedema–telangiectasia syndrome 71.26
   late-onset primary lymphoedema 103.24–103.25
   lymphoedema–distichiasis syndrome 71.25–71.26
   microcephaly with or without chorioretinopathy, lymphoedema and mental retardation 71.27
   with myelodysplasia 71.27–71.28
   pathophysiology 103.19–103.20
   St George's classification algorithm 103.18
   terminology **103.18**
primary (naevoid) congenital hypertrichosis 87.85–87.86
primary neutrophilic cicatricial alopecias 87.48–87.50
primary Raynaud phenomenon 124.10–124.12
primary syphilis 29.6–29.7, 29.17
primary systemic or amyloid light-chain amyloidosis (extravascular) 149.13
primary systemic amyloidosis
   haemorrhagic bulla 56.13
   macroglossia 56.12
   nail dystrophy 56.13
   periorbital bleeding 56.11
primary telangiectasias 101.16, **101.17**, **101.18**
primary tumours, Merkel cell carcinoma 146.6, 146.8
primin allergy 127.71, 127.73
primitive polypoid/non-neural granular cell tumour see dermal non-neural granular cell tumour
Primula dermatitis 127.5, *127.14–127.15*, 127.20–127.22, 127.71, 127.72–127.73
prioritisation, health economics 6.5
PRISMA see Preferred Reporting Items for Systematic Reviews and Meta-analyses
procollagen-lysine, 2-oxoglutarate 5-dioxygenase 3 (*PLOD3*) 69.7–69.8
proctitis/proctocolitis syndrome, lymphogranuloma venereum 30.15, 30.16, 30.17
productivity costs, health economic evaluation 6.3

proflavine, topical therapies 18.10
progeroid laminopathies 77.4
progeroid syndromes see premature ageing syndromes
progesterone-only pill (POP) 87.95
progestins
   acneform reaction 88.13
   acne vulgaris treatment 88.50–88.51
programmed cell death (PDCD) 71.2
progressive bacterial synergistic gangrene 26.77, 26.78
progressive hemifacial atrophy (PHA) 55.23, 55.24–55.25
progressive hyperpigmentation 68.10
progressive macular hypomelanosis (PMH) 86.44–86.45
progressive mucinous histiocytosis 135.23
progressive nodular histiocytosis (PNH) 135.19
progressive symmetrical erythrokeratoderma (PSEK) 63.19–63.20
pro-haptens 127.8
prohormones, transformation into active metabolite 150.7
pro-inflammatory cytokines, antigen-presenting cells 127.7
pro-inflammatory topical treatments, molluscum contagiosum infection 25.18
prolactin
   central nervous system controlled endocrine signalling axis 150.2
   hair follicle 87.11–87.12
prolidase deficiency 70.11–70.12, **72.7**, 79.12–79.13
proliferating trichilemmal tumour 137.5–137.6
proline synthesis defects 79.14–79.15
PROMs see Patient-Reported Outcome Measures
pro-opiomelanocortin deficiency (POMC) **72.7**
   C202T mutation 72.8
   gene structure and post-translational processing 72.8
pro-opiomelanocortin and prohormone convertase deficiency 72.4–72.6
prophylactic dressings, pressure ulcer prevention 123.9
prophylactic phototherapy, PLE management 126.7–126.8
prophylactic skin treatments, papulopustular eruptions 119.4
prophylactic surgical excision of naevi, not recommended to prevent melanoma 142.3
Propionibacterium see *Cutibacterium*
propolis 127.59, 127.74–127.78
propranolol
   burn treatment 125.14
   infantile haemangioma treatment 116.8
propylene glycol (PG) 12.3, 12.5, 127.59
PROS see PIK3CA-related overgrowth spectrum
Prospective Register of Systematic Reviews (PROSPERO) 17.8, 17.9
prostaglandin D2 (PGD2), release in skin 14.1
prostaglandins
   hair disorders 87.94–87.95
   male hair loss 87.62
prosthetic implants, cutaneous reactions 127.19
prosthetics, hair loss cover 87.69, 87.101
protease inhibitor (PI), HAART regimes 98.6–98.7
proteases
   Mas-related G-protein-coupled receptor agonists, endothelin 81.1
   pruritus **81.3**, 81.5
protein contact dermatitis (PCD) 127.10, 127.83, 127.85
protein C/protein S-related disease, purpura 99.15–99.17

protein-energy malnutrition 61.2, 61.3
   hair reddening 61.4
   skin signs of nutritional disease 61.5
protein fibre, types of 2.2
proteins
   in epidermolysis bullosa 69.2–69.8
   skin fragility link 69.5–69.8
proteinuria, nail–patella syndrome 67.16
protein–hyaluronic acid complex
   normal component of the dermal extracellular matrix 57.1
   see also cutaneous mucinoses; mucin
proteoglycans (PGs) 2.36–2.39
   functions of 2.38–2.39
   gene location **2.39**
   molecular characteristics and tissue distribution 2.38, **2.39**
Proteus syndrome 71.10–71.11, **72.10**, 73.6, **101.28**, 103.23–103.24
proton beam therapy 24.2–24.3
protothecosis 32.94
protozoal infestations/infections 33.35–33.55
   eye 107.40
   HIV coinfections 31.29
   oral involvement 108.57
provocation testing, cutaneous photosensitivity diseases 126.4–126.6, 126.12, 126.19, 126.34
proximal subungual onychomycosis 32.48
PRP see pityriasis rubra pilaris; platelet-rich plasma
PRS see polygenic risk score
pruriginosa dystrophic epidermolysis bullosa 69.16
prurigo
   cutaneous manifestations of Hodgkin disease 139.49
   terminology 81.14
prurigo-like morphology, chronic actinic dermatitis 126.17
prurigo nodularis (PN) 81.14–81.18, 84.15–84.18
   clinical features 81.16–81.17, 84.16–84.17
   epidemiology 81.14, 84.16
   investigations 81.17–81.18
   lichen simplex chronicus relationship 84.15
   management 81.18, 84.17–84.18
   pathophysiology 81.15–81.16
   underlying diseases **81.17**
pruritic conditions (pruritus/xerosis/ichthyosis/prurigo)
   hepatitis C 25.76
   HIV 31.12
pruritus 81.1–81.21
   acetylcholine **81.3**, 81.4
   antihistamines 41.27
   atopic eczema 41.12, 81.7–81.8
   brachioradial 81.12, 83.6–83.7
   central transmission of itch 81.3
   chronic 81.1–81.14
   chronic kidney disease related 81.8–81.9
   clinical features 81.6–81.13
   cutaneous induction of itch 81.2–81.3
   cutaneous manifestations of Hodgkin disease 139.49
   definitions/nomenclature 81.1
   diabetes 81.10
   diabetic patients 62.6–62.7
   drug-induced 81.10–81.11, 117.2–117.3
   fibreglass dermatitis 122.21
   friction blisters 122.9
   genital pruritus **109.2**
   gold toxicity 121.4
   hepatobiliary disease/cholestasis 81.9–81.10
   histamine/histamine receptors **81.3**, 81.4
   in ichthyoses 63.46, 63.47
   inflamed skin/dermatoses 81.7
   itching purpura 99.7, 99.8, **99.9**
   lichen simplex 81.18–81.20
   lichen simplex chronicus 84.15
   liver disease association 153.8
   localised 81.12

malignancy manifestation 81.10
mediators of itching in skin diseases **81.3**, 81.4–81.8
methamphetamine-induced 120.5
neoplasia association 148.27
neurological aspects 81.2–81.4, 81.11–81.12
neuropathic 83.5–83.6
neuropathic pruritus 81.11–81.12
non-atopic causes 84.16
notalgia paraesthetica 81.12
opioid peptides **81.3**, 81.4–81.5
peripheral and central neuronal sensation 81.4
phototherapy adverse effects 21.12
polycythaemia vera 81.10
in pregnancy 81.11, 113.13–113.24, **113.20**
prurigo nodularis 81.14–81.18
psoriasis vulgaris 81.8
psychiatric and psychosomatic diseases/psychogenic pruritus 81.12
psychogenic 84.27–84.29
PUVA phototherapy adverse effects 21.13
renal failure and dialysis complications 154.3, *154.4*
scalp 105.14–105.17
scratching 81.3–81.4
senescence 81.11
systemic diseases 81.8–81.10
systemic sclerosis 54.16, **54.26**
tachykinins **81.3**, 81.4
thyrotoxicosis 81.10
trophic syndromes 82.7–82.9
see also itching
pruritus ani 111.3–111.6
   clinical features 111.5–111.6
   epidemiology 111.5
   excoriations and lichenification, idiopathic pruritus 111.6
   management of 111.6
   medicament allergens 127.46
   pathophysiology 111.5
   secondary causes of **111.4–111.5**
PS see potassium sorbate
PSCC see penile squamous cell carcinoma
PSD see penoscrotodynia
PSEK see progressive symmetrical erythrokeratoderma
Pseudallescheria boydii see *Scedosporium apiospermum*
pseudo-ainhum 63.55, 63.56, *63.64*, 94.48
pseudoallergic reactions
   drug hypersensitivity 14.2–14.3
   urticaria 42.5, 42.6, 42.8
pseudochromhidrosis 92.18
pseudocowpox (PCPV) see milker's nodule
pseudocyst, external ear 106.8–106.9
pseudoedematous-appearing striae 94.12
pseudoepitheliomatous hyperplasia 132.9–132.10
pseudoepitheliomatous micaceous and keratotic balanitis (PEMKB) 109.35
pseudofolliculitis 26.27, 91.8–91.10, 93.1–93.2
pseudofolliculitis barbae 91.8, *91.9*, 122.23
pseudohypoaldosteronism, miliaria association 92.13
pseudo-Kaposi syndrome see acroangiodermatitis
pseudologia fantastica 84.37
pseudolymphoma 134.1–134.3
   B-cell/lymphocytoma cutis 134.1, 134.2, 134.8–134.10
   external ear 106.34
   oral involvement 108.72
   pathophysiology 134.1–134.2
   T-cell origin 134.1–134.2
pseudomembranous candidiasis 32.61
Pseudomonas infections 26.51–26.53
   botryomycosis 26.76–26.77
   clinical features and variants 26.52–26.53
   colonisation of wounds, colour *4.14*

Pseudomonas infections (*continued*)
  epidemiology 26.51
  management 26.53
  P. aeruginosa/P. pyocyanea 26.51–26.53
  pathophysiology 26.51
  see also ecthyma gangrenosum;
    Stenotrophomonas maltophilia
pseudomyogenic haemangioendothelioma
  136.34
pseudopelade of Brocq (PB) 87.44–87.46
pseudo-pernia *see* chilblain-like lesions
pseudophotodermatitis 127.72
Pseudophyllidea, infections 33.31,
  33.34–33.35
pseudopods, melanomas 145.7, *145.8*
pseudoporphyria 58.18–58.19
  bullous eruption due to renal
    failure/dialysis 154.4, *154.5*
  drug-induced 126.29
pseudopyogenic granuloma *see* epithelioid
    haemangioma
pseudosarcomatous
    fasciitis/pseudosarcomatous
    fibromatosis *see* nodular fasciitis
pseudosarcomatous
    fibroblastic/myofibroblastic
    proliferations, ischaemic fasciitis
  136.6
pseudoxanthoma elasticum (PXE)
  70.31–70.35, 94.30–94.31, 97.30
  associated diseases 70.31
  of axillary skin *70.32*
  cardiovascular changes 70.33
  'chicken skin' appearance *70.32*
  clinical variants 70.34
  diagnostic criteria **70.32**
  differential diagnosis 70.34
  gastrointestinal changes 70.33
  investigations 70.34
  management of 70.34–70.35
  obstetric risk 70.33–70.34
  ocular changes 70.33
  pathophysiology 70.31–70.32
  skin changes 70.32–70.33
PSI *see* Psoriasis Symptom Inventory
psittacosis 26.79
psoralen photosensitisers
  adverse effects 21.9, 107.43–107.44
  development of PUVA 21.2
  natural sunlight therapies 21.2
  oral and topical regimens 21.9
  photochemotherapy principles 21.1
  used in PUVA 21.9
psoralen and ultraviolet A (PUVA) 86.17,
  126.6
  cutaneous T-cell lymphoma 139.21,
    139.22, 139.23
  development 21.2
  lentigines 86.17, 131.7–131.8
  mastocytosis treatment 46.10
  palmoplantar pustulosis 35.39
  psoriasis treatment 35.23
  UVB phototherapy comparison 21.5–21.6
  see also phototherapy
psoriasiform dermatitis *85.14*
psoriasiform irritant contact dermatitis
  128.4
psoriasiform palmar phenotype,
  Papillon–Lefèvre syndrome *63.69*
psoriasiform plaques, zinc deficiency *61.26*
psoriasiform sarcoidosis 96.13
psoriasis 35.1–35.48
  acute generalised exanthematous
    pustulosis distinction *118.4*
  alcohol misuse relationship 84.40
  alopecia 87.34, 105.3
  ano-genital psoriasis 109.9–109.10
  assessment tools 16.3, **16.3**
  atopic eczema cost comparison *6.10*
  biologic therapies 9.8–9.9
  classification **35.2**
  diagnosis 4.1
  disease associations 5.11
  ear dermatoses **106.23**, *106.25*
  economic burden of 6.8–6.10
  erythrodermic psoriasis 39.32
  eyelid 107.6
  genetic factors 8.1
  global distribution **7.3**
  gold reactions 121.4
  hand dermatitis differentiation 127.22,
    128.5
  HIV 31.15–31.17
  hypopigmentation *86.44*
  infantile psoriasis 115.3–115.4
  inflammation mechanism 9.8
  irritant contact dermatitis 129.1, *129.2*
  keratoderma climactericum 63.72
  male genitalia 109.9–109.10
  mechanical injuries 122.2
  oral lesions 108.35
  perineal and perianal skin 111.8
  peristomal skin *112.9*, 112.10, 112.11
  phototherapy 21.3–21.4
  pityriasis rubra pilaris comparison **36.2**
  polymorphic light eruption 126.2
  in pregnancy 113.10–113.11
  psychodermatology 84.3
  psychological and social factors 15.4
  PUVA-induced lentigines in patient with
    131.7
  quality of life assessment 16.7–16.8
  radiation dermatitis differentiation
    119.14
  recreational drug-related 120.3
  scalp 105.2–105.4
  susceptibility genes and pathways **35.3**
  vitamin D analogue topical treatment
    18.27–18.28
  vulva 110.17–110.18
  see also psoriasis vulgaris (chronic plaque
    psoriasis); psoriatic arthritis;
    pustular psoriasis
Psoriasis Area and Severity Index (PASI)
  16.3, 35.16–35.17, **35.27**
Psoriasis Disability Index (PDI) 16.8
Psoriasis Epidemiology Screening tool
  (PEST) 16.3
Psoriasis Family Impact 16.10
psoriasis gyrata *1.5*
Psoriasis Symptom Inventory (PSI) 16.5
psoriasis vulgaris (chronic plaque psoriasis)
  35.1–35.31
  acute guttate psoriasis 35.12–35.13
  age at onset 35.2
  alcohol misuse 35.4
  atypical forms of 35.14
  Auspitz sign *35.9*
  biologic therapy 35.27–35.31
    adalimumab 35.28
    bimekizumab 35.30
    biosimilars 35.29
    brodalumab 35.30
    certolizumab pegol 35.28–35.29
    etanercept 35.28
    IL-12/IL-23 p40 inhibitor 35.29
    IL-17 inhibitors 35.30
    IL-23p 19 inhibitors 35.30–35.31
    infliximab 35.27–35.28
    ixekizumab 35.30
    registries 35.29
    secukinumab 35.30
    short-term efficacy in randomised trials
      35.27
    TNF-alpha inhibitors 35.27
  cancer association 35.18
  cardiovascular disease 35.19
  in childhood 35.15
  cigarette smoking 35.4
  clinical features 35.6–35.12
  clinical variants 35.12–35.14
  complications and co-morbidities
    35.17–35.19
  differential diagnosis 35.16
  disease course and prognosis 35.19
  drug reactions 35.3–35.4
  elephantine psoriasis 35.14
  environmental factors 35.3–35.4
  epidemiology 35.1–35.2
  epidermal hyperplasia with
    suprapapillary thinning *35.6*
  erythema, scaling and induration, grading
    of **35.17**
  erythrodermic psoriasis 35.14, **35.16**
  flexural psoriasis (inverse psoriasis) 35.8,
    35.9, **35.16**
  follicular psoriasis 35.7, *35.9*
  genetics 35.2–35.3
  genital psoriasis 35.10
  guttate psoriasis 35.15, **35.16**, 35.19
  hepatobiliary disease 35.19
  histopathology 35.5, *35.6*
  history 35.6
  HIV-induced or exacerbated psoriasis
    35.15–35.16
  immune-mediated inflammatory disease
    association 35.18
  incidence and prevalence 35.1–35.2
  infection 35.3, 35.18
  intraepidermal spongiform pustule *35.5*
  investigations 35.19–35.20
  linear psoriasis 35.15
  management 35.20–35.31
  metabolic syndrome association 35.18
  molecular genetics 35.2–35.3
  mucosal lesions 35.11–35.12
  Munro microabscess formation in lesional
    stratum corneum *35.6*
  nail psoriasis 35.10–35.11, *35.12*
  non-pustular palmoplantar psoriasis
    35.10, *35.11*
  in older age groups 35.15
  ostraceous psoriasis 35.14
  pathogenic mechanisms 35.4–35.5
  physical trauma 35.4
  phytotherapy 35.22–35.23
  pityriasis rubra pilaris comparison **36.2**
  plaques
    changes in fully developed plaques
      35.5
    encircled by clear peripheral zone (halo
      or ring of Woronoff) *35.7*
    fiery red plaques of unstable psoriasis
      35.13
    with gross hyperkeratosis *35.14*
    red scaly plaques *35.7*
    silvery white scaling *35.8*
  pregnancy outcomes 35.19
  presentation 35.6
  pruritus 81.8
  psychological distress 35.4
  psychological/psychiatric morbidity
    35.19
  PUVA photochemotherapy 35.23
  remissions from 35.19
  scalp psoriasis 35.7, *35.9*
  seborrhoeic psoriasis (sebopsoriasis)
    35.7–35.8
  segmental psoriasis 35.15
  severity classification 35.16–35.17
  sunlight exposure 35.4
  systemic therapy 35.23–35.27
    acitretin 35.25–35.26
    apremilast 35.26
    ciclosporin 35.25
    fumaric acid esters 35.26
    hydroxycarbamide (hydroxyurea)
      35.26
    methotrexate 35.23–35.25
    properties of **35.24**
    tofacitinib 35.27
    tyrosine kinase 2 inhibitor 35.27
  topical treatment 35.20–35.22
    calcineurin inhibitors 35.22
    coal tar 35.21–35.22
    corticosteroids 35.20, *35.21*
    dithranol 35.21
    novel agents 35.22
    vitamin D analogues 35.20–35.21
  unstable psoriasis 35.13, *35.14*, *35.35*
  vascular bleeding points *35.9*
psoriatic alopecia 87.34, 105.3
psoriatic arthritis 35.41–35.46
  age at onset 35.42
  assessment tools 16.3
  associated diseases 35.42
  biologic treatment 35.45–35.46
  Classification of Psoriatic Arthritis
    (CASPAR) criteria **35.41**
  clinical features 35.43
  distal interphalangeal involvement *35.42*
  epidemiology 35.42
  genetics 35.42
  investigations 35.43
  management *35.44*
  pathophysiology 35.42–35.43
  severity classification 35.43
  systemic therapy 35.44–35.45
  treatment 35.43–35.46
PSS-AD *see* Psychosomatic Scale for Atopic
    Dermatitis
PSSs *see* peeling skin syndromes
psychiatric disorders
  male genitalia 109.44
  oral effects 108.83
  see also anxiety; body dysmorphic
    disorder; depression; stress
psychiatric side-effects of systemic therapies
  19.7, 19.18, *19.19*, 19.20, 19.43, 19.45
psychiatric therapies
  alternative therapies 84.48
  combined somatic/psychological
    disorders 84.47–84.48
  drug therapies 84.43–84.47
  psychological therapies 84.47–84.48
  use in dermatology 84.42–84.43
  see also talk therapies
psychoactive drugs *see* psychotropic drugs
Psychoactive Substances Act 2016 120.4
psychodermatolgy
  atopic eczema 41.19
  urticaria 42.8
psychodermatology 1.8–1.9, 84.1–84.49
  "by proxy" disorders 84.5, 84.14, 84.26,
    84.29, 84.33, 84.37–84.38
  classification 84.2
  deliberate self-harm 84.38–84.39
  delusional beliefs 84.5–84.12
  eating disorders 84.26–84.27, 108.83
  factitious skin disease 84.29–84.38,
    97.48–97.50, *108.61*
  'golden rules' 84.2–84.3
  illicit drug use 120.2
  models of service provision 84.2
  multidisciplinary teams 84.2
  national and international organisations
    84.2
  obsessive–compulsive behaviour
    84.12–84.26
  psoriasis 35.19
  psychoemotional stress role in skin disease
    150.8
  psychogenic itch 84.27–84.29
  psychogenic pruritus 81.12
  quality of life assessment 84.4–84.5
  skin-related health anxieties 84.25–84.26
  stigmatisation 1.9, 5.5, 16.8, 28.1, 28.16,
    84.3–84.4
  therapies for psychological disorders
    84.42–84.48
  treating skin condition concomitantly with
    psychological disease 84.2, 84.14
  see also suicidality
psychoemotional stress, role in skin disease
  150.8
psychogenic itch 84.27–84.29
psychogenic pruritus 81.12, **105.15**
psychological care, stepped approach **15.5**
psychological distress
  acne 88.28–88.29
  morphoea 55.29
  psoriasis vulgaris 35.4
psychological and emotional factors,
  exacerbating cutaneous disorders
  84.1, 84.2
psychological factors, diagnosis 4.5
psychological impacts, measurement
  16.11–16.12
psychological methods, cutaneous wart
  therapy 25.60–25.61
psychological and social factors

atopic eczema 41.19–41.20
  beliefs/emotions/behaviours 15.1–15.3
  childhood and adolescence 15.3, 15.4
  co-morbidities of recreational drug use
    120.8
  holistic management of skin disease
    15.5–15.7
  ichthyoses 63.46
  impacts of long-term conditions
    15.1–15.5
  lymphoedema 103.7
  specific conditions 15.3–15.4
psychopharmacological treatments
  antidepressants 84.43–84.44, **84.44**, **84.45**,
    117.3
  antipsychotics 84.44–84.46
  anxiolytics 84.46
  body dysmorphic disorder 84.14
  mood stabilisers 84.46–84.47
Psychosomatic Scale for Atopic Dermatitis
  (PSS-AD) 16.8
psychotherapies *see* psychiatric therapies
psychotropic drugs
  acneform reaction 88.13
  hypermelanosis 86.26–86.27
  recreational use 120.1
PTBPFR *see*
    para-tert-butylphenolformaldehyde
    resin
PTD *see* (*p*-)phenylenediamine and
    toluene-2,5-diamine
PTEN *see* phosphatase and tensin homologue
PTEN hamartoma tumour syndrome (PHTS)
    71.2, 71.13–71.14, **72.10**, *78.11*, **78.14**,
    148.11–148.12
  oral involvement 108.85
  storiform collagenoma 136.3
  trichilemmoma 137.6
pterygium syndromes 70.37–70.38
PTLD *see* post-transplant
    lymphoproliferative disorder
PTM *see* pretibial myxoedema
ptosis 107.6
ptychotropic porokeratosis 63.74, 85.21,
    85.22, 109.35
pubertal growth striae *94.10*, 94.11
pubic hair
  androgen-stimulated growth 87.10
  male 109.4, 109.27
  trichomycosis 26.41–26.42, 109.27
public health approach, epidemiology 5.2,
    5.4–5.7
pudendal neuropathic pain/neuralgia 83.7,
    83.8
PUFAs *see* polyunsaturated fatty acids
puffy hand syndrome *120.7*
pulley sutures 20.18
pulmonary blastomycosis 32.85
pulmonary disorders
  fungal diseases 32.81–32.88
  interstitial lung disease 52.1, 52.2, 52.7,
    52.11–52.12, 69.15
  junctional epidermolysis bullosa with
    interstitial lung disease 69.15
  Mycobacterium kansasii 27.35
  tuberculosis 27.2, 27.5, 27.6
  tuberous sclerosis complex 78.9
pulmonary involvement
  drug reaction with eosinophilia and
    systemic symptoms 118.9, 118.11
  Erdheim–Chester disease 135.22
  methotrexate toxicity 19.26
  microscopic polyangiitis 100.21–100.22
  systemic lupus erythematosus 51.31
  systemic sclerosis 54.18, **54.26**
pulmonary oedema, inhalation injury
    125.4–125.5
pulmonary sarcoidosis 96.5, 96.15–96.16
pulpitis *128.5*
pulsed dye lasers (PDLs), vascular lesions
    23.6–23.12
punch biopsies 3.3, 20.9–20.10
punctate autosomal dominant porokeratosis
    63.59
punctate keratosis of the palmar creases
    63.60

punctate lesions, palmoplantar keratoderma
    punctata 63.59
punctate palmoplantar porokeratosis
    85.20–85.21
punctuate keratotic projections 63.59
pure diffuse leprosy 28.8
pure neural leprosy 28.10
puritic and dyskeratotic dermatoses (PDD),
    human polyomavirus-6 and -7
    25.48–25.49
purpura 99.1–99.25
  acroangiodermatitis 99.4
  actinic purpura 99.5
  annularis telangiectodes 99.7, 99.8, **99.9**
  antiphospholipid antibody syndrome
    99.17–99.19
  associated diseases **100.4**
  atrophie blanche 99.20–99.21
  bacterial infections 99.14
  blood vessels, abnormal or decreased
    support of 99.5–99.7
  calcific uraemic arteriolopathy 99.23
  cardiac embolus 99.15
  causes **99.2**, **99.5**
  cholesterol embolus 99.14–99.15
  classification 99.1, 99.2
  coagulation disorders **99.2**
  contact allergy **99.9**
  corticosteroid purpura 99.5
  cryogelling/cryoagglutination disorders
    99.11–99.14
  cryoglobulinaemia 124.13
  Degos disease 99.21–99.22
  diagnosis by lesion size of macular
    non-retiform
    haemorrhage/petechiae **99.3**
  drug-induced purpura **99.4**
  dysproteinaemic purpura 99.6–99.7
  emboli 99.14–99.19
  exercise-induced purpura 99.5, **99.9**
  fungal infections 99.14
  gravitational purpura 99.4
  heparin-induced thrombocytopenia
    99.9–99.10
  heparin necrosis 99.9–99.10
  hypergammaglobulinaemic purpura
    99.6–99.7
  infections 99.14
  with inflammation **99.2**
  intravascular causes **99.2**, 99.4–99.5
  itching purpura 99.7, 99.8, **99.9**
  lichen aureus 99.7, 99.8, **99.9**
  livedoid vasculopathy 99.20–99.21
  lupus anticoagulant syndrome
    99.17–99.19
  malignant atrophic papulosis 99.21–99.22
  mechanical vascular causes **99.2**
  microvascular occlusion disorders
    99.9–99.24
  non-thrombocytopenic vascular causes
    99.4–99.7
  oral involvement 108.27
  oxalate ebmolus 99.15
  paroxysmal finger haematoma 99.5–99.6
  physical and artefactual bleeding 99.6
  pigmented purpuric dermatoses
    99.7–99.9
  pigmented purpuric lichenoid dermatosis
    of Gougerot and Blum 99.7, 99.8,
    99.9
  platelet disorders 99.2–99.4
  primary ecchymotic haemorrhage
    syndromes 99.4–99.7
  protein C/protein S-related disease
    99.15–99.17
  purpura fulminans 99.15–99.17
  retiform/stallate 25.111, *53.4*, 99.16
  Schamberg disease 99.7, 99.8, **99.9**
  scurvy 99.6
  in Sjögren syndrome 53.10–53.11
  Sneddon syndrome 99.19–99.20
  solar purpura 99.23–99.24
  systemic coagulopathies 99.15–99.19
  thrombocytopenia 99.2–99.4
  thrombocytosis 99.3–99.4, 99.10–99.11

  trauma injury 99.6
  vascular coagulopathies 99.19–99.24
  Waldenström hypergammaglobulinaemic
    purpura 99.6–99.7
  warfarin-induced necrosis 99.15–99.17
purpura annularis telangiectodes (Majocchi
    disease) 99.7, 99.8, **99.9**
purpura artefact, induced bruising 84.33
purpura fulminans, neonatal 114.21–114.22,
    114.27
purpuric lesions, calciphylaxis 59.7
purpuric macules, Stevens–Johnson
    syndrome/toxic epidermal
    necrolysis *118.14*
purpuric polymorphic light eruption 126.4,
    126.5
purpuric reactions
  allergens 127.20
  COVID-19 infection 25.109, 25.111, *25.112*
  COVID-19 vaccines 25.118
purse string sutures 20.18
PUs *see* polyurethanes
pustular conditions of the scalp
    105.12–105.14
  diagnosis *105.13*
  erosive pustular dermatosis of the scalp
    105.13–105.14
pustular drug rash 118.1
pustular folliculitis 91.3–91.5, 93.8
pustular miliaria 92.13
pustular patch test reactions 127.27
pustular psoriasis 35.31–35.41, 118.4
  acrodermatitis continua of Hallopeau
    35.39–35.41
  diagnosis of **35.32**
  generalised pustular psoriasis
    35.31–35.36
  IL36RN gene 118.2, 118.3
  palmoplantar pustulosis 35.36–35.39
  von Zumbusch variant 35.33–35.34, 118.4
pustular pyoderma gangrenosum 49.4
pustular ulcerative syphilide 29.10
pustules 3.43
  chemical peels, side effect of *160.14*
  rosacea 89.6, *89.7*, 89.12, **89.14**–**89.15**
pustulose exanthemique aiguë generalisés
    (PEAG)
PUVA *see* psoralen and ultraviolet A
PV *see* pemphigus vulgaris; polycythaemia
    vera
P-values, incompatibility of data with a
    statistical model 17.20–17.21
PVD *see* peripheral vascular disease
PVL *see* Panton–Valentine leukocidin
    virulence factor
PWA *see* persons with albinism
PWS *see* port wine stains; Prader–Willi
    syndrome
PXE *see* pseudoxanthoma elasticum
Pyemotes mites 34.51–34.52
pyknosis 3.43
pyloric atresia
  junctional epidermolysis bullosa with
    69.13–69.14
  severe recessive epidermolysis bullosa
    simplex with 69.11
pyoderma, global distribution **7.3**
pyoderma faciale, differential diagnosis
    88.34, *88.36*
pyoderma gangrenosum (PG) 49.1–49.8,
    53.6, 120.5
  acne conglobata association 88.63
  associated diseases 49.2
  associated with liver disease 153.9
  biologic therapy 49.7
  bullous pyoderma gangrenosum
    49.4–49.5
  causative organisms 49.4
  clinical features 49.4
  clinical variants 49.4–49.5
  complications and co-morbidities 49.6
  differential diagnosis 49.5–49.6
  environmental factors 49.4
  epidemiology 49.1–49.2
  extracutaneous pyoderma gangrenosum
    49.5

  genetics 49.3, 49.4
  granulomatous superficial pyoderma
    gangrenosum 49.5, *49.6*
  haematological neoplasms 149.7
  healing ulcer and scarring *49.5*
  immune system activation 49.3
  inflammatory pathways recruitment 49.3
  internal malignancy association 148.23,
    148.24
  intravenous immunoglobulin therapy
    49.7
  investigations 49.6
  lesion appearance *49.4*, *49.5*
  male genitalia 109.9, 109.23
  management 49.6–49.8
  Maverakis diagnostic criteria **49.2**
  neutrophil activation 49.3
  parastomal pyoderma gangrenosum
    49.4, *49.5*
  pathology 49.3
  pathomechanism of 49.3
  peristomal skin *112.10*, 112.13–112.15
  predisposing factors 49.2
  pustular pyoderma gangrenosum 49.4
  sarcoidosis association 96.15
  severity classification 49.6
  tissue destruction 49.3–49.4
  treatment for **49.7**
  vegetative pyoderma gangrenosum 49.5,
    49.6
pyodermatitis-pyostomatitis vegetans
    (PD-PSV) 49.19–49.20
pyoderma vegetans, possible bacterial/viral
    roles 26.88
pyogenic arthritis-pyoderma
    gangrenosum-acne (PAPA)
    syndrome **45.5**, **45.6**, 45.13,
    88.8–88.10, **88.11**, 88.63
pyogenic granuloma (PG) (lobular capillary
    haemangioma) *71.2*, 136.25–136.27
  in acne 88.41
  infants 116.10–116.11
  laser therapies 23.11
  oral *113.3*
  within port-wine stains 136.26
pyogenic infection
  external ear 106.19
  recurrent 80.18
pyogenic sterile arthritis, pyoderma
    gangrenosum and acne syndrome
    see pyogenic arthritis-pyoderma
    gangrenosum-acne syndrome
pyostomatitis vegetans, oral involvement
    108.74
pyrethroids, topical therapies 18.14
pyridoxine (vitamin B6) deficiency
    61.17–61.18
pyrin-associated autoinflammation with
    neutrophilic dermatosis (PAAND)
    45.10–45.11
pyruvic acid (PA), chemical peels 160.2
Pythium insidiosum infection 32.94
PyV *see* polyomaviruses

Q

QALY *see* Quality-Adjusted Life Year
QES *see* Questionnaire on Experience with
    Skin complaints
Q fever 97.46
QoL *see* quality of life
Q-switched lasers, tattoo and pigmented
    lesion treatments 23.12–23.17
Quality-Adjusted Life Year (QALY) *6.3*, *6.4*,
    16.9
quality of life (QoL) assessment 4.5,
    16.5–16.11
  acne 88.38–88.39, **88.40**
  adolescents 16.10
  children 16.9–16.10
  dermatology specific measures 16.6
  disease specific measures 16.7–16.9
  evaluation 6.3
  families 16.10–16.11
  general health measures 16.6
  Harmonising Outcome Measures for
    Eczema 16.3

quality of life (QoL) assessment (*continued*)
  informing clinical decisions 16.6
  meaning 16.5–16.6
  measurement 6.4
  methods 16.6
  occupational skin disease 16.12
  practical use of measures 16.11
  psychodermatology 84.4–84.5
  purpose 16.6
  rosacea 89.5
Quality of Reporting of Meta-analyses (QUOROM), systemic review assessment 17.8
quaternium-15 127.51
quenching effects, patch testing 127.29
Questionnaire on Experience with Skin complaints (QES) 16.8
quinine-induced photo-lichenoid eruption 4.7
quinines, allergic contact dermatitis 127.80
quintana fever *see* trench fever
QUOROM *see* Quality of Reporting of Meta-analyses

R

RA *see* rheumatoid arthritis
Rab GTPase Rab27B, epidermolysis bullosa 69.4
racial factors
  dermatomyositis 52.1
  facial melanoses 86.9
  see also skin of colour
radial streak patterns *see* peripheral streak patterns; starburst patterns
radiation dermatitis *see* radiodermatitis
radiation-induced angiosarcoma, atypical vascular proliferation after radiotherapy comparison 136.38–136.39
radiation-induced carcinogenesis 24.4, 24.21
  latent period 24.4, 24.21
  management 24.21
  rare tumours 24.21
  risk in treatment of benign conditions 24.4, 24.21
  sarcomas 24.21
  tumour risks in immunocompromised people 147.9
radiation reactions
  early/acute 24.18, *24.19*
  late/chronic 24.18–24.20
radiation recall phenomena 119.12–119.13
radiculoneuropathy, primary ano-genital herpes infection 25.25
radiodermatitis 105.5–105.6, 109.12, 119.13–119.15
radiofrequency (RF), skin tightening 161.6
  methods of delivery 161.7
  microneedling devices 161.8
  safety and adverse events 161.7
radiological examination 4.22–4.23
radiological investigations, peripheral vascular disease **101.4**
radio-responsiveness, radiotherapy 24.4
radiotherapy 24.1–24.24
  associated skin side effects 119.13–119.15
  atypical vascular proliferation after radiotherapy 136.38–136.39
  basal cell carcinoma 140.16–140.17
  benign skin conditions 24.4, 24.7
  Bowen disease 141.24
  brachytherapy 24.3
  causing post-ionising radiation keratosis 141.14–141.15
  compared to surgery for skin cancer 24.8, **24.10**
  cutaneous side effects 119.1–119.15
  cutaneous squamous cell carcinoma 141.35, 141.37
  cutaneous T-cell lymphoma 139.15, 139.16, 139.21, 139.22
  dose fractionation and treatment regimens 24.10
  early/acute reactions 24.18, *24.19*

electron beam therapy 24.1–24.2
hypofractionated regimens for melanoma 24.14
indications 24.4, 24.7–24.10
melanoma 144.2
morphoea 55.14
multivoltage X-ray techniques 24.3–24.4
particular skin sites with basal cell or squamous cell carcinomas *24.9*, 24.10–24.12
proton beam therapy 24.2–24.3
radio-curability and radio-responsiveness 24.4
superficial techniques 24.33
tumour recurrence 24.20–24.21
tumours induction *see* radiation induced carcinogenesis
types 24.1–24.3
raised linear bands of infancy 114.18–114.19
Rajka Langeland severity classification, atopic eczema 16.4
RAK *see* reticulate acropigmentation of Kitamura
Ramazzini, Bernadino 1.4
random-effects models, systematic reviews 17.10
randomisation sequence assessment, evidence based medicine 17.12, 17.13
randomised controlled clinical trials (RCTs)
  bullous pemphigoid 50.20–50.21, **50.23**
  mucous membrane pemphigoid 50.30–50.31
  see also evidence based medicine
rapid acoustic pulse (RAP) technology, cellulite treatment 161.9
Rapunzel syndrome 84.24
RAS *see* recurrent aphthous stomatitis
RASA1 mutations *see* RASopathies
rashes *see* exanthems
Ras-MAPK signalling pathway 78.7, *78.8*, **78.9**
RASopathies 78.7, *78.8*, **78.9**
  cardiac and cutaneous malformations 151.3
  lymphatic abnormalities 103.24
  neurofibromatoses 78.7, *78.8*, **78.9**
Ras–mitogen activated protein kinase (Ras-MAPK) signal transduction pathway 78.7, *78.8*
  genetic syndromes of **78.9**
rat-bite fevers 26.75–26.76, 130.5
  Spirillum minus 26.75
  Streptobacillus moniliformis 26.75–26.76
rationalisation, health economics 6.5
rational medicine
  growth of 1.2–1.4
  see also evidence based medicine
rat transitional epithelium, antibody detection 3.20
Raynaud phenomenon (RP) 53.1, 124.10–124.13, 129.15–129.16
  acrocyanosis distinction 124.7
  cannabis-induced 120.4
  causes **54.19**
  clinical features **54.19**
  fingertip rewarming in patient with *54.22*
  fish stings 130.4
  internal malignancy association 148.24–148.25
  investigation and management **54.25**
  in systemic lupus erythematosus 51.26
  systemic sclerosis *54.3*, 54.15, **54.19**
  vibration white finger 122.24
al-Razi, Muhammad ibn Zakariya ('Rhazes') 1.3
RCM *see* reflectance confocal microscopy
RCTs *see* randomised controlled clinical trials
RD *see* Refsum disease
RDD *see* Rosai–Dorfman–Destombes disease
RDTC *see* Regional Dermatology Training Centre, Moshi, Tanzania
reactivation of viruses 25.4
  after COVID-19 vaccination 25.118
  in COVID-19 patients 25.111

human herpesvirus 6 and 7 25.40
immunomodulatory drug effects 19.3
zoster 25.32–25.36
reactive angioendotheliomatosis 136.24–136.25
reactive arthritis (Reiter's syndrome) 155.2, *155.3*
  eye disease **107.35**
  oral involvement 108.68
  vulva 110.18
reactive cutaneous lymphoid hyperplasia *see* lymphocytoma cutis/B-cell pseudolymphoma
reactive diluents, resins 127.69
reactive granulomatous dermatitis (RGD) 53.5
reactive inflammatory erythemas 47.1–47.17
  annular erythema of infancy 47.9, *47.10*
  erythema annulare centrifugum 47.6–47.8
  erythema chronicum migrans 47.9
  erythema gyratum repens 47.11–47.12
  erythema marginatum 47.9–47.11
  erythema multiforme 47.1–47.6
  necrolytic migratory erythema 47.12–47.16
  rheumatic fever, Duckett Jones criteria for diagnosis of **47.11**
reactive material, removal techniques 122.19
reactive oxygen intermediates (ROIs), erythema nodosum 97.21
reactive oxygen species (ROS)
  ageing of skin 156.4, 156.6
  hair pigmentation 87.12–87.13
reactive perforating collagenosis 63.76
  lip lesions 108.64
  renal failure and dialysis complications 154.3–154.4
reactive vascular lesions 136.23–136.25
rebound phenomena, discontinuation of corticosteroids 18.21
recalcitrant irritant dermatitis, excessive hand washing 84.26
recall reaction dermatitis 119.12–119.13
RECAP *see* Recap of Atopic Eczema
Recap of Atopic Eczema (RECAP) 16.3
ReCell 125.6
receptor–effector system, drug action mechanisms 13.5
receptor tyrosine kinases (RTKs), transmembrane drug mechanisms 13.5
recessive dystrophic epidermolysis bullosa 69.5, 69.16–69.18, *69.16*, **78.14**
  cancer and 69.26–69.27
  combined with dominant 69.18
  management of 69.25–69.26
recessive X-linked ichthyosis 63.5–63.7
recombinant human growth hormone (rhGH), burn treatment 125.13
recombinant protein therapy, ectodermal dysplasias 69.27
record keeping, systemic therapy 19.2
recreational drug use 120.1–120.9
  delusional infestation 84.5, 84.6, 84.7, 84.8, 84.9
  olfactory delusions 84.10
  pharmaceutical drug interactions 120.3
recto-vaginal fistula *111.7*
rectum
  ano-rectal abscess 111.27–111.28
  gastrointestinal polyposis 78.11
recurrent angioedema without weals *see* angioedema without weals
recurrent aphthous stomatitis (RAS) 108.37–108.38
recurrent cellulitis *see* erysipelas
recurrent cutaneous necrotising eosinophilic vasculitis 100.10–100.11
recurrent focal palmar peeling 39.16
recurrent genital herpes 25.26
recurrent infundibulofolliculitis 91.14–91.15, 93.6–93.7

recurrent labial HSV infection (RHL) 108.52–108.53
recurrent lymphocytic meningitis, herpes simplex virus 25.23
recurrent melanocytic naevi 131.26–131.27
recurrent oro-facial and cutaneous herpes 25.22–25.24
recurrent toxin-mediated perineal erythema 26.32, *26.33*
recurring digital fibrous tumour of childhood *see* inclusion body (digital) fibromatosis
red ear syndrome **106.23**
redness (erythema) 4.13, 126.1
  acne vulgaris **88.27**, 88.29
  atopic eczema 41.15
  chemical peels, side effect of 160.11–160.12
  chronic venous insufficiency **101.43**
  dermatomyositis 52.3, 52.4, *52.5*, *52.6*
  differential diagnosis 89.7
  disease course 89.11
  drug/chemical photosensitivity *126.29*
  epidermolysis bullosa acquista *50.45*
  grading of in psoriasis vulgaris **35.17**
  hereditary angio-oedema 43.4
  indicator of pressure ulcers 123.4
  irritant contact dermatitis 128.6
  laser therapies 23.9–23.11, *23.12*, *23.13*
  lichen planus *110.12*
  linear IgA disease *50.37*
  morphoea *55.18*
  non-blanchable 123.4, **123.5**, 123.8
  ultraviolet radiation *10.3*, *10.4*
  UVB phototherapy adverse effects 21.11–21.12
  UVR exposure 10.7
  venous leg ulcer *102.5*
  see also erythema...; flushing; rosacea
α5-reductase inhibitors 87.96
Reduviidae (kissing bugs/assassin bugs/cone-nosed bugs) 34.29
Reed naevi 131.34, 131.37, 145.5, 145.6
Reed naevi *see* Spitz naevi
Reed naevus 131.34, *131.37*, *145.2*, 145.5, 145.6
Reed syndrome (hereditary leiomyomatosis and renal cell cancer) **78.14**, *78.15*, 148.12, 154.2
reference listed drug (RLD), topical bioavailability/bioequivalence assessment 12.7, 12.8
reflectance confocal microscopy (RCM) 4.21, *4.22*, 142.9
Refsum disease (RD) 63.30–63.32
refugee camps *see* displaced persons camps
Regional Dermatology Training Centre, Moshi, Tanzania (RDTC) 7.7
RegiSCAR drug reactions **118.9**
regression structures, melanoma 145.7, *145.8*
regressive melanoma 142.14, *142.17*, 142.20
regulations, drug application approval 13.13
regulatory T cells (Tregs) 127.9
Reiter's syndrome *see* reactive arthritis
RELA haploinsufficiency 45.15
relapsing fever (epidemic), *Borelia recurrentis* 26.72
relapsing polychondritis 155.11–155.13
  ear dermatoses **106.23**
  respiratory disease 152.2
relaxed skin tension lines, principles of surgical design 20.20–20.21
REM *see* reticular erythematous mucinosis
Renaissance medicine 1.3
renal abnormalities/dysfunction
  drug reaction with eosinophilia and systemic symptoms 118.9, 118.11
  systemic lupus erythematosus 51.31
renal cancer, syndromes linked with **78.14**
renal cell carcinoma, flushing **104.8**
renal cell carcinoma syndrome, hereditary cutaneous leiomyomatosis links 154.2

renal disorders 154.1–154.7
  calcific arteriolopathy 97.32–97.33
  calciphylaxis involving the penis 109.24
  chronic kidney disease 81.8–81.9
  nail–patella syndrome 67.15, 67.16
  oral involvement 108.83
  skin involvement 154.2, *154.3*
  systemic lupus erythematosus 51.31
  systemic sclerosis 54.18, **54.24**
  see also nephropathy
renal failure, hypermelanosis 86.21–86.22
renal failure and dialysis, cutaneous signs 154.3–154.5
renal failure and dialysis complications, Kyrle disease 154.3–154.4
renal function, drug elimination 13.3
renal transplantation
  dermatological consequences of immunosuppression 154.5–154.6
  see also organ transplant recipients
repeat open application tests (ROATs), allergen testing 127.28, 127.33, 127.49, 127.50
reperfusion injury 123.2
repetitive behaviour disorders 84.22–84.26
repigmentation pattern, piebaldism 68.4
repositioning interventions, pressure ulcers 123.6–123.8, 123.10
reproductive toxicity, methotrexate 19.26
resin contact allergy 127.65–127.66
resins, allergy to 127.68–127.71
resin systems, allergy to 127.18
respiratory fungal diseases 32.82–32.88
respiratory support, SJS/TEN management 118.20
respiratory symptoms
  BSL management 98.15, 98.16
  dermatomyositis 52.7–52.8
  syndromic ichthyoses **63.39**
  yellow nail syndrome 152.6
respiratory syncytial virus (RSV) 25.99–25.100
respiratory system 152.1–152.7
respiratory tract infections, skin features 26.79
restless leg syndrome (RLS) 83.10–83.11
restrictive dermopathy 63.38, 70.24, **77.2**
resuscitation, burn shock 125.2–125.4
resuscitation fluids
  inhalation injuries 125.5
  types 125.3–125.4
resuscitation formulae 125.2–125.3
resveratrol, topical depigmenting agents 18.33
retapamulin, topical therapies 18.11
reticular degeneration 3.40–3.41
reticular dermis, mechanical strength 122.4–122.5
reticular erythematous mucinosis (REM) 57.8–57.9
reticular hyperpigmentation, heat-associated carcinomas *124.15*
reticular pattern naevi
  dermoscopy *145.2*, *145.3*, 145.4
  Spitz naevi 145.6
reticular variant, mid-dermal elastolysis 94.26
reticulate acropigmentation of Kitamura (RAK) 68.13, *68.14*
reticulate hyperpigmentation, drug/chemical photosensitivity 126.3
reticular scarring, congenital erosive and vesicular dermatosis with 94.14
reticuloendothelial system, sarcoidosis 96.5
reticulohistiocytoma 135.22
reticulohistiocytosis 135.25–135.27
retiform haemangioendothelioma 136.32–136.33
retiform parapsoriasis *see* large plaque parapsoriasis
retiform purpura 99.16
  COVID-19 association 25.111
  in patient with mixed connective tissue disease *53.4*

retina, pseudoxanthoma elasticum 70.33
retinal anlage tumour *see* pigmented neuroectodermal tumour of infancy
retinaldehyde, cosmeceutical use of 157.7
retinoic acid (tretinoin) 18.23, 18.24
  chemical peels 160.2
  topical depigmenting agents 18.32
  topical therapies 18.25
retinoids
  acne vulgaris treatment 88.45–88.46, 88.47
  chemical structure *18.24*
  cosmeceutical use of 157.6–157.7
  dermatitis reactions 88.55
  eye, side effects on 107.43
  hidradenitis suppurativa treatment 90.10
  keratinocyte cancer chemoprevention 147.20
  synthetic 19.41–19.42
  topical therapies 18.23–18.26
  use during pregnancy 63.44–63.45, **113.22–113.23**
retinoids (systemic therapy) 19.42–19.44
  cautions 19.44
  contraindications 19.44
  cutaneous T-cell lymphoma 139.16, 139.23
  dermatological uses 19.42
  drug–drug interactions 19.44
  monitoring 19.44
  pharmacological properties 19.42
  potential adverse effects 19.43–19.44, 63.44–63.45
  pre-treatment screening 19.44
retinol (vitamin A)
  cosmeceutical use of 157.7
  deficiency 61.7–61.8, 85.14–85.15, 86.23–86.24
  excess 61.8–61.9
  metabolic production 18.23–18.24
  topical therapies 18.24
retinyl esters, cosmeceutical use of 157.7
retrovirus infections 25.78–25.80
reverse smoking (bidi), keratoses 108.33
revertant mosaicism 8.8
Revesz syndrome 67.15
rexinoid oral therapy, cutaneous T-cell lymphoma 139.15, 139.23
RF *see* radiofrequency
RGD *see* reactive granulomatous dermatitis
rhabdomyocyte (striated muscle cell), microscopic examination of *3.37*
rhabdomyoma 136.55
  oral involvement 108.14
rhabdomyomatous congenital hamartoma 136.55
rhabdovirus infections 25.97
rheumatic diseases
  calluses 122.7
  hyperpigmentation 86.20
rheumatic fever 53.12, 155.3
  cutaneous lesions 151.5, *151.6*
  Duckett Jones criteria for diagnosis of *47.11*
rheumatoid arthritis (RA) 53.3–53.8, 155.5–155.6, *155.7*
  callosities 122.9
  clinical features 53.4, **53.5**
  clinical variants 97.16
  epidemiology 53.4
  fibroblastic rheumatism 53.7–53.8
  gold treatment 121.3–121.4
  interstitial granulomatous dermatitis *53.6*
  investigations 53.8
  leg ulcers 53.7
  management 53.8
  medium vessel vasculitis *53.8*
  oral involvement 108.68
  panniculitis 97.52
  pathophysiology 53.4
  pyoderma gangrenosum 53.6
  reactive granulomatous dermatitis 53.5
  rheumatoid neutrophilic dermatosis 53.5–53.6

rheumatoid nodules 53.5
rheumatoid vasculitis 53.6–53.7
  skin manifestations 155.5–155.6, *155.7*
  systemic lupus erythematosus comparison **51.30**
  vascular lesions associated with 53.6
rheumatoid disease 155.1–155.16
  ear dermatoses **106.23**
  oral involvement 108.67–108.69, **108.68**
rheumatoid neutrophilic dermatosis (RND) 53.5–53.6, 155.6, *155.8*
rheumatoid nodules (RN) 53.5, 97.15–97.17, 155.5–155.6, *155.7*, *155.8*
rheumatoid vasculitis (RV) 53.6–53.7, 155.6
rhGH *see* recombinant human growth hormone
rhinoentomophthoromycosis 32.79–32.80
rhinophyma
  disease course 89.11
  photothermal ablation 23.22
  sex prevalence 89.2
  treatment 89.13
rhinoscleroma, *Klebsiella pneumoniae* subsp. *rhinoscleromatis* 26.56–26.57
rhinosporidiosis 32.79
RHL *see* recurrent labial HSV infection
RHSF *see* European Hidradenitis Suppurativa Foundation
rhytids (wrinkles)
  ablative fractional resurfacing 161.5
  ageing of skin 156.2, 156.5
  cosmeceuticals 157.4–157.7
  dermal fillers, indication for 158.1, **158.3**
  glyphic wrinkles 94.2
  laser-assisted drug delivery 161.5
  mid-dermal elastolysis 94.26
  reduction of by botulinum toxin application 159.5, *159.6*, *159.7*
  smoker's skin *156.4*
riboflavin (vitamin B2) deficiency 61.14–61.15
rickets, hair disorders 87.29
rickettsial infections 26.80–26.84
  scrub typhus group 26.84
  spotted fever group 26.81–26.83
  transitional group 26.83–26.84
  typhus group 26.80–26.81
rickettsialpox 26.83–26.84
Rickettsia prowazekii, epidemic typhus 26.80–26.81
rifamycins 19.47
ring eczema 39.16, 128.3
ringworm of the beard *see* tinea barbae
ringworm of the body *see* tinea corporis
ringworm of the face *see* tinea faciei
ringworm of the foot *see* tinea peddis
ringworm of the groin *see* tinea cruris
ringworm of the hand *see* tinea manuum
ringworm of the nails (onychomycosis caused by dermatophytes) 32.47–32.49
ringworm of the scalp *see* tinea capitis
risk reduction for systemic therapy 19.1–19.2, 19.3
Ritter disease *see* staphylococcal scalded skin syndrome
rituximab 135.29
  mucous membrane pemphigoid, management of 107.31–107.32
  pemphigus treatment 50.9
  systemic sclerosis treatment 54.24–54.25
river blindness *see* onchocerciasis
RLD *see* reference listed drug
RLS *see* restless leg syndrome
RN *see* rheumatoid nodules
RNA editing, dyschromatoses 68.14–68.15
RNA profiling, immune cell analysis 9.2
RNA sequencing, melanoma diagnosis 142.21
RNA viruses 25.78–25.120
  human coronavirus 25.100–25.119
  human retroviruses 25.78–25.80
  paramyxoviruses 25.97–25.100
  pathogenesis 25.2, 25.5
  Picornaviruses/enteroviruses 25.93–25.97

rhabdoviruses 25.97
  togaviruses 25.80, 25.87–25.92
  viral haemorrhagic fevers 25.80–25.87
RND *see* rheumatoid neutrophilic dermatosis
ROATs *see* repeat open application tests
Robles disease *see* onchocerciasis
Rocky Mountain spotted fever, rickettsial infection 26.82
rodent bites 26.75–26.76, 130.5
rodent borne viruses, haemorrhagic fevers 25.81–25.83
rodent flea disease transmission
  plague 26.59–26.60
  rickettsial infection/murine typhus 26.81
roflumilast, psoriasis treatment 35.22
ROIs *see* reactive oxygen intermediates
Roman Empire, rational medicine 1.3
ROS *see* reactive oxygen species
rosacea 89.1–89.20
  causative organisms 89.4
  classification 89.1
  clinical features 89.5
  definition 89.1
  diagnostic features **89.2**, 89.5–89.6, 89.12
  differential diagnosis 88.34
  disease course 89.11
  epidemiology 89.2
  flushing **104.4**
  laser therapies 23.9, *23.12*
  major features **89.2**, 89.6
  management 89.11–89.12
  on mid-face *88.35*
  minor features **89.2**, 89.6–89.7
  pathology 89.3–89.5
  pathophysiology 89.2–89.4
  in pregnancy 113.11–113.12
  prognosis 89.11
  sarcoidosis differential diagnosis 96.3
  treatment **89.13–89.14**
rosacea fulminans 89.16
rosacea-like dermatoses due to medication 89.10
rosacea-like erythema of the face, dermatomyositis 52.3, *52.5*
Rosai–Dorfman disease 3.23, 135.1
Rosai–Dorfman–Destombes disease (RDD) 135.27, *135.28*, 149.17
rose, cosmeceutical use of 157.8
roseola infantum (sixth disease) 25.39–25.40, 115.5–115.6
roseolar rash (macular syphilide) *29.8*, 29.9
Ross River virus (RRV) 25.90
Ross syndrome 92.7, 92.9, 92.12
rotations flaps, surgical reconstruction **20.24**, 20.25
Rothmann–Makai disease 97.8
Rothmund–Thomson syndrome (RTS) 75.4–75.6, **78.12**, 148.12, 148.13
  clinical features **75.2**, 75.5–75.6
  differential diagnosis 75.6
  genetics 75.5
  management 75.6
round cell liposarcoma 136.59
roundworms *see* nematodes
Royal Society of Tropical Medicine and Hygiene (RSTMH) 7.6
RP *see* Raynaud phenomenon
RRV *see* Ross River virus
RSPO4 gene, hereditary anonychia 67.16
RSTMH *see* Royal Society of Tropical Medicine and Hygiene
RSV *see* respiratory syncytial virus
RTKs *see* receptor tyrosine kinases
RTS *see* Rothmund–Thomson syndrome
rubber allergy 127.17, 127.62–65, 127.68; 127.84–127.85
rubber gloves, allergies *39.14*, 127.63
rubber products, genital contact dermatitis **109.13**
rubella 25.91–25.92
  clinical features 25.92
  congenital rubella 114.23
  epidemiology 25.91
  managements 25.92
  pathophysiology 25.91–25.92

rubeosis, diabetic patients 62.2
Rubinstein–Taybi syndrome **72.7**
rufous albinism 68.6
Ruijs–Aalfs syndrome **72.5**
running intradermal suture 20.19
rural versus urban environments, atopic eczema 41.6–41.7
RV *see* rheumatoid vasculitis

S

S-100 protein (melanocyte marker) 3.23, 3.25
SA *see* salicylic acid; sorbic acid
SABR *see* stereotactic ablative radiotherapy
SAC *see* seasonal allergic conjunctivitis
SACD *see* systemic allergic contact dermatitis
sacral herpes zoster 109.28
SADSS *see* Six Area Six Sign Atopic Dermatitis severity score
safety issues
　electrosurgery 20.45–20.46
　phototherapy 21.16
　radiofrequency skin tightening 161.7
　skin surgery 20.6–20.7, 20.11
　treatments in pregnancy 113.19–113.24
SAHA *see* seborrhoea, acne, hirsutism and/or androgenic alopecia syndrome
salbutamol, topical therapies 18.41
salicylic acid (SA) 63.44
　acne vulgaris treatment 88.57
　chemical peels 160.3–160.4, 160.10
salicylism, ichthyoses 63.42
salivary glands 108.4, 108.6
SALT *see* severity of alopecia tool
saltpetre disease 94.31
salt-split human skin substrate, subepithelial blistering disease diagnosis 3.20
salvage therapy, haemophagocytic lymphohistiocytosis 135.13–135.14
sampling errors, epidemiological studies 5.14
SAM syndrome *see* severe dermatitis–multiple allergies–metabolic wasting syndrome
sandflies 33.43, 33.45, *33.52*, 34.3, *34.7*
sand worm eruption, *see also* cutaneous larva migrans
Sanger sequencing 69.22–69.23
San Joaquin valley fever *see* coccidioidomycosis
SAPHO *see* synovitis, acne, pustulosis, hyperostosis and osteitis
saprophytic moulds, superficial mycoses 32.18
sarcoidal granulomas, subcutaneous sarcoidosis 97.54
sarcoidal granulomatous inflammation, tattoos 122.22
sarcoid dactylitis 96.12, 155.7, *155.9*
sarcoidosis 89.10, 89.19, 96.1–96.18, 105.9
　arthropathies 155.7, *155.9*
　cardiac involvement 151.4
　ear dermatoses **106.23**
　erythema nodosum with 97.21–97.22
　eye disease **107.35**
　facial, photothermal ablation 23.22
　foreign body reactions 122.17
　induced by drugs 96.4
　lip lesions 108.64
　metastatic calcinosis cutis 59.5
　neuroendocrinology 150.16
　oral lesions 108.67
　panniculitis 97.53–97.54
　pulmonary involvement 152.5
　systemic manifestations 96.5
sarcomas
　clear cell 136.64
　fat cells 136.58–136.59
　low-grade fibromyxoid sarcoma 136.18–136.19
　malignant vascular tumours 136.34–136.37

　neural origins 136.51–136.52
　non Kaposi in immunocompromised people 147.16
　radiation-induced 24.21
　undifferentiated soft tissue sarcoma 136.17–136.18
　see also dermatofibrosarcoma protuberans; Kaposi sarcomas; myxofibrosarcoma; myxoinflammatory fibroblastic sarcoma; pseudosarcomatous fibroblastic/myofibroblastic proliferations
Sarcoptidae (mites)
　animal 34.50
　human classical scabies 34.41–34.48
　human crusted scabies 34.48–34.50
SARS-CoV-2 spike protein stains perniosis 124.5
　see also COVID-19/SARS-CoV-2
SART3 see Squamous Cell Carcinoma Antigen Recognized by T-cells
Sartorius Score, hidradenitis suppurativa 16.4
SASH *see* Severity and Area Score for Hidradenitis
Sata, Sarachiro 1.7
SAVI *see* STING-associated vasculopathy with onset in infancy
sawah itch *see* cercarial dermatitis
saw-toothing 3.43
sBCC *see* superficial basal cell carcinoma; superficial basal cell carcinomas
SC *see* stratum corneum
scabies 34.41–34.50, 127.22
　animal scabies 34.50
　diagnosis 4.22
　global control measures 7.9
　global distribution **7.3**
　HIV 31.29
　human classical scabies 34.41–34.48
　human crusted scabies 34.48–34.50
　incidence of 7.2
　infants 115.9
　male genitalia 109.29, *109.30*
　in Panama **5.2**, 5.3
　perineal and perianal skin 111.16
　population approach to 5.2
　in pregnancy 113.5–113.6
　pseudolymphoma 134.1, 134.2
　secondary infections 26.10, 26.11
　treatment during pregnancy **113.20**
scabs, wound healing 11.10
scalded mouth syndrome *see* burning mouth syndrome
scaling
　acquired ichthyosis 63.47
　collarette scaling *4.13*
　health economics 6.5
　ichthyosis vulgaris 63.4, *63.5*
　recessive X-linked ichthyosis 63.5, *63.6*
　scalp disorders 105.1–105.6
scalp
　cooling treatments for chemotherapy-induced alopecia 119.6
　microscopic examination of skin 3.33
scalp desquamation, ichthyoses 63.45
scalp disorders 3.45, 105.1–105.18
　allergic contact dermatitis of 127.16
　BAP1-inactivated naevus 131.34
　Brunsting–Perry pemphigoid 50.53
　chronic non-scarring folliculitis 91.13–91.14
　chronic pain/dysaesthesia/tenderness without obvious cause 82.12
　contact dermatitis 105.5
　cutis verticis gyrata 105.10
　dermatomyositis 52.3–52.4, *52.5*
　discoid lupus erythematosus 51.4
　dissecting cellulitis 88.37
　follicular plugging, discoid lupus erythematosus *51.4*
　folliculitis 88.35, 93.5–93.6
　folliculitis keloidalis 93.3

　human immunodeficiency virus infection 105.12
　infections of the scalp 105.12
　lichen planopilaris *37.5*, 37.6
　lichen simplex chronicus 105.5
　linear morphoea en coup de sabre *55.24*
　lipoedema of 98.24–98.25
　melanocytic naevi 131.22–131.23, *131.34*
　mucous membrane pemphigoid 50.29
　pityriasis amiantacea 105.4
　pityriasis amiantacea in psoriasis 35.9
　pruritus 105.14–105.17
　　associated diseases 105.14–105.15
　　causative organisms 105.15–105.16
　　classification *105.16*
　　clinical features 105.16
　　cutaneous sensory receptors and mediators *105.16*
　　epidemiology 105.16
　　investigations *105.16*
　　management 105.16–105.17
　　pathophysiology 105.15
　psoriasis 105.2–105.4
　psoriasis vulgaris 35.7, *35.9*
　pustular conditions 105.12–105.14
　　diagnosis *105.13*
　　erosive pustular dermatosis of the scalp 105.13–105.14
　radiodermatitis 105.5–105.6
　scaling disorders 105.1–105.6
　　contact dermatitis 105.5
　　lichen simplex chronicus 105.5
　　pityriasis amiantacea 105.4
　　psoriasis 105.2–105.4
　　radiodermatitis 105.5–105.6
　　seborrhoeic dermatitis 105.1–105.2
　scalp dyaesthesia 105.17–105.18
　seborrhoeic dermatitis 105.1–105.2
　secondary cicatricial alopecia 87.52–87.53, 105.6–105.9
　　causes **105.6**
　　cicatricial (mucous membrane) pemphigoid 105.6
　　dissecting cellulitis of scalp 105.7–105.8
　　follicular mucinosis 105.8
　　granulomatous conditions 105.9
　　sarcoidosis 105.9
　　sclerosing conditions 105.8–105.9
　syphilis 105.12
　thickened scalp disorders 105.10–105.11
　　cutis verticis gyrata 105.10
　　lipoedematous alopecia 105.10–105.11
　tumours of the scalp 105.11–105.12
　　pilosebaceous unit 105.11
　　scalp metastases 105.11–105.12
　　sebaceous naevus 105.11
　　syringocystadenoma papilliferum 105.11
scalp hair
　anagen phase *87.8*
　cyclical behaviour 87.9
　density 87.3
scalp margin
　necrotising lymphocytic folliculitis 91.12–91.13, 93.4
　varioliform scars 93.4
SCARF syndrome **70.16**
scarlet fever 26.35–26.36
　clinical features 26.35–26.36
　epidemiology 26.35
　management 26.26
　pathophysiology 26.35
scarring
　acne scars, chemical peels 160.5, *160.6*
　acne vulgaris *88.3*, **88.4**, 88.29, 88.39–88.41
　actinic prurigo *126.12*
　chemical peels, side effect of 160.14
　chronic wounds 11.8–11.9
　discoid lupus erythematosus 51.4, *51.5*, *51.7*, *51.8*
　external ear 106.14–106.15
　formation of scar tissue 9.7
　hidradenitis suppurativa 90.4, 90.6, 90.8, *111.11*, *111.12*

　hypertrophic scars 11.9
　initiation of *11.7*
　intermediate recessive epidermolysis bullosa 69.16
　intravenous drug administration 120.6–120.7
　inversa recessive dystrophic epidermolysis bullosa *69.18*
　keloid scars 11.9, 106.14–106.15
　larimal duct scarring, in erosive lichen planus *110.12*
　lichen sclerosus *110.9*
　mimics of acne scarring 88.38
　oral tissues 108.68
　skin folds 93.1
　trichloroacetic acid chemical reconstruction of skin scars *160.6*
　unsatisfactory outcomes of skin surgery **20.41**, 20.42
scarring alopecia 87.13–87.14, 87.36–87.38, 96.13, 98.24
　folliculitis 91.11
　monitoring/assessment *87.19–87.20*
scarring psoriasis 87.34
SCARS *see* self-assessment of clinical acne-related scars; severe cutaneous adverse reactions
scar-sarcoidosis 96.11
SCC *see* squamous cell carcinoma; squamous cell carcinomas
Scedosporium apiospermum (Pseudallescheria boydii) 32.75
SCF *see* stem cell factor
SCFN *see* subcutaneous fat necrosis of the newborn
Schamberg capillaritis 86.49
Schamberg disease 99.7, 99.8, **99.9**
Schaumann bodies, sarcoidosis 96.3
Schilder disease 86.21
Schimmelpenning–Feuerstein–Mims syndrome (SFM) 71.23–71.24, 73.5–73.6
　see also HRAS/KRAS mosaicism; phakomatosis pigmentokeratotica
schistosomes, cercarial dermatitis 33.29–33.30
schistosomiasis (bilharziasis) 33.26–33.29, 111.16
　clinical features 33.27–33.28
　management 33.28–33.29
　pathophysiology 33.26–33.27
Schnitzler syndrome 45.20–45.21
　paraprotein activity 149.12–149.13
　Strasbourg diagnostic criteria **45.20**
Schöpf–Schulz–Passarge syndrome 63.68, **78.13**
Schwann cells, microscopic examination of 3.37
schwannoma 136.44–136.45
Schweninger–Buzzi-type anetoderma 94.23
SCI *see* Skin Cancer Index
SCID *see* severe combined immunodeficiency
SCLE *see* subacute cutaneous lupus erythematosus
sclera, in osteogenesis imperfecta *70.13*
sclerema neonatorum 97.37, 97.59–97.60, 114.17–114.18
scleroderma
　meaning 55.1
　see also morphoea; systemic sclerosis
scleroderma spectrum disorders **54.19**, 55.1
sclerodermatous processes, digestive system 153.6
sclerodermiform basal cell carcinoma *see* morphoeic basal cell carcinoma
sclerodermiform reaction, vitamins K and B$_{12}$ 122.19
scleroedema **54.20**, 57.9–57.11
　diabetic and non-diabetic types 57.9
　diabetic patients 57.9, 57.10, 62.5–62.6, *62.7*
　differences from scleromyxoedema **57.5**
　neonates 97.60
scleroedema of Buschke, paraprotein activity 149.10–149.11

scleroma *see* rhinoscelroma
scleromyxoedema **54.20**, 57.2–57.6
  lung disease 152.6
  paraprotein activity 149.10
sclerosing angioma *see* fibrous histiocytoma
sclerosing cholangitis 63.41
sclerosing collagenoma, Cowden syndrome 78.11
sclerosing epithelial hamartoma *see* desmoplastic trichoepithelioma
sclerosing lipogranuloma 97.49, 97.50
sclerosing lymphangitis, penis 109.8
sclerosing panniculitis 97.30–97.32
sclerosing post-irradiation panniculitis 97.63–97.64, 119.15
sclerosing skin conditions, UVA-1 phototherapy 21.6
sclerosing/syringomatous sweat duct carcinoma *see* microcystic adnexal carcinoma
sclerosis
  causes **55.14**
  localised form *see* morphoea
  systemic *see* systemic sclerosis
  terminology 55.1
sclerotic collagen bundles, deep morphoea 97.13
sclerotic panatrophy 94.19–94.20
Scopulariopsis brevicaulis, onychomycoses 32.53–32.55
SCORing Atopic Dermatitis (SCORAD) 16.3, 16.4
scorpions 34.36–34.37
SCORTEN scoring system, SJS/TEN 118.18
SCPs *see* superficial chemical peels
scratching
  habit reversal therapy 84.37–84.38
  lichen simplex chronicus 81.18–81.20, 84.15
  nodular prurigo 84.16
  prurigo nodularis 81.14–81.18
  pruritus 81.3–81.4
  see also chronic pruritus; pruritus
scratch tests 4.24, 127.86
screening, early melanoma detection 142.18
scRNA-seq *see* single-cell RNA sequencing
scrofuloderma (tuberculosis colliquativa cutis) 27.13–27.16
scrotal calcinosis 59.4, *59.5*, 109.30
scrotal candidiasis 32.64–32.65
scrotal lymphoedema, hidradenitis suppurativa *90.9*
scrotal squamous carcinoma 129.14
scrotal tongue *108.87*
scrotum
  acute scrotum 109.23, 109.25–109.26
  calcinosis 109.30
  carcinoma of 109.39
  eczematous dermatoses 109.11
  examination of 109.4
  Fordyce spots 93.11
  inflammation 109.26
  microscopic examination of skin 3.33
  panniculitis 109.23
  polyarteritis nodosa 109.26
  porokeratosis of Mibelli 109.35
  psoriasis vulgaris 35.10
  scrotal angiokeratoma of Fordyce *109.6*
  squamous cell carcinoma 109.39
  swelling, causes of **109.20**
  tinea 109.27–109.28
scrub typhus group (STG), Rickettsiae 26.80, 26.84
scurvy
  purpura 99.6
  vitamin C deficiency 61.21, *61.22*
Scyphozoa, stings from 130.1
SD *see* seborrhoeic dermatitis
SDGs *see* Sustainable Development Goals
SDRIFE *see* symmetrical drug-related intertriginous and flexural exanthema
SDTI *see* suspected deep tissue injury
sea anemone stings 130.1–130.3
seabather's eruption 130.2

sea-blue histiocytosis 135.22–135.23
sea mat stings 130.4
seasonal allergic conjunctivitis (SAC) 107.16, 107.17, 107.18
seasonal hair shedding 87.9, 87.56
seatworm *see* enterobiasis
sea urchin injuries (SUIs) 130.3
sebaceous adenomas 88.32–88.33
  oral lesions 108.30
  and sebaceomas 137.16–137.17
sebaceous carcinomas 88.33, 137.18, 147.16
  eyelid *107.12*, 107.49
sebaceous cysts *see* epidermoid cysts
sebaceous duct epithelial walled cutaneous cysts 133.6–133.7
sebaceous gland disorders 91.15–91.18
sebaceous gland hyperplasia 88.32, 91.17–91.18, 93.12–93.13
sebaceous gland hypertrophy, neonates 114.4
sebaceous glands 2.43
  changes in during pregnancy 113.2–113.3
  embryonic development 2.5
  eosinophilic pustular folliculitis 93.7
  male genitalia 109.6
  neuropeptide–cytokines/chemokine signalling 88.18
sebaceous gland secretion, neonates 114.3
sebaceous gland tumours 88.32
  carcinomas in immunocompromised people 147.16
  visceral malignancy 148.12
sebaceous hyperplasia, photothermal ablation 23.21–23.22
sebaceous naevus (organoid naevus) *73.5, 73.6, 73.7, 73.8,* 87.30, 88.32, 105.11, *106.33,* 137.19–137.20
sebopsoriasis *see* seborrhoeic psoriasis
seborrhoea 88.41
  in quadriplegic patients 83.19
seborrhoea, acne, hirsutism and/or androgenic alopecia (SAHA) syndrome 88.11
seborrhoeic blepharitis **107.8**
seborrhoeic dermatitis 127.21
  vulva 110.14
seborrhoeic dermatitis (SD) 40.1–40.10, *89.8,* 105.1–105.2
  alcohol misuse relationship 84.40
  causative organisms 40.2–40.4
  clinical features 40.4–40.7
  clinical variants 40.5–40.6
  differential diagnosis 40.6
  drugs inducing or exacerbating condition 40.6–40.7
  ear dermatoses **106.23**
  environment and lifestyle factors 40.4, 40.7
  epidemiology 40.1–40.2
  genetic factors 40.4
  HIV 31.12, 31.15
  HIV association 40.7
  infants 40.5, 41.22, 115.1–115.2
  Langerhans cell histiocytosis 135.6–135.7
  Malassezia yeast 32.14
  male genitalia 109.12, 109.13
  management 40.8–40.9
  pathophysiology 40.2–40.4
  perineal and perianal skin 111.8, *111.9*
  in quadriplegic patients 83.19
  systemic treatments 40.9
  thickened yellow adherent scales *105.2*
  topical antifungals 40.8
  topical keratolytics 40.8
  topical treatment agents 40.8–40.9
  see also infantile seborrhoeic dermatitis
seborrhoeic eczema *see* seborrhoeic dermatitis
seborrhoeic keratosis (SK) 132.1–132.4
  eyelid 107.44
  inverted follicular keratosis 137.2–137.3
  laser therapies 23.16
  malignancy association 132.1–132.2
  management 132.3–132.4
  pathophysiology 132.2–132.3

seborrhoeic melanosis 40.5, *040.6*
seborrhoeic psoriasis (sebopsoriasis) 35.7–35.8, 40.1, 40.6, 40.7
seborrhoeic wart *see* seborrhoeic keratosis
Sebutapes, sebum analysis *88.28, 88.43*
secondary anetoderma 94.23, 94.24–94.25
secondary care 5.13
secondary cicatricial alopecia 87.52–87.53, 105.6–105.9
  causes *105.6*
  dissecting cellulitis of scalp 105.7–105.8
  follicular mucinosis 105.8
  granulomatous conditions 105.9
  linear morphoea ('en coup de sabre) 105.8–105.9
  morphoea 105.8
  mucous membrane pemphigoid 105.6
  sarcoidosis 105.9
  sclerosing conditions 105.8–105.9
secondary cutaneous B-cell lymphomas 139.43–139.45
  intravascular large B-cell lymphoma 139.43–139.44
  lymphomatoid granulomatosis 139.44–139.45
secondary cutaneous mucinoses 57.1, **57.2**, 57.18
secondary cutaneous T-cell lymphoma 139.45
  angioimmunoblastic lymphoma 139.45
secondary erythromelalgia 101.7, 101.8
secondary haemophagocytic lymphohistiocytosis 135.11, 135.14
secondary infections, arthropod bites and stings 34.2
secondary infections of skin lesions, nodular prurigo 84.15
secondary intention healing, skin surgery 20.21, 20.22
secondary livedo reticularis 124.8
secondary localised cutaneous amyloidosis (SLCA) 56.2, **56.3**, 56.9
secondary Raynaud phenomenon 124.10–124.12
secondary syphilis 29.7–29.12, 29.17–29.18
  nephrotic syndrome 154.6
secondary to inflammatory disease/infections 59.1–59.3
second-degree burns 125.6
second primary cancers, increase risk in Merkel cell carcinoma 146.2
secosteroids (vitamin D analogues), topical therapies 18.26–18.29
Secretan's syndrome 97.50
secretory carcinoma 137.40
secretory coil, eccrine glands 92.2, 92.16
secukinumab
  psoriasis treatment 35.30
  psoriatic arthritis treatment 35.45–35.46
sedge pool itch *see* cercarial dermatitis
segmental infantile haemangioma **116.2**, 116.3–116.4
segmental lentiginosis 86.16
segmental odonto-maxillary dysplasia 73.3
segmental psoriasis 35.15
segmental vitiligo 86.34, 86.36, *86.37*, 86.38–86.39, *86.40*
SEI *see* superficial epidermolytic ichthyosis
selective photothermolysis, theory 23.5–23.6
selective serotonin reuptake inhibitors (SSRIs) 84.43, **84.44**, 117.3
selenium deficiency 61.29–61.30
selenium excess (selenosis) 61.30–61.31, 121.6–121.7
Self-Administered Psoriasis Area and Severity Index 16.3
self-assessment, *see also* Patient-Reported Outcome Measures
self-assessment of clinical acne-related scars (SCARS) 16.4
self-esteem 15.1
self-examination, early melanoma detection 142.18

self-healing collodion baby (SHCB) 63.8
self-healing cutaneous mucinosis 57.14
self-help 5.12
self-improving congenital ichthyosis (SICI) 63.7, 63.8, *63.11*, 63.12
self-improving dystrophic epidermolysis bullosa 69.16
self-induced traumatic panniculitis 97.50
self-mutilation, male genitalia 109.9
self-mutilation of the skin
  deliberate self-harm 84.38–84.39
  delusional infestation 84.7
  factitious skin disease 84.29–84.36, 84.37
  malingering 84.36–84.37
  obsessive–compulsive behaviour 84.15–84.22
self-neglect, lack of skin cleaning 84.36
semicircular lipoatrophy (SL) 97.55, 98.9–98.10, 122.15
semi-open tests, allergic contact dermatitis 127.33
senescence, pruritus 81.11
senescent alopecia 87.67–87.68
senile freckle *see* solar lentigo
senile keratosis/senile wart *see* seborrhoeic keratosis
senile purpura *see* actinic purpura
sensitisation 127.6–127.9
  acanthosis facilitation 127.8
  patch testing 127.32
  potential of allergens 127.8–127.9
  risk 127.9
sensitising agents
  antihistamines 18.37
  hair regrowth in alopecia 18.33–18.34
  occupational hazards 129.8–129.11
  reactions to topical therapy 18.5
  use in topical therapies 18.33–18.34
  see also allergic reactions
sensitive skin 128.10–128.11
sensory irritation 128.10–128.11
sensory nerves, anatomy of head and neck 20.2, *20.3*
sensory perception, and skin ageing 2.45
sentinel lymph node biopsy (SLNB) 106.29, 106.32–106.33, 143.4–143.6
sentinel (lymph) node status, melanoma, prognostic markers 142.21, 142.22
sepsis
  burn injuries 125.11
  drug reaction distinction 118.10
  risk for neonates 114.2
  SJS/TEN complications 118.20
  vasculitis 100.7
septal panniculitis 97.11, *97.23*
septicaemia, acute SJS/TEN 118.17
septic arthritis 155.4
serine protease inhibitor Kazal-type 5 (*SPINK5*) 69.6
serine synthesis defects 79.14–79.15
seroconversion, HIV 31.5, 31.6–31.7, 31.11
serological diagnosis, of immunobullous disorders 3.20
serological tests, viral infections 25.5–25.6
seromas 103.32, 103.33
seronegative arthritis 155.5
serotoninergic syndromes, cocaine use 120.3
serpiginous lesions, on foot *4.16*
serpin B8 (*SERPINB8*), skin fragility disorders 69.6
serration pattern analysis, direct immunofluorescence findings 3.17
serum autoantibodies
  bullous pemphigoid 50.14–50.15
  mucous membrane pemphigoid 50.25–50.26
serum protein electrophoresis, cryoglobulinaemic vasculitis *100.17*
serum sickness-like reaction (SSLR), hepatitis B 25.74
Servelle–Martorelle syndrome **101.28**
sesquiterpene lactone mix (SLM) 127.73
sesquiterpene lactones (STLs) 127.71

severe acute respiratory syndrome coronavirus-2 see COVID-19/SARS-CoV-2
severe autosomal recessive epidermolysis bullosa simplex   69.10
severe combined immunodeficiency (SCID)   **80.4**, 80.7–80.9
   skin cancer   147.2
severe cutaneous adverse reactions (SCARs)
   to COVID-19 vaccines   25.119
   to drugs   118.1–118.22
severe dermatitis–multiple allergies–metabolic wasting (SAM) syndrome   63.28, 63.63
severe epidermolysis bullosa simplex   69.9
severe erythroderma, Desmons syndrome   *63.35*
severe junctional epidermolysis bullosa
   management of   69.25
   molecular pathology   *69.13*
severe recessive dystrophic epidermolysis bullosa   69.16–69.18
   management of   69.25–69.26
severe recessive epidermolysis bullosa simplex, with pyloric atresia   69.11
severity of alopecia tool (SALT)   87.24, *87.25*
Severity and Area Score for Hidradenitis (SASH)   16.5
severity rating, types of scales   81.12–81.13
sex chromosome defects   74.3–74.5
   fragile X syndrome   74.5
   Klinefelter syndrome   74.4
   Turner syndrome   74.3–74.4
   XXXXY syndrome   74.4–74.5
   XXYY syndrome   74.4
   XYY syndrome   74.4
sex differences
   burning mouth syndrome   82.2
   dermatomyositis   52.2
   hormone responses in skin/appendages   150.8
   urticarial vasculitis   44.2
sex reversal, palmoplantar keratodermas and   63.67–63.68
sex steroids, and atopic eczema   41.19
sexual abuse of children, ano-genital signs of   109.9
sexual behaviour, ChemSex/drugs with sex   120.2–120.3
sexual development, disorders of   110.5
sexual hair growth   87.2
sexually acquired reactive arthritis (SARA)
   genital chlamydia   30.9, 30.10, 30.11, 30.12, 30.13, 30.14
   gonorrhoea   30.5–30.6
sexually transmitted infections (STIs)
   ano-genital warts   25.61–25.64
   genital herpes   25.24–25.26
   global overview   29.1–29.2
   gonorrhoea   30.1–30.8
   illicit drug-related   120.3
   male genitalia   109.28–109.29
   non-syphilitic bacterial diseases   30.1–30.26
   perineal and perianal skin   111.16–111.17
   recurrent genital herpes increasing risk of HIV and other STIs   25.26
   see also HIV; syphilis
sexual functioning, impact measures   16.12
Sézary syndrome (SS)   139.16–139.25
   clinical features   139.18–139.19
   definition   139.16
   erythroderma in   *39.33*
   management   139.20–139.25
   molecular features   139.19–139.20
   pathophysiology   139.16–139.18
   relationship to mycosis fungoides   139.2, 139.19–139.20
   staging   **139.8**
SFM see Schimmelpenning–Feuerstein–Mims syndrome
SFN see small fibre neuropathy
Shah–Waardenburg syndrome   68.5
shame, emotional effects of skin conditions   15.2

shampoos
   allergic reactions   127.16, 127.50
   alopecia management   87.98
shared decision making, holistic management of skin disease   15.6, 15.7
shared delusions, delusional infestation   84.5
shave biopsy   3.4
   epidermolysis bullosa diagnosis   69.21
   principles   20.10–20.11
shave excisions   20.10–20.11, *20.45*
shaving practices, pseudofolliculitis   91.9–91.11
'shawl-sign', redness on back in dermatomyositis   52.4, *52.6*
SHCB see self-healing collodion baby
shear force, pressure ulcers   123.2, 123.3
shearing stresses   122.3
SHH see sonic hedgehog
SHHis see sonic hedgehog pathway inhibitors
shin
   diabetic bulla on   *62.7*
   diabetic dermopathy   *62.2*
   granuloma annulare   *95.7*
   necrobiosis lipoidica   62.6, *95.9*
shingles see herpes zoster
shiny white line dermoscopy patterns, melanoma   145.7, 145.14, *145.15*
SHML see sinus histiocytosis with massive lymphadenopathy
shockwave therapy, skin tightening   161.6
shoes
   allergic contact dermatitis   127.17, 127.67–127.68
   callosities   122.8
short anagen syndrome   87.53, 87.83
short-arm deletion syndrome, chromosome 4   74.3
short-arm deletion syndrome, chromosome 5   74.3
short stature/lipoedema syndrome   **72.12**
SHORT syndrome   **72.5**
shoulder
   granuloma annulare   95.2
   naevus of Ito   *131.15*
   subcutaneous fat necrosis of the newborn   114.16
SHP see Specific Health Problem
Shulman syndrome (eosinophilic fasciitis)   **54.20**, 55.2, **55.3**, **55.4**, 55.21–55.23, 55.22, **55.27**, 97.13
sialidosis, glycoproteinoses   79.3
Sicariidae (fiddleback/violin spiders)   34.35–34.36
SICI see self-improving congenital ichthyosis
sideroblastic anaemia with B-cell immunodeficiency, periodic fevers and developmental delay (SIFD)   45.19
signalling disorders
   blistering   69.24
   IL-10   45.16
signalling protein mutations, acquired immunodeficiency diseases   **149.20**
signal peptides, cosmeceutical use of   157.5–157.6
signal transducer and activator of transcription (STAT) proteins
   STAT1 gain-of-function mutation, oro-pharyngeal *Candida* infection   80.17
   STAT3 loss of function mutations, hyper-IgE syndrome   80.17
   STAT inhibitor medication for pyoderma gangrenosum treatment   49.7
signal transduction pathway, drug action mechanisms   13.5
sign of Leser–Trélat   148.16
SIL see squamous intraepithelial lesions
sildenafil   124.12
silicone
   reactions to   122.21
   topical therapies   18.41

silicone implants, factitious panniculitis   97.48
silicones, dermal fillers   158.7
Silk Road   1.2
silver, dermatological reactions   121.7–121.8
silver nitrate
   caustic agent for skin surgery   20.47
   topical therapies   18.9
silver sulfadiazine, topical therapies   18.11–18.12
SIM1 deficiency   **72.6**
Simon Broome Register Group, familial hypercholesterolaemia diagnosis   **60.7**
simple interrupted skin sutures   20.14–20.17
Simplified Psoriasis Index (SPI)   16.3, 16.8
simulated skin disease (dermatitis simulata)   84.36
Simuliidae (blackflies)   34.7, 34.9
Simulium species (blackfly), onchocerciasis vector   33.1, 33.2, 33.3
Sinclair scale, hair grading   87.58, 87.65
Sindbis virus (SINV)   25.88
single-cell genomics   8.2
single-cell RNA sequencing (scRNA-seq)   9.2
single-gene disorders   8.2, 8.3, 8.4
single nuclei RNA sequencing (snRNA-seq)   9.2
single nucleotide polymorphisms (SNPs), skin cancer risks   147.6
single-organ small-vessel vasculitis   100.5–100.12
single system Langerhans cell histiocytoses (SS-LCH)   135.2–135.8
sinonasal melanoma   142.14–142.15
sinuses, lips   108.86
sinuses, preauricular, infants   115.12
sinus histiocytosis with massive lymphadenopathy (SHML)   135.27–135.29
sinusoidal haemangioma   136.30–136.31
SINV see Sindbis virus
siphonaptera see fleas
Siphonophora, stings from   130.1
Sipple syndrome see multiple endocrine neoplasia type 2A
sitosterolaemia   60.11
Six Area Six Sign Atopic Dermatitis severity score (SASSAD)   16.4
sixth disease see roseola infantum
SJIA see systemic juvenile idiopathic arthritis
Sjögren syndrome (SS)   53.9–53.11
   classification criteria   **53.10**
   clinical features   53.10
   eye disease   **107.35**
   investigations   53.11
   management   53.11
   mucocutaneous features of   53.10–53.11
   respiratory disease   152.3
Sjögren–Larsson syndrome (SLS)   63.32–63.33
SJS see Stevens–Johnson syndrome
SJS/TEN see Stevens–Johnson syndrome/toxic epidermal necrolysis
SK see seborrhoeic keratosis
skeletal abnormalities   78.3
skeletal muscle tumours   136.55–136.56
skeletal osteomas, familial adenomatous polyposis   78.11
skin ageing see ageing of skin
skin anatomy   9.1, 9.2
skin appendage tumours   137.1–137.49
   immunocompromised people   147.16
skin barrier dysfunction, irritant contact dermatitis   128.2
skin biopsy see biopsy of skin
skin cancer   1.8, 7.2
   acquired immunodeficiency diseases   147.2–147.5
   clinicopathological features, immunocompromised people   147.10–147.16
   direct, mortality and morbidity costs of melanoma   **6.7**

   economic burden of   6.1, 6.5–6.8
   effects of altered healthcare during COVID-19 pandemic   25.120
   factors influencing treatment choice   24.8, **24.10**
   global distribution   **7.3**
   HIV/AIDS   147.2–147.3
   host genetic predisposition, immunocompromised people   147.6
   immunocompromised people   147.1–147.26
   clinicopathological features   147.10–147.16
   drug effects on cancer risk   147.6–147.8
   management   147.16–147.24
   organisations   147.25
   pathogenesis   147.5–147.10
   screening and surveillance   147.24–147.25
   intralesional therapies   20.47–20.48
   management
      immunocompromised people   147.16–147.24
      protocols for organ transplant recipients   **147.22**, **147.23**
      treatment comparisons   20.32–20.33
   see also Mohs micrographic surgery
   occupationally-induced   129.14–129.15
   oculocutaneous albinism   68.7
   pathogenesis, immunocompromised people   147.5–147.10
   persons with albinism   7.10–7.11, 7.12, 7.13
   and photoageing   10.11
   prevalence of   5.10
   primary immunodeficiency diseases/inborn errors of immunity   147.1–147.2
   psychological and social factors   15.4
   quality of life assessment   16.9
   resources used and persons affected by   **6.6**
   screening and surveillance, immunocompromised people   147.24–147.25
   solid-organ transplant recipients   147.3–147.4, **147.22**, **147.23**
   surveillance after phototherapy   21.16–21.17
   ultraviolet radiation effects in immunocompromised people   147.5–147.6
   UVR exposure   10.9–10.10
   xeroderma pigmentosum   76.4, 76.5
Skin Cancer Index (SCI)   16.9
skincare creams, irritant contact dermatitis   129.4
skincare principles, occupational dermatology   **129.4**
skin cleaning neglect   84.36
skin cleansing, neonates   114.2
skin colour   86.1–86.2
   changes as signs of cardiac disease   151.1
   lightening cosmeceuticals   157.3–157.4
   malaria   33.36
   melanoma risk in fair skin   142.3
   see also jaundice; pigmentation
skin of colour (SOC)   4.13–4.15, 86.1–86.2
   acne vulgaris   **88.45**
   acne vulgaris treatment   88.43–88.44
   ageing in   156.1–156.3
   atopic eczema   41.16
   chemical peels   160.15
   discoid lupus erythematosus   *51.7*
   facial melanoses   86.9
   geographic distribution of pigmentation   86.7–86.8
   inherited patterned lentiginosis   86.16
   matching principles in surgical design   20.21
   mucocutaneous manifestations of COVID-19 infection   25.104
   photoageing scale   156.7
   sun exposure responses   86.8

Skindex (dermatology life quality index)   6.4, 15.3, 16.3, 16.6–16.8, 16.12, 35.17
Skindex-Teen   16.10
skin extensibility   122.5
skin folds
  amicrobial pustulosis   49.20–49.21
  scarring   93.1
skin fragility disorders   69.1–69.28
skin grafting
  ectodermal dysplasias   69.27
  full-thickness grafts   20.30, 20.35
skin hydration
  effects on skin bacteria   26.4, 26.5
  pressure ulcers   123.3
skin infections   1.7–1.8
  effects on urinary tract   154.6
  immunosuppressed renal allograft recipients   154.5–154.6
skin injuries, mechanical   122.1–122.29
skin lesions with uncertain/unpredictable malignant potential   141.1–141.18
  actinic keratoses   141.1–141.12
  arsenical keratosis   141.13–141.14
  cutaneous horn   141.12–141.13
  disseminated superficial actinic porokeratosis   141.15–141.18
  post-ionising radiation keratosis   141.14–141.15
skin lightening, cosmeceuticals   157.3–157.4
skin microbiome   2.13, 2.14, 26.2–26.6
  atopic eczema   9.8, 41.9
  erythematotelangiectatic rosacea   89.4
  hair follicle   87.11
  immune system   9.7–9.8, 26.5, 26.6, 103.2, 103.3
  Malassezia yeast species   32.10
  normal   26.3–26.5
skin necrosis, calciphylaxis   154.2, 154.3
skin-only Langerhans cell histiocytoses   135.3–135.4, 135.9–135.10
skin picking disorders   82.7–82.9, 84.19–84.20
  see also acné excoriée; lichen simplex chronicus
'skin popping'   120.6–120.7
skin prick test, contact dermatitis   129.7
skin properties, objective measures   16.5
skin protection, pressure ulcer prevention   123.9
skin-related health anxieties   84.25–84.26
Skin Related NTDs Cross Cutting Group (NNN Skin NTD CCG)   7.6
skin samples, superficial mycoses identification   32.7
skin, structure and function   2.1–2.47
  adherens junctions   2.19–2.20
  adnexal structures   2.5–2.7
  ageing of skin   2.45–2.46
  anchoring fibrils   2.26–2.27
  blood vessels   2.40–2.42
  cellular progression   2.1
  collagens   2.27–2.29
    basement membrane collagen   2.22–2.23
    biosynthesis   2.29–2.31, 2.30
    cross-linking   2.31
    degradation   2.31–2.32
    gene expression   2.29–2.31
    genetic heterogeneity   2.27
    hydroxylation reactions   2.29, 2.30
    periodicity in collagen fibres   2.23
  components of normal skin   2.1–2.3, 2.2
  dermal–epidermal basement membrane zone   2.21–2.22
    basement membrane collagen   2.22–2.23
    hemidesmosomes   2.25–2.26
    laminins   2.23–2.25
  dermis   2.2
    collagen fibres   2.27
    embryonic development   2.5
    immune surveillance   2.15, 2.16
    microvessels in   2.41
    desmosomes   2.18–2.19
    development of skin   2.3–2.5

elastic fibres   2.32–2.33, 2.34
  assembly and cross-linking   2.35
  degradation   2.34–2.35
elastin   2.33–2.35
elastin-associated microfibrils   2.35–2.36
embryonic development of skin   2.3–2.5
epidermis   2.1, 2.2
  cornified cell envelope   2.7
  desmosomes   2.18–2.19
  differentiation   2.6, 2.7, 2.8
  embryonic development   2.3
  hyperproliferation   2.8
  Merkel cells   2.2, 2.11–2.12
  mesenchymal cells   2.4
  nail bed   2.11
  structures of   2.5–2.7
extracellular matrix   2.27–2.28, 2.40
fibroblasts   2.3, 2.39–2.40, 2.45
focal adhesions   2.26
gap junctions   2.20
glabrous skin   2.43
glycosaminoglycans   2.36–2.39
hair-bearing skin   2.43
hair follicles, embryonic development   2.3–2.5, 2.5
hemidesmosomes   2.25–2.26
immune ecosystem   2.12–2.13
immune surveillance   2.15, 2.16
keratinocytes   2.1, 2.7–2.8
laminins   2.23–2.25
Langerhans cells   2.1–2.2, 2.13–2.15
  skin ageing   2.45
lymphatic network   2.42
mast cells   2.15–2.17
melanocytes   2.1, 2.17–2.18
Merkel cells   2.2, 2.11–2.12
  embryonic development   2.5
microbiome   2.13
motor innervation   2.2–2.3
nails   2.10–2.11
physiological functions of skin   2.42–2.43
pilosebaceous units   2.9–2.10
proteoglycans   2.36–2.39
skin homeostasis   2.43–2.45
subcutaneous fat   2.42, 2.43
sweat glands   2.2, 2.8–2.9
tight junctions   2.20–2.21
types of human skin   2.43
skin substitutes, wound healing   11.12, 11.13
skin surface electrical properties, stratum corneum hydration measurement   16.5
skin surgery   20.1–20.52
  anatomical considerations   20.1–20.4
  biopsies   20.8–20.11
  caustic agents   20.47, 20.50
  complications   20.33, 20.40–20.42, **20.41**
    flaps   20.29, 20.33
  cryosurgery   20.46–20.47
  curettage   20.48
  dressings   20.37–20.38
  electrosurgery   20.42–20.46
  equipment, needles and suture materials   20.12
  equipment requirements   20.4–20.5
  flaps   20.22–20.29, **20.24–20.25**, 20.30–20.33
  grafts   20.29–20.30, 20.34, 20.35
  haemostasis for open wounds   20.48
  hygiene and sterilisation   20.5–20.7
  local anaesthetics   20.7–20.8
  Mohs micrographic surgery   20.30–20.37
  pharmacological complications   20.40
  post-operative care   20.37–20.40
  preoperative preparation   20.11
  presurgical procedures and techniques   20.4–20.11
  snip excision   20.48
  specific conditions   20.49–20.50
  suture removal   20.40
  suturing   20.12–20.19
  undermining levels and tissue planes   20.4, **20.6**
  unsatisfactory outcomes   20.42
  see also surgical treatment

skin tags   132.8–132.9
  diabetic patients   62.3
  male genitalia   109.5–109.6
  pre-auricular   106.8
  vulval   **110.32**
skin testing   4.23–4.25
  delayed (4–8 h) tests   4.24
  immediate-weal tests   4.24
  intradermal tests for detection of delayed sensitivity to antigens   4.24–4.25
  techniques   4.23–4.24
skin thickening, lichen simplex chronicus   84.15
skin thickness, irritant contact dermatitis   128.6
skin tightening therapies   161.6–161.8
skin tumours
  immunosuppressed renal allograft recipients   154.6
  occupationally-induced   129.14–129.15
  see also benign proliferations; skin cancer
skin tunnels, hidradenitis suppurativa   90.4, 90.6, 90.11
skin-window technique   4.24
SL *see* semicircular lipoatrophy
slapped cheek syndrome *see* erythema infectiosum (fifth disease)
slaughterhouse eczema   39.15–39.16
SLBN *see* sentinel lymph node biopsy
SLCA *see* secondary localised cutaneous amyloidosis
SLE *see* systemic lupus erythematosus
sleep deprivation, and acne   88.25
sleeping sickness *see* African trypanosomiasis
SLE-like vasculopathy   80.18
sliding flaps, surgical reconstruction   20.23
SLM *see* sesquiterpene lactone mix
SLN *see* speckled lentiginous naevus
SLNB *see* sentinel lymph node biopsy
Slovakia, non-melanoma skin cancer, incidence of   6.1
SLS *see* Sjögren–Larsson syndrome
SM *see* steatocystoma multiplex; systemic mastocytosis
small fibre neuropathy (SFN)   **83.9**
small molecule therapy, epidermolysis bullosa   69.28
small plaque parapsoriasis (SPP)   39.27, 134.6–134.7
smallpox (variola virus)   1.3, 25.6–25.7
small-vessel ANCA-associated vasculitis   100.9, 100.13, 100.20–100.28, 152.3–152.4
small-vessel immune complex-associated vasculitis   100.13–100.20
small-vessel vasculitis, involving respiratory system   152.3–152.4
smartphone apps   5.13
  diagnosis   4.26
  disease outcome measurement and recording   16.2
SMC *see* smooth muscle cell
Smith–Lemli–Opitz syndrome   79.15
smoke, hazards and risks of electrosurgery   20.45–20.46
smoker's melanosis   108.16–108.17
smoking   5.10
  acne   88.19
  ageing of skin   156.4
  dermal connective tissue damage   94.2
  hidradenitis suppurativa association   90.2, 90.9
  keratoses   108.33
  oral hyperpigmentation   108.16–108.17
  oral squamous cell carcinoma   108.46
  penile carcinoma, risk factor for   109.36
  psoriasis association   120.3
  psoriasis vulgaris   35.4
  rosacea risk   89.3
smooth muscle cells (SMCs)   2.40–2.41
  microscopic examination of   3.37
  venous malformations   71.14
smooth muscle hamartoma   73.19, 136.52–136.53

smooth muscle tumours   136.52–136.55
SmPC *see* summary of product characteristics
SMS *see* sodium metabisulphite
snake bites   130.5–130.7
Sneddon syndrome   99.19–99.20
Sneddon–Wilkinson disease   118.4
Snow, John   5.9–5.10
snRNA-seq *see* single nuclei RNA sequencing
snuff dipper's keratosis   108.33
SO *see* superficial onychomycosis
SOC *see* skin of colour
social factors
  diagnosis   4.5
  see also psychological and social factors
social impacts of long-term conditions   15.1–15.4
social inclusion   15.1
social medicine   1.8–1.9
socioeconomic factors, epidemiology   5.10–5.11
sodium bicarbonate, ichthyoses management   63.43
sodium hypochlorite, topical therapies   18.10
sodium metabisulphite (SMS)   127.56
sodium thiosulphate, calciphylaxis treatment   59.8
soft chancre *see* chancroid
soft fibromas *see* skin tags
soft-tissue augmentation *see* dermal fillers
soft-tissue tumours   136.1–136.68
  fat cells   136.56–136.59
  fibrohistiocytic tumours   136.19–136.23
  fibrous/myofibroblastic   136.2–136.19
  lymphatic tumours   136.37–136.39
  muscle tumours   136.52–136.56
  peripheral neuroectodermal tumours   136.42–136.52
  perivascular cells   136.39–136.42
  skeletal muscle cells   136.55–136.56
  smooth muscle cells   136.52–136.55
  uncertain histogenesis   136.59–136.64
  vascular tumours   136.23–136.37
SofWave, ultrasound skin tightening   161.7
SoJIA *see* systemic-onset juvenile idiopathic arthritis
solar cheilitis/cheilosis *see* actinic cheilitis
solar lentigo (actinic lentigo)   131.5–131.7, 160.7
solar purpura   99.23–99.24
solar urticaria (SU)   **42.9**, 42.12, 126.21–126.24, 126.32–126.33
sole of foot
  acral naevi   131.24
  blue rubber bleb naevus syndrome   71.17
  congenital generalised lipodystrophies   72.2
  eccrine poroma   137.25–137.26
  lichen planus of   37.7
  microscopic examination of skin   3.33
  non-pustular palmoplantar psoriasis   35.10, 35.11
  pompholyx eczema   39.14
  recurrent focal palmar peeling   39.16
solid facial (lymph)oedema (Morbihan disease)   88.41, 89.10, 89.16, 89.17, 103.47, 103.48
solid-organ transplant recipients (SOTRs)
  skin cancer risks   147.3–147.4
  see also organ transplant recipients
solitary circumscribed neuroma   136.43–136.44
solitary lichen planus *see* lichenoid keratosis
solitary neurofibroma   136.45–136.46
solitary venous malformations   101.24–101.25
soluble oils   129.1
  irritant contact dermatitis   129.2
solvent fumes, inhaling   120.4
somatic mutation   8.5
somatic RASopathies associated with lymphatic abnormalities   103.24
somatosensory system lesions/disease, neuropathic pain definition   82.5

somatostatin analogue octreotide 97.43
sonic hedgehog pathway inhibitors (SHHis), basal cell carcinoma treatment 140.17–140.18
sonic hedgehog (SHH) pathway, basal cell carcinoma pathogenesis 140.3, *140.5*, 140.17, 140.18
sorbic acid (SA) 127.58
sorbisan sesquioleate 127.44
Sotos syndrome **72.12**
SOTRs *see* solid-organ transplant recipients
South American blastomycosis *see* paracoccidioidomycosis
SOX-10 (transcription factor) 3.24
soya, cosmeceutical use of 157.10
SP *see* substance P
Spain, psoriasis, economic burden of **6.8**, 6.9
Spanish fly *see* cantharidin
sparganosis 33.34–33.35
  clinical features and variants 33.35
  pathophysiology 33.34–33.35
sparganum proliferum 33.35
spastic diplegia, KID syndrome *63.33*
spatial genomics technologies, immune system 9.2
spatial transcriptomics, immune system 9.2–9.3
specialists *see* multidisciplinary teams
Specific Health Problem (SHP) versions, work productivity assessment instruments 16.13
'specimen sign', delusional infestation 84.7–84.8
speckled lentiginous naevus (SLN/naevus spilus) *4.8*, 23.16, 73.15–73.16, 131.15–131.17
speckled leukoplakia, oral lesions *108.34*
spectacle-frame acanthoma 122.14–122.15
spectrophotometric image analysis 4.21
spEDS *see* spondylodysplastic Ehlers–Danlos syndrome
'speedballs' 120.7
SPF *see* sun protection factor
sphincter, anal 111.2–111.3
sphingolipidoses 79.5–79.6
SPI *see* Simplified Psoriasis Index
spice allergies 127.41–127.45
spiders (Araneae) 34.34–34.36
spider telangiectases 101.10–101.12, **101.17**, 153.8
  associated diseases 101.11
  clinical features **101.11**
  investigations for **101.12**
  laser therapies 23.9
  management of **101.12**
  pathophysiology 101.11
Spiegler's tumour *see* cylindroma
Spiegler–Fendt sarcoid *see* lymphocytoma cutis/B-cell pseudolymphoma
spina bifida, tuft hair association *83.18*
spinal cord injury, dermatoses associated with 83.19–83.20
spinal dysraphism 83.17–83.19
  localised hypertrichosis 87.86
spindle cell haemangioma (haemangioendothelioma) *71.20*, 136.31
spindle cell lipoma 136.58
spindle cell naevi *see* Spitz naevi
SPINK5, skin fragility disorders 69.6
spinulosis of the face 85.13
spiny keratoderma 63.59–63.60
spiradenocarcinoma 137.36
spiradenoma 137.31–137.32
  cylindroma relationship 137.30
Spirillum minus (*Spirillum minor*), rat-bite fever 26.75
spirochaetes 26.69–26.76
  Borrelia spp. 26.72–26.74
  Leptospira spp. 26.74–26.75
  non-syphilitic spirochaetal ulcerative balanoposthitis 109.27
  rat-bite fevers 26.75–26.76
  treponemes 26.69–26.72

spironolactone 87.70, 87.95–87.96
  acne vulgaris treatment 88.51
spironolactone treatment, hidradenitis suppurativa 90.10
Spitz naevi 3.36, *3.37*, **131.16**, 131.32–131.37
  atypical Spitz tumours *131.36*, **131.36**
  BAP1-inactivated naevus of the scalp *131.34*
  classic Spitz naevus *131.35*, **131.36**
  clinical features 131.33–131.34
  compound naevus *131.33*
  congenital 73.15
  dermoscopic patterns *145.2*, 145.5, 145.6–145.7
  differential diagnosis 131.34
  disease course and prognosis 131.35
  genetics 131.33
  investigations 131.35–131.37
  management 131.37
  pathology 131.32–131.33
  pigmented Spitz naevus *131.35*
  Reed naevus *131.34*, *131.37*, *145.2*, 145.5, 145.6
Spitzoid melanoma (malignant Spitz tumour/malignant spitzoiid neoplasm) 142.8, 142.20, 142.21
S-plasty, skin surgery 20.21–20.22, *20.23*
split-skin indirect technique, immunofluorescence 3.13–3.14
split-thickness skin grafts 20.30, *20.34*
spondyloarthritis 155.2, 155.5, 155.7, 155.13
spondylodysplastic Ehlers–Danlos syndrome (spEDS) **70.5–70.6**, 70.9
sponge stings 130.3
spongiosis 3.43, 126.14, *126.15*
spontaneous atrophic scarring of cheeks 94.14–94.15
spontaneously regressing tumours, keratoacanthoma 141.38–141.41
spontaneous urticaria
  acute 42.5, 42.15–42.16
  chronic 42.5, *42.6*, 42.7, 42.16, *42.17*
sporadic MMDK 85.18, 85.19
sporadic typhus (Brill–Zinsser disease) 26.81
Sporothrix schenckii 32.72
sporotichosis 32.70–32.72
  clinical features 32.71–32.72
  epidemiology 32.70
  management 32.72
  pathophysiology 32.70–32.71
  systemic form 32.71
sports, traumatic effects 122.16–122.17
spotted fever group (SFG), Rickettsiae 26.80, 26.81–26.83
spot tests, allergic contact dermatitis 127.33–127.34
SPP *see* small plaque parapsoriasis
SPPK *see* striate palmoplantar keratoderma
SPTCL *see* subcutaneous panniculitis T-cell lymphomas
squamoid eccrine ductal carcinoma 137.34–137.35
Squamous Cell Carcinoma Antigen Recognized by T-cells (*SART3*) 85.20
squamous cell carcinoma (SCC) 141.1–141.46
  anal cancer 111.21–111.24
  arsenic poisoning 121.2
  associated conditions 141.1–141.27
  biopsy 3.4
  definitions/nomenclature 141.26
  diagnosis of 3.21
  drug/chemical photosensitivity 126.30
  dyskeratosis congenita 67.14
  ear/auricle 106.27–106.29
  ectodermal dysplasias 69.18, 69.26–69.27
  eyelid 107.47, 107.48
  female genitalia 110.36–110.37
  heat-associated 124.15
  hidradenitis suppurativa co-morbidity 90.7
  incidence compared to basal cell carcinoma

as a keratinocyte cancer 141.1
keratoacanthoma relationship 141.38
KID syndrome *63.34*
lichen sclerosus *110.9*
lip 108.44–108.45
male genitalia 109.35–109.42
metastatic risk 141.26
pilonidal sinus 122.23
possible precursors
  actinic keratoses 141.1–141.12
  arsenical keratosis 141.13–141.14
  cutaneous horn 141.12–141.13
  disseminated superficial actinic porokeratosis 141.15–141.18
  post-ionising radiation keratosis 141.14–141.15
pseudoepitheliomatous hyperplasia mimicking 132.9–132.10
radiotherapy 24.13–24.14
radiotherapy indications 24.8–24.10
well-differentiated/keratoacanthomatous type 141.38
  see also Bowen disease; cutaneous squamous cell carcinoma; *in situ* carcinoma of the skin; oral squamous cell carcinoma
squamous cell epithelioma *see* cutaneous squamous cell carcinoma
squamous hyperplasia, penis 109.34–109.35
squamous intraepithelial lesions (SIL), anal/perianal/genital areas 109.34–109.35, 110.34–110.36, 141.24, 141.26
SRs (systemic retinoids) *see* retinoids (systemic therapy)
SS *see* Sézary syndrome; Sjögren syndrome
SSc *see* systemic sclerosis
SS-LCH *see* single system Langerhans cell histiocytoses
SSLR *see* serum sickness-like reaction
SSM *see* superficial spreading melanoma
SSR *see* sympathetic skin response
SSRIs *see* selective serotonin re-uptake inhibitors
SSSS *see* staphylococcal scalded skin syndrome
staining techniques
  artefacts 3.32
  avidin–biotin staining method *3.16*
  biopsy 3.7–3.10
standardisation of terminology 1.4, *1.5*
standing cutaneous deformity ('cone' or 'dog ear') repair 20.22, *20.23*
staphylococcal infections 26.8–26.10, 26.12–26.32
  ano-genital cellulitis 109.26
  blepharitis **107.8**, *107.9*, 107.10
  cold abscesses of the large folds in neonates 114.25
  external ear 106.19
  female genitalia 110.25
  HIV 31.20–31.21
  non-bullous impetigo 26.13
  Panton–Valentine leukocidin virulence factor 111.13–111.14
  see also methicillin-resistant *Staphylococcus aureus*
staphylococcal scalded skin syndrome (SSSS) 2.19, 26.6, 26.27–26.30
  children 26.27, 26.28, *26.28*
  clinical features 26.28–26.29
  infants 115.7–115.8
  management 26.29, **26.30**
  neonates 114.24–114.25
  pathophysiology 26.28
staphylococcal toxic shock syndrome 26.30–26.32
Staphylococcus spp.
  causing infections 26.8–26.10
  coagulase negative 26.9–26.10
  immune responses 9.7
  normal skin flora 26.3
  S. aureus
    antibiotic resistance, impetigo management 26.16

atopic eczema 41.10
botryomycosis 26.76–26.77
colonisation of skin 26.2, 26.3, 26.4, 26.6
co-pathogen in dermatophytosis 32.22
discoid eczema colonisation *88.56*
EGFR inhibitors 119.3
epidemiology 26.6–26.7
follicular infections 26.22–26.27
folliculitis decalvans 87.48–87.49
folliculitis keloidalis 93.3
genetics 26.9
impetigo 26.14
infections 26.6–26.9
methicillin-resistant 26.8–26.9, 31.21, 31.37, 109.28
necrotising lymphocytic folliculitis 93.4–93.5
pathophysiology 26.7–26.9
perianal cellulitis type dermatitis 26.34
recurrent toxin-mediated perineal erythema 26.32
resident on skin 26.3
scalp itch 105.16
skin infections 26.12–26.13, 26.28–26.29
toxic shock syndrome 26.30–26.32
  see also methicillin-resistant *Staphylococcus aureus*
S. epidermidis 9.7, 26.9–26.10
S. hominis 26.3, 26.9
S. lugdunensis 26.9
S. saccharolyticus 26.3
S. saprophyticus 26.3, 26.9
starburst pattern
  melanoma 145.13, *145.15*
  Reed (Spitz) naevi *145.2*, 145.5, 145.6
'starfish' keratoses, Vohwinkel syndrome *63.64*
starvation
  adiponectin system 97.5
  see also malnutrition
stasis dermatitis/eczema *see* venous eczema
STAT *see* signal transducer and activator of transcription
static friction, laws of 122.6
statin treatment, pachyonychia congenita 63.52, 67.12
statistical methods, clinical research papers 17.20–17.24
statistical summary presentation, clinical research papers 17.18–17.20
Staurozoa, stings from 130.2
steatocystoma multiplex (SM) 88.33–88.34, 133.6, *133.7*
stelae, hair loss 87.64
stellate pseudoscars 94.13, *94.14*
stellate purpura *see* retiform purpura
stem cell factor (SCF) 2.15
  KIT receptor mutations 46.1, 46.2
stem cells 2.43–2.45
  burn treatment 125.8
  epidermal proliferation of *2.43*, 2.44
  epithelial stem cells *2.43*
  hair disorder treatment 87.95
  proliferative potential of 2.44
  wound healing therapy 11.11
Stemmer's sign, lipoedema differential diagnosis 98.22, 98.23
Stenotrophomonas maltophilia 26.55–26.56
stereotactic ablative radiotherapy (SABR), and stereotactic radiosurgery for melanoma 24.14
sterile, *see also* amicrobial
sterile furuncles (abscesses) 26.23
sterile pustules
  eosinophilic pustular folliculitis 93.9, *93.10*
  infantile eosinophilic pustular folliculitis *91.7*
sterilisation, skin surgery 20.5–20.7
steroid hormones
  metabolism and synthesis in skin *150.3*
  signalling effects in skin 150.7
steroid-modified tinea 32.49–32.50

steroids
  colloid milium   94.6–94.9
  rosacea induction   89.17
  withdrawal syndrome   19.18
  see also corticosteroids
Stevens–Johnson syndrome (SJS)
  acute conjunctivitis with mucus discharge   107.33
  erythema multiforme   47.1–47.2
  haemorrhagic crusting of lips   108.61
  history   118.12
  management   107.33–107.34
  musculoskeletal therapy effects   155.10, 155.15
  ocular complications of   107.32–107.33
  oral involvement   108.61, 108.79, 118.20
  T-cell-mediated drug hypersensitivity   14.3, 14.7
  toxic epidermal necrolysis relationship   47.1–47.2, 118.12
  varicella infection/vaccination   25.30
Stevens–Johnson syndrome/toxic epidermal necrolysis (SJS/TEN)   47.1–47.2, 107.32–107.34, 108.79, 118.1–118.2, 118.10, 118.12–118.22
stiff skin syndrome   70.22–70.23
stigma/sigmatization/stigmatisation   1.9, 5.5
  assessment measures   16.8
  leprosy   28.1, 28.16
  psychodermatology   84.3–84.4
  see also Questionnaire on Experience with Skin complaints
stigmata, congenital syphilis   29.26
Still disease   45.21–45.22, 53.8–53.9, 100.29
STING-associated vasculopathy with onset in infancy (SAVI)   **45.5**, **45.6**, 45.13–45.14
stinging potential, sensory irritation   128.10–128.11
stingray stings   130.4
stings
  hymenoptera   34.15–34.18
  marine/aquatic animals   130.1–130.5
stippled calcification, Conradi–Hünermann–Happle syndrome   63.23
STIs see sexually transmitted infections
StK see stucco keratosis
STLs see sesquiterpene lactones
'stocking' distribution, multivoltage X-ray techniques   24.3–24.4, *24.6–24.7*
stomas   112.1–112.16
  allergic contact dermatitis   112.7–112.8
  appliance types   112.1, **112.3**
  assessment of patient   112.1
  corticosteroids for inflammatory peristomal skin diseases   **112.4**
  Crohn ulceration   112.13–112.15
  definition   112.1
  dermatological assessment   **112.3**
  dermatoses associated with underlying bowel disease   112.12–112.15
  infections   112.8–112.10
  irritant skin reactions   112.2–112.7
  lichen sclerosus   112.10
  localised bullous pemphigoid   112.10, 112.12
  nicorandil ulceration   112.10, *112.12*
  pain   *112.6*
  patch test series   **112.9**
  psoriasis   *112.9*, 112.10, 112.11
  pyoderma gangrenosum   *112.10*, 112.13–112.15
  skin complications   153.7
  streptococcal cellulitis   *112.10*
  treatment for   112.1
  types of   112.1, **112.3**
  ulceration   112.10, 112.12–112.15
stomatitis
  angular   32.62–32.63, 108.20, 108.59–108.60
  candidal see acute pseudomembranous candidiasis; chronic erythematous candidiasis

denture-induced   32.62, 108.20–108.21
herpetic   *108.52*
  primary herpetic gingivostomatitis   25.20–25.24
  vesicular stomatitis virus   25.97
stomatodynia see burning mouth syndrome
stored product mites   34.50–34.51
storiform collagenoma   136.3–136.4
storiform patterning   3.43
storiform perineural fibroma see perineurioma
stork bite see naevus flammeus
Stormorken syndrome   63.30
STP see superficial thrombophlebitis
strain   122.3
strangulation of the penis   109.8
Strasbourg diagnostic criteria, Schnitzler syndrome   **45.20**
stratum basale, epidermis   2.5
stratum corneum (SC)   122.4
  black heel   *122.11*
  calluses   122.7
  epidermis   2.1, 2.6
  friction blisters   *122.9*
  function of   12.1, 12.8–12.9
  hydration measurement, surface electrical properties   16.5
  irritant contact dermatitis   128.2
  percutaneous absorption mechanisms   12.1–12.2
  permeability coefficient of water across   12.2
  sampling of by tape-stripping   12.8
  sensitising chemicals   127.6
stratum granulosum, epidermis   2.5–2.6
stratum lucidum, epidermis   2.7
strawberry naevus, eyelid   107.46–107.47
strawberry tongue   108.25
streblodactyly   94.41
Streptobacillus moniliformis   26.75–26.76
streptocerciasis (*Mansonella streptocerca* infection)   33.6–33.7
streptococcal cellulitis
  necrotising   26.78
  perianal   26.33–26.34, 111.14
  peristomal skin   *112.10*
streptococcal impetigo, post-streptococcal glomerulonephritis   154.6
Streptococcal infections of female genitalia   26.33, 110.25–110.26
streptococcal toxic shock-like syndrome (STSLS)   26.30, 26.36–26.37
Streptococcus
  groups   26.12
  infections   26.10–26.12
  S. agalactiae (group B)
    diseases   26.12
    toxic shock-like syndrome   26.36–26.37
  scarlet fever   26.35–26.36
  S. dysgalactiae (group C)
    diseases   26.12
    toxic shock-like syndrome   26.36–26.37
  skin infections   26.13
  S. pyogenes (group A)   26.10–26.12
    antibiotic resistance, impetigo management   26.16
    diseases   26.12
    epidemiology   26.10–26.11
    M antigens   26.35
    pathophysiology   26.11–26.12
    recurrent toxin-mediated perineal erythema   26.32
    toxic shock-like syndrome   26.30, 26.36–26.37
    vulvovaginitis   26.33, 110.25
  S. suis, toxic shock-like syndrome   26.36–26.37
  toxin-mediated disease   26.32, 26.35–26.37
  transients on skin   26.3, 26.4
stress   122.3
  and acne   88.25
  associated hormones   150.8–150.9
  emotional effects of skin conditions   15.2
  relaxation   122.3
  systemic lupus erythematosus   51.21

urticaria   42.8
  see also psychodermatology
stretch marks see striae
striae   *4.9*, *94.7*, *94.8*, 94.9–94.12
striae distensae   94.32
  in pregnancy   *113.2*, 113.3
  sports injuries   122.17
striae of Wickham, penis   *109.19*
striated muscle hamartoma see rhabdomyomatous congenital hamartoma
striate palmoplantar keratoderma (SPPK)   63.56–63.58, 63.62–63.63, 69.7
'strimmer phytophotodermatosis   *4.9*
Strongyloides stercoralis
  ancylostomiasis   33.15–33.17
  perineal and perianal skin   111.16
strongyloidiasis   33.17–33.18
  clinical features   33.17–33.18
  management   33.18
  pathophysiology   33.17
structure of skin see skin, structure and function
strumous bubo see lymphogranuloma venereum
stucco keratosis (StK)   132.4
Sturge–Weber syndrome (SWS)   71.3–71.4, 73.20, **101.28**, 108.27
SU see solar urticaria
subacute annular generalised pustular psoriasis   35.34
subacute cutaneous lupus erythematosus (SCLE)   51.12–51.16
  associated diseases   51.12
  autoantibody status   51.13
  clinical features   51.14
  clinical variants   51.14
  complications and co-morbidities   51.15
  differential diagnosis   **51.15**
  drug-induced SCLE   51.13
  drugs associated with development of   **51.13–51.14**
  epidemiology   51.12
  genetics   51.14
  investigations   51.15
  lesion appearance   *51.15*
  management   51.15–51.16
  pathology   51.14
  pathophysiology   51.12–51.13
  predisposing factors   51.13–51.14
subacute nodular migratory panniculitis   97.25
subacute panniculitis-like T-cell lymphoma   **72.11**
subareolar duct papillomatosis see nipple, adenoma
subcision, cellulite management   98.26
subclinical and latent viral infections
  herpes simplex   25.19–25.20
  human papillomaviruses   25.51–25.52
subcorneal haematoma, black heel   *122.11*
subcorneal pustular dermatosis   49.17–49.19, 118.4
  associated diseases   49.17
  histology   *49.17*
  management   49.18–49.19
  pathophysiology   49.17
  presentation   49.18
  pustule appearance   *49.18*
subcorneal pustules   3.43
subcutaneous atypical smooth muscle tumour (leiomyosarcoma)   136.54–136.55
subcutaneous calcification see calcification of skin and subcutaneous tissues
subcutaneous drug administration, dermatoses induced by   120.6–120.8
subcutaneous fat
  anatomy   97.1–97.5
  necrosis and pancreatic disease   153.6
  physiology   97.1–97.5
  role of   2.43
subcutaneous fat disorders   2.42
  arteries   97.7

fungal infections   97.47
  inflammatory diseases   97.6
  miscellaneous disorders   98.25–98.27
  neonates   97.37, 97.57–97.58, 114.14–114.18, **114.18**
  non-inflammatory disorders   98.1–98.30
subcutaneous fat necrosis of the newborn (SCFN)   97.37, 97.57–97.58, 114.15–114.17, **114.18**
subcutaneous γ/δ T-cell lymphoma   97.61–97.63
subcutaneous glatiramer acetate injections   97.48–97.49
subcutaneous granuloma annulare   97.14–97.15
  rheumatoid nodule differentiation   97.16–97.17
subcutaneous granulomas   97.12, 97.54
subcutaneous lipomatosis   98.15–98.21
subcutaneous mycoses   32.69–32.80
Subcutaneous mycosis due to *Basidiobolus* and *Conidiobolus*   32.79–32.80
subcutaneous necrobiosis lipoidica   97.11
subcutaneous necrotising infections   26.77–26.78
subcutaneous nodules
  autoinflammatory diseases   **80.19**
  progressive nodular histiocytosis   135.19
  rheumatoid arthritis   155.5–155.6
  in systemic lupus erythematosus   51.28
subcutaneous panniculitis-like T-cell lymphoma   97.61–97.63, 139.29–139.31
subcutaneous panniculitis T-cell lymphoma (SPTCL)   97.39–97.40, 97.46, 97.61–97.63, 139.29–139.31
subcutaneous phycomycosis   32.79–32.80
subcutaneous sarcoidosis   96.3, 96.11–96.12, 97.53–97.54
subcutaneous Sweet syndrome   49.12, 97.51
subcutaneous tissue
  anatomy   97.2–97.3
  cellular composition   97.1–97.2
  vascularisation   97.6
subcutaneous tumours, juvenile hyaline fibromatosis   94.42
subcutaneous zygomycosis   32.79–32.80
subepidermal blistering   85.28
  heat-associated diseases   124.15, *124.16*
subepidermal nodular fibrosis see fibrous histiocytoma
subjective sensory irritation   128.10–128.11
sublamina densa blistering, antigen mapping   69.21
submammary flexural psoriasis   35.9
Sub-Saharan Africa, persons with albinism   7.10–7.11, 7.12, *7.13*
substance P (SP), pruritus   **81.3**, 81.4
subungual haematoma, sports injuries   122.16
subungual melanoma, presentation   142.10–142.11, *142.15*
succulent gums, neonates   114.4
suction blisters, neonates   114.4
sudamina see miliaria crystallina
sudoriparous angioma see eccrine angiomatous hamartoma
suicidality
  acne patients   88.39
  body dysmorphic disorder   84.13
  delusional infestation   84.7, 84.8, 84.9
  dermatological patients   84.41–84.42
  eating disorders   84.27
  isotretinoin acne treatment   84.42
  psychodermatology   84.2, 84.41–84.42
  recalcitrant itch   84.28
  risk assessment   84.41–84.42
  risk factors   **84.41**
  self-harm   84.38
  SSRI antidepressants   84.43
SUIs see sea urchin injuries
sulfasalazine, cutaneous adverse effects   155.15
sulphites, allergic reactions   127.56
sulphonamides, urticaria treatment   42.19

sulphonylureas, eczema 117.4
sulphur, acne vulgaris treatment 88.57
summary of product characteristics (SmPC), systemic therapy 19.2, 19.3
sunbed UVR exposure 10.13
  polymorphic light eruption 126.4
sunburn
  melanoma risk 142.6
  xeroderma pigmentosum 76.4
sun-damaged skin, melanomas 145.9, *145.11*, **145.11**
sunlight exposure
  children melanoma risk 142.6
  granuloma annulare 95.2
  infantile eosinophilic pustular folliculitis 91.7
  mechanical injuries 122.5
  melanoma risk 142.5–142.6, 145.9
  Merkel cell carcinoma risk 146.2–146.3
  occupational skin cancer 129.14
  pigmentation response 86.8–86.9, *86.44*, 86.46
  psoriasis vulgaris 35.4
  solar purpura 99.23–99.24
  sun-related dermatoses 7.8
  suppressing immune responses and permitting progression of immunogenic tumours 146.3
  UVR exposure 10.12–10.13
  UVR path lengths *10.3*
  see also ultraviolet radiation
sun protection factor (SPF), sunscreens 10.11–10.12
sunscreens 18.34–18.36
  photoallergic reactions 127.62, 127.79
  photopatch testing *126.31*
  photoprotection 10.11–10.12
  photosensitivity management 126.36–126.37
  porphyria, management of 58.5
superantigen toxins, recurrent perineal erythema 26.32
superficial actinic porokeratosis 85.21, 85.22–85.23
superficial angiomyxoma 136.59–136.60
superficial basal cell carcinoma (sBCC) 140.3, *140.4*, 140.6, *140.8*, 140.9, *140.11*
  mimicking Bowen disease *141.20*
  photodynamic therapy 22.6–22.7
  photothermal ablation 23.21
superficial burn wounds 125.6, 128.12
superficial chemical peels (SCPs) 160.4
superficial epidermolytic ichthyosis (SEI) 63.15–63.16, *63.18*
superficial fibromatoses 94.33
  palmar and plantar fibromatosis 136.12–136.13
superficial folliculitis 91.1–91.8
superficial haemosiderotic lymphovascular malformation *see* hobnail haemangioma
superficial mucocoeles, oral ulceration 108.42
superficial mycoses *see* dermatophytes
superficial onychomycosis (SO)
  caused by dermatophytes 32.47–32.48
  caused by non-dermatophyte moulds 32.54–32.55
superficial papillary adenomatosis *see* nipple, adenoma
superficial radiotherapy, basal cell carcinoma/squamous cell carcinoma 24.8–24.10
superficial spreading melanoma (SSM)
  melanoma classification 142.7, 142.8
  presentation 142.10, *142.11*, *142.12*, 142.20
superficial subcutaneous fat 97.3
superficial thrombophlebitis (STP) 97.8–97.9, *97.10*, 97.24
superficial ulceration, striae 94.8
superficial venous thrombosis 101.34–101.35
  clinical features **101.35**
  investigations for **101.35**

treatment **101.36**
  see also thrombophlebitis migrans
superficial X-ray therapy
  depth dose curves 24.1
  principles 24.1
  techniques and equipment 24.3
superinfections
  ichthyoses 63.46
  mal de Meleda 63.55
supernumerary ribs, Waardenburg syndrome 68.5
support surfaces, pressure ulcer prevention 123.8–123.9, 123.10
suppressor T cells, sensitisation reaction 127.9
suprabasal keratins, gene expression 2.8
suprabulbar region, hair follicles 87.4, 87.6
surfactants, allergies 127.59
surgeons, preoperative preparation 20.11
surgical complications 20.29, 20.33, 20.40–20.42, **20.41**
surgical smoke, hazards and risks of electrosurgery 20.45–20.46
surgical treatment 1.8
  auricle melanoma 106.32
  basal cell carcinoma 140.14–140.16
  body dysmorphic disorder 84.15
  burns 125.8
  compared to radiotherapy for basal cell or squamous cell carcinomas 24.8, **24.10**
  cutaneous squamous cell carcinoma 141.35
  cutaneous tuberculosis 27.10
  cutaneous warts 25.59
  during pregnancy 113.24
  hidradenitis suppurativa 90.10–90.11
  hyperhidrosis 92.9–92.10
  induced non-healing of wounds 84.33, *84.34*, 84.37
  lymphoedema 103.60–103.61
  melanoma 143.1–143.6
  perineal and perianal skin conditions 111.25–111.33
  pressure ulcers 123.11–123.12
  reconstruction principles of design 20.19–20.21
  tissue sampling for molecular genetic profiling of melanoma 144.1
  see also skin surgery
suspected deep tissue injury (SDTI), pressure ulcers **123.6**
Sustainable Development Goals (SDGs) 7.1, 7.6–7.7
sutural alopecia 87.30
sutures
  removal after skin surgery 20.40
  wound healing 11.10
suturing for skin surgery
  knot tying 20.12–20.14
  needles and materials 20.12
  techniques 20.14–20.19
swamp cancer *see Pythium insidiosum* infection
sweat duct carcinoma *see* adnexal carcinoma NOS
sweat gland abscesses, neonates 114.25
sweat gland carcinomas 137.33–137.40
sweat gland cellular inclusions, disorders with 92.15
sweat glands 2.2, 2.8–2.9, 2.43
  apoeccrine glands 2.9, 92.1
  disorders 92.1–92.22
  embryonic development 2.5
  inherited immunodeficiency **80.4–80.6**
  perspiration types 2.9
  tumours of skin appendages 137.1–137.2
  see also apocrine glands; eccrine glands
sweating
  atopic eczema 41.18–41.19
  cholinergic urticaria 42.11–42.12
  mechanical injuries 122.1
  neonates 114.3
  obesity 98.27

thermal 2.9
thermoregulation 92.3, 92.4
  see also hyperhidrosis
Sweden
  health economics, holistic perspective 6.2
  skin cancer, economic burden of 6.6, **6.7**
Sweet syndrome 49.8–49.15, 97.51
  associated diseases 49.8–49.10
  causative organisms 49.10
  classic Sweet syndrome 49.8, *49.11*
  clinical features 49.11–49.12
  clinical variants 49.12
  dermal infiltrate in lesional skin *49.14*
  diagnostic criteria **49.13**
  differential diagnosis 49.13
  disease course and prognosis 49.14
  drug-induced Sweet syndrome 49.8, 49.10–49.11
  drug reactions 49.8, 49.10–49.11, 149.6
  environmental factors 49.10–49.11
  epidemiology 49.8
  erythema nodosum with 97.21–97.23
  on face *49.12*
  genetics 49.10
  histiocytoid Sweet syndrome 49.12, *49.14*, 97.22–97.23, 149.6
  histology *49.11*
  investigations 49.14
  on leg *49.12*
  malignancy association 148.23–148.24, 149.6, 149.7
  management 49.14–49.15
  neutrophilic dermatosis of dorsal hands 49.12, *49.13*
  oral ulceration 108.41
  paraneoplastic forms 149.6–149.7
  pathology 49.10
  predisposing factors 49.10
  pseudovesicles within inflammatory plaques *49.11*
  reactivation in COVID-19 patients 25.112
  sarcoidosis association 96.15
  severity classification 49.14
  subcutaneous Sweet syndrome 49.12
  treatment for 49.14–49.15
  see also VEXAS syndrome
swelling
  eyelids 118.14, *118.16*, 129.6
  face 98.19, 103.46–103.49
  limbs 103.9–103.10, 103.16–103.17, 103.44–103.46
  mouth 95.14, 108.8–108.14, **108.9**, 127.72
  penoscrotal **109.20**
  vulva *95.15*
  see also loiasis; oedema
'swimmer's' itch *see* cercarial dermatitis
'swimmer's shoulder' 122.17
swimming pool granuloma (*Mycobacterium marinum*) 27.32–27.35
'Swiss cheese model', drug-related patient harm *13.10*
Switzerland, psoriasis, economic burden of 6.8
SWS *see* Sturge–Weber syndrome
sycosis 26.26–26.27
symmetrical acrokeratoderma 63.20
symmetrical drug-related intertriginous and flexural exanthema (SDRIFE) 127.46
symmetrical dyschromatoses 68.14–68.15
sympathectomy, hyperhidrosis treatment 92.9–92.10
sympathetic nerve endings, sweat glands 2.9
sympathetic nerve injury 83.20
sympathetic nerves, gustatory hyperhidrosis 92.8
sympathetic skin response (SSR), neurophysiological testing for skin innervation 83.5
symplastic haemangioma 136.31–136.32
symptoms, measurement tools 16.5
synaptophysin 3.23
syndecans 2.38

syndromic congenital ichthyosis 63.22–63.62
syndromic genodermatoses with nail anomalies **67.2–67.3**
syndromic hidradenitis suppurativa 90.2
syndromic ichthyosis **63.3**, 63.22–63.62
syndromic keratodermas 63.62–63.71
syndromic lymphoedema 103.20–103.22
syndromic palmoplantar keratoderma **63.57**
synophrys 107.4
synovitis, acne, pustulosis, hyperostosis and osteitis (SAPHO) syndrome 45.22, 88.7, 88.63
synthetic cannabinoid receptor agonists 120.2
synthetic coolants 129.1
synthetic retinoids 19.41–19.42
syphilis 29.1–29.29
  clinical features 29.5–29.20
  congenital 29.2, 29.22–29.29, 114.27–114.28
  congenital neonatal 114.27–114.28
  definition and nomenclature 29.2
  differential diagnoses 29.17–29.18
  endemic syphilis (bejel) 26.70
  epidemiology 29.2–29.3
  of eyebrows *105.12*
  eye involvement 107.39–107.40
  hair loss 29.10, *29.12*, 87.35
  HIV coinfection 31.21–31.22
  HIV relationship 29.16, 29.17
  investigations and tests 29.18–29.20
  latent stage 29.12
  late skin forms 29.12–29.14
  male genitalia 109.28
  management 29.20–29.22
  nephrotic syndrome 154.6
  ocular syphilis 29.16, 107.39–107.40
  oral involvement 108.34, 108.56
  pathophysiology 29.3–29.5
  perianal skin 111.16
  in pregnancy 113.6
  primary stage 29.6–29.7, 29.17
  pustule 'grape cluster' *1.6*
  rashes 29.7–29.10
  scalp infection 105.12
  secondary stage 29.7–29.12, 29.17–29.18
  sexual contact identification and treatment 29.22
  stages and course 29.5–29.6
  systemic features 29.10, 29.12
  tertiary/late stage 29.12–29.17, 29.18
  treatment for 1.7–1.8
syphilitic alopecia 29.10, *29.12*, 87.35
syphilitic leukoplakia 108.34
syringocystadenoma
  papilliferum 105.11, 137.19–137.20
  in sebaceous naevus 73.8
  see also syringoma
syringocystoma *see* syringoma
syringoid eccrine carcinoma (adnexal carcinoma NOS) 137.37
syringoma 4.8, 4.10, 137.27–137.28
  differential diagnosis 88.30
  malignant *see* microcystic adnexal carcinoma
  vulva **110.32**
syringomyelia 83.16–83.17
systematic reviews, critical appraisal for evidence based medicine 17.8–17.12
systematised linear porokeratosis 85.22
systemic absorption of topical therapies
  adverse effects 18.5
  application quantity 18.3
  corticosteroids 18.19–18.20
systemic allergic contact dermatitis (SACD), drug-induced eczema 117.3–117.5
systemically reactivated contact dermatitis 127.18–127.19
systemic amyloidoses with cutaneous involvement **56.3**, 56.10–56.13
  macroglossia *56.12*
  periorbital bleeding *56.11*

plasmacytoma-associated systemic
   amyloidosis   56.11
 treatment   56.14
systemic antibiotics   19.46–19.48
 hidradenitis suppurativa treatment
   90.9–90.10
systemic antihistamines   19.3–19.4
systemic autoimmune diseases, skin and
   renal involvement   154.6
systemic calcium homeostasis, cutaneous
   metastatic calcification   59.5–59.6
systemic candidiasis   32.92–32.93
systemic capillary leak syndrome (Clarkson
   syndrome)   43.4
systemic chondromalacia, *see also* relapsing
   polychondritis
systemic coagulopathies, purpura
   99.15–99.19
systemic component, histiocytosis
   135.14–135.29
systemic contact dermatitis, medicament
   allergens   127.46
systemic disorders
 acquired ichthyosis   63.48
 cardiac involvement   151.4–151.5
 causing pruritus   81.8–81.10
 changes in microbial ecology of the skin
   26.4
 hypermelanosis   86.19–86.25
 involving respiratory system   152.5–152.6
 liver disease with cutaneous features
   153.7–153.8
 mechanical injuries   122.1–122.2
systemic drug-induced photosensitivity
   126.27–126.28
systemic drug reactions   118.1, 118.4–118.12
systemic drug-related intertriginous and
   flexural exanthema (SDRIFE)
   117.5, 127.18
systemic drug treatment
 antifungal therapy   19.48, 40.9
 follicular eruptions   91.2–91.3
 hyperhidrosis   92.9
 phototherapy combination   21.10
 sarcoidosis   96.17
systemic features
 dermatomyositis   52.7–52.8
 sarcoidosis   96.5
systemic immunotherapy, cutaneous warts
   25.60
systemic juvenile idiopathic arthritis
   (SJIA/Still disease)   45.21–45.22,
   53.8, 53.9
systemic juvenile xanthogranuloma   135.17
systemic lupus erythematosus (SLE)   51.1,
   51.16–51.38, 87.55, 89.8
 age at onset   51.18
 antinuclear antibody (ANA) test
   51.34–51.36
 arthritis   51.30
 assessment of disease activity   51.36
 association with other diseases
   51.32–51.33
 autoantibodies   51.20–51.21
 bone changes   51.30
 bullous lesions   51.28–51.29
 cardiac involvement   151.4
 cardiovascular disease   51.30
 cell appearance   *51.18*
 'chilblain' lesions   *51.9*, 51.25
 in children   51.32
 classification   **51.16**
 clinical features   51.21–51.29
 complications and co-morbidities
   51.30–51.32
 in contraception   51.32
 coronary artery disease   51.30
 cutaneous features   **51.23**
 cutaneous vascular reactions   51.26–51.27
 Degos-like lesions   *51.27*
 diagnosis criteria   *51.17*
 differential diagnosis   51.29–51.30
 discoid lupus erythematosus
   relationship/comparison   51.6,
   51.9

disease course and prognosis   51.34
drug-induced SLE   51.21, **51.22**
dystrophic calcinosis   51.28
ear   51.32
in elderly people   51.32
environmental factors   51.21
epidemiology   51.17–51.18
eye   51.32
gastrointestinal tract   51.31
genetics   51.19–51.20
hair changes   51.25–51.26
hearing loss   51.32
heart   51.30
hepatic lesions   51.31
hormonal factors   51.21
and immune system   51.20–51.21
immunohistology   51.19
infections   51.21
internal malignancy association   148.21
internal organs   51.19
investigations   51.34–51.36
and Kikuchi–Fujimoto disease   51.33
leg ulcers   *51.26*
liver disease   51.31
lungs   51.31
'lupus hair' with diffuse alopecia   *51.26*
lupus nephritis, classification   **51.20**
lupus non-specific changes   51.25
lupus-specific changes   51.23–51.25
macroscopic/microscopic appearances
   51.18, *51.19*
management   51.36–51.38
mucinosis   51.28
mucous membrane lesions   51.29
muscle changes   51.30
nail changes   51.25
neurological disease   51.31–51.32
ocular changes   51.32
oral involvement   108.78
pathological features   **51.18**
pathophysiology   51.18–51.19
pigmentary changes   51.28
in pregnancy   51.32, 113.7–113.8
pulmonary system   51.31
renal changes   51.31
respiratory disease   152.2
rheumatoid arthritis comparison   51.30
skin features   51.19
stress   51.21
subcutaneous nodules   51.28
susceptible genes and pathways   **51.20**
thyroid disease   51.31
treatment of non-renal SLE   *51.37*
ultraviolet radiation   51.21
urticarial lesions   51.27–51.28
vasculitis   51.26
vasculopathy   51.26–51.27
systemic mastocytosis (SM)   46.2, *46.4*, 46.6
systemic mucormycosis   32.93
systemic mycoses   32.80–32.94
 identification   32.80–32.81
 pathophysiology   32.80
systemic neoplasia
 associated skin conditions   148.1–148.28
 see also internal malignancy
systemic non-eczematous reactions to
   allergens   127.21
systemic-onset juvenile idiopathic arthritis
   (SoJIA/Still disease)   45.21–45.22,
   53.8, 53.9
systemic photodynamic therapy   22.2
systemic retinoid therapy *see* retinoids
   (systemic therapy)
systemic sarcoidosis   96.7, 96.15–96.16
systemic sclerosis (SSc)   3.44, 54.1–54.29,
   86.20–86.21, 94.45
 age of onset   54.7–54.8
 associated diseases   54.8–54.10
 autoantibodies
   and clinical associations   **54.5–54.6**
   type and frequency   **54.9**
 calcinosis   54.17, **54.26**
 cancer risk   54.9–54.10
 cardiac involvement   54.17–54.18, **54.23**,
   151.4

cardiopulmonary manifestations
   54.17–54.18
cardiorespiratory pulmonary fibrosis
   54.23
causative organisms   54.13
cellular and molecular pathogenesis
   54.12
chemotherapy   54.25–54.26
classification   54.1–54.2, **54.7**
clinical features   **54.2, 54.5–54.6**,
   54.15–54.18
clinical variants   54.18
complications and co-morbidities   54.21
connective tissue disease   54.8–54.9
critical digital ischaemia/ulceration
   54.25
cutaneous manifestations   54.15–54.17
diagnosis   54.21–54.22
differential diagnosis   54.18–54.20
diffuse cutaneous   **54.2**
digital ulceration   54.17, **54.25**
disease assessment   **54.17**
disease course and prognosis   54.21
disease modifying drugs, targets for
   54.27
dyspigmentation   54.17
dystrophic calcification   59.1, 59.2
endothelial-to-mesenchymal transition
   54.10
environmental and drug-induced
   94.45–94.46
environmental factors   54.14–54.15
epidemiology   54.7–54.8
erectile dysfunction   54.28
fibrosis   54.11–54.13
gastrointestinal manifestations   54.17,
   54.23
genetics   54.13–54.14
histopathology   *54.12*
history   54.15
immune-mediated inflammation
   54.10–54.11
incidence and prevalence   54.7
internal malignancy association   148.21
investigations   54.21, 54.22, **54.23–54.24**,
   54.26
limited cutaneous SSc   **54.2**
localised scleroderma cutaneous
   assessment tool   **55.33–55.34**
lung involvement   **54.26**
malignancy risk   54.9–54.10
management   54.22–54.29, **54.26**, *54.28*
 targets for disease modifying drugs
   54.27
mechanical properties   122.5
modified Rodnan skin score   **54.17**
muscle involvement   54.18
musculoskeletal manifestations   54.18
oral involvement   108.68–108.69
organ-based disease assessment   54.22
pathogenesis   *54.27*
pathophysiology   54.10–54.13
predisposing factors   54.10
presentation   54.15–54.18
pruritus   54.16, **54.26**
pulmonary manifestations   54.18, **54.26**
Raynaud phenomenon   *54.3*, 54.15, *54.22*
 causes and clinical features   **54.19**
 investigation and management   **54.25**
renal manifestations   54.18, **54.24**
respiratory disease   152.2
scleroderma spectrum disorders   **54.19**,
   55.1
scleromyxoedema comparison   57.5
severity classification   54.20–54.21
skin thickening   54.15–54.16
synonyms and inclusions   54.1
telangiectasia   54.16–54.17, **54.26**
tendon friction rubs   54.18
terminology   55.1
vasculopathy   54.10, **54.25**
 see also morphoea; sclerosis
systemic therapy   19.1–19.50
 anti-inflammatory and
   immunomodulatory drugs
   19.2–19.46

drug interactions   19.2
hidradenitis suppurativa   90.9–90.10
ichthyoses   63.44–63.45
melanoma   144.1–144.12
patient education   19.2
patient selection   19.1–19.2
prescribing and monitoring practice   19.2
recessive dystrophic epidermolysis bullosa
   69.26
record keeping   19.2
risk reduction   19.1–19.2, 19.3
standards of care   19.1
versus topical therapy   19.1
vitiligo   86.39–86.40

T

TA *see* tufted angioma
tabanid flies (*Chrysops* species)   33.12
 see also loiasis
tabetic neurosyphilis   29.15–29.16
tacalcitol, topical therapies   18.28
tachykinins, pruritus   **81.3**, 81.4
tachyphylaxis
 corticosteroids   18.20
 systemic glucocorticoid therapy   19.19
tacrolimus
 topical therapies   18.22, **18.23**
 wound healing   11.12
TAD *see* transient acantholytic dermatosis
Taenia solium, cysticercosis   33.32–33.34
TAK *see* transient aquagenic keratoderma
Takayasu arteritis   100.34–100.35
Talaromyces marneffei (penicilliosis)   31.28,
   32.89–32.90
Talimogene laherparepvec (T-vec), oncolytic
   virus therapy   144.1
talk therapies
 body dysmorphic disorder   84.14
 cognitive behavioural therapy   84.47
 combined somatic/psychological
   disorders   84.47–84.48
 habit reversal therapies   84.12, 84.15,
   84.17, 84.18, 84.20, 84.21, 84.25, 84.47
 nodular prurigo   *84.18*
 skin related health anxieties   84.26
tanapox virus (TANV)   25.19
tanning
 ability variation/skin types   2.18, **86.9**,
   142.3
 melanoma risk   142.3
 physiology of   68.1, 86.9
 sunbed use   10.13
 sun-reactive skin types   **86.9**
 UVR exposure   10.7–10.8
TANV *see* tanapox virus
Tanzania, Regional Dermatology Training
   Centre   7.7
tapeworms *see* cestodes
tapinarof, psoriasis treatment   35.22
targeted oncology therapies   87.73,
   144.4–144.5, **144.11**, **144.11**, 144.12
target lesions   *4.15*
targetoid haemosiderotic haemangioma *see*
   hobnail haemangioma
targetoid haemosiderotic naevus
   131.30–131.32
tars, topical therapies   18.36–18.37
tattoo granulomas, photothermal ablation
   23.23
tattoos
 allergic granulomatous reactions   127.21
 amalgam tattoos, mouth   108.15
 body art, mouth   108.15–108.16
 foreign body reactions   122.21–122.22
 hair disorders   87.101
 hypermelanosis   86.53–86.54
 mercury allergy   127.41
 p-phenylenediamine allergy   127.60
 pseudoepitheliomatous hyperplasia
   132.9, *132.10*
 removal by laser treatment   23.12–23.15
tattoo sarcoidosis   96.11
taxane, palmoplantar erythrodysaesthesia
   119.2
tazarotene, topical therapies   18.25–18.26

TBHQ see t-butylhydroquinone
TBI see total body irradiation
TBSA see total body surface area
t-butylhydroquinone (TBHQ) 127.59
TCA CROSS see trichloroacetic acid chemical reconstruction of skin scars
TCDD see 2,3,7,8-Tetrachlorodibenzo-p-dioxin-p-dioxin
T-cell leukaemia–lymphomas, cells of origin 139.3
T-cell lymphoma
  panniculitis-like 97.61–97.63
  positive staining of atypical cells 3.28
  radiotherapy 24.16, 24.18
  see also cutaneous T-cell lymphoma
T-cell-mediated drug hypersensitivity 14.3–14.4
  acute generalised exanthematous pustulosis 14.4
  drug reaction with eosinophilia and systemic symptoms 14.3–14.4, 14.7
  Stevens–Johnson syndrome 14.3, 14.7
  toxic epidermal necrolysis 14.3, 14.7
T-cell pseudolymphoma 134.1–134.2
T-cell receptor gene analysis, mycosis fungoides 139.6–139.8
T-cell recognition of drugs 14.4–14.6
  altered peptide repertoir model 14.6
  hapten/pro-hapten model 14.5–14.6
  MHC–peptide–TCR interaction 14.4, 14.5
  pharmacological interaction model 14.5, 14.6
T cells 9.4, 9.5–9.7, 14.4, 14.5, 50.2, 127.9
T-cells
  activation 2.12, 14.4
  allergens binding to 127.7
  allergic contact dermatitis 9.10
  dermis 2.15
  immune system 9.3–9.6, 103.3
  in pemphigus 50.2
T-cell theory, drug-specific 118.5
TCI see topical calcineurin inhibitors
TDT see thermal damage time
TE see telogen effluvium
tear film, precorneal 107.3
tea tree oil, allergy to 127.71
TEC see toxic erythema of chemotherapy
Technetium-99 bone scintigraphy 124.2, 124.3
Tedania ignis, stings from 130.3
TEE see transepidermal elimination; transepithelial elimination
Teenagers' Quality of Life Index (T-QoL) 16.10
teenagers, see also adolescents
teeth
  anatomy of 108.4
  betel staining 108.15
  congenital syphilis 29.26, 29.28
  dental plaque 108.5
  epidermolysis bullosa presentation 69.17, 69.18
  eruption cyst 108.10
  eruption cyst over a primary tooth 108.10
  incontinentia pigmenti presentation 68.11
  methamphetamine-induced tooth decay 120.5
  pachyonychia congenita presentation 67.12
  periodontal Ehlers–Danlos syndrome 70.5, 70.10
  phantom tooth pain/trigeminal neuropathic pain 82.5–82.7
  tooth decay, methamphetamine-induced 120.5
teething, flushing in children 104.10
telangiectases 101.10–101.22, 101.39, 101.44
  angiokeratomas 101.13–101.14, 101.17
  angioma serpiginosum 101.16, 101.17, 101.18, 101.18
  causes of 101.10
  cherry angiomas 101.12–101.13, 101.17
  facial 23.9–23.10
  generalised essential telangiectasia 101.17, 101.18–101.19

hereditary benign telangiectasia 101.17, 101.20, 101.21
histology 101.10
laser therapies 23.6, 23.9–23.11, 23.12
leg veins 23.11
pathophysiology 101.10
primary telangiectasias 101.16, 101.17, 101.18
spider telangiectases 101.10–101.12, 101.17
unilateral naevoid telangiectasia syndrome 101.20–101.22
venous lakes 101.14–101.16, 101.17
telangiectasia
  atrophic stria with 94.8
  hereditary haemorrhagic telangiectasia 71.12–71.13
  hereditary haemorrhagic telangiectasia (Osler–Rendu–Weber syndrome) 108.26
  metastatic carcinoma 148.3–148.4
  necrobiosis lipoidica 95.11
  oral involvement 108.27
  Rothmund–Thomson syndrome 75.5
  skin lesions associated with gastrointestinal disorders 153.7
  systemic sclerosis 54.16–54.17, 54.26
  see also hereditary haemorrhagic telangiectasia; spider telangiectases
telangiectasia, elevated erythropoietin and erythrocytosis, monoclonal gammopathy, perinephric fluid collections and intrapulmonary shunting (TEMPI) syndrome 149.12
telangiectasia macularis eruptiva perstans (TMEP) 46.1, 46.5
telangiectatic metastatic carcinoma 148.3–148.4
telangiectatic rosacea 89.9
  major features 89.6, 89.7, 89.12
  pathology 89.3
  treatment 89.14
teledermatology 1.9, 4.25–4.26, 5.13, 7.8–7.9
Tel Hashomer criteria, familial Mediterranean fever diagnosis 45.10
telogen effluvium (TE) 87.13, 87.53–87.60
  COVID-19 association 25.113
telogen (hair follicle resting phase) 87.7–87.8, 87.21, 87.57
telogen release, hair fall 87.53
telomeres, dyskeratosis congenita 67.13
telomere shortening, skin ageing 2.45–2.46
'telomeropathies' 67.13
temperature-dependent urticaria 42.9, 42.10–42.11
TEMPI (telangiectasia, elevated erythropoietin and erythrocytosis, monoclonal gammopathy, perinephric fluid collections and intrapulmonary shunting) syndrome 149.12
temporal triangular alopecia (TTA) 87.28
TEN see toxic epidermal necrolysis
tendon friction rubs, systemic sclerosis 54.18
tendon xanthomas 60.2–60.3
tennis toe 122.16
tenosynovial fibroma 136.11
tenosynovial giant cell tumour 136.19
tensile strength, elastic tissue 94.21
teratogenicity
  methotrexate 19.26
  mycophenolate 19.29
  retinoid therapy 19.43, 19.44
  thalidomide 19.45, 19.46
terbinafine, dermatophytosis treatment 32.32
terminology
  commonly used dermatopathological terms 3.38–3.43
  standardisation of 1.4, 1.5
terpenes, allergic contact dermatitis 127.42–127.43

terra firme forme see dermatitis passivata
tertiary syphilis 29.12–29.17, 29.18
'tertiary teledermatology' 4.26
TERT telomerase gene, melanoma risk 142.5
testis, torsion of 109.25
testosterone, hair growth stimulation 87.10
tetanus immunisation, bites 130.6
2,3,7,8-tetrachlorodibenzo-p-dioxin-p-dioxin (TCDD) 129.12
tetracyclines 19.47, 19.48
  hypermelanosis 86.27–86.28
  topical therapies 18.12
tetraethylthiuram disulphide, eczema 117.4
tetraspanins, epidermolysis bullosa 69.4
TEWL see transepidermal water loss
Texier disease 97.50
textile dermatitis 127.65–127.67
textile dyes, genital contact dermatitis 109.13
texture of skin, matching principles in surgical design 20.21
TFIIH see transcription/DNA repair factor IIH
TGF see transforming growth factor
TGF-β binding proteins see latent transforming growth factor beta binding proteins
TGM1 mutations, congenital ichthyosiform erythroderma 63.12
TH2 activity, alopecia areata 87.22
thalidomide 19.44–19.45
  dermatological uses 19.44
  pharmacological properties 19.44–19.45
  potential adverse effects 19.45
  safety considerations 19.45–19.46
  sarcoidosis treatment 96.17
thallium, dermatological reactions 121.8–121.9
theque, definition 3.43
therapeutic relationship between clinician and patient 84.47
therapeutic window, clinical pharmacology 13.2
therapy
  assessing benefit to patients, Patient Benefit Index tool 16.5
  decisions, appraising clinical trials 17.12–17.13
  principles of topical therapy 18.1–18.42
Theridiidae (widow spiders) 34.34–34.35
thermal damage time (TDT), light assisted hair removal 23.5–23.6
thermal relaxation time (TRT), of skin chromophores 23.5
thermal sweating 2.9
thermokinetic selectivity, laser treatments 23.6
thermolipolysis, fat contouring 161.9
thermoplastics, allergic contact dermatitis 127.68
thermoregulation 2.9, 2.42–2.43
thermoregulatory sweating 92.3, 92.4
THET see Tropical Health and Education Trust
thiamine (vitamin B1) deficiency 61.13–61.14
thickening of skin, diabetic patients 62.5–62.6
thigh
  cicatricial pemphigoid 50.52
  cryopyrin-associated periodic syndrome 45.9
  cutaneous small-vessel vasculitis 100.7
  erythema multiforme 47.2
  hemihyperplasia–multiple lipomatosis syndrome 72.11
  lichen striatus 37.18
  linear IgA disease 50.37
  massive localised lymphoedema 103.53
  microtrauma to 98.9
  urticaria pigmentosa 46.4
thiomersal, allergic reactions 127.3–127.5
thiopurine methyl transferase (TPMT), polymorphism affecting

azathioprine metabolism 19.8–19.9, 19.10
thioureas 127.65
thiuram mix (sensitisers) 127.63–127.64
thiurams 127.64
thorax, pulmonary haemorrhage, microscopic polyangiitis 100.21
Thost–Unna keratoderma 63.53
threadworm see enterobiasis
Three Item Severity Score (TIS) 16.4
thrips (Thysanoptera) 34.30
thromboangiitis obliterans 101.3–101.6
  causative organisms 101.6
  clinical features 101.6
  epidemiology 101.4
  investigations for 101.6
  ischaemic toes 101.6
  management of 101.7
  pathophysiology 101.5–101.6
  vascular occlusion and corkscrew collaterals 101.7
thrombocytopenia, purpura 31.12, 31.14, 99.2–99.4
thrombocytosis, purpura 99.3–99.4, 99.10–99.11
thrombophlebitis, neoplasia association 148.26
thrombophlebitis migrans 101.35–101.36
thrombosis see venous thrombosis
thrush see candidiasis
thumbnail, lichen planus 37.12
thymol, traditional topical therapy 18.38
thyroid disease
  myxoedema 57.11–57.14
  systemic lupus erythematosus 51.31
thyroid dysfunction, drug reaction with eosinophilia and systemic symptoms 118.9, 118.11
thyroid dysfunction (hyper/hypothyroidism), dermatoendocrinology 150.7, 150.10, 150.11, 150.19–150.20
thyroiditis, granuloma annulare 95.1
thyroid medullary cancer, flushing 104.7, 148.26
thyrotoxicosis, pruritus 81.10
thyroxine, urticaria treatment 42.19
Thysanoptera (thrips) 34.30
ticks (Acari) 34.37–34.41
  anaphylactic reactions to bites 14.2
  carried diseases 26.66–26.67, 26.72, 26.82–26.83, 34.39–34.41
'tick typhus', rickettsial infections 26.82–26.83
'tiger-tail pattern', trichothiodystrophy 63.37
tight junctions 2.20–2.21
Time Trade-Off (TTO), quality of life assessment 16.9
TIMPs see tissue inhibitors of metalloproteinases
tinea
  allergic reactions 32.50
  granuloma annulare mistaken for 95.5
  penis/scrotum 109.27–109.28
  steroid-modified infections 32.50
  see also dermatophytosis
tinea barbae 32.40–32.41
tinea capitis 32.37–32.40, 87.24
  clinical features 32.38
  clinical variants 32.38–32.39
  epidemiology 32.37–32.38
  infants 115.8–115.9
  infection control 32.31–32.32, 32.40
  late sequelae of radio treatment 24.4, 24.8, 24.21
  management 32.40
  pathophysiology 32.38
tinea circinata see tinea corporis
tinea corporis 4.10, 32.35–32.37
  clinical features 32.35–32.37
  corticosteroid effects 32.49–32.50
  discoid skin lesions 39.10
  infants 115.8

management 32.37
pathophysiology 32.35
tinea cruris 32.45–32.46
    female genitalia 110.28
tinea faciei 32.41–32.42, 89.10
    infants 115.8
tinea incognito, female genitalia 110.28
tinea manuum 32.44–32.45
tinea nigra (pityriasis nigra) 1
tinea nigra (tinea nigra palmaris/pityriasis nigra) 32.14–32.15
tinea nodosa see black piedra
tinea peddis 32.42–32.44
    clinical features 32.43–32.44
    epidemiology 32.42
    management 32.44
    pathophysiology 32.42–32.43
    sports association 122.16
tinea tonsurans see tinea capitis
tinea unguium (onychomycosis caused by dermatophytes) 32.47–32.49
tinea versicolor/tinea flavea see pityriasis versicolor
TIS see Three Item Severity Score
tissue-bound autoantibodies
    bullous pemphigoid 50.13–50.14
    mucous membrane pemphigoid 50.25
tissue cooling, avoiding epidermal heat damage during laser therapies 23.6
tissue engineering, wound healing 11.11–11.13
tissue inhibitors of metalloproteinases (TIMPs) 2.32
    wound healing 11.5
tissue injury, alpha-1 antitrypsin 97.44
tissue macrophages, microscopic examination of 3.36
tissue optics, fate of incident light on skin 23.3–23.4
tissue-processing machine 3.7
tissue tightening therapies 161.6–161.8
tixocortol pivalate, allergic reactions 127.47
TKIs see tyrosine kinase inhibitors
TL-01 UVB see narrow-band UVB
TLR-4 see Toll-like receptor
TMD see transient myeloproliferative disorder
TMEP see telangiectasia macularis eruptiva perstans
TN see trichorrhexis nodosa; trigeminal neuralgia
TNF-α, sarcoidosis 96.4
TNF-α inhibitors
    cutaneous adverse effects 155.15
    psoriasis treatment 35.27
    sarcoidosis treatment 96.17
TNF-inhibitor-associated alopecia 87.34–87.35
TNM (tumour, node, metastases) classification, oral squamous cell carcinoma 108.47, **108.48**
tobacco smoke exposure
    ageing of skin 156.4
    atopic eczema 41.7
tobacco use
    keratoses 108.33
    oral hyperpigmentation 108.16–108.17
    oral squamous cell carcinoma 108.46
    types 108.33
    see also smoking
tocilizumab
    morphoea treatment 55.39
    systemic sclerosis treatment 54.24
tocopherol 127.59
toe
    acquired digital fibrokeratoma 136.4
    acral fibromyxoma 136.59
    bandaging, lymphoedema therapy 103.59
    'chilblain' lesions 51.9
    discoid lupus erythematosus 51.8
    epidermolysis bullosa acquisita 50.45
    fibro-osseous pseudotumour of the digits 136.6

frostbite 124.2, *124.3*
lymphoedema 103.6
neuropathic ulcer 83.14, 83.15
perniosis 124.6
pretibial myxoedema 103.42
primary localised cutaneous amyloidosis 56.8
psoriatic arthritis 35.41
systemic sclerosis 54.4
see also phalanges
toe cleft intertrigo (athletes foot), see also tinea peddis
toe clefts, microbiome 26.3, 26.5
toenail dystrophy 63.51
    epidermolysis bullosa 69.17
    pachyonychia congenita 67.1, *67.11*
toenails
    lichen planus 37.12
    metal poisoning signs 121.1
    see also nails
toe systolic BP, peripheral vascular disease **101.4**
tofacitinib, psoriasis treatment 35.27
togaviruses 25.80, 25.87–25.93
Toll-like receptor 4 (TLR-4) 127.7
Toll-like receptors, transmembrane drug mechanisms 13.5
Toll-like receptor signalling, skin defence against pathogens 26.5, 26.6
tolnaftate, topical therapies 18.12–18.13
toluene-2,5-diamine 127.60–127.61
tombstone comedones, hidradenitis suppurativa 90.5
tongue
    amyloidosis 108.69–108.70
    anatomy of 108.4
    angioedema 108.10
    ankyloglossia 108.87
    black hairy tongue 108.16, *108.17*
    brown tongue 108.16
    candidiasis 108.32
    circumvallate papillae *108.7*
    coated tongue 108.16
    dorsum, examination of 108.7
    examination of 108.7
    fissured tongue 108.87–108.88
    fungiform papillae *108.7*
    furred tongue 108.52
    geographic tongue (benign migratory glossitis/erythema migrans) 108.24
        in patient with psoriasis 35.13
    glossitis 108.22, 108.24–108.25
    herpes simplex lingual recurrence *108.71*
    herpetic stomatitis 108.52
    Kawasaki disease 115.10
    leiomyoma 108.13
    leukoplakia 75.3
    linear IgA disease 50.37
    lingual erythema migrans 108.24
    lingual thyroid 108.11
    lingual tonsil 108.11
    macroglossia 108.11–108.12, *108.69*
        primary systemic amyloidosis 56.12
    median rhomboid glossitis 108.22
    multiple endocrine neoplasia 108.13–108.14, *108.13*, 148.10
    oral lichen planus *108.77*
    osteoma mucosae 108.14
    piercing of (body art) 108.16
    pigmented lesions 108.15
    polyarteritis nodosa 108.69
    scrotal tongue *108.87*
    squamous cell carcinoma *108.46*
    strawberry tongue 108.25
    strawberry tongue, Kawasaki disease *115.10*
    venous malformation 71.15
    ventrum, examination of 108.7
tongue cancer patient, facial lymphoedema *103.48*
tonofilament aggregates, pachyonychia congenita 63.52
'tonotubular' PPK 63.50
tophaceous gout 155.9, *155.10*

topical anaesthetics, biopsy 3.2–3.3
topical calcineurin inhibitors (TCI), atopic eczema treatment 41.27
topical dressings, burn management 125.8
topical drug delivery 12.1–12.9
    absorbed dose 12.4
    advice/instructions for patients 18.4
    application quantity and frequency 18.3–18.4
    bioavailability/bioequivalence assessment 12.7–12.8
        in vitro methods 12.7
        in vivo methods 12.7–12.8
    creams 12.3–12.4
    drug concentration 18.1–18.2
    drug structure/properties and skin permeation 12.2–12.3
    efficacy influences 18.2
    efficiency of 12.4
    flux measurement 12.3, 12.4, 12.5
    formulation design and dosage choice 12.5
    formulation 'metamorphosis' 12.6–12.7
    formulations 12.3–12.4
    hazards 18.4–18.5
    hydrocarbon-based formulations 12.3
    'metamorphosis' of formulation 12.6–12.7
    non-volatile residual phase design 12.6–12.7
    patient-centred optimisation 12.4–12.7
    percutaneous absorption mechanisms 12.1–12.2
    polar gel formulations 12.3
    saturated solutions
        with partitioning and diffusion enhancers 12.6
        with partitioning enhancers 12.5–12.6
        simple solutions 12.5
    skin barrier function 12.1
topical photosensitisation, photodynamic therapy 22.2
topical therapies
    acne 129.12
    actinic keratosis 141.8–141.10
    acute herpetic neuralgia 82.4
    advice/instructions for patients 18.4
    antibiotics 18.10–18.12
    antifungal agents 18.12–18.13, 32.33–32.34, 40.8
    anti-inflammatory agents 40.8–40.9
    antineoplastic agents 18.29–18.31
    antiparasitic agents 18.13–18.14
    antiseptics 18.9–18.10, 123.11
    antiviral agents 18.13, 25.23–25.24
    application frequency 18.3
    application quantity 18.3–18.4
    astringents 18.9
    atopic eczema 41.27
    basal cell carcinoma 140.11, 140.12
    Bowen disease 141.23, 141.24
    calcineurin inhibitors 18.22–18.26, 41.27
    corticosteroids/glucocorticoids 18.14–18.22, 46.10, 129.12
    cutaneous T-cell lymphoma 139.21–139.22
    cutaneous warts 25.59–25.60
    cytotoxic agents 18.29–18.31
    depigmenting agents 18.31–18.33
    drug concentration 18.1–18.2
    efficacy influences 18.2
    emollients 18.8–18.9
    erythema multiforme-like reactions to 47.4–47.5
    formulations 18.5–18.8
    hazards 18.4–18.5
    herpes simplex infections 25.23–25.24
    hidradenitis suppurativa 90.9
    hyperhidrosis 92.8–92.9
    immunotherapy 25.59–25.60
    impetigo 26.16
    keratolytics 40.8
    lidocaine 82.4
    mastocytosis 46.10
    minoxidil 87.70, 87.73, 87.94

occlusion 18.21
phototherapy combination 21.10
potency classification of corticosteroids 18.14–18.15, **18.16**
prescribing 18.1–18.4
pressure ulcers 123.11
primary localised cutaneous amyloidosis 56.13–56.14
principles 18.1–18.42
prostaglandins 87.94–87.95
retinoids 18.23–18.26
seborrhoeic dermatitis 40.8
systemic absorption and effects 18.3, 18.5
traditional remedies 18.38
vehicles 12.3–12.4, 18.2–18.3, 18.5–18.8
vitamin D analogues 18.26–18.29
TORCH syndrome, viral infections 25.221
tori mandibularis 108.7, *108.8*
torso involvement, dermatomyositis 52.4–52.5, *52.6*
torus palatinus 108.7, *108.8*
total body irradiation (TBI), lipodystrophy association 98.8–98.9
total body surface area (TBSA), burn size 125.1–125.2
totally dystrophic onychomycosis 32.48
total skin electron beam therapy (TSEBT)
    cutaneous T-cell lymphoma 139.20–139.21, 139.22
    mycosis fungoides 24.16, *24.17*
touch domes 2.12
touch perception 2.12
Touton cells, juvenile xanthogranuloma 135.15
Touton giant cell 3.36
Townes–Brocks syndrome **106.7**
toxic epidermal necrolysis (TEN) 47.1–47.2
    arsenic 121.2
    management 107.33–107.34
    ocular complications 107.32–107.33
    renal effects 154.6
    and Stevens–Johnson syndrome 47.1–47.2, 107.32–107.34, 108.79, 118.1–118.2, 118.10, 118.12–118.22
    T-cell-mediated drug hypersensitivity 14.3, 14.7
toxic erythema of chemotherapy (TEC) 119.1–119.2
toxic erythema of the newborn 114.5–114.6
Toxicodendron species dermatitis 127.5, 127.11, 127.71–127.72, 127.73–127.74
toxic pustuloderma 118.1
toxic reactions, local anaesthetics 20.7–20.8
toxic shock syndrome (TSS) 26.30–26.32
    clinical features 26.30–26.31
    epidemiology 26.30
    management 26.32
    pathophysiology 26.30
    streptococcal 26.30, 26.36–26.37
    see also streptococcal toxic shock-like syndrome
toxins
    bacterial 26.32, 26.35–26.37, 26.38
    botulinum 26.43, 159.1–159.9
    cutaneous T-cell lymphoma therapy 139.25
    metals 121.1–121.10
    see also cytotoxic agents
Toxocara canis see visceral larva migrans
Toxocara cati see visceral larva migrans
Toxocara malayensis see visceral larva migrans
toxocariasis (visceral larva migrans) 33.20–33.21
toxoplasmosis 33.54–33.55
    clinical features 33.54
    management 33.54–33.55
    pathophysiology 33.54
TPMT see thiopurine methyl transferase
T-QoL see Teenagers' Quality of Life Index
trace elements
    hypermetabolism treatment 125.12
    resuscitation use 125.4
traction alopecia 87.31–87.32, 87.42
traditional remedies see complementary/alternative/traditional therapies; herbals

training programmes/resources
  for dermatologists 7.8
  for dermatology 7.11–7.12
  health care workers 7.8
  teledermatology 7.9
  see also educational partnerships; patient education
tralokinumab, systemic therapy 19.36–19.37
tranexamic acid
  cosmeceutical use of 157.4
  urticaria treatment 42.19
transaldolase deficiency 70.16
transaminitis, haemophagocytic lymphohistiocytosis 135.12
transcription/DNA repair factor IIH (TFIIH) 63.37
transcriptomics
  immune system 9.2–9.3
  skin ageing 2.46
transepidermal elimination (TEE) 94.53–94.55
transepidermal water loss (TEWL) 12.1, 128.2–128.3, 128.6
  atopic eczema 41.23
  irritant contact dermatitis 129.5
  neonates 14.2
  skin barrier function assessment 16.5
  xerosis cutis 85.26
transepithelial elimination (TEE), pseudoxanthoma elasticum 94.30
transforming growth factor (TGF) 71.2
transfusion-associated graft-versus-host disease 149.15
transfusion reactions, skin involvement 149.15
transgender patients, hair loss 87.71
transglutaminase-1, congenital ichthyosiform erythroderma 63.11
transglutaminase 1 deficient skin 63.15
transglutaminase 5 (*TGM5*), skin fragility disorders 69.5
transient acantholytic dermatosis (TAD/Grover disease) 85.23–85.25, 148.17
transient aquagenic keratoderma (TAK) 63.61–63.62
transient erythema *see* flushing
transient myeloproliferative disorder (TMD), neonatal pustulosis of 114.8
transient pustular melanosis, neonates 114.7–114.8
transmission electron microscopy
  dermal–epidermal basement membrane zone 2.22
  elastic fibres 2.34
  epidermolysis bullosa diagnosis 69.21–69.22
  fibroblasts 2.40, 156.9
transplants *see* graft versus host disease; organ transplant recipients
transport media, biopsy 3.4–3.5, **3.5**
transposition flaps, surgical reconstruction **20.24**, 20.26
TRAPS *see* tumour necrosis factor receptor-associated periodic syndrome
trauma
  dystrophic calcification of skin and subcutaneous tissues 59.3
  male genitalia 109.8–109.9
  morphoea association 55.13–55.14
  scratching/manipulating skin, trigeminal trophic syndrome 82.7–82.8
trauma-induced lymphoedema 103.40
traumatic lesions, female genitalia 110.42–110.43
traumatic neuroma 136.43
traumatic panniculitis 97.50, 97.54–97.56
traumatic ulcerative granuloma with stromal eosinophilia (TUGSE), oral ulceration 108.37
travel abroad, cutaneous leishmaniasis 33.51
Treacher Collins syndrome 106.5, **106.7**

treadmill test, peripheral vascular disease **101.4**
tree balsams 127.42
tree moss allergy 127.45, 127.73
tregeminal neuralgia *see* trigeminal neuralgia
Tregs (regulatory T cells) 127.9
trematodes 33.26–33.31
trench fever, *Bartonella quintana* 26.62
trench foot 124.4–124.5
trench mouth *see* acute necrotising (ulcerative) gingivitis and noma
Treponema pallidum
  subsp. *carateum*, pinta 26.71–26.72
  subsp. *endemicum*, endemic syphilis 26.70
  subsp. *pertenue*, yaws 26.70–26.71
Treponema pallidum subsp. *pallidum* 29.2, 29.3–29.5
treponematoses
  differential diagnosis 29.4, 29.12, 29.19
  endemic/non-venereal 26.69–26.72
  eye 107.39–107.40
  microbiology 29.5
  see also syphilis; yaws
tretinoin, *see also* retinoic acid
triangular lunula, nail dysplasia with 67.15, 67.16
triangular shape melanonychia, melanoma involving nail unit 145.13
Triatominae (assassin bugs) 34.29
triazole antifungals 19.48
trichiasis 119.6
trichilemmal carcinoma 137.7
trichilemmal cysts (pilar cysts) 105.11, 133.4–133.5, *133.6*, 137.5–137.6
trichilemmal tumour proliferating 137.5–137.6
trichilemmoma 137.6–137.7
trichinelliasis *see* trichinosis
trichinellosis *see* trichinosis
trichiniasis *see* trichinosis
trichinosis 33.24–33.26
  clinical features 33.25
  management 33.25–33.26
  pathophysiology 33.24–33.25
trichloroacetic acid
  caustic agent for skin surgery 20.47
  chemical peels 160.2–160.3, 160.10
trichloroacetic acid chemical reconstruction of skin scars (TCA CROSS) 160.6
trichoadenoma 137.4–137.5
trichobacteriosis *see* trichomycosis
trichobezoar 84.24
trichoblastic fibroma *see* trichoblastoma
trichoblastoma 137.11–137.12
trichoblastoma spectrum, trichoepithelioma 137.9–137.10
trichochrome B *86.7*
trichochromes 86.5, *86.6*
trichodiscomas 137.15
  histology of *78.15*
trichodynia 87.54
  COVID-19 association 25.113
trichodysplasia spinulosa polyomavirus (TSPyV/TSV/HPyV-8) 25.48, 85.15–85.17, 87.36
trichoepithelioma 105.11, 137.9–137.10
  photothermal ablation 23.21
trichofolliculoma 137.8–137.9
trichogenic fibroma *see* trichoblastoma
trichograms 87.14, 87.55
trichokinesis 105.14
tricholemmal cysts *see* trichilemmal cysts
tricholemmoma *see* trichilemmoma
trichomatricoma *see* pilomatricoma
trichomegaly 107.4
trichomoniasis 33.38–33.39
  clinical features 33.38
  epidemiology 33.38
  management 33.38–33.39
trichomycosis axillaris 26.41–26.42
trichomycosis nodularis (black piedra) 32.15–32.16
trichomycosis pubis 109.27
trichophytide, dermatophytide reaction 32.50

trichophytin test 4.25
Trichophyton spp.
  dermatophytosis 32.18–32.20, **32.19**, 32.26–32.30
  hand eczema 39.17
  T. rubrum 32.27–32.28, 32.29, *32.29*
trichoptilosis 87.75
trichorrexis invaginata 63.27
trichorrhexis invaginata 87.79, *87.80*
trichorrhexis nodosa (TN) 87.75–87.77, 87.93–87.94
  argininosuccinic aciduria 79.13
trichoscopy 4.21, 87.65–87.66, 87.74
Trichosporon yeasts 32.66–32.67, 32.93
trichosporosis nodosa *see* white piedra
trichostasis spinulosa 87.83–87.84
trichothiodystrophy (TTD) 63.36–63.38, 76.5, 76.9–76.10, **77.2**, 87.80
trichotillomania (TTM)/trichotillosis 84.22–84.25, 87.14, 87.24, 87.32–87.34
trichrome stains 3.8
trichrome vitiligo 86.36, *86.38*
triclosan 127.58
triclosan/triclocarban, topical therapies 18.10
tricone ('dog ear') repair 20.22
tricyclic antidepressants 84.44, **84.45**
trifarotene, topical therapies 18.26
trigeminal cranial nerve (CN V), anatomy of head and neck 20.2, *20.3*
trigeminal nerve, ophalmic zoster 25.33
trigeminal neuralgia (TN)/trigeminal neuropathic pain syndrome 82.5–82.7, 108.66–108.67
trigeminal trophic syndrome (TTS) 82.7–82.8, 108.67
triglycerides 97.4
trimethylaminuria (fish odour syndrome) 84.11, 92.17–92.18
tripe palms *see* acanthosis palmaris
triple response of Lewis, testing for skin innervation 83.5
trisomy 8 myelodysplasia, Behçet-like disease association 149.8
trisomy 13 (Patau syndrome) 74.2–74.3
trisomy 18 (Edwards syndrome) 74.2
trisomy 21 *see* Down syndrome
Triton tumour *see* neuromuscular hamartoma
TrkB deficiency **72.6**
trophic syndromes, skin picking disorders 82.8–82.9
tropical bubo *see* lymphogranuloma venereum
Tropical Dermatology: A Syndrome-Based Approach (online course) 7.12
tropical disorders
  actinic lichen planus 37.7
  lymphatic filariasis 103.33–103.36
  neglected tropical diseases 7.2, 7.6, 7.7, 7.11–7.12
tropical elephantiasis *see* lymphatic filariasis
Tropical Health and Education Trust (THET) 7.14
tropical ulcers 26.68–26.69
tropoelastin 2.33
Trousseau sign 97.9
TRT *see* thermal relaxation time
true histiocytic lymphoma 135.30–135.31
Trueperella pyogenes, infection 26.43
trunk
  atrophoderma of Pasini–Pierini 55.19
  bowel-associated dermatitis–arthritis syndrome 49.16
  bullous pemphigoid 50.18
  keratolytic winter erythema lesions 63.73, 63.74
  linear IgA disease 50.36
  linear morphoea trunk/limb variant 55.22
  lithium-induced acne 88.13
  microscopic examination of skin 3.33–3.34
  morphoea 55.5, 55.20
  pansclerotic morphoea 55.21
  pityriasis rubra pilaris, type I *36.4*, 36.6

  plaque morphoea *55.20*
  psoriasis vulgaris *35.7*, *35.13*
  pustules, bowel-associated dermatitis–arthritis syndrome 49.16
toxic erythema of the newborn *114.5*
trypanosomiasis 33.39–33.43
  clinical features 33.40–33.42
  epidemiology 33.39
  investigations 33.42–33.43
  management 33.43
  pathophysiology 33.39–33.40, *33.41*
  see also African trypanosomiasis; American trypanosomiasis
trypsin, pancreatic panniculitis 97.41
TSC *see* tuberous sclerosis complex
TSEBT *see* total skin electron beam therapy
tsetse flies, trypanosomiasis 33.39–33.40, *33.41*, 33.42
TSPyV *see* trichodysplasia spinulosa polyomavirus
TST *see* tuberculosis skin test
TSV *see* trichodysplasia spinulosa polyomavirus
TTA *see* temporal triangular alopecia
TTD *see* trichothiodystrophy
t-test, statistical analysis of clinical studies 17.21
TTM *see* trichotillomania
TTO *see* Time Trade-Off
TTS *see* trigeminal trophic syndrome
tubercles of Montgomery, Fordyce spots 93.12
tuberculids 27.24–27.32
  erythema induratum of Bazin 27.29–27.31
  lichen scrofulosorum 27.25–27.27
  other nodular lesions 27.31–27.32
  papulonecrotic tuberculid 27.27–27.29
tuberculin test 4.24
tuberculoid/borderline tuberculoid leprosy 28.1, 28.2–28.3, 28.4, 28.6, *28.7*, **28.7**, 28.8, 28.9, 28.10
tuberculoid granulomas 96.3
tuberculoid leprosy 94.30
tuberculosis 27.2–27.5
  acute cutaneous miliary 27.17
  BCG vaccination 5.3, 27.3–27.5, 27.10–27.11, 27.20, 27.21, 27.25, 27.27–27.29, 27.40, 80.8
  congenital tuberculosis 114.28
  cutaneous manifestations 152.4
  diagnostic tests 27.4–27.5, 27.8–27.9
  ear dermatoses **106.23**
  epidemiology 27.2–27.4
  erythema induratum of Bazin 97.26, 97.29
  erythema nodosum 97.25
  eye infection 107.39
  oral lesions 108.56
  penis 109.27
  perianal skin 111.15
  sarcoidosis causation 96.4
  see also mycobacterial infections; *Mycobacterium tuberculosis*; tuberculosis of the skin
tuberculosis colliquativa cutis (scrofuloderma) 27.13–27.16
tuberculosis cutis indurativa *see* erythema induratum of Bazin
tuberculosis cutis lichenoides *see* lichen scrofulosorum
tuberculosis cutis miliaris acuta generalisata *see* acute cutaneous miliary tuberculosis
tuberculosis cutis miliaris disseminate *see* acute cutaneous miliary tuberculosis
tuberculosis papulonecrotica (papulonecrotic tuberculid) 27.27–27.29
tuberculosis of the skin (cutaneous tuberculosis) 27.5–27.24
  acute cutaneous miliary tuberculosis 27.17
  classification 27.5–27.6

diagnosis 27.7–27.9
HIV 31.22
lupus vulgaris 27.20–27.24
metastatic tuberculous abscess 27.17–27.19
orificial tuberculosis 27.16–27.17
pathophysiology 27.6–27.7
primary inoculation 27.12–27.13
scrofuloderma 27.13–27.16
treatment 27.9–27.10
warty tuberculosis 27.19–27.20
tuberculosis skin test (TST) 27.4
tuberculosis verrucosa cutis (warty tuberculosis) 27.19–27.20
tuberculous mastitis 27.31–27.32
tuberous sclerosis complex (TSC) 78.7–78.10, 148.10
 cardiac rhabdomyomas 78.9
 clinical features 78.7–78.9
 diagnostic criteria **78.10**
 endocrine disorders 78.9
 investigations 78.10
 management 78.10
 mosaic forms of 78.8
 neurological features 78.8–78.9
 ocular signs 78.9
 oral involvement 108.87
 pulmonary involvement 78.9, 152.5
 renal involvement 154.2
tuberous xanthomas 60.3
tubular adenoma 137.28
tubular apocrine adenoma 137.28
tufted angioma (TA), infants 116.10, *116.11*
tufted folliculitis 87.49, 87.84
TUGSE *see* traumatic ulcerative granuloma with stromal eosinophilia
tularaemia, *Francisella tularensis* 26.57–26.58
tumefactive primary localised cutaneous amyloidosis 56.5
 tumour resemblance *56.8*
tumour classification, melanoma 142.8
tumour necrosis factor, allergic contact dermatitis 127.10
tumour necrosis factor antagonists (systemic therapy) 19.32–19.34
 cautions 19.33–19.34
 contraindications 19.33
 dermatological uses 19.32
 drug–drug interactions 19.34
 pharmacological properties 19.32–19.33
 potential adverse effects 19.33
 pre-treatment screening 19.34
tumour necrosis factor inhibitor-associated alopecia 87.34–87.35
tumour necrosis factor receptor-associated periodic syndrome (TRAPS) **45.5, 45.6**, 45.9
tumour necrosis receptor associated periodic syndrome, renal involvement 154.2
tumours
 acanthosis nigricans association 85.3, 85.4–85.5
 acquired ichthyosis association 85.2
 dystrophic calcification of skin and subcutaneous tissues 59.3–59.4
 spread to skin 148.2–148.7
tumours of ano-genital mammary-like glands 137.40
tumours of fat cells 136.56–136.59
tumour spillage (direct contamination of wounds with tumour cells during a laparoscopy or surgical procedure) 148.3–148.4
tumours of the scalp 105.11–105.12
 pilosebaceous unit tumours 105.11
 scalp metastases 105.11–105.12
 sebaceous naevus 105.11
 syringocystadenoma papilliferum 105.11
tumours of skin appendages 137.1–137.49
 apocrine gland tumours 137.18–137.23
 classification 137.2
 eccrine or apocrine gland/follicular tumours 137.28–137.33
 eccrine gland hamartomas and tumours 137.23–137.28

external root sheath tumours 137.5–137.7
from eccrine and apocrine glands 137.1–137.2
hair follicle mesenchyme lesions 137.15–137.16
hair follicle tumours 137.2–137.5
hair matrix tumours 137.13–137.15
hamartomas and hair germ tumours and cysts 137.7–137.13
miscellaneous 137.40–137.44
sebaceous gland tumours 137.16–137.18
sweat gland carcinomas 137.33–137.40
tumours of uncertain malignancy, keratoacanthoma 141.38
Tunga penetrans (sand flea/jigger/chigoe) 34.15
tungiasis 34.15
tunnel disease *see* ancylostomiasis
turban tumour *see* cylindroma
'turf toe' 122.16
turmeric (curcuminoids), cosmeceutical use of *157.8, 157.9*
Turner, Daniel 1.3, *1.4*
Turner syndrome 74.3–74.4, 86.41, 103.20, **106.7**
 infant with *71.28*
turpentine allergy 127.74–127.78
T-vec *see* Talimogene laherparepvec
'two-hit' hypothesis of genetic disorders, disseminated superficial actinic porokeratosis 141.16
tylosis, oral lesions 108.30
tylosis with oesophageal cancer 63.66, *63.67*, **78.13**
tympanic membrane *106.2*
type 1 interferonopathies 45.13–45.15
 Aicardi–Goutières syndrome (AGS) **45.5, 45.6**, 45.13
 chronic atypical neutrophilic dermatosis with lipodystrophy and elevated temperature **45.5, 45.6**, 45.14–45.15
 STING-associated vasculopathy with onset in infancy **45.5, 45.6**, 45.13–45.14
type I cryoglobulinaemia (intravascular) and perniosis 149.13–149.14
type III hypersensitivity reactions, urticarial vasculitis 44.2
type VII collagen (*COL17A1*) 69.5, 69.16, 69.18–69.19, 69.21, 69.22, 69.27
type XVII collagen (*COL17A1*) 69.5
typhus group Rickettsiae 26.80–26.81
typical (classical) epidermodysplasia verruciformis 25.66, 25.69
tyrosinaemia type II 63.70–63.71, 79.11–79.12
tyrosine 68.1
tyrosine kinase inhibitors (TKIs)
 hair pigmentation 87.73–87.74
 hypertrichoses 119.6
 mastocytosis treatment 46.10
 psoriasis treatment 35.27
Tzanck smears 3.29–3.30

U

UAS *see* urticarial activity scores
ubiquinone *see* coenzyme Q10
UCT *see* urticaria control test
UCTD *see* undifferentiated connective tissue disease
'ugly duckling' sign *see* intra-individual comparative analysis of naevi
UK *see* United Kingdom
ulceration 102.1–102.13
 anal fissure 111.30–111.31
 arterial leg ulcers 102.7–102.10
 Behçet-like syndrome associated with trisomy 8 myelodysplasia 149.8
 calciphylaxis 59.7
 chemical burns 128.12
 dermatomyositis 52.5, 52.6, *52.8*, 52.9, 52.11
 diabetic patients 62.1, 62.2–62.3
 diphtheria 26.38–26.39
 female genitalia 110.18–110.20

herpes simplex virus infection, neonatal *114.22*
human immunodeficiency virus infection **111.17**
hypertensive ischaemic ulcers 102.10–102.13
infantile haemangiomas 116.5, *116.6*
intravenous drug administration 120.6–120.7
ischaemic ulcer *101.44*
male genitalia 109.5, 109.22–109.24, 109.28
melanoma 142.7, 142.10, 142.11, 142.20, 142.21, 142.22, **142.23**, 145.14
mixed leg ulcers 102.4–102.7
Mycobacterium ulcerans infection 27.36–27.40
neuropathic ulcer 83.13–83.19
perineal and perianal skin 111.12–111.13, 111.30–111.31
peripheral vascular disease *101.3*
peristomal skin 112.10, 112.12–112.15
prolidase deficiency 79.13
rheumatoid arthritis-associated 53.7, 155.6
striae 94.8
tropical ulcers 26.68–26.69
venous leg ulcers 102.1–102.4
wound healing 11.2, 11.12
see also granuloma inguinale; leg ulcers; oral ulcers
ulcerative basal cell carcinoma 140.8–140.9
ulcerative colitis (UC)
 Crohn disease distinction 153.1–153.2
 oral involvement 108.74
 psoriasis in 35.18
 skin involvement 153.2, 153.3
ulcerative sarcoidosis 96.13
ulcus molle *see* chancroid
ulerythema ophryogenes 89.8
ulnar-mammary syndrome **72.7**
ultrasound 4.22
 foreign body reactions 122.18
 peripheral vascular disease *101.4*, **101.4**
 psoriatic plaque thickness measurements 16.5
 skin tightening 161.6–161.8
 superficial temporal artery, giant cell arteritis 100.33
ultraviolet filters, allergies 127.62, 127.79, 127.80, 127.82
ultraviolet index (UVI) 10.13
ultraviolet light, Wood's light examination for superficial mycosis 32.6–32.7
ultraviolet radiation (UVR) 10.1–10.14
 absorption spectrum *10.4*
 and acne 88.25–88.26
 action spectroscopy 10.4–10.5
 acute and carcinogenic effects of UVR exposure 10.7
 ageing of skin 10.10–10.11, 156.7–156.8, *156.10*
 allergic contact dermatitis 127.11
 artificial sources 10.2–10.3, 21.1, 21.2–21.3, 142.6
 calibration/dosimetry 21.3, *21.4*
 chronic effects of 10.9–10.11
 clinical effects of 10.7–10.11
 cutaneous squamous cell carcinoma 141.27, 141.30
 damaging effects 86.8
 emission spectra *10.3*
 erythema response 126.1
 Fitzpatrick classification of acute and carcinogenic effects 10.7
 Flegel disease 85.17
 genetic changes 147.5
 history of phototherapy 21.2
 interactions with skin 10.3–10.4
 measurement 10.2
 melanocyte number 2.18
 melanocytes response to 86.5–86.7
 melanoma risk 142.5–142.6
 Merkel cell carcinoma risk 146.2–146.3
 molecular and cellular effects 10.5–10.6

non-solar sources 10.13
normal effects on skin 10.5–10.11
occupational skin cancer 129.14
oral squamous cell carcinoma 108.46
path lengths for differing solar elevations *10.3*
personal and population exposure to 10.12–10.14
photon absorption *10.4*
photoprotection 10.11–10.12
phototherapy 1.8
 use during pregnancy 113.21–113.24
physicochemical aspects 10.3–10.4
pigmentation regulation 86.5–86.7
PLE manifestation 126.3
porokeratosis 85.22–85.23
principles 21.2–21.3
production and sources 10.1–10.2
reduced tumour immune surveillance, skin cancer risks 147.5–147.6
risks versus benefits of population UVR exposure 10.13–10.14
rosacea risk 89.11
skin ageing 2.46
skin cancer risks
 immunocompromised people 147.5–147.6
 occupational 129.14
solar urticaria 126.21–126.24
subcategories 10.2
suppressing immune responses and permitting progression of immunogenic tumours 146.3
systemic lupus erythematosus 51.21
tanning response 86.9
terrestrial UVR 10.2
transient acantholytic dermatosis 85.23
UVA-1 phototherapy 126.7–126.8
UVA/UVB wavelength ranges 21.1
UV index 10.13
xeroderma pigmentosum 76.3–76.5
see also photoageing; photochemotherapy; phototherapy; sunlight
ultraviolet recall reaction 119.11
ultraviolet-sensitive syndrome (UVSS) 76.8
umbilicus
 angiokeratoma corporis diffusum 79.7
 bacterial infections 26.5
 bullous pemphigoid *50.19*
 flexural psoriasis 35.9
 neonatal care 114.2–114.3
UN *see* United Nations
uncinarial dermatitis *see* ancylostomiasis
uncombable hair syndrome 87.46, 87.82, *87.83*
undecenoic acid, topical therapies 18.13
undernutrition *see* malnutrition
undifferentiated connective tissue disease (UCTD) 53.1–53.3
undifferentiated soft tissue sarcoma (USTS) 136.17–136.18
undulant fever *see* brucellosis
Unicararia stenocephala see cutaneous larva migrans
unifocal bone disease, Langerhans cell histiocytosis 135.8
unilateral acanthosis nigricans 85.5
unilateral lentiginosis 86.16
unilateral naevoid telangiectasia syndrome 101.20–101.22
 clinical features **101.21**
 grouped lesions *101.21*
United Kingdom (UK)
 basal cell carcinoma incidence 6.1
 Biobank 8.1
 Ethiopia Residents Programme 7.8
 global health activities 7.14
 skin cancer, economic burden of 6.1
United Nations (UN) 7.4–7.5
United States
 dermatology history 1.7
 economic burden of disease 6.5
 psoriasis, economic burden of **6.8**, 6.9
 skin cancer, economic burden of 6.5, **6.7**
unsatisfactory outcomes of skin surgery **20.41**, 20.42

unstable psoriasis 35.13, *35.14*, *35.35*
upadacitinib, atopic eczema treatment 41.30, **41.31**
upper dermal elastolysis 94.26
upper dermal perivascular lymphohistiocytic infiltrate, chronic actinic dermatitis 126.14, *126.15*
uraemia, cutaneous signs 154.3
uraemic pruritus 81.8–81.9
urban versus rural environments, atopic eczema 41.6–41.7, 41.8
urethral caruncle, vulva 110.32
urethral involvement, Stevens–Johnson syndrome/toxic epidermal necrolysis *118.17*, 118.18
urinary tract
  effects of skin diseases 154.6
  see also renal disorders
urinary tract abnormalities, epidermolysis bullosa 69.26
uro-genital tract examination, SJS/TEN 118.20
urostomy **112.3**
  chronic papillomatous dermatitis *112.8*
  ileal metaplasia *112.7*
  irritant skin reaction *112.2*
  lichen sclerosus *112.11*
urticaria 42.1–42.20
  acute spontaneous urticaria 42.5, 42.15–42.16
  aetiology 42.4–42.5, **42.13**
  aggravating factors **42.7**
  allergic 42.5, 127.82–127.86
  anaphylaxis 42.1
  ancient Chinese medical text 1.2
  anetoderma 94.25
  angioedema swellings 42.1, *42.3*
  antihistamine treatment 42.17–42.18, 42.19
  aquagenic urticaria **42.9**, 42.12, *42.13*
  assessment tools 16.5
  associated diseases 42.3
  atopic eczema association 41.22
  autoallergic reactions 42.5–42.6
  autoimmune disease association 42.3
  autoimmune urticaria 42.6
  autoinflammatory diseases **80.19**
  biopsy 3.45
  burden on patient and society 42.14
  causes 42.4–42.5, **42.13**
  cholinergic urticaria **42.9**, 42.11–42.12
  chronic condition associated with genital herpes 25.26
  chronic spontaneous urticaria 42.5, 42.6, 42.7, 42.16, *42.17*
  classification 42.1, **42.8**
  clinical features 42.7–42.14
  cold contact urticaria **42.9**, 42.10–42.11
  complications and co-morbidities 42.14
  contact urticaria 42.13–42.14
  COVID-19 association 25.109, *25.111*
  delayed pressure urticaria **42.9**, 42.10
  dermal oedema 42.6
  dermographism 42.9–42.10
  and diet **42.6**, 42.8
  dietary pseudoallergens 42.8
  differential diagnosis **42.1**, 42.14
  disease course and prognosis 42.14–42.15
  drug-induced 42.5, 42.8, 117.5–117.7
  environmental factors 42.7
  epidemiology 42.2–42.3
  exercise-induced urticaria 42.12
  genetics 42.7
  heat contact urticaria **42.9**, 42.10
  histology 42.6
  idiopathic urticaria 42.5
  immunological and non-immunological stimuli 42.3–42.4
  immunomodulatory and immunosuppressive treatments 42.19
  inducible urticarias 42.8–42.14
    challenge procedures **42.9**
    classification **42.8**
    infants 115.5
  and infection 42.3, 42.5, 42.6, 42.8
  infestation-related urticaria 42.6
  investigations 42.15–42.16
  malignancy association 42.3, 148.23
  management 42.16–42.19
    adverse effects of antihistamines 42.17–42.18
    first line treatment 42.16–42.17
    second line treatment 42.18
    third line treatment (targeted therapies) 42.19
  mast cell role 42.3–42.4
  mechanical forces, reactions to 42.9–42.10
  and menstrual cycle 42.8
  natural history of urticaria in hospital patients study *42.15*
  non-allergic urticaria 42.5, 42.13–42.14
  non-pharmacological treatments 42.19
  oral allergy syndrome 42.13
  pathology 42.6–42.7
  pathophysiology 42.3–42.4
  pharmacological treatments 42.19
  predisposing factors 42.4
  pregnancy 42.8, 42.18, 113.12
  pseudoallergic reactions 42.5, 42.6, 42.8
  psychological factors 15.4, 42.8
  quality of life assessment 16.9
  reactions to COVID-19 (mRNA) vaccines 25.117
  rescue medication 42.18
  severity classification 42.14
  solar urticaria **42.9**, 42.12
  stress 42.8
  symptomatic dermographism 42.9–42.10
  in systemic lupus erythematosus 51.27–51.28
  temperature-dependent urticaria **42.9**, 42.10–42.11
  terminology 42.1
  UVR exposure 126.21–126.24
  vibratory urticaria **42.9**, 42.10, 45.19
  vulva 110.16
  weals/wealing 42.1, *42.2*, 42.6, 42.7, *42.11*, *42.13*, 94.25
urticaria control test (UCT) 16.5
urticarial activity scores (UAS/UAS7/UAS$_{ID}$) 16.5
urticaria-like follicular mucinosis 57.16–57.17
urticarial like rash, complex and polygenic autoinflammatory diseases presenting with urticarial or maculopapular rash 45.20–45.22
urticarial vasculitis 44.1–44.6
  clinical features 44.3–44.4
  clinical variants 44.3–44.4
  drugs implicated in development 44.3
  epidemiology 44.1–44.2
  genetics 44.3
  histopathology 44.1, *44.5*
  infections implicated in development 44.3
  investigations 44.4–44.5
  leucocytoclastic vasculitis 44.1, 44.3
  management 44.5–44.6
  pathology 44.2–44.3
urticaria pigmentosa
  biopsy 3.2
  in children *46.4*, *46.5*
  Darier's sign 46.5
  maculopapular cutaneous mastocytosis *46.1*
  mast cell infiltrates 46.3
  mastocytomas 46.3
  mastocytosis 46.3–46.5
  treatment 46.10
  wealing 46.5
Uruma fever *see* Mayaro virus
ustekinumab, systemic therapy 19.34–19.35
USTS *see* undifferentiated soft tissue sarcoma
uterine leiomyoma 154.2
  see also hereditary leiomyomatosis and renal cell cancer
utility measures, quality of life assessment 16.9

UV *see* ultraviolet radiation
UVA-1 phototherapy
  administration 21.10–21.11
  adverse effects 21.15
  atopic eczema 21.4, 21.6
  conditions treated 21.6–21.7
  history 21.2
  lupus erythematosus 21.6
  mycosis fungoides 21.7
  principles 21.1, 21.2
  sclerosing skin conditions 21.6
UVA exposure
  allergic contact dermatitis 127.11
  photopatch tests 127.81
UVB exposure, allergic contact dermatitis 127.11
UVB phototherapy
  administration 21.7–21.9
  adverse effects 21.11–21.13
  polymorphic light eruption 126.7–126.8, *126.36*
  principles 21.1
  PUVA comparison 21.5–21.6
  vitiligo 86.39
uveal melanoma
  genetic factors 142.4
  system treatment 144.7–144.8
uveitis, Adamantiades–Behçet disease patients 48.4, *48.6*
UVI *see* ultraviolet index
UV light *see* ultraviolet radiation
UVR *see* ultraviolet radiation
UVSS *see* ultraviolet-sensitive syndrome

V

vaccination
  and atopic eczema 41.8–41.9
  complications 25.8–25.9
  COVID-19 25.117–25.119
  development of vaccinia virus 25.7
  and morphoea 55.13
  mpox 25.12
  recombinant hepatitis B associated skin conditions 25.75
  smallpox 25.6, 25.7
vaccinia virus (VAVC) 25.7–25.8
  cowpox virus relationship 25.7, 25.12
Vagabonds' disease 86.23–86.24
vagina, recto-vaginal fistula *111.7*
vaginal adenosis 110.44
vaginal candidiasis *see* vulvo-vaginal candidiasis
vaginal discharge, diagnosis of 110.24–110.25
vaginal infections
  amoebiasis 33.37
  enterobiasis 33.15
  streptococcal 26.33, 110.25
  trichomoniasis 33.38–33.39
valaciclovir, pharmacological properties 19.49
validation, measurement methods 16.2–16.3
validity of research
  evidence based medicine 17.8–17.10, 17.12–17.16, 17.17
  strengthening validity of trials 17.14–17.15
valley fever *see* coccidioidomycosis
vancomycin, hypersensitivity reactions to 14.6
Van der Woude syndrome 108.87
VAP *see* ventilator-associated pneumonia
variable-vessel vasculitis, involving respiratory system 152.4
varicella infection 25.28–25.32
  clinical features 25.29–25.30
  complications and co-morbidities 25.30–25.31
  epidemiology 25.29
  infants 115.6–115.7
  investigations 25.31
  management 25.31–25.32
  oral involvement 108.51
  pathophysiology 25.29

varicella-zoster virus (VZV) 25.28–25.36, 87.35–87.36
  fetal varicella syndrome 114.23
  HIV 31.23–31.24
  in pregnancy 113.5
  see also varicella; zoster
varicose eczema 39.19–39.22
varicose veins 101.38–101.39, 101.42
  on abdomen, associated with liver disease 153.9
  clinical features **101.40**
  management of **101.40**
  pathogenesis **101.39**
varicosities
  labial veins 110.4
  oral involvement 108.27
variegate porphyria (VP) 58.5, 58.7, 58.9, 58.12, 58.17–58.18
  clinical features 58.17–58.18
  genetic counselling 58.18
  investigations 58.18
variola virus (VARV; smallpox) 25.6–25.7
varioliform atrophy 94.15–94.16
varioliform scars
  hydroa vacciniforme 126.25, *126.26*
  necrotising lymphocytic folliculitis 91.12
  scalp margin *93.4*
VARV *see* variola virus
VAS *see* visual analogue scale
vascular calcification, calcific arteriolopathy 97.32–97.33
vascular changes
  during pregnancy **113.2**, 113.3
  liver disease association 153.8–153.9
vascular coagulopathies, purpura 99.19–99.24
vascular disorders 71.1–71.28
  arteriovenous disorders 71.11–71.14
  capillary disorders 71.3–71.11
  classification of 71.1
  genetic mutations 71.1, *71.2*
  internal malignancy association 148.24–148.26
  lymphatic disorders 71.1, 71.21–71.28
  protein mutations in *71.2*
  venous disorders 71.14–71.21
  see also peripheral vascular disease
vascular Ehlers–Danlos syndrome (vEDS) **70.4**, 70.8–70.9, 70.11
vascular endothelial growth factor receptor (VEGFR) *71.2*
vascular endothelial growth factor (VEGF) *71.2*
  loricrin keratoderma 63.56
  wound healing *11.6*
vascularised composite tissue allografts (VCAs), skin cancer risks 147.4
vascular lasers 23.6–23.12
  complications 23.12
  devices 23.7
  indications 23.7
  light–tissue interactions 23.6
  tests and assessments 23.7–23.8
vascular lesions
  atypical vascular proliferation after radiotherapy 136.38–136.39
  laser therapies 23.6–23.12
  mouth 108.25–108.28
  proliferative 108.27
  rheumatoid arthritis 53.6
vascular malformations
  classification **116.1**
  cutaneous 101.26–101.31
  infantile haemangioma comparison **116.1**
vascular syndromes, ocular features **107.42**
vascular tumours 136.23–136.37
  benign types 136.25–136.32
  intermediate malignancy types 136.32–136.34
  malignant types 136.34–136.37
  reactive lesions 136.23–136.25
vasculature 2.40–2.42
vasculitides *see* vasculitis
vasculitis
  autoinflammatory diseases **80.19**

cardiac involvement 151.4
drug-induced 120.5
erythema induratum 97.28–97.29
erythema nodosum 97.24
gastrointestinal and skin manifestations **153.7**
internal malignancy association 148.25
lupus panniculitis 97.38
nodular as a tuberculid 27.29, 27.31
nomenclature and classification 154.6
oral involvement 108.69
panniculitis 97.6
paraprotein-associated 149.14
relapsing polychondritis 155.11, 155.12
renal and skin involvement 154.6
respiratory system involvement 152.3–152.4
rheumatoid arthritis *53.8*, 155.6, *155.8*
rheumatoid nodules 97.16
in Sjögren syndrome 53.10
in systemic lupus erythematosus 51.26
urticarial 44.1–44.6
see also erythema induratum of Bazin; urticarial vasculitis
vasculitis, cutaneous 100.1–100.37
ANCA-associated vasculitis 100.9, 100.13, 100.20–100.28, 152.3–152.4
antiglomerular basement membrane vasculitis 100.19–100.20
classification **100.2**
clinical features 100.1–100.3
clinical variants 100.3–100.4
cocaine-induced 120.5
cryoglobulinaemic vasculitis 100.15–100.17
cutaneous arteritis 100.28–100.30
cutaneous small-vessel vasculitis 100.5–100.8
due to infection *100.7*
due to sepsis *100.7*
eosinophilic granulomatosis with polyangiitis 100.25–100.28
erythema elevatum diutinum 100.8–100.10
giant cell arteritis 100.32–100.34
granuloma faciale 100.11–100.12
granulomatosis with polyangiitis 100.22–100.25
history 100.1–100.2
hypocomplementaemic urticarial vasculitis 100.18–100.19
IgA vasculitis 100.13–100.15
investigations 100.4
Kawasaki disease 100.30–100.32
large-vessel vasculitis 100.32–100.35
leukocytoclastic *100.6*, 100.8
management 100.5
medium-vessel vasculitis *100.3*, 100.28–100.32
microscopic polyangiitis 100.20–100.22
physical signs **100.3**
polyarteritis nodosa 100.28–100.30
presentation 100.2–100.3
purpura pattern **100.4**
recurrent cutaneous necrotising eosinophilic vasculitis 100.10–100.11
single-organ small-vessel vasculitis 100.5–100.12
small-vessel ANCA-associated vasculitis 100.9, 100.13, 100.20–100.28, 152.3–152.4
small-vessel immune complex-associated vasculitis 100.13–100.20
systemic examination **100.3**
Takayasu arteritis 100.34–100.35
ulcerated necrotic lesions *100.3*
urticarial 100.18–100.19
vasculogenesis 101.1
vasculopathic ulcers, dermatomyositis 52.5, 52.6, *52.8*, 52.9, 52.11
vasculopathy
autoinflammatory diseases **80.19**
calciphylaxis 59.6–59.9
systemic lupus erythematosus 51.26–51.27

systemic sclerosis 54.10, **54.25**
vasoactive intestinal peptide (VIP) 2.9
vasoconstriction, cold-induced 124.1, 124.12
vasoconstriction assay, topical bioavailability/bioequivalence assessment 12.8
vasoconstrictors, Raynaud phenomenon 124.12
vasodilatation, perniosis 124.5
vasodilatory substances, Raynaud phenomenon 124.12
vasomotor symptoms, hand–arm vibration syndrome 122.25
vaso-occlusive disorders, COVID-19 association 25.111
VAT adipocytes *see* visceral adipose tissue adipocytes
VAVC *see* vaccinia virus
VCAs *see* vascularised composite tissue allografts
VDDRIIa *see* vitamin D-dependent rickets type 2a
Vedic writings 1.2
vEDS *see* vascular Ehlers–Danlos syndrome
vegetable oils, topical medication vehicles 18.6
vegetative pyoderma gangrenosum 49.5, *49.6*
VEGF *see* vascular endothelial growth factor
VEGFR *see* vascular endothelial growth factor receptor
vehicles for topical therapies
choice and formulations 18.2–18.3, 18.5–18.8
corticosteroids 18.21
veins
intravenous drug administration 120.7
subcutaneous fat 97.7
superficial thrombophlebitis *97.10*
veins in the periorbital and temple area, laser therapies 23.11, *23.14*
vellus hair cyst 137.8
velocardiofacial syndrome (22q11 deletion syndrome) 108.87
Velpeau, Aristide Auguste Stanislas 90.1
vemurafenib (RAF inhibitor)
causing keratoacanthoma 141.38, 141.41
Langerhans cell histiocytoses therapy 135.9
radiation recall *119.13*
Venezuelan haemorrhagic fever 25.82–25.83
venoms
allergic reactions 34.9, 34.16–34.18
antivenoms 130.3
aquatic and marine animal stings 130.1–130.5
arachnids 34.34–34.37
centipedes/millipedes 34.57
cnidarian stings 130.2
fish stings 130.4
hymenoptera 34.2, 34.9, 34.16–34.18
immunotherapy 34.18
lepidoptera/caterpillars 34.33–34.34
management 34.6
pharmacologically active agents 34.2
snake bites 130.5
venuous oedema 103.10–103.12
venous, venous thrombosis 101.31–101.38
venous disorders 71.14–71.21, 101.31–101.46
anatomy 101.31
arteriovenous malformations 101.22–101.24
blue rubber bleb naevus syndrome 71.2, 71.17–71.18
cerebral cavernous malformation-associated cutaneous lesions 71.2, 71.19
chronic venous insufficiency 101.40–101.46
cutaneo-mucosal venous malformation 71.16–71.17
cutaneous vascular malformations 101.26–101.31

glomuvenous malformation *71.2*, 71.18–71.19
haemangioma 101.26, *101.27*
Klippel–Trenaunay syndrome 101.27–101.30
Maffucci syndrome 71.20–71.21
mixed leg ulcers 102.4–102.7
Parkes Weber syndrome **101.28**, 101.30–101.31
physiology 101.31
telangiectases 101.10–101.22
ulceration *101.44*, 102.1–102.13
varicose veins 101.38–101.39, **101.40**
varicosities, labial veins 110.4
venous macrocirculation 101.31
see also verrucous...
venous eczema
allergic contact dermatitis 127.45
chronic venous insufficiency **101.43**
lower leg eczema 39.19–39.22
venous hypertension 97.30
venous lakes 101.14–101.16, **101.17**
larger venous lake *101.16*
laser therapies 23.11
lip *4.14*, 108.28
small venous lake *101.15*
venous leg ulcers (VLUs) 102.1–102.4
chronic venous disease *102.5*, *102.6*
clinical features 102.3
compression therapy *102.5*
disorders associated with **102.2**
epidemiology 102.2
ethnicity 102.2
histology *102.3*, 102.4
investigations for 102.3–102.4
management of 102.4, *102.6*
pathophysiology 102.2–102.3
post-thrombotic syndrome *102.6*
wound histology 102.4
venous macrocirculation 101.31
venous malformations (VMs) 71.14–71.16, 101.24–101.25
clinical features **101.25**
investigations for **101.25**
management of 101.25
treatment options **101.26**
verrucous 71.19–71.20
venous mucocutaneous malformation (VMCM) 71.16–71.17, 108.28
venous obstruction, neoplasia association 148.27
venous system 101.31
venous thromboembolism *102.6*
venous thrombosis 101.31–101.38
deep-vein thrombosis 101.31–101.34
Mondor disease 101.36–101.37
neoplasia association 148.26–148.27
superficial veins 97.8–97.9
superficial venous thrombosis 101.34–101.35
thrombophlebitis migrans 101.35–101.36
venous ulceration 39.21
ventilator-associated pneumonia (VAP) 125.10–125.11
verapamil 94.52
vermilionectomy, mucosal advancement flap repair 20.22
vermilion (outer lip) 108.3
vernal keratoconjunctivitis (VKC) 107.16, 107.17, *107.18*, 107.22
Verneuil's disease 90.1
vernix caseosa, neonates 114.3, 114.4
verruca plana (plane warts) 25.52, 25.53–25.54
see also cutaneous warts
verruca vulgaris (common warts) 25.52, 25.53, 25.54
see also cutaneous warts
verruciform xanthoma
ear dermatoses **106.23**
male genitalia 109.30–109.31
oral 108.14
vulva **110.32**
verrucous carcinoma 108.48
female genitalia 110.37

verrucous carcinoma of the foot (epithelioma cuniculatum) 141.31
verrucous dermatitis *see* chromoblastomycosis
verrucous epidermal naevus *73.4*, *73.5*
verrucous haemangioma 101.26, *101.27*
verrucous perforating collagenoma 94.55
verrucous sarcoidosis 96.13
verrucous-stage incontinentia pigmenti *68.11*
verrucous venous malformation (VVM) 71.19–71.20
verruga peruana, *Bartonella bacilliformis* 26.65–26.66
versican 2.38, *2.39*
vertebrate vectors of disease
dog/cat bites 130.6
leishmaniasis 33.43, **33.45**
nematode infection from non-human animals 33.18–33.26
rat bites 26.75–26.76, 130.5
vertex binding, pattern hair loss 87.61
vesicating species of beetle 34.30–34.31
vesicular dermatosis with reticulate scarring 94.14
vesicular eczema
allergic contact dermatitis *127.13*
hand 127.38
irritant contact dermatitis 129.6
vesicular stomatitis virus 25.97
vesiculobullous eruptions, COVID-19 association 25.109
vesiculobullous-stage incontinentia pigmenti *68.11*
vestibular papillomatosis, labia minora 110.4
vestibule, structure and function of 110.2–110.3
VEXAS (vacuoles, E1 enzyme, X-linked, autoinflammatory, somatic) syndrome (Sweet syndrome) 45.19, 149.6, 149.7
VHFs *see* viral haemorrhagic fevers
vibration, definition 122.24
vibration white finger 122.24, 129.15–129.16
vibratory angioedema 122.25
vibratory urticaria **42.9**, 42.10, 45.19
Vibrio vulnificus infections 26.66
villi 3.43
vimentin 3.25
VIN *see* vulval intraepithelial neoplasia
Vincent's angina *see* acute necrotising (ulcerative) gingivitis and noma
vinegar treatment, cnidarian stings 130.2–130.3
vinyl chloride-induced osteolysis *94.46*
violaceous (lilac) colouring of the skin, upper eyelids in dermatomyositis 52.3
VIP *see* vasoactive intestinal peptide
viral arthropathies 155.2–155.3
viral carcinogenesis
Kaposi sarcoma 138.1–138.6
lymphoepithelioma-like carcinoma 137.43, 137.44
Merkel cell carcinoma 146.2, *146.3*
possible role in keratoacanthoma 141.39
skin cancer risks in immunocompromised people 147.8–147.9
viral haemorrhagic fevers (VHFs) 25.80–25.87, **25.81**
viral infections 25.1–25.129
burn injuries 125.10
classification 25.3–25.4
diagnosis of 3.29–3.31
DNA viruses 25.2, **25.3**, 25.5, 25.6–25.78
drug-induced exanthems 117.1–117.2
exanthems 25.4–25.5
exanthems in infants 115.5–115.7
external ear 106.20
eyelid 107.34–107.38
female genitalia 110.28–110.31
general pathology 25.2, 25.4–25.6
HIV coinfections 31.23–31.26
iatrogenic immunosuppression 149.20, *149.21*

viral infections (*continued*)
  immunosuppressed renal allograft recipients 154.5
  laboratory diagnosis 25.5
  perineal and perianal skin 111.15–111.16
  persistent infection/latency/reactivation 25.4
  postherpetic neuralgia 82.4–82.5
  psoriasis associated with antiviral immune pathways 31.16
  RNA viruses 25.2, **25.3–25.4**, 25.5, 25.78–25.120
  serological tests 25.5–25.6
  skin infection effects on urinary tract 154.6
  see also COVID-19/SARS-CoV-2; Epstein–Barr virus; HIV infection; human herpesvirus; human papillomavirus
viral warts (verrucae)
  immunosuppressed renal allograft recipients 154.5, *154.6*
  laser therapies 23.12, *23.14*
  male genitalia 109.29
  photodynamic therapy 22.7–22.8
  primary immunodeficiencies 149.19
  see also ano-genital warts; cutaneous warts; human papillomavirus
Virchow, Rudolf 56.1
virilism 87.91
virocyte-like cells, myxoinflammatory fibroblastic sarcoma 136.17
virus-negative Merkel cell carcinoma 146.2, 146.3, *146.4*, 146.5, 146.9
visceral adipose tissue (VAT) adipocytes 97.5
visceral larva migrans
  clinical features 33.21
  management 33.21
  pathophysiology 33.20–33.21
visceral leishmaniasis 33.51–33.54
  clinical features 33.51–33.53
  clinical variants **33.45**, 33.51–33.52
  epidemiology **33.45**, 33.51
  investigations 33.53–33.54
  management 33.54
  pathophysiology 33.51
visceral tumour metastases to skin 24.15, 148.4–148.6
viscoelastic materials 122.3
visual analogue scale (VAS), itch assessment tool 16.5
vitamin D analogues
  psoriasis treatment 35.20–35.21
  topical therapies 18.26–18.29
vitamin D-dependent rickets type 2a (VDDRIIa) 87.29
vitamin K deficiency bleeding (VKDB) 61.12–61.13
vitamin and mineral disorders, inherited metabolic diseases 79.15–79.18
vitamins 61.7–61.24
  ascorbic acid as topical depigmenting agents 18.33
  biochemistry 18.26–18.27
  biotin deficiency 61.22–61.24
  biotin metabolism disorders 79.15
  cosmeceutical use of 157.2–157.3, 157.6–157.7
  deficiencies 61.13–61.19
  disorders **79.2**
  hair loss 87.63
  hypermelanosis 86.23–86.24
  ichthyoses 63.46
  metabolism, metastatic calcinosis cutis 59.5
  niacin deficiency 61.15–61.17, *61.17*
  oral features 108.70
  photosensitivity management 126.37
  phrynoderma *61.8*, 85.14–85.15
  pigmentary disorders 86.8
  resuscitation use 125.3–125.4
  sclerodermiform reaction 122.19
  skin manifestations of impaired absorption 153.1

and sunscreen use 10.12
supplement for hypermetabolism treatment 125.12
topical therapies 18.24, 18.26–18.29
UVR exposure 10.9
vitamin A
  cosmeceutical use of retinol 157.6–157.7
  deficiency 61.7–61.8, 85.14–85.15, 86.23–86.24
  excess 61.8–61.9
  hypermelanosis 86.23–86.24
  metabolic production 18.23–18.24
  topical retinol therapies 18.24
  see also retinoids
vitamin B complex, cosmeceutical use of 157.2
vitamin B1, deficiency 61.13–61.14
vitamin B2
  acneform reaction 88.13
  deficiency 61.14–61.15
vitamin B3, deficiency 61.15–61.17
vitamin B6
  acneform reaction 88.13
  deficiency 61.17–61.18
vitamin B7 (biotin)
  deficiency 61.22–61.24
  metabolism disorders 79.15
vitamin B9 deficiency 61.18–61.19
vitamin B12
  acneform reaction 88.13
  deficiency 61.19–61.21, 86.23–86.24, *108.25*, 108.70
  atrophic glossitis *108.25*
vitamin C
  acne vulgaris treatment 88.57
  ascorbic acid as topical depigmenting agents 18.33
  deficiency 61.21–61.22
vitamin D_3(25-hydroxy), acne vulgaris 88.19
vitamin D
  and acne 88.19
  alopecia areata 87.23
  deficiency 61.9–61.11, 86.8, 87.23, 87.29
vitamin D analogue therapies 18.26–18.29, 35.20–35.21
vitamin deficiencies, folate deficiency 61.18–61.19, 86.23–86.24
vitamin E
  cosmeceutical use of 157.3
  deficiency 61.11–61.12
  excess 61.12
vitamin K_1 panniculitis 97.48
vitamin K
  deficiency 61.12–61.13
  sclerodermiform reaction 122.19
vitiligo 68.4, 86.34–86.41, 87.93
  dermatoendocrinology **150.6**, **150.11**, *150.16*, 150.18
  female genitalia 110.20–110.21
  koebnerisation 127.20–127.21
  mechanical injuries 122.2
  occupational *86.46*
  phototherapy 21.4
  psychological and social factors 15.4
  radiotherapy-associated 119.15
  treatment 86.33, 86.39–86.40
VKC *see* vernal keratoconjunctivitis
VKDB *see* vitamin K deficiency bleeding
VKHS *see* Vogt–Koyanagi–Harada syndrome
VLUs *see* venous leg ulcers
VMCM *see* venous mucocutaneous malformation
VMs *see* venous malformations
Voerner–Unna–Thost keratoderma *63.51*
Vogt–Koyanagi–Harada syndrome (VKHS) 86.42, 87.93
Vohwinkel syndrome 63.63–63.64
Voigt–Futcher lines *86.2*
volar skin of palms and soles, acral melanoma 145.9, 145.11–145.13
volatile substances
  inhaling 120.4
  irritant contact dermatitis 128.4

volumisation, dermal filler injection 158.1, *158.4*
volunteering opportunities 7.13, **7.15**
von Hippel–Lindau syndrome (familial cerebelloretinal angiomatosis) 148.9, 154.2
von Kossa method staining technique 3.9
von Recklinghausen disease *see* neurofibromatosis type 1
von Zumbusch variant, pustular psoriasis 35.33–35.34, 118.4
voriconazole photosensitivity *126.31*
VP *see* variegate porphyria
'V-sign', redness on chest in dermatomyositis 52.4
vulva
  acne 110.45
  bacterial infections 110.25–110.27
  benign tumours 110.31–110.33
  cutaneous Crohn disease *95.15*
  Fordyce spots 93.11
  fungal infections 110.27–110.28
  genital papular acantholytic dyskeratosis 110.45
  graft-versus-host disease 110.43–110.44
  hidradenoma papilliferum 110.31–110.33, 137.20–137.21
  inflammatory dermatoses of 110.6–110.18
  lymphangiectasia 103.31
  malignant neoplasms 110.36–110.40
  melanoma 110.39–110.40, 142.11
  melanosis 110.21–110.22, *131.10*
  microbiome 26.5
  mucous membrane pemphigoid *50.28*
  necrolytic migratory erythema 110.44–110.45
  non-sexually acquired genital ulcers 110.19–110.20
  oedema 110.23–110.24
  pain disorders 110.40–110.42
  premalignant conditions 110.34–110.36
  psoriasis vulgaris 35.10
  structure and function of 110.2–110.3
  tumours, hidradenoma papilliferum 110.31–110.33, 137.20–137.21
  viral infections 110.28–110.31
  warts *110.30*
  see also genitalia, female; vulvo-vaginal
vulval intraepithelial neoplasia (VIN) 110.34, 110.35, 141.26
vulval swelling, cutaneous Crohn disease *95.15*
vulval ulcers
  aphthous ulcers 110.19
  Behçet disease 110.20
  causes of **110.19**
  non-sexually acquired genital ulcers 110.19–110.20
vulvar pemphigoid *50.26*
vulvodynia 82.9–82.11, 110.40–110.42
vulvo-vaginal adenosis 110.44
vulvo-vaginal candidiasis 32.63–32.64, 110.27–110.28
  HIV 31.26
vulvodynia misdiagnosis 82.10
vulvo-vaginal-gingival syndrome *110.12*
vulvovaginitis
  streptococcal/bacterial 26.33, 110.25
  see also vulvo-vaginal candidiasis
VVM *see* verrucous venous malformation
VZV *see* varicella-zoster virus

W
Waardenburg syndrome 68.5, 86.4
Wade–Fite stain 3.9
Wagner foot ulcer classification **83.14**
Waldenström hypergammaglobulinaemic purpura 99.6–99.7
Waldenström macroglobulinaemia, oral involvement 108.72
warfarin-induced necrosis, purpura 99.15–99.17
Wars, Hypogammaglobulinemia, Infections, Myelocathexis syndrome (WHIM) 80.16–80.17

warts (verrucae) 4.7
  eyelid 107.34, *107.36*
  on lip, HIV infection *108.14*
  treatment during pregnancy **113.21**
  see also ano-genital warts; cutaneous warts; genital warts; seborrhoeic keratosis; viral warts
warts, immuno-deficiency, lymphoedema and ano-genital dysplasia (WILD syndrome) 103.22
warty dyskeratoma (WD) 108.30–108.31, 132.5–132.6
warty tuberculosis (tuberculosis verrucosa cutis) 27.19–27.20
wasps 34.16
WAT *see* white adipose tissue
water, light absorption by skin 23.4
water fleas, *Cyclops* species and dracunculiasis 33.13
water hardness, and atopic eczema 41.23
wavelength of laser light, selective photothermolysis 23.5
wax (cerumen), external ear 106.2–106.3
waxes, topical medication vehicles 18.7
waxy keratoses of childhood 63.78–63.79
WBS *see* Williams–Beuren syndrome
WD *see* warty dyskeratoma
weals/wealing
  immediate-weal tests 4.24
  jellyfish stings 130.2
  urticaria 42.1, *42.2*, *42.6*, 42.7, *42.11*, *42.13*
  urticaria pigmentosa *46.5*
weathering of hair 87.6, 87.75–87.80, 87.93
weathering nodules, ear dermatoses **106.23**, *106.26*
Weber–Christian disease 97.8
Weber–Cockayne disease 122.10
wedge excision, lip/eyelid/ear surgery 20.22
weeverfish stings 130.4–130.5
Weibel–Palade bodies 2.41, *2.42*
Weidermann–Rautenstrauch syndrome **72.5**
weight gain, cellulite 98.26
Weil disease 26.74, 26.75
Weisse, Faneuil 1.7
well-differentiated liposarcoma 136.58–136.59
well-differentiated SCC (keratoacanthomatous type) 141.38
  see also keratoacanthoma
Wells syndrome 47.16
Wermer syndrome *see* multiple endocrine neoplasia type 1
Werner syndrome (pangeria) 70.26–70.27, **72.5**, 75.6, 77.1–77.3, **78.12**, 148.12, 148.13
wet beriberi, vitamin B1 deficiency 61.14
wet gangrene of the foot, diabetic patients 62.2
wet-wrap technique, atopic eczema treatment 41.28
WHIM (Wars, Hypogammaglobulinemia, Infections, Myelocathexis) syndrome 80.16–80.17
Whipple disease (*Tropheryma whippelii* infection) 97.47, 153.4, 155.5
whisker hair 87.81
white adipose tissue (WAT) 72.1
white dermographism, atopic eczema 41.17–41.18
white fat 97.1–97.2
white fibrous papulosis of the neck 94.39–94.40
white finger skin patches 129.15–129.16
White, James 1.7
white piedra 32.16–32.17, 32.66–32.67
white shiny line dermoscopy patterns, melanoma 145.7, 145.14, *145.15*
white sponge naevus, oral lesions 108.31
white structures
  melanoma 145.14, *145.15*
  see also blue-white veil

whitlow-like lesions
  inoculation herpes simplex   25.28
  mpox   25.9, 25.10
Whitmore disease *see* melioidosis
WHO *see* World Health Organization
whole body cabins/cabinets, equipment for phototherapy delivery   21.2–21.3, 21.8, *21.9*, 21.10, 21.16
Wickham striae
  lichen planus   37.3, 37.13, 110.11, *111.10*
  penis   *109.19*
wide local excision (WLE), melanoma   143.1–143.4
widow spiders (Theridiidae)   34.34–34.35
Wiedemann–Rautenstrauch syndrome (neonatal progeria syndrome)   **77.2**
wigs   87.28, 87.69, 87.101
Wildemuth ear   106.5
WILD syndrome (warts, immuno-deficiency, lymphoedema and ano-genital dysplasia)   103.22
Wilkinson's triangle (chronic actinic dermatitis)   *4.6*
Willan, Robert   1.4, *1.5*
Williams–Beuren syndrome (WBS)   70.18–70.19, **72.12**
Williams syndrome   2.34
willingness to pay (WTP)
  health economics   6.4
  utility measure   16.9
Wilson disease   79.17
Wilson, Sir Erasmus   1.6, *1.7*
Winchester syndrome   70.23–70.24
Wiskott–Aldrich syndrome   80.9, 148.13
  oral involvement   108.28
  skin cancer   147.2
Wissler–Fanconi syndrome *see* adult-onset Still disease
witchcraft syndrome   84.33
WLE *see* wide local excision
Wnt signalling   2.3, 2.4
Wolff–Chaikoff effect, potassium iodide systemic therapy   19.30
women with HIV/AIDS   31.36
wood allergies   127.74–127.78
wood dust allergy   127.17
Wood's light examination, superficial mycosis identification   4.19–4.20, 32.6–32.7, 32.12
wood tars, topical therapies   18.36
Woolf syndrome   68.9
woolly hair   87.80–87.82
  palmoplantar keratodermas   63.62–63.63
Woringer–Kolopp disease *see* pagetoid reticulosis
work impacts, measures   16.12–16.13
work productivity, impact assessment   16.12–16.13
Work Productivity and Activity Impairment: General Health (WPAI:GH)   16.13
World Health Organization (WHO)   7.5
  classification of cutaneous tumours
    lymphoma   139.1, **139.2**, 139.6, 139.37
    melanoma   142.8
  Global Programme to Eliminate Lymphatic Filariasis   103.35
  neglected tropical diseases roadmap   7.7
Woronoff, halo/ring of, psoriasis vulgaris   35.7
wound care
  bites   130.6, 130.7
  pressure ulcers   123.10–123.11
wound healing   11.1–11.13
  abnormal healing and scarring   11.8–11.9
  acute wounds
    cytokine/growth factor role   **11.5**
    healing stages   *11.1*

age-related changes   11.2, 11.10
angiogenesis   11.5–11.6
chronic wounds   11.2
  abnormal healing and scarring   11.8–11.9
  causes of   11.11
collagenous cross-linking   11.7
cytokines   **11.4**, **11.5**
diabetes   11.9
excessive healing   11.2
fibroblasts   11.6, 11.7–11.8
grafts   11.11–11.12
growth factors   **11.4**, *11.5*, **11.5**, *11.6*, 11.11
hyaluronan role   2.39
impairment of   11.2
inflammatory memory   9.9
inflammatory response   11.2–11.3
keratinocytes   11.4–11.5
lymphangiogenesis   103.3
matrix metalloproteinases   11.4, *11.5*, 11.8, **11.9**
matrix synthesis   11.7–11.8
novel therapies   11.11–11.13
regulation of   11.2
revascularisation of wound   11.6
scarring   11.8–11.9
  initiation of   *11.7*
skin substitutes   11.12, *11.13*
stages of   11.1
stem cell therapy   11.11
tissue engineering   11.11–11.13
tissue homeostasis   9.6–9.7
treatment of   11.10–11.11
wound infection, pressure ulcers   123.10–123.11
wounds, *Pseudomonas* colonisation   4.14
WPAI:GH *see* Work Productivity and Activity Impairment: General Health
wrinkles (rhytids)
  ablative fractional resurfacing   161.5
  ageing of skin   156.2, 156.5
  cosmeceuticals   157.4–157.7
  dermal fillers, indication for   158.1, **158.3**
  glyphic wrinkles   94.2
  laser-assisted drug delivery   161.5
  mid-dermal elastolysis   94.26
  reduction of by botulinum toxin application   159.5, *159.6*, *159.7*
  smoker's skin   156.4
wrist
  anti-p200 pemphigoid   *50.41*
  atopic eczema   41.13
  lichen planus   37.3, 39.17
  Nékam disease   37.11
  psoriasis vulgaris   35.8
WTP *see* willingness to pay

X

xanthelasmas   60.4–60.5, 107.44
xanthoerythroderma perstans *see* small plaque parapsoriasis
xanthogranuloma   97.17–97.18, **106.23**
xanthoma disseminatum (XD)   135.19–135.21
xanthomas   60.2–60.6
  classification   60.2
  colour of   *4.14*
  dyslipidaemic plane (planar) xanthomas   60.4–60.6
  ear dermatoses   **106.23**
  eruptive xanthomas   60.4
  palmar xanthomas   60.5–60.6
  plane xanthomas   60.5
  tendon xanthomas   60.2–60.3
  tuberous xanthomas   60.3
  xanthelasmas   60.4–60.5

xanthomatosis   *60.6*
X chromosome   8.4, 74.3–74.5
XD *see* xanthoma disseminatum
xeroderma pigmentosum/Cockayne syndrome complex (XP/CS)   76.5
xeroderma pigmentosum/trichothiodystrophy (XP/TTD) syndrome   76.5
xeroderma pigmentosum variant (XP-V)   **76.3**, 76.5
xeroderma pigmentosum (XP)   76.1–76.6, **78.12**, 126.32–126.33, 148.9
  clinical features   76.3–76.5
  clinical variants   76.5
  complementation groups   76.1, 76.3
  differential diagnosis   76.5–76.6
  epidemiology   76.2
  exaggerated sunburn and pigmentary changes   76.4–76.5
  genes, chromosomal locations and protein functions   **76.3**
  investigations   76.6
  management   76.6
  neurodegeneration   76.5
  ocular manifestations   76.5
  oral involvement   108.87
  pathophysiology   76.2–76.3
  skin cancer   *76.4*, 76.5
xerosis cutis (dry skin)   85.26–85.28
  atopic eczema association   41.15
  methamphetamine-induced   120.5
  renal failure and dialysis complications   154.3
X-linked agammaglobulinaemia (Bruton disease)   80.5, 80.13
X-linked congenital generalised hypertrichosis   87.85
X-linked dominant (XLD) inheritance   8.4
X-linked keratosis follicularis spinulosa decalvans   63.24–63.25, 85.11, 87.48
X-linked lymphoproliferative diseases   80.10–80.11
X-linked recessive (XLR) inheritance   8.4
X-linked skin disease, linear manifestations of   73.22
X-linked syndromes
  alopecia   63.69
  distal cholesterol biosynthesis   63.22–63.26
XP *see* xeroderma pigmentosum
XP/CS *see* xeroderma pigmentosum/Cockayne syndrome complex
XP/TTD *see* xeroderma pigmentosum/trichothiodystrophy syndrome
XP-V *see* xeroderma pigmentosum variant
X-ray photon beams   24.1
X-ray therapy
  intensity modulated radiotherapy   24.3
  kilovoltage and megavoltage modalities   24.1
  principles   24.1
  superficial treatment causing bone and cartilage necrosis   24.2
XXXXY syndrome   74.4–74.5, **106.7**
XXYY syndrome   74.4
XYY syndrome   74.4

Y

Yao syndrome   45.22
yatapoxviruses   **25.6**, 25.19
  see also tanapox virus
yaws   26.70–26.71
  clinical features   26.71
  epidemiology   26.70–26.71
  male genitalia   109.27
  presentations   29.12
  syphilis similarities   29.5, 29.12

Y chromosome   8.4, 74.3–74.5
years lost due to disability (YLD)   5.6, *5.7*, *5.8*
yeast infections
  burn injuries   125.10
  in pregnancy   113.7
yeasts
  biology   32.2–32.3
  identification of isolates   32.9–32.10
  morphology and diseases   **32.3**
  see also Candida; Malassezia; Trichosporon
yellow fever, filivirus haemorrhagic fever   25.85
yellow-nail syndrome (YNS)   103.21–103.22, 152.6
Yersinia enterocolitica   26.60
Yersinia pestis   26.59–26.60
YLD *see* years lost due to disability
YNS *see* yellow-nail syndrome
Yushchenko, Viktor, dioxin poisoning-induced acne   *88.15*

Z

Zambian haemorrhagic fever   25.82
Zeis, cyst of   107.45
Ziehl–Neelsen method   3.9
Zika virus (ZIKV)   25.87
Zimmermann–Laband syndrome   106.5, **106.7**
zinc
  acne vulgaris treatment   88.51–88.52, 88.57
  telogen effluvium treatment   87.59
zinc deficiency   61.25–61.27
  acrodermatitis enteropathica   108.20
  blistering diseases   69.24
  chronic liver disease   153.9
  hair loss   *87.55*, 87.59
Ziprkowski–Margolis syndrome   68.9
zoon balanoposthitis   109.14–109.15
zoonotic bacterial infections
  anthrax   26.44–26.45
  brucellosis   26.60–26.62
  cat scratch disease   26.62–26.64
  corynebacteria causing diphtheria   26.38
  glanders   26.55
  leptospirosis   26.74–26.75
  Pasteurella multocida   26.59
  rat-bite fevers   26.75–26.76, 130.5
  streptococcal toxic shock-like syndrome   26.37
  tick-borne, ehrlichiosis and anaplasmosis   26.66–26.67
  tularaemia   26.57–26.58
  Yersinia pestis/plague   26.59–26.60
zoonotic viral infections
  foot and mouth disease   25.95
  herpes B virus   25.43
  orthopoxviruses   25.8–25.13
  pseudocowpox/paravaccinia   25.15
  SARS-CoV-2   25.100
  vesicular stomatitis virus infection   25.97
  viral haemorrhagic fevers   25.80
zoon vulvitis   110.13–110.14
zoophilic dermatophytes   32.19, 32.20
zoster *see* herpes zoster
zosteriform lentiginosis   86.16
zosteriform lentiginous naevus *see* speckled lentiginous naevus
z-plasty   20.26–20.27, *20.30*
Zurhausenvirales (papillomaviruses)   25.49
  see also human papillomavirus
zygomycosis *see* mucormycosis